HARRISON'S 15TH EDITION

PRINCIPLES OF INTERNAL MEDICINE

EDITORS OF PREVIOUS EDITIONS

T. R. HARRISON
Editor-in-Chief, Editions 1, 2, 3, 4, 5

W. R. RESNICK
Editor, Editions 1, 2, 3, 4, 5

M. M. WINTROBE
Editor, Editions 1, 2, 3, 4, 5
Editor-in-Chief, Editions 6, 7

G. W. THORN
Editor, Editions 1, 2, 3, 4, 5, 6, 7
Editor-in-Chief, Edition 8

R. D. ADAMS
Editor, Editions 2, 3, 4, 5, 6, 7, 8, 9, 10

P. B. BEESON
Editor, Editions 1, 2

I. L. BENNETT, JR.
Editor, Editions 3, 4, 5, 6

E. BRAUNWALD
Editor, Editions 6, 7, 8, 9, 10, 12, 13, 14
Editor-in-Chief, Edition 11

K. J. ISSELBACHER
Editor, Editions 6, 7, 8, 10, 11, 12, 14
Editor-in-Chief, Editions 9, 13

R. G. PETERSDORF
Editor, Editions 6, 7, 8, 9, 11, 12, 13
Editor-in-Chief, Edition 10

J. D. WILSON
Editor, Editions 9, 10, 11, 13, 14
Editor-in-Chief, Edition 12

J. B. MARTIN
Editor, Editions 10, 11, 12, 13, 14

A. S. FAUCI
Editor, Editions 11, 12, 13
Editor-in-Chief, Edition 14

R. ROOT
Editor, Edition 12

D. L. KASPER
Editor, Editions 13, 14

S. L. HAUSER
Editor, Edition 14

D. L. LONGO
Editor, Edition 14

HARRISON'S 15TH EDITION

PRINCIPLES OF INTERNAL MEDICINE

EDITORS

EUGENE BRAUNWALD, MD, MD(Hon), ScD(Hon)
Distinguished Hersey Professor of Medicine, Faculty Dean for Academic Programs at Brigham and Women's Hospital and Massachusetts General Hospital, Harvard Medical School; Vice-President for Academic Programs, Partners HealthCare Systems, Boston

ANTHONY S. FAUCI, MD, ScD(Hon)
Chief, Laboratory of Immunoregulation; Director, National Institute of Allergy and Infectious Diseases, National Institutes of Health, Bethesda

DENNIS L. KASPER, MD, MA(Hon)
William Ellery Channing Professor of Medicine, Professor of Microbiology and Molecular Genetics, Executive Dean for Academic Programs, Harvard Medical School; Director, Channing Laboratory, Department of Medicine, Brigham and Women's Hospital, Boston

STEPHEN L. HAUSER, MD
Betty Anker Fife Professor and Chairman, Department of Neurology, University of California San Francisco, San Francisco

DAN L. LONGO, MD
Scientific Director, National Institute on Aging, National Institutes of Health, Bethesda and Baltimore

J. LARRY JAMESON, MD, PhD
Irving S. Cutter Professor and Chairman, Department of Medicine, Northwestern University Medical School; Physician-in-Chief, Northwestern Memorial Hospital, Chicago

VOLUME 2

McGraw-Hill
MEDICAL PUBLISHING DIVISION

New York San Francisco Washington, DC Auckland Bogotá Caracas Lisbon London
Madrid Mexico City Milan Montreal New Delhi San Juan Singapore Sydney Tokyo Toronto

McGraw-Hill

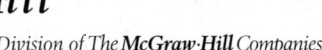

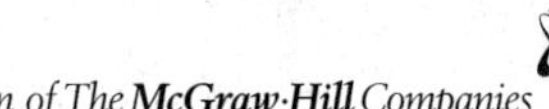

A Division of The **McGraw·Hill** *Companies*

Note: Dr. Fauci and Dr. Longo's works as editors and authors were performed outside the scope of their employment as U.S. government employees. These works represent their personal and professional views and not necessarily those of the U.S. government.

Harrison's
PRINCIPLES OF INTERNAL MEDICINE
Fifteenth Edition

234567890 DOWDOW 098765432
ISBN 0-07-007272-8 (Combo)
0-07-007273-6 (Vol. 1)
0-07-007274-4 (Vol. 2)
0-07-913686-9 (Set)

FOREIGN LANGUAGE EDITIONS

Arabic (13e)—McGraw-Hill Libri Italia srl (est. 1996)
Chinese (12e)—McGraw-Hill Book Company—Singapore © 1994
Croatian (13e)—Placebo, Split, Croatia
French (14e)—McGraw-Hill Publishing Co., Maidenhead, UK © 1999
German (14e)—McGraw-Hill Publishing Co., Maidenhead, UK © 1999
Greek (14e)—Parissianos, Athens, Greece © 2000
Italian (14e)—McGraw-Hill Libri Italia srl, Milan © 1999
Japanese (11e)—Hirokawa © 1991
Polish (14e)—Czelej Publishing Company, Lubin, Poland (est. 2000)
Portuguese (14e)—McGraw-Hill Interamericana do Brasil Ltda © 1998
Romania (14e)—Teora Publishers, Bucharest, Romania (est. 2000)
Spanish (14e)—McGraw-Hill Interamericana de Espana, Madrid © 1998
Turkish (13e)—McGraw-Hill Libri Italia srl (est. 1996)

This book was set in Times Roman by Progressive Information Technologies. The editors were Martin Wonsiewicz and Mariapaz Ramos Englis. The production director was Robert Laffler. The index was prepared by Irving C. Tullar. The text and cover designer was Marsha Cohen/Parallelogram Graphics.

R. R. Donnelley and Sons, Inc. was the printer and binder.

Library of Congress Cataloging-in-Publication Data

Harrison's principles of internal medicine—15th ed./editors, Eugene Braunwald . . . [et al.]. p. cm.
Includes bibliographical references and index.
ISBN 0-07-913686-9 (set)—ISBN 0-07-007273-6 (v. 1)—ISBN 0-07-007274-4 (v. 2)
1. Internal medicine. I. Braunwald, Eugene, date
RC46.H333 2001
616—dc21

00-063809

INTERNATIONAL EDITION ISBN 0-07-118319-1 (Set); 0-07-118320-5 (Vol 1); 0-07-118321-3 (Vol 2)

DEDICATION

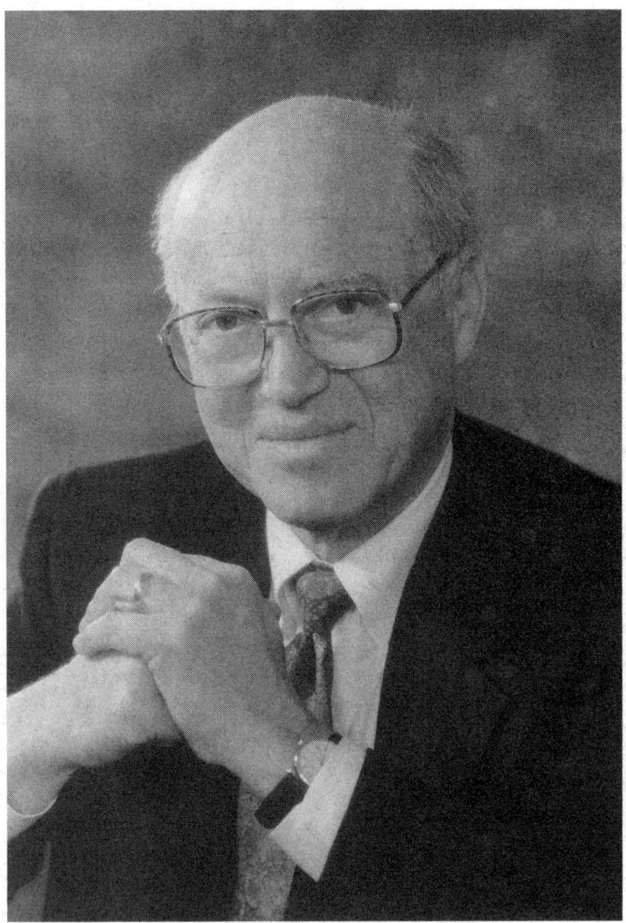

KURT J. ISSELBACHER

With this edition, the editors acknowledge the many contributions of our colleague Kurt J. Isselbacher, who served as an editor of *Harrison's* for nine editions, the sixth through the fourteenth, including Editor-in-Chief of the ninth and thirteenth editions. For more than three decades Dr. Isselbacher played a decisive role in ensuring that *Harrison's* epitomized the state of the art and science of internal medicine and the essence of accuracy and clarity. His indelible contributions to *Harrison's* are felt in the fifteenth edition and will endure into the future.

Dr. Isselbacher is a graduate of Harvard College and of the Harvard Medical School. His further training included a residency in medicine at the Massachusetts General Hospital and a research fellowship at the National Institutes of Health. Chosen to lead the Gastrointestinal Unit of the MGH at the remarkable age of 31, over the ensuing 30 years as Chief of that Unit, he was a leader in advancing both the clinical specialty of gastroenterology and the basic understanding of gastrointestinal disease. Under his leadership, the MGH Gastrointestinal Unit became renowned for its training program in academic gastroenterology as well as for being one of the world's leading centers for clinical and research activities in gastroenterology. In 1987, Dr. Isselbacher undertook new challenges as the first Director of the Cancer Center at the MGH, bringing his characteristic insight and leadership to this new task. In a relatively short time, the MGH Cancer Center has emerged as a premier cancer research institute. Dr. Isselbacher holds the Mallinckrodt Distinguished Professorship of Medicine at Harvard Medical School, and he has been a powerful force for excellence in scholarship at this institution since his graduation. For almost 30 years he served as Chairman of the Executive Committee of Harvard's Departments of Medicine and played a pivotal role in the departments' growth and quest for excellence.

Dr. Isselbacher combines the attributes of an excellent scientist with those of a superb clinician and teacher. He has trained generations of physicians and investigators, including many who are now leaders in academic medicine. As the author of more than 400 scientific articles in leading journals, his research contributions include definition of enzymatic defects in absorptive disorders, and delineation of biochemical mechanisms of absorption, malabsorption, protein synthesis, derangements of metabolism, and immunologic aspects of hepatic gastrointestinal disease. Kurt Isselbacher has been a recipient of many well-earned honors, including the Distinguished Achievement Award and the Friedenwald Medal of the American Gastroenterological Association, the John Phillips Memorial Award for distinguished contributions to clinical medicine from the American College of Physicians, as well as the Kober Medal of the Association of American Physicians. He is a member of the National Academy of Sciences and of its Institute of Medicine and has served as President of the American Gastroenterological Association, the American Association for the Study of Liver Disease, and the Association of American Physicians.

Kurt Isselbacher exemplifies the highest values of medicine. A caring, empathic physician, he consistently combines compassion with incisive analysis in the care of patients. With contributions as a clinician, teacher, scientist, and editor, he has advanced the care of patients with gastrointestinal disorders and cancer while educating generations of physicians.

DEDICATION

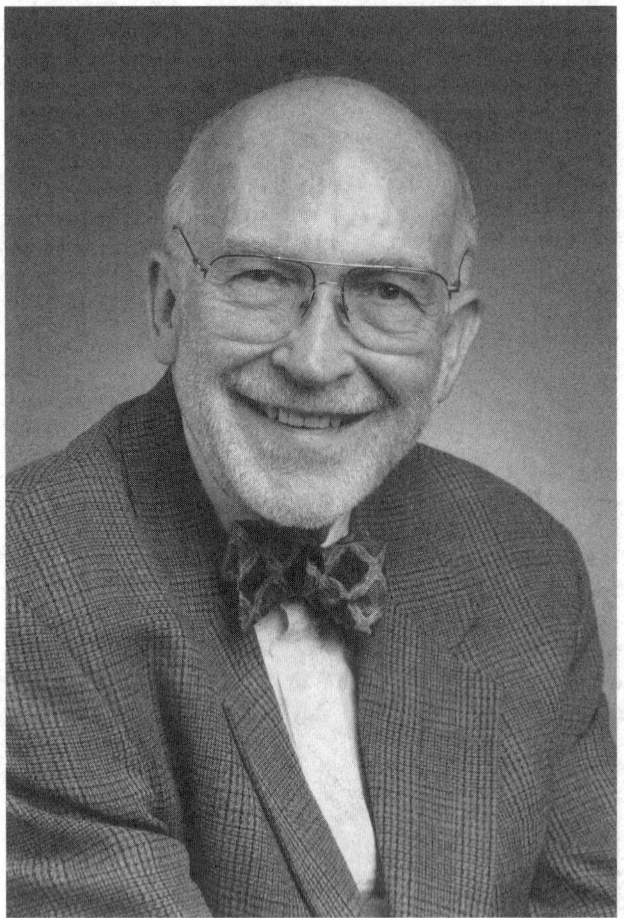

JEAN DONALD WILSON

Jean Wilson served as editor of the ninth through the fourteenth editions of *Harrison's Principles of Internal Medicine* from 1978 to 1998; he was Editor-in-Chief of the twelfth edition. A native of Texas, Jean Wilson attended the University of Texas at Austin and the University of Texas Southwestern Medical School in Dallas. He trained as a resident in internal medicine and as a fellow in endocrinology and metabolism at Parkland Hospital. With the exception of 2 years of research in biochemistry in the intramural program of the National Institutes of Health, Dr. Wilson spent his entire career at the University of Texas Southwestern Medical School, where he now holds the Charles Cameron Sprague Distinguished Chair in Biomedical Science.

Dr. Wilson is one of America's most distinguished biomedical scientists and is largely responsible for working out the mechanism of action and physiology of the male sex hormones from the embryo to the normal and diseased adult. Among his many important discoveries has been the 5α-reductase reaction, whereby male target tissues convert testosterone to the more active androgen, dihydrotestosterone. He has been honored many times for his research, having received the Ernst Oppenheimer Memorial Award of the Endocrine Society, the Amory Prize of the American Academy of Arts and Sciences, the Lita Annenberg Hazen Award for Excellence in Clinical Research, the Henry Dale Medal of the Society for Endocrinology, the Gregory Pincus Award of the Worcester Foundation for Experimental Biology, the Fred Conrad Koch Award of the Endocrine Society, and the Kober Medal of the Association of American Physicians.

Amongst his memberships are the National Academy of Sciences, the Institute of Medicine of the National Academy of Sciences, and the American Academy of Arts and Sciences. He is a Fellow of the Royal College of Physicians. He has served as President of the American Society for Clinical Investigation, the Association of American Physicians, and the Endocrine Society. For two decades, Dr. Wilson directed the enormously successful MD/PhD program and for 8 years, the highly esteemed Endocrine-Metabolism Division at Southwestern.

Perhaps the finest thing that can be said of Jean Wilson is that he is a professor of internal medicine in the complete sense. He is, and always has been, a superb teacher and exemplary clinician while constantly maintaining a sterling career in research. Perhaps nothing describes him better than the enduring image of this renowned academic physician trimming callouses and ulcers in the Diabetic Foot Care Clinic at Parkland Memorial Hospital, his teaching hospital, where the patients are the medically indigent of Dallas.

Dr. Wilson is a man of diverse interests, a true intellectual. One of his great gifts and loves is scientific and medical editing. He served as Editor-in-Chief of the *Journal of Clinical Investigation* and of *Williams Textbook of Endocrinology*. As an editor of *Harrison's* for two decades, Dr. Wilson made ample use of his conspicuous strengths as clinician, teacher, and scientist. His meticulous scholarship and high standards have had an enormous impact, not only on the Endocrinology, Metabolism, and Genetics sections, for which he had primary responsibility, but on the entire book.

DEDICATION

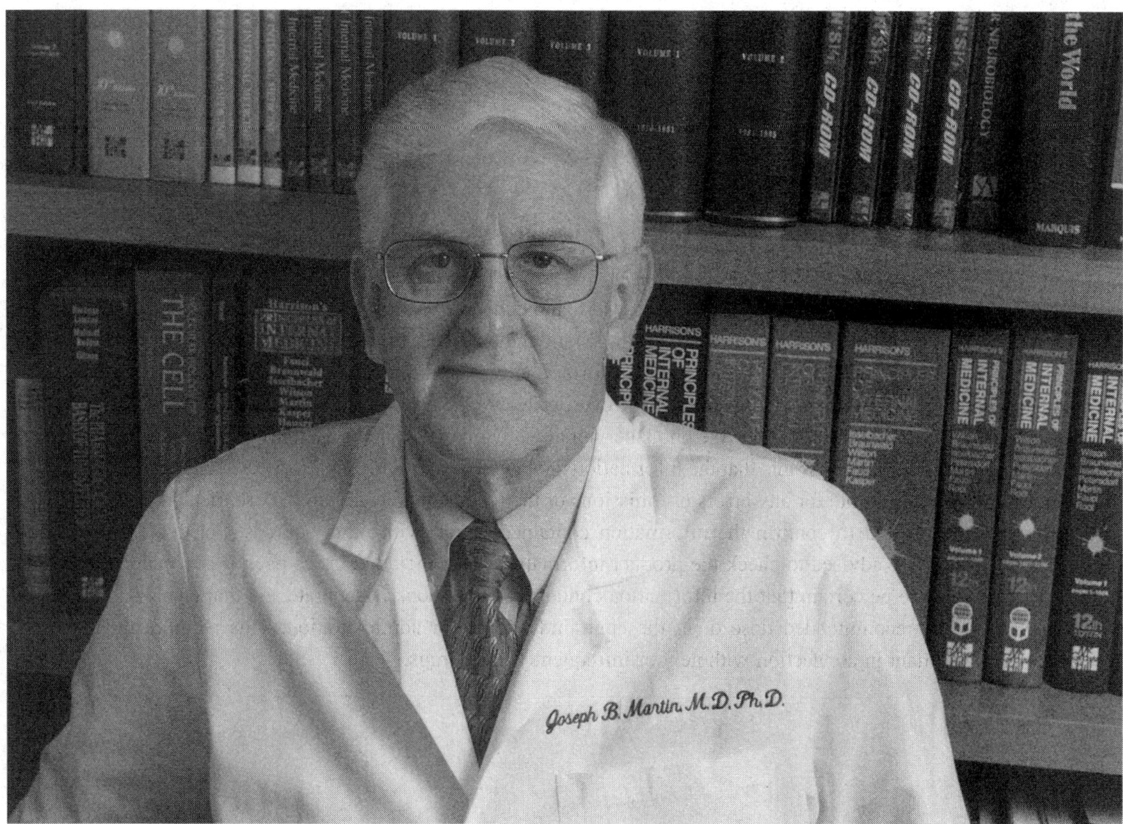

JOSEPH B. MARTIN

The editors wish to acknowledge the enormous contributions made by Joseph B. Martin, who edited the Neurology section of *Harrison's* from the tenth to the fourteenth editions. Dr. Martin followed Dr. Raymond D. Adams as editor of the Neurology section. In retrospect, the choice of Joseph Martin to replace Adams was prescient. It foresaw the transformation of neurology in the 1980s and 1990s from a largely descriptive discipline to one of the most dynamic and rapidly evolving areas of internal medicine. With his appointment as editor, the textbook had secured the foremost leader in the new field of molecular neurology to its ranks. Beginning with the tenth edition, Martin built upon the powerful didactic structure of the "syndromic approach" to neurology created by Adams and emphasized advances in molecular genetics and cell biology that reclassify neurologic diseases, clarify disease mechanisms, and offer new insights into clinical diagnosis and therapy. During his tenure, the neurology section of *Harrison's* became the best resource of its kind for the exposition of new discoveries in neurology and contributed substantially to the growing overall success of the textbook.

Born in Bassano, Alberta, Canada, Dr. Martin received his premedical and medical education at the University of Alberta, Edmonton, trained in neurology at Case Western University, and received the PhD from the University of Rochester. His career in academic medicine began in 1971 at McGill University in Montreal, where he established an independent laboratory focused on hypothalamic regulation of pituitary hormone secretion, and where he quickly rose to become Chair of the Department of Neurology and Neurosurgery. In 1978, he joined the faculty at Harvard Medical School as Bullard (later Julianne Dorn) Professor of Neurology and Chief of the Neurology Service at Massachusetts General Hospital. While at Harvard, he established the Huntington's Disease Center Without Walls, which in 1983 reported the spectacular finding of a genetic marker linked to Huntington's disease, thereby inaugurating the modern era of molecular neurogenetics. In 1989 Dr. Martin joined the University of California, San Francisco, initially serving as Dean of the School of Medicine and subsequently as Chancellor. Among his many achievements at UCSF was the conception of a major new research campus in San Francisco, which is fast becoming a reality. In July 1997, he returned to Harvard as the Caroline Shields Walker Professor of Neurobiology and Clinical Neuroscience and Dean of the Faculty of Medicine. A wonderful teacher and physician, Joe Martin has inspired a generation of housestaff, students, and colleagues at Harvard and UCSF.

Dr. Martin has received many honors, including honorary degrees from five distinguished universities and the Abraham Flexner Award of the Association of American Medical Colleges. He serves or has served on the editorial boards of nineteen medical and neurology journals. He is a member of the Institute of Medicine of the National Academy of Sciences and has served as President of the American Neurological Association.

Dr. Martin's many contributions to this textbook were enhanced by his extraordinary organizational skills and by a clear and direct style of writing and editing that permitted him to distill complex concepts into easily readable prose accessible to a general medical readership. As an example, his chapter on neurogenetics has become an instant classic and a highlight of each new edition of the book. The editors greatly value their friendship with this remarkable man whose integrity and intellectual strengths have served *Harrison's* so well during the past two decades.

CONTENTS

SECTION 2
DISORDERS OF HEMATOPOIESIS

SECTION 3
DISORDERS OF HEMOSTASIS

Part Seven

INFECTIOUS DISEASES

SECTION 1
BASIC CONSIDERATIONS IN INFECTIOUS DISEASES

SECTION 2
CLINICAL SYNDROMES: COMMUNITY-ACQUIRED INFECTIONS

Part Ten

DISORDERS OF THE KIDNEY AND URINARY TRACT

Part Eleven

DISORDERS OF THE GASTROINTESTINAL SYSTEM

SECTION 1
DISORDERS OF THE ALIMENTARY TRACT

SECTION 2
LIVER AND BILIARY TRACT DISEASE

Part Fourteen

NEUROLOGIC DISORDERS

SECTION 1
DIAGNOSIS OF NEUROLOGIC DISORDERS

SECTION 2
DISEASES OF THE CENTRAL NERVOUS SYSTEM

SECTION 3
DISORDERS OF NERVE AND MUSCLES

SECTION 4
CHRONIC FATIGUE SYNDROME

SECTION 5
PSYCHIATRIC DISORDERS

SECTION 6
ALCOHOLISM AND DRUG DEPENDENCY

CONTRIBUTORS

Numbers in brackets refer to chapters written or co-written by the contributor.

ELIAS ABRUTYN, MD
Professor of Medicine and Public Health; Associate Provost and Associate Dean for Faculty Affairs, Department of Medicine, Division of Infectious Diseases, MCP Hahnemann University School of Medicine, Philadelphia [143, 144]

JOHN W. ADAMSON, MD
Director, Blood Research Institute, Blood Center of Southeastern Wisconsin, Milwaukee [61, 105]

DAVID A. AHLQUIST, MD
Professor of Medicine, Mayo Medical School; Consultant in Gastroenterology, Mayo Clinic and Foundation, Rochester [42]

LEENA ALA-KOKKO, MD
Collagen Research Unit, Biocenter Oulu and Department of Medical Biochemistry, University of Oulu, Finland [351]

MUHAMMAD T. AL-LOZI, MBBS
Assistant Professor of Neurology, Washington University, St. Louis [101]

MICHAEL J. AMINOFF, MD
Professor of Neurology, University of California San Francisco, San Francisco [22, 357, 363]

KENNETH C. ANDERSON, MD
Associate Professor of Medicine, Harvard Medical School; Medical Director, Blood Component Laboratory, Dana-Farber Cancer Institute, Boston [114]

ELLIOTT M. ANTMAN, MD
Associate Professor of Medicine, Harvard Medical School; Director, Samuel A. Levine Cardiac Unit, Brigham and Women's Hospital, Boston [243]

FREDERICK R. APPELBAUM, MD
Member and Director, Clinical Research Division Fred Hutchinson Cancer Research Center; Professor and Head, Division of Medical Oncology, University of Washington School of Medicine, Seattle [115]

GORDON L. ARCHER, MD
Chairman, Division of Infectious Diseases, Department of Internal Medicine; Professor of Medicine and Microbiology/Immunology, Medical College of Virginia, Campus of Virginia Commonwealth University, Richmond [137]

JAMES O. ARMITAGE, MD
Dean, College of Medicine, and Professor of Internal Medicine, Section of Oncology/Hematology, University of Nebraska, Omaha [112]

ARTHUR K. ASBURY, MD
Van Meter Professor of Neurology Emeritus, University of Pennsylvania School of Medicine, Philadelphia [23, 377, 378]

JOHN R. ASPLIN, MD
Assistant Professor of Medicine, Section of Nephrology, University of Chicago, Pritzker School of Medicine, Chicago [276, 279]

JOHN C. ATHERTON, MRCP
Lecturer, Department of Medicine, Division of Gastroenterology and Institute of Infections and Immunity, University of Nottingham, Nottingham, England [154]

PAUL S. AUERBACH, MD
Clinical Professor of Surgery, Division of Emergency Medicine, Stanford University School of Medicine, Los Altos [397]

K. FRANK AUSTEN, MD
Theodore Bevier Bayles Professor of Medicine, Harvard Medical School; Director, Inflammation and Allergic Diseases Research Section, Division of Rheumatology, Immunology and Allergy, Brigham and Women's Hospital, Boston [310]

BERNARD M. BABIOR, MD, PhD
Head, Division of Biochemistry, Department of Molecular and Experimental Medicine, The Scripps Research Institute; Professor and Staff Physician, Division of Hematology and Oncology, Department of Medicine, Scripps Clinic and Research Foundation, La Jolla [107]

KAMAL F. BADR, MD
Professor and Chair, Department of Internal Medicine, American University of Beirut (Lebanon); Attending Physician, American University of Beirut Medical Center, Beirut, Lebanon [278]

DONALD S. BAIM, MD
Professor of Medicine, Harvard Medical School; Director, Center for Minimally Invasive Therapy, Brigham and Women's Hospital, Boston [228, 245]

ROBERT L. BARBIERI, MD
Kate Macy Ladd Professor Obstetrics, Gynecology and Reproductive Biology, Harvard Medical School; Chairman, Department of Obstetrics and Gynecology, Brigham and Women's Hospital, Boston [7]

TAMAR F. BARLAM, MD
Assistant Professor of Medicine, Harvard Medical School; Senior Associate Physician, Beth Israel Deaconess Medical Center, Boston; Director, Project on Antibiotic Resistance, Center for Science in the Public Interest, Washington, D.C. [19, 150]

KENNETH J. BART, MD, MPH, MSHPM
Director, Graduate School of Public Health, San Diego State University, San Diego [122]

M. FLINT BEAL, MD
Anne Parrish Titzel Professor and Chairman of Neurology, Weill Medical College; Neurologist-in-Chief, New York Presbyterian Hospital, New York [367, 376]

ROBERT S. BENJAMIN, MD
Internist and Professor of Medicine, Chairman, Department of Melanoma/ Sarcoma Medical Oncology; Medical Director, Multidisciplinary Sarcoma Center, The University of Texas M.D. Anderson Cancer Center, Houston [98]

JOHN E. BENNETT, MD
Head, Clinical Mycology Section, Laboratory of Clinical Investigation, National Institute of Allergy and Infectious Diseases, National Institutes of Health, Potomac [200, 201, 202, 203, 204, 205, 206, 207, 208]

EDWARD J. BENZ, JR., MD
Richard and Susan Smith Professor of Medicine, Professor of Pediatrics and Pathology, Harvard Medical School; President, Dana-Farber Cancer Institute, Boston [106]

PAUL D. BERK, MD
Department of Medicine, Division of Liver Disease, Mount Sinai School of Medicine, New York [294]

DAVID R. BICKERS, MD
Carl Truman Nelson Professor and Chairman, Department of Dermatology, Columbia University, New York [60]

HENRY J. BINDER, MD
Professor of Medicine, Section of Digestive Diseases, Yale University, New Haven [286]

THOMAS D. BIRD, MD
Professor of Neurology, University of Washington; Chief of Neurology, Veterans Affairs Medical Center, Seattle [26, 362, 379]

NEIL R. BLACKLOW, MD
Richard M. Haidack Distinguished Professor of Medicine, Molecular Genetics and Microbiology, University of Massachusetts Medical School, Worcester [187]

MARTIN J. BLASER, MD
Frederick J. King Professor of Internal Medicine, Chairman, Department of Medicine, and Professor of Microbiology, New York University School of Medicine, New York [154, 158]

CLARA D. BLOOMFIELD, MD
Director, The Ohio State University Comprehensive Cancer Center; Deputy Director, The Arthur G. James Cancer Hospital and Richard J. Solove Research Institute; William G. Pace III Endowed Chair in Cancer Research; Director and Professor, Division of Hematology and Oncology, Department of Internal Medicine, College of Medicine and Public Health, The Ohio State University, Columbus [111]

RICHARD S. BLUMBERG, MD
Associate Professor of Medicine, Harvard Medical School; Chief, Division of Gastroenterology, Department of Medicine, Brigham and Women's Hospital, Boston [287]

JEAN L. BOLOGNIA, MD
Professor of Dermatology, Yale University School of Medicine, New Haven [57]

GEORGE J. BOSL, MD
Chairman, Department of Medicine, Memorial Sloan-Kettering Cancer Center; Professor of Medicine, Cornell University Medical College, New York [96]

PATRICK BOSQUE, MD
Assistant Professor of Neurology, Institute for Neurodegenerative Diseases, University of California San Francisco, San Francisco [375]

RICHARD C. BOUCHER, MD
William Rand Kenan Professor of Medicine, University of North Carolina at Chapel Hill; Director, Cystic Fibrosis/Pulmonary Research & Treatment Center, Chapel Hill [257]

KAREN D. BRADSHAW, MD
Associate Professor of Obstetrics and Gynecology, The University of Texas Southwestern Medical Center, Dallas [52, 336]

HUGH R. BRADY, MD, PhD
Professor of Medicine and Therapeutics, University College Dublin; Mater Misericordiae Hospital, Dublin, Ireland [269, 273, 274, 275]

KENNETH D. BRANDT, MD
Professor of Medicine and Head, Rheumatology Division, Indiana University School of Medicine; Director, Indiana University Multipurpose Arthritis and Musculoskeletal Disease Center, Indianapolis [321]

EUGENE BRAUNWALD, MD, MD(Hon), ScD(Hon)
Distinguished Hersey Professor of Medicine; Faculty Dean for Academic Programs at Brigham and Women's Hospital and Massachusetts General Hospital, Harvard Medical School; Vice-President for Academic Programs, Partners HealthCare System, Boston [32, 33, 34, 36, 37, 224, 225, 231, 232, 236, 237, 238, 239, 243, 244]

IRWIN M. BRAVERMAN, MD
Professor of Dermatology, Yale University School of Medicine, New Haven [57]

OTIS W. BRAWLEY, MD
Assistant Director, Office of Special Populations Research, Office of the Director, National Cancer Institute, National Institutes of Health, Bethesda [80]

JOEL G. BREMAN, MD, DTPH
Deputy Director, Division of International Training and Research, Fogarty International Center, National Institutes of Health, Bethesda [214]

BARRY M. BRENNER, MD, DSc(Hon), DMSc(Hon)
Samuel A. Levine Professor of Medicine, Harvard Medical School; Director, Renal Division, Brigham and Women's Hospital, Boston [47, 49, 268, 269, 270, 271, 273, 274, 275, 277, 278, 281]

ROBERT M. BRENNER, MD
Associate Medical Director, Clinical Research, Amgen Inc., Thousand Oaks, California [268]

CHARLES G. D. BROOK, MA, MD
Emeritus Professor of Pediatric Endocrinology, University College London, London, UK [8]

CLAIRE V. BROOME, MD
Senior Advisor to the Director, Integrated Health Information Systems, Centers for Disease Control and Prevention, Atlanta [142]

ROBERT H. BROWN, JR., DPhil, MD
Associate Neurologist, Massachusetts General Hospital; Professor of Neurology, Harvard Medical School, Boston [365, 383]

ROBERT C. BRUNHAM, MD
Professor of Medicine; Director and Medical Director, University of British Columbia Centre for Disease Control, Vancouver, BC, Canada [133]

H. FRANKLIN BUNN, MD
Professor of Medicine, Harvard Medical School; Physician, Brigham and Women's Hospital, Boston [107, 108]

DAVID M. BURNS, MD
Professor of Medicine, University of California San Diego, San Diego [390]

MICHAEL J. BURNS, MD
Instructor of Medicine, Harvard Medical School; Department of Emergency Medicine, Division of Toxicology, Beth Israel Deaconess Medical Center, Boston [396]

JOAN R. BUTTERTON, MD
Assistant Professor of Medicine, Harvard Medical School; Assistant in Medicine, Infectious Disease Division, Massachusetts General Hospital, Boston [131]

JOHN C. BYRD, MD
Director of Clinical Research, Hematology-Oncology Service, Department of Medicine, Walter Reed Army Medical Center, Washington, D.C. [111]

STEPHEN B. CALDERWOOD, MD
Chief, Division of Infectious Diseases, Massachusetts General Hospital; Associate Professor of Medicine (Microbiology and Molecular Genetics), Harvard Medical School, Boston [131]

MICHAEL CAMILLERI, MD
Professor of Medicine and Physiology, Mayo Medical School; Consultant in Gastroenterology, Physiology and Biophysics, Mayo Clinic and Mayo Foundation, Rochester [42]

GRANT L. CAMPBELL, MD, PhD
Division of Vector-Borne Infectious Diseases, National Center for Infectious Diseases, Centers for Disease Control and Prevention, Fort Collins [162, 175]

MARK D. CARLSON, MD
Vice Chair, Department of Medicine, University Hospitals of Cleveland; Associate Professor of Medicine, Case Western Reserve University School of Medicine, Cleveland [21]

CHARLES B. CARPENTER, MD
Professor of Medicine, Harvard Medical School; Senior Physician, Brigham and Women's Hospital, Boston [272]

BRUCE R. CARR, MD
Professor and Director, Division of Reproductive Endocrinology, and Holder, Paul C. MacDonald Distinguished Chair in Obstetrics and Gynecology, The University of Texas Southwestern Medical Center, Dallas [52, 336]

AGUSTIN CASTELLANOS, MD
Professor of Medicine and Director, Clinical Electrophysiology, University of Miami School of Medicine, Miami [39]

PHILLIP F. CHANCE, MD
Professor of Pediatrics and Neurology, University of Washington School of Medicine; Chief, Division of Genetics and Development, Children's Hospital and Regional Medical Center, Seattle [379]

FENG-YEE CHANG, MD, DSc
Associate Professor of Medicine, National Defense Medical Center; Chief, Division of Infectious Diseases, Tri-Service General Hospital, Taipei, Taiwan [151]

YUAN-TSONG CHEN, MD, PhD
Professor of Pediatrics and Genetics, and Chief, Division of Medical Genetics, Duke University Medical Center, Durham [350]

JOHN S. CHILD, MD
Professor of Medicine, University of California, Los Angeles; Co-Chief, Cardiology and Co-Director, Ahmanson/UCLA Adult Congenital Heart Disease Center, UCLA Medical Center, Los Angeles [234]

OLIVIER M. CHOSIDOW, MD
Department of Internal Medicine, Pitie-Salpêtrière Hospital, Paris, France [59]

RAYMOND T. CHUNG, MD
Medical Director, Liver Transplant Program; Director, Liver Service, Gastrointestinal Unit, Massachusetts General Hospital; Assistant Professor of Medicine, Harvard Medical School, Boston [299]

FREDRIC L. COE, MD
Professor of Medicine and Physiology and Director, Clinical Research Training Program, University of Chicago Pritzker School of Medicine, Chicago [276, 279]

ALAN S. COHEN, MD
Distinguished Professor of Medicine in Rheumatology, Emeritus, and Conrad Wesselhoeft Professor of Medicine, Emeritus, Boston University School of Medicine; Chief of Medicine and Director, Emeritus, Thorndike Memorial Laboratory, Boston City Hospital, Boston [319]

JEFFREY I. COHEN, MD
Head, Medical Virology Section, Laboratory of Clinical Investigation, National Institute of Allergy and Infectious Diseases, National Institutes of Health, Bethesda [184, 193]

FRANCIS S. COLLINS, MD, PhD
Director, National Human Genome Research Institute, National Institutes of Health, Bethesda [81]

WILSON S. COLUCCI, MD
Professor of Medicine, and Chief, Cardiovascular Medicine, Boston University School of Medicine, Boston [240]

GERALD A. COLVIN, DO
Assistant Professor of Medicine and Medical Research Scientist, University of Massachusetts Memorial Medical Center, Worcester [104]

MAUREEN T. CONNELLY, MD, MPH
Instructor in Medicine, Harvard Medical School; Harvard Pilgrim Health Care, Boston [10]

MAX D. COOPER, MD
Professor of Medicine, Pediatrics and Howard Hughes Medical Institute Investigator, University of Alabama at Birmingham, Birmingham [308]

LAWRENCE COREY, MD
Professor, Medicine and Laboratory Medicine, and Head, Virology Division, University of Washington; Head, Program in Infectious Diseases, Fred Hutchinson Cancer Research Center, Seattle [182, 197]

FELICIA COSMAN, MD
Associate Professor of Clinical Medicine, Columbia University; Medical Director, Clinical Research Center, Helen Hayes Hospital, West Haverstraw [342]

MARK A. CREAGER, MD
Associate Professor of Medicine, Harvard Medical School; Director, Vascular Center, Brigham and Women's Hospital, Boston [247, 248]

PHILIP E. CRYER, MD
Irene E. and Michael M. Karl Professor of Endocrinology and Metabolism, and Director, Division of Endocrinology, Diabetes and Metabolism, Washington University School of Medicine, St. Louis [334]

RONALD G. CRYSTAL, MD
Bruce Webster Professor of Medicine, Director, Institute of Genetic Medicine, and Director, The Arthur and Rochelle Belfer Gene Therapy Care Facility, Weill Medical College of Cornell University, New York [318]

JOHN J. CUSH, MD
Medical Director, Arthritis Center, Presbyterian Hospital of Dallas, Dallas [320]

CHARLES A. CZEISLER, MD, PhD
Professor of Medicine, Harvard Medical School; Director, Sleep Disorders and Circadian Medicine, Brigham and Women's Hospital, Boston [27]

MARINOS C. DALAKAS, JR., MD
Chief, Neuromuscular Diseases Section, National Institute of Neurological Disorders and Stroke, National Institutes of Health, Bethesda [382]

DANIEL F. DANZL, MD
Professor and Chair, Department of Emergency Medicine, University of Louisville School of Medicine, Floyd Knobs, IN [20]

ROBERT B. DAROFF, MD
Chief of Staff and Senior Vice President for Academic Affairs, University Hospitals of Cleveland; Professor of Neurology and Associate Dean, Case Western Reserve University School of Medicine, Cleveland [21]

MEHUL T. DATTANI, MD
Senior Lecturer/Honorary Consultant in Pediatric Endocrinology, Institute of Child Health and Great Ormond Street Children's Hospital, London, UK [8]

CHARLES E. DAVIS, MD
Professor of Pathology and Medicine, University of California - San Diego School of Medicine; Director Emeritus, Microbiology Laboratory, UCSD Medical Center, San Diego [211]

JOHN DEL VALLE, MD
Professor of Medicine, Division of Gastroenterology, Department of Medicine, University of Michigan School of Medicine, Ann Arbor [285]

BRADLEY M. DENKER, MD
Assistant Professor of Medicine, Harvard Medical School; Associate Physician, Brigham and Women's Hospital, Boston [47]

DAVID T. DENNIS, MD, MPH
Chief, Bacterial Zoonoses Branch, Centers for Disease Control and Prevention, Fort Collins [162, 175]

ROBERT L. DERESIEWICZ, MD
Assistant Professor of Medicine, Harvard Medical School, Boston [139, 159]

ROBERT J. DESNICK, PhD, MD
Professor and Chairman, Department of Human Genetics, Mount Sinai School of Medicine, New York [346]

BETTY DIAMOND, MD
Chief, Division of Rheumatology, Department of Microbiology and Immunology, Albert Einstein College of Medicine, New York [307]

JULES L. DIENSTAG, MD
Associate Professor of Medicine, Harvard Medical School; Physician, Massachusetts General Hospital, Boston [91, 295, 296, 297, 301]

WILLIAM P. DILLON, MD
Professor of Radiology, Neurology and Neurosurgery; Chief, Diagnostic Neuroradiology, University of California San Francisco, San Francisco [358]

CHARLES A. DINARELLO, MD
Professor of Medicine, University of Colorado Health Sciences Center, Denver [17]

ROBERT G. DLUHY, MD
Professor of Medicine, Harvard Medical School, Brigham and Women's Hospital, Boston [331]

RAPHAEL DOLIN, MD
Maxwell Finland Professor of Medicine, and Dean for Clinical Programs, Harvard Medical School, Boston [181, 189, 190]

DANIEL B. DRACHMAN, MD
Professor of Neurology and Neurosciences; Director, Neuromuscular Unit, The Johns Hopkins University School of Medicine, Baltimore [380]

JEFFREY M. DRAZEN, MD
Professor of Medicine, Harvard Medical School; Senior Physician, Brigham and Women's Hospital, Boston [249, 250, 251, 266]

THOMAS D. DUBOSE, JR., MD
Peter T. Bohan Professor and Chairman, Department of Internal Medicine; Professor of Molecular and Integrative Physiology, University of Kansas School of Medicine, Kansas City [50]

J. STEPHEN DUMLER, MD
Associate Professor and Associate Director, Division of Medical Microbiology, Department of Pathology, The Johns Hopkins Medical Institutions, Baltimore [177]

ANDREA E. DUNAIF, MD
Associate Professor of Medicine, Director, Center of Excellence in Women's Health, Harvard Medical School; Chief, Division of Women's Health and Senior Physician, Brigham and Women's Hospital, Boston [6]

MARLENE DURAND, MD
Assistant Professor of Medicine, Harvard Medical School, Boston [30]

JANICE DUTCHER, MD
Professor of Medicine, New York Medical College; Associate Director for Clinical Affairs, Our Lady of Mercy Comprehensive Cancer Center, New York [102]

JOHANNA DWYER, MD
Professor of Medicine and Community Health, Tufts University School of Medicine; Professor, Tufts University School of Nutrition Science and Policy; Senior Scientist, Jean Mayer USDA Human Nutrition Research Center at Tufts University, Boston [73]

VICTOR J. DZAU, MD
Hersey Professor of the Theory and Practice of Physic (Medicine), Harvard Medical School; Chairman, Department of Medicine, and Director of Research, Brigham and Women's Hospital, Boston [247, 248]

JEFFERY S. DZIECZKOWSKI, MD
Assistant Professor, Departments of Pathology and Internal Medicine, Wayne State University School of Medicine, Detroit [114]

J. DONALD EASTON, MD
Professor and Chair, Department of Clinical Neurosciences, Brown University School of Medicine; Neurologist-in-Chief, Rhode Island Hospital, Providence [361]

DAVID A. EHRMANN, MD
Associate Professor, Section of Endocrinology, Department of Medicine, University of Chicago, Chicago [53]

JOHN W. ENGSTROM, MD
Associate Professor of Neurology, and Vice Chairman, Department of Neurology, University of California San Francisco, San Francisco [16, 366]

ALAN EPSTEIN, MD
Assistant Professor of Medicine, Brown University School of Medicine, Providence [289]

ANTHONY S. FAUCI, MD
Chief, Laboratory of Immunoregulation; Director, National Institute of Allergy and Infectious Diseases, National Institutes of Health, Bethesda [191, 305, 309, 317]

MURRAY J. FAVUS, MD
Professor of Medicine, University of Chicago Pritzker School of Medicine; Director, General Clinical Research Center; Director, Bone Program, Chicago [279]

ROBERT G. FENTON, MD, PhD
Associate Professor of Medicine, University of Maryland Greenebaum Cancer Center, Baltimore [82]

HOWARD L. FIELDS, MD, PhD
Professor of Neurology and Physiology, University of California San Francisco, San Francisco [12]

GREGORY A. FILICE, MD
Associate Professor of Medicine, University of Minnesota; Chief, Infectious Disease Section, Veterans Affairs Medical Center, Minneapolis [165]

ROBERT FINBERG, MD
Professor of Medicine, and Chair Department of Medicine, University of Massachusetts Medical School, Worcester [85, 136]

JOYCE D. FINGEROTH, MD
Assistant Professor of Medicine, Harvard Medical School; Physician, Beth Israel Deaconess Medical Center, Boston [136]

JEFFREY S. FLIER, MD
George C. Reisman Professor of Medicine, Harvard Medical School; Vice-Chair for Research, and Chief, Division of Endocrinology, Department of Medicine, Beth Israel Deaconess Medical Center, Boston [77]

JUDAH FOLKMAN, MD
Surgeon-in-Chief, Emeritus, Director, Surgical Research Laboratory, Children's Hospital; Andrus Professor of Pediatric Surgery, Professor of Cell Biology, Department of Surgery, Harvard Medical School, Boston [83]

SONIA FRIEDMAN, MD
Instructor in Medicine, Harvard Medical School; Associate Physician in Medicine, Brigham and Women's Hospital, Boston [287]

WILLIAM F. FRIEDMAN, MD
J.H. Nicholson Professor of Pediatrics (Cardiology); Associate Dean for Academic Affairs, University of California, Los Angeles School of Medicine and UCLA Medical Center, Los Angeles [234]

ADRIANE FUGH-BERMAN, MD
Assistant Clinical Professor, Department of Health Care Sciences, George Washington University School of Medicine, Washington, D.C. [11]

ROBERT F. GAGEL, MD
Chairman, Department of Internal Medicine Specialties, and Chief, Section of Endocrine Neoplasia and Hormonal Disorders, University of Texas M.D. Anderson Cancer Center, Houston [339]

JOHN I. GALLIN, MD
Director, NIH Warren Grant G. Magnuson Clinical Center; NIH Associate Director for Clinical Research; Chief Laboratory of Host Defenses, National Institute of Allergy and Infectious Diseases, National Institutes of Health, Bethesda [64]

ABHIMANYU GARG, MD
Professor, Department of Internal Medicine, Center for Human Nutrition, University of Texas Southwestern Medical Center at Dallas; Director, Diabetes Clinic, Department of Veterans Affairs Medical Center, Dallas [354]

ROBERT H. GELBER, MD
Clinical Professor of Medicine and Dermatology, University of California San Francisco, San Anselmo [170]

JEFFREY A. GELFAND, MD
Visiting Professor of Medicine, Harvard Medical School; Distinguished Professor of Medicine, Tufts University School of Medicine; Attending Physician in Infectious Diseases, Massachusetts General Hospital, Boston [17, 125]

ANNE A. GERSHON, MD
Professor of Pediatrics, and Director of Division of Pediatric Infectious Diseases, Columbia University College of Physicians and Surgeons, New York [194, 195, 196]

MARC GHANY, MD
Medical Staff Fellow, Liver Diseases Section, Digestive Diseases Branch, National Institute of Diabetes and Digestive and Kidney Diseases, National Institutes of Health, Bethesda [292]

RAYMOND J. GIBBONS, MD
Arthur M. and Glady D. Gray Professor of Medicine, Mayo Medical School, Rochester [227]

BRUCE C. GILLILAND, MD
Professor of Medicine and Laboratory Medicine, University of Washington School of Medicine, Seattle [313, 325, 326]

HENRY N. GINSBERG, MD
Irving Professor of Medicine, Columbia University College of Physicians and Surgeons, New York [344]

ELI GLATSTEIN, MD
Vice-Chairman and Clinical Director, Radiation Oncology, University of Pennsylvania Medical Center, Philadelphia [394]

ROBERT M. GLICKMAN, MD
Professor of Medicine and Dean, New York University School of Medicine, New York [46]

IRA J. GOLDBERG, MD
Professor of Medicine, Division of Preventive Medicine and Nutrition, Columbia University College of Physicians and Surgeons, New York [344]

ARY L. GOLDBERGER, MD
Associate Professor of Medicine, Harvard Medical School; Director, Margret and H.A. Rey Laboratory for Nonlinear Dynamics in Medicine, Beth Israel Deaconess Medical Center, Boston [226]

SAMUEL Z. GOLDHABER, MD
Associate Professor of Medicine, Harvard Medical School; Director, Venous Thromboembolism Research Group; Director, Cardiac Center's Anticoagulation Service, Brigham and Women's Hospital, Boston [261]

DONALD E. GOODKIN, MD
San Rafael, California [371]

RAJ K. GOYAL, MD
Associate Chief of Staff for Research and Development, VA Medical Center; Mallinckrodt Professor of Medicine, Harvard Medical School, West Roxbury [40, 284]

GREGORY A. GRABOWSKI, MD
Professor of Pediatrics; Director, Division and Program in Human Genetics, Children's Hospital Research Foundation, Cincinnati [349]

JACOB GREEN, MD
Associate Professor of Medicine, Department of Nephrology, Technion Faculty of Medicine, Haifa, Israel [270]

HARRY B. GREENBERG, MD
Senior Associate Dean for Research, Professor of Medicine, Microbiology and Immunology, and ACOS for Research VAPAHCS, Stanford University, Stanford [192]

NORTON J. GREENBERGER, MD
Professor of Medicine, and Senior Associate Dean for Medical Education, University of Kansas School of Medicine, Kansas City [302, 303, 304]

JOHN S. GREENSPAN, BDS, PhD
Professor and Chair, Department of Stomatology and Director, Oral AIDS Center, School of Dentistry; Professor, Department of Pathology, and Director, AIDS Clinical Research Center, School of Medicine, University of California San Francisco, San Francisco [31]

DARYL R. GRESS, MD
Associate Professor of Neurology and Neurosurgery; Director, Neurovascular Service, University of California San Francisco, San Francisco [376]

JAMES E. GRIFFIN, MD
Diana and Richard C. Strauss Professor in Biomedical Research, and Professor of Internal Medicine, University of Texas Southwestern Medical Center, Dallas [335, 338]

WILLIAM GROSSMAN, MD
Myer Friedman Distinguished Professor of Medicine, University of California San Francisco; Chief of Cardiology, University of California San Francisco Medical Center, San Francisco [228]

RASIM GUCALP, MD
Associate Professor of Medicine, Department of Oncology, Montefiore Medical Center, Albert Einstein College of Medicine, New York [102]

BEVRA HANNAHS HAHN, MD
Professor of Medicine, Chief of Rheumatology, and Vice-Chair, Department of Medicine, University of California, Los Angeles, Los Angeles [311]

STEPHEN M. HAHN, MD
Assistant Professor of Medicine, Department of Radiation Oncology, University of Pennsylvania Medical Center, Philadelphia [394]

JANET E. HALL, MD
Associate Professor of Medicine, Harvard Medical School; Assistant Chief, Reproductive Endocrine Unit, Massachusetts General Hospital, Boston [54]

SCOTT A. HALPERIN, MD
Professor of Pediatrics, and Associate Professor of Microbiology and Immunology, Dalhousie University; Head, Pediatric Infectious Diseases, IWK-Grace Health Center, Halifax, Nova Scotia, Canada [152]

CHARLES H. HALSTED, MD
Professor of Internal Medicine, Division of Clinical Nutrition and Metabolism, University of California-Davis School of Medicine, Davis [74]

ROBERT I. HANDIN, MD
Professor of Medicine, Harvard Medical School; Co-Director, Hematology Division, and Executive Vice Chairman, Department of Medicine, Brigham and Women's Hospital, Boston [62, 116, 117, 118]

GAVIN HART, MD, MPH
Director, STD Services, Royal Adelaide Hospital; Clinical Associate Professor, School of Medicine, Flinders University, Adelaide South Australia, Australia [164]

WILLIAM L. HASLER, MD
Associate Professor of Internal Medicine, Division of Gastroenterology, University of Michigan Medical Center, Ann Arbor [41]

TERRY HASSOLD, PhD
Professor, Department of Genetics, Case Western Reserve University and the Center for Human Genetics, University Hospitals of Cleveland, Cleveland [66]

STEPHEN L. HAUSER, MD
Betty Anker Fife Professor and Chairman, Department of Neurology, University of California San Francisco, San Francisco [355, 356, 361, 367, 368, 371, 378]

BARTON F. HAYNES, MD
Frederic M. Hanes Professor of Medicine, and Chair, Department of Medicine, Duke University Medical Center, Durham [305]

J. CLAUDE HEMPHILL III, MD
Assistant Professor of Neurology, University of California San Francisco; Director, Neurovascular and Neurocritical Care Program, San Francisco General Hospital, San Francisco [376]

PATRICK H. HENRY, MD
Chairman, Department of Medicine, St. John's Mercy Medical Center, St. Louis [63]

BARBARA L. HERWALDT, MD, MPH
Medical Epidemiologist, Division of Parasitic Diseases, Centers for Disease Control Prevention, Atlanta [215]

MARTIN S. HIRSCH, MD
Professor of Medicine, Harvard Medical School; Director, AIDS Clinical Research, Massachusetts General Hospital, Boston [185]

BERNARD HIRSCHEL, MD
Associate Professor of Medicine; Head, HIV/AIDS Section, Division of Infectious Diseases, University Hospital, Geneva [171]

MICHAEL F. HOLICK, MD, PhD
Professor of Medicine, Department of Endocrinology, Diabetes and Metabolism, Boston University School of Medicine, Boston [340]

STEVEN M. HOLLAND, MD
Senior Investigator and Head, Immunopathogenesis Unit, Clinical Pathophysiology Section, Laboratory of Host Defenses, National Institute of Allergy and Infectious Diseases, National Institute of Health, Bethesda [64]

KING K. HOLMES, MD, PhD
Professor of Medicine, and Director, Center for AIDS and Sexually Transmitted Diseases, University of Washington; Head, Infectious Diseases, Harborview Medical Center, Seattle [132, 133]

RANDALL K. HOLMES, MD, PhD
Professor and Chair, Department of Microbiology, University of Colorado School of Medicine, Denver [141]

ERIC G. HONIG, MD
Professor of Medicine, Emory University School of Medicine, Atlanta [258]

JAY H. HOOFNAGLE, MD
Director, Division of Digestive Diseases and Nutrition, National Institute of Diabetes and Digestive and Kidney Diseases, National Institutes of Health, Bethesda [292]

JONATHAN C. HORTON, MD, PhD
Associate Professor of Ophthalmology, Neurology, and Physiology, University of California San Francisco, San Francisco [28]

LYN HOWARD, MB
Professor of Medicine, Associate Professor of Pediatrics, and Head-Division of Clinical Nutrition in Department of Medicine, Albany Medical College, Albany [76]

HOWARD HU, MD, DPH
Associate Professor of Occupational Medicine, Harvard School of Public Health; Assistant Professor of Medicine, Harvard Medical School; Associate Physician, Channing Laboratory, Brigham and Women's Hospital, Boston [5, 391, 395]

GARY W. HUNNINGHAKE, MD
Professor, Department of Internal Medicine, and Director, Division of Pulmonary, Critical Care, and Occupational Medicine, University of Iowa College of Medicine, Iowa City [253]

EDWARD P. INGENITO, MD
Assistant Professor of Medicine, Harvard Medical School; Director, Pulmonary Function Laboratory, Brigham and Women's Hospital, Boston [266]

Roland H. Ingram, Jr., MD
Martha West Looney Professor Emeritus, Emory University School of Medicine, Atlanta [32, 258, 265]

Thomas S. Inui, ScM, MD
President and CEO, The Fetzer Institute, Kalamazoo, Michigan [10]

Mark A. Israel, MD
Professor, Departments of Neurological Surgery and Pediatrics; Director, Preuss Laboratory of Molecular Neuro-Oncology, University of California San Francisco, San Francisco [370]

Kurt J. Isselbacher, MD
Distinguished Mallinckrodt Professor of Medicine, Harvard Medical School; Physician and Director, Massachusetts General Hospital Cancer Center, Boston [91, 282, 289, 295, 296, 297, 345]

Richard F. Jacobs, MD, FAAP
Horace C. Cabe Professor of Pediatrics, University of Arkansas for Medical Sciences; Chief, Pediatric Infectious Diseases, Arkansas Children's Hospital, Little Rock [161]

J. Larry Jameson, MD, PhD
Irving S. Cutter Professor and Chairman, Department of Medicine, Northwestern University Medical School; Physician-in-Chief, Northwestern Memorial Hospital, Chicago [65, 68, 327, 330]

Robert T. Jensen, MD
Digestive Diseases Branch, National Institute of Diabetes and Digestive and Kidney Diseases, National Institutes of Health, Bethesda [93]

Donald R. Johns, MD
Associate Professor of Neurology and Ophthalmology; Harvard Medical School; Director, Division of Neuromuscular Disease, Beth Israel Deaconess Medical Center, Boston [67]

Bruce E. Johnson, MD
Associate Professor of Medicine, Brigham and Women's Hospital and Harvard Medical School; Program Director, Lowe Center for Thoracic Oncology, Dana-Farber Cancer Institute, Boston [100]

Michael Joseph, MD
Physician, Weber Medical Clinic, Ltd., Olney, Illinois [30]

Mark E. Josephson, MD
Professor of Medicine, Harvard Medical School; Director of the Harvard Thorndike Electrophysiology Institute and Arrhythmia Services, Beth Israel Deaconess Medical Center, Boston [229, 230]

Edward L. Kaplan, MD
Professor of Pediatrics, Department of Pediatrics, University of Minnesota Medical School, Minneapolis [235]

Marshall M. Kaplan, MD
Professor of Medicine, Tufts University School of Medicine; Chief, Gastroenterology Department, New England Medical Center, Boston [45, 293]

Adolf W. Karchmer, MD
Chief, Division of Infectious Diseases, Beth Israel Deaconess Medical Center; Professor of Medicine, Harvard Medical School, Boston [126]

Dennis L. Kasper, MD, MA (Hon)
William Ellery Channing Professor of Medicine, Professor of Microbiology and Molecular Genetics, Executive Dean for Academic Programs, Harvard Medical School; Director, Channing Laboratory, Department of Medicine, Brigham and Women's Hospital, Boston [19, 119, 130, 145, 150, 160, 167]

Lloyd H. Kasper, MD
Professor of Medicine (Neurology) and Microbiology, Dartmouth Medical School, Hanover [217]

Mark A. Kay, MD, PhD
Director, Program in Human Gene Therapy, and Associate Professor, Departments of Pediatrics and Genetics, Stanford University School of Medicine, Stanford [69]

Elaine T. Kaye, MD
Clinical Instructor in Dermatology, Harvard Medical School; Assistant in Medicine, Department of Medicine, Children's Hospital Medical Center, Weston [18]

Kenneth M. Kaye, MD
Assistant Professor of Medicine, Harvard Medical School; Associate Physician, Division of Infectious Diseases, Brigham and Women's Hospital, Boston [18]

Gerald T. Keusch, MD
Associate Director for International Research; Director, Fogarty International Center, National Institutes of Health; Professor of Medicine, Tufts University School of Medicine; New England Medical Center, Bethesda [122, 157, 159]

J. S. Keystone, MD
Professor of Medicine, University of Toronto; Centre for Travel and Tropical Medicine, Division of Infectious Disease, Toronto General Hospital, Toronto, Ontario, Canada [123]

Elliott Kieff, MD, PhD
Albee Professor of Medicine and Microbiology and Molecular Genetics, Harvard Medical School, Boston [180]

Talmadge E. King, Jr., MD
Constance B. Wofsy Distinguished Professor and Vice Chairman, Department of Medicine, University of California San Francisco; Chief, Medical Services, San Francisco General Hospital, San Francisco [259]

Louis V. Kirchhoff, MD, MPH
Professor, Department of Internal Medicine, University of Iowa; Staff Physician, Department of Veterans Affairs Medical Center, Iowa City [216]

Joel N. Kline, MD
Assistant Professor, University of Iowa College of Medicine, Iowa City [253]

Howard K. Koh, MD, PhD
Professor of Dermatology, Medicine and Public Health, Boston University Schools of Medicine and Public Health; Co-Director, Skin Oncology Program, Director, Cancer Prevention and Control Center, Boston [86]

Anthony L. Komaroff, MD
Professor of Medicine, Harvard Medical School; Senior Physician, Brigham and Women's Hospital, Boston [6]

Peter Kopp, MD
Assistant Professor of Medicine, Division of Endocrinology, Metabolism and Molecular Medicine, Northwestern University, Chicago [65]

Walter J. Koroshetz, MD
Associate Professor of Neurology and Medicine; Associate Director, Stroke and Clinical Neurology Services, Massachusetts General Hospital, Harvard Medical School, Boston [374]

P. E. Kozarsky, MD
Associate Professor of Medicine, Emory University School of Medicine; Adjunct Assistant Professor of Medicine, Emory University School of Public Health, Atlanta [123]

Barnett S. Kramer, MD, MPH
Director, Office of Medical Applications of Research, National Institutes of Health, Bethesda [80]

Stephen M. Krane, MD
Persis, Cyrus and Marlow B. Harrison Professor of Medicine, Harvard Medical School; Physician and Chief, Arthritis Unit, Massachusetts General Hospital, Boston [340, 343]

Helena Kuivaniemi, MD, PhD
Associate Professor, Wayne State University School of Medicine, Detroit [351]

Loren Laine, MD
Professor of Medicine, University of Southern California School of Medicine, Los Angeles [44]

Anil K. Lalwani, MD
Associate Professor, Department of Otolaryngology- Head and Neck Surgery, University of California San Francisco, San Francisco [29]

Lewis Landsberg, MD
Professor of Medicine, Vice-President for Medical Affairs, and Dean, Northwestern University Medical School, Chicago [72, 332]

H. Clifford Lane, MD
Head, Clinical and Molecular Retrovirology Section, Laboratory of Immunoregulation; Clinical Director, National Institute of Allergy and Infectious Diseases, National Institutes of Health, Bethesda [309]

Thomas J. Lawley, MD
Professor, Department of Dermatology, and Dean, Emory University School of Medicine, Atlanta [55, 56, 58]

Raphael C. Lee, MBME, MD, ScD, PhD(Hon)
Professor of Surgery (Plastic), Professor of Organismal Biology and Anatomy (Biomechanics) and, Director, Electrical Injury Research Program, University of Chicago; Attending Surgeon, Ancilla / St. Mary's Burn Center, Chicago [393]

Thomas H. Lee, MD, MSc
Associate Professor, Harvard Medical School; Medical Director, Partners Community Health Care, Inc., Boston [13]

Cammie F. Lesser, MD, PhD
Infectious Disease Fellow, University of Washington, Seattle [156]

Matthew E. Levison, MD
Professor of Medicine and Public Health, and Chief, Division of Infectious Diseases, Allegheny University of the Health Sciences, Philadelphia [255]

Peter Libby, MD
Mallinckrodt Professor of Medicine, Harvard Medical School; Chief, Cardiovascular Medicine, Brigham and Women's Hospital, Boston [241, 242]

Richard W. Light, MD
Professor of Medicine, Vanderbilt University; Director, Pulmonary Diseases, Saint Thomas Hospital, Nashville [262]

Christopher H. Linden, MD
Associate Professor, Department of Emergency Medicine, University of Massachusetts Medical School, Worcester [396]

Robert Lindsay, MBChB, PhD
Professor of Clinical Medicine, Columbia University College of Physicians and Surgeons; Chief, Internal Medicine, Helen Hayes Hospital, West Haverstraw, New York [342]

Marc E. Lippman, MD
John G. Searle Professor and Chairman, Department of Internal Medicine, University of Michigan Health Science System, Ann Arbor [89]

Peter E. Lipsky, MD
Scientific Director, National Institute of Arthritis and Musculoskeletal and Skin Diseases, National Institutes of Health, Bethesda [307, 312, 315, 320]

Leo X. Liu, MD, DTMH
Assistant Professor of Medicine, Harvard Medical School; Division of Infectious Diseases, Department of Medicine, Beth Israel Deaconess Medical Center, Boston [219]

Bernard Lo, MD
Professor of Medicine and Director, Program in Medical Ethics, University of California San Francisco, San Francisco [2]

Dan L. Longo, MD
Scientific Director, National Institute on Aging, National Institutes of Health, Bethesda and Baltimore [61, 63, 79, 82, 84, 103, 112, 113, 191]

Frank M. Longo, MD, PhD
Professor of Neurology, University of California San Francisco; Chief of Neurology, Veterans Affairs Medical Center, Department of Neurology, San Francisco [359]

Nicola Longo, MD, PhD
Associate Professor, Division of Medical Genetics, Department of Pediatrics, Emory University School of Medicine Atlanta [352, 353]

Daniel H. Lowenstein, MD
Carl W. Walter Professor of Neurology and Dean for Medical Education, Harvard Medical School, Boston [360]

Sheila A. Lukehart, PhD
Research Professor of Medicine, Division of Allergy and Infectious Diseases, University of Washington School of Medicine, Seattle [172, 173]

M. Monir Madkour, DM
Military Hospital, Riyadh, Saudi Arabia; Faculty of Medicine, Ain Shams University, Cairo, Egypt, Riyadh, Saudi Arabia [160]

Lawrence C. Madoff, MD
Assistant Professor of Medicine, Harvard Medical School; Associate Physician, Channing Laboratory and Division of Infectious Diseases, Brigham and Women's Hospital, Boston [119, 127]

James H. Maguire, MD
Associate Professor of Medicine, Harvard Medical School; Department of Immunology and Infectious Diseases, Harvard School of Public Health, Boston [129, 323, 398]

Adel A.F. Mahmoud, MD, PhD
President, Merck Vaccines, Merck & Co., Inc., Whitehouse Station, New Jersey [222]

Ronald V. Maier, MD
Professor and Vice Chairman of Surgery, University of Washington; Surgeon in Chief, Harborview Medical Center, Seattle [38]

Mark E. Mailliard, MD
Associate Professor of Medicine, Division of Gastroenterology and Hepatology, University of Nebraska Medical Center, Omaha [298]

Daniel B. Mark, MD, MPH
Professor of Medicine, Duke University Medical Center; Director, Outcomes Research and Assessment Group, Durham [3, 4]

Thomas Marrie, MD
Professor and Chair, Department of Medicine, University of Alberta, Edmonton, Alberta, Canada [177]

Joseph B. Martin, MD, PhD, MA (Hon)
Dean of the Faculty of Medicine; Caroline Shields Walker Professor of Neurobiology and Clinical Neuroscience, Harvard Medical School, Boston [12, 356, 359, 366]

Janet R. Maurer, MD
Head, Section of Advanced Lung Disease and Lung Transplantation, Division of Pulmonary and Critical Care Medicine, and Medical Director, Transplant Center, The Cleveland Clinic Foundation, Cleveland [267]

Robert J. Mayer, MD
Professor of Medicine, Harvard Medical School; Vice-Chair for Academic Affairs, Department of Adult Oncology, Dana-Farber Cancer Institute, Boston [90, 92]

John D. McConnell, MD
Professor and Chairman, Department of Urology, The University of Texas Southwestern Medical Center, Dallas [48]

William M. McCormack, MD
Professor of Medicine and of Obstetrics and Gynecology, and Chief, Division of Infectious Diseases, State University of New York, New York [178]

E. Regis McFadden, Jr., MD
Argyl J. Beams Professor of Medicine, Director, Division of Pulmonary and Critical Care Medicine, University Hospitals of Cleveland, Cleveland [252]

Kevin T. McVary, MD
Associate Professor, Department of Urology, Northwestern University Medical School, Chicago [51]

Nancy K. Mello, PhD
Professor of Psychology (Neuroscience), Harvard Medical School; Alcohol and Drug Abuse Research Center, McLean Hospital, Belmont [389]

Shlomo Melmed, MD
Professor and Director, Cedars Sinai Research Institute, University of California Los Angeles School of Medicine, Los Angeles [328]

Jerry R. Mendell, MD
Chairman and Professor of Neurology; Director, Neuromuscular Disease Center, The Ohio State University, Columbus [381, 383]

Jack H. Mendelson, MD
Professor of Psychiatry (Neuroscience), Harvard Medical School; Alcohol and Drug Abuse Research Center, McLean Hospital, Belmont [389]

Robert O. Messing, MD
Associate Professor of Neurology, and Associate Director, Ernest Gallo Clinic and Research Center, University of California San Francisco, San Francisco [386]

M. -MARSEL MESULAM, MD
Ruth and Evelyn Dunbar Professor of Neurology and Psychiatry; Director, Center for Behavioral and Cognitive Neurology; Director, Alzheimer's Program, Northwestern University Medical School, Chicago [25]

SUSAN MIESFELDT, MD
Assistant Professor of Medicine, Division of Hematology and Oncology, University of Virginia Health System, Charlottesville [68]

EDGAR L. MILFORD, MD
Associate Professor of Medicine, Harvard Medical School; Director of Renal Transplantation, Brigham and Women's Hospital, Boston [272]

SAMUEL I. MILLER, MD
Professor of Medicine and Microbiology, University of Washington, Seattle [156]

JOHN D. MINNA, MD
Professor, Internal Medicine and Pharmacology; Director, Hamon Center for Therapeutic Oncology Research, University of Texas Southwestern Medical Center, Dallas [88]

JEROME H. MODELL, MD
Associate Vice President for Health Affairs, and Professor of Anesthesiology, College of Medicine, University of Florida, Gainesville [392]

THOMAS A. MOORE, MD
Clinical Assistant Professor, Department of Internal Medicine, University of Kansas School of Medicine, Wichita [212]

MARC MOSS, MD
Assistant Professor of Medicine, Emory University School of Medicine; Director, Medical Intensive Care Unit, Grady Memorial Hospital, Atlanta [265]

ROBERT J. MOTZER, MD
Associate Attending Physician, Division of Solid Tumor Oncology, Department of Medicine, Memorial Sloan-Kettering Cancer Center; Associate Professor of Medicine, Cornell University Medical College, New York [94, 96]

HARALAMPOS M. MOUTSOPOULOS, MD
Professor and Director, Department of Pathophysiology, National University School of Medicine; President of the National Organization for Medicines, Athens, Greece [314, 316]

ROBERT S. MUNFORD, MD
Jan and Henri Bromberg Professor of Internal Medicine, and Professor of Microbiology, University of Texas Southwestern Medical Center, Dallas [124, 146]

TIMOTHY F. MURPHY, MD
Professor of Medicine and Microbiology, and Chief, Division of Infectious Diseases, State University of New York at Buffalo, Buffalo [149]

DANIEL M. MUSHER, MD
Professor of Medicine, and Professor of Molecular Virology, Baylor College of Medicine; Chief, Infectious Diseases, Veterans Affairs Medical Center, Houston [138, 148]

ROBERT J. MYERBURG, MD
Professor of Medicine and Physiology; Director, Division of Cardiology, University of Miami School of Medicine, Miami [39]

GERALD T. NEPOM, MD, PhD
Professor, Department of Immunology, University of Washington School of Medicine; Director, Virginia Mason Research Center, Seattle [306]

RICHARD A. NISHIMURA, MD
Professor of Medicine, Mayo Medical School, Rochester [227]

ROBERT L. NORRIS, MD
Associate Professor of Surgery, Department of Surgery; Chief, Division of Emergency Medicine, Stanford University, Stanford [397]

THOMAS B. NUTMAN, MD
Head, Helminth Immunology Section, Laboratory of Parasitic Diseases, National Institute of Allergy and Infectious Diseases, National Institutes of Health, Bethesda [220, 221]

JOHN A. OATES, MD
The Thomas F. Frist, Sr. Professor of Medicine, and Professor of Pharmacology, Vanderbilt University School of Medicine, Nashville [70]

RICHARD J. O'BRIEN, MD
Chief, Research and Evaluation Branch Division of Tuberculosis Elimination, Centers for Diseases Control and Prevention, Atlanta [169]

PATRICK T. O'GARA, MD
Associate Professor of Medicine, Harvard Medical School; Director, Clinical Cardiology, Brigham & Women's Hospital, Boston [34]

CHRISTOPHER A. OHL, MD
Assistant Professor of Medicine, Section on Infectious Diseases, Wake Forest University School of Medicine; Director, Center for Antimicrobial Utilization, Stewardship and Epidemiology, Baptist Medical Center, Winston-Salem [155]

RICHARD K. OLNEY, MD
Professor of Neurology, University of California San Francisco, San Francisco [22]

YVONNE M. O'MEARA, MD, FRCPI
Senior Lecturer in Medicine, University College Dublin; Consultant Nephrologist, Mater Misericordiae Hospital, Dublin, Ireland [274, 275]

ANDREW B. ONDERDONK, PhD
Professor of Pathology, Harvard Medical School; Director of Clinical Microbiology, Brigham and Women's Hospital, Boston [121]

ROBERT A. O'ROURKE, MD
Charles Conrad Brown Distinguished Professor of Cardiovascular Science, University of Texas Health Science Center at San Antonio, San Antonio [225]

CHUNG OWYANG, MD
Professor of Internal Medicine, H. Marvin Pollard Collegiate Professor and Chief, Division of Gastroenterology, Department of Internal Medicine, University of Michigan Medical Center, Ann Arbor [288]

JEFFREY PARSONNET, MD
Associate Professor of Medicine and of Microbiology, Dartmouth Medical School; Staff Physician, Infectious Diseases Section, Dartmouth-Hitchcock Medical Center, Lebanon [139]

SHREYASKUMAR R. PATEL, MD
Associate Professor of Medicine, Department of Melanoma/Sarcoma, Medical Oncology, University of Texas, MD Anderson Cancer Center, Houston [98]

GUSTAV PAUMGARTNER, MD
Professor of Medicine, Ludwig Maximiliam University of Munich, Durchwal, Germany [302]

STEPHEN J. PEROUTKA, MD
Burlingame, California [15]

MICHAEL C. PERRY, MD, MS
Professor of Internal Medicine; Director, Division of Hematology/Oncology, Nellie B. Smith Professor of Oncology, University of Missouri/Ellis Fischel Cancer Center; Consultant, Harry S. Truman VA Hospital, Columbia [103]

ALAN PESTRONK, MD
Professor of Neurology, Washington University, St. Louis [101]

CLARENCE J. PETERS, MD
Chief, Special Pathogens Branch, Centers for Disease Control and Prevention; Adjunct Professor of Microbiology and Immunology, Emory University, Atlanta [198, 199]

ELIOT A. PHILLIPSON, MD
Sir John and Lady Eaton Professor and Chair, Department of Medicine, University of Toronto, Toronto, Ontario, Canada [263, 264]

GERALD B. PIER, PhD
Professor of Medicine (Microbiology and Molecular Genetics), Harvard Medical School; Microbiologist, Brigham and Women's Hospital, Boston [120]

DANIEL K. PODOLSKY, MD
Mallinckrodt Professor of Medicine, Harvard Medical School; Chief of Gastrointestinal Unit; Director, Center for the Study of Inflammatory Bowel Disease, Massachusetts General Hospital, Boston [282, 299, 300]

RONALD E. POLK, Pharm. D.
Professor, Pharmacy and Medicine, School of Pharmacy Medical College of Virginia Campus, Virginia Commonwealth University, Richmond [137]

MATTHEW POLLACK, MD
Professor of Medicine, Uniformed Services University; F. Edward He'bert School of Medicine; Attending Staff Physician, Internal Medicine and Infectious Diseases, National Naval Medical Center, Bethesda [155]

JOHN T. POTTS, JR., MD
Distinguished Jackson Professor of Clinical Medicine, Harvard Medical School; Director of Research, Massachusetts General Hospital, Boston [341]

LAWRIE W. POWELL, MD, PhD
Professor of Medicine, The University of Queensland and Royal Brisbane Hospital, Brisbane, Queensland, Australia [345]

ALVIN C. POWERS, MD
Associate Professor of Medicine, Molecular Physiology and Biophysics, Vanderbilt University School of Medicine; Chief, Section of Endocrinology and Diabetes, VA Medical Center, Nashville [333]

DANIEL S. PRATT, MD
Assistant Professor of Medicine, Tufts University School of Medicine; Medical Director of Liver Transplantation, New England Medical Center, Boston [45, 293]

DARWIN J. PROCKOP, MD, PhD
Professor and Director, Center for Gene Therapy, Philadelphia [351]

DANIEL T. PRICE, MD
Assistant Professor of Medicine, Boston University School of Medicine; Staff Physician, Boston Veterans Affairs Medical Center, West Roxbury [240]

STANLEY B. PRUSINER, MD
Director, Institute for Neurodegenerative Diseases; Professor, Departments of Neurology, Biochemistry and Biophysics, University of California San Francisco, San Francisco [375]

PETER J. QUESENBERRY, MD
Professor of Medicine, University of Massachusetts School of Medicine, Worcester [104]

SANJAY RAM, MD
Assistant Professor of Medicine, Section of Infectious Diseases, Boston University School of Medicine and Boston Medical Center, Boston [147]

DIDIER RAOULT, MD
Professor of Medicine, Unité des Rickettsies, School of Medicine, University of Aux-Marseille, Marseille, France [177]

NEIL H. RASKIN, MD
Professor of Neurology, University of California San Francisco, San Francisco [15]

MARIO RAVIGLIONE, MD
TB Coordinator, Communicable Disease Programme, World Health Organization, Geneva, Switzerland [169]

SHARON L. REED, MD
Professor of Pathology and Medicine, and Director, Microbiology and Virology Laboratories, University of California, San Diego Medical Center, San Diego [213]

ANTONIO J. REGINATO, MD
Professor of Medicine, and Head, Division of Rheumatology, Cooper University Medical Center, Robert Wood Johnson Medical School at Camden, Camden [322]

RICHARD C. REICHMAN, MD
Professor of Medicine, Microbiology and Immunology, Head Infectious Diseases Unit, Senior Associate Dean for Clinical Research, University of Rochester School of Medicine and Dentistry, Rochester [188]

CAROL M. REIFE, MD
Clinical Assistant Professor of Medicine, Jefferson Medical College, Thomas Jefferson University, Philadelphia [43]

JOHN T. REPKE, MD
Chris J. and Marie A. Olson Professor of Obstetrics and Gynecology, and Chairman, Department of Obstetrics and Gynecology, University of Nebraska Medical Center, Omaha [7]

NEIL M. RESNICK, MD
Professor of Medicine, University of Pittsburgh School of Medicine; Chief, Division of Gerontology and Geriatric Medicine, University of Pittsburgh Healthcare System, Pittsburgh [9]

VICTOR I. REUS, MD
Professor of Psychiatry, University of California San Francisco; Medical Director, Langley Porter Hospital, San Francisco [385]

PETER A. RICE, MD
Professor of Medicine and Chief, Section of Infectious Diseases, Boston University School of Medicine and Boston Medical Center, Boston [147]

STUART RICH, MD
Professor of Medicine, Rush Medical College; Director, Rush Heart Institute Center for Pulmonary Heart Disease, Chicago [260]

GARY S. RICHARDSON, MD
Assistant Professor of Psychiatry, Case Western Reserve University; Senior Research Scientist, Sleep Disorders and Research Center, Henry Ford Hospital, Cleveland [27]

CELESTE ROBB-NICHOLSON, MD
Assistant Professor of Medicine, Harvard Medical School; Assistant Physician, Massachusetts General Hospital, Boston [6]

GARY L. ROBERTSON, MD
Professor of Medicine and Neurology, Northwestern University Medical School, Chicago [329]

DAN M. RODEN, MD
Professor of Medicine and Pharmacology; Director, Division of Clinical Pharmacology, Vanderbilt University School of Medicine, Nashville [70]

KAREN L. ROOS, MD
Professor of Neurology, Indiana University School of Medicine, Indianapolis [372]

ALLAN H. ROPPER, MD
Professor and Chairman of Neurology, Tufts University School of Medicine; Chief, Division of Neurology, St. Elizabeth's Medical Center, Boston [24, 369]

ROGER N. ROSENBERG, MD
Zale Distinguished Chair in Neurology; Professor of Neurology and Physiology, University of Texas Southwestern Medical Center; Attending Neurologist, Parkland Hospital and Zale-Lipsky University Hospital, Dallas [364]

WENDELL ROSSE, MD
Florence Reynaud McAlister Professor of Medicine and Medical Research, Department of Medicine, Duke University Medical School, Durham [108]

DAVID W. RUSSELL, MD, PhD
Associate Professor of Medicine, Division of Hematology University of Washington School of Medicine, Seattle [69]

ROBERT M. RUSSELL, MD
Professor of Medicine and Nutrition, Tufts University; Associate Director, USDA Human Nutrition Research Center, Tufts University, Boston [75]

THOMAS A. RUSSO, MD, CM
Assistant Professor of Medicine, Division of Infectious Diseases, Department of Medicine, State University of New York at Buffalo, Buffalo [153, 166]

STEPHEN M. SAGAR, MD
Professor of Neurology, Case Western Reserve School of Medicine, Cleveland [370]

EDWARD A. SAUSVILLE, MD, PhD
Associate Director, Developmental Therapeutics Program, Division of Cancer Treatment and Diagnosis, National Cancer Institute, Bethesda [84]

MOHAMED H. SAYEGH, MD
Associate Professor of Medicine, Harvard Medical School; Research Director, Laboratory of Immunogenetics and Transplantation, Brigham and Women's Hospital, Boston [272]

I. HERBERT SCHEINBERG, MD
Senior Lecturer in Medicine, College of Physicians and Surgeons, Columbia University, New York [348]

HOWARD I. SCHER, MD
Attending Physician, Chief, Genitourinary Oncology Service, Division of Solid Tumor Oncology, Department of Medicine, Memorial Sloan-Kettering Cancer Center; Professor of Medicine, Department of Medicine, Weill Medical College, New York [94, 95]

ALAN L. SCHILLER, MD
Irene Heinz Given and John LaPorte Given Professor and Chairman of Pathology, Mount Sinai School of Medicine; Chairman of Pathology, The Mount Sinai Hospital, New York [343]

HARRY W. SCHROEDER, JR., MD, PhD
Professor of Medicine and Microbiology, University of Alabama at Birmingham, Birmingham [308]

JOHN S. SCHROEDER, MD
Professor of Medicine, Cardiovascular Medicine, Stanford University School of Medicine, Stanford [233]

ANNE SCHUCHAT, MD
Chief, Respiratory Diseases Branch, Division of Bacterial and Mycotic Diseases, National Center for Infectious Diseases, Centers for Disease Control and Prevention, Atlanta [142]

MARC A. SCHUCKIT, MD
Professor of Psychiatry, University of California San Diego, and Veterans Affairs Medical Center, San Diego [387, 388]

PETER H. SCHUR, MD
Professor of Medicine, Harvard Medical School; Physician, Brigham and Women's Hospital, Boston [324]

STUART SCHWARTZ, PhD
Professor, Department of Genetics, Case Western Reserve University and the Center for Human Genetics, University Hospitals of Cleveland, Cleveland [66]

DAVID S. SEGAL, PhD
Professor of Psychiatry, University of California San Diego, La Jolla [388]

JULIAN L. SEIFTER, MD
Associate Professor of Medicine, Harvard Medical School; Physician, Brigham and Women's Hospital, Boston [281]

ANDREW P. SELWYN, MA, MD
Professor of Medicine, Harvard Medical School, Boston [244]

STEVEN I. SHERMAN, MD
Associate Professor, Section of Endocrine Neoplasia and Hormonal Disorders, University of Texas M.D. Anderson Cancer Center, Houston [339]

KARL SKORECKI, MD
Annie Chutick Professor of Medicine, Bruce Rappaport Faculty of Medicine, Technion-Israel Institute of Technology; Director, Department of Nephrology and Molecular Medicine, Rambam Medical Center, Haifa, Israel [270]

WILLIAM SILEN, MD
Johnson and Johnson Distinguished Professor of Surgery, and Dean for Faculty Development and Diversity, Harvard Medical School; Physician, Brigham and Women's Hospital, Boston [14, 290, 291]

GARY G. SINGER, MD
Assistant Professor of Medicine, Washington University School of Medicine; Associate Director, Transplant Nephrology, Barnes Jewish Hospital, St. Louis [49]

AJAY K. SINGH, MD
Associate Professor of Medicine, Harvard Medical School; Directory of Clinical Nephrology, Brigham and Women's Hospital, Boston [271]

JEAN D. SIPE, PhD
Scientific Review Administrator, Center for Scientific Review, National Institutes of Health; Adjunct Professor, Department of Biochemistry, Boston University School of Medicine, Bethesda [319]

WADE S. SMITH, MD, PhD
Assistant Professor of Neurology; Director, Stroke Service, University of California San Francisco, San Francisco [361]

JAMES B. SNOW, JR., MD
Professor Emeritus, Department of Otorhinolaryngology, University of Pennsylvania; former Director, National Institute on Deafness and Other Communication Disorders, National Institutes of Health, Bethesda [29]

ARTHUR J. SOBER, MD
Associate Professor of Dermatology, Harvard Medical School; Associate Chief of Dermatology, Massachusetts General Hospital, Boston [86]

MICHAEL F. SORRELL, MD
Robert L. Grissom Professor of Medicine; Medical Director, Liver Transplant Program, University of Nebraska Medical Center, Omaha [298]

PETER SPEELMAN, MD
Division of Infectious Diseases, Tropical Medicine and AIDS, Department of Internal Medicine, Academic Medical Center, University of Amsterdam, Amsterdam, The Netherlands [174]

FRANK E. SPEIZER, MD
Edward H. Kass Professor of Medicine, Harvard Medical School; Co-Director, Channing Laboratory, Brigham and Women's Hospital, Boston [5, 254, 391]

ANDREW SPIELMAN, ScD
Professor of Tropical Public Health, Harvard School of Public Health, Boston [398]

JERRY L. SPIVAK, MD
Professor of Medicine and Oncology, The Johns Hopkins University School of Medicine, Baltimore [110]

WALTER E. STAMM, MD
Professor of Medicine and Head, Division of Allergy and Infectious Diseases, University of Washington School of Medicine, Seattle [179, 280]

ALLEN C. STEERE, MD
Zucker Professor of Medicine, Tufts University School of Medicine; Chief, Rheumatology/Immunology, New England Medical Center, Boston [176]

ROBERT S. STERN, MD
Carl J. Herzog Professor of Dermatology, Harvard Medical School; Dermatologist-in-Chief, Beth Israel Deaconess Medical Center, Boston [59]

DENNIS L. STEVENS, MD, PhD
Professor of Medicine, University of Washington School of Medicine, Seattle; Chief, Infectious Diseases, VA Medical Center, Boise [128]

RICHARD M. STONE, MD
Associate Professor of Medicine, Harvard Medical School; Clinical Director, Adult Leukemia Program, Dana-Farber Cancer Institute, Brigham and Women's Hospital, Boston [99]

STEPHEN E. STRAUS, MD
Chief, Laboratory of Clinical Investigation, National Institute of Allergy and Infectious Diseases, National Institutes of Health, Bethesda [384]

MORTON N. SWARTZ, MD
Professor, Department of Medicine, Harvard Medical School; Chief, James Jackson Firm Medical Services, Massachusetts General Hospital, Boston [374]

ROBERT A. SWERLICK, MD
Associate Professor, Department of Dermatology, Emory University School of Medicine, Atlanta [56]

A. JAMIL TAJIK, MD
Thomas J. Walker Jr. Professor of Medicine and Pediatrics, Mayo Medical School; Chair, Division of Cardiovascular Diseases, Mayo Clinic, Rochester [227]

JOEL D. TAUROG, MD
Professor of Internal Medicine, and William M. and Gay Burnett Professor for Arthritis Research, University of Texas Southwestern Medical Center; Interim Chief, Division of Rheumatic Diseases and Interim Director, Harold C. Simmons Arthritis Research Center, Dallas [306, 315]

SCOTT J. THALER, MD
Director, Clinical Monitor, Clinical Research, Vaccines, Merck Research Laboratories, Merck & Co., Inc., Blue Bell [323]

Lucy Stuart Tompkins, MD, PhD
Professor of Medicine (Infectious Diseases and Geographic Medicine), Professor of Microbiology, Immunology and Pathology, Stanford University School of Medicine, Stanford [163]

Mark Topazian, MD
Associate Professor of Medicine, Yale University School of Medicine; Assistant Director, Gastrointestinal Procedure Center, Yale New Haven Hospital, New Haven [283]

Phillip P. Toskes, MD
Professor of Medicine and Director, Division of Gastroenterology, Hepatology and Nutrition; Associate Chairman for Clinical Affairs, Department of Medicine, University of Florida, Gainesville [303, 304]

Jeffrey M. Trent, PhD
Chief, Laboratory of Cancer Genetics; Director, Division of Intramural Research, National Human Genome Research Institute, National Institutes of Health, Bethesda [81]

Gerard Tromp, PhD
Assistant Professor, Wayne State University School of Medicine, Detroit [351]

Kenneth L. Tyler, MD
Vice Chairman and Professor of Neurology, Professor of Medicine, Microbiology and Immunology, University of Colorado Health Sciences Center; Chief, Neurology Service, Denver VA Medical Center, Denver [372, 373]

Everett E. Vokes, MD
Duchossois Professor, Departments of Medicine and Radiation Oncology; Director, Section of Hematology/Oncology, University of Chicago Medical Center, Chicago [87]

Matthew K. Waldor, MD
Assistant Professor of Medicine, New England Medical Center, Tufts University School of Medicine, Boston [159]

David Walker, MD
Professor and Chairman, Department of Pathology, University of Texas Medical Branch, Galveston [177]

Richard J. Wallace, Jr., MD
Professor and Chairman, Department of Microbiology and Research, University of Texas Health Center at Tyler, Tyler [168]

B. Timothy Walsh, MD
William and Joy Ruane Professor of Pediatric Psychopharmacology, Department of Psychiatry, College of Physicians and Surgeons, Columbia University; Director, Eating Disorders Research Unit, New York State Psychiatric Institute, New York [78]

Peter D. Walzer, MD
Professor of Medicine, University of Cincinnati College of Medicine; Chief, Infectious Diseases, VA Medical Center, Cincinnati [209]

Frederick C.S. Wang, MD
Associate Professor of Medicine, Harvard Medical School; Physician, Brigham and Women's Hospital, Boston [180, 186]

Carl V. Washington, Jr., MD
Assistant Professor of Dermatology, Emory University School of Medicine; Director, Mohs Surgery Unit, The Emory Clinic, Atlanta [86]

Anthony P. Weetman, MD, DSC
Professor of Medicine and Dean, University of Sheffield Medical School; Consultant Physician, Northern General Hospital, Sheffield, UK [330]

Steven E. Weinberger, MD
Professor of Medicine, Harvard Medical School; Vice-Chairman, Department of Medicine, Beth Israel Deaconess Medical Center, Boston [33, 249, 250, 251, 256]

Robert A. Weinstein, MD
Professor of Medicine, Rush Medical College; Chairman of Infectious Diseases, Cook County Hospital, Chicago [134]

Peter F. Weller, MD
Professor of Medicine, Harvard Medical School; Co-Chief, Division of Infectious Diseases, Chief, Division of Allergy and Inflammation, Department of Medicine, Beth Israel Deaconess Medical Center, Boston [210, 218, 219, 220, 221, 223]

Michael R. Wessels, MD
Associate Professor of Pediatrics and Medicine, Harvard Medical School; Chief, Division of Infectious Diseases, Children's Hospital; Channing Laboratory, Brigham and Women's Hospital, Boston [140]

Meir Wetzler, MD
Assistant Professor of Medicine, State University of New York at Buffalo, Buffalo [111]

A. Clinton White, Jr., MD
Associate Professor of Medicine, Department of Medicine, Microbiology and Immunology, Baylor College of Medicine, Houston [223]

Nicholas J. White, DSC, MD
Professor of Tropical Medicine, Mahidol University, Thailand and Oxford University, UK, Bangkok, Thailand [214]

Richard J. Whitley, MD
Loeb Eminent Scholar Chair in Pediatrics, Professor of Pediatrics, Microbiology and Medicine, University of Alabama at Birmingham, Birmingham [183]

Grant R. Wilkinson, PhD
Professor of Pharmacology, Vanderbilt University School of Medicine, Nashville [70]

Gordon H. Williams, MD
Professor of Medicine, Harvard Medical School; Chief, Endocrine-Hypertension Division, Brigham & Women's Hospital, Boston [35, 246, 331]

Jean D. Wilson, MD
Charles Cameron Sprague Distinguished Chair and Clinical Professor of Internal Medicine, The University of Texas Southwestern Medical Center, Dallas [335, 337, 338]

John W. Winkelman, MD, PhD
Assistant Professor of Psychiatry, Harvard Medical School; Medical Director, Sleep Health Center, Brigham and Women's Hospital, Boston [27]

Bruce U. Wintroub, MD
Associate Dean, Professor and Chair of Dermatology, University of California at San Francisco, San Francisco [59]

Gregory P. Wittenberg, MD
Rapid City Medical Center, LLP, Rapid City [86]

Allan W. Wolkoff, MD
Department of Medicine and Marion Bessin Liver Center, Albert Einstein College of Medicine, New York [294]

Alastair J.J. Wood, MB, ChB
Assistant Vice Chancellor, Professor of Medicine, Professor of Pharmacology, Vanderbilt University, School of Medicine, Nashville [71]

Robert L. Wortmann, MD
Professor and Chairman, Department of Internal Medicine, University of Oklahoma College of Medicine, Tulsa [347]

Paul W. Wright, MD
Director of Predoctoral Education and Professor of Family Practice, University of Texas Health Center, Tyler [168]

Joshua Wynne, MD, MBA
Professor of Internal Medicine, Wayne State University, Detroit [238]

Kim B. Yancey, MD
Senior Investigator, Dermatology Branch, Division of Clinical Sciences, National Cancer Institute, National Institutes of Health; Adjunct Professor, Department of Dermatology, Uniformed Services University of the Health Sciences, Bethesda [55, 58]

James B. Young, MD
Professor of Medicine, Northwestern University Medical School; Attending Physician, Northwestern Memorial Hospital, Chicago [72, 332]

Neal S. Young, MD
Chief, Hematology Branch, National Heart, Lung and Blood Institute, National Institutes of Health, Bethesda [109]

Robert C. Young, MD
President, Fox Chase Cancer Center, Philadelphia [97]

Alan S.L. Yu, MB, BChir
Assistant Professor of Medicine, Harvard Medical School; Associate Physician, Renal Division, Brigham and Women's Hospital, Boston [277]

Victor L. Yu, MD
Professor of Medicine, University of Pittsburgh; Chief, Infectious Disease Section, VA Medical Center, Pittsburgh [151]

Dori F. Zaleznik, MD
Assistant Professor of Medicine, Harvard Medical School; Senior Physician, Beth Israel Deaconess Medical Center, Wellesley, Boston [130, 135, 145]

Peter Zimetbaum, MD
Instructor in Medicine, Harvard Medical School; Cardiovascular Division, Beth Israel Deaconess Medical Center, Boston [229, 230]

Philippe E. Zimmern, MD
Associate Professor of Urology, The University of Texas Southwestern Medical School, Dallas [48]

PREFACE

The first edition of *Harrison's Principles of Internal Medicine* was published in the middle of the twentieth century, more than 50 years ago. In this fifteenth edition, the first of the new century, the text has undergone major revision to reflect further understanding of the biology and pathophysiology of disease and at the same time to retain those facts that, while not new, remain clinically useful and important. Virtually every chapter in this new edition has been completely or substantially rewritten, and a record 86 are new or have new authors. In this preface, we cannot describe all of these changes; however, we would like to call to the reader's attention those that are particularly noteworthy.

Part One, "Introduction to Clinical Medicine," contains new chapters dealing with decision making and cost awareness in clinical medicine. A growing number of patients are turning to alternative therapies, and these are discussed in a new chapter. New authors describe contemporary approaches to medical problems associated with pregnancy and the peripartum period. The chapters on medical ethics and on segments of the population that often present special problems—adolescents, women, and the elderly—have been revised and updated.

Part Two, "Cardinal Manifestations and Presentation of Disease," serves as a comprehensive introduction to clinical medicine, examining current concepts of the pathophysiology and differential diagnosis to be considered in patients with these manifestations. Major symptoms are reviewed and correlated with specific disease states, and clinical approaches to patients presenting with these symptoms are summarized. New chapters have been prepared on chest discomfort, headache, hypothermia, shock, and disorders of smell, taste, and hearing. A new chapter succinctly outlines a rational approach to the febrile patient presenting to the emergency department. The sections on alterations in gastrointestinal and sexual function are almost entirely new.

Given the explosive advances in human genetics, including the completion of a working draft of the sequence of the entire human genome and its growing relevance to clinical practice, Part Three, "Genetics and Disease," has been expanded and completely rewritten with new chapters on human genetics, chromosomal genetics, genetic defects, mitochondrial dysfunction, genetic screening and counseling, as well as gene therapy.

Part Four, "Clinical Pharmacology," provides a sound theoretical basis for pharmacotherapy, so critical to every aspect of medical practice.

Part Five, "Nutrition," has been extensively revised, with five new authors contributing chapters. This section covers nutritional considerations related to clinical medicine, including nutritional requirements, assessment of nutritional status, protein-energy malnutrition, and enteral and parenteral nutrition. It contains a new chapter on obesity, which incorporates the results of rapidly developing basic research in this important field.

The core of *Harrison's* encompasses the disorders of the organ systems and is contained in Parts Six through Fifteen. These sections include succinct accounts of the pathophysiology of the diseases involving the major organ systems and emphasize clinical manifestations, diagnostic procedures, differential diagnosis, and treatment strategies. The treatment sections of virtually every chapter have been amplified and updated. They are supplemented by the liberal use of algorithms, and are clearly highlighted. Guidelines for disease management prepared by specialty societies are included for the first time.

Part Six, "Oncology and Hematology," includes twelve chapters with new authors, including a new chapter by Judah Folkman on angiogenesis. In addition, a new chapter has been added on the medical problems that can arise in patients cured of cancer, including disease-related and treatment-related sequelae. The chapters on myeloid and lymphoid neoplasms include the new World Health Organization classification schemes. A conscientious effort has been made to provide specific, up-to-date treatment recommendations. Where appropriate, diagnostic and management algorithms have been incorporated.

Changes in Part Seven, "Infectious Diseases," include the latest information on the pathology, genetics, and epidemiology of infectious diseases while focusing sharply on the needs of clinicians who must accurately diagnose and treat infections in their patients. Specific recommendations are offered for therapeutic regimens, including the drug of choice, dose, duration, and alternatives. Current figures and trends in antimicrobial resistance are presented and considered in light of their impact on therapeutic choices. New authors cover the latest advances in the management of diseases such as infective endocarditis, meningococcal and gonococcal infections, and schistosomiasis. The overview of pathogenesis from earlier editions has been expanded to encompass viruses, fungi, and parasites as well as bacteria. The Atlas of Hematology includes a complete diagnostic set of spectacular color plates showing malaria-infected red blood cells.

In Part Eight, "Disorders of the Cardiovascular System," a new chapter on the prevention of atherosclerosis focuses not only on the importance of the traditional risk factors but also on the novel risk factors that influence plaque stability. Global risk assessment and management are described. Both primary and secondary prevention of atherosclerosis are discussed. Myocardial imaging by means of ultrasound or radionuclide techniques, at rest and during stress, plays an ever more critical role in assessment of patients with ischemic heart disease, and a new chapter focuses on the clinical use of these important technologies.

Despite major advances in its diagnosis and therapy, acute myocardial infarction remains the most common cause of death in industrialized nations. The chapter on acute myocardial infarction provides important new information on myocardial reperfusion therapy, thrombolysis, and primary coronary angioplasty and summarizes guidelines for acute coronary care and for risk stratification in the postinfarct patient. Unstable angina and congestive heart failure have emerged as two of the most common conditions leading to hospital admission in Western nations. Important advances in pathophysiology and therapy of these two very important conditions are included.

Enormous strides have been made in the use of lung transplantation for selected patients with end-stage, irreversible, pulmonary parenchymal and vascular disease, and Part Nine, "Disorders of the Respiratory System," provides a chapter that focuses on patient selection for this therapy. New chapters on interstitial and granulomatous lung diseases as well as on sleep apnea provide contemporary views of these conditions at the interface between basic science and clinical pulmonology.

In Part Ten, "Disorders of the Kidney and Urinary Tract," there has been considerable revision, with a new chapter on dialysis, incorporating the most recent advances.

In Part Eleven, "Disorders of the Gastrointestinal System," several new authors have contributed to the section on liver and biliary tract disease, and all chapters have been extensively revised. The section is pivoted by a new chapter on "Approach to the Patient with Liver Disease." Recent advances in the therapy of hepatitis B and C have been highlighted. New authors have contributed chapters on endoscopy, peptic ulcer disease, disorders of absorption, inflammatory bowel disease, and irritable bowel syndrome. Our new contributors include the leaders in gastroenterology and hepatology.

In Part Twelve, "Disorders of the Immune System, Connective Tissue, and Joints," the updating focuses on therapy. The chapter on

"Introduction to the Immune System" has been completely rewritten and provides a comprehensive review of the human immune system, using the modern designations of innate versus adaptive immunity. The chapter on HIV disease and AIDS is comprehensive and up-to-date and includes coverage of the natural history, epidemiology, and immunopathogenic mechanisms of HIV disease. In addition, the chapter contains both an organ system by organ system approach and a delineation of the major complications of HIV disease. The sections on therapy include a state-of-the-art discussion of the striking treatment advances of HIV infection with combinations of antiretroviral agents as well as the complications of such therapy.

Profound changes can be found in Part Thirteen, "Endocrinology and Metabolism." Many new authors have been recruited, and all chapters have been extensively revised under the direction of our new editor, Dr. J. Larry Jameson. Nine of these chapters are completely new, including those on the pituitary, thyroid, diabetes mellitus, and osteoporosis. These clinically demanding topics retain a traditional pathophysiologic approach that characterizes the field of endocrinology. In addition, new insights from genetics permeate this section, and the results of evidence-based medicine provide a firm foundation for medical decision making and treatment.

Part Fourteen, "Neurologic Disorders," has been thoroughly updated and expanded. The theme of genetics is emphasized throughout the section, and new chapters highlight the remarkable progress made during the "decade of the brain" in the 1990s that has elucidated the molecular basis of many neurologic and psychiatric diseases. One of the new chapters, written by 1997 Nobel Laureate Stanley B. Prusiner, summarizes the unique biology of prions and the clinical features of human prion disorders, including "mad cow disease."

The very latest information can be found on treatment of epilepsy, Parkinson's disease, and Alzheimer's disease. Coverage of immune-mediated disorders of the nervous system has been greatly expanded to include the many new insights into pathogenesis and treatment that have appeared since the fourteenth edition. The chapter on cerebrovascular diseases offers state-of-the-art information on prevention and treatment of stroke, the third leading killer in the developed world; this chapter is a mini-textbook of stroke and stroke therapy. Another feature of the fifteenth edition is a discussion of the acute neurologic disorders encountered in the setting of critical illness; this chapter should be of value to all physicians who care for hospitalized patients.

Throughout the book, there is an emphasis on the use of neuroimaging figures to illustrate the various disorders discussed. *Harrison's* exceptional collection of high-quality neuroimaging photographs sets a new standard for textbooks of medicine.

Finally, Part Fifteen, "Environmental and Occupational Hazards," has been expanded and reorganized.

In view of the requirements for continuing education for licensure and relicensure, as well as the emphasis on certification and recertification, a revision of the Pre-Test Self-Assessment and Review will again be published with this edition. It consists of several hundred questions based on *Harrison's*, along with answers and explanations for the answers. The *Companion Handbook* that was pioneered as a supplement to the eleventh edition of *Harrison's* has been updated and will appear shortly after the publication of this edition. A CD-ROM version of *Harrison's* has been available since the thirteenth edition. An expanded CD-ROM version of the fifteenth edition will be available and will be regularly updated. In 1998, *Harrison's* went online to provide a "living" textbook of internal medicine. In addition to providing full search capabilities of the text, *Harrison's Online* offers daily updating, reports of clinical trials, practice guidelines, and concise reviews of timely topics, as well as new references with links to MEDLINE abstracts.

The fifteenth edition of *Harrison's* welcomes a new editor, Dr. J. Larry Jameson, who has taken on principal responsibility for the sections on Nutrition, Genetics, Endocrinology, and Metabolism and whose impact on this edition is already clear. Dr. Kurt J. Isselbacher, Dr. Jean D. Wilson, and Dr. Joseph B. Martin have left the editorial group. Their enormous contributions to *Harrison's* are cited elsewhere. Special thanks go to Dr. Robert F. Schrier who has prepared biographies of Nobel Prize Laureates in Physiology or Medicine. These brief essays remind us how deeply our current knowledge and practice of medicine depends on seminal contributions to biomedical science and informs about the lives of some of the most outstanding contributors.

We wish to express our appreciation to our many associates and colleagues, who, as experts in their fields, have helped us with constructive criticism and helpful suggestions. We acknowledge especially the contributions of:

Donna Ambrosino, Peter Banks, Richard Blumberg, Douglas Brust, Myron Cohen, Jonathan Edlow, Christopher Fanta, Mary Gillam, Douglas Golenbach, Fred Gorelick, Charles Halsted, Lee Kaplan, Peter Kopp, Bruce Levy, Leo Liu, William Lowe, Lawrence Madoff, Josh Meeks, Mark Molitch, Chung Owyang, Eugene Pergament, Alice Pau, Gerald Pier, Peter Rice, Paul Sax, Tom Schnitzer, Julian Seifter, Anushua Sinha, Steven Weinberger, Michael Wessels, and Lee Wetzler.

This book could not have been edited without the dedicated help of our co-workers in the editorial offices of the individual editors. We are especially indebted to Scott Cromer, Pat Duffey, Sarah Anne Matero, Julie McCoy, Elizabeth Robbins, Kathryn Saxon, Marie Scurti, and Julieta Tayco.

Finally, we continue to be indebted to two outstanding members of the McGraw-Hill organization: Mariapaz Ramos Englis, Senior Managing Editor, and Martin J. Wonsiewicz, Publisher. They are an effective team who have given the editors constant encouragement and sage advice and have been of enormous help in bringing this edition to fruition in a timely manner.

The Editors

HARRISON'S 15TH EDITION

PRINCIPLES OF INTERNAL MEDICINE

PART NINE

DISORDERS OF THE RESPIRATORY SYSTEM

Section 1
DIAGNOSIS

249 APPROACH TO THE PATIENT WITH DISEASE OF THE RESPIRATORY SYSTEM

Jeffrey M. Drazen, Steven E. Weinberger

Patients with disease of the respiratory system generally present because of symptoms, an abnormality on a chest radiograph, or both. A set of diagnostic possibilities is often suggested by the initial problems at presentation, including the particular symptom(s) and the appearance of any radiographic abnormalities. The differential diagnosis is then refined on the basis of additional information gleaned from physical examination, pulmonary function testing, additional imaging studies, and bronchoscopic examination. This chapter will consider the approach to the patient based on the major patterns of presentation, focusing on the history, the physical examination, and the chest radiograph. →*For further discussion of pulmonary function testing, see Chap. 250, and of other diagnostic studies, see Chap. 251.*

CLINICAL PRESENTATION

HISTORY Dyspnea (shortness of breath) and cough are the primary presenting symptoms for patients with respiratory system disease. Less common symptoms include hemoptysis (the coughing up of blood) and chest pain, often with a pleuritic quality.

Dyspnea (See also Chap. 32) When evaluating a patient with shortness of breath, one should first determine the time course over which the symptom has become manifest. Patients who were well previously and developed *acute* shortness of breath (over a period of hours to days) can have acute disease affecting the airways (an acute attack of asthma), the pulmonary parenchyma (acute pulmonary edema or an acute infectious process such as a bacterial pneumonia), the pleural space (a pneumothorax), or the pulmonary vasculature (a pulmonary embolus). A *subacute* presentation (over days to weeks) can suggest an exacerbation of preexisting airways disease (asthma or chronic bronchitis), a parenchymal infection or a noninfectious inflammatory process that proceeds at a relatively slow pace (*Pneumocystis carinii* pneumonia in a patient with AIDS, mycobacterial or fungal pneumonia, Wegener's granulomatosis, eosinophilic pneumonia, bronchiolitis obliterans with organizing pneumonia, and many others), neuromuscular disease (Guillain-Barré syndrome, myasthenia gravis), pleural disease (pleural effusion from a variety of possible causes), or chronic cardiac disease (congestive heart failure). A *chronic* presentation (over months to years) often indicates chronic obstructive lung disease, chronic interstitial lung disease, or chronic cardiac disease. Chronic diseases of airways (not only chronic obstructive lung disease but also asthma) are characterized by exacerbations and remissions. Patients often have periods when they are severely limited by shortness of breath, but these may be interspersed with periods in which symptoms are minimal or absent. In contrast, many of the diseases of pulmonary parenchyma are characterized by a slow but inexorable progression.

Other Respiratory Symptoms *Cough* (Chap. 33) may indicate the presence of lung disease, but cough per se is not useful for the differential diagnosis. The presence of sputum accompanying the cough often suggests airway disease and may be seen in asthma, chronic bronchitis, or bronchiectasis.

Hemoptysis (Chap. 33) can originate from disease of the airways, the pulmonary parenchyma, or the vasculature. Diseases of the airways can be inflammatory (acute or chronic bronchitis, bronchiectasis, or cystic fibrosis) or neoplastic (bronchogenic carcinoma or bronchial carcinoid tumors). Parenchymal diseases causing hemoptysis may be either localized (pneumonia, lung abscess, tuberculosis, or infection with *Aspergillus*) or diffuse (Goodpasture's syndrome, idiopathic pulmonary hemosiderosis). Vascular diseases potentially associated with hemoptysis include pulmonary thromboembolic disease and pulmonary arteriovenous malformations.

Chest pain (Chap. 13) caused by diseases of the respiratory system usually originates from involvement of the parietal pleura. As a result, the pain is accentuated by respiratory motion and is often referred to as *pleuritic*. Common examples include primary pleural disorders, such as neoplasm or inflammatory disorders involving the pleura, or pulmonary parenchymal disorders that extend to the pleural surface, such as pneumonia or pulmonary infarction.

Additional Historic Information Information about risk factors for lung disease should be explicitly explored to assure a complete basis of historic data. A history of current and past smoking, especially of cigarettes, should be sought from all patients. The smoking history should include the number of years of smoking, the intensity (i.e., number of packs per day), and, if the patient no longer smokes, the interval since smoking cessation. The risk of lung cancer falls progressively with the interval following discontinuation of smoking, and loss of lung function above the expected age-related decline ceases with the discontinuation of smoking. Even though chronic obstructive lung disease and neoplasia are the two most important respiratory complications of smoking, other respiratory disorders (e.g., spontaneous pneumothorax, respiratory bronchiolitis–interstitial lung disease, eosinophilic granuloma of the lung, and pulmonary hemorrhage with Goodpasture's syndrome) are also associated with smoking. A history of significant secondhand (passive) exposure to smoke, whether in the home or at the workplace, should also be sought as it may be a risk factor for neoplasia or an exacerbating factor for airways disease.

The patient may have been exposed to other inhaled agents associated with lung disease, which act either via direct toxicity or through immune mechanisms (Chaps. 253 and 254). Such exposures can be either occupational or avocational, indicating the importance of detailed occupational and personal histories, the latter stressing exposures related to hobbies or the home environment. Important agents include the inorganic dusts associated with pneumoconiosis (especially asbestos and silica dusts) and organic antigens associated with hypersensitivity pneumonitis (especially antigens from molds and animal proteins). Asthma, which is more common in women than men, is often exacerbated by exposure to environmental allergens (dust mites, pet dander, or cockroach allergens in the home or allergens in the outdoor environment such as pollen and ragweed) or may be caused by occupational exposures (diisocyanates). Exposure to particular infectious agents can be suggested by contacts with individuals with known respiratory infections (especially tuberculosis) or by residence in an area with endemic pathogens (histoplasmosis, coccidioidomycosis, blastomycosis).

A history of coexisting nonrespiratory disease or of risk factors for or previous treatment of such diseases should be sought, as they may

Table 249-1 Typical Chest Examination Findings in Selected Clinical Conditions

Condition	Percussion	Fremitus	Breath Sounds	Voice Transmission	Adventitious Sounds
Normal	Resonant	Normal	Vesicular (at lung bases)	Normal	Absent
Consolidation or atelectasis (with patent airway)	Dull	Increased	Bronchial	Bronchophony, whispered pectoriloquy, egophony	Crackles
Consolidation or atelectasis (with blocked airway)	Dull	Decreased	Decreased	Decreased	Absent
Asthma	Resonant	Normal	Vesicular	Normal	Wheezing
Interstitial lung disease	Resonant	Normal	Vesicular	Normal	Crackles
Emphysema	Hyperresonant	Decreased	Decreased	Decreased	Absent or wheezing
Pneumothorax	Hyperresonant	Decreased	Decreased	Decreased	Absent
Pleural effusion	Dull	Decreased	Decreased[a]	Decreased[a]	Absent or pleural friction rub

[a] May be altered by collapse of underlying lung, which will increase transmission of sound.
SOURCE: Adapted from Weinberger.

predispose a patient to both infectious and noninfectious respiratory system complications. Common examples include systemic rheumatic diseases that are associated with pleural or parenchymal lung disease (Chap. 312), metastatic neoplastic disease in the lung, or impaired host defense mechanisms and secondary infection, which occur in the case of hematologic and lymph node malignancies. Risk factors for AIDS should be sought, as the lungs are not only the most common site of AIDS-defining infection but also can be involved by nonfectious complications of AIDS (Chap. 309). Treatment of nonrespiratory disease can be associated with respiratory complications, either because of effects on host defense mechanisms (immunosuppressive agents, cancer chemotherapy) with resulting infection or because of direct effects on the pulmonary parenchyma (cancer chemotherapy, radiation therapy, or treatment with other agents, such as amiodarone) or on the airways (beta-blocking agents causing airflow obstruction, angiotensin-converting enzyme inhibitors causing cough) (Chap. 253).

Family history is important for evaluating diseases that have a genetic component. These include disorders such as cystic fibrosis, α_1-antitrypsin deficiency, and asthma.

PHYSICAL EXAMINATION The general principles of inspection, palpation, percussion, and auscultation apply to the examination of the respiratory system. However, the physical examination should be directed not only toward ascertaining abnormalities of the lungs and thorax but also toward recognizing other findings that may reflect underlying lung disease.

On *inspection*, the rate and pattern of breathing as well as the depth and symmetry of lung expansion are observed. Breathing that is unusually rapid, labored, or associated with the use of accessory muscles of respiration generally indicates either augmented respiratory demands or an increased work of breathing. Asymmetric expansion of the chest is usually due to an asymmetric process affecting the lungs, such as endobronchial obstruction of a large airway, unilateral parenchymal or pleural disease, or unilateral phrenic nerve paralysis. Visible abnormalities of the thoracic cage include kyphoscoliosis and ankylosing spondylitis, either of which can alter compliance of the thorax, increase the work of breathing, and cause dyspnea.

On *palpation*, the symmetry of lung expansion can be assessed, generally confirming the findings observed by inspection. Vibration produced by spoken sounds is transmitted to the chest wall and is assessed by the presence or absence and symmetry of tactile fremitus. Transmission of vibration is decreased or absent if pleural liquid is interposed between the lung and the chest wall or if an endobronchial obstruction alters sound transmission. In contrast, transmitted vibration may increase over an area of underlying pulmonary consolidation.

The relative resonance or dullness of the tissue underlying the chest wall is assessed by *percussion*. The normal sound of underlying air-containing lung is resonant. In contrast, consolidated lung or a pleural effusion sounds dull, while emphysema or air in the pleural space results in a hyperresonant percussion note.

On *auscultation* of the lungs, the examiner listens for both the quality and intensity of the breath sounds and for the presence of extra, or adventitious, sounds. Normal breath sounds heard through the stethoscope at the periphery of the lung are described as *vesicular breath sounds*, in which inspiration is louder and longer than expiration. If sound transmission is impaired by endobronchial obstruction or by air or liquid in the pleural space, breath sounds are diminished in intensity or absent. When sound transmission is improved through consolidated lung, the resulting *bronchial breath sounds* have a more tubular quality and a more pronounced expiratory phase. Sound transmission can also be assessed by listening to spoken or whispered sounds; when these are transmitted through consolidated lung, *bronchophony* and *whispered pectoriloquy*, respectively, are present. The sound of a spoken E becomes more like an A, though with a nasal or bleating quality, a finding that is termed *egophony*.

The primary adventitious (abnormal) sounds that can be heard include crackles (rales), wheezes, and rhonchi. *Crackles* represent the typically inspiratory sound created when alveoli and small airways open and close with respiration, and they are often associated with interstitial lung disease, microatelectasis, or filling of alveoli by liquid. *Wheezes*, which are generally more prominent during expiration than inspiration, reflect the oscillation of airway walls that occurs when there is airflow limitation, as may be produced by bronchospasm, airway edema or collapse, or intraluminal obstruction by neoplasm or secretions. *Rhonchi* is the term applied to the sounds created when there is free liquid in the airway lumen; the viscous interaction between the free liquid and the moving air creates a low-pitched vibratory sound. Other adventitious sounds include pleural friction rubs and stridor. The gritty sound of a *pleural friction rub* indicates inflamed pleural surfaces rubbing against each other, often during both inspiratory and expiratory phases of the respiratory cycle. *Stridor*, which occurs primarily during inspiration, represents flow through a narrowed upper airway, as occurs in an infant with croup.

A summary of the patterns of physical findings on pulmonary examination in common types of respiratory system disease is shown in Table 249-1.

A meticulous *general physical examination* is mandatory in patients with disorders of the respiratory system. Enlarged lymph nodes in the cervical and supraclavicular regions should be sought. Disturbances of mentation or even coma can occur in patients with acute carbon dioxide retention and hypoxemia. Telltale stains on the fingers point to heavy cigarette smoking; infected teeth and gums may occur in patients with aspiration pneumonitis and lung abscess.

Clubbing of the digits can be found in lung cancer, interstitial lung disease, and chronic infections in the thorax, such as bronchiectasis, lung abscess, and empyema. Clubbing can also be seen with congenital heart disease associated with right-to-left shunting and with a variety of chronic inflammatory or infectious diseases, such as inflammatory bowel disease and endocarditis. A number of systemic diseases, such as systemic lupus erythematosus, scleroderma, and rheumatoid arthritis, may be associated with pulmonary complications, even though their primary clinical manifestations and physical findings are not primarily related to the lungs. Conversely, other diseases that most commonly affect the respiratory system, such as sarcoidosis, can have findings on physical examination not related to the respiratory system, including ocular findings (uveitis, conjunctival granulomas) and skin findings (erythema nodosum, cutaneous granulomas).

CHEST RADIOGRAPHY

Chest radiography is often the initial diagnostic study performed to evaluate patients with respiratory symptoms, but it can also provide the initial evidence of disease in patients who are free of symptoms. Perhaps the most common example of the latter situation is the finding of one or more nodules or masses when the radiograph is performed for a reason other than evaluation of respiratory symptoms.

A number of diagnostic possibilities are often suggested by the radiographic pattern (Figs. 249-1 and 249-2). A localized region of opacification involving the pulmonary parenchyma can be described as a nodule (usually <6 cm in diameter), a mass (usually ≥ 6 cm in diameter), or an infiltrate. Diffuse disease with increased opacification is usually characterized as having an alveolar, an interstitial, or a nodular pattern. In contrast, increased radiolucency can be localized, as seen with a cyst or bulla, or generalized, as occurs with emphysema. The chest radiograph is also particularly useful for the detection of pleural disease, especially if manifested by the presence of air or liquid in the pleural space. An abnormal appearance of the hila and/or the mediastinum can suggest a mass or enlargement of lymph nodes.

A summary of representative diagnoses suggested by these common radiographic patterns is presented in Table 249-2.

Additional Diagnostic Evaluation Further information for clarification of radiographic abnormalities is frequently obtained with computed tomographic scanning of the chest (Chap. 251; see Fig. 265-2). This technique is more sensitive than plain radiography in detecting subtle abnormalities and can suggest specific diagnoses based on the pattern of abnormality. →***For further discussion of the use of other imaging studies, including magnetic resonance imaging, scintigraphic studies, ultrasound, and angiography, see Chap. 251.***

Alteration in the function of the lungs as a result of respiratory system disease is assessed objectively by pulmonary function tests, and effects on gas exchange are evaluated by measurement of arterial blood gases or by oximetry (Chap. 250). As part of pulmonary function testing, quantitation of forced expiratory flow assesses the presence of obstructive physiology, which is consistent with diseases affecting the

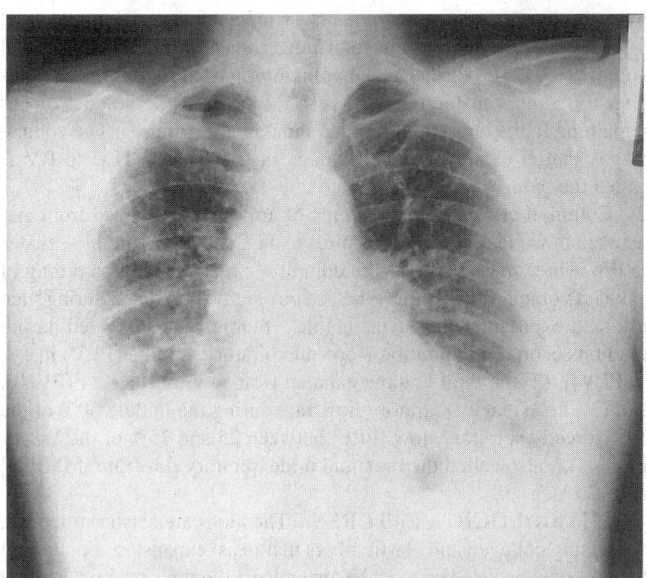

FIGURE 249-1 Posteroanterior (PA) chest radiograph of a patient with diffuse interstitial lung disease due to idiopathic pulmonary fibrosis. (*From Weinberger, Principles of Pulmonary Medicine, 3d ed. Philadelphia, Saunders, 1998, with permission*).

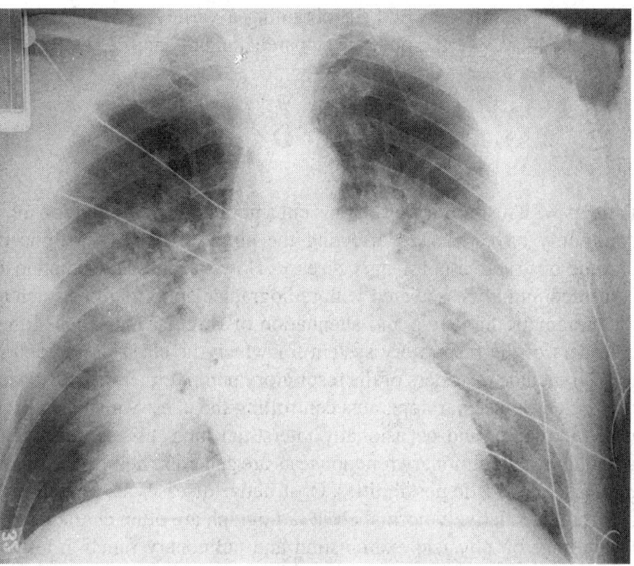

FIGURE 249-2 Anteroposterior (AP) chest radiograph demonstrating a diffuse alveolar filling pattern due to the acute respiratory distress syndrome (ARDS).

structure or function of the airways, such as asthma and chronic obstructive lung disease. Measurement of lung volumes assesses the presence of restrictive disorders, seen with diseases of the pulmonary parenchyma or respiratory pump and with space-occupying processes within the pleura.

Bronchoscopy is useful in some settings for visualizing abnor-

Table 249-2 Major Respiratory Diagnoses with Common Chest Radiographic Patterns

Solitary circumscribed density—nodule (<6 cm) or mass (≥6 cm)
- Primary or metastatic neoplasm
- Localized infection (bacterial abscess, mycobacterial or fungal infection)
- Wegener's granulomatosis (one or several nodules)
- Rheumatoid nodule (one or several nodules)
- Vascular malformation
- Bronchogenic cyst

Localized opacification (infiltrate)
- Pneumonia (bacterial, atypical, mycobacterial, or fungal infection)
- Neoplasm
- Radiation pneumonitis
- Bronchiolitis obliterans with organizing pneumonia
- Bronchocentric granulomatosis
- Pulmonary infarction

Diffuse interstitial disease
- Idiopathic pulmonary fibrosis
- Pulmonary fibrosis with systemic rheumatic disease
- Sarcoidosis
- Drug-induced lung disease
- Pneumoconiosis
- Hypersensitivity pneumonitis
- Infection (*Pneumocystis*, viral pneumonia)
- Eosinophilic granuloma

Diffuse alveolar disease
- Cardiogenic pulmonary edema
- Acute respiratory distress syndrome
- Diffuse alveolar hemorrhage
- Infection (*Pneumocystis*, viral or bacterial pneumonia)
- Sarcoidosis

Diffuse nodular disease
- Metastatic neoplasm
- Hematogenous spread of infection (bacterial, mycobacterial, fungal)
- Pneumoconiosis
- Eosinophilic granuloma

malities of the airways and for obtaining a variety of samples from either the airway or the pulmonary parenchyma (Chap. 251).

INTEGRATION OF THE PRESENTING CLINICAL PATTERN AND DIAGNOSTIC STUDIES

Patients with respiratory symptoms but a normal chest radiograph most commonly have diseases affecting the airways, such as asthma or chronic obstructive pulmonary disease. However, the latter diagnosis is also commonly associated with radiographic abnormalities, such as diaphragmatic flattening and attenuation of vascular markings. Other disorders of the respiratory system for which the chest radiograph is normal include disorders of the respiratory pump (either the chest wall or the neuromuscular apparatus controlling the chest wall) or pulmonary circulation and occasionally interstitial lung disease. Chest examination and pulmonary function tests are generally helpful in sorting out these diagnostic possibilities. Obstructive diseases associated with a normal or relatively normal chest radiograph are often characterized by findings on physical examination and pulmonary function testing that are typical for these conditions. Similarly, diseases of the respiratory pump or interstitial diseases may also be suggested by findings on physical examination or by particular patterns of restrictive disease seen on pulmonary function testing.

When respiratory symptoms are accompanied by radiographic abnormalities, diseases of the pulmonary parenchyma or the pleura are usually present. Either diffuse or localized parenchymal lung disease is generally visualized well on the radiograph, and both air and liquid in the pleural space (pneumothorax and pleural effusion, respectively) are usually readily detected by radiography.

Radiographic findings in the absence of respiratory symptoms often indicate localized disease affecting the airways or the pulmonary parenchyma. One or more nodules or masses can suggest intrathoracic malignancy, but they also can be the manifestation of a current or previous infectious process. Patients with diffuse parenchymal lung disease on radiographic examination may be free of symptoms, as is sometimes the case with pulmonary sarcoidosis.

In approaching the patient with pulmonary disease, consideration must be given to the observation that substantial changes in the relative incidence of diseases affecting the respiratory system have taken place in the United States during the past four decades. The prevalence of chronic infectious disorders such as lung abscess and bronchiectasis has decreased. Tuberculosis declined only to undergo resurgence when two susceptible populations, patients with AIDS and immigrants from Southeast Asia, increased in number. Patients with chronic bronchitis and with emphysema now survive longer and form an increasing fraction of patients with chronic respiratory disease, as do patients with environmental lung disease and with drug-induced pulmonary disease. Modern intercontinental travel has increased the appearance in the western world of parasitic infestations of the lung. Also, the reduction of immune competence that occurs in patients with AIDS and in those with diabetes as well as in patients being treated for a variety of malignancies and those receiving immunosuppressive drugs has led to an increasing incidence of opportunistic infections of the lungs with a variety of microorganisms that were rarely pathogenic in the past.

BIBLIOGRAPHY

ALBERT RK et al (eds): *Comprehensive Respiratory Medicine*. St. Louis, Mosby, 1999

DEGOWIN R et al: *DeGowin & DeGowin's Diagnostic Examination*, 7th ed. New York, McGraw-Hill, 2000

EBI-KRYSTON KL: Respiratory symptoms and pulmonary function as predictors of 10-year mortality from respiratory disease, cardiovascular disease, and all causes in the Whitehall Study. J Clin Epidemiol 41:251, 1988

IRWIN RS, MADISON JM: Anatomical diagnostic protocol in evaluating chronic cough with specific reference to gastroesophageal reflux disease. Am J Med 108:1265, 2000

JUNIPER EF: Impact of upper respiratory allergic diseases on quality of life. J Allergy Clin Immunol 101:5386, 1998

MARTINEZ FD et al: Asthma and wheezing in the first six years of life. N Engl J Med 332:133, 1995

WEINBERGER SE: *Principles of Pulmonary Medicine*, 3d ed. Philadelphia, Saunders, 1998

WELTY C et al: The relationship of airways responsiveness to cold air, cigarette smoking, and atopy to respiratory symptoms and pulmonary function in adults. Am Rev Respir Dis 130:198, 1984

250

Steven E. Weinberger, Jeffrey M. Drazen

DISTURBANCES OF RESPIRATORY FUNCTION

CNS	central nervous system	MIP	maximal inspiratory pressure
ERV	expiratory reserve volume	MMFR	maximal midexpiratory flow rate
FEF	forced expiratory flow	PAP	pulmonary arterial pressure
FEV	forced expiratory volume	PVR	pulmonary vascular resistance
FRC	functional residual capacity	RV	residual volume
FVC	forced vital capacity	TLC	total lung capacity
IC	inspiratory capacity	VC	vital capacity
MEP	maximal expiratory pressure		

The respiratory system includes the lungs, the central nervous system (CNS), the chest wall (with the diaphragm and intercostal muscles), and the pulmonary circulation. The CNS controls the activity of the muscles of the chest wall, which constitute the pump of the respiratory system. Because these components of the respiratory system act in concert to achieve gas exchange, malfunction of an individual component or alteration of the relationships among components can lead to disturbances in function. In this chapter we consider three major aspects of disturbed respiratory function: (1) disturbances in ventilatory function, (2) disturbances in the pulmonary circulation, and (3) disturbances in gas exchange. →*For further discussion of disorders relating to CNS control of ventilation, see Chap. 263.*

DISTURBANCES IN VENTILATORY FUNCTION

Ventilation is the process whereby the lungs replenish the gas in the alveoli. Measurements of ventilatory function in common diagnostic use consist of quantification of the gas volume contained in the lungs under certain circumstances and the rate at which gas can be expelled from the lungs. Two measurements of lung volume commonly used for respiratory diagnosis are total lung capacity (TLC) and residual volume (RV). The former is the volume of gas contained in the lungs after a maximal inspiration, whereas the latter is the volume of gas remaining in the lungs at the end of a maximal expiration. The volume of gas that is exhaled from the lungs in going from TLC to RV is called the *vital capacity* (VC) (Fig. 250-1).

Common clinical measurements of airflow are obtained from maneuvers in which the subject inspires to TLC and then forcibly exhales to RV. Three measurements are commonly made from a recording of exhaled volume versus time—i.e., a spirogram—obtained during such a forced expiratory maneuver: (1) the volume of gas exhaled during the first second of expiration [forced expiratory volume (FEV) in 1 s, or FEV_1], (2) the total volume exhaled [forced vital capacity (FVC)], and (3) the average expiratory flow rate during the middle 50% of the VC [forced expiratory flow (FEF) between 25 and 75% of the VC, or $FEF_{25-75\%}$, also called the maximal midexpiratory flow rate (MMFR)] (Fig. 250-2).

PHYSIOLOGIC FEATURES The lungs are elastic structures, containing collagen and elastic fibers that resist expansion. For normal lungs to contain air, they must be distended either by a positive internal pressure—i.e., by a pressure in the airways and alveolar spaces—or by a negative external pressure—i.e., by a pressure outside the lung. The relationship between the volume of gas contained in the lungs and the distending pressure (the *transpulmonary pressure*, or P_{TP}, defined

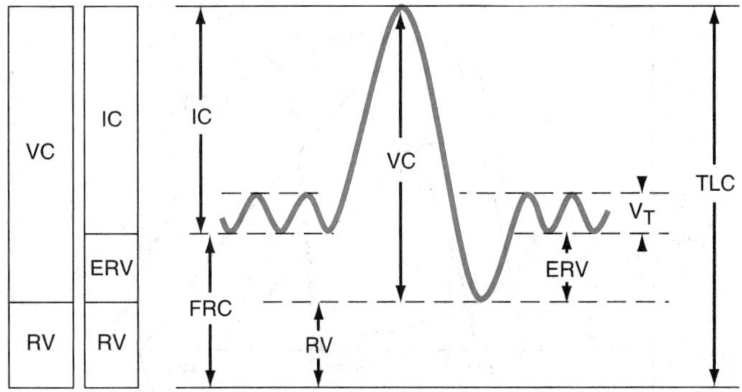

FIGURE 250-1 Lung volumes, shown by block diagrams *(left)* and by a spirographic tracing *(right)*. TLC, total lung capacity; VC, vital capacity; RV, residual volume; IC, inspiratory capacity; ERV, expiratory reserve volume; FRC, functional residual capacity; V_T, tidal volume. *(From Weinberger, with permission.)*

as internal pressure minus external pressure) is described by the pressure-volume curve of the lungs (Fig. 250-3*A*).

The chest wall is also an elastic structure, with properties similar to those of an expandable and compressible spring. The relationship between the volume enclosed by the chest wall and the distending pressure for the chest wall is described by the pressure-volume curve of the chest wall (Fig. 250-3*B*). For the chest wall to assume a volume different from its resting volume, the internal or external pressures acting on it must be altered.

At functional residual capacity (FRC), defined as the volume of gas in the lungs at the end of a normal exhalation, the lungs are partially inflated, so their elastic recoil exerts a force tending to empty the lungs. At the same time, chest wall volume is such that its elastic recoil promotes outward expansion. FRC occurs at the lung volume at which the tendency of the lungs to contract is opposed by the equal and opposite tendency of the chest wall to expand (Fig. 250-3*C*).

For the lungs and the chest wall to achieve a volume other than the resting volume (FRC), either the pressures acting on them must be changed passively—e.g., by a mechanical ventilator that delivers positive pressure to the airways and alveoli—or the respiratory muscles must actively oppose the tendency of the lungs and the chest wall to return to FRC. During inhalation to volumes above FRC, the inspiratory muscles actively overcome the tendency of the respiratory system to decrease volume back to FRC. During active exhalation to volumes below FRC, expiratory muscle activity must overcome the tendency of the respiratory system to increase volume back to FRC.

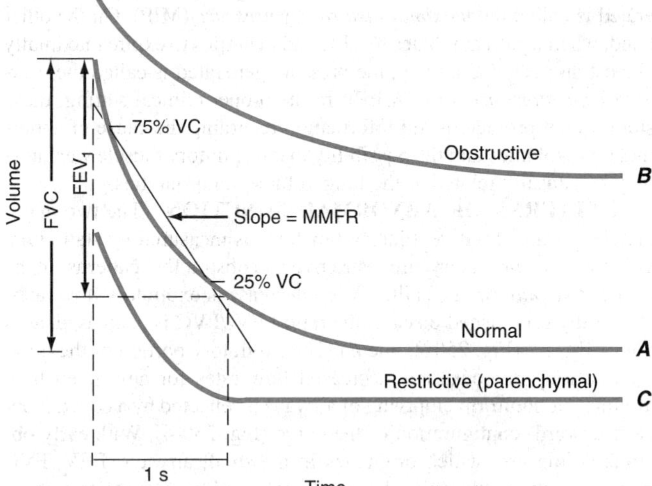

FIGURE 250-2 Spirographic tracings of forced expiration, comparing a normal tracing *(A)* and tracings in obstructive *(B)* and parenchymal restrictive *(C)* disease. Calculations of FVC, FEV_1, and $FEF_{25-75\%}$ are shown only for the normal tracing. Since there is no measure of absolute starting volume with spirometry, the curves are artificially positioned to show the relative starting lung volumes in the different conditions.

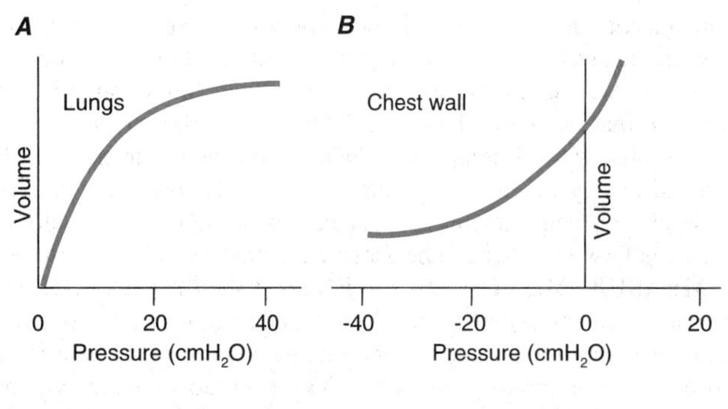

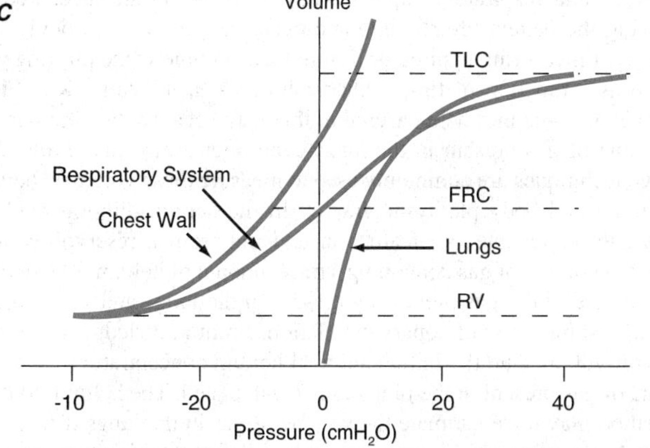

FIGURE 250-3 *A*. Pressure-volume curve of the lungs. *B*. Pressure-volume curve of the chest wall. *C*. Pressure-volume curve of the respiratory system, showing the superimposed component curves of the lungs and the chest wall. RV, residual volume; FRC, functional residual capacity; TLC, total lung capacity. *(From Weinberger, with permission.)*

At TLC, the maximal force applied by the inspiratory muscles to expand the lungs is opposed mainly by the inward recoil of the lungs. As a consequence, the major determinants of TLC are the stiffness of the lungs and inspiratory muscle strength. If the lungs become stiffer—i.e., less compliant—TLC is decreased. If the lungs become less stiff (more compliant), TLC is increased. If the inspiratory muscles are significantly weakened, they are less able to overcome the inward elastic recoil of the lungs, and TLC is lowered.

At RV, the force exerted by the expiratory muscles to decrease lung volume further is balanced by the outward recoil of the chest wall, which becomes extremely stiff at low lung volumes. Two factors influence the volume of gas contained in the lungs at RV. The first is the ability of the subject to exert a prolonged expiratory effort, which is related to muscle strength and the ability to overcome sensory stimuli from the chest wall. The second is the ability of the lungs to empty to a small volume. In normal lungs, as P_{TP} is lowered, lung volume decreases. In lungs with diseased airways, as P_{TP} is lowered, flow limitation or airway closure may limit the amount of gas that can be expired. Consequently, either weak expiratory muscles or intrinsic airways disease can result in an elevation in measured RV.

Dynamic measurements of ventilatory function are made by having the subject inhale to TLC and then perform a forced expiration to RV. If a subject performs a series of such expiratory maneuvers using increasing muscular intensity, expiratory flow rates will increase until a certain level of effort is reached. Beyond this level, additional effort at any given lung volume will not increase the forced expiratory flow rate; this phenomenon is known as the *effort independence* of forced expiratory flow. The physiologic mechanisms determining the flow rates during this effort-independent phase of FEF have been shown to be the elastic recoil of the lung, the airflow resistance of the airways between the alveolar zone and the physical site of flow limitation, and the airway wall compliance at the site of flow limitation. Physical processes that decrease elastic recoil, increase airflow resistance, or increase airway wall compliance decrease the flow rate that can be achieved at any given lung volume. Conversely, processes that increase elastic recoil, decrease resistance, or stiffen airway walls increase the flow rate that can be achieved at any given lung volume.

MEASUREMENT OF VENTILATORY FUNCTION Ventilatory function is measured under static conditions for determination of lung volumes and under dynamic conditions for determination of forced expiratory flow rates. VC, expiratory reserve volume (ERV), and inspiratory capacity (IC) (Fig. 250-1) are measured by having the patient breathe into and out of a spirometer, a device capable of measuring expired or inspired gas volume while plotting volume as a function of time. Other volumes—specifically, RV, FRC, and TLC —cannot be measured in this way because they include the volume of gas present in the lungs even after a maximal expiration. Two techniques are commonly used to measure these volumes: helium dilution and body plethysmography. In the helium dilution method, the subject repeatedly breathes in and out from a reservoir with a known volume of gas containing a trace amount of helium. The helium is diluted by the gas previously present in the lungs and very little is absorbed into the pulmonary circulation. From knowledge of the reservoir volume and the initial and final helium concentrations, the volume of gas present in the lungs can be calculated. The helium dilution method may underestimate the volume of gas in the lungs if there are slowly communicating airspaces, such as bullae. In this situation, lung volumes can be measured more accurately with a body plethysmograph, a sealed box in which the patient sits while panting against a closed mouthpiece. Because there is no airflow into or out of the plethysmograph, the pressure changes in the thorax during panting cause compression and rarefaction of gas in the lungs and simultaneous rarefaction and compression of gas in the plethysmograph. By measuring the pressure changes in the plethysmograph and at the mouthpiece, the volume of gas in the thorax can be calculated using Boyle's law.

Lung volumes and measurements made during forced expiration are interpreted by comparing the values measured with the values expected given the age, height, sex, and race of the patient (Appendix A). Regression curves have been constructed on the basis of data obtained from large numbers of normal, nonsmoking individuals without evidence of lung disease. Predicted values for a given patient can then be obtained by using the patient's age and height in the appropriate regression equation; different equations are used depending on the patient's race and gender. Because there is some variability among normal individuals, values between 80 and 120% of the predicted value have traditionally been considered normal. Increasingly, calculated percentiles are used in determining normality. Specifically, values of individual measurements falling below the fifth percentile are considered to be below normal.

The normal value for the ratio FEV_1/FVC is approximately 0.75 to 0.80, although this value does fall somewhat with advancing age. The $FEF_{25-75\%}$ is often considered a more sensitive measurement of early airflow obstruction, particularly in small airways. However, this measurement must be interpreted cautiously in patients with abnormally small lungs (low TLC and VC). These patients exhale less air during forced expiration, and the $FEF_{25-75\%}$ may appear abnormal relative to the usual predicted value, even though it is normal relative to the size of the patient's lungs.

It is also a common practice to plot expiratory flow rates against lung volume (rather than against time); the close linkage of flow rates to lung volumes produces a typical *flow-volume curve* (Fig. 250-4). In addition, the spirometric values mentioned above can be calculated from the flow-volume curve. Commonly, flow rates during a maximal inspiratory effort performed as rapidly as possible are plotted as well, making the flow-volume curve into a *flow-volume loop*. At TLC, before expiratory flow starts, the flow rate is zero; once forced expiration has begun, a high peak flow rate is rapidly achieved. As expiration continues and lung volume approaches RV, the flow rate falls progressively, in a nearly linear fashion as a function of lung volume for a person with normal lung function. During maximal inspiration from RV to TLC, inspiratory flow is most rapid at the midpoint of inspiration, so the inspiratory portion of the loop is U-shaped or saddle-shaped. The flow rates achieved during maximal expiration can be analyzed quantitatively by comparing the flow rates at specified lung volumes with the predicted values or qualitatively by analyzing the shape of the descending limb of the expiratory curve.

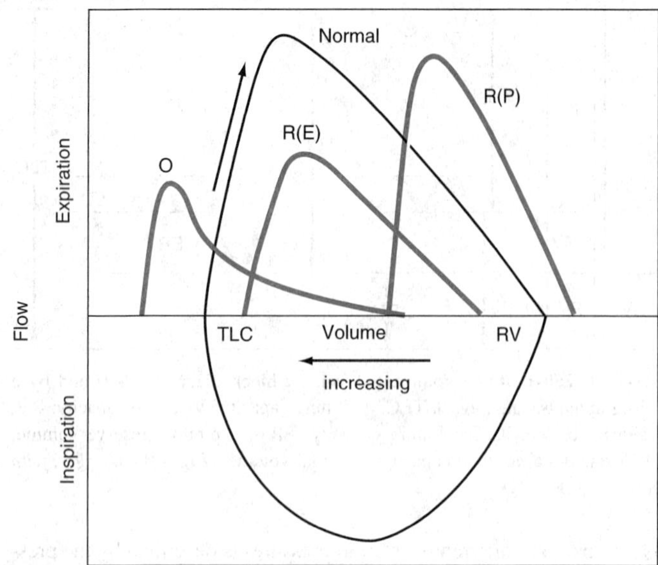

FIGURE 250-4 Flow-volume curves in different conditions: O, obstructive disease; R(P), parenchymal restrictive disease; R(E), extraparenchymal restrictive disease with limitation in inspiration and expiration. Forced expiration is plotted in all conditions; forced inspiration is shown only for the normal curve. TLC, total lung capacity; RV, residual volume. By convention, lung volume increases to the left on the abscissa. The arrow alongside the normal curve indicates the direction of expiration from TLC to RV.

Assessing the strength of respiratory muscles is an additional part of the overall evaluation of some patients with respiratory dysfunction. When a patient exhales completely to RV and then tries to inspire maximally against an occluded airway, the pressure that can be generated is called the *maximal inspiratory pressure* (MIP). On the other hand, when a patient inhales to TLC and then tries to expire maximally against an occluded airway, the pressure generated is called the *maximal expiratory pressure* (MEP). In the proper clinical setting, these studies may provide useful information regarding the cause of abnormal lung volumes and the possibility that respiratory muscle weakness may be causally related to the lung volume abnormalities.

PATTERNS OF ABNORMAL FUNCTION The two major patterns of abnormal ventilatory function, as measured by static lung volumes and spirometry, are restrictive and obstructive patterns. In the *obstructive pattern*, the hallmark is a decrease in expiratory flow rates. With fully established disease, the ratio FEV_1/FVC is decreased, as is the $FEF_{25-75\%}$ (Fig. 250-2, line *B*). The expiratory portion of the flow-volume loop demonstrates decreased flow rates for any given lung volume. Nonuniform emptying of airways is reflected by a coved (concave upward) configuration of the curve (Fig. 250-4). With early obstructive disease, which originates in the small airways, FEV_1/FVC may be normal; the only abnormalities noted on routine testing of pulmonary function may be a depression in $FEF_{25-75\%}$ and an abnormal, i.e., coved, configuration in the terminal portion of the forced expiratory flow-volume curve.

In *obstructive* disease, the TLC is normal or increased. When helium equilibration tests are used to measure lung volumes, the measured volume may be less than the actual volume if helium was not well distributed to all regions of the lung. Residual volume is elevated as a result of airway closure during expiration, and the ratio RV/TLC is increased. VC is frequently decreased in obstructive disease because of the striking elevations in RV with only minor changes in TLC.

Table 250-1 Alterations in Ventilatory Function

	TLC	RV	VC	FEV_1/FVC	MIP	MEP
Obstructive	N to ↑	↑	↓	↓[a]	N	N
Restrictive						
Pulmonary parenchymal	↓	↓	↓	N to ↑	N	N
Extraparenchymal—inspiratory	↓	N to ↓	↓	N	↓/N[b]	N
Extraparenchymal—inspiratory + expiratory	↓	↑	↓	Variable	↓/N[b]	↓/N[b]

[a] Mild obstructive (small airways) disease may have decreased $FEF_{25-75\%}$ with normal FEV_1/FVC.
[b] Reduced if due to respiratory muscle weakness; normal if due to chest wall stiffness.
NOTE: N, normal; for other abbreviations, see text.

A *restrictive pattern* can be broadly divided into two subgroups, depending on the location of the pathology: pulmonary parenchymal and extraparenchymal. For extraparenchymal disease, dysfunction can be predominantly in inspiration or in both inspiration and expiration (Table 250-1). The hallmark of a restrictive pattern, found in all these subcategories, is a decrease in lung volumes, primarily TLC and VC. In pulmonary parenchymal disease, RV is also generally decreased, and forced expiratory flow rates are preserved. In fact, when FEV_1 is considered as a percentage of the FVC, the flow rates are often supranormal, i.e., disproportionately high relative to the size of the lungs (Fig. 250-2, line *C*). The flow-volume curve may graphically demonstrate this disproportionate relationship between flow rates and lung volumes, since the expiratory portion of the curve appears relatively tall (preserved flow rates) but narrow (decreased lung volumes), as shown in Fig. 250-4.

In the extraparenchymal pattern characterized by *inspiratory dysfunction*, caused by either inspiratory muscle weakness or a stiff chest wall, inadequate distending forces are exerted on an otherwise normal lung. As a result, TLC values are less than predicted, RV is often not significantly affected, and expiratory flow rates are preserved. If inspiratory muscle weakness is the cause of this pattern, then MIP is decreased. In the extraparenchymal pattern characterized by *inspiratory and expiratory dysfunction*, the ability to expire to a normal RV is also limited, because of either expiratory muscle weakness or a deformed chest wall that is abnormally rigid at volumes below FRC. Consequently, RV is often elevated, unlike the pattern observed in the other restrictive subcategories. The ratio FEV_1/FVC is variable and depends on expiratory muscle strength. If expiratory muscle strength is significantly decreased, then MEP is decreased, the ability to expire rapidly is impaired, and FEV_1/FVC may be decreased even though there is no airflow obstruction. If expiratory muscle strength is normal but the chest wall is abnormally stiff below FRC, then FEV_1/FVC is normal or increased.

CLINICAL CORRELATIONS Table 250-1 summarizes the expected alterations in ventilatory function as indicated by pulmonary function testing. One reason to establish a ventilatory diagnosis is to categorize the functional disorder. This information can be useful in diagnosis, as outlined in Table 250-2. Note that lung disease such as pulmonary vascular disease or lung nodules can be present without abnormal ventilatory function, but the presence of specific diagnostic findings is an aid in differential diagnosis.

DISTURBANCES IN THE PULMONARY CIRCULATION

PHYSIOLOGIC FEATURES The pulmonary vasculature must handle the entire output of the right ventricle, approximately 5 L/min in a normal adult at rest. The comparatively thin-walled vessels of the pulmonary arterial system provide relatively little resistance to flow and are capable of handling this large volume of blood at perfusion pressures that are low compared with those of the systemic circulation. The normal mean pulmonary artery pressure is 15 mmHg, as compared to approximately 95 mmHg for the normal mean aortic pressure. Regional blood flow in the lung is dependent on hydrostatic forces. In an upright person, pulmonary arterial pressure (PAP) is lowest at the apex of the lung and highest at the lung base. As a result, in the upright position, perfusion is least at the apex and greatest at the base. When cardiac output increases, as occurs during exercise, the pulmonary vasculature is capable of recruiting previously unperfused vessels and distending underperfused vessels, thus responding to the increase in flow with a decrease in pulmonary vascular resistance. In consequence, the increase in mean PAP, even with a three- to fourfold increase in cardiac output, is small.

METHODS OF MEASUREMENT Assessment of circulatory function in the pulmonary vasculature depends on measuring pulmonary vascular pressures and cardiac output. Clinically, these measurements are commonly made in intensive care units capable of invasive monitoring and in cardiac catheterization laboratories. With a flow-directed pulmonary arterial (Swan-Ganz) catheter, PAP and pulmonary capillary wedge pressure can be measured directly, and cardiac output can be obtained by the thermodilution method. Pulmonary vascular resistance (PVR) can then be calculated according to the equation

$$PVR = 80(PAP - PCW)/CO$$

where PVR = pulmonary vascular resistance (dyn·s/cm^5); PAP = mean pulmonary arterial pressure (mmHg); PCW = pulmonary capillary wedge pressure (mmHg); and CO = cardiac output (L/min).

The normal value for pulmonary vascular resistance is approximately 50 to 150 dyn·s/cm^5.

MECHANISMS OF ABNORMAL FUNCTION (See also Chap. 260) PVR may increase by a variety of mechanisms. Pulmonary arterial and arteriolar vasoconstriction is a prominent response to alveolar hypoxia. PVR also increases if intraluminal thrombi or proliferation of smooth muscle in vessel walls diminishes the luminal cross-sectional area. If small pulmonary vessels are destroyed, either

Table 250-2 Common Respiratory Diseases by Diagnostic Categories

OBSTRUCTIVE

- Asthma
- Chronic obstructive lung disease (chronic bronchitis, emphysema)
- Bronchiectasis
- Cystic fibrosis
- Bronchiolitis

RESTRICTIVE—PARENCHYMAL

- Sarcoidosis
- Idiopathic pulmonary fibrosis
- Pneumoconiosis
- Drug- or radiation-induced interstitial lung disease

RESTRICTIVE—EXTRAPARENCHYMAL

- Neuromuscular
  - Diaphragmatic weakness/paralysis
  - Myasthenia gravis[a]
  - Guillain-Barré syndrome[a]
  - Muscular dystrophies[a]
  - Cervical spine injury[a]
- Chest wall
  - Kyphoscoliosis
  - Obesity
  - Ankylosing spondylitis[a]

[a] Can have inspiratory and expiratory limitation (see text).

by scarring or by loss of alveolar walls, the total cross-sectional area of the pulmonary vascular bed diminishes, and PVR increases. When PVR is elevated, either PAP rises to maintain normal cardiac output or cardiac output falls if PAP does not increase.

CLINICAL CORRELATIONS Disturbances in the function of the pulmonary vasculature as a result of primary cardiac disease, either congenital heart disease or conditions that elevate left atrial pressure, such as mitral stenosis, are beyond the scope of this chapter and are discussed in Chaps. 234 and 236, respectively. Instead, the focus will be on the pulmonary vasculature as its function is affected by diseases primarily involving the respiratory system, including the pulmonary vessels themselves.

All diseases of the respiratory system causing hypoxemia are potentially capable of increasing PVR, since alveolar hypoxia is a very potent stimulus for pulmonary vasoconstriction. The more prolonged and intense the hypoxic stimulus, the more likely it is that a significant increase in PVR producing pulmonary hypertension will result. In practice, patients with hypoxemia caused by chronic obstructive lung disease, interstitial lung disease, chest wall disease, and the obesity hypoventilation–sleep apnea syndrome are particularly prone to developing pulmonary hypertension. If there are additional structural changes in the pulmonary vasculature secondary to the underlying process, these will increase the likelihood of developing pulmonary hypertension.

With diseases directly affecting the pulmonary vessels, a decrease in the cross-sectional area of the pulmonary vascular bed is primarily responsible for increased PVR, while hypoxemia generally plays a lesser role. In the case of recurrent pulmonary emboli, parts of the pulmonary arterial system are occluded by intraluminal thrombi originating in the systemic venous system. With primary pulmonary hypertension (Chap. 260) or with pulmonary vascular disease secondary to scleroderma, the small pulmonary arteries and arterioles are affected by a generalized obliterative process that narrows and occludes these vessels. PVR increases, and significant pulmonary hypertension often results.

DISTURBANCES IN GAS EXCHANGE

PHYSIOLOGIC FEATURES The primary functions of the respiratory system are to remove the appropriate amount of CO_2 from blood entering the pulmonary circulation and to provide adequate O_2 to blood leaving the pulmonary circulation. For these functions to be carried out properly, there must be adequate provision of fresh air to the alveoli for delivery of O_2 and removal of CO_2 (ventilation), adequate circulation of blood through the pulmonary vasculature (perfusion), adequate movement of gas between alveoli and pulmonary capillaries (diffusion), and appropriate contact between alveolar gas and pulmonary capillary blood (ventilation-perfusion matching).

A normal individual at rest inspires approximately 12 to 16 times per minute, each breath having a tidal volume of approximately 500 mL. A portion (approximately 30%) of the fresh air inspired with each breath does not reach the alveoli but remains in the conducting airways of the lung. This component of each breath, which is not generally available for gas exchange, is called the *anatomic dead space component*. The remaining 70% reaches the alveolar zone, mixes rapidly with the gas already there, and can participate in gas exchange. In this example, the total ventilation each minute is approximately 7 L, composed of 2 L/min of dead space ventilation and 5 L/min of alveolar ventilation. In certain diseases, some alveoli are ventilated but not perfused, so that some ventilation in addition to the anatomic dead space component is wasted. If total dead space ventilation is increased but total minute ventilation is unchanged, then alveolar ventilation must fall correspondingly.

Gas exchange is dependent on alveolar ventilation rather than total minute ventilation, as outlined below. The partial pressure of CO_2 in arterial blood (Pa_{CO_2}) is directly proportional to the amount of CO_2 produced per minute ($\dot{V}_{CO_2}$) and inversely proportional to alveolar ventilation ($\dot{V}A$), according to the relationship

$$Pa_{CO_2} = 0.863 \times \dot{V}_{CO_2}/\dot{V}A$$

where $\dot{V}_{CO_2}$ is expressed in mL/min, $\dot{V}A$ in L/min, and Pa_{CO_2} in mmHg. At fixed $\dot{V}_{CO_2}$, when alveolar ventilation increases, Pa_{CO_2} falls, and when alveolar ventilation decreases, Pa_{CO_2} rises. Maintaining a normal level of O_2 in the alveoli (and consequently in arterial blood) also depends on provision of adequate alveolar ventilation to replenish alveolar O_2. This principle will become more apparent from consideration of the alveolar gas equation below.

Diffusion of O_2 and CO_2 Both O_2 and CO_2 diffuse readily down their respective concentration gradients through the alveolar wall and pulmonary capillary endothelium. Under normal circumstances, this process is rapid, and equilibration of both gases is complete within one-third of the transit time of erythrocytes through the pulmonary capillary bed. Even in disease states in which diffusion of gases is impaired, the impairment is unlikely to be severe enough to prevent equilibration of CO_2 and O_2. Consequently, a diffusion abnormality rarely results in arterial hypoxemia at rest. If erythrocyte transit time in the pulmonary circulation is shortened, as occurs with exercise, and diffusion is impaired, then diffusion limitation may contribute to hypoxemia. Exercise testing can often demonstrate such physiologically significant abnormalities due to impaired diffusion. Even though diffusion limitation rarely makes a clinically significant contribution to resting hypoxemia, clinical measurements of what is known as *diffusing capacity* (see below) can be a useful measure of the integrity of the alveolar-capillary membrane.

Ventilation-Perfusion Matching In addition to the absolute levels of alveolar ventilation and perfusion, gas exchange depends critically on the proper matching of ventilation and perfusion. The spectrum of possible ventilation-perfusion ($\dot{V}/\dot{Q}$) ratios in an alveolar-capillary unit ranges from zero, in which ventilation is totally absent and the unit behaves as a shunt, to infinity, in which perfusion is totally absent and the unit behaves as dead space. The P_{O_2} and P_{CO_2} of blood leaving each alveolar-capillary unit depend on the gas tension (of blood and air) entering that unit and on the particular $\dot{V}/\dot{Q}$ ratio of the unit. At one extreme, when an alveolar-capillary unit has a $\dot{V}/\dot{Q}$ ratio of 0 and behaves as a shunt, blood leaving the unit has the composition of mixed venous blood entering the pulmonary capillaries, i.e., $P\bar{v}_{O_2} \approx 40$ mmHg and $P\bar{v}_{CO_2} \approx 46$ mmHg. At the other extreme, when an alveolar-capillary unit has a high $\dot{V}/\dot{Q}$ ratio, it behaves almost like dead space, and the small amount of blood leaving the unit has partial pressures of O_2 and CO_2 ($P_{O_2} \approx 150$ mmHg, $P_{CO_2} \approx 0$ mmHg while breathing room air) approaching the composition of inspired gas.

In the ideal situation, all alveolar-capillary units have equal matching of ventilation and perfusion, i.e., a ratio of approximately 1 when each is expressed in L/min. However, even in the normal individual, some $\dot{V}/\dot{Q}$ mismatching is present, since there is normally a gradient of blood flow from the apices to the bases of the lungs. There is a similar gradient of ventilation from the apices to the bases, but it is less marked than the perfusion gradient. As a result, ventilation-perfusion ratios are higher at the lung apices than at the lung bases. Therefore, blood coming from the apices has a higher P_{O_2} and lower P_{CO_2} than blood coming from the bases. The net P_{O_2} and P_{CO_2} of the blood mixture coming from all areas of the lung is a flow-weighted average of the individual components, which reflects both the relative amount of blood from each unit and the O_2 and CO_2 *content* of the blood coming from each unit. Because of the sigmoid shape of the oxyhemoglobin dissociation curve (see Fig. 106-2), it is important to distinguish between the partial pressure and the content of O_2 in blood. Hemoglobin is almost fully (~90%) saturated at a P_{O_2} of 60 mmHg, and little additional O_2 is carried by hemoglobin even with a substantial elevation of P_{O_2} above 60 mmHg. On the other hand, significant O_2 desaturation of hemoglobin occurs once P_{O_2} falls below 60 mmHg and onto the steep descending limb of the curve. As a result, blood coming from regions of the lung with a high $\dot{V}/\dot{Q}$ ratio and a high P_{O_2} has only a small elevation in O_2 content and cannot compensate for blood coming from regions with a low $\dot{V}/\dot{Q}$ ratio and a low P_{O_2}, which has a significantly decreased O_2 content. Although $\dot{V}/\dot{Q}$ mismatching can influence P_{CO_2}, this effect is less marked and is often overcome by an increase in overall minute ventilation.

MEASUREMENT OF GAS EXCHANGE Arterial Blood Gases The most commonly used measures of gas exchange are the partial pressures of O_2 and CO_2 in arterial blood, i.e., Pa_{O_2} and Pa_{CO_2}, respectively. These partial pressures do not measure directly the quantity of O_2 and CO_2 in blood but rather the driving pressure for the gas in blood. The actual quantity or content of a gas in blood also depends on the solubility of the gas in plasma and the ability of any component of blood to react with or bind the gas of interest. Since hemoglobin is capable of binding large amounts of O_2, oxygenated hemoglobin is the primary form in which O_2 is transported in blood. The actual content of O_2 in blood therefore depends both on the hemoglobin concentration and on the Pa_{O_2}. The Pa_{O_2} determines what percentage of hemoglobin is saturated with O_2, based on the position on the oxyhemoglobin dissociation curve. Oxygen content in normal blood (at 37°C, pH 7.4) can be determined by adding the amount of O_2 dissolved in plasma to the amount bound to hemoglobin, according to the equation

$$O_2 \text{ content} = 1.34 \times [\text{hemoglobin}] \times \text{saturation} + 0.0031 \times P_{O_2}$$

since each gram of hemoglobin is capable of carrying 1.34 mL O_2 when fully saturated, and the amount of O_2 that can be dissolved in plasma is proportional to the P_{O_2}, with 0.0031 mL O_2 dissolved per deciliter of blood per mmHg P_{O_2}. In arterial blood, the amount of O_2 transported dissolved in plasma (approximately 0.3 mL O_2 per deciliter of blood) is trivial compared with the amount bound to hemoglobin (approximately 20 mL O_2 per deciliter of blood).

Most commonly, P_{O_2} is the measurement used to assess the effect of respiratory disease on the oxygenation of arterial blood. Direct measurement of O_2 saturation in arterial blood by oximetry is also important in selected clinical conditions. For example, in patients with carbon monoxide intoxication, carbon monoxide preferentially displaces O_2 from hemoglobin, essentially making a portion of hemoglobin unavailable for binding to O_2. In this circumstance, carbon monoxide saturation is high and O_2 saturation is low, even though the driving pressure for O_2 to bind to hemoglobin, reflected by P_{O_2}, is normal. Measurement of O_2 saturation is also important for the determination of O_2 content when mixed venous blood is sampled from a pulmonary arterial catheter to calculate cardiac output by the Fick technique. In mixed venous blood, the P_{O_2} is normally about 40 mmHg, but small changes in P_{O_2} may reflect relatively large changes in O_2 saturation.

A useful calculation in the assessment of oxygenation is the alveolar-arterial O_2 difference ($PA_{O_2} - Pa_{O_2}$), commonly called the *alveolar-arterial O_2 gradient* (or A − a gradient). This calculation takes into account the fact that alveolar and, hence, arterial P_{O_2} can be expected to change depending on the level of alveolar ventilation, reflected by the arterial P_{CO_2}. When a patient hyperventilates and has a low P_{CO_2} in arterial blood and alveolar gas, alveolar and arterial P_{O_2} will rise; conversely, hypoventilation and a high P_{CO_2} are accompanied by a decrease in alveolar and arterial P_{O_2}. These changes in arterial P_{O_2} are independent of abnormalities in O_2 transfer at the alveolar-capillary level and reflect only the dependence of alveolar P_{O_2} on the level of alveolar ventilation.

In order to determine the alveolar-arterial O_2 difference, the alveolar P_{O_2} (PA_{O_2}) must first be calculated. The equation most commonly used for this purpose, a simplified form of the alveolar gas equation, is

$$PA_{O_2} = FI_{O_2} \times (P_B - P_{H_2O}) - Pa_{CO_2}/R$$

where FI_{O_2} = fractional concentration of inspired O_2 (≈0.21 when breathing room air); P_B = barometric pressure (approximately 760 mmHg at sea level); P_{H_2O} = water vapor pressure (47 mmHg when air is fully saturated at 37°C); and R = respiratory quotient (the ratio of CO_2 production to O_2 consumption, usually assumed to be 0.8). If the preceding values are substituted into the equation for the patient breathing air at sea level, the equation becomes

$$PA_{O_2} = 150 - 1.25 \times Pa_{CO_2}$$

The alveolar-arterial O_2 difference can then be calculated by subtracting measured Pa_{O_2} from calculated PA_{O_2}. In a healthy young person breathing room air, the $PA_{O_2} - Pa_{O_2}$ is normally less than 15 mmHg; this value increases with age and may be as high as 30 mmHg in elderly patients.

The adequacy of CO_2 elimination is measured by the partial pressure of CO_2 in arterial blood, i.e., Pa_{CO_2}. A more complete understanding of the mechanisms and chronicity of abnormal levels of P_{CO_2} also requires measurement of pH and/or bicarbonate (HCO_3^-), since P_{CO_2} and the patient's acid-base status are so closely intertwined (Chap. 50).

Pulse Oximetry Because measurement of Pa_{O_2} requires arterial puncture, it is not ideal either for office use or for routine or frequent measurement in the inpatient setting. Additionally, because it provides intermittent rather than continuous data about the patient's oxygenation, it is not ideal for close monitoring of unstable patients. Pulse oximetry, an alternative method for assessing oxygenation, is readily available in many clinical settings. Using a probe usually clipped over a patient's finger, the pulse oximeter calculates oxygen saturation (rather than Pa_{O_2}) based on measurements of absorption of two wavelengths of light by hemoglobin in pulsatile, cutaneous arterial blood. Because of differential absorption of the two wavelengths of light by oxygenated and nonoxygenated hemoglobin, the percentage of hemoglobin that is saturated with oxygen, i.e., the Sa_{O_2}, can be calculated and displayed instantaneously.

Although the pulse oximeter has been a major advance in the noninvasive, continuous monitoring of oxygenation, there are several issues and potential problems concerning its use. First, the clinician must be aware of the relationship between oxygen saturation and tension as shown by the oxyhemoglobin dissociation curve (Fig. 106-2). Because the curve becomes relatively flat above an arterial P_{O_2} of 60 mmHg (corresponding to Sa_{O_2} = 90%), the oximeter is relatively insensitive to changes in Pa_{O_2} above this level. In addition, the position of the curve and therefore the specific relationship between Pa_{O_2} and Sa_{O_2} may change depending on factors such as temperature, pH, and the erythrocyte concentration of 2,3-diphosphoglycerate. Second, when cutaneous perfusion is decreased, e.g., owing to low cardiac output or the use of vasoconstrictors, the signal from the oximeter may be less reliable or even unobtainable. Third, other forms of hemoglobin, such as carboxyhemoglobin and methemoglobin, are not distinguishable from oxyhemoglobin when only two wavelengths of light are used. The Sa_{O_2} values reported by the pulse oximeter are not reliable in the presence of significant amounts of either of these forms of hemoglobin. In contrast, the device used to measure oxygen saturation in samples of arterial blood, called the CO-oximeter, uses at least four wavelengths of light and is capable of distinguishing oxyhemoglobin, deoxygenated hemoglobin, carboxyhemoglobin, and methemoglobin. Finally, the clinician must remember that the often-used goal of $Sa_{O_2} \geq$ 90% does not indicate anything about CO_2 elimination and therefore does not ensure a clinically acceptable P_{CO_2}.

Diffusing Capacity The ability of gas to diffuse across the alveolar-capillary membrane is ordinarily assessed by the diffusing capacity of the lung for carbon monoxide (DL_{CO}). In this test, a small concentration of carbon monoxide (0.3%) is inhaled, usually in a single breath that is held for approximately 10 s. The carbon monoxide is diluted by the gas already present in the alveoli and is also taken up by hemoglobin as the erythrocytes course through the pulmonary capillary system. The concentration of carbon monoxide in exhaled gas is measured, and DL_{CO} is calculated as the quantity of carbon monoxide absorbed per minute per mmHg pressure gradient from the alveoli to the pulmonary capillaries. The value obtained for DL_{CO} depends on the alveolar-capillary surface area available for gas exchange and on the pulmonary capillary blood volume. In addition, the thickness of the alveolar-capillary membrane, the degree of $\dot{V}/\dot{Q}$ mismatching, and the patient's hemoglobin level will affect the measurement. Because of this effect of hemoglobin levels on DL_{CO}, the measured DL_{CO} is frequently corrected to take the patient's hemoglobin level into account. The value for DL_{CO}, ideally corrected for hemoglobin, can then be compared with a predicted value, based either on age, height, and gender or on the alveolar volume (VA) at which the value was obtained. Alternatively, the DL_{CO} can be divided by VA and the resulting value for DL_{CO}/VA compared with a predicted value.

Approach to the Patient

Arterial Blood Gases Hypoxemia is a common manifestation of a variety of diseases affecting the lungs or other parts of the respiratory system. The broad clinical problem of hypoxemia is often best characterized according to the underlying mechanism. The four basic, and not mutually exclusive, mechanisms of hypoxemia are (1) a decrease in inspired P_{O_2}, (2) hypoventilation, (3) shunting, and (4) $\dot{V}/\dot{Q}$ mismatching. Hypoxemia due to decreased diffusion occurs only under selected clinical circumstances and is not usually included among the general categories of hypoxemia. Determining the underlying mechanism for hypoxemia depends on measurement of the Pa_{CO_2}, calculation of $PA_{O_2} - Pa_{O_2}$, and knowledge of the response to supplemental O_2. A flowchart summarizing the approach to the hypoxemic patient is given in Fig. 250-5.

A decrease in the inspired P_{O_2} and hypoventilation both cause hypoxemia by lowering PA_{O_2} and therefore Pa_{O_2}. In each case, gas exchange at the alveolar-capillary level occurs normally, and $PA_{O_2} - Pa_{O_2}$ is not elevated. Hypoxemia due to decreased inspired P_{O_2} can be diagnosed from knowledge of the clinical situation. Inspired P_{O_2} is lowered either because the patient is at a high altitude, where barometric pressure is low, or, much less commonly, because the patient is breathing a gas mixture containing less than 21% O_2. The hallmark of hypoventilation as a cause of hypoxemia is an elevation in Pa_{CO_2}. This is associated with an increase in PA_{CO_2} and a fall in PA_{O_2}. When hypoxemia is due purely to a low inspired P_{O_2} or to alveolar hypoventilation, $PA_{O_2} - Pa_{O_2}$ is normal. If $PA_{O_2} - Pa_{O_2}$ and Pa_{CO_2} are both elevated, then an additional mechanism, such as $\dot{V}/\dot{Q}$ mismatching or shunting, is contributing to hypoxemia.

Shunting is a cause of hypoxemia when desaturated blood effectively bypasses oxygenation at the alveolar-capillary level. This situation occurs either because a structural problem allows desaturated blood to bypass the normal site of gas exchange or because perfused alveoli are not ventilated. Shunting is associated with an elevation in the $PA_{O_2} - Pa_{O_2}$ value. When shunting is an important contributing factor to hypoxemia, the lowered Pa_{O_2} is relatively refractory to improvement by supplemental O_2.

Finally, the largest clinical category of hypoxemia is $\dot{V}/\dot{Q}$ mismatching. With $\dot{V}/\dot{Q}$ mismatching, regions with low $\dot{V}/\dot{Q}$ ratios contribute blood with a low P_{O_2} and a low O_2 content. Corresponding regions with high $\dot{V}/\dot{Q}$ ratios contribute blood with a high P_{O_2}. However, because blood is already almost fully saturated at a normal P_{O_2}, elevation of the P_{O_2} to a high value does not significantly increase O_2 saturation or content and therefore cannot compensate for the reduction of O_2 saturation and content in blood coming from regions with a low $\dot{V}/\dot{Q}$ ratio. When $\dot{V}/\dot{Q}$ mismatch is the primary cause of hypoxemia, $PA_{O_2} - Pa_{O_2}$ is elevated, and P_{CO_2} generally is normal. Supplemental O_2 corrects the hypoxemia by raising the P_{O_2} in blood coming from regions with a low $\dot{V}/\dot{Q}$ ratio; this response distinguishes hypoxemia due to $\dot{V}/\dot{Q}$ mismatching from that due to true shunt.

The essential mechanism underlying all cases of hypercapnia is alveolar ventilation that is inadequate for the amount of CO_2 produced. It is conceptually useful to characterize CO_2 retention further, based on a more detailed examination of the potential contributing factors. These include (1) increased CO_2 production; (2) decreased ventilatory drive ("won't breathe"); (3) malfunction of the respiratory pump or increased airways resistance, which makes it more difficult to sustain adequate ventilation ("can't breathe"); and (4) inefficiency of gas exchange (increased dead space or $\dot{V}/\dot{Q}$ mismatch) necessitating a compensatory increase in overall minute ventilation. In practice, more than one of these mechanisms is commonly responsible for hypercapnia, since increased minute ventilation is capable of compensating for increased CO_2 production and for inefficiencies of gas exchange.

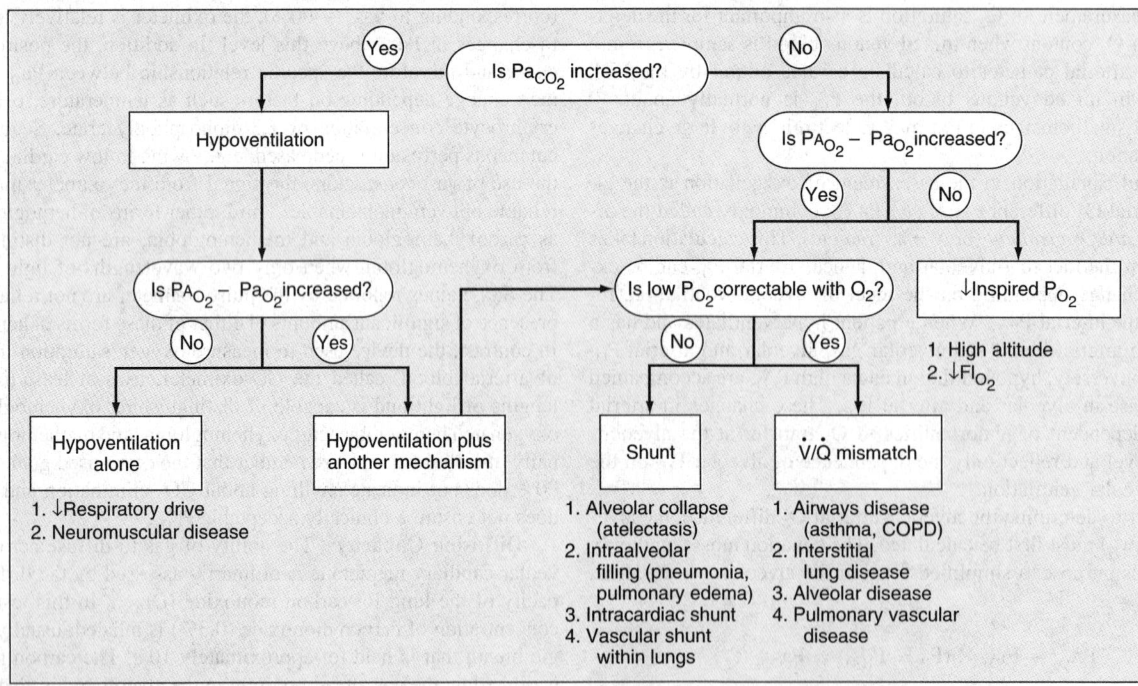

FIGURE 250-5 Flow diagram outlining the diagnostic approach to the patient with hypoxemia (Pa_{O_2} < 80 mmHg). $PA_{O_2} - Pa_{O_2}$ is usually < 15 mmHg for subjects ≤30 years old and increases by ~3 mmHg per decade after age 30.

Diffusing Capacity Although abnormalities in diffusion are rarely responsible for hypoxemia, clinical measurement of diffusing capacity is frequently used to assess the functional integrity of the alveolar-capillary membrane, which includes the pulmonary capillary bed. Diseases that affect solely the airways generally do not lower DL_{CO}, whereas diseases that affect the alveolar walls or the pulmonary capillary bed will have an effect on DL_{CO}. Even though DL_{CO} is a useful marker for assessing whether disease affecting the alveolar-capillary bed is present, an abnormal DL_{CO} does not necessarily imply that diffusion limitation is responsible for hypoxemia in a particular patient.

CLINICAL CORRELATIONS Useful clinical correlations can be made with the mechanisms underlying hypoxemia (Fig. 250-5). A lowered inspired P_{O_2}contributes to hypoxemia if either the patient is at high altitude or if the concentration of inspired O_2 is less than 21%. The latter problem occurs if a patient receiving anesthesia or ventilatory support is inadvertently given a gas mixture to breathe containing less than 21% O_2 or if O_2 is consumed from the ambient gas, as can occur during smoke inhalation from a fire. The primary feature of hypoventilation as a cause of hypoxemia is an elevation in arterial P_{CO_2}. →*For further discussion of the clinical correlations with hypoventilation, see Chap. 263.*

Shunting as a cause of hypoxemia can reflect transfer of blood from the right to the left side of the heart without passage through the pulmonary circulation, as occurs with an intracardiac shunt. This problem is most common in the setting of cyanotic congenital heart disease, when an interatrial or interventricular septal defect is associated with pulmonary hypertension so that shunting is in the right-to-left rather than the left-to-right direction. Shunting of blood through the pulmonary parenchyma is most frequently due to disease causing absence of ventilation to perfused alveoli. This can occur if the alveoli are atelectatic or if they are filled with fluid, as in pulmonary edema (both cardiogenic and noncardiogenic), or with extensive intraalveolar exudation of fluid due to pneumonia. Less commonly, vascular anomalies with arteriovenous shunting in the lung can cause hypoxemia. These anomalies can be hereditary, as found with hereditary hemorrhagic telangiectasia (Osler-Rendu-Weber syndrome), or acquired, as in pulmonary vascular malformations secondary to hepatic cirrhosis, which are similar to the commonly recognized cutaneous vascular malformations ("spider hemangiomas").

Ventilation-perfusion mismatch is the most common cause of hypoxemia clinically. Most of the processes affecting either the airways or the pulmonary parenchyma are distributed unevenly throughout the lungs and do not necessarily affect ventilation and perfusion equally. Some areas of lung may have good perfusion and poor ventilation, whereas others may have poor perfusion and relatively good ventilation. Important examples of airways diseases in which $\dot{V}/\dot{Q}$ mismatch causes hypoxemia are asthma and chronic obstructive lung disease. Parenchymal lung diseases causing $\dot{V}/\dot{Q}$ mismatch and hypoxemia include interstitial lung disease and pneumonia.

Clinically important alterations in CO_2 elimination range from excessive ventilation and hypocapnia to inadequate CO_2 elimination and hypercapnia. →*For further discussion of these clinical problems, see Chap. 263.*

Diffusing Capacity Measurement of DL_{CO} may be useful for assessing disease affecting the alveolar-capillary bed or the pulmonary vasculature. In practice, three main categories of disease are associated with lowered DL_{CO}: interstitial lung disease, emphysema, and pulmonary vascular disease. With interstitial lung disease, scarring of alveolar-capillary units diminishes the area of the alveolar-capillary bed as well as pulmonary blood volume. With emphysema, alveolar walls are destroyed, so the surface area of the alveolar-capillary bed is again diminished. In patients with disease causing a decrease in the cross-sectional area and volume of the pulmonary vascular bed, such as recurrent pulmonary emboli or primary pulmonary hypertension, DL_{CO} is commonly diminished.

Diffusing capacity may be elevated if pulmonary blood volume is increased, as may be seen in congestive heart failure. However, once interstitial and alveolar edema ensue, the net DL_{CO} depends on the opposing influences of increased pulmonary capillary blood volume elevating DL_{CO} and pulmonary edema decreasing it. Finding an elevated DL_{CO} may be useful in the diagnosis of alveolar hemorrhage, as in Goodpasture's syndrome. Hemoglobin contained in erythrocytes in the alveolar lumen is capable of binding carbon monoxide, so the exhaled carbon monoxide concentration is diminished and the measured DL_{CO} is increased.

BIBLIOGRAPHY

AMERICAN THORACIC SOCIETY: Lung function testing: Selection of reference values and interpretative strategies. Am Rev Respir Dis 144:1202, 1991

CELLI BR: The importance of spirometry in COPD and asthma: effect on approach to management. Chest 117:15S, 2000

CRAPO RO: Pulmonary-function testing. N Engl J Med 331:25, 1994

———, FORSTER RE II: Carbon monoxide diffusing capacity. Clin Chest Med 10:187, 1989

LEVITZKY MG: Pulmonary Physiology, 5th ed. New York, McGraw-Hill, 1999

QUANJER PH et al: Lung volumes and forced ventilatory flows. Report Working Party Standardization of Lung Function Tests, European Community for Steel and Coal. Official Statement of the European Respiratory Society. Eur Respir J [Suppl] 16:5, 1993

SHAPIRO BA et al: *Clinical Application of Blood Gases*, 5th ed. St. Louis, Mosby, 1994

SOCIETY OF CRITICAL CARE MEDICINE: A model for technology assessment applied to pulse oximetry. Crit Care Med 21:615, 1993

WEINBERGER SE: *Principles of Pulmonary Medicine*, 3d ed. Philadelphia, Saunders, 1998

WEST JB, WAGNER PD: Pulmonary gas exchange. Am J Respir Crit Care Med 157 (Pt 2): S82, 1998

251

Steven E. Weinberger, Jeffrey M. Drazen

DIAGNOSTIC PROCEDURES IN RESPIRATORY DISEASE

The diagnostic modalities available for assessing the patient with suspected or known respiratory system disease include imaging studies and techniques for acquiring biologic specimens, some of which involve direct visualization of part of the respiratory system. →*Methods used to characterize the functional changes developing as a result of disease, including pulmonary function tests and measurements of gas exchange, are discussed in Chap. 250.*

IMAGING STUDIES

ROUTINE RADIOGRAPHY Routine chest radiography, which generally includes both posteroanterior and lateral views, is an integral part of the diagnostic evaluation of diseases involving the pulmonary parenchyma, the pleura, and, to a lesser extent, the airways and the mediastinum (see Figs. 249-1 and 249-2). Lateral decubitus views are often useful for determining whether pleural abnormalities represent freely flowing fluid, whereas apical lordotic views can often visualize disease at the lung apices better than the standard posteroanterior view. Portable equipment, which is often used for acutely ill patients who either cannot be transported to a radiology suite or cannot stand up for posteroanterior and lateral views, generally yields just a single radiograph taken in the anteroposterior direction. →*Common radiographic patterns and their clinical correlates are reviewed in Chap. 249.*

COMPUTED TOMOGRAPHY Computed tomography (CT) offers several advantages over routine chest radiography. First, the use of cross-sectional images often makes it possible to distinguish between densities that would be superimposed on plain radiographs. Second, CT is far better than routine radiographic studies at characterizing tissue density, distinguishing subtle differences in density between adjacent structures, and providing accurate size assessment of lesions. As a result, CT is particularly valuable in assessing hilar and mediastinal disease (which is often poorly characterized by plain radiography), in identifying and characterizing disease adjacent to the chest wall or spine (including pleural disease), and in identifying areas of fat density or calcification in pulmonary nodules (Fig. 251-1). Its utility in the assessment of mediastinal disease has made CT an important tool in the staging of lung cancer (Chap. 88), as an assessment of tumor involvement of mediastinal lymph nodes is critical to proper staging. With the additional use of contrast material, CT also makes it possible to distinguish vascular from nonvascular structures, which is particularly important in distinguishing lymph nodes and masses from vascular structures.

Helical CT scanning allows the collection of continuous data over a larger volume of lung during a single breath-holding maneuver than is possible with conventional CT. With CT angiography, in which intravenous contrast is administered and images are acquired rapidly by helical scanning, pulmonary emboli can be detected in segmental and larger pulmonary arteries. With high-resolution CT (HRCT), the thickness of individual cross-sectional images is approximately 1 to 2 mm, rather than the usual 10 mm, and the images are reconstructed with high-spatial-resolution algorithms. The detail that can be seen on HRCT scans allows better recognition of subtle parenchymal and airway disease, such as bronchiectasis, emphysema, and diffuse parenchymal disease (Fig. 251-2). Certain nearly pathognomonic patterns have now been recognized for many of the interstitial lung diseases, such as lymphangitic carcinoma, idiopathic pulmonary fibrosis, sarcoidosis, and eosinophilic granuloma; at present it is not yet clear in what settings these patterns will obviate the need for obtaining lung tissue.

MAGNETIC RESONANCE IMAGING The role of magnetic resonance imaging (MRI) in the evaluation of respiratory system disease is less well defined than that of CT. Because MRI generally provides a less detailed view of the pulmonary parenchyma as well as poorer spatial resolution, its usefulness in the evaluation of parenchymal lung disease is limited at present. However, MRI has advantages over CT in certain clinical settings. Because its images can be reconstructed in sagittal and coronal as well as transverse planes, MRI may be better for imaging abnormalities near the lung apex, the spine, and the thoracoabdominal junction. In addition, vascular structures can be distinguished from nonvascular structures without the need for contrast. Flowing blood does not produce a signal on MRI, so vessels appear as hollow tubular structures. This feature can be useful in determining whether abnormal hilar or mediastinal densities are vascular in origin and in defining aortic lesions such as aneurysms or dissection.

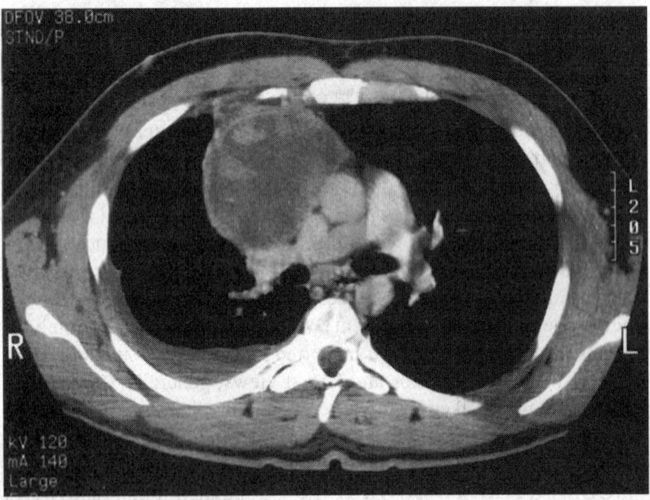

FIGURE 251-1 CT scan demonstrating a mediastinal mass of heterogeneous density. CT is superior to plain radiography for the detection of abnormal mediastinal densities and the distinction of masses from adjacent vascular structures.

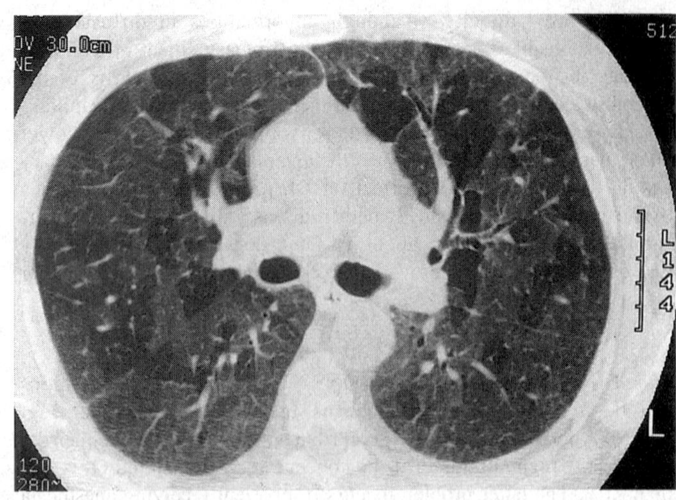

FIGURE 251-2 High-resolution CT scan demonstrating pulmonary parenchyma with a heterogeneous appearance. Most of the parenchyma has a subtle "ground-glass" pattern of increased density, best recognized by comparison with the intervening areas of normal lung, which have irregular but well-defined borders. The ground-glass pattern in this patient was due to hypersensitivity pneumonitis. *(From Weinberger, with permission.)*

SCINTIGRAPHIC IMAGING Radioactive isotopes, administered by either intravenous or inhaled routes, allow the lungs to be imaged with a gamma camera. The most common use of such imaging is ventilation-perfusion lung scanning performed for evaluation of pulmonary embolism. When injected intravenously, albumin macroaggregates labeled with technetium 99m become lodged in pulmonary capillaries; therefore, the distribution of the trapped radioisotope follows the distribution of blood flow. When inhaled, radiolabeled xenon gas can be used to demonstrate the distribution of ventilation. For example, pulmonary thromboembolism usually produces one or more regions of ventilation-perfusion mismatch—that is, regions in which there is a defect in perfusion that follows the distribution of a vessel and that is not accompanied by a corresponding defect in ventilation (Chap. 261). Another common use of such radioisotope scans is in a patient with impaired lung function who is being considered for lung resection. The distribution of the isotope(s) can be used to assess the regional distribution of blood flow and ventilation, allowing the physician to estimate the level of postoperative lung function.

Another scintigraphic imaging technique, gallium imaging, has been of diagnostic value in patients with *Pneumocystis carinii* pneumonia and other opportunistic infections. Use of gallium imaging may provide clues to sort out the differential diagnosis of pulmonary infiltrates in immunosuppressed patients, especially patients with AIDS.

PULMONARY ANGIOGRAPHY The pulmonary arterial system can be visualized by pulmonary angiography, in which radiopaque contrast medium is injected through a catheter previously threaded into the pulmonary artery. When performed in cases of pulmonary embolism, pulmonary angiography demonstrates the consequences of an intravascular clot—either a defect in the lumen of a vessel (a "filling defect") or an abrupt termination ("cutoff") of the vessel. Other, less common indications for pulmonary angiography include visualization of a suspected pulmonary arteriovenous malformation and assessment of pulmonary arterial invasion by a neoplasm.

ULTRASOUND Because ultrasound energy is rapidly dissipated in air, ultrasound imaging is not useful for evaluation of the pulmonary parenchyma. However, it is helpful in the detection and localization of pleural abnormalities and is often used as a guide to placement of a needle for sampling of pleural liquid (i.e., for thoracentesis).

TECHNIQUES FOR OBTAINING BIOLOGIC SPECIMENS

COLLECTION OF SPUTUM Sputum can be collected either by spontaneous expectoration or after inhalation of an irritating aerosol, such as hypertonic saline. The latter method, called *sputum induction*, is commonly used to obtain sputum for diagnostic studies, either because sputum is not spontaneously being produced or because of an expected higher yield of certain types of findings. Knowledge of the appearance and quality of the sputum specimen obtained is especially important when one is interested in Gram's staining and culture. Because sputum consists mainly of secretions from the tracheobronchial tree rather than the upper airway, the finding of alveolar macrophages and other inflammatory cells is consistent with a lower respiratory tract origin of the sample, whereas the presence of squamous epithelial cells in a "sputum" sample indicates contamination by secretions from the upper airways.

Besides processing for routine bacterial pathogens by Gram's staining and culture, sputum can be processed for a variety of other pathogens, including staining and culture for mycobacteria or fungi, culture for viruses, and staining for *P. carinii*. In the specific case of sputum obtained for evaluation of *P. carinii* pneumonia in a patient infected with HIV, for example, sputum should be collected by induction, rather than spontaneous expectoration, and an immunofluorescent stain should be used to detect the organisms. Cytologic staining of sputum for malignant cells, using the traditional Papanicolaou method, allows noninvasive evaluation for suspected lung cancer. Traditional stains and cultures are now also being supplemented in some cases by immunologic techniques and by molecular biologic methods, including the use of polymerase chain reaction amplification and DNA probes.

PERCUTANEOUS NEEDLE ASPIRATION A needle can be inserted through the chest wall into a pulmonary lesion for the purpose of aspirating material for analysis by cytologic or microbiologic techniques. The procedure is usually carried out under CT guidance, which assists in the positioning of the needle and assures that it is localized in the lesion. Although the potential risks of this procedure include intrapulmonary bleeding and creation of a pneumothorax with collapse of the underlying lung, the low risk of complication in experienced hands is usually worth the information obtained. However, a limitation of the technique is sampling error due to the small amount of material obtained. Thus, findings other than a specific cytologic or microbiologic diagnosis are of limited clinical value.

THORACENTESIS Sampling of pleural liquid by thoracentesis is commonly performed for diagnostic purposes or, in the case of a large effusion, for palliation of dyspnea. Diagnostic sampling, either by blind needle aspiration or after localization by ultrasound, allows the collection of liquid for microbiologic and cytologic studies. Analysis of the fluid obtained for its cellular composition and chemical constituents, including glucose, protein, and lactate dehydrogenase, allows the effusion to be classified as either exudative or transudative (Chap. 262). In some cases, particularly in the setting of possible tuberculous involvement of the pleura (tuberculous pleuritis), closed biopsy of the parietal pleura is also performed, using a cutting needle (either an Abrams or a Cope biopsy needle) to sample tissue for histopathologic examination and culture.

BRONCHOSCOPY Bronchoscopy is the process of direct visualization of the tracheobronchial tree. Bronchoscopy with a rigid bronchoscope is generally performed in an operating room on a patient under general anesthesia. The development of a flexible fiberoptic bronchoscope has revolutionized the diagnostic use of bronchoscopy. Although bronchoscopy is now performed almost exclusively with fiberoptic instruments, rigid bronchoscopes still have a role in selected circumstances, primarily because of their larger suction channel and the fact that the patient can be ventilated through the bronchoscope channel. These situations include the retrieval of a foreign body and the suctioning of a massive hemorrhage, for which the small suction channel of the bronchoscope may be insufficient.

Flexible Fiberoptic Bronchoscopy This is an outpatient procedure that is usually performed in an awake but sedated patient. The bronchoscope is passed through either the mouth or the nose, between the vocal cords, and into the trachea. The ability to flex the scope makes it possible to visualize virtually all airways to the level of subsegmental bronchi. The bronchoscopist is able to identify endobronchial pathology, including tumors, granulomas, bronchitis, foreign bodies, and sites of bleeding. Samples from airway lesions can be taken by several methods, including washing, brushing, and biopsy. Washing involves instillation of sterile saline through a channel of the bronchoscope and onto the surface of a lesion. A portion of the liquid is collected by suctioning through the bronchoscope, and the recovered material can be analyzed for cells (cytology) or organisms (by standard stains and cultures). Brushing or biopsy of the surface of the lesion, using a small brush or biopsy forceps at the end of a long cable inserted through a channel of the bronchoscope, allows recovery of cellular material or tissue for analysis by standard cytologic and histopathologic methods.

The bronchoscope can be used to sample material not only from the regions that can be directly visualized (i.e., the airways) but also from the more distal pulmonary parenchyma. With the bronchoscope wedged into a subsegmental airway, aliquots of sterile saline can be instilled through the scope, allowing sampling of cells and organisms even from alveolar spaces. This procedure, called *bronchoalveolar lavage*, has been particularly useful for the recovery of organisms such as *P. carinii* in patients with HIV infection.

Brushing and biopsy of the distal lung parenchyma can also be performed with the same instruments that are used for endobronchial sampling. These instruments can be passed through the scope into small airways, where they penetrate the airway wall, allowing biopsy of peribronchial alveolar tissue. This procedure, called *transbronchial biopsy*, is used when there is either relatively diffuse disease or a localized lesion of adequate size. With the aid of fluoroscopic imaging, the bronchoscopist is able to determine not only whether and when the instrument is in the area of abnormality, but also the proximity of the instrument to the pleural surface. If the forceps are too close to the pleural surface, there is a risk of violating the visceral pleura and creating a pneumothorax; the other potential complication of transbronchial biopsy is pulmonary hemorrhage. The incidence of these complications is less than several percent.

Another procedure involves use of a hollow-bore needle passed through the bronchoscope for sampling of tissue adjacent to the trachea or a large bronchus. The needle is passed through the airway wall, and cellular material can be aspirated from mass lesions or enlarged lymph nodes, generally in a search for malignant cells. This procedure can facilitate the staging of lung cancer by identifying mediastinal lymph node involvement and in some cases obviates the need for a more invasive procedure.

The bronchoscope may provide the opportunity for treatment as well as diagnosis. For example, an aspirated foreign body may be retrieved with an instrument passed through the scope, and bleeding may be controlled with a balloon catheter similarly introduced. Newer interventional techniques performed through a bronchoscope include methods for achieving and maintaining patency of airways that are partially or completely occluded, especially by tumors. These techniques include laser therapy, cryotherapy, electrocautery, and stent placement.

VIDEO-ASSISTED THORACIC SURGERY Recent advances in video technology have allowed the development of thoracoscopy, or video-assisted thoracic surgery (VATS), for the diagnosis and management of pleural as well as parenchymal lung disease. This procedure, done under general anesthesia, involves the passage of a rigid scope with a distal lens through a trocar inserted into the pleura. A high-quality image is shown on a monitor screen, allowing the operator to manipulate instruments passed into the pleural space through separate small intercostal incisions. With these instruments, the operator can biopsy lesions of the pleura under direct vision, which provides an obvious advantage over closed pleural biopsy. In addition, this procedure is now used commonly to biopsy peripheral lung tissue or to remove peripheral nodules, for both diagnostic and therapeutic purposes. Because this procedure is much less invasive than the traditional thoracotomy performed for lung biopsy, it has largely supplanted "open lung biopsy."

THORACOTOMY Although frequently replaced by VATS, thoracotomy remains an option for the diagnostic sampling of lung tissue. It provides the largest amount of material, and it can be used to biopsy and/or excise lesions that are too deep or too close to vital structures for removal by VATS. The choice between VATS and thoracotomy needs to be made on a case-by-case basis, and the relative indications for each are still evolving as more experience is being gained with VATS.

MEDIASTINOSCOPY AND MEDIASTINOTOMY Tissue biopsy is often critical for the diagnosis of mediastinal masses or enlarged mediastinal lymph nodes. Although CT is useful for determining the size of mediastinal lymph nodes as part of the staging of lung cancer, confirmation that enlarged lymph nodes are actually involved with tumor generally requires biopsy and histopathologic examination. The two major procedures used to obtain specimens from masses or nodes in the mediastinum are mediastinoscopy (via a suprasternal approach) and mediastinotomy (via a parasternal approach). Both procedures are performed under general anesthesia by a qualified surgeon. In the case of suprasternal mediastinoscopy, a rigid mediastinoscope is inserted at the suprasternal notch and passed into the mediastinum along a pathway just anterior to the trachea. Tissue can be obtained with biopsy forceps passed through the scope, sampling masses or nodes that are in a paratracheal or pretracheal position. Left paratracheal and aortopulmonary lymph nodes are not accessible by this route and thus are commonly sampled by parasternal mediastinotomy (the Chamberlain procedure). This approach involves either a right or left parasternal incision and dissection directly down to a mass or node that requires biopsy.

BIBLIOGRAPHY

ALBERT RK et al (eds): *Comprehensive Respiratory Medicine*. Philadelphia, Mosby, 1999

DICHTER JR et al: Approach to the immunocompromised host with pulmonary symptoms. Hematol Oncol Clin North Am 7:887, 1993

ETTINGER NA: Invasive diagnostic approaches to pulmonary infiltrates. Semin Respir Infect 8:168, 1993

HARRIS RJ et al: The diagnostic and therapeutic utility of thoracoscopy. A review. Chest 108:828, 1995

MCELVEIN RB: Procedures in the evaluation of chest disease. Clin Chest Med 13:1, 1992

WANG K-P, MEHTA AC: *Flexible Bronchoscopy*, Cambridge, MA, Blackwell, 1995

WEBB WR et al: *High-Resolution CT of the Lung*, 2d ed. Philadelphia, Lippincott-Raven, 1996

WEINBERGER SE: *Principles of Pulmonary Medicine*, 3d ed. Philadelphia, Saunders, 1998

Section 2
DISEASES OF THE RESPIRATORY SYSTEM

252 ASTHMA

E. R. McFadden, Jr.

DEFINITION Asthma is defined as a chronic inflammatory disease of airways that is characterized by increased responsiveness of the tracheobronchial tree to a multiplicity of stimuli. It is manifested physiologically by a widespread narrowing of the air passages, which may be relieved spontaneously or as a result of therapy, and clinically by paroxysms of dyspnea, cough, and wheezing. Asthma is an episodic disease, with acute exacerbations interspersed with symptom-free periods. Typically, most attacks are short-lived, lasting minutes to hours, and clinically the patient seems to recover completely after an attack. However, there can be a phase in which the patient experiences some degree of airway obstruction daily. This phase can be mild, with or without superimposed severe episodes, or much more serious, with severe obstruction persisting for days or weeks; the latter condition is known as *status asthmaticus*. In unusual circumstances, acute episodes can cause death.

PREVALENCE AND ETIOLOGY Asthma is very common; it is estimated that 4 to 5% of the population of the United States is affected. Similar figures have been reported from other countries. Bronchial asthma occurs at all ages but predominantly in early life. About one-half of cases develop before age 10, and another third occur before age 40. In childhood, there is a 2:1 male/female preponderance, but the sex ratio equalizes by age 30.

From an etiologic standpoint, asthma is a heterogeneous disease. It is useful for epidemiologic and clinical purposes to classify asthma by the principal stimuli that incite or are associated with acute episodes. However, it is important to emphasize that this distinction may often be artificial, and the response of a given subclassification usually can be initiated by more than one type of stimulus. Furthermore, the application of molecular and cell biologic techniques to asthma pathogenesis is also beginning to blur this type of classification. With these reservations in mind, one can describe two broad types of asthma: allergic and idiosyncratic.

Atopy is the single largest risk factor for the development of asthma. *Allergic asthma* is often associated with a personal and/or family history of allergic diseases such as rhinitis, urticaria, and eczema, with positive wheal-and-flare skin reactions to intradermal injection of extracts of airborne antigens, with increased levels of IgE in the serum, and/or with a positive response to provocation tests involving the inhalation of specific antigen.

A significant fraction of patients with asthma present with no personal or family history of allergy, with negative skin tests, and with normal serum levels of IgE, and therefore have disease that cannot be classified on the basis of defined immunologic mechanisms. These patients are said to have *idiosyncratic asthma*. Many develop a typical symptom complex on contracting an upper respiratory illness. The initial insult may be little more than a common cold, but after several days the patient begins to develop paroxysms of wheezing and dyspnea that can last for days to months. These individuals should not be confused with persons in whom the symptoms of bronchospasm are superimposed on chronic bronchitis or bronchiectasis (Chaps. 256 and 258).

Many patients have disease that does not fit clearly into either of the preceding categories but instead falls into a mixed group with features of each. In general, asthma that has its onset in early life tends to have a strong allergic component, whereas asthma that develops late tends to be nonallergic or to have a mixed etiology.

PATHOGENESIS OF ASTHMA The common denominator underlying the asthmatic diathesis is a nonspecific hyperirritability of the tracheobronchial tree. When airway reactivity is high, symptoms are more severe and persistent, and the amount of therapy required to control the patient's complaints is greater. In addition, the magnitude of diurnal fluctuations in lung function is greater, and the patient tends to awaken at night or in the early morning with breathlessness.

In both normal and asthmatic individuals, airway reactivity rises after viral infections of the respiratory tract and exposure to oxidant air pollutants such as ozone and nitrogen dioxide (but not sulfur dioxide). Viral infections have more profound consequences, and airway responsiveness may remain elevated for many weeks after a seemingly trivial upper respiratory tract infection. In contrast, airway reactivity remains high for only a few days after exposure to ozone. Allergens can cause airway responsiveness to rise within minutes and to remain elevated for weeks. If the dose of antigen is high enough, acute episodes of obstruction may occur daily for a prolonged period after a single exposure.

The most popular hypothesis at present for the pathogenesis of asthma is that it derives from a state of persistent subacute inflammation of the airways. An active inflammatory process is frequently observed in endobronchial biopsy specimens even from asymptomatic patients. The airways can be edematous and infiltrated with eosinophils, neutrophils, and lymphocytes, with or without an increase in the collagen content of the epithelial basement membrane. There may also be glandular hypertrophy. The most ubiquitous finding is a generalized increase in cellularity associated with an elevated capillary density. Occasionally, denudation of the epithelium may also be observed.

Although the translation of these histologic observations into a disease process is still incomplete, it is widely believed that the physiologic and clinical features of asthma derive from an interaction among the resident and infiltrating inflammatory cells in the airway surface epithelium, inflammatory mediators, and cytokines. The cells thought to play important parts in the inflammatory response are mast cells, eosinophils, lymphocytes, and epithelial cells. The roles of neutrophils and macrophages are less well defined. Each of these cell types can contribute mediators and cytokines to initiate and amplify both acute inflammation and the long-term pathologic changes described above. The mediators released—histamine; bradykinin; the leukotrienes C, D, and E; platelet-activating factor; and prostaglandins (PGs) E_2, $F_2\alpha$, and D_2—produce an intense, immediate inflammatory reaction involving bronchoconstriction, vascular congestion, and edema formation. In addition to their ability to evoke prolonged contraction of airway smooth muscle and mucosal edema, the leukotrienes may also account for some of the other pathophysiologic features of asthma, such as increased mucus production and impaired mucociliary transport. This intense local event can then be followed by a more chronic one. The chemotactic factors elaborated (eosinophil and neutrophil chemotactic factors of anaphylaxis and leukotriene B_4) bring eosinophils, platelets, and polymorphonuclear leukocytes to the site of the reaction. These infiltrating cells as well as resident macrophages and the airway epithelium itself potentially are an additional source of mediators to enhance both the immediate and the cellular phase. The airway epithelium is both the target of, and a contributor to, the inflammatory cascade. These cells amplify bronchoconstriction by elaborating endothelin-1 and promoting vasodilatation through the release of nitric oxide, PGE_2 and the 15-hydroxyeicosatetraenoic acid (15-HETE) products of arachidonic acid metabolism. They also generate cytokines such as granulocyte-macrophage colony stimulating factor (GM-CSF), interleukin (IL)8, Rantes, and eotaxin.

Like the mast cell in the early reaction, the eosinophil appears to play an important part in the infiltrative component. The granular proteins in this cell (major basic protein and eosinophilic cationic protein) and oxygen-derived free radical are capable of destroying the airway epithelium, which then is sloughed into the bronchial lumen in the form of Creola bodies. Besides resulting in a loss of barrier and secretory function, such damage elicits the production of chemotactic cytokines, leading to further inflammation. In theory, it also can expose sensory nerve endings, thus initiating neurogenic inflammatory pathways. That, in turn, could convert a primary local event into a generalized reaction via a reflex mechanism.

T lymphocytes also appear to be important in the inflammatory response. These cells are present in increased numbers in asthmatic airways and produce cytokines that activate cell-mediated immunity, as well as humoral (IgE) immune responses. Activated T cells recovered from the lungs of persons with asthma express messenger RNA for the cytokines known to play a part in the recruitment and activation of mast cells and eosinophils. Furthermore, the T_H1 and T_H2 lymphocyte subtypes have functions that may influence the asthmatic response. The T_H1 cytokines IL-2 and interferon (IFN) γ can promote the growth and differentiation of B cells and the activation of macrophages, respectively. The T_H2 cytokines IL-4 and IL-5 stimulate B-cell growth and immunoglobulin secretion, and IL-5 promotes eosinophil proliferation, differentiation, and activation. It can also facilitate granule release from basophils.

Cytokine production is another central component of the inflammation of asthma. Cytokines are synthesized and released from many of the inflammatory cells mentioned above, as well as from epithelial cells, fibroblasts, endothelial cells, and airway smooth muscle. Cytokines activate specific cell-surface receptors that are coupled to signal transduction pathways, which often result in alterations of gene regulation and enzyme production. The cytokines that are particularly relevant to asthma are secreted by T lymphocytes and include IL-3 enhanced (mast cell survival), IL-4 and IL-13 (switching of B lymphocytes to IgE production and expression of adhesion molecules), and IL-5 (differentiation and enhanced survival of eosinophils). Other cytokines, such as IL-1B, IL-6, IL-11, tumor necrosis factor α (TNF-α) and GM-CSF, are proinflammatory and may amplify the inflammatory response.

The relative roles of each of the above elements in the production of heightened airway reactivity and clinical asthma have yet to be determined. Although inflammation is clearly important, recent evidence indicates that the intensity of the cellular infiltrate in the airways is not related either to the severity of the disease state or to the level of airway reactivity. Furthermore, it is unlikely that any one cell type or mediator accounts for every feature. For example, mast cell–derived mediators cannot explain the whole picture, for they have been found in the blood of individuals with mast cell–related diseases such as cold-induced and cholinergic-induced urticaria and in the airways of atopic individuals without asthma. Since these individuals had no lower respiratory illness or complaints, these alleged mediators of asthma would appear to need a unique background from which to exhibit their effects. Similarly, the inflammatory cells believed to be relevant to asthma are also found in the airways of atopic individuals without asthma, raising the possibility that they are merely nonspecific markers of atopy rather than specific indexes of asthma. Finally, the therapeutic administration of IL-2 and GM-CSF to patients with cancer results in eosinophilia with cell activation but not in asthma.

Genetic Considerations Although there is little doubt that asthma has a strong familial component, the identification of the genetic mechanisms underlying the illness has proven difficult for multiple reasons, including such fundamental issues as a lack of uniform agreement on the definition of the disease, the inability to define a single phenotype, non-Mendelian modes of inheritance, and an incomplete understanding of how environmental factors modify genetic expression. Screening families for candidate genes has identified multiple chromosomal regions that relate to atopy, elevated IgE levels, and airway hyperresponsiveness. Evidence for genetic linkage of high total serum IgE levels and atopy has been observed on chromosomes 5q, 11q, and 12q in a number of populations scattered throughout the world. Regions of the genome demonstrating evidence for linkage to bronchial hyperreactivity also typically show evidence for linkage to elevated total serum IgE levels. Excellent candidate genes exist for specific abnormalities in asthma within the regions that were identified in the linkage studies. For example, chromosome 5q contains cytokine clusters including IL-4, IL-5, IL-9, and IL-13. Other regions on chromosome 5q also contain the beta-adrenergic receptors and the glucocorticoid receptors. Chromosome 6p contains regions that are important in antigen presentation and mediation of the inflammatory response. Chromosome 12q contains two genes that could influence atopy and airway hyperresponsiveness, including nitric oxide synthase. ■

The stimuli that interact with airway responsiveness and incite acute episodes of asthma can be grouped into seven major categories: allergenic, pharmacologic, environmental, occupational, infectious, exercise-related, and emotional.

Allergens Allergic asthma is dependent on an IgE response controlled by T and B lymphocytes and activated by the interaction of antigen with mast cell–bound IgE molecules. The airway epithelium and submucosa contain dendritic cells that capture and process antigen. After taking up an immunogen, these cells migrate to the local lymph nodes where they present the material to T cell receptors. In the appropriate genetic setting, the interaction of antigen with a naïve T cell T_H0 in the presence of IL-4 leads to the differentiation of the cell to a T_H2 subset. This process not only helps facilitate the inflammation of asthma but also causes B lymphocytes to switch their antibody production from IgG and IgM to IgE. Most of the allergens that provoke asthma are airborne, and to induce a state of sensitivity they must be reasonably abundant for considerable periods of time. Once sensitization has occurred, however, the patient can exhibit exquisite responsivity, so that minute amounts of the offending agent can produce significant exacerbations of the disease. Immune mechanisms appear to be causally related to the development of asthma in 25 to 35% of all cases and to be contributory in perhaps another third. Higher prevalences have been suggested, but it is difficult to know how to interpret the data because of confounding factors. Allergic asthma is frequently seasonal, and it is most often observed in children and young adults. A nonseasonal form may result from allergy to feathers, animal danders, dust mites, molds, and other antigens that are present continuously in the environment. Exposure to antigen typically produces an immediate response in which airway obstruction develops in minutes and then resolves. In 30 to 50% of patients, a second wave of bronchoconstriction, the so-called late reaction, develops 6 to 10 h later. In a minority, only a late reaction occurs. It was formerly thought that the late reaction was essential to the development of the increase in airway reactivity that follows antigen exposure. Recent data show that not to be the case.

The mechanism by which an inhaled allergen provokes an acute episode of asthma depends in part on antigen-antibody interactions on the surface of pulmonary mast cells, with the subsequent generation and release of the mediators of immediate hypersensitivity. Current hypotheses hold that very small antigenic particles penetrate the lung's defenses and come in contact with mast cells that interdigitate with the epithelium at the luminal surface of the central airways. The subsequent elaboration of mediators and cytokines then produces the sequence outlined above.

Pharmacologic Stimuli The drugs most commonly associated with the induction of acute episodes of asthma are aspirin, coloring agents such as tartrazine, β-adrenergic antagonists, and sulfiting agents. It is important to recognize drug-induced bronchial narrowing because its presence is often associated with great morbidity. Furthermore, death sometimes has followed the ingestion of aspirin (or other nonsteroidal anti-inflammatory agents) or β-adrenergic antagonists. The typical aspirin-sensitive respiratory syndrome primarily affects adults, although the condition may occur in childhood. This problem usually begins with perennial vasomotor rhinitis that is followed by a hyperplastic rhinosinusitis with nasal polyps. Progressive asthma then appears. On exposure to even very small quantities of aspirin, affected individuals typically develop ocular and nasal congestion and acute, often severe episodes of airways obstruction. The prevalence of aspirin sensitivity in patients with asthma varies from study to study, but many authorities feel that 10% is a reasonable figure. There is a great deal of cross reactivity between aspirin and other nonsteroidal anti-inflammatory compounds that inhibit prostaglandin G/H synthase 1 (cyclooxygenase type 1). Indomethacin, fenoprofen, naproxen, zomepirac sodium, ibuprofen, mefenamic acid, and phenylbutazone are particularly important in this regard. However, acetaminophen, sodium salicylate, choline salicylate, salicylamide, and propoxyphene are well tolerated. The exact frequency of cross reactivity to tartrazine and other dyes in aspirin-sensitive individuals with asthma is also controversial; again, 10% is the commonly accepted figure. This peculiar complication of aspirin-sensitive asthma is particularly insidious, however, in that tartrazine and other potentially troublesome dyes are widely present in the environment and may be unknowingly ingested by sensitive patients.

Patients with aspirin sensitivity can be desensitized by daily administration of the drug. After this form of therapy, cross tolerance also develops to other nonsteroidal anti-inflammatory agents. The mechanism by which aspirin and other such drugs produce bronchospasm appears to be a chronic overexcretion of cysteinyl leukotrienes, which activate mast cells. The adverse reaction to aspirin can be inhibited with the use of leukotriene synthesis blockers or receptor antagonists.

Beta-adrenergic antagonists regularly obstruct the airways in individuals with asthma as well as in others with heightened airway reactivity and should be avoided by such individuals. Even the selective $beta_1$ agents have this propensity, particularly at higher doses. In fact, the local use of $beta_1$ blockers in the eye for the treatment of glaucoma has been associated with worsening asthma.

Sulfiting agents, such as potassium metabisulfite, potassium and sodium bisulfite, sodium sulfite, and sulfur dioxide, which are widely used in the food and pharmaceutical industries as sanitizing and preserving agents, also can produce acute airway obstruction in sensitive individuals. Exposure usually follows ingestion of food or beverages containing these compounds, e.g., salads, fresh fruit, potatoes, shellfish, and wine. Exacerbation of asthma has been reported after the use of sulfite-containing topical ophthalmic solutions, intravenous glucocorticoids, and some inhalational bronchodilator solutions. The incidence and mechanism of action of this phenomenon are unknown. When suspected, the diagnosis can be confirmed by either oral or inhalational provocations.

Environment and Air Pollution (See also Chap. 254) Environmental causes of asthma are usually related to climatic conditions that promote the concentration of atmospheric pollutants and antigens. These conditions tend to develop in heavily industrial or densely populated urban areas and are frequently associated with thermal inversions or other situations creating stagnant air masses. In these circumstances, although the general population can develop respiratory symptoms, patients with asthma and other respiratory diseases tend to be more severely affected. The air pollutants known to have this effect are ozone, nitrogen dioxide, and sulfur dioxide. Sulfur dioxide needs to be present in high concentrations and produces its greatest effects during periods of high ventilation. In some regions of North America, seasonal concentrations of airborne antigens such as pollen can rise high enough to result in epidemics of asthma admissions to hospitals and an increase in the death rate. These events may be ameliorated by treating patients prophylactically with anti-inflammatory drugs before the allergy season begins.

Occupational Factors (See also Chap. 254) Occupation-related asthma is a significant health problem, and acute and chronic airway obstruction has been reported to follow exposure to a large number of compounds used in many types of industrial processes. Bronchoconstriction can result from working with or being exposed to *metal salts* (e.g., platinum, chrome, and nickel), *wood and vegetable dusts* (e.g., those of oak, western red cedar, grain, flour, castor bean, green coffee bean, mako, gum acacia, karay gum, and tragacanth), *pharmaceutical agents* (e.g., antibiotics, piperazine, and cimetidine), *industrial chemicals and plastics* (e.g., toluene diisocyanate, phthalic acid anhydride, trimellitic anhydride, persulfates, ethylenediamine, *p*-phenylenediamine, and various dyes), *biologic enzymes* (e.g., laundry detergents and pancreatic enzymes), and *animal and insect dusts, serums, and secretions.* It is important to recognize that exposure to sensitizing chemicals, particularly those used in paints, solvents, and plastics, also can occur during leisure or non-work-related activities.

There seem to be three underlying mechanisms for this airway obstruction: (1) In some cases, the offending agent results in the formation of a specific IgE, and the cause seems immunologic (the immunologic reaction can be immediate, late, or dual); (2) in other cases, the substance causes a direct liberation of bronchoconstrictor substances; and (3) in other instances, the substance causes direct or reflex stimulation of the airways of individuals with either latent or frank asthma. If the occupational agent causes an immediate or dual immunologic reaction, the history is similar to that which occurs with exposure to other antigens. Often, however, patients will give a characteristic cyclic history. They are well when they arrive at work, and symptoms develop toward the end of the shift, progress after the work site is left, and then regress. Absence from work during weekends or vacations brings about remission. Frequently, there are similar symptoms in fellow employees.

Infections Respiratory infections are the most common of the stimuli that evoke acute exacerbations of asthma. Well-controlled investigations have demonstrated that respiratory viruses and not bacteria or allergy to microorganisms are the major etiologic factors. In young children, the most important infectious agents are respiratory syncytial virus and parainfluenza virus. In older children and adults, rhinovirus and influenza virus predominate as pathogens. Simple colonization of the tracheobronchial tree is insufficient to evoke acute episodes of bronchospasm, and attacks of asthma occur only when symptoms of an ongoing respiratory tract infection are, or have been, present. Viral infections can actively and chronically destabilize asthma, and they are perhaps the only stimuli that can produce constant symptoms for weeks. The mechanism by which viruses induce exacerbations of asthma may be related to the production of T cell–derived cytokines that potentiate the infiltration of inflammatory cells into already susceptible airways.

Exercise Exercise is a very common precipitant of acute episodes of asthma. This stimulus differs from other naturally occurring provocations, such as antigens, viral infections, and air pollutants, in that it does not evoke any long-term sequelae, nor does it increase airway reactivity. Exercise can be made to provoke bronchospasm in every patient with asthma, and in some it is the only trigger that produces symptoms. When such patients are followed for sufficient periods, however, they often develop recurring episodes of airway obstruction independent of exercise; thus, the onset of this problem frequently is the first manifestation of the full-blown asthmatic syndrome. The critical variables that determine the severity of the postexertional airway obstruction are the levels of ventilation achieved and the temperature and humidity of the inspired air. The higher the ventilation and the lower the heat content of the air, the greater the response. For the same inspired air conditions, running produces a more severe attack of asthma than walking. Conversely, for a given task, the inhalation of cold air markedly enhances the response, while warm, humid air blunts or abolishes it. Consequently, activities such as ice hockey, cross-country skiing, and ice skating are more provocative than is swimming in an indoor, heated pool. The mechanism by which exercise produces obstruction may be related to a thermally produced hyperemia and engorgement of the microvasculature of the bronchial wall and does not appear to involve smooth-muscle contraction.

Emotional Stress Abundant objective data demonstrate that psychological factors can interact with the asthmatic diathesis to worsen or ameliorate the disease process. The pathways and nature of the interactions are complex but are operational to some extent in almost half the patients studied. Changes in airway caliber seem to be mediated through modification of vagal efferent activity, but endorphins also may play a role. The most frequently studied variable has been that of suggestion, and the weight of current evidence indicates that it can be quite important in selected individuals with asthma. When psychically responsive individuals are given the appropriate suggestion, they can actually decrease or increase the pharmacologic effects of adrenergic and cholinergic stimuli on their airways. The extent to which psychological factors participate in the induction and/or continuation of any given acute exacerbation is not established but probably varies from patient to patient and in the same patient from episode to episode.

PATHOLOGY In a patient who has died of acute asthma, the most striking feature of the lungs at necropsy is their gross overdistention and failure to collapse when the pleural cavities are opened. When the lungs are cut, numerous gelatinous plugs of exudate are found in most of the bronchial branches down to the terminal bronchioles. Histologic examination shows hypertrophy of the bronchial smooth muscle, hyperplasia of mucosal and submucosal vessels, mucosal edema, denudation of the surface epithelium, pronounced thickening of the basement membrane, and eosinophilic infiltrates in the bronchial wall. There is an absence of any of the well-recognized forms of destructive emphysema.

PATHOPHYSIOLOGY The pathophysiologic hallmark of asthma is a reduction in airway diameter brought about by contraction of smooth muscle, vascular congestion, edema of the bronchial wall, and thick, tenacious secretions. The net result is an increase in airway resistance, a decrease in forced expiratory volumes and flow rates, hyperinflation of the lungs and thorax, increased work of breathing, alterations in respiratory muscle function, changes in elastic recoil, abnormal distribution of both ventilation and pulmonary blood flow with mismatched ratios, and altered arterial blood gas concentrations. Thus, although asthma is considered to be primarily a disease of airways, virtually all aspects of pulmonary function are compromised during an acute attack. In addition, in very symptomatic patients there frequently is electrocardiographic evidence of right ventricular hypertrophy and pulmonary hypertension. When a patient presents for therapy, his or her forced vital capacity tends to be ≤50% of normal. The 1-s forced expiratory volume (FEV_1) averages 30% or less of predicted, while the maximum and minimum midexpiratory flow rates are reduced to 20% or less of expected. In keeping with the alterations in mechanics, the associated air trapping is substantial. In acutely ill patients, residual volume (RV) frequently approaches 400% of normal, while functional residual capacity doubles. The patient tends to report that the attack has ended clinically when the RV has fallen to 200% of its predicted value and the FEV_1 reaches 50% of the predicted level.

Hypoxia is a universal finding during acute exacerbations, but frank ventilatory failure is relatively uncommon, being observed in 10 to 15% of patients presenting for therapy. Most individuals with asthma have hypocapnia and a respiratory alkalosis. In acutely ill patients, the finding of a normal arterial carbon dioxide tension tends to be associated with quite severe levels of obstruction. Consequently, when found in a symptomatic individual, it should be viewed as representing impending respiratory failure, and the patient should be treated accordingly. Equally, the presence of metabolic acidosis in the setting of acute asthma signifies severe obstruction. Usually, there are no clinical counterparts to the derangements in blood gases. Cyanosis is a very late sign. Hence, a dangerous level of hypoxia can go undetected. Likewise, signs attributable to carbon dioxide retention, such as sweating, tachycardia, and wide pulse pressure, or to acidosis, such as tachypnea, tend not to be of great value in predicting the presence of hypercapnia or hydrogen ion excess in individual patients, because they are too frequently seen in anxious patients with more moderate disease. Trying to judge the state of an acutely ill patient's ventilatory status on clinical grounds alone can be extremely hazardous, and clinical indicators should not be relied on with any confidence. Therefore, in patients with suspected alveolar hypoventilation, arterial blood gas tensions must be measured.

CLINICAL FEATURES The symptoms of asthma consist of a triad of dyspnea, cough, and wheezing, the last often being regarded as the *sine qua non.* In its most typical form, asthma is an episodic disease, and all three symptoms coexist. At the onset of an attack, patients experience a sense of constriction in the chest, often with a nonproductive cough. Respiration becomes audibly harsh, wheezing in both phases of respiration becomes prominent, expiration becomes prolonged, and patients frequently have tachypnea, tachycardia, and mild systolic hypertension. The lungs rapidly become overinflated, and the anteroposterior diameter of the thorax increases. If the attack is severe or prolonged, there may be a loss of adventitial breath sounds, and wheezing becomes very high pitched. Furthermore, the accessory muscles become visibly active, and a paradoxical pulse often develops. These two signs are extremely valuable in indicating the severity of the obstruction. In the presence of either, pulmonary function tends to be significantly more impaired than in their absence. It is important to note that the development of a paradoxical pulse depends on the generation of large negative intrathoracic pressures. Thus, if the patient's breathing is shallow, this sign and/or the use of accessory muscles could be absent even though obstruction is quite severe. The other signs and symptoms of asthma only imperfectly reflect the physiologic alterations that are present. Indeed, if the disappearance of subjective complaints or even of wheezing is used as the end point at which therapy for an acute attack is terminated, an enormous reservoir of residual disease will be missed.

The end of an episode is frequently marked by a cough that produces thick, stringy mucus, which often takes the form of casts of the distal airways (Curschmann's spirals) and, when examined microscopically, often shows eosinophils and Charcot-Leyden crystals. In extreme situations, wheezing may lessen markedly or even disappear, cough may become extremely ineffective, and the patient may begin a gasping type of respiratory pattern. These findings imply extensive mucus plugging and impending suffocation. Ventilatory assistance by mechanical means may be required. Atelectasis due to inspissated secretions occasionally occurs with asthmatic attacks. Spontaneous pneumothorax and/or pneumomediastinum occur but are rare.

Less typically, a patient with asthma may complain of intermittent episodes of nonproductive cough or exertional dyspnea. Unlike other individuals with asthma, when these patients are examined during symptomatic periods, they tend to have normal breath sounds but may wheeze after repeated forced exhalations and/or may show ventilatory impairments when tested in the laboratory. In the absence of both these signs, a bronchoprovocation test may be required to make the diagnosis.

DIFFERENTIAL DIAGNOSIS The differentiation of asthma from other diseases associated with dyspnea and wheezing is usually not difficult, particularly if the patient is seen during an acute episode. The physical findings and symptoms listed above and the history of periodic attacks are quite characteristic. A personal or family history of allergic diseases such as eczema, rhinitis, or urticaria is valuable contributory evidence. An extremely common feature of asthma is nocturnal awakening with dyspnea and/or wheezing. In fact, this phenomenon is so prevalent that its absence raises doubt about the diagnosis. *Upper airway obstruction by tumor* or *laryngeal edema* can occasionally be confused with asthma. Typically, a patient with such a condition will present with stridor, and the harsh respiratory sounds can be localized to the area of the trachea. Diffuse wheezing throughout both lung fields is usually absent. However, differentiation can sometimes be difficult, and indirect laryngoscopy or bronchoscopy may be required. Asthma-like symptoms have been described in patients with glottic dysfunction. These individuals narrow their glottis during inspiration and expiration, producing episodic attacks of severe airway obstruction. Occasionally, carbon dioxide retention develops. However, unlike asthma, the arterial oxygen tension is well preserved, and the alveolar-arterial gradient for oxygen narrows during the episode, instead of widening as with lower airway obstruction. To establish the diagnosis of glottic dysfunction, the glottis should be examined when the patient is symptomatic. Normal findings at such a time exclude the diagnosis; normal findings during asymptomatic periods do not.

Persistent wheezing localized to one area of the chest in association with paroxysms of coughing indicates *endobronchial disease* such as foreign-body aspiration, a neoplasm, or bronchial stenosis.

The signs and symptoms of *acute left ventricular failure* occasionally mimic asthma, but the findings of moist basilar rales, gallop rhythms, blood-tinged sputum, and other signs of heart failure (Chap. 232) allow the appropriate diagnosis to be reached.

Recurrent episodes of bronchospasm can occur with *carcinoid tumors* (Chap. 93), *recurrent pulmonary emboli* (Chap. 261), and *chronic bronchitis* (Chap. 258). In chronic bronchitis there are no true symptom-free periods, and one can usually obtain a history of chronic cough and sputum production as a background on which acute attacks of wheezing are superimposed. Recurrent emboli can be very difficult to separate from asthma. Frequently, patients with this condition present with episodes of breathlessness, particularly on exertion, and they sometimes wheeze. Pulmonary function studies may show evidence of peripheral airway obstruction (Chap. 250); when these changes are present, lung scans also may be abnormal. The therapeutic response to bronchodilators and to the institution of anticoagulant therapy may be helpful, but pulmonary angiography may be necessary to establish the correct diagnosis.

Eosinophilic pneumonias (Chap. 253) are often associated with asthmatic symptoms, as are various chemical pneumonias and exposures to insecticides and cholinergic drugs. Bronchospasm occasionally is a manifestation of *systemic vasculitis* with pulmonary involvement.

DIAGNOSIS The diagnosis of asthma is established by demonstrating reversible airway obstruction. *Reversibility* is traditionally defined as a 15% or greater increase in FEV_1 after two puffs of a β-adrenergic agonist. When the spirometry results are normal at presentation, the diagnosis can be made by showing heightened airway responsiveness to challenges with histamine, methacholine, or isocapnic hyperventilation of cold air. Once the diagnosis is confirmed, the course of the illness and the effectiveness of therapy can be followed by measuring peak expiratory flow rates (PEFRs) at home and/or the FEV_1 in the laboratory. Positive wheal-and-flare reactions to skin tests can be demonstrated to various allergens, but such findings do not necessarily correlate with the intrapulmonary events. Sputum and blood eosinophilia and measurement of serum IgE levels are also helpful but are not specific for asthma. Chest roentgenograms showing hyperinflation are also nondiagnostic.

℞ **TREATMENT** Elimination of the causative agent(s) from the environment of an allergic individual with asthma is the most successful means available for treating this condition (for details on avoidance, see Chap. 310). Desensitization or immunotherapy with extracts of the suspected allergens has enjoyed widespread favor, but controlled studies are limited and have not proved it to be highly effective.

Drug Treatment The available agents for treating asthma can be divided into two general categories: drugs that inhibit smooth muscle contraction, i.e., the so-called "quick relief medications" (beta-adrenergic agonists, methylxanthines, and anticholinergics) and agents that prevent and/or reverse inflammation, i.e., the "long-term control medications" (glucocorticoids, leukotriene inhibitors and receptor antagonists, and mast cell–stabilizing agents).

Adrenergic stimulants The drugs in this category consist of the catecholamines, resorcinols, and saligenins. These agents are analogues and produce airway dilation through stimulation of beta-adrenergic receptors and activation of G proteins with the resultant formation of cyclic adenosine monophosphate (AMP). They also decrease release of mediators and improve mucociliary transport. The catecholamines available for clinical use are epinephrine, isoproterenol, and isoetharine. As a group, these compounds are short-acting (30 to 90 min) and are effective only when administered by inhalational or parenteral routes. Epinephrine and isoproterenol are not β_2-selective and have considerable chronotropic and inotropic cardiac effects. Epinephrine also has substantial alpha-stimulating effects. The usual dose is 0.3 to 0.5 mL of a 1:1000 solution administered subcutaneously. Isoproterenol is devoid of alpha activity and is the most potent agent of this group. It is usually administered in a 1:200 solution by inhalation. Isoetharine is the most β_2-selective compound of this class, but it is a relatively weak bronchodilator. It is employed as an aerosol and supplied as a 1% solution. The use of these agents in treating asthma has been superceded by longer acting selective β_2 agonists.

The commonly used resorcinols are metaproterenol, terbutaline, and fenoterol, and the most widely known saligenin is albuterol (salbutamol). With the exception of metaproterenol, these drugs are highly selective for the respiratory tract and virtually devoid of significant cardiac effects except at high doses. Their major side effect is tremor. They are active by all routes of administration, and because their chemical structures allow them to bypass the metabolic processes used to degrade the catecholamines, their effects are relatively long-lasting (4 to 6 h). Differences in potency and duration among agents can be eliminated by adjusting doses and/or administration schedules.

Inhalation is the preferred route of administration because it allows maximal bronchodilation with fewer side effects. In the past it was fashionable to treat episodes of severe asthma with intravenous sympathomimetics such as isoproterenol. This approach no longer appears justifiable. Isoproterenol infusions clearly can induce myocardial damage, and even for the β_2-selective agents such as terbutaline and albuterol, intravenous administration offers no advantages over the inhaled route.

Salmeterol is a very long-lasting (9 to 12 h) congener of albuterol. When given every 12 h, it is effective in providing sustained symptomatic relief. It is particularly helpful for conditions such as nocturnal and exercise-induced asthma. It is not recommended for the treatment of acute episodes because of its relatively slow onset of action (approximately 30 min), nor is it intended as a rescue drug for breakthrough symptoms. In addition, its long half-life means that administration of extra doses can cause cumulative side effects.

Methylxanthines Theophylline and its various salts are medium-potency bronchodilators that work by increasing cyclic AMP by the inhibition of phosphodiesterase. The therapeutic plasma concentrations of theophylline traditionally have been thought to lie between 10 and 20 μg/mL. Some sources, however, recommend a lower target range between 5 and 15 μg/mL to avoid toxicity. The dose required to achieve the desired level varies widely from patient to patient owing to differences in the metabolism of the drug. Theophylline clearance, and thus the dosage requirement, is decreased substantially in neonates and the elderly and those with acute and chronic hepatic dysfunction, cardiac decompensation, and cor pulmonale. Clearance is also decreased during febrile illnesses. Clearance is increased in children. In addition, a number of important drug interactions can alter theophylline metabolism. Clearance falls with the concurrent use of erythromycin and other macrolide antibiotics, the quinolone antibiotics, and troleandomycin, allopurinol, cimetidine, and propranolol. It rises with use of cigarettes, marijuana, phenobarbital, phenytoin, or any other drug that is capable of inducing hepatic microsomal enzymes.

For maintenance therapy, long-acting theophylline compounds are available and are usually given once or twice daily. The dose is adjusted on the basis of the clinical response with the aid of serum theophylline measurements. Single-dose administration in the evening reduces nocturnal symptoms and helps keep the patient complaint-free during the day. Aminophylline and theophylline are available for intravenous use. The recommendations for intravenous therapy in children aged 9 to 16 and in young adult smokers not currently receiving theophylline products are a loading dose of 6 mg/kg followed by an infusion of 1 mg/kg per hour for the next 12 h and then 0.8 mg/kg per hour thereafter. In nonsmoking adults, older patients, and those with cor pulmonale, congestive heart failure, and liver disease, the loading dose remains the same, but the maintenance dose is reduced to between 0.1 and 0.5 mg/kg per hour. In patients already receiving theophylline, the loading dose is frequently withheld or, in extreme situations, reduced to 0.5 mg/kg.

The most common side effects of theophylline are nervousness, nausea, vomiting, anorexia, and headache. At plasma levels greater than 30 μg/mL there is a risk of seizures and cardiac arrhythmias.

Anticholinergics Anticholinergic drugs such as atropine sulfate produce bronchodilation in patients with asthma, but their use is limited by systemic side effects. Nonabsorbable quaternary ammonium congeners (atropine methylnitrate and ipratropium bromide) have been found to be both effective and free of untoward effects. They may be of particular benefit for patients with coexistent heart disease, in whom the use of methylxanthines and β-adrenergic stimulants may be dangerous. The major disadvantages of the anticholinergics are that they are slow to act (60 to 90 min may be required before peak bronchodilation is achieved) and they are only of modest potency.

Glucocorticoids Glucocorticoids are the most potent and most effective anti-inflammatory medications available. Systemic or oral steroids are most beneficial in acute illness when severe airway obstruction is not resolving or is worsening despite intense optimal bronchodilator therapy, and in chronic disease when there has been failure of a previously optimal regimen with frequent recurrences of symptoms of increasing severity. Inhaled glucocorticoids are used in the long-term control of asthma.

Glucocorticoids are not bronchodilators and the correct dose to use in acute situations is a matter of debate. The available data indicate that very high doses do not offer any advantage over more conventional amounts. In the United States, a usual starting dose is 40 to 60 mg of methylprednisolone intravenously every 6 h. Since intravenous and oral administration produce the same effects, prednisone, 60 mg every 6 h, can be substituted. Clinical impressions suggest that smaller quantities may work as effectively, but there are no confirmatory data. In the United Kingdom and elsewhere, acute asthma both in and out of hospital is frequently treated with doses of prednisolone ranging from 30 to 40 mg given once daily. It should be emphasized that the effects of steroids in acute asthma are not immediate and may not be seen for 6 h or more after the initial administration. Consequently, it is mandatory to continue vigorous bronchodilator therapy during this interval. Irrespective of the regimen chosen, it is important to appreciate that rapid tapering of glucocorticoids frequently results in recurrent obstruction. Most authorities recommend reducing the dose by one-half every third to fifth day after an acute episode. In situations in which it appears that continued steroid therapy will be needed, an alternate-day schedule should be instituted to minimize side effects. This is particularly important in children, since continuous glucocorticoid administration interrupts growth. Long-acting preparations such as dexamethasone should not be used in this approach, for they defeat the purpose of alternate-day schedules by causing prolonged suppression of the pituitary-adrenal axis. The availability of inhaled agents has all but eliminated the need for this form of therapy.

Inhaled Glucocorticoids These drugs are indicated in patients with persistent symptoms. The agents currently available in the United States are beclomethasone, budesonide, flunisolide, fluticasone propionate, and triamcinolone acetonide. Each has relative advantages and disadvantages, and they are not absolutely interchangeable on either a microgram or a per puff basis. However, all of these drugs share the ability to control inflammation, facilitate the long-term prevention of symptoms, and reduce the need for oral glucocorticoids.

There is no fixed dose of inhaled steroid that works for all patients. Requirements are dictated by the response of the individual and wax and wane in concert with progression of the disease. Generally, the worse the patient's condition, the more inhaled steroid is needed to gain control. Once achieved, however, remission can often be maintained with quantities as low as one or two puffs/day. Inhaled steroids can take up to a week or more to produce improvements; consequently, in rapidly deteriorating situations, it is best to prescribe oral preparations and initiate inhaled drugs as the dose of the former is reduced. In less emergent circumstances, the quantity of inhaled drug can be increased up to 2 to 2.5 times the recommended starting doses. It is critical to remember that the side effects increase in proportion to the dose-time product. In addition to thrush and dysphonia, the increased systemic absorption that accompanies larger doses of inhaled steroids has been reported to produce adrenal suppression, cataract formation, decreased growth in children, interference with bone metabolism, and purpura. As is the case with oral agents, suppression of inflammation, per se, cannot be relied upon to provide optimal results. It is essential to continue adrenergic or methylxanthine bronchodilators if the patient's disease is unstable.

Mast cell–stabilizing agents Cromolyn sodium and nedocromil sodium do not influence airway tone. Their major therapeutic effect is to inhibit the degranulation of mast cells, thereby preventing the release of the chemical mediators of anaphylaxis.

Cromolyn sodium and nedocromil, like the inhaled steroids, improve lung function, reduce symptoms, and lower airway reactivity in persons with asthma. They are most effective in atopic patients who have either seasonal disease or perennial airway stimulation. A therapeutic trial of two puffs four times daily for 4 to 6 weeks frequently is necessary before the beneficial effects of the drug appear. Unlike steroids, nedocromil and cromolyn sodium, when given prophylactically, block the acute obstructive effects of exposure to antigen, industrial chemicals, exercise, or cold air. With antigen, the late response is also abolished. Therefore, a patient who has intermittent exposure to either antigenic or nonantigenic stimuli that provoke acute episodes of asthma need not use these drugs continuously but instead can obtain protection by taking the drug only 15 to 20 min before contact with the precipitant.

Leukotriene modifiers As mentioned earlier, the cysteinyl leukotrienes (LTC_4, LTD_4, and LTE_4) produce many of the critical elements of asthma, and drugs have been developed to either reduce the synthesis of all of the leukotrienes by inhibiting 5-lipoxygenase (5-LO), the enzyme involved in their production, or competitively antagonizing the principal moiety (LTD_4). Zileuton is the only 5-lipoxygenase synthesis inhibitor that is available in the United States. It is a modest bronchodilator that reduces asthma morbidity, provides protection against exercise-induced asthma, and diminishes nocturnal symptoms, but it has limited effectiveness against allergens. Hepatic enzyme levels can be elevated after its use, and there are significant interactions with other drugs metabolized in the liver. The LTD_4 receptor antagonists (zafirlukast and montelukast) have therapeutic and toxicologic profiles similar to that of zileuton but are long acting and permit twice to single daily dose schedules.

This class of drugs does not appear to be uniformly effective in all patients with asthma. Although precise figures are lacking, most authorities put the number of positive responders at less than 50%. As yet, there is no way of determining prospectively who will benefit, so clinical trials are required. Typically, if there is no improvement after one month, treatment can be discontinued.

Miscellaneous agents It has been suggested that steroid-dependent patients might benefit from the use of immunosuppressant agents such as methotrexate or gold salts. The effects of these agents on steroid dosage and disease activity are minor, and side effects can be considerable. Consequently, this form of treatment can be viewed only as experimental. Opiates, sedatives, and tranquilizers should be absolutely avoided in the acutely ill patient with asthma because the risk of depressing alveolar ventilation is great, and respiratory arrest has been reported to occur shortly after their use. Admittedly, most individuals are anxious and frightened, but experience has shown that they can be calmed equally well by the physician's presence and reassurances. β-Adrenergic blockers and parasympathetic agonists are contraindicated because they can cause marked deterioration in lung function.

Expectorants and mucolytic agents have enjoyed great vogue in the past, but they do not add significantly to the treatment of the acute or chronic phases of this disease. Mucolytic agents such as acetylcysteine may actually produce bronchospasm when administered to susceptible patients with asthma. This effect can be overcome by aerosolizing them in solution with a β-adrenergic agent. The use of intravenous fluids in the treatment of acute asthma also has been advocated. There is little evidence that this adjunct hastens recovery. Nonstandard bronchodilators, such as intravenous magnesium sulfate, for the treatment of acute asthma attacks are not yet warranted in clinical practice because of the controversy surrounding their efficacy.

Special instructions The treatment of patients with asthma who have coexisting conditions such as heart disease or pregnancy does not differ materially from that outlined above. Therapy with inhaled β_2-selective and anti-inflammatory agents is the mainstay. The lowest doses of adrenergics that produce the desired effects should be used.

FRAMEWORK FOR MANAGEMENT **Emergency Situations** The most effective treatment for acute episodes of asthma requires a systematic approach based on the aggressive use of sympathomimetic agents and serial monitoring of key indices of improvement. Reliance on empirism and subjective assessment is no longer acceptable. Multiple inhalations of a short-acting sympathomimetic, such as albuterol, are the cornerstone of most regimens. These drugs provide three to four times more relief than does intravenous aminophylline. Anticholinergic drugs are not first-line therapy because of their long lag time to onset (~ 30 to 40 min) and their relatively modest bronchodilator properties. In emergency situations, β_2 agonists can be given every 20 min by handheld nebulizer for 2 to 3 doses. The optimum cumulative dose of albuterol appears to lie between 5 and 10 mg. It does not matter how the adrenergic agonists are inhaled. Treatment with albuterol administered by jet nebulizer, metered dose inhaler, or dry powder inhaler all provide equal resolution in acute situations. Aminophylline or ipratropium can be added to the regimen after the first hour in an attempt to speed resolution. Recent studies in a large series of patients demonstrate that β_2 agonists alone terminate attacks in approximately two-thirds of patients, and that another 5 to 10% benefit from a methylxanthine or ipratropium in combination with a sympathomimetic. The remainder have a poor acute response to all forms of therapy.

Acute episodes of bronchial asthma are one of the most common respiratory emergencies seen in the practice of medicine, and it is essential that the physician recognize which episodes of airway obstruction are life-threatening and which patients demand what level of care. These distinctions can be made readily by assessing selected clinical parameters in combination with measures of expiratory flow and gas exchange. The presence of a paradoxical pulse, use of accessory muscles, and marked hyperinflation of the thorax signify severe airways obstruction, and failure of these signs to remit promptly after aggressive therapy mandates objective monitoring of the patient with measurements of arterial blood gases and the peak expiratory flow rate (PEFR) or FEV_1.

In general, there is a correlation between the severity of the obstruction with which the patient presents and the time it takes to resolve it. Those individuals with the most impairment typically require the most extensive therapy for resolution. If the PEFR or FEV_1 is equal to or less than 20% of predicted on presentation and does not double within an hour of receiving the preceding therapy, the patient is likely to require extensive treatment including glucocorticoids before the obstruction dissipates. This group represents approximately 20% of all the patients who present for acute care. They generally require 3 to 4 days of inpatient treatment before becoming asymptomatic. In such individuals, if the clinical signs of a paradoxical pulse and accessory muscle use are diminishing, and/or if PEFR is increasing, there is no need to change medications or doses; the patient need only be followed. However, if the PEFR falls by more than 20% of its previous value or if the magnitude of the pulsus paradoxicus is increasing, serial measures of arterial blood gases are required, as well as a reconsideration of the therapeutic modalities being employed. If the patient has hypocarbia, one can afford to continue the current approaches a while longer. On the other hand, if the Pa_{CO_2} is within the normal range or is elevated, the patient should be monitored in an intensive care setting, and therapy should be intensified to reverse or arrest the patient's respiratory failure.

Chronic Treatment The goal of chronic therapy is to achieve a stable, asymptomatic state with the best pulmonary function possible using the least amount of medication. The first step is to educate patients to function as partners in their management. The severity of the illness needs to be assessed and monitored with objective measures of lung function. Asthma triggers should be avoided or controlled, and plans should be made for both chronic management and treatment of exacerbations. Regular follow-up care is mandatory. With respect to pharmacologic interventions, in general, the simplest approach works best. Infrequent symptoms require only the use of an inhaled sympathomimetic on an "as needed" basis. When the disease worsens, as manifested by nocturnal awakenings and daytime symptoms, inhaled steroids and/or mast cell–stabilizing agents should be added. If symptoms do not abate, the dose of inhaled steroids can be increased. An upper limit has not yet been established, but side effects of glucocorticoid excess begin to appear more frequently when the dose exceeds 2.0 mg/d. Persistent asthma complaints can be treated with long-acting inhaled β_2 agonists, sustained-release theophylline, and/or parasympatholytics. In patients with recurrent or perennial symptoms and unstable lung function, oral steroids in a single daily dose are added to the regimen. Once control is reached and sustained for several weeks, a step-down reduction in therapy should be undertaken, beginning with the most toxic drug, to find the minimum amount of medication required to keep the patient well. During this process, the PEFR should be monitored and medication adjustments should be based on objective changes in lung function as well as on the patient's symptoms.

PROGNOSIS AND CLINICAL COURSE The mortality rate from asthma is small. The most recent figures indicate fewer than 5000 deaths per year out of a population of approximately 10 million patients at risk. Death rates, however, appear to be rising in inner-city areas where there is limited availability of health care.

Information on the clinical course of asthma suggests a good prognosis particularly for those whose disease is mild and develops in childhood. The number of children who still have asthma 7 to 10 years after the initial diagnosis varies from 26 to 78%, averaging 46%; however, the percentage who continue to have severe disease is relatively low (6 to 19%).

Although there are reports of patients with asthma developing irreversible changes in lung function, these individuals frequently have comorbid stimuli such as cigarette smoking that could account for these findings. Even when untreated, individuals with asthma do not continuously move from mild to severe disease with time. Rather, their clinical course is characterized by exacerbations and remissions. Some studies suggest that spontaneous remissions occur in approximately 20% of those who develop the disease as adults and that 40% or so can be expected to experience improvement, with less frequent and severe attacks, as they grow older.

BIBLIOGRAPHY

AMERICAN THORACIC SOCIETY: Guidelines for the evaluation of impairment/disability in patients with asthma. Am Rev Respir Dis 147:1056, 1993

———: Progress of the interface of inflammation and asthma. Am J Respir Crit Care Med 152:385, 1995

BARNES PJ, ADCOCK IM: Transcription factors and asthma. Eur Respir J 12:221, 1998

BURR ML: Epidemiology of asthma. Monogr Allergy 31:80, 1993

HOLGATE ST: The cellular and mediator basis of asthma in relation to natural history. Lancet 350 (Suppl 2):5, 1997

MCFADDEN ER JR: Evolving concepts in the pathogenesis and management of asthma. Adv Intern Med 39:357, 1994

———, GILBERT IA: Exercise-induced asthma. N Engl J Med 330:1362, 1994

——— et al: Protocol therapy for acute asthma: Therapeutic benefits and cost savings. Am J Med 99:651, 1995

——— et al: Comparison of two dose regimens of albuterol in acute asthma. Am J Med 105:12, 1998

SANDFORD A et al: The genetics of asthma. Am J Respir Crit Care Med 153:1749, 1996

SHEFFER AL, TAGGART VS: The National Asthma Education Program. Expert panel report guidelines for the diagnosis and management of asthma. Med Care 31:MS20, 1993

WARDLAW AJ: The role of air pollution in asthma. Clin Exp Allergy 23:81, 1993

253

Joel N. Kline, Gary W. Hunninghake

HYPERSENSITIVITY PNEUMONITIS AND PULMONARY INFILTRATES WITH EOSINOPHILIA

HYPERSENSITIVITY PNEUMONITIS

Hypersensitivity pneumonitis (HP), or extrinsic allergic alveolitis, is an immunologically induced inflammatory disorder of the lung parenchyma, involving alveolar walls and terminal airways, secondary to repeated inhalation of a variety of organic agents by a susceptible host. Causes of HP are typically designated with colorful names denoting the occupational or avocational risk associated with the disease; "farmer's lung" is the term most commonly used for HP due to inhalation of antigens present in moldy hay, such as thermophilic actinomyces, *Micropolyspora faeni*, and *Aspergillus* species. The prevalence of HP is unknown but varies with the environmental exposure and the specific antigen involved. The prevalence of farmer's lung among Wisconsin dairy farmers has been reported as 4.2 per 1000. The diagnosis of HP requires a constellation of clinical, radiographic, physiologic, pathologic, and immunologic criteria, each of which is rarely pathognomonic alone; and the preferred treatment is avoidance of the causative antigen when practical.

ETIOLOGY Agents implicated as causes of HP include those listed in Table 253-1. Many cases of HP occurring in various occupations involve exposure to similar agents, particularly the thermophilic actinomycetes. In the United States, the most common types of HP are farmer's lung, bird fancier's lung, and chemical worker's lung. In *farmer's lung*, inhalation of proteins such as thermophilic bacteria and fungal spores that are present in moldy bedding and feed are most commonly responsible for the development of HP. These antigens are probably also responsible for the etiology of *mushroom worker's disease* (moldy composted growth medium is the source of the proteins) and *bagassosis* (moldy sugar cane is the source). *Bird fancier's lung* (and the related disorders of duck fever, turkey handler's lung, and dove pillow's lung) is a response to inhalation of bird proteins from feathers and droppings. *Chemical worker's lung* is an example of how simple chemicals, such as isocyanates, may also cause immune-mediated diseases. In this case, antihapten antibodies may be responsible for the development of HP.

PATHOGENESIS The finding that precipitating antibodies against extracts of moldy hay were demonstrable in most patients with farmer's lung led to the early conclusion that HP was an immune-complex–mediated reaction. Subsequent investigations of HP in humans and animal models provided evidence for the importance of cell-mediated hypersensitivity. The very early (acute) reaction is characterized by an increase in polymorphonuclear leukocytes in the alveoli and small airways. This early lesion is followed by an influx of mononuclear cells into the lung and the formation of granulomas that appear to be the result of a classic delayed (T cell mediated) hypersensitivity reaction to repeated inhalation of antigen and adjuvant-active materials. Recent studies in animal models suggest that the disease is mediated as a classic T_H1 cell-mediated immune response to antigen.

Bronchoalveolar lavage in patients with HP consistently demonstrates an increase in the number of T lymphocytes in lavage fluid (a finding that is also observed in patients with other granulomatous lung disorders). Patients with recent or continual exposure to antigen may have an increase in the number of polymorphonuclear leukocytes in lavage fluid. Increased numbers of mast cells have also been reported. In most patients examined during recovery from acute disease, the T lymphocytes in lavage fluid are predominantly the CD8+ T cell subset.

Table 253-1 Selected Examples of Hypersensitivity Pneumonitis (HP)

Disease	Antigen	Source of Antigen
Bagassosis	Thermophilic actinomycetes[a]	"Moldy" bagasse (sugar cane)
Bird fancier's, breeder's, or handler's lung[b]	Parakeet, pigeon, chicken, turkey proteins	Avian droppings or feathers
Cephalosporium HP	Contaminated basement (sewage)	*Cephalosporium*
Cheese washer's lung	*Penicillium casei*	Moldy cheese
Chemical worker's lung[b]	Isocyanates	Polyurethane foam, varnishes, lacquer
Coffee worker's lung	Coffee bean dust	Coffee beans
Compost lung	*Aspergillus*	Compost
Detergent worker's disease	*Bacillus subtilis* enzymes	Detergent
Familial HP	*B. subtilis*	Contaminated wood dust in walls
Farmer's lung[b]	Thermophilic actinomycetes[a]	"Moldy" hay, grain, silage
Fish meal worker's lung	Fish meal dust	Fish meal
Furrier's lung	Animal fur dust	Animal pelts
Hot tub lung	*Cladosporium* sp.	Mold on ceiling
Humidifier or air-conditioner lung (ventilation pneumonitis)	*Aureobasidium pullulans* or other microorganisms	Contaminated water in humidification or forced-air air-conditioning systems
Japanese summer house HP	*Trichosporon cutaneum*	House dust? Bird droppings
Laboratory worker's HP	Male rat urine	Laboratory rat
Lycoperdonosis	*Lycoperdon* puffballs	Puffball spores
Malt worker's lung	*A. fumigatus* or *A. clavatus*	Moldy barley
Maple bark disease	*Cryptostroma corticale*	Maple bark
Miller's lung	*Sitophilus granarius* (wheat weevil)	Infested wheat flour
Mushroom worker's lung	Thermophilic actinomycetes,[a] other	Mushroom compost
Paulis HP	Paulis reagent	Laboratory reagent
Pituitary snuff taker's lung	Animal proteins	Heterologous pituitary snuff
Potato riddler's lung	Thermophilic actinomycetes,[a] *Aspergillus*	"Moldy" hay around potatoes
Sauna taker's lung	*Aureobasidium* sp., other	Contaminated sauna water
Sequoiosis	*Aureobasidium, Graphium* sp.	Redwood sawdust
Streptomyces albus HP	*Streptomyces albus*	Contaminated fertilizer
Suberosis	Cork dust mold	Cork dust
Tap water lung	Unknown	Contaminated tap water
Thatched roof disease	*Sacchoromonospora viridis*	Dried grasses and leaves
Tobacco worker's disease	*Aspergillus* sp.	Mold on tobacco
Winegrower's lung	*Botrytis cinerea*	Mold on grapes
Wood trimmer's disease	*Rhizopus* sp., *Mucor* sp.	Contaminated wood trimmings
Woodman's disease	*Penicillium* sp.	Oak and maple trees
Woodworker's lung	Wood dust, *Alternaria*	Oak, cedar, pine, and mahogany dusts

[a] Thermophilic actinomycetes species include *Micropolyspora faeni, Thermoactinomyces vulgaris, T. saccharrii, T. viridis,* and *T. candidus.*

[b] Most common causes of hypersensitivity pneumonitis in the United States.

In patients with very recent exposure to antigen, however, the numbers of CD4+ T cells may increase in lavage fluid. Similar findings may be present in similarly exposed, asymptomatic individuals. These observations and others in animal models suggest that there is an active modulation of granuloma formation in the lung by immunoregulatory T cells and associated cytokines in this disorder.

CLINICAL PRESENTATION The clinical picture is that of an interstitial pneumonitis, although it varies from patient to patient and seems related to the frequency and intensity of exposure to the causative antigen and perhaps other host factors. The presentation can be *acute, subacute,* or *chronic.* In the *acute form,* symptoms such as cough, fever, chills, malaise, and dyspnea may occur 6 to 8 h after exposure to the antigen and usually clear within a few days if there is no further exposure to antigen. The *subacute form* often appears insidiously over a period of weeks marked by cough and dyspnea and may progress to cyanosis and severe dyspnea requiring hospitalization. In some patients, a subacute form of the disease may persist after an acute presentation of the disorder, especially if there is continued exposure to antigen. In most patients with the acute or subacute form of HP, the symptoms, signs, and other manifestations of HP disappear within days, weeks, or months if the causative agent is no longer inhaled. Transformation to a chronic form of the disease may occur in patients with continued antigen exposure, but the frequency of such progression is uncertain. The *chronic form* of HP may be clinically indistinguishable from pulmonary fibrosis due to a wide variety of causes. Physical examination may reveal clubbing. This stage may progressively worsen, resulting in dependence on supplemental O_2, pulmonary hypertension, and death from respiratory failure. An indolent gradually progressive form of the disease can be associated with cough and exertional dyspnea without a prior history consistent with acute or subacute manifestations. Such a gradual onset frequently occurs with low-dose exposure to the antigen.

Because strict definitions of acute, subacute, and chronic stages of HP have not been generally agreed on, interpretation of epidemiologic and clinical studies can be difficult. Therefore, it has been proposed that HP be described as recently diagnosed, recurrent or progressive, or residual disease. For these categories, required diagnostic criteria include the presence of an appropriate exposure; exertional dyspnea; inspiratory crackles; and, if performed, lymphocytic alveolitis on bronchoalveolar lavage. Supportive criteria include recurrent febrile episodes, radiographic infiltrates, diminished pulmonary diffusing capacity, precipitating antibodies to appropriate antigens, histopathologic demonstration of granulomas, and improvement in symptoms with avoidance of exposure.

DIAGNOSIS After acute exposure to antigen, neutrophilia and lymphopenia are frequently present. Eosinophilia is not a feature. All forms of the disease may be associated with elevations in erythrocyte sedimentation rate, C-reactive protein, rheumatoid factor, and serum immunoglobulins. Antinuclear antibodies are rarely present and appear to have no pathogenic role. Examination for *serum precipitins* against suspected antigens, such as those listed in Table 253-1, is an important part of the diagnostic workup and should be performed on any patient with interstitial lung disease, especially if a suggestive exposure history is elicited. If found, precipitins indicate sufficient exposure to the causative agent for generation of an immunologic response. The diagnosis of HP is not established solely by the presence of precipitins, however, as precipitins are found in sera of many individuals exposed to appropriate antigens who demonstrate no other evidence of HP. False-negative results may occur because of poor-quality antigens or an inappropriate choice of antigens. Extraction of antigens from the suspected source may at times be helpful.

No specific or distinctive *chest roentgenogram* occurs in HP. It can be normal even in symptomatic patients. The acute or subacute phase may be associated with poorly defined, patchy, or diffuse infiltrates or with discrete, nodular infiltrates (Fig. 253-1). In the chronic phase, the chest x-ray usually shows a diffuse reticulonodular infiltrate. Honeycombing may eventually develop as the condition progresses. Apical sparing is common, suggesting that disease severity correlates with inhaled antigen load, but no particular distribution or pattern is classic for HP. Abnormalities rarely seen in HP include pleural effusion or thickening, and hilar adenopathy. High-resolution chest computed tomography (CT) has been reported to show a characteristic constellation of abnormalities, including (1) global lung involvement with increased lung density, (2) prominence of medium-sized bronchial walls, (3) patchy air space opacification with reticular and nodular patterns and midzone prominence, and (4) absence of hilar lymph node enlargement. No pathognomonic CT features of HP have been described (Fig. 253-2).

Pulmonary function studies in all forms of HP may show a restrictive or obstructive pattern with loss of lung volumes, impaired diffusion capacity, decreased compliance, and an exercise-induced hypoxemia. Resting hypoxemia may also be found. Bronchospasm and bronchial hyperreactivity are sometimes found in acute HP. With antigen avoidance, the pulmonary function abnormalities are usually reversible, but they may gradually increase in severity or may occur rapidly after acute or subacute exposure to antigen.

Bronchoalveolar lavage is used in some centers to aid in diagnostic evaluation. A marked lymphocytic alveolitis on bronchoalveolar lavage is almost universal, although not pathognomonic. Lymphocytes typically have a decreased helper/suppressor ratio and are activated. Alveolar neutrophilia is also prominent acutely but tends to fade in the absence of recurrent exposure. Bronchoalveolar mastocytosis may correlate with disease activity. *Lung biopsy*, obtained through flexible bronchoscopy, open-lung procedures, or thoracoscopy, may be diagnostic. Although the histopathology is distinctive, it may not be pathognomonic of HP. When the biopsy is taken during the active phase of disease, typical findings include an interstitial alveolar infiltrate consisting of plasma cells, lymphocytes, and occasional eosinophils and neutrophils, usually with accompanying granulomas. Interstitial fibrosis may be present but most often is mild in earlier stages of the disease. Some degree of bronchiolitis is found in about half the cases, whereas vasculitis is not a feature of the disorder. The triad of mononuclear bronchiolitis; interstitial infiltrates of lymphocytes and plasma cells; and single, nonnecrotizing, and randomly scattered parenchymal granulomas without mural vascular involvement is consistent with but not specific for HP.

Inhalation challenge studies have been described as useful to differentiate between HP and other interstitial lung diseases. These tests should be performed in a center that specializes in provocation testing for reasons of both safety and accuracy. Moveover, because the antigens used for provocation testing are not standardized, interpretation of these tests is difficult. In general, these tests may be used to support a diagnosis of HP, but they are not sufficiently accepted to either confirm or deny the diagnosis. The lack of standardized, nonirritating antigens and of proven controlled protocols makes *skin testing* useful only for research purposes. Similarly, in vitro tests of cell-mediated (delayed) hypersensitivity have not consistently been shown to correlate with clinical HP and have no place in the routine diagnostic workup.

In summary, the diagnosis in most cases is established by (1) consistent history, physical findings, pulmonary function tests, and chest x-ray; (2) exposure to a recognized antigen; and (3) finding an antibody to that antigen. In a few circumstances, bronchoalveolar lavage and/or lung biopsy may be needed. Provocation tests may be useful but are not essential for the diagnosis.

DIFFERENTIAL DIAGNOSIS Chronic HP may often be difficult to distinguish from a number of other interstitial lung disorders such as idiopathic pulmonary fibrosis, sarcoidosis, interstitial lung disease associated with a collagen vascular disorder, and drug-induced lung diseases. A negative history for use of relevant drugs and no evidence of a systemic disorder usually exclude the presence of drug-induced lung disease or a collagen vascular disorder. Bronchoalveolar lavage often shows predominance of neutrophils in idiopathic pulmonary fibrosis and a predominance of CD4+ lymphocytes in sarcoidosis. Hilar/paratracheal lymphadenopathy or evidence of multisystem involvement also favors the diagnosis of sarcoidosis. In some patients, a lung biopsy may be required to differentiate chronic HP from other interstitial diseases. The lung disease associated with acute or subacute HP may clinically resemble other disorders that present with systemic symptoms and recurrent pulmonary infiltrates, including the allergic bronchopulmonary mycoses and other eosinophilic pneumonias.

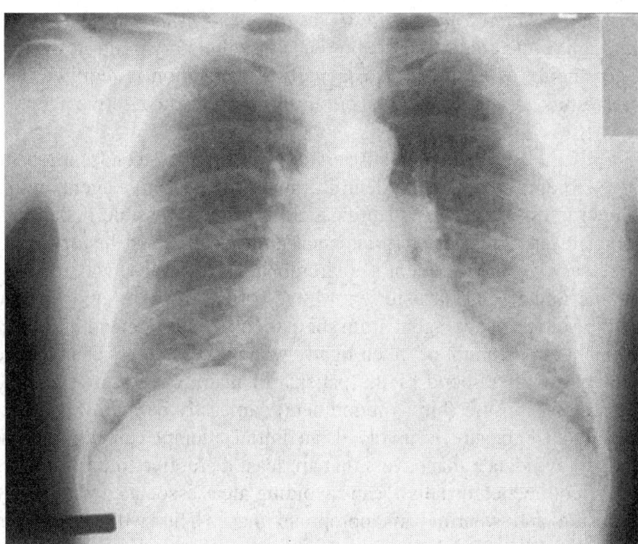

FIGURE 253-1 Chest X-ray of acute HP demonstrating interstitial infiltrates most prominently in the lower lung fields bilaterally. *(Courtesy of JS Wilson.)*

Eosinophilic pneumonia is often associated with asthma and is typified by peripheral eosinophilia; neither of these is a feature of HP. Allergic bronchopulmonary aspergillosis (ABPA) is the most common example of the allergic bronchopulmonary mycoses and is sometimes confused with HP because of the presence of precipitating antibodies to *A. fumigatus*. ABPA is associated with allergic (atopic) asthma. Acute HP may be confused with *organic dust toxic syndrome* (ODTS), a condition that is more common than HP. ODTS follows heavy exposure to organic dusts and is characterized by transient fever and muscle aches, with or without dyspnea and cough. Serum precipitins are absent, and the chest x-ray is usually normal. Studies have shown no immunologic basis for ODTS, and endotoxin is suspected to be involved in its pathogenesis. This distinction is important, as ODTS is a self-limited disorder without significant long-term sequellae, whereas continued antigen exposure in HP can result in permanent disability. Massive exposure to moldy silage may result in a syndrome

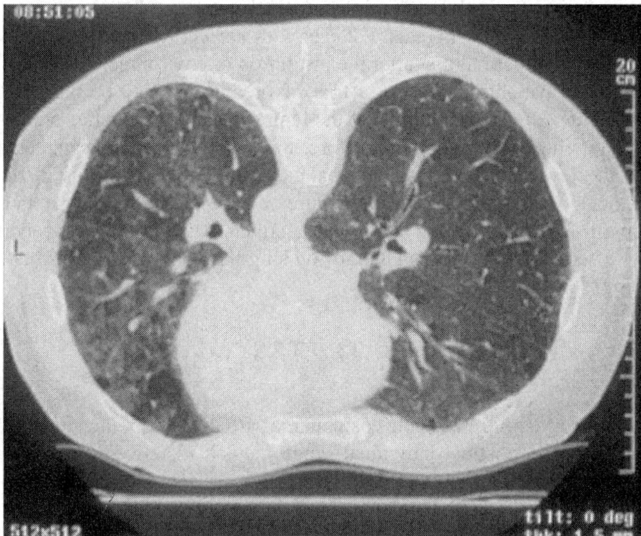

FIGURE 253-2 Chest CT scan of a case of acute hypersensitivity pneumonitis in which scattered regions of ground glass and nodular infiltrates are seen bilaterally. *(Courtesy of JS Wilson.)*

termed *pulmonary mycotoxicosis*, or *atypical farmer's lung*, with fever, chills, and cough and the presence of pulmonary infiltrates within a few hours of exposure. No previous sensitization is required, and precipitins are absent to *Aspergillus*, the suspected causative agent.

℞ **TREATMENT** Because effective treatment depends largely on avoiding the antigen, identification of the causative agent and its source is essential. This identification is usually possible if the physician takes a careful environmental and occupational history or, if necessary, visits the patient's environment. The simplest way to avoid the incriminated agent is to remove the patient from the environment or the source of the agent from the patient's environment. This recommendation cannot be taken lightly when it completely changes the life-style or livelihood of the patient. In many cases, however, the source of exposure (birds, humidifiers) can easily be removed. If occupational exposure is involved, an initial attempt can be made at antigen avoidance maneuvers that are least disruptive to the patient's livelihood, which usually means avoiding areas associated with heavy exposure and wearing an appropriate mask. This will not protect against small-molecular-weight agents such as isocyanates, which require more elaborate respiratory systems. Pollen masks, personal dust respirators, airstream helmets, and ventilated helmets with a supply of fresh air are increasingly efficient means of purifying inhaled air. If symptoms recur or physiologic abnormalities progress in spite of these measures, then more effective measures to avoid antigen exposure must be pursued. Compromises with environmental control pertain primarily to the acute, recurrent, transient clinical form of HP and must be accompanied by careful follow-up. Subacute forms are ordinarily the result of a heavy, sustained exposure. The chronic form typically results from low-grade or recurrent exposure over many months or years, and the lung disease may already be partially irreversible. These patients are usually advised to avoid completely all possible contact with the offending agent, although follow-up studies of individuals with farmer's lung and bird fancier's lung have found resolution of the disease despite continued exposure in some patients.

Patients with the *acute*, recurrent form of HP usually recover without need for glucocorticoids. *Subacute* HP may be associated with severe symptoms and marked physiologic impairment and may continue to progress for several days despite hospitalization. Urgent establishment of the diagnosis and prompt institution of glucocorticoid treatment are indicated in such patients. Such therapy may also hasten recovery in patients with lesser involvement. Prednisone at a dosage of 1 mg/kg per day or its equivalent is continued for 7 to 14 days and then tapered over the ensuing 2 to 6 weeks at a rate that depends on the patient's clinical status. Patients with *chronic* HP may gradually recover without therapy after the institution of environmental control. In many patients, however, a trial of prednisone may be useful to obtain maximal reversibility of the lung disease. After initial prednisone therapy (1 mg/kg per day for 2 to 4 weeks), the drug is tapered to the lowest dosage that will maintain the functional status of the patient. Many patients will not require or benefit from long-term therapy if there is no further exposure to antigen. Available studies report no effect of glucocorticoid therapy on long-term prognosis of farmer's lung.

PULMONARY INFILTRATES WITH EOSINOPHILIA

Pulmonary infiltrates with eosinophilia (PIE, eosinophilic pneumonias) include distinct individual syndromes characterized by eosinophilic pulmonary infiltrates and, commonly, peripheral blood eosinophilia. Since Loeffler's initial description of a transient, benign syndrome of migratory pulmonary infiltrates and peripheral blood eosinophilia of unknown cause, this group of disorders has been enlarged to include several diseases of both known and unknown etiology (Table 253-2). These diseases may be considered as putative hypersensitivity lung diseases but are not to be confused with HP (extrinsic allergic alveolitis), in which eosinophilia is not a feature. When an eosinophilic pneumonia is associated with bronchial asthma, it is important to determine if the patient has atopic asthma and has wheal-and-flare skin reactivity to *Aspergillus* or other relevant fungal antigens. If so, other criteria should be sought for diagnosis of ABPA (Table 253-3) or other, rarer examples of allergic bronchopulmonary mycosis such as those caused by *Penicillium*, *Candida*, *Curvularia*, or *Helminthosporium* spp. *A. fumigatus* is the most common cause of ABPA, although other *Aspergillus* species have also been implicated. ABPA has been reported to complicate cystic fibrosis. The chest roentgenogram in ABPA may show transient, recurrent infiltrates or may suggest the presence of proximal bronchiectasis. High-resolution chest CT is a sensitive, noninvasive technique for the recognition of proximal bronchiectasis. The bronchial asthma of ABPA likely involves an IgE-mediated hypersensitivity, whereas the bronchiectasis associated with this disorder is thought to result from a deposition of immune complexes in proximal airways. Treatment usually requires the long-term use of systemic glucocorticoids.

Table 253-2 Pulmonary Infiltrates with Eosinophilia

ETIOLOGY KNOWN
Allergic bronchopulmonary mycoses
Parasitic infestations
Drug reactions
Eosinophilia-myalgia syndrome
IDIOPATHIC
Loeffler's syndrome
Acute eosinophilic pneumonia
Chronic eosinophilic pneumonia
Allergic granulomatosis of Churg and Strauss
Hypereosinophilic syndrome

Tropical eosinophilia is usually caused by filarial infection; however, eosinophilic pneumonias also occur with other parasites such as *Ascaris*, *Ancyclostoma* sp., *Toxocara* sp., and *Strongyloides stercoralis*. Tropical eosinophilia due to *Wuchereria bancrofti* or *W. malayi* occurs most commonly in southern Asia, Africa, and South America, and is treated successfully with diethylcarbamazine.

Drug-induced eosinophilic pneumonias are exemplified by acute reactions to nitrofurantoin, which may begin 2 h to 10 days after nitrofurantoin is started, with symptoms of dry cough, fever, chills, and dyspnea; an eosinophilic pleural effusion accompanying patchy or diffuse pulmonary infiltrates may also occur. Other drugs associated with eosinophilic pneumonias include sulfonamides, penicillin, chlorpropamide, thiazides, tricyclic antidepressants, hydralazine, mephenesin, mecamylamine, nickel carbonyl vapor, gold salts, isoniazid, para-aminosalicylic acid, and others. Treatment consists of withdrawal of the incriminated drugs and the use of glucocorticoids, if necessary. The eosinophilia-myalgia syndrome, caused by dietary supplements of L-tryptophan, is occasionally associated with pulmonary infiltrates.

Table 253-3 Diagnostic Features of Allergic Bronchopulmonary Aspergillosis (ABPA)

MAIN DIAGNOSTIC CRITERIA
Bronchial asthma
Pulmonary infiltrates
Peripheral eosinophilia ($>1000/\mu L$)
Immediate wheal-and-flare response to *A. fumigatus*
Serum precipitins to *A. fumigatus*
Elevated serum IgE
Central bronchiectasis
OTHER DIAGNOSTIC FEATURES
History of brownish plugs in sputum
Culture of *A. fumigatus* from sputum
Elevated IgE (and IgG) class antibodies specific for *A. fumigatus*

The group of idiopathic eosinophilic pneumonias consists of diseases of varying severity. *Loeffler's syndrome* was originally reported as a benign, acute eosinophilic pneumonia of unknown cause characterized by migrating pulmonary infiltrates and minimal clinical manifestations. In some patients, these clinical characteristics may prove to be secondary to parasites or drugs. *Acute eosinophilic pneumonia* has been described recently as an idiopathic acute febrile illness lasting less than 7 days with severe hypoxemia, pulmonary infiltrates, and no history of asthma. *Chronic eosinophilic pneumonia* presents with significant systemic symptoms including fever, chills, night sweats, cough, anorexia, and weight loss lasting for several weeks to months. The chest x-ray classically shows peripheral infiltrates resembling a photographic negative of pulmonary edema. Some patients also have bronchial asthma of the intrinsic or nonallergic type. Dramatic clearing of symptoms and chest x-rays is often noted within 48 h after initiation of glucocorticoid therapy.

Allergic angiitis and granulomatosis of Churg and Strauss is a multisystem vasculitic disorder that frequently involves the skin, kidney, and nervous system in addition to the lung. The disorder may occur at any age and favors persons with a history of bronchial asthma. The asthma often is progressive until the onset of fever and exaggerated eosinophilia, at which time the symptoms of asthma may ease. The illness may be fulminating and the prognosis grave unless treated aggressively with glucocorticoids and, at times, immunosuppressive therapy. The recent introduction of leukotriene-modifying agents (zafirlukast, zyleuton, and montelukast) has unmasked a number of cases of unrecognized Churg-Strauss syndrome when individuals with asthma have been weaned from glucocorticoids with the use of these antigens.

The *hypereosinophilic syndrome* is characterized by the presence of more than 1500 eosinophils per microliter of peripheral blood for 6 months or longer; lack of evidence for parasitic, allergic, or other known causes of eosinophilia; and signs or symptoms of multisystem organ dysfunction. Consistent features are blood and bone marrow eosinophilia with tissue infiltration by relatively mature eosinophils. The heart may be involved with tricuspid valve abnormalities or endomyocardial fibrosis and a restrictive, biventricular cardiomyopathy. Other organs affected typically include the lungs, liver, spleen, skin, and nervous system. Treatment consists of glucocorticoids and/or hydroxyurea, plus treatment as needed for cardiac dysfunction, which is frequently responsible for much of the morbidity and mortality in this syndrome.

BIBLIOGRAPHY

Hypersensitivity Pneumonitis

Denis M: Proinflammatory cytokines in hypersensitivity pneumonitis. Am J Respir Crit Care Med 151:164, 1995

Gudmundsson G et al: IL-12 modulates expression of hypersensitivity pneumonitis. J Immunol 161:991, 1998

Gurney JW et al: Agricultural disorders of the lung. Radiographics 11:625, 1991

Kokkarinen JI et al: Recovery of pulmonary function in farmer's lung. A five-year followup study. Am Rev Respir Dis 147:793, 1993

Marx JJ et al: Cohort studies of immunologic lung disease among Wisconsin dairy farmers. Am J Int Med 18:263, 1990

Ramirez-Venegas A et al: Utility of a provocation test for diagnosis of chronic pigeon breeder's disease. Am J Respir Crit Care Med 158:862, 1998

Richerson HB et al: Guidelines for the clinical evaluation of hypersensitivity pneumonitis. J Allergy Clin Immunol 84:839, 1989

Rose CS: Hypersensitivity pneumonitis, in *Textbook of Respiratory Medicine*, Murray JF, Nadel JA (eds). Philadelphia, Saunders, 2000, pp 1867–1884

Rose C, King TE: Controversies in hypersensitivity pneumonitis. Am Rev Respir Dis 145:1, 1992

Eosinophilic Pneumonia

Mroueh S, Spock A: Allergic bronchopulmonary aspergillosis in patients with cystic fibrosis. Chest 105:32, 1994

Patterson R, Greenberger PA, Roberts ML (eds): *Allergic Bronchopulmonary Aspergillosis*. Providence, RI, OceanSide Pub, 1995

Rosenow EC III et al: Drug-induced pulmonary disease: An update. Chest 102:239, 1992

Shintani H et al: Acute eosinophilic pneumonia caused by cigarette smoking. Intern Med 39:66, 2000

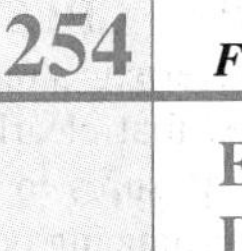

Frank E. Speizer

254 ENVIRONMENTAL LUNG DISEASES

This chapter provides perspectives on ways to assess pulmonary diseases for which environmental causes are suspected. This assessment is important because removal of the patient from a harmful environment is often the only intervention that might prevent further significant deterioration or lead to improvement in a patient's condition. Furthermore, the identification of an environment-associated disease in a single patient may lead to primary preventive strategies affecting other similarly exposed people who have not yet developed disease.

The exact magnitude of the problem is unknown, but there is no question that large numbers of people are at risk for developing serious respiratory disease as a result of occupational or environmental exposures. For example, recent estimates suggest that approximately 2.4 million workers in the United States have been exposed to crystalline silica or asbestos dust in mining and nonmining industries. Even if only 5% of these workers (a conservative estimate) are to suffer from respiratory disease as a result of their exposure, this figure represents more than 100,000 individuals.

Although industries are required to spend substantial amounts of capital in efforts to protect their workers, occupationally related respiratory diseases continue to occur. These diseases are often attributed to exposures in the past, at a time when we were not aware of the risk incurred and the need for worker protection to the degree that we are today.

HISTORY AND PHYSICAL EXAMINATION The patient's history is of paramount importance in assessing any potential occupational or environmental exposure, and the physician must ask the patient to describe a suspected environmental exposure in detail.

Inquiry into specific work practices should include questions about specific contaminants involved, the availability and use of personal respiratory protection devices, the size and ventilation of workspaces, and whether coworkers have similar complaints. In addition, the patient must be questioned about alternative sources for potentially toxic exposures, including hobbies or other environmental exposures at home. Short-term exposures to potential toxic agents in the distant past must also be considered (Chap. 391).

Many people are aware of the potential hazards in their workplaces, and many states require that employees be informed about potentially hazardous exposures. These requirements include the provision of specific educational materials (including Material Safety Data Sheets), personal protective equipment and instructions in its use, and information on environmental control procedures. Reminders posted in the workplace may warn workers about hazardous substances. Protective clothing, lockers, and shower facilities may be considered necessary parts of the job. However, even in these more progressive industries, the introduction of new processes, particularly when related to the use of new chemical compounds, may change exposure significantly, and often only the employee on the production line is aware of the change. For the physician who regularly sees patients from a particular industry, a visit to the work site can be very instructive. Alternatively, physicians can request inspections by appropriate federal and/or state authorities.

The physical examination of patients with environment-related lung diseases may help to determine the nature and severity of the pulmonary condition. Unfortunately, the pulmonary response to most injurious agents is the development of a limited number of nonspecific physical signs. These findings do not point to the specific causative agent, and other types of information must be used to arrive at an etiologic diagnosis.

PULMONARY FUNCTION TESTS AND CHEST RADIOGRAPHY Many mineral dusts produce characteristic alterations in the mechanics of breathing and lung volumes that clearly indicate a restrictive pattern (Chaps. 250 and 259). Exposures to a number of organic dusts or chemical agents capable of producing occupational asthma result in pronounced obstructive patterns of pulmonary dysfunction that may be reversible (Chap. 252). Measurement of change in forced expiratory volume (FEV_1) before and after a working shift can be used to detect an acute inflammatory or bronchoconstrictive response. An acute decrement of FEV_1 over the first work shift of the week is a characteristic feature of cotton textile workers with byssinosis.

The chest radiograph is useful in detecting and monitoring the pulmonary response to mineral dusts. The International Labour Organization (ILO) International Classification of Radiographs of Pneumoconioses classifies chest radiographs according to the nature and size of opacities seen and the extent of involvement of the parenchyma. In general, opacities may be round or irregular, small (<10 mm in diameter) or large. They may be few in number, with visible normal lung markings, partially obscure normal markings, or totally obscure normal markings. Although useful for screening large numbers of workers, the ILO system lacks specificity and may over- or underestimate the functional impact of pneumoconiosis. With dusts causing rounded, regular opacities like those evident in coal worker's pneumoconiosis, the degree of involvement on the chest radiograph may be extensive, while pulmonary function may be only minimally impaired.

In contrast, in pneumoconiosis causing linear, irregular opacities like those seen in asbestosis, the radiograph may lead to underestimation of the severity of the impairment. It is possible for a patient to have a history of exposure, a moderately reduced forced vital capacity (FVC), and a reduced diffusion capacity in asbestosis with a relatively normal chest radiograph. The radiographic findings of irregular or linear opacities are simply more difficult to separate from normal markings until relatively late in the disease. When shadows become large, as shown in Fig. 254-1, the condition is termed *complicated pneumoconiosis*, sometimes called progressive massive fibrosis (PMF). For the individual patient with a history of exposure, conventional computed tomography (CT) and high-resolution computed tomography (HRCT) have improved the sensitivity of identifying diffuse parenchymal abnormalities of the lung. The procedures have been shown to provide earlier detection of silicosis and asbestosis.

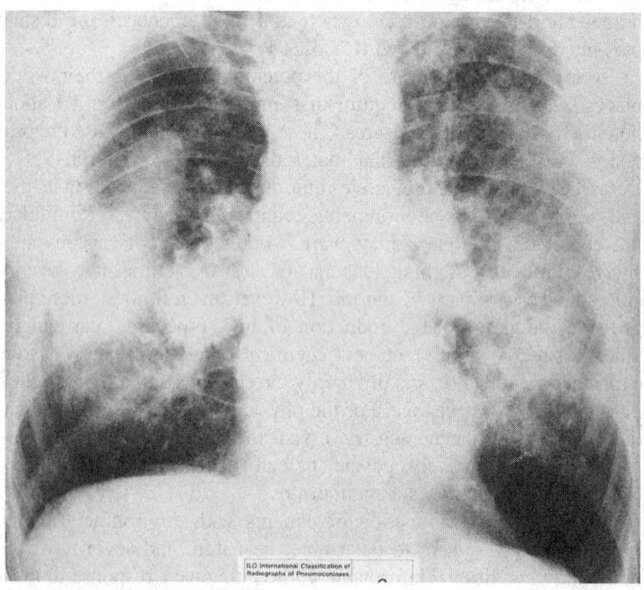

FIGURE 254-1 Progressive Massive Fibrosis ILO Classification C. Lesions are bilateral relatively homogeneous, symmetric and stable over at least one year. *(With permission of the ILO International Classification of Radiographs of Pneumoconiosis–revised 1980.)*

Other diagnostic procedures of use in identifying environment-induced lung disease include evaluation of heavy metal concentrations in urine (arsenic in smelter workers, cadmium in battery plant workers); bacteriologic studies (tuberculosis in medical care personnel, anthrax in wool sorters); fungal studies (coccidioidomycosis in southwestern farm workers, histoplasmosis in poultry or pigeon handlers); and serologic studies (psittacosis in pet shop workers or owners of sick birds, Q fever in tanners or slaughterhouse workers). Ultimately, a lung biopsy may be required both for morphologic diagnosis of the underlying pulmonary disease and for attempted identification of the specific etiologic agent.

MEASUREMENT OF EXPOSURE If reliable environmental sampling data are available, this information should be used in assessing a patient's exposure. Since many of the chronic diseases result from exposure over many years, current environmental measurements should be combined with work histories to arrive at estimates of past exposure. Even in acute conditions, when monitoring of exposure may be possible, little may be known about the actual dose received by the lung. Most of the research on health effects of air pollutants (discussed later in this chapter) has relied on fixed-station monitoring of outdoor air, often at locations somewhat distant from the residences of the people being studied. In addition, most people spend less than 20% of their time outdoors. Therefore, outdoor measurements can be used only in a relative sense, and they cannot be relied on to estimate actual dose.

In situations where individual exposure to specific agents—either in a work setting or via ambient air pollutants—has been determined, transport of these agents through the airways may be an important factor affecting dose. Highly soluble gases such as sulfur dioxide are absorbed in the upper airway and presumably produce their effects by reflex response of sensitive neural fibrils in the trachea or larger airways. In contrast, nitrogen dioxide, which is less soluble, may reach the bronchioles and alveoli in sufficient quantities to result in an acute life-threatening disease in farmers exposed even briefly to the gas evolved from moldy hay in silos (silo-filler's disease).

Particle size and chemistry of air contaminants also must be considered. Particles above 10 to 15 μm in diameter, because of their settling velocities in air, do not penetrate beyond the upper airways. These larger particles are often referred to as "fugitive dusts" and include pollens, other windblown dusts, and dusts resulting from mechanical industrial processes. They have little or no role in chronic respiratory disease except perhaps as related to cancer (see below).

Particles below 10 μm in size are created by the burning of fossil fuels or high-temperature industrial processes resulting in condensation products from gases, fumes, or vapors. These particles are divided into two size fractions on the basis of their chemical characteristics. Particles of approximately 2.5 to 10 μm (coarse-mode fraction) contain crustal elements, such as silica, aluminum, and iron. These particles mostly deposit relatively high in the tracheobronchial tree. Although the total mass of an ambient sample is dominated by these larger respirable particles, the number of particles, and therefore the surface area on which potential toxic agents can deposit and be carried to the lower airways, is dominated by particles smaller than 2.5 μm (fine-mode fraction or accumulation mode). The smallest particles, those less than 0.1 μm in size, remain in the airstream and deposit in the lung only on a random basis as they come into contact with the alveolar walls.

Besides the size characteristics of particles and the solubility of gases, the actual chemical composition, mechanical properties, and immunogenicity or infectivity of inhaled material determine in large part the nature of the diseases found among exposed persons. Few studies to date have directly measured those characteristics. However, they are of increasing concern as management strategies for environmental and occupational exposures are developed.

OCCUPATIONAL EXPOSURES AND PULMONARY DISEASE

ASBESTOSIS Except in localized regions with single industrial exposures, such as coal-mining or granite-quarrying regions, the most frequent inorganic dust-related chronic pulmonary diseases are associated with industries using *asbestiform fibers*. *Asbestos* is a generic term for several different mineral silicates, including chrysolite, amosite, anthophyllite, and crocidolite. Besides workers involved in the mining, milling, and manufacturing of asbestos products, workers in the building trades, including pipe fitters and boilermakers, were exposed to asbestos, which was widely used in construction because of its exceptional thermal and electric insulation properties. In addition, asbestos was used in the manufacture of fire-smothering blankets and safety garments, as filler for plastic materials, in cement and floor tiles, and in friction materials, such as brake and clutch linings.

Exposure to asbestos is not limited to persons who directly handle the material. Cases of asbestos-related diseases have been encountered in individuals with only moderate exposure, such as the painter or electrician who works alongside the insulation worker in a shipyard or the housewife who does no more than shake out and wash her husband's work clothes. Community exposure has probably resulted from the use of asbestos-containing material sprayed on steel girders in many large buildings as a safety feature to prevent buckling in case of fire.

Asbestos was first used extensively in the 1940s. Starting in 1975 it was mostly replaced with synthetic mineral fibers, such as fiberglass or slag wool. However, asbestos is still used in the manufacture of brake linings and remains as pipe and boiler insulation in hundreds of thousands of workplaces and homes. Despite current regulations mandating adequate training for any worker potentially exposed to asbestos, exposure probably continues among inexperienced demolition workers. The major health effects from exposure to asbestos are pulmonary fibrosis (asbestosis) and cancers of the respiratory tract, the pleura, and (in rare cases) the peritoneum.

Asbestosis is a diffuse interstitial fibrosing disease of the lung that is directly related to the intensity and duration of exposure. Except for its association with a history of exposure to asbestos (generally in a work setting), asbestosis resembles the other forms of diffuse interstitial fibrosis (Chap. 259). Usually, moderate to severe exposure has taken place for at least 10 years before the disease becomes manifest.

Physiologic studies reveal a restrictive pattern with a decrease in lung volumes. Flow rates are commonly reduced less than would be predicted on the basis of the volume reduction. An early sign of severe disease may be a reduction in diffusing capacity.

Pulmonary fibrosis may occur following sufficient exposure to any of the asbestiform fiber types. The fibrotic lesions do not appear to relate to either shape or chemical composition of any fiber type. During phagocytosis of the asbestos fiber, the membrane of the macrophage is damaged and this damage results in the release of lysosomes containing enzymes that may act to damage the lung parenchyma. The clinical manifestations are typical of those physical findings in any patient with pulmonary fibrosis (Chap. 259).

Diagnosis The chest radiograph can be used to detect a number of manifestations of asbestos exposure as well as to identify specific lesions. Past exposure is specifically indicated by pleural plaques, which are characterized by either thickening or calcification along the parietal pleura, particularly along the lower lung fields, the diaphragm, and the cardiac border. Without additional manifestations, pleural plaques imply only exposure, not pulmonary impairment. Benign pleural effusions may occur, particularly in patients with asbestosis, but are not necessarily restricted to those with overt disease. The fluid is sterile but may be a serous or blood-stained exudate and may occur bilaterally. The effusion may be slowly progressive or may resolve spontaneously.

The radiographic diagnosis of asbestosis depends on the presence of irregular or linear opacities, usually first noted in the lower lung fields and spreading into the middle and upper lung fields as the disease progresses. An indistinct heart border or a "ground glass" appearance in the lung fields is seen in some cases. As the fibrotic changes in the parenchyma begin to coalesce, the patient develops obliteration of entire acinar units, with eventual formation of the classical honeycombed lung, which appears on chest radiographs as coarse infiltrates with small (about 7- to 10-μm) air spaces. In cases in which the x-ray changes are less obvious, HRCT may show distinct changes of subpleural curvilinear lines 5 to 10 cm in length that appear to be parallel to the pleural surface; these alterations increase the positive predictive value of radiographic evidence from approximately 85% to about 100%.

In general, newly diagnosed cases will have resulted from exposure levels that were present many years before and, in spite of the patients' having left the industry, are attributable to that former exposure. Since the patient may be eligible for compensation within a specific time frame after the diagnosis of an asbestos-related disease is made, the physician making the diagnosis should be certain to inform the patient promptly. On occasion, the physician may have reason to suspect ongoing exposure from a patient's current job description or actual monitoring data. In such cases, federal or state health authorities may need to be notified. Present-day occupational safety and health regulations, if followed properly, protect workers from exposure.

Casual, nonoccupational exposure to undisturbed sources of asbestos-containing materials—e.g., in walls of schools or other buildings—represents little if any hazard to people who inhabit or work in such buildings. Because the association of smoking and asbestos exposure increases the risk of developing lung cancer (see below), it is extremely important to advise patients with a history of exposure to asbestos to stop smoking. No specific therapy is available in the management of patients with asbestosis. The supportive care is the same as that given to any patient with diffuse interstitial fibrosis from any cause.

Lung cancer (Chap. 88), either squamous cell carcinoma or adenocarcinoma, is the most frequent cancer associated with asbestos exposure. The excess frequency of lung cancer in asbestos workers is associated with a minimum lapse of 15 to 19 years between first exposure and development of the disease. Persons with more exposure are at greater risk of disease. In addition, there appears to be a significant multiplicative effect that leads to a far greater risk of lung cancer in persons who are cigarette smokers and have asbestos exposure than would be expected from the additive risk of each factor. To date, efforts to consider these high-risk individuals for special surveillance studies, including sputum cytologic examinations and repeated chest x-rays as frequently as every 4 to 6 months, have resulted in neither significant early detection nor prolonged survival once the lung cancer is found.

Mesotheliomas (Chap. 262), both pleural and peritoneal, are also associated with asbestos exposure. In contrast to lung cancers, these tumors do not appear to be associated with smoking. Relatively short-term asbestos exposures of 1 to 2 years or less occurring some 20 to 25 years in the past have been associated with the development of mesotheliomas (an observation that emphasizes the importance of obtaining a complete environmental exposure history). The risk for this type of tumor peaks 30 to 35 years after initial exposure. Since maximum exposure took place in the United States between 1930 and 1960, peak incidence of disease in men occurred in 1997, with a total of 2300 cases. Incidence is expected to decline over the next 30+ years to about 500 cases per year.

Although approximately 50% of mesotheliomas metastasize, the tumor generally is locally invasive, and death usually results from local extension. Most patients present with effusions that may obscure the underlying pleural tumor. In contrast to the findings in effusion due to other causes, because of the restriction placed on the chest wall, no shift of mediastinal structures toward the opposite side of the chest will be seen. The major diagnostic problem is differentiation from peripherally spreading pulmonary adenocarcinoma or from adenocarcinoma metastasized to pleura from an extrathoracic primary site. Although a needle biopsy may be diagnostic, an open biopsy is often necessary, and even the latter procedure may not provide a definitive diagnosis of the origin of the tumor.

Since epidemiologic studies have shown that more than 80% of mesotheliomas may be associated with asbestos exposure, documented mesothelioma in a worker with occupational exposure to asbestos may be compensable in many parts of the United States.

SILICOSIS In spite of the technical adequacy of existing protective equipment, *free silica* (SiO_2), or crystalline quartz, is still a major occupational hazard. In the United States, estimates of potential numbers of exposed workers range between 1.2 and 3 million people. The major occupational exposures include: mining; stonecutting; employment in abrasive industries, such as stone, clay, glass, and cement manufacturing; foundry work; packing of silica flour; and quarrying, particularly of granite. Most often, progressive pulmonary fibrosis (silicosis) occurs in a dose-response fashion after many years of exposure.

Workers exposed through sandblasting in confined spaces, tunneling through rock with high quartz content (15 to 25%), or the manufacture of abrasive soaps may develop acute silicosis with as little as 10 months' exposure. The disease may be rapidly fatal in less than 2 years, despite the discontinuation of exposure. A radiographic picture of profuse miliary infiltration or consolidation is characteristic of acute silicosis.

In long-term, less intense exposure, small rounded opacities in the upper lobes, with retraction and hilar adenopathy, classically appear on the radiograph after 15 to 20 years. Calcification of hilar nodes may occur in as many as 20% of cases and produces the characteristic "eggshell" pattern. These changes may be preceded by or associated with a reticular pattern of irregular densities that are uniformly present throughout the upper lung zones.

The nodular fibrosis may be progressive in the absence of further exposure, with coalescence and formation of nonsegmental conglomerates of irregular masses in excess of 1 cm in diameter. These masses become quite large and are characteristic of PMF (Figure 254-1). Significant functional impairment with both restrictive and obstructive components may be associated with this form of silicosis. In the late stages of the disease, ventilatory failure may develop. In more subtle cases, CT may be helpful both in identifying nodules, which are preferentially located in the posterior aspect of the upper lobes, as well as in identifying larger opacities and more coalescence than might be noted on regular chest x-rays. Patients with silicosis are at greater risk of acquiring *Mycobacterium tuberculosis* infections (silicotuberculosis) and atypical mycobacterial infections. Because the frequency with which tuberculosis has been found at autopsy in patients with PMF exceeds considerably the frequency of premorbid diagnosis, treatment for tuberculosis is indicated in any patient with silicosis and a positive tuberculin test.

Other less hazardous silicates include Fuller's earth, kaolin, mica, diatomaceous earths, silica gel, soapstone, carbonate dusts, and cement dusts. The production of fibrosis in workers exposed to these agents is believed to be related either to the free silica content of these dusts or, for substances that contain no free silica, to the potentially large dust loads to which these workers may be exposed.

Other silicates, including *talc dusts*, may be contaminated with asbestos and/or free silica. Accidental exposure to significant quantities of talc may result in an acute syndrome with cough, cyanosis, and labored breathing (acute talcosis). Severe progressive fibrosis with respiratory failure may ensue within a few years. Far more common is the fibrosis and/or pleural or lung cancer associated with chronic exposure in rubber workers who use commercial talc as a lubricant in tire molds. Pure talc does not produce fibrosis; thus, it is difficult to sort out whether the effects are due to the contamination of commercial talc by asbestos or by free silica.

COAL WORKER'S PNEUMOCONIOSIS (CWP) *Coal dust* is associated with CWP, which has enormous social, economic, and medical significance in every nation in which coal mining is an important industry. Simple radiographically identified CWP is seen in 12% of all miners and in as many as 50% of anthracite miners with more than 20 years' work on the coal face. The prevalence of disease is lower in workers in bituminous coal mines. Since much western U.S. coal is bituminous, CWP is less prevalent in that region.

Much of the symptomatology associated with simple CWP appears to be similar and additive to the effects of cigarette smoking on the development of chronic bronchitis and obstructive lung disease (Chap. 258). In the early stages of simple CWP, radiographic abnormalities consist of small, irregular opacities (reticular pattern). With prolonged exposure, one sees small, rounded, regular opacities, 1 to 5 mm in diameter (nodular pattern). Calcification is generally not seen, although approximately 10% of older anthracite miners have calcified nodules.

Complicated CWP is manifested by the appearance on the chest radiograph of nodules ranging from 1 cm in diameter to the size of an entire lobe, generally confined to the upper half of the lungs. This condition, considered a form of PMF, is accompanied by a significant reduction in diffusing capacity and is associated with premature mortality. In contrast to patients with silicosis, underground miners with simple CWP develop PMF at a rate of only 5 to 15%, depending on the type of coal.

The mechanism whereby PMF occurs in CWP is not fully understood. Several hypotheses have been proposed, including: (1) sufficient free silica is present in the dust; (2) normal clearance mechanisms are unable to clear the excessive dust loads; and (3) atypical reactions to *M. tuberculosis* occur. As previously described, PMF in silicosis is associated with prolonged duration and high intensity of exposure to free silica. Heavy exposure to carbon particles free of silica occurs in carbon black, graphite, and charcoal workers. The prolonged exposure of these workers may result in sufficient accumulation of carbon in the lung to produce PMF. The mechanism appears to relate to a breakdown of the clearance capacity of the airways.

Caplan's syndrome (Chap. 312), first described in coal miners but subsequently found in patients with a variety of pneumoconioses, includes seropositive rheumatoid arthritis with characteristic PMF. The syndrome suggests an immunopathologic mechanism. Over the last decade, the mechanisms by which the chronic inhalation of mineral dusts produce an increase in inflammatory cells (including macrophages and neutrophils), which in turn causes PMF, have been explored. Coal dust can: (1) be a source of reactive oxygen species causing lung injury; (2) result in stimulation of macrophages to produce cytokines and enhance production of (anti)fibrogenic factors such as TNF-α; (3) increase protease activity; and (4) increase inactivation of α_1-antitrypsin and leukocyte elastase activity. The final pathologic pathway may be fibrosis resulting from the interactions of a variety of these mechanisms.

BERYLLIOSIS Beryllium may produce an acute pneumonitis or, far more commonly, a chronic interstitial pneumonitis. Unless one inquires specifically about occupational exposures to beryllium in the manufacture of alloys, ceramics, high-technology electronics, and (before the 1950s) the production of fluorescent lights, one may miss entirely the etiologic relationship to an occupational exposure. Nonspecific pulmonary function tests may be normal or may indicate evidence of restrictive disease. Between 2 and 15 years of exposure, depending on its intensity, are required for the disease to become manifest. On open lung biopsy, granulomatous formation similar to that seen in sarcoidosis (Chap. 318) may make differentiation impossible unless tissue levels of beryllium are measured.

Other hard metals, including aluminum powders, chromium, cobalt, titanium dioxide, and tungsten, may produce an interstitial pneumonitis, but this is rare.

OTHER INORGANIC DUSTS Other dusts are considered *nuisance dusts* because their major environmental and health effects seem to be reduction in visibility and irritation of eyes, ears, nasal passages, and other mucous membranes, respectively. If they penetrate to the lower airways, these dusts do not affect the architecture of the terminal bronchioles or acinar spaces nor do they destroy collagen. Generally, clinical effects are reversible. Pulmonary function tests are usually normal unless another disease process coexists. If the dusts are radiodense, macular collections may produce striking radiographic pictures that are so characteristic that patients with a history of significant exposure are easily diagnosed as having the condition that bears the name reflecting the nature of the dust. Examples of radiodense dusts include iron and iron oxides from welding or silver finishing (*siderosis*); tin oxide used in metallurgy, color stabilization, printing, and the manufacture of porcelain, glass, and fabric (*stannosis*); and barium sulfate used as a catalyst for organic reactions, drilling mud components, and electroplating (*baritosis*). Other metal dusts producing similar radiodense pictures include *cerium dioxide* and *antimony salts*.

Most of the inorganic dusts discussed thus far are associated with the production of either dust macules or interstitial fibrotic changes in the lung. Another set of dusts (Table 254-1), along with some of the dusts previously discussed, is associated with chronic mucous hypersecretion (chronic bronchitis), with or without reduction of expiratory flow rates. These conditions are caused by cigarette smoking, and any effort to attribute some component of the disease to occupational and environmental exposures must take cigarette smoking into account. Most studies suggest an additive effect of dust exposure and smoking. The pattern of the effect is similar to that of cigarette smoking, suggesting that small airway inflammation may be the initial site of pathologic response in those cases associated with the development of obstructive lung disease. Cigarette smoke is usually the more noxious agent, and dust effects may be discernible only in nonsmokers.

ORGANIC DUSTS Some of the specific diseases associated with organic dusts are discussed in detail in the chapters on asthma (Chap. 252) and hypersensitivity pneumonitis (Chap. 253). Many of these diseases are named for the specific setting in which they are found, e.g., farmer's lung, malt worker's disease, or mushroom worker's disease. Occupational and other environmental exposures must be sought when these conditions are suspected. Often the temporal relation of symptoms to exposure furnishes the best evidence for the diagnosis. Three occupational groups are singled out for discussion because they represent the largest proportion of people affected by the diseases resulting from organic dusts.

Cotton Dust (Byssinosis) Estimates of the number of exposed persons in the United States vary, but probably over 800,000 persons are exposed occupationally to cotton, flax, or hemp in the production of yarns for cotton, linen, and rope making. Although this discussion focuses on cotton, the same syndrome—albeit somewhat less severe—has been reported in association with exposure to flax, hemp, and jute.

Exposure occurs throughout the manufacturing process but is most pronounced in those portions of the factory involved with the treatment of the cotton prior to spinning—i.e., blowing, mixing, and carding (straightening of fibers). Attempts to control dust levels by use of exhaust hoods, general increases in ventilation, and wetting procedures in some settings have been highly successful. However, respiratory protective equipment appears to be required during certain operations to prevent workers from being exposed to levels of dust that exceed the current U.S. cotton dust standard.

Byssinosis is characterized clinically as occasional (early stage) and then regular (late stage) chest tightness toward the end of the first day of the workweek ("Monday chest tightness"). In epidemiologic studies, depending on the level of exposure via the carding room air, up to 80% of employees may show a significant drop in their FEV_1 over the course of a Monday shift.

Initially the symptoms do not recur on subsequent days of the week. However, in 10 to 25% of workers, the disease may be progressive, with chest tightness recurring or persisting throughout the workweek. After more than 10 years of exposure, workers with recurrent symptoms are more likely to have an obstructive pattern on pulmonary function testing. These higher grades of impairment are seen in workers exposed both to high levels of dust and for greater

Table 254-1 Selected Occupational Dusts Believed to Be Associated with Mucous Hypersecretion and/or Obstructive Airway Disease and Other Respiratory Diseases[a]

Agent (Exposure)	Mucous Hypersecretion	Obstruction	Other Conditions[b]
INORGANIC DUSTS			
Antimony (storage batteries, solder, ceramics, glass, plastics)	X		P
Arsenic (manufacture of pesticides, pigments, glass, alloys)	X		C
Barium and compounds including BaO, $BaSO_4$, $BaCO_3$ (catalysts, drilling mud, electroplating)	X		P
Cadmium dust (electroplating, battery manufacture, welding, smelting, aluminum soldering)	X	X	P
Cement dust (construction trades, manufacture of cement blocks)	X	X	
Chromium and CrO_3, CrF_2 (corrosion inhibitor pigment, metallurgy, electroplating)	X		C
Coal dust (mining)	X		P
Coke oven emissions (retort house, coke ovens)	X	X	P, C
Graphite (steelmaking, lubricants, pencils, paints, stove polish)	X	X	P
Iron dust (steel and nonferrous foundry workers, welding)	X		P
Mica (insulation, roofing shingles, oil refining, rubber manufacturing)	X		P
Phosphorus, elemental chlorides, sulfides (manufacture of fireworks, agricultural chemicals, insecticides, pesticides)	X	X	
Rock dusts (miners, tunnelers, quarry workers)	X		P
Vanadium pentoxide (welding electrodes, additive to steel, by-product in ash from oil burning)	X	X	
ORGANIC DUSTS (see Chap. 253)			
Cotton dust, flax, hemp (manufacture of yarns for linen, rope, cotton; ginning, cottonseed crushing; waste fiber processing)	X	X	
Grain dusts (farmers, workers in grain elevators, barge and grain ship crew members)	X	X	
Moldy hay (farmers, other animal attendants)	X		HP

[a] The table excludes agents associated with asthma as the primary disease (see Chap. 252).
[b] Other conditions include hypersensitivity pneumonitis (HP), pneumoconiosis (P), and cancers (C).
NOTE: X indicates that mucous hypersecretion or obstruction is associated with exposure.

durations. There is an additive effect of cotton dust exposure plus cigarette smoking. The highest grades of impairment are generally seen in smokers.

Treatment in the early stages of the disease is directed toward reversing the bronchospasm with bronchodilators; however, the chest tightness appears to relate, at least in part, to histamine release, and antihistamines have been shown to lessen the anticipated fall in FEV_1 the first day of the week. Clearly, reduction of dust exposure is of primary importance. All workers with persistent symptoms or significantly reduced levels of pulmonary function should be moved to areas of lower risk of exposure. Regular surveillance of pulmonary function in the industry has made it easier to identify affected persons. Persons with reduced pulmonary function, a personal history of respiratory allergy, and a history of continued cigarette smoking should be considered at increased risk of developing byssinosis in association with work in the cotton industry.

Grain Dust Although the exact number of workers at risk in the United States is not known, at least 500,000 people work in grain elevators, and over 2 million farmers are potentially exposed to grain dust. The presentation of disease in grain elevator employees or in workers in flour or feed mills is virtually identical to the characteristic findings in cigarette smokers, i.e., persistent cough, mucous hypersecretion, wheeze and dyspnea on exertion, and reduced FEV_1 and FEV_1/FVC ratio (Chap. 250).

Dust concentrations in grain elevators vary greatly but appear to be in excess of 10,000 $\mu g/m^3$; approximately one-third of the particles, by weight, are in the respirable range. The effect of grain dust exposure is additive to that of cigarette smoking, with approximately 50% of workers who smoke having symptoms. Among nonsmoking grain elevator operators, approximately one-quarter have mucous hypersecretion, about five times the number that would be expected in unexposed nonsmokers. However, evidence of obstruction on pulmonary function studies is observed only in workers who smoke. It is not clear whether the reason is an enhancement of the cigarette smoking effect in exposed workers or a greater susceptibility of smokers to the effects of grain dust.

Farmer's Lung This condition results from exposure to moldy hay containing spores of thermophilic actinomycetes that produce a hypersensitivity pneumonitis (Chap. 253). There are few good population-based estimates of the frequency of occurrence of this condition in the United States. However, among farmers in Great Britain, the rate of disease ranges from approximately 10 to 50 per 1000. The prevalence of disease varies in association with rainfall, which determines the amount of fungal growth, and with differences in agricultural practices related to turning and stacking hay.

The patient with acute farmer's lung presents 4 to 8 h after exposure with fever, chills, malaise, cough, and dyspnea without wheezing. The history of exposure is obviously essential to distinguish this disease from influenza or pneumonia with similar symptoms. In the chronic form of the disease, the history of repeated attacks after similar exposure is important in differentiating this syndrome from other causes of patchy fibrosis (e.g., sarcoidosis).

A wide variety of other organic dusts are associated with the occurrence of hypersensitivity pneumonitis (Chap. 253). For those patients who present with hypersensitivity pneumonitis, specific and careful inquiry about occupations, hobbies, or other home environmental exposures will, in most cases, reveal the source of the etiologic agent.

ASSESSMENT OF DISABILITY Significant reduction of dust levels in coal mines has resulted from federal legislation, enacted in the United States in 1969, that requires that respirable dust levels in underground mines be reduced to less than 2000 $\mu g/m^3$. This same legislation authorizes payment to coal miners (or their survivors) totally disabled by CWP. The criteria for disability from CWP remain unclear and arbitrary. It is critical that physicians involved in occupational lung disease claim cases be aware of detailed exposure histories of their patients, in terms of both occupational exposures and other environmental exposures (cigarette smoking). To assess disability properly may require input not only from physicians but also from experts in ergonomics and vocational rehabilitation, lawyers, and employer and employee representatives.

Most commonly, the patient presents with asthma, and it is the physician's task to decide whether the asthma is occupation-induced or work-aggravated asthma. The distinction is important not only because of the implications for disability compensation but also because the longer one is exposed to an inciting agent, the worse the prognosis for recovery from occupation-induced asthma. The clinical evaluation of such a patient requires adherence to a prescribed protocol that may include not only the components of the evaluation previously described but also rechallenge of the patient in a controlled setting or under a carefully monitored program in a work setting.

TOXIC CHEMICALS Exposure to toxic chemicals affecting the lung generally involves gases and vapors. A common accident is one in which the victim is trapped in a confined space where the chemicals have accumulated to toxic levels. In addition to the specific toxic effects of the chemical, the victim will often sustain considerable anoxia, which can play a dominant role in determining whether the individual survives.

Table 254-2 lists a variety of toxic agents that can produce acute and sometimes life-threatening reactions in the lung. All these agents in sufficient concentrations have been demonstrated, at least in animal studies, to affect the lower airways and disrupt alveolar architecture, either acutely or as a result of chronic exposure. Some of these agents may be generated acutely in the environment. For example, when plastics burn, a number of compounds, including hydrogen cyanide and hydrochloric acid, may be formed and released. →*The effects and treatment of exposure to these toxic gases are discussed in Chap. 391.*

Firefighters and fire victims are at risk of *smoke inhalation*, a numerically important cause of acute cardiorespiratory failure. Smoke inhalation kills more fire victims than does thermal injury. Carbon monoxide poisoning with resulting significant hypoxemia can be life-threatening (Chap. 396). Firefighters may inappropriately use the "blackness" of the smoke to indicate the degree of incomplete combustion and thus of carbon monoxide elevation. The use of synthetic materials (plastic, polyurethanes), which, when burned, may release a variety of other toxic agents, must be considered when evaluating smoke inhalation victims. Exposed victims may suffer some degree of lower respiratory tract inflammation, similar to that seen with exposure to other irritant gases (e.g., chlorine). Severe cases may include pulmonary edema.

Firefighters and victims also may be exposed to large quantities of particulate smoke. Significant long-term effects are not clearly associated with this particulate exposure except as related to the production of irritating effects on the upper airways; however, increased airway responsiveness in firefighters with repeated episodes of smoke inhalation has been demonstrated.

Some agents used in the manufacture of synthetic materials such as plastics, polyurethanes, and other polymers have resulted in some workers' being sensitized to extremely low levels of *isocyanates*, *aromatic amines*, or *aldehydes*. Repeated exposure to these agents causes some workers to develop chronic cough and sputum production, asthma, or episodes of low-grade fever and malaise.

Exposure occurs by an unusual route in *polymer fume fever*. Polymers, notably fluorocarbons, which at normal temperatures produce no reaction, may be transmitted from a worker's hands to his or her cigarettes. As the cigarette burns, the polymer is volatilized, and the inhaled agent causes a characteristic syndrome of fever, chills, malaise, and occasionally mild wheezing. The same scenario applies when workers are exposed to heated polymers without cigarette use—*meat wrappers' asthma*. A similar self-limited, influenza-like syndrome—*metal fume fever*—results from acute exposure to fumes or smoke of zinc, copper, magnesium, and other volatilized metals. The syndrome may begin several hours after work and resolves within 24 h, only to

Table 254-2 Selected Common Toxic Chemical Agents Affecting the Lung

Agent(s)	Selected Exposures	Acute Effects from High or Accidental Exposure	Chronic Effects from Relatively Low Exposure
Acid fumes; H_2SO_4, HNO_3	Manufacture of fertilizers, chlorinated organic compounds, dyes, explosives, rubber products, metal etching, plastics	Mucous membrane irritation, followed by chemical pneumonitis 2–3 days later	Bronchitis and suggestion of mildly reduced pulmonary function in children with lifelong residential exposure to high levels; clinical significance unknown
Ammonia	Refrigeration; petroleum refining; manufacture of fertilizers, explosives, plastics, and other chemicals	Same as for acid fumes	Chronic bronchitis
Cyanides	Electroplating; extraction of gold or silver; manufacture of mirrors, fumigants, photo supplies	Increase in respiratory rate followed by respiratory arrest, lactic acidosis, pulmonary edema, death	No data
Diazomethane	Methylating agent for acid compounds; laboratory workers	Violent coughing, dyspnea, wheezing, pulmonary edema	No data
Formaldehyde	Manufacture of resins, leathers, rubber, metals, and woods; laboratory workers, embalmers; emission from urethane foam insulation	Same as for acid fumes	Cancers in one species; no data on humans
Halides (Cl, Br, F)	Bleaching in pulp, paper, textile industry; manufacture of chemical compounds; synthetic rubber, plastics, disinfectant, rocket fuel, gasoline	Mucous membrane irritation, pulmonary edema; possible reduced FVC 1–2 yrs after exposure	Dryness of mucous membrane, epistaxis, dental fluorosis, tracheobronchitis
Hydrogen sulfide	By-product of many industrial processes, oil, other petroleum processes and storage	Respiratory paralysis similar to cyanides	Conjunctival irritation, chronic bronchitis, recurrent pneumonitis
Isocyanates (TDI, HDI, MDI)	Production of polyurethane foams, plastics, adhesives, surface coatings	Mucous membrane irritation, dyspnea, cough, wheeze, pulmonary edema	Upper respiratory tract irritation, cough, asthma, allergic alveolitis
Nitrogen dioxide	Silage, metal etching, explosives, rocket fuels, welding, by-product of burning fossil fuels	Cough, dyspnea, pulmonary edema may be delayed 4–12 h; possible result from acute exposure: bronchiolitis obliterans in 2–6 wks	Emphysema in animals, ?chronic bronchitis, associated with reduced lung function in children with lifelong residential exposure, clinical significance unknown
Ozone	Arc welding, flour bleaching, deodorizing, emissions from copying equipment, photochemical air pollutant	Mucous membrane irritant, pulmonary hemorrhage and edema, reduced pulmonary function transiently in children and adults exposed to summer haze	Chronic eye irritation
Phosgene	Organic compound, metallurgy, volatilization of chlorine-containing compounds	Delayed onset of bronchiolitis and pulmonary edema	Chronic bronchitis
Phthalic anhydride	Manufacture of resin esters, polyester resins, thermoactivated adhesives	Nasal irritation, cough	Asthma, chronic bronchitis
Sulfur dioxide	Manufacture of sulfuric acid, bleaches, coating of nonferrous metals, food processing, refrigerant, burning of fossil fuels, wood pulp industry	Mucous membrane irritant, epistaxis	?Chronic bronchitis

return on repeated exposure. A proper occupational history should make the diagnosis evident.

ENVIRONMENTAL RESPIRATORY CARCINOGENS Historically, it has been the astute clinician who has recognized a higher incidence of malignant tumors associated with certain environmental exposures. When these observations are linked to an occupational setting, they must be pursued by epidemiologic studies of relatively large groups of both current and former workers. Often the concentration and/or exact nature of the substances involved in the putative exposures cannot be determined. Rarely, the possibility that a substance can play an etiologic role in cancer is supported by observing that a few cases of a very rare tumor in a particular group represent "an epidemic." Examples are nasal sinus and lung cancer in nickel workers, angiosarcomas of the liver in vinyl chloride workers, and adenocarcinomas of the nose in woodworkers.

Only in those few cases in which animal studies have been carried out can one confirm that a given suspected agent is really a carcinogen. For example, bis(chloromethyl)ether (BCME) has been shown to produce tumors in animals and oat cell cancer of the lung in humans. In this particular case, BCME, used as a chemical intermediary in the manufacture of a number of organic compounds, was found to produce tumors in animals at about the same time as the substance was introduced into industry.

In addition to asbestos exposures, other occupational exposures associated with either proven or suspected respiratory carcinogens include those to acrylonitrile, arsenic compounds, beryllium (animal studies only), BCME, chromium, polycyclic hydrocarbons (through coke oven emissions), iron oxide, isopropyl oil (nasal sinuses), mustard gas, the various ores used to produce pure nickel, talc (possible asbestos contamination in both mining and milling), vinyl chloride, welding materials, wood used in woodworking (nasal cancer only), and uranium. The occurrence of excess cancers in uranium miners raises the possibility that a large number of workers are at risk by virtue of exposure to similar radiation hazards. This number includes not only workers involved in processing uranium but also workers exposed in underground mining operations where radon daughters may be emitted from rock formations.

GENERAL ENVIRONMENTAL EXPOSURES

AIR POLLUTION Dramatic and disastrous episodes of air pollution inversion have been documented in many industrialized centers in the world. Each of these episodes has been associated with excess acute mortality in the very old, the very young, and those with chronic cardiopulmonary diseases. The most dramatic event was the London fog of 1952, in which approximately 4000 excess deaths occurred over a 2-week period following 5 days of severe cold and dense fog. Similar episodes in the United States, although less dramatic in terms of total deaths, occurred in Donora, Pennsylvania, in 1948 and in New York City in the 1960s. In these episodes, which were generally associated with cold temperature and air stagnation, patients with underlying cardiopulmonary disease were most severely affected.

In addition to significant excess mortality during these episodes, a large number of people required medical care for cardiorespiratory complaints. Subsequent follow-up studies failed to implicate these episodic disasters in the etiology of chronic respiratory disease in adults. On the other hand, many epidemiologic studies of both international and regional differences in the prevalences of chronic respiratory disease suggest that long-term exposures in polluted areas in the early to middle part of the twentieth century were associated with excess chronic respiratory disease.

In 1970, the U.S. government established air quality standards for several pollutants believed to be responsible for excess cardiorespiratory diseases. Primary standards regulated by the Environmental Protection Agency (EPA) designed to protect the public health with an adequate margin of safety exist for sulfur dioxide, particulates $<10\ \mu m$ in size, nitrogen dioxide, ozone, lead, and carbon monoxide. Standards for each of these pollutants are updated regularly through an extensive review process conducted by the EPA. In 1997, a new standard was added for particles less than 2.5 μm; however, the standard does not become effective until year 2002.

Pollutants are generated from both stationary sources (power plants and industrial complexes) and mobile sources (automobiles), and none of the pollutants occurs in isolation. Thus, except for the change in carboxyhemoglobin from carbon monoxide exposure, it becomes extremely difficult to relate any specific health effect to any single pollutant. Furthermore, pollutants may be changed by chemical reactions after being emitted. For example, reducing agents, such as sulfur dioxide and particulate matter from a power plant stack, may react in air to produce acid sulfates and aerosols, the precursors of acid rain, which can be transported long distances in the atmosphere. Oxidizing substances, such as oxides of nitrogen and oxidants from automobile exhaust, may react with sunlight to produce ozone. Although originally a problem confined to the southwestern part of the United States, in recent years, at least during the summertime, elevated ozone and acid aerosol levels have been documented throughout the United States. Both acute and chronic effects of these exposures are currently under investigation.

The symptoms and diseases associated with air pollution are the same as the noncancerogenic conditions commonly associated with cigarette smoking. In addition, respiratory illness in early childhood has been associated with chronic exposure to only modestly elevated levels of SO_2 and respirable particles. Recent population-based studies comparing cities that have relatively high levels of particulate exposures with less polluted communities suggest excess morbidity and mortality from cardiorespiratory conditions in long-term residents of the former communities. This finding, in part, has led to greater emphasis on publicizing pollution alert levels. One can only advise individuals with significant cardiopulmonary impairment to stay indoors during periods when pollution exceeds current standards.

INDOOR EXPOSURE Because of increased concern about energy costs, efforts to become energy efficient have led to reduced air-exchange rates in indoor environments. The unintentional effect of these efforts has been to increase exposures to a variety of air contaminants heretofore not considered important.

Until relatively recently, little attention was given to the effects of *passive cigarette smoking* (Chap. 390). Several studies have shown that the respirable particulate load in any household is directly proportional to the number of cigarette smokers living in the home. Increases in prevalence of respiratory illnesses and reduced levels of pulmonary function measured with simple spirometry have been found in children of smoking parents in a number of studies.

Evidence from numerous case-control and cohort studies shows modest excess disease associations for cardiopulmonary diseases and lung cancer. Because most of these excess relative risks appear to be below 50%, it is virtually impossible for any one of the studies to be considered definitive. Thus, the techniques of meta-analysis have been used effectively to combine data from the best of these studies. The most recent meta-analyses for lung cancer, cardiac disease, and respiratory disease in terms of excess mortality suggest an approximately 25% increase for each condition, even after adjustment for major potential confounders. According to measures of plasma cotinine, a metabolite of nicotine, a nonsmoker living with a smoker is exposed to approximately 1% of the level of tobacco smoke to which a smoker of 20 cigarettes a day is exposed. In spite of some prominent detractors, these combined relative risks appear to be consistent with the estimated exposure levels and suggest a consensus that the associations are causal.

Radon gas is believed to be a risk factor for lung cancer. The main radon product (radon 222) is a gas that results from the decay series of uranium 238, with the immediate precursor being radium 226. The amount of radium in earth materials determines how much radon gas will be emitted. Outdoors, the concentrations are trivial. Indoors, levels are dependent on the ventilation rate and the size of the space into which the gas is emitted. Levels associated with excess lung cancer risk may be present in as many as 10% of the houses in the United States. When smokers reside in the household, the problem is potentially greater, since the molecular size of radon particles allows them to readily attach to smoke particles that are inhaled. Fortunately, technology is available for assessing and reducing the level of exposure.

Other indoor exposures associated with an increased risk of atopy and asthma include those to such specific recognized putative biologic agents as cockroach antigen, dust mites, and pet danders. Other indoor chemical agents include formaldehyde, perfumes, and latex particles. Of recent interest are the nonspecific responses associated with "tight-building syndrome," in which no particular agent has been implicated; the affected individuals suffer from a wide variety of complaints, including respiratory symptoms, that are relieved only by avoiding exposure in the building in question. The degree to which "smells" or other sensory stimuli are involved in the triggering of potentially incapacitating psychological or physical responses has yet to be determined, and the long-term consequences of such environmental exposures are as yet unknown.

PORTAL OF ENTRY The lung is a primary point of entry into the body for a number of toxic agents that affect other organ systems. For example, the lung is a route of entry for benzene (bone marrow), carbon disulfide (cardiovascular and nervous systems), cadmium (kidney), and metallic mercury (kidney, central nervous system). Thus, in any disease state of obscure origin, it is important to consider the possibility of inhaled environmental agents. Such consideration can sometimes furnish the clue needed to identify a specific external cause for a disorder that might otherwise be labeled "idiopathic."

BIBLIOGRAPHY

BALAAN MR et al: Clinical aspects of coal workers' pneumoconiosis and silicosis. Occup Med 8:19, 1993

BECKLAKE MR et al: The relationship between acute and chronic airway responses to occupational exposures. Curr Pulmonol 9:25, 1988

BLANC PD: Acute pulmonary responses to toxic exposures. In *Textbook of Respiratory Medicine*, 3d ed. Murray JF, Nadel JA (eds). Philadelphia, WB Saunders, 2000, pp 1903–1914

CHAN-YEUNG M, MALO J-L: Occupational asthma. N Engl J Med 333: 107, 1995

CHECKOWAY H, FRANZBLAU A: Is silicosis required for silica-associated lung cancer? Am J Indust Med 37:252, 2000

COCHRANE AL, MOORE FA: A 20-year follow-up of men aged 55–64 including coal miners and foundry workers in Staveley. Br J Ind Med 37:226, 1980

Guidelines for the Use of International Labour Office Classification of Radiographs of Pneumoconiosis. Occupational Safety and Health Sciences 22 (Revised 1980). Geneva, ILO, 1980

HACKSHAW AK et al: The accumulated evidence on lung cancer and environmental tobacco smoke. Br Med J 315:980, 1997

HE J et al: Passive smoking and the risk of coronary heart disease—a meta-analysis of epidemiologic studies. New Engl J Med 340:920, 1999

LEONARD JF, TEMPLETON PA: Pulmonary imaging techniques in the diagnosis of occupational interstitial lung disease, in *Occupational Medicine: State of the Art Reviews*, vol 7, no 2, WS Beckett, R Bascon (eds). Philadelphia, Hanley and Belfus, 1992, pp 241–260

MULLOY KB et al: Use of chest radiographs in epidemiological investigations of pneumoconioses. Br J Ind Med 50:273, 1993

PARKES WR: *Occupational Lung Disorders*, 3d ed. Oxford, Butterworth-Heinemann, 1994

PRICE B: Analysis of current trends in United States mesothelioma incidence. Am J Epidemiol 145:211, 1997

ROSENMAN KD et al: Silicosis in the 1990s. Chest 111:779, 1997

SAMET JM, SPENGLER JD: *Indoor Air Pollution: A Health Perspective*, Baltimore, The Johns Hopkins University, 1991, Chaps. 2 and 15

SCHENKER MB: Regulatory and policy issues, in *Occupational and Environmental Respiratory Disease*, P Harber et al: (eds). St Louis, Mosby Year Books, 1996

SCHINS RP, BORM PJ: Mechanisms and mediators in coal dust induced toxicity: A review. Ann Occup Hyg 43:7, 1999

255

Matthew E. Levison

PNEUMONIA, INCLUDING NECROTIZING PULMONARY INFECTIONS (LUNG ABSCESS)

BAL bronchoalveolar lavage	PCP *P. carinii* pneumonia
CFU colony-forming units	PORT Pneumonia Patient Outcomes Research Team
HPS hantavirus pulmonary syndrome	PSB protected double-sheathed brush
ICU intensive care unit	TMP-SMZ trimethoprim-sulfamethoxazole
IDSA Infectious Diseases Society of America	TTA transtracheal aspiration
MIC minimal inhibitory concentration	

Pneumonia is an infection of the pulmonary parenchyma that can be caused by various bacterial species, including mycoplasmas, chlamydiae, and rickettsiae; viruses; fungi; and parasites (Table 255-1). Thus pneumonia is not a single disease but a group of specific infections, each with a different epidemiology, pathogenesis, clinical presentation, and clinical course. Identification of the etiologic microorganism is of primary importance, since this is the key to appropriate antimicrobial therapy. However, because of the serious nature of the infection, antimicrobial therapy generally needs to be started immediately, often before laboratory confirmation of the causative agent. The specific microbial etiology remains elusive in more than one-third of cases—e.g., when no sputum is available for examination, blood cultures are sterile, and there is no pleural fluid. Serologic confirmation requires weeks because of the late formation of specific antibody.

Thus initial antimicrobial therapy is often empirical and is based on the setting in which the infection was acquired, the clinical presentation, patterns of abnormality on chest radiography, results of staining of sputum or other infected body fluids, and current patterns of susceptibility of the suspected pathogens to antimicrobial agents. After the etiologic agent is identified, specific antimicrobial therapy can be chosen.

DEFENSE MECHANISMS The lung is a complex structure composed of aggregates of units that are formed by the progressive branching of the airways. Approximately 80% of the cells lining the central airways are ciliated, pseudostratified, columnar epithelial cells; the percentage decreases in the peripheral airways. Each ciliated cell contains about 200 cilia that beat in coordinated waves ~1000 times per minute, with a fast forward stroke and a slower backward recovery. Ciliary motion is also coordinated between adjacent cells so that each wave is propagated toward the oropharynx. The cilia are covered by a liquid film that is ~5 to 10 μm thick and is composed of two layers. The outer, or gel, layer is viscous and traps deposited particles. The cilia beat in the less viscous inner, or sol, layer. During the forward stroke, the tips of the cilia just touch the viscous gel and propel it toward the oropharynx. During recovery, the cilia move entirely within

Table 255-1 Microbial Pathogens That Cause Pneumonia

Community-Acquired	Hospital-Acquired	HIV Infection–Associated
Mycoplasma pneumoniae	Enteric aerobic gram-negative bacilli	*Pneumocystis carinii*
Streptococcus pneumoniae	*Pseudomonas aeruginosa*	*M. tuberculosis*
Haemophilus influenzae	*S. aureus*	*S. pneumoniae*
Chlamydia pneumoniae	Oral anaerobes	*H. influenzae*
Legionella pneumophila		
Oral anaerobes		
Moraxella catarrhalis		
Staphylococcus aureus		
Nocardia spp.		
Viruses[a]		
Fungi[b]		
Mycobacterium tuberculosis		
Chlamydia psittaci		

[a] Influenza virus, cytomegalovirus, respiratory syncytial virus, measles virus, varicella-zoster virus, and hantavirus.
[b] *Histoplasma*, *Coccidioides*, and *Blastomyces* spp.

the low-resistance sol layer. Ciliated cells are interspersed with mucus-secreting cells in the trachea and bronchi but not in the bronchioles.

The alveolar walls, from blood to air, consist of the endothelium that lines the network of anastomotic capillaries, the capillary basement membrane, the interstitial tissue, the alveolar basement membrane, the alveolar lining epithelial cells (which are either flattened type I pneumocytes that cover 95% of the alveolar surface or rounded, granular, surfactant-producing type II pneumocytes), and epithelial lining fluid. The epithelial lining fluid contains surfactant, fibronectin, and immunoglobulin, which may opsonize or—in the presence of complement—lyse microbial pathogens deposited on the alveolar surface. Loosely attached to the lining cells or lying free within the lumen are the alveolar macrophages, lymphocytes, and a few polymorphonuclear leukocytes.

The lower respiratory tract is normally sterile, despite being adjacent to enormous numbers of microorganisms that reside in the oropharynx and being exposed to environmental microorganisms in inhaled air. This sterility is the result of efficient filtering and clearance mechanisms.

Infectious particles deposited on the squamous epithelium of distal nasal surfaces normally are removed by sneezing, while those deposited on the more proximal ciliated surfaces are swept posteriorly in the mucus lining into the nasopharynx, where they are swallowed or expectorated. Reflex closure of the glottis and cough protect the lower respiratory tract. Those particles deposited on the tracheobronchial surface are swept by ciliary motion toward the oropharynx. Infectious particles that bypass defenses in the airways and are deposited on the alveolar surface are cleared by phagocytic cells and humoral factors. Alveolar macrophages are the major phagocytes in the lower respiratory tract. Some phagocytosed microorganisms are killed by the phagocyte's oxygen-dependent systems, lysosomal enzymes, and cationic proteins. Other microorganisms can evade microbicidal mechanisms and persist within the macrophage. For example, *Mycobacterium tuberculosis* persists within the lysosome, while *Legionella* resides within intracellular inclusions that fail to fuse with lysosomes. Intracellular pathogens can then be transported to the ciliated surfaces and into the oropharynx or via the lymphatics to regional lymph nodes. The alveolar macrophages process and present microbial antigens to the lymphocyte and also secrete cytokines (e.g., tumor necrosis factor and interleukin 1) that modulate the immune process in T and B lymphocytes. Cytokines facilitate the generation of an inflammatory response, activate alveolar macrophages, and recruit additional phagocytes and other immunologic factors from plasma. The inflammatory exudate is responsible for many of the local signs of pulmonary consolidation and for the systemic manifestations of pneumonia, such as fever, chills, myalgias, and malaise.

TRANSMISSION Microbial pathogens may enter the lung by one of several routes.

Aspiration of Organisms That Colonize the Oropharynx Most pulmonary pathogens originate in the oropharyngeal flora. Aspiration of these pathogens is the most common mechanism for the production of pneumonia. At various times during the year, healthy individuals transiently carry common pulmonary pathogens in the nasopharynx; these pathogens include *Streptococcus pneumoniae*, *S. pyogenes*, *Mycoplasma pneumoniae*, *Haemophilus influenzae*, and *Moraxella catarrhalis*. The sources of anaerobic pulmonary pathogens, such as *Porphyromonas gingivalis*, *Prevotella melaninogenica*, *Fusobacterium nucleatum*, *Actinomyces* spp., spirochetes, and anaerobic streptococci, are the gingival crevice and dental plaque, which contain more than 10^{11} colony-forming units (CFU) of microorganisms per gram. The frequency of aerobic gram-negative bacillary colonization of the oropharyngeal mucosa, which is unusual in healthy persons (<2%), increases with hospitalization, worsening debility, severe underlying illness, alcoholism, diabetes, and advanced age. This change may be a consequence of increased salivary proteolytic activity, which destroys fibronectin, a glycoprotein coating the surface of the mucosa. Fibronectin is the receptor for the normal gram-positive flora of the oropharynx. Loss of fibronectin exposes the receptors for aerobic gram-negative bacilli on the epithelial cell surface. The source of aerobic gram-negative bacilli may be the patient's own stomach (which can become colonized with these organisms as the result of an increase in gastric pH with atrophic gastritis or after the use of H_2-blocking agents or antacids), contaminated respiratory equipment, hands of health care workers, or contaminated food and water. Nasogastric tubes can facilitate the transfer of gastric bacteria to the pharynx.

About 50% of healthy adults aspirate oropharyngeal secretions into the lower respiratory tract during sleep. Aspiration occurs more frequently and may be more pronounced in individuals with an impaired level of consciousness (e.g., alcoholics; drug abusers; and patients who have had seizures, strokes, or general anesthesia), neurologic dysfunction of the oropharynx, and swallowing disorders or mechanical impediments (e.g., nasogastric or endotracheal tubes). Pneumonia due to anaerobes is an especially likely outcome if the aspirated material is large in volume or contains virulent components of the anaerobic microbial flora or foreign bodies, such as aspirated food or necrotic tissue. Impairment of the cough reflex increases the risk of pneumonia, as does mucociliary or alveolar macrophage dysfunction.

Inhalation of Infectious Aerosols Deposition of inhaled particles within the respiratory tract is determined primarily by particle size. Particles >10 μm in diameter are deposited mostly in the nose and upper airways. Particles <5 μm in diameter (also called *airborne droplet nuclei*) and containing one or perhaps two microorganisms fail to settle out by gravity but rather remain suspended in the atmosphere for long periods unless removed by ventilation or by filtration in the lungs of the individual breathing the contaminated air. Transmission of an infectious agent in the form of an aerosol is particularly efficient. These infectious aerosols are small enough to bypass host defenses in the upper respiratory tract and airways. A greater percentage of particles are deposited in small bronchioles and alveoli as particle size decreases below 5 μm. One inhaled particle of appropriate size may be sufficient to reach the alveolus and initiate infection. The etiologies of pneumonia typically acquired by inhalation of infectious aerosols include tuberculosis, influenza, legionellosis, psittacosis, histoplasmosis, Q fever, and hantavirus pulmonary syndrome (HPS).

Hematogenous Dissemination from an Extrapulmonary Site Infection, usually with *Staphylococcus aureus*, disseminates hematogenously to the lungs in patients (such as intravenous drug users) who have either right- or left-sided bacterial endocarditis and in patients with intravenous catheter infections. *Fusobacterium* infections of the retropharyngeal tissues (Lemierre's syndrome—i.e., retropharyngeal abscess and jugular venous thrombophlebitis) also disseminate hematogenously to the lungs.

Direct Inoculation and Contiguous Spread Two additional routes of transmission of bacteria to the lungs are direct inoculation (as a result of either tracheal intubation or stab wounds to the chest) and contiguous spread from an adjacent site of infection.

PATHOLOGY The pneumonic process may involve primarily the interstitium or the alveoli. Involvement of an entire lobe is called *lobar pneumonia*. When the process is restricted to alveoli contiguous to bronchi, it is called *bronchopneumonia*. Confluent bronchopneumonia may be indistinguishable from lobar pneumonia. Cavities develop when necrotic lung tissue is discharged into communicating airways, resulting in either necrotizing pneumonia (multiple small cavities, each <2 cm in diameter, in one or more bronchopulmonary segments or lobes) or lung abscess (one or more cavities >2 cm in diameter). The classification of pneumonia is best based upon the causative microorganism rather than upon these anatomic characteristics (the criteria used in the past).

EPIDEMIOLOGY The patient's living circumstances, occupation, travel history, pet or animal exposure history, and contacts with other ill individuals as well as the physician's knowledge of the epidemic curve of community outbreaks provide clues to the microbial etiology of a given case of pneumonia (Table 255-1). The relative frequency of various pulmonary pathogens varies with the setting in which the infection was acquired—e.g., community, nursing home, or hospital. In patients hospitalized with community-acquired pneumonia, the most frequent pathogens are *S. pneumoniae*, *H. influenzae*, *Chlamydia pneumoniae*, and *Legionella pneumophila*. *C. pneumoniae* is often found in association with other pathogens, including *S. pneumoniae*, and the associated pathogen appears to influence the course of the pneumonia. *M. pneumoniae*, which usually causes mild illness, is common among outpatients with community-acquired pneumonia, but may also be an underappreciated cause in all age groups of severe pneumonia that requires hospitalization. In contrast, enteric aerobic gram-negative bacilli and *Pseudomonas aeruginosa*, uncommon causes of community-acquired pneumonia, are estimated to account for >50% of cases of hospital-acquired pneumonia, while *S. aureus* is responsible for >10%. The relative frequencies of pathogens in pneumonia acquired in nursing homes fall somewhere between those of community- and hospital-acquired pneumonia. Enteric aerobic gram-negative bacilli and *P. aeruginosa* are more common among nursing home residents than among patients who acquire pneumonia in noninstitutional settings.

The season of the year and the geographic location are other predictors of etiology. The frequency of influenza virus as a cause of both community-acquired and institutionally acquired pneumonia increases during the winter months. Moreover, influenza virus infection causes an increase in the frequency of secondary bacterial pneumonia due to *S. pneumoniae*, *S. aureus*, and *H. influenzae*. Outbreaks of influenza in a community tend to be explosive and widespread, with many secondary cases resulting from the short incubation period of several days and the high degree of communicability. *Legionella* colonizes hot-water storage systems that provide favorable conditions for its proliferation, such as warm temperature, stagnation, and sediment accumulation. Acquisition of *Legionella* pneumonia requires exposure to aerosols generated from these contaminated water supplies—e.g., during an overnight stay in a hotel with a faulty air-handling system or after repair of domestic plumbing in buildings with contaminated water supplies. Legionellosis also occurs in explosive outbreaks when large numbers of susceptible people are exposed to an infectious aerosol; however, no secondary cases occur because of the low level of communicability of *L. pneumophila*. *Mycoplasma* causes outbreaks, usually in relatively closed populations such as those at military bases, at colleges, or in households; however, because of its long incubation period (2 to 3 weeks) and its relatively low degree of communicability, *Mycoplasma* infection moves through the community slowly, affecting another person as the first is recovering. In communities where infection with HIV type 1 is endemic, *Pneumocystis carinii* and *M. tuberculosis* are more prominent causes of community-acquired pneumonia. *Chlamydia psittaci* produces illness in bird handlers. Histoplasmosis, blastomycosis, and coccidioidomycosis are causes of pneumonia that have specific geographic distributions.

HPS is a newly described, frequently fatal disease caused by one of several hantaviruses. Most cases in the United States have been reported from the Four Corners area (New Mexico, Arizona, Utah, and Colorado), where the pathogen is the Sin Nombre virus. The primary hosts are rodents, which apparently remain healthy but excrete the virus in urine, feces, and saliva. Hantavirus infection is acquired by inhalation of infectious aerosols when rodent nests are disturbed by human domestic, occupational, or recreational activities. The appearance of HPS in the southwestern United States is thought to have occurred because of increased rainfall in the region, which increased the rodent food supply and thus the rodent population. No person-to-person transmission of HPS is thought to have taken place, except perhaps in an outbreak in southern Argentina in 1996.

AGE AND COMORBIDITY Age is an important predictor of the infecting agent in pneumonia. *Chlamydia trachomatis* and respiratory syncytial virus are common among infants < 6 months of age; *H. influenzae* among children 6 months to 5 years of age; *M. pneumoniae*, *C. pneumoniae*, and hantavirus among young adults; *H. influenzae* and *M. catarrhalis* among elderly individuals with chronic lung disease; and *L. pneumophila* among elderly persons, smokers, and persons with compromised cell-mediated immunity (e.g., transplant recipients), renal or hepatic failure, diabetes, or systemic malignancy.

Oral anaerobes, frequently in combination with aerobic bacterial components of the human flora (e.g., viridans streptococci), are causes of community-acquired pneumonia and anaerobic lung abscess in patients who are prone to aspiration. Edentulous persons, who have lower numbers of oral anaerobes, are less likely to develop pneumonia due to anaerobes. When the etiology of community-acquired pneumonia in unselected hospitalized patients has been studied by methods that entail strict anaerobic bacteriology and that avoid contamination of lower respiratory tract secretions by the oral flora, anaerobic bacteria have been found to account for as many as 20 to 30% of cases. In hospital-acquired pneumonia, anaerobes are the pathogens—with or without aerobic copathogens—in about one-third of cases. However, the aerobic copathogens in hospital-acquired pneumonia are frequently virulent microorganisms in their own right (e.g., enteric aerobic gram-negative bacilli, *P. aeruginosa*, and *S. aureus*).

The patient's underlying disease may be characterized by specific immunologic or inflammatory defects that predispose to pneumonia due to specific pathogens (Table 255-2). For example, immunoglobulin deficiencies—especially those involving IgG subtypes 2 and 4, which are important in the immune response to encapsulated organisms (e.g., *S. pneumoniae* and *H. influenzae*)—may be associated with recurrent sinopulmonary infections. Immunoglobulin deficiencies may be inherited, or they may be acquired (i.e., as a result of either decreased production, as in lymphoproliferative malignancies, or excessive protein loss, as in nephrosis or protein-losing enteropathy). Inherited immunoglobulin deficiencies may be global or selective. Patients with recurrent sinopulmonary infections and a selective deficiency of IgG2 and/or IgG4 may have a total plasma IgG level within the normal range, as these particular IgG subtypes constitute only 25% of total IgG. HIV-infected patients may also exhibit ineffective antibody formation, which predisposes to infection with these encapsulated bacteria. Severe neutropenia (<500 neutrophils/μL) increases the risk of infections due to *P. aeruginosa*, Enterobacteriaceae, *S. aureus*, and (if neutropenia is prolonged) *Aspergillus*. The risk is unusually high for infections due to *M. tuberculosis* among HIV-infected patients with circulating CD4+ lymphocyte counts of <500/μL; for infections due to *P. carinii*, *Histoplasma capsulatum*, and *Cryptococcus neoformans* among those with CD4+ counts of <200/μL; and for infections due to *M. avium-intracellulare* and cytomegalovirus among those with counts of <50/μL. Long-term glucocorticoid therapy increases the risk of tuberculosis and nocardiosis.

Table 255-2 Pulmonary Pathogens Associated with Specific Defects in Host Defenses

Defect	Pathogens
Severe hypogammaglobulinemia	Encapsulated bacteria: *Streptococcus pneumoniae*, *Haemophilus influenzae*
Severe neutropenia	*Pseudomonas aeruginosa*, Enterobacteriaceae, *Staphylococcus aureus*, *Aspergillus*
Defective cell-mediated immunity	
CD4+ lymphocyte count	
<500/μL	*Mycobacterium tuberculosis*
<200/μL	*Pneumocystis carinii*, *Histoplasma capsulatum*, *Cryptococcus neoformans*
<50/μL	*Mycobacterium avium-intracellulare*, cytomegalovirus
Long-term glucocorticoid therapy	*M. tuberculosis*, *Nocardia*

CLINICAL MANIFESTATIONS **Community-Acquired Pneumonia** Community-acquired pneumonia has traditionally been thought to present as either of two syndromes: the typical presentation or the atypical presentation. Although current data suggest that these two syndromes may be less distinct than was once thought, the characteristics of the clinical presentation may nevertheless have some diagnostic value.

The "typical" pneumonia syndrome is characterized by the sudden onset of fever, cough productive of purulent sputum, shortness of breath, and (in some cases) pleuritic chest pain; signs of pulmonary consolidation (dullness, increased fremitus, egophony, bronchial breath sounds, and rales) may be found on physical examination in areas of radiographic abnormality. The typical pneumonia syndrome is usually caused by the most common bacterial pathogen in community-acquired pneumonia, *S. pneumoniae*, but can also be due to other bacterial pathogens, such as *H. influenzae* and mixed anaerobic and aerobic components of the oral flora.

The "atypical" pneumonia syndrome is characterized by a more gradual onset, a dry cough, shortness of breath, a prominence of extrapulmonary symptoms (such as headache, myalgias, fatigue, sore throat, nausea, vomiting, and diarrhea), and abnormalities on chest radiographs despite minimal signs of pulmonary involvement (other than rales) on physical examination. Atypical pneumonia is classically produced by *M. pneumoniae* but can also be caused by *L. pneumophila*, *C. pneumoniae*, oral anaerobes, and *P. carinii* as well as by *S. pneumoniae* and the less frequently encountered pathogens *C. psittaci*, *Coxiella burnetii*, *Francisella tularensis*, *H. capsulatum*, and *Coccidioides immitis*. *Mycoplasma* pneumonia (Chap. 178) may be complicated by erythema multiforme, hemolytic anemia, bullous myringitis, encephalitis, and transverse myelitis. *Legionella* pneumonia (Chap. 151) is frequently associated with deterioration in mental status, renal and hepatic abnormalities, and marked hyponatremia; pneumonia due to *H. capsulatum* (Chap. 201) or *C. immitis* (Chap. 202) is often accompanied by erythema nodosum. In *C. pneumoniae* pneumonia (Chap. 179), sore throat, hoarseness, and wheezing are relatively common. The atypical pneumonia syndrome in patients whose behavioral history places them at risk of HIV infection suggests *Pneumocystis* infection. These patients may have concurrent infections caused by other opportunistic pathogens, such as pulmonary (and frequently extrapulmonary) tuberculosis, oral thrush due to *Candida albicans*, or extensive perineal ulcers due to herpes simplex virus.

Certain viruses also produce pneumonia that is usually characterized by an atypical presentation—i.e., chills, fever, shortness of breath, dry nonproductive cough, and predominance of extrapulmonary symptoms. Primary viral pneumonia can be caused by influenza virus (usually as part of a community outbreak in winter), by respiratory syncytial virus (in children and immunosuppressed individuals), by measles or varicella-zoster virus (accompanied by the characteristic rash), and by cytomegalovirus (in patients immunocompromised by HIV infection or by therapy given in association with organ transplantation). Hantavirus causes an initial nonspecific febrile prodrome, after which the patient develops rapidly progressive respiratory failure and diffuse pulmonary infiltrates on chest radiographs as a result of exudation into the pulmonary interstitium and alveoli, with thrombocytopenia, neutrophilic leukocytosis, circulating immunoblasts, and laboratory evidence of hemoconcentration. In addition, influenza and measles can predispose to secondary bacterial pneumonia as a result of the destruction of the mucociliary barrier of the airways. Secondary bacterial infection may either follow the viral infection without interruption or be separated from the viral infection by several days of transient relief of symptoms. Bacterial infection may be heralded by sudden worsening of the patient's clinical condition, with persisting or renewed chills, fever, and cough productive of purulent sputum, possibly accompanied by pleuritic chest pain.

Patients with hematogenous *S. aureus* pneumonia may present with fever and dyspnea only. In these cases the inflammatory response is initially confined to the pulmonary interstitium. Cough, sputum production, and signs of pulmonary consolidation develop only after the infection extends into the bronchi. These patients are usually gravely ill, with intravascular infection as well as pneumonia, and may have signs of endocarditis (Chap. 126).

Nocardiosis (Chap. 165) is frequently complicated by metastasis of lesions to the skin and central nervous system. Signs of pulmonary consolidation, cough, and sputum production may be lacking in patients who are unable to mount an inflammatory response, such as those with agranulocytosis. The major manifestations in these patients may be limited to fever, tachypnea, agitation, and altered mental status. Elderly or severely ill patients may fail to develop fever.

Tuberculosis also produces an atypical presentation that is characterized by fever, night sweats, cough, and shortness of breath and sometimes by pleuritic chest pain and blood-streaked sputum. Several weeks usually elapse before the patient seeks medical attention because of the gradual worsening of these symptoms, by which time he or she will have lost considerable weight.

Nosocomial Pneumonia Patients with nosocomial pneumonia often pose a diagnostic challenge. The differential diagnosis of acute respiratory disease in critically ill, hospitalized patients is diverse and includes noninfectious entities, such as congestive heart failure, acute respiratory distress syndrome, preexisting lung disease, atelectasis, and oxygen- or drug-related toxicities, that may be difficult to distinguish clinically or radiologically from pneumonia. The usual criteria for nosocomial pneumonia, which include new or progressive pulmonary infiltrates, purulent tracheobronchial secretions, fever, and leukocytosis, are frequently unreliable in these patients, who often have preexisting pulmonary disease, endotracheal tubes that irritate the tracheal mucosa and may elicit an inflammatory exudate in respiratory secretions, or multiple other problems likely to produce fever and leukocytosis. Patients with nosocomial pneumonia complicating an underlying illness associated with significant neutropenia often have no purulent respiratory tract secretions or pulmonary infiltrates, and patients with nosocomial pneumonia complicating uremia or cirrhosis often remain afebrile. In addition, the patients at greatest risk for nosocomial pneumonia are most likely to be heavily colonized with potential pulmonary pathogens in the oropharyngeal or tracheobronchial mucosa; thus the presence of these organisms in gram-stained preparations or cultures of respiratory tract secretions does not necessarily confirm the diagnosis of pneumonia.

Aspiration Pneumonia and Anaerobic Lung Abscess Aspiration of a sufficient volume of gastric acid produces a chemical pneumonitis characterized by acute dyspnea and wheezing with hypoxemia and infiltrates on chest radiographs in one or both lower lobes. Clinical findings following aspiration of particulate matter depend on the extent of endobronchial obstruction and range from acute apnea to persistent cough with or without recurrent infection. Although the aspiration of oral anaerobes can initially lead to an infiltrative process, it ultimately results in putrid sputum, tissue necrosis, and pulmonary cavities. In about three-quarters of cases, the clinical course of an abscess of anaerobic polymicrobial etiology is indolent and mimics that of pulmonary tuberculosis, with cough, shortness of breath, chills, fever, night sweats, weight loss, pleuritic chest pain, and blood-streaked sputum lasting for several weeks or more. In other patients the disease may present more acutely. Patients with anaerobic abscesses are usually prone to aspiration of oropharyngeal contents and have periodontal disease. One genus of oral anaerobes, *Actinomyces*, produces a chronic fibrotic necrotizing process that crosses tissue planes and may involve the pleural space, ribs, vertebrae, and subcutaneous tissue, with eventual discharge of sulfur granules (macroscopic bacterial masses) through the skin (empyema necessitatis).

DIAGNOSIS Radiography Chest radiography is more sensitive than physical examination for detection of pulmonary infiltrates. Indeed, *P. carinii* pneumonia (PCP) is the only relatively common form of pneumonia associated with false-negative chest radiographs; up to 30% of patients with PCP have false-negative results. Chest radiographs can confirm the presence and location of the pulmonary infiltrate; assess the extent of the pulmonary infection; detect pleural involvement, pulmonary cavitation, or hilar lymphadenopathy; and gauge the response to antimicrobial therapy. However, chest radiographs may be normal when the patient is unable to mount an inflammatory response (e.g., in agranulocytosis) or is in the early stage of an infiltrative process (e.g., in hematogenous *S. aureus* pneumonia or PCP associated with AIDS). High-resolution computed tomography of the lungs can improve the accuracy of diagnosis of pneumonia, especially when the process involves lung obscured by the diaphragm, liver, ribs and clavicles, or heart.

The anatomic localization of the inflammatory process, as visualized in chest radiographs, occasionally has diagnostic implications. Most pulmonary pathogens produce focal lesions. A multicentric distribution suggests hematogenous infection, in which case the remote location of the primary infection (e.g., endocarditis or thrombophlebitis) should be sought. Hematogenous pneumonia, which results from septic embolization in patients with thrombophlebitis or right-sided endocarditis and from bacteremia in patients with left-sided endocarditis, appears on the chest radiograph as multiple areas of pulmonary infiltration that subsequently may cavitate. A diffuse distribution suggests the involvement of *P. carinii*, cytomegalovirus, hantavirus, measles virus, or herpes zoster virus (with pneumonia due to the last two pathogens diagnosed by the characteristic accompanying rash). Pleurisy and hilar nodal enlargement are unusual with PCP and cytomegalovirus pneumonia; their presence suggests another etiology. Diffuse lesions in immunocompromised patients also suggest legionellosis, tuberculosis, histoplasmosis, *Mycoplasma* infection, or disseminated strongyloidiasis.

Oral anaerobes, *S. aureus, S. pneumoniae* serotype III, aerobic gram-negative bacilli, *M. tuberculosis*, and fungi as well as certain noninfectious conditions can produce tissue necrosis and pulmonary cavities (Table 255-3). In contrast, *H. influenzae*, *M. pneumoniae*, viruses, and most other serotypes of *S. pneumoniae* almost never cause cavities. Apical disease, with or without cavities, suggests reactivation tuberculosis. Anaerobic abscesses are located in dependent, poorly ventilated, and poorly draining bronchopulmonary segments and characteristically have air-fluid levels, unlike the well-ventilated, well-

Table 255-3 Causes of Pulmonary Cavities

INFECTIOUS
Bacteria: Oral anaerobes (*Bacteroides* spp., fusobacteria, *Actinomyces* spp., anaerobic and microaerophilic cocci), enteric aerobic gram-negative bacilli, *Pseudomonas aeruginosa*, *Legionella* spp., *Staphylococcus aureus*, *Streptococcus pneumoniae* serotype III, *Mycobacterium tuberculosis*, *Nocardia* spp.
Fungi: *Histoplasma capsulatum*, *Coccidioides immitis*, *Blastomyces* spp.
NONINFECTIOUS
Neoplasms, Wegener's granulomatosis, infarction, infected bullae and cysts

drained upper-lobe cavities caused by *M. tuberculosis*, an obligate aerobe. Air-fluid levels may also be present in cavities due to pulmonary necrosis of other infectious etiologies, such as *S. aureus* and aerobic gram-negative bacilli. *Mucor* and *Aspergillus* invade blood vessels and cause pleural-based, wedge-shaped areas of pulmonary infarction; these infarcts may subsequently cavitate.

In the patient with an uncomplicated course, chest radiographs need not be repeated before discharge, since the resolution of infiltrates may take up to 6 weeks after initial presentation. However, patients who do not respond clinically, who have a pleural effusion on admission, who may have postobstructive pneumonia, or who are infected with certain pathogens (e.g., *S. aureus*, aerobic gram-negative bacilli, or oral anaerobes) need more intensive surveillance. At times, computed tomography may be especially helpful in distinguishing different processes—e.g., pleural effusion versus underlying pulmonary consolidation, hilar adenopathy versus pulmonary mass, and pulmonary abscess versus empyema with an air-fluid level.

Sputum Examination Examination of the sputum remains the mainstay of the evaluation of a patient with acute bacterial pneumonia. Unfortunately, expectorated material is frequently contaminated by potentially pathogenic bacteria that colonize the upper respiratory tract (and sometimes the lower respiratory tract) without actually causing disease. This contamination reduces the diagnostic specificity of any lower respiratory tract specimen. In addition, it has been estimated that the usual laboratory processing methods detect the pulmonary pathogen in fewer than 50% of expectorated sputum samples from patients with bacteremic *S. pneumoniae* pneumonia. This low sensitivity may be due to misidentification of the α-hemolytic colonies of *S. pneumoniae* as nonpathogenic α-hemolytic streptococci ("normal flora"), overgrowth of the cultures by hardier colonizing organisms, or loss of more fastidious organisms due to slow transport or improper processing. In addition, certain common pulmonary pathogens, such as anaerobes, mycoplasmas, chlamydiae, *Pneumocystis*, mycobacteria, fungi, and legionellae, cannot be cultured by routine methods.

Since expectorated material is routinely contaminated by oral anaerobes, the diagnosis of anaerobic pulmonary infection is frequently inferred. Confirmation of such a diagnosis requires the culture of anaerobes from pulmonary secretions that are uncontaminated by oropharyngeal secretions, which in turn requires the collection of pulmonary secretions by special techniques, such as transtracheal aspiration (TTA), transthoracic lung puncture, and protected brush via bronchoscopy. These procedures are invasive and are usually not used unless the patient fails to respond to empirical therapy.

Gram's staining of sputum specimens, screened initially under low-power magnification (10× objective and 10× eyepiece) to determine the degree of contamination with squamous epithelial cells, is of utmost diagnostic importance. In patients with the typical pneumonia syndrome who produce purulent sputum, the sensitivity and specificity of Gram's staining of sputum minimally contaminated by upper respiratory tract secretions ($>$25 polymorphonuclear leukocytes and $<$10 epithelial cells per low-power field) in identifying the pathogen as *S. pneumoniae* are 62 and 85%, respectively. Gram's staining in this case is more specific and probably more sensitive than the accompanying sputum culture. The finding of mixed flora on Gram's staining of an uncontaminated sputum specimen suggests an anaerobic infection. Acid-fast staining of sputum should be undertaken when mycobacterial infection is suspected. Examination by an experienced pathologist of Giemsa-stained expectorated respiratory secretions from patients with AIDS has given satisfactory results in the diagnosis of PCP. The sensitivity of sputum examination is enhanced by the use of monoclonal antibodies to *Pneumocystis* and is diminished by prior prophylactic use of inhaled pentamidine. Blastomycosis can be diagnosed by the examination of wet preparations of sputum. Sputum stained directly with fluorescent antibody can be examined for *Legionella*, but this test yields false-negative results relatively often. Thus sputum should also be cultured for *Legionella* on special media.

Expectorated sputum usually is easily collected from patients with a vigorous cough but may be scant in patients with an atypical syndrome, in the elderly, and in persons with altered mental status. If the patient is not producing sputum and can cooperate, respiratory secretions should be induced with ultrasonic nebulization of 3% saline. An attempt to obtain lower respiratory secretions by passage of a catheter through the nose or mouth rarely achieves the desired results in an alert patient and is discouraged; usually the catheter can be found coiled in the oropharynx.

In some cases that do not require the patient's hospitalization (see "Decision to Hospitalize," below), an accurate microbial diagnosis may not be crucial, and empirical therapy can be started on the basis of clinical and epidemiologic evidence alone. This approach may also be appropriate for hospitalized patients who are not severely ill and who are unable to produce an induced sputum specimen. Use of invasive procedures to establish a microbial diagnosis carries risks that must be weighed against potential benefits. However, the decision to initiate empirical therapy without an evaluation of induced sputum should be undertaken with caution and, in the case of hospitalized patients, should always be accompanied by the culture of several blood samples. The ability to understand the cause of a poor response to empirical antimicrobial therapy (Table 255-4) may be compromised by the lack of initial sputum and blood cultures. Establishing a specific microbial etiology in the individual patient is important, for it allows institution of specific pathogen–directed antimicrobial therapy and reduces the use of broad-spectrum combination regimens to cover multiple possible pathogens. Use of a single narrow-spectrum antimicrobial agent exposes the patient to fewer potential adverse drug reactions and reduces the pressure for selection of antimicrobial resistance. Emergence of antimicrobial resistance is a type of adverse drug reaction unlike others, because it is "contagious." In addition, establishing a microbial diagnosis can help define local community outbreaks and antimicrobial resistance patterns.

Invasive Procedures The sensitivities and specificities of the invasive procedures described below for obtaining pulmonary material vary with the type of immunocompromised patient, the type of pulmonary lesion, and the degree of prior exposure to therapeutic or prophylactic antimicrobial agents.

Transtracheal aspiration Popular several decades ago, TTA is rarely performed today. Although the sensitivity of the procedure is high (approaching 90%), the specificity is low. The material obtained by TTA (from a catheter inserted through the cricothyroid cartilage and advanced toward the carina) is not contaminated by upper respiratory tract secretions but can contain organisms that colonize the tracheobronchial tree without necessarily causing pneumonia. Significant morbidity and even death have attended the use of TTA. Contraindicated in patients with a bleeding diathesis, TTA may cause infection at the puncture site and may lead to severe subcutaneous and mediastinal emphysema in patients who are coughing vigorously.

Percutaneous transthoracic lung puncture This procedure employs a skinny (small-gauge) needle that is advanced into the area of pulmonary consolidation with computed tomographic guidance. It requires that the patient cooperate, have good hemostasis, and be able to tolerate a possible associated pulmonary hemorrhage or pneumothorax. Patients on mechanical ventilation cannot undergo lung puncture because of the high incidence of complicating pneumothorax.

Table 255-4 Factors Involved in Poor Response to Empirical Antimicrobial Therapy

Incorrect microbiologic diagnosis
Inappropriate antimicrobial agent or dosing regimen
Drug hypersensitivity or other adverse effect (e.g., *Clostridium difficile* colitis)
Infectious complication: empyema, metastatic spread, superinfection
Atelectasis, parapneumonic effusion, phlebitis
Poor host defenses (e.g., endobronchial obstruction, life-threatening comorbidity)

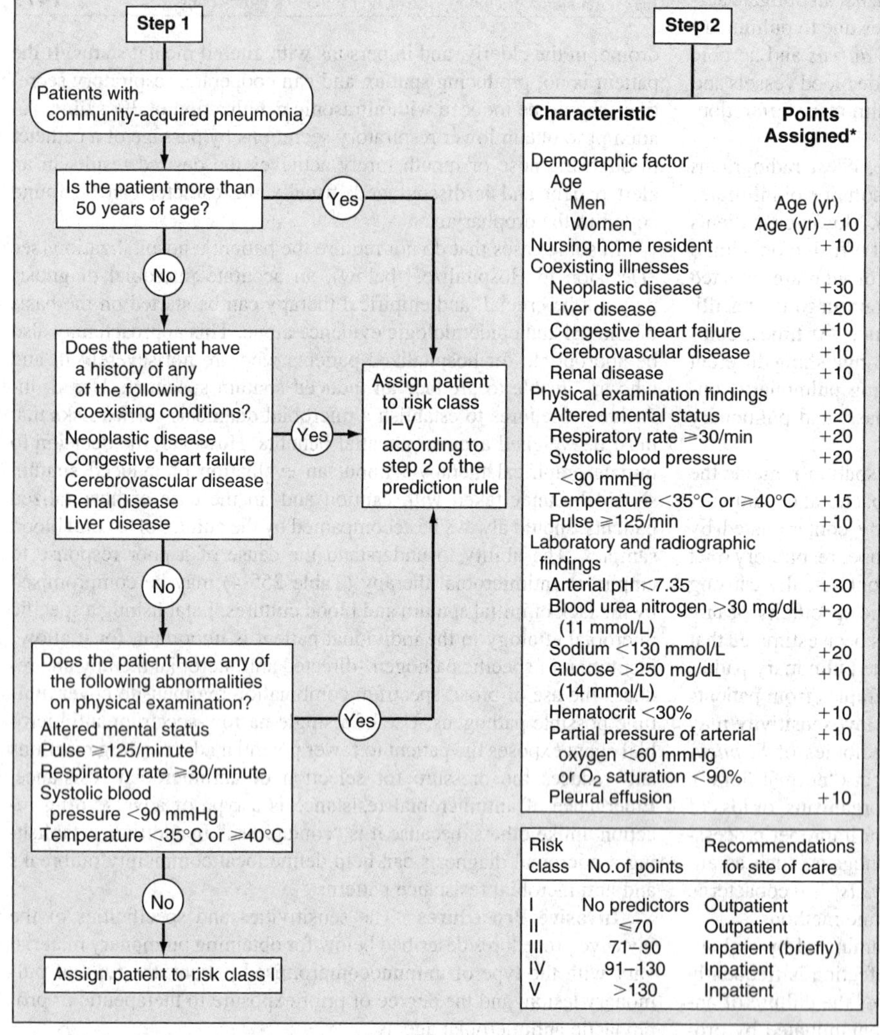

Step 1
Patients with community-acquired pneumonia
Is the patient more than 50 years of age?
Yes
No
Does the patient have a history of any of the following coexisting conditions?
Neoplastic disease
Congestive heart failure
Cerebrovascular disease
Renal disease
Liver disease
Yes
No
Does the patient have any of the following abnormalities on physical examination?
Altered mental status
Pulse ≥125/minute
Respiratory rate ≥30/minute
Systolic blood pressure <90 mmHg
Temperature <35°C or ≥40°C
Yes
No
Assign patient to risk class I
Assign patient to risk class II–V according to step 2 of the prediction rule
Step 2
Characteristic | Points Assigned*
Demographic factor
Age
Men | Age (yr)
Women | Age (yr) − 10
Nursing home resident | +10
Coexisting illnesses
Neoplastic disease | +30
Liver disease | +20
Congestive heart failure | +10
Cerebrovascular disease | +10
Renal disease | +10
Physical examination findings
Altered mental status | +20
Respiratory rate ≥30/min | +20
Systolic blood pressure <90 mmHg | +20
Temperature <35°C or ≥40°C | +15
Pulse ≥125/min | +10
Laboratory and radiographic findings
Arterial pH <7.35 | +30
Blood urea nitrogen >30 mg/dL (11 mmol/L) | +20
Sodium <130 mmol/L | +20
Glucose >250 mg/dL (14 mmol/L) | +10
Hematocrit <30% | +10
Partial pressure of arterial oxygen <60 mmHg or O2 saturation <90% | +10
Pleural effusion | +10
Risk class | No.of points | Recommendations for site of care
I | No predictors | Outpatient
II | ≤70 | Outpatient
III | 71–90 | Inpatient (briefly)
IV | 91–130 | Inpatient
V | >130 | Inpatient

FIGURE 255-1 Criteria for hospitalization of patients with pneumonia: the PORT score. *A risk score (total point score) for a given patient is obtained by summing the patient's age in years (age minus 10 for females) and the points for each applicable patient characteristic. †Oxygen saturation of <90% is also considered abnormal. *(Adapted from Fine et al. and Bartlett et al.)*

Fiberoptic bronchoscopy Fiberoptic bronchoscopy is safe and relatively well tolerated and has become the standard invasive procedure used to obtain lower respiratory tract secretions from seriously ill or immunocompromised patients with complex or progressive pneumonia. This technique provides a direct view of the lower airways. Specimens obtained by bronchoscopy should be subjected to Gram's, acid-fast, *Legionella* direct fluorescent antibody, and Gomori's methenamine silver staining and should be cultured for routine aerobic and anaerobic bacteria, legionellae, mycobacteria, and fungi. Samples are collected with a protected double-sheathed brush (PSB), by bronchoalveolar lavage (BAL), or by transbronchial biopsy (TBB) at the site of pulmonary consolidation. The PSB sample is usually contaminated by oropharyngeal flora; quantitative cultures of the 1 mL of sterile culture medium into which the brush is placed after withdrawal from the inner catheter must be performed to differentiate contamination (<1000 CFU/mL) from infection (≥1000 CFU/mL). The results of PSB are highly specific and highly sensitive, especially when the patient has not received antibiotics before culture. BAL is usually performed with 150 to 200 mL of sterile, nonbacteriostatic saline. When used to facilitate endoscopy, local anesthetic agents with antibacterial activity can lower the sensitivity of culture results. Quantitative bacteriologic evaluation of BAL fluid has given results similar to those obtained with the PSB technique. Gram's staining of the cytocentrifuged BAL fluid specimen can serve as an immediate guide in the selection of antimicrobial therapy to be administered while culture results are awaited.

Open-lung biopsy This procedure is most commonly needed when specimens obtained bronchoscopically from an immunocompromised patient with progressive pneumonia have been unrevealing. Limitations on the performance of an open-lung biopsy include hypoxemia and a bleeding diathesis, which may supervene while the physician is deciding whether to undertake this procedure. Results of an open-lung biopsy are considered diagnostic because of the large size of the tissue sample. The diagnostic yield of this procedure is greatest in focal lesions, whereas bronchoscopic evaluation is most useful in diffuse lesions.

Other Diagnostic Tests In the initial evaluation of a patient with pneumonia, at least two blood samples for culture should be obtained from different venipuncture sites; if empyema is a clinical consideration, diagnostic thoracentesis is indicated. Positive blood or pleural fluid culture is generally considered diagnostic of the etiology of pneumonia. However, bacteremia and empyema each occur in fewer than 10 to 30% of patients with pneumonia.

Serologic studies are sometimes helpful in defining the etiology of certain types of pneumonia, although serologic diagnosis—because it is often delayed by the need to demonstrate at least a fourfold rise in convalescent-phase antibody titer—is usually retrospective. A single IgM antibody titer of >1:16, a single IgG antibody titer of >1:128, or a fourfold or greater rise in the IgG titer obtained by indirect immunofluorescence is diagnostic of *M. pneumoniae* infection. A single IgM antibody titer of ≥1:20, a single IgG antibody titer of ≥1:128, or a fourfold or greater rise in the IgG titer obtained by micro-indirect immunofluorescence is diagnostic of *C. pneumoniae* infection. A single *Legionella* antibody titer of ≥1:256 or a fourfold rise to a titer of ≥1:128 suggests acute legionellosis. A highly sensitive and specific urinary antigen test is available to detect *L. pneumophila* serogroup 1 in patients with pneumonia; this organism accounts for ~70% of *L. pneumophila* infections. The diagnosis of hantavirus infection is confirmed by detection of IgM serum antibodies, a rising titer of IgG serum antibodies, hantavirus-specific RNA by polymerase chain reaction in clinical specimens, and hantavirus-specific antigen by immunohistochemistry.

DECISION TO HOSPITALIZE Approximately 20% of patients with community-acquired pneumonia are hospitalized, some perhaps unnecessarily. Use of inpatient hospital services is costly and at times poses risks to the patient (e.g., the risk of nosocomial infections). Thus hospitalization must be justified by anticipation of a poor outcome if the case is managed in an outpatient setting.

The Pneumonia Patient Outcomes Research Team (PORT) has attempted to quantify the risk of death and other adverse outcomes of community-acquired pneumonia by assignment of points to 19 variables (Fig. 255-1), with stratification of patients into five classes based on cumulative point score. This prediction rule was derived and validated in a large number of patients. On the basis of their observations, the PORT investigators suggest that outpatient management is appropriate for many patients in classes I and II, in whom the risks of subsequent hospitalization (≤8.2%) and of death (<0.6%) are low. They suggest outpatient management after a short hospital stay for patients in class III, whose risk of subsequent hospitalization if initially treated at home is 16.7% but whose risk of admission to the intensive care unit (ICU) is 5.9%—similar to that for patients in classes I and II. The PORT investigators further suggest that patients in classes IV and V (risk of death, 8.2 and 29.2%, respectively; risk of ICU admission, 11.4 and 17.3%, respectively) should receive traditional inpatient care. An expert panel from the Infectious Diseases Society of America (IDSA) endorses the PORT recommendations.

Other characteristics that favor a decision to hospitalize the patient include the known presence of certain etiologic microorganisms (e.g., *S. aureus*) that are associated with a poor prognosis, multilobe pulmonary involvement, suppurative complications (e.g., empyema or septic arthritis), evidence of poor functional status (e.g., hypotension or hypoxemia on presentation in patients otherwise in classes I, II, and III), evidence of a patient's inability to comply with treatment recommendations, anticipated difficulty in assessing the response to outpatient treatment, and an inadequate home support system that may compromise outpatient care. Discharge from the hospital should be guided by similar considerations.

℞ TREATMENT **Community-Acquired Pneumonia: Outpatient Management** Most cases of community-acquired pneumonia in otherwise-healthy adults do not require hospitalization. Although desirable, it is often impractical in the outpatient setting to obtain a chest radiograph and sputum Gram's stain and culture in order to confirm the clinical diagnosis of pneumonia and its microbial etiology before starting antimicrobial therapy. Consequently, the oral antimicrobial treatment administered in the outpatient setting is frequently empirical (Table 255-5). The pathogen in such a situation is likely to be *M. pneumoniae*, *S. pneumoniae*, or *C. pneumoniae*. In older patients with underlying chronic respiratory disease, *L. pneumophila*, *H. influenzae*, or *M. catarrhalis* should also be considered. In patients at risk of aspiration, oral anaerobes may be involved. Few oral antimicrobial drugs have a reliable spectrum encompassing all of these pathogens (Table 255-5). Whatever regimen is chosen, its antimicrobial activity should encompass *S. pneumoniae*, the most common cause of pneumonia. Increasing resistance among pneumococci to all the available oral antimicrobial agents precludes the designation of any one agent as the clear drug of choice.

Strains of *S. pneumoniae* for which the minimal inhibitory concentration (MIC) of penicillin (as determined by the broth dilution method) is 0.1 to 1.0 μg/mL are considered to have intermediate-level resistance, while strains whose MIC is >1.0 μg/mL are considered to have high-level resistance. The current, less time-consuming method to screen for penicillin resistance is the use of a 1-μg oxacillin disk in a disk diffusion assay. Penicillin resistance (i.e., an MIC ≥0.1 μg/mL) is indicated by a zone of growth inhibition of ≤19 mm. Antimicrobial gradient paper strips (the E-test), which yield the exact MIC, are as accurate as the broth dilution technique, can be performed as rapidly as the oxacillin disk diffusion assay, and have replaced the oxacillin disk test in many institutions.

The resistance of *S. pneumoniae* to penicillin varies greatly with the source of the clinical sample tested (e.g., strains isolated from middle-ear fluid are most often resistant), the age of the patient (e.g., resistance is more frequent among children than among adults), the setting (e.g., resistance is more common in day-care centers), the patient's socioeconomic status (the frequency of resistance is highest in samples from suburban and white patients), and the geographic region in which the specimen was collected. Caution must be exercised in the interpretation of surveys of antimicrobial resistance among pneumococci in the United States, which can be strongly affected by these types of sampling bias. In a national survey of clinical isolates from normally sterile body sites that was conducted in 1997 in various surveillance areas throughout the United States by the Centers for Disease Control and Prevention (CDC), 11% (range, 6 to 19%) of 3110 isolates of *S. pneumoniae* exhibited intermediate-level resistance to penicillin, and 14% (range, 8 to 26%) displayed high-level resistance. However, in another national survey of the antimicrobial susceptibility of clinical isolates obtained from respiratory tract sites between February and June 1997 at 27 U.S. medical centers (SENTRY surveillance program), 28% of 845 isolates (with a range of 11 to 52% at the various medical centers) displayed intermediate-level penicillin resistance, and an additional 16% (with a range of 0 to 33%) displayed high-level penicillin resistance.

As a consequence of the production of altered penicillin-binding proteins with decreased β-lactam affinity, penicillin-resistant *S. pneumoniae* exhibits at least some degree of cross-resistance to all β-lactams, including the extended-spectrum third- and fourth-generation cephalosporins. Since the mechanism of penicillin resistance does not involve β-lactamase production, β-lactam/β-lactamase inhibitor combinations (e.g., amoxicillin/clavulanate) offer no advantage. Indeed, the MICs of penicillin and amoxicillin are nearly identical, but the serum levels after equivalent doses are much higher for amoxicillin than for penicillin, a difference that may reflect a therapeutic advantage of amoxicillin. Among the oral cephalosporins, cefaclor, cefadroxil, and cephalexin have variable activity against penicillin-sensitive strains; cefuroxime and cefpodoxime have activity against penicillin-susceptible strains but variable activity against penicillin-intermediate strains and no activity against highly penicillin-resistant strains.

Table 255-5 Empirical Oral Antimicrobial Therapy for Outpatient Management of Community-Acquired Pneumonia

	Value of Indicated Antimicrobial[a]							
Pathogen	**Penicillin G**	**Amoxicillin/ Clavulanate**	**Cefuroxime**	**Trimethoprim-Sulfamethoxazole**	**Doxycycline**	**Erythromycin**	**Ciprofloxacin**	**Newer Fluoroquinolones[b]**
Streptococcus pneumoniae	±[c]	±[c]	±[c]	±[c]	+[c]	±[c]	±	+[c]
Haemophilus influenzae	−	+	+	+	+	−[d]	+	+
Moraxella catarrhalis	−	+	+	+	+	+	+	+
Anaerobes	±	+	±	−	−	−	−	±
Mycoplasma pneumoniae	−	−	−	−	+	+	+	+
Chlamydia pneumoniae	−	−	−	−	+	+	+	+
Legionella pneumophila	−	−	−	±	±	+	+	+

[a] +, effective; −, ineffective; ±, sometimes effective.
[b] Levofloxacin, gatifloxacin, moxifloxacin, and sparfloxacin.
[c] In the United States, about 42% of strains are currently resistant to penicillin (15% with high-level penicillin resistance), 20% to amoxicillin and cefuroxime, 20–30% to trimethoprim-sulfamethoxazole, 7–10% to doxycycline (tetracycline), 14% to erythromycin, and <4% to the newer fluoroquinolones.
[d] The new macrolides azithromycin and clarithromycin are more active against *H. influenzae* than erythromycin and are equally or more active against other respiratory pathogens.

Resistance to other antimicrobial agents, such as the macrolides (erythromycin, clarithromycin, and azithromycin), clindamycin, tetracycline and doxycycline, and trimethoprim-sulfamethoxazole (TMP-SMZ), is also more common among penicillin-intermediate strains than among penicillin-susceptible strains, and it is most common among highly penicillin-resistant strains. Overall rates of resistance among *S. pneumoniae* strains are ~14% for the macrolides, 4% for clindamycin, up to 10% for tetracyclines, and 20 to 30% for TMP-SMZ. Rates of resistance to the newer fluoroquinolones levofloxacin, gatifloxacin, moxifloxacin, and sparfloxacin are <4%, regardless of penicillin susceptibility. At best, the older fluoroquinolones (e.g., ciprofloxacin) have borderline activity, as judged by serum levels in relation to MICs of these drugs against the pneumococcus.

Optimally, the choice of antimicrobial drugs for empirical therapy should be guided by local resistance patterns, if known. Options for empirical antimicrobial therapy should be modified in light of continually evolving antimicrobial resistance patterns resulting from the introduction of new resistant clones into the community from other regions or the emergence of resistant mutants under the selective pressure of local patterns of antimicrobial use. The IDSA has published guidelines for the treatment of community-acquired pneumonia. These guidelines emphasize the need for a chest radiograph when pneumonia is suspected and for the establishment of a microbial diagnosis (e.g., by sputum Gram's stain with or without culture) whenever possible. Doxycycline and the newer fluoroquinolones are recommended alternatives for initial empirical oral therapy, especially when penicillin-resistant pneumococci are suspected. The utility of the macrolides and amoxicillin depends on susceptibility of pneumococci in the local community.

The regimen should be modified for patients with particular epidemiologic factors or comorbidities related to specific pathogens—e.g., structural lung disease or suspected aspiration. Aspiration pneumonia can be treated with amoxicillin/clavulanate, clindamycin, or amoxicillin plus metronidazole because these regimens are active against oral anaerobes. Metronidazole alone has inadequate activity against microaerophilic gram-positive cocci and must be supplemented with a β-lactam agent that compensates for this defect in spectrum. If macrolides are used and *H. influenzae* is suspected, azithromycin or clarithromycin is preferred because of erythromycin's poor activity against this organism. Alternative agents for *H. influenzae* include amoxicillin/clavulanate, doxycycline, or a fluoroquinolone. The β-lactams are not active against pathogens causing atypical pneumonia (e.g., *Mycoplasma, C. pneumoniae*, or *Legionella*), in which case doxycycline, a macrolide, or a fluoroquinolone is preferred.

The IDSA guidelines recommend that pneumococcal pneumonia be treated for 7 to 10 days or until the patient has been afebrile for 72 h. Pneumonia caused by *Legionella, C. pneumoniae*, or *Mycoplasma* should be treated for 2 to 3 weeks unless azithromycin is used, in which case a 5-day course is acceptable because of the drug's prolonged half-life in tissues.

Community-Acquired Pneumonia: Inpatient Management Patients who have community-acquired pneumonia and are ill enough to be hospitalized (Fig. 255-1) must have a chest radiograph to establish the diagnosis of pneumonia, must undergo prompt microbiologic evaluation (including Gram's staining and culture of sputum and culture of two blood samples drawn by separate venipuncture), and must receive empirical antimicrobial therapy based on Gram's staining of sputum and knowledge of the current antimicrobial sensitivities of the pulmonary pathogens in the local geographic area (Tables 255-6 and 255-7). Antimicrobial therapy should be initiated promptly (e.g., within 8 h of admission). Parenteral antimicrobial therapy in the hospitalized patient is usually mandatory. A lack of sputum production, an atypical clinical presentation, the presence of diffuse radiographic infiltrates, a rapidly progressive downhill course, and a poor response to prior empirical therapy are among the indications for the use of invasive procedures to detect the pulmonary pathogen, especially in the immunocompromised patient. Although broad-spectrum antibacterial therapy should be started during a full evaluation in severely ill patients with rapidly progressing illness, these empirical regimens cannot encompass all the possible pathogens without producing unnecessary toxicity and expense. Indeed, in immunocompromised patients (including those with neutropenia or HIV infection), the number of microbial and noninfectious causes of pulmonary disease is large and increasing. Since failure to provide specific treatment can prove rapidly fatal, a diagnosis should be sought aggressively so that optimal therapy can be started promptly.

Penicillin or ampicillin remains the drug of choice for infection due to penicillin-susceptible pneumococci. Studies suggest that high-

Table 255-6 Empirical Antimicrobial Therapy for the Management of Hospitalized Patients with Community-Acquired Pneumonia

	Value of Indicated Antimicrobial[a]							
Pathogen	Penicillin G	Second-Generation Cephalosporins	Third- and Fourth-Generation Cephalosporins[b]	Metronidazole	Trimethoprim-Sulfamethoxazole	Erythromycin	Ampicillin/ Sulbactam	Newer Fluoro-quinolones[c]
Streptococcus pneumoniae	±[d]	±[d]	+[d]	−	±[d]	±[d]	±[d]	+[d]
Staphylococcus aureus	−	+	+	−	+	+	+	+
Haemophilus influenzae	−	+	+	−	+	−	+	+
Moraxella catarrhalis	−	+	+	−	+	+	+	+
Anaerobic gram-positive cocci	+	+	+	±	−	±	+	±
Anaerobic gram-negative bacilli	−	−	−	+	−	−	+	±
Chlamydia pneumoniae	−	−	−	−	−	+	−	+
Legionella pneumophila	−	−	−	−	±	+	−	+
Mycoplasma pneumoniae	−	−	−	−	−	+	−	+

[a] +, effective; −, ineffective; ±, sometimes effective.
[b] Ceftriaxone, cefotaxime, and cefepime.
[c] Levofloxacin, gatifloxacin, moxifloxacin, and sparfloxacin.
[d] In the United States, about 42% of strains are currently resistant to penicillin (15% with high-level penicillin resistance; ampicillin slightly less active than penicillin), 20% are resistant to cefuroxime (similar activity displayed by the first-generation cephalosporin cephalothin), 4–5% are highly resistant to third- or fourth-generation cephalosporins, 20–30% are resistant to trimethoprim-sulfamethoxazole, 7–10% are resistant to doxycycline (tetracycline), 14% are resistant to erythromycin, and <4% are resistant to the newer fluoroquinolones.

Table 255-7 Dosage of Antimicrobial Agents for the Treatment of Pneumonia in Hospitalized Patients[a]

Drug	Dosage
Ampicillin/sulbactam	3 g IV q6h
Aztreonam	2 g IV q8h
Cefazolin	1–2 g IV q8h
Cefepime	2 g IV q8h
Cefotaxime, ceftizoxime	1–2 g IV q8–12h
Ceftazidime	2 g IV q8h
Ceftriaxone	1–2 g IV q12h
Cefuroxime	750 mg IV q8h
Ciprofloxacin	400 mg IV or 750 mg PO q12h
Clindamycin	600–900 mg IV q8h
Erythromycin	0.5–1.0 g IV q6h
Gentamicin (or tobramycin)	5 mg/kg/d in 3 equally divided doses IV q8h
Imipenem	500 mg IV q6h
Levofloxacin	500 mg IV or PO q24h
Metronidazole	500 mg IV or PO q6h
Nafcillin	2 g IV q4h
Penicillin G	3 million units IV q4–6h
Piperacillin/tazobactam	4.5 g IV q6h
Ticarcillin/clavulanate	3.1 g IV q4h
Vancomycin	1 g (15 mg/kg) IV q12h

[a] Dosage must be modified for patients with renal failure. Guidelines on the duration of therapy for each pathogen are given in the text of this chapter and of chapters on specific infecting agents.

dose intravenous penicillin G (e.g., 10 to 20 million units daily), ampicillin (2 g every 6 h), ceftriaxone (1 or 2 g every 24 h), or cefotaxime (1 to 2 g every 6 h) constitutes adequate therapy for pneumonia due to strains exhibiting intermediate resistance to penicillin (MIC, 0.1 to 1 μg/mL). The effectiveness of high-dose intravenous penicillin against pneumonia due to highly resistant pneumococcal strains is unknown, but MICs of cefotaxime and ceftriaxone for these strains are usually lower than those of penicillin or ampicillin and most other β-lactam antibiotics. Ceftriaxone or cefotaxime may be effective when the MIC of penicillin is $\geq$1 μg/mL and those of ceftriaxone and cefotaxime are $\leq$2 μg/mL. However, highly cephalosporin-resistant strains have become a problem in certain geographic areas. Since all penicillin resistant strains are sensitive to vancomycin, initial empirical therapy should include this antibiotic (1 g intravenously every 12 h) when the patient with pneumococcal pneumonia is severely ill, has significant comorbidity, and lives in a region where highly penicillin- or cephalosporin-resistant strains have become common.

If the result of Gram's staining of sputum is not interpretable or not available, then the IDSA guidelines recommend empirical therapy for patients hospitalized on a general medical unit with a β-lactam (e.g., ceftriaxone, cefotaxime) or a β-lactam/β-lactamase inhibitor combination, with or without a macrolide, or with one of the fluoroquinolones alone. Seriously ill patients who are hospitalized in the ICU should always receive a macrolide or a newer fluoroquinolone in addition to the β-lactam to cover *Legionella*. The therapeutic regimens should be modified further in the following situations: structural disease of the lung (e.g., bronchiectasis) requires treatment with an anti-*Pseudomonas* β-lactam plus a macrolide or with a newer fluoroquinolone plus an aminoglycoside; penicillin allergy requires treatment with a newer fluoroquinolone, with or without clindamycin; and suspected aspiration requires treatment with a newer fluoroquinolone plus either clindamycin or metronidazole or with a β-lactam/β-lactamase inhibitor combination alone. A recent study of almost 13,000 elderly hospitalized patients with pneumonia, which controlled for severity of illness, baseline differences in patient characteristics, and processes of care, documented 30-day mortality that was 26 to 36% lower among those treated initially with a fluoroquinolone alone or a macrolide combined with a second- or nonpseudomonal third-generation cephalosporin than among those initially given a nonpseudomonal third-generation cephalosporin alone. This result may reflect the importance of pathogens such as *Mycoplasma*, *Legionella*, and *C. pneumoniae* in these patients.

Therapy can be switched from intravenous to oral agents within 3 days to complete a 7- to 10-day course if the patient's clinical condition improves rapidly and if antimicrobial agents that are readily absorbed after oral administration and that reach tissue levels above the MIC are available. The presence of *S. aureus* or aerobic gram-negative bacilli or the development of suppurative complications requires a more prolonged course of therapy. Pneumonia caused by *Legionella*, *C. pneumoniae*, or *Mycoplasma* should be treated for 2 to 3 weeks unless azithromycin is used. Anaerobic lung abscess should be treated with the regimens suggested for aspiration pneumonia until a chest radiograph (with radiography performed at 2-week intervals) is clear or shows only a small stable scar. Therapy is prolonged for $\geq$6 weeks to prevent relapse, although shorter courses are probably sufficient for many patients. Surgery is rarely required for lung abscess; indications for surgery include massive hemoptysis and suspected neoplasm. Supportive measures include the administration of supplemental oxygen and intravenous fluids, assistance in clearing secretions, fiberoptic bronchoscopy, and (if necessary) ventilatory support. Caution should be exercised in bronchoscopic drainage of large, fluid-filled lung abscesses because of the potential for sudden massive spillage of large collections of pus into the airways.

Patients with risk factors for HIV infection and an atypical pneumonia syndrome should be evaluated for PCP because of its frequency as an index diagnosis in HIV infection and its potential severity. Tuberculosis and other causes of atypical pneumonia must be excluded as part of the evaluation of these patients. Empirical therapy can consist of either TMP-SMZ (15 to 20 mg of trimethoprim per kg, given daily in four divided doses intravenously or by mouth) or pentamidine (3 to 4 mg/kg daily, given intravenously), and therapy is continued for 3 weeks in confirmed cases of PCP. Although some data suggest that TMP-SMZ is more effective than pentamidine, further studies directly comparing the two agents are needed. The frequency and severity of the adverse effects of the two drugs are generally thought to be equivalent. The addition of glucocorticoids (prednisone, 40 mg twice daily, with subsequent tapering of the dose) early in the course of PCP in patients with an arterial P_{O_2} of <70 mmHg decreases the need for mechanical ventilation and improves the patient's chances of survival and functional status. Prophylaxis for recurrent PCP must be started at the end of therapy.

Institutionally Acquired Pneumonia Pneumonia acquired in institutions such as nursing homes or hospitals is frequently caused by enteric aerobic gram-negative bacilli, *P. aeruginosa*, or *S. aureus*, with or without oral anaerobes. Again, the selection of empirical antimicrobial therapy should be guided by Gram's staining of sputum (Tables 255-7 and 255-8) and knowledge of the prevalent nosocomial pathogens and their current in vitro antimicrobial sensitivity patterns in the institution involved. An aggressive diagnostic approach is needed in some circumstances, especially for the immunocompromised patient (as outlined above).

S. aureus acquired in some institutions is frequently methicillin resistant. Such strains are resistant to all β-lactam antibiotics and may also be resistant to clindamycin, erythromycin, and the fluoroquinolones. Only vancomycin is predictably active against these organisms, and this drug should be added to the empirical regimen when methicillin-resistant organisms may be involved in pneumonia.

When multiantibiotic resistance is a problem, pneumonia due to gram-negative bacilli in the institutionalized patient can be treated initially with a β-lactam active against *P. aeruginosa* (ceftazidime, cefepime, piperacillin/tazobactam, ticarcillin/clavulanate, aztreonam, or imipenem) or with a parenterally administered fluoroquinolone (ciprofloxacin, ofloxacin, gatifloxacin, or levofloxacin). Among the fluoroquinolones, ciprofloxacin remains the most potent antipseudomonal agent. Ticarcillin/clavulanate and piperacillin/tazobactam are preferred over other penicillins with activity against *P. aeruginosa* (e.g., ticarcillin or piperacillin alone), which are not sufficiently active against *Klebsiella pneumoniae*, a relatively common pathogen. However, for

Table 255-8 Empirical Antimicrobial Therapy, Based on Gram's Staining of Sputum, for Institutionally Acquired Pneumonia

Etiology	Regimen
Presumptive *Staphylococcus aureus*	Nafcillin or vancomycin[a]
Presumptive enteric aerobic gram-negative bacilli or *Pseudomonas aeruginosa*	1. Ceftazidime or cefepime ± aminoglycoside 2. Ticarcillin/clavulanate or piperacillin/tazobactam ± aminoglycoside 3. Aztreonam ± aminoglycoside 4. Imipenem[b,c] ± aminoglycoside 5. Fluoroquinolone[c] ± aminoglycoside or β-lactam
Mixed flora	1. Ceftazidime or cefepime + clindamycin (or metronidazole) ± aminoglycoside[e] 2. Ticarcillin/clavulanate or piperacillin/tazobactam ± aminoglycoside[e] 3. Aztreonam + clindamycin (or metronidazole[d]) ± aminoglycoside[e] 4. Imipenem[b,c] ± aminoglycoside[e] 5. Fluoroquinolone[c] + clindamycin (or metronidazole[d,e]) ± aminoglycoside or β-lactam

[a] If methicillin-resistant *S. aureus* is known to exist in the institution, use vancomycin; otherwise, use an antistaphylococcal β-lactam such as nafcillin or cefazolin.
[b] Use when extended-spectrum β-lactamase producers are endemic in the institution.
[c] Use when chromosomally encoded, inducible β-lactamase producers are endemic in the institution.
[d] Metronidazole must be combined with vancomycin or another antimicrobial that covers microaerophilic and anaerobic gram-positive cocci.
[e] Add vancomycin if methicillin-resistant *S. aureus* is present in the institution.

infection suspected to be due to *P. aeruginosa*, the higher dose recommended by the package insert is required; a lower dose contains less piperacillin or ticarcillin than is needed to be effective against this organism. Ampicillin/sulbactam, the other parenterally administered β-lactam/β-lactamase inhibitor combination, is not active against many nosocomial pathogens, such as *P. aeruginosa*, *Enterobacter* spp., and *Serratia* spp., and therefore is inappropriate as empirical therapy for nosocomial pneumonia.

In seriously ill patients, especially those infected with organisms in which resistance frequently emerges during therapy (e.g., *P. aeruginosa*), use of a β-lactam/aminoglycoside or β-lactam/fluoroquinolone combination is prudent. Combinations of a β-lactam plus an aminoglycoside are used for bactericidal synergy. Combinations of a β-lactam or an aminoglycoside with a fluoroquinolone are not expected to enhance the already-rapid bactericidal activity of the fluoroquinolone alone. However, such combinations are also used to broaden the spectrum of antibacterial activity, to cover the possibility of infection with resistant pathogens, to treat polymicrobial infection, and to prevent the emergence of antimicrobial resistance.

Pneumonia due to possible coinfection with aerobic gram-negative bacilli and anaerobes, as reflected by a polymicrobial flora on Gram's staining of sputum, can usually be treated with any of the following regimens: (1) cefepime or ceftazidime plus metronidazole or clindamycin, (2) aztreonam or a fluoroquinolone plus clindamycin, or (3) imipenem, piperacillin/tazobactam, or ticarcillin/clavulanate. The regimens should include double coverage for *P. aeruginosa* when this organism is suspected (Table 255-8).

The production of chromosomally encoded, inducible β-lactamases by some aerobic gram-negative bacilli, including *Serratia marcescens*, *Enterobacter cloacae*, *Citrobacter freundii*, *Morganella morganii*, *P. aeruginosa*, and *Acinetobacter calcoaceticus*, has important implications for the treatment of nosocomial pneumonia in institutions where these organisms are common nosocomial pathogens. Antibiotic resistance in these pathogens has been attributed to two related mechanisms: inducible production of chromosomally encoded β-lactamases and selection of mutants that have lost the genes that control expression of β-lactamase production. The control genes repress β-lactamase production in the absence of a β-lactam agent and allow β-lactamase production in the presence of a β-lactam agent. This group of organisms has a relatively high mutation rate for loss of these control genes, and their loss results in continuous production of large amounts of β-lactamase (*stable derepression*). The derepressed mutants are resistant to third-generation cephalosporins, aztreonam, and broad-spectrum penicillins. These chromosomally encoded, inducible β-lactamases are not inhibited by clavulanic acid, tazobactam, or sulbactam.

Selection by the β-lactam antibiotic of the derepressed mutants present in the dense bacterial populations of infected pulmonary tissue at the initiation of antibiotic therapy apparently accounts for the emergence of resistance during therapy, which is especially problematic in severely compromised patients whose defective host defenses are unable to control the growth of a few resistant mutants. The only β-lactam agents that maintain activity against the derepressed mutants are the fourth-generation cephalosporin cefepime and the carbapenem imipenem. The fluoroquinolones and aminoglycosides may also retain activity against these mutants. TMP-SMZ may remain active against all of these gram-negative bacilli except *P. aeruginosa*, which is inherently resistant to this agent. Some clinicians have questioned the efficacy of aminoglycosides alone for the treatment of gram-negative bacillary pneumonia. The poor clinical efficacy of aminoglycosides has been attributed to the low drug levels attained in bronchial secretions and to a loss of antimicrobial activity due to the relative acidity of purulent secretions, the anaerobic conditions in infected lung, and (in the case of *P. aeruginosa*) the divalent cations calcium and magnesium. The nephrotoxicity and ototoxicity of aminoglycosides frequently lead to underdosing with these agents. These problems are compounded by unpredictable pharmacokinetics that necessitate measurement of serum levels of aminoglycosides. If multiantibiotic-resistant nosocomial organisms are likely to be the pathogens infecting severely compromised patients, reliable empirical agents may be fluoroquinolones, cefepime, and imipenem—unless resistance to these drugs is also endemic in the institution. Some strains of *K. pneumoniae* and *Escherichia coli* have acquired a plasmid encoding the production of an extended-spectrum β-lactamase that can be detected as in vitro resistance to ceftazidime or aztreonam. The presence of an extended-spectrum β-lactamase confers resistance to all third-generation cephalosporins and aztreonam. Some of these strains may also be resistant to piperacillin/tazobactam and cefepime, and many are also resistant to the fluoroquinolones. The only reliable agents are the carbapenems, such as imipenem. Up-to-date knowledge of the antimicrobial sensitivities of an institution's nosocomial pathogens and use of various preventive practices are mandatory.

Amantadine (200 mg/d for most adults and 100 mg/d for persons >65 years of age) is effective for the prevention of influenza A virus infection in the unimmunized patient during an influenza A outbreak and for the treatment (for 5 to 7 days) of early influenza A virus infection. Ribavirin is effective for respiratory syncytial virus infection. Intravenous acyclovir (5 to 10 mg/kg every 8 h for 7 to 14 days) is appropriate for varicella pneumonia. Treatment of cytomegalovirus pneumonia has yielded unsatisfactory results, but intravenous immunoglobulin combined with ganciclovir may be effective in some instances. Therapy for hantavirus pulmonary syndrome is supportive, and overall mortality has been 55%.

PREVENTION The prevention of pneumonia involves either (1) decreasing the likelihood of encountering the pathogen or (2) strengthening the host's response once the pathogen is encountered. The first approach can include measures such as hand washing and glove use by persons who care for patients infected with contact-transmitted pathogens (e.g., aerobic gram-negative bacilli); use of face masks or negative-pressure isolation rooms for patients with pneumonia due to pathogens spread by the aerosol route (e.g., *M. tuberculosis*); prompt institution of effective chemotherapy for patients with contagious illnesses; and correction of conditions that facilitate aspiration. The second approach includes the use of chemoprophylaxis or immunization for patients at risk. Chemoprophylaxis may be administered to patients who have encountered or are likely to encounter the pathogen before they become symptomatic (e.g., amantadine during a community outbreak of influenza A, as mentioned above; isoniazid for tuberculosis; or TMP-SMZ for pneumocystosis) or to patients who are likely to have a recurrence following recovery from a symptomatic episode (e.g., TMP-SMZ for pneumocystosis in patients with HIV infection). The prevention of nosocomial pneumonia requires good infection control practices, judicious use of broad-spectrum antimicrobial agents, and maintenance of patients' gastric acidity—a major factor that prevents colonization of the gastrointestinal tract by nosocomial gram-negative bacillary pathogens. To prevent stress ulceration, it is preferable to use sucralfate, which maintains gastric acidity, rather than H_2-blocking agents. To prevent ventilator-associated nosocomial pneumonia, the following strategies have been proposed: use of the semirecumbent position, of endotracheal tubes that allow continuous aspiration of secretions accumulating above the cuff, and of heat and moisture exchangers that reduce the formation of condensate within the tubing circuitry. Vaccines (Chaps. 122, 138, 149, 190, and 194) are available for immunization against *S. pneumoniae*, *H. influenzae* type b, influenza viruses A and B, and measles virus. Influenza vaccine is strongly recommended for individuals >55 years old and pneumococcal vaccine for those >65 years old; these vaccines should be administered to persons of any age who are at risk of adverse consequences of influenza or pneumonia because of underlying conditions. Pneumococcal, *Haemophilus*, and influenza vaccines are recommended for HIV-infected patients who are still capable of responding to a vaccine challenge. The currently available 23-valent pneumococcal vaccine covers 88% of the serotypes causing systemic disease as well as 8% of related serotypes. The increasing prevalence of multiantibiotic resistance among pneumococci makes pneumococcal immunization of high-risk individuals of utmost importance. Immune serum globulin is available for intravenous replacement therapy in those patients with congenital or acquired hypogammaglobulinemia. Some patients who have selective IgG2 subtype deficiency and recurrent sinopulmonary infections and who are immunologically unresponsive to capsular polysaccharide vaccines may nevertheless have an antibody response to the capsular polysaccharide that is covalently linked to a protein, as it is in the conjugate *H. influenzae* type b vaccine and a similar experimental conjugate pneumococcal vaccine.

BIBLIOGRAPHY

BARTLETT JG et al: Community-acquired pneumonia in adults: Guidelines for management. Clin Infect Dis 26:811, 1998

BOWTON DL: Nosocomial pneumonia in the ICU—year 2000 and beyond. Chest 115: 28S, 1999

DOERN GV et al: Prevalence of antimicrobial resistance among respiratory tract isolates of *Streptococcus pneumoniae* in North America: 1997 results from the SENTRY Antimicrobial Surveillance Program. Clin Infect Dis 27:764, 1998

FINE MJ et al: A prediction rule to identify low risk patients with community-acquired pneumonia. N Engl J Med 236:243, 1987

GLEASON PP et al: Associations between initial antimicrobial therapy and the medical outcomes for hospitalized elderly patients with pneumonia. Arch Intern Med 159: 2562, 1999

HAHN DL et al: Association of *Chlamydia pneumoniae* (strain TWAR) infection with wheezing, asthmatic bronchitis and adult-onset asthma. JAMA 266:225, 1991

JACOBS MR: Treatment and diagnosis of infections caused by drug-resistant *Streptococcus pneumoniae*. Clin Infect Dis 15:119, 1992

LEVISON ME, BUSH L: Pharmacodynamics of antimicrobial agents. Bactericidal and postantibiotic effects. Infect Dis Clin North Am 3:415, 1989

——— et al: Clindamycin compared with penicillin for the treatment of anaerobic lung abscess. Ann Intern Med 98:466, 1983

MEEHAN TP et al: Quality of care, process and outcome in elderly patients with pneumonia. JAMA 278:2080, 1997

PALLARES R et al: Resistance to penicillin and cephalosporin and mortality from severe pneumococcal pneumonia in Barcelona, Spain. N Engl J Med 333:474, 1995

RAMIREZ JA et al: Early switch from intravenous to oral cephalosporins in the treatment of hospitalized patients with community-acquired pneumonia. Arch Intern Med 155: 1273, 1995

SANDERS CC, SANDERS WE JR: Clinical significance of inducible β-lactamase in gram-negative bacteria. Eur J Clin Microbiol 6:435, 1987

SHELHAMER JH et al: NIH Conference: Respiratory disease in the immunosuppressed patient. Ann Intern Med 117:415, 1992

STEINHOFF D et al: *Chlamydia pneumoniae* as a cause of community-acquired pneumonia in hospitalized patients in Berlin. Clin Infect Dis 22:958, 1996

WOODHEAD MA et al: Prospective study of the aetiology and outcome of pneumonia in the community. Lancet 1:671, 1987

256

Steven E. Weinberger

BRONCHIECTASIS

DEFINITION Bronchiectasis is an abnormal and permanent dilatation of bronchi. It may be either focal, involving airways supplying a limited region of pulmonary parenchyma, or diffuse, involving airways in a more widespread distribution. Although this definition is based on pathologic changes in the bronchi, diagnosis is often suggested by the clinical consequences of chronic or recurrent infection in the dilated airways and the associated secretions that pool within these airways.

PATHOLOGY The bronchial dilatation of bronchiectasis is associated with destructive and inflammatory changes in the walls of medium-sized airways, often at the level of segmental or subsegmental bronchi. The normal structural components of the wall, including cartilage, muscle, and elastic tissue, are destroyed and may be replaced by fibrous tissue. The dilated airways frequently contain pools of thick, purulent material, while more peripheral airways are often occluded by secretions or obliterated and replaced by fibrous tissue. Additional microscopic features include bronchial and peribronchial inflammation and fibrosis, ulceration of the bronchial wall, squamous metaplasia, and mucous gland hyperplasia. The parenchyma normally supplied by the affected airways is abnormal, containing varying combinations of fibrosis, emphysema, bronchopneumonia, and atelectasis. As a result of the inflammation, vascularity of the bronchial wall increases, with associated enlargement of the bronchial arteries and anastomoses between the bronchial and pulmonary arterial circulations.

Three different patterns of bronchiectasis were described by Reid in 1950. In *cylindrical bronchiectasis* the bronchi appear as uniformly dilated tubes that end abruptly at the point that smaller airways are obstructed by secretions. In *varicose bronchiectasis* the affected bronchi have an irregular or beaded pattern of dilatation resembling varicose veins. In *saccular (cystic) bronchiectasis* the bronchi have a ballooned appearance at the periphery, ending in blind sacs without recognizable bronchial structures distal to the sacs.

ETIOLOGY AND PATHOGENESIS Bronchiectasis is a consequence of inflammation and destruction of the structural components of the bronchial wall. Infection is the usual cause of the inflammation; microorganisms such as *Pseudomonas aeruginosa* and *Haemophilus influenzae* produce pigments, proteases, and other toxins that injure the respiratory epithelium and impair mucociliary clearance. The host inflammatory response induces epithelial injury, largely as a result of mediators released from neutrophils. As protection against infection is compromised, the dilated airways become more susceptible to colonization and growth of bacteria. Thus, a reinforcing cycle can result, with inflammation producing airway damage, impaired clearance of microorganisms, and further infection, which then completes the cycle by inciting more inflammation.

Infectious Causes Adenovirus and influenza virus are the main viruses that cause bronchiectasis in association with lower respiratory tract involvement. Virulent bacterial infections, especially with potentially necrotizing organisms such as *Staphylococcus aureus*, *Kleb-*

siella, and anaerobes, remain important causes of bronchiectasis when antibiotic treatment of a pneumonia is not given or is significantly delayed. Bronchiectasis has been reported in patients with HIV infection, perhaps at least partly due to recurrent bacterial infection. Tuberculosis can produce bronchiectasis by a necrotizing effect on pulmonary parenchyma and airways and indirectly as a consequence of airway obstruction from bronchostenosis or extrinsic compression by lymph nodes. Nontuberculous mycobacteria are frequently cultured from patients with bronchiectasis, often as secondary infections or colonizing organisms. However, it has now also been recognized that these organisms, especially those of the *Mycobacterium avium* complex, can serve as primary pathogens associated with the development and/or progression of bronchiectasis. Mycoplasmal and necrotizing fungal infections are rare causes of bronchiectasis.

Impaired host defense mechanisms are often involved in the predisposition to recurrent infections. The major cause of localized impairment of host defenses is endobronchial obstruction. Bacteria and secretions cannot be cleared adequately from the obstructed airway, which develops recurrent or chronic infection. Slowly growing endobronchial neoplasms such as carcinoid tumors may be associated with bronchiectasis. Foreign-body aspiration is another important cause of endobronchial obstruction, particularly in children. Airway obstruction can also result from bronchostenosis, from impacted secretions, or from extrinsic compression by enlarged lymph nodes.

Generalized impairment of pulmonary defense mechanisms occurs with immunoglobulin deficiency, primary ciliary disorders, or cystic fibrosis. Infections and bronchiectasis are therefore often more diffuse. With panhypogammaglobulinemia, the best described of the immunoglobulin disorders associated with recurrent infection and bronchiectasis, patients often also have a history of sinus or skin infections. Selective deficiency of an IgG subclass, especially IgG2, has also been described in a small number of patients with bronchiectasis.

The primary disorders associated with ciliary dysfunction, termed *primary ciliary dyskinesia*, are responsible for 5 to 10% of cases of bronchiectasis. Numerous defects are encompassed under this category, including structural abnormalities of the dynein arms, radial spokes, and microtubules. The cilia become dyskinetic; their coordinated, propulsive action is diminished, and bacterial clearance is impaired. The clinical effects include recurrent upper and lower respiratory tract infections, such as sinusitis, otitis media, and bronchiectasis. Because normal sperm motility also depends on proper ciliary function, males are generally infertile (Chap. 335). Approximately half of patients with primary ciliary dyskinesia fall into the subgroup of *Kartagener's syndrome*, in which situs inversus accompanies bronchiectasis and sinusitis.

In cystic fibrosis (Chap. 257), the tenacious secretions in the bronchi are associated with impaired bacterial clearance, resulting in colonization and recurrent infection with a variety of organisms, particularly mucoid strains of *P. aeruginosa* but also *S. aureus*, *H. influenzae*, *Escherichia coli*, and *Burkholderia cepacia*.

Noninfectious Causes Some cases of bronchiectasis are associated with exposure to a toxic substance that incites a severe inflammatory response. Examples include inhalation of a toxic gas such as ammonia or aspiration of acidic gastric contents, though the latter problem is often also complicated by aspiration of bacteria. An immune response in the airway may also trigger inflammation, destructive changes, and bronchial dilatation. This mechanism is presumably responsible at least in part for bronchiectasis with allergic bronchopulmonary aspergillosis (ABPA), which is due to an immune response to *Aspergillus* organisms that have colonized the airway (Chap. 253). Bronchiectasis accompanying ABPA often involves proximal airways and is associated with mucoid impaction. Bronchiectasis also occurs rarely in ulcerative colitis, rheumatoid arthritis, and Sjögren's syndrome, but it is not known whether an immune response triggers airway inflammation in these patients.

In α_1-antitrypsin deficiency, the usual respiratory complication is the early development of panacinar emphysema, but affected individuals may occasionally have bronchiectasis. In the *yellow nail syndrome*, which is due to hypoplastic lymphatics, the triad of lymphedema, pleural effusion, and yellow discoloration of the nails is accompanied by bronchiectasis in approximately 40% of patients.

CLINICAL MANIFESTATIONS Patients typically present with persistent or recurrent cough and purulent sputum production. Hemoptysis occurs in 50 to 70% of cases and can be due to bleeding from friable, inflamed airway mucosa. More significant, even massive bleeding is often a consequence of bleeding from hypertrophied bronchial arteries.

When a specific infectious episode initiates bronchiectasis, patients may describe a severe pneumonia followed by chronic cough and sputum production. Alternatively, patients without a dramatic initiating event often describe the insidious onset of symptoms. In some cases, patients are either asymptomatic or have a nonproductive cough, often associated with "dry" bronchiectasis in an upper lobe. Dyspnea or wheezing generally reflects either widespread bronchiectasis or underlying chronic obstructive pulmonary disease. With exacerbations of infection, the amount of sputum increases, it becomes more purulent and often more bloody, and patients may become febrile. Such episodes may be due solely to exacerbations of the airway infection, but associated parenchymal infiltrates sometimes reflect an adjacent pneumonia.

Physical examination of the chest overlying an area of bronchiectasis is quite variable. Any combination of crackles, rhonchi, and wheezes may be heard, all of which reflect the damaged airways containing significant secretions. As with other types of chronic intrathoracic infection, clubbing may be present. Patients with severe, diffuse disease, particularly those with chronic hypoxemia, may have associated cor pulmonale and right ventricular failure. Amyloidosis can result from chronic infection and inflammation but is now seldom seen.

RADIOGRAPHIC AND LABORATORY FINDINGS Though the chest radiograph is important in the evaluation of suspected bronchiectasis, the findings are often nonspecific. At one extreme, the radiograph may be normal with mild disease. Alternatively, patients with saccular bronchiectasis may have prominent cystic spaces, either with or without air-liquid levels, corresponding to the dilated airways. These may be difficult to distinguish from enlarged airspaces due to bullous emphysema or from regions of honeycombing in patients with severe interstitial lung disease. Other findings are due to dilated airways with thickened walls, which result from peribronchial inflammation. Because of decreased aeration and atelectasis of the associated pulmonary parenchyma, these dilated airways are often crowded together in parallel. When seen longitudinally, the airways appear as "tram tracks"; when seen in cross-section, they produce "ring shadows." Because the dilated airways may be filled with secretions, the lumen may appear dense rather than radiolucent, producing an opaque tubular or branched tubular structure.

Bronchography, which involves coating the airways with a radiopaque, iodinated lipid dye instilled through a catheter or bronchoscope, can provide excellent visualization of bronchiectatic airways. However, this technique has now been replaced by computed tomography (CT), which also provides an excellent view of dilated airways as seen in cross-sectional images (Fig. 256-1). With the advent of high-resolution CT scanning, in which the images are 1.0 to 1.5 mm thick, the sensitivity for detecting bronchiectasis has improved even further. Other features on high-resolution CT scanning can suggest a specific etiology of the bronchiectasis. For example, bronchiectasis of relatively proximal airways suggests ABPA, whereas the presence of multiple small pulmonary nodules (nodular bronchiectasis) suggests infection with *M. avium* complex.

Examination of sputum often reveals an abundance of neutrophils and colonization or infection with a variety of possible organisms. Appropriate staining and culturing of sputum often provide a guide to antibiotic therapy.

Additional evaluation is aimed at diagnosing the cause for the bronchiectasis. When bronchiectasis is focal, fiberoptic bronchoscopy

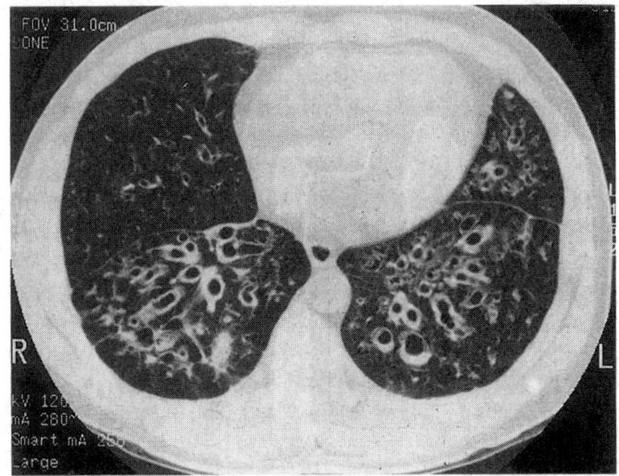

FIGURE 256-1 High-resolution CT scan of bronchiectasis showing dilated airways in both lower lobes and in the lingula. When seen in cross section, the dilated airways have a ringlike appearance. *(From Weinberger, with permission).*

may reveal an underlying endobronchial obstruction. In other cases, upper lobe involvement may be suggestive of either tuberculosis or ABPA. With more widespread disease, measurement of sweat chloride levels for cystic fibrosis, structural or functional assessment of nasal or bronchial cilia or sperm for primary ciliary dyskinesia, and quantitative assessment of immunoglobulins may explain recurrent airway infection. In an asthmatic person with proximal bronchiectasis or other historical features to suggest ABPA, skin testing, serology, and sputum culture for *Aspergillus* are helpful in confirming the diagnosis.

Pulmonary function tests may demonstrate airflow obstruction as a consequence of diffuse bronchiectasis or associated chronic obstructive lung disease. Bronchial hyperreactivity, e.g., to methacholine challenge, and some reversibility of the airflow obstruction with inhaled bronchodilators are relatively common.

℞ TREATMENT Therapy has four major goals: (1) elimination of an identifiable underlying problem; (2) improved clearance of tracheobronchial secretions; (3) control of infection, particularly during acute exacerbations; and (4) reversal of airflow obstruction. Appropriate treatment should be instituted when a treatable cause is found, for example, treatment of hypogammaglobulinemia with immunoglobulin replacement, tuberculosis with antituberculous agents, and ABPA with glucocorticoids.

Secretions are typically copious and thick and contribute to the symptoms. Chest physical therapy with vibration, percussion, and postural drainage frequently helps patients with copious secretions. Mucolytic agents to thin secretions and allow better clearance are controversial. Aerosolized recombinant DNase, which decreases viscosity of sputum by breaking down DNA released from neutrophils, has been shown to improve pulmonary function in cystic fibrosis, but similar benefits have not been found with bronchiectasis due to other etiologies.

Antibiotics have an important role in management. For patients with infrequent exacerbations characterized by an increase in quantity and purulence of the sputum, antibiotics are commonly used only during acute episodes. Although choice of an antibiotic may be guided by Gram's stain and culture of sputum, empiric coverage (e.g., with ampicillin, amoxicillin, trimethoprim-sulfamethoxazole, or cefaclor) is often given initially. When *P. aeruginosa* is present, oral therapy with a quinolone or parenteral therapy with an aminoglycoside or third-generation cephalosporin may be appropriate. In patients with chronic purulent sputum despite short courses of antibiotics, more prolonged courses, e.g., with oral amoxicillin or inhaled aminoglycosides, or intermittent but regular courses of single or rotating antibiotics have been used.

Bronchodilators to improve obstruction and aid clearance of secretions are particularly useful in patients with airway hyperreactivity and reversible airflow obstruction. Although surgical therapy was common in the past, more effective antibiotic and supportive therapy has largely replaced surgery. However, when bronchiectasis is localized and the morbidity is substantial despite adequate medical therapy, surgical resection of the involved region of lung should be considered.

When massive hemoptysis, often originating from the hypertrophied bronchial circulation, does not resolve with conservative therapy, including rest and antibiotics, therapeutic options are either surgical resection or bronchial arterial embolization (Chap. 33). Although resection may be successful if disease is localized, embolization is preferable with widespread disease. In patients with extensive disease, chronic hypoxemia and cor pulmonale may indicate the need for long-term supplemental oxygen. For selected patients who are disabled despite maximal therapy, lung transplantation is a therapeutic option.

BIBLIOGRAPHY

AFZELIUS BA: Immotile cilia syndrome: Past, present, and prospects for the future. Thorax 53:894, 1998

JONES A, ROWE BH: Bronchopulmonary hygiene physical therapy in bronchiectasis and chronic obstructive pulmonary disease: a systemic review. Heart & Lung 29:125, 2000

KANG EY et al: Bronchiectasis: Comparison of preoperative thin-section CT and pathologic findings in resected specimens. Radiology 195:649, 1995

KING MA et al: Bronchial dilatation in patients with HIV infection: CT assessment and correlation with pulmonary function tests and findings at bronchoalveolar lavage. AJR Am J Roentgenol 168:1535, 1997

LUCE JM: Bronchiectasis, in *Textbook of Respiratory Medicine*, 3[d] ed, JF Murray, JA Nadel (eds). Philadelphia, Saunders, 2000, pp 1325–1342

NICOTRA MB et al: Clinical, pathophysiologic, and microbiologic characterization of bronchiectasis in an aging cohort. Chest 108:955, 1995

WALLACE RJ JR et al: Polyclonal *Mycobacterium avium* complex infections in patients with nodular bronchiectasis. Am J Respir Crit Care Med 158:1235, 1998

WEINBERGER SE: *Principles of Pulmonary Medicine*, 3d ed. Philadelphia, Saunders, 1998

257 CYSTIC FIBROSIS

Richard C. Boucher

Cystic fibrosis (CF) is a monogenetic disorder that presents as a multisystem disease. The first signs and symptoms typically occur in childhood, but about 7% of patients in the United States are diagnosed as adults. Due to improvements in therapy, more than 36% of patients are now adults ≥18 years of age and 12% are past the age of 30. The median survival is over 32 years for males and 29 years for females with CF. Thus, CF is no longer only a pediatric disease, and internists must be prepared to recognize and treat its many complications. This disease is characterized by chronic airways infection that ultimately leads to bronchiectasis and bronchiolectasis, exocrine pancreatic insufficiency and intestinal dysfunction, abnormal sweat gland function, and urogenital dysfunction.

PATHOGENESIS

GENETIC CONSIDERATIONS CF is an autosomal recessive disease resulting from mutations in a gene located on chromosome 7. The prevalence of CF varies with the ethnic origin of a population. CF is detected in approximately 1 in 3000 live births in the Caucasian population of North America and northern Europe, 1 in 17,000 live births of African-Americans, and 1 in 90,000 live births of the Asian population of Hawaii. The most common mutation in the CF gene (~70% of CF chromosomes) is a 3-bp deletion that results in an absence of phenylalanine at amino acid position 508 (ΔF_{508}) of the CF gene protein product, known as the CF transmembrane regulator (CFTR). The large number (>800) of relatively uncommon (<2%) mutations identified in the CF gene makes it difficult to use DNA diagnostic technologies for identifying heterozygotes in populations at large, and no simple physiologic measurements allow heterozygote detection. ■

CFTR PROTEIN The CFTR protein is a single polypeptide chain containing 1480 amino acids that appears to function both as a cyclic AMP–regulated Cl^- channel and, as its name implies, a regulator of other ion channels. The fully processed form of CFTR is found in the plasma membrane in normal epithelia (Fig. 257-1). Biochemical studies indicate that the ΔF_{508} mutation leads to improper processing and intracellular degradation of the CFTR protein. Thus, absence of CFTR at appropriate cellular sites is often part of the pathophysiology of CF. However, other mutations in the CF gene produce CFTR proteins that are fully processed but are nonfunctional or only partially functional at the appropriate cellular sites.

EPITHELIAL DYSFUNCTION The epithelia affected by CF exhibit different functions in their native state; i.e., some are volume-absorbing (airways and distal intestinal epithelia), some are salt-absorbing but not volume absorbing (sweat duct), and others are volume-secretory (proximal intestine and pancreas). Given this diverse array of native activities, it should not be surprising that CF produces very different effects on patterns of electrolyte and water transport. However, the unifying concept is that all affected tissues express abnormal ion transport function.

ORGAN-SPECIFIC PATHOPHYSIOLOGY **Lung** The diagnostic biophysical hallmark of CF is the raised transepithelial electric potential difference (PD) detected in airway epithelia. The transepithelial PD reflects components of both the rate of active ion transport and the resistance to ion flow of the superficial epithelium. CF airway epithelia exhibit both raised transport rates (Na^+) and decreased Cl^- permeability (Fig. 257-2). The Cl^- permeability defect reflects at least in part the absence of cyclic AMP–dependent kinase and protein kinase C–regulated Cl^- transport that is mediated by the Cl^- channel functions of CFTR. An important observation is that there is an alternative Cl^- channel expressed in airway epithelia. This "alternative" Cl^- channel (Cl_a^-) is different from CFTR and is regulated by intracellular Ca^{2+} levels. This channel can substitute for CFTR with regard to net Cl^- transport and may be a potential therapeutic target.

Raised Na^+ absorption is a routine feature of CF airway epithelia. Na^+ transport abnormalities in CF are not a widespread feature of the CF epithelial phenotype and appear confined to volume-absorbing epithelia. Recent studies demonstrate that the increased Na^+ transport reflects the absence of CFTR's tonic inhibitory regulatory function on Na^+ channel activity. It appears that CFTR inhibits Na^+ channel activity as a part of its general function to act as a "switch" that coordinates the balance between Na^+ absorption and Cl^- secretion.

The central hypothesis of CF airways pathophysiology has been that an abnormally high rate of Na^+ absorption and low rate of Cl^- secretion reduce the salt and water content of mucus and deplete the volume of the perciliary liquid (PCL). Both the thickening of mucins and the depletion of the PCL lead to a failure to clear mucus normally from the airways by either ciliary or airflow-dependent (cough) mechanisms. An alternative hypothesis suggests that the central defect in CF airways is raised salt concentration in secretions that inhibits the function of antimicrobial substances. Direct measurements of salt concentration *in vivo* have, however, provided no evidence that there are differences in salt concentration in CF versus normal airway secretions.

The unique predisposition of CF airways to chronic infection by *Staphylococcus aureus* and *Pseudomonas aeruginosa* raises the issue that other as yet undefined abnormalities in airway surface liquids also may contribute to the failure of lung defense. However, it may be that *Pseudomonas* is selected by its propensity to grow in biofilm

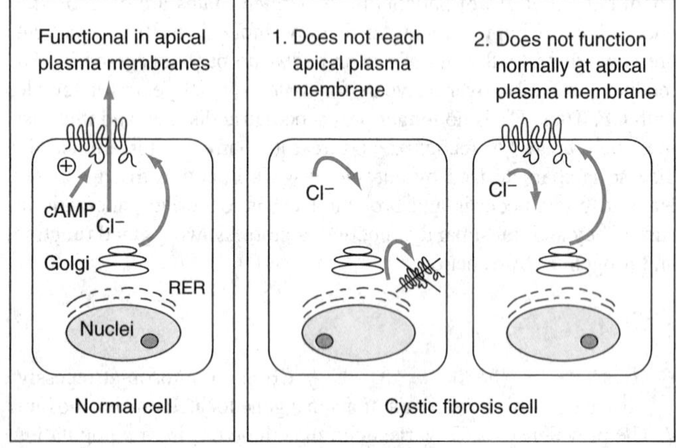

FIGURE 257-1 Cellular metabolism of the CFTR protein. In a normal cell (*left*), CFTR is synthesized in the rough endoplasmic reticulum (RER), is glycosylated in the Golgi apparatus, and functions as a Cl^- channel and regulator of other ion channels when located in the plasma membrane. Two possible outcomes of mutations in the CF gene are shown (*right*). (1) If a mutation disturbs protein folding, e.g., the ΔF_{508} mutation, CFTR is degraded intracellularly so that no protein is transported to the plasma membrane. (2) With other mutations, the abnormal protein is processed and trafficks to the plasma membrane but functions abnormally at that site.

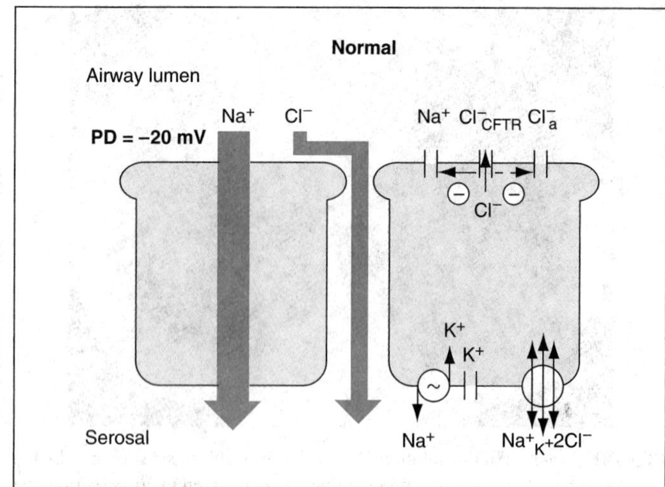

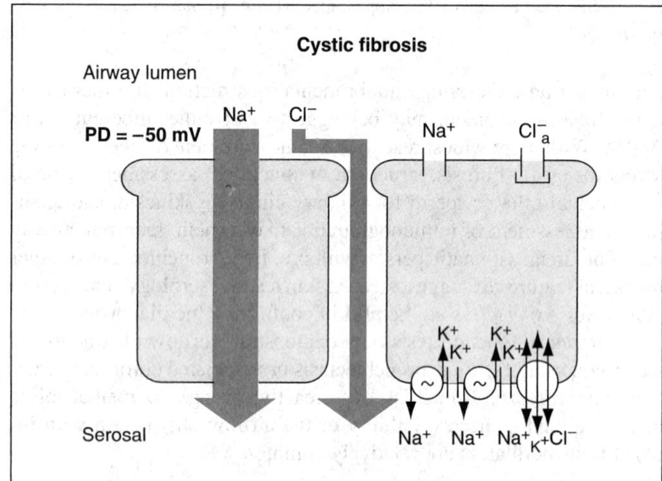

FIGURE 257-2 Comparison of ion transport properties of normal (*top*) and CF (*bottom*) airway epithelia. The vectors describe routes and magnitudes of Na^+ and Cl^- transport. The normal basal pattern for ion transport is absorption of Na^+ from the lumen via an amiloride-sensitive Na^+ channel. This process is accelerated in CF. The capacity to initiate cyclic AMP–mediated Cl^- secretion is diminished in CF airway epithelia due to absence/dysfunction of the CFTR Cl^- channel. The accelerated Na^+ absorption in CF reflects the absence of CFTR inhibitory effects on Na^+ channels. Cl_a^-, alternative Cl^- channel; PD, potential difference; CFTR, cystic fibrosis transmembrane regulator.

colonies on the surfaces of thickened, retained mucus plaques in CF airways.

Gastrointestinal Tract The gastrointestinal effects of CF are diverse. In the exocrine pancreas, the absence of the CFTR Cl^- channel in the apical membrane of pancreatic ductal epithelia limits the function of an apical membrane Cl^--HCO_3^- exchanger to secrete HCO_3^- and Na^+ (by a passive process) into the duct. The failure to secrete Na^+-HCO_3^- and water leads to retention of enzymes in the pancreas and ultimately destruction of virtually all pancreatic tissue. The CF intestinal epithelium, because of the lack of Cl^- and water secretion, fails to flush the secreted mucins and other macromolecules from intestinal crypts. The diminished CFTR-mediated secretion of liquid may be exacerbated by excessive absorption of liquid in the distal intestine, reflecting abnormalities of CFTR-mediated regulation of Na^+ absorption (both mediated by Na^+ channels and possibly other Na^+ transporters, e.g., Na^+-H^+ exchangers). Both dysfunctions lead to dessicated intraluminal contents and obstruction of both the small and large intestines. In the hepatobiliary system, defective hepatic ductal Cl^- and water secretion causes retention of biliary secretions and focal biliary cirrhosis and bile duct proliferation in approximately 25 to 30% of patients with CF. The inability of the CF gallbladder epithelium to secrete salt and water can lead to both chronic cholecystitis and cholelithiasis.

Sweat Gland Patients with CF secrete nearly normal volumes of sweat in the sweat acinus. However, they are not able to absorb NaCl from sweat as it moves through the sweat duct due to the inability to absorb Cl^- across the ductal epithelial cells.

CLINICAL FEATURES

Most patients with CF present with signs and symptoms of the disease in childhood. Approximately 15% of patients present within the first 24 h of life with gastrointestinal obstruction, termed *meconium ileus*. Other common presentations within the first year or two of life include respiratory tract symptoms, most prominently cough and/or recurrent pulmonary infiltrates, and failure to thrive. A significant proportion of patients (~7%), however, are diagnosed after age 18.

RESPIRATORY TRACT Upper respiratory tract disease is almost universal in patients with CF. Chronic sinusitis is common in childhood and leads to nasal obstruction and rhinorrhea. The occurrence of nasal polyps approaches 25% and often requires surgery.

In the lower respiratory tract, the first symptom of CF is cough. With time, the cough becomes persistent and produces viscous, purulent, often greenish colored sputum. Inevitably, periods of clinical stability are interrupted by "exacerbations," defined by increased cough, weight loss, increased sputum volume, and decrements in pulmonary function. These exacerbations require aggressive therapy, including frequent postural drainage and oral antibiotics, and often intravenous antibiotics (see below), with the goal being recovery of lung function. Over the course of years, the exacerbations become more frequent and the recovery of lost lung function incomplete, leading to respiratory failure.

Patients with CF exhibit a characteristic sputum microbiology. *Haemophilus influenzae* and *S. aureus* are often the first organisms recovered from samples of lung secretions in newly diagnosed patients with CF. *P. aeruginosa* is typically cultured from lower respiratory tract secretions thereafter. After repetitive antibiotic exposure, *P. aeruginosa*, often in a mucoid form, is usually the predominant organism recovered from sputum and may be present as several strains with different antibiotic sensitivities. *Burkholderia* (formerly *Pseudomonas*) *cepacia* has been recovered from CF sputum and is pathogenic. Patient-to-patient spread of certain strains of this organism indicates that infection control in the hospital should be practiced. Other gram-negative rods recovered from CF sputum include *Xanthomonas zylosoxida* and *P. gladioli*, and occasionally, mucoid forms of *Proteus*, *Escherichia coli*, and *Klebsiella*. Up to 50% of patients with CF have *Aspergillus fumigatus* in their sputum, and up to 10% of these patients exhibit the syndrome of allergic bronchopulmonary aspergillosis. *Mycobacterium tuberculosis* is rare in patients with CF. However, 10 to 20% of adult patients with CF have sputum cultures positive for nontuberculous mycobacteria, and in some patients these microorganisms are associated with disease.

The first lung function abnormalities observed in children with CF, increased ratios of residual volume to total lung capacity, suggest that small airways disease is the first functional lung abnormality in CF. As the disease progresses, both reversible and irreversible changes in forced vital capacity and forced expiratory volume in 1 s are noted. The reversible component reflects the accumulation of intraluminal secretions and/or airway reactivity, which occurs in 40 to 60% of patients with CF. The irreversible component reflects chronic destruction of the airway wall and bronchiolitis.

The earliest chest x-ray change in CF lungs is hyperinflation, reflecting small airways obstruction. Later, signs of luminal mucus impaction, bronchial cuffing, and finally, bronchiectasis, e.g., ring shadows, are noted. For reasons that are still unknown, the right upper lobe displays the earliest and most severe changes. Neither CT nor MRI scanning is routinely performed on patients with CF.

CF pulmonary disease is associated with many intermittent complications. Pneumothorax is common (>10% of patients). The production of small amounts of blood in sputum is common in CF patients with advanced pulmonary disease and appears to be associated with lung infection. Massive hemoptysis is life-threatening and difficult to localize bronchoscopically. With advanced lung disease, digital clubbing becomes evident in virtually all patients with CF. As late events, respiratory failure and cor pulmonale are prominent features of CF.

GASTROINTESTINAL TRACT The syndrome of meconium ileus in infants presents with abdominal distention, failure to pass stool, and emesis. The abdominal flat plate can be diagnostic with small intestinal air fluid levels, a granular appearance representing meconium, and a small colon. In children and young adults, a syndrome termed *meconium ileus equivalent* or distal intestinal obstruction occurs. The syndrome presents with right lower quadrant pain, loss of appetite, occasional emesis, and often a palpable mass. The syndrome can be confused with appendicitis, which occurs frequently in patients with CF. The characteristic intestinal abnormalities are complicated by exocrine pancreatic insufficiency in more than 90% of patients with CF. Insufficient pancreatic enzyme release yields the typical pattern of protein and fat malabsorption, with frequent, bulky, foul-smelling stools. Signs and symptoms of malabsorption of fat-soluble vitamins, including vitamins E and K, are also noted. Pancreatic beta cells are typically spared, but function decreases with age, causing hyperglycemia and increasing requirements for insulin in older patients with CF.

GENITOURINARY SYSTEM Late onset of puberty is common in both males and females with CF. The delayed maturational pattern is likely secondary to the effects of chronic lung disease and inadequate nutrition on reproductive endocrine function. More than 95% of male patients with CF are azoospermic, reflecting obliteration of the vas deferens that probably reflects defective liquid secretion. Twenty percent of women with CF are infertile due to effects of chronic lung disease on the menstrual cycle; thick, tenacious cervical mucus that blocks sperm migration; and possibly fallopian tube/uterine wall abnormalities in liquid transport. More than 90% of completed pregnancies produce viable infants, and women with CF are generally able to breast-feed infants normally.

DIAGNOSIS

Because of the large number of CF mutations, DNA analysis is not used for primary diagnosis. The primary diagnosis of CF rests on a combination of clinical criteria and analyses of sweat Cl^- values. The values for the Na^+ and Cl^- concentration in sweat vary with age, but typically in adults a Cl^- concentration of >70 mEq/L discriminates between patients with CF and patients with other lung diseases.

DNA analyses are being performed increasingly in patients with CF. Comprehensive genotype-phenotype relationships have not yet been established sufficiently for prognosis. A relationship between ΔF_{508} homozygosity and pancreatic insufficiency has been established, but no predictive relationship holds for ΔF_{508} homozygosity and lung disease.

Between 1 and 2% of patients with the clinical syndrome of CF have normal sweat Cl^- values. In most of these patients, the nasal transepithelial PD is raised into the diagnostic range for CF, and sweat acini do not secrete in response to injected beta-adrenergic agonists. A single mutation of the CFTR gene, 3849 + 10 kb C → T, is associated with approximately 50% of CF patients with normal sweat Cl^- values.

℞ **TREATMENT** The major objectives of therapy for CF are to promote clearance of secretions and control infection in the lung, provide adequate nutrition, and prevent intestinal obstruction. Ultimately, gene therapy may become the treatment of choice.

Lung Disease The principal techniques for clearing pulmonary secretions are breathing exercises, flutter valves, and chest percussion. Regular use of these maneuvers is effective in preserving lung function. There is increasing interest in the use of hypertonic saline (3 to 7%) aerosols to augment the clearance of secretions.

More than 95% of patients with CF die of complications resulting from lung infection. Antibiotics are the principal agents available for treating lung infection, and their use should be guided by sputum culture results. Early intervention with antibiotics is useful, and long courses of treatment are the rule. Because of increased total-body clearance and volume of distribution of antibiotics in patients with CF, the required doses are higher for patients with CF than for patients with similar chest infections who do not have CF.

Increased cough and mucus production are treated with antibiotics given orally. Typical oral agents used to treat *Staphylococcus* include a semisynthetic penicillin or a cephalosporin. Oral ciprofloxacin may reduce pseudomonal bacterial counts and control symptoms. However, its clinical usefulness may be limited by rapid emergence of resistant organisms, and accordingly, courses should be intermittent (2 to 3 weeks) and not chronic. More severe exacerbations, or exacerbations associated with bacteria resistant to oral antibiotics, require intravenous antibiotics. Traditionally, intravenous therapy has been given in the hospital, but outpatient intravenous antibiotic administration has gained widespread acceptance. Usually, two drugs, often one of them an aminoglycoside, are used to treat *P. aeruginosa* to hinder emergence of resistant organisms. Drug dosage should be monitored so that levels for gentamicin or tobramycin peak at ranges of $\sim$10 μg/mL and exhibit troughs of $<$2 μg/mL. Usually, a cephalosporin, e.g., ceftazadime, and/or a penicillin derivative is used as the second drug. Antibiotics directed at *Staphylococcus* and/or *H. influenzae* are added depending on the results of the culture. Aerosolization of antibiotics also may have an important role in treating CF lung infection. Large doses of aminoglycosides, e.g., 600 mg tobramycin twice daily, via aerosol may be effective at delaying exacerbations. Aerosol administration also permits the use of other drugs, e.g., colistin, that are relatively ineffective by the intravenous route.

A number of pharmacologic agents for promoting mucus clearance are in use. *N*-acetyl-cysteine, which solubilizes mucus glycoproteins, has not been shown to have clinically significant effects on mucus clearance and/or lung function. Recombinant human DNAse, however, degrades the concentrated DNA in CF sputum, decreases sputum viscosity, and increases airflow during short-term administration. Long-term (6 months) DNAse treatment increases the time between pulmonary exacerbations. Most patients receive a therapeutic trial of DNAse to test for efficacy, and a sizeable minority appear to demonstrate persistent objective benefits. Clinical trials of experimental drugs aimed at restoring salt and water content of secretions are underway. The most promising may be long-acting nucleotide (UTP)-based compounds that appear active in inducing liquid secretion in CF airways.

Inhaled β-adrenergic agonists can be useful to control airways constriction. They achieve a short-term increase in airflow, but long-term benefit has not been shown. Inhaled anticholinergics provide an alternative. Oral steroids are not first-line agents for controlling airways constriction and are of no use in improving the nonreversible component of lung function. Steroids may be useful for treating allergic bronchopulmonary aspergillosis.

The chronic damage to airway walls reflects to some extent the destructive activities of inflammatory enzymes generated in part by inflammatory cells. To date, specific therapies with antiproteases have not been successfully developed. However, a subset of adolescents with CF appears to benefit from long-term, high-dose non-steroidal (ibuprofen) therapy.

A number of pulmonary complications require acute interventions. Atelectasis is best treated with chest physiotherapy and antibiotic therapy. Pneumothoraces involving 10% or less of the lung can be observed without intervention. The use of chest tubes to expand collapsed, diseased lung often requires long periods of time, and sclerosing agents should be used with caution because of possible limitations for subsequent lung transplantation. Small-volume hemoptysis requires no specific therapy other than treatment of lung infection and assessment of coagulation and vitamin K status. If massive hemoptysis occurs, bronchial artery embolization can be successful. The most ominous complications of CF are respiratory failure and cor pulmonale. The most effective conventional therapy for these conditions is vigorous medical management of the lung disease and O_2 supplementation. Noninvasive positive pressure ventilation through a face mask may be an effective adjunctive therapy. Ultimately, the only effective treatment for respiratory failure in CF is lung transplantation (Chap. 267). The 2-year survival for lung transplantation exceeds 60%, and deaths in transplant patients result principally from graft rejection, often involving obliterative bronchiolitis. The transplanted lungs do not develop a CF-specific phenotype.

Gastrointestinal Disease Maintenance of adequate nutrition is critical for the health of the patient with CF. Most ($>$90%) of patients with CF benefit from pancreatic enzyme replacement. Capsules generally contain between 4000 and 29,000 units of lipase. The dose of enzymes (typically no more than 20,000 units/kg per meal) should be adjusted on the basis of weight gain, abdominal symptomatology, and character of stools. Replacement of fat-soluble vitamins, particularly vitamins E and K, is usually required. Hyperglycemia most often becomes manifest in the adult and typically requires insulin treatment.

For treatment of acute obstruction due to meconium ileus equivalent, megalodiatrizoate or other hypertonic radiocontrast materials delivered by enema to the terminal ileum are utilized. For control of symptoms, adjustment of pancreatic enzymes and the supplementation of intake by salt solutions containing osmotically active agents, e.g., propyleneglycol or lactulose, are utilized. Persistent symptoms may indicate a diagnosis of gastrointestinal malignancy, which is increased in incidence in patients with CF. Hepatic and gallbladder complications are treated as for patients without CF. End-stage liver disease can be treated by transplantation, which has a 2-year survival rate exceeding 50%.

Psychosocial Factors CF imposes a tremendous burden on patients. Health insurance, career options, family planning, and life expectancy become major issues. Thus, assisting patients with the psychosocial adjustments required by CF is critical.

BIBLIOGRAPHY

BEAR CE et al: Purification and functional reconstitution of the cystic fibrosis transmembrane conductance regulator (CFTR). Cell 68:809, 1992

BOUCHER RC et al: Cystic fibrosis, in *Textbook of Respiratory Medicine*, 3[d] ed, JF Murray, JA Nadel (eds). Philadelphia, Saunders, 2000, pp 1291–1324

CHENG SH et al: Defective intracellular transport and processing of CFTR is the molecular basis of most cystic fibrosis. Cell 63:827, 1990

DINWIDDIE R: Pathogenesis of lung disease in cystic fibrosis. Respiration 67:3, 2000

DRUMM M: What happens to DeltaF508 *in vivo*? J Clin Invest 103:1369, 1999

FITZSIMMONS SC: *CFF Patient Registry. 1997 Annual Report.* Bethesda, MD, Cystic Fibrosis Foundation, 1998

HIGHSMITH WE et al: A novel mutation in the cystic fibrosis gene in patients with pulmonary disease but normal sweat chloride concentrations. N Engl J Med 331:974, 1994

HULL J et al: Elemental content of airway surface liquid from infants with cystic fibrosis. Am J Respir Crit Care Med 157:10, 1998

KNOWLES MR et al: Ion compositon of airway surface liquid of patients with cystic fibrosis as compared to normal and disease-control subjects. J Clin Invest 100:2588, 1997

KONSTAN MW, BERGER M: Current understanding of the inflammatory process in cystic fibrosis: Onset and etiology. Pediatr Pulmonol 24:137, 1997

——— et al: Effect of high-dose ibuprofen in patients with cystic fibrosis. N Engl J Med 332:848, 1995

MATSUI H et al: Evidence for perciliary liquid layer depletion, not abnormal ion composition, in the pathogenesis of cystic fibrosis airways disease. Cell 95:1005, 1998

O'LOUGHLIN EV et al: Abnormal epithelial transport in cystic fibrosis jejunum. Am J Physiol 260:G758, 1991

RAMSEY BW et al: Efficacy of aerosolized tobramycin in patients with cystic fibrosis. N Engl J Med 328:1740, 1993

SMITH JJ et al: Cystic fibrosis airway epithelia fail to kill bacteria because of abnormal airway surface fluid. Cell 85:229, 1996

ZIELENSKI J, TSUI LC: Cystic fibrosis: Genotypic and phenotypic variations. Annu Rev Genet 29:777, 1995

258

Eric G. Honig, Roland H. Ingram, Jr.

CHRONIC BRONCHITIS, EMPHYSEMA, AND AIRWAYS OBSTRUCTION

DEFINITION Chronic obstructive pulmonary disease (COPD) is the name of a group of chronic and slowly progressive respiratory disorders characterized by reduced maximal expiratory flow during forced exhalation. Most of the airflow obstruction is fixed, but a variable degree of reversibility and bronchial hyperreactivity may be seen. COPD may coexist with asthma and, when abnormal airway reactivity is present, differentiation between these disorders can be challenging. COPD comprises emphysema and chronic bronchitis, two distinct processes, although most often present in combination. The definition excludes other causes of chronic airflow obstruction such as cystic fibrosis (Chap. 257), bronchiolitis obliterans (Chap. 259), and bronchiectasis (Chap. 256).

Emphysema is defined anatomically as a permanent and destructive enlargement of airspaces distal to the terminal bronchioles without obvious fibrosis and with loss of normal architecture. *Chronic bronchitis* is defined clinically as the presence of a cough productive of sputum not attributable to other causes on most days for at least 3 months over 2 consecutive years. Chronic bronchitis may be present in the absence of airflow limitation, but COPD always involves clinically significant airflow limitation.

EPIDEMIOLOGY COPD is a common medical problem affecting an estimated 16 million Americans. Males are more frequently affected than females, and Caucasians more frequently than African Americans. There is a higher prevalence of COPD among persons with a lower socioeconomic status and in those with a history of low birth weight. COPD is the fourth leading cause of death in the United States and is the only one of the 10 leading causes of death for which mortality rates are still rising. Prevalence peaks in the seventh and eighth decades, then levels off, largely due to mortality.

DISEASE MECHANISMS

PATHOGENESIS COPD evolves from an inflammatory process involving the airways and distal airspaces. Increased activity of

oxidants combined with decreased activity of antioxidants, termed *oxidative stress*, have been implicated in the development of inflammation and COPD. Cigarette smoke produces high concentrations of oxygen free radicals including superoxide, hydrogen peroxide, and hypochlorous acid. Cigarette smoke is an independent source of Fe^{2+}, releases Fe^{2+} from ferritin, and catalyzes the formation of the highly active hydroxyl radical from O_2^- and H_2O_2 by eosinophils, neutrophils, and alveolar macrophages. Cigarette tar contains nitric oxide and induces nitric oxide synthase. In the presence of oxidants, NO is metabolized to cytotoxic peroxynitrates. In order for elastase to degrade elastin, α_1 antitrypsin (α_1AT) must be inactivated. Cigarette smoke, oxidants, activated neutrophils, and type II alveolar pneumocytes are all capable of inactivating α_1AT as well as matrix metalloproteinase inhibitors. Oxidant stress is also capable of inducing mucus hypersecretion. Cigarette smoke also acts as a chemoattractant and upregulates adhesion molecules. Smoke increases neutrophil transit time through the pulmonary circulation, increases adhesion, and decreases deformability. Smoke and elastase both increase the expression of the proinflammatory nuclear transcription factor κB (NfκB) as well as interleukin 8, a chemokine found to be elevated in COPD patients, that recruits neutrophils, basophils, eosinophils, and T lymphocytes.

The submucosa of the small airway in patients with COPD has increased numbers of CD8 lymphocytes and eosinophils, macrophages, and mast cells. Neutrophils are increased in smokers, but their numbers do not correlate with the presence of airflow obstruction. Patients with chronic airflow obstruction show higher levels of myeloperoxidase and eosinophilic cationic protein than do patients with normal airflow. Macrophages and mast cells produce transforming growth factor β (TGF-β), a peptide related to fibrogenesis. Patients with chronic airflow obstruction show a twofold elevation of TGF-β in lavage liquid; the amount of TGF-β shows a significant negative correlation with FEV_1 (the forced expiratory volume in 1 s). Smoke also leads to lipid peroxidation and to DNA damage. Widespread point mutations of the p53 gene locus have been identified in patients with lung cancer and precancerous dysplasia. These may predispose to the development of lung cancer.

RISK FACTORS COPD is characterized by a reduced FEV_1 and an accelerated rate of decline of FEV_1. The reduction in FEV_1 can occur by any of three pathways: (1) impaired childhood growth and development, with a lower peak in early adulthood and a normal rate of decline with aging (e.g., early childhood infection and passive smoke exposure); (2) normal growth and development with a premature peak but normal subsequent decline (e.g., asthma and passive smoking); and (3) normal growth and development and peak with accelerated decline (e.g., active smoking and, to a lesser degree, environmental exposures).

Smoking Cigarette smoking is the most commonly identified correlate with both chronic bronchitis during life and extent of emphysema at postmortem. The prevalence of COPD shows a dose-response relationship with the number of pack-years of tobacco consumed. Some 90% of all COPD patients are current or former tobacco smokers. Experimental studies have shown that prolonged cigarette smoking impairs respiratory epithelial ciliary movement, inhibits function of alveolar macrophages, and leads to hypertrophy and hyperplasia of mucus-secreting glands; massive exposure in dogs can produce emphysematous changes. Cigarette smoke also inhibits antiproteases and causes polymorphonuclear leukocytes to release proteolytic enzymes acutely. Cigarette smoke can produce an acute increase in airways resistance due to vagally mediated smooth-muscle constriction by stimulating submucosal irritant receptors. Increased airways responsiveness is associated with more rapid progression in patients with chronic airways obstruction. Obstruction of small airways is the earliest demonstrable mechanical defect in young cigarette smokers and may disappear completely after cessation of smoking.

Although smoking cessation does not result in complete reversal of more pronounced obstruction, there is a significant slowing of the decline in lung function in all smokers who give up cigarettes. Passive exposure to tobacco smoke correlates with respiratory symptoms such as cough, wheeze, and sputum production. Not only is cigarette smoking the most common single factor leading to chronic airways obstruction, it also adds to the effects of every other contributory factor to be discussed below.

Air Pollution The incidence and mortality rates of both chronic bronchitis and emphysema may be higher in heavily industrialized urban areas. Exacerbations of bronchitis are clearly related to periods of heavy pollution with sulfur dioxide (SO_2) and particulate matter. While nitrogen dioxide (NO_2) can produce small-airways obstruction (bronchiolitis) in experimental animals exposed to high concentrations, there are no data convincingly implicating NO_2, at even the highest pollutant levels, in the pathogenesis or worsening of airways obstruction in humans (Chap. 254).

Occupation Chronic bronchitis is more prevalent in workers who engage in occupations exposing them to either inorganic or organic dusts or to noxious gases. Epidemiologic surveys have succeeded in demonstrating an accelerated decline in lung function in many such workers—e.g., workers in plastics plants exposed to toluene diisocyanate, and carding room workers in cotton mills (Chap. 254)—suggesting that their occupational exposure contributes to their future disability.

Infection Morbidity, mortality, and frequency of acute respiratory illnesses are higher in patients with chronic bronchitis. Many attempts have been made to relate these illnesses to infection with viruses, mycoplasmas, and bacteria. However, only the rhinovirus is found more often during exacerbations; that is to say, pathogenic bacteria, mycoplasmas, and viruses other than rhinovirus are found just as often between as during exacerbations. Epidemiologic studies, however, implicate acute respiratory illness as one of the major factors associated with the etiology as well as the progression of chronic airways obstruction. Cigarette smokers may either transitorily develop or worsen small-airways obstruction in association with even mild viral respiratory infections. There is also some evidence that severe viral pneumonia early in life may lead to chronic obstruction, predominantly in small airways.

GENETIC CONSIDERATIONS Despite the strong etiologic association between smoking and COPD, only 15 to 20% of smokers lose FEV_1 at a rate fast enough to manifest COPD. Epidemiologic evidence of familial clustering of COPD cases is strong and repeated, suggesting that susceptibility to the effects of tobacco smoke has genetic determinants. Twin studies show that even after controlling for active and passive smoking, FEV_1 correlated more closely in monozygotic than dizygotic twins and more than in other family members with a lesser percentage of shared genotype. In first-degree relatives of a cohort of COPD patients with normal α_1AT levels, FEV_1 was reduced compared to controls but only among current or ex-smokers. Smoking and nonsmoking relatives of control subjects both had normal FEV_1. These data suggest genetic risk factors that are expressed in response to smoking.

α_1 Antitrypsin Deficiency Thus far, deficiency of α_1AT is the only genetic abnormality that has been specifically linked to COPD. α_1AT is a 394–amino acid serine proteinase inhibitor whose synthesis is governed by a 12.2-kB 7-exon gene located at 14q32.1. α_1AT synthesis is expressed primarily in the liver and to a lesser degree in neutrophils and monocytes. Hepatic α_1AT escapes into the general circulation, where it counteracts neutrophil elastase. Normal levels of α_1AT are 20 to 48 μmol/L; levels above 11 μmol/L (35% of normal) are considered protective. There are 75 known alleles of α_1AT, which are inherited in an autosomal codominant manner and are generally classified as normal (MM), deficient, null, or dysfunctional. The most common deficient allele, termed ZZ (or Pi^{ZZ} phenotype), results from a single amino acid substitution ^{342}Glu → Lys, which causes spontaneous polymerization of the polypeptide, markedly impeding its release into the circulation from the liver. What does escape is vulnerable to oxidation and spontaneous polymerization, further impeding its function. The retained material is associated with hepatic cirrhosis (Chap. 299), while diminished circulating levels (2.5 to 7 μmol/L, averaging 16% of normal) lead to antiprotease deficiency. Pi^{ZZ}, the most common disease-related α_1AT abnormality, occurs in 1:2000 to 1:7000 persons of European descent and is rare in those of Oriental and African lineage. Pi^{SS} phenotypes are associated with α_1AT levels of 15 to 33 μmol (mean 52% of normal). Pi^{null} have no detectable antiprotease levels. Heterozygotes have intermediate levels of antiprotease.

Clinically significant deficiency of α_1AT, with levels below 11 μmol/L, has been associated with homozygous Pi^{ZZ}, $Pi^{nullnull}$, or Pi^{nullZ} and the premature development of severe emphysema, chronic bronchitis, or bronchiectasis. α_1AT deficiency accounts for 2% of observed cases of emphysema. Rare below age 25, the disease usually presents as dyspnea and cough in patients in their fourth decade. Although not a true population-based study, a large national registry of 1129 severe α_1AT-deficiency cases indicated that the typical patient was in the mid-forties, with an FEV_1 and a pulmonary diffusing capacity at or below 50% of the predicted levels. Most had exertional dyspnea and wheezing, but fewer than half reported a chronic cough. Nearly 80% had a positive family history of lung disease, and 25% reported a positive family history for liver disease. The average rate of decline of FEV_1 is reported to be 100 to 130 mL per year for smokers and 50 to 80 mL per year for ex-smokers or lifetime nonsmokers with α_1AT deficiency.

Pathologically, panacinar emphysema predominates, and radiographically, changes are more marked in the lower lobes. It is becoming increasingly apparent that tobacco smoking is an extremely important cofactor for the development of disease in α_1AT-deficient individuals. Only a few lifetime nonsmokers with Pi^{ZZ} develop emphysema. Most never have symptoms, have a normal rate of decline of FEV_1, and live a normal life span. Many cases are discovered only as a consequence of family screening of emphysema patients. Because the total number of Pi^{ZZ} individuals is unknown, the risk of disease for smokers is difficult to ascertain accurately. The risk of disease is lower still for heterozygotes with one M or S allele. Smoking is again an important cofactor. ■

PATHOLOGY The pathologic changes of COPD involve large and small airways and the terminal respiratory unit. Airway narrowing is seen in large and small airways and is caused by changes in their normal constituents in response to persistent inflammation.

The airway epithelium is characterized by squamous metaplasia, atrophy of ciliated cells, and hypertrophy of mucus glands. The remodeled epithelium actively produces cytokines that amplify and sustain the inflammatory process. The small airways are the major site of airflow limitation. Small airways show a variety of lesions narrowing their lumina, including goblet cell hyperplasia, mucosal and submucosal inflammatory cells, edema, peribronchial fibrosis, intraluminal mucus plugs, and increased smooth muscle. CD8+ T lymphocytes and B lymphocytes characterize the inflammatory infiltrate. The marked thickening of the subepithelial lamina reticularis, characteristic of asthma, is absent in COPD.

In the central airways, subepithelial inflammation is present with increased numbers of eosinophils and CD8+ T lymphocytes. Unlike asthma, the eosinophils are not activated and do not degranulate. Neutrophils are present in the epithelium but not in the subepithelial layers. In larger cartilaginous airways, chronic bronchitis is associated with hypertrophy of submucosal mucus-producing glands. Quantitation of this anatomic change, known as the *Reid index*, is based on the ratio of the thickness of the submucosal glands to that of the bronchial wall. In persons without a history of chronic bronchitis, the mean ratio is 0.44 ± 0.09, whereas in those with such a history, the mean ratio is 0.52 ± 0.08. Although a low index is rarely associated with symptoms and a high index is commonly associated with symptoms during life, there is a great deal of overlap. Therefore, many persons will have morphologic changes in large airways without having had chronic bronchitis.

Emphysema begins as an increase in the number and size of alveolar fenestrae and results in the eventual destruction of alveolar septae and their attachments to terminal and respiratory bronchioles. Emphysema is classified according to the pattern of involvement of the gas-exchanging units (acini) of the lung distal to the terminal bronchiole. With *centriacinar emphysema*, the distention and destruction are mainly limited to the respiratory bronchioles with relatively less change peripherally in the acinus. Because of the large functional reserve in the lung, many units must be involved in order for overall dysfunction to be detectable. The centrally destroyed regions of the acinus have a high ventilation/perfusion ratio because the capillaries are missing, yet ventilation continues. This results in a deficit of perfusion relative to ventilation, while the peripheral portions of the acinus have crowded and small alveoli with intact, perfused capillaries giving a low ventilation/perfusion ratio. This results in a deficit of ventilation relative to blood flow, giving a high alveolar-arterial P_{O_2} difference ($PA_{O_2} - Pa_{O_2}$) (Chap. 250).

During normal aging, airspaces enlarge and alveolar ducts increase in diameter. These changes are extremely common in lungs from persons over age 50 and may be misidentified as emphysema.

Panacinar emphysema involves both the central and peripheral portions of the acinus, which results, if the process is extensive, in a reduction of the alveolar-capillary gas exchange surface and loss of elastic recoil properties. When emphysema is severe, it may be difficult to distinguish between the two types, which most often coexist in the same lung.

PATHOPHYSIOLOGY **Airflow Limitation** Although both chronic bronchitis and emphysema can exist without evidence of obstruction, by the time a patient begins to experience dyspnea as a result of these processes, obstruction is always demonstrable. Airflow limitation and increased airways resistance may be caused by loss of elastic recoil driving passive exhalation due to emphysema, by increased collapsibility of small airways through loss of radial traction on airways, or to increased resistance due to intrinsic narrowing of small airways.

In addition to providing radial support to airways during quiet breathing, the elastic recoil properties of the lung serve as a major determinant of maximal expiratory flow rates. The static recoil pressure of the lung is the difference between alveolar and intrapleural pressure. During forced exhalations, when alveolar and intrapleural pressures are high, there are points in the airway at which bronchial pressure equals pleural pressure. Flow does not increase with higher pleural pressure after these points become fixed, so that the effective driving pressure between alveoli and such points is the elastic recoil pressure of the lung (Fig. 258-1). Hence maximal expiratory flow rates represent a complex and dynamic interplay among airways caliber, elastic recoil pressures, and collapsibility of airways. Correlative studies of structure and function suggest that small-airway narrowing is the most important correlate of airflow obstruction, followed by loss of elastic recoil. Collapsibility is probably a less important factor. As a direct consequence of the altered pressure-airflow relationships, the work of breathing is increased in bronchitis and emphysema. Since flow-resistive work is flow rate-dependent, there is a disproportionate increase in the work of breathing when ventilation must be increased, as in exercise.

Hyperinflation The designated subdivisions of the lung volume outlined in Chap. 250 are abnormal to varying degrees in both bronchitis and emphysema. The residual volume and functional residual capacity (FRC) are almost always higher than normal. Since the normal FRC is the volume at which the inward recoil of the lung is balanced by the outward recoil of the chest wall, loss of elastic recoil of the lung results in a higher FRC. In addition, prolongation of expiration in association with obstruction would lead to a dynamic increase in FRC (dynamic hyperinflation) if inspiration is initiated before the respiratory system reaches its static balance point. Dynamic hyperinflation contributes additionally to the discomfort associated with airflow obstruction by flattening the diaphragm and placing it at a mechanical disadvantage due to shortened diaphragmatic fiber length and a perpendicular insertion with the lower ribs. The exertional increase in end-expiratory lung volume and consequent decrease in inspiratory capacity have been strongly associated with the degree of dyspnea. Elevations of total lung capacity (TLC) are frequent. The exact cause is uncertain, but increases in total lung capacity are often found in association with decreases in the elastic recoil of the lung. Although the vital capacity is frequently reduced, significant airways obstruction can be present with a normal to near-normal vital capacity.

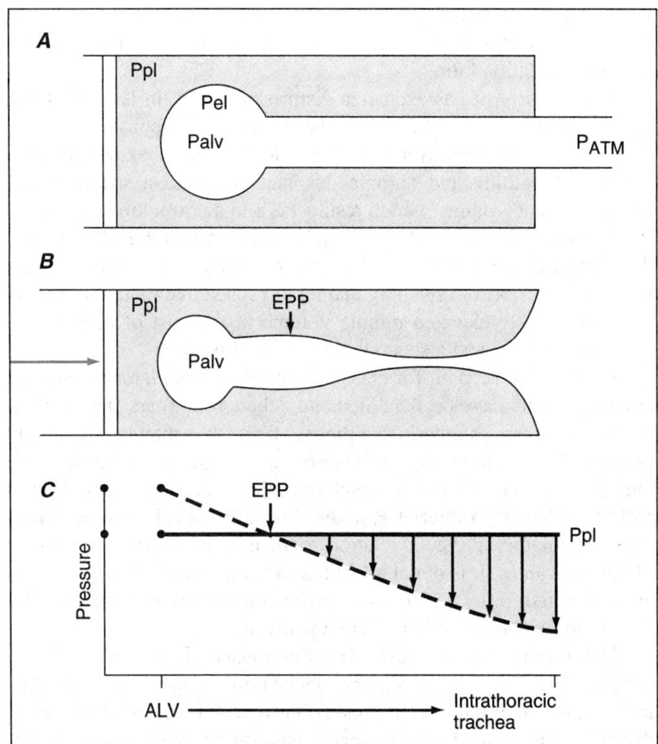

FIGURE 258-1 *A.* A schematic diagram of the lung and intrathoracic airways with no airflow. The alveolar pressure (Palv) is greater than pleural pressure (Ppl) by an amount equal to the elastic recoil pressure of the lung (Pel)—i.e., Palv is the algebraic sum of Ppl + Pel. With no airflow Palv equals atmospheric pressure (P_{ATM}), and for all of the intrathoracic airways, pressure outside is less than the pressure inside due to the Pel. *B.* The same schematic lung during forced exhalation when pleural pressure becomes quite positive (*arrow*). Palv is still greater than Ppl by an amount equal to Pel. However, there is a pressure drop along the airway associated with flow, and at some point Ppl equals local bronchial pressure (so called equal pressure point, EPP). Mouthward from this point, Ppl exceeds local bronchial pressure and hence acts to compress the airways. *C.* Pressure within the airways from alveoli to the intrathoracic trachea is shown as a dashed line (---) and Ppl is shown as a constant (—). Therefore, the driving pressure from alveoli to EPP is equal to Pel, and a decrease in Pel (i.e., loss of elastic recoil) would mean a smaller driving pressure and smaller flow rates.

Impaired Gas Exchange Maldistribution of inspired gas and blood flow is always present to some extent. When the mismatching is severe, impairment of gas exchange is reflected in abnormalities of arterial blood gases. Small-airway narrowing causes a decrease in ventilation of their distal alveolar acini. When alveolar capillaries remain intact, this results in mismatching of ventilation and blood flow, reduced ventilation-perfusion ratios, and mild to moderate hypoxemia. With emphysema, destruction of alveolar walls may decrease alveolar capillary perfusion as well, better preserving ventilation-perfusion matching, and Pa_{O_2}. Shunt hypoxemia is unusual. There are regions of the lung with a deficit of perfusion in relation to ventilation that increase the wasted ventilation ratio (i.e., V_d/V_t; Chap. 250). At a normal resting CO_2 production, the net effective alveolar ventilation, as reflected by the arterial P_{CO_2}, may be excessive, normal, or insufficient, depending on the relationship of the overall minute volume to the wasted ventilation ratio.

The severity of gas exchange disturbances and, in large part, the clinical manifestations depend on the ventilatory response to the disordered lung function. Some patients, at the cost of extremely high effort of breathing and chronic dyspnea, maintain a strikingly increased minute volume, which results both in a normal to low arterial P_{CO_2}, despite the high V_d/V_t, and a relatively high arterial P_{O_2}, despite the high difference, $PA_{O_2} - Pa_{O_2}$. Other patients with only modest increases in effort of breathing and less dyspnea maintain a normal to only moderately elevated minute volume at the cost of accepting a high arterial P_{CO_2} and a severely depressed arterial P_{O_2}.

Factors that account for clear differences in ventilatory responses among patients have been studied and debated for years. The bulk of available evidence suggests that those patients who maintain relatively normal or low arterial P_{CO_2} levels are those with an increased ventilatory drive relative to their blood gas values, and those who chronically maintain high arterial P_{CO_2} and lower P_{O_2} levels have a diminished ventilatory drive in relation to their more severely deranged blood gas values. It is not at all certain whether individual differences are accounted for by variations in peripheral or central chemoreceptor sensitivity or through other afferent pathways.

Pulmonary Circulation The pulmonary circulation malfunctions not only in terms of regional distribution of blood flow but also in terms of abnormal overall pressure-flow relationships. In advanced disease, there is often mild to severe pulmonary hypertension at rest, with further increases disproportionate to cardiac output elevations during exercise. A reduction in the total cross-sectional area of the pulmonary vascular bed can be attributed to thickening of medium and large muscular pulmonary arteries, to enhanced contraction of vascular smooth muscle in pulmonary arteries and arterioles, as well as to destruction of alveolar septa with loss of capillaries. Rarely does loss of capillaries alone lead to severe pulmonary hypertension with cor pulmonale, except as a near-terminal event (Chap. 237). Of more importance is the constriction of pulmonary vessels in response to alveolar hypoxia. The pulmonary arteries of patients with severe hypoxemia COPD have been shown to exhibit increased contractility and impaired relaxation in response to pharmacologic stimuli in vitro. These differences between the pulmonary arteries of COPD patients and normal individuals are abolished by inhibition of NO synthase, suggesting that patients develop an endothelial defect in NO synthesis. The constriction is somewhat reversible by an increase in alveolar P_{O_2} with therapy.

There is a synergism between hypoxia and acidosis that assumes importance during episodes of acute or chronic respiratory insufficiency. Chronic hypoxia, especially in concert with carboxyhemoglobinemia, often seen with heavy cigarette smoking, leads not only to pulmonary vascular constriction but also to secondary erythrocytosis. The latter, although not proved to be a significant contributor to pulmonary hypertension, could add to pulmonary vascular resistance. As discussed in Chap. 237, chronic afterload on the right ventricle leads to hypertrophy and, in association with disordered blood gases, ultimately to failure. Hypoventilation may occur during rapid eye movement sleep and lead to desaturation, which may be severe. Repeated desaturation may cause pulmonary hypertension.

Renal and Hormonal Dysfunction Chronic hypoxemia and hypercapnia have been shown to cause increased circulating levels of norepinephrine, renin, and aldosterone and decreased levels of antidiuretic hormone. Renal arterial endothelium in COPD patients exhibits defects similar to those seen in the pulmonary arteries, shifting renal blood flow from the cortex to the medulla and impairing renal functional reserve. The combination of hemodynamic and hormonal disturbances leads to defective excretion of salt and water loads and, together with right ventricular dysfunction, to the plethoric and cyanotic manifestations of some patients with COPD.

Cachexia Weight loss sometimes occurs in patients with advanced COPD. A body-mass index (BMI) < 25 kg/m^2 is associated with increased frequency of exacerbations and with significantly reduced survival. Cachexia has been attributed to caloric intake failing to keep pace with energy expenditures associated with increased work of breathing, but more recent evidence suggests that a biochemical basis is more likely. Hypoxemia leads to increased circulating levels of tumor necrosis factor α (TNF-α), and weight loss has now been correlated with levels of the latter.

Peripheral Muscle Dysfunction Protein and muscle are lost as part of wasting in advanced COPD. Skeletal muscle bulk is lost with proportional reductions in strength. Proximal limb girdle muscles of the upper and lower extremities are particularly affected, contributing to dyspnea with activities of daily living. Fiber composition in skeletal muscle changes, favoring endurance over strength. These changes occur in parallel with FEV_1 and independently of glucocorticoid use, which can also cause myopathy and muscle weakness.

Osteoporosis Loss of bone density is common in advanced disease. Over half of COPD patients lose more than 1 SD of bony density, and more than one-third have values more than 2 SDs below normal. Vertebral fractures are especially common. These changes are even more severe in patients receiving chronic glucocorticoid therapy.

NATURAL HISTORY COPD is identified by the presence of an abnormal FEV_1 in middle age, usually early in the fifth decade, and is characterized by an accelerated decline of FEV_1 with aging. In normal individuals, FEV_1 normally reaches a lifetime peak at age 25 and undergoes a linear decline of about 35 mL per year thereafter. Annual loss of FEV_1 among susceptible individuals who develop COPD is between 50 and 100 mL per year. Greater rates of decline have been associated with mucus hypersecretion, especially in men, and with bronchial hyperreactivity. Acute exacerbations do not alter the rate of decline. Dyspnea and impairment of physical work capacity are characteristic only of moderately severe to severe airways obstruction. There is considerable variation among individual patients. The majority of patients usually experience exertional dyspnea when FEV_1 falls below 40% of predicted and have dyspnea at rest when the FEV_1 <25% of predicted. In addition to dyspnea at rest, CO_2 retention and cor pulmonale frequently occur when the FEV_1 falls to 25% of predicted. With a respiratory infection, small changes in the degree of obstruction can make a large difference in symptoms and gas exchange. Thus small therapeutic gains may have rewarding results.

Exacerbation The clinical course of COPD can be characterized as one of slow progression and relative stability punctuated by episodic exacerbations occurring, on average, a little more than once per year. Exacerbations are generally described as a worsening of previously stable disease characterized by increased dyspnea, wheeze, and cough and sputum volume, tenacity, and purulence, with variable degrees of water retention and with worsening gas exchange and ventilation-perfusion relationships. Hyperinflation and work of breathing are increased. To the extent that diaphragmatic function and neuromuscular drive can compensate for the increased work, Pa_{CO_2} will not rise, but when work demands exceed respiratory pump capacity, hypercapnia and respiratory acidemia ensue. Cardiac output often does not increase sufficiently to compensate for the increased oxygen consumption from respiratory muscles, thereby compounding the hypoxemia due to $\dot{V}/\dot{Q}$ mismatching and hypercapnia.

Most COPD exacerbations are thought to be a consequence of acute tracheobronchitis, usually infectious. Most infections are primarily bacterial or the consequence of bacterial superinfection of a primary viral process. Exacerbations may also be triggered by, and must be distinguished from, left ventricular failure, cardiac arrhythmias, pneumothorax, pneumonia, and pulmonary thromboembolism. Upper airway obstruction, aspiration, rhinitis or sinusitis, asthma, or gastroesophageal reflux should be excluded. Although COPD exacerbations are individually serious and potentially life-threatening, they do not cause accelerated declines of FEV_1 over time.

CLINICAL MANIFESTATIONS

HISTORY Patients with COPD are most often tobacco smokers with a history of at least one pack per day for at least 20 years. The disease is only rarely seen in nonsmokers. Onset is typically in the fifth decade and often comes to attention as a productive cough or acute chest illness. Exertional dyspnea is usually not encountered until the sixth or seventh decade. The patient's perception of dyspnea correlates poorly with physiologic measurements, especially among older patients. A morning "smoker's cough" is frequent, usually mucoid in character but becoming purulent during exacerbations, which in early disease are intermittent and infrequent. Volume is generally small. Production of more than 60 mL/d should prompt investigation for bronchiectasis. The frequency and severity of cough generally do not correlate with the degree of functional impairment. Wheezing may be present but does not indicate severity of illness. As COPD progresses, exacerbations become more severe and more frequent. Gas exchange disturbances, worsen and dyspnea becomes progressive. Exercise tolerance becomes progressively limited. With worsening hypoxemia, erythrocytosis and cyanosis may occur. The development of morning headache may indicate the onset of significant CO_2 retention. In advanced disease, weight loss is frequent and correlates with an adverse prognosis. When blood gas derangements are severe, cor pulmonale may manifest itself by peripheral edema and water retention. Anxiety, depression, and sleep disturbances are not infrequent.

PHYSICAL FINDINGS The physical examination has poor sensitivity and variable reproducibility in COPD. Findings may be minimal or even normal in mild disease, requiring objective laboratory data for confirmation. In early disease, the only abnormal findings may be wheezes on forced expiration and a forced expiratory time prolonged beyond 6 s. With progressive disease, findings of hyperinflation become more apparent. These include an increased anteroposterior diameter of the chest, inspiratory retraction of the lower rib margins (Hoover's sign), decreased cardiac dullness, and distant heart and breath sounds. Coarse inspiratory crackles and rhonchi may be heard, especially at the bases. To gain better mechanical advantage for their compromised respiratory muscles, patients with severe airflow obstruction may adopt a characteristic tripod sitting posture with the neck angled forward and the upper torso supported on the elbows and arms. Breathing through pursed lips prolongs expiratory time and may help reduce dynamic hyperinflation.

Cor pulmonale and right heart failure may be evidenced by dependent edema and an enlarged, tender liver (Chap. 237). With pulmonary hypertension, a loud pulmonic component of the second heart sound may be audible, along with a right ventricular heave and a murmur of tricuspid regurgitation; these findings may be obscured by hyperinflation. If right-sided pressures are sufficiently high, neck veins may elevate instead of collapse with inspiration (Kussmaul's sign). Cyanosis is a somewhat unreliable manifestation of severe hypoxemia and is seen when severe hypoxemia and erythrocytosis are present.

Radiographic Findings A posteroanterior and lateral chest film should be obtained primarily to exclude competing diagnoses. They may be entirely normal in mild disease. As COPD progresses, abnormalities reflect emphysema, hyperinflation, and pulmonary hypertension. Emphysema is manifested by an increased lucency of the lungs. In smokers, these changes are more prominent in the upper lobes, while in α_1AT deficiency, they are more likely in basal zones. Local radiolucencies >1 cm in diameter and surrounded by hairline arcuate shadows indicate the presence of bullae and are highly specific for emphysema. With hyperinflation, the chest becomes vertically elongated with low flattened diaphragms. The heart shadow is also vertical and narrow. The retrosternal airspace is increased on the lateral view, and the sternal-diaphragmatic angle exceeds 90°. In the presence of pulmonary hypertension, the pulmonary arteries become enlarged and taper rapidly. The right heart border may become prominent and impinge on the retrosternal airspace. The presence of "dirty lung fields" may reflect the presence of bronchiolitis.

Computed tomography has greater sensitivity and specificity for emphysema than the plain film but is rarely necessary except for the diagnosis of bronchiectasis and evaluation of bullous disease. Nonhomogeneous distribution of emphysema is thought by some to be an indicator of suitability for lung volume reduction surgery (LVRS).

PULMONARY FUNCTION TESTING (See also Chap. 250) Because of the imprecision of clinical findings, objective evaluation of the presence, severity, and reversibility of airflow obstruction is essential in the diagnostic evaluation of COPD. A normal FEV_1 essentially excludes the diagnosis. The spirogram in COPD shows decreased volume changes with time and a failure to reach a plateau after 3 to 5 s. Continued airflow may be evident for 10 s or more on forced exhalation. The flow-volume curve shows diminished expiratory flow at all lung volumes. Expiratory flow is concave to the volume axis. When flow is plotted against absolute lung volume, the entire curve is shifted to higher volumes, reflecting hyperinflation. Serial spirometry is important in assessing the rate of decline of FEV_1.

Reversibility is assessed by spirometry before and after administration of an inhaled bronchodilator, most often a short-acting β_2-adrenergic agonist. Testing should be performed when the patient is clinically stable. Short-acting bronchodilators should be withheld for 6 h, long-acting dilators for 12 h, and theophylline for 24 h prior to testing. A significant response is an increase of at least 12% and 200 mL in either FEV_1 or forced vital capacity (FVC). Postbronchodilator FEV_1 is useful for prognostication. Although only one-third of COPD patients show a significant response to an inhaled bronchodilator in the pulmonary function laboratory on any one day, two-thirds will show a significant response when tested with different bronchodilators on several different occasions. The degree of bronchodilator response at any one testing session does not predict the degree of clinical benefit to the patient. Therefore, bronchodilators are given irrespective of the acute response obtained in the pulmonary function laboratory. The American Thoracic Society recommends staging COPD by FEV_1. Stage I, mild disease, is defined as $FEV_1 \geq 50\%$ predicted; stage II, moderate disease, 35 to 49% predicted; and stage III, severe disease, <35% predicted.

Lung volumes are useful for the assessment of hyperinflation. Transfer factor for carbon monoxide (DL_{CO}) correlates negatively with the degree of emphysema but is not specific and may miss mild disease. Neither test is indicated routinely, but DL_{CO} may help distinguish chronic asthma from emphysema.

Measurements for arterial blood gas are not needed for mild disease, but they should be assessed routinely for stage II or stage III COPD. Patients with pulmonary hypertension or cor pulmonale with normal daytime blood gases should be evaluated for nocturnal desaturation by overnight oximetry. Polysomnography to exclude concurrent sleep apnea should be obtained for patients who also complain of excessive daytime somnolence or who have a history of snoring.

α_1AT levels are not needed routinely but should be obtained for chronic airflow obstruction or chronic bronchitis in nonsmokers, as well as in COPD patients with bronchiectasis, cirrhosis without apparent risks, premature emphysema, or basilar emphysema; in patients under age 50 with unremitting asthma; and in individuals with a family history of α_1AT deficiency.

℞ **TREATMENT** Treatment of COPD is based on the principles of prevention of further evolution of disease, preservation of airflow, preservation and enhancement of functional capacity, management of physiologic complications, and avoidance of exacerbations.

Smoking Cessation (See also Chap. 390) The Lung Health Study has demonstrated that elimination of tobacco smoking confers significant survival benefit to patients with COPD. Prolonged survival is associated with reduced rates of malignancy and cardiovascular disease as well as with a significant increment in FEV_1 in the first year after smoking cessation. The rate of decline of FEV_1 reverts back to that of a nonsmoker. Although bronchodilator therapy produces similar first-year gains in FEV_1, pharmacotherapy alone does not modify the decline of airflow over time. Even unsuccessful quitters show significant benefits when compared to continuing smokers.

Despite the demonstrated benefits of smoking cessation, sustained quitting is difficult to achieve. Overall, only 6% of smokers succeed in quitting long term, and 70 to 80% of short-term quitters start smoking again. Successful quitting requires concerted active and continuing intervention by the physician. The physician should address the issue in regular patient visits, assess the patient's readiness to quit, advise the patient as to the best methods for smoking cessation, provide emotional and pharmacologic support, and arrange close follow-up of the patient's efforts. The concept of "lung age" may be helpful in promoting smoking cessation by determining the age at which the observed FEV_1 would be a normal finding. Lungs of 50- to 60-year-old smokers may be "normal" for a 70- to 80-year-old individual. Nicotine patches and nicotine polacrilex gum improve quit rates, especially among nicotine-dependent smokers. The addition of oral bupropion at 150 mg twice daily produces significant additional benefit, with a 1-year sustained abstinence rate of 22.5% compared to 6% for placebo. Smoking cessation is typically associated with weight gain of 3 to 4 kg. To minimize weight gain, reluctance to quit, and relapse, prospective quitters should be counseled to reduce caloric intake and to increase physical activity.

Bronchodilators These drugs improve dyspnea and exercise tolerance by improving airflow and by reducing end-expiratory lung volume and air-trapping. Although airflow limitation is relatively fixed, some degree of response to bronchodilator medication is usually present. Bronchodilator medication is available in metered-dose inhaler (and some dry-powder inhalers) and in nebulizable and oral forms. Inhalers deliver medications directly to the airways and have limited systemic absorption and side effects. Proper use requires timing and coordination of inspiration and inhaler actuation and presents frequent difficulties for chronic lung patients. These problems can usually be overcome with education and with the use of holding chambers. Aerosol nebulizers have no pharmacologic advantage over metered-dose inhalers. Their use should be limited to patients who remain unable to master metered dose inhalers adequately. Oral medication is associated with higher rates of adherence than inhalers but shows higher rates of systemic side effects without superior bronchodilation.

Three major classes of bronchodilators are commonly employed in the treatment of patients with COPD: short- and long-acting β_2-adrenergic agonists, anticholinergics, and theophylline derivatives. Short-acting β_2-agonists (albuterol, pirbuterol, terbutaline, metaproterenol) are relatively bronchoselective with minimal effects on heart rate and blood pressure. They produce significant bronchodilation at 5 to 15 min and remain effective for 4 to 6 h. Long-acting β_2-agonists (oral sustained-release albuterol and inhaled salmeterol) have an onset of action of 15 to 30 min and a 12-h duration of action. Anticholinergic agents (ipratropium bromide) have a 30- to 60-min onset of action and a 4- to 6-h duration. Theophyllines are generally administered orally in 12- or 24-h preparations. Recommended bronchodilator regimens are shown in Table 258-1.

Regular use of ipratropium may lead to improvements in baseline FEV_1 when compared with short-acting β_2-agonists. When used together, ipratropium and short-acting β_2-agents show greater clinical efficacy than either agent alone, without an increase in side effects. Salmeterol as a single agent produces longer lasting bronchodilation than ipratropium, improves baseline FEV_1 over time, and is not associated with loss of efficacy over a period of several months. Salmeterol, however, has not yet been evaluated as a component of combination therapy.

Table 258-1 Recommended Bronchodilator Therapy for Chronic Obstructive Pulmonary Disease

Stage	FEV_1, % predicted	Treatment
I	> 50	β_2-agonist prn
II	35–49	Combined anticholinergic and β_2-agonist
III	<35	Above plus long-acting β_2-agonist and/or sustained release theophylline Consider oral glucocorticoid trial

SOURCE: Celli et al, 1995, and Pearson et al, 1997.

Theophylline is a weak bronchodilator with a narrow therapeutic window. Much of its clinical benefit derives from effects other than bronchodilation; therapeutic doses of theophylline increase ventilatory drive, enhance diaphragmatic contractility, and increase cardiac output. About 20% of COPD patients respond to theophylline with improved airflow, exercise tolerance, and quality of life. Theophylline produces additional benefits in exercise capacity and quality of life when used in combination with short-acting β_2-adrenergic agonists. The therapeutic range for theophylline is commonly given as 10 to 20 μg/mL, with greater efficacy but greater toxicity seen at higher serum levels. The risk of toxicity is greater in older patients and in those with heart and kidney disease. Optimal dosing must balance the competing considerations of risk and benefit for each individual patient.

Glucocorticoids Because COPD, like asthma, is a disease associated with airway inflammation, glucocorticoids are an intuitively attractive therapeutic modality. Nevertheless, results of clinical trials of glucocorticoid therapy in COPD patients have shown less impressive benefits when compared to patients with asthma. The degree of response to glucocorticoids appears to correlate with the presence of asthmatic features, but data supporting their use is limited. Only 10% more patients show subjective benefit and increase their FEV_1 or forced vital capacity by at least 20% when compared to those on placebo. Responders cannot be reliably identified on clinical grounds, although response to an inhaled β_2-agonist is commonly used as a predictor. The benefits of a 10- to 14-day trial of 30 to 40 mg/d of prednisone for patients with stage III disease who have not responded adequately to mixed bronchodilator therapy remain to be proven. Long-term systemic glucocorticoid use is associated with multiple side effects. In particular, they have been associated with worsened osteoporosis and increased risk of vertebral fracture. If systemic steroids are used, the lowest effective dose should be employed and alternate-day dosing used whenever possible. The use of inhaled glucocorticoids ameliorates systemic side effects. Three large clinical trials have shown that inhaled glucocorticoids do not alter the rate of decline of FEV_1. While an inhaled glucocorticoid does not decrease the number or frequency of COPD exacerbations, it may decrease their severity and reduce the need for hospitalization. Symptoms and exercise tolerance improve on inhaled glucocorticoids.

Management of α_1AT Deficiency Given the central role of smoking in the pathogenesis of disease, smoking cessation is an important cornerstone in the management of α_1AT deficiency. Exogenous α_1AT derived from pooled human plasma administered intravenously in a weekly dose of 60 mg/kg has been shown to induce protective levels of α_1AT in deficient individuals. Because of the expense and inconvenience of the treatment, replacement of α_1AT is used only for patients over age 18 with α_1AT levels below 11 μmol/L who have stopped smoking and who have airflow obstruction. A recently published large nonrandomized trial showed that augmentation therapy significantly decreased 5-year mortality (RR 0.64) for patients receiving replacement. The rate of decline of FEV_1 also decreased with augmentation therapy. In both instances, benefit was largely restricted to those patients with FEV_1 35 to 49% of predicted. These findings require confirmation in randomized controlled trials.

Oxygen Severe and progressive hypoxemia is often seen in advanced COPD and may result in cellular hypoxia with deleterious physiologic consequences. The establishment of adequate systemic oxygen transport is essential to the prevention of tissue hypoxia and requires attention to cardiac output and hemoglobin concentration as well as to arterial O_2 saturation (Sa_{O_2}). Long-term O_2 therapy has been shown to reverse secondary polycythemia; improve body weight; ameliorate cor pulmonale; and enhance neuropsychiatric function, exercise tolerance, and activities of daily living. Two major studies, one in the United States and one in the United Kingdom, established a survival benefit for long-term O_2 therapy that increased with the number of hours per day that O_2 was used. The mechanism for this benefit has not been conclusively elucidated, but it appears to be related to the stabilization of pulmonary hemodynamics.

The need for long-term O_2 therapy should be documented with measurement of arterial blood gases obtained at rest and confirmed by a separate determination of resting arterial blood gases during a period of medical stability after 30 to 90 days of optimum medical therapy. Once the need for O_2 has been demonstrated in a stable patient, the requirement is generally for the duration of the patient's life. Patients with a $Pa_{O_2} \leq 55$ mmHg or $Sa_{O_2} \leq 88\%$ should be provided with oxygen titrated to raise Sa_{O_2} to $\geq 90\%$. Oxygen is likewise indicated for patients who have a PaO_2 of 56 to 59 mmHg with $Sa_{O_2} \geq 89\%$ when hematocrit is 55% or when cor pulmonale or other objective evidence of pulmonary hypertension is present. Oxygen may be appropriate for patients whose resting awake $Pa_{O_2} \geq 60$ mmHg with $Sa_{O_2} \geq 90\%$ if they become hypoxic during exercise or sleep. Once oxygen is prescribed, the dose should be titrated to maintain $Sa_{O_2} \geq 90\%$ during sleep and normal walking, as well as at rest, and it should be used for a minimum of 15 h a day to realize a survival benefit.

Oxygen is most frequently delivered through a nasal cannula at rates of 2 to 5 L/min. Oxygen-sparing cannulae are available. Transtracheal administration provides further O_2-sparing benefits but requires scrupulous attention to catheter maintenance and hygiene and is not suitable for all patients. Oxygen is packaged as compressed gas or compressed liquid or can be delivered from an O_2concentrator, a molecular sieve that enriches O_2 by removing nitrogen from ambient air. O_2 should be prescribed from sources that are appropriate to the individual patient's life-style and needs. It is customary to provide a stationary O_2 source, either an O_2 concentrator, which is dependent on a reliable source of electricity, or 100-kg (200-lb) H cylinders of compressed O_2. Flow resistance imposes a 15-m (50-ft) practical limit to the length of tubing connecting the O_2 source to the patient's cannula. For patients whose activities of daily living require ambulation beyond this limit, ambulatory or portable systems should be provided. Ambulatory O_2 needs may be met with rolling 10-kg (22-lb) E cylinders of compressed O_2, or with portable 2-kg (4.5-lb) aluminum cylinders or 3-kg (6.6-lb) liquid oxygen packs. The duration of O_2 availability from an O_2 concentrator is unlimited. For compressed gas and liquid sources, the amount of available oxygen is determined by the size of the system and the patient's liter flow needs. Portable systems generally provide 4 to 5 h of O_2 flow.

Oxygen therapy is generally safe. Cylinders should be secured to prevent tipping over or potentially explosive disconnection of the regulator valve. Oxygen should be stored away from open flames or other source of heat, and patients and family members should be educated to be especially scrupulous about avoiding smoking in the presence of flowing O_2.

Prophylaxis No evidence supports the prophylactic use of antibiotics in stable COPD. Yearly influenza vaccination is recommended for all patients with chronic cardiopulmonary disease, although objective benefit has not been conclusively demonstrated. Pneumococcal vaccination with 23-valent polysaccharide is also recommended. Amantadine should be used for unvaccinated patients who are placed at risk by an outbreak of influenza A.

Rehabilitation Airflow limitation, dyspnea, and muscle loss and deconditioning all compromise cardiopulmonary fitness and contribute to a progressively constrained daily life and unsatisfactory quality of life. Pulmonary rehabilitation is a multidisciplinary program of care for patients with chronic respiratory impairments that is individually tailored and designed to optimize physical and social performance. A pulmonary rehabilitation program consists of exercise training, patient education, psychosocial and behavioral intervention, and regular assessment of outcomes and is designed to minimize the disability and handicap imposed by the physiologic impairments consequent to COPD. Rehabilitation in COPD should be considered for patients with persistent symptoms and disability despite optimal medical management. Spirometric criteria should not be the primary basis for referral into rehabilitation programs. Exercise consists of 20 to 30 min of upper and lower extremity exercise at 60 to 75% maximum $\dot{V}_{O_2}$ or heart rate two to five times a week. Both strength and endurance exercises are provided. Education covers pursed lip and other breathing strategies to minimize dyspnea, energy-conservation skills, principles of medications and proper use of metered-dose inhalers, nutrition, and end-of-life decision-making. Behavioral interventions focus on dyspnea, depression, and self-sufficiency and on issues of control, coping, and role function. Dyspnea, exercise tolerance, activity level, and quality of life are followed at regular intervals. Pulmonary rehabilitation programs have been shown to improve endurance time for submaximal exercise by 38 to 80% and 6-min walking distance by 80 to 113 m. Clinically meaningful reduction in dyspnea and improvement of quality of life have been reported. No clinical trials have been adequately designed to address the issue of survival benefit. Reductions in costs of care and resource consumption have not reached statistical significance.

Despite maximal medical therapy, when COPD progresses to stage III and is complicated by hypercapnia or pulmonary hypertension, surgical approaches to treatment may be considered.

Transplantation (See also Chap. 267) Owing to its frequency in the general population, emphysema is the most common indication for lung transplantation. Transplantation should be actively considered for end-stage COPD patients when the prognosis from the disease is worse than the survival statistics for the surgery. Lung transplantation should be considered for COPD patients who, despite maximal medical therapy, have an $FEV_1 < 25\%$ predicted and with pulmonary hypertension or cor pulmonale. Precedence is given to those patients with a Pa_{CO_2} of 55 mmHg and progressive deterioration. Asthma and other reversible airflow limitation must be excluded. Rehabilitation and long-term O_2 therapy, where appropriate, should be provided prior to transplant evaluation.

Lung Volume Reduction Surgery LVRS, or pneumectomy, is designed to relieve dyspnea and improve exercise function in severely disabled patients with stage III emphysema. At operation, severely emphysematous lung tissue is resected, leading to improvement in elastic recoil in the remaining pulmonary parenchyma. This decreases hyperinflation and enhances diaphragmatic function, with consequent 25 to 50% improvement of airflow and exercise capacity. In early uncontrolled studies, hospital mortality for LVRS ranged from 5 to 18% and hospital stays averaged 9 to 18 days, with frequent significant air leaks. Cost of LVRS was $33,000 to $70,000 per case. Because of the large number of potential candidates, the high cost involved, and unanswered questions about the benefits of the operation, use of LVRS in the United States has been restricted to a multicenter randomized controlled trial, the National Emphysema Treatment Trial (NETT), comparing LVRS with best medical therapy. Stage III emphysema patients accepted for evaluation into NETT are under age 75, are severely hyperinflated, and have severe dyspnea despite optimal medical therapy. Contraindications to LVRS are similar to those for lung transplantation, including active smoking, marked obesity or cachexia, and inability to undertake pulmonary rehabilitation successfully. There has been little consensus regarding features identifying ideal and suboptimal candidates for the surgery. Radiographic heterogeneity of disease and the absence of significant intrinsic airway disease have been suggested characteristics of patients likely to benefit. Results from the NETT suggest that physiologic benefits from LVRS may begin to be lost as early as 1 year after surgery. Accelerated declines of FEV_1 have been reported, averaging 100 mL per year and particularly marked in those patients with the greatest postoperative gains in airflow. Improvements in dyspnea and exercise tolerance may be sustained for as long as 3 years but may decline thereafter. Until these issues are satisfactorily resolved, LVRS will remain an experimental procedure.

Treatment of Exacerbations • ***Triage*** The initial decision in the management of an exacerbation of COPD is whether hospitalization is necessary. Rapidity of evolution of symptoms and response to initial therapy, level of consciousness, presence or absence of respiratory distress, severity of gas exchange disturbance, and arterial blood gas deviation from the patient's stable baseline should influence the decision to hospitalize. The patient's ability to manage at home and the resources available for home care should weigh heavily in the decision-making process.

Home therapy For patients with mild exacerbations for whom outpatient therapy is appropriate, a combination of anticholinergic and short-acting β_2-adrenergic agonist bronchodilators should be prescribed. Although β_2-agonists may be given as frequently as once an hour, there is no advantage to administering anticholinergic bronchodilators more frequently than every 4 to 6 h. Metered-dose inhalers should be used with spacers. There is no evidence that the use of nebulizers provides any improvement in outcome.

The presence of increased sputum volume or purulence suggest an infectious cause of an exacerbation. With either of these features is present in conjunction with increased breathlessness or when both are present, antibiotics should be prescribed. The organisms most frequently associated with mild COPD exacerbations include *Streptococcus pneumoniae*, *Haemophilus influenzae*, and *Moraxella catarrhalis*. Trimethoprim/sulfamethoxazole, doxycycline, or amoxicillin is an appropriate management option, although choices may be modified by local antibiotic sensitivity data.

There is a need for well-controlled studies on the utility of glucocorticoids in the outpatient management of COPD exacerbations. Oral glucocorticoids may be continued in patients already receiving such treatment or given to patients who do not show a satisfactory response to bronchodilator therapy. The usual dose is 20 to 40 mg daily for 7 to 10 days. Short-term glucocorticoid therapy lasting less than 3 weeks may be discontinued without the use of a tapering dose.

Hospital management For patients with exacerbations of sufficient severity to warrant hospitalization, improvement of airflow, gas exchange, and acid-base status are of central importance. Hospitalized patients should receive bronchodilators, antibiotics, oral glucocorticoids, and sufficient O_2 to keep the $Sa_{O_2} \geq 90\%$. β_2-agonists and anticholinergic agents should be given together every 4 to 6 h. The frequency of sympathomimetic bronchodilator administration may be increased as needed to as often as every 20 min. Because high doses of β_2-agonists may cause hypokalemia, serum potassium levels and heart rate should be monitored closely for patients receiving frequent doses of these agents. Data are contradictory regarding the addition of theophylline to the bronchodilator regiment of patients showing an inadequate initial response, yet the current American and British Thoracic Societies' guidelines recommend consideration of its use to produce plasma theophylline levels between 10 and 20 μg/mL. Oral glucocorticoids have been shown to produce modest improvements in FEV_1 and in the duration of hospitalization for COPD exacerbations. Recent data indicate that more severe COPD exacerbations are associated with the recovery of enterobacteriaciae in respiratory secretions. For this reason, a second- or third-generation cephalosporin, a fluoroquinolone, a second-generation macrolide, or an extended-spectrum penicillin is now recommended as initial therapy. Attempts to obtain diagnostically adequate sputum should be made, and, when available, sputum results should be used to individualize therapy in the light of local microbial sensitivity spectra. Oxygen therapy is an important component of the management of a severe exacerbation of COPD. It is important to maintain the $Sa_{O_2} > 90\%$ and Pa_{O_2} between 60 and 65 mmHg for most patients. In many cases, administration of O_2 will result in worsening hypercapnia, although rarely to a clinically significant degree if the O_2 is used only in amounts to achieve the minimal goals. The elevation of Pa_{CO_2} is multifactorial, resulting from increased dead space due to reduced tidal volume as well as from the Haldane effect, i.e., a right wave shift of the CO_2 dissociation curve in the presence of increased saturated hemoglobin. The lower the initial Pa_{O_2} and the greater the increase, the larger the increase in Pa_{CO_2} observed. Patients whose pH on presentation is below 7.25 and with $Pa_{O_2} < 50$ mmHg are at particular risk and should be observed closely.

For patients at increased risk of hypercapnia, administration of controlled concentrations of O_2 through a Venturi mask is reasonable. Inspired O_2 concentrations (FI_{O_2}) of 0.24 to 0.28 are usually sufficient to keep $Sa_{O_2} \geq 90\%$.

Mechanical Ventilation (See also Chap. 266) Patients with impaired consciousness, respiratory distress evidenced by tachypnea with a respiratory rate greater than 35 breaths per minute and/or abdominal paradox, severe hypoxemia, or significant respiratory acidosis with pH < 7.25 and who deteriorate despite treatment are candidates for immediate ventilatory support using either noninvasive (mask) or invasive (intubation) approaches. The goals are to buy time for medical treatments to take effect, to rest the respiratory muscles, and to improve gas exchange abnormalities while avoiding the major complications of mechanical ventilatory support.

Noninvasive positive-pressure ventilation (NIPPV) delivered by nasal mask should be considered in units that have experience with the technique for patients who remain alert and cooperative, who are not heavily sedated, who are hemodynamically stable, and who are able to clear their airways by coughing up secretions. In these circumstances, NIPPV has been shown to be successful in avoiding the need for endotracheal intubation in up to 70% of cases. Success, as evidenced by improved Pa_{CO_2} and pH, should be evident within the first 60 min. Part-time NIPPV for 6 to 8 h per day may afford sufficient respiratory muscle rest to avert the need for invasive conventional ventilation. Failed attempts at NIPPV can be followed by intubation and conventional ventilation and do not appear to carry a worse prognosis. Successful application of NIPPV has been associated with a decrease in intensive care and hospital stays, incidence of nosocomial pneumonia, and costs.

Before committing to endotracheal intubation and conventional ventilatory support, the patient's wishes for such support, the patient's quality of life, and the benefits and costs of care should be thoroughly reviewed. Where the patient's wishes cannot be clearly ascertained or there is uncertainty about the appropriateness of the intervention, intubation and ventilation should proceed. If mechanical ventilatory support is subsequently determined to be inappropriate, support may then be withdrawn.

Once intubation is accomplished, the patient can be ventilated in the controlled ventilation, assist-control, intermittent mandatory ventilation, or pressure support modes. FI_{O_2} should be sufficient to obtain $Sa_{O_2} \geq 90\%$ and Pa_{O_2} of 60 to 65 mmHg. An FI_{O_2} of 0.24 to 0.40 is usually adequate for the purpose. Minute volume should be adequate to keep pH ≥ 7.25, but one should not strive to achieve a "normal" Pa_{CO_2}. It is important to try to avoid overventilation and hyperinflation in ventilated COPD patients. Because the time constant for exhalation is abnormally prolonged, it is essential to allow adequate expiratory time to permit as complete emptying of each breath as possible, preferably at least 3 to 4 s. This is best accomplished by minimizing tidal volume and respiratory rate. Lesser gains in expiratory (E) time can be obtained by high inspiratory (I) flow rates and I:E ratios of 1:2 or higher. Inadequate expiratory time leads to dynamic hyperinflation and in turn to the development of intrinsic positive end-expiratory pressure (PEEPi). PEEPi is just as capable of producing hypotension as extrinsically applied PEEP. When a mechanically ventilated patient with obstructive lung disease abruptly develops hypotension, PEEPi should be excluded, either by direct measurement or by disconnecting the patient from the ventilator for 30 to 60 s. PEEPi and dynamic hyperinflation increase the work of breathing, place the diaphragm at mechanical disadvantage, and contribute significantly to difficulties in weaning from ventilatory support. Over a period of days, as the underlying precipitants of the exacerbation are controlled, airway obstruction gradually remits and gas exchange improves and it becomes appropriate to consider removal from mechanical ventilatory support.

The principles of weaning from mechanical ventilation are discussed in detail in Chap. 266.

Prognosis after exacerbation The hospital mortality rate for an episode of respiratory failure in COPD ranges from 11 to 25% and depends on the severity of the episode, the patient's chronic health and nutritional status, and the presence of cor pulmonale or congestive heart failure. Data regarding subsequent course may be helpful in educating COPD patients and in guiding their subsequent management decisions. Among survivors of mechanical ventilation, the 6-month mortality rate is approximately 40%. Two-thirds of survivors have frequent recurrences of exacerbations, and functional status thereafter is often poor.

BIBLIOGRAPHY

BERNARD S et al: Peripheral muscle weakness in patients with chronic obstructive pulmonary disease. Am J Respir Crit Care Med 158:629, 1998

BROCHARD L et al: Noninvasive ventilation for acute exacerbations of chronic obstructive pulmonary disease. N Engl J Med 333:817, 1995

CELLI B et al: Standards for the diagnosis and care of patients with chronic obstructive pulmonary disease. Am J Respir Crit Care Med 152:S77, 1995

CONNORS AF et al: Outcomes following acute exacerbation of severe chronic obstructive lung disease. The SUPPORT investigators (Study to Understand Prognoses and Preferences for Outcomes and Risks of Treatments). Am J Respir Crit Care Med 154: 959, 1996

FEIN A: Lung volume reduction surgery: Answering the crucial questions. Chest 113: 277S, 1998.

HOGG JC: Chronic bronchitis: The role of viruses. Semin Respir Infect 15:32, 2000

LAREAU SC et al: Pulmonary rehabilitation 1999. Am J Respir Crit Care Med 159:1666, 1999

MADISON J, IRWIN R: Chronic obstructive pulmonary disease. Lancet 352:467, 1998

NIEWOEHNER DE et al: Effect of systemic glucocorticoids on exacerbations of chronic obstructive pulmonary disease. N Engl J Med 340:1941, 1999

O'BYRNE PM, POSTMA DS: The many faces of airway inflammation. Asthma and chronic obstructive pulmonary disease. Am J Respir Crit Care Med 159:S1, 1999

PEARSON M et al: BTS Guidelines for the management of chronic obstructive pulmonary disease. Thorax 52(Suppl 5):S1, 1997

PIQUETTE CA et al: Chronic bronchitis and emphysema, in *Textbook of Respiratory Medicine*, 3[d] ed, JF Murray, JA Nadel (eds). Philadelphia, Saunders, 2000, pp 1187–1246

SCHOLS AM: Nutrition in chronic obstructive pulmonary disease. Curr Opin Pulm Med 6:110, 2000

SETHI JM, ROCHESTER CL: Smoking and chronic obstructive pulmonary disease. Clin Chest Med 21:67, 2000

259 INTERSTITIAL LUNG DISEASES

Talmadge E. King, Jr.

AIP acute interstitial pneumonia	FEV_1 forced expiratory volume in one second
ARDS acute respiratory distress syndrome	FVC forced vital capacity
BAL bronchoalveolar lavage	GM-CSF granulocyte-macrophage colony stimulating factor
BG bronchocentric granulomatosis	HRCT high-resolution computed tomography
BOOP bronchiolitis obliterans with organizing pneumonia	ILDs interstitial lung diseases
COP cryptogenic organizing pneumonia	IPF idiopathic pulmonary fibrosis
CTDs connective tissue diseases	LAM lymphangioleiomyomatosis
DAHs diffuse alveolar hemorrhage syndromes	NSIP nonspecific interstitial pneumonia
DIP desquamative interstitial pneumonitis	PAP pulmonary alveolar proteinosis
D_{LCO} diffusing capacity of the lung for carbon monoxide	PLCH pulmonary Langerhans cell histiocytosis
DTPA diethylenetriamene pentaacetate	SLE systemic lupus erythematosus
	TLC total lung capacity
	UIP usual interstitial pneumonia

The interstitial lung diseases (ILDs) represent a large number of conditions that involve the parenchyma of the lung—the alveoli, the alveolar epithelium, the capillary endothelium, and the spaces between these structures, as well as the perivascular and lymphatic tissues. This heterogeneous group of disorders is classified together because of similar clinical, roentgenographic, physiologic, or pathologic manifestations. These disorders are often associated with considerable morbidity and mortality, and there is little consensus regarding the best management of most of them.

ILDs have been difficult to classify because more than 200 known individual diseases are characterized by diffuse parenchymal lung involvement, either as the primary condition or as a significant part of a multiorgan process, as may occur in the connective tissue diseases (CTDs). One useful approach to classification is to separate the ILDs into two groups, those of known and those of unknown causes (Table 259-1). Each of these groups can be subdivided into subgroups according to the presence or absence of histologic evidence of granulomas in interstitial or vascular areas. For each ILD there may be an acute phase, and there is usually a chronic one as well. Rarely, some are recurrent, with intervals of subclinical disease.

Sarcoidosis (Chap. 318), idiopathic pulmonary fibrosis (IPF), and pulmonary fibrosis associated with CTDs (Chaps. 311 to 317) are the

Table 259-1 Major Categories of Alveolar and Interstitial Inflammatory Lung Disease

Lung Response: Alveolitis, Interstitial Inflammation, and Fibrosis	
KNOWN CAUSE	
Asbestos	Radiation
Fumes, gases	Aspiration pneumonia
Drugs (antibiotics, amiodarone, gold) and chemotherapy drugs	Residual of adult respiratory distress syndrome
UNKNOWN CAUSE	
Idiopathic interstitial pneumonias	Pulmonary alveolar proteinosis
Idiopathic pulmonary fibrosis (usual interstitial pneumonia)	Lymphocytic infiltrative disorders (lymphocytic interstitial pneumonitis associated with connective tissue disease)
Desquamative interstitial pneumonia	Eosinophilic pneumonias
Respiratory bronchiolitis-associated interstitial lung disease	Lymphangioleiomyomatosis
Acute interstitial pneumonia (diffuse alveolar damage)	Amyloidosis
Cryptogenic organizing pneumonia (bronchiolitis obliterans with organizing pneumonia)	Inherited diseases
Nonspecific interstitial pneumonia	Tuberous sclerosis, neurofibromatosis, Niemann-Pick disease, Gaucher's disease, Hermansky-Pudlak syndrome
Connective tissue diseases	Gastrointestinal or liver diseases (Crohn's disease, primary biliary cirrhosis, chronic active hepatitis, ulcerative colitis)
Systemic lupus erythematosus, rheumatoid arthritis, ankylosing spondylitis, systemic sclerosis, Sjögren's syndrome, polymyositis-dermatomyositis	Graft-vs.-host disease (bone marrow transplantation; solid organ transplantation)
Pulmonary hemorrhage syndromes	
Goodpasture's syndrome, idiopathic pulmonary hemosiderosis, isolated pulmonary capillaritis	
Lung Response: Granulomatous	
KNOWN CAUSE	
Hypersensitivity pneumonitis (organic dusts)	Inorganic dusts: beryllium silica
UNKNOWN CAUSE	
Sarcoidosis	Bronchocentric granulomatosis
Langerhans cell granulomatosis (eosinophilic granuloma of the lung)	Lymphomatoid granulomatosis
Granulomatous vasculitides	
Wegener's granulomatosis, allergic granulomatosis of Churg-Strauss	

most common ILDs of unknown etiology. Among the ILDs of known cause, the largest group comprises occupational and environmental exposures, especially the inhalation of inorganic dusts, organic dusts, and various fumes or gases (Chaps. 253 and 254). A clinical diagnosis is possible for many forms of ILD, especially if an occupational and environmental history is aggressively pursued. For other forms, tissue examination, usually obtained by thoracoscopic or open lung biopsy is critical to confirmation of the diagnosis. High-resolution computed tomography (HRCT) scanning promises to improve diagnostic accuracy further as histologic-image correlation is perfected.

PATHOGENESIS

The ILDs are nonmalignant disorders and are not caused by identified infectious agents. The precise pathway(s) leading from injury to fibrosis is not known. Although there are multiple initiating agent(s) of injury, the immunopathogenic responses of lung tissue are limited, and the mechanisms of repair have common features. Two major histopathologic patterns are found in patients with ILD: a granulomatous pattern (Fig. 259-1) and a pattern in which inflammation and fibrosis predominate.

GRANULOMATOUS LUNG DISEASE This process is characterized by an accumulation of T lymphocytes, macrophages, and epithelioid cells organized into discrete structures (granulomas) in the lung parenchyma. The granulomatous lesions can progress to fibrosis. Many patients with granulomatous lung disease remain free of severe impairment of lung function, or, when symptomatic, they improve after treatment. The main differential diagnosis is between sarcoidosis (Chap. 318) and hypersensitivity pneumonitis (Chap. 253).

INFLAMMATION AND FIBROSIS The initial insult is an injury to the epithelial surface causing inflammation in the air spaces and alveolar walls. If the disease becomes chronic, inflammation spreads to adjacent portions of the interstitium and vasculature and eventually causes interstitial fibrosis. Other important histopathologic patterns in ILDs include diffuse alveolar damage (acute or organizing), desquamative interstitial pneumonia, respiratory bronchiolitis, lymphocytic interstitial pneumonia, and an organizing pneumonia [bronchiolitis obliterans with organizing pneumonia (BOOP) pattern]. The development of irreversible scarring (fibrosis) of alveolar walls, airways, or vasculature is the most feared outcome in all of these conditions because it is often progressive and leads to significant derangement of ventilatory function and gas exchange.

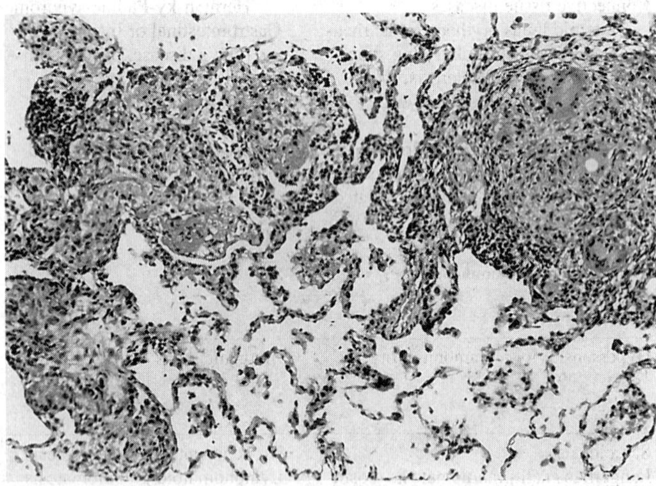

FIGURE 259-1 Hypersensitivity pneumonitis. Granulomatous inflammation with scattered, small, ill-formed granulomas, which in this case manifest primarily as clusters of giant cells.

INITIAL EVALUATION

Patients with ILDs come to medical attention mainly because of the onset of progressive exertional dyspnea or a persistent, nonproductive cough. Hemoptysis, wheezing, and chest pain may be present. Often, the identification of interstitial opacities on chest x-ray focuses the diagnostic approach toward one of the ILDs.

HISTORY **Duration of Illness** *Acute presentation* (days to weeks), while unusual, occurs with allergy (drugs, fungi, helminths), acute idiopathic interstitial pneumonia, eosinophilic pneumonia, and hypersensitivity pneumonitis. These conditions may be confused with atypical pneumonias because of diffuse alveolar opacities on chest x-ray. *Subacute presentation* (weeks to months) may occur in all ILDs but is seen especially in sarcoidosis, drug-induced ILDs, the alveolar hemorrhage syndromes, cryptogenic organizing pneumonia (COP), and the acute immunologic pneumonia that complicates systemic lupus erythematosus (SLE) or polymyositis. In most ILDs the symptoms and signs are *chronic* (months to years). Examples include IPF, sarcoidosis, pulmonary Langerhans cell histiocytosis (PLCH) (also known as Langerhans cell granulomatosis, eosinophilic granuloma, and histiocytosis X), pneumoconioses, and CTDs. *Episodic presentations* are unusual and include eosinophilic pneumonia, hypersensitivity pneumonitis, cryptogenic organizing pneumonia, vasculitides, pulmonary hemorrhage, and Churg-Strauss syndrome.

Age Most patients with sarcoidosis, ILD associated with CTD, lymphangioleiomyomatosis (LAM), PLCH, inherited forms of ILD (familial IPF, Gaucher's disease, Hermansky-Pudlak syndrome) present between the ages of 20 and 40 years. Most patients with IPF are older than 50 years.

Gender LAM and pulmonary involvement in tuberous sclerosis occur exclusively in premenopausal women. Also, ILD in Hermansky-Pudlak syndrome and in the CTDs is more common in women; an exception is ILD in rheumatoid arthritis, which is more common in men. Because of occupational exposures, pneumoconioses also occur more frequently in men.

Family History Family history is occasionally helpful because familial associations (with an autosomal dominant pattern) have been identified in tuberous sclerosis and neurofibromatosis. An autosomal recessive pattern of inheritance occurs in Niemann-Pick disease, Gaucher's disease, and the Hermansky-Pudlak syndrome. Familial clustering has been increasingly identified in sarcoidosis and familial pulmonary fibrosis, a process similar to IPF.

Smoking History Patients with PLCH, desquamative interstitial pneumonia (DIP), Goodpasture's syndrome, and respiratory bronchiolitis are almost always current or former smokers. Two-thirds to 75% of patients with IPF have a history of smoking.

Occupation and Environmental History A strict chronological listing of the patient's lifelong employment must be sought, including specific duties and known exposures. In hypersensitivity pneumonitis (Fig. 259-1), respiratory symptoms, fever, chills, and an abnormal chest roentgenogram are often temporally related to a hobby (pigeon breeder's disease) or to the workplace (Farmer's lung) (Chap. 253). Symptoms may diminish or disappear after the patient leaves the site of exposure for several days; similarly, symptoms may reappear on returning to the exposure site.

Other Important Past History Parasitic infections may cause pulmonary eosinophilia, and therefore a travel history should be taken in patients with known or suspected ILD. History of risk factors for HIV infection should be elicited from all patients with ILD because several processes may occur at the time of initial presentation or during the clinical course, e.g., HIV infection, BOOP, acute interstitial pneumonia, lymphocytic interstitial pneumonitis, or diffuse alveolar hemorrhage.

RESPIRATORY SYMPTOMS AND SIGNS Dyspnea is a common and prominent complaint in patients with ILD, especially the idiopathic interstitial pneumonias, hypersensitivity pneumonitis, COP, sarcoidosis, eosinophilic pneumonias, and PLCH. Some patients, especially patients with sarcoidosis, silicosis, PLCH, hypersensitivity pneumonitis, lipoid pneumonia, or lymphangitis carcinomatosis may have extensive parenchymal lung disease on chest x-ray without significant dyspnea, especially early in the course of the illness. Wheezing is an uncommon manifestation of ILD but has been described in patients with chronic eosinophilic pneumonia, Churg-Strauss syndrome, respiratory bronchiolitis, and sarcoidosis. Clinically significant chest pain is uncommon in most ILDs. However, substernal discomfort is common in sarcoidosis. Sudden worsening of dyspnea, especially if associated with acute chest pain, may indicate a spontaneous pneumothorax, which occurs in PLCH, tuberous sclerosis, LAM, and neurofibromatosis. Frank hemoptysis and blood-streaked sputum are rarely presenting manifestations of ILD but can be seen in the diffuse alveolar hemorrhage syndromes (DAHs), LAM, tuberous sclerosis, and the granulomatous vasculitides. Fatigue and weight loss are common in all ILDs.

PHYSICAL EXAMINATION The findings are usually not specific. Most commonly, physical examination reveals tachypnea, and bibasilar end-inspiratory dry crackles, which are common in most forms of ILD associated with inflammation but are less likely to be heard in the granulomatous lung diseases. Crackles may be present in the absence of radiographic abnormalities on the chest radiograph. Scattered late inspiratory high-pitched rhonchi—so-called inspiratory squeaks—are heard in patients with bronchiolitis. The cardiac examination is usually normal except in the mid or late stages of the disease when findings of pulmonary hypertension and cor pulmonale may become evident (Chap. 237). Cyanosis and clubbing of the digits occurs in some patients with advanced disease.

LABORATORY Antinuclear antibodies, anti-immunoglobulin antibodies (rheumatoid factors), and circulating immune complexes are identified in some patients, even in the absence of a defined CTD. A raised LDH is a nonspecific finding common to ILDs. Elevation of the serum angiotensin-converting enzyme level is common in sarcoidosis. Serum precipitins confirm exposure when hypersensitivity pneumonitis is suspected, although they are not diagnostic of the process. Antineutrophil cytoplasmic or anti-basement membrane antibodies are useful if vasculitis is suspected. The electrocardiogram is usually normal unless pulmonary hypertension is present; then it demonstrates right-axis deviation or right ventricular hypertrophy. Echocardiography also reveals right ventricular dilatation and/or hypertrophy in the presence of pulmonary hypertension.

CHEST IMAGING STUDIES **Chest X-ray** ILD may be first suspected on the basis of an abnormal chest radiograph, which most commonly reveals a bibasilar reticular pattern. A nodular or mixed pattern of alveolar filling and increased reticular markings may also be present (see Fig. 249-1). A subgroup of ILDs exhibit nodular opacities with a predilection for the upper lung zones [sarcoidosis, PLCH, chronic hypersensitivity pneumonitis, silicosis, berylliosis, rheumatoid arthritis (necrobiotic nodular form), ankylosing spondylitis]. The chest x-ray correlates poorly with the clinical or histopathologic stage of the disease. The radiographic finding of honeycombing correlates with pathologic findings of small cystic spaces and progressive fibrosis; when present, it portends a poor prognosis. In most cases, the chest radiograph is nonspecific and usually does not allow a specific diagnosis.

Computed Tomography HRCT is superior to the plain chest x-ray for early detection and confirmation of suspected ILD. Also, HRCT allows better assessment of the extent and distribution of disease, and it is especially useful in the investigation of patients with a normal chest radiograph. Coexisting disease is often best recognized on HRCT scanning, e.g., mediastinal adenopathy, carcinoma, or emphysema. In the appropriate clinical setting HRCT may be sufficiently characteristic to preclude the need for lung biopsy in IPF, sarcoidosis, hypersensitivity pneumonitis, asbestosis, lymphangitic carcinoma, and PLCH. When a lung biopsy is required, HRCT scanning is useful for determining the most appropriate area from which biopsy samples should be taken.

Radionuclide Scanning Gallium-67 lung scanning is of limited value in evaluating the inflammatory component of ILD. An accelerated clearance from the lung of soluble aerosolized hydrophilic radionuclides such as ^{99m}Tc-diethylenetriamene pentaacetate (DTPA) is an index of pulmonary epithelial permeability that results from inflammation. This test may provide a means of assessing the activity of ILD. Normal ^{99m}Tc-DTPA clearance in IPF predicts stable disease, while rapid clearance identifies patients at risk for deterioration.

PULMONARY FUNCTION TESTING **Spirometry and Lung Volumes** Measurement of lung function is important in assessing the extent of pulmonary involvement in patients with ILD. Most forms of ILD produce a restrictive defect with reduced total lung capacity (TLC), functional residual capacity, and residual volume (Chap. 250). Forced expiratory volume in one second (FEV_1) and forced vital capacity (FVC) are reduced, but these changes are related to the decreased TLC. The FEV_1/FVC ratio is usually normal or increased. Reductions in lung volumes increase as lung stiffness worsens with disease progression. A few disorders (uncommon in sarcoidosis and hypersensitivity pneumonitis, while common in tuberous sclerosis and LAM) produce interstitial opacities on chest x-ray and obstructive airflow limitation on lung function testing.

Diffusing Capacity A reduction in the diffusing capacity of the lung for carbon monoxide D_{LCO} is a common but nonspecific finding in most ILDs. This decrease is due, in part, to effacement of the alveolar capillary units but, more importantly, to mismatching of ventilation and perfusion ($\dot{V}/\dot{Q}$). Lung regions with reduced compliance due to either fibrosis or cellular infiltration may be poorly ventilated but may still maintain adequate blood flow and $\dot{V}/\dot{Q}$ in these regions act like true venous admixture. The severity of the reduction in D_{LCO} does not correlate with disease stage.

Arterial Blood Gas The resting arterial blood gas may be normal or reveal hypoxemia (secondary to a mismatching of ventilation to perfusion) and respiratory alkalosis. A normal arterial O_2 tension (or saturation by oximetry) at rest does not rule out significant hypoxemia during exercise or sleep. CO_2 retention is rare and is usually a manifestation of end-stage disease.

Cardiopulmonary Exercise Testing Because hypoxemia at rest is not always present and because severe exercise-induced hypoxemia may go undetected, it is useful to perform exercise testing with measurement of arterial blood gases to detect abnormalities of gas exchange. Arterial oxygen desaturation, a failure to decrease dead space appropriately with exercise [i.e., a high V_D/V_T ratio (Chap. 250)], and an excessive increase in respiratory rate with a lower-than-expected recruitment of tidal volume provide useful information about physiologic abnormalities and extent of disease. Serial assessment of resting and exercise gas exchange is an excellent method for following disease activity and responsiveness to treatment, especially in patients with IPF.

FIBEROPTIC BRONCHOSCOPY AND BRONCHOALVEOLAR LAVAGE (BAL) In selected diseases (e.g., sarcoidosis, hypersensitivity pneumonitis, DAHs, cancer, pulmonary alveolar proteinosis), cellular analysis of BAL fluid may be useful in narrowing the differential diagnostic possibilities among various types of ILD. The role for BAL in defining the stage of disease and assessment of disease progression or response to therapy remains poorly understood, and the usefulness of BAL in the clinical assessment and management remains to be established.

TISSUE AND CELLULAR EXAMINATION Lung biopsy is the most effective method for confirming the diagnosis and assessing disease activity. The findings may identify a more treatable process than originally suspected, particularly chronic hypersensitivity pneumonitis, COP, respiratory bronchiolitis-associated ILD, or sarcoidosis. Biopsy should be obtained before initiation of treatment. A definitive diagnosis avoids confusion and anxiety later in the clinical course if the patient does not respond to therapy or suffers serious side effects from it.

Fiberoptic bronchoscopy with multiple transbronchial lung biopsies (4 to 8 biopsy samples) is often the initial procedure of choice, especially when sarcoidosis, lymphangitic carcinomatosis, eosinophilic pneumonia, Goodpasture's syndrome, or infection are suspected. If a specific diagnosis is not made by transbronchial biopsy, then surgical lung biopsy by video-assisted thoracic surgery or open thoracotomy is indicated. Adequate-sized biopsies from multiple sites, usually from two lobes, should be obtained. Relative contraindications to lung biopsy include serious cardiovascular disease, "honeycombing" and other roentgenographic evidence of diffuse end-stage disease, severe pulmonary dysfunction, or other major operative risks, especially in the elderly.

℞ TREATMENT Although the course of ILD is variable, progression is common and often insidious. All treatable possibilities should be carefully considered. Since therapy does not reverse fibrosis, the major goals of treatment are permanent removal of the offending agent when known and early identification and aggressive suppression of the acute and chronic inflammatory process, thereby reducing further lung damage.

Hypoxemia (PaO_2 <55 mmHg) at rest and/or with exercise should be managed by supplemental oxygen. If cor pulmonale develops, diuretic therapy and phlebotomy may occasionally be required (Chap. 237).

Drug Therapy Glucocorticoids are the mainstay of therapy for suppression of the alveolitis present in ILD, but the success rate is low. There have been no placebo-controlled trials of glucocorticoids in ILD, so there is no direct evidence that steroids improve survival in many of the diseases for which they are commonly used. Glucocorticoid therapy is recommended for symptomatic ILD patients with idiopathic interstitial pneumonias, eosinophilic pneumonias, COP, CTD, sarcoidosis, acute inorganic dust exposures, acute radiation pneumonitis, DAH, and drug-induced ILD. In organic dust disease, glucocorticoids are recommended for both the acute and chronic stages.

The optimal dose and proper length of therapy with glucocorticoids in the treatment of most ILDs is not known. A common starting dose is prednisone, 0.5 to 1 mg/kg in a once-daily oral dose (based on the patient's lean body weight). This dose is continued for 4 to 12 weeks, at which time the patient is reevaluated. If the patient is stable or improved, the dose is tapered to 0.25 to 0.5 mg/kg and is maintained at this level for an additional 4 to 12 weeks depending on the course. Rapid tapering or a shortened course of glucocorticoid treatment can result in recurrence. If the patient's condition continues to decline while on glucocorticoids, a second agent (see below) is often added and the prednisone dose is lowered to or maintained at 0.25 mg/kg per day.

Cyclophosphamide and azathioprine (1 to 2 mg/kg lean body weight per day) with or without glucocorticoids, have been tried with variable success in IPF, vasculitis, and other ILDs. An objective response usually requires at least 8 to 12 weeks to occur. In situations in which these drugs have failed or could not be tolerated, other agents, including methotrexate, colchicine, penicillamine, and cyclosporine, have been tried. However, their role in the treatment of ILDs remains to be determined.

Many cases of ILD are chronic and irreversible despite the therapy discussed above, and lung transplantation may then be considered (Chap. 267).

INDIVIDUAL FORMS OF ILD

IDIOPATHIC PULMONARY FIBROSIS Several risk factors appear to be associated with the development of IPF, a common ILD of unknown etiology. These include cigarette smoking; exposure to antidepressants; a history of chronic aspiration secondary to gastroesophageal reflux; and exposures to metal dust, wood dust, and solvents. Numerous viruses have been implicated in the pathogenesis of IPF, but no clear evidence for a viral etiology has been confirmed. The most compelling evidence for participation of genetic factors is the description fo familial cases of pulmonary fibrosis, which is transmitted as an autosomal dominant trait with variable penetrance. An association has been reported between IPF and α_1 antitrypsin inhibition (Pi) alleles on chromosome 14.

Clinical Manifestations Exertional dyspnea, a nonproductive cough, and inspiratory crackles with or without digital clubbing may be present on physical examination. The chest roentgenogram and HRCT typically show patchy, predominantly peripheral, subpleural, reticular opacities in the lower lung zones. There may also be a ground-glass opacity usually associated with traction bronchiectasis and bronchiolectasis or subpleural honeycombing. Pulmonary function tests often reveal a restrictive pattern, a reduced D_{LCO}, and arterial hypoxemia that is exaggerated or elicited by exercise.

Histologic Findings Confirmation of the presence of the usual interstitial pneumonia (UIP) pattern on histologic examination is essential to confirm this diagnosis (Fig. 259-2). Transbronchial biopsies are not helpful in making the diagnosis of UIP, and surgical biopsy is usually required. The histologic hallmark and chief diagnostic criterion of UIP is a heterogeneous appearance at low magnification with alternating areas of normal lung, interstitial inflammation, fibrosis, and honeycomb changes. The latter are composed of cystic fibrotic air spaces that are frequently lined by bronchiolar epithelium and filled with mucin. Smooth muscle hyperplasia is commonly present in areas of fibrosis and honeycomb change. Biopsies taken from patients during an accelerated phase of their illness may show a combination of UIP and diffuse alveolar damage. These histologic abnormalities affect the peripheral, subpleural parenchyma most severely. The interstitial inflammation is usually patchy and consists of a lymphoplasmacytic infiltrate in the alveolar septa, associated with hyperplasia of type 2 pneumocytes. The fibrotic zones are composed mainly of dense collagen, although scattered foci of proliferating fibroblasts are a consistent finding. The extent of fibroblastic proliferation is predictive of disease progression. A UIP-like pattern can also be seen with CTDs, pneumoconioses (e.g., asbestosis), radiation injury, certain drug-induced lung diseases (e.g., nitrofurantoin), and chronic aspiration. Also, a fibrotic pattern may be found in the chronic stage of several specific disorders such as sarcoidosis, chronic hypersensitivity pneumonitis, organized chronic eosinophilic pneumonia, and PLCH. Since other histopathologic features are frequently present in these syndromes, the term UIP is used for those patients in whom the lesion is idiopathic and not associated with another condition.

℞ TREATMENT The clinical course is variable with a 5-year survival rate of 30 to 50% after diagnosis. Treatment options in-

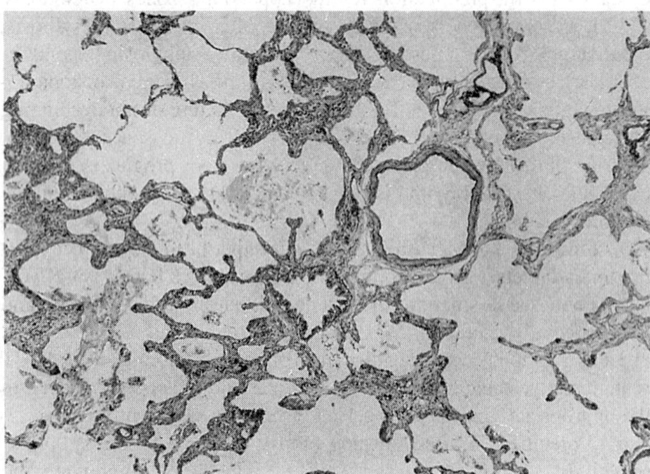

FIGURE 259-2 Usual interstitial pneumonia (UIP). Interstitial fibrous thickening emanates from peribronchiolar regions. Microhoneycombing is present. Few discernable normal alveolar walls are present. The bronchiole and vessel are unaffected.

clude glucocorticoids, cytotoxic agents (e.g., azathioprine, cyclophosphamide), and antifibrotic agents (e.g., colchicine, pirfenidone, or interferon gamma-1b), alone or in combination with glucocorticoids. However, there is no firm evidence that any of these treatment approaches improves survival or the quality of life. Because of the poor prognosis in untreated patients, a therapeutic trial may be tried. If therapy is recommended, it should be started at the first identification of clinical or physiologic evidence of impairment of lung function. Lung transplantation should be considered for those patients who experience progressive deterioration despite optimal medical management and who meet the established criteria (Chap. 267).

DESQUAMATIVE INTERSTITIAL PNEUMONIA DIP is a rare but distinct clinical and pathologic entity found exclusively in cigarette smokers. The histologic hallmark is the extensive accumulation of macrophages in intraalveolar spaces with minimal interstitial fibrosis. The peak incidence is in the fourth and fifth decades. Most patients present with dyspnea. Lung function testing shows a restrictive pattern with reduced DL_{CO} and arterial hypoxemia. The chest x-ray usually shows diffuse hazy opacities. Clinical recognition of DIP is important because the process is associated with a better prognosis (10-year survival rate is ~70%) and a better response to smoking cessation and systemic glucocorticoids than the more common IPF. Respiratory bronchiolitis-associated ILD is considered to be a subset of DIP and is characterized by the accumulation of macrophages in peribronchical alveoli.

ACUTE INTERSTITIAL PNEUMONIA (AIP) (HAMMAN-RICH SYNDROME) This is a rare, fulminant form of lung injury characterized by diffuse alveolar damage on lung biopsy. Most patients are older than 40 years. AIP is similar in presentation to the acute respiratory distress syndrome (ARDS) (Chap. 265) and probably corresponds to the subset of cases of idiopathic ARDS. The onset is usually abrupt in a previously healthy individual. A prodromal illness, usually lasting 7 to 14 days before presentation, is common. Fever, cough, and dyspnea are frequent manifestations at presentation. Diffuse, bilateral, air-space opacification is present on chest radiograph. HRCT scans show bilateral, patchy, symmetric areas of ground-glass attenuation. Bilateral areas of air-space consolidation may also be present. A predominantly subpleural distribution may be seen. The diagnosis of AIP requires the presence of a clinical syndrome of idiopathic ARDS and pathologic confirmation of organizing diffuse alveolar damage. Therefore, lung biopsy is required to confirm the diagnosis. Most patients have moderate to severe hypoxemia and develop respiratory failure. Mechanical ventilation is often required. The mortality rate is high (>60%), with most patients dying within 6 months of presentation. Recurrences have been reported. However, those who recover often have substantial improvement in lung function. The main treatment is supportive. It is not clear that glucocorticoid therapy is effective.

NONSPECIFIC INTERSTITIAL PNEUMONIA (NSIP) This condition defines a subgroup of the idiopathic interstitial pneumonias that can be distinguished clinically and pathologically from UIP, DIP, AIP, and idiopathic BOOP. Lung biopsy shows varying proportions of chronic interstitial inflammation and fibrosis. NSIP is a subacute restrictive process that usually occurs at a younger age than UIP. It is often associated with a febrile illness, relative lack of clubbing, and HRCT findings that show ground-glass opacities and areas of consolidation. Unlike patients with IPF, most patients with NSIP have a good prognosis, and most show improvement after treatment with glucocorticoids.

ILD ASSOCIATED WITH CONNECTIVE TISSUE DISORDERS Clinical findings suggestive of a CTD (musculoskeletal pain, weakness, fatigue, fever, joint pains or swelling, photosensitivity, Raynaud's phenomenon, pleuritis, dry eyes, dry mouth) should be sought in any patient with ILD. The CTDs may be difficult to rule out since the pulmonary manifestations occasionally precede the more typical systemic manifestations by months or years. The most common form of pulmonary involvement is a chronic interstitial pat-

tern similar to that in patients with IPF. However, determining the precise nature of lung involvement in most of the CTDs is difficult due to the high incidence of lung involvement caused by disease-associated complications of esophageal dysfunction (predisposing to aspiration and secondary infections), respiratory muscle weakness (atelectasis and secondary infections), complications of therapy (opportunistic infections), and associated malignancies.

Progressive Systemic Sclerosis (PSS) (See also Chap. 313) Clinical evidence of ILD is present in about one-half of patients with progressive systemic sclerosis, and pathologic evidence in three-quarters. Pulmonary function tests show a restrictive pattern and impaired diffusing capacity, often before any clinical or radiographic evidence of lung disease appears. Pulmonary vascular disease alone or in association with pulmonary fibrosis, pleuritis, or recurrent aspiration pneumonitis is strikingly resistant to current modes of therapy.

Rheumatoid Arthritis (RA) (See also Chap. 312) ILD associated with rheumatoid arthritis is more common in men. Pulmonary manifestations of rheumatoid arthritis include pleurisy with or without effusion, ILD in up to 20% of cases, necrobiotic nodules (nonpneumoconiotic intrapulmonary rheumatoid nodules) with or without cavities, Caplan's syndrome (rheumatoid pneumoconiosis), pulmonary hypertension secondary to rheumatoid pulmonary vasculitis, BOOP, and upper airway obstruction due to arytenoid arthritis.

Systemic Lupus Erythematosus (See also Chap. 311) Lung disease is a common complication in SLE. Pleuritis with or without effusion is the most common pulmonary manifestation. Other lung manifestations include the following: atelectasis, diaphragmatic dysfunction with loss of lung volumes, pulmonary vascular disease, pulmonary hemorrhage, uremic pulmonary edema, infectious pneumonia, and BOOP. Acute lupus pneumonitis characterized by pulmonary capillaritis leading to alveolar hemorrhage is common. Chronic, progressive ILD is uncommon. It is important to exclude pulmonary infection. Although pleuropulmonary involvement may not be evident clinically, pulmonary function testing, particularly D_{LCO} reveals abnormalities in many patients with SLE.

Polymyositis and Dermatomyositis (PM/DM) (See also Chap. 382) ILD occurs in ~10% of patients with polymyositis and dermatomyositis, and the clinical features are similar to those of IPF. Diffuse reticular or nodular opacities with or without an alveolar component occur radiographically, with a predilection for the lung bases. ILD occurs more commonly in the subgroup of patients with an anti-Jo-1 antibody that is directed to histidyl tRNA synthetase. Weakness of respiratory muscles contributing to aspiration pneumonia may be present. A rapidly progressive illness characterized by diffuse alveolar damage may cause respiratory failure.

Sjögren's Syndrome (See also Chap. 314) General dryness and lack of airways secretion cause the major problems of hoarseness, cough, and bronchitis. Lymphocytic interstitial pneumonitis, lymphoma, pseudolymphoma, bronchiolitis, and bronchiolitis obliterans are associated with this condition. Lung biopsy is frequently required to establish a precise pulmonary diagnosis. Glucocorticoids have been used in the management of ILD associated with Sjögren's syndrome with some degree of clinical success.

DRUG-INDUCED ILD (See also Chap. 71) Many classes of drugs have the potential to induce diffuse ILD, which is manifest most commonly as exertional dyspnea and nonproductive cough. A detailed history of the medications taken by the patient is needed to identify drug-induced disease, including over-the-counter medications, oily nose drops, or petroleum products (mineral oil). In most cases, the pathogenesis is unknown, although a combination of direct toxic effects of the drug (or its metabolite) and indirect inflammatory and immunologic events is likely. The onset of the illness may be abrupt and fulminant, or it may be insidious, extending over weeks to months. The drug may have been taken for several years before a reaction develops (e.g., amiodarone), or the lung disease may occur weeks to years after the drug has been discontinued (e.g., carmustine). The extent and severity of disease are usually dose related. Treatment consists of discontinuation of any possible offending drug and supportive care.

CRYPTOGENIC ORGANIZING PNEUMONIA (COP) Also known as idiopathic BOOP, COP is a clinicopathologic syndrome of unknown etiology. The onset is usually in the fifth and sixth decades. The presentation may be of a flu-like illness with cough, fever, malaise, fatigue, and weight loss. Inspiratory crackles are frequently present on examination. Pulmonary function is usually impaired, with a restrictive defect and arterial hypoxemia being most common. The roentgenographic manifestations are distinctive, revealing bilateral, patchy, or diffuse alveolar opacities in the presence of normal lung volume. Recurrent and migratory pulmonary opacities are common. HRCT shows areas of air-space consolidation, ground-glass opacities, small nodular opacities and bronchial wall thickening and dilation. These changes occur more frequently in the periphery of the lung and in the lower lung zone. Lung biopsy shows granulation tissue within small airways, alveolar ducts, and airspaces, with chronic inflammation in the surrounding alveoli. Glucocorticoid therapy induces clinical recovery in two-thirds of patients. A few patients have rapidly progressive courses with fatal outcomes despite glucocorticoids.

Foci of organizing pneumonia (i.e., a "BOOP pattern") is a nonspecific reaction to lung injury found adjacent to other pathologic processes or as a component of other primary pulmonary disorders (e.g., cryptococcosis, Wegener's granulomatosis, lymphoma, hypersensitivity pneumonitis, and eosinophilic pneumonia). Consequently, the clinician must carefully reevaluate any patient found to have this histopathologic lesion to rule out these possibilities.

EOSINOPHILIC PNEUMONIA See Chap. 253

PULMONARY ALVEOLAR PROTEINOSIS Although not strictly an ILD, pulmonary alveolar proteinosis (PAP) resembles and is therefore considered with these conditions. It has been proposed that a defect in macrophage function, more specifically an impaired ability to process surfactant, may play a role in the pathogenesis of PAP. This diffuse disease is characterized by the accumulation of an amorphous, periodic acid-Schiff–positive lipoproteinaceous material in the distal air spaces. There is little or no lung inflammation, and the underlying lung architecture is preserved. Mutant mice lacking the gene for granulocyte-macrophage colony stimulating factor (GM-CSF) have a similar accumulation of surfactant and surfactant apoprotein in the alveolar spaces. Moreover, reconstitution of the respiratory epithelium of GM-CSF knockout mice with the GM-CSF gene completely corrects the alveolar proteinosis. Data from BAL studies in patients suggest that PAP is an autoimmune disease with neutralizing antibody of immunoglobulin G isotype against GM-CSF. These findings suggest that neutralization of GM-CSF bioactivity by the antibody causes dysfunction of alveolar macrophages, which results in reduced surfactant clearance.

The typical age of presentation is 30 to 50 years, and males predominate. The clinical presentation is usually insidious and manifested by progressive exertional dyspnea, fatigue, weight loss, and low-grade fever. A nonproductive cough is common, but occasionally expectoration of "chunky" gelatinous material may occur. Polycythemia, hypergammaglobulinemia, and increased LDH levels are frequent. Markedly elevated serum levels of lung surfactant proteins A and D have been found in PAP. Radiographically, bilateral symmetrical alveolar opacities located centrally in mid and lower lung zones result in a "bat-wing" distribution. HRCT shows a ground-glass opacification and thickened intralobular structures and interlobular septa. Whole lung lavage(s) through a double-lumen endotracheal tube provides relief to many patients with dyspnea or progressive hypoxemia and also may provide long-term benefit.

PULMONARY LYMPHANGIOLEIOMYOMATOSIS Pulmonary LAM is a rare condition that afflicts premenopausal women and should be suspected in young women with emphysema, recurrent pneumothorax, or chylous pleural effusion. It is often misdiagnosed as asthma or chronic obstructive pulmonary disease. Pathologically, LAM is characterized by the proliferation of atypical pulmonary interstitial smooth muscle and cyst formation. The immature-appearing smooth-muscle cells react with monoclonal antibody HMB45, which recognizes a 100-kDa glycoprotein (gp100) originally found in human melanoma cells. Caucasians are affected much more commonly than members of other racial groups. The disease accelerates during pregnancy and abates after oopherectomy. Common complaints at presentation are dyspnea, cough, and chest pain. Hemoptysis may be life threatening. Spontaneous pneumothorax occurs in 50% of patients; it may be bilateral and necessitate pleurodesis. Chylothorax, chyloperitonium (chylous ascites), chyluria, and chylopericardium are other complications. Pulmonary function testing usually reveals an obstructive or mixed obstructive-restrictive pattern, and gas exchange is often abnormal. HRCT shows thin-walled cysts surrounded by normal lung without zonal predominance. Progression is common, with a median survival of 8 to 10 years from diagnosis. Oophorectomy, progesterone (10 mg/d), and, more recently, tamoxifen and luteinizing hormone-releasing hormone analogs have been used. Lung transplantation offers the only hope for cure despite reports of recurrent disease in the transplanted lung.

SYNDROMES OF ILD WITH DIFFUSE ALVEOLAR HEMORRHAGE Injury to arterioles, venules, and the alveolar septal (alveolar wall or interstitial) capillaries can result in hemoptysis secondary to disruption of the alveolar-capillary basement membrane. This results in bleeding into the alveolar spaces, which characterizes DAH. Pulmonary capillaritis, characterized by a neutrophilic infiltration of the alveolar septae, may lead to necrosis of these structures, loss of capillary structural integrity, and the pouring of red blood cells into the alveolar space. Fibrinoid necrosis of the interstitium and red blood cells within the interstitial space are sometimes seen. Bland pulmonary hemorrhage (i.e., DAH without inflammation of the alveolar structures) may also occur.

The clinical onset is often abrupt, with cough, fever, and dyspnea. Severe respiratory distress requiring ventilatory support may be evident at initial presentation. Although hemoptysis is expected, it can be absent at the time of presentation in one-third of the cases. For patients without hemoptysis, new alveolar opacities, a falling hemoglobin level, and hemorrhagic BAL fluid point to the diagnosis. The chest radiograph is nonspecific and most commonly shows new patchy or diffuse alveolar opacities. Recurrent episodes of DAH may lead to pulmonary fibrosis, resulting in interstitial opacities on the chest radiograph. An elevated white blood cell count and falling hematocrit are frequent. Evidence for impaired renal function caused by focal segmental necrotizing glomerulonephritis, usually with crescent formation, may also be present.

Varying degrees of hypoxemia may occur and often are severe enough to require ventilatory support. The D_{LCO} may be increased, resulting from the increased hemoglobin within the alveoli compartment. Evaluation of either lung or renal tissue by immunofluorescent techniques indicates an absence of immune complexes (pauci-immune) in Wegener's granulomatosis, microscopic polyangiitis pauci-immune glomerulonephritis, and isolated pulmonary capillaritis. A granular pattern is found in the CTDs, particularly SLE, and a characteristic linear deposition is found in Goodpasture's syndrome. Granular deposition of IgA-containing immune complexes are present in Henoch-Schönlein purpura.

The mainstay of therapy for the DAH associated with systemic vasculitis, CTD, Goodpasture's syndrome, and isolated pulmonary capillaritis is intravenous methylprenisolone, 0.5 to 2.0 g daily in divided doses for up to 5 days, followed by a gradual tapering, and then maintenance on an oral preparation. Prompt initiation of therapy is important, particularly in the face of renal insufficiency, since early initiation of therapy has the best chance of preserving renal function. The decision to start other immunosuppressive therapy (cyclophosphamide or azathioprine) acutely depends on the severity of illness.

Goodpasture's Syndrome Pulmonary hemorrhage and glomerulonephritis are features in most patients with this disease (Chap. 275). Autoantibodies to renal glomerular and lung alveolar basement membranes are present. This syndrome can present and recur as DAH without an associated glomerulonephritis. In such case, circulating anti-basement membrane antibody is often absent, and the only way to establish the diagnosis is by demonstrating linear immunofluorescence in lung tissue. The underlying histology may be bland hemorrhage or DAH associated with capillaritis. Plasmapheresis has been recommended as adjunctive treatment.

Idiopathic Pulmonary Hemosiderosis This condition is a diagnosis of exclusion. Only 20% of reported cases occur in adults. In children, the condition is associated with celiac disease, and elevated IgA levels are found in 50% of patients. These associations are lacking in most adults. A lung biopsy is usually necessary to document the lack of inflammatory injury in the lung tissues and to exclude other diseases with confidence.

INHERITED DISORDERS ASSOCIATED WITH ILD Pulmonary opacities and respiratory symptoms typical of ILD can develop in related family members and in several inherited diseases. These include the phakomatoses, tuberous sclerosis and neurofibromatosis (Chap. 370), and the lysosomal storage diseases, Niemann-Pick disease and Gaucher's disease (Chap. 349). The Hermansky-Pudlak syndrome (Chap. 116) is an autosomal recessive disorder in which granulomatous colitis and ILD may occur. It is characterized by oculocutaneous albinism, bleeding diathesis secondary to platelet dysfunction, and the accumulation of a chromolipid, lipofuscin material in cells of the reticuloendothelial system. The pulmonary fibrosis is similar to IPF, but the alveolar macrophages may contain cytoplasmic ceroid-like inclusions.

ILD WITH A GRANULOMATOUS RESPONSE IN LUNG TISSUE OR VASCULAR STRUCTURES Inhalation of organic dusts, which cause hypersensitivity pneumonitis, or of inorganic dust, such as silica, which elicits a granulomatous inflammatory reaction leading to ILD, produces diseases of known etiology (Table 259-1) that are discussed in Chaps. 253 and 254. Sarcoidosis (Chap. 318) is prominent among granulomatous diseases of unknown cause in which ILD is an important feature.

Pulmonary Langerhans Cell Histiocytosis (PLCH, Pulmonary Histiocytosis X, Langerhans Cell Granulomatosis, or Eosinophilic Granuloma PLCH is a rare, smoking-related, diffuse lung disease that primarily affects men between the ages of 20 and 40 years. The clinical presentation varies from an asymptomatic state to a rapidly progressive condition. The most common clinical manifestations at presentation are cough, dyspnea, chest pain, weight loss, and fever. Pneumothorax occurs in about 25% of patients. Hemoptysis and diabetes insipidus are rare manifestations. The radiographic features vary with the stage of the disease. The combination of ill-defined or stellate nodules (2 to 10 mm in diameter), reticular or nodular opacities, bizarre-shaped upper zone cysts, preservation of lung volume, and sparing of the costophrenic angles are characteristics of PLCH. HRCT that reveals a combination of nodules and thin-walled cysts is virtually diagnostic of PLCH. The most frequent pulmonary function abnormality is a markedly reduced D_{LCO}, although varying degrees of restrictive disease, airflow limitation, and diminished exercise capacity may occur. Discontinuance of smoking is the key treatment, resulting in clinical improvement in one-third of patients. Most patients with PLCH suffer persistent or progressive disease. Death due to respiratory failure occurs in ~10% of patients.

Granulomatous Vasculitides (See also Chap. 317) The granulomatous vasculitides are characterized by pulmonary angiitis (i.e., inflammation and necrosis of blood vessels) with associated granuloma formation (i.e., infiltrates of lymphocytes, plasma cells, epithelioid cells, or histiocytes, with or without the presence of multinucleated giant cells, sometimes with tissue necrosis). The lungs are almost always involved, although any organ system may be affected. Wegener's granulomatosis and allergic angiitis and granulomatosis (Churg-

Strauss syndrome) primarily affect the lung but are associated with a systemic vasculitis as well. The granulomatous vasculitides generally limited to the lung include necrotizing sarcoid granulomatosis and benign lymphocytic angiitis and granulomatosis. Granulomatous infection and pulmonary angiitis due to irritating embolic material (e.g., talc) are important known causes of pulmonary vasculitis.

LYMPHOCYTIC INFILTRATIVE DISORDERS This group of disorders features lymphocyte and plasma cell infiltration of the lung parenchyma. The disorders either are benign or can behave as low-grade lymphomas. Included are angioimmunoblastic lymphadenopathy with dysproteinemia, a rare lymphoproliferative disorder characterized by diffuse lymphadenopathy, fever, hepatosplenomegaly, and hemolytic anemia, with ILD in some cases.

Lymphocytic Interstitial Pneumonitis This rare form of ILD occurs in adults, some of whom have an autoimmune disease or dysproteinemia. It has been reported in patients with Sjögren's syndrome and HIV infection.

Lymphomatoid Granulomatosis This multisystem disorder of unknown etiology is an angiocentric malignant (T cell) lymphoma characterized by a polymorphic lymphoid infiltrate, an angiitis, and granulomatosis. Although it may affect virtually any organ, it is most frequently characterized by pulmonary, skin, and central nervous system involvement.

BRONCHOCENTRIC GRANULOMATOSIS Rather than a specific clinical entity, bronchocentric granulomatosis (BG) is a descriptive histologic term that describes an uncommon and nonspecific pathologic response to a variety of airway injuries. There is evidence that BG is caused by a hypersensitivity reaction to *Aspergillus* or other fungi in patients with asthma. About half of the patients described have chronic asthma with severe wheezing and peripheral blood eosinophilia. In patients with asthma, BG probably represents one pathologic manifestation of allergic bronchopulmonary aspergillosis, or another allergic mycosis. In patients without asthma, BG has been associated with rheumatoid arthritis and a variety of infections, including tuberculosis, echinococcosis, histoplasmosis, coccidiodomycosis, and nocardiosis. The chest roentgenogram reveals irregularly shaped nodular or mass lesions with ill-defined margins, which are usually unilateral and solitary, with an upper-lobe predominance. Glucocorticoids are the treatment of choice, often with excellent outcome, although recurrences may occur as therapy is tapered or stopped.

BIBLIOGRAPHY

AMERICAN THORACIC SOCIETY: Idiopathic pulmonary fibrosis: Diagnosis and treatment. International Consensus Statement. Am J Resp Crit Care Med 161:646, 2000

BJORAKER JA et al: Prognostic significance of histiopathologic subsets in idiopathic pulmonary fibrosis. Am J Respir Crit Care Med 157:199, 1998

BRITISH THORACIC SOCIETY: The Diagnosis, Assessment and Treatment of Diffuse Parenchymal Lung Disease in Adults. Thorax 54 (Suppl 1):S1-S28, 1999

GOLDSTEIN LS et al: Pulmonary alveolar proteinosis: Clinical features and outcomes. Chest 114:1357, 1998

JENNINGS CA et al: Pauci-immune pulmonary capillaritis and diffuse alveolar hemorrhage: A vasculitic process limited to the lungs. Am J Respir Crit Care Med 155:1101, 1997

KALASSIAN KG, RAFFIN TA: Lymphangioleiomyomatosis, in *Textbook of Respiratory Medicine*, 3d ed, JF Murray, JA Nadel (eds). Philadelphia, Saunders, 2000, pp 1775–1788

KATZENSTEIN ALA, MYERS JL: Idiopathic pulmonary fibrosis. Clinical relevance of pathologic classification. Am J Respir Crit Care Med 157:1310, 1998

KING TE Jr: Connective tissue disease, *Interstitial Lung Diseases*, 3d ed, MI Schwarz, TE King, Jr. (eds). Hamilton, BC Decker, 1998, 451-505

LIMPER AH, ROSENOW III EC: Drug-induced interstitial lung disease. Curr Opin Pulm Med 2:396, 1996

NAGAI S et al: Idiopathic nonspecific interstitial pneumonia/fibrosis: Comparison with idiopathic pulmonary fibrosis and BOOP. Europ Respir J 12:1010, 1998

TAZI A et al: Adult pulmonary Langerhans' cell histiocytosis. Thorax 55:405, 2000

260 PRIMARY PULMONARY HYPERTENSION

Stuart Rich

Primary pulmonary hypertension is an uncommon disease characterized by increased pulmonary artery pressure and pulmonary vascular resistance. The incidence has been estimated at approximately 2 cases per million. There is a female-to-male preponderance (1.7:1), with patients most commonly presenting in the third and fourth decades, although the age range is from infancy to greater than 60 years. Because the predominant symptom of primary pulmonary hypertension is dyspnea, which can have an insidious onset in an otherwise healthy person, the disease is typically diagnosed late in its course. By that time, the clinical and laboratory findings of severe pulmonary hypertension are usually present.

PATHOLOGY The histopathology of primary pulmonary hypertension is not pathognomonic for the disease but represents a pulmonary arteriopathy that is observed in pulmonary hypertension from a variety of causes. A wide spectrum of vascular abnormalities involving the endothelium, smooth muscle cells, and extracellular matrix is present. Heterogeneity with respect to these abnormalities is often seen from patient to patient, and within patients. The most common features noted are medial hypertrophy, concentric and eccentric intimal fibrosis, recanalized thrombi appearing as fibrous webs, and plexiform lesions. In most patients, varying degrees of these abnormalities can be found. Rare variant forms of primary pulmonary hypertension also exist.

Pulmonary venoocclusive disease is a rare and distinct pathologic entity, found in fewer than 10% of patients with primary pulmonary hypertension. Histologically, it is manifest by widespread intimal proliferation and fibrosis of the intrapulmonary veins and venules, occasionally extending to the arteriolar bed. The pulmonary venous obstruction explains the increased pulmonary capillary wedge pressure observed in patients with advanced disease. These patients may develop orthopnea that can mimic left ventricular failure.

Pulmonary capillary hemangiomatosis is also a very rare form of primary pulmonary hypertension. Histologically, it is characterized by infiltrating thin-walled blood vessels that are widespread throughout the pulmonary interstitium and walls of the pulmonary arteries and veins. These patients often have hemoptysis as a clinical feature.

ETIOLOGY It is likely that there are several pathobiologic processes that result in pulmonary hypertension as a final common pathway. These include inhibition of the voltage-regulated (Kv) potassium channel producing vasoconstriction secondary to contraction of the pulmonary artery smooth muscle cells, an imbalance in vasoconstricting and vasodilating mediators that are involved in the control of pulmonary vascular tone (including prostacyclin and thromboxane), reduced expression of nitric oxide synthase in the endothelium of the pulmonary arterial bed, inflammation, thrombosis in situ of the pulmonary vascular bed from a procoagulant state, and persistent matrix protein synthesis in the pulmonary arteries. The types of abnormalities that occur are likely influenced by the patient's genotype and exposure to risk factors that serve to trigger these processes. Risk factors that have been linked to the development of pulmonary hypertension include anorexigens, collagen vascular diseases, congenital systemic to pulmonary shunts, portal hypertension, and HIV infection.

Recently, a marked increase in the incidence of primary pulmonary hypertension occurred in Europe and the United States as a result of the widespread use of the fenfluramine appetite suppressants. The clinical and pathologic features of these cases were identical to patients with primary pulmonary hypertension who were unexposed. Atlhough very limited exposure to the fenfluramines can cause primary pulmonary hypertension, the risk increased dramatically with prolonged use. Like the experience with aminorex, an anorexigen that produced a similar epidemic in the 1960s, the incidence of primary pulmonary hypertension fell when the drugs were withdrawn from the market. The mechanism by which these agents produce pulmonary hypertension is unknown.

GENETIC CONSIDERATIONS The locus of a gene linked to familial primary pulmonary hypertension has been identified on chromosome 2q31-32. Familial primary pulmonary hypertension occurs in approximately 6 to 12% of cases and is characterized by autosomal dominant inheritance, variable age of onset, and incomplete penetrance. The clinical and pathologic features of familial and sporadic primary pulmonary hypertension are virtually identical. Genetic anticipation, which relates to offspring of subsequent generations manifesting the disease at younger ages or with greater severity, is also a feature. Trinucleotide repeat expansion, originally described in several neurologic disorders, remains the only biologic explanation for genetic anticipation and raises the possibility that the pathogenesis of familial primary pulmonary hypertension may have a neurologic basis. Patients who present with sporadic disease probably possess a genetic predisposition that becomes expressed following exposure to an external trigger or risk factor. ■

PATHOPHYSIOLOGY The underlying hemodynamic derangement in primary pulmonary hypertension is an increased resistance to pulmonary blood flow. Early in the disease there is a marked elevation in pulmonary artery pressure with relatively normal cardiac function. Over time the cardiac output becomes progressively reduced rather than the pulmonary artery pressure becoming progressively increased. Initially, the pulmonary arteries may respond to vasodilators, but as the disease progresses, the elevated pulmonary vascular resistance becomes fixed. The pulmonary capillary wedge pressure remains normal until the late stages, when it tends to rise in response to impaired diastolic filling of the left ventricle due to the altered configuration of the intraventricular septum. Eventually, as the right ventricle fails, the right atrial and right ventricular end-diastolic pressures rise in an attempt to compensate for the myocardial depression that has developed in response to chronic severe right ventricular pressure overload.

Pulmonary function is usually normal in primary pulmonary hypertension, although a mild restrictive pattern (Chap. 250) is sometimes seen. Hypoxemia is common and is believed to be due to a mismatch between pulmonary ventilation and perfusion, magnified by a low cardiac output. Occasional patients with a patent foramen ovale may develop right-to-left shunting, which can also contribute to systemic arterial desaturation.

DIAGNOSIS Primary pulmonary hypertension refers to pulmonary arterial hypertension wihtout an identifiable risk factor. Clinically, primary pulmonary arterial hypertension should be distinguished from pulmonary venous hypertension, pulmonary hypertension associated with disorders of the respiratory system and/or hypoxema, and pulmonary hypertension due to chronic thrombotic and/or embolic disease (Chap. 261).

A thorough diagnostic evaluation to look for all potential causes should be undertaken (Fig. 260-1). The history usually reveals the gradual onset of shortness of breath with effort, progressing until the patient is dyspneic with minimal activity. The average duration from symptom onset until diagnosis is 2.5 years. Other common symptoms are fatigue, angina pectoris that likely represents right ventricular ischemia, syncope, near syncope, and peripheral edema.

The physical examination is characteristic. Increased jugular venous pressure, a reduced carotid pulse, and an easily palpable right ventricular lift are typical. Most patients have an increased pulmonic component of the second heart sound and right-sided third and fourth heart sounds. Tricuspid regurgitation is a clinical feature of right ventricular failure. Peripheral cyanosis and/or edema tend to occur in later stages of the disease. Clubbing is not a feature.

The chest x-ray generally shows enlarged central pulmonary arteries and clear lung fields. The electrocardiogram usually reveals right axis deviation and right ventricular hypertrophy. The echocardiogram

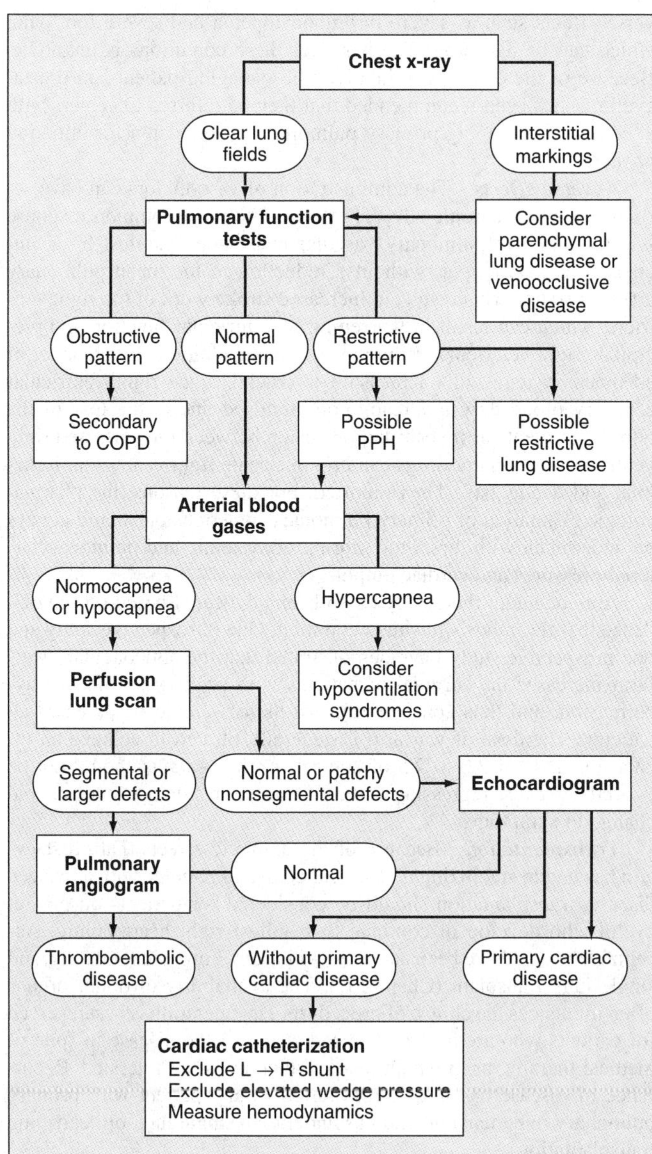

FIGURE 260-1 An algorithm for the workup of a patient with unexplained pulmonary hypertension.

demonstrates right ventricular enlargement, a reduction in left ventricular cavity size, and abnormal septal configuration consistent with right ventricular pressure overload. Doppler studies have revealed a marked dependence on atrial systole for ventricular filling. Hypoxemia, hypocapnia, and an abnormal diffusing capacity for carbon monoxide are almost invariable findings. A mild restrictive pattern on pulmonary function is sometimes observed, but evidence of airways obstruction suggests a secondary etiology for the pulmonary hypertension. The presence of significant restrictive changes on pulmonary function testing (Chap. 250) should prompt a high-resolution computed tomographic scan to look for interstitial lung disease, which may otherwise not be obvious. A perfusion lung scan may be normal or abnormal with multiple diffuse patchy filling defects of a nonsegmental nature and not suggestive of pulmonary thromboembolism. If the lung scan reveals perfusion defects of a segmental or subsegmental nature, a pulmonary angiogram must be done. Severe pulmonary hypertension in a patient with a high-probability lung scan should suggest a chronic process and *not* acute pulmonary embolism, since the nonconditioned right ventricle is unable to generate high systolic pressures acutely in the face of pulmonary thromboembolism. Chronic thromboembolic obstruction of the large pulmonary arteries (Chap. 261) can mimic primary pulmonary hypertension but can be amenable to treatment with surgical thromboendarterectomy.

There is risk in performing pulmonary angiography in patients with primary pulmonary hypertension, and it is recommended that selective or subselective injections with small amounts of low-osmolar, nonionic contrast material be made following the pretreatment with 1 mg atropine to prevent vagally mediated bradycardia.

Cardiac catheterization is mandatory to characterize the disease and exclude an underlying cardiac shunt as the cause. The use of balloon-flotation catheters, especially those with removable guidewires, can facilitate right heart catheterization. A right-to-left shunt might be attributable to a patent foramen ovale, but any left-to-right shunting implies the presence of a congenital defect. Although it may be difficult to obtain, the pulmonary capillary wedge pressure is normal. If it is increased, left heart catheterization should also be performed to exclude mitral stenosis or increased left ventricular end-diastolic pressures as the cause of the pulmonary hypertension. Although the diagnostic evaluation of these patients can be hazardous, experience from a national multicenter study revealed no mortality or serious morbidity in more than 300 patients whose evaluation included pulmonary angiography and cardiac catheterization. It is not necessary to perform an open lung biopsy in these patients to make an accurate diagnosis. Laboratory tests should also be performed, including antinuclear antibody and HIV testing.

On occasion, a patient may have marked elevations in pulmonary artery pressure in association with mild obstructive or interstitial lung disease, essential hypertension, ischemic heart disease, or valvular heart disease. Although it may appear that the pulmonary hypertension is out of proportion to the underlying associated condition, it likely represents a pulmonary vasoconstrictive response to the associated condition, which is serving as a trigger of pulmonary arterial hypertension. Thus severe pulmonary hypertension can coexist with mild chronic obstructive pulmonary disease, small intracardiac shunts, mild mitral stenosis, and even ischemic heart disease. The distinction is important because the treatment of pulmonary hypertension should always include treating the underlying associated cause.

NATURAL HISTORY The natural history of primary pulmonary hypertension is unknown because initially the disease is largely asymptomatic. Several older series have reported a mean survival of 2 to 3 years for patients from the time of diagnosis. Functional class is a strong predictor of survival, since patients who are New York Heart Association functional classes II and III have a mean survival of 3.5 years compared with those who are functional class IV, in whom the mean survival is 6 months. The cause of death is usually right ventricular failure or sudden death; sudden death appears to be a late feature of the disease. Increased right atrial pressure above 15 mmHg and reduced cardiac index below 2 (L/min)/m^2 are hemodynamic predictors of a poor prognosis.

℞ **TREATMENT** Because the pulmonary vascular resistance increases dramatically with exercise, patients should be cautioned against participating in activities that demand increased physical stress. Digoxin may increase cardiac output and lower circulating levels of norepinephrine. Diuretic therapy relieves dyspnea and peripheral edema and may be useful in reducing right ventricular volume overload in the presence of tricuspid regurgitation.

It is recommended that all patients in whom primary pulmonary hypertension is confirmed undergo acute drug testing with short-acting pulmonary vasodilators to determine the extent of pulmonary vasodilator reserve or reactivity (Fig. 260-2). Intravenous adenosine, inhaled nitric oxide, and intravenous prostacyclin all appear to have similar effects in reducing pulmonary vascular resistance acutely with little effect on the systemic vascular bed. Adenosine is given as a constant infusion in doses of 50 (μg/kg)/min and increased every 2 min until side effects develop. Similarly, prostacyclin is given in doses of 2 (ng/kg)/min and increased every 30 min until side effects develop. Maximal physiologic effectiveness of the therapy is determined at the highest tolerated dose. Nitric oxide is generally administered via in-

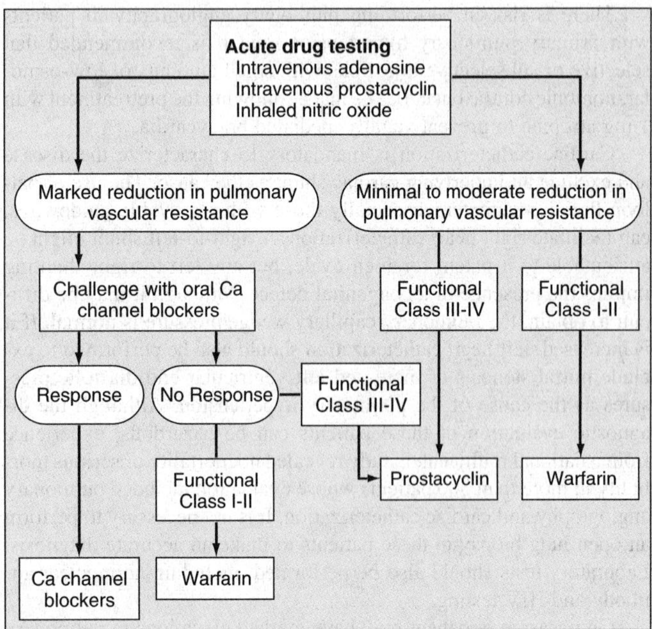

FIGURE 260-2 An algorithm for the evaluation and drug treatment of a patient with primary pulmonary hypertension.

halation in 5 to 10 parts per million and increased every few minutes until no further effectiveness is obtained.

Calcium channel antagonists Patients who have substantial reductions in pulmonary vascular resistance from the short-acting vasodilators may be candidates to receive oral calcium channel blockers. These drugs should be administered under direct hemodynamic guidance in order to determine effectiveness and safety. Typically, patients will require high doses (e.g., nifedipine, 120 to 240 mg/d, or diltiazem, 540 to 900 mg/d*). Patients who manifest significant reductions in mean pulmonary artery pressure and pulmonary vascular resistance should demonstrate improved symptoms, regression of right ventricular hypertrophy, and improved survival with chronic therapy. However, fewer than half the patients who are responsive to the short-acting vasodilators will respond to this regimen. It is unknown whether the response to calcium blockers depends on the histologic subtype, but the therapy appears to be more successful in patients who are diagnosed early and have less advanced disease.

Prostacyclin This agent has been approved as a treatment of primary pulmonary hypertension for patients who are functional class III or IV and unresponsive to conventional therapy. Clinical trials have demonstrated that patients realize an improvement in symptoms and exercise tolerance and reduction in mortality, even if no acute hemodynamic response to drug challenge occurs. The drug can only be administered intravenously and requires placement of a permanent central venous catheter and continuous dose titration, as tolerance develops in all patients over a short period of time. The optimal dose has not been determined. Patients may deteriorate clinically from too much or too little drug. The side effects of prostacyclin, which include flushing, jaw pain, and diarrhea, are generally tolerated by most patients. The major problems with this therapy have been infections related to the venous catheter, which requires close monitoring and diligence on behalf of the patient. Recent data suggest that prostacyclin, in addition to its vasodilator and antithrombotic properties, may lead to reversal of the vascular remodeling that occurs in primary pulmonary hypertension. Long-term use of prostacyclin has been associated with adverse effects such as severe thrombocytopenia and severe foot pain, which can be disabling. The basis for these conditions is unknown. Because of the complexity involved in managing patients on prostacyclin, it has been recommended that they be referred to centers with expertise in managing primary pulmonary hypertension for initiation of therapy.

*These agents have not been approved for the treatment of primary pulmonary hypertension by the U.S. Food and Drug Administration.

Adverse effects The administration of vasodilators can have serious acute and chronic adverse effects. The most common response is a reduction in pulmonary vascular resistance, manifest by an increased cardiac output, without a reduction in the mean pulmonary artery pressure. This results in increased stroke work of the right ventricle, which can result in worsening of ventricular function and precipitate right ventricular failure over time. In addition, maintenance of adequate systemic blood pressure is crucial, since right ventricular coronary blood flow is already compromised due to the loss of the normal gradient for myocardial perfusion between the aorta and right ventricle. Vasodilator drugs can provoke acute right ventricular ischemia, and deaths have been reported. For these reasons, the pharmacologic evaluation of primary pulmonary hypertension should always be undertaken with direct monitoring of systemic and pulmonary arterial pressures and cardiac output.

Anticoagulant therapy has also been advocated based on the evidence that thrombosis in situ is common. One retrospective study and one prospective study have demonstrated that the anticoagulant warfarin increases the survival of patients with primary pulmonary hypertension, and thus consideration for its use should be given to all patients. The dose of warfarin is generally titrated to achieve an increase in INR of 2.0 to 2.5 of control. Anticoagulants should not be expected to cause regression of the disease and result in any substantial change in symptoms.

Transplantation Because of the dramatic effects that prostacyclin has had in stabilizing the clinical course of patients with advanced disease, transplantation should be considered for patients on prostacyclin who develop or continue to manifest right heart failure. Acceptable results have been achieved with heart-lung, bilateral lung, and single lung transplant (Chap. 267). The availability of donor organs often influences the choice of procedure. The operation is best reserved for patients who are in the advanced stages of the disease in spite of medical therapy, or in whom medical therapy is not tolerated. Recurrence of disease has not been reported in any patient with primary pulmonary hypertension who has undergone single lung or heart-lung transplantation.

BIBLIOGRAPHY

ARROLIGA AC et al: Primary pulmonary hypertension: Update on pathogenesis and novel therapies. Cleve Clin J Med 67:175, 181, 189, 2000

MCLAUGHLIN VV et al: Reduction in pulmonary vascular resistance with long-term prostacyclin therapy in primary pulmonary hypertension. N Engl J Med 338:273, 1998

RICH S, BRAUNWALD E: Pulmonary hypertension, in *Heart Disease*, 6th ed, E Braunwald (ed). Philadelphia, Saunders, 2001, Chap. 53

RICH S (ed): Primary Pulmonary Hypertension: Executive Summary from the World Symposium—Primary Pulmonary Hypertension 1998. Available from the World Health Organization via the Internet (www.who.int/ncd/cvd/pph.html)

RUBIN LJ et al: Pulmonary vasculitis and primary pulmonary hypertension, in *Textbook of Respiratory Medicine*, 3d ed, JF Murray, JA Nadel (eds). Philadelphia, Saunders, 2000, pp 1533–1556

261 PULMONARY THROMBOEMBOLISM

Samuel Z. Goldhaber

GENETIC CONSIDERATIONS Rudolf Virchow postulated more than a century ago that three potentially overlapping factors predisposed to venous thrombosis: (1) local trauma to the vessel wall; (2) hypercoagulability; and (3) stasis. We now believe that many patients who suffer pulmonary thromboembolism (PTE) have an under-

Table 261-1 Stressors That May Precipitate Pulmonary Thromboembolism

Surgery, trauma
Obesity
Oral contraceptives, pregnancy, postpartum, postmenopausal hormone replacement
Cancer (sometimes occult) or cancer chemotherapy
Immobilization (stroke or intensive care unit patients)
Indwelling central venous catheter

lying inherited predisposition that remains clinically silent until an acquired stressor occurs such as surgery, obesity, or pregnancy (Table 261-1). When PTE is identified, a detailed family history for venous thromboembolism should be obtained.

Factor V Leiden The most frequent inherited predisposition to hypercoagulability is resistance to the endogenous anticoagulant protein, activated protein C. The phenotype of activated protein C resistance is associated with a single point mutation, designated *factor V Leiden*, in the factor V gene. This missense mutation—a single nucleotide substitution of adenine for guanine 1691—causes an amino acid substitution of glutamine for arginine at position 506.

The prevalence of the heterozygous state was about 6% in healthy American male physicians participating in the Physicians' Health Study and was three times higher among those physicians who subsequently developed venous thrombosis. Furthermore, after anticoagulation (for at least 3 months) was completed and discontinued, those participants with factor V Leiden had a much higher rate of recurrent venous thrombosis than those without. A single-point mutation in the 3′ untranslated region of the prothrombin gene (G-to-A transition at nucleotide position 20210) appears to be associated with increased levels of prothrombin (factor II), the precursor of thrombin. In the Physicians' Health Study, the prevalence of the prothrombin gene mutation among control subjects was 3.9%. The G20210A mutation conferred an approximate doubling of the risk of venous thrombosis. Nevertheless, factor V Leiden is more common than all other (identified) inherited hypercoagulable states, including the prothrombin gene mutation, deficiencies in protein C, protein S, antithrombin III, and disorders of plasminogen (Chap. 117). ■

PATHOPHYSIOLOGY

EMBOLIZATION When venous thrombi become dislodged from their site of formation, they embolize to the pulmonary arterial circulation or, paradoxically, to the arterial circulation through a patent foramen ovale or atrial septal defect. About half of patients with pelvic vein thrombosis or proximal leg deep venous thrombosis (DVT) have PTE, which is usually asymptomatic. Isolated calf vein or upper extremity venous thromboses also pose a risk (albeit lower) of PTE. Isolated calf vein thrombi are the most common source of paradoxical embolism.

PHYSIOLOGY Pulmonary embolism can have the following effects:

1. *Increased pulmonary vascular resistance* due to vascular obstruction or neurohumoral agents including serotonin
2. *Impaired gas exchange* due to increased alveolar dead space from vascular obstruction and hypoxemia from alveolar hypoventilation in the nonobstructed lung, right-to-left shunting, and impaired carbon monoxide transfer due to loss of gas exchange surface
3. *Alveolar hyperventilation* due to reflex stimulation of irritant receptors
4. *Increased airway resistance* due to bronchoconstriction
5. *Decreased pulmonary compliance* due to lung edema, lung hemorrhage, or loss of surfactant

Right Ventricular Dysfunction Progressive right heart failure is the usual cause of death from PTE. In the International Cooperative Pulmonary Embolism Registry (ICOPER), the presence of right ventricular dysfunction on baseline echocardiography of PTE patients was associated with a doubling of the 3-month mortality rate. As pulmonary vascular resistance increases, right ventricular wall tension rises and perpetuates further right ventricular dilatation and dysfunction. Consequently, the interventricular septum bulges into and compresses an intrinsically normal left ventricle. Increased right ventricular wall tension also compresses the right coronary artery and may precipitate myocardial ischemia and right ventricular infarction. Underfilling of the left ventricle may lead to a fall in left ventricular output and systemic arterial pressure, thereby provoking myocardial ischemia due to compromised coronary artery perfusion. Eventually, circulatory collapse and death may ensue.

DIAGNOSIS

The clinical setting can be immensely helpful in suggesting the diagnosis of PTE. Patients with prior venous thromboembolism are at increased risk of recurrence (Table 261-1).

CLINICAL SYNDROMES Patients with *massive PTE* present with systemic arterial hypotension and usually have anatomically widespread thromboembolism. Primary therapy with thrombolysis or embolectomy offers the greatest chance of survival. Those with *moderate to large PTE* have right ventricular hypokinesis on echocardiography but normal systemic arterial pressure. Optimal management is controversial; such patients may benefit from primary therapy to prevent recurrent embolism. Patients with *small to moderate PTE* have both normal right heart function and normal systemic arterial pressure. They have a good prognosis with either adequate anticoagulation or an inferior vena caval filter. The presence of *pulmonary infarction* usually indicates a small PTE, but one that is exquisitely painful, because it lodges near the innervation of pleural nerves.

Nonthrombotic pulmonary embolism may be easily overlooked. Possible etiologies include fat embolism after blunt trauma and long bone fractures, tumor embolism, or air embolism. Intravenous drug users may inject themselves with a wide array of substances, such as hair, talc, or cotton. *Amniotic fluid embolism* occurs when fetal membranes leak or tear at the placental margin. The pulmonary edema seen in this syndrome is probably due primarily to alveolar capillary leakage.

SYMPTOMS AND SIGNS Dyspnea is the most frequent symptom of PTE, and tachypnea is its most frequent sign. Whereas dyspnea, syncope, hypotension, or cyanosis indicate a massive PTE, pleuritic pain, cough, or hemoptysis often suggest a small embolism located distally near the pleura. On *physical examination*, young and previously healthy individuals may simply appear anxious but otherwise seem deceptively well, even with an anatomically large PTE. They need not have "classic" signs such as tachycardia, low-grade fever, neck vein distention, or an accentuated pulmonic component of the second heart sound. Sometimes, a paradoxical bradycardia occurs.

In older patients who complain of vague chest discomfort, the diagnosis of PTE may not be apparent unless signs of right heart failure are present. Unfortunately, because acute coronary ischemic syndromes are so common, one may overlook the possibility of life-threatening PTE and may inadvertently discharge these patients from the hospital after the exclusion of myocardial infarction with serial cardiac enzyme measurements and electrocardiograms.

DIFFERENTIAL DIAGNOSIS The differential diagnosis of PTE is broad (Table 261-2). Although PTE is known as "the great masquerader," quite often another illness simulates PTE. For example, when the proposed diagnosis of PTE is supposedly confirmed with a combination of dyspnea, chest pain, and an abnormal lung scan, the correct diagnosis of pneumonia might become apparent 12 h later when an infiltrate blossoms on chest x-ray, purulent sputum is first produced, and high fever and shaking chills develop.

Some patients have PTE and a coexisting illness such as pneumonia or heart failure. In such circumstances, clinical improvement

Table 261-2 Differential Diagnosis of Pulmonary Thromboembolism

Myocardial infarction, unstable angina
Pneumonia, bronchitis, COPD exacerbation
Congestive heart failure
Asthma
Pericarditis
Primary pulmonary hypertension
Rib fracture, pneumothorax
Costochondritis, ''musculoskeletal pain,'' anxiety

NOTE: COPD, chronic obstructive pulmonary disease.

will often fail to occur despite standard medical treatment of the concomitant illness. This situation can serve as a clinical clue to the possible coexistence of PTE.

NONIMAGING DIAGNOSTIC MODALITIES These are generally safer, less expensive, but also less specific than diagnostic modalities that employ imaging.

Blood Tests The quantitative *plasma D-dimer enzyme-linked immunosorbent assay (ELISA)* level is elevated (>500 ng/mL) in more than 90% of patients with PTE, reflecting plasmin's breakdown of fibrin and indicating endogenous (though clinically ineffective) thrombolysis. A qualitative latex agglutination D-dimer assay, which is more readily available and less expensive than an ELISA, can be obtained initially; if elevated, the ELISA will also be elevated. However, if the latex agglutination is normal, a D-dimer ELISA should be obtained, because the ELISA is much more sensitive than the latex agglutination D-dimer assay, which cannot be used to exclude PTE. The plasma D-dimer ELISA has a high negative predictive value and can be used to help exclude PTE. However, neither D-dimer assay is specific. Levels increase in patients with myocardial infarction, sepsis, or almost any systemic illness.

Data from the Prospective Investigation of Pulmonary Embolism Diagnosis (PIOPED) indicate that, contrary to classic teaching, *arterial blood gases* lack diagnostic utility for PTE. Among patients suspected of PTE, neither the room air arterial P_{O_2} nor calculation of the alveolar-arterial oxygen gradient can reliably differentiate or triage patients who actually have PTE at angiography.

Electrocardiogram Classic abnormalities include sinus tachycardia; new-onset atrial fibrillation or flutter; and an S wave in lead I, a Q wave in lead III, and an inverted T wave in lead III (Chap. 226). Often, the QRS axis is greater than 90°. T-wave inversion in leads V_1 to V_4 reflects right ventricular strain.

NONINVASIVE IMAGING MODALITIES **Chest Roentgenography** A normal or near-normal chest x-ray in a dyspneic patient suggests PTE. Well-established abnormalities include focal oligemia (Westermark's sign), a peripheral wedged-shaped density above the diaphragm (Hampton's hump), or an enlarged right descending pulmonary artery (Palla's sign).

Venous Ultrasonography Confirmed DVT is usually an adequate surrogate for PTE. Ultrasonography of the deep venous system relies upon loss of vein compressibility as the primary criterion for DVT. About one-third of patients with PTE have no imaging evidence of DVT. In these situations, the clot may have already embolized to the lung or is in the pelvic veins, where ultrasonography is usually inadequate. Therefore, the workup for PTE should continue if there is high clinical suspicion, despite a normal ultrasound examination.

Lung Scanning (See also Chap. 251) Lung scanning is the principal imaging test for the diagnosis of PTE. Small particulate aggregates of albumin labeled with a gamma-emitting radionuclide are injected intravenously and are trapped in the pulmonary capillary bed. A perfusion scan defect indicates absent or decreased blood flow, possibly due to PTE. Ventilation scans, obtained with radiolabeled inhaled gases such as xenon or krypton, improve the specificity of the perfusion scan. Abnormal ventilation scans indicate abnormal nonventilated lung, thereby providing possible explanations for perfusion defects other than acute PTE. A high probability scan for PTE is defined as having two or more segmental perfusion defects in the presence of normal ventilation (Fig. 261-1).

Lung scanning is particularly useful if the results are normal or near-normal, or if there is a high probability for PTE. The diagnosis of PTE is very unlikely in patients with normal and near-normal scans but, in contrast, is about 90% certain in patients with high-probability scans. Unfortunately, fewer than half of patients with angiographically confirmed PTE have a high-probability scan. Importantly, as many as 40% of patients with high clinical suspicion for PTE and "low-probability" scans do, in fact, have PTE at angiography.

Chest CT Computed tomography (CT) of the chest with intravenous contrast effectively diagnoses large, central PTE but may fail to detect more peripherally located thrombi that are clinically important. In a comparison with standard contrast pulmonary angiography at Massachusetts General Hospital, the sensitivity of chest CT for PTE was only 60%.

Echocardiography This technique is useful for rapid triage of acutely ill patients who may have PTE. Bedside echocardiography can usually reliably differentiate among illnesses that have radically different treatment, including acute myocardial infarction, pericardial tamponade, dissection of the aorta, and PTE complicated by right heart failure. Detection of right ventricular dysfunction due to PTE helps to stratify the risk, delineate the prognosis, and plan optimal management.

INVASIVE DIAGNOSTIC MODALITIES **Pulmonary Angiography** Selective pulmonary angiography is the most specific examination available for establishing the definitive diagnosis of PTE and can detect emboli as small as 1 to 2 mm. A definitive diagnosis of PTE depends upon visualization of an intraluminal filling defect in more than one projection. Secondary signs of PTE include abrupt occlusion ("cut-off") of vessels; segmental oligemia or avascularity; a prolonged arterial phase with slow filling; or tortuous, tapering peripheral vessels.

Pulmonary angiography can be carried out safely among properly selected patients at hospitals that perform at least several studies per month. In PIOPED, the procedure resulted in death in five patients (0.5%), two of whom had severe heart failure prior to the procedure. Angiography is most useful when the clinical likelihood of PTE differs substantially from the lung scan result or when the lung scan is of intermediate probability for PTE.

Contrast Phlebography This technique has been mostly replaced by ultra-

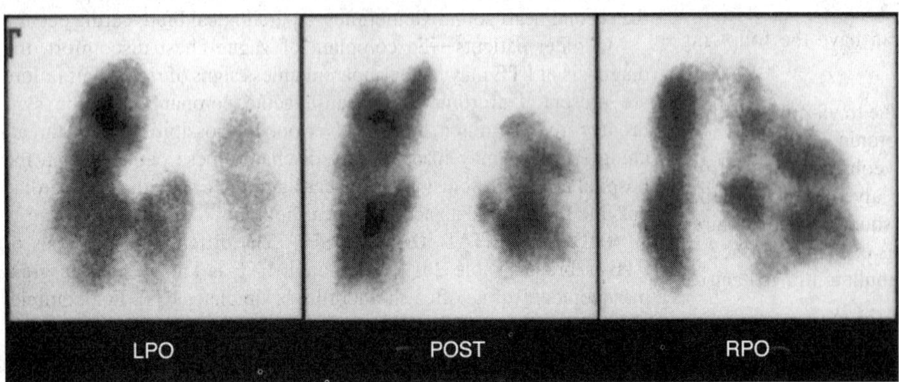

FIGURE 261-1 These three views of the pulmonary perfusion scan illustrate multiple segmental perfusion defects in both lung fields. The ventilation scan, which is normal, is not shown. The marked mismatch between normal ventilation and abnormal perfusion makes this lung scan *high probability for PTE*. LPO, left posterior oblique; POST, posterior; RPO, right posterior oblique.

sonography. Venography is costly, uncomfortable, and occasionally results in contrast allergy or contrast-induced phlebitis. Contrast phlebography is worthwhile when there is a discrepancy between the clinical suspicion and the ultrasound result. Phlebography is also useful for diagnosing isolated calf vein thrombosis or recurrent DVT. A recently approved nuclear medicine test utilizing a synthetic peptide that binds preferentially to the glycoprotein IIb/IIIa receptors on activated platelets may eventually replace contrast phlebography in clinical practice. This radiopharmaceutical permits scintigraphic imaging of acute DVT and may be especially useful for differentiating acute from chronic DVT.

INTEGRATED DIAGNOSTIC APPROACH We advocate an integrated diagnostic approach to streamline the workup of PTE (Fig. 261-2). This strategy combines the clinical likelihood of PTE with the results of noninvasive testing especially D-dimer ELISA, venous ultrasonography, and lung scanning to determine whether pulmonary angiography is warranted.

℞ TREATMENT Consensus guidelines from the American College of Chest Physicians are summarized as follows.

Primary versus Secondary Therapy Primary therapy consists of clot dissolution with thrombolysis or removal of PTE by embolectomy. Anticoagulation with heparin and warfarin or placement of an inferior vena caval filter constitutes secondary prevention of recurrent PTE rather than primary therapy.

Primary therapy should be reserved for patients at high risk of an adverse clinical outcome. When right ventricular function remains normal, patients typically have good clinical outcomes with anticoagulation alone (Fig. 261-3).

Adjunctive Therapy Important adjunctive measures include pain relief (especially with nonsteroidal anti-inflammatory agents), supplemental oxygenation, and psychological support. Dobutamine—a β-adrenergic agonist with positive inotropic and pulmonary vasodilating effects—may successfully treat right heart failure and cardiogenic shock. Volume loading should be undertaken cautiously because increased right ventricular dilatation can lead to even further reductions in left ventricular forward output.

Heparin Heparin binds to and accelerates the activity of antithrombin III, an enzyme that inhibits the coagulation factors thrombin (factor IIa), Xa, IXa, XIa, and XIIa. Heparin thus prevents additional thrombus formation and permits endogenous fibrinolytic mechanisms to lyse clot that has already formed. After 5 to 7 days of heparin, residual thrombus begins to stabilize in the endothelium of the vein

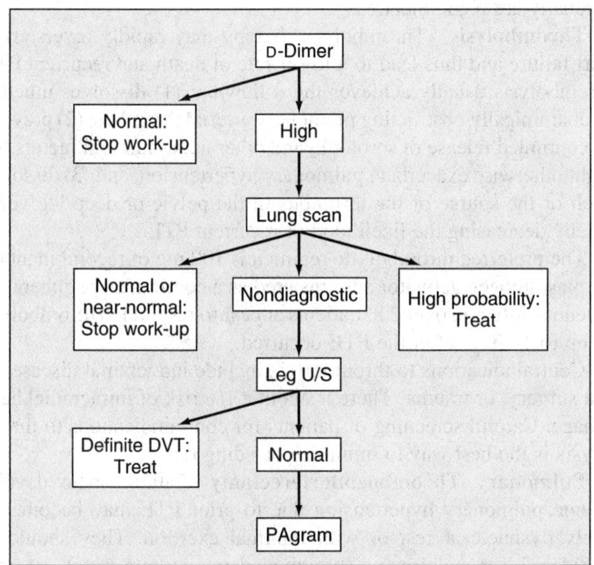

FIGURE 261-2 PTE diagnosis strategy: An integrated diagnostic approach. U/S, ultrasound; PAgram, pulmonary arteriogram.

Guidelines for the Treatment of Pulmonary Embolism

1. Treat DVT or PTE with therapeutic levels of unfractionated intravenous heparin, adjusted subcutaneous heparin, or low-molecular-weight heparin for at least 5 days and overlap with oral anticoagulation for at least 4 to 5 days. Consider a longer course of heparin for massive PTE or severe iliofemoral DVT.
2. For most patients, heparin and oral anticoagulation can be started together and heparin discontinued on day 5 or 6 if the INR has been therapeutic for two consecutive days.
3. Continue oral anticoagulant therapy for at least 3 months with a target INR of 2.5 (range 2.0 to 3.0).
4. Patients with reversible or time-limited risk factors can be treated for 3 to 6 months. Patients with a first episode of idiopathic DVT should be treated for at least 6 months. Patients with recurrent venous thrombosis or a continuing risk factor such as cancer, inhibitor deficiency states, or antiphospholipid antibody syndrome should be treated indefinitely.
5. Isolated calf vein DVT should be treated with anticoagulation for at least 3 months.
6. The use of thrombolytic agents continues to be highly individualized, and clinicians should have some latitude in using these agents. Patients with hemodynamically unstable PTE or massive iliofemoral thrombosis are the best candidates.
7. Inferior vena caval filter placement is recommended when there is a contraindication to or failure of anticoagulation, for chronic recurrent embolism with pulmonary hypertension, and with concurrent performance of surgical pulmonary embolectomy or pulmonary endarterectomy.

* Modified from TM Hyers et al: Antithrombotic therapy for venous thromboembolic disease Chest 114:561S, 1998.

or pulmonary artery. However, heparin does *not* directly dissolve thrombus that already exists.

Low-molecular-weight heparins These fragments of unfractionated heparin exhibit less binding to plasma proteins and endothelial cells and consequently have greater bioavailability, a more predictable dose response, and a longer half-life than unfractionated heparin. No laboratory monitoring or dose adjustment is needed unless the patient is markedly obese or has renal insufficiency. Therefore, low-molecular-weight heparins are far more convenient to use than unfractionated heparin.

A meta-analysis of more than 3,500 acute DVT patients showed that those treated with low-molecular-weight heparin had an overall 29% reduction in mortality and major bleeding compared with the unfractionated heparin group. *Enoxaparin*, originally approved for prophylaxis, has recently received Food and Drug Administration approval for treatment of PTE in the presence of DVT with a once-daily dose of 1.5 mg/kg subcutaneously. However, it is almost always ad-

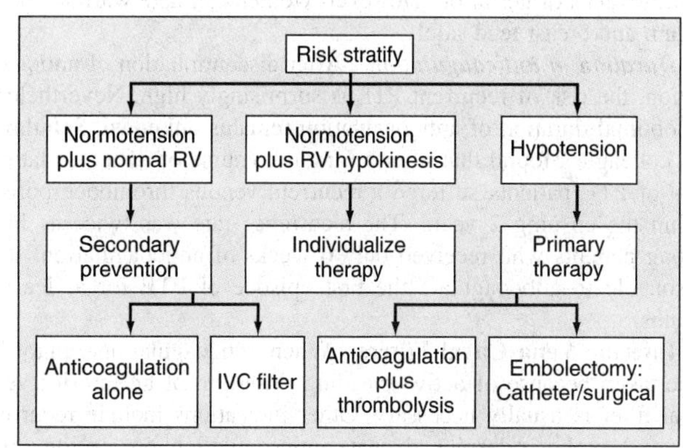

FIGURE 261-3 Acute PTE management: Risk stratification. RV, right ventricular; IVC, inferior vena cava.

ministered as 1 mg/kg twice daily. *Dalteparin* is approved for prophylaxis but not for treatment of venous thromboembolism.

Dosing For unfractionated heparin, a typical bolus is 5000 to 10,000 units followed by a continuous infusion of 1000 to 1500 units/h. An activated partial thromboplastin time that is at least twice the control value should provide a therapeutic level of heparin. Nomograms based upon a patient's weight may assist in adjusting the infusion rate of heparin.

Complications The most important adverse effect of heparin is hemorrhage. For life-threatening or intracranial hemorrhage, protamine sulfate can be administered. Heparin-associated thrombocytopenia and osteopenia are far less common with low-molecular-weight heparins than with unfractionated heparin. Heparin-associated elevations in transaminase levels occur commonly but are rarely associated with clinical toxicity.

Warfarin This vitamin K antagonist prevents γ carboxylation activation of coagulation factors II, VII, IX, and X. The full effect of warfarin often requires 5 days, even if the prothrombin time, used for monitoring, becomes elevated more rapidly. When warfarin is initiated during an active thrombotic state, the levels of protein C and S decline, thus creating a thrombogenic potential. By overlapping heparin and warfarin for 5 days, the procoagulant effect of unopposed warfarin can be counteracted. Thus, heparin acts as a "bridge" until the full anticoagulant effect of warfarin is obtained.

Dosing In an average-sized adult, warfarin is usually initiated in a dose of 5 mg. Doses of 7.5 or 10 mg can be used in obese or large framed young patients who are otherwise healthy. Patients who are malnourished or who have received prolonged courses of antibiotics are probably deficient in vitamin K and should receive smaller initial doses of warfarin, such as 2.5 mg. The prothrombin time is standardized by using the International Normalized Ratio (INR) to assess the anticoagulant effect of warfarin (Chap. 118). The target INR should be approximately 2.5–3.0.

Complications As with heparin, bleeding is the most important and common complication associated with warfarin administration. Life-threatening bleeding can be treated with cryoprecipitate or fresh frozen plasma (usually 2 units) to achieve immediate hemostasis. For less serious bleeding, or an excessively high INR in the absence of bleeding, vitamin K may be administered. An initial dose of 5 to 10 mg subcutaneously will help lower the INR toward the upper portion of the therapeutic range within about 6 h. Reversing excessive INRs with oral rather than subcutaneous vitamin K will facilitate reestablishing a stable dose of warfarin.

Warfarin-induced skin necrosis is a rare complication that may be related to warfarin-induced reduction of protein C. It is usually associated with administration of a high initial dose of warfarin during an acute thrombotic state in which heparin is withheld. During pregnancy, warfarin should be avoided if possible because of warfarin embryopathy, which is most common with exposure during the sixth through twelfth weeks of gestation. However, women can take warfarin postpartum and breast feed safely.

Duration of anticoagulation After discontinuation of anticoagulation, the risk of recurrent PTE is surprisingly high. Nevertheless, the optimal duration of anticoagulation remains unknown. Schulman and colleagues found that after a 6-month course of anticoagulation, 14% of PTE patients suffered a recurrent venous thromboembolism within the ensuing 2 years. The recurrence rate was twice as high among patients who received only 6 weeks of anticoagulation. It is reasonable to anticoagulate the first episode of PTE for at least 6 months.

Inferior Vena Caval Filters When anticoagulation cannot be undertaken because of active bleeding, insertion of an inferior vena caval filter is usually necessary. Other indications include recurrent venous thrombosis despite adequate anticoagulation, prevention of recurrent PTE in patients with right heart failure who are not candidates for thrombolysis, or prophylaxis of extremely high risk patients. The Bird's Nest filter infrarenally or, if necessary, a Greenfield filter suprarenally are recommended.

Table 261-3 Prevention of Pulmonary Thromboembolism

Condition	Strategy
Total hip or knee replacement; hip or pelvis fracture	Warfarin (Coumadin) (target INR 2.0–2.5) × 4–6 weeks Low-molecular-weight heparin [e.g., enoxaparin (Lovenox), 30 mg SC twice daily] IPC ± warfarin (Coumadin)
Gynecologic cancer surgery	Warfarin (Coumadin) (target INR 2.0–2.5) ± IPC Unfractionated heparin, 5000 U q8 h ± IPC Dalteparin (Fragmin) 2500 U once daily ± IPC Enoxaparin 40 mg SC once daily
Urologic surgery	Warfarin (Coumadin) (target INR 2.0–2.5) ± IPC
Thoracic surgery	IPC *plus* unfractionated heparin, 5000 U q8 h
High-risk general surgery (e.g., prior VTE, current cancer, or obesity)	IPC *or* graded-compression stockings *plus* unfractionated heparin, 5000 U q8 h Dalteparin (Fragmin) 5000 U SC or Enoxaparin (Lovenox), 40 mg SC once daily
General, gynecologic, or urologic surgery (without prior VTE) for noncancerous conditions	Graded-compression stockings *plus* unfractionated heparin 5000 U q12h Dalteparin 2500 U SC once daily Enoxaparin 40 mg SC once daily IPC alone
Neurosurgery, eye surgery, or other surgery when prophylactic anticoagulation is contraindicated	Graded-compression stockings ± IPC
Medical conditions	Graded-compression stockings ± heparin, 5000 U q8–12h IPC alone Enoxaparin (Lovenox) 40 mg SC once daily

NOTE: IPC, intermittent pneumatic compression; VTE, venous thromboembolism.

Thrombolysis Thrombolytic therapy may rapidly reverse right heart failure and thus lead to a lower rate of death and recurrent PTE. Thrombolysis usually achieves the following: (1) dissolves much of the anatomically obstructing pulmonary arterial thrombus; (2) prevents the continued release of serotonin and other neurohumoral factors that might otherwise exacerbate pulmonary hypertension; and (3) dissolves much of the source of the thrombus in the pelvic or deep leg veins, thereby decreasing the likelihood of recurrent PTE.

The preferred thrombolytic regimen is 100 mg of recombinant tissue plasminogen activator administered as a continuous peripheral intravenous infusion over 2 h. Patients appear to respond to thrombolysis for up to 14 days after the PTE occurred.

Contraindications to thrombolysis include intracranial disease, recent surgery, or trauma. There is about a 1% risk of intracranial hemorrhage. Careful screening of patients for contraindications to thrombolysis is the best way to minimize bleeding risk.

Pulmonary Thromboendarterectomy Patients who develop chronic pulmonary hypertension due to prior PTE may become severely dyspneic at rest or with minimal exertion. They should be considered for pulmonary thromboendarterectomy which, if successful, can markedly reduce and at times even cure pulmonary hypertension.

Prevention Prevention of PTE is of paramount importance because it is both difficult to recognize and expensive to treat. Fortunately, effective mechanical and pharmacologic prophylaxis modalities are widely available and usually effective (Table 261-3).

BIBLIOGRAPHY

DECOUSUS H et al: A clinical trial of vena caval filters in the prevention of pulmonary embolism in patients with proximal deep-vein thrombosis. N Engl J Med 338:409, 1998

FEDULLO PF: Pulmonary thromboembolism, in *Textbook of Respiratory Medicine*, 3d ed, JF Murray, JA Nadel (eds). Philadelphia, Saunders, 2000, pp 1503–1532

GOLDHABER SZ et al: Acute pulmonary embolism: Clinical outcomes in the International Cooperative Pulmonary Embolism Registry (ICOPER). Lancet 353:1386, 1999

GOLDHABER SZ: Contemporary pulmonary embolism thrombolysis. Chest 107:45S, 1995

GOULD MK et al: Low-molecular-weight heparins compared with unfractionated heparin for treatment of acute deep venous thrombosis. A meta-analysis of randomized, controlled trials. Ann Intern Med 130:800, 1999

INDIK JH, ALPERT JS: Detection of pulmonary embolism by D-dimer assay, spiral computed tomography, and magnetic resonance imaging. Progr Cardiovasc Dis 42:261, 2000

KEARON C et al: A comparison of three months of anticoagulation with extended anticoagulation for a first episode of idiopathic venuos thromboembolism. N Engl J Med 340:901, 1999

LUALDI JC, GOLDHABER SZ: Right ventricular dysfunction after acute pulmonary embolism: Pathophysiologic factors, detection, and therapeutic implications. Am Heart J 130:1276, 1995

MULLINS MD et al: The role of spiral volumetric computed tomography in the diagnosis of pulmonary embolism. Arch Intern Med 160:293, 2000

PERRIER A et al: Noninvasive diagnosis of venous thromboembolism in outpatients. Lancet 353:190, 1999

RIDKER P et al: G20210A mutation in prothrombin gene and risk of myocardial infarction, stroke, and venous thrombosis in a large cohort of US Men. Circulation 99:999, 1999

RIDKER PM et al: Mutation in the gene coding for coagulation factor V and risks of future myocardial infarction, stroke, and venous thrombosis in apparently healthy men. N Engl J Med 332:912, 1995

262

Richard W. Light

DISORDERS OF THE PLEURA, MEDIASTINUM, AND DIAPHRAGM

DISORDERS OF THE PLEURA

PLEURAL EFFUSION The pleural space lies between the lung and chest wall and normally contains a very thin layer of fluid, which serves as a coupling system. A pleural effusion is present when there is an excess quantity of fluid in the pleural space.

Etiology Pleural fluid accumulates when pleural fluid formation exceeds pleural fluid absorption. Normally, fluid enters the pleural space from the capillaries in the parietal pleura and is removed via the lymphatics situated in the parietal pleura. Fluid also can enter the pleural space from the interstitial spaces of the lung via the visceral pleura or from the peritoneal cavity via small holes in the diaphragm. The lymphatics have the capacity to absorb 20 times more fluid than is normally formed. Accordingly, a pleural effusion may develop when there is excess pleural fluid formation (from the parietal pleura, the interstitial spaces of the lung, or the peritoneal cavity) or when there is decreased fluid removal by the lymphatics.

Diagnostic Approach When a patient is found to have a pleural effusion, an effort should be made to determine the cause (Fig. 262-1). The first step is to determine whether the effusion is a transudate or an exudate. A *transudative* pleural effusion occurs when *systemic factors* that influence the formation and absorption of pleural fluid are altered. The leading causes of transudative pleural effusions in the United States are left ventricular failure, pulmonary embolism, and cirrhosis. An *exudative* pleural effusion occurs when *local factors* that influence the formation and absorption of pleural fluid are altered. The leading causes of exudative pleural effusions are bacterial pneumonia,

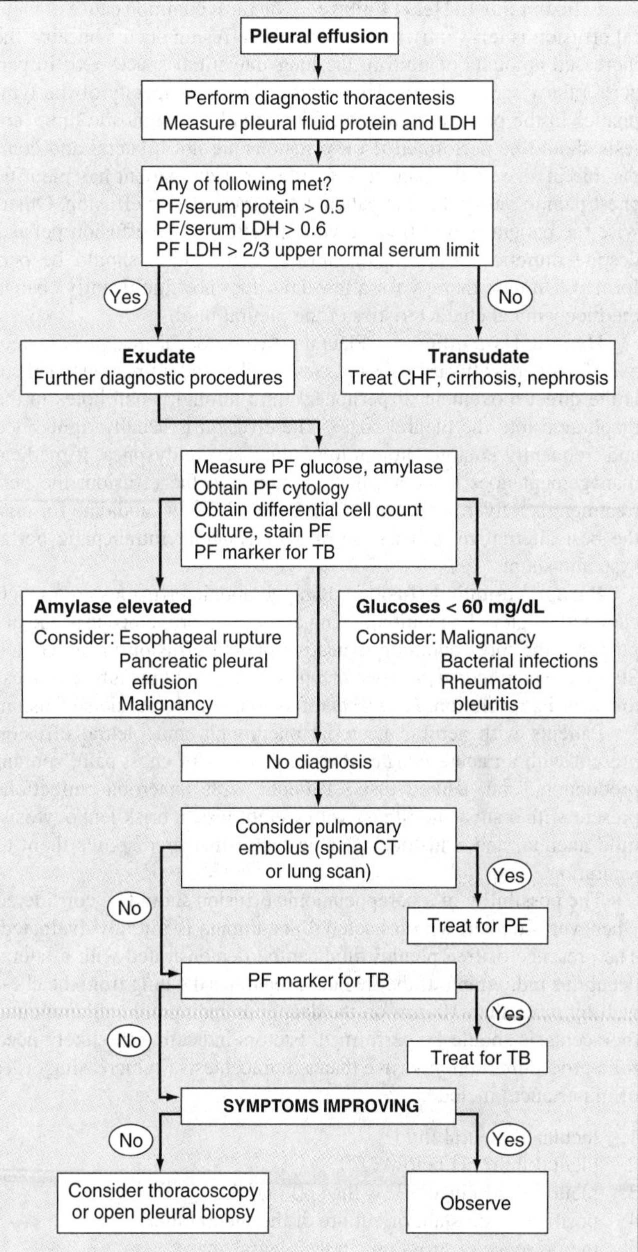

FIGURE 262-1 Approach to the diagnosis of pleural effusions; PF, pleural fluid.

malignancy, viral infection, and pulmonary embolism. The primary reason to make this differentiation is that additional diagnostic procedures are indicated with exudative effusions to define the cause of the local disease.

Transudative and exudative pleural effusions are distinguished by measuring the lactate dehydrogenase (LDH) and protein levels in the pleural fluid. Exudative pleural effusions meet at least one of the following criteria, whereas transudative pleural effusions meet none:

1. pleural fluid protein/serum protein >0.5
2. pleural fluid LDH/serum LDH >0.6
3. pleural fluid LDH more than two-thirds normal upper limit for serum

If a patient has an exudative pleural effusion, the following tests on the pleural fluid should be obtained: description of the fluid, glucose level, amylase level, differential cell count, microbiologic studies, and cytology.

Effusion due to Heart Failure The most common cause of pleural effusion is left ventricular failure. The effusion occurs because the increased amounts of fluid in the lung interstitial spaces exit in part across the visceral pleura. This overwhelms the capacity of the lymphatics in the parietal pleura to remove fluid. A diagnostic thoracentesis should be performed if the effusions are not bilateral and comparable in size, if the patient is febrile, or if the patient has pleuritic chest pain to verify that the patient has a transudative effusion. Otherwise the patient is best treated with diuretics. If the effusion persists despite diuretic therapy, a diagnostic thoracentesis should be performed. Diuretic therapy for a few days does not significantly change the biochemical characteristics of the pleural fluid.

Hepatic Hydrothorax Pleural effusions occur in approximately 5% of patients with cirrhosis and ascites. The predominant mechanism is the direct movement of peritoneal fluid through small holes in the diaphragm into the pleural space. The effusion is usually right-sided and frequently is large enough to produce severe dyspnea. If medical management does not control the ascites and the effusion, the best treatment is a liver transplant. If the patient is not a candidate for this, the best alternative is insertion of a transjugular intrahepatic portal systemic shunt.

Parapneumonic Effusion Parapneumonic effusions are associated with bacterial pneumonia, lung abscess, or bronchiectasis and are probably the most common exudative pleural effusion in the United States. A *complicated parapneumonic effusion* requires tube thoracostomy for its resolution. *Empyema* refers to a grossly purulent effusion.

Patients with aerobic bacterial pneumonia and pleural effusion present with an acute febrile illness consisting of chest pain, sputum production, and leukocytosis. Patients with anaerobic infections present with a subacute illness with weight loss, a brisk leukocytosis, mild anemia, and a history of some factor that predisposes them to aspiration.

The possibility of a parapneumonic effusion should be considered whenever a patient with a bacterial pneumonia is initially evaluated. The presence of free pleural fluid can be demonstrated with a lateral decubitus radiograph. If the free fluid separates the lung from the chest wall by more than 10 mm on the decubitus radiograph, a therapeutic thoracentesis should be performed. Factors indicating the likely need for a procedure more invasive than a thoracentesis (in increasing order of importance) include:

1. loculated pleural fluid
2. pleural fluid pH below 7.20
3. pleural fluid glucose less than 60 mg/dL
4. positive Gram stain or culture of the pleural fluid
5. the presence of gross pus in the pleural space

If the fluid recurs after the initial therapeutic thoracentesis, a repeat thoracentesis should be performed if any of the above characteristics are present. If the fluid recurs a second time, tube thoracostomy should be performed if any of the poor prognostic factors are present. If the fluid cannot be completely removed with the therapeutic thoracentesis, consideration should be given to inserting a chest tube and instilling a thrombolytic (streptokinase, 250,000 units or urokinase, 100,000 units) or performing thoracoscopy with the breakdown of adhesions. Decortication should be considered when the above are ineffective.

Effusion Secondary to Malignancy Malignant pleural effusions secondary to metastatic disease are the second most common type of exudative pleural effusion. The three tumors that cause approximately 75% of all malignant pleural effusions are lung carcinoma, breast carcinoma, and lymphoma. Most patients complain of dyspnea, which is frequently out of proportion to the size of the effusion. The pleural fluid is an exudate, and its glucose level may be reduced if the tumor burden in the pleural space is high.

The diagnosis is usually made via cytology of the pleural fluid. If the initial cytologic examination is negative, then thoracoscopy is the best next procedure if malignancy is strongly suspected. At the time of thoracoscopy, talc or some similar agent should be instilled into the pleural space to effect a pleurodesis. If thoracoscopy is unavailable, then needle biopsy of the pleura should be performed.

Patients with a malignant pleural effusion are treated symptomatically for the most part, since the presence of the effusion indicates disseminated disease and most malignancies associated with pleural effusion are not curable with chemotherapy. The only symptom that can be attributed to the effusion itself is dyspnea. If the patient's lifestyle is compromised by dyspnea, and if the dyspnea is relieved with a therapeutic thoracentesis, then one of the following procedures should be performed: (1) tube thoracostomy with the instillation of a sclerosing agent such as talc, 5 g in a slurry, or doxycycline, 500 mg; (2) outpatient insertion of a small indwelling catheter; or (3) thoracoscopy with pleural abrasion or the insufflation of talc.

Mesothelioma Malignant mesotheliomas are primary tumors that arise from the mesothelial cells that line the pleural cavities. Most are related to asbestos exposure. Patients with mesothelioma present with chest pain and shortness of breath. The chest radiograph reveals a pleural effusion, generalized pleural thickening, and a shrunken hemithorax. Thoracoscopy or open pleural biopsy is usually necessary to establish the diagnosis. Various treatment modalities, including radical surgery, chemotherapy, and radiation therapy, have been tried, but none has been proven to be more effective than symptomatic therapy. It is recommended that chest pain be treated with opiates and that shortness of breath be treated with oxygen and/or opiates.

Effusion Secondary to Pulmonary Embolization The diagnosis most commonly overlooked in the differential diagnosis of a patient with an undiagnosed pleural effusion is pulmonary embolism. Dyspnea is the most common symptom. The pleural fluid can be either transudative or exudative. The diagnosis is suggested by spiral CT scans, perfusion lung scanning and/or pulmonary arteriography (Chap. 261). Treatment of the patient with a pleural effusion secondary to pulmonary embolism is the same as for any patient with pulmonary emboli. If the pleural effusion increases in size after anticoagulation, the patient probably has recurrent emboli or another complication such as a hemothorax or a pleural infection.

Tuberculous Pleuritis (See also Chap. 169) In many parts of the world, the most common cause of an exudative pleural effusion is tuberculosis, but this is relatively uncommon in the United States. Tuberculous pleural effusions are thought to be due primarily to a hypersensitivity reaction to tuberculous protein in the pleural space. Patients with tuberculous pleuritis present with fever, weight loss, dyspnea, and/or pleuritic chest pain. The pleural fluid is an exudate with predominantly small lymphocytes. The diagnosis is established by demonstrating high levels of TB markers in the pleural fluid (adenosine deaminase $>$ 45 IU/L, gamma interferon $>$ 140 pg/mL, or positive PCR for tuberculous DNA). Alternatively, the diagnosis can be established by culture of the pleural fluid, needle biopsy of the pleura, or thoracoscopy. The recommended treatment of pleural and pulmonary tuberculosis is identical (Chap. 169).

Effusion Secondary to Viral Infection Viral infections are probably responsible for a sizable percentage of undiagnosed exudative pleural effusions. In many series, no diagnosis is established for approximately 20% of exudative effusions, and these effusions resolve spontaneously with no long-term residua. The importance of these effusions is that one should not be too aggressive in trying to establish a diagnosis for the undiagnosed effusion, particularly if the patient is improving clinically.

AIDS Pleural effusions are uncommon in such patients. The most common cause is Kaposi's sarcoma, followed by parapneumonic effusion. Other common causes are tuberculosis, cryptococcosis, and lymphoma. Pleural effusions are very uncommon with *Pneumocystis carinii* infection.

Chylothorax A chylothorax occurs when the thoracic duct is disrupted and chyle accumulates in the pleural space. The most common cause of chylothorax is trauma, but it also may result from tumors in the mediastinum. Patients with chylothorax present with dyspnea, and a large pleural effusion is present on the chest radiograph. Thoracentesis reveals milky fluid, and biochemical analysis reveals a triglyceride level that exceeds 110 mg/dL. Patients with chylothorax and no obvious trauma should have a lymphangiogram and a mediastinal computed tomographic (CT) scan to assess the mediastinum for lymph nodes. The treatment of choice for most chylothoraces is implantation of a pleuroperitoneal shunt. Patients with chylothoraces should not undergo prolonged tube thoracostomy with chest tube drainage because this will lead to malnutrition and immunologic incompetence.

Hemothorax When a diagnostic thoracentesis reveals bloody pleural fluid, a hematocrit should be obtained on the pleural fluid. If the hematocrit is >50% that of the peripheral blood, the patient has a hemothorax. Most hemothoraces are the result of trauma; other causes include rupture of a blood vessel or tumor. Most patients with hemothorax should be treated with tube thoracostomy, which allows continuous quantification of bleeding. If the bleeding emanates from a laceration of the pleura, apposition of the two pleural surfaces is likely to stop the bleeding. If the pleural hemorrhage exceeds 200 mL/h, consideration should be given to thoracotomy.

Miscellaneous Causes of Pleural Effusion There are many other causes of pleural effusion (Table 262-1). Key features of some of these conditions are as follows: If the pleural fluid amylase level is elevated, the diagnosis of esophageal rupture or pancreatic disease is likely. If the patient is febrile, has predominantly polymorphonuclear cells in the pleural fluid, and has no pulmonary parenchymal abnormalities, an intraabdominal abscess should be considered. The diagnosis of an asbestos pleural effusion is one of exclusion. Benign ovarian tumors can produce ascites and a pleural effusion (Meigs' syndrome), as can the ovarian hyperstimulation syndrome. Several drugs can cause pleural effusion; the associated fluid is usually eosinophilic. Pleural effusions commonly occur following coronary artery bypass surgery. Effusions occurring within the first weeks are typically left-sided and bloody, with large numbers of eosinophils, and respond to one or two therapeutic thoracenteses. Effusions occurring after the first few weeks are typically left-sided and clear yellow, with predominantly small lymphocytes, and tend to recur. Other medical manipulations that induce pleural effusions include abdominal surgery, endoscopic variceal sclerotherapy, radiation therapy, liver or lung transplantation, or the intravascular insertion of central lines.

Table 262-1 Differential Diagnoses of Pleural Effusions

TRANSUDATIVE PLEURAL EFFUSIONS	
1. Congestive heart failure	5. Peritoneal dialysis
2. Cirrhosis	6. Superior vena cava obstruction
3. Pulmonary embolization	7. Myxedema
4. Nephrotic syndrome	8. Urinothorax
EXUDATIVE PLEURAL EFFUSIONS	
1. Neoplastic diseases	6. Post-coronary artery bypass surgery
a. Metastatic disease	7. Asbestos exposure
b. Mesothelioma	8. Sarcoidosis
2. Infectious diseases	9. Uremia
a. Bacterial infections	10. Meigs' syndrome
b. Tuberculosis	11. Yellow nail syndrome
c. Fungal infections	12. Drug-induced pleural disease
d. Viral infections	a. Nitrofurantoin
e. Parasitic infections	b. Dantrolene
3. Pulmonary embolization	c. Methysergide
4. Gastrointestinal disease	d. Bromocriptine
a. Esophageal perforation	e. Procarbazine
b. Pancreatic disease	f. Amiodarone
c. Intraabdominal abscesses	13. Trapped lung
d. Diaphragmatic hernia	14. Radiation therapy
e. After abdominal surgery	15. Post-cardiac injury syndrome
f. Endoscopic variceal sclerotherapy	16. Hemothorax
g. After liver transplant	17. Iatrogenic injury
5. Collagen-vascular diseases	18. Ovarian hyperstimulation syndrome
a. Rheumatoid pleuritis	19. Pericardial disease
b. Systemic lupus erythematosus	20. Chylothorax
c. Drug-induced lupus	
d. Immunoblastic lymphadenopathy	
e. Sjögren's syndrome	
f. Wegener's granulomatosis	
g. Churg-Strauss syndrome	

PNEUMOTHORAX Pneumothorax is the presence of gas in the pleural space. A *spontaneous pneumothorax* is one that occurs without antecedent trauma to the thorax. A *primary spontaneous pneumothorax* occurs in the absence of underlying lung disease, while a *secondary spontaneous pneumothorax* occurs in its presence. A *traumatic pneumothorax* results from penetrating or nonpenetrating chest injuries. A *tension pneumothorax* is a pneumothorax in which the pressure in the pleural space is positive throughout the respiratory cycle.

Primary Spontaneous Pneumothorax Primary spontaneous pneumothoraces are usually due to rupture of apical pleural blebs, small cystic spaces that lie within or immediately under the visceral pleura. Primary spontaneous pneumothoraces occur almost exclusively in smokers, which suggests that these patients have subclinical lung disease. Approximately one-half of patients with an initial primary spontaneous pneumothorax will have a recurrence. The initial recommended treatment for primary spontaneous pneumothorax is simple aspiration. If the lung does not expand with aspiration, or if the patient has a recurrent pneumothorax, thoracoscopy with stapling of blebs and pleural abrasion is indicated. Thoracoscopy or thoracotomy with pleural abrasion is almost 100% successful in preventing recurrences.

Secondary Spontaneous Pneumothorax Most secondary spontaneous pneumothoraces are due to chronic obstructive pulmonary disease, but pneumothoraces have been reported with virtually every lung disease. Pneumothorax in patients with lung disease is more life-threatening than it is in normal individuals because of the lack of pulmonary reserve in these patients. Nearly all patients with secondary spontaneous pneumothorax should be treated with tube thoracostomy and the instillation of a sclerosing agent such as doxycycline or talc. Patients with secondary spontaneous pneumothoraces who have a persistent air leak, an unexpanded lung after 3 days of tube thoracostomy, or a recurrent pneumothorax should be subjected to thoracoscopy with bleb resection and pleural abrasion.

Traumatic Pneumothorax Traumatic pneumothoraces can result from both penetrating and nonpenetrating chest trauma. Traumatic pneumothoraces should be treated with tube thoracostomy unless they are very small. If a hemopneumothorax is present, one chest tube should be placed in the superior part of the hemithorax to evacuate the air, and another should be placed in the inferior part of the hemithorax to remove the blood. Iatrogenic pneumothorax is a type of traumatic pneumothorax which is becoming more common. The leading causes are transthoracic needle aspiration, thoracentesis, and the insertion of central intravenous catheters. The treatment differs according to the degree of distress and can be observation, supplemental oxygen, aspiration, or tube thoracostomy.

Tension Pneumothorax This condition usually occurs during mechanical ventilation or resuscitative efforts. The positive pleural pressure is life-threatening both because ventilation is severely compromised and because the positive pressure is transmitted to the mediastinum, which results in decreased venous return to the heart and reduced cardiac output.

Difficulty in ventilation during resuscitation or high peak inspiratory pressures during mechanical ventilation strongly suggest the diagnosis. The diagnosis is made by the finding of an enlarged hemithorax with no breath sounds and shift of the mediastinum to the contralateral side. Tension pneumothorax must be treated as a medical emergency. If the tension in the pleural space is not relieved, the patient is likely to die from inadequate cardiac output or marked hypoxemia. A large-bore needle should be inserted into the pleural space through the second anterior intercostal space. If large amounts of gas escape from the needle after insertion, the diagnosis is confirmed. The needle should be left in place until a thoracostomy tube can be inserted.

DISORDERS OF THE MEDIASTINUM

The mediastinum is the region between the pleural sacs. It is separated into three compartments. The *anterior mediastinum* extends from the sternum anteriorly to the pericardium and brachiocephalic vessels posteriorly. It contains the thymus gland; the anterior mediastinal lymph nodes; and the internal mammary arteries and veins. The *middle mediastinum* lies between the anterior and posterior mediastina and contains the heart; the ascending and transverse arches of the aorta; the venae cavae; the brachiocephalic arteries and veins; the phrenic nerves; the trachea, main bronchi, and their contiguous lymph nodes; and the pulmonary arteries and veins. The *posterior mediastinum* is bounded by the pericardium and trachea anteriorly and the vertebral column posteriorly. It contains the descending thoracic aorta; esophagus; thoracic duct; azygos and hemiazygos veins; and the posterior group of mediastinal lymph nodes.

MEDIASTINAL MASSES The first step in evaluating a mediastinal mass lesion is to place it in one of the three mediastinal compartments, since each has different characteristic lesions. The most common lesions in the anterior mediastinum are thymomas, lymphomas, teratomatous neoplasms, and thyroid masses. The most common masses in the middle mediastinum are vascular masses, lymph node enlargement from metastases or granulomatous disease, and pleuropericardial and bronchogenic cysts. In the posterior mediastinum, neurogenic tumors, meningoceles, meningomyeloceles, gastroenteric cysts, and esophageal diverticula are commonly found.

CT scanning is the most valuable imaging technique for evaluating mediastinal masses and is the only imaging technique that should be done in most instances. Barium studies of the gastrointestinal tract are indicated in many patients with posterior mediastinal lesions, since hernias, diverticula, and achalasia are readily diagnosed in this manner. An ^{131}I nuclear medicine scan can efficiently establish the diagnosis of intrathoracic goiter.

A definite diagnosis can be obtained with mediastinoscopy or anterior mediastinotomy in many patients with masses in the anterior or middle mediastinal compartments. A diagnosis can be established without thoracotomy via percutaneous fine-needle aspiration biopsy of mediastinal masses in any of the mediastinal compartments. In many cases the diagnosis can be established and the mediastinal mass removed with video-assisted thoracoscopy.

ACUTE MEDIASTINITIS Most cases of acute mediastinitis are either due to esophageal perforation or occur after median sternotomy for cardiac surgery. Patients with esophageal rupture are acutely ill with chest pain and dyspnea due to the mediastinal infection. The esophageal rupture can occur spontaneously or as a complication of esophagoscopy or the insertion of a Blakemore tube. Appropriate treatment is exploration of the mediastinum with primary repair of the esophageal tear and drainage of the pleural space and the mediastinum.

The incidence of mediastinitis following median sternotomy is 0.4 to 5.0%. Patients most commonly present with wound drainage. Other presentations include sepsis or a widened mediastinum. The diagnosis is usually established with mediastinal needle aspiration. Treatment includes immediate drainage, debridement, and parenteral antibiotic therapy, but the mortality still exceeds 20%.

CHRONIC MEDIASTINITIS The spectrum of chronic mediastinitis ranges from granulomatous inflammation of the lymph nodes in the mediastinum to fibrosing mediastinitis. Most cases are due to tuberculosis or histoplasmosis, but sarcoidosis, silicosis, and other fungal diseases are at times causative. Patients with granulomatous mediastinitis are usually asymptomatic. Those with fibrosing mediastinitis usually have signs of compression of some mediastinal structure such as the superior vena cava or large airways, phrenic or recurrent laryngeal nerve paralysis, or obstruction of the pulmonary artery or proximal pulmonary veins. Other than antituberculous therapy for tuberculous mediastinitis, no medical or surgical therapy has been demonstrated to be effective for mediastinal fibrosis.

PNEUMOMEDIASTINUM In this condition, there is gas in the interstices of the mediastinum. The three main causes are: (1) alveolar rupture with dissection of air into the mediastinum; (2) perforation or rupture of the esophagus, trachea, or main bronchi; and (3) dissection of air from the neck or the abdomen into the mediastinum. Typically, there is severe substernal chest pain with or without radiation into the neck and arms. The physical examination usually reveals subcutaneous emphysema in the suprasternal notch and *Hamman's sign*, which is a crunching or clicking noise synchronous with the heartbeat and best heard in the left lateral decubitus position. The diagnosis is confirmed with the chest radiograph. Usually no treatment is required, but the mediastinal air will be absorbed faster if the patient inspires high concentrations of oxygen. If mediastinal structures are compressed, the compression can be relieved with needle aspiration.

DISORDERS OF THE DIAPHRAGM

DIAPHRAGMATIC PARALYSIS The presence of bilateral diaphragmatic paralysis almost always causes severe morbidity in adults. The most common causes include high spinal cord injury, thoracic trauma (including cardiac surgery), multiple sclerosis, anterior horn disease, and muscular dystrophy. Most patients with severe diaphragmatic weakness present with hypercapnic respiratory failure, frequently complicated by cor pulmonale and right ventricular failure, atelectasis, and pneumonia.

The degree of diaphragmatic weakness is best quantitated by measuring transdiaphragmatic pressures. The treatment of choice is assisted ventilation for all or part of each day. This is best accomplished without tracheostomy using nasal intermittent positive airway pressure. If the nerve to the diaphragm is intact, diaphragmatic pacing may be a viable alternative. If the paralysis occurs during open heart surgery, recovery frequently occurs, but it may take 6 months or more.

Unilateral paralysis of the diaphragm is much more common than is bilateral paralysis. The most common cause is nerve invasion from malignancy, usually a bronchogenic carcinoma. If the patient does not have malignancy, then usually no cause for the paralysis is found. The diagnosis is suggested by finding an elevated hemidiaphragm on the chest roentgenogram. Confirmation is best established with the "sniff test." When a patient is observed with fluoroscopy while sniffing, the paralyzed diaphragm will move paradoxically upward due to the negative intrathoracic pressure. Patients with a unilateral paralyzed diaphragm are usually asymptomatic. Their vital capacity and total lung capacity are each reduced about 25%. If a patient has a mediastinal mass in conjunction with the diaphragmatic paralysis, further workup should be done. However, if the patient is asymptomatic with a normal chest radiograph, no invasive procedures are warranted.

BIBLIOGRAPHY

GIERADA D et al: Imaging evaluation of the diaphragm. Chest Surg Clin N Am 8:237, 1998

HAMM H et al: Parapneumonic effusion and empyema. Eur Respir J 10:1150, 1997

LIGHT RW et al: Pleural sclerosis for the treatment of pneumothorax and pleural effusion. Lung 175:213, 1997

LIGHT RW, BROADDUS VC: Pleural Effusion, in *Textbook of Respiratory Medicine*, 3d ed, JF Murray, JA Nadel (eds). Saunders, Philadelphia, 2000, pp 2013–2042

SAHN SA, HEFFNER JE: Spontaneous pneumothorax. N Engl J Med 342:868, 2000

STROLLO DC et al: Primary mediastinal tumors. Tumors of the anterior mediastinum. Chest 112:511, 1997

STROLLO DC et al: Primary mediastinal tumors, Part II. Tumors of the middle and posterior mediastinum. Chest 112:1344, 1997

263 DISORDERS OF VENTILATION

Eliot A. Phillipson

HYPOVENTILATION

DEFINITION AND ETIOLOGY Alveolar hypoventilation exists by definition when arterial P_{CO_2} (Pa_{CO_2}) increases above the normal range of 37 to 43 mmHg, but in clinically important hypoventilation syndromes Pa_{CO_2} is generally in the range of 50 to 80 mmHg. Hypoventilation disorders can be acute or chronic. The acute disorders, which represent life-threatening emergencies, are discussed in Chap. 265; this chapter deals with chronic hypoventilation syndromes.

Chronic hypoventilation can result from numerous disease entities (Table 263-1), but in all cases the underlying mechanism involves a defect in either the metabolic respiratory control system, the respiratory neuromuscular system, or the ventilatory apparatus. Disorders associated with impaired respiratory drive, defects in the respiratory neuromuscular system, some chest wall disorders such as obesity, and upper airway obstruction produce an increase in Pa_{CO_2}, despite normal lungs, because of a reduction in overall minute volume of ventilation and hence in alveolar ventilation. In contrast, most disorders of the chest wall and disorders of the lower airways and lungs may produce an increase in Pa_{CO_2}, despite a normal or even increased minute volume of ventilation, because of severe ventilation-perfusion mismatching that results in net alveolar hypoventilation.

Several hypoventilation syndromes involve combined disturbances in two elements of the respiratory system. For example, patients with chronic obstructive pulmonary disease may hypoventilate not simply because of impaired ventilatory mechanics but also because of a reduced central respiratory drive, which can be inherent or secondary to a coexisting metabolic alkalosis (related to diuretic and steroid therapy).

PHYSIOLOGIC AND CLINICAL FEATURES Regardless of cause, the hallmark of all alveolar hypoventilation syndromes is an increase in alveolar P_{CO_2} (PA_{CO_2}) and therefore in Pa_{CO_2} (Fig. 263-1). The resulting respiratory acidosis eventually leads to a compensatory increase in plasma HCO_3^- concentration and a decrease in Cl^- concentration. The increase in PA_{CO_2} produces an obligatory decrease in PA_{O_2}, resulting in hypoxemia. If severe, the hypoxemia manifests clinically as cyanosis and can stimulate erythropoiesis and induce secondary polycythemia. The combination of chronic hypoxemia and hypercapnia may also induce pulmonary vasoconstriction, leading eventually to pulmonary hypertension, right ventricular hypertrophy, and congestive heart failure. The disturbances in arterial blood gases are typically magnified during sleep because of a further reduction in central respiratory drive. The resulting increased nocturnal hypercapnia may cause cerebral vasodilation leading to morning headache; sleep quality may also be severely impaired, resulting in morning fatigue, daytime somnolence, mental confusion, and intellectual impairment. Other clinical features associated with hypoventilation syndromes are related to the specific underlying disease (Table 263-1).

DIAGNOSIS Investigation of the patient with chronic hypoventilation involves several laboratory tests that will usually localize the disorder to either the metabolic respiratory control system, the neuromuscular system, or the ventilatory apparatus (Fig. 263-2). Defects in the control system impair responses to chemical stimuli, including ventilatory, occlusion pressure, and diaphragmatic electromyographic (EMG) responses. During sleep, hypoventilation is usually more marked, and central apneas and hypopneas are common. However, because the behavioral respiratory control system (which is anatomically distinct from the metabolic control system), the neuromuscular system, and the ventilatory apparatus are intact, such patients can usually hyperventilate voluntarily, generate normal inspiratory and expiratory muscle pressures (PI_{max}, PE_{max}, respectively) against an occluded airway, generate normal lung volumes and flow rates on routine spirometry, and have normal respiratory system resistance and compliance and a normal alveolar-arterial P_{O_2}[$(A - a)P_{O_2}$] difference. Patients with defects in the respiratory neuromuscular system also have impaired responses to chemical stimuli but in addition are unable to hyperventilate voluntarily or to generate normal static respiratory muscle pressures, lung volumes, and flow rates. However, at least in the early stages of the disease, the resistance and compliance of the respiratory system and the alveolar-arterial oxygen difference are normal.

Table 263-1 Chronic Hypoventilation Syndromes

Mechanism	Site of Defect	Disorder
Impaired respiratory drive	Peripheral and central chemoreceptors	Carotid body dysfunction, trauma
		Prolonged hypoxia
		Metabolic alkalosis
	Brainstem respiratory neurons	Bulbar poliomyelitis, encephalitis
		Brainstem infarction, hemorrhage, trauma
		Brainstem demyelination, degeneration
		Chronic drug administration
		Primary alveolar hypoventilation syndrome
Defective respiratory neuromuscular system	Spinal cord and peripheral nerves	High cervical trauma
		Poliomyelitis
		Motor neuron disease
		Peripheral neuropathy
	Respiratory muscles	Myasthenia gravis
		Muscular dystrophy
		Chronic myopathy
Impaired ventilatory apparatus	Chest wall	Kyphoscoliosis
		Fibrothorax
		Thoracoplasty
		Ankylosing spondylitis
		Obesity hypoventilation
	Airways and lungs	Laryngeal and tracheal stenosis
		Obstructive sleep apnea
		Cystic fibrosis
		Chronic obstructive pulmonary disease

SOURCE: From Phillipson, with permission.

In contrast to patients with disorders of the respiratory control or neuromuscular systems, patients with disorders of the chest wall, lungs, and airways typically demonstrate abnormalities of respiratory system resistance and compliance and have a widened $(A - a)P_{O_2}$. Because of the impaired mechanics of breathing, routine spirometric tests are abnormal, as is the ventilatory response to chemical stimuli. However, because the neuromuscular system is intact, tests that are independent of resistance and compliance are usually normal, including tests of respiratory muscle strength and of respiratory control that do not involve airflow.

℞ **TREATMENT** The management of chronic hypoventilation must be individualized to the patient's particular disorder, circumstances, and needs and should include measures directed toward the underlying disease. Coexistent metabolic alkalosis should be corrected, including elevations of HCO_3^- that are inappropriately high for the degree of chronic hypercapnia. Administration of supplemental oxygen is effective in attenuating hypoxemia, polycythemia, and pulmonary hypertension, but can aggravate CO_2 retention and the associated neurologic symptoms. For this reason, supplemental oxygen must be prescribed judiciously and the results monitored carefully. Pharmacologic agents that stimulate respiration (particularly progesterone) are of benefit in some patients, but generally, results are disappointing.

Most patients with chronic hypoventilation related to impairment of respiratory drive or neuromuscular disease eventually require me-

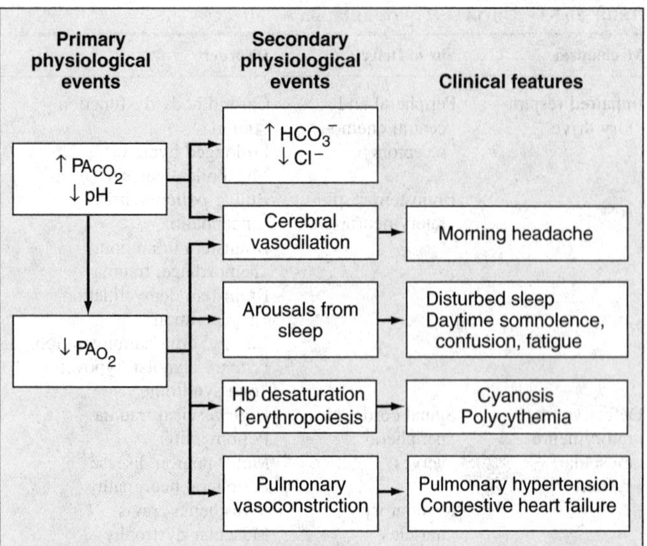

FIGURE 263-1 Physiologic and clinical features of alveolar hypoventilation. Hb, hemoglobin; PA_{CO_2}, alveolar P_{CO_2}; PA_{O_2}, alveolar P_{O_2}. *(After Phillipson.)*

chanical ventilatory assistance for effective management. When hypoventilation is severe, treatment may be required on a 24-h basis, but in most patients ventilatory assistance only during sleep produces dramatic clinical improvement and lowering of daytime Pa_{CO_2}. In patients with reduced respiratory drive but intact respiratory lower motor neurons, phrenic nerves, and respiratory muscles, diaphragmatic pacing through an implanted phrenic electrode can be very effective. However, for patients with defects in the respiratory nerves and muscles, electrophrenic pacing is contraindicated. Such patients can usually be managed effectively with either intermittent negative-pressure ventilation in a cuirass or intermittent positive-pressure ventilation delivered through a tracheostomy or nose mask. For patients who require ventilatory assistance only during sleep, positive-pressure ventilation through a nose mask is the preferred method because it obviates a tracheostomy and avoids the problem of upper airway occlusion that can arise in a negative-pressure ventilator. Hypoventilation related to restrictive disorders of the chest wall (Table 263-1) can also be managed effectively with nocturnal intermittent positive-pressure ventilation through a nose mask or tracheostomy.

HYPOVENTILATION SYNDROMES

PRIMARY ALVEOLAR HYPOVENTILATION Primary alveolar hypoventilation (PAH) is a disorder of unknown cause characterized by chronic hypercapnia and hypoxemia in the absence of identifiable neuromuscular disease or mechanical ventilatory impairment. The disorder is thought to arise from a defect in the metabolic respiratory control system, but few neuropathologic studies have been reported in such patients. Recent studies in animals suggest an important role for genetic factors in the pathogenesis of hypoventilation. Isolated PAH is relatively rare, and although it occurs in all age groups, the majority of reported cases have been in males aged 20 to 50 years. The disorder typically develops insidiously and often first comes to attention when severe respiratory depression follows administration of standard doses of sedatives or anesthetics. As the degree of hypoventilation increases, patients typically develop lethargy, fatigue, daytime somnolence, disturbed sleep, and morning headaches; eventually cyanosis, polycythemia, pulmonary hypertension, and congestive heart failure occur (Fig. 263-1). Despite severe arterial blood gas derangements, dyspnea is uncommon, presumably because of impaired chemoreception and ventilatory drive. If left untreated, PAH is usually progressive over a period of months to years and ultimately fatal.

The key diagnostic finding in PAH is a chronic respiratory acidosis in the absence of respiratory muscle weakness or impaired ventilatory mechanics (Fig. 263-2). Because patients can hyperventilate voluntarily and reduce Pa_{CO_2} to normal or even hypocapnic levels, hypercapnia may not be demonstrable in a single arterial blood sample, but the presence of an elevated plasma HCO_3^- level should draw attention to the underlying chronic disturbance. Despite normal ventilatory mechanics and respiratory muscle strength, ventilatory responses to chemical stimuli are reduced or absent (Fig. 263-2), and breath-holding time may be markedly prolonged without any sensation of dyspnea.

Patients with PAH maintain rhythmic respiration when awake, although the level of ventilation is below normal. However, during sleep, when breathing is critically dependent on the metabolic control system, there is typically a further deterioration in ventilation with frequent episodes of central hypopnea or apnea.

PAH must be distinguished from other central hypoventilation

Site of defect	Responses to CO_2, hypoxia: Ventil.	P.1	EMGdi	Sleep studies	Voluntary hyperventil.	PI_{max} PE_{max}	Volume flow rates	Resistance, compliance	(A-a) P_{O_2}
Metabolic control system (chemoreceptors, brainstem integrating neurons)	↓	↓	↓	↑ Hypoventil, central apneas	N	N	N	N	N
Respiratory neuromuscular system (brainstem motoneurons, spinal cord, respiratory nerves and muscles)	↓	↓	↓	↑ Hypoventil, central apneas	↓	↓	↓	N	N
Ventilatory apparatus (chest wall, lungs, airways)	↓	N	N	Variable	↓	N	Abnormal	Abnormal	↑

FIGURE 263-2 Pattern of laboratory test results in alveolar hypoventilation syndromes, based on the site of defect. Ventil, ventilation; P.1, mouth pressure generated after 0.1 s of inspiration against an occluded airway; EMGdi, diaphragmatic EMG; PI_{max}, PE_{max}, maximum inspiratory or expiratory pressure that can be generated against an occluded airway; (A − a) P_{O_2}, alveolar-arterial P_{O_2} difference; N, normal. Defects in the metabolic control system impair central respiratory drive in response to chemical stimuli (CO_2 or hypoxia); therefore responses of EMGdi, P.1, and minute volume of ventilation are reduced and hypoventilation during sleep is aggravated. In contrast, tests of voluntary respiratory control, muscle strength, lung mechanics, and gas exchange [(A − a)P_{O_2}] are normal. Defects in the respiratory neuromuscular system impair muscle strength; therefore all tests dependent on muscular activity (voluntary or in response to metabolic stimuli) are abnormal, but lung resistance, lung compliance, and gas exchange are normal. Defects in the ventilatory apparatus usually impair gas exchange. Because resistance and compliance are also impaired, all tests dependent on ventilation (whether voluntary or in response to chemical stimuli) are abnormal; in contrast, tests of muscle activity or strength that do not involve airflow (i.e., P.1, EMGdi, PI_{max}, PE_{max}) are normal. *(After Phillipson.)*

syndromes that are secondary to underlying neurologic disease of the brainstem or chemoreceptors (Table 263-1). This distinction requires a careful neurologic investigation for evidence of brainstem or autonomic disturbances. Unrecognized respiratory neuromuscular disorders, particularly those that produce diaphragmatic weakness, are often misdiagnosed as PAH. However, such disorders can usually be suspected on clinical grounds (see below) and can be confirmed by the finding of reduced voluntary hyperventilation, as well as PI_{max} and PE_{max}.

Some patients with PAH respond favorably to respiratory stimulant medications and to supplemental oxygen. However, the majority eventually require mechanical ventilatory assistance. Excellent long-term benefits can be achieved with diaphragmatic pacing by electrophrenic stimulation or with negative- or positive-pressure mechanical ventilation. The administration of such treatment only during sleep is sufficient in most patients.

RESPIRATORY NEUROMUSCULAR DISORDERS Several primary disorders of the spinal cord, peripheral respiratory nerves, and respiratory muscles produce a chronic hypoventilation syndrome (Table 263-1). Hypoventilation usually develops gradually over a period of months to years and often first comes to attention when a relatively trivial increase in mechanical ventilatory load (such as mild airways obstruction) produces severe respiratory failure. In some of the disorders (such as motor neuron disease, myasthenia gravis, and muscular dystrophy), involvement of the respiratory nerves or muscles is usually a later feature of a more widespread disease. In other disorders, respiratory involvement can be an early or even isolated feature, and hence the underlying problem is often not suspected. Included in this category are the postpolio syndrome (a form of chronic respiratory insufficiency that develops 20 to 30 years following recovery from poliomyelitis), the myopathy associated with adult acid maltase deficiency, and idiopathic diaphragmatic paralysis.

Generally, respiratory neuromuscular disorders do not result in chronic hypoventilation unless there is significant weakness of the diaphragm. Distinguishing features of bilateral diaphragmatic weakness include orthopnea, paradoxical movement of the abdomen in the supine posture, and paradoxical diaphragmatic movement under fluoroscopy. However, the absence of these features does not exclude diaphragmatic weakness. Important laboratory features are a rapid deterioration of ventilation during a maximum voluntary ventilation maneuver and reduced PI_{max} and PE_{max} (Fig. 263-2). More sophisticated investigations reveal reduced or absent transdiaphragmatic pressures, calculated from simultaneous measurement of esophageal and gastric pressures; reduced diaphragmatic EMG responses (recorded from an esophageal electrode) to transcutaneous phrenic nerve stimulation; and marked hypopnea and arterial oxygen desaturation during rapid eye movement sleep, when there is normally a physiologic inhibition of all nondiaphragmatic respiratory muscles and breathing becomes critically dependent on diaphragmatic activity.

The management of chronic alveolar hypoventilation due to respiratory neuromuscular disease involves treatment of the underlying disorder, where feasible, and mechanical ventilatory assistance as described for the primary alveolar hypoventilation syndrome. However, electrophrenic diaphragmatic pacing is contraindicated in these disorders, except for high cervical spinal cord lesions in which the phrenic lower motor neurons and nerves are intact.

OBESITY-HYPOVENTILATION SYNDROME Massive obesity represents a mechanical load to the respiratory system because the added weight on the rib cage and abdomen serves to reduce the compliance of the chest wall. As a result, the functional residual capacity (i.e., end-expiratory lung volume) is reduced, particularly in the recumbent posture. An important consequence of breathing at a low lung volume is that some airways, particularly those in the lung bases, may be closed throughout part or even all of each tidal breath, resulting in underventilation of the lung bases and widening of the $(A - a)P_{O_2}$. Nevertheless, in the majority of obese individuals, central respiratory drive is increased sufficiently to maintain a normal Pa_{CO_2}. However, a small proportion of obese patients develop chronic hypercapnia, hypoxemia, and eventually polycythemia, pulmonary hypertension, and

right-sided heart failure. Recent studies in mice demonstrate that genetically obese mice lacking circulating leptin also develop chronic hypoventilation that can be reversed by leptin infusions. Those patients who also develop daytime somnolence have been designated as having the *Pickwickian syndrome* (Chap. 27). In many such patients, obstructive sleep apnea is a prominent feature, and even in those patients without sleep apnea, sleep-induced hypoventilation is an important element of the disorder and contributes to its progression. Most patients demonstrate a decrease in central respiratory drive, which may be inherent or acquired, and many have mild to moderate degrees of airflow obstruction, usually related to smoking. Based on these considerations, several therapeutic measures can be of considerable benefit, including weight loss, cessation of smoking, elimination of obstructive sleep apnea, and enhancement of respiratory drive by medications such as progesterone.

HYPERVENTILATION AND ITS SYNDROMES

DEFINITION AND ETIOLOGY Alveolar hyperventilation exists when Pa_{CO_2} decreases below the normal range of 37 to 43 mmHg. *Hyperventilation* is not synonymous with *hyperpnea*, which refers to an increased minute volume of ventilation without reference to Pa_{CO_2}. Although hyperventilation is frequently associated with dyspnea, patients who are hyperventilating do not necessarily complain of shortness of breath; and conversely, patients with dyspnea need not be hyperventilating.

Numerous disease entities can be associated with alveolar hyperventilation (Table 263-2), but in all cases the underlying mechanism involves an increase in respiratory drive that is mediated through either the behavioral or the metabolic respiratory control systems (Fig. 263-3). Thus hypoxemia drives ventilation by stimulating the peripheral chemoreceptors, and several pulmonary disorders and congestive heart failure drive ventilation by stimulating afferent vagal receptors in the lungs and airways. Low cardiac output and hypotension stimulate the peripheral chemoreceptors and inhibit the baroreceptors, both of which increase ventilation. Metabolic acidosis, a potent respiratory stimulant, excites both the peripheral and central chemoreceptors and increases the sensitivity of the peripheral chemoreceptors to coexistent hypoxemia. Hepatic failure can also produce hyperventilation, presumably as a result of metabolic stimuli acting on the peripheral and central chemoreceptors.

Several neurologic and psychological disorders are thought to drive ventilation through the behavioral respiratory control system. Included in this category are psychogenic or anxiety hyperventilation and severe cerebrovascular insufficiency, which may interfere with the inhibitory influence normally exerted by cortical structures on the

Table 263-2 Hyperventilation Syndromes

1. Hypoxemia
   a. High altitude
   b. Pulmonary disease
   c. Cardiac shunts
2. Pulmonary disorders
   a. Pneumonia
   b. Interstitial pneumonitis, fibrosis, edema
   c. Pulmonary emboli, vascular disease
   d. Bronchial asthma
   e. Pneumothorax
   f. Chest wall disorders
3. Cardiovascular disorders
   a. Congestive heart failure
   b. Hypotension
4. Metabolic disorders
   a. Acidosis (diabetic, renal, lactic)
   b. Hepatic failure
5. Neurologic and psychogenic disorders
   a. Psychogenic or anxiety hyperventilation
   b. Central nervous system infection, tumors
6. Drug-induced
   a. Salicylates
   b. Methylxanthine derivatives
   c. β-Adrenergic agonists
   d. Progesterone
7. Miscellaneous
   a. Fever, sepsis
   b. Pain
   c. Pregnancy

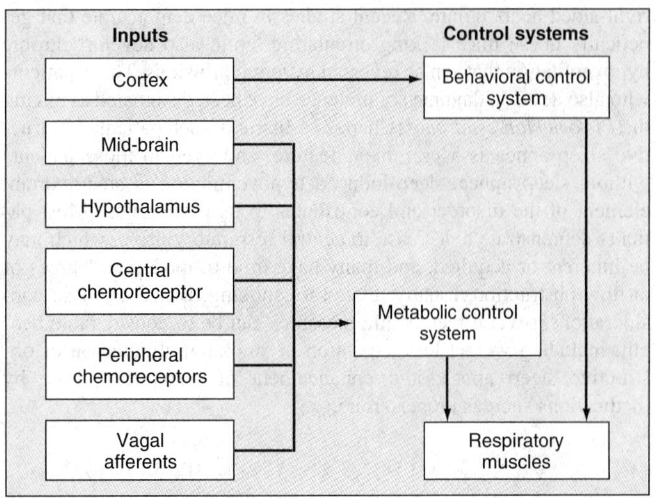

FIGURE 263-3 Schematic diagram of the mechanisms involved in alveolar hyperventilation. *(From Slutsky and Phillipson.)*

brainstem respiratory neurons. Rarely, disorders of the midbrain and hypothalamus induce hyperventilation, and it is conceivable that fever and sepsis also cause hyperventilation through effects on these structures. Several drugs cause hyperventilation by stimulating the central or peripheral chemoreceptors or by direct action on the brainstem respiratory neurons. Chronic hyperventilation is a normal feature of pregnancy and results from the effects of progesterone and other hormones acting on the respiratory neurons.

PHYSIOLOGIC AND CLINICAL FEATURES Because hyperventilation is associated with increased respiratory drive, muscle effort, and minute volume of ventilation, the most frequent symptom associated with hyperventilation is dyspnea. However, there is considerable discrepancy between the degree of hyperventilation, as measured by Pa_{CO_2}, and the degree of associated dyspnea. From a physiologic standpoint, hyperventilation is beneficial in patients who are hypoxemic, because the alveolar hypocapnia is associated with an increase in alveolar and arterial P_{O_2}. Conversely, hyperventilation can also be detrimental. In particular, the alkalemia associated with hypocapnia may produce neurologic symptoms, including dizziness, visual impairment, syncope, and seizure activity (secondary to cerebral vasoconstriction); parasthesia, carpopedal spasm, and tetany (secondary to decreased free serum calcium); and muscle weakness (secondary to hypophosphatemia). Severe alkalemia can also induce cardiac arrhythmias and evidence of myocardial ischemia. Patients with a primary respiratory alkalosis are also prone to periodic breathing and central sleep apnea (Chap. 264).

DIAGNOSIS In most patients with a hyperventilation syndrome, the cause is readily apparent on the basis of history, physical examination, and knowledge of coexisting medical disorders (Table 263-2). In patients in whom the cause is not clinically apparent, investigation begins with arterial blood gas analysis, which establishes the presence of alveolar hyperventilation (decreased Pa_{CO_2}) and its severity. Equally important is the arterial pH, which generally allows the disorder to be classified as either a primary respiratory alkalosis (elevated pH) or a primary metabolic acidosis (decreased pH). Also of importance is the Pa_{O_2} and calculation of the $(A - a)P_{O_2}$, since a widened alveolar-arterial oxygen difference suggests a pulmonary disorder as the underlying cause. The finding of a reduced plasma HCO_3^- level establishes the chronic nature of the disorder and points toward an organic cause. Measurements of ventilation and arterial or transcutaneous P_{CO_2} during sleep are very useful in suspected psychogenic hyperventilation, since such patients do not maintain the hyperventilation during sleep.

The disorders that most frequently give rise to unexplained hyperventilation are pulmonary vascular disease (particularly chronic or recurrent thromboembolism) and psychogenic or anxiety hyperventilation. Hyperventilation due to pulmonary vascular disease is associated with exertional dyspnea, a widened $(A - a)P_{O_2}$ and maintenance of hyperventilation during exercise. In contrast, patients with psychogenic hyperventilation typically complain of dyspnea at rest and not during mild exercise and of the need to sigh frequently. They are also more likely to complain of dizziness, sweating, palpitations, and paresthesia. During mild to moderate exercise, their hyperventilation tends to disappear and $(A - a)P_{O_2}$ is normal, but heart rate and cardiac output may be increased relative to metabolic rate.

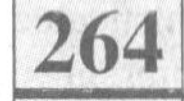
TREATMENT Alveolar hyperventilation is usually of relatively minor clinical consequence and therefore is generally managed by appropriate treatment of the underlying cause. In the few patients in whom alkalemia is thought to be inducing significant cerebral vasoconstriction, paresthesia, tetany, or cardiac disturbances, inhalation of a low concentration of CO_2 can be very beneficial. For patients with disabling psychogenic hyperventilation, careful explanation of the basis of their symptoms can be reassuring and is often sufficient. Others have benefited from β-adrenergic antagonists or an exercise program. Specific treatment for anxiety may also be indicated.

BIBLIOGRAPHY

FANBURG BL, SICILIAN L (eds): Respiratory dysfunction in neuromuscular disease. Clin Chest Med 15:(4)607, 1994

KATZ ES et al: Late-onset central hypoventilation with hypothalmic dysfunction: A distinct clinical syndrome. Pediatr Pulmonol 29:62, 2000

O'DONNELL CP et al: Leptin prevents respiratory depression in obesity. Am J Respir Crit Care Med 159:1477, 1999

PHILLIPSON EA, SLUTSKY AS: Hypoventilation and hyperventilation syndromes, in *Textbook of Respiratory Medicine*, 3d ed, JF Murray, JA Nadel (eds). Philadelphia, Saunders, 2000, pp 2139–2152

SLUTSKY AS, PHILLIPSON EA: Hyperventilation syndromes, in *Textbook of Respiratory Medicine*, JF Murray, JA Nadel (eds). Philadelphia, Saunders, 1994, chap 85, pp 2325–2332

TANKERSLEY CG et al: Genetic control of differential baseline breathing pattern. J Appl Physiol 82:874, 1997

264

Eliot A. Phillipson

SLEEP APNEA

DEFINITION AND CLASSIFICATION *Sleep apnea* is defined as an intermittent cessation of airflow at the nose and mouth during sleep. By convention, apneas of at least 10 s duration have been considered important, but in most patients the apneas are 20 to 30 s in duration and may be as long as 2 to 3 min. *Sleep apnea syndrome* refers to a clinical disorder that arises from recurrent apneas during sleep. The clinical importance of sleep apnea arises from the fact that it is one of the leading causes of excessive daytime sleepiness. Indeed, epidemiologic studies have established a prevalence of clinically important sleep apnea of at least 2% in middle-aged women and 4% in middle-aged men.

Sleep apneas can be central or obstructive in type. In central sleep apnea (CSA) the neural drive to all the respiratory muscles is transiently abolished. In contrast, in obstructive sleep apnea (OSA) airflow ceases despite continuing respiratory drive because of occlusion of the oropharyngeal airway.

OBSTRUCTIVE SLEEP APNEA **Pathogenesis** The definitive event in OSA is occlusion of the upper airway usually at the level of the oropharynx. The resulting apnea leads to progressive asphyxia until there is a brief arousal from sleep, whereupon airway patency is restored and airflow resumes. The patient then returns to sleep, and the sequence of events is repeated, often up to 400 to 500 times per night, resulting in marked fragmentation of sleep.

The immediate factor leading to collapse of the upper airway in OSA is the generation of a critical subatmospheric pressure during inspiration that exceeds the ability of the airway dilator and abductor muscles to maintain airway stability. During wakefulness, upper airway muscle activity is greater than normal in patients with OSA, presumably to compensate for airway narrowing (see below) and a high upper airway resistance. Sleep plays a permissive but crucial role by reducing the activity of the muscles and their protective reflex response to subatmospheric airway pressures. Alcohol is frequently an important cofactor because of its selective depressant influence on the upper airway muscles and on the arousal response that terminates each apnea. In most patients the patency of the airway is also compromised structurally and therefore predisposed to occlusion. In a minority of patients the structural compromise is due to obvious anatomic disturbances, such as adenotonsillar hypertrophy, retrognathia, and macroglossia. However, in the majority of patients the structural defect is simply a subtle reduction in airway size that can often be appreciated clinically as "pharyngeal crowding" and that can usually be demonstrated by imaging and acoustic reflection techniques. Obesity frequently contributes to the reduction in size of the upper airways, either by increasing fat deposition in the soft tissues of the pharynx or by compressing the pharynx by superficial fat masses in the neck. More sophisticated studies also demonstrate a high airway compliance—i.e., the airway is "floppy" and therefore prone to collapse.

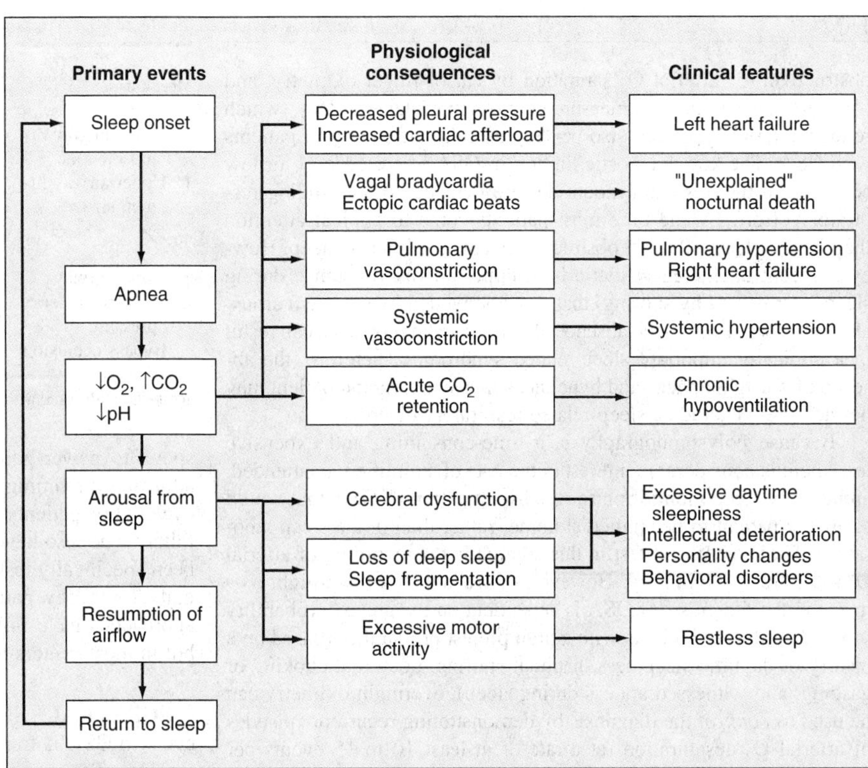

FIGURE 264-1 The primary sequence of events, physiologic responses, and clinical features of obstructive sleep apnea.

Pathophysiologic and Clinical Features The narrowing of the upper airways during sleep, which predisposes to OSA, inevitably results in snoring. In most patients, snoring antedates the development of obstructive events by many years. However, the majority of snoring individuals do not have an OSA disorder, nor is there definitive evidence that snoring per se is associated with long-term health risks. Hence, in the absence of other symptoms, snoring alone does not warrant an investigation for OSA but does call for preventive counselling, particularly with regard to weight gain and alcohol consumption.

The recurrent episodes of nocturnal asphyxia and of arousal from sleep that characterize OSA lead to a series of secondary physiologic events, which in turn give rise in some patients to the clinical complications of the syndrome (Fig. 264-1). The most common manifestations are neuropsychiatric and behavioral disturbances that are thought to arise from the fragmentation of sleep and loss of slow-wave sleep induced by the recurrent arousal responses. Nocturnal cerebral hypoxia may also play an important role. The most pervasive manifestation is excessive daytime sleepiness. Initially, daytime sleepiness manifests under passive conditions, such as reading or watching television; but as the disorder progresses, sleepiness encroaches into all daily activities and can become disabling and dangerous. Several studies have demonstrated two to seven times more motor vehicle accidents in patients with OSA compared with other drivers. Other related symptoms include intellectual impairment, memory loss, and personality disturbances.

The other major manifestations of OSA are cardiorespiratory in nature and are thought to arise from the recurrent episodes of nocturnal asphyxia and of negative intrathoracic pressure, which increases left ventricular afterload (Fig. 264-1). Many patients demonstrate a cyclical slowing of the heart during the apneas to 30 to 50 beats per minute, followed by a tachycardia of 90 to 120 beats per minute during the ventilatory phase. A small number of patients develop severe bradycardia or dangerous tachyarrhythmias, leading to the notion that OSA may result in sudden death during sleep, but firm corroborative data are lacking. Unlike in healthy subjects, in patients with OSA systemic blood pressure fails to decrease during sleep. In fact, blood pressure typically rises abruptly at the termination of each obstructive event as a result of sympathetic nervous activation and reflex vasoconstriction. Furthermore, over 50% of patients with OSA have systemic hypertension. Several epidemiologic studies have implicated OSA as a risk factor for the development of systemic hypertension, and recent studies in an animal model demonstrate directly that OSA can cause sustained increases in daytime blood pressure. Emerging data also suggest that OSA can precipitate myocardial ischemia in patients with coronary artery disease and can adversely affect left ventricular function, both acutely and chronically, in patients with congestive heart failure. This complication is probably due to the combined effects of increased left ventricular afterload during each obstructive event, secondary to increased negative intrathoracic pressure (Fig. 264-1), recurrent nocturnal hypoxemia, and chronically elevated sympathoadrenal activity. Treatment of OSA in such patients often results in dramatic improvement in left ventricular function and in clinical cardiac status. Finally, up to 20% of patients with OSA develop mild pulmonary hypertension (in the absence of intrinsic lung disease), and a small proportion (<10%) develop pulmonary hypertension, right ventricular failure, polycythemia, and chronic hypercapnia and hypoxemia. All such patients have evidence of sustained daytime hypoxemia in addition to the nocturnal ventilatory disturbance, usually as a result of reduced ventilatory drive and/or diffuse airways obstruction.

Diagnosis Although OSA occurs at any age, and is more prevalent in women than was previously thought, the typical patient is a male aged 30 to 60 years who presents with a history of snoring, excessive daytime sleepiness, nocturnal choking or gasping, witnessed apneas during sleep, moderate obesity, and often mild to moderate hypertension. The definitive investigation for suspected OSA is polysomnography, a detailed overnight sleep study that includes recording of (1) electrographic variables (electroencephalogram, electrooculogram, and submental electromyogram) that permit the identification of sleep and its various stages, (2) ventilatory variables that permit the identification of apneas and their classification as central or obstructive, (3) arterial O_2 saturation by ear or finger oximetry, and (4) heart rate. Continuous measurement of transcutaneous P_{CO_2} (which reflects arterial P_{CO_2}) can also be very useful, particularly in patients with CSA. The key diagnostic finding in OSA is episodes of airflow cessation at the nose and mouth despite evidence of continuing respiratory effort. By the time most patients come to clinical attention they have at least 10 to 15 obstructive events per hour of sleep. However, recent data suggest that a high upper airway resistance during sleep (manifested by snoring) that is accompanied by recurrent arousals from sleep, even in the absence of apneas and hypopneas, can result in a clinically important sleep-related syndrome. Therefore, the absence of outright apneas and hypopneas in a symptomatic patient may not definitely exclude a sleep-related respiratory disorder.

Because polysomnography is a time-consuming and expensive test, there is considerable interest in the role of simplified, unattended, ambulatory sleep monitoring for the investigation of OSA that would allow the patient to be studied at home, rather than in the sleep laboratory. The most useful test in this context is the recording of arterial O_2 saturation by oximetry. However, the reliability of overnight oximetry in the diagnosis of OSA is dependent on the pretest probability of the disorder. In patients with a high pretest probability (based on a history of daytime sleepiness, habitual snoring, nocturnal choking or gasping, and witnessed apneas during sleep), overnight oximetry can be used to *confirm* the diagnosis by demonstrating recurrent episodes of arterial O_2 desaturation (at a rate of at least 10 to 15 events per hour). Such findings obviate the need for full polysomnography and allow initiation of treatment with nasal continuous positive airway pressure (CPAP) during sleep (see "Treatment"). However, negative results in a patient with a high clinical probability of OSA do not exclude the diagnosis but mandate that the patient proceed to polysomnography to investigate the cause of the daytime sleepiness. In contrast, when the pretest probability of OSA is low (such as the patient with only occasional snoring, few witnessed apneas, and no daytime sleepiness), the absence of arterial O_2 desaturation can be used to *exclude* the diagnosis and thereby obviate the need for full polysomnography.

Studies suggest that overnight oximetry can obviate the need for polysomnography in about one-third of clinic patients referred for consideration of OSA, either by *confirming* the diagnosis in patients with a *high* pretest probability of the disorder, or by *excluding* the diagnosis in patients with a *low* pretest probability. In the remaining two-thirds of patients with an intermediate pretest probability of OSA, overnight oximetry alone will not be definitive; hence such patients will require polysomnography.

℞ **TREATMENT** (Table 264-1) Several approaches to treatment of OSA have been advocated, based on an understanding of the mechanisms underlying the disorder. Mild to moderate OSA can often be managed effectively by modest weight reduction, avoidance of alcohol, improvement of nasal patency, and avoidance of sleeping in the supine posture. Intraoral appliances, designed to keep the mandible and tongue forward, are also effective in 55 to 80% of patients. The most widely used treatments in severe OSA are uvulopalatopharyngoplasty and nasal CPAP during sleep. Uvulopalatopharyngoplasty is a surgical procedure designed to increase the pharyngeal lumen by resecting redundant soft tissue. When applied to unselected patients with OSA, it produces long-term cure in fewer than 50% but more discriminating selection of patients yields a higher rate of success. Other surgical approaches, including mandibular advancement and hyoid osteotomy have a more limited application but higher rate of success in selected patients. Nasal CPAP, which prevents upper airway occlusion by splinting the pharyngeal airway with a positive pressure delivered through a nose mask, is currently the most successful long-term approach to treatment, being well tolerated and effective in over 80% of patients, provided that they have received proper training. Patients who are unable to tolerate conventional nasal CPAP may respond to newer generation devices that provide more flexibility in adjusting the timing and levels of inspiratory and expiratory pressure cycles. For patients with ischemic heart disease or congestive heart failure who also have OSA, nasal CPAP is the only treatment that has been specifically tested and is considered the treatment of choice. Finally, for the few patients with severe OSA in whom all other treatment approaches have failed, tracheostomy can provide immediate relief, but in most centers is performed only very rarely.

Table 264-1 Management of Obstructive Sleep Apnea (OSA)

Mechanism	Mild to Moderate OSA	Moderate to Severe OSA
↑ Upper airway muscle tone	Avoidance of alcohol, sedatives	—
↑ Upper airway lumen size	Weight reduction Avoidance of supine posture Oral prosthesis	Uvulopalatopharyngoplasty
↓ Upper airway subatmospheric pressure	Improved nasal patency	Nasal continuous positive airway pressure
Bypass occlusion		Tracheostomy

SOURCE: Phillipson, with permission.

CENTRAL SLEEP APNEA Pathogenesis The definitive event in CSA is transient abolition of central drive to the ventilatory muscles. The resulting apnea leads to a primary sequence of events similar to those of OSA (Fig. 264-1). Several underlying mechanisms can result in cessation of respiratory drive during sleep (Table 264-2). First are defects in the metabolic respiratory control system and respiratory neuromuscular apparatus. Such defects usually produce a chronic alveolar hypoventilation syndrome (in addition to CSA) that becomes more severe during sleep when the stimulatory effect of wakefulness on breathing is abolished. In contrast are CSA disorders that arise from transient instabilities in an otherwise intact respiratory control system. Common to all these disorders is a P_{CO_2} level during sleep that falls transiently below the critical P_{CO_2} required for respiratory rhythm generation. The most frequent instability of this type occurs at sleep onset, because the P_{CO_2} level of wakefulness is often lower than that required for rhythm generation in sleep; hence with loss of the stimulatory effect of wakefulness on breathing (referred to as the *waking neural drive*), an apnea develops at sleep onset until P_{CO_2} rises to the critical level (Fig. 264-2). However, if the central nervous system state fluctuates at sleep onset between "asleep" and "awake," a pattern of periodic breathing develops as respiration follows the changes in state. During each cycle, the waning phase of ventilation includes an hypopnea or outright central apnea (Cheyne-Stokes respiration). In most patients with CSA, the tendency to develop periodic breathing and central apneas during sleep is enhanced by some degree of chronic hyperventilation during wakefulness that

Table 264-2 Mechanisms Underlying Central Sleep Apnea

Underlying Mechanism	Clinical Example
Defects in metabolic control system or respiratory muscles	Primary and secondary central alveolar hypoventilation syndromes Respiratory muscle weakness
Transient instabilities in central respiratory drive	Sleep onset Hyperventilation-induced hypocapnia Idiopathic Hypoxia (high altitude, pulmonary disease) Cardiovascular disease, pulmonary congestion Central nervous system disease Prolonged circulation time

SOURCE: Phillipson, with permission.

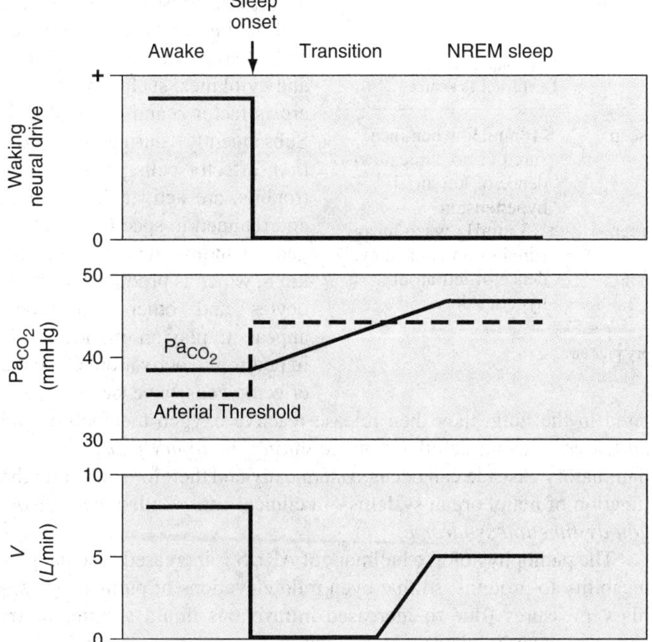

FIGURE 264-2 Schematic diagram of the mechanisms underlying central sleep apnea at sleep onset. With loss of the waking neural drive to breathing, the arterial threshold P_{CO_2} for rhythm generation increases above the Pa_{CO_2} present during wakefulness; ventilation (V) falls to zero and apnea ensues until Pa_{CO_2} rises above the threshold for rhythm generation during sleep. NREM, non-rapid eye movement. *(From TD Bradley, EA Phillipson, Clin Chest Med 13:439, 1992.)*

drives the P_{CO_2} level below the threshold required for rhythm generation during sleep. Such hyperventilation is frequently idiopathic in nature. Hypoxia, whether due to high altitude or to underlying cardiorespiratory disease, also enhances the tendency to periodic breathing and CSA for the same reasons. Periodic breathing and CSA are also common in patients with congestive heart failure. In such patients the decreases in Pa_{CO_2} that trigger transient abolition of central respiratory drive are associated with higher left ventricular end-diastolic volume and filling pressure than in congestive heart failure patients without CSA. The hyperventilation probably results, therefore, from pulmonary congestion and stimulation of pulmonary vagal receptors.

Pathophysiologic and Clinical Features Many healthy individuals demonstrate a small number of central apneas during sleep, particularly at sleep onset and in rapid eye movement sleep. These apneas are not associated with any physiologic or clinical disturbances. In patients with clinically important CSA, the primary sequence of events that characterizes the disorder leads to prominent physiologic and clinical consequences (Fig. 264-1). In those patients whose CSA is a component of an alveolar hypoventilation syndrome, daytime hypercapnia and hypoxemia are usually evident, and the clinical picture is dominated by a history of recurrent respiratory failure, polycythemia, pulmonary hypertension, and right-sided heart failure. Complaints of sleeping poorly, morning headache, and daytime fatigue and sleepiness are also prominent. In contrast, in patients whose CSA results from an instability in respiratory drive, the clinical picture is dominated by features related to sleep disturbance, including recurrent nocturnal awakenings, morning fatigue, and daytime sleepiness. In patients with congestive heart failure, CSA can be an important (and frequently overlooked) cause of daytime sleepiness and fatigue. Recent studies also indicate that CSA can trigger sympathetic nervous activation in patients with heart failure and thereby exert a secondary deleterious effect on the underlying cardiac disorder.

Diagnosis Initially, many patients with CSA are suspected clinically of having OSA because of a history of snoring, sleep disturbance, and daytime sleepiness. However, obesity and hypertension are less prominent in CSA than in OSA. Definitive diagnosis of CSA requires a polysomnographic study, with the *key observation being recurrent apneas that are not accompanied by respiratory effort*. Measurements of transcutaneous P_{CO_2} are particularly useful in CSA. Those patients with a defect in respiratory control or neuromuscular function typically demonstrate an elevated P_{CO_2} that tends to increase progressively during the night, particularly during rapid eye movement sleep. In contrast, patients with instabilities in the respiratory control system typically demonstrate a mild degree of hypocapnia, which is an integral pathogenetic feature of their disorder (see above).

℞ TREATMENT The management of patients whose CSA is a component of an alveolar hypoventilation syndrome is essentially the same as management of the underlying hypoventilation disorder (Chap. 263). Management of patients whose CSA arises from an instability of respiratory drive is more problematic. Patients with hypoxemia usually respond favorably to nocturnal supplemental oxygen. Others have responded to acidification with acetazolamide, and recent reports indicate a good response to nasal CPAP (as for OSA). The mechanism by which CPAP abolishes central apneas probably involves a small increase in Pa_{CO_2} as a result of the added expiratory mechanical load. In patients whose CSA is secondary to congestive heart failure, CPAP is particularly effective in improving sleep quality and daytime cardiac function. In fact, recent randomized trials have demonstrated that CPAP has a beneficial effect on several surrogate markers of mortality in patients with congestive heart failure, including left ventricular ejection fraction, functional mitral regurgitation, and norepinephrine concentrations.

BIBLIOGRAPHY

AMERICAN THORACIC SOCIETY: Indications and standards for use of nasal continuous positive airway pressure (CPAP) in sleep apnea syndromes. Am J Respir Crit Care Med 150:1738, 1994

BRADLEY TD, PHILLIPSON EA: Sleep disorders, in *Textbook of Respiratory Medicine*, 3d ed, JF Murray, JA Nadel (eds). Philadelphia, Saunders, 2000, pp 2153–2170

BROOKS D et al: Obstructive sleep apnea as a cause of systemic hypertension: Evidence from a canine model. J Clin Invest 99:106, 1997

DEEGAN PC, MCNICHOLAS WT: Pathophysiology of obstructive sleep apnoea. Eur Respir J 8:1161, 1995

JAVAHERI S et al: Sleep apnea in 81 ambulatory male patients with stable heart failure. Circulation 97:2154, 1998

PHILLIPS BG, SOMERS VK: Neural and humeral mechanisms mediating cardiovascular responses to obstructive sleep apnea. Resp Physiol 119:181, 2000

TERAN-SANTOS J et al: The association between sleep apnea and the risk of traffic accidents. N Engl J Med 340:847, 1999

YOUNG T et al: Population-based study of sleep-disordered breathing as a risk factor for hypertension. Arch Intern Med 157:1746, 1997

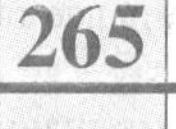

Marc Moss, Roland H. Ingram, Jr.

265 ACUTE RESPIRATORY DISTRESS SYNDROME

Lung injury in acute respiratory distress syndrome (ARDS) is characterized by increased permeability of the alveolar-capillary membrane, diffuse alveolar damage, and the accumulation of proteinaceous pulmonary edema. This clinical syndrome was first described in the archival literature by military physicians when respiratory failure occurred in battlefield casualties during World Wars I and II. However, it was not until the 1960s, when mechanical ventilation was used for patients with acute respiratory failure, that ARDS was first officially named. Initially the "A" in ARDS stood for "adult" to differentiate this syndrome from the infantile respiratory distress syndrome. With the more recent recognition that ARDS occurs in all age groups, the "A" now stands for "acute."

Table 265-1 Recommended Criteria for Acute Lung Injury (ALI) and Acute Respiratory Distress Syndrome (ARDS)

	Timing	Oxygenation	Chest Radiograph	Pulmonary Arterial Occlusion Pressure
ALI Criteria	Acute onset	$Pa_{O_2}/FI_{O_2} \leq 300$ mmHg (regardless of PEEP level)	Bilateral infiltrates seen on frontal chest radiograph	≤18mmHg when measured or no clinical evidence of left atrial hypertension
ARDS Criteria	Acute onset	$Pa_{O_2}/FI_{O_2} \leq 200$ mmHg (regardless of PEEP level)	Bilateral infiltrates seen on frontal chest radiograph	≤18 mmHg when measured or no clinical evidence of left atrial hypertension

NOTE: Pa_{O_2}, arterial oxygen tension; FI_{O_2}, inspiratory O_2 fraction; PEEP, positive end-expiratory pressure.
SOURCE: From Bernard et al.

The diagnostic criteria used to define ARDS have evolved over the past three decades. Originally, most definitions required three general criteria: severe hypoxemia, decreased pulmonary compliance, and diffuse pulmonary infiltrates on chest radiograph. With the increasing utilization of pulmonary arterial catheters in the intensive care unit, ARDS was noted to be a "noncardiogenic" form of pulmonary edema (Chap. 32). Subsequently, some proposed definitions of ARDS required documentation of a normal pulmonary arterial occlusion pressure. However, due to the lack of an established definition and the recognition that ARDS is the severe form of a wide spectrum of lung injury, an American-European Consensus Conference proposed a new definition of ARDS that is now uniformly accepted (Table 265-1). Acute lung injury, which is a mild form of ARDS, was also defined and differs from ARDS based on less severe hypoxemia (Table 265-1).

CLINICAL CHARACTERISTICS Many predisposing factors are associated with the development of ARDS, including conditions that injure the lung directly and those that produce damage through indirect mechanisms via the hematogenous delivery of inflammatory mediators (Table 265-2). The most common of these at-risk conditions are severe sepsis, major trauma, and aspiration of gastric contents. In general, 30 to 40% of individuals with at least one of these diagnoses will eventually develop ARDS. This incidence increases in patients with more than one at-risk condition. A history of chronic alcohol abuse is also associated with an increased risk of developing ARDS in critically ill patients with an at-risk diagnosis.

ARDS occurs within 5 days of the initial at-risk diagnosis in the majority of patients, and over 50% will develop ARDS in the first 24 h. The earliest clinical sign is often an increase in the respiratory frequency, followed by dyspnea. There are no characteristic laboratory abnormalities for ARDS patients except those related to a specific underlying condition, such as leukocytosis in sepsis or an elevated serum amylase level in pancreatitis. Radiographically, the lung fields may be clear initially; diffuse bilateral interstitial or alveolar infiltrates occur as ARDS develops (Fig. 265-1). Though these radiographic changes appear homogeneous on chest radiograph, computed tomography demonstrates a heterogeneous pattern with a predominance of infiltrates in the dependent regions of the lung (Fig. 265-2).

PATHOPHYSIOLOGY ARDS may be the pulmonary manifestation of a systemic process and is the consequence of an overexpression of the normal inflammatory response. This inflammatory cascade has been divided into three overlapping phases—initiation, amplification, and injury. During *initiation*, a precipitating event, such as sepsis, causes both immune and nonimmune cells to produce and release a variety of mediators and cytokines, such as tumor necrosis factor α and interleukin 1. Subsequently, during *amplification*, effector cells, such as neutrophils, are activated, recruited, and retained in specific target organs including the lung. Interleukin 8, which is produced by monocytes and other cell types, appears to play an important role in neutrophil activation. Once the effector cells have been sequestered in the lung, they then release reactive oxygen metabolites and proteases, causing cellular damage during the *injury phase*. This inflammatory cascade can occur systemically and therefore may alter the function of many organ systems—a clinical entity called *multiple organ dysfunction syndrome*.

The pathophysiologic hallmark of ARDS is increased vascular permeability to proteins, so that even mild elevations of pulmonary capillary pressures (due to increased intravenous liquid administration and/or myocardial depression, which may occur in sepsis) greatly increase interstitial and alveolar edema. Alveolar damage is further exaggerated by the quantitative reduction is surfactant synthesis due to injury to type II pneumocytes as well as to further qualitative abnormalities in the size, composition, and metabolism of the remaining surfactant pool, leading to alveolar collapse. Although these atelectatic and liquid-filled regions of the lung contribute to a reduction in the compliance of the lung as a whole, significant regions of nondependent lung have relatively normal mechanical and gas-exchanging properties. However, the decreased overall pulmonary compliance requires large inspiratory pressures to be generated by the respiratory muscles, resulting in an increase in the work of breathing.

Though ARDS is not routinely considered a disease of the airways, airway resistance may be increased due to bronchial wall edema and cytokine-mediated bronchospasm. Pulmonary vascular resistance and pulmonary arterial pressures may also be elevated as a result of in-

Table 265-2 Conditions That May Lead to the Acute Respiratory Distress Syndrome

Direct injury to alveolar epithelium	Indirect lung injury
Aspiration of gastric contents	Sepsis syndrome
Diffuse pulmonary infection	Severe nonthoracic trauma
Near drowning	Hypertransfusion
Pulmonary contusion	Pancreatitis
Toxic inhalation	Cardiopulmonary bypass

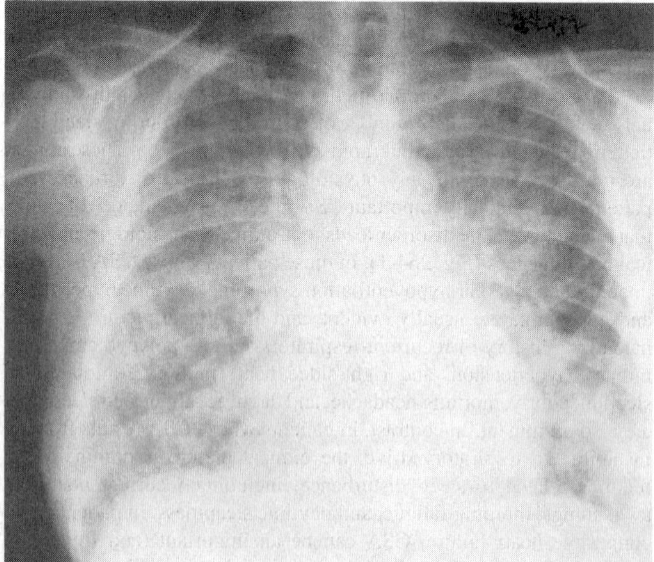

FIGURE 265-1 A standard posteroanterior chest radiograph from a patient with acute respiratory distress syndrome secondary to a severe viral pneumonitis. Such a diffuse radiographic change is typical of all conditions listed in Table 265-2 when they are severe enough to cause acute hypoxemic respiratory failure. A similar radiographic picture is also seen in pulmonary edema due to left ventricular failure (Chap. 32).

creased pulmonary vascular smooth-muscle tone, perivascular edema, microvascular thrombosis, and the production of humoral factors such as leukotrienes and thromboxane A_2, which can directly cause vasoconstriction.

PATHOLOGY During the initial exudative phase, covering the first few days after lung injury, the following occur: (1) epithelial cell injury represented by extensive necrosis of type I pneumocytes and a denuded basement membrane, (2) swelling of endothelial cells with the widening of intercellular junctions, (3) the formation of hyaline membranes composed of fibrin and other matrix proteins in alveolar ducts and airspaces, and (4) a neutrophilic inflammation. Fibrin thrombi may be seen in the alveolar capillaries and smaller pulmonary arteries. The second pathologic phase of ARDS is characterized by proliferation of a variety of cells and resolution of the neutrophilic inflammation. Cuboidal type II cells and squamous epithelium cover denuded alveolar basement membranes. Over the ensuing days to weeks, architectural restoration of lung tissue is usually observed in survivors of ARDS. However, interstitial fibrosis and extensive restructuring of the lung parenchyma may occur with cystic and honeycomb changes in some ARDS patients, resulting in chronic pulmonary dysfunction or death.

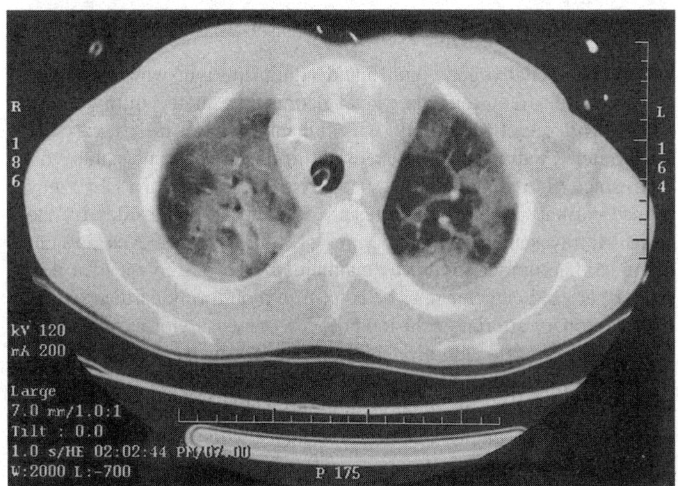

FIGURE 265-2 Computed tomographic image of a patient with acute respiratory distress syndrome demonstrating marked heterogeneity of pulmonary infiltrates with increased density in dependent regions.

℞ **TREATMENT** Currently there are no specific therapies that correct the underlying abnormalities in the permeability of the alveolar-capillary membrane or control the activated inflammatory response in patients with ARDS. However, the use of physiologically targeted strategies of mechanical ventilation and intensive care unit management have led to a more favorable outcome for these critically ill patients.

Mechanical Ventilatory Support In the presence of ARDS, adequate oxygenation is not usually maintained when oxygen is supplied through noninvasive measures. Therefore, most ARDS patients require mechanical ventilation during their hospitalization. The primary goal of the ventilatory management in ARDS is to achieve ventilation and oxygenation that are adequate to support organ function. The major complications of mechanical ventilation are oxygen toxicity and barotrauma, which include not only pneumothorax, pneumomedistinum, and subcutaneous emphysema but also primary alveolar damage. As demonstrated on computed tomography images of the lungs in ARDS patients (Fig. 265-2), a large portion of the alveoli are atelectatic or liquid-filled. However, some nondependent regions of the lung remain radiographically unaffected, and due to their greater compliance they receive a greater proportion of the tidal volume. When large tidal volumes (10 to 12 mL/kg of ideal body weight) are forced into these smaller areas, damage may occur in epithelial and endothelial cells. The sequelae of this injury include alterations in lung liquid balance, increases in permeability, and severe alveolar damage. The deleterious effects of these large tidal volumes and subsequent high alveolar pressures has been termed *volutrauma*.

The currently recommended ventilatory strategies for ARDS patients focus on the limitation of airway pressures to a maximum inflation pressure that should not exceed 30 to 35 cmH_2O, rather than on strategies that attempt to achieve a normal Pa_{CO_2}. Because of the decreased overall lung compliance in ARDS patients, the use of low tidal volumes (~ 6 mL/kg of ideal body weight) is usually required. The subsequent decrease in minute ventilation may result in hypercapnia and respiratory acidosis. This ventilatory strategy, which emphasizes the limitation of transpulmonary pressures at the expense of hypercapnia, has been termed *permissive hypercapnia*.

After intubation, the inspired oxygen fraction (FI_{O_2}) is initially set at 1.0 and then decreased in steps to the lowest FI_{O_2} that will maintain an arterial oxygen tension (Pa_{O_2}) of approximately 60 mmHg. If Pa_{O_2} cannot be maintained at 60 mmHg by an $FI_{O_2} \leq 0.6$, positive end-expiratory pressure (PEEP) may be added (Chap. 266). PEEP improves oxygenation by elevating mean alveolar pressure, thereby recruiting atelectatic alveoli and preventing end-expiratory airway and alveolar closure. In addition, PEEP may prevent alveolar damage by reducing the repetitive and cyclical reopening of closed alveoli during the respiratory cycle. Because PEEP may also overdistend uninvolved alveoli, it should be added cautiously, starting at 5 cmH_2O and increasing in increments of 3 to 5 cmH_2O to a maximum of 20 to 24 cmH_2O. Because airway pressure is transmitted to the pleural space, cardiac output may be adversely affected by the addition of PEEP. In general, the optimal level of PEEP is the amount that achieves an acceptable arterial O_2 saturation (≥90%) with nontoxic FI_{O_2} levels (≤0.6) but without significantly compromising cardiac output. The comprehensive ventilatory strategy that combines low tidal volumes with adequate levels of PEEP has been termed a *lung-protective strategy*. ARDS patients ventilated with this technique have improved 28-day survival and require less time on mechanical ventilation when compared with ARDS patients treated with conventional ventilation using large tidal volumes achieving normal Pa_{CO_2} levels.

Several other ventilatory strategies have been examined with the goal of improving oxygenation. However, none of these techniques has definitively been proven to be beneficial for ARDS patients. When turned from a supine to prone position, ARDS patients develop a more uniform distribution of pleural pressures, with an improvement in ventilation/perfusion matching and better postural drainage of secretions. Prone positioning may improve oxygenation in >75% of ARDS patients. However, the turning of these critically ill patients from the supine to the prone position is not without potential complications, such as unplanned extubation and removal of central venous catheters. The term *inverse ratio ventilation* is defined when the inspiratory (I) time exceeds the expiratory (E) time (i.e., > one-half of the respiratory cycle; I:E ratio > 1:1). This mode of ventilation is able to maintain a higher mean airway pressure, a major determinant of oxygenation, with lower peak airway pressures than conventional ventilation. However, due to the decrease in expiratory time, inverse ratio ventilation is potentially associated with dynamic hyperinflation and increases in end-expiratory pressure. Finally, partial liquid ventilation with perfluorocarbon, a radiopaque, inert, colorless liquid that carries a large quantity of O_2, and CO_2, has been studied in patients with severe ARDS. When perfluorocarbon is administered into the trachea of intubated patients, patients can be safely and adequately oxygenated and ventilated with routine mechanical ventilation.

Intravascular volume management Although pulmonary edema in ARDS patients is a consequence of increased permeability of the alveolar-capillary membrane, elevations in the intravascular hydrostatic pressure may also contribute to the accumulation of alveolar liquid and result in worsening oxygenation. Therefore, the optimal fluid management for patients with ARDS requires a balancing between liquid restriction, which may cause hypotension and decreased perfusion to vital organs, and liquid administration, which may increase oxygen requirements. Small decrements in the intravascular volume with diuretic use produce significant decreases in extravascular lung water. Caution must be exercised in reducing intravascular volume, since vigorous diuresis, especially in the setting of PEEP, may reduce cardiac output and perfusion of critical organs. Ideally, the lowest intravascular hydrostatic pressure that also achieves an adequate cardiac output should be maintained. The placement of a pulmonary arterial catheter may be helpful in monitoring cardiac output and pulmonary arterial occlusion pressure (a measure of intravascular volume) in order to optimize the fluid management of patients with ARDS. However, the placement of a pulmonary arterial catheter and the clinical decisions based upon information derived from the catheter do not appear to improve and may actually worsen the outcome of general intensive care unit patients. Therefore the role of the pulmonary arterial catheter for ARDS patients is presently unclear.

Pharmacologic Therapies Due to their anti-inflammatory properties, glucocorticoids have been used in patients with ARDS, but when administered in high doses (30 mg/kg intravenously every 6 h for a total of four doses), they are not beneficial in the early course of the disease. In contrast, one small randomized study reported an improvement in mortality when glucocorticoids were given after 7 days of unresolving ARDS. In this study, active surveillance for infection was required before enrollment, and glucocorticoids were administered for up to 32 days. Future recommendations regarding the use of these drugs for ARDS patients will be based upon the results of an ongoing multicenter study.

Patients with ARDS have both quantitative and qualitative abnormalities in surfactant, rendering surfactant-replacement therapy an attractive therapeutic modality. In one large randomized study of sepsis-induced ARDS, the administration of synthetic surfactant in an aerosolized form had no significant effect on outcome. Due to concerns with the efficacy of the delivery technique and the lack of essential surfactant-associated proteins in this particular replacement therapy, further studies of different surfactant preparations and modes of administration are presently ongoing.

When inhaled, nitric oxide vasodilates the pulmonary vasculature adjacent to well-ventilated alveoli, thereby improving ventilation-perfusion mismatching. Because of its subsequent inactivation by hemoglobin, nitric oxide produces a selective pulmonary vasodilation without systemic hemodynamic effects. Though inhaled nitric oxide appears to improve oxygenation initially, it is presently unknown whether this therapy will reduce mortality rates in ARDS patients.

PROGNOSIS Since the initial descriptions of ARDS, mortality rates have ranged from 50 to 70%, although they may now be declining with optimal therapy. Mortality rates are higher in patients over 65 years of age, in those with an at-risk diagnosis of sepsis, and when associated with dysfunction of other organ systems. The cause of death for patients with ARDS has been traditionally divided into early causes (within 72 h) and late causes (after 3 days). Most early deaths are attributed to the original presenting illness or injury. Secondary infection and sepsis, persistent respiratory failure, and multiple-organ dysfunction are the most common causes of death in those ARDS patients who live at least 3 days.

In survivors of ARDS, abnormalities in pulmonary function normally improve considerably by 3 months and reach maximum levels of correction by 6 months after extubation. Although pulmonary function markedly recovers in many survivors, over 50% of these patients will continue to have abnormalities, including restrictive impairment or decreased diffusing capacity. Patients with severe ARDS, characterized by extreme hypoxemia and a longer duration of illness, usually have more pulmonary dysfunction than individuals with mild ARDS. Survivors of ARDS also have significant reductions in their quality of life, specifically in regard to physical functioning when compared to other previously critically ill patients.

BIBLIOGRAPHY

ABRAHAM E et al: Consensus conference definitions for sepsis, septic shock, acute lung injury, and acute respiratory distress syndrome: Time for a reevaluation. Crit Care Med 28:232, 2000

AMATO MBP et al: Effect of a protective-ventilatory strategy on mortality in the acute respiratory distress syndrome. N Engl J Med 338:347, 1998

BERNARD GR et al: The American-European consensus conference on ARDS: Definitions, mechanisms, relevant outcomes, and clinical trial coordination. Am J Respir Crit Care Med 149:818, 1994

DAVIDSON TA et al: Reduced quality of life in survivors of acute respiratory distress syndrome compared with critically ill control patients. JAMA 281:354, 1999

DREYFUSS D, SAUMON G: Ventilator-induced lung injury: Lessons from experimental studies. Am J Respir Crit Care Med 157:294, 1998

FLICK MR, MATTHAY MA: Pulmonary edema and acute lung injury, in *Textbook of Respiratory Medicine*, 3d ed, JF Murray, JA Nadel (eds). Philadelphia, Saunders, 2000

MILBERG JA et al: Improved survival of patients with acute respiratory distress syndrome (ARDS):1983–1993. JAMA 273:306, 1995

WARE LB, MATTHAY MA: The acute respiratory distress syndrome. N Engl J Med 342: 1334, 2000

266 MECHANICAL VENTILATORY SUPPORT

Edward P. Ingenito, Jeffrey M. Drazen

ACMV assist control mode ventilation
ARDS acute respiratory distress syndrome
CPAP continuous positive airway pressure
ECMO extracorporeal membrane oxygenation
IRV inverse inspiratory-to-expiratory ratio ventilation
NIV noninvasive ventilation
OLV open lung ventilation
PCV pressure-control ventilation
PEEP positive end-expiratory pressure
PSV pressure-support ventilation
Sa_{O_2} arterial O_2 saturation
SIMV synchronized intermittent mandatory ventilation
$\dot{V}/\dot{Q}$ ventilation perfusion

Ventilators are specially designed pumps that can support the ventilatory function of the respiratory system and improve oxygenation through application of high oxygen content gas and positive pressure. They are a mainstay of physiologic supportive care and are used to stabilize patients with respiratory failure as the underlying disease process is definitively treated.

INDICATIONS FOR MECHANICAL VENTILATION

Respiratory failure is the primary indication for initiation of mechanical ventilation. There are two basic types of respiratory failure.

Hypoxemic respiratory failure most commonly results from pulmonary conditions such as severe pneumonia, pulmonary edema, pulmonary hemorrhage, and respiratory distress syndrome causing ventilation-perfusion ($\dot{V}/\dot{Q}$) mismatch and shunt. Hypoxemic respiratory failure is present when arterial O_2 saturation (Sa_{O_2}) $< 90\%$ is observed despite an inspired O_2 fraction (FI_{O_2}) > 0.6. The goal of ventilator treatment in this setting is to provide adequate Sa_{O_2} through a combination of supplemental O_2 and specific patterns of ventilation that enhance oxygenation.

Hypercarbic respiratory failure results from disease states causing either a decrease in minute ventilation or an increase in physiologic dead space such that, despite adequate total minute ventilation, alveolar ventilation is inadequate to meet metabolic demands. Common clinical conditions associated with hypercarbic respiratory failure include neuromuscular diseases, such as myasthenia gravis, ascending polyradiculopathy, and myopathies, as well as diseases that cause respiratory muscle fatigue due to increased workload, such as asthma, chronic obstructive pulmonary disease, and restrictive lung disease. *Acute* hypercarbic respiratory failure is characterized by arterial P_{CO_2} values of greater than 50 mmHg and an arterial pH above 7.30.

Mechanical ventilation generally should be instituted in acute hypercarbic respiratory failure. In contrast, the decision to institute mechanical ventilation when components of both acute and chronic hypercarbic respiratory failure are present depends on blood gas parameters and clinical evaluation. In particular, if a patient is not in respiratory distress and is not mentally impaired by CO_2 accumulation, it is not mandatory to initiate mechanical ventilation while other forms of treatment are being administered. The goal of ventilator treatment in hypercarbic respiratory failure is to normalize arterial pH through changes in CO_2 tensions. In patients with severe obstructive or restrictive lung disease, elevation in airway pressures may limit tidal volumes to the extent that normalization of pH is not possible, a situation known as *permissive hypercapnia*. Hypoxemic and hypercarbic respiratory failure may coexist in a given individual; in such cases, the indications for and goals of mechanical ventilation are similar to those in these two individual entities.

Accepted therapeutic applications of mechanical ventilation include controlled hyperventilation to reduce cerebral blood flow in patients with increased intracranial pressure or to improve pulmonary hemodynamics in patients with postoperative pulmonary hypertension. Mechanical ventilation also has been used to reduce the work of breathing in patients with congestive heart failure, especially in the presence of myocardial ischemia. Ventilator support is also frequently used in conjunction with endotracheal intubation to prevent aspiration of gastric contents in otherwise unstable patients during gastric lavage for suspected drug overdose or during upper gastrointestinal endoscopy. In the critically ill patient, intubation and mechanical ventilation are indicated before essential diagnostic or therapeutic studies if it appears that respiratory failure may occur during these maneuvers.

PHYSIOLOGIC ASPECTS OF MECHANICAL VENTILATION

Most modern mechanical ventilators function by providing warmed and humidified gas to the airway opening in conformance with various specific volume, pressure, and time patterns. The ventilator serves as the energy source for inspiration, replacing the muscles of the diaphragm and chest wall. Expiration is passive, driven by the recoil of the lungs and chest wall; at the completion of inspiration, internal ventilator circuitry vents the airway to atmospheric pressure or a specified level of positive end-expiratory pressure (PEEP).

PEEP helps maintain alveolar patency in the presence of destabilizing factors and therefore reverses hypoxemia and atelectasis by improving $\dot{V}/\dot{Q}$ matching of ventilation and perfusion. PEEP levels between 0 and 10 cmH_2O are generally safe and effective; higher levels are recommended only in the management of significant refractory hypoxemia unresponsive to increments in FI_{O_2} up to 0.6.

ESTABLISHING AND MAINTAINING AN AIRWAY A cuffed endotracheal tube must be inserted to allow positive-pressure ventilators to deliver conditioned gas, at pressures above atmospheric pressure, to the lungs in a controlled fashion. If neuromuscular paralysis is to be induced during intubation, the use of agents whose mechanism of action includes depolarization at the neuromuscular junction, such as succinylcholine chloride, should be avoided in patients with renal failure, tumor lysis syndrome, crush injuries, medical conditions associated with elevated serum potassium levels, and muscular dystrophy syndromes. Opiates and benzodiazepines can have a deleterious effect on hemodynamics in patients with depressed cardiac function or low systemic vascular resistance and should be used cautiously in this setting. Morphine can promote histamine release from tissue mast cells and may worsen bronchospasm in patients with asthma; fentanyl, sufentanil, and alfentanil are acceptable alternatives to morphine. Ketamine may increase systemic arterial pressure as well as intracranial pressure and has been associated with dramatic hallucinatory responses; it should be used with caution in patients with hypertensive crisis, increased intracranial pressures, or a history of psychiatric disorders.

Patients who require ventilator support for extended periods of time may be candidates for tracheostomy. Although definitive guidelines for performing a tracheostomy in the ventilated patient have not been established, in current clinical practice patients who are anticipated to require ventilator therapy for more than 3 weeks should be considered for this procedure. While it does not clearly reduce the incidence of laryngeal injury or tracheal stenosis, tracheostomy has been associated with improved patient comfort and enhanced ability to partake in rehabilitation-oriented activities.

VENTILATOR MODES This setting specifies the manner in which ventilator breaths are triggered, cycled, and limited; commonly used modes of mechanical ventilation are given in Table 266-1. The *trigger*, either an inspiratory effort or a time-based signal, defines what the ventilator senses to initiate an assisted cycle. *Cycle* refers to the factors that determine the end of inspiration. For example, in volume-cycled ventilation, inspiration ends when a specific tidal volume is delivered to the patient. Other types of cycling include pressure cycling, time cycling, and flow cycling. *Limiting factors* are operator-specified values, such as airway pressure, that are monitored by transducers internal to the ventilator circuit throughout the respiratory cycle; if the specified values are exceeded, inspiratory flow is immediately stopped, and the ventilator circuit is vented to atmospheric pressure or the specified PEEP.

Assist Control Mode Ventilation (ACMV) An inspiratory cycle is initiated either by the patient's inspiratory effort or, if no patient effort is detected within a specified time window, by a timer signal within the ventilator. Every breath delivered consists of the operator-specified tidal volume. Ventilatory rate is determined either by the patient or by the operator-specified backup rate, whichever is of higher frequency (Fig. 266-1*A*). ACMV is the recommended mode for initiation of mechanical ventilation because it ensures a backup minute ventilation in the absence of an intact respiratory drive and allows for synchronization of the ventilator cycle with the patient's inspiratory effort.

Problems can arise when ACMV is used in patients with tachypnea due to nonrespiratory or nonmetabolic factors such as anxiety, pain, or airway irritation. Respiratory alkalemia may develop and trigger myoclonus or seizures. Dynamic hyperinflation (so-called auto-PEEP) may occur if the patient's respiratory mechanics are such that inadequate time is available for complete exhalation between inspiratory cycles. Auto-PEEP can limit venous return, decrease cardiac output, and increase airway pressures, predisposing to barotrauma. ACMV is not effective for weaning patients from mechanical ventilation because it provides full ventilator assistance on each patient-initiated breath.

Synchronized Intermittent Mandatory Ventilation (SIMV) The major difference between SIMV and ACMV is that in the former the patient is allowed to breathe spontaneously, i.e., without ventilator assist, between delivered ventilator breaths. However, mandatory breaths are delivered in synchrony with the patient's inspiratory efforts at a frequency determined by the operator. If the patient fails to initiate a breath, the ventilator delivers a fixed-tidal-volume breath and resets the internal timer for the next inspiratory cycle (Fig. 266-1*B*). SIMV differs from ACMV in that only the preset number of breaths is ventilator-assisted.

SIMV allows patients with an intact respiratory drive to exercise inspiratory muscles between assisted breaths. This characteristic makes SIMV a useful mode of ventilation for both supporting and weaning intubated patients. SIMV may be difficult to use in patients with tachypnea because they may attempt to exhale during the ventilator-programmed inspiratory cycle. When this occurs, the airway pressure may exceed the inspiratory pressure limit, the ventilator-assisted breath will be aborted, and minute volume may drop below that programmed by the operator. In this setting, if the tachypnea is in response to respiratory or metabolic acidosis, a change to ACMV will increase minute ventilation and help normalize the pH while the underlying process is further evaluated.

Continuous Positive Airway Pressure (CPAP) This is not a true support-mode of ventilation, inasmuch as all ventilation occurs

Table 266-1 Clinical Characteristics of Commonly Used Modes of Mechanical Ventilation

Ventilator Mode	Independent Variables (Set by User)	Dependent Variables (Monitored by User)	Trigger/Cycle Limit	Advantages	Disadvantages	Initial Settings
ACMV[a]	FI_{O_2} Tidal volume Ventilator rate Level of PEEP Inspiratory flow pattern Peak inspiratory flow Pressure limit	Peak airway pressure, Pa_{O_2}, Pa_{CO_2} Mean airway pressure I/E ratio	Patient/timer Pressure limit	Timer backup Patient-vent synchrony Patient controls minute ventilation	Not useful for weaning Potential for dangerous respiratory alkalosis	FI_{O_2} = 1.0[b] V_t = 10–15 mL/kg[a] f = 12–15/min PEEP = 0–5 cmH_2O Inspiratory flow = 60 L/min
SIMV[a]	Same as for ACMV	Same as for ACMV	Same as for ACMV	Timer backup useful for weaning	Potential dysynchrony	Same as for ACMV[a]
CPAP	FI_{O_2} Level of CPAP	Tidal volume Rate, flow pattern Airway pressure Pa_{O_2}, Pa_{CO_2}, I/E ratio	No trigger Pressure limit	Allows assessment of spontaneous function Helps prevent atelectasis	No backup	FI_{O_2} = 0.5–1.0[b] CPAP = 5–15 cmH_2O
PCV[a]	FI_{O_2} Inspiratory pressure level Ventilator rate Level of PEEP Pressure limit I/E ratio	Tidal volume Flow rate, pattern Minute ventilation Pa_{O_2}, Pa_{CO_2}	Timer/patient Timer/pressure limit	System pressures regulated Useful for barotrauma treatment Timer backup	Requires heavy sedation Not useful for weaning	FI_{O_2} = 1.0[b] PC = 20–40 cmH_2O[a] PEEP = 5–10 cmH_2O f = 12–15/min I/E = 0.7/1–4/1
PSV	FI_{O_2} Inspiratory pressure level PEEP Pressure limit	Same as for PCV + I/E ratio	Inspiratory flow Pressure limit	Assures synchrony Good for weaning	No timer backup	FI_{O_2} = 0.5–1.0[b] PS = 10–30 cmH_2O 5 cmH_2O usually the level used PEEP = 0–5 cmH_2O

[a] Open lung ventilation (OLV) involves the use of any of these specific modes with tidal volumes (or applied pressures) to achieve 5–6 mL/kg, and positive end expiratory pressures achieve maximal alveolar recruitment.
[b] FIO_2 is usually set to 1.0 initially, unless there is a specific clinical indication to minimize FIO_2, such as history of chemotherapy with bleomycin. Once adequate oxygenation is documented by blood gas analysis, FIO_2 should be decreased in decrements of 0.1–0.2 as tolerated, until the lowest FIO_2 required for an Sa_{O_2} >90% is achieved.
ABBREVIATIONS: f, frequency; I/E, inspiration/expiration.

through the patient's spontaneous efforts. The ventilator provides fresh gas to the breathing circuit with each inspiration and charges the circuit to a constant, operator-specified pressure that can range from 0 to 20 cmH_2O (Fig. 266-1*C*). CPAP is used to assess extubation potential in patients who have been effectively weaned and are requiring little ventilator support and in patients with intact respiratory system function who require an endotracheal tube for airway protection.

Pressure-Control Ventilation (PCV) This form of ventilation is time triggered, time cycled, and pressure limited. During the inspiratory phase, a given pressure is imposed at the airway opening, and the pressure remains at this user-specified level throughout inspiration (Fig. 266-2*A*). Since inspiratory airway pressure is specified by the operator, tidal volume and inspiratory flow rate are *dependent* rather than *independent* variables and are not user specified. PCV is the preferred mode of ventilation for patients with documented barotrauma, because airway pressures can be limited, and for postoperative thoracic surgical patients, in whom the shear forces across a fresh suture line should be limited. When PCV is used, minute ventilation and tidal volume must be monitored; minute ventilation is altered through changes in rate or in the pressure-control value.

The major practical limitation of PCV is patient-ventilator asynchrony related to its time-cycled and time-triggered characteristics. Because PCV requires that the patient passively accept ventilator breaths, most patients require heavy sedation to be maintained on this ventilatory mode, which may be hazardous in the hemodynamically unstable patient.

PCV with the use of a prolonged inspiratory time is frequently applied to patients with severe hypoxemic respiratory failure. This approach, called inverse inspiratory-to-expiratory ratio ventilation (IRV), increases mean distending pressures without increasing peak airway pressures. It is thought to work in conjunction with PEEP to open collapsed alveoli and improve oxygenation. IRV may be associated with fewer deleterious effects than conventional volume-cycled ventilation, which requires higher peak airway pressures to achieve an equivalent reduction in shunt fraction.

Pressure-Support Ventilation (PSV) This form of ventilation is patient triggered, flow cycled, and pressure limited; it is specifically designed for use in the weaning process. During PSV, the inspiratory phase is terminated when inspiratory airflow falls below a certain level; in most ventilators this flow rate cannot be adjusted by the operator. When PSV is used, patients receive ventilator assist only when the ventilator detects an inspiratory effort (Fig. 266-2*B*). PSV also can be used in combination with SIMV to ensure volume-cycled backup for patients whose respiratory drive is depressed either spontaneously or as a result of various therapeutic maneuvers.

PSV is well tolerated by most patients who are being weaned; PSV parameters can be set to provide fully or nearly fully ventilatory support and can be withdrawn slowly over a period of days in a systematic fashion to gradually load the respiratory muscles.

Open Lung Ventilation (OLV) OLV is not a distinct mode of ventilation, but rather a strategy for applying either volume-cycled or pressure-control ventilation to patients with severe respiratory failure. In OLV, the primary objectives of ventilator support are maintenance of adequate oxygenation and avoidance of cyclic opening and closing of alveolar units by selecting a level of PEEP that allows the majority of units to remain inflated during tidal ventilation. Achievement of eucapnia and normal blood pH through adjustments in ventilator tidal volume and breathing frequency are of lower priority. Clinical and

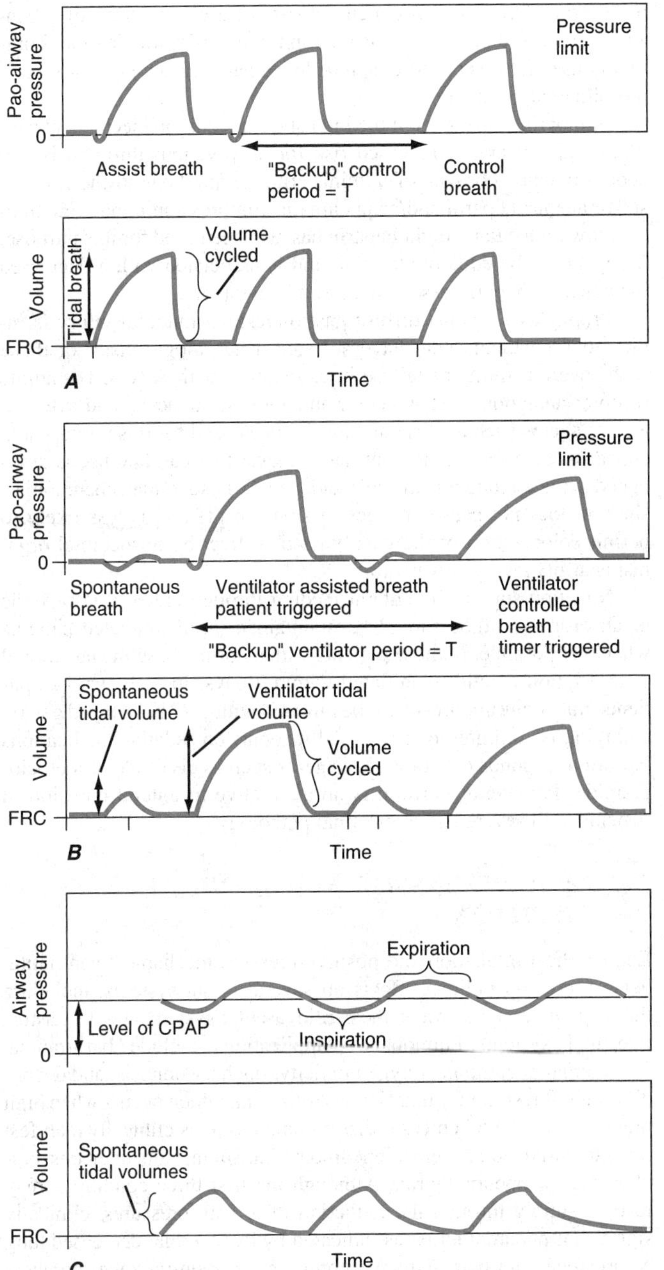

FIGURE 266-1 *A.* Airway pressure and lung volume versus time profile during ACMV. Assisted breaths are triggered by the patient's effort. Controlled breaths are triggered by the ventilator timer. Every breath, whether triggered by the patient or by the timer, is a complete volume-cycled breath, with airway pressure as a dependent variable. The pressure limit is set above the peak inspiratory pressure. *B.* Airway pressure and lung volume versus time profiles during SIMV. Spontaneous breaths occur between patient-triggered assisted breaths and timer-triggered breaths. The tidal volume of the spontaneous breaths is determined by the patient's effort and lung impedance. Assisted and controlled breaths are volume cycled. *C.* Airway pressure and lung volume versus time profiles during CPAP. Breathing is spontaneous, and no ventilator assist is provided. The spontaneous profile is superimposed on an elevated mean airway pressure that the user specifies. FRC, functional residual capacity.

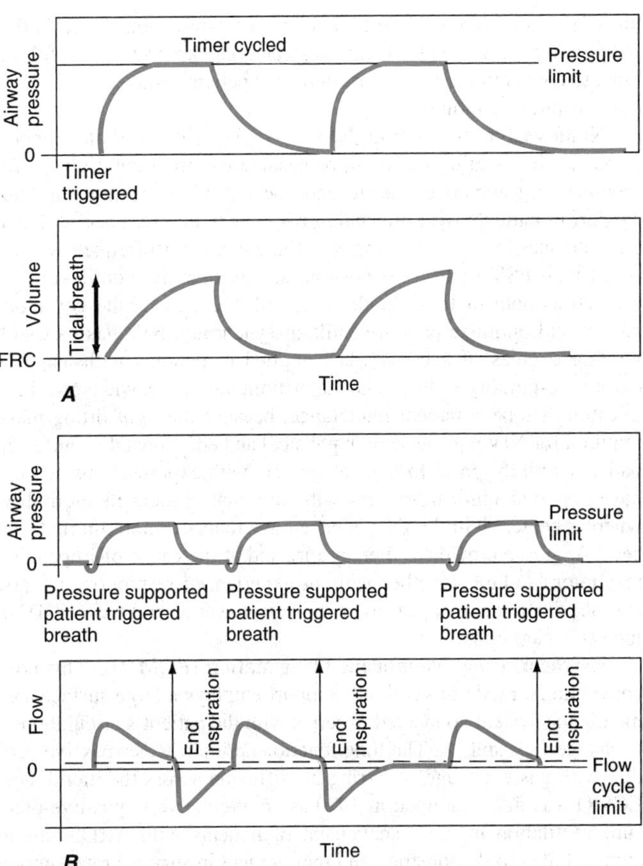

FIGURE 266-2 *A.* Airway pressure and lung volume versus time profiles during PCV. All breaths are timer triggered, timer cycled, and pressure limited. Peak airway pressure is set by the operator, and tidal volume is a dependent variable. The profiles shown here display the pressure limit as slightly higher than pressure-control level. This need not be the case, but it is appropriate to set the pressure limit only slightly above the pressure-control level when using this mode of ventilation for management of the patient with barotrauma. *B.* Airway pressure and airway flow versus time profiles during PSV. All breaths are patient triggered and flow cycled. Inspiration is cycled off when the inspiratory flow drops below a predetermined threshold internally set in the ventilator circuit. In the example shown, the pressure limit is slightly greater than the pressure-support level. Since each can be set independently, this need not be the case. FRC, functional residual capacity.

experimental observations indicate that high airway pressures and repeated opening and closing of alveoli can cause microstructural lung damage, propagation of lung injury through generation of inflammatory cytokines, and direct barotrauma. Current data suggest that a small tidal volume (i.e., 6 mL/kg) provides adequate ventilatory support with a lower incidence of adverse effects than more conventional tidal volumes of 10-15 mL/kg. These potential complications can have dire consequences in patients with respiratory failure. Alternatively, hypercapnia and consequent respiratory acidosis tend to be well tolerated physiologically, except in patients with significant hemodynamic compromise, ventricular dysfunction, cardiac dysrrhythmias, or increased intracranial pressure. OLV has been used most extensively in the management of patients with hypoxemic respiratory failure due to acute lung injury. Although few randomized clinical trials of OLV have been performed, available data suggest that OLV reduces the morality rate and improves gas exhange in patients with acute lung injury.

Prone Positioning during Mechanical Ventilation Patients with acute respiratory distress syndrome (ARDS) experience hypoxemia as a result of intrapulmonary shunt due to regional atelectasis. Recent studies in patients with ARDS have demonstrated that collapse occurs most extensively in the dependent regions of the lung. Increasing airway pressures to counterbalance the compressive effects of the surrounding lung in these collapsed regions improves gas exchange but may result in potentially dangerous peak airway pressures. Prone positioning, in both experimental and clinical studies, reduces shunt and improves oxygenation by causing regional improvements in transpulmonary distending pressures wtihout overexpanding already patent alveoli. In clinical practice, prone positioning has been used in conjunction with both volume-cycled and pressure-control ventilation with equivalent clinical effectiveness and appears to be a useful adjunct to conventional ventilator support in patients with severe hypoxemic respiratory failure.

Noninvasive Ventilation (NIV) Noninvasive ventilator support through a tight-fitting facemask or nasal mask, traditionally used for treatment of sleep apnea, has recently been used as primary ventilator support in patients with impending respiratory failure. Facemask and nasal devices for administering NIV therapy are most frequently combined with PSV or bi-level positive airway pressure ventilation, inasmuch as both of these modes are well tolerated by the conscious patient and optimize patient-ventilator synchrony. NIV has met with varying degrees of success when applied to patients with acute or chronic respiratory failure. The major limitation to its widespread application has been patient intolerance, because the tight-fitting mask required for NIV can cause both physical and emotional discomfort in patients with dyspnea. In general, centers with experience using NIV have reported clinical success with minimal associated morbidity, whereas centers with less experience have reported more limited success. Aggressive medical therapy directed at the cause of impending respiratory failure, together with an experienced respiratory therapy and physician team, appear to be the keys to successful use of NIV in intensive care units.

Extracorporeal Membrane Oxygenation (ECMO) This nonconventional mode of ventilator support employs a large surface area membrane system connected in series with the patient's circulation to exchange CO_2 and O_2. The lung functions primarily as a passive conduit with gas exchange occurring by diffusion across the membrane. ECMO was first examined in 1970 as an alternative to positive-pressure ventilation in the management of patients with ARDS. Initial studies failed to demonstrate an improvement in survival rates among patients treated with ECMO. Although several uncontrolled trials have since suggested that ECMO does improve outcome among patients with ARDS, a 1993 study comparing survival rates of patients with ARDS treated with ECMO and those treated with conventional ventilator therapy showed no difference in mortality rates, but the morbidity rates and hospital costs were increased among ECMO-treated patients. Presently, the use of ECMO in patients with ARDS is not recommended.

Guidelines for Managing the Ventilated Patient

Most patients who are started on ventilator support receive ACMV or SIMV, because these modes ensure user-specified backup minute ventilation in the event that the patient fails to initiate respiratory efforts. Once the intubated patient has been stabilized with respect to oxygenation, definitive therapy for the underlying process responsible for respiratory failure is formulated and initiated. Subsequent modifications in ventilator therapy must be provided in parallel with changes in the patient's clinical status. As improvement in respiratory function is noted, the first priorities are to reduce PEEP and supplemental O_2. Once a patient can achieve adequate arterial saturation with an $F\text{I}_{O_2} \leq 0.5$ and 5 cmH_2O PEEP, attempts should be made to reduce the level of mechanical ventilatory support. Patients previously on full ventilator support should be switched to a ventilator mode that allows for weaning, such as SIMV, PSV, or SIMV combined with PSV. Ventilator therapy can then be gradually removed, as outlined in the section on weaning. Patients whose condition continues to deteriorate after ventilator support is initiated may require increased O_2, PEEP, and alternative modes of ventilation such as IRV.

GENERAL SUPPORT IN THE VENTILATED PATIENT

Patients who are started on mechanical ventilation usually require some form of sedation and analgesia to maintain an acceptable level of comfort. Often, this regimen consists of a combination of a benzodiazepine and opiate administered intravenously. Medications commonly used for this purpose include lorazepam, midazolam, diazepam, morphine, and fentanyl.

Immobilized patients in the intensive care unit on mechanical ventilator support are at increased risk for deep venous thrombosis; accepted practice consists of administering prophylaxis in the form of subcutaneous heparin and/or pneumatic compression boots. Fractionated low molecular weight heparin has also been used for this purpose; it appears to be equally effective and is associated with a decreased incidence of heparin-associated thrombocytopenia.

Prophylaxis against diffuse gastrointestinal mucosal injury is indicated for patients who have suffered a neurologic insult or those with severe respiratory failure in association with ARDS. Histamine receptor antagonists (H_2-receptor antagonists), antacids, and cytoprotective agents such as carafate have all been used for this purpose and appear to be effective. Recent data suggest that carafate use is associated with a reduction in the incidence of nosocomial pneumonias, since it does not cause changes in stomach pH and is less likely to permit colonization of the gastrointestinal tract by nosocomial organisms at pH levels near neutral.

Nutrition support by enteral feeding through either a nasogastric or an orogastric tube should be maintained in all intubated patients whenever possible. In those patients with a normal baseline nutritional state, support should be initiated within 7 days. In malnourished patients, nutrition support should be initiated within 72 h. Delayed gastric emptying is common in critically ill patients on sedative medications but often responds to promotility agents such as cisapride or metoclopramide. Parenteral nutrition is an alternative to enteral nutrition in patients with severe gastrointestinal pathology.

COMPLICATIONS OF MECHANICAL VENTILATION

Endotracheal intubation and positive-pressure mechanical ventilation have direct and indirect effects on several organ systems, including the lung and upper airways, the cardiovascular system, and the gastrointestinal system. Pulmonary complications include barotrauma, nosocomial pneumonia, oxygen toxicity, tracheal stenosis, and deconditioning of respiratory muscles. *Barotrauma*, which occurs when high pressures (i.e., > 50 cmH_2O) disrupt lung tissue, is clinically manifest by interstitial emphysema, pneumomediastinum, subcutaneous emphysema, or pneumothorax. Although the first three conditions may resolve simply through the reduction of airway pressures, clinically significant pneumothorax, as indicated by hypoxemia, decreased lung compliance, and hemodynamic compromise, requires tube thoracostomy.

Patients intubated for longer than 72 h are at high risk for *nosocomial pneumonia* as a result of aspiration from the upper airways through small leaks around the endotracheal tube cuff; the most common organisms responsible for this condition are enteric gram-negative rods, *Staphylococcus aureus*, and anaerobic bacteria. Because the endotracheal tube and upper airways of patients on mechanical ventilation are commonly colonized with bacteria, the diagnosis of nosocomial pneumonia requires "protected brush" bronchoscopic sampling of airway secretions coupled with quantitative microbiologic techniques to differentiate colonization from infection.

Oxygen toxicity is a potential complication when an $F\text{I}_{O_2} \geq 0.6$ is required for more than 72 h. The condition can be prevented in some cases through the use of PEEP to allow for $F\text{I}_{O_2}$ values to go below 0.6 while primary therapy for the underlying condition is instituted. Although O_2 toxicity is thought to result from the effects of oxygen free radical on the lung interstitium, the therapeutic use of antioxidants such as superoxide dismutase, catalase, selenium, and vitamin E remains experimental.

Hypotension resulting from elevated intrathoracic pressures with decreased venous return is almost always responsive to intravascular volume repletion. In patients judged to have hypotension or respiratory failure on the basis of alveolar edema, hemodynamic monitoring with a pulmonary arterial catheter may be of value in optimizing O_2 delivery via manipulation of intravascular volume and $F_{I_{O_2}}$ and PEEP levels.

Gastrointestinal effects of positive-pressure ventilation include *stress ulceration* and *mild to moderate cholestasis*. It is common practice to provide prophylaxis with H_2-receptor antagonists or sucralfate for stress-related ulcers. Mild cholestasis (i.e., total bilirubin values ≤4.0) attributable to the effects of increased intrathoracic pressures on portal vein pressures is common and generally self-limited. Cholestasis of a more severe degree should not be attributed to a positive-pressure ventilation response and is more likely due to a primary hepatic process.

WEANING FROM MECHANICAL VENTILATION

Removal of mechanical ventilator support requires that a number of criteria be met. Upper airway function must be intact for a patient to remain extubated but is difficult to assess in the intubated patient. Therefore, if a patient can breathe on his or her own through an endotracheal tube but develops stridor or recurrent aspiration once the tube is removed, upper airway dysfunction or an abnormal swallowing mechanism should be suspected and plans for achieving a stable airway developed. An intact cough during suctioning is a good indicator of a patient's ability to mobilize secretions. Respiratory drive and chest wall function are assessed by observation of respiratory rate, tidal volume, inspiratory pressure, and vital capacity. The weaning index, defined as the ratio of breathing frequency to tidal volume (breaths per minute per liter), is both sensitive and specific for predicting the likelihood of successful extubation. When this ratio is less than 105 with the patient breathing without mechanical assistance through an endotracheal tube, successful extubation is likely. An inspiratory pressure of more than −30 cmH_2O and a vital capacity of greater than 10 mL/kg are considered indicators of acceptable chest wall and diaphragm function. Alveolar ventilation is generally adequate when elimination of CO_2 is sufficient to maintain arterial pH in the range of 7.35 to 7.40, and an $Sa_{O_2} > 90\%$ can be achieved with an $F_{I_{O_2}} < 0.5$ and a PEEP ≤ 5 cmH_2O. Although many patients may not meet all criteria for weaning, the likelihood that a patient will tolerate extubation without difficulty increases as more criteria are met.

Many approaches to weaning patients from ventilator support have been advocated. T-piece and CPAP weaning are best tolerated by patients who have undergone mechanical ventilation for brief periods and require little respiratory muscle reconditioning, whereas SIMV and PSV are best for patients who have been intubated for extended periods and require gradual respiratory-muscle reconditioning.

T-piece weaning involves brief spontaneous breathing trials with supplemental O_2. These trials are usually initiated for 5 min/h followed by a 1-h interval of rest. T-piece trials are increased in 5- to 10-min increments until the patient can remain ventilator independent for periods of several hours. Extubation can then be attempted. CPAP weaning is similar to T-piece weaning except that trials of spontaneous breathing are conducted on the ventilator in CPAP mode.

Weaning by means of SIMV involves gradually tapering the mandatory backup rate in increments of 2 to 4 breaths per minute while monitoring blood gas parameters and respiratory rates. Rates of greater than 25 breaths per minute on withdrawal of mandatory ventilator breaths generally indicate respiratory muscle fatigue and the need to combine periods of exercise with periods of rest. Exercise periods are gradually increased until a patient remains stable on SIMV at 4 breaths per minute or less without needing rest at higher SIMV rates. A CPAP or T-piece trial can then be attempted before planned extubation.

PSV, as described in detail above, is used primarily for weaning from mechanical ventilation. PSV is usually initiated at a level adequate for full ventilator support (PSV_{max}); i.e., PSV is set slightly below the peak inspiratory pressures required by the patient during volume-cycled ventilation. The level of pressure support is then gradually withdrawn in increments of 5 cmH_2O until a level is reached at which the respiratory rate increases to 25 breaths per minute. At this point, intermittent periods of higher-pressure support are alternated with periods of lower-pressure support to provide muscle reconditioning without causing diaphragmatic fatigue. Gradual withdrawal of PSV continues until the level of support is just adequate to overcome the resistance of the endotracheal tube (approximately 5 to 10 cmH_2O). Support can be discontinued and the patient extubated.

BIBLIOGRAPHY

AMATO MBP et al: Effect of a protective-ventilation strategy on mortality in the acute respiratory distress syndrome. N Engl J Med 338:347, 1998

ESTEBAN A et al: A comparison of four methods of weaning patients from mechanical ventilation. N Engl J Med 332:345, 1995

HILL LL, PEARL RG: Flow triggering, pressure-triggering, and autotriggering during mechanical ventilation. Crit Care Med 28:579, 2000

HINSON JR, MARINI JJ: Principles of mechanical ventilator use in respiratory failure. Annu Rev Med 43:341, 1992

INGENITO EP, DRAZEN JM: Mechanical ventilators, in *Principles of Critical Care*, 2d ed., JB Hall, GA Schmidt, LDH Wood (eds). New York, McGraw-Hill, 1997, pp 142–154

MACINTYRE NR: Principles of mechanical ventilation, in *Textbook of Respiratory Medicine*, 3d ed, JF Murray, JA Nadel (eds). Philadelphia, Saunders, 2000, pp 2471–2486

MORRIS AH et al: Randomized clinical trial of pressure control inverse ratio ventilation and extracorporeal membrane oxygenation for adult respiratory distress syndrome. Am J Resp Crit Care Med 149:295, 1994

RANIERI VM et al: Physiologic effects of positive end expiratory pressure in patients with chronic obstructive pulmonary disease during acute ventilatory failure and controlled mechanical ventilation. Am Rev Respir Dis 147:5, 1993

YOUNES M: Proportional assist ventilation: A new approach to ventilatory support. Am Rev Respir Dis 45:114, 1992

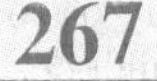

Janet R. Maurer

267 LUNG TRANSPLANTATION

Lung transplantation for end-stage lung disease has been a therapeutic option since the 1980s. Several transplant options are available for carefully selected patients: unilateral lung transplant, bilateral lung transplant, heart-lung transplant (Chap. 233), and living lobar transplant. The first successful type of lung transplant was heart-lung, which was performed for a variety of indications and in increasing numbers until 1989. Beginning in 1989, the numbers of both unilateral and bilateral lung transplants performed increased dramatically and, along with the increasing demand for heart donors, greatly reduced the number of donor organs available for heart-lung procedures. By the mid-1990s, unilateral and bilateral lung transplant numbers also had plateaued because of donor shortages and have remained relatively stable at approximately 1250 operations worldwide per year. Of these, 60% are unilateral lung transplants and 40% are bilateral. Heart-lung transplants have leveled off at between 100 and 150 per year. In its 1999 report, the Registry of the International Society for Heart and Lung Transplantation, in conjunction with the United Network for Organ Sharing, had recorded a cumulative total of 8997 isolated lung transplants and 2350 heart-lung transplants.

INDICATIONS Emphysema, either smoking-induced or secondary to α_1-antitrypsin deficiency, has been the single largest indication for lung transplantation. This diagnosis accounts for about 55% of unilateral lung transplants, 29% of bilateral, and 6% of heart-lung transplants. Other major indications for unilateral lung transplants include idiopathic pulmonary fibrosis (21%) and primary pulmonary hypertension (5%). Patients with cystic fibrosis comprise the largest group of bilateral lung recipients, approximately 34% of the total, followed by patients with emphysema, patients with primary pulmonary hypertension (10%), and those with idiopathic pulmonary fibrosis (7.5%). The major diagnoses among heart-lung recipients are primary and secondary pulmonary hypertension (54%) and cystic fibrosis (16%). With the widespread use of unilateral and bilateral lung transplants, the indications for heart-lung transplant have become very circumscribed, so that now most candidates for this type of transplant have either concomitant left ventricular disease and end-stage lung disease or irreparable congenital heart disease with Eisenmenger's syndrome. Patients receiving living lobar donations have been either children or young adults, and most have suffered from cystic fibrosis. In most of these operations, a lower lobe is donated from each of two adults, who are often, but not always, related to the recipient. Living donation is performed in a limited number of lung transplant programs, and the donor morbidity rate has been acceptable.

RECIPIENT SELECTION Because donor lungs are the scarcest of the common solid organs transplanted, patients with end-stage lung disease undergo extensive evaluation to select the best potential candidates. In 1998, this process was further standardized with the publication of the International Guidelines for the Selection of Lung Transplant Candidates. Approximate age limits of 65 years for unilateral lung, 60 years for bilateral lung, and 55 years for heart-lung transplants were set. Chronic medical conditions that can be adequately controlled and have not resulted in end-organ damage, e.g., systemic hypertension, are acceptable in lung transplant candidates. However, in a case where a chronic illness is often associated with nonpulmonary organ damage, e.g., diabetes mellitus, a careful assessment of target organ function is necessary.

Absolute contraindications to lung transplantation include dysfunction of major organs (other than lung), infection with HIV, active malignancy within 2 years with the exception of basal cell and squamous cell skin cancer, hepatitis B antigen positivity, and hepatitis C with biopsy-proven histologic evidence of liver disease. Conditions that represent relative contraindications include symptomatic osteoporosis; severe musculoskeletal disease affecting the thorax; high-dose corticosteroid use; weight less than 70% or greater than 130% of ideal body weight; alcohol, cigarette, or narcotic abuse/addiction within 6 months before evaluation; psychosocial problems, including noncompliance, that cannot be adequately resolved through pharmacologic treatment or counseling; requirement for invasive ventilation; and colonization with fungi or atypical mycobacteria. Colonization is of particular concern when a unilateral lung transplant is being considered. Disease-specific guidelines (Table 267-1) are chosen to identify candidates who are within the transplant "window"—that is, patients who are ill enough to fit within the category of "end-stage" and have progressive disease, yet are able to survive the pre-transplant waiting and perioperative time periods. In the past few years, increasing experience with large numbers of patients with end-stage disease has made it much easier to estimate life expectancies; however, patients with diagnoses of emphysema and Eisenmenger's type pulmonary hypertension remain problematic in this regard because posttransplant statistical analysis does not show a clear survival benefit for recipients within the first 2 years. In these types of patient, selection usually includes consideration of quality-of-life issues as well as survival rates.

SELECTION OF TRANSPLANT PROCEDURE The only diseases that currently mandate a specific procedure are (1) irreparable congenital cardiac defects with Eisenmenger's syndrome (heart-lung transplant); (2) advanced lung disease with concomitant left ventricular dysfunction (heart-lung transplant); and (3) bronchiectatic lung disease, e.g., cystic fibrosis (bilateral lung transplant or bilobar living donor lung transplant). In essentially all other circumstances unilateral lung transplantation can be performed with acceptable early and mid-term results. Bilateral lung transplantation, however, is often preferred if difficulty is anticipated in postoperative management, especially in patients with pulmonary hypertension; if significant bullous disease in present in emphysema; if a patient is very young; or if there are specific individual recipient considerations. As noted below, the long-term survival rates of bilateral lung recipients may be superior; nevertheless, transplant centers have generally chosen to maximize the donor organ resource by performing unilateral lung transplants whenever possible, rather than opting for potentially slightly increased survival periods.

Table 267-1 Disease-specific Selection Guidelines

Emphysema/chronic obstructive pulmonary disease FEV$_1$ < 25% predicted And/or $Pa_{CO_2} \geq 55$ mmHg And/or ↑ Pulmonary artery pressures (PAP) Cystic fibrosis/bronchiectasis FEV$_1$ < 30% predicted or FEV$_1$ > 30% predicted and any of the following: Rapid decrease in FEV$_1$ Massive hemoptysis Cachexia Frequent hospitalizations Useful adjunctive criteria $Pa_{CO_2} \geq 50$ mmHg $Pa_{O_2} \leq 55$ mmHg	Idiopathic pulmonary fibrosis Symptomatic, progressive disease despite drug therapy: Reassess every 3 months Rest or exercise desaturation "Symptomatic" often corresponds to VC < 60-70% predicted DLCO < 50-60% predicted Pulmonary hypertension Symptomatic, progressive disease despite optimal medical treatment; usually New York Heart Association functional class III or IV; gold standard medical treatment considered to be prostacyclin Useful hemodynamic predictors Cardiac index < 2 L/min/m^2 Right atrial pressure > 15 mmHg Mean pulmonary artery pressure > 55 mmHg

NOTE: VC, vital capacity; DLCO, lung diffusing capacity measured with carbon monoxide.
SOURCE: Adapted from the Joint Statement of the ASTP/ATS/ERS/ISHCT.

PROGNOSIS The 1- and 2-year survival rates for unilateral and bilateral lung transplant recipients are 67 and 62%, respectively. Longer term data show a divergence in survival rates by 5 years, with the half-life of bilateral transplant recipients (4.9 years) significantly longer than that of unilateral transplant recipients (3.6 years). Among unilateral graft recipients, patients with emphysema appear to have the best early survival rate (nearly 80% at one year), and patients with idiopathic pulmonary fibrosis and those with pulmonary hypertension have the worst (60 to 65%). Living lobar recipients have early survival rates that are between the rates of these groups, but long-term data are not available for this population.

FUNCTIONAL OUTCOMES Arterial blood gas levels improve markedly in unilateral and bilateral lung transplant recipients by 3 months posttransplant. In both groups, Pa_{CO_2} normalizes; in bilateral lung transplant recipients, Pa_{O_2} also normalizes. Unilateral lung recipients may continue to have mild hypoxemia but rarely require supplemental oxygen. Pulmonary function studies usually reach their maximum values for both groups between 3 and 12 months postoperatively. Unilateral graft recipients who had a preoperative diagnosis of parenchymal lung disease attain 60 to 65% of their predicted FVC and FEV$_1$ values. The values for bilateral lung recipients often approach normal predicted values, but these patients can have mild restrictive physiology. Diffusing capacities are usually slightly decreased in all groups. Airway hyperresponsiveness without clinically relevant asthma can be demonstrated in the majority of lung transplant recipients.

Exercise capacity has been the most interesting functional outcome observed in lung transplant recipients. With respect to nongraded exercise capacity, usually measured by 6- or 12-min walk studies, unilateral and bilateral graft recipients demonstrate marked and similar improvement in distances covered after transplantation. Typically, transplant recipients can walk 100 to 120 m/min within 6 months of transplant and are generally able to sustain this rate over time. On graded exercise studies, however, both groups achieve only 40 to 60% of predicted maximum values, with bilateral lung recipients usually performing slightly better than unilateral lung recipients. This exercise limitation has been extensively studied particularly in bilateral lung recipients. The limitation appears not to be cardiac or ventilatory but rather related to muscle deconditioning and abnormalities in skeletal muscle oxidative capacity. Rarely is the exercise limitation in these patients enough to impact on their normal daily activities or their quality of life.

POSTTRANSPLANT MANAGEMENT ISSUES **Airway Complications** Technical improvements and surgical experience have greatly reduced significant anastomotic complications in lung transplant recipients. It is not uncommon to see small dehiscences of the airway in the first weeks posttransplant, but these generally heal without significant stricture. Probably fewer than 10% of patients will have stenosis severe enough to require balloon dilatation, laser resection, or a stent. When required, wire stents are most often used and are well tolerated. Late-occurring bronchomalacia, often at the anastomotic site, has also been treated with stents.

Acute Rejection A three-pronged immunosuppressive approach, which is used in most lung transplant programs, includes either cyclosporine or tacrolimus, either azathioprine or mycophenolate mofetil, and prednisone. Cytolytic induction is rarely used in these patients because of the risk of infection. Most lung transplant recipients experience at least one episode of acute rejection, usually within the first 3 months, although episodes have been reported to occur up to several years after transplantation. From 10 to 15% of patients have recurrent acute or persistent acute rejection, which predisposes them to chronic rejection. Symptoms include a general feeling of malaise, dyspnea, and sometimes cough. Findings may include low grade fever, rales, mild hypoxemia, decreasing FVC and FEV_1 values, increased white blood cell count, and ill-defined infiltrates with or without pleural effusion on chest x-ray. If a patient presents early in an episode of acute rejection, as most do, the findings are minimal and the chest radiogram is clear. Histologic diagnosis, which is the "gold standard," is routinely made by transbronchial biopsy, with a sensitivity of about 80% and a specificity approaching 100%. Bronchoscopy is also helpful in this setting to rule out infections that may have similar presentations.

Acute rejection episodes occurring early after transplantation respond in at least 80% of patients to bolus methylprednisolone. Late episodes and recurrent or persistent episodes often require both intensification of immunosuppression and changes in immunosuppressive drugs. Up to 20% of asymptomatic patients have at least one episode of acute rejection detected by surveillance transbronchial biopsy in the first 2 years posttransplant. It is not clear whether asymptomatic rejection requires therapy, as the impact on outcome is unknown. Thus, the use of surveillance bronchoscopy and the treatment of asymptomatic rejection vary considerably from institution to institution, and there are at present no clear guidelines in this area.

Bronchiolitis Obliterans Bronchiolitis obliterans is both the primary manifestation of chronic rejection and the most feared complication in lung transplant recipients. It occurs to some degree in at least 50% of survivors by 5 years posttransplant and is a factor in more than one-third of late deaths. Although it can occur as early as 2 months posttransplant, the onset is more often at least 6 months and the mean onset is from 1 to 2 years after surgery. The precipitating factors and initiating events in bronchiolitis obliterans are topics of intensive research both in transplant recipients and in several animal models. Those factors most consistently associated with the process include the numbers and severity of acute rejection episodes and episodes of cytomegalovirus (CMV) pneumonia, but not clearly CMV infection alone. Other factors with weaker associations include HLA mismatches, other viral infections, and the development of anti-HLA antibodies. Clinically, the onset of this process is often subacute, with a very gradual onset of dyspnea and fatigue or malaise, often accompanied by viral-type symptoms or dry cough. It can also be asymptomatic and detected by routine pulmonary function studies that show, initially, a decrease in the FEF_{25-75}, often followed one to several months later by decreasing FEV_1. This insidious development of small airway obstruction is often well established before it is clinically recognized, and for that reason frequent pulmonary function testing is recommended for lung transplant recipients. Chest radiograms are usually normal, but even early in the disease expiratory computed tomography (CT) scans show a mottled appearance with peripheral hyperlucency. Transbronchial biopsy is very specific but not sensitive in diagnosis, but patients usually undergo at least one bronchoscopy at the onset of disease to attempt histologic documentation and to rule out possible infections. Because of the difficulty in histologic diagnosis, a typical clinical picture in the absence of other etiology is considered sufficient to establish a diagnosis of *bronchiolitis obliterans syndrome*. The progression of this complication can be very rapid, with early death; but more often it is one of a gradually decreasing FEV_1 over months to years, which in the later stages is frequently accompanied by bronchomalacia, proximal bronchiectasis, and recurrent pseudomonal or other infections.

Effective treatment remains evasive. A few immunosuppressive protocols tried in small numbers of patients have been found to "stabilize" pulmonary function, but improved function is unusual. Likely, by the time the process is recognized in most patients, fibrotic obliteration of the airway is already present; the key to treatment may lie in identifying markers of incipient disease and much earlier intervention.

Infections Infections rank second only to rejection as a cause of morbidity in lung transplant recipients and are the most common cause of mortality, accounting for one-third of all deaths in both the early and the late posttransplant periods. The transplanted lung may be uniquely vulnerable to infection because of impaired mucociliary clearance, loss of cough reflex, and other poorly defined local factors. In addition, the donor lungs are often colonized with organisms that are transmitted directly to the immunosuppressed recipient. Early series reported that at least 60% of lung recipients early in their course develop infections requiring treatment. Now the extensive use of broad antibacterial, antifungal, anti-*pneumocystis*, and antiviral prophylaxis, often maintained for at least 3 months postoperatively, seems to have reduced the early infective morbidity and mortality.

Infections with paramyxoviral organisms, adenovirus, and influenza A have now been well documented and have an overall death rate of about 20%. The role of antiviral therapy is unclear. The most lethal infections are those with invasive fungal organisms, particularly those caused by *Aspergillus* species, which have been reported to colonize in 20 to 50% of recipients. Invasive disease caused by these organisms can vary from ulcerative bronchitis to localized parenchymal infiltrates to empyema to disseminated disease. *Aspergillus* is particularly likely to be problematic when patients require increased immunosuppression or have other complications; one study has reported an increased rate of invasive disease in the native lung of unilateral lung transplant recipients.

The highest risk periods for infection are in the first few months posttransplant and late after transplant if bronchiolitis obliterans or other vital organ dysfunction, e.g., renal failure, develops. Since it may be very difficult to distinguish infection from rejection in the early posttransplant period, bronchoscopy with appropriate biopsies and cultures is often necessary to establish a diagnosis.

Immunosuppressive and Medical Complications Medical complications related to immunosuppression, to the underlying diagnosis, or to aging are major causes of morbidity in long-term survivors of lung transplantation and account for up to 10% of late deaths. Current immunosuppressive regimens with cyclosporine or tacrolimus cause some nephrotoxicity in virtually all patients. Although few progress to renal failure, hypertension and hyperlipidemia are common. Neurotoxicity, including delirium, headaches, seizures, and, occasionally, strokes, has been reported in up to 20% of patients. Osteoporosis occurs in more than half the patients, and vertebral compression fractures are common. Other problems include thromboembolic disease, gastric complications (especially gastroparesis), hyperglycemia, and increased rates of malignancy.

Posttransplant lymphoproliferative disorders associated with Epstein-Barr virus occur in 5 to 10% of lung transplant recipients. Nearly all occur within the first year after transplant. Recent data suggest a much higher incidence of this disease in patients who are Epstein-Barr naïve and who receive an Epstein-Barr positive graft. Treatment for this disorder, reported to have an approximate 50% survival rate, is usually reduced immunosuppression and antiviral and anti-B lymphocyte drugs. Survivors often develop bronchiolitis obliterans.

Recurrence of Underlying Disease Several different underlying diseases may recur in lung transplant recipients. These diseases include sarcoidosis, lymphangioleiomyomatosis, giant cell interstitial pneumonia, panbronchiolitis, eosinophilic granuloma, bronchoalveolar cell carcinoma, and desquamative interstitial pneumonia.

BIBLIOGRAPHY

BOEHLER A et al: Bronchiolitis obliterans after lung transplantation: A review. Chest 114: 1411, 1998

BOEHLER A, ESTENNE M: Obliterative bronchiolitis after lung transplantation. Curr Opin Pulm Med 6:133, 2000

HOSENPUD JD et al: The Registry of the International Society for Heart and Lung Transplantation. Fifteenth official report–1998. J Heart Lung Transplant 17:656, 1998

JOINT STATEMENT OF THE AMERICAN SOCIETY FOR TRANSPLANT PHYSICIANS (ASTP)/AMERICAN THORACIC SOCIETY (ATS)/EUROPEAN RESPIRATORY SOCIETY (ERS); INTERNATIONAL SOCIETY FOR HEART AND LUNG TRANSPLANTATION (ISHLT): International guidelines for the selection of lung transplant candidates. Am J Respir Crit Care Med 158:335, 1998

MAURER JR (ed): Surgical approaches to end-stage disease: Lung transplantation and volume reduction. Clin Chest Med 18(2), 1997

NOBEL PRIZE IN PHYSIOLOGY OR MEDICINE, 1985

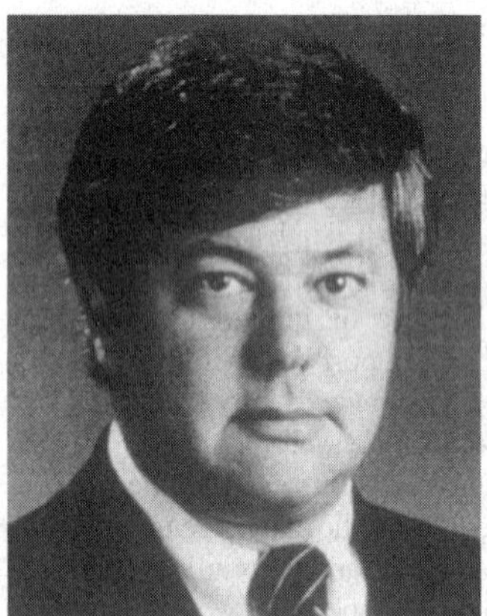

Michael Stuart Brown was born in New York on April 13, 1941, the eldest child of Harry and Evelyn Brown, who moved their family to Elkins Park, Pennsylvania, in 1952. Michael Brown attended high school there and then went to the University of Pennsylvania where he received his B.S. in chemistry in 1962 and his M.D. in 1966 as an honors graduate.

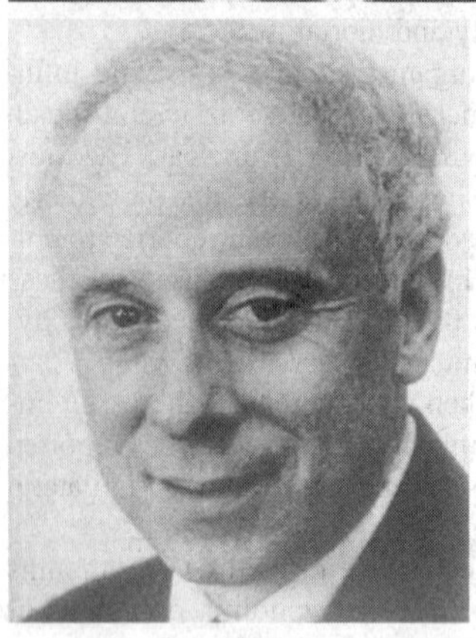

Joseph Leonard Goldstein was born on April 18, 1940, in Sumter, South Carolina, the only child of Isadore and Fannie Goldstein. The family owned a clothing store in Kingstree, South Carolina, a town of five thousand, where Goldstein attended public school. He earned his B.S. in chemistry, graduating *summa cum laude* from Washington and Lee University in Lexington, Virginia, in 1962. He attended medical school at the University of Texas at Dallas where on graduation he received the Outstanding Medical School Graduate Award.

Brown and Goldstein both entered internship in internal medicine at Massachusetts General Hospital in 1966, became good friends, and both went on to the National Institutes of Health (NIH) as Clinical Associates. Brown specialized in digestive and hereditary diseases and worked in Earl Stadtman's Laboratory of Biochemistry; Goldstein worked in Marshall Nirenberg's Laboratory of Biochemical Genetics, where he saw patients with lipid disorders. Goldstein convinced Brown to join the Gastroenterology Division at Texas Southwestern Medical School in 1971. Goldstein arrived at the same institution in 1972 after 2 years in Arno Motulsky's laboratory at the University of Washington in Seattle. Goldstein was appointed head of a new Division of Medical Genetics on his return to Texas Southwestern Medical School, a promise that Donald Seldin, the chair of Internal Medicine, had made to him in 1966 at the time of his graduation from medical school.

Brown and Goldstein decided to combine their laboratories, and so began one of the most distinguished dual scientific careers in the history of medicine. Goldstein had seen patients at the NIH with familial hypercholesterolemia (FH) who developed skin deposits of cholesterol, atherosclerosis, and heart attacks at a young age. Brown and Goldstein decided to work on this problem, particularly since they had access to some of these patients in Texas. Goldstein then established a culture technique for skin from both normal individuals and patients with FH. The cells were then analyzed biochemically by Brown. In 1973 Brown and Goldstein discovered a key enzyme in cholesterol production, HMG-coenzyme A (CoA) reductase, which could be regulated in normal skin fibroblasts by the amount of low-density lipoprotein (LDL) in the medium. Adding LDL to the normal cells switched off HMG-CoA reductase, and the cells ceased making cholesterol. However, the skin cells from FH patients continued to make cholesterol with even very high levels of LDL in the medium. Because LDL in alcohol entered these normal cells from FH patients and switched off HMG-CoA reductase, Brown and Goldstein concluded that the genetic mutation must involve a receptor that would bind the LDL and facilitate its entry into the cell. In 1976, using radiolabeled LDL and electron microscopy, Brown and Goldstein, along with R.G.W. Anderson, localized the LDL receptor on coated pits in normal skin fibroblasts; the receptors were absent in the FH skin cultures. A further defect relating to impaired internalization of the receptor after LDL binding was then described. Normally the LDL receptor recycled back to the cell surface within 10 min after lysosomal-induced release of the cholesterol and inhibition of HMG-CoA reductase. Drugs were then developed that would inhibit HMG-CoA reductase and thus decrease the cellular production of cholesterol. Lovastatin (mevalin) was the first such drug marketed to block the synthesis of cholesterol in order to decrease the occurrence of heart attacks.

In 1984 the LDL receptor gene was localized on chromosome 19, and the nucleotide sequence of the gene that produces HMG-CoA reductase was established. The human LDL receptor gene was then sequenced, and one domain was shown to be homologous to the gene sequence for epidermal growth factor.

In 1985 Brown and Goldstein received both the Albert D. Lasker Award in Basic Medical Research, and the Nobel Prize in Physiology or Medicine. Their discoveries of the entry process of cholesterol into the cell and the regulation of cellular synthesis of cholesterol were monumental and have implications for millions of people worldwide who have or will have atherosclerotic cardiovascular disease.

REFERENCES

1. Magill FN (ed): *Nobel Prize Winners: Physiology or Medicine*, vol 3. Pasadena, Salem Press, 1993
2. Schrier RW: *A Salute to Nobel Laureates in Physiology and Medicine*, Proceedings of the Association of American Physicians 108(1): Jan 1996

Robert W. Schrier, MD

268 DISTURBANCES OF RENAL FUNCTION

Robert M. Brenner, Barry M. Brenner

Near constancy of the composition of the internal environment, including the volume, tonicity, and compartmental distribution of the body fluids, is essential to survival. With normal day-to-day variations in the intake of food and water, preservation of the internal environment requires the excretion of these substances in amounts that balance the quantities ingested. Although losses from intestines, lungs, and skin contribute to this excretory capacity, the greatest responsibility for solute and water excretion is borne by the kidneys.

The kidneys regulate the composition and volume of the plasma water. This, in turn, determines the composition and volume of the entire *extracellular* fluid compartment. Through the continuous exchange of water and solutes across all cell membranes, the kidneys influence the *intracellular* fluid compartment as well. These functions are served by a variety of physiologic mechanisms that enable individuals to excrete excesses of water and nonmetabolized solutes contained in the diet, as well as the nonvolatile end products of nitrogen metabolism, such as urea and creatinine. Conversely, when faced with deficits of water or solute, excretion of water or specific solute(s) is curtailed via appropriate mechanisms for renal conservation, reducing the likelihood of volume or solute depletion. The purpose of this chapter is to review the excretory functions of the kidney and to examine how these functions are affected by chronic renal disease.

EFFECTS OF NEPHRON LOSS ON RENAL EXCRETORY MECHANISMS

The volume of urine excreted (averaging 1.5 L/d or roughly 1 mL/min) represents the sum of two large, directionally opposite processes—namely, *ultrafiltration* of 180 L/d or more of plasma water (or 125 mL/min) and *reabsorption* of more than 99% of this filtrate by transport processes in the renal tubules. While renal blood flow accounts for about 20% of resting cardiac output, the kidneys comprise only about 1% of total body weight. This disproportionate allocation of cardiac output, greatly exceeding blood flow per gram of brain, heart or liver, is required for the process of ultrafiltration.

GLOMERULAR ULTRAFILTRATION Urine production begins at the glomerulus where an ultrafiltrate of plasma is formed. The rate of glomerular ultrafiltration (glomerular filtration rate, GFR) is governed chiefly by forces favoring filtration on the one hand (hydraulic pressure in the glomerular capillaries) and forces opposing filtration on the other (the sum of hydraulic pressure in Bowman's space and colloid osmotic pressure in the glomerular capillaries). The rate of glomerular plasma flow and the total surface area of the glomerular capillaries are also determinants of GFR. Decreased GFR can therefore be expected when (1) glomerular hydraulic pressure is reduced (as in circulatory shock); (2) tubule (hence Bowman's space) hydraulic pressure is elevated, as in urinary tract obstruction; (3) plasma colloid osmotic pressure rises to high levels (hemoconcentration due to severe volume depletion, myeloma, or other dysproteinemias); (4) renal, and hence glomerular, blood flow is reduced (severe hypovolemia, cardiac failure); (5) permeability is reduced (diffuse glomerular disease); or (6) filtration surface area is diminished, through focal or diffuse nephron loss in progressive renal failure.

The glomerular capillary wall is specially adapted to allow passage of extremely large volumes of water while retaining all but the smallest solute molecules. Molecules the size of inulin (approximately 5200 mol wt) pass freely across the glomerular filtration barrier, appearing at approximately the same concentration in Bowman's space as in plasma. The passage of solutes across the glomerular barrier decreases progressively with increasing molecular size such that, as the molecular weight of albumin is approached, most of the solute is retained in the plasma. Albumin, a polyanionic molecule in plasma, is further retarded at the glomerular filtration barrier by *electrostatic forces* imparted by negatively charged cell-surface molecules on the epithelial foot processes that form the *filtration slits* and the *slit diaphragms*. With disruption of these structural and electrostatic barriers, as in many forms of glomerular injury (Chaps. 273 to 275), large quantities of plasma proteins gain access to the glomerular filtrate.

Glomerular Adaptations to Nephron Loss With loss of nephron mass, the remaining functional (or least injured) nephrons tend to hypertrophy and take on an increased workload so that the overall loss of function is minimized. For example, a patient with a unilateral nephrectomy loses one-half of the nephron mass, resulting in a 50% reduction in GFR at the time of surgery. However, the GFR in the remaining kidney begins to increase after 1 or 2 weeks, and within several months GFR may rise to 80% of the preoperative value. This indicates that the GFR of the individual remaining nephrons has increased above normal, a state known as *hyperfiltration.* Increases in single-nephron GFR may be achieved by renal hemodynamic adjustments (increased glomerular plasma flow and increased glomerular capillary hydraulic pressure), which augment the forces driving ultrafiltration, and by glomerular hypertrophy, which increases the maximum surface area available for filtration. These structural adaptations are evident from the enlargement of glomeruli (and tubules) seen on histologic sections from people with single kidneys. Similar structural changes are observed in kidneys damaged by chronic disease processes; foci of hypertrophied glomeruli and tubules are interspersed with areas of atrophic or scarred parenchyma. Although direct measurements of single-nephron GFR cannot be made in humans, it is reasonable to conclude that focal nephron enlargement as occurs in chronically diseased kidneys generally signifies focally increased single-nephron GFR, and that these dynamic adaptations represent compensatory adjustments for the effects of nephron loss through disease.

Glomerulotubular Balance The close integration of glomerular and tubular functions (*glomerulotubular balance*) seen in chronic renal failure (CRF) supports the notion that progressive nephron obliteration is the usual mode of GFR reduction in CRF. Preservation of glomerulotubular balance until the terminal stages of CRF is fundamental to the *intact-nephron hypothesis*, which states that as CRF advances, kidney function is supported by a diminishing pool of functioning (or hyperfunctioning) nephrons, rather than relatively constant numbers of nephrons, each with diminishing function. This concept has important implications for the mechanisms of disease progression in CRF. A considerable amount of evidence suggests that nephrons subjected to increased excretory burdens for prolonged periods actually sustain injury as a result of these adaptations: thus the cost of these compensatory adaptations to nephron loss may ultimately be relentless destruction of the remaining nephron pool.

The magnitude of the single-nephron hyperfiltration induced by loss of 50% of the total nephron mass usually has no serious adverse clinical consequences, even when sustained over two to three decades. When more than 50% of the total nephron mass is lost, however, as in renal-sparing surgery for bilateral trauma or neoplasm or from a renal disease whose activity has abated, the remaining nephrons are forced to the limits of their compensatory capacity. While these adaptations achieve remarkable short-term success at offsetting the tendency for GFR to fall, over time, proteinuria and focal and segmental glomerulosclerosis develop, the more so where greater amounts of nephrons are lost or removed. As a result, a progressive decline in GFR ensues. Experimental study of the processes that advance glomerular injury show that the adverse long-term consequences of severe nephron deficits are invariably preceded by increases in glomerular capillary hydraulic pressure (glomerular capillary hypertension), glomerular hyperperfusion, and hypertrophy. Interventions directed against these compensatory and maladaptive responses can greatly ameliorate the subsequent development of renal failure. In particular, drugs (e.g., angiotensin-converting enzyme inhibitors and angiotensin II receptor blockers) and other interventions (such as dietary protein restriction) that lower glomerular pressure can slow the rate of progression of experimental and human renal disease. In the absence of such interventions, more and more glomeruli cease to function through advancing glomerulosclerosis and disruption of tubule structure and function, leading eventually to total loss of GFR (i.e., end-stage renal disease). This *final common pathway* for chronic renal injury helps to explain the observed progressive nature of chronic renal failure resulting from many different kidney diseases.

Biologic Consequences of Sustained Reductions in GFR Although nephron loss can proceed, to some extent, without equivalent loss of GFR due to the compensatory mechanisms described above, determination of the total GFR of both kidneys remains the most reliable clinical index of overall excretory function. The effects of impaired GFR are to reduce the total rate of delivery of solute into the glomerular filtrate. When accompanied by comparably reduced rates of urinary excretion, *retention* and *accumulation* of the unexcreted solute occurs, resulting in increased concentrations of the substance in the plasma and other body fluids.

Figure 268-1 depicts the major types of response to impaired GFR. The degree of reduction in total GFR is plotted on the abscissa, expressed as a percentage of normal (100%). The renal handling of most solutes normally present in glomerular filtrate conforms to one of three patterns. Curve *A* describes the pattern with substances such as creatinine and urea that normally depend largely on glomerular filtration for urinary excretion; i.e., secretion contributes little to overall excretion. Therefore, as illustrated, gradual reductions in GFR are accompanied by progressive increases in plasma levels of creatinine, urea, and other substances normally excreted primarily by filtration.

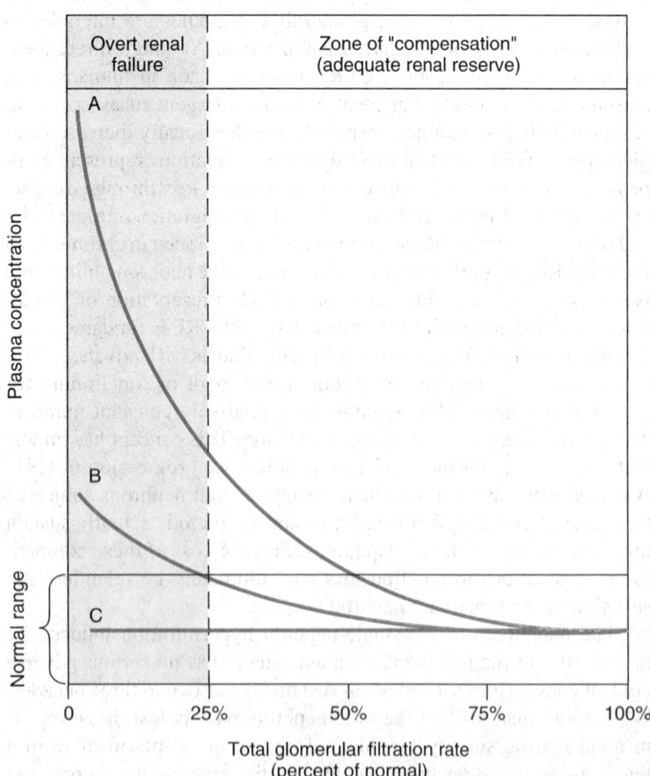

FIGURE 268-1 Representative patterns of adaptation for different types of solutes in body fluids in chronic renal failure. *(After NS Bricker et al, in BM Brenner, 2000.)*

The clinical course of CRF usually also approximates the pattern described by curve *A*. Patients with CRF usually pass from a long asymptomatic period of "compensation" to a more accelerated and clinically overt terminal phase. In other words, despite chronic injury leading to destruction of more than 50% of nephrons, plasma elevations of creatinine and urea may still lie within the normal limits for these substances. With further nephron loss and reduction in GFR, however, the limits of renal reserve are exceeded and continued accumulations of curve *A*–type solutes lead to abnormally elevated plasma concentrations (Fig. 268-1). Because some of these retained solutes are thought to exert "toxic" effects on all organ systems, clinical manifestations of CRF may now become apparent. Consequently, in patients with substantial reductions in nephron mass but near-normal plasma creatinine, overt uremia may be precipitated by a modest additional decline in GFR.

The accumulation of curve *A*–type solutes with chronic loss of renal function proceeds until external balance is restored, i.e., intake and/or production rates exactly match excretion rates. In the case of creatinine, for example, assuming a constant rate of creatinine production, a 50% reduction in GFR results in an approximate doubling of the plasma creatinine concentration. The latter restores the filtered load of creatinine (i.e., the product of GFR and plasma creatinine concentration) to normal, and the urinary excretion rate once again is equivalent to creatinine production. Since creatinine secretion contributes only slightly, elimination of the retained creatinine is not possible and the plasma concentration remains twice normal. With further loss of GFR, elevations in plasma creatinine are compounded by loss of nephron excretory function and creatinine retained as the result of earlier nephron destruction (Fig. 268-1). *In practice, so long as the net rates of acquisition and production (i.e., liver function and muscle mass) remain reasonably constant, the inverse relationship between plasma concentrations of solutes such as creatinine and urea and GFR is sufficiently reliable to serve as clinical indices of GFR.* However, where muscle mass is low, as with severe weight loss, unremarkable plasma levels of creatinine may belie substantial reductions in GFR.

In contrast to solutes of the curve *A* type, plasma levels of phosphate (PO_4^{3-}), urate, and potassium (K^+) and hydrogen (H^+) ions usually do not rise until the GFR falls to a small percentage of normal. With progressive renal failure this pattern of response (curve *B* in Fig. 268-1) reflects the participation of tubule transport mechanisms in the excretion of these substances. In other words, *as GFR declines, the tubules facilitate greater elimination of these substances, by enhancing secretion and/or by diminishing reabsorption, so that a greater fraction of the filtered load is excreted.* Plasma levels of curve *B*–type solutes, therefore, rise less than those of curve *A* because, with progressive reductions in GFR, *excretion rate per nephron* and therefore *fractional excretion* both increase. Eventually, however, with further loss of GFR, enhanced fractional excretion can no longer mitigate the reduction in net filtered load of these solutes and plasma levels rise (Fig. 268-1). For urate, PO_4^{3-}, and K^+, at least, increased fractional excretion serves to maintain normal plasma levels until GFR falls to less than one-fourth of normal.

Finally, for certain solutes, such as sodium chloride (NaCl), plasma concentrations remain normal throughout the course of CRF, despite unrestricted intake of these substances (curve *C* in Fig. 268-1). The compensatory mechanism required to achieve this represents a fundamental adaptation to chronic renal injury. To illustrate the magnitude of this adaptation, it is useful to compare the excretion of sodium (Na^+) in a normal individual (GFR of 125 mL/min) with that of a patient with advanced renal failure (GFR of 2 mL/min). Both individuals consume a conventional diet containing 7 g/d of salt (120 mmol Na^+). With a normal serum Na^+ concentration of 140 mmol/L, external Na^+ balance is achieved by excreting approximately 0.5% of the filtered load. By contrast, for external balance to be maintained in the patient with CRF, fractional excretion of Na^+ must rise to 30%. In other words, *to maintain external Na^+* balance, the same amount of Na^+ must be excreted into the urine each day in the patient with CRF as in the normal individual. Given the drastic reduction in GFR in CRF, external balance can only be maintained by marked adaptations in the reabsorptive processes in surviving tubules. In this manner, a progressively larger fraction of the filtered load escapes reabsorption and appears in the final urine. In short, *the rate of excretion of Na^+* per surviving nephron increases in inverse proportion to the composite GFR in surviving nephrons.

ADAPTATIONS IN TUBULE TRANSPORT MECHANISMS IN RESPONSE TO NEPHRON LOSS

Despite progressive nephron loss, many mechanisms that regulate renal solute and water balance differ only quantitatively, and not qualitatively, from those that operate normally. Thus, glomerulotubular balance is maintained. The most important of these mechanisms are considered below.

TUBULAR TRANSPORT OF SODIUM CHLORIDE AND WATER Most of the filtered water and sodium salts are reabsorbed by the tubules, leaving small and variable amounts, equivalent on average to the quantities ingested, to reach the final urine. About two-thirds of the glomerular ultrafiltrate is reabsorbed in the *proximal tubule* with little change in the osmolality or Na^+ concentration of the unreabsorbed fraction (Fig. 268-2). In other words, fluid reabsorption in the proximal tubule is nearly *isosmotic* and is coupled to the active transport of Na^+. Since chloride (Cl^-) and bicarbonate (HCO_3^-) are the primary anions in the extracellular fluid, they constitute the main solutes that accompany Na^+ reabsorption in the renal tubules. In the earliest portion of the proximal tubule, bicarbonate is the principal anion that accompanies the reabsorption of Na^+. This process occurs via a Na^+/H^+ exchanger at the luminal brush border and is dependent on the activity of carbonic anhydrase. Glucose, amino acids, and other organic solutes (e.g., lactate) are also extensively reabsorbed in the proximal tubule by cotransport mechanisms that link the cellular entry of these organic molecules with Na^+. The coupling of water absorption (i.e., volume) with solute absorption appears to be dependent upon three processes. First, given the remarkably high water permeability of this segment, very small transepithelial osmolality differences, i.e., *luminal hypotonicity* of the order of 2 to 3 mosmol/L produced by solute absorption, could drive water absorption. Second, due to preferential absorption of HCO_3^- and organic solutes in the early portions of the proximal tubule, the concentrations of these substances decrease along the proximal tubule while that of chloride increases. Volume reabsorption would then occur if the diffusion of Na^+ and Cl^- down their respective electrochemical gradients across the proximal tubule epithelium occurred more easily than the back-diffusion of sodium bicarbonate into the lumen, creating an *effective osmotic pressure gradient*. Finally, *lateral interstitial space hypertonicity* produced by differences in the rates at which solutes are transported into the spaces or exit them by diffusion may also contribute to the coupling of water and solute reabsorption.

Reabsorption of Fluid from Proximal Convoluted Tubules This is sensitive to *Starling forces*, i.e., the hydraulic and colloid osmotic (or oncotic) pressures acting across the walls of the peritubular capillaries. Because the plasma proteins in glomerular capillaries are concentrated by ultrafiltration, oncotic pressure rises along the glomerular capillary network. This step-up in oncotic pressure is transmitted largely unchanged to the first branches of the peritubular capillaries via the efferent arterioles. These resistance vessels cause a substantial drop in hydraulic pressure, however, so that when the plasma reaches the peritubular capillaries, oncotic pressure greatly exceeds hydraulic pressure. The Starling forces are therefore oriented in an *uptake* mode, in contrast to their configuration at the glomerulus where hydraulic pressure exceeds oncotic pressure, favoring *filtration*.

The extent to which oncotic pressure exceeds hydraulic pressure in the peritubular capillary network modulates the overall rate of fluid absorption by the peritubular capillaries. Therefore, when peritubular capillary oncotic pressure falls, or hydraulic pressure rises, uptake of fluid by these capillaries is reduced. As a result, fluid is retained in the interstitial space, tending to increase hydraulic pressure, ultimately retarding the egress of fluid from the lateral intercellular channels. Without an adequate route of drainage, fluid in the intercellular channels leaks back into the tubule lumen, thereby *diminishing net fluid reabsorption* from this tubule segment. The opposite occurs in states where peritubular oncotic pressure is increased (increased filtration fraction) or hydraulic pressure is decreased (enhanced efferent arteriolar tone). Under these circumstances, peritubular capillary uptake of reabsorbate is augmented, leading ultimately to *enhanced net fluid reabsorption* by the proximal tubule. Although physical factors appear to be the major determinants of fluid reabsorption in the proximal tubule, hormones (e.g., angiotensin II) may also modulate fluid reabsorption directly, by enhancing luminal Na^+ entry into proximal tubule cells via an apical Na^+/H^+ exchanger.

The Limbs of Henle's Loop In contrast to the proximal tubule, active outward transport of Na has not been established for the *thin ascending limb of Henle's loop*. However, passive outward salt transport does occur, as indicated in Fig. 268-2. In the next nephron segment, the *medullary thick ascending limb of Henle*, the concentration of NaCl is reduced as fluid traverses this segment. Here Cl^- absorption occurs by an active process involving a Na^+:K^+:$2Cl^-$ cotransport mechanism in the luminal membrane, with one-half of Na^+ absorption proceeding passively, driven by the lumen positive transepithelial voltage difference. This cotransporter is the site of action of the powerful loop diuretics and mutations give rise to Bartter's syndrome. Since the ascending limb of Henle is impermeable to water, net NaCl reabsorption generates a hypotonic tubule fluid and gives rise to the high NaCl concentration of the outer medullary interstitium (Fig. 268-2). In certain animals, arginine vasopressin (AVP; also called ADH) enhances NaCl absorption in the medullary portion of the thick ascending limb, but whether this occurs in humans is uncertain.

Distal Tubule The fluid leaving the thick ascending limb of Henle is normally of low NaCl concentration, a characteristic independent of the organism's hydration or dietary status. In the *distal tubule*, water reabsorption is variable, depending on the state of hydration or, specifically, on the presence or absence ofAVP in plasma. In the absence of AVP, this and more distal nephron segments are impermeable to water, so that hypotonic fluid entering this segment is excreted as *dilute urine*. Indeed, continued salt reabsorption along the distal convoluted tubule (DCT) and connecting tubule segments, a process that can be inhibited by the thiazide classes of diuretics, results in further dilution of the urine. In the presence of AVP, the permeability of these nephron segments to water increases. This is made possible by the insertion of proteins known as *aquaporins* into the luminal cell membrane of DCT cells. These proteins facilitate water movement from the low osmolality environment of the DCT lumen into the higher osmolality of the medullary interstitium, thereby contributing to the creation of a concentrated final urine. NaCl continues to be reabsorbed from the tubule lumen against moderately steep chemical and electrical gradients. The reabsorption of NaCl at the collecting tubule is enhanced by *aldosterone*.

Collecting Tubules and Ducts The *cortical collecting tubule* possesses a low permeability to water in the absence of AVP, whereas permeability increases in the presence of this hormone. The sensitivity of this segment to AVP appears to be more pronounced than that of the DCT. As with the DCT, the cortical collecting tubule is capable of active reabsorption of NaCl and its stimulation by aldosterone.

The terminal segment of the distal nephron is the highly branched *papillary collecting duct*. Continued electrolyte transport in this segment results in the large ion concentration differences that normally exist between urine and plasma. As in the cortical collecting tubule,

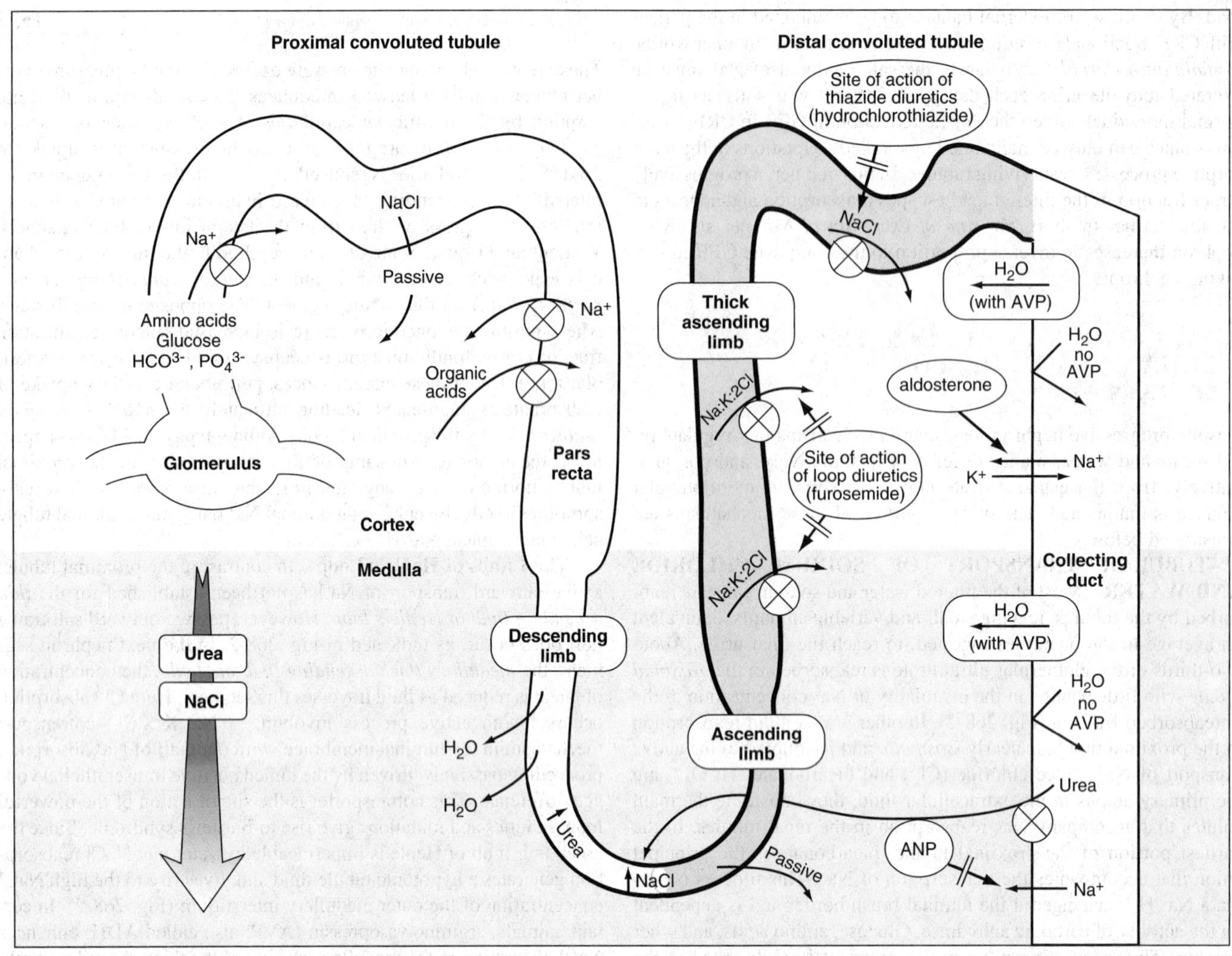

FIGURE 268-2 Transport functions of the various anatomic segments of the mammalian nephron. Fluid reabsorption across the proximal tubule is isosmotic and accounts for reabsorption of approximately two-thirds of the filtered Na^+ and H_2O. The major portions of the filtered HCO_3^-, amino acids, glucose, and phosphate are reabsorbed in the early proximal convoluted tubule. Reabsorption of glucose and amino acids is coupled to Na^+ transport and thereby generates a negative potential difference within the tubule lumen. At the same time, HCO_3^- is reabsorbed by a nonelectrogenic mechanism, via H^+ secretion. The active transport of these solutes results in transepithelial concentration and effective osmotic pressure gradients promoting H_2O flow across the proximal tubule, into the peritubular capillaries. The rise in tubule fluid Cl^- concentration is a necessary reciprocal consequence of the decreased luminal HCO_3^- concentration. The resultant high concentration of Cl^- becomes an important force for the outward passive transport of Cl^- down its concentration gradient, resulting in a lumen-positive potential difference in the late proximal convoluted tubule. The pars recta of the proximal tubule is capable of active electrogenic transport of Na^+ independent of organic solute transport. Under normal conditions, approximately one-third of the glomerular filtrate enters the descending limb of Henle's loop. Because the thin descending limb is incapable of active outward NaCl transport and is characterized by low permeability to Na^+ but high H_2O permeability, H_2O is abstracted passively as the fluid approaches the bend of Henle's loop. Hypertonic fluid with a greater NaCl concentration but lower urea concentration than the surrounding medullary interstitium thus enters the thin ascending limb of Henle, which is largely impermeable to H_2O and urea but highly permeable to NaCl. This permits passive outward diffusion of NaCl. Active Na:K:2Cl transport across the water-impermeable thick ascending limb of Henle allows for separation of solute and water. In consequence, tubule fluid becomes dilute and the medullary interstitium hypertonic. Irrespective of the final osmolality of the urine, the fluid that enters the distal convoluted tubule is always hypoosmotic. This segment exhibits active Na^+ reabsorption. All but the terminal portion of the distal convoluted tubule is water-impermeable, even in the presence of AVP. Aldosterone exerts its effect in this segment by enhancing Na^+ reabsorption, which is variably coupled to K^+ and H^+ secretion. The cortical and papillary portions of the collecting duct are sites where AVP exerts its principal effect. The permeability of these segments to H_2O in the absence of AVP is very low but can be greatly enhanced in the presence of AVP. These segments are also characterized by active Na^+ reabsorption, which appears to depend on the presence of mineralocorticoid. In the absence of AVP, the collecting tubule is water-impermeable so that hypotonic tubule fluid courses through it. However, in the presence of AVP, water is avidly reabsorbed here, resulting in hypertonic final urine. Sites of action of furosemide and thiazide diuretics and of aldosterone and atrial natriuretic peptide (ANP) are shown.

Na^+ transport appears to be active, since reabsorption proceeds against sizeable electrochemical gradients. The rate of Na^+ transport in this segment depends on the load of Na^+ delivered from more proximal segments and is also affected by aldosterone. The permeability to water is also increased markedly in the presence of AVP.

Effects of Nephron Loss on Sodium Chloride Transport in Surviving Nephrons With progressive nephron loss, *maintenance of external balance for NaCl requires that fractional salt excretion increases in concert with the decline in GFR.* Several mechanisms contribute to this adaptive increase in fractional Na^+ excretion. With loss of functioning nephron units, peritubular capillary Starling forces are presumably altered in directions that serve to reduce proximal tubule reabsorption of NaCl and water. For example, a rise in peritubular capillary hydraulic pressure, which tends to inhibit net proximal fluid reabsorption, might be anticipated with systemic hypertension, a common feature of chronic renal failure. Similarly, reductions in peritubular capillary oncotic pressures may be anticipated due to reductions in both filtration fraction and hypoalbuminemia.

Aldosterone, which normally exerts a potent influence on tubule transport, probably does not figure prominently in reducing fractional Na^+ excretion, since aldosterone levels are seldom reduced in CRF. Furthermore, external Na^+ balance is preserved in bilaterally adrenalectomized dogs on fixed replacement doses of mineralocorticoid. Yet another factor contributing to the suppression of fractional NaCl reabsorption in CRF may relate to the retention of various organic solutes as GFR declines.

Several factors that regulate NaCl transport across tubules under resting conditions are also likely to contribute to the enhanced fractional excretion of salt in renal insufficiency. Atrial natriuretic peptides are released from the heart in response to elevated cardiac (atrial) filling pressures as seen with increased plasma volume or atrial tachyarrhythmias. These peptides affect natriuresis by reducing net Na^+ reabsorption through complementary actions on Na^+ transport in the collecting duct and by altering Starling forces in the adjacent vasa recta. The vascular actions of natriuretic peptides may also extend to glomerular hemodynamics, with afferent arteriolar vasodilatation contributing to increased single-nephron GFR and hence an increase in the amount of Na^+ filtered. Other modulators of tubule transport processes may also contribute to increased single-nephron natriuresis in the setting of reduced renal mass or nephron loss. Vasodilator prostaglandins are present at increased plasma levels in CRF, as are other inhibitors of transport, including inhibitor(s) of the Na^+,K^+-ATPase. This latter factor has not yet been fully characterized; whether its presence represents a homeostatic adaptation for maintenance of fluid balance or an unregulated accumulation of a toxin remains uncertain.

Serum and urine from patients with uremia contain factors capable of experimentally inhibiting NaCl transport across frog skin, toad bladder, and rat renal tubule. Accumulation of natriuretic factors in uremia may not be without cost; the "trade-off" for maintenance of external Na^+ balance is the possibility of generalized abnormalities occurring in Na^+ transport across cell membranes, which often occur in advanced renal failure (Chap. 270).

The obligatory high rate of solute excretion per surviving nephron (so-called osmotic diuresis due to urea and other retained solutes) also contributes to enhancing fractional NaCl excretion, much as occurs in normal individuals after the administration of mannitol or other nonreabsorbable solutes. Finally, certain forms of CRF are associated with unusually large losses of salt in the urine. These *salt-wasting nephropathies* include chronic pyelonephritis and other tubulointerstitial diseases (Chap. 277) as well as polycystic and medullary cystic diseases. These disorders have in common greater destruction of medullary and tubulointerstitial, rather than cortical and glomerular, portions of the renal parenchyma. Preferential impairment of tubule reabsorptive function, rather than a primary reduction in glomerular filtration, may, therefore, underlie the salt-losing tendency in these disorders. Clinical derangements that alter renal handling of NaCl in CRF (including hypo- and hypervolemia, hypertension, etc.) are considered in Chap. 270.

EFFECTS OF NEPHRON LOSS ON WATER REABSORPTION IN SURVIVING NEPHRONS As with NaCl, there is a progressive increase in the fractional excretion of water with advancing renal insufficiency, so that external water balance can be maintained even with a total GFR of 5 mL/min or less. The adaptations of water handling by the diseased kidney are of importance in the defects in urinary concentration and dilution and hence the polyuria, nocturia, and tendency to develop water overload encountered in CRF (Chap. 47). To appreciate the mechanisms involved, the responses of a normal and a uremic individual maintaining external water balance need to be considered. Assuming both individuals have the same dietary and fluid intakes, total solute and volume excretion in both should be identical as well. If the *obligatory solute load* to be excreted by each is 600 mmol/d (600 mosmol/d) and the urine osmolality is 300 mmol/kg water (300 mosmol/kg), a urine volume of 2 L/d will be required to excrete the total solute. If the GFR in normal and uremic individuals totals 180 and 4 L/d, respectively, urinary volume excretion of 2 L/d represents excretion of slightly more than 1% of the total glomerular filtrate in the normal subject compared with 50% in the uremic patient. Since the range of urine osmolalities that the diseased kidney can achieve [250 to 350 mmol/kg (250 to 350 mosmol/kg)] is narrower than in the normal kidney [40 to 1200 mmol/kg (40 to 1200 mosmol/kg)], the individual with normal function is able to excrete the obligatory daily solute load of 600 mmol (600 mosmol) in as little as 500 mL urine per day or as much as 15 L/d, compared with the narrower range in renal insufficiency, from about 1.7 to 2.4 L/d.

In CRF, the limited capacity to concentrate the urine often correlates with other measures of impaired renal function. Isosthenuria (urine of similar osmolality to plasma) is therefore an almost universal finding when the GFR falls below 25 mL/min. At this level of GFR and below, urine osmolality does not rise even when supraphysiologic doses of AVP are administered, suggesting that the concentrating defect relates to impaired concentrating capacity in surviving nephrons. The associated increased fractional excretion per nephron of a variety of solutes produces an obligatory water loss (solute diuresis) at roughly isotonic proportions. Consequently, formation of a concentrated urine is prevented. Disease-induced abnormalities of the architecture of the renal medulla (loops of Henle, vasa recta), aberrations in medullary blood flow, and defective transport of NaCl in the ascending limb of Henle also contribute to this defect in urine concentration.

Since patients with CRF are unable to excrete concentrated or dilute urine, they must have access to adequate, and to some extent, relatively constant amounts of water per day to ensure that they have adequate water to eliminate total daily solute loads. For this reason, restriction of fluid intake may be hazardous in patients with CRF. Likewise, impairment of diluting capacity may prevent many patients from excreting excess ingested fluid. The consequences of the abnormal patterns of water excretion, and the attendant susceptibilities to develop hypo- and hypernatremia, are considered in Chaps. 49 and 270.

TUBULE TRANSPORT OF PHOSPHATE WITH NORMAL AND REDUCED NEPHRON MASS Under normal physiologic conditions, about 80 to 90% of phosphate is reabsorbed, mainly in the proximal tubule. *Parathyroid hormone* (PTH), by augmenting phosphate excretion via inhibition of this proximal reabsorptive process (Chap. 340), plays a central role in phosphate homeostasis. When dietary phosphate intake increases, a *transient* rise in plasma phosphate concentration is usually observed. This results in a similarly transient reduction in the plasma ionized calcium level (due largely to deposition of calcium phosphate in bone), which is sensed by a specific receptor on parathyroid cells, stimulating PTH secretion. By enhancing fractional phosphate excretion, PTH restores external phosphate balance and normophosphatemia. This enables plasma ionized calcium levels to return to normal, thereby removing the stimulus to PTH release and restoring the phosphate control system to the original steady state.

With advancing renal failure and constant dietary intake of phosphate, external phosphate balance is achieved by progressive reduction in fractional phosphate reabsorption. Enhanced PTH secretion is an important determinant of this phosphaturic response. With succeeding decrements in total GFR, the amount of phosphate filtered by surviving glomeruli is reduced, leading to transient phosphate retention and, therefore, a rise (albeit small) in plasma phosphate concentration. This leads to a small, reciprocal decline in plasma levels of ionized calcium and a corresponding increase in PTH secretion. Although the phosphaturic response of surviving tubules to this elevation in circulating PTH restores plasma phosphate and calcium to normal levels (at least in the "compensated" stage of CRF described by curve *B* in Fig. 268-1), the new steady-state conditions are only achieved at the cost of *persistently elevated plasma PTH levels*. With progressive reductions in GFR, the process is repeated, resulting in substantially elevated PTH levels.

Alterations in Vitamin D Metabolism These alterations also contribute to elevated PTH levels in CRF. The kidney is normally the major site of *conversion of vitamin D to its active metabolites.* As discussed in Chap. 340, vitamin D, synthesized in skin or acquired in the diet, undergoes initial hydroxylation in the liver to form 25-hydroxyvitamin D [25(OH)D]. The kidney is the site of a second important conversion to 1,25-hydroxyvitamin D [1,25(OH$_2$)D]. This active form of vitamin D acts directly on the parathyroid gland to suppress PTH secretion as well as to enhance intestinal absorption of calcium and phosphate resorption and promote resorption of these ions from bone. In addition, 1,25(OH)D$_2$ probably opposes the phosphaturic actions of PTH in the renal tubule by augmenting, rather than diminishing, phosphate reabsorption. With advancing renal disease, nephron loss reduces the renal capacity for vitamin D hydroxylation; phosphate retention also impairs this reaction. Not only are the circulating levels of 1,25(OH)D$_2$ diminished in uremia, but the receptors that mediate its action at the parathyroid gland are also diminished. These two effects remove inhibitory influences on PTH secretion, leading again to increased plasma PTH levels. Reduction in circulating 1,25(OH)D$_2$ levels, by suppressing intestinal calcium absorption, contributes to the development of the hypocalcemia and hyperparathyroidism of CRF (Chap. 270).

Hyperparathyroidism in Chronic Renal Failure At least two additional processes are thought to contribute to hyperparathyroidism in CRF. One relates to resistance of bone to the calcemic effect of PTH in uremia. This resistance necessitates a higher level of PTH to demineralize bone and maintain the plasma calcium concentration. The other derives from the finding that reductions in renal mass impair the kidneys' capacity to degrade circulating PTH. Ultimately, however, phosphate conforms more to a curve *B*– rather than a curve *C*–type pattern in Fig. 268-1, and phosphate retention occurs when the GFR falls below about 25 mL/min, signifying that these latter forms of adaptation play limited roles.

Since PTH exerts major effects on bone as well as renal tubules, the external balance of phosphate in CRF is achieved at the expense of elevated PTH levels, which, in turn, account for many of the bone changes of renal osteodystrophy (i.e., *secondary hyperparathyroidism*; Fig. 270-1). In support of this *trade-off hypothesis*, when dietary phosphate intake is reduced in proportion to the reduction in GFR in animals with CRF, external balance of phosphate no longer requires augmentation of fractional phosphate excretion in surviving nephrons. Accordingly, circulating levels of PTH no longer rise, and the bone changes of secondary hyperparathyroidism are diminished, if not prevented.

HYDROGEN AND BICARBONATE TRANSPORT WITH NORMAL AND REDUCED RENAL MASS As discussed in Chap. 50, the pH of extracellular fluid is normally maintained within a narrow range (7.36 to 7.44) despite day-to-day fluctuations in the quantity of acids added to the extracellular fluid from dietary and metabolic sources (approximately 1 mmol H^+ per kilogram of body weight per day). These acids consume buffers from both extracellular and intracellular fluid, of which HCO_3^- is the most important in the intracellular compartment. Such buffering minimizes changes in pH. Long-term effectiveness of the HCO_3^- buffer system, however, requires mechanisms for replenishment, otherwise unrelenting acquisition of nonvolatile acids from dietary and metabolic sources would ultimately exhaust buffering capacity, culminating in fatal acidosis. The kidneys normally function to prevent this eventuality by *regenerating* bicarbonate, thereby maintaining plasma concentrations of HCO_3^-. In addition, the kidneys also *reclaim* HCO_3^- in the glomerular ultrafiltrate. Reclamation of filtered HCO_3^- takes place largely in the proximal tubule and, under normal circumstances, is virtually complete below a critical plasma HCO_3^- concentration—the threshold concentration—which in humans is normally about 26 mmol/L, identical to the concentration of HCO_3^- in plasma. As a consequence, HCO_3^- wastage is prevented. Alternatively, when plasma HCO_3^- rises above this threshold, reabsorption becomes less complete, allowing escape of excess HCO_3^- into the final urine, which restores the plasma HCO_3^- towards normal levels. Despite complete reabsorption of HCO_3^-, metabolic acidosis would still ensue if HCO_3^- consumed in buffering nonvolatile acids were not constantly regenerated.

The *reabsorption* of filtered HCO_3^- occurs by the following mechanism. Filtered bicarbonate combines with H^+ secreted from proximal tubule cells via the Na^+/H^+ exchange, to form carbonic acid (H_2CO_3). Dehydration of carbonic acid under the influence of *luminal* carbonic anhydrase yields H_2O and CO_2, which is free to diffuse from lumen to peritubular blood. In the proximal tubule cell, the OH^- left behind by the H^+ secretion reacts with CO_2, under the influence of *intracellular* carbonic anhydrase, forming HCO_3^-. This ion is transported across the contraluminal proximal tubule cell membrane, via an electrogenic Na/HCO_3^- cotransporter, to reenter the extracellular HCO_3^- pool. The net result is *reclamation of a filtered bicarbonate ion.* Secreted H^+ is also free to react with nonbicarbonate buffers [e.g., phosphate or ammonia (NH_4^+)] in the tubule lumen, and hydrogen ions are excreted in these forms in the final urine. Again, the OH^- left behind in the proximal tubule cell from H^+ secretion reacts with CO_2, forming bicarbonate—also representing *regeneration of an HCO_3^- ion.*

Hydrogen ions in the urine are bound to filtered buffers (e.g., phosphate) in amounts equivalent to the amounts of alkali required to titrate the pH of the urine up to the pH of the blood (the so-called titratable acid). It is not usually possible to excrete all the daily acid load in the form of titratable acid due to limits of urinary pH. Metabolism of glutamine by proximal tubule cells to yield ammonium (ammoniagenesis) serves as an additional mechanism for H^+ elimination and bicarbonate regeneration. Glutamine metabolism forms not only NH_4^+ (i.e., NH_3 plus H^+) but also HCO_3^-, which is transported across the proximal tubule (HCO_3^- regeneration). The NH_4^+ must be excreted in the urine for this process to be effective in bicarbonate regeneration. The excretion of ammonium involves secretion by proximal tubule cells (possibly by the Na^+/H^+ exchanger as Na^+/NH_4^+), generation of high medullary interstitial NH_4^+ concentration by an elaborate countercurrent multiplication/exchange system, and finally, secretion of the interstitial NH_4^+ by the collecting duct by a combination of H^+ secretion and passive NH_3 diffusion. *Ammoniagenesis* is responsive to the acid-base needs of the individual. When faced with an acute acid burden and an increased need for HCO_3^- regeneration, the rate of renal ammonia synthesis increases sharply.

The quantity of hydrogen ions excreted as titratable acid and NH_4^+ is equal to the quantity of HCO_3^- regenerated in tubule cells and added to plasma. Under steady-state conditions, the net quantity of acid excreted into the urine (the sum of titratable acid and NH_4^+ less HCO_3^-) must equal the quantity of acid gained by the extracellular fluid from all sources. Metabolic acidosis and alkalosis result when this delicate balance is perturbed, the former the result of insufficient net acid excretion, and the latter due to excessive acid excretion.

Progressive loss of renal function usually causes little or no change in arterial pH, plasma bicarbonate concentration, or arterial carbon dioxide tension (P_{CO_2}) until GFR falls below 25% of normal. Thereafter, all three tend to decline as *metabolic acidosis* ensues. In general, the metabolic acidosis of CRF is not due to overproduction of acids but is rather a reflection of nephron loss, which limits the amount of NH_3 (and therefore also HCO_3^-) that can be generated. Although surviving nephrons appear to be capable of generating supranormal amounts of NH_3 *per nephron*, the diminished nephron population causes overall production to be reduced to an extent that is insufficient to permit adequate buffering of H^+ in urine. As a result, although patients with CRF may be able to acidify their urine normally (i.e., urine pH as low as 4.5), the defect in NH_3 production limits daily net acid excretion to 30 to 40 mmol, or one-half to two-thirds the quantity of nonvolatile acid added to the extracellular fluid in the same time period. Metabolic acidosis resulting from this daily positive balance of H^+ is seldom florid in CRF of mild to moderate severity. Relative stability of plasma bicarbonate (albeit at reduced levels of 14 to 18 mmol/L) is maintained at the expense of buffering by bone. Because it contains large reserves of alkaline salts (calcium phosphate and calcium bicarbonate), bone constitutes a major reserve of buffering capacity. Dissolution of these buffers contributes to the osteodystrophy of CRF (Fig. 270-1).

Although the acidosis of CRF is due to loss of tubule mass, it nevertheless depends to a large part on the level of GFR. When GFR is reduced to only a moderate extent (i.e., to about 50% of normal), retention of anions, principally sulfates and phosphates, is not pronounced. Therefore, as the plasma HCO_3^- falls owing to dysfunction or loss of tubules, retention of Cl^- by the kidneys leads to a *hyperchloremic acidosis.* At this stage *the anion gap is normal.* With further reductions in GFR and progressive azotemia, however, the retention of phosphates, sulfates, and other *unmeasured* anions ensues and plasma Cl^- falls to normal levels despite the reduction in plasma HCO_3^- concentration. *An elevated anion gap therefore develops.*

TUBULE POTASSIUM TRANSPORT WITH NORMAL AND REDUCED NEPHRON MASS As with H^+, the concentration of K^+ in extracellular fluid is normally maintained within a relatively narrow range, 4 to 5 mmol/L. At least 95% of total-body K^+ is in the intracellular compartment, where the intracellular concentration is approximately 160 mmol/L. Normal individuals maintain external K^+ balance by excreting amounts into the urine that equal the intake, less the relatively small losses in stool and sweat. K^+ is freely filtered at the glomerulus, although the amount excreted usually represents no more than about 20% of the quantity filtered. The great bulk of the K^+ filtered is reabsorbed in the early portions of the nephron, about two-thirds in the proximal tubule, and an additional 20 to 25% in the loop of Henle. A *K^+ secretory process* operates in the distal tubule and terminal nephron segments. This process is largely dependent on Na^+ reabsorption and the accompanying lumen-negative voltage creating an electrical gradient across the tubule wall, favoring K^+ secretion into the lumen of the distal tubule and collecting duct.

The ability to maintain external K^+ balance and normal plasma K^+ concentration until relatively late in the course of CRF is a consequence primarily of a progressive increase in fractional excretion of K^+. Greatly enhanced rates of K^+ secretion occur in distal portions of surviving tubules. The augmented secretion rate of aldosterone contributes to enhanced tubule secretion of K^+. In addition, both the increased distal tubule flow rates in surviving nephrons, due to the osmotic diuresis, and enhanced luminal electronegativity, created by the increased presence of highly impermeable anions such as phosphate and sulfate, enhance K^+ secretion. Aldosterone also stimulates net entry of K^+ into the lumen of the colon, a mechanism known to be enhanced in CRF. →*More detailed discussions of abnormal K^+ homeostasis in acute and chronic forms of renal failure are given in Chaps. 269 and 270.*

ACKNOWLEDGMENT

Harald S. MacKenzie was a co-author of this chapter in the 14th edition and some of the content of that chapter is carried forward to the present edition.

BIBLIOGRAPHY

BRENNER BM: Nephron adaptation to renal injury or ablation. Am J Physiol 249:F324, 1985

——— (ed): *Brenner and Rector's The Kidney*, 6th ed. Philadelphia, Saunders, 2000

——— et al: Diverse biological actions of atrial natriuretic peptides. Physiol Rev 70:665, 1990

BUSHINSKY DA: The contribution of acidosis to renal osteodystrophy. Kidney Int 47:1816, 1995

KAJI D, KAHN T: Na^+-K^+ pump in chronic renal failure. Am J Physiol 252:F785, 1987

PRICE SR, MITCH WE: Metabolic acidosis and uremic toxicity: Protein and amino acid metabolism. Semin Nephrol 14:232, 1994

269

Hugh R. Brady, Barry M. Brenner

ACUTE RENAL FAILURE

Acute renal failure (ARF) is a syndrome characterized by rapid decline in glomerular filtration rate (hours to days), retention of nitrogenous waste products, and perturbation of extracellular fluid volume and electrolyte and acid-base homeostasis. ARF complicates approximately 5% of hospital admissions and up to 30% of admissions to intensive care units. Oliguria (urine output < 500 mL/d) is a frequent but not invariable clinical feature (~50%). ARF is usually asymptomatic and is diagnosed when biochemical screening of hospitalized patients reveals a recent increase in plasma urea and creatinine concentrations. It may complicate a wide range of diseases, which for purposes of diagnosis and management are conveniently divided into three categories: (1) diseases that cause renal hypoperfusion without compromising the integrity of renal parenchyma (*prerenal ARF*, prerenal azotemia) (~55%); (2) diseases that directly involve renal parenchyma (*intrinsic renal ARF*, renal azotemia) (~40%); and (3) diseases associated with urinary tract obstruction (*postrenal ARF*, postrenal azotemia) (~5%). Most ARF is reversible, the kidney being relatively unique among major organs in its ability to recover from almost complete loss of function. Nevertheless, ARF is associated with major in-hospital morbidity and mortality, in large part due to the serious nature of the illnesses that precipitate the ARF.

ETIOLOGY AND PATHOPHYSIOLOGY

PRERENAL ARF (PRERENAL AZOTEMIA) Prerenal ARF is the most common form of ARF and represents a physiologic response to mild to moderate renal hypoperfusion. Prerenal ARF is rapidly reversible upon restoration of renal blood flow and glomerular ultrafiltration pressure. Renal parenchymal tissue is not damaged; indeed, kidneys from individuals with prerenal ARF function well when transplanted into recipients with normal cardiovascular function. More severe hypoperfusion may lead to ischemic injury of renal parenchyma and intrinsic renal ARF. Thus, prerenal ARF and intrinsic renal ARF due to ischemia are part of a spectrum of manifestations of renal hypoperfusion. As shown in Table 269-1, prerenal ARF can complicate any disease that induces hypovolemia, low cardiac output, systemic vasodilatation, or selective renal vasoconstriction.

Hypovolemia leads to a fall in mean systemic arterial pressure, which is detected as reduced stretch by arterial (e.g., carotid sinus) and cardiac baroreceptors. Activated baroreceptors trigger a coordinated series of neural and humoral responses designed to restore blood volume and arterial pressure. These include activation of the sympathetic nervous system and renin-angiotensin-aldosterone system and release of arginine vasopressin (AVP; formerly called antidiuretic hormone). Norepinephrine, angiotensin II, and AVP act in concert in an attempt to preserve cardiac and cerebral perfusion by stimulating vasoconstriction in relatively "nonessential" vascular beds, such as the musculocutaneous and splanchnic circulations, by inhibiting salt loss through sweat glands, by stimulating thirst and salt appetite, and by promoting renal salt and water retention. Glomerular perfusion, ultrafiltration pressure, and filtration rate are preserved during mild hypoperfusion through several compensatory mechanisms. Stretch receptors in afferent arterioles, in response to a reduction in perfusion pressure, trigger afferent arteriolar vasodilatation through a local myogenic reflex (autoregulation). Biosynthesis of vasodilator prostaglandins (e.g., prostaglandin F_2 and prostacyclin) is also enhanced, and these compounds preferentially dilate afferent arterioles. In addition, angiotensin II induces preferential constriction of efferent arterioles.

Table 269-1 Classification and Major Causes of Acute Renal Failure (ARF)

PRERENAL ARF

I. Hypovolemia
  A. Hemorrhage, burns, dehydration
  B. Gastrointestinal fluid loss: vomiting, surgical drainage, diarrhea
  C. Renal fluid loss: diuretics, osmotic diuresis (e.g., diabetes mellitus), hypoadrenalism
  D. Sequestration in extravascular space: pancreatitis, peritonitis, trauma, burns, severe hypoalbuminemia
II. Low cardiac output
  A. Diseases of myocardium, valves, and pericardium; arrhythmias; tamponade
  B. Other: pulmonary hypertension, massive pulmonary embolus, positive pressure mechanical ventilation
III. Altered renal systemic vascular resistance ratio
  A. Systemic vasodilatation: sepsis, antihypertensives, afterload reducers, anesthesia, anaphylaxis
  B. Renal vasoconstriction: hypercalcemia, norepinephrine, epinephrine, cyclosporine, FK506, amphotericin B
  C. Cirrhosis with ascites (hepatorenal syndrome)
IV. Renal hypoperfusion with impairment of renal autoregulatory responses
  Cyclooxygenase inhibitors, angiotensin-converting enzyme inhibitors
V. Hyperviscosity syndrome (rare)
  Multiple myeloma, macroglobulinemia, polycythemia

INTRINSIC RENAL ARF

I. Renovascular obstruction (bilateral or unilateral in the setting of one functioning kidney)
  A. Renal artery obstruction: atherosclerotic plaque, thrombosis, embolism, dissecting aneurysm, vasculitis
  B. Renal vein obstruction: thrombosis, compression
II. Disease of glomeruli or renal microvasculature
  A. Glomerulonephritis and vasculitis
  B. Hemolytic uremic syndrome, thrombotic thrombocytopenic purpura, disseminated intravascular coagulation, toxemia of pregnancy, accelerated hypertension, radiation nephritis, systemic lupus erythematosus, scleroderma
III. Acute tubular necrosis
  A. Ischemia: as for prerenal ARF (hypovolemia, low cardiac output, renal vasoconstriction, systemic vasodilatation), obstetric complications (abruptio placentae, postpartum hemorrhage)
  B. Toxins
    1. Exogenous: radiocontrast, cyclosporine, antibiotics (e.g., aminoglycosides), chemotherapy (e.g., cisplatin), organic solvents (e.g., ethylene glycol), acetaminophen, illegal abortifacients
    2. Endogenous: rhabdomyolysis, hemolysis, uric acid, oxalate, plasma cell dyscrasia (e.g., myeloma)
IV. Interstitial nephritis
  A. Allergic: antibiotics (e.g., β-lactams, sulfonamides, trimethoprim, rifampicin), nonsteroidal anti-inflammatory agents, diuretics, captopril
  B. Infection: bacterial (e.g., acute pyelonephritis, leptospirosis), viral (e.g., cytomegalovirus), fungal (e.g., candidiasis)
  C. Infiltration: lymphoma, leukemia, sarcoidosis
  D. Idiopathic
V. Intratubular deposition and obstruction
  Myeloma proteins, uric acid, oxalate, acyclovir, methotrexate, sulphonamides
VI. Renal allograft rejection

POSTRENAL ARF (OBSTRUCTION)

I. Ureteric
  Calculi, blood clot, sloughed papillae, cancer, external compression (e.g., retroperitoneal fibrosis)
II. Bladder neck
  Neurogenic bladder, prostatic hypertrophy, calculi, cancer, blood clot
III. Urethra
  Stricture, congenital valve, phimosis

As a result, intraglomerular pressure is maintained, the fraction of plasma flowing through glomerular capillaries that is filtered is increased (filtration fraction), and glomerular filtration rate (GFR) is preserved. During states of more severe hypoperfusion, these compensatory responses are overwhelmed and GFR falls, leading to prerenal ARF.

Autoregulatory dilatation of afferent arterioles is maximal at mean systemic arterial blood pressures of ~80 mmHg, and hypotension below this level is associated with a precipitous decline in GFR. Lesser degrees of hypotension may provoke prerenal ARF in the elderly and in patients with diseases affecting the integrity of afferent arterioles (e.g., hypertensive nephrosclerosis, diabetic vasculopathy). In addition, drugs that interfere with adaptive responses in the renal microcirculation may convert compensated renal hypoperfusion into overt prerenal ARF or trigger progression of prerenal ARF to ischemic intrinsic renal ARF (see below). Pharmacologic inhibitors of either renal prostaglandin biosynthesis [*cyclooxygenase inhibitors*; nonsteroidal anti-inflammatory drugs (NSAIDs)] or angiotensin-converting enzyme (ACE) activity (ACE inhibitors) are the major culprits and should be used judiciously in the setting of suspected renal hypoperfusion. NSAIDs do not compromise GFR in healthy individuals but may precipitate prerenal ARF in patients with volume depletion or in those with chronic renal insufficiency in whom GFR is maintained, in part, through prostaglandin-mediated hyperfiltration through the remaining functional nephrons. ACE inhibitors can also compromise GFR in individuals with renal hypoperfusion and should be used with special care in patients with bilateral renal artery stenosis or unilateral stenosis in a solitary functioning kidney. Glomerular perfusion and filtration may be exquisitely dependent on the actions of angiotensin II under the latter circumstances. Angiotensin II preserves glomerular filtration pressure distal to stenoses by elevating systemic arterial pressure and by triggering selective constriction of efferent arterioles. ACE inhibitors blunt these responses and precipitate ARF, usually reversible, in ~30% of these patients.

Hepatorenal Syndrome This is a particularly aggressive form of ARF that frequently complicates hepatic failure due to advanced cirrhosis or other liver diseases, including malignancy, hepatic resection, and biliary obstruction. Intrarenal vasoconstriction and avid sodium retention are early sequelae of these diseases and may be detected before changes in systemic hemodynamics. Patients with advanced liver disease, portal hypertension, and ascites also have increased plasma volume but reduced "effective" arterial blood volume as a consequence of systemic vasodilatation and pooling of blood in the portal circulation. Renal failure typically develops slowly over weeks or months in parallel with deteriorating hepatic function but may accelerate dramatically following a variety of hemodynamic insults, including hemorrhage, paracentesis, and overzealous use of diuretics, vasodilators, or cyclooxygenase inhibitors. In full-blown hepatorenal syndrome, ARF progresses even after optimization of systemic hemodynamics and systemic arterial blood volume and removal of nephrotoxins, probably as a result of ongoing intrarenal vasoconstriction, hypoperfusion, and ischemia triggered by circulating factors or neural impulses originating in the failing liver. Indeed, it must be remembered that patients with liver disease may develop other forms of ARF (e.g., sepsis, nephrotoxic medications), and a diagnosis of hepatorenal syndrome should be made only after exclusion of other possible reversible causes.

INTRINSIC RENAL ARF (INTRINSIC RENAL AZOTEMIA) Intrinsic renal ARF can complicate many diverse diseases of the renal parenchyma. From a clinicopathologic viewpoint, it is useful to divide the causes of intrinsic renal ARF into (1) diseases of large renal vessels, (2) diseases of the renal microcirculation and glomeruli, (3) ischemic and nephrotoxic ARF, and (4) tubulointerstitial diseases (Table 269-1). Most intrinsic renal ARF is triggered by ischemia (ischemic ARF) or nephrotoxins (nephrotoxic ARF), insults that classically induce acute tubular necrosis (ATN). Accordingly, the terms ARF and ATN are usually used interchangeably in these settings. However, as many as 20 to 30% of patients with ischemic or nephrotoxic ARF do not have clinical (granular or tubular cell urinary casts) or morphologic evidence of tubular necrosis, underscoring the role of sublethal injury to tubular epithelium and injury to other renal cells (e.g., endothelial cells) in the pathophysiology of this syndrome.

Etiology and Pathophysiology of Ischemic ARF Prerenal ARF and ischemic ARF are part of a spectrum of manifestations of renal hypoperfusion. Ischemic ARF differs from prerenal ARF in that the hypoperfusion induces ischemic injury to renal parenchymal cells, particularly tubular epithelium, and recovery typically takes 1 to 2 weeks after normalization of renal perfusion as it requires repair and regeneration of renal cells. In its most extreme form, ischemia leads to bilateral renal cortical necrosis and irreversible renal failure. Ischemic ARF occurs most frequently in patients undergoing major cardiovascular surgery or suffering severe trauma, hemorrhage, sepsis, and/or volume depletion (Table 269-1). Ischemic ARF can also complicate milder forms of true hypovolemia or reduced "effective" arterial blood volume if they occur in the presence of other insults (e.g., nephrotoxins or sepsis) or in patients with compromised autoregulatory defense mechanisms or preexisting renal disease.

The course of ischemic ARF is typically characterized by three phases: the initiation, maintenance, and recovery phases. The *initiation phase* (hours to days) is the initial period of renal hypoperfusion during which ischemic injury is evolving. GFR declines because (1) glomerular ultrafiltration pressure is reduced as a consequence of the fall in renal blood flow, (2) the flow of glomerular filtrate within tubules is obstructed by casts comprising epithelial cells and necrotic debris derived from ischemic tubule epithelium, and (3) there is backleak of glomerular filtrate through injured tubular epithelium (Fig. 269-1). Ischemic injury is most prominent in the terminal medullary portion of the proximal tubule (S_3 segment, pars recta) and the medullary portion of the thick ascending limb of the loop of Henle. Both segments have high rates of active (ATP-dependent) solute transport and oxygen consumption and are located in a zone of the kidney (the outer medulla) that is relatively ischemic, even under basal conditions, by virtue of the unique countercurrent arrangement of the medullary vasculature. Cellular ischemia results in a series of alterations in energetics, ion transport, and membrane integrity that ultimately lead to cell injury and, if severe, cell apoptosis or necrosis. These alterations include depletion of ATP, inhibition of active sodium transport and transport of other solutes, impairment of cell volume regulation and cell swelling, cytoskeletal disruption and loss of cell polarity, cell-cell and cell-matrix attachment, accumulation of intracellular calcium, altered phospholipid metabolism, oxygen free radical formation, and peroxidation of membrane lipids. Importantly, renal injury can be limited by restoration of renal blood flow during this period.

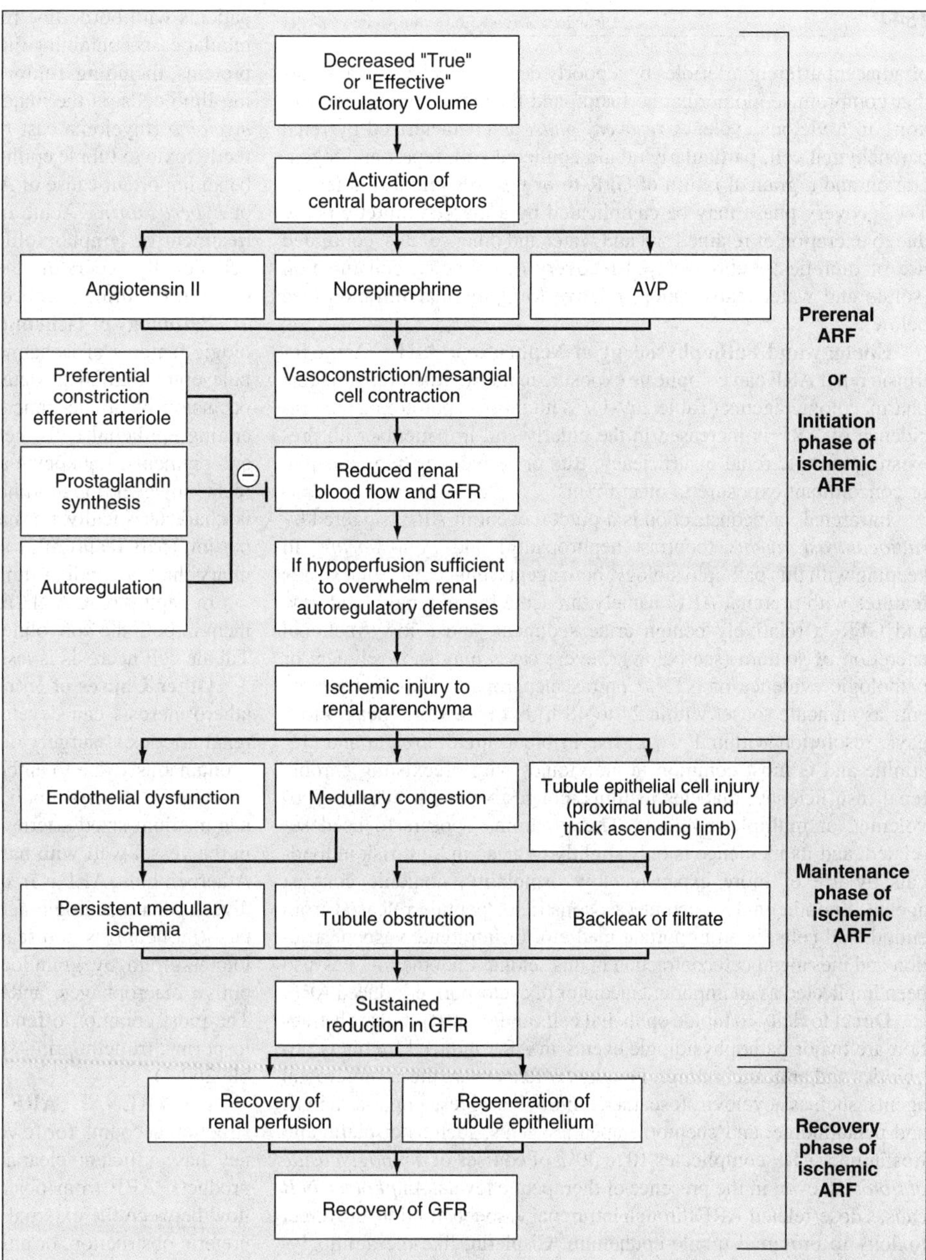

FIGURE 269-1 Overview of the pathophysiology of prerenal ARF and ischemic intrinsic renal ARF: A spectrum of manifestations of renal hypoperfusion (ARF, acute renal failure; AVP, arginine vasopressin; GFR, glomerular filtration rate.)

The initiation phase is followed by a *maintenance phase* (typically 1 to 2 weeks) during which renal cell injury is established, GFR stabilizes at its nadir (typically 5 to 10 mL/min), urine output is lowest, and uremic complications arise (see below). The reasons why the GFR remains low during this phase, despite correction of systemic hemodynamics, are still being defined. Putative mechanisms include persistent intrarenal vasoconstriction and medullary ischemia triggered by dysregulated release of vasoactive mediators from injured endothelial cells (e.g., decreased nitric oxide, increased endothelin-1 and platelet-activating factor), congestion of medullary blood vessels, and reperfusion injury induced by reactive oxygen species and other mediators derived from leukocytes or renal parenchymal cells (Fig. 269-1). In addition, epithelial cell injury per se may contribute to persistent intrarenal vasoconstriction by a process termed *tubuloglomerular feedback*. Specialized epithelial cells in the macula densa region of distal tubules detect increases in distal salt (probably chloride) delivery that occur as a consequence of impaired reabsorption by more proximal nephron segments. Macula densa cells in turn stimulate constriction of adjacent afferent arterioles by a poorly defined mechanism and further compromise glomerular perfusion and filtration, thereby contributing to a vicious cycle. A *recovery phase* is characterized by renal parenchymal cell, particularly tubule epithelial cell, repair and regeneration and a gradual return of GFR to or towards premorbid levels. The recovery phase may be complicated by a marked diuretic phase due to excretion of retained salt and water and other solutes, continued use of diuretics, and/or delayed recovery of epithelial cell function (solute and water reabsorption) relative to glomerular filtration (see below).

Etiology and Pathophysiology of Nephrotoxic ARF Acute intrinsic renal ARF can complicate exposure to many structurally diverse pharmacologic agents (Table 269-1). With most nephrotoxins, the incidence of ARF is increased in the elderly and in patients with preexisting chronic renal insufficiency, true or "effective" hypovolemia, or concomitant exposure to other toxins.

Intrarenal vasoconstriction is a pivotal event in ARF triggered by *radiocontrast agents* (contrast nephropathy) and *cyclosporine*. In keeping with this pathophysiology, both agents induce ARF that shares features with prerenal ARF: namely, an acute fall in renal blood flow and GFR, a relatively benign urine sediment, and a low fractional excretion of sodium (see below). Severe cases may show clinical or pathologic evidence of ATN. Contrast nephropathy classically presents as an acute (onset within 24 to 48 h) but reversible (peak 3 to 5 days, resolution within 1 week) rise in blood urea nitrogen and creatinine and is most common in individuals with preexisting chronic renal insufficiency, diabetes mellitus, congestive heart failure, hypovolemia, or multiple myeloma. The syndrome appears to be dose-related, and its incidence is only slightly reduced in high-risk individuals by use of more expensive low osmolality, nonionic contrast agents. Endothelin-1, a potent vasoconstrictor peptide released from endothelial cells, is an important mediator of intrarenal vasoconstriction and mesangial cell contraction in this setting. Endothelin-1 has also been implicated as an important mediator of cyclosporine-induced ARF.

Direct toxicity to tubule epithelial cells and/or intratubular obstruction are major pathophysiologic events in ARF induced by many antibiotics and anticancer drugs. Frequent offenders are the antimicrobial agents, such as acyclovir, foscarnet, aminoglycosides, amphotericin B, and pentamidine, and chemotherapeutic agents, such as cisplatin and ifosfamide. ARF complicates 10 to 30% of courses of *aminoglycoside antibiotics*, even in the presence of therapeutic levels. *Amphotericin B* causes dose-related ARF through intrarenal vasoconstriction and direct toxicity to proximal tubule epithelium. Cisplatin, like the aminoglycosides, is accumulated by proximal tubule cells and typically provokes ARF after 7 to 10 days of exposure by inducing mitochondrial injury, inhibition of ATPase activity and solute transport, free radical–mediated injury to cell membranes, apoptosis and/or necrosis.

The most common endogenous nephrotoxins are calcium, myoglobin, hemoglobin, urate, oxalate, and myeloma light chains. Hypercalcemia can compromise GFR, predominantly by inducing intrarenal vasoconstriction. Calcium phosphate deposition within the kidney may also contribute. Both *rhabdomyolysis* and *hemolysis* can induce ARF, particularly in hypovolemic or acidotic individuals. Myoglobinuric ARF complicates approximately 30% of cases of rhabdomyolysis. Common causes of the latter include traumatic crush injury, acute muscle ischemia, seizures, excessive exercise, heat stroke or malignant hyperthermia, intoxications (e.g., alcohol, cocaine), and infectious or metabolic disorders. ARF due to hemolysis is relatively rare and is observed following massive blood transfusion reactions. It has been postulated that myoglobin and hemoglobin or other compounds released from muscle or red blood cells cause ARF via toxic effects on tubule epithelial cells or by inducing intratubular cast formation. Hypovolemia or acidosis may contribute to the pathogenesis of ARF in this setting by promoting intratubular cast formation. In addition, both hemoglobin and myoglobin are potent inhibitors of nitric oxide bioactivity and may trigger intrarenal vasoconstriction and ischemia in patients with borderline renal hypoperfusion. The formation of intratubular casts containing filtered immunoglobulin light chains and other proteins, including Tamm-Horsfall protein produced by thick ascending limb cells, is the major trigger for ARF in patients with *multiple myeloma* (myeloma cast nephropathy). Light chains may also be directly toxic to tubule epithelial cells. Intratubular obstruction may also be an important cause of ARF in patients with severe *hyperuricosuria* or *hyperoxaluria*. Acute uric acid nephropathy typically complicates treatment of lymphoproliferative or myeloproliferative disorders but occasionally occurs in other forms of primary or secondary hyperuricemia if the urine is concentrated.

Pathology of Ischemic and Nephrotoxic ARF The classic pathologic features of ischemic ARF are patchy and focal necrosis of tubule epithelium with detachment from its basement membrane and occlusion of tubule lumens with casts composed of intact or degenerating epithelial cells, cellular debris, Tamm-Horsfall mucoprotein, and pigments. Leukocyte accumulation is frequently observed in vasa recta; however, the morphology of the glomeruli and renal vasculature is characteristically normal. Necrosis is most severe in the straight portion (pars recta) of proximal tubules but may also affect the medullary thick ascending limb of the loop of Henle.

In nephrotoxic ARF, morphologic changes tend to be most prominent in both the convoluted and straight portions of proximal tubules. Tubule cell necrosis is less pronounced than in ischemic ARF.

Other Causes of Intrinsic Renal ARF Patients with advanced atherosclerosis can develop ARF after manipulation of the aorta or renal arteries at surgery or angiography, following trauma, or, rarely, spontaneously due to embolization of cholesterol crystals to the renal vasculature (atheroembolic ARF). Cholesterol crystals lodge in small- and medium-sized arteries and incite a giant cell and fibrotic reaction in the vessel wall with narrowing or obstruction of the vessel lumen. Atheroembolic ARF is frequently irreversible. A myriad of structurally diverse pharmacologic agents induce ARF by triggering allergic interstitial nephritis, a disease characterized by infiltration of the tubulointerstitium by granulocytes (typically but not invariably eosinophils), macrophages, and/or lymphocytes and by interstitial edema. The most common offenders are antibiotics (e.g., penicillins, cephalosporins, trimethoprim, sulfonamides, rifampicin) and NSAIDs (Table 269-1).

POSTRENAL ARF (See also Chap. 281) Urinary tract obstruction accounts for fewer than 5% of cases of ARF. Since one kidney has sufficient clearance capacity to excrete nitrogenous waste products, ARF from obstruction requires either obstruction to urine flow between the external urethral meatus and bladder neck, bilateral ureteric obstruction, or unilateral ureteric obstruction in a patient with one functioning kidney or preexisting chronic renal insufficiency. Bladder neck obstruction represents the most common cause of postrenal ARF and is usually due to prostatic disease (e.g., hypertrophy, neoplasia, or infection), neurogenic bladder, or therapy with anticholinergic drugs. Less common causes of acute lower urinary tract obstruction include blood clots, calculi, and urethritis with spasm. Ureteric obstruction may result from intraluminal obstruction (e.g., calculi, blood clots, sloughed renal papillae), infiltration of the ureteric wall (e.g., neoplasia), or external compression (e.g., retroperitoneal fibrosis, neoplasia or abscess, inadvertent surgical ligature). During the early stages of obstruction (hours to days), continued glomerular filtration leads to increased intraluminal pressure upstream to the site of obstruction. As a result there are gradual distention of proximal ureter, renal pelvis, and calyces and a fall in GFR. Acute obstruction is initially associated with modest increase in renal blood flow, but arteriolar vasoconstriction soon supervenes, leading to a further decline in glomerular filtration.

CLINICAL FEATURES AND DIFFERENTIAL DIAGNOSIS

Patients presenting with renal failure should be assessed initially to determine if the decline in GFR is acute or chronic. An acute process is easily established if a review of laboratory records reveals a recent rise in blood urea and creatinine levels, but previous measurements are not always available. Findings that suggest chronic renal failure (Chap. 270) include anemia, neuropathy, and radiologic evidence of renal osteodystrophy or small scarred kidneys. However, it should be noted that anemia may also complicate ARF (see below), and renal size may be normal or increased in several chronic renal diseases (e.g., diabetic nephropathy, amyloidosis, polycystic kidney disease). Once a diagnosis of ARF has been established, several issues should be addressed promptly: (1) the identification of the cause of ARF, (2) the elimination of the triggering insult (e.g., nephrotoxin) and/or institution of disease-specific therapies, and (3) the prevention and management of uremic complications.

CLINICAL ASSESSMENT Clinical clues to *prerenal* ARF are symptoms of thirst and orthostatic dizziness and physical evidence of orthostatic hypotension and tachycardia, reduced jugular venous pressure, decreased skin turgor, dry mucous membranes, and reduced axillary sweating. Case records should be reviewed for documentation of a progressive fall in urine output and body weight and treatment with NSAIDs or ACE inhibitors. Careful clinical examination may reveal stigmata of chronic liver disease and portal hypertension, advanced cardiac failure, sepsis, or other causes of reduced "effective" arterial blood volume (Table 269-1).

Intrinsic renal ARF due to ischemia is likely following severe renal hypoperfusion complicating hypovolemic or septic shock or following major surgery. The likelihood of ischemic ARF is increased further if ARF persists despite normalization of systemic hemodynamics. Diagnosis of nephrotoxic ARF requires careful review of the clinical data and pharmacy, nursing, and radiology records for evidence of recent exposure to nephrotoxic medications or radiocontrast agents or to endogenous toxins (e.g., myoglobin, hemoglobin, uric acid, myeloma protein, or elevated levels of serum calcium).

Although ischemic and nephrotoxic ARF account for more than 90% of cases of intrinsic renal ARF, other renal parenchymal diseases must be considered (Table 269-2). Flank pain may be a prominent symptom following occlusion of a renal artery or vein and with other parenchymal diseases distending the renal capsule (e.g., severe glomerulonephritis or pyelonephritis). Subcutaneous nodules, livido reticularis, bright orange retinal arteriolar plaques, and digital ischemia, despite palpable pedal pulses, are clues to atheroembolization. ARF in association with oliguria, edema, hypertension, and an "active" urine sediment (nephritic syndrome) suggests acute glomerulonephritis or vasculitis. Malignant hypertension is a likely cause of ARF in patients with severe hypertension and evidence of hypertensive injury to other organs (e.g., left ventricular hypertrophy and failure, hypertensive retinopathy and papilledema, neurologic dysfunction). Fever, arthralgias, and a pruritic erythematous rash following exposure to a new drug suggest allergic interstitial nephritis, although systemic features of hypersensitivity are frequently absent.

Postrenal ARF presents with suprapubic and flank pain due to distention of the bladder and of the renal collecting system and capsule, respectively. Colicky flank pain radiating to the groin suggests acute ureteric obstruction. Prostatic disease is likely if there is a history of nocturia, frequency, and hesitancy and enlargement or induration of the prostate on rectal examination. Neurogenic bladder should be suspected in patients receiving anticholinergic medications or with physical evidence of autonomic dysfunction. Definitive diagnosis of postrenal ARF hinges on judicious use of radiologic investigations and rapid improvement in renal function following relief of obstruction.

URINALYSIS Anuria suggests complete urinary tract obstruction but may complicate severe cases of prerenal or intrinsic renal ARF. Wide fluctuations in urine output raise the possibility of intermittent obstruction, whereas patients with partial urinary tract obstruction can present with polyuria due to impairment of urine concentrating mechanisms.

In prerenal ARF, the sediment is characteristically acellular and contains transparent hyaline casts ("bland," "benign," "inactive" urine sediment). Hyaline casts are formed in concentrated urine from normal constitutents of urine—principally Tamm-Horsfall protein, which is secreted by epithelial cells of the loop of Henle. Postrenal ARF may also present with an inactive sediment, although hematuria and pyuria are common in patients with intraluminal obstruction or prostatic disease. Pigmented "muddy brown" granular casts and casts containing tubule epithelial cells are characteristic of ATN and suggest ischemic or nephrotoxic ARF. They are usually found in association with microscopic hematuria and mild "tubular" proteinuria (<1 g/d); the latter reflects impaired reabsorption and processing of filtered proteins by injured proximal tubules. Casts are absent, however, in 20 to 30% of patients with ischemic or nephrotoxic ARF and are not a requisite for diagnosis. In general, red blood cell casts indicate glomerular injury or, less often, acute tubulointerstitial nephritis. White cell casts and nonpigmented granular casts suggest interstitial nephritis, whereas broad granular casts are characteristic of chronic renal disease and probably reflect interstitial fibrosis and dilatation of tubules. Eosinophiluria (>5% of urine leukocytes) is a common finding (~90%) in antibiotic-induced allergic interstitial nephritis when studied using Hansel's stain; however, lymphocytes may predominate in allergic interstitial nephritis induced by NSAIDs. Eosinophiluria is also a feature of atheroembolic ARF. Occasional uric acid crystals (pleomorphic in shape) are common in the concentrated urine of prerenal ARF but suggest acute urate nephropathy if seen in abundance. Oxalate (envelope-shaped) and hippurate (needle-shaped) crystals raise the possibility of ethylene glycol ingestion and toxicity.

Increased urine protein excretion, but <1 g/d, is common in ATN due to failure of injured proximal tubules to reabsorb filtered protein and excretion of cellular debris ("tubular proteinuria"). Proteinuria of >1 g/d suggests injury to the glomerular ultrafiltration barrier ("glomerular proteinuria") or excretion of myeloma light chains. The latter are not detected by conventional dipsticks (which detect albumin) and must be sought by other means (e.g., sulfosalicylic acid test, immunoelectrophoresis). Heavy proteinuria is also a frequent finding (~80%) in patients who develop combined allergic interstitial nephritis and minimal change glomerulopathy when treated with NSAIDs. A similar syndrome can be triggered by ampicillin, rifampicin, or interferon α. Hemoglobinuria or myoglobinuria should be suspected if urine is strongly positive for heme by dipstick, but contains few red cells, and if the supernatant of centrifuged urine is positive for free heme. Bilirubinuria may provide a clue to the presence of hepatorenal syndrome.

RENAL FAILURE INDICES Analysis of urine and blood biochemistry is particularly useful for distinguishing prerenal ARF from ischemic or nephrotoxic intrinsic renal ARF (Table 269-3). The fractional excretion of sodium (FE_{Na}) is most useful in this regard. The FE_{Na} relates sodium clearance to creatinine clearance. Sodium is reabsorbed avidly from glomerular filtrate in patients with prerenal ARF, in an attempt to restore intravascular volume, but not in patients with ischemic or nephrotoxic intrinsic ARF, as a result of tubular epithelial cell injury. In contrast, creatinine is not reabsorbed in either setting. Consequently, patients with prerenal ARF typically have a FE_{Na} of <1.0% (frequently <0.1%), whereas the FE_{Na} in patients with ischemic or nephrotoxic ARF is usually >1.0%. The *renal failure index* (Table 269-3) provides comparable information, since clinical variations in serum sodium concentration are relatively small. *Urine sodium concentration* is a less sensitive index for distinguishing prerenal ARF from ischemic and nephrotoxic ARF as values overlap between groups. Similarly, indices of urinary concentrating ability such as urine specific gravity, urine osmolality, urine-to-plasma urea ratio, and blood urea-to-creatinine ratio are of limited value in differential diagnosis.

Many caveats apply when interpreting biochemical renal failure indices. FE_{Na} may be >1.0% in prerenal ARF if patients are receiving diuretics or have bicarbonaturia (accompanied by sodium to maintain electroneutrality), preexisting chronic renal failure complicated by salt wasting, or adrenal insufficiency. In contrast, the FE_{Na} is <1.0% in

Table 269-2 Useful Clinical Features, Urinary Findings, and Confirmatory Tests in the Differential Diagnosis of Major Causes of ARF

Cause of Acute Renal Failure	Suggestive Clinical Features	Typical Urinalysis	Some Confirmatory Tests
I. Prerenal ARF	Evidence of true volume depletion (thirst, postural or absolute hypotension and tachycardia, low jugular venous pressure, dry mucous membranes/axillae, weight loss, fluid output > input) or decreased "effective" circulatory volume (e.g., heart failure, liver failure), treatment with NSAIDs or ACE inhibitors	Hyaline casts FE_{Na} <1% U_{Na} <10 mmol/L SG >1.018	Occasionally requires invasive hemodynamic monitoring; rapid resolution of ARF upon restoration of renal perfusion
II. Intrinsic renal ARF			
A. Diseases involving large renal vessels			
1. Renal artery thrombosis	History of atrial fibrillation or recent myocardial infarct; flank or abdominal pain	Mild proteinuria Occasionally red cells	Elevated LDH with normal transaminases, renal arteriogram
2. Atheroembolism	Age usually > 50 years, recent manipulation of aorta, retinal plaques, subcutaneous nodules, palpable purpura, livedo reticularis, vasculopathy, hypertension, anticoagulation	Often normal, eosinophiluria, rarely casts	Eosinophilia, hypocomplementemia, skin biopsy, renal biopsy
3. Renal vein thrombosis	Evidence of nephrotic syndrome or pulmonary embolism, flank pain	Proteinuria, hematuria	Inferior vena cavagram and selective renal venogram
B. Diseases of small vessels and glomeruli			
1. Glomerulonephritis/vasculitis	Compatible clinical history (e.g., recent infection) sinusitis, lung hemorrhage, skin rash or ulcers, arthralgias, new cardiac murmur, history of hepatitis B or C infection	Red cell or granular casts, red cells, white cells, mild proteinuria	Low C3, ANCA, anti-GBM Ab, ANA, ASO, anti-DNAse, cryoglobulins, blood cultures, renal biopsy
2. Hemolytic-uremic syndrome/ thrombotic thrombocytopenic purpura	Compatible clinical history (e.g., recent gastrointestinal infection, cyclosporine, anovulants), fever, pallor, ecchymoses, neurologic abnormalities	May be normal, red cells, mild proteinuria, rarely red cell/granular casts	Anemia, thrombocytopenia, schistocytes on blood smear, increased LDH, renal biopsy
3. Malignant hypertension	Severe hypertension with headaches, cardiac failure, retinopathy, neurologic dysfunction, papilledema	Red cells, red cell casts, proteinuria	LVH by echocardiography/ECG, resolution of ARF with control of blood pressure
C. ARF mediated by ischemia or toxins (ATN)			
1. Ischemia	Recent hemorrhage, hypotension (e.g., cardiac arrest), surgery	Muddy brown granular or tubular epithelial cell casts FE_{Na} >1% U_{Na} >20 mmol/L SG <1.015	Clinical assessment and urinalysis usually sufficient for diagnosis
2. Exogenous toxins	Recent radiocontrast study, nephrotoxic antibiotics or anticancer agents often coexistent with volume depletion, sepsis, or chronic renal insufficiency	Muddy brown granular or tubular epithelial cell casts FE_{Na} >1% U_{Na} >20 mmol/L SG <1.015	Clinical assessment and urinalysis usually sufficient for diagnosis
3. Endogenous toxins	History suggestive of rhabdomyolysis (seizures, coma, ethanol abuse, trauma)	Urine supernatant positive for heme	Hyperkalemia, hyperphosphatemia, hypocalcemia, increased circulating myoglobin, CPK (MM), and uric acid
	History suggestive of hemolysis (blood transfusion)	Urine supernatant pink and positive for heme	Hyperkalemia, hyperphosphatemia, hypocalcemia, hyperuricemia, pink plasma positive for hemoglobin
	History suggestive of tumor lysis (recent chemotherapy), myeloma (bone pain), or ethylene glycol ingestion	Urate crystals, dipstick-negative proteinuria, oxalate crystals, respectively	Hyperuricemia, hyperkalemia, hyperphosphatemia (for tumor lysis); circulating or urinary monoclonal spike (for myeloma); toxicology screen, acidosis, osmolal gap (for ethylene glycol)

(continued)

Cause of Acute Renal Failure	Suggestive Clinical Features	Typical Urinalysis	Some Confirmatory
D. Acute diseases of the tubulo-interstitium			
1. Allergic interstitial nephritis	Recent ingestion of drug, and fever, rash, or arthralgias	White cell casts, white cells (frequently eosinphiluria), red cells, rarely red cell casts, proteinuria (occasionally nephrotic)	Systemic eosinophilia, skin biopsy of rash (leukocytoclastic vasculitis), renal biopsy
2. Acute bilateral pyelonephritis	Flank pain and tenderness, toxic, febrile	Leukocytes, proteinuria, red cells, bacteria	Urine and blood cultures
III. Postrenal ARF	Abdominal or flank pain, palpable bladder	Frequently normal, hematuria if stones, hemorrhage, malignancy, or prostatic hypertrophy	Plain film, renal ultrasound, IVP, retrograde or anterograde pyelography, CT scan

NOTE: NSAIDs, nonsteroidal anti-inflammatory drugs; U_{Na}, urine sodium concentration; SG, specific gravity; LDH, lactate dehydrogenase; C3, complement component; ANCA, antineutrophil cytoplasmic autoantibody; anti-GBM Ab, anti-glomerular basement membrane antibody; ANA, antinuclear antibody; ASO, antistreptolysin O; LVH, left ventricular hypertrophy; ECG, electrocardiogram; CK, creatine kinase; IVP, intravenous pyelogram; CT, computed tomography.

SOURCE: Adapted with permission from Brady et al.

approximately 15% of patients with nonoliguric ischemic or nephrotoxic ARF. The FE_{Na} is often <1.0% in ARF due to urinary tract obstruction, glomerulonephritis, and vascular diseases.

LABORATORY FINDINGS Serial measurements of serum creatinine can provide useful pointers to the cause of ARF. Prerenal ARF is typified by fluctuating levels that parallel changes in hemodynamic function. Creatinine rises rapidly (within 24 to 48 h) in patients with ARF following renal ischemia, atheroembolization, and radiocontrast exposure. Peak creatinine levels are observed after 3 to 5 days with contrast nephropathy and return to baseline after 5 to 7 days. In contrast, creatinine levels typically peak later (7 to 10 days) in ischemic ARF and atheroembolic disease. The initial rise in serum creatinine is characteristically delayed until the second week of therapy with many tubule epithelial cell toxins (e.g., aminoglycosides, cisplatin) and probably reflects the need for accumulation of these agents within cells before GFR falls.

Hyperkalemia, hyperphosphatemia, hypocalcemia, and elevations in serum uric acid and creatine kinase (MM isoenzyme) levels at presentation suggest a diagnosis of rhabdomyolysis. Hyperuricemia [>890 μmol/L (>15 mg/dL)] in association with hyperkalemia, hyperphosphatemia, and increased circulating levels of intracellular enzymes such as lactate dehydrogenase may indicate acute urate nephropathy and tumor lysis syndrome following cancer chemotherapy. A wide serum anion and osmolal gap (measured serum osmolality minus the serum osmolality calculated from serum sodium, glucose, and urea concentrations) indicate the presence of an unusual anion or osmole in the circulation and are clues to diagnosis of ethylene glycol or methanol ingestion. Severe anemia in the absence of hemorrhage raises the possibility of hemolysis, multiple myeloma, or thrombotic microangiopathy. Systemic eosinophilia suggests allergic interstitial nephritis but is also a feature of atheroembolic disease and polyangiitis nodosa.

Table 269-3 Urine Diagnostic Indices in Differentiation of Prerenal versus Intrinsic Renal ARF

Diagnostic Index	Typical Findings	
	Prerenal ARF	Intrinsic Renal ARF
Fractional excretion of sodium (%)[a] $\frac{U_{Na} \times P_{Cr}}{P_{Na} \times U_{Cr}} \times 100$	<1	>1
Urine sodium concentration (mmol/L)	<10	>20
Urine creatinine to plasma creatinine ratio	>40	<20
Urine urea nitrogen to plasma urea nitrogen ratio	>8	<3
Urine specific gravity	>1.020	~1.010
Urine osmolality (mosmol/kg H_2O)	>500	~300
Plasma BUN/creatinine ratio	>20	<10–15
Renal failure index[a] $\frac{U_{Na}}{U_{Cr}/P_{Cr}}$	<1	>1
Urinary sediment	Hyaline casts	Muddy brown granular casts

[a] Most sensitive indices.

NOTE: ARF, acute renal failure; U_{Na}, urine sodium concentration; P_{Cr}, plasma creatinine concentration; P_{Na}, plasma sodium concentration; U_{Cr}, urine creatinine concentration; BUN, blood urea nitrogen.

RADIOLOGIC FINDINGS Imaging of the urinary tract by ultrasonography is useful to exclude postrenal ARF. Computed tomography and magnetic resonance imaging are alternative imaging modalities. Whereas pelvicalyceal dilatation is usual with urinary tract obstruction (98% sensitivity), dilatation may be absent immediately following obstruction or in patients with ureteric encasement (e.g., retroperitoneal fibrosis, neoplasia). Retrograde or anterograde pyelography are more definitive investigations in complex cases and provide precise localization of the site of obstruction. A plain film of the abdomen, with tomography if necessary, is a valuable initial screening technique in patients with suspected nephrolithiasis. Doppler ultrasonography and magnetic resonance flow imaging appear promising for assessment of patency of renal arteries and veins in patients with suspected vascular obstruction; however, contrast angiography is usually required for definitive diagnosis.

RENAL BIOPSY Biopsy is reserved for patients in whom prerenal and postrenal ARF have been excluded and the cause of intrinsic renal ARF is unclear. Renal biopsy is particularly useful when clinical assessment and laboratory investigations suggest diagnoses other than ischemic or nephrotoxic injury that may respond to disease-specific therapy. Examples include glomerulonephritis, vasculitis, hemolytic-uremic syndrome, thrombotic thrombocytopenic purpura, and allergic interstitial nephritis.

COMPLICATIONS

ARF impairs renal excretion of sodium, potassium, and water and perturbs divalent cation homeostasis and urinary acidification mechanisms. As a result, ARF is frequently complicated by intravascular volume overload, hyponatremia, hyperkalemia, hyperphosphatemia, hypocalcemia, hypermagnesemia, and metabolic acidosis. In addition, patients are unable to excrete nitrogenous waste products and are prone to develop the uremic syndrome (Chap. 270). The speed of development and the severity of these complications reflect the degree of renal impairment and catabolic state of the patient.

Expansion of extracellular fluid volume is an inevitable consequence of diminished salt and water excretion in oliguric or anuric individuals. Whereas milder forms are characterized by weight gain, bibasilar lung rales, raised jugular venous pressure, and dependent edema, continued volume expansion may precipitate life-threatening pulmonary edema. Hypervolemia may be particularly problematic in patients receiving multiple intravenous medications and enteral or parenteral nutrition. Excessive administration of free water either through ingestion and nasogastric administration or as hypotonic saline or isotonic dextrose solutions (dextrose being metabolized) can induce *hypoosmolality* and *hyponatremia*, which, if severe, lead to cerebral edema and neurologic abnormalities, including seizures.

Hyperkalemia is a frequent complication of ARF. Serum potassium typically rises by 0.5 mmol/L per day in oliguric and anuric patients due to impaired excretion of ingested or infused potassium and potassium released from injured tissue. Coexistent metabolic acidosis may exacerbate hyperkalemia by promoting potassium efflux from cells. Hyperkalemia may be particularly severe, even at the time of diagnosis, in patients with rhabdomyolysis, hemolysis, and tumor lysis syndrome. Mild hyperkalemia (<6.0 mmol/L) is usually asymptomatic. Higher levels are typically associated with electrocardiographic abnormalities and/or increased cardiac excitability (Chap. 226).

Metabolism of dietary protein yields between 50 and 100 mmol/d of fixed nonvolatile acids that are normally excreted by the kidneys. Consequently, ARF is typically complicated by *metabolic acidosis*, often with an increased serum anion gap (Chap. 50). Acidosis can be particularly severe when endogenous production of hydrogen ions is increased by other mechanisms (e.g., diabetic or fasting ketoacidosis; lactic acidosis complicating generalized tissue hypoperfusion, liver disease, or sepsis; metabolism of ethylene glycol or methanol).

Mild *hyperphosphatemia* is an almost invariable complication of ARF. Severe hyperphosphatemia may develop in highly catabolic patients or following rhabdomyolysis, hemolysis, or tumor lysis. Metastatic deposition of calcium phosphate can lead to *hypocalcemia*, particularly when the product of serum calcium (mg/dL) and phosphate (mg/dL) concentrations exceeds 70. Other factors that contribute to hypocalcemia include tissue resistance to the actions of parathyroid hormone and reduced levels of 1,25-dihydroxyvitamin D. Hypocalcemia is often asymptomatic but can cause perioral paresthesias, muscle cramps, seizures, hallucinations and confusion, and prolongation of the QT interval and nonspecific T-wave changes on electrocardiography (Chap. 341).

Anemia develops rapidly in ARF and is usually mild and multifactorial in origin. Contributing factors include impaired erythropoiesis, hemolysis, bleeding, hemodilution, and reduced red cell survival time. Prolongation of the *bleeding time* and *leukocytosis* are also common. Common contributors to the bleeding diathesis include mild thrombocytopenia, platelet dysfunction, and/or clotting factor abnormalities (e.g., factor VIII dysfunction), whereas leukocytosis usually reflects sepsis, a stress response, or other concurrent illness. *Infection* is a common and serious complication of ARF, occurring in 50 to 90% of cases and accounting for up to 75% of deaths. It is unclear whether patients with ARF have a clinically significant defect in host immune responses or whether the high incidence of infection reflects repeated breaches of mucocutaneous barriers (e.g., intravenous cannulae, mechanical ventilation, bladder catheterization). *Cardiopulmonary complications* of ARF include arrhythmias, myocardial infarction, pericarditis and pericardial effusion, pulmonary edema, and pulmonary embolism. Mild *gastrointestinal bleeding* is common (10 to 30%) and is usually due to stress ulceration of gastric or small intestinal mucosa.

Protracted periods of severe ARF are invariably associated with the development of the *uremic syndrome* (Chap. 270).

A *vigorous diuresis* can occur during the recovery phase of ARF (see above) and lead to intravascular volume depletion and delayed recovery of GFR by causing secondary prerenal ARF. *Hypernatremia* can also complicate recovery if water losses via hypotonic urine are not replaced or if losses are inappropriately replaced by relatively hypertonic saline solutions. *Hypokalemia*, *hypomagnesemia*, *hypophosphatemia*, and *hypocalcemia* are less common metabolic complications during this period.

℞ TREATMENT **Prevention** Because there are no specific therapies for ischemic or nephrotoxic ARF, prevention is of paramount importance. Many cases of ischemic ARF can be avoided by close attention to cardiovascular function and intravascular volume in high-risk patients, such as the elderly and those with preexisting renal insufficiency. Indeed, aggressive restoration of intravascular volume has been shown to reduce the incidence of ischemic ARF dramatically after major surgery or trauma, burns, or cholera. The incidence of nephrotoxic ARF can be reduced by tailoring the dosage of potential nephrotoxins to body size and GFR; for example, reducing the dose or frequency of administration of drugs in patients with preexisting renal impairment. In this regard, it should be noted that serum creatinine is a relatively insensitive index of GFR and may overestimate GFR considerably in small or elderly patients. For purposes of drug dosing, it is advisable to estimate the GFR using the Cockcroft-Gault formula, which factors in the variables of age and weight (Chap. 47). Adjusting drug dosage according to circulating drug levels also appears to limit renal injury in patients receiving aminoglycoside antibiotics or cyclosporine. Diuretics, cyclooxygenase inhibitors, ACE inhibitors, and other vasodilators should be used with caution in patients with suspected true or "effective" hypovolemia or renovascular disease as they may precipitate prerenal ARF or convert the latter to ischemic ARF. Hypovolemia should be avoided in patients receiving nephrotoxic medications as renal hypoperfusion potentiates the toxicity of most nephrotoxins. Allopurinol and forced alkaline diuresis are useful in patients at high risk for acute urate nephropathy (e.g., cancer chemotherapy in hematologic malignancies) to limit uric acid generation and prevent precipitation of urate crystals in renal tubules. Forced alkaline diuresis may also prevent or attenuate ARF in patients receiving high-dose methotrexate or suffering from rhabdomyolysis. *N*-acetylcysteine limits acetaminophen-induced renal injury if given within 24 h of ingestion. Dimercaprol, a chelating agent, may prevent heavy metal nephrotoxicity. Ethanol inhibits ethylene glycol metabolism to oxalic acid and other toxic metabolites and is an important adjunct to hemodialysis in the emergency management of ethylene glycol intoxication.

Specific Therapies By definition, prerenal ARF is rapidly reversible upon correction of the primary hemodynamic abnormality, and postrenal ARF resolves upon relief of obstruction. To date, there are no specific therapies for established intrinsic renal ARF due to ischemia or nephrotoxicity. Management of these disorders should focus on elimination of the causative hemodynamic abnormality or toxin, avoidance of additional insults, and prevention and treatment of complications. Specific treatment of other causes of intrinsic renal ARF depends on the underlying pathology.

Prerenal ARF The composition of replacement fluids for treatment of prerenal ARF due to hypovolemia must be tailored according to the composition of the lost fluid. Severe hypovolemia due to hemorrhage should be corrected with packed red blood cells, whereas isotonic saline is usually appropriate replacement for mild to moderate hemorrhage or plasma loss (e.g., burns, pancreatitis). Urinary and gastrointestinal fluids can vary greatly in composition but are usually hypotonic. Hypotonic solutions (e.g., 0.45% saline) are usually recommended as initial replacement in patients with prerenal ARF due to increased urinary or gastrointestinal fluid losses, although isotonic saline may be more appropriate in severe cases. Subsequent therapy should be based on measurements of the volume and ionic content of excreted or drained fluids. Serum potassium and acid-base status should be monitored carefully, and potassium and bicarbonate supplemented as appropriate. Cardiac failure may require aggressive management with positive inotropes, preload and afterload reducing agents, antiarrhythmic drugs, and mechanical aids such as intraaortic balloon pumps. Invasive hemodynamic monitoring may be required to guide therapy for complicated conditions in patients in whom clinical assessment of cardiovascular function and intravascular volume proves unreliable.

Fluid management may be particularly difficult in patients with cirrhosis complicated by ascites. In this setting, it is important to distinguish between full-blown hepatorenal syndrome (Chap. 299), which carries a grave prognosis, and reversible ARF due to true or "effective" hypovolemia induced by overzealous use of diuretics or sepsis (e.g., spontaneous bacterial peritonitis). The contribution of hypovolemia to ARF can be definitively assessed only by administration of a fluid challenge. Fluids should be administered slowly and titrated against jugular venous pressure and, if necessary, central venous and pulmonary capillary wedge pressure, abdominal girth, and urine output. Patients with a reversible prerenal component typically have an increase in urine output and fall in serum creatinine, whereas patients with hepatorenal syndrome do not and may suffer increased ascites formation and pulmonary compromise if not monitored closely. Large volumes of ascitic fluid can usually be drained by paracentesis without deterioration in renal function if intravenous albumin is administered simultaneously. Indeed, "large-volume paracentesis" may afford an increase in GFR, possibly by lowering intraabdominal pressure and improving flow in renal veins. Shunting of ascitic fluid from the peritoneum to a central vein (peritoneojugular shunt, LeVeen or Denver shunts) is an alternative approach in refractory cases but has not been shown to improve survival in controlled trials. The efficacy of the newer technique of transjugular intrahepatic portosystemic shunting (TIPS procedure) is currently undergoing rigorous clinical assessment. Shunting can also improve GFR and sodium excretion transiently, probably because the increase in central blood volume stimulates release of atrial natriuretic peptides and inhibits secretion of aldosterone and norepinephrine.

Intrinsic renal ARF Many different approaches have been tested for their ability to attenuate injury or hasten recovery in ischemic and nephrotoxic ARF. These include atrial natriuretic peptide (ANP), low-dose dopamine, loop-blocking diuretics, calcium channel blockers, α-adrenoreceptor blockers, prostaglandin analogues, antioxidants, antibodies against leukocyte adhesion molecules, and insulin-like growth factor. Whereas many of these are beneficial in experimental models of ischemic or nephrotoxic ARF, they have either failed to confer consistent benefit or proved ineffective in humans.

ARF due to other intrinsic renal diseases such as acute glomerulonephritis or vasculitis may respond to glucocorticoids, alkylating agents, and/or plasmapheresis, depending on the primary pathology. Glucocorticoids also hasten remission in some cases of allergic interstitial nephritis. Aggressive control of systemic arterial pressure is of paramount importance in limiting renal injury in malignant hypertensive nephrosclerosis, toxemia of pregnancy, and other vascular diseases. Hypertension and ARF due to scleroderma may be exquisitely sensitive to treatment with ACE inhibitors.

Postrenal ARF Management of postrenal ARF requires close collaboration between nephrologist, urologist, and radiologist. Obstruction of the urethra or bladder neck is usually managed initially by transurethral or suprapubic placement of a bladder catheter, which provides temporary relief while the obstructing lesion is identified and treated definitively. Similarly, ureteric obstruction may be treated initially by percutaneous catheterization of the dilated renal pelvis or ureter. Indeed, obstructing lesions can often be removed percutaneously (e.g., calculus, sloughed papilla) or bypassed by insertion of a ureteric stent (e.g., carcinoma). Most patients experience an appropriate diuresis for several days following relief of obstruction. Approximately 5% of patients develop a transient salt-wasting syndrome that may require administration of intravenous saline to maintain blood pressure.

Supportive Measures (Table 269-4) Following correction of hypovolemia, salt and water intake are tailored to match losses. Hypervolemia can usually be managed by restriction of salt and water

Table 269-4 Management of Ischemic and Nephrotoxic Acute Renal Failure[a]

Management Issue	Therapy
REVERSE CAUSATIVE RENAL INSULT	
Ischemic ARF	Restore systemic hemodynamics and renal perfusion
Nephrotoxic ARF	Eliminate nephrotoxins Consider specific measures (e.g., forced alkaline diuresis, chelators: see text)
PREVENTION AND TREATMENT OF COMPLICATIONS	
Intravascular volume overload	Salt (1–2 g/d) and water (usually <1 L/d) restriction Diuretics (usually loop blockers ± thiazide) Ultrafiltration or dialysis
Hyponatremia	Restriction of enteral free water intake (<1 L/d) Avoid hypotonic intravenous solutions (including dextrose solutions)
Hyperkalemia	Restriction of dietary K^+ intake (usually <40 mmol/d) Eliminate K^+ supplements and K^+-sparing diuretics Potassium-binding ion-exchange resins (e.g., sodium polystyrene sulphonate) Glucose (50 mL of 50% dextrose) and insulin (10 units regular) Sodium bicarbonate (usually 50–100 mmol) Calcium gluconate (10 mL of 10% solution over 5 min) Dialysis (with low K^+ dialysate)
Metabolic acidosis	Restriction of dietary protein (usually 0.6 g/kg per day of high biologic value) Sodium bicarbonate (maintain serum bicarbonate >15 mmol/L or arterial pH >7.2) Dialysis
Hyperphosphatemia	Restriction of dietary phosphate intake (usually <800 mg/d) Phosphate binding agents (calcium carbonate, aluminum hydroxide)
Hypocalcemia	Calcium carbonate (if symptomatic or if sodium bicarbonate to be administered) Calcium gluconate (10–20 mL of 10% solution)
Hypermagnesemia	Discontinue Mg^{2+}-containing antacids
Hyperuricemia	Treatment usually not necessary [if <890 μmol/L (<15 mg/dL)]
Nutrition	Restriction of dietary protein (~0.6 g/kg per day) Carbohydrate (~100 g/d) Enteral or parenteral nutrition (if recovery prolonged or patient very catabolic)
Indications for dialysis	Clinical evidence (symptoms or signs) of uremia Intractable intravascular volume overload Hyperkalemia or severe acidosis resistant to conservative measures ?Prophylactic dialysis when urea >100–150 mg/dL or creatinine >8–10 mg/dL
PRESCRIBING OF MEDICATIONS	
Choice of agents	Avoid other nephrotoxins, ACE inhibitors, cyclooxygenase inhibitors, and radiocontrast unless absolute indication and no alternative agent
Drug dosing	Adjust doses and frequency of administration for degree of renal impairment

[a] These are general recommendations and must be tailored to needs of individual patients.

intake and diuretics. Indeed, there is, as yet, no proven rationale for administration of diuretics in ARF except to treat this complication. High doses of loop-blocking diuretics such as furosemide (up to 200 to 400 mg intravenously) or bumetanide (up to 10 mg intravenously administered as a bolus or by continuous infusion) may promote diuresis in patients who fail to respond to conventional doses. Subpressor doses of dopamine are claimed to promote salt and water excretion by increasing renal blood flow and GFR and by inhibiting tubule sodium reabsorption; however, subpressor ("low-dose," "renal-dose,") dopamine has proved ineffective in clinical trials and may trigger arrythmias and sudden cardiac death in critically ill patients. Ultrafiltration or dialysis is used to treat severe hypervolemia when conservative measures fail. Hyponatremia and hypoosmolality can usually be controlled by restriction of free water intake. Conversely, hypernatremia is treated by administration of water or intravenous hypotonic saline or isotonic dextrose–containing solutions.

→***The management of hyperkalemia is described in Chap. 49.***

Metabolic acidosis is not treated unless serum bicarbonate concentration falls below 15 mmol/L or arterial pH falls below 7.2. More severe acidosis is corrected by oral or intravenous sodium bicarbonate. Initial rates of replacement are guided by estimates of bicarbonate deficit and adjusted thereafter according to serum levels (Chap. 50). Patients are monitored for complications of bicarbonate administration such as hypervolemia, metabolic alkalosis, hypocalcemia, and hypokalemia. From a practical point of view, most patients requiring sodium bicarbonate need emergency dialysis within days. Hyperphosphatemia is usually controlled by restriction of dietary phosphate and by oral aluminum hydroxide or calcium carbonate, which reduce gastrointestinal absorption of phosphate. Hypocalcemia does not usually require treatment unless severe, as may occur with rhabdomyolysis or pancreatitis or following admininstration of bicarbonate. Hyperuricemia is typically mild [<890 μmol/L (< 15 mg/dL)] and does not require intervention.

The objective of *nutritional management* during the maintenance phase of ARF is to provide sufficient calories to avoid catabolism and starvation ketoacidosis, while minimizing production of nitrogenous waste. This is best achieved by restricting dietary protein to approximately 0.6 g/kg per day of protein of high biologic value (i.e., rich in essential amino acids) and to provide most calories as carbohydrate (approximately 100 g daily). Nutritional management is easier in nonoliguric patients and following institution of dialysis. Vigorous parenteral hyperalimentation is claimed to improve prognosis; however, convincing benefit has yet to be demonstrated in controlled trials.

Anemia may necessitate blood transfusion if severe or if recovery is delayed. In contrast to chronic renal failure, recombinant human erythropoietin is rarely used in ARF because bone marrow resistance to erythropoietin is common, more immediate treatment of anemia (if any) is required, and renal failure is usually self-limiting. Uremic bleeding usually responds to correction of anemia, administration of desmopressin or estrogens, or dialysis. Regular doses of antacids appear to reduce the incidence of gastrointestinal hemorrhage significantly and may be more effective in this regard than H_2 antagonists, or proton pump inhibitors. Meticulous care of intravenous cannulae, bladder catheters, and other invasive devices is mandatory to avoid infections. Unfortunately, prophylactic antibiotics have not been shown to reduce the incidence of infection in these high-risk patients.

Indications and modalities of dialysis Dialysis replaces renal function until regeneration and repair restore renal function. Hemodialysis and peritoneal dialysis appear equally effective for management of ARF. Thus, the dialysis modality is chosen according to the needs of individual patients (e.g., peritoneal dialysis may be preferable if the patient is hemodynamically unstable, and hemodialysis after abdominal surgery involving the peritoneum), the expertise of the nephrologist, and the facilities of the institution. Vascular access for conventional intermittent hemodialysis is best achieved by insertion of a temporary double-lumen hemodialysis catheter into the internal jugular vein. The subclavian and femoral veins are alternative access sites. Peritoneal dialysis is achieved by insertion of a single-lumen cuffed catheter into the peritoneal cavity. Absolute indications for dialysis include symptoms or signs of the uremic syndrome and management of refractory hypervolemia, hyperkalemia, or acidosis. Many nephrologists also initiate dialysis empirically for blood urea levels of >100 mg/dL, even in the absence of clinical uremia; however, this approach has yet to be validated in controlled clinical trials. Nor is it clear whether intensive dialysis prescribed to maintain blood urea and creatinine below a certain level is beneficial. The latter are important issues since unnecessary or intensive hemodialysis can exacerbate ATN and delay renal recovery by triggering hypotension and repeated renal hypoperfusion. Moreover, an expanding body of evidence suggests that leukocytes, activated directly by contact with hemodialysis membranes or as a result of membrane-triggered complement activation, then travel to the already-compromised renal microcirculation where they further exacerbate renal injury.

Continuous arteriovenous hemodiafiltration (CAVH) and continuous venovenous hemodiafiltration (CVVH) are alternatives to conventional intermittent hemodialysis techniques for treatment of ARF. They are particularly valuable techniques in patients in whom intermittent hemodialysis fails to control hypervolemia or uremia and for those who do not tolerate intermittent hemodialysis and in whom peritoneal dialysis is not possible. CAVH requires both arterial and venous access. The patient's own blood pressure generates an ultrafiltrate of plasma across a porous biocompatible dialysis membrane. A physiologic crystalloid solution is passed along the other side of the membrane to achieve diffusive clearance. CVVH, in contrast, requires only a double-lumen venous catheter as a blood pump generates ultrafiltration pressure across the dialysis membrane. These newer continuous techniques have not been compared to conventional intermittent hemodialysis in prospective, adequately controlled trials, and the choice of technique is currently tailored to the specific needs of the patient, the resources of the institution, and the expertise of the physician. Potential disadvantages of continuous hemodialysis techniques are the need for prolonged immobilization in bed, systemic anticoagulation, arterial cannulation (in CAVH), and prolonged exposure of blood to synthetic, albeit relatively biocompatible, dialysis membranes.

OUTCOME AND LONG-TERM PROGNOSIS

The mortality rate among patients with ARF approximates 50% and has changed little over the past 30 years. It should be stressed, however, that patients usually die from sequelae of the primary illness that induced ARF and not from ARF itself. Indeed, the kidney is one of the few organs whose function can be replaced artificially (i.e., by dialysis) for protracted periods of time. In agreement with this interpretation, mortality rates vary greatly depending on the cause of ARF: ~15% in obstetric patients, ~30% in toxin-related ARF, and ~60% following trauma or major surgery. Oliguria (<400 mL/d) at time of presentation and a rise in serum creatinine of >265 μmol/L (>3 mg/dL) are associated with a poor prognosis and probably reflect the severity of renal injury and of the primary illness. Mortality rates are higher in older debilitated patients and in those with multiple organ failure. Most patients who survive an episode of ARF recover sufficient renal function to live normal lives. However, 50% have subclinical impairment of renal function or residual scarring on renal biopsy. Approximately 5% of patients never recover function and require long-term renal replacement with dialysis or transplantation. An additional 5% suffer progressive decline in GFR, following an initial recovery phase, probably due to hemodynamic stress and sclerosis of remnant glomeruli (Chap. 273).

BIBLIOGRAPHY

BRADY HR, WILCOX CS (eds): *Therapy in Nephrology and Hypertension.* Philadelphia, Saunders, 1999

——— et al: Acute renal failure, in *Brenner and Rector's The Kidney*, 6th ed., BM Brenner (ed). Philadelphia, Saunders, 2000, pp 1201–1262

DENTON MD et al: "Renal-dose" dopamine for the treatment of acute renal failure: Scientific rationale, experimental studies and clinical trials. Kidney Int 49:4, 1996

HAKIM RM et al: Effect of dialysis membrane in the treatment of patients with acute renal failure. N Engl J Med 334:1338, 1994

HIMMELFARB J et al: Mutlicenter comparison of dialysis membranes in the treatment of acute renal failure requiring dialysis. J Am Soc Nephrol 9:257, 1998

MEYER MM: Renal Replacement therapies. Crit Care Clinics 16:29, 2000

OLSEN S, SOLEZ K: Acute tubular necrosis and toxic renal injury, in *Renal Pathology with Clinical and Functional Correlations*, 2d ed, CC Tisher, BM Brenner (eds). Philadelphia, Lippincott, 1994, pp 769–809

STAR RA: Treatment of acute renal failure. Kidney Int 54:1817, 1998

THADHANI R et al: Acute renal failure. N Engl J Med 334:1448, 1996

270

Karl Skorecki, Jacob Green, Barry M. Brenner

CHRONIC RENAL FAILURE

MECHANISMS OF CHRONIC RENAL FAILURE

DEFINITIONS *Chronic renal disease (CRD)* is a pathophysiologic process with multiple etiologies, resulting in the inexorable attrition of nephron number and function, and frequently leading to *end-stage renal disease (ESRD)*. In turn, ESRD represents a clinical state or condition in which there has been an irreversible loss of endogenous renal function, of a degree sufficient to render the patient permanently dependent upon renal replacement therapy (dialysis or transplantation) in order to avoid life-threatening *uremia*. Uremia is the clinical and laboratory syndrome, reflecting dysfunction of all organ systems as a result of untreated or undertreated acute or chronic renal failure. Given the capacity of the kidneys to regain function following acute injury (Chap. 269), the vast majority (>90%) of patients with ESRD have reached this state as a result of CRD.

PATHOPHYSIOLOGY OF CRD The pathophysiology of CRD involves initiating mechanisms specific to the underlying etiology as well as a set of progressive mechanisms that are a common consequence following long-term reduction of renal mass, irrespective of etiology. Such reduction of renal mass causes structural and functional hypertrophy of surviving nephrons. This compensatory hypertrophy is mediated by vasoactive molecules, cytokines, and growth factors and is due initially to adaptive hyperfiltration, in turn mediated by increases in glomerular capillary pressure and flow. Eventually, these short-term adaptations prove maladaptive, in that they predispose to sclerosis of the remaining viable nephron population. This final common pathway for inexorable attrition of residual nephron function may persist even after the initiating or underlying disease process has become inactive. Increased intrarenal activity of the renin-angiotensin axis appears to contribute both to the initial adaptive hyperfiltration and to the subsequent maladaptive hypertrophy and sclerosis. These maladaptive long-term actions of renin-angiotensin axis activation are mediated in part through downstream growth factors such as transforming growth factor β. Interindividual variability in the risk and rate of CRD progression can be explained in part by variations in the genes encoding components of these and other pathways involved in glomerular and tubulointerstitial fibrosis and sclerosis (see "Genetic Considerations in the Progression of CRD," below).

The earliest stage common to all forms of CRD is a loss of renal reserve. When kidney function is entirely normal, glomerular filtration rate (GFR) can be augmented by 20 to 30% in response to the stimulus of a protein challenge. During the earliest stage of loss of renal reserve, basal GFR may be normal or even elevated (hyperfiltration), but the expected further rise in response to a protein challenge is attenuated. This early stage is particularly well documented in diabetic nephropathy. At this stage, the only clue may be at the level of laboratory measurements, which estimate GFR. The most commonly utilized laboratory measurements are the serum urea and creatinine concentrations. By the time serum urea and creatinine concentrations are even mildly elevated, substantial chronic nephron injury has already occurred.

Table 270-1 Prevalence and Incidence Counts by Major Etiology for U.S. Medicare–Treated End-Stage Renal Disease for 1997

	Prevalence, n = 304,083		Incidence, n = 79.102	
	Count	Percent	Count	Percent
Diabetes	100,892	33.2	33,096	41.8
Hypertension	72,961	24.0	20,066	25.4
Glomerulonephritis	52,229	17.2	7,390	9.3
Cystic disease	13,992	4.6	1,772	2.2

SOURCE: From United States Renal Data System 1999 Annual Report Preliminary Data, U.S. Department of Health and Human Services, Health Care Financing Administration (www.med.umich.edu/usrds/).

As GFR declines to levels as low as 30% of normal, patients may remain asymptomatic with only biochemical evidence of the decline in GFR, i.e., rise in serum concentrations of urea and creatinine. However, careful scrutiny usually reveals early additional clinical and laboratory manifestations of renal insufficiency. These may include nocturia, mild anemia and loss of energy, decreasing appetite and early disturbances in nutritional status, and abnormalities in calcium and phosphorus metabolism (*moderate renal insufficiency*). As GFR falls to below 30% of normal, an increasing number and severity of uremic clinical manifestations and biochemical abnormalities supervene (*severe renal insufficiency*). At the stages of mild and moderate renal insufficiency, intercurrent clinical stress may compromise renal function still further, inducing signs and symptoms of overt uremia. Such intercurrent clinical conditions to which patients with CRD may be particularly susceptible include infection (urinary, respiratory, or gastrointestinal), poorly controlled hypertension, hyper- or hypovolemia, and drug or radiocontrast nephrotoxicity, among others. When GFR falls below 5 to 10% of normal (ESRD), continued survival without renal replacement therapy becomes impossible.

ETIOLOGY There has been a dramatic increase in the incidence of ESRD as well as a shift in the relative incidence of etiologies of CRD during the past two decades. Whereas glomerulonephritis was the leading cause of CRD in the past, diabetic and hypertensive nephropathy are now much more frequent underlying etiologies (Table 270-1). This may be a consequence of more effective prevention and treatment of glomerulonephritis or of diminished mortality from other causes among individuals with diabetes and hypertension. Greater overall longevity and diminished premature cardiovascular mortality have also increased the mean age of patients presenting with ESRD. Hypertension is a particularly common cause of CRD in the elderly, in whom chronic renal ischemia due to renovascular disease may be an underrecognized additional contribution to the pathophysiologic process. Many patients present at an advanced stage of CRD, precluding definitive determination of etiology.

GENETIC CONSIDERATIONS **Progression of CRD** Disorders with clear-cut monogenic inheritance comprise a small but important component among the etiologies of CRD. Among these, autosomal dominant polycystic kidney disease is the most common on a world-wide basis (Chap. 276). Alport's hereditary nephritis (Chap. 275) is a less common cause of both benign hematuria without progression to CRD and more severe nephron injury with progression to ESRD, and it usually displays an X-linked pattern of inheritance. In contrast, the two most common etiologies of CRD (Table 270-1), namely diabetes mellitus (both types 1 and 2) and essential hypertension, display complex polygenic patterns of inheritance. Both candidate locus and genome-wide strategies have been used to pinpoint genes that contribute to the risks for development of these disorders.

Recent evidence also suggests that reflux nephropathy may have a heritable basis, again involving the contribution of several genetic loci.

Striking interindividual variability in the rate of progression to ESRD is a characteristic feature among patients with either inherited or acquired causes of CRD, irrespective of underlying etiology. This interindividual variability has an important heritable component, clarification of which may help guide therapeutic approaches. A number of genetic loci that contribute to the progression of CRD have been identified. Most extensively studied has been an insertion/deletion polymorphism of the angiotensin-converting enzyme (ACE) gene, previously shown to contribute to cardiovascular disease risk. Studies in a wide variety of disorders, including diabetic nephropathy, glomerulonephritis, polycystic kidney disease, and CRD caused by urologic abnormalities, have revealed an important contribution of this locus to progressive deterioration of renal function. The two different alleles defined by this polymorphism of the ACE gene are associated with corresponding differences in the endogenous activity of the encoded enzyme. The homozygous deletion (D/D) variant is associated with the highest expression of endogenous ACE activity and a greater risk of CRD progression. This finding has important therapeutic implications and leads to the prediction that ACE inhibitor therapy might be most effective in patients who are homozygous for the "at-risk" allele. Similar conclusions have been reached with respect to genes encoding other components of the renin-angiotensin axis, including the angiotensinogen gene, and the angiotensin receptor. These findings are consistent with the important role of intraglomerular hemodynamic perturbations in progressive renal injury. ■

PATHOPHYSIOLOGY AND BIOCHEMISTRY OF UREMIA The uremic syndrome results from functional derangements of many organ systems, although the prominence of specific symptoms varies among patients. *Azotemia* refers to the retention of nitrogenous waste products as renal insufficiency develops. *Uremia* refers to the more advanced stages of progressive renal insufficiency when the complex, multiorgan system derangements become clinically manifest. The term uremia was adopted originally because of the presumption that all of the abnormalities result from retention in the blood of end products of metabolism normally excreted in the urine. The most likely candidates as toxins in uremia are the by-products of protein and amino acid metabolism. Unlike fats and carbohydrates, which are eventually metabolized to carbon dioxide and water—substances readily excreted even in uremic subjects via lungs and skin—the products of protein and amino acid metabolism depend primarily on the kidneys for excretion. Although a number of such products have been identified (Table 270-2), the clinical symptoms of uremia correlate poorly with the blood levels of these products. This is because uremia involves more than renal excretory failure alone. A host of metabolic and endocrine functions normally subserved by the kidney are also impaired, resulting in anemia; malnutrition; impaired metabolism of carbohydrates, fats, and proteins; defective utilization of energy; and metabolic bone disease. Thus, the pathophysiology of the uremic syndrome can be divided into those sets of abnormalities consequent to the accumulation of products of protein metabolism on the one hand, and on the other hand, abnormalities consequent to the loss of other renal functions, such as fluid and electrolyte homeostasis and synthesis of certain hormones [e.g., erythropoietin (EPO), 1.25-dihydroxycholecalciferol].

Although not the major cause of overt uremic toxicity, urea may contribute to some of the clinical abnormalities, including anorexia, malaise, vomiting, and headache. Elevated levels of plasma *guanidinosuccinic acid*, by interfering with activation of platelet factor III by ADP, contribute to the impaired platelet function in CRD. *Creatinine* may cause adverse effects following conversion to metabolites such as sarcosine and methylguanidine. Nitrogenous compounds with a molecular mass of 500 to 12,000 Da (so-called middle molecules) are also

Table 270-2 Uremic "Toxins"

By-products of protein and amino acid metabolism
- Urea—80% of total (excreted nitrogen)
- Guanidino compounds
  - Guanidine
  - Methylguanidine
  - Dimethylguanidine
  - Creatinine
  - Creatine
  - Guanidinosuccinic acid
- Urates and hippurates
- End products of nucleic acid metabolism
- End products of aliphatic amine metabolism
- End products of aromatic amino acid metabolism
  - Tryptophan
  - Tyrosine
  - Phenylalanine
- Other nitrogenous substances
  - Polyamines
  - Myoinositol
  - Phenols
  - Benzoates
  - Indoles
- Advanced glycation end products

Inhibitors of ligand-protein binding
Glucuronoconjugates and aglycones
Inhibitors of somatomedin and insulin action

retained in CRD and similarly are believed to contribute to morbidity and mortality in uremic subjects. Decreased renal excretion is not the only reason why such middle-sized molecules, along with various cytokines and growth factors, accumulate in uremic plasma. The kidney normally catabolizes a number of circulating plasma proteins and polypeptides; with reduced renal mass, this capacity is impaired. Furthermore, plasma levels of many polypeptide hormones, including parathyroid hormone (PTH) insulin, glucagon, luteinizing hormone, and prolactin, rise with renal failure, not only because of impaired renal catabolism but also because of enhanced glandular secretion. Of these, excessive PTH has been suggested to be an important uremic "toxin" because of its adverse effect of elevating cellular cytosolic Ca^{2+} levels in several tissues and organs.

CLINICAL AND LABORATORY MANIFESTATIONS OF CHRONIC RENAL FAILURE AND UREMIA

Uremia leads to disturbances in the function of every organ system. Chronic dialysis (Chap. 271) reduces the incidence and severity of these disturbances, so that, where modern medicine is practiced, the overt and florid manifestations of uremia have largely disappeared. Unfortunately, as indicated in Table 270-3, even optimal dialysis therapy is not a panacea, because some disturbances resulting from impaired renal function fail to respond fully, while others continue to progress.

FLUID, ELECTROLYTE, AND ACID-BASE DISORDERS (See also Chaps. 49 and 50) **Sodium and Water Homeostasis** When the GFR is normal, >24,000 mmol of Na^+ are filtered per day. An overwhelming fraction of this Na^+ load is reabsorbed by the tubules, leaving only a small fraction (usually <1%) to be excreted. Thus, even when the GFR falls markedly to levels as low as 10% of normal, the filtered load of Na^+ still far exceeds daily requirements for urinary Na^+ excretion. Therefore, any abnormalities in overall Na^+ balance will reflect the relationship between the filtered load and fractional reabsorption (glomerulotubular balance). Progressive nephron injury can be associated with a tendency to Na^+ retention, Na^+ wasting, or maintenance of Na^+ balance, depending in part on the underlying etiology (glomerular vs. tubulointerstitial disease), ongoing diuretic treatment, and comorbid conditions that affect Na^+ balance, such as cardiac failure or cirrhosis. Osmotic regulation of vasopressin release and of thirst are also preserved. Even when tubule response to vasopressin is diminished, normal thirst mechanisms and access to H_2O generally prevent hypernatremia. However, a compromised capacity to excrete a maximally dilute urine with progressive CRD may lead to hyponatremia.

In most patients with stable CRD, the total body contents of Na^+ and H_2O are increased modestly, although this may not be clinically apparent. The underlying etiologic disease process may itself disrupt glomerulotubular balance and promote Na^+ retention (e.g., glomerulonephitis), or excessive Na^+ ingestion may lead to cumulative positive Na^+ balance and attendant extracellular fluid volume (ECFV) expansion. Such ECFV expansion contributes to hypertension, which in turn accelerates further the progression of nephron injury. As long as water intake does not exceed the capacity for free water clearance, the ECFV expansion will be isotonic and the patient will remain normonatremic. On the other hand, hyponatremia will be the consequence of excessive water ingestion. However, in view of the concomitant impairment in urinary concentrating mechanism, severe hyponatremia is not usual in predialysis patients, and water restriction is only necessary when hyponatremia is documented. In such patients, a daily intake of fluid equal to the urine volume per day plus about 500 mL usually maintains the serum Na^+ concentration at normal levels.

Table 270-3 Clinical Abnormalities in Uremia[a]

Fluid and electrolyte disturbances Volume expansion and contraction (I) Hypernatremia and hyponatremia (I) Hyperkalemia and hypokalemia (I) Metabolic acidosis (I) Hyperphosphatemia (I) Hypocalcemia (I) Endocrine-metabolic disturbances Secondary hyperparathyroidism (I or P) Adynamic osteomalacia (D) Vitamin D–deficient osteomalacia (I) Carbohydrate intolerance (I) Hyperuricemia (I or P) Hypertriglyceridemia (I or P) Increased Lp(a) level (P) Decreased high-density lipoprotein level (P) Protein-calorie malnutrition (I or P) Impaired growth and development (P) Infertility and sexual dysfunction (P) Amenorrhea (P) Hypothermia (I) Dialysis-induced β_2-microglobulin Amyloidosis (P)	Neuromuscular disturbances Fatigue (I)[b] Sleep disorders (P) Headache (I or P) Impaired mentation (I)[b] Lethargy (I)[b] Asterixis (I) Muscular irritability (I) Peripheral neuropathy (I or P) Restless legs syndrome (I or P) Paralysis (I or P) Myoclonus (I) Seizures (I or P) Coma (I) Muscle cramps (D) Dialysis disequilibrium syndrome (D) Myopathy (P or D) Cardiovascular and pulmonary disturbances Arterial hypertension (I or P) Congestive heart failure or pulmonary edema (I) Pericarditis (I) Cardiomyopathy (I or P) Uremic lung (I) Accelerated atherosclerosis (P or D) Hypotension and arrhythmias (D) Vascular calcification (P or D)	Dermatologic disturbances Pallor (I)[b] Hyperpigmentation (I, P, or D) Pruritus (P) Ecchymoses (I) Uremic frost (I) Gastrointestinal disturbances Anorexia (I) Nausea and vomiting (I) Uremic fetor (I) Gastroenteritis (I) Peptic ulcer (I or P) Gastrointestinal bleeding (I, P, or D) Hepatitis (D) Idiopathic ascites (D) Peritonitis (D) Hematologic and immunologic disturbances Anemia (I)[b] Lymphocytopenia (P) Bleeding diathesis (I or D)[b] Increased susceptibility to infection (I or P) Splenomegaly and hypersplenism (P) Leukopenia (D) Hypocomplementemia (D)

[a] Virtually all abnormalities in this table are completely reversed in time by successful renal transplantation. The response of these abnormalities to hemodialysis or peritoneal dialysis therapy is more variable. (I) denotes an abnormality that usually improves with an optimal program of dialysis and related therapy; (P) denotes one that tends to persist or even progress, despite an optimal program; (D) denotes one that develops only after initiation of dialysis therapy.

[b] Improves with dialysis and erythropoietin therapy.

Weight gain usually associated with volume expansion may be offset in patients with CRD by concomitant loss of lean body mass. In the CRD patient who is not yet on dialysis but has clear evidence of ECFV expansion, administration of loop diuretics coupled with restriction of salt intake are the mainstays of therapy. It should be noted that resistance to loop diuretics in renal failure often mandates use of higher doses than those usually used when GFR is well preserved. The combination of loop diuretics with metalozone, which inhibits the Na-Cl cotransporter of the distal convoluted tubule, can sometimes overcome diuretic resistance. When the GFR falls to <5 to 10 mL/min, even high doses of combination diuretics are ineffective. ECFV expansion under these circumstances usually means that dialysis is indicated. In dialysis patients with volume expansion, management should include ultrafiltration and restriction of salt and water intake between dialysis treatments.

Patients with CRD also have impaired renal mechanisms for conserving Na^+ and H_2O (Chap. 268). When an *extrarenal* cause for fluid loss is present (e.g., vomiting, diarrhea, sweating, fever), these patients are prone to volume depletion. Depletion of ECFV may compromise residual renal function with resulting signs and symptoms of overt uremia. Because of impaired renal Na^+ and H_2O conservation mechanisms, the usual indices of prerenal azotemia (oliguria, high urine osmolality, low urinary Na^+ concentration, and low fractional excretion of Na^+) are not useful. Cautious volume repletion, usually with normal saline, returns ECFV to normal and usually restores renal function to prior levels.

Potassium Homeostasis (See also Chap. 49) When GFR is normal, the approximate daily filtered load of K^+ is 700 mmol. The majority of this filtered load is reabsorbed in tubule segments prior to the cortical collecting tubule, and most of the K^+ excreted in the final urine reflects events governing K^+ handling at the level of the cortical collecting tubule and beyond. These factors include the flow of luminal fluid and the delivery and reabsorption of Na^+, which generates the lumen-negative electromotive force for K^+ secretion at the aldosterone-responsive distal nephron sites. In CRD, these factors may be well preserved, such that a decline in GFR is not necessarily accompanied by a concomitant and proportionate decline in urinary K^+ excretion. In addition, K^+ excretion in the gastrointestinal tract is augmented in patients with CRD. However, hyperkalemia may be precipitated in a number of clinical situations, including augmented dietary intake, protein catabolism, hemolysis, hemorrhage, transfusion of stored red blood cells, metabolic acidosis, and following the exposure to a variety of medications that inhibit K^+ entry into cells or K^+ secretion in the distal nephron. Most commonly encountered medications in this regard are beta blockers, ACE inhibitors, K^+-sparing diuretics (amiloride, triamterene, spironolactone), and nonsteroidal anti-inflammatory drugs (NSAIDs). In addition, certain etiologies of CRD may be associated with earlier and more severe disruption of K^+ secretory mechanisms in the distal nephron, relative to the reduction in GFR. Most important are conditions associated with hyporeninemic hypoaldosteronism (e.g., diabetic nephropathy and certain forms of distal renal tubular acidosis; Chap. 49).

Most commonly, clinically significant hyperkalemia does not occur until the GFR falls to below 10 mL/min or unless there is exposure to a K^+ load, either endogenous (e.g., hemolysis, trauma, infection) or exogenous (e.g., administration of stored blood, K^+-containing medications, K^+-containing dietary salt substitute). In kidney transplant re-

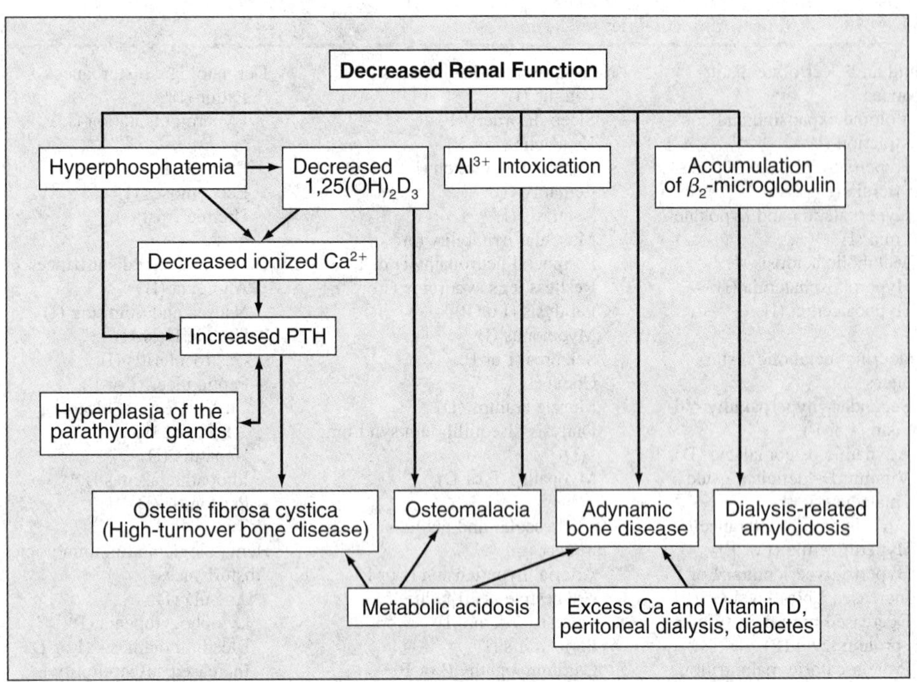

FIGURE 270-1 Flowchart for the development of bone, phosphate, and calcium abnormalities in chronic renal disease. (PTH, parathyroid hormone; PD, peritoneal dialysis.)

cipients, cyclosporine is another common cause of increased plasma K^+ concentration. Hyperkalemia in CRD patients may also be induced by abrupt falls in plasma pH, since acidosis is associated with efflux of K^+ from the intracellular to the extracellular fluid compartment.

Although total-body K^+ is frequently reduced in CRD, *hypokalemia* is uncommon. The occurrence of hypokalemia usually reflects markedly reduced dietary K^+ intake, in association with excessive diuretic therapy or gastrointestinal losses. Hypokalemia occurs as a result of primary renal K^+ wasting in association with other solute transport abnormalities, as in Fanconi's syndrome, renal tubular acidosis, or other forms of hereditary or acquired tubulointerstitial diseases. However, even under these circumstances, as GFR declines, the tendency to hypokalemia diminishes and hyperkalemia may supervene. Accordingly, K^+ supplementation and K^+-sparing diuretics should be used with caution as GFR declines.

Metabolic Acidosis (See also Chap. 50) In adults, the metabolism of dietary protein generates approximately 1 mmol/kg per day of H^+. The H^+ must be excreted, primarily by renal mechanisms, if neutral acid-base balance is to be maintained. Acidosis is a common disturbance during the advanced stages of CRD. Although in a majority of patients with CRD the urine can be acidified normally, these patients have a reduced ability to produce ammonia. In part this is a consequence of limited ATP utilization, resulting from diminished Na^+ reabsorption in the proximal tubule. As a result, the use of glutamine as an energy source is limited, which in turn limits proximal tubule ammonia production. Hyperkalemia, when present, further depresses urinary ammonium excretion. The combination of hyperkalemia and hyperchloremic metabolic acidosis (known as type IV renal tubular acidosis or hyporeninemic hypoaldosteronism) is most characteristically seen in patients with diabetes or in those with predominantly tubulointerstitial disease. Treatment of the hyperkalemia frequently improves the acidosis as well.

With advancing renal failure, total urinary net daily acid excretion is usually limited to 30 to 40 mmol; thus, throughout the remainder of their course of CRD, many patients may be in a positive H^+ balance of 20 to 40 mmol/d. The retained H^+ is buffered by bone salts. In the early stages, the accompanying organic anions are excreted in the urine, and the metabolic acidosis is of the non-anion gap variety. However, with advanced renal failure, a fairly large "anion gap" may develop (to approximately 20 mmol/L) with a reciprocal fall in plasma HCO_3^- concentration. In most patients, the metabolic acidosis is mild and the pH is rarely less than 7.35. The metabolic acidosis can usually be corrected by treating the patient with 20 to 30 mmol of sodium bicarbonate or sodium citrate daily. However, the concomitant Na^+ load mandates careful attention to volume status and the potential need for diuretic agents. Also, citrate enhances aluminum absorption in the large bowel, and citrate-containing antacids should be avoided if aluminum-containing drugs are also administered. As with other abnormalities in CRD, severe symptomatic manifestations of acid-base imbalance occur when the patient is challenged with an excessive endogenous or exogenous acid load or loses excessive alkali (e.g., with diarrhea).

BONE, PHOSPHATE, AND CALCIUM ABNORMALITIES (Fig. 270-1) (See also Chap. 340) Although clinical symptoms of bone disease are present before dialysis in fewer than 10% of patients with ESRD, radiologic and histologic abnormalities are observed in about 35 and 90%, respectively. Two principal types of bone disorders are observed in patients with ESRD: a high-turnover osteodystrophy, known as *osteitis fibrosa cystica*, and a low-turnover state characterized initially by *osteomalacia* and subsequently by *adynamic bone disease*. In osteitis fibrosa, the number and size of the osteoclasts are increased, as are the number and depth of the osteoclastic resorption lacunae. Collagen deposition is less ordered, and the rate of bone turnover is markedly increased. In osteomalacia, the rate of mineralization is slower than that of collagen synthesis, resulting in excessive accumulation of unmineralized osteoid and widened osteoid seams. In adynamic uremic osteodystrophy, a parallel marked reduction in the rate of mineralization and collagen synthesis results in osteoid seams of normal width. While these disorders are often discussed as if they were distinct, they commonly overlap in a given patient with ESRD.

High-Turnover Uremic Osteodystrophy This condition is associated with elevated PTH levels. The hyperparathyroid state is attributable both to hyperplastic growth of the parathyroid glands and to augmented release of hormone from each individual parathyroid cell. The main factors responsible for deranged PTH synthesis in CRD are related to altered metabolism of phosphate, calcitrol [$1,25(OH)_2D_3$], and Ca^{2+}.

Phosphate (PO_4^{3-}) Hyperphosphatemia is a feature of advanced renal failure. The serum phosphate concentration rises in patients with a GFR < 20 mL/min, but retention of PO_4^{3-} can be documented in balance studies with even less severe declines in GFR. The retained PO_4^{3-} is a major cause of the development of secondary hyperparathyroidism in CRD. PO_4^{3-} exerts indirect effects on PTH secretion by decreasing renal production of calcitriol (see below) and by lowering plasma ionized Ca^{2+}. Recent studies also suggest a direct stimulatory role of PO_4^{3-} at the level of the parathyroid gland, in the absence of changes in serum Ca^{2+} or calcitriol levels. Dietary restriction of PO_4^{3-} as well as gastrointestinal PO_4^{3-} binders may prevent hyperphosphatemia, thereby mitigating the rise in PTH levels.

Calcitriol Under normal conditions, calcitriol exerts negative feedback control on the parathyroid gland through both direct (i.e., diminished transcription of pre-proPTH mRNA) and indirect mechanisms. The latter act through stimulation of intestinal absorption of Ca^{2+} and the skeletal mobilization of Ca^{2+}, thereby increasing plasma Ca^{2+} and inhibiting PTH secretion. Therefore, reduced synthesis of $1,25(OH)_2D_3$ during CRD plays a key role in the pathogenesis of hyperparathyroidism, both directly and through hypocalcemia. The abnormal vitamin D metabolism may be related to the renal disease itself (since the active vitamin D metabolite is normally produced in the proximal tubule) and to the hyperphosphatemia, which has a suppressive effect on the renal 1α-hydroxylase enzyme. Furthermore, a decrease in the number of calcitriol receptors in the parathyroid tissue of uremic patients has been reported by several groups. Recent studies have demonstrated a marked decrease in vitamin D–receptor expression in areas of nodular transformation within hyperplastic parathyroid tissue but revealed no such receptor downregulation in diffuse hyperplastic parathyroid tissue. Since vitamin D also has an antiproliferative effect on parathyroid cells, this phenomenon may provide an explanation for the marked PTH secretion as well as the abnormal glandular growth pattern characteristic of nodular hyperparathyroidism.

Calcium The total plasma Ca^{2+} concentration in patients with CRD is often significantly lower than normal. Patients with CRD tolerate the hypocalcemia quite well; rarely is a patient symptomatic from the decreased Ca^{2+} concentration. This may partly be due to the frequent concomitant acidosis, which offsets some of the neuromuscular effects of hypocalcemia. The hypocalcemia in CRD results from decreased intestinal absorption of Ca^{2+} due to vitamin D deficiency (see above). Also, with the increasing serum PO_4^{3-} level, Ca^{2+} phosphate is deposited in soft tissues and serum Ca^{2+} concentration (both total and ionized) declines. In addition, patients with CRD are resistant to the action of PTH. Hypocalcemia is a potent stimulus to PTH secretion and leads to hyperplasia of the parathyroid gland. Ca^{2+} binds to a specific Ca^{2+}-sensing receptor protein located in the cell membrane. The Ca^{2+}-sensing receptor is linked to several cytoplasmic messenger systems by one or more GTP-binding proteins. These signaling pathways are responsible for either enhanced or suppressed release of PTH during acute hypo- and hypercalcemia, respectively. Several studies have demonstrated the mRNA and protein expression of the Ca^{2+}-sensing receptor to be reduced in primary (adenomas) and secondary hyperparathyroidism (hyperplasia) compared to the expression in normal parathyroid tissue. In secondary hyperparathyroidism, expression of the Ca^{2+}-sensing receptor is often depressed in nodular areas compared with adjacent nonnodular hyperplasia. Thus, decreased Ca^{2+} receptor expression in hyperparathyroidism is compatible with a less efficient control of PTH synthesis and release, in response to varying plasma Ca^{2+} concentration.

In addition to excessive release of PTH from individual parathyroid cells, the size of the glands also increases as renal failure progresses. This abnormal growth of the parathyroid glands may assume one of the following patterns: (1) diffuse hyperplasia (polyclonal growth), (2) nodular growth (monoclonal growth) within diffuse hyperplastic tissue, or (3) diffuse monoclonal hyperplasia ("adenoma," or tertiary autonomous hyperparathyroidism). Patients with monoclonal ("autonomous") hyperplasia are especially prone to develop hypercalcemia following successful kidney transplantation, often necessitating parathyroidectomy.

During the initial phase of CRD, the elevated PTH levels may normalize serum levels of Ca^{2+}, PO_4^{3-}, and vitamin D. Therefore hypocalcemia, hyperphosphatemia, and reduced $1,25(OH)_2D_3$ are observed only as CRD progresses. However, even at the earliest stages of CRD, the elevated PTH levels adversely affect bone metabolism, causing increased osteoclastic and osteoblastic activity (high-turnover bone disease). Additional detrimental factors include the chronic uremic acidosis, which inhibits osteoblastic bone formation and stimulates osteoclastic bone resorption.

Low-Turnover Uremic Osteodystrophy Originally thought to result solely from vitamin D deficiency, *osteomalacia* (Chap. 342) has now been more closely associated with aluminum toxicity. Aluminum was first identified as a presumed cause of dialysis dementia in dialysis patients, and shortly thereafter aluminum deposition in bone was shown to be associated with osteomalacia. The sources of aluminum were phosphate binders and the water used in preparing dialysate. Aluminum is no longer present as a contaminant in dialysate, but it still is widely utilized as a phosphate binder in some settings. Approximately one-third of dialysis and CRD patients ingest at least some aluminum. Aluminum deposition adversely affects mineral deposition at the mineralization front.

Aplastic renal osteodystrophy occurs in many patients who have no evidence of excess aluminum accumulation. These patients have relatively low levels of PTH. The disorder is associated with the use of supraphysiologic Ca^{2+} concentrations in peritoneal dialysate and the excessive use of oral Ca^{2+} and vitamin D preparations in both hemodialysis and peritoneal dialysis patients. These sources of exogenous Ca^{2+} might lower serum PTH to levels that are inadequate for maintaining normal bone turnover.

Yet another type of skeletal lesion that occurs in ESRD patients after many years of dialysis therapy results from *amyloid deposition* related to the accumulation of β_2-microglobulin. This syndrome presents as carpal tunnel syndrome, tenosynovitis of the hands, shoulder arthropathy, bone cysts, cervical spondyloarthropathy, and cervical pseudotumors. It is characterized on x-ray films by cysts in the carpal bones and femoral neck. Amyloid tumoral masses may be best appreciated by ultrasound examination or computed tomography.

With high-turnover osteitis fibrosa cystica, vitamin D–deficient and aluminum-induced osteomalacia, and dialysis-related amyloidosis, ESRD patients are prone to spontaneous fractures, which are slow to heal. The ribs are most commonly involved in the case of osteitis fibrosa cystica. The femoral neck is a frequent site of aluminum-induced osteomalacia and dialysis-related amyloidosis and is also prone to pathologic fractures. Bone pain, even in the absence of fractures, is common. In osteitis fibrosa cystica, a proximal myopathy often coexists, giving rise to gait abnormalities and to impairment of ambulation. Similarly, a myopathy may also accompany amyloid arthropathy. In CRD, there is a tendency to extraosseous or metastatic calcification when the calcium-phosphate product is very high ($>$70 when expressed as mg/dL). Medium-sized blood vessels; subcutaneous, articular, and periarticular tissues; myocardium; eyes; and lungs are common sites of metastatic calcification. *Calciphylaxis* refers to devastating necrotic extremity soft tissue lesions related to vascular occlusion and metastatic calcification.

The Effect of Uremic Acidosis on Bone Disease As previously noted, in patients with CRD, a decrease in acid excretion leads to unremitting positive H^+ balance. If extracellular fluid HCO_3^- were the only H^+ buffer available, it would become progressively depleted and the concentration of serum HCO_3^-, and thus pH, would fall to levels incompatible with life. However, during CRD, extracellular fluid HCO_3^- and pH remain stable, although reduced, for long periods; thus, either non-HCO_3^- buffers must neutralize the retained hydrogen ions or acid production must decrease. Acid production does not appear to diminish in patients with renal failure; yet such patients excrete only approximately two-thirds of their daily hydrogen ion production. Thus substantial buffering of the retained hydrogen ions almost certainly occurs. Because of its mass and potential buffering capacity, bone is a likely site for the chronic hydrogen ion buffering.

℞ TREATMENT *Secondary hyperparathyroidism* and *osteitis fibrosa* are best prevented and treated by reducing serum PO_4^{3-} concentration through the use of a PO_4^{3-} restricted diet as well as oral PO_4^{3-}-binding agents. Calcium carbonate and calcium acetate are the preferred PO_4^{3-} binding agents, but in some rare circumstances a combination of short-term aluminum hydroxide and calcium carbonate is necessary. In such cases, aluminum levels should be monitored, and citrate antacids, which enhance aluminum absorption, should be avoided. Daily oral calcitriol, or intermittent oral or intravenous pulses, appear to exert a direct suppressive effect on PTH secretion, in addition to the indirect effect mediated through raising Ca^{2+} levels. Intravenous pulses are especially convenient for patients on hemodialysis. The use of calcitriol and Ca^{2+} preparations in the predialysis population must take into account potential effects of increased phosphate and Ca^{2+} on the rate of progression of CRD. In the dialysis population, dialysate Ca^{2+}, calcium carbonate, calcium acetate, aluminum hydroxide, and calcitriol must be properly balanced to maintain the serum PO_4^{3-} concentration at approximately 1.4 mmol/L (4.5 mg/dL) and the serum Ca^{2+} at approximately 2.5 mmol/L (10 mg/dL) in an attempt to suppress parathyroid hyperplasia, thus avoiding or reversing osteitis fibrosa cystica, osteomalacia, and myopathy. It is particularly important to maintain the Ca^{2+}-PO_4^{3-} product in the normal range to avoid metastatic calcification. Several analogues of calcitriol are now being evaluated. Such analogues would be beneficial if they had the same effect on PTH mRNA as calcitriol and increased the margin of safety and efficacy by having less hyperphosphatemic and hypercalcemic effects. In this manner, it might be possible to have a greater suppressive effect on PTH transcription because a higher dose could be used safely.

Adynamic bone disease is often a consequence of overzealous treatment of secondary hyperparathyroidism. Therefore, suppression of PTH levels to less than 120 pg/mL in uremic patients may not be desirable. The incidence of aluminum-induced osteomalacia has been greatly reduced with the recognition of aluminum as the principal culprit. Therapy for this disorder is continued avoidance of aluminum, with possible use of a chelating agent such as desferoxamine along with high-flux dialysis. Management of metabolic acidosis should aim to maintain a nearly normal level of plasma HCO_3^-, with the administration of calcium acetate or calcium carbonate in the first instance, and with the addition of $NaHCO_3$ if necessary. Excessive administration of alkali should be avoided to minimize risk of urinary precipitation of calcium phosphate.

At present, there is no good therapy for *dialysis-related amyloidosis*. Local physical therapy, glucocorticoid injections, and NSAIDs constitute current options.

Other Solutes *Uric acid* retention is a common feature of CRD but rarely leads to symptomatic gout. Treatment of hyperuricemia is not necessary unless recurrent gout becomes a problem. When recurrent symptomatic gout occurs, a reduced dose of allopurinol (100 to 200 mg/d) is usually sufficient to inhibit uric acid synthesis. Hypophosphatemia is rare and, when it occurs, is usually a consequence of overzealous oral administration of phosphate-binding gels. Because serum magnesium levels tend to rise in CRD, magnesium-containing antacids and cathartics should be avoided.

CARDIOVASCULAR AND PULMONARY ABNORMALITIES **Congestive Heart Failure** (See also Chap. 232) Salt and water retention in uremia often result in congestive heart failure and/or pulmonary edema. A unique form of pulmonary congestion and edema may occur even in the absence of volume overload and is associated with normal or mildly elevated intracardiac and pulmonary capillary wedge pressures. This entity, characterized radiologically by peripheral vascular congestion giving rise to a "butterfly wing" distribution, is due to increased permeability of alveolar capillary membranes. This "low-pressure" pulmonary edema as well as cardiopulmonary abnormalities associated with circulatory overload usually respond promptly to vigorous dialysis.

Hypertension and Left Ventricular Hypertrophy (See also Chap. 246) Hypertension is the most common complication of CRD and ESRD. When it is not found, the patient may have a salt-wasting form of renal disease (e.g., medullary cystic disease, chronic tubulointerstitial disease, or papillary necrosis), may be receiving antihypertensive therapy, or be volume-depleted, the last condition usually due to excessive gastrointestinal fluid losses or overzealous diuretic therapy. Since volume overload is the major cause of hypertension in uremia, the normotensive state can often be restored by appropriate use of diuretics in the predialysis patient or with aggressive ultrafiltration in dialysis patients. Nevertheless, because of hyperreninemia, some patients remain hypertensive despite rigorous salt and water restriction and ultrafiltration. Rarely, patients develop accelerated or malignant hypertension. Intravenous nitroprusside, labetolol, or more recently approved agents such as fenoldopam or urapidil, together with control of ECFV, generally controls such hypertension. Subsequently, such patients usually require more than one oral antihypertensive drug. Enalaprilat or other ACE inhibitors may also be considered, but in the face of bilateral renovascular disease they have the potential to further reduce GFR abruptly. Administration of erythropoietin (EPO) (p. 1557) may raise blood pressure and increase the requirement for antihypertensive drugs. A high percentage of patients with CRD present with left ventricular hypertrophy or dilated cardiomyopathy. These are among the most ominous risk factors for excess cardiovascular morbidity and mortality in patients with CRD and ESRD and are thought to be related primarily to prolonged hypertension and ECFV overload. In addition, anemia and the surgical placement of an arteriovenous anastomosis for future or ongoing dialysis access may generate a high cardiac output state, which also intensifies the burden placed on the left ventricle.

℞ TREATMENT Management of hypertension in CRD can be considered in terms of two overall goals: to slow the progression of CRD itself and to prevent the extrarenal complications of hypertension, such as cardiovascular disease and stroke. In all patients with CRD, blood pressure should be controlled to at least the level established in the guidelines of the Joint National Commission on Hypertension Detection Education and Follow-up Program (130/80–85 mmHg). In the elderly, levels of 140 mmHg may be a more realistic target. In predialysis patients with proteinuria $>$ 1 g per 24 hr, blood pressure should be further reduced to a mean arterial pressure of 92 mmHg (equivalent to 125/75 mmHg), where possible. Volume control is the mainstay of therapy, with addition of antihypertensive agents as needed when hypertension persists despite achievement of a normovolemic state. When salt retention and hypervolemia contribute to hypertension, salt restriction and diuretics are indicated as initial therapy. The choice of additional agents to slow the progression of CRD based upon reduction of intraglomerular hypertension and proteinuria is considered below. In ESRD patients, considerations related to slowing of nephron injury are less important, and the main goal is to prevent cardiac hypertrophy and stroke. The choice of antihypertensive agents may come from all the major classes, with careful consideration of comorbid conditions. However, powerful direct-acting vasodilators, such as hydralazine or minoxidil, may perpetuate the tendency to cardiac hypertrophy, despite the lowering of blood pressure. Therefore, prolonged use of such agents should be reserved for those very rare patients in whom severe refractory hypertension persists, despite adequate volume reduction and compliance with all other classes of antihypertensives.

Atherosclerotic Coronary and Peripheral Vascular Disease Hypertension, hyperhomocysteinemia, and lipid abnormalities promote atherosclerosis but are potentially treatable complications of CRD. Ongoing or prior nephrotic syndrome is also associated with hyperlipidemia and hypercoagulability, which increase the risk of occlusive vascular disease. Since diabetes mellitus and hypertension are themselves the two most frequent etiologies of CRD, it is not surprising that cardiovascular disease is the most frequent cause of death in ESRD patients. Therefore, accepted life-style changes and therapeutic measures for cardiac risk reduction (Chap. 242) are especially important in this group of patients. The approach to managing hypertension has been outlined above. Hyperhomocysteinemia may respond to vitamin therapy, which includes folate supplementation to between 1 and 5 mg/d. Hyperlipidemia in patients with CRD and ESRD should be managed aggressively according to the guidelines of the National Cholesterol Education Program (Chaps. 242 and 344). If dietary measures are inadequate, the preferred lipid-lowering medications are gemfibrozil and an HMG-CoA reductase inhibitor. However, these two classes of agents ordinarily should not be combined because of an increased risk of myositis and rhabomyolysis in CRD and ESRD patients.

Abnormalities in Ca^{2+} and PO_4^{3-} metabolism (see above) may lead to metastatic vascular calcification and markedly increase the propensity to coronary, cerebral, and peripheral occlusive vascular disease. By careful attention to the guidelines noted above for the management of divalent ion metabolism and bone disease, avoidance of an elevated Ca^{2+}-PO_4^{3-} product may mitigate this effect.

Pericarditis (See also Chap. 239) With the advent of early initiation of renal replacement therapy, pericarditis is now observed more often in underdialyzed patients than in patients with CRD in whom dialysis has not yet been initiated. Pericardial pain with respiratory accentuation, accompanied by a friction rub, are the hallmarks of uremic pericarditis. The finding of a multicomponent friction rub strongly supports the diagnosis. Furthermore, the usual occurrence of multiple cardiac murmurs, S_3 and S_4 heart sounds, and transmitted bruits from arteriovenous access devices may render precordial auscultation more challenging in this group of patients. Classic electrocardiographic abnormalities include PR-interval shortening and diffuse ST-segment elevation. Pericarditis may be accompanied by the accumulation of pericardial fluid, readily detected by echocardiography, sometimes leading to cardiac tamponade. Pericardial fluid in uremic pericarditis is more often hemorrhagic than in viral pericarditis.

℞ TREATMENT Uremic pericarditis is an absolute indication for initiation of dialysis or for intensification of the dialysis prescription in those already on dialysis. Because of the propensity to hemorrhagic pericardial fluid, heparin-free dialysis is indicated. Pericardiectomy should be considered only if more conservative measures fail. Nonuremic causes of pericarditis and pericardial effusion include viral, malignant, and tuberculous pericarditis and pericarditis associated with myocardial infarction; these are also more frequent in patients with ESRD and should be managed according to the dictates of the underlying disease process.

HEMATOLOGIC ABNORMALITIES Anemia of CRD (See also Chap. 105) A normocytic, normochromic anemia is present in the majority of patients with CRD. It is usually observed when the GFR falls below 30 mL/min. When untreated, the anemia of CRD is associated with a number of physiologic abnormalities, including decreased tissue oxygen delivery and utilization, increased cardiac output, cardiac enlargement, ventricular hypertrophy, angina, congestive heart failure, decreased cognition and mental acuity, altered menstrual cycles, and impaired immune responsiveness. In addition, anemia may play a role in growth retardation in children. The primary cause of anemia in patients with CRD is insufficient production of EPO by the diseased kidneys. Additional factors include the following: iron deficiency, either related to or independent of blood loss from repeated laboratory testing, needle punctures, blood retention in the dialyzer and tubing, or gastrointestinal bleeding; severe hyperparathyroidism; acute and chronic inflammatory conditions; aluminum toxicity; folate deficiency; shortened red cell survival; hypothyroidism; and underlying hemoglobinopathies. These potential contributing factors should be considered and addressed.

Before 1989, the EPO-deficient condition characteristic of CRD could only be treated with blood transfusions and anabolic steroids, with limited success and substantial complications. The availability of recombinant human EPO, approved by the U.S. Food and Drug Administration in 1989, has been one of the most significant advances in the care of renal patients in the past decade. Considerable debate continues regarding the optimal target hematocrit in dialysis patients receiving EPO. Mortality and hospitalization studies support the National Kidney Foundation Dialysis Outcomes Quality Initiative target hematocrit range of 33 to 36% as providing the best associated outcomes. EPO can be administered either intravenously or subcutaneously. Most studies have shown that administering EPO by the subcutaneous route has a sparing effect, with the target hematocrit achieved at a lower EPO dose. Management guidelines for the correction of anemia in CRD are as follows.

Management Guidelines—Correction of Anemia in CRD

ERYTHROPOIETIN	
SC	80–120 units/kg per week (divided into × 2–3/week)
IV	120–180 units/kg per week (divided into × 3/week)
Target Hct/Hb	33–36%/11–12 g/dL
Optimal rate of correction[a]	Increase Hct by 4–6% over 4-week period (achieve goal values within 2–3 months)

IRON

Monitor iron stores by percent transferrin saturation (TSAT) and serum ferritin.

If patient is iron-deficient [TSAT < 20% ferritin < 100 ng/mL (<100 mg/L)] administer iron 50–100 mg IV twice per week for 5 weeks (or for 10 successive dialysis sessions). If iron indices are still low, repeat the same course.

If iron indices are normal yet Hct/Hb are still inadequate, administer IV iron as outlined above. Monitor Hct/Hb, TSAT, and ferritin.

Withhold iron therapy when TSAT > 50% and/or ferritin > 800 ng/mL (>800 μg/L)

[a] If correction of anemia is inadequate, consider causes for refractoriness as outlined in text.

The iron status of the patient with CRD must be assessed, and adequate iron stores should be available before treatment with EPO is initiated. Iron supplementation is usually essential to ensure an adequate response to EPO in patients with CRD, because the demands for iron by the erythroid marrow frequently exceed the amount of iron that is immediately available for erythropoiesis (as measured by percent transferrin saturation) as well as iron stores (as measured by serum ferritin). In most cases, intravenous iron will be required to achieve and/or maintain adequate iron. However, excessive iron therapy may be associated with a number of complications, including hemosiderosis, accelerated atherosclerosis, increased susceptibility to infection, and possibly an increased propensity to the emergence of malignancies. In addition to iron, an adequate supply of the other major substrates and cofactors for erythrocyte production must be assured, especially vitamin B_{12} and folate. Anemia resistant to recommended doses of EPO in the face of adequate availability of iron and vitamin factors often suggests inadequate dialysis; uncontrolled hyperparathyroidism; aluminum toxicity; chronic blood loss or hemolysis; and associated hemoglobinopathy, malnutrition, chronic infection, multiple myeloma, or another malignancy. Blood transfusions may contribute to suppression of erythropoiesis in CRD; because they increase the risk of hepatitis, hemosiderosis, and transplant sensitization, they should be avoided unless the anemia fails to respond to EPO and the patient is symptomatic.

Abnormal Hemostasis Abnormal hemostasis is common in CRD and is characterized by a tendency to abnormal bleeding and bruising. Bleeding from surgical wounds and spontaneous bleeding into the gastrointestinal tract, pericardial sac, or intracranial vault (in the form of subdural hematoma or intracerebral hemorrhage) are of greatest concern. Prolongation of bleeding time, decreased activity of platelet factor III, abnormal platelet aggregation and adhesiveness, and impaired prothrombin consumption contribute to the clotting defects. The abnormality in platelet factor III correlates with increased plasma levels of guanidinosuccinic acid and can be corrected by dialysis. Prolongation of the bleeding time is common even in well-dialyzed patients. Abnormal bleeding times and coagulopathy in patients with renal failure may be reversed with desmopressin, cryoprecipitate, conjugated estrogens, and blood transfusions, as well as by the use of EPO.

Enhanced Susceptibility to Infection Changes in leukocyte formation and function in uremia lead to enhanced susceptibility to infection. Lymphocytopenia and atrophy of lymphoid structures occur, whereas neutrophil production is relatively unimpaired. Nevertheless, the function of all leukocyte cell types may be affected adversely by uremic serum. Alterations in monocyte, lymphocyte, and neutrophil function cause impairment of acute inflammatory responses, decreased delayed hypersensitivity, and altered late immune function.

There is a tendency for uremic patients to have less fever in response to infection, perhaps because of the effects of uremia on the hypothalamic temperature control center. Leukocyte function may also be impaired in patients with CRD because of coexisting acidosis, hyperglycemia, protein-calorie malnutrition, and serum and tissue hyperosmolarity (due to azotemia). In patients treated with hemodialysis, leukocyte function is disturbed because of the effects of the bioincompatibility of various dialysis membranes. Activation of cytokine and complement cascades likewise occurs when blood comes in contact with dialysis membranes. These substances in turn alter inflammatory and immune responses of the uremic patient. Mucosal barriers to infection may also be defective, and, in dialysis patients, vascular and peritoneal access devices are common portals of entry for pathogens, especially staphylococci. Glucocorticoids and immunosuppressive drugs used for various renal diseases and renal transplantation further increase the risk of infection.

NEUROMUSCULAR ABNORMALITIES Subtle disturbances of central nervous system function, including inability to concentrate, drowsiness, and insomnia, are among the early symptoms of uremia. Mild behavioral changes, loss of memory, and errors in judgment soon follow and may be associated with neuromuscular irritability, including hiccoughs, cramps, and fasciculations/twitching of muscles. Asterixis, myoclonus, and chorea are common in terminal uremia, as are stupor, seizures, and coma. Peripheral neuropathy is also common in advanced CRD. Initially, sensory nerves are involved more than motor nerves, lower extremities more than upper, and distal portions of the extremities more than proximal. The "restless legs syndrome" is characterized by ill-defined sensations of discomfort in the feet and lower legs requiring frequent leg movement. If dialysis is not instituted soon after onset of sensory abnormalities, motor involvement follows, including loss of deep tendon reflexes, weakness, peroneal nerve palsy (foot drop), and, eventually, flaccid quadriplegia. Accordingly, evidence of peripheral neuropathy is a firm indication for the initiation of dialysis or transplantation. Some of the central nervous system and neuromuscular complications of advanced uremia resolve with dialysis, although nonspecific electroencephalographic abnormalities may persist (Table 270-3). Successful transplantation may reverse residual peripheral neuropathy.

Two types of neurologic disturbances are unique to patients on chronic dialysis (Chap. 271). *Dialysis dementia* may occur in patients who have been on dialysis for many years and is characterized by speech dyspraxia, myoclonus, dementia, and eventually seizures and death. Aluminum intoxication is probably the major contributor to this syndrome, but other factors, such as viral infections, may play a role since not all patients with aluminum exposure develop the syndrome. *Dialysis disequilibrium*, which occurs during the first few dialyses in association with rapid reduction of blood urea levels, manifests clinically with nausea, vomiting, drowsiness, headache, and, rarely, seizures. The syndrome has been attributed to cerebral edema and increased intracranial pressure due to the rapid (dialysis-induced) shifts of omsolality and pH between extracellular and intracellular fluids. This complication can often be anticipated and prevented in patients who present with markedly elevated concentrations of plasma urea, by prescribing an initial dialysis regimen that produces slower solute removal.

GASTROINTESTINAL ABNORMALITIES Anorexia, hiccoughs, nausea, and vomiting are common early manifestations of uremia. Protein restriction is useful in diminishing nausea and vomiting late in the course of renal failure. However, protein restriction should not be implemented in patients with early signs of protein-calorie malnutrition. *Uremic fetor*, a uriniferous odor to the breath, derives from the breakdown of urea to ammonia in saliva and is often associated with an unpleasant metallic taste sensation. Mucosal ulcerations leading to blood loss can occur at any level of the gastrointestinal tract in the very late stages of CRD. Peptic ulcer disease is common in uremic patients. Whether this high incidence is related to altered gastric acidity, enhanced colonization by *Helicobacter pylori*, or hypersecretion of gastrin is unknown. Patients with CRD, particularly those with polycystic kidney disease, have an increased incidence of diverticulosis. Pancreatitis and angiodysplasia of the large bowel with chronic bleeding have been noted more commonly in dialysis patients. Hepatitis B antigenemia was very common in the past, but it is much less so now because of the implementation of universal precautions, the use of hepatitis B vaccine, and the diminished need for blood transfusions resulting from the introduction of EPO. There is a higher incidence of hepatitis C virus infection in patients treated with chronic hemodialysis. Unlike hepatitis B, this infection is most often persistent. Although it does not seem to cause significant liver disease in most patients, it is a definite concern in patients who subsequently undergo transplantation and immunosuppression, in whom the incidence of active chronic hepatitis and cirrhosis is considerably higher than in those without hepatitis C infection. →*The role of interferon and antiviral treatment in both hepatitis B and C infections is discussed in Chap. 295.*

ENDOCRINE-METABOLIC DISTURBANCES Disturbances in parathyroid function, protein-calorie and lipid metabolism, and overall nutritional abnormalities of uremia have already been considered.

Glucose metabolism is impaired, as evidenced by a slowing of the rate at which blood glucose levels decline after a glucose load. Fasting blood glucose is usually normal or only slightly elevated, and the mild glucose intolerance related to uremia per se, when present, does not require specific therapy. Because the kidney contributes significantly to insulin removal from the circulation, plasma levels of insulin are slightly to moderately elevated in most uremic subjects, both in the fasting and post-prandial states. However, the response to insulin and glucose utilization is impaired in CRD. Many renal hypoglycemic drugs require dose reduction in renal failure, and some, such as metformin, are contraindicated when GFR has diminished by more than approximately 25 to 50%.

In women, *estrogen levels* are low, and amenorrhea and inability to carry pregnancies to term are common manifestations of uremia. When GFR has declined by approximately 30%, pregnancy may hasten the progression of CRD. In women with ESRD, the reappearance of menses is a sign of efficient renal replacement therapy and is a frequent occurrence after an adequate chronic dialysis regimen has been established. Successful pregnancies are rare. In men with CRD, including those receiving chronic dialysis, impotence, oligospermia, and germinal cell dysplasia are common, as are reduced plasma testosterone levels. Like growth, sexual maturation is often impaired in adolescent children with CRD, even among those treated with chronic dialysis. Many of these abnormalities improve or reverse with successful renal transplantation.

DERMATOLOGIC ABNORMALITIES The skin may show evidence of anemia (pallor), defective hemostasis (ecchymoses and hematomas), calcium deposition and secondary hyperparathyroidism (pruritus, excoriations), dehydration (poor skin turgor, dry mucous membranes), and the general cutaneous consequences of protein-calorie malnutrition. A sallow, yellow cast may reflect the combined influences of anemia and retention of a variety of pigmented metabolites, or *urochromes*. The gray to bronze discoloration of the skin related to transfusional hemochromatosis has now become uncommon with the availability and usage of EPO. In advanced uremia, the concentration of urea in sweat may be so high that, after evaporation, a fine white powder can be found on the skin surface—so-called uremic (urea) frost. Although many of these cutaneous abnormalities improve with dialysis, *uremic pruritus* often remains a problem. The first lines of management are to rule out unrelated skin disorders, to adjust the dialysis prescription so as to ensure adequacy of dialysis, and to control PO_4^{3-}concentration with avoidance of an elevated Ca^{2+}-PO_4^{3-} product. Occasionally, pruritus remains refractory to these measures and to other nonspecific systemic and topical therapies. The latter has itself been reported to improve pruritus. Skin necrosis can occur as part of the calciphylaxis syndrome, which also includes subcutaneous, vascular, joint, and visceral calcification in patients with poorly controlled calcium-phosphate product.

DIAGNOSTIC APPROACH

The most important initial step in the evaluation of a patient presenting de novo with biochemical or clinical evidence of renal failure is to distinguish CRD, which may be first coming to clinical attention, from true acute renal failure. The demonstration of evidence of chronic metabolic bone disease and anemia and the finding of bilaterally reduced kidney size by imaging studies strongly favor a long-standing process consistent with CRD. However, these findings do not rule out the superimposition of an acute and reversible exacerbating factor that has accelerated the decline in GFR (see below). Having established that the patient suffers from CRD, in the early stages it is often possible to establish the underlying etiology. However, when the CRD process is quite advanced, then definitively establishing an underlying etiology becomes less feasible in many cases and also of less therapeutic significance.

ESTABLISHING THE ETIOLOGY Of special importance in establishing the etiology of CRD are a history of hypertension; diabetes; systemic infectious, inflammatory, or metabolic diseases; exposure to drugs and toxins; and a family history of renal and urologic disease. Drugs of particular importance include analgesics (usage frequently underestimated or denied by the patient), NSAIDs, gold, penicillamine, antimicrobials, lithium, and ACE inhibitors. In evaluating the uremic syndrome, questions about appetite, diet, nausea, vomiting, hiccoughing, shortness of breath, edema, weight change, muscle cramps, bone pain, mental acuity, and activities of daily living are especially helpful.

Physical Examination Particular attention should be paid to blood pressure, fundoscopy, precordial examination, examination of the abdomen for bruits and palpable renal masses, extremity examination for edema, and neurologic examination for the presence of asterixis, muscle weakness, and neuropathy. In addition, the evaluation of prostate size in men and potential pelvic masses in women should be undertaken by appropriate physical examination.

Laboratory Investigations These should also focus on a search for clues to an underlying disease process and its continued activity. Therefore, if the history and physical examination warrant, immunologic tests for systemic lupus erythematosus and vasculitis might be considered. Serum and urinary protein electrophoresis should be undertaken in all patients over the age of 40 with unexplained CRD and anemia, to rule out paraproteinemia. Other tests to determine the severity and chronicity of the disease include serial measurements of serum creatinine and blood urea nitrogen, hemoglobin, calcium, phosphate, and alkaline phosphatase to assess metabolic bone disease. Urine analysis may be helpful in assessing the presence of ongoing activity of the underlying inflammatory or proteinuric disease process, and when indicated should be supplemented by a 24-h urine collection for quantifying protein excretion. The latter is particularly helpful in guiding management strategies aimed at ameliorating the progression of CRD. The presence of *broad casts* on examination of the urinary sediment is a nonspecific finding seen with all diverse etiologies and reflects chronic tubulointerstitial scarring and tubular atrophy with widened tubule diameter, usually signifying an advanced stage of CRD.

Imaging Studies The most useful among these is renal sonography. An ultrasound examination of the kidneys verifies the presence of two symmetric kidneys, provides an estimate of kidney size, and rules out renal masses and obstructive uropathy. The documentation of symmetric small kidneys supports the diagnosis of progressive CRD with an irreversible component of scarring. The occurrence of normal kidney size suggests the possibility of an acute rather than chronic process. However, polycystic kidney disease, amyloidosis, and diabetes may lead to CRD with normal-sized or even enlarged kidneys. Documentation of asymmetric kidney size suggests either a unilateral developmental or urologic abnormality or chronic renovascular disease. In the latter case, a vascular imaging procedure, such as duplex Doppler sonography of the renal arteries, radionuclide scintigraphy, or magnetic resonance angiography should be considered. A computed tomographic scan without contrast may be useful in assessing kidney stone activity, in the appropriate clinical context. Voiding cystourethrography to rule out reflux may be indicated in some younger patients with a history of enuresis or with a family history of reflux. However, in most cases, by the time CRD is established, reflux has resolved; even if present, its repair may not stabilize renal function. In any case, imaging studies should avoid exposure to intravenous radiocontrast dye where possible because of its nephrotoxicity.

Differentiation of CRD from Acute Renal Failure The most classic constellation of laboratory and imaging findings that distinguishes progressive CRD from acute renal failure are bilaterally small (<8.5 cm) kidneys, anemia, hyperphosphatemia and hypocalcemia with elevated PTH levels, and a urinary sediment that is inactive or reveals proteinuria and broad casts. Furthermore, integration of a particular constellation of clinical, laboratory, and imaging findings based on the approach noted above strongly supports a particular presumed underlying etiologic disease process. For example, in a patient with insulin-dependent type 1 diabetes mellitus of 15 to 20 years' duration, diabetic retinopathy, and nephrotic-range albuminuria without hematuria, the diagnosis of diabetic nephropathy is likely. The diagnosis of chronic hypertensive nephrosclerosis (Chap. 278) requires a history of long-standing hypertension, in the absence of evidence for another renal disease process, and hence is usually a diagnosis of exclusion. Usually, proteinuria is mild to moderate (<3 g/d) and the urine sediment inactive. In many cases of presumed hypertensive nephrosclerosis, renovascular disease may not only be the cause of hypertension but also may cause ischemic renal damage. Bilateral renovascular ischemic disease may be a greatly underdiagnosed cause of CRD. This is of therapeutic significance from two points of view: (1) documentation of ischemic renal disease may prompt revascularization therapy in some patients, with occasional dramatic stabilization or improvement in renal function; and (2) renovascular ischemic disease is a contraindication to ACE inhibitor therapy in most cases. Analgesic-associated chronic tubulointerstitial nephropathy is also an underdiagnosed cause of CRD. Imaging studies, including computed tomography, often reveal pathognomonic features such as papillary calcification and necrosis. Under such circumstances, cessation of analgesic exposure may dramatically stabilize renal function.

Kidney Biopsy This procedure should be reserved for patients with near-normal kidney size, in whom a clear-cut diagnosis cannot be made by less invasive means, and when the possibility of a reversible underlying disease process remains tenable so that clarification of the underlying etiology may alter management. The extent of tubulointerstitial scarring on kidney biopsy generally provides the most reliable pathologic correlate indicating prognosis for continued deterioration toward ESRD. Contraindications to renal biopsy include bilateral small kidneys, polycystic kidney disease, uncontrolled hypertension, urinary tract or perinephric infection, bleeding diathesis, respiratory distress, and morbid obesity.

℞ TREATMENT This refers to all of the preventive and therapeutic measures that precede and aim to prevent or postpone ESRD and renal replacement therapy.

Specific Therapy The optimal time for specific therapy aimed at the underlying disease process is usually well before there has been a measurable decline in baseline GFR, and usually well before CRD is established. When kidney size remains well preserved, renal biopsy results may provide an index of chronicity versus disease activity, which might help in guiding therapeutic decisions. In contrast, by the time CRD is established and GFR has irreversibly declined to less than 20 to 30% of normal, the risks of immunomodulatory and other therapies aimed at treating an underlying past or ongoing disease process may outweigh the benefits.

Superimposed Factors It is of benefit to follow and plot the rate of decline in GFR in patients with CRD. Any acceleration in the rate of decline should prompt a search for a superimposed acute process. The differential diagnosis should be developed in a systematic manner, as for any patient with acute renal failure (Chap. 269). Particular attention should be directed to factors that more commonly lead to an acute and reversible decline in GFR in patients with CRD. These include superimposed volume depletion, accelerated and uncontrolled hypertension, urinary tract infection, superimposed obstructive uropathy (e.g., due to stone disease, papillary necrosis), nephrotoxic effect of medications (e.g., NSAIDs) and radiocontrast agents, and reactivation or flare of the original underlying etiologic disease process.

Measures to Mitigate Hyperfiltration Injury The two major therapeutic tools currently available in the mitigation of hyperfiltration injury are: (1) dietary protein restriction, and (2) pharmacologic management of intraglomerular hypertension.

Protein Restriction in CRD Management guidelines for protein restriction in CRD are shown in the following table. In contrast to fat and carbohydrates, protein in excess of the daily requirement is not stored but is degraded to form urea and other nitrogenous wastes, which are principally excreted by the kidney. In addition, protein-rich foods contain hydrogen ions, PO_4^{3-}, sulfates, and other inorganic ions that are also eliminated by the kidney. Therefore, when patients with CRD consume excessive dietary protein, nitrogenous wastes and inorganic ions accumulate, resulting in the clinical and metabolic disturbances characteristic of uremia. Restricting dietary protein can ameliorate many uremic symptoms and may slow the actual rate of nephron injury. The effectiveness of protein restriction in slowing the progression of CRD has been evaluated in a number of controlled clinical trials. The Modification of Diet in Renal Disease (MDRD) Study was the most extensive trial devoted to this question, but it nevertheless yielded an ambiguous result, although positive trends emerged when it ended after an average follow-up of only 2.2 years. In a separate study of patients with insulin-dependent diabetic nephropathy, protein restriction was shown to slow progression significantly in one well-controlled study. Two meta-analyses of studies of the effects of protein restriction on progression concluded that low-protein diets slow progression of both diabetic and nondiabetic renal disease.

Management Guidelines—Dietary Protein Restriction in CRD

GFR, mL/min	Protein, g/kg per d	Phosphorus, g/kg per d
>60	Protein restriction not usually recommended	No restriction
25–60	0.6 g/kg per d including ≥0.35 g/kg per d of HBV	≤10
5–25	0.6 g/kg per d including ≥0.35 g/kg per d of HBV	≤10
	or	
	0.3 g/kg per d supplemented with EAA or KA	≤9
<60 (nephrotic syndrome)	0.8 g/kg per d (plus 1 g protein/g proteinuria) *or*	≤12
	0.3 g/kg per d supplemented with EAA or KA (plus 1 g protein/g proteinuria)	≤9

NOTE: GFR, glomerular filtration rate; HBV, high biologic value protein; EAA, essential amino acid supplement; KA, ketoanalogue supplement.

It is crucial that protein restriction be carried out in the context of an overall dietary program that optimizes nutritional status and avoids malnutrition, especially as patients near dialysis or transplantation. Measurements of urinary nitrogen appearance, anthropometric and biochemical measurements, as well as dietary consultation are mandatory to preempt malnutrition. Among the most readily available and useful indices of malnutrition are plasma concentrations of albumin (<3.8 g/dL), pre-albumin (<18 mg/dL), and transferrin (<180 μg/dL). Metabolic and nutritional studies indicate that protein requirements for patients with CRD are similar to those for normal adults, approximately 0.6 g/kg per day. However, there is a particular requirement in patients with CRD that the composition of dietary protein be higher in essential amino acids, and that this be combined with an overall energy supply sufficient to mitigate a catabolic state. Energy requirements in the range of 35 kcal/kg per day are recommended.

Fortunately, even patients with advanced CRD are able to activate the same adaptive responses to dietary protein restriction as healthy individuals, i.e., a postprandial suppression of whole-body protein degradation and a marked inhibition of amino acid oxidation. After at least 1 year of therapy with a low-protein diet (range 12 to 24 months) these same adaptive responses persist, indicating that the compensatory responses to dietary protein restriction are sustained during long-term therapy. Further evidence that low-protein diets are safe in CRD patients is provided by the finding that nutritional indices remain normal during long-term therapy.

Pharmacologic management of intraglomerular hypertension In addition to reduction of cardiovascular disease risk, antihypertensive therapy in patients with CRD also aims to slow the progression of nephron injury by ameliorating intraglomerular hypertension and hypertrophy. Progressive renal injury in CRD appears to be most closely related to the height of intraglomerular pressure and/or the extent of glomerular hypertrophy. The MDRD and other studies demonstrated that control of hypertension is as important as dietary protein restriction in slowing the progression of CRD. Furthermore, the target for pharmacologic therapy was highly dependent on the level of proteinuria. Indeed, proteinuria is now considered a risk factor for progressive nephron injury; the prior level of proteinuria correlates with the subsequent rate of GFR decline. Elevated blood pressure increases proteinuria due to the transmission to the glomeruli of the elevated systemic pressure. Conversely, the protective effect of antihypertensive medications is evident through the curtailment of proteinuria. Thus, the more effective a given treatment is in lowering proteinuria, the greater the subsequent impact on protection from GFR decline.

Some antihypertensive agents, particularly the ACE inhibitors, may be superior to others in affording renal protection. The advantage of this pharmacologic class is thought to relate to salutary modulation of intraglomerular hemodynamics over and above effects on systemic blood pressure. Several well-designed studies have now established favorable outcomes for ACE inhibitors in slowing the progression of diabetic nephropathy. ACE inhibitors have been shown to be more effective than diuretics, beta blockers, and calcium antagonists in reducing urinary albumin excretion in both hypertensive and diabetic patients. Furthermore, these drugs have been shown to facilitate the regression of remodeling more generally in the cardiovascular system and to improve endothelial function in resistance arterioles of humans with hypertension. In nondiabetic CRD, the European AIPRI trial documented a 53% additional reduction in the risk of doubling serum creatinine levels with ACE inhibitor therapy compared to conventional regimens that did not include ACE inhibitors. The reduction in the risk was greater in patients with mild renal insufficiency and in those with proteinuria >1g/d. In a recent meta-analysis, information from all the randomized ACE inhibitor trials in patients with nondiabetic renal disease was combined; the conclusion is that ACE inhibitors are more effective than other antihypertensive agents in reducing the development of ESRD. A similar salutary effect on kidney function as observed with ACE inhibitors has been observed recently with the angiotensin II receptor antagonists, which also possess significant antiproteinuric properties.

Among the calcium channel blockers, diltiazem and verapamil appear to exhibit antiproteinuric and renal protective effects not shared by the dihydropyridines. As a group, these drugs do not adversely affect renal function in patients with nondiabetic renal insufficiency, and they may be more effective in preventing or ameliorating progressive renal injury than some other classes of antihypertensive drugs in this group of patients. Thus, it appears that at least two different categories of responses may exist: one in which progression is strongly associated with systemic and intraglomerular hypertension and with proteinuria (e.g., diabetic nephropathy, glomerular diseases) and in which ACE inhibitors and angiotensin-receptor blockers are likely to be the first choice; and the second in which proteinuria is mild or absent (e.g., adult polycystic kidney disease), probably with a less prominent role for intraglomerular hypertension, and which might respond as well to calcium channel blockers. The level of blood pressure lowering is also of crucial importance in achieving a significant renal protective effect. Clinical practice guidelines are summarized below.

Use of Drugs (See also Chaps. 70 and 71) Although the loading dose of most drugs is not affected by CRD, maintenance doses of many drugs need to be adjusted. One exception is digoxin, whose volume of distribution is decreased in CRD, mandating a concomitant reduction in the loading dose in addition to adjustment of the maintenance dose. For those drugs in which >70% excretion is by a nonrenal (e.g., hepatic or intestinal) route, dosage adjustment may not be needed. Some drugs that should be entirely avoided include meperidine, metformin, and other oral hypoglycemics with a renal route of elimination. Commonly used medications that require either a reduction in dosage or interval include allopurinol, many antibiotics, several hypertensives, and anti-arrhythmics. For a comprehensive detailed and authoritative listing of the recommended dose adjustment for most of the commonly used medications, the reader is referred to the American College of Physicians handbook of "Drug Prescribing in Renal Failure" (see www.acponline.org).

Preparation for Renal Replacement Therapy Over the past 35 years, renal replacement therapy using dialysis and transplantation has prolonged the lives of hundreds of thousands of patients with ESRD. Renal replacement therapy should *not* be initiated when the patient is totally asymptomatic; however, dialysis and/or transplantation should be started sufficiently early to prevent serious complications of the uremic state. Clear indications for initiation of renal replacement therapy include pericarditis, progressive neuropathy attributable to uremia, encephalopathy, muscle irritability, anorexia and nausea that is not

Management Guidelines for BP Control in CRD

• Target BP in CRD	130/80–85 mmHg
• With proteinuria (>1 g/d)	125/75 mmHg (MAP 92 mmHg)
• Recommended medications	• Diuretics to achieve normovolemia • In diabetic nephropathy or CRD with proteinuria—ACE inhibitor or angiotensin receptor antagonists alone or in combination with diuretic. • In other causes of CRD, calcium entry blocker alpha and beta blockers considered as alternatives

NOTE: MAP, mean arterial pressure.

ameliorated by reasonable protein restriction, and fluid and electrolyte abnormalities that are refractory to conservative measures. The latter include volume overload unresponsive to diuretic therapy, hyperkalemia unresponsive to dietary potassium restriction, and progressive metabolic acidosis that cannot be managed with alkali therapy. Clinical clues indicating the imminent development of uremic complications are a history of hiccoughing, intractable pruritus, morning nausea and vomiting, muscle twitching and cramps, and the presence of asterixis on physical examination. In addition, the patient whose follow-up and compliance with conservative management are questionable should be considered for earlier initiation of renal replacement therapy, lest potentially life-threatening uremic complications or electrolyte disturbances supervene.

The correlation of uremic symptoms with renal function varies from patient to patient depending on the cause of renal disease (earlier onset of symptoms in patients with diabetes mellitus), muscle mass (large, muscular patients tolerate high levels of azotemia), diet, nutritional status, and coexisting conditions. Therefore, it is ill-advised to assign a certain "usual" level of blood urea nitrogen, serum creatinine, or GFR to the need to start dialysis. Nevertheless, in the United States, the Health Care Financing Administration has assigned levels of serum creatinine and creatinine clearance to qualify for reimbursement from Medicare for patients receiving dialysis. Serum creatinine must be ≥700 μmol/L (≥8.0 mg/dL) and the creatinine clearance must be ≤0.17 mL/s (≤10 mL/min).

Patient education Social, psychological, and physical preparation for the transition to renal replacement therapy and choice of the optimal initial modality is best accomplished with a gradual approach involving a multidisciplinary team. While conservative measures are being carried out in patients with CRD, it is important to prepare them with an intensive educational program, explaining the likelihood and timing of initiation of renal replacement therapy and the various forms of therapy available. The more knowledgeable patients are concerning hemodialysis, peritoneal dialysis, and transplantation, the easier and more appropriate will be their decisions at a later time. Exploration of social service support resources is of great importance. In those who may perform home dialysis or undergo transplantation, early education of family members for selection and preparation as a home dialysis helper or a related donor for transplantation should occur long before the onset of symptomatic renal failure.

Selection of patients to be treated with various modalities of dialysis or transplantation is a matter of some debate, with considerable variation in different parts of the world. In general, in the United States and some other countries, nearly all patients who have reached ESRD are accepted for dialysis if they or their families desire prolongation of life, irrespective of age.

In terms of dialysis treatment modalities (Chap. 271), large multicenter studies have not shown a consistent or convincing advantage in terms of morbidity or mortality, of one modality over another.

Only kidney transplantation (Chap. 272) offers the potential for nearly complete rehabilitation. This is because dialysis techniques replace only 10 to 15% of normal kidney function at the level of small-solute removal and are even less efficient at the removal of larger solutes. Generally, kidney transplantation follows a prior period of dialysis treatment. All patients in whom an acute reversible component of renal failure has not been completely excluded should be supported with dialysis first, at least for some period of time, to allow for possible return of renal function before consideration of transplantation. Recovery of endogenous renal function in patients treated with dialysis for more than 6 months is a rare occurrence. Usually these are patients in whom the underlying disease process has been acute or subacute—such as one of the thrombotic microangiopathies, rapidly progressive glomerulonephritis, or obstructive uropathy. Patients approaching ESRD in whom a reversible component has been excluded, and who have a good antigenic match with a willing donor, may occasionally be considered for primary transplantation without intervening dialysis.

ACKNOWLEDGMENT

Dr. J. Michael Lazarus was a co-author of this chapter in the 14th edition, and some of the material in that chapter is carried forward to the present edition.

BIBLIOGRAPHY

ARONOFF GR et al: *Drug Prescribing in Renal Failure*, 4th ed. American College of Physicians, 1999

BAILIE GR et al: Parenteral iron use in the management of anemia in end-stage renal disease patients. Am J Kid Dis 35:1, 2000

BURTON C, HARRIS KP: The role of proteinuria in the progression of chronic renal failure. Am J Kidney Dis 27:765, 1996

BUSHINSKY DA: The contribution of acidosis to renal osteodystrophy. Kidney Int 47: 1816, 1995

HAKIM RM, LAZARUS JM: Initiation of dialysis. J Am Soc Nephrol 6:1319, 1995

LEVEY AS et al: A more accurate method to estimate glomerular filtration rate from serum creatinine: A new prediction equation. Ann Intern Med 130:461, 1999

LEWIS EJ et al: The effect of angiotensin-converting-enzyme inhibition on diabetic nephropathy. N Engl J Med 329:1456, 1993

MASCHIO G et al: Effect of the ACE inhibitor benazepril on the progression of chronic renal insufficiency. N Engl J Med 334:939, 1996

PEDRINI MT et al: The effect of dietary protein restriction on the progression of diabetic and nondiabetic renal diseases: A meta-analysis. Ann Intern Med 124:627, 1996

TOTO RD et al: "Strict" blood pressure control and progression of renal disease in hypertensive nephrosclerosis. Kidney Int 48:851, 1995

WALSER M et al: Should protein intake be restricted in predialysis patients? Kidney Int 55:771, 1999

271 *Ajay K. Singh, Barry M. Brenner*

DIALYSIS IN THE TREATMENT OF RENAL FAILURE

With the widespread availability of dialysis, the lives of hundreds of thousands of patients with end-stage renal disease (ESRD) have been prolonged. In the United States alone, there are now approximately 300,000 patients with ESRD. The overall incidence of ESRD is 242 cases per million population per year. The incident population of patients with ESRD is increasing at approximately 8% each year. The incidence of ESRD is disproportionately higher in African Americans (758 per million population per year) as compared with white Americans (180 per million population per year). In the United States, the leading cause of ESRD is diabetes mellitus, accounting for more than 40% of newly diagnosed cases of ESRD. The second most common cause is hypertension, which is estimated to cause 30% of ESRD cases. Other causes of ESRD include glomerulonephritis, polycystic kidney disease, and obstructive uropathy.

Dialysis care in the United States is funded through the Medicare End-Stage Renal Dialysis program; the cost was approximately $13.5 billion in 1997. Although the total program expense has increased dramatically, the cost for treating individual patients in inflation-adjusted terms has gone down. In addition, quality and outcomes have improved through better management of dialysis dose, improved nutrition, management of anemia, and control of hypertension. The cost of dialysis, which ranges from $45,000 to $65,000 per year, has been demonstrated to vary according to the presence or absence of diabetes mellitus and whether the treatment modality is hemodialysis or peritoneal dialysis. The mortality of patients with ESRD is lowest in Europe and Japan but is very high in the developing world because of the limited availability of dialysis. In the United States, the mortality rate of patients on dialysis is approximately 18% per year. Deaths are due mainly to cardiovascular diseases and infections (approximately 50% and 15% of deaths, respectively).

TREATMENT OPTIONS FOR ESRD PATIENTS

Commonly accepted criteria for putting patients on dialysis include: the presence of the uremic syndrome; the presence of hyperkalemia unresponsive to conservative measures; extracellular volume expansion; acidosis refractory to medical therapy; a bleeding diathesis; and a creatinine clearance of <10 cc/min per 1.73m². There is emerging consensus that patients with ESRD should be started on dialysis early. Although vigorous protein restriction can maintain the blood urea nitrogen at an acceptable level in these patients, it may come at the price of significant malnutrition, which in turn correlates with mortality on dialysis. In addition to carefully evaluating patients for the onset of uremia (Chap. 270), regular measurement of renal function is important.

Renal function can be assessed by measurement of serum creatinine and blood urea nitrogen or of creatinine and urea clearance, or the direct measurement of glomerular filtration rate (GFR) using a radioisotope such as iothalamate. Creatinine clearance usually overestimates glomerular filtration rate because a substantial fraction of creatinine excretion in advanced renal failure occurs as a consequence of proximal tubular secretion. On the other hand, urea clearance invariably underestimates GFR because urea is reabsorbed in the distal nephron. Thus, when measurement of GFR by a direct test is not available, the average of the sum of the creatinine and urea clearance, or a cimetidine-blocked creatinine clearance (cimetidine blocks proximal tubular secretion), is recommended. Early referral to a nephrologist for advanced planning and creation of a dialysis access, education about ESRD treatment options, and the aggressive management of the complications of chronic renal failure, including acidosis, anemia, and hyperparathyroidism, are important.

The treatment options available for patients with renal failure depend on whether it is acute or chronic (Fig. 271-1). In acute renal failure, treatments include hemodialysis, continuous renal replacement therapies (see p. 1565), and peritoneal dialysis. In chronic renal failure (ESRD) the options include hemodialysis (in center or at home); peritoneal dialysis, either as continuous ambulatory peritoneal dialysis (CAPD) or continuous cyclic peritoneal dialysis (CCPD); or transplantation (Chap. 272). Although there are geographic variations, hemodialysis remains the most common therapeutic modality for ESRD (>80% of patients in the United States). The choice between hemodialysis and peritoneal dialysis involves the interplay of various factors that include the patient's age, the presence of comorbid conditions, the ability to perform the procedure, and the patient's own conceptions

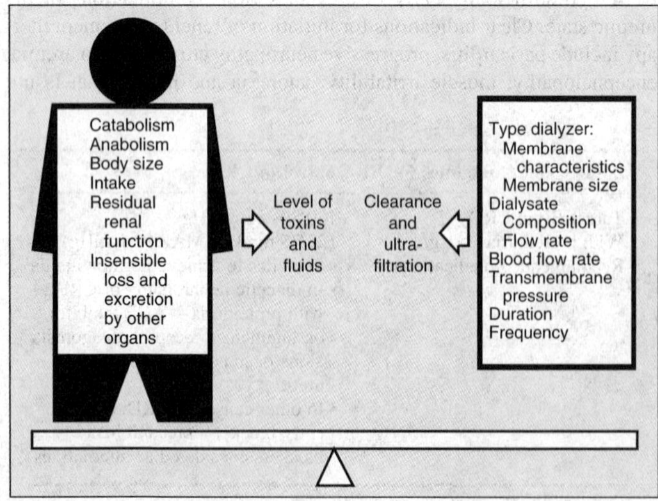

FIGURE 271-1 Factors in the development of the uremic syndrome and considerations in its treatment.

about the therapy. Peritoneal dialysis is favored in younger patients because of their better manual dexterity and greater visual acuity, and because younger patients prefer the independence and flexibility of home-based peritoneal dialysis treatment. In contrast, larger patients (>80 kg), patients with no residual renal function, and patients who have truncal obesity with or without prior abdominal surgery are more suited to hemodialysis. Larger patients with no residual renal function are more appropriate for hemodialysis because these patients have a large volume of distribution of urea and require significantly higher amounts of peritoneal dialysis, which may be difficult to achieve because of the limited willingness of patients to perform more than four exchanges each day. In some patients, the inability to obtain vascular access predicates a switch from hemodialysis to peritoneal dialysis.

HEMODIALYSIS

This consists of diffusion that occurs bi-directionally across a semipermeable membrane. Movement of metabolic waste products takes place down a concentration gradient from the circulation into the dialysate, and in the reverse direction. The rate of diffusive transport increases in response to several factors, including the magnitude of the concentration gradient, the membrane surface area, and the mass transfer coefficient of the membrane. The latter is a function of the porosity and thickness of the membrane, the size of the solute molecule, and the conditions of flow on the two sides of the membrane. According to the laws of diffusion, the larger the molecule, the slower its rate of transfer across the membrane. A small molecule such as urea (60 Da) undergoes substantial clearance, whereas a larger molecule such as creatinine (113 Da), is cleared much less efficiently. In addition to diffusive clearance, movement of toxic materials such as urea from the circulation into the dialysate may occur as a result of ultrafiltration. Convective clearance occurs because of solvent drag

with solutes getting swept along with water across the semipermeable dialysis membrane.

THE DIALYZER There are three essential components to dialysis: the dialyzer, the composition and delivery of the dialysate, and the blood delivery system (Fig. 271-2). The dialyzer consists of a plastic device with the facility to perfuse blood and dialysate compartments at very high flow rates. The surface area of dialysis membranes in adult patients is usually in the range of 0.8 to 1.2 m^2.

There are currently two geometric configurations for dialyzers: hollow fiber and flat plate. The hollow fiber dialyzer is the most common in use in the United States. These dialyzers are composed of bundles of capillary tubes through which blood circulates while dialysate travels on the outside of the fiber bundle. In contrast, the less frequently utilized flat plate dialyzers are composed of sandwiched sheets of membrane in a parallel plate configuration. The advantage of the hollow fiber construction is the lower priming volume (60 to 90 mL vs 100 to 120 mL for the flat plate) and easier reprocessing of the filter for reuse in future dialysis treatments.

Recent advances have led to the development of many different types of membrane material. Broadly, there are four categories of dialysis membranes: cellulose, substituted cellulose, cellulosynthetic, and synthetic. Over the past two decades, there has been a gradual switch from cellulose-derived to synthetic membranes, because the latter are more biocompatible. Bioincompatibility may be defined as the ability of the membrane to activate the complement cascade. Cellulosic membranes are bioincompatible because of the presence of free hydroxyl groups on the membrane surface. In contrast, with the substituted cellulose membranes (e.g., cellulose acetate) or the cellulosynthetic membranes, the hydroxyl groups are chemically bonded to either acetate or tertiary amino groups, resulting in limited complement

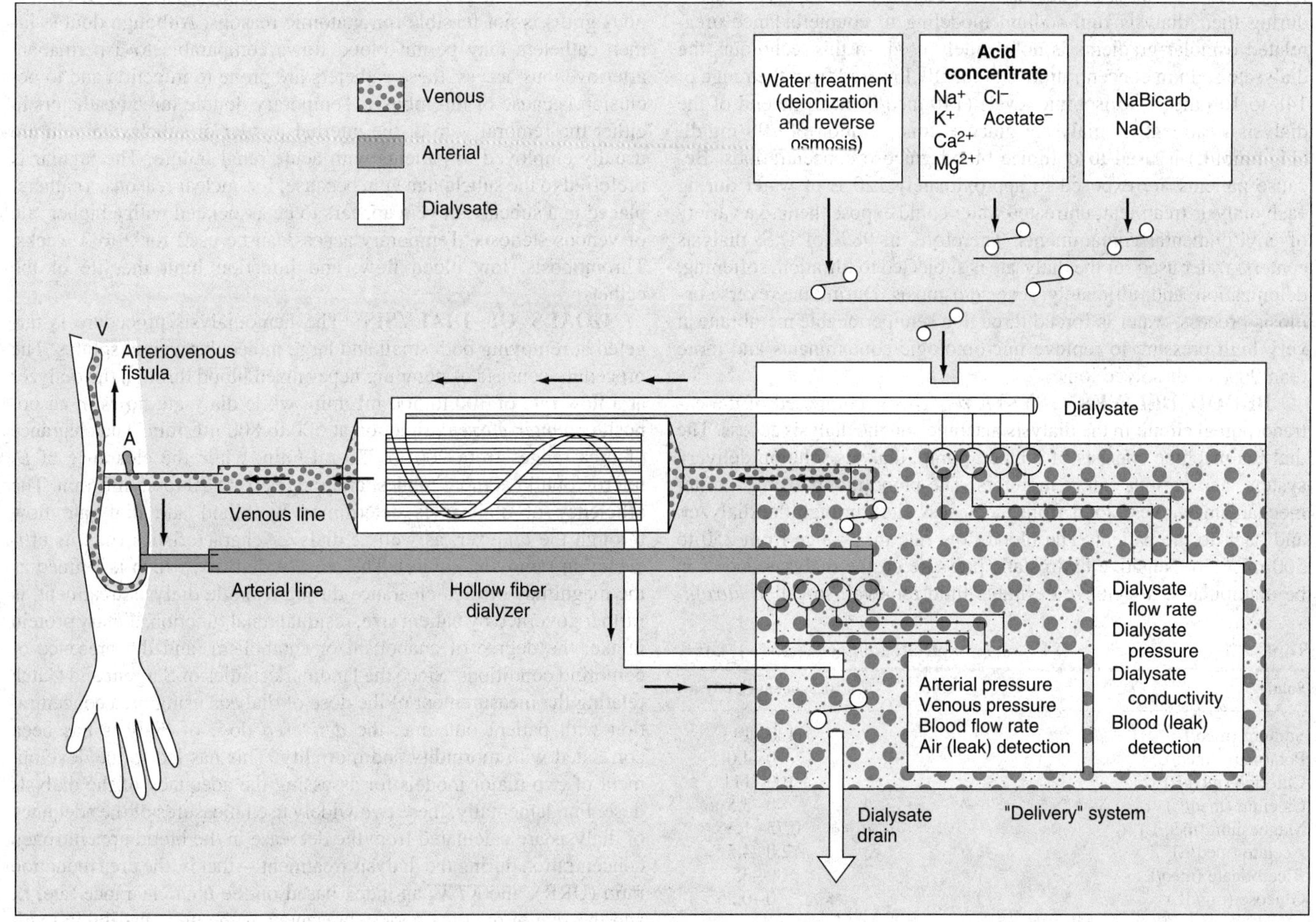

FIGURE 271-2 Schema for hemodialysis.

activation. Synthetic membranes, such as polysulfone, polymethylmethacrylate, and polyacrylonitrile membranes are more biocompatible because of the absence of these hydroxyl groups. Polysulfone membranes are now used in over 60% of the dialysis treatments in the United States.

Reprocessing and reuse of hemodialyzers is employed for patients on chronic hemodialysis in nearly 80% of dialysis centers in the United States, in large part because of the expense of individual dialyzers. Evidence also suggests that reuse reduces complement activation, the incidence of anaphylactoid reactions to the membrane (first-use syndrome), and, in some studies, mortality rates among dialysis patients. In most centers, only the dialyzer unit is reprocessed and reused, whereas in the developing world blood lines are also frequently reused. The reprocessing procedure can be either manual or automated. It consists of the sequential rinsing of the blood and dialysate compartments with water, a chemical cleansing step with reverse ultrafiltration from the dialysate to the blood compartment, the testing of the patency of the dialyzer, and, finally, disinfection of the dialyzer. Formaldehyde, peracetic acid–hydrogen peroxide, and glutaraldehyde are the most frequently used reprocessing agents, with peracetic acid–hydrogen peroxide being the most common.

DIALYSATE The composition of dialysate is listed in Table 271-1. Bicarbonate has replaced acetate as the preferred buffer in the United States. This change has resulted in fewer episodes of hypotension during dialysis. The potassium concentration of dialysate may be varied from 0 to 4 mmol/L depending on the predialysis plasma potassium concentration. The usual dialysate calcium concentration is 1.25 mmol/L (2.5 meq/L). The usual dialysate sodium concentration is 140 mmol/L. Lower dialysate sodium concentrations are associated with a higher frequency of hypotension, cramping, nausea, vomiting, fatigue, and dizziness. In patients who frequently develop hypotension during their dialysis run, sodium modeling to counterbalance urea-related osmolar gradients is now widely used. In this technique, the dialysate sodium concentration is gradually lowered from the range of 148 to 160 meq/L to isotonic levels (140 meq/L) near the end of the dialysis treatment. A dialysate glucose concentration of 200 mg/dL (11 mmol/L) is used to optimize blood glucose concentrations. Because patients are exposed to approximately 120 L of water during each dialysis treatment, untreated water could expose them to a variety of environmental contaminants. Therefore, in 98% of U.S. dialysis centers, water used for the dialysate is subjected to filtration, softening, deionization, and, ultimately, reverse osmosis. During the reverse osmosis process, water is forced through a semipermeable membrane at very high pressure to remove microbiologic contaminants and more than 90% of dissolved ions.

BLOOD DELIVERY SYSTEM This is composed of the extracorporeal circuit in the dialysis machine and the dialysis access. The dialysis machine consists of a blood pump, dialysis solution delivery system, and various safety monitors. The blood pump, using a roller mechanism, moves blood from the access site, through the dialyzer, and back to the patient. The blood flow rate may range from 250 to 500 mL/min. Negative hydrostatic pressure on the dialysate side can be manipulated to achieve desirable fluid removal, so-called *ultrafiltration*. Dialysis membranes have different ultrafiltration coefficients (i.e., mL removed/min per mmHg) so that along with hydrostatic changes, fluid removal can be varied. The dialysis solution delivery system dilutes the dialysate concentrate with water, and monitors the temperature, conductivity, and flow of dialysate. The dialysate may be delivered to the dialyzer from a storage tank or a proportioning system that manufactures dialysate online.

Table 271-1 Composition of Commercial Dialysate for Hemodialysate

Solute	Bicarbonate Dialysate
Sodium (meq/L)	137–143
Potassium (meq/L)	0–4.0
Chloride (meq/L)	100–111
Calcium (meq/L)	0–3.5
Magnesium (meq/L)	0.75–1.5
Acetate (meq/L)	2.0–4.5
Bicarbonate (meq/L)	30–35
Glucose (mg/dL)	0–0.25

Dialysis Access The fistula, graft, or catheter through which blood is obtained for hemodialysis is often referred to as a *dialysis access*. A native fistula created by the anastomosis of an artery to a vein (e.g., the Cimino-Breschia fistula, in which the cephalic vein is anastomosed to the radial artery) results in arterialization of the vein. This faciliates its subsequent use in the placement of large needles (typically 15 gauge) to access the circulation. Although fistulas have a high patency rate (approximately 80% are patent at 3 years following creation), fistulas are created in only approximately 30% of patients in the United States. In the majority of U.S. dialysis patients, the dialysis access consists of an arteriovenous graft which interposes prosthetic material, such as polytetrafluoroethylene, between an artery and a vein. Such grafts have a 3-year patency rate of only 20%. Reasons for the higher rates of graft placement include the late referral of patients to vascular access surgeons so that by the time surgery is planned, the patient's arm veins have already been obliterated through multiple blood draws; the high prevalence of patients with diabetes mellitus and its associated microvascular disease; and the greater surgical skill required in creating a fistula. The most common access-related complication is thrombosis due to intimal hyperplasia, which results in stenosis proximal to the venous anastomosis.

A double lumen cuffed catheter may be a reasonable alternative to either a native arteriovenous fistula or a graft in selected patients in whom dialysis is required relatively urgently, such as patients who manifest delayed recovery from acute renal failure, or where a further permanent access procedure (e.g., arteriovenous fistula or arteriovenous graft) is not feasible for anatomic reasons. Although double lumen catheters may permit blood flows comparable to a permanent arteriovenous access, these catheters are prone to infection and to occlusion because of thrombosis. Temporary double lumen catheters in either the femoral vein or the internal jugular or subclavian vein are usually employed in patients with acute renal failure. The jugular is preferred to the subclavian vein because, for unclear reasons, a catheter placed in a subclavian vein appears to be associated with a higher rate of venous stenosis. Temporary access can be used for 2 to 3 weeks. Thromobosis, low blood flow, and infection limit the life of the catheter.

GOALS OF DIALYSIS The hemodialysis procedure is targeted at removing both small and large molecular weight solutes. The procedure consists of pumping heparinized blood through the dialyzer at a flow rate of 300 to 500 mL/min, while dialysate flows in an opposite *counter-current* direction at 500 to 800 mL/min. The clearance of urea ranges from 200 to 350 mL/min, while the clearance of β_2 microglobulin is more modest and ranges from 20 to 25 mL/min. The efficiency of dialysis is determined by blood and dialysate flow through the dialyzer, as well as dialyzer characteristics (i.e., its efficiency in removing solute). The *dose* of dialysis, which is defined as the magnitude of urea clearance during a single dialysis treatment, is further governed by patient size, residual renal function, dietary protein intake, the degree of anabolism or catabolism, and the presence of comorbid conditions. Since the landmark studies of Sargent and Gatch relating the measurement of the dose of dialysis using urea concentration with patient outcome, the *delivered* dose of dialysis has been correlated with morbidity and mortality. This has led to the development of two major models for assessing the adequacy of the dialysis dose. Fundamentally, these two widely used measures of the adequacy of dialysis are calculated from the decrease in the blood urea nitrogen concentration during the dialysis treatment—that is, the urea reduction ratio (URR), and *KT/V*, an index based on the urea clearance rate, *K*, and the size of the urea pool, represented as the urea distribution volume, V. K, which is the sum of clearance by the dialyzer plus renal clearance, is multiplied by the time spent on dialysis, T. Increasingly, KT/V has become the preferred marker for dialysis adequacy. Currently, a URR of 65% and a KT/V of 1.2 per treatment are minimal standards for adequacy; lower levels of dialysis treatment are associated with increased morbidity and mortality.

For the majority of patients with chronic renal failure, between 9 and 12 h of dialysis is required each week, usually divided into three equal sessions. However, the dialysis dose must be individualized. The measurement of dialysis adequacy using KT/V or the URR serve only as a guide; body size, residual renal function, dietary intake, complicating illness, degree of anabolism or catabolism, and the presence of large interdialytic fluid gains are important factors in consideration of the dialysis prescription.

COMPLICATIONS DURING HEMODIALYSIS Hypotension is the most common acute complication of hemodialysis. Numerous factors appear to increase the risk of hypotension, including excessive ultrafiltration with inadequate compensatory vascular filling, impaired vasoactive or autonomic responses, osmolar shifts, food ingestion, impaired cardiac reserve, the use of antihypertensive drugs, and vasodilation due to the use of warm dialysate. Because of the vasodilatory and cardiodepressive effects of acetate, the use of acetate as the buffer in dialysate was once a common cause of hypotension. Since the introduction of bicarbonate-containing dialysate, dialysis-associated hypotension has become common. The management of hypotension during dialysis consists of discontinuing ultrafiltration, the administration of 100 to 250 cc of isotonic saline, and, in patients with hypoalbuminemia, administration of salt-poor albumin. Hypotension during dialysis can frequently be prevented by careful evaluation of the dry weight, holding of antihypertensive medications on the day prior to and on the day of dialysis, and avoiding heavy meals during dialysis. Additional maneuvers include the performance of sequential ultrafiltration followed by dialysis and cooling of the dialysate during dialysis treatment.

Muscle cramps during dialysis are also a common complication of the procedure. However, since the introduction of volumetric controls on dialysis machines and sodium modelling, the incidence of cramps has fallen. The etiology of dialysis-associated cramps remains obscure. Changes in muscle perfusion because of excessively aggressive volume removal, particularly below the estimated dry weight and the use of low sodium containing dialysate, have been proposed as precipitants of dialysis-associated cramps. Strategies that may be used to prevent cramps include reducing volume removal during dialysis, the use of higher concentrations of sodium in the dialysate, and the use of quinine sulfate (260 mg 2 h before treatment).

Anaphylactoid reactions to the dialyzer, particularly on its first use, have been reported most frequently with the bioincompatible cellulosic-containing membranes. With the gradual phasing out of cuprophane membranes in the United States, the first use syndrome has become relatively uncommon. The first use syndrome consists of either an intermediate hypersensitivity reaction due to an IgE mediated reaction to ethylene oxide used in the sterilization of new dialyzers, or a symptom complex of nonspecific chest and back pain, which appears to result from complement activation and cytokine release.

The major cause of death in patients with ESRD receiving chronic dialysis is cardiovascular disease. The rate of death from cardiac disease is higher in patients on hemodialysis as compared to patients on peritoneal dialysis and renal transplantation. The underlying cause of cardiovascular disease is unclear but may be related to the inadequate treatment of hypertension; the presence of hyperlipidemia, homocystinemia and anemia; the calcification of coronary arteries in patients with an elevated calcium-phosphorus product; and perhaps alterations in cardiovascular dynamics during the dialysis treatment. Intensive investigation of the mechanisms and potential interventions that could impact on reducing the mortality from cardiovascular causes is currently underway.

CONTINUOUS RENAL REPLACEMENT THERAPY Continuous renal replacement therapies (CRRT) have become increasingly prevalent in the intensive care unit setting for management of acute renal failure. The advantages of CRRT over intermittent hemodialysis are that it is usually better tolerated hemodynamically; it facilitates gradual correction of biochemical abnormalities; it is highly effective in removing fluid; and it is technically simple to perform. Clearance of toxic materials (using urea as the marker) can occur with CRRT from convective clearance alone if the ultrafiltration rate is high and with diffusive clearance if dialysis accompanies ultrafiltration. CRRT techniques include continuous arteriovenous hemodiafiltration (CAVH/D) with or without dialysis, and continuous veno-venous hemodiafiltration (CVVH/D) with or without dialysis. Veno-venous therapies differ fundamentally from arteriovenous therapies in that veno-venous therapies do not require arterial access. This allows obtaining less risky and easier vascular access. However, because there is no systemic arterial pressure to drive hemofiltration, veno-venous therapies require a blood pump in the extracorporeal circuit. Veno-venous therapies such as CVVH provide substantial flexibility because changing the blood flow rate in the pump can change the ultrafiltration and clearance rates. In contrast, arterio-venous therapies such as CAVH are associated with variable efficiency because the systemic blood pressure is frequently low or unstable in patients with acute renal failure. Furthermore, low blood flow with CAVH may also result in clotting of the extracorporeal circuit. CAVH often results in clearance rates as low as 10 to 15 mL/min, whereas CVVH may generate clearances in the range of 30 to 40 mL/min. Thus, in light of these advantages of CVVH, many centers have completely switched from arteriovenous to veno-venous therapies in patients with acute renal failure in the ICU setting.

Vascular access in patients on CVVH is usually achieved by the insertion of a double-lumen catheter into the femoral vein. The blood pump is typically set to deliver approximately 150 to 180 mL/min. In automated systems, (e.g., the Cobe Prisma system), the treatment is volumetrically governed by continuously weighing the effluent and replacement solutions and using a servomechanism to drive the replacement fluid pump at a rate computed either to balance the inflow and loss of fluid or to maintain a predetermined rate of fluid loss. Anticoagulation of the extracorporeal circuit is via a heparin infusion (200 to 1600 U/h) through the inflow side of the circuit. Alternatively, citrate can be used to chelate calcium in the extracorporeal circuit to provide regional anticoagulation in selected patients who cannot undergo systemic heparinization. The replacement solution in continuous therapies is designed specifically to replace calcium, magnesium, and bicarbonate. In place of bicarbonate, lactate or citrate is the buffer in the replacement solution. However, bicarbonate-based replacement fluid is the preferred option in patients with liver failure because of the impaired ability of the liver to metabolize either lactate or acetate into bicarbonate.

PERITONEAL DIALYSIS

This consists of infusing 1 to 3 L of a dextrose-containing solution into the peritoneal cavity and allowing the fluid to dwell for 2 to 4 h. As with hemodialysis, toxic materials are removed through a combination of convective clearance generated through ultrafiltration, and diffusive clearance down a concentration gradient. The clearance of solute and water during a peritoneal dialysis exchange depends on the balance between the movement of solute and water into the peritoneal cavity versus absorption from the peritoneal cavity. The rate of diffusion diminishes with time and eventually stops when equilibriation between plasma and dialysate is reached. Absorption of solutes and water from the peritoneal cavity occurs across the peritoneal membrane into the peritoneal capillary circulation and via peritoneal lymphatics into the lymphatic circulation. The rate of peritoneal solute transport varies from patient to patient and may be altered by the presence of infection (peritonitis), drugs such as beta blockers and calcium channel blockers, and by physical factors such as position and exercise.

FORMS OF PERITONEAL DIALYSIS Peritoneal dialysis may be carried out as continuous ambulatory peritoneal dialysis (CAPD), continuous cyclic peritoneal dialysis (CCPD), or nocturnal intermittent peritoneal dialysis (NIPD). In CAPD, dialysis solution is manually infused into the peritoneal cavity during the day and exchanged 3 to 4 times daily. A nighttime dwell is frequently instilled at bedtime and remains in the peritoneal cavity through the night. The drainage of spent dialysate (effluence) is performed manually with the assistance of gravity to move fluid out of the abdomen. In CCPD, exchanges are performed in an automated fashion, usually at night; the patient is connected to the automated cycler, which then performs 4 to 5 exchange cycles while the patient sleeps. Peritoneal dialysis cyclers automatically cycle dialysate in and out of the abdominal cavity. In the morning the patient, with the last exchange remaining in the abdomen, is disconnected from the cycler and goes about his regular daily activities. In NIPD, the patient is given approximately 10 h of cycling each night, with the abdomen left dry during the day.

Peritoneal dialysis solutions are available in various volumes ranging from 0.5 to 3.0 L. The electrolyte composition is shown in Table 271-2. Lactate is the preferred buffer in peritoneal dialysis solutions. Acetate in peritoneal dialysis solutions appears to accelerate peritoneal sclerosis, whereas use of bicarbonte results in precipitation of calcium and caramelization of glucose. The most common additives to peritoneal dialysis solutions are heparin and antibiotics during an episode of acute peritonitis. Insulin may also be added in patients with diabetes mellitus.

ACCESS TO THE PERITONEAL CAVITY This is obtained through a peritoneal catheter. These are either *acute* catheters, used to perform acute continuous peritoneal dialysis, usually in an emergency setting, or *chronic* catheters, which have either one or two Dacron cuffs and are tunneled under the skin into the peritoneal cavity. An acute catheter consists of a straight or slightly curved rigid tube with several holes at its distal end. Catheters can be inserted at the bedside by making a small incision in the anterior abdominal wall; the catheter is inserted with the assistance of a guidewire or stylet. Acute catheters are anchored externally with adhesives or sutures and are usually reserved for temporary use because of the risk of infection, which increases after 72 h of use. In contrast, chronic catheters are flexible and made of silicon rubber with numerous side holes at the distal end. These chronic catheters usually have two Dacron cuffs to promote fibroblast proliferation, granulation and invasion of the cuff. The scarring that occurs around the cuffs anchors the catheter and seals it from bacteria tracking from the skin surface into the peritoneal cavity; it also prevents the external leakage of fluid from the peritoneal cavity. The cuffs are placed in the preperitoneal plane and approximately 2 cm from the skin surface. The most common chronic peritoneal dialysis catheter in use is the Tenckhoff catheter, which contains two cuffs.

Table 271-2 Composition of Peritoneal Dialysate

Solute	Dianeal (PD-2)
Sodium (meq/L)	132
Potassium (meq/L)	0
Chloride (meq/L)	96
Calcium (meq/L)	3.5
Magnesium (meq/L)	0.5
D,L-Lactate (meq/L)	40
Glucose (g%)	
1.5	
2.5	
4.25	
pH	5.2

The initial CAPD prescription consists of the infusion of a 2-L volume of a 1.5% dextrose concentration peritoneal dialysis solution into the peritoneal cavity over 10 min and allowing it to dwell for 2.5 h. The effluent solution is then drained over 20 min before the next exchange. Three daytime exchanges are accompanied by a 2 L nighttime dwell as the standard prescription. Because peritoneal membrane characteristics vary from one individual to another, the peritoneal equilibrium test should be employed within 2 months of a patient initiating peritoneal dialysis. This test measures the peritoneal membrane transfer rate for solutes (usually urea and creatinine) based on the ratio of their concentration in dialysate and plasma at specific times during the dialysate dwell. It allows patients to be classified as low, low–average, high–average, and high transporters. Approximately 10 to 17% of patients are high transporters, 50% high–average transporters, 25 to 30% low–average transporters, and 1 to 5% low transporters. Identifying the high transporters early is important, since these patients not only demonstrate excellent solute removal, they also absorb glucose rapidly; maximum ultrafiltration occurs early in the dwell, followed by reabsorption of water back into the circulation over the course of the dwell. Such patients benefit from either NIPD or CAPD without a nighttime dwell.

The dose of peritoneal dialysis required to provide adequate or optimal dialysis as measured by patient outcomes is not known. However, there is emerging consensus that the weekly KT/V should be >2.0 and the creatinine clearance >65 L/week per 1.73 m^2. The most frequently utilized approach to calculating a weekly KT/V and creatinine clearance is by collecting the spent dialysate and urine over a 24-h period. The peritoneal dialysis prescription can be tailored to improve suboptimal clearance values by either increasing the volume of individual exchanges, increasing the number of exchanges, or by combining the CAPD and CCPD techniques. In combining these techniques, the CAPD patient hooks up to a cycler at night and the machine automatically performs one or two nocturnal exchanges, whereas the CCPD patient makes an additional manual daytime exchange.

ACKNOWLEDGMENT

Dr. J. Michael Lazarus was a co-author of this chapter in the 14th edition; some of his material has been carried forward to the present edition.

BIBLIOGRAPHY

BRENNER BM (ed): *Brenner and Rector's The Kidney*, 6th ed. Philadelphia, Saunders, 2000

BURKART JM: Peritoneal dialysis, in *Brenner and Rector's The Kidney*, 6th ed, BM Brenner (ed). Philadelphia, Saunders, 2000

DENKER BM et al: Hemodialysis, in *Brenner and Rector's The Kidney*, 6th ed, BM Brenner (ed). Philadelphia, Saunders, 2000

DEPNER TA: *Prescribing Hemodialysis: A Guide to Urea Modeling*. Boston, Kluwer Academic, 1991

DIAZ-BUXO JA: Early referral and selection of peritoneal dialysis as a treatment modality. Nephrol Dialy Transplant 15:147, 2000

GOTCH FA, SARGENT JA: A mechanistic analysis of the National Cooperative Dialysis Study (NCDS). Kidney Int 28:526, 1985

HAKIM RM: Clinical implications of hemodialysis membrane bioincompatibility. Kidney Int 44:484, 1993

FORNI LG, HILTON PJ: Current concepts: Continuous hemofiltration in the treatment of acute renal failure. N Engl J Med 336:1303, 1997

KESHAVIAH P: Technology and clinical application of hemodialysis, in *The Principles and Practice of Nephrology*, HR Jacobson et al (eds). St. Louis, Mosby-Year Book, 1995

MEYER MM: Renal replacement therapies. Crit Care Clin 16:29, 2000

PASTAN S, BAILEY J: Dialysis therapy. N Engl J Med 338:1428, 1998

RENAL DATA SYSTEM: USRDS 1997 annual data report. Bethesda, MD, National Institutes of Diabetes and Digestive and Kidney Disease, 1997

SANG GL et al: Sodium ramping in hemodialysis: A study of beneficial and adverse effect. Am J Kidney Dis 29:669 1997

SHULMAN G, JAKIM RM: Complications of hemodialysis, *The Principles and Practice of Nephrology*, HR Jacobson et al (eds.). St. Louis, Mosby-Year Book, p 673, 1995

TASK FORCE ON REUSE OF DIALYZERS, COUNCIL ON DIALYSIS, NATIONAL KIDNEY FOUNDATION: National Kidney Foundation report on dialyzer reuse. Am J Kidney Dis 30:859, 1997

272 Charles B. Carpenter, Edgar L. Milford, Mohamed H. Sayegh

TRANSPLANTATION IN THE TREATMENT OF RENAL FAILURE

Transplantation of the human kidney is frequently the most effective treatment of advanced chronic renal failure. Worldwide, tens of thousands of such procedures have been performed. When azathioprine and prednisone were initially used as immunosuppressive drugs in the 1960s, the results with properly matched familial donors were superior to those with organs from cadaveric donors, namely, 75 to 90% compared with 50 to 60% graft survival rates at 1 year. During the 1970s and 1980s, the success rate at the 1-year mark for cadaveric transplants rose progressively. By the time cyclosporine was introduced in the early 1980s, cadaveric donor grafts had a 70% 1-year survival and reached the 80 to 85% level in the mid 1990s (Fig. 272-1). After the first year, graft survival curves show an exponential decline in numbers of functioning grafts from which a half-life ($t_{1/2}$) in years is calculated (Fig. 272-1). Mortality rates after transplantation are highest in the first year and are age-related: 2% for ages 6 to 45 years, 7% for ages 46 to 60 years, and 10% for ages over 60 years, and lower thereafter. These rates compare favorably to those in the chronic dialysis population, even after risk adjustments for age, diabetes, and cardiovascular status. Occasionally, acute irreversible rejection may occur after many months of good function, especially if the patient neglects to take the immunosuppressive drugs. Most grafts, however, succumb at varying rates to a chronic vascular and interstitial obliterative process termed *chronic rejection*, although its pathogenesis is incompletely understood. Overall, transplantation returns the majority of patients to an improved life-style and an improved life expectancy, as compared to patients on dialysis; however, careful prospective cohort studies have yet to be reported.

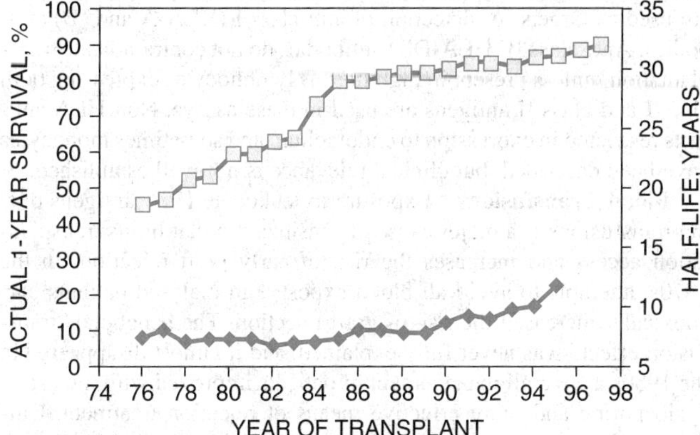

FIGURE 272-1 Graft survival of first cadaveric renal transplant cohorts since 1976. These are registry data from the United States. The upper curve is the actual 1-year graft survival (-□-), which has reached almost 90% for the patients transplanted in 1997. Note the moderate annual rise in the early years up to 1983, when cyclosporine was introduced and 1-year graft survivals increased for 2 years. Since 1985 there has been a slow (1%/year) improvement. The lower curve is a representation of long-term graft survival, expressed as a half-life in years (-◆-) of those grafts functioning at 1 year. With thousands of cases in each cohort and a minimum of 3 years follow-up, an accurate half-life can be determined from a log-linear plot. The last calculated value of 11.6 years, although tentative because of the 2-year follow-up, is close to the historic value for haplotype-matched family donors (Table 272-1). The trend in the rise in half-life during the previous 5 years from 6 to 9 years is certainly meaningful and represents improved clinical management, as well as the introduction of mandatory sharing of HLA-matched cadaveric kidneys through the United Network for Organ Sharing. *[Drawn from data of JM Cecka, in JM Cecka and PI Terasaki (eds): Clinical Transplants, 1997, UCLA Tissue Typing Laboratory Los Angeles, 1998, pp 1–14. Updated from the UNOS web site.]*

RECIPIENT SELECTION Transplantation should be undertaken only when there is a state of irreversible renal failure. When a living donor is available, a period of chronic dialysis may be avoided. When end-stage renal disease is the result of diabetes mellitus, there is special merit in having a transplant before it is necessary to initiate maintenance dialysis in order to minimize progression of cardiovascular complications of diabetes, which are frequently accelerated during chronic dialysis. In patients who must wait for a cadaveric donor kidney, a dialysis program must be established since the waiting time will be in the 3 to 4 year range for most patients. Each candidate must have a careful risk/benefit evaluation. Elderly patients over age 70, patients with metastatic malignancy, or those with advanced cardiopulmonary disease are generally poor operative risks and are also more susceptible to infections in the setting of immunosuppressive medications. Coronary artery revascularization may be indicated in select patients prior to transplantation. Because of the growing shortage of available cadaveric organs in relation to the expanding chronic dialysis population, patients who do not have a life expectancy of at least 5 years are generally not placed on the national waiting list in the United States.

DONOR SELECTION Donors can be cadavers or volunteer living donors. The latter are usually family members selected to have at least partial compatibility for HLA antigens. Living volunteer donors should be normal on physical examination and of the same major ABO blood group, because crossing major blood group barriers prejudices survival of the allograft. It is possible, however, to transplant a kidney of a type O donor into an A, B, or AB recipient. Selective renal arteriography should be performed on donors to rule out the presence of multiple or abnormal renal arteries, because the surgical procedure is difficult and the ischemic time of the transplanted kidney long when vascular abnormalities exist. Cadaveric donors should be free of malignant neoplastic disease, hepatitis, and HIV because of possible transmission to the recipient. Increased risk of graft failure exists when the donor is elderly or has renal failure and when the kidney has a prolonged period of ischemia and storage.

In the United States, there is a coordinated national system (United Network for Organ Sharing) of regulations, allocation support, and outcomes analysis for kidney transplantation. It is now possible to remove cadaver kidneys and to maintain them for up to 48 h on cold pulsatile perfusion or simple flushing and cooling. This permits adequate time for typing, cross-matching, transportation, and selection problems to be solved.

TISSUE TYPING AND CLINICAL IMMUNOGENETICS Matching for antigens of the HLA major histocompatibility gene complex (Chap. 306) is an important criterion for selection of donors for renal allografts. Each mammalian species has a single chromosomal region that encodes the strong, or major, transplantation antigens, and this region on the human sixth chromosome is called *HLA*. HLA antigens have been classically defined by serologic techniques, but methods to define specific nucleotide sequences in genomic DNA are increasingly being used. Other antigens, called "minor," may nevertheless play crucial roles, in addition to the ABH(O) blood groups and endothelial antigens that are not shared with lymphocytes. The Rh system is not expressed on graft tissue. Evidence for designation of HLA as the genetic region encoding major transplantation antigens comes from the success rate in living related donor renal and bone marrow transplantation, with superior results in HLA-identical sibling pairs. Nevertheless, 5% of HLA-identical renal allografts are rejected, often within the first weeks after transplantation. These failures represent states of prior sensitization to non-HLA antigens. Non-HLA antigens are relatively weak when initially encountered and are therefore suppressible by conventional immunosuppressive therapy. Once priming has occurred, however, secondary responses are much more refractory to treatment. ABO incompatibilities are hazardous because of the presence of natural anti-A and anti-B antibodies in recipients and the normal expression of A and B blood group substances on endothelium, resulting in immediate vascular injury.

Living Donors When first-degree relatives are donors, graft survival rates at 1 year are slightly greater than those for cadaver grafts, with the exception of HLA-identical donors where 1-year results are approximately 95%. After the first year, the long-term survival rates as defined by the $t_{1/2}$ still favor the partially matched (one HLA haplotype) family donor over a randomly selected cadaver donor (Table 272-1). In addition, living donors provide the advantage of immediate availability. Waiting lists for cadaveric kidneys have grown faster than the available organ supply, to the point where most new patients with end-stage renal disease wait for more than 4 years. In response to this increasing disparity between cadaver donor supply and patient demand, living unrelated volunteers, usually spouses or close friends, are being accepted as donors in increasing numbers. It is illegal in the United States to purchase organs for transplantation. The results of transplantation using living unrelated donors have been most satisfactory, with initial and long-term survival rates the same as for partial HLA-matched family donors and better than for partially matched cadaveric donors (Table 272-1).

Concern has been expressed regarding the potential risk to a volunteer kidney donor of premature renal failure after several years of increased blood flow and hyperfiltration per nephron in the remaining kidney. There are a few reports of the development of hypertension, proteinuria, and even lesions of focal segmental sclerosis in donors under long-term follow-up. Difficulties in donors followed for 20 or more years are unusual, however, and it may be that having a single kidney becomes significant only when another condition, such as hypertension, is superimposed. It is also desirable to consider the risk of development of type 1 diabetes mellitus in a family member who is a potential donor to a diabetic renal failure patient. Anti-insulin and anti-islet antibodies should be measured, and glucose tolerance tests should be performed in such donors to rule out a prediabetic state.

HLA Matching and Cadaveric Donors The question of whether matching of HLA antigens in unrelated donor-recipient pairs would approximate the high initial success rates and slow rates of subsequent graft loss with HLA-identical sib pairs could not be answered until the late 1980s when reliable class II histocompatibility (DR) typing became widely available. Now that pooled data on tens of thousands of cadaveric renal transplants from all over the world are available, the HLA-matching effect can be clearly seen, especially in the long-term $t_{1/2}$ half-life survival figures. It is shown in Table 272-1 that there is an overall beneficial effect of HLA matching in first cadaveric grafts. When compared with HLA-identical transplants, in which the 1-year graft survival rate is 95% and the subsequent half-life is 25 years, one-HLA-haplotype–matched family donor transplants have 1-year survival rates of 85% with a 12-year half-life (Table 272-1). With increasing numbers of mismatches for cadaveric donors, the half-life decreases from 20 to 7.7 years. The survival rates at the 10-year mark are projected to range from 65 (zero mismatches) to 34% (six mismatches). Many centers now report 1-year graft survival rates in the 85 to 90% range for all renal transplants (Fig. 272-1), possibly the result of heavy initial immunosuppression, but the subsequent half-lives are similar to those above. There is controversy regarding the value of cadaveric organ-sharing rules that are based entirely upon the numbers of HLA mismatches. Avoidance of mismatching for six antigens Table 272-1) is a top priority in the United States, however, and 20% of kidneys are transplanted on this basis. Table 272-1 also shows the interaction of HLA matching and graft ischemia on results; namely, kidneys from HLA-incompatible spousal donors do better than those from similarly mismatched cadaver donors, suggesting that the additional ischemic injury of organ storage is important. When such a cadaveric donor is HLA-compatible, however, ischemia and storage do not impede the matching benefit.

Table 272-1 Effect of HLA-A, -B, -DR Mismatching on Kidney Graft Survival[a]

Donor Mismatches	Half-Life of Graft Survival, years	10-Year Graft Survival, %
Living related donor (HLA-identical sib = none)	24.0	74
Cadaver (none for 6 antigens)	20.3	65
Living related donor (1 haplotype = 3)	12.0	54
Living unrelated donor (average 4)	12.0	54
Cadaver (overall)	9.0	40
Cadaver (1 or 2)	10.4	45
Cadaver (3 or 4)	8.4	38
Cadaver (5 or 6)	7.7	34

[a] HLA antigens are codominantly inherited: each person has two A, two B, and two DR antigens, for a total of six.

Presensitization A positive cross match of recipient serum with donor T lymphocytes representing anti-HLA class I is usually predictive of an acute vasculitic event termed *hyperacute rejection*. Patients with anti-HLA antibodies can be safely transplanted if careful cross matching of donor blood lymphocytes with recipient serum is performed. Patients sustained by dialysis often show fluctuating antibody titers and specificity patterns. At the time of assignment of a cadaveric kidney, cross matches are performed with at least a current serum. Previously analyzed antibody specificities and additional cross matches are performed accordingly. Techniques for cross matching are not universally standardized; however, at least two techniques are employed in most laboratories. The minimal purpose for the cross match is avoidance of hyperacute rejection mediated by recipient antibodies to donor HLA class I antigens. Sensitive tests, such as the use of flow cytometry, can be useful for avoidance of accelerated, and often untreatable, early graft rejection in patients receiving second or third transplants. Donor T lymphocytes, which express only class I antigens, are used as targets for detection of anti-class I (HLA-A and -B) antibodies. Anti-class II (HLA-DR) antibodies do not contraindicate transplantation, unless present in high titer. B lymphocytes expressing both class I and class II antigens are used in these assays. Non-HLA antigens restricted in expression to endothelium and sometimes monocytes have been described, but clinical relevance is not well established.

Blood Transfusions Exposure to leukocyte HLA antigens during transfusions is a major cause of sensitization that limits transplantation access and increases the risk of early graft rejection. In the 1970s, attempts to avoid all blood exposure in dialysed patients paradoxically increased the risk of graft rejection. The beneficial "transfusion effect" was never fully explained, and it almost disappeared in the 1980s as overall management of patients improved with the use of cyclosporine and more effective means of rejection treatment. Currently, with the use of erythropoietin the need for transfusion is much reduced. It has been noted, however, that nontransfused patients do have more rejection activity.

IMMUNOLOGY OF REJECTION Knowledge of the immunology of tissue transplantation stems largely from animal experimentation. However, enough evidence has accumulated in humans to indicate that the mechanisms are not qualitatively different from those found in other areas of immunology (Chap. 305). Early rejection is associated with activation of T lymphocytes having direct specificity against donor antigens. These may be cytotoxic cells (CD8+ or CD4+) or cells that mediate delayed hypersensitivity (CD4+); however, significant numbers of B lymphocytes, natural killer cells, and macrophages appear in the early infiltrate, and cells capable of mediating antibody-dependent cell-mediated cytotoxicity are also present. Many of the B lymphocytes produce immunoglobulins. The spectrum of cellular and humoral response and graft injury is quite varied, depending on specific genetic differences between donor and recipient and states of presensitization. The greater the degree of presensitization, the more likely it is that one will find antibody-mediated vascular lesions. All the processes shown in Fig. 272-2 are possible, but their relative contribution varies from case to case. Monitoring of peripheral blood lymphocyte subsets utilizing monoclonal antibodies to functionally related surface molecules, such as CD4 (T helper cells) and CD8 (T cytotoxic cells), has been related to the degree of rejection activity in some surveys. Since the principal role of the CD4 molecule is to promote interaction of T cells with class II HLA molecules on antigen-presenting cells and similarly CD8 interacts with class I HLA (Chap. 305), it is not surprising that both types of T cells are usually present. Finally, the cytokine mediators of the cellular immune response [interleukin (IL) 1 to IL-4, IL-6, IL-10, IL-12, tumor necrosis factor (TNF), and interferon γ] are involved in the control and expression of the alloimmune rejection response. For example, T cell production of interferon γ causes increased expression of HLA antigens on endothelial cells. In normal immunobiology this effect may be to promote more efficient presentation of foreign antigen, while in transplantation it enhances the immunogenicity of the vascularized transplant. Also, IL-2, the major growth factor for expansion of effector T cells, is the product of a major subset of CD4 cells (Th1), while other CD4 cells (Th2) produce B cell growth factors, such as IL-4.

The failure of transplanted kidneys after several years of adequate function is said to be due to "chronic rejection." In such kidneys, the development of nephrosclerosis, with proliferation of the vascular intima of renal vessels, and intimal fibrosis, with marked decrease in the lumen of the vessels, takes place (Fig. 272-3). The result is renal ischemia, hypertension, tubular atrophy, interstitial fibrosis, and glomerular atrophy with eventual renal failure. It is not established, however, whether slow deterioration of graft function over years is due to the same mechanisms in all cases. In addition to the established influence of HLA incompatibility, the age, number of nephrons, and ischemic history of a donor kidney may contribute to ultimate progressive renal failure in transplanted patients.

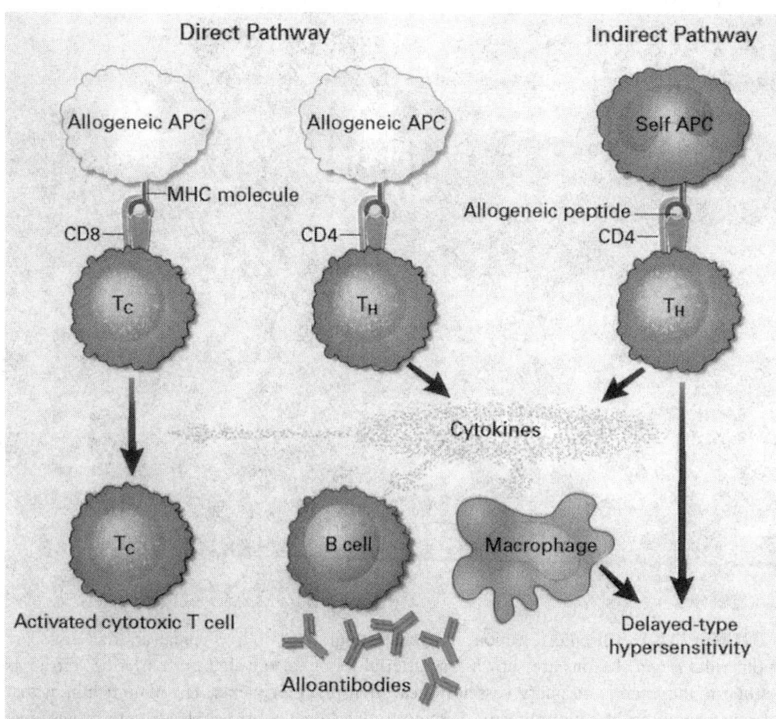

FIGURE 272-2 Recognition pathways for major histocompatibility complex (MHC) antigens. Graft rejection is initiated by CD4 helper T lymphocytes (T_H) having antigen receptors that bind to specific complexes of peptides and MHC class II molecules on antigen-presenting cells (APC). In transplantation, in contrast to other immunologic responses, there are two sets of T cell clones involved in rejection. In the direct pathway the class II MHC of donor allogeneic APCs is recognized by CD4 T_H cells that bind to the intact MHC molecule, and class I MHC allogeneic cells are recognized by CD8 T cells. The latter generally proliferate into cytotoxic cells (T_C). In the indirect pathway, the incompatible MHC molecules are processed into peptides that are presented by the self-APCs of the recipient. The indirect, but not the direct, pathway is the normal physiologic process in T cell recognition of foreign antigens. Once T_H cells are activated, they proliferate, and by secretion of cytokines and direct contact exert strong helper effects on macrophages, T_C, and B cells. *(From Sayegh and Turka, Copyright 1998, Massachusetts Medical Society. All rights reserved.)*

IMMUNOSUPPRESSIVE TREATMENT Immunosuppressive therapy, as presently available, generally suppresses all immune responses, including those to bacteria, fungi, and even malignant tumors. In the 1950s when clinical renal transplantation began, sublethal total-body irradiation was employed. We have now reached the point where sophisticated pharmacologic immunosuppression is available, but it still has the hazard of promoting infection and malignancy. In general, all clinically useful drugs are more selective to primary than to memory immune responses. Agents to suppress the immune response are discussed in the following paragraphs, and those currently in clinical use are listed in Table 272-2.

Drugs *Azathioprine*, an analogue of mercaptopurine, was for two decades the keystone to immunosuppressive therapy in humans. This agent can inhibit synthesis of DNA, RNA, or both. Because cell division and proliferation are a necessary part of the immune response to antigenic stimulation, suppression by this agent may be mediated by the inhibition of mitosis of immunologically competent lymphoid cells, interfering with synthesis of DNA. Alternatively, immunosuppression may be brought about by blocking the synthesis of RNA (possibly messenger RNA), inhibiting processing of antigens prior to lymphocyte stimulation. Therapy with azathioprine in doses of 1.5 to 2.0 mg/kg per day is generally added to cyclosporine as a means of decreasing the requirements for the latter. Because azathioprine is rapidly metabolized by the liver, its dosage need not be varied directly in relation to renal function, even though renal failure results in retention of the metabolites of azathioprine. Reduction in dosage is required because of leukopenia and occasionally thrombocytopenia. Excessive amounts of azathioprine may also cause jaundice, anemia, and alopecia. If it is essential to administer allopurinol concurrently, the azathioprine dose must be reduced, since inhibition of xanthine oxidase delays degradation. This combination is best avoided.

Mycophenolate mofetil is now used in place of azathioprine in many centers. It has a similar mode of action and a mild degree of gastrointestinal toxicity but produces minimal bone marrow suppression. Its advantage is its increased potency in preventing or reversing rejection.

Glucocorticoids are important adjuncts to immunosuppressive therapy. Of all the agents employed, prednisone has effects that are easiest to assess, and in large doses it is usually effective for the reversal of rejection. In general, 200 to 300 mg prednisone is given immediately prior to or at the time of transplantation, and the dosage is reduced to 30 mg within a week. The side effects of the glucocorticoids, particularly impairment of wound healing and predisposition to infection, make it desirable to taper the dose as rapidly as possible in the immediate postoperative period. Customarily, methylprednisolone, 0.5 to 1.0 g intravenously, is administered immediately upon diagnosis of beginning rejection and continued once daily for 3 days. When the drug is effective, the results are usually apparent within 96 h. Such "pulse" doses are not effective in chronic rejection. Most patients whose renal function is stable after 6 months or a year do not require large doses of prednisone; maintenance doses of 10 to 15 mg/d are the rule. Many patients tolerate an alternate-day course of steroids without an increased risk of rejection.

A major effect of steroids is on the monocyte-macrophage system, preventing the release of IL-6 and IL-1. Lymphopenia after large doses of glucocorticoids is primarily due to sequestration of recirculating blood lymphocytes to lymphoid tissue.

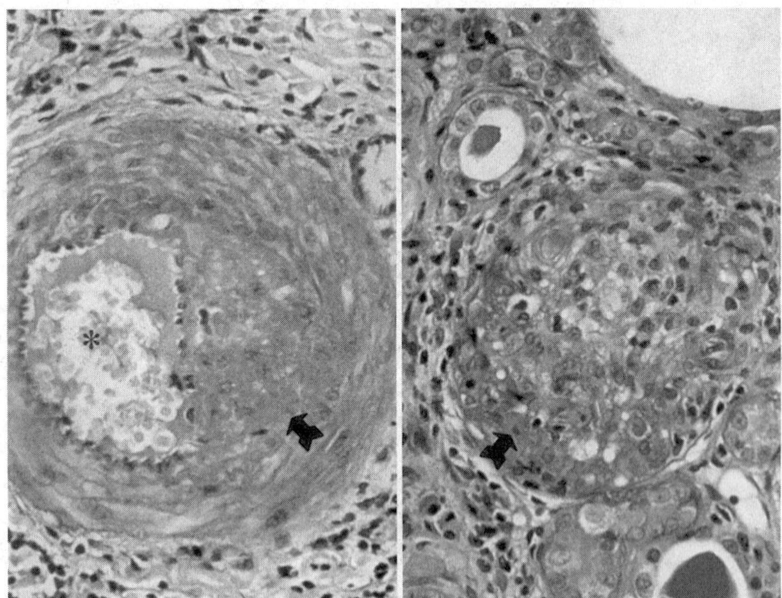

FIGURE 272-3 Chronic rejection in a renal allograft (×400). Typical arterial *(left)* and glomerular *(right)* lesions are shown. The arterial lesion, also called graft arteriosclerosis, is similar to that seen in coronary vessels of heart transplant recipients. The main feature is that of myointimal proliferation, mostly of smooth muscle cells (arrow), leading to progressive luminal narrowing (*) with resultant ischemia. The glomerular lesion consists of mesangial proliferation with occlusion of capillary spaces, leading ultimately to glomerulosclerosis (arrow). The net result of these lesions in the vasculature is interstitial atrophy and fibrosis. *(From Sayegh and Turka, Copyright 1998, Massachusetts Medical Society. All rights reserved.)*

Cyclosporine is a fungal peptide with potent immunosuppressive activity. It acts on the calcineurin pathway to block transcription of mRNA for IL-2 and other proinflammatory cytokines, thereby inhibiting T cell proliferation. Although it works alone, cyclosporine is more effective in conjunction with glucocorticoids. Since cyclosporine blocks production of IL-2 by T cells, its combination with steroids is expected to produce a double block in the macrophage → IL-6/IL-1 → T cell → IL-2 sequence. As noted, clinical results with tens of thousands of renal transplants have been impressive. Of its toxic effects (nephrotoxicity, hepatoxicity, hirsutism, tremor, gingival hyperplasia, diabetes), only nephrotoxicity presents a serious management problem and is further discussed below.

Tacrolimus (FK-506) is a fungal macrolide that has the same mode of action, and a similar side effect profile, as cyclosporine. It does not produce hirsutism or gingival hyperplasia, however. De novo induction of diabetes mellitus is more common with tacrolimus. The drug was first used in liver transplantation, and may substitute for cyclosporine entirely, or be tried as an alternative in renal patients whose rejections are poorly controlled by cyclosporine.

Sirolimus (previously called rapamycin) is another fungal macrolide but has a different mode of action: namely, it inhibits T cell growth factor pathways, preventing the response to IL-2 and other cytokines. It shows some promise in clinical trials in combination with cyclosporine.

Antibodies to Lymphocytes When serum from animals made immune to host lymphocytes is injected into the recipient, a marked suppression of cellular immunity to the tissue graft results. The action on cell-mediated immunity is greater than on humoral immunity. A globulin fraction of serum [antilymphocyte globulin (ALG)] is the agent generally employed. For use in humans, peripheral human lymphocytes, thymocytes, or lymphocytes from spleens or thoracic duct fistulas have been injected into horses, rabbits, or goats to produce antilymphocyte serum, from which the globulin fraction is then separated. Monoclonal antibodies against defined lymphocyte subsets offer a more precise and standardized form of therapy. OKT3 is directed to the CD3 molecules that form a portion of the T cell antigen-receptor complex; hence CD3 is expressed on all mature T cells. CD4 or CD8 molecules also form part of the fully activated cluster of molecules, and monoclonal antibodies to these offer the potential for more selective targeting of T cell subsets. Another approach to more selective therapy is to target the 55-kDa alpha chain of the IL-2 receptor, expressed only on T cells that have been recently activated. The problem with such mouse antibodies is the potential for developing human antimouse antibodies (HAMA), an event that limits the effective period of use. Genetically engineered monoclonal antibodies can solve this problem. Two such antibodies to the IL-2 receptor, in which either a chimeric protein has been made between mouse Fab with human Fc (basiliximab) or "humanized" by splicing the combining sites of the mouse into a molecule that is 90% human IgG (daclizumab), have been approved for use, after clinical evidence of reduction of rejection episodes. Their precise clinical role is under study.

Table 272-2 Maintenance Immunosuppressive Drugs

Agent	Pharmacology	Mechanisms	Side Effects
Glucocorticoids	Increased bioavailability with hypoalbuminemia and liver disease; prednisone/prednisolone generally used	Binds cytosolic receptors and heat shock proteins. Blocks transcription of IL-1,-2,-3,-6, TNF-α, and IFN-γ	Hypertension, glucose intolerance, dyslipidemia, osteoporosis
Cyclosporine (CsA)	Lipid-soluble polypeptide, variable absorption, microemulsion more predictable	Trimolecular complex with cyclophilin and calcineurin → block in cytokine (e.g., IL-2) production; however, stimulates TGF-β production	Nephrotoxicity, hypertension, dyslipidemia, glucose intolerance, hirsutism/hyperplasia of gums
Tacrolimus (FK506)	Macrolide, well absorbed	Trimolecular complex with FKBP-12 and calcineurin → block in cytokine (e.g., IL-2) production; may stimulate TGF-β production	Similar to CsA, but hirsutism/hyperplasia of gums unusual, and diabetes more likely
Azathioprine	Mercaptopurine analogue	Hepatic metabolites inhibit purine synthesis	Marrow suppression (WBC > RBC > platelets)
Mycophenolate Mofetil (MMF)	Metabolized to mycophenolic acid	Inhibits purine synthesis via inosine monophosphate dehydrogenase	Diarrhea/cramps; dose-related liver and marrow suppression is uncommon
Sirolimus	Macrolide, poor oral bioavailability	Complexes with FKBP-12 and then blocks p70 S6 kinase in the IL-2 receptor pathway for proliferation	Hyperlipidemia, thrombocytopenia

NOTE: IL, interleukin; TNF, tumor necrosis factor; IFN, interferon; TGF, transforming growth factor; FKBP-12, FK506 binding protein 12; WBC, white blood cells; RBC, red blood cells.

CLINICAL COURSE AND MANAGEMENT OF THE RECIPIENT Adequate hemodialysis should be performed within 48 h of surgery, and care should be taken that the serum potassium level is not markedly elevated so that intraoperative cardiac arrhythmias can be averted. The diuresis that commonly occurs postoperatively must be carefully monitored; in some instances it may be massive, reflecting the inability of ischemic tubules to regulate sodium and water excretion; with large diureses, massive potassium losses may occur. Most chronically uremic patients have some excess of extracellular fluid, and it is useful to maintain an expanded fluid volume in the immediate postoperative period. Acute tubular necrosis (ATN) may cause immediate oliguria or may follow an initial short period of graft function. ATN is most likely when cadaveric donors have been hypotensive or if the interval between cessation of blood flow and organ harvest (warm ischemic time) is more than a few minutes. Recovery usually occurs within 3 weeks, although periods as long as 6 weeks have been reported. Superimposition of rejection on ATN is common, and the differential diagnosis may be difficult without a graft biopsy. Cyclosporine therapy prolongs ATN, and some patients do not diurese until the dose is drastically reduced. Many centers avoid starting cyclosporine for the first several days, using ALG or a monoclonal antibody along with mycophenolate mofetil and prednisone until renal function is established.

The Rejection Episode Early diagnosis of rejection allows prompt institution of therapy to preserve renal function and prevent irreversible damage. Clinical evidence of rejection is rarely characterized by fever, swelling, and tenderness over the allograft. Rejection may present only with a rise in serum creatinine, with or without a reduction in urine volume. The focus should be on ruling out other causes of functional deterioration.

Arteriography and radioactive iodohippurate sodium renograms of the transplanted kidney may be useful in ascertaining changes in the renal vasculature and in renal blood flow, even in the absence of urinary flow. Thrombosis of the renal vein occurs rarely; it may be reversible if caused by technical factors and intervention is prompt. Diagnostic ultrasound is the procedure of choice to rule out urinary obstruction or to confirm the presence of perirenal collections of urine, blood, or lymph. When renal function has been good initially, a rise in the serum creatinine level is the most sensitive and reliable indicator of possible rejection and may be the only sign.

Calcineurin inhibitors (cyclosporine or tacrolimus) may cause deterioration in renal function in a manner similar to a rejection episode. In fact, rejection processes tend to be more indolent with these inhibitors, and the only way to make a diagnosis may be by renal biopsy. Calcineurin inhibitors have an afferent arteriolar constrictor effect on the kidney and may produce permanent vascular and interstitial injury after sustained high-dose therapy. Addition of angiotensin-converting enzyme (ACE) inhibitors or nonsteroidal anti-inflammatory drugs are likely to raise serum creatinine levels. The former are generally safe to use after the early months, while the latter are best avoided in all renal transplant patients. There is no universally accepted lesion(s) that makes a diagnosis of calcineurin inhibitor toxicity, although interstitial fibrosis, isometric tubular vacuolization, and thickening of arteriolar walls have been noted by some. Basically, if the biopsy does not reveal moderate and active cellular rejection activity, the serum creatinine will most likely respond to a reduction in dose. Blood levels of drug can be useful if very high or very low but do not correlate precisely with renal function, although serial changes in a patient can be useful. If rejection activity is present in the biopsy, appropriate therapy is indicated. The first rejection episode is usually treated with intravenous administration of methylprednisolone, 500 to 1000 mg daily for 3 days. Failure to respond is indication for antibody therapy, usually with OKT3.

OKT3 monoclonal antibody, given intravenously for 10 to 14 days, is effective in more than 90% of first rejections, and less so if methylprednisolone pulses have failed and in cases of severe recurrent rejection activity. A major problem with OKT3 is that severe systemic reactions may be produced during the first day or two of therapy. Chills, fever, hypotension, and headache are the direct result of the antibody effects on the targeted T cells, most likely related to the known potential of OKT3 to activate T cells nonspecifically with release of cytokines, especially TNF-α. If the antibody is administered to overhydrated oliguric patients, pulmonary edema may be induced. These reactions are not characteristic of other monoclonal antibodies, such as those to the IL-2 receptor. Recurrent or rebound rejection activity may require additional therapy. In such circumstances, methylprednisolone may be effective even though it failed initially. Second courses of OKT3 may be given in spite of HAMA generated in response to the first course if the titers are low and the human antibodies are not directed to the combining-site region (idiotype) of the OKT3.

Management Problems The usual clinical manifestations of infection in the posttransplant period are blunted by immunosuppressive therapy. The major toxic effect of azathioprine is bone marrow suppression, which is less likely with mycophenolate mofetil, while calcineurin inhibitors have no marrow effects. All drugs predispose to unusual opportunistic infections, however. The signs and symptoms of infection may be masked and distorted, and fever without obvious cause is common. Only after days or weeks it may become apparent that it has a viral or fungal origin. Bacterial infections are most common during the first month after transplantation. The importance of blood cultures in such patients cannot be overemphasized, because systemic infection without obvious foci is frequent, although wound infections with or without urinary fistulas are most common. Particularly ominous are rapidly occurring pulmonary lesions, which may result in death within 5 days of onset. When these become apparent, immunosuppressive agents should be discontinued, except for maintenance doses of prednisone. Aggressive diagnostic procedures, including transbronchial and open lung biopsy, are frequently indicated. In the case of *Pneumocystis carinii* (Chap. 209) infection, trimethoprim-sulfamethoxazole is the treatment of choice; amphotericin B has been used effectively in systemic fungal infections. Prophylaxis against *P. carinii* with daily, or alternate day, low-dose trimethoprim-sulfamethoxazole is very effective. Involvement of the oropharynx with *Candida* (Chap. 205) may be treated with local nystatin. Tissue-invasive fungal infections require treatment with systemic agents such as fluconazole. Small doses (a total of 300 mg) of amphotericin given over a period of 2 weeks may be effective in fungal infections refractory to fluconazole. Macrolide antibiotics, especially ketoconazole and erythromycin, and some calcium channel blockers (diltiazem, verapamil) compete with calcineurin inhibitors for P450 catabolism and cause elevated levels of these immunosuppressive drugs. Analeptics, such as phenytoin and carbamazepine, will increase catabolism to result in low levels. *Aspergillus* (Chap. 206), *Nocardia* (Chap. 165), and cytomegalovirus (CMV) (Chap. 185) infections also occur.

CMV is a common and dangerous infection in transplant recipients. It does not generally appear until the end of the first posttransplant month. Active CMV infection is sometimes associated, or occasionally confused, with rejection episodes. Patients at highest risk for severe CMV disease are those without anti-CMV antibodies who receive a graft from a CMV antibody–positive donor (15% mortality). Serial intravenous administration of high-titer CMV immune globulin is effective in reducing this risk. Prophylactic use of ganciclovir is an effective alternative. Early diagnosis in a febrile patient can be made by detecting CMV antigens in the blood. A rise in IgM antibodies to CMV is also diagnostic. Culture of CMV from blood may be less sensitive. Tissue invasion of CMV is common in the gastrointestinal tract and lungs. CMV retinopathy occurs late in the course, if untreated. Treatment of active CMV disease with ganciclovir is always indicated. Many patients immune to CMV can activate the virus after heavy immunosuppression, such as with OKT3. Concurrent treatment with ganciclovir during OKT3 administration appears to be effective for prophylaxis of CMV activation. The complications of glucocorticoid therapy are well known and include gastrointestinal bleeding, impairment of wound healing, osteoporosis, diabetes mellitus, cataract formation, and hemorrhagic pancreatitis. The treatment of unexplained jaundice in transplant patients should include cessation or reduction of immunosuppressive drugs if hepatitis or drug toxicity is suspected. It is surprising that cessation of azathioprine or calcineurin inhibitor therapy in such circumstances often does not result in rejection of a graft, at least for several weeks. Acyclovir is effective in therapy of herpes simplex virus infections.

Antiplatelet agents and anticoagulants, although effective in theory, have not been successful in the prevention of the "chronic rejection" vascular lesions. Persistent elevation of serum creatinine levels above 220 μmol/L (2.5 mg/dL) in patients on calcineurin inhibitor is an indication for dose reduction, particularly if calcineurin inhibitor blood levels are elevated. The risk of long-term cumulative toxicity to the kidney now seems to be low. In general, minimal or no rejection during the first 6 months after transplantation is a predictor of safety in reducing immunosuppression therapy over subsequent months to years, but chronic progressive vasculopathy may still occur.

Despite the potential teratogenic effects of immunosuppressive agents, both women and men have become parents after transplantation. The incidence of congenital abnormalities in the offspring is not increased.

Glomerular Lesions Glomerular lesions occur in 10 to 15% of allografts, even when the original disease was accidental removal of a solitary kidney. The pathogenesis is related to a chronic rejection process. In some cases the lesions resemble those of the original glomerular disease. In most instances, the recurrence of the original renal lesions represents no threat to the immediate prognosis, and a primary diagnosis of glomerulonephritis is rarely a contraindication to transplantation. Focal segmental glomerulosclerosis may recur up to 30% of the time, with one-third of these patients losing graft function. Hemolytic uremic syndrome also has a high recurrence rate.

Malignancy The incidence of tumors in patients on immunosuppressive therapy is 5 to 6%, or approximately 100 times greater than that in the general population of the same age range. The most common lesions are cancer of the skin and lips and carcinoma in situ of the cervix, as well as lymphomas, such as non-Hodgkin's lymphomas. The risks are increased in proportion to the total immunosuppressive load administered and time elapsed since transplantation. Surveillance for skin and cervical cancers is necessary.

Other Complications *Hypercalcemia* after transplantation may indicate failure of hyperplastic parathyroid glands to regress. Aseptic necrosis of the head of the femur is probably due to preexisting hyperparathyroidism, with aggravation by glucocorticoid treatment. With improved management of calcium and phosphorus metabolism during chronic dialysis, the incidence of parathyroid-related complications has fallen dramatically. Persistent hyperparathyroid activity may require subtotal parathyroidectomy.

Hypertension may be caused by (1) native kidneys; (2) rejection activity in the transplant; (3) renal artery stenosis, if an end-to-end anastomosis was constructed with an iliac artery branch; and (4) renal calcineurin inhibitor toxicity. The latter may improve with reduction in dose. Whereas ACE inhibitors may be useful, calcium channel blockers are more frequently used initially. Amelioration of hypertension to the 120–130/70–80 mmHg range should be the goal in all patients.

Chronic hepatitis, particularly when due to hepatitis B virus, can be a progressive, fatal disease over a decade or so. Patients who are persistently hepatitis B surface antigen–positive are at higher risk, according to some studies, but the presence of hepatitis C virus is also a concern when one embarks on a course of immunosuppression in a transplant recipient.

Both chronic dialysis and renal transplant patients have a higher incidence of death from myocardial infarction and stroke than in the population at large, and this is particularly true in diabetic patients. Contributing factors are the use of glucocorticoids, hypertension, and hypertriglyceridemia. Increased low-density lipoprotein cholesterol and depressed high-density lipoprotein cholesterol concentrations may be exaggerated after transplantation and require treatment. Recipients of renal transplants have a high prevalence of coronary artery and peripheral vascular diseases. The percentage of deaths from these causes has been slowly rising as the numbers of transplanted diabetic patients and the average age of all recipients increase. More than 50% of renal recipient mortality is attributable to cardiovascular disease. In addition to strict control of blood pressure and blood lipid levels, close monitoring of patients for indications of further medical or surgical intervention is an important part of management.

BIBLIOGRAPHY

COSIO FG et al: Relationships between arterial hypertension and renal allograft survival in African-American patients. Am J Kidney Dis 29:419, 1997

MASSY AZ, KASISKE BL: Post-transplant hyperlipidemia: Mechanisms and management. J Am Soc Nephrol 7:971, 1996

MCKAY DB et al: Clinical renal transplantation, in *Brenner and Rector's The Kidney*, 6th ed, B Brenner (ed). Philadelphia, Saunders 2000, pp 2542–2605

PIRSCH J et al: A comparison of tacrolimus (FK506) and cyclosporine for immunosuppression after cadaveric renal transplantation. FK506 Kidney Transplant Study Group. Transplantation 63:977, 1997

SAYEGH MH, TURKA LA: The role of T-cell costimulatory activation pathways in transplant rejection. N Engl J Med 338:1813, 1998

——— et al: Transplantation immunobiology, in *Brenner and Rector's The Kidney*, 6th ed, B Brenner (ed). Philadelphia, Saunders, 2000, pp 2518–2541

STEWART G et al: Ischemic heart disease following renal transplantation. Nephrol Dial Transplant 15:269, 2000

273

Hugh R. Brady, Barry M. Brenner

PATHOGENESIS OF GLOMERULAR INJURY

The glomerulus is a modified capillary network that delivers an ultrafiltrate of plasma to Bowman's space, the most proximal portion of the renal tubule. Approximately 1.6 million glomeruli are present in two mature kidneys (range 0.5 to 2.4 million) and collectively they produce 120 to 180 L of ultrafiltrate daily. Glomerular filtration rate (GFR) is dependent on glomerular blood flow, ultrafiltration pressure, and surface area. These parameters are tightly regulated through changes in afferent and efferent arteriolar tone (for blood flow and ultrafiltration pressure) and mesangial cell contractility (for filtration surface area). Arteriolar tone and mesangial cell contractility are, in turn, modulated by neurohumoral factors, local myenteric reflexes, and endothelium-derived vasoactive substances, such as nitric oxide, prostacyclin, and endothelins. In health, glomerular endothelium is also antithrombotic and antiadhesive for leukocytes and platelets, thereby preventing inappropriate vascular thrombosis and inflammation during the filtration process. Filtration of most plasma proteins and all blood cells is normally prevented as a consequence of the physiochemical and electrostatic charge characteristics of the glomerular filtration barrier, the latter being composed of fenestrated glomerular endothelium, basement membrane, and the foot processes and slit diaphragms of visceral epithelial cells (podocytes). Parietal epithelium facilitates glomerular filtration by maintaining the integrity of Bowman's space. In keeping with the physiologic functions of the glomerulus outlined above, virtually all glomerular injury results in impairment of glomerular filtration and/or the inappropriate appearance of plasma proteins and blood cells in the urine.

CLINICOPATHOLOGIC CORRELATES IN GLOMERULAR DISEASE

The major glomerulopathies are described in Chap. 274, and major morphologic patterns of glomerular disease and their clinical features are summarized in Table 273-1. These clinicopathologic entities can be induced by a variety of different pathogenetic mechanisms. Thus, prompt diagnosis, optimal management, and accurate prognostication is a multistep process that requires (1) recognition of the presenting clinical syndrome, (2) delineation of the underlying morphologic pat-

Table 273-1 Major Clinicopathologic Presentation of Glomerular Disease

Structural Pattern	Typical Clinical Presentation	Typical Pathology Findings	Most Common Etiologies[a]
Diffuse proliferative GN	Acute nephritic syndrome: Acute renal failure over days to weeks, hypertension, edema, oliguria, active urine sediment, subnephrotic proteinuria	Diffuse increase in cellularity of tufts of most glomeruli due to infiltration by neutrophils and monocytes, and proliferation of glomerular endothelial and mesangial cells	Immune complex GN: idiopathic, postinfectious, SLE, SBE, cryoglobulinemia, HSP Pauci-immune GN and anti-GBM disease (crescentic GN common—see below)
Crescentic GN	Rapidly progressive glomerulonephritis (RPGN): Subacute renal failure over weeks to months, active urine sediment, variable amount of hypertension, edema, oliguria, and proteinuria	Majority of glomeruli contain areas of fibrinoid necrosis and crescents in Bowman's space, composed of proliferating parietal epithelial cells, infiltrating macrophages, and fibrin	Immune complex GN (as above) Pauci-immune GN: Wegener's granulomatosis, microscopic polyarteritis nodosa, renal-limited crescentic GN Anti-GBM disease (Goodpasture's syndrome if lung hemorrhage)
Focal proliferative GN	Mild to moderate glomerular inflammation: Active urine sediment and mild to moderate decline in GFR	Segmental areas of proliferation and necrosis in less than 50% of glomeruli, occasionally with crescent formation	Early and milder forms, or recovery phase of most diseases causing diffuse proliferative and crescentic GN IgA nephropathy/HSP
Mesangial proliferative GN	Chronic glomerular inflammation: Proteinuria, hematuria, hypertension, variable effect on GFR	Proliferation of mesangial cells and matrix	IgA nephropathy/HSP Early and milder forms, or recovery phases of most diseases that cause diffuse proliferative and crescentic GN (see above) In association with minimal change glomerulopathy and FSGS
Membranoproliferative GN	Variable combination of nephritic and nephrotic features: Acute or subacute decline in GFR, active urine sediment, proteinuria often in nephrotic range	Diffuse proliferation of mesangial cells and infiltration of glomeruli by macrophages; increased mesangial matrix and thickening and reduplication of glomerular basement membrane	Immune complex GN (as for diffuse proliferative GN) In association with thrombotic microangiopathies (see below) In association with deposition diseases (see below) Postrenal or -marrow transplantation
Minimal change GN	Nephrotic syndrome: Proteinuria of >3–3.5 g/d, hypoalbuminemia, edema, hyperlipidemia, lipiduria, thrombotic diathesis, slow decline in GFR in 10–30%.	Light microscopy normal, but electron microscopy (EM) shows foot process effacement	Idiopathic In association with drug-induced interstitial nephritis, HIV infection, heroin, Hodgkin's and other lymphomas
Focal segmental glomerulosclerosis	Nephrotic syndrome: Proteinuria of >3–3.5 g/d, hypoalbuminemia, edema, hyperlipidemia, lipiduria, thrombotic diathesis, slow decline in GFR in 10–30%.	Segmental capillary collapse affecting <50% of glomeruli with entrapment of amorphous hyaline material. EM shows foot process effacement	Primary FSGS: idiopathic, HIV, heroin, lysosomal diseases, Charcot-Marie-Tooth Secondary response to reduction in nephron number from any cause (hyperfiltration injury)
Nodular or global sclerosis	Proteinuria and chronic renal failure	Sclerosis of most glomeruli with interstitial fibrosis	Diabetic nephropathy Potential long-term consequence of most glomerulopathies listed above
Membranous GN	Nephrotic syndrome: Proteinuria of >3–3.5 g/d, hypoalbuminemia, edema, hyperlipidemia, lipiduria, thrombotic diathesis, slow decline in GFR in 10–30%	Diffuse thickening of the glomerular basement membrane with subepithelial projections (''spikes'') around immune deposits	Idiopathic Infections (e.g., Hepatitis B & C, syphilis, schistasomiasis, malaria, leprosy) Drugs (e.g., gold, penicillamine, captopril) Autoimmune diseases (SLE, rheumatoid arthritis) Paraneoplastic
Deposition diseases	Combination of nephritic and nephrotic features: Renal failure over months to years, proteinuria, hematuria, and hypertension.	Mesangial expansion and thickening of glomerular capillary wall; variable cellular proliferation and crescent formation	Amyloid Cryoglobulinemia Light chain deposition disease Fibrillary/immunotactoid GN

(continued)

tern of glomerular injury, and (3) elucidation of the specific renal-limited or systemic disease that triggered glomerular dysfunction.

NOMENCLATURE The terms *glomerulonephritis* and *glomerulopathy* are usually used interchangeably to denote glomerular injury, although some authorities reserve the former term for injury with evidence of inflammation such as leukocyte infiltration, antibody deposition, and/or complement activation. Glomerular diseases are classified as *primary* when the pathology is confined to the kidney and any

Table 273-1 Major Clinicopathologic Presentation of Glomerular Disease—*(continued)*

Structural Pattern	Typical Clinical Presentation	Typical Pathology Findings	Most Common Etiologies[a]
Thrombotic microangiopathy	Acute or subacute renal failure: Variable degree of hypertension, edema and proteinuria, urine sediment usually contains red blood cells, but less activity than patients with nephritic syndrome or RPGN	Microthrombi in glomerular capillaries ± endothelial injury	Idiopathic In association with gastrointestinal infections, or drugs such as anovulants, mitomycin C, cyclosporine Other diseases: SLE, scleroderma, toxemia, malignant hypertension
Nonimmune basement membrane abnormalities	Asymptomatic hematuria and variable renal failure	Alport's syndrome—mesangial hypercellularity with focal sclerosis and interstitial fibrosis; splintering of GBM on EM.	Alport's syndrome, Thin basement membrane disease. Nail patella syndrome, Lecithin–cholesterol acyltransferase deficiency

[a] Includes most common etiologies: For complete list, see Chap. 274.

NOTE: Diffuse, affecting ≥50% of glomeruli; focal, affecting <50% of glomeruli; global, affecting ≥50% of glomerular tuft; segmental, affecting <50% of glomerular tuft; GN, glomerulonephritis; FSGS, focal segmental glomerulosclerosis; HSP, Henoch-Schönlein purpura; SLE, systemic lupus erythematosus; SBE, subacute bacterial endocarditis; GBM, glomerular basement membrane; GFR, glomerular filtration rate.

systemic features are a direct consequence of glomerular dysfunction (e.g., pulmonary edema, hypertension, the uremic syndrome). Usually, but not always, the term primary is synonymous with *idiopathic*. Glomerular diseases are classified as *secondary* when part of a multisystem disorder. In general, *acute* refers to glomerular injury occurring over days or weeks, *subacute* or *rapidly progressive* over weeks or a few months, and *chronic* over many months or years. Lesions are classified as *focal* or *diffuse* when they involve the minority (<50%) or majority (≥50%) of glomeruli, respectively. Lesions are termed *segmental* or *global* when they involve part of or almost all of the glomerular tuft, respectively. *Proliferative* is used to describe an increase in glomerular cell number, which can be due to infiltration by leukocytes or proliferation of resident glomerular cells. Proliferation of resident glomerular cells is classified as *intracapillary* or *endocapillary* when referring to endothelial or mesangial cells and *extracapillary* when referring to cells in Bowman's space. A *crescent* is a half-moon-shaped collection of cells in Bowman's space, usually composed of proliferating parietal epithelial cells and infiltrating monocytes. Because crescentic glomerulonephritis is often associated with renal failure that progresses rapidly over week to months, the clinical term *rapidly progressive glomerulonephritis* and pathologic term *crescentic glomerulonephritis* are often used interchangeably. The description *membranous* is applied to glomerulonephritis dominated by expansion of the glomerular basement membrane (GBM) by immune deposits. *Sclerosis* refers to an increase in the amount of homogeneous nonfibrillar extracellular material of the same ultrastructural appearance and chemical composition as GBM and mesangial matrix. This process is distinct from *fibrosis*, which involves deposition of collagens type I and III and is more commonly a consequence of healing of crescents or tubulointerstitial inflammation.

MAJOR CLINICOPATHOLOGIC ENTITIES Most glomerulopathies are still classified and named according to their morphologic features (Table 273-1). The major *inflammatory glomerulopathies* are focal proliferative glomerulonephritis (termed *mesangial proliferative* if the proliferating cells are predominantly mesangial cells), diffuse proliferative glomerulonephritis, and crescentic glomerulonephritis. These diseases typically present with a *nephritic-type* "active" urine sediment characterized by the presence of red blood cells, red blood cell casts, leukocytes, and *subnephrotic* proteinuria of <3 g/24 h. The severity of renal insufficiency varies in proportion to the degree of proliferation and necrosis.

The major morphologic patterns affecting the glomerular filtration barrier for proteins, namely the GBM and visceral epithelial cells, are membranous glomerulopathy, minimal change disease, and focal and segmental glomerulosclerosis. These entities typically present with *nephrotic-range* proteinuria of >3 g/24 h and the presence of few red blood cells, leukocytes, or cellular casts. As a consequence of the heavy proteinuria, nephrotic syndrome is associated with hypoalbuminemia, edema, hyperlipidemia, and lipiduria. Membranoproliferative glomerulonephritis, as the name suggests, is a hybrid lesion that presents with a combination of nephritic and nephrotic features.

The *glomerular deposition diseases* are a group of disorders characterized by prominent extravascular deposition of a paraprotein or fibrillar material. These diseases can also trigger nephritic-type and nephrotic-type responses (or a combination of both) and thus show marked clinical and morphologic overlap with the entities described above.

The *thrombotic microangiopathies* are a family of diseases in which the pathologic presentation is dominated by thrombi within the renal microvasculature, often leading to renal insufficiency.

MAJOR DETERMINANTS OF GLOMERULAR INJURY

Important determinants of the severity of glomerular injury include (1) the nature of the primary insult and the secondary mediator systems that it invokes, (2) the site of injury within the glomerulus; and (3) the speed of onset, extent, and intensity of disease.

PRIMARY INSULT Glomeruli are susceptible to a variety of inflammatory, metabolic, hemodynamic, toxic, and infectious insults (Table 273-2). Most human glomerular disease is triggered by immune attack, diabetes mellitus, or hypertension. Diverse insults can induce similar clinicopathologic presentations, suggesting marked overlap among downstream molecular and cellular responses. For example, infections (e.g., streptococcal pharyngitis, bacterial endocarditis) and vasculitides (e.g., Henoch-Schönlein purpura, microscopic polyarteritis) can each trigger acute proliferative glomerulonephritis with the nephritic syndrome. Similarly, metabolic (e.g., diabetes mellitus) and deposition diseases (e.g., amyloid) can each induce glomerulosclerosis with nephrotic syndrome. An important corollary is that pharmacologic agents that inhibit common secondary mediator systems may prove effective in treating glomerular diseases of diverse etiologies (see below).

SITE OF INJURY The consequences of injury at different sites within the glomerulus can be predicted from the physiologic functions of the cells within the local milieu (Table 273-3). The major sequelae of injury to the *endothelium* and *subendothelial aspect of the GBM* are (1) recruitment of leukocytes leading to inflammatory glomerulonephritis, (2) perturbed hemostasis leading to thrombotic microangiopathy, and (3) vasoconstriction and mesangial cell contraction leading to acute renal failure. It is usual for one of these phenotypes to dominate the presentation of specific diseases. *Mesangial* injury is usually immunologic in origin and, being more localized, induces less dramatic impairment of glomerular filtration. Patients typically present with asymptomatic abnormalities of the urinary sediment and mild renal insufficiency. Proteinuria dominates the clinical presentation of injury to the *subepithelial aspect of the GBM* and *visceral epithelial* *cells*. As with mesangial injury, GFR is often only mildly compromised in this setting. The classic pathologic manifestation of *parietal epithelial cell* injury is crescent formation. Crescents can be the dominant morphologic presentation of glomerular disease or complicate proliferative or membranous lesions.

SPEED OF ONSET, INTENSITY, AND EXTENT OF INJURY To illustrate the importance of the speed of onset, extent, and intensity of glomerular injury, it is instructive to compare two forms of immune complex glomerulonephritis, namely, acute postinfectious glomerulonephritis and IgA nephropathy. Postinfectious glomerulonephritis is characterized by rapid and extensive formation of immune complexes throughout the glomerular capillary wall, which often provokes acute renal failure with the classic hallmarks of acute inflammation: complement activation, leukocyte recruitment, lysosomal enzyme release, free radical generation, and perturbation of vascular tone and permeability. In contrast, IgA nephropathy is characterized by slow, but sustained, formation of immune complexes, largely confined to the mesangium; less dramatic activation of complement and other secondary mediator systems; and either stability of GFR or progressive renal insufficiency over 10 to 20 years.

Table 273-2 Primary Mechanisms of Glomerular Injury

Mechanism of Injury	Some Renal Insults/Defects	Glomerular Disease
Immunologic[a]	Immunoglobulin[b]	Immune complex–mediated glomerulonephritis
	Cell-mediated injury[b]	Pauci-immune glomerulonephritis
	Cytokine (or other soluble factor)	Primary focal segmental glomerulosclerosis
	Persistent complement activation	Membranoproliferative glomerulonephritis (type II)
Metabolic[a]	Hyperglycemia[b]	Diabetic nephropathy
	Fabry's disease and sialidosis	Focal segmental glomerulosclerosis
Hemodynamic[a]	Systemic hypertension[b]	Hypertensive nephrosclerosis
	Intraglomerular hypertension[b]	Secondary focal segmental glomerulosclerosis
Toxic	*E. coli*–derived verotoxin	Thrombotic microangiopathy
	Therapeutic drugs (e.g., NSAIDs)	Minimal change disease
	Recreational drugs (heroin)	Focal segmental glomerulosclerosis
Deposition	Amyloid fibrils	Amyloid nephropathy
Infectious	HIV	HIV nephropathy
	Subacute bacterial endocarditis	Immune complex glomerulonephritis
Inherited	Defect in gene for $\alpha5$ chain of type IV collagen	Alport's syndrome
	Abnormally thin basement membrane	Thin basement membrane disease

[a] Most common categories.
[b] Most common insults within these categories.
NOTE: NSAIDs, nonsteroidal anti-inflammatory drugs.

IMMUNOLOGIC GLOMERULAR INJURY

Immune-mediated glomerulonephritis (Chaps. 274 and 275) accounts for a large fraction of acquired renal disease. The majority of cases are associated with the deposition of antibodies, often autoantibodies, within the glomerular tuft, indicating dysregulation of humoral immunity. Cellular immune mechanisms also contribute to the pathogenesis of antibody-mediated glomerulonephritis by modulating antibody production and through antibody-dependent cell cytotoxicity (see below). In addition, cellular immune mechanisms probably play a primary role in the pathophysiology of "pauci-immune" glomerulonephritides, notable for robust glomerular inflammation in the absence of immunoglobulin deposition.

ANTIBODY-MEDIATED INJURY (Fig. 273-1) Most antibody-mediated glomerulonephritis in humans is initiated by reactivity of circulating antibodies with auto- or "planted" antigens within the glomerulus. The major mechanisms of antibody deposition within the glomerulus are (1) reactivity of circulating autoantibodies with intrinsic autoantigens that are components of normal glomerular parenchyma, (2) in situ formation of immune complexes through interaction of circulating antibodies with extrinsic antigens that have been planted within the glomerulus, and (3) intraglomerular trapping of immune complexes that have formed in the systemic circulation. Autoantibodies against neutrophil cytoplasmic antigens in the circulation may represent an additional mechanism of antibody-mediated glomerular injury in patients without discernible immune complexes in the glomerular parenchyma (see below).

Generation of Nephritogenic Antibodies Exposure of the host to a foreign antigen (e.g., a prodromal infection) has been implicated as the trigger for the generation of nephritogenic autoantibodies in several forms of glomerulonephritis. Foreign antigens can provoke autoantibody formation through several mechanisms. First, a foreign antigen, whose structure resembles that of a host glomerular antigen, may stimulate the production of autoantibodies that cross-react with the intrinsic glomerular antigen ("molecular mimickry"). Second, the foreign antigen may trigger aberrant expression of major histocompatibility complex class II molecules on glomerular cells which present previously "invisible" autoantigens to T lymphocytes and thereby generate an autoimmune response. Third, the foreign antigen can trigger polyclonal activation of B lymphocytes, some of which generate nephritogenic antibodies. Alternatively, individuals may suffer a breakdown of immune tolerance through other mechanisms (e.g., genetically programmed). Autoreactive B cells are usually deleted in the thymus during development (clonal deletion) or rendered anergic in peripheral lymphoid tissue (clonal anergy). Similar tolerogenic mechanisms exist for deleting or anergizing autoreactive T helper cells that modulate immunoglobulin production by autoreactive B cells. Perturbation of either of these tolerogenic mechanisms could drive immunoglobulin production in some forms of autoimmune glomerulonephritis. Indeed, defective clonal deletion of autoreactive T cells has been demonstrated in experimental lupus nephritis due to defective synthesis of Fas, a cell-surface receptor that modulates T cell deletion through apoptosis (programmed cell death) within the thymus.

Table 273-3 Correlation between Site of Glomerular Injury and Clinicopathologic Presentation

Target of Injury	Physiologic Role	Response to Injury	Representative Glomerular Disease
Endothelial cell	Maintains glomerular perfusion	Vasoconstriction	Acute renal failure
	Prevents leukocyte adhesion	Leukocyte infiltration	Focal or diffuse proliferative GN
	Prevents platelet aggregation and clotting	Intravascular microthrombi	Thrombotic microangiopathies
Mesangial cell	Controls glomerular filtration surface area	Proliferation/increased matrix	Mesangioproliferative GN/glomerulosclerosis
Basement membrane	Prevents filtration of plasma proteins	Proteinuria	Membranous nephropathy
Visceral epithelial cell	Prevents filtration of plasma proteins	Proteinuria	Minimal change disease and FSGS
Parietal epithelial cell	Maintains Bowman's space	Crescent formation	Crescentic GN

NOTE: GN, glomerulonephritis; FSGS, focal segmental glomerulosclerosis.

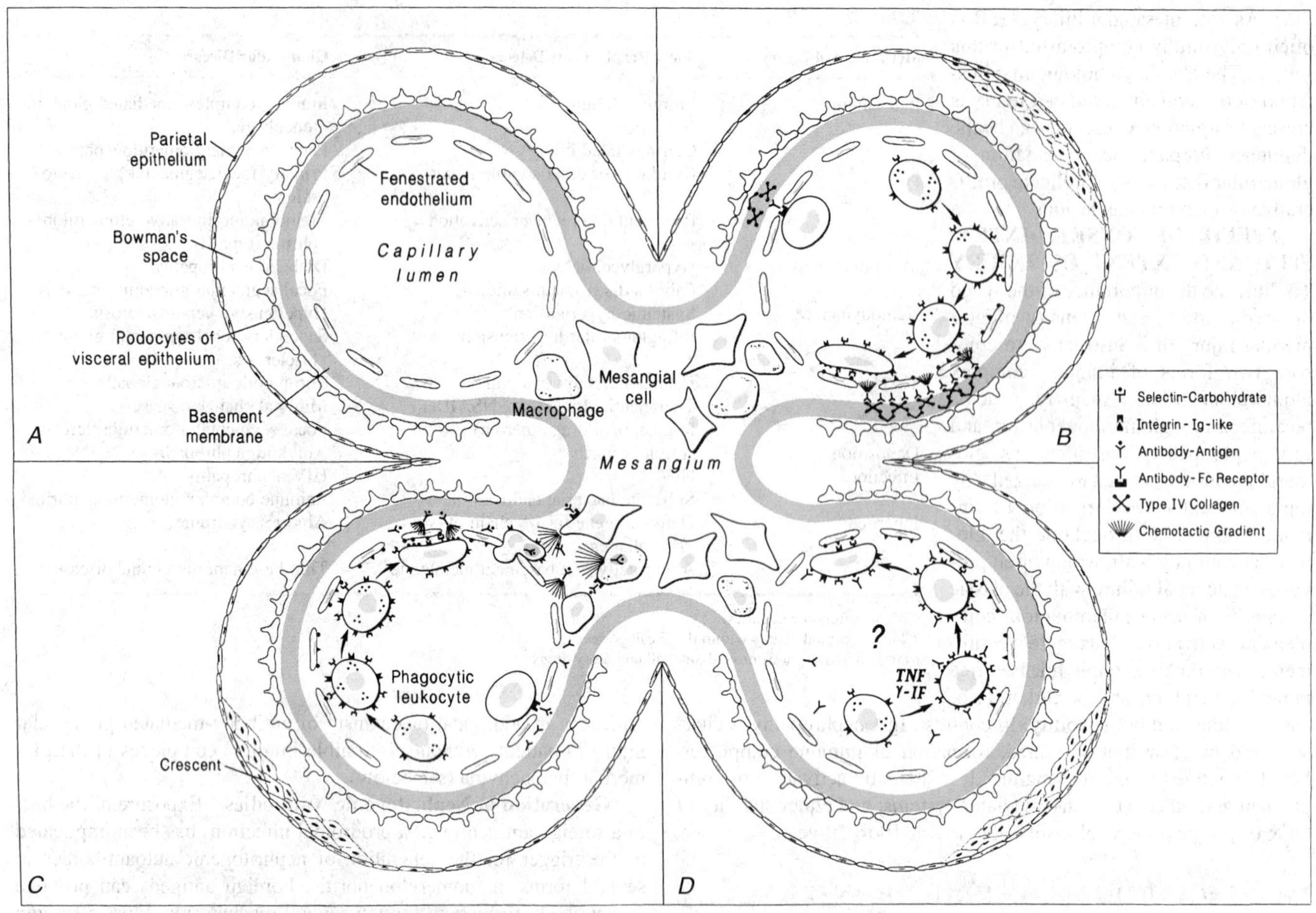

FIGURE 273-1 Major mechanisms of antibody-mediated injury in glomerulonephritis. *A*. Normal glomerulus. Key components of "healthy" glomerular capillary loop. *B*. Antiglomerular basement membrane antibody-mediated glomerulonephritis. Linear deposition of IgG against the Goodpasture antigen. The latter autoantigen is a normal constituent of the noncollagenous domain of $\alpha3$ chain of type IV collagen, whose "chicken wire"–like structure is essential for maintenance of normal glomerular basement membrane architecture and function. *C*. Immune complex-mediated glomerulonephritis. Immune complexes scattered throughout the glomerular capillary wall, e.g., as can occur in lupus nephritis or postinfectious glomerulonephritis. In mechanisms *B* and *C*, leukocyte chemotaxis is triggered by complement components, chemokines, and other inflammatory mediators. Leukocyte–endothelial cell adhesion is supported by four major classes of adhesion molecules: the selectins and their diverse carbohydrate-bearing ligands, the leukocyte integrins, and immunoglobulin-like molecules such as intercellular adhesion molecule-1. Leukocytes also adhere through binding of their Fc receptors to the Fc domains of immunoglobulin. *D*. Antineutrophil cytoplasmic antibody (ANCA)-associated glomerulonephritis. In diseases such as Wegener's granulomatosis, ANCA are postulated to induce glomerular injury by interacting with neutrophil granule components that have migrated to the cell surface following priming of neutrophils by cytokines, as may occur during a prodromal viral illness. Reactivity of ANCA with neutrophil granule components in vitro triggers neutrophil activation and endothelial cell injury. This mechanism of glomerular injury remains to be established definitively in vivo, however, hence the symbol "?" in the cartoon. Crescents are formed by proliferation of parietal epithelial cells and migration of monocyte-macrophages into the glomerulus from the glomerular capillary lumen and tubulointerstitial space. As they expand, crescents compress the glomerular capillary tuft and are a rich source of mediators that further amplify the inflammatory response. TNF, tumor necrosis factor; γ-IF, interferon-γ.

Deposition of Nephritogenic Antibodies within the Glomerulus (Fig. 273-1) Anti-GBM antibody disease (p. 1583) is the classic nephritis initiated by interaction of autoantibody with intrinsic glomerular antigen. Afflicted patients have a circulating antibody directed at a 28-kDa antigen (Goodpasture antigen) located in the noncollagenous NC1 domain of the $\alpha3$ chain of type IV collagen. This type of collagen is preferentially expressed in glomerular and pulmonary alveolar basement membranes. Autoantibodies against mesangial cell antigens have been detected in the serum of patients with IgA nephropathy, the most common form of glomerulonephritis in humans; however, the pathogenicity of these autoantibodies has yet to be defined. Poststreptococcal glomerulonephritis and lupus nephritis are examples of glomerulonephritides that are probably initiated by interaction of circulating antibodies with planted antigens. Several streptococcal antigens have been isolated from immune deposits of kidneys with poststreptococcal glomerulonephritis, including nephritis strain–associated antigen and a cytoplasmic protein endostreptosin. In addition, patients with poststreptococcal glomerulonephritis can have circulating antibodies against laminin, type IV collagen, and heparan sulphate proteoglycans, suggesting that molecular mimickry may also contribute. Similar findings have been reported in experimental and human lupus nephritis. Here, circulating anti-DNA antibodies may potentially induce immune complex glomerulonephritis by reacting with DNA bound to GBM or with planted DNA-histone complexes (nucleosomes). However, it should be noted that patients with systemic lupus erythematosus have a variety of circulating autoantibodies, and the pathogenetic culprit(s) in lupus nephritis have yet to be identified definitively. Cryoglobulinemia, due to chronic hepatitis C infection, is an example of glomerulonephritis initiated by trapping of immune complexes. These patients have circulating and intraglomerular immune complexes composed of hepatitis C antigens, polyclonal antihepatitis C IgG, and a second antibody, usually a monoclonal IgM, directed against the IgG. In support of the pathogenicity of circulating cryoglobulins, their injection into laboratory mice induces glomerulonephritis with many of the hallmarks of human disease.

Site of Antibody Deposition The site of antibody deposition within the glomerulus is a critical determinant of the clinicopathologic presentation. Among the factors that determine the site of deposition are the avidity, affinity, and quantity of the antibody; the size, charge, and site of the antigen; the size of the immune complexes; the efficiency of the clearance mechanisms for immune complexes; and local hemodynamic factors. Relatively anionic antigens are repelled by the GBM, which is negatively charged, and tend to be trapped in the subendothelial cell space and mesangium. In contrast, relatively cationic antigens tend to permeate the GBM and deposit within the GBM or in the subepithelial space. Acute deposition of antibody in the subendothelial cell space or mesangium typically triggers a nephritic-type response characterized by rapid recruitment of leukocytes and platelets, probably because inflammatory mediators generated at these sites are strategically positioned to activate endothelial and hematogenous cells. Inflammation is more severe when antibody is deposited in the subendothelial space, as compared with mesangium, at least in part because the mesangium abuts only 25 to 33% of the capillary wall. Antibody deposition in the subepithelial cell space typically induces a nephrotic-type response characterized by proteinuria without a pronounced inflammatory cell infiltrate, probably because the immune complexes are shielded from circulating inflammatory cells by the GBM and because the large fluid flux from blood to Bowman's space minimizes back-diffusion of inflammatory mediators towards the endothelium and vascular lumen.

Recruitment of Inflammatory Cells (Fig. 273-1) Leukocytes and platelets are important mediators of injury in most forms of acute and subacute glomerulonephritis. Immunoglobulin can provoke recruitment of leukocytes through several mechanisms. Many antibody subclasses activate the complement cascade, and complement proteins such as C3a, C5a, and C5b-9 (membrane attack complex) are potent stimuli for leukocyte recruitment, either through their direct effects on leukocytes (C3a, C5a) or by increasing endothelial cell adhesiveness for leukocytes (C5b-9). Complement-independent mechanisms also contribute. Leukocytes express Fc receptors that can directly engage the Fc portion of immunoglobulin. Resident glomerular macrophages, endothelial cells, and mesangial cells also express Fc receptors, engagement of which can trigger release of an array of inflammatory mediators and chemotactic cytokines (chemokines) that promote directed locomotion of leukocytes (chemotaxis), binding of leukocytes to inflamed endothelium through cell surface leukocyte adhesion molecules, and diapedesis of leukocytes to the extravascular space.

The mechanisms of platelet recruitment in glomerulonephritis are less well defined. Potential mechanisms include direct binding of platelet Fc receptors with immunoglobulin, and interactions of platelets with endothelium, trapped leukocytes, collagen, and other components of exposed GBM, and with products of the coagulation cascade such as fibrin.

Mediators of Glomerular Injury (Fig. 273-2) *Nephritic-type antibody-mediated glomerular injury* is a vivid example of host defense gone awry. In normal host defense, leukocytes engulf microorganisms into phagosomes, which then fuse with intracellular lysosomes. Microorganisms are destroyed within phagolysosomes through the actions of free radicals, proteolytic enzymes, and other toxic molecules. This process facilitates killing with relative protection and preservation of host tissue. When host defense is inappropriately activated in autoimmune diseases, the inciting antigens are often fixed to (planted antigens) or are a component of host tissue (autoantigen). As a result, phagocytosis is less efficient ("frustrated phagocytosis"), and there is release of toxic moieties such as oxidants and proteases into the parenchyma where they destroy host cells and matrix components. In addition, cytotoxic T lymphocytes and natural killer cells can damage resident glomerular cells by releasing toxic compounds, such as perforins, a process that is facilitated by binding of these cytotoxic cells to glomerular cells through HLA molecules, Fc portions of immunoglobulin (antibody-dependent cell cytotoxicity), and other immune recognition systems. Platelets promote nephritic injury by promoting leukocyte recruitment and intrarenal vasoconstriction and by triggering microthrombi formation. Cytokines, such as tumor necrosis factor α, interleukin 1β, and interferon γ, play a key role in the amplification and maintenance of glomerular inflammation by induc-

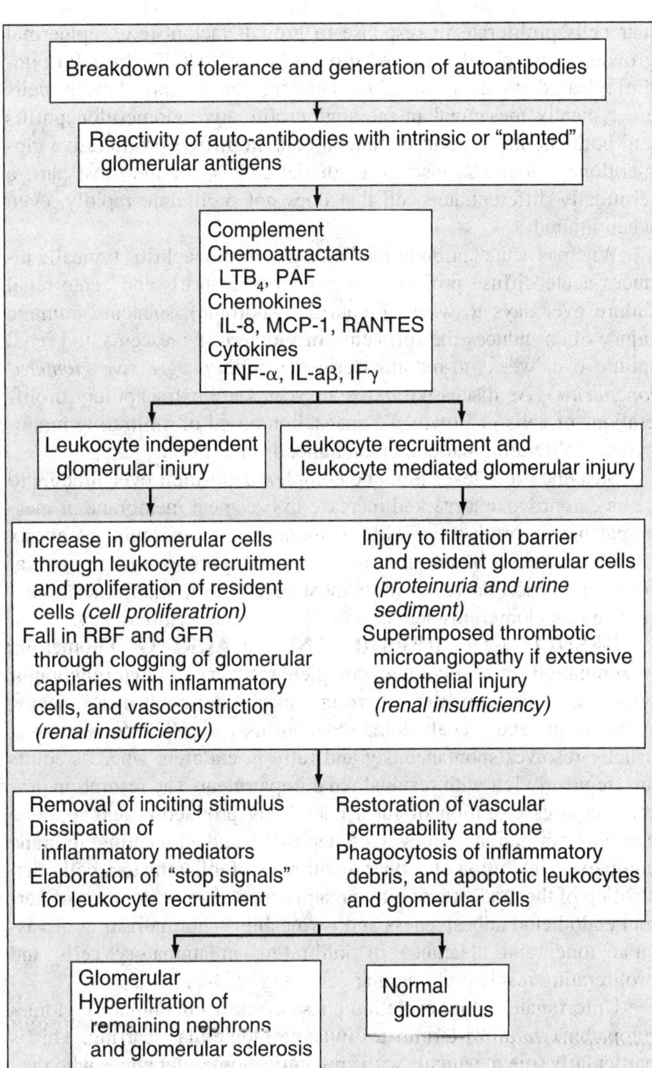

FIGURE 273-2 Mediator systems in acute immune complex–mediated glomerulonephritis: A paradigm of renal inflammation. Abbreviations: LTB_4, leukotriene B_4; PAF, platelet-activating factor; IL, interleukin; MCP-1, monocyte chemotactic peptide-1; TNF-α, tumor necrosis factor α; Ifγ, interferon γ; RBF, renal blood flow; GFR, glomerular filtration rate.

ing de novo synthesis of leukocyte adhesion molecules, chemokines, and other inflammatory mediators.

Leukocytes play a lesser role in *nephrotic-type antibody-mediated glomerular injury* (Chap. 274). Membranous glomerulopathy is the prototypic entity and is initiated by the formation of subepithelial immune complexes; these provoke production of "spikes" of new basement membrane that eventually encircle and incorporate the immune complexes into the GBM. The antigenic targets in human membranous glomerulopathy have not been determined but may be planted antigens or autoantigens shed from parietal epithelial cells. The frequent association with infections, malignancies, and drugs suggests involvement of planted antigens or molecular mimickry (see above); however, many cases may represent a true loss of tolerance against autoantigens. The membrane attack complex of complement (C5b-9) appears to be a major effector of injury to the glomerular filtration barrier in this setting.

CELL PROLIFERATION AND ACCUMULATION OF EXTRACELLULAR MATRIX A hallmark of the nephritic-type proliferative glomerulopathies is an increase in glomerular cell number. Initially, this hypercellularity is due predominantly to infiltration of the glomerular tuft by leukocytes. Subsequently, resident glomerular cells proliferate in response to growth factors [e.g., epidermal growth factor, platelet-derived growth factor (PDGF), thrombospondin] released into the local inflammatory milieu. The proliferating cells are typically mesangial in mesangioproliferative glomerulonephritis and both endothelial and mesangial cells in diffuse proliferative glomerulonephritis. The visceral epithelial cell is, for the most part, a terminally differentiated cell that does not proliferate rapidly, even when injured.

Whereas acute antibody-mediated glomerulonephritis typically induces acute diffuse proliferative glomerulonephritis and acute renal failure over days to weeks (nephritic syndrome), subacute immune injury often induces the formation of glomerular crescents and renal failure over weeks-to-months (termed *rapidly progressive glomerulonephritis*). As discussed above, crescents are extracapillary proliferations of cells in Bowman's space, composed of infiltrating monocytes, proliferating parietal epithelial cells, and fibrin.

Sustained low level immune complex deposition over months to years can provoke a marked increase in basement membrane or mesangial matrix production. Mild to moderate accumulation of matrix usually manifests as proteinuria due to disruption of the glomerular filtration barrier; however, in its most severe form, matrix accumulation causes glomerulosclerosis and chronic renal insufficiency.

RESOLUTION, REPAIR, AND SCARRING Glomerular inflammation can resolve with complete recovery of renal function or with a variable amount of scarring and chronic renal insufficiency. Acute poststreptococcal glomerulonephritis (p. 1582), for example, usually resolves spontaneously and fully in children, whereas adults are frequently left with residual renal impairment. The resolution process requires cessation of further antibody production and immune complex formation, removal of deposited and circulating immune complexes, inhibition of further recruitment of inflammatory cells, dissipation of the gradients of inflammatory mediators, restoration of normal endothelial adhesiveness and permeability, normalization of vascular tone, and clearance of infiltrating inflammatory cells and proliferating resident glomerular cells (Fig. 273-1).

Unfortunately, the resolution phase of most inflammatory glomerulopathies in adults terminates in some glomerular scarring. This is particularly true in patients with crescentic glomerulopathies who may be left with end-stage renal failure requiring dialysis or transplantation. Transforming growth factor (TGF) β, a cytokine, stimulates production of extracellular matrix by most glomerular cells, inhibits synthesis of tissue proteases that normally degrade matrix proteins, and is a potent stimulus for scar formation immediately following glomerular injury.

Moderate-to-severe glomerulonephritis is usually associated with a variable degree of tubulointerstitial inflammation and scarring in addition to glomerular injury. Indeed, the severity of tubulointerstitial injury usually correlates closely with long-term impairment of renal function. The pathogenesis of tubulointerstitial inflammation in this setting is unclear. Potential mechanisms include: (1) primary involvement of both the glomeruli and the tubulointerstitium in autoimmune disease; (2) induction of tubulointerstitial inflammation by mediators generated by diseased glomeruli which then diffuse into the tubulointerstitium via blood, tubular fluid, or the interstitial space; (3) injury to tubule epithelial cells by excessive filtered proteins ("protein overload" hypothesis); and (4) ischemia to areas of the tubulointerstitium downstream to areas of robust glomerular inflammation or severe glomerulosclerosis.

OTHER MECHANISMS OF ANTIBODY-MEDIATED INJURY Several other autoantibodies have been implicated as mediators of renal injury in patients with glomerulonephritis.

Antineutrophil Cytoplasmic Antibodies (ANCA) Immunoglobulin is not detected in the glomerulus in approximately 40% of patients with rapidly progressive glomerulonephritis ("pauci-immune crescentic glomerulonephritis"). The majority of these patients have Wegener's granulomatosis, microscopic polyangiitis nodosa, or renal-limited crescentic glomerulonephritis and have autoantibodies against neutrophil cytoplasmic antigens in their circulation. When reactive with ethanol-fixed neutrophils isolated from healthy volunteers, ANCA stain results in either a cytoplasmic pattern (c-ANCA) or perinuclear pattern (p-ANCA). In the case of c-ANCA, the neutrophil antigen is usually proteinase-3, a constituent of neutrophil primary granules. In the case of p-ANCA, the antigen is usually myeloperoxidase, another granule constituent that migrates to the perinuclear area upon ethanol fixation. Whereas a greater number of patients with Wegener's granulomatosis have c-ANCA and a greater proportion of patients with renal-limited disease have p-ANCA, the morphologic features, response to treatment, and overall prognosis appear to be similar in patients with either c-ANCA or p-ANCA. ANCA stimulate cytokine-primed human neutrophils to generate reactive oxygen species and injure endothelium in vitro. These findings raise the possibility that ANCA may be pathogenetic in vivo in the presence of circulating cytokines, as may occur following a prodromal infection.

Antiendothelial Cell Antibodies Circulating antibodies against endothelial antigens have been reported in several inflammatory vasculitides and glomerulonephritides. Their titers tend to correlate with disease activity, and some activate endothelial cells and increase their adhesiveness for leukocytes, suggesting a pathogenetic role.

C3 Nephritic Factor Some patients with membranoproliferative glomerulonephritis (Chap. 273) have large deposits of electron-dense material within the GBM that does not stain for immunoglobulin (dense deposit disease; membranoproliferative glomerulonephritis type II). Intriguingly, most of these patients have a circulating IgG, termed the *C3 nephritic factor*, directed at C3bBb (C3 convertase) of the alternative pathway of complement.

CELL-MEDIATED INJURY Although cell-mediated injury is, as yet, less well defined than antibody-mediated glomerular injury, T cells have also been implicated as independent mediators of glomerular injury and as modulators of the production of nephritogenic antibodies. T cells may be particularly important as initiators of injury in pauci-immune glomerulonephritis. T cells interact, through their cell-surface T cell receptor/CD3 complex, with antigens presented in the groove of major histocompatibility complex molecules of resident glomerular endothelial, mesangial, and epithelial cells, a process that is facilitated by cell-cell adhesion and costimulatory molecules. Cytokines and other mediators released by activated T cells are potent stimuli for further leukocyte recruitment, cytotoxicity, and fibrogenesis. CD4 T lymphocytes are important recruiters of macrophages and trigger clonal expansion of autoreactive B cells; they also promote glomerular cell injury by CD8 cytotoxic T lymphocytes and natural killer cells and through antibody-dependent cell cytotoxicity. Soluble factors derived from T cells have also been implicated in the pathogenesis of proteinuria in minimal change disease and primary focal segmental glomerulosclerosis. The identity and molecular characterization of these nonimmunoglobulin circulating permeability factors remain to be determined.

NONIMMUNOLOGIC GLOMERULAR INJURY

METABOLIC **Diabetic Nephropathy** (See also Chaps. 275 and 333) Nephropathy complicates approximately 30% of cases of type 1 and type 2 diabetes mellitus and is characterized clinically by proteinuria and progressive renal insufficiency. The typical glomerular lesion is glomerulosclerosis due to thickening of the GBM and expansion of the mesangium with extracellular matrix. Factors implicated as triggers for increased matrix production include glomerular hypertension; the direct effects of hyperglycemia on mesangial cells; advanced glycosylation end-products; growth factors such as growth hormone, insulin-like growth factor 1, and angiotensin II; cytokines such as TGF-β; hyperlipidemia; and cell sorbitol accumulation.

Complementary clinical and laboratory approaches suggest a central role for hemodynamic factors. Glomerular hydrostatic pressure and GFR increase within months of the development of hyperglycemia. The mechanism by which diabetes mellitus induces glomerular hypertension is still being defined but appears to involve atrial natriuretic peptide. In this framework, glycosuria triggers increased reabsorption of glucose coupled to sodium in the proximal tubule, thereby increasing total-body sodium and extracellular fluid volume. As a compensatory response, atrial natriuretic peptide is released from cardiac myocytes and induces natriuresis in part by triggering afferent arteriolar dilatation and thereby increasing intraglomerular pressure and GFR. Whereas this compensatory response is appropriate in the short term, sustained glomerular hypertension provokes thickening of the GBM, increased mesangial matrix production, and glomerulosclerosis and disruption of barrier function. In keeping with a central role for intraglomerular pressure in the pathogenesis of diabetic nephropathy, angiotensin-converting enzyme inhibitors, which lower intraglomerular pressure, slow the progression of diabetic nephropathy, even in normotensive patients. It remains to be determined why diabetes mellitus and glomerular hypertension include glomerulosclerosis in some but not all individuals. Epidemiologic studies and studies of disease concordance in identical twins suggest that important, but as yet unidentified, genetic factors may play a role. It is likely that hemodynamic and metabolic factors act in concert to generate the final glomerulosclerotic phenotype in genetically predisposed patients.

Other Metabolic Diseases Several rare inherited lysosomal enzyme defects induce focal segmental glomerulosclerosis, probably by allowing accumulation of toxic metabolites in renal cells. *Fabry's disease* (α-galactosidase deficiency; Chap. 349) and *sialidosis* (*N*-acetylneuraminic acid hydrolase deficiency; Chap. 349) are the major culprits in this regard. Both tend to induce focal segmental or global glomerulosclerosis by preferentially affecting visceral epithelial cells, probably because these are terminally differentiated cells with a very slow replication rate. *Partial lipodystrophy* is a rare metabolic disorder characterized by lipoatrophy affecting the arms, neck, and chest, often with redistribution of fat to the hips and legs. Approximately one-third of patients develop glomerular disease, usually type II membranoproliferative glomerulopathy (dense deposit disease; Chap. 274).

HEMODYNAMIC GLOMERULAR INJURY High intraglomerular pressure is a major cause of glomerular injury in humans and can result from systemic hypertension or a local change in glomerular hemodynamics (glomerular hypertension).

Systemic Hypertension (See also Chap. 246) Although the kidneys have evolved sophisticated mechanisms for autoregulating glomerular blood flow and pressure, marked or sustained increments in systemic blood pressure can overwhelm these compensatory systems and perturb glomerular morphology and function. In its most dramatic form, namely malignant hypertension, hemodynamic stress causes massive fibrinoid necrosis of afferent arterioles and glomeruli, thrombotic microangiopathy, acute renal failure, and a nephritic urinary sediment. Chronic sustained hypertension typically leads to arteriolar vasoconstriction and sclerosis, which, in turn, cause secondary atrophy and sclerosis of glomeruli and the tubulointerstitium. A variety of molecular signals appear to couple elevations in intravascular pressure to myointimal proliferation and eventually sclerosis of the vessel wall. These include growth factors such as angiotensin II, epidermal growth factor, and PDGF; cytokines such as TGF-β; and activation of stretch activated ion channels and early response genes.

Glomerular Hypertension The pathophysiology of diabetic nephropathy, discussed above, illustrates the importance of intraglomerular pressure as a stimulus for mesangial matrix production and glomerulosclerosis. Glomerular hypertension is also a key factor in the pathogenesis of the progressive glomerulosclerosis and renal failure that complicate the adaptive response of remnant nephrons to increased workload following loss of the other nephrons from any cause, including chronic allograft failure (see below). Importantly, these changes in glomerular hemodynamics and pressure appear to precede the development of systemic hypertension and are independent risk factors for glomerular injury.

TOXIC GLOMERULOPATHIES The renal microvasculature is a relatively uncommon site for toxic injury, by comparison with the tubular interstitium; however, there are a few important exceptions. Verotoxin, derived from *Escherichia coli* during bouts of infective diarrhea, is directly toxic to renal endothelium and induces the hemolytic-uremic syndrome. In this setting, verotoxin interacts with a specific cell membrane receptor, perturbs the antithrombotic phenotype of endothelium, and triggers the development of thrombotic microangiopathy. Irradiation, mitomycin, cyclosporine, and anovulants can also induce thrombotic microangiopathy through poorly defined mechanisms. Nonsteroidal anti-inflammatory drugs, rifampin, ampicillin, and interferon-α can induce an unusual combination of acute renal failure with nephrotic syndrome. The characteristic pathologic correlates of this syndrome are allergic interstitial nephritis and fusion of the foot processes of the visceral epithelial cells, the latter accounting for the marked proteinuria. How these structurally diverse agents induce epithelial cell injury is unclear.

DEPOSITION DISEASES The glomerular deposition diseases are a group of diverse conditions in which abnormal proteins are deposited in glomeruli, where they provoke an inflammatory reaction and/or glomerulosclerosis. The major glomerular deposition diseases are cryoglobulinemia, amyloidosis, light and heavy chain deposition disease, and fibrillary/immunotactoid glomerulopathy. *Cryoglobulins* (Chap. 317) are immunoglobulins that precipitate in the cold and can be composed of either monoclonal immunoglobulin, usually generated by a lymphoproliferative malignancy (type I); a mixture of polyclonal immunoglobulin (usually IgG) and monoclonal immunoglobulin (usually IgM) directed to epitopes on polyclonal IgG (type II); or a mixture of polyclonal antibodies, one or more having anti-IgG activity (type III). As discussed above, cryoglobulins can induce nephritic-type and nephrotic-type injury depending on the rapidity, severity, and site of immunoglobulin deposition. Most cryoglobulinemic glomerulopathy is associated with type II cryoglobulins, the majority of which are now recognized to be triggered by chronic hepatitis B or C infection. *Glomerular amyloidosis* (Chaps. 275 and 319) is one of the five most common causes of nephrotic syndrome in adults and is characterized by extracellular deposition of amyloid fibrils composed, in part, of fragments of immunoglobulin light chains (AL amyloid) or serum amyloid A, the acute-phase reactant (AA amyloid). In light chain deposition diseases, intact immunoglobulin light chains, usually kappa, are deposited in a granular, rather than fibrillary, pattern. The composition of the deposits in *fibrillary/immunotactoid glomerulopathy* is still being defined and may also include immunoglobulin and/or fibronectin-containing cryoglobulins. These different types of deposits, in addition to directly disrupting glomerular architecture, provoke mesangial matrix production and glomerulosclerosis. Fibrillary/immunotactoid glomerulopathy can also present as acute or subacute glomerular inflammation. How these diverse deposits trigger glomerular matrix production and recruitment of inflammatory cells has yet to be determined.

INFECTIOUS CAUSES OF GLOMERULAR DISEASE Infectious organisms can induce glomerular disease through several different mechanisms: (1) by direct infection of renal cells, (2) by elaborating nephrotoxins such as *E. coli*–derived verotoxin, (3) by inciting intraglomerular deposition of immune complexes (e.g., postinfectious glomerulonephritis) or cryoglobulins (e.g., hepatitis B or C), and (4) by providing a chronic stimulus for amyloid fibril formation, as in AA amyloidosis. Direct infection of glomerular cells is a relatively rare mechanism of injury but has been implicated in the pathogenesis of nephropathy associated with HIV. This entity is characterized histologically by an aggressive form of focal segmental glomerulosclerosis, microcystic tubular dilatation, and interstitial fibrosis. Viral genome and several proteins have been detected in glomerular and tubular cells in this disease, and infection of glomerular cells induces expression of TGF-β, a major stimulus for mesangial matrix production and sclerosis.

INHERITED GLOMERULAR DISEASES *Alport's syndrome* (hereditary nephritis; Chap. 275), the prototypical inherited glomerular disease, is usually transmitted as an X-linked dominant trait, although autosomal recessive forms have been reported. Patients afflicted with the classic X-linked form have a mutation in the COL4A5 gene that encodes the $\alpha5$ chain of type IV collagen located on the X chromosome. As a result, the GBM is irregular with longitudinal layering, splitting, or thickening, and patients develop hematuria, progressive glomerulosclerosis, and renal failure. *Thin basement membrane disease* is another relatively common disorder of the GBM. In contrast to Alport's syndrome, this entity is usually inherited as an autosomal dominant or recessive trait and appears to be relatively benign. As the name suggests, the basement membrane is thin but otherwise ultrastructurally normal. Patients typically experience recurrent benign hematuria. The molecular basis for thin basement membrane disease has yet to be elucidated fully; however, defects in the gene encoding the $\alpha4$ chain of type IV collagen have been reported in some families. Rarer hereditary glomerular diseases include *nail-patella syndrome* (osteoonychodysplasia), which is associated with a relatively benign mottling of the basement membrane with lucent rarefractions; *partial lipodystrophy*, which is associated with type II membranoproliferative glomerulonephritis (dense deposit disease); and *familial lecithin–cholesterol acyltransferase deficiency*, which is associated with distortion of the basement membrane by irregular rounded lucent zones, increased mesangial matrix production, and progressive sclerosis and renal insufficiency.

GLOMERULAR ADAPTATION TO NEPHRON LOSS

Nephron loss, from any cause, is followed by compensatory hyperfiltration in the remaining functional glomeruli. This adaptive response is appropriate in the short-term and maintains GFR. Over years, however, the hyperfiltering remnant nephrons develop focal and segmental glomerulosclerosis, and eventually global sclerosis, that manifests clinically as proteinuria, hypertension, and progressive renal insufficiency. Sustained glomerular capillary hypertension has been implicated as a major stimulus for glomerulosclerosis in this setting. Increased glomerular blood flow and ultrafiltration pressure are early findings in remnant nephrons in most experimental models in which the function of more than 50% of nephron mass has been lost through surgical ablation, immunologic or toxic injury, or other mechanisms. Sustained glomerular hypertension is thought to stimulate the accumulation of extracellular matrix by perturbing the function of visceral epithelial and mesangial cells, either directly or by increasing the flux of circulating macromolecules through the glomerular capillary wall. As with most forms of glomerulosclerosis, TGF-β may be an important regulator of matrix accumulation in remnant nephrons. Angiotensin II, PDGF, and endothelins are other potential modulators of this process. Maneuvers that lower intraglomerular pressure, such as low-protein diet or treatment with angiotensin-converting enzyme inhibitors, slow the development of glomerulosclerosis and renal failure. Glomerular hypertrophy, intracapillary microthrombi, recruited macrophages, and hyperlipidemia are other potential stimuli for glomerulosclerosis. Indeed, glomerular capillary hypertension and hypertrophy appear to be independent risk factors that could act synergistically to cause progressive renal insufficiency. Intriguingly, angiotensin II may trigger TGF-β production in remnant nephrons, suggesting that angiotensin-converting enzyme inhibitors may be renoprotective through complementary effects on glomerular hemodynamics and matrix production.

BIBLIOGRAPHY

APPEL G, RISHNAM JR: Secondary glomerular diseases, in *Brenner & Rector's The Kidney*, 6th ed, BM Brenner (ed). Philadelphia, Saunders, 2000, pp 1350–1448

BRADY HR: Leukocyte adhesion molecules and kidney diseases. Kidney Int 45:1285, 1994

BERDEN JH: Lupus nephritis. Kidney Int 52:538, 1997

FALK R et al: Primary glomerular diseases, in *Brenner & Rector's The Kidney*, 6th ed, BM Brenner (ed). Philadelphia, Saunders, 2000, pp 1263–1349

HOFFMAN GS, SPECKS U: Antineutrophil cytoplasmic antibodies. Arthritis Rheum 41: 1521, 1998

HOLDSWORTH SR et al: Th1 and Th2 T helper cell subsets affect patterns of injury and outcomes in glomerulonephritis. Kidney Int 55:1198, 1999

KASHTAN CE: Alport syndrome and thin glomerular basement membrane disease. J Am Soc Nephrol 9:1736, 1998

KELLY PT, HAPONIK EF: Goodpasture's syndrome: Molecular and clinical advances. Medicine (Baltimore) 73:171, 1994

KITAMURA M, FINE LH: The concept of glomerular self-defense. Kidney Int 55:1639, 1999

KROWLEWSKI AS: Genetics of diabetic nephropathy: Evidence for major and minor gene effects. Kidney Int 55:1582, 1999

MACKENZIE HS et al: Adaptation to nephron loss, in *Brenner & Rector's The Kidney*, 6th ed, BM Brenner (ed). Philadelphia, Saunders, 2000, pp 1901–1942

SAVIN NJ et al: Circulating factor associated with increased glomerular permeability to albumin in recurrent focal segmental glomerulosclerosis. N Engl J Med 334:878, 1996

STEHMAN-BREEN C, JOHNSON RJ: Hepatitis C virus–associated glomerulonephritis. Adv Intern Med 43:79, 1998

274 *Hugh R. Brady, Yvonne M. O'Meara, Barry M. Brenner*

THE MAJOR GLOMERULOPATHIES

ACE angiotensin-converting enzyme	MPGN membranoproliferative glomerulonephritis
ANCA antineutrophil cytoplasmic antibody	NSAIDs nonsteroidal anti-inflammatory drugs
ESRD end-stage renal disease	PAS periodic acid–Schiff
FSGS focal and segmental glomerulosclerosis	RPGN rapidly progressive glomerulonephritis
GBM glomerular basement membrane	SLE systemic lupus erythematosus
GFR glomerular filtration rate	TBM thin basement membrane
MCD minimal change disease	

Glomerular injury can arise from diverse renal-limited and systemic diseases and is the major cause of end-stage renal disease (ESRD) requiring dialysis and transplantation. In this chapter, we describe the epidemiology, clinical presentations, pathology, and treatment of the major glomerulopathies. We focus on the *primary glomerulopathies*, glomerular diseases in which the pathologic process is confined to the kidney and in which systemic features are a direct consequence of impaired glomerular filtration (e.g., hypervolemia, hypertension, uremic syndrome). Considered here are the five major clinical presentations of glomerulopathy: acute nephritic syndrome, rapidly progressive glomerulonephritis (RPGN), nephrotic syndrome, asymptomatic abnormalities of the urinary sediment (hematuria, proteinuria), and chronic glomerulonephritis. ***→Glomerulopathies associated with systemic diseases (*****secondary glomerulopathies*****) are discussed in Chap. 275. The nomenclature pertaining to the classification and clinicopathologic description of glomerular disease and the pathogenetic mechanisms of glomerular injury are reviewed in Chap. 273.***

ACUTE NEPHRITIC SYNDROME AND RAPIDLY PROGRESSIVE GLOMERULONEPHRITIS

CLINICAL FEATURES AND CLINICOPATHOLOGIC CORRELATES The *acute nephritic syndrome* is the clinical correlate of acute glomerular inflammation. In its most dramatic form, the acute nephritic syndrome is characterized by sudden onset (i.e., over days to weeks) of *acute renal failure* and *oliguria* (<400 mL of urine per day). Renal blood flow and glomerular filtration rate (GFR) fall as a result of obstruction of the glomerular capillary lumen by infiltrating inflammatory cells and proliferating resident glomerular cells. Renal blood flow and GFR are further compromised by intrarenal vasoconstriction and mesangial cell contraction that result from local imbalances of vasoconstrictor (e.g., leukotrienes, platelet-activating factor, thromboxanes, endothelins) and vasodilator substances (e.g., nitric oxide, prostacyclin) within the renal microcirculation. *Extracellular fluid volume expansion*, *edema*, and *hypertension* develop because of impaired GFR and enhanced tubular reabsorption of salt and water. As a result of injury to the glomerular capillary wall, urinalysis typically reveals *red blood cell casts*, dysmorphic red blood cells, leukocytes, and subnephrotic proteinuria of <3.5 g per 24 h ("nephritic urinary sediment"). *Hematuria* is often macroscopic.

The classic pathologic correlate of the nephritic syndrome is *proliferative glomerulonephritis*. The proliferation of glomerular cells is due initially to infiltration of the glomerular tuft by neutrophils and monocytes and subsequently to proliferation of resident glomerular endothelial and mesangial cells (endocapillary proliferation). In its most severe form, the nephritic syndrome is associated with acute inflammation of most glomeruli, i.e., *acute diffuse proliferative glomerulonephritis*. When less vigorous, fewer than 50% of glomeruli may be involved, i.e., *focal proliferative glomerulonephritis*. In milder forms of nephritic injury, cellular proliferation may be confined to the mesangium, i.e., *mesangioproliferative glomerulonephritis*.

RPGN is the clinical correlate of more *subacute glomerular inflammation*. Patients develop renal failure over weeks to months in association with a nephritic urinary sediment, subnephrotic proteinuria and variable oliguria, hypervolemia, edema, and hypertension. The classic pathologic correlate of RPGN is crescent formation involving most glomeruli (*crescentic glomerulonephritis*), crescents being half-moon-shaped lesions in Bowman's space composed of proliferating parietal epithelial cells and infiltrating monocytes (*extracapillary proliferation*). In practice, the clinical term *rapidly progressive glomerulonephritis* and the pathologic term *crescentic glomerulonephritis* are often used interchangeably. In addition to classic crescentic glomerulonephritis, in which crescents dominate the glomerular pathology, crescents can also develop concomitantly with proliferative glomerulonephritis or as a complication of membranous glomerulopathy and other more indolent forms of glomerular inflammation.

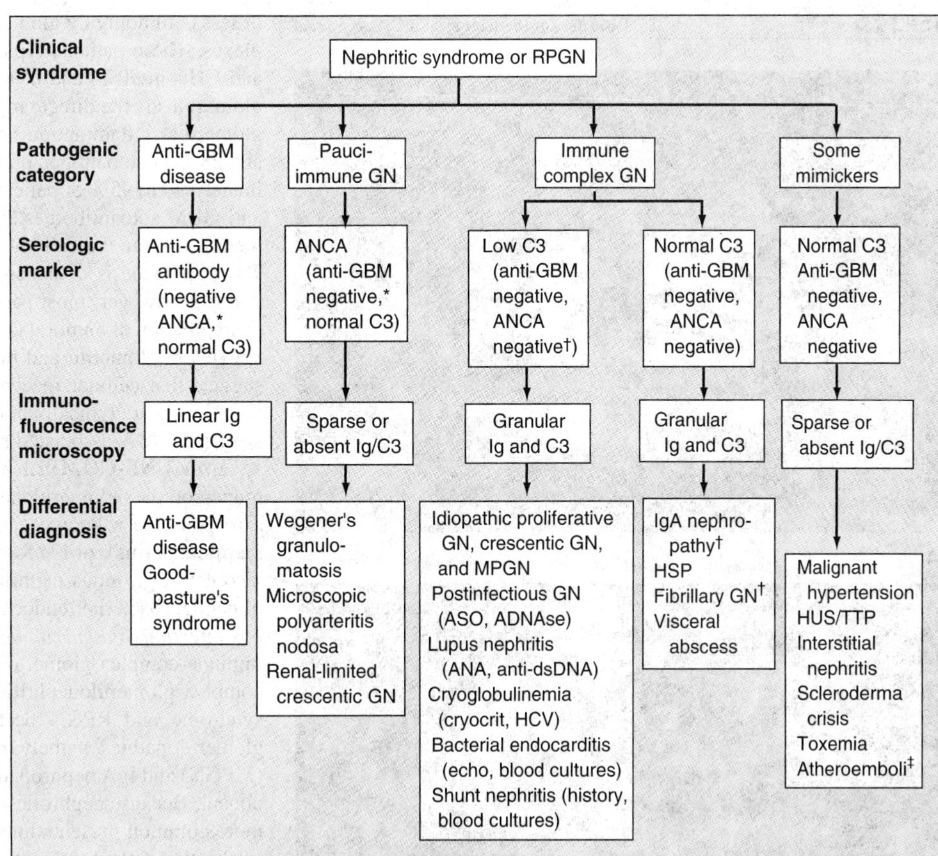

FIGURE 274-1 Differential diagnosis of nephritic syndrome and rapidly progressive glomerulonephritis.

Abbreviations: GN, glomerulonephritis; RPGN, rapidly progressive glomerulonephritis; MPGN, membranoproliferative glomerulonephritis; GBM, glomerular basement membrane; ANCA, antineutrophil cytoplasmic antibodies; Ig, immunoglobulin; C3, third component of complement; ASO, antistreptolysin O antibody titer; ADNAse, anti-deoxyribonuclease antibody titer; ANA, antinuclear antibody; anti-dsDNA, anti-double-stranded DNA antibody; HCV, hepatitis C virus; echo, echocardiogram; HSP, Henoch-Schönlein purpura; HUS, hemolytic-uremic syndrome; TTP, thrombotic thrombocytopenic purpura.

*Approximately 20% of patients with anti-GBM disease have ANCA, which may portend a better prognosis.

†Nephritic syndrome and RPGN are unusual presentations of IgA nephropathy and fibrillary GN.

‡Atheroembolic renal disease may cause transient hypocomplementemia.

The acute nephritic syndrome and RPGN are part of a spectrum of presentations of immunologically mediated proliferative glomerulonephritis. Studies of experimental models suggest that nephritic syndrome and diffuse proliferative glomerulonephritis represent an acute immune response to a sudden large antigen load, whereas RPGN and crescentic glomerulonephritis represent a more subacute immune response to a smaller antigen load in presensitized individuals. At the other end of the spectrum, chronic low-grade immune injury presents with slowly progressive renal insufficiency or asymptomatic hematuria in association with focal proliferative or mesangioproliferative glomerulonephritis. These more indolent forms of immune-mediated glomerulonephritis are discussed later in this chapter.

ETIOLOGY AND DIFFERENTIAL DIAGNOSIS Acute nephritic syndrome and RPGN can result from renal-limited *primary* glomerulopathy or from *secondary* glomerulopathy complicating systemic disease. Figure 274-1 highlights the histopathologic and serologic features that help distinguish among the major causes of nephritic syndrome and RPGN (see also Fig. 274-2). In general, rapid diagnosis and prompt treatment are critical to avoid the development of irreversible renal failure. Renal biopsy remains the "gold standard" for diagnosis. *Immunofluorescence microscopy* is particularly helpful and identifies three major patterns of deposition of immunoglobulin that define three broad diagnostic categories: (1) *granular* deposits of immunoglobulin, a hallmark of *immune-complex glomerulonephritis*; (2) *linear* deposition of immunoglobulin along the glomerular basement membrane (GBM), characteristic of anti-GBM disease; and (3) paucity or absence of immunoglobulin, so-called *pauci-immune glomerulonephritis* (Figs. 273-1 and 274-2). Most patients (>70%) with full-blown acute nephritic syndrome have immune-complex glomerulonephritis. Pauci-immune glomerulonephritis is less common in this setting (<30%) and anti-GBM disease is rare (<1%). Among patients with RPGN, immune-complex glomerulonephritis and pauci-immune glomerulonephritis are equally prevalent (~45% each), whereas anti-GBM disease again accounts for a minority of cases (<10%).

Three *serologic markers* often predict the immunofluorescence microscopy findings in nephritic syndrome and RPGN and may obviate the need for renal biopsy in classic cases. They are the serum C3 level and titers of anti-GBM antibody and antineutrophil cytoplasmic antibody (ANCA) (Fig. 274-1). As discussed in Chap. 273, the kidney is host to immune attack in immune-complex glomerulonephritis, most cases being initiated either by in situ formation of immune complexes

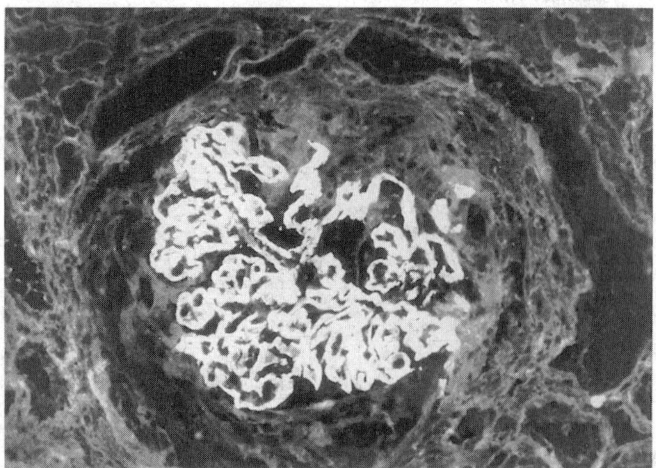

A

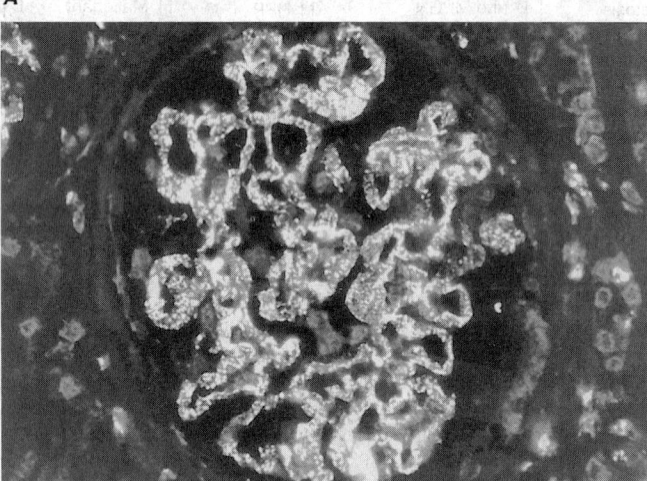

B

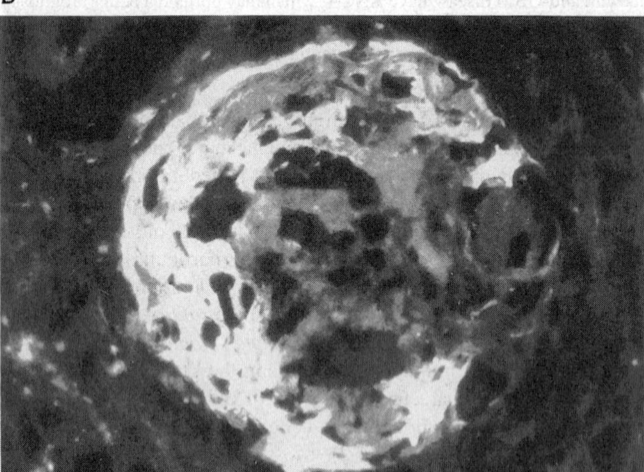

C

FIGURE 274-2 Typical findings on immunofluorescence microscopy of renal biopsy specimens from patients with anti-glomerular basement membrane antibody disease, immune-complex–mediated glomerulonephritis, and pauci-immune glomerulonephritis. Specimens in the upper and middle panels were stained for immunoglobulin and show the classical linear "ribbon-like" pattern of anti-GBM disease (*A*) and granular pattern of immune-complex–mediated glomerulonephritis (*B*). Immunoglobulin is sparse or absent in patients with pauci-immune glomerulonephritis (not shown); however, abundant fibrin is detected in crescents (*C*). *(Micrographs courtesy of Dr. Helmut Rennke).*

or less commonly by glomerular trapping of circulating immune complexes. These patients typically have hypocomplementemia (low C3 and CH_{50} in 90%) and negative anti-GBM and ANCA serology. The glomerulus is the direct target of immune attack in anti-GBM disease, glomerular inflammation being initiated by an autoantibody directed at a 28-kDa autoantigen on the α3 chain of type IV collagen. Approximately 90 to 95% of patients with anti-GBM disease have circulating anti-GBM autoantibodies detectable by immunoassay; serum complement levels are typically normal, and ANCA are usually not detected. The pathogenesis of pauci-immune glomerulonephritis is still being defined; however, most patients have circulating ANCA, implicating dysregulation of humoral immunity. The presence of mononuclear leukocytes in glomeruli and the paucity of glomerular immune deposits suggest that cellular mechanisms are also involved. Serum complement levels are typically normal, and anti-GBM titers are usually negative in ANCA-associated renal disease.

IMMUNE-COMPLEX GLOMERULONEPHRITIS Immune-complex glomerulonephritis may (1) be idiopathic, (2) represent a response to a known antigenic stimulus (e.g., postinfectious glomerulonephritis), or (3) form part of a multisystem immune-complex disorder (e.g., lupus nephritis, Henoch-Schönlein purpura, cryoglobulinemia, bacterial endocarditis; Fig. 274-1). Here, we focus on *postinfectious glomerulonephritis*, the best characterized *primary* immune-complex glomerulonephritis. The major *secondary* immune-complex glomerulonephritides are discussed in Chap. 275. Nephritic syndrome and RPGN occasionally complicate two other primary glomerulopathies, namely, membranoproliferative glomerulonephritis (MPGN) and IgA nephropathy when there is a florid proliferative component. Because nephrotic syndrome and asymptomatic hematuria are more common presentations of MPGN and IgA nephropathy, respectively, these glomerulopathies are discussed in later sections on nephrotic syndrome and asymptomatic urinary abnormalities.

POSTSTREPTOCOCCAL GLOMERULONEPHRITIS This is the prototypical postinfectious glomerulonephritis and a leading cause of acute nephritic syndrome. Most cases are sporadic, though the disease can occur as an epidemic. Glomerulonephritis develops, on average, 10 days after pharyngitis or 2 weeks after a skin infection (impetigo) with a nephritogenic strain of group A β-hemolytic streptococcus. The known nephritic strains include M types 1, 2, 4, 12, 18, 25, 49, 55, 57, and 60. Immunity to these strains is type-specific and long-lasting, and repeated infection and nephritis are rare. Epidemic poststreptococcal glomerulonephritis is most commonly encountered in children of 2 to 6 years of age with pharyngitis during the winter months. This entity appears to be decreasing in frequency, possibly due to more widespread and prompt use of antibiotics. Poststreptococcal glomerulonephritis in association with cutaneous infections usually occurs in a setting of poor personal hygiene or streptococcal superinfection of another skin disease.

The classic clinical presentation of poststreptococcal glomerulonephritis is full-blown nephritic syndrome with oliguric acute renal failure; however, most patients have milder disease. Indeed, subclinical cases outnumber overt cases by four- to tenfold during epidemics. Patients with overt disease present with gross hematuria (red or "smoky" urine), headache, and generalized symptoms such as anorexia, nausea, vomiting, and malaise. Swelling of the renal capsule can cause flank or back pain. Physical examination reveals hypervolemia, edema, and hypertension. The urinary sediment is nephritic, with dysmorphic red blood cells, red cell casts, leukocytes, occasionally leukocyte casts, and subnephrotic proteinuria. Fewer than 5% of patients develop nephrotic-range proteinuria. The latter may only manifest as acute nephritis resolves and renal blood flow and GFR recover. Coexistent rheumatic fever is extremely rare.

The serum creatinine is often mildly elevated at presentation. Serum C3 levels and CH_{50} are depressed within 2 weeks in ~90% of cases. C4 levels are characteristically normal, indicating activation of the alternate pathway of complement. Complement levels usually return to normal within 6 to 8 weeks. Persistently depressed levels after this period should suggest another cause, such as the presence of a C3 nephritic factor (see "Membranoproliferative Glomerulonephritis"). The majority of patients (>75%) have transient hypergammaglobulinemia and mixed cryoglobulinemia. The antecedent streptococcal infection may still be evident or may have resolved either spontaneously or in response to antibiotic therapy. Most patients (>90%) have circulating antibodies against streptococcal exoenzymes such as antistreptolysin O (ASO), anti-deoxyribonuclease B (anti-DNAse B), antistreptokinase (ASKase), anti-nicotinyl adenine dinucleotidase (anti-NADase), and antihyaluronidase (AHase). ASO, anti-DNAse B, anti-NAD, and AHase are most useful after pharyngeal infection, whereas anti-DNAse B and AHase are more sensitive indices of streptococcal skin infection. Antibody titers tend to rise after 7 days, peak after 1 month, and return to normal levels after 3 to 4 months. These tests are relatively specific, with a false-positive rate of <5%. Early antibiotic therapy may prevent the development of an antibody response.

Acute poststreptococcal glomerulonephritis is usually diagnosed on clinical and serologic grounds, without resort to renal biopsy, especially in children with a typical antecedent history. The characteristic lesion on light microscopy is diffuse proliferative glomerulonephritis. Crescents are uncommon, and extraglomerular involvement is usually mild. Immunofluorescence microscopy reveals diffuse granular deposition of IgG and C3, giving rise to a "starry sky" appearance (Fig. 274-2). More extensive immunoglobulin deposition throughout the glomerular capillary wall ("garland pattern") is associated with a worse prognosis. The characteristic finding on electron microscopy is the presence of large electron-dense immune deposits in the subendothelial, subepithelial, and mesangial areas. The acute inflammatory reaction is initiated, in large part, by the subendothelial and mesangial deposits, which activate complement and trigger leukocyte recruitment and glomerular injury. Subepithelial deposits are often more prominent on electron microscopy, however, probably because the subendothelial and mesangial deposits are scavenged more efficiently by invading phagocytes. Extensive subepithelial immune deposits, or "humps," tend to be associated with worse proteinuria, being juxtaposed to the glomerular filtration barrier for protein. →*The pathogenesis of immune-complex glomerulonephritis is discussed extensively in Chap. 273.*

In addition to poststreptococcal glomerulonephritis, the nephritic syndrome and RPGN can complicate acute immune-complex glomerulonephritis due to other viral, bacterial, fungal, and parasitic infections. Several warrant specific mention. Diffuse proliferative immune-complex glomerulonephritis is a well-described complication of acute and subacute bacterial endocarditis and is usually associated with hypocomplementemia. The glomerular lesion typically resolves following eradication of the cardiac infection. *Shunt nephritis* is a syndrome characterized by immune-complex glomerulonephritis secondary to infection of ventriculoatrial shunts inserted for treatment of childhood hydrocephalus. The most common offending organism is coagulase-negative staphylococcus. Renal impairment is usually mild and associated with hypocomplementemia. Nephrotic syndrome complicates 30% of cases. Acute proliferative glomerulonephritis can also complicate *chronic suppurative infections* and *visceral abscesses*. Patients typically present with a fever of unknown origin and an active urine sediment. Although immune deposits containing IgG and C3 are detected on renal biopsy, serum complement levels are usually normal.

℞ **TREATMENT** Treatment of poststreptococcal glomerulonephritis focuses on eliminating the streptococcal infection with antibiotics and providing supportive therapy until spontaneous resolution of glomerular inflammation occurs. Patients are usually confined to bed during the acute inflammatory phase. Diuretics and antihypertensive agents are employed to control extracellular fluid volume and blood pressure. Dialysis is rarely needed to control hypervolemia or the uremic syndrome. Poststreptococcal glomerulonephritis carries an excellent prognosis and rarely causes ESRD. Microscopic hematuria may persist for as long as 1 year after the acute episode but eventually

resolves. Whereas complete recovery is the rule in children, adults may occasionally be left with residual renal impairment.

Antiglomerular Basement Membrane Disease Anti-GBM disease is an autoimmune disease in which autoantibodies directed against type IV collagen induce RPGN and crescentic glomerulonephritis (Figs. 273-1, 274-1, and 274-2). Acute nephritic syndrome is rare. Between 50 and 70% of patients have lung hemorrhage; the clinical complex of anti-GBM nephritis and lung hemorrhage is referred to as *Goodpasture's syndrome*. Anti-GBM disease is a rare disorder of unknown etiology with an annual incidence of 0.5 per million. There is a bimodal peak in incidence. Patients with Goodpasture's syndrome are typically young males (5 to 40 years; male-female ratio of 6:1). In contrast, patients presenting during the second peak in the sixth decade rarely suffer lung hemorrhage and have an almost equal sex distribution. The target antigen is a component of the noncollagenous (NCI) domain of the $\alpha 3$ chain of type IV collagen, the $\alpha 3$ chain being preferentially expressed in glomerular and pulmonary alveolar basement membrane. The trigger(s) for loss of self-tolerance to this Goodpasture antigen has not been well defined. A genetic predisposition is suggested by an association with HLA-DRw2 and occasional occurrence in identical twins. Patients with lung hemorrhage are more likely to be cigarette smokers and to have suffered a recent upper respiratory tract infection or exposure to volatile hydrocarbon solvents. These observations suggest that diverse insults to the alveolar basement membrane may render previously sequestered Goodpasture antigens available for interaction with circulating autoantibodies. It is not clear whether environmental factors also trigger the onset of nephritis. Binding of anti-GBM antibodies to the GBM induces activation of complement, leukocyte recruitment, necrotizing proliferative glomerulonephritis, disruption of the glomerular capillary wall, leakage of fibrin into Bowman's space, and crescent formation (Chap. 273). A similar sequence of events in the lung leads to disruption of the alveolar capillary wall and pulmonary hemorrhage.

Anti-GBM disease commonly presents with hematuria, nephritic urinary sediment, subnephrotic proteinuria, and rapidly progressive renal failure over weeks, with or without pulmonary hemorrhage. When pulmonary hemorrhage occurs, it usually predates nephritis by weeks or months. Hemoptysis can vary from fluffy pulmonary infiltrates on chest x-ray and mild dyspnea on exertion to life-threatening pulmonary hemorrhage. Hypertension is unusual and occurs in fewer than 20% of cases.

The diagnostic serologic marker is circulating anti-GBM antibodies with a specificity for the NCI domain of the $\alpha 3$ chain of type IV collagen (Fig. 274-1). Anti-GBM antibodies are detected in the serum of >90% of patients with anti-GBM nephritis by specific immunoassay. If immunoassays are not available, circulating anti-GBM antibodies can be detected in 60 to 80% of patients by indirect immunofluorescence, i.e., by incubating the patient's serum with stored sections of normal human kidneys. Complement levels are normal. About 20% of patients have low titers of ANCA, usually a perinuclear ANCA (Chap. 275), the pathophysiologic significance of which is unclear. Occasional patients have a positive cytoplasmic ANCA, which may signal the presence of coexistent extraglomerular renal vasculitis. Patients with lung involvement frequently have microcytic, hypochromic, iron-deficiency anemia from alveolar hemorrhage, and abnormal bilateral hilar and basilar interstitial shadowing on chest x-ray that may be difficult to distinguish from pulmonary edema or infection. The diffusion capacity for carbon dioxide is a useful tool for distinguishing among the latter diagnoses, being increased in patients with lung hemorrhage due to uptake of carbon monoxide by alveolar blood, and reduced in patients with infection or pulmonary edema.

Renal biopsy is the gold standard for diagnosis of anti-GBM nephritis. The typical morphologic pattern on light microscopy is diffuse proliferative glomerulonephritis, with focal necrotizing lesions and crescents in >50% of glomeruli (crescentic glomerulonephritis). Immunofluorescence microscopy reveals linear ribbon-like deposition of IgG along the GBM (Fig. 274-2). C3 is present in the same distribution in 70% of patients. Prominent IgG deposition along the tubule basement membrane and tubulointerstitial inflammation is found occasionally. Electron microscopy reveals nonspecific inflammatory changes without immune deposits. Typical features on lung biopsy include alveolar hemorrhage, disruption of alveolar septa, hemosiderin-laden macrophages, and linear staining of IgG along the alveolar capillary basement membrane.

It should be noted that Goodpasture's syndrome is not the only cause of the pulmonary-renal syndrome (i.e., renal failure and lung hemorrhage). Other important causes of this clinical complex include severe cardiac failure complicated by pulmonary edema (often blood-tinged) and prerenal azotemia; renal failure from any cause complicated by hypervolemia and pulmonary edema; immune complex–mediated vasculitides such as systemic lupus erythematosus (SLE), Henoch-Schönlein purpura, and cryoglobulinemia; pauci-immune vasculitides such as Wegener's granulomatosis and polyarteritis nodosa; infections such as Legionnaire's disease; and renal vein thrombosis with pulmonary embolism. In general, these disorders can be differentiated by astute analysis of the clinical, serologic, and histopathologic findings.

℞ TREATMENT Prior to the introduction of immunosuppressive therapy, greater than 80% of patients with anti-GBM nephritis developed ESRD within 1 year, and many patients died from pulmonary hemorrhage or complications of uremia. With early and aggressive use of plasmapheresis, glucocorticoids, cyclophosphamide, and azathioprine, renal and patient survival have improved dramatically. In general, emergency plasmapheresis is performed daily or on alternate days until anti-GBM antibodies are not detected in the circulation (usually 1 to 2 weeks). Prednisone (1 mg/kg per day) is started simultaneously, in combination with either cyclophosphamide (2 to 3 mg/kg per day) or azathioprine (1 to 2 mg/kg per day) to suppress new synthesis of anti-GBM antibodies. The speed of initiation of therapy is a critical determinant of outcome. One-year renal survival approaches 90% if treatment is started before serum creatinine exceeds 442 μmol/L (5 mg/dL) and falls to about 10% if renal failure is more advanced. Patients who require dialysis at presentation rarely recover renal function. Serial anti-GBM titers are monitored to gauge response to therapy. Relapses are not unusual and are often heralded by rising antibody titers. In patients with ESRD, renal transplantation is a viable treatment option. Recurrence of anti-GBM nephritis in the allograft is extremely unusual provided that anti-GBM antibody titers have been consistently negative for 2 to 3 months prior to transplantation. However, in occasional patients with Alport's syndrome, when the allograft presents normal GBM components to the immune system of the recipient for the first time, anti-GBM nephritis can occur de novo in renal allografts.

Pauci-Immune Glomerulonephritis The major pauci-immune glomerulonephritides are *idiopathic renal-limited crescentic glomerulonephritis, microscopic polyarteritis nodosa,* and *Wegener's granulomatosis* (Fig. 274-1). RPGN is a more common clinical presentation than acute nephritic syndrome, and the usual pathology is necrotizing glomerulonephritis with crescents affecting >50% of glomeruli (crescentic glomerulonephritis). The marked overlap of clinical features and glomerular histopathology, and the presence of circulating ANCA in most patients, suggest that these entities are a spectrum of a single disease. Here, we focus on idiopathic renal-limited crescentic glomerulonephritis. →***The ANCA-associated glomerulopathies with extrarenal features, namely Wegener's granulomatosis, Churg-Strauss syndrome, and microscopic polyarteritis nodosa, are discussed in Chap. 275.***

Idiopathic Renal-Limited Crescentic Glomerulonephritis This is more common in middle-aged and older patients and shows a slight male preponderance. Patients typically present with RPGN, nephritic syndrome being rare. ANCA, usually a perinuclear ANCA IgG with specificity for myeloperoxidase (Chap. 275), are detected in 70 to 90% of patients (Fig. 274-1). The erythrocyte sedimentation rate and C-reactive protein levels may be elevated; however, C3 levels are typically normal, and circulating immune complexes, cryoglobulins, and anti-GBM antibodies are not detected. Most patients have crescents on light microscopy, often associated with necrotizing glomerulonephritis. Immune deposits are scanty or absent. Immunofluorescence microscopy reveals abundant fibrin deposits within crescents (Fig. 274-2). Most cases are treated aggressively with glucocorticoids, with or without cyclophosphamide or azathioprine (Chap. 275).

NEPHROTIC SYNDROME

GENERAL FEATURES AND COMPLICATIONS The *nephrotic syndrome* is a clinical complex characterized by a number of renal and extrarenal features, the most prominent of which are proteinuria of >3.5 g per 1.73 m^2 per 24 h (in practice, >3.0 to 3.5 g per 24 h), hypoalbuminemia, edema, hyperlipidemia, lipiduria, and hypercoagulability. It should be stressed that the key component is *proteinuria,* which results from altered permeability of the glomerular filtration barrier for protein, namely the GBM and the podocytes and their slit diaphragms. The other components of the nephrotic syndrome and the ensuing metabolic complications are all secondary to urine protein loss and can occur with lesser degrees of proteinuria or may be absent even in patients with massive proteinuria.

In general, the greater the proteinuria, the lower the serum albumin level. *Hypoalbuminemia* is compounded further by increased renal catabolism and inadequate, albeit usually increased, hepatic synthesis of albumin. The pathophysiology of *edema* formation in nephrotic syndrome is poorly understood. The *underfilling hypothesis* postulates that hypoalbuminemia results in decreased intravascular oncotic pressure, leading to leakage of extracellular fluid from blood to the interstitium. Intravascular volume falls, thereby stimulating activation of the renin-angiotensin-aldosterone axis and the sympathetic nervous system and release of vasopressin (antidiuretic hormone), and suppressing atrial natriuretic peptide release. These neural and hormonal responses promote renal salt and water retention, thereby restoring intravascular volume and triggering further leakage of fluid to the interstitium. This hypothesis does not, however, explain the occurrence of edema in many patients in whom plasma volume is expanded and the renin-angiotensin-aldosterone axis is suppressed. The latter finding suggests that *primary renal salt and water retention* may also contribute to edema formation in some cases.

Hyperlipidemia is believed to be a consequence of increased hepatic lipoprotein synthesis that is triggered by reduced oncotic pressure and may be compounded by increased urinary loss of proteins that regulate lipid homeostasis. Low-density lipoproteins and cholesterol are increased in the majority of patients, whereas very low density lipoproteins and triglycerides tend to rise in patients with severe disease. Although not proven conclusively, hyperlipidemia may accelerate atherosclerosis and progression of renal disease.

Hypercoagulability is probably multifactorial in origin and is caused, at least in part, by increased urinary loss of antithrombin III, altered levels and/or activity of proteins C and S, hyperfibrinogenemia due to increased hepatic synthesis, impaired fibrinolysis, and increased platelet aggregability. As a consequence of these perturbations, patients can develop spontaneous *peripheral arterial or venous thrombosis, renal vein thrombosis,* and *pulmonary embolism.* Clinical features that suggest acute renal vein thrombosis include sudden onset of flank or abdominal pain, gross hematuria, a left-sided varicocele (the left testicular vein drains into the renal vein), increased proteinuria, and an acute decline in GFR. Chronic renal vein thrombosis is usually asymptomatic. Renal vein thrombosis is particularly common (up to

40%) in patients with nephrotic syndrome due to membranous glomerulopathy, membranoproliferative glomerulonephritis, and amyloidosis.

Other metabolic complications of nephrotic syndrome include *protein malnutrition* and iron-resistant *microcytic hypochromic anemia* due to transferrin loss. *Hypocalcemia* and secondary hyperparathyroidism can occur as a consequence of vitamin D deficiency due to enhanced urinary excretion of cholecalciferol-binding protein, whereas loss of thyroxine-binding globulin can result in *depressed thyroxine levels*. An increased susceptibility to *infection* may reflect low levels of IgG that result from urinary loss and increased catabolism. In addition, patients are prone to unpredictable changes in the *pharmacokinetics* of therapeutic agents that are normally bound to plasma proteins.

ETIOLOGY AND DIFFERENTIAL DIAGNOSIS Proteinuria >150 mg per 24 h is abnormal and can result from a number of mechanisms. *Glomerular proteinuria* results from leakage of plasma proteins through a perturbed glomerular filtration barrier; *tubular proteinuria* results from failure of tubular reabsorption of low-molecular-weight plasma proteins that are normally filtered and then reabsorbed and metabolized by tubular epithelium; *overflow proteinuria* results from filtration of proteins, usually immunoglobulin light chains, that are present in excess in the circulation. Tubular proteinuria virtually never exceeds 2 g per 24 h and thus, by definition, never causes nephrotic syndrome. Overflow proteinuria should be suspected in patients with clinical or laboratory evidence of multiple myeloma or other lymphoproliferative malignancy. Suspicion is heightened when there is a discrepancy between proteinuria detected by dipsticks, which are sensitive to albumin but not light chains, and the sulfosalicylic acid precipitation method, which detects both.

Nephrotic syndrome can complicate any disease that perturbs the negative electrostatic charge or architecture of the GBM and the podocytes and their slit diaphragms. Six entities account for greater than 90% of cases of nephrotic syndrome in adults: minimal change disease (MCD), focal and segmental glomerulosclerosis (FSGS), membranous glomerulopathy, MPGN, diabetic nephropathy, and amyloidosis. Diabetic nephropathy and amyloidosis, being manifestations of systemic diseases, are discussed in Chap. 275. *Renal biopsy* is a valuable tool in adults with nephrotic syndrome for establishing a definitive diagnosis, guiding therapy, and estimating prognosis. Renal biopsy is not required in the majority of children with nephrotic syndrome as most cases are due to MCD and respond to empiric treatment with glucocorticoids.

MINIMAL CHANGE DISEASE This glomerulopathy accounts for about 80% of nephrotic syndrome in children of younger than 16 years and 20% in adults (Table 274-1). The peak incidence is between 6 and 8 years. Patients typically present with nephrotic syndrome and benign urinary sediment. Microscopic hematuria is present in 20 to 30%. Hypertension and renal insufficiency are very rare.

MCD (also called nil disease, lipoid nephrosis, or foot process disease) is so named because glomerular size and architecture are normal by light microscopy. Immunofluorescence studies are typically negative for immunoglobulin and C3. Mild mesangial hypercellularity and sparse deposits of C3 and IgM may be detected. Occasionally, mesangial proliferation is associated with scanty IgA deposits, similar to those found in IgA nephropathy. However, the natural history of this variant and response to therapy resemble classic MCD. Electron microscopy reveals characteristic *diffuse effacement of the foot processes of visceral epithelial cells* (Fig. 274-3). This morphologic finding is referred to as foot process fusion in the older literature.

Table 274-1 Major Causes of Minimal Change Disease (Nil Disease, Lipoid Nephrosis)

Idiopathic (majority)
In association with systemic diseases or drugs
- Drug-induced interstitial nephritis induced by NSAIDs, rifampin, interferon α
- Hodgkin's disease and other lymphoproliferative malignancy
- HIV infection

NOTE: NSAIDs, nonsteroidal anti-inflammatory drugs.

The etiology of MCD is unknown and the vast majority of cases are idiopathic (Table 274-1). MCD occasionally develops after upper respiratory tract infection, immunizations, and atopic attacks. Patients with atopy and MCD have an increased incidence of HLA-B12, suggesting a genetic predisposition. MCD, often in association with interstitial nephritis, is a rare side effect of nonsteroidal anti-inflammatory drugs (NSAIDs), rifampin, and interferon-α. The occasional association with lymphoproliferative malignancies (such as Hodgkin's lymphoma), the tendency for idiopathic MCD to remit during intercurrent viral infection such as measles, and the good response of idiopathic forms to immunosuppressive agents (see below) suggest an immune etiology. In children, the urine contains albumin principally and minimal amounts of higher molecular weight proteins such as IgG and α_2-macroglobulin. This *selective proteinuria* in conjunction with foot process effacement suggests injury to podocytes and loss of the fixed *negative charge* in the glomerular filtration barrier for protein. Proteinuria is typically nonselective in adults, suggesting more extensive perturbation of membrane permeability.

℞ **TREATMENT** MCD is highly steroid-responsive and carries an excellent prognosis. Spontaneous remission occurs in 30 to 40% of childhood cases but is less common in adults. Approximately 90% of children and 50% of adults enter remission following 8 weeks of high-dose oral glucocorticoids. In a typical regimen using prednisone, children receive 60 mg/m^2 of body surface area daily for 4 weeks, followed by 40 mg/m^2 on alternate days for an additional 4 weeks; adults receive 1 to 1.5 mg/kg body weight per day for 4 weeks, followed by 1 mg/kg per day on alternate days for 4 weeks. Up to 90% of adults enter remission if therapy is extended for 20 to 24 weeks. Nephrotic syndrome relapses in over 50% of cases following withdrawal of glucocorticoids. Alkylating agents are reserved for the small number of patients who fail to achieve lasting remission. These include patients who relapse during or shortly after withdrawal of steroids (steroid-dependent) and those who relapse more than three times per year (frequently relapsing). In these settings, cyclophosphamide (2 to 3 mg/kg per day) or chlorambucil (0.1 to 0.2 mg/kg per day) is started after steroid-induced remission and continued for 8 to 12 weeks. Cytotoxic agents may also induce remission in occasional steroid-resistant cases. These benefits must be balanced against the risk of infertility, cystitis, alopecia, infection, and secondary malignancies, particularly in children and young adults. Azathioprine has not been proven to be a useful adjunct to steroid therapy. Cyclosporine induces remission in 60 to 80% of patients; it is an alternative to cytotoxic agents and an option in patients who are resistant to cytotoxic agents. Unfortunately, relapse is usual when cyclosporine is withdrawn, and long-term therapy carries the risk of nephrotoxicity and other side effects. Long-term renal and patient survival is excellent in MCD.

FOCAL AND SEGMENTAL GLOMERULOSCLEROSIS WITH HYALINOSIS The pathognomonic morphologic lesion in FSGS is sclerosis with hyalinosis involving portions (segmental) of fewer than 50% (focal) of glomeruli on a tissue section. The incidence of idiopathic (primary) FSGS has increased over the past two decades so that it now accounts for about one-third of cases of nephrotic syndrome in adults and as many as one-half of cases of nephrotic syndrome in blacks. FSGS can complicate a number of systemic diseases and sustained glomerular capillary hypertension following nephron loss from any cause (Table 274-2 and Chap. 273).

Idiopathic FSGS typically presents as nephrotic syndrome (~66%) or subnephrotic proteinuria (~33%) in association with hypertension, mild renal insufficiency, and an abnormal urine sediment that contains

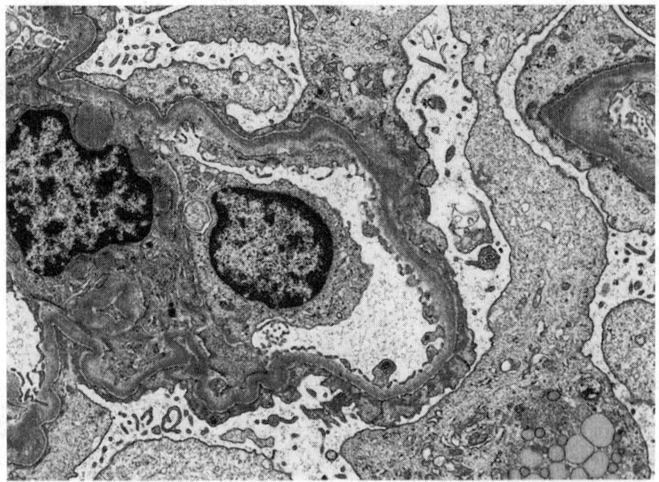

A

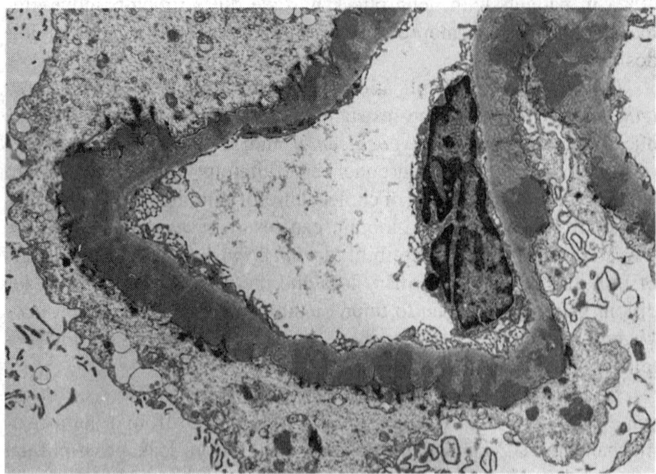

B

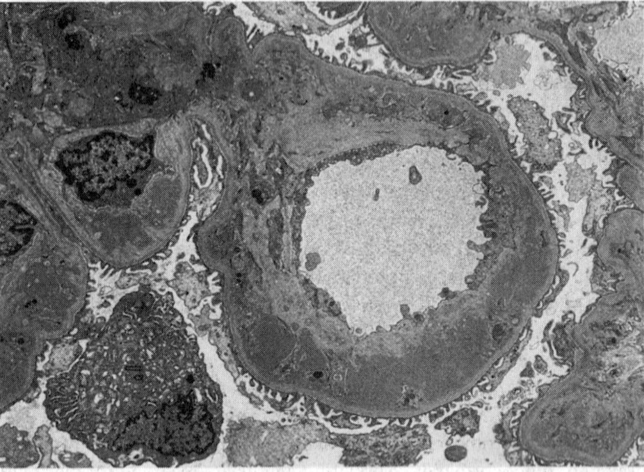

C

FIGURE 274-3 Typical findings on electron microscopy of renal biopsy specimens from patients with minimal change glomerulopathy, membranous glomerulopathy, and membranoproliferative glomerulonephritis. The pathognomonic feature of minimal change glomerulopathy (*A*) is effacement of foot processes of visceral epithelial cells (podocytes), giving the impression of foot process fusion. Foot process effacement is also evident in focal and segmental glomerulosclerosis (not shown here); in addition, there is typically detachment of podocytes from basement membrane, areas of glomerular capillary collapse, deposits of hyaline material, and sclerosis. Membranous nephropathy (*B*) is characterized by immune complexes in the subepithelial space. These electron-dense immune deposits stimulate production of new GBM, which eventually surrounds and incorporates the immune deposits into the GBM. The hallmarks of type I membranoproliferative glomerulonephritis (*C*) are increased mesangial cellularity and matrix and thickening and reduplication of the GBM. The latter is initiated by formation of electron-dense immune complexes on the subendothelial aspect of the GBM, which are subsequently covered by a new layer of GBM, probably produced by regenerating endothelial cells. *(Micrographs courtesy of Dr. Helmut Rennke.)*

red blood cells and leukocytes. Proteinuria is nonselective in most cases.

Light microscopy of renal biopsy tissue reveals FSGS with entrapment of amorphous hyaline material, a process that shows a predilection for juxtamedullary glomeruli. The sclerotic scars contain areas of glomerular capillary collapse and hyaline material composed of collagen types I, III, and IV. Adhesions occur between areas of capillary collapse and Bowman's capsule. Immunofluorescence studies are usually negative. Electron microscopy reveals evidence of damage to visceral epithelial cells, including swelling and detachment of podocytes from the GBM, effacement of foot processes, transition to foam cells, and overt cell degeneration and necrosis.

The etiology of primary FSGS is unclear (Table 274-2). There is evidence that a circulating nonimmunoglobulin permeability factor triggers FSGS in at least a subgroup of patients. The latter individuals tend to be young and prone to develop early recurrence of FSGS following renal transplantation. Plasmapharesis has been employed with variable success to control the nephrotic syndrome in this group. The overlap of clinical and morphologic features between MCD and FSGS has prompted some authorities to speculate that they are a spectrum of morphologic manifestations of a single pathogenetic process. FSGS is a potential long-term consequence of nephron loss from any cause. It can complicate congenital renal diseases such as congenital oligomeganephronia, in which both kidneys have a reduced complement of nephrons, and congenital unilateral agenesis. In addition, FSGS may develop following acquired loss of nephrons from extensive surgical ablation of renal mass; reflux nephropathy; glomerulonephritis; interstitial nephritis; sickle cell disease; and the combined effects of ischemia, cyclosporine nephrotoxicity, and rejection on renal allograft function (Table 274-2). It appears that >50% of nephrons must be lost for development of secondary FSGS.

℞ **TREATMENT** In contrast to MCD, spontaneous remission of primary FSGS is rare and renal prognosis is relatively poor. Proteinuria remits in only 20 to 40% of patients treated with glucocorticoids for 8 weeks. Uncontrolled studies suggest that up to 70% respond

Table 274-2 Etiology of Focal and Segmental Glomerulosclerosis

Idiopathic (majority)
In association with systemic diseases or drugs
- HIV infection
- Diabetes mellitus
- Fabry's disease
- Sialidosis
- Charcot-Marie-Tooth disease

As consequence of sustained glomerular capillary hypertension
- Congenital oligonephropathies
  - Unilateral renal agenesis
  - Oligomeganephronia
- Acquired nephron loss
  - Surgical resection
  - Reflux nephropathy
  - Glomerulonephritis or tubulointerstitial nephritis
- Other adaptive responses
  - Sickle cell nephropathy
  - Obesity with sleep apnea syndrome
  - Familial dysautonomia
- Miscellaneous
  - Heroin use

when steroid therapy is prolonged for 16 to 24 weeks. Cyclophosphamide and cyclosporine, when used at doses described above for MCD, induce partial or complete remission in 50 to 60% of steroid-responsive patients but are generally ineffective in steroid-resistant cases. Poor prognostic factors at presentation include hypertension, abnormal renal function, black race, and persistent heavy proteinuria. Renal transplantation is complicated by recurrence of FSGS in the allograft in about 50% of cases and graft loss in about 10%. Factors associated with an increased risk of recurrence include a short time interval between the onset of the FSGS and ESRD, young age at onset, and possibly the presence of mesangial hypercellularity on renal biopsy.

MEMBRANOUS GLOMERULOPATHY This lesion is a leading cause of idiopathic nephrotic syndrome in adults (30 to 40%) and a rare cause in children (<5%). It has a peak incidence between the ages of 30 to 50 years and a male-female ratio of 2:1 (Table 274-3). Membranous glomerulopathy derives its name from the characteristic light-microscopic appearance on renal biopsy, namely diffuse thickening of the GBM, which is most apparent upon staining with periodic acid–Schiff (PAS). Most patients (>80%) present with nephrotic syndrome, proteinuria usually being nonselective. Microscopic hematuria is present in up to 50% of cases, but red blood cells casts, macroscopic hematuria, and leukocytes are extremely rare. Hypertension is documented in only 10 to 30% of patients at the outset but is common later in patients with progressive renal failure. Serologic tests such as antinuclear antibody, ANCA, anti-GBM antibody, cryoglobulin titers, and complement levels are normal in the idiopathic form.

Light microscopy of renal biopsy sections reveals diffuse thickening of the GBM without evidence of inflammation or cellular proliferation. Silver staining demonstrates characteristic *spikes* along the GBM, which represent projections of new basement membrane engulfing subepithelial immune deposits. Immunofluorescence reveals granular deposition of IgG, C3, and the terminal components of complement (C5b–9) along the glomerular capillary wall. Electron-microscopic appearances vary depending on the stage of disease. The earliest finding is the presence of subepithelial immune deposits (Fig. 274-3). As these deposits enlarge, spikes of new basement membrane extend out between the immune deposits and begin to engulf them. With time, the deposits are completely surrounded and incorporated into the basement membrane.

The pathogenesis of idiopathic human membranous glomerulopathy is incompletely understood. The presence of electron-dense immune deposits that contain IgG and C3 suggest an immune process. About one-third of adult membranous nephropathy occurs in association with systemic diseases such as SLE, infections such as hepatitis B, malignancy, and drug therapy with gold and penicillamine (Table 274-3).

Table 274-3 Conditions Associated with Membranous Glomerulopathy

Idiopathic (majority)	
In association with systemic diseases or drugs	
Infection	Hepatitis B and C, secondary and congenital syphilis, malaria, schistosomiasis, leprosy, hydatid disease, filariasis, enterococcal endocarditis
Systemic autoimmune diseases	SLE, rheumatoid disease, Sjögren's syndrome, Hashimoto's disease, Graves' disease, mixed connective tissue disease, primary biliary cirrhosis, ankylosing spondylitis, dermatitis herpetiformis, bullous pemphigoid, myasthenia gravis
Neoplasia	Carcinoma of the breast, lung, colon, stomach, and esophagus; melanoma; renal cell carcinoma; neuroblastoma; carotid body tumor
Drugs	Gold, penicillamine, captopril, NSAIDs, probenecid, trimethadione, chlormethiazole, mercury
Miscellaneous	Sarcoidosis, diabetes mellitus, sickle cell disease, Crohn's disease, Guillain-Barré syndrome, Weber-Christian disease, Fanconi's syndrome, α_1 antitrypsin deficiency, angiofollicular lymph node hyperplasia

NOTE: SLE, systemic lupus erythematosus; NSAIDs, nonsteroidal anti-inflammatory drugs.

Table 274-4 Causes of Membranoproliferative (Mesangiocapillary) Glomerulonephritis (MPGN)

Idiopathic	
Type I	With subendothelial and mesangial immune deposits
Type II	With intramembranous dense deposits containing sparse or no Ig; associated with C3 nephritic factor
Type III	Features of type I MPGN and membranous nephropathy
In association with systemic diseases or drugs[a]	
Systemic immune-complex disease	SLE, mixed cryoglobulinemia, Sjögren's syndrome
Chronic infections	Hepatitis B and C, HIV, bacterial endocarditis, ventriculoatrial shunts, visceral abscess
Malignancy	Leukemias, lymphomas
Liver disease	Chronic active hepatitis and cirrhosis (usually associated with hepatitis B or C)
Miscellaneous	Partial lipodystrophy, heroin use, sarcoidosis, inherited C2 deficiency, thrombotic microangiopathies

[a] Usual with morphologic features of idiopathic type I MPGN (see above).
NOTE: SLE, systemic lupus erythematosus.

Nephrotic syndrome remits spontaneously and completely in up to 40% of patients with membranous glomerulopathy. The natural history of another 30 to 40% is characterized by repeated relapses and remissions. The final 10 to 20% suffer a slow progressive decline in GFR that typically culminates in ESRD after 10 to 15 years. Presenting features that predict a poor prognosis include male gender, older age, hypertension, severe proteinuria and hyperlipidemia, and impaired renal function. Controlled trials of glucocorticoids have failed to show consistent improvement in proteinuria or renal protection. Cyclophosphamide, chlorambucil, and cyclosporine have each been shown to reduce proteinuria and/or slow the decline in GFR in patients with progressive disease in small or uncontrolled studies. These observations need to be confirmed in controlled prospective studies. Transplantation is a successful treatment option for patients who reach ESRD.

MEMBRANOPROLIFERATIVE GLOMERULONEPHRITIS This morphologic entity, also known as mesangiocapillary glomerulonephritis, is characterized by thickening of the GBM and proliferative changes on light microscopy (Table 274-4). Two major types are identified; both are characterized by a diffuse increase in mesangial cellularity and matrix, and by thickening and reduplication of the GBM such that the lobular pattern of the glomerular tuft is exaggerated. The hallmark of type I MPGN is the presence of subendothelial and mesangial deposits on electron microscopy that contain C3 and IgG or IgM; rarely, IgA deposits are demonstrated by immunofluorescence microscopy (Fig. 274-3). The hallmark of type II MPGN (dense deposit disease) is the presence of electron-dense deposits within the GBM and other renal basement membranes (shown by electron microscopy) that stain for C3, but little or no immunoglobulin.

Most patients with type I MPGN present with heavy proteinuria or nephrotic syndrome, active urinary sediment, and normal or mildly impaired GFR. C3 levels are usually depressed, and C1q and C4 levels are borderline or low. Type I MPGN is an immune-complex glomerulonephritis and can be associated with a variety of chronic infections (e.g., bacterial endocarditis, HIV, hepatitis B and C), systemic immune-complex diseases (e.g., SLE, cryoglobulinemia), and malignancies (e.g., leukemias, lymphomas). Type I MPGN is a relatively benign disease, and 70 to 85% of patients survive without clinically significant impairment of GFR. There is no proven therapy for patients with progressive disease beyond eradicating the underlying infection, malignancy, or systemic disease, when possible. The incidence of type I MPGN appears to be falling, possibly because the overall incidence of hepatitis C infection has fallen dramatically in western society over the past decade.

Type II MPGN can also present with proteinuria and nephrotic syndrome; however, some patients present with nephritic syndrome, RPGN, or recurrent macroscopic hematuria. Type II MPGN is an autoimmune disease in which patients have an IgG autoantibody, termed *C3 nephritic factor*, that binds to C3 convertase, the enzyme that metabolizes C3, and renders it resistant to inactivation (Chap. 273). Type II MPGN runs a variable course; the GFR remains stable in some patients and declines gradually to ESRD over 5 to 10 years in others. There is no effective therapy for this disease.

FIBRILLARY-IMMUNOTACTOID GLOMERULOPATHY This emerging clinicopathologic entity accounts for 1% of diagnoses in most large renal biopsy series. Virtually all patients present with proteinuria, and >50% have nephrotic syndrome. The majority of patients also have hematuria, hypertension, and renal insufficiency. The light-microscopic appearances vary from mesangial expansion and basement membrane thickening with PAS-positive material to proliferative and crescentic glomerulonephritis. On electron microscopy, this PAS-positive material is observed to be composed of randomly arranged (fibrillary glomerulopathy) or organized bundles (immunotactoid glomerulopathy) of microfibrils and microtubules, the compositon of which has yet to be defined. The etiology of fibrillary-immunotactoid glomerulopathy remains to be determined. Patients with the immunotactoid variant have an increased incidence of lymphoproliferative malignancy. There is no proven therapy for fibrillary-immunotactoid glomerulopathy, and many patients progress to ESRD over 1 to 10 years. Transplantation appears to be a viable option in the latter setting.

MESANGIAL PROLIFERATIVE GLOMERULONEPHRITIS In 5 to 10% of patients with idiopathic nephrotic syndrome, renal biopsy reveals a diffuse increase in glomerular cellularity, predominantly due to proliferation of mesangial and endothelial cells, and infiltration by monocytes. Findings on immunofluorescence microscopy vary and include deposits of IgA, IgG, IgM, and/or complement, or absence of immune reactants. It is likely that this morphologic entity is, in fact, a heterogeneous group of diseases that includes atypical forms of MCD and FSGS and milder or resolving forms of the immune-complex and pauci-immune glomerulopathies described above under nephritic syndrome and RPGN. In keeping with the heterogeneity of this diagnosis, the prognosis is variable. In general, persistent nephrotic-range proteinuria signals a poor prognosis, with many patients progressing to ESRD over 10 to 20 years despite immunosuppressive therapy.

℞ TREATMENT **Nephrotic Syndrome and Complications** The treatment of nephrotic syndrome involves (1) specific treatment of the underlying morphologic entity and, when possible, causative disease (see above); (2) general measures to control proteinuria if remission is not achieved through immunosuppressive therapy and other specific measures; and (3) general measures to control nephrotic complications.

General measures may be warranted to control proteinuria in nephrotic syndrome if patients do not respond to immunosuppressive therapy and other specific measures and suffer progressive renal failure or severe nephrotic complications. Nonspecific measures that may reduce proteinuria include *angiotensin-converting enzyme (ACE) inhibitors*, and *NSAIDs*. The first of these measures aim to reduce proteinuria and slow the rate of progression of renal failure by lowering intraglomerular pressure and preventing the development of hemodynamically mediated focal segmental glomerulosclerosis. There is conclusive evidence that ACE inhibitors are renoprotective in human diabetic nephropathy (Chap. 275) and that ACE inhibitors slow the development of secondary FSGS in experimental animals. Their role in the treatment of nephrotic syndrome in other settings is unproven. NSAIDs also reduce proteinuria in some patients with nephrotic syndrome, probably by altering glomerular hemodynamics and GBM permeability characteristics. This potential benefit must be balanced against the risk of inducing acute renal failure, hyperkalemia, salt and water retention, and other side effects.

Complications of nephrotic syndrome that may require treatment include edema, hyperlipidemia, thromboembolism, malnutrition, and vitamin D deficiency. Edema should be managed cautiously by moderate *salt restriction*, usually 1 to 2 g/day, and the judicious use of *loop diuretics*. It is unwise to remove >1.0 kg of edema per day as more aggressive diuresis may precipitate intravascular volume depletion and prerenal azotemia. Administration of salt-poor albumin is not recommended as most is excreted within 24 to 48 h. Whereas many nephrologists advocate lowering low-density lipoproteins and cholesterol levels with *lipid-lowering drugs* to prevent accelerated atherosclerosis and slow the rate of decline of GFR, the value of such interventions in this setting has not been conclusively shown. *Anticoagulation* is indicated for patients with deep venous thrombosis, arterial thrombosis, and pulmonary embolism. Patients may be relatively resistant to heparin as a consequence of antithrombin III deficiency. Renal vein and vena caval angiography are probably indicated only when embolization occurs on anticoagulation and insertion of a caval filter is contemplated. There is no consensus regarding the optimal *diet* for patients with nephrotic syndrome. High-protein diets to prevent protein malnutrition are now in disfavor, since protein supplements have little, if any, effect on serum albumin levels and may hasten the progression of renal disease by increasing urinary protein excretion. The potential value of dietary protein restriction for reducing proteinuria must be balanced against the risk of contributing to malnutrition. *Vitamin D* supplementation is advisable in patients with clinical or biochemical evidence of vitamin D deficiency.

ASYMPTOMATIC ABNORMALITIES OF THE URINARY SEDIMENT

HEMATURIA Most asymptomatic glomerular hematuria is due to *IgA nephropathy* (Berger's disease) or *thin basement membrane (TBM) disease* (benign hematuria). A rarer but more ominous cause of isolated hematuria is *Alport's syndrome*. The latter is the most common form of hereditary nephritis, is usually transmitted as an X-linked dominant trait, and is associated with sensorineural deafness, ophthalmologic abnormalities, and progressive renal insufficiency (Chap. 275). TBM disease is sometimes familial but, in contrast to Alport's syndrome, is usually a benign disorder. Asymptomatic hematuria may also be the presenting feature of indolent forms of most other primary and secondary proliferative glomerulopathies (Fig. 274-1). Glomerular hematuria must be distinguished from a variety of renal parenchymal and extrarenal causes of hematuria. It is particularly important to exclude malignancy of the kidney or urinary tract, particularly in older male patients (Chap. 94). Other potential diagnoses include vascular, cystic, and tubulointerstitial diseases; papillary necrosis; hypercalciuria and hyperuricosuria; benign prostatic hypertrophy; and renal calculi. Important clues to the presence of glomerular hematuria are the presence of urinary red blood cell casts, dysmorphic urinary red blood cells, proteinuria of greater than 2.0 g per 24 h, and clinical or serologic evidence of nephritic syndrome, RPGN, or a compatible systemic disease.

IgA Nephropathy (Berger's Disease) IgA nephropathy is the most common glomerulopathy worldwide and accounts for 10 to 40% of glomerulonephritis in most series (Table 274-5). The disease is particularly common in southern Europe and Asia and appears to be more common in blacks than whites. Familial clustering has been reported but is rare. No consistent HLA association has emerged, although HLA-B35 appears to be more common in French patients. Most cases are idiopathic. The renal and serologic abnormalities in IgA nephropathy and Henoch-Schönlein purpura (Chap. 275) are indistinguishable, and most authorities consider these to be a spectrum

Table 274-5 Diseases Associated with IgA Nephropathy

Idiopathic (majority)	
Renal-limited or as component of Henoch-Schönlein purpura	
In association with systemic diseases or drugs[a]	
Liver	Chronic liver disease with involvement of biliary tree
Gastrointestinal	Celiac disease, Crohn's disease, adenocarcinoma
Respiratory	Idiopathic interstitial pneumonitis, obstructive bronchiolitis, adenocarcinoma
Skin	Dermatitis herpetiformis, mycosis fungoides, leprosy
Eyes	Episcleritis, anterior uveitis
Miscellaneous	Ankylosing spondylitis, relapsing polychondritis, Sjögren's syndrome, monoclonal IgA gammopathy, schistosomiasis

[a] Although prominent deposition of IgA has been reported with each of these conditions, significant glomerular inflammation and dysfunction are rare.

of a single disease. Less commonly, IgA nephropathy is found in association with systemic diseases, including chronic liver disease, Crohn's disease, gastrointestinal adenocarcinoma, chronic obstructive bronchiolitis, idiopathic interstitial pneumonia, dermatitis herpetiformis, mycosis fungoides, leprosy, ankylosing spondylitis, relapsing polychondritis, and Sjögren's syndrome. In many of these conditions, IgA is deposited in the glomerulus without inducing inflammation, and this may be a clinically insignificant consequence of perturbed IgA homeostasis.

Patients with IgA nephropathy typically present with gross hematuria, often 24 to 48 h after a pharyngeal or gastrointestinal infection, vaccination, or strenuous exercise. Other cases are diagnosed upon detection of microscopic hematuria during routine physical examinations. Hypertension (20 to 30%) and nephrotic syndrome (~10%) are unusual at presentation. Light microscopy of renal biopsy specimens typically shows mesangial expansion by increased matrix and cells. Diffuse proliferation, cellular crescents, interstitial inflammation, and areas of glomerulosclerosis may be evident in severe cases. The diagnostic finding, for which the disease is named, is mesangial deposition of IgA, detected by immunofluorescence microscopy. C3 is usually detected in the area of immune deposits, and IgG is observed in 50% of cases. Electron microscopy reveals electron-dense deposits in the mesangium and, in severe cases, these extend into the paramesangial subendothelial space. The pathogenesis of IgA nephropathy is incompletely understood.

℞ TREATMENT There is no proven therapy for IgA nephropathy. A recent, relatively large randomized controlled trial suggested a benefit of fish oils in patients with progressive disease and heavy proteinuria; however, this experience has not been universal. Some authorities advocate a trial of high-dose glucocorticoids with or without cytotoxic agents in patients with severe nephrotic syndrome and those with nephritic syndrome or RPGN and evidence of active inflammation on renal biopsy.

IgA nephropathy typically smolders for decades, with patients often suffering exacerbations of hematuria and renal impairment during intercurrent infections. As many as 20 to 50% of patients develop ESRD within 20 years. Clinical predictors of a poor prognosis include older age, male sex, hypertension, nephrotic-range proteinuria, and renal insufficiency at presentation. Histologic features that predict an aggressive course include diffuse severe disease, extracapillary proliferation (crescents), extension of immune attack into the paramesangial subendothelial space, glomerulosclerosis, interstitial fibrosis, and arteriolar hyalinosis.

Thin Basement Membrane Disease (Benign Hematuria) This disorder can be heredofamilial or sporadic and is as common as IgA nephropathy in some series of asymptomatic hematuria. When familial, it is usually inherited as an autosomal dominant trait and is due to a defect in the gene encoding the α4 chain of type IV collagen. TBM disease typically manifests in childhood as persistent hematuria. Intermittent hematuria and exacerbation of hematuria during upper respiratory tract infections have also been reported. The kidney is normal on light and immunofluorescence microscopy. The GBM is thin (usually <275 nm in children and <300 nm in adults) by comparison with normal subjects. TBM disease is usually a benign condition, and progressive renal impairment or proteinuria should prompt a search for an alternative diagnosis. A small proportion of patients do, however, appear to develop hypertension and focal glomerulosclerosis upon long-term follow-up. The molecular basis for the sporadic form of TBM disease has not been determined.

PROTEINURIA Between 0.5 and 10% of the population have isolated proteinuria, defined as proteinuria in the presence of an otherwise normal urinary sediment, a radiologically normal urinary tract, and the absence of known renal disease. The majority of these patients excrete <2 g of protein per day, and more than 80% have an excellent prognosis (*benign isolated proteinuria*). A minority (10 to 25%) are found to have persistent proteinuria (*persistent isolated proteinuria*), some of whom develop progressive renal insufficiency over 10 to 20 years.

Benign Isolated Proteinuria The major categories of benign isolated proteinuria are idiopathic transient proteinuria, functional proteinuria, intermittent proteinuria, and postural proteinuria. *Idiopathic transient proteinuria* is usually observed in young adults and refers to dipstick-positive proteinuria in an otherwise healthy individual that disappears spontaneously by the next clinic visit. *Functional proteinuria* refers to transient proteinuria during fever, exposure to cold, emotional stress, congestive cardiac failure, or obstructive sleep apnea. This phenomenon is presumed to be mediated through changes in glomerular ultrafiltration pressure and/or membrane permeability. Patients with *intermittent proteinuria* have proteinuria in approximately half of their urine samples in the absence of other renal or systemic abnormalities. *Postural proteinuria* is proteinuria (usually <2.0 g per 24 h) that is evident only in the upright position. This disorder affects 2 to 5% of adolescents and may be transient (~80%) or fixed (~20%). Fixed postural proteinuria resolves within 10 to 20 years in most cases. In each of these conditions, renal biopsy reveals either normal renal parenchyma or mild and nonspecific changes involving podocytes or the mesangium. All carry an excellent prognosis.

Persistent Isolated Proteinuria Isolated proteinuria detected on multiple ambulatory clinic visits in both the recumbent and upright position usually signals a structural renal lesion. Virtually all glomerulopathies that induce nephrotic syndrome (see above) can cause persistent isolated proteinuria. The most common lesion on renal biopsy is mild mesangial proliferative glomerulonephritis with or without focal and segmental glomerulosclerosis (30 to 70%), followed by focal or diffuse proliferative glomerulonephritis (~15%) and interstitial nephritis (~5%). Although this clinical entity carries a worse prognosis than benign isolated proteinuria, the prognosis is still relatively good, with only 20 to 40% of patients developing renal insufficiency after 20 years. Furthermore, progression to ESRD is extremely rare. It is wise to exclude monoclonal gammopathy by urinary electrophoresis in older patients.

CHRONIC GLOMERULONEPHRITIS

This syndrome is characterized by persistent proteinuria and/or hematuria and renal insufficiency that progresses slowly over years. Chronic glomerulonephritis usually comes to light (1) upon routine urinalysis, (2) when routine blood tests reveal unexplained anemia or elevated blood urea nitrogen and creatinine, (3) following discovery of bilateral small kidneys on abdominal imaging, (4) during evaluation for secondary causes of hypertension, or (5) during a clinical exacerbation of glomerulonephritis triggered by pharyngitis (synpharyngitic) or other infections. Chronic glomerulonephritis can be a manifestation of virtually all of the major glomerulopathies. Renal biopsy typically reveals a variable combination of proliferative, membranous, and sclerotic changes, depending on the causative glomerulopathy. Arteriosclerosis, induced by secondary hypertension, is a common finding in the renal vasculature. Tubulointerstitial inflammation and scarring are frequent additional findings and portend a poor prognosis. Glomerular hypertension and hyperfiltration through remnant functioning nephrons can hasten progression to ESRD (Chap. 273). Treatment is directed at lowering systemic and glomerular hypertension, usually with an ACE inhibitor, and controlling extracellular fluid volume, anemia, metabolic abnormalities, and the uremic syndrome through judicious use of diuretics, erythropoietin, and dietary modification (Chap. 270). Some patients develop ESRD and require renal replacement therapy with dialysis or transplantation.

BIBLIOGRAPHY

BOLTON WK: Goodpasture's syndrome. Kidney Int 50:1753, 1996

BRADY HR: Fibrillary glomerulopathy. Kidney Int 53:1421, 1998

———, WILCOX CS (eds): *Therapy in Nephrology and Hypertension*. Philadelphia, Saunders, 1999

COUSER WG: Glomerulonephritis. Lancet 353:1509, 1999

D'AMICO G: Pathogenesis of immunoglobulin A nephropathy. Curr Opin Nephrol Hypertens 7:247, 1998

FALK R et al: Primary glomerular diseases, in *Brenner & Rector's The Kidney*, 6th ed, BM Brenner (ed). Philadelphia, Saunders, 2000, pp 1263–1349

HAAS M et al: Changing etiologies of unexplained adult nephrotic syndrome: A comparison of renal biopsy findings from 1976–1979 and 1995–1997. Am J Kidney Dis 30:621, 1997

HRICIK DE et al: Glomerulonephritis. N Engl J Med 339:889, 1998

JENNETTE C, FALK R: Small-vessel vasculitides. N Engl J Med 337:1512, 1997

MACKENZIE HS et al: Adaptation to nephron loss, in *Brenner & Rector's The Kidney*, 6th ed, BM Brenner (ed). Philadelphia, Saunders, 2000, 1901–1942

ORTH SR, RITZ E: The nephrotic syndrome. N Engl J Med 338:1202, 1998

275

Yvonne M. O'Meara, Hugh R. Brady, Barry M. Brenner

GLOMERULOPATHIES ASSOCIATED WITH MULTISYSTEM DISEASES

AA	amyloid A	HBV	hepatitis B virus
ACE	Angiotensin-converting enzyme	HCV	hepatitis C virus
AL	amyloid L	HIVAN	HIV-associated nephropathy
ANA	antinuclear antibody	LCDD	light chain deposition disease
ANCA	antineutrophil cytoplasmic antibodies	MPGN	membranoproliferative glomerulonephritis
DM	diabetes mellitus	NSAIDs	nonsteroidal anti-inflammatory drugs
EMC	"essential" mixed cryoglobulinemia	PAN	polyarteritis nodosa
ESRD	end-stage renal disease	RPGN	rapidly progressive glomerulonephritis
GBM	glomerular basement membrane	SLE	systemic lupus erythematosus
GFR	glomerular filtration rate		

An array of multisystem diseases can cause glomerular injury, with glomerulopathy being either the dominant presenting feature or a relatively benign and clinically insignificant manifestation that is overshadowed by involvement of other organs. Glomerulopathies associated with multisystem diseases are often classified as *secondary* glomerulopathies to distinguish them from the *primary* glomerulopathies (Chap. 274) in which the pathology is limited to the kidneys. It should be emphasized, however, that most morphologic patterns of glomerular injury (see Table 273-1) can manifest as a renal-limited process (i.e., primary) or as part of a systemic disease (i.e., secondary). The diagnostic approach to glomerular disease involves identifying the presenting clinical syndrome (e.g., nephritic, nephrotic), defining the pathologic features (e.g., proliferative, crescentic, membranous), and attempting to establish the specific disease that provoked glomerular injury [e.g., systemic lupus erythematosus (SLE), Henoch-Schönlein purpura].

In this chapter, we focus on the epidemiology, clinicopathologic features, and management of the major glomerulopathies associated with systemic diseases. →*The pathogenesis of glomerular injury is discussed in Chap. 273, and the overall place of the major glomerulopathies in the differential diagnosis of the major renal syndromes is described in Chap. 274.*

DIABETIC NEPHROPATHY

(See also Chaps. 273 and 333)

Diabetic nephropathy is the leading cause of end-stage renal disease (ESRD) in western societies and accounts for 30 to 35% of patients on renal replacement therapy in North America. Type 1 diabetes mellitus (type 1 DM; formerly, insulin-dependent diabetes mellitus) and type 2 diabetes mellitus (type 2 DM; formerly, non-insulin-dependent diabetes mellitus) affect 0.5 and 4% of the population, respectively. Nephropathy complicates 30% of cases of type 1 DM and approximately 20% of cases of type 2 DM. However, most diabetic patients with ESRD have type 2 DM because of the greater prevalence of type 2 DM worldwide (90% of all individuals with diabetes). Risk factors for the development of diabetic nephropathy include hyperglycemia, systemic hypertension, glomerular hypertension and hyperfiltration, proteinuria, and possibly cigarette smoking, hyperlipidemia, and gene polymorphisms affecting the activity of the renin-angiotensin-aldosterone axis. For reasons that are unclear, ESRD from diabetic nephropathy is more common in blacks with type 2 DM than in whites (4:1 ratio), whereas the reverse is true for type 1 DM.

The pathophysiology, clinical features, and morphology of diabetic nephropathy are similar in type 1 and type 2 DM, although the time course may be condensed in type 2 DM. Glomerular hypertension and hyperfiltration are the earliest renal abnormalities in experimental and human diabetes and are observed within days to weeks of diagnosis. Microalbuminuria, so named because the abnormal albumin excretion of 30 to 300 mg/24 h is below the limits of detection of standard dipsticks, develops after approximately 5 years of sustained glomerular hypertension and hyperfiltration in type 1 DM. Microalbuminuria is the first manifestation of injury to the glomerular filtration barrier and predicts the development of overt nephropathy. Dipstick-positive proteinuria, ultimately reaching nephrotic levels, typically develops 5 to 10 years after the onset of microalbuminuria (i.e., 10 to 15 years after the onset of diabetes) and is associated with hypertension and progressive loss of renal function. In addition, patients can display features of tubulointerstitial disease such as hyperkalemia and type IV renal tubular acidosis. ESRD typically develops 5 to 10 years after the development of overt nephropathy. As noted above, the course of diabetic nephropathy may be shorter in type 2 DM, and many patients present with established nephropathy and hypertension. Diabetic nephropathy is usually diagnosed on clinical grounds without a renal biopsy. Supportive clues are the presence of normal sized or enlarged kidneys, evidence of proliferative diabetic retinopathy, and a bland urinary sediment. Retinopathy is found in 90 and 60% of patients with type 1 and type 2 DM, respectively, who develop nephropathy.

The earliest morphologic abnormalities in diabetic nephropathy are thickening of the glomerular basement membrane (GBM) and expansion of the mesangium due to accumulation of extracellular matrix. With time, matrix accumulation becomes diffuse and is evident as eosinophilic, periodic acid Schiff–positive glomerulosclerosis on renal biopsy. Prominent areas of nodular matrix expansion (nodular glomerulosclerosis, the classic Kimmelsteil-Wilson lesion) are often superimposed on this background. The glomeruli and kidneys are typically normal or increased in size, distinguishing diabetic nephropathy from most other forms of chronic renal insufficiency (renal amyloidosis and polycystic kidney disease being other important exceptions). Immunofluorescence microscopy may reveal deposition of IgG along the GBM in a linear pattern, but this does not appear to be immunopathogenetic as in anti-GBM disease. Immune deposits are not seen.

The renal vasculature typically displays evidence of atherosclerosis, as a consequence of hyperlipidemia, and hypertensive arteriosclerosis.

℞ TREATMENT Therapy is aimed at retarding the progression of nephropathy through control of blood sugar, systemic blood pressure, and glomerular capillary pressure. Glycemic control is achieved through regulation of diet and administration of oral hypoglycemic agents and insulin (Chap. 333). Angiotensin-converting enzyme (ACE) inhibitors are the drugs of choice as they control both systemic hypertension and intraglomerular hypertension by inhibiting the actions of angiotensin II on the systemic vasculature and renal efferent arterioles. ACE inhibitors also attenuate the stimulatory effect of angiotensin II on glomerular cell growth and matrix production. Because ACE inhibitors have been shown conclusively to delay the time to ESRD by 50% in patients with type 1 DM in a large randomized controlled trial and to delay progression significantly in type 2 DM, it is felt that all patients with diabetes should receive an ACE inhibitor on the development of microalbuminuria, even in the absence of systemic hypertension (Fig. 275-1). However, approximately 80% of patients with diabetes require more than one drug to control systemic hypertension, and aggressive lowering of blood pressure in these patients retards not only the rate of progression of nephropathy, but also the rate of progression of other complications of DM.

Diabetic nephropathy is the most common cause of ESRD requiring renal replacement therapy, and patients with diabetes have the highest annual mortality rate (20 to 30%) of any group on dialysis, in large part as a result of accelerated atherosclerosis. The survival rates of younger patients undergoing either peritoneal dialysis or hemodialysis are comparable; however, older patients with diabetes appear to have a higher mortality rate on peritoneal dialysis. Transplantation is the preferred mode of renal replacement therapy in patients who are otherwise medically suitable.

IMMUNOLOGICALLY MEDIATED MULTISYSTEM DISEASES

The glomerulus is a frequent target of injury in a variety of immunologically mediated multisystem diseases, particularly systemic vasculitis and SLE. Systemic vasculitis is usually classified according to the size of the inflamed vessel (Chap. 317). The major *large vessel* vasculitides are Takayasu's disease and giant cell arteritis. Glomerular injury is exceedingly rare in these diseases.

CLASSIC POLYARTERITIS NODOSA(See also Chap. 317) The typical glomerular lesion in classic polyarteritis nodosa (PAN) is ischemic collapse and obsolescence. Characteristic clinical and serologic features are hypertension, a bland urine sediment with subnephrotic proteinuria, slowly progressive renal insufficiency, normal serum complement levels, and absence of antineutrophil cytoplasmic antibodies (ANCA). Treatment with glucocorticoids and immunosuppressive agents, such as cyclophosphamide, affords a 5-year patient survival of approximately 80%, as compared with 10% in untreated cases.

ANCA-ASSOCIATED SMALL-VESSEL VASCULITIS The ANCA-associated small-vessel vasculitides are Wegener's granulomatosis, the microscopic and Churg-Strauss variants of polyarteritis nodosa, and pauci-immune renal-limited glomerulonephritis. These diseases share a number of clinicopathologic and serologic features and may represent a spectrum of manifestations of a single disease. They are more common in whites and older patients (mean age 57 years) and show a slight male preponderance. Their incidence peaks in the winter months, and many patients have a viral-like prodrome, suggesting a pathogenetic role for an infective agent. Patients typically present with nonspecific constitutional symptoms and signs such as lethargy, malaise, anorexia, weight loss, fever, arthralgias, and myalgias. Nonspecific laboratory abnormalities include a rapid sedimentation rate, elevated C-reactive protein, leukocytosis, thrombocytosis, and normochromic, normocytic anemia. Serum complement levels are typically normal.

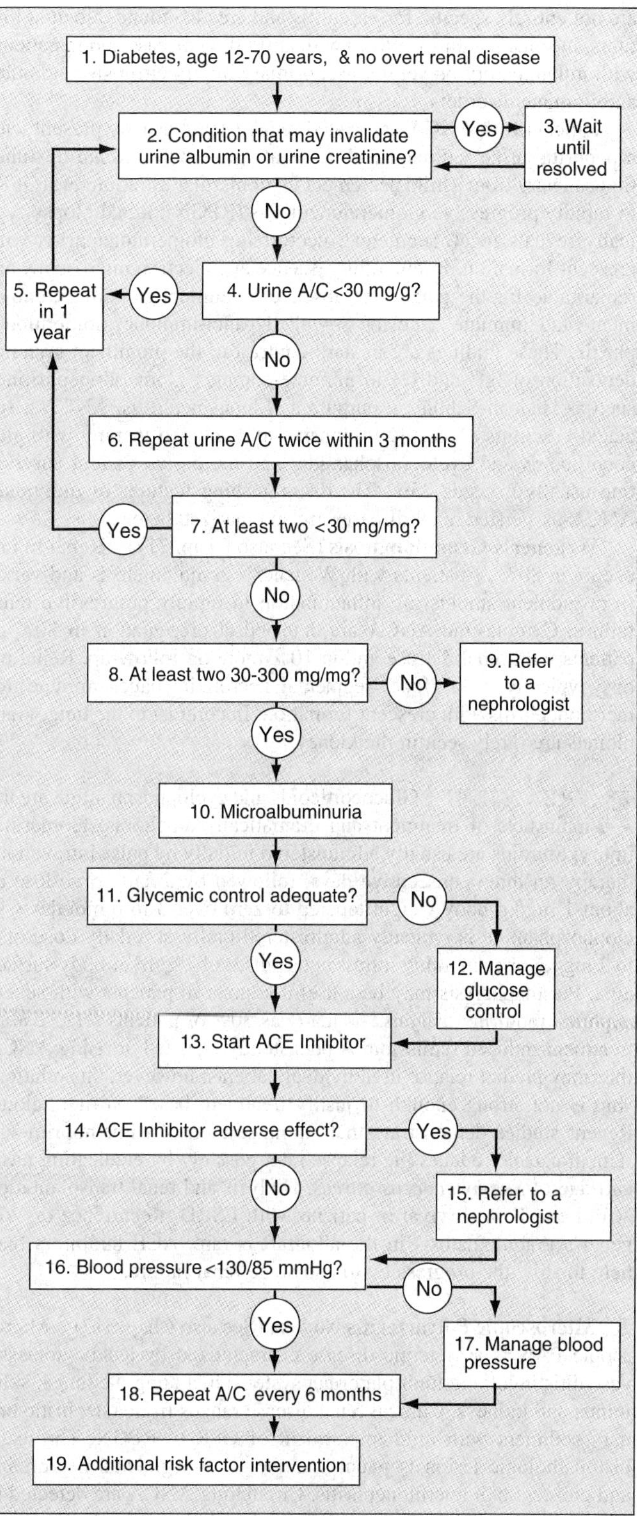

FIGURE 275-1 Algorithm for screening and management of microalbuminuria in patients with diabetes mellitus. A/C, albumin (in mg)/creatinine (in mg) in a spot urine sample. *(Reproduced from Bennett et al, with permission.)*

The majority of patients with these conditions have circulating ANCA. It is not clear whether ANCA are involved in the pathogenesis of vasculitis or merely represent an epiphenomenon of the vasculitic process, and there is debate whether serial ANCA titers are useful for monitoring disease activity and predicting relapse. Some ANCA activate cytokine-primed neutrophils in vitro and provoke them to injure endothelial cells, suggesting a pathogenetic role (Chap. 273). ANCA are not entirely specific for vasculitis and are also found, albeit at low titers, in some patients (~20%) with anti-GBM disease and in patients with inflammatory bowel disease, primary biliary cirrhosis, and other autoimmune disorders.

Patients with ANCA-associated renal disease usually present with a nephritic urine sediment and moderate proteinuria. Renal dysfunction can vary from a mild decrement in glomerular filtration rate (GFR) to rapidly progressive glomerulonephritis (RPGN). Renal biopsy typically reveals focal, segmental, necrotizing glomerulonephritis with crescent formation. Immunofluorescence and electron microscopy are remarkable for the paucity or absence of immunoglobulin, complement, and immune deposits: so-called pauci-immune glomerulonephritis. These findings are in stark contrast to the prominent granular deposition of IgG and C3 in immune-complex glomerulonephritides such as Henoch-Schönlein purpura and lupus nephritis. ANCA-associated vasculitis is usually responsive to combined therapy with glucocorticoids and cyclophosphamide, and the 5-year patient survival rate usually exceeds 75%. The distinguishing features of individual ANCA-associated renal diseases are summarized below.

Wegener's Granulomatosis (See also Chap. 317) Renal injury occurs in 80% of patients with Wegener's granulomatosis and varies from indolent smoldering inflammation to rapidly progressive renal failure. Cytoplasmic ANCA are detected at presentation in 80% of patients with renal disease and in 10% more on follow-up. Renal biopsy typically reveals focal, segmental, necrotizing pauci-immune glomerulonephritis with crescent formation. In contrast to the lung, granulomas are rarely seen in the kidney.

℞ TREATMENT Glucocorticoids and cyclophosphamide are the mainstays of treatment and dramatically ameliorate glomerular injury. Steroids are usually administered initially by pulse intravenous therapy on three consecutive days, followed by a daily oral dose of about 1 mg/kg body weight tapered to zero over 3 to 6 months. Cyclophosphamide is typically administered orally at a daily dose of 1 to 2 mg/kg or as monthly intravenous pulses of 1 g/m^2 of body surface area. Plasmapheresis may be a useful adjunct in patients with severe nephritis requiring dialysis. As many as 30% of patients relapse after treatment-induced remission. A persistently elevated or rising ANCA titer may predict relapse in individual patients; however, this relationship is not strong enough to justify treatment based on titers alone. Recent studies demonstrate that administration of trimethoprim-sulfamethoxazole reduces the relapse rate, possibly by eradicating nasal carriage of *Staphylococcus aureus*. Dialysis and renal transplantation afford excellent survival in patients with ESRD. Recurrence of Wegener's granulomatosis in the allograft is rare. ACE inhibitors may help to slow the progression to end-stage renal failure.

Microscopic Polyarteritis Nodosa (See also Chap. 317) Microscopic PAN is a systemic disease characterized by leukocytoclastic vasculitis involving multiple organ systems including the lungs, skin, joints, and kidneys. Clinical renal disease ranges from a nephritic urinary sediment with mild impairment of GFR to RPGN. The usual histopathologic lesion is pauci-immune focal segmental necrotizing and crescentic glomerulonephritis. Circulating ANCA are detected in 70 to 80% of patients at presentation, with cytoplasmic and perinuclear ANCA being equally prevalent. The treatment of microscopic PAN involves glucocorticoids and cyclophosphamide, as for Wegener's granulomatosis. Plasmapheresis may benefit patients with severe acute renal failure or massive pulmonary hemorrhage.

Churg-Strauss Syndrome (See also Chap. 317) Clinical renal involvement in Churg-Strauss syndrome is relatively infrequent and usually limited to mild proteinuria and hematuria. Evolution to chronic renal failure is rare. Renal biopsy most frequently reveals extraglomerular pathology, with involvement of the renal vasculature and tubulointerstitium by granulomatous vasculitis. Focal segmental glomerulonephritis with crescents is also seen. A minority of patients have focal segmental necrotizing glomerulonephritis.

Henoch-Schönlein Purpura (See also Chap. 317) Extrarenal features of Henoch-Schönlein purpura include a petechial rash on the extremities, arthropathy, and abdominal pain. Nephritis is present in 80% of patients and manifests as a nephritic urine sediment and moderate proteinuria. Macroscopic hematuria and nephrotic-range proteinuria are uncommon. Light-microscopic appearances can vary from mild mesangial proliferation and expansion to diffuse proliferation with glomerular crescents. The glomerular lesion is identical to that found in IgA nephropathy (Berger's disease; see Chap. 274), suggesting that Henoch-Schönlein nephritis and IgA nephropathy are a spectrum of manifestations of a single disease. The *sine qua non* for diagnosis is the presence of mesangial IgA deposition on immunofluorescence microscopy. IgG and C3 are also detected. Electron microscopy reveals mesangial immune deposits. Immune complexes may also be present in the peripheral glomerular capillary wall and paramesangial areas. Biopsy of involved skin reveals dermal IgA deposition and leukocytoclastic vasculitis. IgA deposition is also seen in areas of uninvolved skin.

℞ TREATMENT Since there is no proven therapy for Henoch-Schönlein nephritis, treatment is supportive. Steroids and/or cytotoxic agents are often tried in patients with severe disease, but without compelling scientific evidence to support their use. The disease typically undergoes clinical exacerbations and remissions in the first year and then enters long-term remission. The prognosis is generally excellent; chronic renal failure and persistent hypertension occur in fewer than 10% of patients.

ESSENTIAL MIXED CRYOGLOBULINEMIA (See also Chap. 317) Renal involvement is most common with the mixed cryoglobulinemias (types II and III), which are more common in females and usually begin in the sixth decade. Most patients present with a variable combination of leukocytoclastic vasculitis, skin ulcerations, arthralgias, fatigue, and Raynaud's phenomenon. Renal disease is a complication in 50% of patients and usually develops after 12 to 24 months. The typical clinical renal manifestations are nephrotic-range proteinuria, microscopic hematuria, and hypertension. Acute nephritic syndrome occurs in 20 to 30%, and oliguric acute renal failure in about 5% of patients with renal disease. The characteristic morphologic lesions are diffuse mesangial proliferative or membranoproliferative glomerulonephritis. The glomerular capillaries frequently contain eosinophilic hyaline "pseudothrombi" composed of precipitated immunoglobulins. Granular deposition of IgG, IgM, and C3 is usually prominent on immunofluorescence microscopy. Electron microscopy typically reveals subendothelial deposits containing microfibrils and microtubules that display a characteristic "thumbprint" appearance.

Circulating levels of C3, C4, and CH50 are depressed in about 80% of patients with renal involvement, and a transient antinuclear antibody (ANA) (speckled pattern) is sometimes detected. Abnormal liver function tests are found in about 15% of patients at presentation and in up to 50% subsequently. It now appears that most patients with "essential" mixed cryoglobulinemia (EMC) (i.e., idiopathic) are chronically infected with hepatitis C virus (HCV). In keeping with a pathogenetic role for this virus, HCV RNA has been isolated from the serum of patients with EMC, indicating active infection, and anti-HCV antibodies have been detected in both the serum and cryoprecipitates in association with viral antigens.

℞ TREATMENT Traditionally, glucocorticoids, with or without cyclophosphamide, and plasmapheresis were the standard treatment for EMC. Recent reports indicate that interferon α controls viral replication and stabilizes renal function in most patients infected with EMC and HCV. Unfortunately, most patients relapse when interferon α is discontinued, a major problem given the prohibitive cost of the drug. In general, patient and renal survival are good in EMC, with 75% of patients being alive at 10 years.

SYSTEMIC LUPUS ERYTHEMATOSUS (See also Chap. 311) Renal involvement is clinically evident in 40 to 85% of patients with SLE; it varies from isolated abnormalities of the urinary sediment to full-blown nephritic or nephrotic syndrome or chronic renal failure. Most glomerular injury is triggered by the formation of immune complexes within the glomerular capillary wall; however, thrombotic microangiopathy may be the dominant reason for renal dysfunction in a small subset of patients with the antiphospholipid antibody syndrome.

Immune-Complex–Mediated Lupus Nephritis The renal biopsy has proven very useful for identifying the different patterns of immune-complex glomerulonephritis in SLE, which are diverse, portend different prognoses, and do not necessarily correlate with the clinical findings. Indeed, clinically silent lupus nephritis is well described in which the urinalysis is virtually normal but renal biopsy demonstrates varying degrees of injury.

The World Health Organization categorizes lupus nephritis into six histologic classes. *Class I* consists of a normal biopsy on light microscopy with occasional mesangial deposits on immunofluorescence microscopy. Patients in this category usually do not have clinical renal disease. Patients with *class II* or mesangial lupus nephritis have prominent mesangial deposits of IgG, IgM, and C3 on immunofluorescence and electron microscopy. Mesangial lupus nephritis is designated as class IIA when the glomeruli are normal by light microscopy and class IIB when there is mesangial hypercellularity. Microscopic hematuria is common with this lesion, and 25 to 50% of patients have moderate proteinuria. Nephrotic syndrome is not seen, and renal survival is excellent (>90% at 5 years). *Class III* describes focal segmental proliferative lupus nephritis with necrosis or sclerosis affecting fewer than 50% of glomeruli. Up to one-third of patients have nephrotic syndrome, and glomerular filtration is impaired in 15 to 25%. In *class IV* or diffuse proliferative lupus nephritis, most glomeruli show cell proliferation, often with crescent formation. Other features on light microscopy include fibrinoid necrosis and "wire loops," which are caused by basement membrane thickening and mesangial interposition between basement membrane and endothelial cells. Deposits of IgG, IgM, IgA, and C3 are evident by immunofluorescence, and crescents stain positive for fibrin. Electron microscopy reveals numerous immune deposits in mesangial, subepithelial, and subendothelial locations. Tubuloreticular structures are frequently seen in endothelial cells. These are not specific for lupus nephritis and also occur in HIV-associated nephropathy. Electron microscopy may also reveal curvilinear parallel arrays of microfibrils, measuring approximately 10 to 15 nm in diameter, with "thumbprinting," similar to those seen in cryoglobulinemia. Nephrotic syndrome and renal insufficiency are present in at least 50% of patients with class IV disease. Diffuse proliferative lupus nephritis is the most aggressive renal lesion in SLE, and as many as 30% of these patients progress to terminal renal failure. *Class V* is termed membranous lupus nephritis because of its similarity to idiopathic membranous glomerulopathy. Thickening of the GBM is evident by light microscopy. Electron microscopy reveals predominant subepithelial deposits in addition to subendothelial and mesangial deposits. Proliferative changes may also be evident, but the predominant pattern is that of membranous glomerulopathy. Most patients present with nephrotic syndrome (90%), but significant impairment of GFR is relatively unusual (10%). Tubulointerstitial changes such as active infiltration by inflammatory cells, tubular atrophy, and interstitial fibrosis are seen to varying degrees in lupus nephritis and are most severe in classes III and IV, especially in patients with long-standing disease. *Class VI* probably represents the end stages of proliferative lupus nephritis and is characterized by diffuse glomerulosclerosis and advanced tubulointerstitial disease. These patients are often hypertensive, may have nephrotic syndrome, and usually have impaired GFR.

Transformation from one class to another is relatively frequent. For example, class III often progresses to class IV spontaneously, and

class IV can transform to class II or class V after treatment. Class II and class V lupus nephritis may predate other manifestations of lupus, whereas class III and class IV usually occur in patients who have systemic features of SLE. A semiquantitative analysis can be performed by using a variety of features on renal biopsy, scored 0 to 3+, to derive indices of disease activity and chronicity. Features that suggest active inflammation include endocapillary proliferation, glomerular leukocyte infiltration, wire loop deposits, cellular crescents, and interstitial inflammation. In contrast, features that suggest chronicity include glomerulosclerosis, fibrous crescents, tubular atrophy, and interstitital fibrosis. In some, but not all, studies, these indices have been useful in predicting response to therapy and renal prognosis.

Patients with active lupus nephritis have a range of serologic abnormalities. Hypocomplementemia is present in 75 to 90% of patients and is most striking with diffuse proliferative glomerulonephritis. ANA are usually detected (95 to 99%), although not specific for SLE. ANA titers tend to fall with treatment, and ANA may not be detected during remissions. Anti-double-stranded DNA (dsDNA) antibodies are highly specific for SLE, and changes in their titers correlate with the activity of lupus nephritis. Almost 100% of patients taking procainamide and 65% of patients taking hydralazine develop ANA; however, overt lupus, including nephritis, occurs in fewer than 10% of these patients, and anti-DNA antibodies are not usually detected. Other antibodies found in patients with SLE include anti-Sm (17 to 30%; highly specific, but not sensitive); anti-RNP, which frequently accompanies anti-Sm in low titer; anti-Ro (35%); anti-La (15%); and anti-histone antibodies (70% of patients with SLE and 95% of patients with drug-induced lupus).

Rx **TREATMENT** The treatment of lupus nephritis is controversial and based largely on the class of injury and disease activity. Because there is relatively poor correlation between clinical features (urinalysis findings, serum creatinine) and histologic class, the renal biopsy findings are an important guide to therapy. Treatment is not indicated for class I and most cases of class II lupus nephritis, as these histologic patterns portend an excellent prognosis (100% and >90% 5-year survival rates, respectively). Extrarenal manifestations may warrant treatment with glucocorticoids, salicylates, or antimalarials. Glucocorticoids and cyclophosphamide are the mainstays of therapy for patients with proliferative nephritis (classes III and IV). High-dose steroids given as intravenous boluses (pulse therapy) are usually effective at rapidly controlling acute glomerular inflammation. Cyclophosphamide and azathioprine are important adjuncts to steroid therapy and appear to afford better long-term preservation of renal function than steroids alone. Intravenous pulse cyclophosphamide is as efficacious as oral therapy and appears to be less toxic. Most authorities advocate an initial regimen of monthly intravenous boluses of cyclophosphamide for 6 months. Subsequent therapy is tailored to disease activity and typically involves dosing every 3 to 6 months for a total treatment period of 18 to 24 months. The initial dose of cyclophosphamide is 0.5 g/m^2, and the dose is increased gradually to a maximum of 1 g/m^2 unless patients develop leukopenia or other side effects. Steroids are usually started simultaneously at 1 mg/kg per day and are tapered over the first 6 months to a maintenance dose of 5 to 10 mg/d for the duration of cyclophosphamide therapy. Five-year renal survival rates of 60 to 90% have been obtained with this and similar regimens. A large randomized, prospective trial indicated that plasmapheresis does not offer additional benefit in patients with severe proliferative lupus nephritis. Mycophenolate mofetil has recently been used to treat patients with lupus nephritis that is resistant to steroids and cyclophosphamide.

The management of membranous lupus nephritis is less well defined. As with idiopathic membranous glomerulopathy, the incidence of spontaneous remission approaches 50% in membranous lupus nephritis, and the course of the disease is generally indolent, with a 70-

to 90% renal survival rate at 5 years. Some authorities advocate steroids and ACE inhibitors at the time of diagnosis, whereas others reserve them for patients with progressive renal insufficiency or severe nephrotic syndrome. Useful parameters for monitoring the response to therapy and predicting relapse include the activity of the urine sediment, proteinuria, GFR, serum complement levels, and anti-dsDNA titers. Despite maximal immunosuppressive therapy, about 20% of patients with aggressive lupus nephritis develop ESRD requiring dialysis. SLE tends to become quiescent with advanced uremia, and patients rarely develop systemic flares once they commence dialysis. Recurrence of nephritis and systemic flares are also very uncommon after renal transplantation, and allograft survival rates are comparable to those in patients with other causes of ESRD.

ANTIPHOSPHOLIPID ANTIBODY SYNDROME AND THROMBOTIC MICROANGIOPATHY Patients with this syndrome can develop a variable degree of renal impairment due to thrombotic microangiopathy. The latter typically affects the interlobular arteries, arterioles, and glomerular capillaries and is characterized by intravascular microthrombi and swelling of endothelial cells. Decreased levels of tissue plasminogen activator and increased level of α_2-antiplasmin, both of which would tend to promote thrombosis, have been described in this syndrome. Anticoagulation to maintain the Internalized Normal Ratio (INR) >3.0 may be beneficial in reducing the incidence of recurrent thromboses. There are uncontrolled reports of a benefit of plasmapheresis in the setting of acute renal failure secondary to thrombotic microangiopathy.

RHEUMATOID ARTHRITIS (See also Chap. 312) Although extra-articular manifestations are present in 35% of patients with rheumatoid arthritis, direct involvement of the kidney by rheumatoid disease is rare, and glomerular injury is usually secondary to amyloid A (AA) amyloidosis or a side effect of drug therapy. AA amyloidosis is a complication experienced by 10 to 20% of patients with rheumatoid arthritis, and renal involvement is evident clinically in 3 to 10% of these patients (nephrotic syndrome, renal insufficiency). Amyloidosis is more frequent in patients with rheumatoid arthritis of long duration (>10 years), with circulating rheumatoid factor, and with destructive arthropathy. Less frequent glomerular lesions include mesangial proliferative glomerulonephritis and basement membrane thickening by subepithelial immune deposits. Gold and penicillamine may cause nephrotic syndrome by inducing membranous glomerulopathy, whereas nonsteroidal anti-inflammatory drugs (NSAIDs) can trigger the nephrotic syndrome by inducing minimal change nephropathy, usually in association with acute interstitial nephritis (see below).

SJÖGREN'S SYNDROME (See also Chap. 314) Tubulointerstitial injury is the most common form of renal involvement in Sjögren's syndrome and usually presents as either Fanconi's syndrome, distal renal tubular acidosis, or impairment of renal concentrating ability. Glomerulonephritis is relatively rare and should prompt a search for evidence of secondary causes. Membranous glomerulopathy and membranoproliferative glomerulonephritis (MPGN) are the most common lesions. Anecdotal reports describe successful therapy with glucocorticoids and cytotoxic agents.

POLYMYOSITIS AND DERMATOMYOSITIS (See also Chap. 382) Occasional cases of focal mesangial proliferative glomerulonephritis with mesangial deposition of IgG and complement have been described in polymyositis/dermatomyositis. Membranous glomerulopathy has also been reported, particularly when polymyositis/dermatomyositis is associated with malignancy.

MIXED CONNECTIVE TISSUE DISEASE (See also Chap. 313) Mixed connective tissue disease is a syndrome that includes features of SLE, scleroderma, and polymyositis and is associated with high titers of antiribonucleoprotein antibodies and negative antismooth muscle antibodies. Renal involvement occurs in fewer than 15% of patients and manifests as hematuria and subnephrotic proteinuria. The usual pathologic lesion is membranous glomerulopathy or MPGN. The prognosis is usually excellent, and steroid therapy may be useful in rare patients with progressive renal disease.

GLOMERULAR DEPOSITION DISEASES

The glomerular deposition diseases are characterized by deposition of abnormal proteins, usually immunoglobulins or fragments thereof, within the glomerulus. They include amyloidosis, light and heavy chain deposition disease, cryoglobulinemia, and fibrillary/immunotactoid glomerulonephritis. Here, we focus on amyloidosis and light chain deposition disease (LCDD). Cryoglobulinemic nephropathy is described above in the discussion on systemic vasculitis. →***Fibrillary and immunotactoid glomerulopathy are discussed in Chap. 274.***

AMYLOIDOSIS (See also Chap. 319) Amyloidosis is classified according to the major component of its fibrils: for example, immunoglobulin light chains in amyloid L (AL) amyloidosis, serum amyloid A in AA amyloidosis, β_2-microglobulin in dialysis-associated amyloidosis, and amyloid β protein in Alzheimer's disease and Down's syndrome. Amyloid deposits also contain a nonfibrillar component called the P component, a serum α_1 glycoprotein with a high affinity for the fibrillar components of all forms of amyloid. AL and AA amyloidosis frequently involve the kidneys, whereas involvement by other forms of amyloidosis is very rare.

There is substantial overlap in the renal clinicopathologic presentations of AL and AA amyloidosis. Glomeruli are involved in 75 to 90% of patients, usually in association with involvement of other organs. The clinical correlate of glomerular amyloid deposition is nephrotic-range proteinuria. In addition, over 50% of patients have impaired glomerular filtration at diagnosis. Hypertension is present in about 20 to 25%. Renal size is usually normal or slightly enlarged. A minority of patients present with renal failure due to amyloid deposition in the renal vasculature or with Fanconi's syndrome, nephrogenic diabetes insipidus, or renal tubular acidosis due to involvement of the tubulointerstitium. Rectal biopsy and abdominal fat pad biopsy reveal amyloid deposits in about 70% of patients and may obviate the need for renal biopsy.

Renal biopsy gives a very high yield if there is clinical evidence of renal involvement. The earliest pathologic changes are mesangial expansion by amorphous hyaline material and thickening of the GBM. Further amyloid deposition results in the development of large nodular eosinophilic masses. When stained with Congo red, these deposits show apple-green birefringence under polarized light. Immunofluorescence microscopy is usually only weakly positive for immunoglobulin light chains because amyloid fibrils are usually derived from the variable region of light chains. Electron microscopy reveals the characteristic nonbranching extracellular amyloid fibrils of 7.5 to 10 nm in diameter. Tubulointerstitial and vascular deposits of amyloid are also seen and may occasionally be more prominent than glomerular deposits.

℞ **TREATMENT** Most patients with renal involvement by AL amyloidosis develop ESRD within 2 to 5 years. No treatment has been shown consistently to improve this prognosis; however, some success has been reported with a combination of melphalan and prednisone. Preliminary studies have reported a benefit of high-dose melphelan with autologous stem cell transplantation. Colchicine delays the onset of nephropathy in patients with familial Mediterranean fever but has not proved useful in patients with established disease or with other forms of amyloid. Remissions may be achieved in AA amyloidosis by eradication of the underlying cause. Renal replacement therapy is offered to patients who reach ESRD; however, the 1-year survival rate on dialysis is low (~66%) by comparison with other causes of ESRD. Most patients die from extrarenal complications, particularly cardiovascular disease. Renal transplantation is a viable option in patients with AA amyloidosis whose primary disease has been eradicated. Transplantation is also an option for patients with AL amyloidosis, although a poor prognosis because of extrarenal organ involvement may preclude them as candidates. Here again, the survival rate is lower by comparison with other causes of ESRD; most of the excess mortality is due to infectious and cardiovascular complications. Recurrence of amyloidosis in the allograft is common but rarely leads to graft loss.

LIGHT CHAIN DEPOSITION DISEASE (See also Chap. 113) Renal involvement is a complication in 90% of patients with LCDD and is often the dominant feature. Nephrotic syndrome and renal impairment are the usual presenting features. Microscopic hematuria occurs in about 20% of patients. Defective hydrogen ion and potassium excretion and urinary concentration may be evident if light chains are deposited predominantly in the tubules. The most common pathologic lesion on renal biopsy is ribbon-like thickening of the tubular basement membrane due to light chain deposition. Mesangial expansion and nodular glomerulosclerosis are found in about 33% of patients. This light-microscopic appearance resembles that of idiopathic MPGN and diabetic nephropathy. Superimposed crescentic change is occasionally seen. Immunofluorescence studies are strongly positive for monoclonal light chains, in contrast to AL amyloid, because the constant region of the immunoglobulin is typically deposited. The tissue deposits in LCDD are granular rather than fibrillar on electron microscopy, appear more amorphous in character, do not stain with Congo red, and seem to have a greater affinity for basement membranes.

The prognosis of LCDD is poor when it is associated with multiple myeloma, and most patients progess rapidly to ESRD. Treatment with melphalan and prednisone has been reported to reduce proteinuria and stabilize renal function in uncontrolled studies. In the absence of myeloma, the prognosis is somewhat more variable, and several patients have undergone successful renal transplantation.

WALDENSTRÖM'S MACROGLOBULINEMIA (See also Chap. 113) This disorder is characterized by monoclonal proliferation of an IgM-secreting clone of plasma cells. The circulating IgM paraprotein frequently gives rise to the hyperviscosity syndrome, which may compromise renal blood flow and GFR. Direct renal involvement is rare and, when present, involves deposition of large amorphous deposits of eosinophilic material in the glomerular capillaries. Renal amyloidosis can also occur.

DRUG-INDUCED GLOMERULAR DISEASE

A variety of drugs damage the glomerular filtration barrier and induce proteinuria and nephrotic syndrome. In contrast, drug-induced proliferative glomerulonephritis is rare. The more common drug-induced glomerulopathies are discussed here. Additional associations are included in Table 275-1 and Table 71-1.

NSAIDs have a variety of renal side effects, including hemodynamically mediated acute renal failure, salt and water retention, hyponatremia, hyperkalemia, papillary necrosis, acute interstitial nephritis, nephrotic syndrome, and ESRD. Nephrotic syndrome and acute renal failure frequently coexist due to a combination of acute interstitial nephritis and a glomerular lesion that is identical to that of minimal change disease. This entity occurs most commonly in patients on propionic acid derivatives such as fenoprofen, ibuprofen, and naproxen but can occur with other NSAIDs, ampicillin, rifampin, and interferon α. Withdrawal of the drug usually results in resolution of renal disease. Membranous nephropathy is also described as an idiosyncratic reaction to NSAIDs.

Gold therapy, administered by injection or orally, induces proteinuria in 5 to 25% of patients with rheumatoid arthritis. Proteinuria develops after 4 to 6 months of therapy, and up to 33% of patients develop full-blown nephrotic syndrome. Renal biopsy typically reveals membranous glomerulopathy, though minimal change disease or mesangial proliferative lesions have also been described. Progressive renal impairment is rare. Nephrotic syndrome is more common in patients who are HLA-B8/DR3 positive, suggesting a genetic susceptibility. Withdrawal of the drug leads to gradual resolution of the proteinuria.

Penicillamine also induces proteinuria in 5 to 30% of patients. As with gold, the underlying glomerular lesion is usually membranous glomerulopathy, and proteinuria gradually resolves after withdrawal of the drug. Acute renal failure secondary to crescentic glomerulonephritis with immune deposits has also been described.

Table 275-1 Drug-Induced Glomerular Disease

Morphologic Lesion	Causative Agent
Minimal change diseases (usually with interstitial nephritis)	Nonsteroidal anti-inflammatory agents Recombinant interferon α Rifampin Ampicillin
Membranous nephropathy	Penicillamine Gold Mercury Trimethadione Captopril Chlormethiazole
Focal segmental glomerulosclerosis	Heroin
Pauci-immune necrotizing GN	Ciprofloxacin Hydralazine
Proliferative GN with vasculitis	Allopurinol Penicillin Sulfonamides Thiazides Intravenous amphetamines
RPGN	Rifampin Warfarin Carbimazole Amoxicillin Penicillamine

NOTE: GN, glomerulonephritis; RPGN, rapidly progressive glomerulonephritis.

Intravenous heroin use is associated with an increased incidence of focal and segmental glomerulosclerosis (heroin-associated nephropathy). It is not clear whether the nephrotoxin in this setting is heroin itself or a contaminant. Heroin-associated nephropathy occurs predominantly in blacks and is characterized by nephrotic syndrome, hypertension, and a gradual progression to ESRD over a period of 3 to 5 years. The pathologic features are similar to those of idiopathic focal segmental glomerulosclerosis, although mesangial deposition of IgM and C3 may be more prominent. The incidence of this disease appears to be declining steadily. Potential reasons for the decline include increased purity of street heroin and a bias to attribute focal segmental glomerulosclerosis to HIV infection when both risk factors coexist. Intravenous *amphetamine* abuse is a rare cause of systemic necrotizing vasculitis.

HEREDITARY DISEASES WITH GLOMERULAR INVOLVEMENT

ALPORT'S SYNDROME (See also Chap. 351) Alport's syndrome is the most common hereditary nephritis and is usually transmitted as an X-linked dominant trait. The genetic defect resides in the gene for the $\alpha5$ chain of type IV collagen located on the long arm of the X chromosome; type IV collagen is a major structural component of the GBM. Numerous genetic mutations have been detected, ranging from major deletions to point mutations, and this genetic heterogeneity is reflected in the phenotypic variations of the disease. In the X-linked forms, males usually present with microscopic hematuria, proteinuria (nephrotic-range in 30%), and progressive renal insufficiency. Common extrarenal manifestations include sensorineural hearing loss (~60%), bilateral anterior lenticonus (~15 to 30%), and recurrent corneal erosions. Platelet defects are described but are rare. Female carriers usually have mild disease and do not develop renal insufficiency. Autosomal dominant and recessive forms also exist in which there are mutations in the gene for the $\alpha3$ chain of type IV collagen, and males and females are equally affected. Genetic analysis to detect mutations in the genes encoding the $\alpha3$ and $\alpha5$ chains of type IV collagen may become the diagnostic method of choice.

Typical light-microscopic features on renal biopsy include mesangial hypercellularity, focal and segmental glomerulosclerosis, chronic tubulointerstitial fibrosis, atrophy, and accumulation of foam cells. Electron microscopy reveals thickening, fragmentation, and lamellation of the lamina densa of the GBM. Patchy thinning of the GBM may also be seen, especially early in the course of the disease and in female carriers.

Males with the disease tend to progress to ESRD and are suitable candidates for dialysis and transplantation. About 5% of transplant recipients develop anti-GBM disease in the renal allograft; their immune system recognizes normal GBM of the transplanted kidney as a foreign antigen. These patients can have antibodies against the $\alpha3$ (Goodpasture antigen) or $\alpha5$ chains of type IV collagen, probably because defective synthesis of the $\alpha5$ chain results in defective incorporation or orientation of the $\alpha3$ chain in the GBM.

SICKLE CELL DISEASE (See also Chap. 106) Glomerular disease is common (15 to 30%) in homozygotes for sickle cell disease. Glomerular hyperfiltration and hypertrophy occur within the first 5 years of life. Approximately 15 to 30% of patients develop proteinuria in the first three decades, and 5% develop ESRD. The glomerular pathology is usually focal segmental glomerulosclerosis, probably due to sustained glomerular capillary hypertension. MPGN is also seen on occasion. Predictors of chronic renal failure are worsening anemia, proteinuria, nephrotic syndrome, and hypertension. ACE inhibitors may slow the progression of renal disease by lowering systemic and glomerular capillary hypertension.

FABRY'S DISEASE (See also Chap. 349) In patients with Fabry's disease, renal biopsy reveals accumulation of neutral glycosphingolipids with terminal α-galactosyl moieties in lysosomes of glomerular, tubular, vascular, and interstitial cells. Focal and global glomerulosclerosis are later features. Electron microscopy reveals stacked, concentric lamellar profiles known as "myeloid" bodies, which are characteristic. Renal disease manifests in the late teens to early twenties with lipiduria, proteinuria with minimal hematuria, nephrotic syndrome, hypertension, and progressive renal insufficiency. The most striking systemic manifestations are skin lesions (angiokeratomas), corneal and lens opacities, painful dysesthesias of the extremities, and arthropathy of the terminal interphalangeal joints. The diagnosis of Fabry's disease can often be made by careful physical examination, especially if many of the typical clinical features are present. Measurement of urinary glycosphingolipids and estimation of peripheral leukocyte α-galactosidase levels help confirm the diagnosis. The renal lesion is progressive, and these patients often tolerate hemodynamic changes during dialysis poorly because of progressive vascular disease. Successful renal transplantation has been reported despite recurrence in the allograft.

NAIL-PATELLA SYNDROME The nail-patella syndrome is a rare hereditary disorder transmitted as an autosomal dominant trait. The abnormal gene is located on the long arm of chromosome 9, and candidate genes include the $\alpha1$ chain of type V collagen and the LIM homeodomain protein Lmxlb. The phenotype is characterized by multiple osseous abnormalities, primarily affecting the elbows and knees, and nail dysplasia. About 50% of patients have clinically evident nephropathy. The light-microscopic features on renal biopsy include local GBM thickening, tubular atrophy, interstitial fibrosis, and varying degrees of glomerular sclerosis. Electron microscopy reveals irregular thickening of the GBM, with electrolucent areas giving it a "moth-eaten" appearance. Cross-striated fibrils with the periodicity of collagen can be identified in the mesangium and basement membrane. The disease usually manifests clinically as asymptomatic hematuria and proteinuria, occasionally in the nephrotic range, but it may be silent. The renal lesion is relatively benign, and progression to ESRD occurs in 10 to 30% of patients.

LIPODYSTROPHY MPGN type II (dense deposit disease) is the most frequent glomerular lesion in patients with lipodystrophy (80%), whereas MPGN type I affects the remainder (20%). The disease occurs mostly in females between the ages of 5 and 15 years, and the clinical presentation and course are similar to those of idiopathic MPGN, namely nephrotic-range proteinuria and progressive renal insufficiency. Low C3 levels are common in association with C3 nephritic factor (Chap. 274).

LECITHIN-CHOLESTEROL ACYLTRANSFERASE DEFICIENCY (See also Chap. 344) Renal manifestations of this disease include proteinuria, microscopic hematuria, and progressive renal insufficiency. Renal biopsy typically reveals focal and segmental glomerulosclerosis. Electron-microscopic findings include irregular rounded, lucent lacunae that contain solid or laminated dense structures in the GBM, mesangial matrix, and Bowman's capsular and renal tubular basement membranes. Endothelial cell detachment is also evident, and capillary lumens may be occluded by vacuolated foam cells. Recurrence of the disease has been documented in the renal allograft but without marked impairment of graft function.

GLOMERULAR LESIONS ASSOCIATED WITH INFECTIOUS DISEASES

VIRAL INFECTIONS Hepatitis B, hepatitis C, and HIV are strongly associated with glomerular disease (Table 275-2). Glomerular lesions associated with *hepatitis B virus* (HBV) infection include

Table 275-2 Glomerular Lesions Associated with Infectious Diseases

Morphologic Lesion	Common Disease or Inciting Organism
Diffuse proliferative glomerulonephritis (classic postinfectious glomerulonephritis)	Streptococcal pharyngitis Acute/subacute bacterial endocarditis Visceral sepsis Typhoid fever Syphilis Leptospirosis (*Mycobacterium leprae*) Toxoplasmosis Falciparum malaria *Plasmodium falciparum* Varicella, mumps, echovirus, coxsackievirus, measles Infectious mononucleosis Hepatitis B and C
Membranoproliferative glomerulonephritis	Subacute bacterial endocarditis Ventriculoatrial shunt infection Visceral sepsis Hepatitis C infection Hepatitis B infection *P. falciparum* Schistosomiasis
Mesangial proliferative glomerulonephritis	Recovery phase of postinfectious glomerulonephritis
Membranous nephropathy	Hepatitis C infection Hepatitis B infection Syphilis Filiariasis Hydatid disease Schistosomiasis *Plasmodium malariae* Leprosy Enterococcal endocarditis
Focal segmental glomerulosclerosis	HIV infection Schistosomiasis
Renal amyloidosis	Any chronic infection

membranous glomerulopathy, MPGN, IgA nephropathy, essential mixed cryoglobulinemia, and polyarteritis nodosa. Membranous glomerulopathy is most common. In endemic areas, such as Asia and Africa, 80 to 100% of children and 30 to 45% of adults with membranous glomerulopathy have HBV surface antigenemia. HBV antigens have been identified in renal immune deposits, suggesting in situ immune-complex formation after planting of HBV antigens or trapping of circulating immune complexes containing HBV antigens. Patients typically present with nephrotic syndrome and microscopic hematuria. Hypertension and renal impairment are rare. The most common associated hepatic lesion is chronic persistent or chronic active hepatitis. In nonendemic areas there is a male preponderance, and many patients are intravenous drug users or have other risk factor for acquisition of HBV. The asymptomatic carrier state of HBV is frequently associated with MPGN in endemic areas. Hypertension and azotemia are more common with this morphologic pattern than with membranous glomerulopathy. Children with HBV-associated membranous glomerulonephritis have a good prognosis, and almost two-thirds enter spontaneous remission within 3 years. ESRD is rare. In contrast, 30% of adults develop progressive renal failure within 5 years, with 10% reaching ESRD. Steroids and cytotoxic agents are contraindicated as they may lead to increased viral replication and worsening of liver disease. Interferon α may reduce proteinuria and stabilize renal function in patients with progressive disease.

HCV infection (Chap. 295) should be considered in all patients with cryoglobulinemic proliferative glomerulonephritis, MPGN, and membranous glomerulopathy. These three clinocopathologic entities may represent a spectrum of morphologic manifestations of the same pathogenetic process, namely HCV-induced immune-complex disease. Up to 30% of patients with chronic HCV infection have an abnormal urinary sediment. HCV infection accounts for 10 to 20% of type I MPGN and is a major cause of essential mixed cryoglobulinemia. Renal biopsy reveals typical features of type I MPGN and IgG, IgM, C3, and/or cryoglobulin deposits. Most patients present with nephrotic syndrome and microscopic hematuria and may have red blood cell casts. Liver function tests are usually abnormal, and C3 levels are typically depressed. Anti-HCV antibodies are detected in most patients, and viral RNA has been documented in blood and cryoglobulins. Various treatments have been reported to be useful in HCV-induced renal disease including steroids, cytotoxic agents, and plasmapheresis; however, controlled trials to support their use are lacking. Interferon α has been demonstrated to clear antigenemia, lower cryoglobulin levels, and stabilize renal disease. Unfortunately, relapse is usual once the drug is discontinued.

HIV infection (Chap. 309) has been associated with focal segmental glomerulosclerosis, acute diffuse proliferative glomerulonephritis, and mesangioproliferative glomerulonephritis, including IgA nephropathy, MPGN, and membranous glomerulopathy. The classic and most common HIV-associated glomerulopathy is an aggressive form of focal segmental glomerulosclerosis, an entity that is termed *HIV-associated nephropathy (HIVAN)*. This disease may be the first manifestation of infection in otherwise asymptomatic patients. HIVAN is more common in blacks than in other ethnic groups and is more frequent in intravenous drug abusers with HIV infection than in homosexuals. The disease has been described in all high-risk groups, however, including infants of HIV-positive mothers. Renal biopsy typically reveals visceral epithelial cell swelling, collapse of the glomerular capillary tuft, severe tubulointerstitial inflammation, and microcystic dilatation of renal tubules. Electron microscopy characteristically reveals severe visceral epithelial cell injury and tubuloreticular inclusions in glomerular endothelial cells, tubular cells and infiltrating leukocytes. This constellation of findings has been termed collapsing glomerulopathy, but it should be emphasized that a similar picture can be seen in the absence of HIV infection. The presence of tubuloreticular inclusions and the aggressive clinical course distinguish HIVAN from idiopathic focal segmental glomerulosclerosis. The mechanisms of renal cell injury are still being defined. Viral DNA has been demonstrated in the renal epithelia of HIV-infected patients with and without nephropathy,

suggesting that pathogenetic factors, other than infection of cells, are required for induction of disease. The typical clinical correlates of HIVAN are severe nephrotic syndrome and rapid progression to ESRD, occurring in weeks to months. Despite early reports of poor survival of patients on dialysis, more recent studies indicate improved survival for both asymptomatic patients with HIV and patients with full-blown AIDS. There is no proven therapy for HIVAN. The initial experience with combined highly active antiretroviral therapy (triple therapy) suggests that these regimens have reduced the incidence of nephropathy in HIV-infected patients and improved prognosis in patients with established nephropathy.

BACTERIAL INFECTIONS (Table 275-2) Immune-complex glomerulonephritis is a relatively frequent complication of infective *endocarditis* (Chap. 126). Other mechanisms of renal injury in bacterial endocarditis include embolic renal infarction, septic abscesses, acute tubular necrosis secondary to septicemia and drug therapy, disseminated intravascular coagulation, and antibiotic-induced acute interstitial nephritis. Patients typically present with microscopic hematuria, urinary red blood cell casts, pyuria and modest proteinuria (nephrotic range in 25% of patients), and variable degrees of renal failure. Rheumatoid factor is present in 10 to 70%, and circulating immune complexes in 90%. Serum complement levels are usually depressed. Renal biopsy reveals mild focal proliferative glomerulonephritis with mesangial and capillary wall deposition of IgG and C3 by immunofluorescence microscopy and subendothelial, mesangial, and subepithelial electron-dense deposits by electron microscopy. Occasional patients develop diffuse necrotizing glomerulonephritis with crescent formation and present with nephritic syndrome or RPGN. Endocarditis-associated glomerulonephritis typically has a good prognosis and resolves with eradication of the underlying infection.

Immune-complex glomerulonephritis is a complication in 1 to 4% of patients with *infected ventriculoatrial shunts*. Nephritis can manifest weeks to years after shunt insertion and usually presents with microscopic hematuria. Nephrotic syndrome occurs in 30 to 50%. The usual renal pathology is a membranoproliferative pattern, although diffuse proliferation can also occur. Immunofluorescence reveals IgM and C3 in the capillary wall and mesangial area, while subendothelial deposits and mesangial interposition are seen by electron microscopy. Up to one-third of patients may have residual renal impairment despite removal of the infected shunt and resolution of the infection.

Suppurative infections such as intrathoracic and intraabdominal abscesses, osteomyelitis, and dental abscesses have been associated with glomerulonephritis. The usual presentation is hematuria, urinary red blood cell casts, proteinuria, and acute renal failure. Oliguria and hypertension are common. Pathologic renal lesions include mesangial proliferative, membranoproliferative, and diffuse proliferative glomerulonephritis with crescents. Immunofluorescence reveals mesangial and capillary wall deposition predominantly of C3, although IgG and IgM may also be seen.

Nephrotic syndrome is a complication in 0.3% of patients with secondary *syphilis* and 8% of patients with congenital syphilis. The usual pathology is membranous glomerulopathy; however, mild mesangial and endocapillary proliferation can occur. IgG and IgM are evident in affected regions by immunofluorescence microscopy, and treponemal antigens have been identified in diseased glomeruli. C3 and C4 are typically depressed in congenital syphilis. The treatment consists of penicillin to eradicate the infection.

Leprosy most commonly causes AA amyloidosis; however, a syndrome resembling acute poststreptococcal glomerulonephritis has also been described.

PROTOZOAN AND PARASITIC INFECTIONS Transient proteinuria (50% of patients) and nephrotic syndrome (<1% of patients) are complications of infection with *Plasmodium falciparum*. Membranoproliferative glomerulonephritis is the usual pathologic lesion and may respond to eradication of infection. *Plasmodium malariae* has been associated with diffuse or focal proliferative glomerulonephritis, membranous glomerulopathy, and minimal change disease. Eradication of the malarial infection does not consistently induce remission of the nephrotic syndrome. *Schistosoma mansoni* causes nephrotic syndrome in 5 to 10% of patients, and progression to ESRD is common. The usual pathology is MPGN or mesangial proliferative glomerulonephritis, although membranous glomerulonephritis and amyloidosis are occasionally seen. *Filiariasis* can trigger membranous glomerulonephritis (*Loa loa*) and occasionally induces proliferative glomerulonephritis (*Onchocerca volvulus*). *Congenital toxoplasmosis* infection occasionally induces immune-complex glomerulonephritis characterized by mesangial and subendothelial immune deposits that contain *Toxoplasma* antigens. Membranous glomerulopathy and proliferative glomerulonephritis are occasional complications of *hydatid disease* and *trichinosis*, respectively.

GLOMERULAR LESIONS ASSOCIATED WITH NEOPLASIA

Glomerulopathies associated with neoplasia include membranous glomerulopathy, minimal change disease, focal segmental glomerulosclerosis, immune-complex glomerulonephritis, fibrillary/immunotactoid glomerulonephritis, LCDD, and amyloidosis. Mild proteinuria is common in patients with *solid tumors*, but overt glomerulonephritis is rare. Occasional patients with solid tumors of the lung, gastrointestinal tract, breast, kidney, and ovary develop full-blown nephrotic syndrome, usually due to a membranous glomerulopathy. Estimates of the incidence of occult malignancy in patients presenting with membranous glomerulopathy range from 0.1 to 10%. Most authorities agree that an extensive search for malignancy is not indicated, unless there are other suggestive clinical features. As many as 35% of patients with renal cell carcinoma have mesangial deposition of IgG and C3 visible on immunofluorescence; however, morphologic abnormalities are detected in only 50% of these patients, and clinically significant glomerulopathy is rare. Glomerular amyloidosis has also been described in association with this tumor.

An array of glomerular disease has been reported in patients with lymphoproliferative malignancy. Nephrotic syndrome is a recognized complication of *Hodgkin's lymphoma*, with 70% of cases due to minimal change disease. The latter may occur concurrently with (40 to 45%), precede (10 to 15%), or follow (40 to 50%) diagnosis of the malignancy. It is postulated that a lymphokine or other mediator released by malignant T lymphocytes perturbs podocyte function and alters glomerular permeability in this setting. Nephrotic syndrome typically resolves with successful treatment and relapses with recurrence of disease. Less frequent associations with Hodgkin's lymphoma include focal segmental glomerulosclerosis, membranous glomerulopathy, MPGN, proliferative glomerulonephritis, and crescentic glomerulonephritis. Minimal change disease, membranous glomerulopathy, MPGN, and crescentic glomerulonephritis have also been reported in patients with *non-Hodgkin's lymphoma*. Glomerulopathy in the context of leukemia is rare. MPGN can complicate *chronic lymphatic leukemia* and related *B cell lymphomas*, particularly when associated with cryoglobulinemia. Other glomerular lesions associated with *paraproteinemia* include primary amyloid, LCDD, proliferative glomerulonephritis induced by cryoglobulinemia, and fibrillary/immunotactoid glomerulopathy. Here again, the renal lesion frequently improves or resolves with successful treatment of the underlying malignancy.

BIBLIOGRAPHY

APPEL G, RISHNAM JR: Secondary glomerular diseases, in *Brenner & Rector's The Kidney*, 6th ed, BM Brenner (ed). Philadelphia, Saunders, 2000, pp 1350–1448

AUSTIN HA: Natural history and treatment of lupus nephritis. Seminar Nephrol 19:2, 1999

BENNETT PH et al: Screening and management of microalbuminuria in patients with diabetes mellitus: Recommendations to the Scientific Advisory Board of the National Kidney Foundation from an ad hoc committee of the Council on Diabetes Mellitus of the National Kidney Foundation. Am J Kidney Dis 25:107, 1995

BRADY HR, WILCOX CS (eds): *Therapy in Nephrology and Hypertension*. Philadelphia, Saunders, 1999

D'AGATI V et al: HIV infection and the kidney. J Am Soc Nephrol 8:139, 1997

DAGHESTANI L et al: Renal manifestations of hepatitis C infection. Am J Med 106:347, 1999

FALK RH, SKINNER M: The systemic amyloidoses: an overview. Adv Intern Med 45:107, 2000

KASHTAN CE: Alport syndrome and thin glomerular basement membrane disease. J Am Soc Nephrol 9:1736, 1998

PARVING HH et al: Diabetic nephropathy, in *Brenner & Rector's The Kidney*, 6th ed, BM Brenner (ed). Philadelphia, Saunders, 2000, pp 1731–1773

STEGALL MD et al: Pancreas transplantation for the prevention of diabetic nephropathy. Mayo Clin Proc 75:49, 2000

STEHMAN-BREEN C, JOHNSON RJ: Hepatitis C virus-associated glomerulonephritis. Adv Intern Med 43:79, 1998

276

John R. Asplin, Fredric L. Coe

HEREDITARY TUBULAR DISORDERS

The hereditary renal tubular disorders and their morphologic and functional abnormalities, mode of inheritance, and associated abnormalities are summarized in Table 276-1. The individual disorders are discussed in detail below.

AUTOSOMAL DOMINANT POLYCYSTIC KIDNEY DISEASE

ETIOLOGY AND PATHOLOGY Autosomal dominant polycystic kidney disease (ADPKD) has a prevalence of 1:300 to 1:1000 and accounts for approximately 10% of end-stage renal disease (ESRD) in the United States. Some 90% of cases are inherited as an autosomal dominant trait, and approximately 10% are spontaneous mutations.

GENETIC CONSIDERATIONS Three forms of ADPKD have been identified. ADPKD-1 accounts for 90% of cases, and the gene has been localized to the short arm of chromosome 16. The gene for ADPKD-2 has been mapped to the long arm of chromosome 4. The protein products of the two genes form the polycystin complex, which may regulate cell-cell or cell-matrix interactions. A defect in either of these proteins interrupts the normal function of the polycystin complex, resulting in the same phenotype for two distinct genetic abnormalities. ADPKD-2 appears to have a later age of onset of symptoms and renal failure than ADPKD-1. A third form has been documented but has not been mapped to a gene at this point. ■

The kidneys are grossly enlarged, with multiple cysts studding the surface of the kidney. The cysts contain straw-colored fluid that may become hemorrhagic. The cysts are spherical, vary in size from a few millimeters to centimeters, and are distributed evenly throughout the cortex and medulla. Only 1 to 5% of nephrons will develop cysts. Cysts form when a "second hit" causes a somatic mutation in the normal allele of a tubule cell, leading to monoclonal proliferation of the tubular epithelium. The remaining renal parenchyma reveals varying degrees of tubular atrophy, interstitial fibrosis, and nephrosclerosis.

CLINICAL FEATURES The disease may present at any age but most frequently causes symptoms in the third or fourth decade. Patients may develop chronic flank pain from the mass effect of the enlarged kidneys. Acute pain indicates infection, urinary tract obstruction by clot or stone, or sudden hemorrhage into a cyst. Gross and microscopic hematuria are common, and impaired renal concentrating ability frequently leads to nocturia. Nephrolithiasis occurs in 15 to 20% of patients, calcium oxalate and uric acid stones being most common. Low urine pH, low urine citrate, and urinary stasis from distortion of the collecting system by cysts all play a role in stone formation. Hypertension is found in 20 to 30% of children and up to 75% of adults. It is secondary to intrarenal ischemia from distortion of the renal architecture, leading to activation of the renin-angiotensin system. Patients with hypertension have a much more rapid progression to ESRD. Urinary tract infection is common and may involve the bladder or renal interstitium (pyelonephritis) or infect a cyst (pyocyst). Pyocysts can be difficult to diagnose but are more likely to be present if the patient has positive blood cultures, new renal pain, or failed to improve clinically after a standard course of antibiotic therapy.

Progressive decline in renal function is common, with approximately 50% of patients developing ESRD by age 60. However, there is considerable variation in age of onset of renal failure, even within the same family. Hypertension, recurrent infections, male sex, and early age of diagnosis are related to early onset renal failure. Renal failure usually progresses slowly; if a sudden decrement in kidney function occurs, ureteral obstruction from stone, clot, or compression by a cyst are likely causes. Patients usually have high hematocrits for their level of renal function, as erythropoietin production is high. Fluid overload is uncommon because of a tendency for renal salt wasting.

Extrarenal manifestations of this disease are frequent and underscore the systemic nature of the defect. Hepatic cysts occur in 50 to 70% of patients. Cysts are generally asymptomatic, and liver function

Table 276-1 Renal Tubule Defects

Disease	Renal Morphologic Abnormalities	Renal Functional Abnormalities	Mode of Inheritance	Associated Abnormalities
Autosomal dominant polycystic disease	Cortical and medullary cysts	Chronic renal failure, >20 yr	AD	Hepatic cysts, intracranial aneurysms, colonic diverticula
Autosomal recessive polycystic disease	Distal tubule and collecting duct cysts	Chronic renal failure, <20 yr	AR	Congenital hepatic fibrosis
Tuberous sclerosis	Renal cysts and angiomyolipomas	None	AD	Skin lesions, hamartomas of the central nervous system
Von Hippel–Lindau disease	Renal cysts, increased risk of renal cell cancer	None	AD	Hemangioblastoma of the retina and central nervous system
Medullary sponge kidney	Dilated collecting ducts	Nephrocalcinosis, hematuria	AD, S	None
Juvenile nephronophthisis	Medullary cysts, small kidneys	Chronic renal failure, <20 yr polyuria, salt wasting	AR	Hepatic fibrosis, retinal abnormalities
Medullary cystic disease	Medullary cysts, small kidneys	Chronic renal failure, >20 yr polyuria, salt wasting	AD	None
Liddle's syndrome	None	Hypokalemia, alkalosis, low aldosterone levels	AR	Hypertension
Bartter's syndrome	Juxtaglomerular apparatus hyperplasia	Hypokalemia, alkalosis, high aldosterone levels	AR, S	None
Congenital nephrogenic diabetes insipidus	None	Vasopressin renal concentrating defect	XL, AR	None
Renal tubular acidosis, type 1	Nephrocalcinosis	Impaired proton secretion in distal tubule, non-anion-gap metabolic acidosis	AD, AR, XL, S, ACQ	Rickets, osteomalacia, nephrolithiasis
Renal tubular acidosis, type 2	None	Reduced bicarbonate reabsorption, non-anion-gap metabolic acidosis	AR, AD, XL, ACQ	Fanconi syndrome, rickets
Renal tubular acidosis, type 4	Chronic renal insufficiency	Reduced proton and potassium secretion	ACQ	Renal insufficiency
X-linked hypophosphatemia	None	Reduced phosphate reabsorption	XL	Rickets, osteomalacia, normal serum $1,25(OH)_2D_3$
Vitamin D–dependent rickets, type 1	None	Defective renal $1,25(OH)_2D_3$ production	AR	Rickets, osteomalacia, low serum $1,25(OH)_2D_3$
Vitamin D–dependent rickets, type 2	None	Renal resistance to $1,25(OH)_2D_3$	AR, S	Rickets, osteomalacia, high serum $1,25(OH)_2D_3$
Oncogenic osteomalacia	None	Reduced phosphate reabsorption	ACQ	Osteomalacia, mesenchymal tumors
X-linked recessive nephrolithiasis	Interstitial fibrosis, medullary calcifications	Hypercalciuria, low-molecular-weight proteinuria	XL	Renal failure
Isolated hyperuricemia	None	Reduced urate reabsorption	AR	Variable hypercalciuria
Hartnup disorder	None	Reduced reabsorption of neutral amino acids	AR	Dermatitis, diarrhea, dementia
Cystinuria	Cystine stones	Reduced reabsorption of dibasic amino acids	AR	Short stature
Iminoglycinuria	None	Reduced reabsorption of proline, hydroxyproline, and glycine	AR	None
Fanconi syndrome	Swan neck deformity of proximal tubule	Reduced reabsorption of bicarbonate, glucose, phosphate, uric acid, and amino acids	AR	Rickets, osteomalacia, hypokalemia, metabolic acidosis

NOTE: AD, autosomal dominant; AR, autosomal recessive; XL, X-linked; ACQ, acquired; S, sporadic is normal, though women may develop massive hepatic cystic disease on occasion. Cyst formation has also been observed in the spleen, pancreas, and ovaries. Intracranial aneurysms are present in 5 to 10% of asymptomatic patients, with potential for permanent neurologic injury or death from subarachnoid hemorrhage. Screening of all ADPKD patients for aneurysms is not recommended, but patients with a family history of subarachnoid hemorrhage should be studied noninvasively with magnetic resonance imaging angiography. Colonic diverticular disease is the most common extrarenal abnormality, and patients are more likely to develop perforation than the general population with colonic diverticula. Mitral valve prolapse is found in 25% of patients, and the prevalence of aortic and tricuspid valve insufficiency is increased.

DIAGNOSIS Ultrasound is the preferred technique for diagnosis of symptomatic patients and for screening asymptomatic family members. The ability to detect cysts increases with the subject's age: 80 to 90% of ADPKD patients over the age of 20 will have detectable cysts, and almost 100% over the age of 30 will have cysts. At least three to five cysts in each kidney is the standard diagnostic criteria for ADPKD. Computed tomography (CT) scan may be more sensitive than ultrasound in detection of small cysts. Genetic linkage analysis is now available for diagnosis of ADPKD but is reserved for cases where radiographic imaging is negative and the need for definitive diagnosis critical, such as screening family members for potential kidney donation.

℞ TREATMENT The goals of treatment are to slow the rate of progression of renal disease and minimize symptoms. Hypertension and renal infection should be treated aggressively to maintain renal function. Converting enzyme inhibitors are effective antihypertensive agents, though patients should be closely monitored as some develop renal insufficiency and hyperkalemia. Urinary infection is treated in a standard manner unless a pyocyst is suspected, in which case antibiotics that penetrate cysts should be used, such as trimethoprim-sulfamethoxazole, ciprofloxacin, and chloramphenicol. Chronic pain from cysts can be managed by cyst puncture and sclerosis with ethanol.

AUTOSOMAL RECESSIVE POLYCYSTIC KIDNEY DISEASE

GENETIC CONSIDERATIONS Autosomal recessive polycystic kidney disease (ARPKD) is a rare genetic disease that has an incidence between 1:10,000 and 1:40,000. The gene for ARPKD has been localized to chromosome 6. In the past, ARPKD was considered to be a family of disorders, categorized as neonatal, infantile, and childhood forms depending on the age of onset and the relative degree of involvement of the kidneys and liver. However, variable clinical presentations within siblings in the same family, as well as the localization of the disease to chromosome 6 in multiple families, support the premise that this is a single genetic disease with variable phenotypic presentation. ■

At birth the kidneys are enlarged with a smooth external surface. The distal tubules and collecting ducts are dilated into elongated cysts that are arranged in a radial fashion. As the patient ages, the cysts may become more spherical and the disease can be confused with ADPKD. Interstitial fibrosis is also seen as renal function deteriorates. Liver involvement includes proliferation and dilation of small intrahepatic bile ducts as well as periportal fibrosis.

CLINICAL FEATURES The majority of cases are diagnosed in the first year of life, presenting as bilateral abdominal masses. Death in the neonatal period is most commonly due to pulmonary hypoplasia. Hypertension and impaired urinary concentrating ability are common. The time course to ESRD is variable, though many children maintain adequate kidney function for years. Older children present with complications secondary to congenital hepatic fibrosis and generally have less severe kidney disease. Hepatosplenomegaly, portal hypertension, and esophageal varices are frequent complications of ARPKD.

DIAGNOSIS Ultrasound is the most common technique used to diagnose ARPKD, prenatally and in childhood. Ultrasound examination reveals enlarged kidneys with increased echogenicity. At times spherical cysts may be seen, potentially leading to an incorrect diagnosis of ADPKD. A thorough family history and imaging the kidneys of the parents aids in differentiation from other cystic diseases. The recent mapping of the gene should allow linkage studies to be used in diagnosis.

℞ TREATMENT Aggressive treatment of hypertension and urinary tract infection are the major goals of therapy in order to maintain native renal function as long as possible. Dialysis and transplant are appropriate when kidney failure occurs. Hepatic fibrosis may lead to life-threatening variceal hemorrhage, requiring sclerotherapy or portocaval shunting.

TUBEROUS SCLEROSIS

Patients with this multisystem disease most commonly present with skin lesions and benign tumors of the central nervous system (Chap. 370). Renal involvement is common; angiomyolipomas are the most frequent abnormality and are usually bilateral. Renal cysts may be present as well and can give an appearance similar to that of ADPKD. Histologically, the cysts are unique—the cyst lining cells are large with an eosinophilic staining cytoplasm and may form hyperplastic nodules that can fill the cyst space.

GENETIC CONSIDERATIONS One-third of cases are inherited as an autosomal dominant trait, the rest are due to sporadic mutations. Mutations of tumor-suppression genes have been identified on chromosomes 9 (*TSC1*) and 16 (*TSC2*). Mutations of *TSC2* account for the majority of cases and are more likely to be associated with mental retardation and polycystic kidneys. Tuberous sclerosis may be confused with ADPKD if extrarenal manifestations are minimal. ■

VON HIPPEL–LINDAU DISEASE

This autosomal dominant disease is characterized by hemangioblastomas of the retina and the central nervous system (Chap. 370). Renal cysts occur in the majority of cases and are usually bilateral. The *VHL* gene is a tumor-suppressor gene and has been localized to chromosome 3. It is the same gene that is mutated in sporadic renal cell carcinoma, which may be found in up to 25% of patients with von Hippel–Lindau disease and is frequently multifocal. Yearly screening of adults using CT scans has been recommended in an attempt to diagnose renal cell cancers at an early stage.

MEDULLARY SPONGE KIDNEY

ETIOLOGY AND PATHOLOGY Medullary sponge kidney (MSK) is a congenital disorder. Although some cases have apparent autosomal dominant inheritance, most are sporadic. It is found in 0.5 to 1% of all intravenous pyelograms. Males and females are affected equally. The pathologic lesion is cystic dilation of the inner medullary and papillary collecting ducts, with collecting diameters ranging from 1 to 5 mm. Bilateral renal involvement is present in 70% of cases, but not all papillae are equally affected. The dilated ducts are lined by cuboidal epithelium with areas of pseudostratified and stratified squamous epithelium. Calculi are frequently found in the dilated collecting ducts.

CLINICAL FEATURES Patients generally present in the third or fourth decade with kidney stones, infection, or recurrent hematuria. The disease is most commonly diagnosed by intravenous pyelogram,

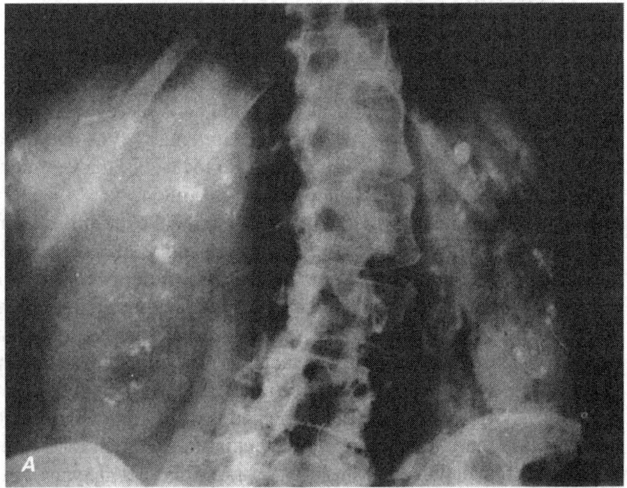

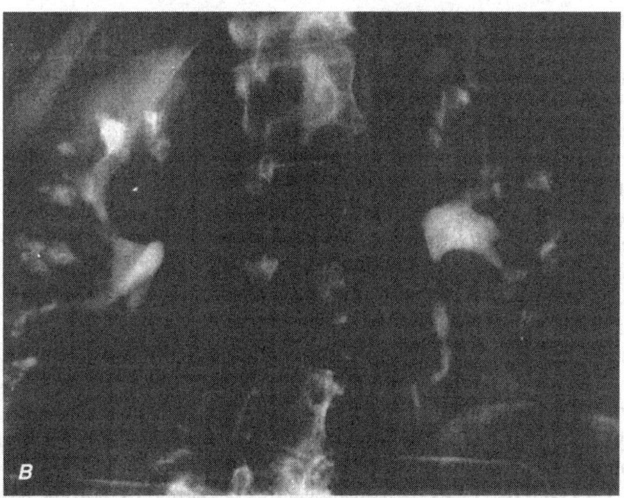

FIGURE 276-1 *A.* Radiographic appearance of medullary sponge kidney. Abdominal flat plate reveals multiple bilateral calcifications. *B.* Radiographic contrast material accumulates in the dilated and cystic terminal collecting ducts and obscures the calcifications.

which shows linear striations radiating into the renal papillae or small cystic collections of contrast in the dilated ducts (Fig. 276-1). Approximately 60% of patients with MSK have stones, and 12% of all stone formers will have MSK. Hypercalciuria occurs with the same frequency in MSK as it does in random stone formers. Papillary nephrocalcinosis occurs more frequently in patients with MSK than in the random stone former. Proteinuria is minimal, if present at all, and renal function is normally preserved unless there is renal damage from recurrent infection or severe stone disease.

℞ **TREATMENT** Asymptomatic patients require no specific therapy except to maintain high fluid intake to reduce the risk of nephrolithiasis. If stones are present, standard laboratory evaluation should be done and metabolic abnormalities treated as in any stone former (Chap. 279). Infection should be treated aggressively, and instrumentation of the urinary tract should be minimized to avoid introducing infection.

JUVENILE NEPHRONOPHTHISIS/MEDULLARY CYSTIC DISEASE

ETIOLOGY AND PATHOLOGY Juvenile nephronophthisis (JN) and medullary cystic disease (MCD) have similar pathologic findings but differ in inheritance pattern and age of onset.

GENETIC CONSIDERATIONS JN is inherited as an autosomal recessive disease; linkage studies have shown 70% of the cases to map to a gene (*NPH1*) on the short arm of chromosome 2. MCD is an autosomal dominant disease. Linkage analysis has identified genes on chromosomes 1 and 16 as being associated with MCD. In both conditions, the kidneys tend to be small, with cysts throughout the medulla; the cortex and papilla rarely have cysts. The cysts originate in the collecting ducts, distal convoluted tubules, and loops of Henle and range in size from 1 to 10 mm. Sclerotic glomeruli, tubule atrophy, and interstitial fibrosis are frequent findings on biopsy. ■

CLINICAL FEATURES Patients with JN present during childhood with symptoms of polyuria, growth retardation, anemia, and progressive renal insufficiency. Most patients develop ESRD prior to the age of 20; JN accounts for 2 to 10% of renal failure in children. Hepatic fibrosis and cerebellar ataxia has been reported in association with JN. JN with retinal degeneration is termed the *Senior-Loken syndrome*; it does not link to the *NPH1* gene at chromosome 2. MCD presents in the third or fourth decade, though some cases may be diagnosed in the elderly population. Presenting symptoms in MCD are the same as in JN except for growth retardation. In addition, MCD does not have extrarenal abnormalities. Severe salt wasting can be seen, though this is usually a transient phase that resolves as the disease progresses to ESRD. Other features of tubule damage are often found, including hyperkalemia and hyperchloremic metabolic acidosis. Proteinuria is mild, and hematuria is rare.

DIAGNOSIS The diagnosis is suggested by a family history of renal disease. The pattern of inheritance and age of onset aid in distinguishing JN/MCD from other inherited diseases. Radiographic studies show small kidneys, loss of the corticomedullary junction, and multiple cysts in the medulla. CT scan is more sensitive than ultrasound in making the diagnosis. Open renal biopsy, including medullary tissue, may be required for diagnosis in some cases.

℞ **TREATMENT** Treatment is mainly supportive, as there is no specific therapy to prevent loss of renal function. Patients with salt wasting require a large oral intake of salt and water to maintain adequate extracellular volume. Alkali replacement and erythropoietin are required for acidosis and anemia, respectively. Renal transplantation has been performed in numerous patients, and the disease does not recur.

LIDDLE'S SYNDROME

Liddle's syndrome is a rare familial disease with a clinical presentation of hyperaldosteronism, consisting of hypertension, hypokalemia, and metabolic alkalosis. However, aldosterone levels are undetectable in these patients, and a nonaldosterone mineralocorticoid has not been isolated. Increased distal tubule sodium reabsorption, due to activating mutations in the amiloride-sensitive sodium channel, has been described in multiple families. Pharmacologic agents that block distal tubule sodium uptake, such as amiloride and triamterene, are effective in treating the hypertension and electrolyte abnormalities. As expected, spironolactone is ineffective, since the disease is not mediated via the aldosterone receptor.

BARTTER'S SYNDROME

CLINICAL FEATURES Hypokalemia secondary to renal potassium wasting, metabolic alkalosis, and normal to low blood pressure are the clinical features of Bartter's syndrome. Three phenotypes of Bartter's syndrome have now been recognized. *Antenatal Bartter's syndrome* is characterized by polyhydramnios and premature delivery. During infancy, episodes of fever and dehydration are common and can lead to growth retardation. Nephrocalcinosis secondary to hypercalciuria is frequent. The infants also have a characteristic facies consisting of a triangular face with prominent eyes and ears. Prostaglandin E production is very high. Most cases of *classic Bartter's syndrome* present during childhood. Symptoms such as weakness and cramps are secondary to the hypokalemia. Polyuria and nocturia are common due to the hypokalemia-induced nephrogenic diabetes insipidus. Growth retardation may be seen. The *Gitelman's variant of Bartter's syndrome* presents during adolescence or adulthood and generally has a milder course than Bartter's syndrome. The dominant features are fatigue and weakness. It is distinguished from Bartter's syndrome by hypocalciuria, hypomagnesemia with hypermagnesuria, and normal prostaglandin production. All three forms are inherited as autosomal recessive traits. Although rarely required for diagnosis, renal biopsy reveals hyperplasia of the juxtaglomerular apparatus and prominence of medullary interstitial cells, with variable degrees of interstitial fibrosis, though these are not pathognomonic for the syndrome.

PATHOGENESIS The pathogenesis of Bartter's syndrome has long been a matter of debate as the distinction of the primary disorder from the secondary phenomena induced by volume depletion and hypokalemia is difficult.

GENETIC CONSIDERATIONS Recently, mutations in several renal tubule transport proteins have been shown to be responsible for the syndrome. In antenatal and classic Bartter's syndrome, impaired Cl^- reabsorption in the thick ascending limb of the loop of Henle is the underlying defect. Inadequate Cl^- reabsorption causes volume depletion and activates the renin-angiotensin system. Distal delivery of NaCl and water are high in the presence of high aldosterone, promoting secretion of K^+ and H^+ ions. Prostaglandin overproduction is mediated by volume depletion, hypokalemia, and high angiotensin II and kallikrein levels. Increased prostaglandin production contributes to the severity of disease by inducing resistance to the pressor effects of angiotensin II and reducing reabsorption in the thick ascending limb of the loop of Henle. Mutations in the bumetanide-sensitive Na:K:2Cl channel, the apical ATP-regulated K^+ channel, and the basolateral Cl^- channel have been described in classic and antenatal Bartter's. All of these mutations would lead to a loss of Cl^- reabsorption in the loop of Henle. In Gitelman's syndrome, mutations have been found in the thiazide-sensitive NaCl transporter. The reduced Na^+ reabsorption in the distal convoluted tubule leads to volume depletion and hypokalemia, though not as severe as would result from a lesion in the loop of Henle. Loss of activity of the thiazide-sensitive transporter increases tubule calcium reabsorption, leading to the classic finding of hypocalciuria in Gitelman's syndrome. ■

DIAGNOSIS Hypokalemia, metabolic alkalosis, and normal to low blood pressure are the clinical findings characteristic of Bartter's syndrome. The differential diagnosis includes vomiting, surreptitious diuretic abuse, and magnesium deficiency. Chronic vomiting can be diagnosed by a low urine Cl^- concentration. Magnesium deficiency causes kaluresis and alkalosis, simulating Bartter's syndrome. Serum and urine magnesium will be low in such cases. Diuretic abuse produces metabolic abnormalities indistinguishable from Bartter's syndrome. Urine should be screened for diuretics multiple times before the diagnosis of Bartter's is made in a patient without a family history of the disorder.

℞ TREATMENT Dietary intake of sodium and potassium should be liberal. Potassium supplements are usually required. Magnesium supplements are needed in patients with Gitelman's syndrome. Spironolactone will reduce potassium wasting. Prostaglandin synthetase inhibitors are useful in patients with antenatal and classic Bartter's syndrome but are of no benefit in Gitelman's syndrome. Angiotensin-converting enzyme inhibitors may be beneficial in some patients.

CONGENITAL NEPHROGENIC DIABETES INSIPIDUS

GENETIC CONSIDERATIONS This rare genetic disorder is most commonly inherited as an X-linked disease, with full expression in males and variable penetrance in females. Vasopressin acts through two receptors; type 1 receptors are located in the vasculature, while type 2 receptors are found in the collecting ducts of the kidney. In nephrogenic diabetes insipidus (NDI), only the actions requiring type 2 receptors are abnormal. Inactivating mutations of the type 2 vasopressin receptor, located on the long arm of the X chromosome, are responsible for the renal resistance to vasopressin. Less frequently, NDI may be inherited as an autosomal recessive trait, in which mutations in the gene for the water channels in collecting duct cells (aquaporin 2) lead to abnormal cell routing of aquaporin 2. ■

CLINICAL FEATURES The clinical presentation is that of persistent polyuria, dehydration, and hypotonic urine in the presence of hypernatremia. Vasopressin levels are appropriately elevated in the hypertonic state, but renal response is lacking. The onset of the disorder is in infancy. The recurrent hypernatremia may lead to seizures or mental retardation. Once old enough to satisfy their thirst, children will be clinically stable though in a chronic state of polyuria and polydypsia. Renal function is normal, and radiographic studies of the urinary system reveal dilated ureters and bladder secondary to the chronically high urine flow. Since the most common form of the disease is X-linked, most patients are male. Heterozygous females generally have mild concentrating defects, though a few have phenotypic expression similar to males due to skewed X-chromosome inactivation. In the autosomal recessive form, males and females are affected equally.

℞ TREATMENT Treatment is aimed at maintaining adequate hydration. In the infant, low-solute feedings and high water intake are generally adequate. Addition of a thiazide diuretic reduces urine flow by inhibiting sodium reabsorption in the distal convoluted tubule. This lowers free water production and, by causing extracellular volume contraction, increases proximal salt and water reabsorption, reducing delivery to the distal nephron. Administration of vasopressin and its analogues has no role in the management of this disorder.

RENAL TUBULAR ACIDOSIS

Renal tubular acidosis (RTA) is a disorder of renal acidification out of proportion to the reduction in glomerular filtration rate. RTA is characterized by hyperchloremic metabolic acidosis with a normal serum anion gap $[Na^+ - (Cl^- + HCO_3^-)]$. There are multiple forms of RTA, depending on which aspects of renal acid handling have been affected. Defective bicarbonate reabsorption in the proximal tubule, suppressed renal ammoniagenesis, and inadequate distal tublule proton secretion are the abnormalities that produce RTA. Three types of RTA exist (Table 276-2). Types 1 and 2 may be inherited or acquired. Type 4 is acquired and is associated with either hypoaldosteronism or tubular hyporesponsiveness to mineralocorticoids. Type 3 was formerly used to define distal RTA with bicarbonate wasting in children; however, the bicarbonaturia resolves with age and is not truly part of a pathologic process. The term *type 3 RTA* is no longer used.

TYPE 1 (DISTAL) RTA In this disorder the distal nephron does not lower urine pH normally, either because the collecting ducts permit excessive back-diffusion of hydrogen ions from lumen to blood or because there is inadequate transport of hydrogen ions. Excretion of titratable acid is low, as inadequate proton secretion prevents titration of urinary buffers such as phosphate. Urine ammonium excretion is inappropriately low for the level of acidosis, as the defect in acidification reduces the ion trapping required for ammonium excretion. Urinary concentration and potassium conservation also tend to be impaired.

Chronic acidosis lowers tubule reabsorption of calcium, causing renal hypercalciuria and mild secondary hyperparathyroidism. Buffering of bone by the daily metabolic acid load contributes to hypercalciuria. Urine citrate excretion is low, as acidosis and hypokalemia stimulate proximal tubule reabsorption of citrate. The hypercalciuria, alkaline urine, and low levels of urine citrate, which normally complexes about 40% of urine calcium, cause calcium phosphate stones and nephrocalcinosis. Growth in children is stunted because of rickets; this growth defect responds to amelioration of the acidosis with alkali. In the adult, osteomalacia occurs. In both children and adults, bone diseases may result, in part, from acidosis-induced loss of bone material and inadequate production of 1,25-dihydroxyvitamin D_3 [$1,25(OH)_2D_3$]. Since the kidney does not conserve potassium or concentrate the urine normally, polyuria and hypokalemia occur. With the stress of an intercurrent illness, acidosis and hypokalemia can be life-threatening.

Table 276-2 Comparison of Normal Anion-Gap Acidoses

Finding	Type 1 RTA	Type 2 RTA	Type 4 RTA	GI Bicarbonate Loss
Normal anion-gap acidosis	Yes	Yes	Yes	Yes
Minimum urine pH	>5.5	<5.5	<5.5	5 to 6
% filtered bicarbonate excreted	<10	>15	<10	<10
Serum potassium	Low	Low	High	Low
Fanconi syndrome	No	Yes	No	No
Stones/nephrocalcinosis	Yes	No	No	No
Daily acid excretion	Low	Normal	Low	High
Urine anion gap	Positive	Positive	Positive	Negative
Daily bicarbonate replacement needs	<4 mmol/kg	>4 mmol/kg	<4 mmol/kg	Variable

NOTE: RTA, renal tubular acidosis.

GENETIC CONSIDERATIONS Type 1 RTA can be familial, with autosomal dominant as the most common form of inheritance. X-linked, autosomal recessive, and sporadic cases have been reported. Mutations in the chloride-bicarbonate exchange gene (*AE1*) have been found in the autosomal dominant form. The cause of the autosomal recessive form is not known at this time. Other hereditary diseases that cause type 1 RTA include galactosemia, Ehler-Danlos syndrome, Fabry's disease, MSK, Wilson's disease, and hereditary elliptocytosis. The majority of cases of type 1 RTA are secondary to a systemic disorder such as Sjögren's syndrome, hypergammaglobulinemia, chronic active hepatitis, or lupus. ■

Diagnosis The diagnosis of type 1 RTA is suggested by a normal anion gap metabolic acidosis with a simultaneous urine pH greater than 5.5. Osteomalacia or rickets and calcium phosphate stones or nephrocalcinosis support the diagnosis, though they are not present in all cases. Bicarbonaturia is not present, which distinguishes this disorder from type 2 RTA. If acidosis is not severe and urine pH is equivocal, the oral ammonium chloride (NH_4Cl) loading test should be carried out: 0.1 g (1.9 mmol) NH_4Cl per kilogram of body weight is administered, and blood and urine pH are measured repeatedly over the next 6 h. Although systemic acidosis worsens, urine pH does not fall below 5.5. Urinary tract infection must not be present during this test because bacteria may possess urease, which hydrolyzes urea to ammonia and produces an alkaline urine.

Chronic diarrheal states cause normal anion gap acidosis and hypokalemia; urine pH may be >5.5 if ammonium production is very high. The urine anion gap ($Na^+ + K^+ - Cl^-$) can be used to estimate renal ammonium production and distinguish RTA from gastrointestinal bicarbonate loss. Normally the urine anion gap is positive, as unmeasured anions exceed unmeasured cations. If urine ammonium levels are high, urine chloride concentration increases to balance the charge. Unmeasured cation (predominantly ammonium) now exceeds unmeasured anion, and the urine anion gap is negative. During metabolic acidosis, a negative urine anion gap suggests an extrarenal cause of acidosis, whereas a positive urine anion gap suggests RTA. The urine anion gap cannot be used if there are large amounts of unmeasured anions, such as bicarbonate or ketones, in the urine.

℞ **TREATMENT** Alkali supplements are the standard therapy. Enough alkali is prescribed to titrate the daily metabolic acid production, usually in the range of 0.5 to 2.0 mmol/kg body weight in four to six divided doses per day. Sodium bicarbonate and Shohl's solution (1 mmol sodium citrate and 1 mmol citric acid per mL) are common treatments. Potassium alkali salts can be used if hypokalemia is a persistent problem. Citrate requires less frequent dosing than bicarbonate salts as it is metabolized to bicarbonate after absorption. The dose of alkali should be raised until acidosis and hypercalciuria are both eliminated, and the patients should be followed by measurements of serum potassium, chloride, and CO_2 content approximately twice yearly. Requirements for alkali usually rise during intercurrent illnesses but are usually below 4 mmol/kg body weight per day. The relatives of patients with idiopathic type 1 RTA should be screened for this disorder, as timely treatment can prevent growth retardation in children. Incomplete RTA secondary to idiopathic hypercalciuria is best treated using thiazide diuretics in conjunction with potassium citrate (Chap. 279).

TYPE 2 (PROXIMAL) RTA Type 2 RTA usually occurs as part of a generalized disorder of proximal tubule function, presenting as hyperchloremic acidosis with other features of Fanconi syndrome. Bicarbonate reabsorption in the proximal tubule is defective. At normal concentrations of plasma bicarbonate, large amounts of bicarbonate are delivered to the distal tubule, overwhelming the absorptive capacity of the distal tubule and resulting in bicarbonaturia. As plasma bicarbonate levels fall, the lower filtered load of bicarbonate can be reabsorbed by the proximal tubule, resulting in normal distal delivery of bicarbonate. At this point the distal nephron can acidify the urine normally, resulting in normal excretion of daily metabolic acid production, albeit at a low serum bicarbonate level. Hypophosphatemia and low calcitriol levels are common and may lead to rickets or osteomalacia. Hypercalciuria occurs, but stone formation is unusual since urine citrate levels are normal or high because of reduced proximal tubule citrate reabsorption. Type 2 RTA may be inherited as autosomal dominant, autosomal recessive, or X-linked disorder. It may be acquired in association with other diseases (see "Fanconi Syndrome") or be secondary to drugs that inhibit carbonic anhydrase activity, such as acetazolamide.

Type 2 RTA may be distinguished from type 1 RTA by the ability to normally acidify urine during spontaneous or ammonium chloride–induced acidosis. Correction of acidosis with bicarbonate will result in bicarbonaturia in type 2 RTA but not type 1 RTA. Fractional excretion of bicarbonate is >15% at normal or near-normal serum bicarbonate levels. In distal RTA it is <10%. It is unusual for serum bicarbonate levels to fall below 15 mmol/L in proximal RTA. The urine anion gap will be positive, as ammonium excretion is normal to handle daily acid production but is not elevated as in nonrenal causes of acidosis.

℞ **TREATMENT** Children should be treated to prevent growth retardation. Alkali must be given in large amounts daily, 5 to 15 mmol/kg body weight per day, because bicarbonate is rapidly excreted in the urine. A thiazide diuretic can be used in conjunction with a low-salt diet to reduce the amount of bicarbonate required. Potassium supplementation is often required.

TYPE 4 RTA In type 4 RTA, also called *hyperkalemic distal RTA*, distal tubule secretion of both potassium and hydrogen ions is abnormal, resulting in hyperchloremic acidosis with hyperkalemia. Type 4 RTA is an acquired disorder; a moderate degree of renal insufficiency is present in the majority of patients. Patients with type 4 RTA can be differentiated from patients with type 1 since they have an acid urine (pH $<$ 5.5) during periods of acidosis (Table 276-2) and hyperkalemia. They differ from type 2 patients by having a fractional excretion of bicarbonate $<$10% and a daily bicarbonate requirement of 1 to 3 mmol/kg body weight per day. Because potassium and hydrogen ion excretion are abnormal, such patients are considered to have generalized distal nephron dysfunction due to either insufficient aldosterone production or intrinsic renal disease causing aldosterone resistance. The resulting hyperkalemia reduces proximal tubule ammonia production, in addition to the inadequate proton secretion, leading to inadequate excretion of the daily metabolic proton load. These patients have an acid urine despite reduced proton secretion because there is inadequate ammonia to buffer protons in the distal tubule. If buffer delivery to the distal nephron is increased, urine pH will rise despite persistent acidosis.

Type 4 RTA due to inadequate aldosterone production has multiple etiologies. Hyporeninemic hypoaldosteronism is the most common cause of type 4 RTA. Plasma levels of renin and aldosterone are subnormal, even during extracellular volume depletion, and the most common causes of this are diabetic nephropathy and chronic tubulointerstitial nephropathies. Nonsteroidal anti-inflammatory drugs, angiotensin-converting enzyme inhibitors, trimethoprim, and heparin can reduce aldosterone production and produce a type 4 RTA. Drug-induced type 4 RTA is usually seen in patients with preexisting renal insufficiency. Reduced aldosterone production may be due to adrenal disease, either occurring as an isolated defect or as part of a more generalized adrenal disorder (Chap. 331). Renin levels are normal to high in adrenal disorders.

Patients with tubular resistance to aldosterone present with the same clinical features as those with hyporeninemic hypoaldosteronism. A tubulointerstitial process damages the distal tubule, restricting potassium and hydrogen ion excretion, despite adequate aldosterone levels. Obstructive uropathy and sickle cell disease are the most common causes of acquired tubular resistance to aldosterone. Hyporeninemic hypoaldosteronism can be found in addition to tubular aldosterone resistance in many patients. Spironolactone, a competitive inhibitor of the aldosterone receptor, produces an aldosterone-resistant state. Amiloride and triamterene are diuretics that block sodium transport in the distal nephron, blunting the effect of aldosterone on the distal tubule.

℞ TREATMENT This is aimed mainly at reducing serum potassium, as acidosis will usually improve once the hyperkalemic block of ammonium production is removed. All patients should be placed on a low-potassium diet. Any drug that suppresses aldosterone production or blocks aldosterone effect should be discontinued. Mineralocorticoid supplementation with fludrocortisone, 0.1 to 0.2 mg/d, will improve hyperkalemia and acidosis; however, the patients who also have a partial tubule resistance to mineralocorticoid will require a higher dose. Mineralocorticoid replacement may not be appropriate for patients with hypertension or a history of heart failure. In such situations, a loop diuretic with a liberal sodium intake can usually promote adequate potassium excretion. Exchange resins will reduce potassium levels but are usually not tolerated well enough to be used for long-term treatment.

PSEUDOHYPOALDOSTERONISM

GENETIC CONSIDERATIONS This rare inherited disorder is transmitted as either an autosomal dominant or recessive trait. The autosomal dominant form is caused by mutations in the mineralocorticoid receptor gene; the autosomal recessive disease is caused by inactivating mutations in the amiloride-sensitive epithelial sodium channel. The inability to respond to aldosterone leads to hyperkalemia, metabolic acidosis, salt wasting, and volume depletion, which present during childhood. Plasma renin and aldosterone levels are elevated. Treatment includes salt supplements, alkali, and potassium restriction. ■

VITAMIN D DISORDERS

X-LINKED HYPOPHOSPHATEMIC RICKETS (See also Chap. 342) This disorder, also called *vitamin D–resistant rickets*, is an X-linked dominant disorder characterized by hypophosphatemia with renal phosphate wasting, rickets, and short stature. Hypophosphatemia is present soon after birth; rachitic bowing of the legs develops when the child begins to walk. Children have growth retardation, which is limited almost entirely to the lower extremities. Dentition is delayed, and skull abnormalities are common. Females generally have less severe disease than males. Presentation in adults ranges from disabling bone pain to no active symptoms, but generally some physical sign of childhood disease, such as short stature or bowed legs, is present. Overgrowth of bone at joints or sites of muscle attachment may reduce the mobility of the joint or cause nerve entrapment.

Hypophosphatemia secondary to reduced renal phosphate reabsorption is the hallmark of the disease. Intestinal phosphate absorption is low, worsening hypophosphatemia. Serum calcium levels are usually normal, with low intestinal absorption and renal excretion of calcium. Serum alkaline phosphatase and osteocalcin levels are elevated. Parathyroid hormone levels are normal, as would be expected with normal serum calcium. $1,25(OH)_2D_3$ levels are usually normal, though in the setting of hypophosphatemia $1,25(OH)_2D_3$ levels should be elevated. Inadequate 1α-hydroxylase activity appears to play some role in the disease. Linkage analysis has localized the gene to the Xp22.1 region of the X chromosome. The gene has been identified and appears to be related to a family of endopeptidase genes.

℞ TREATMENT The goal of therapy is to raise serum phosphorous to normal or near-normal levels to improve bone mineralization. Oral neutral phosphate, 1 to 4 g/d in four to six doses, combined with calcitriol is an effective therapy that improves growth rate, reduces bone pain, and leads to radiographically evident improvement of the bone disease. Patients should be closely monitored during therapy as they may develop nephrocalcinosis and renal insufficiency.

VITAMIN D–DEPENDENT RICKETS TYPE I

GENETIC CONSIDERATIONS This is an autosomal recessive disorder in which $1,25(OH)_2D_3$ levels are very low but 25-hydroxyvitamin D levels are normal. The disease is caused by inactivating mutations in the gene encoding the 1α-hydroxylase enzyme, leading to a clinical syndrome of vitamin D deficiency. ■

Symptoms usually appear before the age of 2, including rickets and growth retardation. Levels of serum calcium and phosphorous are low, but that of alkaline phosphatase is elevated. Intestinal calcium absorption and urinary calcium excretion are low. Parathyroid hormone is elevated in response to the hypocalcemia, resulting in increased urinary phosphate losses.

℞ TREATMENT Calcitriol (0.5 to 1 μg/d) leads to rapid correction of the biochemical abnormalities and resolution of the bone disease. Calcium and phosphorous supplementation are usually not required.

VITAMIN D–DEPENDENT RICKETS TYPE II (See also Chap. 342) End-organ resistance to $1,25(OH)_2D_3$ is the pathogenesis of this disorder. Serum calcium and phosphate levels are low, secondary hyperparathyroidism is present, and $1,25(OH)_2D_3$ levels are elevated. Inheritance is usually autosomal recessive, though sporadic cases have been reported. Most patients present during childhood with rickets, though some have a milder form of disease not recognized until adulthood. Alopecia is common and tends to be associated with the more severe childhood form of the disease. Multiple defects have been detected in $1,25(OH)_2D_3$ receptor interaction, including absent hormone binding to the receptor, decreased receptor affinity, abnormal hormone-receptor localization, and abnormalities of the DNA-binding domain of the receptor. Pharmacologic doses of calcitriol (5 to 30 μg/d) along with mineral supplementation will improve the biochemical disorders and bone disease, though some patients have no response to massive doses of calcitriol.

ONCOGENIC OSTEOMALACIA This syndrome generally occurs in adults with highly vascular mesenchymal tumors. Patients present with bone pain and muscle weakness. Symptoms may be present for years before the correct diagnosis is made. Over 90% of the tumors are benign, and most are found in the extremities or maxillofacial region. Hypophosphatemia secondary to renal phosphate wasting and low levels of $1,25(OH)_2D_3$ are the major biochemical abnormalities. Serum calcium and parathyroid hormone levels are normal. It appears the tumor produces a humoral agent that reduces proximal tubule phosphate reabsorption and 1α-hydroxylase activity. Removal of the tumor leads to rapid resolution of the disease.

X-LINKED RECESSIVE NEPHROLITHIASIS

This disorder presents as calcium nephrolithiasis in male children and progresses to nephrocalcinosis and renal failure. Low-molecular-weight proteinuria and hypercalciuria are also prominent features of the disease. Kidney biopsy reveals tubular atrophy, interstitial fibrosis, and medullary calcifications. The gene has been mapped to the short arm of the X chromosome and encodes a voltage-gated chloride channel (CLC-5). Dent's disease has been mapped to the same gene and has a similar presentation, except for an increased incidence of rickets.

ISOLATED HYPOURICEMIA (See also Chap. 353)

This disorder is generally inherited as an autosomal recessive trait. Most commonly there is deficient urate reabsorption in the proximal tubule, though some patients have been demonstrated to oversecrete urate. Serum uric acid is usually <120 μmol/L (2 mg/dL) and hyperuricosuria is common, possibly due to decreased intestinal urate excretion. Hypouricemia is usually an incidental finding, as patients with this disorder are asymptomatic except for an increased risk of nephrolithiasis. Other disorders associated with hypouricemia include Fanconi syndrome, Wilson's disease, Hodgkin's disease, and Hartnup disease. No treatment is required except for high fluid intake to prevent kidney stones. Alkali and allopurinol may be used to prevent stones if fluids alone are not sufficient. Hypercalciuria has been associated with isolated hypouricemia in some families.

SELECTED DISORDERS OF AMINO ACID TRANSPORT

HARTNUP DISEASE This disorder is characterized by reduced intestinal absorption and renal reabsorption of neutral amino acids. The defect involves an amino acid transporter on the brush border of the jejunum and the proximal tubule. Intestinal absorption of free amino acids is reduced, though the neutral amino acids can be absorbed when present in di- and tripeptides. Degradation of unabsorbed tryptophan by intestinal bacteria produces indolic acids that are absorbed and subsequently excreted at high levels in the urine of these patients. The disorder is inherited as an autosomal recessive trait, affecting males and females equally. Widespread screening of newborns has estimated an incidence of 1 in 24,000 live births.

The majority of individuals with this disorder are asymptomatic. Approximately 10 to 20% present with clinical symptoms similar to those seen in pellagra, including a photosensitive erythematous scaly rash, intermittent cerebral ataxia, delirium, and diarrhea. Short stature is noted in some patients. The symptoms are thought to be due to deficiency in the essential amino acid tryptophan and resultant inadequate synthesis of nicotinamide. Though the inheritance of the disorder is Mendelian autosomal recessive, the development of symptomatic disease appears to be multifactorial. Diet, environment, and polygenic traits controlling plasma amino acid levels all contribute to development of symptoms.

Clinically affected patients can be differentiated from patients with pellagra by dietary history and the presence of aminoaciduria. Diagnosis is made by the characteristic finding of large amounts of neutral amino acids in the urine. It can easily be distinguished from generalized aminoaciduria by the normal excretion of proline. There are no other renal tubule defects as in Fanconi syndrome. Heterozygotes have normal urinary amino acid excretion.

℞ **TREATMENT** Symptomatic individuals should receive oral nicotinamide, 40 to 200 mg/d, and a high-protein diet to compensate for the poor amino acid absorption. Some patients who do not respond to nicotinamide may improve with tryptophan ethyl ester, which is lipid soluble and can be absorbed without an active transport system.

FANCONI SYNDROME

GENETIC CONSIDERATIONS Fanconi syndrome is a generalized defect in proximal tubule transport involving amino acids, glucose, phosphate, uric acid, sodium, potassium, bicarbonate, and proteins. Idiopathic Fanconi syndrome may be inherited as an autosomal dominant, autosomal recessive, or X-linked trait. Sporadic cases are also seen. A variety of inherited systemic disorders are also associated with Fanconi syndrome including Wilson's disease, galactosemia, tyrosinemia, cystinosis, fructose intolerance, and Lowe's oculocerebral syndrome. The syndrome may be acquired in multiple myeloma, amyloid, and heavy metal toxicity. ■

The patients may present with a wide array of laboratory abnormalities including proximal renal tubular acidosis, glucosuria with a normal serum glucose, hypophosphatemia, hypouricemia, hypokalemia, generalized aminoaciduria, and low-molecular-weight proteinuria. Some patients do not have abnormalities in all proximal tubule transporters and may present with only a few of the laboratory findings. Rickets and osteomalacia are common findings secondary to the hypophosphatemia; production of calcitriol may also be abnormal. Metabolic acidosis also contributes to the bone disease. Polyuria, salt wasting, and hypokalemia may be quite severe.

℞ **TREATMENT** Treatment includes phosphate supplements and calcitriol to heal the bone lesions, alkali for the acidosis, and liberal intake of salt and water. Alkali in the form of potassium salts may be particularly useful in the patient with RTA and hypokalemia. Aminoaciduria, glucosuria, hypouricemia, and low-molecular-weight proteinuria do not require treatment.

BIBLIOGRAPHY

DELIYSKA B et al: Association of Bartter's syndrome with vasculitis. Nephrol Dial Transplant 15:102, 2000

DEVUYST O et al: Intrarenal and subcellular distribution of the human chloride channel CLC-5 reveals a pathophysiologic basis for Dent's disease. Hum Mol Genet 8:247, 1999

DIXON PH et al: Mutational analysis of the PHEX gene in X-linked hypophosphatemia. J Clin Endocrinol Metab 83:3615, 1998

GELLER DS et al: Mutations in the mineralocorticoid receptor gene cause autosomal dominant pseudohypoaldosteronism type 1. Nat Genet 19:279, 1998

KARET FE et al: Mutations in the chloride-bicarbonate exchanger gene AE1 cause autosomal dominant but not autosomal recessive distal renal acidosis. Proc Natl Acad Sci 95:6337, 1998

KONRAD M et al: Familial juvenile nephronophthisis. J Mol Med 76:310, 1998

MONKAWA T et al: Novel mutations in thiazide-sensitive Na-Cl cotransporter gene of patients with Gitelman's syndrome. J Am Soc Nephrol 11:65, 2000

SCHEINMAN SJ et al: Genetic disorders of renal electrolyte transport. N Engl J Med 340: 1177, 1999

VAN ADELSBERG J: Polycystin-1 interacts with E-cadherin and the catenins—clues to the pathogenesis of cyst formation in ADPKD? Nephrol Dial Transplant 15:1, 2000

WANG JT et al: Genetics of vitamin D 1α-hydroxylase deficiency in 17 families. Am J Hum Genet 63:1694, 1998

WARNOCK DG: Liddle syndrome: An autosomal dominant form of human hypertension. Kidney Int 53:18, 1998

277 TUBULOINTERSTITIAL DISEASES OF THE KIDNEY

Alan S. L. Yu, Barry M. Brenner

Primary tubulointerstitial diseases of the kidney, as distinct from the disorders considered in Chaps. 274 and 275, are characterized by histologic and functional abnormalities that involve the tubules and interstitium to a greater degree than the glomeruli and renal vasculature (Table 277-1). Secondary tubulointerstitial disease occurs as a consequence of progressive glomerular or vascular injury. These disorders can be further divided into acute and chronic forms. The chronic group may be due to sustained insults by a factor or factors that initially cause acute disease or to a slower, progressive, cumulative insult without an identifiable acute episode. Morphologically, acute forms of these disorders are characterized by interstitial edema, often associated with cortical and medullary infiltration by both mononuclear cells and polymorphonuclear leukocytes, and patchy areas of tubule cell necrosis. In more chronic forms, interstitial fibrosis predominates, inflammatory cells are typically mononuclear, and abnormalities of the tubules tend to be more widespread, as evidenced by atrophy, luminal dilatation, and thickening of tubule basement membranes. Because of the nonspecific nature of the histology, particularly in chronic tubulointerstitial diseases, biopsy specimens rarely provide a specific diagnosis. The urine sediment is also unlikely to be diagnostic, except in allergic forms of acute tubulointerstitial disease, in which eosinophils may predominate in the urinary sediment.

Defects in renal function often accompany these alterations of tubule and interstitial structure (Table 277-2). Proximal tubule dysfunction may be manifested as selective reabsorptive defects leading to hypokalemia, aminoaciduria, glycosuria, phosphaturia, uricosuria, or bicarbonaturia (proximal or type II renal tubular acidosis; Chap. 276). In combination, these defects constitute the *Fanconi syndrome*. Proteinuria, predominantly of low-molecular-weight proteins, is usually modest, rarely exceeding 2 g/d.

Defects in urinary acidification and concentrating ability often represent the most troublesome of the tubule dysfunctions encountered in patients with tubulointerstitial disease. Hyperchloremic metabolic acidosis often develops at a relatively early stage in the course. Patients with this finding generally elaborate urine of maximal acidity (pH $\leq$ 5.3). In such patients the defect in acid excretion is usually caused by a reduced capacity to generate and excrete ammonia due to the reduction in renal mass. Preferential damage to the collecting ducts, as in amyloidosis or chronic obstructive uropathy, may also predispose to distal or type I renal tubular acidosis (RTA), characterized by high urine pH ($\geq$5.5) during spontaneous or NH_4Cl-induced metabolic acidosis. Patients with tubulointerstitial diseases affecting predominantly medullary and papillary structures may also exhibit concentrating de-

Table 277-1 Principal Causes of Tubulointerstitial Disease of the Kidney

ACUTE INTERSTITIAL NEPHRITIS

- Drugs[a]
  - Antibiotics (β-lactams, sulfonamides, quinolones, vancomycin, erythromycin, minocycline, rifampin, ethambutol, acyclovir)
  - Nonsteroidal anti-inflammatory drugs
  - Diuretics (thiazides, furosemide, triamterene)
  - Anticonvulsants (phenytoin, phenobarbital, carbamazepine, valproic acid)
  - Miscellaneous (captopril, H_2 receptor blockers, omeprazole, mesalazine, indinavir, allopurinol)
- Infection
  - Bacteria (*Streptococcus, Staphylococcus, Legionella, Salmonella, Brucella, Yersinia, Corynebacterium diphtheriae*)
  - Viruses (Epstein-Barr virus, cytomegalovirus, Hantavirus, HIV)
  - Miscellaneous (*Leptospira, Rickettsia, Mycoplasma*)
- Idiopathic
  - Tubulointerstitial nephritis-uveitis syndrome
  - Anti-tubule basement membrane disease
  - Sarcoidosis

CHRONIC TUBULOINTERSTITIAL DISEASES

- Hereditary renal diseases
  - Polycystic kidney disease[a] (Chap. 276)
  - Medullary cystic disease (Chap. 276)
  - Medullary sponge kidney (Chap. 276)
- Exogenous toxins
  - Analgesic nephropathy[a]
  - Lead nephropathy
  - Miscellaneous nephrotoxins (e.g. lithium[a], cyclosporine[a], heavy metals, slimming regimens with Chinese herbs)
- Metabolic toxins
  - Hyperuricemia[a]
  - Hypercalcemia
  - Miscellaneous metabolic toxins (e.g., hypokalemia, hyperoxaluria, cystinosis, Fabry's disease)
- Autoimmune disorders
  - Sjögren's syndrome
- Neoplastic disorders
  - Leukemia
  - Lymphoma
  - Multiple myeloma[a]
- Miscellaneous disorders
  - Sickle cell nephropathy
  - Chronic pyelonephritis
  - Chronic urinary tract obstruction
  - Vesicoureteral reflux[a]
  - Radiation nephritis
  - Balkan nephropathy
  - Tubulointerstitial disease secondary to glomerular and vascular disease

[a] Common

Table 277-2 Functional Consequences of Tubulointerstitial Disease

Defect	Cause(s)
Reduced glomerular filtration rate[a]	Obliteration of microvasculature and obstruction of tubules
Fanconi syndrome	Damage to proximal tubular reabsorption of glucose, amino acids, phosphate, and bicarbonate
Hyperchloremic acidosis[a]	1. Reduced ammonia production 2. Inability to acidify the collecting duct fluid (distal renal tubular acidosis) 3. Proximal bicarbonate wasting
Tubular or small-molecular-weight proteinuria[a]	Failure of proximal tubule protein reabsorption
Polyuria, isothenuria[a]	Damage to medullary tubules and vasculature
Hyperkalemia[a]	Potassium secretory defects including aldosterone resistance
Salt wasting	Distal tubular damage with impaired sodium reabsorption

[a] Common

fects, with resultant nocturia and polyuria. Analgesic nephropathy and sickle cell disease are prototypes of this form of injury.

TOXINS

Although the kidneys constitute less than 1% of total body mass, they receive approximately 20% of the cardiac output, and 90% or more of renal blood flow is distributed to the renal cortex. Exposure of tubules and interstitium of the renal cortex to circulating toxins is therefore greater than for most other tissues. Transport processes in renal tubules contribute further to the intrarenal accumulation of toxins, enhancing local concentrations of noxious agents. The urinary concentrating mechanism can also establish high levels of toxins within medullary and papillary portions of the kidney, predisposing these regions to chemical injury. Finally, the relatively acid pH of the fluid within most nephron segments may affect the ionization characteristics of potentially toxic compounds and thereby influence local concentration and solubility. Although these processes render the kidney vulnerable to toxic injury, the role of nephrotoxins in renal damage often goes unrecognized because the manifestations of such injury are usually nonspecific in nature and insidious in onset. Diagnosis largely depends on a history of exposure to a certain toxin. Particular attention should be paid to the occupational history, as well as to an assessment of exposure—current and remote—to drugs, especially antibiotics and analgesics, and to dietary supplements or herbal remedies. The recognition of a potential association between a patient's renal disease and exposure to a nephrotoxin is crucial, because, unlike many other forms of renal disease, progression of the functional and morphologic abnormalities associated with toxin-induced nephropathies may be prevented, and even reversed, by eliminating additional exposure.

EXOGENOUS TOXINS **Analgesic Nephropathy** A distinct clinicopathologic syndrome has been described in heavy users of analgesic mixtures containing phenacetin in combination with aspirin, acetaminophen, or caffeine. These individuals have an approximately 20-fold increased risk of end-stage renal disease (ESRD). Analgesic nephropathy has been an important cause of chronic renal failure in Australia, Switzerland, Sweden, Belgium, and the southeastern United States.

Morphologically, analgesic nephropathy is characterized by papillary necrosis and tubulointerstitial inflammation. At an early stage, damage to the vascular supply of the inner medulla (vasa recta) leads to a local interstitial inflammatory reaction and, eventually, to papillary ischemia, necrosis, fibrosis, and calcification. The susceptibility of the renal papillae to damage by phenacetin is believed to be related to the establishment of a renal gradient for its acetaminophen metabolite, resulting in papillary tip concentrations tenfold higher than those in renal cortex. Hydration dissipates this gradient and may explain the protective effect of this maneuver in preventing phenacetin-induced papillary necrosis in animals. Aspirin in these analgesic compounds contributes to renal injury by uncoupling oxidative phosphorylation in renal mitochondria and by inhibiting the synthesis of renal prostaglandins, which are potent endogenous renal vasodilator hormones.

Analgesic nephropathy occurs some three to five times more commonly in women than in men. A direct relationship exists between the total amount of analgesic compounds ingested and the degree of renal impairment. The intake of 1.0 g phenacetin per day for 1 to 3 years or the total ingestion of 2 kg phenacetin in combination with other analgesics appears to represent minimum requirements for the development of analgesic nephropathy.

Whether single-ingredient analgesics other than phenacetin, when used alone, cause renal disease is controversial. Recent reports have suggested a two- to threefold increase in the risk of ESRD among regular users of acetaminophen, and perhaps nonsteroidal anti-inflammatory drugs (NSAIDs), but not among regular users of aspirin. Until conclusive evidence is available, physicians should consider screening regular users of acetaminophen and NSAIDs for evidence of renal disease.

In analgesic nephropathy, renal function usually declines gradually, in association with chronic necrosis of papillae and diffuse tubulointerstitial damage to the renal cortex. Occasionally, papillary necrosis may be associated with hematuria and even renal colic owing to obstruction of a ureter by necrotic tissue. More than half of patients with analgesic nephropathy have pyuria, which, if persistently associated with sterile urine, provides an important clue to the diagnosis. Nonetheless, active pyelonephritis may coexist in patients with analgesic nephropathy. Proteinuria, if present, is typically mild (< 1 g/d). Patients with analgesic nephropathy are usually unable to generate maximally concentrated urine, reflecting the underlying medullary and papillary damage. An acquired form of distal RTA may contribute to the development of *nephrocalcinosis.* The occurrence of anemia out of proportion to the degree of azotemia also may provide a clue to the diagnosis of analgesic nephropathy. When analgesic nephropathy has progressed to renal insufficiency, the kidneys usually appear bilaterally shrunken on intravenous pyelography, and the calyces are deformed. A "ring sign" on the pyelogram is pathognomonic of papillary necrosis and represents the radiolucent sloughed papilla surrounded by the radiodense contrast material in the calyx. Renal sonography may reveal papillary calcifications surrounding the central sinus complex in a "garland" pattern. Transitional cell carcinoma may develop in the urinary pelvis or ureters as a late complication of analgesic abuse.

Rx TREATMENT Every effort must be made to convince the patient who ingests excessive amounts of analgesic combinations to discontinue this hazardous practice. When renal damage is at an early stage, cessation of abuse usually arrests the progression of the nephrotoxic process; not infrequently, overall renal function improves with time. With continued abuse, however, progressive renal damage leads invariably to chronic renal failure.

Lead Nephropathy (See also Chap. 395) Lead intoxication may produce a chronic tubulointerstitial renal disease. Children who repeatedly ingest lead-based paints may develop kidney disease as adults. Significant occupational exposure may occur in a diverse variety of workplaces where lead containing metals or paints are heated to high temperatures, such as battery factories, smelters, salvage yards, and firing ranges. Alcohol, illegally distilled in an apparatus constructed from automobile radiators (so-called moonshine), is another cause of lead poisoning. Environmental lead exposure, particularly in industrial regions, may be great enough to produce changes in renal function.

Tubule transport processes enhance the accumulation of lead within renal cells, particularly in the proximal convoluted tubule, leading to cell degeneration, mitochondrial swelling, and eosinophilic intranuclear inclusion bodies rich in lead. In addition to tubule degeneration and atrophy, lead nephropathy is associated with ischemic changes in the glomeruli, fibrosis of the adventitia of small renal arterioles, and focal areas of cortical scarring. Eventually, the kidneys become atrophic. Urinary excretion of lead, porphyrin precursors such as δ-aminolevulinic acid and coproporphyrin, and urobilinogen, may be increased. Patients with chronic lead nephropathy are characteristically *hyperuricemic*, a consequence of enhanced reabsorption of filtered urate. Acute gouty arthritis (so-called saturnine gout) develops in about 50% of patients with lead nephropathy, in striking contrast to other forms of chronic renal failure in which de novo gout is rare (Chap. 347). Hypertension is also a complication. Therefore, in any patient with slowly progressive renal failure, atrophic kidneys, gout, and hypertension, the diagnosis of lead intoxication should be considered. Features of acute lead intoxication (abdominal colic, anemia, peripheral neuropathy, and encephalopathy) are usually absent.

The diagnosis may be suspected by finding elevated serum levels of lead. However, because blood levels may not be elevated even in the presence of a toxic total-body burden of lead, the quantitation of lead excretion following infusion of the chelating agent calcium disodium edetate is a more reliable indicator of serious lead exposure. While urinary excretion of more than 0.6 mg/d of lead is generally considered to be indicative of overt or potential toxicity, recent evidence suggests that even lead burdens of 0.15 to 0.6 mg/d may cause progressive loss of renal function.

℞ TREATMENT Treatment includes removing the patient from the source of exposure and augmenting lead excretion with a chelating agent such as calcium disodium edetate.

Miscellaneous Nephrotoxins Use of *lithium salts* for bipolar disorder has been associated with polyuria and polydipsia caused by tubulointerstitial disease. There are only rare reports of chronic renal insufficiency attributable to this agent. Renal function should be followed in patients taking this drug, and caution should be exercised if lithium is employed in patients with underlying renal disease.

The immunosuppressant *cyclosporine* causes both acute and chronic renal injury. The acute injury and the use of cyclosporine in transplantation are discussed in Chap. 272. The chronic injury results in an irreversible reduction in glomerular filtration rate (GFR), with mild proteinuria and arterial hypertension. Hyperkalemia is a relatively common complication and results in part from tubule resistance to aldosterone. Hypomagnesemia due to urinary magnesium wasting is less common but can cause hypocalcemia. The histologic changes in renal tissue include patchy interstitial fibrosis and tubular atrophy. In addition, the intrarenal vasculature often demonstrates hyalinosis, and focal segmental glomerular sclerosis can be present as well. Fibrosis may be the result of a cyclosporine-induced increase in renal collagen production. Vasoconstrictive mediators, such as angiotensin II, or vasoconstriction itself may also play a role in chronic cyclosporine toxicity. In patients receiving this drug for renal transplantation (Chap. 272), chronic rejection and recurrence of the primary disease may coincide with chronic cyclosporine injury, and on clinical grounds, distinction among these may be difficult. Although most patients experience stable, albeit reduced, renal function, progressive renal injury can occur without a progressive reduction in GFR. Dose reduction appears to mitigate cyclosporine-associated renal fibrosis but may increase the risk of rejection and graft loss. The optimal dosage of cyclosporine in renal transplantation remains controversial. Treatment of any associated arterial hypertension may lessen renal injury.

Many agents that commonly lead to acute renal failure are also capable of producing tubulointerstitial injury (Chap. 269). These include antibiotics (e.g., aminoglycosides, amphotericin B), radiographic contrast agents, various hydrocarbons (e.g., carbon tetrachloride), and heavy metals (e.g., mercury, cadmium, and bismuth).

METABOLIC TOXINS Acute Uric Acid Nephropathy (See also Chap. 322) Acute overproduction of uric acid and extreme hyperuricemia often lead to a rapidly progressive renal insufficiency, so-called acute uric acid nephropathy. This tubulointerstitial disease is usually seen as part of the tumor lysis syndrome in patients given cytotoxic drugs for the treatment of lymphoproliferative or myeloproliferative disorders but may also occur in these patients before such treatment is begun. The pathologic changes are largely the result of deposition of uric acid crystals in the kidneys and their collecting systems, leading to partial or complete obstruction of collecting ducts, renal pelvis, or ureter. Since obstruction is often bilateral, patients typically show the clinical course of acute renal failure, characterized by oliguria and rapidly rising serum creatinine concentration. In the early phase uric acid crystals can be found in urine, usually in association with microscopic or gross hematuria. Hyperuricemia can also be a consequence of renal failure of any etiology. The finding of a urine uric acid–creatinine ratio greater than 1 mg/mg (0.7 mol/mol) distinguishes acute uric acid nephropathy from other causes of renal failure.

Prevention of hyperuricemia in patients at risk by treatment with allopurinol in doses of 200 to 800 mg/d prior to cytotoxic therapy reduces the danger of acute uric acid nephropathy. Once hyperuricemia develops, however, efforts should be directed to preventing deposition of uric acid within the urinary tract. Increasing urine volume with potent diuretics (furosemide or mannitol) effectively lowers intratubular uric acid concentrations, and alkalinization of the urine to pH 7 or greater with sodium bicarbonate and/or a carbonic anhydrase inhibitor (acetazolamide) enhances uric acid solubility. If these efforts, together with allopurinol therapy, are ineffective in preventing acute renal failure, dialysis should be instituted to lower the serum uric acid concentration as well as to treat the acute manifestations of uremia.

Gouty Nephropathy (See also Chap. 322) Patients with less severe but prolonged forms of hyperuricemia are predisposed to a more chronic tubulointerstitial disorder, often referred to as *gouty nephropathy*. The severity of renal involvement correlates with the duration and magnitude of the elevation of the serum uric acid concentration. Histologically, the distinctive feature of gouty nephropathy is the presence of crystalline deposits of uric acid and monosodium urate salts in kidney parenchyma. These deposits not only cause intrarenal obstruction but also incite an inflammatory response, leading to lymphocytic infiltration, foreign-body giant cell reaction, and eventual fibrosis, especially of medullary and papillary regions of the kidney. Bacteriuria and pyelonephritis occur in about one-fourth of cases, presumably as complications of intrarenal urinary stasis. Since patients with gout frequently suffer from hypertension and hyperlipidemia, degenerative changes of the renal arterioles may constitute a striking feature of the histologic abnormality, often out of proportion to other morphologic defects. Clinically, gouty nephropathy is an insidious cause of renal insufficiency. Early in its course, GFR may be near normal, often despite focal morphologic changes in medullary and cortical interstitium, proteinuria, and diminished urinary concentrating ability. Whether reducing serum uric acid levels with allopurinol exerts a beneficial effect on the kidney remains to be demonstrated. Although such undesirable consequences of hyperuricemia as gout and uric acid stones respond well to allopurinol, use of this drug in asymptomatic hyperuricemia has not been shown to improve renal function consistently. On the other hand, uricosuric agents such as probenecid, which may increase uric acid stone production, clearly have no role in the treatment of renal disease associated with hyperuricemia.

Hypercalcemic Nephropathy (See also Chap. 341) Chronic hypercalcemia, as occurs in primary hyperparathyroidism, sarcoidosis, multiple myeloma, vitamin D intoxication, or metastatic bone disease, can cause tubulointerstitial damage and progressive renal insufficiency. The earliest lesion is a focal degenerative change in renal epithelia, primarily in collecting ducts, distal convoluted tubules, and loops of Henle. Tubule cell necrosis leads to nephron obstruction and stasis of intrarenal urine, favoring local precipitation of calcium salts and infection. Dilatation and atrophy of tubules eventually occur, as do interstitial fibrosis, mononuclear leukocyte infiltration, and interstitial calcium deposition (nephrocalcinosis). Calcium deposition also may occur in glomeruli and the walls of renal arterioles.

Clinically, the most striking defect is an inability to concentrate the urine maximally, resulting in polyuria and nocturia. Defective transport of NaCl in the ascending limb of Henle's loop is responsible, at least in part, for this concentrating defect. Additionally, reduced collecting duct responsiveness to vasopressin may contribute. Reductions in GFR and renal blood flow also occur, both in acute severe hypercalcemia and with prolonged hypercalcemia of lesser severity. Distal RTA and sodium and potassium wasting also have been described in these chronic states. Eventually, uncontrolled hypercalcemia leads to severe tubulointerstitial damage and overt renal failure. Abdominal x-rays may demonstrate nephrocalcinosis as well as nephrolithiasis, the latter due to the hypercalciuria that often accompanies hypercalcemia.

℞ TREATMENT This consists of reducing the serum calcium concentration toward normal and correcting the primary abnormality of calcium metabolism. The management of hypercalcemia is discussed in Chap. 341. Prognosis for recovery of renal function depends on the severity of the renal lesion at the time hypercalcemia is corrected. Renal dysfunction of acute hypercalcemia may be completely reversible. Gradual, progressive renal insufficiency related to chronic hypercalcemia, however, may not improve with correction of the calcium disorder. Nonetheless, every effort should be made to return serum calcium concentration to normal to minimize further loss of renal function.

Hypokalemic Nephropathy (See also Chap. 49) Disturbances of renal structure and function occur commonly in patients with moderate to severe potassium depletion of at least several weeks' duration. Histologically, renal epithelial cells are often seen to contain numerous vacuoles, most marked in proximal tubules. Glomeruli are reduced in size and may become sclerotic. Whether prolonged or recurrent potassium deficiency results in irreversible tubulointerstitial fibrosis, scarring, and atrophy is unresolved. Loss of urinary concentrating ability is the most commonly encountered functional defect and may be due to defective operation of the countercurrent multiplier system and elevated intrarenal prostaglandins. Nocturia, polyuria, and polydipsia are frequent symptoms. Urinalysis often reveals no abnormalities except for mild proteinuria. Serum creatinine and urea nitrogen concentrations usually remain within normal limits.

Miscellaneous Metabolic Toxins Urinary oxalate, derived from the metabolism of glycine and, to a variable extent, from ingested oxalate, may deposit as insoluble intratubular calcium oxalate crystals and result in chronic tubulointerstitial damage in patients with hereditary or acquired forms of *hyperoxaluria*. *Cystinosis* and *Fabry's disease* are other hereditary depositional disorders affecting the renal tubules and interstitium (Chap. 276).

RENAL PARENCHYMAL DISEASE ASSOCIATED WITH EXTRARENAL NEOPLASM

Except for the glomerulopathies associated with lymphomas and several solid tumors (Chap. 275), the renal manifestations of primary extrarenal neoplastic processes are confined mainly to the interstitium and tubules. Although metastatic renal involvement by solid tumors is unusual, the kidneys are often invaded by neoplastic cells in various lymphomas and leukemias and in multiple myeloma. In postmortem studies of patients with *lymphoma*, renal involvement is found in approximately half. The involvement may be focal, in the form of multiple discrete nodules, or diffuse, with lymphomatous infiltration throughout the renal parenchyma. Diffuse infiltration is seen most commonly in lymphomas other than Hodgkin's disease. There may be flank pain related to massive renal infiltration, and x-rays may show enlargement of one or both kidneys. Renal insufficiency occurs in a minority of cases, and overt uremia is rare. Treatment of the primary disease may improve renal function in these cases.

The kidneys are also commonly involved in various forms of *leukemia*. At postmortem examination, bilateral renal involvement is present in approximately 50% of cases. As with lymphoma, uremia is rarely, if ever, a consequence of leukemic infiltration of the kidneys. The kidneys can also be involved in leukemias because of the associated high incidence of hyperuricemia, hypercalcemia, and lysozymuria. The myelogenous leukemias, particularly of the monocytic type, may be complicated by tubule defects involving potassium and magnesium wasting.

PLASMA CELL DYSCRASIAS Several glomerular and tubulointerstitial disorders may occur in association with plasma cell dyscrasias (Table 277-3; Chap. 113). Infiltration of the kidneys with myeloma cells is infrequent. When it occurs, the process is usually focal, so renal insufficiency from this cause is also uncommon. The more usual lesion is *myeloma kidney*, characterized histologically by atrophic tubules, many with eosinophilic intraluminal casts, and numerous multinucleated giant cells within tubule walls and in the interstitium. The frequent occurrence of myeloma kidney in patients with

Table 277-3 Renal Diseases Associated with Plasma Cell Dyscrasias

Disease	Clinical Manifestations
Plasma cell infiltration (Chap. 113)	None
Hypercalcemia[a] (Chap. 341)	Acute renal failure, diabetes insipidus
Myeloma kidney[a] (Chap. 113)	Acute renal failure, Fanconi syndrome, diabetes insipidus
Amyloidosis[a] (Chaps. 275 and 319)	Nephrotic syndrome, distal renal tubular acidosis, diabetes insipidus, renal failure
Light chain deposition disease (Chap. 275)	Nephrotic syndrome, renal failure
Type I/II cryoglobulinemia (Chaps. 273 and 317)	Hematuria, proteinuria, vasculitis, renal failure
Immunotactoid glomerulopathy (Chap. 273)	Nephrotic syndrome, hypertension, renal failure

[a] Common

Bence Jones proteinuria has suggested a causal relation. Bence Jones proteins are thought to cause myeloma kidney through direct toxicity to renal tubule cells. In addition, Bence Jones proteins may precipitate within the distal nephron where the high concentrations of these proteins and the acid composition of the tubule fluid favor intraluminal cast formation and intrarenal obstruction. Occasionally, acute renal failure occurs after intravenous pyelography in patients with multiple myeloma and is believed to result from the further precipitation of Bence Jones proteins induced by dehydration prior to radiographic study. Dehydration of the patient with myeloma in preparation for intravenous pyelography should therefore be avoided. Multiple myeloma may also affect the kidneys indirectly. Hypercalcemia or hyperuricemia may lead to the nephropathies described above. Proximal tubule disorders are also seen occasionally, including type II proximal RTA and the Fanconi syndrome.

AMYLOIDOSIS (See also Chaps. 275 and 319) Glomerular pathology usually predominates and leads to heavy proteinuria and azotemia. However, tubule function may also be deranged, giving rise to a nephrogenic diabetes insipidus and to distal (type I) RTA. In several cases these functional abnormalities correlated with peritubular deposition of amyloid, particularly in areas surrounding vasa rectae, loops of Henle, and collecting ducts. Bilateral enlargement of the kidneys, especially in a patient with massive proteinuria and tubule dysfunction, should raise the possibility of amyloid renal disease.

IMMUNE DISORDERS

ALLERGIC INTERSTITIAL NEPHRITIS An acute diffuse tubulointerstitial reaction may result from hypersensitivity to a number of drugs, including sulfonamides, many penicillins and cephalosporins, the fluoroquinolone antibiotics ciprofloxacin and norfloxacin, and the antituberculous drugs isoniazid and rifampin. Acute tubulointerstitial damage has also occurred after use of thiazide and loop diuretics, antiulcer medications (cimetidine, ranitidine, and omeprazole), and NSAIDs. Of note, the tubulointerstitial nephropathy that develops in some patients taking NSAIDs may be associated with nephrotic-range proteinuria and histologic evidence of either minimal change or membranous glomerulopathy. Grossly, the kidneys are usually enlarged. Histologically, the glomeruli appear normal. The principal pathologic abnormalities are in the interstitium of the kidney, which reveals pronounced edema and infiltration with polymorphonuclear leukocytes, lymphocytes, plasma cells, and, in some cases, large numbers of eosinophils. If the process is severe, tubule cell necrosis and regeneration may also be apparent. Immunofluorescence studies have either been unrevealing or demonstrated a linear pattern of immunoglobulin and complement deposition along tubule basement membranes. In a few cases of methicillin-induced acute tubulointerstitial disease, circulating anti-tubule basement membrane antibodies have also been found, suggesting that autoantibody formation may have been induced by the penicilloyl hapten of methicillin (by conjugation of hapten with tubule basement membrane proteins, thereby altering the native antigenicity of the basement membrane).

Most patients require several weeks of drug exposure before developing evidence of renal injury. Rare cases have occurred after only a few doses or after a year of more of use. Azotemia is usually present; a diagnostic triad of fever, skin rash, and peripheral blood eosinophilia is highly suggestive of acute tubulointerstitial nephritis but is often absent. Examination of the urine sediment reveals hematuria and often pyuria; occasionally, eosinophils may be present. Proteinuria is usually mild to moderate, except in cases of NSAID-induced tubulointerstitial nephritis with minimal change glomerulopathy. The clinical picture may be confused with acute glomerulonephritis, but when acute azotemia and hematuria are accompanied by eosinophilia, skin rash, and a history of drug exposure, a hypersensitivity reaction leading to acute tubulointerstitial nephritis should be regarded as the leading diagnostic possibility. Discontinuation of the drug usually results in complete reversal of the renal injury; rarely, renal damage may be irreversible. Glucocorticoids may accelerate renal recovery, but their value has not been definitively established.

SJÖGREN'S SYNDROME (See also Chap. 314) When the kidneys are involved in this disorder, the predominant histologic findings are those of chronic tubulointerstitial disease. Interstitial infiltrates are composed primarily of lymphocytes, causing the histology of the renal parenchyma in these patients to resemble that of the salivary and lacrimal glands. Renal functional defects include diminished urinary concentrating ability and distal (type I) RTA. Urinalysis may show pyuria (predominantly lymphocyturia) and mild proteinuria.

TUBULOINTERSTITIAL ABNORMALITIES ASSOCIATED WITH GLOMERULONEPHRITIS Primary glomerulopathies are often associated with damage to tubules and the interstitium. Occasionally, the primary disorder may affect glomeruli and tubules directly. For example, in more than half of patients with the nephropathy of systemic lupus erythematosus, deposits of immune complexes can be identified in tubule basement membranes, usually accompanied by an interstitial mononuclear inflammatory reaction. Similarly, in many patients with glomerulonephritis associated with anti-glomerular basement membrane antibody, the same antibody is reactive against tubule basement membranes as well. More frequently, tubulointerstitial damage is a secondary consequence of glomerular dysfunction. The extent of tubulointerstitial fibrosis correlates closely with the degree of renal impairment. Potential mechanisms by which glomerular disease might cause tublointerstitial injury include glomerular leak of plasma proteins toxic to epithelial cells, activation of tubule epithelial cells by glomerulus-derived cytokines, reduced peritubular blood flow leading to downstream tubulointerstitial ischemia, and hyperfunction of remnant tubules.

MISCELLANEOUS DISORDERS

VESICOURETERAL REFLUX (See also Chap. 281) When the function of the ureterovesical junction is impaired, urine may reflux into the ureters due to the high intravesical pressure that develops during voiding. Clinically, reflux is often detected on the voiding and postvoiding films obtained during intravenous pyelography, although voiding cystourethrography may be required for definitive diagnosis. Bladder infection may ascend the urinary tract to the kidneys through incompetent ureterovesical sphincters. Not surprisingly, therefore, reflux is often discovered in patients with acute and/or chronic urinary tract infections. With more severe degrees of reflux, characterized by dilatation of ureters and renal pelves, progressive renal damage often appears, and although active infection may also be present, uncertainty exists as to the necessity of infection in producing the scarred kidney of reflux nephropathy. Substantial proteinuria is often present, and glomerular lesions similar to those of idiopathic focal glomerulosclerosis (Chap. 274) are often found in addition to the changes of chronic tubulointerstitial disease. Surgical correction of reflux is usually necessary only with the more severe degrees of reflux since renal damage correlates with the extent of reflux. Obviously, if extensive glomerulosclerosis already exists, urologic repair may no longer be warranted.

RADIATION NEPHRITIS Renal dysfunction can be expected to occur if 23 Gy (2300 rad) or more of x-ray irradiation is administered to both kidneys during a period of 5 weeks or less. Histologic examination of the kidneys reveals hyalinized glomeruli, atrophic tubules, extensive interstitial fibrosis, and hyalinization of the media of renal arterioles. Radiation-induced renal ischemia is believed to be the main pathogenic factor responsible for the tubulointerstitial damage, which may not become evident clinically for months after completion of radiation. The presentation of acute radiation nephritis includes rapidly progressive azotemia, moderate to malignant hypertension, anemia, and proteinuria that may reach the nephrotic range. More than 50% progress to chronic renal failure. A more insidious form is characterized by slower development of azotemia, anemia, and nephrotic syndrome. Malignant hypertension may follow unilateral renal irradiation and resolve with ipsilateral nephrectomy. Radiation nephritis has all but vanished because of heightened awareness of its pathogenesis by radiotherapists.

ACKNOWLEDGMENT

Dr. Elliott Levy and Dr. Thomas H. Hostetter were co-authors of this chapter in the 14th edition and some of the material in that chapter is carried forward to the present edition.

BIBLIOGRAPHY

ADLER SG et al: Hypersensitivity phenomena and the kidney: Role of drugs and environmental agents. Am J Kidney Dis 5:75, 1985

ARANT BS: Reflux nephropathy. Kidney 21:19, 1989

BENNETT WM: Lead nephropathy. Kidney Int 28:218, 1985

———, DEBROE ME: Analgesic nephropathy. A preventable renal disease. N Engl J Med 320:1269, 1989

BOTON R et al: Prevalence, pathogenesis, and treatment of renal dysfunction associated with chronic lithium therapy. Am J Kidney Dis 10:329, 1987

BRUZZI I et al: Role of increased glomerular protein traffic in the progression of renal failure. Kidney Int 52(Suppl 62):S-29, 1997

CAMERON JS: Immunologically mediated interstitial nephritis: Primary and secondary. Adv Nephrol 18:207, 1989

DELZELL E, SHAPIRO S: A review of epidemiologic studies of nonnarcotic analgesics and chronic renal disease. Medicine 77:102, 1998

KELLY CJ, NEILSON EG: Tubulointerstitial diseases, in *Brenner and Rector's The Kidney*, 6th ed, BM Brenner (ed). Philadelphia, Saunders, 2000 pp 1509–1536

KYLE RA: Monoclonal proteins and renal disease. Annu Rev Med 45:71, 1994

LIN J et al: Chelation therapy for patients with elevated body lead burden and progressive renal insufficiency: A randomized, controlled trial. Ann Intern Med 130:7, 1999

MYERS BD et al: The long-term course of cyclosporine-associated chronic nephropathy. Kidney Int 33:590, 1988

278

Kamal F. Badr, Barry M. Brenner

VASCULAR INJURY TO THE KIDNEY

ACE angiotensin-converting enzyme	MRA magnetic resonance angiography
AST aspartate aminotransferase	MRI magnetic resonance imaging
BUN blood urea nitrogen	PRA plasma renin activity
FGS focal segmental sclerosis	RVT renal vein thrombosis
GFR glomerular filtration rate	TTP thrombotic thrombocytopenic purpura
HUS hemolytic uremic syndrome	VCAM-1 vascular cell adhesion molecule-1
LDH lactic dehydrogenase	

Adequate delivery of blood to the glomerular capillary network is crucial for glomerular filtration and overall salt and water balance. Thus,

Table 278-1 Clinical Presentations of Ischemic Renal Disease

Acute renal failure
Progressive azotemia in a patient with known renovascular hypertension (usually on medical therapy)
Unexplained progressive azotemia in an elderly patient with or without refractory hypertension
Hypertension and azotemia in a renal transplant patient

in addition to the threat to the viability of renal tissue, vascular injury to the kidney may compromise the maintenance of body fluid volume and composition. Involvement of the renal vessels by atherosclerotic, hypertensive, embolic, inflammatory, and hematologic disorders is usually a manifestation of generalized vascular pathology. The morphologic and clinical responses to these insults and the unique renal vasculopathy associated with the toxemias of pregnancy are considered in this chapter.

THROMBOEMBOLIC DISEASES OF THE RENAL ARTERIES Thrombosis of the major renal arteries or their branches is an important cause of deterioration of renal function, especially in the elderly. It is often difficult to diagnose and therefore requires a high index of suspicion. Thrombosis may occur as a result of intrinsic pathology in the renal vessels (posttraumatic, atherosclerotic, or inflammatory) or as a result of emboli originating in distant vessels, most commonly fat emboli, emboli originating in the left heart (mural thrombi following myocardial infarction, bacterial endocarditis, or aseptic vegetations), or "paradoxical" emboli passing from the right side of the circulation via a patent foramen ovale or atrial septal defect. Renal emboli are bilateral in 15 to 30% of cases.

The clinical presentation is variable, depending on the time course and the extent of the occlusive event. Acute thrombosis and infarction, such as follows embolization, may result in sudden onset of flank pain and tenderness, fever, hematuria, leukocytosis, nausea, and vomiting. If infarction occurs, renal enzymes may be elevated, namely aspartate aminotransferase (AST), lactic dehydrogenase (LDH; most reliable), and alkaline phosphatase, which rise and fall in the order listed. Urinary lactic dehydrogenase and alkaline phosphatase also may increase after infarction. Renal function deteriorates acutely, leading in bilateral thrombosis to acute oliguric renal failure. More gradual (i.e., atherosclerotic) occlusion of a single renal artery may go undetected. A spectrum of clinical presentations lies between these two extremes (Table 278-1). Hypertension usually follows renal infarction and results from renin release in the peri-infarction zone. Hypertension is usually transient but may be persistent. Diagnosis is established by renal arteriography.

℞ TREATMENT Management of *acute* renal arterial thrombosis includes surgical intervention, anticoagulant therapy, conservative and supportive therapy, and control of hypertension. The choice of treatment depends mainly on (1) the condition of the patient, in particular the patient's ability to withstand major surgery, and (2) the extent of renovascular occlusion and amount of renal mass at risk of infarction. In general, supportive care and anticoagulant therapy are indicated in unilateral disease. In bilateral thrombosis, medical and surgical therapies yield comparable results. Twenty-five percent of patients die during the acute episode, usually from extrarenal complications. In *chronic* ischemic renal disease, surgical revascularization is more likely to preserve and improve renal function and to control the hypertension (see below).

ATHEROEMBOLIC DISEASE OF THE RENAL ARTERIES Atheroembolic disease typically results from multiple showers of cholesterol-containing microemboli dislodged from atheromatous plaques in large arteries. Such emboli occlude small (150- to 200-μm diameter) vessels in the kidneys and in other organs (retina, brain, pancreas, muscles, skin, and extremities). Atheroembolic disease usually occurs in an elderly individual with atherosclerotic disease elsewhere and usually follows aortic surgery or renal or coronary arteriography. Spontaneous atheroembolic disease has also been reported. Manifestations include deterioration of renal function (sudden or gradual), mild proteinuria, microscopic hematuria, and leukocyturia. Urine volume may remain normal or fall to oliguric levels depending on severity. Renal ischemia can induce or exacerbate preexisting hypertension. In elderly patients with mild to moderate cholesterol embolization, the remaining nephrons may subsequently undergo injury, likely a result of hyperfiltration, which may lead to nephrotic-range proteinuria. Renal biopsy reveals "focal segmental sclerosis" (FGS). Renal function deteriorates at a slower rate in these individuals than in patients with more substantial embolic burdens, and they would be expected to benefit from angiotensin-converting enzyme (ACE) inhibitor therapy aimed at lowering intraglomerular pressures in remnant nephrons, even if their systemic blood pressure is in the "normal" range.

Antemortem diagnosis of atherosclerotic renal emboli is difficult. The demonstration of cholesterol emboli in the retina is helpful, but a firm diagnosis is established only by demonstration of cholesterol crystals in the smaller arteries and arterioles in renal biopsy or autopsy specimens. These also may be seen in asymptomatic skeletal muscle or skin. No specific treatment is available.

RENAL VEIN THROMBOSIS (RVT) Thrombosis of one or both main renal veins occurs in a variety of settings (Table 278-2). The pathogenesis is not always clear, particularly when it occurs in so-called hypercoagulable states such as may develop in pregnant women, users of oral contraceptives, subjects with nephrotic syndrome, or dehydrated infants. Nephrotic syndrome accompanying membranous glomerulopathy and certain carcinomas seems to predispose to the development of RVT, which occurs in 10 to 50% of patients with these disorders. RVT may exacerbate preexisting proteinuria but is infrequently the cause of the nephrotic syndrome.

The clinical manifestations depend on the severity and abruptness of its occurrence. Acute cases occur typically in children and are characterized by sudden loss of renal function, often accompanied by fever, chills, lumbar tenderness (with kidney enlargement), leukocytosis, and hematuria. Hemorrhagic infarction and renal rupture may lead to hypovolemic shock. In young adults RVT is usually suspected from an unexpected and relatively acute or subacute deterioration of renal function and/or exacerbation of proteinuria and hematuria in the appropriate clinical setting (underlying nephrotic syndrome, trauma, pregnancy, oral contraceptive use). In cases of gradual thrombosis, usually occurring in the elderly, the only manifestation may be recurrent pulmonary emboli or development of hypertension. A Fanconi-like syndrome and proximal renal tubular acidosis have been described.

The definitive diagnosis can only be established through selective renal venography with visualization of the occluding thrombus. Short of angiography, magnetic resonance imaging (MRI) often provides definitive evidence of thrombus.

℞ TREATMENT Treatment consists of anticoagulation, the main purpose of which is prevention of pulmonary embolization, although some authors have also claimed improvement in renal function and proteinuria. Encouraging reports have appeared concerning the use of streptokinase. Spontaneous recanalization with clinical improvement also has been observed. Anticoagulant therapy is more rewarding in the acute thrombosis seen in younger individuals. Nephrectomy is

Table 278-2 Conditions Associated with Renal Vein Thrombosis

Trauma
Extrinsic compression (lymph nodes, aortic aneurysm, tumor)
Invasion by renal cell carcinoma
Dehydration (infants)
Nephrotic syndrome
Pregnancy or oral contraceptives

advocated in infants with life-threatening renal infarction. Thrombectomy is effective in some cases.

RENAL ARTERY STENOSIS/ISCHEMIC RENAL DISEASE Stenosis of the main renal artery and/or its major branches accounts for 2 to 5% of hypertension (see Chap. 246). The common cause in the middle-aged and elderly is an atheromatous plaque at the origin of the renal artery. In a large unselected autopsy series, stenosis producing > 50% renal artery diameter reduction was found in 18% of those between 65 and 74 years of age and in 42% of those older than 75 years. Bilateral involvement was found in half of the affected cases in both age groups. Ischemic renal disease has emerged as an important cause of end-stage renal disease. It should be considered seriously in elderly individuals, particularly in those with evidence of atherosclerotic arterial disease elsewhere. In elderly patients with myocardial infarction or symptomatic peripheral vascular disease, the incidence of renal arterial stenosis can be up to 40%. In younger women, stenosis is due to intrinsic structural abnormalities of the arterial wall caused by a heterogeneous group of lesions termed *fibromuscular dysplasia*.

Renal artery stenosis should be suspected when hypertension develops in a previously normotensive individual over 50 years of age or in the young (under 30 years) with suggestive features: symptoms of vascular insufficiency to other organs, high-pitched epigastric bruit on physical examination, symptoms of hypokalemia secondary to hyperaldosteronism (muscle weakness, tetany, polyuria), and metabolic alkalosis. If renal arterial stenosis is suspected, the best initial screening test is a renal ultrasound, which may reveal unilateral renal hypotrophy (but normal cortical echogenicity). Absence of compensatory hypertrophy in the contralateral kidney should raise the suspicion of bilateral stensosis or superimposed intrinsic (structural) renal disease, most commonly hypertensive or diabetic nephropathy. A positive captopril test, which has a sensitivity and specificity of greater than 95%, constitutes an excellent follow-up procedure to assess the need for more invasive radiographic evaluation. The test relies on the exaggerated increase in plasma renin activity (PRA) after administration of captopril to patients with renovascular hypertension as compared with those with essential hypertension. It is considered positive when all the following criteria are satisfied: stimulated PRA of 12 (μg/L)/h, absolute increase in PRA of 10 (μg/L)/h or more, and increase in PRA of >150% [or 400% if baseline PRA is <3 (μg/L)/h]. Because ACE inhibitors magnify the impairment in renal blood flow and glomerular filtration rate (GFR) caused by functionally significant renal artery stenosis, use of these drugs in association with ^{99m}Tc-DTPA or ^{99m}MAG$_3$ renography greatly enhances the predictive value of radionuclide renography (90% sensitivity and specificity). Magnetic resonance angiography (MRA) has replaced previous modalities as the most sensitive (100%) and specific (95%) test for the diagnosis of renal arterial stenosis. The most definitive diagnostic procedure is bilateral arteriography with repeated bilateral renal vein and systemic renin determinations. If renal vein renin measurements from the two kidneys differ by a factor of 1.5:1 or more (higher value from the affected kidney) in a patient with radiographic unilateral renal artery stenosis, the chance of cure of hypertension by surgical reconstruction or angioplasty is almost 90%, particularly if the renal vein renin level from the unaffected kidney is equal to or less than systemic levels (suppressible). A ratio of less than 1.5:1, however, does not exclude the diagnosis of renovascular hypertension, particularly in the presence of bilateral disease.

℞ **TREATMENT** The aims of treatment are control of the blood pressure and restoration of perfusion to the ischemic kidney. In general, it is now firmly established that interventional therapy (i.e., surgery or angioplasty) is superior to medical therapy, which, while controlling blood pressure, does little to salvage renal mass lost to ischemic injury. Success rates with percutaneous transluminal angioplasty in young patients with fibromuscular dysplasia are 50% cure and improvement in blood pressure control in another 30%. Angioplasty is best suited for noncalcified, segmental short lesions and is also useful in some elderly patients who are poor surgical risks. About half of elderly individuals with reduced renal function as a result of renal arterial stenosis improve following angioplasty or surgery, even when preintervention arteriography shows little evidence of cortical perfusion. Despite the risks associated with surgery, long-term follow-up studies demonstrate an advantage of surgery over angioplasty both with regard to the incidence of restenosis and to the preservation or improvement in GFR. As with coronary angioplasty, stenting of renal arteries following balloon angioplasty is being used increasingly. Initial results are highly encouraging, with restenosis rates less than 15% at 6 months. Renal functional recovery or stabilization of renal function is seen in approximately 70% of patients. An illustrative example of renal artery stenting is shown in Fig. 278-1.

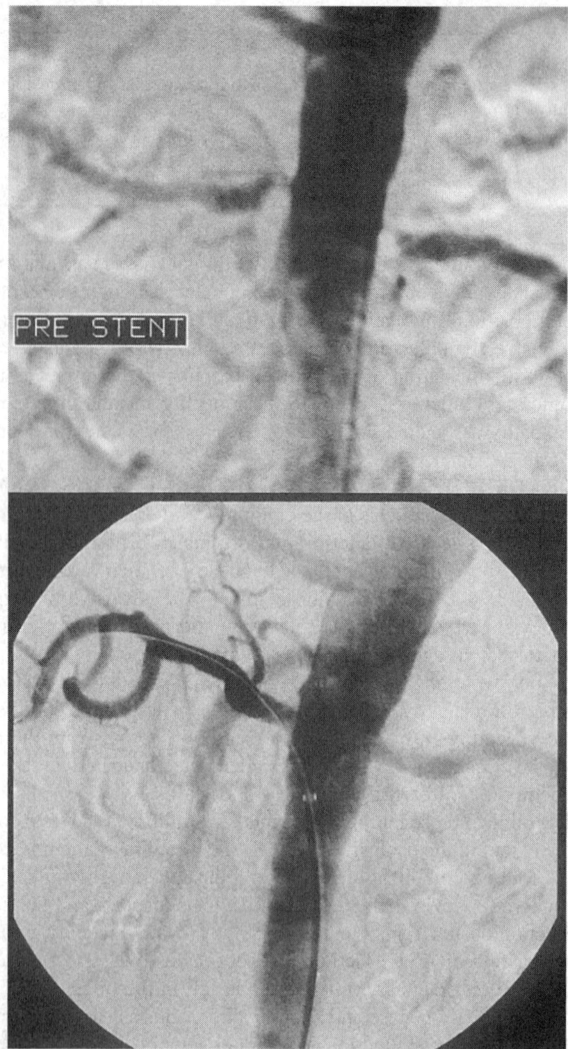

FIGURE 278-1 Bilateral severe ostial renal arterial stenosis prior to and following balloon dilatation and stent placement in a patient with severe hypertension and renal insufficiency.

Renal artery stenosis, particularly if atherosclerotic, is a progressive disease that may lead to gradual and silent loss of renal functional tissue (ischemic renal disease). Progression of ipsilateral atherosclerotic narrowing can be expected in nearly 50% of individuals, resulting in complete occlusion in about 10%. Thus, these patients need careful follow-up of initially nonclinically significant narrowing (<70%) for the possibility of further occlusion or the development of contralateral disease (30%). Compensatory contralateral hypertrophy may maintain renal function until affected by superimposed pathologic processes, at which time azotemia supervenes. Ischemic renal disease is now recognized as a significant cause of end-stage renal disease in patients over 50 years of age (approximately 15%). Even if angioplasty or surgery fail to return blood pressure to normal, these procedures usually render medical therapy easier.

HEMOLYTIC UREMIC SYNDROME (HUS) AND THROMBOTIC THROMBOCYTOPENIC PURPURA (TTP) (See also Chap. 116) HUS and TTP, consumptive coagulopathies characterized by microangiopathic hemolytic anemia and thrombocytopenia, have a particular predilection for the kidney and the central nervous system, the latter especially in TTP. The kidneys of patients with HUS or TTP often exhibit a "flea-bitten" appearance, the result of multiple cortical hemorrhagic infarcts. The major sites of pathology are the small renal arteries and afferent arterioles, which are nearly occluded as a result of marked intimal hyperplasia (particularly in TTP) and fibrin deposits in the subintimal regions. When the vasoocclusive process is extensive, bilateral cortical necrosis may occur. In addition, arteriolar microaneurysms, glomerular infarction, or nonspecific focal changes may be seen. In keeping with the focal nature of the vascular lesions, patchy areas of interstitial edema, tubular necrosis, and, eventually, fibrosis occur. By immunofluorescence staining, complement components and immunoglobulins may be demonstrated in the arterioles, and fibrinogen deposits are present in arteries, arterioles, and glomerular capillary loops.

Several mechanisms have been implicated in the etiology of the intravascular coagulopathy seen in HUS and TTP, including induction of a generalized Shwartzman phenomenon by microorganisms or endotoxin, genetic predisposition, and deficiency of platelet antiaggregatory substance(s) (e.g., prostacyclin). Some patients improve after exchange transfusion or plasmapheresis, suggesting accumulation of an as yet unidentified toxin.

Renal failure is common in both HUS and TTP, usually manifested by azotemia, mild proteinuria, microscopic and/or gross hematuria, and cylindruria. Patients with HUS have more severe renal failure, often marked by oligoanuria and hypertension and commonly progressing to chronic renal failure. The prognosis in HUS is better in children than in adults. In TTP, the course of which may span days to months, renal failure is usually less severe.

℞ TREATMENT In the management of TTP, high-dose glucocorticoids and plasma exchange often provide complete remission or cure. Plasma exchange should be initiated as early as possible, and the treatment cycles can be repeated if thrombocytopenia recurs. Splenectomy and antiplatelet therapy also have been used with varying degrees of success in patients with TTP. The success of plasma exchange in adult HUS is less well established than in TTP.

ARTERIOLAR NEPHROSCLEROSIS (See also Chaps. 241 and 246) Whether hypertension is "essential" or of known etiology, persistent exposure of the renal circulation to elevated intraluminal pressures results in development of intrinsic lesions of the renal arterioles (hyaline arteriolosclerosis) that eventually lead to loss of function (nephrosclerosis). Nephrosclerosis is divided into two distinct entities: "benign" and "malignant" (or accelerated).

Benign Arteriolar Nephrosclerosis Benign arteriolar nephrosclerosis is seen in patients who are hypertensive for an extended period of time (blood pressure more than 150/90 mmHg) but whose hypertension has not progressed to a malignant form (described below). Such patients, usually in the older age group, are often discovered to be hypertensive on routine physical examination or as a result of nonspecific symptomatology (e.g., headaches, weakness, palpitations).

Kidney size is normal to reduced, with loss of cortical mass leading to a fine granularity. Although the larger arteries may show atherosclerotic changes, the characteristic pathology is in the afferent arterioles, which have thickened walls due to deposition of homogeneous eosinophilic material (hyaline arteriolosclerosis). This material is composed of plasma proteins and fats that have been deposited in the arteriolar wall due to injury to the endothelium, probably secondary to the elevated intraluminal hydraulic pressure. Narrowing of vascular lumina results, with consequent ischemic injury to glomeruli and tubules.

Nephrosclerosis accompanying long-standing systemic arterial hypertension is only one manifestation of a generalized process affecting the cardiovascular system. Physical examination, therefore, may reveal changes in retinal vessels (arteriolar narrowing and/or flame-shaped hemorrhages), cardiac hypertrophy, and possibly signs of congestive heart failure. Renal disease may manifest as a mild to moderate elevation of serum creatinine concentration, microscopic hematuria, and/or mild proteinuria. In general, clinical evaluation does not reveal significant renal abnormalities. More specialized examination may disclose elevated urinary albumin excretion, tapering and loss of caliber of intrarenal vessels on arteriography, and an exaggerated natriuresis in response to a fluid challenge. Patients with benign nephrosclerosis maintain a near-normal GFR despite a reduction in renal blood flow.

Malignant Arteriolar Nephrosclerosis Patients with long-standing benign hypertension or patients not known to be hypertensive previously may develop malignant hypertension characterized by a sudden (accelerated) elevation of blood pressure (diastolic often above 130 mmHg) accompanied by papilledema, central nervous system manifestations, cardiac decompensation, and acute progressive deterioration of renal function. The absence of papilledema does not rule out the diagnosis in a patient with markedly elevated blood pressure and rapidly declining renal function. The kidneys are characterized by a flea-bitten appearance resulting from hemorrhages in surface capillaries. Histologically, two distinct vascular lesions can be seen. The first, affecting arterioles, is fibrinoid necrosis, i.e., infiltration of arteriolar walls with eosinophilic material including fibrin. There is thickening of vessel walls and, occasionally, an inflammatory infiltrate (necrotizing arteriolitis). The second lesion, involving the interlobular arteries, is a concentric hyperplastic proliferation of the cellular elements of the vascular wall with deposition of collagen to form a hyperplastic arteriolitis (onion-skin lesion). Fibrinoid necrosis occasionally extends into the glomeruli, which also may undergo proliferative changes or total necrosis. Most glomerular and tubular changes are secondary to ischemia and infarction. The sequence of events leading to the development of malignant hypertension is poorly defined. Two pathophysiologic alterations appear central in its initiation and/or perpetuation: (1) increased permeability of vessel walls to invasion by plasma components, particularly fibrin, which activates clotting mechanisms leading to a microangiopathic hemolytic anemia, thus perpetuating the vascular pathology; and (2) activation of the renin-angiotensin-aldosterone system at some point in the disease process, which contributes to the acceleration and maintenance of blood pressure elevation and, in turn, to vascular injury.

Malignant hypertension is most likely to develop in a previously hypertensive individual, usually in the third or fourth decade of life. There is a higher incidence among men, particularly black men. The presenting symptoms are usually neurologic (dizziness, headache, blurring of vision, altered states of consciousness, and focal or generalized seizures). Cardiac decompensation and renal failure appear thereafter. Renal abnormalities include a rapid rise in serum creatinine, hematuria (at times macroscopic), proteinuria, and red and white blood cell casts in the sediment. Nephrotic syndrome may be present. Elevated plasma aldosterone levels cause hypokalemic metabolic alkalosis in the early phase. Uremic acidosis and hyperkalemia eventually obscure these early findings. Hematologic indices of microangiopathic hemolytic anemia (i.e., schistocytes) are often seen.

℞ TREATMENT Control of hypertension is the principal goal of therapy for both benign and malignant forms. The time of initiation of therapy, its effectiveness, and patient compliance are crucial factors in arresting the progression of benign nephrosclerosis. Untreated, most of these patients succumb to the extrarenal complications of hypertension. In contrast, malignant hypertension is a medical emergency; its natural course includes a death rate of 80 to 90% within 1 year of onset, almost always due to uremia. Supportive measures should be instituted to control the neurologic, cardiac, and other complications of acute renal failure, but the mainstay of therapy is prompt and aggressive reduction of blood pressure, which, if successful, can reverse all complications in the majority of patients. Presently, 5-year survival is 50%, and some patients have evidence of partial reversal of the vascular lesions and a return of renal function to near-normal levels.

SCLERODERMA (PROGRESSIVE SYSTEMIC SCLEROSIS) (See also Chap. 313) Renal vascular involvement in scleroderma is characterized by a distinctive lesion of the small arteries (diameters of 150 to 500 μm) consisting of intimal proliferation, medial thinning, and increased collagen deposition in the adventitial layer. Fibrinoid changes in the walls of afferent arterioles and microinfarcts may occur. Glomerular changes are generally nonspecific and secondary to ischemic damage. Tubules are often atrophic. As part of a generalized increase in vasomotor tone, a vasospastic (Raynaud-like) phenomenon at the level of the renal vasculature contributes to the renal insufficiency. Reduction in renal blood flow is the major mechanism underlying the deterioration in kidney function, being present in 80% of patients, even in the absence of other clinical abnormalities. As vascular narrowing progresses, hypertension, azotemia, and proteinuria eventually develop. Plasma renin rises in response to sustained renal ischemia. The resulting hypertension causes further renal injury and may play a role in the ultimate destruction of nephrons. As more and more nephrons are lost to the combined insults of ischemia and hypertension, development of azotemia heralds a particularly grim prognosis. Proteinuria, usually mild, is a consequence of ischemic and hypertensive glomerular injury.

Although most patients with scleroderma present with extrarenal manifestations, renal involvement is eventually manifested in half of patients followed for up to 20 years. Renal involvement can present in one of two ways, depending on whether malignant hypertension is superimposed on the renal pathology: (1) *Persistent urinary abnormalities* with or without hypertension tend to follow an indolent course with mild proteinuria, occasional casts, cellular elements in the urinary sediment, and a propensity for development of hypertension. Azotemia is absent initially, but when it develops, dialysis is required within 1 year. (2) *Scleroderma renal crisis* is a rapid deterioration in renal function, usually accompanied by malignant hypertension, oliguria, fluid retention, microangiopathic hemolytic anemia, and central nervous system involvement. It may occur in patients with previously undemonstrable or slowly progressive renal disease. Untreated, it leads to chronic renal failure within days to months.

The prognosis of scleroderma renal disease is generally poor, particularly following the onset of azotemia. Aggressive antihypertensive therapy may be effective in delaying the progression of renal failure. In scleroderma renal crisis, prompt treatment with beta blockers, minoxidil, and particularly ACE inhibitors may reverse acute renal failure. The effect of these interventions on renal function over the long term is uncertain.

SICKLE CELL NEPHROPATHY (See also Chaps. 106 and 275) Sickle cell disease causes renal complications that arise mainly as a result of sickling of red blood cells in the microvasculature. The hypertonic and relatively hypoxic environment of the renal medulla, coupled with the slow blood flow in the vasa recta, favors the sickling of red blood cells, with resultant local infarction (papillary necrosis). Functional tubule defects in patients with sickle cell disease are likely the result of partial ischemic injury to the renal tubules.

In addition to the intrarenal microvascular pathology described above, young patients with sickle cell disease are characterized by renal hyperperfusion, glomerular hypertrophy, and hyperfiltration. Many of these individuals eventually develop a glomerulopathy leading to glomerular proteinuria (present in as many as 30%) and, in some, the nephrotic syndrome. In recent studies, the mechanisms underlying proteinuria in sickle cell nephropathy have been characterized as an early increase in pore radius, followed, as renal failure supervenes, with a reduction in pore number, but the onset of a dramatic loss of size-selectivity. Mild azotemia and hyperuricemia also can develop, but advanced renal failure and uremia are rare. Pathologic examination reveals the typical lesion of "hyperfiltration nephropathy," namely, focal segmental glomerular sclerosis. This finding has led to the suggestion that anemia-induced hyperfiltration in childhood is the principal cause of the adult glomerulopathy. Nephron loss secondary to ischemic injury also contributes to the development of azotemia in these patients.

In addition to the glomerulopathy described above, renal complications of sickle cell disease include the following: *Cortical infarcts* can cause loss of function, persistent hematuria, and perinephric hematomas. *Papillary infarcts*, demonstrated radiographically in 50% of patients with sickle trait, lead to an increased risk of bacterial infection in the scarred renal tissues and functional tubule abnormalities. Painless gross hematuria occurs with a higher frequency in sickle trait than in sickle cell disease and likely results from infarctive episodes in the renal medulla. *Functional tubule abnormalities* such as nephrogenic diabetes insipidus result from marked reduction in vasa recta blood flow, combined with ischemic tubule injury. This concentrating defect places these patients at increased risk of dehydration and, hence, sickling crises. The concentrating defect also occurs in individuals with sickle trait. Other tubule defects involve potassium and hydrogen ion excretion, occasionally leading to hyperkalemic metabolic acidosis and a defect in uric acid excretion which, combined with increased purine synthesis in the bone marrow, results in hyperuricemia.

Management of sickle nephropathy is not separate from that of overall patient management (Chap. 106). In addition, however, the use of ACE inhibitors has been associated with improvement of the hyperfiltration glomerulopathy.

TOXEMIAS OF PREGNANCY (See also Chap. 7) Renal function is "reset" at a higher level during normal pregnancy. Renal plasma flow and GFR both increase by 30 to 50%. Therefore, serum creatinine levels above 70 μmol/L (0.8 mg/dL) or blood urea nitrogen (BUN) levels above 4.6 mmol/L (13 mg/dL) are abnormal in pregnant women and should be investigated. Systolic and diastolic blood pressures decrease by an average of 10 to 15 mmHg below pregravid values. A diastolic pressure above 75 mmHg during the second trimester or above 85 mmHg during the third trimester is therefore abnormal. Vasodilation in the uterine, renal, and cutaneous beds, vasodilator prostaglandin release from the uteroplacental unit, and a decrease in arteriolar sensitivity to angiotensin II all play a role in the decline of blood pressure during pregnancy.

Preeclampsia-Eclampsia The toxemia syndrome, usually occurring in the third trimester of primigravidas, includes hypertension, proteinuria, edema, consumptive coagulopathy, sodium retention, hyperreflexia (preeclampsia), and, if uncontrolled, convulsions (eclampsia). In pure preeclampsia (i.e., not superimposed on previously existing hypertensive or renal disease), the primary sites of pathology are the glomerular endothelial cells. These cells show marked swelling due to an increase in cytoplasmic volume with vacuolization (endotheliosis) and encroach on the vascular lumen, rendering the enlarged glomeruli ischemic. The glomerular basement membrane and the extraglomerular blood vessels are intact. The pathogenesis is unknown. Coagulation abnormalities, hormonal factors, uteroplacental ischemia, and immune mechanisms have all been implicated. Increased microvascular reactivity may be a result of endothelial cell damage, which, in turn, alters the balance of endothelium-derived vasodilator/vasoconstrictor autacoids. Recent evidence suggests that preeclampsia may be characterized by selective dysregulation of vascular cell adhesion molecule-1 (VCAM-1) (but not other leukocyte adhesion molecules). This abnormality is not present in non-proteinuric gestational hypertension, and subsides post-partum. Induction of VCAM-1 expression in preeclampsia may contribute to leukocyte-mediated tissue injury in this condition or may reflect perturbation of other, previously unrecognized functions of this molecule in pregnancy. Despite sodium retention, intravascular volume is contracted as compared with pregravid values. An increased sensitivity to angiotensin II is the basis for the "roll-over test" (an increase in diastolic blood pressure of 20 mmHg or more on changing the patient's position from lateral recumbent to supine, presumably due to alterations in circulating angiotensin levels). In the supine position, the reduction in venous return due to compression by the gravid uterus increases circulating levels of angiotensin II. This increase results in a hypertensive response in preeclamptic patients, who are hyperresponsive to angiotensin II, but not in normal women, in whom pregnancy leads to a relative resistance to the pressor effects of this hormone.

A diagnosis of preeclampsia-related hypertension can be made when repeated measurements over a 4- to 6-h period show a blood pressure of 140/85 mmHg or more. The rise in blood pressure tends to be more severe at night. When preeclampsia occurs in a previously hypertensive patient, a rapid acceleration of the blood pressure elevation is accompanied by an increase in proteinuria, oliguria, edema, and coagulopathy. This is a life-threatening syndrome and tends to recur with future pregnancies. In addition to proteinuria, which correlates with the severity of the renal lesion, GFR and renal plasma flow are depressed. In view of the preexisting high levels, however, GFR in preeclamptic women often remains above nonpregnant levels. Uric acid clearance also falls, resulting in hyperuricemia. In the postpartum period, these patients are particularly susceptible to the development of "postpartum renal failure," which is thought to be a form of adult HUS.

℞ TREATMENT Treatment consists of bed rest in a quiet environment and control of neurologic manifestations and blood pressure, the former with magnesium sulfate and the latter usually with vasodilators such as hydralazine and methyldopa. Diuretics are avoided. The ultimate "treatment" is delivery, which should be induced if fetal maturity is adequate or if life-threatening coagulopathy or renal failure occur. The long-term prognosis is generally favorable.

Development of acute renal failure/preeclampsia in a pregnant woman should alert the physician to potential preexisting renal disease and/or hypertension. The latter is particularly likely if systolic blood pressure is greater than 200 mmHg. Hypertension and preexisting proteinuria tend to worsen in 50% of women during pregnancy. In addition, these abnormalities may be unmasked during pregnancy as the first manifestations of an underlying glomerulopathy. Conversely, patients with established underlying renal disease should be followed closely during pregnancy, with monthly measurements of 24-h urinary protein excretion and GFR. Sudden deterioration should raise suspicion of superimposed preeclampsia. There is no convincing evidence that pregnancy has an adverse effect on the long-term outcome of immunologic glomerular diseases or diabetic nephropathy. In all situations, control of blood pressure should be the primary therapeutic goal in view of its established beneficial effects on the progression of renal injury.

Bilateral Cortical Necrosis Acute bilateral cortical necrosis is associated with septic abortions, abruptio placentae, and preeclampsia. Coagulation in cortical vessels and arterioles leads to renal tissue necrosis. Anuria and renal failure ensue and may be irreversible. In other cases, renal function returns partially, but on long-term follow-up most patients slowly progress to uremia.

BIBLIOGRAPHY

CAREY RM et al: Role of the angiotensin type 2 receptor in the regulation of blood pressure and renal function. Hypertension 35:155, 2000

CHATZIANTONIOU C, DUSSAULE JC: Endothelin and renal vascular fibrosis: of mice and men. Curr Opin Nephrol Hypertens 9:31, 2000

GHANIOUS VE et al: Evaluating patients with renal failure for renal artery stenosis with gadolinium-enhanced magnetic resonance angiography. Am J Kidney Dis 33:36, 1999

GREENBERG A et al: Focal segmental glomerulosclerosis associated with nephrotic syndrome in cholesterol atheroembolism. Clinicopathologic correlations. Am J Kidney Dis 29:344, 1997

GRIST TM: Magnetic resonance angiography of renal artery stenosis. Am J Kidney Dis 24:700, 1994

HARDEN RN et al: Effect of renal artery stenting on progression of renovascular renal failure. Lancet 349:1133, 1997

REDMAN CWG: Hypertension in pregnancy, in *Medical Disorders in Obstetric Practice*, M DeSwiet (ed). Oxford, Blackwell Scientific, 1995

SYMPOSIUM ON ISCHEMIC RENAL DISEASE: Am J Kidney Dis 24:614, 1994

TUTTLE KR, RAABE RD: Endovascular stents for renal artery revascularization. Curr Opin Nephrol Hypertens 7:695, 1998

UZO T et al: Prevalence and predictions of renal artery stenosis in patients with myocardial infarction. Am J Kidney Dis 29:733, 1997

YADED M, LLACH F: Vascular complications involving the renal vessels, in *The Kidney*, 6th ed, BM Brenner (ed). Philadelphia, Saunders, 2001

279

John R. Asplin, Fredric L. Coe, Murray J. Favus

NEPHROLITHIASIS

TYPES OF STONES

Calcium salts, uric acid, cystine, and struvite ($MgNH_4PO_4$) are the basic constituents of most kidney stones in the western hemisphere. Calcium oxalate and calcium phosphate stones make up 75 to 85% of the total (Table 279-1) and may be admixed in the same stone. Calcium phosphate in stones is usually hydroxyapatite [$Ca_5(PO_4)_3OH$] or, less commonly, brushite ($CaHPO_4 \cdot H_2O$).

Calcium stones are more common in men; the average age of onset is the third decade. Approximately 60% of people who form a single calcium stone eventually form another within the next 10 years. The average rate of new stone formation in patients who have had a previous stone is about one stone every 2 or 3 years. Calcium stone disease is frequently familial.

In the urine, calcium oxalate monohydrate crystals (whewellite) usually grow as biconcave ovals that resemble red blood cells in shape and size but may occur in a larger, "dumbbell" form. In polarized light the crystals appear bright against a dark background, with an intensity that is dependent on orientation, a property known as *birefringence*. Calcium oxalate dihydrate crystals (weddellite) are bipyramidal. Apatite crystals do not exhibit birefringence and appear amorphous because the actual crystals are too small to be resolved by light microscopy.

Uric acid stones (Table 279-1) are radiolucent and are also more common in men. Half of patients with uric acid stones have gout; uric acid lithiasis is usually familial whether or not gout is present. In urine, uric acid crystals are red-orange in color because they absorb the pigment uricine. Anhydrous uric acid produces small crystals that appear amorphous by light microscopy. They are indistinguishable from apatite crystals, except for their birefringence. Uric acid dihydrate tends to form teardrop-shaped crystals as well as flat, rhomboid plates; both are strongly birefringent. Uric acid gravel appears like red dust, and the stones are also orange or red on some occasions. *Cystine stones* are uncommon (Table 279-1), lemon yellow, and sparkle; radiopacity is due to the sulfur content. Cystine crystals appear in the urine as flat, hexagonal plates.

Struvite stones are common (Table 279-1) and potentially dangerous. These stones occur mainly in women or patients who require chronic bladder catheterization and result from urinary tract infection with urease-producing bacteria, usually *Proteus* species. The stones

Table 279-1 Major Causes of Renal Stones

Stone Type and Causes	Percent of all Stones[a]	Percent Occurrence of Specific Causes[a]	Ratio of Males to Females	Etiology	Diagnosis	Treatment
Calcium stones	75–85		2:1 to 3:1			
Idiopathic hypercalciuria		50–55	2:1	Hereditary (?)	Normocalcemia, unexplained hypercalciuria[b]	Thiazide diuretic agents
Hyperuricosuria		20	4:1	Diet	Urine uric acid >750 mg per 24 h (women), >800 mg per 24 h (men)	Allopurinol or diet
Primary hyperparathyroidism		5	3:10	Neoplasia	Unexplained hypercalcemia	Surgery
Distal renal tubular acidosis		Rare	1:1	Hereditary	Hyperchloremic acidosis, minimum urine pH >5.5	Alkali replacement
Intestinal hyperoxaluria		~1–2	1:1	Bowel surgery	Urine oxalate >50 mg per 24 h	Cholestyramine or oral calcium loading
Hereditary hyperoxaluria		Rare	1:1	Hereditary	Urine oxalate and glycolic or l-glyceric acid increased	Fluids and pyridoxine
Hypocitraturia		15–60	2:1 to 5:1	Hereditary (?), diet	Urine citrate <320 mg per 24 h	Alkali supplements
Idiopathic stone disease		20	2:1	Unknown	None of the above present	Oral phosphate, fluids
Uric acid stones	5–8					
Gout		~50	3:1 to 4:1	Hereditary	Clinical diagnosis	Alkali and allopurinol
Idiopathic		~50	1:1	Hereditary (?)	Uric acid stones, no gout	Alkali and allopurinol if daily urine uric acid above 1000 mg
Dehydration		?	1:1	Intestinal, habit	History, intestinal fluid loss	Alkali, fluids, reversal of cause
Lesch-Nyhan syndrome		Rare	Males only	Hereditary	Reduced hypoxanthine-guanine phosphoribosyltransferase level	Allopurinol
Malignant tumors		Rare	1:1	Neoplasia	Clinical diagnosis	Allopurinol
Cystine stones	1		1:1	Hereditary	Stone type; elevated cystine excretion	Massive fluids, alkali, D-penicillamine if needed
Struvite stones	10–15		2:10	Infection	Stone type	Antimicrobial agents and judicious surgery

[a] Values are percent of patients who form a particular type of stone and who display each specific cause of stones.
[b] Urine calcium above 300 mg per 24 h (men), 250 mg per 24 h (women), or 4 mg/kg per 24 h either sex. Hyperthyroidism, Cushing syndrome, sarcoidosis, malignant tumors, immobilization, vitamin D intoxication, rapidly progressive bone disease, and Paget's disease all cause hypercalciuria and must be excluded in diagnosis of idiopathic hypercalciuria.

can grow to a large size and fill the renal pelvis and calyces to produce a "staghorn" appearance. They are radiopaque and have a variable internal density. In urine, struvite crystals are rectangular prisms said to resemble coffin lids.

MANIFESTATIONS OF STONES

As stones grow on the surfaces of the renal papillae or within the collecting system, they need not produce symptoms. Asymptomatic stones may be discovered during the course of radiographic studies undertaken for unrelated reasons. Stones rank, along with benign and malignant neoplasms, renal cysts, and genitourinary tuberculosis, among the common causes of isolated hematuria. Much of the time, however, stones break loose and enter the ureter or occlude the ureteropelvic junction, causing pain and obstruction.

STONE PASSAGE A stone can traverse the ureter without symptoms, but passage usually produces pain and bleeding. The pain begins gradually, usually in the flank, but increases over the next 20 to 60 min to become so severe that narcotic drugs may be needed for its control. The pain may remain in the flank or spread downward and anteriorly toward the ipsilateral loin, testis, or vulva. Pain that migrates downward indicates that the stone has passed to the lower third of the ureter, but if the pain does not migrate, the position of the stone cannot be predicted. A stone in the portion of the ureter within the bladder wall causes frequency, urgency, and dysuria that may be confused with urinary tract infection. The vast majority of ureteral stones less than 0.5 cm in diameter will pass spontaneously.

It has been standard practice to diagnose acute renal colic by intravenous pyelography; however, helical computed tomography (CT) scan without radiocontrast enhancement is now the preferred procedure. CT has the advantage of detecting uric acid stones in addition to the traditional radioopaque stones, and CT does not expose the patient to the risk of radio-contrast agents.

OTHER SYNDROMES **Staghorn Calculi** Struvite, cystine, and uric acid stones often grow too large to enter the ureter. They gradually fill the renal pelvis and may extend outward through the infundibula to the calyces themselves.

Nephrocalcinosis Calcium stones grow on the papillae. Most break loose and cause colic, but they may remain in place so that multiple papillary calcifications are found by x-ray, a condition termed *nephrocalcinosis*. Papillary nephrocalcinosis is common in hereditary distal renal tubular acidosis (RTA) and in other types of severe hypercalciuria. In medullary sponge kidney disease (Chap. 276) calcification may occur in dilated distal collecting ducts.

Sludge Sufficient uric acid or cystine in the urine may plug both ureters with precipitate. Calcium oxalate crystals do not do this because less than 100 mg oxalate usually is excreted daily in the urine even in severe hyperoxaluric states, compared with 1000 mg uric acid in patients with hyperuricosuria and 400 to 800 mg cystine in patients with cystinuria. Calcium phosphate crystals can render the urine milky but do not plug the urinary tract.

INFECTION Although urinary tract infection is not a direct consequence of stone disease, it can occur after instrumentation and surgery of the urinary tract, which are frequent in the treatment of stone disease. Stone disease and urinary tract infection can enhance their respective seriousness and interfere with treatment. Obstruction of an infected kidney by a stone may lead to sepsis and extensive damage of renal tissue, since it converts the urinary tract proximal to the obstruction into a closed, or partially closed, space that can become an abscess. Stones may harbor bacteria in the stone matrix, leading to recurrent urinary tract infection. On the other hand, infection due to bacteria that possess the enzyme urease can cause stones composed of struvite.

ACTIVITY OF STONE DISEASE Active disease means that new stones are forming or that preformed stones are growing. Sequential radiographs of the renal areas are needed to document the growth or appearance of new stones and to ensure that passed stones are actually newly formed, not preexistent ones.

PATHOGENESIS OF STONES

Urinary stones usually arise because of the breakdown of a delicate balance. The kidneys must conserve water, but they must excrete materials that have a low solubility. These two opposing requirements must be balanced during adaptation to diet, climate, and activity. The problem is mitigated to some extent by the fact that urine contains substances that inhibit crystallization of calcium salts and others that bind calcium in soluble complexes. These protective mechanisms are less than perfect. When the urine becomes supersaturated with insoluble materials, because excretion rates are excessive and/or because water conservation is extreme, crystals form and may grow and aggregate to form a stone.

SUPERSATURATION In a solution in equilibrium with crystals of calcium oxalate, the product of the chemical activities of the calcium and oxalate ions in the solution is termed the *equilibrium solubility product*. If crystals are removed, and if either calcium or oxalate ions are added to the solution, the activity product increases, but the solution may remain clear; no new crystals form. Such a solution is *metastably supersaturated*. If new calcium oxalate seed crystals are now added, they will grow in size. Ultimately, the activity product reaches a critical value at which a solid phase begins to develop spontaneously. This value is called the *upper limit of metastability*, or the *formation product*. Stone growth in the urinary tract requires a urine that, on average, is above the equilibrium solubility product. Excessive supersaturation is common in stone formation.

Calcium, oxalate, and phosphate form many stable soluble complexes among themselves and with other substances in urine, such as citrate. As a result, their free ion activities are below their chemical concentrations and can be measured only by indirect techniques. Reduction in ligands such as citrate can increase ion activity without changing total urinary calcium. Urine supersaturation can be increased by dehydration or by overexcretion of calcium, oxalate, phosphate, cystine, or uric acid. Urine pH is also important; phosphate and uric acid are weak acids that dissociate readily over the physiologic range of urine pH. Alkaline urine contains more dibasic phosphate, favoring deposits of brushite, and apatite. Below a urine pH of 5.5, uric acid crystals (pK 5.47) predominate, whereas phosphate crystals are rare. The solubility of calcium oxalate, on the other hand, is not influenced by changes in urine pH. Measurements of supersaturation in a pooled 24-h urine sample probably underestimate the risk of precipitation. Transient dehydration, variation of urine pH, and postprandial bursts of overexcretion may cause values considerably above average.

NUCLEATION **Homogeneous Nucleation** In urine that is supersaturated with respect to calcium oxalate, these two ions form clusters. Most small clusters eventually disperse because the internal forces that hold them together are too weak to overcome the random tendency of ions to move away. Clusters of over 100 ions can remain stable because attractive forces balance surface losses. Once they are stable, nuclei can grow at levels of supersaturation below that needed for their creation. The formation product marks the point at which stable nuclei become frequent enough to create a permanent solid phase.

Heterogeneous Nucleation If a supersaturated urine is seeded with preformed nuclei of a crystal that is similar in structure to calcium oxalate, calcium and oxalate ions in solution will bind to the crystal's surface as they would on a seed crystal of calcium oxalate itself. The seeding of a supersaturated solution by foreign nuclei is called *heterogeneous nucleation*. Cell debris, calcifications on the renal papillae, as well as other urinary crystals, can serve as heterogeneous nuclei that permit calcium oxalate stones to form, even though urine calcium oxalate supersaturation never exceeds the metastable limit for homogenous nucleation.

INHIBITORS OF CRYSTAL FORMATION Stable nuclei must grow and aggregate to produce a stone of clinical significance. Urine contains potent inhibitors of nucleation, growth, and aggregation for calcium oxalate and calcium phosphate but not for uric acid, cystine, or struvite. Inorganic pyrophosphate is a potent inhibitor that appears to affect calcium phosphate more than calcium oxalate crystals. Citrate inhibits crystal growth and nucleation, though most of the stone inhibitory activity of citrate is due to lowering urine supersaturation via complexation of calcium. Other urine components such as glycoproteins inhibit all three processes of calcium oxalate stone formation. Slowing of crystal growth increases the apparent upper limit of metastability because the critical growth of ion clusters into stable nuclei is hindered. As a consequence of the presence of these inhibitors, crystal growth in urine is slow compared with growth in simple salt solutions, and the upper limit of metastability is higher.

EVALUATION AND TREATMENT OF PATIENTS WITH NEPHROLITHIASIS

Most patients with nephrolithiasis have remediable metabolic disorders that cause stones and can be detected by chemical analyses of serum and urine. Adults with recurrent kidney stones and children with even a single kidney stone should be evaluated. A practical outpatient evaluation consists of two or three 24-h urine collections, each with a corresponding blood sample; measurements of serum and urine calcium, uric acid, electrolytes and creatinine, urine pH, volume, oxalate, and citrate should be made. Since stone risks vary with diet, activity, and environment, at least one urine collection should be made on a weekend when the patient is at home and another on a work day. When possible, the composition of kidney stones should be determined because treatment depends on stone type (Table 279-1). No matter what disorders are found, every patient should be counseled to avoid dehydration and to drink sufficient water so that they excrete at least 2 L of urine every day. Since treatment is prolonged, the use of medications must be justified by the activity and severity of stone disease and the importance of protection against new stones.

Rx **TREATMENT** The management of stones already present in the kidneys or urinary tract requires a combined medical and surgical approach. The specific treatment depends on the location of the stone, the extent of obstruction, the function of the affected and unaffected kidney, the presence or absence of urinary tract infection, the progress of stone passage, and the risks of operation or anesthesia given the clinical state of the patient. In general, severe obstruction, infection, intractable pain, and serious bleeding are indications for removal of a stone.

In the past, stones were removed by operation or by passing a flexible basket retrograde up the ureter from the bladder during cystoscopy. There are now three alternatives. *Extracorporeal lithotripsy* causes the in situ fragmentation of stones in the kidney, renal pelvis, or ureter by exposing them to shock waves. The kidney stone is centered at a focal point of parabolic reflectors, and high-intensity shock waves are created by high-voltage discharge. The waves are transmitted to the patient using water as a conduction medium, either by placing the patient in a water tank or by placing water-filled cushions between the patient and the shock wave generators. After multiple discharges, most stones are reduced to powder that moves through the ureter into the bladder. *Percutaneous ultrasonic lithotripsy* requires the passage of a rigid cystoscope-like instrument into the renal pelvis through a small incision in the flank. Stones can be disrupted by a small ultrasound transducer, and fragments can be removed directly. The last method is *laser lithotripsy via a ureteroscope* for removal of ureteral stones. These various forms of lithotripsy have largely replaced pyelolithotomy and ureterolithotomy.

CALCIUM STONES **Idiopathic Hypercalciuria** (See also Chap. 341) This condition appears to be hereditary, and its diagnosis is straightforward (Table 279-1). In some patients, primary intestinal hyperabsorption of calcium causes transient postprandial hypercalcemia that suppresses secretion of parathyroid hormone. The renal tubules are deprived of the normal stimulus to reabsorb calcium at the same time that the filtered load of calcium is increased. In other patients, reabsorption of calcium by the renal tubules appears to be defective, and secondary hyperparathyroidism is evoked by urinary losses of calcium. Renal synthesis of 1,25-dihydroxyvitamin D is increased, enhancing intestinal absorption of calcium. In the past, the separation of "absorptive" and "renal" forms of hypercalciuria was used to guide treatment. However, these may not be distinct entities but the extremes of a continuum of behavior. Vitamin D overactivity, either through high vitamin D levels or excess vitamin D receptor, is a likely explanation for the hypercalciuria in many of these patients. Hypercalciuria contributes to stone formation by raising urine saturation with respect to calcium oxalate and calcium phosphate.

℞ TREATMENT Thiazide diuretics lower urine calcium in idiopathic hypercalciuria and are effective in preventing the formation of stones. Three 3-year randomized trials have shown a 50% decrease in stone formation in the thiazide-treated group as compared to the placebo-treated controls. The drug effect requires slight contraction of the extracellular fluid volume, and massive use of NaCl reduces its therapeutic effect. Thiazide-induced hypokalemia should be aggressively treated since hypokalemia will reduce urine citrate, increasing urine calcium ion levels.

Hyperuricosuria About 20% of calcium oxalate stone formers are hyperuricosuric, primarily because of an excessive intake of purine from meat, fish, and poultry. The mechanism of stone formation is probably due to salting out calcium oxalate by urate. A low-purine diet is desirable but difficult for many patients to achieve. The alternative is allopurinol, which has been shown to be effective in a randomized controlled trial. A dose of 100 mg bid is usually sufficient.

Primary Hyperparathyroidism (See also Chap. 341) The diagnosis of this condition is established by documenting that hypercalcemia that cannot be otherwise explained is accompanied by inappropriately elevated serum concentrations of parathyroid hormone. Hypercalciuria, usually present, raises the urine supersaturation of calcium phosphate and/or calcium oxalate (Table 279-1). Prompt diagnosis is important because parathyroidectomy should be carried out before renal damage or bone disease occurs.

Distal Renal Tubular Acidosis (See also Chap. 276) The defect in this condition seems to reside in the distal nephron, which cannot establish a normal pH gradient between urine and blood, leading to hyperchloremic acidosis. The diagnosis is suggested by a minimum urine pH in the presence of systemic acidosis above 5.5. If the diagnosis is in doubt because metabolic abnormalities are mild, oral challenge with NH_4Cl, 1.9 mmol/kg of body weight, will not lower urine pH below 5.5 in patients with distal RTA. Hypercalciuria, an alkaline urine, and a low urine citrate level cause supersaturation with respect to calcium phosphate. Calcium phosphate stones form, nephrocalcinosis is common, and osteomalacia or rickets may occur. Renal damage is frequent, and glomerular filtration rate falls gradually. Treatment with supplemental alkali reverses hypercalciuria and limits the production of new stones. The usual dose of sodium bicarbonate is 0.5 to 2.0 mmol/kg of body weight per day in four to six divided doses. An alternative is potassium citrate supplementation, given at the same dose per day but needing to be given only three to four times per day. In incomplete distal RTA, systemic acidosis is absent, but urine pH cannot be lowered below 5.5 after an exogenous acid load such as ammonium chloride. Incomplete RTA may develop in some patients who form calcium oxalate stones because of idiopathic hypercalciuria; the importance of RTA in producing stones in this situation is uncertain, and thiazide treatment is a reasonable alternative. Some patients with incomplete RTA form calcium phosphate stones because of low urine citrate and an alkaline urine and are best treated with alkali as if RTA were complete.

Hyperoxaluria Overabsorption of dietary oxalate and consequent oxaluria, i.e., so-called intestinal oxaluria, is one consequence of fat malabsorption (Chap. 286). The latter can be caused by a variety of conditions, including bacterial overgrowth syndromes, chronic disease of the pancreas and biliary tract, jejunoileal bypass in treatment of obesity, or ileal resection for inflammatory bowel disease. With fat malabsorption, calcium in the bowel lumen is bound by fatty acids instead of oxalate, which is left free for absorption in the colon. Delivery of unabsorbed fatty acids and bile salts to the colon may injure the colonic mucosa and enhance oxalate absorption. Dietary excess of oxalate in patients with normal intestinal function is a common cause of mild elevation of urine oxalate, but seldom to the level seen in patients with enteric hyperoxaluria. Hereditary hyperoxaluria states are rare causes of severe hyperoxaluria; patients usually present with recurrent calcium oxalate stones during childhood. Type I hereditary hyperoxaluria is inherited as an autosomal recessive trait and is due to a deficiency in the peroxisomal enzyme alanine:glyoxylate aminotransferase. Type II is due to a deficiency of D-glyceric dehydrogenase. Ethylene glycol intoxication and methoxyflurane also can cause oxalate overproduction and hyperoxaluria. Hyperoxaluria from any cause can produce tubulointerstitial nephropathy (Chap. 277) and lead to stone formation.

℞ TREATMENT The oxalate-binding resin cholestyramine at a dose of 8 to 16 g/d, correction of fat malabsorption, and a low-fat, low oxalate diet are effective treatments for oxaluria secondary to intestinal overabsorption. Calcium supplements, given with meals, precipitate oxalate in the gut lumen providing an alternative form of therapy. Treatment for hereditary hyperoxaluria includes a high fluid intake, neutral phosphate, and pyridoxine (25 to 200 mg/d). Citrate supplementation may also have some benefit. Even with aggressive therapy, irreversible renal failure secondary to recurrent stone formation often occurs. Segmental liver transplant, to correct the enzyme defect, combined with a kidney transplant have been successfully utilized in patients with hereditary hyperoxaluria.

Hypocitraturia Urine citrate prevents calcium stone formation by creating a soluble complex with calcium, effectively reducing free urine calcium. Hypocitraturia is found in 15 to 60% of stone formers, either as a single disorder or in combination with other metabolic abnormalities. It can be secondary to systemic disorders, such as RTA, chronic diarrheal illness, or hypokalemia, or it may be a primary disorder, in which case it is called *idiopathic hypocitraturia.*

℞ TREATMENT Treatment is with alkali, which increases urine citrate excretion; generally bicarbonate or citrate salts are used. Potassium salts are preferred as sodium loading increases urinary excretion of calcium, reducing the effectiveness of treatment. A recent randomized, placebo-controlled trial has demonstrated the effectiveness of potassium citrate in idiopathic hypocitraturia.

Idiopathic Calcium Lithiasis Some patients have no metabolic cause for stones despite a thorough metabolic evaluation (Table 279-1). The best treatment appears to be high fluid intake so that the urine specific gravity remains at 1.005 or below throughout the day and night. Oral phosphate at a dose of 2 g phosphorus daily may lower urine calcium and increase urine pyrophosphate and thereby reduce the rate of recurrence. Orthophosphate causes mild nausea and diarrhea initially, but tolerance may improve with continued intake. Thiazide treatment to reduce calcium excretion and allopurinol to diminish uric acid output also may be helpful.

URIC ACID STONES These stones form because the urine becomes supersaturated with undissociated uric acid that is protonated at its N-9 position. In gout, idiopathic uric acid lithiasis, and dehydration, the average pH is usually below 5.4 and often below 5.0. Undissociated uric acid therefore predominates and is soluble in urine only in concentrations of 100 mg/L. Concentrations above this level represent supersaturation that causes crystals and stones to form. Hyperuricosuria, when present, increases supersaturation, but urine of low pH can be supersaturated with undissociated uric acid even though the daily excretion rate is normal. Myeloproliferative syndromes, chemotherapy of malignant tumors, and the Lesch-Nyhan syndrome cause such massive production of uric acid and consequent hyperuricosuria that stones and uric acid sludge form even at a normal urine pH. Plugging of the renal collecting tubules by uric acid crystals can cause acute renal failure.

℞ TREATMENT The two goals of treatment are to raise urine pH and to lower excessive urine uric acid excretion to less than 1 g/d. Supplemental alkali, 1 to 3 mmol/kg of body weight per day, should be given in three or four evenly spaced, divided doses, one of which should be given at bedtime. The form of the alkali may be important. Potassium citrate may reduce the risk of calcium salts crystallizing when urine pH is increased, whereas sodium citrate or sodium bicarbonate may increase the risk. If the overnight urine pH is below 5.5, the evening dose of alkali may be raised or 250 mg acetazolamide added at bedtime. A low-purine diet should be instituted in those uric acid stone formers with hyperuricosuria. Patients who continue to form uric acid stones despite treatment with fluids, alkali, and a low-purine diet should have allopurinol added to their regimen. If hypercalciuria is also present, it should be specifically treated, as alkali alone could lead to calcium phosphate stone formation.

CYSTINURIA AND CYSTINE STONES (See also Chap. 352) In this disorder, proximal tubular and jejunal transport of the dibasic amino acids cystine, lysine, arginine, and ornithine are defective, and excessive amounts are lost in the urine. Clinical disease is due solely to the insolubility of cystine, which forms stones.

Pathogenesis Cystinuria occurs because of defective transport of amino acids by the brush borders of renal tubule and intestinal epithelial cells. Cystine, lysine, arginine, and ornithine appear to share a common renal transport pathway, since infusion of lysine decreases tubular reabsorption of the other three. However, cystine is also transported by a separate transport mechanism, because cystinuria and dibasic aminoaciduria can occur independently. The intestinal defects are not similar in all patients who are homozygous for cystinuria, and the extent of aminoaciduria in individuals who are heterozygous carriers of the defect varies from family to family. Three types of inheritance have been described (Chap. 352). A gene located on chromosome 2 and designated SLC3A1, codes for a dibasic amino acid transporter and has been found to be abnormal in Type I cystinuria. Linkage analysis has mapped Type III cystinuria to chromosome 19.

Diagnosis Cystine stones are formed only by patients with cystinuria, but 10% of stones in cystinuric patients do not contain cystine; therefore, every stone former should be screened for the disease. The sediment from a first morning urine specimen in many patients with homozygous cystinuria reveals typical flat, hexagonal, platelike cystine crystals. Cystinuria also can be detected using the urine sodium nitroprusside test. The test is positive with 75 to 125 mg cystine per gram of creatinine, a concentration lower than that in the urine of patients with cystinuria but above the levels in normal urine. Because the test is sensitive, it is positive in many asymptomatic heterozygotes for cystinuria. A positive nitroprusside test or the finding of cystine crystals in the urine sediment should be evaluated by measurement of daily cystine excretion. Normal adults excrete 40 to 60 mg cystine per gram of creatinine, heterozygotes usually excrete less than 300 mg/g, and homozygotes almost always excrete above 250 mg/g.

℞ TREATMENT This consists of a high fluid intake, even at night. Daily urine volume should exceed 3 L. Raising urine pH with alkali is helpful, provided the urine pH exceeds 7.5. A low-salt diet (100 mmol/d) can reduce cystine excretion up to 40%. Because side effects are frequent, drugs such as penicillamine and tiopronin, which form the soluble disulfide cysteine-drug complexes, should be used only when fluid loading, salt reduction, and alkali therapy are ineffective. Captopril, which has a free sulfhydryl group to bind cysteine, has been used in a limited number of patients with some success. Low-methionine diets have not proved to be practical for clinical use, but patients should avoid protein gluttony.

STRUVITE STONES These stones are a result of urinary infection with bacteria, usually *Proteus* species, which possess urease, an enzyme that degrades urea to NH_3 and CO_2. The NH_3 hydrolyzes to NH_4^+ and raises urine pH to 8 or 9. The CO_2 hydrates to H_2CO_3 and then dissociates to CO_3^{2-} which precipitates with calcium as $CaCO_3$. The NH_4^+ precipitates PO_4^{3-} and Mg^{2+} to form $MgNH_4PO_4$ (struvite). The result is a stone of calcium carbonate admixed with struvite. Struvite does not form in urine in the absence of infection, because NH_4^+ concentration is low in urine that is alkaline in response to physiologic stimuli. Chronic *Proteus* infection can occur because of impaired urinary drainage, urologic instrumentation or surgery, and especially with chronic antibiotic treatment, which can favor the dominance of *Proteus* in the urinary tract.

℞ TREATMENT Complete removal of the stone with subsequent sterilization of the urinary tract is the treatment of choice for patients who can tolerate the procedures. Open surgery is successful in debulking the stone and improving renal function if obstruction is present; however, there is recurrence of stone in 25% of the patients. Irrigation of the renal pelvis and calyces with hemiacidrin, a solution that dissolves struvite, can reduce recurrence after surgery. Newer procedures such as lithotripsy and percutaneous nephrolithotomy, alone or in combination, have largely replaced open surgery. Stone-free rates of 50 to 90% have been reported after these procedures. Antimicrobial treatment is best reserved for dealing with acute infection and for maintenance of a sterile urine after surgery, in the hope of preventing recurrence or minimizing stone growth. Urine cultures and culture of stone fragments removed at surgery should guide the choice of antibiotic. Methenamine mandelate, which lowers urine pH and liberates formaldehyde, can be used for chronic suppression of infection when a stone is present. For patients who are not candidates for surgical removal of stone, acetohydroxamic acid, an inhibitor of urease, can be used. Though effective in treating the stones, acetohydroxamic acid has many side effects, such as headache, tremor, and thrombophlebitis, which limits its use. Lowering urine pH with chronic administration of NH_4Cl may retard stone growth but also may raise urine calcium level and promote the formation of calcium oxalate stones.

BIBLIOGRAPHY

BORGHI L et al: Urinary volume, water and recurrences in idiopathic calcium nephrolithiasis: A 5 year randomized prospective study. J Urol 155:839, 1996

BRUNO M, MARANGELLA M: Cystinuria: Recent advances in pathophysiology and genetics. Contrib Nephrol 122:173, 1997

COE FL, PARKS JH: New insights into the pathophysiology of and treatment of nephrolithiasis: New research venues. J Bone Miner Res 12:522, 1997

CONSENSUS CONFERENCE: Prevention and treatment of kidney stones. JAMA 260:977, 1988

CURHAN GC et al: Comparison of dietary calcium with supplemental calcium and other nutrients as factors affecting the risk of kidney stones in women. Ann Intern Med 126:497, 1997

HEILBERG IP: Update on dietary recommendations and medical treatment of renal stone disease. Nephrol Dial Transplant 15:117, 2000

KRAMER G et al: Role of bacteria in the development of kidney stones. Curr Opin Urol 10:35, 2000

RODMAN JS: Struvite stones. Nephron 81(Suppl 1):50, 1999

SEGURA JW et al: Ureteral Stones Clinical Guidelines Panel summary report on the management of ureteral calculi. J Urol 158:1915, 1997

280

Walter E. Stamm

URINARY TRACT INFECTIONS AND PYELONEPHRITIS

DEFINITIONS Acute infections of the urinary tract can be subdivided into two general anatomic categories: lower tract infection (urethritis and cystitis) and upper tract infection (acute pyelonephritis, prostatitis, and intrarenal and perinephric abscesses). Infections at these various sites may occur together or independently and may either be asymptomatic or present as one of the clinical syndromes described below. Infections of the urethra and bladder are often considered superficial (or mucosal) infections, while prostatitis, pyelonephritis, and renal suppuration signify tissue invasion.

From a microbiologic perspective, urinary tract infection (UTI) exists when pathogenic microorganisms are detected in the urine, urethra, bladder, kidney, or prostate. In most instances, growth of more than 10^5 organisms per milliliter from a properly collected midstream "clean-catch" urine sample indicates infection. However, significant bacteriuria is lacking in some cases of true UTI. Especially in symptomatic patients, a smaller number of bacteria (10^2 to 10^4/mL) may signify infection. In urine specimens obtained by suprapubic aspiration or "in-and-out" catheterization and in samples from a patient with an indwelling catheter, colony counts of 10^2 to 10^4/mL generally indicate infection. Conversely, colony counts of $>10^5$/mL of midstream urine are occasionally due to specimen contamination, which is especially likely when multiple species are found.

Infections that recur after antibiotic therapy can be due to the persistence of the originally infecting strain (as judged by species, antibiogram, serotype, and molecular type) or to reinfection with a new strain. "Same-strain" recurrent infections that become evident within 2 weeks of cessation of therapy can be the result of unresolved renal or prostatic infection (termed *relapse*) or of persistent vaginal or intestinal colonization leading to rapid reinfection of the bladder.

Symptoms of dysuria, urgency, and frequency that are unaccompanied by significant bacteriuria have been termed the *acute urethral syndrome*. Although widely used, this term lacks anatomic precision because many cases so designated are actually bladder infections. Moreover, since the causative agent can usually be identified in these patients, the term *syndrome*—implying unknown causation—is inappropriate.

Chronic pyelonephritis refers to chronic interstitial nephritis believed to result from bacterial infection of the kidney (Chap. 277). Many noninfectious diseases also cause an interstitial nephritis that is indistinguishable pathologically from chronic pyelonephritis.

ACUTE UTIs: URETHRITIS, CYSTITIS, AND PYELONEPHRITIS

EPIDEMIOLOGY Epidemiologically, UTIs are subdivided into catheter-associated (or nosocomial) infections and non-catheter-associated (or community-acquired) infections. Infections in either category may be symptomatic or asymptomatic. Acute community-acquired infections are very common and account for more than 7 million office visits annually in the United States. These infections occur in 1 to 3% of schoolgirls and then increase markedly in incidence with the onset of sexual activity in adolescence. The vast majority of acute symptomatic infections involve young women; a prospective study demonstrated an annual incidence of 0.5 to 0.7 infections per patient-year in this group. Acute symptomatic UTIs are unusual in men under the age of 50. The development of asymptomatic bacteriuria parallels that of symptomatic infection and is rare among men under 50 but common among women between 20 and 50. Asymptomatic bacteriuria is more common among elderly men and women, with rates as high as 40 to 50% in some studies.

ETIOLOGY Many different microorganisms can infect the urinary tract, but by far the most common agents are the gram-negative bacilli. *Escherichia coli* causes approximately 80% of acute infections in patients without catheters, urologic abnormalities, or calculi. Other gram-negative rods, especially *Proteus* and *Klebsiella* and occasionally *Enterobacter*, account for a smaller proportion of uncomplicated infections. These organisms, plus *Serratia* and *Pseudomonas*, assume increasing importance in recurrent infections and in infections associated with urologic manipulation, calculi, or obstruction. They play a major role in nosocomial, catheter-associated infections (see below). *Proteus* spp., by virtue of urease production, and *Klebsiella* spp., through the production of extracellular slime and polysaccharides, predispose to stone formation and are isolated more frequently from patients with calculi.

Gram-positive cocci play a lesser role in UTIs. However, *Staphylococcus saprophyticus*—a novobiocin-resistant, coagulase-negative species—accounts for 10 to 15% of acute symptomatic UTIs in young females. Enterococci occasionally cause acute uncomplicated cystitis in women. More commonly, enterococci and *Staphylococcus aureus* cause infections in patients with renal stones or previous instrumentation or surgery. Isolation of *S. aureus* from the urine should arouse suspicion of bacteremic infection of the kidney.

About one-third of women with dysuria and frequency have either an insignificant number of bacteria in midstream urine cultures or completely sterile cultures and have been previously defined as having the urethral syndrome. About three-quarters of these women have pyuria, while one-quarter have no pyuria and little objective evidence of infection. In the women with pyuria, two groups of pathogens account for most infections. Low quantities (10^2 to 10^4 bacteria per milliliter) of typical bacterial uropathogens such as *E. coli*, *S. saprophyticus*, *Klebsiella*, or *Proteus* are found in midstream urine specimens from most of these women. These bacteria are probably the causative agents in these infections because they can usually be isolated from a suprapubic aspirate, are associated with pyuria, and respond to appropriate antimicrobial therapy. In other women with acute urinary symptoms, pyuria, and urine that is sterile (even when obtained by suprapubic aspiration), sexually transmitted urethritis-producing agents such as *Chlamydia trachomatis*, *Neisseria gonorrhoeae*, and herpes simplex virus are etiologically important. These agents are found most frequently in young, sexually active women with new sexual partners.

The causative role of nonbacterial pathogens in UTIs remains poorly defined. *Ureaplasma urealyticum* has frequently been isolated from the urethra and urine of patients with acute dysuria and frequency but is also found in specimens from many patients without urinary symptoms. Ureaplasmas probably account for some cases of urethritis and cystitis. *U. urealyticum* and *Mycoplasma hominis* have been isolated from prostatic and renal tissues of patients with acute prostatitis and pyelonephritis, respectively, and are probably responsible for some of these infections as well. Adenoviruses cause acute hemorrhagic cystitis in children and in some young adults, often in epidemics. Although other viruses can be isolated from urine (e.g., cytomegalovirus), they are thought not to cause UTI. Colonization of the urine of catheterized or diabetic patients by *Candida* and other fungal species is common and sometimes progresses to symptomatic invasive infection (Chap. 205). →*Mycobacterial infection of the genitourinary tract is discussed in Chap. 169.*

PATHOGENESIS AND SOURCES OF INFECTION The urinary tract should be viewed as a single anatomic unit that is united by a continuous column of urine extending from the urethra to the kidney. In the vast majority of UTIs, bacteria gain access to the bladder via the urethra. Ascent of bacteria from the bladder may follow and is probably the pathway for most renal parenchymal infections.

The vaginal introitus and distal urethra are normally colonized by diphtheroids, streptococcal species, lactobacilli, and staphylococcal species but not by the enteric gram-negative bacilli that commonly cause UTIs. In females prone to the development of cystitis, however, enteric gram-negative organisms residing in the bowel colonize the introitus, the periurethral skin, and the distal urethra before and during episodes of bacteriuria. The factors that predispose to periurethral colonization with gram-negative bacilli remain poorly understood, but alteration of the normal vaginal flora by antibiotics, other genital infections, or contraceptives (especially spermicide) appears to play an important role. Loss of the normally dominant H_2O_2-producing lactobacilli in the vaginal flora appears to facilitate colonization by *E. coli*. Small numbers of periurethral bacteria probably gain entry to the bladder frequently, a process that is facilitated in some cases by urethral massage during intercourse. Whether bladder infection ensues depends on interacting effects of the pathogenicity of the strain, the inoculum size, and the local and systemic host defense mechanisms.

Under normal circumstances, bacteria placed in the bladder are rapidly cleared, partly through the flushing and dilutional effects of voiding but also as a result of the antibacterial properties of urine and the bladder mucosa. Owing mostly to a high urea concentration and high osmolarity, the bladder urine of many normal persons inhibits or kills bacteria. Prostatic secretions possess antibacterial properties as well. Polymorphonuclear leukocytes enter the bladder epithelium and the urine soon after infection arises and play a role in clearing bacteriuria. The role of locally produced antibody remains unclear.

Hematogenous pyelonephritis occurs most often in debilitated patients who are either chronically ill or receiving immunosuppressive therapy. Metastatic staphylococcal or candidal infections of the kidney may follow bacteremia or fungemia, spreading from distant foci of infection in the bone, skin, vasculature, or elsewhere.

CONDITIONS AFFECTING PATHOGENESIS **Gender and Sexual Activity** The female urethra appears to be particularly prone to colonization with colonic gram-negative bacilli because of its proximity to the anus, its short length (about 4 cm), and its termination beneath the labia. Sexual intercourse causes the introduction of bacteria into the bladder and is temporally associated with the onset of cystitis; it thus appears to be important in the pathogenesis of UTIs in younger women. Voiding after intercourse reduces the risk of cystitis, probably because it promotes the clearance of bacteria introduced during intercourse. In addition, use of spermicidal compounds with a diaphragm or cervical cap or of spermicide-coated condoms dramatically alters the normal introital bacterial flora and has been associated with marked increases in vaginal colonization with *E. coli* and in the risk of UTI.

In males who are <50 years old and who have no history of heterosexual or homosexual rectal intercourse, UTI is exceedingly uncommon, and this diagnosis should be questioned in the absence of clear documentation. An important factor predisposing to bacteriuria in men is urethral obstruction due to prostatic hypertrophy. Homosexuality is also associated with an increased risk of cystitis in men, probably related to rectal intercourse. Men (and women) who are infected with HIV and who have CD4+ T cell counts of $<200/\mu L$ are at increased risk of both bacteriuria and symptomatic UTI. Finally, lack of circumcision has been identified as a risk factor for UTI in both neonates and young men.

Pregnancy UTIs are detected in 2 to 8% of pregnant women. Symptomatic upper tract infections, in particular, are unusually common during pregnancy; fully 20 to 30% of pregnant women with asymptomatic bacteriuria subsequently develop pyelonephritis. This

predisposition to upper tract infection during pregnancy results from decreased ureteral tone, decreased ureteral peristalsis, and temporary incompetence of the vesicoureteral valves. Bladder catheterization during or after delivery causes additional infections. Increased incidences of low-birth-weight infants, premature delivery, and newborn mortality result from UTIs during pregnancy, particularly those infections involving the upper tract.

Obstruction Any impediment to the free flow of urine—tumor, stricture, stone, or prostatic hypertrophy—results in hydronephrosis and a greatly increased frequency of UTI. Infection superimposed on urinary tract obstruction may lead to rapid destruction of renal tissue. It is of utmost importance, therefore, when infection is present, to identify and repair obstructive lesions. On the other hand, when an obstruction is minor and is not progressive or associated with infection, great caution should be exercised in attempting surgical correction. The introduction of infection in such cases may be more damaging than an uncorrected minor obstruction that does not significantly impair renal function.

Neurogenic Bladder Dysfunction Interference with the nerve supply to the bladder, as in spinal cord injury, tabes dorsalis, multiple sclerosis, diabetes, and other diseases, may be associated with UTI. The infection may be initiated by the use of catheters for bladder drainage and is favored by the prolonged stasis of urine in the bladder. An additional factor often operative in these cases is bone demineralization due to immobilization, which causes hypercalciuria, calculus formation, and obstructive uropathy.

Vesicoureteral Reflux Defined as reflux of urine from the bladder cavity up into the ureters and sometimes into the renal pelvis, vesicoureteral reflux occurs during voiding or with elevation of pressure in the bladder. In practice, this condition is demonstrated by the finding of retrograde movement of radiopaque or radioactive material during a voiding cystourethrogram. An anatomically impaired vesicoureteral junction facilitates reflux of bacteria and thus upper tract infection. However, since a fluid connection between the bladder and the kidney always exists, even in the normal urinary system, some retrograde movement of bacteria probably takes place during infection but is not detected by radiologic techniques.

Vesicoureteral reflux is common among children with anatomic abnormalities of the urinary tract as well as among children with anatomically normal but infected urinary tracts. In the latter group, reflux disappears with advancing age and is probably attributable to factors other than UTI. Long-term follow-up of children with UTI who have reflux has established that renal damage correlates with marked reflux, not with infection.

The routine search for reflux would be aided by the development of noninvasive tests applicable to young children, in whom the need for an effective technique is greatest. In the meantime, it appears reasonable to search for reflux in anyone with unexplained failure of renal growth or with renal scarring, because UTI per se is an insufficient explanation for these abnormalities. On the other hand, it is doubtful that all children who have recurrent UTIs but whose urinary tract appears normal on pyelography should be subjected to voiding cystoureterography merely for the detection of the rare patient with marked reflux not revealed by the intravenous pyelogram.

Bacterial Virulence Factors Not all strains of *E. coli* are equally capable of infecting the intact urinary tract. Bacterial virulence factors markedly influence the likelihood that a given strain, once introduced into the bladder, will cause UTI. Most *E. coli* strains that cause symptomatic UTIs in noncatheterized patients belong to a small number of specific O, K, and H serogroups. These uropathogenic clones have accumulated a number of virulence genes that are often closely linked on the bacterial chromosome in "virulence islands." Adherence of bacteria to uroepithelial cells is a critical first step in the initiation of infection. For both *E. coli* and *Proteus*, fimbriae (hairlike proteinaceous surface appendages) mediate the attachment of bacteria to specific receptors on epithelial cells. The attachment of bacteria to uroepithelial cells initiates a number of important events in the mucosal epithelial cell, including secretion of interleukin (IL) 6 and IL-8 and induction of both apoptosis and epithelial cell desquamation. Besides fimbriae, uropathogenic *E. coli* strains usually produce hemolysin and aerobactin (a siderophore for scavenging iron) and are resistant to the bactericidal action of human serum. Nearly all *E. coli* strains causing acute pyelonephritis and most of those causing acute cystitis are uropathogenic. In contrast, infections in patients with structural or functional abnormalities of the urinary tract are generally caused by bacterial strains that lack these uropathogenic properties; the implication is that these properties are not needed for infection of the compromised urinary tract.

Genetic Factors Increasing evidence suggests that host genetic factors influence susceptibility to UTI. A maternal history of UTI is more often found among women who have experienced recurrent UTIs than among controls. The number and type of receptors on uroepithelial cells to which bacteria may attach are at least in part genetically determined. Many of these structures are components of blood group antigens and are present on both erythrocytes and uroepithelial cells. For example, P fimbriae mediate attachment of *E. coli* to P-positive erythrocytes and are found on nearly all strains causing acute uncomplicated pyelonephritis. Conversely, P blood group–negative individuals, who lack these receptors, have a decreased likelihood of pyelonephritis. It has also been demonstrated that nonsecretors of blood group antigens are at increased risk of recurrent UTI; this predisposition may relate to a different profile of genetically determined glycolipids on uroepithelial cells.

LOCALIZATION OF INFECTION Unfortunately, currently available methods of distinguishing renal parenchymal infection from cystitis are neither reliable nor convenient enough for routine clinical use. Fever or an elevated level of C-reactive protein often accompanies acute pyelonephritis and is found in rare cases of cystitis but may also occur in infections other than pyelonephritis.

CLINICAL PRESENTATION **Cystitis** Patients with cystitis usually report dysuria, frequency, urgency, and suprapubic pain. The urine often becomes grossly cloudy and malodorous, and it is bloody in about 30% of cases. White cells and bacteria can be detected by examination of unspun urine in most cases. However, some women with cystitis have only 10^2 to 10^4 bacteria per milliliter of urine, and in these instances bacteria cannot be seen in a Gram-stained preparation of unspun urine. Physical examination generally reveals only tenderness of the urethra or the suprapubic area. If a genital lesion or a vaginal discharge is evident, especially in conjunction with fewer than 10^5 bacteria per milliliter on urine culture, then pathogens that may cause urethritis, vaginitis, or cervicitis, such as *C. trachomatis*, *N. gonorrhoeae*, *Trichomonas*, *Candida*, and herpes simplex virus, should be considered. Prominent systemic manifestations such as a temperature of >38.3°C (>101°F), nausea, and vomiting usually indicate concomitant renal infection, as does costovertebral angle tenderness. However, the absence of these findings does not ensure that infection is limited to the bladder and urethra.

Acute Pyelonephritis Symptoms of acute pyelonephritis generally develop rapidly over a few hours or a day and include a fever, shaking chills, nausea, vomiting, and diarrhea. Symptoms of cystitis may or may not be present. Besides fever, tachycardia, and generalized muscle tenderness, physical examination reveals marked tenderness on deep pressure in one or both costovertebral angles or on deep abdominal palpation. In some patients, signs and symptoms of gram-negative sepsis predominate. Most patients have significant leukocytosis and bacteria detectable in Gram-stained unspun urine. Leukocyte casts are present in the urine of some patients, and the detection of these casts is pathognomonic. Hematuria may be demonstrated during the acute phase of the disease; if it persists after acute manifestations of infection have subsided, a stone, a tumor, or tuberculosis should be considered.

Except in individuals with papillary necrosis, abscess formation, or urinary obstruction, the manifestations of acute pyelonephritis usually respond to therapy within 48 to 72 h. However, despite the absence of symptoms, bacteriuria or pyuria may persist. In severe pyelonephritis, fever subsides more slowly and may not disappear for several days, even after appropriate antibiotic treatment has been instituted.

Urethritis Approximately 30% of women with acute dysuria, frequency, and pyuria have midstream urine cultures that show either no growth or insignificant bacterial growth. Clinically, these women cannot always be readily distinguished from those with cystitis. In this situation, a distinction should be made between women infected with sexually transmitted pathogens, such as *C. trachomatis*, *N. gonorrhoeae*, or herpes simplex virus, and those with low-count *E. coli* or staphylococcal infection of the urethra and bladder. Chlamydial or gonococcal infection should be suspected in women with a gradual onset of illness, no hematuria, no suprapubic pain, and >7 days of symptoms. The additional history of a recent sex-partner change, especially if the patient's partner has recently had chlamydial or gonococcal urethritis, should heighten the suspicion of a sexually transmitted infection, as should the finding of mucopurulent cervicitis (Chaps. 132 and 133). Gross hematuria, suprapubic pain, an abrupt onset of illness, a duration of illness of <3 days, and a history of UTIs favor the diagnosis of *E. coli* UTI.

Catheter-Associated UTIs (See also Chap. 135) Bacteriuria develops in at least 10 to 15% of hospitalized patients with indwelling urethral catheters. The risk of infection is about 3 to 5% per day of catheterization. *E. coli*, *Proteus*, *Pseudomonas*, *Klebsiella*, *Serratia*, staphylococci, enterococci, and *Candida* usually cause these infections. Many infecting strains display markedly greater antimicrobial resistance than organisms that cause community-acquired UTIs. Factors associated with an increased risk of catheter-associated UTI include female sex, prolonged catheterization, severe underlying illness, disconnection of the catheter and drainage tube, other types of faulty catheter care, and lack of systemic antimicrobial therapy.

Infection occurs when bacteria reach the bladder by one of two routes: by migrating through the column of urine in the catheter lumen (intraluminal route) or by moving up the mucous sheath outside the catheter (periurethral route). Hospital-acquired pathogens reach the patient's catheter or urine-collecting system on the hands of hospital personnel, in contaminated solutions or irrigants, and via contaminated instruments or disinfectants. Bacteria usually enter the catheter system at the catheter–collecting tube junction or at the drainage bag portal. The organisms then ascend intraluminally into the bladder within 24 to 72 h. Alternatively, the patient's own bowel flora may colonize the perineal skin and periurethral area and reach the bladder via the external surface of the catheter. This route is particularly common in women. Studies have demonstrated the importance of the attachment and growth of bacteria on the surfaces of the catheter in the pathogenesis of catheter-associated UTI. Such bacteria growing in biofilms on the catheter eventually produce encrustations consisting of bacteria, bacterial glycocalyces, host urinary proteins, and urinary salts. These encrustations provide a refuge for bacteria and may protect them from antimicrobial agents and phagocytes.

Clinically, most catheter-associated infections cause minimal symptoms and no fever and often resolve after withdrawal of the catheter. The frequency of upper tract infection associated with catheter-induced bacteriuria is unknown. Gram-negative bacteremia, which follows catheter-associated bacteriuria in 1 to 2% of cases, is the most significant recognized complication of catheter-induced UTIs. The catheterized urinary tract has repeatedly been demonstrated to be the most common source of gram-negative bacteremia in hospitalized patients, generally accounting for about 30% of cases.

Catheter-associated UTIs can sometimes be prevented in patients catheterized for <2 weeks by use of a sterile closed collecting system, by attention to aseptic technique during insertion and care of the catheter, and by measures to minimize cross-infection. Other preventive approaches, including short courses of systemic antimicrobial therapy, topical application of periurethral antimicrobial ointments, use of preconnected catheter–drainage tube units, use of catheters impregnated with antimicrobial agents, and addition of antimicrobial drugs to the drainage bag, have all been protective in at least one controlled trial but are not recommended for general use. Despite precautions, the majority of patients catheterized for >2 weeks eventually develop bacteriuria. The need for treatment as well as the optimal type and duration of treatment for such patients with asymptomatic bacteriuria have not been established. Removal of the catheter in conjunction with a short course of antibiotics to which the organism is susceptible probably constitutes the best course of action and nearly always eradicates bacteriuria. Treatment of asymptomatic catheter-associated bacteriuria may be of greatest benefit to elderly women, who most often develop symptoms if left untreated. If the catheter cannot be removed, antibiotic therapy usually proves to be unsuccessful and may in fact result in infection with a more resistant strain. In this situation, the bacteriuria should be ignored unless the patient develops symptoms or is at high risk of developing bacteremia. In these cases, use of systemic antibiotics or urinary bladder antiseptics may reduce the degree of bacteriuria and the likelihood of bacteremia. Because of spinal cord injury, incontinence, or other factors, some patients in hospitals or nursing homes require long-term or semipermanent bladder catheterization. Measures intended to prevent infection have been largely unsuccessful, and essentially all such chronically catheterized patients develop bacteriuria. If feasible, intermittent catheterization by a nurse or by the patient appears to reduce the incidence of bacteriuria and associated complications in such patients. Treatment should be provided when symptomatic infections arise, but treatment of asymptomatic bacteriuria in such patients has no apparent benefit.

DIAGNOSTIC TESTING Determination of the number and type of bacteria in the urine is an extremely important diagnostic procedure. In symptomatic patients, bacteria are usually present in the urine in large numbers ($\geq 10^5$/mL). In asymptomatic patients, two consecutive urine specimens should be examined bacteriologically before therapy is instituted, and $\geq 10^5$ bacteria of a single species per milliliter should be demonstrable in both specimens. Since the large number of bacteria in the bladder urine is due in part to bacterial multiplication during residence in the bladder cavity, samples of urine from the ureters or renal pelvis may contain $<10^5$ bacteria per milliliter and yet indicate infection. Similarly, the presence of bacteriuria of any degree in suprapubic aspirates or of $\geq 10^2$ bacteria per milliliter of urine obtained by catheterization usually indicates infection. In some circumstances (antibiotic treatment, high urea concentration, high osmolarity, low pH), urine inhibits bacterial multiplication, resulting in relatively low bacterial colony counts despite infection. For this reason, antiseptic solutions should not be used in washing the periurethral area before collection of the urine specimen. Water diuresis or recent voiding also reduces bacterial counts in urine.

Rapid methods of detection of bacteriuria have been developed as alternatives to standard culture methods. These methods detect bacterial growth by photometry, bioluminescence, or other means and provide results rapidly, usually in 1 to 2 h. Compared with urine cultures, these techniques generally exhibit a sensitivity of 95 to 98% and a negative predictive value of >99% when bacteriuria is defined as 10^5 colony-forming units per milliliter. However, the sensitivity of these tests falls to 60 to 80% when 10^2 to 10^4 colony-forming units per milliliter is the standard of comparison.

Microscopy of urine from symptomatic patients can be of great diagnostic value. Microscopic bacteriuria, which is best assessed with Gram-stained uncentrifuged urine, is found in more than 90% of specimens from patients whose infections are associated with colony counts of at least 10^5/mL, and this finding is very specific. However, bacteria cannot usually be detected microscopically in infections with lower colony counts (10^2 to 10^4/mL). The detection of bacteria by urinary microscopy thus constitutes firm evidence of infection, but the absence of microscopically detectable bacteria does not exclude the diagnosis. When carefully sought by means of chamber-count microscopy, pyuria is a highly sensitive indicator of UTI in symptomatic patients. Pyuria is demonstrated in nearly all acute bacterial UTIs, and its absence calls the diagnosis into question. The leukocyte esterase "dipstick" method is less sensitive than microscopy in identifying pyuria but is a useful alternative where microscopy is not feasible. Pyuria in the absence of bacteriuria (sterile pyuria) may indicate infection with unusual bacterial agents such as *C. trachomatis*, *U. urealyticum*, and *Mycobacterium tuberculosis* or with fungi. Alternatively, sterile pyuria may be demonstrated in noninfectious urologic conditions such as calculi, anatomic abnormality, nephrocalcinosis, vesicoureteral reflux, interstitial nephritis, or polycystic disease.

Although many authorities have recommended that urine culture and antimicrobial susceptibility testing be performed for any patient with a suspected UTI, it may be more practical and cost-effective to manage women who have symptoms characteristic of acute uncomplicated cystitis without an initial urine culture. Two approaches to presumptive therapy have generally been used. In the first, treatment is initiated solely on the basis of a typical history and/or typical findings on physical examination. In the second, women with symptoms and signs of acute cystitis and without complicating factors are managed with urinary microscopy (or, alternatively, with a leukocyte esterase test). A positive result for pyuria and/or bacteriuria provides enough evidence of infection to indicate that urine culture and susceptibility testing can be omitted and the patient treated empirically. Urine should be cultured, however, when a woman's symptoms and urine-examination findings leave the diagnosis of cystitis in question. Pretherapy cultures and susceptibility testing are also essential in the management of all patients with suspected upper tract infections and of those with complicating factors, as in these situations any of a variety of pathogens may be involved and antibiotic therapy is best tailored to the individual organism.

℞ **TREATMENT** The following principles underlie the treatment of UTIs:

1. Except in acute uncomplicated cystitis in women, a quantitative urine culture, a Gram stain, or an alternative rapid diagnostic test should be performed to confirm infection before treatment is begun. When culture results become available, antimicrobial sensitivity testing should be used to direct therapy.
2. Factors predisposing to infection, such as obstruction and calculi, should be identified and corrected if possible.
3. Relief of clinical symptoms does not always indicate bacteriologic cure.
4. Each course of treatment should be classified after its completion as a failure (symptoms and/or bacteriuria not eradicated during therapy or in the immediate posttreatment culture) or a cure (resolution of symptoms and elimination of bacteriuria). Recurrent infections should be classified as same-strain or different-strain and as early (occurring within 2 weeks of the end of therapy) or late.
5. In general, uncomplicated infections confined to the lower urinary tract respond to short courses of therapy, while upper tract infections require longer treatment. After therapy, early recurrences due to the same strain may result from an unresolved upper tract focus of infection but often (especially after short-course therapy for cystitis) result from persistent vaginal colonization. Recurrences >2 weeks after the cessation of therapy nearly always represent reinfection with a new strain or with the previously infecting strain that has persisted in the vaginal and rectal flora.
6. Despite increasing resistance, community-acquired infections, especially initial infections, are usually due to more antibiotic-sensitive strains.
7. In patients with repeated infections, instrumentation, or recent hospitalization, the presence of antibiotic-resistant strains should be suspected.

The anatomic location of a UTI greatly influences the success or failure of a therapeutic regimen. Bladder bacteriuria (cystitis) can usually be eliminated with nearly any antimicrobial agent to which the infecting strain is sensitive; in the past, it was demonstrated that as little as a single dose of 500 mg of intramuscular kanamycin eliminated bladder bacteriuria in most cases. With upper tract infections, however, single-dose therapy fails in the majority of cases, and even a 7-day course is unsuccessful in many instances. Longer periods of treatment (2 to 6 weeks) aimed at eradicating a persistent focus of infection may be necessary in some cases.

In *acute uncomplicated cystitis*, more than 90 to 95% of infections are due to one of two organisms: *E. coli* or *S. saprophyticus*. Although resistance patterns vary geographically and resistance has increased in many areas, most strains are sensitive to many antibiotics. In most parts of the United States, more than one-quarter of *E. coli* strains causing acute cystitis are resistant to amoxicillin, sulfa drugs, and cephalexin, and resistance to trimethoprim (TMP) and trimethoprim-sulfamethoxazole (TMP-SMZ) is now approaching these levels as well.

Many have advocated single-dose treatment for acute cystitis. The advantages of single-dose therapy include less expense, ensured compliance, fewer side effects, and perhaps less intense pressure favoring the selection of resistant organisms in the intestinal, vaginal, or perineal flora. However, more frequent recurrences develop shortly after single-dose therapy than after 3-day treatment, and single-dose therapy does not eradicate vaginal colonization with *E. coli* as effectively as do longer regimens. A 3-day course of therapy with TMP-SMZ, TMP, norfloxacin, ciprofloxacin, or ofloxacin appears to preserve the low rate of side effects of single-dose therapy while improving efficacy (Table 280-1); thus 3-day regimens are currently preferred for acute cystitis. Neither single-dose nor 3-day therapy should be used for women with symptoms or signs of pyelonephritis, urologic abnormalities or stones, or previous infections due to antibiotic-resistant organisms. Males with UTI often have urologic abnormalities or prostatic involvement and hence are not candidates for single-dose or 3-day therapy. For empirical therapy, they should generally receive a 7- to 14-day course of a fluoroquinolone (Table 280-1).

The choice of treatment for women with acute urethritis depends on the etiologic agent involved. In chlamydial infection, azithromycin (1 g in a single oral dose) or doxycycline (100 mg orally bid for 7 days) should be used. Women with acute dysuria and frequency, negative urine cultures, and no pyuria usually do not respond to antimicrobial agents.

In women, *acute uncomplicated pyelonephritis* without accompanying clinical evidence of calculi or urologic disease is due to *E. coli* in most cases. Although the optimal route and duration of therapy have not been established, a 7- to 14-day course of a fluoroquinolone, an aminoglycoside, or a third-generation cephalosporin is usually adequate. Neither ampicillin nor TMP-SMZ should be used as initial therapy because >25% of strains of *E. coli* causing pyelonephritis are now resistant to these drugs in vitro. For at least the first few days of treatment, antibiotics should probably be given intravenously to most patients, but patients with mild symptoms can be treated for 7 to 14 days with an oral antibiotic (usually ciprofloxacin or ofloxacin), with or without an initial single parenteral dose (Table 280-1). Patients who fail to respond to treatment within 72 h or who relapse after therapy should be evaluated for unrecognized suppurative foci, calculi, or urologic disease.

Complicated UTIs (those arising in a setting of catheterization, instrumentation, urologic anatomic or functional abnormalities, stones, obstruction, immunosuppression, renal disease, or diabetes) are typically due to hospital-acquired bacteria, including *E. coli*, *Klebsiella*, *Proteus*, *Serratia*, *Pseudomonas*, enterococci, and staphylococci. Many of the infecting strains are antibiotic-resistant. Empirical antibiotic therapy ideally provides broad-spectrum coverage against these

Table 280-1 Treatment Regimens for Bacterial Urinary Tract Infections

Condition	Characteristic Pathogens	Mitigating Circumstances	Recommended Empirical Treatment[a]
Acute uncomplicated cystitis in women	*Escherichia coli, Staphylococcus saprophyticus, Proteus mirabilis, Klebsiella pneumoniae*	None	3-Day regimens: oral TMP-SMZ, TMP, quinolone; 7-day regimen: macrocrystalline nitrofurantoin[b]
		Diabetes, symptoms for >7 d, recent UTI, use of diaphragm, age >65 years	Consider 7-day regimen: oral TMP-SMZ, TMP, quinolone[b]
		Pregnancy	Consider 7-day regimen: oral amoxicillin, macrocrystalline nitrofurantoin, cefpodoxime proxetil, or TMP-SMZ[b]
Acute uncomplicated pyelonephritis in women	*E. coli, P. mirabilis, S. saprophyticus*	Mild to moderate illness, no nausea or vomiting; outpatient therapy	Oral[c] quinolone for 7–14 d (initial dose given IV if desired); or single-dose ceftriaxone[d] or gentamicin[d] IV followed by oral TMP-SMZ[b] for 14 d
		Severe illness or possible urosepsis: hospitalization required	Parenteral[d] ceftriaxone, quinolone, gentamicin (± ampicillin), or aztreonam until defervescence; then oral[c] quinolone, cephalosporin, or TMP-SMZ for 14 d
Complicated UTI in men and women	*E. coli, Proteus, Klebsiella, Pseudomonas, Serratia,* enterococci, staphylococci	Mild to moderate illness, no nausea or vomiting: outpatient therapy	Oral[c] quinolone for 10–14 d
		Severe illness or possible urosepsis: hospitalization required	Parenteral[d] ampicillin and gentamicin, quinolone, ceftriaxone, aztreonam, ticarcillin/clavulanate, or imipenem-cilastatin until defervescence; then oral[c] quinolone or TMP-SMZ for 10–21 d

[a] Treatments listed are those to be prescribed before the etiologic agent is known; Gram's staining can be helpful in the selection of empirical therapy. Such therapy can be modified once the infecting agent has been identified. Fluoroquinolones should not be used in pregnancy. TMP-SMZ, although not approved for use in pregnancy, has been widely used. Gentamicin should be used with caution in pregnancy because of its possible toxicity to eighth-nerve development in the fetus.

[b] Multiday oral regimens for cystitis are as follows: TMP-SMZ, 160/800 mg q12h; TMP, 100 mg q12h; norfloxacin, 400 mg q12h; ciprofloxacin, 250 mg q12h; ofloxacin, 200 mg q12h; lomefloxacin, 400 mg/d; enoxacin, 400 mg q12h; macrocrystalline nitrofurantoin, 100 mg qid; amoxicillin, 250 mg q8h; cefpodoxime proxetil, 100 mg q12h.

[c] Oral regimens for pyelonephritis and complicated UTI are as follows: TMP-SMZ, 160/800 mg q12h; ciprofloxacin, 500 mg q12h; ofloxacin, 200–300 mg q12h; lomefloxacin, 400 mg/d; enoxacin, 400 mg q12h; amoxicillin, 500 mg q8h; cefpodoxime proxetil, 200 mg q12h.

[d] Parenteral regimens are as follows: ciprofloxacin, 200–400 mg q12h; ofloxacin, 200–400 mg q12h; gentamicin, 1 mg/kg q8h; ceftriaxone, 1–2 g/d; ampicillin, 1 g q6h; imipenem-cilastatin, 250–500 mg q6-8h; ticarcillin/clavulanate, 3.2 g q8h; aztreonam, 1 g q8–12h.

NOTE: UTI, urinary tract infection; TMP, trimethoprim; TMP-SMZ, trimethoprim-sulfamethoxazole.

pathogens. In patients with minimal or mild symptoms, oral therapy with a fluoroquinolone, such as ciprofloxacin or ofloxacin, can be administered until culture results and antibiotic sensitivities are known. In patients with more severe illness, including acute pyelonephritis or suspected urosepsis, hospitalization and parenteral therapy should be undertaken. Commonly used empirical regimens include imipenem alone, a penicillin or cephalosporin plus an aminoglycoside, and (when the involvement of enterococci is unlikely) ceftriaxone or ceftazidime. When information on the antimicrobial sensitivity pattern of the infecting strain becomes available, a more specific antimicrobial regimen can be selected. Therapy should generally be administered for 10 to 21 days, with the exact duration depending on the severity of the infection and the susceptibility of the infecting strain. Follow-up cultures 2 to 4 weeks after cessation of therapy should be performed to demonstrate cure.

In *pregnancy*, acute cystitis can be managed with 7 days of treatment with amoxicillin, nitrofurantoin, or a cephalosporin. All pregnant women should be screened for asymptomatic bacteriuria during the first trimester and, if bacteriuric, should be treated with one of the regimens listed in Table 280-1. After treatment, a culture should be performed to ensure cure, and cultures should be repeated monthly thereafter until delivery. Acute pyelonephritis in pregnancy should be managed with hospitalization and parenteral antibiotic therapy, generally with a cephalosporin or an extended-spectrum penicillin. Continuous low-dose prophylaxis with nitrofurantoin should be given to women who have recurrent infections during pregnancy.

Asymptomatic bacteriuria is common, especially among elderly patients, but has not been linked to adverse outcomes in most circumstances other than pregnancy (see above). Thus antimicrobial therapy is unnecessary and may in fact promote the emergence of resistant strains in most patients with asymptomatic bacteriuria. High-risk patients with neutropenia, renal transplants, obstruction, or other complicating conditions may require treatment when asymptomatic bacteriuria occurs. Seven days of therapy with an oral agent to which the organism is sensitive should be given initially. If bacteriuria persists, it can be monitored without further treatment in most patients. Longer-term therapy (4 to 6 weeks) may be necessary in high-risk patients with persistent asymptomatic bacteriuria.

UROLOGIC EVALUATION Very few women with recurrent UTIs have correctable lesions discovered at cystoscopy or upon intravenous pyelography, and these procedures should not be undertaken routinely in such cases. Urologic evaluation should be performed in selected instances—namely, in women with relapsing infection, a history of childhood infections, stones or painless hematuria, or recurrent pyelonephritis. Most males with UTI should be considered to have complicated infection and thus should be evaluated urologically. Possible exceptions include young men who have cystitis associated with sexual activity, who are uncircumcised, or who have AIDS. Men or women presenting with acute infection and signs or symptoms suggestive of an obstruction or stones should undergo prompt urologic evaluation, generally by means of ultrasound.

PROGNOSIS In patients with uncomplicated cystitis or pyelonephritis, treatment ordinarily results in complete resolution of symptoms. Lower tract infections in women are of concern mainly because they cause discomfort, morbidity, loss of time from work, and substantial health-care costs. Cystitis may also result in upper tract infection or in bacteremia (especially during instrumentation), but little evidence suggests that renal impairment follows. When repeated episodes of cystitis occur, they are nearly always reinfections, not relapses.

Acute uncomplicated pyelonephritis in adults rarely progresses to renal functional impairment and chronic renal disease. Repeated upper tract infections often represent relapse rather than reinfection, and a vigorous search for renal calculi or an underlying urologic abnormality should be undertaken. If neither is found, 6 weeks of chemotherapy may be useful in eradicating an unresolved focus of infection.

Repeated symptomatic UTIs in children and in adults with obstructive uropathy, neurogenic bladder, structural renal disease, or diabetes progress to chronic renal disease with unusual frequency. Asymptomatic bacteriuria in these groups as well as in adults without urologic disease or obstruction predisposes to increased numbers of episodes of symptomatic infection but does not result in renal impairment in most instances.

PREVENTION Women who experience frequent symptomatic UTIs (≥3 per year on average) are candidates for long-term administration of low-dose antibiotics directed at preventing recurrences. Such women should be advised to avoid spermicide use and to void soon after intercourse. Daily or thrice-weekly administration of a single dose of TMP-SMZ (80/400 mg), TMP alone (100 mg), or nitrofurantoin (50 mg) has been particularly effective. Norfloxacin and other fluoroquinolones have also been used for prophylaxis. Prophylaxis should be initiated only after bacteriuria has been eradicated with a full-dose treatment regimen. The same prophylactic regimens can be used after sexual intercourse to prevent episodes of symptomatic infection in women in whom UTIs are temporally related to intercourse. Other patients for whom prophylaxis appears to have some merit include men with chronic prostatitis; patients undergoing prostatectomy, both during the operation and in the postoperative period; and pregnant women with asymptomatic bacteriuria. All pregnant women should be screened for bacteriuria in the first trimester and should be treated if bacteriuria is demonstrated.

PAPILLARY NECROSIS

When infection of the renal pyramids develops in association with vascular diseases of the kidney or with urinary tract obstruction, renal papillary necrosis is likely to result. Patients with diabetes, sickle cell disease, chronic alcoholism, and vascular disease seem peculiarly susceptible to this complication. Hematuria, pain in the flank or abdomen, and chills and fever are the most common presenting symptoms. Acute renal failure with oliguria or anuria sometimes develops. Rarely, sloughing of a pyramid may take place without symptoms in a patient with chronic UTI, and the diagnosis is made when the necrotic tissue is passed in the urine or identified as a "ring shadow" on pyelography. If renal function deteriorates suddenly in a diabetic individual or a patient with chronic obstruction, the diagnosis of renal papillary necrosis should be entertained, even in the absence of fever or pain. Renal papillary necrosis is often bilateral; when it is unilateral, however, nephrectomy may be a life-saving approach to the management of overwhelming infection.

EMPHYSEMATOUS PYELONEPHRITIS AND CYSTITIS

These unusual clinical entities almost always occur in diabetic patients, often in concert with urinary obstruction and chronic infection. Emphysematous pyelonephritis is usually characterized by a rapidly progressive clinical course, with high fever, leukocytosis, renal parenchymal necrosis, and accumulation of fermentative gases in the kidney and perinephric tissues. Most patients also have pyuria and glucosuria. *E. coli* causes most cases, but occasionally other Enterobacteriaceae are isolated. Gas in tissues can often be seen on plain films and can best be confirmed and localized by computed tomography. Surgical resection of the involved tissue in addition to systemic antimicrobial therapy is usually needed to prevent mortality in emphysematous pyelonephritis.

Emphysematous cystitis also occurs primarily in diabetic patients, usually in association with *E. coli* or other facultative gram-negative rods and often in relation to bladder outlet obstruction. Patients with this condition are generally less severely ill and have less rapidly progressive disease than those with emphysematous pyelonephritis. The patient typically reports abdominal pain, dysuria, frequency, and (in some cases) pneumaturia. Computed tomography shows gas within both the bladder lumen and the bladder wall. Generally, conservative therapy with systemic antimicrobial agents and relief of outlet obstruction are effective, but some patients do not respond to these measures and require cystectomy.

RENAL AND PERINEPHRIC ABSCESS

See Chap. 130.

PROSTATITIS

The term *prostatitis* has been used for various inflammatory conditions affecting the prostate, including acute and chronic infections with specific bacteria and, more commonly, instances in which signs and symptoms of prostatic inflammation are present but no specific organisms can be detected. Patients with acute bacterial prostatitis can usually be identified on the basis of typical symptoms and signs, pyuria, and bacteriuria. To classify a patient with suspected chronic prostatitis correctly, first-void and midstream urine specimens, a prostatic expressate, and a postmassage urine specimen should be quantitatively cultured and evaluated for numbers of leukocytes. On the basis of the results of these studies, patients can be classified as having chronic bacterial prostatitis, chronic nonbacterial prostatitis, or prostatodynia. Patients with suspected chronic prostatitis usually have low back pain, perineal or testicular discomfort, mild dysuria, and lower urinary obstructive symptoms. Microscopic pyuria may be the only objective manifestation of prostatic disease.

ACUTE BACTERIAL PROSTATITIS When it occurs spontaneously, this disease generally affects young men; however, it may also be associated with an indwelling urethral catheter. It is characterized by fever, chills, dysuria, and a tense or boggy, extremely tender prostate. Although prostatic massage usually produces purulent secretions with a large number of bacteria on culture, bacteremia may result from manipulation of the inflamed gland. For this reason and because the etiologic agent can usually be identified by Gram's staining and culture of urine, vigorous prostatic massage should be avoided. In non-catheter-associated cases, the infection is generally due to common gram-negative urinary tract pathogens (*E. coli* or *Klebsiella*). Initially, an intravenous fluoroquinolone, third-generation cephalosporin, or aminoglycoside can be administered if gram-negative rods are visible in urine, and a cephalosporin or nafcillin can be given if gram-positive cocci are detected. Although many of these drugs do not readily diffuse into the noninflamed prostate gland, the response to antibiotics in acute bacterial prostatitis is usually prompt, perhaps because drugs penetrate more readily into the acutely inflamed prostate. In catheter-associated cases, the spectrum of etiologic agents is broader, including hospital-acquired gram-negative rods and enterococci. The urinary Gram stain may be particularly helpful in such cases. Imipenem, an aminoglycoside, a fluoroquinolone, or a third-generation cephalosporin should be used for initial therapy until the organism has been isolated and its susceptibilities have been determined. The long-term prognosis is good, although in some instances acute infection may result in abscess formation, epididymoorchitis, seminal vesiculitis, septicemia, and residual chronic bacterial prostatitis. Since the advent of antibiotics, the frequency of acute bacterial prostatitis has diminished markedly. In many instances, infections diagnosed as acute prostatitis are probably cases of posterior urethritis.

CHRONIC BACTERIAL PROSTATITIS This entity is now infrequent but should be considered in men with a history of recurrent bacteriuria. Symptoms are often lacking between episodes, and the prostate usually feels normal on palpation. Obstructive symptoms or perineal pain develops in some patients. Intermittently, infection spreads to the bladder, producing frequency, urgency, and dysuria. A pattern of relapsing infection in a middle-aged man strongly suggests chronic bacterial prostatitis. Classically, the diagnosis is established by culture of *E. coli*, *Klebsiella*, *Proteus*, or other uropathogenic bacteria from the expressed prostatic secretion or postmassage urine in higher quantities than are found in first-void or midstream urine. Antibiotics promptly relieve the symptoms associated with acute exacerbations but have been less effective in eradicating the focus of chronic infection in the prostate. The relative ineffectiveness of antimicrobial agents for long-term cure results in part from the poor penetration of the prostate by most of these drugs; the low pH that prevails in this organ precludes the passage of most agents. Fluoroquinolones, including ciprofloxacin and ofloxacin, have been considerably more successful than other antimicrobials, but they must generally be given for at least 12 weeks to be effective. Patients with frequent episodes of acute cystitis in whom attempts at curative therapy fail can be managed with prolonged courses of antimicrobials (usually a sulfonamide, TMP, or nitrofurantoin), with a view toward suppressing symptoms and keeping the bladder urine sterile. Total prostatectomy obviously results in the cure of chronic prostatitis but is associated with considerable morbidity. Transurethral prostatectomy is safer but cures only one-third of patients.

NONBACTERIAL PROSTATITIS Patients who present with symptoms and signs of prostatitis, increased numbers of leukocytes in expressed prostatic secretion and postmassage urine, no bacterial growth in cultures, and no history of recurrent episodes of bacterial prostatitis are classified as having nonbacterial prostatitis. Prostatic inflammation can be considered present when the expressed prostatic secretion and postmassage urine contain at least tenfold more leukocytes than the first-void and midstream urine specimens or when the expressed prostatic secretion contains ≥1000 leukocytes per microliter.

The presumably infectious etiology of this condition remains unidentified. Evidence for a causative role of both *U. urealyticum* and *C. trachomatis* has been presented but is not conclusive. Since most cases of nonbacterial prostatitis occur in young, sexually active men and since many cases follow an episode of nonspecific urethritis, the causative agent may well be sexually transmitted. The effectiveness of antimicrobial agents in this condition remains uncertain. Some patients benefit from a 4- to 6-week course of treatment with erythromycin, doxycycline, TMP-SMZ, or a fluoroquinolone, but controlled trials are lacking.

PROSTATODYNIA Patients who have symptoms and signs of prostatitis but who have no evidence of prostatic inflammation (normal leukocyte counts) and negative urine cultures are classified as having prostatodynia. Despite their symptoms, these patients most likely do not have prostatic infection and should not be given antimicrobial agents.

BIBLIOGRAPHY

AGACE W et al: Host resistance to urinary tract infection, in *Molecular Pathogenesis and Clinical Management*, HLT Mobley, JW Warren (eds). Washington, DC, ASM Press, 1996, pp 221–245

EISENSTADT J, WASHINGTON JA: Diagnostic microbiology for bacteria and yeasts causing urinary tract infections, in *Molecular Pathogenesis and Clinical Management*, HLT Mobley, JW Warren (eds). Washington, DC, ASM Press, 1996, pp 29–67

GRATACOS E et al: Screening and treatment of asymptomatic bacteriuria in pregnancy prevent pyelonephritis. J Infect Dis 169:1390, 1994

GUPTA K et al: Increasing prevalence of antimicrobial resistance among uropathogens causing acute uncomplicated cystitis in women. JAMA 281:736, 1999

HOOTON TM, STAMM WE: Diagnosis and treatment of uncomplicated urinary tract infection. Infect Dis Clin North Am 11:551, 1997

——— et al: Randomized comparative trial and cost analysis of 3-day antimicrobial regimens for treatment of acute cystitis in women. JAMA 273:41, 1995

——— et al: A prospective study of risk factors for symptomatic urinary tract infection in young women. N Engl J Med 335:468, 1996

JOHNSON JR: Treatment and prevention of urinary tract infections, in *Urinary Tract Infections: Molecular Pathogenesis and Clinical Management*, HLT Mobley, JW Warren (eds). Washington, DC, ASM Press, 1996, pp 95–118

SCHAEFFER AJ: Urinary tract infection in men—state of the art. Infection (Suppl 1):S19, 1994

STAMM WE, HOOTON TM: Catheter-associated urinary tract infections: Epidemiology, pathogenesis, prevention. Am J Med 91(Suppl 3B):655, 1991

———, ———: Management of urinary tract infections in adults. N Engl J Med 329: 1328, 1993

WARREN JW et al: Guidelines for antimicrobial therapy of uncomplicated acute bacterial cystitis and acute pyelonephritis in women. Clin Infect Dis 29:745, 1999

281 URINARY TRACT OBSTRUCTION

Julian L. Seifter, Barry M. Brenner

Obstruction to the flow of urine, with attendant stasis and elevation in urinary tract pressure, impairs renal and urinary conduit functions and is a common cause of acute and chronic renal failure. With early relief of obstruction, the defects in function usually disappear completely. However, chronic obstruction may produce permanent loss of renal mass (renal atrophy) and excretory capability, as well as enhanced susceptibility to local infection and stone formation. Early diagnosis and prompt therapy are therefore essential to minimize the otherwise devastating effects of obstruction on kidney structure and function.

ETIOLOGY Obstruction to urine flow can result from *intrinsic* or *extrinsic mechanical blockade* as well as from *functional defects* not associated with fixed occlusion of the urinary drainage system. Mechanical obstruction can occur at any level of the urinary tract, from the renal calyces to the external urethral meatus. Normal points of narrowing, such as the ureteropelvic and ureterovesical junctions, bladder neck, and urethral meatus, are common sites of obstruction. When blockage is above the level of the bladder, unilateral dilatation of the ureter (*hydroureter*) and renal pyelocalyceal system (*hydronephrosis*) occur; lesions at or below the level of the bladder cause bilateral involvement.

Common forms of obstruction are listed in Table 281-1. In childhood, *congenital malformations*, including marked narrowing of the ureteropelvic junction, anomalous (retrocaval) location of the ureter, and posterior urethral valves, predominate. The latter defect is the most common cause of bilateral hydronephrosis in boys. Children may also have bladder dysfunction secondary to congenital urethral stricture, urethral meatal stenosis, or bladder neck obstruction. In adults, urinary tract obstruction is due mainly to *acquired defects*. Pelvic tumors, calculi, and urethral stricture predominate. Ligation of, or injury to, the ureter during pelvic or colonic surgery can lead to hydronephrosis which, if unilateral, may remain relatively silent and undetected. *Schistosoma haematobium* and genitourinary tuberculosis are infectious causes of ureteral obstruction. Obstructive uropathy may also result from extrinsic neoplastic (carcinoma of cervix or colon, retroperitoneal lymphoma) or inflammatory disorders. One such inflammatory disorder is retroperitoneal fibrosis, a process of unknown cause seen most commonly in middle-aged men, which occasionally leads to bilateral ureteral obstruction. Retroperitoneal fibrosis must be distinguished from other retroperitoneal causes of ureteral obstruction, particularly lymphomas and pelvic neoplasms.

Functional impairment of urine flow usually results from disorders that involve both the ureter and bladder. Common functional lesions include neurogenic bladder, often with adynamic ureter, and vesicoureteral reflux. Reflux of urine from bladder to ureter(s) is more common in children than in adults and may result in severe unilateral or bilateral hydroureter and hydronephrosis. Abnormal insertion of the ureter into the bladder is the most common cause of vesicoureteral reflux in children. Reflux in the absence of urinary tract infection or bladder neck obstruction usually does not lead to renal parenchymal damage and often resolves spontaneously as the child matures. Surgical reinsertion of the ureter into the bladder is indicated if reflux is severe and unlikely to improve spontaneously, if renal function deteriorates, or if urinary tract infections recur despite chronic antimicrobial therapy. Hydronephrosis, usually more marked on the right than on the left, is common in pregnancy, due both to ureteral compression by the enlarged uterus and to functional effects of progesterone.

CLINICAL FEATURES The pathophysiology and clinical features of urinary tract obstruction are summarized in Table 281-2. *Pain* is the symptom that most commonly provokes the need for medical attention. The pain of urinary tract obstruction is due to distention of the collecting system or renal capsule. The severity of the pain is influenced more by the rate at which distention develops than by the degree of distention. Acute supravesical obstruction, as from a stone lodged in a ureter (Chap. 279), is associated with excruciatingly severe pain, usually called *renal colic*. This pain is relatively steady and continuous, with little fluctuation in intensity, and often radiates to the lower abdomen, testes, or labia. By contrast, more insidious causes of obstruction, such as chronic narrowing of the ureteropelvic junction, may produce little or no pain yet result in total destruction of the affected kidney. Flank pain that occurs only with micturition is pathognomonic of vesicoureteral reflux.

Azotemia develops in urinary tract obstruction when overall excretory function is impaired. This may occur in the setting of bladder outlet obstruction, bilateral renal pelvic or ureteric obstruction, or unilateral disease in a patient with a solitary functioning kidney. Complete bilateral obstruction should be suspected when acute renal failure is accompanied by anuria. Any patient with renal failure otherwise unexplained or with a history of nephrolithiasis, hematuria, diabetes mellitus, prostatic enlargement, pelvic surgery, trauma, or tumor should be evaluated for urinary tract obstruction.

In the acute setting, bilateral obstruction may result in sodium and water retention that may mimic prerenal azotemia. However, with more prolonged obstruction, symptoms of *polyuria* and *nocturia* commonly accompany partial urinary tract obstruction and result from impaired renal concentrating ability. This defect usually does not improve with administration of vasopressin and is therefore a form of acquired nephrogenic diabetes insipidus. Disturbances in sodium chloride transport in the ascending limb of Henle and, in azotemic patients, the

Table 281-1 Common Mechanical Causes of Urinary Tract Obstruction

Ureter	Bladder Outlet	Urethra
CONGENITAL		
Ureteropelvic junction narrowing or obstruction	Bladder neck obstruction	Posterior urethral valves
Ureterovesical junction narrowing or obstruction	Ureterocele	Anterior urethral valves
Ureterocele		Stricture
Retrocaval ureter		Meatal stenosis
		Phimosis
ACQUIRED INTRINSIC DEFECTS		
Calculi	Benign prostatic hyperplasia	Stricture
Inflammation	Cancer of prostate	Tumor
Trauma	Cancer of bladder	Calculi
Sloughed papillae	Calculi	Trauma
Tumor	Diabetic neuropathy	Phimosis
Blood clots	Spinal cord disease	
Uric acid crystals	Anticholinergic drugs and α-adrenergic antagonists	
ACQUIRED EXTRINSIC DEFECTS		
Pregnant uterus	Carcinoma of cervix, colon	Trauma
Retroperitoneal fibrosis	Trauma	
Aortic aneurysm		
Uterine leiomyomata		
Carcinoma of uterus, prostate, bladder, colon, rectum		
Lymphoma, pelvic inflammatory disease		
Accidental surgical ligation		

Table 281-2 Pathophysiology of Bilateral Ureteral Obstruction

Hemodynamic Effects	Tubule Effects	Clinical Features
ACUTE		
↑ Renal blood flow ↓ GFR ↓ Medullary blood flow ↑ Vasodilator prostaglandins	↑ Ureteral and tubule pressures ↑ Reabsorption of Na^+, urea, water	Pain (capsule distention) Azotemia Oliguria or anuria
CHRONIC		
↓ Renal blood flow ↓ ↓ GFR ↑ Vasoconstrictor prostaglandins ↑ Renin-angiotensin production	↓ Medullary osmolarity ↓ Concentrating ability Structural damage; parenchymal atrophy ↓ Transport functions for Na^+, K^+, H^+	Azotemia Hypertension ADH-insensitive polyuria Natriuresis Hyperkalemic, hyperchloremic acidosis
RELEASE OF OBSTRUCTION		
Slow ↑ in GFR (variable)	↓ Tubule pressure ↑ Solute load per nephron (urea, NaCl) Natriuretic factors present	Postobstructive diuresis Potential for volume depletion and electrolyte imbalance due to losses of Na^+, K^+, PO_4^{2-}, Mg^{2+}, and water

NOTE: GFR, glomerular filtration rate.

osmotic (urea) diuresis per nephron lead to decreased medullary hypertonicity and hence a concentrating defect. Partial obstruction, therefore, may be associated with increased rather than decreased urine output. Indeed, wide fluctuations in urine output in a patient with azotemia should always raise the possibility of intermittent or partial urinary tract obstruction. If fluid intake is inadequate, severe dehydration and hypernatremia may develop. Hesitancy and straining to initiate the urinary stream, postvoid dribbling, urinary frequency, and (overflow) incontinence are common with obstruction at or below the level of the bladder.

In addition to loss of urinary concentrating ability and azotemia, partial bilateral urinary tract obstruction often results in other derangements of renal function, including *acquired distal renal tubular acidosis, hyperkalemia*, and *renal salt wasting*. These defects in tubule function are often accompanied by renal tubulointerstitial damage. Morphologic abnormalities appear early in the course of obstruction; initially the interstitium becomes edematous and infiltrated with mononuclear inflammatory cells. With continued obstruction, the interstitium becomes fibrotic; scarring and atrophy of the papillae and medulla occur and precede these processes in the cortex.

The possibility of urinary tract obstruction must always be considered in patients with urinary tract infections or urolithiasis. Urinary stasis encourages the growth of organisms as well as the formation of crystals, especially magnesium ammonium phosphate (struvite). *Hypertension* is frequent in acute and subacute unilateral obstruction and is usually a consequence of increased release of renin by the involved kidney. Chronic unilateral or bilateral hydronephrosis, in the presence of extracellular volume expansion or other renal disease, may result in significant hypertension. *Erythrocytosis*, an infrequent complication of obstructive uropathy, is probably secondary to increased erythropoietin production by the obstructed kidney.

DIAGNOSIS A history of difficulty in voiding, pain, infection, or changes in urinary volume is common. Evidence for distention of the kidney or urinary bladder can often be obtained by palpation and percussion of the abdomen. A careful rectal examination may reveal enlargement or nodularity of the prostate, abnormal rectal sphincter tone, or a rectal or pelvic mass. The penis should be inspected for evidence of meatal stenosis or phimosis. In the female, vaginal, uterine, and rectal lesions responsible for urinary tract obstruction are usually revealed by inspection and palpation.

Urinalysis and examination of the urine sediment may reveal hematuria, pyuria, and bacteriuria. Often, however, the urine sediment is normal, even when obstruction leads to marked azotemia and extensive structural damage. An abdominal scout film should be obtained to evaluate the possibility of nephrocalcinosis or a radiopaque stone at any level of the urinary collecting system. As indicated in Fig. 281-1, if urinary tract obstruction is suspected, a bladder catheter should be inserted. If diuresis does not follow, then abdominal ultrasonography should be performed to evaluate renal and bladder size, as well as pyelocalyceal contour. Ultrasonography is approximately 90% specific and sensitive for detection of hydronephrosis. False-positive results are associated with diuresis, renal cysts, or presence of an extrarenal pelvis, a normal congenital variant. Hydronephrosis may be absent on ultrasound when obstruction is associated with volume contraction, staghorn calculi, retroperitoneal fibrosis, or infiltrative renal disease.

In some cases, the intravenous urogram may define the site of obstruction. In the presence of obstruction, the appearance time of the nephrogram is often delayed. Eventually, however, the renal image becomes more dense than normal because of slow tubular fluid flow rate, which results in enhanced water reabsorption by the nephrons and greater concentration of contrast medium within tubules. The kidney involved by an acute obstructive process is usually slightly enlarged, and there is dilatation of the calyces, renal pelvis, and ureter above the obstruction. The ureter, however, is not tortuous, as is the case when the obstruction is chronic. In comparison with the nephrogram, the urogram may be extremely faint, especially if the dilated renal pelvis is voluminous, causing dilution of the contrast medium. The radiographic study

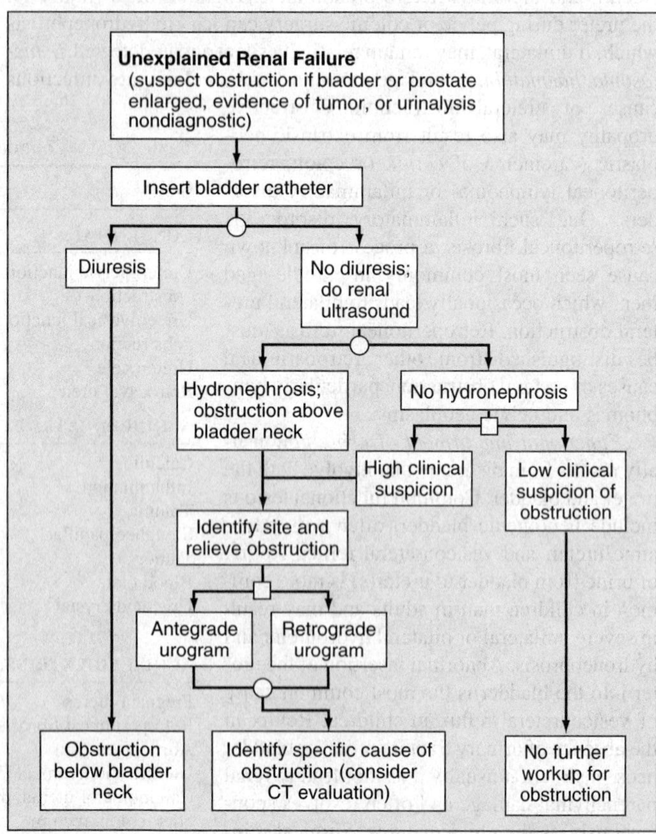

FIGURE 281-1 Diagnostic approach for urinary tract obstruction in unexplained renal failure. Circles represent diagnostic procedures, and squares indicate clinical decisions based on available data. CT, computed tomography.

should be continued until the site of obstruction is determined or the contrast medium is excreted. Radionuclide scans define less anatomic detail than intravenous urography and, like the urogram, are of limited value when renal function is poor. Nonetheless, such scans are sensitive for the detection of obstruction and provide a substitute test in some patients at high risk for reaction to intravenous contrast.

To facilitate visualization of a suspected lesion in a ureter or renal pelvis, *retrograde* or *antegrade urography* should be attempted. These diagnostic studies may be preferable to the intravenous urogram in the azotemic patient, in whom poor excretory function precludes adequate visualization of the collecting system. Furthermore, intravenous urography carries the risk of contrast-induced acute renal failure in patients with proteinuria, renal insufficiency, diabetes mellitus, or multiple myeloma, particularly when performed under conditions of dehydration. The retrograde approach involves catheterization of the involved ureter under cystoscopic control, while the antegrade technique necessitates placement of a catheter into the renal pelvis via a needle inserted percutaneously under ultrasonic or fluoroscopic guidance. While the antegrade approach carries the added advantage of providing immediate decompression of a unilateral obstructing lesion, many urologists initially attempt the retrograde approach and resort to the antegrade method only when attempts at retrograde catheterization are unsuccessful or when cystoscopy or general anesthesia is contraindicated.

Patients suspected of having intermittent ureteropelvic obstruction (whether functional or mechanical) should have radiologic evaluation while they are in pain, since a normal urogram is commonly seen during asymptomatic periods. Hydration often helps to provoke a symptomatic attack. Voiding cystourethrography is of great value in the diagnosis of vesicoureteral reflux and bladder neck and urethral obstructions. Patients with obstruction at or below the level of the bladder exhibit thickening, trabeculation, and diverticula of the bladder wall. Postvoiding films reveal residual urine. If these radiographic studies fail to provide adequate information for diagnosis, endoscopic visualization by the urologist often permits precise identification of lesions involving the urethra, prostate, bladder, and ureteral orifices.

Computed tomography is useful in the diagnosis of specific intra-abdominal and retroperitoneal causes of obstruction but is less practical as an initial test to establish the presence of obstruction. Magnetic resonance imaging may also be useful in the identification of specific obstructive causes.

℞ **TREATMENT** An individual with any form of urinary tract obstruction complicated by infection requires relief of obstruction as soon as possible to prevent development of generalized sepsis and progressive renal damage. On a temporary basis, depending on the site of obstruction, drainage is often satisfactorily achieved by nephrostomy; ureterostomy; or ureteral, urethral, or suprapubic catheterization. The patient with acute urinary tract infection and obstruction should be given appropriate antibiotics based on in vitro bacterial sensitivity and ability of the drug to concentrate in the kidney and urine. Treatment may be required for 3 to 4 weeks. Chronic or recurrent infections in an obstructed kidney with poor intrinsic function may necessitate nephrectomy. When infection is not present, immediate surgery often is not required, even in the presence of complete obstruction and anuria (because of the availability of dialysis), at least until acid-base, fluid and electrolyte, and cardiovascular status are restored to normal. Nevertheless, the site of obstruction should be ascertained as soon as feasible, in part because of the possibility that sepsis may occur and necessitate prompt urologic intervention. Elective relief of obstruction is usually recommended in patients with urinary retention, recurrent urinary tract infections, persistent pain, or progressive loss of renal function. Infrequently, mechanical obstruction can be alleviated by nonsurgical means, as with radiation therapy for retroperitoneal lymphoma. Likewise, functional obstruction secondary to neurogenic bladder may be decreased with the combination of frequent voiding and cholinergic drugs. →*The approach to obstruction secondary to renal stones is discussed in Chap. 279.*

PROGNOSIS With relief of obstruction, the prognosis regarding return of renal function depends largely on whether irreversible renal damage has occurred. When obstruction is not relieved, the course will depend mainly on whether the obstruction is complete or incomplete, bilateral or unilateral, and whether urinary tract infection is also present. Complete obstruction with infection can lead to total destruction of the kidney within days. In dogs, relief of complete obstruction of 1 and 2 weeks' duration restores glomerular filtration rate to 60 and 30% of normal, respectively; after 8 weeks of obstruction, recovery does not occur. Nevertheless, in the absence of definitive evidence of irreversibility, every effort should be made to decompress in the hope of restoring renal function at least partially. A renal radionuclide scan, performed after a prolonged period of decompression, may be used to predict reversible renal function.

POSTOBSTRUCTIVE DIURESIS Relief of bilateral, but not unilateral, complete urinary tract obstruction commonly leads to a postobstructive diuresis, characterized by polyuria, which may be massive. The urine is usually hypotonic and may contain large amounts of sodium chloride, potassium, and magnesium. The natriuresis is due, at least in part, to the excretion of retained urea, which acts as a poorly reabsorbable solute and diminishes salt and water reabsorption in the tubules (osmotic diuresis). The increase in intratubular pressure very likely also contributes to the impairment in net sodium chloride reabsorption, especially in the terminal nephron segments. Natriuretic factors (other than urea) may also accumulate during uremia induced by obstruction and depress salt and water reabsorption when urine flow is reestablished. In the majority of patients this diuresis is physiologic, resulting in the *appropriate* excretion of the excesses of salt and water retained during the period of obstruction. When extracellular volume and composition return to normal, the diuresis usually abates spontaneously. Therefore, replacement of urinary losses should serve only to prevent hypovolemia, hypotension, or disturbances in serum electrolyte concentrations. Occasionally, iatrogenic expansion of extracellular volume, secondary to administration of excessive quantities of intravenous fluids, is responsible for, or sustains, the diuresis observed in the postobstructive period. Replacement of no more than two-thirds of urinary volume losses per day is usually effective in avoiding this complication. The loss of electrolyte-free water with urea may result in hypernatremia. Serum and urine sodium and osmolal concentrations should guide the use of appropriate intravenous replacement. Often replacement with 0.45% saline is required. In a rare patient, relief of obstruction may be followed by urinary salt and water losses severe enough to provoke profound dehydration and vascular collapse. In these patients, an intrinsic defect in tubule reabsorptive function is probably responsible for the marked diuresis. Appropriate therapy in such patients includes intravenous administration of salt-containing solutions to replace sodium and volume deficits.

BIBLIOGRAPHY

CURHAN GC et al: Urinary tract obstruction, in *Brenner and Rector's The Kidney*, 6th ed, BM Brenner (ed). Philadelphia, Saunders, 2000, pp 1820–1843

GULMI FA et al: Pathophysiology of urinary tract obstruction, in *Campbell's Urology*, 7th ed, PC Walsh et al (eds). Philadelphia, Saunders, 1998, pp 342–385

KAYE AD, POLLACK HM: Diagnostic imaging approach to the patient with obstructive uropathy. Semin Nephrol 2:55, 1982

KLAHR S: Urinary tract obstruction, in *Diseases of the Kidney*, 6th ed, RW Schrier, CW Gottschalk (eds). Boston, Little, Brown, 1997, pp 709–738

WILSON DR: Renal function during and following obstruction. Annu Rev Med 28:329, 1977

NOBEL PRIZE IN PHYSIOLOGY OR MEDICINE, 1956

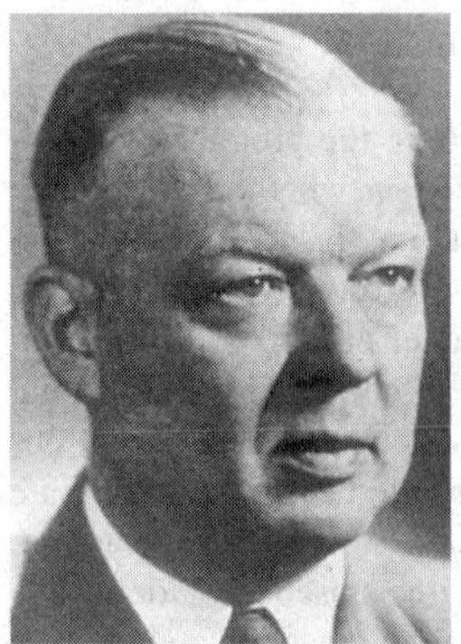

Werner Theodor Otto Forssmann was born August 29, 1904, in Berlin, Germany, the son of Julius and Emmy Forssmann. His father was an attorney who was killed in World War I in 1916. Forssmann received a broad liberal arts education early in life and then in 1922 entered Friedrich Wilhelm University in Berlin to study medicine. After graduation in 1929, he received further training by working with surgeons and urologists at several different hospitals. During that time he worked with Richard Schneider in Eberswalde, a small Prussian town north of Berlin. Forssmann had become fascinated with the results of earlier animal work and asked Schneider if he could perform cardiac catheterization in humans. Schneider forbade Forssmann from conducting such experiments either on patients or himself. Nevertheless, Forssmann decided to perform the heart experiment on himself. With local anesthesia, he inserted a needle in his left arm antecubital vein through which he inserted a catheter and then went to the x-ray room where he placed himself in front of the fluoroscope. Forssmann used a mirror and saw that the catheter was at the level of his humerus. Despite the urging to stop by a young colleague who had just entered the room, Forssmann advanced the catheter into the right side of the heart. He then documented his success by taking some x-rays. At first Schneider was furious but then congratulated Forssmann and urged him to publish his results immediately. This paper, entitled "Probing the Right Ventricle of the Heart," was published on November 5, 1929, in *Klinische Wochenschrift*.

To further his research, with the help of Schneider he obtained a position at the "Mecca of German Surgery" with Ferdinand Sauerbruch at Charité Hospital in Berlin. Immediately after publication of his article, Forssmann became a celebrity and was besieged by reporters. Although unfounded, Ernst Unger claimed priority on the basis of his intraarterial therapy. This controversy, combined with professional jealousy that described Forssmann's experiment as a "circus stunt," led Sauerbruch to dismiss him only 3 months after his arrival at Charité. Forssmann then returned to work with Schneider, who encouraged him to continue his work on cardiac catheterization in a systematic manner. He found better x-ray equipment, used contrast material, and worked on dogs that were kept in his mother's apartment. Forssmann also performed further cardiac catheterization experiments on himself, demonstrating the first use of contrast material in humans. Altogether, he performed nine cardiac catheterizations on himself. His contrast medium results were published in the *Münchner Medizinische Wochenschrift*.

Forssmann's experiments had long been forgotten in his own country when André Cournand and Dickinson Richards, over a decade later, began their development of cardiac catheterization at Columbia Physicians and Surgeons Medical School and Bellevue Hospital in New York. In their first journal article they recognized Forssmann's contributions to the development of cardiac catheterization. Unfortunately, because of the events of World War II, Forssmann was unable to participate in this further development of cardiac catheterization in New York City. Nevertheless, because of the courageous experiments on himself, Forssmann demonstrated the safety and potential of cardiac catheterization and contrast radiography and provided the foundation for modern cardiology.

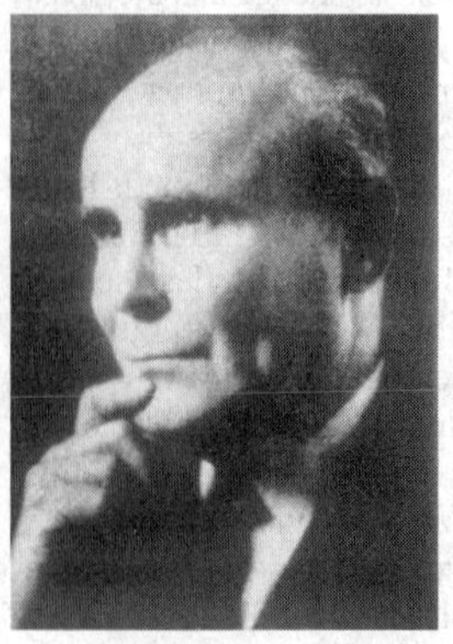

André Frédéric Cournand was born in Paris, France, to Jules and Marguerite Weber Cournand on September 24, 1895. His father was a dentist and inventor who had twenty-five patents. Cournand's early education was at the Lycée Condorcet; he then obtained his baccalauréat at the Faculté des Lettres of the University of Sorbonne in 1913 and a diploma in physics, chemistry, and biology from the Faculté des Sciences in 1914. After his first year in medical school, he volunteered for the French Army and toward the end of World War I was wounded and gassed. He received the Croix de Guerre with three bronze stars. After the war he completed his thesis and received his medical degree from the University of Paris in 1930. He then traveled to the United States with the intent to spend a year on the chest (tuberculosis) service at Bellevue Hospital in the Columbia University Division. He decided to stay in the United States when he was offered a chief residency and an opportunity to work with Dickinson Richards on the physiology and pathophysiology of respiration. Thus, Cournand and Richards commenced the collaborative research in 1932 that changed the future of cardiology.

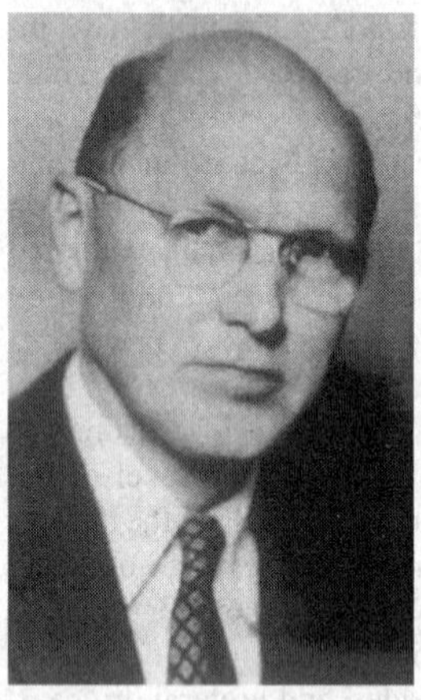

Dickinson Woodruff Richards, Jr., was born on October 30, 1895, to Dickinson Woodruff and Sally Lambert Richards. After his early education at Hotchkiss School in Connecticut, where he studied the humanities, Richards entered Yale University and graduated in 1917. He then entered the United States Army as a lieutenant with an artillery unit. After the war, he attended medical school at the College of Physicians and Surgeons at Columbia University, followed, in 1923, by a residency in internal medicine at Presbyterian Hospital. During this time, Lawrence J. Henderson at Harvard University became his mentor, and they published three papers in the area of pulmonary and cardiovascular circulation. Following his residency, he had a fellowship at the National Institute of Medical Research in London from 1927 to 1928 under his other mentor, Henry Hollet Dale. Richards once said, "A man's mind and his actions are chiefly molded by a very few. For me, in the early years, there were Lawrence J. Henderson and Henry Hollet Dale." Richards returned from his fellowship in London and joined the faculty of the College of Physicians and Surgeons at Columbia University. His collaborative research with Cournand began in 1932. In his autobiography, Cournand wrote that "Modesty and greatness seldom harmonize in an individual," but cited Richards as ". . .one of those few in whom these apparently opposite qualities balanced one another."

Cournand and Richards considered themselves primarily as pulmonary rather than cardiac physiologists. They developed a series of pulmonary function tests that were then applied to patients with pulmonary tuberculosis, chronic emphysema, and lung fibrosis. After 4 years of experimental work with dogs and a chimpanzee, they undertook cardiac catheterization in humans in 1940—some 11 years after Forssmann's original publication.

They investigated systemic hypertension, heart failure, and acquired and congenital heart disease. Pulmonary heart disease was characterized as ". . .cardiac hypertrophy and dilatation secondary to disease of the lung." The research of Cournand and Richards was a brilliant demonstration of basic research translated to clinical medicine, including the diagnosis and treatment of disease. On the basis of their research, cardiac surgery for correction of congenital and acquired defects became possible.

REFERENCES

1. Magill FN (ed): *Nobel Prize Winners: Physiology or Medicine*, vol 2. Pasadena, Salem Press, 1993
2. Schrier RW: *A Salute to Nobel Laureates in Physiology and Medicine*, Proceedings of the Association of American Physicians 108(1): Jan 1996
3. Sourkes TL: *Nobel Prize Winners in Medicine and Physiology 1901–1965*. London: Abelard-Schuman, 1967

Robert W. Schrier, MD

PART ELEVEN

DISORDERS OF THE GASTROINTESTINAL SYSTEM

Section 1
DISORDERS OF THE ALIMENTARY TRACT

282

Daniel K. Podolsky, Kurt J. Isselbacher

APPROACH TO THE PATIENT WITH GASTROINTESTINAL DISEASE

BIOLOGIC CONSIDERATIONS The mucosal surface of the gastrointestinal (GI) tract is composed of a highly dynamic population of epithelial cells that are specialized for transmembrane absorption and secretion. These secretory and absorptive abilities facilitate digestion and nutrient uptake, which must be accomplished while keeping out potentially harmful pathogens and mutagens in the lumen. The barrier function is accomplished through both the physical integrity of the mucosal surface and the extensive population of resident immune cells.

The intestinal lymphoid system reflects a balance between dampening immune reactivity at the mucosal surface to prevent the constant and unrestrained activation of immune and inflammatory processes and immune response amplification in the underlying lamina propria and submucosa ready to respond when surface defenses have been breached. Derangements in the balance of suppression and stimulation predispose the GI tract to numerous inflammatory conditions.

The epithelial cells of the mucosal surface turn over very rapidly; the entire surface is regenerated every 24 to 72 h. This rapid turnover may permit rapid recovery of function following an acute insult and protect the cells against many mutagens in the lumen. Indeed, the small intestine rarely develops epithelial cancers. The slower turnover of colonic epithelium, the slower movement of the luminal contents, and differences in the mutagens in the luminal contents appear to foster colon cancers. Another fundamental feature of the GI mucosa is the spatial segregation of the proliferative compartment from the terminally differentiated cells, especially in the small intestine, where a gradient of differentiation exists from the depths of the crypts of Lieberkühn to the villus tip. This organization has a strong effect on the histology and pathophysiology of many mucosal disorders, such as celiac sprue.

Diseases of the GI tract produce clinical consequences through physical disruption of the mucosal layer (e.g., blood loss, fluid loss, pathogenic invasion) or nutritional derangements caused by impaired digestion and nutrient absorption. Focal or localized disease processes are more likely to disrupt mucosa; diffuse processes are more likely to alter absorption.

While the essential roles of the GI tract—the absorption of nutrients and the excretion of the products—are accomplished in large part at the luminal surface, GI function also depends on the coordinated propulsion of food through the lumen by smooth-muscle contraction. The local and distant neural and endocrine factors that contribute to the regulation of intestinal motility are complex. Disruption of normal motility is common, with alterations in frequency of bowel movements, abdominal distention, abdominal pain, and nausea, individually or in varying combinations (so-called functional bowel complaints), affecting as many as 15% of adults. Such symptoms may result from dysmotility related to the *direct* effects of an obstructing lesion or to the *indirect* actions of substances released by a primary mucosal disorder (e.g., inflammatory mediators such as arachidonic acid metabolites that also affect smooth-muscle activity).

The spectrum of diseases affecting the GI tract and their clinical manifestations are related to the component organ(s) involved (Table 282-1). Thus, esophageal disorders manifest themselves mainly through their effects on swallowing; gastric disorders are dominated by features relating to acid secretion; and diseases of the small and large intestine demonstrate disruption of nutrition and alterations of bowel movements. The GI tract may also be affected by systemic disorders, including vascular, inflammatory, infectious, and neoplastic conditions leading to focal or diffuse structural lesions. Metabolic and endocrine abnormalities as well as some drugs can disrupt normal bowel motility. When no structural lesion can be identified to explain GI symptoms, the disorder is termed *functional.* Table 282-2 summarizes criteria that may be used to distinguish functional from organic or structural diseases of the GI tract.

CLINICAL CONSIDERATIONS **History** A thorough clinical history is essential in directing the clinician's attention to appropriate diagnostic considerations in the patient with GI symptoms (Table 282-1). The most common complaints include pain and alterations in bowel habit, especially diarrhea or constipation. *Abdominal pain* is the most frequent and variable complaint and may reflect a broad spectrum of problems, from self-limited to urgent (Chap. 14). The intensity should be assessed and an initial distinction should be made between pain of acute onset and more chronic discomfort. Pain of abrupt onset more often reflects serious illness requiring urgent intervention, while a history of chronic discomfort is most often related to an indolent disorder. Dyspepsia, an ill-defined upper abdominal discomfort, is especially common and is often accompanied by varying degrees of nausea, bloating, and distention. Dyspepsia may be associated with peptic ulceration, but non-ulcer dyspepsia (NUD) is more common. A change in the pattern or character of pain may signify disease progression. Ascertaining the location of the pain (upper or lower, localized or diffuse), its character (sharp, burning, cramping), and its relationship to meals will often provide clues into the most important diagnostic considerations. Discomfort while the patient is eating suggests an esophageal disorder. Pain occurring shortly after the meal may signify biliary tract disease or abdominal angina; pain 30 to 90 min later is typical of peptic disease. Pain that is not affected by eating suggests a process outside of the bowel lumen, such as abscess, peritonitis, pancreatitis, and some malignancies. Conversely, factors that relieve the symptom are also helpful. For example, eating or antacid use typically relieves pain in peptic ulcer disease or gastritis. A relationship to bowel movement, especially together with an altered bowel habit, should focus attention on a disorder of the small or large bowel, such as inflammatory bowel disease.

Alterations in bowel habit can result from either disruption of normal intestinal motility or significant structural pathology. The temporal evolution of the change, the nature of the alteration, and the presence of other constitutional symptoms such as weight loss, fever, or anorexia are important. Temporary variation in bowel habit in association with some life stress and in the absence of signs of systemic illness suggests the common "irritable bowel syndrome," especially when the alteration varies between diarrhea and constipation. Small, pellet-like stools associated with symptoms of dyspepsia (bloating, nausea, and "gas") are common. This diagnosis can essentially be made on the basis of a thorough history and physical examination and very limited laboratory testing, to exclude structural disease.

Constipation is a common complaint and may reflect an obstructing process but is more often due to impaired motility; though often

Table 282-1 Overview of Approach to Patients with Common Gastrointestinal Disorders

Site of Disorder	Common Symptoms	Possible Physical Signs	Potential Procedures or Laboratory Studies
Esophagus	Dysphagia Odynophagia Heartburn, chest pain Hematemesis/melena		Esophagoscopy Barium swallow Manometry Bernstein test
Stomach	Nausea and vomiting Epigastric pain Hematemesis/melena Early satiety	Distention Tenderness Succussion splash Mass	Gastroscopy Upper GI x-ray series Nasogastric aspiration Gastric emptying
Small Intestine			
Duodenum	Pain Nausea/vomiting Hematemesis	Tenderness Altered bowel sounds Distention Mass	Duodenoscopy Small bowel follow-through, enteroclysis Kidney-ureter-bladder x-ray series D-Xylose absorption tests
Jejunum	Pain Diarrhea	Altered bowel sounds Distention Mass	CT Stool cultures, stool examination for ova and parasites Small bowel biopsy
Ileum	Pain Diarrhea	Altered bowel sounds Distention Mass	Colonoscopy
Colon	Diarrhea Pain Blood Constipation	Tenderness Mass Distention Altered bowel sounds	Sigmoidoscopy Colonoscopy Barium enema Stool culture, stool examination for ova and parasites *Clostridium difficile* toxin assay
Anus/Rectum	Pain Urgency Hematochezia Pruritus Constipation Incontinence Tenesmus	Tenderness Altered sphincter tone Perianal abnormality	Sigmoidoscopy Anoscopy Anorectal manometry
Nonspecific	Weight loss Fever Anorexia Nausea and vomiting		Complete blood count Erythrocyte sedimentation rate Fecal occult blood test

NOTE: GI, gastrointestinal; CT, computed tomography.

tory may clarify that "constipation" actually reflects more an unrealized expectation of regularity than significant pathology. In contrast, progressively worsening constipation and weight loss in an adult with previously regular habits suggests the possible presence of an underlying obstructing process, particularly malignancy.

Although *diarrhea* refers to an increased frequency of movements, patients often use the term to describe loose or watery stools. If diarrhea is described, the daily average number of stools, their consistency, their pattern, and the presence of blood should be defined. The occurrence of nocturnal or true bloody diarrhea almost always reflects structural rather than functional bowel disease. A pungent stool odor or the presence of undigested meat in the movement is suggestive of pancreatic insufficiency. An alteration in color can be seen in cholestasis or steatorrhea (light-colored) or hemorrhage (melenic to maroon or bright red). Mucus in the movement is usually a sign of a functional bowel syndrome, while pus suggests infectious or inflammatory disease. Less common but more dramatic are the symptoms of acute GI bleeding, including hematemesis, melena, and hematochezia, which usually lead to prompt seeking of medical attention but should always be enquired after by the clinician.

functional in nature, drugs (e.g., anticholinergics), neurologic processes (e.g., Hirschsprung's disease), or smooth-muscle diseases (e.g., scleroderma) may cause decreased motility. The history and physical examination may provide evidence of a more generalized disorder such as hypothyroidism or depression. Pain associated with constipation may suggest an anal or perianal process with stool retention. The his-

In the evaluation of male patients, especially those with diarrhea or dysphagia, a tactful inquiry into sexual activity is essential. Homosexual males are at increased risk for a large variety of GI disorders as well as AIDS, which may first manifest itself with GI symptoms. AIDS patients are susceptible to a wide range of infections and neoplastic disorders of the GI tract, liver, and biliary tract (Chap. 308).

Table 282-2 Distinguishing between Functional and Organic/Structural Disease of Gastrointestinal Tract

	Functional	Organic: Neoplastic	Organic: Inflammatory
Symptoms			
Weight loss	None	Common	Sometimes
Diarrhea	Daytime only	Day ± night	Day and night
Blood loss	None	Frequent	Frequent
Fever	None	Rare	Frequent
Pain	Cramping, relieved by defecation	Minor to severe	May be localized; may be severe
Bowel habit (diarrhea or constipation)	Alternating diarrhea/constipation Pellet-like stools	Constipation (rarely diarrhea) Change in caliber	Diarrhea or normal
Laboratory tests			
Hematocrit	Normal	Often decreased	May be decreased
White blood cell count	Normal	Usually normal	Often elevated
Erythrocyte sedimentation rate	Normal	Usually increased	Usually increased

Finally, careful attention must be given to a general medical history with an emphasis on present or past use of medications or nonprescription drugs. Thyroid and other metabolic disorders, especially those affecting calcium metabolism, can cause a variety of GI symptoms. Unless asked, patients may forget to mention that they take aspirin almost daily for headache, and this may account for occult blood found in the stool. The use of daily laxatives may explain chronic diarrhea.

Physical Examination, Endoscopy, and Radiology All of the cardinal methods of examination are helpful in evaluating the patient with GI symptoms (Table 282-1). *Inspection* may disclose signs of cholestasis or nutritional deficiencies. Examination of the abdomen for an abnormal contour or inspection of the perianal region may reveal signs of a mass or a draining fistula. *Auscultation* may elicit a succussion splash in patients with symptoms of gastric outlet obstruction. The absence of bowel sounds or an alteration in pitch can lead to recognition of an evolving ileus or an obstructing process. A bruit may be noted when symptoms of ischemic bowel disease are present. Careful *palpation* of the abdomen is especially important in detecting tenderness and masses, which can lead to the recognition of cholecystitis, Crohn's disease, periappendiceal abscess, and many other disorders. Findings on abdominal palpation will often be complemented by *percussion*, which is essential to assessing liver and spleen size.

Elicitation of *rebound tenderness*, either direct or referred, after abrupt removal of the examining hand provides an important clue to localized or more generalized peritonitis, which may suggest abdominal emergencies, such as a perforated viscus, intraabdominal abscess, or bowel infarction. Typically, the patient will remain immobile to avoid the accentuation of pain that may follow even slight movement or jarring of the abdomen. By contrast, patients with severe pain deriving from visceral disease, such as intestinal ischemia, are sometimes frantic to find a comfortable position. In these disorders, the absence of findings on palpation may be in striking contrast to the evident distress of the patient. Only when the process progresses to tissue destruction (e.g., intestinal infarction) and secondary peritonitis will the abdominal examination prove remarkable, often in concert with striking signs of systemic illness, including hemodynamic instability.

In addition to the examination of the abdomen, a digital rectal examination is also essential. In the patient with complaints of stool incontinence, the integrity of the sphincter can be assessed. Masses intrinsic to the rectum as well as abnormalities in the pelvis or the pouch of Douglas may only be detected by this examination. The presence of frank or occult blood in the stool is always important diagnostic information. Sigmoidoscopy should be viewed as a routine part of the physical examination in the patient with diarrhea, constipation, or frank or occult fecal blood. Sigmoidoscopy performed with either a rigid or a flexible fiberoptic instrument allows for direct inspection of the rectosigmoid mucosa, permitting the detection of cancers and polyps in this lower bowel segment that could be missed by barium x-rays. Inflammatory changes of the mucosa can help identify patients with infectious dysentery or other forms of colitis. Edema, granularity, diffuse friability (easily induced mucosal bleeding), and superficial ulcerations are characteristic of ulcerative colitis. Fresh stool samples for microbiologic studies and superficial mucosal biopsies obtained at the time of sigmoidoscopy can also yield crucial diagnostic information. The presence of polyps is an indication for colonoscopy (Chap. 283).

Many upper and lower GI tract disorders are accessible to inspection via fiberoptic instruments. As a result, endoscopy has supplanted conventional contrast x-ray studies for many clinical problems, both because of its heightened precision for diagnosis and the opportunity in many instances to accomplish meaningful therapeutic intervention. However, it should be emphasized that *no procedure should be considered routine* and used indiscriminately; there must be a rational basis for its use in the individual patient. These techniques are discussed in detail in Chap. 283. Upper GI endoscopy permits evaluation of the esophagus, stomach, duodenum, and, with specially designed instruments, proximal jejunum. Side-viewing scopes permit inspection and cannulation of the ampulla of Vater, facilitating retrograde cholangiopancreatography. Evaluation of some patients will be further benefited by endoscopic ultrasound (US), which can delineate submucosal mass lesions and abnormalities in the pancreas. The colonoscope can be used to visualize the entire colon and often the terminal ileum, resulting in more accurate diagnosis of inflammatory bowel disease and mass lesions. Colonic polyps can almost always be removed at the time of their initial identification.

Endoscopic techniques are relatively precise in defining many problems, but the limitations of these tools, as well as the continued advantages of x-ray studies in some situations, should be recognized. Endoscopic tools are not useful in assessing GI motility, which may be assessed more accurately by barium studies. In addition, the small intestine remains largely inaccessible to fiberoptic instruments. In hospitals where endoscopy is not feasible, the upper GI series and barium enema remain good diagnostic modalities to evaluate the upper and lower GI tract, especially when air-contrast techniques are employed. However, they should generally be avoided in patients with GI bleeding or suspected bowel obstruction. In addition, the cathartics used to prepare the bowel may markedly worsen the condition of a patient with obstructing lesions or colitis.

Although endoscopy has obviated the need for many conventional GI x-rays, other radiologic imaging modalities, including US, computed tomography (CT), and magnetic resonance imaging (MRI), have assumed a larger role in patients with GI symptoms. Both US and CT are useful in the delineation of abdominal masses. CT, though more expensive, is often more effective in the evaluation of the lower abdomen, where inflammatory masses in patients with Crohn's disease or complications of diverticular disease may be accurately imaged. However, US is an effective and less expensive tool for the evaluation of the right upper quadrant, including the gall bladder and biliary tract. MRI may give exquisitely accurate information on the anatomic extent of invasive rectal cancers and blood flow in patients with vascular disorders, but the full range of its uses in GI disorders remains to be delineated. More sophisticated CT and MRI equipment can actually permit the performance of digital angiography without the invasive catheterization necessary in conventional visceral angiography. CT "virtual colonoscopy," a nonendoscopic method of visualizing the colon, is developing rapidly.

Radionuclide scans can be used to localize a site of bleeding in the GI tract. Radiolabeled technetium can detect a Meckel's diverticulum, which is an occasional source of bleeding.

DIAGNOSTIC APPROACHES (Table 282-1) **Abdominal Pain** Determining the cause of abdominal pain is frequently a clinical challenge (Chap. 14). Differential diagnostic considerations may encompass diseases extrinsic to the GI tract, such as disorders of the genitourinary tract (e.g., pelvic inflammatory disease) and the peritoneum. The initial goal is to distinguish between an urgent problem and a nonacute disorder. Initial clinical impressions based on the history and physical examination can be further refined through routine laboratory tests such as a complete blood count and differential as well as plain films of the abdomen. Specific features will dictate the appropriateness of urgent US or CT examination or the need to proceed promptly with surgery. In the patient with a long-standing and relatively stable problem, diagnostic evaluation can be more deliberate. A functional basis for the complaint may be established on the strength of the history and physical examination alone. Radiologic contrast studies, other imaging modalities (e.g., US, CT), or endoscopic examination may be appropriate. If these approaches do not determine the cause of the patient's symptoms, more unusual causes of abdominal pain such as acute intermittent porphyria may have to be excluded through specific urine or blood tests (Chap. 346).

Problems of Swallowing Dysphagia nearly always signifies the presence of structural pathology. The approach should be as follows:

1. *Thorough determination of the nature of dysphagia*. Is the difficulty primarily in swallowing liquids, solids, or both? The location of the difficulty from the patient's perspective and presence or absence of accompanying *odynophagia* (pain on swallowing) are important to ascertain. These historic clues are complemented by careful visual and neurologic examination of the oropharynx.

2. *Routine esophageal x-rays* in the upright and lateral or Trendelenburg position. The horizontal views are essential for demonstration of the swallowing mechanism, unaided by gravity, and of the esophagogastric junction. For details of the pharyngoesophageal area, cineradiography is necessary because of the rapidity with which the

contrast medium passes through. Hiatus hernia is extremely common (in 15 to 35% of persons over 50) and is often asymptomatic. Careful attention is usually needed to detect lower esophageal rings or webs, which may be visible as indentations in the barium column only from a limited angle.

3. *Esophagoscopy.* This procedure is desirable to biopsy masses or abnormal mucosa and to obtain washings for exfoliative cytologic study. The diagnoses of peptic esophagitis and Barrett's esophagus are made endoscopically. Endoscopy is the most sensitive technique for identifying esophageal or gastric varices, although they are seldom important in the absence of hemorrhage. Endoscopic instruments with a US probe at the tip (endoscopic ultrasound) are useful diagnostic and staging tools for certain problems of the esophagus (and other sites of the GI tract).

4. *Manometric studies* of the upper esophagus, particularly in conjunction with cineradiography. This procedure offers the best means of differentiating among disorders originating in the central nervous system, primary pharyngeal muscular disease, and cricopharyngeal dystonia. Manometry of the lower esophagus is useful in the diagnosis of diffuse esophageal spasm, achalasia, and infiltrative diseases that alter esophageal motility.

5. *24-Hour monitoring of esophageal pH* may be used to document esophageal reflux.

Peptic or Digestive Disorders The approaches to these disorders include the following:

1. *Insertion of a nasogastric tube.* This approach is used to establish whether significant gastric retention (more than 75 mL of gastric contents in the fasting state) exists and whether acid, bile, blood, or other materials are present. If pyloric obstruction or gastric atony is present, the tube is used to maintain suction while the patient's electrolyte and fluid balance is restored to normal; the stomach is kept as clean as possible so that diagnostic investigation may be carried out.

2. *Upper gastrointestinal endoscopy* (Chap. 283). This procedure is most helpful in assessing the mucosa in gastritis or, together with biopsy and brushings for cytology, in differentiating between peptic and neoplastic ulcerating lesions. It may identify a specific bleeding site in clinical situations where several potential bleeding sites could exist, as in the patient with portal hypertension. In addition, it may be possible to cauterize or otherwise intervene to control hemorrhage via the endoscope (e.g., by injections of vasoconstricting agents such as epinephrine). *Helicobacter pylori* is a frequent cause of gastritis in patients with peptic ulceration and non-ulcer dyspepsia. Although *H. pylori* infection can be confirmed by endoscopy and biopsy, the diagnosis is more commonly made by breath and serologic tests (Chap. 285). Endoscopy is the diagnostic method of choice in the setting of upper GI bleeding (Chap. 44). Endoscopy can detect a number of potential sources of upper GI bleeding that are often missed by x-ray studies (e.g., erosive gastritis, Mallory-Weiss tear). Gastroscopy is particularly helpful in inspecting the postoperative stomach, especially in detecting stomal ulceration or so-called alkaline reflux gastritis. The first and second portions of the duodenum can also be routinely examined, and important information about ulcers and other lesions can be obtained. Radiologic studies may be useful when endoscopy is not readily available or in the assessment of suspected motility disorders (e.g., gastroparesis). In addition, radiologic examination may be preferred when there are contraindications to safe endoscopy.

3. *Gastric acid secretory studies.* Although not routinely necessary, these studies are useful in the diagnosis of the Zollinger-Ellison syndrome or atrophic gastritis and for determination of completeness of vagotomy. They should not be performed for the routine diagnosis of uncomplicated duodenal ulcer or to influence the choice of surgery for peptic ulcer.

Obstructive and Vascular Disorders of the Small Intestine (See also Chaps. 289 and 290) The plain x-ray film of the abdomen is the most important diagnostic adjunct to careful physical examination in patients with symptoms of obstruction. Patterns of dilation of individual loops of intestine may be characteristic, as in volvulus or acute pancreatitis; erect and decubitus views will often show fluid levels in the affected segments. Motility disorders of the small intestine (temporary ileus or chronic intestinal pseudoobstruction) may also present with obstructive symptoms and similar x-ray findings but must be managed medically without surgical intervention. Air under the diaphragm is diagnostic of a perforated viscus; air in the portal vein usually results from intestinal necrosis from mesenteric vascular occlusion. The diagnostic accuracy of the plain x-ray film in all types of intestinal obstruction is about 75%. In patients with symptoms of incomplete obstruction, the radiographic small-bowel series will often be diagnostic in defining the site and degree of obstruction. Infrequently, in this setting, all conventional x-ray studies are unremarkable. In such cases, the radiologist may perform a small-bowel enteroclysis study by passing a special tube into the proximal jejunum; the rapid instillation of barium through the tube will distend the intestine and often reveal subtle lesions missed by other tests.

Vascular diseases of the small intestine are among the most difficult diseases to diagnose. In chronic mesenteric ischemia, radiographic, endoscopic, and laboratory tests are usually normal. Early in the course of acute mesenteric ischemia, the plain film of the abdomen may be unremarkable despite complaints of severe abdominal pain. In these settings, prompt mesenteric angiography is essential to confirm the diagnosis of vascular disease.

Inflammatory and Neoplastic Diseases of Small and Large Intestine Patients with these conditions are usually identified by history, physical examination, and careful examination of the stools for exudate and blood. Examination of fresh stool samples for common bacterial pathogens and parasites by laboratories skilled in these techniques is important in identifying or excluding infectious causes of diarrhea, particularly in the patient with colitis. Sigmoidoscopy is valuable in identifying mucosal and neoplastic lesions of the rectum and distal colon. The mucosal surface of the entire colon and terminal ileum can be examined directly and biopsied through the fiberoptic sigmoidoscope or colonoscope. The radiologic examination of the small intestine is highly reliable in identifying the prestenotic and stenotic lesions of Crohn's disease. In the colon, a single barium enema examination in a well-prepared patient has a diagnostic accuracy of 80 to 85%; the addition of air-contrast technique brings the accuracy up over 90%. Accuracy is greatly limited if the patient is poorly prepared for the examination. Colonoscopy may be preferable because of its greater accuracy and the fact that it enables the operator to remove any polyps that are encountered and to obtain preoperative tissue confirmation in the patient who probably has cancer.

Peroral biopsy of the small intestine (now most often accomplished during endoscopy) and forceps biopsy of the rectosigmoid are of considerable importance in revealing mucosal disease. Rectal biopsy is an excellent means of demonstrating amyloidosis, schistosomiasis, and amebiasis. Submucosal disease is not seen in these superficial biopsies. Hirschsprung's disease is diagnosed histologically by a deep surgical biopsy of the lower part of the rectum.

Malabsorption Syndromes Malabsorption may be suspected on the basis of history and physical examination and confirmed by examination of the stool. Radiologic examination is helpful to rule out local lesions and to suggest motor and secretory dysfunction, but it is rarely diagnostic unless an abnormal small-bowel mucosa or fistulas between the intestine and stomach are demonstrated.

Microscopic examination of a stool specimen stained with Sudan is a simple screening test for steatorrhea. Chemical analysis of 3-day stool collection for fat, with the patient on a standard diet, is used to establish the diagnosis of steatorrhea. The D-xylose absorption test is about 90% accurate in distinguishing mucosal disease from pancreatic insufficiency. Peroral biopsy of the small intestine via the endoscope or a specialized biopsy device is of value in the diagnosis of celiac disease, and it may show the less common infiltrations of the mucosa by amyloid or bacterial mucoproteins (Whipple's disease). Leakage of protein into the intestinal lumen may cause hypoproteinemia and can be demonstrated by the recovery in stools of the serum protein α_1-antitrypsin or intravenously administrated markers such as iodine- or chromium-labeled isotopes. →*The tests useful in the diagnosis of malabsorption are discussed in Chap. 286.*

GI Bleeding (See also Chap. 44) Acute bleeding in the GI tract is a common clinical problem. The history usually provides a reliable distinction between lower and upper tract sources. Once the patient with upper tract bleeding is hemodynamically stable, a nasogastric tube is placed to confirm the site of blood loss and to empty the stomach. Endoscopy is then performed to define the cause and often to treat it. In patients with acute lower tract bleeding, sigmoidosopy may permit detection of distal sites of bleeding. Colonoscopy may also be of value, but visualization may be limited by active bleeding and poor bowel preparation. Barium studies should be avoided in the acute setting. They are usually nondiagnostic and the persistent contrast may interfere with interpretation of angiographic studies, which can often define a site of bleeding that is otherwise obscure. Radionuclide bleeding scan can locate the bleeding site. A Meckel's scan can be diagnostic when active bleeding arises distal to the duodenum in the absence of an identifiable source in the colon.

BIBLIOGRAPHY

JOHNSON LR et al: *Physiology of the Gastrointestinal Tract,* 3d ed. New York, Raven, 1995

FELDMAN M et al: *Gastrointestinal and Liver Disease,* 6th ed. Philadelphia, Saunders, 1998

YAMADA T et al: *Textbook of Gastroenterology,* 3d ed. Philadelphia, Lippincott Williams & Wilkins, 1999

283 GASTROINTESTINAL ENDOSCOPY

Mark Topazian

Gastrointestinal endoscopy has been attempted for over 200 years, but the introduction of semi-rigid gastroscopes in the middle of the twentieth century marked the dawn of the modern endoscopic era. Since then, rapid advances in endoscopic technology have led to dramatic changes in the diagnosis and treatment of many digestive diseases. Innovative endoscopic devices and new endoscopic treatment modalities continue to expand the use of endoscopy in patient care.

Flexible endoscopes provide either an optical image (transmitted over fiberoptic bundles) or an electronic video image (generated by a charge-coupled device in the tip of the endoscope; see **Color Atlas, Section III**). Operator controls permit deflection of the endoscope tip; fiberoptic bundles bring light to the tip of the endoscope; and working channels allow washing, suctioning, and the passage of instruments. Progressive changes in the diameter and stiffness of endoscopes have improved the ease and patient tolerance of endoscopy.

ENDOSCOPIC PROCEDURES

Upper Endoscopy Upper endoscopy, also referred to as esophagogastroduodenoscopy (EGD), is performed by passing a flexible endoscope through the mouth into the esophagus, stomach, bulb, and second duodenum. The procedure is the best method of examining the upper gastrointestinal mucosa. While the upper gastrointestinal radiographic series has similar accuracy for diagnosis of duodenal ulcer, EGD is superior for detection of gastric ulcers and permits directed biopsy and endoscopic therapy, if needed. Topical pharyngeal anesthesia is used, and intravenous conscious sedation is given to most patients in the United States to ease the anxiety and discomfort of the procedure, although in many countries EGD is routinely performed without sedation. The recent development of ultrathin, 5-mm diameter endoscopes for transnasal, unsedated EGD may decrease the use of sedation for EGD in the United States, also decreasing the costs and risks of the procedure.

Colonoscopy Colonoscopy is performed by passing a flexible colonoscope through the anal canal into the rectum and colon. The cecum is reached in over 95% of cases, and the terminal ileum can often be examined. Colonoscopy is the "gold standard" for diagnosis of colonic mucosal disease. Barium enema is more accurate for evaluation of diverticula and for accurate measurement of colonic strictures, but colonoscopy has greater sensitivity for polyps and cancers. Colonoscopy is more uncomfortable than EGD for most patients, and conscious sedation is usually given before colonoscopy in the United States, although a willing patient and a skilled examiner can complete the procedure without sedation in many cases.

Flexible Sigmoidoscopy Flexible sigmoidoscopy is similar to colonoscopy but visualizes only the rectum and a variable portion of the left colon, typically to 60 cm from the anal verge. This procedure causes abdominal cramping, but it is brief and is almost always performed without sedation. Flexible sigmoidoscopy is primarily used to screen asymptomatic, average-risk patients for colonic polyps and may also be used for evaluation of diarrhea and hematochezia.

Enteroscopy Enteroscopy is the relatively new field of small-bowel endoscopy. Two techniques are currently used. "Push" enteroscopy is performed with a long endoscope similar in design to an upper endoscope. The enteroscope is pushed down the small bowel with the help of a stiffening overtube that extends from the mouth to the duodenum. The mid-jejunum can often be reached; an instrument channel is present for biopsies or endoscopic therapy. "Sonde" enteroscopy uses a very thin, long, flexible endoscope with a weighted tip and no biopsy capability. The sonde enteroscope is passed through the nose, dragged to the duodenum by a standard endoscope, then slowly propelled forward by intestinal peristalsis for several hours. The cecum or distal ileum is reached in most cases. The small-bowel mucosa is examined during sonde enteroscope withdrawal, although parts of the mucosa may be missed when the endoscope is pulled back around turns. The major indication for these procedures is unexplained small-bowel bleeding.

Endoscopic Retrograde Cholangiopancreatography (ERCP) During ERCP, a side-viewing endoscope is passed through the mouth to the duodenum, the ampulla of Vater is identified and cannulated with a thin plastic catheter, and radiographic contrast material is injected into the bile duct and pancreatic duct under fluoroscopic guidance (Fig. 283-1). When indicated, the sphincter of Oddi can be opened using the technique of endoscopic sphincterotomy (Fig. 283-2). Stones can be retrieved from the ducts, and strictures of the ducts can be biopsied, dilated, and stented. ERCP is often performed for therapy but remains an important diagnostic tool, especially for bile duct stones.

Endoscopic Ultrasound (EUS) EUS utilizes high-frequency ultrasound transducers incorporated into the tip of a flexible endoscope. Ultrasound images are obtained of the gut wall and adjacent organs, vessels, and lymph nodes. By sacrificing depth of ultrasound penetration and bringing the ultrasound transducer close to the area of interest via endoscopy, very high resolution images are obtained. EUS provides the most accurate preoperative local staging of esophageal, pancreatic, and rectal malignancies, although it does not detect most distant metastases. Examples of EUS tumor staging are shown in Fig. 283-3. EUS is also highly sensitive for diagnosis of bile duct stones, gallbladder disease, submucosal gastrointestinal lesions, and chronic pancreatitis. Fine-needle aspiration of masses and lymph nodes in the posterior mediastinum, abdomen, and pelvis can be performed under EUS guidance.

RISKS OF ENDOSCOPY

All endoscopic procedures carry some risk of bleeding and gastrointestinal perforation. These risks are quite low with diagnostic upper

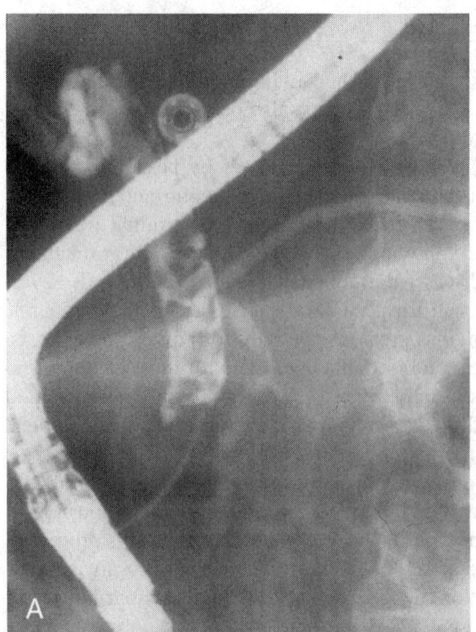

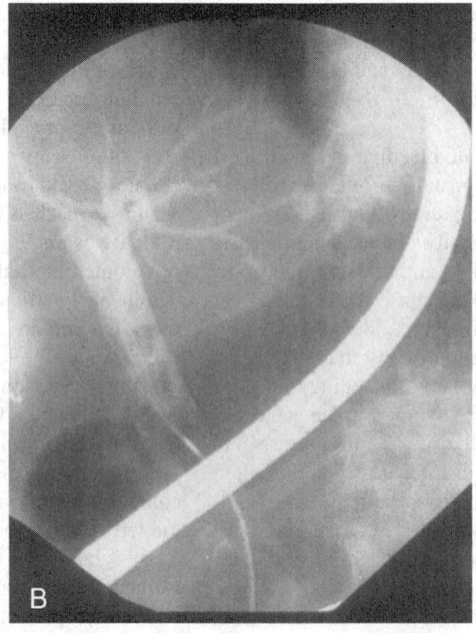

FIGURE 283-1 Endoscopic retrograde cholangiopancreatography (ERCP) for bile duct stones with cholangitis. *A.* Faceted bile duct stones are demonstrated in the common bile duct. *B.* After endoscopic sphincterotomy, the stones are extracted with a Dormia basket. A small abscess communicates with the left intrahepatic duct.

endoscopy and colonoscopy (<1:1000 procedures), although the risk is as high as 1:100 when therapeutic procedures such as polypectomy, control of hemorrhage, or stricture dilation are performed. Bleeding and perforation are rare with flexible sigmoidoscopy. The risks for diagnostic EUS are similar to the risks for diagnostic upper endoscopy.

Infectious complications are unusual with most endoscopic procedures. Stricture dilation, variceal sclerotherapy, and ERCP for biliary obstruction all carry a higher incidence of postprocedure bacteremia, and prophylactic antibiotics may be indicated for these procedures in some patients (Table 283-1).

ERCP carries additional risks. Pancreatitis occurs in about 5% of patients undergoing ERCP and is seen in up to 25% of patients with sphincter of Oddi dysfunction. Post-ERCP pancreatitis is usually mild and self-limited but may infrequently result in prolonged hospitalization, surgery, diabetes, or death. Bleeding occurs after 1% of endoscopic sphincterotomies. Ascending cholangitis, pseudocyst infection, and retroperitoneal perforation and abscess may all occur as a result of ERCP.

The conscious sedation administered during endoscopy may cause respiratory depression or allergic reactions. Percutaneous gastrostomy tube placement during EGD is associated with a 10 to 15% incidence of complications, most often wound infections. Fasciitis, pneumonia, bleeding, and colonic injury may result from gastrostomy placement.

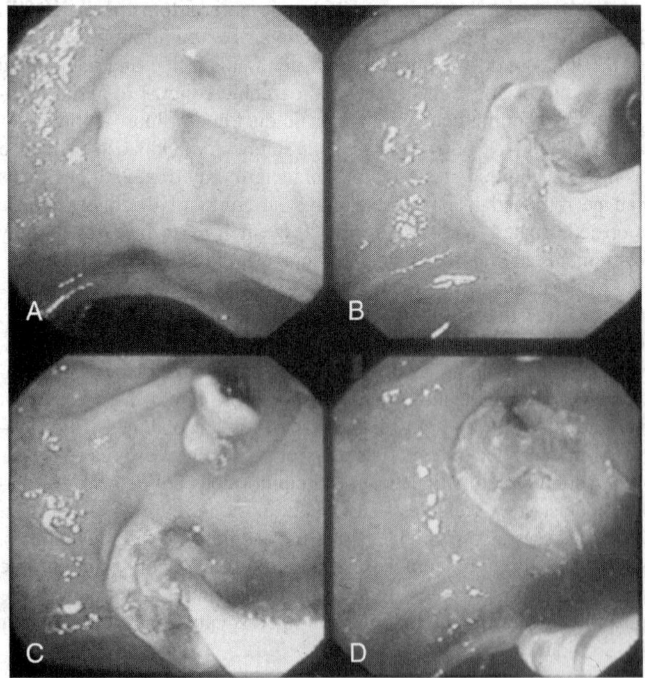

FIGURE 283-2 Endoscopic sphincterotomy. *A.* A normal-appearing ampulla of Vater. *B.* Sphincterotomy is performed with electrocautery. *C.* Bile duct stones are extracted with a balloon catheter. *D.* Final appearance of the sphincterotomy.

URGENT ENDOSCOPY

ACUTE GASTROINTESTINAL HEMORRHAGE Endoscopy is an important diagnostic and therapeutic technique for patients with acute gastrointestinal hemorrhage. Although most gastrointestinal bleeding stops spontaneously, a minority of patients will have persistent or recurrent hemorrhage that may be life-threatening. Clinical predictors of rebleeding help identify patients most likely to benefit from urgent endoscopy and endoscopic, angiographic, or surgical hemostasis.

Initial Evaluation The initial evaluation of the bleeding patient focuses on the magnitude of hemorrhage as reflected by the postural vital signs, the frequency of hematemesis or melena, and (in some cases) findings on nasogastric lavage. The measured values of hematocrit and hemoglobin lag the clinical course and are not reliable gauges of the magnitude of acute bleeding. This initial evaluation, completed well before the bleeding source is confidently identified, guides immediate supportive care of the patient and helps determine the timing of endoscopy. The magnitude of the initial hemorrhage is probably the most important indication for urgent endoscopy, since a large initial bleed increases the likelihood of ongoing or recurrent bleeding. Patients with resting hypotension, repeated hematemesis, nasogastric aspirate that does not clear with repeated lavage, or those requiring blood transfusions should be considered for urgent endoscopy. In addition, patients with cirrhosis, coagulopathy, or respiratory or renal failure and those over 70 years of age are more likely to have significant rebleeding.

Bedside evaluation also suggests an upper or lower gastrointestinal source of bleeding in most patients. About 90% of patients with melena are bleeding proximal to the ligament of Treitz, and about 90% of patients with hematochezia are bleeding from the colon. It is important to note, however, that melena can result from bleeding in the small bowel or right colon, especially in older patients with slow colonic transit, so colonoscopy should be performed in patients with melena when upper endoscopy is unrevealing. Similarly, a minority of patients with massive hematochezia are bleeding from a duodenal ulcer, with rapid intestinal transit. Hence early upper endoscopy should be considered in patients with massive hematochezia.

Endoscopy should be performed after the patient has been resuscitated with intravenous fluids and transfusions as necessary. Marked coagulopathy or thrombocytopenia is usually treated before endoscopy, since correction of these abnormalities may lead to resolution of bleeding, and techniques for endoscopic hemostasis are limited in such patients. Metabolic derangements should also be addressed. Tracheal intubation for airway protection should be considered before upper endoscopy in patients with repeated hematemesis and suspected variceal hemorrhage.

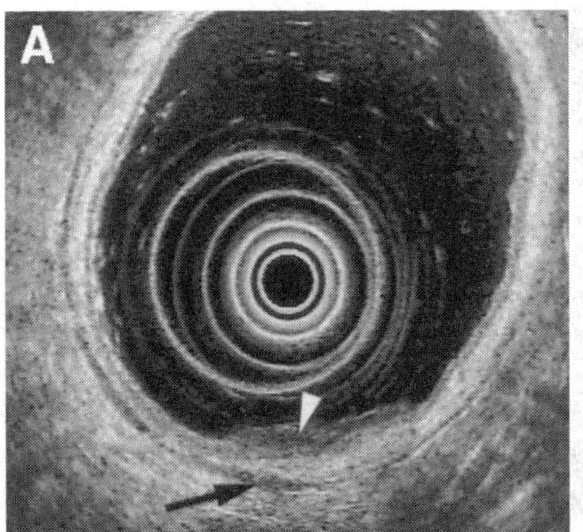

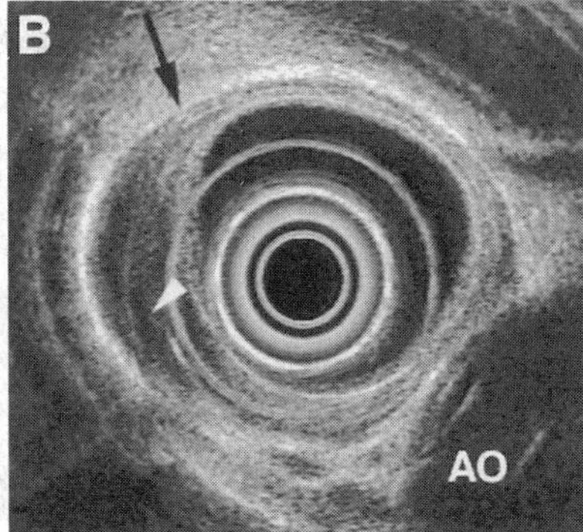

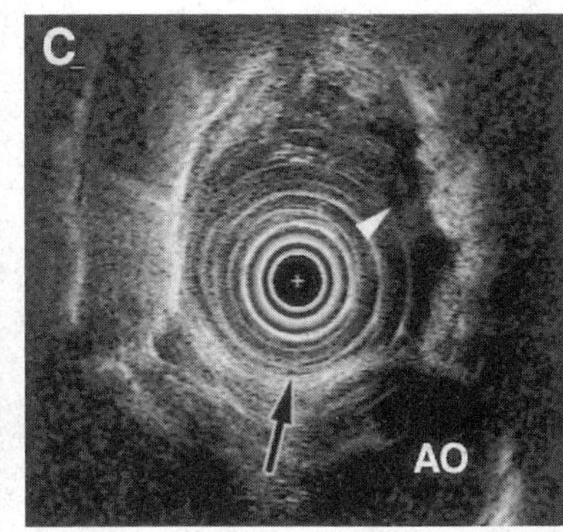

FIGURE 283-3 Local staging of gastrointestinal cancers with endoscopic ultrasound. In each example the white arrowhead marks the primary tumor and the black arrow indicates the muscularis propria (mp) of the intestinal wall. "AO" indicates aorta. *A.* T1 gastric cancer. The tumor does not invade the mp. *B.* T2 esophageal cancer. The tumor invades the mp. *C.* T3 esophageal cancer. The tumor extends through the mp into the surrounding tissue, and focally abuts the aorta.

Most patients with impressive hematochezia can undergo colonoscopy after a rapid colonic purge with a polyethylene glycol solution; the preparation fluid is often administered via a nasogastric tube. In a minority of cases, persistent bleeding and recurrent hemodynamic instability prevent endoscopic visualization of the colonic mucosa, and other techniques (such as bleeding scans, angiography, or emergency subtotal colectomy) must be employed. Even in these cases, however, the anal and rectal mucosa should be visualized endoscopically early in the course, since bleeding lesions in or close to the anal canal are generally amenable to surgical transanal hemostatic techniques; and upper endoscopy should be performed to exclude duodenal ulcer.

Peptic Ulcer The endoscopic appearance of peptic ulcers provides useful prognostic information in patients with acute hemorrhage. When a platelet plug is seen protruding from a vessel wall in the base of an ulcer (a so-called sentinel clot or visible vessel), there is a 40% chance of major rebleeding from the ulcer. This finding often leads to local endoscopic therapy to decrease the rebleeding rate. A clean-based ulcer, on the other hand, is associated with low (3 to 5%) risk of rebleeding; patients with melena and a clean-based duodenal ulcer are often discharged to home from the emergency department or endoscopy suite if they are young, reliable, and otherwise healthy. Other findings have an intermediate risk of rebleeding: flat red or purple spots in the ulcer base have a 10% risk, and large adherent clots covering the ulcer base have a 20% risk. Occasionally, active spurting from an ulcer is seen (with >90% risk of ongoing bleeding). Examples of endoscopic stigmata of recent hemorrhage are shown in Fig. 283-4.

Patients with a visible vessel or active bleeding are usually treated endoscopically, decreasing rebleeding rates by about half. Hemostatic techniques include "coaptive coagulation" of the vessel in the base of the ulcer, using a thermal probe that is pressed against the site of bleeding, or injection of epinephrine or sclerosant into and around the vessel.

Varices Two complementary strategies guide therapy of bleeding varices: local treatment of the bleeding vessel and treatment of underlying portal hypertension. Local therapies (including endoscopic sclerotherapy, endoscopic band ligation, and balloon tamponade with a Sengstaken-Blakemore tube) effectively control acute hemorrhage in most patients and are the mainstay of acute treatment, although therapies that decrease portal pressures (pharmacologic treatment, surgical shunts, or radiologically placed intrahepatic shunts) also play an important role.

Endoscopic band ligation is the preferred local therapy for bleeding esophageal varices. In this technique a varix is suctioned into a cap fitted on the end of the endoscope, and a rubber band is then released from the cap, ligating the varix. Acute hemorrhage can be controlled in up to 90% of patients, and complications (such as sepsis, symptomatic esophageal ulceration, or esophageal stenosis) are uncommon. Endoscopic sclerotherapy is an older technique in which a sclerosing, thrombogenic solution is injected into or next to esophageal varices. Sclerotherapy also controls acute hemorrhage in most patients but has higher complication rates. These techniques are used when varices are actively bleeding during endoscopy or (more commonly) when varices are the only identifiable cause of acute hemorrhage.

After treatment of the acute hemorrhage, an elective course of endoscopic therapy can be undertaken with the goal of eradicating esophageal varices and preventing rebleeding months to years later. This chronic therapy is less successful, preventing long term rebleeding in about 50% of patients. Pharmacologic therapies that decrease portal pressure have similar efficacy, and the two modalities may be combined.

Gastric varices are less amenable to endoscopic therapy and are usually treated with a portal decompressive procedure (surgical portosystemic shunt or radiologic transjugular portosystemic shunt). Endoscopic therapy of gastric varices is usually reserved for actively bleeding varices or for patients with thrombosis of the portal venous system.

Dieulafoy's Lesion This lesion, also called *persistent caliber artery*, is a large-caliber arteriole that runs immediately beneath the gastrointestinal mucosa and bleeds through a pinpoint mucosal erosion. Dieulafoy's lesion is seen most commonly on the lesser curvature of the proximal stomach, causes impressive arterial hemorrhage, and is

Table 283-1 Antibiotic Prophylaxis for Selected Endoscopic Procedures

Patient Condition	Procedure Contemplated	Antibiotic Prophylaxis[a]
Prosthetic valve, history of endocarditis, systemic-pulmonary shunt, Synthetic vascular graft (<1 year old)	High risk[b]	Recommended
	Low risk[c]	Optional (insufficient data)
Rheumatic valvular disease, mitral valve prolapse with insufficiency, congenital cardiac malformations, hypertrophic cardiomyopathy	High risk	Optional (insufficient data)
	Low risk	Not recommended
Pacemakers, implantable defibrillators, Prior coronary artery bypass grafts; prosthetic joints	High or low risk	Not recommended

[a] Acceptable antibiotic regimens for esophageal procedures include amoxicillin, 2 g PO, 1 h before or ampicillin, 2 g IV, 30 min before upper endoscopy; clindamycin, 600 mg PO, may be substituted in penicillin-allergic patients. Acceptable regimens for colonic procedures in high-risk patients include gentamicin, 1.5 mg/kg (not to exceed 120 mg), and ampicillin, 2 g IV, within 30 min of colonoscopy, with amoxicillin, 1 g orally, 6 h later; vancomycin, 1 g IV, may be substituted for penicillins in penicillin-allergic patients. For colonic procedures in moderate-risk patients, amoxicillin, 2 g PO, 1 h before the procedure or vancomycin, 1 g IV, are sufficient.

[b] High-risk endoscopic procedures: stricture dilation, variceal sclerosis, endoscopic retrograde cholangiopancreatography with an obstructed biliary tree.

[c] Low-risk endoscopic procedures: upper endoscopy and colonoscopy with or without biopsy and polyp removal, variceal ligation.

SOURCE: Adapted from *Antibiotic Prophylaxis for Endoscopic Procedures*, American Society for Gastrointestinal Endoscopy, 1998.

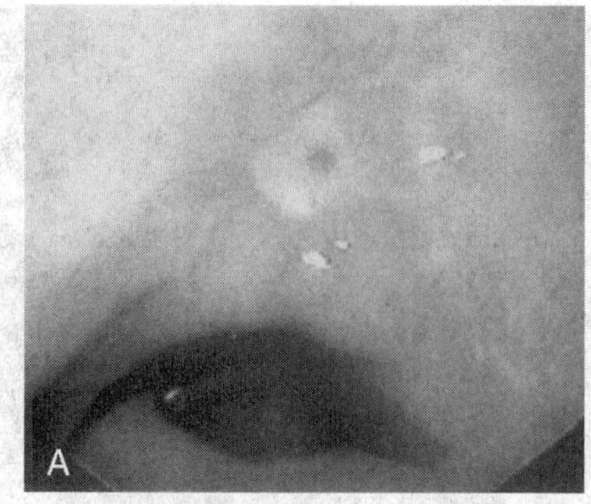

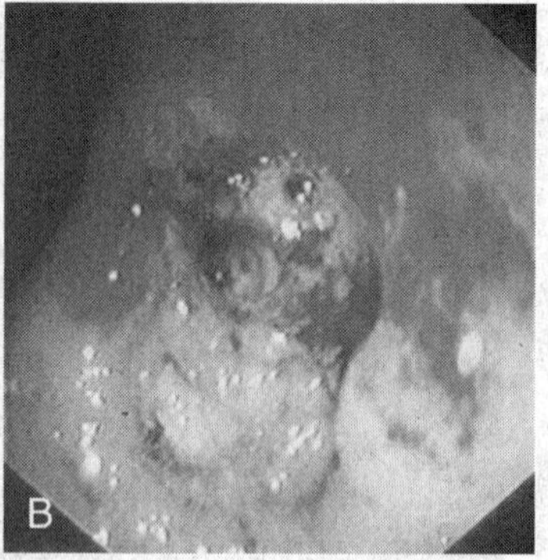

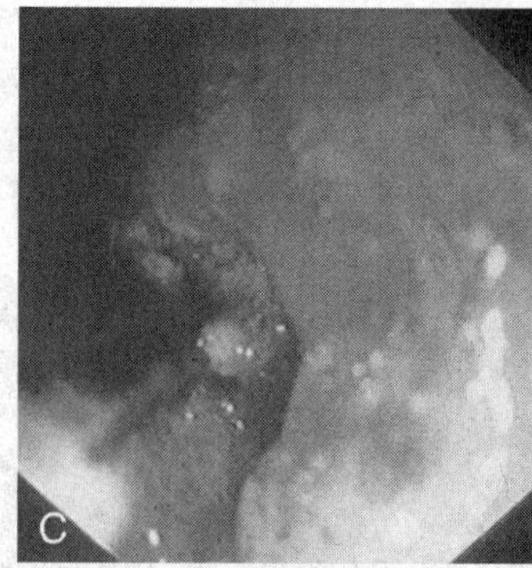

FIGURE 283-4 Endoscopic stigmata of recent bleeding in peptic ulcers. *A.* A flat red spot in an ulcer base. *B.* A sentinel clot protruding from an ulcer base. *C.* Coagulation of the sentinel clot shown in (*B*) with a thermal probe. (*Courtesy of American Society for Gastrointestinal Endoscopy.*)

difficult to diagnose; it is often recognized only after repeated endoscopy for recurrent bleeding. Endoscopic therapy with a thermal probe usually controls acute bleeding and successfully ablates the underlying vessel once the bleeding site has been identified. Embolization or surgical oversewing are sometimes required.

Mallory-Weiss Tear A Mallory-Weiss tear is a linear mucosal rent near or across the gastroesophageal junction that is often associated with retching or vomiting. When the tear disrupts a submucosal arteriole, brisk hemorrhage may result. Endoscopy is the best method of diagnosis, and an actively bleeding tear can be treated endoscopically with coaptive coagulation using a thermal probe or by injection of dilute epinephrine. Since Mallory-Weiss tears only rarely rebleed, a sentinel clot in the base of the tear is usually not treated endoscopically.

Vascular Ectasias Vascular ectasias are flat mucosal vascular anomalies best diagnosed by endoscopy. They usually cause slow intestinal blood loss and have several characteristic distributions in the gastrointestinal tract. When limited to the cecum, where they occur as senile lesions, or the gastric antrum (gastric antral vascular ectasias, or "watermelon stomach"), ectasias are often responsive to local endoscopic ablative therapy. Patients with diffuse small-bowel vascular ectasias (associated with chronic renal failure and with hereditary hemorrhagic telangiectasia) often continue to bleed despite endoscopic treatment of accessible lesions and require systemic therapy.

Colonic Diverticula Diverticula form where nutrient arteries penetrate the muscular wall of the colon en route to the colonic mucosa. The artery found in the base of a diverticulum may bleed, causing painless and impressive hematochezia. Colonoscopy is indicated in patients with hematochezia and suspected diverticular hemorrhage, since other causes of bleeding (such as vascular ectasias, colitis, and colonic malignancy) must be excluded. In addition, an actively bleeding diverticulum is occasionally seen and treated during colonoscopy.

GASTROINTESTINAL OBSTRUCTION AND PSEUDO-OBSTRUCTION Endoscopy is useful for evaluation and treatment of some forms of gastrointestinal obstruction. An important exception is small-bowel obstruction, which is generally not diagnosed by endoscopy or amenable to endoscopic therapy. Esophageal, gastroduodenal, and colonic obstruction or pseudoobstruction can all be diagnosed endoscopically and are often managed endoscopically as well.

Acute Esophageal Obstruction Esophageal obstruction by impacted food or an ingested foreign body is a potentially life-threatening event. Left untreated, the patient may develop esophageal ulceration, ischemia, and perforation. Patients with persistent esophageal obstruction often have hypersalivation and are usually unable to swallow water; endoscopy is generally the best initial test in such patients, since endoscopic removal of the obstructing material is usually possible, and the presence of an underlying esophageal stricture can often be determined. Radiographs of the chest and neck should be considered before endoscopy in patients with fever, obstruction for ≥24 h, or ingestion of a sharp object such as a fishbone. Radiographic contrast studies interfere with subsequent endoscopy and are not advisable in patients with a clinical picture of persistent obstruction, unless an esophageal perforation is suspected. Occasionally, sublingual nifedipine or nitrates, or intravenous glucagon, may resolve an esophageal food impaction, but in most patients there is an underlying web, ring, or stricture and endoscopic removal of the obstructing food bolus is necessary.

Gastric Outlet Obstruction Obstruction of the gastric outlet is commonly caused by malignancy of the prepyloric gastric antrum or chronic peptic ulceration with stenosis of the pylorus. Patients vomit partially digested food many hours after eating. Gastric decompression with a nasogastric tube and subsequent lavage for removal of retained material is the first step in treatment. The diagnosis can then be confirmed with a saline load test, if desired. Endoscopy is useful for diagnosis and treatment. Patients with pyloric stenosis may be treated with endoscopic balloon dilation of the pylorus, and a course of endoscopic dilation results in long-term relief of symptoms in about 50% of patients. Malignant pyloric obstruction can be treated with endoscopically placed expandable stents if the patient is deemed a poor surgical candidate.

Colonic Obstruction and Pseudoobstruction These both present with abdominal distention and discomfort; tympany; and a dilated, air-filled colon on plain abdominal radiography. Both conditions may lead to colonic perforation if untreated. Acute colonic pseudoobstruction is a form of colonic ileus that is usually attributable to electrolyte disorders, narcotic and anticholinergic medications, immobility (as after surgery), and retroperitoneal hemorrhage or mass. Multiple causative factors are often present. Either colonoscopy or a water-soluble contrast enema may be used to look for an obstructing lesion and differentiate obstruction from pseudoobstruction. One of these diagnostic studies should be strongly considered if the patient does not have clear risk factors for pseudoobstruction, if radiographs do not show air in the rectum and sigmoid, or if the patient fails to improve when the underlying causes of pseudoobstruction have been addressed. The risk of cecal perforation in pseudoobstruction rises when the cecal diameter exceeds 12 cm, and in such patients decompression of the colon may be achieved using intravenous neostigmine, colonoscopic decompression, or placement of a cecostomy tube. Most patients should receive a trial of conservative therapy (with correction of electrolyte disorders, removal of offending medications, and increased mobilization) before undergoing an invasive decompressive procedure.

Colonic obstruction is an indication for urgent surgery. In poor operative candidates or those with symptomatic partial obstruction from malignancy, a colonoscopically placed expandable stent can relieve obstruction and permit preparation of the bowel for elective surgery.

ACUTE BILIARY OBSTRUCTION The steady, severe pain that occurs when a gallstone acutely obstructs the common bile duct often brings patients to a hospital. The diagnosis of a ductal stone is suspected when the patient is jaundiced or when serum liver tests or pancreatic enzyme levels are elevated, and it is confirmed by direct

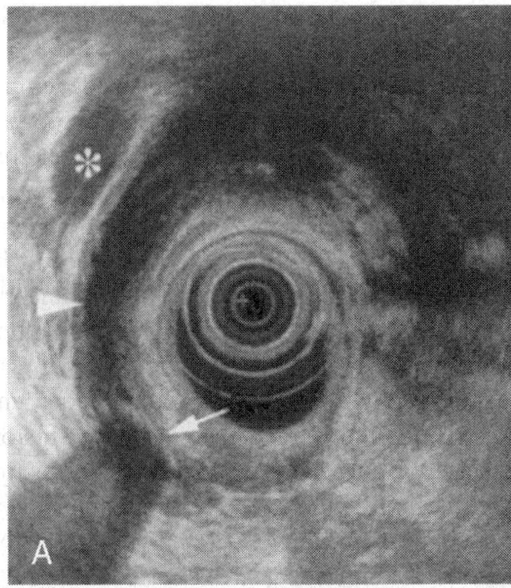

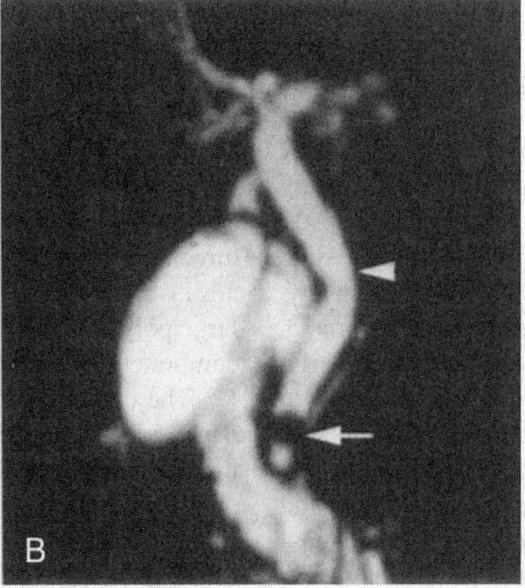

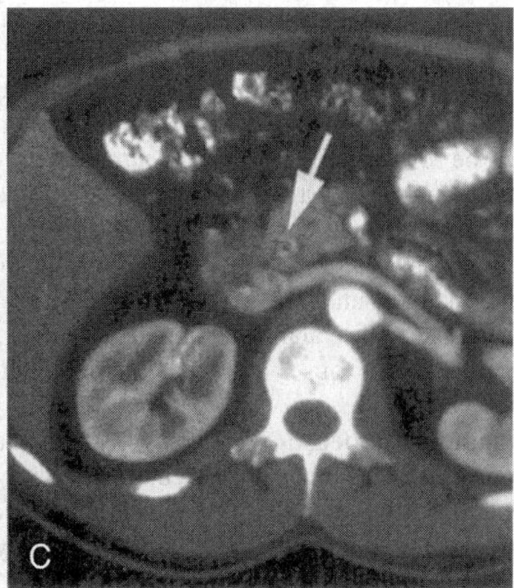

FIGURE 283-5 New methods of bile duct imaging. Arrows mark bile duct stones. Arrowheads indicate the common bile duct, and the asterisk marks the portal vein. *A.* Endoscopic ultrasonography (EUS). *B.* Magnetic resonance cholangiography (MRCP). *C.* Helical computed tomography.

cholangiography (performed endoscopically, percutaneously, or during surgery). ERCP is currently the primary means of diagnosing and treating common bile duct stones in most hospitals in the United States.

Bile Duct Imaging While traditional noninvasive imaging tests such as ultrasound and biliary scintigraphy are not sufficiently accurate for reliable diagnosis of bile duct stones, newer imaging modalities such as spiral computed tomography (CT), magnetic resonance cholangiopancreatography (MRCP), and EUS are more accurate and have an emerging role in diagnosis. Examples of these modalities are shown in Fig. 283-5. During MRCP, images are obtained that demonstrate stagnant or slowly flowing fluid and subtract all other tissue. The resulting images of the right upper quadrant are strikingly similar to a direct cholangiogram, although with less resolution. MRCP can be performed rapidly without sedation and does not require any radiographic contrast. When an echo-endoscope is passed into the duodenum, detailed EUS views of the adjacent bile duct are readily obtained. While this procedure requires intravenous sedation, it has a very low incidence of complications, in contradistinction to ERCP. Spiral CT has a sensitivity of 85% for diagnosis of bile duct stones, MRCP has a sensitivity of 85 to 95%, and EUS has a sensitivity of 88 to 98%. EUS is more accurate than ERCP in some hands.

The clinical role of these new imaging techniques is evolving. When a bile duct stone is highly likely and urgent treatment is required (as in a patient with jaundice and biliary sepsis), ERCP is the procedure of choice, since it remains the gold standard for diagnosis and provides immediate treatment. When a persistent bile duct stone is relatively unlikely (as in a patient with gallstone pancreatitis), less-invasive imaging techniques may supplant ERCP or intraoperative cholangiography.

Ascending Cholangitis Charcot's triad of jaundice, abdominal pain, and fever is present in about 70% of patients with ascending cholangitis and biliary sepsis. Initially, such patients are managed with fluid resuscitation and intravenous antibiotics. Abdominal ultrasound is often done early in the course, to look for gallbladder stones and bile duct dilation. The bile duct may not be dilated early in the course of acute biliary obstruction, however. Medical management usually improves the patient's clinical status, providing a window of approximately 24 h during which biliary drainage should be established, typically by ERCP. Undue delay can result in recrudesence of overt sepsis and increased morbidity. If, in addition to Charcot's triad, shock and confusion are present (Reynolds's pentad), urgent attempts to restore biliary drainage are usually indicated.

Gallstone Pancreatitis Gallstones may cause acute pancreatitis as they pass through the ampulla of Vater, where they obstruct the pancreatic duct (and sometimes cause reflux of bile into the pancreas). The occurrence of gallstone pancreatitis usually implies passage of a stone into the duodenum, and only about 20% of patients harbor a persistent stone in the ampulla or the common bile duct. Retained stones are more common in the subset of patients with jaundice, severe pancreatitis, or superimposed ascending cholangitis.

Urgent ERCP decreases the morbidity of gallstone pancreatitis in some subsets of patients, but it remains unclear whether the benefit of ERCP is mainly attributable to treatment and prevention of ascending cholangitis or to relief of pancreatic duct obstruction. ERCP is warranted early in the course of gallstone pancreatitis if ascending cholangitis is also suspected, especially in a jaundiced patient. Urgent ERCP may also be indicated in the minority of patients predicted to have severe pancreatitis using a multifactorial index of severity such as the Glasgow, Ranson's, or Apache II score.

ELECTIVE ENDOSCOPY

Dyspepsia and Reflux Dyspepsia is a burning discomfort in the upper abdomen that may be caused by diverse processes such as gastroesophageal reflux, peptic ulcer disease, and "nonulcer dyspepsia," a heterogeneous category that includes disorders of motility, sensation, and somatization. Gastric and esophageal malignancies are less common causes of dyspepsia. Careful history taking allows accurate differential diagnosis of dyspepsia in only about half of patients. In the remainder, endoscopy can be a useful diagnostic tool, especially in those patients whose symptoms are not resolved by an empirical trial of symptomatic treatment.

Gastroesophageal Reflux Disease (GERD) When classic symptoms of gastroesophageal reflux are present, such as water brash and substernal heartburn, presumptive diagnosis and empirical treatment are often sufficient. Although endoscopy is sensitive for diagnosis of esophagitis, it misses some cases of reflux, since some patients have symptomatic reflux without esophagitis. The most sensitive test for diagnosis of GERD is 24-h ambulatory pH monitoring. Endoscopy is nevertheless indicated in patients with resistant reflux symptoms and in those with recurrent dyspepsia after treatment that is not clearly due to reflux on clinical grounds alone, to assess the esophagus and exclude other diseases. Endoscopy is also advised in a patient with reflux and dysphagia, to look for a stricture or malignancy. Endoscopy is probably also indicated in patients with long-standing ($\geq$10 years) frequent heartburn, who are at sixfold increased risk of Barrett's esophagus compared to a patient with $<$1 year of reflux symptoms. Patients with Barrett's esophagus usually enter a program of periodic endoscopy with biopsies, to detect dysplasia or early carcinoma.

Peptic Ulcer Peptic ulcer classically causes epigastric gnawing or burning, often occurring nocturnally and promptly relieved by food or antacids. Although endoscopy is the most sensitive diagnostic test for peptic ulcer, immediate endoscopy is not a cost-effective strategy in young patients with ulcer-like dyspeptic symptoms unless endoscopy is available at low cost. Patients with suspected peptic ulcer should be evaluated for *Helicobacter pylori* infection. Serology (which documents past or present infection) and urea breath testing (which demonstrates current infection) are less invasive and costly than endoscopy with biopsy. Patients with ulcer-like symptoms despite treatment should undergo endoscopy to exclude gastric malignancy, and patients with "alarm symptoms" (early satiety or anorexia, early recurrence of symptoms, anemia) should also undergo endoscopy.

Nonulcer Dyspepsia This may be associated with bloating and, unlike peptic ulcer, tends not to remit and recur. Most patients do not respond to acid-reducing, prokinetic, or anti-*Helicobacter* therapy and are referred for endoscopy to exclude a refractory ulcer. While endoscopy usefully excludes other diagnoses, it generally does little to improve the treatment of patients with nonulcer dyspepsia.

Dysphagia About 50% of patients with difficulty swallowing have a mechanical obstruction; the remainder have a motor disorder. Careful history taking often suggests a diagnosis and leads to the appropriate use of diagnostic tests. Esophageal strictures typically cause progressive dysphagia, first for solids, then liquids; esophageal motor disorders often cause intermittent dysphagia for both solids and liquids. Some underlying disorders have characteristic historical features: Schatzki's ring causes episodic dysphagia for solids, typically at the beginning of a meal; pharyngeal motor disorders are associated with difficulty initiating deglutition ("transfer dysphagia") and nasal reflux with swallowing; and achalasia may cause nocturnal regurgitation of undigested food particles.

When mechanical obstruction is suspected, endoscopy is a useful initial diagnostic test, since it permits immediate biopsy and dilation of strictures, masses, or rings. Blind or forceful passage of an endoscope may lead to perforation in a patient with stenosis of the cervical esophagus or a Zencker's diverticulum, but gentle passage of an endoscope under direct visual guidance is reasonably safe even in these patients. Endoscopy can miss a subtle stricture or ring in some patients.

When a motor disorder is suspected, esophageal radiography is the best initial diagnostic test. The pharyngeal swallowing mechanism, esophageal peristalsis, and the lower esophageal sphincter can all be assessed. In some disorders, subsequent esophageal manometry may also be important for diagnosis.

Anemia and Occult Blood in the Stool Iron-deficiency anemia may be attributed to poor iron absorption (as in celiac sprue) or, more commonly, chronic blood loss. Intestinal bleeding should be strongly suspected in men and postmenopausal women with iron-deficiency anemia, and colonoscopy is indicated in such patients, even in the absence of detectable occult blood in the stool. About 30% will have large colonic polyps, 10% will have colorectal cancer, and additional patients will have colonic vascular lesions. When a convincing source of blood loss is not found in the colon, upper gastrointestinal endoscopy should also be performed; if no lesion is found, duodenal biopsies should be obtained to exclude sprue. Evaluation of the small bowel may be appropriate if both EGD and colonoscopy are unrevealing.

Tests for occult blood in the stool detect hemoglobin or the heme moiety and are most sensitive for colonic blood loss, although they will also detect larger amounts of upper gastrointestinal bleeding. Patients with occult blood in normal-appearing stool should undergo colonoscopy to diagnose or exclude colorectal neoplasia. The diagnostic yield is lower than in iron-deficiency anemia. Whether upper endoscopy is also indicated largely depends on the patient's symptoms.

The small intestine may be the source of chronic intestinal bleeding, especially if colonoscopy and upper endoscopy are not diagnostic. The utility of small-bowel evaluation varies with the clinical setting and is most important in patients whose bleeding causes chronic or recurrent anemia. While small-bowel radiography is usually normal, partial or total small-bowel enteroscopy yields a specific diagnosis in about 50% of such patients. The commonest finding is mucosal vascular ectasias or telangiectasias.

Colorectal Cancer Screening Most colon cancers develop from preexisting colonic adenomas, and colorectal cancer can be largely prevented by the detection and removal of colonic adenomatous polyps. Screening for polyps and early, asymptomatic cancers can be accomplished both by testing stool specimens for occult blood and by directly examining the colonic mucosa. Since tests for occult blood are insensitive, detecting only about one-fourth of colon cancers and large polyps, visualization of at least a part of the colon is an important component of colorectal cancer screening.

The choice of screening strategy for an asymptomatic patient depends in part on their personal and family history. A past history of inflammatory bowel disease or colorectal polyps, a family history of two or more first-degree family members with adenomatous polyps or cancer, certain familial cancer syndromes, or the finding of occult blood in the stool all place an individual at increased risk and alter screening recommendations. An individual without these factors is generally considered at average risk, and screening flexible sigmoidoscopy every 5 years beginning at age 50 is recommended. Screening strategies for higher risk patients are in Table 283-2. Screening strategies for the patient with one family member with colorectal cancer are debated. When the index case occurred at a young age (<60 years), screening colonoscopy should be offered when the patient is 10 years younger than the affected relative was when diagnosed.

Flexible sigmoidoscopy is an effective screening tool for two reasons: (1) the majority of colorectal cancers have traditionally occurred in the rectum and left colon, and (2) many right-sided colon cancers are associated with synchronous left-sided adenomas. The detection of an adenoma during sigmoidoscopy generally leads to full colonoscopy and detection of right-sided cancers, if present. Over the past several decades, however, there has been a gradual change in the distribution of colon cancers, with proportionally fewer rectal and left-sided can-

Table 283-2 Colorectal Cancer Screening Strategies for Patients at Increased Risk

	Recommendation
PERSONAL HISTORY	
History of colon cancer	Evaluate entire colon around the time of resection, then colonoscopy every 3 to 5 years
History of colonic adenomas	Colonoscopy every 3 to 5 years
Ulcerative pancolitis of 8 years duration, left-sided colitis >15 years' duration	Colonoscopy with biopsies every 1 to 3 years
FAMILY HISTORY	
Familial adenomatous polyposis	Consider genetic testing Annual sigmoidoscopy beginning at age 10 to 12, consider colectomy when polyps develop; if no polyps, annual sigmoidoscopy until age 40, then every 3 to 5 years
Hereditary non-polyposis colorectal cancer (HNPCC)	Consider genetic testing Colonoscopy every 2 years beginning at 25 or when 5 years younger than the youngest affected relative; annual colonoscopy after age 40
Two first-degree relatives with colorectal cancer or adenomas	Colonoscopy every 3 to 5 years, beginning when 10 years younger than the youngest affected relative
One first-degree relative with sporadic colorectal cancer or adenoma before age 60	Same as above

SOURCE: Adapted from *Screening and Surveillance Colonoscopy in Individuals at Increased Risk for Colorectal Cancer*, American Society for Gastrointestinal Endoscopy, 1998.

cers than in the past. This has spurred interest in evaluating the entire colon during a single screening examination. Barium enema has been advocated but requires flexible sigmoidoscopy also, to exclude missed rectal lesions. Large studies of colonoscopy for screening of average-risk individuals are currently underway. In addition, the new imaging technique of "virtual colonoscopy" holds considerable promise. This modality uses data from helical CT to generate a graphical display of a "flight" down the colonic lumen. While this technique is not yet sufficiently sensitive for routine clinical use, further refinement may result in a useful noninvasive screening method.

Diarrhea Most cases of diarrhea are acute, self-limited, and due to infections or medication. Chronic diarrhea (lasting >6 weeks) is more often due to a primary inflammatory or malabsorptive disorder, is less likely to resolve spontaneously, and generally requires diagnostic evaluation. Patients with chronic diarrhea or severe, unexplained acute diarrhea often undergo endoscopy if stool tests for pathogens are unrevealing. The choice of endoscopic test depends on the clinical setting.

Patients with colonic symptoms and findings such as bloody diarrhea, tenesmus, fever, or leukocytes in stool generally undergo sigmoidoscopy or colonoscopy to look for colitis. Sigmoidoscopy is often adequate and is the best initial test in most such patients. On the other hand, patients with symptoms and findings suggesting small-bowel disease such as large-volume watery stools; substantial weight loss; and malabsorption of iron, calcium, or fat may undergo upper endoscopy with duodenal biopsies.

Many patients with chronic diarrhea do not fit either of these patterns. When there is a long-standing history of alternating constipation and diarrhea dating to early adulthood, without findings such as blood in the stool or anemia, a diagnosis of irritable bowel syndrome may be made without direct visualization of the bowel. Steatorrhea and upper abdominal pain may prompt evaluation of the pancreas rather than the gut. Patients whose chronic diarrhea is not easily categorized often undergo initial colonoscopy to examine the entire colon (and terminal ileum) for inflammatory or neoplastic disease.

Minor Hematochezia Bright red blood passed with or on formed brown stool usually has a rectal, anal, or distal sigmoid source. Patients with even trivial amounts of hematochezia should be investigated with flexible sigmoidoscopy to exclude large polyps or cancers in the distal bowel. Patients who report red blood on the toilet tissue only, without blood in the toilet or on the stool, are bleeding from a lesion in the anal canal, and careful external and digital examinations and anoscopy are sufficient for diagnosis in most cases.

Unexplained Pancreatitis About 20% of patients with pancreatitis have no identified cause after routine clinical investigation (including a review of medication and alcohol use, measurement of serum triglyceride and calcium levels, abdominal ultrasonography, and CT). Endoscopic techniques lead to a specific diagnosis in the majority of such patients, often altering clinical management. Endoscopic investigation is particularly appropriate if the patient has had more than one episode of pancreatitis.

Microlithiasis, or the presence of microscopic crystals in bile, is a leading cause of previously unexplained acute pancreatitis and is sometimes seen during abdominal ultrasonography as layering sludge or flecks of floating, echogenic material in the gallbladder. Gallbladder bile can be obtained for microscopic analysis by administering a cholecystokinin analogue during endoscopy, causing contraction of the gallbladder. Bile is suctioned from the duodenum as it drains from the papilla, and the darkest fraction is examined for cholesterol crystals or bilirubinate granules. Alternatively, bile can be aspirated from the bile duct during ERCP or the gallbladder can be examined for sludge or crystals by EUS before administering cholecystokinin. The latter strategy is probably the most sensitive means of diagnosing microlithiasis.

Previously undetected chronic pancreatitis, pancreatic malignancy, or pancreas divisum may be diagnosed by either ERCP or EUS. Although ERCP remains the gold standard imaging test for chronic pan-

creatitis, EUS has good sensitivity and less risk than ERCP. Sphincter of Oddi dysfunction probably causes some cases of pancreatitis and can be diagnosed by manometric studies performed during ERCP.

OPEN-ACCESS ENDOSCOPY

While gastroenterologists have traditionally seen patients in consultation before arranging an endoscopic procedure, direct scheduling of endoscopic procedures by primary care physicians, or *open-access endoscopy*, is an increasingly common practice. When the indications for endoscopy are clear cut and appropriate, the procedural risks are low, and the patient understands what to expect, open-access endoscopy streamlines patient care and decreases costs.

Patients referred for open-access endoscopy should have a recent history, physical examination, and medication review. A copy of such an evaluation should be available when the patient comes to the endoscopy suite. Patients with unstable cardiovascular or respiratory conditions should not be referred directly for open-access endoscopy. Patients with selected cardiac conditions undergoing certain procedures should be prescribed prophylactic antibiotics prior to endoscopy, as described in Table 283-1. In addition, patients taking anticoagulants may need changes in treatment before endoscopy, as detailed in Table 283-3. While many endoscopists recommend discontinuing aspirin for 5 days before elective endoscopic procedures, most evidence suggests that in the absence of a preexisting bleeding disorder it is safe to perform endoscopic procedures in patients taking aspirin and nonsteroidal anti-inflammatory drugs.

Common indications for open-access EGD include dyspepsia resistant to a trial of appropriate therapy; dysphagia or odynophagia; gastrointestinal bleeding; and persistent vomiting, anorexia, or early satiety. Open-access colonoscopy is often requested in men or postmenopausal women with iron-deficiency anemia, patients with occult blood in the stool, patients with a previous history of colorectal adenomatous polyps or cancer, and for screening in patients with above-average risk for colon cancer, as described in Table 283-2. Flexible sigmoidoscopy is commonly performed as an open-access procedure for cancer screening in asymptomatic persons over 50 and for patients with hematochezia.

Table 283-3 Management of Anticoagulation before Endoscopic Procedures

	High Patient Risk of Thromboembolism[a]	Low Patient Risk of Thromboembolism[b]
High-risk procedure[c]	Stop warfarin 3–5 days before the procedure; consider heparin when INR is below the therapeutic range	Stop warfarin 3–5 days before the procedure; restart warfarin after the procedure
Low-risk procedure[d]	No change in anticoagulation; elective procedures should be delayed while INR is above the therapeutic range	No change in anticoagulation; elective procedures should be delayed while INR is above the therapeutic range

[a] High-risk conditions: atrial fibrillation associated with valvular heart disease, mechanical valve in the mitral position, mechanical valve and prior thromboembolic event.
[b] Low-risk conditions: Uncomplicated or paroxysmal nonvalvular atrial fibrillation, mechanical valve in the aortic position, bioprosthetic valve, deep vein thrombosis.
[c] High-risk procedures: Polypectomy, stricture dilation, treatment of varices, gastrostomy placement, biliary sphincterotomy, endoscopic ultrasound with needle aspiration.
[d] Low-risk procedures: Diagnostic upper endoscopy, colonoscopy, sigmoidoscopy with or without biopsy, diagnostic endoscopic retrograde cholangiopancreatography, endoscopic ultrasound without needle aspiration.

NOTE: INR, international normalized ratio.

SOURCE: Adapted from *The Management of Anticoagulants and Anti-Inflammatory Medications in Patients Undergoing Endoscopic Procedures*, American Society for Gastrointestinal Endoscopy, 1998.

When patients are referred for open-access colonoscopy, the primary care provider may need to choose a colonic preparation. Commonly used oral preparations include polyethelene glycol lavage solution and sodium phosphate. Sodium phosphate may cause fluid and electrolyte abnormalities, especially in patients with renal failure, congestive heart failure, and patients over 70 years of age.

BIBLIOGRAPHY

Caletti G, Fusaroli P: Endoscopic ultrasonography. Endoscopy 31:95, 1999

Dajani AS et al: Prevention of bacterial endocarditis: Recommendations by the American Heart Association. Clin Infect Dis 25:1448, 1997

Ofman JJ, Rabeneck L: The effectiveness of endoscopy in the management of dyspepsia: A qualitative systematic review. Am J Med 106:335, 1999

Stanley AJ, Hayes PC: Portal hypertension and variceal haemorrhage. Lancet 350: 1235, 1997

Steele RJ: The preprocedural care of the patient with gastrointestinal bleeding. Gastrointest Endosc Clin N Am 7:551, 1997

Zuccaro G Jr: Management of the adult patient with acute lower gastrointestinal bleeding. Am J Gastroenterol 93:1202, 1998

284

Raj K. Goyal

DISEASES OF THE ESOPHAGUS

The two major functions of the esophagus are the transport of the food bolus from the mouth to the stomach and the prevention of retrograde flow of gastrointestinal contents. The transport function is achieved by peristaltic contractions in the pharynx and esophagus associated with relaxation of upper and lower esophageal sphincters (Chap. 40). Retrograde flow is prevented by the two esophageal sphincters, which remain closed between swallows. The upper esophageal sphincter (UES) consists of the cricopharyngeus and inferior pharyngeal constrictor muscles, striated muscles innervated by excitatory somatic lower motor neurons. These muscles exhibit no myogenic tone and receive no inhibitory innervation. The UES remains closed owing to the elastic properties of its wall and to neurogenic tonic contraction of the sphincter muscles. It is opened by central inhibition of the sphincter muscles in concert with forward displacement of the larynx by the suprahyoid muscles. In contrast, the lower esophageal sphincter (LES) is composed of smooth muscle and is innervated by parallel sets of parasympathetic excitatory and inhibitory pathways. It remains closed because of its intrinsic myogenic tone, which is modulated by the excitatory and inhibitory nerves. It opens in response to the activity of the inhibitory nerves. The neurotransmitters of the excitatory nerves are acetylcholine and substance P, and those of the inhibitory nerves are vasoactive intestinal peptide (VIP) and nitric oxide. The function of the LES is supplemented by the striated muscle of the diaphragmatic crura, which surrounds the LES and acts as an external LES. Relaxation of the LES without esophageal contraction occurs during belching and gastric distention. Gastric distention–evoked transient lower esophageal sphincter relaxation (tLESR) is a vasovagal reflex. Fatty meals, smoking, and beverages with a high xanthine content (tea, coffee, cola) also cause a reduction in sphincter pressure. Many hormones and neurotransmitters can modify LES pressure. Muscarinic M_2 and M_3 receptor agonists, α-adrenergic agonists, gastrin, substance P, and prostaglandin $F_{2\alpha}$ cause contraction. Nicotine, β-adrenergic agonists, dopamine, cholecystokinin, secretin, VIP, calcitonin gene–related peptide (CGRP), adenosine, prostaglandin E, and nitric oxide donors such as nitrates reduce sphincter pressure.

SYMPTOMS

DYSPHAGIA See Chap. 40.

ESOPHAGEAL PAIN *Heartburn*, or pyrosis, is characterized by burning retrosternal discomfort that may move up and down the chest like a wave. When severe, it may radiate to the sides of the chest, the neck, and the angles of the jaw. Heartburn is a characteristic symptom of reflux esophagitis and may be associated with regurgitation or a feeling of warm fluid climbing up the throat. It is aggravated by bending forward, straining, or lying recumbent and is worse after meals. It is relieved by an upright posture, by the swallowing of saliva or water, and, more reliably, by antacids. Heartburn is produced by heightened mucosal sensitivity and can be reproduced by infusion of dilute (0.1 *N*) hydrochloric acid (Bernstein test) or neutral hyperosmolar solutions into the esophagus.

Odynophagia, or painful swallowing, is characteristic of nonreflux esophagitis, particularly monilial and herpes esophagitis. Odynophagia may occur with peptic ulcer of the esophagus (Barrett's ulcer), carcinoma with periesophageal involvement, caustic damage of the esophagus, and esophageal perforation. Odynophagia is unusual in uncomplicated reflux esophagitis. Crampy chest pain associated with impaction of a food bolus should be distinguished from odynophagia.

Atypical chest pain other than heartburn and odynophagia occurs in reflux esophagitis or esophageal motility disorders such as diffuse esophageal spasm. Spasm may occur spontaneously or during a meal. Chest pain due to periesophageal involvement with carcinoma or peptic ulcer may be constant and agonizing. Sometimes different types of esophageal pains exist together in the same patient, and frequently patients are not able to describe the pain accurately enough to allow its classification. Coronary artery disease should always be excluded before the esophagus is considered as the cause of atypical chest pain. The most frequent esophageal cause of chest pain is reflux esophagitis. Some patients with atypical chest pain have nonspecific esophageal motor abnormalities of uncertain significance. Many of these patients have behavioral abnormalities, psychosomatic disorders, depression, anxiety, panic reactions, and other psychological disorders.

REGURGITATION *Regurgitation* is the effortless appearance of gastric or esophageal contents in the mouth. In distal esophageal obstruction and stasis, as in achalasia or the presence of a large diverticulum, the regurgitated material consists of tasteless mucoid fluid or undigested food. Regurgitation of sour or bitter-tasting material occurs in severe gastroesophageal reflux and is associated with incompetence of both the UES and the LES. Regurgitation may result in laryngeal aspiration, with spells of coughing and choking that awaken the patient from sleep, and in aspiration pneumonia. Water brash is reflex salivary hypersecretion that occurs in response to peptic esophagitis and should not be confused with regurgitation.

DIAGNOSTIC TESTS

RADIOLOGIC STUDIES Barium swallow with fluoroscopy and an esophagogram is a widely used test for the diagnosis of esophageal disease and can be used to evaluate both structural and motor disorders. Spontaneous reflux of barium from the stomach into the esophagus suggests gastroesophageal reflux. Esophageal peristalsis is best studied in the recumbent position, because in the upright position barium passage occurs largely by gravity alone. A double-contrast esophagogram, obtained by coating the esophageal mucosa with barium and distending the esophageal lumen with air using effervescent granules, is particularly useful in demonstrating mucosal ulcers and early cancers. A barium-soaked piece of bread or a 13-mm barium tablet is sometimes used to demonstrate an obstructive lesion. Figures 284-1 and 284-2 illustrate the radiographic appearance of some esophageal disorders. Since the oropharyngeal phase of swallowing lasts no more than a second, videofluoroscopy is necessary to permit detection and analysis of abnormalities of oral and pharyngeal function. The pharynx is examined to detect stasis of barium in the valleculae and

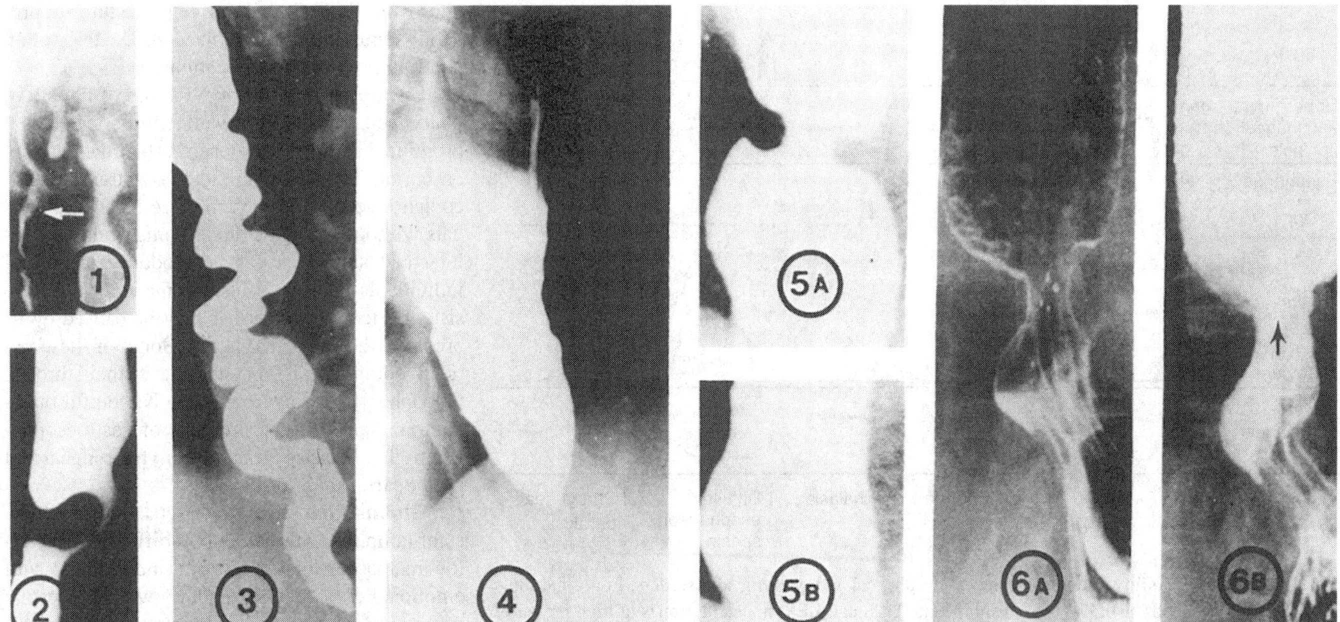

FIGURE 284-1 Radiographic appearance of some motor disorders of the pharynx and esophagus. (1) Pharyngeal paralysis with tracheal aspiration (*arrow*). (2) Cricopharyngeal achalasia. Note the prominent cricopharyngeus, which is recognized by its smoothness and location in the posterior wall. (3) Diffuse esophageal spasm. Note typical corkscrew appearance of the lower part of the esophagus. (4) Achalasia, showing a dilated esophageal body with an air-fluid level and a closed lower esophageal sphincter. (5) Muscular (contractile) lower esophageal ring. The asymmetric contraction visible in (5A) has disappeared in (5B), obtained during the same examination. (6) Scleroderma esophagus showing dilated esophagus with a stricture (6A) and reflux of barium from the stomach into the esophagus (6B). *(Courtesy of Dr. Harvey Goldstein.)*

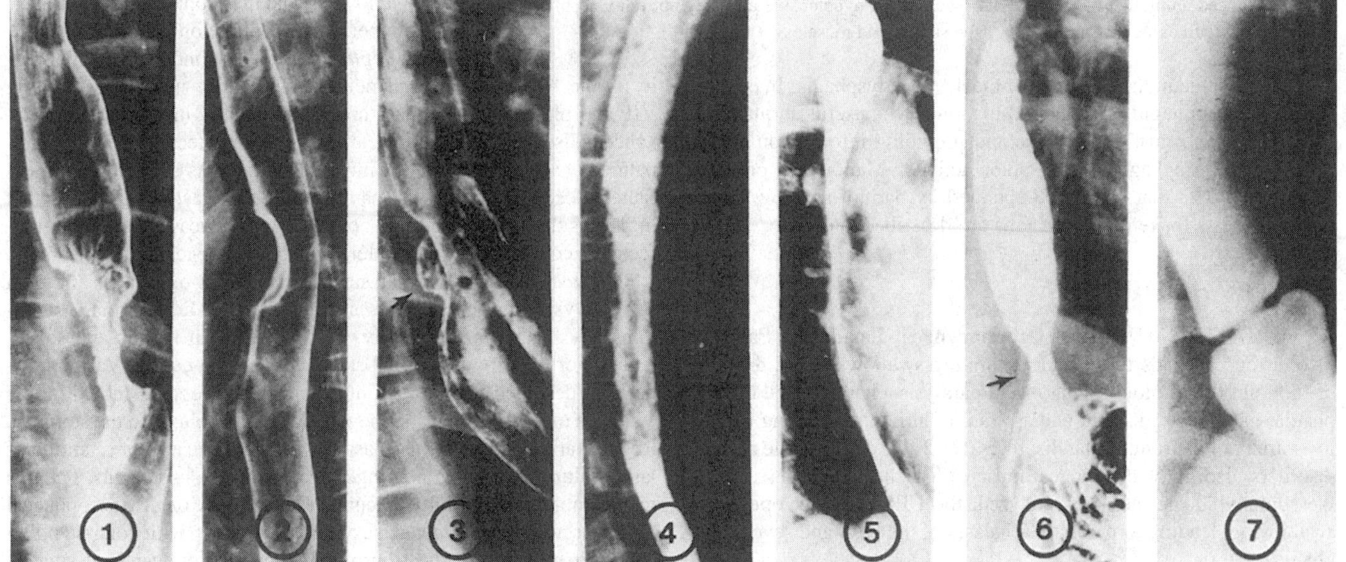

FIGURE 284-2 Selected structural lesions of the esophagus. (1) Carcinoma of the esophagus, with typical annular narrowing with overhanging margins and destruction of the mucosa. (2) Leiomyoma of the esophagus, with a smooth filling defect and right angles of origin from the esophageal wall. (3) Esophageal ulcer in columnar-cell-lined esophagus (Barrett's esophagus). (4) Monilial esophagitis, with irregular plaquelike filling defects. (5) Long stricture secondary to lye ingestion. (6) Peptic stricture, short and tubular, with associated hiatus hernia. (7) Lower esophageal mucosal (Schatzki) ring. A thin, weblike annular constriction at the esophagogastric junction is associated with a small hiatal hernia. *(Courtesy of Dr. Harvey Goldstein.)*

piriform sinuses and regurgitation of barium into the nose and tracheobronchial tree.

ESOPHAGOSCOPY Esophagoscopy is the direct method of establishing the cause of mechanical dysphagia and of identifying mucosal lesions that may not be identified by the usual barium swallow. If the lumen is markedly narrowed, use of a smaller-caliber endoscope may be needed; on occasion a stricture must be dilated before the examination can be completed. Endoscopic biopsies are useful in diagnosing carcinoma, reflux esophagitis, and other mucosal diseases. Cells obtained by a cytology balloon or brushing the mucosa can be evaluated for carcinoma. Endoscopic ultrasonography permits evaluation of intramural masses and staging of esophageal cancer.

ESOPHAGEAL MOTILITY The study of esophageal motility entails simultaneous recording of pressures from different sites in the esophageal lumen with an assembly of pressure sensors positioned 5 cm apart. The UES and LES appear as zones of high pressure that relax on swallowing. The pharynx and esophagus normally show peristaltic waves with each swallow.

Esophageal motility studies are helpful in the diagnosis of esophageal motor disorders (achalasia, spasm, scleroderma) (Fig. 284-3) but

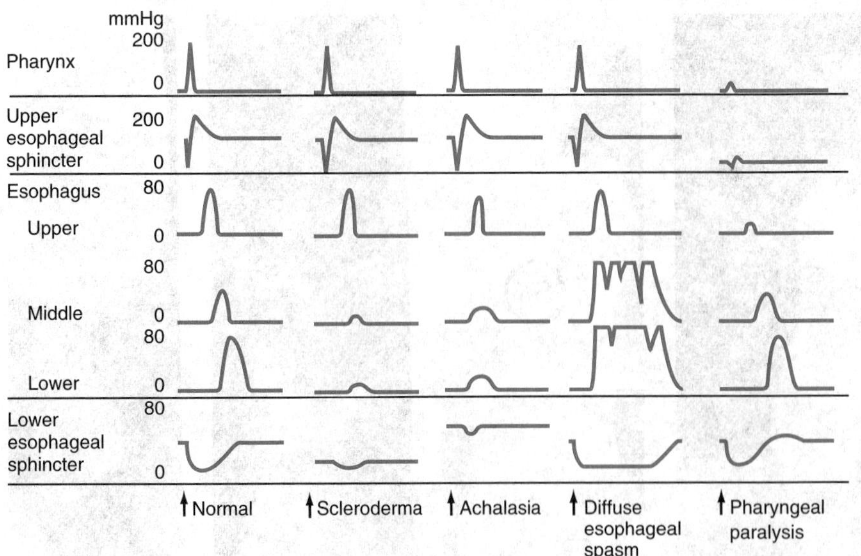

FIGURE 284-3 Motility patterns in selected esophageal and pharyngeal disorders. In normal individuals, the upper and lower esophageal sphincters (UES and LES) appear as zones of high pressure. With a swallow (indicated by ↑), pressure in the sphincters falls and a contraction wave starts in the pharynx and progresses down the esophagus. In scleroderma, the lower part of the esophagus (smooth muscle) shows a reduced amplitude of contractions, which may be peristaltic or simultaneous in onset, and hypotension of the LES. In achalasia, the lower part of the esophagus shows contractions that are reduced in amplitude and simultaneous in onset. In contrast to scleroderma, the LES in achalasia is hypertensive and fails to relax in response to a swallow. In diffuse esophageal spasm, the lower part of the esophagus shows simultaneous-onset, large-amplitude, prolonged, repetitive contractions. In pharyngeal paralysis, the smooth-muscle part of the esophagus is normal. The skeletal muscle part shows a reduced amplitude of contractions. The UES is hypotensive and may not relax normally on swallowing due to associated weakness of the suprahyoid muscles.

are of little value in the diagnosis of mechanical dysphagia. In patients with reflux esophagitis, esophageal manometry is useful in quantitating lower esophageal competence and providing information on the status of the esophageal body motor activity. Manometry provides quantitative data that cannot be obtained by barium swallow or endoscopy. Tests for reflux esophagitis are described later.

MOTOR DISORDERS

STRIATED MUSCLE Oropharyngeal Paralysis Paralysis of oral muscle leads to difficulty initiating swallowing and drooling of food out of the mouth. Pharyngeal paralysis, characterized by dysphagia, nasal regurgitation, and aspiration during swallowing, occurs in a variety of neuromuscular disorders (see Table 40-1). Some of these disorders also involve laryngeal muscles, causing hoarseness. When the suprahyoid muscles are paralyzed, the UES does not open with swallowing, leading to paralytic achalasia of the UES and severe dysphagia.

Videofluoroscopy with barium of various consistencies may reveal difficulties in the oral phase of swallowing. The test may show barium in the valleculae and piriform sinuses, nasal and tracheal aspiration, failure of the upper sphincter to open, and/or abnormal movement of the hyoid bone and the larynx with a swallow (Fig. 284-1). Motility studies demonstrate a reduced amplitude of pharyngeal and upper esophageal contractions and reduced basal upper esophageal sphincter pressure without further relaxation on swallowing (Fig. 284-3). Patients with myasthenia gravis (Chap. 380) and polymyositis (Chap. 382) respond to treatment. Dysphagia resulting from a cerebrovascular accident improves with time, although often not completely. Treatment consists of maneuvers to reduce pharyngeal stasis and enhance airway protection under the direction of a trained swallow therapist. Feeding by a nasogastric tube or an endoscopically placed gastrostomy tube may be necessary for nutritional support; however, these maneuvers do not provide protection against aspiration of salivary secretions. Cricopharyngeal myotomy is sometimes performed, but its usefulness is unproven. Extensive operative procedures to prevent aspiration are rarely needed. Death is often due to pulmonary complications.

Cricopharyngeal Bar Failure of the cricopharyngeus to relax on swallowing appears as a prominent bar on the posterior wall of the pharynx on barium swallow (Fig. 284-1). A transient cricopharyngeal bar is seen in up to 5% of individuals without dysphagia undergoing upper gastrointestinal studies; it can be produced in normal individuals during a Valsalva maneuver. A persistent cricopharyngeal bar may be caused by fibrosis in the cricopharyngeus. Some of these patients complain of food sticking in their throats. Cricopharyngeal myotomy may be helpful but is contraindicated in the presence of gastroesophageal reflux because it may lead to pharyngeal and pulmonary aspiration.

Globus Pharyngeus A sensation of a constant lump in the throat, but no difficulty in swallowing, occurs especially in individuals with emotional disorders, particularly women. Results of barium studies and manometry are normal. Treatment consists primarily of reassurance. Some patients with globus pharyngeus have associated reflux esophagitis, and they may respond to treatment of the esophagitis.

SMOOTH MUSCLE Achalasia Achalasia is a motor disorder of the esophageal smooth muscle in which the LES does not relax normally with swallowing, and the esophageal body undergoes nonperistaltic contractions.

Pathophysiology The underlying abnormality is the loss of intramural neurons. Inhibitory neurons containing VIP and nitric oxide synthase are predominantly involved, but in advanced disease cholinergic neurons are also affected. Primary idiopathic achalasia accounts for most of the patients seen in the United States. Secondary achalasia may be caused by gastric carcinoma that infiltrates the esophagus, lymphoma, Chagas' disease, certain viral infections, eosinophilic gastroenteritis, and neurodegenerative disorders.

Clinical features Achalasia affects patients of all ages and both sexes. Dysphagia, chest pain, and regurgitation are the main symptoms. Dysphagia appears early, occurs with both liquids and solids, and is worsened by emotional stress and hurried eating. Various maneuvers designed to increase intraesophageal pressure, including the Valsalva maneuver, may aid the passage of the bolus into the stomach. Regurgitation and pulmonary aspiration occur because of retention of large volumes of saliva and ingested food in the esophagus. Patients may complain of difficulty belching. The presence of gastroesophageal reflux argues against achalasia; and in patients with long-standing heartburn, cessation of heartburn and appearance of dysphagia suggest development of achalasia on top of reflux esophagitis. The course is usually chronic, with progressive dysphagia and weight loss over months to years. Achalasia associated with carcinoma is characterized by severe weight loss and a rapid downhill course if untreated.

Diagnosis A chest x-ray shows absence of the gastric air bubble and sometimes a tubular mediastinal mass beside the aorta. An air-fluid level in the mediastinum in the upright position represents retained food in the esophagus. Barium swallow shows esophageal dilation, and in advanced cases the esophagus may become sigmoid. On fluoroscopy, normal peristalsis is lost in the lower two-thirds of the esophagus. The terminal part of the esophagus shows a persistent beak-like narrowing representing the nonrelaxing LES (Fig. 284-1).

Manometry shows the basal LES pressure to be normal or elevated, and swallow-induced relaxation either does not occur or is reduced in degree, duration, and consistency. The esophageal body shows an elevated resting pressure. In response to swallows, primary peristaltic waves are replaced by simultaneous-onset contractions (Fig. 284-3).

These contractions may be of poor amplitude (classic achalasia) or of large amplitude and long duration (vigorous achalasia). Cholecystokinin (CCK), which normally causes a fall in the sphincter pressure, paradoxically causes contraction of the LES (the CCK test). This paradoxical response occurs because, in achalasia, the neurally transmitted inhibitory effect of CCK is absent owing to the loss of inhibitory neurons. Endoscopy is helpful in excluding the secondary causes of achalasia, particularly gastric carcinoma.

℞ TREATMENT Treatment with soft foods, sedatives, and anticholinergic drugs is usually unsatisfactory. Nitrates and calcium channel blockers provide short-term benefit, but their use may be limited by side effects. Nitroglycerin, 0.3 to 0.6 mg, is used sublingually before meals and as needed for chest pain. Isosorbide dinitrate, 2.5 to 5 mg sublingually or 10 to 20 mg orally, is used before meals. Nitrates are associated with headache and postural hypotension. The calcium channel blocker nifedipine, 10 to 20 mg orally or sublingually before meals, is also effective. Endoscopic intrasphincteric injection of botulinum toxin is effective over a short period in some patients. Repeated injections may lead to fibrosis, complicating further operative therapy. Botulinum toxin acts by blocking cholinergic excitatory nerves in the sphincter. Balloon dilatation reduces the basal LES pressure by tearing muscle fibers. In experienced hands, this technique is effective in ~85% of patients. Perforation and bleeding are potential complications. Heller's extramucosal myotomy of the LES, in which the circular muscle layer is incised, is equally effective. Laparoscopic myotomy is the procedure of choice. Reflux esophagitis and peptic stricture may follow successful treatment (more often with myotomy than with balloon dilatation).

Diffuse Esophageal Spasm and Related Motor Disorders These disorders present with clinical symptoms of chest pain and dysphagia and are recognized by their manometric features. In pure form, they all show normal relaxation to swallows. Diffuse esophageal spasm is characterized by nonperistaltic contractions, usually of large amplitude and long duration. An esophageal motility pattern showing hypertensive but peristaltic contractions has been called "nutcracker esophagus."

Pathophysiology Nonperistaltic contractions are due to dysfunction of inhibitory nerves. Histopathologic studies show patchy neural degeneration localized to nerve processes, rather than the prominent degeneration of nerve cell bodies seen in achalasia. Diffuse esophageal spasm may progress to achlasia. Hypertensive peristaltic contractions and hypertensive or hypercontracting LES may represent cholinergic or myogenic hyperactivity.

Clinical features Diffuse spasm and related motor disorders cannot be distinguished clinically. They all present with chest pain, dysphagia, or both. Chest pain is particularly marked in patients with esophageal contractions of large amplitude and long duration. Chest pain usually occurs at rest but may be brought on by swallowing or by emotional stress. The pain is retrosternal; it may radiate to the back, the sides of the chest, both arms, or the sides of the jaw and may last from a few seconds to several minutes. It may be acute and severe, mimicking the pain of myocardial ischemia. Dysphagia for solids and liquids may occur with or without chest pain and is correlated particularly with simultaneous-onset contractions.

Diffuse esophageal spasm and related esophageal motor disorders must be differentiated from other causes of chest pain, particularly ischemic heart disease with atypical angina. A complete cardiac workup should be done before a noncardiac etiology is considered seriously. The presence of dysphagia in association with pain should point to the esophagus as the site of disease. Esophageal motility disorders are an uncommon cause of noncardiac chest pain, which is more commonly due to reflux esophagitis or visceral hypersensitivity.

Diagnosis In diffuse esophageal spasm, barium swallow shows that normal sequential peristalsis below the aortic arch is replaced by uncoordinated simultaneous contractions that produce the appearance of curling or multiple ripples in the wall, sacculations, and pseudodiverticula—the "corkscrew" esophagus (Fig. 284-1). Sometimes an esophageal contraction obliterates the lumen, and barium is pushed away in both directions. The barium swallow is frequently normal in diffuse esophageal spasm and mostly normal in the related disorders.

Diffuse esophageal spasm (Fig. 284-3) and related motor disorders (hypertensive peristaltic contraction, hypertensive LES and hypercontracting LES) are manometric diagnoses. Because these abnormalities may be episodic, the results of manometry may be normal at the time of the study. Several techniques are used to provoke esophageal spasm. Cold swallows produce the chest pain but do not produce spasm on manometric studies. Solid boluses and pharmacologic agents, particularly edrophonium, induce both chest pain and motor abnormalities. However, correlation between induction of pain and motility changes is poor. The usefulness of pharmacologic provocative tests is limited.

℞ TREATMENT Anticholinergics are usually of limited value. Agents that relax smooth muscle, such as sublingual nitroglycerin (0.3 to 0.6 mg) or longer-acting agents such as isosorbide dinitrate (10 to 30 mg orally before meals) and nifedipine (10 to 20 mg orally before meals) are helpful. Sublingual forms of these agents can also be used. Reassurance and tranquilizers are helpful in allaying apprehension.

Scleroderma Esophagus The esophageal lesions in systemic sclerosis consist of atrophy of smooth muscle, manifested by weakness in the lower two-thirds of the esophageal body and incompetence of the LES. The esophageal wall is thin and atrophic and may exhibit areas of patchy fibrosis. Patients usually present with dysphagia to solids. Liquids may cause dysphagia when the patient is recumbent. These patients usually also complain of heartburn, regurgitation, and other symptoms of gastroesophageal reflux disease (GERD). Barium swallow shows dilation and loss of peristaltic contractions in the middle and distal portions of the esophagus. The LES is patulous, and gastroesophageal reflux may occur freely (Fig. 284-1). Mucosal changes due to esophageal ulceration and esophageal stricture may be present. Motility studies show a marked reduction in the amplitude of smooth-muscle contractions, which may be peristaltic or nonperistaltic. The resting pressure of the LES is subnormal, but sphincter relaxation is normal (Fig. 284-3). Similar esophageal motor abnormalities are found in other collagen vascular diseases and in Raynaud's syndrome alone. Dietary adjustments with the use of soft foods are helpful in management. GERD and its complications should be treated aggressively.

GASTROESOPHAGEAL REFLUX DISEASE

GERD is one of the most prevalent gastrointestinal disorders. Population-based studies show that up to 15% of individuals have heartburn at least once a week and about 7% have heartburn daily. Symptoms are caused by back flow of gastric acid and other gastric contents into the esophagus due to incompetent barriers at the gastroesophageal junction.

Pathophysiology The normal antireflux mechanisms consist of the LES, the crural diaphragm, and the anatomic location of the gastroesophageal junction below the diaphragmatic hiatus. Reflux occurs only when the gradient of pressure between the LES and the stomach is lost. It can be caused by a sustained or transient decrease in LES tone. A sustained hypotension of the LES may be due to muscle weakness that is often without apparent cause. Secondary causes of LES incompetence include scleroderma-like diseases, myopathy associated with chronic intestinal pseudo-obstruction, pregnancy, smoking, anticholinergic drugs, smooth-muscle relaxants [β-adrenergic agents, aminophylline, nitrates, calcium channel blockers, phosphodiesterase inhibitors that increase cyclic AMP or cyclic GMP (including sildenofil)], surgical destruction of the LES, and esophagitis. tLESR without associated esophageal contraction is due to a vagal reflex in which LES relaxation is elicited by gastric distention. Increased tLESR is associated with GERD. A similar reflex operates during belching. Apart from incompetent barriers, gastric contents are most likely to reflux (1) when gastric volume is increased (after meals, in pyloric obstruction, in gastric stasis, during acid hypersecretion states), (2) when gastric contents are near the gastroesophageal junction (in recumbency, bending down, hiatus hernia), and (3) when gastric pressure is increased (obesity, pregnancy, ascites, tight clothes). Incompetence of the diaphragmatic crural muscle, which surrounds the esophageal hiatus in the diaphragm and functions as an external LES, also predisposes to GERD.

The total exposure of the esophagus to refluxed acid correlates with potential for mucosal damage. Exposure depends on the amount of refluxed material per episode, frequency of episodes, and rate of clearing the esophagus by gravity and peristaltic contractions. When peristaltic contractions are impaired, esophageal clearance is impaired. Acid refluxed into the esophagus is neutralized by saliva. Thus, impaired salivary secretion also increases esophageal exposure time. If the refluxed material extends to the cervical esophagus and breaches the upper sphincter, it can enter the pharynx, larynx, and trachea, causing chronic cough, bronchoconstriction, pharyngitis, laryngitis, or bronchitis.

Reflux esophagitis is a complication of reflux and develops when mucosal defenses are unable to counteract the damage done by acid, pepsin, and bile. *Mild esophagitis* involves microscopic changes of mucosal infiltration with granulocytes or eosinophils, hyperplasia of basal cells, and elongation of dermal pegs. Endoscopic appearance may be normal. *Erosive esophagitis* involves endoscopically apparent mucosal damage, redness, friability, bleeding, superficial, linear ulcers, and exudates. *Peptic stricture* results from fibrosis that causes lumenal constriction. These strictures occur in ~10% of patients with untreated GERD. Short strictures caused by spontaneous reflux are usually 1 to 3 cm long and are present in the distal esophagus near the squamocolumnar junction (Fig. 284-2). Long, tubular peptic strictures can result from persistent vomiting or prolonged nasogastric intubation. Erosive esophagitis may cause bleeding and heal by intestinal metaplasia (*Barrett's esophagus*) that is a risk factor for adenocarcinoma.

Clinical Features Regurgitation of sour material in the mouth and heartburn are the characteristic symptoms of GERD. Heartburn is produced by the contact of refluxed material with the inflamed or sensitized esophageal mucosa. Angina-like or atypical chest pain occurs in some patients, while others experience no heartburn or chest pain. Persistent dysphagia suggests development of a peptic stricture. Most patients with peptic stricture have a history of several years of heartburn preceding dysphagia. However, in one-third of patients, dysphagia is the presenting symptom. Rapidly progressive dysphagia and weight loss may indicate the development of adenocarcinoma in Barrett's esophagus. Bleeding occurs due to mucosal erosions or Barrett's ulcer. Severe reflux may reach the pharynx and mouth and result in laryngitis, morning hoarseness, and pulmonary aspiration. Recurrent pulmonary aspiration can cause aspiration pneumonia, pulmonary fibrosis, or chronic asthma. By contrast, many patients with GERD remain asymptomatic or self-treated and do not seek attention until severe complications occur.

Diagnosis The diagnostic approach to GERD can be divided into three categories:

1. documentation of mucosal injury,
2. documentation and quantitation of reflux, and
3. definition of the pathophysiology.

Reflux esophagitis and its complications are documented by the use of barium swallow, esophagoscopy, and mucosal biopsy. The results of barium swallow are usually normal in uncomplicated esophagitis but may reveal a stricture or ulcer. A high esophageal peptic stricture, a deep ulcer, or adenocarcinoma suggest Barrett's esophagus. Uncomplicated Barrett's esophagus is not diagnosed reliably by barium studies. Esophagoscopy may reveal the presence of erosive esophagitis, distal peptic stricture, or a columnar-cell-lined lower esophagus with or without a proximally located peptic stricture, ulcer, or adenocarcinoma. Results of esophagoscopy may be normal in many patients with esophagitis; in such patients, mucosal biopsies and the Bernstein test are helpful. The mucosal biopsies should be performed at least 5 cm above the LES, because the esophageal mucosal changes of chronic esophagitis are quite frequent in the most distal esophagus in otherwise normal individuals. About 10% of biopsies yield a false-positive or false-negative result. The Bernstein test involves the infusion of solutions of 0.1 *N* HCl and normal saline into the esophagus. It is useful in diagnosing reflux esophagitis that is not endoscopically obvious. In patients with reflux esophagitis, infusion of acid, but not of saline, reproduces the symptoms of heartburn. Infusion of acid in normal individuals usually produces no symptoms. Supraesophageal manifestations are diagnosed by careful otolaryngological exam.

A therapeutic trial with a proton pump inhibitor (such as omeprazole, 40 mg bid) for 1 week provides strong support for the diagnosis of GERD.

Documentation and quantitation of reflux when necessary can be done by ambulatory long-term (24-h) esophageal pH recording. For evaluation of pharyngeal reflux, a system of recording simultaneously from pharyngeal and esophageal sites may be useful. The pH recordings are helpful only in the evaluation of acid reflux. The presence of bile or intestinal alkaline secretions is suggested by the occurrence of reflux symptoms in the absence of gastric acid and demonstration of bile in an aspirate of esophageal reflux fluid. Documentation of reflux is necessary only when the role of reflux in the symptom complex is unclear, particularly in evaluation of supraesophageal symptoms and chest pain without endoscopic evidence of esophagitis.

Definition of pathophysiologic factors in GERD is sometimes indicated for management decisions such as antireflex surgery. Esophageal motility studies may provide useful quantitative information on the competence of the LES and on esophageal motor function.

Rx TREATMENT The goals of treatment are to decrease gastroesophageal reflux, render the refluxate harmless, improve esophageal clearance, and protect the esophageal mucosa. The management of uncomplicated cases generally includes weight reduction, sleeping with the head of the bed elevated by about 4 to 6 in. with blocks, and elimination of factors that increase abdominal pressure. Patients should not smoke and should avoid consuming fatty foods, coffee, chocolate, alcohol, mint, orange juice, and certain medications (such as anticholinergic drugs, calcium channel blockers, and other smooth-muscle relaxants). They should also avoid ingesting large quantities of fluids with meals. In mild cases, life-style changes and over-the-counter antisecretory agents may be adequate. In moderate cases, H_2 receptor blocking agents (cimetidine, 300 mg; ranitidine, 150 mg bid; famotidine, 20 mg bid; nizatidine 150 mg bid) for 6 to 12 weeks are effective in symptom relief. Higher doses are necessary for healing erosive esophagitis, but proton pump inhibitors (PPIs) are more effective in this setting.

In cases resistant to H_2 receptor blockers and severe cases, rigorous acid suppression with a PPI is recommended. The PPIs are comparably effective: omeprazole (40 mg/d), lansoprazole (30 mg/d), pantoprazole (40 mg/d), and rabeprazole (20 mg/d) for 8 weeks can heal erosive esophagitis in up to 90% of patients. Reflux esophagitis requires prolonged therapy, for 3 to 6 months or longer if the disease recurs quickly. After initial therapy, a lower maintenance dose of PPI is used. Side effects are minimal. Aggressive acid suppression causes hypergastrinemia but does not increase the risk for carcinoid tumors or gastrinomas. Vitamin B_{12} absorption is compromised by the treatment. Patients with reflux esophagitis who have complications, such as Barrett's esophagus with concomitant esophagitis, should be treated vigorously. Patients who have an associated peptic stricture are treated with dilators to relieve dysphagia as well as provided with vigorous treatment for reflux.

Antireflux surgery, in which the gastric fundus is wrapped around the esophagus (fundoplication), increases the LES pressure and should be considered for patients with resistant and complicated reflux esophagitis that does not respond fully to medical therapy or for patients for whom long-term medical therapy is not desirable. Laparoscopic fundoplication is the surgery of choice. Ideal candidates for fundoplication are those in whom motility studies show persistently inadequate LES pressure but normal peristaltic contractions in the esophageal body.

Patients with alkaline esophagitis are treated with general antireflux measures and neutralization of bile salts with cholestyramine, aluminum hydroxide, or sucralfate. Sucralfate is particularly useful in these cases, as it also serves as a mucosal protector.

BARRETT'S ESOPHAGUS The metaplasia of esophageal squamous epithelium to columnar epithelium (Barrett's esophagus) is a complication of severe reflux esophagitis, and it is a risk factor for esophageal adenocarcinoma (Chap. 90). Metaplastic columnar epithelium develops during healing of erosive esophagitis with continued acid reflux because columnar epithelium is more resistant to acid-pepsin damage than squamous epithelium. The metaplastic epithelium is a mosaic of different epithelial types including goblet cells and columnar cells that have features of both secretory and absorptive cells (incomplete or type III metaplasia). Barrett's epithelium progresses through a dysplastic stage before developing into adenocarcinoma. The rate of cancer development is 1 in 200 patient years; those with longer than 2 to 3 cm of intestinal metaplasia have a risk of developing esophageal cancer that is 30 to 125 times the risk of the general population.

Given the natural history, reflux esophagitis should be aggressively treated with drugs, and erosive esophagitis should be treated with drugs and surgery, if necessary, to prevent Barrett's esophagus. The prevalence of intestinal metaplasia is estimated at 4 to 10% of patients with significant heartburn. Barrett's esophagus is more common in men, particularly white men, and prevalence increases with age. A one-time esophagoscopy is recommended in patients with persistent GERD symptoms at age 50. Established metaplasia does not regress with treatment; thus, acid suppression and fundoplication are indicated only when active esophagitis is also present.

The need and frequency of surveillance endoscopies in patients with established Barrett's esophagus are debated. The risk of developing esophageal adenocarcinoma is related to the length of involved esophageal mucosa. People with short segments of Barrett's esophagus (distal 2 to 3 cm) account for up to 25% of unselected patients undergoing endoscopy with or without GERD symptoms and appear to be at low risk. They are not routinely surveyed. However, those with long-segment Barrett's esophagus (>3 cm) are advised to have endoscopic surveillance at 1-year intervals for 2 years and then every 2 to 3 years. The frequency is increased if dysplasia is detected independent of the length of the metaplasia. Optical methods of recognizing dysplasia during the endoscopy (laser-induced fluorescence spectroscopy, optical coherence tomography) are being developed. Once high-grade dysplasia is detected, treatment of choice is esophagectomy of the Barrett's segment. Photodynamic laser or thermocoagulative mucosal ablation and endoscopic mucosal resection are being evaluated as alternatives.

Barrett's esophagus can also lead to chronic peptic ulcer of the esophagus with high (midesophageal) and long strictures.

INFLAMMATORY DISORDERS

INFECTIOUS ESOPHAGITIS Infectious esophagitis can be due to viral, bacterial, fungal, or parasitic organisms. In severely immunocompromised patients, multiple organisms may coexist.

Viral Esophagitis *Herpes simplex virus* (HSV) type 1 occasionally causes esophagitis in immunocompetent individuals, but either HSV type 1 or HSV type 2 may afflict patients who are immunosuppressed (Chap. 182). Patients complain of an acute onset of chest pain, odynophagia, and dysphagia. Bleeding may occur in severe cases; and systemic manifestations such as nausea, vomiting, fever, chills, and mild leukocytosis may be present. Herpetic vesicles on the nose and

lips may provide a clue to the diagnosis. Barium swallow is inadequate to detect early lesions and cannot reliably distinguish HSV infection from other types of infections. Endoscopy shows vesicles and small, discrete, punched-out superficial ulcerations with or without a fibrinous exudate. In later stages, a diffuse erosive esophagitis develops from enlargement and coalescence of the ulcers. Mucosal cells from a biopsy sample taken at the edge of an ulcer or from a cytologic smear show ballooning degeneration, ground-glass changes in the nuclei with eosinophilic intranuclear inclusions (Cowdry type A), and giant cell formation on routine stains. Culture for HSV becomes positive within days and is helpful in diagnosis. In patients with severe odynophagia, intravenous acyclovir, 400 mg five times a day, is usually initiated. Symptoms usually resolve in 1 week, but large ulcerations may take longer to heal. Foscarnet (90 mg/kg intravenously every 8 h) is used if resistance to acyclovir occurs.

Varicella-zoster virus (VZV) (Chap. 183) sometimes produces esophagitis in children with chickenpox and adults with herpes zoster. Esophageal VZV also can be the source of disseminated VZV infection without skin involvement. In an immunocompromised host, VZV esophagitis causes vesicles and confluent ulcers and usually resolves spontaneously, but it may cause necrotizing esophagitis in a severely compromised host. On routine histologic examination of mucosal biopsy samples or cytology specimens, VZV is difficult to distinguish from HSV, but the distinction can be made immunohistologically or by culture. Acyclovir reduces the duration of symptoms in VZV esophagitis.

Cytomegalovirus (CMV) infections (Chap. 185) occur only in immunocompromised patients. CMV is usually activated from a latent stage or may be acquired from blood product transfusions. CMV lesions initially appear as serpiginous ulcers in an otherwise normal mucosa. These may coalesce to form giant ulcers, particularly in the distal esophagus.

Patients present with odynophagia, chest pain, hematemesis, nausea, and vomiting. Diagnosis requires endoscopy and biopsies of the ulcer. Mucosal brushings are not useful. Routine histologic examination shows intranuclear and small intracytoplasmic inclusions in large fibroblasts and endothelial cells. Immunohistology with monoclonal antibodies to CMV and in situ hybridization of CMV DNA on centrifugation culture and are useful for early diagnosis. Ganciclovir, 5 mg/kg every 12 h intravenously, is the treatment of choice. Foscarnet (90 mg/kg every 12 h intravenously) is used in resistant cases. Therapy is continued until healing occurs, which may take 2 to 4 weeks.

HIV (Chap. 309) may be associated with a self-limited syndrome of acute esophageal ulceration associated with oral ulcers and a maculopapular skin rash, which occurs at the time of HIV seroconversion. Some patients with advanced disease have deep, persistent esophageal ulcers requiring treatment with oral glucocorticoids or thalidomide. Some ulcers respond to local steroid injection.

Bacterial Esophagitis *Bacterial esophagitis* is unusual, but esophagitis caused by *Lactobacillus* and β-hemolytic streptococci can occur in the immunocompromised host. In patients with profound granulocytopenia and patients with cancer, bacterial esophagitis is often missed because it is commonly present with other organisms, including viruses and fungi. In patients with AIDS, infection with *Cryptosporidium* or *Pneumocystis carinii* may cause nonspecific inflammation, and *Mycobacterium tuberculosis* infection may cause deep ulcerations of the distal esophagus.

***Candida* Esophagitis** *Candida* species are normal commensals in the throat but become pathogenic and produce esophagitis in immunodeficiency states. *Candida* esophagitis can occur without any predisposing factors. Patients may be asymptomatic or complain of odynophagia and dysphagia. Oral thrush or other evidence of mucocutaneous candidiasis may be absent. Rarely, *Candida* esophagitis is complicated by esophageal bleeding, perforation, and stricture or by systemic invasion. Barium swallow may be normal or show multiple nodular filling defects of various sizes (Fig. 284-2). Large nodular defects may resemble grape clusters. Endoscopy shows small, yellow-white raised plaques with surrounding erythema in mild disease. Confluent linear and nodular plaques reflect extensive disease. Diagnosis is made by demonstration of yeast or hyphal forms in plaque smears and exudate stained with periodic acid–Schiff or Gomori silver stains. Histologic examination is often negative. Culture is not useful in diagnosis but may define the species and the drug sensitivities of the yeast (Chap. 205). Fluconazole (200 mg on the first day, followed by 100 mg daily) is the preferred treatment of esophageal candidiasis because it is effective and its absorption is not affected by high gastric pH. Fluconazole is available in oral and intravenous formulations. Ketoconazole (200 to 400 mg in a single daily oral dose) is also effective treatment, and the higher dose is used in severely immunocompromised hosts; however, its bioavailability is severely reduced at increased gastric pH. Patients who respond poorly are treated with amphotericin, 10 to 15 mg as an intravenous infusion for 6 h daily to a total dose of 300 to 500 mg. Nystatin oral suspension (100,000 units per ml) in doses of 10 to 20 mL every 6 h is effective for oral thrush. In resistant cases, amphotericin lozenges are used for 7 to 10 days followed by nystatin or fluconazole for as long as the host resistance remains low.

OTHER TYPES OF ESOPHAGITIS *Radiation esophagitis* is a common occurrence during radiation treatment for thoracic cancers. The frequency and severity of esophagitis increase with the amount of radiation delivered and may be enhanced by radiosensitizing drugs like doxorubicin, bleomycin, cyclophosphamide, and cisplatin. Dysphagia and odynophagia may last several weeks to several months after therapy. The esophageal mucosa becomes erythematous, edematous, and friable. Superficial erosions coalesce to form larger superficial ulcers. Submucosal fibrosis and degenerative changes in the blood vessels, muscles, and myenteric neurons may occur. The treatment is relief of pain with viscous lidocaine during the acute phase; indomethacin treatment may reduce radiation damage. Esophageal stricture may develop.

Corrosive esophagitis is caused by the ingestion of caustic agents, such as strong alkali or acid. Severe corrosive injury may lead to esophageal perforation, bleeding, and death. Glucocorticoids are not useful in acute corrosive esophagitis. Healing is usually associated with stricture formation. Caustic strictures are usually long and rigid (Fig. 284-2) and generally require dilatation with dilators passed over a guidewire through the stricture. *Pill-induced esophagitis* is associated with the ingestion of certain types of pills and occurs most often in bedridden patients. Antibiotics such as doxycycline, tetracycline, oxytetracycline, minocycline, penicillin, and clindamycin account for more than half the cases. Nonsteroidal anti-inflammatory agents such as aspirin, indomethacin, and ibuprofen may cause injury. Other commonly prescribed pills that cause esophageal injury include potassium chloride, ferrous sulfate or succinate, quinidine, alprenolol, theophylline, ascorbic acid, pinaverum bromide, alendronate, and pamidronate. Pill esophagitis can be prevented by avoiding the offending agents or by having patients take pills in the upright position and wash them down with copious amounts of fluids.

Sclerotherapy for bleeding esophageal varices usually produces transient retrosternal chest pain and dysphagia; esophageal ulcer, stricture, hematoma, or perforation may occur. Variceal banding causes similar complications but less frequently. *Esophagitis associated with mucocutaneous and systemic diseases* is usually associated with blister and bulla formation, epithelial desquamation, and thin, weblike, or dense esophageal strictures. Pemphigus vulgaris and bullous pemphigoid form intraepithelial and subepithelial bullae, respectively, and can be distinguished by specific immunohistology; both are characterized by sloughing of epithelium or the presence of esophageal casts. Glucocorticoid treatment is usually effective. Cicatricial pemphigoid, Stevens-Johnson syndrome, and toxic epidermolysis bullosa can produce esophageal bullous lesions and strictures requiring gentle dilatation. Graft-versus-host disease occurs in patients who have received allogeneic bone marrow transplants and is associated with generalized desquamation and esophageal strictures. Behçet's disease and eosinophilic gastroenteritis may involve the esophagus and may respond to glucocorticoid therapy. An erosive lichen planus also can involve the esophagus. Crohn's disease may cause inflammatory strictures, sinus tracts, filiform polyps, and fistulas in the esophagus.

OTHER ESOPHAGEAL DISORDERS

DIVERTICULA Diverticula are outpouchings of the wall of the esophagus. A *Zenker's diverticulum* appears in the natural zone of weakness in the posterior hypopharyngeal wall (Killian's triangle) and causes halitosis and regurgitation of saliva and food particles consumed several days previously. When it becomes large and filled with food, such a diverticulum can compress the esophagus and cause dysphagia or complete obstruction. Nasogastric intubation and endoscopy should be performed with utmost care in these patients, since they may cause perforation of the diverticulum. A *midesophageal diverticulum* may be caused by traction from old adhesions or by propulsion associated with esophageal motor abnormalities. An *epiphrenic diverticulum* may be associated with achalasia. Small or medium-sized diverticula and midesophageal and epiphrenic diverticula are usually asymptomatic. *Diffuse intramural diverticulosis* of the esophagus is due to dilation of the deep esophageal glands and may lead to chronic candidiasis or to the development of a stricture high up in the esophagus. These patients may present with dysphagia. Symptomatic Zenker's diverticula are treated by cricopharyngeal myotomy with or without diverticulectomy. Very large symptomatic esophageal diverticula are removed surgically. When they are associated with motor abnormalities, distal myotomy is performed. Strictures associated with diffuse intramural diverticulosis are treated with rubber dilators.

WEBS AND RINGS Weblike constrictions of the esophagus are usually congenital or inflammatory in origin. Asymptomatic hypopharyngeal webs are demonstrated in <10% of normal individuals. When concentric, they cause intermittent dysphagia to solids. The combination of symptomatic hypopharyngeal webs and iron-deficiency anemia in middle-aged women constitutes *Plummer-Vinson syndrome*. The clinical importance of this syndrome is uncertain. Midesophageal webs are rare. A *lower esophageal mucosal ring* (Schatzki ring) is a thin, weblike constriction located at the squamocolumnar mucosal junction at or near the border of the LES (Fig. 284-2). It invariably produces dysphagia when the lumen diameter is <1.3 cm. Dysphagia to solids is the only symptom, and it is usually episodic. Asymptomatic rings may be present in ~10% of normal individuals. A lower esophageal ring is one of the common causes of dysphagia. Symptomatic webs and mucosal lower esophageal rings are easily treated by dilatation. A *lower esophageal muscular ring* (contractile ring) is located proximal to the site of mucosal rings and may represent an abnormal uppermost segment of the LES. These rings can be recognized by the fact that they are not constant in size and shape. They also may cause dysphagia and should be differentiated from peptic strictures, achalasia, and lower esophageal mucosal ring. Muscular rings do not respond well to dilatation.

HIATAL HERNIA A *hiatal hernia* is a herniation of part of the stomach into the thoracic cavity through the esophageal hiatus in the diaphragm. A *sliding hiatal hernia* is one in which the gastroesophageal junction and fundus of the stomach slide upward. A sliding hernia may result from weakening of the anchors of the gastroesophageal junction to the diaphragm, from longitudinal contraction of the esophagus, or from increased intraabdominal pressure. Small sliding hernias can be demonstrated commonly during barium studies if intraabdominal pressure is increased. Incidence increases with age; in individuals in the sixth decade of life, the prevalence of such hernias is ~60%. Small sliding hiatal hernias alone probably produce no symptoms but can contribute to reflux esophagitis. A *paraesophageal hernia* is one in which the esophagogastric junction remains fixed in its normal location and a pouch of stomach is herniated beside the gastroesophageal junction through the esophageal hiatus. A paraesophageal or mixed paraesophageal and sliding hernia may become incarcerated and strangulate, leading to acute chest pain, dysphagia, and a mediastinal mass and requiring surgery. A herniated gastric pouch may cause dysphagia, develop gastritis, or ulcerate, causing chronic blood loss. Large paraesophageal hernias should be surgically repaired.

MECHANICAL TRAUMA *Esophageal rupture* may be caused by (1) iatrogenic damage from instrumentation of the esophagus or external trauma, (2) increased intraesophageal pressure associated with forceful vomiting or retching (*spontaneous rupture* or *Boerhaave's syndrome*), or (3) diseases of the esophagus such as corrosive esophagitis, esophageal ulcer, and neoplasm. The site of perforation depends on the cause. Instrumental perforation usually occurs in the pharynx or lower esophagus, just above the diaphragm in the posterolateral wall. Esophageal perforation causes severe retrosternal chest pain, which may be worsened by swallowing and breathing. Free air enters the mediastinum and spreads to neighboring structures, causing palpable subcutaneous emphysema in the neck, mediastinal crackling sounds on auscultation, and pneumothorax. With time, secondary infection supervenes, and mediastinal abscess may develop. Esophageal perforation associated with vomiting usually deposits gastric contents in the mediastinum and causes severe mediastinal complications. By contrast, instrumental perforation may be clinically mild and free of severe complications. Spontaneous rupture of the esophagus may mimic myocardial infarction, pancreatitis, or rupture of an abdominal viscus. Symptoms of chest pain may be mild, particularly in the elderly. Mediastinal emphysema may develop late. An x-ray of the chest shows abnormalities in most patients, but computed tomography of the chest is more sensitive in detecting mediastinal air. Fluid from pleural effusions may have a high content of (salivary) amylase. The diagnosis is confirmed by swallow of radiopaque contrast material. Gastrograffin is used initially, and if no leak is found, a small amount of thin barium is used to confirm the diagnosis. Treatment includes esophageal and gastric suction and parenteral broad-spectrum antibiotics. Surgical drainage and repair of the laceration should be performed as soon as possible. In patients with terminal carcinoma, surgical repair may not be feasible, and patients with minor instrumental perforation can be treated conservatively. Extensive corrosive damage may require esophageal diversion and excision of the damaged portion.

Mucosal Tear (Mallory-Weiss Syndrome) This tear is usually caused by vomiting, retching, or vigorous coughing. The tear usually involves the gastric mucosa near the squamocolumnar mucosal junction. Patients present with upper gastrointestinal bleeding, which may be severe. In most patients bleeding ceases spontaneously; continued bleeding may respond to vasopressin therapy or angiographic embolization. Surgery is rarely needed.

Intramural Hematoma Emetogenic injury, particularly in patients with bleeding abnormalities, can cause bleeding between the mucosal and muscle layers of the esophagus. The patients develop sudden dysphagia. The diagnosis is made by barium swallow and computed tomography. Resolution is usually spontaneous.

FOREIGN BODIES Foreign bodies may lodge in the cervical esophagus just beyond the UES, near the aortic arch, or above the LES. Impaction of a bolus of food, particularly a piece of meat or bread, may occur when the esophageal lumen is narrowed due to stricture, carcinoma, or a lower esophageal ring. Acute impaction causes a complete inability to swallow and severe chest pain. Both foreign bodies and food boluses may be removed endoscopically. Use of a meat tenderizer to facilitate passage of a meat bolus is discouraged because of potential esophageal perforation and aspiration pneumonia.

BIBLIOGRAPHY

COOK IJ, KHARILAS PJ: AGA technical review on management of oropharyngeal dysphagia. Gastroenterology 116:455, 1999

GOYAL RK, HAMILTON FA: Columna lined (Barrett's) esophagus: Highlights of the NIDDK/VHA conference. Clinician 17 (6):1, 1999

GOYAL RK, SIVARAO DV: Functional anatomy and physiology of swallowing and esophageal motility, in *The Esophagus*, DO Castell, JE Richter (eds). Philadelphia, Lippincott, Williams and Wilkins, 1999, pp 1–31

HEUDERBERT GR et al: Choice of long-term strategy for the management of patients with severe esophagitis: A cost-utility analysis. Gastroenterology 112:1078, 1997

KIRKENDALL JW: Pill-induced esophageal injury, in *The Esophagus*, DO Castell, JE Richter (eds). Philadelphia, Lippincott, Williams and Wilkins, 1999, pp 527–37

SAMPLINER RE: The Practice Parameters Committee of the American College of Gastroenterology: Practice guidelines on the diagnosis, surveillance, and therapy of Barrett's esophagus. Am J Gastroenterol 93:1028, 1998

SHAKER R (guest ed): First multidisciplinary international symposium on supraesophageal complications of reflux disease. Am J Med 103:1S, 1997

SPECHLER SJ: AGA technical review on treatment of patients with dysphagia caused by benign disorders of the distal esophagus. Gastroenterology 117:233, 1999

285 *John Del Valle*

PEPTIC ULCER DISEASE AND RELATED DISORDERS

PEPTIC ULCER DISEASE

Burning epigastric pain exacerbated by fasting and improved with meals is a symptom complex associated with peptic ulcer disease (PUD). An *ulcer* is defined as disruption of the mucosal integrity of the stomach and/or duodenum leading to a local defect or excavation due to active inflammation. Ulcers occur within the stomach and/or duodenum and are often chronic in nature. Acid peptic disorders are very common in the United States, with 4 million individuals (new cases and recurrences) affected per year. Lifetime prevalence of PUD in the United States is approximately 12% in men and 10% in women. Moreover, an estimated 15,000 deaths per year occur as a consequence of complicated PUD. The financial impact of these common disorders has been substantial, with an estimated burden on health care costs of >$15 billion per year in the United States.

GASTRIC PHYSIOLOGY Despite the constant attack on the gastroduodenal mucosa by a host of noxious agents (acid, pepsin, bile acids, pancreatic enzymes, drugs, and bacteria), integrity is maintained by an intricate system that provides mucosal defense and repair.

Gastric Anatomy The gastric epithelial lining consists of rugae that contain microscopic gastric pits, each branching into four or five gastric glands made up of highly specialized epithelial cells. The makeup of gastric glands varies with their anatomic location. Glands within the gastric cardia comprise <5% of the gastric gland area and contain mucous and endocrine cells. The majority of gastric glands (75%) are found within the oxyntic mucosa and contain mucous neck, parietal, chief, endocrine, and enterochromaffin cells (Fig. 285-1). Pyloric glands contain mucous and endocrine cells (including gastrin cells) and are found in the antrum.

The parietal cell, also known as the oxyntic cell, is usually found in the neck, or isthmus, or the oxyntic gland. The resting, or unstimulated, parietal cell has prominent cytoplasmic tubulovesicles and intracellular canaliculi containing short microvilli along its apical surface (Fig. 285-2). H^+, K^+-ATPase is expressed in the tubulovesicle membrane; upon cell stimulation, this membrane, along with apical membranes, transforms into a dense network of apical intracellular canaliculi containing long microvilli. Acid secretion, a process requiring high energy, occurs at the apical canalicular surface. Numerous mitochondria (30 to 40% of total cell volume) generate the energy required for secretion.

Gastroduodenal Mucosal Defense The gastric epithelium is under a constant assault by a series of endogenous noxious factors including HCl, pepsinogen/pepsin, and bile salts. In addition, a steady flow of exogenous substances such as medications, alcohol, and bacteria encounter the gastric mucosa. A highly intricate biologic system is in place to provide defense from mucosal injury and to repair any injury that may occur.

The mucosal defense system can be envisioned as a three-level

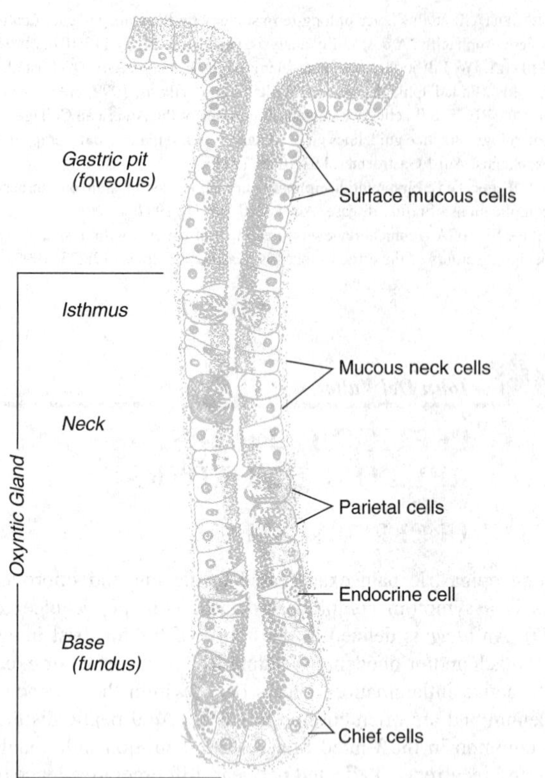

FIGURE 285-1 Diagramatic representation of the oxyntic gastric gland. *(Adapted from S Ito, RJ Winchester: Cell Biol 16:541, 1963.)*

barrier, composed of preepithelial, epithelial, and subepithelial elements (Fig. 285-3). The first line of defense is a mucus-bicarbonate layer, which serves as a physicochemical barrier to multiple molecules including hydrogen ions. Mucus is secreted in a regulated fashion by gastroduodenal surface epithelial cells. It consists primarily of water (95%) and a mixture of lipids and glycoproteins. Mucin is the constituent glycoprotein that, in combination with phospholipids (also secreted by gastric mucous cells), forms a hydrophobic surface with fatty acids that extend into the lumen from the cell membrane. The mucous gel functions as a nonstirred water layer impeding diffusion of ions and molecules such as pepsin. Bicarbonate, secreted by surface epithelial cells of the gastroduodenal mucosa into the mucous gel, forms a pH gradient ranging from 1 to 2 at the gastric luminal surface and reaching 6 to 7 along the epithelial cell surface. Bicarbonate secretion

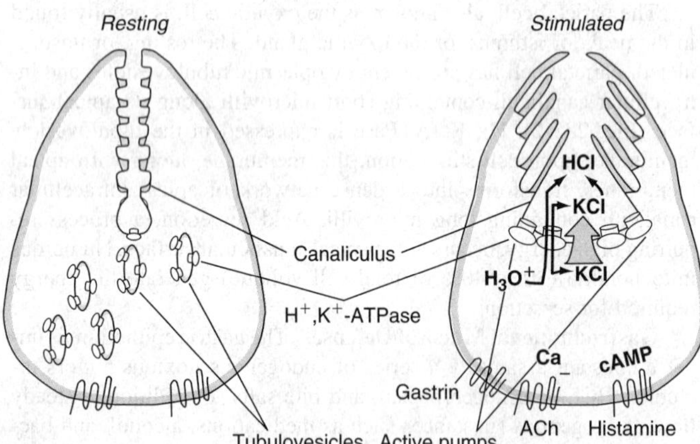

FIGURE 285-2 Gastric parietal cell undergoing transformation after secretagogue-mediated stimulation. *(Adapted from SJ Hersey, G Sachs: Physiol Rev 75:155, 1995.)*

is stimulated by calcium, prostaglandins, cholinergic input, and luminal acidification.

Surface epithelial cells provide the next line of defense through several factors, including mucus production, epithelial cell ionic transporters that maintain intracellular pH and bicarbonate production, and intracellular tight junctions. If the preepithelial barrier were breached, gastric epithelial cells bordering a site of injury can migrate to restore a damaged region (*restitution*). This process occurs independent of cell division and requires uninterrupted blood flow and an alkaline pH in the surrounding environment. Several growth factors including epidermal growth factor (EGF), transforming growth factor (TGF) α, and basic fibroblast growth factor (FGF) modulate the process of restitution. Larger defects that are not effectively repaired by restitution require cell proliferation. Epithelial cell regeneration is regulated by prostaglandins and growth factors such as EGF and TGF-α. In tandem with epithelial cell renewal, formation of new vessels (*angiogenesis*) within the injured microvascular bed occurs. Both FGF and vascular endothelial growth factor (VEGF) are important in regulating angiogenesis in the gastric mucosa.

An elaborate microvascular system within the gastric submucosal layer is the key component of the subepithelial defense/repair system. A rich submucosal circulatory bed provides HCO_3^-, which neutralizes the acid generated by parietal cell secretion of HCl. Moreover, this microcirculatory bed provides an adequate supply of micronutrients and oxygen while removing toxic metabolic by-products.

Prostaglandins play a central role in gastric epithelial defense/repair (Fig. 285-4). The gastric mucosa contains abundant levels of prostaglandins. These metabolites of arachidonic acid regulate the release of mucosal bicarbonate and mucus, inhibit parietal cell secretion, and are important in maintaining mucosal blood flow and epithelial cell restitution. Prostaglandins are derived from esterified arachidonic acid, which is formed from phospholipids (cell membrane) by the action of phospholipase A_2. A key enzyme that controls the rate-limiting step in prostaglandin synthesis is cyclooxygenase (COX), which is present in two isoforms (COX-1, COX-2), each having distinct characteristics regarding structure, tissue distribution, and expression. COX-1 is expressed in a host of tissues including the stomach, platelets, kidneys, and endothelial cells. This isoform is expressed in a constitutive manner and plays an important role in maintaining the integrity of renal function, platelet aggregation, and gastrointestinal mucosal integrity. In contrast, the expression of COX-2 is inducible by inflammatory stimuli, and it is expressed in macrophages, leukocytes, fibroblasts, and synovial cells. The beneficial effects of nonsteroidal anti-inflammatory drugs (NSAIDs) on tissue inflammation are due to inhibition of COX-2; the toxicity of these drugs (e.g., gastrointestinal mucosal ulceration and renal dysfunction) is related to inhibition of the COX-1 isoform. The highly COX-2-selective NSAIDs have the potential to provide the beneficial effect of decreasing tissue inflammation while minimizing toxicity in the gastrointestinal tract (see below).

Physiology of Gastric Secretion Hydrochloric acid and pepsinogen are the two principal gastric secretory products capable of inducing mucosal injury. Acid secretion should be viewed as occurring under basal and stimulated conditions. Basal acid production occurs in a circadian pattern, with highest levels occurring during the night and lowest levels during the morning hours. Cholinergic input via the vagus nerve and histaminergic input from local gastric sources (see below) are the principal contributors to basal acid secretion. Stimulated gastric acid secretion occurs primarily in three phases based on the site where the signal originates (cephalic, gastric, and intestinal). Sight, smell, and taste of food are the components of the cephalic phase, which stimulates gastric secretion via the vagus nerve. The gastric phase is activated once food enters the stomach. This component of secretion is driven by nutrients (amino acids and amines) that directly stimulate the G cell to release gastrin, which in turn activates the parietal cell via direct and indirect mechanisms (see below). Distention of the stomach wall also leads to gastrin release and acid production. The last phase of gastric acid secretion is initiated as food enters the intestine and is mediated by luminal distention and nutrient assimilation. A series of pathways that inhibit gastric acid production are also set into motion during these phases. The gastrointestinal hormone somatostatin is released from endocrine cells found in the gastric mucosa (D cells) in response to HCl. Somatostatin can inhibit acid production by both direct (parietal cell) and indirect mechanisms [decreased histamine release from enterochromaffin-like (ECL) cells and gastrin release from G cells]. Additional neural (central and peripheral) and hormonal (secretin, cholecystokinin) factors play a role in counterbalancing acid secretion. Under physiologic circumstances, these phases are occurring simultaneously.

The acid-secreting parietal cell is located in the oxyntic gland, adjacent to other cellular elements (ECL cell, D cell) important in the gastric secretory process (Fig. 285-5). This unique cell also secretes intrinsic factor. The parietal cell expresses receptors for several stimulants of acid secretion including histamine (H_2), gastrin (cholecystokinin B/gastrin receptor) and acetylcholine (muscarinic, M_3). Each of these are G protein–linked, seven transmembrane–spanning receptors. Binding of histamine to the H_2 receptor leads to activation of adenylate cyclase and an increase in cyclic AMP. Activation of the gastrin and muscarinic receptors results in activation of the protein kinase C/phosphoinositide signaling pathway. Each of these signaling pathways in turn regulates a series of downstream kinase cascades, which control the acid-secreting pump, H^+, K^+-ATPase. The discovery that different ligands and their corresponding receptors lead to activation of different signaling pathways explains the potentiation of acid secretion that occurs when histamine and gastrin or acetylcholine are combined. More importantly, this observation explains why blocking one receptor type (H_2) decreases acid secretion stimulated by agents that activate a different pathway (gastrin, acetylcholine). Parietal cells also express receptors for ligands that inhibit acid production (prostaglandins, somatostatin, and EGF).

The enzyme H^+, K^+-ATPase is responsible for generating the large concentration of H^+. It is a membrane-bound protein that consists of two subunits, α and β. The active catalytic site is found within the α subunit; the function of the β subunit is unclear. This enzyme uses the chemical energy of ATP to transfer H^+ ions from parietal cell cytoplasm to the secretory canaliculi in exchange for K^+. The H^+,K^+-ATPase is located within the secretory canaliculus and in nonsecretory cytoplasmic tubulovesicles. The tubulovesicles are impermeable to K^+, which leads to an inactive pump in this location. The distribution of pumps between the nonsecretory vesicles and the secretory canaliculus varies according to parietal cell activity (Fig. 285-2). Under resting conditions, only 5% of pumps are within the secretory canaliculus, whereas upon parietal cell stimulation, tubulovesicles are immediately transferred to the secretory canalicular membrane, where 60 to 70% of the pumps are activated. Proton pumps are recycled back to the inactive state in cytoplasmic vesicles once parietal cell activation ceases.

The chief cell, found primarily in the gastric fundus, synthesizes and secretes pepsinogen, the inactive precursor of the proteolytic enzyme pepsin. The acid environment within the stomach leads to cleavage of the inactive precursor to pepsin and provides the low pH (<2.0) required for pepsin activity. Pepsin activity is significantly diminished at a pH of 4 and irreversibly inactivated and denatured at a pH of ≥7. Many of the secretagogues that stimulate acid secretion also stimulate pepsinogen release. The precise role of pepsin in the pathogenesis of PUD remains to be established.

PATHOPHYSIOLOGIC BASIS OF PEPTIC ULCER DISEASE PUD encompasses both gastric and duodenal ulcers. Ulcers are defined as a break in the mucosal surface >5 mm in size, with depth to the submucosa. Duodenal (DU) and gastric ulcers (GU) share many common features in terms of pathogenesis, diagnosis, and treatment, but several factors distinguish them from one another.

Epidemiology • ***Duodenal ulcers*** DUs are estimated to occur in 6 to 15% of the western population. The incidence of DUs declined steadily from 1960 to 1980 and has remained stable since then. The death rates, need for surgery, and physician visits have decreased by >50% over the past 30 years. The reason for the reduction in the frequency of DUs is likely related to the decreasing frequency of *Helicobacter pylori*. Before the discovery of *H. pylori*, the natural history of DUs was typified by frequent recurrences after initial therapy. Eradication of *H. pylori* has greatly reduced these recurrence rates.

Gastric ulcers GUs tend to occur later in life than duodenal lesions, with a peak incidence reported in the sixth decade. More than half of GUs occur in males and are less common than DUs, perhaps due to the higher likelihood of GUs being silent and presenting only after a complication develops. Autopsy studies suggest a similar incidence of DUs and GUs.

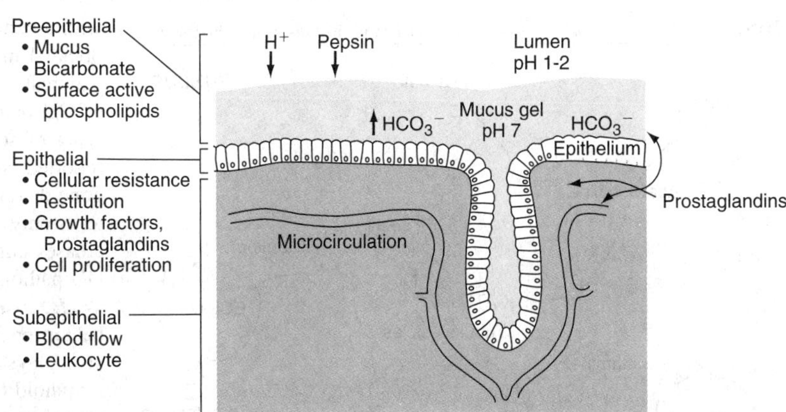

FIGURE 285-3 Components involved in providing gastroduodenal mucosal defense and repair.

Pathology • ***Duodenal ulcers*** DUs occur most often in the first portion of duodenum (>95%), with ~90% located within 3 cm of the pylorus. They are usually ≤1 cm in diameter but can occasionally reach 3 to 6 cm (giant ulcer). Ulcers are sharply demarcated, with depth at times reaching the muscularis propria. The base of the ulcer often consists of a zone of eosinophilic necrosis with surrounding fibrosis. Malignant duodenal ulcers are extremely rare.

Gastric ulcers In contrast to DUs, GUs can represent a malignancy. Benign GUs are most often found distal to the junction between the antrum and the acid secretory mucosa. This junction is variable, but in general the antral mucosa extends about two thirds of the distance of the lesser curvature and one third the way up the greater curvature. Benign GUs are quite rare in the gastric fundus and are histologically similar to DUs. Benign GUs associated with *H. pylori* are associated with antral gastritis. In contrast, NSAID-related GUs

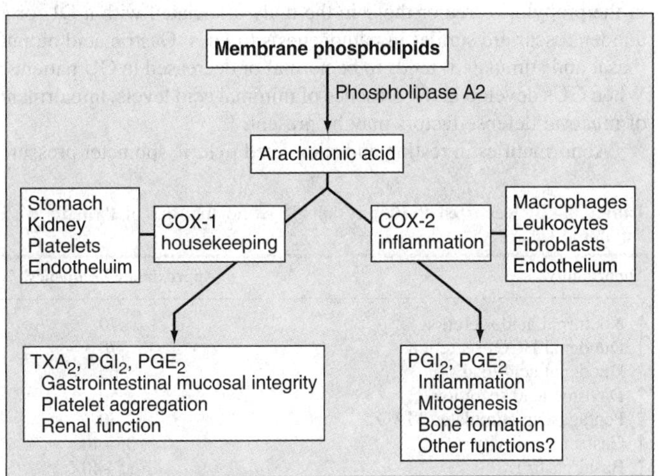

FIGURE 285-4 Schematic representation of the steps involved in synthesis of prostaglandin E_2 (PGE_2) and prostacyclin (PGI_2). Characteristics and distribution of the cyclooxgenase (COX) enzymes 1 and 2 are also shown. TXA_2, thromboxane A_2.

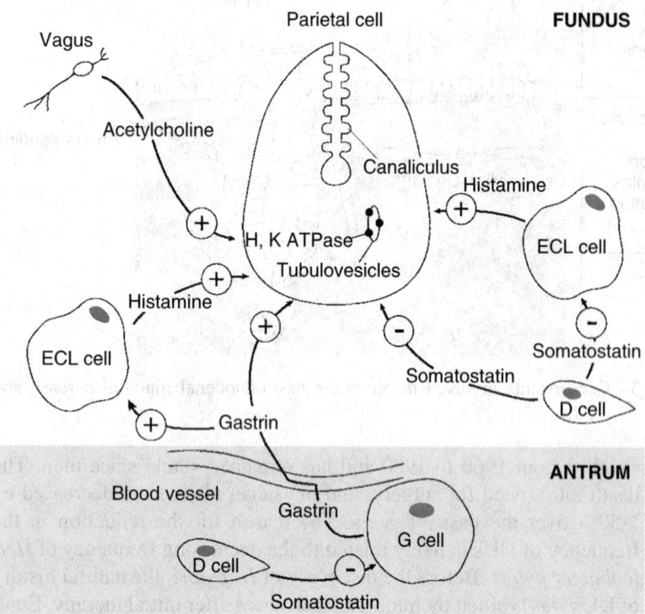

FIGURE 285-5 Regulation of gastric acid secretion at the cellular level. ECL cell, enterochromaffin-like cell.

are not accompanied by chronic active gastritis but may instead have evidence of a chemical gastropathy.

Pathophysiology It is now clear that *H. pylori* and NSAID-induced injury account for the majority of DUs. Gastric acid contributes to mucosal injury but does not play a primary role.

Duodenal ulcers Many acid secretory abnormalities have been described in DU patients (Table 285-1). Of these, average basal and nocturnal gastric acid secretion appear to be increased in DU patients as compared to control; however, the level of overlap between DU patients and control subjects is substantial. The reason for this altered secretory process is unclear, but *H. pylori* infection may contribute to this finding. Accelerated gastric emptying of liquids has been noted in some DU patients but is not consistently observed; its role in DU formation, if any, is unclear. Bicarbonate secretion is significantly decreased in the duodenal bulb of patients with an active DU as compared to control subjects. *H. pylori* infection may also play a role in this process.

Gastric ulcer As in DUs, the majority of GUs can be attributed to either *H. pylori* or NSAID-induced mucosal damage. GUs that occur in the prepyloric area or those in the body associated with a DU or a duodenal scar are similar in pathogenesis to DUs. Gastric acid output (basal and stimulated) tends to be normal or decreased in GU patients. When GUs develop in the presence of minimal acid levels, impairment of mucosal defense factors may be present.

Abnormalities in resting and stimulated pyloric sphincter pressure with a concomitant increase in duodenal gastric reflux have been implicated in some GU patients. Although bile acids, lysolecithin, and pancreatic enzymes may injure gastric mucosa, a definite role for these in GU pathogenesis has not been established. Delayed gastric emptying of solids has been described in GU patients but has not been reported consistently. The observation that patients who have undergone disruption of the normal pyloric barrier (pyloroplasty, gastroenterostomy) often have superficial gastritis without frank ulceration decreases enthusiasm for duodenal gastric reflux as an explanation for GU pathogenesis.

Table 285-1 Reported Pathophysiologic Abnormalities in Patients with Duodenal Ulcers

Abnormality	Approximate Frequency, %
↑ Nocturnal acid secretion	70
↓ Duodenal HCO_3 secretion	70
↑ Duodenal acid load	65
↑ Daytime acid secretion	50
↑ Pentagastrin-stimulated MAO	40
↑ Gastrin sensitivity	35–40
↑ Basal gastrin	35–40
↑ Gastric emptying	30
↓ pH inhibition of gastrin release	25
↑ Postprandial gastrin release	25

NOTE: MAO, maximal acid output.

H. pylori and acid peptic disorders Gastric infection with the bacterium *H. pylori* accounts for the majority of PUD. This organism also plays a role in the development of gastric mucosal-associated lymphoid tissue (MALT) lymphoma and gastric adenocarcinoma. Although the entire genome of *H. pylori* has been sequenced, it is still not clear how this organism, which is in the stomach, causes ulceration in the duodenum, or whether its eradication will lead to a decrease in gastric cancer.

THE BACTERIUM The bacterium, initially named *Campylobacter pyloridis*, is a gram-negative microaerophilic rod found most commonly in the deeper portions of the mucous gel coating the gastric mucosa or between the mucous layer and the gastric epithelium. It may attach to gastric epithelium but under normal circumstances does not appear to invade cells. It is strategically designed to live within the aggressive environment of the stomach. It is S-shaped (~0.5 × 3 μm in size) and contains multiple sheathed flagella. Initially, *H. pylori* resides in the antrum but, over time, migrates towards the more proximal segments of the stomach. The organism is capable of transforming into a coccoid form, which represents a dormant state that may facilitate survival in adverse conditions. The bacterium expresses a host of factors that contribute to its ability to colonize the gastric mucosa and produce mucosal injury. Several of the key bacterial factors include urease (converting urea to NH_3 and water, thus alkalinizing the surrounding acidic environment), catalase, lipase, adhesins, platelet-activating factor, cytotoxin-associated gene protein (Cag A), pic B (induces cytokines), and vacuolating cytotoxin (Vac A). Multiple strains of *H. pylori* exist and are characterized by their ability to express several of these factors (Cag A, Vac A, etc.). It is possible that the different diseases related to *H. pylori* infection can be attributed to different strains of the organism with distinct pathogenic features.

EPIDEMIOLOGY The prevalence of *H. pylori* varies throughout the world and depends to a great extent on the overall standard of living in the region. In developing parts of the world, 80% of the population may be infected by the age of 20. In contrast, in the United States, this organism is rare in childhood. The overall prevalence of *H. pylori* in the United States is ~30%, with individuals born before 1950 having a higher rate of infection than those born later. About 10% of Americans <30 are colonized with the bacteria. This rate of colonization increases with age, with about 50% of individuals age 50 being infected. Factors that predispose to higher colonization rates include poor socioeconomic status and less education. These factors, not race, are responsible for the rate of *H. pylori* infection in blacks and Hispanic Americans being double the rate seen in whites of comparable age. A summary of risk factors for *H. pylori* infection is shown in Table 285-2.

Transmission of *H. pylori* occurs from person to person, following an oral-oral or fecal-oral route. The risk of *H. pylori* infection is declining in developing countries. The rate of infection in the United States has fallen by >50% when compared to 30 years ago.

Table 285-2 Risk Factors for *H. pylori* Infection

Birth or residence in a developing country
Low socioeconomic status
Domestic crowding
Unsanitary living conditions
Unclean food or water
Exposure to gastric contents of infected individual

Pathophysiology *H. pylori* infection is virtually always associated with a chronic active gastritis, but only 10 to 15% of infected individuals develop frank peptic ulceration. The basis for this difference is unknown. Initial studies suggested that >90% of all DUs were associated with *H. pylori*, but *H. pylori* is present in only 30 to 60% of individuals with DU and 70% of patients with GU. The pathophysiology of ulcers not associated with *H. pylori* or NSAID ingestion [or the rare Zollinger-Ellison syndrome (ZES)] is unclear.

The particular end result of *H. pylori* infection (gastritis, PUD, gastric MALT lymphoma, gastric cancer) is determined by a complex interplay between bacterial and host factors (Fig. 285-6).

1. *Bacterial factors*: *H. pylori* is able to facilitate gastric residence, induce mucosal injury, and avoid host defense. Different strains of *H. pylori* produce different virulence factors. A specific region of the bacterial genome, the pathogenicity island, encodes the virulence factors Cag A and pic B. Vac A also contributes to pathogenicity, though it is not encoded within the pathogenicity island. These virulence factors, in conjunction with additional bacterial constituents, can cause mucosal damage. Urease, which allows the bacteria to reside in the acidic stomach, generates NH_3, which can damage epithelial cells. The bacteria produce surface factors that are chemotactic for neutrophils and monocytes, which in turn contribute to epithelial cell injury (see below). *H. pylori* makes proteases and phospholipases that break down the glycoprotein lipid complex of the mucous gel, thus reducing the efficacy of this first line of mucosal defense. *H. pylori* expresses adhesins, which facilitate attachment of the bacteria to gastric epithelial cells. Although lipopolysaccharide (LPS) of gram-negative bacteria often plays an important role in the infection, *H. pylori* LPS has low immunologic activity compared to that of other organisms. It may promote a smoldering chronic inflammation.

2. *Host factors*: The host responds to *H. pylori* infection by mounting an inflammatory response, which contributes to gastric epithelial cell damage without providing immunity against infection. The neutrophil response is strong both in acute and chronic infection. In addition, T lymphocytes and plasma cells are components of the chronic inflammatory infiltrate, supporting the involvement of antigen-specific cellular and humoral responses. A number of cytokines are released from both epithelial and immune modulatory cells in response to *H. pylori* infection including the proinflammatory cytokines tumor necrosis factor (TNF)α, interleukin (IL)1α/β, IL-6, interferon (IFN)γ, and granulocyte-macrophage colony stimulating factor. Several chemokines such as IL-8 and growth-regulated oncogene (GRO) α, involved in neutrophil recruitment/activation, and RANTES, which recruits mononuclear cells, have been observed in *H. pylori*-infected mucosa.

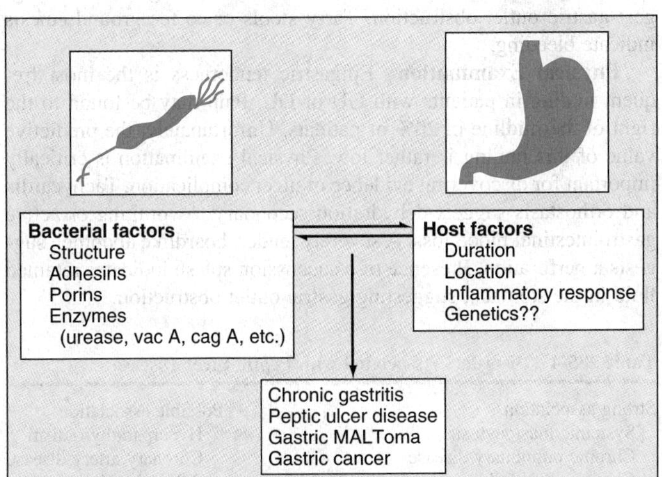

FIGURE 285-6 Outline of the bacterial and host factors important in determining *H. pylori*–induced gastrointestinal disease. MALT, mucosal-associated lymphoid tissue.

The reason for *H. pylori*-mediated duodenal ulceration remains unclear. One potential explanation is that gastric metaplasia in the duodenum of DU patients permits *H. pylori* to bind to it and produce local injury secondary to the host response. Another hypothesis is that *H. pylori* antral infection could lead to increased acid production, increased duodenal acid, and mucosal injury. Basal and stimulated [meal, gastrin-releasing peptide (GRP)] gastrin release are increased in *H. pylori*–infected individuals, and somatostatin-secreting D cells may be decreased. *H. pylori* infection might induce increased acid secretion through both direct and indirect actions of *H. pylori* and proinflammatory cytokines (IL-8, TNF, and IL-1) on G, D, and parietal cells (Fig. 285-7). *H. pylori* infection has also been associated with decreased duodenal mucosal bicarbonate production. Data supporting and contradicting each of these interesting theories have been demonstrated. Thus, the mechanism by which *H pylori* infection of the stomach leads to duodenal ulceration remains to be established.

NSAIDs-induced disease • *Epidemiology* NSAIDs represent one of the most commonly used medications in the United States. More than 30 billion over-the-counter tablets and 70 million prescriptions are sold yearly in the United States alone. The spectrum of NSAID-induced morbidity ranges from nausea and dyspepsia (prevalence reported as high as 50 to 60%) to a serious gastrointestinal complication such as frank peptic ulceration complicated by bleeding or perforation in as many as 3 to 4% of users per year. About 20,000 patients die each year from serious gastrointestinal complications from NSAIDs. Unfortunately, dyspeptic symptoms do not correlate with NSAID-induced pathology. Over 80% of patients with serious NSAID-related complications did not have preceding dyspepsia. In view of the lack of warning signs, it is important to identify patients who are at increased risk for morbidity and mortality related to NSAID usage. A summary of established and possible risk factors is presented in Table 285-3.

Pathophysiology Prostaglandins play a critical role in maintaining gastroduodenal mucosal integrity and repair. It therefore follows that interruption of prostaglandin synthesis can impair mucosal defense and repair, thus facilitating mucosal injury via a systemic mechanism. A summary of the pathogenetic pathways by which systemically administered NSAIDs may lead to mucosal injury is shown in Fig. 285-8.

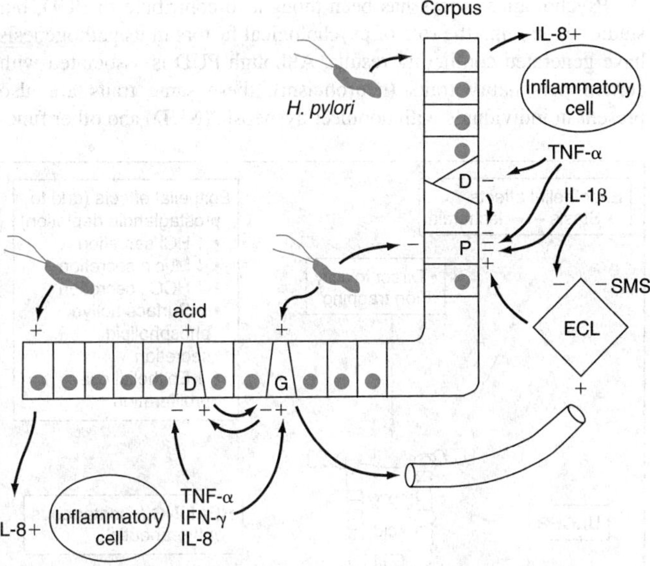

FIGURE 285-7 Summary of potential mechanisms by which *H. pylori* may lead to gastric secretory abnormalities. D, somatostatin cell; ECL, enterochromaffin-like; G, G cell; IFN, interferon; IL, interleukin; P, parietal cell; SMS, somatostatin; TNF, tumor necrosis factor. *(Adapted from J Calam et al: Gastroenterology 113:543, 1997.)*

Table 285-3 Risk Factors for NSAID-Induced Gastroduodenal Ulceration

Established	Possible
Advanced age	Concomitant infection with *H. pylori*
History of ulcer	Cigarette smoking
Concomitant use of glucocorticoids	Alcohol consumption
High-dose NSAIDs	
Multiple NSAIDs	
Concomitant use of anticoagulants	
Serious or multisystem disease	

Injury to the mucosa also occurs as a result of the topical encounter with NSAIDs. Aspirin and many NSAIDs are weak acids that remain in a nonionized lipophilic form when found within the acid environment of the stomach. Under these conditions, NSAIDs migrate across lipid membranes of epithelial cells, leading to cell injury once trapped intracellularly in an ionized form. Topical NSAIDs can also alter the surface mucous layer, permitting back diffusion of H^+ and pepsin, leading to further epithelial cell damage.

Miscellaneous pathogenetic factors in acid peptic disease Cigarette smoking has been implicated in the pathogenesis of PUD. Not only have smokers been found to have ulcers more frequently than do nonsmokers, but smoking appears to decrease healing rates, impair response to therapy, and increase ulcer-related complications such as perforation. The mechanism responsible for increased ulcer diathesis in smokers is unknown. Theories have included altered gastric emptying, decreased proximal duodenal bicarbonate production, and cigarette-induced generation of noxious mucosal free radicals. Acid secretion is *not* abnormal in smokers. Despite these interesting theories, a unifying mechanism for cigarette-induced peptic ulcer diathesis has not been established.

Genetic predisposition has also been considered to play a role in ulcer development. First-degree relatives of DU patients are three times as likely to develop an ulcer; however, the potential role of *H. pylori* infection in contacts is a major consideration. Increased frequency of blood group O and of the nonsecretor status have also been implicated as genetic risk factors for peptic diathesis. However, *H. pylori* preferentially binds to group O antigens. Therefore, the role of genetic predisposition in common PUD has not been established.

Psychological stress has been thought to contribute to PUD, but studies examining the role of psychological factors in its pathogenesis have generated conflicting results. Although PUD is associated with certain personality traits (neuroticism), these same traits are also present in individuals with nonulcer dyspepsia (NUD) and other functional and organic disorders. Although more work in this area is needed, no typical PUD personality has been found.

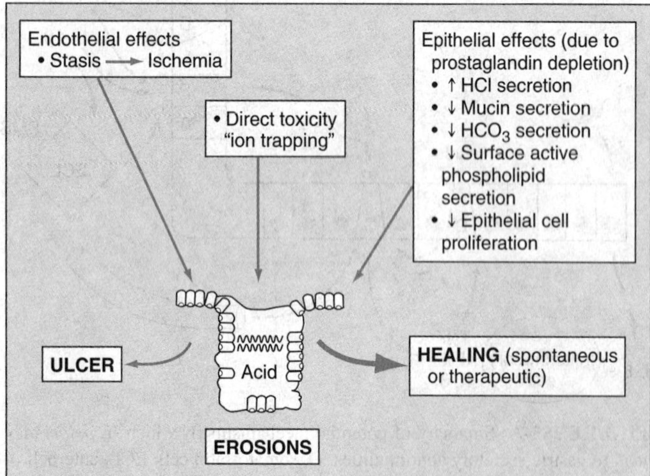

FIGURE 285-8 Mechanisms by which NSAIDs may induce mucosal injury. *(Adapted from J Scheiman et al: J Clin Outcomes Management 3:23, 1996.)*

Diet has also been thought to play a role in peptic diseases. Certain foods can cause dyspepsia, but no convincing studies indicate an association between ulcer formation and a specific diet. This is also true for beverages containing alcohol and caffeine. Specific chronic disorders have been associated with PUD (Table 285-4).

Multiple factors play a role in the pathogenesis of PUD. The two predominant causes are *H. pylori* infection and NSAID ingestion. PUD not related to *H. pylori* or NSAIDs may be increasing. Independent of the inciting or injurious agent, peptic ulcers develop as a result of an imbalance between mucosal protection/repair and aggressive factors. Gastric acid plays an essential role in mucosal injury.

CLINICAL FEATURES **History** Abdominal pain is common to many gastrointestinal disorders, including DU and GU, but has a poor predictive value for the presence of either DU or GU. Up to 10% of patients with NSAID-induced mucosal disease can present with a complication (bleeding, perforation, and obstruction) without antecedent symptoms. Despite this poor correlation, a careful history and physical examination are essential components of the approach to a patient suspected of having peptic ulcers.

Epigastric pain described as a burning or gnawing discomfort can be present in both DU and GU. The discomfort is also described as an ill-defined, aching sensation or as hunger pain. The typical pain pattern in DU occurs 90 min to 3 h after a meal and is frequently relieved by antacids or food. Pain that awakes the patient from sleep (between midnight and 3 A.M.) is the most discriminating symptom, with two-thirds of DU patients describing this complaint. Unfortunately, this symptom is also present in one-third of patients with NUD. The pain pattern in GU patients may be different from that in DU patients, where discomfort may actually be precipitated by food. Nausea and weight loss occur more commonly in GU patients. In the United States, endoscopy detects ulcers in <30% of patients who have dyspepsia. Despite this, 40% of these individuals with typical ulcer symptoms had an ulcer crater, and 40% had gastroduodenitis on endoscopic examination.

The mechanism for development of abdominal pain in ulcer patients is unknown. Several possible explanations include acid-induced activation of chemical receptors in the duodenum, enhanced duodenal sensitivity to bile acids and pepsin, or altered gastroduodenal motility.

Variation in the intensity or distribution of the abdominal pain, as well as the onset of associated symptoms such as nausea and/or vomiting, may be indicative of an ulcer complication. Dyspepsia that becomes constant, is no longer relieved by food or antacids, or radiates to the back may indicate a penetrating ulcer (pancreas). Sudden onset of severe, generalized abdominal pain may indicate perforation. Pain worsening with meals, nausea, and vomiting of undigested food suggest gastric outlet obstruction. Tarry stools or coffee ground emesis indicate bleeding.

Physical Examination Epigastric tenderness is the most frequent finding in patients with GU or DU. Pain may be found to the right of the midline in 20% of patients. Unfortunately, the predictive value of this finding is rather low. Physical examination is critically important for discovering evidence of ulcer complication. Tachycardia and orthostasis suggest dehydration secondary to vomiting or active gastrointestinal blood loss. A severely tender, boardlike abdomen suggests a perforation. Presence of a succussion splash indicates retained fluid in the stomach, suggesting gastric outlet obstruction.

Table 285-4 Disorders Associated with Peptic Ulcer Disease

Strong association	Possible association
Systemic mastocytosis	Hyperparathyroidism
Chronic pulmonary disease	Coronary artery disease
Chronic renal failure	Polycythemia vera
Cirrhosis	Chronic pancreatitis
Nephrolithiasis	
α Antitrypsin deficiency	

PUD-Related Complications • ***Gastrointestinal bleeding*** Gastrointestinal bleeding is the most common complication observed in PUD. It occurs in ~15% of patients and more often in individuals >60 years old. The higher incidence in the elderly is likely due to the increased use of NSAIDs in this group. As many as 20% of patients with ulcer-related hemorrhage bleed without any preceding warning signs or symptoms.

Perforation The second most common ulcer-related complication is perforation, being reported in as many as 6 to 7% of PUD patients. As in the case of bleeding, the incidence of perforation in the elderly appears to be increasing secondary to increased use of NSAIDs. Penetration is a form of perforation in which the ulcer bed tunnels into an adjacent organ. DUs tend to penetrate posteriorly into the pancreas, leading to pancreatitis, whereas GUs tend to penetrate into the left hepatic lobe. Gastrocolic fistulas associated with GUs have also been described.

Gastric outlet obstruction Gastric outlet obstruction is the least common ulcer-related complication, occurring in 1 to 2% of patients. A patient may have relative obstruction secondary to ulcer-related inflammation and edema in the peripyloric region. This process often resolves with ulcer healing. A fixed, mechanical obstruction secondary to scar formation in the peripyloric areas is also possible. The latter requires endoscopic (balloon dilation) or surgical intervention. Signs and symptoms relative to mechanical obstruction may develop insidiously. New onset of early satiety, nausea, vomiting, increase of postprandial abdominal pain, and weight loss should make gastric outlet obstruction a possible diagnosis.

Differential Diagnosis The list of gastrointestinal and nongastrointestinal disorders that can mimic ulceration of the stomach or duodenum is quite extensive. The most commonly encountered diagnosis among patients seen for upper abdominal discomfort is NUD. NUD, also known as *functional dyspepsia* or *essential dyspepsia*, refers to a group of heterogeneous disorders typified by upper abdominal pain without the presence of an ulcer. Dyspepsia has been reported to occur in up to 30% of the U.S. population. Up to 60% of patients seeking medical care for dyspepsia have a negative diagnostic evaluation. The etiology of NUD is not established, and the potential role of *H. pylori* in NUD remains controversial.

Several additional disease processes that may present with "ulcer-like" symptoms include proximal gastrointestinal tumors, gastroesophageal reflux, vascular disease, pancreaticobiliary disease (biliary colic, chronic pancreatitis), and gastroduodenal Crohn's disease.

Diagnostic Evaluation In view of the poor predictive value of abdominal pain for the presence of a gastroduodenal ulcer and the multiple disease processes that can mimic this disease, the clinician is often confronted with having to establish the presence of an ulcer. Documentation of an ulcer requires either a radiographic (barium study) or an endoscopic procedure.

Barium studies of the proximal gastrointestinal tract are still commonly used as a first test for documenting an ulcer. The sensitivity of older single-contrast barium meals for detecting a DU is as high as 80%, with a double-contrast study providing detection rates as high as 90%. Sensitivity for detection is decreased in small ulcers (<0.5 cm), presence of previous scarring, or in postoperative patients. A DU appears as a well-demarcated crater, most often seen in the bulb. A GU may represent benign or malignant disease. Typically, a benign GU also appears as a discrete crater with radiating mucosal folds originating from the ulcer margin. Ulcers >3 cm in size or those associated with a mass are more often malignant. Unfortunately, up to 8% of GUs that appear to be benign by radiographic appearance are malignant by endoscopy or surgery. Radiographic studies that show a GU must be followed by endoscopy and biopsy.

Endoscopy provides the most sensitive and specific approach for examining the upper gastrointestinal tract. In addition to permitting direct visualization of the mucosa, endoscopy facilitates photographic documentation of a mucosal defect and tissue biopsy to rule out malignancy (GU) or *H. pylori*. Endoscopic examination is particularly helpful in identifying lesions too small to detect by radiographic examination, for evaluation of atypical radiographic abnormalities, or to determine if an ulcer is a source of blood loss.

Although the methods for diagnosing *H. pylori* are outlined in Chap. 154, a brief summary will be included here (Table 285-5). PyloriTek, a biopsy urease test, has a sensitivity and specificity of >90 to 95%. In the interest of making a diagnosis of *H. pylori* without the need for performing endoscopy, several noninvasive methods for detecting this organism have been developed. Three types of studies routinely used include serologic testing, the ^{13}C- or ^{14}C-urea breath test, and the fecal *H. pylori* antigen test.

Occasionally, specialized testing such as serum gastrin and gastric acid analysis or sham feeding may be needed in individuals with complicated or refractory PUD (see "Zollinger-Ellison Syndrome," below). Screening for aspirin or NSAIDS (blood or urine) may also be necessary in refractory, *H. pylori*–negative PUD patients.

℞ **TREATMENT** Before the discovery of *H. pylori*, the therapy of PUD disease was centered on the old dictum by Schwartz of "no acid, no ulcer." Although acid secretion is still important in the pathogenesis of PUD, eradication of *H. pylori* and therapy/prevention of NSAID-induced disease is the mainstay. A summary of commonly used drugs for treatment of acid peptic disorders is shown in Table 285-6.

Acid Neutralizing/Inhibitory Drugs • ***Antacids*** Before we understood the important role of histamine in stimulating parietal cell activity, neutralization of secreted acid with antacids constituted the main form of therapy for peptic ulcers. They are now rarely, if ever, used as the primary therapeutic agent but instead are often used by patients for symptomatic relief of dyspepsia. The most commonly used agents are mixtures of aluminum hydroxide and magnesium hydroxide. Aluminum hydroxide can produce constipation and phosphate depletion; magnesium hydroxide may cause loose stools. Many of the commonly used antacids (e.g., Maalox, Mylanta) have a combination of both aluminum and magnesium hydroxide in order to avoid these side effects. The magnesium-containing preparation should not be used in chronic renal failure patients because of possible hypermagnesemia, and aluminum may cause chronic neurotoxicity in these patients.

Calcium carbonate and sodium bicarbonate are potent antacids with varying levels of potential problems. The long-term use of calcium carbonate (converts to calcium chloride in the stomach) can lead to milk-alkali syndrome (hypercalcemia, hyperphosphatemia with possible renal calcinosis and progression to renal insufficiency). Sodium bicarbonate may induce systemic alkalosis.

Table 285-5 Tests for Detection of *H. pylori*

Test	Sensitivity/Specificity, %	Comments
INVASIVE (ENDOSCOPY/BIOPSY REQUIRED)		
Rapid urease	80–95/95–100	Simple; false negative with recent use of PPIs, antibiotics, or bismuth compounds
Histology	80–90/>95	Requires pathology processing and staining; provides histologic information
Culture	—/—	Time-consuming, expensive, dependent on experience; allows determination of antibiotic susceptibility
NON-INVASIVE		
Serology	>80/>90	Inexpensive, convenient; not useful for early follow-up
Urea breath test	>90/>90	Simple, rapid; useful for early follow-up; false negative with recent therapy (see rapid urease test)

NOTE: PPI, proton pump inhibitor.

Table 285-6 Drugs Used in the Treatment of Peptic Ulcer Disease

Drug Type/Mechanism	Examples	Dose
Acid-suppressing drugs		
Antacids	Mylanta, Maalox, Tums, Gaviscon	100–140 meq/L 1 and 3 h after meals and hs
H_2 receptor antagonists	Cimetidine	800 mg hs
	Ranitidine	300 mg hs
	Famotidine	40 mg hs
	Nizatidine	300 mg hs
Proton pump inhibitors	Omeprazole	20 mg/d
	Lansoprazole	30 mg/d
	Rabeprazole	20 mg/d
	Pantoprazole	40 mg/d
Mucosal protective agents		
Sucralfate	Sucralfate	1 g qid
Prostaglandin analogue	Misoprostol	200 μg qid
Bismuth-containing compounds	Bismuth subsalicylate (BSS)	See anti-*H. Pylori* regimens (Table 285-7)

H_2 receptor antagonists Four of these agents are presently available (cimetidine, ranitidine, famotidine, and nizatidine), and their structures share homology with histamine (Fig. 285-9). Although each has different potency, all will significantly inhibit basal and stimulated acid secretion to comparable levels when used at therapeutic doses. Moreover, similar ulcer-healing rates are achieved with each drug when used at the correct dosage. Presently, this class of drug is often used for treatment of active ulcers (4 to 6 weeks) in combination with antibiotics directed at eradicating *H. pylori* (see below).

Cimetidine was the first H_2 receptor antagonist used for the treatment of acid peptic disorders. The initial recommended dosing profile for cimetidine was 300 mg four times per day. Subsequent studies have documented the efficacy of using 800 mg at bedtime for treatment of active ulcer, with healing rates approaching 80% at 4 weeks. Cimetidine may have weak antiandrogenic side effects resulting in reversible gynecomastia and impotence, primarily in patients receiving high doses for prolonged periods of time (months to years, as in ZES).

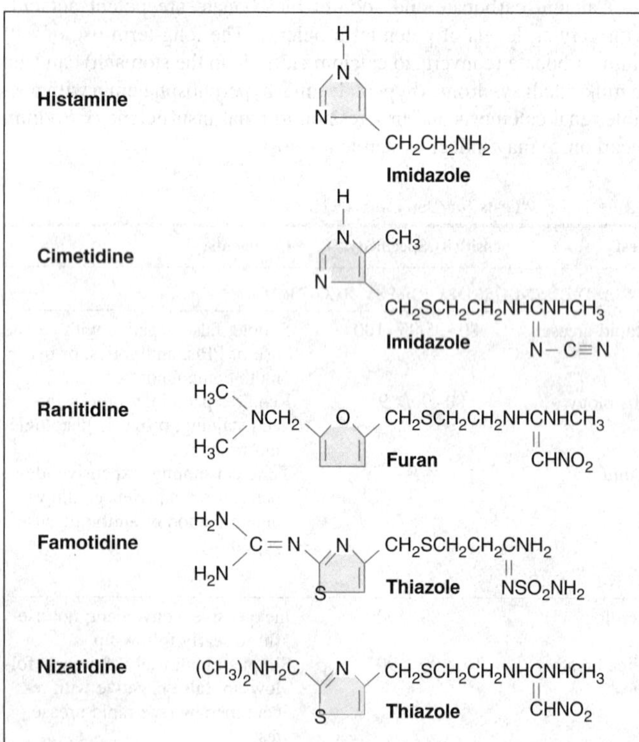

FIGURE 285-9 Structure of H_2 receptor antagonists.

In view of cimetidine's ability to inhibit cytochrome P450, careful monitoring of drugs such as warfarin, phenytoin, and theophylline is indicated with long-term usage. Other rare reversible adverse effects reported with cimetidine include confusion and elevated levels of serum aminotransferases, creatinine, and serum prolactin. Ranitidine, famotidine, and nizatidine are more potent H_2 receptor antagonists than cimetidine. Each can be used once a day at bedtime. Comparable nighttime dosing regimens are ranitidine, 300 mg, famotidine, 40 mg, and nizatidine, 300 mg.

Additional rare, reversible systemic toxicities reported with H_2 receptor antagonists include pancytopenia, neutropenia, anemia, and thrombocytopenia, with a prevalence rate varying from 0.01 to 0.2%. Cimetidine and rantidine (to a lesser extent) can bind to hepatic cytochrome P450, whereas the newer agents, famotidine and nizatidine, do not.

Proton pump (H^+,K^+-ATPase) inhibitors Omeprazole, lansoprazole, and the newest additions, rabeprazole and pantoprazole, are substituted benzimidazole derivatives that covalently bind and irreversibly inhibit H^+,K^+-ATPase. These are the most potent acid inhibitory agents available. Omeprazole and lansoprazole are the proton pump inhibitors (PPIs) that have been used for the longest time. Both are acid labile and are administered as enteric-coated granules in a sustained-release capsule that dissolves within the small intestine at a pH of 6. These agents are lipophilic compounds; upon entering the parietal cell, they are protonated and trapped within the acid environment of the tubulovesicular and canalicular system. These agents potently inhibit all phases of gastric acid secretion. Onset of action is rapid, with a maximum acid inhibitory effect between 2 and 6 h after administration and duration of inhibition lasting up to 72 to 96 h. With repeated daily dosing, progressive acid inhibitory effects are observed, with basal and secretagogue-stimulated acid production being inhibited by >95% after 1 week of therapy. The half-life of PPIs is approximately 18 h, thus it can take between 2 and 5 days for gastric acid secretion to return to normal levels once these drugs have been discontinued. Because the pumps need to be activated for these agents to be effective, their efficacy is maximized if they are administered before a meal (e.g., in the morning before breakfast). Standard dosing for omeprazole and lansoprazole is 20 mg and 30 mg once per day, respectively. Mild to moderate hypergastrinemia has been observed in patients taking these drugs. Carcinoid tumors developed in some animals given the drugs preclinically; however, extensive experience has failed to demonstrate gastric carcinoid tumor development in humans. Serum gastrin levels return to normal levels within 1 to 2 weeks after drug cessation. As with any agent that leads to significant hypochlorhydria, PPIs may interfere with absorption of drugs such as ketoconazole, ampicillin, iron, and digoxin. Hepatic cytochrome P450 can be inhibited by these agents, but the overall clinical significance of this observation is not definitely established. Caution should be taken when using warfarin, diazepam, and phenytoin concomitantly with PPIs.

Cytoprotective Agents • ***Sucralfate*** Sucralfate is a complex sucrose salt in which the hydroxyl groups have been substituted by aluminum hydroxide and sulfate. This compound is insoluble in water and becomes a viscous paste within the stomach and duodenum, binding primarily to sites of active ulceration. Sucralfate may act by several mechanisms. In the gastric environment, aluminum hydroxide dissociates, leaving the polar sulfate anion, which can bind to positively charged tissue proteins found within the ulcer bed, and providing a physicochemical barrier impeding further tissue injury by acid and pepsin. Sucralfate may also induce a trophic effect by binding growth factors such as EGF, enhance prostaglandin synthesis, stimulate mucous and bicarbonate secretion, and enhance mucosal defense and repair. Toxicity from this drug is rare, with constipation being the most common one reported (2 to 3%). It should be avoided in patients with chronic renal insufficiency to prevent aluminum-induced neurotoxicity. Hypophosphatemia and gastric bezoar formation have also been rarely reported. Standard dosing of sucralfate is 1 g four times per day.

Bismuth-containing preparations Sir William Osler considered bismuth-containing compounds the drug of choice for treating PUD.

The resurgence in the use of these agents is due to their effect against *H. pylori*. Colloidal bismuth subcitrate (CBS) and bismuth subsalicylate (BSS, Pepto-Bismol) are the most widely used preparations. The mechanism by which these agents induce ulcer healing is unclear. Potential mechanisms include ulcer coating; prevention of further pepsin/HCl-induced damage; binding of pepsin; and stimulation of prostaglandins, bicarbonate, and mucous secretion. Adverse effects with short-term usage are rare with bismuth compounds. Long-term usage with high doses, especially with the avidly absorbed CBS, may lead to neurotoxicity. These compounds are commonly used as one of the agents in an anti-*H. pylori* regimen (see below).

Prostaglandin analogues In view of their central role in maintaining mucosal integrity and repair, stable prostaglandin analogues were developed for the treatment of PUD. The prostaglandin E_1 derivative misoprostal is the only agent of this class approved by the U.S. Food and Drug Administration for clinical use in the prevention of NSAID-induced gastroduodenal mucosal injury (see below). The mechanism by which this rapidly absorbed drug provides its therapeutic effect is through enhancement of mucosal defense and repair. Prostaglandin analogues enhance mucous bicarbonate secretion, stimulate mucosal blood flow, and decrease mucosal cell turnover. The most common toxicity noted with this drug is diarrhea (10 to 30% incidence). Other major toxicities include uterine bleeding and contractions; misoprostal is contraindicated in women who may be pregnant, and women of childbearing age must be made clearly aware of this potential drug toxicity. The standard therapeutic dose is 200 μg four times per day.

Miscellaneous drugs A number of drugs aimed at treating acid peptic disorders have been developed over the years. In view of their limited utilization in the United States, if any, they will only be listed briefly. Anticholinergics, designed to inhibit activation of the muscarinic receptor in parietal cells, met with limited success due to their relatively weak acid-inhibiting effect and significant side effects (dry eyes, dry mouth, urinary retention). Tricyclic antidepressants have been suggested by some, but again the toxicity of these agents in comparison to the safe, effective drugs already described, precludes their utility. Finally, the licorice extract carbenoxolone has aldosterone like side effects with fluid retention and hypokalemia, making it an undesirable therapeutic option.

Therapy of *H. pylori* Extensive effort has been placed into determining who of the many individuals with *H. pylori* infection should be treated. The common conclusion arrived at by multiple consensus conferences (National Institutes of Health Consensus Development, American Digestive Health Foundation International Update Conference, European Maastricht Consensus, and Asia Pacific Consensus Conference) is that *H. pylori* should be eradicated in patients with documented PUD. This holds true independent of time of presentation (first episode or not), severity of symptoms, presence of confounding factors such as ingestion of NSAIDs, or whether the ulcer is in remission. Some have advocated treating patients with a history of documented PUD who are found to be *H. pylori*–positive by serology or breath testing. Over half of patients with gastric MALT lymphoma experience complete remission of the tumor in response to *H. pylori* eradication. Treating patients with NUD or to prevent gastric cancer remains controversial.

Multiple drugs have been evaluated in the therapy of *H. pylori*. No single agent is effective in eradicating the organism. Combination therapy for 14 days provides the greatest efficacy. A short-time course administration (7 to 10 days), although attractive, has not proven as successful as the 14-day regimens. The agents used with the greatest frequency include amoxicillin, metronidazole, tetracycline, clarithromycin, and bismuth compounds.

The physician's goal in treating PUD is to provide relief of symptoms (pain or dyspepsia), promote ulcer healing, and ultimately prevent ulcer recurrence and complications. The greatest impact of understanding the role of *H. pylori* in peptic disease has been the ability to prevent recurrence of what was often a recurring disease. Documented eradication of *H. pylori* in patients with PUD is associated with a dramatic decrease in ulcer recurrence to 4% (as compared to 59%) in GU patients and 6% (compared to 67%) in DU patients. Eradication of the organism may lead to diminished recurrent ulcer bleeding. The impact of its eradication on ulcer perforation is unclear.

Suggested treatment regimens for *H. pylori* are outlined in Table 285-7. Choice of a particular regimen will be influenced by several factors including efficacy, patient tolerance, existing antibiotic resistance, and cost of the drugs. The aim for initial eradication rates should be 85 to 90%. Dual therapy [PPI plus amoxicillin, PPI plus clarithromycin, ranitidine bismuth citrate (Tritec) plus clarithromycin] are not recommended in view of studies demonstrating eradication rates of <80 to 85%. The combination of bismuth, metronidazole, and tetracycline was the first triple regimen found effective against *H. pylori*. The combination of two antibiotics plus either a PPI, H_2 blocker, or bismuth compound has comparable success rates. Addition of acid suppression assists in providing early symptom relief and may enhance bacterial eradication.

Triple therapy, although effective, has several drawbacks, including the potential for poor patient compliance and drug-induced side effects. Compliance is being addressed somewhat by simplifying the regimens so that patients can take the medications twice a day. Simpler (dual therapy) and shorter regimens (7 and 10 days) are not as effective as triple therapy for 14 days. Two anti-*H. pylori* regimens are available in prepackaged formulation: Prevpac (lansoprazole, clarithromycin, and amoxicillin) and Helidac (bismuth subsalicylate, tetracycline, and metronidazole). The contents of the Prevpac are to be taken twice per day for 14 days, whereas Helidac constituents are taken four times per day with an antisecretory agent (PPI or H_2 blocker), also taken for at least 14 days.

Side effects have been reported in up to 20 to 30% of patients on triple therapy. Bismuth may cause black stools, constipation, or darkening of the tongue. The most feared complication with amoxicillin is pseudomembranous colitis, but this occurs in <1 to 2% of patients. Amoxicillin can also lead to antibiotic-associated diarrhea, nausea, vomiting, skin rash, and allergic reaction. Tetracycline has been reported to cause rashes and very rarely hepatotoxicity and anaphylaxis.

One important concern with treating patients who may not need treatment is the potential for development of antibiotic-resistant strains. The incidence and type of antibiotic-resistant *H. pylori* strains vary worldwide. Strains resistant to metronidazole, clarithromycin, amoxicillin, and tetracycline have been described, with the latter two being uncommon. Antibiotic-resistant strains are the most common

Table 285-7 Regimens Recommended for Eradication of *H. pylori* Infection

Drug	Dose
TRIPLE THERAPY	
1. Bismuth subsalicylate *plus*	2 tablets qid
Metronidazole *plus*	250 mg qid
Tetracycline[a]	500 mg qid
2. Ranitidine bismuth citrate *plus*	400 mg bid
Tetracycline *plus*	500 mg bid
Clarithromycin *or* metronidazole	500 mg bid
3. Omeprazole (lansoprazole) *plus*	20 mg bid (30 mg bid)
Clarithromycin *plus*	250 or 500 mg bid
Metronidazole[b] *or*	500 mg bid
Amoxicillin[c]	1 g bid
QUADRUPLE THERAPY	
Omeprazole (lansoprazole)	20 mg (30 mg) daily
Bismuth subsalicylate	2 tablets qid
Metronidazole	250 mg qid
Tetracycline	500 mg qid

[a] Alternative: use prepacked Helidac (see text).
[b] Alternative: use prepacked Prevpac (see text).
[c] Use either metronidazole or amoxicillin, but not both.

cause for treatment failure in compliant patients. Unfortunately, in vitro resistance does not predict outcome in patients. Culture and sensitivity testing of *H. pylori* is not performed routinely. Although resistance to metronidazole has been found in as many as 30% and 95% of isolates in North America and Asia, respectively, triple therapy is effective in eradicating the organism in >50% of patients infected with a resistant strain.

Failure of *H. pylori* eradication with triple therapy is usually due to infection with a resistant organism. Quadruple therapy (Table 285-7) where clarithromycin is substituted for metronidazole (or vice versa) should be the next step. If eradication is still not achieved in a compliant patient, then culture and sensitivity of the organism should be considered.

Reinfection after successful eradication of *H. pylori* is rare in the United States (<1%/year). If recurrent infection occurs within the first 6 months after completing therapy, the most likely explanation is recrudescence as opposed to reinfection, which occurs later in time.

Therapy of NSAID-Related Gastric or Duodenal Injury Medical intervention for NSAID-related mucosal injury includes treatment of an active ulcer and prevention of future injury. Recommendations for the treatment and prevention of NSAID-related mucosal injury are in Table 285-8. Ideally the injurious agent should be stopped as the first step in the therapy of an active NSAID-induced ulcer. If that is possible, then treatment with one of the acid inhibitory agents (H_2 blockers, PPIs) is indicated. Cessation of NSAIDs is not always possible because of the patient's severe underlying disease. Only PPIs can heal GUs or DUs, independent of whether NSAIDs are discontinued.

Prevention of NSAID-induced ulceration can be accomplished by misoprostol (200 μg qid) or a PPI. High-dose H_2 blockers (famotidine, 40 mg bid) have also shown some promise. The use of COX-2-selective NSAIDs may also reduce injury to gastric mucosa. Two highly selective COX-2 inhibitors, celecoxib and rofecoxib, are 100 times more selective inhibitors of COX-2 than standard NSAIDs, leading to gastric or duodenal mucosal injury that is comparable to placebo. However, evaluation of possible drug toxicities, such as altered renal function and induction of thrombosis, requires more data.

Approach and Therapy: Summary Controversy continues regarding the best approach to the patient who presents with dyspepsia (Chap. 41). The discovery of *H. pylori* and its role in pathogenesis of ulcers has added a new variable to the equation. Previously, if a patient <50 presented with dyspepsia and without alarming signs or symptoms suggestive of an ulcer complication or malignancy, an empirical therapeutic trial with acid suppression was commonly recommended. Although this approach is practiced by some today, an approach presently gaining approval for the treatment of patients with dyspepsia is outlined in Fig. 285-10. The referral to a gastroenterologist is for the potential need of endoscopy and subsequent evaluation and treatment if the endoscopy is negative.

Once an ulcer (GU or DU) is documented, then the main issue at stake is whether *H. pylori* or an NSAID is involved. With *H. pylori* present, independent of the NSAID status, triple therapy is recommended for 14 days, followed by continued acid-suppressing drugs (H_2 receptor antagonist or PPIs) for a total of 4 to 6 weeks. Selection of patients for documentation of *H. pylori* eradication is an area of some debate. The test of choice for documenting eradication is the urea breath test (UBT). The stool antigen study may also hold promise for this purpose and should certainly be performed if UBT is not available. Serologic testing is not useful for the purpose of documenting eradication since antibody titers fall slowly and often do not become undetectable. Two approaches toward documentation of eradication exist: (1) test for eradication only in individuals with a complicated course or in individuals who are frail or with multisystem disease who would do poorly with an ulcer recurrence, and (2) test all patients for successful eradication. Some recommend that patients with complicated ulcer disease or who are frail should be treated with long-term acid suppression, thus making documentation of *H. pylori* eradication a moot point. In view of this discrepancy in practice, it would be best to discuss with the patient the different options available.

Table 285-8 Recommendations for Treatment of NSAID-Related Mucosal Injury

Clinical Setting	Recommendation
Active ulcer	
NSAID discontinued	H_2 receptor antagonist or PPI
NSAID continued	PPI
Prophylactic therapy	Misoprostol
	PPI
	Selective COX-2 inhibitor
H. pylori infection	Eradication if active ulcer present or there is a past history of peptic ulcer disease

NOTE: PPI, proton pump inhibitor; COX-2, isoenzyme of cyclooxygenase.

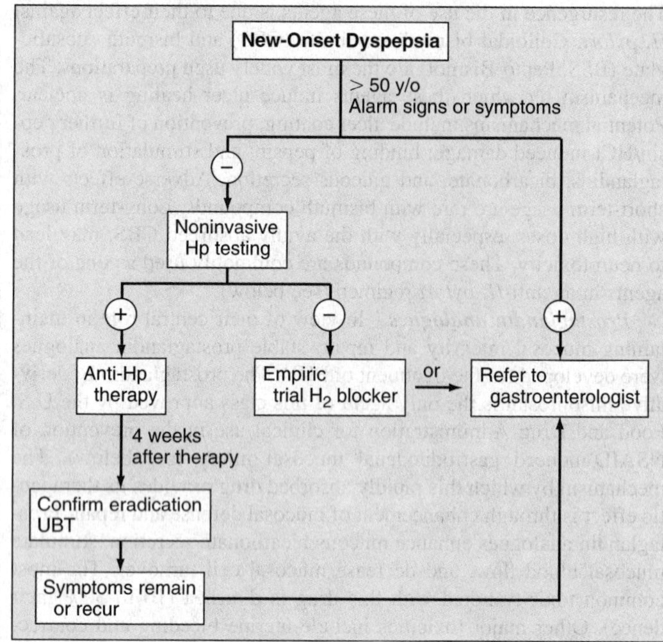

FIGURE 285-10 Overview of new-onset dyspepsia. Hp, *H. pylori*; UBT, urea breath test. *(Adapted from BS Anand and DY Graham: Endoscopy 31: 215, 1999.)*

Several issues differentiate the approach to a GU versus a DU. GUs, especially of the body and fundus, have the potential of being malignant. Multiple biopsies of a GU should be taken initially; even if these are negative for neoplasm, repeat endoscopy to document healing at 8 to 12 weeks should be performed, with biopsy if the ulcer is still present. About 70% of GUs eventually found to be malignant undergo significant (usually incomplete) healing.

The majority (>90%) of GUs and DUs heal with the conventional therapy outlined above. A GU that fails to heal after 12 weeks and a DU that doesn't heal after 8 weeks of therapy should be considered refractory. Once poor compliance and persistent *H. pylori* infection have been excluded, NSAID use, either inadvertent or surreptitious, must be excluded. In addition, cigarette smoking must be eliminated. For a GU, malignancy must be meticulously excluded. Next, consideration should be given to a gastric hypersecretory state, which can be excluded with gastric acid analysis. Although a subset of patients have gastric acid hypersecretion of unclear etiology as a contributing factor to refractory ulcers, ZES should be excluded with a fasting gastrin or secretin stimulation test (see below). More than 90% of refractory ulcers (either DUs or GUs) heal after 8 weeks of treatment with higher doses of PPI (omeprazole, 40 mg/d). This higher dose is also effective in maintaining remission. Surgical intervention may be a consideration at this point; however, other rare causes of refractory ulcers must be excluded before recommending surgery. Rare etiologies of refractory ulcers that may be diagnosed by gastric or duodenal biopsies include: ischemia, Crohn's disease, amyloidosis, sarcoidosis, lymphoma, eosinophilic gastroenteritis, or infection [cytomegalovirus (CMV), tuberculosis, or syphilis].

Surgical Therapy Surgical intervention in PUD can be viewed as being either elective, for treatment of medically refractory disease, or as urgent/emergent, for the treatment of an ulcer-related complication. Refractory ulcers are an exceedingly rare occurrence. Surgery is more often required for treatment of an ulcer-related complication. Gastrointestinal bleeding (Chap. 44), perforation, and gastric outlet obstruction are the three complications that may require surgical intervention.

Hemorrhage is the most common ulcer-related complication, occurring in ~15 to 25% of patients. Bleeding may occur in any age group but is most often seen in older patients (sixth decade or beyond). The majority of patients stop bleeding spontaneously, but in some, endoscopic therapy (Chap. 283) is necessary. Patients unresponsive or refractory to endoscopic intervention will require surgery (~5% of transfusion-requiring patients).

Free peritoneal perforation occurs in ~2 to 3% of DU patients. As in the case of bleeding, up to 10% of these patients will not have antecedent ulcer symptoms. Concomitant bleeding may occur in up to 10% of patients with perforation, with mortality being increased substantially. Peptic ulcer can also penetrate into adjacent organs, especially with a posterior DU, which can penetrate into the pancreas, colon, liver, or biliary tree.

Pyloric channel ulcers or DUs can lead to gastric outlet obstruction in ~2 to 3% of patients. This can result from chronic scarring or from impaired motility due to inflammation and/or edema with pylorospasm. Patients may present with early satiety, nausea, vomiting of undigested food, and weight loss. Conservative management with nasogastric suction, intravenous hydration/nutrition, and antisecretory agents is indicated for 7 to 10 days with the hope that a functional obstruction will reverse. If a mechanical obstruction persists, endoscopic intervention with balloon dilation may be effective. Surgery should be considered if all else fails.

Specific Operations for Duodenal Ulcers Surgical treatment is designed to decrease gastric acid secretion. Operations most commonly performed include vagotomy and drainage (by pyloroplasty, gastroduodenostomy, or gastrojejunostomy), highly selective vagotomy (which does not require a drainage procedure), and vagotomy with antrectomy. The specific procedure performed is dictated by the underlying circumstances: elective vs. emergency, the degree and extent of duodenal ulceration, and the expertise of the surgeon.

Vagotomy is a component of each of these procedures and is aimed at decreasing acid secretion through ablating cholinergic input to the stomach. Unfortunately, both truncal and selective vagotomy (preserves the celiac and hepatic branches) result in gastric atony despite successful reduction of both basal acid output (BAO, decreased by 85%) and maximal acid output (MAO, decreased by 50%). Drainage procedure through pyloroplasty or gastroduodenostomy is required in an effort to compensate for the vagotomy-induced gastric motility disorder. To minimize gastric dysmotility, highly selective vagotomy (also known as parietal cell, super selective, and proximal vagotomy) was developed. Only the vagal fibers innervating the portion of the stomach that contains parietal cells is transected, thus leaving fibers important for regulating gastric motility intact. Although this procedure leads to an immediate decrease in both BAO and stimulated acid output, acid secretion recovers over time. By the end of the first postoperative year, basal and stimulated acid output are ~30 and 50%, respectively, of preoperative levels. Ulcer recurrence rates are higher with highly selective vagotomy, although the overall complication rates are lower (Table 285-9).

The procedure that provides the lowest rates of ulcer recurrence but has the highest complication rate is vagotomy (truncal or selective) in combination with antrectomy. Antrectomy is aimed at eliminating an additional stimulant of gastric acid secretion, gastrin. Gastrin orig-

Table 285-9 Outcome in Patients After Acid-Reducing Gastric Surgery

Operation	Ulcer Recurrence Rates, %	Complication Rates
Vagotomy and antrectomy (Billroth I or II)	1	Highest
Vagotomy and pyloroplasty	10	Intermediate
Highly selective vagotomy	≥10	Lowest

inates from G cells found in the antrum. Two principal types of reanastomoses are used after antrectomy, gastroduodenostomy (Billroth I) or gastrojejunostomy (Billroth II) (Fig. 285-11). Although Billroth I is often preferred over II, severe duodenal inflammation or scarring may preclude its performance.

Of these procedures, highly selective vagotomy may be the one of choice in the elective setting, except in situations where ulcer recurrence rates are high (prepyloric ulcers and those refractory to H_2 therapy). Selection of vagotomy and antrectomy may be more appropriate in these circumstances.

These procedures have been traditionally performed by standard laparotomy. The advent of laparoscopic surgery has led several surgical teams to successfully perform highly selective vagotomy, truncal vagotomy/pyloroplasty, and truncal vagotomy/antrectomy through this approach. An increase in the number of laparoscopic procedures for treatment of PUD is expected.

Specific Operations for Gastric Ulcers The location and the presence of a concomitant DU dictate the operative procedure performed for a GU. Antrectomy (including the ulcer) with a Billroth I anastomosis is the treatment of choice for an antral ulcer. Vagotomy is performed only if a DU is present. Although ulcer excision with vagotomy and drainage procedure has been proposed, the higher incidence of ulcer recurrence makes this a less desirable approach. Ulcers located near the esophagogastric junction may require a more radical approach, a subtotal gastrectomy with a Roux-en-Y esophagogastrojejunostomy (Csende's procedure). A less aggressive approach including antrectomy, intraoperative ulcer biopsy, and vagotomy (Kelling-Madlener procedure) may be indicated in fragile patients with a high GU. Ulcer recurrence approaches 30% with this procedure.

Surgery-Related Complications Complications seen after surgery for PUD are related primarily to the extent of the anatomical modification performed. Minimal alteration (highly selective vagot-

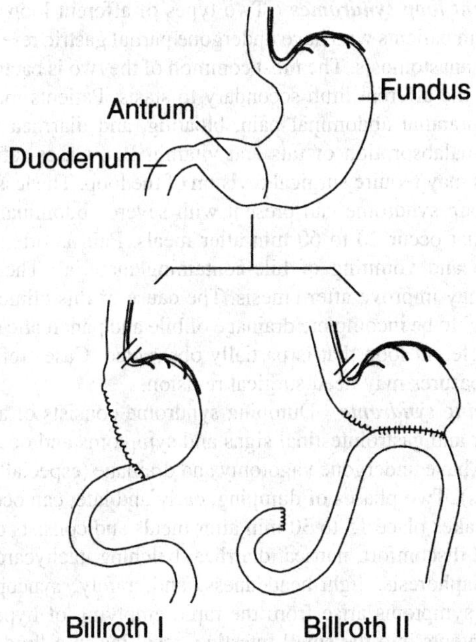

FIGURE 285-11 Schematic representation of Billroth I and II procedures.

omy) is associated with higher rates of ulcer recurrence and less gastrointestinal disturbance. More aggressive surgical procedures have a lower rate of ulcer recurrence but a greater incidence of gastrointestinal dysfunction. Overall, morbidity and mortality related to these procedures are quite low. Morbidity associated with vagotomy and antrectomy or pyloroplasty is $\leq$5%, with mortality ~1%. Highly selective vagotomy has lower morbidity and mortality rates of 1 and 0.3%, respectively.

In addition to the potential early consequences of any intraabdominal procedure (bleeding, infection, thromboembolism), gastroparesis, duodenal stump leak, and efferent loop obstruction can be observed.

Recurrent ulceration The risk of ulcer recurrence is directly related to the procedure performed (Table 285-9). Ulcers that recur after partial gastric resection tend to develop at the anastomosis (stomal or marginal ulcer). Epigastric abdominal pain is the most frequent presenting complaint. Severity and duration of pain tend to be more progressive than observed with DUs before surgery.

Ulcers may recur for several reasons including incomplete vagotomy, retained antrum, and, less likely, persistent or recurrent *H. pylori* infection. ZES should have been excluded preoperatively. More recently, surreptitious use of NSAIDs has been found to be a reason for recurrent ulcers after surgery, especially if the initial procedure was done for an NSAID-induced ulcer. Once *H. pylori* and NSAIDs have been excluded as etiologic factors, the question of incomplete vagotomy or retained gastric antrum should be explored. For the latter, fasting plasma gastrin levels should be determined. If elevated, retained antrum or ZES (see below) should be considered. A combination of acid secretory analysis and secretin stimulation (see below) can assist in this differential diagnosis. Incomplete vagotomy can be ruled out by gastric acid analysis coupled with sham feeding. In this test, gastric acid output is measured while the patient sees, smells, and chews a meal (without swallowing). The cephalic phase of gastric secretion, which is mediated by the vagus, is being assessed with this study. An increase in gastric acid output in response to sham feeding is evidence that the vagus nerve is intact.

Medical therapy with H_2 blockers will heal postoperative ulceration in 70 to 90% of patients. The efficacy of PPIs has not been fully assessed in this group, but one may anticipate greater rates of ulcer healing compared to those obtained with H_2 blockers. Repeat operation (complete vagotomy, partial gastrectomy) may be required in a small subgroup of patients who have not responded to aggressive medical management.

Afferent loop syndromes Two types of afferent loop syndrome can occur in patients who have undergone partial gastric resection with Billroth II anastomosis. The most common of the two is bacterial overgrowth in the afferent limb secondary to stasis. Patients may experience postprandial abdominal pain, bloating, and diarrhea with concomitant malabsorption of fats and vitamin B_{12}. Cases refractory to antibiotics may require surgical revision of the loop. The less common afferent loop syndrome can present with severe abdominal pain and bloating that occur 20 to 60 min after meals. Pain is often followed by nausea and vomiting of bile-containing material. The pain and bloating may improve after emesis. The cause of this clinical picture is theorized to be incomplete drainage of bile and pancreatic secretions from an afferent loop that is partially obstructed. Cases refractory to dietary measures may need surgical revision.

Dumping syndrome Dumping syndrome consists of a series of vasomotor and gastrointestinal signs and symptoms and occurs in patients who have undergone vagotomy and drainage (especially Billroth procedures). Two phases of dumping, early and late, can occur. Early dumping takes place 15 to 30 min after meals and consists of crampy abdominal discomfort, nausea, diarrhea, belching, tachycardia, palpitations, diaphoresis, light-headedness, and, rarely, syncope. These signs and symptoms arise from the rapid emptying of hyperosmolar gastric contents into the small intestine, resulting in a fluid shift into the gut lumen with plasma volume contraction and acute intestinal distention. Release of vasoactive gastrointestinal hormones (vasoactive intestinal polypeptide, neurotensin, motilin) is also theorized to play a role in early dumping.

The late phase of dumping typically occurs 90 min to 3 h after meals. Vasomotor symptoms (light-headedness, diaphoresis, palpitations, tachycardia, and syncope) predominate during this phase. This component of dumping is thought to be secondary to hypoglycemia from excessive insulin release.

Dumping syndrome is most noticeable after meals rich in simple carbohydrates (especially sucrose) and high osmolarity. Ingestion of large amounts of fluids may also contribute. Up to 50% of post-vagotomy and drainage patients will experience dumping syndrome to some degree. Signs and symptoms often improve with time, but a severe protracted picture can occur in up to 1% of patients.

Dietary modification is the cornerstone of therapy for patients with dumping syndrome. Small, multiple (six) meals devoid of simple carbohydrates coupled with elimination of liquids during meals is important. Antidiarrheals and anticholinergic agents are complimentary to diet. The somatostatin analogue octreotide has been successful in diet refractory cases. This drug is administered subcutaneously (50 μg tid), titrated according to clinical response. Recently a long-acting formulation has become available, but its use in dumping syndrome has not been examined.

Postvagotomy diarrhea Up to 10% of patients may seek medical attention for the treatment of postvagotomy diarrhea. This complication is most commonly observed after truncal vagotomy. Patients may complain of intermittent diarrhea that occurs typically 1 to 2 h after meals. Occasionally the symptoms may be severe and relentless. This is due to a motility disorder from interruption of the vagal fibers supplying the luminal gut. Other contributing factors may include decreased absorption of nutrients (see below), increased excretion of bile acids, and release of luminal factors that promote secretion. Diphenoxylate or loperamide is often useful in symptom control. The bile salt–binding agent cholestyramine may be helpful in severe cases. Surgical reversal of a 10-cm segment of jejunum may yield a substantial improvement in bowel frequency in a subset of patients.

Bile reflux gastropathy A subset of post-partial gastrectomy patients will present with abdominal pain, early satiety, nausea, and vomiting, who have as the only finding mucosal erythema of the gastric remnant. Histologic examination of the gastric mucosa reveals minimal inflammation but the presence of epithelial cell injury. This clinical picture is categorized as bile or alkaline reflux gastropathy/gastritis. Although reflux of bile is implicated as the reason for this disorder, the mechanism is unknown. Prokinetic agents (cisapride, 10 to 20 mg before meals and at bedtime) and cholestyramine have been effective treatments. Cisapride may cause cardiac arrhythmias. Severe refractory symptoms may require using either nuclear scanning with ^{99m}Tc-HIDA, to document reflux, or an alkaline challenge test, where 0.1 *N* NaOH is infused into the stomach in an effort to reproduce the patient's symptoms. Surgical diversion of pancreaticobiliary secretions away from the gastric remnant with a Roux-en-Y gastrojejunostomy consisting of a long (50 to 60 cm) Roux limb has been used in severe cases. Bilious vomiting improves, but early satiety and bloating may persist in up to 50% of patients.

Maldigestion and malabsorption Weight loss can be observed in up to 60% of patients after partial gastric resection. A significant component of this weight reduction is due to decreased oral intake. However, mild steatorrhea can also develop. Reasons for maldigestion/malabsorption include decreased gastric acid production, rapid gastric emptying, decreased food dispersion in the stomach, reduced luminal bile concentration, reduced pancreatic secretory response to feeding, and rapid intestinal transit.

Decreased serum vitamin B_{12} levels can be observed after partial gastrectomy. This is usually not due to deficiency of intrinsic factor (IF), since a minimal amount of parietal cells (source of IF) are removed during antrectomy. Reduced vitamin B_{12} may be due to competition for the vitamin by bacterial overgrowth or inability to split the vitamin from its protein-bound source due to hypochlorhydria.

Iron-deficiency anemia may be a consequence of impaired absorption of dietary iron in patients with a Billroth II gastrojejunotomy. Absorption of iron salts is normal in these individuals; thus a favorable response to oral iron supplementation can be anticipated. Folate deficiency with concomitant anemia can also develop in these patients. This deficiency may be secondary to decreased absorption or diminished oral intake.

Malabsorption of vitamin D and calcium resulting in osteoporosis and osteomalacia is common after partial gastrectomy and gastrojejunostomy (Billroth II). Osteomalacia can occur as a late complication in up to 25% of post-partial gastrectomy patients. Bone fractures occur twice as commonly in men after gastric surgery as in a control population. It may take years before x-ray findings demonstrate diminished bone density. Elevated alkaline phosphatase, reduced serum calcium, bone pain, and pathologic fractures may be seen in patients with osteomalacia. The high incidence of these abnormalities in this subgroup of patients justifies treating them with vitamin D and calcium supplementation indefinitely. Therapy is especially important in females.

Gastric adenocarcinoma The incidence of adenocarcinoma in the gastric stump is increased 15 years after resection. Some have reported a four- to fivefold increase in gastric cancer 20 to 25 years after resection. The pathogenesis is unclear but may involve alkaline reflux, bacterial proliferation, or hypochlorhydria. Endoscopic screening every other year may detect surgically treatable disease.

RELATED CONDITIONS

ZOLLINGER–ELLISON SYNDROME Severe peptic ulcer diathesis secondary to gastric acid hypersecretion due to unregulated gastrin release from a non-β cell endocrine tumor (gastrinoma) defines the components of the ZES. Initially, ZES was typified by aggressive and refractory ulceration in which total gastrectomy provided the only chance for enhancing survival. Today ZES can be cured by surgical resection in up to 30% of patients.

Epidemiology The incidence of ZES varies from 0.1 to 1% of individuals presenting with PUD. Males are more commonly affected than females, and the majority of patients are diagnosed between ages 30 and 50. Gastrinomas are classified into sporadic tumors (more common) and those associated with multiple endocrine neoplasia (MEN) type I (see below).

Pathophysiology Hypergastremia originating from an autonomous neoplasm is the driving force responsible for the clinical manifestations in ZES. Gastrin stimulates acid secretion through gastrin receptors on parietal cells and by inducing histamine release from ECL cells. Gastrin also has a trophic action on gastric epithelial cells. Longstanding hypergastrinemia leads to markedly increased gastric acid secretion through both parietal cell stimulation and increased parietal cell mass. The increased gastric acid output leads to the peptic ulcer diathesis, erosive esophagitis, and diarrhea.

Tumor Distribution Although early studies suggested that the vast majority of gastrinomas occurred within the pancreas, a significant number of these lesions are extrapancreatic. Over 80% of these tumors are found within the hypothetical gastrinoma triangle (confluence of the cystic and common bile ducts superiorly, junction of the second and third portions of the duodenum inferiorly, and junction of the neck and body of the pancreas medially). Duodenal tumors constitute the most common nonpancreatic lesion; up to 50% of gastrinomas are found here. Less common extrapancreatic sites include stomach, bones, ovaries, heart, liver, and lymph nodes. More than 60% of tumors are considered malignant, with up to 30 to 50% of patients having multiple lesions or metastatic disease at presentation. Histologically, gastrin-producing cells appear well differentiated, expressing markers typically found in endocrine neoplasms (chromogranin, neuron-specific enolase).

Clinical Manifestations Gastric acid hypersecretion is responsible for the signs and symptoms observed in patients with ZES. Peptic ulcer is the most common clinical manifestation, occurring in >90% of gastrinoma patients. Initial presentation and ulcer location (duodenal bulb) may be indistinguishable from common PUD. Clinical situations that should create suspicion of gastrinoma are ulcers in unusual locations (second part of the duodenum and beyond), ulcers refractory to standard medical therapy, ulcer recurrence after acid-reducing surgery, or ulcers presenting with frank complications (bleeding, obstruction, and perforation). Symptoms of esophageal origin are present in up to two-thirds of patients with ZES, with a spectrum ranging from mild esophagitis to frank ulceration with stricture and Barrett's mucosa.

Diarrhea is the next most common clinical manifestation in up to 50% of patients. Although diarrhea often occurs concomitantly with acid peptic disease, it may also occur independent of an ulcer. Etiology of the diarrhea is multifactorial, resulting from marked volume overload to the small bowel, pancreatic enzyme inactivation by acid, and damage of the intestinal epithelial surface by acid. The epithelial damage can lead to a mild degree of maldigestion and malabsorption of nutrients. The diarrhea may also have a secretory component due to the direct stimulatory effect of gastrin on enterocytes or the cosecretion of additional hormones from the tumor, such as vasoactive intestinal peptide.

Gastrinomas can develop in the presence of MEN I syndrome (Chap. 93) in approximately 25% of patients. This autosomal dominant disorder involves primarily three organ sites: the parathyroid glands (80 to 90%), pancreas (40 to 80%), and pituitary gland (30 to 60%). The genetic defect in MEN I is in the long arm of chromosome 11 (11q11-q13). In view of the stimulatory effect of calcium on gastric secretion, the hyperparathyroidism and hypercalcemia seen in MEN I patients may have a direct effect on ulcer disease. Resolution of hypercalcemia by parathyroidectomy reduces gastrin and gastric acid output in gastrinoma patients. An additional distinguishing feature in ZES patients with MEN I is the higher incidence of gastric carcinoid tumor development (as compared to patients with sporadic gastrinomas). Gastrinomas tend to be smaller, multiple, and located in the duodenal wall more often than is seen in patients with sporadic ZES. Establishing the diagnosis of MEN I is critical not only from the standpoint of providing genetic counseling to the patient and his or her family but also from the surgical approach recommended.

Diagnosis The first step in the evaluation of a patient suspected of having ZES is to obtain a fasting gastrin level. A list of clinical scenarios that should arouse suspicion regarding this diagnosis is shown in Table 285-10. Fasting gastrin levels are usually <150 pg/mL. Virtually all gastrinoma patients will have a gastrin level >150 to 200 pg/mL. Measurement of fasting gastrin should be repeated to confirm the clinical suspicion.

Multiple processes can lead to an elevated fasting gastrin level (Table 285-11), with gastric hypochlorhydria or achlorhydria being the most frequent causes. Gastric acid induces feedback inhibition of gastrin release. A decrease in acid production will subsequently lead to failure of the feedback inhibitory pathway, resulting in net hypergastrinemia. Gastrin levels will thus be high in patients using antisecretory agents for the treatment of acid peptic disorders and dyspepsia. *H. pylori* infection can also cause hypergastrinemia.

Table 285-10 When to Obtain a Fasting Serum Gastrin Level

Multiple ulcers
Ulcers in unusual locations
Ulcers associated with severe esophagitis
Ulcers resistant to therapy, with frequent recurrences
Ulcer patients awaiting surgery
Extensive family history of peptic ulcer disease
Postoperative ulcer recurrence
Basal hyperchlorhydria
Unexplained diarrhea or steatorrhea
Hypercalcemia
Family history of pancreatic islet, pituitary, or parathyroid tumor
Prominent gastric or duodenal folds

Table 285-11 Differential Diagnosis of Hypergastrinemia

Hypochlorhydria or achlorhydria with or without pernicious anemia
Retained gastric antrum
G cell hyperplasia
Gastric outlet obstruction
Renal insufficiency
Massive small-bowel obstruction
Others: rheumatoid arthritis, vitiligo, diabetes, pheochromocytoma

The next step in establishing a biochemical diagnosis of gastrinoma is to assess acid secretion. Nothing further needs to be done if decreased acid output is observed. In contrast, normal or elevated gastric acid output suggests a need for additional tests. Gastric acid analysis is performed by placing a nasogastric tube in the stomach and drawing samples at 15-min intervals for 1 h during unstimulated or basal state (BAO), followed by continued sampling after administration of intravenous pentagastrin (MAO). Up to 90% of gastrinoma patients may have a BAO of ≥15 meq/h (normal <4 meq/h). Up to 12% of patients with common PUD may have comparable levels of acid secretion. A BAO/MAO ratio >0.6 is highly suggestive of ZES, but a ratio <0.6 does not exclude the diagnosis.

Gastrin provocative tests have been developed in an effort to differentiate between the causes of hypergastrinemia and are especially helpful in patients with indeterminant acid secretory studies. The tests are the secretin stimulation test, the calcium infusion study, and a standard meal test. In each of these, a fasted patient has an indwelling intravenous catheter in place for serial blood sampling and an intravenous line in place for secretin or calcium infusion. The patient receives either secretion (intravenous bolus of 2 μg/kg) or calcium (calcium gluconate, 5 mg/kg body weight over 3 h) or is fed a meal. Blood is then drawn at predetermined intervals (10 min and 1 min before and at 2, 5, 10, 15, 20, and 30 min after injection for secretin stimulation and at 30-min intervals during the calcium infusion). The most sensitive and specific gastrin provocative test for the diagnosis of gastrinoma is the secretin study. An increase in gastrin of ≥200 pg within 15 min of secretin injection has a sensitivity and specificity of >90% for ZES. The calcium infusion study is less sensitive and specific than the secretin test, with a rise of >400 pg/mL observed in ~80% of gastrinoma patients. The lower accuracy, coupled with it being a more cumbersome study with greater potential for adverse effects, makes calcium infusion less useful and therefore rarely, if ever, utilized. Rarely, one may observe increased BAO and hypergastrinemia in a patient who in the past has been categorized as having G cell hyperplasia or hyperfunction. This set of findings may have been due to *H. pylori*. The standard meal test was devised to assist in making the diagnosis of G cell–related hyperactivity, by observing a dramatic increase in gastrin after a meal (>200%). This test is not useful in differentiating between G cell hyperfunction and ZES.

Tumor Localization Once the biochemical diagnosis of gastrinoma has been confirmed, the tumor must be located. Multiple imaging studies have been utilized in an effort to enhance tumor localization (Table 285-12). The broad range of sensitivity is due to the variable success rates achieved by the different investigative groups. Endoscopic ultrasound (EUS) permits imaging of the pancreas with a high degree of resolution (<5 mm). This modality is particularly helpful in excluding small neoplasms within the pancreas and in assessing the presence of surrounding lymph nodes and vascular involvement. Several types of endocrine tumors express cell-surface receptors for somatostatin. This permits the localization of gastrinomas by measuring the uptake of the stable somatostatin analogue, ^{111}In-pentriotide (*octreoscan*) with sensitivity and specificity rates of >75%.

Up to 50% of patients have metastatic disease at diagnosis. Success in controlling gastric acid hypersecretion has shifted the emphasis of therapy towards providing a surgical cure. Detecting the primary tumor and excluding metastatic disease are critical in view of this paradigm shift. Once a biochemical diagnosis has been confirmed, the patient should first undergo an abdominal computed tomographic scan, magnetic resonance imaging, or octreoscan (depending on availability) to exclude metastatic disease. Once metastatic disease has been excluded, an experienced endocrine surgeon may opt for exploratory laparotomy with intraoperative ultrasound or transillumination. In other centers, careful examination of the peripancreatic area with EUS, accompanied by endoscopic exploration of the duodenum for primary tumors, will be performed before surgery. Selective arterial secretin injection (SASI) may be a useful adjuvant for localizing tumors in a subset of patients.

Table 285-12 Sensitivity of Imaging Studies in Zollinger-Ellison Syndrome

	Sensitivity, %	
Study	Primary Gastrinoma	Metastatic Gastrinoma
Ultrasound	21–28	14
CT scan	35–59	35–72
Selective angiography	35–68	33–86
Portal venous sampling	70–90	N/A
SASI	55–78	41
MRI	30–60	71
Otreoscan	67–86	80–100
EUS	80–100	N/A

NOTE: CT, computed tomography; SASI, selective arterial secretin injection; MRI, magnetic resonance imaging; Octreoscan, imaging with indium-111-labeled pentriotide; EUS, endoscopic ultrasonography.

TREATMENT Treatment of functional endocrine tumors is directed at ameliorating the signs and symptoms related to hormone overproduction, curative resection of the neoplasm, and attempts to control tumor growth in metastatic disease.

PPIs are the treatment of choice and have decreased the need for total gastrectomy. Initial doses of omeprazole or lansoprazole should be in the range of 60 mg/d. Dosing can be adjusted to achieve a BAO <10 meq/h (at the drug trough) in surgery-naive patients and to <5 meq/h in individuals who have previously undergone an acid-reducing operation. Although the somatostatin analogue has inhibitory effects on gastrin release from receptor-bearing tumors and inhibits gastric acid secretion to some extent, PPIs have the advantage of reducing parietal cell activity to a greater degree.

The ultimate goal of surgery would be to provide a definitive cure. Improved understanding of tumor distribution has led to 10-year disease-free intervals as high as 34% in sporadic gastrinoma patients undergoing surgery. A positive outcome is highly dependent on the experience of the surgical team treating these rare tumors. Surgical therapy of gastrinoma patients with MEN I remains controversial because of the difficulty in rendering these patients disease free with surgery. In contrast to the encouraging postoperative results observed in patients with sporadic disease, only 6% of MEN I patients are disease free 5 years after an operation. Some groups suggest surgery only if a clearly identifiable, nonmetastatic lesion is documented by structural studies. Others advocate a more aggressive approach, where all patients free of hepatic metastasis are explored and all detected tumors in the duodenum are resected; this is followed by enucleation of lesions in the pancreatic head, with a distal pancreatectomy to follow. The outcome of the two approaches has not been clearly defined.

Therapy of metastatic endocrine tumors in general remains suboptimal; gastrinomas are no exception. A host of medical therapeutic approaches including chemotherapy (streptozotocin, 5-fluorouracil, and doxorubicin), IFN-α, and hepatic artery embolization lead to significant toxicity without a substantial improvement in overall survival. Surgical approaches including debulking surgery and liver transplantation for hepatic metastasis have also produced limited benefit. Therefore, early recognition and surgery are the only chances for curing this disease.

The 5- and 10-year survival rates for gastrinoma patients are 62 to

75% and 47 to 53%, respectively. Individuals with the entire tumor resected or those with a negative laparotomy have 5- and 10-year survival rates >90%. Patients with incompletely resected tumors have 5- and 10-year survival of 43% and 25%, respectively. Patients with hepatic metastasis have <20% survival at 5 years. Favorable prognostic indicators include primary duodenal wall tumors, isolated lymph node tumor, and undetectable tumor upon surgical exploration. Poor prognostic indicators include hepatic metastases or the presence of Cushing's syndrome in a sporadic gastrinoma patient.

STRESS-RELATED MUCOSAL INJURY Patients suffering from shock, sepsis, massive burns, severe trauma, or head injury can develop acute erosive gastric mucosal changes or frank ulceration with bleeding. Classified as stress-induced gastritis or ulcers, injury is most commonly observed in the acid-producing (fundus and body) portions of the stomach. The most common presentation is gastrointestinal bleeding, which is usually minimal but can occasionally be life-threatening. Respiratory failure requiring mechanical ventilation and underlying coagulopathy are risk factors for bleeding, which tends to occur 48 to 72 h after the acute injury or insult.

Histologically, stress injury does not contain inflammation or *H. pylori*; thus "gastritis" is a misnomer. Although elevated gastric acid secretion may be noted in patients with stress ulceration after head trauma (Cushing's ulcer) and severe burns (Curling's ulcer), mucosal ischemia and breakdown of the normal protective barriers of the stomach also play an important role in the pathogenesis. Acid must contribute to injury in view of the significant drop in bleeding noted when acid inhibitors are used as a prophylactic measure for stress gastritis.

Improvement in the general management of intensive care unit patients has led to a significant decrease in the incidence of gastrointestinal bleeding due to stress ulceration. The estimated decrease in bleeding is from 20 to 30% to <15%. This improvement has led to some debate regarding the need for prophylactic therapy. The limited benefit of medical (endoscopic, angiographic) and surgical therapy in a patient with hemodynamically compromising bleeding associated with stress ulcer/gastritis supports the use of preventive measures in high-risk patients (mechanically ventilated, coagulopathy, multiorgan failure, or severe burns). Maintenance of gastric pH >3.5 with continuous infusion of H_2 blockers or liquid antacids administered every 2 to 3 h are viable options. Sucralfate slurry (1 g every 4 to 6 h) has also been successful. If bleeding occurs despite these measures, endoscopy, intraarterial vasopressin, or embolization are options. If all else fails, then surgery should be considered. Although vagotomy and antrectomy may be used, the better approach would be a total gastrectomy, which has an exceedingly high mortality rate in this setting.

GASTRITIS The term *gastritis* should be reserved for histologically documented inflammation of the gastric mucosa. Gastritis is *not* the mucosal erythema seen during endoscopy and is *not* interchangeable with "dyspepsia." The etiologic factors leading to gastritis are broad and heterogeneous. Gastritis has been classified based on time course (acute vs. chronic), histologic features, and anatomic distribution or proposed pathogenic mechanism (Table 285-13).

Table 285-13 Classification of Gastritis

I. Acute gastritis	II. Chronic Atrophic Gastritis
A. Acute *H. pylori* infection	A. Type A: Autoimmune, body-predominant
B. Other acute infectious gastritides	B. Type B: *H. pylori*–related, antral predominant
1. Bacterial (other than *H. pylori*)	C. Indeterminant
2. *Helicobacter helmanni*	III. Uncommon Forms of Gastritis
3. Phlegmonous	A. Lymphocytic
4. Mycobacterial	B. Eosinophilic
5. Syphilitic	C. Crohn's disease
6. Viral	D. Sarcoidosis
7. Parasitic	E. Isolated granulomatous gastritis
8. Fungal	

The correlation between the histologic findings of gastritis, the clinical picture of abdominal pain or dyspepsia, and endoscopic findings noted on gross inspection of the gastric mucosa is poor. Therefore, there is no typical clinical manifestation of gastritis.

Acute Gastritis The most common causes of acute gastritis are infectious. Acute infection with *H. pylori* induces gastritis. However, *H. pylori* acute gastritis has not been extensively studied. Reported as presenting with sudden onset of epigastric pain, nausea, and vomiting, limited mucosal histologic studies demonstrate a marked infiltrate of neutrophils with edema and hyperemia. If not treated, this picture will evolve into one of chronic gastritis. Hypochlorhydria lasting for up to 1 year may follow acute *H. pylori* infection.

The highly acidic gastric environment may be one reason why infectious processes of the stomach are rare. Bacterial infection of the stomach or phlegmonous gastritis is a rare potentially life-threatening disorder, characterized by marked and diffuse acute inflammatory infiltrates of the entire gastric wall, at times accompanied by necrosis. Elderly individuals, alcoholics, and AIDS patients may be affected. Potential iatrogenic causes include polypectomy and mucosal injection with India ink. Organisms associated with this entity include streptococci, staphylococci, *Escherichia coli*, *Proteus*, and *Haemophilus*. Failure of supportive measures and antibiotics may result in gastrectomy.

Other types of infectious gastritis may occur in immunocompromised individuals such as AIDS patients. Examples include herpetic (herpes simplex) or CMV gastritis. The histologic finding of intranuclear inclusions would be observed in the latter.

Chronic Gastritis Chronic gastritis is identified histologically by an inflammatory cell infiltrate consisting primarily of lymphocytes and plasma cells, with very scant neutrophil involvement. Distribution of the inflammation may be patchy, initially involving superficial and glandular portions of the gastric mucosa. This picture may progress to more severe glandular destruction, with atrophy and metaplasia. Chronic gastritis has been classified according to histologic characteristics. These include superficial atrophic changes and gastric atrophy.

The early phase of chronic gastritis is *superficial gastritis*. The inflammatory changes are limited to the lamina propria of the surface mucosa, with edema and cellular infiltrates separating intact gastric glands. Additional findings may include decreased mucus in the mucous cells and decreased mitotic figures in the glandular cells. The next stage is *atrophic gastritis*. The inflammatory infiltrate extends deeper into the mucosa, with progressive distortion and destruction of the glands. The final stage of chronic gastritis is *gastric atrophy*. Glandular structures are lost; there is a paucity of inflammatory infiltrates. Endoscopically the mucosa may be substantially thin, permitting clear visualization of the underlying blood vessels.

Gastric glands may undergo morphologic transformation in chronic gastritis. Intestinal metaplasia denotes the conversion of gastric glands to a small intestinal phenotype with small-bowel mucosal glands containing goblet cells. The metaplastic changes may vary in distribution from patchy to fairly extensive gastric involvement. Intestinal metaplasia is an important predisposing factor for gastric cancer (Chap. 90).

Chronic gastritis is also classified according to the predominant site of involvement. Type A refers to the body-predominant form (autoimmune) and type B is the central-predominant form (*H. pylori*–related). This classification is artificial in view of the difficulty in distinguishing these two entities. The term *AB gastritis* has been used to refer to a mixed antral/body picture.

Type A Gastritis The less common of the two forms involves primarily the fundus and body, with antral sparing. Traditionally, this form of gastritis has been associated with pernicious anemia (Chap. 107) in the presence of circulating antibodies against parietal cells and intrinsic factor; thus it is also called *autoimmune gastritis*. *H. pylori* infection can lead to a similar distribution of gastritis. The characteristics of an autoimmune picture are not always present.

Antibodies to parietal cells have been detected in >90% of patients with pernicious anemia and in up to 50% of patients with type A gastritis. Anti-parietal cell antibodies are cytotoxic for gastric mucous cells. The parietal cell antibody is directed against H^+,K^+-ATPase. T cells are also implicated in the injury pattern of this form of gastritis.

Parietal cell antibodies and atrophic gastritis are observed in family members of patients with pernicious anemia. These antibodies are observed in up to 20% of individuals over age 60 and in ~20% of patients with vitiligo and Addison's disease. About half of patients with pernicious anemia have antibodies to thyroid antigens, and about 30% of patients with thyroid disease have circulating anti-parietal cell antibodies. Anti-intrinsic factor antibodies are more specific than parietal cell antibodies for type A gastritis, being present in ~40% of patients with pernicious anemia. Another parameter consistent with this form of gastritis being autoimmune in origin is the higher incidence of specific familial histocompatibility haplotypes such as HLA-B8 and -DR3.

The parietal cell–containing gastric gland is preferentially targeted in this form of gastritis, and achlorhydria results. Parietal cells are the source of intrinsic factor, lack of which will lead to vitamin B_{12} deficiency and its sequelae (megaloblastic anemia, neurologic dysfunction).

Gastric acid plays an important role in feedback inhibition of gastrin release from G cells. Achlorhydria, coupled with relative sparing of the antral mucosa (site of G cells), leads to hypergastrinemia. Gastrin levels can be markedly elevated (>500 pg/mL) in patients with pernicious anemia. ECL cell hyperplasia with frank development of gastric carcinoid tumors may result from gastrin trophic effects. The role of gastrin in carcinoid development is confirmed by the observation that antrectomy leads to regression of these lesions. Hypergastrinemia and achlorhydria may also be seen in non-pernicious anemia-associated type A gastritis.

Type B gastritis Type B, or antral-predominant, gastritis is the more common form of chronic gastritis. *H. pylori* infection is the cause of this entity. Although described as "antral-predominant," this is likely a misnomer in view of studies documenting the progression of the inflammatory process towards the body and fundus of infected individuals. The conversion to a pan-gastritis is time-dependent—estimated to require 15 to 20 years. This form of gastritis increases with age, being present in up to 100% of people over age 70. Histology improves after *H. pylori* eradication. The number of *H. pylori* organisms decreases dramatically with progression to gastric atrophy, and the degree of inflammation correlates with the level of these organisms. Early on, with antral-predominant findings, the quantity of *H. pylori* is highest and a dense chronic inflammatory infiltrate of the lamina propria is noted accompanied by epithelial cell infiltration with polymorphonuclear leukocytes (Fig. 285-12).

Multifocal atrophic gastritis, gastric atrophy with subsequent metaplasia, has been observed in chronic *H. pylori*–induced gastritis. This may ultimately lead to development of gastric adenocarcinoma (Fig. 285-13; Chap. 90). *H. pylori* infection is now considered an independent risk factor for gastric cancer. Worldwide epidemiologic studies have documented a higher incidence of *H. pylori* infection in patients with adenocarcinoma of the stomach as compared to control subjects. Seropositivity for *H. pylori* is associated with a three- to sixfold increased risk of gastric cancer. This risk may be as high as ninefold after adjusting for the inaccuracy of serologic testing in the elderly. The mechanism by which *H. pylori* infection leads to cancer is unknown. However, eradication of *H. pylori* as a general preventative measure for gastric cancer is not recommended.

Infection with *H. pylori* is also associated with development of a low grade B cell lymphoma, gastric MALT lymphoma (Chap. 112). The chronic T cell stimulation caused by the infection leads to production of cytokines that promote the B cell tumor. Tumor growth remains dependent upon the presence of *H. pylori* in that its eradication is often associated with complete regression of the tumor. The tumor may take more than a year to regress after treating the infection. Such patients should be followed by EUS every 2 to 3 months. If the tumor is stable or decreasing in size, no other therapy is necessary. If the tumor grows, it may have become a high-grade B cell lymphoma. When the tumor becomes a high-grade aggressive lymphoma histologically, it loses responsiveness to *H. pylori* eradication.

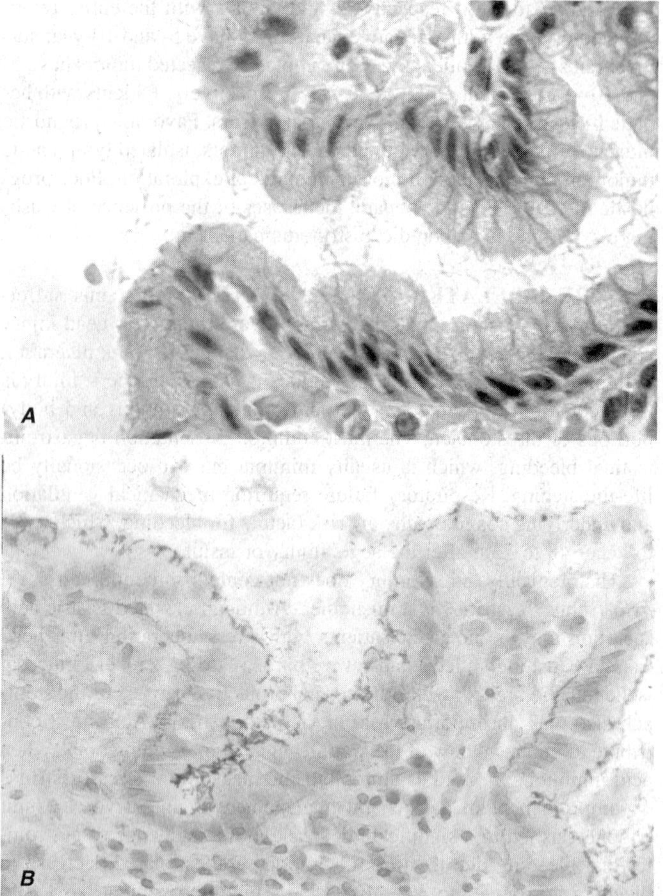

FIGURE 285-12 Chronic gastritis and *Helicobacter pylori* organisms. *A.* H&E stain of gastric mucosa showing surface foveolar cells, adherent mucus, and scattered bacillary forms within the mucus. *B.* Steiner silver stain of superficial gastric mucosa, showing abundant darkly staining microorganisms layered over the apical portion of the surface epithelium. Note that there is no tissue invasion. *[Courtesy of James M. Crawford, M.D., Ph.D. Reprinted with permission from JM Crawford, in V Kumar et al (eds): Basic Pathology. Philadelphia, Saunders, 1997]*

℞ **TREATMENT** Treatment in chronic gastritis is aimed at the sequelae and not the underlying inflammation. Patients with pernicious anemia will require parenteral vitamin B_{12} supplementation on a long-term basis. Eradication of *H. pylori* is not routinely recommended unless PUD or a low-grade MALT lymphoma is present.

Miscellaneous Forms of Gastritis *Lymphocytic gastritis* is characterized histologically by intense infiltration of the surface epithelium with lymphocytes. The infiltrative process is primarily in the body of the stomach and consists of mature T cells and plasmacytes. The etiology of this form of chronic gastritis is unknown. It has been described in patients with celiac sprue, but whether there is a common factor associating these two entities is unknown. No specific symptoms suggest lymphocytic gastritis. A subgroup of patients has thickened folds noted on endoscopy. These folds are often capped by small nodules that contain a central depression or erosion; this form of the disease is called *varioliform gastritis. H. pylori* probably plays no significant role in lymphocytic gastritis. Therapy with glucocorticoids or sodium cromoglycate has obtained unclear results.

Marked eosinophilic infiltration involving any layer of the stomach (mucosa, muscularis propria, and serosa) is characteristic of *eosinophilic gastritis*. Affected individuals will often have circulating eosinophilia with clinical manifestation of systemic allergy. Involvement may range from isolated gastric disease to diffuse eosinophilic gastroenteritis. Antral involvement predominates, with prominent edematous folds being observed on endoscopy. These prominent antral folds can lead to outlet obstruction. Patients can present with epigastric discomfort, nausea, and vomiting. Treatment with glucocorticoids has been successful.

Several systemic disorders may be associated with *granulomatous gastritis*. Gastric involvement has been observed in Crohn's disease. Involvement may range from granulomatous infiltrates noted only on gastric biopsies to frank ulceration and stricture formation. Gastric Crohn's disease usually occurs in the presence of small-intestinal disease. Several rare infectious processes can lead to granulomatous gastritis, including histoplasmosis, candidiasis, syphilis, and tuberculosis. Other unusual causes of this form of gastritis include sarcoidosis, idiopathic granulomatous gastritis, and eosinophilic granulomas involving the stomach. Establishing the specific etiologic agent in this form of gastritis can be difficult, at times requiring repeat endoscopy with biopsy and cytology. Occasionally, a surgically obtained full-thickness biopsy of the stomach may be required to exclude malignancy.

MÉNÉTRIER'S DISEASE Ménétrier's disease is a rare entity characterized by large, tortuous gastric mucosal folds. The differential diagnosis of large gastric folds includes ZES, malignancy, infectious etiologies (CMV, histoplasmosis, syphilis), and infiltrative disorders such as sarcoidosis. The mucosal folds in Ménétrier's disease are often most prominent in the body and fundus. Histologically, massive foveolar hyperplasia (hyperplasia of surface and glandular mucous cells) is noted, which replaces most of the chief and parietal cells. This hyperplasia produces the prominent folds observed. The pits of the gastric glands elongate and may become extremely tortuous. Although the lamina propria may contain a mild chronic inflammatory infiltrate, Ménétrier's disease is *not* considered a form of gastritis. The etiology of this unusual clinical picture is unknown. Overexpression of growth factors such as TGF-α may be involved in the process.

Epigastric pain at times accompanied by nausea, vomiting, anorexia, and weight loss are signs and symptoms in patients with Ménétrier's disease. Occult gastrointestinal bleeding may occur, but overt bleeding is unusual and, when present, is due to superficial mucosal erosions. Between 20 and 100% of patients (depending on time of presentation) develop a protein-losing gastropathy accompanied by hypoalbuminemia and edema. Gastric acid secretion is usually reduced or absent because of the replacement of parietal cells. Large gastric folds are readily detectable by either radiographic (barium meal) or endoscopic methods. Endoscopy with deep mucosal biopsy (and cytology) is required to establish the diagnosis and exclude the other entities that may present in a similar manner. A nondiagnostic biopsy may lead to a surgically obtained full-thickness biopsy to exclude malignancy.

℞ **TREATMENT** Medical therapy with anticholinergic agents, prostaglandins, PPIs, prednisone, and H_2 receptor antagonists has obtained varying results. Anticholinergics decrease protein loss. A high-protein diet should be recommended to replace protein loss in patients with hypoalbuminemia. Ulcers should be treated with a standard approach. Severe disease with persistent and substantial protein loss may require total gastrectomy. Subtotal gastrectomy is performed by some; it may be associated with higher morbidity and mortality secondary to the difficulty in obtaining a patent and long-lasting anastomosis between normal and hyperplastic tissues.

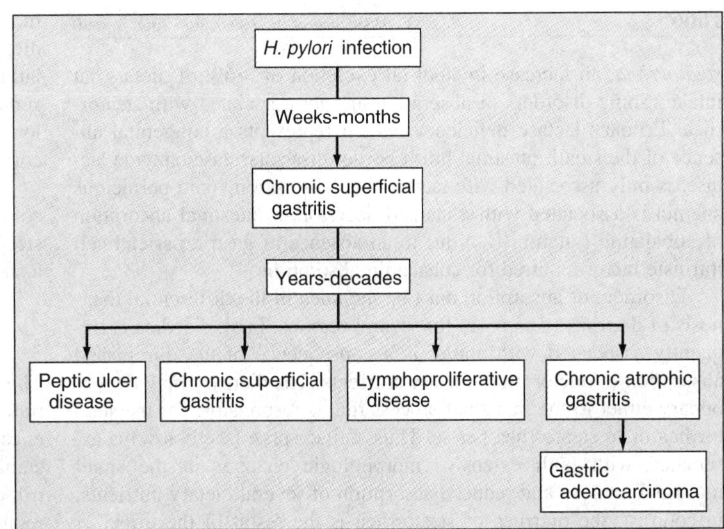

FIGURE 285-13 Potential long-term consequences of *H. pylori* infection.

ACKNOWLEDGMENT

The author acknowledges the contribution of material to this chapter by Dr. Lawrence Friedman and Dr. Walter Peterson from their chapter on this subject in the 14th edition and is grateful to Pamela Glazer for typing this manuscript.

BIBLIOGRAPHY

AGREUS L, TALLEY NJ: Dyspepsia: Current understanding and management. Annu Rev Med 49:475, 1997

BERARDI RR, WELAGE LS: Proton-pump inhibitors in acid-related diseases. Am J Health Syst Pharm 55:2249, 1998

CAPPELL MS, SCHEIN JR: Diagnosis and treatment of nonsteroidal anti-inflammatory drug-associated upper gastrointestinal toxicity. Gastroenterol Clin North Am 29:97, 2000

GRAHAM DY et al: Practical advice on eradicating *Helicobacter pylori* infection. Postgrad Med 105:137, 1999

KALANTAR J et al: Chronic gastritis and nonulcer dyspepsia. Curr Top Microbiol Immunol 241:31, 1999

MCCOLL KE et al: Interactions between *H. pylori* infection, gastric acid secretion and antisecretory therapy. Br Med Bull 54:121, 1998

MITCHELL HM: The epidemiology of *Helicobacter pylori*. Curr Top Microbiol Immunol 241:11, 1999

NORTON JA et al: Surgery to cure the Zollinger-Ellison syndrome. N Engl J Med 341: 635, 1999

PEEK RM JR, BLASER MJ: Pathophysiology of *Helicobacter pylori*–induced gastritis and peptic ulcer disease. Am J Med 102:200, 1997

WOLFE MM et al: Gastrointestinal toxicity of nonsteroidal antiinflammatory drugs. N Engl J Med 340:1888, 1999

286

Henry J. Binder

DISORDERS OF ABSORPTION

Disorders of absorption represent a broad spectrum of conditions with multiple etiologies and varied clinical manifestations. Almost all of these clinical problems are associated with *diminished* intestinal absorption of one or more dietary nutrients and are often referred to as the *malabsorption syndrome*. This latter term is not ideal as it represents a pathophysiologic state, does *not* provide an etiologic explanation for the underlying problem, and should not be considered an adequate final diagnosis. The only clinical situations in which absorption is *increased* are hemochromatosis and Wilson's disease, in which there is increased absorption of iron and copper, respectively.

Most, but not all, of these clinical conditions are associated with *steatorrhea*, an increase in stool fat excretion of >6% of dietary fat intake. Some disorders of absorption are not associated with steatorrhea: Primary lactase deficiency, which represents a congenital absence of the small intestinal brush border disaccharidase enzyme lactase, is only associated with lactose "malabsorption," and pernicious anemia is associated with a marked decrease in intestinal absorption of cobalamin (vitamin B_{12}) due to an absence of gastric parietal cell intrinsic factor required for cobalamin absorption.

Disorders of absorption must be included in the differential diagnosis of diarrhea (Chap. 42) for several reasons. First, diarrhea is frequently associated with and/or is a consequence of the diminished absorption of one or more dietary nutrients. The diarrhea may be secondary either to the intestinal process that is responsible for the steatorrhea or to steatorrhea per se. Thus, celiac sprue (see below) is associated with both extensive morphologic changes in the small intestinal mucosa and reduced absorption of several dietary nutrients; in contrast, the diarrhea of steatorrhea is the result of the effect of nonabsorbed dietary fatty acids on intestinal, usually colonic, ion transport. For example, oleic acid and ricinoleic acid (a bacterially hydroxylated fatty acid that is also the active ingredient in castor oil, a widely used laxative) induce active colonic Cl secretion, most likely secondary to increasing intracellular Ca. In addition, diarrhea per se may result in mild steatorrhea (<11 g fat excretion while on a 100-g fat diet). Second, as diarrhea is both a symptom and a sign, most patients will indicate that they have diarrhea, not that they have fat malabsorption. Third, many intestinal disorders that have diarrhea as a prominent symptom (e.g., ulcerative colitis, traveler's diarrhea secondary to an enterotoxin produced by *Escherichia coli*) do not necessarily have diminished absorption of any dietary nutrient.

Diarrhea as a *symptom* (i.e., when used by patients to describe their bowel movement pattern) may be either a decrease in stool consistency, an increase in stool volume, an increase in number of bowel movements, or any combination of these three changes. In contrast, diarrhea as a *sign* is a quantitative increase in stool water or weight of >200 to 225 mL, or g per 24 h, when a western-type diet is consumed. Individuals consuming a diet with a higher fiber content may normally have a stool weight of up to 400 g/24 h. Thus, it is essential that the clinician clarify what an individual patient means by diarrhea, especially since 10% of patients referred to gastroenterologists for further evaluation of unexplained diarrhea do not have an increase in stool water when it is determined quantitatively. Such patients may have small, frequent, somewhat loose bowel movements with stool urgency that is indicative of proctitis but do not have an increase in stool weight or volume.

It is also critical to establish whether a patient's diarrhea is secondary to diminished absorption of one or more dietary nutrients, in contrast to diarrhea that is due to small- and/or large-intestinal fluid and electrolyte secretion. The former has often been termed *osmotic diarrhea*, while the latter has been referred to as *secretory diarrhea*. Unfortunately, as there can be both secretory and osmotic elements present simultaneously in the same disorder, this separation is not always precise. Nonetheless, two studies, determination of stool electrolytes, and observation of the effect of a fast on stool output can help make this distinction.

The demonstration of the effect of prolonged (>24 h) fasting on stool output can be very effective in suggesting that a *dietary nutrient* is responsible for the individual's diarrhea. A secretory diarrhea associated with enterotoxin-induced traveler's diarrhea would not be affected by prolonged fasting, as enterotoxin-induced stimulation of intestinal fluid and electrolyte secretion is not altered by eating. In contrast, diarrhea secondary to lactose malabsorption in primary lactase deficiency would undoubtedly cease during a prolonged fast. Thus, a substantial decrease in stool output while fasting during a quantitative stool collection of at least 24 h is presumptive evidence that the diarrhea is related to malabsorption of a dietary nutrient. The persistence of stool output while fasting indicates the likelihood that the diarrhea is secretory and that the cause of diarrhea is *not* due to a dietary nutrient. Either a luminal (e.g., *E. coli* enterotoxin) or circulating (e.g., vasoactive intestinal peptide) secretogogue could be responsible for the patient's diarrhea persisting unaltered during a prolonged fast. The observed effects of fasting can be compared and correlated with stool electrolyte and osmolality determinations.

Measurement of stool electrolytes and osmolality requires the comparison of stool Na^+ and K^+ concentrations determined in liquid stool to the stool osmolality to determine the presence or absence of a so-called stool osmotic gap. The following formula is used:

$$2 \times (\text{stool } [Na^+] + \text{stool } [K^+]) \geq \text{stool osmolality}$$

The cation concentrations are doubled to estimate stool anion concentrations. The presence of a significant osmotic gap suggests the presence in stool water of a substance(s) other than Na/K/anions that presumably is responsible for the patient's diarrhea. Originally, stool osmolality was measured, but it is almost invariably greater than the required 290 to 300 mosmol/kg H_2O, reflecting bacterial degradation of nonabsorbed carbohydrate either immediately before defecation or in the stool jar while awaiting chemical analysis, even when the stool is refrigerated. As a result, the stool osmolality should be assumed to be 300 mosmol/kg H_2O. When the calculated difference is >50, an osmotic gap is present, suggesting that the diarrhea is due to a nonabsorbed dietary nutrient, e.g., a fatty acid and/or carbohydrate. When this difference is <25 to 50, it is presumed that a dietary nutrient is not responsible for the diarrhea. Since elements of both osmotic (i.e., malabsorption of a dietary nutrient) and secretory diarrhea may be present simultaneously, this separation at times is less clear-cut at the bedside than when used as a teaching example. Ideally, the presence of an osmotic gap will be associated with a marked decrease in stool output during a prolonged fast, while the absence of an osmotic gap will likely be present in an individual whose stool output had not been reduced substantially during a period of fasting.

NUTRIENT DIGESTION AND ABSORPTION

The lengths of the small intestine and colon are ~300 cm and ~80 cm, respectively. However, the effective functional surface area is approximately 600-fold greater than that of a hollow tube as a result of the presence of folds, villi (in the small intestine), and microvilli. The functional surface area of the small intestine is somewhat greater than that of a doubles tennis court. In addition to nutrient digestion and absorption, the intestinal epithelia have several other functions:

1. *Barrier and immune defense*. The intestine is exposed to a large number of potential antigens, enteric and invasive microorganisms, and is extremely effective preventing the entry of almost all these agents. The intestinal mucosa also synthesizes and secretes secretory IgA globulin.
2. *Fluid and electrolyte absorption and secretion*. The intestine absorbs approximately 7 to 8 L of fluid daily, comprising dietary fluid intake (1 to 2 L/d) and salivary, gastric, pancreatic, biliary, and intestinal fluid (6 to 7 L/d). The intestine also responds to several stimuli, especially bacteria and bacterial enterotoxins, that induce fluid and electrolyte secretion, often leading to diarrhea (Chap. 131).
3. *Synthesis and secretion of several proteins*. The intestinal mucosa is a major site for the production of proteins, including apolipoproteins.
4. *Production of several bioactive amines and peptides*. The intestine presents one of the largest endocrine organs in the body and produces several amines and peptides that serve as paracrine and hormonal mediators of intestinal function.

The small and large intestine are anatomically distinct in that villi are present in the small intestine but are absent in the colon and functionally distinct in that nutrient digestion and absorption take place in the small intestine but not in the colon. No precise anatomic characteristics separate duodenum, jejunum, and ileum, although certain nutrients are absorbed exclusively in specific areas of the small intestine. However, villus cells in the small intestine (and surface epithelial cells in the colon) and crypt cells have distinct anatomic and functional characteristics. Intestinal epithelial cells are continuously renewed, with new proliferating epithelial cells at the base of the crypt migrating over 48 to 72 h to the tip of the villus (or surface of the colon), where they are well-developed epithelial cells with digestive and absorptive function. This high rate of cell turnover explains the relatively rapid resolution of diarrhea and other digestive tract side effects during chemotherapy as new cells not exposed to these toxic agents are produced. Equally important is the paradigm of separation of villus/surface cell and crypt cell function: digestive hydrolytic enzymes are present primarily in the brush border of villus epithelial cells. Absorptive and secretory functions are also separated, with villus/surface cells largely being the site for absorptive function, while secretory function is present in crypts of both the small and large intestine.

Nutrients, minerals, and vitamins are absorbed by one or more active transport mechanisms. (The mechanisms of intestinal fluid and electrolyte absorption and secretion are discussed in Chap. 42.) Active transport mechanisms are energy-dependent and mediated by membrane transport proteins. These transport processes will result in the *net* movement of a substance against or in the absence of an electrochemical concentration gradient. Intestinal absorption of amino acids and monosaccharides, e.g., glucose, is also a specialized form of active transport—*secondary active transport*. The movement of these actively transported nutrients against a concentration gradient is Na^+-dependent and is due to a Na^+ gradient across the apical membrane. The Na^+ gradient is maintained by Na^+,K^+-ATPase, the so-called Na^+ pump located on the basolateral membrane, which extrudes Na^+ and maintains a low intracellular [Na] as well as the Na^+ gradient across the apical membrane. As a result, active glucose absorption and glucose-stimulated Na^+ absorption require both the apical membrane transport protein, SGLT, and the basolateral Na^+,K^+-ATPase. In addition to glucose absorption being Na^+-dependent, glucose also stimulates Na^+ and fluid absorption, which is the physiologic basis of oral rehydration therapy for the treatment of diarrhea (Chap. 42).

Although the intestinal epithelial cells are crucial mediators of absorption and ion and water flow, the several cell types in the lamina propria (e.g., mast cells, macrophages, myofibroblasts) and the enteric nervous system interact with the epithelium to regulate mucosal cell function. The function of the intestine is the result of the integrated responses of and interactions between both intestinal epithelial cells and intestinal muscle.

ENTEROHEPATIC CIRCULATION OF BILE ACIDS

Bile acids are not present in the diet but are synthesized in the liver by a series of enzymatic steps that also represent cholesterol catabolism. Indeed, interruption of the enterohepatic circulation of bile acids can reduce serum cholesterol levels by 10% before a new steady state is established. Bile acids are either primary or secondary: primary bile acids are synthesized in the liver from cholesterol, and secondary bile acids are synthesized from primary bile acids in the intestine by colonic bacterial enzymes. The two primary bile acids are cholic acid and chenodeoxycholic acid; the two most abundant secondary bile acids are deoxycholic acid and lithocholic acid. Approximately 500 mg bile acids are synthesized in the liver daily, conjugated to either taurine or glycine to form tauro-conjugated or glyco-conjugated bile acids, respectively, that are secreted into the duodenum in bile. The primary functions of bile acids are (1) to promote bile flow, (2) to solubilize cholesterol and phospholipid in the gall bladder by mixed micelle formation, and (3) to enhance dietary lipid digestion and absorption by forming mixed micelles in the proximal small intestine.

Bile acids are primarily absorbed by an active, Na^+-dependent process that is located exclusively in the ileum, though bile acids can also be absorbed to a lesser extent by non-carrier-mediated transport processes in the jejunum, ileum, and colon. Conjugated bile acids that enter the colon are deconjugated by colonic bacterial enzymes to un-

conjugated bile acids and are rapidly absorbed. Colonic bacterial enzymes also dehydroxylate bile acids to secondary bile acids.

Bile acids absorbed from the intestine return to the liver via the portal vein where they are resecreted (Fig. 286-1). Bile acid synthesis is largely autoregulated by 7α-hydroxylase, the initial enzyme in cholesterol degradation. A decrease in the amount of bile acids returning to the liver from the intestine is associated with an increase in bile acid synthesis/cholesterol catabolism, which helps maintain the bile acid pool size relatively constant. However, there is a relatively limited capacity for an increase in bile acid synthesis—about two to two and one-half times (see below). The bile acid pool size is approximately 4 g and is circulated via the enterohepatic circulation about twice during each meal, or six to eight times during a 24-h period. A relatively small quantity of bile acids is not absorbed and is excreted in stool daily; this fecal loss is matched by hepatic bile acid synthesis.

Defects in any of the steps of the enterohepatic circulation of bile acids can result in a decrease in duodenal concentration of conjugated bile acids and, as a result, steatorrhea. Thus, steatorrhea can be caused by abnormalities in bile acid synthesis and excretion, their physical state in the intestinal lumen, and reabsorption (Table 286-1).

Synthesis Decreased bile acid synthesis and steatorrhea have been demonstrated in chronic liver disease, but steatorrhea is often not a major component of the illness of these patients.

Secretion Although bile acid secretion may be reduced or absent in biliary obstruction, steatorrhea is rarely a significant medical problem in these patients. In contrast, primary biliary cirrhosis represents a defect in canalicular excretion of organic anions, including bile acids, and not infrequently is associated with steatorrhea and its consequences, e.g., chronic bone disease. Thus, the osteomalacia and other chronic bone abnormalities often present in patients with primary biliary cirrhosis and other cholestatic syndromes are secondary to steatorrhea that then leads to calcium and vitamin D malabsorption.

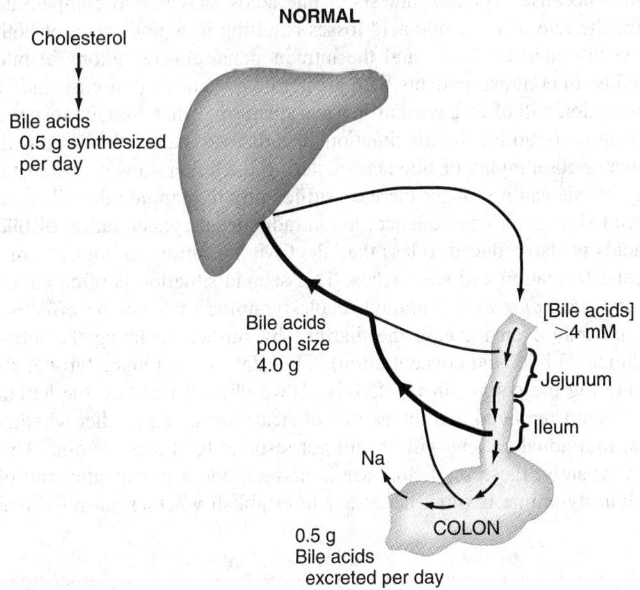

FIGURE 286-1 Schematic representation of the enterohepatic circulation of bile acids. Bile acid synthesis is cholesterol catabolism and occurs in the liver. Bile acids are secreted in bile and are stored in the gall bladder between meals and at night. Food in the duodenum induces the release of cholecystokinin, which is a potent stimulus for gall bladder contraction resulting in bile acid entry into the duodenum. Bile acids are primarily absorbed via a Na-dependent transport process that is located only in the ileum. A relatively small quantity of bile acids (~500 mg) are not absorbed in a 24-h period and are lost in stool. Fecal bile acid losses are matched by bile acid synthesis. The bile acid pool, i.e., the total amount of bile acids in the body at any time, is ~4 g and is circulated twice during each meal or six to eight times in a 24-h period.

Table 286-1 Defects in Enterohepatic Circulation of Bile Acids

Process	Pathophysiologic Defect	Disease Example
Synthesis	Decreased hepatic function	Cirrhosis
Biliary secretion	Altered canalicular function	Primary biliary cirrhosis
Maintenance of conjugated bile acids	Bacterial overgrowth	Jejunal diverticulosis
Reabsorption	Abnormal ileal function	Crohn's disease

Maintenance of Conjugated Bile Acids In bacterial overgrowth syndromes associated with diarrhea, steatorrhea, and macrocytic anemia, there is an increase in a colonic-type of bacterial flora in the small intestine. The steatorrhea is primarily a result of the decrease in conjugated bile acids secondary to their deconjugation by colonic-type bacteria. Two complementary explanations account for the resulting impairment of micelle formation: (1) unconjugated bile acids are rapidly absorbed in the jejunum by nonionic diffusion resulting in a reduced concentration of duodenal bile acids; and (2) the critical micellar concentration (CMC) of unconjugated bile acids is higher than that of conjugated bile acids, and therefore unconjugated bile acids are less effective than conjugated bile acids in micelle formation.

Reabsorption Ileal dysfunction caused by either Crohn's disease or surgical resection results in a decrease in bile acid reabsorption in the ileum and an *increase* in the delivery of bile acids to the large intestine. The resulting clinical consequences—diarrhea with or without steatorrhea—is determined by the *degree* of ileal dysfunction and the *response* of the enterohepatic circulation to bile acid losses (Table 286-2). Patients with limited ileal disease or resection will often have diarrhea, but not steatorrhea. The diarrhea, a result of bile acids in the colon stimulating active Cl secretion, has been called *bile acid diarrhea*, or cholorrheic enteropathy, and responds promptly to cholestyramine, an anion-binding resin. Such patients do not develop steatorrhea because hepatic synthesis of bile acids increases to compensate for the rate of fecal bile acid losses resulting in maintenance of both the bile acid pool size and the intraduodenal concentrations of bile acids. In contrast, patients with greater degrees of ileal disease and/or resection will often have diarrhea and steatorrhea that does not respond to cholestyramine. In this situation, ileal disease is also associated with increased amounts of bile acids entering the colon; however, hepatic synthesis can no longer increase sufficiently to maintain the bile acid pool size. As a consequence, the intraduodenal concentration of bile acids is also reduced to less than the CMC, resulting in impaired micelle formation and steatorrhea. This second situation is often called *fatty acid diarrhea*. Although cholestyramine may not be effective (and may even increase the diarrhea by further depleting the intraduodenal bile acid concentration), a low-fat diet to reduce fatty acids entering the colon can be effective. Two clinical features, the length of ileum removed and the degree of steatorrhea, can predict whether an individual patient will or will not respond to cholestyramine. Unfortunately, these predictors are imperfect, and a therapeutic trial of cholestyramine is often necessary to establish whether an individual patient will benefit from cholestyramine. Table 286-2 contrasts the characteristics of bile acid diarrhea (small ileal dysfunction) and fatty acid diarrhea (large ileal dysfunction).

Table 286-2 Comparison of Bile Acid and Fatty Acid Diarrhea

	Bile Acid Diarrhea	Fatty Acid Diarrhea
Extent of ileal disease	Limited	Extensive
Ileal bile acid absorption	Reduced	Reduced
Fecal bile acid excretion	Increased	Increased
Fecal bile acid loss compensated by hepatic synthesis	Yes	No
Bile acid pool size	Normal	Reduced
Intraduodenal [bile acid]	Normal	Reduced
Steatorrhea	None or mild	>20 g
Response to cholestyramine	Yes	No
Response to low-fat diet	No	Yes

LIPIDS Steatorrhea is caused by one or more defects in the digestion and absorption of dietary fat. Average intake of dietary fat in the United States is approximately 120 to 150 g/d, and fat absorption is linear to dietary fat intake. The total load of fat presented to the small intestine is considerably greater, as substantial amounts of lipid are secreted in bile each day. (See above for discussion of enterohepatic circulation of bile acids.) Three types of fatty acids compose fats: long-chain fatty acids (LCFAs), medium-chain fatty acids (MCFAs), and short-chain fatty acids (SCFAs) (Table 286-3). Dietary fat is exclusively composed of long-chain triglycerides (LCTs), i.e., glycerol that is bound via ester-linkages to three LCFAs. While the majority of dietary LCFAs have carbon chain lengths of 16 or 18, fatty acids of carbon chain length >12 are metabolized in the same manner; saturated and unsaturated fatty acids are handled identically.

Assimilation of dietary lipid requires several integrated processes that can be divided into (1) an intraluminal, or digestive, phase; (2) a mucosal, or absorptive, phase; and (3) a delivery, or postabsorptive, phase. An abnormality at any site of this process can cause steatorrhea (Table 286-4). Therefore, it is essential that any patient with steatorrhea be evaluated to identify the specific physiologic defect in overall lipid digestion-absorption as therapy will be determined by the specific cause responsible for the steatorrhea.

The digestive phase has two components, *lipolysis* and *micellar formation*. Although dietary lipid is in the form of LCTs, the intestinal mucosa does not absorb triglycerides; they must first be hydrolyzed (Fig. 286-2). The initial step in lipid digestion is the formation of emulsions of finely dispersed lipid, which is accomplished by mastication and gastric contractions. Lipolysis, the hydrolysis of triglycerides to free fatty acids, monoglycerides, and glycerol by lipase, is initiated in the stomach by a gastric lipase that has a pH optimum of 4.5 to 6.0. About 20 to 30% of total lipolysis occurs in the stomach. Lipolysis is completed in the duodenum and proximal jejunal by pancreatic lipase, which is inactivated by pH <7.0. Pancreatic lipolysis is greatly enhanced by the presence of a second pancreatic enzyme, colipase, which facilitates the movement of lipase to the triglyceride.

Impaired lipolysis can lead to steatorrhea and can occur in the presence of pancreatic insufficiency due to chronic pancreatitis in adults or cystic fibrosis in children and adolescents. Normal lipolysis can be maintained by approximately 5% of maximal pancreatic lipase secretion; thus, steatorrhea is a late manifestation of these disorders. A reduction in intraduodenal pH can also result in altered lipolysis as pancreatic lipase is inactivated at pH <7. Thus, ~15% of patients with gastrinoma (Chap. 285) with substantial increases in gastric acid secretion from ectopic production of gastrin (usually from an islet cell

Table 286-3 Comparison of Different Types of Fatty Acids

	Long-Chain	Medium-Chain	Short-Chain
Carbon chain length	>12	8–12	<8
Present in diet	In large amounts	In small amounts	No
Origin	In diet as triglycerides	Only in small amounts in diet as triglycerides	Bacterial degradation in colon of nonabsorbed carbohydrate to fatty acids
Primary site of absorption	Small intestine	Small intestine	Colon
Requires pancreatic lipolysis	Yes	No	No
Requires micelle formation	Yes	No	No
Presence in stool	Minimal	No	Substantial

Table 286-4 Defects in Lipid Digestion and Absorption in Steatorrhea

Phase: Process	Pathophysiologic Defect	Disease Example
Digestive		
Lipolysis formation	Decrease lipase secretion	Chronic pancreatitis
Micelle formation	Decreased intraduodenal [bile acids]	See Table 286-1
Absorptive		
Mucosal uptake and resterification	Mucosal dysfunction	Celiac sprue
Post-absorptive		
Chylomicron formation	Absent betalipoproteins	Abetalipoproteinemia
Delivery from intestine	Abnormal lymphatics	Intestinal lymphangiectasia

adenoma) have diarrhea, and some will have steatorrhea believed secondary to acid-inactivation of pancreatic lipase. Similarly, patients with chronic pancreatitis (who have reduced lipase secretion) often have a decrease in pancreatic bicarbonate secretion, which will also result in a decrease in intraduodenal pH and inactivation of endogenous pancreatic lipase or of therapeutically administered lipase.

Overlying the microvillus membrane of the small intestine is the so-called unstirred water layer, a relatively stagnant aqueous phase that must be traversed by the products of lipolysis that are primarily water-insoluble. Water-soluble mixed micelles provide a mechanism for the water-insoluble products of lipolysis to reach the luminal plasma membrane of villus epithelial cells, the site for lipid absorption. Mixed micelles are molecular aggregates composed of fatty acids, monoglycerides, phospholipids, cholesterol, and conjugated bile acids. Mixed micelles are formed when the concentration of conjugated bile acids is greater than its CMC, which differs among the several bile acids present in the small intestinal lumen. Conjugated bile acids, synthesized in the liver and excreted into the duodenum in bile, are regulated by the enterohepatic circulation (see above). Steatorrhea can result from impaired movement of fatty acids across the unstirred aqueous fluid layer in two situations: (1) an increase in the relative thickness of the unstirred water layer that occurs in bacterial overgrowth syndromes (see below) secondary to functional stasis (e.g., scleroderma), and (2) a decrease in the *duodenal* concentration of conjugated bile acids below its CMC, resulting in impaired micelle formation. Thus, steatorrhea can be caused by one or more defects in the enterohepatic circulation of bile acids.

Uptake and reesterification represent the *absorptive phase* of lipid digestion-absorption. Although passive diffusion has been thought responsible, a carrier-mediated process may mediate fatty acid and monoglyceride uptake. Regardless of the uptake process, fatty acids and monoglycerides are reesterified by a series of enzymatic steps in the endoplasmic reticulum and Golgi to form triglycerides, the form in which lipid exits from the intestinal epithelial cell. Impaired lipid absorption as a result of either mucosal inflammation (e.g., celiac sprue) and/or intestinal resection can also lead to steatorrhea.

The reesterified triglycerides require the formation of *chylomicrons* to permit their exit from the small-intestinal epithelial cell and their delivery to the liver via the *lymphatics*. Chylomicrons are composed of β-lipoprotein and contain triglycerides, cholesterol, cholesterol esters, and phospholipids and enter the lymphatics, not the portal vein. Defects in the *postabsorptive phase* of lipid digestion-absorption can also result in steatorrhea, but these disorders are uncommon. Abetalipoproteinemia, or acanthocytosis, is a rare disorder of impaired synthesis of β-lipoprotein associated with abnormal erythrocytes (acanthocytes), neurologic problems, and steatorrhea. Lipolysis, micelle formation, and lipid uptake are all normal in patients with abetalipoproteinemia, but the reesterified triglyceride cannot exit from the epithelial cell because of the failure to produce chylomicrons. Small-intestinal biopsies of these rare patients in the postprandial state reveal lipid-laden small-intestinal epithelial cells that become perfectly normal in appearance following a 72- to 96-fast. Similarly, abnormalities of intestinal lymphatics (e.g., intestinal lymphangiectasia) may also be associated with steatorrhea as well as protein loss (see below). Steatorrhea can result from defects at any of the several steps in lipid digestion-absorption. The mechanism of lipid digestion-absorption outlined above is limited to *dietary* lipid that is almost exclusively in the form of LCTs (Table 286-3). Medium-chain triglycerides (MCTs), composed of fatty acids with carbon chain lengths of 8 to 10, are present in large amounts in coconut oil and are used as a nutritional supplement. MCTs can be digested and absorbed by a different pathway from LCTs and at one time held promise as an important treatment of steatorrhea of almost all etiologies. Unfortunately, their therapeutic effects have been less than expected because their use is often not associated with an increase in body weight for reasons that are not completely understood.

MCTs, in contrast to LCTs, do not require pancreatic lipolysis as the triglyceride can be absorbed intact by the intestinal epithelial cell. Further, micelle formation is not necessary for the absorption of MCTs or medium-chain fatty acids, if hydrolyzed by pancreatic lipase. MCTs are absorbed more efficiently than LCTs for the following reasons: (1) the rate of MCT absorption is greater than that of long-chain fatty acids; (2) medium-chain fatty acids following absorption are not reesterified; (3) following absorption, MCTs are hydrolyzed to medium-chain fatty acids; (4) MCTs do not require chylomicron formation for their exit from the intestinal epithelial cells; and (5) their route of exit is via the portal vein and not via lymphatics. Thus, the absorption of MCTs is greater than that of LCTs in pancreatic insufficiency, conditions with reduced intraduodenal bile acid concentrations, small-intestinal mucosal disease, abetalipoproteinemia, and intestinal lymphangiectasia.

SCFAs are not dietary lipids but are synthesized by colonic bacterial enzymes from nonabsorbed carbohydrate and are the anions in highest concentration in stool (between 80 and 130 m*M*). The SCFAs present in stool are primarily acetate, propionate, and butyrate whose carbon chain lengths are 2, 3, and 4, respectively. Butyrate is the primary nutrient for colonic epithelial cells, and its deficiency may be associated with one or more colitides. SCFAs conserve calories and carbohydrate, because carbohydrates not completely absorbed in the small intestine will not be absorbed in the large intestine due to the absence of both disaccharidases and SGLT, the transport protein that

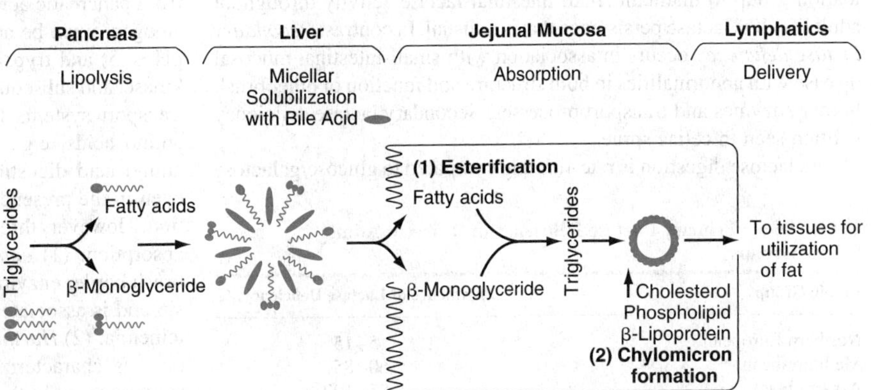

FIGURE 286-2 Schematic representation of lipid digestion and absorption. Dietary lipid is in the form of long-chain triglycerides (LCT). The overall process can be divided into (1) a digestive phase that includes both lipolysis and micelle formation requiring pancreatic lipase and conjugated bile acids, respectively, in the duodenum; (2) an absorptive phase for mucosal uptake and reesterification; and (3) a postabsorptive phase that includes chylomicron formation and exit from the intestinal epithelial cell via lymphatics. *(Courtesy of John M. Dietschy, MD.)*

mediates monosaccharide absorption. In contrast, SCFAs are rapidly absorbed and stimulate colonic Na-Cl and fluid absorption. Most non-*Clostridium difficile* antibiotic-associated diarrhea is due to antibiotic suppression of colonic microflora, with a resulting decrease in SCFA production. As *C. difficile* accounts for about 10 to 15% of all antibiotic-associated diarrhea, a relative decrease in colonic production of SCFAs is the cause of most antibiotic-associated diarrhea.

The clinical manifestations of steatorrhea are a consequence of both the underlying disorder responsible for the development of steatorrhea and steatorrhea per se. Depending on the degree of steatorrhea and the level of dietary intake, significant fat malabsorption may lead to weight loss. Steatorrhea per se can be responsible for diarrhea; if the primary cause of the steatorrhea has not been identified, a low-fat diet can often ameliorate the diarrhea by decreasing fecal fat excretion. Steatorrhea is often associated with fat-soluble vitamin deficiency, which will require replacement with water-soluble preparations of these vitamins.

Disorders of absorption may also be associated with malabsorption of other dietary nutrients, most often carbohydrates, with or without a decrease in dietary lipid digestion and absorption. Therefore, knowledge of the mechanism of the digestion and absorption of carbohydrates, proteins, and other minerals and vitamins is useful in the evaluation of patients with altered intestinal nutrient absorption.

CARBOHYDRATES Carbohydrates in the diet are present in the form of starch, disaccharides (sucrose and lactose), and glucose. Carbohydrates are absorbed only in the small intestine and only in the form of monosaccharides. Therefore, before their absorption, starch and disaccharides must first be digested by pancreatic amylase and intestinal brush border disaccharidases to monosaccharides. Monosaccharide absorption occurs by a Na-dependent process mediated by the brush border transport protein, SGLT.

Lactose malabsorption is the only clinically important disorder of carbohydrate absorption. Lactose, the disaccharide present in milk, requires digestion by brush border lactase to its two constituent monosaccharides, glucose and galactose. Lactase is present in almost all species in the postnatal period but then disappears throughout the animal kingdom, except in humans. Lactase activity persists in many individuals throughout life. Two different types of lactase deficiency exist—primary and secondary. In *primary lactase deficiency*, a genetically determined decrease or absence of lactase is noted, while all other aspects of both intestinal absorption and brush border enzymes are normal. In a number of non-Caucasian groups, primary lactase deficiency is common in adulthood. Table 286-5 presents the incidence of primary lactase deficiency in several different ethnic groups. Northern European and North American Caucasians are the only population group to maintain small-intestinal lactase activity throughout adult life. It is lactase persistence that is unusual. In contrast, *secondary lactase deficiency* occurs in association with small-intestinal mucosal disease with abnormalities in both structure and function of other brush border enzymes and transport processes. Secondary lactase deficiency is often seen in celiac sprue.

As lactose digestion is rate-limiting compared to glucose/galactose absorption, lactase deficiency is associated with significant lactose malabsorption. Some individuals with lactose malabsorption develop symptoms such as diarrhea, abdominal pain, cramps, and/or flatus. Most individuals with primary lactase deficiency do not have symptoms. Since lactose intolerance may be associated with symptoms suggestive of an irritable bowel syndrome, persistence of such symptoms in an individual with lactose intolerance while on a strict lactose-free diet would suggest that the individual's symptoms were related to irritable bowel syndrome.

Table 286-5 Primary Lactase Deficiency in Different Adult Ethnic Groups

Ethnic Group	Prevalence of Lactase Deficiency, %
Northern European	5–15
Mediterranean	60–85
African black	85–100
American black	45–80
American Caucasian	10–25
Native American	50–95
Mexican American	40–75
Asian	90–100

SOURCE: From FJ Simons: Am J Dig Dis 23:963, 1978.

Development of symptoms of lactose intolerance is related to several factors:

1. *Amount of lactose in the diet.*
2. *Rate of gastric emptying.* Symptoms are more likely when gastric emptying is rapid than when gastric emptying is slower. Therefore, it is more likely that skim milk will be associated with symptoms of lactose intolerance than whole milk as the rate of gastric emptying following skim milk intake is more rapid. Similarly, the diarrhea observed following subtotal gastrectomy is often a result of lactose intolerance as gastric emptying is accelerated in patients with a gastrojejunostomy.
3. *Small-intestinal transit time.* Although both the small and large intestine contribute to the development of symptoms, many of the symptoms of lactase deficiency are related to the interaction of colonic bacteria and nonabsorbed lactose. More rapid small-intestinal transit makes symptoms more likely.
4. *Colonic compensation by production of SCFAs* from nonabsorbed lactose. Reduced levels of colonic microflora, which can occur following antibiotic use, will also be associated with increased symptoms following lactose ingestion, especially in a lactase-deficient individual.

Glucose-galactose or monosaccharide malabsorption may also be associated with diarrhea and is due to a congenital absence of SGLT. Diarrhea is present when these individuals ingest carbohydrates that contain actively transported monosaccharides (e.g., glucose, galactose) but not monosaccharides that are not actively transported (e.g., fructose). Fructose is absorbed by the brush border transport protein, GLUT 5, a facilitated diffusion process that is not Na-dependent and is distinct from SGLT. In contrast, some individuals develop diarrhea as a result of consuming large quantities of sorbitol, a sugar used in diabetic candy; sorbitol is only minimally absorbed due to the absence of an intestinal absorptive transport mechanism for sorbitol.

PROTEINS Protein is present in food almost exclusively as polypeptides and requires extensive hydrolysis to di- and tripeptides and amino acids before absorption. Proteolysis occurs in both the stomach and small intestine; it is mediated by pepsin secreted as pepsinogen by gastric chief cells and trypsinogen and other peptidases from pancreatic acinar cells. These proenzymes, pepsinogen and trypsinogen, must be activated to pepsin (by pepsin in the presence of a $pH < 5$) and trypsin (by the intestinal brush border enzyme, enterokinase, and subsequently by trypsin). Proteins are absorbed by separate transport systems for di- and tripeptides and for different types of amino acids, e.g., neutral, dibasic. Alterations in either protein or amino acid digestion and absorption are rarely observed clinically, even in the presence of extensive small-intestinal mucosal inflammation. However, three rare genetic disorders involve protein digestion-absorption: (1) *enterokinase deficiency* is due to an absence of the brush border enzyme that converts the proenzyme trypsinogen to trypsin and is associated with diarrhea, growth retardation, and hypoproteinemia; (2) *Hartnup syndrome*, a defect in neutral amino acid transport, is characterized by a pellagra-like rash and neuropsychiatric symptoms; and (3) *cystinuria*, a defect in dibasic amino acid transport, is associated with renal calculi and chronic pancreatitis.

EVALUATION OF MALABSORPTION

The clues provided by the history, symptoms, and initial preliminary observations will serve to limit extensive, ill-focused, and expensive laboratory and imaging studies. For example, a clinician evaluating a patient with symptoms suggestive of malabsorption who recently had extensive small-intestinal resection for mesenteric ischemia should direct the initial assessment almost exclusively to define whether a short-bowel syndrome might explain the entire clinical picture. Similarly, the development of a pattern of bowel movements suggestive of steatorrhea in a patient with long-standing alcohol abuse and chronic pancreatitis should lead toward assessing pancreatic exocrine function.

The classic picture of malabsorption described in textbooks ≥30 years ago is rarely seen today in most parts of the United States. As a consequence, diseases with malabsorption must be suspected in individuals with less severe symptoms and signs and with subtle evidence of the altered absorption of only a *single* nutrient rather than obvious evidence of the malabsorption of multiple nutrients.

Although diarrhea can be caused by changes in fluid and electrolyte movement in either the small or the large intestine, dietary nutrients are absorbed almost exclusively in the small intestine. Therefore, the demonstration of diminished absorption of a dietary nutrient provides unequivocal evidence of small-intestinal disease, although colonic dysfunction may also be present (e.g., Crohn's disease may involve both small and large intestine). Dietary nutrient absorption may be segmental or heterogeneous along the small intestine and is site-specific. Thus, for example, calcium, iron, and folic acid are exclusively absorbed by active transport processes in the proximal small intestine, especially the duodenum; in contrast, the active transport mechanisms for both cobalamin and bile acids are present only in the ileum. Therefore, in an individual who years previously had had an intestinal resection, the details of which are not presently available, a presentation with evidence of calcium, folic acid, and iron malabsorption but without cobalamin deficiency would make it likely that the duodenum and jejunum, but not ileum, had been resected.

Some nutrients, e.g., glucose, amino acids, and lipids, are absorbed throughout the small intestine, though there is evidence that their rate of absorption is greater in the proximal than in the distal segments. However, following segmental resection of the small intestine, the remaining segments will undergo both morphologic and functional "adaptation" to enhance absorption. Such adaptation is secondary to both the presence of luminal nutrients and hormonal stimuli and may not be complete in humans for several months following the resection. Adaptation is critical for individuals who have undergone massive resection of the small intestine and/or colon to help ensure survival.

Establishing the presence of steatorrhea and identifying its specific cause are often quite difficult for several reasons. Despite attempts to develop tests that do *not* require the collection of stool to document the presence of steatorrhea, the "gold standard" still remains a timed, quantitative stool fat determination. On a practical basis, stool collections are invariably difficult and often incomplete as nobody wants to handle stool. A qualitative test—Sudan III stain—has long been available to establish the presence of an increase in stool fat. This test is rapid and inexpensive but, as a qualitative test, does not establish the degree of fat malabsorption and is best used as a preliminary screening study. Many of the blood, breath, and isotopic tests that have been developed either: (1) do not directly measure fat absorption, (2) have excellent sensitivity when steatorrhea is obvious and severe but have poor sensitivity when steatorrhea is mild, or (3) have not survived the transition from their development in a laboratory to commercial utilization and dissemination.

Despite this situation, the use of routine laboratory studies (i.e., complete blood count, prothrombin time, serum protein determination, alkaline phosphatase) may suggest the presence of dietary nutrient depletion, especially iron, folate, cobalamin, and vitamins D and K. Additional studies include measurement of serum carotene, cholesterol, albumin, iron, folate, and cobalamin levels. The serum carotene level can also be reduced if the patient has poor dietary intake of leafy vegetables.

If steatorrhea and/or altered absorption of other nutrients are suspected, the history, clinical observations, and laboratory testing can help detect deficiency of a dietary nutrient, especially the fat-soluble vitamins A, D, E, or K. Thus, evidence of metabolic bone disease with elevated alkaline phosphatase and/or reduced serum calcium levels would suggest vitamin D malabsorption. A deficiency of vitamin K would be suggested by an elevated prothrombin time in an individual without liver disease who was not taking anticoagulants. Macrocytic anemia would lead to evaluation of whether cobalamin or folic acid malabsorption was present. The presence of iron-deficiency anemia in the absence of occult bleeding from the gastrointestinal tract in either a male or a nonmenstruating female would require evaluation of iron malabsorption and the exclusion of celiac sprue, as iron is absorbed exclusively in the proximal small intestine.

At times, however, a timed (72-h) quantitative stool collection, preferably on a defined diet, must be obtained to determine stool fat content and establish the presence of steatorrhea. The presence of steatorrhea then requires further assessment to establish the pathophysiologic process(es) responsible for the defect in dietary lipid digestion-absorption (Table 286-4). Some of the other studies include the Schilling test, D-xylose test, duodenal mucosal biopsy, small-intestinal radiologic examination, and tests of pancreatic exocrine function.

THE SCHILLING TEST This test is performed to determine the cause for cobalamin malabsorption. Since cobalamin absorption requires multiple steps, including gastric, pancreatic, and ileal processes, the Schilling test can also be used to assess the integrity of these other organs (Chap. 107). Cobalamin is present primarily in meat. Except in strict vegans, *dietary* cobalamin deficiency is exceedingly uncommon. Dietary cobalamin is bound in the stomach to a glycoprotein called *R-binder protein*, which is synthesized in both the stomach and salivary glands. This cobalamin–R binder complex is formed in the acid milieu of the stomach. Cobalamin absorption has an absolute requirement for intrinsic factor, another glycoprotein synthesized and released by gastric parietal cells, to promote its uptake by specific cobalamin receptors on the brush border of ileal enterocytes. Pancreatic protease enzymes split the cobalamin–R binder complex to release cobalamin in the proximal small intestine, where cobalamin is then bound by intrinsic factor.

As a consequence, cobalamin absorption may be abnormal in the following:

1. Pernicious anemia, a disease in which immunologically mediated atrophy of gastric parietal cells leads to an absence of both gastric acid and intrinsic factor secretion.
2. Chronic pancreatitis as a result of deficiency of pancreatic proteases to split the cobalamin–R binder complex. Although 50% of patients with chronic pancreatitis have been reported to have an abnormal Schilling test that was corrected by pancreatic enzyme replacement, the presence of a cobalamin-responsive macrocytic anemia in chronic pancreatitis is extremely rare. Although this probably reflects a difference in the digestion/absorption of cobalamin in food versus that in a crystalline form, the Schilling test can still be used to assess pancreatic exocrine function.
3. Achlorhydria or absence of another factor secreted with acid that is responsible for splitting cobalamin away from the proteins in food to which it is bound can lead to vitamin B_{12} malabsorption. Up to one-third of individuals over >60 years have marginal vitamin B_{12} absorption because of the inability to release cobalamin from food; these people have no defects in absorbing crystalline vitamin B_{12}.
4. Bacterial overgrowth syndromes, which are most often secondary to stasis in the small intestine, produce cobalamin deficiency from bacterial utilization of cobalamin (often referred to as *stagnant bowel syndrome*) (see below).
5. Ileal dysfunction (either as a result of inflammation or prior intestinal resection) due to impaired function of the mechanism of cobalamin–intrinsic factor uptake by ileal intestinal epithelial cells.

The Schilling test is performed by administering ^{58}Co-labeled cobalamin and collecting urine for 24 h and is dependent upon normal

Table 286-6 Differential Results of Schilling Test in Several Diseases Associated with Cobalamin (Cbl) Malabsorption

	^{58}Co-Cbl	With IF	With Pancreatic Enzymes	After 5 Days of Antibiotics
Pernicious anemia	Reduced	Normal	Reduced	Reduced
Chronic pancreatitis	Reduced	Reduced	Normal	Reduced
Bacterial overgrowth	Reduced	Reduced	Reduced	Normal
Ileal disease	Reduced	Reduced	Reduced	Reduced

NOTE: IF, intrinsic factor.

renal and bladder function. Urinary excretion of cobalamin will reflect cobalamin absorption provided that intrahepatic binding sites for cobalamin are fully occupied. To ensure saturation of hepatic cobalamin binding sites so that all absorbed radiolabeled cobalamin will be excreted in urine, 1 mg cobalamin is administered intramuscularly 1 h following ingestion of the radiolabeled cobalamin. The Schilling test may be abnormal (usually defined as <10% excretion in 24 h) in pernicious anemia, chronic pancreatitis, blind loop syndrome, and ileal disease (Table 286-6). Therefore, whenever an abnormal Schilling test is found, ^{58}Co-labeled cobalamin should be administered on another occasion either bound to intrinsic factor, with pancreatic enzymes, or following a 5-day course of antibiotics (often tetracycline). A variation of the Schilling test can detect failure to split cobalamin from food proteins. The labeled cobalamin is cooked together with a scrambled egg and administered orally. People with achlorydria will excrete <10% of the labeled cobalamin in the urine. In addition to establishing the etiology for cobalamin deficiency, the Schilling test can be used to help delineate the pathologic process responsible for steatorrhea by assessing ileal, pancreatic, and small-intestinal luminal function.

URINARY D-XYLOSE TEST The urinary D-xylose test for carbohydrate absorption provides an assessment of proximal small-intestinal mucosal function. D-Xylose, a pentose, is absorbed almost exclusively in the proximal small intestine. The D-xylose test is usually performed by giving 25 g D-xylose and collecting urine for 5 h. An abnormal test (<4.5 g excretion) primarily reflects the presence of duodenal/jejunal mucosal disease. The D-xylose test can also be abnormal in patients with blind loop syndrome (as a consequence primarily of abnormal intestinal mucosa) and, as a false-positive study, in patients with large collections of fluid in a third space (i.e., ascites, pleural fluid). The ease of obtaining a mucosal biopsy of the small intestine by endoscopy and the false-negative rate of the D-xylose test have led to its diminished use. When small-intestinal mucosal disease is suspected, a small-intestinal mucosal biopsy should be performed.

RADIOLOGIC EXAMINATION Radiologic examination of the small intestine using barium contrast (small-bowel series or study) can provide important information in the evaluation of the patient with presumed or suspected malabsorption. These studies are most often performed in conjunction with the examination of the esophagus, stomach, and duodenal bulb, and insufficient barium is given the patient to permit an adequate examination of the small-intestinal mucosa, especially the ileum. As a result, many gastrointestinal radiologists alter the procedure of a barium contrast examination of the small intestine by performing either a small-bowel series in which a large amount of barium is given by mouth without concurrent examination of the esophagus and stomach or an enteroclysis study in which a large amount of barium is introduced into the duodenum via a fluoroscopically placed tube. In addition, many of the diagnostic features initially described by radiologists to denote the presence of small-intestinal disease (e.g., flocculation, segmentation) are rarely seen with current barium suspensions. Nonetheless, in skilled hands barium contrast examination of the small intestine can yield important information. For example, with extensive mucosal disease, dilatation of intestine can be seen as well as dilution of barium from increased intestinal fluid secretion (Fig. 286-3). A normal barium contrast study does *not* exclude the possibility of small-intestinal disease. However, a small-bowel series remains a very useful examination to assess for the presence of anatomic abnormalities, such as strictures and fistulas (as in Crohn's disease) or blind loop syndrome (e.g., multiple jejunal diverticula), and to define the extent of a previous surgical resection.

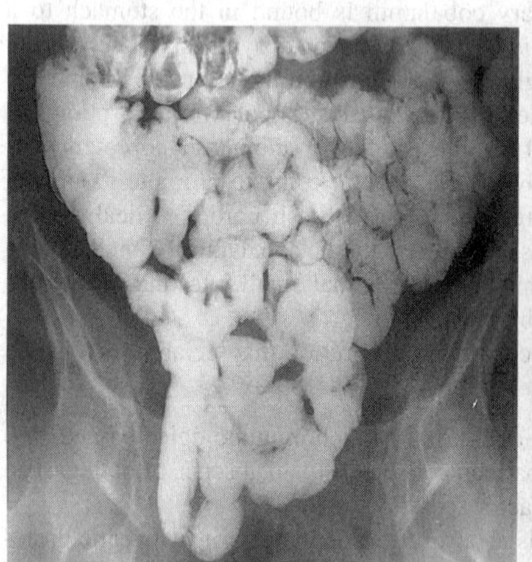
A

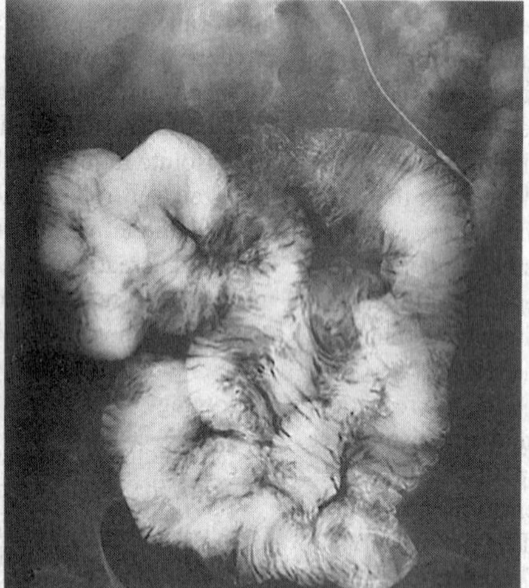
B

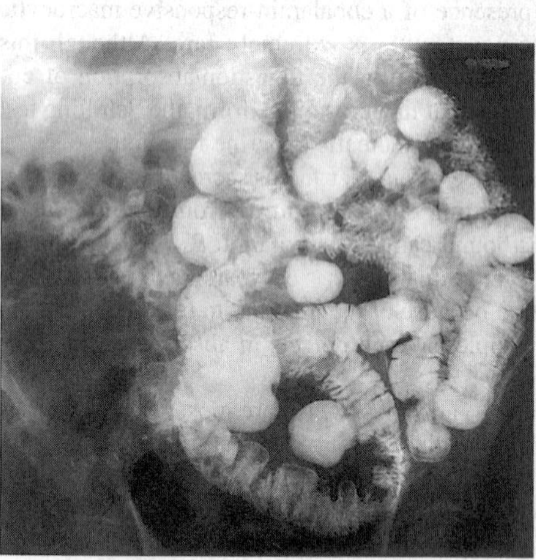
C

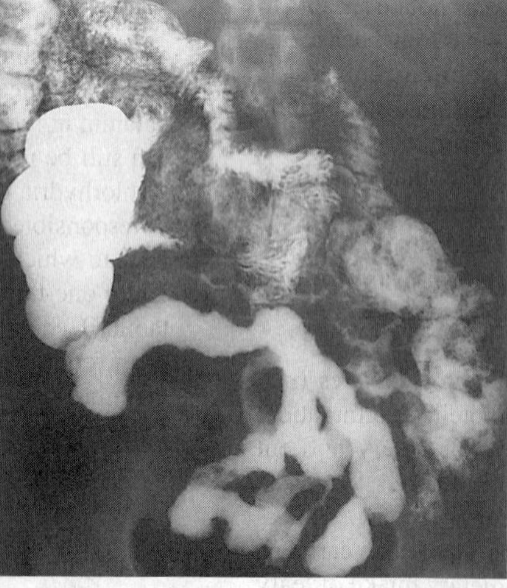
D

FIGURE 286-3 Barium contrast small-intestinal radiologic examinations. *A.* Normal individual. *B.* Celiac sprue. *C.* Jejunal diverticulosis. *D.* Crohn's disease. *(Courtesy of Morton Burrell, MD, Yale University.)*

BIOPSY OF SMALL-INTESTINAL MUCOSA A small-intestinal mucosal biopsy is essential in the evaluation of a patient with documented steatorrhea or chronic diarrhea (lasting >3 weeks) (Chap. 42). The ready availability of endoscopic equipment to examine the stomach and duodenum has led to their almost uniform use as the preferred method to obtain histologic material of proximal small-intestinal mucosa. The primary indications for a small-intestinal biopsy are (1) evaluation of a patient either with documented or suspected steatorrhea or with chronic diarrhea, and (2) diffuse or focal abnormalities of the small intestine defined on a small-intestinal series. Lesions seen on small-bowel biopsy can be classified into three different categories (Table 286-7): (1) diffuse, specific; (2) patchy, specific; and (3) diffuse, nonspecific.

1. *Diffuse, specific lesions.* There are relatively few diseases associated with altered nutrient absorption that have specific histopathologic abnormalities on small-intestinal mucosal biopsy, and they are uncommon. *Whipple's disease* is characterized by the presence of periodic acid–Schiff (PAS)-positive macrophages in the lamina propria, while the bacilli that are also present may require electron-microscopic examination for identification (Fig. 286-4). *Abetalipoproteinemia* is characterized by a normal mucosal appearance except for the presence of mucosal absorptive cells that contain lipid postprandially and disappear following a prolonged period of either fat-free intake or fasting. *Immune globulin deficiency* is associated with a variety of histopathologic findings on small-intestinal mucosal biopsy. The characteristic feature is the absence or substantial reduction in the number of plasma cells in the lamina propria; the mucosal architecture may be either perfectly normal or flat, i.e., villus atrophy. As patients with immune globulin deficiency are often infected with *Giardia lamblia, Giardia* trophozoites may also be seen in the biopsy.

2. *Patchy, specific lesions.* Several diseases are associated with abnormal small-intestinal mucosal biopsies, but the characteristic features that are present have a patchy distribution. As a result, biopsies

Table 286-7 Disease that Can be Diagnosed by Small-Intestinal Mucosal Biopsies

Lesions	Pathologic Findings
Diffuse, specific	
Whipple's disease	Lamina propria contains macrophages containing PAS + material
Agammaglobulinemia	No plasma cells; either normal or absent villi ("flat mucosa");
Abetalipoproteinemia	Normal villi; epithelial cells vacuolated with fat
Patchy, specific	
Intestinal lymphoma	Malignant cells in lamina propria and submucosa
Intestinal lymphangiectasia	Dilated lymphatics; clubbed villi
Eosinophilic gastroenteritis	Eosinophil infiltration of lamina propria and mucosa
Amyloidosis	Amyloid deposits
Crohn's disease	Noncaseating granulomas
Infection by one or more microorganisms (see text)	Specific organisms
Mastocytosis	Mast cell infiltration of lamina propria
Diffuse, nonspecific	
Celiac sprue	Short or absent villi; mononuclear infiltrate; epithelial cell damage; hypertrophy of crypts
Tropical sprue	Similar to celiac sprue
Bacterial overgrowth	Patchy damage to villi; lymphocyte infiltration
Folate deficiency	Short villi; decreased mitosis in crypts; megalocytosis
Vitamin B_{12} deficiency	Similar to folate deficiency
Radiation enteritis	Similar to folate deficiency
Zollinger-Ellison syndrome	Mucosal ulceration and erosion from acid
Protein-calorie malnutrition	Villus atrophy; secondary bacterial overgrowth
Drug-induced enteritis	Variable histology

NOTE: PAS+, periodic acid–Schiff positive.

obtained randomly or in the absence of abnormalities visualized endoscopically may not reveal these diagnostic features. Intestinal *lymphoma* can at times be diagnosed on mucosal biopsy by the identification of malignant lymphoma cells in the lamina propria and submucosa (Chap. 112). The presence of dilated lymphatics in the submucosa and sometimes in the lamina propria indicates the presence of *lymphangiectasia* associated with hypoproteinemia secondary to protein loss into the intestine. *Eosinophilic gastroenteritis* represents a heterogeneous group of disorders with a spectrum of presentations and symptoms with a eosinophilic infiltrate of the lamina propria, with or without peripheral eosinophilia. The patchy nature of the infiltrate as well as its presence in the submucosa often leads to an absence of histopathologic findings on mucosal biopsy. As the involvement of the duodenum in *Crohn's disease* is also submucosal and not necessarily continuous, mucosal biopsies are not the most direct approach to the diagnosis of duodenal Crohn's disease (Chap. 287). Amyloid deposition can be identified by Congo Red stain in some patients with *amyloidosis* involving the duodenum (Chap. 319).

Several microorganisms can be identified on small-intestinal biopsies, establishing a correct diagnosis. Many of these microorganisms are associated with diarrhea that occurs in immunodeficient individuals, especially those with HIV infection, and include *Cryptosporidium, Isospora belli*, cytomegalovirus, *Mycobacterium avium intracellulare*, and *G. lamblia*.

3. *Diffuse, nonspecific lesions. Celiac sprue* presents with a characteristic mucosal appearance on duodenal/proximal jejunal mucosal biopsy that is not diagnostic of the disease. The diagnosis of celiac sprue is established by clinical, histologic, and immunologic response to a gluten-free diet. *Tropical sprue* is associated with histopathologic findings similar to those of celiac sprue after a tropical or subtropical exposure but does not respond to gluten restriction; most often symptoms improve with antibiotics and folate administration.

Patients with steatorrhea require assessment of *pancreatic exocrine function*, which is often abnormal in chronic pancreatitis. No test assesses pancreatic exocrine function well. Endoscopic approaches provide excellent assessment of pancreatic duct anatomy but do not assess exocrine function (Chap. 303). One noninvasive study (bentiromide test) of pancreatic exocrine function is based on the feeding of a tripeptide containing *p*-aminobenzoic acid (PABA). Following splitting of PABA by pancreatic proteases, PABA is liberated, absorbed, and excreted in urine. Reduced proteolysis results in reduced urinary excretion of PABA. This test is neither sensitive nor specific.

Table 286-8 summarizes the results of the D-xylose test, Schilling test, and small-intestinal mucosal biopsy in patients with five different causes of steatorrhea.

SPECIFIC DISEASE ENTITIES

CELIAC SPRUE Celiac sprue is a not uncommon cause of malabsorption of one or more nutrients in Caucasians, especially those of European descent. Celiac sprue has had several other names including nontropical sprue, celiac disease (in children), adult celiac disease, and gluten-sensitive enteropathy. The etiology of celiac sprue is not known, but environmental, genetic, and immunologic factors are important. Celiac sprue has protean manifestations, almost all of which are secondary to nutrient malabsorption, and a varied natural history, with the onset of symptoms occurring at ages ranging from the first year of life through the eighth decade.

The hallmark of celiac sprue is the presence of an abnormal small-intestinal biopsy (Fig. 286-4) and the response of both symptoms, evidence of malabsorption and the histopathologic changes on the small-intestinal biopsy, to the elimination of gluten from the diet. The histopathologic changes have a proximal to distal intestinal distribution of severity, which probably reflects the exposure of the intestinal mucosa to varied amounts of dietary gluten; the degree of symptoms is related to the extent of these histopathologic changes.

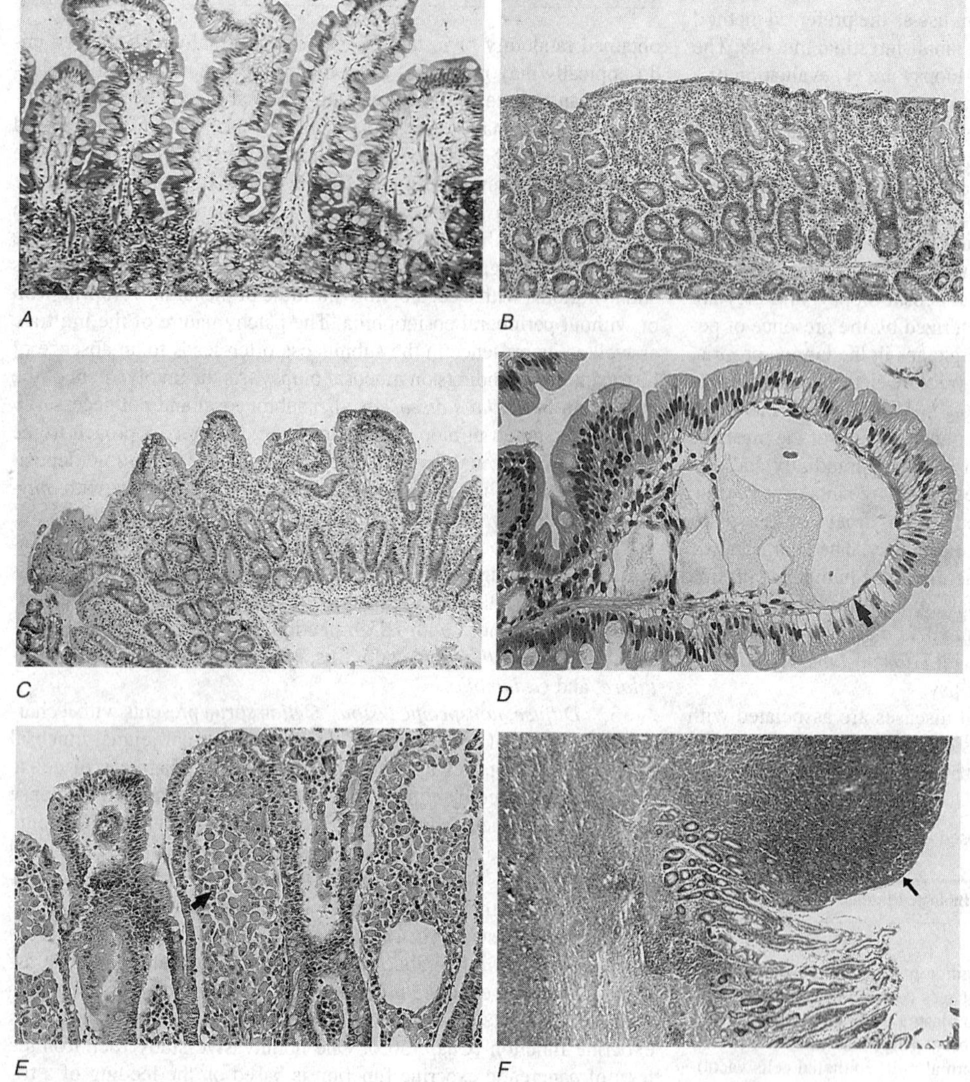

FIGURE 286-4 Small-intestinal mucosal biopsies. *A*. Normal individual. *B*. Untreated celiac sprue. *C*. Treated celiac sprue. *D*. Intestinal lymphangiectasia. *E*. Whipple's disease. *F*. Lymphoma. *(Courtesy of Marie Robert, MD, Yale University.)*

The symptoms of celiac sprue may appear with the introduction of cereals in an infant's diet, although there is frequently a spontaneous remission during the second decade of life that may be either permanent or followed by the reappearance of symptoms over several years. Alternatively, the symptoms of celiac sprue may first become evident at almost any age throughout adulthood. In many patients, frequent spontaneous remissions and exacerbations occur. The symptoms range from significant malabsorption of multiple nutrients with diarrhea, steatorrhea, weight loss, and the consequences of nutrient depletion (i.e., anemia and metabolic bone disease) to the absence of any gastrointestinal symptoms but with evidence of the depletion of a single nutrient (e.g., folate deficiency, osteomalacia, edema from protein loss). Asymptomatic relatives of patients with celiac sprue have been identified as having this disease either by small-intestinal biopsy or by serologic studies (e.g., antiendomysial antibodies).

Etiology The etiology of celiac sprue is not known, but environmental, genetic, and immunologic factors all appear to contribute to the disease.

One *environmental* factor is the clear association of the disease with gliadin, a component of gluten that is present in wheat, barley, rye, and, in smaller amounts, oats. In addition to the role of gluten restriction in treatment, the instillation of gluten into both normal-appearing rectum and distal ileum of patients with celiac sprue results within hours in morphologic changes.

An *immunologic* component to etiology is suspected for three reasons. First, serum antibodies, IgA antigliadin and antiendomysial antibodies, are present, but it is also not known whether such antibodies are primary or secondary to the tissue damage. The antiendomysial antibody has 90 to 95% sensitivity and 90 to 95% specificity, and the antigen recognized by the antiendomysial antibody test is tissue transglutaminase. The relationship of this autoantibody to pathogenetic mechanism(s) responsible for celiac sprue remains to be established. Nonetheless, this antibody will undoubtedly prove extremely useful in establishing the true prevalence of celiac sprue in the general population and may provide important clues to its etiology. Second, treatment with prednisolone for 4 weeks of a patient with celiac sprue who continues to eat gluten will induce a remission and convert the "flat" abnormal duodenal biopsy to a more normal appearing one. Third, gliadin peptides may interact with gliadin-specific T cells that may either mediate tissue injury or induce the release of one or more cytokines that are responsible for the tissue injury.

Genetic factor(s) also appear to be involved in celiac sprue. The incidence of celiac sprue varies widely in different population groups (high in Caucasians, low in blacks and orientals) and is 10% in first-degree relatives of celiac sprue patients. Furthermore, about 95% of patients with celiac sprue express the HLA-DQ2 allele, though only a minority of all persons expressing DQ2 have celiac sprue.

Diagnosis A small-intestinal biopsy is required to establish a diagnosis of celiac sprue (Fig. 286-4). A biopsy should be performed in patients with symptoms and laboratory findings suggestive of nutrient malabsorption and/or deficiency.

Table 286-8 Results of Diagnostic Studies in Different Causes of Steatorrhea

	D-Xylose Test	Schilling Test	Duodenal Mucosal Biopsy
Chronic pancreatitis	Normal	50% abnormal; if abnormal, normal with pancreatic enzymes	Normal
Bacterial overgrowth syndrome	Normal or only modestly abnormal	Often abnormal; if abnormal, normal after antibiotics	Usually normal
Ileal disease	Normal	Abnormal	Normal
Celiac sprue	Decreased	Normal	Abnormal: probably "flat"
Intestinal lymphangiectasia	Normal	Normal	Abnormal: "dilated lymphatics"

Since the presentation of celiac sprue is often subtle, without overt evidence of malabsorption or nutrient deficiency, it is important to have a relatively low threshold to perform a biopsy. It is more prudent to perform a biopsy than to obtain another test of intestinal absorption, which can never completely exclude or establish this diagnosis.

The diagnosis of celiac sprue requires the presence of characteristic histopathologic changes on small-intestinal biopsy together with a prompt clinical and histopathologic response following the institution of a gluten-free diet. If serologic studies have detected the presence of IgA antiendomysial antibodies, they too should disappear after a gluten-free diet is started. The changes seen on duodenal/jejunal biopsy are restricted to the mucosa and include: (1) absence or reduced height of villi, resulting in a "flat" appearance; (2) increased loss of villus cells in association with increased crypt cell proliferation resulting in crypt hyperplasia and loss of villus structure, with consequent villus, but not mucosal, atrophy; (3) cuboidal appearance and nuclei that are no longer oriented basally in surface epithelial cells and increased intraepithelial lymphocytes; and (4) increased lymphocytes and plasma cells in the lamina propria. Although these histopathologic features are characteristic of celiac sprue, they are *not* diagnostic because a similar appearance can be seen in tropical sprue, eosinophilic enteritis, and milk-protein intolerance in children and occasionally in lymphoma, bacterial overgrowth, Crohn's disease, and gastrinoma with acid hypersecretion. However, the presence of a characteristic histopathologic appearance that reverts to normal following the initiation of a gluten-free diet establishes the diagnosis of celiac sprue. Readministration of gluten with or without an additional small-intestinal biopsy is not necessary.

Failure to Respond to Gluten Restriction The most common cause of persistent symptoms in a patient who fulfills all the criteria of the diagnosis of celiac sprue is continued intake of gluten. Gluten is ubiquitous, and significant effort must be made to exclude all gluten from the diet. Use of rice in place of wheat flour is very helpful, and several support groups provide important aid to patients with celiac sprue and to their families. About 90% of patients who have the characteristic findings of celiac sprue will respond to complete dietary gluten restriction. The remainder represent a heterogeneous group (whose condition is often called *refractory sprue*) that includes some patients who (1) respond to restriction of other dietary protein, e.g., soy; (2) respond to glucocorticoids; (3) are "temporary," i.e., the clinical and morphologic findings disappear after several months or years; or (4) fail to respond to all measures and have a fatal outcome, with or without documented complications of celiac sprue.

Mechanism of Diarrhea The diarrhea in celiac sprue has several pathogenetic mechanisms. Diarrhea may be secondary to (1) steatorrhea, which is primarily a result of the changes in jejunal mucosal function; (2) secondary lactase deficiency, a consequence of changes in jejunal brush border enzymatic function; (3) bile acid malabsorption resulting in bile acid–induced fluid secretion in the colon, in cases with more extensive disease involving the ileum; and (4) endogenous fluid secretion resulting from the crypt hyperplasia. Patients with more severe involvement with celiac sprue may obtain temporary improvement with *dietary lactose and fat restriction* while awaiting the full effects of total gluten restriction, which represents primary therapy.

Associated Diseases Celiac sprue is associated with dermatitis herpetiformis (DH), though the association has not been explained. Patients with DH have characteristic papulovesicular lesions that respond to dapsone. Almost all patients with DH have histopathologic changes in the small intestine consistent with celiac sprue, although usually much milder and less diffuse in distribution. Most patients with DH have mild, or no, gastrointestinal symptoms. In contrast, relatively few patients with celiac sprue have DH.

Celiac sprue is also associated with insulin-dependent diabetes mellitus and IgA globulin deficiency. The clinical importance of the former association is that although severe watery diarrhea without evidence of malabsorption is most often seen in patients with "diabetic diarrhea" (Chap. 333), a small-intestinal biopsy must at times be considered to exclude this association.

Complications The most important complication of celiac sprue is the development of a malignancy. An increased incidence of both gastrointestinal and nongastrointestinal neoplasms as well as intestinal lymphoma exists in patients with celiac sprue. For unexplained reasons the occurrence of lymphoma in patients with celiac sprue is higher in Ireland and the United Kingdom than in the United States. The possibility of lymphoma must be considered whenever a patient with celiac sprue previously doing well on a gluten-free diet is no longer responsive to gluten restriction or a patient who presents with clinical and histopathologic features consistent with celiac sprue does not respond to a gluten-free diet. Other complications of celiac sprue include the development of intestinal ulceration independent of lymphoma and so-called refractory sprue (see above) and collagenous sprue. In *collagenous sprue*, a layer of collagen-like material is present beneath the basement membrane; these patients generally do not respond to a gluten-free diet and often have a poor prognosis.

TROPICAL SPRUE Tropical sprue is a poorly understood syndrome that affects both expatriates and natives in certain but not all tropical areas and is manifested by chronic diarrhea, steatorrhea, weight loss, and nutritional deficiencies, including those of both folate and cobalamin. This disease affects 5 to 10% of the population in some tropical areas.

Chronic diarrhea in a tropical environment is most often caused by infectious agents including *G. lamblia*, *Yersinia enterocolitica*, *C. difficile*, *Cryptosporidium parvum*, and *Cyclospora cayetanensis*, among other organisms. Tropical sprue should not be entertained as a possible diagnosis until the presence of cysts and trophozoites has been excluded in three stool samples. →***Chronic infections of the gastrointestinal tract and diarrhea in patients with or without AIDS are discussed in Chaps. 309 and 131.***

The small-intestinal mucosa in individuals living in tropical areas is not identical to that of individuals who reside in temperate climates. Biopsies reveal a mild alteration of villus architecture with a modest increase in mononuclear cells in the lamina propria, which on occasion can be as severe as that seen in celiac sprue. These changes are observed both in native residents and in expatriates living in tropical regions, are usually associated with mild decreases in absorptive function, but revert to "normal" when an individual moves or returns to a temperate area. Some have suggested that the changes seen in tropical enteropathy and in tropical sprue represent different ends of the spectrum of a single entity, but convincing evidence to support this concept is lacking.

Etiology The etiology of tropical sprue is not known, though because tropical sprue responds to antibiotics, the consensus is that tropical sprue may be caused by one or more infectious agents. Nonetheless, multiple uncertainties regarding the etiology and pathogenesis of tropical sprue exist. First, its occurrence is not evenly distributed in all tropical areas; rather, it is found in specific locations including South India, the Philippines, and several Caribbean islands (e.g., Puerto Rico, Haiti) but is rarely observed in Africa, Jamaica, or Southeast Asia. Second, an occasional individual will not develop symptoms of tropical sprue until long after having left an endemic area. This is the reason why the original term for celiac sprue was *nontropical sprue* to distinguish it from tropical sprue. Third, multiple microorganisms have been identified on jejunal aspirate with relatively little consistency among studies. *Klebsiella pneumoniae*, *Enterobacter cloacae*, or *E. coli* have been implicated in some studies of tropical sprue, while other investigations have favored a role for a toxin produced by one or more of these bacteria. Fourth, the incidence of tropical sprue appears to have decreased substantially during the past decade. One speculation for this reduced occurrence of tropical sprue is the wider use of antibiotics in acute diarrhea especially in travelers to tropical areas from temperate countries. Fifth, the role of folic acid deficiency in the pathogenesis of tropical sprue requires clarification. Folic acid is absorbed exclusively in the duodenum and proximal jejunum, and most patients with tropical sprue have evidence of folate malabsorption and depletion. Although folate deficiency can cause changes in small-intestinal mucosa that are corrected by folate replacement, the several earlier studies reporting that tropical sprue could be cured by folic acid did not provide an explanation for the "insult" that was initially responsible for folate malabsorption.

The clinical pattern of tropical sprue varies in different areas of the world (e.g., India vs. Puerto Rico). Not infrequently, individuals in India initially will report the occurrence of an acute enteritis before the development of steatorrhea and malabsorption. In contrast, in Puerto Rico, a most insidious onset of symptoms and a more dramatic response to antibiotics is seen than in some other locations. Tropical sprue in different areas of the world may not be the same disease; there may be similar clinical entities but with different etiologies.

Diagnosis The diagnosis of tropical sprue is best made by the presence of an abnormal small-intestinal mucosal biopsy in an individual with chronic diarrhea and evidence of malabsorption who is either residing or has recently lived in a tropic country. The small-intestinal biopsy in tropical sprue does not have pathognomonic features but resembles, and can often be indistinguishable from, that seen in celiac sprue (Fig. 286-4). The biopsy in tropical sprue will have less villus architectural alteration and more mononuclear cell infiltrate in the lamina propria. In contrast to celiac sprue, the histopathologic features of tropical sprue are present with a similar degree of severity throughout the small intestine, and a gluten-free diet does not result in either clinical or histopathologic improvement in tropical sprue.

℞ TREATMENT Broad-spectrum antibiotics and folic acid are most often curative, especially if the patient leaves the tropical area and does not return. Tetracycline should be used for up to 6 months and may be associated with improvement within 1 to 2 weeks. Folic acid alone will induce a hematologic remission as well as improvement in appetite, weight gain, and some morphologic changes in small intestinal biopsy. Because of the presence of marked folate deficiency, folic acid is most often given together with antibiotics.

SHORT BOWEL SYNDROME This is a descriptive term for the myriad clinical problems that often occur following resection of varying lengths of small intestine. The factors that determine both the type and degree of symptoms include: (1) the specific segment (jejunum vs. ileum) resected, (2) the length of the resected segment, (3) the integrity of the ileocecal valve, (4) whether any large intestine has also been removed, (5) residual disease in the remaining small and/or large intestine (e.g., Crohn's disease, mesenteric artery disease), and (6) the degree of adaptation in the remaining intestine. Short bowel syndrome can occur at any age from neonates through the elderly.

Three different situations in adults demand intestinal resections: (1) mesenteric vascular disease including both atherosclerosis, thrombotic phenomena, and vasculitidies; (2) primary mucosal and submucosal disease, e.g., Crohn's disease; and (3) operations without preexisting small intestinal disease, such as trauma and jejunoileal bypass for obesity.

Following resection of the small intestine, the residual intestine undergoes adaptation of both structure and function that may last for up to 6 to 12 months. Adaptation requires the continued intake of dietary nutrients and calories to stimulate it via direct contact with ileal mucosa, the release of one or more intestinal hormones, and pancreatic and biliary secretions. Thus, enteral nutrition and calorie administration must be maintained, especially in the early postoperative period, even if an extensive intestinal resection requiring total parenteral nutrition (TPN) was required. The subsequent ability of such patients to absorb nutrients will not be known for several months until after adaptation is completed.

Multiple factors besides the absence of intestinal mucosa (required for both lipid and fluid and electrolyte absorption) contribute to the diarrhea and steatorrhea in these patients. Removal of the ileum and especially the ileocecal valve is often associated with more severe diarrhea than jejunal resection. Without part or all of the ileum, diarrhea can be caused by an increase in bile acids entering the colon, leading to their stimulation of colonic fluid and electrolyte secretion. Absence of the ileocecal valve is also associated with a decrease in intestinal transit time and bacterial overgrowth from the colon. Lactose intolerance as a result of the removal of lactase-containing mucosa as well as gastric hypersecretion will also contribute to the diarrhea.

In addition to diarrhea and/or steatorrhea, a range of nonintestinal symptoms are also observed in some patients. A significant increase in renal calcium oxalate calculi is observed in patients with a small-intestinal resection with an intact colon and is due to an increase in oxalate absorption by the large intestine, with subsequent hyperoxaluria. Since oxalate is high in relatively few foods (e.g., spinach, rhubarb, tea), dietary restrictions alone are not adequate treatment. Cholestyramine, an anion-binding resin, and calcium have proved useful in reducing the hyperoxaluria. Similarly, an increase in cholesterol gall stones is seen that is related to a decrease in the bile acid pool size, which results in the generation of cholesterol supersaturation in gall bladder bile. Gastric hypersecretion of acid occurs in many patients following large resections of the small intestine. The etiology is unclear but may be related to either reduced hormonal inhibition of acid secretion or increased gastrin levels due to reduced small-intestinal catabolism of circulating gastrin. The resulting gastric acid secretion may be an important factor contributing to the diarrhea and steatorrhea. A reduced pH in the duodenum can inactivate pancreatic lipase and/or precipitate duodenal bile acids, thereby increasing steatorrhea, and an increase in gastric secretion can create a volume overload relative to the reduced small-intestinal absorptive capacity. Inhibition of gastric acid secretion with either proton pump inhibitors or H_2 receptor antagonists can help in reducing the diarrhea and steatorrhea.

℞ TREATMENT Treatment of short bowel syndrome depends on the severity of symptoms and whether the individual is able to maintain caloric and electrolyte balance with oral intake alone. Initial treatment includes judicious use of opiates to reduce stool output and to establish an effective diet. An initial diet should be low-fat, high-carbohydrate to minimize the diarrhea from fatty acid stimulation of colonic fluid secretion. Both MCT (see above), a low-lactose diet, and various fiber-containing diets should also be tried. In the absence of an ileocecal valve, the possibility of bacterial overgrowth must be considered and treated. If gastric acid hypersecretion is contributing to the diarrhea and steatorrhea, a proton pump inhibitor may be helpful. Usually none of these therapeutic approaches will provide an instant solution but will reduce disabling diarrhea.

The patient's vitamin and mineral status must also be monitored, and replacement therapy initiated, if indicated. Fat-soluble vitamins, folate, cobalamin, calcium, iron, magnesium, and zinc are the most critical factors to monitor on a regular basis. If these approaches are not successful, home TPN represents an established therapy that can be maintained for many years. Intestinal transplantation is beginning to become established as a possible approach for individuals with extensive intestinal resection who cannot be maintained without TPN.

BACTERIAL OVERGROWTH SYNDROME Bacterial overgrowth syndrome comprises a group of disorders with diarrhea, steatorrhea, and macrocytic anemia whose common feature is the proliferation of colon-type bacteria within the small intestine. This bacterial proliferation is due to stasis caused by impaired peristalsis (i.e., *functional stasis*), changes in intestinal anatomy (i.e., *anatomic stasis*), or direct communication between the small and large intestine. These conditions have also been referred to as *stagnant bowel syndrome* or *blind loop syndrome*.

Pathogenesis The manifestations of bacterial overgrowth syndromes are a direct consequence of the presence of increased amounts of a colonic-type bacterial flora, such as *E. coli* or *Bacteroides*, in the small intestine. *Macrocytic anemia* is due to cobalamin, not folate, deficiency. Most bacteria require cobalamin for growth, and increasing concentrations of bacteria use up the relatively small amounts of dietary cobalamin. *Steatorrhea* is due to impaired micelle formation as a consequence of a reduced intraduodenal concentration of bile acids and the presence of unconjugated bile acids. Certain bacteria, e.g., *Bacteroides*, deconjugate conjugated bile acids to unconjugated bile acids. In the presence of bacterial overgrowth, unconjugated bile acids will be absorbed more rapidly than conjugated bile acids, and, as a result, the intraduodenal concentration of bile acids will be reduced. In addition, the CMC of unconjugated bile acids is higher than that of conjugated bile acids, resulting in a decrease in micelle formation. *Diarrhea* is due, at least in part, to the steatorrhea, when it is present. However, some patients manifest diarrhea *without* steatorrhea, and it is assumed that the colonic-type bacteria in these patients are producing one or more bacterial enterotoxins that are responsible for fluid secretion and diarrhea.

Etiology The etiology of these different disorders is bacterial proliferation in the small intestinal lumen secondary to either anatomic or functional stasis or to a communication between the relatively sterile small intestine and the colon with its high levels of aerobic and anaerobic bacteria. Several examples of anatomic stasis have been identified: (1) one or more diverticula (both duodenal and jejunal) (Figure 286-3C); (2) fistulas and strictures related to Crohn's disease (Figure 286-3D); (3) a proximal duodenal afferent loop following a subtotal gastrectomy and gastrojejunostomy; (4) a bypass of the intestine, e.g., jejunoileal bypass for obesity; and (5) dilatation at the site of a previous intestinal anastomosis. The common feature of all of these anatomic derangements is the presence of a segment(s) of intestine that is out of continuity of propagated peristalsis, resulting in stasis and bacterial proliferation. Bacterial overgrowth syndromes can also occur in the absence of an anatomic blind loop when functional stasis is present. The best example of impaired peristalsis and bacterial overgrowth in the absence of a blind loop is scleroderma, where motility abnormalities exist in both the esophagus and small intestine (Chap. 313). Functional stasis and bacterial overgrowth can also occur in association with diabetes mellitus and in the small intestine when a direct connection exists between the small and large intestine, including an ileocolonic resection, or occasionally following an enterocolic anastomosis that permits entry of bacteria into the small intestine as a result of bypassing the ileocecal valve.

Diagnosis The diagnosis may be suspected from the combination of a low serum cobalamin level and an elevated serum folate level as enteric bacteria frequently produce folate compounds that will be absorbed in the duodenum. Ideally, the diagnosis of the bacterial overgrowth syndrome is the demonstration of increased levels of aerobic and/or anaerobic colonic-type bacteria in a jejunal aspirate obtained by intubation. This specialized test is rarely available, and bacterial overgrowth is best established by a Schilling test (Table 286-6), which should be abnormal following the administration of ^{58}Co-labeled cobalamin, with or without the administration of intrinsic factor. Following the administration of tetracycline for 5 days, the Schilling test will become normal, confirming the diagnosis of bacterial overgrowth.

℞ TREATMENT Primary treatment should be directed, if at all possible, to the surgical correction of an anatomic blind loop. In the absence of functional stasis, it is important to define the anatomic relationships responsible for stasis and bacterial overgrowth. For example, bacterial overgrowth secondary to strictures, one or more diverticula, or a proximal afferent loop can potentially be cured by surgical correction of the anatomic state. In contrast, the functional stasis of scleroderma or certain anatomic stasis states (e.g., multiple jejunal diverticula), cannot be corrected surgically, and these conditions should be treated with broad-spectrum antibiotics. Tetracycline used to be the initial treatment of choice but with increasing resistance, other antibiotics such as metronidazole, amoxicillin/clavulinic acid (Augmentin), and cephalosporin have been employed. The antibiotic should be given for approximately 3 weeks or until symptoms remit. Since the natural history of these conditions is chronic, antibiotics should not be given continuously, and symptoms usually remit within 2 to 3 weeks of initial antibiotic therapy. Therapy need not be repeated until symptoms recur. In the presence of frequent recurrences several treatment strategies exist, but the use of antibiotics for 1 week per month whether or not symptoms are present is often most effective.

Unfortunately, therapy for bacterial overgrowth syndrome is largely empirical, with an absence of clinical trials on which to base decisions regarding the antibiotic to be used, the duration of treatment, and/or the best approach for treating recurrences. Bacterial overgrowth may also occur as a component of another chronic disease, e.g., Crohn's disease, radiation enteritis, or short bowel syndrome. Treatment of the bacterial overgrowth in these settings will not cure the underlying problem but may be very important in ameliorating a subset of clinical problems that are related to bacterial overgrowth.

WHIPPLE'S DISEASE Whipple's disease is a chronic multisystem disease associated with diarrhea, steatorrhea, weight loss, arthralgia, and central nervous system and cardiac problems that is caused by the bacteria *Tropheryma whippelii*. Until the identification of *T. whippelii* by polymerase chain reaction during the past decade, the hallmark of Whipple's disease had been the presence of PAS-positive macrophages in the small intestine and other organs with evidence of disease. Long before the establishment of *T. whippelii* as the causative agent of Whipple's disease, gram-positive bacilli had been identified both within and outside of macrophages.

Etiology Whipple's disease is caused by a small gram-positive bacillus, *T. whippelii*. The bacillus, an actinobacterium, has low virulence but high infectivity, and relatively minimal symptoms are observed compared to the extent of the bacilli in multiple tissues.

Clinical Presentation The onset of Whipple's disease is insidious and is characterized by diarrhea, steatorrhea, abdominal pain, weight loss, migratory large-joint arthropathy, and fever as well as ophthalmologic and central nervous system symptoms. The development of dementia is a relatively late symptom and is an extremely poor prognostic sign, especially in patients who relapse following the induction of a remission with antibiotics. For unexplained reasons, the disease occurs primarily in middle-aged (50-year old) Caucasian men. The steatorrhea in these patients is generally believed secondary to both small-intestinal mucosal injury and lymphatic obstruction secondary to the increased number of PAS-positive macrophages in the lamina propria of the small intestine.

Diagnosis The diagnosis of Whipple's disease is suggested by a multisystem disease in a 50-year-old Caucasian male with diarrhea and steatorrhea. Obtaining tissue biopsies from the small intestine and/or other organs that may be involved (e.g., liver, lymph nodes, heart, eyes, central nervous system, or synovial membranes), based on the patient's symptoms, is the primary approach to establish the diagnosis of Whipple's disease. The presence of PAS-positive macrophages containing the characteristic small (0.25×1 to $2\ \mu m$) bacilli is suggestive of this diagnosis. However, Whipple's disease can be confused with the PAS-positive macrophages containing *M. avian* complex, which may be a cause of diarrhea in AIDS. The presence of the *T. whippelii* bacillus outside of macrophages is a more important indicator of active disease than their presence within the macrophages. *T. whippelii* has now been successfully grown in culture.

℞ TREATMENT The treatment for Whipple's disease is prolonged use of antibiotics. At the present time the drug of choice is double-strength trimethoprim/sulfamethoxazole for approximately 1 year. PAS-positive macrophages can persist following successful treatment, and the presence of bacilli outside of macrophages is indicative of persistent infection or an early sign of recurrence. Recurrence of disease activity, especially with dementia, is an extremely poor prognostic sign and requires an antibiotic that crosses the blood-brain barrier. If trimethoprim/sulfamethoxazole is not tolerated, chloramphenicol is an appropriate second choice.

PROTEIN-LOSING ENTEROPATHY Protein-losing enteropathy is not a specific disease but rather describes a group of gastrointestinal and nongastrointestinal disorders with hypoproteinemia and edema in the absence of either proteinuria or defects in protein synthesis, e.g., chronic liver disease. These diseases are characterized by excess protein loss into the gastrointestinal tract. Normally, about 10% of the total protein catabolism occurs via the gastrointestinal tract. Evidence of increased protein loss into the gastrointestinal tract has been established in >65 different diseases, which can be classified into three primary groups: (1) mucosal ulceration such that the protein loss primarily represents exudation across damaged mucosa, e.g., ulcerative colitis, gastrointestinal carcinomas, peptic ulcer; (2) nonulcerated mucosa but with evidence of mucosal damage so that the protein loss represents loss across epithelia with altered permeability, e.g., celiac sprue and Ménétrier's disease in the small intestine and stomach, respectively; (3) lymphatic dysfunction, either representing primary lymphatic disease or secondary to partial lymphatic obstruction that may occur as a result of enlarged lymph nodes or cardiac disease.

Diagnosis The diagnosis of protein-losing enteropathy is suggested by the presence of peripheral edema and low serum albumin and globulin levels in the absence of renal and hepatic disease. It is extremely rare for an individual with protein-losing enteropathy to have selective loss of *only* albumin or *only* globulins. Therefore, marked reduction of serum albumin with normal serum globulins should not initiate an evaluation for protein-losing enteropathy but should suggest the presence of renal and/or hepatic disease. Likewise, reduced serum globulins with normal serum albumin levels is more likely a result of reduced globulin synthesis rather than enhanced globulin loss into the intestine. Documentation of an increase in protein loss into the gastrointestinal tract has been established by the administration of one of several radiolabeled proteins and its quantitation in stool during a 24- or 48-h period. Unfortunately, none of these radiolabeled proteins are available for routine clinical use. α_1-Antitrypsin, a protein that represents approximately 4% of total serum proteins and is resistant to proteolysis, can be used to document enhanced rates of serum protein loss into the intestinal tract but cannot be used to assess gastric protein loss due to its degradation in an acid milieu. α_1-Antitrypsin clearance is measured by determining stool volume and both stool and plasma α_1-antitrypsin concentrations. In addition to the loss of protein via abnormal and distended lymphatics, peripheral lymphocytes may also be lost via lymphatics, resulting in a relative lymphopenia. Thus, the presence of lymphopenia in a patient with hypoproteinemia supports the presence of increased loss of protein into the gastrointestinal tract.

Patients with increased protein loss into the gastrointestinal tract from lymphatic obstruction often have steatorrhea and diarrhea. The steatorrhea is a result of altered lymphatic flow as lipid-containing chylomicrons exit from intestinal epithelial cells via intestinal lymphatics (Table 286-4; Fig. 286-4). In the absence of mechanical or anatomic lymphatic obstruction, instrinsic intestinal lymphatic dysfunction, with or without lymphatic dysfunction in the peripheral extremities, has been named *intestinal lymphangiectasia*. Similarly, about 50% of individuals with intrinsic peripheral lymphatic disease (Milroy's disease) will also have intestinal lymphangiectasia and hypoproteinemia. Other than steatorrhea and enhanced protein loss into the gastrointestinal tract, all other aspects of intestinal absorptive function are normal in intestinal lymphangiectasia.

Other Causes Patients who appear to have idiopathic protein-losing enteropathy without any evidence of gastrointestinal disease should be examined for cardiac disease and especially right-sided valvular disease and chronic pericarditis (Chap. 236). On occasion, hypoproteinemia can be the only presentation for these two types of heart disease. Ménétrier's disease (also called *hypertrophic gastropathy*) is an uncommon entity that involves the body and fundus of the stomach and is characterized by large gastric folds, reduced gastric acid secretion, and, at times, enhanced protein loss into the stomach.

Table 286-9 Classification of Malabsorption Syndromes

- Inadequate digestion
  - Postgastrectomy[a]
  - Deficiency or inactivation of pancreatic lipase
    - Exocrine pancreatic insufficiency
      - Chronic pancreatitis
      - Pancreatic carcinoma
      - Cystic fibrosis
      - Pancreatic insufficiency—congenital or acquired
    - Gastrinoma—acid inactivation of lipase[a]
    - Drugs—orlistat

- Reduced intraduodenal bile acid concentration/impaired micelle formation
  - Liver disease
    - Parenchymal liver disease
    - Cholestatic liver disease
  - Bacterial overgrowth in small intestine:
    - Anatomic stasis
      - Afferent loop stasis/blind loop/strictures/fistulae
    - Functional stasis
      - Diabetes[a]
      - Scleroderma[a]
      - Intestinal pseudoobstruction
  - Interrupted enterohepatic circulation of bile salts
    - Ileal resection
    - Crohn's disease[a]
  - Drugs (bind or precipitate bile salts)—neomycin, cholestyramine, calcium carbonate

- Impaired mucosal absorption/mucosal loss or defect
  - Intestinal resection or bypass
  - Inflammation, infiltration, or infection:

Crohn's disease[a]	Celiac disease
Amyloidosis	Collagenous sprue
Scleroderma[a]	Whipple's disease
Lymphoma[a]	Radiation enteritis
Eosinophilic enteritis	Folate and vitamin B_{12} deficiency
Mastocytosis	Infections—salmonellosis, giardiasis
Tropical sprue	Graft-vs.-host disease

  - Genetic disorders
    - Disaccharidase deficiency
    - Agammaglobulinemia
    - Abetalipoproteinemia
    - Hartnup disease
    - Cystinuria

- Impaired nutrient delivery to and/or from intestine:
  - Lymphatic obstruction
    - Lymphoma[a]
    - Lymphangiectasia
  - Circulatory disorders
    - Congestive heart failure
    - Constrictive pericarditis
    - Mesenteric artery atherosclerosis
    - Vasculitis

- Endocrine and metabolic disorders
  - Diabetes[a]
  - Hypoparathyroidism
  - Adrenal insufficiency
  - Hyperthyroidism
  - Carcinoid syndrome

[a] Malabsorption caused by more than one mechanism.

℞ **TREATMENT** As excess protein loss into the gastrointestinal tract is most often secondary to a specific disease, treatment should be directed primarily to the underlying disease process and not to the hypoproteinemia. For example, if significant hypoproteinemia with resulting peripheral edema is present secondary to either celiac sprue or ulcerative colitis, a gluten-free diet or mesalamine, respectively, would be the initial therapy. When enhanced protein loss is secondary to lymphatic obstruction, it is critical to establish the nature of this obstruction. Identification of mesenteric nodes or lymphoma may be possible by imaging studies. Similarly, it is important to exclude cardiac disease as a cause of protein-losing enteropathy either by echosonography or, on occasion, by a right-heart catheterization.

The increased protein loss that occurs in intestinal lymphangiectasia is a result of distended lymphatics associated with lipid malabsorption. Treatment of the hypoproteinemia is accomplished by a low-

Table 286-10 Pathophysiology of Clinical Manifestations of Malabsorption Disorders

Symptom or Sign	Mechanism
Weight loss/malnutrition	Anorexia, malabsorption of nutrients
Diarrhea	Impaired absorption or secretion of water and electrolytes; unabsorbed dihydroxy bile acids and fatty acids
Flatus	Bacterial fermentation of unabsorbed carbohydrate
Glossitis, cheilosis, stomatitis	Deficiency of iron, vitamin B_{12}, folate, and vitamin A
Abdominal pain	Bowel distention or inflammation, pancreatitis
Bone pain	Calcium, vitamin D malabsorption, protein deficiency, osteoporosis
Tetany, paresthesia	Calcium and magnesium malabsorption
Weakness	Anemia, electrolyte depletion (particularly K^+)
Nocturia	Delayed absorption of water, hypokalemia
Azotemia, hypotension	Fluid and electrolyte depletion
Amenorrhea, decreased libido	Protein depletion, decreased calories, secondary hypopituitarism
Anemia	Impaired absorption of iron, folate, vitamin B_{12}
Bleeding	Vitamin K malabsorption, hypoprothrombinemia
Night blindness/xerophthalmia	Vitamin A malabsorption
Peripheral neuropathy	Vitamin B_{12} and thiamine deficiency
Dermatitis	Deficiency of vitamin A, zinc, and essential fatty acid

fat diet and the administration of MCTs (Table 286-3), which do not exit from the intestinal epithelial cells via lymphatics but are delivered to the body via the portal vein.

SUMMARY

A pathophysiologic classification of the many conditions that can produce malabsorption is given in Table 286-9. A summary of the pathophysiology of the various clinical manifestations of malabsorption is given in Table 286-10.

BIBLIOGRAPHY

American Gastroenterological Association: Technical review on the evaluation and management of chronic diarrhea. Gastroenterology 116:1464, 1999

Cook SI, Sellin JH: Short chain fatty acids in health and disease. Aliment Pharmacol Ther 12:499, 1998

Craig RM, Ehrenpreis ED: D-Xylose testing. J Clin Gastroenterol 29:143, 1999

Greenberger NJ: Enzymatic therapy in patients with chronic pancreatitis. Gastroenterol Clin North Am 28:687, 1999

Harewood GC, Murray JA: Approaching the patient with chronic malabsorption syndrome. Semin Gastrointest Dis 14:138, 1999

Ramaiah C, Boynton RF: Whipple's disease. Gastroenterol Clin North Am 27:683, 1998

Shaw AD, Davies GJ: Lactose intolerance: Problems in diagnosis and treatment. J Clin Gastroenterol 28:208, 1999

Trier JS: Diagnosis of celiac sprue. Gastroenterology 115:211, 1998

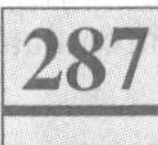

Sonia Friedman, Richard S. Blumberg

287 INFLAMMATORY BOWEL DISEASE

Inflammatory bowel disease (IBD) is an idiopathic and chronic intestinal inflammation. Ulcerative colitis (UC) and Crohn's disease (CD) are the two major types of IBD.

EPIDEMIOLOGY

The incidence of IBD varies within different geographic areas. Northern countries, such as the United States, United Kingdom, Norway, and Sweden, have the highest rates. The incidence rates of UC and CD in the United States are about 11 per 100,000 and 7 per 100,000, respectively (Table 287-1). Countries in southern Europe, South Africa, and Australia have lower incidence rates: 2 to 6.3 per 100,000 for UC, and 0.9 to 3.1 per 100,000 for CD. In Asia and South America, IBD is rare; incidence rates of UC and CD are 0.5 and 0.08 per 100,000, respectively. The highest mortality in IBD patients is during the first years of disease and in long duration disease due to the risk of colon cancer. In a Swedish population study, the standardized mortality ratios for CD and UC were 1.51 and 1.37, respectively.

Table 287-1 Epidemiology of IBD

	Ulcerative Colitis	Crohn's Disease
Incidence (U.S.)	11/100,000	7/100,000
Age of onset	15–30 & 60–80	15–30 & 60–80
Ethnicity	Jewish > Non-Jewish Caucasian > African American > Hispanic > Asian	
Male:female ratio	1:1	1.1–1.8:1
Smoking	May prevent disease	May cause disease
Oral contraceptives	No increased risk	Relative risk 1.9
Appendectomy	Protective	Not protective
Monozygotic twins	8% concordance	67% concordance
Dizygotic twins	0% concordance	20% concordance

The peak age of onset of UC and CD is between 15 and 30 years. A second peak occurs between the ages of 60 and 80. The male to female ratio for UC is 1:1 and for CD is 1.1 to 1.8:1. A two- to fourfold increased frequency of UC and CD in Jewish populations has been described in the United States, Europe, and South Africa. Furthermore, disease frequency differs within the Jewish populations. The prevalence of IBD in Ashkenazi Jews is about twice that of Israeli-born, Sephardic, or Oriental Jews. The prevalence decreases progressively in non-Jewish Caucasian, African-American, Hispanic, and Asian populations. Urban areas have a higher prevalence of IBD than rural areas and high socioeconomic classes have a higher prevalence than lower socioeconomic classes.

The effects of cigarette smoking are different in UC and CD. The risk of UC in smokers is 40% that of nonsmokers. Additionally, former smokers have a 1.7-fold increased risk for UC than people who have never smoked. In contrast, smoking is associated with a twofold increased risk of CD. Oral contraceptives are also linked to CD; the relative risk of CD for oral contraceptive users is about 1.9. Appendectomy appears to be protective against UC but further studies are needed.

IBD runs in families. If a patient has IBD, the lifetime risk that a first-degree relative will be affected is ~10%. If two parents have IBD, each child has a 36% chance of being affected. In twin studies, 67% of monozygotic twins are concordant for CD and 20% are concordant for UC, whereas 8% of dizygotic twins are concordant for CD and none are concordant for UC. There is also concordance for anatomic site and clinical type of CD within families.

Additional evidence for genetic predisposition to IBD comes from its association with certain genetic syndromes. UC and CD are both associated with Turner's syndrome, and Hermansky-Pudlak syndrome is associated with a granulomatous colitis. Glycogen storage disease type 1b can present with Crohn's-like lesions of the large and small bowel. Other immunodeficiency disorders, such as hypogammaglobulinemia, selective IgA deficiency, and hereditary angioedema, also exhibit an increased association with IBD.

ETIOLOGY AND PATHOGENESIS

Although IBD has been described as a clinical entity for over 100 years, its etiology and pathogenesis have not been definitively elaborated. Various studies have led to a consensus hypothesis that in genetically predisposed individuals, both exogenous factors (e.g., infectious agents, normal lumenal flora) and host factors (e.g., intestinal epithelial cell barrier function, vascular supply, neuronal activity) together cause a chronic state of dysregulated mucosal immune function that is further modified by specific environmental factors (e.g., smoking). Although it is possible that the chronic activation of the mucosal immune system may represent an appropriate response to a chronic unidentified infectious agent, a search for such an agent has thus far been unrewarding. As such, IBD must currently be considered an inappropriate response to either the endogenous microbial flora within the intestine, with or without some component of autoimmunity. Importantly, the normal intestine contains a significant concentration of immune cells in a chronic state of so-called *physiologic inflammation*, in which the gut is poised for, but actively restrained from, full immunologic responses. During the course of infections in the normal host, full activation of the gut-associated lymphoid tissue occurs but is rapidly superceded by downregulation of the immune response and tissue repair. In IBD this process is not regulated normally.

GENETIC CONSIDERATIONS IBD is a polygenic disorder that gives rise to multiple clinical subgroups within UC and CD. Genome-wide searches have shown that potential disease-associated loci are present on chromosomes 16, 12, 7, 3, and 1, although the specific gene associations are undefined. HLA alleles may play a role. UC patients disproportionately express DR2-related alleles, whereas in CD an increased use of the DR5 DQ1 haplotype or the DRB*0301 allele has been described. In UC patients with pancolitis undergoing total proctocolectomy, 14.3% versus 3.2% of non-IBD controls express the HLA DRB1*0103 allele. This allele is associated with extensive disease and extraintestinal manifestations such as mouth ulcers, arthritis, and uveitis. Other associations with immunoregulatory genes include the intercellular adhesion molecule R241 allele in UC and CD and the interleukin (IL) 1 receptor antagonist allele 2 in UC patients that is associated with total colonic inflammation. Although not proven at the genetic level, patients with IBD and their first-degree relatives may exhibit diminished intestinal epithelial cell barrier function. ■

DEFECTIVE IMMUNE REGULATION IN IBD The normal state of the mucosal immune system is one of inhibited immune responses to lumenal contents due to oral tolerance that occurs in the normal individual. When soluble antigens are administered orally rather than subcutaneously or intramuscularly, antigen-specific nonresponsiveness is induced. Multiple mechanisms are involved in the induction of oral tolerance and include deletion or anergy of antigen-reactive T cells or activation of CD4+ T cells that suppress gut inflammation through secretion of inhibitory cytokines (IL-10, TGF-β). Oral tolerance may be responsible for the lack of immune responsiveness to dietary antigens and the commensal flora in the intestinal lumen. In IBD this tightly regulated state of suppression of inflammation is altered, leading to uncontrolled inflammation. The mechanisms that maintain this regulated state of immune suppression are unknown.

Gene knockout (-/-) or transgenic (Tg) mouse models of colitis have revealed that deleting specific cytokines (e.g., IL-2, IL-10, TGF-β) or their receptors, deleting molecules associated with T-cell antigen recognition (e.g., T-cell antigen receptors, MHC class II), or interfering with intestinal epithelial cell barrier function (e.g., blocking N-cadherin, deleting multidrug resistance gene 1a or trefoil factor) leads to colitis. Thus, a variety of specific alterations can lead to unregulated autoimmunity directed at the colon in mice.

In both UC and CD, activated CD4+ T cells present in the lamina propria and peripheral blood secrete inflammatory cytokines. Some directly activate other inflammatory cells (macrophages and B cells) and others act indirectly to recruit other lymphocytes, inflammatory leukocytes, and mononuclear cells from the peripheral vasculature into the gut through interactions between homing receptors on leukocytes (e.g., $\alpha 4\beta 7$ integrin) and addressins on vascular endothelium (e.g., MadCAM1). CD4+ T cells can be subdivided into two major categories both of which may be associated with colitis in animal models and humans: T_H1 cells (IFN-γ, TNF) and T_H2 cells (IL-4, IL-5, IL-13). T_H1 cells appear to induce transmural granulomatous inflammation that resembles CD, and T_H2 cells appear to induce superficial mucosal inflammation more characteristic of UC. The T_H1 cytokine pathway is initiated by IL-12, a key cytokine in the pathogenesis of experimental models of mucosal inflammation. Thus, use of antibodies to block proinflammatory cytokines (e.g., anti-TNF-α, anti-IL-12) or molecules associated with leukocyte recruitment (e.g., anti-$\alpha 4\beta 7$) or use of cytokines that inhibit inflammation (e.g., IL-10) or promote intestinal barrier function (e.g., IL-11) may be beneficial to humans with colitis.

THE INFLAMMATORY CASCADE IN IBD Once initiated in IBD, the immune inflammatory response is perpetuated as a consequence of T-cell activation. A sequential cascade of inflammatory mediators acts to extend the response; each step is a potential target for therapy. Inflammatory cytokines, such as IL-1, IL-6, and tumor necrosis factor (TNF) have diverse effects on tissue. They promote fibrogenesis, collagen production, activation of tissue metalloproteinases, and the production of other inflammatory mediators; they also activate the coagulation cascade in local blood vessels (e.g., increased production of von Willebrand's factor). These cytokines are normally produced in response to infection, but are usually turned off or inhibited at the appropriate time to limit tissue damage. In IBD their activity is not regulated, resulting in an imbalance between the proinflammatory and anti-inflammatory mediators. Therapies such as the 5-ASA compounds are potent inhibitors of these inflammatory mediators through inhibition of transcription factors such as NF-κB that regulate their expression.

EXOGENOUS FACTORS IBD may have an as yet undefined infectious etiology. Three specific agents have received the greatest attention, *Mycobacterium paratuberculosis*, *Paramyxovirus*, and *Helicobacter* species. The immune response to a specific organism could be expressed differently, depending upon the individual's genetic background. Although *M. paratuberculosis* had initially been identified in CD patients, further studies have not confirmed a disease association. In addition, antimycobacterial agents have not been effective in treating CD. A role for the measles virus or paramyxoviruses in the development of CD has been suggested based on an increase in the incidence of CD in England that paralleled use of the measles vaccine. However, studies in the United States have not substantiated this finding. In an animal model of IBD, *Helicobacter hepaticus* has been implicated as a trigger for the inflammatory response; evidence in people is lacking.

Multiple pathogens (e.g., *Salmonella, Shigella sp., Campylobacter sp.*) may initiate IBD by triggering an inflammatory response that the mucosal immune system may fail to control. However, in an IBD patient the normal flora is likely perceived as if it were a pathogen. Anaerobic organisms, particularly *Bacteroides* species, may be responsible for the induction of inflammation. Such a notion is supported by the response in patients with CD to agents that alter the intestinal flora, such as metronidazole, ciprofloxacin, and elemental diets. CD also responds to fecal diversion, demonstrating the ability of lumenal contents to exacerbate disease. On the other hand, other bacterial organisms, so-called probiotics such as *Lactobacillus sp.*, downregulate inflammation in animal models and humans.

Psychosocial factors can contribute to clinical exacerbation of symptoms. Major life events such as illness or death in the family, divorce or separation, interpersonal conflict, or other major loss, are associated with an increase in IBD symptoms such as pain, bowel dysfunction, and bleeding. Acute daily stress can exacerbate bowel symptoms even after controlling for major life events. When the *sickness impact profile*, a measurement of overall psychological and physical functioning is used, IBD patients have functional impairment greater than that of a health maintenance organization population but less than that of patients with chronic back pain or amyotrophic lateral sclerosis. IBD patients have been hypothesized to have a characteristic personality that renders them susceptible to emotional stresses. However, emotional dysfunction could also be the result of chronic illness and should be considered when treating these patients.

PATHOLOGY

ULCERATIVE COLITIS: MACROSCOPIC FEATURES UC is a mucosal disease that usually involves the rectum and extends proximally to involve all or part of the colon. Approximately 40 to 50% of patients have disease limited to the rectum and rectosigmoid, 30 to 40% have disease extending beyond the sigmoid but not involving the whole colon, and 20% have a total colitis. Proximal spread occurs in continuity without areas of uninvolved mucosa. When the whole colon is involved, the inflammation extends 1 to 2 cm into the terminal ileum in 10 to 20% of patients. This is called *backwash ileitis* and has little clinical significance. Although variations in macroscopic activity may suggest skip areas, biopsies from normal-appearing mucosa are usually abnormal. Thus, it is important to obtain multiple biopsies from apparently uninvolved mucosa, whether proximal or distal, during endoscopy.

With mild inflammation, the mucosa is erythematous and has a fine granular surface that looks like sandpaper. In more severe disease, the mucosa is hemorrhagic, edematous, and ulcerated (Fig. 287-1). In long-standing disease, inflammatory polyps (pseudopolyps) may be present as a result of epithelial regeneration. The mucosa may appear normal in remission but in patients with many years of disease it appears atrophic and featureless and the entire colon becomes narrowed and foreshortened. Patients with fulminant disease can develop a toxic colitis or a toxic megacolon where the bowel wall becomes very thin and the mucosa is severely ulcerated, which may lead to perforation.

ULCERATIVE COLITIS: MICROSCOPIC FEATURES Histologic findings correlate well with the endoscopic appearance and clinical course of UC. The process is limited to the mucosa and superficial submucosa with deeper layers unaffected except in fulminant disease. In UC, two major histologic features are indicative of chronicity and help distinguish it from infectious or acute self-limited colitis. First, the crypt architecture of the colon is distorted; crypts may be bifid and reduced in number, often with a gap between the crypt bases and the muscularis mucosae. Second, some patients have basal plasma cells and multiple basal lymphoid aggregates. Mucosal vascular congestion with edema and focal hemorrhage, and an inflammatory cell infiltrate of neutrophils, lymphocytes, plasma cells, and macrophages may be present. The neutrophils invade the epithelium, usually in the crypts, and give rise to cryptitis and, ultimately, to crypt abscesses (Fig. 287-2). The cryptitis is associated with mucus discharge from goblet cells and increased epithelial cell turnover. Histologically, this results in goblet cell depletion. Other chronic changes that are sometimes seen are neuronal hypertrophy and fibromuscular hyperplasia of the muscularis mucosae.

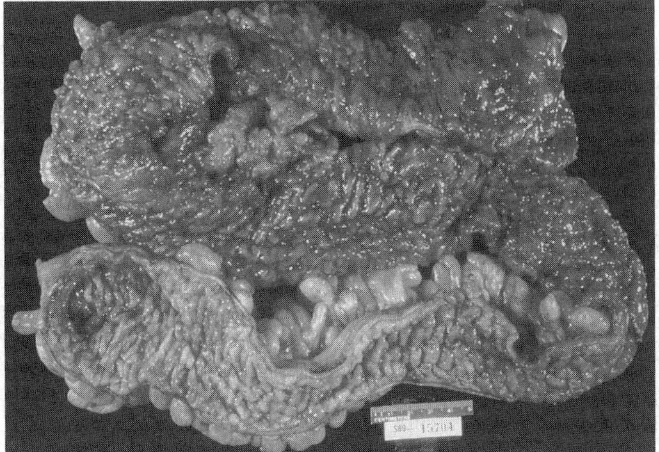

FIGURE 287-1 Pan-ulcerative colitis. Mucosa has a lumpy, bumpy appearance because of areas of inflamed but intact mucosa separated by ulcerated areas. *(Courtesy of Dr. EK Rosado and Dr. CA Perkos, Division of Gastrointestinal Pathology, Department of Pathology, Emory University, Atlanta, Georgia.)*

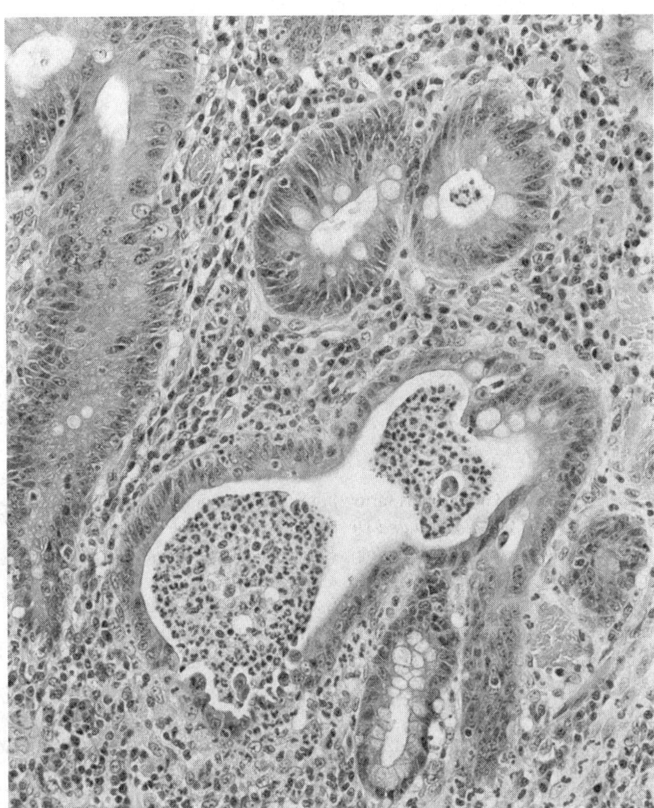

FIGURE 287-2 Characteristic findings of IBD in a case of ulcerative colitis: crypt distortion, cryptitis, and crypt abscess. *(Courtesy of Dr. EK Rosado and Dr. CA Perkos, Division of Gastrointestinal Pathology, Department of Pathology, Emory University, Atlanta, Georgia.)*

CROHN'S DISEASE: MACROSCOPIC FEATURES CD can affect any part of the gastrointestinal tract from the mouth to the anus. Some 30 to 40% of patients have small bowel disease alone, 40 to 55% have disease involving both the small and large intestines, and 15 to 25% have colitis alone. In the 75% of patients with small intestinal disease, the terminal ileum is involved in 90%. Unlike UC, which almost always involves the rectum, the rectum is often spared in CD. CD is segmental, with skip areas in the midst of diseased intestine (Fig. 287-3). Perirectal fistulas, fissures, abscesses, and anal stenosis are present in one-third of patients with CD, particularly those with colonic involvement. CD may also involve the liver and the pancreas.

Unlike UC, CD is a transmural process. Endoscopically, aphthous or small superficial ulcerations characterize mild disease; in more ac-

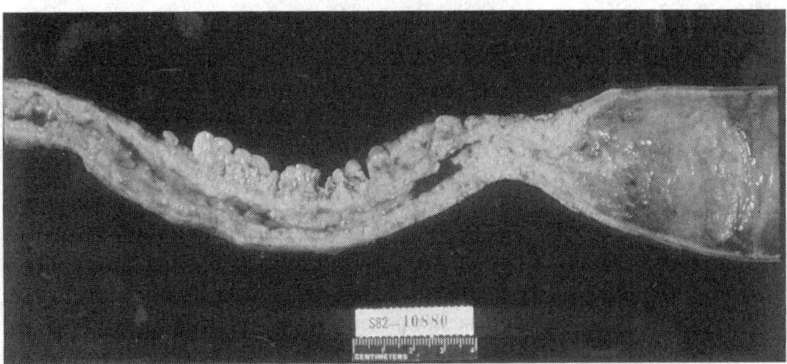

FIGURE 287-3 Portion of colon with stricture in patient with CD. *(Courtesy of Dr. EK Rosado and Dr. CA Perkos, Division of Gastrointestinal Pathology, Department of Pathology, Emory University, Atlanta, Georgia.)*

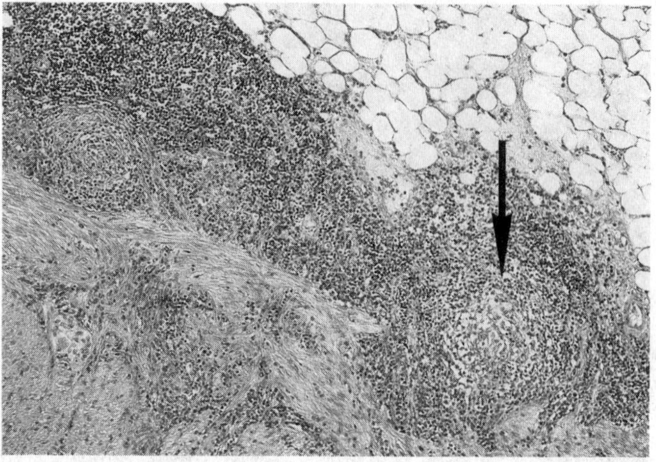

FIGURE 287-4 Granulomas (arrow) in bowel wall and serosa of colon, CD. *(Courtesy of Dr. EK Rosado and Dr. CA Perkos, Division of Gastrointestinal Pathology, Department of Pathology, Emory University, Atlanta, Georgia.)*

tive disease, stellate ulcerations fuse longitudinally and transversely to demarcate islands of mucosa that frequently are histologically normal. This "cobblestone" appearance is characteristic of CD, both endoscopically and by barium radiography. As in UC, pseudopolyps can form in CD.

Active CD is characterized by focal inflammation and formation of fistula tracts, which resolve by fibrosis and stricturing of the bowel. The bowel wall thickens and becomes narrowed and fibrotic, leading to chronic, recurrent bowel obstructions. Projections of thickened mesentery encase the bowel ("creeping fat") and serosal and mesenteric inflammation promote adhesions and fistula formation.

CROHN'S DISEASE: MICROSCOPIC FEATURES The earliest lesions are aphthoid ulcerations and focal crypt abscesses with loose aggregations of macrophages, which form noncaseating granulomas in all layers of the bowel wall from mucosa to serosa (Fig. 287-4). Granulomas can be seen in lymph nodes, mesentery, peritoneum, liver, and pancreas. Although granulomas are a pathognomonic feature of CD, only half of cases reveal granulomas on surgical or endoscopic biopsy specimens. Other histologic features of CD include submucosal or subserosal lymphoid aggregates, particularly away from areas of ulceration, gross and microscopic skip areas, and transmural inflammation that is accompanied by fissures that penetrate deeply into the bowel wall and sometimes form fistulous tracts or local abscesses.

CLINICAL PRESENTATION

ULCERATIVE COLITIS Signs and Symptoms The major symptoms of UC are diarrhea, rectal bleeding, tenesmus, passage of mucus, and crampy abdominal pain. The severity of symptoms correlates with the extent of disease. Although UC can present acutely, symptoms usually have been present for weeks to months. Occasionally, diarrhea and bleeding are so intermittent and mild that the patient does not seek medical attention.

Patients with proctitis usually pass fresh blood or blood-stained mucus, either mixed with stool or streaked onto the surface of a normal or hard stool. They also have tenesmus, or urgency with a feeling of incomplete evacuation. They rarely have abdominal pain. With proctitis or proctosigmoiditis, proximal transit slows, which may account for the constipation that is commonly seen in patients with distal disease.

When the disease extends beyond the rectum, blood is usually mixed with stool, or grossly bloody diarrhea may be noted. Colonic motility is altered by inflammation with rapid transit through the inflamed intestine. When the disease is severe, patients pass a liquid stool containing blood, pus, and fecal matter. Diarrhea is often nocturnal and/or postprandial. Although severe pain is not a prominent symptom, some patients with active disease may experience vague lower abdominal discomfort or mild central abdominal cramping. Severe cramping and abdominal pain can occur in association with severe attacks of the disease. Other symptoms in moderate to severe disease include anorexia, nausea, vomiting, fever, and weight loss.

Physical signs of proctitis include a tender anal canal and blood on rectal exam. With more extensive disease, patients have tenderness to palpation directly over the colon. Patients with a toxic colitis have severe pain and bleeding, and those with megacolon have hepatic tympany. Both may have signs of peritonitis if a perforation has occurred. The classification of disease activity is shown in Table 287-2.

Laboratory, Endoscopic, and Radiographic Features Active disease can be associated with a rise in acute phase reactants (C-reactive protein, orosomucoid levels), platelet count, erythrocyte sedimentation rate (ESR) and a decrease in hemoglobin. In severely ill patients, the serum albumin level will fall rather quickly. Leukocytosis may be present but is not a specific indicator of disease activity. Proctitis or proctosigmoiditis rarely causes a rise in C-reactive protein. Diagnosis relies upon the patient's history; clinical symptoms, negative stool examination for bacteria, *Clostridium difficile* toxin, and ova and parasites; sigmoidoscopic appearance; and histology of rectal or colonic biopsy specimens.

Sigmoidoscopy is used to assess disease activity and is often performed before treatment. Histologic features change more slowly than clinical features but can also be used to grade disease activity.

Patients with a severe attack of UC should have a plain, supine film of the abdomen. In the presence of severe disease, the margin of the colon becomes edematous and irregular (Fig. 287-5). Colonic thickening and toxic dilation can both be seen on a plain radiograph.

The earliest radiologic change of UC seen on single-contrast barium enema is a fine mucosal granularity. With increasing severity, the mucosa becomes thickened and superficial ulcers are seen. Deep ulcerations can appear as "collar-button" ulcers, which indicate that the ulceration has penetrated the mucosa. Haustral folds may be normal in mild disease, but as activity progresses they become edematous and thickened. Loss of haustration can occur, especially in patients with long-standing disease. In addition, the colon becomes shortened and narrowed. Polyps in the colon may be postinflammatory polyps or pseudopolyps, adenomatous polyps, or carcinoma.

Computed tomography (CT) scanning is not as helpful as endoscopy and barium enema in making the diagnosis of UC, but typical findings include mild mural thickening (<1.5 cm), inhomogeneous wall density, absence of small bowel thickening, increased perirectal and presacral fat, target appearance of the rectum, and adenopathy.

Complications Only 15% of patients with UC present initially with catastrophic illness. Massive hemorrhage occurs with severe

Table 287-2 Ulcerative Colitis: Disease Presentation

	Mild	Moderate	Severe
Bowel movements	<4 per day	4–6 per day	>6 per day
Blood in stool	Small	Moderate	Severe
Fever	None	<37.5°C mean	>37.5°C mean
Tachycardia	None	<90 mean pulse	>90 mean pulse
Anemia	Mild	>75%	≤75%
Sedimentation rate	<30 mm		>30 mm
Endoscopic appearance	Erythema, decreased vascular pattern, fine granularity	Marked erythema, coarse granularity, absent vascular markings, contact bleeding, no ulcerations	Spontaneous bleeding, ulcerations

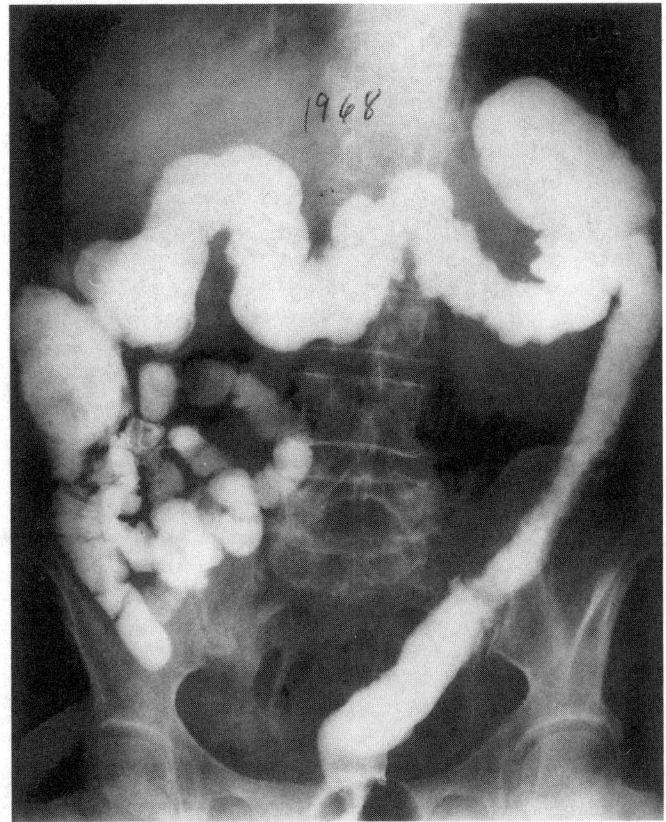

FIGURE 287-5 Barium enema in a patient with acute ulcerative colitis: inflammation of the entire colon. *(Courtesy of Dr. JM Braver, Gastrointestinal Radiology, Department of Radiology, Brigham and Women's Hospital, Boston, Massachusetts.)*

attacks of disease in 1% of patients and treatment for the disease usually stops the bleeding. However, if patients require 6 to 8 units of blood within 24 to 48 h, colectomy is indicated. Toxic megacolon is defined as a transverse colon with a diameter of more than 5.0 cm to 6.0 cm, with loss of haustration in patients with severe attacks of UC. It occurs in about 5% of attacks and can be triggered by electrolyte abnormalities and narcotics. Approximately 50% of acute dilations will resolve with medical therapy alone, but urgent colectomy is required for those that do not improve. Perforation is the most dangerous of the local complications, and the physical signs of peritonitis may not be obvious, especially if the patient is receiving glucocorticoids. Although perforation is rare, the mortality rate for perforation complicating a toxic megacolon is about 15%. In addition, patients can develop a toxic colitis and such severe ulcerations that the bowel may perforate without first dilating.

Obstructions caused by benign stricture formation occur in 10% of patients, with one-third of the strictures occurring in the rectum. These should be surveyed endoscopically for carcinoma. UC patients occasionally develop anal fissures, perianal abscesses, or hemorrhoids but the occurrence of extensive perianal lesions should suggest CD.

CROHN'S DISEASE Signs and Symptoms Although CD usually presents as acute or chronic bowel inflammation, the inflammatory process evolves toward one of two patterns of disease: a fibrostenotic-obstructing pattern or a penetrating-fistulous pattern, each with different treatments and prognoses. The site of disease influences the clinical manifestations.

Ileocolitis Because the most common site of inflammation is the terminal ileum, the usual presentation of ileocolitis is a chronic history of recurrent episodes of right lower quadrant pain and diarrhea. Sometimes the initial presentation mimics acute appendicitis with pronounced right lower quadrant pain, a palpable mass, fever, and leukocytosis. Only at laparotomy, when the appendix is found to be normal, is the ileitis discovered. Pain is usually colicky; it precedes and is relieved by defecation. A low-grade fever is usually noted. High-spiking fever suggests intraabdominal abscess formation. Weight loss is common—typically 10 to 20% of body weight—and develops as a consequence of diarrhea, anorexia, and fear of eating.

An inflammatory mass may be palpated in the right lower quadrant of the abdomen. The mass is composed of inflamed bowel, adherent and indurated mesentery, and enlarged abdominal lymph nodes. Extension of the mass can cause obstruction of the right ureter or bladder inflammation, manifested by dysuria and fever. Edema, bowel wall thickening, and fibrosis of the bowel wall within the mass account for the radiographic "string sign" of a narrowed intestinal lumen.

Bowel obstruction may take several forms. In the early stages of the disease, bowel wall edema and spasm produce intermittent obstructive manifestations and increasing symptoms of postprandial pain. Over several years, this persistent inflammation gradually progresses to fibrostenotic narrowing and stricture. Diarrhea will decrease and eventually lead to chronic bowel obstruction and obstipation. Acute episodes of obstruction occur as well, precipitated by bowel inflammation and spasm or sometimes by impaction of undigested food. These episodes usually resolve with intravenous fluids and gastric decompression.

Severe inflammation of the ileocecal region may lead to localized wall thinning, with microperforation and fistula formation to the adjacent bowel, the skin, the urinary bladder, or to an abscess cavity in the mesentery. Enterovesical fistulas typically present as dysuria or recurrent bladder infections or less commonly as pneumaturia or fecaluria. Enterocutaneous fistulas follow tissue planes of least resistance, usually draining through abdominal surgical scars. Enterovaginal fistulas are rare and present as dyspareunia or as a feculent or foul-smelling, often painful vaginal discharge. They are unlikely to develop without a prior hysterectomy.

Jejunoileitis Extensive inflammatory disease is associated with a loss of digestive and absorptive surface, resulting in malabsorption and steatorrhea. Nutritional deficiencies can also result from poor intake and enteric losses and protein and other nutrients. Intestinal malabsorption can cause hypoalbuminemia, hypocalcemia, hypomagnesemia, coagulopathy, and hyperoxaluria with nephrolithiasis. Vertebral fractures are caused by a combination of vitamin D deficiency, hypocalcemia, and prolonged glucocorticoid use. Pellagra from niacin deficiency has been reported in extensive small bowel disease, and malabsorption of vitamin B12 can lead to a megaloblastic anemia.

Diarrhea is characteristic of active disease; its causes include: (1) bacterial overgrowth in obstructive stasis or fistulization, (2) bile-acid malabsorption due to a diseased or resected terminal ileum, (3) intestinal inflammation with decreased water absorption and increased secretion of electrolytes.

Colitis and Perianal Disease Patients with colitis present with low-grade fevers, malaise, diarrhea, crampy abdominal pain, and sometimes hematochezia. Gross bleeding due to deep colonic ulceration is not as common as in UC and appears in about half of patients with exclusively colonic disease. Only 1 to 2% bleed massively. Pain is caused by passage of fecal material through narrowed and inflamed segments of large bowel. Decreased rectal compliance is another cause for diarrhea in Crohn's colitis patients. Toxic megacolon has been associated with severe inflammation and short-duration disease.

Stricturing can occur in the colon, and patients can develop fibrous strictures with symptoms of bowel obstruction. Also, colonic disease may fistulize into the stomach or duodenum, causing feculent vomiting, or to the proximal or mid small bowel, causing malabsorption by "short circuiting" and bacterial overgrowth. Approximately 10% of women with Crohn's colitis will develop a rectovaginal fistula.

Perianal disease affects about one-third of patients with Crohn's colitis and is manifested by incontinence, large hemorrhoidal tags, anal strictures, anorectal fistulae, and perirectal abscesses. Not all patients with perianal fistula will have endoscopic evidence of colonic inflammation.

Gastroduodenal Disease Symptoms and signs of upper gastrointestinal tract disease include nausea, vomiting, and epigastric pain. Patients usually have a *H. pylori*-negative gastritis. The second portion of the duodenum is more commonly involved than the bulb. Fistulas involving the stomach or duodenum arise from the small or large bowel and do not necessarily signify the presence of upper gastrointestinal tract involvement. Patients with advanced gastroduodenal CD may develop a chronic gastric outlet obstruction.

Laboratory, Endoscopic, and Radiographic Features Laboratory abnormalities include elevated sedimentation rate and C-reactive protein. In more severe disease, findings include hypoalbuminemia, anemia, and leukocytosis.

Endoscopic features of CD include rectal sparing, aphthous ulcerations, fistulas, and skip lesions. Endoscopy is useful for biopsy of mass lesions or strictures, or for visualization of filling defects seen on barium enema. Colonoscopy allows examination and biopsy of the terminal ileum, and upper endoscopy is useful in diagnosing gastroduodenal involvement in patients with upper tract symptoms. Ileal or colonic strictures may be dilated with balloons introduced through the colonoscope. Endoscopic appearance correlates poorly with clinical remission; thus, repeated endoscopy is not used to monitor the inflammation.

In CD early radiographic findings in the small bowel include thickened folds and aphthous ulcerations. "Cobblestoning" from longitudinal and transverse ulcerations most frequently involves the small bowel (Fig. 287-6). In more advanced disease, strictures, fistulas (Fig. 287-7), inflammatory masses, and abscesses may be detected. The earliest macroscopic findings of colonic CD are aphthous ulcers. These small ulcers are often multiple and separated by normal intervening mucosa. As more severe disease develops, aphthous ulcers become enlarged, deeper, and occasionally connected to one another, forming longitudinal stellate, serpiginous, and linear ulcers.

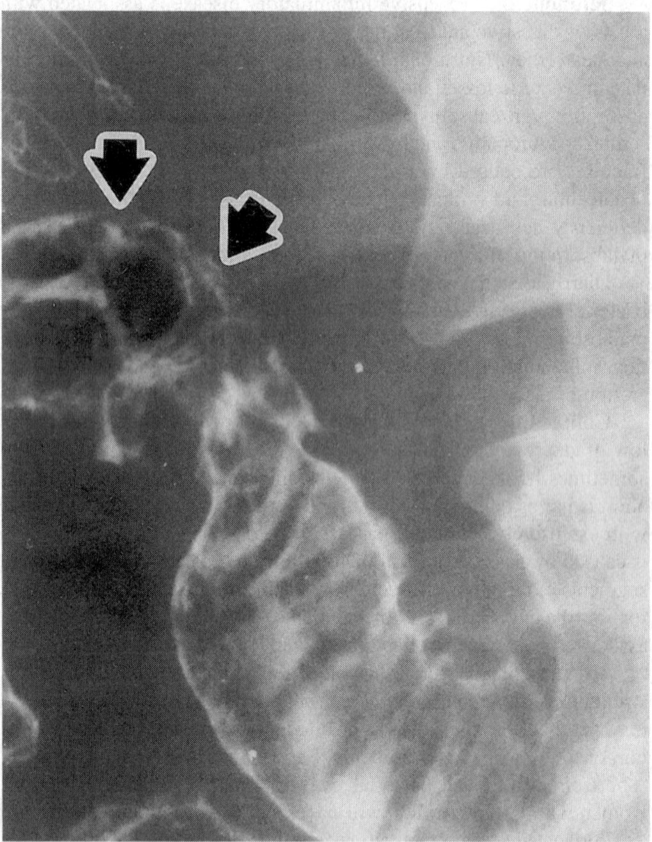

FIGURE 287-6 Crohn's disease: small bowel series demonstrating "cobblestoning" of the terminal ileum (arrows). *(Courtesy of Dr. JM Braver, Gastrointestinal Radiology, Department of Radiology, Brigham and Women's Hospital, Boston, Massachusetts.)*

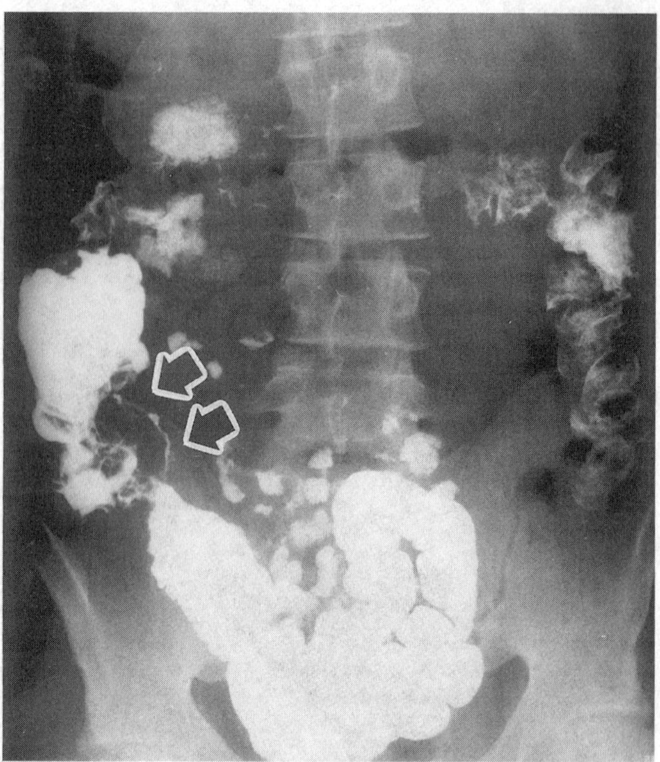

FIGURE 287-7 Small bowel series demonstrating distal ileal inflammation and fistulization (arrows) in a patient with CD. *(Courtesy of Dr. JM Braver, Gastrointestinal Radiology, Department of Radiology, Brigham and Women's Hospital, Boston, Massachusetts.)*

The transmural inflammation of CD leads to decreased luminal diameter and limited distensibility. As ulcers progress deeper, they can lead to fistula formation. The radiographic "string sign" represents long areas of circumferential inflammation and fibrosis, resulting in long segments of luminal narrowing. The segmental nature of CD results in wide gaps of normal or dilated bowel between involved segments.

CT findings include mural thickening >2 cm, homogeneous wall density, mural thickening of small bowel, mesenteric fat stranding, perianal disease, and adenopathy. CT scanning can help identify abscesses, fistulas, and sinus tracts. Magnetic resonance imaging (MRI) may prove superior for demonstrating pelvic lesions such as ischiorectal abscesses.

Complications Because CD is a transmural process, serosal adhesions develop that provide direct pathways for fistula formation and reduce the incidence of free perforation. Free perforation occurs in 1 to 2% of patients, usually in the ileum but occasionally in the jejunum or as a complication of toxic megacolon. The peritonitis of free perforation, especially colonic, may be fatal. Generalized peritonitis may also result from the rupture of an intraabdominal abscess. Other complications include intestinal obstruction in 40%, massive hemorrhage, malabsorption, and severe perianal disease.

Serologic Markers Several serologic markers may be used to differentiate between CD and UC and help to predict the course of disease. Two antibodies that can be detected in the serum of IBD patients are perinuclear antineutrophil cytoplasmic antibody (pANCA) and anti-*Saccharomyces cerevisiae* antibodies (ASCA). A distinct set of antineutrophil cytoplasmic antibodies with perinuclear staining by indirect immunofluorescence is associated with UC. The antigens to which these antibodies are directed have not been identified, but they are distinct from those associated with vasculitis and may be related to histones. pANCA positivity is found in about 60 to 70% of UC patients and 5 to 10% of CD patients; 5 to 15% of first-degree relatives of UC patients are pANCA positive, whereas only 2 to 3% of the general population is pANCA positive. pANCA may also identify specific disease phenotypes. pANCA positivity is more often associated with pancolitis, early surgery, pouchitis, or inflammation of the pouch after ileal pouch-anal anastamosis (IPAA) and primary sclerosing cholangitis. pANCA in CD is associated with colonic disease that resembles UC.

ASCA antibodies recognize mannose sequences in the cell wall mannan of *S. cerevisiae*; 60 to 70% of CD patients, 10 to 15% of UC patients, and up to 5% of non-IBD controls are ASCA positive. The combined measurement of pANCA and ASCA has been advocated as a valuable diagnostic approach to IBD. In one report, pANCA positivity with ASCA negativity yielded a 57% sensitivity and 97% specificity for UC, whereas pANCA negativity with ASCA positivity yielded a 49% sensitivity and 97% specificity for CD. ASCA was associated with small bowel CD. These antibody tests may help decide whether a patient with indeterminate colitis should undergo an IPAA, because patients with predominant features of CD often have a more difficult postoperative course.

Anti-goblet cell autoantibodies (GABs)—autoantibodies against two target antigens in colonic epithelial cells—are present in 39% of UC patients, 30% of CD patients, 21% of first-degree relatives of UC patients, 19% of first-degree relatives of CD patients, and 2% of healthy controls. An anti-colon antibody is found in 36% of UC patients and 13% of CD patients and healthy controls. In addition, 31% of CD patients and 4% of UC patients have serum antibodies against pancreatic acinar cells or pancreatic autoantibodies (PABs). Antibodies to red cell membrane antigens that cross-react with enteropathogens such as *Campylobacter sp.* may be associated with hemolytic anemia in CD. None of these antibodies are useful in the diagnosis and management of patients with IBD.

DIFFERENTIAL DIAGNOSIS OF UC AND CD

UC and CD have similar features to many other diseases. In the absence of a key diagnostic test, a combination of clinical, laboratory, histopathologic, radiographic, and therapeutic observations is required (Table 287-3). Once a diagnosis of IBD is made, distinguishing between UC and CD is impossible in 10 to 20% of cases. These are termed *indeterminate* colitis.

INFECTIOUS DISEASE Infections of the small intestines and colon can mimic CD or UC. They may be bacterial, fungal, viral, or protozoal in origin (Table 287-4). *Campylobacter* colitis can mimic the endoscopic appearance of severe UC and can cause a relapse of established UC. *Salmonella* can cause watery or bloody diarrhea, nausea, and vomiting. Shigellosis causes watery diarrhea, abdominal pain, and fever followed by rectal tenesmus and by the passage of blood and mucus per rectum. All three are usually self-limited but 1% of patients infected with *Salmonella* become asymptomatic carriers. *Yersinia enterocolitica* infection occurs mainly in the terminal ileum and causes mucosal ulceration, neutrophil invasion, and thickening of the ileal wall. Other bacterial infections that may mimic IBD include *C. difficile*, which presents with watery diarrhea, tenesmus, nausea, and vomiting, and *Escherichia coli*, three categories of which can cause colitis. These are enterohemorrhagic, enteroinvasive, and enteroadherent *E. coli*, all of which can cause bloody diarrhea and abdominal tenderness. Diagnosis of bacterial colitis is made by sending stool specimens for bacterial culture and *C. difficile* toxin analysis. Gonorrhea, *Chlamydia*, and syphilis can also cause proctitis

Gastrointestinal involvement with mycobacterial infection occurs primarily in the immunosuppressed patient but may occur in patients with normal immunity. Distal ileal and cecal involvement predominates and patients present with symptoms of small bowel obstruction and a tender abdominal mass. The diagnosis is made most directly by colonoscopy with biopsy and culture. *Mycobacterium avium intracellulare* complex infection occurs in advanced stages of HIV infection and in other profoundly immunocompromised states, and usually manifests as a systemic infection with diarrhea, abdominal pain, weight

Table 287-3 Different Clinical, Endoscopic, and Radiographic Features

	Ulcerative Colitis	Crohn's Disease
CLINICAL		
Gross blood in stool	Yes	Occasionally
Mucus	Yes	Occasionally
Systemic symptoms	Occasionally	Frequently
Pain	Occasionally	Frequently
Abdominal mass	Rarely	Yes
Significant perineal disease	No	Frequently
Fistulas	No	Yes
Small intestinal obstruction	No	Frequently
Colonic obstruction	Rarely	Frequently
Response to antibiotics	No	Yes
Recurrence after surgery	No	Yes
ANCA-positive	Frequently	Rarely
ENDOSCOPIC		
Rectal sparing	Rarely	Frequently
Continuous disease	Yes	Occasionally
"Cobblestoning"	No	Yes
Granuloma on biopsy	No	Occasionally
RADIOGRAPHIC		
Small bowel significantly abnormal	No	Yes
Abnormal terminal ileum	Occasionally	Yes
Segmental colitis	No	Yes
Asymmetrical colitis	No	Yes
Stricture	Occasionally	Frequently

NOTE: ANCA, antineutrophil cytoplasm antibody

loss, fever, and malabsorption. Diagnosis is established by acid-fast smear and culture of mucosal biopsies.

Although most of the patients with viral colitis are immunosuppressed, cytomegalovirus (CMV) and herpes simplex proctitis may occur in immunocompetent individuals. CMV occurs most commonly

Table 287-4 Diseases That Mimic IBD

INFECTIOUS ETIOLOGIES		
Bacterial	**Mycobacterial**	**Viral**
Salmonella	Tuberculosis	Cytomegalovirus
Shigella	*Mycobacterium avium*	Herpes simplex
Toxigenic *Escherichia coli*		HIV
	Parasitic	**Fungal**
Campylobacter	Amebiasis	Histoplasmosis
Yersinia	*Isospora*	*Candida*
Clostridium difficile	*Trichuris trichura*	*Aspergillus*
	Hookworm	
Gonorrhea	*Strongyloides*	
Chlamydia trachomatis		
NONINFECTIOUS ETIOLOGIES		
Inflammatory	**Neoplastic**	**Drugs and Chemicals**
Appendicitis	Lymphoma	NSAIDs
Diverticulitis	Metastatic carcinoma	Phosphasoda
Diversion colitis	Carcinoma of the ileum	Cathartic colon
Collagenous/lymphocytic colitis		Gold
Ischemic colitis	Carcinoid	Oral contraceptives
Radiation colitis/enteritis	Familial polyposis	Cocaine
		Chemotherapy
Solitary rectal ulcer		
Eosinophilc gastroenteritis		
Neutropenic colitis		
Bechet's syndrome		
Graft-versus-host disease		

NOTE: NSAIDs, nonsteroidal anti-inflammatory drugs

in the esophagus, colon, and rectum, but may also involve the small intestine. Symptoms include abdominal pain, bloody diarrhea, fever, and weight loss. With severe disease, necrosis and perforation can occur. Diagnosis is made by identification of intranuclear inclusions in mucosal cells on biopsy. Herpes simplex infection of the gastrointestinal tract is limited to the oropharynx, anorectum, and perianal areas. Symptoms include anorectal pain, tenesmus, constipation, inguinal adenopathy, difficulty with urinary voiding, and sacral paresthesias. Diagnosis is made by rectal biopsy. HIV itself can cause diarrhea, nausea, vomiting, and anorexia. Small intestinal biopsies show partial villus atrophy; small bowel bacterial overgrowth and fat malabsorption may also be noted.

Protozoan parasites include *Isospora belli*, which can cause a self-limited infection in healthy hosts but causes a chronic profuse, watery diarrhea and weight loss in AIDS patients. *Entamoeba histolytica* or related species infect about 10% of the world's population; symptoms include abdominal pain, tenesmus, frequent loose stool containing blood and mucus, and abdominal tenderness. Colonoscopy reveals focal punctate ulcers with normal intervening mucosa; diagnosis is made by biopsy or serum amebic antibodies. Fulminant amebic colitis is rare but has a mortality rate of >50%.

Other parasitic infections that may mimic IBD include hookworm (*Necator americanus*), whipworm (*Trichuris trichiura*), and *Strongyloides stercoralis*. In severely immunocompromised patients *Candida* or *Aspergillus* can be identified in the submucosa. Disseminated histoplasmosis can involve the ileocecal area.

NONINFECTIOUS DISEASE Many diseases may mimic IBD (Table 287-4). Diverticulitis can be confused with CD clinically and radiographically. Both diseases cause fever, abdominal pain, tender abdominal mass, leukocytosis, elevated ESR, partial obstruction, and fistulas. Perianal disease or ileitis on small bowel series favors the diagnosis of CD. Significant endoscopic mucosal abnormalities are more likely in CD than in diverticulitis. Endoscopic or clinical recurrence following segmental resection favors CD. Diverticular-associated colitis is similar to CD, but mucosal abnormalities are limited to the sigmoid and descending colon.

Ischemic colitis is commonly confused with IBD. The ischemic process can be chronic and diffuse as in UC, or segmental as in CD. Colonic inflammation due to ischemia may resolve quickly or may persist and result in transmural scarring and stricture formation. Ischemic bowel disease should be considered in the elderly following abdominal aortic aneurysm repair or when a patient has a hypercoagulable state or a severe cardiac or peripheral vascular disorder. Patients usually present with sudden onset of left lower quadrant pain, urgency to defecate, and the passage of bright red blood per rectum. Endoscopic examination often demonstrates a normal-appearing rectum and a sharp transition to an area of inflammation in the descending colon and splenic flexure.

The effects of radiation therapy on the gastrointestinal tract can be difficult to distinguish from IBD. Acute symptoms can occur within 1 to 2 weeks of starting radiotherapy. When the rectum and sigmoid are irradiated, patients develop bloody, mucoid diarrhea and tenesmus, as in distal UC. With small bowel involvement, diarrhea is common. Late symptoms include malabsorption and weight loss. Stricturing with obstruction and bacterial overgrowth may occur. Fistulas can penetrate the bladder, vagina, or abdominal wall. Flexible sigmoidoscopy reveals mucosal granularity, friability, numerous telangiectasias, and occasionally discrete ulcerations. Biopsy can be diagnostic.

Solitary rectal ulcer syndrome is uncommon and can be confused with IBD. It occurs in mostly young females and may be caused by impaired evacuation and failure of relaxation of the puborectalis muscle. Ulceration may arise from anal sphincter overactivity, higher intrarectal pressures during defecation, and digital removal of stool. Patients complain of constipation with straining and pass blood and mucus per rectum. Other symptoms include abdominal pain, diarrhea, tenesmus, and perineal pain. The ulceration, which can be as large as 5 cm in diameter, is usually seen anteriorly or anteriorlaterally 3 to 15 cm from the anal verge. Biopsies can be diagnostic.

Several types of colitis have been associated with nonsteroidal anti-inflammatory drugs (NSAID), including de novo colitis, reactivation of IBD, and proctitis caused by use of suppositories. Most patients with NSAID-related colitis present with diarrhea and abdominal pain and complications include stricture, bleeding, obstruction, perforation, and fistulization. Withdrawal of these agents is crucial, and in cases of reactivated IBD, standard therapies are indicated.

INDETERMINITE COLITIS Cases of IBD that cannot be categorized as UC or CD are called *indeterminate* colitis. Long-term follow-up reduces the number of patients labeled indeterminate to about 10%. The disease course of indeterminate colitis is unclear and surgical recommendations are difficult, especially since up to 20% of pouches fail, requiring ileosotomy. A multistage ileal pouch-anal anastamosis (the initial stage consisting of a subtotal colectomy with Hartman pouch) with careful histologic evaluation of the resected specimen to exclude CD is advised. Medical therapy is similar to UC and CD; most clinicians use 5-ASA drugs, glucocorticoids, and immunomodulators as necessary.

THE ATYPICAL COLITIDIES Two atypical colitides—collagenous colitis and lymphocytic colitis—have completely normal endoscopic appearances. Collagenous colitis has two main histologic components: increased subepithelial collagen deposition and colitis with increased intraepithelial lymphocytes. Female to male ratio is 9:1, and most patients present in the sixth or seventh decades of life. The main symptom is chronic watery diarrhea. Treatments range from sulfasalazine and lomotil to bismuth to glucocorticoids for refractory disease.

Lymphocytic colitis has features similar to collagenous colitis including age at onset and clinical presentation, but it has almost equal incidence in men and women and no subepithelial collagen deposition on pathologic section. However, intraepithelial lymphocytes are increased. Diarrhea stops in the majority of patients treated with sulfasalazine or prednisone.

Diversion colitis is an inflammatory process that arises in segments of the large intestine that are excluded from the fecal stream. It usually occurs in patients with ileostomy or colostomy when a mucus fistula or a Hartman's pouch has been created. Diversion colitis is reversible by surgical reanastamosis. Clinically, patients have mucus or bloody discharge from the rectum. Erythema, granularity, friability, and, in more severe cases, ulceration can be seen on endoscopy. Histopathology shows areas of active inflammation with foci of cryptitis and crypt abscesses. Crypt architecture is normal and this differentiates it from UC. It may be impossible to distinguish from CD. Short-chain fatty acid enemas will help in diversion colitis, but the definitive therapy is surgical reanastamosis.

EXTRAINTESTINAL MANIFESTATIONS

IBD is associated with a variety of extraintestinal manifestations; up to one-third of patients have at least one. Patients with perianal CD are at higher risk for developing extraintestinal manifestations than other IBD patients.

DERMATOLOGIC Erythema nodosum (EN) occurs in up to 15% of CD patients and 10% of UC patients. Attacks usually correlate with bowel activity; skin lesions develop after the onset of bowel symptoms, and patients frequently have concomitant active peripheral arthritis. The lesions of EN are hot, red, tender nodules measuring 1 to 5 cm in diameter and are found on the anterior surface of the lower legs, ankles, calves, thighs, and arms. Therapy is directed toward the underlying bowel disease.

Pyoderma gangrenosum (PG) is seen in 1 to 12% of UC patients and less commonly in CD colitis. Although it usually presents after the diagnosis of IBD, PG may occur years before the onset of bowel symptoms, run a course independent of the bowel disease, respond poorly to colectomy, and even develop years after proctocolectomy. It is usually associated with severe disease. Lesions are commonly found on the dorsal surface of the feet and legs but may occur on the arms, chest, stoma, and even the face. PG usually begins as a pustule and then spreads concentrically to rapidly undermine healthy skin. Lesions then ulcerate with violaceous edges surrounded by a margin of erythema. Centrally, they contain necrotic tissue with blood and exudates. Lesions may be single or multiple and grow as large as 30 cm. They are sometimes very difficult to treat and often require intravenous antibiotics, intravenous glucocorticoids, dapsone, purinethinol, thalidomide, or intravenous cyclosporine.

Other dermatologic manifestations include pyoderma vegetans that occurs in intertriginous areas, pyostomatitis vegetans that involves the mucous membranes, and metastatic CD, a rare disorder defined by cutaneous granuloma formation. Psoriasis affects 5 to 10% of patients with IBD and is unrelated to bowel activity. Perianal skin tags are found in 75 to 80% of patients with CD, especially those with colonic involvement. Oral mucosal lesions are seen often in CD and rarely in UC and include aphthous stomatitis and "cobblestone" lesions of the buccal mucosa.

RHEUMATOLOGIC Peripheral arthritis develops in 15 to 20% of IBD patients, is more common in CD, and worsens with exacerbations of bowel activity. It is asymmetric, polyarticular, and migratory, and most often affects large joints of the upper and lower extremities. Treatment is directed at reducing bowel inflammation. In severe UC, colectomy frequently cures the arthritis.

Ankylosing spondylitis (AS) occurs in about 10% of IBD patients and is more common in CD than UC. About two-thirds of IBD patients with AS test positive for the HLA-B27 antigen. The activity of AS is not related to bowel activity and does not remit with glucocorticoids or colectomy. It most often affects the spine and pelvis, producing symptoms of diffuse low-back pain, buttock pain, and morning stiffness. The course is continuous and progressive leading to permanent skeletal damage and deformity.

Sacroiliitis is symmetrical, occurs equally in UC and CD, is often asymptomatic, does not correlate with bowel activity, and does not necessarily progress to AS. Other rheumatic manifestations include hypertrophic osteoarthropathy, osteoporosis and osteomalacia secondary to malabsorption of calcium and vitamin D as well as glucocorticoid therapy, pelvic/femoral osteomyelitis, and relapsing polychondritis.

OCULAR The incidence of ocular complications in IBD patients is 1 to 10%. The most common are conjunctivitis, anterior uveitis/iritis, and episcleritis. Uveitis is associated with both UC and CD colitis, may be found during periods of remission, and may develop in patients following bowel resection. Symptoms include ocular pain, photophobia, blurred vision, and headache. Prompt intervention, sometimes with systemic glucocorticoids, is required to prevent scarring and visual impairment. Episcleritis is a benign disorder that presents with symptoms of mild ocular burning. It occurs in 3 to 4% of IBD patients, more commonly in CD colitis, and is treated with topical glucocorticoids.

HEPATOBILIARY Hepatic steatosis is detectable in about half of the abnormal liver biopsies from patients with CD and UC; patients usually present with hepatomegaly. Fatty liver usually results from a combination of chronic debilitating illness, malnutrition, and glucocorticoid therapy. Cholelithiasis is more common in CD than UC and occurs in 10 to 35% of patients with ileitis or ileal resection. Gallstone formation is caused by malabsorption of bile acids resulting in depletion of the bile salt pool and the secretion of lithogenic bile.

Primary sclerosing cholangitis (PSC) is characterized by both intrahepatic and extrahepatic bile duct inflammation and fibrosis, frequently leading to biliary cirrhosis and hepatic failure; 1 to 5% of patients with IBD have PSC, but 50 to 75% of patients with PSC have IBD. Although it can be recognized after the diagnosis of IBD, PSC can be detected earlier or even years after proctocolectomy. Most patients have no symptoms at the time of diagnosis; when symptoms are present they consist of fatigue, jaundice, abdominal pain, fever, anorexia, and malaise. Diagnosis is made by endoscopic retrograde cholangiopancreatography (ERCP), which demonstrates multiple bile duct strictures alternating with relatively normal segments. The bile acid ursodeoxycholic acid (ursodiol) may reduce alkaline phosphatase and serum aminotransferase levels, but histologic improvement has been marginal and it has no definitive long-term benefit. Endoscopic stenting may be palliative for cholestasis secondary to bile duct obstruction. Patients with symptomatic disease develop cirrhosis and liver failure over 5 to 10 years and eventually require liver transplantation. Ten percent of PSC patients develop cholangiocarcinoma and cannot be transplanted. Pericholangitis is a subset of PSC found in about 30% of IBD patients; it is confined to small bile ducts and is usually benign.

UROLOGIC The most frequent genitourinary complications are calculi, ureteral obstruction, and fistulas. The highest frequency of nephrolithiasis (10 to 20%) occurs in patients with CD following small bowel resection or ileostomy. Calcium oxalate stones develop secondary to hyperoxaluria, which results from increased absorption of dietary oxalate. Normally, dietary calcium combines with luminal oxalate to form insoluble calcium oxalate, which is eliminated in the stool. In patients with ileal dysfunction, however, nonabsorbed fatty acids bind calcium and leave oxalate unbound. The unbound oxalate is then delivered to the colon, where it is readily absorbed, especially in the presence of colonic inflammation.

OTHER The risk of thromboembolic disease increases when IBD becomes active, and patients may present with deep vein thrombosis, pulmonary embolism, cerebrovascular accidents, and arterial emboli. Factors responsible for the hypercoagulable state include reactive thrombocytosis, increased levels of fibrinopeptide A, factor V, factor VIII, fibrinogen, accelerated thromboplastin generation, antithrombin III deficiency secondary to increased gut losses or increased catabolism, and free protein S deficiency. A spectrum of vasculitidies involving small, medium, and large vessels has also been observed in IBD patients.

Patients with IBD have an increased prevalence of osteoporosis secondary to vitamin D deficiency, calcium malabsorption, malnutrition, and corticosteroid use. Deficiencies of vitamin B12 and fat-soluble vitamins may occur after ileal resection or with ileal disease.

More common cardiopulmonary manifestations include endocarditis, myocarditis, pleuropericarditis, and interstitial lung disease. A secondary or reactive amyloidosis can occur in patients with longstanding IBD, especially in patients with CD. Amyloid material is deposited systemically and can cause diarrhea, constipation, and renal failure. The renal disease can be successfully treated with colchicine. Pancreatitis is a rare extra-intestinal manifestation of IBD and results from duodenal fistulas, ampullary CD, gallstones, PSC, drugs such as 6-mercaptopurine or azathioprine, autoimmune pancreatitis, and primary CD of the pancreas.

℞ TREATMENT **5-ASA Agents** The mainstay of therapy for mild to moderate UC and CD colitis is sulfasalazine and the other 5-ASA agents. Sulfasalazine was originally developed to deliver both antibacterial (sulfapyridine) and anti-inflammatory (5-aminosalicylic acid, 5-ASA) therapy into the connective tissues of joints and the colonic mucosa. The molecular structure provides a convenient delivery system to the colon by allowing the intact molecule to pass through the small intestine after only partial absorption, and to be broken down in the colon by bacterial azo reductases that cleave the azo bond linking the sulfa and 5-ASA moieties. Sulfasalazine is effective in inducing and maintaining remission in mild to moderate UC and CD ileocolitis and colitis, but its high rate of side effects limits its use. Although sulfasalazine is more effective at higher doses, at 6 or 8 g/d up to 30% of patients experience allergic reactions or intolerable side effects such as headache, anorexia, nausea, and vomiting that are attributable to the sulfapyridine moiety. Hypersensitivity reactions, independent of sulfapyridine levels, include rash, fever, hepatitis, agranulocytosis, hypersensitivity pneumonitis, pancreatitis, worsening of colitis, and reversible sperm abnormalities. Sulfasalazine can also impair folate absorption and patients should be supplemented with folic acid.

Table 287-5 Oral 5-ASA Preparations

Preparation	Formulation	Delivery	Dosing, g/d
AZO-BOND			
Sulfasalazine (500 mg)	Sulfapyridine-5-ASA	Colon	3–6 (acute) 2–4 (maintenance)
Olsalazine (250 mg)	5-ASA-5-ASA	Colon	1–3
Balsalazide (500–750 mg)	Aminobenzoyl-alanine-5-ASA	Colon	2–6
DELAYED-RELEASE			
Asacol (400 mg)	Eudragit S (pH 7)	Distal ileum-colon	2.4–4.8 (acute) 0.8–4.8 (maintenance)
Claversal (250–500 mg)	Eudragit L (pH 6)	Ileum-colon	1.5–3 (acute) 0.75–3 (maintenance)
SUSTAINED-RELEASE			
Pentasa (250 mg)	Ethylcellulose micro-granules	Stomach-colon	2–4 (acute) 1.5–4 (maintenance)

Newer sulfa-free aminosalicylate preparations deliver increased amounts of the pharmacologically active ingredient of sulfasalazine (5-ASA, mesalamine) to the site of active bowel disease while limiting systemic toxicity. 5-ASA may function through inhibition of NF-κB activity. Sulfa-free aminosalicylate formulations include alternative azo-bonded carriers, 5-ASA dimers, pH-dependent tablets, and continuous-release preparations. Each has the same efficacy as sulfasalazine when equimolar concentrations are used. Olsalazine is composed of two 5-ASA radicals linked by an azo bond which is split in the colon by bacterial reduction and two 5-ASA molecules are released. Olsalazine is similar in effectiveness to sulfasalazine in treating CD and UC, but up to 17% of patients experience non-bloody diarrhea caused by increased secretion of fluid in the small bowel. Balsalazide contains an azo bond binding mesalamine to the carrier molecule 4-amino benzoyl β alanine; it is effective in the colon. Claversal is an enteric-coated form of 5-ASA that consists of mesalamine surrounded by an acrylic-based polymer resin and a cellulose coating that releases mesalamine at pH $>$ 6.0, a level that is present from the mid-jejunum continuously to the distal colon.

The most commonly used drugs besides sulfasalazine in the United States are Asacol and Pentasa. Asacol is also an enteric-coated form of mesalamine, but it has a slightly different release pattern, with 5-ASA liberated at pH $>$ 7.0. The disintegration of Asacol is variable with complete break-up of the tablet occurring in many different parts of the gut ranging from the small intestine to the splenic flexure; it has increased gastric residence when taken with a meal. Asacol is used to induce and maintain remission in UC and in CD ileitis, ileocolitis, and colitis. Appropriate doses of Asacol and the other 5-ASA compounds are shown in (Table 287-5). Some 50 to 75% of patients with mild to moderate UC and CD improve when treated with 2 g/d of 5-ASA; the dose response continues up to at least 4.8 g/d. Doses of 1.5-4 g/d maintain remission in 50 to 75% of patients with UC and CD.

Pentasa is another mesalamine formulation that uses an ethylcellulose coating to allow water absorption into small beads containing the mesalamine. Water dissolves the 5-ASA, which then diffuses out of the bead into the lumen. Disintegration of the capsule occurs in the stomach. The microspheres then disperse throughout the entire gastrointestinal tract from the small intestine through the distal colon in both fasted or fed conditions. Controlled trials of Pentasa and Asacol in active CD demonstrate a 40 to 60% clinical improvement or remission, and meta-analyses demonstrate maintenance of CD remission with 1.5 to 3 g/d of 5-ASA in 68 to 95% of patients. Pentasa at a dose of 2 g/d is more effective than placebo in postoperative prophylaxis of CD.

Topical mesalamine enemas are effective in mild-to-moderate distal UC and CD. Clinical response occurs in up to 80% of UC patients with colitis distal to the splenic flexure. Mesalamine suppositories, which are no longer available in the United States but are available in Canada, at doses of 500 mg twice a day are effective in treating proctitis.

Glucocorticoids The majority of patients with moderate to severe UC benefit from oral or parenteral glucocorticoids. Prednisone is usually started at doses of 40 to 60 mg/d for active UC that is unresponsive to 5-ASA therapy. Parenteral glucocorticoids may be administered as intravenous hydrocortisone 300 mg/d or methylprednisolone 40 to 60 mg/d. Adrenocorticotropic hormone (ACTH) is occasionally preferred for glucocorticoid-naïve patients despite a risk of adrenal hemorrhage. ACTH has equivalent efficacy to intravenous hydrocortisone in both glucocorticoid-naïve and -experienced CD patients.

Topically applied glucocorticoids are also beneficial for distal colitis and may serve as an adjunct in those who have rectal involvement plus more proximal disease. Hydrocortisone enemas or foam may control active disease, although they have no proven role as maintenance therapy. These glucocorticoids are significantly absorbed from the rectum and can lead to adrenal suppression with prolonged administration. The systemic effects of standard glucocorticoid formulations have led to the development of more potent formulations that are less well absorbed and have increased first-pass metabolism. Budesonide is being used in enema form with favorable preliminary results in distal UC.

Glucocorticoids are also effective for treatment of moderate-to-severe CD and induce a 60 to 70% remission rate compared to a 30% placebo response. Controlled ileal-release budesonide has been nearly equal to prednisone for ileocolonic CD at a dose of 9 mg/d.

Glucocorticoids play no role in maintenance therapy in either UC or CD. Once clinical remission has been induced, they should be tapered according to the clinical activity, normally at a rate of no more than 5 mg per week. They can usually be tapered to 20 mg/d within 4 to 5 weeks but often take several months to be discontinued altogether. The side effects are numerous, including fluid retention, abdominal striae, fat redistribution, hyperglycemia, subcapsular cataracts, osteonecrosis, myopathy, emotional disturbances, and withdrawal symptoms. Most of these side effects, aside from osteonecrosis, are related to the dose and duration of therapy.

Antibiotics Despite numerous trials, antibiotics have no role in the treatment of active or quiescent UC. However, pouchitis, which occurs in about a third of UC patients after colectomy and ileal pouch-anal anastamosis, usually responds to treatment with metronidazole or ciprofloxacin.

Metronidazole is effective in active inflammatory, fistulous, and perianal CD and may prevent recurrence after ileal resection. The most effective dose is 15 to 20 mg/kg per day in three divided doses; it is usually continued for several months. Common side effects include nausea, metallic taste, and disulfiram-like reaction. Peripheral neuropathy can occur with prolonged administration (several months) and on rare occasions is permanent despite discontinuation. Ciprofloxacin (500 mg bid) is also beneficial for inflammatory, perianal, and fistulous CD. These two antibiotics should be used as second-line drugs in active CD after 5-ASA agents and as first-line drugs in perianal and fistulous CD.

Azathioprine and 6-Mercaptopurine Azathioprine and 6-mercaptopurine (6-MP) are purine analogues commonly employed in the management of glucocorticoid-dependent IBD. Azathioprine is rapidly absorbed and converted to 6-MP, which is then metabolized to the active end product, thioinosinic acid, an inhibitor of purine ribonucleotide synthesis and cell proliferation. These agents also inhibit the immune response. Efficacy is seen at 3 to 4 weeks. Compliance can be monitored by measuring the level of 6-thioguanine, an end product of 6-MP metabolism. Azathioprine (2.0 to 2.5 mg/kg per day) or 6-MP (1.0-1.5 mg/kg per day) have been employed successfully as glucocorticoid-sparing agents in up to two-thirds of UC and CD patients previously unable to be weaned from glucocorticoids. The role of these immunomodulators as maintenance therapy in UC and CD and for treating active perianal disease and fistulas in CD appears promising. In addition, 6-MP at a dose of 50 mg/d is more effective than Pentasa or placebo for post-operative prophylaxis of CD.

Although azathioprine and 6-MP are usually well tolerated, pancreatitis occurs in 3 to 4% of patients, typically presents within the first few weeks of therapy, and is always completely reversible when the drug is stopped. Other side effects include nausea, fever, rash, and hepatitis. Bone marrow suppression (particularly leukopenia) is dose-related and often delayed, necessitating regular monitoring of the complete blood count. Additionally, 1 in 300 individuals lacks thiopurine methyltransferase, the enzyme responsible for drug metabolism; an additional 11% of the population are heterozygotes with intermediate enzyme activity. Both are at increased risk of toxicity because of increased accumulation of thioguanine metabolites. No increased risk of cancer has been documented in IBD patients taking these medications long-term.

Methotrexate Methotrexate (MTX) inhibits dihydrofolate reductase, resulting in impaired DNA synthesis. Additional anti-inflammatory properties may be related to decreased IL-1 production. Intramuscular or subcutaneous MTX (25 mg per week) is effective in inducing remission and reducing glucocorticoid dosage and 15 mg per week is effective in maintaining remission in active CD. Potential toxicities include leukopenia and hepatic fibrosis, necessitating periodic evaluation of complete blood counts and liver enzymes. The role of liver biopsy in patients on long-term MTX is uncertain. Hypersensitivity pneumonitis is a rare but serious complication of therapy. MTX should only be used when either 6-MP or azathioprine are ineffective or poorly tolerated.

Table 287-6 Medical Management of IBD

Ulcerative Colitis: Active Disease

	Mild	Moderate	Severe	Fulminant
Distal	5-ASA oral and/or enema	5-ASA oral and/or enema Glucocorticoid enema Oral glucocorticoid	5-ASA oral and/or enema Glucocorticoid enema Oral or IV glucocorticoid	Intravenous glucocorticoid Intravenous CSA
Extensive	5-ASA oral or enema	5-ASA oral and/or enema Glucocorticoid enema Oral glucocorticoid	5-ASA oral and/or enema Glucocorticoid enema Oral or IV glucocorticoid	Intravenous glucocorticoid Intravenous CSA

Ulcerative Colitis: Maintenance Therapy

Distal	5-ASA oral and/or enema 6-MP or azathioprine
Extensive	5-ASA oral and/or enema 6-MP or azathioprine

Crohn's Disease: Active Disease

Mild–Moderate	Severe	Perianal or Fistulizing Disease
5-ASA oral or enema Metronidazole and/or ciprofloxacin Oral glucocorticoids Azathioprine or 6-MP Infliximab	5-ASA oral or enema Metronidazole and/or ciprofloxacin Oral or IV glucocorticoids Azathioprine or 6-MP Infliximab TPN or elemental diet Intravenous cyclosporine	Metronidazole and/or ciprofloxacin Azathioprine or 6-MP Infliximab Intravenous CSA

Crohn's Disease: Maintenance Therapy

Inflammatory	Perianal or Fistulizing Disease
5-ASA oral or enema Metronidazole and/or ciprofloxacin Azathioprine or 6-MP	Metronidazole and/or ciprofloxacin Azathioprine or 6-MP

NOTE: CSA, cyclosporine; 6-MP, 6-mercaptopurine; TPN, total parenteral nutrition

Cyclosporine Cyclosporine (CSA) alters the immune response by acting as a potent inhibitor of T cell-mediated responses. Although CSA acts primarily via inhibition of IL-2 production from T helper cells, it also decreases recruitment of cytotoxic T cells and blocks other cytokines, including IL-3, IL-4, interferon α, and TNF. It has a more rapid onset of action than 6-MP and azathioprine.

CSA is most effective given at 4 mg/kg per day IV in severe UC that is refractory to intravenous glucocorticoids, with 82% of patients responding. CSA can be an alternative to colectomy. The long-term success of oral CSA is not as dramatic, but if patients are started on 6-MP or azathioprine at the time of hospital discharge, remission can be maintained. Intravenous CSA is effective in 80% of patients with refractory fistulas, but 6-MP or azathioprine must be used to maintain remission. Oral CSA alone is only effective at a higher dose (7.5 mg/kg per day) in active disease but is not effective in maintaining remission without 6-MP/azathioprine. Serum levels should be monitored and kept in the range of 200 to 400 ng/mL.

CSA has the potential for significant toxicity, and renal function should be frequently monitored. Hypertension, gingival hyperplasia, hypertrichosis, paresthesias, tremors, headaches, and electrolyte abnormalities are common side effects. Creatinine elevation calls for dose reduction or discontinuation. Seizures may also complicate therapy, especially if serum cholesterol levels are less than 120 mg/dL. Opportunistic infections, most notably *Pneumocystis carinii* pneumonia, have occurred with combination immunosuppressive treatment; prophylaxis should then be given.

Nutritional Therapies Dietary antigens may act as stimuli of the mucosal immune response. Patients with active CD respond to bowel rest, along with total enteral or total parenteral nutrition (TPN). Bowel rest and TPN are as effective as glucocorticoids for inducing remission of active CD but are not as effective as maintenance therapy. Enteral nutrition in the form of elemental or peptide-based preparations are also as effective as glucocorticiods or TPN, but these diets are not palatable. Enteral diets may provide the small intestine with nutrients vital to cell growth and do not have the complications of TPN. In contrast to CD, active UC is not effectively treated with either elemental diets or TPN. Standard medical management of UC and CD is reviewed in (Table 287-6).

Newer Medical Therapies • *Anti-tumor necrosis factor antibody* TNF is a key inflammatory cytokine and mediator of intestinal inflammation. The expression of TNF is increased in IBD. Infliximab is a chimeric mouse-human monoclonal antibody against TNF that is extremely effective in CD. It blocks TNF in the serum and at the cell surface and likely lyses TNF-producing macrophages and T cells through complement fixation and antibody-dependent cytotoxicity. Of active CD patients refractory to glucocorticoids, 6-MP, or 5-ASA, 65% will respond to intravenous infliximab (5 mg/kg); one-third will enter complete remission. Patients who experience an initial response will respond again to repeated infusions of infliximab every 8 weeks up to 44 weeks. Thus infliximab may be also be efficacious in maintaining remission. However, more trials need to be completed on remission maintenance after infliximab therapy.

Infliximab is also effective in CD patients with refractory perianal and enterocutaneous fistulas, with a 68% response rate (50% reduction in fistula drainage) and a 50% complete remission rate. The effects of infliximab for both inflammatory and fistulous disease last 12 weeks on average but longer in some patients.

The incidence of antibodies to infliximab (25% of the molecule is murine) is 13%. One side effect is a lupus-like syndrome, which is rare and reversible after stopping the drug. Anti-double-stranded DNA antibodies occur in 9% but are not associated with clinical lupus.

Among more than 1000 patients treated with infliximab, four developed lymphoma: one patient with CD, two with rheumatoid arthritis, and one with AIDS. Since the risk of lymphoma is already increased in these conditions, it is unclear whether infliximab is the cause. Thus, infliximab is extremely effective in refractory inflammatory and fistulous CD, but should be used only when necessary. Results on the efficacy of infliximab in UC are mixed.

Newer immunosuppressive agents Tacrolimus has a mechanism of action similar to cyclosporine. It has shown efficacy in children with refractory IBD and in adults with extensive involvement of the small bowel.

Mycophenolate mofetil inhibits the de novo pathway of purine synthesis in lymphocytes, disrupting the conversion of inosine monophosphate to guanosine monophosphate (GMP) by reversible inhibition of inosine monophosphate dehydrogenase. The resulting depletion of intracellular GMP suppresses the generation of cytotoxic T cells and formation of antibodies by activated B cells. Patients with CD or UC who received either 500 mg twice a day or 15 mg/kg per day in two divided doses have tolerated the drug well and have experienced benefit with reduction of glucocorticoid requirements.

Thalidomide has been shown to inhibit TNF production by monocytes and other cells. Thalidomide is effective in glucocorticoid refractory and fistulous CD, but randomized controlled trials still need to be performed.

The anti-inflammatory cytokines IL-10 is an anti-inflammatory and immunosuppressive cytokine produced by subsets of T and B cells, macrophages, and monocytes. It decreases T_H1 production of IL-2 and interferon γ, and limits production of IL-1, IL-6, IL-8, TNF, IL-12, and granulocyte-macrophage colony-stimulating factor. IL-10 has a moderate benefit in active CD.

IL-11 is a cytokine with thrombopoietic activity and mucosal protective effects that is effective in reducing inflammation in animal models of colitis. It seems to be effective in active CD, but more trials are needed.

Surgical Therapy • ***Ulcerative colitis*** Nearly half of patients with extensive chronic UC undergo surgery within the first 10 years of their illness. The indications for surgery are listed in (Table 287-7). Morbidity is about 20% in elective, 30% for urgent, and 40% for emergency proctocolectomy. The risks are primarily hemorrhage, contamination and sepsis, and neural injury. Although single-stage total proctocolectomy with ileostomy has been the operation of choice, newer operations maintain continence while surgically removing the involved rectal mucosa.

The IPAA is the most frequent continence-preserving operation performed. Because UC is a mucosal disease, the rectal mucosa can be dissected out and removed down to the dentate line of the anus or about 2 cm proximal to it. The ileum is fashioned into a pouch that serves as a neorectum. This ileal pouch is then sutured circumferentially to the anus in an end-to-end fashion. If performed carefully, this operation preserves the anal sphincter and maintains continence. The overall operative morbidity is 10%, with the major complication being bowel obstruction. Pouch failure necessitating conversion to permanent ileostomy occurs in 5 to 10% of patients. Some inflamed rectal mucosa is usually left behind, and thus endoscopic surveillance is necessary. Primary dysplasia of the ileal mucosa of the pouch has occurred rarely.

Table 287-7 Indications for Surgery

Ulcerative Colitis	Crohn's Disease
Intractable disease	CD of Small Intestine
Fulminant disease	Stricture and obstruction unresponsive to medical therapy
Toxic megacolon	Massive hemorrhage
Colonic perforation	Refractory fistula
Massive colonic hemorrhage	Abscess
Extracolonic disease	CD of Colon and Rectum
Colonic obstruction	Intractable disease
Colon cancer prophylaxis	Fulminant disease
Colon dysplasia or cancer	Perianal disease unresponsive to medical therapy
	Refractory fistula
	Colonic obstruction
	Cancer prophylaxis
	Colon dysplasia or cancer

Patients with IPAAs usually have about six to eight bowel movements a day. On validated quality of life indices, they report better performance in sports and sexual activities than ileostomy patients. The most frequent late complication of IPAA is pouchitis in about one-third of patients with UC. This syndrome consists of increased stool frequency, watery stools, cramping, urgency, nocturnal leakage of stool, arthralgias, malaise, and fever. Although it usually responds to antibiotics, in 3% of patients it is refractory and requires pouch take-down.

Crohn's disease Most patients with CD require at least one operation in their lifetime. The need for surgery is related to duration of disease and the site of involvement. Patients with small bowel disease have an 80% chance of requiring surgery. Those with colitis alone have a 50% chance. The indications for surgery are shown in (Table 287-7).

Small Intestinal Disease Because CD is chronic and recurrent with no clear surgical cure, as little intestine as possible is resected. Current surgical alternatives for treatment of obstructing CD include resection of the diseased segment and strictureplasty. Surgical resection of the diseased segment is the most frequently performed operation, and in most cases primary anastomosis can be done to restore continuity. If much of the small bowel has already been resected and the strictures are short with intervening areas of normal mucosa, strictureplasties should be done to avoid a functionally insufficient length of bowel. The strictured area of intestine is incised longitudinally and the incision sutured transversely, thus widening the narrowed area. Complications of strictureplasty include prolonged ileus, hemorrhage, fistula, abscess, leak, and restricture.

Colorectal disease A greater percentage of patients with CD colitis require surgery for intractability, fulminant disease, and anorectal disease. Several alternatives are available, ranging from the use of a temporary loop ileostomy to resection of segments of diseased colon or even the entire colon and rectum. For patients with segmental involvement, segmental colon resection with primary anastomosis can be performed. In 20 to 25% of patients with extensive colitis, the rectum is spared sufficiently to consider rectal preservation. Most surgeons believe that an IPAA is contraindicated in CD due to the high incidence of pouch failure. A diverting colostomy may help heal severe perianal disease or rectovaginal fistulas, but disease almost always recurs with reanastomosis. Often, these patients require a total proctocolectomy and ileostomy.

INFLAMMATORY BOWEL DISEASE AND PREGNANCY

When adjusted for patient age, the fertility rate in UC is probably normal. In contrast, fertility is reduced in CD in proportion to disease activity and can be restored when remission is induced. The ovaries and fallopian tubes can be affected by the inflammatory process of CD, especially on the right side because of the proximity of the terminal ileum. In addition, perirectal, perineal, rectovaginal abscesses, and fistulae can result in dyspareunia. Infertility in men can be caused by sulfasalazine but reverses when treatment is stopped.

In UC, fetal outcome approximates that in the normal population. In CD, spontaneous abortions, stillbirths, and developmental defects are increased with increased disease activity, not medications. The courses of CD and UC during pregnancy mostly correlate with disease activity at the time of conception. Most CD patients can deliver vaginally, but cesarean section may be the preferred route of delivery for patients with anorectal and perirectal abscesses and fistulas to reduce the likelihood of fistulas developing or extending into the episiotomy scar.

Sulfasalazine, mesalamine, and olsalazine are safe for use in pregnancy, but folate supplementation must be given with sulfasalazine. No adverse affects have been reported from sulfasalazine in nursing infants. Topical 5-ASA agents are also safe during pregnancy. Glucocorticoids are generally safe for use during pregnancy and are indicated for patients with moderate to severe disease activity. The amount of glucocorticoids received by the nursing infant is minimal. The safest antibiotics to use for CD in pregnancy are ampicillin, cephalosporin, or ciprofloxicin. Flagyl is teratogenic and tumorigenic in high doses, passes into breast milk, and should be avoided.

6-MP and azathioprine pose minimal or no risk during pregnancy, but experience is limited. If the patient cannot be weaned from the drug or has an exacerbation that requires 6-MP/azathioprine during pregnancy, she should continue the drug with informed consent. Their effects during nursing are unknown.

There is little data on cyclosporine in pregnancy. In a small number of patients with severe IBD treated with intravenous cyclosporine during pregnancy, 80% of pregnancies were successfully completed without development of renal toxicity, congenital malformations, or developmental defects. However, because of the lack of data, cyclosporine should probably be avoided unless the patient would otherwise require surgery. Methotrexate is contraindicated in pregnancy and nursing.

Surgery in UC should be performed only for emergency indications, including severe hemorrhage, perforation, and megacolon refractory to medical therapy. Total colectomy and ileostomy carries a 60% risk of postoperative spontaneous abortion. Fetal mortality is also high in CD requiring surgery. Patients with ileostomies and IPAAs tolerate pregnancy well.

INFLAMMATORY BOWEL DISEASE IN THE ELDERLY

The most common presenting symptoms in the elderly are diarrhea, weight loss, and abdominal pain. CD in the elderly is mostly colonic with a distal distribution and occurs predominantly in women. Proctitis has been documented in 50% of elderly patients and the diagnosis is often delayed. Diseases that can mimic CD in the elderly are ischemic colitis, diverticular disease, irritable bowel, infectious colitides, and malignancies, including carcinoma, lymphoma, and carcinoid. The incidence of surgery is high in elderly patients, with up to 50% of patients with ileitis, ileocolitis, or extensive colitis requiring urgent or early surgery for first-time disease. In addition, surgery has a much higher morbidity than in younger patients, although the rate of post-

operative recurrence is less. Most elderly patients respond as well as younger individuals to medical management.

UC in the elderly is more common in men, presents usually with diarrhea and weight loss, and may have a more distal distribution than in younger patients. Most elderly patients have a favorable response to medical therapy, especially 5-ASA agents, and immunosuppressives used in conjunction with low doses of glucocorticoids. Cyclosporine has been used more frequently in the elderly, but the age-related decreases in renal clearance may affect dosing. Glucocorticoid complications such as osteoporosis and hyperglycemia are also increased in the elderly. 6-MP and azathioprine are well tolerated in the elderly. Surgery also has a higher morbidity and mortality in UC, and elderly patients have a longer hospital stay than younger patients. The risk of colon cancer in UC and CD colitis is no greater than that in the general population since the duration of disease is short and the extent of disease is often distal.

CANCER IN INFLAMMATORY BOWEL DISEASE

ULCERATIVE COLITIS Patients with long-standing UC are at increased risk for developing colonic epithelial dysplasia and carcinoma (Fig. 287-8). Several features distinguish sporadic (SCC) and colitis-associated (CAC) colon cancers. First, SCC usually arise from an adenomatous polyp; CAC typically arise from either flat dysplasia or a dysplasia-associated lesion or mass (DALM). Second, multiple synchronous colon cancers occur in 3 to 5% of SCC but in 12% of CAC. Third, the mean age of individuals with SCC is in the sixties; the mean age of those with CAC is in the thirties. Fourth, SCC exhibits a left-sided predominance, whereas CAC is distributed more uniformly

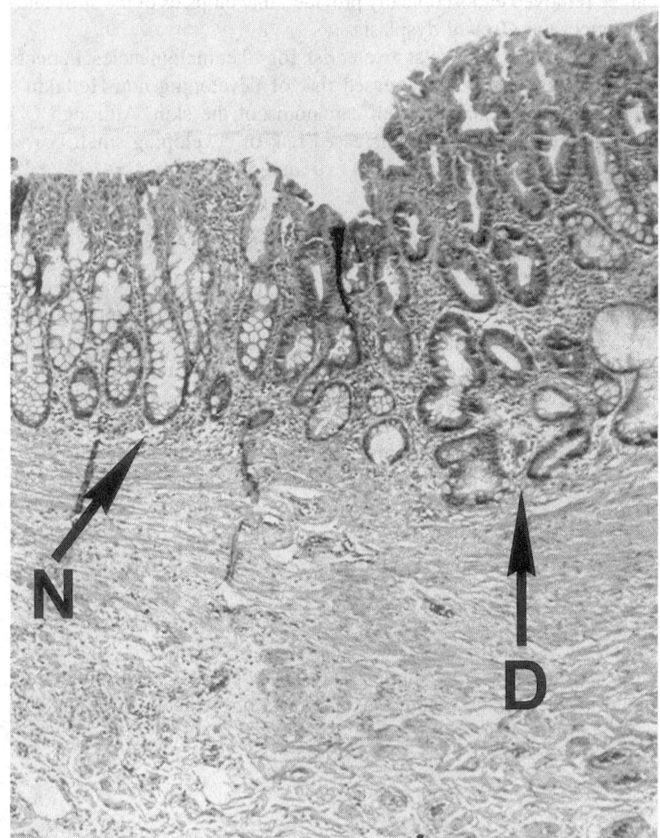

FIGURE 287-8 Low power transition between dysplasia (D) and non-dysplastic (N) mucosa in a case of ulcerative colitis. *(Courtesy of Dr. EK Rosado and Dr. CA Perkos, Division of Gastrointestinal Pathology, Department of Pathology, Emory University, Atlanta, Georgia.)*

throughout the colon. Fifth, mucinous and anaplastic cancers are more common in CAC than SCC. At the molecular level, p53 mutations occur much earlier and *APC* gene mutations much later in CAC than SCC.

The risk of neoplasia in chronic UC increases with duration and extent of disease. For patients with pancolitis, the risk of cancer rises 0.5 to 1% per year after 8 to 10 years of disease. This observed increase in cancer rates has led to the endorsement of surveillance colonoscopies with biopsies for patients with chronic UC as the standard of care. Annual or biennial colonoscopy with multiple biopsies has been advocated for patients with more than 8 to 10 years of pancolitis or 12 to 15 years of left-sided colitis and has been widely employed to screen and survey for subsequent dysplasia and carcinoma.

CROHN'S DISEASE Risk factors for developing colorectal cancer in CD are a history of colonic (or ileocolonic) involvement and long disease duration. The cancer risks in CD and UC are probably equivalent for similar extent and duration of disease. In patients with extensive colonic involvement, the overall risk is increased 18-fold and the cumulative risk is 8% at 22 years. Thus, the same endoscopic surveillance strategy used for UC is recommended for patients with chronic CD colitis. A pediatric colonoscope can be used to pass narrow strictures in CD patients and impassable strictures can be surveyed with annual barium enemas. A colon resection should be performed if there is evidence of malignancy.

MANAGEMENT OF DYSPLASIA AND CANCER If high grade dysplasia (HGD) is encountered on colonoscopic surveillance, the usual treatment for UC is colectomy and for CD is either colectomy or segmental resection. If low grade dysplasia (LGD) is found, the management is controversial. Many investigators recommend immediate colectomy, but some repeat the colonoscopy in 1 to 6 months and search for recurrent dysplasia. Polyps in chronic colitis can be removed endoscopically provided that biopsies of the surrounding mucosa are free of dysplasia.

IBD patients are also at greater risk for other malignancies. Patients with CD may have an increased risk of developing non-Hodgkin's lymphoma and squamous cell carcinoma of the skin. Although CD patients have a twelvefold increased risk of developing small bowel cancer, this type of carcinoma is extremely rare.

QUALITY OF LIFE IN INFLAMMATORY BOWEL DISEASE

The assessment of health-related quality of life plays an important role in the evaluation and treatment of IBD patients. Although clinical trials have generally relied upon traditional disease activity indices such as the Crohn's Disease Activity Index (CDAI) to measure therapeutic efficacy, these measures do not reflect quality of life. The Inflammatory Bowel Disease Questionnaire (IBDQ) is a validated, disease-specific instrument that has been used to measure quality of life. It is a 32-item questionnaire that measures global function, systemic and bowel symptoms, functional and social impairment, and emotional function. When compared to the general population, IBD patients have an impaired quality of life in all six categories. The most frequent concerns of UC patients are having an ostomy bag, developing cancer, effects of medication, the uncertain nature of the disease, and having surgery. The most frequent concerns of CD patients are the uncertain nature of the disease, energy level, effects of medication, having surgery, and having an ostomy bag.

BIBLIOGRAPHY

BLUMBERG RS et al: Animal models of mucosal inflammation and their relation to human inflammatory bowel disease. Curr Opin Immunol 111:648, 1999

FEAGAN BG et al: A comparison of methotrexate with placebo for the maintenance of remission in Crohn's disease. N Engl J Med 342:1627, 2000

HANAUER SB, MEYERS S: Management of Crohn's disease in adults. Am J Gastroenterol 92:559, 1997

IRVINE EJ: Quality of life issues in patients with inflammatory bowel disease. Am J Gastroenterol 92:18S, 1997

ITZKOWITZ S: Inflammatory bowel disease and cancer. Gastroenterol Clin North Am 26: 129, 1997

KIRSNER JB (ed): *Inflammatory Bowel Disease*, 5th ed. Philadelphia, Saunders, 2000

KORELITZ BI: Inflammatory bowel disease and pregnancy. Gastroenterol Clin North Am 27:213, 1998

KORNBLUTH A, SACHAR DB: Ulcerative colitis practice guidelines in adults. Am J Gastroenterol 92:204, 1997

SHANAHAN F et al: Neutrophil autoantibodies in ulcerative colitis: Familial aggregation and genetic heterogeneity. Gastroenterology 103:456, 1992

TARGAN SR et al: A short-term study of chimeric monoclonal cA2 to tumor necrosis factor alpha for Crohn's disease. N Engl J Med 337:1029, 1997

288 IRRITABLE BOWEL SYNDROME

Chung Owyang

Irritable bowel syndrome (IBS) is a gastrointestinal (GI) disorder characterized by altered bowel habits and abdominal pain in the absence of detectable structural abnormalities. No clear diagnostic markers exist for IBS, so all definitions of the disease are based on the clinical presentation. The Rome criteria for the diagnosis of IBS are summarized in Table 288-1. IBS is one of the most common conditions encountered in clinical practice but one of the least well understood. Until recently, many physicians did not consider IBS to be a disease at all; they viewed it as nothing more than a somatic manifestation of psychological stress. With the availability of better techniques to study colonic and GI motility and visceral sensory function, along with the development of newer concepts about the importance of the brain in regulating gut function, significant progress has been made toward a better understanding of the pathogenesis of IBS. Improved methods of treatment may result from these insights.

CLINICAL FEATURES IBS is a disorder of young people, with most new cases presenting before age 45. However, some reports suggest that the elderly are troubled by IBS symptoms up to 92% as often as middle-aged persons. Indeed, many of the diagnoses of "painful diverticular disease" given the elderly patients may represent IBS. Women are diagnosed with IBS two to three times as often as men and make up 80% of the population with severe IBS. Patients with IBS may fall into two broad clinical groups. Most commonly, patients have abdominal pain associated with altered bowel habits that include constipation, diarrhea, or both. In the second group, patients have painless diarrhea. This latter group accounts for <20% of patients with IBS; their condition may be a separate entity but is generally considered a variant of IBS.

Abdominal Pain Abdominal pain in IBS is highly variable in intensity and location. Pain in IBS is localized to the hypogastrum in 25%, the right side in 20%, to the left side in 20%, and the epigastrum in 10% of patients. Pain is frequently episodic and crampy but may be superimposed on a background of constant ache. Pain may be mild enough to be ignored or it may interfere with daily activities. Despite this, malnutrition due to inadequate caloric intake is exceedingly rare with IBS. Sleep deprivation is also unusual because abdominal pain

Table 288-1 Rome Criteria for the Diagnosis of IBS

Abdominal Pain/Discomfort[a]	AND	Two or More at Least 25% of the Time[a]
Relieved with defecation		Change in stool frequency
and/or		Change in consistency
With change in stool frequency		Difficult stool passage
and/or		Sense of incomplete evacuation
With change in stool consistency		Presence of mucus in stool

[a] Symptoms must have been present for > 3 months.

is almost uniformly present only during waking hours. Pain is often exacerbated by eating or emotional stress and relieved by passage of flatus or stools.

Altered Bowel Habits Alteration in bowel habits is the most consistent clinical feature in IBS. Symptoms usually begin in adult life. The most common pattern is constipation alternating with diarrhea, usually with one of these symptoms predominating. At first, constipation may be episodic, but eventually it becomes continuous and increasingly intractable to treatment with laxatives. Stools are usually hard with narrowed caliber, possibly reflecting excessive dehydration caused by prolonged colonic retention and spasm. Most patients also experience a sense of incomplete evacuation, thus leading to repeated attempts at defecation in a short time span. Patients whose predominant symptom is constipation may have weeks or months of constipation interrupted with brief periods of diarrhea. In other patients, diarrhea may be the predominant symptom. Diarrhea resulting from IBS usually consists of small volumes of loose stools, and most patients have stool volumes of <200 mL. Nocturnal diarrhea does not occur in IBS. Diarrhea may be aggravated by emotional stress or eating. Stool may be accompanied by passage of large amounts of mucus; hence, the term *mucous colitis* has been used to describe IBS. This is a misnomer, since inflammation is not present. Bleeding is not a feature of IBS unless hemorrhoids are present, and malabsorption or weight loss does not occur.

Gas and Flatulence Patients with IBS frequently complain of abdominal distention and increased belching or flatulence, all of which they attribute to increased gas. Although some patients with these symptoms actually may have a larger amount of gas, quantitative measurements reveal that most patients who complain of increased gas generate no more than a normal amount of intestinal gas. Most IBS patients develop symptoms even with minimal gut distention, suggesting that the basis of their complaints is reduced tolerance of distention rather than an abnormal quantity of intraluminal gas. In addition, patients with IBS tend to reflux gas from the distal to the more proximal intestine, which may explain the belching.

Upper Gastrointestinal Symptoms Between 25 and 50% of patients with IBS complain of dyspepsia, heartburn, nausea, and vomiting. This suggests that areas of the gut other than the colon may be involved. Prolonged ambulant recordings of small bowel motility in patients with IBS show a high incidence of abnormalities in the small bowel during the waking period; nocturnal motor patterns are no different from those of healthy controls. A characteristic finding is the frequent occurrence of episodes of clustered contractions recurring at 0- to 9-min intervals. These episodes have a mean duration of 46 min and are often associated with transient abdominal pain and discomfort. A similar pattern has been observed in patients with IBS by the application of psychological stressors and by intravenous neostigmine. In addition, temporary abolition of migrating motor complexes is observed in IBS patients under mental stress. Thus, IBS appears to be a paroxysmal motor disorder that may be detected in the small bowel.

PATHOPHYSIOLOGY The pathogenesis of IBS is poorly understood, although roles for abnormal gut motor and sensory activity, central neural dysfunction, psychological disturbances, stress, and luminal factors have been proposed.

Colonic myoelectrical and motor activity under unstimulated conditions are generally normal, but abnormalities are more prominent under stimulated conditions in IBS. IBS patients may exhibit increased rectosigmoid motor activity for up to 3 h after eating. Provocative stimuli also induce exaggerated colonic motor responses in IBS patients compared to healthy volunteers. For example, inflation of rectal balloons both in diarrhea- and constipation-predominant IBS patients leads to marked distention-evoked contractile activity, which may be prolonged.

As with studies of motor activity, IBS patients frequently exhibit exaggerated sensory responses to visceral stimulation. Postprandial pain has been temporally related to entry of food bolus into the cecum in 74% of patients. Exaggerated symptoms can be induced by visceral distention in IBS patients. Rectal balloon inflation produces both nonpainful and painful sensations at lower volumes in IBS patients than in healthy controls without altering rectal tension, suggestive of visceral afferent dysfunction in IBS. The visceral hyperalgesia of IBS appears to be selective for mechanoreceptor-activated stimuli, as perception of intestinal mucosal electrical stimulation is normal in IBS. Similar studies show gastric and esophageal hypersensitivity in patients with nonulcer dyspepsia and noncardiac chest pain, raising the possibility that these conditions have a similar pathophysiologic basis. In contrast to their enhanced gut sensitivity, IBS patients do not exhibit heightened sensitivity elsewhere in the body. Thus the afferent pathway disturbances in IBS appear to be selective for visceral innervation, with sparing of somatic pathways. The mechanisms responsible for visceral hypersensitivity are unclear. These exaggerated responses may be due to: (1) increased end organ sensitivity with recruitment of "silent" nociceptors; (2) spinal hyperexcitability with activation of nitric oxide and possibly other neurotransmitters; (3) endogenous (cortical and brainstem) modulation of caudad nociceptive transmission; and (4) over time, the possible development of long-term hyperalgesia due to development of neuroplasticity, resulting in permanent or semipermanent changes in neural responses to chronic or recurrent visceral stimulation.

The role of central nervous system (CNS) factors in the pathogenesis of IBS is strongly suggested by (1) the clinical association of emotional disorders and stress with symptom exacerbation, and (2) the therapeutic response to therapies that act on cerebral cortical sites. Positron emission tomography has shown alterations in regional cerebral blood flow in IBS patients. In healthy individuals, rectal distention increases blood flow in the anterior cingulate cortex, a region with an abundance of opiate receptors, which, when activated, may help to reduce sensory input. In contrast, IBS patients exhibit no increased blood flow in the anterior cingulate gyrus but show activation of the prefrontal cortex, either in response to rectal activation or in anticipation of rectal distention. Activation of the frontal lobes may activate a vigilance network within the brain that increases alertness. The anterior cingulate cortex and the prefrontal cortex appear to have reciprocal inhibitory associations. In patients with IBS, the preferential activation of the prefrontal lobe without activation of the anterior cingulate cortex may represent a form of cerebral dysfunction leading to the increased perception of visceral pain.

Abnormal psychiatric features are recorded in up to 80% of IBS patients; however, no single psychiatric diagnosis predominates. An association between prior sexual or physical abuse and development of IBS has been reported. Forms of sexual abuse associated with IBS include verbal aggression, exhibitionism, sexual harassment, sexual touching, and rape. The pathophysiologic relationship between IBS and sexual or physical abuse is unknown. However, physical and sexual abuse may result in hypervigilence to body sensations at the CNS level and visceral hypersensitivity at the gut level.

Thus patients with IBS frequently demonstrate increased motor reactivity of the colon and small bowel to a variety of stimuli and altered visceral sensation associated with lowered sensation thresholds. These may result from CNS (enteric nervous system) dysregulation.

Approach to the Patient

Because IBS is a disorder for which no pathognomonic abnormalities have been identified, its diagnosis relies on recognition of positive clinical features and elimination of other organic diseases. A careful history and physical examination are frequently helpful in establishing the diagnosis. Clinical features suggestive of IBS include the following: recurrence of lower abdominal pain with altered bowel habits over a period of time without progressive deterioration, onset of symptoms during periods of stress or emotional upset, absence of other systemic symptoms such as fever and weight loss, and small-volume stool without any evidence of blood.

On the other hand, the appearance of the disorder for the first time in old age, progressive course from time of onset, persistent diarrhea after a 48-h fast, and presence of nocturnal diarrhea or steatorrheal stools argue against the diagnosis of IBS.

Because the major symptoms of IBS—abdominal pain, abdominal bloating, and alteration in bowel habits—are common complaints of many GI organic disorders, the list of differential diagnoses is long. The quality, location, and timing of pain may be helpful in suggesting specific disorders. Pain due to IBS that occurs in the epigastric or periumbilical area must be differentiated from biliary tract disease, peptic ulcer disorders, intestinal ischemia, and carcinoma of the stomach and pancreas. If pain occurs mainly in the lower abdomen, the possibility of diverticular disease of the colon, inflammatory bowel disease (including ulcerative colitis and Crohn's disease), and carcinoma of the colon must be considered. Postprandial pain accompanied by bloating, nausea, and vomiting suggests gastroparesis or partial intestinal obstruction. Intestinal infestation with *Giardia lamblia* or other parasites may cause similar symptoms. When diarrhea is the major complaint, the possibility of lactase deficiency, laxative abuse, malabsorption, hyperthyroidism, inflammatory bowel disease, and infectious diarrhea must be ruled out. On the other hand, constipation may be a side effect of many different drugs, such as anticholinergic, antihypertensive, and antidepressant medications. Endocrinopathies such as hypothyroidism and hypoparathyroidism must also be considered in the differential diagnosis of constipation, particularly if other systemic signs or symptoms of these endocrinopathies are present. In addition, acute intermittent porphyria and lead poisoning may present in a fashion similar to IBS, with painful constipation as the major complaint. These possibilities are suspected on the basis of their clinical presentations and are confirmed by appropriate serum and urine tests.

Because IBS is in part a diagnosis of exclusion, certain diagnostic tests should be performed routinely; others may be required depending on the specific presenting symptoms. Factors to be considered when determining the aggressiveness of the diagnostic evaluation include the duration of symptoms, the change in symptoms over time, the age and sex of the patient, the referral status of the patient, prior diagnostic studies, a family history of colorectal malignancy, and the degree of psychosocial dysfunction. Thus a younger individual with mild symptoms requires a minimal diagnostic evaluation, while an older person or an individual with rapidly progressive symptoms should undergo a more thorough exclusion of organic disease. In general most patients should have a complete blood count and sigmoidoscopic examination; in addition, stool specimens should be examined for ova and parasites. In those >40 years, an air-contrast barium enema or colonoscopy should also be done. In patients whose main symptoms are diarrhea and increased gas, the possibility of lactase deficiency should be ruled out with a hydrogen breath test or a lactose-free diet should be prescribed for 3 weeks. In patients with concurrent symptoms of dyspepsia, upper GI radiographs or esophagogastroduodenoscopy may be advisable. In patients with postprandial right upper quadrant pain, ultrasound of the gallbladder should be obtained. Laboratory features that argue against IBS include evidence of anemia, elevated sedimentation rate, presence of leukocytes or blood in stool, and stool volume >200 to 300 mL/d. These findings suggest other diagnostic considerations.

℞ TREATMENT **Patient Counseling and Dietary Alterations** Reassurance and careful explanation of the functional nature of the disorder and of how to avoid obvious food precipitants are important first steps in patient counseling and dietary change. Occasionally, a meticulous dietary history may reveal substances (such as coffee, disaccharides, legumes, and cabbage) that aggravate symptoms. As a therapeutic trial, patients should be encouraged to eliminate any foodstuffs that appear to produce symptoms.

Stool Bulking Agents High-fiber diets and bulking agents, such as bran or hydrophilic colloid, are frequently used in treating IBS. Dietary fiber has multiple effects on colonic physiology. The water-holding action of fibers may contribute to increased stool bulk. Fiber also speeds up colonic transit in most people. In diarrhea-prone patients, whole-colonic transit is faster than average; however, dietary fiber can delay transit. Furthermore, because of their hydrophilic properties, stool-bulking agents bind water and thus prevent both excessive hydration or dehydration of stool. A high-fiber diet relieves diarrhea in some IBS patients. Dietary fiber has also been shown to lower pressures in the sigmoid colon in IBS patients. The effects of fiber on pressure in the rest of the colon are unknown; however, the whole colon is affected by IBS, and the pain of colon spasm often originates from the ascending and transverse segments. Fiber supplementation with psyllium reduces the perception of rectal distention, indicating that fiber may have an effect on visceral afferent function.

The beneficial effects of dietary fiber on colonic physiology suggest that dietary fiber should be an effective treatment for IBS patients, but controlled trials of dietary fiber have produced variable results. IBS is not purely a colonic disorder; many patients may have symptoms originating from the upper gut. Despite the equivocal data regarding efficacy, most gastroenterologists consider stool-bulking agents worth trying in patients with IBS. Patients should be advised to take increasing quantities of bran supplements, such as whole-meal bread, high-bran cereal, or raw bran, until they are passing one or two soft stools daily. Alternatively, psyllium preparations may be used. About 20% of patients, however, complain that a high-fiber diet aggravates such symptoms as bloating and distention. These undesirable effects usually disappear spontaneously after several weeks.

Antispasmodics Anticholinergic drugs may provide temporary relief for symptoms such as painful cramps related to intestinal spasm. Although controlled clinical trials have produced mixed results, evidence generally supports use of anticholinergic drugs for pain. Meta-analysis of 26 double-blind clinical trials of antispasmodic agents in IBS showed better global improvement (62%) and abdominal pain reduction (64%) compared to placebo (35% and 45%, respectively). The drugs are most effective when prescribed in anticipation of predictable pain. Physiologic studies demonstrate that anticholinergic drugs inhibit the gastrocolic reflex; hence, postprandial pain is best managed by giving antispasmodics 30 min before meals so that effective blood levels are achieved shortly before the anticipated onset of pain. Most anticholinergics contain natural belladonna alkaloids, which may cause xerostomia, urinary hesitancy and retention, blurred vision, and drowsiness. Some physicians prefer to use synthetic anticholinergics, such as dicyclomine, that have less effect on mucous membrane secretions and therefore produce fewer undesirable side effects.

Antidiarrheal Agents When diarrhea is severe, especially in the painless diarrhea variant of IBS, small doses of diphenoxylate (Lomotil), 2.5 to 5 mg every 4 to 6 h, can be prescribed. These agents are less addictive than paregoric, codeine, or tincture of opium. In general, the intestines do not become tolerant of the antidiarrheal effect of opiates, and increasing doses are not required to maintain antidiarrheal potency. These agents are most useful if taken before anticipated stressful events that are known to cause diarrhea. Treatment with antidiarrheals, however, should be considered only as temporary management; the final goal of treatment is gradual withdrawal of medication with substitution of a high-fiber diet.

Drug Antidepressants In addition to their mood-elevating effects, antidepressent medications have several physiologic effects that may be beneficial in IBS. In diarrhea-predominant IBS patients, the tricyclic antidepressant imipramine slows jejunal migrating motor complex transit propagation and delays orocecal and whole-gut transit, indicative of a motor inhibitory effect. Tricyclic agents may alter visceral afferent neural function.

Tricyclic antidepressants may be effective in some IBS patients. In a 2-month study of desipramine, abdominal pain improved in 86% of patients compared to 59% given a placebo. Another study of desipramine in 28 IBS patients showed improvement in stool frequency, diarrhea, pain, and depression. Improvements were mainly observed in diarrhea-predominant patients, with no improvement noted in constipated patients. The efficacy of other antidepressant agents is less well evaluated. An uncontrolled review of antidepressant therapy in 138 patients with IBS, including both tricyclic agents and the newer selective serotonin reuptake inhibitors (e.g., fluxetine, paroxetine, and sertraline), reported symptomatic improvement in 89% of individuals, especially those in the pain-predominant subtype. However, no placebo-controlled trials of the selective serotonin inhibitors have been reported in IBS to date.

Antiflatulence Therapy The management of excessive gas is seldom satisfactory, except in cases of obvious aerophagia or disaccharidase deficiency. Patients should be advised to eat slowly; not chew gum or drink carbonated beverages; and avoid artificial sweeteners, legumes, and foods of the cabbage family. Simethicone, antacids, and activated charcoal have all been tried, usually with disappointing results.

FUTURE DIRECTIONS IN MEDICAL TREATMENT OF IBS Medications that blunt the visceral hyperalgesia of IBS are in development. Such "antiafferent" agents might act via one or more mechanisms, including (1) modification of release of pain-inducing mediators in the gut wall, (2) blockade or activation of peripheral afferent nerve receptors, (3) inhibition of afferent nerve transmission, or (4) modification of afferent activity in the CNS. These include the kappa opioid compounds and serotonin receptor ($5HT_3$) antagonists such as alosetron and octreotide.

Such compounds have been shown to reduce perception of painful mechanical visceral stimulation in patients with IBS. Furthermore, placebo-controlled trials with IBS patients have shown that alosetron or fedotozine, a kappa opioid analogue, reduces both pain and the severity of disease. Additional clinical studies of this group of compounds may lead to new therapeutic approaches for the treatment of IBS.

BIBLIOGRAPHY

BUENO L et al: Mediators and pharmacology of visceral sensitivity: From basic to clinical investigations. Gastroenterology 112:1714, 1997

DROSSMAN DA et al: American Gastroenterological Association technical review on irritable bowel syndrome. Gastroenterology 112:2120, 1997

HASLER WL, OWYANG C: Irritable bowel syndrome, in T Yamada (ed): *Textbook of Gastroenterology*, Philadelphia, Lippincott, Williams & Wilkins, p 1884, 1999

LYNN RB, FRIEDMAN LS: Irritable bowel syndrome. N Engl J Med 329:1940, 1993

MAYER AE, GEDHART GF: Basic and clinical aspects of visceral hyperalgesia. Gastroenterology 107:271, 1994

SILVERMAN DHS et al: Regional cerebral activity in normal and pathologic perception of visceral pain. Gastroenterology 112:64, 1997

289

Kurt J. Isselbacher, Alan Epstein

DIVERTICULAR, VASCULAR, AND OTHER DISORDERS OF THE INTESTINE AND PERITONEUM

DIVERTICULAR DISEASE

Diverticula may be either congenital or acquired and may affect either the small or large intestine. Congenital diverticula are herniations of the entire thickness of intestinal wall, while the more common acquired diverticula consist of herniations of the mucosa through the muscularis, generally at the site of a nutrient artery.

SMALL-INTESTINAL DIVERTICULA Diverticula may occur in any portion of the small intestine; however, with the exception of Meckel's diverticulum, the most common locations are in the duodenum and jejunum. Most often diverticula are asymptomatic and discovered incidentally on upper gastrointestinal x-rays. On occasion, however, they may cause symptoms either because of their anatomic proximity to other structures or rarely from inflammation or bleeding.

Duodenal diverticula arise singly from the medial surface of the second portion of the duodenum. In most patients they cause no symptoms. Rarely, they may present as acute diverticulitis with abdominal pain, fever, gastrointestinal bleeding, or, most rarely, perforation. Periampullary diverticula are occasionally associated with cholangitis or pancreatitis. Jejunal diverticula, while less common, may also be the site of acute inflammation, bleeding, or perforation with resulting abscess or peritonitis.

Multiple jejunal diverticula may be associated with malabsorption related to bacterial overgrowth within the diverticula, similar to other situations where intestinal stasis (e.g., blind loops) permits bacterial proliferation. →***The consequences of bacterial proliferation with resultant mucosal damage, deconjugation of bile salts, and vitamin B_{12} malabsorption are discussed in Chap. 286.***

Meckel's diverticulum, a persistent omphalomesenteric duct, is the most frequent congenital anomaly of the digestive tract, occurring in ~2% of autopsied adults. The diverticulum is wide-mouthed, about 5 cm long, and arises from the antimesenteric border of the ileum, usually within 100 cm of the ileocecal valve. The sac may be lined with normal ileal mucosa (approximately half) or contain gastric, duodenal, pancreatic, or colonic mucosa. While rarely symptomatic after age 5, Meckel's diverticulum may produce hemorrhage, inflammation, and obstruction in children and teenagers.

Hemorrhage occurs almost exclusively before age 10 and invariably results from peptic ulceration of ileal mucosa adjacent to a Meckel's diverticulum lined with gastric mucosa. The diagnosis may be established by isotope scanning of the abdomen after injection of technetium-99, which is taken up by the ectopic gastric mucosa in the diverticulum. False-negative and false-positive Meckel's scans are not uncommon; thus, other clinical and laboratory features must be assessed carefully before recommending surgery. In older children and young adults, inflammation of the diverticulum may mimic acute appendicitis. Mechanical obstruction may also occur if the diverticulum intussuscepts into the lumen of the bowel or twists on a fibrous remnant of the omphalomesenteric duct that extends from the diverticulum to the abdominal wall. The treatment of any of these complications of Meckel's diverticulum is surgical excision.

COLONIC DIVERTICULA Diverticula of the colon are herniations or saclike protrusions of the mucosa through the muscularis, at the point where a nutrient artery penetrates the muscularis. Diverticula occur most commonly in the sigmoid colon and decrease in frequency in the proximal colon. They increase with age; the incidence is 20 to 50% in western populations over age 50. The exact mechanism for their formation is unknown but may be related to an increase in intraluminal pressure. Thickening of the muscle coat of the colon in most patients with diverticula suggests that herniations of mucosa are caused by increased pressure produced by colonic muscle contractions. The rarity of colonic diverticula in underdeveloped nations has led to the speculation that diverticula result from the highly refined western diet, which is deficient in dietary fiber or roughage. It is proposed that such diets result in decreased fecal bulk, narrowing of the colon, and an increase in intraluminal pressure in order to move the smaller fecal mass. However, the role of dietary fiber in the etiology and treatment of diverticular disease remains to be determined.

Colonic diverticula are usually asymptomatic and are an incidental finding on barium enema or colonoscopy. The major complications of inflammation, both acute and chronic, and hemorrhage occur in only a small percentage of individuals with diverticulosis. Since diverticulosis is quite common in older patients, one must avoid the temptation of attributing pain or bleeding to the diverticula unless other conditions, especially colon cancer, have been excluded.

DIVERTICULITIS Inflammation can occur in or around the diverticular sac. The cause of diverticulitis is probably mechanical, related to retention in the diverticula of undigested food residue and bacteria, which may form a hard mass called a *fecalith*. This compromises the blood supply to the thin-walled sac (made up solely of mucosa and serosa) and renders it susceptible to invasion by colonic bacteria. The inflammatory process may vary from a small intramural or pericolic abscess to generalized peritonitis. Some attacks are accompanied by minimal symptoms and seem to heal spontaneously. Studies of resected specimens indicate that most perforations of the diverticular sac are small and result in inflammation of the sac itself and the adjacent serosal surface. Diverticulitis occurs more often in men than in women and three times as often in the left as in the right colon. This suggests that diverticulitis may be related to the higher intraluminal pressures and the more solid fecal material in the sigmoid and descending colon.

Acute colonic diverticulitis is a disease of variable severity characterized by fever, left lower quadrant abdominal pain, and signs of peritoneal irritation—muscle spasm, guarding, rebound tenderness. Rectal examination may reveal a tender mass if the area of inflammation is close to the rectum. Although constipation may not have been noted before onset of the illness, the inflammation around the colon often results in some degree of acute constipation or obstipation. Rectal bleeding, usually microscopic, is noted in 25% of cases; it is rarely massive. Polymorphonuclear leukocytosis is common. Complications include free perforation, which results in acute peritonitis, sepsis, and shock, particularly in the elderly. The perforation may be walled off by adherent omentum or neighboring structures such as the bladder or small bowel. Abscess formation or fistulas then occur as the inflammatory mass burrows into other organs. Severe pericolitis may cause a fibrous stricture around the bowel, which can be associated with colonic obstruction and may mimic a neoplasm.

Diagnosis During the acute phase of diverticulitis, barium enema and sigmoidoscopy may be hazardous, since contrast material or air under pressure may lead to rupture of an inflamed diverticulum and convert a walled-off inflammatory lesion to a free perforation. These examinations are usually safe after adequate treatment and healing of the diverticulitis. The radiologic findings on barium enema suggestive of diverticulitis are leakage of barium from a diverticular sac, stricture formation, and the presence of a pericolic inflammatory mass. In many patients the distortion caused by inflammation prevents a clear distinction between cancer and diverticulitis. In these cases, colonoscopy or surgical excision may be required for accurate diagnosis. Abdominal computed tomography scan may demonstrate the presence of a pericolic abscess.

℞ TREATMENT Most patients with acute diverticulitis require bowel rest, intravenous fluids, and broad-spectrum antibiotics. Repeated attacks of diverticulitis in the same area generally require surgical resection. Severe attacks with acute peritoneal signs, suspected abscess, or perforation require intravenous antibiotics directed against gram-negative anaerobic bacteria, followed by surgical drainage or resection. The usual procedure is a diverting colostomy with resection of the involved colon; reanastomosis is then performed at a second operation.

PAINFUL DIVERTICULAR DISEASE WITHOUT DIVERTICULITIS Some patients with diverticulosis develop recurrent left lower quadrant colicky pain without clinical or pathologic evidence of acute diverticulitis. They often have bouts of alternating constipation and diarrhea; the pain may be relieved by defecation or passage of flatus. These features suggest the coexistence of the irritable bowel syndrome. Examination during a bout of pain reveals tenderness of the sigmoid colon, but signs of peritoneal inflammation such as rebound tenderness, muscle guarding, fever, and leukocytosis are absent. Barium enema shows typical diverticula without evidence of inflammation and stricture, plus a "sawtooth" irregularity of the lumen, reflecting muscle hypertrophy and spasm. In some patients the pain is severe enough to warrant observation in a hospital and restriction of food, since feeding aggravates the pain by causing colonic contraction. Anticholinergics, which reduce sigmoid contractions, and mild sedation are usually all that is required. After recovery, the patient should be started on a high-residue diet or given a bulk laxative such as hemicellulose, unprocessed bran, or psyllium extract. Surgical excision is usually not indicated unless acute diverticulitis or its complications occur.

HEMORRHAGE FROM DIVERTICULA Massive hemorrhage from colonic diverticula is one of the most common causes of hematochezia in patients over age 60. This complication of diverticulosis is caused by erosion of a vessel by a fecalith within the diverticular sac. The bleeding is painless and not accompanied by signs or symptoms of diverticulitis. Most cases of mild or moderate hemorrhage stop spontaneously with bed rest and blood transfusion. Localization of bleeding can be obtained by bleeding scan or angiography. In patients with severe hemorrhage, mesenteric angiography can be both diagnostic in localizing the bleeding site and therapeutic, since vasoconstrictive drugs or artificial blood clot infused intraarterially can sometimes effectively control hemorrhage. Colonoscopy is also useful in evaluating acute hematochezia, and the endoscopist may be able to cauterize angiodysplasias (Chap. 44). The location of bleeding diverticula is more commonly in the right colon, particularly the ascending colon, in contrast to the sigmoid colon, where diverticula are more numerous.

MOTILITY DISORDERS

Normal intestinal motility involves the delicate interplay of the gut motor system, neural influences of the autonomic and central nervous system, as well as hormonal factors, specifically gut neuropeptides. In addition, many drugs used in the treatment of disease (e.g., opioids, antibiotics) affect and influence intestinal motility directly or indirectly. Table 289-1 lists some of the disorders of the enteric motor and neural system. Only the more clinically relevant ones are discussed.

MEGACOLON Megacolon, or giant colon, is characterized by massive distention of the colon, usually accompanied by severe constipation or obstipation. This condition can be either congenital or acquired and is seen in all age groups. Acute toxic megacolon is a severe complication of ulcerative colitis (Chap. 287).

Aganglionic Megacolon (Hirschsprung's Disease) This is a congenital disorder due to absence of enteric neurons (ganglions) in the distal colon and rectum. This aganglionic segment loses its neural inhibition and remains contracted. Hirschsprung's disease is a heterogeneous genetic disorder—some patients have an autosomal dominant form of the disease with mutations in the *RET* gene; many have an autosomal recessive form with a mutation in the endothelin-B receptor gene. Hirschsprung's disease is a multigenic trait; genes on 9q31 affect the phenotype of the *RET* gene mutations. These defects result in the gestational failure of neural crest cells to migrate to the distal colon. The disease manifests in early infancy, occurring more frequently in males, and is often familial. These infants have massive abdominal distention, absent bowel movements, and impaired nutrition due to chronic obstruction of the colon. In some individuals with less severe symptoms, the disease may not be diagnosed until adolescence or early adulthood. The aganglionic and contracted segment of bowel is unable to relax to permit passage of stool, causing the normal proximal colon to become greatly dilated. On rectal examination the ampulla is empty of feces and the anal sphincter is normal. Barium enema reveals a narrowed segment in the rectosigmoid, with massive dilation above. Diagnosis is made by full-thickness surgical biopsy under anesthesia and demonstration of absent ganglion cells in the diseased segment. In most patients the aganglionic segment is in the rectosigmoid colon. The treatment of choice is a pull-through procedure in which normally innervated colon is anastomosed to the distal rectum just above the

Table 289-1 Some Motility Disorders of the Enteric Nervous System

Disorder	Comment
Intestinal pseudoobstruction	
Visceral neuropathy	Autosomal dominant disorder characterized by dilatation of jejunum and ileum and degeneration and loss of neurons.
Visceral neuropathy with basal ganglia calcifications	Autosomal recessive disorder with dilatation of duodenum and small bowel and mental retardation. Calcification of basal ganglia and degeneration of myenteric plexus.
Megacolon	
Hirschsprung's disease	Congenital disorder characterized by colonic dilatation proximal to an aganglionic, contracted distal colon and rectum. Caused by gestational failure of neural crest cells to migrate to distal colon. An autosomal dominant form is associated with mutations of the *RET* gene, and an autosomal recessive form with mutation of the endothelin, B-receptor gene.
Multiple endocrine neoplasia type 2A (MEN-2A)	Features similar to those of Hirschsprung's disease. Medullary thyroid cancer, parathyroid hyperplasia, and pheochromocytoma are characteristic. ? Mutation of *RET* gene.
Generalized, with hyperganglionosis	
MEN-2B (Sipple's syndrome)	Achalasia and pseudoobstruction reported with ganglioneuromatosis of myenteric and submucosal plexuses. Medullary thyroid cancer, pheochromocytoma, and mucosal neuromas are characteristic. Mutation of *RET* gene reported.
Neurofibromatosis (von Recklinghausen's disease)	Achalasia and megacolon reported, with neuronal dysplasia of the myenteric plexus. Central nervous system tumors, neurofibromas, pigmented iris, hamartomas, café au lait spots, and mental retardation are characteristic.
Generalized, with hypoganglionosis	
Chagas' disease	Achalasia, intestinal, and colonic pseudoobstruction; megaloureter; and myocarditis due to infection with *Trypanosoma cruzi*. Possible autoimmune response to parasitic antigen.
Paraneoplastic syndrome	Achalasia, gastroparesis, and intestinal pseudoobstruction reported in some patients with small-cell lung cancer and carcinoid tumors. Serum antibodies reactive to enteric neurons.
Cytomegalovirus infection	Esophageal dysmotility, delayed gastric emptying, achalasia, and pseudoobstruction reported, with intranuclear neuronal viral inclusions and loss of myenteric neurons.
Myotonic dystrophy	Autosomal dominant disorder with impaired esophageal and gastric transit and intestinal pseudoobstruction, selective loss of substance P– and enkephalin-containing enteric neurons and preservation of neurons containing neuropeptide Y or vasoactive intestinal polypeptide. Myotonia, weakness, cataracts, cardiac abnormalities, gonadal atrophy, and mental retardation are characteristic.
Generalized, other	
Parkinson's disease	Achalasia, pseudoobstruction, and megacolon reported in some patients, with Lewy bodies in the myenteric plexus of the esophagus and colon.
Diabetes mellitus	Gastroparesis and intestinal and colonic dysmotility, with generalized autonomic neuropathy. Myenteric plexus morphologically intact.
Amyloidosis	Achalasia, gastroparesis, and pseudoobstruction, with amyloid deposits in both smooth muscle and the myenteric plexus.
Fabry's disease	Impaired gastric emptying, jejunal and colonic diverticulosis, and malabsorption, with glycolipid deposition in neurons of the myenteric plexus and decreased numbers of enlarged ganglion cells. Cutaneous angiokeratoma, renal insufficiency, and cardiovascular and central nervous system damage are also seen.
Disorders caused by exogenous neural toxins	Intestinal and colonic pseudoobstruction, with increased argyrophilia of the myenteric plexus.

SOURCE: Modified from Goyal and Hirano, with permission.

internal sphincter, thus bypassing the contracted aganglionic segment and restoring normal defecation.

Acquired Megacolon In Central and South America, infection with *Trypanosoma cruzi* (Chagas' disease) can result in destruction of the ganglion cells of the colon, producing a clinical picture similar to congenital megacolon, except that the onset is in adult life rather than in childhood. A number of other diseases are associated with megacolon in adults. Patients with schizophrenia or depression, particularly institutionalized patients, may have obstipation and massive colonic dilatation. Severe neurologic disorders, including cerebral atrophy, spinal cord injury, and parkinsonism, also may cause megacolon. Myxedema, infiltrative diseases such as amyloidosis, and primary systemic sclerosis also can reduce colonic motility and produce marked colonic distention. Narcotic drugs, particularly morphine and codeine, can cause severe constipation, especially when administered to bedridden patients. Digital rectal examination of adults with acquired megacolon reveals a rectum distended with feces, as opposed to the empty rectum in aganglionic megacolon. Treatment is aimed at the underlying disease, as well as the careful use of enemas and cathartics.

Intestinal Pseudoobstruction Intestinal pseudoobstruction is an acute or chronic motility disorder characterized by distention or dilation of the small and large intestine. Abdominal pain, nausea, and vomiting may lead to diagnostic confusion with mechanical obstruction; but as the name of this condition implies, the underlying cause is not obstruction but rather a severe dysmotility resulting in distention. Pseudoobstruction may be primary or secondary and acute or chronic. In primary or idiopathic pseudoobstruction no other contributing condition can be identified, and the motility disorder is attributed to abnormalities of sympathetic innervation or of the muscle layers of the intestine. Secondary pseudoobstruction may result from primary systemic sclerosis, diabetes, amyloidosis, neurologic diseases, drugs, or sepsis.

Chronic or Intermittent Secondary Pseudoobstruction Numerous medical conditions can cause chronic dilation of the large and small bowel. Some of these may involve the intestinal smooth muscle, such as primary systemic sclerosis, amyloidosis, or muscular dystrophy. Endocrine disorders, including myxedema and diabetes mellitus, may result in chronic distention, which in the diabetic patient results from autonomic visceral neuropathy. Chronic neurologic diseases, including Parkinson's disease and stroke, may be complicated by chronic pseudoobstruction; in these patients drugs and relative immobility are contributing features. Finally, institutionalized psychotic patients may suffer from prolonged megacolon.

The symptoms of chronic secondary pseudoobstruction are chronic or intermittent constipation, crampy abdominal pain, anorexia, and bloating. Gastric distention and disordered swallowing may be present. Abdominal x-rays reveal gaseous distention of the large and small bowel and occasionally of the stomach. Air-fluid levels are unusual and should raise the possibility of mechanical obstruction. Upper gastrointestinal series and barium enema do not reveal specific abnormalities of the intestine such as tumor, stricture, or volvulus. The presence of an autoimmune disorder or endocrinopathy may require confirmation by serologic or blood tests; biopsy may be needed as in amyloidosis or muscular dystrophy.

The treatment of chronic intestinal pseudoobstruction is made difficult by the complexity and chronicity of the underlying systemic disease. Patients with primary systemic sclerosis may respond to broad-spectrum antibiotics if intestinal bacterial overgrowth is suspected. Metoclopramide may benefit gastric dysmotility in the diabetic patient. Discontinuation of psychotropic or anti-Parkinson drugs may occasionally result in improvement. Cathartics and enemas may be required to relieve fecal impaction, and the regular use of stool softeners and a high-fiber diet may help prevent recurrences.

Idiopathic Intestinal Pseudoobstruction This term describes the condition of patients with signs and symptoms of pseudoobstruction in whom no systemic disease can be identified. The typical patient has recurrent attacks of abdominal pain and distention with nausea and vomiting. The small intestine is primarily involved, and chronic constipation is much less frequent than in secondary pseudoobstruction. Steatorrhea secondary to bacterial overgrowth of the small intestine is common and may lead to chronic diarrhea and malnutrition. Many patients exhibit abnormalities of motility in the esophagus and urinary bladder, in addition to the small and large intestine. Neuromuscular defects have been described in patients with this syndrome, including abnormalities of the mesenteric plexus and myopathy of the intestinal and urinary bladder smooth muscle (so-called hollow visceral myopathy). Elevated prostaglandin E levels have been reported in some patients.

Management of idiopathic pseudoobstruction is unsatisfactory. Surgery to relieve "obstruction" is to be avoided, since the condition is often worsened by abdominal surgery. Medical therapy with metoclopramide and cholinergic agents has been unsuccessful. Nutritional support in the form of low-residue elemental diets or parenteral hyperalimentation may be helpful. Unfortunately, the lack of effective therapy and the progressive nature of the illness make the prognosis of idiopathic pseudoobstruction rather poor. Death from malnutrition and steatorrhea are common. The long-term impact of total parenteral nutrition on this disease is not yet clear.

Acute Intestinal Pseudoobstruction This entity, sometimes referred to as *Ogilvie's syndrome*, is characterized by acute intestinal dilation involving primarily the colon but occasionally also the small intestine. As in other forms of pseudoobstruction, the clinical features are difficult to distinguish from mechanical obstruction. The patient may complain of colicky lower abdominal pain and acute constipation. Examination reveals a distended, tympanitic abdomen, with reduced or absent bowel sounds. Localized tenderness over the distended colon is common, but diffuse abdominal tenderness, rigidity, or rebound tenderness are unusual. Abdominal films reveal massive dilation of the colon and small intestine, occasionally with the presence of air-fluid levels. The cecum, being the most capacious part of the colon, is often massively dilated and tender. The onset of these symptoms usually occurs in patients who have recently undergone severe surgical or medical stress, such as major surgery, myocardial infarction, sepsis, or respiratory failure. Patients with acute pseudoobstruction are frequently on respirators, have received narcotics or sedatives, and have metabolic and electrolyte disturbances. Ogilvie's syndrome may also be due to paraneoplastic obstruction.

Management of acute pseudoobstruction requires careful correction of fluid and electrolyte abnormalities, intubation of the stomach or small intestine for decompression, and avoidance of drugs that depress intestinal motility. Barium enema may be hazardous because of the risk of perforating the already dilated bowel. Decompressive colonoscopy is beneficial in some patients, and cecostomy may be required in some patients with massive cecal dilation. The outcome depends in large part on the prognosis of the associated medical or surgical conditions. Patients who recover from the underlying medical or surgical conditions usually have a return of normal colonic function.

IRRITABLE BOWEL SYNDROME See Chap. 288.

CHRONIC CONSTIPATION Chronic constipation is widespread in western society, with ~10% of the population taking laxatives on a regular basis. Most cases of chronic constipation arise from habitual neglect of afferent impulses, failure to initiate defecation, and accumulation of large, dry fecal masses in the rectum. This voluntary suppression of the call to stool may arise during the period of toilet training in childhood or later in life because of a sense of social impropriety, unaccustomed surroundings, uncomfortable toilet facilities, or illnesses that require confinement to bed. Chronic constipation is much more common in women, with onset typically in late adolescence or early adulthood. As constant distention of the rectum with feces becomes chronic, the patient grows less aware of rectal fullness. Bowel movements become progressively more difficult, and painful hemorrhoids or anal fissures reinforce suppression of the urge to defecate. To avoid these problems the patient begins the chronic use of laxatives or enemas, without which defecation becomes impossible.
→*The mechanism of defecation is discussed in Chap. 42.*

℞ TREATMENT The physician should make every attempt to educate the patient about the chain of events that has led to chronic constipation. Attempts should be made to alter patterns of many years' duration, and the patient must recognize the importance of responding to, rather than suppressing, the urge to defecate. Defecation should be attempted at a given time each day. In most individuals the call to stool occurs in the morning after breakfast. Physical exercise such as a brisk walk just before attempts at defecation may be helpful. Patients are instructed to increase dietary bulk with foods rich in fiber, such as green vegetables and unprocessed cereal grains, or by the regular use of bulk laxatives, such as hemicellulose, psyllium extract, and powdered unprocessed bran. The success of such a regimen depends to some extent on the duration of symptoms. Elderly patients with long-standing constipation and reliance on enemas or laxatives are more resistant to these measures than younger patients whose bowel patterns are less established. Moreover, poor muscle tone, reduced physical activity, and increased incidence of other medical conditions make the problem more difficult in the older age group. Bedridden elderly patients often develop severe constipation and even fecal impaction unless preventive measures are taken. This applies not only to patients with previous constipation but also to those with regular bowel movements before their confining illness. Regular administration of stool softeners, bulk laxatives, or mild cathartics is necessary until full ambulation and a normal diet are resumed. The onset of fecal impaction in bedridden patients is heralded by a feeling of rectal distention, urgency of defecation, or tenesmus. Occasionally, the fecal impaction will result in low-grade chronic obstruction with dilation and increased fluid content proximal to the impaction; "paradoxical diarrhea" may thus occur as fluid moves past the obstructing fecal mass. This situation will be aggravated if antidiarrheal drugs are given because the underlying constipation will be worsened. The appropriate maneuver is to disimpact the rectum manually or to administer gentle enemas if the impaction is beyond the reach of the finger.

DISORDERS OF THE MESENTERIC CIRCULATION

Ischemia of the intestine is the end result of interruption or reduction of its blood supply. However, the clinical manifestations of intestinal ischemia range from mild chronic symptoms to a catastrophic acute episode, depending on the vascular supply involved, the extent of the occlusion or ischemia, and the rapidity of the process. The clinician should be aware of the spectrum of clinical manifestations (Table 289-2). The gut derives its arterial blood supply from the celiac axis and the superior and inferior mesenteric arteries. The small intestine

Table 289-2 Patterns of Intestinal Ischemia

Condition	Etiology	Clinical Features	Management
Mesenteric artery embolus	Arterial embolus associated with atrial fibrillation or rheumatic heart disease	Acute central abdominal pain, shock, peritonitis	Immediate angiography and embolectomy if possible
Abdominal angina	Atherosclerosis of celiac and superior mesenteric arteries	Chronic postprandial pain, weight loss	Angiography and surgery in selected cases
Ischemic colitis	Low-flow state	Acute lower abdominal pain, rectal bleeding	Sigmoidoscopy; surgery only for peritonitis

is supplied by the celiac and superior mesenteric arteries, the colon by branches of the superior and inferior mesenteric arteries. A rich network of anastomotic vessels and the possible development of collateral circulation determine the clinical picture of acute or chronic intestinal arterial insufficiency.

MESENTERIC ISCHEMIA AND INFARCTION Acute intestinal ischemia may be classified as occlusive or nonocclusive. *Occlusion* accounts for about 75% of acute intestinal ischemia and may result from an arterial thrombus (one-third of arterial occlusions) or embolus (two-thirds of arterial occlusions) of the celiac or superior mesenteric arteries, or from venous occlusion (<5% of occlusions) in the same distribution. Arterial embolus occurs most commonly in patients with chronic or recurrent atrial fibrillation, artificial heart valves, or valvular heart disease; arterial thrombosis is usually associated with extensive atherosclerosis or low cardiac output. Venous occlusion is rare; it is occasionally seen in women taking oral contraceptives. Approximately one-fourth of patients with mesenteric ischemia have no definite occlusion of a major vessel, a condition referred to as *nonocclusive ischemia*. The exact cause of nonocclusive disease is obscure; systemic arterial hypotension, cardiac arrhythmias, prolonged heart failure, digitalis therapy, dehydration, and endotoxemia can be contributing factors.

The major clinical feature of acute mesenteric ischemia is severe abdominal pain, often colicky and periumbilical at the onset, later becoming diffuse and constant. Vomiting, anorexia, diarrhea, and constipation are also frequent but of little diagnostic help. Examination of the abdomen may reveal tenderness and distention. Bowel sounds are often normal even in the face of severe infarction. Some patients have a surprisingly normal abdominal examination in spite of severe pain. Mild gastrointestinal bleeding is often detected by examination of stool for occult blood; gross hemorrhage is unusual except in ischemic colitis. Leukocytosis is often present. Late in the course of the disease (24 to 72 h), gangrene of the bowel occurs with diffuse peritonitis, sepsis, and shock. Abdominal plain films in patients with mesenteric ischemia may reveal air-fluid levels and distention. Barium study of the small intestine reveals nonspecific dilation, poor motility, and evidence of thick mucosal folds ("thumbprinting") (Fig. 289-1).

Acute mesenteric ischemia is a grave condition with a high morbidity and mortality. Patients suspected of having acute arterial embolus should undergo immediate celiac and mesenteric angiography to localize the embolus, followed by embolectomy. Restoration of normal circulation may allow complete recovery if performed before irreversible necrosis or gangrene has occurred. Unfortunately, infarction and transmural necrosis are frequently found at surgery, necessitating resection. Arterial or venous thrombosis is not generally amenable to surgical removal of the thrombus, and resection of the affected bowel is required. Similarly, patients with nonocclusive ischemia are not candidates for corrective vascular surgery (as major vessels are patent). These individuals often have extensive necrosis of the small or large intestine because of the widespread nature of the ischemic event. The decision to operate when mesenteric ischemia is suspected is often difficult, because the typical patient is a poor surgical risk owing to

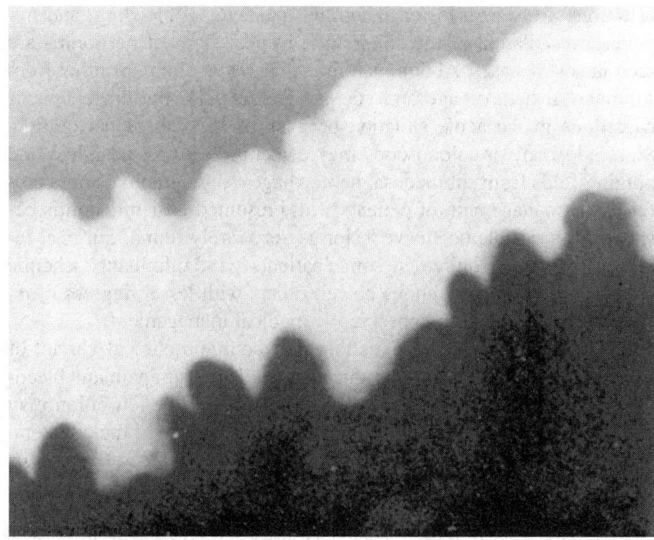

FIGURE 289-1 Barium enema showing "thumbprinting" or submucosal edema of the inferior margin of the transverse colon in a patient with acute ischemic colitis.

advanced age, dehydration, sepsis, and other serious medical conditions.

Chronic arterial insufficiency may precede acute vascular insufficiency, producing so-called abdominal angina. As in angina pectoris, the pain of chronic mesenteric insufficiency occurs under conditions of increased demand for splanchnic blood flow. The patient complains of intermittent dull or cramping midabdominal pain 15 to 30 min after a meal, lasting for several hours postprandially. Significant weight loss due to decreased food intake may be present. Chronic intestinal ischemia also may produce mucosal damage and malabsorption, which in turn aggravates the weight loss. Since abdominal angina may progress to bowel infarction, arteriographic studies should be performed to confirm the diagnosis in those patients who are candidates for abdominal vascular surgery. The only definitive treatment is vascular surgery or balloon angioplasty to remove the thrombus or the construction of bypass arterial grafts to the ischemic bowel.

A number of systemic conditions are associated with *vasculitis* of the large and small arteries supplying the intestine. Most often these disorders can be recognized by the associated extraintestinal manifestations, as in polyarteritis nodosa, lupus erythematosus, dermatomyositis, Henoch-Schönlein purpura (allergic vasculitis), and rheumatoid vasculitis. When larger arteries are involved, as in polyarteritis nodosa, the picture of acute intestinal infarction is similar to that of embolic or atherosclerotic vascular occlusion. Often the involvement of smaller vessels leads to areas of intramural hemorrhage and edema resulting in abdominal pain, variable degrees of intestinal obstruction, and bleeding. Barium enema may show "thumbprinting" and "spiculation" due to localized edema, hemorrhage, and ulceration (Fig. 289-1). In many instances, treatment of the underlying disorder may lead to regression of symptoms. If signs of an acute abdomen develop, surgical exploration is usually indicated.

Intramural small-intestinal hemorrhage may occur with vasculitis, trauma, or impaired coagulation, especially in patients receiving anticoagulants. The clinical and radiologic features resemble those seen with vasculitis and local mucosal hemorrhage.

ISCHEMIC COLITIS Ischemia of the colon most often affects the elderly because of their greater frequency of vascular disease. Ischemic colitis is almost always nonocclusive. Shunting of blood away from the mucosa may contribute to this condition, but the mechanism of ischemia is not known.

The clinical picture depends on the degree of ischemia and its rate of development. In *acute fulminant ischemic colitis*, the major manifestations are severe lower abdominal pain, rectal bleeding, and hypotension. Dilation of the colon and physical signs of peritonitis are seen in severe cases. Abdominal films may reveal thumbprinting from submucosal hemorrhage and edema (Fig. 289-1). Barium enema is hazardous in the acute situation because of the risk of perforation. Sigmoidoscopy or colonoscopy may detect ulcerations, friability, and bulging folds from submucosal hemorrhage. Angiography is not helpful in the management of patients with presumed ischemic colitis because a remediable occlusive lesion is very rarely found. Surgical resection may be required in some patients with fulminant ischemic colitis to remove gangrenous bowel; others with lesser degrees of ischemia may respond to conservative medical management.

Subacute ischemic colitis is the most common clinical variant of ischemic colonic disease. It produces lesser degrees of pain and bleeding, often occurring over several days or weeks. The left colon may be involved, but the rectum is usually spared because of the collateral blood supply, a feature distinguishing it from acute ulcerative colitis. Barium enema reveals edema, cobblestoning, thumbprinting, and occasionally superficial ulceration. Angiography is not indicated because almost all cases are nonocclusive. Occasionally, *stricture formation* may follow a bout of ischemic colitis or may present de novo without a history of antecedent pain or bloody diarrhea. Most cases of nonocclusive ischemic colitis resolve in 2 to 4 weeks and do not recur. Surgery is not required except for obstruction secondary to postischemic stricture.

ANGIODYSPLASIA OF THE COLON These are vascular ectasias or arteriovenous malformations (AVMs) that occur in the right colon of many older individuals and may cause bleeding (Chap. 44). Angiodysplasia is a degenerative lesion consisting of dilated, distorted, thin-walled vessels lined by vascular endothelium. It may result from partial obstruction of the submucosal venous plexus by the tension generated in the cecal wall during muscular contraction. Grossly, angiodysplasias look similar to spider angiomas of the skin and on colonoscopy appear as star-shaped branching vessels in the submucosa measuring from 2 mm to 1 cm in diameter. The lesions are usually multiple and are found primarily in the cecum and ascending colon, but in some patients they may be distributed from the stomach to rectum.

Cecal angiodysplasia is important because of the likelihood of bleeding, either massively or chronically. In patients over age 60, ~1/4 of colonic bleeding episodes are secondary to angiodysplasia. The diagnosis is easiest to establish by colonoscopy, which allows treatment by laser photocoagulation, electrocautery, or injection with sclerosant. Some patients with massive uncontrolled bleeding or multiple sites of angiodysplasia may require right hemicolectomy. Angiodysplasias may also respond to chronic estrogen-progesterone therapy.

ANORECTAL PROBLEMS

HEMORRHOIDS The internal hemorrhoidal plexus of veins is located in the submucosal space above the valves of Morgagni. The anal canal separates it from the external hemorrhoidal venous plexus, but the two spaces communicate under the anal canal, the submucosa of which is attached to underlying tissue to form the interhemorrhoidal depression. Whenever the internal hemorrhoidal plexus is enlarged, the associated supporting tissue mass is increased, and the resultant venous swelling is called an *internal hemorrhoid*. When veins in the external hemorrhoidal plexus become enlarged or thrombosed, the resultant bluish mass is called an *external hemorrhoid*.

Both types of hemorrhoids are very common and are associated with increased hydrostatic pressure in the portal venous system, such as during pregnancy, straining at stool, or with cirrhosis. When internal hemorrhoids enlarge, pain is not a usual feature until the situation is complicated by thrombosis, infection, or erosion of the overlying mucosal surface. Most persons complain of bright red blood on the toilet tissue or coating the stool, with a feeling of vague anal discomfort. The discomfort is increased when the hemorrhoid enlarges or prolapses through the anus; prolapse is often accompanied by edema and sphincteric spasm. If not treated, prolapse usually becomes chronic as the muscularis stays stretched, and the patient complains of constant soiling of underclothing with very little pain. Prolapsed hemorrhoids may become thrombosed; the overlying mucous membrane may bleed profusely from the trauma of defecation.

Because they lie under the skin, external hemorrhoids are quite often painful, particularly if there is a sudden increase in their mass. These episodes result in a tender blue swelling at the anal verge due to thrombosis of a vein in the external plexus and need not be associated with enlargement of the internal veins. Since the thrombus usually lies at the level of the sphincteric muscles, anal spasm often occurs.

The diagnosis of internal and external hemorrhoids is made by inspection, digital examination, and direct vision through the anoscope and proctoscope. Since such lesions are very common, they must not be regarded as the cause of rectal bleeding or iron deficiency anemia until a thorough investigation has been made of the more proximal gastrointestinal tract. Acute blood loss can occasionally be attributed to internal hemorrhoids. Chronic anemia or occult blood in the stool in the presence of large but not definitely bleeding hemorrhoids requires a search for a polyp, cancer, or ulcer.

℞ **TREATMENT** Most hemorrhoids respond to conservative therapy such as sitz baths or other forms of moist heat, suppositories, stool softeners, and bed rest. Internal hemorrhoids that remain permanently prolapsed are best treated surgically; milder degrees of prolapse or enlargement with pruritus ani or intermittent bleeding can be handled successfully by banding or injection of sclerosing solutions. External hemorrhoids that become acutely thrombosed are treated by incision, extraction of the clot, and compression of the incised area following clot removal. No surgical procedure should be carried out in the presence of acute inflammation of the anus, ulcerative proctitis, or ulcerative colitis. Proctoscopy or colonoscopy should always be performed before a patient undergoes hemorrhoidectomy.

ANAL INFLAMMATION Perianal inflammatory lesions may be primary or may be associated with inflammatory bowel disease or diverticular disease. *Anal fissures* are superficial erosions of the anal canal which usually heal rapidly with conservative therapy. *Anal ulcers* are more chronic and deep and give symptoms largely as the result of painful spasm of the external anal sphincter during and after defecation. Bleeding may occur with either fissure or ulcer; healing of the ulcer is often associated with a hypertrophied anal papilla and some degrees of anal contracture. The spasm associated with chronic anal fissure/ulcer can be managed with oral nifedipine or local botulinum toxin. *Fistula in ano*, a tract leading from the rectal lumen to the perianal skin, usually results from local crypt abscesses. The fistula is a chronically inflamed canal made up of fibrous tissue surrounding granulation tissue, the lumen of which may be difficult to demonstrate. *Perirectal abscesses* often represent the tracking down into the anal area of purulent material escaping from the rectosigmoid; diverticulitis, Crohn's disease, ulcerative colitis, or previous surgery may be the underlying cause. Fistulas between the rectum and vagina or the rectum and bladder represent serious complications of granulomatous, septic, or malignant disorders and require the patient to be hospitalized for definitive diagnostic and therapeutic procedures.

PERITONEAL AND MESENTERIC DISEASES

ACUTE PERITONITIS Peritonitis is a localized or generalized inflammatory process of the peritoneum that may appear in both acute and chronic forms. In the acute form the motor activity of the intestine is decreased, and the intestinal lumen becomes distended with gas and fluid. Fluid accumulates as a result of failure to reabsorb the 7 or 8 L normally secreted daily into the lumen and absorbed from the distal small bowel and colon. Because of accumulation of fluid in the peritoneal cavity as well as decreased oral intake, rapid depletion of the plasma volume with impaired cardiac and renal function may occur.

Etiology *Bacterial peritonitis* may be due to entry of bacteria into the peritoneal cavity from a perforation in the gastrointestinal tract or from an external penetrating wound. *Chemical peritonitis* results from spillage of pancreatic enzymes, gastric acid, or bile as a result of injury or perforation of the intestine or biliary tract. *Sterile peritonitis* occurs in patients with systemic lupus erythematosus, porphyria, and familial Mediterranean fever (FMF) during disease attacks.

The most common causes of bacterial peritonitis are appendicitis; perforations associated with diverticulitis; peptic ulcer; gangrenous gallbladder; and gangrenous obstruction of the small bowel from adhesive bands, incarcerated hernia, or volvulus. Any lesion leading to the escape of intestinal bacteria may be a source, including a perforating carcinoma, foreign body, and ulcerative colitis. The peritoneal cavity is remarkably resistant to contamination, and unless continuing contamination occurs, the peritonitis remains localized. Patients with alcoholic cirrhosis and ascites have an increased susceptibility to *spontaneous bacterial peritonitis*, usually from enteric pathogens. This complication occurs in the absence of recognizable perforation of a viscus and may be due to leakage of bacteria through the intestinal wall (Chap. 299).

Clinical Features The cardinal manifestations of peritonitis are acute abdominal pain and tenderness. The location of the pain and tenderness depends on the underlying cause and whether the inflammation is localized or generalized. In *localized peritonitis*, as seen in uncomplicated appendicitis or diverticulitis, the physical findings are limited to the area of inflammation. With widespread peritoneal inflammation there is *generalized peritonitis* with diffuse abdominal tenderness and rebound. Rigidity of the abdominal wall is a common finding in peritonitis and may be localized or generalized.

Peristalsis may be present initially but usually disappears as the illness progresses and bowel sounds disappear. Hypotension, tachycardia, oliguria, and leukocytosis with cell counts $>20{,}000/\mu L$, are common, especially in generalized peritonitis. Plain abdominal films may reveal dilation of the large and small bowel with edema of the small-bowel wall, as evidenced by the distance between adjacent loops of gas-filled small intestine. Diagnostic paracentesis is sometimes valuable in determining the nature of the exudate as well as whether bacteria can be demonstrated or cultured.

GONOCOCCAL PERITONITIS This usually involves an extension of gonococcal infection from a primary focus in the female reproductive tract. The signs of inflammation usually are limited to the pelvis, but there may be findings of a mild generalized peritonitis. Occasionally, the patient has right upper quadrant pain and tenderness caused by gonococcal perihepatitis involving the liver capsule and adjacent peritoneum (Fitz-Hugh–Curtis syndrome) (Chap. 147).

STARCH PERITONITIS An acute granulomatous peritonitis can develop in some patients as a foreign-body reaction to cornstarch used to powder surgical gloves. The clinical picture is that of acute abdominal pain and fever 10 to 30 days after an abdominal operation. The diagnosis can be made by paracentesis and demonstration of starch granules in monocytes. However, most patients are reexplored because of the fear of abscess or bacterial peritonitis, with the finding of foreign-body granuloma studding the peritoneum.

PSEUDOMYXOMA PERITONEI This is a rare condition resulting from rupture of a mucocele of the appendix, a mucinous ovarian cyst, or mucin-secreting intestinal or ovarian adenocarcinoma. The abdomen becomes filled with masses of jelly-like mucus. Occasional patients are cured with removal of the mucocele or the ovarian cyst and most of the myxomatous material. In other cases, however, the mucoid material recurs, leading to progressive wasting and eventual

death. Colloid carcinoma arising from the stomach or colon with peritoneal implants may resemble pseudomyxoma at laparotomy. The course of this type of highly malignant tumor is one of rapid cachexia and early death. The diagnosis usually can be made by the appearance of many highly malignant cells in the peritoneal implants.

PNEUMATOSIS CYSTOIDES INTESTINALIS This is a condition in which multiple gas-filled blebs or cysts accumulate in the intestinal wall beneath the serosal surface of the bowel. The exact source of the gas has not been explained satisfactorily. In some instances, this disease is associated with specific ulceration of the intestinal mucosa, in particular peptic ulcer with outlet obstruction. Cysts in the wall of the small bowel are seen as an occasional complication of mesenteric vascular occlusion. In the large bowel, these cysts are usually benign, may be seen with a variety of other disorders, and usually disappear over time.

Physical findings are not specific and the diagnosis is made either by x-ray or at laparotomy. Occasionally, the subserosal cysts may rupture, resulting in pneumoperitoneum.

CHYLOUS ASCITES See Chap. 46.

MESENTERIC LIPODYSTROPHY This is a rare disorder usually affecting middle-aged women and characterized pathologically by infiltration of the mesentery with lipid-laden macrophages and fibrous tissue. These patients present with ill-defined abdominal pain and occasionally an abdominal mass. The diagnosis is made at laparotomy by demonstration of thick fibrofatty masses at the root of the mesentery with retraction and distortion of the bowel loops.

FAMILIAL MEDITERRANEAN FEVER

Familial Mediterranean fever (FMF, familial paroxysmal polyserositis) is an inherited disorder, characterized by recurrent episodes of fever, peritonitis, and/or pleuritis. Arthritis, skin lesions, and amyloidosis are seen in some patients.

FMF occurs predominantly in patients of non-Ashkenazi (Sephardic) Jewish, Armenian, and Arabic ancestry. However, the disease has been seen in patients of Italian, Ashkenazi Jewish, and Anglo-Saxon descent as well as others.

ETIOLOGY FMF is an autosomal recessive trait characterized by mutations in the *MEFV* gene located on 16p. The gene encodes a 781-amino acid protein called *pyrin* expressed in cells of the myeloid lineage. The gene is in the *RoRet* family, and the product appears to function as a transcription factor based on the presence of a nuclear localization signal, a zinc finger, and a coiled-coil domain. Its expression in granulocytes is increased by proinflammatory cytokines and reduced by anti-inflammatory cytokines. Mutations associated with FMF cluster in exon 10. Different mutations appear to be associated with distinct disease manifestations; replacement of methionine 694 by valine is common in patients who have amyloidosis as a feature of the disease. Valine 726 replacement by alanine is rarely associated with amyloidosis. Other as yet unknown genes may modify the phenotype or be responsible for FMF in non-Mediterranean populations.

PATHOLOGY Despite the striking clinical manifestations during an acute attack of FMF, no specific pathologic alterations have been found. At laparotomy there is acute peritoneal inflammation with an exudate that contains a predominance of polymorphonuclear leukocytes. A disproportionately large number of male patients develop gallbladder disease with and without cholelithiasis. Pleural and joint inflammation are also nonspecific.

In the amyloidosis that accompanies FMF, amyloid is deposited in the intima and media of the arterioles, the subendothelial region of venules, the glomeruli, and the spleen. Aside from their vessels, the heart and liver are uninvolved.

MANIFESTATIONS The symptoms of FMF often begin between the ages of 5 and 15, although attacks sometimes commence during infancy and onset has occurred as late as age 50. The duration and frequency of attacks vary greatly in the same patient, and their occurrence follows no set pattern. The usual acute episode lasts 1 to 2 days, but some may be prolonged for 7 to 10 days. The attacks range in frequency from twice weekly to once a year, but 2 to 4 weeks is the most common interval. Spontaneous remissions lasting years have been seen. The severity and frequency of the attacks decrease with age or with development of amyloidosis.

Fever Fever is a cardinal manifestation and is present during most attacks. Rarely, fever may be present without serositis. The temperature may be preceded by a chill and will peak in 12 to 24 h. Defervescence is often accompanied by diaphoresis. The fever ranges from 38.5° to 40°C but is quite variable.

Abdominal Pain Abdominal pain occurs in >95% of patients and may vary in severity in the same patient. Minor premonitory discomfort may precede an acute episode by 24 to 48 h. The pain usually starts in one quadrant and then spreads to involve the whole abdomen. The initial site is usually very tender. Tenderness may remain localized with referred pain in other areas, and may radiate to the back. Diaphragmatic irritation may lead to splinting of the chest and pain in one or both shoulders. Nausea and vomiting sometimes occur. The abdomen is usually distended and may become rigid, with decreased or absent bowel sounds. On x-ray the wall of the small intestine may appear edematous, transit of barium is slowed, and fluid levels may be seen. An abdominal operation may precipitate an acute attack of FMF, which may be confused with other postoperative complications.

Chest Pain Most patients with abdominal attacks have referred chest pain at one time or another, and 75% also develop acute pleuritic pain with or without abdominal symptoms. In 30%, the attacks of pleuritis precede the onset of abdominal attacks by varying periods of time, and a small number of patients never develop abdominal attacks. Chest pain is usually unilateral and is associated with diminished breath sounds, a friction rub, or a transient pleural effusion.

Joint Pain In Israel, 75% of patients report at least one episode of acute arthritis. Arthritis can be distinct from abdominal or pleural attacks, can be acute or, rarely, chronic, and may involve one or several joints. Effusions are common, with large joints most frequently involved. Radiologic findings are nonspecific. Despite careful search, frank arthritis rarely has been seen in the United States. Some patients have a history of rheumatic fever-like illness in childhood, but in a large series of patients, including 30 from the Middle East, acute arthritis was not observed. Mild arthralgia is common during acute attacks but is nonspecific.

Skin Manifestations Skin involvement occurs in one-third of patients. These lesions consist of painful, erythematous areas of swelling from 5 to 20 cm in diameter, usually located on the lower legs, the medial malleolus, or the dorsum of the foot. They may occur without abdominal or pleural pain and subside within 24 to 48 h.

Other Signs and Symptoms Involvement of other serosal membranes has been reported, but pericarditis and meningitis are rare. Hematuria, splenomegaly, and small white dots called *colloid bodies* in the ocular fundus are findings of questionable significance. Rarely, migraine-like headaches accompany acute abdominal attacks, and some patients have become somewhat irrational or show extreme emotional lability during attacks. Whether these are primary manifestations of FMF or secondary effects of pain and fever is unclear.

Complications Depression and lack of motivation are common, and patients with FMF require considerable support. A striking number of patients have developed gallbladder disease.

Amyloidosis has been reported in Israel, North Africa, and elsewhere in the Middle East, but its occurrence is rare in the United States. These findings are even more striking because there are probably as many known FMF patients in the United States as in Israel. Thus, environmental or nutritional, as well as genetic, factors may play a role in the development of amyloidosis in FMF.

LABORATORY FINDINGS Polymorphonuclear leukocytosis ranging from 10,000 to 30,000 cells/μL is almost invariable during acute attacks. The erythrocyte sedimentation rate is elevated during attacks but returns to normal between attacks. Plasma fibrinogen, serum haptoglobin, ceruloplasmin, and C-reactive protein increase during the episodes. Plasma lipids are normal, and no consistent abnormalities of hepatic or renal function are seen. When amyloidosis is present, laboratory findings are typical of a nephrotic syndrome followed by renal insufficiency.

DIAGNOSIS When the typical acute attacks of FMF occur in an individual of appropriate ethnic background with a family history of FMF, the diagnosis is easy. When a patient is seen for the first time, a variety of other febrile illnesses must be excluded, such as acute appendicitis, pancreatitis, porphyria, cholecystitis, intestinal obstruction, and other major abdominal catastrophes.

Some inherited hyperlipidemias may mimic the clinical picture of FMF, but lipid analysis will eliminate them from consideration. The FMF patient is not immune to other diseases, and when an attack differs from the usual pattern or is more prolonged, consideration should be given to other diagnostic possibilities. The pleural form of the disease is sometimes difficult to differentiate from acute pulmonary infection or infarction, but the rapid disappearance of signs and symptoms resolves the problem. The erythema is sometimes difficult to differentiate from superficial thrombophlebitis or cellulitis.

The most difficult diagnostic problem in FMF is the patient who presents with fever alone. In this situation an extensive diagnostic workup for fever of unknown origin may be required. Fortunately, such patients are rare, and all eventually develop serosal involvement. Until specific diagnostic tests for FMF are available, patients with recurrent fever but without signs of inflammation of one of the serosal membranes should not be categorized as having FMF.

PROGNOSIS Despite the severity of the symptoms during some acute attacks, most patients are remarkably free of debilitation between attacks and are able to lead fairly normal lives. The greatest hazard to patients is prolonged periods of hospitalization due to erroneous diagnoses or failure to understand the disease. In the United States, the prognosis of patients with FMF does not seem to be different from that of patients with other chronic nonfatal illnesses. Death usually results from causes unrelated to the underlying disease.

In the past, ~25% of FMF patients in Israel developed amyloidosis, and this complication usually led to death. However, the widespread use of colchicine has resulted in a dramatic decrease in the incidence of amyloidosis.

℞ **TREATMENT** During the past 25 years, the outlook of patients with FMF has been altered dramatically. Chronic administration of colchicine greatly reduces the number of acute attacks of FMF. It is recommended that 0.6 mg colchicine be taken by mouth three times a day. If patients develop gastrointestinal side effects with this dose, it should be reduced to 0.6 mg taken twice a day. Although an occasional patient will respond to 0.6 mg taken only once a day, this amount is less likely to be beneficial. Most FMF patients will respond favorably to colchicine prophylaxis.

BIBLIOGRAPHY

DiLorenzo C: Pseudo-obstruction: Current approaches. Gastroenterology 116:980, 1999

Ferzoco LB et al: Acute diverticulitis. N Engl J Med 338:1521, 1998

Foutch PG: Colonic angiodysplasia. Gastroenterologist 5:148, 1997

Goyal RK, Hirano I: Mechanisms of disease: The enteric nervous system. N Engl J Med 334:1106, 1996

International FMF Consortium: Ancient missense mutations in a new member of the *RoRet* gene family are likely to cause Familial Mediterranean Fever. Cell 90:797, 1997

Jensen DM et al: Urgent colonoscopy for the diagnosis and treatment of severe diverticular hemorrhage. N Engl J Med 342:78, 2000

Kellow JE, Malcolm A: Motility. Curr Opin Gastroenterol 12:134, 1996

Maria G, Brisinda G: Nonoperative management of chronic anal fissure. Dis Colon Rectum 43:721, 2000

McKinsey JF, Gewertz BL: Acute mesenteric ischemia. Surg Clin North Am 77:307, 1997

290 ACUTE INTESTINAL OBSTRUCTION

William Silen

ETIOLOGY AND CLASSIFICATION Intestinal obstruction may be *mechanical* or *nonmechanical* (resulting from neuromuscular disturbances that produce either adynamic or dynamic ileus). The causes of mechanical obstruction of the lumen are conveniently divided into (1) lesions *extrinsic* to the intestine, e.g., adhesive bands, internal and external hernias; (2) lesions *intrinsic* to the wall of the intestine, e.g., diverticulitis, carcinoma, regional enteritis; and (3) obturation of the lumen, e.g., gallstone obstruction, intussusception. Clinically, however, it is most useful to consider whether the obstructive mechanism involves the small or large intestine, because the causes, symptoms, and treatments are different (see below). Adhesions and external hernias are the most common causes of obstruction of the small intestine, constituting 70 to 75% of cases of this type. Adhesions, however, almost never produce obstruction of the colon, where carcinoma, sigmoid diverticulitis, and volvulus, in that order, are the most common causes and together account for about 90% of the cases. Primary intestinal pseudoobstruction (Chap. 289) is a chronic motility disorder that frequently mimics mechanical obstruction. Unnecessary operations in such patients should be avoided.

Adynamic ileus is probably the most common overall cause of obstruction. The development of this condition is mediated via the hormonal component of the sympathoadrenal system. Adynamic ileus may occur after any peritoneal insult, and its severity and duration will be dependent to some degree on the type of peritoneal injury. Hydrochloric acid, colonic contents, and pancreatic enzymes are among the most irritating substances, whereas blood and urine are less so. Adynamic ileus occurs to some degree after any abdominal operation. Retroperitoneal hematomas, particularly associated with vertebral fracture, commonly cause severe adynamic ileus, and the latter may occur with other retroperitoneal conditions, such as ureteral calculus or severe pyelonephritis. Thoracic diseases, including lower-lobe pneumonia, fractured ribs, and myocardial infarction, frequently produce adynamic ileus, as do electrolyte disturbances, particularly potassium depletion. Finally, intestinal ischemia, whether the result of vascular occlusion or intestinal distention itself, may perpetuate an adynamic ileus.

Spastic ileus or *dynamic ileus* is very uncommon and results from extreme and prolonged contraction of the intestine. It has been observed in heavy metal poisoning, uremia, porphyria, and extensive intestinal ulcerations.

PATHOPHYSIOLOGY Distention of the intestine is caused by the accumulation of gas and fluid proximal to and within the obstructed segment. Between 70 and 80% of intestinal gas consists of swallowed air, and because this is composed mainly of nitrogen, which is poorly absorbed from the intestinal lumen, removal of air by continuous gastric suction is a useful adjunct in the treatment of intestinal distention. The accumulation of fluid proximal to the obstructing mechanism results not only from ingested fluid, swallowed saliva, gastric juice, and biliary and pancreatic secretions but also from interference with normal sodium and water transport. During the first 12 to 24 h of obstruction, there is a marked depression of flux from lumen to blood of sodium and consequently water in the distended proximal intestine. After 24 h, there is movement of sodium and water into the lumen, contributing further to the distention and fluid losses. Intraluminal pressure rises from a normal of 2 to 4 cmH_2O to 8 to 10 cmH_2O. During peristalsis, when simple obstruction or a "closed loop" is present, pressures reach 30 to 60 cmH_2O. Closed-loop obstruction of the small intestine results when the lumen is occluded at two points by a single mechanism such as a hernial ring or adhesive band, thus producing a closed loop whose blood supply is often obstructed at the same time. Strangulation of the loop itself is thus common in association with marked distention proximal to the involved loop. A form of closed-loop obstruction is encountered when complete obstruction of the colon exists in the presence of a competent ileocecal valve (85% of individuals). Although the blood supply of the colon is not entrapped within the obstructing mechanism, distention of the cecum is extreme because of its greater diameter (Laplace's law), and impairment of the intramural blood supply is considerable with consequent gangrene of the cecal wall, usually anteriorly. Necrosis of the small intestine may occur by the same mechanism of interference with intramural blood flow when distention is extreme, but this sequence is uncommon in the small intestine. Once impairment of blood supply occurs, bacterial invasion supervenes, and peritonitis develops. The systemic effects of extreme distention include elevation of the diaphragm with restricted ventilation and subsequent atelectasis. Venous return via the inferior vena cava may also be impaired.

The loss of fluids and electrolytes may be extreme and, unless replacement is prompt, leads to hemoconcentration, hypovolemia, renal insufficiency, shock, and death. Vomiting, accumulation of fluids within the lumen by the mechanisms described above, and the sequestration of fluid into the edematous intestinal wall and peritoneal cavity as a result of impairment of venous return from the intestine all contribute to massive loss of fluid and electrolytes, especially potassium. As soon as significant impedance to venous return is present, the intestine becomes severely congested, and blood begins to seep into the intestinal lumen. Blood loss may reach significant levels when long segments of intestine are involved.

SYMPTOMS *Mechanical small-intestinal obstruction* is characterized by cramping midabdominal pain, which tends to be more severe the higher the obstruction. The pain occurs in paroxysms, and the patient is relatively comfortable in the intervals between the pains. Audible borborygmi are often noted by the patient simultaneously with the paroxysms of pain. The pain may become less severe as distention progresses, probably because motility is impaired in the edematous intestine. When strangulation is present, the pain is usually more localized and may be steady and severe without a colicky component, a fact that often causes delay in diagnosis of obstruction. Vomiting is almost invariable, and it is earlier and more profuse the higher the obstruction. The vomitus initially contains bile and mucus and remains as such if the obstruction is high in the intestine. With low ileal obstruction, the vomitus becomes feculent, i.e., orange-brown in color with a foul odor, which results from the overgrowth of bacteria proximal to the obstruction. Hiccups (singultus) are common. Obstipation and failure to pass gas by rectum are invariably present when the obstruction is complete, although some stool and gas may be passed spontaneously or after an enema shortly after onset of the complete obstruction. Diarrhea is occasionally observed in partial obstruction. Blood in the stool is rare but does occur in cases of intussusception. Other than some minor but inconsistent differences in pain patterns noted above, the symptoms of strangulating obstructions cannot be distinguished from those of nonstrangulating obstructions.

Mechanical colonic obstruction produces colicky abdominal pain similar in quality to that of small-intestinal obstruction but of much lower intensity. Complaints of pain are occasionally absent in stoic elderly patients. Vomiting occurs late, if at all, particularly if the ileocecal valve is competent. Paradoxically, feculent vomitus is very rare. A history of recent alterations in bowel habits and blood in the stool is common because carcinoma and diverticulitis are the most frequent causes. Constipation becomes progressive, and obstipation with failure to pass gas ensues. Acute symptoms may develop over a period of a week. Cecal volvulus more closely resembles obstruction of the small intestine clinically, whereas patients with sigmoid volvulus more typically have the picture of colonic obstruction in which marked distention predominates, with relatively less pain.

In *adynamic ileus*, colicky pain is absent, and only discomfort from distention is evident. Vomiting may be frequent but is rarely profuse. It usually consists of gastric contents and bile and is almost never feculent. Complete obstipation may or may not occur. Singultus (hiccups) is common.

PHYSICAL FINDINGS *Abdominal distention* is the hallmark of all forms of intestinal obstruction. It is least marked in cases of obstruction high in the small intestine and most marked in colonic obstruction. Early, especially in closed-loop strangulating small-bowel obstruction, distention may be barely perceptible or absent. Tenderness and rigidity are usually minimal; the temperature is rarely above 37.8°C (100°F) in nonstrangulating obstruction of the small and large intestine. Contrary to popular belief, the same is true of strangulating obstruction until very late, a fact that has often resulted in unfortunate delay in treatment. Signs and symptoms of shock also occur *very late* in strangulating obstruction. The appearance of shock, tenderness, rigidity, and fever often means that contamination of the peritoneum with infected intestinal content has occurred. Hernial orifices should always be carefully examined for the presence of a mass. The presence of a palpable abdominal mass usually signifies a closed-loop strangulating small-bowel obstruction because the tense fluid-filled loop is the palpable lesion. Auscultation may reveal loud, high-pitched borborygmi coincident with the colicky pain, but this finding is often absent late in strangulating or nonstrangulating obstruction. A quiet abdomen does not eliminate the possibility of obstruction, nor does it necessarily establish the diagnosis of adynamic ileus.

LABORATORY AND X-RAY FINDINGS Leukocytosis, with shift to the left, usually occurs when strangulation is present, but a normal white blood cell count does not exclude strangulation. Elevation of the serum amylase level is encountered occasionally in all forms of intestinal obstruction, especially the strangulating variety.

The x-ray is extremely valuable but under certain circumstances may also be misleading. In nonstrangulating complete small-bowel obstruction, x-rays are almost completely reliable. Distention of fluid- and gas-filled loops of small intestine usually arranged in a "stepladder" pattern with air-fluid levels and an absence or paucity of colonic gas are pathognomonic (Fig. 290-1). These findings, however, are absent in slightly over half the cases of strangulating small-bowel obstruction, especially early in the disease. A general haze due to peritoneal fluid and sometimes a "coffee bean"–shaped mass are seen in strangulating obstruction. Occasionally, the films are normal, but when symptoms are consistent with obstruction of the small intestine, a normal film should suggest strangulation. In these circumstances, computed tomography may be very useful. Roentgenographic differentiation of partial mechanical small-bowel obstruction from adynamic ileus may be impossible because gas is present in both the small and large intestines; however, colonic distention is usually more prominent in adynamic ileus. A radiopaque dye given by mouth is useful in making this distinction.

Colonic obstruction with a competent ileocecal valve is easily recognized because distention with gas is mainly confined to the colon. Barium enema, sigmoidoscopy, or colonoscopy, depending on the suspected site of obstruction, is usually advisable to determine the nature of the lesion, except when concomitant perforation is suspected, a rare occurrence. Sigmoidoscopy may be therapeutic in cases of sigmoid volvulus. When the ileocecal valve is incompetent, the films resemble those of partial small-bowel obstruction or adynamic ileus, and barium enema or colonoscopy is necessary to establish the correct diagnosis. Barium given by mouth is perfectly safe when obstruction is in the small intestine, since the barium sulfate does not become inspissated in this location. *Barium should never be given by mouth to a patient with possible colonic obstruction* until that possibility has been excluded by barium enema.

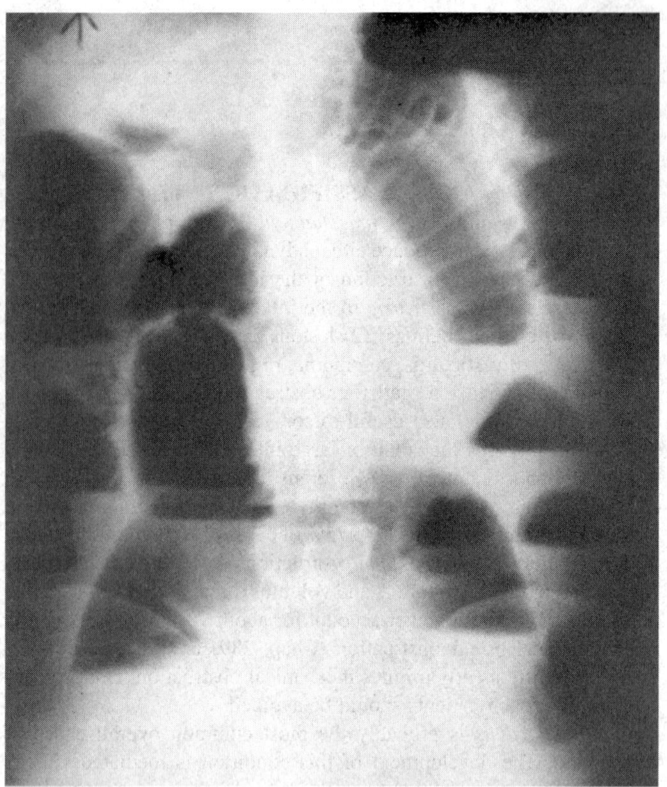

FIGURE 290-1 Acute mechanical obstruction of small intestine (upright film). Note air-fluid levels, marked distention of bowel loops, and absence of colonic gas.

℞ TREATMENT **Small-Intestinal Obstruction** The overall mortality rate for obstruction of the small intestine is about 10%, even under the most optimal conditions. While the mortality rate for nonstrangulating obstruction is as low as 5 to 8%, that for strangulating obstruction has been reported to be between 20 and 75%. Well over half the deaths from small-bowel obstruction occur in those with strangulation; however, the latter constitute only one-fourth to one-third of the cases. Careful studies indicate that the clinical, laboratory, and x-ray findings are not reliable in distinguishing strangulating from nonstrangulating obstruction when obstruction is complete. Complete obstruction is suggested when passage of gas or stool per rectum has ceased and when gas is absent in the distal intestine by x-ray. Since strangulating small-bowel obstruction is always complete, operation should always be undertaken in such patients after suitable preparation. Before operation, fluid and electrolyte balance should be restored and decompression instituted by means of a nasogastric tube. Replacement of potassium is especially important because intake is nil and losses in vomitus are large. From 6 to 8 h of preparation may be necessary. During this period, broad-spectrum antibiotics are indicated if strangulation is felt to be likely, but operation should not be delayed unless there is unequivocal clinical and roentgenographic evidence of resolution of the obstruction during the period of preparation. Attempts to pass a long tube into the small intestine usually fail while putting the patient through uncomfortable, unproductive manipulations that delay appropriate fluid replacement and decompression. *There are few, if any, indications for the use of a long intestinal tube.* Procrastination of operation because of improvement in well-being of the patient during resuscitation and gastric decompression usually leads to unnecessary and hazardous delay in proper treatment. Purely nonoperative therapy is safe only in the presence of incomplete obstruction and is best utilized in patients with (1) repeated episodes of partial obstruction, (2) recent postoperative partial obstruction, and (3) partial obstruction following a recent episode of diffuse peritonitis.

Colonic Obstruction The mortality rate for colonic obstruction is about 20%. As in small-bowel obstruction, nonoperative treatment is contraindicated unless the obstruction is incomplete. Occasionally, but not always, when the obstruction is incomplete, nonoperative therapy may result in sufficient decompression that a definitive operative procedure can be undertaken at a later date. This can usually be accomplished by discontinuation of all oral intake and perhaps by nasogastric suction, although attempts to decompress a *completely* obstructed colon by intubation are almost invariably futile. A long intestinal tube will not decompress an obstructed colon with a competent ileocecal valve. When obstruction is complete, early operation is mandatory, especially when the ileocecal valve is competent; cecal gangrene is likely if the cecal diameter exceeds 10 cm on plain abdominal film. For obstruction on the left side of the colon, the most common site, preliminary operative decompression by cecostomy or transverse colostomy followed by definitive resection of the primary lesion has been the treatment of choice. Recently, primary resection of obstructing left-sided lesions with on-table washout of the colon has been accomplished safely. For a lesion of the right or transverse colon, primary resection and anastomosis can be performed safely because distention of the ileum with consequent discrepancy in size and hazard in suture are not present.

Adynamic Ileus This type of ileus usually responds to nonoperative continuous decompression and adequate treatment of the primary disease. The prognosis is usually good. Successful decompression of severe colonic ileus has been accomplished by colonoscopy, but this should be avoided if tenderness in the right lower quadrant suggests possible cecal gangrene. Neostigmine is effective in cases of colonic ileus that have not responded to other conservative treatment. Rarely, adynamic colonic distention may become so great that cecostomy is required if cecal gangrene is feared. Spastic ileus usually responds to treatment of the primary disease.

BIBLIOGRAPHY

BULKLEY GB et al: Intraoperative determination of small intestinal viability following ischemic injury: Prospective controlled trial of two adjuvant methods (Doppler and fluorescein) compared with standard clinical judgement. Ann Surg 193:628, 1981

DUBOIS A et al: Postoperative ileus: Physiopathology, etiology and treatment. Ann Surg 178:781, 1973

ESKELINEN M et al: Contributions of history-taking, physical examination, and computer assistance to diagnosis of acute small-bowel obstruction. A prospective study of 1333 patients with acute abdominal pain. Scand J Gastroenterol 29:715, 1994

HOFSETTER SR: Acute adhesive obstruction of the small intestine. Surg Gynecol Obstet 152:141, 1981

JACKSON BR: The diagnosis of colonic obstruction. Dis Colon Rectum 25:603, 1982

PESCHIERA JL, BEERMAN SP: Intestinal dysfunction associated with acute thoracolumbar fractures. Orthop Rev 19:284, 1990

PONEC RJ et al: Neostigmine for the treatment of acute colonic pseudo-obstruction. N Engl J Med 341:137, 1999

SILEN W: *Cope's Early Diagnosis of the Acute Abdomen*, 18th ed. London, Oxford, 1991

291

William Silen

ACUTE APPENDICITIS

INCIDENCE AND EPIDEMIOLOGY The peak incidence of acute appendicitis is in the second and third decades of life; it is relatively rare at the extremes of age. Males and females are equally affected, except between puberty and age 25, when males predominate in a 3:2 ratio. Perforation is more common in infancy and in the aged, during which periods mortality rates are highest. The mortality rate has decreased steadily in Europe and the United States from 8.1 per 100,000 of the population in 1941 to less than 1 per 100,000 in 1970 and subsequently. The absolute incidence of the disease also decreased by about 40% between 1940 and 1960 but since then has remained unchanged. Although various factors such as changing dietary habits, altered intestinal flora, and better nutrition and intake of vitamins have been suggested to explain the reduced incidence, the exact reasons have not been elucidated. The overall incidence of appendicitis is much lower in underdeveloped countries, especially parts of Africa, and in lower socioeconomic groups.

PATHOGENESIS Luminal obstruction has long been considered the pathogenetic hallmark. However, obstruction can be identified in only 30 to 40% of cases; ulceration of the mucosa is the initial event in the majority. The cause of the ulceration is unknown, although a viral etiology has been postulated. Infection with *Yersinia* organisms may cause the disease, since high complement fixation antibody titers have been found in up to 30% of cases of proven appendicitis. Whether the inflammatory reaction seen with ulceration is sufficient to obstruct the tiny appendiceal lumen even transiently is not clear. Obstruction, when present, is most commonly caused by a fecalith, which results from accumulation and inspissation of fecal matter around vegetable fibers. Enlarged lymphoid follicles associated with viral infections (e.g., measles), inspissated barium, worms (e.g., pinworms, *Ascaris*, and *Taenia*), and tumors (e.g., carcinoid or carcinoma) may also obstruct the lumen. Secretion of mucus distends the organ, which has a capacity of only 0.1 to 0.2 mL, and luminal pressures rise as high as 60 cmH_2O. Luminal bacteria multiply and invade the appendiceal wall as venous engorgement and subsequent arterial compromise result from the high intraluminal pressures. Finally, gangrene and perforation occur. If the process evolves slowly, adjacent organs such as the terminal ileum, cecum, and omentum may wall off the appendiceal area so that a localized abscess will develop, whereas rapid progression of vascular impairment may cause perforation with free access to the peritoneal cavity. Subsequent rupture of primary appendiceal abscesses may produce fistulas between the appendix and bladder, small intestine, sigmoid, or cecum. Occasionally, acute appendicitis may be the first manifestation of Crohn's disease.

While chronic infection of the appendix with tuberculosis, amebiasis, and actinomycosis may occur, a useful clinical aphorism states that *chronic appendiceal inflammation is not usually the cause of prolonged abdominal pain of weeks' or months' duration.* In contrast, recurrent acute appendicitis does occur, often with complete resolution of inflammation and symptoms between attacks. Recurrent acute appendicitis may become more frequent as antibiotics are dispensed more freely and if a long appendiceal stump is left after laparoscopic appendectomy.

CLINICAL MANIFESTATIONS The history and sequence of symptoms are important diagnostic features of appendicitis. The initial symptom is almost invariably *abdominal pain* of the visceral type, resulting from appendiceal contractions or distention of the lumen. It is usually poorly localized in the periumbilical or epigastric region with an accompanying urge to defecate or pass flatus, neither of which relieves the distress. This visceral pain is mild, often cramping, and rarely catastrophic in nature, usually lasting 4 to 6 h, but it may not be noted by stoic individuals or by some patients during sleep. As inflammation spreads to the parietal peritoneal surfaces, the pain becomes somatic, steady, and more severe, aggravated by motion or cough, and usually located in the *right lower quadrant. Anorexia* is nearly universal; a hungry patient does not have acute appendicitis. *Nausea* and *vomiting* occur in 50 to 60% of cases, but vomiting is usually self-limited. The development of nausea and vomiting before the onset of pain is extremely rare. Change in bowel habit is of little diagnostic value, since any or no alteration may be observed, although the presence of diarrhea caused by an inflamed appendix in juxtaposition to the sigmoid may cause serious diagnostic difficulties. Urinary frequency and dysuria occur if the appendix lies adjacent to the bladder. The typical sequence of symptoms (poorly localized periumbilical pain followed by nausea and vomiting with subsequent shift of pain to the right lower quadrant) occurs in only 50 to 60% of patients.

Physical findings vary with time after onset of the illness and according to the location of the appendix, which may be situated deep in the pelvic cul-de-sac; in the right lower quadrant in any relation to the peritoneum, cecum, and small intestine; in the right upper quadrant (especially during pregnancy); or even in the left lower quadrant. *The diagnosis cannot be established unless tenderness can be elicited.* While tenderness is sometimes absent in the early visceral stage of the disease, it ultimately always develops and is found in any location corresponding to the position of the appendix. Abdominal tenderness may be completely absent if a retrocecal or pelvic appendix is present, in which case the sole physical finding may be tenderness in the flank or on rectal or pelvic examination. Percussion, rebound tenderness, and referred rebound tenderness are often, but not invariably, present; they are most likely to be absent early in the illness. Flexion of the right hip and guarded movement by the patient are due to parietal peritoneal involvement. Hyperesthesia of the skin of the right lower quadrant and a positive psoas or obturator sign are often late findings and are rarely of diagnostic value. When the inflamed appendix is in close proximity to the anterior parietal peritoneum, muscular rigidity is present yet is often minimal early.

The temperature is usually normal or slightly elevated [37.2 to 38°C (99 to 100.5°F)], but a temperature > 38.3°C (101°F) should suggest perforation. Tachycardia is commensurate with the elevation of the temperature. Rigidity and tenderness become more marked as the disease progresses to perforation and localized or diffuse peritonitis. Distention is rare unless severe diffuse peritonitis has developed. The disappearance of pain and tenderness just before perforation is extremely unusual. A mass may develop if localized perforation has occurred but usually will not be detectable before 3 days after onset. Earlier presence of a mass suggests carcinoma of the cecum or Crohn's disease. Perforation is rare before 24 h after onset of symptoms, but the rate may be as high as 80% after 48 h.

Diagnosis is based primarily on clinical grounds. Although moderate leukocytosis of 10,000 to 18,000 cells/μL is frequent (with a concomitant left shift), the absence of leukocytosis does not rule out acute appendicitis. Leukocytosis of >20,000 cells/μL suggests probable perforation. Anemia and blood in the stool suggest a primary diagnosis of carcinoma of the cecum, especially in elderly individuals. The urine may contain a few white or red blood cells without bacteria if the appendix lies close to the right ureter or bladder. Urinalysis is most useful in excluding genitourinary conditions that may mimic acute appendicitis.

Radiographs are rarely of value except when an opaque fecalith (5% of patients) is observed in the right lower quadrant (especially in children). Consequently, abdominal films are not routinely obtained unless other conditions such as intestinal obstruction or ureteral calculus may be present. In some patients with recurrent or prolonged symptoms, a careful barium enema or computed tomography (CT) scan may reveal an extrinsic defect on the medial wall of the cecum or a calcified fecalith. The value of CT scan in acute appendicitis is being evaluated. The diagnosis may also be established by the ultrasonic demonstration of an enlarged and thick-walled appendix. Ultrasound is most useful to exclude ovarian cysts, ectopic pregnancy, or tuboovarian abscess.

While the typical historic sequence and physical findings are present in 50 to 60% of cases, a wide variety of atypical patterns of disease are encountered, especially at the age extremes and during pregnancy. Infants under 2 years of age have a 70 to 80% incidence of perforation and generalized peritonitis. Any infant or child with diarrhea, vomiting, and abdominal pain is highly suspect. Fever is much more common in this age group, and abdominal distention is often the only physical finding. In the elderly, pain and tenderness are often blunted, and thus the diagnosis is frequently delayed and leads to a 30% incidence of perforation in patients over 70. Elderly patients often present initially with a slightly painful mass (a primary appendiceal abscess) or with adhesive intestinal obstruction 5 or 6 days after a previously undetected perforated appendix.

Appendicitis occurs about once in every 1000 pregnancies and is the most common extrauterine condition requiring abdominal operation. The diagnosis may be missed or delayed because of the frequent occurrence of mild abdominal discomfort and nausea and vomiting during pregnancy. During the last trimester, when the mortality rate from appendicitis is highest, uterine displacement of the appendix to the right upper quadrant and laterally leads to confusion in diagnosis because pain and tenderness are similarly displaced.

DIFFERENTIAL DIAGNOSIS Appendicitis can be confused with any condition that causes abdominal pain. Diagnostic accuracy is about 75 to 80% for experienced clinicians and must be based solely on the clinical criteria outlined. It is probably better to err slightly in the direction of overdiagnosis, since delay is associated with perforation and increased morbidity and mortality. In unperforated appendicitis, the mortality rate is 0.1%, little more than that associated with general anesthesia; for perforated appendicitis, overall mortality is 3%, (15% in the elderly). In doubtful cases, 4 to 6 h of observation is always more beneficial than harmful. The most common conditions discovered at operation when acute appendicitis is erroneously diagnosed are, in order of frequency, mesenteric lymphadenitis, no organic disease, acute pelvic inflammatory disease, ruptured graafian follicle or corpus luteum cyst, and acute gastroenteritis. In addition, acute cholecystitis, perforated ulcer, acute pancreatitis, acute diverticulitis, strangulating intestinal obstruction, ureteral calculus, and pyelonephritis may present diagnostic difficulties.

Differentiation of *pelvic inflammatory disease* from acute appendicitis on clinical grounds may be virtually impossible. Gram-negative intracellular diplococci on cervical smear are not pathognomonic unless *Neisseria gonorrhoeae* can be cultured. Pain on movement of the cervix is not specific and may occur in appendicitis if perforation has occurred or if the appendix lies adjacent to the uterus or adnexa. *Rupture of a graafian follicle* (mittelschmerz) occurs at midcycle and will spill off blood and fluid to produce pain and tenderness more diffuse and usually of a less severe degree than in appendicitis. Fever and leukocytosis are usually absent. *Rupture of a corpus luteum cyst* is identical clinically to rupture of a graafian follicle but develops about the time of menstruation. The presence of an adnexal mass, evidence of blood loss, and a positive pregnancy test help differentiate *ruptured tubal pregnancy*, but a negative pregnancy test is present when tubal abortion has occurred. *Twisted ovarian cyst* and *endometriosis* are occasionally difficult to distinguish from appendicitis. In all these female conditions, ultrasonography, laparoscopy, and occasionally CT may be of great value.

Acute mesenteric lymphadenitis is the diagnosis usually given when enlarged, slightly reddened lymph nodes at the root of the mesentery and a normal appendix are encountered at operation in a patient who usually has right lower quadrant tenderness. Whether this is a single, discrete entity is unclear, since the causative factor is not known. Some of these patients have infection with *Y. pseudotuberculosis* or *Y. enterocolytica*, in which case the diagnosis can be established by culture of the mesenteric nodes or by serologic titers (Chap. 162). The diagnosis is essentially impossible clinically, although retrospectively these patients may have a higher temperature and more diffuse pain and tenderness. Children seem to be affected more frequently than adults. *Acute gastroenteritis* usually causes profuse watery diarrhea, often with nausea and vomiting, but without localized findings. Between cramps, the abdomen is completely relaxed. In *Salmonella* gastroenteritis, the abdominal findings are similar, although the pain may be more severe and more localized, and fever and chills are common. The occurrence of similar symptoms among other members of the family may be helpful. When the diagnosis of acute pelvic appendicitis with perforation has been missed, gastroenteritis is the most common previous working diagnosis. Persistent abdominal or rectal tenderness should eliminate the diagnosis of gastroenteritis. *Regional enteritis* (Crohn's disease) is usually associated with a more prolonged history, often with previous exacerbations regarded as episodes of gastroenteritis unless the diagnosis has been established previously. *Meckel's diverticulitis* usually cannot be distinguished from acute appendicitis but is very rare.

℞ **TREATMENT** Cathartics and enemas should be avoided if appendicitis is under consideration, and antibiotics should not be administered when the diagnosis is in question, since they will only mask the perforation. The treatment is early operation and appendectomy as soon as the patient can be prepared. Appendectomy is increasingly accomplished laparoscopically and may have some benefits over the open technique. Preparation for operation rarely takes more than 1 to 2 h in early appendicitis but may require 6 to 8 h in cases of severe sepsis and dehydration associated with late perforation. The *only* circumstance in which operation is *not* indicated is the presence of a palpable mass 3 to 5 days after the onset of symptoms. Should operation be undertaken at that time, a phlegmon rather than a definitive abscess will be found, and complications from its dissection are frequent. Such patients treated with broad-spectrum antibiotics, parenteral fluids, and rest usually show resolution of the mass and symptoms within 1 week. *Interval appendectomy* should be done safely 3 months later. Should the mass enlarge or the patient become more toxic, drainage of the abscess is necessary. The complications of sub-

phrenic, pelvic, or other intraabdominal abscesses usually follow perforation with generalized peritonitis and can be avoided by early diagnosis of the disease.

BIBLIOGRAPHY

GRONROOS JM, GRONROOS P: Leucocyte count and C-reactive protein in the diagnosis of acute appendicitis. Br J Surg 86:501, 1999

NGUYEN DB et al: Appendectomy in the pre- and postlaparoscopic areas. J Gastrointest Surg 3:67, 1999

RAO P et al: Effect of computed tomography of the appendix on treatment of patients and use of hospital resources. N Engl J Med 338:141, 1998

WADE DS et al: Accuracy of ultrasound in the diagnosis of acute appendicitis compared with the surgeon's clinical impression. Arch Surg 128:1039, 1993

Section 2
LIVER AND BILIARY TRACT DISEASE

292

Marc Ghany, Jay H. Hoofnagle

APPROACH TO THE PATIENT WITH LIVER DISEASE

In most instances, a diagnosis of liver disease can be made accurately by a careful history, physical examination, and application of a few laboratory tests. In some instances, radiologic examinations are helpful or, indeed, diagnostic. Liver biopsy is considered the "gold standard" in evaluation of liver disease but is now needed less for diagnosis than for grading and staging disease. This chapter provides an introduction to diagnosis and management of liver disease, briefly reviewing the structure and function of the liver; the major clinical manifestations of liver disease; and the use of clinical history, physical examination, laboratory tests, imaging studies, and liver biopsy.

LIVER STRUCTURE AND FUNCTION The liver is the largest organ of the body, weighing 1 to 1.5 kg and representing 1.5 to 2.5% of the lean body mass. The size and shape of the liver vary and generally match the general body shape—long and lean or squat and square. The liver is located in the right upper quadrant of the abdomen under the right lower rib cage against the diaphragm and projects for a variable extent into the left upper quadrant. The liver is held in place by ligamentous attachments to the diaphragm, peritoneum, great vessels, and upper gastrointestinal organs. It receives a dual blood supply; approximately 20% of the blood flow is oxygen-rich blood from the hepatic artery, and 80% is nutrient-rich blood from the portal vein arising from the stomach, intestines, and spleen.

The majority of cells in the liver are hepatocytes, which constitute two-thirds of the mass of the liver. The remaining cell types are Kupffer cells (members of the reticuloendothelial system), stellate (Ito or fat-storing) cells, endothelial cells and blood vessels, bile ductular cells, and supporting structures. Viewed by light microscopy, the liver appears to be organized in lobules, with portal areas at the periphery and central veins in the center of each lobule. However, from a functional point of view, the liver is organized into acini, with both hepatic arterial and portal venous blood entering the acinus from the portal areas and then flowing through the sinusoids to the terminal hepatic veins. The advantage of viewing the acinus as the physiologic unit of the liver is that it helps to explain the morphologic patterns of many vascular and biliary diseases not explained by the lobular arrangement.

Portal areas of the liver consist of small veins, arteries, bile ducts, and lymphatics organized in a loose stroma of supporting matrix and small amounts of collagen. Blood flowing into the portal areas is distributed through the sinusoids, passing from zone 1 to zone 3 of the acinus and draining into the terminal hepatic veins ("central veins"). The sinusoids are lined by unique endothelial cells that have prominent fenestrae of variable size, allowing the free flow of plasma but not cellular elements. The plasma is thus in direct contact with hepatocytes in the subendothelial space of Disse.

Hepatocytes have distinct polarity. The basolateral side of the hepatocyte lines the space of Disse and is richly lined with microvilli; it demonstrates endocytotic and pinocytotic activity, with passive and active uptake of nutrients, proteins, and other molecules. The apical pole of the hepatocyte forms the cannicular membranes through which bile components are secreted. The canniculi of hepatocytes form a fine network, which fuses into the bile ductular elements near the portal areas. Kupffer cells usually lie within the sinusoidal vascular space and represent the largest group of fixed macrophages in the body. The stellate cells are located in the space of Disse but are not usually prominent unless activated, when they produce collagen and matrix. Red blood cells stay in the sinusoidal space as blood flows through the lobules, but white blood cells can migrate through or around endothelial cells into the space of Disse and from there to portal areas, where they can return to the circulation through lymphatics.

Hepatocytes perform numerous and vital roles in maintaining homeostasis and health. These functions include the synthesis of most essential serum proteins (albumin, carrier proteins, coagulation factors, many hormonal and growth factors), the production of bile and its carriers (bile acids, cholesterol, lecithin, phospholipids), the regulation of nutrients (glucose, glycogen, lipids, cholesterol, amino acids), and metabolism and conjugation of lipophilic compounds (bilirubin, cations, drugs) for excretion in the bile or urine. Measurement of these activities to assess liver function is complicated by the multiplicity and variability of these functions. The most commonly used liver "function" tests are measurements of serum bilirubin, albumin, and prothrombin time. The serum bilirubin level is a measure of hepatic conjugation and excretion, and the serum albumin level and prothrombin time are measures of protein synthesis. Abnormalities of bilirubin, albumin, and prothrombin time are typical of hepatic dysfunction. Frank liver failure is incompatible with life, and the functions of the liver are too complex and diverse to be subserved by a mechanical pump; dialysis membrane; or concoction of infused hormones, proteins, and growth factors.

LIVER DISEASES While there are many causes of liver disease (Table 292-1), they generally present clinically in a few distinct patterns, usually classified as either hepatocellular or cholestatic (obstructive). In *hepatocellular diseases* (such as viral hepatitis or alcoholic liver disease), features of liver injury, inflammation, and necrosis

Table 292-1 Liver Diseases

Inherited hyperbilirubinemia	Liver involvement in systemic diseases
Gilbert's syndrome	Sarcoidosis
Crigler-Najjar syndrome, types I and II	Amyloidosis
Dubin-Johnson syndrome	Glycogen storage diseases
Rotor syndrome	Celiac disease
Viral hepatitis	Tuberculosis
Hepatitis A	*Myobacterium avium intracellulare*
Hepatitis B	Cholestatic syndromes
Hepatitis C	Benign postoperative cholestasis
Hepatitis D	Jaundice of sepsis
Hepatitis E	Total parenteral nutrition (TPN)–induced jaundice
Others (mononucleosis, herpes, adenovirus hepatitis)	Cholestasis of pregnancy
Cryptogenic hepatitis	Cholangitis and cholecystitis
Immune and autoimmune liver diseases	Extrahepatic biliary obstruction (stone, stricture, cancer)
Primary biliary cirrhosis	Biliary atresia
Autoimmune hepatitis	Caroli's disease
Sclerosing cholangitis	Cryptosporidiosis
Overlap syndromes	Drug-induced liver disease
Graft-vs-host disease	Hepatocellular patterns (isoniazid, acetaminophen)
Allograft rejection	Cholestatic patterns (methyltestosterone)
Genetic liver diseases	Mixed patterns (sulfonamides, phenytoin)
α_1 Antitrypsin deficiency	Micro- and macrovesicular steatosis (methotrexate, fialuridine)
Hemochromatosis	Vascular injury
Wilson's disease	Venoocclusive disease
Benign recurrent intrahepatic cholestasis (BRIC)	Budd-Chiari syndrome
Familial intrahepatic cholestasis (FIC), types I–III	Ischemic hepatitis
Others (galactosemia, tyrosinemia, cystic fibrosis, Niemann-Pick disease, Gaucher's disease)	Passive congestion
Alcoholic liver disease	Portal vein thrombosis
Acute fatty liver	Nodular regenerative hyperplasia
Acute alcoholic hepatitis	Mass lesions
Laennec's cirrhosis	Hepatocellular carcinoma
Nonalcoholic fatty liver	Cholangiocarcinoma
Steatosis	Adenoma
Steatohepatitis	Focal nodular hyperplasia
Acute fatty liver of pregnancy	Metastatic tumors
	Abscess
	Cysts

predominate. In *cholestatic diseases* (such as gall stone or malignant obstruction, primary biliary cirrhosis, many drug-induced liver diseases), features of inhibition of bile flow predominate. The pattern of onset and prominence of symptoms can rapidly suggest a diagnosis, particularly if major risk factors are considered, such as the age and sex of the patient and a history of exposure or risk behaviors.

Typical presenting symptoms of liver disease include jaundice, fatigue, itching, right upper quadrant pain, abdominal distention, and intestinal bleeding. At present, however, many patients are diagnosed with liver disease who have no symptoms and who have been found to have abnormalities in biochemical liver tests as a part of a routine physical examination or screening for blood donation or for insurance or employment. The wide availability of batteries of liver tests makes it relatively simple to demonstrate the presence of liver injury as well as to rule it out in someone suspected of liver disease.

Evaluation of patients with liver disease should be directed at (1) establishing the etiologic diagnosis, (2) estimating the disease severity (grading), and (3) establishing the disease stage (staging). *Diagnosis* should focus on the category of disease, such as hepatocellular versus cholestatic injury, as well as on the specific etiologic diagnosis. *Grading* refers to assessing the severity or activity of disease—active or inactive, and mild, moderate, or severe. *Staging* refers to estimating the place in the course of the natural history of the disease, whether acute or chronic; early or late; precirrhotic, cirrhotic, or end-stage.

The goal of this chapter is to introduce general, salient concepts in the evaluation of patients with liver disease that help lead to the diagnoses discussed in subsequent chapters.

CLINICAL HISTORY The clinical history should focus on the symptoms of liver disease—their nature, pattern of onset, and progression—and on potential risk factors for liver disease. The symptoms of liver disease include constitutional symptoms such as fatigue, weakness, nausea, poor appetite, and malaise and the more liver-specific symptoms of jaundice, dark urine, light stools, itching, abdominal pain, and bloating. Symptoms can also suggest the presence of cirrhosis, end-stage liver disease, or complications of cirrhosis such as portal hypertension. Generally, the constellation of symptoms and their pattern of onset rather than a specific symptom points to an etiology.

Fatigue is the most common and most characteristic symptom of liver disease. It is variously described as lethargy, weakness, listlessness, malaise, increased need for sleep, lack of stamina, and poor energy. The fatigue of liver disease typically arises after activity or exercise and is rarely present or severe in the morning after adequate rest (afternoon versus morning fatigue). Fatigue in liver disease is often intermittent and variable in severity from hour to hour and day to day. In some patients, it may not be clear whether fatigue is due to the liver disease or to other problems such as stress, anxiety, sleep disturbance, or a concurrent illness.

Nausea occurs with more severe liver disease and may accompany fatigue or be provoked by odors of food or eating fatty foods. Vomiting can occur but is rarely persistent or prominent. Poor appetite with weight loss occurs commonly in acute liver diseases but is rare in chronic disease, except when cirrhosis is present and advanced. Diarrhea is uncommon in liver disease, except with severe jaundice, in which case lack of bile acids reaching the intestine can lead to steatorrhea.

Right upper quadrant discomfort or ache ("liver pain") occurs in many liver diseases and is usually marked by tenderness over the liver area. The pain arises from stretching or irritation of Glisson's capsule, which surrounds the liver and is rich in nerve endings. Severe pain is most typical of gall bladder disease, liver abscess, and severe venoocclusive disease but is an occasional accompaniment of acute hepatitis.

Itching occurs with acute liver disease, appearing early in obstructive jaundice (from biliary obstruction or drug-induced cholestasis) and somewhat later in hepatocellular disease (acute hepatitis). Itching also occurs in chronic liver diseases, typically the cholestatic forms such as primary biliary cirrhosis and sclerosing cholangitis where it is often the presenting symptom, occurring before the onset of jaundice. However, itching can occur in any liver disease, particularly once cirrhosis is present.

Jaundice is the hallmark symptom of liver disease and perhaps the most reliable marker of severity. Patients usually report darkening of the urine before they notice scleral icterus. Jaundice is rarely detectable with a bilirubin level less than 43 μmol/L (2.5 mg/dL). With severe cholestasis there will also be lightening of the color of the stools and steatorrhea. Jaundice without dark urine usually indicates indirect (unconjugated) hyperbilirubinemia and is typical of hemolytic anemia and the genetic disorders of bilirubin conjugation, the common and benign form being Gilbert's syndrome and the rare and severe form being Crigler-Najjar syndrome. Gilbert's syndrome affects up to 5% of the population; the jaundice is more noticeable after fasting and with stress.

Major risk factors for liver disease that should be sought in the clinical history include details of alcohol use, medications (including herbal compounds, birth control pills, and over-the-counter medications), personal habits, sexual activity, travel, exposure to jaundiced or other high-risk persons, injection drug use, recent surgery, remote or recent transfusion with blood and blood products, occupation, accidental exposure to blood or needlestick, and familial history of liver disease.

For assessing the risk of viral hepatitis, a careful history of sexual activity is of particular importance and should include life-time number of sexual partners and, for men, a history of having sex with men. Sexual exposure is a common mode of spread of hepatitis B but is rare for hepatitis C. Maternal-infant transmission occurs with both hepatitis B and C. Vertical spread of hepatitis B can now be prevented by passive and active immunization of the infant at birth. Vertical spread of hepatitis C is uncommon, but there are no known means of prevention. A history of injection drug use, even in the remote past, is of great importance in assessing the risk for hepatitis B and C. Injection drug use is now the single most common risk factor for hepatitis C. Transfusion with blood or blood products is no longer an important risk factor for acute viral hepatitis. However, blood transfusions received before the introduction of sensitive enzyme immunoassays for antibody to hepatitis C virus (anti-HCV) in 1992 is an important risk factor for chronic hepatitis C. Blood transfusion before 1986, when screening for antibody to hepatitis B core antigen (anti-HBc) was introduced, is also a risk factor for hepatitis B. Travel to an underdeveloped area of the world, exposure to persons with jaundice, and exposure to young children in day-care centers are risk factors for hepatitis A. Tattooing and body piercing (for hepatitis B and C) and eating shellfish (for hepatitis A) are frequently mentioned but actually quite rate types of exposure for acquiring hepatitis.

A history of alcohol intake is important in assessing the cause of liver disease and also in planning management and recommendations. In the United States, for example, at least 70% of adults drink alcohol to some degree, but significant alcohol intake is less common; in population-based surveys, only 5% have more than two drinks per day, the average drink representing 11 to 15 g alcohol. Alcohol consumption associated with an increased rate of alcoholic liver disease is probably more than two drinks (22 to 30 g) per day in women and three drinks (33 to 45 g) in men. Most patients with alcoholic cirrhosis have a much higher daily intake and have drunk excessively for 10 years or more before onset of liver disease. In assessing alcohol intake, the history should also focus upon whether alcohol abuse or dependence is present. Alcoholism is usually defined on the behavioral patterns and consequences of alcohol intake, not on the basis of the amount of alcohol intake. *Abuse* is defined by a repetitive pattern of drinking alcohol that has adverse effects on social, family, occupational, or health status. *Dependence* is defined by alcohol-seeking behavior, despite its adverse effects. Many alcoholics demonstrate both dependence and abuse, and dependence is considered the more serious and advanced form of alcoholism. A clinically helpful approach to diagnosis of alcohol dependence and abuse is the use of the CAGE questionnaire (Table 292-2), which is recommended in all medical history taking.

Family history can be helpful in assessing liver disease. Familial causes of liver disease include Wilson's disease; hemochromatosis and α_1-antitrypsin (α_1AT) deficiency; and the more uncommon inherited pediatric liver diseases of familial intrahepatic cholestasis (FIC), benign recurrent intrahepatic cholestasis (BRIC), and Alagille's syndrome. Onset of severe liver disease in childhood or adolescence with a family history of liver disease or neuropsychiatric disturbance should lead to investigation for Wilson's disease. A family history of cirrhosis, diabetes, or endocrine failure and the appearance of liver disease in adulthood should suggest hemochromatosis and lead to investigation of iron status. Patients with abnormal iron studies warrant genotyping of the HFE gene for the C282Y and H63D mutations typical of genetic hemochromatosis. A family history of emphysema should provoke investigation of α_1AT levels and, if low, for Pi genotype.

Table 292-2 CAGE Questions[a]

Acronym	Question
C	Have you ever felt you ought to *C*ut down on your drinking?
A	Have people *A*nnoyed you by criticizing your drinking?
G	Have you ever felt *G*uilty or bad about your drinking?
E	Have you ever had a drink first thing in the morning to steady your nerves or get rid of a hangover (*E*yeopener)?

[a] One "yes" response should raise suspicion of an alcohol use problem, and more than one is a strong indication that abuse or dependence exists.

PHYSICAL EXAMINATION The physical examination rarely demonstrates evidence of liver dysfunction in a patient without symptoms or laboratory findings, nor are most signs of liver disease specific to one diagnosis. Thus, the physical examination usually complements rather than replaces the need for other diagnostic approaches. In many patients, the physical examination is normal unless the disease is acute or severe and advanced. Nevertheless, the physical examination is important in that it can be the first evidence for the presence of hepatic failure, portal hypertension, and liver decompensation. In addition, the physical examination can reveal signs that point to a specific diagnosis, either in risk factors or in associated diseases or findings.

Typical physical findings in liver disease are icterus, hepatomegaly, hepatic tenderness, splenomegaly, spider angiomata, palmar erythema, and excoriations. Signs of advanced disease include muscle-wasting, ascites, edema, dilated abdominal veins, hepatic fetor, asterixis, mental confusion, stupor, and coma.

Icterus is best appreciated by inspecting the sclera under natural light. In fair-skinned individuals, a yellow color of the skin may be obvious. In dark-skinned individuals, the mucous membranes below the tongue can demonstrate jaundice. Jaundice is rarely detectable if the serum bilirubin level is <43 μmol/L (2.5 μg/dL) but may remain detectable below this level during recovery from jaundice (because of protein and tissue binding of conjugated bilirubin).

Spider angiomata and palmar erythema occur in both acute and chronic liver disease and may be especially prominent in persons with cirrhosis, but they can occur in normal individuals and are frequently present during pregnancy. Spider angiomata are superficial, tortuous arterioles and, unlike simple telangiectases, typically fill from the center outwards. Spider angiomata occur only on the arms, face, and upper torso; they can be pulsatile and may be difficult to detect in dark-skinned individuals.

Hepatomegaly is not a very reliable sign of liver disease, because of the variability of the size and shape of the liver and the physical impediments to assessing liver size by percussion and palpation. Marked hepatomegaly is typical of cirrhosis, venoocclusive disease, metastatic or primary cancers of the liver, and alcoholic hepatitis. Careful assessment of the liver edge may also demonstrate unusual firmness, irregularity of the surface, or frank nodules. Perhaps the most reliable physical finding in examining the liver is hepatic tenderness. Discomfort on touching or pressing on the liver should be carefully sought with percussive comparison of the right and left upper quadrants.

Splenomegaly occurs in many medical conditions but can be a subtle but significant physical finding in liver disease. The availability of ultrasound (US) assessment of the spleen allows for confirmation of the physical finding.

Signs of advanced liver disease include muscle-wasting and weight loss as well as hepatomegaly, bruising, ascites, and edema. Ascites is best appreciated by attempts to detect shifting dullness by careful percussion. US examination will confirm the finding of ascites in equivocal cases. Peripheral edema can occur with or without ascites. In patients with advanced liver disease, other factors frequently contribute to edema formation, including hypoalbuminemia, venous insufficiency, heart failure, and medications.

Hepatic failure is defined as the occurrence of signs or symptoms of hepatic encephalopathy in a person with severe acute or chronic liver disease. The first signs of hepatic encephalopathy can be subtle and nonspecific—change in sleep patterns, change in personality, irritability, and mental dullness. Thereafter, confusion, disorientation, stupor, and eventually coma supervene. Physical findings include asterixis and flapping tremors of the body and tongue. *Fetor hepaticus* refers to the slightly sweet, ammoniacal odor that is common in patients with liver failure, particularly if there is portal-venous shunting of blood around the liver. Other causes of coma and confusion should be excluded, mainly electrolyte imbalances, sedative use, and renal or respiratory failure. A helpful measure of hepatic encephalopathy is a careful mental status examination and use of the trail-making test, which consists of a series of 20 numbered circles that the patient is asked to connect as rapidly as possible using a pencil. The normal range for the connect-the-dot test is 15 to 30 s; it is considerably delayed in patients with early hepatic encephalopathy. Other tests include drawing abstract objects or comparison of a signature to previous examples.

Other signs of advanced liver disease include umbilical hernia from ascites, prominent veins over the abdomen, and *caput medusa*, which consists of collateral veins seen radiating from the umbilicus and resulting from the recanulation of the umbilical vein. Widened pulse pressure and signs of a hyperdynamic circulation can occur in patients with cirrhosis as a result of fluid and sodium retention, increased cardiac output, and reduced peripheral resistance. Patients with long-standing cirrhosis are prone to develop the hepatopulmonary syndrome with hypoxemia due to pulmonary arteriovenous shunting, characterized by hypoxia that worsens when lying flat.

Several skin disorders and changes occur commonly in liver disease. Hyperpigmentation is typical of advanced chronic cholestatic diseases such as primary biliary cirrhosis and sclerosing cholangitis. In these same conditions, xanthelasma and tendon xanthomata occur as a result of retention and high serum levels of lipids and cholesterol. A slate-gray pigmentation to the skin also occurs with hemochromatosis if iron levels are high for a prolonged period. Mucocutaneous vasculitis with palpable purpura, especially on the lower extremities, is typical of cryoglobulinemia of chronic hepatitis C but can also occur in chronic hepatitis B.

Some physical signs point to specific liver diseases. Kayser-Fleischer rings occur in Wilson's disease and consist of a golden-brown copper pigment deposited at the periphery of the cornea; they are best seen by slit-lamp examination. In metastatic liver disease or primary hepatocellular carcinoma, signs of cachexia and wasting may be prominent, as well as firm hepatomegaly and a hepatic bruit.

LABORATORY TESTING Diagnosis in liver disease is greatly aided by the availability of reliable and sensitive tests of liver injury and function. Use and interpretation of liver function tests is summarized in Chap. 293. A typical battery of blood tests used for initial assessment of liver disease includes measuring levels of serum alanine and aspartate aminotransferases (ALT and AST), alkaline phosphatase, direct and total serum bilirubin, and albumin and assessing prothrombin time. The pattern of abnormalities generally points to hepatocellular versus cholestatic liver disease and will help to decide whether the disease is acute or chronic and whether cirrhosis and hepatic failure are present. Based on these results, further testing over time may be necessary. Other laboratory tests may be helpful, such as γ-glutamyl transpeptidase (GGT) to define whether alkaline phosphatase elevations are due to liver disease; hepatitis serology to define the type of viral hepatitis; and autoimmune markers to diagnose primary biliary cirrhosis (antimitochondrial antibody; AMA), sclerosing cholangitis (peripheral antineutrophil cytoplasmic antibody; pANCA), autoimmune hepatitis (antinuclear, smooth-muscle, and liver-kidney microsomal antibody). A simple delineation of laboratory abnormalities and common liver diseases is given in Table 292-3.

Table 292-3 Important Diagnostic Tests in Common Liver Diseases

Disease	Diagnostic Test
Hepatitis A	Anti-HAV IgM
Hepatitis B	
Acute	HBsAg and anti-HBc IgM
Chronic	HBsAg and HBeAg and/or HBV DNA
Hepatitis C	Anti-HCV and HCV RNA
Hepatitis D (delta)	HBsAg and anti-HDV
Hepatitis E	Anti-HEV
Autoimmune hepatitis	ANA or SMA, elevated IgG levels, and compatible histology
Primary biliary cirrhosis	Mitochondrial antibody, elevated IgM levels, and compatible histology
Primary sclerosing cholangitis	p-ANCA, cholangiography
Drug-induced liver disease	History of drug ingestion
Alcoholic liver disease	History of excessive alcohol intake and compatible histology
Nonalcoholic steatohepatitis	Ultrasound or CT evidence of fatty liver and compatible histology
α_1 Antitrypsin disease	Reduced α_1 antitrypsin levels, phenotypes PiZZ or PiSZ
Wilson's disease	Decreased serum ceruloplasmin and increased urinary copper; increased hepatic copper level
Hemochromatosis	Elevated iron saturation and serum ferritin; genetic testing for HFE gene mutations
Hepatocellular cancer	Elevated α-fetoprotein level >500; ultrasound or CT image of mass

NOTE: HAV, HBV, HCV, HDV, HEV: hepatitis A, B, C, D, or E virus; HBsAg, hepatitis B surface antigen; HBc, hepatitis B core (antigen); HBeAg, hepatitis e antigen; ANA, antinuclear antibodies; SMA, smooth muscle antibody; p-ANCA, peripheral antineutrophil cytoplasmic antibody; CT, computed tomography.

DIAGNOSTIC IMAGING There have been great advances made in hepatic imaging, although no method is suitably accurate in demonstrating underlying cirrhosis. There are many modalities available for imaging the liver. US, computed tomography (CT), and magnetic resonance imaging (MRI) are the most commonly employed and are complementary to each other. In general, US and CT have a high sensitivity for detecting biliary duct dilatation and are the first-line options for investigating the patient with suspected obstructive jaundice. Both US and CT can detect a fatty liver, which appears bright on both studies. Endoscopic retrograde cholangiopancreatography (ERCP) is the procedure of choice for visualization of the biliary tree. ERCP also provides several therapeutic options in patients with obstructive jaundice, such as sphincterotomy, stone extraction, and placement of nasobiliary catheters and biliary stents. Doppler US and MRI are used to assess hepatic vasculature and hemodynamics and to monitor surgically or radiologically placed vascular shunts such as transjugular intrahepatic portosystemic shunts (TIPS). CT and MRI are indicated for the identification and evaluation of hepatic masses, staging of liver tumors, and preoperative assessment. With regard to mass lesions, sensitivity of hepatic imaging continues to increase; unfortunately, specificity remains a problem, and often two and sometimes three studies are needed before a diagnosis can be reached. Finally, interventional radiologic techniques allow the biopsy of solitary lesions, insertion of drains into hepatic abscesses, and creation of vascular shunts in patients with portal hypertension. Which modality to use depends on factors such as availability, cost, and experience of the radiologist with each technique.

LIVER BIOPSY Liver biopsy remains the gold standard in the evaluation of patients with liver disease, particularly in patients with chronic liver diseases. In selected instances, liver biopsy is necessary for diagnosis but is more often useful in assessing the severity (grade) and stage of liver damage, in predicting prognosis, and in monitoring response to treatment.

Diagnosis of Liver Disease The major causes of liver disease and key diagnostic features are outlined in Table 292-3 (specifics of diagnosis are discussed in later chapters). The most common causes of acute liver disease are viral hepatitis (particularly hepatitis A, B, and C), drug-induced liver injury, cholangitis, and alcoholic liver disease. Liver biopsy is usually not needed in the diagnosis and management of acute liver disease, exceptions being situations where the diagnosis remains unclear despite thorough clinical and laboratory investigation. Liver biopsy can be helpful in the diagnosis of drug-induced liver disease and in establishing the diagnosis of acute alcoholic hepatitis.

The most common causes of chronic liver disease in general order of frequency are chronic hepatitis C, alcoholic liver disease, nonalcoholic steatohepatitis, chronic hepatitis B, autoimmune hepatitis, sclerosing cholangitis, primary biliary cirrhosis, hemochromatosis, and Wilson's disease. Strict diagnostic criteria have not been developed for most liver diseases, but liver biopsy plays an important role in the diagnosis of autoimmune hepatitis, primary biliary cirrhosis, nonalcoholic and alcoholic steatohepatitis, and Wilson's disease (with a quantitative hepatic copper level).

Grading and Staging of Liver Disease Grading refers to an assessment of the severity or activity of liver disease, whether acute or chronic; active or inactive; and mild, moderate, or severe. Liver biopsy is the most accurate means of assessing severity, particularly in chronic liver disease. Serum aminotransferase levels are used as a convenient and noninvasive means to follow disease activity, but aminotransferases are not always reliable in reflecting disease severity. Thus, normal serum aminotransferases in patients with hepatitis B surface antigen (HBsAg) in serum may indicate the inactive HBsAg carrier state or may reflect mild chronic hepatitis B or hepatitis B with fluctuating disease activity. Serum testing for hepatitis B e antigen and hepatitis B virus DNA can help resolve these different patterns, but these markers can also fluctuate and change over time. Similarly, in chronic hepatitis C, serum aminotransferases can be normal despite moderate activity of disease. Finally, in both alcoholic and nonalcoholic steatohepatitis, aminotransferases are quite unreliable in reflecting severity. In these conditions, liver biopsy is helpful in guiding management and recommending therapy, particularly if therapy is difficult, prolonged, and expensive as is often the case in chronic viral hepatitis. There are several well-verified numerical scales for grading activity in chronic liver disease, the most common being the histology activity index and the Ishak histology scale.

Liver biopsy is also the most accurate means of assessing stage of disease as early or advanced, precirrhotic, and cirrhotic. Staging of disease pertains largely to chronic liver diseases in which progression to cirrhosis and end-stage liver disease can occur, but which may require years or decades to develop. Clinical features, biochemical tests, and hepatic imaging studies are helpful in assessing stage but generally become abnormal only in the middle to late stages of cirrhosis. Early stages of cirrhosis are generally detectable only by liver biopsy. In assessing stage, the degree of fibrosis is usually used as its quantitative measure. The amount of fibrosis is generally staged on a 0 to 4+ (histology activity index) or 0 to 6+ scale (Ishak scale).

Cirrhosis can also be staged clinically. A reliable staging system is the modified Child-Pugh classification with a scoring system of 5 to 15: scores of 5 and 6 being Child-Pugh class A (consistent with "compensated cirrhosis"), scores of 7 to 9 indicating class B, and 10 to 15 class C (Table 292-4). This scoring system was initially devised to stratify patients into risk groups prior to undergoing portal decompressive surgery. It is now used to assess prognosis in cirrhosis and provides the standard criteria for listing for liver transplantation (Child-Pugh class B). The Child-Pugh score is a reasonably reliable predictor of survival in many liver diseases and predicts the likelihood of major complications of cirrhosis such as bleeding from varices and spontaneous bacterial peritonitis. Other means of assessing stage and survival have been developed for primary biliary cirrhosis and sclerosing cholangitis (Mayo Risk scores), which are somewhat more accurate but which actually rely mostly on the same measurements as the Child-Pugh score.

Table 292-4 Child-Pugh Classification of Cirrhosis

Factor	1	2	3
Serum bilirubin, μmol/L (mg/dL)	<34(<2.0)	34–51(2.0–3.0)	>51(>3.0)
Serum albumin, g/L(g/dL)	>35(>3.5)	30–35(3.0–3.5)	<30(<3.0)
Ascites	None	Easily controlled	Poorly controlled
Neurologic disorder	None	Minimal	Advanced coma
Prothrombin time (second prolonged) (INR)	0–4 <1.7	4–6 1.7–2.3	>6 >2.3

NOTE: The Child-Pugh score is calculated by adding the scores of the five factors and can range from 5 to 15. Child-Pugh class is either A (a score of 5 to 6), B (7 to 9), or C (10 and above). In general, "decompensation" indicates cirrhosis with a Child-Pugh score of ≥7 (Child-Pugh class B), and this level is an accepted criterion for listing for liver transplantation.

Thus, liver biopsy is helpful not only in diagnosis but also in management of chronic liver disease and assessment of prognosis. Because liver biopsy is an invasive procedure and not without complications, it should be used only when it will contribute materially to management and therapeutic decisions.

BIBLIOGRAPHY

BACON BR, DI BISCEGLIE AM (eds): *Liver Disease: Diagnosis and Management*. Philadelphia, Churchill Livingstone, 1999

BELLENTANI S et al: Prevalence of chronic liver disease in the general population of Northern Italy: The Dionysos Study. Hepatology 20:1442, 1994

BENNETT WF et al: Review of hepatic imaging and a problem-oriented approach to liver masses. Hepatology 12:761, 1990

DESMET VJ et al: Classification of chronic hepatitis: Diagnosis, grading and staging. Hepatology 19:1513, 1994

DICKSON ER et al: Prognosis in primary biliary cirrhosis: Model for decision making. Hepatology 10:1, 1989. Also available at www.mayo.edu/int-med/gi/model/mayomodl.htm

EWING JA: Detecting alcoholism, the CAGE questionnaire. JAMA 252:1905, 1984

ISHAK K et al: Histological grading and staging of chronic hepatitis. J Hepatol 22:696, 1995

SCHIFF ER et al (eds): *Schiff's Diseases of the Liver*, 8th ed. Philadelphia, Lippincott-Raven, 1999

ZAKIM D, BOYER TD (eds): *Hepatology: A Textbook of Liver Disease*, 3d ed. Philadelphia, Saunders, 1996

293

Daniel S. Pratt, Marshall M. Kaplan

EVALUATION OF LIVER FUNCTION

Several biochemical tests are useful in the evaluation and management of patients with hepatic dysfunction. These tests can be used to (1) detect the presence of liver disease; (2) distinguish among different types of liver disorders; (3) gauge the extent of known liver damage; and (4) follow the response to treatment.

Liver tests have shortcomings. They can be normal in patients with serious liver disease and abnormal in patients with diseases that do not affect the liver. Liver tests rarely suggest a specific diagnosis; rather, they suggest a general category of liver disease, such as hepatocellular or cholestatic, which then further directs the evaluation.

The liver carries out thousands of biochemical functions, most of which cannot be easily measured by blood tests. Laboratory tests measure only a limited number of these functions. In fact, many tests, such as the aminotransferases or alkaline phosphatase, do not measure liver function at all. Rather, they detect liver cell damage or interference

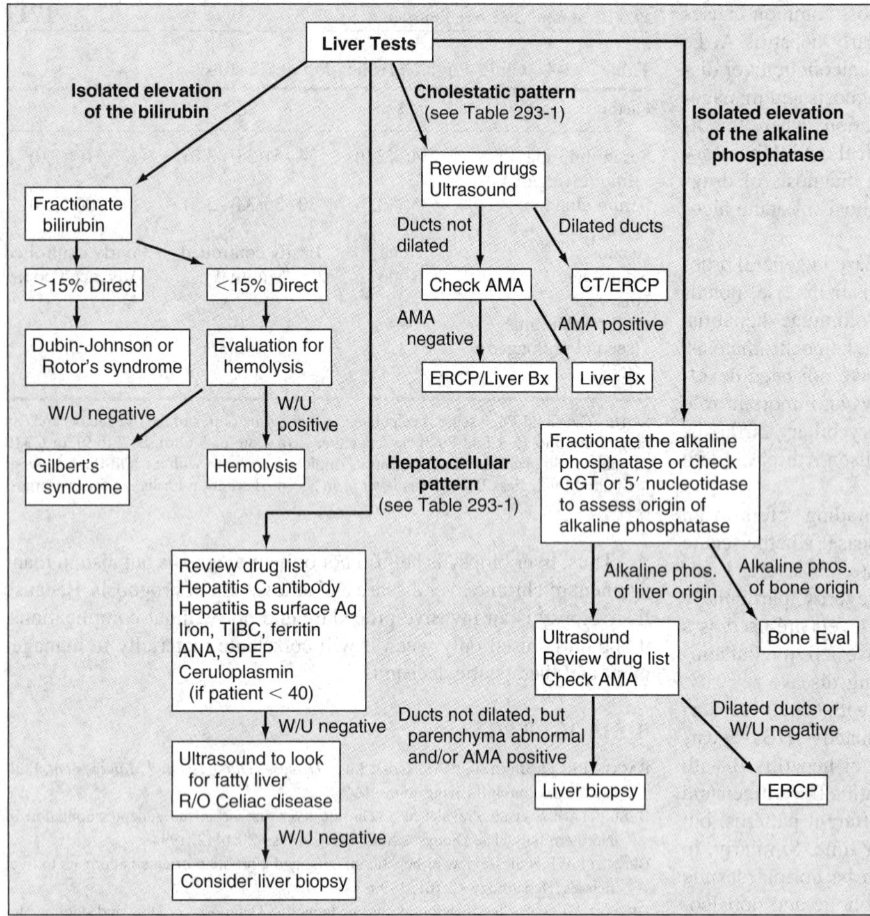

FIGURE 293-1 ERCP, endoscopic retrograde cholangiopancreatography; CT, computerized tomography; AMA, antimitochondrial antibody; ANA, antinuclear antibody; SPEP, serum protein electrophoresis; TIBC, total iron binding capacity; GGT, gamma glutamyl transpeptidase.

with bile flow. Thus, no one test enables the clinician to accurately assess the liver's total functional capacity.

To increase both the sensitivity and the specificity of laboratory tests in the detection of liver disease, it is best to use them as a battery. Those tests usually employed in clinical practice include the bilirubin, aminotransferases, alkaline phosphatase, albumin, and prothrombin time tests. When more than one of these tests provide abnormal findings, or the findings are persistently abnormal on serial determinations, the probability of liver disease is high. When all test results are normal, the probability of missing occult liver disease is low.

When evaluating patients with liver disorders, it is helpful to group these tests into general categories. The classification we have found most useful is given below.

TESTS BASED ON DETOXIFICATION AND EXCRETORY FUNCTIONS **Serum Bilirubin** Bilirubin, a breakdown product of the porphyrin ring of heme-containing proteins, is found in the blood in two fractions—conjugated and unconjugated. The *van den Bergh assay*, or a variation of it, is still used in most clinical chemistry laboratories to determine the total serum bilirubin level and what amount is conjugated or unconjugated bilirubin. In this assay, the direct fraction provides an approximate determination of the conjugated bilirubin in serum. The total serum bilirubin is the amount that reacts after the addition of alcohol. The indirect fraction is the difference between the total and the direct bilirubin and provides an estimate of the unconjugated bilirubin in serum. The unconjugated fraction, also termed the indirect fraction, is insoluble in water and is bound to albumin in the blood. The conjugated (direct) bilirubin fraction is water soluble and can therefore be excreted by the kidney. When measured by the original van den Bergh method, the normal total serum bilirubin concentration is less than 1 mg/dL. Up to 30%, or 0.3 mg/dL, of the total is direct-reacting (or conjugated) bilirubin.

Elevation of the unconjugated fraction of bilirubin is rarely due to liver disease. An isolated elevation of unconjugated bilirubin is seen primarily in hemolytic disorders and in a number of genetic conditions such as Crigler-Najjar and Gilbert's syndromes. *Gilbert's syndrome* is a common, benign condition with a reported incidence in 3 to 7% of the population. It is marked by the impaired conjugation of bilirubin due to reduced bilirubin uridine diphosphate (UDP) glucuronosyltransferase activity. This results in mild unconjugated hyperbilirubinemia, which is marked by considerable fluctuations and is sometimes only identified during periods of fasting. One molecular defect that has been identified in patients with Gilbert's syndrome is in the TATAA element in the 5′ promoter region of the bilirubin UDP-glucuronosyltransferase gene upstream of exon 1. This defect alone is not necessarily sufficient for producing the clinical syndrome of Gilbert's, as there are patients who are homozygous for this defect yet do not have the levels of hyperbilirubinemia typically seen in Gilbert's syndrome. Isolated unconjugated hyperbilirubinemia (bilirubin elevated, but less than 15% direct) should prompt a workup for hemolysis (Fig. 293-1). In the absence of hemolysis, an isolated unconjugated hyperbilirubinemia can be attributed to Gilbert's syndrome and no further evaluation is required.

In contrast, conjugated hyperbilirubinemia almost always implies liver or biliary tract disease. The rate-limiting step in bilirubin metabolism is not conjugation of bilirubin, but rather the transport of conjugated bilirubin into the bile canaliculi. Thus, elevation of the conjugated fraction may be seen in any type of liver disease. In most liver diseases, both conjugated and unconjugated fractions of the bilirubin tend to be elevated. Except in the presence of a purely unconjugated hyperbilirubinemia, fractionation of the bilirubin is rarely helpful in determining the cause of jaundice.

Concern may be generated by a slower than expected decline of the serum bilirubin during convalescence from certain liver diseases. This can be attributed to the covalent binding of conjugated bilirubin to serum albumin that occurs when there is a prolonged episode of conjugated hyperbilirubinemia. The serum half-life of the albumin-bilirubin complex (15 days) is much longer than that of conjugated bilirubin and closer to that of albumin.

Urine Bilirubin Unconjugated bilirubin always binds to albumin in the serum and is not filtered by the kidney. Therefore, any bilirubin found in the urine is conjugated bilirubin; the presence of bilirubinuria implies the presence of liver disease. A urine dipstick test can theoretically give the same information as fractionation of the serum bilirubin. This test is almost 100% accurate. Phenothiazines may give a false positive reading with the Ictotest tablet.

Blood Ammonia Ammonia is produced in the body during normal protein metabolism and by intestinal bacteria, primarily those in the colon. The liver plays a role in the detoxification of ammonia by converting it to urea, which is excreted by the kidneys. Striated muscle also plays a role in detoxification of ammonia, which is combined with glutamic acid to form glutamine. Patients with advanced liver disease typically have significant muscle wasting, which likely contributes to hyperammonemia in these patients. Some physicians use the blood ammonia for detecting encephalopathy or for monitoring hepatic synthetic function, although its use for either of these indications has problems. There is very poor correlation between either the presence or the degree of acute encephalopathy and elevation of blood ammonia; it can be occasionally useful for identifying the occult liver disease in patients with mental status changes. There is also a poor correlation of the blood serum ammonia and hepatic function. The ammonia can be elevated in patients with severe portal hypertension and portal blood shunting around the liver even in the presence of normal or near normal hepatic function.

Serum Enzymes The liver contains thousands of enzymes, some of which are also present in the serum in very low concentrations. These enzymes have no known function in the serum and behave like other serum proteins. They are distributed in the plasma and in interstitial fluid and have characteristic half-lives, usually measured in days. Very little is known about the catabolism of serum enzymes, although they are probably cleared by cells in the reticuloendothelial system. The elevation of a given enzyme activity in the serum is thought to primarily reflect its increased rate of entrance into serum from damaged liver cells.

Serum enzyme tests can be grouped into three categories: (1) enzymes whose elevation in serum reflects damage to hepatocytes; (2) enzymes whose elevation in serum reflects cholestasis; and (3) enzyme tests that do not fit precisely into either pattern.

Enzymes that reflect damage to hepatocytes The aminotransferases (transaminases) are sensitive indicators of liver cell injury and are most helpful in recognizing acute hepatocellular diseases such as hepatitis. They include the aspartate aminotransferase (AST) and the alanine aminotransferase (ALT). AST is found in the liver, cardiac muscle, skeletal muscle, kidneys, brain, pancreas, lungs, leukocytes, and erythrocytes in decreasing order of concentration. ALT is found primarily in the liver. The aminotransferases are normally present in the serum in low concentrations. These enzymes are released into the blood in greater amounts when there is damage to the liver cell membrane resulting in increased permeability. Liver cell necrosis is not required for the release of the aminotransferases and there is a poor correlation between the degree of liver cell damage and the level of the aminotransferases. Thus, the absolute elevation of the aminotransferases is of no prognostic significance in acute hepatocellular disorders.

Any type of liver cell injury can cause modest elevations in the serum aminotransferases. Levels of up to 300 U/L are nonspecific and may be found in any type of liver disorder. Striking elevations—i.e., aminotransferases >1000 U/L—occur almost exclusively in disorders associated with extensive hepatocellular injury such as (1) viral hepatitis, (2) ischemic liver injury (prolonged hypotension or acute heart failure), or (3) toxin or drug-induced liver injury.

The pattern of the aminotransferase elevation can be helpful diagnostically. In most acute hepatocellular disorders, the ALT is higher than or equal to the AST. An AST:ALT ratio >2:1 is suggestive while a ratio >3:1 is highly suggestive of alcoholic liver disease. The AST in alcoholic liver disease is rarely >300 U/L and the ALT is often normal. A low level of ALT in the serum is due to an alcohol-induced deficiency of pyridoxal phosphate.

The aminotransferases are usually not greatly elevated in obstructive jaundice. One notable exception occurs during the acute phase of biliary obstruction caused by the passage of a gallstone into the common bile duct. In this setting, the aminotransferases can briefly be in the 1,000 to 2,000 U/L range. However, aminotransferase levels decrease quickly and the liver function tests rapidly evolve into one typical of cholestasis.

Enzymes that reflect cholestasis The activities of three enzymes—alkaline phosphatase, 5′-nucleotidase, and gamma glutamyl transpeptidase (GGT)—are usually elevated in cholestasis. Alkaline phosphatase and 5′-nucleotidase are found in or near the bile canalicular membrane of hepatocytes, while GGT is located in the endoplasmic reticulum and in bile duct epithelial cells. Reflecting its more diffuse localization in the liver, GGT elevation in serum is less specific for cholestasis than are elevations of alkaline phosphatase or 5′-nucleotidase. Some have advocated the use of GGT to identify patients

with occult alcohol use. Its lack of specificity makes its use in this setting questionable.

The normal serum alkaline phosphatase consists of many distinct isoenzymes found in the liver, bone, placenta, and, less commonly, small intestine. Patients over age 60 can have a mildly elevated alkaline phosphatase (1 to 1½ times normal), while individuals with blood types O and B can have an elevation of the serum alkaline phosphatase after eating a fatty meal due to the influx of intestinal alkaline phosphatase into the blood. It is also nonpathologically elevated in children and adolescents undergoing rapid bone growth because of bone alkaline phosphatase, and late in normal pregnancies due to the influx of placental alkaline phosphatase.

Elevation of liver-derived alkaline phosphatase is not totally specific for cholestasis and a less than threefold elevation can be seen in almost any type of liver disease. Alkaline phosphatase elevations greater than four times normal occur primarily in patients with cholestatic liver disorders, infiltrative liver diseases such as cancer, and bone conditions characterized by rapid bone turnover (e.g., Paget's disease). In bone diseases, the elevation is due to increased amounts of the bone isoenzymes. In liver diseases, the elevation is almost always due to increased amounts of the liver isoenzyme.

If an elevated serum alkaline phosphatase is the only abnormal finding in an apparently healthy person, or if the degree of elevation is higher than expected in the clinical setting, identification of the source of elevated isoenzymes is helpful (Fig. 293-1). This problem can be approached in several ways. First, and most precise, is the fractionation of the alkaline phosphatase by electrophoresis. The second approach is based on the observation that alkaline phosphatases from individual tissues differ in susceptibility to inactivation by heat. The finding of an elevated serum alkaline phosphatase level in a patient with a heat-stable fraction strongly suggests that the placenta or a tumor is the source of the elevated enzyme in serum. Susceptibility to inactivation by heat increases, respectively, for the intestinal, liver, and bone alkaline phosphatases, bone being by far the most sensitive. The third, best substantiated, and most available approach involves the measurement of serum 5′-nucleotidase or GGT. These enzymes are rarely elevated in conditions other than liver disease.

In the absence of jaundice or elevated aminotransferases, an elevated alkaline phosphatase of liver origin often, but not always, suggests early cholestasis and, less often, hepatic infiltration by tumor or granulomata. Other conditions that cause isolated elevations of the alkaline phosphatase include Hodgkin's disease, diabetes, hyperthyroidism, congestive heart failure, and inflammatory bowel disease.

The level of serum alkaline phosphatase elevation is not helpful in distinguishing between intrahepatic and extrahepatic cholestasis. There is essentially no difference among the values found in obstructive jaundice due to cancer, common duct stone, sclerosing cholangitis, or bile duct stricture. Values are similarly increased in patients with intrahepatic cholestasis due to drug-induced hepatitis, primary biliary cirrhosis, rejection of transplanted livers, and, rarely, alcohol-induced steatonecrosis. Values are also greatly elevated in hepatobiliary disorders seen in patients with AIDS (e.g., AIDS cholangiopathy due to cytomegalovirus or cryptosporidial infection and tuberculosis with hepatic involvement).

TESTS THAT MEASURE BIOSYNTHETIC FUNCTION OF THE LIVER **Serum Albumin** Serum albumin is synthesized exclusively by hepatocytes. Serum albumin has a long half-life: 15 to 20 days, with approximately 4% degraded per day. Because of this slow turnover, the serum albumin is not a good indicator of acute or mild hepatic dysfunction; only minimal changes in the serum albumin are seen in acute liver conditions such as viral hepatitis, drug-related hepatoxicity, and obstructive jaundice. In hepatitis, albumin levels below 3 g/dL should raise the possibility of chronic liver disease. Hypoalbuminemia is more common in chronic liver disorders such as cirrhosis and usually reflects severe liver damage and decreased albumin synthesis. One exception is the patient with ascites

Table 293-1 Liver Test Patterns in Hepatobiliary Disorders

Type of Disorder	Bilirubin	Aminotransferases	Alkaline Phosphatase	Albumin	Prothrombin Time
Hemolysis/Gilbert's syndrome	Normal to 5 mg/dl 85% due to indirect fractions No bilirubinuria	Normal	Normal	Normal	Normal
Acute hepatocellular necrosis (viral and drug hepatitis, hepatotoxins, acute heart failure)	Both fractions may be elevated Peak usually follows aminotransferases Bilirubinuria	Elevated, often >500 IU ALT >AST	Normal to <3 times normal elevation	Normal	Usually normal. If >5X above control and not corrected by parenteral vitamin K, suggests poor prognosis
Chronic hepatocellular disorders	Both fractions may be elevated Bilirubinuria	Elevated, but usually <300 IU	Normal to <3 times normal elevation	Often decreased	Often prolonged Fails to correct with parenteral vitamin K
Alcoholic hepatitis Cirrhosis	Both fractions may be elevated Bilirubinuria	AST:ALT >2 suggests alcoholic hepatitis or cirrhosis	Normal to <3 times normal elevation	Often decreased	Often prolonged Fails to correct with parenteral vitamin K
Intra- and extra-hepatic cholestasis (Obstructive jaundice)	Both fractions may be elevated Bilirubinuria	Normal to moderate elevation Rarely >500 IU	Elevated, often >4 times normal elevation	Normal, unless chronic	Normal If prolonged, will correct with parenteral vitamin K
Infiltrative diseases (tumor, granulomata); partial bile duct obstruction	Usually normal	Normal to slight elevation	Elevated, often > 4 times normal elevation Fractionate, or confirm liver origin with 5′ nucleotidase or gamma glutamyl transpeptidase	Normal	Normal

in whom synthesis may be normal or even increased, but levels are low because of the increased volume of distribution. However, hypoalbuminemia is not specific for liver disease and may occur in protein malnutrition of any cause, as well as protein-losing enteropathies, nephrotic syndrome, and chronic infections that are associated with prolonged increases in serum interleukin-1 and/or tumor necrosis factor levels that inhibit albumin synthesis. Serum albumin should not be measured for screening in patients in whom there is no suspicion of liver disease. A general medical clinic study of consecutive patients in whom no indications were present for albumin measurement showed that while 12% of patients had abnormal test results, the finding was of clinical importance in only 0.4%.

Serum Globulins Serum globulins are a group of proteins made up of gamma globulins (immunoglobulins) produced by B lymphocytes and alpha and beta globulins produced primarily in hepatocytes. Gamma globulins are increased in chronic liver disease, such as chronic hepatitis and cirrhosis. In cirrhosis, the increased serum gamma globulin concentration is due to the increased synthesis of antibodies, some of which are directed against intestinal bacteria. This occurs because the cirrhotic liver fails to clear bacterial antigens that normally reach the liver through the hepatic circulation.

Increases in the concentration of specific isotypes of gamma globulins are often helpful in the recognition of certain chronic liver diseases. Diffuse polyclonal increases in IgG levels are common in autoimmune hepatitis; increases greater than 100% should alert the clinician to this possibility. Increases in the IgM levels are common in primary biliary cirrhosis, while increases in the IgA levels occur in alcoholic liver disease.

Coagulation Factors With the exception of factor VIII, the blood clotting factors are made exclusively in hepatocytes. Their serum half-lives are much shorter than albumin, ranging from 6 hours for factor VII to 5 days for fibrinogen. Because of their rapid turnover, measurement of the clotting factors is the single best acute measure of hepatic synthetic function and helpful in both the diagnosis and assessing the prognosis of acute parenchymal liver disease. Useful for this purpose is the *serum prothrombin time*, which collectively measures factors II, V, VII, and X. Biosynthesis of factors II, VII, IX, and X depends on vitamin K. The prothrombin time may be elevated in hepatitis and cirrhosis as well as in disorders that lead to vitamin K deficiency such as obstructive jaundice or fat malabsorption of any kind. Marked prolongation of the prothrombin time, >5 s above control and not corrected by parenteral vitamin K administration, is a poor prognostic sign in acute viral hepatitis and other acute and chronic liver diseases.

OTHER DIAGNOSTIC TESTS While tests may direct the physician to a category of liver disease, additional radiologic testing and procedures are often necessary to make the proper diagnosis, as shown in Fig. 293-1. The two most commonly-used ancillary tests are reviewed here.

Percutaneous Liver Biopsy Percutaneous biopsy of the liver is a safe procedure that can be easily performed at the bedside with local anesthesia. Liver biopsy is of proven value in the following situations: (1) hepatocellular disease of uncertain cause; (2) prolonged hepatitis with the possibility of chronic active hepatitis; (3) unexplained hepatomegaly; (4) unexplained splenomegaly; (5) hepatic filling defects by radiologic imaging; (6) fever of unknown origin; (7) staging of malignant lymphoma. Liver biopsy is most accurate in disorders causing diffuse changes throughout the liver and is subject to sampling error in focal infiltrative disorders such as hepatic metastases. Liver biopsy should not be the initial procedure in the diagnosis of cholestasis. The biliary tree should first be assessed for signs of obstruction.

Ultrasonography Ultrasonography is the first diagnostic test to use in patients whose liver tests suggest cholestasis, to look for the presence of a dilated intrahepatic or extrahepatic biliary tree, or to identify gallstones. In addition, it shows space-occupying lesions within the liver, enables the clinician to distinguish between cystic and solid masses, and helps direct percutaneous biopsies. Ultrasound with Doppler imaging can detect the patency of the portal vein, hepatic artery, and hepatic veins and determine the direction of blood flow. This is the first test ordered in patients suspected of having Budd-Chiari syndrome.

USE OF LIVER TESTS As previously noted, the best way to increase the sensitivity and specificity of laboratory tests in the detection of liver disease is to employ a battery of tests that include the aminotransferases, alkaline phosphatase, bilirubin, albumin, and prothrombin time along with the judicious use of the other tests described in this chapter. Table 293-1 shows how patterns of liver tests can lead the clinician to a category of disease which will direct further evaluation. However, it is important to remember that no single set of liver tests will necessarily provide a diagnosis. It is often necessary to repeat these tests on several occasions over days to weeks for a diagnostic pattern to emerge. Figure 293-1 is an algorithm for the evaluation of chronically abnormal liver tests.

BIBLIOGRAPHY

Bosma PJ et al: The genetic basis of the reduced expression of bilirubin UDP-glucoronosyltransferase 1 in Gilbert's syndrome. New Engl J Med 333:1171, 1995

Brensilver HL, Kaplan MM: Significance of elevated liver alkaline phosphatase in serum. Gastroenterology 68:1556, 1975

Cohen JA, Kaplan MM: The SGOT/SGPT ratio: an indicator of alcoholic liver disease. Dig Dis Sci 24:835, 1979

Pratt DS, Kaplan MM: Laboratory tests, in *Schiff's Diseases of the Liver*, 8th ed, ER Schiff et al (eds). Philadelphia, Lippincott, 1999

Weiss JS et al: The clinical importance of a protein bound fraction of serum bilirubin in patients with hyperbilirubinemia. N Engl J Med 309:147, 1983

294

Paul D. Berk, Allan W. Wolkoff

BILIRUBIN METABOLISM AND THE HYPERBILIRUBINEMIAS

BILIRUBIN METABOLISM

SOURCES OF BILIRUBIN Bilirubin is the end-product of the metabolic degradation of heme, the prosthetic group of hemoglobin, myoglobin, the cytochrome P450s, and various other hemoproteins. The first step in the conversion of heme to bilirubin is the stereospecific oxidative opening of the heme molecule at its α-bridge carbon by the microsomal enzyme *heme oxygenase*, resulting in the formation of equimolar quantities of carbon monoxide and of the green tetrapyrrole biliverdin. Biliverdin is then reduced by a second enzyme, biliverdin reductase, to bilirubin. Between 70 and 90% of bilirubin is derived from degradation of the hemoglobin of senescent or injured circulating red blood cells. The remainder has several sources, including hemoglobin produced during the process of ineffective erythropoiesis within the bone marrow and the turnover of nonhemoglobin hemoproteins in cells throughout the body. Degradation of red-cell hemoglobin occurs principally in the spleen but also throughout the rest of the peripheral reticuloendothelial system, including the Kupffer cells within the liver. Bilirubin produced in the periphery is transported to the liver within the plasma, where, due to its insolubility in aqueous solutions, it is tightly bound to albumin.

The anatomy of the hepatic acinus is highly specialized to facilitate the extraction of such tightly protein-bound compounds (Fig. 294-1). Cuboidal hepatocytes within the hepatic cell plates are immediately adjacent to sinusoids on two surfaces. The endothelial cells of the sinusoids are fenestrated, allowing ready exchange of plasma between the sinusoidal blood and the extracellular space of Disse and affording direct access of the bilirubin-albumin complex to the surface of the hepatocyte, which is greatly expanded by the elaboration of microvilli.

HEPATIC DISPOSITION OF BILIRUBIN Since bilirubin is a potentially toxic waste product, hepatic handling is designed to

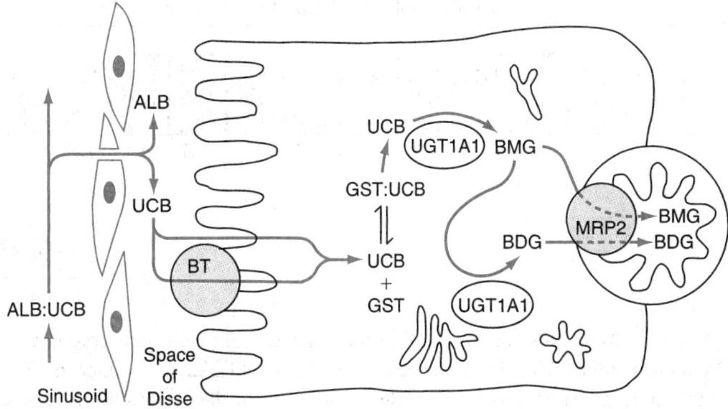

FIGURE 294-1 Hepatocellular bilirubin transport. Albumin-bound bilirubin in sinusoidal blood passes through endothelial cell fenestrae to reach the hepatocyte surface, entering the cell by both facilitated and simple diffusional processes. Within the cell it is bound to glutathione-S-transferases and conjugated by bilirubin-UDP-glucuronosyltransferase (UGT1A1) to mono- and diglucuronides, which are actively transported across the canalicular membrane into the bile. ALB, albumin; UCB, unconjugated bilirubin, UGT1A1, bilirubin-UDP-glucuronosyltransferase; BMG, bilirubin monoglucuronide; GST, glutathione-S-transferase; MRP2, multidrug resistance-associated protein 2; BDG, bilirubin diglucuronide; BT, proposed bilirubin transporter.

eliminate it from the body via the biliary tract. Transfer of bilirubin from blood to bile involves four distinct but interrelated steps, described below (Fig. 294-1).

Hepatocellular Uptake Bilirubin most likely enters the hepatocyte both by a facilitated transport mechanism and by passive diffusion. While kinetic data suggest that facilitated transport is the predominant process and several putative bilirubin transporters have been identified, none has been cloned successfully. Cloned transporters such as *organic anion transport protein* (OATP) and *sodium taurocholate co-transporting polypeptide* (NTCP), which are responsible for the hepatocellular uptake of other organic substrates, including sulfobromophthalein and bile acids, specifically do not transport bilirubin. Therefore, the precise mechanism of bilirubin uptake remains to be determined.

Intracellular Binding Having crossed the plasma membrane to enter the cell, bilirubin partitions between the lipid environment of intracellular membranes and the aqueous cytosol, in which it is kept in solution by binding as a nonsubstrate ligand to several of the glutathione-S-transferases, formerly called ligandins.

Conjugation The aqueous insolubility of bilirubin reflects a rigid, highly ordered molecular structure in which internal hydrogen bonding involving the propionic acid carboxyl groups of one dipyrrolic half of the molecule and the imino and lactam groups of the opposite half blocks solvent access to these polar residues. When the carboxyl groups are esterified by conjugation with glucuronic acid residues, the internal hydrogen bonding is disrupted, rendering the resulting mono- and diglucuronide conjugates highly soluble in aqueous solution.

Bilirubin glucuronidation is catalyzed by a specific UDP-glucuronosyltransferase. The UDP-glucuronosyltransferases have been classified into gene families based on the degree of homology between the various protein isoforms. Those that conjugate bilirubin and certain other substrates have been designated the *UGT1* family and have been shown to be expressed from a single gene complex by alternative splicing. This gene complex contains multiple substrate-specific first exons, designated A1, A2, . . . (Fig. 294-2), each with its own promoter and each encoding the amino-terminal end of a specific isoform, as well as four common exons (exons 2 to 5) that encode the shared carboxyl-terminal end of all of the *UGT1* isoforms. The various first exons encode the specific substrate-binding sites for each isoform, while the shared exons encode common glycosylation, UDP-glucuronic acid-binding, transmembrane, and stop transfer domains. Exon

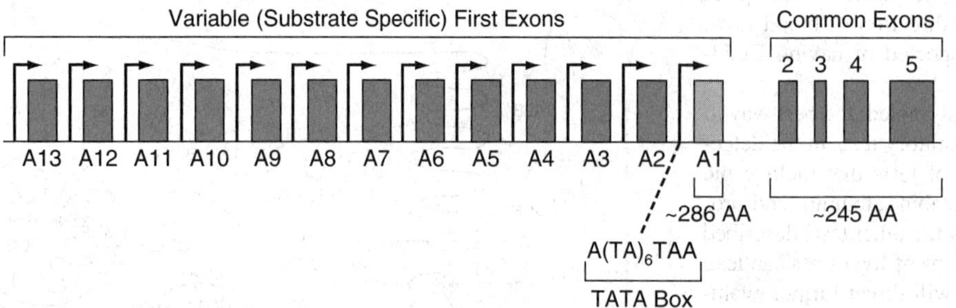

FIGURE 294-2 Structural organization of the human *UGT1* gene complex. This large complex on chromosome 2 contains at least 13 substrate-specific first exons (A1, A2, . . .), each with its own promoter, that encode the amino-terminal substrate-specific 286 amino acids of the various *UGT1* encoded isoforms, and common exons 2 to 5, that encode the 245 carboxyl-terminal amino acids common to all of the isoforms. mRNAs for specific isoforms are assembled by splicing a particular first exon such as the bilirubin-specific exon A1 to exons 2 to 5. The resulting message encodes a complete enzyme, in this particular case bilirubin-UDP-glucuronosyltransferase (UGT1A1). Mutations in a first exon affect only a single isoform. Those in exons 2 to 5 affect all enzymes encoded by the UGT1 complex.

A1 and the four common exons, collectively designated the *UGT1A1* gene (Fig. 294-2), encode the physiologically critical enzyme bilirubin-UDP-glucuronosyltransferase (UGT1A1). A critical corollary of the organization of the *UGT1* gene is that a mutation in one of the first exons will affect only a single enzyme isoform. By contrast, a mutation in exons 2 to 5 will alter all isoforms encoded by the *UGT1* gene complex.

Biliary Excretion Normal bile typically contains less than 5% unconjugated bilirubin, an average of 7% bilirubin monoconjugates, and 90% bilirubin diconjugates. The proportion of monoconjugates increases in the presence of an increased bilirubin load (hemolysis) or a reduced bilirubin-conjugating capacity. Bilirubin mono- and diglucuronides are excreted across the canalicular plasma membrane into the canaliculus by an ATP-dependent transport process mediated by a canalicular membrane protein called *multidrug resistance-associated protein 2* (MRP2). MRP2 is a member of the MRP gene family, other members of which pump certain types of drug conjugates, as well as unmodified anticancer drugs, out of cells. It is also a member of the ATP-binding cassette (ABC) superfamily. Mutations in the rat homologue of MRP2 result in conjugated hyperbilirubinemia in several jaundiced strains that serve as models of the Dubin-Johnson syndrome. It has recently been established that the Dubin-Johnson syndrome in humans also results from mutations in MRP2 (see below).

BILIRUBIN IN PLASMA Although physicians equate the direct-reacting fraction of bilirubin in plasma with conjugated bilirubin and the indirect fraction with unconjugated bilirubin, modern analytical methods document that normal plasma contains virtually no bilirubin conjugates. The 10 to 20% of bilirubin in normal plasma that gives a prompt (direct) diazo reaction is an artifact of the kinetics of the van den Bergh reaction, which, along with various modifications, is the method most commonly used to quantitate bilirubin in clinical laboratories. Indeed, when the direct-reacting fraction is less than 15% of total bilirubin at virtually any total bilirubin concentration, the bilirubin in the sample can be considered as essentially all unconjugated. The canalicular transport mechanism for excretion of bilirubin conjugates is very sensitive to injury. Accordingly, in hepatocellular disease, as well as with either cholestasis or mechanical obstruction to the bile ducts, bilirubin conjugates within the hepatocyte, prevented from taking their normal path into the canaliculi and down the bile ducts, may reflux into the bloodstream, resulting in a mixed or, less often, a truly conjugated hyperbilirubinemia.

EXTRAHEPATIC ASPECTS OF BILIRUBIN DISPOSITION **Bilirubin in the Gut** Following secretion into bile, conjugated bilirubin reaches the duodenum and passes down the gastrointestinal tract without reabsorption by the intestinal mucosa. Although some reaches the feces unaltered, an appreciable fraction is converted to urobilinogen and related compounds by bacterial metabolism within the ileum and colon. Urobilinogen is reabsorbed from these sites, reaches the liver via the portal circulation, and is reexcreted into bile, undergoing an enterohepatic circulation. Urobilinogen not taken up by the liver reaches the systemic circulation, from which some is cleared by the kidneys. Urinary urobilinogen excretion normally does not exceed 4 mg/d. In the presence of hemolysis, which increases the amount of bilirubin entering the gut (and hence the amount of urobilinogen formed and reabsorbed), or in the presence of hepatic disease, which decreases hepatic extraction of urobilinogen, plasma urobilinogen levels rise, as does the amount excreted in the urine. Severe cholestasis, bile duct obstruction, or administration of broad-spectrum antibiotics that eliminate the enteric flora required for the conversion of bilirubin to urobilinogens, markedly decrease formation of urobilinogen and its urinary excretion.

Unconjugated bilirubin ordinarily does not reach the gut except in neonates or, by ill-defined alternative pathways, in the presence of severe unconjugated hyperbilirubinemia (e.g., Crigler-Najjar syndrome type I). In these circumstances, however, unconjugated bilirubin is readily reabsorbed from the gut lumen, amplifying the underlying hyperbilirubinemia.

Renal Excretion of Bilirubin Conjugates Unconjugated bilirubin is not excreted in urine no matter how high its plasma concentration, since it is too tightly bound to albumin for effective glomerular filtration and there is no tubular mechanism for its renal secretion. By contrast, the polar bilirubin conjugates are far less tightly bound to albumin and are readily filtered at the glomerulus. Bilirubin conjugates are not secreted by the renal tubules but may be minimally reabsorbed. Since normal plasma contains virtually exclusively unconjugated bilirubin, no bilirubin normally appears in the urine. Indeed, bilirubinuria indicates the presence of conjugated bilirubin in plasma and, therefore, hepatobiliary dysfunction.

CLINICAL PHYSIOLOGY The plasma concentration of unconjugated bilirubin ([Br]) is determined by the rate at which newly synthesized bilirubin enters the plasma (plasma bilirubin turnover, BrT) and hepatic bilirubin clearance (C_{Br}), according to the following relationship:

$$[\text{Br}] = \frac{\text{k}\cdot\text{BrT(mg/kg body weight per day)}}{C_{Br}\text{(mL/min per kg body weight)}} \qquad (1)$$

where k is a constant related to the different units of time employed in the conventional expression of BrT and C_{Br}. BrT closely reflects total bilirubin production; C_{Br}, analogous to the creatinine clearance test widely used to assess kidney function, is a measure of the rate at which bilirubin is extracted from plasma and is a true quantitative test of liver function. While not easily quantified in routine clinical settings, investigative measurements of BrT and C_{Br} have yielded useful pathophysiologic insights into the unconjugated hyperbilirubinemias.

Equation (1) indicates that the unconjugated bilirubin concentration will increase in the presence of either an increase in BrT or a reduction in hepatic C_{Br}. This equation therefore provides a basis for classifying unconjugated hyperbilirubinemias according to pathogenesis. Furthermore, for an individual with a given value for C_{Br}, or for a population in which C_{Br} varies within a narrow range, [Br] will increase as a linear function of BrT, with a slope relating increases in the plasma [Br] to increased BrT equal to k/C_{Br}. For individuals or populations with reduced bilirubin clearance (e.g., in Gilbert's syndrome, see below), this slope will be steeper than in normal individuals. Conversely, for a given BrT, the relationship between [Br] and

C_{Br} is hyperbolic, like the relation between serum creatinine concentration and creatinine clearance. In any patient, if C_{Br} is reduced from its baseline value, [Br] will be increased in consequence, in direct proportion to the extent of the decrease in C_{Br}.

DISORDERS OF BILIRUBIN METABOLISM LEADING TO UNCONJUGATED HYPERBILIRUBINEMIA

INCREASED BILIRUBIN PRODUCTION **Hemolysis** Increased destruction of erythrocytes leads to increased bilirubin turnover and unconjugated hyperbilirubinemia. With normal liver function, the hyperbilirubinemia is usually modest. In particular, since the bone marrow is only capable of a sustained eightfold increase in erythrocyte production in response to a hemolytic stress, hemolysis alone cannot result in a sustained hyperbilirubinemia of more than approximately 68 μmol/L (4 mg/dL). Higher values imply concomitant hepatic dysfunction.

The causes of hemolysis are numerous. Besides specific hemolytic disorders, mild hemolytic processes accompany many acquired systemic diseases. When hemolysis is the only abnormality in an otherwise healthy individual, the result is a purely unconjugated hyperbilirubinemia, with the direct-reacting fraction as measured in a typical clinical laboratory being ≤15% of the total serum bilirubin. In the presence of systemic disease, which may include a degree of hepatic dysfunction, hemolysis may produce a component of conjugated hyperbilirubinemia in addition to an elevated unconjugated bilirubin concentration.

Prolonged hemolysis may lead to the precipitation of bilirubin salts within the gall bladder or biliary tree, resulting in the formation of gallstones in which bilirubin, rather than cholesterol, is the major component. Such pigment stones may lead to acute or chronic cholecystitis, biliary obstruction, or any other biliary tract consequence of calculous disease.

Ineffective Erythropoiesis During erythroid maturation, small amounts of hemoglobin may be lost during nuclear extrusion, and a fraction of developing erythroid cells is destroyed within the marrow. These processes normally account for 10 to 15% of bilirubin produced. In various disorders, including thalassemia major, frankly megaloblastic anemias due to folate or vitamin B_{12} deficiency, congenital erythropoietic porphyria, lead poisoning, and various congenital and acquired dyserythropoietic anemias, the fraction of total bilirubin production derived from ineffective erythropoiesis is increased, reaching as much as 70% of the total, and may be sufficient to produce modest degrees of unconjugated hyperbilirubinemia.

Miscellaneous Degradation of the hemoglobin of extravascular collections of erythrocytes, such as those seen in massive tissue infarctions or large hematomas, may lead transiently to unconjugated hyperbilirubinemia.

DECREASED HEPATIC BILIRUBIN CLEARANCE **Decreased Hepatic Uptake** As noted above, the mechanisms by which bilirubin enters hepatocytes are not fully defined but probably include both diffusion and facilitated transport. Decreased hepatic bilirubin uptake is believed to contribute to the unconjugated hyperbilirubinemia of Gilbert's syndrome (GS), although the molecular basis for this finding remains unclear (see below). Several drugs, including flavispidic acid, novobiocin, and various cholecystographic contrast agents, have been reported to inhibit bilirubin uptake. The resulting unconjugated hyperbilirubinemia resolves with cessation of the medication.

Impaired Conjugation • ***Physiologic neonatal jaundice*** Bilirubin produced by the fetus is cleared by the placenta and eliminated by the maternal liver. Consequently, bilirubin concentrations in normal neonates at birth are low. The presence of jaundice at birth is pathologic and requires investigation. Immediately after birth, the neonatal liver must assume responsibility for bilirubin clearance and excretion. However, many aspects of hepatic physiology are incompletely developed at birth. Levels of UGT1A1 are low, and alternative pathways allow passage of unconjugated bilirubin into the gut. Since the intestinal flora that converts bilirubin to urobilinogen is also undeveloped, an enterohepatic circulation of unconjugated bilirubin ensues. In consequence, most neonates develop mild unconjugated hyperbilirubinemia between days 2 and 5 after birth. Peak levels are typically less than 85 to 170 μmol/L (5 to 10 mg/dL) and decline to normal adult concentrations within 2 weeks, as mechanisms required for bilirubin disposition mature.

Prematurity, with more profound immaturity of hepatic function, or hemolysis, such as occurs with erythroblastosis fetalis, results in higher levels of unconjugated hyperbilirubinemia. A rapidly rising unconjugated bilirubin concentration, or absolute levels in excess of 340 μmol/L (20 mg/dL), puts the infant at risk for bilirubin encephalopathy, or *kernicterus*, in which bilirubin crosses an immature blood-brain barrier and precipitates in the basal ganglia and other areas of the brain. The consequences range from appreciable neurologic deficits to death. Principal treatment options include phototherapy, which converts bilirubin into photoisomers that are soluble in aqueous media and readily excretable in bile without conjugation, and exchange transfusion.

The canalicular mechanisms responsible for bilirubin excretion are also immature at birth, and their maturation may, on occasion, lag behind that of UGT1A1. This may lead to transient conjugated neonatal hyperbilirubinemia, especially in infants with hemolysis.

Acquired conjugation defects A modest reduction in bilirubin-conjugating capacity may be observed in advanced hepatitis or cirrhosis. However, in this setting, conjugation is better preserved than other aspects of bilirubin disposition, such as canalicular excretion. Various drugs, including pregnanediol, novobiocin, chloramphenicol, and gentamicin, may produce unconjugated hyperbilirubinemia by inhibiting UGT1A1 activity. Finally, certain fatty acids and the progestational steroid 3α,20β-pregnanediol, identified in the breast milk but not the serum of mothers whose infants have excessive neonatal hyperbilirubinemia (*breast milk jaundice*), inhibit bilirubin conjugation. The pathogenesis of breast milk jaundice appears to differ from that of transient familial neonatal hyperbilirubinemia (Lucey-Driscoll syndrome), in which a UGT1A1 inhibitor is found in maternal serum.

HEREDITARY DEFECTS IN BILIRUBIN CONJUGATION Three familial disorders characterized by differing degrees of unconjugated hyperbilirubinemia have long been recognized. The defining clinical features of each are described below (Table 294-1). While these disorders have been recognized for decades to reflect differing degrees of deficiency in the ability to conjugate bilirubin, recent advances in the molecular biology of the *UGT1* gene complex have elucidated their interrelationships and clarified previously puzzling features.

Crigler-Najjar Syndrome, Type I (CN-I) This disorder is characterized by striking unconjugated hyperbilirubinemia of about 340 to 765 μmol/L (20 to 45 mg/dL) that appears in the neonatal period and persists for life. Other conventional hepatic biochemical tests such as serum aminotransferases and alkaline phosphatase are normal, and there is no evidence of hemolysis. Hepatic histology is also essentially normal except for the occasional presence of bile plugs within canaliculi.

Bilirubin glucuronides are markedly reduced or absent from the nearly colorless bile, and there is no detectable constitutive expression of UGT1A1 activity in hepatic tissue. Neither UGT1A1 activity nor the serum bilirubin concentration responds to administration of phenobarbital or other enzyme inducers. In the absence of conjugation, unconjugated bilirubin accumulates in plasma, from which it is eliminated very slowly by alternative pathways that include direct passage into the bile and small intestine. These account for the small amounts of urobilinogen found in feces. No bilirubin is found in the urine.

First described in 1952, the disorder is rare (estimated prevalence of 0.6 to 1.0 per million). Many patients are from geographically or socially isolated communities in which consanguinity is common, and pedigree analyses suggest an autosomal recessive pattern of inheritance. The majority of patients (type IA) exhibit defects in the glu-

Table 294-1 Principal Differential Characteristics of Gilbert's and Crigler-Najjar Syndromes

Feature	Crigler-Najjar Syndrome Type I	Crigler-Najjar Syndrome Type II	Gilbert's Syndrome
Total serum bilirubin, μmol/L [mg/dL]	310–755 (usually >345) [18–45 (usually >20)]	100–430 (usually ≤345) [6–25 (usually ≤20)]	Typically ≤70 μmol/L [≤4 mg/dL] in absence of fasting or hemolysis
Routine liver tests	Normal	Normal	Normal
Response to phenobarbital	None	Decreases bilirubin by >25%	Decreases bilirubin to normal
Kernicterus	Usual	Rare	No
Hepatic histology	Normal	Normal	Usually normal; increased lipofuscin pigment in some
Bile characteristics			
Color:	Pale or colorless	Pigmented	Normal dark color
Bilirubin fractions:	>90% unconjugated	Largest fraction (mean:57%) monoconjugates	Mainly diconjugates but monoconjugates increased (mean 23%)
Bilirubin UDP-glucuronosyl-transferase activity	Typically absent; traces in some patients.	Markedly reduced: 0 to 10% of normal	Reduced: typically 10–33% of normal
Inheritance (all autosomal)	Recessive	Predominantly recessive	Promoter mutation: recessive Missense mutations: 7 of 8 dominant; 1 reportedly recessive

curonide conjugation of a spectrum of substrates in addition to bilirubin, including various drugs and other xenobiotics. These individuals have mutations in one of the common exons (2 to 5) of the *UGT1* gene (Fig. 294-2). In a smaller subset (type IB), the defect is limited largely to bilirubin conjugation, and the causative mutation is in the bilirubin-specific exon A1. More than 30 different *UGT1A1* mutations responsible for CN-I have been identified, including deletions, frameshifts, alterations in intronic splice donor and acceptor sites, and point mutations that introduce premature stop codons or alter critical aminoacids. Their common feature is that they all encode proteins with absent or, at most, traces of bilirubin-UDP-glucuronosyltransferase enzymatic activity.

Prior to the availability of phototherapy, most patients with CN-I died of bilirubin encephalopathy (kernicterus) in infancy or early childhood. A few lived as long as early adult life without overt neurologic damage, although more subtle testing usually indicated mild but progressive brain damage. In all such cases, in the absence of liver transplantation, death eventually supervened from late-onset bilirubin encephalopathy, which often followed a nonspecific febrile illness. Recent data suggest that the best hope for survival of a neurologically intact patient involves the following regimen: (1) about 12 h/d of phototherapy from birth throughout childhood, perhaps supplemented by exchange transfusion in the immediate neonatal period; (2) use of tin-protoporphyrin to blunt transient episodes of increased hyperbilirubinemia; and (3) early liver transplantation, prior to the onset of brain damage. In a single patient, transplantation with isolated allogeneic hepatocytes produced a clinically significant reduction in serum bilirubin concentration.

Crigler-Najjar Syndrome, Type II (CN-II) Characterized by marked unconjugated hyperbilirubinemia in the absence of abnormalities of other conventional hepatic biochemical tests, hepatic histology, or hemolysis, this condition was recognized as a distinct entity in 1962. It differs from CN-I in several specific ways (Table 294-1). (1) Although there is considerable overlap, average bilirubin concentrations are lower in CN-II; (2) accordingly, CN-II is only infrequently associated with kernicterus; (3) bile is deeply colored and bilirubin glucuronides are present, with a striking, characteristic increase in monoglucuronides; (4) UGT1A1 in liver is usually present at reduced levels (typically ≤10% of normal) but may be undetectable by less sensitive older assays; (5) while typically detected in infancy, hyperbilirubinemia was not recognized in some cases until later in life, and in one instance, until age 34. As with CN-I, most CN-II cases exhibit abnormalities in the conjugation of other compounds, such as salicylamide and menthol, but in some instances the defect appears limited to bilirubin.

Reduction of serum bilirubin concentrations by more than 25% in response to enzyme inducers such as phenobarbital distinguishes CN-II from CN-I, although this response may not be elicited in early infancy and often is not accompanied by measurable UGT1A1 induction. Bilirubin concentrations during phenobarbital administration do not return to normal but are typically in the range of 51 to 86 μmol/L (3 to 5 mg/dL). Although the incidence of kernicterus in CN-II is low, instances have occurred, not only in infants but in adolescents and adults, often in the setting of an intercurrent illness, fasting, or any other factor that temporarily raises the serum bilirubin concentration above baseline. For this reason, phenobarbital therapy is widely recommended, a single bedtime dose often sufficing to maintain clinically safe plasma bilirubin concentrations.

At least 10 different mutations of *UGT1* associated with CN-II have been identified. Their common feature is that they encode for a bilirubin-UDP-glucuronosyltransferase with markedly reduced but detectable enzymatic activity. The spectrum of residual enzyme activity explains the spectrum of phenotypic severity of the resulting hyperbilirubinemia. Molecular analysis has established that a large majority of CN-II patients are either homozygotes or compound heterozygotes for CN-II mutations and that individuals carrying one mutated and one entirely normal allele have normal bilirubin concentrations. Possible inheritance in one case as a dominant negative mutation remains to be confirmed.

Gilbert's Syndrome This syndrome is characterized by mild unconjugated hyperbilirubinemia, normal values for standard hepatic biochemical tests, and normal hepatic histology other than a modest increase of lipofuscin pigment in some patients. Serum bilirubin concentrations are most often <51 μmol/L (<3 mg/dL), although both higher and lower values are frequent. The spectrum of hyperbilirubinemia fades into that of CN-II at serum bilirubin concentrations of 86 to 136 μmol/L (5 to 8 mg/dL). At the other end of the scale, the distinction between mild cases of GS and a normal state is often blurred. Bilirubin concentrations may fluctuate substantially in any given individual, and at least 25% of patients will exhibit temporarily normal values during prolonged follow-up. More elevated values are associated with stress, fatigue, alcohol use, reduced caloric intake, and intercurrent illness, while increased caloric intake or administration of enzyme-inducing agents produce lower bilirubin levels. GS is most often diagnosed at or shortly after puberty or in adult life during routine examinations that include multichannel biochemical analyses.

UGT1A1 activity is typically reduced to 10 to 35% of normal, and bile pigments in bile exhibit a characteristic increase in bilirubin monoglucuronides. Studies of radiobilirubin kinetics indicate that hepatic bilirubin clearance is reduced to an average of one-third of normal. Administration of phenobarbital normalizes both the serum bilirubin concentration and hepatic bilirubin clearance. However, failure of UGT1A1 activity to improve in many such instances suggests the possible coexistence of an additional defect. Compartmental analysis of bilirubin kinetic data suggests that GS patients have a defect in bilirubin uptake as well as in conjugation. Defect(s) in the hepatic uptake of other organic anions that at least partially share an uptake mechanism with bilirubin, such as sulfobromophthalein and indocyanine green, are observed in some, but not all, patients. The disposition of bile acids, which do not utilize the bilirubin uptake mechanism, is normal.

The magnitude of changes in the plasma bilirubin concentration induced by provocation tests such as 48 h of fasting or the intravenous administration of nicotinic acid have been reported to be of help in separating GS patients from normal individuals. Other studies dispute this assertion. Moreover, on theoretical grounds, the results of such studies should provide no more information than simple measurements of the baseline plasma bilirubin concentration.

Family studies indicate that GS and hereditary hemolytic anemias such as hereditary spherocytosis, glucose-6-phosphate dehydrogenase deficiency, and β-thalassemia trait sort independently. Reports of hemolysis in up to 50% of GS patients are believed to reflect better case finding, since patients with both GS and hemolysis have higher bilirubin concentrations, and are more likely to be jaundiced, than patients with either defect alone.

GS is common, with many series placing its prevalence at 8% or more. Males predominate over females by reported ratios ranging from 1.5:1 to more than 7:1. However, these ratios may have a large artifactual component since normal males have higher mean bilirubin levels than normal females, but the diagnosis of GS is often based on comparison to normal ranges established in men. The high prevalence of GS in the general population may explain the reported frequency of mild unconjugated hyperbilirubinemia in liver transplant recipients.

The disposition of most xenobiotics metabolized by glucuronidation appears to be normal in GS, as is oxidative drug metabolism in the majority of reported studies. The principal exception is the metabolism of the anti-tumor agent irinotecan (CPT-11). Its active metabolite (SN-38) is glucuronidated specifically by bilirubin-UDP-glucuronosyltransferase. Administration of CPT-11 to patients with GS has resulted in several toxicities, including intractable diarrhea and myelosuppression. Some reports also suggest abnormal disposition of menthol, estradiol benzoate, acetaminophen, tolbutamide, and rifamycin SV. Although some of these studies have been disputed, and there have been no reports of clinical complications from use of these agents in GS, prudence should be exercised in prescribing them, or any agents metabolized primarily by glucuronidation, in this condition.

Most older pedigree studies of GS were consistent with autosomal dominant inheritance with variable expressivity. However, studies of the *UGT1* gene in GS have indicated a variety of molecular genetic bases for the phenotypic picture and several different patterns of inheritance. Studies in European and U.S. patients found that the majority of GS patients had normal coding regions for UGT1A1 but were homozygous for an abnormality consisting of an extra TA (i.e., A[TA]$_7$TAA rather than A[TA]$_6$TAA) in the promoter region of the first exon. This appeared to be a necessary but not a sufficient genetic basis for clinically expressed GS, since 15% of normal controls were also homozygous for this variant. While normal by standard criteria, these individuals had somewhat higher bilirubin concentrations than the rest of the controls studied. Heterozygotes for this abnormality had bilirubin concentrations identical to those homozygous for the A[TA]$_6$TAA allele. The prevalence of the A[TA]$_7$TAA allele in a general western population is 30%, in which case 9% would be homozygotes. This is slightly higher than the prevalence of GS based on purely phenotypic parameters. It was suggested that additional variables, such as mild hemolysis or a defect in bilirubin uptake, might be among the factors enhancing phenotypic expression of the defect. Phenotypic expression of GS due solely to the A[TA]$_7$TAA promoter abnormality is inherited as an autosomal recessive trait.

A number of CN-II kindreds have been identified in which there is also an allele containing a normal coding region but the A[TA]$_7$TAA

promoter abnormality. CN-II heterozygotes who have the A[TA]$_6$TAA promoter are phenotypically normal, whereas those with the A[TA]$_7$TAA promoter express the phenotypic picture of GS. GS in such kindreds may also result from homozygosity for the A[TA]$_7$TAA promoter abnormality.

Seven different missense mutations in the *UGT1* gene that reportedly cause GS with dominant inheritance have been found in Japanese individuals. Another Japanese patient with mild unconjugated hyperbilirubinemia was homozygous for a missense mutation in exon 5. GS in her family appeared to be recessive. Missense mutations causing GS have not been reported outside of Japan.

DISORDERS OF BILIRUBIN METABOLISM LEADING TO MIXED OR PREDOMINANTLY CONJUGATED HYPERBILIRUBINEMIA

In hyperbilirubinemia due to acquired liver disease (e.g., acute hepatitis, common bile duct stone), there are usually elevations in the serum concentrations of both conjugated and unconjugated bilirubin. Although biliary tract obstruction or hepatocellular cholestatic injury may present on occasion with a predominantly conjugated hyperbilirubinemia, it is generally not possible to differentiate intrahepatic from extrahepatic causes of jaundice based upon the serum levels or relative proportions of unconjugated and conjugated bilirubin. The major reason for determining the amounts of conjugated and unconjugated bilirubin in the serum is for the initial differentiation of hepatic parenchymal and obstructive disorders (mixed conjugated and unconjugated hyperbilirubinemia) from the inheritable and hemolytic disorders discussed above that are associated with unconjugated hyperbilirubinemia.

FAMILIAL DEFECTS IN HEPATIC EXCRETORY FUNCTION Dubin-Johnson Syndrome This benign, relatively rare disorder is characterized by low-grade, predominantly conjugated hyperbilirubinemia. Total bilirubin concentrations are typically between 34 and 85 μmol/L (2 and 5 mg/dL) but on occasion can be in the normal range or as high as 340 to 430 μmol/L (20 to 25 mg/dL) and can fluctuate widely in any given patient. The degree of hyperbilirubinemia may be increased by intercurrent illness, oral contraceptive use, and pregnancy. As the hyperbilirubinemia is due to a predominant rise in conjugated bilirubin, bilirubinuria is characteristically present. Aside from elevated serum bilirubin levels, other routine laboratory tests are normal. Physical examination is usually normal except for jaundice, although an occasional patient may have hepatosplenomegaly.

Patients with Dubin-Johnson syndrome are usually asymptomatic, although some may have vague constitutional symptoms. These latter patients have usually undergone extensive and often unnecessary diagnostic examinations for unexplained jaundice and have high levels of anxiety. In women, the condition may be subclinical until the patient becomes pregnant or receives oral contraceptives, at which time chemical hyperbilirubinemia becomes frank jaundice. Even in these situations, other routine liver function tests, including serum alkaline phosphatase and transaminase activities, are normal.

A cardinal feature of Dubin-Johnson syndrome is the accumulation in the lysosomes of centrilobular hepatocytes of dark, coarsely granular pigment. As a result, the liver may be grossly black in appearance. This pigment is thought to be derived from epinephrine metabolites that are not excreted normally. The pigment may disappear during bouts of viral hepatitis, only to reaccumulate slowly after recovery.

Biliary excretion of a number of anionic compounds is compromised in Dubin-Johnson syndrome. These include various cholecystographic agents, as well as sulfobromophthalein (Bromsulphalein, BSP), a synthetic dye formerly used in a test of liver function. In this test, the rate of disappearance of BSP from plasma was determined following bolus intravenous administration. BSP is conjugated with glutathione in the hepatocyte; the resulting conjugate is normally excreted rapidly into the canaliculus. Patients with Dubin-Johnson syndrome exhibit a characteristic rise in its plasma concentration at 90 min after injection, due to reflux of conjugated BSP into the circulation from the hepatocyte. Dyes such as indocyanine green (ICG) that are taken up by hepatocytes but are not further metabolized prior to biliary excretion do not show this reflux phenomenon. Continuous BSP infusion studies suggest a reduction in the t_{max} for biliary excretion. Bile acid disposition, including hepatocellular uptake and biliary excretion, are normal in Dubin-Johnson syndrome. These patients have normal serum and biliary bile acid concentrations and do not have pruritus.

By analogy with findings in several mutant rat strains, the selective defect in biliary excretion of bilirubin conjugates and certain other classes of organic compounds, but not of bile acids, that characterizes the Dubin-Johnson syndrome was found to reflect defective expression of MRP2, an ATP-dependent canalicular membrane transporter. Several different mutations in the *MRP2* gene produce the Dubin-Johnson phenotype, which has an autosomal recessive pattern of inheritance. Although MRP2 is undoubtedly important in the biliary excretion of conjugated bilirubin, the fact that this pigment is still excreted in the absence of MRP2 suggests that other, as yet uncharacterized, transport proteins may serve in a secondary role in this process.

Patients with Dubin-Johnson syndrome also have a diagnostic abnormality in urinary coproporphyrin excretion. There are two naturally occurring coproporphyrin isomers, I and III. Normally, approximately 75% of the coproporphyrin in urine is isomer III. In urine from Dubin-Johnson syndrome patients, total coproporphyrin content is normal, but more than 80% is isomer I. Heterozygotes for the syndrome show an intermediate pattern. The molecular basis for this phenomenon remains unclear.

Rotor Syndrome This benign, autosomal recessive disorder is clinically similar to the Dubin-Johnson syndrome, although it is seen even less frequently. A major phenotypic difference is that the liver in patients with Rotor syndrome has no increased pigmentation and appears totally normal. The only abnormality in routine laboratory tests is an elevation of total serum bilirubin, due to a predominant rise in conjugated bilirubin. This is accompanied by bilirubinuria. Several additional features differentiate Rotor and Dubin-Johnson syndromes. In Rotor syndrome, the gallbladder is usually visualized on oral cholecystography, in contrast to the nonvisualization that is typical of Dubin-Johnson syndrome. The pattern of urinary coproporphyrin excretion also differs. The pattern in Rotor syndrome resembles that of many acquired disorders of hepatobiliary function, in which coproporphyrin I, the major coproporphyrin isomer in bile, refluxes from the hepatocyte back into the circulation and is excreted in urine. Thus, total urinary coproporphyrin excretion is substantially increased in Rotor syndrome, in contrast to the normal levels seen in Dubin-Johnson syndrome. Although the fraction of coproporphyrin I in urine is elevated, it is usually less than 70% of the total, as compared to 80% or more in Dubin-Johnson syndrome. The disorders also can be distinguished by their patterns of BSP excretion. Although clearance of BSP from plasma is delayed in Rotor syndrome, there is no reflux of conjugated BSP back into the circulation as seen in Dubin-Johnson syndrome. Kinetic analysis of plasma BSP infusion studies suggests the presence of a defect in intrahepatocellular storage of this compound. This has never been demonstrated directly, and the molecular basis of Rotor syndrome remains unknown.

Benign Recurrent Intrahepatic Cholestasis (BRIC) This rare disorder is characterized by recurrent attacks of pruritus and jaundice. The typical episode begins with mild malaise and elevations in serum aminotransferase levels, followed rapidly by rises in alkaline phosphatase and bilirubin and onset of jaundice and itching. The first one or two episodes may be misdiagnosed as acute viral hepatitis. The cholestatic episodes, which may begin in childhood or adulthood, can vary in duration from several weeks to months, following which there is complete clinical and biochemical resolution. Intervals between attacks may vary from several months to years. Between episodes, physical examination is normal, as are serum levels of bile acids, bilirubin, transaminases, and alkaline phosphatase. The disorder is familial and has an autosomal recessive pattern of inheritance. BRIC is considered a benign disorder in that it does not lead to cirrhosis or end-stage liver disease. However, the episodes of jaundice and pruritus can be prolonged and debilitating, and some patients have undergone liver transplantation to relieve the intractable and disabling symptoms. Treatment during the cholestatic episodes is symptomatic; there is no specific treatment to prevent or shorten the occurrence of episodes.

A gene termed *FIC1* was recently identified and found to be mutated in patients with BRIC. Curiously, this gene is expressed strongly in the small intestine but only weakly in the liver. The protein encoded by *FIC1* shows little similarity to genes that have been shown to play a role in bile canalicular excretion of various compounds. Rather, it appears to be a member of a P-type ATPase family that transports aminophospholipids from the outer to the inner leaflet of a variety of cell membranes.

Progressive Familial Intrahepatic Cholestasis (FIC) This name is applied to three phenotypically related syndromes. Progressive FIC type 1 (Byler disease) presents in early infancy as cholestasis that may be initially episodic. However, in contrast to BRIC, Byler disease progresses to malnutrition, growth retardation, and end-stage liver disease during childhood. This disorder is also a consequence of an FIC1 mutation. The functional relationship of the *FIC1* protein to the pathogenesis of cholestasis in these disorders is unknown. Two other types of progressive FIC (types 2 and 3) have been described. Type 2 is associated with a mutation in the protein named *sister of p-glycoprotein*, which is the major bile canalicular exporter of bile acids. Type 3 has been associated with a mutation of MDR3, a protein that is essential for normal bile canalicular excretion of phospholipids. Although all three types of progressive FIC have similar clinical phenotypes, only type 3 is associated with high serum levels of γ-glutamyltransferase activity. In contrast, activity of this enzyme is normal or only mildly elevated in symptomatic BRIC and progressive FIC types 1 and 2.

BIBLIOGRAPHY

AONO S et al: Analysis of genes for bilirubin UDP-glucuronosyltransferase in Gilbert's syndrome. Lancet 345:959, 1995

BERK PD, NOYER C: Bilirubin metabolism and the hereditary hyperbilirubinemias. Semin in Liver Dis 14:323, 1994

BOSMA P et al: The genetic basis of the reduced expression of bilirubin-UDP-glucuronosyltransferase 1 in Gilbert's syndrome. N Engl J Med 333:1171, 1995

CLARKE DJ et al: Genetic defects of the UDP-glucuronosyltransferase 1 (*UGT1*) gene that cause familial non-haemolytic unconjugated hyperbilirubinaemias. Clin Chim Acta 266:63, 1997

IYANAGI T et al: Biochemical and molecular aspects of genetic disorders of bilirubin metabolism. Biochim Biophys Acta 1407:173, 1998

KARTENBECK J et al: Absence of the canalicular isoform of the *MRP* gene-encoded conjugate export pump from the hepatocytes in the Dubin-Johnson syndrome. Hepatology 23:1061, 1996

PAULUSMA CC et al: A mutation in the human canalicular multispecific organic anion transporter gene causes the Dubin-Johnson syndrome. Hepatology 25:1539, 1997

ROY CHOWDHURY J et al: Hereditary jaundice and disorders of bilirubin metabolism, in *The Metabolic and Molecular Bases of Inherited Disease*, 7th ed, CR Scriver et al (eds.) New York, McGraw-Hill, 1995, pp 2161–2208

ROY CHOWDHURY J et al: Bilirubin metabolism and its disorders, in *Hepatology*, 3d ed. D Zakim, T Boyer (eds.) Philadelphia, Saunders, 1996, pp 323–347

SEPPEN J et al: Discrimination between Crigler-Najjar type I and II by expression of mutant bilirubin uridine diphosphate-glucuronosyltransferase. J Clin Invest 94:2385, 1994

VAN DER VEERE CN et al: Current therapy for Crigler-Najjar syndrome Type 1: Report of a world registry. Hepatology 24:311, 1996

295

Jules L. Dienstag, Kurt J. Isselbacher

ACUTE VIRAL HEPATITIS

ALT alanine aminotransferase	HBV hepatitis B virus
AST aspartate aminotransferase	HBxAg hepatitis B x antigen
bDNA branched-chain complementary DNA	HCV hepatitis C virus
	HDV hepatitis D virus
ELU enzyme-linked immunoassay units	HEV hepatitis E virus
	IG immune globulin
EMC essential mixed cryoglobulinemia	LKM liver-kidney microsomes
	NS nonstructural
HAV hepatitis A virus	PCR polymerase chain reaction
HBcAg hepatitis B core antigen	PT prothrombin time
HBeAg hepatitis B e antigen	RIBA recombinant immunoblot assay
HBIG hepatitis B immune globulin	
HBsAg hepatitis B surface antigen	

Acute viral hepatitis is a systemic infection affecting the liver predominantly. Almost all cases of acute viral hepatitis are caused by one of five viral agents: hepatitis A virus (HAV), hepatitis B virus (HBV), hepatitis C virus (HCV), the HBV-associated delta agent or hepatitis D virus (HDV), and hepatitis E virus (HEV). Other transfusion-transmitted agents, e.g., "hepatitis G" virus and "TT" virus, have been identified but do not cause hepatitis. All these human hepatitis viruses are RNA viruses, except for hepatitis B, which is a DNA virus. Although these agents can be distinguished by their molecular and antigenic properties, all types of viral hepatitis produce clinically similar illnesses. These range from asymptomatic and inapparent to fulminant and fatal acute infections common to all types, on the one hand, and from subclinical persistent infections to rapidly progressive chronic liver disease with cirrhosis and even hepatocellular carcinoma, common to the bloodborne types (HBV, HCV, and HDV), on the other.

VIROLOGY AND ETIOLOGY **Hepatitis A** Hepatitis A virus is a nonenveloped 27-nm, heat-, acid-, and ether-resistant RNA virus in the hepatovirus genus of the picornavirus family (Fig. 295-1). Its virion contains four capsid polypeptides, designated VP1 to VP4, which are cleaved posttranslationally from the polyprotein product of a 7500-nucleotide genome. Inactivation of viral activity can be achieved by boiling for 1 min, by contact with formaldehyde and chlorine, or by ultraviolet irradiation. Despite nucleotide sequence variation of up to 20% among isolates of HAV, all strains of this virus are immunologically indistinguishable and belong to one serotype. Hepatitis A has an incubation period of approximately 4 weeks. Its replication is limited to the liver, but the virus is present in the liver, bile, stools, and blood during the late incubation period and acute preicteric phase of illness. Despite persistence of virus in the liver, viral shedding in feces, viremia, and infectivity diminish rapidly once jaundice becomes apparent. HAV is the only one of the human hepatitis viruses that can be cultivated reproducibly in vitro.

Antibodies to HAV (anti-HAV) can be detected during acute illness when serum aminotransferase activity is elevated and fecal HAV shedding is still occurring. This early antibody response is predominantly of the IgM class and persists for several months, rarely for 6 to 12 months. During convalescence, however, anti-HAV of the IgG class becomes the predominant antibody (Fig. 295-2). Therefore, the diagnosis of hepatitis A is made during acute illness by demonstrating anti-HAV of the IgM class. After acute illness, anti-HAV of the IgG class remains detectable indefinitely, and patients with serum anti-HAV are immune to reinfection. Neutralizing antibody activity parallels the appearance of anti-HAV, and the IgG anti-HAV present in immune globulin accounts for the protection it affords against HAV infection.

Hepatitis B Hepatitis B virus is a DNA virus with a remarkably compact genomic structure; despite its small, circular, 3200-basepair size, HBV DNA codes for four sets of viral products and has a complex, multiparticle structure. HBV achieves its genomic economy by relying on an efficient strategy of encoding proteins from four overlapping genes: S, C, P, and X (Fig. 295-3), as detailed below. Once thought to be unique among viruses, HBV is now recognized as one of a family of animal viruses, hepadnaviruses (hepatotropic DNA viruses), and is classified as hepadnavirus type 1. Similar viruses infect certain species of woodchucks, ground and tree squirrels, and Pekin ducks, to mention the most carefully characterized. Like HBV, all have the same distinctive three morphologic forms, have counterparts to the envelope and nucleocapsid virus antigens of HBV, replicate in the liver but exist in extrahepatic sites, contain their own endogenous DNA polymerase, have partially double-stranded and partially single-stranded genomes, are associated with acute and chronic hepatitis and hepatocellular carcinoma, and rely on a replicative strategy unique among DNA viruses but typical of retroviruses. Instead of DNA replication directly from a DNA template, hepadnaviruses rely on reverse transcription (effected by the DNA polymerase) of minus-strand DNA from a "pregenomic" RNA intermediate. Then plus-strand DNA is transcribed from the minus-strand DNA template by the DNA-dependent DNA polymerase. Viral proteins are translated by the pregenomic RNA, and the proteins and genome are packaged into virions and secreted from the hepatocyte. Although HBV is difficult to cultivate in vitro in the conventional sense from clinical material, several cell lines have been transfected with HBV DNA. Such transfected cells support in vitro replication of the intact virus and its component proteins.

Viral proteins and particles Three particulate forms of HBV (Table 295-1) can be demonstrated by electron microscopy (Fig. 295-1). The most numerous are the 22-nm particles, which appear as spherical or long filamentous forms; these are antigenically indistinguishable from the outer surface or envelope protein of HBV and are thought to represent excess viral envelope protein. Outnumbered in serum by a factor of 100 or 1000 to 1 compared with the spheres and tubules are large, 42-nm, double-shelled spherical particles, which represent the intact hepatitis B virion. The envelope protein expressed on the outer surface of the virion and on the smaller spherical and tubular structures is referred to as *hepatitis B surface antigen* (HBsAg). The concentration of HBsAg and virus particles in the blood may reach 500 μg/mL and 10 trillion particles per milliliter, respectively. The envelope protein, HBsAg, is the product of the S gene of HBV.

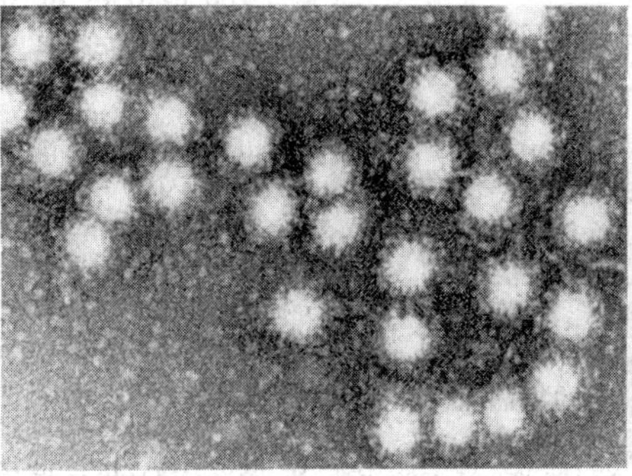

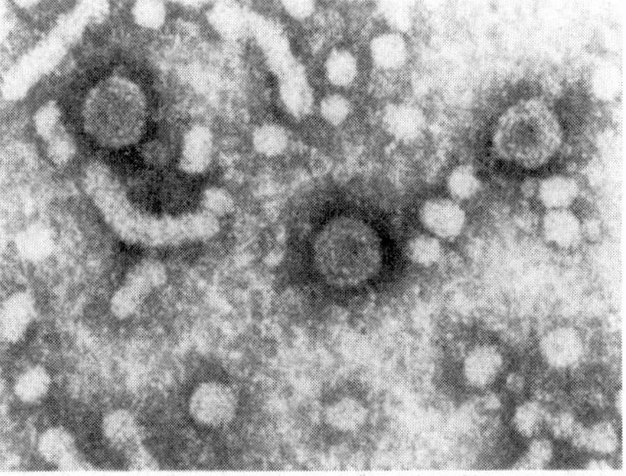

FIGURE 295-1 *A.* Electron micrograph of 27-nm hepatitis A virus particles purified from stool of a patient with acute hepatitis A virus infection and aggregated by hepatitis A antibody. *B.* Electron micrograph of concentrated serum from a patient with hepatitis B infection, demonstrating the 42-nm virions, tubular forms, and spherical 22-nm particles of hepatitis B surface antigen. 132,000×. (Hepatitis D resembles 42-nm virions of hepatitis B but is smaller, 35 to 37 nm; hepatitis E resembles hepatitis A virus but is slightly larger, 32 to 34 nm; hepatitis C has not been visualized definitively.)

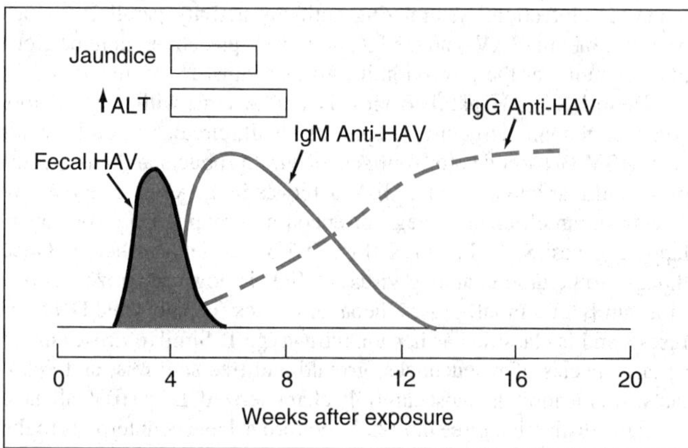

FIGURE 295-2 Scheme of typical clinical and laboratory features of viral hepatitis A.

A number of different HBsAg subdeterminants have been identified. There is a common group-reactive antigen, *a*, shared by all HBsAg isolates. In addition, HBsAg may contain one of several subtype-specific antigens, namely, *d* or *y*, *w* or *r*, as well as other more recently characterized specificities. Hepatitis B isolates fall into one of at least eight subtypes and six genotypes (A–F); however, clinical course and outcome are independent of subtype and genotype [except for an increase in "precore" mutations (see below) in certain genotypes].

Upstream of the S gene are the pre-S genes (Fig. 295-3), which code for pre-S gene products, including receptors on the HBV surface for polymerized human serum albumin and for hepatocyte membrane proteins. The pre-S region actually consists of both pre-S1 and pre-S2. Depending on where translation is initiated, three potential HBsAg gene products are synthesized. The protein product of the S gene is HBsAg (*major protein*), the product of the S region plus the adjacent pre-S2 region is the *middle protein*, and the product of the pre-S1 plus pre-S2 plus S regions is the *large protein*. Compared with the smaller spherical and tubular particles of HBV, complete 42-nm virions are enriched in the large protein. Both pre-S proteins and their respective antibodies can be detected during HBV infection, and the period of pre-S antigenemia appears to coincide with other markers of virus replication, as detailed below.

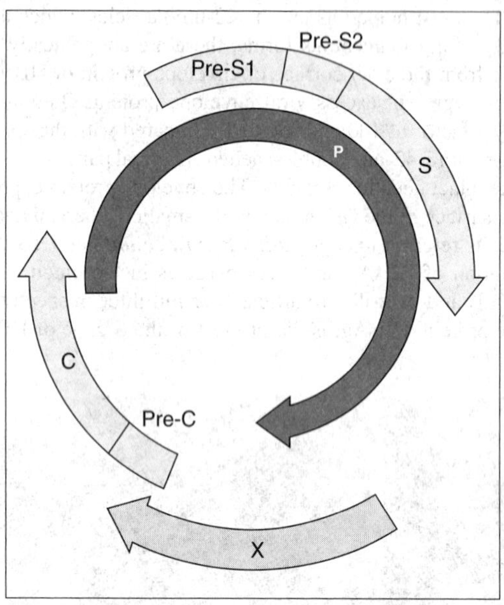

FIGURE 295-3 Its compact genomic structure, with overlapping genes, permits HBV to code for multiple proteins. The S gene codes for the "major" envelope protein, HBsAg. Pre-S1 and pre-S2, upstream of S, combine with S to code for two larger proteins, "middle" protein, the product of pre-S2 + S, and "large" protein, the product of pre-S1 + pre-S2 + S. The largest gene, P, codes for DNA polymerase. The C gene codes for two nucleocapsid proteins, HBeAg, a soluble, secreted protein (initiation from the pre-C region of the gene) and HBcAg, the intracellular core protein (initiation after pre-C). The X gene codes for HBxAg, which can transactivate the transcription of cellular and viral genes; its clinical relevance is not known, but it may contribute to carcinogenesis by binding to p53.

The intact 42-nm virion can be disrupted by mild detergents, and the 27-nm nucleocapsid core particle isolated. Nucleocapsid proteins are coded for by the C gene. The antigen expressed on the surface of the nucleocapsid core is referred to as *hepatitis B core antigen* (HBcAg), and its corresponding antibody is anti-HBc. A third HBV antigen is *hepatitis B e antigen* (HBeAg), a soluble, nonparticulate, nucleocapsid protein that is immunologically distinct from intact HBcAg but is a product of the same C gene. The C gene has two initiation codons, a precore and a core region (Fig. 295-3). If translation is initiated at the precore region, the protein product is HBeAg, which has a signal peptide that binds it to the smooth endoplasmic reticulum and leads to its secretion into the circulation. If translation begins with the core region, HBcAg is the protein product; it has no signal peptide, it is not secreted, but it assembles into nucleocapsid particles, which bind to and incorporate RNA and which, ultimately, contain HBV DNA. Also packaged within the nucleocapsid core is a DNA polymerase, which directs replication and repair of HBV DNA. When packaging within viral proteins is complete, synthesis of the incomplete plus strand stops; this accounts for the single-stranded gap and for differences in the size of the gap. HBcAg particles remain in the hepatocyte, where they are readily detectable by immunohistochemical staining, and are exported after encapsidation by an envelope of HBsAg. Therefore, naked core particles do not circulate in the serum. The secreted nucleocapsid protein, HBeAg, provides a convenient, readily detectable, qualitative marker of HBV replication and relative infectivity.

HBsAg-positive serum containing HBeAg is more likely to be highly infectious and to be associated with the presence of hepatitis B virions (and detectable HBV DNA, see below) than HBeAg-negative or anti-HBe-positive serum. For example, HBsAg carrier mothers who are HBeAg-positive almost invariably (>90%) transmit hepatitis B infection to their offspring, whereas HBsAg carrier mothers with anti-HBe rarely (10 to 15%) infect their offspring.

Early during the course of acute hepatitis B, HBeAg appears transiently; its disappearance may be a harbinger of clinical improvement and resolution of infection. Persistence of HBeAg in serum beyond the first 3 months of acute infection may be predictive of the development of chronic infection, and the presence of HBeAg during chronic hepatitis B is associated with ongoing viral replication, infectivity, and inflammatory liver injury.

The third of the HBV genes is the largest, the P gene (Fig. 295-3), which codes for the DNA polymerase; as noted above, this enzyme has both DNA-dependent DNA polymerase and RNA-dependent reverse transcriptase activities. The fourth gene, X, codes for a small, nonparticulate protein that is capable of transactivating the transcription of both viral and cellular genes (Fig. 295-3). Such transactivation may enhance the replication of HBV, leading to the clinical association observed between the expression of the product of the X gene, hepatitis B x antigen (HBxAg), and antibodies to it in patients with severe chronic hepatitis and hepatocellular carcinoma. The trans-activating activity can enhance the transcription and replication of other viruses besides HBV, such as HIV. Cellular processes transactivated by X include the human interferon γ gene and class I major histocompatibility genes; potentially, these effects could contribute to enhanced susceptibility of HBV-infected hepatocytes to cytolytic T cells. The expression of X can also induce programmed cell death (apoptosis). The X gene and its protein product, however, are absent in nonmammalian hepadnaviruses; therefore, X is not essential for hepadnavirus replication.

Table 295-1 Nomenclature and Features of Hepatitis Viruses

Hepatitis Type	Virus Particle	Morphology	Genome[a]	Classification	Antigen(s)	Antibodies	Remarks
HAV	27 nm	Icosahedral nonenveloped	7.5-kb RNA, linear, ss, +	Hepatovirus	HAV	anti-HAV	Early fecal shedding Diagnosis: IgM anti-HAV Previous infection: IgG anti-HAV
HBV	42 nm	Double-shelled virion (surface and core) spherical	3.2-kb DNA, circular, ss/ds	Hepadnavirus	HBsAg HBcAg HBeAg	anti-HBs anti-HBc anti-HBe	Bloodborne virus; carrier state Acute diagnosis: HBsAg, IgM anti-HBc Chronic diagnosis: IgG anti-HBc, HBsAg Markers of replication: HBeAg, HBV DNA Liver, lymphocytes, other organs
	27 nm	Nucleocapsid core			HBcAg HBeAg	anti-HBc anti-HBe	Nucleocapsid contains DNA and DNA polymerase; present in hepatocyte nucleus; HBcAg does not circulate; HBeAg (soluble, nonparticulate) and HBV DNA circulate—correlate with infectivity and complete virions
	22 nm	Spherical and filamentous; represents excess virus coat material			HBsAg	anti-HBs	HBsAg detectable in >95% of patients with acute hepatitis B; found in serum, body fluids, hepatocyte cytoplasm; anti-HBs appears following infection—protective antibody
HCV	Approx. 40–60 nm	Enveloped	9.4-kb RNA, linear, ss, +	Flavivirus-like	HCV C100-3 C33c C22-3 NS5	anti-HCV	Bloodborne agent, formerly labeled non-A, non-B hepatitis Acute diagnosis: anti-HCV (C33c, C22-3, NS5), HCV RNA Chronic diagnosis: anti-HCV (C100-3, C33c, C22-3, NS5) and HCV RNA; cytoplasmic location in hepatocytes
HDV	35–37 nm	Enveloped hybrid particle with HBsAg coat and HDV core	1.7-kb RNA, circular, ss, −	Resembles viroids and plant satellite viruses	HBsAg HDV antigen	anti-HBs anti-HDV	Defective RNA virus, requires helper function of HBV (hepadnaviruses); HDV antigen present in hepatocyte nucleus Diagnosis: anti-HDV, HDV RNA; HBV/HDV coinfection—IgM anti-HBc and anti-HDV; HDV superinfection—IgG anti-HBc and anti-HDV
HEV	32–34 nm	Nonenveloped icosahedral	7.6-kb RNA, linear, ss, +	Alphavirus-like	HEV antigen	anti-HEV	Agent of enterically transmitted hepatitis; rare in USA; occurs in Asia, Mediterranean countries, Central America Diagnosis: IgM/IgG anti-HEV (assays being developed); virus in stool, bile, hepatocyte cytoplasm

[a] ss, single-stranded; ss/ds, partially single-stranded, partially double-stranded; −, minus-stranded; +, plus-stranded.

Serologic and virologic markers After infection with HBV, the first virologic marker detectable in serum is HBsAg (Fig. 295-4). Circulating HBsAg precedes elevations of serum aminotransferase activity and clinical symptoms and remains detectable during the entire icteric or symptomatic phase of acute hepatitis B and beyond. In typical cases, HBsAg becomes undetectable 1 to 2 months after the onset of jaundice and rarely persists beyond 6 months. After HBsAg disappears, antibody to HBsAg (anti-HBs) becomes detectable in serum and remains detectable indefinitely thereafter. Because HBcAg is sequestered within an HBsAg coat, HBcAg is not detectable routinely in the serum of patients with HBV infection. By contrast, anti-HBc is readily demonstrable in serum, beginning within the first 1 to 2 weeks after the appearance of HBsAg and preceding detectable levels of anti-HBs by weeks to months. Because variability exists in the time of appearance of anti-HBs after HBV infection, occasionally a gap of several weeks or longer may separate the disappearance of HBsAg and the appearance of anti-HBs. During this "gap" or "window" period, anti-HBc may represent serologic evidence of current or recent HBV infection, and blood containing anti-HBc in the absence of HBsAg and anti-HBs has been implicated in the development of transfusion-associated hepatitis B. In part because the sensitivity of immunoassays for HBsAg and anti-HBs has increased, however, this window period is rarely encountered. In some persons, years after HBV infection, anti-HBc may persist in the circulation longer than anti-HBs. Therefore, isolated anti-HBc does not necessarily indicate active virus replication; most instances of isolated anti-HBc represent hepatitis B infection in the remote past. Rarely, however, isolated anti-HBc represents low-level hepatitis B viremia, with HBsAg below the detection threshold; occasionally, isolated anti-HBc represents a cross-reacting or false-positive immunologic specificity. Recent and remote HBV infections can be distinguished by determination of the immunoglobulin class of anti-HBc. Anti-HBc of the IgM class (IgM anti-HBc) predominates

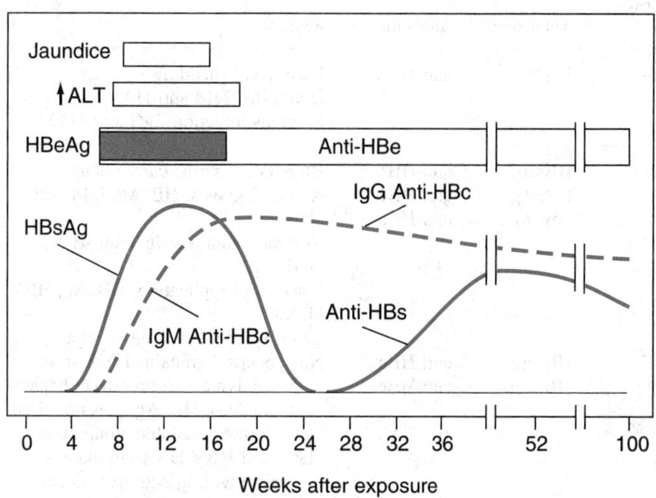

FIGURE 295-4 Scheme of typical clinical and laboratory features of acute viral hepatitis B.

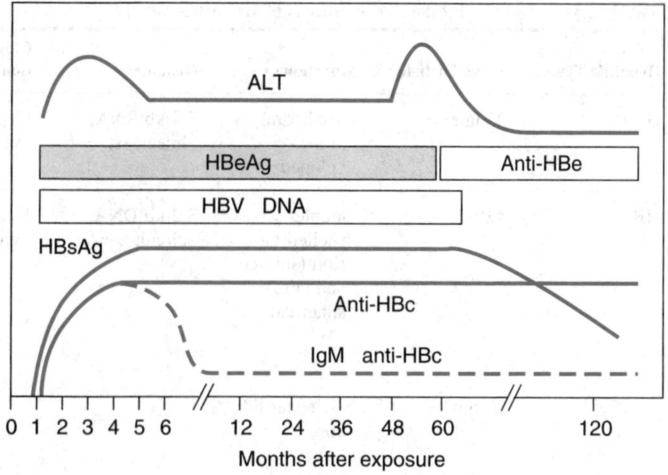

FIGURE 295-5 Scheme of typical laboratory features of chronic viral hepatitis B. HBeAg and HBV DNA can be detected in serum during the *replicative phase* of chronic infection, which is associated with infectivity and liver injury. Seroconversion from the replicative phase to the *nonreplicative phase* occurs at a rate of approximately 10 to 15% per year and is heralded by an acute hepatitis–like elevation of ALT activity; during the nonreplicative phase, infectivity and liver injury are limited.

during the first 6 months after acute infection, whereas IgG anti-HBc is the predominant class of anti-HBc beyond 6 months. Therefore, patients with current or recent acute hepatitis B, including those in the anti-HBc window, have IgM anti-HBc in their serum. In patients who have recovered from hepatitis B in the remote past as well as those with chronic HBV infection, anti-HBc is predominantly of the IgG class. Infrequently, in no more than 1 to 5% of patients with acute HBV infection, levels of HBsAg are too low to be detected; in such cases, the presence of IgM anti-HBc establishes the diagnosis of acute hepatitis B. When isolated anti-HBc occurs in the rare patient with chronic hepatitis B whose HBsAg level is below the sensitivity threshold of contemporary immunoassays (a low-level carrier), the anti-HBc is of the IgG class. Generally, in persons who have recovered from hepatitis B, anti-HBs and anti-HBc persist indefinitely.

The temporal association between the appearance of anti-HBs and resolution of HBV infection as well as the observation that persons with anti-HBs in serum are protected against reinfection with HBV suggest that *anti-HBs is the protective antibody*. Therefore, strategies for prevention of HBV infection are based on providing susceptible persons with circulating anti-HBs (see below). Occasionally, in 10 to 20% of patients with chronic hepatitis B, low-level, low-affinity anti-HBs can be detected. This antibody is directed against a subtype determinant different from that represented by the patient's HBsAg; its presence is thought to reflect the stimulation of a related clone of antibody-forming cells, but it has no clinical relevance and does not signal imminent clearance of hepatitis B.

The other readily detectable serologic marker of HBV infection, HBeAg, appears concurrently with or shortly after HBsAg. Its appearance coincides temporally with high levels of virus replication and reflects the presence of circulating intact virions and detectable HBV DNA. Pre-S1 and pre-S2 proteins are also expressed during periods of peak replication, but assays for these gene products are not routinely available. In self-limited HBV infections, HBeAg becomes undetectable shortly after peak elevations in aminotransferase activity, before the disappearance of HBsAg, and anti-HBe then becomes detectable, coinciding with a period of relatively lower infectivity (Fig. 295-4). Because markers of HBV replication appear transiently during acute infection, testing for such markers is of little clinical utility in typical cases of acute HBV infection. In contrast, markers of HBV replication provide valuable information in patients with protracted infections.

Departing from the pattern typical of acute HBV infections, in chronic HBV infection, HBsAg remains detectable beyond 6 months, anti-HBc is primarily of the IgG class, and anti-HBs is either undetectable or detectable at low levels (see "Laboratory Features," below) (Fig. 295-5). During early chronic HBV infection, HBV DNA can be detected both in serum and in hepatocyte nuclei, where it is present in free or episomal form. This *replicative stage* of HBV infection is the time of maximal infectivity and liver injury; HBeAg is a qualitative marker and HBV DNA a quantitative marker of this replicative phase, during which all three forms of HBV circulate, including intact virions. Over time, the replicative phase of chronic HBV infection gives way to a relatively *nonreplicative phase*. This occurs at a rate of approximately 10% per year and is accompanied by seroconversion from HBeAg-positive to anti-HBe-positive. In most cases, this seroconversion coincides with a transient, acute hepatitis-like elevation in aminotransferase activity, believed to reflect cell-mediated clearance of virus-infected hepatocytes. In the nonreplicative phase of chronic infection, when HBV DNA is demonstrable in hepatocyte nuclei, it tends to be integrated into the host genome. In this phase, only spherical and tubular forms of HBV, *not intact virions*, circulate, and liver injury tends to subside. Most such patients would be characterized as asymptomatic HBV *carriers*. In reality, the designations *replicative* and *nonreplicative* are only relative; even in the so-called nonreplicative phase, HBV replication can be detected with highly sensitive amplification probes such as the polymerase chain reaction. Still, the distinctions are pathophysiologically and clinically meaningful. Occasionally, nonreplicative HBV infection converts back to replicative infection. Such spontaneous reactivations are accompanied by reexpression of HBeAg and HBV DNA, and sometimes of IgM anti-HBc, as well as by exacerbations of liver injury.

Molecular variants Variation occurs throughout the HBV genome, and clinical isolates of HBV that do not express typical viral proteins have been attributed to mutations in individual or even multiple gene locations. For example, variants have been described that lack nucleocapsid proteins, envelope proteins, or both. Two categories of HBV have attracted the most attention. One of these was identified initially in Mediterranean countries among patients with an unusual serologic-clinical profile. They have severe chronic HBV infection and detectable HBV DNA but with anti-HBe instead of HBeAg. These patients were found to be infected with an HBV mutant that contained an alteration in the precore region rendering the virus incapable of encoding HBeAg. Although several potential mutation sites exist in the pre-C region, the region of the C gene necessary for the expression of HBeAg (see "Virology and Etiology," above), the most commonly encountered in such patients is a single base substitution, from G to A, which occurs in the second to last codon of the pre-C gene at nucleotide 1896. This substitution results in the replacement of the

TGG tryptophan codon by a stop codon (TAG), which prevents the translation of HBeAg. Another mutation in the core promoter region prevents transcription of the coding region for HBeAg and yields an HBeAg-negative phenotype. Patients with such precore mutants that are unable to secrete HBeAg tend to have severe liver disease that progresses rapidly to cirrhosis and that does not respond readily to antiviral therapy. Both "wild-type" HBV and precore mutant HBV can coexist in the same patient, or mutant HBV may arise during wild-type HBV infection. In addition, clusters of fulminant hepatitis B in Israel and Japan have been attributed to common-source infection with a precore mutant. Fulminant hepatitis B in North America and western Europe, however, occurs in patients infected with wild-type HBV, in the absence of precore mutants, and both precore mutants and other mutations throughout the HBV genome occur commonly even in patients with typical, self-limited, milder forms of HBV infection. In areas where chronic HBV infection is common, precore mutations are more frequent and may reflect viral evolution driven by immune selection. Additional investigation is necessary to define the effect of precore mutants on the pathogenicity and natural history of HBV infection.

The second important category of HBV mutants consists of *escape mutants*, in which a single amino acid substitution, from glycine to arginine, occurs at position 145 of the immunodominant *a* determinant common to all subtypes of HBsAg. This change in HBsAg leads to a critical conformational change that results in a loss of neutralizing activity by anti-HBs. This specific HBV/*a* mutant has been observed in two situations, active and passive immunization, in which humoral immunologic pressure may favor evolutionary change ("escape") in the virus—in a small number of hepatitis B vaccine recipients who acquired HBV infection despite the prior appearance of neutralizing anti-HBs and in liver transplant recipients who underwent the procedure for hepatitis B and who were treated with a high-potency human monoclonal anti-HBs preparation. Although such mutants have not been recognized frequently, their existence raises a concern that may complicate vaccination strategies and serologic diagnosis.

Extrahepatic sites Hepatitis B antigens and HBV DNA have been identified in extrahepatic sites, including lymph nodes, bone marrow, circulating lymphocytes, spleen, and pancreas. Although the virus does not appear to be associated with tissue injury in any of these extrahepatic sites, its presence in these "remote" reservoirs has been invoked to explain the recurrence of HBV infection after orthotopic liver transplantation. A more complete understanding of the clinical relevance of extrahepatic HBV remains to be defined.

Hepatitis D The delta hepatitis agent, or HDV, is a defective RNA virus that coinfects with and requires the helper function of HBV (or other hepadnaviruses) for its replication and expression. Slightly smaller than HBV, delta is a formalin-sensitive, 35- to 37-nm virus with a hybrid structure. Its nucleocapsid expresses delta antigen, which bears no antigenic homology with any of the HBV antigens, and contains the virus genome. The delta core is "encapsidated" by an outer envelope of HBsAg, indistinguishable from that of HBV except in its relative compositions of major, middle, and large HBsAg component proteins. The genome is a small, 1700-nucleotide, circular, single-stranded RNA (minus strand) that is nonhomologous with HBV DNA (except for a small area of the polymerase gene) but that has features and the rolling circle model of replication common to genomes of plant satellite viruses or viroids. HDV RNA contains many areas of internal complementarity; therefore, it can fold on itself by internal base pairing to form an unusual, very stable, rodlike structure. HDV RNA replicates via RNA-directed RNA synthesis by transcription of genomic RNA to a complementary antigenomic (plus strand) RNA; the antigenomic RNA, in turn, serves as a template for subsequent genomic RNA synthesis. Between the genomic and antigenomic RNAs of HDV, there are coding regions for nine proteins. Delta antigen, which is a product of the antigenomic strand, exists in two forms, a small, 195-amino-acid species, which plays a role in facilitating HDV RNA replication, and a large, 214-amino-acid species, which appears to suppress replication but is required for assembly of the antigen into virions.

Although complete hepatitis D virions and liver injury require the cooperative helper function of HBV, intracellular replication of HDV RNA can occur without HBV. Genomic heterogeneity among HDV isolates has been described; however, pathophysiologic and clinical consequences of this genetic diversity have not been recognized.

HDV can either infect a person simultaneously with HBV (*coinfection*) or superinfect a person already infected with HBV (*superinfection*); when HDV infection is transmitted from a donor with one HBsAg subtype to an HBsAg-positive recipient with a different subtype, the HDV agent assumes the HBsAg subtype of the recipient, rather than the donor. Because HDV relies absolutely on HBV, the duration of HDV infection is determined by the duration of (and cannot outlast) HBV infection. HDV antigen is expressed primarily in hepatocyte nuclei and is occasionally detectable in serum. During acute HDV infection, anti-HDV of the IgM class predominates, and 30 to 40 days may elapse after symptoms appear before anti-HDV can be detected. In self-limited infection, anti-HDV is low titer and transient, rarely remaining detectable beyond the clearance of HBsAg and HDV antigen. In chronic HDV infection, anti-HDV circulates in high titer, and both IgM and IgG anti-HDV can be detected. HDV antigen in the liver and HDV RNA in serum and liver can be detected during HDV replication.

Hepatitis C Hepatitis C virus, which, before its identification was labeled "non-A, non-B hepatitis," is a linear, single-stranded, positive-sense, 9400-nucleotide RNA virus, the genome of which is similar in organization to that of flaviviruses and pestiviruses; HCV constitutes its own genus in the family Flaviviridae. The HCV genome contains a single large open reading frame (gene) that codes for a virus polyprotein of approximately 3000 amino acids. The 5′ end of the genome consists of an untranslated region adjacent to the genes for structural proteins, the nucleocapsid core protein and two envelope glycoproteins, E1 and E2/NS1. The 5′ untranslated region and core gene are highly conserved among genotypes, but the envelope proteins are coded for by the hypervariable region, which varies from isolate to isolate and may allow the virus to evade host immunologic containment directed at accessible virus-envelope proteins. The 3′ end of the genome contains the genes for nonstructural (NS) proteins. The first reported HCV clone, 5-1-1, and the nucleotide sequence coding for C100-3, the recombinant virus protein used in the first immunoassay for antibodies to HCV, reside within the NS4 gene, and the RNA-dependent RNA polymerase, through which HCV replicates, is encoded by the NS5 region (Fig. 295-6). Because HCV does not rep-

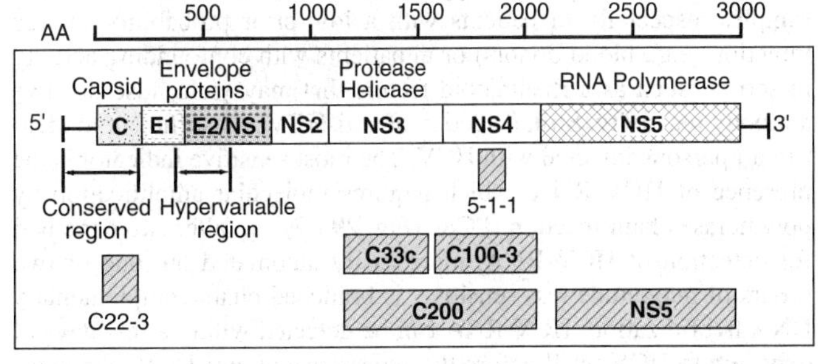

FIGURE 295-6 Organization of the hepatitis C virus genome and its associated proteins. Structural genes at the 5′ end include the nucleocapsid region, C, and the envelope regions, E1 and E2. The 5′ untranslated region and the C region are highly conserved among isolates, while the envelope domain E2/NS1 contains the hypervariable region. At the 3′ end are five nonstructural (NS) regions. Viral proteins included in the first-generation (C100-3), second-generation (C200, a fusion protein of C100-3 and C33c, and C22-3), and third-generation (C22-3, C200, or C33c and C100-3, and NS5) immunoassays and in the recombinant immunoblot assay (5-1-1, C100-3, C33c, C22-3, NS5) are presented below their corresponding genes (AA = amino acid).

licate via a DNA intermediate, it does not integrate into the host genome. Because HCV tends to circulate in very low titer, visualization of virus particles, estimated to be 40 to 60 nm in diameter, has been difficult. Although in vitro HCV replication remains difficult to accomplish convincingly, the chimpanzee has proven to be an invaluable experimental animal model.

At least six distinct genotypes, as well as subtypes within genotypes, of HCV have been identified by nucleotide sequencing. Genotypes differ one from another in sequence homology by ≥30%. Because divergence of HCV isolates within a genotype or subtype, and within the same host, may vary insufficiently to define a distinct genotype, these intragenotypic differences are referred to as *quasispecies* and differ in sequence homology by only a few percent. The genotypic and quasispecies diversity of HCV, resulting from its high mutation rate, interferes with effective humoral immunity. Neutralizing antibodies to HCV have been demonstrated, but they tend to be short-lived; and HCV infection does not induce lasting immunity against reinfection with different virus isolates or even the same virus isolate. Thus, neither *heterologous* nor *homologous* immunity appears to develop after acute HCV infection. Some HCV genotypes are distributed worldwide, while others are more geographically confined. In addition, differences in pathogenicity and responsiveness to antiviral therapy have been reported among genotypes; however, the biologic impact of genotype and quasispecies differences remains incompletely defined.

As noted above, the first assay detected antibodies to C100-3, a recombinant polypeptide derived from the NS4 region of the genome. In most patients with acute hepatitis C, antibody detected with this assay appears between 1 to 3 months after the onset of acute hepatitis but sometimes not for a year or longer. Second-generation assays incorporate recombinant proteins from the nucleocapsid core region, C22-3, and the NS3 region, C33c (expressed in combination with C100-3 as C200); these assays are more sensitive (by approximately 20%) and detect anti-HCV 30 to 90 days earlier, during the period of acute hepatitis. A third-generation immunoassay, which incorporates proteins from the NS5 region and replaces some recombinant proteins with synthetic peptides, may detect anti-HCV even earlier. Because nonspecificity has been encountered in clinical samples tested for anti-HCV, a supplementary recombinant immunoblot assay was introduced. Reactivity in an immunoassay is "confirmed" by incubation with a nitrocellulose strip that contains individual bands of recombinant or synthetic HCV proteins. This approach allows the demonstration of individual antibodies to nonstructural and structural viral proteins and identifies false-positive reactivity associated with nonviral specificities. It is useful to support the validity of anti-HCV-reactive samples, especially in patients with a low prior probability of true infection (e.g., blood donors) or in patients with confounding activity in serum (such as a rheumatoid factor) that may yield false-positive antibody reactivity. Still, detection of anti-HCV is insufficient to identify all persons infected with HCV. The most sensitive indicator is the presence of HCV RNA, which requires molecular amplification by polymerase chain reaction (PCR) (Fig. 295-7). An alternative method for detection of HCV RNA, more easily automated but one or two orders of magnitude less sensitive, is branched-chain complementary DNA hybridization. HCV RNA can be detected within a few days of exposure to HCV, well before the appearance of anti-HCV, and tends to persist for the duration of HCV infection; however, in patients with chronic HCV infection, occasionally, HCV RNA may be detectable only intermittently. Application of sensitive molecular probes for HCV RNA has revealed the presence of replicative HCV in peripheral blood lymphocytes of infected persons; however, as is the case for HBV in lymphocytes, the clinical relevance of HCV lymphocyte infection is not known.

Hepatitis E Previously labeled *epidemic* or *enterically transmitted non-A, non-B hepatitis*, HEV is an enterically transmitted virus that occurs primarily in India, Asia, Africa, and Central America. This agent, with epidemiologic features resembling those of hepatitis A, is a 32- to 34-nm, nonenveloped, HAV-like virus with a 7600-nucleotide, single-stranded, positive-sense RNA genome. HEV has three open reading frames (genes), the largest of which encodes nonstructural proteins involved in virus replication. A middle-sized gene encodes the nucleocapsid protein, and the smallest, whose function is not known, encodes protein specificities to which antibodies appear in human serum. All HEV isolates appear to belong to a single serotype, despite genomic heterogeneity of up to 25%. There is no genomic or antigenic homology, however, between HEV and HAV or other picornaviruses; and HEV, although resembling calciviruses, appears to be sufficiently distinct from any known agent to merit a new classification of its own within the alphavirus group. The virus has been detected in stool, bile, and liver and is excreted in the stool during the late incubation period; immune responses to viral antigens occur very early during the course of acute infection. Both IgM anti-HEV and IgG anti-HEV can be detected, but both fall rapidly after acute infection, reaching low levels within 9 to 12 months. Currently, serologic testing for HEV infection is not available routinely.

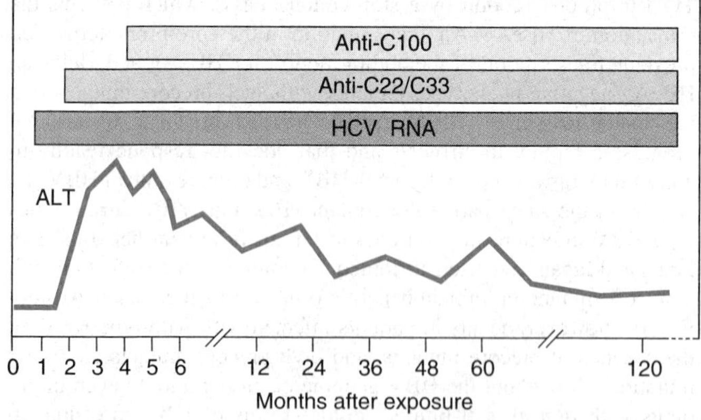

FIGURE 295-7 Scheme of typical laboratory features during acute hepatitis C progressing to chronicity. HCV RNA is the first detectable event, preceding ALT elevation and the appearance of anti-HCV. The appearance of antibody to C100, detectable with first-generation assays, is delayed from 1 to 3 months after the appearance of antibody to C22 and C33, antibodies that are included in second-generation immunoassays. Anti-HCV detectable with second-generation assays appears during acute hepatitis C.

PATHOGENESIS Under ordinary circumstances, none of the hepatitis viruses is known to be directly cytopathic to hepatocytes. Evidence suggests that the clinical manifestations and outcomes after acute liver injury associated with viral hepatitis are determined by the immunologic responses of the host.

Hepatitis B Among the viral hepatitides, the immunopathogenesis of hepatitis B has been studied most extensively. Certainly for this agent, the existence of asymptomatic hepatitis B carriers with normal liver histology and function suggests that the virus is not directly cytopathic. The fact that patients with defects in cellular immune competence are more likely to remain chronically infected rather than to clear the virus is cited to support the role of cellular immune responses in the pathogenesis of hepatitis B–related liver injury. The model that has the most experimental support involves cytolytic T cells sensitized specifically to recognize host and hepatitis B viral antigens on the liver cell surface. Recent laboratory observations suggest that nucleocapsid proteins (HBcAg and possibly HBeAg), present on the cell membrane in minute quantities, are the viral target antigens that, with host antigens, invite cytolytic T cells to destroy HBV-infected hepatocytes. Differences in the robustness of cytolytic T cell responsiveness and in the elaboration of antiviral cytokines by T cells have been invoked to explain differences in outcomes between those who recover after acute hepatitis and those who progress to chronic hepatitis or between those with mild and those with severe (fulminant) acute HBV infection.

A recent observation provides further insight into the mechanism of viral clearance in acute hepatitis B. Although a robust cytolytic T cell response occurs and eliminates virus-infected liver cells during acute hepatitis B, more than 90% of HBV DNA has been found in experimentally infected chimpanzees to disappear from the liver and blood before maximal T cell infiltration of the liver and before most of the biochemical and histologic evidence of liver injury. This observation suggests that inflammatory cytokines, independent of cytopathic antiviral mechanisms, participate in early viral clearance; this effect has been shown to represent elimination of HBV replicative intermediates from the cytoplasm and covalently closed circular viral DNA from the nucleus of infected hepatocytes.

Debate continues over the relative importance of viral and host factors in the pathogenesis of HBV-associated liver injury and its outcome. As noted above, precore genetic mutants of HBV have been associated with the more severe outcomes of HBV infection (severe chronic and fulminant hepatitis), suggesting that, under certain circumstances, relative pathogenicity is a property of the virus, not the host. The fact that concomitant HDV and HBV infections are associated with more severe liver injury than HBV infection alone and the fact that cells transfected in vitro with the gene for HDV (delta) antigen express HDV antigen and then become necrotic in the absence of any immunologic influences are also consistent with a viral effect on pathogenicity. Similarly, in patients who undergo liver transplantation for end-stage chronic hepatitis B, occasionally, rapidly progressive liver injury appears in the new liver. This clinical pattern is associated with an unusual histologic pattern in the new liver, *fibrosing cholestatic hepatitis*, which, ultrastructurally, appears to represent a choking of the cell with overwhelming quantities of HBsAg. This observation suggests that under the influence of the potent immunosuppressive agents required to prevent allograft rejection, HBV may have a direct cytopathic effect on liver cells, independent of the immune system.

Although the precise mechanism of liver injury in HBV infection remains elusive, studies of nucleocapsid proteins have shed light on the profound immunologic tolerance to HBV of babies born to mothers with highly replicative (HBeAg-positive), chronic HBV infection. In HBeAg-expressing transgenic mice, in utero exposure to HBeAg, which is sufficiently small to traverse the placenta, induces T cell tolerance to both nucleocapsid proteins. This, in turn, may explain why, when infection occurs so early in life, immunologic clearance does not occur, and protracted, lifelong infection ensues.

Hepatitis C Undoubtedly, cell-mediated immune responses and elaboration by T cells of antiviral cytokines contribute to the containment of infection and pathogenesis of liver injury associated with hepatitis C. Perhaps HCV infection of lymphoid cells plays a role in moderating immune responsiveness to the virus, as well. Intrahepatic HLA class-I-restricted cytolytic T cells directed at nucleocapsid, envelope, and NS viral protein antigens have been demonstrated in patients with chronic hepatitis C. Such virus-specific cytolytic T cell responses, however, do not correlate adequately with the degree of liver injury or with recovery. Several HLA alleles have been linked with self-limited hepatitis C, but such associations do not apply universally. Finally, cross-reactivity between viral and host autoantigens has been invoked to explain the association between hepatitis C and a subset of patients with autoimmune hepatitis and antibodies to liver kidney microsomal antigen (anti-LKM) (Chap. 297).

Extrahepatic Manifestations Immune complex–mediated tissue damage appears to play a pathogenetic role in the extrahepatic manifestations of acute hepatitis B. The occasional prodromal serum sickness–like syndrome observed in acute hepatitis B appears to be related to the deposition in tissue blood vessel walls of circulating immune complexes leading to activation of the complement system. The clinical consequences are urticarial rash, angioedema, fever, and arthritis. During the early prodrome of HBV infection in these patients, HBsAg in high titer in association with small amounts of anti-HBs leads to the formation of soluble, circulating immune complexes (in antigen excess). Complement components in the serum are depressed during the arthritic phase of the illness and are also detectable in the circulating immune complexes, which also contain HBsAg, anti-HBs, IgG, IgM, IgA, and fibrin.

In patients with chronic hepatitis B, other types of immune-complex disease may be seen. Glomerulonephritis with the nephrotic syndrome is occasionally observed; HBsAg, immunoglobulin, and C3 deposition has been found in the glomerular basement membrane. While polyarteritis nodosa develops in considerably fewer than 1% of patients with HBV infection, 20 to 30% of patients with polyarteritis nodosa have HBsAg in serum (Chap. 317). In these patients, the affected small and medium-sized arterioles have been shown to contain HBsAg, immunoglobulins, and complement components. Another extrahepatic manifestation of viral hepatitis, essential mixed cryoglobulinemia (EMC), was reported initially to be associated with hepatitis B. The disorder is characterized clinically by arthritis and cutaneous vasculitis (palpable purpura) and serologically by the presence of circulating cryoprecipitable immune complexes of more than one immunoglobulin class (Chap. 275). Many patients with this syndrome have chronic liver disease, but the association with HBV infection is limited; instead, a substantial proportion have chronic HCV infection. Their circulating immune complexes contain HCV RNA at a concentration that exceeds its serum concentration, favoring a primary role for the virus in the pathogenesis of EMC.

PATHOLOGY The typical morphologic lesions of all types of viral hepatitis are similar and consist of panlobular infiltration with mononuclear cells, hepatic cell necrosis, hyperplasia of Kupffer cells, and variable degrees of cholestasis. Hepatic cell regeneration is present, as evidenced by numerous mitotic figures, multinucleated cells, and "rosette" or "pseudoacinar" formation. The mononuclear infiltration consists primarily of small lymphocytes, although plasma cells and eosinophils occasionally are present. Liver cell damage consists of hepatic cell degeneration and necrosis, cell dropout, ballooning of cells, and acidophilic degeneration of hepatocytes (forming so-called Councilman bodies). Large hepatocytes with a ground glass appearance of the cytoplasm may be seen in chronic but not in acute HBV infection; these cells contain HBsAg and can be identified histochemically with orcein or aldehyde fuchsin. In uncomplicated viral hepatitis, the reticulin framework is preserved.

In hepatitis C, the histologic lesion is often remarkable for a relative paucity of inflammation, a marked increase in activation of sinusoidal lining cells, lymphoid aggregates, the presence of fat, and, occasionally, bile duct lesions in which biliary epithelial cells appear to be piled up without interruption of the basement membrane. Occasionally, microvesicular steatosis occurs in hepatitis D. In hepatitis E, a common histologic feature is marked cholestasis. A cholestatic variant of slowly resolving acute hepatitis A also has been described.

A more severe histologic lesion, *bridging hepatic necrosis*, also termed *subacute* or *confluent necrosis*, is occasionally observed in some patients with acute hepatitis. "Bridging" between lobules results from large areas of hepatic cell dropout, with collapse of the reticulin framework. Characteristically, the bridge consists of condensed reticulum, inflammatory debris, and degenerating liver cells that span adjacent portal areas, portal to central veins, or central vein to central vein. This lesion had been thought to have prognostic significance; in many of the originally described patients with this lesion, a subacute course terminated in death within several weeks to months, or severe chronic hepatitis and postnecrotic cirrhosis developed. More recent investigations have failed to uphold the association between bridging necrosis and such a poor prognosis in patients with acute hepatitis. Although the frequency of bridging may be higher among hospitalized patients with severe acute hepatitis, and although cirrhosis, chronic hepatitis, and even death have occurred in this group, the frequency of bridging necrosis in uncomplicated acute viral hepatitis is probably on the order of 1 to 5%. Prospective studies have failed to demonstrate a difference in prognosis between patients with acute hepatitis who have bridging necrosis and those who do not. Therefore, although demonstration of this lesion in patients with chronic hepatitis has prognostic significance (Chap. 297), its demonstration during acute hepatitis is less meaningful, and liver biopsies to identify this lesion are no longer undertaken routinely in patients with acute hepatitis. In *massive hepatic necrosis* (fulminant hepatitis, acute yellow atrophy), the striking feature at postmortem examination is the finding of a small, shrunken, soft liver. Histologic examination reveals massive necrosis and dropout of liver cells of most lobules with extensive collapse and condensation of the reticulin framework.

Immunofluorescence and immunoperoxidase antibody studies have localized HBsAg to the cytoplasm and plasma membrane of infected liver cells. In contrast, HBcAg predominates in the nucleus, but occasionally, scant amounts are also seen in the cytoplasm and on the cell membrane. Electron-microscopic studies of liver biopsy material have demonstrated the presence of HBsAg particles in the cytoplasm and HBcAg particles in the nucleus of liver cells during hepatitis B infection. These morphologic observations suggest that DNA is synthesized and packaged within core particles in the nucleus, while the envelope is assembled in the cytoplasm, resulting in the formation of intact hepatitis B virus. HDV antigen is localized to the hepatocyte nucleus, while HAV, HCV, and HEV antigens are localized to the cytoplasm.

EPIDEMIOLOGY Before the availability of serologic tests for hepatitis viruses, all viral hepatitis cases were labeled either as "infectious" or "serum" hepatitis. Modes of transmission overlap, however, and *a clear distinction among the different types of viral hepatitis cannot be made solely on the basis of clinical or epidemiologic features* (Table 295-2). The most accurate means to distinguish the various types of viral hepatitis involves specific serologic testing.

Hepatitis A *This agent is transmitted almost exclusively by the fecal-oral route.* Person-to-person spread of HAV is enhanced by poor personal hygiene and overcrowding; large outbreaks as well as sporadic cases have been traced to contaminated food, water, milk, frozen raspberries and strawberries, and shellfish. Intrafamily and intrainstitutional spread are also common. Early epidemiologic observations suggested that there is a predilection for hepatitis A to occur in late fall and early winter. In temperate zones, epidemic waves have been recorded every 5 to 20 years as new segments of nonimmune population appeared; however, in developed countries, the incidence of type A hepatitis has been declining, presumably as a function of improved sanitation, and these cyclic patterns are no longer being observed. No HAV carrier state has been identified after acute type A hepatitis; perpetuation of the virus in nature depends presumably on nonepidemic, inapparent subclinical infection.

In the general population, anti-HAV, an excellent marker for previous HAV infection, increases in prevalence as a function of increasing age and of decreasing socioeconomic status. In the 1970s, serologic evidence of prior hepatitis A infection occurred in about 40% of urban populations in the United States, most of whose members never recalled having had a symptomatic case of hepatitis. In subsequent decades, however, the prevalence of anti-HAV has been declining in the United States. In developing countries, exposure, infection, and subsequent immunity are almost universal in childhood. As the frequency of subclinical childhood infections declines in developed countries, a susceptible cohort of adults emerges. Hepatitis A tends to be more symptomatic in adults; therefore, paradoxically, as the frequency of HAV infection declines, the likelihood of clinically apparent, even severe, HAV illnesses increases in the susceptible adult population. Travel to endemic areas is a common source of infection for adults from nonendemic areas. More recently recognized epidemiologic foci of HAV infection include child-care centers, neonatal intensive care units, promiscuous homosexual men, and injection drug users. Although hepatitis A is rarely bloodborne, several outbreaks have been recognized in recipients of clotting factor concentrates.

Hepatitis B Percutaneous inoculation has long been recognized as a major route of hepatitis B transmission, but the outmoded designation "serum hepatitis" is an inaccurate label for the epidemiologic spectrum of HBV infection recognized today. As detailed below, most of the hepatitis transmitted by blood transfusion is not caused by HBV; moreover, in approximately two-thirds of patients with acute type B hepatitis, there is no history of an identifiable percutaneous exposure. We now recognize that many cases of type B hepatitis result from less obvious modes of nonpercutaneous or covert percutaneous transmis-

Table 295-2 Clinical and Epidemiologic Features of Viral Hepatitis

Feature	HAV	HBV	HCV	HDV	HEV
Incubation (days)	15–45, mean 30	30–180, mean 60–90	15–160, mean 50	30–180, mean 60–90	14–60, mean 40
Onset	Acute	Insidious or acute	Insidious	Insidious or acute	Acute
Age preference	Children, young adults	Young adults (sexual and percutaneous), babies, toddlers	Any age, but more common in adults	Any age (similar to HBV)	Young adults (20–40 years)
Transmission					
Fecal-oral	+++	–	–	–	+++
Percutaneous	Unusual	+++	+++	+++	–
Perinatal	–	+++	±[a]	+	–
Sexual	±	++	±[a]	++	–
Clinical					
Severity	Mild	Occasionally severe	Moderate	Occasionally severe	Mild
Fulminant	0.1%	0.1–1%	0.1%	5–20%[b]	1–2%[e]
Progression to chronicity	None	Occasional (1–10%) (90% of neonates)	Common (50–70% chronic hepatitis; 80–90% chronic infection)	Common[d]	None
Carrier	None	0.1–30%[c]	1.5–3.2%	Variable[f]	None
Cancer	None	+ (neonatal infection)	+	±	None
Prognosis	Excellent	Worse with age, debility	Moderate	Acute, good Chronic, poor	Good
Prophylaxis	IG Inactivated vaccine	HBIG Recombinant vaccine	None	HBV vaccine (none for HBV carriers)	Unknown
Therapy	None	Interferon Lamivudine	Interferon plus ribavirin	Interferon ±	None

[a] Primarily with HIV coinfection and high-level viremia in index case; risk approximately 5%.
[b] Up to 5% in acute HBV/HDV coinfection; up to 20% in HDV superinfection of chronic HBV infection.
[c] Varies considerably throughout the world and in subpopulations within countries; see text.
[d] In acute HBV/HDV coinfection, the frequency of chronicity is the same as that for HBV; in HDV superinfection, chronicity is invariable.
[e] 10–20% in pregnant women.
[f] Common in Mediterranean countries, rare in North America and western Europe.

sion. HBsAg has been identified in almost every body fluid from infected persons, and at least some of these body fluids—most notably semen and saliva—are infectious, albeit less so than serum, when administered percutaneously or nonpercutaneously to experimental animals. Among the nonpercutaneous modes of HBV transmission, oral ingestion has been documented as a potential but inefficient route of exposure. By contrast, the two nonpercutaneous routes considered to have the greatest impact are intimate (especially sexual) contact and perinatal transmission.

In sub-Saharan Africa, intimate contact among toddlers is considered instrumental in contributing to the maintenance of the high frequency of hepatitis B in the population. Perinatal transmission occurs primarily in infants born to HBsAg carrier mothers or mothers with acute hepatitis B during the third trimester of pregnancy or during the early postpartum period. Perinatal transmission is uncommon in North America and western Europe but occurs with great frequency and is the most important mode of HBV perpetuation in the Far East and developing countries. Although the precise mode of perinatal transmission is unknown, and although approximately 10% of infections may be acquired in utero, epidemiologic evidence suggests that most infections occur approximately at the time of delivery and are not related to breast feeding. The likelihood of perinatal transmission of HBV correlates with the presence of HBeAg; 90% of HBeAg-positive mothers but only 10 to 15% of anti-HBe-positive mothers transmit HBV infection to their offspring. In most cases, acute infection in the neonate is clinically asymptomatic, but the child is very likely to become an HBsAg carrier.

The more than 350 million HBsAg carriers in the world constitute the main reservoir of hepatitis B in human beings. Serum HBsAg is infrequent (0.1 to 0.5%) in normal populations in the United States and western Europe. However, a prevalence of up to 5 to 20% has been found in the Far East and in some tropical countries; in persons with Down's syndrome, lepromatous leprosy, leukemia, Hodgkin's disease, polyarteritis nodosa; in patients with chronic renal disease on hemodialysis; and in injection drug users.

Other groups with high rates of HBV infection include spouses of acutely infected persons, sexually promiscuous persons (especially promiscuous homosexual men), health care workers exposed to blood, persons who require repeated transfusions especially with pooled blood product concentrates (e.g., hemophiliacs), residents and staff of custodial institutions for the mentally retarded, prisoners, and, to a lesser extent, family members of chronically infected patients. In volunteer blood donors, the prevalence of anti-HBs, a reflection of previous HBV infection, ranges from 5 to 10%, but the prevalence is higher in lower socioeconomic strata, older age groups, and persons—including those mentioned above—exposed to blood products.

Prevalence of infection, modes of transmission, and human behavior conspire to mold geographically different epidemiologic patterns of HBV infection. In the Far East and Africa, hepatitis B, a disease of the newborn and young children, is perpetuated by a cycle of maternal-neonatal spread. In North America and western Europe, hepatitis B is primarily a disease of adolescence and early adulthood, the time of life when intimate sexual contact as well as recreational and occupational percutaneous exposures tend to occur.

Hepatitis D Infection with HDV has a worldwide distribution, but two epidemiologic patterns exist. In Mediterranean countries (northern Africa, southern Europe, the Middle East), HDV infection is endemic among those with hepatitis B, and the disease is transmitted predominantly by nonpercutaneous means, especially close personal contact. In nonendemic areas, such as the United States and northern Europe, HDV infection is confined to persons exposed frequently to blood and blood products, primarily injection drug users and hemophiliacs. HDV infection can be introduced into a population through drug users or by migration of persons from endemic to nonendemic areas. Thus, patterns of population migration and human behavior facilitating percutaneous contact play important roles in the introduction and amplification of HDV infection. Occasionally, the migrating epidemiology of hepatitis D is expressed in explosive outbreaks of severe hepatitis, such as those that have occurred in remote South American villages as well as in urban centers in the United States. Ultimately, such outbreaks of hepatitis D—either of coinfections with acute hepatitis B or of superinfections in those already infected with HBV—may blur the distinctions between endemic and nonendemic areas.

Hepatitis C Routine screening of blood donors for HBsAg and the elimination of commercial blood sources in the early 1970s reduced the frequency of, but did not eliminate, transfusion-associated hepatitis. During the 1970s, the likelihood of acquiring hepatitis after transfusion of voluntarily donated, HBsAg-screened blood was approximately 10% per patient (up to 0.9% per unit transfused); 90 to 95% of these cases were classified, based on serologic exclusion of hepatitis A and B, as "non-A, non-B" hepatitis. For patients requiring transfusion of pooled products, such as clotting factor concentrates, the risk was even higher, up to 20 to 30%, while for those receiving such products as albumin and immune globulin, because of prior treatment of these materials by heating to 60°C or cold ethanol fractionation, there was no risk of hepatitis.

During the 1980s, voluntary self-exclusion of blood donors with risk factors for AIDS and then the introduction of donor screening for anti-HIV reduced further the likelihood of transfusion-associated hepatitis to under 5%. During the late 1980s and early 1990s, the introduction first of "surrogate" screening tests for non-A, non-B hepatitis [alanine aminotransferase (ALT) and anti-HBc, both shown to identify blood donors with a higher likelihood of transmitting non-A, non-B hepatitis to recipients] and, subsequently, after the discovery of HCV, first-generation immunoassays for anti-HCV reduced the frequency of transfusion-associated hepatitis even further. A prospective analysis of transfusion-associated hepatitis conducted between 1986 and 1990 showed that the incidence of transfusion-associated hepatitis at one urban university hospital fell from a baseline of 3.8% per patient (0.45% per unit transfused) to 1.5% per patient (0.19% per unit) after the introduction of surrogate testing and to 0.6% per patient (0.03% per unit) after the introduction of first-generation anti-HCV assays. The introduction of second-generation anti-HCV assays has reduced the frequency of transfusion-associated hepatitis C to almost imperceptible levels, 1 in 100,000.

In addition to being transmitted by transfusion, hepatitis C can be transmitted by other percutaneous routes, such as self-injection with intravenous drugs. In addition, this virus can be transmitted by occupational exposure to blood, and the likelihood of infection is increased in hemodialysis units. Although the frequency of transfusion-associated hepatitis C fell as a result of blood donor screening, the overall frequency of hepatitis C remained the same until the early 1990s, when the overall frequency fell by 80%, in parallel with a reduction in the number of new cases in injection drug users. After the exclusion of anti-HCV-positive plasma units from the donor pool, rare, sporadic instances have occurred of hepatitis C among recipients of immune globulin preparations for intravenous (but not intramuscular) use.

Serologic evidence for HCV infection occurs in 90% of patients with a history of transfusion-associated hepatitis (almost all occurring before 1992, when second-generation HCV-screening tests were introduced), hemophiliacs and others treated with clotting factors, and injection-drug users; 60 to 70% of patients with sporadic "non-A, non-B" hepatitis who lack identifiable risk factors; 0.5% of volunteer blood donors; and 1.8% of the general population in the United States, which translates into 4 million persons. Comparable frequencies of HCV infection occur in most countries around the world, but extraordinarily high prevalences of HCV infection occur in certain countries, such as Egypt, where more than 20% of the population in some cities is infected. In the United States, African Americans and Mexican Americans have higher frequencies of HCV infection than whites, and 30- to 49-year-old adult males have the highest frequencies of infection. Chronic hepatitis C accounts for 20% of sporadic acute hepatitis and 40% of chronic liver disease, is the most frequent indication for liver transplantation, and is estimated to account for 8000 to 10,000 deaths per year in the United States.

Most asymptomatic blood donors found to have anti-HCV and approximately 40% of persons with reported cases of acute hepatitis C do not fall into a recognized risk group; however, many such blood donors do recall risk-associated behaviors when questioned carefully, and most patients with acute hepatitis C in the absence of clear-cut risk factors tend to be of lower socioeconomic backgrounds. Thorough questioning of anti-HCV-reactive blood donors has identified nasal cocaine inhalation, with shared equipment, as a potential risk factor for acquiring HCV infection.

As a bloodborne infection, HCV potentially can be transmitted sexually and perinatally; however, both of these modes of transmission are inefficient for hepatitis C. Although 10 to 15% of patients with acute hepatitis C report having potential sexual sources of infection, most studies have failed to identify sexual transmission of this agent. The chances of sexual and perinatal transmission have been estimated to be approximately 5%, well below comparable rates for HIV and HBV infections. Moreover, sexual transmission appears to be confined to such subgroups as persons with multiple sexual partners and sexually transmitted diseases; transmission of HCV infection is rare between stable, monogamous sexual partners. Breast feeding does not increase the risk of HCV infection between an infected mother and her infant. Infection of health workers is not dramatically higher than among the general population; however, health workers are more likely to acquire HCV infection through accidental needle punctures, the efficiency of which ranges between 3 and 10%. Infection of household contacts is rare as well.

Other groups with an increased frequency of HCV infection include patients who require hemodialysis and organ transplantation and those who require transfusions in the setting of cancer chemotherapy. In immunosuppressed individuals, levels of anti-HCV may be undetectable, and a diagnosis may require testing for HCV RNA. Although new acute cases of hepatitis C are rare, newly diagnosed cases are common among otherwise healthy persons who experimented briefly with injection drugs two or three decades earlier. Such instances usually remain unrecognized for years, until unearthed by laboratory screening for routine medical examinations, insurance applications, and attempted blood donation.

Hepatitis E The enteric form of non-A, non-B hepatitis identified in India, Asia, Africa, and Central America resembles hepatitis A in its primarily enteric mode of spread. The commonly recognized cases occur after contamination of water supplies such as after monsoon flooding, but sporadic, isolated cases occur. An epidemiologic feature that distinguishes HEV from other enteric agents is the rarity of secondary person-to-person spread from infected persons to their close contacts. Infections arise in populations that are immune to HAV and favor young adults. It is not known if hepatitis E occurs outside of recognized endemic areas, for example, in the United States, but preliminary studies suggest that HEV does not account for any of the sporadic "non-A, non-B" cases in nonendemic areas. Cases imported from endemic areas have been found in the United States.

CLINICAL AND LABORATORY FEATURES **Symptoms and Signs** Acute viral hepatitis occurs after an incubation period that varies according to the responsible agent. Generally, incubation periods for hepatitis A range from 15 to 45 days (mean 4 weeks), for hepatitis B and D from 30 to 180 days (mean 4 to 12 weeks), for hepatitis C from 15 to 160 days (mean 7 weeks), and for hepatitis E from 14 to 60 days (mean 5 to 6 weeks). The *prodromal symptoms* of acute viral hepatitis are systemic and quite variable. Constitutional symptoms of anorexia, nausea and vomiting, fatigue, malaise, arthralgias, myalgias, headache, photophobia, pharyngitis, cough, and coryza may precede the onset of jaundice by 1 to 2 weeks. The nausea, vomiting, and anorexia are frequently associated with alterations in olfaction and taste. A low-grade fever between 38 and 39°C (100 to 102°F) is more often present in hepatitis A and E than in hepatitis B or C, except when hepatitis B is heralded by a serum sicknesslike syndrome; rarely, a fever of 39.5 to 40°C (103 to 104°F) may accompany the constitutional symptoms. Dark urine and clay-colored stools may be noticed by the patient from 1 to 5 days before the onset of clinical jaundice.

With the onset of *clinical jaundice*, the constitutional prodromal symptoms usually diminish, but in some patients mild weight loss (2.5 to 5 kg) is common and may continue during the entire icteric phase. The liver becomes enlarged and tender and may be associated with right upper quadrant pain and discomfort. Infrequently, patients present with a cholestatic picture, suggesting extrahepatic biliary obstruction. Splenomegaly and cervical adenopathy are present in 10 to 20% of patients with acute hepatitis. Rarely, a few spider angiomas appear during the icteric phase and disappear during convalescence. During the *recovery phase*, constitutional symptoms disappear, but usually some liver enlargement and abnormalities in liver biochemical tests are still evident. The duration of the posticteric phase is variable, ranging from 2 to 12 weeks, and usually is more prolonged in acute hepatitis B and C. Complete clinical and biochemical recovery is to be expected 1 to 2 months after all cases of hepatitis A and E and 3 to 4 months after the onset of jaundice in three-quarters of uncomplicated cases of hepatitis B and C. In the remainder, biochemical recovery may be delayed. A substantial proportion of patients with viral hepatitis never become icteric.

Infection with HDV can occur in the presence of acute or chronic HBV infection; the duration of HBV infection determines the duration of HDV infection. When acute HDV and HBV infection occur simultaneously, clinical and biochemical features may be indistinguishable from those of HBV infection alone, although occasionally they are more severe. As opposed to patients with *acute* HBV infection, patients with *chronic* HBV infection can support HDV replication indefinitely. This can happen when acute HDV infection occurs in the presence of a nonresolving acute HBV infection. More commonly, acute HDV infection becomes chronic when it is superimposed on an underlying chronic HBV infection. In such cases, the HDV superinfection appears as a clinical exacerbation or an episode resembling acute viral hepatitis in someone already chronically infected with HBV. Superinfection with HDV in a patient with chronic hepatitis B often leads to clinical deterioration (see below).

In addition to superinfections with other hepatitis agents, acute hepatitis-like clinical events in persons with chronic hepatitis B may accompany spontaneous HBeAg–to–anti-HBe seroconversion or spontaneous reactivation, i.e., reversion from nonreplicative to replicative infection. Such reactivations can occur as well in therapeutically immunosuppressed patients with chronic HBV infection when cytotoxic-immunosuppressive drugs are withdrawn; in these cases, restoration of immune competence is thought to allow resumption of previously checked cell-mediated cytolysis of HBV-infected hepatocytes. Occasionally, acute clinical exacerbations of chronic hepatitis B may represent the emergence of a precore mutant (see "Virology and Etiology," above).

Laboratory Features The serum aminotransferases aspartate aminotransferase (AST) and ALT (previously designated SGOT and SGPT) show a variable increase during the prodromal phase of acute viral hepatitis and precede the rise in bilirubin level (Figs. 295-2 and 295-4). The acute level of these enzymes, however, does not correlate well with the degree of liver cell damage. Peak levels vary from 400 to 4000 IU or more; these levels are usually reached at the time the patient is clinically icteric and diminish progressively during the recovery phase of acute hepatitis. The diagnosis of anicteric hepatitis is difficult and requires a high index of suspicion; it is based on clinical features and on aminotransferase elevations, although mild increases in conjugated bilirubin also may be found.

Jaundice is usually visible in the sclera or skin when the serum bilirubin value exceeds 43 μmol/L (2.5 mg/dL). When jaundice appears, the serum bilirubin typically rises to levels ranging from 85 to 340 μmol/L (5 to 20 mg/dL). The serum bilirubin may continue to rise despite falling serum aminotransferase levels. In most instances, the total bilirubin is equally divided between the conjugated and unconjugated fractions. Bilirubin levels above 340 μmol/L (20 mg/dL) extending and persisting late into the course of viral hepatitis are more likely to be associated with severe disease. In certain patients with underlying hemolytic anemia, however, such as glucose-6-phosphate dehydrogenase deficiency and sickle cell anemia, a high serum bilirubin level is common, resulting from superimposed hemolysis. In such patients, bilirubin levels greater than 513 μmol/L (30 mg/dL) have been observed and are not necessarily associated with a poor prognosis.

Neutropenia and lymphopenia are transient and are followed by a relative lymphocytosis. Atypical lymphocytes (varying between 2 and 20%) are common during the acute phase. These atypical lymphocytes are indistinguishable from those seen in infectious mononucleosis. Measurement of the prothrombin time (PT) is important in patients with acute viral hepatitis, for a prolonged value may reflect a severe synthetic defect, signify extensive hepatocellular necrosis, and indicate a worse prognosis. Occasionally, a prolonged PT may occur with only mild increases in the serum bilirubin and aminotransferase levels. Prolonged nausea and vomiting, inadequate carbohydrate intake, and poor hepatic glycogen reserves may contribute to hypoglycemia noted occasionally in patients with severe viral hepatitis. Serum alkaline phosphatase may be normal or only mildly elevated, while a fall in serum albumin is uncommon in uncomplicated acute viral hepatitis. In some patients, mild and transient steatorrhea has been noted as well as slight microscopic hematuria and minimal proteinuria.

A diffuse but mild elevation of the gamma globulin fraction is common during acute viral hepatitis. Serum IgG and IgM levels are elevated in about one-third of patients during the acute phase of viral hepatitis, but the serum IgM level is elevated more characteristically during acute hepatitis A. During the acute phase of viral hepatitis, antibodies to smooth muscle and other cell constituents may be present, and low titers of rheumatoid factor, nuclear antibody, and heterophil antibody also can be found occasionally. In hepatitis C and D, antibodies to liver-kidney microsomes (LKM) may occur; however, the species of LKM antibodies in the two types of hepatitis are different from each other as well as from the LKM antibody species characteristic of autoimmune chronic hepatitis type 2 (Chap. 297). The autoantibodies in viral hepatitis are nonspecific and also can be associated with other viral and systemic diseases. In contrast, virus-specific antibodies, which appear during and after hepatitis virus infection, are serologic markers of diagnostic importance.

As described above, serologic tests are available with which to establish a diagnosis of hepatitis A, B, D, and C. Tests for fecal or serum HAV are not routinely available. Therefore, a diagnosis of type A hepatitis is based on detection of IgM anti-HAV during acute illness (Fig. 295-2). Rheumatoid factor can give rise to false-positive results in this test.

A diagnosis of HBV infection can usually be made by detection of HBsAg in serum. Infrequently, levels of HBsAg are too low to be detected during acute HBV infection, even with the current generation of highly sensitive immunoassays. In such cases, the diagnosis can be established by the presence of IgM anti-HBc.

The titer of HBsAg bears little relation to the severity of clinical disease. Indeed, there may be an inverse correlation between the serum concentration of HBsAg and the degree of liver cell damage. For example, titers are highest in immunosuppressed patients, lower in patients with chronic liver disease (but higher in mild chronic than in severe chronic hepatitis), and very low in patients with acute fulminant hepatitis. These observations suggest that in hepatitis B the degree of liver cell damage and the clinical course are probably related to variations in the patient's immune response to HBV rather than to the amount of circulating HBsAg. In immunocompetent persons, however, there is a correlation between markers of HBV *replication* and liver injury (see below).

Another serologic marker that may be of value in patients with hepatitis B is HBeAg. Its principal clinical usefulness is as an indicator of relative infectivity. Because HBeAg is invariably present during early acute hepatitis B, HBeAg testing is indicated primarily during follow-up of chronic infection.

In patients with hepatitis B surface antigenemia of unknown duration, e.g., blood donors found to be HBsAg-positive and referred to a physician for evaluation, testing for IgM anti-HBc may be useful to distinguish between acute or recent infection (IgM anti-HBc-positive) and chronic HBV infection (IgM anti-HBc-negative, IgG anti-HBc-positive). A false-positive test for IgM anti-HBc may be encountered in patients with high-titer rheumatoid factor.

Anti-HBs is rarely detectable in the presence of HBsAg in patients with *acute* hepatitis B, but 10 to 20% of persons with *chronic* HBV infection may harbor low-level anti-HBs. This antibody is directed not against the common group determinant, *a*, but against the heterotypic subtype determinant (e.g., HBsAg of subtype *ad* with anti-HBs of subtype *y*). In most cases, this serologic pattern cannot be attributed to infection with two different HBV subtypes, and the presence of this antibody is not a harbinger of imminent HBsAg clearance. When such antibody is detected, its presence is of no recognized clinical significance (see "Virology and Etiology," above).

After immunization with hepatitis B vaccine, which consists of HBsAg alone, anti-HBs is the only serologic marker to appear. The commonly encountered serologic patterns of hepatitis B and their interpretations are summarized in Table 295-3. Tests for the detection of HBV DNA in liver and serum are now available. Like HBeAg, serum HBV DNA is an indicator of HBV replication, but tests for HBV DNA are more sensitive and quantitative. Hybridization assays for HBV DNA have a sensitivity of approximately 10^5 to 10^6 virions/mL, a relative threshold below which infectivity and liver injury are limited and HBeAg is usually undetectable. Currently, testing for HBV DNA has shifted from insensitive hybridization assays to amplification assays, e.g., the polymerase chain reaction–based assay, which can detect as few as 100 or 1000 virions/mL. With increased sensitivity,

Table 295-3 Commonly Encountered Serologic Patterns of Hepatitis B Infection

HBsAg	Anti-HBs	Anti-HBc	HBeAg	Anti-HBe	Interpretation
+	−	IgM	+	−	Acute HBV infection, high infectivity
+	−	IgG	+	−	Chronic HBV infection, high infectivity
+	−	IgG	−	+	Late-acute or chronic HBV infection, low infectivity
+	+	+	+/−	+/−	1. HBsAg of one subtype and heterotypic anti-HBs (common) 2. Process of seroconversion from HBsAg to anti-HBs (rare)
−	−	IgM	+/−	+/−	1. Acute HBV infection 2. Anti-HBc window
−	−	IgG	−	+/−	1. Low-level HBsAg carrier 2. Remote past infection
−	+	IgG	−	+/−	Recovery from HBV infection
−	+	−	−	−	1. Immunization with HBsAg (after vaccination) 2. Remote past infection (?) 3. False-positive

amplification assays remain reactive well below the threshold for infectivity and liver injury. These markers are useful in following the course of HBV replication in patients with chronic hepatitis B receiving antiviral chemotherapy, e.g., with interferon or lamivudine (Chap. 297). In immunocompetent persons, a general correlation does appear to exist between the level of HBV replication, as reflected by the level of HBV DNA in serum, and the degree of liver injury. High serum HBV DNA levels, increased expression of viral antigens, and necroinflammatory activity in the liver go hand in hand unless immunosuppression interferes with cytolytic T cell responses to virus-infected cells; reduction of HBV replication with antiviral drugs tends to be accompanied by an improvement in liver histology.

In patients with hepatitis C, an episodic pattern of aminotransferase elevation is common. A specific serologic diagnosis of hepatitis C can be made by demonstrating the presence in serum of anti-HCV. When a second- or third-generation immunoassay (that detects antibodies to nonstructural and nucleocapsid proteins) is used, anti-HCV can be detected in acute hepatitis C during the initial phase of elevated aminotransferase activity. This antibody may never become detectable in 5 to 10% of patients with acute hepatitis C, and levels of anti-HCV may become undetectable after recovery from acute hepatitis C. In patients with chronic hepatitis C, anti-HCV is detectable in >95% of cases. Nonspecificity can confound immunoassays for anti-HCV, especially in persons with a low prior probability of infection, such as volunteer blood donors, or in persons with circulating rheumatoid factor, which can bind nonspecifically to assay reagents. A supplementary recombinant immunoblot assay (RIBA), in which serum is incubated with a nitrocellulose strip containing viral protein bands, can be used to establish the specific viral proteins to which anti-HCV is directed (see "Virology and Etiology," above). Such RIBA determinations are used routinely to confirm anti-HCV reactivity in blood donors, but determinations of HCV RNA have supplanted RIBA in many clinical settings. Assays for HCV RNA are the most sensitive tests for HCV infection and represent the "gold standard" in establishing a diagnosis of hepatitis C. HCV RNA can be detected even before acute elevation of aminotransferase activity and before the appearance of anti-HCV in patients with acute hepatitis C. In addition, HCV RNA remains detectable indefinitely, continuously in most but intermittently in some, in patients with chronic hepatitis C (even detectable in some persons with normal liver tests, i.e., asymptomatic carriers). In the small minority of patients with hepatitis C who lack anti-HCV, a diagnosis can be supported by detection of HCV RNA. If all these tests are negative and the patient has a well-characterized case of hepatitis after percutaneous exposure to blood or blood products, a diagnosis of hepatitis caused by another agent, as yet unidentified, can be entertained.

Amplification techniques are required to detect HCV RNA, and two are available. One is a branched-chain complementary DNA (bDNA) assay, in which the detection signal (a colorimetrically detectable enzyme bound to a complementary DNA probe) is amplified. The other is a PCR assay, in which the viral RNA is reverse transcribed to complementary DNA and then amplified by repeated cycles of DNA synthesis and polymerization. Both can be used as quantitative assays and a measurement of relative "viral load"; PCR, with a sensitivity of 10^2 to 10^3 virions per milliliter is more sensitive than bDNA, with a sensitivity of 2×10^5. Determination of viral load is not a reliable marker of disease severity or prognosis but is helpful in predicting relative responsiveness to antiviral therapy. The same is true for determinations of HCV genotype (Chap. 297).

A proportion of patients with hepatitis C have isolated anti-HBc in their blood, a reflection of a common risk in certain populations to multiple bloodborne hepatitis agents. The anti-HBc in such cases is almost invariably of the IgG class and usually represents HBV infection in the remote past, rarely current HBV infection with low-level virus carriage.

The presence of HDV infection can be identified by demonstrating intrahepatic HDV antigen or, more practically, an anti-HDV seroconversion (a rise in titer of anti-HDV or de novo appearance of anti-HDV). Circulating HDV antigen, also diagnostic of acute infection, is detectable only briefly, if at all. Because anti-HDV is often undetectable once HBsAg disappears, retrospective serodiagnosis of acute self-limited, simultaneous HBV and HDV infection is difficult. Early diagnosis of acute infection may be hampered by a delay of up to 30 to 40 days in the appearance of anti-HDV.

When a patient presents with acute hepatitis and has HBsAg and anti-HDV in serum, determination of the class of anti-HBc is helpful in establishing the relationship between infection with HBV and HDV. Although IgM anti-HBc does not distinguish *absolutely* between acute and chronic HBV infection, its presence is a reliable indicator of recent infection and its absence a reliable indicator of infection in the remote past. In simultaneous acute HBV and HDV infections, IgM anti-HBc will be detectable, while in acute HDV infection superimposed on chronic HBV infection, anti-HBc will be of the IgG class.

Tests for the presence of HDV RNA are useful for determining the presence of ongoing HDV replication and relative infectivity. Currently, probes for this marker are restricted to a limited number of research laboratories. Similarly, diagnostic tests for hepatitis E are confined to a small number of research laboratories.

Liver biopsy is rarely necessary or indicated in acute viral hepatitis, except when there is a question about the diagnosis or when there is clinical evidence suggesting a diagnosis of chronic hepatitis.

A diagnostic algorithm can be applied in the evaluation of cases of acute viral hepatitis. A patient with acute hepatitis should undergo four serologic tests, HBsAg, IgM anti-HAV, IgM anti-HBc, and anti-HCV (Table 295-4). The presence of HBsAg, with or without IgM anti-HBc, represents HBV infection. If IgM anti-HBc is present, the HBV infection is considered acute; if IgM anti-HBc is absent, the HBV infection is considered chronic. A diagnosis of acute hepatitis B can be made in the absence of HBsAg when IgM anti-HBc is detectable. A diagnosis of acute hepatitis A is based on the presence of IgM anti-HAV. If IgM anti-HAV coexists with HBsAg, a diagnosis of simultaneous HAV and HBV infections can be made; if IgM anti-HBc (with or without HBsAg) is detectable, the patient has simultaneous acute hepatitis A and B, and if IgM anti-HBc is undetectable, the patient has acute hepatitis A superimposed on chronic HBV infection. The presence of anti-HCV, if confirmable, supports a diagnosis of acute hepatitis C. Occasionally, testing for HCV RNA or repeat anti-HCV testing later during the illness is necessary to establish the diagnosis. Absence of all serologic markers is consistent with a diagnosis of "non-A, non-B, non-C" hepatitis, if the epidemiologic setting is appropriate.

In patients with chronic hepatitis, initial testing should consist of HBsAg and anti-HCV. Anti-HCV supports and HCV RNA testing establishes the diagnosis of chronic hepatitis C. If a serologic diagnosis

Table 295-4 Simplified Diagnostic Approach in Patients Presenting with Acute Hepatitis

Serologic Tests of Patient's Serum				
HBsAg	IgM Anti-HAV	IgM Anti-HBc	Anti-HCV	Diagnostic Interpretation
+	−	+	−	Acute hepatitis B
+	−	−	−	Chronic hepatitis B
+	+	−	−	Acute hepatitis A superimposed on chronic hepatitis B
+	+	+	−	Acute hepatitis A and B
−	+	−	−	Acute hepatitis A
−	+	+	−	Acute hepatitis A and B (HBsAg below detection threshold)
−	−	+	−	Acute hepatitis B (HBsAg below detection threshold)
−	−	−	+	Acute hepatitis C

of chronic hepatitis B is made, testing for HBeAg and anti-HBe is indicated to evaluate relative infectivity. Testing for HBV DNA in such patients provides a more quantitative and sensitive measure of the level of virus replication and, therefore, is very helpful during antiviral therapy (Chap. 297). In patients with hepatitis B, testing for anti-HDV is useful under the following circumstances: patients with severe and fulminant diseases, patients with severe chronic disease, patients with chronic hepatitis B who have acute hepatitis-like exacerbations, persons with frequent percutaneous exposures, and persons from areas where HDV infection is endemic.

PROGNOSIS Virtually all previously healthy patients with hepatitis A recover completely from their illness with no clinical sequelae. Similarly, in acute hepatitis B, 95 to 99% of previously healthy adults have a favorable course and recover completely. There are, however, certain clinical and laboratory features that suggest a more complicated and protracted course. Patients of advanced age and with serious underlying medical disorders may have a prolonged course and are more likely to experience severe hepatitis. Initial presenting features such as ascites, peripheral edema, and symptoms of hepatic encephalopathy suggest a poorer prognosis. In addition, a prolonged PT, low serum albumin level, hypoglycemia, and very high serum bilirubin values suggest severe hepatocellular disease. Patients with these clinical and laboratory features deserve prompt hospital admission. The case-fatality rate in hepatitis A and B is very low (approximately 0.1%) but is increased by advanced age and underlying debilitating disorders. Among patients ill enough to be hospitalized for acute hepatitis B, the fatality rate is 1%. Hepatitis C occurring after transfusion is less severe during the acute phase than hepatitis B and is more likely to be anicteric; fatalities are rare, but the precise case-fatality rate is not known. In outbreaks of waterborne hepatitis E in India and Asia, the case-fatality rate is 1 to 2% and up to 10 to 20% in pregnant women. Patients with simultaneous acute hepatitis B and hepatitis D do not necessarily experience a higher mortality rate than do patients with acute hepatitis B alone; however, in several recent outbreaks of acute simultaneous HBV and HDV infection among injection drug users, the case-fatality rate has been approximately 5%. In the case of HDV superinfection of a person with chronic hepatitis B, the likelihood of fulminant hepatitis and death is increased substantially. Although the case-fatality rate for hepatitis D has not been defined adequately, in outbreaks of severe HDV superinfection in isolated populations with a high hepatitis B carrier rate, the mortality rate has been recorded in excess of 20%.

COMPLICATIONS AND SEQUELAE A small proportion of patients with hepatitis A experience *relapsing hepatitis* weeks to months after apparent recovery from acute hepatitis. Relapses are characterized by recurrence of symptoms, aminotransferase elevations, occasionally jaundice, and fecal excretion of HAV. Another unusual variant of acute hepatitis A is *cholestatic hepatitis*, characterized by protracted cholestatic jaundice and pruritus. Rarely, liver test abnormalities persist for many months, even up to a year. Even when these complications occur, hepatitis A remains self-limited and does not progress to chronic liver disease. During the prodromal phase of acute hepatitis B, a serum sickness–like syndrome characterized by arthralgia or arthritis, rash, angioedema, and rarely hematuria and proteinuria may develop in 5 to 10% of patients. This syndrome occurs before the onset of clinical jaundice, and these patients are often erroneously diagnosed as having rheumatologic diseases. The diagnosis can be established by measuring serum aminotransferase levels, which are almost invariably elevated, and serum HBsAg. As noted above, EMC is an immune-complex disease that can complicate hepatitis C. Attention has been drawn as well to associations between hepatitis C and such cutaneous disorders as porphyria cutanea tarda and lichen planus. A mechanism for these associations is unknown.

The most feared complication of viral hepatitis is *fulminant hepatitis* (massive hepatic necrosis); fortunately, this is a rare event. Fulminant hepatitis is primarily seen in hepatitis B and D, as well as hepatitis E, but rare fulminant cases of hepatitis A occur primarily in older adults and in persons with underlying chronic liver disease. Hepatitis B accounts for more than 50% of fulminant hepatitis cases, a sizable proportion of which are associated with HDV infection. Participation of HDV can be documented in approximately one-third of patients with acute fulminant hepatitis B and two-thirds of patients with fulminant hepatitis superimposed on chronic hepatitis B. Fulminant hepatitis is seen rarely in hepatitis C, but hepatitis E, as noted above, can be complicated by fatal fulminant hepatitis in 1 to 2% of all cases and in up to 20% of cases occurring in pregnant women. Patients usually present with signs and symptoms of encephalopathy that may evolve to deep coma. The liver is usually small and the PT excessively prolonged. The combination of rapidly shrinking liver size, rapidly rising bilirubin level, and marked prolongation of the PT, even as aminotransferase levels fall, together with clinical signs of confusion, disorientation, somnolence, ascites, and edema, indicates that the patient has hepatic failure with encephalopathy. Cerebral edema is common; brainstem compression, gastrointestinal bleeding, sepsis, respiratory failure, cardiovascular collapse, and renal failure are terminal events. The mortality rate is exceedingly high (greater than 80% in patients with deep coma), but patients who survive may have a complete biochemical and histologic recovery. If a donor liver can be located in time, liver transplantation may be life-saving in patients with fulminant hepatitis.

It is particularly important to document the disappearance of HBsAg after apparent clinical recovery from acute hepatitis B. Before laboratory methods were available to distinguish between acute hepatitis and acute hepatitis–like exacerbations (*spontaneous reactivations*) of chronic hepatitis B, observations suggested that approximately 10% of patients remained HBsAg-positive for longer than 6 months after the onset of clinically apparent acute hepatitis B. Half these persons cleared the antigen from their circulations during the next several years, but the other 5% remained chronically HBsAg-positive. More recent observations suggest that the true rate of chronic infection after clinically apparent acute hepatitis B is as low as 1% in normal, immunocompetent, young adults. Earlier, higher estimates may have been biased by inadvertent inclusion of acute exacerbations in chronically infected patients; these patients, chronically HBsAg-positive before exacerbation, were unlikely to seroconvert to HBsAg-negative thereafter. Whether the rate of chronicity is 10 or 1%, such patients have anti-HBc in serum; anti-HBs is either undetected or detected at low titer against the opposite subtype specificity of the antigen (see "Laboratory Features," above). These patients may (1) be asymptomatic carriers, (2) have low-grade, mild chronic hepatitis, or (3) have moderate to severe chronic hepatitis with or without cirrhosis. The likelihood of becoming an HBsAg carrier after acute HBV infection is especially high among neonates, persons with Down's syndrome, chronically hemodialyzed patients, and immunosuppressed patients, including persons with HIV infection.

Chronic hepatitis is an important late complication of acute hepatitis B occurring in a small proportion of patients with acute disease but more common in those who present with chronic infection without having experienced an acute illness (Chap. 297). Certain clinical and laboratory features suggest progression of acute hepatitis to chronic hepatitis: (1) lack of complete resolution of clinical symptoms of anorexia, weight loss, and fatigue and the persistence of hepatomegaly; (2) the presence of bridging or multilobular hepatic necrosis on liver biopsy during protracted, severe acute viral hepatitis; (3) failure of the serum aminotransferase, bilirubin, and globulin levels to return to normal within 6 to 12 months after the acute illness; and (4) the persistence of HBeAg beyond 3 months or HBsAg beyond 6 months after acute hepatitis.

Although acute hepatitis D infection does not increase the likelihood of chronicity of simultaneous acute hepatitis B, hepatitis D has the potential for contributing to the severity of chronic hepatitis B. Hepatitis D superinfection can transform asymptomatic or mild chronic hepatitis B into severe, progressive chronic hepatitis and cirrhosis; it also can accelerate the course of chronic hepatitis B. Some

HDV superinfections in patients with chronic hepatitis B lead to fulminant hepatitis. Although HDV and HBV infections are associated with severe liver disease, mild hepatitis and even asymptomatic carriage have been identified in some patients, and the disease may become indolent beyond the early years of infection. After transfusion-associated acute hepatitis C, at least 50% of patients have abnormal biochemical liver tests for more than a year. In some experiences, the frequency of progression to chronicity after acute hepatitis C is as high as 70%. In most of these patients, liver histology is consistent with moderate to severe chronic hepatitis. Even among those who recover biochemically, the likelihood of retaining circulating HCV RNA is high. Thus, after acute HCV infection, the likelihood of remaining chronically *infected* approaches 85 to 90%. Although many patients with chronic hepatitis C have no symptoms, cirrhosis may develop in as many as 20% within 10 to 20 years of acute illness; in some series of cases, cirrhosis has been reported in as many as 50% of patients with chronic hepatitis C. Although chronic hepatitis C accounts for at least a quarter of cases of chronic liver disease and a quarter of patients undergoing liver transplantation for end-stage liver disease in the United States and Europe, in the majority of patients with chronic hepatitis C, morbidity and mortality are limited during the initial 20 years after the onset of infection. Progression of chronic hepatitis C may be influenced by hepatitis C genotype, age of acquisition, duration of infection, and immunosuppression, as well as by coexisting excessive alcohol use or other hepatitis virus infection. In contrast, neither HAV nor HEV causes chronic liver disease.

Rare complications of viral hepatitis include pancreatitis, myocarditis, atypical pneumonia, aplastic anemia, transverse myelitis, and peripheral neuropathy. *Carriers* of HBsAg, particularly those infected in infancy or early childhood, have an enhanced risk of hepatocellular carcinoma. The risk of hepatocellular carcinoma is increased as well in patients with chronic hepatitis C, almost exclusively in patients with cirrhosis, and almost always after at least several decades, usually after three decades of disease (see Chap. 91). In children, hepatitis B may present rarely with anicteric hepatitis, a nonpruritic papular rash of the face, buttocks, and limbs, and lymphadenopathy (papular acrodermatitis of childhood or Gianotti-Crosti syndrome).

DIFFERENTIAL DIAGNOSIS Viral diseases such as infectious mononucleosis; those due to cytomegalovirus, herpes simplex, and coxsackieviruses; and toxoplasmosis may share certain clinical features with viral hepatitis and cause elevations in serum aminotransferase and less commonly in serum bilirubin levels. Tests such as the differential heterophile and serologic tests for these agents may be helpful in the differential diagnosis if HBsAg, anti-HBc, IgM anti-HAV, and anti-HCV determinations are negative. Aminotransferase elevations can accompany almost any systemic viral infection; other rare causes of liver injury confused with viral hepatitis are infections with *Leptospira*, *Candida*, *Brucella*, *Mycobacteria*, and *Pneumocystis*. A complete drug history is particularly important, for many drugs and certain anesthetic agents can produce a picture of either acute hepatitis or cholestasis (Chap. 296). Equally important is a past history of unexplained "repeated episodes" of acute hepatitis. This history should alert the physician to the possibility that the underlying disorder is chronic hepatitis. Alcoholic hepatitis also must be considered, but usually the serum aminotransferase levels are not as markedly elevated and other stigmata of alcoholism may be present. The finding on liver biopsy of fatty infiltration, a neutrophilic inflammatory reaction, and "alcoholic hyaline" would be consistent with alcohol-induced rather than viral liver injury. Because acute hepatitis may present with right upper quadrant abdominal pain, nausea and vomiting, fever, and icterus, it is often confused with acute cholecystitis, common duct stone, or ascending cholangitis. Patients with acute viral hepatitis may tolerate surgery poorly; therefore, it is important to exclude this diagnosis, and in confusing cases, a percutaneous liver biopsy may be necessary before laparotomy. Viral hepatitis in the elderly is often misdiagnosed as obstructive jaundice resulting from a common duct stone or carcinoma of the pancreas. Because acute hepatitis in the elderly may be quite severe and the operative mortality high, a thorough evaluation including biochemical tests, radiographic studies of the biliary tree, and even liver biopsy may be necessary to exclude primary parenchymal liver disease. Another clinical constellation that may mimic acute hepatitis is right ventricular failure with passive hepatic congestion or hypoperfusion syndromes, such as those associated with shock, severe hypotension, and severe left ventricular failure. Also included in this general category is any disorder that interferes with venous return to the heart, such as right atrial myxoma, constrictive pericarditis, hepatic vein occlusion (Budd-Chiari syndrome), or venoocclusive disease. Clinical features are usually sufficient to distinguish between these vascular disorders and viral hepatitis. Acute fatty liver of pregnancy, cholestasis of pregnancy, eclampsia, and the HELLP syndrome (hemolysis, elevated liver tests, and low platelets) can be confused with viral hepatitis during pregnancy. Very rarely, malignancies metastatic to the liver can mimic acute or even fulminant viral hepatitis. Occasionally, genetic or metabolic liver disorders (e.g., Wilson's disease, α_1-antitrypsin deficiency) are confused with viral hepatitis.

℞ TREATMENT **Treatment of Acute Attack** Although therapy has been developed for chronic hepatitis B and C (Chap. 297), opportunities for treating acute hepatitis caused by HBV or HCV are limited. In hepatitis B, among previously healthy adults who present with clinically apparent acute hepatitis, recovery occurs in approximately 99%; therefore, antiviral therapy is not likely to improve the rate of recovery and is not required. In rare instances of severe acute hepatitis B, treatment with a nucleoside analogue, such as lamivudine, at the 100-mg/d oral dose used to treat chronic hepatitis B (Chap. 297), has been attempted successfully. However, clinical trials have not been done to establish the efficacy of this approach, severe acute hepatitis B is not an approved indication for therapy, and the duration of therapy has not been determined. In typical cases of acute hepatitis C, recovery is rare, progression to chronic hepatitis is the rule, occurring in 85 to 90% of patients, and meta-analyses of small clinical trials suggest that antiviral therapy with interferon alpha (3 million units subcutaneously three times a week) is beneficial, reducing the rate of chronicity considerably by inducing sustained responses in 40% of patients. The duration of therapy and whether to add the nucleoside analogue ribavirin remain to be determined, but the most reasonable approach is to follow recommendations for treatment of chronic hepatitis C (Chap 297). Because of the marked reduction over the last two decades in the frequency of acute hepatitis C, opportunities to identify and treat patients with acute hepatitis C are rare indeed. Hospital epidemiologists, however, will encounter health workers who sustain hepatitis C-contaminated needle sticks; when monitoring for ALT elevations and HCV RNA after these accidents identifies acute hepatitis C, therapy should be initiated.

Notwithstanding these specific therapeutic considerations, in most cases of typical acute viral hepatitis, specific treatment generally is not necessary. Although hospitalization may be required for clinically severe illness, most patients do not require hospital care. Forced and prolonged bed rest is not essential for full recovery, but many patients will feel better with restricted physical activity. A high-calorie diet is desirable, and because many patients may experience nausea late in the day, the major caloric intake is best tolerated in the morning. Intravenous feeding is necessary in the acute stage if the patient has persistent vomiting and cannot maintain oral intake. Drugs capable of producing adverse reactions such as cholestasis and drugs metabolized by the liver should be avoided. If severe pruritus is present, the use of the bile salt–sequestering resin cholestyramine will usually alleviate this symptom. Glucocorticoid therapy has no value in acute viral hepatitis. Even in severe cases associated with *bridging necrosis*, controlled trials have failed to demonstrate the efficacy of steroids. In fact, such therapy may be hazardous.

Physical isolation of patients with hepatitis to a single room and bathroom is rarely necessary except in the case of fecal incontinence for hepatitis A and E or uncontrolled, voluminous bleeding for hepatitis B (with or without concomitant hepatitis D) and hepatitis C. Because most patients hospitalized with hepatitis A excrete little if any HAV, the likelihood of HAV transmission from these patients during their hospitalization is low. Therefore, burdensome *enteric precautions are no longer recommended.* Although gloves should be worn when the bedpans or fecal material of patients with hepatitis A are handled, these precautions do not represent a departure from sensible procedure for all hospitalized patients. For patients with hepatitis B and hepatitis C, emphasis should be placed on blood precautions, i.e., avoiding direct, ungloved hand contact with blood and other body fluids. Enteric precautions are unnecessary. The importance of simple hygienic precautions, such as hand washing, cannot be overemphasized. Universal precautions that have been adopted for all patients apply to patients with viral hepatitis.

Hospitalized patients may be discharged when there is substantial symptomatic improvement, a significant downward trend in the serum aminotransferase and bilirubin values, and a return to normal of the PT. Mild aminotransferase elevations should not be considered contraindications to the gradual resumption of normal activity.

In *fulminant hepatitis,* the goal of therapy is to support the patient by maintenance of fluid balance, support of circulation and respiration, control of bleeding, correction of hypoglycemia, and treatment of other complications of the comatose state in anticipation of liver regeneration and repair. Protein intake should be restricted, and oral lactulose or neomycin administered. Glucocorticoid therapy has been shown in controlled trials to be ineffective. Likewise, exchange transfusion, plasmapheresis, human cross-circulation, porcine liver cross-perfusion, and hemoperfusion have not been proven to enhance survival. Meticulous intensive care is the one factor that does appear to improve survival. Orthotopic liver transplantation is resorted to with increasing frequency, with excellent results, in patients with fulminant hepatitis (Chap. 301).

PROPHYLAXIS Because application of therapy for acute viral hepatitis is limited, and because antiviral therapy for chronic viral hepatitis is effective in only a proportion of patients (Chap. 297), emphasis is placed on prevention through immunization. The prophylactic approach differs for each of the types of viral hepatitis. In the past, immunoprophylaxis relied exclusively on passive immunization with antibody-containing globulin preparations purified by cold ethanol fractionation from the plasma of hundreds of normal donors. Currently, for hepatitis A and B, active immunization with vaccines is available as well.

Hepatitis A Both passive immunization with immune globulin (IG) and active immunization with a killed vaccine are available. All preparations of IG contain anti-HAV concentrations sufficient to be protective. When administered before exposure or during the early incubation period, IG is effective in preventing clinically apparent hepatitis A. In some cases, IG does not abort infection but, by attenuating it, renders it inapparent. As a result, long-lasting "passive-active" immunity occurs; however, this is now considered to be the exception rather than the rule. For postexposure prophylaxis of intimate contacts (household, institutional) of persons with hepatitis A, the administration of 0.02 mL/kg is recommended as early after exposure as possible; it may be effective even when administered as late as 2 weeks after exposure. Prophylaxis is not necessary for casual contacts (office, factory, school, or hospital), for most elderly persons, who are very likely to be immune, or for those known to have anti-HAV in their serum. In day-care centers, recognition of hepatitis A in children or staff should provide a stimulus for immunoprophylaxis in the center and in the children's family members. By the time most common-source outbreaks of hepatitis A are recognized, it is usually too late in the incubation period for IG to be effective; however, prophylaxis may limit the frequency of secondary cases. For travelers to tropical countries, developing countries, and other areas outside standard tourist routes, IG prophylaxis had been recommended, before a vaccine became available. When such travel lasted less than 3 months, 0.02 mL/kg was given; for longer travel or residence in these areas, a dose of 0.06 mL/kg every 4 to 6 months was recommended. Administration of plasma-derived globulin is safe; it has not been associated with transmission of AIDS to recipients, and the AIDS virus (HIV) is inactivated by 25% alcohol, to which plasma is subjected during the cold ethanol fractionation process.

Formalin-inactivated vaccines made from strains of HAV attenuated in tissue culture have been shown to be safe, immunogenic, and effective in preventing hepatitis A. Hepatitis A vaccines are approved for use in persons who are at least 2 years old and appear to provide adequate protection 4 weeks after a primary inoculation. If it can be given within 4 weeks of an expected exposure, such as by travel to an endemic area, hepatitis A vaccine is the preferred approach to *preexposure* immunoprophylaxis. If travel is more imminent, IG (0.02 mL/kg) should be administered at a different injection site, along with the first dose of vaccine. Because vaccination provides long-lasting protection (protective levels of anti-HAV should last 20 years after vaccination), persons whose risk will be sustained (e.g., frequent travelers or those remaining in endemic areas for prolonged periods) should be vaccinated, and vaccine should supplant the need for repeated IG injections. Other groups who are candidates for hepatitis A vaccination include military personnel, populations with cyclic outbreaks of hepatitis A (e.g., Alaskan natives), employees of day-care centers, primate handlers, laboratory workers exposed to hepatitis A or fecal specimens, children in communities with a high frequency of hepatitis A, and patients with chronic liver disease. Because of an increased risk of fulminant hepatitis A—observed in some experiences but not confirmed in others—among patients with chronic hepatitis C, patients with chronic hepatitis C have been singled out as candidates for hepatitis A vaccination. Other populations whose recognized risk of hepatitis A is increased should be vaccinated, including men who have sex with men, injection drug users, and persons with clotting disorders who require frequent administration of clotting-factor concentrates. Recommendations for dose and frequency differ for the two approved vaccine preparations; all injections are intramuscular. For the hepatitis A vaccine manufactured by SmithKline Beecham (Havrix), adults (older than 18 years) should receive two 1.0-mL injections containing 1440 enzyme-linked immunoassay units (ELU) 6 to 12 months apart. Children age 2 to 18 years should receive three 0.5-mL injections containing 360 ELU at time zero, 6, and 12 months or two 0.5-mL injections containing 720 ELU 6 to 12 months apart. For the hepatitis A vaccine manufactured by Merck (Vaqta), adults (older than 17 years) should receive two 1.0-mL injections containing 50 units 6 months apart; children age 2 to 17 years should receive two 0.5-mL doses containing 25 units 6 to 18 months apart. Hepatitis A vaccine has been reported to be effective in preventing secondary household cases of acute hepatitis A, but its role in other instances of postexposure prophylaxis remains to be demonstrated.

Hepatitis B Until 1982, prevention of hepatitis B was based on *passive* immunoprophylaxis either with standard IG, containing modest levels of anti-HBs, or hepatitis B immune globulin (HBIG), containing high-titer anti-HBs. The efficacy of standard IG has never been established and remains questionable; even the efficacy of HBIG, demonstrated in several clinical trials, has been challenged, and its contribution appears to be in reducing the frequency of clinical *illness,* not in preventing *infection.* The first vaccine for *active* immunization, introduced in 1982, was prepared from purified, noninfectious 22-nm spherical forms of HBsAg derived from the plasma of healthy HBsAg carriers. In 1987, the plasma-derived vaccine was supplanted by a genetically engineered vaccine derived from recombinant yeast. The latter vaccine consists of HBsAg particles that are nonglycosylated but are otherwise indistinguishable from natural HBsAg; two recombinant vaccines are licensed for use in the United States. Current recommendations can be divided into those for preexposure and postexposure prophylaxis.

For *preexposure* prophylaxis against hepatitis B in settings of frequent exposure (health workers exposed to blood, hemodialysis patients and staff, residents and staff of custodial institutions for the developmentally handicapped, injection drug users, inmates of long-term correctional facilities, promiscuous homosexual men as well as promiscuous heterosexual individuals, persons such as hemophiliacs who require long-term, high-volume therapy with blood derivatives, household and sexual contacts of HBsAg carriers, persons living in or traveling extensively in endemic areas, unvaccinated children under the age of 18, and unvaccinated children who are Alaskan natives, Pacific Islanders, or residents in households of first-generation immigrants from endemic countries), three intramuscular (deltoid, not gluteal) injections of hepatitis B vaccine are recommended at 0, 1, and 6 months. Pregnancy is *not* a contraindication to vaccination. In areas of low HBV endemicity such as the United States, despite the availability of safe and effective hepatitis B vaccines, a strategy of vaccinating persons in high-risk groups has not been effective. The incidence of new hepatitis B cases continued to increase in the United States after introduction of vaccines; fewer than 10% of all targeted persons in high-risk groups have actually been vaccinated, and approximately 30% of persons with sporadic acute hepatitis B do not fall into any high-risk-group category. Therefore, to have an impact on the frequency of HBV infection in an area of low endemicity such as the United States, universal hepatitis B vaccination in childhood has been recommended. For unvaccinated children born after the implementation of universal infant vaccination, vaccination during early adolescence, at age 11 to 12 years, was recommended, and this recommendation has been extended to include all unvaccinated children age 0 to 18 years.

The two available recombinant hepatitis B vaccines are comparable, one containing 10 μg of HBsAg (Recombivax-HB) and the other containing 20 μg of HBsAg (Engerix-B), and recommended doses for each injection vary for the two preparations. For Recombivax-HB, 2.5 μg is recommended for children $<$11 years of age born to HBsAg-negative mothers, 5 μg for infants born to HBsAg-positive mothers (see below) and for children and adolescents 11 to 19 years of age; 10 μg for immunocompetent adults; and 40 μg for dialysis patients and other immunosuppressed persons. For Engerix-B, 10 μg is recommended for children aged 10 and under, 20 μg for immunocompetent children older than 10 years of age and adults, and 40 μg for dialysis patients and other immunocompromised persons.

For unvaccinated persons sustaining an exposure to HBV, *postexposure* prophylaxis with a combination of HBIG (for rapid achievement of high-titer circulating anti-HBs) and hepatitis B vaccine (for achievement of long-lasting immunity as well as its apparent efficacy in attenuating clinical illness after exposure) is recommended. For *perinatal* exposure of infants born to HBsAg-positive mothers, a single dose of HBIG, 0.5 mL, should be administered intramuscularly in the thigh *immediately after birth*, followed by a complete course of three injections of recombinant hepatitis B vaccine (see doses above) to be started within the first 12 h of life. For those experiencing a direct percutaneous inoculation or transmucosal exposure to HBsAg-positive blood or body fluids (e.g., accidental *needle stick*, other mucosal penetration, or ingestion), a single intramuscular dose of HBIG, 0.06 mL/kg, administered as soon after exposure as possible, is followed by a complete course of hepatitis B vaccine to begin within the first week. For those exposed by *sexual* contact to a patient with acute hepatitis B, a single intramuscular dose of HBIG, 0.06 mL/kg, should be given within 14 days of exposure, to be followed by a complete course of hepatitis B vaccine. When both HBIG and hepatitis B vaccine are recommended, they may be given at the same time but at separate sites.

The precise duration of protection afforded by hepatitis B vaccine is unknown; however, approximately 80 to 90% of immunocompetent vaccinees retain protective levels of anti-HBs for at least 5 years, and 60 to 80% for 10 years. Thereafter and even after anti-HBs becomes undetectable, protection persists against clinical hepatitis B, hepatitis B surface antigenemia, and chronic HBV infection. Currently, *booster* immunizations are not recommended routinely, except in immunosuppressed persons who have lost detectable anti-HBs or immunocompetent persons who sustain percutaneous HBsAg-positive inoculations after losing detectable antibody. Specifically, for hemodialysis patients, annual anti-HBs testing is recommended after vaccination; booster doses are recommended when anti-HBs levels fall below 10 mIU/mL.

Hepatitis D Infection with hepatitis D can be prevented by vaccinating susceptible persons with hepatitis B vaccine. No product is available for immunoprophylaxis to prevent HDV superinfection in HBsAg carriers; for them, avoidance of percutaneous exposures and limitation of intimate contact with persons who have HDV infection are recommended.

Hepatitis C IG is ineffective in preventing hepatitis C and is no longer recommended for postexposure prophylaxis in cases of perinatal, needle stick, or sexual exposure. Although a prototype vaccine that induces antibodies to HCV envelope protein has been developed, currently, hepatitis C vaccination is not feasible practically. Genotype and quasispecies viral heterogeneity, as well as rapid evasion of neutralizing antibodies by this rapidly mutating virus, conspire to render HCV a difficult target for immunoprophylaxis with a vaccine. Prevention of transfusion-associated hepatitis C has been accomplished by the following successively introduced measures: Exclusion of commercial blood donors and reliance on a volunteer blood supply; screening donor blood with surrogate markers such as ALT (no longer recommended) and anti-HBc, markers that identify segments of the blood donor population with an increased risk of bloodborne infections; exclusion of blood donors in high-risk groups for AIDS and the introduction of anti-HIV screening tests; and progressively sensitive serologic screening tests for anti-HCV. Chemical and heat treatment of blood products used for large-pool and concentrated blood derivates are being pursued.

In the absence of active or passive immunization, prevention of hepatitis C includes behavior changes and precautions to limit exposures to infected persons. Recommendations designed to identify patients with clinically inapparent hepatitis as candidates for medical management have as a secondary benefit the identification of persons whose contacts could be at risk of becoming infected. A so-called "look-back" program has been recommended to identify persons who were transfused before 1992 with blood from a donor found subsequently to have hepatitis C. In addition, anti-HCV testing is recommended for anyone who received a blood transfusion or a transplanted organ before the introduction of second-generation screening tests in 1992, people who ever used injection drugs, chronically hemodialyzed patients, persons with clotting disorders who received clotting factors made before 1987 from pooled blood products, persons with elevated aminotransferase levels, health workers exposed to HCV-positive blood or contaminated needles, and children born to HCV-positive mothers.

For stable, monogamous sexual partners, sexual transmission of hepatitis C is unlikely, and sexual barrier precautions are not recommended. For persons with multiple sexual partners or with sexually transmitted diseases, the risk of sexual transmission of hepatitis C is increased, and barrier precautions (latex condoms) are recommended. A person with hepatitis C should avoid sharing such items as razors, toothbrushes, and nail clippers with sexual partners and family members. No special precautions are recommended for babies born to mothers with hepatitis C, and breast feeding does not have to be restricted.

Hepatitis E Whether IG prevents hepatitis E remains undetermined. Development of a vaccine is in progress.

BIBLIOGRAPHY

ALTER MJ et al: The epidemiology of viral hepatitis in the United States. Gastroenterol Clin North Am 23:437, 1994

ALTER MJ et al: The prevalence of hepatitis C virus infection in the United States, 1988 through 1994. N Engl J Med 341:556, 1999

BARRERA JM et al: Persistent hepatitis C viremia after acute self-limiting posttransfusion hepatitis C. Hepatology 21:639, 1995

Carman W et al: Viral genetic variation: Hepatitis B virus as a clinical example. Lancet 341:349, 1993

Centers for Disease Control and Prevention: Hepatitis B virus: A comprehensive strategy for eliminating transmission in the United States through universal childhood vaccination: Recommendations of the Immunization Practices Advisory Committee (ACIP). MMWR 40 (No. RR-13):1, 1991

———: Update: Recommendations to prevent hepatitis B virus transmission—United States. MMWR 44:574, 1995

———: Prevention of hepatitis A through active or passive immunization: Recommendations of the Advisory Committee on Immunization Practices (ACIP). MMWR 48 (No. RR-12):1, 1999

———: Recommendations for prevention and control of hepatitis C virus (HCV) infection and HCV-related chronic disease. MMWR 47:1, 1998

Conry-Cantilena C et al: Routes of infection, viremia, and liver disease in blood donors found to have hepatitis C virus infection. N Engl J Med 334:1691, 1996

Consensus Statement: EASL international consensus conference on hepatitis C. J Hepatol 30:956, 1999

Dienstag JL: Non-A, non-B hepatitis. I. Recognition, epidemiology, and clinical features. II. Experimental transmission, putative virus agents and markers, and prevention. Gastroenterology 85:439, 743, 1983

Donahue JG et al: The declining risk of post-transfusion hepatitis C virus infection. N Engl J Med 327:369, 1992

Farci P et al: Lack of protective immunity against reinfection with hepatitis C virus. Science 258:135, 1992

Guidotti LG et al: Viral clearance without destruction of infected cells during acute HBV infection. Science 284:825, 1999

Hoofnagle JH: Type D (delta) hepatitis. JAMA 261:1321, 1989

Houghton M et al: Molecular biology of the hepatitis C viruses: Implications for diagnosis, development and control of viral disease. Hepatology 14:381, 1991

Hutin YJF et al: A multistate, foodborne outbreak of hepatitis A. N Engl J Med 340:595, 1999

Koff RS: Hepatitis A. Lancet 341:1643, 1998

Krawczynski K: Hepatitis E. Hepatology 17:932, 1993

Major ME et al: The molecular virology of hepatitis C. Hepatology 25:1527, 1997

Margolis HS et al: Prevention of hepatitis B virus transmission by immunization: An economic analysis of current recommendations. JAMA 274:1201, 1995

Marinos G et al: Hepatitis B virus variants with core gene deletions in the evolution of chronic hepatitis B infection. Gastroenterology 111:183, 1996

Martell M et al: Hepatitis C virus (HCV) circulates as a population of different but closely related genomes: Quasispecies nature of HCV genome distribution. J Virol 66:3225, 1992

National Institutes of Health Consensus Development Conference: Management of hepatitis C. Hepatology 26 (Suppl 1):1S, 1997

Okamoto H et al: Superinfection of chimpanzees carrying hepatitis C virus of genotype II/1b with that of genotype III/2a or I/1a. Hepatology 20:1131, 1994

Purcell RH: Hepatitis viruses: Changing patterns of human disease. Proc Natl Acad Sci USA 91:2401, 1994

Reherman B et al: Cytotoxic T lymphocyte responsiveness after resolution of chronic hepatitis B virus infection. J Clin Invest 67:1655, 1996

Sato S et al: Hepatitis B virus strains with mutations in the core promoter in patients with fulminant hepatitis. Ann Intern Med 122:241, 1995

Schreiber GB et al: The risk of transfusion-transmitted viral infection. N Engl J Med 334:1685, 1996

Seeff LB: Natural history of viral hepatitis, type C. Semin Gastrointest Dis 6:20, 1995

——— et al: A serologic follow-up of the 1942 epidemic of post-vaccination hepatitis in the United States Army. N Engl J Med 316:965, 1987

——— et al: Long-term mortality after transfusion-association non-A, non-B hepatitis. N Engl J Med 327:1906, 1992

Shakil AO et al: Volunteer blood donors with antibody to hepatitis C virus: Clinical, biochemical, virologic, and histologic features. Ann Intern Med 123:330, 1995

Simmonds P: Variability of hepatitis C virus. Hepatology 21:570, 1995

Takahashi M et al: Natural history of chronic hepatitis C. Am J Gastroenterol 88:240, 1993

Tong MJ et al: Clinical outcomes after transfusion-associated hepatitis C. N Engl J Med 332:1463, 1995

van der Poel CL et al: Hepatitis C virus six years on. Lancet 344:1475, 1994

Vento S et al: Fulminant hepatitis associated with hepatitis A virus superinfection in patients with chronic hepatitis C. N Engl J Med 338:286, 1998

Werzberger A et al: A controlled trial of formalin-inactivated hepatitis A vaccine in healthy children. N Engl J Med 327:453, 1992

Wilner IR et al: Serious hepatitis A: An analysis of patients hospitalized during an urban epidemic in the United States. Ann Intern Med 128:111, 1998

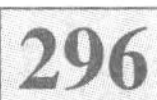

296

Jules L. Dienstag, Kurt J. Isselbacher

TOXIC AND DRUG-INDUCED HEPATITIS

Liver injury may follow the inhalation, ingestion, or parenteral administration of a number of pharmacologic and chemical agents. These include industrial toxins (e.g., carbon tetrachloride, trichloroethylene, and yellow phosphorus), the heat-stable toxic bicyclic octapeptides of certain species of *Amanita* and *Galerina* (hepatotoxic mushroom poisoning), and, more commonly, pharmacologic agents used in medical therapy. It is essential that any patient presenting with jaundice or altered biochemical liver tests be questioned carefully about exposure to chemicals used in work or at home and drugs taken by prescription or bought "over the counter." Hepatotoxic drugs can injure the hepatocyte directly, e.g., via a free-radical or metabolic intermediate that causes peroxidation of membrane lipids and that results in liver cell injury. Alternatively, the drug or its metabolite can distort cell membranes or other cellular molecules or block biochemical pathways or cellular integrity. Such injuries, in turn, may lead to necrosis of hepatocytes; injure bile ducts, producing cholestasis; or block pathways of lipid movement, inhibit protein synthesis, or impair mitochondrial oxidation of fatty acids, resulting in fat accumulation (steatosis). In general, two major types of chemical hepatotoxicity have been recognized: (1) direct toxic type and (2) idiosyncratic type.

Most drugs, which are water-insoluble, undergo a series of metabolic transformation steps, culminating in a water-soluble form appropriate for renal or biliary excretion. This process begins with oxidation or methylation initially mediated by the mixed-function oxygenases cytochrome P450 (phase I reaction), followed by glucuronidation or sulfation (phase II reaction) or inactivation by glutathione. Most drug hepatotoxicity is mediated by a phase I toxic metabolite, but glutathione depletion, precluding inactivation of harmful compounds by glutathione S-transferase, can contribute as well.

As shown in Table 296-1, direct toxic hepatitis occurs with predictable regularity in individuals exposed to the offending agent and is dose-dependent. The latent period between exposure and liver injury is usually short (often several hours), although clinical manifestations may be delayed for 24 to 48 h. Agents producing toxic hepatitis are generally systemic poisons or are converted in the liver to toxic metabolites. The direct hepatotoxins result in morphologic abnormalities that are reasonably characteristic and reproducible for each toxin. For example, carbon tetrachloride and trichloroethylene characteristically produce a centrilobular zonal necrosis, whereas yellow phosphorus poisoning typically results in periportal injury. The hepatotoxic octapeptides of *Amanita phalloides* usually produce massive hepatic necrosis. The lethal dose of the toxin is about 10 mg, the amount found in a single deathcap mushroom. Tetracycline, when administered in intravenous doses >1.5 g daily, leads to microvesicular fat deposits in the liver. Liver injury, which is often only one facet of the toxicity produced by the direct hepatotoxins, may go unrecognized until jaundice appears.

In idiosyncratic drug reactions the occurrence of hepatitis is usually infrequent and unpredictable, the response is not dose-dependent, and it may occur at any time during or shortly after exposure to the drug. Extrahepatic manifestations of hypersensitivity, such as rash, arthralgias, fever, leukocytosis, and eosinophilia, occur in about one-quarter of patients with idiosyncratic hepatotoxic drug reactions; this observation and the unpredictability of idiosyncratic drug hepatotoxicity contributed to the hypothesis that this category of drug reactions is immunologically mediated. More recent evidence, however, suggests that, in most cases, even idiosyncratic reactions represent direct hepatotoxicity but are caused by drug metabolites rather than by the intact compound. Even the prototype of idiosyncratic hepatotoxicity re-

Table 296-1 Some Features of Toxic and Drug-Induced Hepatic Injury

Features	Direct Toxic Effect[a] (Carbon Tetrachloride)	(Acetaminophen)	Idiosyncratic[a] (Halothane)	(Isoniazid)	(Chlorpromazine)	Other[a] (Oral Contraceptive Agents)
Predictable and dose-related toxicity	+	+	0	0	0	+
Latent period	Short	Short	Variable	Variable	Variable	Variable
Arthralgia, fever, rash, eosinophilia	0	0	+	0	+	0
Liver morphology	Necrosis, fatty infiltration	Centrilobular necrosis	Similar to viral hepatitis	Similar to viral hepatitis	Cholestasis *with* portal inflammation	Cholestasis *without* portal inflammation, vascular lesions

[a] The drugs listed are typical samples.

actions, halothane hepatitis, and isoniazid hepatotoxicity, associated frequently with hypersensitivity manifestations, are now recognized to be mediated by toxic metabolites that damage liver cells directly. Currently, most idiosyncratic reactions are thought to result from differences in metabolic reactivity to specific agents; host susceptibility is mediated by the kinetics of toxic metabolite generation, which differs among individuals. Occasionally, however, the clinical features of an allergic reaction (prominent tissue eosinophilia, autoantibodies, etc.) are difficult to ignore. In vitro models have been described in which lymphocyte cytotoxicity can be demonstrated against rabbit hepatocytes altered by incubation with the potential offending drug. Furthermore, several instances of drug hepatotoxicity are associated with the appearance of autoantibodies, including a class of antibodies to liver-kidney microsomes, anti-LKM2, directed against a cytochrome P450 enzyme. Similarly, in selected cases, a drug or its metabolite has been shown to bind to a host cellular component forming a hapten; the immune response to this "neoantigen" is postulated to play a role in the pathogenesis of liver injury. Therefore, some authorities subdivide idiosyncratic drug hepatotoxicity into hypersensitivity (allergic) and "metabolic" categories. Several unusual exceptions notwithstanding, true drug allergy is difficult to support in most cases of idiosyncratic drug-induced liver injury.

Idiosyncratic reactions lead to a morphologic pattern that is more variable than those produced by direct toxins; a single agent is often capable of causing a variety of lesions, although certain patterns tend to predominate. Depending on the agent involved, idiosyncratic hepatitis may result in a clinical and morphologic picture indistinguishable from that of viral hepatitis (e.g., halothane) or may simulate extrahepatic bile duct obstruction clinically with morphologic evidence of cholestasis. Drug-induced cholestasis ranges from mild to increasingly severe: (1) bland cholestasis with limited hepatocellular injury (e.g., estrogens, 17, α-substituted androgens); (2) inflammatory cholestasis (e.g., phenothiazines, amoxicillin–clavulanic acid, oxacillin, erythromcyin estolate); (3) sclerosing cholangitis (e.g., after intrahepatic infusion of the chemotherapeutic agent floxuridine for hepatic metastases from a primary colonic carcinoma); (4) disappearance of bile ducts, "ductopenic" cholestasis, similar to that observed in chronic rejection following liver transplantation (e.g., carbamazine, chlorpromazine, tricyclic antidepressant agents). Morphologic alterations may also include bridging hepatic necrosis (e.g., methyldopa), or, infrequently, hepatic granulomas (e.g., sulfonamides). Some drugs result in macrovesicular or microvesicular steatosis or steatohepatitis, which in some cases has been linked to mitochondrial dysfunciton and lipid peroxidation. Severe hepatotoxicity associated with steatohepatitis, most likely a result of mitochondrial toxicity, is being recognized with increasing frequency among patients receiving antiretroviral therapy with reverse transcriptase inhibitors (e.g., zidovudine, didanosine) or protease inhibitors (e.g., indinavir, ritonavir) for HIV infection.

Not all adverse hepatic drug reactions can be classified as either toxic or idiosyncratic in type. For example, oral contraceptives, which combine estrogenic and progestational compounds, may result in impairment of hepatic tests and occasionally in jaundice. However, they do not produce necrosis or fatty change, manifestations of hypersensitivity are generally absent, and susceptibility to the development of oral contraceptive–induced cholestasis appears to be genetically determined. Other instances of genetically determined drug hepatotoxicity have been identified. For example, approximately 10% of the population have an autosomally recessive trait associated with the absence of cytochrome P450 enzyme 2D6 and have impaired debrisoquine-4-hydroxylase enzyme activity. As a result, they cannot metabolize, and are at increased risk of hepatotoxicity resulting from, certain compounds such as desipramine, propranolol, and quinidine.

Because drug-induced hepatitis is often a presumptive diagnosis and many other disorders produce a similar clinicopathologic picture, evidence of a causal relationship between the use of a drug and subsequent liver injury may be difficult to establish. The relationship is most convincing for the direct hepatotoxins, which lead to a high frequency of hepatic impairment after a short latent period. Idiosyncratic reactions may be reproduced, in some instances, when rechallenge, after an asymptomatic period, results in a recurrence of signs, symptoms, and morphologic and biochemical abnormalities. Rechallenge, however, is often ethically unfeasible, because severe reactions may occur.

℞ **TREATMENT** Treatment of toxic and drug-induced hepatic disease is largely supportive, except in acetaminophen hepatotoxicity (see below). In patients with fulminant hepatitis resulting from drug hepatotoxicity, liver transplantation may be life-saving (Chap. 301). Withdrawal of the suspected agent is indicated at the first sign of an adverse reaction. In the case of the direct toxins, liver involvement should not divert attention from renal or other organ involvement, which may also threaten survival.

In Table 296-2, several classes of chemical agents are listed, together with examples of the pattern of liver injury produced by them. Certain drugs appear to be responsible for the development of chronic as well as acute hepatic injury. For example, oxyphenisatin, methyldopa, and isoniazid have been associated with moderate to severe chronic hepatitis, and halothane and methotrexate have been implicated in the development of cirrhosis. A syndrome resembling primary biliary cirrhosis has been described following treatment with chlorpromazine, methyl testosterone, tolbutamide, and other drugs. Portal hypertension in the absence of cirrhosis may result from alterations in hepatic architecture produced by vitamin A or arsenic intoxication, industrial exposure to vinyl chloride, or administration of thorium dioxide. The latter three agents have also been associated with angiosarcoma of the liver. Oral contraceptives have been implicated in the development of hepatic adenoma and, rarely, hepatocellular carcinoma and occlusion of the hepatic vein (Budd-Chiari syndrome). Another unusual lesion, peliosis hepatis (blood cysts of the liver), has been observed in some patients treated with anabolic steroids. The existence of these hepatic disorders expands the spectrum of liver injury induced by chemical agents and emphasizes the need for a thorough drug history in all patients with liver dysfunction.

Table 296-2 Principal Alterations of Hepatic Morphology Produced by Some Commonly Used Drugs and Chemicals[a]

Principal Morphologic Change	Class of Agent	Example
Cholestasis	Anabolic steroid	Methyl testosterone
	Anti-inflammatory	Sulindac
	Antithyroid	Methimazole
	Antibiotic	Erythromycin estolate, nitrofurantoin, rifampin, amoxicillin–clavulinic acid, oxacillin
	Oral contraceptive	Norethynodrel with mestranol
	Oral hypoglycemic	Chlorpropamide
	Tranquilizer	Chlorpromazine[b]
	Oncotherapeutic	Anabolic steroids, busulfan, tamoxifen
	Immunosuppressive	Cyclosporine
	Anticonvulsant	Carbamazine
	Calcium channel blocker	Nifedipine, verapamil
Fatty liver	Antibiotic	Tetracycline
	Anticonvulsant	Sodium valproate
	Antiarrhythmic	Amiodarone
	Antiviral	Dideoxynucleosides (e.g., zidovudine) protease inhibitors (e.g., indinavir, ritonavir)
	Oncotherapeutic	Asparaginase, methotrexate
Hepatitis	Anesthetic	Halothane[c]
	Anticonvulsant	Phenytoin, carbamazine
	Antihypertensive	Methyldopa,[c] captopril, enalapril
	Antibiotic	Isoniazid,[c] rifampin, nitrofurantoin
	Diuretic	Chlorothiazide
	Laxative	Oxyphenisatin[c]
	Antidepressant	Iproniazid, amitriptyline, imipramine
	Anti-inflammatory	Ibuprofen, indomethacin, diclofenac, sulindac
	Antifungal	Ketoconazole, fluconazole, itraconazole
	Antiviral	Zidovudine, dideoxy inosine
	Calcium channel blocker	Nifedipine, verapamil, diltiazem
	Antiandrogen	Flutamide
Mixed hepatitis/cholestatic	Immunosuppressive	Azathioprine
	Lipid-lowering	Nicotinic acid, lovastatin
Toxic (necrosis)	Hydrocarbon	Carbon tetrachloride
	Metal	Yellow phosphorus
	Mushroom	*Amanita phalloides*
	Analgesic	Acetaminophen
	Solvent	Dimethylformamide
Granulomas	Anti-inflammatory	Phenylbutazone
	Antibiotic	Sulfanomides
	Xanthine oxidase inhibitor	Allopurinol
	Antiarrhythmic	Quinidine
	Anticonvulsant	Carbamazine

[a] Several agents cause more than one type of liver lesion and appear under more than one category.
[b] Rarely associated with primary biliary cirrhosis–like lesion.
[c] Occasionally associated with chronic hepatitis or bridging hepatic necrosis or cirrhosis.

The following are the patterns of adverse hepatic reactions for some prototypic agents.

ACETAMINOPHEN HEPATOTOXICITY (DIRECT TOXIN) Acetaminophen has caused severe centrilobular hepatic necrosis when ingested in large amounts in suicide attempts or accidentally by children. A single dose of 10 to 15 g, occasionally less, may produce clinical evidence of liver injury. Fatal fulminant disease is usually (although not invariably) associated with ingestion of 25 g or more. Blood levels of acetaminophen correlate with the severity of hepatic injury (levels >300 μg/mL 4 h after ingestion are predictive of the development of severe damage; levels <150 μg/mL suggest that hepatic injury is highly unlikely). Nausea, vomiting, diarrhea, abdominal pain, and shock are early manifestations occurring 4 to 12 h after ingestion. Then 24 to 48 h later, when these features are abating, hepatic injury becomes apparent. Maximal abnormalities and hepatic failure may not be evident until 4 to 6 days after ingestion, and aminotransferase levels approaching 10,000 units are not uncommon. Renal failure and myocardial injury may be present.

Acetaminophen is metabolized predominantly by a phase II reaction to innocuous sulfate and glucuronide metabolites; however, a small proportion of acetaminophen is metabolized by a phase I reaction to a hepatotoxic metabolite formed from the parent compound by the cytochrome P450 2E1. This metabolite, *N*-acetyl-benzoquinone-imide (NAPQI), is detoxified by binding to "hepatoprotective" glutathione to become harmless, water-soluble mercapturic acid, which undergoes renal excretion. When excessive amounts of NAPQI are formed, or when glutathione levels are low, glutathione levels are depleted and overwhelmed, permitting covalent binding to nucleophilic hepatocyte macromolecules. This process is believed to lead to hepatocyte necrosis; the precise sequence and mechanism are unknown. Hepatic injury may be potentiated by prior administration of alcohol or other drugs, by conditions that stimulate the mixed-function oxidase system, or by conditions such as starvation that reduce hepatic glutathione levels. Cimetidine, which inhibits P450 enzymes, has the potential to reduce generation of the toxic metabolite. Alcohol induces cytochrome P450 2E1; consequently, increased levels of the toxic metabolite NAPQI are produced in chronic alcoholics after acetaminophen ingestion. In addition, alcohol suppresses hepatic glutathione production. Therefore, in chronic alcoholics, the toxic dose of acetaminophen may be as low as 2 g, and alcoholic patients should be warned specifically about the dangers of even standard doses of this commonly used drug. Such "therapeutic misadventures" also occur occasionally in patients with severe, febrile illnesses or pain syndromes; in such a setting, several days of anorexia and near-fasting coupled with regular administration of extra-strength acetaminophen formulations result in a combination of glutathione depletion and relatively high NAPQI levels in the absence of a history of recognized acetaminophen overdose.

℞ **TREATMENT** Treatment of acetaminophen overdosage includes gastric lavage, supportive measures, and oral administration of activated charcoal or cholestyramine to prevent absorption of residual drug. Neither of these agents appears to be effective if given more than 30 min after acetaminophen ingestion; if they are used, the stomach lavage should be done before other agents are administered orally. The chances of possible-, probable-, and high-risk hepatotoxicity can be derived from a nomogram plot (see Fig. 396-2), readily available in emergency departments, of acetaminophen plasma levels as a function of hours after ingestion. In patients with high acetaminophen blood levels (>200 μg/mL measured at 4 h or >100 μg/mL at 8 h after ingestion), the administration of sulfhydryl compounds (e.g., cysteamine, cysteine, or *N*-acetylcysteine) appears to reduce the severity of hepatic necrosis. These agents appear to act by providing a reservoir of sulfhydryl groups to bind the toxic metabolites or by stimulating synthesis and repletion of hepatic glutathione. Therapy should be begun within 8 h of ingestion but may be effective even if given as late as 24 to 36 h after overdose. Later administration of sulfhydryl compounds is of uncertain value. Routine use of *N*-acetylcysteine has reduced substantially the occurrence of fatal acetaminophen hepatotoxicity. When given orally, *N*-acetylcysteine is diluted to yield a 5% solution. A loading dose of 140 mg/kg is given, followed by 70 mg/kg every 4 h for 15 to 20 doses. Whenever a patient with potential acetaminophen hepatotoxicity is encountered, a local poison control center should be contacted. Treatment can be stopped when plasma acetominophen levels indicate that the risk of liver damage is low.

Survivors of acute acetaminophen overdose usually have no evidence of hepatic sequelae. In a few patients, prolonged or repeated administration of acetaminophen in therapeutic doses appears to have led to the development of chronic hepatitis and cirrhosis.

HALOTHANE HEPATOTOXICITY (IDIOSYNCRATIC REACTION) Administration of halothane, a nonexplosive fluorinated hydrocarbon anesthetic agent that is structurally similar to chloroform, results in severe hepatic necrosis in a small number of individuals, many of whom have previously been exposed to this agent. The failure to produce similar hepatic lesions reliably in animals, the rarity of hepatic impairment in human beings, and the delayed appearance of hepatic injury suggest that halothane is not a direct hepatotoxin but rather a sensitizing agent. However, manifestations of hypersensitivity are seen in <25% of cases. A genetic predisposition leading to an idiosyncratic metabolic reactivity has been postulated and appears to be the most likely mechanism of halothane hepatotoxicity. Adults (rather than children), obese people, and women appear to be particularly susceptible. Fever, moderate leukocytosis, and eosinophilia may occur in the first week following halothane administration. Jaundice is usually noted 7 to 10 days after exposure but may occur earlier in previously exposed patients. Nausea and vomiting may precede the onset of jaundice. Hepatomegaly is often mild, but liver tenderness is common. The serum aminotransferase levels are elevated. The pathologic changes at autopsy are indistinguishable from massive hepatic necrosis resulting from viral hepatitis. The case-fatality rate of halothane hepatitis is not known but may vary from 20 to 40% in cases with severe liver involvement. It is strongly suggested that patients in whom unexplained spiking fever, especially delayed fever, or jaundice develops after halothane anesthesia not receive this agent again. Because cross-reactions between halothane and methoxyfluorane have been reported, the latter agent should not be used after halothane reactions. Later-generation halogenated hydrocarbon anesthetics, which have supplanted halothane except in rare instances, are felt to be associated with a lower risk of hepatotoxicity.

METHYLDOPA HEPATOTOXICITY (TOXIC AND IDIOSYNCRATIC REACTION) Minor alterations in liver tests are reported in about 5% of patients treated with this antihypertensive agent. These trivial abnormalities typically resolve despite continued drug administration. In <1% of patients, acute liver injury resembling viral or chronic hepatitis or, rarely, a cholestatic reaction is seen 1 to 20 weeks after methyldopa is started. In 50% of cases the interval is <4 weeks. A prodrome of fever, anorexia, and malaise may be noted for a few days before the onset of jaundice. Rash, lymphadenopathy, arthralgia, and eosinophilia are rare. Serologic markers of autoimmunity are detected infrequently, and <5% of patients have a Coombs-positive hemolytic anemia. In about 15% of patients with methyldopa hepatotoxicity, the clinical, biochemical, and histologic features are those of moderate to severe chronic hepatitis, with or without bridging necrosis and macronodular cirrhosis. With discontinuation of the drug, the disorder usually resolves.

ISONIAZID HEPATOTOXICITY (TOXIC AND IDIOSYNCRATIC REACTION) In approximately 10% of adults treated with the antituberculosis agent isoniazid, elevated serum aminotransferase levels develop during the first few weeks of therapy; this appears to represent an adaptive response to a toxic metabolite of the drug. Whether or not isoniazid is continued, these values (usually <200 units) return to normal in a few weeks. In about 1% of treated patients, an illness develops that is indistinguishable from viral hepatitis; approximately half of these cases occur within the first 2 months of treatment, while in the remainder, clinical disease may be delayed for many months. Liver biopsy reveals morphologic changes similar to those of viral hepatitis or bridging hepatic necrosis. The disease may be severe, with a case-fatality rate of 10%. Important liver injury appears to be age-related, increasing substantially after age 35; the highest frequency is in patients over age 50, the lowest under the age of 20. Even for patients >50 years of age monitored carefully during therapy, hepatotoxicity occurs in only approximately 2%, well below the risk estimate derived from earlier experiences. Isoniazid hepatotoxicity is enhanced by alcohol and rifampicin. Fever, rash, eosinophilia, and other manifestations of drug allergy are distinctly unusual. A reactive metabolite of acetylhydrazine, a metabolite of isoniazid, may be responsible for liver injury, and patients who are rapid acetylators would be more prone to such injury. A picture resembling chronic hepatitis has been observed in a few patients.

SODIUM VALPROATE HEPATOTOXICITY (TOXIC AND IDIOSYNCRATIC REACTION) Sodium valproate, an anticonvulsant useful in the treatment of petit mal and other seizure disorders, has been associated with the development of severe hepatic toxicity and, rarely, fatalities, predominantly in children but also in adults. Asymptomatic elevations of serum aminotransferase levels have been recognized in as many as 45% of treated patients. These "adaptive" changes, however, appear to have no clinical importance, for major hepatotoxicity is not seen in the majority of patients despite continuation of drug therapy. In those rare patients in whom jaundice, encephalopathy, and evidence of hepatic failure are found, examination of liver tissue reveals microvesicular fat and bridging hepatic necrosis, predominantly in the centrilobular zone. Bile duct injury may also be apparent. It seems likely that sodium valproate is not directly hepatotoxic but that its metabolite, 4-pentenoic acid, may be responsible for hepatic injury.

PHENYTOIN HEPATOTOXICITY (IDIOSYNCRATIC REACTION) Phenytoin, formerly diphenylhydantoin, a mainstay in the treatment of seizure disorders, has been associated in rare instances with the development of severe hepatitis-like liver injury leading to fulminant hepatic failure. In many patients the hepatitis is associated with striking fever, lymphadenopathy, rash (Stevens-Johnson syndrome or exfoliative dermatitis), leukocytosis, and eosinophilia, suggesting an immunologically mediated hypersensitivity mechanism. Despite these observations, there is also evidence that metabolic idiosyncrasy may be responsible for hepatic injury. In the liver, phenytoin is converted by the cytochrome P450 system to metabolites, which include the highly reactive electrophilic arene oxides. These metabolites are normally metabolized further by epoxide hydrolases. A defect (genetic or acquired) in epoxide hydrolase activity could permit covalent binding of arene oxides to hepatic macromolecules, thereby leading to hepatic injury. Regardless of the mechanism, hepatic injury is usually manifest within the first 2 months after beginning phenytoin therapy. With the exception of an abundance of eosinophils in the liver, the clinical, biochemical, and histologic picture resembles that of viral hepatitis. In rare instances, bile duct injury may be the salient feature of phenytoin hepatotoxicity, with striking features of intrahepatic cholestasis. Asymptomatic elevations of aminotransferase and alkaline phosphatase levels have been observed in a sizable proportion of patients receiving long-term phenytoin therapy. These liver changes are believed by some authorities to represent the potent hepatic enzyme–inducing properties of phenytoin and are accompanied histologically by swelling of hepatocytes in the absence of necroinflammatory activity or evidence of chronic liver disease.

CHLORPROMAZINE HEPATOTOXICITY (CHOLESTATIC IDIOSYNCRATIC REACTION) In about 1% of patients receiving chlorpromazine, intrahepatic cholestasis with jaundice develops after 1 to 4 weeks of treatment. In rare instances, jaundice has been reported after a single exposure. Anicteric reactions are frequent. The onset may be abrupt, with fever, rash, arthralgias, lymphadenopathy, nausea, vomiting, and epigastric or right upper quadrant pain. Pruritus may precede the appearance of jaundice, dark urine, and light stools. Eosinophilia with or without mild leukocytosis may be present, and conjugated hyperbilirubinemia, moderately elevated serum alkaline phosphatase, and mildly elevated serum aminotransferase levels (100 to 200 units) are noted. Liver biopsy reveals cholestasis, bile plugs in dilated bile canaliculi, and a dense portal infiltrate of polymorphonuclear, eosinophilic, and mononuclear leukocytes. Occasionally, scattered foci of hepatic parenchymal necrosis may be evident. Jaundice and pruritus usually subside within 4 to 8 weeks following cessation of therapy, without sequelae, and fatalities are rare. Cholestyramine may be of value in relieving severe pruritus. In a small number of patients, jaundice is prolonged for several months to years; rarely, a disorder resembling but distinct from primary biliary cirrhosis may develop.

AMIODARONE HEPATOTOXICITY (TOXIC AND IDIOSYNCRATIC REACTION) Therapy with this potent antiarrhythmic drug is accompanied in 15 to 50% of patients by modest elevations of serum aminotransferase levels that may remain stable or diminish despite continuation of the drug. Such abnormalities may appear days to many months after beginning therapy. A proportion of those with elevated aminotransferase levels have detectable hepatomegaly, and clinically important liver disease develops in <5% of patients. Features that represent a direct effect of the drug on the liver and that are common to the majority of long-term recipients are ultrastructural phospholipidosis, unaccompanied by clinical liver disease, and interference with hepatic mixed-function oxidase metabolism of other drugs. The cationic amphiphilic drug and its major metabolite desethylamiodarone accumulate in hepatocyte lysosomes and mitochondria and in bile duct epithelium. The relatively common elevations in aminotransferase levels are also considered a predictable, dose-dependent, direct hepatotoxic effect. On the other hand, in the rare patient with clinically apparent, symptomatic liver disease, liver injury resembling that seen in alcoholic liver disease is observed. The so-called pseudoalcoholic liver injury can range from steatosis, to alcoholic hepatitis-like neutrophilic infiltration and Mallory's hyaline, to cirrhosis. Electron-microscopic demonstration of phospholipid-laden lysosomal lamellar bodies can help to distinguish amiodarone hepatotoxicity from typical alcoholic hepatitis. This category of liver injury appears to be a metabolic idiosyncracy that allows hepatotoxic metabolites to be generated. Rarely, an acute idiosyncratic hepatocellular injury resembling viral hepatitis or cholestatic hepatitis occurs. Hepatic granulomas have occasionally been observed. Because amiodarone has a long half-life, liver injury may persist for months after the drug is stopped.

ERYTHROMYCIN HEPATOTOXICITY (CHOLESTATIC IDIOSYNCRATIC REACTION) The most important adverse effect associated with erythromycin, more common in children than adults, is the infrequent occurrence of a cholestatic reaction. Although most of these reactions have been associated with erythromycin estolate, other erythromycins may also be responsible. The reaction usually begins during the first 2 or 3 weeks of therapy and includes nausea, vomiting, fever, right upper quadrant abdominal pain, jaundice, leukocytosis, and moderately elevated aminotransferase levels. The clinical picture can resemble acute cholecystitis or bacterial cholangitis. Liver biopsy reveals variable cholestasis; portal inflammation comprising lymphocytes, polymorphonuclear leukocytes, and eosinophils; and scattered foci of hepatocyte necrosis. Symptoms and laboratory findings usually subside within a few days of drug withdrawal, and evidence of chronic liver disease has not been found on follow-up. The precise mechanism remains ill-defined.

ORAL CONTRACEPTIVE HEPATOTOXICITY (CHOLESTATIC REACTION) The administration of oral contraceptive combinations of estrogenic and progestational steroids leads to intrahepatic cholestasis with pruritus and jaundice in a small number of patients weeks to months after taking these agents. Especially susceptible seem to be patients with recurrent idiopathic jaundice of pregnancy, severe pruritus of pregnancy, or a family history of these disorders. With the exception of liver biochemical tests, laboratory studies are normal, and extrahepatic manifestations of hypersensitivity are absent. Liver biopsy reveals cholestasis with bile plugs in dilated canaliculi and striking bilirubin staining of liver cells. In contrast to chlorpromazine-induced cholestasis, portal inflammation is absent. The lesion is reversible on withdrawal of the agent. The two steroid components appear to act synergistically on hepatic function, although the estrogen may be primarily responsible. Oral contraceptives are contraindicated in patients with a history of recurrent jaundice of pregnancy. Primarily benign, but rarely malignant, neoplasms of the liver, hepatic vein occlusion, and peripheral sinusoidal dilatation have also been associated with oral contraceptive therapy.

17,α-ALKYL-SUBSTITUTED ANABOLIC STEROIDS (CHOLESTATIC REACTION) In the majority of patients receiving these agents, used therapeutically mainly in the treatment of bone marrow failure but used surreptitiously and without medical indication by athletes to improve their performance, mild hepatic dysfunction develops. Impaired excretory function is the predominant defect, but the precise mechanism is uncertain. Jaundice, which appears to be dose-related, develops in only a minority of patients and may be the sole clinical manifestation of hepatotoxicity, although anorexia, nausea, and malaise may occur. Pruritus is not a prominent feature. Serum aminotransferase levels are usually <100 units, and serum alkaline phosphatase levels are normal, mildly elevated, or, in <5% of patients, three or more times the upper limit of normal. Examination of liver tissue reveals cholestasis without inflammation or necrosis. Hepatic sinusoidal dilatation and peliosis hepatis have been found in a few patients. The cholestatic disorder is usually reversible on cessation of treatment, although fatalities have been linked to peliosis. An association with hepatic adenoma and hepatocellular carcinoma has been reported.

TRIMETHOPRIM-SULFAMETHOXAZOLE HEPATOTOXICITY (IDIOSYNCRATIC REACTION) This antibiotic combination is used routinely for urinary tract infections in immunocompetent persons and for prophylaxis against and therapy of *Pneumocystis carinii* pneumonia in immunosuppressed persons (transplant recipients, patients with AIDS). With its increasing use, its occasional hepatotoxicity is being recognized with growing frequency. Its likelihood is unpredictable, but when it occurs, trimethoprim-sulfamethoxazole hepatotoxicity follows a relatively uniform latency period of several weeks and is often accompanied by eosinophilia, rash, and other features of a hypersensitivity reaction. Biochemically and histologically, acute hepatocellular necrosis predominates, but cholestatic features are quite frequent. Occasionally, cholestasis without necrosis occurs, and very rarely, a severe cholangiolytic pattern of liver injury is observed. In most cases, liver injury is self-limited, but rare fatalities have been recorded. The hepatotoxicity is attributable to the sulfamethoxazole component of the drug and is similar in features to that seen with other sulfonamides; tissue eosinophilia and granulomas may be seen.

HYDROXYMETHYLGLUTARYL-COENZYME (HMG-COA) REDUCTASE INHIBITORS ("STATINS") (IDIOSYNCRATIC MIXED HEPATOCELLULAR AND CHOLESTATIC REACTION) Between 1 and 2% of patients taking lovastatin, simvastatin, pravastatin, fluvastatin, or one of the newer "statin" drugs for the treatment of hypercholesterolemia experience asymptomatic, reversible elevations (> threefold) of aminotransferase activity. Acute hepatitis-like histologic changes, centrilobular necrosis, and centrilobular cholestasis have been described in several cases. In a larger proportion, minor aminotrasferase elevations appear during the first several weeks of therapy. Careful laboratory monitoring can distinguish between patients with minor, transitory changes, who may continue therapy, and those with more profound and sustained abnormalities, who should discontinue therapy.

TOTAL PARENTERAL NUTRITION (STEATOSIS, CHOLESTASIS) Total parenteral nutrition (TPN) is often complicated by cholestatic hepatitis attributable to either steatosis, cholestasis, or gallstones (or gallbladder sludge). Steatosis or steatohepatitis may result from the excess carbohydrate calories in these nutritional supplements and is the predominant form of TPN-associated liver disorder in adults. The frequency of this complication has been reduced substantially by the introduction of balanced TPN formulas that rely on lipid as an alternative caloric source. Cholestasis and cholelithiasis, caused by the absence of stimulation of bile flow and secretion resulting from the lack of oral intake, is the predominant form of TPN-associated liver disease in infants, especially in premature neonates. Often, cholestasis in such neonates is multifactorial, contributed to by other factors such as sepsis, hypoxemia, and hypotension; occasionally, TPN-induced cholestasis in neonates culminates in chronic liver disease and liver failure. When TPN-associated liver test abnormalities occur in adults, balancing the TPN formula with more lipid is the intervention of first recourse. In infants with TPN-associated cholestasis, the addition of oral feeding may ameliorate the problem. Therapeutic interventions suggested, but not yet shown to be of proven benefit, include CCK, ursodeoxycholic acid, *S*-adenosyl methionine, and taurine.

"ALTERNATIVE MEDICINES" (IDIOSYNCRATIC HEPATITIS, STEATOSIS) The misguided popularity of herbal medications that are of scientifically unproven efficacy and that lack prospective safety oversight by regulatory agencies has resulted in occasional instances of hepatotoxicity. Included among the herbal remedies associated with toxic hepatitis are jin bu huan (Chap. 11), xiao-chai-hu-tang, germander, chaparral, senna, mistletoe, skullcap, gentian, comfrey (containing pyrrolizidine alkaloids), and herbal teas. Recently well characterized are the acute hepatitis-like histologic lesions following jin bu huan use: focal hepatocellular necrosis, mixed mononuclear portal tract infiltration, coagulative necrosis, apoptotic hepatocyte degeneration, tissue eosinophilia, and microvesicular steatosis. Megadoses of vitamin A can injure the liver, as can pyrrolizidine alkaloids, which often contaminate Chinese herbal preparations and can cause a venoocclusive injury leading to sinusoidal hepatic vein obstruction. Given the widespread use of such poorly defined herbal preparations, hepatotoxicity is likely to be encountered with increasing frequency; therefore, a drug history in patients with acute and chronic liver disease should include use of "alternative medicines" and other nonprescription preparations sold in so-called health food stores.

BIBLIOGRAPHY

BLACK M et al: Isoniazid-associated hepatitis in 114 patients. Gastroenterology 69:389, 1975

——— et al: Acetaminophen hepatotoxicity. Ann Rev Med 35:577, 1984

BERSON A et al: Steatohepatitis-inducing drugs cause mitochondrial dysfunction and lipid peroxidation in rat hepatocytes. Gastroenterology 114:764, 1998

FARRELL GC: Drug-induced hepatic injury. J Gastroenterol Hepatol 12(Suppl):S242, 1997

GRIMBERT S et al: Acute hepatitis induced by HMG-CoA reductase inhibitor, lovastatin. Dig Dis Sci 39:2032, 1994

KAPLOWITZ N (ed): Recent advances in drug metabolism and hepatotoxicity. Semin Liver Dis 10:233, 1990

LEE WM: Drug-induced hepatotoxicity. N Engl J Med 333:1118, 1995

LEWIS JH et al: Amiodarone hepatotoxicity: Prevalence and clinicopathologic correlations among 104 patients. Hepatology 9:679, 1989

LUDWIG J, AXELSEN R: Drug effects on the liver: An updated tabular compilation of drugs and drug-related hepatic diseases. Dig Dis Sci 28:651, 1983

MALKIN A et al: A seven year experience of severe acetaminophen-induced hepatotoxicity (1987–1993). Gastroenterology 109:1907, 1995

MORGAN DJ, SMALLWOOD RA: Drug-induced liver disease. Curr Opinion Gastroenterol 12:246, 1996

NOLAN CM et al: Hepatotoxicity associated with isoniazid preventive therapy. JAMA 281:1014, 1999

QUIGLEY EMM et al: Hepatobiliary complications of total parenteral nutrition. Gastroenterology 104:786, 1993

RABINOVITZ M et al: Hepatotoxicity of nonsteroidal anti-inflammatory drugs. Am J Gastroenterol 87:1696, 1992

RUMACK BH et al: Acetaminophen overdose. JAMA 141:380, 1981

SALPETER SR et al: Monitored isoniazid prophylaxis for low-risk tuberculin reactors older than 35 years of age. Ann Intern Med 127:1051, 1997

SCHIODT FV et al: Acetaminophen toxicity in an urban county hospital. N Engl J Med 337:1112, 1997

SEEFF LB et al: Acetaminophen hepatotoxicity in alcoholics: A therapeutic misadventure. Ann Intern Med 104:399, 1986

SMILKSTEIN MJ et al: Efficacy of *N*-acetylcysteine in the treatment of acetaminophen overdose. N Engl J Med 319:1557, 1988

TARAZI EM et al: Sulindac-associated hepatic injury: Analysis of 91 cases reported to the Food and Drug Administration. Gastroenterology 104:569, 1993

WHITCOMB DC et al: Association of acetaminophen hepatotoxicity with fasting and ethanol use. JAMA 272:1845, 1994

WOOLF GM et al: Acute hepatitis associated with the Chinese herbal product Jin Bu Huan. Ann Intern Med 121:729, 1994

ZIMMERMAN HJ: Drug-induced liver disease, in *Schiff's Diseases of the Liver*, 8th ed. E Schiff et al (eds). Philadelphia, Lippincott-Raven, 1999, p 973

———, ISHAK KG: Valproate-induced hepatic injury: Analysis of 23 fatal cases. Hepatology 2:591, 1982

———, MADDREY WC: Acetaminophen (paracetamol) hepatotoxicity with regular intake of alcohol: Analysis of instances of therapeutic misadventure. Hepatology 22:767, 1995

297 CHRONIC HEPATITIS

Jules L. Dienstag, Kurt J. Isselbacher

ALT, or SGPT alanine aminotransferase	HBV hepatitis B virus
anti-LKM antibodies to liver-kidney microsomes	HCV hepatitis C virus
	HDV chronic hepatitis D virus
	HCC hepatocellular carcinoma
ANA antinuclear antibodies	HAI histologic activity index
AST, or SGOT aspartate aminotransferase	IFN-α interferon α
	PEG polyethylene glycol
HBcAg hepatitis B core antigen	PCR polymerase chain reaction
HBeAg hepatitis B e antigen	YMDD tyrosine-methionine-aspartate-aspartate
HBsAg hepatitis B surface antigen	

Chronic hepatitis represents a series of liver disorders of varying causes and severity in which hepatic inflammation and necrosis continue for at least 6 months. Milder forms are nonprogressive or only slowly progressive, while more severe forms may be associated with scarring and architectural reorganization, which, when advanced, lead ultimately to cirrhosis. Several categories of chronic hepatitis have been recognized. These include chronic viral hepatitis (Chap. 295), drug-induced chronic hepatitis (Chap. 296), and autoimmune chronic hepatitis. In many cases, clinical and laboratory features are insufficient to allow assignment into one of these three categories; these "idiopathic" cases are also believed to represent autoimmune chronic hepatitis. Finally, clinical and laboratory features of chronic hepatitis are observed occasionally in patients with such hereditary/metabolic disorders as Wilson's disease (copper overload) and even occasionally in patients with alcoholic liver injury (Chap. 298). Although all types of chronic hepatitis share certain clinical, laboratory, and histopathologic features, chronic viral and chronic autoimmune hepatitis are sufficiently distinct to merit separate discussions.

CLASSIFICATION OF CHRONIC HEPATITIS Common to all forms of chronic hepatitis are histopathologic distinctions based on localization and extent of liver injury. These vary from the milder forms, previously labeled chronic persistent hepatitis and chronic lobular hepatitis, to the more severe form, formerly called chronic active hepatitis. When first defined, these designations were felt to have prognostic implications, which have been challenged by more recent observations. Compared to the time more than two decades ago when the histologic designations chronic persistent, chronic lobular, and chronic active hepatitis were adopted, much more information is currently available about the causes, natural history, pathogenesis, serologic features, and therapy of chronic hepatitis. Therefore, categorization of chronic hepatitis based primarily upon histopathologic features has been replaced by a more informative classification based upon a combination of clinical, serologic, and histologic variables. Classification of chronic hepatitis is based upon (1) its *cause*, (2) its histologic activity, or *grade*, and (3) its degree of progression, or *stage*. Thus, neither clinical features alone nor histologic features—requiring liver biopsy—alone are sufficient to characterize and distinguish among the several categories of chronic hepatitis.

Classification by Cause Clinical and serologic features allow the establishment of a diagnosis of *chronic viral hepatitis*, caused by hepatitis B, hepatitis B plus D, hepatitis C, or potentially other unknown viruses; *autoimmune hepatitis*, including several subcategories, types 1, 2, and 3, based on serologic distinctions; *drug-associated chronic hepatitis*; and a category of unknown cause, or *cryptogenic* chronic hepatitis (Table 297-1). These are addressed in more detail below.

Classification by Grade Grade, a histologic assessment of necroinflammatory activity, is based upon examination of the liver biopsy. An assessment of important histologic features includes the degree of *periportal necrosis* and the disruption of the limiting plate of periportal hepatocytes by inflammatory cells (so-called *piecemeal necrosis* or *interface hepatitis*); the degree of confluent necrosis that links or forms bridges between vascular structures—between portal tract and portal tract or even more important bridges between portal tract and central vein—referred to as *bridging necrosis*; the degree of hepatocyte degeneration and focal necrosis within the lobule; and the degree of *portal inflammation*. Several scoring systems that take these histologic features into account have been devised, and the most popular is the numerical histologic activity index (HAI), based on the work of Knodell and Ishak (Table 297-2). Technically, the HAI, which is primarily a measure of *grade*, also includes an assessment of fibrosis, which is currently used to categorize *stage* of the disease, as described below. Such precise HAI scoring tends to be used more in measuring disease activity before and after therapy in clinical studies. In clinical practice, more qualitative grading suffices. Based on the presence and degree of these features of histologic activity, chronic hepatitis can be graded as mild, moderate, or severe.

Classification by Stage The stage of chronic hepatitis, which reflects the level of progression of the disease, is based on the degree of fibrosis. When fibrosis is so extensive that fibrous septa surround parenchymal nodules and alter the normal architecture of the liver lobule, the histologic lesion is defined as cirrhosis. Staging is based on the degree of fibrosis as follows:

0 = no fibrosis
1 = mild fibrosis
2 = moderate fibrosis
3 = severe fibrosis, including bridging fibrosis
4 = cirrhosis

Reconciliation between Histologic Classification and New Classification For historical purposes, and to provide the basis for navigating several decades worth of literature on chronic hepatitis, the histologic categories of chronic persistent hepatitis, chronic lobular hepatitis, and chronic active hepatitis are worth reviewing and linking with their new-classification counterparts (Table 297-3).

Table 297-1 Clinical and Laboratory Features of Chronic Hepatitis

Type of Hepatitis	Diagnostic Test(s)	Autoantibodies	Therapy
Chronic hepatitis B	HBsAg, IgG anti-HBc, HBeAg, HBV DNA	Uncommon	INF-α, lamivudine
Chronic hepatitis C	Anti-HCV (EIA and RIBA), HCV RNA	Anti-LKM1[a]	INF-α plus ribavirin
Chronic hepatitis D	Anti-HDV, HDV RNA, HBsAg, IgG anti-HBc	Anti-LKM3	INF-α (?)
Autoimmune hepatitis	ANA[b] (homogeneous), anti-LKM1(±), hyperglobulinemia	ANA, anti-LKM1, anti-SLA[c]	Prednisone, azathioprine
Drug-associated	—	Uncommon	Withdraw drug
Cryptogenic	All negative	None	Prednisone (?), azathioprine (?)

[a] Antibodies to liver-kidney microsomes type 1 (autoimmune hepatitis type II and some cases of hepatitis C).
[b] Antinuclear antibody (autoimmune hepatitis type I).
[c] Antibodies to soluble liver antigen (autoimmune hepatitis type III).
NOTE: HBsAg, hepatitis B surface antigen; EIA, enzyme immunoassay; RIBA, recombinant immunoblot assay; INF-α, interferon α.

Table 297-2 Histologic Activity Index (Knodell-Ishak Score) in Chronic Hepatitis

Histologic Feature	Severity	Score
1. Periportal necrosis, including piecemeal necrosis (PN), and/or bridging necrosis (BN)	None	0
	Mild PN	1
	Moderate PN	3
	Marked PN	4
	Moderate PN + BN	5
	Marked PN + BN	6
	Multilobular necrosis	10
2. Intralobular necrosis	None	0
	Mild	1
	Moderate	3
	Marked	4
3. Portal inflammation	None	0
	Mild	1
	Moderate	3
	Marked	4
4. Fibrosis	None	0
	Expanding portal tract	1
	Bridging fibrosis	3
	Cirrhosis	4
Maximum score		22

In *chronic persistent hepatitis*, a mononuclear inflammatory infiltrate expands, but is localized to and contained within, portal tracts. The "limiting plate" of periportal hepatocytes is intact, and there is no extension of the necroinflammatory process into the liver lobule. A "cobblestone" arrangement of liver cells, indicative of hepatic regenerative activity, is a common feature, and although minimal periportal fibrosis may be present, *cirrhosis is absent*. As a general rule, patients with chronic persistent hepatitis are asymptomatic or have relatively mild constitutional symptoms (e.g., fatigue, anorexia, nausea); have normal physical findings, except perhaps for liver enlargement, without the usual stigmata of chronic liver disease (see below); and have modest elevations of aminotransferase activities. Progression to more severe lesions (chronic active hepatitis and cirrhosis) was felt to be very unlikely, especially in patients with autoimmune or idiopathic chronic persistent hepatitis; however, progressive disease occurs in patients with chronic persistent *viral* hepatitis and in those with chronic persistent hepatitis following spontaneous or therapeutic remission of autoimmune hepatitis. In the new nomenclature, chronic persistent hepatitis would be classified by *grade* as minimal or mild chronic hepatitis and by *stage* as absent or mild fibrosis.

In patients with *chronic lobular hepatitis*, in addition to portal inflammation, histologic examination of the liver reveals foci of necrosis and inflammation in the liver lobule. Morphologically, chronic lobular hepatitis resembles slowly resolving acute hepatitis. The limiting plate remains intact, periportal fibrosis is absent or limited, lobular architecture is preserved, and progression to chronic active hepatitis and cirrhosis was felt to be rare. Thus chronic lobular hepatitis can be considered a variant of chronic persistent hepatitis with a lobular component, and clinical/laboratory features are comparable. Occasionally, the clinical activity of chronic lobular hepatitis may increase spontaneously; elevation of aminotransferase activity may resemble that seen in acute hepatitis, and transient histologic deterioration can be documented. The same qualifications in prognostic import mentioned above for chronic persistent hepatitis apply to chronic lobular hepatitis. Chronic lobular hepatitis corresponds in the new nomenclature to a mild or moderate *grade* and a *stage* of absent or minimal fibrosis.

Chronic active hepatitis is characterized clinically by continuing hepatic necrosis, portal/periportal and, to a lesser extent, lobular in-

Table 297-3 Correlation Between Earlier and Contemporary Nomenclature of Chronic Hepatitis

	Contemporary Classification	
Old Classification	Grade (Activity)	Stage (Fibrosis)
Chronic persistent hepatitis	Minimal or mild	None or mild
Chronic lobular hepatitis	Mild or moderate	Mild
Chronic active hepatitis	Mild, moderate, or severe	Mild, moderate, or severe

flammation, and fibrosis. Varying in severity from mild to severe, chronic active hepatitis was recognized to be a progressive disorder that can lead to cirrhosis, liver failure, and death. Morphologic characteristics of chronic active hepatitis include (1) a dense mononuclear infiltrate of the portal tracts, which are substantially expanded into the liver lobule (in the autoimmune type, plasma cells represent a component of the infiltrate); (2) destruction of the hepatocytes at the periphery of the lobule, with erosion of the limiting plate of hepatocytes surrounding the portal triads (piecemeal necrosis or interface hepatitis); (3) connective tissue septa surrounding portal tracts and extending from the portal zones into the lobule, isolating parenchymal cells into clusters and enveloping bile ducts; and (4) evidence of hepatocellular regeneration—"rosette" formation, thickened liver cell plates, and regenerative "pseudolobules." This process may be patchy, with individual liver lobules spared, or it may be diffuse. Histologic evidence of single-cell coagulative necrosis, Councilman or acidophilic bodies, appear in the periportal areas. Piecemeal necrosis is the minimal histologic requirement to establish a diagnosis of chronic active hepatitis, but this change is seen even in mild, relatively nonprogressive forms of chronic active hepatitis. A more severe lesion, *bridging hepatic necrosis* (originally termed *subacute hepatic necrosis*), characterizes a more severe and progressive form of chronic active hepatitis. Although bridging necrosis can be seen occasionally in patients with acute hepatitis, in whom it carries no prognostic importance, in chronic active hepatitis this lesion is associated with progression to cirrhosis. Bridging necrosis is characterized by hepatocellular dropout that spans lobules (i.e., between portal tracts—the periphery of the lobule—or between portal tracts and central veins—the centrizonal part of the lobule). Collapse of the reticulin network is a hallmark of bridging necrosis, and bridging fibrosis follows, leading ultimately to architectural reorganization by nodular regeneration, i.e., cirrhosis. A more extensive and ominous variant of bridging necrosis is multilobular collapse, in which bridging necrosis is widespread throughout the liver and which is associated clinically with rapid deterioration and even acute liver failure.

Although progression to cirrhosis is difficult to demonstrate in patients with chronic active hepatitis who have isolated piecemeal necrosis, in more severe forms of chronic active hepatitis, progression to cirrhosis is common. Among patients with chronic active hepatitis on liver biopsy, 20 to 50% also have cirrhosis, even early during the course of the disease. Ordinarily, chronic active hepatitis is more severe clinically than chronic persistent and lobular hepatitis. Although a sizable proportion of patients with chronic active hepatitis are asymptomatic, the majority tend to have mild to severe constitutional symptoms, especially fatigue. Generally, physical findings associated with chronic liver disease and portal hypertension are more common, aminotransferase levels tend to be higher, and jaundice and hyperbilirubinemia are more frequent in this form of chronic hepatitis.

In the new nomenclature for chronic hepatitis, what used to be called chronic active hepatitis spans the entire spectrum of activity *grade* from minimal, to mild, to severe chronic hepatitis, based on the degree of periportal and piecemeal necrosis, on the degree of lobular inflammation and injury, and on the degree of portal inflammation. Similarly, *stage* in chronic active hepatitis can translate to mild, moderate, or severe fibrosis as well as to cirrhosis.

CHRONIC VIRAL HEPATITIS Both the enterically transmitted forms of viral hepatitis, hepatitis A and E, are self-limited and do not cause chronic hepatitis (rare reports notwithstanding in which acute hepatitis A serves as a trigger for the onset of autoimmune hepatitis in genetically susceptible patients). In contrast, the entire clinicopathologic spectrum of chronic hepatitis occurs in patients with chronic viral hepatitis B and C as well as in patients with chronic hepatitis D superimposed on chronic hepatitis B.

Chronic Hepatitis B The likelihood of chronicity after acute hepatitis B varies as a function of age. Infection at birth is associated with a clinically silent acute infection but a 90% chance of chronic infection, while infection in young adulthood in immunocompetent persons is typically associated with clinically apparent acute hepatitis but a risk of chronicity of only approximately 1%. Most cases of chronic hepatitis B among adults, however, occur in patients who never had a recognized episode of clinically apparent acute viral hepatitis. The degree of liver injury (grade) in patients with chronic hepatitis B is variable, ranging from none in asymptomatic carriers, to mild, to severe. Among adults with chronic hepatitis B, histologic features are of prognostic importance. In one long-term study of patients with chronic hepatitis B, investigators found a 5-year survival of 97% for patients with chronic persistent hepatitis (mild chronic hepatitis), of 86% for patients with chronic active hepatitis (moderate to severe chronic hepatitis), and of only 55% for patients with chronic active hepatitis and postnecrotic cirrhosis. The 15-year survival in these cohorts were 77, 66, and 40%, respectively. On the other hand, more recent observations do not allow us to be so sanguine about the prognosis in patients with mild chronic hepatitis; among patients with what used to be labeled chronic persistent hepatitis followed for 1 to 13 years, progression to more severe chronic hepatitis and cirrhosis has been observed in more than a quarter of cases.

Probably more important to consider than histology alone in patients with chronic hepatitis B is the degree of hepatitis B virus (HBV) replication. As reviewed in Chap. 295, chronic hepatitis B can be divided into two phases based on the relative level of HBV replication. The relatively *replicative phase* is characterized by the presence in the serum of markers of HBV replication [hepatitis B e antigen (HBeAg) HBV DNA], by the presence in the liver of detectable intrahepatocyte nucleocapsid antigens [primarily hepatitis B core antigen (HBcAg)], by high infectivity, and by accompanying liver injury; HBV DNA can be detected in the liver but is extrachromosomal. In contrast, the relatively *nonreplicative phase* is characterized by the absence of conventional markers of HBV replication (HBeAg and HBV DNA detectable by hybridization) but an association with anti-HBe, the absence of intrahepatocytic HBcAg, limited infectivity, and minimal liver injury; HBV DNA can be detected in the liver but is integrated into the host genome. Those in the replicative phase tend to have more severe chronic hepatitis, while those in the nonreplicative phase tend to have minimal or mild chronic hepatitis or to be asymptomatic hepatitis B carriers; however, distinctions in HBV replication and in histologic category do not always coincide. The likelihood of converting spontaneously from relatively replicative to nonreplicative chronic HBV infection is approximately 10 to 15% per year. As noted in Chap. 295, the conversion from replicative to nonreplicative chronic hepatitis B is associated with a transient elevation in aminotransferase activity resembling acute hepatitis; occasionally, spontaneous resumptions of replicative activity occur in nonreplicative infection; and occasionally, HBV variants occur in which serologic markers of replication (HBeAg) are absent, despite the presence of replicative infection. Chronic HBV infection, especially when acquired at birth or in early childhood, is associated with an increased risk of hepatocellular carcinoma (Chap. 91). →***A discussion of the pathogenesis of liver injury in patients with chronic hepatitis B appears in Chap. 295.***

The spectrum of *clinical features* of chronic hepatitis B is broad, ranging from asymptomatic infection to debilitating disease or even end-stage, fatal hepatic failure. As noted above, the onset of the disease tends to be insidious in most patients, with the exception of the very few in whom chronic disease follows failure of resolution of clinically apparent acute hepatitis B. The clinical and laboratory features associated with progression from acute to chronic hepatitis B are discussed in Chap. 295. *Fatigue* is a common symptom, and persistent or intermittent *jaundice* is a common feature in severe or advanced cases. Intermittent deepening of jaundice and recurrence of malaise and anorexia, as well as worsening fatigue, are reminiscent of acute hepatitis; such exacerbations may occur spontaneously, often coinciding with evidence of virologic reactivation, may lead to progressive liver injury, and, when superimposed on well-established cirrhosis, may cause hepatic decompensation. Complications of cirrhosis occur in end-stage chronic hepatitis and include ascites, edema, bleeding gastroesophageal varices, hepatic encephalopathy, coagulopathy, or hypersplenism. Occasionally, these complications bring the patient to initial clinical attention. Extrahepatic complications of chronic hepatitis B, similar to those seen during the prodromal phase of acute hepatitis B, are associated with deposition of circulating hepatitis B antigen–antibody immune complexes. These include arthralgias and arthritis, which are common, and the more rare purpuric cutaneous lesions (leukocytoclastic vasculitis), immune-complex glomerulonephritis, and generalized vasculitis (polyarteritis nodosa) (Chaps. 295 and 317).

Laboratory features of chronic hepatitis B do not distinguish adequately between histologically mild and severe hepatitis. Aminotransferase elevations tend to be modest for chronic hepatitis B but may fluctuate in the range of 100 to 1000 units. As is true for acute viral hepatitis B, alanine aminotransferase (ALT, or SGPT) tends to be more elevated than aspartate aminotransferase (AST, or SGOT); however, once cirrhosis is established, AST tends to exceed ALT. Levels of alkaline phosphatase activity tend to be normal or only marginally elevated. In severe cases, moderate elevations in serum bilirubin [51.3 to 171 μmol/L (3 to 10 mg/dL)] occur. Hypoalbuminemia and prolongation of the prothrombin time occur in severe or end-stage cases. Hyperglobulinemia and detectable circulating autoantibodies are distinctly absent in chronic hepatitis B (in contrast to autoimmune hepatitis). →***Viral markers of chronic HBV infection are discussed in Chap. 295.***

℞ TREATMENT Management of chronic hepatitis B depends on the level of virus replication. Although progression to cirrhosis is more likely in severe chronic than in mild or moderate chronic hepatitis B, all forms of chronic viral hepatitis can be progressive. Interferon α (IFN-α) was the first approved therapy for chronic hepatitis B, but the recently approved dideoxynucleoside lamivudine expands the options for treatment. The most common indication for treatment is chronic "replicative" hepatitis B, with detectable HBeAg and HBV DNA (by hybridization assay), elevated ALT activity, and histologic evidence of chronic hepatitis on liver biopsy in an immunocompetent adult. A 16-week course of INF-α given by subcutaneous injection at a daily dose of 5 million units, or three times a week at a dose of 10 million units, results in seroconversion from "replicative" (detectable HBeAg and HBV DNA) to "nonreplicative" (undetectable HBeAg and HBV DNA by hybridization assay) HBV infection in approximately 35% of patients, with a concomitant improvement in liver histologic features. As a result of INF-α therapy, approximately 20% of patients acquire anti-HBe, and in early trials, approximately 8% lost hepatitis B surface antigen (HBsAg). Successful interferon therapy and seroconversion is often accompanied by an acute hepatitis-like elevation in aminotransferase activity, which has been postulated to result from enhanced cytolytic T cell clearance of HBV-infected hepatocytes. Relapse after successful therapy is rare (1 or 2%). The likelihood of responding to interferon is higher in patients with lower levels of HBV DNA and substantial elevations of ALT. Although children can respond as well as adults, interferon therapy has not been effective in very young children infected at birth. Similarly, interferon therapy has not been effective in immunosuppressed persons, Asian patients with minimal-to-mild ALT elevations, patients with pre-core mutant HBV infection (Chap. 295), or in patients with decompensated chronic hepatitis B (in whom such therapy can actually be detrimental, sometimes precipitating decompensation, often associated with severe adverse effects). Among patients with HBeAg loss during therapy, long-term follow-up has demonstrated that 80% experience eventual loss of HBsAg, i.e., all serologic markers of infection, and normalization of ALT over a 9-year posttreatment period. In addition, improved long-term and complication-free survival as well as a reduction in the frequency of hepatocellular carcinoma have been documented among interferon responders, supporting the conclusion that successful interferon therapy improves the natural history of chronic hepatitis B. Indications for interferon therapy in patients with chronic hepatitis B are summarized in Table 297-4.

Complications of interferon therapy include systemic "flulike" symptoms, marrow suppression, emotional lability (irritability commonly, depression rarely), autoimmune reactions (especially autoimmune thyroiditis), and miscellaneous side effects such as alopecia, rashes, diarrhea, and numbness and tingling of the extremities. With the possible exception of autoimmune thyroiditis, all these side effects are reversible upon dose lowering or cessation of therapy.

In patients with chronic hepatitis B, long-term therapy with glucocorticoids is not only ineffective but also detrimental. Short-term glucocorticoid therapy, however, has been advocated as a potential antiviral approach. Glucocorticoids increase HBV replication and expression in hepatocytes and depress cytolytic T cells. When glucocorticoids are administered for a brief time and then withdrawn abruptly, cytolytic T cells, suppressed while HBV replication was enhanced by the drug, resume their presteroid function. These restored cytolytic T cells attack hepatocytes, the HBV expression of which had been enhanced by the brief pulse of glucocorticoid therapy. An acute hepatitis-like flare of aminotransferase activity follows and may be accompanied by a dramatic drop, or even loss of, HBV replication. Such glucocorticoid "priming" prior to interferon therapy has not been shown to be more effective than interferon alone and has been abandoned.

Several nucleoside analogues active against HBV are being evaluated and developed. Famciclovir and ganciclovir have only limited activity against hepatitis B; however, lamivudine, which inhibits reverse transcriptase activity of both HIV and HBV, is a potent and effective agent for patients with chronic hepatitis B. Lamivudine suppresses HBV DNA by a median of four orders of magnitude at oral daily doses of 100 mg. In clinical trials conducted in Asia, North America, Europe, and Australia, lamivudine therapy for 12 months was associated with almost universal suppression of HBV DNA detectable by hybridization assays; loss of HBeAg in 32 to 33%; HBeAg seroconversion (i.e., conversion from HBeAg-reactive to anti-HBe-reactive) in 16 to 20%; normalization of ALT in approximately 40%; improvement in histology in over 50%; and retardation in fibrosis in 20%. Among patients who experienced HBeAg responses during therapy, 70 to 80% maintained the response over longer than a year of follow-up monitoring. Because maintenance of the response to lamivudine occurs in almost all patients with an HBeAg response, the achievement of an HBeAg response may be a viable stopping point in therapy. If

Table 297-4 Patients with Chronic Hepatitis B Who Are Candidates for Antiviral Therapy

	Interferon	Lamivudine
Detectable markers of HBV replication	Yes	Yes
Elevated ALT activity	Yes	Yes
Chronic hepatitis on liver biopsy	Yes	Yes
Immunocompetence	Yes	Yes
Immunosuppression	No	Yes
Acquisition of infection in adulthood (Western)	Yes	Yes
Acquisition of infection in childhood (Asian)	No	Yes
Compensated liver disease	Yes	Yes
Decompensated liver disease	No	Yes
"Wild-type" chronic hepatitis B	Yes	Yes
Pre-core mutant hepatitis B	No	Yes
Prior nonreponse to interferon	No	Yes

HBeAg is unaffected by lamivudine therapy, the current approach is to continue therapy until an HBeAg response occurs, but long-term therapy may be required to suppress HBV replication and, in turn, limit liver injury. Preliminary observations indicate that HBeAg seroconversions can increase to a level of 27% after 2 years and 44% after 3 years of therapy.

Losses of HBsAg have been few during lamivudine therapy, and this observation had been cited as an advantage of interferon over lamivudine; however, in head-to-head comparisons between interferon and lamivudine monotherapy, HBsAg losses were rare in both groups. Trials in which lamivudine and interferon were administered in combination failed to show a benefit of combination therapy over lamivudine monotherapy for either treatment-naive patients or prior interferon nonresponders.

Among patients with HBeAg and HBV DNA but with normal ALT activity, lamivudine suppresses liver injury during therapy but rarely achieves an HBeAg response. In patients with pre-core HBV mutations, who lack HBeAg but who have detectable HBV DNA and liver injury, lamivudine suppresses HBV DNA and normalizes ALT in 65% and improves liver histology in 60%. When therapy is discontinued, reactivation is common, and these patients require long-term therapy.

Clinical and laboratory side effects of lamivudine are negligible, indistinguishable from those observed in placebo recipients. During lamivudine therapy, transient ALT elevations, resembling those seen during interferon therapy and during spontaneous HBeAg-to-anti-HBe seroconversions, occur in a quarter of patients. These ALT elevations may result from restored cytolytic T cell activation permitted by suppression of HBV replication. Similar ALT elevations, however, occur at an identical frequency in placebo recipients, but ALT elevations associated with HBeAg seroconversion are confined to lamivudine-treated patients. When therapy is stopped after a year of therapy, 2- to 3-fold ALT elevations occur in 20 to 30% of lamivudine-treated patients, representing renewed liver-cell injury as HBV replication returns. Although these posttreatment flares are almost always transient and mild, rare severe exacerbations have been observed, mandating close and careful clinical and virologic monitoring after discontinuation of treatment.

Long-term monotherapy with lamivudine is associated with methionine-to-valine or methionine-to-isoleucine mutations in the YMDD (tyrosine-methionine-aspartate-aspartate) motif of HBV DNA polymerase, analogous to mutations that occur in patients with HIV infection treated with this drug. During a year of therapy, YMDD mutations occur in 15 to 30% of patients; the frequency increases at year two to 38% and at year three to almost 50%. Although transient elevations in ALT and HBV DNA levels occur when such variants emerge, YMDD-variant HBV appears to be less replicatively competent and a less robust pathogen. Even after YMDD mutations occur, HBV DNA and ALT levels as well as histologic scores tend to remain lower than baseline levels in immunocompetent patients. In immunosuppressed patients, a proportion of patients with YMDD mutations experience hepatic decompensation. Until other antivirals are developed, the approach to YMDD variants emerging during lamivudine treatment is to continue therapy. Other antiviral drugs, such as the experimental agent adefovir dipivoxil, inhibit YMDD-variant HBV. In the future, combination antiviral therapy will almost invariably become the norm as new agents are introduced.

Because lamivudine monotherapy can result universally in the rapid emergence of YMDD variants in persons with HIV infection, patients with chronic hepatitis B should be tested for anti-HIV prior to therapy; if HIV infection is identified, lamivudine monotherapy at the HBV daily dose of 100 mg is contraindicated. These patients should be treated with triple-drug antiretroviral therapy, including a lamivudine daily dose of 300 mg (Chap. 309). The safety of lamivudine during pregnancy has not been established.

No treatment is indicated or available for asymptomatic "nonreplicative" hepatitis B carriers. Whereas patients with decompensated chronic hepatitis B are not candidates for interferon therapy, they may respond to lamivudine, with reversal of the signs of decompensation.

Table 297-4 summarizes the indications in patients with chronic hepatitis B for antiviral therapy with lamivudine, as compared with interferon. Both drugs are quite comparable in efficacy as first-line therapy for chronic hepatitis B (Table 297-5). Interferon requires only brief-duration therapy, too limited in duration to support viral variants, but requires subcutaneous injections and is associated with a high level of intolerability. Lamivudine requires long-term therapy in most patients and, when used alone, fosters the emergence of viral variants. On the other hand, lamivudine is taken orally, is very well tolerated, leads to improved histology even in the absence of HBeAg responses, and is effective even in patients who fail to respond to interferon. Although some prefer to begin with interferon, most physicians and patients prefer lamivudine as first-line therapy.

For patients with end-stage chronic hepatitis B, liver transplantation is the only potential lifesaving intervention. Reinfection of the new liver is almost universal; however, the likelihood of liver injury associated with hepatitis B in the new liver is variable. The majority of patients become high-level viremic carriers with minimal liver injury. Unfortunately, an unpredictable proportion experience severe hepatitis B–related liver injury, sometimes a fulminant-like hepatitis, sometimes a rapid recapitulation of the original severe chronic hepatitis B (Chap. 301). Prevention of recurrent hepatitis B after liver transplantation has been achieved by *prophylaxis* with hepatitis B immune globulin and with nucleoside analogues such as lamivudine; in addition, nucleoside analogues have been used successfully to *reverse* posttransplantation liver injury associated with recurrent hepatitis B (Chap. 301).

Chronic Hepatitis D (Delta Hepatitis) The clinical and laboratory features of chronic hepatitis D virus (HDV) infection are summarized in Chap. 295. Chronic hepatitis D may follow acute coinfection with HBV but at a rate no higher than the rate of chronicity of hepatitis B. That is, although HDV coinfection can increase the severity of acute hepatitis B, HDV does not increase the likelihood of progression to chronic hepatitis B. However, when HDV superinfection occurs in a person who is already chronically infected with HBV, long-term HDV infection is the rule and a worsening of the liver disease the expected consequence. Except for severity, chronic hepatitis

Table 297-5 Comparison of Interferon and Lamivudine Therapy for Chronic Hepatitis B

	Interferon	Lamivudine
Route of administration	Injection	Oral
Duration of therapy	4 months	≥1 year
Tolerability	Poorly tolerated	Well tolerated
HBeAg loss	33%	32-33%
HBeAg seroconversion	18-20%	16-20%
Normalization of ALT	Confined to HBeAg responders	>40%
HBsAg loss during therapy	3-8%	2-4%
HBsAg loss after therapy	80% over 9 years	To be determined
Histologic improvement	Confined to HBeAg responders	>50%
Retardation of fibrosis	Not demonstrated	20%
Viral resistance	None	15-30% during 1 year
Natural history	Reduced mortality, decompensation, HCC	To be determined
Pre-core mutant hepatitis B	Limited response	>60% response
Candidate range[a]	Narrow	Broad

[a] See Table 297-4

B plus D has similar clinical and laboratory features to those seen in chronic hepatitis B alone. Relatively severe chronic hepatitis, with or without cirrhosis, is the rule, and mild chronic hepatitis the exception. A distinguishing serologic feature of chronic hepatitis D is the presence in the circulation of antibodies to liver-kidney microsomes (anti-LKM); however, the anti-LKM seen in hepatitis D are designated anti-LKM3, are directed against uridine diphosphate glucuronosyltransferase, and are distinct from anti-LKM1 seen in patients with autoimmune hepatitis and in a subset of patients with chronic hepatitis C (see below).

℞ **TREATMENT** Management is not well defined. Glucocorticoids are ineffective and are not used. Preliminary experimental trials of interferon α suggested that conventional doses and durations of therapy lower levels of HDV RNA and aminotransferase activity only transiently during treatment but have no impact on the natural history of the disease. Although high-dose IFN-α (9 million units) three times a week for 12 months may be associated with a sustained loss of HDV replication and clinical improvement in up to 50% of patients, ultimately recurrent HDV replication becomes universal after cessation of therapy. Antiviral therapy for chronic hepatitis D remains the subject of experimental trials; early observations suggest that lamivudine is not effective. In patients with end-stage liver disease secondary to chronic hepatitis D, liver transplantation has been effective. If hepatitis D recurs in the new liver without the expression of hepatitis B (an unusual serologic profile in immunocompetent persons, but common in transplant patients), liver injury is limited. In fact, the outcome of transplantation for chronic hepatitis D is superior to that for chronic hepatitis B (Chap. 301).

Chronic Hepatitis C Regardless of the epidemiologic mode of acquisition of hepatitis C virus (HCV) infection, chronic hepatitis follows acute hepatitis C in 50 to 70% of cases; even in those with a return to normal in aminotransferase levels after acute hepatitis C, chronic infection is common, adding up to an 85 to 90% likelihood of chronic HCV infection after acute hepatitis C. Furthermore, in patients with chronic transfusion-associated hepatitis followed for 10 to 20 years, progression to cirrhosis occurs in about 20%. Such is the case even for patients with relatively clinically mild chronic hepatitis, including those without symptoms, with only modest elevations of aminotransferase activity, and with mild chronic hepatitis on liver biopsy. Even in cohorts of well-compensated patients with chronic hepatitis C (no complications of chronic liver disease and with normal hepatic synthetic function), the prevalence of cirrhosis may be as high as 50%. Many cases of hepatitis C are identified in asymptomatic patients who have no history of acute hepatitis C, e.g., those discovered while attempting to donate blood or as a result of routine laboratory screening tests. The source of HCV infection in most of these cases is not defined, although a long-forgotten percutaneous exposure in the remote past can be elicited in a substantial proportion. The natural history of chronic hepatitis C identified under these circumstances remains to be determined. Among asymptomatic persons with anti-HCV, even when aminotransferase levels are normal, between a third and a half have been reported to have chronic hepatitis on liver biopsy, although mild in most cases. In these asymptomatic persons with normal aminotransferase levels, the presence of detectable circulating HCV RNA appears to distinguish those with chronic hepatitis on biopsy from those with normal liver histology.

Despite this substantial rate of progression of chronic hepatitis C, and despite the fact that liver failure can result from end-stage chronic hepatitis C, the long-term prognosis for chronic hepatitis C in a majority of patients is relatively benign. Mortality over 10 to 20 years among patients with transfusion-associated chronic hepatitis C has been shown not to differ from mortality in a matched population of transfused patients in whom hepatitis C did not develop. Although death in the hepatitis group is more likely to result from liver failure, and although hepatic decompensation may occur in approximately 15% of such patients over the course of a decade, the majority (almost

60%) of patients remain asymptomatic and well compensated, with no clinical sequelae of chronic liver disease. Overall, then, chronic hepatitis C tends to be very slowly and insidiously progressive, if at all, in the vast majority of patients, while in approximately a quarter of cases, chronic hepatitis C will progress eventually to end-stage cirrhosis. Referral bias may account for the more severe outcomes described in cohorts of patients reported from tertiary-care centers versus the more benign outcomes in cohorts of patients monitored from initial blood-product-associated acute hepatitis. Still unexplained, however, are the wide ranges in reported progression to cirrhosis, from 2% over 17 years in a population of women with hepatitis C infection acquired from contaminated anti-D immune globulin to 30% over ≤11 years in recipients of contaminated intravenous immune globulin.

Progression of liver disease in patients with chronic hepatitis C has been reported to be more likely in patients with older age, longer duration of infection, advanced histologic stage and grade, genotype 1 (especially type 1b), more complex quasispecies diversity, and increased hepatic iron. Among these variables, however, duration of infection appears to be the most important, and many of the others probably reflect disease duration to some extent (e.g., quasispecies diversity, hepatic iron accumulation).

Perhaps the best prognostic indicator in chronic hepatitis C is liver histology. Patients with mild necrosis and inflammation as well as those with limited fibrosis have an excellent prognosis and limited progression to cirrhosis. In contrast, among patients with moderate to severe necroinflammatory activity or fibrosis, including septal or bridging fibrosis, progression to cirrhosis is highly likely over the course of 10 to 20 years. Among patients with compensated cirrhosis associated with hepatitis C, the 10-year survival is close to 80 percent; mortality occurs at a rate of 2 to 6% per year, decompensation at a rate of 4 to 5% per year, and hepatocellular carcinoma at a rate of 1 to 3% per year.

In addition, severity of chronic hepatitis is greater and progression of chronic liver disease is more accelerated in patients who have chronic hepatitis C as well as other liver processes, including alcoholic liver disease, chronic hepatitis B, hemochromatosis, and α_1-antitrypsin deficiency. No other epidemiologic or clinical features of chronic hepatitis C (e.g., severity of acute hepatitis, level of aminotransferase activity, level of HCV RNA, presence or absence of jaundice) are predictive of eventual outcome. Despite the relative benignity of chronic hepatitis C over time, cirrhosis following chronic hepatitis C has been associated with the late development, after several decades, of hepatocellular carcinoma (HCC) (Chap. 91). As noted above, the annual rate of HCC in cirrhotic patients with hepatitis C is 1 to 3%.

Clinical features of chronic hepatitis C are similar to those described above for chronic hepatitis B. Generally, *fatigue* is the most common symptom; jaundice is rare. Immune-complex mediated extrahepatic complications of chronic hepatitis C are less common than in chronic hepatitis B, with the exception of essential mixed cryoglobulinemia (Chap. 295). This is the case despite the fact that assays for immune-complex–like activity are often positive in patients with chronic hepatitis C. In addition, chronic hepatitis C has been associated with extrahepatic complications unrelated to immune-complex injury. These include Sjögren's syndrome, lichen planus, and porphyria cutanea tarda. *Laboratory features* of chronic hepatitis C are similar to those in patients with chronic hepatitis B, but aminotransferase levels tend to fluctuate more (the characteristic episodic pattern of aminotransferase activity) and to be lower, especially in patients with long-standing disease. An interesting and occasionally confusing finding in patients with chronic hepatitis C is the presence of autoantibodies. Rarely, patients with autoimmune hepatitis (see below) and hyperglobulinemia have false-positive enzyme immunoassays for anti-HCV. On the other hand, some patients with serologically confirmable chronic hepatitis C have circulating anti-LKM. These antibodies are anti-LKM1, as seen in patients with autoimmune hepatitis *type 2* (see below), and are directed against a 33-amino-acid sequence of P450

IID6. The occurrence of anti-LKM1 in some patients with chronic hepatitis C may result from the partial sequence homology between the epitope recognized by anti-LKM1 and two segments of the HCV polyprotein. In addition, the presence of this autoantibody in some patients with chronic hepatitis C suggests that autoimmunity may be playing a role in the pathogenesis of chronic hepatitis C. *→Histopathologic features of chronic hepatitis C, especially those that distinguish hepatitis C from hepatitis B, are described in Chap. 295.*

℞ **TREATMENT** Two approaches to antiviral therapy of chronic hepatitis C have been approved: *monotherapy* with interferon and *combination therapy* with interferon plus ribavirin. According to a National Institutes of Health Consensus Development Conference in March 1997, responses measured at the end of treatment are referred to as end-treatment responses, and responses sustained for at least 6 months after discontinuation of therapy are referred to as sustained responses.

Interferon Monotherapy Interferon α, administered by subcutaneous injection three times a week for 6 months yields end-treatment biochemical responses (return to normal of ALT levels) as high as approximately 50% and virologic responses (undetectable HCV RNA) by polymerase chain reaction (PCR) of approximately 30%. Unfortunately, because of a relapse rate as high as 90% in end-treatment responders, these responses are not maintained after discontinuation of therapy except in a small minority of patients; after 6 months of interferon monotherapy, the likelihood of a sustained biochemical and virologic response is only approximately 10%. Even in the absence of a biochemical/virologic response, however, end-treatment histologic responses—primarily reductions in periportal and lobular activity—occur in three-fourths of treated patients. Unlike the case in hepatitis B, in chronic hepatitis C successful responses to therapy are not accompanied by transient, acute-hepatitis–like elevations in aminotransferase activity; instead, ALT levels fall precipitously. Between 85 to 90% of responses occur within the first 3 months of therapy; responses thereafter are rare.

In a proportion of cases, markers of HCV replication can be eradicated by interferon therapy, and durable responses with normal ALT, improved histology, and absence of HCV RNA in serum and liver have been documented many years after successful therapy. A small proportion of patients, approximately 10%, experience biochemical "breakthrough" *during* interferon therapy and are classified as nonresponders. In general, they remain refractory to retreatment thereafter; some such breakthroughs are associated with interferon antibodies, while others may reflect mutations in the HCV genome that render HCV nonresponsive to interferon.

Levels of HCV RNA fall in tandem with ALT levels during interferon therapy, but loss of detectable HCV RNA does not preclude relapse. When a patient experiences an apparently sustained biochemical response after discontinuing interferon but continues to remain viremic, as reflected by the persistence of detectable HCV RNA, future biochemical relapse is likely. Patient variables that tend to correlate with *sustained* responsiveness to interferon include a low baseline level of HCV RNA and histologically mild hepatitis. Patients with cirrhosis can respond, but they are less likely to do so and especially unlikely to have a *sustained* response. Patients with HCV genotype 1 are less likely to respond than patients with other genotypes. Other variables reported to correlate with increased responsiveness include brief duration of infection, low HCV quasispecies diversity, immunocompetence, and low liver iron levels. High levels of HCV RNA, more histologically advanced liver disease, and high quasispecies diversity all go hand in hand with advanced duration of infection, which may be the single most important variable determining interferon responsiveness. The ironic fact, then, is that patients whose disease is *least* likely to progress are the ones *most* likely to respond to interferon and vice versa. Finally, among patients with genotype 1b, responsiveness to interferon is enhanced in those with amino-acid-substitution mutations in the nonstructural protein 5A gene.

The most effective approach to increasing responsiveness to interferon monotherapy is to increase the duration of therapy to 12 months or longer, a regimen associated with a sustained biochemical and virologic response of approximately 20%. Higher doses of interferon (e.g., 5 to 10 million units) or daily injections increase response rates only marginally and at a substantial cost in intolerability. Thus, if interferon monotherapy is selected, the consensus is that 3 million units for at least 12 months is the preferred regimen. Currently, three types of IFN-α are approved in the United States; for the two recombinant products, the recommended dose is 3 million units, and for the one synthetic consensus interferon (synthesized to represent the amino acids at each position that occur most frequently among the multiple, natural interferon α subspecies), the dose is 9μg. Several other types of INF-α, including lymphoblastoid interferon, are available in Europe and Asia. A review of the different types of INF-α during the NIH Consensus Development Conference in 1997 led to the conclusion that they are all equivalent in efficacy.

Studies of viral kinetics have shown that despite a virion half life in serum of only 2 to 3 h, the level of HCV is maintained by a high replication rate of 10^{12} hepatitis C virions per day. Interferon α blocks virion production or release with an efficacy that increases with increasing drug doses; moreover, the calculated death rate for infected cells during interferon therapy is inversely related to viral load; patients with the most rapid death rate of infected hepatocytes are more likely to achieve undetectable HCV RNA at 3 months; achieving this landmark is predictive of a subsequent sustained response. Therefore, to achieve rapid viral clearance from serum and the liver, *high-dose induction therapy* has been advocated. In practice, high-dose induction therapy has not yielded higher sustained response rates. Other approaches that have been suggested include tapering therapy slowly, rather than discontinuing therapy abruptly, and, because high liver iron levels are associated with nonresponsiveness, the addition of phlebotomy to interferon therapy. None of these approaches has been shown to be effective.

Long-acting interferons bound to polyethylene glycol (PEG) have several advantages. Such "pegylated" interferons, with elimination times seven-fold longer than standard interferons, achieve prolonged concentration peaks and can be administered once, rather than three times, a week. Instead of the frequent drug peaks and troughs associated with frequent administration of short-acting interferons, administration of pegylated interferons results in drug concentrations that are more stable and sustained over time. Preliminary studies suggest that once-a-week injections of pegylated interferons are at least as effective as standard interferons given three times a week and may result in sustained responses comparable to those achieved with combination interferon-ribavirin therapy (see below).

If a patient relapses after a course of interferon monotherapy, repeating a course of interferon monotherapy is unlikely to achieve a sustained response unless the dose or preferably the duration of therapy is increased. Under these circumstances, sustained response rates as high as 40% can be realized. Although a small proportion of interferon nonresponders can respond to a repeat course of interferon monotherapy, and although a 13% sustained response rate has been reported for prior interferon nonresponders treated with high-dose (15 μg) consensus interferon, the likelihood of responding is not increased substantially by retreating interferon nonresponders with interferon monotherapy.

Combination Interferon-Ribavirin Therapy The most effective way to increase the efficacy of interferon therapy is to add ribavirin, an oral guanoside nucleoside. When used as monotherapy, ribavirin is ineffective and does not reduce HCV RNA levels. In contrast, the combination of interferon at standard doses with ribavirin at doses of 1000 mg (for patients weighing $<$75 kg) to 1200 mg (for patients weighing $\geq$75 kg) per day increases both end-treatment responses and sustained responses in previously untreated patients. Large, international, multicenter trials have shown that end-treatment responses at 6 months or 12 months exceed 50% and sustained responses as high as 33% at 6 months and 41% at 12 months have been achieved. Thus, a full year of combination therapy is twice as effective as a year of interferon monotherapy. Sustained responses were more likely in patients with low viral loads (below 2 million copies/mL), genotypes other than 1, minimal fibrosis, age <40, and females. In patients with low viral loads and non-1 genotypes, sustained response rates can be as high as 95%, and combination therapy for 24 weeks suffices, achieving the same end as continuing therapy for a full year. Therefore, for patients with low viral loads and non-1 genotypes, therapy need last only 6 months. Unless contraindications to the use of combination therapy exist (see below), combination interferon-ribavirin is the treatment of choice for chronic hepatitis C (Table 297-6).

For those who relapse after a 6-month course of interferon monotherapy, a 6-month course of combination therapy results in a sustained response rate of 50%, and retreatment of relapsers is another approved indication for combination therapy. Unfortunately, combination therapy has been disappointing in interferon nonresponders.

Side effects of combination therapy are similar to those of interferon monotherapy; however, ribavirin causes hemolysis; a reduction in hemoglobin of up to 2 to 3 gm or in hematocrit of up 5 to 10% can be anticipated. A small, unpredictable proportion of patients will experience profound, brisk hemolysis, resulting in symptomatic anemia. Therefore, close monitoring of blood counts is crucial, and combination therapy should be avoided in patients with anemia or hemoglobinopathies and in patients with coronary artery disease or cerebrovascular disease, in whom anemia can precipitate an ischemic event. Ribavirin, which is renally excreted, should not be used by patients with renal insufficiency; the drug is teratogenic, precluding its use during pregnancy and mandating the use of efficient contraception during therapy.

Ribavirin therapy has also been characterized by nasal congestion, pruritus, and precipitation of gout; the combination is more difficult to tolerate than interferon monotherapy. In one large clinical trial of combination therapy versus monotherapy among patients treated for a year, 21% of the combination group (but only 14% of the monotherapy group) had to discontinue treatment, while 26% of the combination group (but only 9% of the monotherapy group) required dose reductions.

Indications for Antiviral Therapy Patients with chronic hepatitis C who have elevated ALT levels, detectable HCV RNA, and chronic hepatitis of at least moderate grade and stage are candidates for antiviral therapy with interferon and ribavirin, unless ribavirin is contraindicated (Table 297-6). Preliminary retrospective analyses have shown that interferon treatment improves survival and complication-free survival. One year of combination therapy is standard, but 6 months suffice for patients with non-1 genotypes and low viral loads. For patients treated with interferon monotherapy, 12 months is the standard duration in all cases, regardless of genotype and viral load. According to the NIH Consensus Development Conference in 1997, therapy should be discontinued in patients who have not achieved a normal ALT and an undetectable HCV RNA by month three. Although the vast majority of patients treated with combination therapy who become sustained responders will have achieved an early biochemical and virologic response, a proportion of sustained responders experienced late viral clearance. In addition, even in biochemical and virologic nonresponders, histologic improvement is common. Therefore, recommendations for early cessation of therapy based on interim assessments of biochemical and virologic responsiveness require reevaluation. Although response rates are lower in patients with certain pretreatment variables, selection for treatment should not be based on symptoms, genotype, viral load, or the mode of acquisition of infection.

Patients who have relapsed after an initial course of interferon monotherapy are candidates for a 6-month course of combination interferon-ribavirin therapy; if they cannot tolerate ribavirin, they should be retreated with interferon monotherapy, but the course should be longer. It remains to be determined whether long-term (even indefinite) maintenance therapy will be necessary or effective in patients who relapse repeatedly whenever therapy is discontinued. For interferon nonresponders, retreatment with interferon monotherapy or combination therapy is unlikely to achieve a sustained response. Clinical trials are in progress to determine whether long-term suppression of virus-induced liver injury with antiviral therapy will be of benefit in this population.

In patients with acute hepatitis C, a course of interferon has been shown to reduce the likelihood of chronicity by one-half (Chapter 295). In patients with normal ALT levels, long-term monitoring studies have shown absence of histologic progression, and clinical trials of antiviral therapy have shown no benefit; therefore, treatment of such patients is not recommended. Because hepatitis C can reactivate in patients with normal ALT levels, laboratory monitoring several times a year should be done, and therapy should be considered for sustained elevations in ALT levels. Patients with mild hepatitis on liver biopsy are not routine candidates for antiviral therapy, but treatment decisions should be individualized between physician and patient. Most authorities would recommend a pretreatment liver biopsy to help in the decision-making about therapy.

Table 297-6 Indications and Recommendations for Antiviral Therapy of Chronic Hepatitis C

STANDARD INDICATIONS FOR THERAPY
Elevated ALT activity Fibrosis or moderate to severe hepatitis on liver biopsy Detectable HCV RNA
RETREATMENT RECOMMENDED
Relapsers after an initial course of interferon A 6-month course of combination interferon-ribavirin or a course of interferon monotherapy longer in duration than the original course
ANTIVIRAL THERAPY NOT RECOMMENDED ROUTINELY BUT MANAGEMENT DECISIONS MADE ON AN INDIVIDUAL BASIS
Children (age <18 years) Age >60 Mild hepatitis on liver biopsy Compensated cirrhosis Patients with HIV infection and normal CD4 counts Maintenance therapy in repeated relapsers Nonreponders to a course of recombinant interferon—can be offered a 48-week course of consensus interferon, 15 μg three times a week (clinical trials underway to assess benefit of long-term "suppressive" therapy with other regimens)
LONG-TERM THERAPY RECOMMENDED
Cutaneous vasculitis and glomerulonephritis associated with chronic hepatitis C
ANTIVIRAL THERAPY NOT RECOMMENDED
Decompensated cirrhosis Normal ALT activity
THERAPEUTIC REGIMENS
First-line treatment: INF-α 3 million units subcutaneously three times a week plus ribavirin 1000 mg/d (weight <75 Kg) to 1200 mg/d (weight ≥75 kg) orally Duration of therapy: Genotype 1: 48 weeks Genotypes 2 and 3: 24 weeks *Alternative regimen:* INF-α monotherapy 3 million units (of recombinant interferon alfa-2a or alfa-2b or 9 μg of consensus interferon) subcutaneously three times a week for 48 weeks (primarily for patients in whom combination therapy is contraindicated or not tolerated)
FEATURES ASSOCIATED WITH REDUCED RESPONSIVENESS
Advanced histologic lesion (e.g., advanced cirrhosis) Long-duration disease Genotype 1 High-level HCV RNA (>2 million copies/mL) High HCV quasispecies diversity

Patients with compensated cirrhosis can respond to therapy, although their likelihood of a sustained response is lower than in noncirrhotics. Combination therapy brings sustained response rates in cirrhotics up to the level achieved with interferon monotherapy in noncirrhotics. Retrospective analyses generally have not demonstrated an improvement in survival among interferon-treated cirrhotic patients. Similarly, several studies have suggested that treatment of cirrhotics with hepatitis C reduces the frequency of HCC; however, logistic regression analyses have shown that patient characteristics at the time of therapy (e.g., less advanced disease), not treatment itself, accounted for the reduced frequency of HCC observed in the treated cohort. Patients with decompensated cirrhosis are not candidates for antiviral therapy but should be referred for liver transplantation. After liver transplantation, recurrent hepatitis C is the rule. Most patients who undergo liver transplantation for chronic hepatitis C experience little, if any, morbidity, allograft loss, or mortality associated with recurrent hepatitis C during the early postoperative years (Chapter 301); studies are in progress to determine how best to treat hepatitis C after liver transplantation. The cutaneous and renal vasculitis of HCV-associated essential mixed cryoglobulinemia (Chap. 295) may respond to interferon, but sustained responses are rare after discontinuation of therapy; therefore, prolonged, perhaps indefinite, therapy is recommended in this group.

Anecdotal reports suggest that antiviral therapy may be effective in porphyria cutanea tarda or lichen planus associated with hepatitis C. In patients with HIV infection, responses similar to those seen in other groups have been reported in patients with normal CD4 counts.

AUTOIMMUNE HEPATITIS **Definition** Autoimmune hepatitis (formerly called autoimmune chronic active hepatitis) is a chronic disorder characterized by continuing hepatocellular necrosis and inflammation, usually with fibrosis, which tends to progress to cirrhosis and liver failure. When fulfilling criteria of severity, this type of chronic hepatitis may have a 6-month mortality of as high as 40%. The prominence of extrahepatic features of autoimmunity as well as seroimmunologic abnormalities in this disorder supports an autoimmune process in its pathogenesis; this concept is reflected in the labels "lupoid," plasma cell, or autoimmune hepatitis. Because autoantibodies and other typical features of autoimmunity do not occur in all cases, however, a broader, more appropriate designation for this type of chronic hepatitis is "idiopathic" or cryptogenic. Cases in which hepatotropic viruses, metabolic/genetic derangements, and hepatotoxic drugs have been excluded merit this designation and probably include a spectrum of heterogeneous liver disorders of unknown cause, a proportion of which have characteristic autoimmune features.

Immunopathogenesis The weight of evidence suggests that the progressive liver injury in patients with idiopathic/autoimmune hepatitis is the result of a cell-mediated immunologic attack directed against liver cells; in all likelihood, predisposition to autoimmunity is inherited, while the liver specificity of this injury is triggered by environmental (e.g., chemical or viral) factors. For example, patients have been described in whom apparently self-limited cases of acute hepatitis A or B led to autoimmune hepatitis, presumably because of genetic susceptibility or predisposition. Evidence to support an autoimmune pathogenesis in this type of hepatitis includes the following: (1) In the liver, the histopathologic lesions are composed predominantly of cytotoxic T cells and plasma cells; (2) circulating autoantibodies (nuclear, smooth muscle, thyroid, etc.; see below), rheumatoid factor, and hyperglobulinemia are common; (3) other autoimmune disorders—such as thyroiditis, rheumatoid arthritis, autoimmune hemolytic anemia, ulcerative colitis, proliferative glomerulonephritis, juvenile diabetes mellitus, and Sjögren's syndrome—occur with increased frequency in patients who have autoimmune hepatitis and in their relatives; (4) histocompatibility haplotypes associated with autoimmune diseases, such as HLA-B1, -B8, -DR3, and -DR4, are common in patients with autoimmune hepatitis; and (5) this type of chronic hepatitis is responsive to glucocorticoid/immunosuppressive therapy, effective in a variety of autoimmune disorders.

Cellular immune mechanisms appear to be important in the pathogenesis of autoimmune hepatitis. In vitro studies have suggested that in patients with this disorder, lymphocytes are capable of becoming sensitized to hepatocyte membrane proteins and of destroying liver cells. Abnormalities of immunoregulatory control over cytotoxic lymphocytes (impaired suppressor cell influences) may play a role as well. Studies of genetic predisposition to autoimmune hepatitis demonstrate that certain haplotypes are associated with the disorder, as enumerated above. The precise triggering factors, genetic influences, and cytotoxic and immunoregulatory mechanisms involved in this type of liver injury remain poorly defined.

Intriguing clues into the pathogenesis of autoimmune hepatitis come from the observation that circulating autoantibodies are prevalent in patients with this disorder. Among the autoantibodies described in these patients are antibodies to nuclei [so-called antinuclear antibodies (ANA), primarily in a homogeneous pattern] and smooth muscle (so-called anti-smooth-muscle antibodies, directed at actin), anti-LKM (see below), antibodies to "soluble liver antigen" (directed at a member of the glutathione S-transferase gene family), as well as antibodies to the liver-specific asialoglycoprotein receptor (or "hepatic lectin") and other hepatocyte membrane proteins. Although some of these provide helpful diagnostic markers, their involvement in the pathogenesis of autoimmune hepatitis has not been established.

Humoral immune mechanisms have been shown to play a role in the extrahepatic manifestations of autoimmune/idiopathic hepatitis. Arthralgias, arthritis, cutaneous vasculitis, and glomerulonephritis occurring in patients with autoimmune hepatitis appear to be mediated by the deposition in affected tissue vessels of circulating immune complexes, followed by complement activation, inflammation, and tissue injury. While specific viral antigen-antibody complexes can be identified in acute and chronic viral hepatitis, the nature of the immune complexes in autoimmune hepatitis has not been defined.

Many of the *clinical features* of autoimmune hepatitis are similar to those described for chronic viral hepatitis. The onset of disease may be insidious or abrupt; the disease may present initially like, and be confused with, acute viral hepatitis; a history of recurrent bouts of what had been labeled acute hepatitis is not uncommon. A subset of patients with autoimmune hepatitis has distinct features. Such patients are predominantly young to middle-aged women with marked hyperglobulinemia and high-titer circulating ANA. This is the group with positive LE preparations (initially labeled "lupoid" hepatitis) in whom other autoimmune features are common. Fatigue, malaise, anorexia, amenorrhea, acne, arthralgias, and jaundice are common. Occasionally, arthritis, maculopapular eruptions (including cutaneous vasculitis), erythema nodosum, colitis, pleurisy, pericarditis, anemia, azotemia, and sicca syndrome (keratoconjunctivitis, xerostomia) occur. In some patients, complications of cirrhosis, such as ascites and edema (associated with hypoalbuminemia), encephalopathy, hypersplenism, coagulopathy, or variceal bleeding may bring the patient to initial medical attention.

The course of autoimmune hepatitis may be variable. In those with mild disease or limited histologic lesions (e.g., piecemeal necrosis without bridging), progression to cirrhosis is limited. In those with severe symptomatic autoimmune hepatitis (aminotransferase levels >10 times normal, marked hyperglobulinemia, "aggressive" histologic lesions—bridging necrosis or multilobular collapse, cirrhosis), the 6-month mortality without therapy may be as high as 40%. Such severe disease accounts for only 20% of cases; the natural history of milder disease is variable, often accentuated by spontaneous remissions and exacerbations. Especially poor prognostic signs include multilobular collapse at the time of initial presentation and failure of the bilirubin to improve after 2 weeks of therapy. Death may result from hepatic failure, hepatic coma, other complications of cirrhosis (e.g., variceal hemorrhage), and intercurrent infection. In patients with established cirrhosis, hepatocellular carcinoma may be a late complication (Chap. 91).

Laboratory features of autoimmune hepatitis are similar to those seen in chronic viral hepatitis. Liver biochemical tests are invariably abnormal but may not correlate with the clinical severity or histopathologic features in individual cases. Many patients with autoimmune hepatitis have normal serum bilirubin, alkaline phosphatase, and globulin levels with only minimal aminotransferase elevations. Serum AST and ALT levels are increased and fluctuate in the range of 100 to 1000 units. In severe cases, the serum bilirubin level is moderately elevated [51 to 171 μmol/L (3 to 10 mg/dL)]. Hypoalbuminemia occurs in patients with very active or advanced disease. Serum alkaline phosphatase levels may be moderately elevated or near normal. In a small proportion of patients, marked elevations of alkaline phosphatase activity occur; in such patients, clinical and laboratory features overlap with those of primary biliary cirrhosis (Chap. 299). The prothrombin time is often prolonged, particularly late in the disease or during active phases.

Hypergammaglobulinemia (>2.5 g/dL) is common in autoimmune hepatitis. Rheumatoid factor is common as well. As noted above, circulating autoantibodies are also common. The most characteristic are ANA in a homogeneous staining pattern. Smooth-muscle antibodies are less specific, seen just as frequently in chronic viral hepatitis. Because of the high levels of globulins achieved in the circulation of some patients with autoimmune hepatitis, occasionally the globulins may bind nonspecifically in solid-phase binding immunoassays for viral antibodies. This has been recognized most commonly in tests for antibodies to hepatitis C virus, as noted above. In fact, studies of autoantibodies in autoimmune hepatitis have led to the recognition of new categories of autoimmune hepatitis. *Type I autoimmune hepatitis* is the classic syndrome occurring in young women, associated with marked hyperglobulinemia, lupoid features, and circulating ANA. *Type II autoimmune hepatitis*, often seen in children and more common in Mediterranean populations, is associated not with ANA but with anti-LKM. Actually, anti-LKM represent a heterogeneous group of antibodies. In type II autoimmune hepatitis, the antibody is anti-LKM1, directed against P450 IID6. This is the same anti-LKM seen in some patients with chronic hepatitis C. Anti-LKM2 is seen in drug-induced hepatitis, and anti-LKM3 is seen in patients with chronic hepatitis D. Type II autoimmune hepatitis has been subdivided by some authorities into two categories, one more typically autoimmune and the other associated with viral hepatitis type C. Autoimmune hepatitis type IIa is felt to be autoimmune, is more likely to occur in young women, is associated with hyperglobulinemia, is associated with high-titer anti-LKM1, responds to glucocorticoid therapy, and is seen commonly in western Europe and the United Kingdom. Type IIb autoimmune hepatitis is associated with hepatitis C virus infection, tends to occur in older men, is associated with normal globulin levels and low-titer anti-LKM1, responds to interferon, and occurs most commonly in Mediterranean countries. In addition, another type of autoimmune hepatitis has been recognized, *autoimmune hepatitis type III*. These patients lack ANA and anti-LKM1 and have circulating antibodies to soluble liver antigen, which are directed at hepatocyte cytoplasmic cytokeratins 8 and 18. Most of these patients are women and have clinical features similar to those of patients with type I autoimmune hepatitis.

℞ **TREATMENT** The mainstay of management in autoimmune or idiopathic (nonviral) hepatitis is glucocorticoid therapy. Several controlled clinical trials have documented that such therapy leads to symptomatic, clinical, biochemical, and histologic improvement as well as increased survival. A therapeutic response can be expected in up to 80% of patients. Unfortunately, therapy has not been shown to prevent ultimate progression to cirrhosis. Although some advocate the use of prednisolone (the hepatic metabolite of prednisone), prednisone is just as effective and is favored by most authorities. Therapy may be initiated at 20 mg/d, but a popular regimen in the United States relies on an initiation dose of 60 mg/d. This high dose is tapered successively over the course of a month down to a maintenance level of 20 mg/d. An alternative but equally effective approach is to begin with half the prednisone dose (30 mg/d) along with azathioprine (50 mg/d). With azathioprine maintained at 50 mg/d, the prednisone dose is tapered over the course of a month down to a maintenance level of 10 mg/d. The advantage of the combination approach is a reduction, over the span of an 18-month course of therapy, in serious, life-threatening complications of steroid therapy from 66% down to under 20%. Azathioprine alone, however, is not effective in achieving remission, nor is alternate-day glucocorticoid therapy. Although therapy has been shown to be effective for severe autoimmune hepatitis, therapy is not indicated for mild forms of chronic hepatitis (which used to be labeled chronic persistent hepatitis or chronic lobular hepatitis), and the efficacy of therapy in mild or asymptomatic autoimmune hepatitis has not been established.

Improvement of fatigue, anorexia, malaise, and jaundice tends to occur within days to several weeks; biochemical improvement occurs over the course of several weeks to months, with a fall in serum bilirubin and globulin levels and an increase in serum albumin. Serum aminotransferase levels usually drop promptly, but improvements in AST and ALT alone do not appear to be a reliable marker of recovery in individual patients; histologic improvement, characterized by a decrease in mononuclear infiltration and in hepatocellular necrosis may be delayed for 6 to 24 months. Still, if interpreted cautiously, aminotransferase levels are valuable indicators of relative disease activity, and many authorities do *not* advocate serial liver biopsies to assess therapeutic success or to guide decisions to alter or stop therapy. Therapy should continue for at least 12 to 18 months. After tapering and cessation of therapy, the likelihood of relapse is at least 50%, even if posttreatment histology has improved to show mild chronic hepatitis, and the majority of patients require therapy at maintenance doses indefinitely. Continuing azathioprine alone after cessation of prednisone therapy may reduce the frequency of relapse.

If medical therapy fails, or when chronic hepatitis progresses to cirrhosis and is associated with life-threatening complications of liver decompensation, liver transplantation is the only recourse (Chap. 301). Recurrence of autoimmune hepatitis in the new liver occurs rarely, if at all.

DIFFERENTIAL DIAGNOSIS Early during the course of chronic hepatitis, the disease may resemble typical *acute viral hepatitis*. Without histologic assessment, severe chronic hepatitis cannot be readily distinguished based on clinical or biochemical criteria from mild chronic hepatitis. In adolescence, *Wilson's disease* may present with features of chronic hepatitis long before neurologic manifestations become apparent and before the formation of Kayser-Fleischer rings; in this age group, serum ceruloplasmin and serum and urinary copper determinations plus measurement of liver copper levels will establish the correct diagnosis. *Postnecrotic* or *cryptogenic cirrhosis* and *primary biliary cirrhosis* share clinical features with autoimmune hepatitis; biochemical, serologic, and histologic assessments are usually sufficient to allow these entities to be distinguished from autoimmune hepatitis. Of course, the distinction between autoimmune ("idiopathic") and chronic viral hepatitis is not always straightforward, especially when viral antibodies occur in patients with autoimmune disease or when autoantibodies occur in patients with viral disease. Finally, the presence of extrahepatic features such as arthritis, cutaneous vasculitis, or pleuritis—not to mention the presence of circulating autoantibodies—may cause confusion with *rheumatologic disorders* such as rheumatoid arthritis and systemic lupus erythematosus. The existence of clinical and biochemical features of progressive necroinflammatory liver disease distinguishes chronic hepatitis from these other disorders, which are not associated with severe liver disease.

BIBLIOGRAPHY

Allen MI et al: Identification and characterization of mutations in hepatitis B virus resistant to lamivudine. Hepatology 27:1670, 1998

BONI C et al: Lamivudine treatment can restore T cell responsiveness in chronic hepatitis B. J Clin Invest 102:968, 1998

CHAYAMA K et al: Emergence and takeover of YMDD mutant hepatitis B virus during long-term lamivudine therapy and re-takeover by wild type after cessation of therapy. Hepatology 27:1711, 1998

CONSENSUS STATEMENT: EASL international consensus conference on hepatitis C. J Hepatol 30:956, 1999

CZAJA AJ et al: Autoimmune hepatitis: Evolving concepts and treatment strategies. Dig Dis Sci 40:435, 1995

CZAJA AJ et al: Associations between alleles of the major histocompatibility complex and type I autoimmune hepatitis. Hepatology 25:317, 1997

DAVIS GL et al: Interferon alfa-2b alone or in combination with ribavirin for the treatment of relapse of chronic hepatitis C. N Engl J Med 339:1493, 1998

DESMET VJ et al: Classification of chronic hepatitis: Diagnosis, grading, and staging. Hepatology 19:1513, 1994

DI BISCEGLIE AM: Hepatitis C. Lancet 351:351, 1998

DI BISCEGLIE AM (guest editor): Treatment advances in chronic hepatitis C. Semin Liver Dis 19(Suppl 1):1, 1999

DIENSTAG JL et al: Lamivudine as initial treatment for chronic hepatitis B in the United States. N Engl J Med 341:1256, 1999

DONALDSON P et al: The molecular genetics of autoimmune liver disease. Hepatology 20:225, 1994

ENOMOTO N et al: Mutations in the nonstructural protein 5A gene and response to interferon in patients with chronic hepatitis C virus 1b infection. N Engl J Med 334:77, 1996

FARCI P et al: Treatment of chronic hepatitis D with interferon alfa-2a. N Engl J Med 330:88, 1994

FATTOVICH G et al: Morbidity and mortality in compensated cirrhosis type C: A retrospective follow-up study of 384 patients. Gastroenterology 112:463, 1997

HOOFNAGLE JH, DIBISCEGLIE AM: The treatment of chronic viral hepatitis. N Engl J Med 336:347, 1997

HU K-Q et al: The long-term outcomes of patients with compensated hepatitis C virus-related cirrhosis and history of parenteral exposure in the United States. Hepatology 29:1311, 1999

ISHAK K et al: Histologic grading and staging of chronic hepatitis. J Hepatol 22:696, 1995

JOHNSON PJ et al: Meeting report: International autoimmune hepatitis group. Hepatology 18:998, 1993

JOHNSON PJ et al: Azathioprine for long-term maintenance of remission in autoimmune hepatitis. N Engl J Med 333:958, 1995

KENNY-WALSH E et al: Clinical outcomes after hepatitis C infection from contaminated anti-D immune globulin. N Engl J Med 340:1228, 1999

KRAWITT EL: Autoimmune hepatitis. N Engl J Med 334:897, 1996

LAI C-L et al: A one-year trial of lamivudine for chronic hepatitis B. N Engl J Med 339:61, 1998

LAU DT-Y et al: Long-term follow up of patients with chronic hepatitis B treated with interferon alfa. Gastroenterology 113:1660, 1997

LIN S-M et al: Long-term beneficial effect of interferon therapy in patients with chronic hepatitis B virus infection. Hepatology 29:971, 1999

MARCELLIN P et al: Long-term histologic improvement and loss of detectable intrahepatic HCV RNA in patients with chronic hepatitis C and sustained response to interferon alpha therapy. Ann Intern Med 127:875, 1997

MCHUTCHISON JG et al: Interferon alfa-2b alone or in combination with ribavirin as initial treatment for chronic hepatitis C. N Engl J Med 339:1485, 1998

NATIONAL INSTITUTES OF HEALTH CONSENSUS DEVELOPMENT CONFERENCE: Management of hepatitis C. Hepatology 26(Suppl 1):1S, 1997

NATIONAL DIGESTIVE DISEASES INFORMATION CLEARINGHOUSE: Chronic hepatitis C: Current disease management. NIH Publication No. 99-4230, 1999 (www.niddk.nih.gov/health/digest/pubs/chrnhepc.htm)

NEUMANN AU et al: Hepatitis C viral dynamics in vivo and the antiviral efficacy of interferon-α therapy. Science 282:103, 1998

NIEDERAU C et al: Long-term follow-up of HBeAg-positive patients treated with interferon alfa for chronic hepatitis B. N Engl J Med 334:1422, 1996

NIEDERAU C et al: Prognosis of chronic hepatitis C: Results of a large, prospective cohort study. Hepatology 28:1687, 1998

PAYEN J-L et al: Better efficacy of a 12-month interferon alfa-2b retreatment in patients with chronic hepatitis C relapsing after a 6-month treatment: A multicenter, controlled, randomized trial. Hepatology 28:1680, 1998

POYNARD T et al: Natural history of liver fibrosis progression in patients with chronic hepatitis C. Lancet 349:825, 1997

POYNARD T et al: Randomized trial of interferon α2b plus ribavirin for 48 weeks or for 24 weeks versus interferon α2b plus placebo for 48 weeks for treatment of chronic infection with hepatitis C virus. Lancet 352:1426, 1998

ROSENBERG PM et al: Therapy with nucleoside analogues for hepatitis B virus infection. Clin Liver Dis 3:349, 1999

SEEFF LB: Natural history of viral hepatitis, type C. Semin Gastrointest Dis 6:20, 1995

SERFATY L et al: Determinants of outcome of compensated hepatitis C virus-related cirrhosis. Hepatology 27:1435, 1998

TASSOPOULOS NC et al: Efficacy of lamivudine in patients with hepatitis B e antigen-negative/hepatitis B virus DNA-positive (precore mutant) chronic hepatitis B. Hepatology 29:889, 1999

TONG MJ et al: Clinical outcomes after transfusion-associated hepatitis C. N Engl J Med 332:1463, 1995

WESIERSKA-GADEL J et al: Members of the glutathione S-transferase gene family are antigens in autoimmune hepatitis. Gastroenterology 105:1502, 1998

WONG JB et al: Cost-effectiveness of interferon-α2b treatment for hepatitis B e antigen-positive chronic hepatitis B. Ann Intern Med 122:664, 1995

YANO M et al: The long-term pathological evolution of chronic hepatitis C. Hepatology 23:1334, 1996

298

Mark E. Mailliard, Michael F. Sorrell

ALCOHOLIC LIVER DISEASE

Chronic and excessive alcohol ingestion is one of the major causes of liver disease in the western world. Classically, alcoholic liver injury comprises three major forms: (1) fatty liver, (2) alcoholic hepatitis, and (3) cirrhosis. Although cirrhosis is discussed in Chap. 299, it is important to emphasize that rarely does a pure form of liver injury exist by itself. Fatty liver is present in over 90% of binge and heavy drinkers. A much smaller percentage of drinkers progress to alcoholic hepatitis, thought to be a precursor to cirrhosis. Although alcohol is considered a direct hepatotoxin, only 10 to 20% of alcoholics develop alcoholic hepatitis. The explanation for this apparent paradox is unclear but involves complex factors such as gender and heredity.

ETIOLOGY AND PATHOGENESIS Quantity and duration of alcohol intake are the most important risk factors involved in the development of alcoholic liver disease (Table 298-1). The roles of beverage type and pattern of drinking are less clear. Progress of the hepatic injury beyond the fatty liver stage seems to require additional risk factors that remain incompletely defined. Women are more susceptible to alcoholic liver injury than men; they develop advanced liver disease with substantially less alcohol intake. In general, the time it takes to develop liver disease is directly related to the amount of alcohol consumed. It is useful in estimating alcohol consumption to understand that one beer, four ounces of wine, or one ounce of 80% spirits all contain approximately 12 g of alcohol. The threshold for developing severe alcoholic liver disease in men is an intake of >60 to 80 g/d of alcohol for 10 years, while women are at increased risk for developing similar degrees of liver injury by consuming 20 to 40 g/d. Gender-dependent differences in the gastric and hepatic metabolism of alcohol, in addition to poorly understood hormonal factors, likely contribute to the increased susceptibility of women to alcohol-

Table 298-1 Risk Factors for Alcoholic Liver Disease

Risk Factor	Comment
Quantity	In men, 40–80 g/d of ethanol produces fatty liver; 80–160 g/d for 10–20 years causes hepatitis or cirrhosis. Only 15% of alcoholics develop alcoholic liver disease.
Gender	Women exhibit increased susceptibility to alcoholic liver disease at quantities >20 g/d.
Hepatitis C	HCV infection concurrent with alcoholic liver disease is associated with accelerated disease progression, more advanced histology, and decreased survival rates.
Genetics	The genetics of alcohol dehydrogenase, acetaldehyde dehydrogenase, and polymorphisms of cytochrome P4502E1 need confirmation.
Malnutrition	A common misconception. Alcohol hepatoxicity does not require malnutrition. Patients with alcohol hepatitis should receive aggressive attention to nutritional requirements.

induced liver injury. Social, nutritional, immunologic, and host factors have all been postulated to play a part in the development of the pathogenic process.

Chronic infection with hepatitis C (HCV) (Chap. 297) is an important risk factor in the progression and acceleration of alcoholic liver disease. The presence of HCV in patients with severe alcoholic liver disease is increased five- to tenfold above that in a matched control alcoholic population. Patients with both alcoholic liver injury and HCV develop decompensated liver disease at a younger age and have poorer overall survival rates. As a consequence of the overlapping injurious processes secondary to alcohol abuse and HCV infection, patients can develop an increased liver iron burden and rarely, porphyria cutanea tarda.

Our understanding of the pathogenesis of alcoholic liver injury is incomplete. Alcohol is a direct hepatotoxin, but ingestion of alcohol initiates a variety of metabolic responses that influence the final hepatotoxic response. The initial concept of malnutrition as the major pathogenic mechanism has given way to the present understanding that the metabolism of alcohol by the hepatocyte initiates a cascade of events involving production of protein-aldehyde adducts, lipid peroxidation, immunologic events, and cytokine release (Fig. 298-1). The production of cytokines is in large measure responsible for the systemic manifestations of alcoholic hepatitis, e.g., fever, leukocytosis, and anorexia. The degree of fibrosis stimulated by these complex events determines the extent of architectural derangement of the liver after chronic alcohol ingestion.

PATHOLOGY The liver has a limited repertoire in response to injury. Fatty liver is the initial and most common histologic response to increased alcohol ingestion. The accumulation of fat in the perivenular hepatocytes coincides with the location of alcohol dehydrogenase, the major enzyme responsible for alcohol metabolism. Continuing alcohol ingestion results in fat accumulation throughout the entire hepatic lobule. Despite extensive fatty changes and distortion of the hepatocytes with macrovesicular fat, the cessation of drinking results in normalization of hepatic architecture and fat content in the liver. Alcoholic fatty liver has traditionally been regarded as entirely benign; but similar to the spectrum of non-alcoholic steatohepatitis, certain pathologic features such as giant mitochondria, perivenular fibrosis,

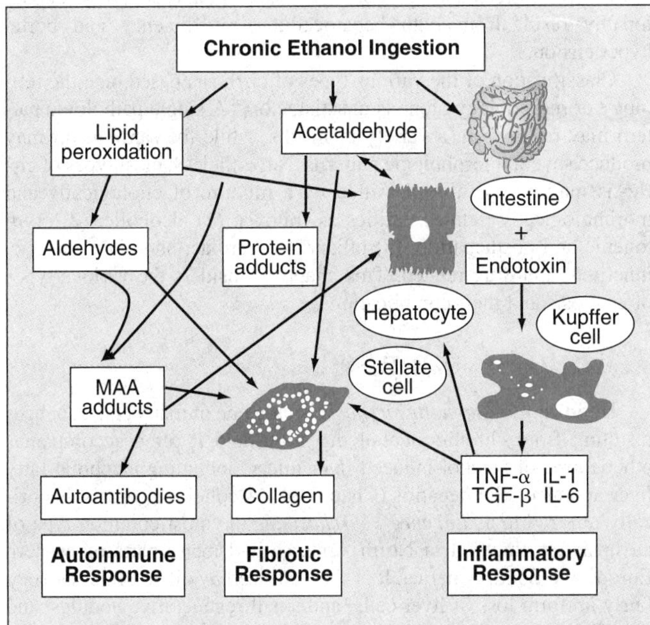

FIGURE 298-1 Biomedical and cellular pathogenesis of liver injury secondary to chronic ethanol ingestion. MAA, malondialdehyde-acetaldehyde; TNF-α, tumor necrosis factor α; TGF-β, transforming growth factor β; IL, interleukin.

and macrovesicular fat may be associated with progressive liver injury.

The transition between fatty liver and the development of alcoholic hepatitis is blurred. The hallmark of alcoholic hepatitis is hepatocyte injury characterized by ballooning degeneration, spotty necrosis, polymorphonuclear infiltration, and fibrosis in the perivenular and perisinusoidal space of Disse. Mallory bodies are often present in florid cases but are neither specific nor necessary to establishing the diagnosis. Alcoholic hepatitis is thought to be a precursor to the development of cirrhosis. However, like fatty liver, it is potentially reversible with cessation of drinking. Cirrhosis is present in up to 50% of patients with biopsy-proven alcoholic hepatitis.

CLINICAL FEATURES The clinical manifestations of alcoholic fatty liver are subtle and characteristically detected as a consequence of the patient's visit for a seemingly unrelated matter. Previously unsuspected hepatomegaly is often the only clinical finding. Occasionally, patients with fatty liver present with right upper quadrant discomfort, tender hepatomegaly, nausea, and jaundice. Differentiation of alcoholic fatty liver from non-alcoholic fatty liver is difficult unless an accurate drinking history is verified. Alcoholism does not respect social and economic class. In every instance where liver disease is present, a thoughtful and sensitive drinking history should be obtained. Alcoholic hepatitis is associated with a wide gamut of clinical features. Fever, spider nevi, jaundice, and abdominal pain simulating an acute abdomen represent the extreme end of the spectrum; but many patients are entirely asymptomatic. Recognition of the clinical features of alcoholic hepatitis is central to the initiation of an effective and appropriate diagnostic and therapeutic strategy.

LABORATORY FEATURES Patients with alcoholic fatty liver are often identified through routine screening tests. The typical laboratory abnormalities are nonspecific and include modest elevations of the aspartate aminotransferase (AST) and alanine aminotransferase (ALT) accompanied by hypertriglyceridemia, hypercholesterolemia, and, occasionally, hyperbilirubinemia. In alcoholic hepatitis and in contrast to other causes of fatty liver, the AST and ALT are usually elevated two- to sevenfold. They rarely are above 400 IU, and the AST/ALT ratio is >1 (Table 298-2). Hyperbilirubinemia is common and is accompanied by modest increases in the alkaline phosphatase. Derangement in hepatocyte synthetic function indicates more serious disease. Hypoalbuminemia and coagulopathy are common in advanced liver injury. The mean corpuscular volume (MCV) and uric acid level are commonly elevated in chronic alcohol abuse. Measurement of the carbohydrate-deficient transferrin (CDT) is superior to the measurement of the gamma-glutamyl transpeptidase (GGTP) or MCV in identifying excessive drinking. Ultrasonography is useful in detecting fatty infiltration of the liver and determining liver size. The demonstration by ultrasound of portal vein flow reversal, ascites, and intra-abdominal collaterals indicates serious liver injury with less potential for complete reversal of liver disease.

PROGNOSIS Critically ill patients with alcoholic hepatitis have short-term mortality rates approaching 70%. Severe alcoholic hepatitis

Table 298-2 Laboratory Diagnosis of Alcoholic Fatty Liver and Alcoholic Hepatitis

Test	Comment
AST	Increased two- to seven-fold, less than 400 U/L, greater than ALT
ALT	Increased two- to seven-fold, less than 400 U/L
AST/ALT	Usually > 1
GGT	Not specific to alcohol, easily inducible, elevated in all forms of fatty liver
CDT	Increased in alcoholism, irrespective of liver disease
MCV	Macrocytosis specific, but insensitive marker of alcoholism

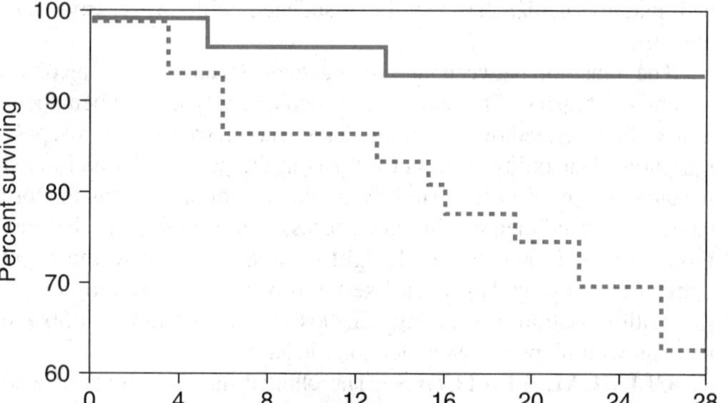

FIGURE 298-2 Effect of glucocorticoid therapy of severe alcoholic hepatitis on short-term survival. Prednisolone, solid line; placebo, broken line. *(Adapted from Carithers et al.)*

is heralded by coagulopathy (prothrombin time >5 s), anemia, serum albumin concentrations below 2.5 mg/dL, serum bilirubin levels >8 mg/dL, renal failure, and ascites. A discriminant function calculated as 4.6 × [prothrombin time − control(seconds)] + serum bilirubin (mg/dL) can identify patients with a poor prognosis (discriminant function >32). The presence of ascites, variceal hemorrhage, deep encephalopathy, or hepatorenal syndrome predicts a dismal prognosis. The pathologic stage of the injury can be helpful in predicting prognosis. Liver biopsy should be performed whenever possible to confirm the diagnosis, to establish potential reversibility of the liver disease, and to guide the therapeutic decisions.

TREATMENT Complete abstinence from alcohol is the cornerstone in the treatment of alcoholic liver disease. Improved survival rates and the potential for reversal of histologic injury regardless of the initial clinical presentation are associated with total avoidance of alcoholic ingestion. Referral of patients to experienced alcohol counselors and/or alcohol treatment programs should be routine in the management of patients with alcoholic liver disease. Attention should be directed to the nutritional and psychosocial states during the evaluation and treatment periods. Because of data suggesting that the pathogenic mechanisms in alcoholic hepatitis involve cytokine release and the perpetuation of injury by immunologic processes, glucocorticoids have been extensively evaluated in the treatment of alcoholic hepatitis. Patients with severe alcoholic hepatitis, defined as a discriminant function >32, were given prednisone, 40 mg/d, or prednisolone, 32 mg/d, for 4 weeks followed by a steroid taper (Fig. 298-2). Exclusion criteria included active gastrointestinal bleeding, sepsis, renal failure, or pancreatitis. Because of inordinate surgical mortality rates and the high rates of recidivism after transplantation, patients with alcoholic hepatitis are not candidates for immediate liver transplantation. The transplant candidacy of these patients should be reevaluated after a defined period of sobriety.

BIBLIOGRAPHY

CARITHERS RL et al: Methylprednisolone therapy in patients with severe alcoholic hepatitis. Ann Intern Med 110:685, 1989

LEEVY CM: Fatty liver: A study of 270 patients with biopsy proven fatty liver and a review of the literature. Medicine 41:249, 1962

SCHIFF ER: Hepatitis C and alcohol. Hepatology 26(3, Suppl 1):395, 1997

TELI MR et al: Determinants of progression to cirrhosis or fibrosis in pure alcoholic fatty liver. Lancet 346:987, 1995

299

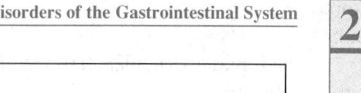

Raymond T. Chung, Daniel K. Podolsky

CIRRHOSIS AND ITS COMPLICATIONS

ALT alanine aminotransferase
AMA antimitochondrial antibody
AST asparate aminotransferase
BCKDC branched chain–ketoacid dehydrogenase complex
CNS central nervous system
CREST calcinosis, Raynaud's phenomenon, esophageal dysmotility, sclerodactyly, telangiectasia
GABA γ-aminobutyric acid
HBV hepatitis B virus
HCV hepatitis C virus
KGDC α-ketoglutarate dehydrogenase complex
PBC primary biliary cirrhosis
PDC pyruvate dehydrogenase complex
SAAG serum-ascites albumin gradient
SBC secondary biliary cirrhosis
SBP spontaneous bacterial peritonitis
TIPS transjugular intrahepatic portosystemic shunt

Cirrhosis is a pathologically defined entity that is associated with a spectrum of characteristic clinical manifestations. The cardinal pathologic features reflect irreversible chronic injury of the hepatic parenchyma and include extensive fibrosis in association with the formation of regenerative nodules. These features result from hepatocyte necrosis, collapse of the supporting reticulin network with subsequent connective tissue deposition, distortion of the vascular bed, and nodular regeneration of remaining liver parenchyma. The central event leading to hepatic fibrosis is activation of the hepatic stellate cell. Upon activation by factors released by hepatocytes and Kupffer cells, the stellate cell assumes a myofibroblast-like conformation and, under the influence of cytokines such as transforming growth factor β (TGF-β), produces fibril-forming type I collagen. The precise point at which fibrosis becomes irreversible is unclear. The pathologic process should be viewed as a final common pathway of many types of chronic liver injury. Clinical features of cirrhosis derive from the morphologic alterations and often reflect the severity of hepatic damage rather than the etiology of the underlying liver disease. Loss of functioning hepatocellular mass may lead to jaundice, edema, coagulopathy, and a variety of metabolic abnormalities; fibrosis and distorted vasculature lead to portal hypertension and its sequelae, including gastroesophageal varices and splenomegaly. Ascites and hepatic encephalopathy result from both hepatocellular insufficiency and portal hypertension.

Classification of the various types of cirrhosis based on either etiology or morphology alone is unsatisfactory. A single pathologic pattern may result from a variety of insults, while the same insult may produce several morphologic patterns. Nevertheless, most types of cirrhosis may be usefully classified by a mixture of etiologically and morphologically defined entities as follows: (1) alcoholic; (2) cryptogenic and posthepatitic; (3) biliary; (4) cardiac; and (5) metabolic, inherited, and drug-related. This chapter considers the various types of cirrhosis and their complications.

ALCOHOLIC CIRRHOSIS

Definition *Alcoholic cirrhosis* is only one of many consequences resulting from chronic alcohol ingestion, and it often accompanies other forms of alcohol-induced liver injury, including alcoholic fatty liver and alcoholic hepatitis (Chap. 298). Alcoholic cirrhosis, historically referred to as *Laennec's cirrhosis*, is the most common type of cirrhosis encountered in North America and many parts of western Europe and South America. It is characterized by diffuse fine scarring, fairly uniform loss of liver cells, and small regenerative nodules, and therefore it is sometimes referred to as *micronodular cirrhosis*. However, micronodular cirrhosis may also result from other types of liver injury (e.g., following jejunoileal bypass), and thus alcoholic cirrhosis and micronodular cirrhosis are not necessarily synonymous. Conversely, alcoholic cirrhosis may progress to macronodular cirrhosis with time.

Etiology See Chap. 298, "Alcoholic Liver Disease."

Pathology and Pathogenesis With continued alcohol intake and destruction of hepatocytes, fibroblasts (including activated hepatic stellate cells that have transformed into myofibroblasts with contractile properties) appear at the site of injury and deposit collagen. Weblike septa of connective tissue appear in periportal and pericentral zones and eventually connect portal triads and central veins. This fine connective tissue network surrounds small masses of remaining liver cells, which regenerate and form nodules. Although regeneration occurs within the small remnants of parenchyma, cell loss generally exceeds replacement. With continuing hepatocyte destruction and collagen deposition, the liver shrinks in size, acquires a nodular appearance, and becomes hard as "end-stage" cirrhosis develops. Although alcoholic cirrhosis is usually a progressive disease, appropriate therapy and strict avoidance of alcohol may arrest the disease at most stages and permit functional improvement. In addition, there is strong evidence that concomitant chronic hepatitis C virus (HCV) infection significantly accelerates development of alcoholic cirrhosis.

Clinical Features • *Signs and symptoms* Alcoholic cirrhosis may be clinically silent, and many cases (10 to 40%) are discovered incidentally at laparotomy or autopsy. In many cases symptoms are insidious in onset, occurring usually after 10 or more years of excessive alcohol use and progressing slowly over subsequent weeks and months. Anorexia and malnutrition lead to weight loss and a reduction in skeletal muscle mass. The patient may experience easy bruising, increasing weakness, and fatigue. Eventually the clinical manifestations of hepatocellular dysfunction and portal hypertension ensue, including progressive jaundice, bleeding from gastroesophageal varices, ascites, and encephalopathy. The abrupt onset of one of these complications may be the first event prompting the patient to seek medical attention. In other cases, cirrhosis first becomes evident when the patient requires treatment of symptoms related to alcoholic hepatitis.

A firm, nodular liver may be an early sign of disease; the liver may be either enlarged, normal, or decreased in size. Other frequent findings include jaundice, palmar erythema, spider angiomas, parotid and lacrimal gland enlargement, clubbing of fingers, splenomegaly, muscle wasting, and ascites with or without peripheral edema. Men may have decreased body hair and/or gynecomastia and testicular atrophy, which, like the cutaneous findings, result from disturbances in hormonal metabolism, including increased peripheral formation of estrogen due to diminished hepatic clearance of the precursor androstenedione. Testicular atrophy may reflect hormonal abnormalities or the toxic effect of alcohol on the testes. In women, signs of virilization or menstrual irregularities may occasionally be encountered. Dupuytren's contractures resulting from fibrosis of the palmar fascia with resulting flexion contracture of the digits are associated with alcoholism but are not specifically related to cirrhosis.

Although the cirrhotic patient may stabilize if drinking is discontinued, over a period of years, the patient may become emaciated, weak, and chronically jaundiced. Ascites and other signs of portal hypertension may become increasingly prominent. Ultimately, most patients with advanced cirrhosis die in hepatic coma, commonly precipitated by hemorrhage from esophageal varices or intercurrent infection. Progressive renal dysfunction often complicates the terminal phase of the illness.

Laboratory findings In advanced alcoholic liver disease, abnormalities of laboratory tests are more common. Anemia may result from acute and chronic gastrointestinal blood loss, coexistent nutritional deficiency (notably of folic acid and vitamin B_{12}), hypersplenism, and a direct suppressive effect of alcohol on the bone marrow. Hemolytic anemia, presumably due to effects of hypercholesterolemia or erythrocyte membranes resulting in unusual spurlike projections (acanthocytosis), has been described in some alcoholics with cirrhosis. Mild or pronounced hyperbilirubinemia may be found, usually in association with varying elevations of serum alkaline phosphatase levels. Levels of serum AST (asparate aminotransferase) are frequently elevated, but levels $>5\mu$kat (300 units) are unusual and should prompt one to look for other coincident or complicating factors. In contrast to viral hepatitis, the serum AST is usually disproportionately elevated relative to ALT (alanine aminotransferase), i.e., AST/ALT ratio >2. This discrepancy in alcoholic liver disease may result from the proportionally greater inhibition of ALT synthesis by ethanol, which may be partially reversed by pyridoxal phosphate.

The serum prothrombin time is frequently prolonged, reflecting reduced synthesis of clotting proteins, most notably the vitamin K–dependent factors (see "Coagulopathy," below). The serum albumin level is usually depressed, while serum globulins are increased. Hypoalbuminemia reflects in part overall impairment in hepatic protein synthesis, while hyperglobulinemia is thought to result from nonspecific stimulation of the reticuloendothelial system. Elevated blood ammonia levels in patients with hepatic encephalopathy reflect diminished hepatic clearance because of impaired liver function and shunting of portal venous blood around the cirrhotic liver into the systemic circulation (see "Hepatic Encephalopathy," below).

A variety of metabolic disturbances may be detected. Glucose intolerance due to endogenous insulin resistance may be present; however, clinical diabetes is uncommon. Central hyperventilation may lead to respiratory alkalosis in patients with cirrhosis. Dietary deficiency and increased urinary losses lead to hypomagnesemia and hypophosphatemia. In patients with ascites and dilutional hyponatremia, hypokalemia may occur from increased urinary potassium losses due in part to hyperaldosteronism. Prerenal azotemia is also observed in such patients.

Diagnosis Alcoholic cirrhosis should be strongly suspected in patients with a history of prolonged or excessive alcohol intake and physical signs of chronic liver disease. However, since only 10 to 15% of individuals with excessive alcohol intake develop cirrhosis, other causes and types of liver disease may have to be excluded. The clinical features and laboratory findings are usually sufficient to provide reasonable indication of the presence and extent of hepatic injury. Although a percutaneous needle biopsy of the liver is not usually necessary to confirm the typical findings of alcoholic hepatitis or cirrhosis, it may be helpful in distinguishing patients with less advanced liver disease from those with cirrhosis and in excluding other forms of liver injury such as viral hepatitis. Biopsy may also be helpful as a diagnostic tool in evaluating patients with clinical findings suggestive of alcoholic liver disease who deny alcohol intake. In patients with features of cholestasis, ultrasonography may be appropriate to exclude the presence of extrahepatic biliary obstruction. When the clinical status of an otherwise stable cirrhotic patient deteriorates without an obvious explanation, complicating conditions, such as infection, portal vein thrombosis, and hepatocellular carcinoma, should be sought.

Prognosis Abstinence from alcohol as well as early and appropriate medical care can decrease long-term morbidity and mortality and delay or prevent the appearance of further complications. Patients who have had a major complication of cirrhosis and who continue to drink have a 5-year survival of less than 50%. However, those patients who remain abstinent have a substantially better prognosis. In general, the overall outlook in patients with advanced liver disease remains poor; most of these patients eventually die as a result of massive variceal hemorrhage and/or profound hepatic encephalopathy.

℞ TREATMENT Alcoholic cirrhosis is a serious illness that requires long-term medical supervision and careful management. Therapy of the underlying liver disease is largely supportive. Specific treatment is directed at particular complications such as variceal bleeding and ascites (see below). While some studies suggest that administration of glucocorticoids in moderately large doses for 4 weeks is helpful in patients with severe alcoholic hepatitis and encephalopathy, these drugs have no role in the treatment of established alcoholic cirrhosis. While one study suggested a mortality benefit for the antifibrotic agent colchicine in alcoholic cirrhosis, it has not yet been reproduced; thus colchicine cannot be routinely recommended.

The patient should be made to realize that there is no medication that will protect the liver against the effects of further alcohol ingestion. Therefore, alcohol should be absolutely forbidden. An important component of the complete care of such patients is encouragement to become involved in an appropriate alcohol counseling program.

All medicines must be administered with caution in the patient with cirrhosis, especially those eliminated or modified through hepatic metabolism or biliary pathways. In particular, care must be taken to avoid overzealous use of drugs that may directly or indirectly precipitate complications of cirrhosis. For example, vigorous treatment of ascites with diuretics may result in electrolyte abnormalities or hypovolemia, which can lead to coma. Similarly, even modest doses of sedatives can lead to deepening encephalopathy. Aspirin should be avoided in patients with cirrhosis because of its effects on coagulation and gastric mucosa. Acetaminophen should be used with caution and in doses of less than 2 g/day. Patients who drink alcohol are more sensitive to the hepatotoxic effects of acetaminophen, probably due to increased metabolism of the drug to toxic intermediates and decreased glutathione levels.

POSTHEPATITIC AND CRYPTOGENIC CIRRHOSIS

Definition Posthepatitic or postnecrotic cirrhosis represents the final common pathway of many types of chronic liver disease. *Coarsely nodular* and *multilobular cirrhosis* are terms synonymous with posthepatitic cirrhosis. The term *cryptogenic cirrhosis* has been used interchangeably with postpathepatitic cirrhosis, but this designation should be reserved for those cases in which the etiology of cirrhosis is unknown (approximately 10% of all patients with cirrhosis).

Etiology *Posthepatitic cirrhosis* is a morphologic term referring to a defined stage of advanced chronic liver injury of both specific and unknown (cryptogenic) causes. Epidemiologic and serologic evidence suggest that viral hepatitis (hepatitis B or hepatitis C) may be an antecedent factor in from one-fourth to three-fourths of cases of apparently cryptogenic posthepatitic cirrhosis. In areas where hepatitis B virus (HBV) infection is endemic (e.g., Southeast Asia, sub-Saharan Africa), up to 15% of the population may acquire the infection in early childhood, and cirrhosis may ultimately develop in one-fourth of these chronic carriers. Although HBV infection is much less prevalent in the United States, it is relatively common among certain high-risk groups (e.g., persons with multiple sexual partners, especially men who have sex with men, injection drug users) and contributes to an increased incidence of cirrhosis. In the United States, HCV infection accounts for many cases of cirrhosis following blood transfusions. Before routine screening of blood donors was introduced, hepatitis C occurred in 5 to 10% of blood recipients. Following infection, cirrhosis may ultimately develop in more than 20% of individuals after 20 years. More than half of patients who would previously have been designated as having cryptogenic chronic liver disease have evidence of HCV infection. Increasing recognition of the progressive nature of nonalcoholic steatohepatitis has revealed that a large portion of cases previously designated cryptogenic cirrhosis may be attributable to this disorder (Chap. 300). Posthepatitic cirrhosis may also develop in patients with autoimmune hepatitis (Chap. 297).

The most common causes of cirrhosis in the United States, which ultimately lead to liver transplantation, include chronic HCV infection, alcohol, primary biliary cirrhosis, primary sclerosing cholangitis, and nonalcoholic steatohepatitis (NASH). Less common causes of posthepatitic cirrhosis, including drugs and toxins, are listed in Table 299-1.

Pathology The posthepatitic liver is typically shrunken in size, distorted in shape, and composed of nodules of liver cells separated by dense and broad bands of fibrosis. The microscopic picture is consistent with the gross impression. Posthepatitic cirrhosis is characterized morphologically by (1) extensive confluent loss of liver cells, (2) stromal collapse and fibrosis resulting in broad bands of connective tissue containing the remains of many portal triads, and (3) irregular nodules of regenerating hepatocytes, varying in size from microscopic to several centimeters in diameter.

Table 299-1 Causes of Cirrhosis and/or Chronic Liver Disease

Infectious Diseases	**Drugs and Toxins** (Chap. 296)
Brucellosis (Chap. 160)	Alcohol (Chap. 298)
Capillariasis (Chap. 220)	Amioradone
Echinococcosis (Chap. 223)	Arsenicals
Schistosomiasis (Chap. 222)	Oral contraceptives (Budd-Chiari)
Toxoplasmosis (Chap. 217)	Pyrrolidizine alkaloids (venoocclusive disease)
Viral hepatitis [hepatitis B, C, D; cytomegalovirus; Epstein-Barr virus (Chaps. 295, 184, 185)]	**Other Causes**
Inherited and Metabolic Disorders (See Chap. 300)	Biliary obstruction (chronic) (Chap. 302)
α_1-Antitrypsin deficiency (Chap. 300)	Cystic fibrosis (Chap. 257)
Alagille's syndrome (Chap. 292)	Graft-versus-host disease (Chap. 115)
Biliary atresia (Chap. 302)	Jejunoileal bypass (Chap. 43)
Familial intrahepatic cholestasis (FIC) types 1-3 (Chap. 302)	Nonalcoholic steatohepatitis (Chap. 300)
Fanconi's syndrome (Chap. 349)	Primary biliary cirrhosis
Galactosemia (Chap. 350)	Primary sclerosing cholangitis (Chap. 302)
Gaucher's disease (Chap. 349)	Sarcoidosis (Chap. 318)
Glycogen storage disease (Chap. 350)	
Hemochromatosis (Chap. 345)	
Hereditary fructose intolerance (Chap. 350)	
Hereditary tyrosinemia (Chap. 352)	
Wilson's disease (Chap. 348)	

Clinical Features In patients with cirrhosis of known etiology in whom there is progression to a posthepatitic stage, the clinical manifestations are an extension of those resulting from the initial disease process. Usually clinical symptoms are related to portal hypertension and its sequelae, such as ascites, splenomegaly, hypersplenism, encephalopathy, and bleeding gastroesophageal varices. The hematologic and liver function abnormalities resemble those seen with other types of cirrhosis. In a few patients with posthepatitic cirrhosis, the diagnosis may be made incidentally at operation, at postmortem, or by a needle biopsy of the liver performed to investigate abnormal liver function tests or hepatomegaly.

Diagnosis and Prognosis Posthepatitic cirrhosis should be suspected in patients with signs and symptoms of cirrhosis or portal hypertension. Needle or operative liver biopsies confirm the diagnosis, although nonuniformity of the pathologic process may result in sampling errors. The diagnosis of cryptogenic cirrhosis is reserved for those patients in whom no known etiology can be demonstrated. About 75% of patients have progressive disease despite supportive therapy and die within 1 to 5 years from complications, including variceal hemorrhage, hepatic encephalopathy, or superimposed hepatocellular carcinoma.

℞ TREATMENT Management is usually limited to treatment of the complications of portal hypertension, including control of ascites, avoidance of drugs or excessive protein intake that may induce hepatic coma, and prompt treatment of infections (see below). In patients with asymptomatic cirrhosis, expectant management alone is appropriate. In those patients in whom posthepatitic cirrhosis has developed as a result of a treatable condition, therapy directed at the primary disorder may limit further progression (e.g., Wilson's disease, hemochromatosis).

BILIARY CIRRHOSIS

Biliary cirrhosis results from injury to or prolonged obstruction of either the intrahepatic or extrahepatic biliary system. It is associated with impaired biliary excretion, destruction of hepatic parenchyma, and progressive fibrosis. Primary biliary cirrhosis (PBC) is characterized by chronic inflammation and fibrous obliteration of intrahepatic bile ductules. Secondary biliary cirrhosis (SBC) is the result of longstanding obstruction of the larger extrahepatic ducts. Although primary and secondary biliary cirrhosis are separate pathophysiologic entities with respect to the initial insult, many clinical features are similar.

PRIMARY BILIARY CIRRHOSIS Etiology and Pathogenesis The cause of PBC remains unknown. Several observations suggest that a disordered immune response may be involved. PBC is frequently associated with a variety of disorders presumed to be autoimmune in nature, such as the syndrome of *c*alcinosis, *R*aynaud's phenomenon, *e*sophageal dysmotility, *s*clerodactyly, *t*elangiectasia (CREST); the sicca syndrome (dry eyes and dry mouth); autoimmune thyroiditis; type 1 diabetes mellitus; and IgA deficiency.

Most important, a circulating IgG antimitochondrial antibody (AMA) is detected in more than 90% of patients with PBC and only rarely in other forms of liver disease. It has been demonstrated that these autoantibodies recognize three to five inner mitochondrial membrane proteins identified as enzymes of the pyruvate dehydrogenase complex (PDC), the branched chain–ketoacid dehydrogenase complex (BCKDC), and the α-ketoglutarate dehydrogenase complex (KGDC). The major autoantigen in PBC (found in 90% of patients) has been identified as the 74-kDa E2 component of the PDC, dihydrolipoamide acetyltransferase. The antibodies are directed to a region essential for binding of a lipoic acid cofactor and inhibit the overall enzymatic activity of the PDC. Other AMA autoantibodies in PNC patients are directed to similar constituents of BCKDC and KGDC and also inhibit their enzymatic function. It remains unclear whether these properties have a direct pathogenetic role in the development of PBC. In addition to AMA, elevated serum levels of IgM and cryoproteins consisting of immune complexes capable of activating the alternative complement pathway are found in 80 to 90% of patients. Aberrant expression of major histocompatibility complex class II molecules has been found on biliary epithelium in association with PBC, suggesting that these cells may serve as antigen-presenting cells in this setting. Lymphocytes are prominent in the portal regions and surround damaged bile ducts. These histologic findings resemble those noted in graft-versus-host disease following bone marrow transplantation and suggest that damage to bile ducts may be immunologically mediated, perhaps reflecting a defect in a suppressor cell population.

Pathology PBC is divided into four stages based on morphologic findings. The earliest recognizable lesion (stage I), termed *chronic nonsuppurative destructive cholangitis*, is a necrotizing inflammatory process of the portal triads. It is characterized by destruction of medium and small bile ducts, a dense infiltrate of acute and chronic inflammatory cells, mild fibrosis, and occasionally, bile stasis. At times, periductal granulomas and lymph follicles are found adjacent to affected bile ducts. Subsequently, the inflammatory infiltrate becomes less prominent, the number of bile ducts is reduced, and smaller bile ductules proliferate (stage II). Progression over a period of months to years leads to a decrease in interlobular ducts, loss of liver cells, and expansion of periportal fibrosis into a network of connective tissue scars (stage III). Ultimately, cirrhosis, which may be micronodular or macronodular, develops (stage IV).

Clinical Features • ***Signs and symptoms*** Many patients with PBC are asymptomatic, and the disease is initially detected on the basis of elevated serum alkaline phosphatase levels during routine screening. The majority of such patients remain asymptomatic for prolonged periods, although most ultimately develop progressive liver injury.

Among patients with symptomatic disease, 90% are women age 35 to 60. Often the earliest symptom is pruritus, which may be either generalized or limited initially to the palms and soles. In addition, fatigue is commonly a prominent early symptom. After several months or years, jaundice and gradual darkening of the exposed areas of the skin (melanosis) may ensue. Other early clinical manifestations of PBC reflect impaired bile excretion. These include steatorrhea and the malabsorption of lipid-soluble vitamins. Protracted elevation of serum lipids, especially cholesterol, leads to subcutaneous lipid deposition around the eyes (xanthelasmas) and over joints and tendons (xanthomas). Over a period of months to years, the itching, jaundice, and hyperpigmentation slowly worsen. Eventually, signs of hepatocellular failure and portal hypertension develop and ascites appears. Progression may be quite variable. Whereas a proportion of asymptomatic patients may show no signs of progression for a decade or longer, in others, death due to hepatic insufficiency may occur within 5 to 10 years after the first signs of the illness. Such decompensation is often precipitated by uncontrolled variceal hemorrhage or infection.

Physical examination may be entirely normal in the early phase of the disease, when patients are asymptomatic or pruritus is the sole complaint. Later, there may be jaundice of varying intensity, hyperpigmentation of the exposed skin areas, xanthelasmas and tendinous and planar xanthomas, moderate to striking hepatomegaly, splenomegaly, and clubbing of the fingers. Bone tenderness, signs of vertebral compression, ecchymoses, glossitis, and dermatitis may all be noted. Clinical evidence of the sicca syndrome can be found in as many as 75% of patients, and serologic evidence of autoimmune thyroid disease in 25%. Other conditions encountered with increased frequency include rheumatoid arthritis, CREST syndrome, keratoconjunctivitis sicca, IgA deficiency, type 1 diabetes mellitus, scleroderma, pernicious anemia, and renal tubular acidosis. Bone disease is often a significant problem encountered over the course of the disease. While osteomalacia occurs due to diminished vitamin D absorption, accelerated osteoporosis in this patient population (the majority of whom are postmenopausal women) is even more common.

Laboratory findings PBC is increasingly diagnosed at a presymptomatic stage, prompted by the finding of a twofold or greater elevation of the serum alkaline phosphatase during routine screening. Serum 5′-nucleotidase activity and γ-glutamyl transpeptidase levels are also elevated. In this setting, serum bilirubin is usually normal and aminotransferase levels minimally increased. The diagnosis is supported by a positive AMA test (titer $>$ 1:40). The latter is both relatively specific and sensitive; a positive test is found in over 90% of symptomatic patients and is present in fewer than 5% of patients with other liver diseases. As the disease evolves, the serum bilirubin level rises progressively and may reach 510 μmol/L (30 mg/dL) or more in the final stages. Serum aminotransferase values rarely exceed 2.5 to 3.3 μkat (150 to 200 units). Hyperlipidemia is common, and a striking increase of the serum unesterified cholesterol is often noted. An abnormal serum lipoprotein (lipoprotein X) may be present in PBC but is not specific and appears in other cholestatic conditions. A deficiency of bile salts in the intestine leads to moderate steatorrhea and impaired absorption of the fat-soluble vitamins and hypoprothrombinemia. Patients with PBC have elevated liver copper levels, but this finding is not specific and is found in all disorders in which there is prolonged cholestasis.

Diagnosis PBC should be considered in middle-aged women with unexplained pruritus or an elevated serum alkaline phosphatase and in whom there may be other clinical or laboratory features of protracted impairment of biliary excretion. Although a positive serum AMA determination provides important diagnostic evidence, false-positive results do occur; therefore, liver biopsy should be performed to confirm the diagnosis. Rarely, the AMA test may be negative in patients with histologic features of PBC. Frequently, patients have antibodies to the E2 protein in tests using these specific antigens. In some cases with histologic features of PBC and a negative AMA, antinuclear or smooth-muscle antibodies are present (as in autoimmune hepatitis), and the designation *autoimmune cholangitis* is applied. The natural history of this entity, however, appears to resemble that of PBC. If the AMA test is negative, the biliary tract should be evaluated to exclude primary sclerosing cholangitis and remediable extrahepatic biliary tract obstruction, especially in view of the frequent presence of coexisting cholelithiasis.

℞ TREATMENT While there is no specific therapy for PBC, ursodiol has shown to improve biochemical and histologic features and might improve survival, particularly liver transplantation–free survival (although this remains unproven). Ursodiol should be given in doses of 10 to 15 mg/kg per day, but lower doses are sometimes just as effective in reducing serum alkaline phosphatase and aminotransferase levels. Ursodiol should be given with food and can be taken in a single dose daily. Side effects are rare: gastrointestinal intolerance (bloating, indigestion) and skin rashes occur but are uncommon. Isolated instances of severe exacerbation of pruritus have been reported in patients with advanced disease. Ursodiol probably works by replacing the endogenously produced hydrophobic bile acids with urosdeoxycholate, a hydrophilic and relatively nontoxic bile acid.

Unfortunately, ursodiol does not prevent ultimate progression of PBC, and the only established "cure" is liver transplantation. Results of liver transplantation for PBC are excellent, survival exceeding that for patients receiving transplantation for most other forms of end-stage liver disease. Recurrence of PBC after liver transplantation has been reported but is uncommon, and the recurrent disease is only slowly progressive. Most patients remain AMA positive after transplantation, and as many as 25% will have histologic features of PBC on liver biopsy after 5 years. Other therapies such as glucocorticoids, colchicine, methotrexate, azathioprine, cyclosporine, and tacrolimus have been reported as effective in small cases series, but none have shown to be effective in adequately controlled trials.

Relief of symptoms is also an important part of management of PBC. As noted, ursodiol may be helpful in controlling symptoms and improving the patient's sense of well-being. Although the mechanism of the protracted pruritus is not entirely clear, cholestyramine, an oral bile salt–sequestering resin, may be helpful in doses of 8 to 12 g/d to decrease both pruritus and hypercholesterolemia. Rifampin, opiate antagonists, ondansetron, plasmapheresis, and ultraviolet light have all been tried for control of pruritus, with varying results. Steatorrhea can be reduced by a low-fat diet and substituting medium-chain triglycerides for dietary long-chain triglycerides. Fat-soluble vitamins A and K should be given by parenteral injection at regular intervals to prevent or correct night blindness and hypoprothrombinemia, respectively. Zinc supplementation may be necessary if night blindness is refractory to vitamin A therapy. An important part of management of PBC and any cholestatic liver disease is assessment and treatment of osteoporosis and osteomalacia. Patients should be screened periodically by bone densitometry and treated as needed with calcium supplements, estrogen, and/or the newer bisphosphonate agents (e.g., alendronate). Progression of PBC leads to the typical complications of advanced liver disease (see below).

SECONDARY BILIARY CIRRHOSIS **Etiology** SBC results from prolonged partial or total obstruction of the common bile duct or its major branches. In adults, obstruction is most frequently caused by postoperative strictures or gallstones, usually with superimposed infectious cholangitis. Chronic pancreatitis may lead to biliary stricture and secondary cirrhosis. SBC is also an important complication of primary sclerosing cholangitis, a progressive immunologic disorder of the intrahepatic and extrahepatic biliary tree (Chap. 302). Patients with malignant tumors of the common bile duct or pancreas rarely survive long enough to develop SBC. In children, congenital biliary atresia and cystic fibrosis are common causes of SBC. Choledochal cysts, if unrecognized, may also be a rare cause of SBC.

Pathology and Pathogenesis Unrelieved obstruction of the extrahepatic bile ducts leads to (1) bile stasis and focal areas of centrilobular necrosis followed by periportal necrosis, (2) proliferation and dilatation of the portal bile ducts and ductules, (3) sterile or infected cholangitis with accumulation of polymorphonuclear infiltrates around bile ducts, and (4) progressive expansion of portal tracts by edema and fibrosis. Extravasation of bile from ruptured interlobular bile ducts into areas of periportal necrosis leads to the formation of "bile lakes" surrounded by cholesterol-rich pseudoxanthomatous cells. As in other forms of cirrhosis, injury is accompanied by regeneration in residual parenchyma. These changes gradually lead to a finely nodular cirrhosis. In general, at least 3 to 12 months is required for biliary obstruction to result in cirrhosis. Relief of the obstruction is frequently accompanied by biochemical and morphologic improvement.

Clinical Features The symptoms, signs, and biochemical findings of SBC are similar to those of PBC. Jaundice and pruritus are usually the most prominent features. In addition, fever and/or right upper quadrant pain, reflecting bouts of cholangitis or biliary colic, are typical. The manifestations of portal hypertension are found only in advanced cases. SBC should be considered in any patient with clinical and laboratory evidence of prolonged obstruction to bile flow, especially when there is a history of previous biliary tract surgery or gallstones, bouts of ascending cholangitis, or right upper quadrant pain. Cholangiography (either percutaneous or endoscopic) usually demonstrates the underlying pathologic process. Liver biopsy, although not always necessary from a clinical standpoint, can document the development of cirrhosis.

℞ TREATMENT Relief of obstruction to bile flow, by either endoscopic or surgical means, is the most important step in the prevention and therapy of SBC. Effective decompression of the biliary tract results in a significant improvement in both symptoms and survival, even in patients with established cirrhosis. When obstruction cannot be relieved, as in sclerosing cholangitis, antibiotics may be helpful acutely in controlling superimposed infection or, when administered on a chronic basis, as prophylactic therapy in suppressing recurring episodes of ascending cholangitis. Without relief of obstruction, there is a steady progression to end-stage cirrhosis and its terminal manifestations.

CARDIAC CIRRHOSIS

Definition Prolonged, severe right-sided congestive heart failure may lead to chronic liver injury and cardiac cirrhosis. The characteristic pathologic features of fibrosis and regenerative nodules distinguish cardiac cirrhosis from both reversible passive congestion of the liver due to acute heart failure and acute hepatocellular necrosis ("ischemic hepatitis" or "shock liver") resulting from systemic hypotension and hypoperfusion of the liver.

Etiology and Pathology In right-sided heart failure, retrograde transmission of elevated venous pressure via the inferior vena cava and hepatic veins leads to congestion of the liver. Hepatic sinusoids become dilated and engorged with blood, and the liver becomes tensely swollen. With prolonged passive congestion and ischemia from poor perfusion secondary to reduced cardiac output, necrosis of centrilobular hepatocytes ensues and leads to fibrosis in these central areas. Ultimately, centrilobular fibrosis develops, with collagen extending outward in a characteristic stellate pattern from the central vein. Gross examination of the liver shows alternating red (congested) and pale (fibrotic) areas, a pattern often referred to as "nutmeg liver." Improvement in management of cardiac disorders, particularly advances in surgical treatment, has reduced the frequency of cardiac cirrhosis.

Clinical Features A range of abnormalities of liver function tests may be found, though none is uniformly present. The serum bilirubin is usually only mildly increased and may be predominantly either conjugated or unconjugated. Mild to moderate elevation in alkaline phosphatase level and prothrombin time prolongation are sometimes present. The AST level is typically mildly elevated but may be transiently very high following a period of marked systemic hypotension (shock liver), when the clinical picture can mimic acute viral or drug-induced hepatitis. In cases of tricuspid insufficiency the liver may be pulsatile, but this finding disappears as cirrhosis develops. With prolonged right-sided heart failure the liver becomes enlarged, firm, and usually nontender. The signs and symptoms of heart failure usually overshadow the liver disease. Bleeding from esophageal varices is rare, but chronic encephalopathy may be prominent, with a waxing and waning course reflecting variations in the severity of right-sided heart failure. Ascites and peripheral edema, often primarily related to the underlying cardiac dysfunction, may be worsened by the superimposed liver disease.

Diagnosis The presence of a firm, enlarged liver with signs of chronic liver disease in a patient with valvular heart disease, constrictive pericarditis, or cor pulmonale of long duration (>10 years) should suggest cardiac cirrhosis. Liver biopsy can confirm the diagnosis but is usually contraindicated because of coagulopathy or ascites. Coexistent chronic heart and liver disease should also raise the possibility of hemochromatosis (Chap. 345), amyloidosis (Chap. 319), or other infiltrative diseases.

Budd-Chiari syndrome resulting from the occlusion of the hepatic veins or inferior vena cava may be confused with acute congestive hepatomegaly. In this condition the liver is grossly enlarged and tender, and severe intractable ascites is present. However, signs and symptoms of heart failure are notably absent. The most common cause is thrombosis of the hepatic veins, often in the setting of polycythemia rubra vera, myeloproliferative syndromes, paroxysmal nocturnal hemoglobinuria, oral contraceptive use, or other hypercoagulable states; it may also result from invasion of the inferior vena cava by tumor, such as renal cell or hepatocellular carcinoma. Idiopathic membranous obstruction of the inferior vena cava is the most common cause of this syndrome in Japan. Hepatic venography or liver biopsy showing centrilobular congestion and sinusoidal dilatation in the absence of right-sided heart failure establishes the diagnosis of Budd-Chiari syndrome. Venocclusive disease affecting the sublobular branches of the hepatic veins and the hepatic venues may result from hepatic irradiation, treatment with certain antineoplastic agents, or ingestion of pyrrolidizine alkaloids present in some herbal teas ("bush tea disease") and can mimic congestive hepatomegaly.

℞ TREATMENT Prevention or treatment of cardiac cirrhosis depends on the diagnosis and therapy of the underlying cardiovascular disorder. Improvement in cardiac function frequently results in improvement of liver function and stabilization of the liver disease.

METABOLIC, HEREDITARY, DRUG-RELATED, AND OTHER TYPES OF CIRRHOSIS (See Table 299-1)

Cirrhosis or hepatitis may result from a wide variety of other processes encompassing the spectrum of etiologic factors listed in Table 299-2. Although some of these disorders have distinctive clinical or morphologic features, the manifestations of cirrhosis are largely independent of the underlying pathogenic mechanism.

NONCIRRHOTIC FIBROSIS OF THE LIVER

Several diseases, either congenital or acquired, may be associated with localized or generalized hepatic fibrosis. They are distinguished from cirrhosis by the absence of hepatocellular damage and the lack of nodular regenerative activity. The clinical manifestations in such cases are largely secondary to portal hypertension. The different types of these disorders are indicated in Table 299-2; with the exception of schistosomiasis in some regions of the world, all these conditions are relatively rare.

Table 299-2 Some Causes of Noncirrhotic Hepatic Fibrosis

Idiopathic portal hypertension (noncirrhotic portal fibrosis, Banti's syndrome); three variants:
- Intrahepatic phlebosclerosis and fibrosis
- Portal and splenic vein sclerosis
- Portal and splenic vein thrombosis

Schistosomiasis ("pipe-stem" fibrosis with presinusoidal portal hypertension)
Congenital hepatic fibrosis (may be associated with polycystic disease of liver and kidneys)

MAJOR COMPLICATIONS OF CIRRHOSIS

The clinical course of patients with advanced cirrhosis is often complicated by a number of important sequelae that are independent of the etiology of the underlying liver disease. These include portal hypertension and its consequences (e.g., gastroesophageal varices and splenomegaly), ascites, hepatic encephalopathy, spontaneous bacterial peritonitis, hepatorenal syndrome, and hepatocellular carcinoma.

PORTAL HYPERTENSION Definition and Pathogenesis Normal pressure in the portal vein is low (5 to 10 mmHg) because vascular resistance in the hepatic sinusoids is minimal. Portal hypertension (>10 mmHg) most commonly results from increased resistance to portal blood flow. Because the portal venous system lacks valves, resistance at any level between the right side of the heart and splanchnic vessels results in retrograde transmission of an elevated pressure. Increased resistance can occur at three levels relative to the hepatic sinusoids: (1) presinusoidal, (2) sinusoidal, and (3) postsinudoidal. Obstruction in the *presinusoidal* venous compartment may be anatomically outside the liver (e.g., portal vein thrombosis) or within the liver itself but at a functional level proximal to the hepatic sinusoids so that the liver parenchyma is not exposed to the elevated venous pressure (e.g., schistosomiasis).

Postsinusoidal obstruction may also occur outside the liver at the level of the hepatic veins (e.g., Budd-Chiari syndrome), the inferior vena cava, or, less commonly, within the liver (e.g., venocclusive disease). When cirrhosis is complicated by portal hypertension, the increased resistance is usually *sinusoidal*. While distinctions between pre-, post-, and sinusoidal processes are conceptually appealing, functional resistance to portal flow in a given patient may occur at more than one level. Portal hypertension may also arise from increased blood flow (e.g., massive splenomegaly or arteriovenous fistulas), but the low outflow resistance of the normal liver makes this a rare clinical problem.

Cirrhosis is the most common cause of portal hypertension in the United States. Clinically significant portal hypertension is present in >60% of patients with cirrhosis. *Portal vein obstruction* is the second most common cause; it may be idiopathic or occur in association with cirrhosis, infection, pancreatitis, or abdominal trauma. Portal vein thrombosis may develop in a variety of hypercoagulable states including polycythemia vera; essential thrombocythemia; deficiencies of protein C, protein S, or antithrombin III; resistance to activated protein C (factor V Leiden); and a mutation of the prothrombin gene (G20210A). Portal vein thrombosis may be idiopathic, though some of these patients may have a subclinical myeloproliferative disorder. Hepatic vein thrombosis (Budd-Chiari syndrome) and hepatic venoocclusive disease are relatively infrequent causes of portal hypertension (see above). Portal vein occlusion may result in massive hematemesis from gastroesophageal varices, but ascites is usually found only when cirrhosis is present. Noncirrhotic portal fibrosis (Table 299-2) accounts for only a few cases of portal hypertension.

Clinical Features The major clinical manifestations of portal hypertension include hemorrhage from gastroesophageal varices, splenomegaly with hypersplenism, ascites, and acute and chronic hepatic encephalopathy. These are related, at least in part, to the development of portal-systemic collateral channels. The absence of valves in the portal venous system facilitates retrograde (hepatofugal) blood flow from the high-pressure portal venous system to the lower-pressure systemic venous circulation. Major sites of collateral flow involve the veins around cardioesophageal junction (esophagogastric varices), the rectum (hemorrhoids), retroperitoneal space, and the falciform ligament of the liver (periumbilical or abdominal wall collaterals). Abdominal wall collaterals appear as tortuous epigastric vessels that radiate from the umbilicus toward the xiphoid and rib margins (caput medusae).

A frequent marker of the presence of cirrhosis in a patient being followed for chronic liver disease is a progressive decrease in platelet count. A low-normal platelet count can be the first clue to progression to cirrhosis. Ultimately, a marked decrease in platelets (to 30,000 to 60,000/μL) and white blood cells can occur.

Diagnosis In patients with known liver disease, the development of portal hypertension is usually revealed by the appearance of splenomegaly, ascites, encephalopathy, and/or esophageal varices. Conversely, the finding of any of these features should prompt evaluation of the patient for the presence of underlying portal hypertension and liver disease. Varices are most reliably documented by fiberoptic esophagoscopy; their presence lends indirect support to the diagnosis of portal hypertension. Although rarely necessary, portal venous pressure may be measured directly by percutaneous transhepatic "skinny needle" catheterization or indirectly through transjugular cannulation of the hepatic veins. Both free and wedged hepatic vein pressure should be measured. While the latter is elevated in sinusoidal and postsinusoidal portal hypertension, including cirrhosis, this measurement is usually normal in presinusoidal portal hypertension. In patients in whom additional information is necessary (e.g., preoperative evaluation before portal-systemic shunt surgery) or when percutaneous catheterization is not feasible, mesenteric and hepatic angiography may be helpful. Particular attention should be directed to the venous phase to assess the patency of the portal vein and the direction of portal blood flow.

℞ TREATMENT Although treatment is usually directed toward a specific complication of portal hypertension, attempts are sometimes made to reduce the pressure in the portal venous system. Surgical decompression procedures have been used for many years to lower portal pressure in patients with bleeding esophageal varices (see below). However, portal-systemic shunt surgery does not result in improved survival rates in patients with cirrhosis. Decompression can now be accomplished without surgery through the percutaneous placement of a portal-systemic shunt, termed a *transjugular intrahepatic portosystemic shunt* (TIPS). β-Adrenergic blockade with propranolol or nadolol reduces portal pressure through vasodilatory effects on both the splanchnic arterial bed and the portal venous system in combination with reduced cardiac output. Such therapy has been shown to be effective in preventing both a first variceal bleed and subsequent episodes after an initial bleed. Treatment of patients with clinically significant sequelae of portal hypertension, especially variceal bleeding, with doses of propranolol titrated to reduce the resting pulse by 25% is reasonable if no contraindications exist.

Vigorous treatment of patients with alcoholic hepatitis and cirrhosis, chronic active hepatitis, or other liver diseases may lead to a fall in portal pressure and to a reduction in variceal size. In general, however, portal hypertension due to cirrhosis is not reversible. In appropriately selected patients, hepatic transplantation will be beneficial.

VARICEAL BLEEDING **Pathogenesis** While vigorous hemorrhage may arise from any portal-systemic venous collaterals, bleeding is most common from varices in the region of the gastroesophageal junction. The factors contributing to bleeding from gastroesophageal varices are not entirely understood but include the degree of portal hypertension (>12 mmHg) and the size of the varices.

Clinical Features and Diagnosis Variceal bleeding often occurs without obvious precipitating factors and usually presents with painless but massive hematemesis with or without melena. Associated signs range from mild postural tachycardia to profound shock, depending on the extent of blood loss and degree of hypovolemia. Because patients with varices may bleed just as frequently from other gastrointestinal lesions (e.g., peptic ulcer, gastritis), exclusion of other bleeding sources is important even in patients with prior variceal hemorrhage. Endoscopy is the best approach to evaluate upper gastrointestinal hemorrhage in patients with known or suspected portal hypertension.

℞ TREATMENT (See Fig. 299-1) Variceal bleeding is a life-threatening emergency. Prompt estimation and vigorous replacement of blood loss to maintain intravascular volume are essential and take precedence over diagnostic studies and more specific intervention to stop the bleeding. However, excessive fluid administration can increase portal pressure with resultant further bleeding and should therefore be avoided. Replacement of clotting factors with fresh-frozen plasma is important in patients with coagulopathy. Patients are best managed in an intensive care unit and require close monitoring of central venous or pulmonary capillary wedge pressures, urine output, and mental status. Only when the patient is hemodynamically stable should attention be directed toward specific diagnostic studies (especially endoscopy) and other therapeutic modalities to prevent further or recurrent bleeding.

About half of all episodes of variceal hemorrhage cease without intervention, although the risk of rebleeding is very high. The medical management of acute variceal hemorrhage includes the use of vasoconstrictors (somatostatin/octreotide or vasopressin), balloon tamponade, and endoscopic banding of varices or endoscopic sclerosis of varices (sclerotherapy). Intravenous infusion of *vasopressin* at a rate of 0.1 to 0.4 U/min results in generalized vasoconstriction leading to diminished blood flow in the portal venous system. Intravenous infusion of vasopressin is as effective as selective intraarterial administration. Control of bleeding can be achieved in up to 80% of cases, but bleeding recurs in more than half after the vasopressin is tapered and discontinued. Furthermore, a number of serious side effects, including cardiac and gastrointestinal tract ischemia, acute renal failure, and hyponatremia, may be associated with vasopressin therapy. Concurrent use of venodilators such as nitroglycerin as an intravenous infusion or isosorbide dinitrate sublingually may enhance the effectiveness of vasopressin and reduce complications. *Somatostatin* and its analogue, *octreotide*, are direct splanchnic vasoconstrictors. In some studies somatostatin, given as an initial 250-μg bolus followed by constant infusion (250 μg/h), has been found to be as effective as vasopressin. Octreotide at doses of 50 to 100 μg/h is also effective. These agents are preferable to vasopressin, offering equivalent efficacy with fewer complications. If bleeding is too vigorous or endoscopy is not available, *balloon tamponade* of the bleeding varices may be accomplished

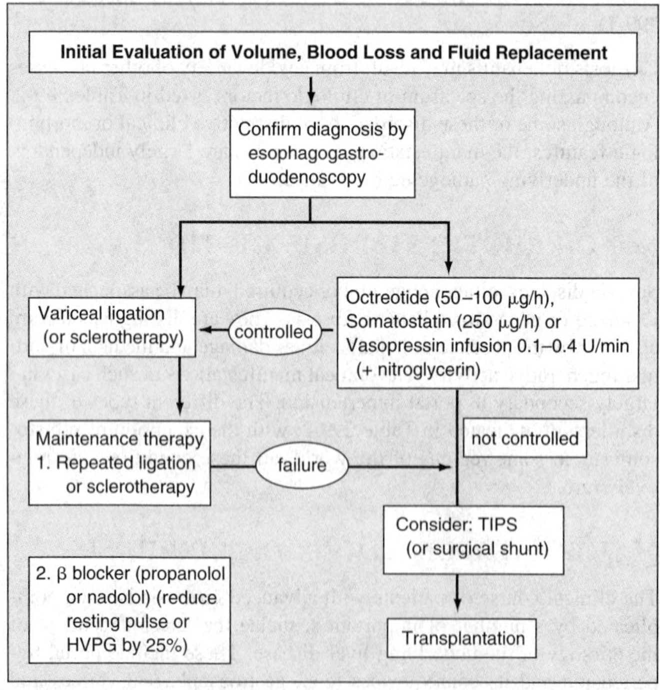

FIGURE 299-1 Approach to the patient with bleeding esophageal varices. Use of a beta blocker is the only intervention demonstrated to offer prophylactic benefit in a patient who has never bled. TIPS, transjugular intrahepatic portosystemic shunt.

with a triple-lumen (Sengstaken-Blakemore) or four-lumen (Minnesota) tube with esophageal and gastric balloons. Because of the high risk of aspiration, endotracheal intubation should be performed prior to placing one of these tubes. After the tube is introduced into the stomach, the gastric balloon is inflated and pulled back into the cardia of the stomach. If bleeding does not stop, the esophageal balloon is inflated for additional tamponade. Complications occur in 15% or more of patients and include aspiration pneumonitis as well as esophageal rupture.

Where available, *endoscopic intervention* should be employed as the first line of treatment to control bleeding acutely (Chaps. 44 and 283). Over the past 18 years, endoscopic sclerosis of esophageal varices has been extensively employed. In this procedure, the varices are injected with one of several sclerosing agents via a needle-tipped catheter passed through the endoscope. After endoscopic identification of varices as the presumed source of bleeding, sclerotherapy controls acute bleeding in up to 90% of cases. In addition, repeated sclerotherapy can be performed until obliteration of all varices is accomplished in an effort to prevent recurrent bleeding. While available data support the efficacy of sclerotherapy in controlling bleeding acutely and in decreasing rebleeding rates, repeated sclerotherapy has not been documented to prolong survival. Mucosal ulceration resulting from injection of the caustic sclerosant may occur and result in further hemorrhage or stenosis. More recently, endoscopic band ligation, in which esophageal varices are ligated and strangulated with endoscopically placed small elastic O-rings, has gained favor. Band ligation has proven to be at least as effective as sclerotherapy in controlling acute variceal bleeding and preventing rebleeding. Because it has been associated with fewer treatment-related complications, band ligation is recommended for long-term obliteration of varices that have bled. Although prophylactic sclerosis or banding of esophageal varices in the absence of proven bleeding cannot yet be recommended, one report suggests that banding may be more effective than beta-blockade in primary prevention of variceal bleeding in high-risk patients.

The effectiveness of *nonselective β-adrenergic blocking agents* (e.g., propranolol) in the management of acute variceal bleeding is limited due to concomitant hypotension resulting from hypovolemia. However, a number of studies suggest they may be of value in secondary prevention of recurrent variceal hemorrhage. Moreover, prophylactic treatment with nonselective beta blockers (propranolol or nadolol) in patients with large ("high-risk") varices that have never bled appears to decrease the incidence of bleeding and prolong survival. Thus, endoscopic screening for varices in patients with cirrhosis is desirable; some have suggested this should be repeated every other year. Patients with portal hypertension without specific contraindications should be given propranolol in doses that produce a 25% reduction in the resting heart rate or the hepatic venous pressure gradient (HVPG), where available. Propranolol may also prevent recurrent bleeding from severe portal hypertensive gastropathy in patients with cirrhosis. The optimal combination of endoscopic and pharmacologic therapy for prevention of recurrent hemorrhage remains to be established and is the subject of ongoing trials.

Surgical treatment of portal hypertension and variceal bleeding involves the creation of a portal-systemic shunt to permit decompression of the portal system. Two types of portal systemic shunts have been used: *nonselective shunts*, to decompress the entire portal system, and *selective shunts*, intended to decompress only the varices while maintaining blood flow to the liver itself. Nonselective shunts include end-to-side or side-to-side portacaval and proximal splenorenal anastomoses; selective shunts include the distal splenorenal shunt. Nonselective shunts are more likely to be complicated by encephalopathy than selective shunts. Emergency portal-systemic nonselective shunts may control acute hemorrhage, but such surgery is usually used only as a last resort because early operative mortality can be high. The role of portal-systemic shunt surgery after initial control of bleeding by nonoperative means is also uncertain. Surgically created shunts effectively reduce the risk of recurrent hemorrhage, but the overall mortality of patients undergoing such surgery is comparable to that of unoperated patients. Although patients who have undergone portal-systemic surgery succumb to recurrent bleeding less commonly than unoperated patients, this improvement is counterbalanced by increased morbidity from encephalopathy and death from progressive liver failure. Increasingly, therapeutic portal-systemic shunts have been reserved for patients who experience further bleeding despite serial endoscopic sclerotherapy or band ligation.

In TIPS, a technique developed to create a portal-systemic shunt by a percutaneous approach, an expandable metal stent is advanced to the hepatic veins under angiographic guidance and then through the substance of the liver to create a direct portacaval channel. This technique offers an alternative to surgery for refractory bleeding due to portal hypertension. However, stents frequently undergo stenosis or occlude over a period of months, prompting the need for a second TIPS or an alternative approach. Encephalopathy may be encountered after TIPS just as in the surgical shunts and is especially problematic in the elderly and those patients with preexisting encephalopathy. TIPS should be reserved for those individuals who fail endoscopic or medical management and are poor surgical risks. TIPS may have a useful role as a "bridge" for those patients with end-stage cirrhosis awaiting liver transplantation. Procedures such as esophageal transection have also been advocated for the management of acute variceal bleeding, but their efficacy remains unproven. Even though recent trials found that esophageal transection was as effective as endoscopic sclerotherapy, transection is usually considered a last resort.

The management of bleeding gastric fundal varices, either alone or in conjunction with esophageal varices, is more problematic, since sclerotherapy and banding are generally not effective. Vasoactive pharmacologic therapy should be instituted, but TIPS or shunt surgery should be considered because of high failure and rebleeding rates. For isolated gastric varices, splenic vein thrombosis should be specifically sought, since splenectomy is curative.

Portal Hypertensive Gastropathy Although variceal hemorrhage is the most commonly encountered bleeding complication of portal hypertension, many patients will develop a congestive gastropathy due to the venous hypertension. In this condition, identified by endoscopic examination, the mucosa appears engorged and friable. Indolent mucosal bleeding occurs rather than the brisk hemorrhage typical of a variceal source. β-Adrenergic blockade with propranolol (reducing splanchnic arterial pressure as well as portal pressure) is sometimes effective in ameliorating this condition. H_2 receptor antagonists or other agents useful in the treatment of peptic disease are usually not helpful.

SPLENOMEGALY Definition and Pathogenesis Congestive splenomegaly is common in patients with severe portal hypertension. Rarely, massive splenomegaly from nonhepatic disease leads to portal hypertension due to increased blood flow in the splenic vein.

Clinical Features Although usually asymptomatic, splenomegaly may be massive and contribute to the thrombocytopenia or pancytopenia of cirrhosis. In the absence of cirrhosis, splenomegaly in association with variceal hemorrhage should suggest the possibility of splenic vein thrombosis.

℞ **TREATMENT** Splenomegaly usually requires no specific treatment, although massive enlargement of the spleen may occasionally necessitate splenectomy at the time of shunt surgery. However, it should be noted that splenectomy without an accompanying shunt may actually increase portal pressure, and portal vein thrombosis may result from splenectomy. Splenectomy may also be indicated if splenomegaly is the cause rather than the result of portal hypertension (as in splenic vein thrombosis). Thrombcytopenia alone is rarely severe enough to necessitate removal of the spleen. Splenectomy should be avoided in a patient eligible for liver transplantation.

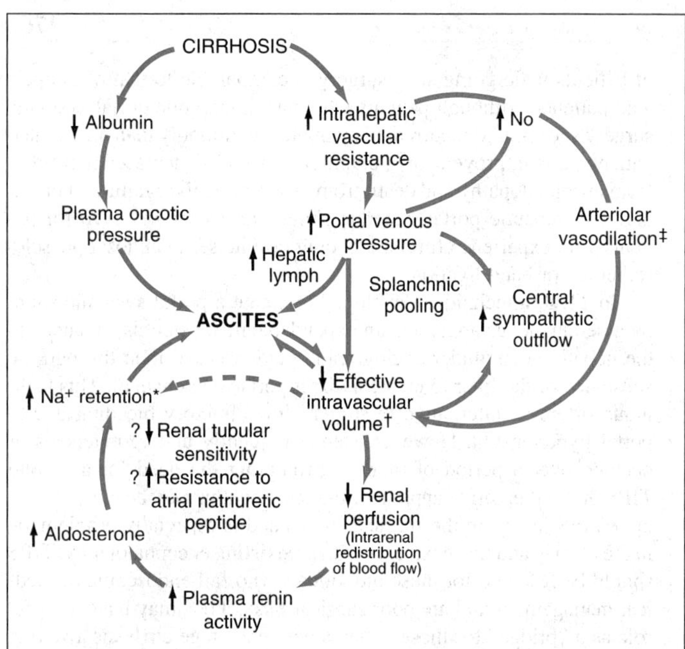

FIGURE 299-2 Multiple factors involved in development of ascites. Current concepts suggest that initiating factor may be primary sodium retention (*"overflow"), diminished effective intravascular volume (†"underfilling"), or arteriolar vasodilation (‡"vasodilation").

ASCITES Definition Ascites is the accumulation of excess fluid within the peritoneal cavity. It is most frequently encountered in patients with cirrhosis and other forms of severe liver disease, but a number of other disorders may lead to either transudative or exudative ascites (Chap. 46).

Pathogenesis The accumulation of ascitic fluid represents a state of total-body sodium and water excess, but the event that initiates this imbalance is unclear. Three theories have been proposed (Fig. 299-2). The "underfilling" theory suggests that the primary abnormality is inappropriate sequestration of fluid within the splanchnic vascular bed due to portal hypertension and a consequent decrease in effective circulating blood volume. According to this theory, an apparent decrease in intravascular volume (underfilling) is sensed by the kidney, which responds by retaining salt and water. The "overflow" theory suggests that the primary abnormality is inappropriate renal retention of salt and water in the absence of volume depletion. A third and more recent theory, the peripheral arterial vasodilation hypothesis, may unify the earlier theories and accounts for the constellation of arterial hypotension and increased cardiac output in association with high levels of vasoconstrictor substances that are routinely found in patients with cirrhosis and ascites. Again, sodium retention is considered secondary to arterial vascular underfilling and the result of a disproportionate increase of the vascular compartment due to arteriolar vasodilation rather than from decreased intravascular volume. According to this theory, portal hypertension results in splanchnic arteriolar vasodilation, mediated by nitric oxide, and leading to underfilling of the arterial vascular space and baroreceptor-mediated stimulation of renin-angiotensin, sympathetic output, and antidiuretic hormone release.

Regardless of the initiating event, a number of factors contribute to accumulation of fluid in the abdominal cavity (Fig. 299-2). Elevated levels of serum epinephrine and norepinephrine have been well documented. *Increased central sympathetic outflow* is found in patients with cirrhosis and ascites but not in those with cirrhosis alone. Increased sympathetic output results in diminished natriuresis by activation of the renin-angiotensin system and diminished sensitivity to atrial natriuretic peptide. *Portal hypertension* plays an important role in the formation of ascites by raising hydrostatic pressure within the splanchnic capillary bed. *Hypoalbuminemia* and *reduced plasma oncotic pressure* also favor the extravasation of fluid from plasma to the peritoneal cavity, and thus ascites is infrequent in patients with cirrhosis unless both portal hypertension and hypoalbuminemia are present. Hepatic lymph may weep freely from the surface of the cirrhotic liver due to distortion and obstruction of hepatic sinusoids and lymphatics and contributes to ascites formation. In contrast to the contribution of transudative fluid from the portal vascular bed, hepatic lymph may weep into the peritoneal cavity even in the absence of marked hypoproteinemia because the endothelial lining of the hepatic sinusoids is discontinuous. This mechanism may account for the high protein concentration present in the ascitic fluid of some patients with venoocclusive disease or the Budd-Chiari syndrome.

Renal factors also play an important role in perpetuating ascites. Patients with ascites fail to excrete a water load in a normal fashion. They have increased renal sodium reabsorption by both proximal and distal tubules, the latter due largely to increased plasma renin activity and secondary hyperaldosteronism. Insensitivity to circulating atrial natriuretic peptide, often present in elevated concentrations in patients with cirrhosis and ascites, may be an important contributory factor in many patients. This insensitivity has been documented in those patients with the most severely impaired sodium excretion, who typically also exhibit low arterial pressure and marked overactivity of the renin-aldosterone axis. Renal vasoconstriction, perhaps resulting from increased serum prostaglandin or catecholamine levels, may also contribute to sodium retention. Recently a role for endothelin, a potent vasoconstrictor peptide, has been proposed. While elevated levels have been reported by some, this has not been observed by others.

As discussed in Chap. 46, ascites may arise in a number of clinical settings in addition to cirrhosis and portal hypertension. Although historically ascites was classified as either transudative or exudative, similar to the characterization of pleural fluids, this schema has limitations. Instead, the serum-ascites albumin gradient (SAAG) provides a better classification than total protein content or other parameters. In cirrhosis, the serum albumin concentration is usually at least 10 g/L (1 g/dL) higher than that of the ascitic fluid, thus yielding a high SAAG [≥11 g/L (≥1.1 g/dL)], reflecting indirectly the abnormally high hydrostatic pressure gradient between the portal bed and the ascitic compartment. Conversely, the presence of a low SAAG [<11 g/L (<1.1 g/dL)] will usually exclude cirrhosis and portal hypertension.

Clinical Features and Diagnosis Usually ascites is first noticed by the patient because of increasing abdominal girth. More pronounced accumulation of fluid may cause shortness of breath because of elevation of the diaphragm. When peritoneal fluid accumulation exceeds 500 mL, ascites may be demonstrated on physical examination by the presence of shifting dullness, a fluid wave, or bulging flanks. Ultrasound examination, preferably with a Doppler study, can detect smaller quantities of ascites and should be performed when physical examination is equivocal or when the cause of the recent onset of ascites is not clear (e.g., exclude Budd-Chiari syndrome or portal vein thrombosis).

℞ **TREATMENT** (See Fig. 299-3) A thorough search should be made for precipitating factors in the patient with recent onset of or worsening ascites, e.g., excessive salt intake, medication noncompliance, superimposed infection, worsening liver disease, portal vein thrombosis, or development of hepatocellular carcinoma. When ascites develops in the setting of severe, acute liver disease, resolution of ascites is likely to follow improvement in liver function. More commonly, ascites develops in patients with stable or steadily worsening liver function. Paracentesis should usually be performed with a small-gauge needle at the time of initial evaluation or at the time of any clinical deterioration of a cirrhotic patient with ascites. A small amount of fluid (<200 mL) should be obtained and examined for evidence of infection, tumor, or other possible causes and complications of ascites. Therapeutic intervention is indicated both to prevent potential complications and to control progressive increase in ascites, which may

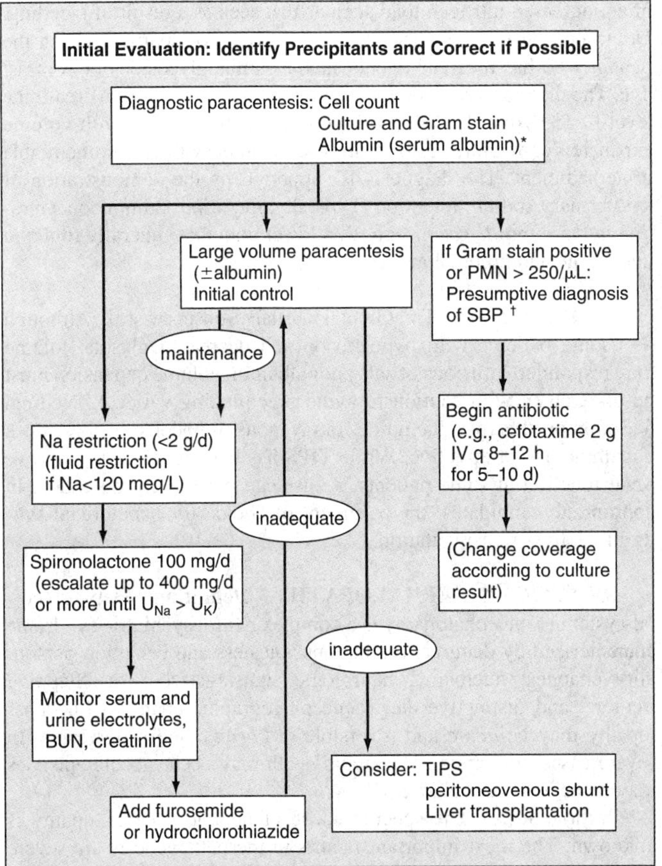

FIGURE 299-3 Approach to the patient with ascites [and spontaneous bacterial peritonitis (SBP)]. PMN, polymorphonuclear leukocytes; TIPS, transjugular intrahepatic portosystemic shunt. *Calculate SAAG [serum ascites albumin gradient = serum albumin − ascites albumin (g/dL)] to confirm high gradient (>1.1 g/dL) in portal hypertension. †If PMN >250/μL but culture is negative = culture negative neutrocytic ascites; begin empirical antibiotic and retap at 48 h; if culture is positive but PMN < 250/μL normal = monomicrobial nonneutrocytic bacterascites; retap; treat if PMN > 250/μL: if polymicrobial infection, exclude secondary peritonitis. U_{Na}, urinary sodium; U_{Ka}, urinary potassium; BUN, blood urea nitrogen.

become pronounced enough to cause physical discomfort. For the patient with a modest accumulation, therapy can be undertaken as an outpatient and should be gentle and incremental (see below). The goal is the loss of no more than 1.0 kg/d if both ascites and peripheral edema are present and no more than 0.5 kg/d in patients with ascites alone. In some patients, particularly those with a large accumulation of fluid, it may be desirable to hospitalize the patient so that daily weights and frequent serum electrolyte levels can be monitored and compliance ensured. Although abdominal girth measurements are frequently used as an index of fluid loss, they tend to be unreliable.

Salt restriction is the cornerstone of therapy. A diet containing 800 mg sodium (2 g NaCl) is often adequate to induce a negative sodium balance and permit diuresis. Response to salt restriction alone is more likely to occur if the ascites is of recent onset, the underlying liver disease is reversible, a precipitating factor can be corrected, or the patient has a high urinary sodium excretion (>25 mmol/d) and normal renal function. Fluid restriction of approximately 1000 mL/d does little to enhance diuresis but may be necessary to correct hyponatremia. If sodium restriction alone fails to result in diuresis and weight loss, diuretics should be prescribed. Because of the role of hyperaldosteronism in sustaining salt retention, spironolactone or other distal tubule–acting diuretics (triamterene, amiloride) are the drugs of choice. These agents are also preferred because of their gentle action and specific potassium-sparing properties. Spironolactone is initially given in a dose of 100 mg a day and is increased as needed by 100 mg/d every several days to a maximum dose that should rarely exceed 400 mg/d. An indication of the minimum effective dose of spironolactone may be obtained by monitoring urinary electrolyte concentrations for a rise in sodium and fall in potassium levels, reflecting effective competitive inhibition of aldosterone. Conversely, the development of azotemia or hyperkalemia may be dose-limiting or even warrant a reduction in the amount of this medication. In some patients, diuresis cannot be initiated despite maximal doses of distal tubule–acting agents (e.g., 400 mg spironolactone) because of avid proximal tubular sodium absorption. More potent and proximally acting diuretics (furosemide, thiazide, or ethacrynic acid) may then be added cautiously to the regimen. Spironolactone plus furosemide, 40 or 80 mg/d, is usually sufficient to initiate a diuresis in most patients. However, such aggressive therapy must be used with great caution to avoid plasma volume depletion, azotemia, and hypokalemia, which may lead to encephalopathy.

In patients with pronounced ascites, particularly those requiring hospitalization, large-volume paracentesis has proven to be an effective and less costly approach to initial management than prolonged bed rest and conventional diuretic treatment. In this approach, ascitic fluid is removed by peritoneal cannula using strict aseptic techniques and monitoring hemodynamic and renal function. This can be safely accomplished in a single session. The need for concomitant albumin replacement by intravenous infusion remains controversial but may be prudent in the patient without peripheral edema, to avoid depleting the intravascular space and precipitating hypotension. Maintenance diuretic therapy in conjunction with sodium restriction may then be instituted to avoid recurrent ascites.

A minority of patients with advanced cirrhosis has "refractory ascites" or rapidly reaccumulate fluid after control by paracentesis. In some patients, a side-to-side *portacaval shunt* may result in improvement in ascites, although generally these patients are extremely poor surgical risks. In the past, intractable ascites has also been treated with the surgical implantation of a plastic *peritoneovenous shunt*, which has a pressure-sensitive, one-way valve allowing ascitic fluid to flow from the abdominal cavity to the superior vena cava. However, the usefulness of this technique is limited by a high rate of complications such as infection, disseminated intravascular coagulation, and thrombosis of the shunt. More recently, in selected patients TIPS has been used effectively to control refractory ascites, although portal decompression, while mobilizing ascitic fluid, has precipitated severe hepatic encephalopathy in some patients. TIPS remains a promising but unproven treatment for refractory ascites. None of these shunts has been shown to extend life expectancy.

SPONTANEOUS BACTERIAL PERITONITIS (SBP) Patients with ascites and cirrhosis may develop acute bacterial peritonitis without an obvious primary source of infection. Patients with very advanced liver disease are particularly susceptible to SBP. The ascitic fluid in these patients typically has especially low concentrations of albumin and other so-called opsonic proteins, which normally may provide some protection against bacteria. Although key steps in the pathogenesis of SBP remain to be elucidated, it is clear that most bacteria contributing to SBP derive from the bowel and eventually are spread to ascitic fluid by the hematogenous route after transmigration through the bowel wall and transversing the lymphatics. Clinical features can include abrupt onset of fever, chills, generalized abdominal pain, and, rarely, rebound abdominal tenderness. However, the clinical symptoms *may be minimal*, and some patients manifest only worsening jaundice or encephalopathy in the absence of localizing abdominal complaints. The diagnosis is based on careful examination of the ascitic fluid. An ascitic fluid leukocyte count of >500 cells/L (with a proportion of polymorphonuclear leukocytes of ≥50%) or more than 250 polymorphonuclear leukocytes should suggest the possibility of bacterial peritonitis while results of bacterial cultures of ascitic fluid are pending. Other measurements such as fluid pH or determination of gradients between serum and fluid pH or lactate are generally not necessary. The presence of more than 10,000 leukocytes per liter, multiple organisms, or failure to improve after standard therapy for 48 h suggest that the peritonitis may be secondary to an infection elsewhere in the body.

A variant of SBP, designated *monomicrobial nonneutrocytic bacterascites*, is sometimes seen. In these patients, culture of ascitic fluid yields bacteria, but the neutrophil count is less than 250/L. These patients often have less severe liver disease than those found initially to have typical SBP. While many patients with this variant have cleared the bacterascites at the time of a subsequent paracentesis, nearly 40% will develop typical SBP; thus follow-up paracentesis is usually warranted in this setting.

Rx TREATMENT Empirical therapy with cefotaxime or ampicillin and an aminoglycoside should be initiated when the diagnosis is first suspected because enteric gram-negative bacilli are found in the majority of cases; less frequently, the infection is caused by pneumococci and other gram-positive bacteria. Cefotaxime is preferable due to the lower rate of renal toxicity. Specific antibiotic therapy can be selected once the specific organism is identified. Therapy is usually administered for 10 to 14 days, although one controlled study has suggested that a 5-day course of intravenous antibiotics may be as effective when repeat paracentesis at 48 h demonstrates a decline in the ascitic polymorphonuclear leukocytes count by more than 50% and negative cultures.

While appropriate antibiotic therapy is usually effective in the treatment of an episode of SBP, recurrent episodes are relatively common; as many as 70% of patients will experience at least one recurrence within a year of the first episode. The risk of recurrence likely reflects the predisposing role of the underlying advanced liver disease that contributed to the development of the first episode of SBP. Recent trials have demonstrated that prophylactic maintenance therapy with norfloxacin (400 mg/d) can reduce the frequency of recurrent SBP. This agent presumably causes selective decontamination of the intestine, eliminating many aerobic gram-negative bacilli. Trimethoprim-sulfamethoxazole given for 5 days a week has also proven effective. Antibiotics may be administered as infrequently as once a week (e.g., ciprofoxacin, 750 mg once weekly). While maintenance therapy reduces the frequency of SBP and need for hospitalization, it is unclear whether this is associated with prolonged survival. Primary prevention of SBP in a subset of high-risk cirrhotic patients [ascitic fluid protein $<$10 g/L ($<$1.0 g/dL)] also appears to be warranted, as is prophylaxis for SBP during variceal hemorrhage.

HEPATORENAL SYNDROME **Definition and Pathogenesis** Hepatorenal syndrome is a serious complication in the patient with cirrhosis and ascites and is characterized by worsening azotemia with avid sodium retention and oliguria in the absence of identifiable specific causes of renal dysfunction. The exact basis for this syndrome is not clear, but altered renal hemodynamics appear to be involved. The kidneys are structurally intact; urinalysis and pyelography are usually normal. Renal biopsy, although rarely needed, is also normal, and in fact, kidneys from such patients have been used successfully for renal transplantation. There are indications that an imbalance in certain metabolites of arachidonic acid (prostaglandins and thromboxane) may play a pathogenetic role.

Clinical Features and Diagnosis Worsening azotemia, hyponatremia, progressive oliguria, and hypotension are the hallmarks of the hepatorenal syndrome. This syndrome, which is distinct from prerenal azotemia, may be precipitated by severe gastrointestinal bleeding, sepsis, or overly vigorous attempts at diuresis or paracentesis; it may also occur without an obvious cause. It is essential to exclude other causes of renal impairment often seen in these patients. These include prerenal azotemia or acute tubular necrosis due to hypovolemia (e.g., secondary to gastrointestinal bleeding or diuretic therapy) or an increased nitrogen load such as that seen as a result of bleeding. Drug nephrotoxicity is also often a consideration, particularly in the patient who has received agents such as aminoglycosides or contrast dye. The diagnosis rests on the finding of an elevated serum creatinine level [$>$133 μmol/L ($>$1.5 g/dL)] that fails to improve with volume expansion or withdrawal of diuretics, together with an unremarkable urine sediment. The diagnosis is supported by the demonstration of avid urinary sodium retention. Typically, the urine sodium concentration is $<$5 mmol/L, a concentration lower than that generally found in uncomplicated prerenal azotemia.

Rx TREATMENT Treatment is usually unsuccessful. Although some patients with hypotension and decreased plasma volume may respond to infusions of salt-poor albumin, volume expansion must be undertaken with caution to avoid precipitating variceal bleeding. Vasodilator therapy, including intravenous infusions of low dose dopamine, is not effective. While TIPS has been reported to improve renal function in some patients, its use can not be recommended. In appropriate candidates, the treatment of choice for hepatorenal syndrome is liver transplantation.

HEPATIC ENCEPHALOPATHY **Definition** Hepatic (portal-systemic) encephalopathy is a complex neuropsychiatric syndrome characterized by disturbances in consciousness and behavior, personality changes, fluctuating neurologic signs, asterixis or "flapping tremor," and distinctive electroencephalographic changes. Encephalopathy may be *acute* and reversible or *chronic* and progressive. In severe cases, irreversible coma and death may occur. Acute episodes may recur with variable frequency.

Pathogenesis The specific cause of hepatic encephalopathy is unknown. The most important factors in the pathogenesis are severe hepatocellular dysfunction and/or intrahepatic and extrahepatic shunting of portal venous blood into the systemic circulation so that the liver is largely bypassed. As a result of these processes, various toxic substances absorbed from the intestine are not detoxified by the liver and lead to metabolic abnormalities in the central nervous system (CNS). *Ammonia* is the substance most often incriminated in the pathogenesis of encephalopathy. Many, but not all, patients with hepatic encephalopathy have elevated blood ammonia levels, and recovery from encephalopathy is often accompanied by declining blood ammonia levels. Other compounds and metabolites that may contribute to the development of encephalopathy include mercaptans (derived from intestinal metabolism of methionine), short-chain fatty acids, and phenol. *False neurochemical transmitters* (e.g., octopamine), resulting in part from alterations in plasma levels of aromatic and branched-chain amino acids, may also play a role. An increase in the permeability of the blood-brain barrier to some of these substances may be an additional factor involved in the pathogenesis of hepatic encephalopathy. Several observations suggest that excessive concentrations of γ-aminobutyric acid (GABA), an inhibitory neurotransmitter, in the CNS are important in the reduced levels of consciousness seen in hepatic encephalopathy. Increased CNS GABA may reflect failure of the liver to extract precursor amino acids efficiently or to remove GABA produced in the intestine. In support of this, there is also evidence to suggest that endogenous benzodiazepines, which act through the GABA receptor, may contribute to the development of hepatic encephalopathy. This evidence includes isolation of 1,4-benzodiazepines from brain tissue of patients with fulminant hepatic failure as well as the partial response observed in some patients and experimental animals after administration of flumazenil, a benzodiazepine antagonist. However, the inconsistent effect of flumazenil in patients with encephalopathy, as well as potential methodologic pitfalls in the measurement of endogenous benzodiazepines, preclude definitive attribution of a role to these substances in the pathogenesis of hepatic encephalopathy. The finding of direct enhancement of GABA receptor activation by ammonia suggests that several of the factors described above may be operating via a final common pathway to produce the neuronal depression of hepatic encephalopathy. Finally, the observation of hyperintensity in the basal ganglia by magnetic resonance imaging in cirrhotic patients suggests that excessive *manganese* deposition may also contribute to the pathogenesis of hepatic encephalopathy. Further studies are needed to determine whether chelation therapy exerts long-term benefit.

In the patient with otherwise stable cirrhosis, hepatic encephalopathy often follows a clearly identifiable precipitating event (Table 299-3). Perhaps the most common predisposing factor is *gastrointestinal bleeding*, which leads to an increase in the production of ammonia and other nitrogenous substances, which are then absorbed. Similarly, *increased dietary protein* may precipitate encephalopathy as a result of increased production of nitrogenous substances by colonic bacteria. *Electrolyte disturbances*, particularly hypokalemic alkalosis secondary to overzealous use of diuretics, vigorous paracentesis, or vomiting, may precipitate hepatic encephalopathy. Systemic alkalosis causes an increase in the amount of nonionic ammonia (NH_3) relative to ammonium ions NH_4^+). Only nonionic (uncharged) ammonia readily crosses the blood-brain barrier and accumulates in the CNS. Hypokalemia also directly stimulates renal ammonia production. Injudicious use of CNS-depressing drugs (e.g., barbiturates, benzodiazepines) and acute infection may trigger or aggravate hepatic encephalopathy, although the mechanisms involved are not clear. Other potential precipitating factors include superimposed acute viral hepatitis, alcoholic hepatitis, extrahepatic bile duct obstruction, constipation, surgery, and other coincidental medical complications.

Hepatic encephalopathy has protean manifestations, and any neurologic abnormality, including focal deficits, may be encountered. In patients with acute encephalopathy, neurologic deficits are completely reversible upon correction of underlying precipitating factors and/or improvement in liver function, but in patients with chronic encephalopathy, the deficits may be irreversible and progressive. Cerebral edema is frequently present and contributes to the clinical picture and overall mortality in patients with both acute and chronic encephalopathy.

The diagnosis of hepatic encephalopathy should be considered when four major factors are present: (1) acute or chronic hepatocellular disease and/or extensive portal-systemic collateral shunts (the latter may be either spontaneous, e.g., secondary to portal hypertension, or surgically created, e.g., portacaval anastomosis); (2) disturbances of awareness and mentation, which may progress from forgetfulness and confusion to stupor and finally coma; (3) shifting combinations of neurologic signs, including asterixis, rigidity, hyperreflexia, extensor plantar signs, and rarely, seizures; and (4) a characteristic (but nonspecific) symmetric, high-voltage, triphasic slow-wave (2 to 5 per second) pattern on the electroencephalogram. Asterixis ("liver flap," "flapping tremor") is a nonrhythmic asymmetric lapse in voluntary sustained position of the extremities, head, and trunk. It is best demonstrated by having the patient extend the arms and dorsiflex the hands. Because elicitation of asterixis depends on sustained voluntary muscle contraction, it is not present in the comatose patient. Asterixis is nonspecific and also occurs in patients with other forms of metabolic brain disease. Disturbances of sleep with reversal of sleep/wake cycles are among the earliest signs of encephalopathy. Alterations in personality, mood disturbances, confusion, deterioration in self-care and handwriting, and daytime somnolence are additional clinical features of encephalopathy. *Fetor hepaticus*, a unique musty odor of the breath and urine believed to be due to mercaptans, may be noted in patients with varying stages of hepatic encephalopathy.

Table 299-3 Common Precipitants of Hepatic Encephalopathy

Increased nitrogen load	Drugs
Gastrointestinal bleeding	Narcotics, tranquilizers, sedatives
Excess dietary protein	Diuretics (see "Electrolyte imbalance")
Azotemia	Miscellaneous
Constipation	Infection
Electrolyte and metabolic imbalance	Surgery
Hypokalemia	Superimposed acute liver disease
Alkalosis	Progressive liver disease
Hypoxia	Portal-systemic shunts
Hyponatremia	
Hypovolemia	

Table 299-4 Clinical Stages of Hepatic Encephalopathy

Stage	Mental Status	Asterixis	EEG
I	Euphoria or depression, mild confusion, slurred speech, disordered sleep	+/−	Triphasic waves
II	Lethargy, moderate confusion	+	Triphasic waves
III	Marked confusion, incoherent speech, sleeping but arousable	+	Triphasic waves
IV	Coma; initially responsive to noxious stimuli, later unresponsive	−	Delta activity

Grading or classifying the stages of hepatic encephalopathy is often helpful in following the course of the illness and assessing response to therapy. One useful classification is shown in Table 299-4.

The diagnosis of hepatic encephalopathy is usually one of exclusion. There are no diagnostic liver function test abnormalities, although an elevated serum ammonia level in the appropriate clinical setting is highly suggestive of the diagnosis. Examination of the cerebrospinal fluid is unremarkable, and computed tomography of the brain shows no characteristic abnormalities until late in stage IV when cerebral edema may supervene. A number of conditions, particularly disorders related to acute and chronic alcoholism, can mimic the clinical features of hepatic encephalopathy. These include acute alcohol intoxication, sedative overdose, delirium tremens, Wernicke's encephalopathy, and Korsakoff's psychosis (Chap. 373). Subdural hematoma, meningitis, and hypoglycemia or other metabolic encephalopathies must also be considered, especially in patients with alcoholic cirrhosis. In young patients with liver disease and neurologic abnormalities, Wilson's disease should be excluded.

℞ **TREATMENT** (See Fig. 299-4) Early recognition and prompt treatment of hepatic encephalopathy are essential. Patients with acute, severe hepatic encephalopathy (stage IV) require the usual supportive measures for the comatose patient. Specific treatment of hepatic encephalopathy is aimed at (1) elimination or treatment of precipitating factors and (2) lowering of blood ammonia (and other toxin) levels by decreasing the absorption of protein and nitrogenous products from the intestine. In the setting of acute gastrointestinal bleeding, blood in the bowel should be promptly evacuated with laxatives (and enemas if necessary) in order to reduce the nitrogen load. Protein should be excluded from the diet, and constipation should be avoided. Ammonia absorption can be decreased by the administration of lactulose, a nonabsorbable disaccharide that acts as an osmotic laxative. Metabolism of lactulose by colonic bacteria may also result in an acid pH that favors conversion of ammonia to the poorly absorbed ammonium ion. In addition, lactulose may actually diminish ammonia production through its direct effects on bacterial metabolism. Acutely, lactulose syrup can be administered in a dose of 30 to 60 mL every hour until diarrhea occurs; thereafter the dose is adjusted (usually 15 to 30 mL three times daily) so that the patient has two to four soft stools daily. Intestinal ammonia production by bacteria can also be decreased by oral administration of a "nonabsorbable" antibiotic such as neomycin (0.5 to 1.0 g every 6 h). However, despite poor absorption, neomycin may reach sufficient concentrations in the bloodstream to cause renal toxicity. Equal benefits may be achieved with broad-spectrum antibiotics such as metronidazole. The use of agents such as levodopa, bromocriptine, keto analogues of essential amino acids, and intravenous amino acid formulations rich in branched-chain amino acids in the treatment of acute hepatic encephalopathy remains of unproven benefit. Flumazenil, a short-acting benzodiazepine antagonist,

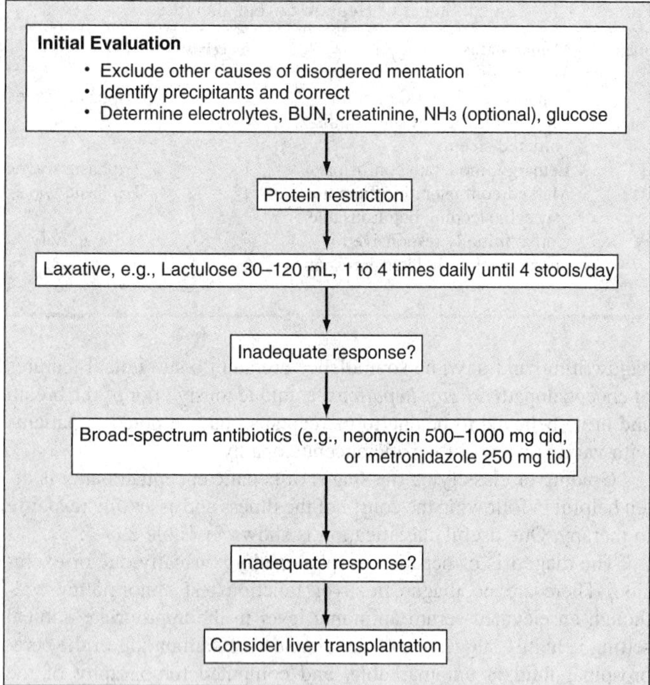
Initial Evaluation
• Exclude other causes of disordered mentation
• Identify precipitants and correct
• Determine electrolytes, BUN, creatinine, NH3 (optional), glucose
Protein restriction
Laxative, e.g., Lactulose 30–120 mL, 1 to 4 times daily until 4 stools/day
Inadequate response?
Broad-spectrum antibiotics (e.g., neomycin 500–1000 mg qid, or metronidazole 250 mg tid)
Inadequate response?
Consider liver transplantation

FIGURE 299-4 Approach to the patient with hepatic encephalopathy. BUN, blood urea nitrogen.

may have a role in management of hepatic encephalopathy precipitated by use of benzodiazepines, if there is a need for urgent therapy. Hemoperfusion to remove toxic substances and therapy directed primarily toward coincident cerebral edema in acute encephalopathy are also of unproven value. The efficacy of extracorporeal liver assist devices employing hepatocytes of porcine or human origin to bridge patients to recovery or transplantation is as yet unproven but is currently being studied.

Chronic encephalopathy may be effectively controlled by administration of lactulose. Management of patients with chronic encephalopathy should include dietary protein restriction (usually to 60 g/d) in combination with low doses of lactulose or neomycin. Nephrotoxicity or ototoxicity may be limiting in prolonged usage of neomycin. There are suggestions that vegetable protein may be preferable to animal protein.

OTHER SEQUELAE OF CIRRHOSIS **Coagulopathy** Patients with cirrhosis often demonstrate a variety of abnormalities in both cellular and humoral clotting function. Thrombocytopenia may result from hypersplenism. In the alcoholic patient, there may be direct bone marrow suppression by ethanol. Diminished protein synthesis may lead to reduced production of fibrinogen (factor I), prothrombin (factor II), and factors V, VII, IX, and X. Reduction in levels of all factors except factor V may be worsened by the coincident malabsorption of the fat-soluble cofactor vitamin K due to cholestasis (Chap. 286). Of these, factor VII appears to be pivotal. In cirrhosis, it is the first of the factors to become depleted and, because of its short half-life, replacement with plasma often fails to correct an elevated prothrombin time. Preliminary studies suggest that selective replacement of factor VII can correct the prothrombin time in patients with cirrhosis.

Hepatocellular Carcinoma See Chap. 91.

HYPOXEMIA AND HEPATOPULMONARY SYNDROME **Definition and Pathogenesis** Mild hypoxemia occurs in approximately one-third of patients with chronic liver disease. The hepatopulmonary syndrome is typically manifest by hypoxemia, platypnea, and orthodeoxia. Hypoxemia usually results from right-to-left intrapulmonary shunts through dilatations in intrapulmonary vessels that can be detected by contrast-enhanced echocardiography or a macroaggregated albumin lung perfusion scan. The mechanisms of shunt formation are unclear, but one animal model suggests that endothelin-1 levels and pulmonary nitric oxide, raised in cirrhosis, correlate with degree of shunting.

℞ **TREATMENT** No specific treatment is consistently effective, though large arteriovenous shunts may be embolized. It is now increasingly recognized that liver transplantation may eventually lead to amelioration of the hepatopulmonary syndrome in cases that have not yet been complicated by advanced pulmonary hypertension.

BIBLIOGRAPHY

Alcoholic, Postnecrotic, and Cryptogenic Cirrhosis

Arroyo V, Ginés P: Arteriolar vasodilation and the pathogenesis of the hyperdynamic circulation and renal sodium and water retention in cirrhosis. Gastroenterology 102: 1077, 1992

Bacon BR et al: Nonalcoholic steatohepatitis: An expanded clinical entity. Gastroenterology 107:1103, 1994

Caldwell H et al: Cryptogenic cirrhosis: Clinical characterization and risk factors for underlying disease. Hepatology 29:664, 1999

Carithers RL et al: Methylprednisolone therapy in patients with severe alcoholic hepatitis. A randomized multicenter trial. Ann Intern Med 110:685, 1989

Friedman SL: The cellular basis of hepatic fibrosis. N Engl J Med 328:1828, 1993

McCullough AJ, O'Connor JFB: Alcoholic liver disease: Recommendations for the American College of Gastroenterology. Am J Gastroenterol 93:2022, 1998

Ramond M-J et al: A randomized trial of prednisolone in patients with severe alcoholic hepatitis. N Engl J Med 326:507, 1992

Sheth SG et al: Nonalcoholic steatohepatitis. Ann Intern Med 126:137, 1997

Biliary and Cardiac Cirrhosis

Beuers U et al: Ursodeoxycholic acid in cholestasis: Potential mechanisms of action and therapeutic applications. Hepatology 28:1449, 1998

Bonnand AM et al: Clinical significance of serum bilirubin levels under ursodeoxycholic acid therapy in patients with primary biliary cirrhosis. Hepatology 29:39, 1999

Combes B et al: A randomized, double-blind, placebo-controlled trial of ursodeoxycholic acid in primary biliary cirrhosis. Hepatology 22:759, 1995

Kaplan MM et al: Medical progress: Primary biliary cirrhosis. N Engl J Med 335:1570, 1996

Locke GR III et al: Time course of histological progression in primary biliary cirrhosis. Hepatology 23:52, 1996

Metcalf JV et al: Natural history of the early primary biliary cirrhosis. Lancet 348:1399, 1996

Poupon RE et al: Ursodiol for the long-term treatment of primary biliary cirrhosis. N Engl J Med 330:1342, 1994

——— et al: Combined analysis of randomized controlled trials of ursodeoxycholic acid in primary biliary cirrhosis. Gastroenterology 113:884, 1997

Wolfhagen FH et al: Oral naltrexone treatment for cholestatic pruritus: A double-blind, placebo-controlled study. Gastroenterology 113:1264, 1997

Hepatic Encephalopathy

Basile AS, Jones EA: Ammonia and GABAergic neurotransmission: Interrelated factors in the pathogenesis of hepatic encephalopathy. Hepatology 25:1303, 1997

Jalan R et al: Review article: Pathogenesis and treatment of chronic hepatic encephalopathy. Aliment Pharmacol Ther 10:681, 1996

Krieger D et al: Manganese and chronic hepatic encephalopathy. Lancet 346:270, 1995

Riordan SM, Williams R: Treatment of hepatic encephalopathy. N Engl J Med 337: 473, 1997

Variceal Hemorrhage

Cello JP et al: Endoscopic sclerotherapy compared with percutaneous transjugular intrahepatic portosystemic shunt after initial sclerotherapy in patients with acute variceal hemorrhage. Ann Intern Med 126:858, 1997

Garcia-Villarreal L et al: Transjugular intrahepatic portosystemic shunt versus endoscopic sclerotherapy for the prevention of variceal rebleeding after recent variceal hemorrhage. Hepatology 29:27, 1999

Grace ND: Diagnosis and treatment of gastrointestinal bleeding secondary to portal hypertension. Am J Gastroenterol 92:1081, 1997

Laine L et al: Endoscopic ligation compared with sclerotherapy for treatment of esophageal variceal bleeding: A meta-analysis. Ann Intern Med 123:280, 1995

Pagliaro L et al: Prevention of first bleeding in cirrhosis: A meta-analysis of randomized trials of nonsurgical treatment. Ann Intern Med 117:59, 1992

Planas R et al: A prospective randomized trial comparing somatostatin and sclerotherapy in the treatment of acute variceal bleeding. Hepatology 20:370, 1994

Sanyal AJ et al: Transjugular intrahepatic portosystemic shunts compared with endoscopic sclerotherapy for the prevention of recurrent variceal hemorrhage. Ann Intern Med 126:849, 1997

STIEGMANN GV et al: Endoscopic sclerotherapy as compared with endoscopic ligation for bleeding esophageal varices. N Engl J Med 326:1527, 1992

SUNG JJY et al: Octreotide infusion or emergency sclerotherapy for variceal haemorrhage. Lancet 342:637, 1993

PORTAL HYPERTENSION AND ASCITES

CHUNG RT et al: Complications of chronic liver disease. Crit Care Clin 11:431, 1995

D'AMICO G et al: The treatment of portal hypertension: A meta-analytic review. Hepatology 22:332, 1995

GINÉS P et al: Paracentesis with intravenous infusion of albumin as compared wtih peritoneovenous shunting in cirrhosis with refractory ascites. N Engl J Med 325:829, 1991

MARTIN P-Y et al: Nitric oxide as a mediator of hemodynamic abnormalities and salt and water retention in cirrhosis. N Engl J Med 339:533, 1998

OCHS A et al: The transjugular intrahepatic portosystemic stent-shunt procedure for refractory ascites. N Engl J Med 332:1192, 1995

POYNARD T et al: Beta-adrenergic-antagonist drugs in the prevention of gastrointestinal bleeding in patients with cirrhosis and esophageal varices. N Engl J Med 324:1532, 1991

RUNYON BA et al: Management of adult patients with ascites caused by cirrhosis. Hepatology 27:264, 1998

SHIFFMAN ML et al: The role of transjugular intrahepatic portosystemic shunt for treatment of portal hypertension and its complications: A conference sponsored by the National Digestive Diseases Advisory Board. Hepatology 22:1591, 1995

STANLEY AJ et al: Long-term follow of transjugular intrahepatic portosystemic stent shunt (TIPS) for the treatment of portal hypertension: Results in 130 patients. Gut 39:479, 1996

SPONTANEOUS BACTERIAL PERITONITIS

NAVASA M et al: Randomized, comparative study of oral ofloxacin versus intravenous cefotaxime in spontaneous bacterial peritonitis. Gastroenterology 111:1011, 1996

ROLACHON A et al: Ciprofloxacin and long-term prevention of spontaneous bacterial peritonitis: Results of a prospective controlled trial. Hepatology 22:1171, 1995

RUNYON BA et al: Short-course versus long-course antibiotic treatment of spontaneous bacterial peritonitis: A randomized controlled study of 100 patients. Gastroenterology 100:1737, 1991

OTHER COMPLICATIONS OF CIRRHOSIS

ABRAMS GA et al: Use of macroaggregated albumin lung scan to diagnose hepatopulmonary syndrome: A new approach. Gastroenterology 114:305, 1998

BERNSTEIN DE et al: Recombinant factor VIIa corrects prothrombin time in cirrhotic patients: A preliminary study. Gastroenterology 113:1930, 1997

300

Daniel K. Podolsky

INFILTRATIVE, GENETIC, AND METABOLIC DISEASES AFFECTING THE LIVER

Many disseminated, systemic, or metabolic diseases involve the liver in a diffuse manner by the infiltration of abnormal cells or the accumulation of chemical substances or metabolites. Chemical accumulation may be extracellular or intracellular and may involve hepatocytes, Kupffer cells, or other elements of the reticuloendothelial system. Although infiltrative diseases may vary widely in cause and extrahepatic manifestations, the findings in the liver may be quite similar. Generalized enlargement and firmness of the liver, gradual and nonspecific deterioration of liver function, and, less often, signs of portal hypertension or ascites are typical features of this group of diseases. Differential diagnosis by clinical means may be difficult on occasion, but in patients in whom ancillary clinical findings do not establish the diagnosis, the diffusely infiltrated liver provides an excellent source of tissue for diagnostic purposes.

HEPATIC STEATOSIS (FATTY LIVER) AND NONALCOHOLIC STEATOHEPATITIS

Slight to moderate enlargement of the liver due to a diffuse accumulation of neutral fat (triglycerides) in hepatocytes is an important clinical and pathologic finding. Imaging techniques such as computed tomography (CT), ultrasound, and magnetic resonance imaging (MRI) may each yield alterations suggesting increased fat in the liver. Several mechanisms can contribute to lipid accumulation in the liver. Fatty liver can be separated into two categories based on whether the fat droplets in the hepatocytes are macrovesicular or microvesicular (Table 300-1). In addition, fatty infiltration may be accompanied by necroinflammatory activity, a condition designated *nonalcoholic steatohepatitis (NASH)*.

MACROVESICULAR FATTY LIVER This is the most common type of fatty liver and is seen most frequently in alcoholism or alcoholic liver disease, diabetes mellitus, obesity, and prolonged parenteral nutrition. Hematoxylin and eosin-stained liver sections show hepatocytes with large, empty vacuoles with the nucleus "pushed" to the periphery of the cell. In general, fat in the liver is not damaging per se, and the fat will disappear with improvement or elimination of the predisposing condition.

Etiology The major causes of fatty liver with macrovesicular fat depend on the age, geographic location, and metabolic-nutritional status of the patient population. *Chronic alcoholism* is the most common cause of hepatic steatosis in this country and in other countries with a high alcohol intake. The severity of fatty involvement is roughly proportional to the duration and degree of alcoholic excess. In addition, in western countries NASH is associated with obesity. Many of these patients (up to one-third) have type 2 diabetes and/or hyperlipidemia. Inflammatory activity when present may reflect the combined effects of oxidative stress, subsequent lipid peroxidation and abnormal cytokine expression, especially increased tumor necrosis factor (TNF).

Protein malnutrition, especially in infancy and early childhood, accounts for most cases of severe fatty liver in the tropical zones of Africa, South America, and Asia. The hepatic changes may be associated with other clinical and pathologic features of kwashiorkor. *Jejunoileal bypass* for surgical treatment of morbid obesity was sometimes associated with severe fatty liver and hepatic failure that could be fatal. In patients with Cushing's syndrome and in those receiving large doses of glucocorticoids, fatty infiltration of the liver may occur. In many *chronic illnesses*, especially those complicated by impaired nutrition or malabsorption, increased fat is found in liver cells. For example, patients with severe ulcerative colitis, chronic pancreatitis, or protracted heart failure frequently have moderate hepatic steatosis at the time of death. Patients maintained on prolonged *total parenteral nutrition* also may develop a fatty liver. In some cases, fatty infiltration and steatohepatitis may occur in the absence of an identifiable cause.

Acute fatty liver is caused by a number of hepatotoxins and is frequently accompanied by signs and symptoms of liver failure. Carbon tetrachloride intoxication, DDT poisoning, and ingestion of substances containing yellow phosphorus result in severe hepatic steatosis. Acute and prolonged alcohol ingestion may also be considered in this category and may be associated with a rapidly enlarging and fat-laden liver.

Table 300-1 Causes of Hepatic Steatosis

Macrovesicular (Large Fat Droplets in Hepatocytes)
Alcohol, alcoholic liver disease[a]
Diabetes mellitus[a]
Obesity[a]
Protein-calorie malnutrition
Total parenteral nutrition[a], jejunoileal bypass
Drugs[a], e.g., methotrexate, aspirin, vitamin A, glucocorticoids, amiodarone, and synthetic estrogen, nucleoside analogues (ddI, AZT)
Microvesicular (Small Fat Droplets in Hepatocytes)
Reye's syndrome
Acute fatty liver of pregnancy
Jamaican vomiting sickness
Drugs, e.g., valproic acid, tetracycline, nucleoside analogues

[a] May also be associated with necroinflammatory activity

Clinical Features The signs and symptoms of hepatic steatosis are related to the degree of fat infiltration, the time course of its accumulation, and the underlying cause. The obese or diabetic patient with a chronic fatty liver is usually asymptomatic and has only mild tenderness over the enlarged liver. The liver function tests are normal or show mild elevations of alkaline phosphatase or aminotransferases. In contrast, the rapid accumulation of fat seen in the setting of hyperalimentation may lead to marked tenderness, presumably resulting from stretching of Glisson's capsule. Similarly, alcoholic patients with acute fatty liver following a bout of heavy drinking may have right upper quadrant pain and tenderness, often with laboratory evidence of cholestasis. The clinical presentation of fatty liver from hepatotoxins is similar to that of fulminant hepatic failure arising from any cause, with evidence of hepatic encephalopathy, marked elevations of prothrombin time and aminotransferases, and variable degrees of jaundice. Although steatohepatitis is generally thought to have a benign clinical course with improvement following elimination of the associated precipitant, in some individuals it may result in significant fibrosis and even cirrhosis. Recent studies indicate that substantial fibrosis or cirrhosis may be present in 15 to 50% of patients with NASH. In the only long-term follow-up study, 30% of patients with fibrosis had cirrhosis after 10 years. It is possible that some cases of "cryptogenic" cirrhosis are due to longstanding NASH and that the fat leaves the liver as endstage liver disease develops.

Diagnosis The findings of a firm, nontender, and generally enlarged liver with minimal hepatic dysfunction in a patient with chronic alcoholism, malnutrition, poorly controlled diabetes mellitus, or obesity should suggest hepatic steatosis. This can usually be detected by CT, MRI, or ultrasound. Modest elevations of aminotransferases are often found in association with hepatic steatohepatitis. A disproportional elevation in AST leading to an AST/ALT ratio greater than 2 is generally associated with alcoholic hepatitis. When diagnostic uncertainty exists, needle biopsy of the liver will demonstrate the increased fat content, the presence of any fibrosis, and possibly the underlying primary disorder.

℞ TREATMENT Adequate nutritional intake, removal of alcohol or offending toxins, and correction of any associated metabolic disorders usually result in recovery. There is no clinical rationale for the use of lipotropic agents such as choline. When indicated, attention should be directed to abstinence from alcohol, careful control of diabetes, weight loss, or correction of intestinal absorptive defects. In the alcoholic fatty liver, there is gradual disappearance of fat from the liver after 4 to 8 weeks of adequate diet and abstinence from alcohol. Similarly, fatty infiltration usually resolves within 2 weeks after discontinuation of parenteral hyperalimentation. Pilot studies in patients with NASH have suggested benefits from vitamin E and phlebotomy. Troglitazone has shown some benefit in those patients with concomitant insulin resistance.

MICROVESICULAR FATTY LIVER This is the less common form of fatty liver. On microscopic examination, the fat is present in many small vacuoles. Although the droplets consist of triglycerides in both the macrovesicular and microvesicular forms, the reason for this difference in morphologic appearance is not clear.

Acute fatty liver of pregnancy (AFLP) is a syndrome that occurs late in pregnancy and is often associated with jaundice and hepatic failure. The liver is typically small. AFLP is more common when the mother is carrying a male fetus and may be associated with a deficiency of long-chain-3-hydroxy acyl COH dehydrogenase. Preeclampsia or the HELLP syndrome, which may complicate eclampsia, presents in a similar fashion and progresses to severe liver dysfunction, though typically with a normal size liver. Aminotransferase elevations are typically modest in all of these conditions (generally <500). If diagnosed in time, the disease usually resolves with termination of the pregnancy. Recurrence in subsequent pregnancies is rare.

Microvesicular fat accumulation also may be seen as a toxic reaction to *valproic acid* and with excessive doses of *tetracycline*. It is a typical finding in *Jamaican vomiting sickness*, which is caused by hypoglycin A present in unripened ackee fruit. Lactic acidosis and severe liver injury with microvesicular fat has been described as a complication of nucleoside analogue therapy.

REYE'S SYNDROME (FATTY LIVER WITH ENCEPHALOPATHY) This acute illness is encountered exclusively in children below 15 years of age. It is characterized clinically by vomiting and signs of progressive central nervous system damage, signs of hepatic injury, and hypoglycemia. Morphologically, there is extensive fatty vacuolization of the liver and renal tubules. There is mitochondrial dysfunction with decreased activity of hepatic mitochondrial enzymes. The cause is unknown, although viral agents and drugs, especially salicylates, have been implicated. Increased aspirin use and much higher serum salicylate levels in children with this illness than in the general population have been described during outbreaks of Reye's syndrome. Recognition of this relationship and reduced aspirin use in this setting may account for the decreasing incidence of Reye's syndrome. However, this illness may occur in the absence of exposure to salicylates. In fatal cases, the liver is enlarged and yellow with striking diffuse fatty microvacuolization of cells. Peripheral zonal hepatic necrosis also has been present in some cases. Fatty changes of the renal tubular cells, cerebral edema, and neuronal degeneration of the brain are the major extrahepatic changes. Electron-microscopic studies show structural alterations of mitochondria in liver, brain, and muscle.

The onset usually follows an upper respiratory tract infection, especially influenza or chickenpox. Within 1 to 3 days, persistent vomiting occurs, together with stupor, which usually progresses rapidly to generalized convulsions and coma. The liver is enlarged, but *jaundice is characteristically absent or minimal*. Elevations in serum aminotransferases and prothrombin time, hypoglycemia, metabolic acidosis, and elevated serum ammonia levels are the major laboratory findings. The mortality rate in Reye's syndrome is approximately 50%. Therapy consists of infusions of 20% glucose and fresh frozen plasma, as well as intravenous mannitol to reduce the cerebral edema. Chronic liver disease has not been reported in survivors.

STORAGE DISEASES

Lipid storage diseases include the hereditary disorders of Gaucher's and Niemann-Pick disease. Other rare diseases associated with increased fat in the liver include abetalipoproteinemia, Tangier disease, Fabry's disease, and types I and V hyperlipoproteinemia (see Chap. 344 for details). Hepatic enlargement caused by distention of liver cells with glycogen is present in some poorly controlled diabetics and frequently in juvenile diabetes. More often, however, hepatomegaly is due to fatty infiltration (see above). Ketoacidosis and vigorous insulin therapy may further enhance hepatic enlargement.

HEPATIC MINERAL ACCUMULATION

WILSON'S DISEASE This is an uncommon inherited disorder of copper metabolism. Wilson's disease presents clinically in adolescence or young adulthood by which time there is excess copper accumulation in the liver and other tissues. Deficiency of the plasma copper protein ceruloplasmin is a characteristic feature. The accumulation appears to result from impaired copper excretion due to a mutation in a gene that encodes a P-type ATPase copper transporter. Clinically, patients may present in teenage or early adult years with chronic hepatitis, cirrhosis, or their complications. A small number of patients will present with fulminant hepatitis. Liver disease is often accompanied by softening and degeneration of the basal ganglia (hepatolenticular degeneration) due to copper deposition, which results in extrapyramidal neurologic and psychiatric symptoms. Brownish pigmentation of Descemet's membrane in the cornea (Kayser-Fleischer rings) is frequently present. Hemolytic anemia is also common, especially with fulminant disease. Liver biopsy may reveal findings ranging from fulminant hepatitis to chronic hepatitis and macronodular cirrhosis, in addition to excess copper levels. Typically, liver cells are ballooned and show increased glycogen with glycogen vacuolization in the nuclei. All patients under age 40 with unexplained chronic hepatitis or cirrhosis should be evaluated for possible Wilson's disease. Prompt diagnosis is important; treatment, which must be continued throughout life, can prevent progression of end-organ damage. →*For further discussion, see Chap. 348.*

HEMOCHROMATOSIS Hemochromatosis may be the most common genetic disorder of humans; it involves accumulation of abnormal amounts of iron due to inappropriate absorption from the intestine. Between 85 and 95% of patients with genetic hemochromatosis are homozygous for a point mutation (cystine to tyrosine at codon 282:C282). The liver, as a primary site of iron storage, is affected most directly. There is diffuse deposition of excess iron in hepatocytes, in contrast to the characteristic accumulation of iron in the reticuloendothelial compartment typical of secondary iron overload and hemosiderosis. Excess hepatic iron commonly results in hepatomegaly. Although liver function is initially well preserved, if the disease is untreated, progressive impairment is followed by the development of cirrhosis. Prompt diagnosis can permit the institution of effective lifelong therapy to reduce the iron load and halt progression of the disease. → *For further discussion, see Chap. 345.*

OTHER INFILTRATIVE AND METABOLIC DISEASES

α_1-ANTITRYPSIN DEFICIENCY Patients with homozygous deficiency of serum α_1-antitrypsin (α_1AT) are prone to develop emphysema in adult life. The disease is suggested by the absence of alpha$_1$ globulin on serum electrophoresis (α_1AT makes up 90% of this fraction normally) and confirmed by direct measurement of α_1AT. The exact phenotype can then be determined by starch electrophoresis. Although there are approximately 75 recognized alleles, only PiZ and PiS are associated with clinical disease. The molecular bases of these altered products have been related to single nucleic acid substitutions—e.g., PiZ is caused by a G (guanine) to A (adenine) transposition, which results in a substitution of a glutamic acid for lysine at residue 292 in the α_1AT protein. Hepatocytes of some patients with this deficiency contain globules positive with the periodic acid Schiff reaction. Approximately 10% of children with homozygous deficiency (PiZZ phenotype) of α_1AT will develop significant liver disease, including neonatal hepatitis and progressive cirrhosis. It has been suggested that 15 to 20 percent of all chronic liver disease in infancy may be attributed to α_1AT deficiency. In adults, the most common manifestation of α_1AT deficiency is asymptomatic cirrhosis, which may progress from a micronodular to a macronodular state and may be complicated by the development of hepatocellular carcinoma. The occurrence of liver disease in these patients is not dependent on the development of lung disease. →*For further discussion, see Chap. 258.*

HURLER'S SYNDROME This is an uncommon hereditary disease that is characterized by the widespread tissue deposition of mucopolysaccharide (chondroitin sulfate B and heparan sulfate) in many tissues. The liver is frequently enlarged and firm. Microscopically, Kupffer cells and other macrophages are enlarged and filled with metachromatic granular material. Cirrhosis may be a late complication. →*For further discussion, see Chap. 349.*

PORPHYRIAS See Chap. 346.

RETICULOENDOTHELIAL DISORDERS (See also Chaps. 61 and 113)

Moderate to massive hepatomegaly and splenomegaly occur frequently in the various types of *leukemia* and *lymphoma*. Jaundice, when present, is usually slight and results from hemolysis, although cholestasis may occasionally be associated with lymphoma as a paraneoplastic syndrome. Deep and protracted jaundice is distinctly rare and is caused by obstruction of the intrahepatic or extrahepatic bile ducts by tumor. Liver biopsy specimens reveal portal and sinusoidal infiltrates in most cases of leukemia, but the cellular pattern may be mixed and nonspecific. Liver biopsy is diagnostic in only 5% of patients with *Hodgkin's disease*. This percentage is increased in those with advanced disease or splenomegaly. Directed biopsy at laparoscopy or laparotomy is more likely to be positive than "blind" needle biopsy. Nonspecific histologic changes in the liver have been described in patients with lymphoma and may contribute to the abnormal liver function tests.

Myeloid metaplasia and other myeloproliferative disorders associated with extramedullary hematopoiesis produce hepatomegaly which may reach huge proportions, especially following splenectomy. Serum alkaline phosphatase elevations are often found. Ascites and portal hypertension, resulting from diffuse involvement of portal venules and lymphatics, are rare complications.

GRANULOMATOUS INFILTRATIONS

Perhaps as a result of the large population of mononuclear phagocytes, a number of systemic granulomatous diseases involve the liver, including sarcoidosis, miliary tuberculosis, histoplasmosis, brucellosis, schistosomiasis, berylliosis, and drug reactions (Table 300-2). In addition, isolated granulomas of no diagnostic importance may be found occasionally in patients with various forms of cirrhosis and hepatitis. The liver infiltrated by granulomas may be slightly enlarged and firm, but hepatic dysfunction is usually limited. Increases in serum alkaline phosphatase are common and may range from mild to marked. Occasionally, mild serum elevations in aminotransferases are also present. In a few patients with sarcoidosis or brucellosis, portal hypertension may develop, and extensive postnecrotic scarring or postnecrotic cirrhosis may follow healing of the granulomatous lesions, as in schistosomiasis.

Needle biopsy of the liver often provides the first definite evidence of a systemic or disseminated granulomatous disease. In patients with sarcoidosis who have neither clinical nor laboratory evidence of hepatic involvement, needle biopsy shows sarcoid granulomas in about 80% of cases. In cases of suspected miliary tuberculosis, a portion of the biopsy should be cultured and stained for mycobacteria. The organism can be detected in the majority of cases, particularly when caseating granulomas are present. Serial sections of the biopsy specimen should be examined if granulomas are not apparent. Individual granulomas are rarely specific in their microscopic appearance, and final diagnosis usually requires other clinical, laboratory, or histologic data.

In approximately 20% of patients, it is not possible to identify a

Table 300-2 Some Causes of Hepatic Granulomas

SYSTEMIC DISEASE	
Sarcoidosis	Berylliosis
Hodgkin's and non-Hodgkin's lymphoma	Crohn's disease
	Wegener's granulomatosis
Primary biliary cirrhosis	Granulomatous hepatitis, idiopathic
INFECTIONS	
Bacterial	Parasitic
Tuberculosis	Schistosomiasis
Mycobacterium avium intracellulare	Rickettsial
	Q fever
Brucellosis	Spirochetes
Leprosy	Syphilis
Viral	Drugs
Epstein-Barr virus	Sulfonamides
Cytomegalovirus	Isoniazid
Chicken pox	Allopurinol

cause for the granulomatous infiltration. When these infiltrates are accompanied by fever of unknown origin, the diagnosis of *granulomatous hepatitis* should be considered. This is an uncommon disorder of unknown cause and is diagnosed by exclusion. While granulomatous hepatitis invariably responds to moderate doses of glucocorticoids, relapses are frequent, and such therapy should never be undertaken unless tuberculous disease or other causes of granulomatous infiltration have been excluded. This may include an initial empiric trial of antituberculous therapy.

AMYLOIDOSIS (See also Chap. 319) Systemic amyloidosis, whether primary and idiopathic, familial, or secondary to chronic inflammatory or neoplastic diseases, often involves the liver. Grossly, the liver infiltrated with amyloid is enlarged and pale and rubbery in consistency. Microscopically, the birefringent amyloid deposits appear as homogeneous waxy material within the space of Disse, often being concentrated in the periportal areas and associated with atrophy of adjacent liver cell plates. Selective involvement of the walls of blood vessels, especially of the hepatic arterioles, may be a striking feature of primary amyloidosis. With this possible exception, however, the hepatic lesions are the same in all forms of amyloidosis and are present in 60 to 90% of cases.

An enlarged and firm liver is found in about 60% of patients, and ascites occurs in advanced stages of the disease in about 20%. Jaundice, portal hypertension, and other signs of chronic liver disease are usually absent. Liver function changes, although frequent, correlate poorly with the extent of liver infiltration. Hypoalbuminemia and elevated serum alkaline phosphatase are common. Hypoalbuminemia, however, may be related to the presence of nephrosis; the prothrombin time is usually normal. The diagnosis is established by biopsy of rectum, skin, liver, or other involved organs and demonstration of the characteristic Congo red-staining deposits by polarizing microscopy.

AIDS-RELATED LIVER DISEASE

In AIDS, evidence of liver disease is quite common but is usually mild with minimal morbidity. In these patients, hepatic granulomatous disease is often present and may be caused by opportunistic infections, with *Mycobacterium avium-intracellulare* being the most frequent pathogen. Cytomegalovirus hepatitis and hepatic mycoses are less common. These patients are frequently being treated for *Pneumocystis carinii* infections with sulfonamides, which also may cause hepatic granulomatous disease. AIDS cholangiopathy has become a well recognized entity. It exhibits features similar to those found in primary sclerosing cholangitis and is typically associated with cryptosporidia, microsporidia, and/or cytomegalovirus infection in the biliary tract. Papillary stenosis is frequently present. In addition, AIDS patients are vulnerable to hepatic injury resulting from drugs used to treat HIV, most notably nucleoside analogues.

ACKNOWLEDGMENT

This chapter represents a revised version of a chapter by Dr. Kurt J. Isselbacher and Dr. Daniel K. Podolsky that has appeared in previous editions of this textbook.

BIBLIOGRAPHY

ADAMS PC, CHAKRABARATI S: Genotypic/phenotypic correlations in genetic hemochromatosis: Evolution of diagnostic criteria. Gastroenterology 114:319, 1998

BACON BR et al: Molecular medicine and hemochromatosis: At the crossroads. Gastroenterology 116:193, 1999

CRYSTAL RG: Alpha 1-antitrypsin deficiency, emphysema and liver disease: Genetic basis and strategy for therapy. J Clin Invest 85:1343, 1990

HURWITZ ES et al: Public Health Service Study on Reye's syndrome and medications. N Engl J Med 313:842, 1985

HUTCHISON DC: Natural history of alpha 1-protease inhibitor deficiency. Am J Med 84: 3, 1988

JAMES O, DAY C: Non-alcoholic steatohepatitis: Another disease of affluence. Lancet 353:1634, 1999

KNOX TA, OLANS LB: Liver disease in pregnancy. N Engl J Med 335(8):569, 1996

MATTEONI CA: et al: Nonalcoholic fatty liver disease: A spectrum of clinical and pathological severity. Gastroenterology 116:1414, 1999

MINAKAMI H et al: Pre-eclampsia: A microvesicular fat disease of the liver. Am J Obstet Gynecol 159:1043, 1988

PERLMUTTER DH: The cellular basis for liver injury in alpha 1-antitrypsin deficiency. Hepatology 13:172, 1991

SCHIFF ER et al: *Diseases of the Liver*, 8th ed. Philadelphia, Lippincott, 1999

SCRIVER CR et al (eds): *The Metabolic and Molecular Bases of Inherited Disease*, 8th ed. New York, McGraw-Hill, 2001

STEINDL P et al: Wilson's disease in patients with liver disease: A diagnostic challenge. Gastroenterology 113:212, 1997

STERNLIEB I: Perspectives on Wilson's disease. Hepatology 12:1234, 1990

ZAKIM D, BOYER TD: *Hepatology: A Textbook of Liver Disease*, 3d ed. Philadelphia, Saunders, 1996

301 LIVER TRANSPLANTATION

Jules L. Dienstag

Liver transplantation—the replacement of the native, diseased liver by a normal organ (allograft) recovered from a brain-dead donor—has matured from an experimental procedure reserved for desperately ill patients to an accepted, lifesaving operation applied much earlier in the natural history of end-stage liver disease. The preferred and technically most advanced approach is *orthotopic transplantation*, in which the native organ is removed and the donor organ is inserted in the same anatomic location. Pioneered in the 1960s by Starzl at the University of Colorado and, later, at the University of Pittsburgh and by Calne in Cambridge, England, liver transplantation is now performed routinely by dozens of centers throughout North America and western Europe. Success and survival have improved from approximately 30% in the 1970s to >80% today. These improved prospects for prolonged survival, dating back to the early 1980s, resulted from refinements in operative technique (including the introduction of venovenous bypass to allow venous return from the extremities and visceral circulation during clamping of the inferior vena cava), improvements in organ procurement and preservation, advances in immunosuppressive therapy, and, perhaps most influentially, more enlightened patient selection and timing. Despite the perioperative morbidity and mortality, the technical and management challenges of the procedure, and its costs, liver transplantation has become the approach of choice for selected patients whose chronic or acute liver disease is progressive, life-threatening, and unresponsive to medical therapy. Based on the current level of success, the number of liver transplants has continued to grow each year; in 1999, >4000 patients received liver allografts in the United States. Still, the demand for new livers continues to outpace availability; in 1999, >6000 patients in the United States were on a waiting list for a donor liver.

INDICATIONS Potential candidates for liver transplantation are children and adults who, in the absence of contraindications (see below), suffer from severe, irreversible liver disease for which alternative medical or surgical treatments have been exhausted or are unavailable. *Timing of the operation is of critical importance.* Indeed, improved timing and better patient selection are felt to have contributed more to the increased success of liver transplantation in the 1980s and beyond than all the impressive technical and immunologic advances combined. Although the disease should be advanced, and although opportunities for spontaneous or medically induced stabilization or recovery should be allowed, the procedure should be done sufficiently early to give the surgical procedure a fair chance for success. Ideally, transplantation should be considered in patients with end-stage liver disease who are experiencing or have experienced a life-threatening complication of hepatic decompensation, whose quality of life has deteriorated to unacceptable levels, or whose liver disease will result predictably in irreversible damage to the central nervous system

(CNS). If this is done sufficiently early, the patient will not have developed any contraindications or extrahepatic systemic deterioration. Although patients with well-compensated cirrhosis can survive for many years, many patients with quasi-stable chronic liver disease have much more advanced disease than may be apparent. As discussed below, the better the status of the patient prior to transplantation, the higher will be the anticipated success rate of transplantation. The decision about *when* to transplant is complex and requires the combined judgment of an experienced team of hepatologists, transplant surgeons, anesthesiologists, and specialists in support services, not to mention the well-informed consent of the patient and the patient's family.

Transplantation in Children Indications for transplantation in children are listed in Table 301-1. The most common is *biliary atresia. Inherited or genetic disorders of metabolism* associated with liver failure constitute another major indication for transplantation in children and adolescents. In Crigler-Najjar disease type I and in certain hereditary disorders of the urea cycle and of amino acid or lactate-pyruvate metabolism, transplantation may be the only way to prevent impending deterioration of CNS function, despite the fact that the native liver is structurally normal. Combined heart and liver transplantation has yielded dramatic improvement in cardiac function and in cholesterol levels in children with homozygous familial hypercholesterolemia; combined liver and kidney transplantation has been successful in patients with hereditary oxalosis. In hemophiliacs with transfusion-associated hepatitis and liver failure, liver transplantation has been associated with recovery of normal factor VIII synthesis.

Transplantation in Adults Liver transplantation is indicated for end-stage *cirrhosis* of all causes (Table 301-1). In sclerosing cholangitis and *Caroli's disease* (multiple cystic dilatations of the intrahepatic biliary tree), recurrent infections and sepsis associated with inflammatory and fibrotic obstruction of the biliary tree may be an indication for transplantation. Because prior biliary surgery complicates, and is a relative contraindication for, liver transplantation, surgical diversion of the biliary tree has been all but abandoned for patients with sclerosing cholangitis. In patients who undergo transplantation for *hepatic vein thrombosis (Budd-Chiari syndrome)*, postoperative anticoagulation is essential; underlying myeloproliferative disorders may have to be treated but are not a contraindication to liver transplantation. If a donor organ can be located quickly, before life-threatening complications—including cerebral edema—set in, patients with *fulminant hepatitis* are candidates for liver transplantation. More controversial as candidates for liver transplantation are patients with *alcoholic cirrhosis*, *chronic viral hepatitis*, and *primary hepatocellular malignancies*. Although all three of these categories are considered to be high risk, liver transplantation can be offered to carefully selected patients. Patients with alcoholic cirrhosis can be considered as candidates for transplantation if they meet strict criteria for abstinence and reform. Patients with chronic hepatitis C have done as well as any other subset of patients after transplantation, despite the fact that recurrent infection in the donor organ is the rule. In patients with chronic hepatitis B, in the absence of measures to prevent recurrent hepatitis B, survival after transplantation is reduced by approximately 10 to 20%; however, prophylactic use of hepatitis B immune globulin (HBIG) during and after transplantation increases the success of transplantation to a level comparable to that seen in patients with nonviral causes of liver decompensation. Specific antiviral drugs, such as lamivudine, that can be used for both prophylaxis against and treatment of recurrent hepatitis B will facilitate further the management of patients undergoing liver transplantation for end-stage hepatitis B. Issues of disease recurrence are discussed in more detail below. Patients with nonmetastatic primary hepatobiliary tumors—primary hepatocellular carcinoma, cholangiocarcinoma, hepatoblastoma, angiosarcoma, epithelioid hemangioendothelioma, and multiple or massive hepatic adenomata—have undergone liver transplantation; however, for hepatobiliary malignancies, overall survival is significantly lower than that for other categories of liver disease. To minimize the very high likelihood of recurrent tumor after transplantation, some centers are evaluating experimental adjuvant chemotherapy protocols. Some transplantation centers have reported excellent long-term, recurrence-free survival in patients with unresectable hepatocellular carcinoma for single tumors <5 cm in diameter or for three or fewer lesions all <3 cm. Consequently, most centers restrict liver transplanation to patients whose hepatic malignancies are confined to these limits. Because the likelihood of recurrent cholangiocarcinoma is almost universal, this tumor is no longer considered an indication for transplantation.

CONTRAINDICATIONS *Absolute contraindications* for transplantation include life-threatening systemic diseases, uncontrolled extrahepatic bacterial or fungal infections, preexisting advanced cardiovascular or pulmonary disease, multiple uncorrectable life-threatening congenital anomalies, metastatic malignancy, active drug or alcohol abuse, and HIV infection (Table 301-2). Because carefully selected patients in their sixties and even seventies have undergone transplantation successfully, advanced age per se is no longer considered an absolute contraindication; however, in older patients, a more thorough preoperative evaluation should be undertaken to exclude ischemic cardiac disease. Advanced age (>70 years), however, may be considered a *relative contraindication*—that is, a factor to be taken into account with other relative contraindications. Other relative contraindications include highly replicative hepatitis B, portal vein thrombosis, preexisting renal disease not associated with liver disease, intrahepatic or biliary sepsis, severe hypoxemia resulting from right-to-left intrapulmonary shunts, previous extensive hepatobiliary sur-

Table 301-1 Indications for Liver Transplantation

Children	Adults
Biliary atresia	Primary biliary cirrhosis
Neonatal hepatitis	Secondary biliary cirrhosis
Congenital hepatic fibrosis	Primary sclerosing cholangitis
Alagille's disease[a]	Caroli's disease[c]
Byler's disease[b]	Cryptogenic cirrhosis
α_1-Antitrypsin deficiency	Chronic hepatitis with cirrhosis
Inherited disorders of metabolism	Hepatic vein thrombosis
Wilson's disease	Fulminant hepatitis
Tyrosinemia	Alcoholic cirrhosis
Glycogen storage diseases	Chronic viral hepatitis
Lysosomal storage diseases	Primary hepatocellular malignancies
Protoporphyria	Hepatic adenomas
Crigler-Najjar disease type I	
Familial hypercholesterolemia	
Hereditary oxalosis	
Hemophilia	

[a] Arteriohepatic dysplasia, with paucity of bile ducts, and congenital malformations, including pulmonary stenosis.
[b] Intrahepatic cholestasis, progressive liver failure, mental and growth retardation.
[c] Multiple cystic dilatations of the intrahepatic biliary tree.

Table 301-2 Contraindications to Liver Transplantation

Absolute	Relative
Uncontrolled extrahepatobiliary infection	Age >70
Uncorrectable, life-limiting congenital anomalies	Portal vein thrombosis
Active substance or alcohol abuse	HIV seropositivity
Advanced cardiopulmonary disease	Previous extrahepatic malignancy
Extrahepatobiliary malignancy	Severe obesity
Metastatic malignancy to the liver	Severe malnutrition/wasting
Cholangiocarcinoma	Medical noncompliance
AIDS	Renal failure
Life-threatening systemic diseases	Intrahepatic sepsis
	Primary hepatic malignancy
	Prior extensive hepatobiliary surgery
	Severe hypoxemia secondary to right-to-left intrapulmonary shunts
	Uncontrolled psychiatric disorder

gery, and any uncontrolled serious psychiatric disorder. Any one of these relative contraindications is insufficient in and of itself to preclude transplantation. For example, the problem of portal vein thrombosis can be overcome by constructing a graft from the donor liver portal vein to the recipient's superior mesenteric vein.

TECHNICAL CONSIDERATIONS **Donor Selection** Donor livers for transplantation are procured primarily from victims of head trauma. Organs from brain-dead donors up to age 60 are acceptable if the following criteria are met: hemodynamic stability; adequate oxygenation; absence of bacterial or fungal infection; serologic exclusion of hepatitis B and C viruses and HIV; absence of abdominal trauma; and absence of hepatic dysfunction. Cardiovascular and respiratory functions are maintained artificially until the liver can be removed. Compatibility in ABO blood group and organ size between donor and recipient are important considerations in donor selection; however, ABO-incompatible or reduced-donor-organ transplants can be performed in emergency or marked donor-scarcity situations. Tissue typing for HLA matching is not required, and preformed cytotoxic HLA antibodies do not preclude liver transplantation. Following perfusion with cold electrolyte solution, the donor liver is removed and packed in ice. The use of University of Wisconsin (UW) solution, rich in lactobionate and raffinose, has permitted the extension of cold ischemic time up to 20 h; however, 12 h may be a more reasonable limit. Improved techniques for harvesting multiple organs from the same donor have increased the availability of donor livers, but the availability of donor livers is far outstripped by the demand. Currently, in the United States, all donor livers are distributed through a nationwide organ-sharing network (United Network of Organ Sharing) designed to allocate available organs based on regional considerations and recipient acuity. Recipients who require the highest level of care (intensive care) have the highest priority, as outlined in Table 301-3.

Surgical Technique Removal of the recipient's native liver is technically difficult, particularly in the presence of portal hypertension with its associated collateral circulation and extensive varices, and even more so in the presence of scarring from previous abdominal operations. The combination of portal hypertension and coagulopathy (elevated prothrombin time and thrombocytopenia) translates into large blood product transfusion requirements. After the portal vein and infrahepatic and suprahepatic inferior vena cavae are dissected, a pump-driven venovenous bypass system is applied to reroute blood from the portal vein and inferior vena cava, preventing congestion of visceral organs. After the hepatic artery and common bile duct are dissected, the native liver is removed and the donor organ inserted. During the anhepatic phase, coagulopathy, hypoglycemia, hypocalcemia, and hypothermia are encountered and must be managed by the anesthesiology team. Caval, portal vein, hepatic artery, and bile duct anastomoses are performed in succession, the last by end-to-end suturing of the donor and recipient common bile ducts or by choledochojejunostomy to a Roux en Y loop if the recipient common bile duct cannot be used for reconstruction (e.g., in sclerosing cholangitis). A typical transplant operation lasts 8 h, with a range of 6 to 18 h. Because of excessive bleeding, large volumes of blood, blood products, and volume expanders may be required during surgery.

Emerging alternatives to orthotopic liver transplantation include split-liver grafts, in which one donor organ is divided and inserted into two recipients; and living-related-donor procedures, in which the left lobe of the liver is harvested from a living-related donor for transplantation into the recipient. Heterotopic liver transplantation, in which the donor liver is inserted without removal of the native liver, has met with very limited success and acceptance, except in a very small number of centers. To support desperately ill patients until a suitable donor organ can be identified, several transplantation centers are studying extracorporeal perfusion with bioartificial liver cartridges constructed from hepatocytes bound to hollow fiber systems and used as temporary hepatic-assist devices, but their efficacy remains to be established. Areas of research with the potential to overcome the shortage of donor organs include hepatocyte transplantation and xenotransplantation with genetically modified organs of nonhuman origin (e.g., swine).

Table 301-3 Liver Transplantation Waiting List Criteria (in Order of Descending Urgency)

Status 1	Fulminant hepatic failure (including primary graft nonfunction and hepatic artery thrombosis within 7 days after transplantation as well as acute decompensated Wilson's disease)[a]
Status 2A	Chronic liver disease with CTP[b] score ≥10, in intensive care unit, predicted <7 days to live, plus one of following: hepatic encephalopathy ≥ stage III; variceal bleeding; heptorenal syndrome; refractory ascites or hepatic hydrothorax; coagulopathy with ongoing bleeding (cannot have extrahepatic sepsis, high-dose or double pressor dependency, or multiorgan failure)
Status 2B	Chronic liver disease with CTP score ≥ 10 or CTP score ≥7 plus one of following: variceal bleeding; hepatorenal syndrome; history of spontaneous bacterial periotonitis; refractory ascites or hepatic hydrothorax; refractory bleeding
Status 3	CTP score ≥7
Status 7	Inactive

[a] For children < 18 years of age, Status 1 includes acute or chronic liver failure plus hospitalization in an intensive care unit or inborn errors of metabolism.

[b] Child-Turcotte-Pugh score components

Points	1	2	3
Encephalopathy	None	Stages I–II	Stages III–IV
Ascites	Absent	Slight, responsive	Moderate-severe
Bilirubin (mg/dL)	<2	2–3	>3
Albumin (g/dL)	>3.5	2.8–3.5	<2.8
Prothrombin time	<15 s	15–17 s	>17 s

The CTP score is calculated by assigning 1 point for any feature in column 1, 2 points for any feature in column 2, and 3 points for any feature in column 3. Class A = ≤6; Class B = 7–9; Class C = ≥10. For cholestatis disorders, such as primary biliary cirrhosis, primary sclerosing cholangitis, etc., the bilirubin categories are <4, 4–10, and >10.

POSTOPERATIVE COURSE AND MANAGEMENT **Immunosuppressive Therapy** The introduction in 1980 of cyclosporine as an immunosuppressive agent contributed substantially to the improvement in survival after liver transplantation. Cyclosporine inhibits early activation of T cells and is specific for T cell functions that result from the interaction of the T cell with its receptor and that involve the calcium-dependent signal transduction pathway. As a result, the activity of cyclosporine leads to inhibition of lymphokine gene activation, blocking interleukins 2, 3, and 4, tumor necrosis factor α, as well as other lymphokines. Cyclosporine also inhibits B cell functions. This process occurs without affecting rapidly dividing cells in the bone marrow, which may account for the reduced frequency of posttransplantation systemic infections. The most common and important side effect of cyclosporine therapy is nephrotoxicity. Cyclosporine causes dose-dependent renal tubular injury and direct renal artery vasospasm. Following renal function, therefore, is important in monitoring cyclosporine therapy, perhaps even a more reliable indicator than blood levels of the drug. Nephrotoxicity is reversible and can be managed by dose reduction. Other adverse effects of cyclosporine therapy include hypertension, hyperkalemia, tremor, hirsutism, glucose intolerance, and gum hyperplasia.

Tacrolimus (originally labeled FK 506) is a macrolide lactone antibiotic isolated from a Japanese soil fungus, *Streptomyces tsukubaensis*. It has the same mechanism of action as cyclosporine but is 10 to 100 times more potent. Initially applied as "rescue" therapy for patients in whom rejection occurred despite the use of cyclosporine, tacrolimus has been shown in two large, multicenter, randomized trials to be associated with a reduced frequency of acute rejection, refractory rejection, and chronic rejection. Although patient and graft survival are the same with these two drugs, the advantage of tacrolimus in minimizing episodes of rejection, reducing the need for additional glucocorticoid doses, and reducing the likelihood of bacterial and cytomegalovirus infection has simplified the management of patients undergoing liver transplantation. In addition, the oral absorption of tacrolimus is more predictable than that of cyclosporine, especially during the early postoperative period when T-tube drainage interferes with the enterohepatic circulation of cyclosporine. As a result, in most transplantation centers, tacrolimus has now supplanted cyclosporine for primary immunosuppression, and many centers rely on oral, rather than intravenous, administration from the outset. For transplantation centers that prefer cyclosporine, a new, better-absorbed, microemulsion preparation is now available.

Although tacrolimus is more potent than cyclosporine, it is also more toxic and more likely to be discontinued for adverse events. The toxicity of tacrolimus is similar to that of cyclosporine; nephrotoxicity and neurotoxicity are the most commonly encountered adverse effects, and neurotoxicity (tremor, seizures, hallucinations, psychoses, coma) is more likely and more severe in tacrolimus-treated patients. Both drugs can cause diabetes mellitus, but tacrolimus does not cause hirsutism or gingival hyperplasia. Because of overlapping toxicity between cyclosporine and tacrolimus, especially nephrotoxicity, and because tacrolimus reduces cyclosporine clearance, these two drugs should not be used together. Because 99% of tacrolimus is metabolized by the liver, hepatic dysfunction reduces its clearance; in primary graft nonfunction (when, for technical reasons or because of ischemic damage prior to its insertion, the allograft is defective and does not function normally from the outset) tacrolimus doses have to be reduced substantially, especially in children. Both cyclosporine and tacrolimus are metabolized by the cytochrome P450 IIIA system, and, therefore, drugs that induce cytochrome P450 (e.g., phenytoin, phenobarbital, carbamazepine, rifampin) reduce available levels of cyclosporine and tacrolimus; drugs that inhibit cytochrome P450 (e.g., erythromycin, fluconazole, ketoconazole, clotrimazole, itraconazole, verapamil, diltiazem, nicardipine, cimetidine, danazol, metoclopramide, bromocriptine) increase cyclosporine and tacrolimus blood levels. Like azathioprine, cyclosporine and tacrolimus appear to be associated with a risk of lymphoproliferative malignancies (see below), which may occur earlier after cyclosporine or tacrolimus than after azathioprine therapy. Because of these side effects, combinations of cyclosporine or tacrolimus with prednisone and azathioprine—all at reduced doses—are preferable regimens for immunosuppressive therapy.

In patients with pretransplant renal dysfunction or renal deterioration that occurs intraoperatively or immediately postoperatively, tacrolimus or cyclosporine therapy may not be practical; under these circumstances, induction or maintenance of immunosuppression with monoclonal antibodies to T cells, OKT3, may be appropriate. Therapy with OKT3 has been especially effective in reversing acute rejection in the posttransplant period and is the standard treatment for acute rejection that fails to respond to methylprednisolone boluses. Intravenous infusions of OKT3 may be complicated by transient fever, chills, and diarrhea. When this drug is used to induce immunosuppression initially or to provide "rescue" in those who reject despite "conventional" therapy, the incidence of bacterial, fungal, and especially cytomegalovirus infections is increased during and after such therapy. In some centers, ganciclovir antiviral therapy is initiated prophylactically as a routine along with OKT3. Another immunosuppressive drug that is likely to be used in the future for patients undergoing liver transplantation is mycophenolic acid, a nonnucleoside purine metabolism inhibitor derived as a fermentation product from several *Penicillium* species. Mycophenolate has been shown to be better than azathioprine, when used with other standard immunosuppressive drugs, in preventing rejection after renal transplantation and has been approved for use in renal transplantation. Rapamycin, an inhibitor of later events in T cell activation, is yet another drug undergoing experimental evaluation as an immunosuppressive agent.

The most important principle of immunosuppression is that the ideal approach strikes a balance between immunosuppression and immunologic competence. Given sufficient immunosuppression, acute liver allograft rejection is always reversible; however, if the cumulative dose of immunosuppressive therapy is too large, the patient will succumb to opportunistic infection. Therefore, immunosuppressive drugs must be used judiciously, with strict attention to the infectious consequences of such therapy.

Postoperative Complications Complications of liver transplantation can be divided into hepatic and nonhepatic categories (Tables 301-4 and 301-5). In addition, both immediately postoperative and late complications are encountered. Patients who undergo liver transplantation as a rule have been chronically ill for protracted periods and may be malnourished and wasted. The impact of such chronic illness and the multisystem failure that accompanies liver failure continues to require attention in the postoperative period. Because of the massive fluid losses and fluid shifts that occur during the operation, patients may remain fluid overloaded during the immediate postoperative period, straining cardiovascular reserve; this effect can be amplified in the face of transient renal dysfunction and pulmonary capillary vascular permeability. Continuous monitoring of cardiovascular and pulmonary function, measures to maintain the integrity of the intravascular compartment and to treat extravascular volume overload, and scrupulous attention to potential sources of and sites of infection are of paramount importance. Cardiovascular instability may also result from the electrolyte imbalance that may accompany reperfusion of the donor liver. Pulmonary function may be compromised further by paralysis of the right hemidiaphragm associated with phrenic nerve injury. The hyperdynamic state with increased cardiac output that is characteristic of patients with liver failure reverses rapidly after successful liver transplantation.

Other immediate management issues include renal dysfunction; prerenal azotemia, acute kidney injury associated with hypoperfusion (acute tubular necrosis), and renal toxicity caused by antibiotics, tacrolimus, or cyclosporine are frequently encountered in the postoperative period, sometimes necessitating dialysis. Occasionally, postoperative intraperitoneal bleeding may be sufficient to increase intraabdominal pressure, which, in turn, may reduce renal blood flow; this effect is rapidly reversible when abdominal distention is relieved by exploratory laparotomy to identify and ligate the bleeding site and to remove intraperitoneal clot. Anemia also may result from acute upper gastrointestinal bleeding or from transient hemolytic anemia, which may be autoimmune, especially when blood group O livers are transplanted into blood group A or B recipients. This autoimmune hemolytic anemia is mediated by donor intrahepatic lymphocytes that recognize red blood cell A or B antigens on recipient erythrocytes. Transient in nature, this process resolves once the donor liver is repopulated by recipient bone marrow–derived lymphocytes; the hemolysis can be treated by transfusing blood group O red blood cells and/or by administering higher doses of glucocorticoids. Transient thrombocytopenia is also commonly encountered. Aplastic anemia, a late occurrence, is rare but has been reported in almost 30% of patients who underwent liver transplantation for acute, severe hepatitis of unknown cause.

Bacterial, fungal, or viral infections are common and may be life-threatening postoperatively. Early after transplant surgery, common postoperative infections predominate—pneumonia, wound infections, infected intraabdominal collections, urinary tract infections, and intravenous line infections—rather than opportunistic infections; these infections may involve the biliary tree and liver as well. Beyond the first postoperative month, the toll of immunosuppression becomes evident, and opportunistic infections—cytomegalovirus, herpes viruses, fungal infections (*Aspergillus*, *Candida*, cryptococcal disease), mycobacterial infections, parasitic infections (*Pneumocystis*, *Toxoplasma*), bacterial infections (*Nocardia*, *Legionella*, and *Listeria*)—predominate. Rarely, early infections represent those transmitted with the donor liver, either infections present in the donor or infections acquired during procurement processing. De novo viral hepatitis infections acquired from the donor organ or from transfused blood products occur after typical incubation periods for these agents (well beyond the first month). Obviously, infections in an immunosuppressed host demand early recognition and prompt management; prophylactic antibiotic therapy is

Table 301-4 Nonhepatic Complications of Liver Transplantation

Fluid overload	
Cardiovascular instability	Arrhythmias
	Congestive heart failure
	Cardiomyopathy
Pulmonary compromise	Pneumonia
	Pulmonary capillary vascular permeability
	Fluid overload
Renal dysfunction	Prerenal azotemia
	Hypoperfusion injury (acute tubular necrosis)
	Drug nephrotoxicity
	↓ renal blood flow secondary to ↑ intraabdominal pressure
Hematologic	Anemia 2° to gastrointestinal and/or intraabdominal bleeding
	Hemolytic anemia, aplastic anemia
	Thrombocytopenia
Infection	Bacterial: early, common postoperative infections
	Fungal/parasitic: late, opportunistic infections
	Viral: late, opportunistic infections, recurrent hepatitis
Neuropsychiatric	Seizures
	Encephalopathy
	Depression
	Difficult Psychosocial Adjustment
Diseases of donor	Infectious
	Malignant
Malignancy	B-cell lymphoma

administered routinely in the immediate postoperative period. Use of sulfamethoxazole with trimethoprim reduces the incidence of postoperative *Pneumocystis carinii* pneumonia.

Neuropsychiatric complications include seizures (commonly associated with cyclosporine and tacrolimus toxicity), encephalopathy, depression, and difficult psychosocial adjustment. Rarely, diseases are transmitted by the allograft from the donor to the recipient. In addition to viral and bacterial infections, malignancies of donor origin have occurred. Lymphoproliferative malignancies, especially B cell lymphoma, are a recognized complication associated with immunosuppressive drugs such as azathioprine, tacrolimus, and cyclosporine (see above). Epstein-Barr virus has been shown to play a contributory role in some of these tumors, which may regress when immunosuppressive therapy is reduced.

Hepatic Complications Hepatic dysfunction after liver transplantation is similar to the hepatic complications encountered after major abdominal and cardiothoracic surgery; however, in addition, there may be complications such as primary graft failure, vascular compromise, failure or obstruction of the biliary anastomoses, and rejection. As in nontransplant surgery, postoperative jaundice may result from prehepatic, intrahepatic, and posthepatic sources. *Prehepatic* sources represent the massive hemoglobin pigment load from transfusions, hemolysis, hematomas, ecchymoses, and other collections of blood. *Early intrahepatic* liver injury includes effects of hepatotoxic drugs and anesthesia; hypoperfusion injury associated with hypotension, sepsis, and shock; and benign postoperative cholestasis. *Late intrahepatic* sources of liver injury include posttransfusion hepatitis and exacerbation of primary disease. *Posthepatic* sources of hepatic dysfunction include biliary obstruction and reduced renal clearance of conjugated bilirubin. Hepatic complications unique to liver transplantation include primary graft failure associated with ischemic injury to the organ during harvesting; vascular compromise associated with thrombosis or stenosis of the portal vein or hepatic artery anastomoses; vascular anastomotic leak; stenosis, obstruction, or leakage of the anastomosed common bile duct; recurrence of primary hepatic disorder (see below); and rejection.

Transplant Rejection Despite the use of immunosuppressive drugs, rejection of the transplanted liver still occurs in a majority of patients, beginning 1 to 2 weeks after surgery. Clinical signs suggesting rejection are fever, right upper quadrant pain, and reduced bile pigment and volume. Leukocytosis may occur, but the most reliable indicators are increases in serum bilirubin and aminotransferase levels. Because these tests lack specificity, distinguishing among rejection and biliary obstruction, primary graft nonfunction, vascular compromise, viral hepatitis, cytomegalovirus infection, drug hepatotoxicity, and recurrent primary disease may be difficult. Radiographic visualization of the biliary tree and/or percutaneous liver biopsy often help to establish the correct diagnosis. Morphologic features of acute rejection include portal infiltration, bile duct injury, and/or endothelial inflammation ("endothelialitis"); some of these findings are reminiscent of graft-versus-host disease and primary biliary cirrhosis. As soon as transplant rejection is suspected, treatment consists of intravenous methylprednisolone in repeated boluses; if this fails to abort rejection, many centers use antibodies to lymphocytes, such as OKT3, or polyclonal antilymphocyte globulin.

Table 301-5 Hepatic Complications of Liver Transplantation

HEPATIC DYSFUNCTION COMMON AFTER MAJOR SURGERY	
Prehepatic	Pigment load
	Hemolysis
	Blood collections (hematomas, abdominal collections)
Intrahepatic	
Early	Hepatotoxic drugs and anesthesia
	Hypoperfusion (hypotension, shock, sepsis)
	Benign postoperative cholestasis
Late	Transfusion-associated hepatitis
	Exacerbation of primary hepatic disease
Posthepatic	Biliary obstruction
	↓ Renal clearance of conjugated bilirubin (renal dysfunction)
HEPATIC DYSFUNCTION UNIQUE TO LIVER TRANSPLANTATION	
Primary graft nonfunction	
Vascular compromise	Portal vein obstruction
	Hepatic artery thrombosis
	Anastomotic leak with intraabdominal bleeding
Bile duct disorder	Stenosis, obstruction, leak
Rejection	
Recurrent primary hepatic disease	

Chronic rejection is a relatively rare outcome that may follow repeated bouts of acute rejection or that occurs unrelated to preceding rejection episodes. Morphologically, chronic rejection is characterized by progressive cholestasis, focal parenchymal necrosis, mononuclear infiltration, vascular lesions (intimal fibrosis, subintimal foam cells, fibrinoid necrosis), and fibrosis. This process may be reflected as ductopenia—the vanishing bile duct syndrome. Some of the histologic hallmarks of chronic rejection may be so similar to those of chronic viral hepatitis that differentiation between the two may be difficult. Reversibility of chronic rejection is limited; in patients with therapy-resistant chronic rejection, retransplantation has yielded encouraging results.

OUTCOME Survival The survival rate for patients undergoing liver transplantation has improved steadily since 1983. One-year survival rates have increased from approximately 70% in the early 1980s to 80 to 90% in the late 1990s. Currently, the 5-year survival rate exceeds 60%. An important observation is the relation between clinical status before transplantation and outcome. For patients who undergo liver transplantation when their level of compensation is high (e.g., still working or only partially disabled), a 1-year survival rate of 85% is common. For those whose level of decompensation mandates continuous in-hospital care prior to transplantation, the 1-year survival rate is about 70%, while for those who are so decompensated that they require life support in an intensive care unit, the 1-year survival rate is approximately 50%. Indeed, the trend toward transplantation earlier in the natural history of end-stage liver disease is a major factor in the increased success of liver transplantation during the 1980s and 1990s. Another important distinction in survival has been drawn between high-risk and low-risk patient categories. For patients who do not fit any "high-risk" designations, 1-year and 5-year survival rates of 85 and 80%, respectively, have been recorded. In contrast, among patients in high-risk categories—cancer, fulminant hepatitis, hepatitis B, age >65, concurrent renal failure, respirator dependence, portal vein thrombosis, and history of a portacaval shunt or multiple right upper quadrant operations—survival statistics fall into the range of 60% at 1 year and 35% at 5 years. Survival after retransplantation for primary graft nonfunction is approximately 50%. Causes of failure of liver transplantation vary with time. Failures within the first 3 months result primarily from technical complications, postoperative infections, and hemorrhage. Transplant failures after the first 3 months are more likely to result from infection, rejection, or recurrent disease (such as malignancy or viral hepatitis).

Recurrence of Primary Disease The recurrence of autoimmune hepatitis or primary sclerosing cholangitis has not been reported. There have been reports of recurrent primary biliary cirrhosis after liver transplantation; however, the histologic features of primary biliary cirrhosis and acute rejection are virtually indistinguishable and occur as frequently in patients with primary biliary cirrhosis as in patients undergoing transplantation for other reasons. Hereditary disorders such as Wilson's disease and α_1-antitrypsin deficiency have not recurred after liver transplantation; however, recurrence of disordered iron metabolism has been observed in some patients with hemochromatosis. Hepatic vein thrombosis (Budd-Chiari syndrome) may recur; this can be minimized by treating underlying lymphoproliferative disorders and by anticoagulation. Cholangiocarcinoma recurs almost invariably; therefore, few centers now transplant such patients. In patients with hepatocellular carcinoma, tumor recurrence in the liver is common after approximately 1 year, although better success has been reported in patients with an unresectable isolated lesion <5 cm or with three or fewer lesions all <3 cm. Trials are underway to assess the benefit of adjuvant chemotherapy.

Hepatitis A can recur after transplantation for fulminant hepatitis A, but such acute reinfection has no serious clinical sequelae. In fulminant hepatitis B, recurrence is not the rule; however, in the absence of any prophylactic measures, hepatitis B usually recurs after transplantation for end-stage chronic hepatitis B. With sufficient immunosuppressive therapy to prevent allograft rejection, levels of hepatitis B viremia increase markedly, regardless of pretransplantation values. A majority of patients undergoing transplantation for chronic hepatitis B become carriers of hepatitis B virus (HBV) with high levels of virus replication but without liver injury; however, some patients experience a rapid recapitulation of severe injury—severe chronic hepatitis or even fulminant hepatitis—after transplantation. *Fibrosing cholestatic hepatitis* is a histologic feature linked to rapidly progressive liver injury in approximately 10% of patients who undergo liver transplantation for hepatitis B. These patients experience marked hyperbilirubinemia, substantial prolongation of the prothrombin time (both out of proportion to relatively modest elevations of aminotransferase activity), and rapidly progressive liver failure. This lesion has been suggested to represent a "choking off" of the hepatocyte by an overwhelming density of HBV proteins. Complications such as sepsis and pancreatitis have also been observed more frequently in patients undergoing liver transplantation for hepatitis B. Although the risk of recurrent hepatitis B is approximately 20% higher in patients with pretransplantation markers of HBV replication (hepatitis B e antigen and HBV DNA), recurrent hepatitis B occurs in at least 60% of patients whose replicative markers were undetectable prior to transplantation, probably because of the enhancing impact of immunosuppressive drugs on HBV replication. Most transplantation centers will not undertake liver transplantation in patients with hepatitis B unless immunoprophylaxis with HBIG is used. Neither preoperative hepatitis B vaccination, preoperative or postoperative interferon therapy, nor short-term (≤2 months) HBIG prophylaxis has been shown to be effective, but a retrospective analysis of data from several hundred European patients followed for 3 years after transplantation has shown that long-term (≥6 months) prophylaxis with HBIG is associated with a lowering of the risk of HBV reinfection from approximately 75% to 35% and a reduction in mortality from approximately 50 percent to 20%.

As a result of long-term HBIG use following liver transplantation for chronic hepatitis B, similar improvements in outcome have been observed in the United States, with 1-year survival rates between 75 and 90%. Currently, with HBIG prophylaxis, the outcome of liver transplantation for chronic hepatitis B is indistinguishable from that for chronic liver disease unassociated with chronic hepatitis B; essentially, medical concerns regarding liver transplantation for chronic hepatitis B have been eliminated. Passive immunoprophylaxis with HBIG is begun during the anhepatic stage of surgery, repeated daily for the first 6 postoperative days, then continued with infusions that are given either at regular intervals of 4 to 6 weeks or, alternatively, when anti-HBs levels fall below a threshold of 100 mIU/mL. In all likelihood, indefinite HBIG infusions will be required, and, occasionally "breakthrough" HBV infection occurs. This approach is very expensive, approximately $20,000 per year, and involves the intravenous administration of a globulin preparation designed for intramuscular injection. Although this approach is now practiced universally, it has not been approved officially by the U.S. Food and Drug Administration; clinical trials of HBIG preparations produced specifically for intravenous administration are in progress.

An alternative and promising but still experimental approach to the prophylaxis of patients with chronic hepatitis B undergoing liver transplantation is the use of nucleoside analogues such as lamivudine (Chap. 297). Limited evidence available to date suggests that lamivudine can be used to prevent recurrence of HBV infection when administered *prior* to transplantation, to treat hepatitis B that recurs *after* transplantation, including in patients who break through HBIG prophylaxis, and to reverse the course of otherwise fatal fibrosing cholestatic hepatitis. Clinical trials have shown that lamivudine monotherapy reduces the level of HBV replication substantially, sometimes even resulting in clearance of HBsAg; reduces ALT levels; and improves histologic features of necrosis and inflammation. Long-term use of lamivudine is safe and effective, but, after several months, a proportion of patients become resistant to lamivudine, resulting from "YMDD" mutations in the HBV polymerase motif (Chap. 297). In approximately half of such resistant patients, hepatic deterioration may ensue. Perhaps the best results with currently available antiviral approaches can be achieved by combining HBIG and lamivudine. In addition, new nucleoside analogues and related drugs are being assessed as antiviral agents against HBV infection. Some of these are effective against lamivudine-associated YMDD variants of HBV; these novel agents also are likely to be used in patients undergoing liver transplantation. Clinical trials are underway to define the optimal application of these antiviral agents in the management of patients undergoing liver transplantation for chronic hepatitis B.

Patients who undergo liver transplantation for chronic hepatitis B plus D have a better survival rate than patients undergoing transplantation for hepatitis B alone. Accounting for up to 40% of all liver transplantation procedures, the most common indication for liver transplantation is end-stage liver disease resulting from chronic hepatitis C. Recurrence of hepatitis C virus (HCV) after liver transplantation can be documented in almost every patient, if sufficiently sensitive virus markers are used. Although acute and chronic liver injury occur after transplantation in patients with chronic hepatitis C, clinical consequences of recurrent hepatitis C are limited during the first 5 years after transplantation. Nonetheless, despite the relative clinical benignity of recurrent hepatitis C in the early years after liver transplantation, and despite the negligible impact on patient survival during these early years, histologic studies have documented the presence of moderate to severe chronic hepatitis in more than half of all patients and bridging fibrosis or cirrhosis in approximately 10%. Ultimately, such histologic evidence of chronic hepatitis and cirrhosis will be expressed clinically as well, and the expectation is that the 10-year outcome will not be as favorable as the 5-year statistics suggest. In a proportion of patients, even during the early posttransplantation period, recurrent hepatitis C may be sufficiently severe biochemically and histologically to merit antiviral therapy. Treatment with interferon monotherapy, which can *suppress* HCV-associated liver injury in approximately half of patients but rarely leads to *sustained* benefit, has been disappointing. The addition of the nucleoside analogue ribavirin to interferon has resulted in improved responses to antiviral therapy, and many centers have adopted some form of combination therapy for their patients with recurrent chronic hepatitis C; however, the efficacy of such combination therapy remains the subject of clinical trials. Of interest is the preliminary observation that the immunosuppressive agent mycophenolate may have a suppressive effect on HCV. A small number succumb to early HCV-associated liver injury, and a syndrome reminiscent of fibrosing cholestatic hepatitis (see above) has been observed rarely. Because patients with more episodes of rejection receive more immunosuppressive therapy, and because immunosuppressive therapy enhances HCV replication, patients with severe or multiple episodes of rejection are more likely to experience early recurrence of hepatitis C after transplantation. Both HCV genotype 1b and high viral load have been linked to recurrent HCV-induced liver disease and to earlier disease recurrence after transplantation; however, the association between genotype and recurrence of HCV-associated liver injury has not been supported by more recent reports.

Patients who undergo liver transplantation for end-stage alcoholic cirrhosis are at risk of resorting to drinking again after transplantation, a potential source of recurrent alcoholic liver injury. Currently, alcoholic liver disease is one of the more common indications for liver transplantation, accounting for 20 to 25% of all liver transplantation procedures, and most transplantation centers screen candidates carefully for predictors of continued abstinence. Recidivism is more likely in patients whose sobriety prior to transplantation was shorter than 6 months. For abstinent patients with alcoholic cirrhosis, liver transplantation can be undertaken successfully, with outcomes comparable to those for other categories of patients with chronic liver disease, when coordinated by a team approach that includes substance abuse counseling.

Posttransplantation Quality of Life Full rehabilitation is achieved in the majority of patients who survive the early postoperative months and escape chronic rejection or unmanageable infection. Psychosocial maladjustment interferes with medical compliance in a small number of patients, but most manage to adhere to immunosuppressive regimens, which must be continued indefinitely. In one study, 85% of patients who survived their transplants returned to gainful activities. In fact, some women have conceived and carried pregnancies to term after transplantation without demonstrable injury to their infants.

BIBLIOGRAPHY

ARAYA V et al: Hepatitis C after orthotopic liver transplantation. Gastroenterology 112:575, 1997

BATTS KP: Acute and chronic hepatic allograft rejection: Pathology and classification. Liver Transpl Surg 5(Suppl 1):S21, 1999

BISMUTH H (ed): Consensus conference on indications of liver transplantation. Hepatology 20(Supp):1, 1994

BIZOLLON T et al: Pilot study of the combination of interferon alfa and ribavirin as therapy of recurrent hepatitis C after liver transplantation. Hepatology 26:500, 1997

CHARLTON M et al: Predictors of patient and graft survival following liver transplantation for hepatitis C. Hepatology 28:823, 1998

DAVIES SE et al: Hepatic histological findings after transplantation for chronic hepatitis B virus infection, including a unique pattern of fibrosing cholestatic hepatitis. Hepatology 13:150, 1991

EUROPEAN FK506 MULTICENTRE LIVER STUDY GROUP: Randomised trial comparing tacrolimus (FK506) and cyclosporin in prevention of liver allograft rejection. Lancet 344:423, 1994

FÉRAY C et al: The course of hepatitis C virus infection after liver transplantation. Hepatology 20:1137, 1994

——— et al: Influence of the genotype of hepatitis C virus on the severity of recurrent liver disease after liver transplantation. Gastroenterology 108:1088, 1995

——— et al: European collaborative study on factors influencing outcome after liver transplantation for hepatitis C. Gastroenterology 117:619, 1999

GANE EJ et al: Long-term outcome of hepatitis C infection after liver transplantation. N Engl J Med 334:815, 1996

GRELLIER L et al: Lamivudine prophylaxis against reinfection in liver transplantation for hepatitis B cirrhosis. Lancet 348:1212, 1996

HOOFNAGLE JH et al: Liver transplantation for alcoholic liver disease: Executive statement and recommendations. Liver Transpl Surg 3:347, 1997

MARKOWITZ JS et al: Prophylaxis against hepatitis B recurrence following liver transplantation using combination lamivudine and hepatitis B immune globulin. Hepatology 28:585, 1998

MAZZAFERRO V et al: Liver transplantation for the treatment of small hepatocellular carcinoma in patients with cirrhosis. N Engl J Med 334:693, 1996

OSORIO RW et al: Predicting recidivism after orthotopic liver transplantation for alcoholic liver disease. Hepatology 20:105, 1994

PERRILLO R et al: Multicenter study of lamivudine therapy for hepatitis B after liver transplantation. Hepatology 29:1581, 1999

POTERUCHA JJ et al: Liver transplantation and hepatitis B. Ann Intern Med 126:805, 1997

PRUETT TL: Improved clinical outcomes with liver transplantation for hepatitis B-induced chronic liver failure using passive immunization. Ann Surg 227:841, 1998

SAMUEL D et al: Liver transplantation in European patients with the hepatitis B surface antigen. N Engl J Med 329:1842, 1993

STARZL TE et al: Liver transplantation. N Engl J Med 321:1014, 1989

TIPPLES GA et al: Mutation in HBV RNA-dependent DNA polymerase confers resistance to lamivudine in vivo. Hepatology 24:714, 1996

U.S. MULTICENTER FK506 LIVER STUDY GROUP: A comparison of tacrolimus (FK506) and cyclosporine for immunosuppression in liver transplantation. N Engl J Med 331:1110, 1994

WADE JJ et al: Bacterial and fungal infections after liver transplantation: An analysis of 284 patients. Hepatology 21:1328, 1995

WRIGHT TL et al: Interferon-α therapy for hepatitis C infection after liver transplantation. Hepatology 20:773, 1994

ZETTERMAN RK (guest ed): Long-term management of the liver transplant patient. Semin Liver Dis 15:123, 1995

302

Norton J. Greenberger, Gustav Paumgartner

DISEASES OF THE GALLBLADDER AND BILE DUCTS

BSEP bile salt export pump	OCG oral cholecystography
CBD common bile duct	PFIC progressive familial intrahepatic cholestasis
CCK cholecystokinin	PTHC percutaneous transhepatic cholangiography
CDCA chenodeoxycholic acid	RUQ right upper quadrant
CT computed tomography	UDCA ursodeoxycholic acid
EBS endoscopic biliary sphincterotomy	
ERCP endoscopic retrograde cholangiopancreatography	

PHYSIOLOGY OF BILE PRODUCTION AND FLOW

Bile Secretion and Composition Bile formed in the hepatic lobules is secreted into a complex network of canaliculi, small bile ductules, and larger bile ducts that run with lymphatics and branches of the portal vein and hepatic artery in portal tracts situated between hepatic lobules. These interlobular bile ducts coalesce to form larger septal bile ducts that join to form the right and left hepatic ducts, which in turn unite to form the common hepatic duct. The common hepatic duct is joined by the cystic duct of the gallbladder to form the common bile duct (CBD), which enters the duodenum (often after joining the main pancreatic duct) through the ampulla of Vater.

Hepatic bile is an isotonic fluid with an electrolyte composition resembling blood plasma. The electrolyte composition of gallbladder bile differs from that of hepatic bile because most of the inorganic anions, chloride and bicarbonate, have been removed by reabsorption across the gallbladder epithelium.

Major components of bile by weight include water (82%), bile acids (12%), lecithin and other phospholipids (4%), and unesterified cholesterol (0.7%). Other constituents include conjugated bilirubin, proteins (IgA, metabolites of hormones, and other proteins metabolized in the liver), electrolytes, mucus, and, often, drugs and their metabolites.

The total daily basal secretion of hepatic bile is approximately 500 to 600 mL. Many substances taken up or synthesized by the hepatocyte are secreted into the bile canalculi. The canalicular membrane forms microvilli and is associated with microfilaments of actin, microtubules, and other contractile elements. Prior to their secretion into the bile, many substances that are taken up into the hepatocyte are conjugated, while others such as phospholipids, a portion of primary bile acids, and some cholesterol are synthesized de novo in the hepatocyte. Three mechanisms are important in regulating bile flow: (1) active transport of bile acids from hepatocytes into the bile canaliculi, (2) active transport of other organic anions, and (3) cholangiocellular secretion. The last is a secretin-mediated and cyclic AMP–dependent mechanism that ultimately results in the secretion of a sodium- and bicarbonate-rich fluid into the bile ducts.

Active vectorial secretion of biliary constituents from the portal blood into the bile canaliculi is driven by a distinct set of polarized transport systems at the basolateral (sinusoidal) and the canalicular plasma membrane domains of the hepatocyte. Two sinusoidal bile salt uptake systems have been cloned in humans, the Na^+/taurocholate cotransporter and the organic anion transporting protein, which also transports a large variety of non-bile salt organic anions. Four ATP-dependent canalicular transport systems ("export pumps") have been identified: a bile salt export pump (BSEP), which was formerly called "sister of P-glycoprotein"; a conjugate export pump (MRP2), also called the canalicular multispecific organic anion transporter, which mediates the canalicular excretion of various amphiphilic conjugates formed by phase II conjugation (e.g., bilirubin diglucuronide); a multidrug export pump (MDR1) for hydrophobic cationic compounds; and a phospholipid export pump (MDR3). The canalicular membrane also contains ATP-independent transport systems such as the Cl^-/HCO_3^- anion exchanger isoform 2 for canalicular bicarbonate secretion. For some of these transporters, genetic defects have been identified that are associated with various forms of cholestasis or defects of biliary excretion. BSEP is defective in progressive familial intrahepatic cholestasis (PFIC) type 2. Mutations of MRP2 cause the Dubin-Johnson syndrome, an inherited form of conjugated hyperbilirubinemia. A defective MDR3 results in PFIC-3. The cystic fibrosis transmembrane regulator located on bile duct epithelial cells is defective in cystic fibrosis, which may be associated with impaired cholangiocellular bile formation and chronic cholestatic liver disease.

The Bile Acids The primary bile acids, cholic acid and chenodeoxycholic acid (CDCA), are synthesized from cholesterol in the liver, conjugated with glycine or taurine, and excreted into the bile. Secondary bile acids, including deoxycholate and lithocholate, are formed in the colon as bacterial metabolites of the primary bile acids. However, lithocholic acid is much less efficiently absorbed from the colon than deoxycholic acid. Another secondary bile acid, found in low concentration is ursodeoxycholic acid (UDCA), a stereoisomer of CDCA. In normal bile, the ratio of glycine to taurine conjugates is about 3:1.

Bile acids are detergents that in aqueous solutions and above a critical concentration of about 2 m*M* form molecular aggregates called *micelles*. Cholesterol alone is poorly soluble in aqueous environments, and its solubility in bile depends on both the total lipid concentration and the relative molar percentages of bile acids and lecithin. Normal ratios of these constituents favor the formation of solubilizing *mixed micelles*, while abnormal ratios promote the precipitation of cholesterol crystals in bile.

In addition to facilitating the biliary excretion of cholesterol, bile acids are necessary for the normal intestinal absorption of dietary fats via a micellar transport mechanism (Chap. 286). Bile acids also serve as a major physiologic driving force for hepatic bile flow and aid in water and electrolyte transport in the small bowel and colon.

Enterohepatic Circulation Bile acids are efficiently conserved under normal conditions. Unconjugated, and to a lesser degree also conjugated, bile acids are absorbed by *passive diffusion* along the entire gut. Quantitatively much more important for bile salt recirculation, however, is the *active transport* mechanism for conjugated bile acids in the distal ileum (Chap. 286). The reabsorbed bile acids enter the portal bloodstream and are taken up rapidly by hepatocytes, reconjugated, and resecreted into bile (enterohepatic circulation).

The normal bile acid pool size is approximately 2 to 4 g. During digestion of a meal, the bile acid pool undergoes at least one or more enterohepatic cycles, depending on the size and composition of the meal. Normally, the bile acid pool circulates approximately 5 to 10 times daily. Intestinal absorption of the pool is about 95% efficient, so fecal loss of bile acids is in the range of 0.3 to 0.6 g/d. This fecal loss is compensated by an equal daily synthesis of bile acids by the liver, and thus the size of the bile acid pool is maintained. Bile acids returning to the liver suppress de novo hepatic synthesis of primary bile acids from cholesterol by inhibiting the rate-limiting enzyme cholesterol 7α-hydroxylase. While the loss of bile salts in stool is usually matched by increased hepatic synthesis, the maximum rate of synthesis is approximately 5 g/d, which may be insufficient to replete the bile acid pool size when there is pronounced impairment of intestinal bile salt reabsorption.

Gallbladder and Sphincteric Functions In the fasting state, the sphincter of Oddi offers a high-pressure zone of resistance to bile flow from the common bile duct into the duodenum. This tonic contraction serves to (1) prevent reflux of duodenal contents into the pancreatic and bile ducts and (2) promote bile filling of the gallbladder. The major factor controlling the evacuation of the gallbladder is the peptide hormone cholecystokinin (CCK), which is released from the duodenal mucosa in response to the ingestion of fats and amino acids. CCK produces (1) powerful contraction of the gallbladder, (2) decreased resistance of the sphincter of Oddi, (3) increased hepatic secretion of bile, and thus (4) enhanced flow of biliary contents into the duodenum.

Hepatic bile is "concentrated" within the gallbladder by energy-dependent transmucosal absorption of water and electrolytes. Almost the entire bile acid pool may be sequestered in the gallbladder following an overnight fast for delivery into the duodenum with the first meal of the day. The normal capacity of the gallbladder is 30 to 50 mL of bile.

DISEASES OF THE GALLBLADDER

CONGENITAL ANOMALIES Anomalies of the biliary tract may be found in 10 to 20% of the population, including abnormalities in number, size, and shape (e.g., agenesis of the gallbladder, duplications, rudimentary or oversized "giant" gallbladders, and diverticula). Phrygian cap is a clinically innocuous entity in which a partial or complete septum (or fold) separates the fundus from the body. Anomalies of position or suspension are not uncommon and include left-sided gallbladder, intrahepatic gallbladder, retrodisplacement of the gallbladder, and "floating" gallbladder. The latter condition predisposes to acute torsion, volvulus, or herniation of the gallbladder.

GALLSTONES Pathogenesis Gallstones are quite prevalent in most western countries. In the United States, autopsy series have shown gallstones in at least 20% of women and in 8% of men over the age of 40. It is estimated that 16 to 20 million persons in the United States have gallstones and that approximately 1 million new cases of cholelithiasis develop each year.

Gallstones are formed by concretion or accretion of normal or abnormal bile constituents. They are divided into three major types; cholesterol and mixed stones account for 80% of the total, with pigment stones comprising the remaining 20%. Mixed and cholesterol gallstones usually contain more than 50% cholesterol monohydrate plus an admixture of calcium salts, bile pigments, proteins, and fatty acids. Pigment stones are composed primarily of calcium bilirubinate; they contain less than 20% cholesterol.

Cholesterol and mixed stones and biliary sludge Cholesterol is essentially water insoluble and requires aqueous dispersion into either micelles or vesicles, both of which require the presence of a second lipid to "liquefy" the cholesterol. Cholesterol and phospholipids are secreted into bile as unilamellar bilayered vesicles, which are converted into mixed micelles consisting of bile acids, phospholipids, and cholesterol by the action of bile acids. If there is an excess of cholesterol in relation to phospholipids and bile acids, unstable cholesterol-rich vesicles remain, which aggregate into large multilamellar vesicles from which cholesterol crystals precipitate (Fig. 302-1).

There are several important mechanisms in the formation of lithogenic (stone-forming) bile. The most important is increased biliary secretion of cholesterol. This may occur in association with obesity, high-caloric and cholesterol-rich diets, or drugs (e.g., clofibrate) and may result from increased activity of HMG-CoA reductase, the rate-limiting enzyme of hepatic cholesterol synthesis, and increased hepatic uptake of cholesterol from blood. In patients with gallstones, dietary cholesterol *increases* biliary cholesterol secretion. This does not occur in non-gallstone patients on high-cholesterol diets. In addition to environmental factors such as high-caloric and cholesterol-rich diets, genetic factors play an important role in cholesterol hypersecretion and gallstone formation. A high prevalence of gallstones is found among first-degree relatives of gallstone carriers and in certain ethnic populations such as American Indians as well as Chilean Indians and Chilean Hispanics. A common genetic trait has been identified for some of these populations by mitochondrial DNA analysis. A genetic defect in the control of cholesterol secretion also exists in certain strains of inbred mice who develop gallstones under a lithogenic diet. In some patients, impaired hepatic conversion of cholesterol to bile acids may also occur, resulting in an increase of the lithogenic cholesterol/bile acid ratio. Lithogenic bile may also result from conditions affecting the enterohepatic circulation of bile acids (e.g., prolonged parenteral alimentation or ileal disease or resection). In addition, most patients with gallstones may have reduced activity of hepatic cholesterol 7α-hydroxylase, the rate-limiting enzyme for primary bile acid synthesis.

Thus an excess of biliary cholesterol in relation to bile acids and phospholipids is primarily due to hypersecretion of cholesterol, but hyposecretion of bile acids may contribute. Two additional disturbances of bile acid metabolism that are likely to contribute to supersaturation of bile with cholesterol are (1) reduction of the bile acid pool and (2) enhanced conversion of cholic acid to deoxycholic acid, with replacement of the cholic acid pool by an expanded deoxycholic acid pool. The first disorder may be caused by more rapid loss of primary bile acid from the small intestine into the colon. The second disturbance may result from enhanced dehydroxylation of cholic acid and increased absorption of newly formed deoxycholic acid. An increased deoxycholate secretion is associated with hypersecretion of cholesterol into bile. While supersaturation of bile with cholesterol is an important prerequisite for gallstone formation, it is not sufficient by itself to produce cholesterol precipitation in vivo. Most people with supersaturated bile do not develop stones because the time required for cholesterol crystals to nucleate and grow is longer than the time bile spends in the gallbladder.

A second important mechanism is *nucleation* of cholesterol monohydrate crystals, which is greatly accelerated in human lithogenic bile; it is this feature rather than the degree of cholesterol supersaturation that distinguishes lithogenic from normal gallbladder bile. Accelerated nucleation of cholesterol monohydrate in bile may be due to either an *excess of pronucleating factors* or a *deficiency of antinucleating factors*. Mucin and certain non-mucin glycoproteins appear to be pronucleating factors, while apolipoproteins AI and AII and other glycoproteins appear to be antinucleating factors. Cholesterol monohydrate

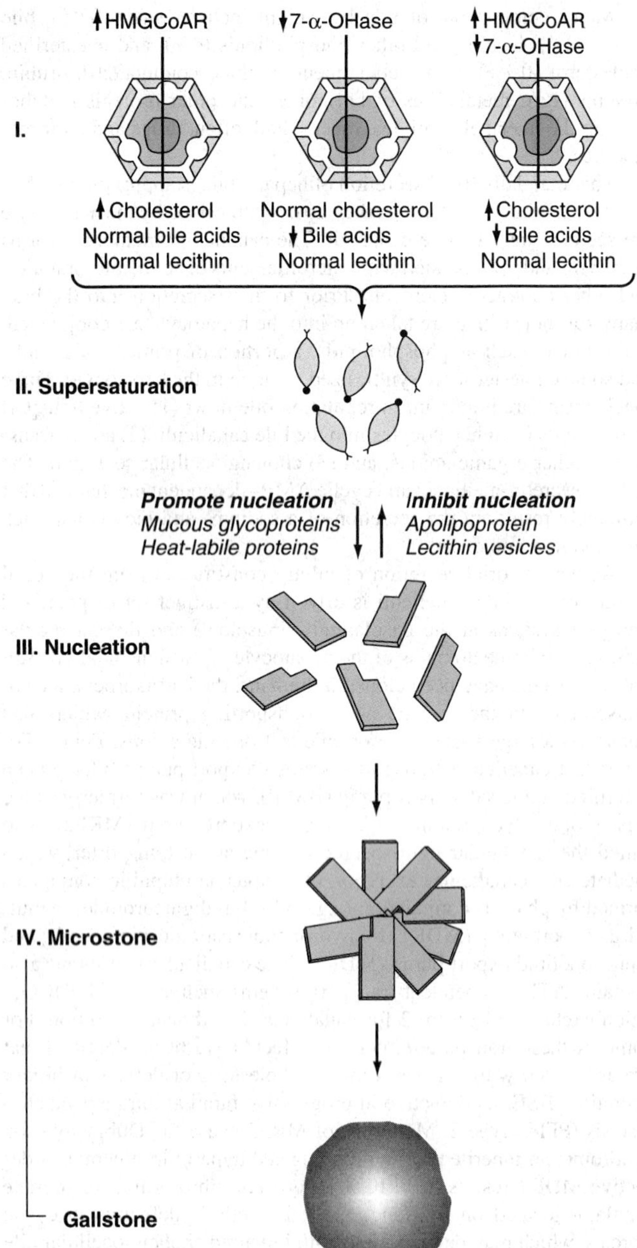

FIGURE 302-1 Scheme showing pathogenesis of gallstone formation. Conditions or factors that increase the ratio of cholesterol to bile acids and lecithin favor gallstone formation (HMG-CoAR, hydroxymethylglutaryl–coenzyme A reductase; 7-α-OHase, cholesterol, 7α-hydroxylase).

crystal nucleation and crystal growth probably occur within the mucin gel layer. Vesicle fusion leads to liquid crystals, which, in turn, nucleate into solid cholesterol monohydrate crystals. Continued growth of the crystals occurs by direct nucleation of cholesterol molecules from supersaturated unilamellar or multilamellar biliary vesicles.

A third important mechanism in cholesterol gallstone formation is *gallbladder hypomotility*. If the gallbladder emptied all supersaturated or crystal-containing bile completely, stones would not be able to grow. A high percentage of patients with gallstones exhibits abnormalities of gallbladder emptying. Ultrasonographic studies show that gallstone patients have an increased gallbladder volume during fasting and also after a test meal (residual volume) and that fractional emptying after gallbladder stimulation is decreased. Gallbladder emptying is a major determinant of gallstone recurrence in patients who underwent biliary lithotripsy. Within 3 years, only 13% of patients with good but 53% of patients with poor gallbladder emptying form recurrent stones.

Table 302-1 Predisposing Factors for Cholesterol and Pigment Gallstone Formation

Cholesterol and Mixed Stones

1. Demographic/genetic factors
   a. Prevalence highest in North American Indians, Chilean Indians, and Chilean Hispanics, greater in Northern Europe and North America than in Asia, lowest in Japan; familial disposition; hereditary aspects
2. Obesity
   a. Normal bile acid pool and secretion but increased biliary secretion of cholesterol
3. Weight loss
   a. Mobilization of tissue cholesterol leads to increased biliary cholesterol secretion while enterohepatic circulation of bile acids is decreased
4. Female sex hormones
   a. Estrogens stimulate hepatic lipoprotein receptors, increase uptake of dietary cholesterol, and increase biliary cholesterol secretion
   b. Natural estrogens, other estrogens, and oral contraceptives lead to decreased bile salt secretion and decreased conversion of cholesterol to cholesteryl esters
5. Ileal disease or resection
   a. Malabsorption of bile acids leads to decreased bile acid pool, and decreased biliary secretion of bile salts
6. Increasing age
   a. Increased biliary secretion of cholesterol, decreased size of bile acid pool, decreased biliary secretion of bile salts
7. Gallbladder hypomotility leading to stasis and formation of sludge
   a. Prolonged parenteral nutrition
   b. Fasting
   c. Pregnancy
   d. Drugs such as octreotide
8. Clofibrate therapy
   a. Increased biliary secretion of cholesterol
9. Decreased bile acid secretion
   a. Primary biliary cirrhosis
   b. Chronic intrahepatic cholestasis
10. Miscellaneous
   a. High-calorie, high-fat diet
   b. Spinal cord injury

Pigment Stones

1. Demographic/genetic factors: Asia, rural setting
2. Chronic hemolysis
3. Alcoholic cirrhosis
4. Chronic biliary tract infection, parasite infestation
5. Increasing age

Biliary sludge is a thick mucous material that upon microscopic examination reveals lecithin-cholesterol crystals, cholesterol monohydrate crystals, calcium bilirubinate, and mucin thread or mucous gels. Biliary sludge typically forms a crescent-like layer in the most dependent portion of the gallbladder and is recognized by characteristic echoes on ultrasonography (see below). The presence of biliary sludge implies two abnormalities: (1) the normal balance between gallbladder mucin secretion and elimination has become deranged and (2) nucleation of biliary solutes has occurred. That biliary sludge may be a precursor form of gallstone disease is evident from several observations. In one study, 96 patients with gallbladder sludge were followed prospectively by serial ultrasound studies. In 18%, biliary sludge disappeared and did not recur for at least 2 years. In 60%, biliary sludge disappeared and reappeared; in 14%, gallstones (8% asymptomatic, 6% symptomatic) developed, and in 6%, severe biliary pain with or without acute pancreatitis occurred. In 12 patients, cholecystectomies were performed, 6 for gallstone-associated biliary pain and 3 in symptomatic patients with sludge but without gallstones who had prior attacks of pancreatitis; the latter did not recur after cholecystectomy. It should be emphasized that biliary sludge can develop with disorders that cause gallbladder hypomotility, i.e., surgery, burns, total parenteral nutrition, pregnancy, and oral contraceptives—all of which are associated with gallstone formation.

Two other conditions are associated with cholesterol stone or biliary sludge formation: pregnancy and very low calorie diet. There appear to be two key changes during pregnancy that contribute to a "cholelithogenic state." First, the composition of the bile acid pool and the cholesterol-carrying capacity of bile change, with a resultant marked increase in cholesterol saturation during the third trimester. Second, ultrasonographic studies have demonstrated that gallbladder contraction in response to a standard meal is sluggish, resulting in impaired gallbladder emptying. That these changes are related to pregnancy per se is supported by several studies that show reversal of these abnormalities after delivery. During pregnancy, gallbladder sludge develops in 20 to 30% of women and gallstones in 5 to 12%. While biliary sludge is a common finding during pregnancy, it is usually asymptomatic and often resolves spontaneously after delivery. Gallstones, which are less common than sludge and frequently associated with biliary colic, may also disappear after delivery because of spontaneous dissolution related to bile becoming unsaturated with cholesterol post partum.

From 10 to 20% of people having rapid weight reduction through very low calorie dieting develop gallstones. In a study involving 600 patients who completed a 16-week, 520-kcal/d diet, UDCA in a dosage of 600 mg/d proved highly effective in preventing gallstone formation; gallstones developed in only 3% of UDCA recipients compared to 28% of placebo-treated patients.

To summarize, cholesterol gallstone disease occurs because of several defects, which include (1) bile supersaturation with cholesterol, (2) nucleation of cholesterol monohydrate with subsequent crystal retention and stone growth, and (3) abnormal gallbladder motor function with delayed emptying and stasis. Other important factors known to predispose to cholesterol stone formation are summarized in Table 302-1.

Pigment stones Gallstones composed largely of calcium bilirubinate are much more common in the Far East than in western countries. The presence of increased amounts of unconjugated, insoluble bilirubin in bile results in the precipitation of bilirubin, which may aggregate to form pigment stones or may form the nidus for growth of mixed cholesterol gallstones. In western countries, chronic hemolytic states (with increased conjugated bilirubin in bile) or alcoholic liver disease are associated with an increased incidence of pigment stones. Deconjugation of an excess of soluble bilirubin mono- and diglucuronide may be mediated by endogenous β-glucuronidase but may also occur by spontaneous alkaline hydrolysis. Sometimes, the enzyme is also produced when bile is chronically infected by bacteria. Pigment stone formation is especially prominent in Asians and is often associated with infections in the biliary tree (Table 302-1).

Diagnosis Procedures of potential use in the diagnosis of cholelithiasis and other diseases of the gallbladder are detailed in Table 302-2. The plain abdominal film may detect gallstones containing sufficient calcium to be radiopaque (10 to 15% of cholesterol and mixed stones and approximately 50% of pigment stones). Plain radiography may also be of use in the diagnosis of emphysematous cholecystitis, porcelain gallbladder, limey bile, and gallstone ileus.

Ultrasonography of the gallbladder is very accurate in the identification of cholelithiasis and has several advantages over oral cholecystography (Fig. 302-2*A*). The gallbladder is easily visualized with the technique, and in fact, failure to image the gallbladder successfully in a fasting patient correlates well with the presence of underlying gallbladder disease. Stones as small as 2 mm in diameter may be confidently identified provided that firm criteria are used [e.g., acoustic "shadowing" of opacities that are within the gallbladder lumen and that change with the patient's position (by gravity)]. In major medical centers, the false-negative and false-positive rates for ultrasound in gallstone patients are about 2 to 4%. Biliary sludge is material of low echogenic activity that typically forms a layer in the most dependent position of the gallbladder. This layer shifts with postural changes but fails to produce acoustic shadowing; these two characteristics distinguish sludges from gallstones. Ultrasound can also be used to assess the emptying function of the gallbladder.

Oral cholecystography (OCG) is a useful procedure for the diag-

Table 302-2 Diagnostic Evaluation of the Gallbladder

Diagnostic Advantages	Diagnostic Limitations	Comment
PLAIN ABDOMINAL X-RAY		
Low cost Readily available	Relatively low yield ?Contraindicated in pregnancy	Pathognomonic findings in: Calcified gallstones Limey bile, porcelain GB Emphysematous cholecystitis Gallstone ileus
GALLBLADDER ULTRASOUND		
Rapid Accurate identification of gallstones (>95%) Simultaneous scanning of GB, liver, bile ducts, pancreas "Real-time" scanning allows assessment of GB volume, contractility Not limited by jaundice, pregnancy May detect very small stones	Bowel gas Massive obesity Ascites Recent barium study	Procedure of choice for detection of stones
RADIOISOTOPE SCANS (HIDA, DIDA, ETC.)		
Accurate identification of cystic duct obstruction Simultaneous assessment of bile ducts	?Contraindicated in pregnancy Serum bilirubin >103–205 μmol/L (6–12 mg/dL) Cholecystogram of low resolution	Indicated for confirmation of suspected acute cholecystitis; less sensitive and less specific in chronic cholecystitis; useful in diagnosis of acalculous cholecystopathy, especially if given with CCK to assess gallbladder emptying
ORAL CHOLECYSTOGRAM		
Low cost Readily available Accurate identification of gallstones (90–95%) Identification of GB anomalies, hyperplastic cholecystoses Identification of chronic GB disease after nonvisualization on double dose	?Contraindicated in pregnancy ?Contraindicated with history of reaction to iodinated contrast Nonvisualization with: Serum bilirubin >34–68 μmol/L (2–4 mg/dL) Failure to ingest or absorb tablets Impaired hepatic excretion Very small stones may be undetected More time-consuming than GBUS	Largely replaced by GBUS A useful procedure in identification of gallstones if diagnostic limitations prevent GBUS Patency of cystic duct can be evaluated prior to nonsurgical therapy

NOTE: GB, gallbladder; CCK, cholecystokinin; GBUS, gallbladder ultrasound.

nosis of gallstones but has been largely replaced by ultrasound. However, OCG is still useful for the selection of patients for nonsurgical therapy of gallstone disease such as lithotripsy or bile acid dissolution therapy. In both these settings, OCG is used to assess the patency of the cystic duct and gallbladder emptying function. Further, OCG can also delineate the size and number of gallstones and determine whether they are calcified. Factors that may produce nonvisualization of the OCG are summarized in Table 302-2.

Radiopharmaceuticals such as ^{99m}Tc-labeled *N*-substituted iminodiacetic acids (HIDA, DIDA, DISIDA, etc.) are rapidly extracted from the blood and are excreted into the biliary tree in high concentration even in the presence of mild to moderate serum bilirubin elevations. Failure to image the gallbladder in the presence of biliary ductal visualization may indicate cystic duct obstruction, acute or chronic cholecystitis, or surgical absence of the organ. Such scans have their greatest application in the diagnosis of acute cholecystitis.

Symptoms of Gallstone Disease Gallstones usually produce symptoms by causing inflammation or obstruction following their migration into the cystic duct or CBD. The most specific and characteristic symptom of gallstone disease is biliary colic. Obstruction of the cystic duct or CBD by a stone produces increased intraluminal pressure and distention of the viscus that cannot be relieved by repetitive biliary contractions. The resultant visceral pain is characteristically a severe, steady ache or pressure in the epigastrium or right upper quadrant (RUQ) of the abdomen with frequent radiation to the interscapular area, right scapula, or shoulder.

Biliary colic begins quite suddenly and may persist with severe intensity for 30 min to 5 h, subsiding gradually or rapidly. An episode of biliary pain is sometimes followed by a residual mild ache or soreness in the RUQ, which may persist for 24 h or so. Nausea and vomiting frequently accompany episodes of biliary colic. An elevated level of serum bilirubin and/or alkaline phosphatase suggests a common duct stone. Fever or chills (rigors) with biliary colic usually imply a complication, i.e., cholecystitis, pancreatitis, or cholangitis. Complaints of vague epigastric fullness, dyspepsia, eructation, or flatulence, especially following a fatty meal, should not be confused with biliary colic. Such symptoms are frequently elicited from patients with gallstone disease but are not specific for biliary calculi. Biliary colic may be precipitated by eating a fatty meal, by consumption of a large meal following a period of prolonged fasting, or by eating a normal meal.

Natural History Gallstone disease discovered in an asymptomatic patient or in a patient whose symptoms are not referable to cholelithiasis is a common clinical problem. The natural history of "silent" or asymptomatic gallstones has occasioned much debate. A study of predominantly male silent gallstone patients suggests that the cumulative risk for the development of symptoms or complications requiring surgery is relatively low—10% at 5 years, 15% at 10 years, and 18% at 15 years. Patients remaining asymptomatic for 15 years were found to be unlikely to develop symptoms during further follow-up, and most patients who did develop complications from their gallstones experienced *prior* warning symptoms. Similar conclusions apply to diabetic patients with silent gallstones. Decision analysis has suggested that (1) the cumulative risk of death due to gallstone disease while on expectant management is small, and (2) prophylactic cholecystectomy is not warranted.

Complications requiring cholecystectomy are much more common in gallstone patients who have developed symptoms of biliary colic. Patients found to have gallstones at a young age are more likely to develop symptoms from cholelithiasis than are patients older than 60 years at the time of initial diagnosis. Patients with diabetes mellitus and gallstones may be somewhat more susceptible to septic compli-

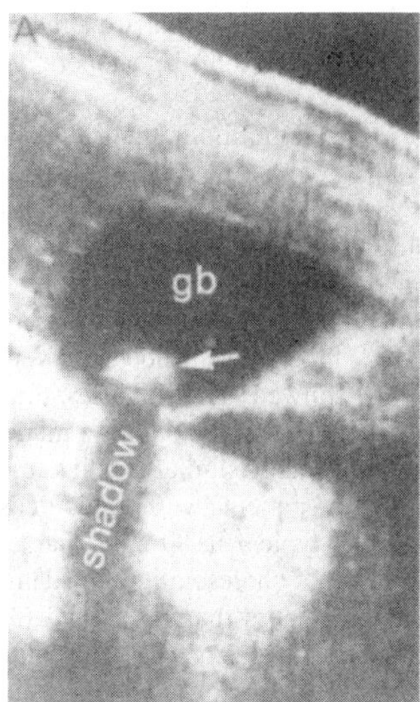

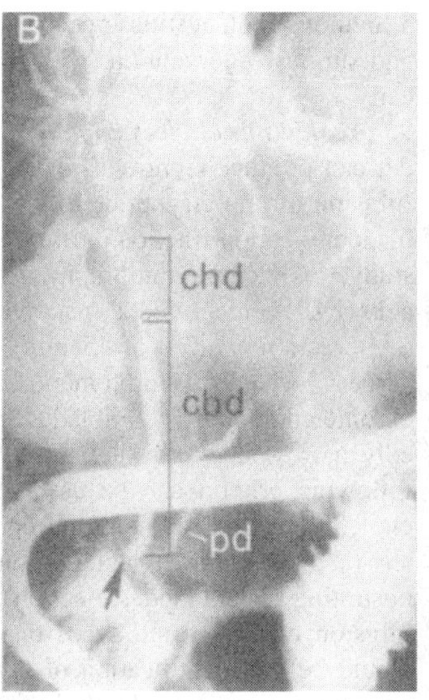

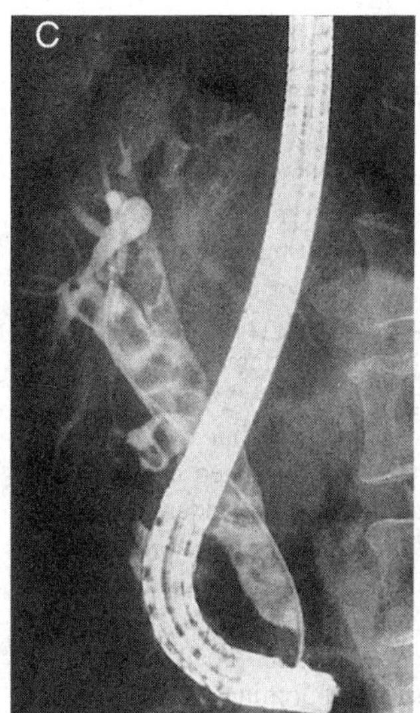

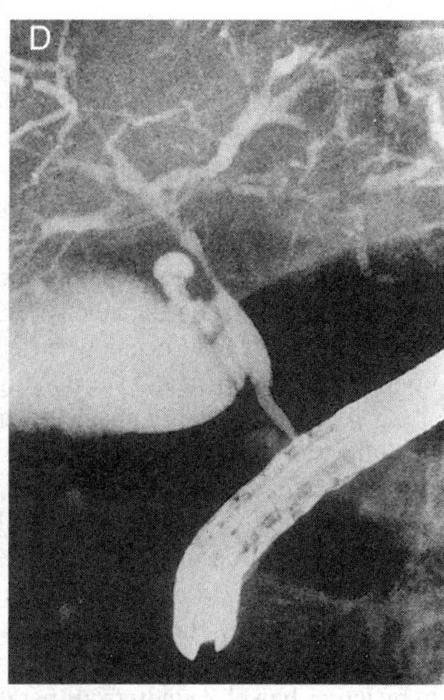

FIGURE 302-2 Examples of ultrasound and radiologic studies of the biliary tract. *A.* An ultrasound study showing a distended gallbladder containing a single large stone (*arrow*) which casts an acoustic shadow. *B.* Endoscopic retrograde cholangiopancreatogram (ERCP) showing normal biliary tract anatomy. In addition to the endoscope and large vertical gallbladder filled with contrast dye, the common hepatic duct (chd), common bile duct (cbd), and pancreatic duct (pd) are shown. The arrow points to the ampulla of Vater. *C.* Percutaneous transhepatic cholangiogram (PTHC) showing choledocholithiasis. The biliary tract is dilatated and contains multiple radiolucent calculi. *D.* ERCP showing sclerosing cholangitis. The common bile duct shows areas that are strictured and narrowed.

cations, but the magnitude of risk of septic biliary complications in diabetic patients is incompletely defined. In addition, asymptomatic gallstone patients with nonvisualization of the gallbladder on OCG appear to have an increased tendency to develop symptoms and complications.

℞ TREATMENT **Surgical Therapy** In asymptomatic gallstone patients, the risk of developing symptoms or complications requiring surgery is quite small (in the range of 1 to 2% per year). Thus a recommendation for cholecystectomy in a patient with gallstones should probably be based on assessment of three factors: (1) the presence of symptoms that are frequent enough or severe enough to interfere with the patient's general routine; (2) the presence of a prior complication of gallstone disease, i.e., history of acute cholecystitis, pancreatitis, gallstone fistula, etc.; or (3) the presence of an underlying condition predisposing the patient to increased risk of gallstone complications (e.g., calcified or porcelain gallbladder and/or a previous attack of acute cholecystitis regardless of current symptomatic status). Patients with very large gallstones (over 2 cm in diameter) and patients having gallstones in a congenitally anomalous gallbladder might also be considered for prophylactic cholecystectomy. Although age under 50 years is a worrisome factor in asymptomatic gallstone patients, few authorities would now recommend routine cholecystectomy in all young patients with silent stones. Laparoscopic cholecystectomy is a minimal-access approach for the removal of the gallbladder together with its stones. Its advantages include a markedly shortened hospital stay as well as decreased cost, and it is the procedure of choice for most patients referred for elective cholecystectomy.

From several studies involving over 4000 patients undergoing laparoscopic cholecystectomy, the following key points emerge: (1) complications develop in about 4% of patients, (2) conversion to laparotomy occurs in 5%, (3) the death rate is remarkably low (i.e., <0.1%), and (4) bile duct injuries are unusual (i.e., 0.2 to 0.5%). These data indicate why laparoscopic cholecystectomy has become the "gold standard" for treating symptomatic cholelithiasis.

Medical Therapy—Gallstone Dissolution UDCA decreases cholesterol saturation of bile and also appears to produce a lamellar liquid crystalline phase in bile that allows a dispersion of cholesterol from stones by physiochemical means. UDCA may also retard cholesterol crystal nucleation. In carefully selected patients with a functioning gallbladder and with radiolucent stones <10 mm in diameter, complete dissolution can be achieved in about 50% of patients within 6 months to 2 years with UDCA at a dose of 8 to 10 mg/kg per day. The highest success rate (i.e., >70%) occurs in patients with small (<5 mm) floating radiolucent gallstones. Probably no more than 10% of patients with *symptomatic* cholelithiasis are candidates for such treatment. However, in addition to the vexing problem of recurrent stones (30 to 50% over 3 to 5 years of follow-up), there is also the factor of taking an expensive drug for an indefinite period of time. The advantages and success of laparoscopic cholecystectomy have largely reduced the role of gallstone dissolution to patients who wish to avoid or are not candidates for elective cholecystectomy.

Gallbladder stones may be fragmented by extracorporeal shock waves. While such shock wave lithotripsy combined with medical litholytic therapy is safe and effective in carefully selected patients with gallbladder calculi (radiolucent, solitary stone <2 cm in well-contracting gallbladder), the procedure is employed infrequently because of the emergence of laparoscopic cholystectomy as the procedure of choice for symptomatic cholelithiasis, the recurrence of gallstones in 30% of patients within 5 years after lithotripsy combined with medical litholytic therapy, and the cost of taking UDCA for a variable period after the procedure.

ACUTE AND CHRONIC CHOLECYSTITIS **Acute Cholecystitis** Acute inflammation of the gallbladder wall usually follows obstruction of the cystic duct by a stone. Inflammatory response can be evoked by three factors: (1) *mechanical inflammation* produced by increased intraluminal pressure and distention with resulting ischemia of the gallbladder mucosa and wall, (2) *chemical inflammation* caused by the release of lysolecithin (due to the action of phospholipase on lecithin in bile) and other local tissue factors, and (3) *bacterial inflammation*, which may play a role in 50 to 85% of patients with acute cholecystitis. The organisms most frequently isolated by culture of gallbladder bile in these patients include *Escherichia coli*, *Klebsiella* spp., group D *Streptococcus*, *Staphylococcus* spp., and *Clostridium* spp.

Acute cholecystitis often begins as an attack of biliary colic that progressively worsens. Approximately 60 to 70% of patients report having experienced prior attacks that resolved spontaneously. As the episode progresses, however, the pain of acute cholecystitis becomes more generalized in the right upper abdomen. As with biliary colic, the pain of cholecystitis may radiate to the interscapular area, right scapula, or shoulder. Peritoneal signs of inflammation such as increased pain with jarring or on deep respiration may be apparent. The patient is anorectic and often nauseated. Vomiting is relatively common and may produce symptoms and signs of vascular and extracellular volume depletion. Jaundice is unusual early in the course of acute cholecystitis but may occur when edematous inflammatory changes involve the bile ducts and surrounding lymph nodes.

A low-grade fever is characteristically present, but shaking chills or rigors are not uncommon. The RUQ of the abdomen is almost invariably tender to palpation. An enlarged, tense gallbladder is palpable in one-quarter to one-half of patients. Deep inspiration or cough during subcostal palpation of the RUQ usually produces increased pain and inspiratory arrest (Murphy's sign). A light blow delivered to the right subcostal area may elicit a marked increase in pain. Localized rebound tenderness in the RUQ is common, as are abdominal distention and hypoactive bowel sounds from paralytic ileus, but generalized peritoneal signs and abdominal rigidity are usually lacking, absent perforation.

The diagnosis of acute cholecystitis is usually made on the basis of a characteristic history and physical examination. The triad of sudden onset of RUQ tenderness, fever, and leukocytosis is highly suggestive. Typically, leukocytosis in the range of 10,000 to 15,000 cells per microliter with a left shift on differential count is found. The serum bilirubin is mildly elevated [<85.5 μmol/L (5 mg/dL)] in 45% of patients, while 25% have modest elevations in serum aminotransferases (usually less than a fivefold elevation). The radionuclide (e.g., HIDA) biliary scan may be confirmatory if bile duct imaging is seen without visualization of the gallbladder. Ultrasound will demonstrate calculi in 90 to 95% of cases.

Approximately 75% of patients treated medically have remission of acute symptoms within 2 to 7 days following hospitalization. In 25%, however, a complication of acute cholecystitis will occur despite conservative treatment (see below). In this setting, prompt surgical intervention is required. Of the 75% of patients with acute cholecystitis who undergo remission of symptoms, approximately one-quarter will experience a recurrence of cholecystitis within 1 year, and 60% will have at least one recurrent bout within 6 years. In view of the natural history of the disease, acute cholecystitis is best treated by early surgery whenever possible.

Acalculous cholecystitis In 5 to 10% of patients with acute cholecystitis, calculi obstructing the cystic duct are not found at surgery. In over 50% of such cases, an underlying explanation for acalculous inflammation is not found. An increased risk for the development of acalculous cholecystitis is especially associated with serious trauma or burns, with the postpartum period following prolonged labor, and with orthopedic and other nonbiliary major surgical operations in the postoperative period. Other precipitating factors include vasculitis, obstructing adenocarcinoma of the gallbladder, diabetes mellitus, torsion of the gallbladder, "unusual" bacterial infections of the gallbladder (e.g., *Leptospira*, *Streptococcus*, *Salmonella*, or *Vibrio cholerae*), and parasitic infestation of the gallbladder. Acalculous cholecystitis may also be seen with a variety of other systemic disease processes (sarcoidosis, cardiovascular disease, tuberculosis, syphilis, actinomycosis, etc.) and may possibly complicate periods of prolonged parenteral hyperalimentation.

Although the clinical manifestations of acalculous cholecystitis are indistinguishable from those of calculous cholecystitis, the setting of acute gallbladder inflammation complicating severe underlying illness is characteristic of acalculous disease. Ultrasound, computed tomography (CT) scanning, or radionuclide examinations demonstrating a large, tense, static gallbladder without stones and with evidence of poor emptying over a prolonged period may be diagnostically useful in some cases. The complication rate for acalculous cholecystitis exceeds that for calculous cholecystitis. Successful management of acute acalculous cholecystitis appears to depend primarily on early diagnosis and surgical intervention, with meticulous attention to postoperative care.

Acalculous cholecystopathy Disordered motility of the gallbladder can produce recurrent biliary pain in patients without gallstones. Infusion of an octapeptide of CCK can be used to measure the gallbladder ejection fraction during cholescintigraphy. In a representative study, CCK cholescintigraphy using ^{99m}Tc-diisopropyl iminodiacetic acid (DIDA) identified 21 patients with an abnormal gallbladder ejection fraction (<40% at 45 min); 10 of 11 patients who underwent surgery became asymptomatic; all 10 showed abnormalities, i.e., chronic cholecystitis, gallbladder muscle hypertrophy, and/or a markedly narrowed cystic duct. From this and other similar studies, the following criteria can be used to identify patients with acalculous cholecystopathy: (1) recurrent episodes of typical RUQ pain characteristic of biliary tract pain, (2) abnormal CCK cholescintigraphy demonstrating a gallbladder ejection fraction of less than 40%, and (3) infusion of CCK reproduces the patient's pain. An additional clue would be the identification of a large gallbladder on ultrasound examination. Finally, it should be noted that sphincter of Oddi dysfunction can also give rise to recurrent RUQ pain and CCK-scintigraphic abnormalities.

Emphysematous cholecystitis So-called emphysematous cholecystitis is thought to begin with acute cholecystitis (calculous or acalculous) followed by ischemia or gangrene of the gallbladder wall and infection by gas-producing organisms. Bacteria most frequently cultured in this setting include anaerobes, such as *C. welchii* or *C. perfringens*, and aerobes, such as *E. coli*. This condition occurs most frequently in elderly men and in patients with diabetes mellitus. The clinical manifestations are essentially indistinguishable from those of nongaseous cholecystitis. The diagnosis is usually made on plain abdominal film by the finding of gas within the gallbladder lumen, dissecting within the gallbladder wall to form a gaseous ring, or in the pericholecystic tissues. The morbidity and mortality rates with emphysematous cholecystitis are considerable. Prompt surgical intervention coupled with appropriate antibiotics is mandatory.

Chronic Cholecystitis Chronic inflammation of the gallbladder wall is almost always associated with the presence of gallstones and is thought to result from repeated bouts of subacute or acute cholecystitis or from persistent mechanical irritation of the gallbladder wall. The presence of bacteria in the bile occurs in more than one-quarter of patients with chronic cholecystitis. Although the presence of infected bile in a patient with *chronic* cholecystitis undergoing elective cholecystectomy probably adds little to the operative risk, intraoperative Gram's staining and routine culturing of bile have been advocated to identify those patients whose gallbladder is colonized with *Clostridium* spp. Appropriate antibiotics intra- and postoperatively are recommended in such patients because colonization with these organisms may be associated with devastating septic complications following surgery. Chronic cholecystitis may be asymptomatic for years, may progress to symptomatic gallbladder disease or to acute cholecystitis, or may present with complications (see below).

Complications of Cholecystitis • ***Empyema and hydrops*** Empyema of the gallbladder usually results from progression of acute cholecystitis with persistent cystic duct obstruction to superinfection of the stagnant bile with a pus-forming bacterial organism. The clinical picture resembles that of cholangitis with high fever, severe RUQ pain, marked leukocytosis, and often, prostration. Empyema of the gallbladder carries a high risk of gram-negative sepsis and/or perforation. Emergency surgical intervention with proper antibiotic coverage is required as soon as the diagnosis is suspected.

Hydrops or mucocele of the gallbladder may also result from prolonged obstruction of the cystic duct, usually by a large solitary calculus. In this instance, the obstructed gallbladder lumen is progressively distended, over a period of time, by mucus (mucocele) or by a clear transudate (hydrops) produced by mucosal epithelial cells. A visible, easily palpable, nontender mass sometimes extending from the RUQ into the right iliac fossa may be found on physical examination.

The patient with hydrops of the gallbladder frequently remains asymptomatic, although chronic RUQ pain may also occur. Cholecystectomy is indicated, since empyema, perforation, or gangrene may complicate the condition.

Gangrene and perforation Gangrene of the gallbladder results from ischemia of the wall and patchy or complete tissue necrosis. Underlying conditions often include marked distention of the gallbladder, vasculitis, diabetes mellitus, empyema, or torsion resulting in arterial occlusion. Gangrene usually predisposes to perforation of the gallbladder, but perforation may also occur in chronic cholecystitis without premonitory warning symptoms. *Localized perforations* are usually contained by the omentum or by adhesions produced by recurrent inflammation of the gallbladder. Bacterial superinfection of the walled-off gallbladder contents results in abscess formation. Most patients are best treated with cholecystectomy, but some seriously ill patients may be managed with cholecystostomy and drainage of the abscess. *Free perforation* is less common but is associated with a mortality rate of approximately 30%. Such patients may experience a sudden transient relief of RUQ pain as the distended gallbladder decompresses; this is followed by signs of generalized peritonitis.

Fistula formation and gallstone ileus *Fistulization* into an adjacent organ adherent to the gallbladder wall may result from inflammation and adhesion formation. Fistulas into the duodenum are most common, followed in frequency by those involving the hepatic flexure of the colon, stomach or jejunum, abdominal wall, and renal pelvis. Clinically "silent" biliary-enteric fistulas occurring as a complication of chronic cholecystitis have been found in up to 5% of patients undergoing cholecystectomy. Asymptomatic cholecystoenteric fistulas may sometimes be diagnosed by finding gas in the biliary tree on plain abdominal films. Barium contrast studies or endoscopy of the upper gastrointestinal tract or colon may demonstrate the fistula. Treatment in the symptomatic patient usually consists of cholecystectomy, CBD exploration, and closure of the fistulous tract.

Gallstone ileus refers to mechanical intestinal obstruction resulting from the passage of a large gallstone into the bowel lumen. The stone customarily enters the duodenum through a cholecystoenteric fistula at that level. The site of obstruction by the impacted gallstone is usually at the ileocecal valve, provided that the more proximal small bowel is of normal caliber. The majority of patients do not give a history of either prior biliary tract symptoms or complaints suggestive of acute cholecystitis or fistulization. Large stones over 2.5 cm in diameter are thought to predispose to fistula formation by gradual erosion through the gallbladder fundus. Diagnostic confirmation may occasionally be found on the plain abdominal film (e.g., small-intestinal obstruction with gas in the biliary tree and a calcified, ectopic gallstone) or following an upper gastrointestinal series (cholecystoduodenal fistula with small-bowel obstruction at the ileocecal valve). Laparotomy with stone extraction (or propulsion into the colon) remains the procedure of choice to relieve obstruction. Evacuation of large stones within the gallbladder should also be performed. In general, the gallbladder and its attachment to the intestines should be left alone.

Limey (milk of calcium) bile and porcelain gallbladder Calcium salts may be secreted into the lumen of the gallbladder in sufficient concentration to produce calcium precipitation and diffuse, hazy opacification of bile or a layering effect on plain abdominal roentgenography. This so-called limey bile, or milk of calcium bile, is usually clinically innocuous, but cholecystectomy is recommended because limey bile most often occurs in a hydropic gallbladder. In the entity called *porcelain gallbladder*, calcium salt deposition within the wall of a chronically inflamed gallbladder may be detected on the plain abdominal film. Cholecystectomy is advised in all patients with porcelain gallbladder because in a high percentage of cases this finding appears to be associated with the development of carcinoma of the gallbladder.

℞ TREATMENT **Medical Therapy** Although surgical intervention remains the mainstay of therapy for acute cholecystitis and its complications, a period of in-hospital stabilization may be required before cholecystectomy. Oral intake is eliminated, nasogastric suction may be indicated, and extracellular volume depletion and electrolyte abnormalities are repaired. Meperidine or nonsteroidal antiinflammatory drugs (NSAIDs) are usually employed for analgesia because they may produce less spasm of the sphincter of Oddi than drugs such as morphine. Intravenous antibiotic therapy is usually indicated in patients with severe acute cholecystitis even though bacterial superinfection of bile may not have occurred in the early stages of the inflammatory process. Postoperative complications of wound infection, abscess formation, or sepsis are reduced in antibiotic-treated patients. Effective antibiotics include ureidopenicillins, ampicillin, metronidazole, and cephalosporins. Combination with an aminoglycoside or other antibiotics may be considered in diabetic or debilitated patients and in those with signs of gram-negative sepsis (Chap. 134).

Surgical Therapy The optimal timing of surgical intervention in patients with acute cholecystitis depends on stabilization of the patient. The clear trend is toward earlier surgery, and this is due in part to requirements for shorter hospital stays. Urgent (emergency) cholecystectomy or cholecystostomy is probably appropriate in most patients in whom a complication of acute cholecystitis such as empyema, emphysematous cholecystitis, or perforation is suspected or confirmed. In uncomplicated cases of acute cholecystitis, up to 30% of patients fail to resolve their symptoms on appropriate medical therapy, and progression of the attack or a supervening complication leads to the performance of early operation (within 24 to 72 h). The technical complications of surgery are not increased in patients undergoing early as opposed to delayed cholecystectomy. Delayed surgical intervention is probably best reserved for (1) patients in whom the overall medical condition imposes an unacceptable risk for early surgery and (2) patients in whom the diagnosis of acute cholecystitis is in doubt. Early cholecystectomy is the treatment of choice for most patients with acute cholecystitis. Mortality figures for emergency cholecystectomy in most centers approach 3%, while the mortality risk for elective or early cholecystectomy approximates 0.5% in patients under age 60. Of course, the operative risks increase with age-related diseases of other organ systems and with the presence of long- or short-term complications of gallbladder disease. Seriously ill or debilitated patients with cholecystitis may be managed with cholecystostomy and tube drainage of the gallbladder. Elective cholecystectomy may then be done at a later date.

Postcholecystectomy Complications Early complications following cholecystectomy include atelectasis and other pulmonary disorders, abscess formation (often subphrenic), external or internal hemorrhage, biliary-enteric fistula, and bile leaks. Jaundice may indicate absorption of bile from an intraabdominal collection following a biliary leak or mechanical obstruction of the CBD by retained calculi, intraductal blood clots, or extrinsic compression. Routine performance of intraoperative cholangiography during cholecystectomy has helped to reduce the incidence of these early complications.

Overall, cholecystectomy is a very successful operation that provides total or near-total relief of preoperative symptoms in 75 to 90% of patients. The most common cause of persistent postcholecystectomy symptoms is an overlooked extrabiliary disorder (e.g., reflux esophagitis, peptic ulceration, pancreatitis, or—most often—irritable bowel syndrome). In a small percentage of patients, however, a disorder of the extrahepatic bile ducts may result in persistent symptomatology. These so-called postcholecystectomy syndromes may be due to (1) biliary strictures, (2) retained biliary calculi, (3) cystic duct stump syndrome, (4) stenosis or dyskinesia of the sphincter of Oddi, or (5) bile salt–induced diarrhea or gastritis.

Cystic duct stump syndrome In the absence of cholangiographically demonstrable retained stones, symptoms resembling biliary colic or cholecystitis in the postcholecystectomy patient have frequently been attributed to disease in a long (>1 cm) cystic duct remnant (cystic duct stump syndrome). Careful analysis, however, reveals that postcholecystectomy complaints are attributable to other causes in almost all patients in whom the symptom complex was originally thought to result from the existence of a long cystic duct stump. Accordingly, considerable care should be taken to investigate the possible role of other factors in the production of postcholecystectomy symptoms before attributing them to cystic duct stump syndrome.

Papillary dysfunction, papillary stenosis, spasm of the sphincter of Oddi, and biliary dyskinesia Symptoms of biliary colic accompanied by signs of recurrent, intermittent biliary obstruction may be produced by papillary stenosis, papillary dysfunction, spasm of the sphincter of Oddi, and biliary dyskinesia. Papillary stenosis is thought to result from acute or chronic inflammation of the papilla of Vater or from glandular hyperplasia of the papillary segment. Five criteria have been used to define papillary stenosis: (1) upper abdominal pain, usually RUQ or epigastric; (2) abnormal liver tests; (3) dilatation of the common bile duct upon endoscopic retrograde cholangiopancreatography (ERCP) examination; (4) delayed (>45 min) drainage of contrast material from the duct; and (5) increased basal pressure of the sphincter of Oddi, a finding that may be of only minor significance. An alternative to ERCP is magnetic resonance cholangiography if ERCP and/or biliary manometry are either unavailable or not feasible. In patients with papillary stenosis, quantitative hepatobiliary scintigraphy has revealed delayed transit from the common bile duct to the bowel, ductal dilatation, and abnormal time-activity dynamics. This technique can also be used before and after sphincterotomy to document improvement in biliary emptying. Treatment consists of endoscopic or surgical sphincteroplasty to ensure wide patency of the distal portions of both the bile and pancreatic ducts. The greater the number of the preceding criteria present, the greater the likelihood that a patient does have a degree of papillary stenosis sufficient to justify correction. The factors usually considered as indications for sphincterotomy include (1) prolonged duration of symptoms, (2) lack of response to symptomatic treatment, (3) presence of severe disability, and (4) the patient's choice of sphincterotomy over surgery (given a clear understanding on his or her part of the risks involved in both procedures).

Criteria for diagnosing dyskinesia of the sphincter of Oddi are even more controversial than those for papillary stenosis. Proposed mechanisms include spasm of the sphincter, denervation sensitivity resulting in hypertonicity, and abnormalities of the sequencing or frequency rates of sphincteric contraction waves. When thorough evaluation has failed to demonstrate another cause for the pain, and when cholangiographic and manometric criteria suggest a diagnosis of biliary dyskinesia, medical treatment with nitrites or anticholinergics to attempt pharmacologic relaxation of the sphincter has been proposed. Endoscopic biliary sphincterotomy (EBS) or surgical sphincteroplasty may be indicated in patients who fail to respond to a 2- to 3-month trial of medical therapy, especially if basal sphincter of Oddi pressures are elevated. EBS has become a well-established procedure for removing bile duct stones and for other biliary and pancreatic problems. Approximately 150,000 such procedures are performed annually in the United States. Key findings in a recent study of EBS include: (1) Dysfunction of the sphincter of Oddi was the most frequent patient-related risk factor for complications; (2) pancreatitis was more frequent in young patients; (3) difficulty in cannulating the bile duct and the use of "precut" sphincterotomy were important technique-related risk factors for complications; and (4) experience in the volume of procedures proved to be important; endoscopists who perform more than one EBS per week had lower complication rates than endoscopists who performed a smaller number of procedures.

Bile salt–induced diarrhea and gastritis Postcholecystectomy patients may develop symptoms and signs of gastritis, which has been attributed to duodenogastric reflux of bile. However, firm data linking an increased incidence of bile gastritis with surgical removal of the gallbladder are lacking. Cholecystectomy induces persistent changes in gut transit, and these changes effect a noticeable modification of bowel habits. Cholecystectomy shortens gut transit time by accelerating passage of the fecal bolus through the colon with marked acceleration in the right colon, thus causing an increase in colonic bile acid output and a shift in bile acid composition toward the more diarrheagenic secondary bile acids. Diarrhea that is severe enough, i.e., three or more watery movements per day, can be classified as postcholecystectomy diarrhea, and this occurs in 8 to 12% of patients undergoing elective cholecystectomy. Treatment with a bile acid sequestering agent, such as cholestyramine, is often effective in ameliorating troublesome diarrhea.

THE HYPERPLASTIC CHOLECYSTOSES The term *hyperplastic cholecystoses* is used to denote a group of disorders of the gallbladder characterized by excessive proliferation of normal tissue components.

Adenomyomatosis is characterized by a benign proliferation of gallbladder surface epithelium with glandlike formations, extramural sinuses, transverse strictures, and/or fundal nodule ("adenoma" or "adenomyoma") formation. Outpouchings of mucosa termed *Rokitansky-Aschoff sinuses* may be seen on oral cholecystography in conjunction with hyperconcentration of contrast medium. Characteristic dimpled filling defects also may be seen.

Cholesterolosis is characterized by abnormal deposition of lipid, especially cholesterol esters, in the lamina propria of the gallbladder wall. In its diffuse form ("strawberry gallbladder"), the gallbladder mucosa is brick red and speckled with bright yellow flecks of lipid. The localized form shows solitary or multiple "cholesterol polyps" studding the gallbladder wall. Cholesterol stones of the gallbladder are found in nearly half the cases. Cholecystectomy is indicated in both adenomyomatosis and cholesterolosis when symptomatic or when cholelithiasis is present.

DISEASES OF THE BILE DUCTS

CONGENITAL ANOMALIES **Biliary Atresia and Hypoplasia** Atretic and hypoplastic lesions of the extrahepatic and major intrahepatic bile ducts are the most common biliary anomalies of clinical relevance encountered in infancy. The clinical picture is one of severe obstructive jaundice during the first month of life, with pale stools. The diagnosis is confirmed by surgical exploration with operative cholangiography. Approximately 10% of cases of biliary atresia are treatable with roux-en-Y choledochojejunostomy, with the Kasai procedure (hepatic portoenterostomy) being attempted in the remainder in an effort to restore some bile flow. Most patients, even those having successful biliary-enteric anastomoses, eventually develop chronic cholangitis, extensive hepatic fibrosis, and portal hypertension.

Choledochal Cysts Cystic dilatation may involve the free portion of the CBD, i.e., choledochal cyst, or may present as diverticulum formation in the intraduodenal segment. In the latter situation, chronic reflux of pancreatic juice into the biliary tree can produce inflammation and stenosis of the extrahepatic bile ducts leading to cholangitis or biliary obstruction. Because the process may be gradual, approximately 50% of patients present with onset of symptoms after age 10. The diagnosis may be made by ultrasound, abdominal CT, or cholangiography. Only one-third of patients show the classic triad of abdominal pain, jaundice, and an abdominal mass. Ultrasonographic detection of a cyst separate from the gallbladder should suggest the diagnosis of choledochal cyst, which can be confirmed by demonstrating the entrance of extrahepatic bile ducts into the cyst. Surgical treatment involves excision of the "cyst" and biliary-enteric anastomosis. Patients with choledochal cysts are at increased risk for the subsequent development of cholangiocarcinoma.

Congenital Biliary Ectasia Cystic dilatation of the intrahepatic bile ducts may involve either the major intrahepatic radicles (Caroli's disease), the inter- and intralobular ducts (congenital hepatic fibrosis), or both. In Caroli's disease, clinical manifestations include recurrent cholangitis, abscess formation in and around the affected ducts, and, sometimes, gallstone formation within portions of ectatic intrahepatic biliary radicles. The CT scan and cholangiographic patterns are usually diagnostic, and treatment with ongoing antibiotic therapy is usually undertaken in an effort to limit the frequency and severity of recurrent bouts of cholangitis. Progression to secondary biliary cirrhosis with portal hypertension, amyloidosis, extrahepatic biliary obstruction, cholangiocarcinoma, or recurrent episodes of sepsis with hepatic abscess formation is common.

CHOLEDOCHOLITHIASIS Pathophysiology and Clinical Manifestations Passage of gallstones into the CBD occurs in approximately 10 to 15% of patients with cholelithiasis. The incidence of common duct stones increases with increasing age of the patient, so that up to 25% of elderly patients may have calculi in the common duct at the time of cholecystectomy. Undetected duct stones are left behind in approximately 1 to 5% of cholecystectomy patients. The overwhelming majority of bile duct stones are cholesterol or mixed stones formed in the gallbladder, which then migrate into the extrahepatic biliary tree through the cystic duct. Primary calculi arising de novo in the ducts are usually pigment stones developing in patients with (1) chronic hemolytic diseases; (2) hepatobiliary parasitism or chronic, recurrent cholangitis; (3) congenital anomalies of the bile ducts (especially Caroli's disease); or (4) dilated, sclerosed, or strictured ducts. Common duct stones may remain asymptomatic for years, may pass spontaneously into the duodenum, or (most often) may present with biliary colic or a complication.

Complications • *Cholangitis* Cholangitis may be acute or chronic, and symptoms result from inflammation, which usually requires at least partial obstruction to the flow of bile. Bacteria are present on bile culture in approximately 75% of patients with acute cholangitis early in the symptomatic course. The characteristic presentation of acute cholangitis involves biliary colic, jaundice, and spiking fevers with chills (Charcot's triad). Blood cultures are frequently positive, and leukocytosis is typical. *Nonsuppurative* acute cholangitis is most common and may respond relatively rapidly to supportive measures and to treatment with antibiotics. In *suppurative* acute cholangitis, however, the presence of pus under pressure in a completely obstructed ductal system leads to symptoms of severe toxicity—mental confusion, bacteremia, and septic shock. Response to antibiotics alone in this setting is relatively poor, multiple hepatic abscesses are often present, and the mortality rate approaches 100% unless prompt endoscopic or surgical relief of the obstruction and drainage of infected bile are carried out. Endoscopic management of bacterial cholangitis is as effective as surgical intervention. ERCP with endoscopic sphincterotomy is safe and the preferred initial procedure for both establishing a definitive diagnosis and providing effective therapy.

Obstructive jaundice Gradual obstruction of the CBD over a period of weeks or months usually leads to initial manifestations of jaundice or pruritus without associated symptoms of biliary colic or cholangitis. Painless jaundice may occur in patients with choledocholithiasis, but this manifestation is much more characteristic of biliary obstruction secondary to malignancy of the head of the pancreas, bile ducts, or ampulla of Vater.

In patients whose obstruction is secondary to choledocholithiasis, associated chronic calculous cholecystitis is very common, and the gallbladder in this setting may be relatively indistensible. The absence of a palpable gallbladder in most patients with biliary obstruction from duct stones is the basis for *Courvoisier's law*, i.e., that the presence of a palpably enlarged gallbladder suggests that the biliary obstruction is secondary to an underlying malignancy rather than to calculous disease. Biliary obstruction causes progressive dilatation of the intrahepatic bile ducts as intrabiliary pressures rise. Hepatic bile flow is suppressed, and regurgitation of conjugated bilirubin into the bloodstream leads to jaundice accompanied by dark urine (bilirubinuria) and light-colored (acholic) stools.

CBD stones should be suspected in any patient with cholecystitis whose serum bilirubin level exceeds 85.5 μmol/L (5 mg/dL). The maximum bilirubin level is seldom over 256.5 μmol/L (15.0 mg/dL) in patients with choledocholithiasis unless concomitant hepatic disease or another factor leading to marked hyperbilirubinemia exists. Serum bilirubin levels of 342.0 μmol/L (20 mg/dL) or more should suggest the possibility of neoplastic obstruction. The serum alkaline phosphatase level is almost always elevated in biliary obstruction. A rise in alkaline phosphatase often precedes clinical jaundice and may be the only abnormality in routine liver function tests. There may be a two- to tenfold elevation of serum aminotransferases, especially in association with acute obstruction. Following relief of the obstructing process, serum aminotransferase elevations usually return rapidly to normal, while the serum bilirubin level may take 1 to 2 weeks to return to normal. The alkaline phosphatase level usually falls slowly, lagging behind the decrease in serum bilirubin.

Pancreatitis The most common associated entity discovered in patients with nonalcoholic acute pancreatitis is biliary tract disease. Biochemical evidence of pancreatic inflammation complicates acute cholecystitis in 15% of cases and choledocholithiasis in over 30%, and the common factor appears to be the passage of gallstones through the common duct. Coexisting pancreatitis should be suspected in patients with symptoms of cholecystitis who develop (1) back pain or pain to the left of the abdominal midline, (2) prolonged vomiting with paralytic ileus, or (3) a pleural effusion, especially on the left side. Surgical treatment of gallstone disease is usually associated with resolution of the pancreatitis.

Secondary biliary cirrhosis Secondary biliary cirrhosis may complicate prolonged or intermittent duct obstruction with or without recurrent cholangitis. Although this complication may be seen in patients with choledocholithiasis, it is more common in cases of prolonged obstruction from stricture or neoplasm. Once established, secondary biliary cirrhosis may be progressive even after correction of the obstructing process, and increasingly severe hepatic cirrhosis may lead to portal hypertension or to hepatic failure and death. Prolonged biliary obstruction may also be associated with clinically relevant deficiencies of the fat-soluble vitamins A, D, and K.

Diagnosis and Treatment The diagnosis of choledocholithiasis is usually made by cholangiography (Table 302-3), either preoperatively by ERCP or intraoperatively at the time of cholecystectomy. As many as 15% of patients undergoing cholecystectomy will prove to have CBD stones. With the advent of laparoscopic cholecystectomy, the management of CBD stones in the presence of gallstones is gradually being clarified. Preoperative ERCP with endoscopic papillotomy and stone extraction is the preferred approach. It not only provides stone clearance but also defines the anatomy of the biliary tree in relationship to the cystic duct. ERCP is indicated in gallstone patients who have any of the following risk factors: (1) a history of jaundice or pancreatitis, (2) abnormal tests of liver function, and (3) ultrasonographic evidence of a dilated CBD or stones in the duct. Alternatively, if intraoperative cholangiography reveals retained stones, postoperative ERCP can be carried out. The need for preoperative ERCP is expected to decrease further as laparoscopic techniques improve.

The widespread use of laparoscopic cholecystectomy and ERCP has decreased the incidence of complicated biliary tract disease and the need for choledocholithotomy and T-tube drainage of the bile ducts. EBS followed by spontaneous passage or stone extraction is the treatment of choice in the management of patients with common duct stones, especially in elderly or poor-risk patients.

TRAUMA, STRICTURES, AND HEMOBILIA Benign strictures of the extrahepatic bile ducts result from surgical trauma in approximately 95% of cases and occur in about 1 in 500 cholecystectomies. Strictures may present with bile leak or abscess formation in the immediate postoperative period or with biliary obstruction or cholangitis as long as 2 years or more following the inciting trauma. The diagnosis is established by percutaneous or endoscopic cholangiography. Endoscopic brushing of biliary strictures is an effective way to establish the nature of the lesion and is more accurate than bile cytology alone. When positive exfoliative cytology is obtained, the diagnosis of a neoplastic stricture is established. This procedure is especially important in patients with primary sclerosing cholangitis who are predisposed to the development of cholangiocarcinomas. Successful operative correction by a skillful surgeon with duct-to-bowel anas-

Table 302-3 Diagnostic Evaluation of the Bile Ducts

Diagnostic Advantages	Diagnostic Limitations	Contraindications	Complications	Comment
HEPATOBILIARY ULTRASOUND				
Rapid Simultaneous scanning of GB, liver, bile ducts, pancreas Accurate identification of dilated bile ducts Not limited by jaundice, pregnancy Guidance for fine-needle biopsy	Bowel gas Massive obesity Ascites Barium Partial bile duct obstruction Poor visualization of distal CBD	None	None	Initial procedure of choice in investigating possible biliary tract obstruction
COMPUTED TOMOGRAPHY				
Simultaneous scanning of GB, liver, bile ducts, pancreas Accurate identification of dilated bile ducts, masses Not limited by jaundice, gas, obesity, ascites High-resolution image Guidance for fine-needle biopsy	Extreme cachexia Movement artifact Ileus Partial bile duct obstruction High cost May not be readily available	Pregnancy	Reaction to iodinated contrast, if used	Indicated for evaluation of hepatic or pancreatic masses Procedure of choice in investigating possible biliary obstruction if diagnostic limitations prevent HBUS
MAGNETIC RESONANCE CHOLANGIOPANCREATOGRAPHY				
Useful modality for visualizing pancreatic and biliary ducts Can identify pancreatic duct dilatation or stricture, pancreatic duct stenosis, and pancreas divisum Has excellent sensitivity for bile duct dilatation, biliary stricture, and intraductal abnormalities	Cannot offer therapeutic intervention			
PERCUTANEOUS TRANSHEPATIC CHOLANGIOGRAM				
Extremely successful when bile ducts dilated Best visualization of proximal biliary tract Possible separate visualization of obstructed left ductal system Bile cytology/culture Percutaneous transhepatic drainage	Nondilated or sclerosed ducts	Pregnancy Uncorrectable coagulopathy Massive ascites ? Hepatic abscess	Bleeding Hemobilia Bile peritonitis Bacteremia, sepsis	Usually, initial cholangiogram of choice when bile ducts are dilated
ENDOSCOPIC RETROGRADE CHOLANGIOPANCREATOGRAM				
Simultaneous pancreatography Visualization/biopsy of ampulla and duodenum Best visualization of distal biliary tract Bile or pancreatic cytology Endoscopic sphincterotomy and stone removal Biliary manometry Not limited by ascites, coagulopathy, abscess	Gastroduodenal obstruction ? Roux en Y biliary-enteric anastomosis	Pregnancy ? Acute pancreatitis ? Severe cardiopulmonary disease	Pancreatitis Cholangitis, sepsis Infected pancreatic pseudocyst Perforation (rare) Hypoxemia, aspiration	Cholangiogram of choice in: Absence of dilated ducts ? Pancreatic, ampullary or gastroduodenal disease Prior biliary surgery PTHC contraindicated or failed Endoscopic sphincterotomy a treatment possibility

NOTE: GB, gallbladder; CBD, common bile duct; HBUS, hepatobiliary ultrasound; PTHC, percutaneous transhepatic cholangiogram. Intravenous cholangiography is an obsolete technique because 40% of common duct stones are missed and there is poor resolution even with tomography. There are few indications for its use, especially since other cholangiographic techniques are usually available.

tomosis is usually possible, although mortality rates from surgical complications, recurrent cholangitis, or secondary biliary cirrhosis are high.

Hemobilia may follow traumatic or operative injury to the liver or bile ducts, intraductal rupture of a hepatic abscess or aneurysm of the hepatic artery, biliary or hepatic tumor hemorrhage, or mechanical complications of choledocholithiasis or hepatobiliary parasitism. Diagnostic procedures such as liver biopsy, percutaneous transhepatic cholangiography (PTHC), and transhepatic biliary drainage catheter placement may also be complicated by hemobilia. Patients often present with a classic triad of biliary colic, obstructive jaundice, and melena or occult blood in the stools. The diagnosis is sometimes made by cholangiographic evidence of blood clot in the biliary tree, but selective angiographic verification may be required. Although minor episodes of hemobilia may resolve without operative intervention, surgical ligation of the bleeding vessel is frequently required.

EXTRINSIC COMPRESSION OF THE BILE DUCTS Partial or complete biliary obstruction may sometimes be produced by extrinsic compression of the ducts. The most common cause of this form of obstructive jaundice is carcinoma of the head of the pancreas. Biliary obstruction may also occur as a complication of either acute or chronic pancreatitis or involvement of lymph nodes in the porta hepatis by lymphoma or metastatic carcinoma. The latter should be distinguished from cholestasis resulting from massive replacement of the liver by tumor.

HEPATOBILIARY PARASITISM Infestation of the biliary tract by adult helminths or their ova may produce a chronic, recurrent pyogenic cholangitis with or without multiple hepatic abscesses, ductal stones, or biliary obstruction. This condition is relatively rare but does occur in inhabitants of southern China and elsewhere in Southeast Asia. The organisms most commonly involved are trematodes or flukes, including *Clonorchis sinensis*, *Opisthorchis viverrini* or *O. felineus*, and *Fasciola hepatica*. The biliary tract also may be involved by intraductal migration of adult *Ascaris lumbricoides* from the duodenum or by intrabiliary rupture of hydatid cysts of the liver produced by *Echinococcus* spp. The diagnosis is made by cholangiography and the presence of characteristic ova on stool examination. When obstruction is present, the treatment of choice is laparotomy under antibiotic coverage, with common duct exploration and a biliary drainage procedure. It should be emphasized that in the Far East, one also sees cholangiohepatitis associated with pigment lithiasis, which may, in fact, be more common than cholangitis due to parasites.

SCLEROSING CHOLANGITIS Primary or idiopathic sclerosing cholangitis is characterized by a progressive, inflammatory, sclerosing, and obliterative process affecting the extrahepatic and/or the intrahepatic bile ducts. The disorder occurs in about 70% in association with inflammatory bowel disease, especially ulcerative colitis. It may also be associated (albeit rarely) with multifocal fibrosclerosis syndromes such as retroperitoneal, mediastinal, and/or periureteral fibrosis; Riedel's struma; or pseudotumor of the orbit. In patients with AIDS, cholangiopancreatography may demonstrate a broad range of biliary tract changes as well as pancreatic duct obstruction and occasionally pancreatitis (Chap. 309). Further, biliary tract lesions in AIDS include infection and cholangiopancreatographic changes similar to primary sclerosing cholangitis. Changes noted include: (1) diffuse involvement of intrahepatic bile ducts alone, (2) involvement of both intra- and extrahepatic bile ducts, (3) ampullary stenosis, (4) stricture of the intrapancreatic portion of the common bile duct, and (5) pancreatic duct involvement. Associated infectious organisms include *Cryptosporidium*, *Mycobacterium avium-intracellulare*, cytomegalovirus, *Microsporidia*, and *Isospora*. In addition, acalculous cholecystitis occurs in up to 10% of patients. ERCP sphincterotomy, while not without risk, provides significant pain reduction in patients with AIDS-associated papillary stenosis. Secondary sclerosing cholangitis may occur as a long-term complication of choledocholithiasis, cholangiocarcinoma, operative or traumatic biliary injury, or contiguous inflammatory processes.

Patients with primary sclerosing cholangitis often present with signs and symptoms of chronic or intermittent biliary obstruction: jaundice, pruritus, RUQ abdominal pain, or acute cholangitis. Late in the course, complete biliary obstruction, secondary biliary cirrhosis, hepatic failure, or portal hypertension with bleeding varices may occur. The diagnosis is usually established by finding multifocal, diffusely distributed strictures with intervening segments of normal or dilated ducts, producing a beaded appearance on cholangiography (Fig. 302-2*D*). The cholangiographic technique of choice in suspected cases is ERCP, since intrahepatic ductal involvement may make PTHC difficult. When a diagnosis of sclerosing cholangitis has been established, a search for associated diseases, especially for chronic inflammatory bowel disease, should be carried out.

A recent study describes the natural history and outcome for 305 patients of Swedish descent with primary sclerosing cholangitis; 134 (44%) of the patients were asymptomatic at the time of diagnosis and, not surprisingly, had a significantly higher survival rate with a median follow-up time of 63 months. The independent predictors of a bad prognosis were age, serum bilirubin concentration, and liver histologic changes. Cholangiocarcinoma was found in 24 patients (8%). Inflammatory bowel disease was closely associated with primary sclerosing cholangitis and had a prevalence of 81% in this study population.

℞ **TREATMENT** Therapy with cholestyramine may help control symptoms of pruritus, and antibiotics are useful when cholangitis complicates the clinical picture. Vitamin D and calcium supplementation may help prevent the loss of bone mass frequently seen in patients with chronic cholestasis. Glucocorticoids, methotrexate, and cyclosporine have not been shown to be efficacious. UDCA improves serum liver tests, but an effect on survival has not been documented. In cases where complete or high-grade biliary obstruction (dominant strictures) has occurred, balloon dilatation, stenting, or (rarely) surgical intervention may be appropriate. Efforts at biliary-enteric anastomosis or stent placement may, however, be complicated by recurrent cholangitis and further progression of the stenosing process. The role of colectomy in patients with sclerosing cholangitis complicating chronic ulcerative colitis is uncertain. The prognosis is unfavorable, with a median survival of 9 to 12 years following the diagnosis, regardless of therapy. Four variables (age, serum bilirubin level, histologic stage, and splenomegaly) predict survival in patients with primary sclerosing cholangitis and serve as the basis for a risk score. Primary sclerosing cholangitis is one of the most common indications for liver transplantation.

In two large studies involving 627 and 3147 patients, the prevalence of gallbladder polyps was 6.7 and 6.9%, respectively, with a marked male predominance. Few significant changes occurred over a 5-year period in asymptomatic patients in whom gallbladder polyps <10 mm in diameter were found. If polyps >10 mm are present and show rapid growth, cholecystectomy should be considered.

ACKNOWLEDGMENT

This chapter was written by Dr. Norton J. Greenberger and Dr. Kurt J. Isselbacher in the previous edition.

BIBLIOGRAPHY

AFDHAL NH et al: Mucin-vesicle interaction in model bile: Evidence for vesicle aggregation and fusion before cholesterol crystal formation. Hepatology 22:856, 1995

APSETEIN MD, CAREY MC: Pathogenesis of cholesterol gallstones: A parsimonious hypothesis. Eur J Clin Invest 26:343, 1996

BERR F et al: 7-Alpha-dehydroxylating bacteria enhance deoxycholic acid input and cholesterol saturation of bile in patients with gallstones. Gastroenterology 111:1611, 1996

BROOME V et al: Natural history and prognostic factors in 305 Swedish patients with primary sclerosing cholangitis. Gut 38:610, 1996

DICKSON ER: Primary sclerosing cholangitis: Refinement and validation of survival models. Gastroenterology 103:1893, 1992

FORT JM et al: Bowel habit after cholecystectomy: Physiologic changes and clinical implications. Gastroenterology 111:617, 1996

FREEMAN ML et al: Complications of endoscopic biliary sphincterotomy. N Engl J Med 335:909, 1996

GEENEN JE et al: The efficacy of endoscopic sphincterotomy after cholecystectomy in patients with sphincter-of-Oddi dysfunction. N Engl J Med 320:82, 1989

HOLZKNECHT N et al: Breath-hold MR cholangiography using snapshot techniques: A prospective comparison with endoscopic cholangiography. Radiology 206:657, 1998

JOHNSTON DE, KAPLAN MM: Medical progress: Pathogenesis and treatment of gallstones. N Engl J Med 328:412, 1993

MARINGHINI A et al: Gallstones, gallbladder cancer, and other gastrointestinal malignancies: An epidemiologic study in Rochester, Minnesota. Ann Intern Med 107:30, 1987

MAY GR et al: Efficacy of bile acid therapy for gallstone dissolution: A meta-analysis of randomized trials. Aliment Pharmacol Ther 7:139, 1993

MCMAHON AG et al: Laparoscopic versus minilaparotomy cholecystectomy: A randomized trial. Lancet 343:135, 1994

MIQUEL JF et al: Genetic epidemiology of cholesterol cholelithiasis among Chilean Hispanics, American Indians and Maoris. Gastroenterology 115:937, 1998

PAULETZKI J et al: Gallbladder emptying and gallstone formation: A prospective study on gallstone recurrence. Gastroenterology 111:765, 1996

RANSOHOFF DF, GRACIE WA: Treatment of gallstones. Ann Intern Med 119:606, 1993

SARIN SK et al: High familial prevalence of gallstones in the first degree relatives of gallstone patients. Hepatology 22:138, 1995

SHIFFMAN M et al: Prophylaxis against gallstone formation with ursodeoxycholic acid in patients. Ann Intern Med 122:999, 1995

STRASBERG SM: Cholelithiasis and acute cholecystitis. Baillieres Clin Gastroenterol 22: 643, 1997

TRAUNER M et al: Molecular pathogenesis of cholestasis. N Engl J Med 339:1217, 1998

Section 3
DISORDERS OF THE PANCREAS

303

Phillip P. Toskes, Norton J. Greenberger

APPROACH TO THE PATIENT WITH PANCREATIC DISEASE

GENERAL CONSIDERATIONS

Inflammatory disease of the pancreas may be acute or chronic. Although good data exist concerning the frequency of acute pancreatitis (about 5000 new cases per year in the United States, with a mortality rate of about 10%), the number of patients who suffer with recurrent acute pancreatitis or chronic pancreatitis is largely undefined. Only one prospective study on the incidence of chronic pancreatitis is available; it showed an incidence of 8.2 new cases per 100,000 per year and a prevalence of 26.4 cases per 100,000. These numbers probably underestimate considerably the true incidence and prevalence, because non-alcohol-induced pancreatitis was largely ignored. At autopsy, the prevalence of chronic pancreatitis ranges from 0.04 to 5%. The relative inaccessibility of the pancreas to direct examination and the nonspecificity of the abdominal pain associated with pancreatitis make the diagnosis of pancreatitis difficult and usually dependent on elevation of blood amylase levels. Many patients with chronic pancreatitis do not have elevated blood amylase levels. Some patients with chronic pancreatitis develop signs and symptoms of pancreatic exocrine insufficiency, and thus objective evidence for pancreatic disease can be demonstrated. However, there is a very large reservoir of pancreatic exocrine function. More than 90% of the pancreas must be damaged before maldigestion of fat and protein is manifested. Even the secretin stimulation test, which is the most sensitive method of assessing pancreatic exocrine function, is probably abnormal only when more than 60% of exocrine function has been lost. Noninvasive, indirect tests of pancreatic exocrine function (bentiromide, serum trypsinogen) are much more likely to give abnormal results in patients with obvious pancreatic disease, i.e., pancreatic calcification, steatorrhea, or diabetes mellitus, than in patients with occult disease. Thus, the number of patients who have subclinical exocrine dysfunction (less than 90% loss of function) is unknown.

The clinical manifestations of acute and chronic pancreatitis and pancreatic insufficiency are protean. Thus, patients may present with hypertriglyceridemia, vitamin B_{12} malabsorption, hypercalcemia, hypocalcemia, hyperglycemia, ascites, pleural effusions, and chronic abdominal pain with normal blood amylase levels. Indeed, if the clinician considers pancreatitis as a possible diagnosis only when presented with a patient having classic symptoms (i.e., severe, constant epigastric pain that radiates through to the back, along with an elevated blood amylase level), only a minority of patients with pancreatitis will be diagnosed correctly.

As emphasized in Chap. 304, the etiologies as well as the clinical manifestations of pancreatitis are quite varied. Although it is well appreciated that pancreatitis is frequently secondary to alcohol abuse and biliary tract disease, it can also be caused by drugs, trauma, and viral infections and is associated with metabolic and connective tissue disorders. In approximately 30% of patients with acute pancreatitis and 25 to 40% of patients with chronic pancreatitis, the etiology is obscure.

TESTS USEFUL IN THE DIAGNOSIS OF PANCREATIC DISEASE

Several tests have proved of value in the evaluation of pancreatic exocrine function. Examples of specific tests and their usefulness in the diagnosis of acute and chronic pancreatitis are summarized in Table 303-1. At most institutions, pancreatic function tests are performed if the diagnosis of pancreatic disease remains a possibility after noninvasive tests [ultrasound, computed tomography (CT)] and invasive tests [endoscopic retrograde cholangiopancreatography (ERCP)] have given normal or inconclusive results. In this regard, tests employing *direct* stimulation of the pancreas are the most sensitive.

PANCREATIC ENZYMES IN BODY FLUIDS The serum amylase level is widely used as a screening test for acute pancreatitis in the patient with acute abdominal pain or back pain. A value greater than 65 U/L should raise the question of acute pancreatitis. Levels greater than 130 U/L make the diagnosis more likely, and values greater than three times normal virtually clinch the diagnosis if gut perforation or infarction is excluded. In acute pancreatitis, the serum amylase is usually elevated within 24 h of onset and remains so for 1 to 3 days. Levels return to normal within 3 to 5 days unless there is extensive pancreatic necrosis, incomplete ductal obstruction, or pseudocyst formation. Approximately 85% of patients with acute pancreatitis have an elevated serum amylase level. This index may be normal, however, if (1) there is a delay (of 2 to 5 days) before blood samples are obtained, (2) the underlying disorder is chronic pancreatitis rather than acute pancreatitis, or (3) hypertriglyceridemia is present. Patients with hypertriglyceridemia and proven pancreatitis have been found to have spuriously low levels of amylase and lipase activity.

The serum amylase is often elevated in other conditions (Table 303-2), in part because the enzyme is found in many organs in addition to the pancreas (salivary glands, liver, small intestine, kidney, fallopian tube) and can be produced by various tumors (carcinomas of the lung, esophagus, breast, and ovary). Isoenzymes of amylase fall into two general categories: those arising from the pancreas (P isoamylases) and those arising from nonpancreatic sources (S isoamylases). The measurement of serum isoamylases is of clinical importance. In normal serum, about 35 to 45% of the amylase is of pancreatic origin. For example, in patients with acute pancreatitis, the total serum amylase level returns to normal more rapidly than the level of pancreatic isoamylase. Thus, in patients seen after the first day, the pancreatic isoamylase level is a more sensitive indicator of pancreatitis than the total serum amylase level. In the past, elevations in serum amylase seen in certain conditions, such as the postoperative state, acute alcohol intoxication, and diabetic ketoacidosis, were assumed to indicate acute

Table 303-1 Tests Useful in the Diagnosis of Acute and Chronic Pancreatitis and Pancreatic Tumors

Test	Principle	Comment
PANCREATIC ENZYMES IN BODY FLUIDS		
Amylase		
1. Serum	Pancreatic inflammation leads to increased enzyme levels	Simple; 20–40% false negatives and positives; reliable if test results are three times the upper limit of normal
2. Urine	Renal clearance of amylase is increased in acute pancreatitis	May be abnormal when serum levels normal; false negatives and positives
3. Amylase/creatinine clearance ratio (C_{am}/C_{cr})	Renal clearance of amylase greater than clearance of creatinine	No more sensitive than serum amylase; many false positives
4. Ascitic fluid	Disruption of gland or main pancreatic duct leads to increased amylase concentration	Can establish diagnosis of pancreatitis; false positives occur with intestinal obstruction and perforated ulcer
5. Pleural fluid	Exudative pleural effusion with pancreatitis	False positives occur with carcinoma of the lung and esophageal perforation
6. Isoenzymes	P isoamylases arise from the pancreas; S isoamylases are from other sources	More sensitive than total serum amylase in diagnosis of acute pancreatitis; useful in identifying nonpancreatic causes of hyperamylasemia
Serum lipase	Pancreatic inflammation leads to increased enzyme levels	New methods have greatly simplified determination; positive in 70–85% of cases.
Serum trypsinogen	Pancreatic inflammation leads to increased levels	*Elevated* in acute pancreatitis; *decreased* in chronic pancreatitis *with* steatorrhea; normal in chronic pancreatitis *without* steatorrhea and in steatorrhea with normal pancreatic function
Pancreatic polypeptide (PP)	PP confined almost totally to the pancreas; release stimulated by nutrients and hormones; such release parallels pancreatic enzyme secretion	Basal, meal-simulated, and hormone-stimulated (by secretin or CCK) PP levels *decreased* in chronic pancreatitis; a fasting PP level >125 pg/mL argues against chronic pancreatitis and pancreatic cancer; increased levels in pancreatic endocrine tumors
STUDIES PERTAINING TO PANCREATIC STRUCTURE		
Radiologic and radionuclide tests		
1. Plain film of the abdomen	Abnormal in acute and chronic pancreatitis	Simple; normal in >50% of cases of both acute and chronic pancreatitis
2. Upper gastrointestinal x-rays	Abnormally thickened duodenal folds; displacement of stomach or widening of duodenal loop suggests a pancreatic mass (inflammatory, neoplastic, cystic)	Simple; frequently normal; largely superseded by US and CT scanning
3. Ultrasonography (US)	Can provide information on edema, inflammation, calcification, pseudocysts, and mass lesions	Simple, noninvasive; sequential studies quite feasible; useful in diagnosis of pseudocyst
4. CT scan	Permits detailed visualization of pancreas and surrounding structures	Useful in the diagnosis of pancreatic calcification, dilated pancreatic ducts, and pancreatic tumors; may not be able to distinguish between inflammatory and neoplastic mass lesions
5. Selective angiography	Can identify pancreatic neoplasms (1) by sheathing of celiac or superior mesenteric branches by tumor or (2) by tumor staining; displacement of vessels by tumor	Indicated (1) in suspected islet cell tumors and (2) before pancreatic or duodenal resection; most reliable features reflect nonresectable pancreatic cancer
6. Endoscopic retrograde cholangiopancreatography (ERCP)	Cannulation of pancreatic and common bile duct permits visualization of pancreatic-biliary ductal system	Provides diagnostic data in 60–85% of cases; differentiation of chronic pancreatitis from pancreatic carcinoma may be difficult
7. Endoscopic ultrasonography (EUS)	High-frequency transducer employed with EUS can produce very high-resolution images and depict changes in the pancreatic duct and parenchyma with better detail	Exact role of EUS versus ERCP and CT not yet fully defined; sensitivity and specificity under study
8. Magnetic resonance cholangiopancreatography	Three dimensional rendering has been used to produce very good images of the pancreatic duct by a noninvasive technique	May be used to evaluate patients judged to be at high risk for ERCP, such as the elderly; may replace ERCP as a diagnostic test, although large controlled studies need to be done
Pancreatic biopsy with US or CT guidance	Percutaneous biopsy with skinny needle and localization of lesion by US	High diagnostic yield; laparotomy avoided; requires special technical skills
TESTS OF EXOCRINE PANCREATIC FUNCTION		
Direct stimulation of the pancreas with analysis of duodenal contents		
1. Secretin-pancreozymin (CCK) test	Secretin leads to increased output of pancreatic juice and HCO_3^-; CCK leads to increased output of pancreatic enzymes; pancreatic secretory response is related to the functional mass of pancreatic tissue	Sensitive enough to detect occult disease; involves duodenal intubation and fluoroscopy; poorly defined normal enzyme response; overlap in chronic pancreatitis; large secretory reserve capacity of the pancreas

(continued)

Table 303-1 Tests Useful in the Diagnosis of Acute and Chronic Pancreatitis and Pancreatic Tumors—(*continued*)

Test	Principle	Comment
Indirect stimulation of pancreas with measurement of pancreatic enzymes		
1. Lundh test meal	Test meal (fat, carbohydrate, and protein) causes increased release of CCK, which causes increased enzyme output; trypsin concentration measured	Useful in pancreatic exocrine insufficiency; false negatives with delayed gastric emptying; false positives in primary mucosal disease of the gut and choledocholithiasis; does not measure secretory capacity
2. Benzoyl-tyrosyl-*p*-aminobenzoic acid (Bz-Ty-PABA, bentiromide) test	Synthetic peptide (Bz-Ty-PABA) is specifically cleaved by chymotrypsin, liberating PABA, which is absorbed; PABA metabolite is excreted in the urine	Simple and reliable test of pancreatic exocrine function; measurement of blood PABA level increases sensitivity; not available in the United States
3. Pancreolauryl test	Fluorescein dilaurate is hydrolyzed by pancreatic elastase and absorbed; fluorescein is measured in urine	Sensitivity and specificity similar to those of serum trypsinogen; not available in the United States
Measurement of intraluminal digestion products		
1. Microscopic examination of stool for undigested meat fibers and fat	Lack of proteolytic and lipolytic enzymes causes decreased digestion of meat fibers and triglycerides	Simple, reliable; not sensitive enough to detect milder cases of pancreatic insufficiency
2. Quantitative stool fat determination	Lack of lipolytic enzymes brings about impaired fat digestion	Reliable, reference standard for defining severity of malabsorption; does not distinguish between maldigestion and malabsorption
3. Fecal nitrogen	Lack of proteolytic enzymes leads to impaired protein digestion, resulting in an increase in stool nitrogen	Does not distinguish between maldigestion and malabsorption; low sensitivity
Measurement of pancreatic enzymes in feces		
1. Elastase	Pancreatic secretion of proteolytic enzymes	Excellent specificity; sensitivity similar to that of serum trypsinogen
Miscellaneous tests		
1. Dual-labeled Schilling test	Intrinsic factor [^{57}Co]cobalamin and Hog R protein [^{58}Co]cobalamin are given together. Since proteases are necessary to cleave R protein, the ratio of labeled cobalamin excreted in urine is an index of exocrine dysfunction.	Time-consuming and expensive

pancreatitis. However, the elevation of serum amylase in such conditions has been shown to be due to an elevation of the S isoamylase. Simple tests to distinguish pancreatic from nonpancreatic amylase are no longer readily available, and such tests are often not reliable when the total amylase is minimally to moderately elevated. An assay of serum trypsinogen (performed by several commercial laboratories) is quite helpful in this regard. Since this enzyme is secreted specifically by the pancreas, a normal serum trypsinogen level in a patient with minimal elevation of serum amylase essentially rules out acute pancreatitis. Urinary amylase measurements, including the amylase/creatinine clearance ratio, are no more sensitive or specific than blood amylase levels.

Elevation of ascitic fluid amylase occurs in acute pancreatitis as well as in (1) pancreatogenous ascites due to disruption of the main pancreatic duct or a leaking pseudocyst and (2) other abdominal disorders that simulate pancreatitis (e.g., intestinal obstruction, intestinal infarction, and perforated peptic ulcer). Elevation of pleural fluid amylase occurs in acute pancreatitis, chronic pancreatitis, carcinoma of the lung, and esophageal perforation.

Lipase may now be the single best enzyme to measure for the diagnosis of acute pancreatitis. Improvements in substrates and technology offer clinicians improved options, especially when a turbidimetric assay is used. The newer lipase assays have colipase as a cofactor and are fully automated.

An assay for trypsinogen (or for trypsin-like immunoreactivity) has a theoretical advantage over amylase and lipase determinations in that the pancreas is the only organ that contains this enzyme. The test appears to be useful in the diagnosis of both acute and chronic pancreatitis. Sensitivity and specificity are comparable to those of amylase and lipase determinations. Since trypsinogen is also excreted by the kidney, elevated serum values are found in renal failure, as is the case with serum amylase and lipase levels. *No single blood test is reliable for the diagnosis of acute pancreatitis in patients with renal failure.* Determining whether a patient with renal failure and abdominal pain has pancreatitis remains a difficult clinical problem. A recent study found that serum amylase levels were elevated in patients with renal dysfunction only when creatinine clearance was less than 50 mL/min.

Table 303-2 Causes of Hyperamylasemia and Hyperamylasuria

PANCREATIC DISEASE

I. Pancreatitis
   A. Acute
   B. Chronic: ductal obstruction
   C. Complications of pancreatitis
      1. Pancreatic pseudocyst
      2. Pancreatogenous ascites
      3. Pancreatic abscess
II. Pancreatic trauma
III. Pancreatic carcinoma

NONPANCREATIC DISORDERS

I. Renal insufficiency
II. Salivary gland lesions
   A. Mumps
   B. Calculus
   C. Irradiation sialadenitis
   D. Maxillofacial surgery
III. "Tumor" hyperamylasemia
   A. Carcinoma of the lung
   B. Carcinoma of the esophagus
   C. Breast carcinoma, ovarian carcinoma
IV. Macroamylasemia
V. Burns
VI. Diabetic ketoacidosis
VII. Pregnancy
VIII. Renal transplantation
IX. Cerebral trauma
X. Drugs: morphine

OTHER ABDOMINAL DISORDERS

I. Biliary tract disease: cholecystitis, choledocholithiasis
II. Intraabdominal disease
   A. Perforated or penetrating peptic ulcer
   B. Intestinal obstruction or infarction
   C. Ruptured ectopic pregnancy
   D. Peritonitis
   E. Aortic aneurysm
   F. Chronic liver disease
   G. Postoperative hyperamylasemia

In such patients, the serum amylase level was invariably less than 500 IU/L in the absence of objective evidence of acute pancreatitis. In that study, serum lipase and trypsin levels paralleled serum amylase values.

A recent study evaluated the sensitivity and specificity of five assays used to diagnose acute pancreatitis: two for amylase, one for lipase, one for trypsin-like immunoreactivity (TLI), and one for pancreatic isoamylase. The data obtained (1) show that, if the best cutoff level is used, all these assays have similar specificities and (2) suggest that total serum amylase is as good an indicator of acute pancreatitis as any of the alternatives. However, inherent in many such studies is the problem that the recognition and diagnosis of acute pancreatitis hinge on the finding of an elevated serum amylase level. The question arises as to whether any diagnostic test result can be proved superior to the total serum amylase level if hyperamylasemia is required for the diagnosis. In other studies, when "objective" confirmation of the clinical diagnosis of pancreatitis was required (ultrasonography, CT, laparotomy), the sensitivity of the serum amylase has been found to be as low as 68%. With these limitations in mind, the recommended screening tests for acute pancreatitis are *total serum amylase* and *serum lipase activities*. Serum amylase values greater than three times normal are highly specific.

STUDIES PERTAINING TO PANCREATIC STRUCTURE

Radiologic Tests Plain films of the abdomen provide useful information in 30 to 50% of patients with acute pancreatitis. The most frequent abnormalities include (1) a localized ileus, usually involving the jejunum ("sentinel loop"); (2) a generalized ileus with air-fluid levels; (3) the "colon cutoff sign," which results from isolated distention of the transverse colon; (4) duodenal distention with air-fluid levels; and (5) a mass, which is frequently a pseudocyst. In chronic pancreatitis, an important radiographic finding is pancreatic calcification, which characteristically is localized adjacent to and superimposed on the second lumbar vertebra (see Fig. 304-3*A*).

Upper gastrointestinal x-rays may reveal displacement of the stomach by the retroperitoneal mass (see Fig. 304-2*A*) or widening and effacement of the duodenal C loop, which also suggest the presence of a pancreatic mass, which could be inflammatory, cystic, or neoplastic. However, the use of x-ray films has been largely superseded by ultrasound.

Ultrasonography can provide important information in patients with acute pancreatitis, chronic pancreatitis, pancreatic calcification, pseudocyst, and pancreatic carcinoma. Echographic appearances can indicate the presence of edema, inflammation, and calcification (not obvious on plain films of the abdomen), as well as pseudocysts, mass lesions, and gallstones (see Figs. 304-2*B* and 304-3*B*). In acute pancreatitis, the pancreas is characteristically enlarged. In pancreatic pseudocyst, the usual appearance is that of an echo-free, smooth, round fluid collection. Pancreatic carcinoma distorts the usual landmarks, and mass lesions greater than 3.0 cm are usually detected as localized, echo-free solid lesions. Ultrasound is often the initial investigation for most patients with suspected pancreatic disease. However, obesity, excess small- and large-bowel gas, and recently performed barium contrast examinations can interfere with ultrasound studies.

CT is the best imaging study for initial evaluation of a suspected chronic pancreatic disorder and for the complications of acute and chronic pancreatitis. It is especially useful in the detection of pancreatic tumors, fluid-containing lesions such as pseudocysts and abscesses, and calcium deposits (see Figs. 304-3*C* and 304-4*A*). Most lesions are characterized by (1) enlargement of the pancreatic outline, (2) distortion of the pancreatic contour, and/or (3) a fluid filling that has a different attenuation coefficient than normal pancreas. However, it is occasionally difficult to distinguish between inflammatory and neoplastic lesions. Oral water-soluble contrast agents may be used to opacify the stomach and duodenum during CT scans; this strategy permits more precise delineation of various organs as well as mass lesions. Dynamic CT (using rapid intravenous administration of contrast) is useful in estimating the degree of pancreatic necrosis and in predicting morbidity and mortality. Spiral (helical) CT provides clear images much more rapidly and essentially negates artifact caused by patient movement (see Fig. 304-2*D*).

Endoscopic ultrasonography (*EUS*) produces high-resolution images of the pancreatic parenchyma and pancreatic duct with a transducer fixed to an endoscope that can be directed onto the surface of the pancreas through the stomach or duodenum. Although criteria for abnormalities on EUS in severe pancreatic disease have been developed, the true sensitivity and specificity of this procedure has yet to be determined. In particular, it is not clear whether EUS can detect early pancreatic disease before abnormalities appear on more conventional radiograph tests such as ultrasonography or CT. The exact role of EUS versus ERCP and CT has yet to be defined.

Magnetic resonance cholangiopancreatography (*MRCP*) is now being used to view both the bile duct and the pancreatic duct. Nonbreath-hold and 3D turbo spin-echo techniques are being utilized to produce superb MRCP images. The main pancreatic duct and common bile duct can be seen well, but there is still a question as to whether changes can be detected consistently in the secondary ducts. MRCP may be particularly useful to evaluate the pancreatic duct in high-risk patients such as the elderly because this is a noninvasive procedure.

Both EUS and MRCP may replace ERCP in some patients. As these techniques become more refined, they may well be the diagnostic tests of choice to evaluate the pancreatic duct. ERCP is still needed to perform therapy of bile duct and pancreatic duct lesions.

Selective catheterization of the celiac and superior mesenteric arteries combined with superselective catheterization of others arteries, such as the hepatic, splenic, and gastroduodenal arteries permits visualization of the pancreas and detection of pancreatic neoplasms and pseudocysts. Pancreatic neoplasms can be identified by the sheathing of blood vessels by a mass lesion (see Fig. 304-1*D*). Hormone-producing pancreatic tumors are especially likely to exhibit increased vascularity and tumor staining. Angiographic abnormalities are noted in many patients with pancreatic carcinoma but are uncommon in patients without pancreatic disease. Angiography complements ultrasonography and ERCP in the study of patients with a suspected pancreatic lesion and may be carried out if ERCP is either unsuccessful or nondiagnostic.

ERCP may provide useful information on the status of the pancreatic ductal system and thus aid in the differential diagnosis of pancreatic disease (see Figs. 304-1*C*, 304-3*D*, and 304-4*B*). Pancreatic carcinoma is characterized by stenosis or obstruction of either the pancreatic duct or the common bile duct; both ductal systems are often abnormal. In chronic pancreatitis, ERCP abnormalities include (1) luminal narrowing, (2) irregularities in the ductal system with stenosis, dilation, sacculation, and ectasia, and (3) blockage of the pancreatic duct by calcium deposits. The presence of ductal stenosis and irregularity can make it difficult to distinguish chronic pancreatitis from carcinoma. It is important to be aware that ERCP changes interpreted as indicating chronic pancreatitis actually may be due to the effects of aging on the pancreatic duct or to the fact that the procedure was performed within several weeks of an attack of acute pancreatitis. Although aging may cause impressive ductal alterations, it does not affect the results of pancreatic function tests (i.e., the secretin test). Elevated serum and/or urine amylase levels after ERCP have been reported in 25 to 75% of patients, but clinical pancreatitis is uncommon. In a series of 300 patients, pancreatitis occurred in only 5 patients after ERCP. If no lesion is found in the biliary and/or pancreatic ducts in a patient with repeated attacks of acute pancreatitis, manometric studies of the sphincter of Oddi may be indicated. Such studies, however, do increase the risk of post-ERCP/manometry acute pancreatitis. Such pancreatitis appears to be more common in patients with a nondilated pancreatic duct.

Pancreatic Biopsy with Radiologic Guidance Percutaneous aspiration biopsy of a pancreatic mass often distinguishes a pancreatic inflammatory mass from a pancreatic neoplasm.

TESTS OF EXOCRINE PANCREATIC FUNCTION

Pancreatic function tests (Table 303-1) can be divided into the following:

1. *Direct stimulation of the pancreas* by intravenous infusion of secretin or secretin plus cholecystokinin (CCK) followed by collection and measurement of duodenal contents
2. *Indirect stimulation of the pancreas* using nutrients or amino acids, fatty acids, and synthetic peptides followed by assays of proteolytic, lipolytic, and amylolytic enzymes
3. Study of *intraluminal digestion products*, such as undigested meat fibers, stool fat, and fecal nitrogen
4. *Measurement of fecal pancreatic enzymes* such as elastase

The secretin test, used to detect diffuse pancreatic disease, is based on the physiologic principle that the pancreatic secretory response is directly related to the functional mass of pancreatic tissue. In the standard assay, secretin is given intravenously in a dose of 1 clinical unit (CU) per kilogram, as either a bolus or a continuous infusion. The results will vary with the secretin preparation used, the dose, the mode of administration, and the completeness with which the duodenal contents are collected. Normal values for the standard secretin test are (1) volume output >2.0 mL/kg per hour, (2) bicarbonate (HCO_3^-) concentration >80 meql/L, and (3) HCO_3^- output >10 meq/L in 1 h. The most reproducible measurement, giving the highest level of discrimination between normal subjects and patients with chronic pancreatitis, appears to be the maximal bicarbonate concentration.

The *combined secretin-CCK test* permits measurement of pancreatic amylase, lipase, trypsin, and chymotrypsin. Although there is overlap in the distributions of enzyme output in normal subjects and patients with pancreatitis in response to this test, markedly low enzyme outputs suggest advanced damage and destruction of acinar cells. With frank exocrine pancreatic insufficiency, there is usually an overall reduction in both HCO_3^- concentration and output of several enzymes. However, with lesser degrees of pancreatic damage there may be a dissociation between HCO_3^- concentration and enzyme output. There also may be a dissociation between the results of the secretin test and those of tests of absorptive function. For example, patients with chronic pancreatitis often have abnormally low outputs of HCO_3^- after secretin but have normal fecal fat excretion. Thus the secretin test measures the secretory capacity of ductular epithelium, while fecal fat excretion indirectly reflects intraluminal lipolytic activity. Steatorrhea does not occur until intraluminal levels of lipase are markedly reduced, underscoring the fact that only small amounts of enzymes are necessary for intraluminal digestive activities. An abnormal secretin test result suggests only that chronic pancreatic damage is present; it will not consistently distinguish between chronic pancreatitis and pancreatic carcinoma.

Another test of exocrine pancreatic function is the *bentiromide test*. This test is an indirect measure of pancreatic function and reflects intraluminal chymotrypsin activity. The test has excellent specificity but is not very sensitive. It no longer is available for clinical use in the United States.

The *serum trypsinogen level*, which is determined by radioimmunoassay, also has excellent specificity but is not very sensitive. It is a simple blood test that can detect severe damage to the exocrine pancreas. The normal values are 28 to 58 ng/mL, and any value below 20 ng/mL reflects pancreatic steatorrhea.

Measurement of *intraluminal digestion products*, i.e., undigested muscle fibers, stool fat, and fecal nitrogen, is discussed in Chap. 286. The amount of elastase in stool reflects the pancreatic output of this proteolytic enzyme. Decreased elastase activity in stool has been reported in patients with chronic pancreatitis and cystic fibrosis. →*Tests useful in the diagnosis of exocrine pancreatic insufficiency and the differential diagnosis of malabsorption are also discussed in Chaps. 286 and 304.*

304

Norton J. Greenberger, Phillip P. Toskes

ACUTE AND CHRONIC PANCREATITIS

APACHE II acute physiology and chronic health evaluation scoring system	HIDA hepatic 2,6-dimethyliminodiacetic acid
AST aspartate aminotransferase	KUB kidney, ureter, and bladder
CCK cholecystokinin	LDH lactic dehydrogenase
CCK-RF CCK releasing factor	NSAIDs nonsteroidal anti-inflammatory drugs
CECT contrast-enhanced dynamic CT	PIPIDA *N-p*-isopropylacetanilide-iminodiacetic acid
CFTR cystic fibrosis transmembrane conductance regulator	TAP trypsinogen activation peptide
CT computed tomography	VIP vasoactive intestinal peptide
ERCP endoscopic retrograde cholangiopancreatography	

BIOCHEMISTRY AND PHYSIOLOGY OF PANCREATIC EXOCRINE SECRETION

GENERAL CONSIDERATIONS The pancreas secretes 1500 to 3000 mL of isosmotic alkaline (pH >8.0) fluid per day containing about 20 enzymes and zymogens. The pancreatic secretions provide the enzymes needed to effect the major digestive activity of the gastrointestinal tract and provide an optimal pH for the function of these enzymes.

REGULATION OF PANCREATIC SECRETION The exocrine pancreas is influenced by intimately interacting hormonal and neural systems. *Gastric acid* is the stimulus for the release of secretin, a peptide with 27 amino acids. Sensitive radioimmunoassay studies for secretin suggest that the pH threshold for its release from the duodenum and jejunum is 4.5. Secretin stimulates the secretion of pancreatic juice rich in *water and electrolytes*. Release of cholecystokinin (CCK) from the duodenum and jejunum is largely triggered by long-chain fatty acids, certain essential amino acids (tryptophan, phenylalanine, valine, methionine), and gastric acid itself. CCK evokes an *enzyme-rich secretion from the pancreas*. Gastrin, although it has the same terminal tetrapeptide as CCK, is a weak stimulus for pancreatic enzyme output. The *parasympathetic nervous system* (via the vagus nerve) exerts significant control over pancreatic secretion. Secretion evoked by secretin and CCK depends on permissive roles of vagal afferent and efferent pathways. This is particularly true for enzyme secretion, whereas water and bicarbonate secretion is heavily dependent on the hormonal effects of secretin and CCK. Also, vagal stimulation effects the release of vasoactive intestinal peptide (VIP), a secretin agonist. Bile salts also stimulate pancreatic secretion, thereby integrating the functions of the biliary tract, pancreas, and small intestine.

Somatostatin acts on multiple sites to induce inhibition of pancreatic secretion. The appropriate roles of other peptides, such as peptide YY, pancreastatin, gastrin-releasing peptide, pituitary adenylate cyclase–activating polypeptide, calcitonin gene–related peptide, and galanin are still being defined. Nitric oxide is an important neurotransmitter in the regulation of pancreatic exocrine secretion, although its mechanism of action has not been fully elucidated.

WATER AND ELECTROLYTE SECRETION Although sodium, potassium, chloride, calcium, zinc, phosphate, and sulfate are found in pancreatic secretions, *bicarbonate is the ion of primary physiologic importance*. In the acini and in the ducts, secretin causes the cells to add water and bicarbonate to the fluid. In the ducts, an exchange occurs between bicarbonate and chloride. There is a good correlation between the maximal bicarbonate output after stimulation with secretin and the pancreatic mass. The bicarbonate output of 120 to 300 mmol/d helps neutralize gastric acid and creates the appropriate pH for the activity of the pancreatic enzymes.

ENZYME SECRETION The pancreas secretes amylolytic, lipolytic, and proteolytic enzymes. *Amylolytic enzymes*, such as amylase, hydrolyze starch to oligosaccharides and to the disaccharide maltose. The *lipolytic enzymes* include lipase, phospholipase A, and cholesterol esterase. Bile salts *inhibit* lipase in isolation; but colipase, another constituent of pancreatic secretion, binds to lipase and prevents this inhibition. Bile salts *activate* phospholipase A and cholesterol esterase. *Proteolytic enzymes* include *endopeptidases* (trypsin, chymotrypsin), which act on internal peptide bonds of proteins and polypeptides; *exopeptidases* (carboxypeptidases, aminopeptidases), which act on the free carboxyl- and amino-terminal ends of peptides, respectively; and elastase. The proteolytic enzymes are secreted as inactive precursors (zymogens). Ribonucleases (deoxyribonucleases, ribonuclease) are also secreted. Although pancreatic enzymes usually are secreted in parallel, nonparallel secretion can occur as a result of exocytosis from heterogeneous sources in the pancreas. *Enterokinase*, an enzyme found in the duodenal mucosa, cleaves the lysine-isoleucine bond of trypsinogen to form trypsin. Trypsin then activates the other proteolytic zymogens in a cascade phenomenon. All pancreatic enzymes have pH optima in the alkaline range.

AUTOPROTECTION OF THE PANCREAS Autodigestion of the pancreas is prevented by the packaging of proteases in precursor form and by the synthesis of protease inhibitors. These protease inhibitors are found in the acinar cell, the pancreatic secretions, and the $alpha_1$- and $alpha_2$-globulin fractions of plasma.

Table 304-1 Causes of Acute Pancreatitis

- Alcohol ingestion (acute and chronic alcoholism)
- Biliary tract disease (gallstones)
- Postoperative state (after abdominal or nonabdominal operation)
- Endoscopic retrograde cholangiopancreatography (ERCP), especially manometric studies of sphincter of Oddi
- Trauma (especially blunt abdominal type)
- Metabolic causes
  - Hypertriglyceridemia
  - Apolipoprotein CII deficiency syndrome
  - Hypercalcemia (e.g., hyperparathyroidism), drug-induced
  - Renal failure
  - After renal transplantation[a]
  - Acute fatty liver of pregnancy[b]
- Hereditary pancreatitis
- Infections
  - Mumps
  - Viral hepatitis
  - Other viral infections (coxsackievirus, echovirus, cytomegalovirus)
  - Ascariasis
  - Infections with *Mycoplasma*, *Campylobacter*, *Mycobacterium avium* complex, other bacteria
- Drugs
  - Drugs for which association is definite
    - Azathioprine, 6-mercaptopurine
    - Sulfonamides
    - Thiazide diuretics
    - Furosemide
    - Estrogens (oral contraceptives)
    - Tetracycline
    - Valproic acid
    - Pentamidine
    - Dideoxyinosine (ddI)
  - Drugs for which association is probable
    - Acetaminophen
    - Nitrofurantoin
    - Methyldopa
    - Erythromycin
    - Salicylates
    - Metronidazole
    - Nonsteroidal anti-inflammatory drugs
    - Angiotensin-converting enzyme (ACE) inhibitors
- Vascular causes and vasculitis
  - Vascular
    - Ischemic-hypoperfusion state (after cardiac surgery)
    - Atherosclerotic emboli
    - Aneurysm of celiac axis/hepatic artery
  - Connective tissue disorders with vasculitis
    - Systemic lupus erythematosus
    - Necrotizing angiitis
    - Thrombotic thrombocytopenic purpura
- Penetrating peptic ulcer
- Obstruction of the ampulla of Vater
  - Regional enteritis
  - Duodenal diverticulum
- Pancreas divisum
- Causes to be considered in patients having recurrent bouts of acute pancreatitis without an obvious cause
  - Occult disease of the biliary tree or pancreatic ducts, especially occult gallstones (microlithiasis, sludge)
  - Drugs
  - Hypertriglyceridemia
  - Pancreas divisum
  - Pancreatic cancer
  - Sphincter of Oddi dysfunction
  - Cystic fibrosis
  - Truly idiopathic

[a] Pancreatitis occurs in 3% of renal transplant patients and is due to many factors, including surgery, hypercalcemia, drugs (glucocorticoids, azathioprine, L-asparaginase, diuretics), and viral infections.

[b] Pancreatitis also occurs in otherwise uncomplicated pregnancy and is most often associated with cholelithiasis.

EXOCRINE-ENDOCRINE RELATIONSHIPS Insulin appears to be needed locally for secretin and CCK to promote exocrine secretion; thus, it acts in a permissive role for these two hormones.

ENTEROPANCREATIC AXIS AND FEEDBACK INHIBITION Pancreatic enzyme secretion is controlled, at least in part, by a negative feedback mechanism induced by the presence of active serine proteases in the duodenum. To illustrate, perfusion of the duodenal lumen with phenylalanine causes a prompt increase in plasma CCK levels as well as increased secretion of chymotrypsin. However, simultaneous perfusion with trypsin blunts both responses. Conversely, perfusion of the duodenal lumen with protease inhibitors actually leads to enzyme hypersecretion. The available evidence supports the concept that the duodenum contains a peptide called CCK releasing factor (CCK-RF) that is involved in stimulating CCK release. Two peptides, luminal CCK-RF and diazepam-binding inhibitor, have been found that may be the CCK-RF. Serine proteases inhibit pancreatic secretion by acting on CCK-RF. It appears that serine proteases inhibit pancreatic secretion by acting on a CCK-releasing peptide in the lumen of the small intestine.

ACUTE PANCREATITIS

GENERAL CONSIDERATIONS Pancreatic inflammatory disease may be classified as (1) acute pancreatitis and (2) chronic pancreatitis. The pathologic spectrum of acute pancreatitis varies from *edematous pancreatitis*, which is usually a mild and self-limited disorder, to *necrotizing pancreatitis*, in which the degree of pancreatic necrosis correlates with the severity of the attack and its systemic manifestations. The term *hemorrhagic pancreatitis* is less meaningful in a clinical sense because variable amounts of interstitial hemorrhage can be found in pancreatitis as well as in other disorders such as pancreatic trauma, pancreatic carcinoma, and severe congestive heart failure.

The incidence of pancreatitis varies in different countries and depends on cause, e.g., alcohol, gallstones, metabolic factors, and drugs (Table 304-1). In the United States, for example, acute pancreatitis is related to alcohol ingestion more commonly than to gallstones; in England, the opposite obtains. There are 185,000 new cases of acute pancreatitis per year in the United States.

ETIOLOGY AND PATHOGENESIS There are many causes of acute pancreatitis (Table 304-1), but the mechanisms by which these conditions trigger pancreatic inflammation have not been identified. Alcoholic patients with pancreatitis may represent a special subset, since most alcoholics do not develop pancreatitis. The list of identifiable causes is growing, and it is likely that pancreatitis related to viral infections, drugs, and as yet undefined factors is more common than heretofore recognized.

Approximately 2 to 5% of cases of acute pancreatitis are drug-related (Table 304-1). Drugs cause pancreatitis either by a hypersensitivity reaction or by the generation of a toxic metabolite, although in some cases it is not clear which of these mechanisms is operative.

Autodigestion is one pathogenetic theory, according to which pancreatitis results when proteolytic enzymes (e.g., trypsinogen, chymotrypsinogen, proelastase, and phospholipase A) are activated in the pancreas rather than in the intestinal lumen. A number of factors (e.g., endotoxins, exotoxins, viral infections, ischemia, anoxia, and direct trauma) are believed to activate these proenzymes. Activated proteolytic enzymes, especially trypsin, not only digest pancreatic and peripancreatic tissues but also can activate other enzymes, such as elastase and phospholipase. The active enzymes then digest cellular membranes and cause proteolysis, edema, interstitial hemorrhage, vascular damage, coagulation necrosis, fat necrosis, and parenchymal cell necrosis. Cellular injury and death result in the liberation of activated enzymes. In addition, activation and release of bradykinin peptides and vasoactive substances (e.g., histamine) are believed to produce vasodilation, increased vascular permeability, and edema. Thus, a cascade of events culminates in the development of acute necrotizing pancreatitis.

The autodigestion theory has largely eclipsed two older theories. First, according to the "common channel" theory, the existence of a common anatomic channel for pancreatic secretions and bile permits reflux of bile into the pancreatic duct, which results in activation of pancreatic enzymes. (Actually, a common channel with free communication between the common bile duct and the main pancreatic duct is infrequently encountered.) The second theory is that obstruction and hypersecretion are pivotal in the development of pancreatitis. Obstruction of the main pancreatic duct, however, produces pancreatic edema but generally not pancreatitis.

A recent hypothesis to explain the intrapancreatic activation of zymogens is that they become activated by *lysosomal hydrolases* in the pancreatic acinar cell itself. In two different types of experimental pancreatitis, it has been demonstrated that digestive enzymes and lysosomal hydrolases become admixed; as a result, the latter can activate the former in the acinar cell. In vitro, lysosomal enzymes such as cathepsin B can activate trypsinogen, and trypsin can activate the other protease precursors. It is still not clear, however, whether the human acinar cell can provide the pH (about 3.0) necessary for activation of trypsinogen by lysosomal hydrolases. It is now believed that ischemia/hypoperfusion can alone result in activation of trypsinogen and pancreatic injury.

CLINICAL FEATURES *Abdominal pain* is the major symptom of acute pancreatitis. Pain may vary from a mild and tolerable discomfort to severe, constant, and incapacitating distress. Characteristically, the pain, which is steady and boring in character, is located in the epigastrium and periumbilical region and often radiates to the back as well as to the chest, flanks, and lower abdomen. The pain is frequently more intense when the patient is supine, and patients often obtain relief by sitting with the trunk flexed and knees drawn up. Nausea, vomiting, and abdominal distention due to gastric and intestinal hypomotility and chemical peritonitis are also frequent complaints.

Physical examination frequently reveals a distressed and anxious patient. Low-grade fever, tachycardia, and hypotension are fairly common. Shock is not unusual and may result from (1) hypovolemia secondary to exudation of blood and plasma proteins into the retroperitoneal space (a "retroperitoneal burn"); (2) increased formation and release of kinin peptides, which cause vasodilation and increased vascular permeability; and (3) systemic effects of proteolytic and lipolytic enzymes released into the circulation. Jaundice occurs infrequently; when present, it usually is due to edema of the head of the pancreas with compression of the intrapancreatic portion of the common bile duct. Erythematous skin nodules due to subcutaneous fat necrosis may occur. In 10 to 20% of patients, there are pulmonary findings, including basilar rales, atelectasis, and pleural effusion, the latter most frequently left-sided. Abdominal tenderness and muscle rigidity are present to a variable degree, but, compared with the intense pain, these signs may be unimpressive. Bowel sounds are usually diminished or absent. A pancreatic pseudocyst may be palpable in the upper abdomen. A faint blue discoloration around the umbilicus (Cullen's sign) may occur as the result of hemoperitoneum, and a blue-red-purple or green-brown discoloration of the flanks (Turner's sign) reflects tissue catabolism of hemoglobin. The latter two findings, which are uncommon, indicate the presence of a severe necrotizing pancreatitis.

LABORATORY DATA The diagnosis of acute pancreatitis is usually established by the detection of an increased level of serum amylase. Values threefold or more above normal virtually clinch the diagnosis if overt salivary gland disease and gut perforation or infarction are excluded. However, there appears to be no definite correlation between the severity of pancreatitis and the degree of serum amylase elevation. After 48 to 72 h, even with continuing evidence of pancreatitis, total serum amylase values tend to return to normal. However, pancreatic isoamylase and lipase levels may remain elevated for 7 to 14 days. It will be recalled that amylase elevations in serum and urine occur in many conditions other than pancreatitis (see Table 303-2). Importantly, patients with *acidemia* (arterial pH $\leq$7.32) may have spurious elevations in serum amylase. In one study, 12 of 33 patients with acidemia had elevated serum amylase, but only 1 had an elevated lipase value; in 9, salivary-type amylase was the predominant serum isoamylase. This finding explains why patients with diabetic ketoacidosis may have marked elevations in serum amylase without any other evidence of acute pancreatitis. Serum lipase activity increases in parallel with amylase activity, and measurement of both enzymes increases the diagnostic yield. An elevated serum lipase or trypsin value is usually diagnostic of acute pancreatitis; these tests are especially helpful in patients with nonpancreatic causes of hyperamylasemia (see Table 303-2). Markedly increased levels of peritoneal or pleural fluid amylase [1500 nmol/L (> 5000 U/dL)] are also helpful, if present, in establishing the diagnosis.

Leukocytosis (15,000 to 20,000 leukocytes per microliter) occurs frequently. Patients with more severe disease may show hemoconcentration with hematocrit values exceeding 50% because of loss of plasma into the retroperitoneal space and peritoneal cavity. *Hyperglycemia* is common and is due to multiple factors, including decreased insulin release, increased glucagon release, and an increased output of adrenal glucocorticoids and catecholamines. *Hypocalcemia* occurs in approximately 25% of patients, and its pathogenesis is incompletely understood. Although earlier studies suggested that the response of the parathyroid gland to a decrease in serum calcium is impaired, subsequent observations have failed to confirm this idea. Intraperitoneal saponification of calcium by fatty acids in areas of fat necrosis occurs occasionally, with large amounts (up to 6.0 g) dissolved or suspended in ascitic fluid. Such "soap formation" also may be significant in patients with pancreatitis, mild hypocalcemia, and little or no obvious ascites. *Hyperbilirubinemia* [serum bilirubin >68 μmol/L (> 4.0 mg/dL)] occurs in approximately 10% of patients. However, jaundice is transient, and serum bilirubin levels return to normal in 4 to 7 days. Serum alkaline phosphatase and aspartate aminotransferase (AST) levels are also transiently elevated and parallel serum bilirubin values. Markedly elevated serum lactic dehydrogenase (LDH) levels [>8.5 μmol/L (> 500 U/dL)] suggest a poor prognosis. Serum albumin is decreased to $\leq$30 g/L ($\leq$3.0 g/dL) in about 10% of patients; this sign is associated with more severe pancreatitis and a higher mortality rate (Table 304-2). *Hypertriglyceridemia* occurs in 15 to 20% of patients, and serum amylase levels in these individuals are often spuriously normal (Chap. 303). Most patients with hypertriglyceridemia and pancreatitis, when subsequently examined, show evidence of an underlying derangement in lipid metabolism which probably antedated the pancreatitis (see below). Approximately 25% of patients have *hypoxemia* (arterial $P_{O_2} \leq 60$ mmHg), which may herald the onset of adult respiratory distress syndrome. Finally, the electrocardiogram is occasionally abnormal in acute pancreatitis with ST-segment and T-wave abnormalities simulating myocardial ischemia.

Although one or more radiologic abnormalities are found in over 50% of patients, the findings are inconstant and nonspecific. The chief value of conventional x-rays [chest films; kidney, ureter, and bladder (KUB) studies] in acute pancreatitis is to help exclude other diagnoses, especially a perforated viscus. Upper gastrointestinal tract x-rays have been superseded by ultrasonography and computed tomography (CT). A CT scan may confirm the clinical impression of acute pancreatitis even in the face of normal serum amylase levels. Importantly, CT is quite helpful in indicating the severity of acute pancreatitis and the

Table 304-2 Factors That Adversely Affect Survival in Acute Pancreatitis

Ranson/Imrie criteria
- At admission or diagnosis
  - Age >55 years
  - Leukocytosis >16,000/μL
  - Hyperglycemia >11 mmol/L (>200 mg/dL)
  - Serum LDH >400 IU/L
  - Serum AST >250 IU/L
- During initial 48 h
  - Fall in hematocrit by >10 percent
  - Fluid deficit of >4000 mL
  - Hypocalcemia [calcium concentration <1.9 mmol/L (<8.0 mg/dL)]
  - Hypoxemia (P_{O_2} <60 mmHg)
  - Increase in BUN to >1.8 mmol/L (>5 mg/dL) after IV fluid administration
  - Hypoalbuminemia [albumin level <32 g/L (<3.2 g/dL)]

Acute physiology and chronic health evaluation (APACHE II) score > 12

Hemorrhagic peritoneal fluid

Obesity [body mass index (BMI) > 29]

Key indicators of organ failure
- Hypotension (blood pressure <90 mmHg) or tachycardia >130 beats per minute
- P_{O_2} <60 mmHg
- Oliguria (<50 mL/h) or increasing blood urea nitrogen (BUN), creatinine
- Metabolic indicators: serum calcium <1.9 mmol/L (<8.0 mg/dL) or serum albumin <32 g/L (<3.2 g/dL)

risk of morbidity and mortality (see below). Sonography and radionuclide scanning [*N-p*-isopropylacetanilide-iminodiacetic acid (PIPIDA) scan; hepatic 2,6-dimethyliminodiacetic acid (HIDA) scan] are useful in acute pancreatitis to evaluate the gallbladder and biliary tree. →*Radiologic studies useful in the diagnosis of acute pancreatitis are discussed in Chap. 303 and listed in Table 303-1.*

DIAGNOSIS Any severe acute pain in the abdomen or back should suggest acute pancreatitis. The diagnosis is usually entertained when a patient with a possible predisposition to pancreatitis presents with severe and constant abdominal pain, nausea, emesis, fever, tachycardia, and abnormal findings on abdominal examination. Laboratory studies frequently reveal leukocytosis, an abnormal appearance on x-rays of the abdomen and chest, hypocalcemia, and hyperglycemia. The diagnosis is usually confirmed by the finding of an elevated level of serum amylase and/or lipase. Not all the above features have to be present for the diagnosis to be established.

The *differential diagnosis* should include the following disorders: (1) perforated viscus, especially peptic ulcer; (2) acute cholecystitis and biliary colic; (3) acute intestinal obstruction; (4) mesenteric vascular occlusion; (5) renal colic; (6) myocardial infarction; (7) dissecting aortic aneurysm; (8) connective tissue disorders with vasculitis; (9) pneumonia; and (10) diabetic ketoacidosis. A penetrating duodenal ulcer usually can be identified by upper gastrointestinal x-rays and/or endoscopy. A perforated duodenal ulcer is readily diagnosed by the presence of free intraperitoneal air. It may be difficult to differentiate acute cholecystitis from acute pancreatitis, since an elevated serum amylase may be found in both disorders. Pain of biliary tract origin is more right-sided and gradual in onset, and ileus is usually absent; sonography and radionuclide scanning are helpful in establishing the diagnosis of cholelithiasis and cholecystitis. Intestinal obstruction due to mechanical factors can be differentiated from pancreatitis by the history of colicky pain, findings on abdominal examination, and x-rays of the abdomen showing changes characteristic of mechanical obstruction. Acute mesenteric vascular occlusion is usually evident in elderly debilitated patients with brisk leukocytosis, abdominal distention, and bloody diarrhea, in whom paracentesis shows sanguineous fluid and arteriography shows vascular occlusion. Serum as well as peritoneal fluid amylase levels are increased, however, in patients with intestinal infarction. Systemic lupus erythematosus and polyarteritis nodosa may be confused with pancreatitis, especially since pancreatitis may develop as a complication of these diseases. Diabetic ketoacidosis is often accompanied by abdominal pain and elevated total serum amylase levels, thus closely mimicking acute pancreatitis. However, the serum lipase and pancreatic isoamylase levels are not elevated in diabetic ketoacidosis.

COURSE OF THE DISEASE AND COMPLICATIONS It is important to identify patients with acute pancreatitis who have an increased risk of dying. Ranson and Imrie have used multiple prognostic criteria and have demonstrated that there is an increased mortality rate when three or more risk factors are identifiable either at the time of admission to the hospital or during the initial 48 h of hospitalization (Table 304-2). Recent studies indicate that obesity is a major risk factor for severe pancreatitis, presumably because the increased deposits of peripancreatic fat in such patients may predispose them to more extensive pancreatic and peripancreatic necrosis. The acute physiology and chronic health evaluation scoring system (APACHE II) uses the worst values of 12 physiologic measurements plus age and previous health status and provides a good description of illness severity for a wide range of common diseases; this score also correlates with outcome. Prospective studies have compared APACHE II with multiple prognostic criteria, i.e., Ranson and Imrie scores, in predicting the severity of acute pancreatitis. On admission, APACHE II identified approximately two-thirds of severe attacks, and after 48 h, the prognostic accuracy of APACHE II is comparable with that of Ranson and Imrie's scoring system. The drawbacks of APACHE II are (1) its complexity, (2) the requirement of a computer for scoring, and (3) standardization regarding peak values and cutoff scores. McMahon and colleagues have shown that the presence of a "toxic broth" or dark (hemorrhagic) fluid in abdominal pancreatitis is also an important prognostic indicator in acute pancreatitis. These multiple-factor scoring systems are difficult to use and have not been embraced consistently by clinicians. There is a great need for a reliable, simple biochemical test that consistently predicts outcome in patients with acute pancreatitis. Three candidate markers that show great promise are C-reactive protein, serum granulocyte elastase, and urinary trypsinogen activation peptide (TAP). The key indicators of a severe attack of acute pancreatitis are also listed in Table 304-2. Importantly, the presence of any one of these factors is associated with an increased risk of complications, and the presence of any two, with a 20 to 30% mortality rate. The high mortality rate of such severely ill patients is due in large part to infection and warrants intensive radiologic intervention and monitoring and/or a combination of radiologic and surgical means, as discussed in detail below.

The local and systemic complications of acute pancreatitis are listed in Table 304-3. In the first 2 to 3 weeks after pancreatitis patients frequently develop an inflammatory mass, which may be due to pancreatic necrosis (with or without infection) or may represent an abscess or pseudocyst (see below). Systemic complications include pulmonary, cardiovascular, hematologic, renal, metabolic, and central nervous system abnormalities. Pancreatitis and hypertriglyceridemia constitute an association in which cause and effect remain incompletely understood. However, several reasonable conclusions can be drawn. First, hypertriglyceridemia can precede and apparently cause pancreatitis. Second, the vast majority (>80%) of patients with acute pancreatitis do not have hypertriglyceridemia. Third, almost all patients with pancreatitis and hypertriglyceridemia have preexisting abnormalities in lipoprotein metabolism. Fourth, many of the patients with this association have persistent hypertriglyceridemia after recovery from pancreatitis and are prone to recurrent episodes of pancreatitis. Fifth, any factor (e.g., drugs or alcohol) that causes an abrupt increase in serum triglycerides to levels greater than 11 mmol/L (1000 mg/dL) can precipitate a bout of pancreatitis that can be associated with significant complications and even become fulminant. To avert the risk of triggering pancreatitis, a fasting serum triglyceride measurement should be obtained before estrogen replacement therapy is begun in postmenopausal women. Fasting levels less than 300 mg/dL pose no risk, whereas levels greater than 750 mg/dL are associated with a high probability of developing pancreatitis. Finally, patients with a defi-

Table 304-3 Complications of Acute Pancreatitis

LOCAL	
Necrosis	Pancreatic ascites
Sterile	Disruption of main pancreatic duct
Infected	Leaking pseudocyst
Pancreatic fluid collections	Involvement of contiguous organs by necrotizing pancreatitis
Pancreatic abscess	Massive intraperitoneal hemorrhage
Pancreatic pseudocyst	Thrombosis of blood vessels (splenic vein, portal vein)
Pain	Bowel infarction
Rupture	Obstructive jaundice
Hemorrhage	
Infection	
Obstruction of gastrointestinal tract (stomach, duodenum, colon)	
SYSTEMIC	
Pulmonary	Renal
Pleural effusion	Oliguria
Atelectasis	Azotemia
Mediastinal abscess	Renal artery and/or renal vein thrombosis
Pneumonitis	Acute tubular necrosis
Adult respiratory distress syndrome	Metabolic
Cardiovascular	Hyperglycemia
Hypotension	Hypertriglyceridemia
Hypovolemia	Hypocalcemia
Hypoalbuminemia	Encephalopathy
Sudden death	Sudden blindness (Purtscher's retinopathy)
Nonspecific ST-T changes in electrocardiogram simulating myocardial infarction	Central nervous system
Pericardial effusion	Psychosis
Hematologic	Fat emboli
Disseminated intravascular coagulation	Fat necrosis
Gastrointestinal hemorrhage[a]	Subcutaneous tissues (erythematous nodules)
Peptic ulcer disease	Bone
Erosive gastritis	Miscellaneous (mediastinum, pleura, nervous system)
Hemorrhagic pancreatic necrosis with erosion into major blood vessels	
Portal vein thrombosis, variceal hemorrhage	

[a] Aggravated by coagulation abnormalities (disseminated intravascular coagulation).

ciency of apolipoprotein CII have an increased incidence of pancreatitis; apolipoprotein CII activates lipoprotein lipase, which is important in clearing chylomicrons from the bloodstream.

Purtscher's retinopathy, a relatively unusual complication, is manifested by a sudden and severe loss of vision in a patient with acute pancreatitis. It is characterized by a peculiar funduscopic appearance with cotton-wool spots and hemorrhages confined to an area limited by the optic disk and macula; it is believed to be due to occlusion of the posterior retinal artery with aggregated granulocytes.

The two most common causes of acute pancreatitis are alcoholism and biliary tract disease; other causes are listed in Table 304-1. The risk of acute pancreatitis in patients with at least one gallstone smaller than 5 mm in diameter is fourfold greater than that in patients with larger stones. However, after a conventional workup, a specific cause is not identified in about 30% of patients. It is important to note that ultrasound examinations fail to detect gallstones, especially microlithiasis and/or sludge, in 4 to 7% of patients. In one series of 31 patients diagnosed initially as having idiopathic acute pancreatitis, 23 were found to have occult gallstone disease. Thus, approximately two-thirds of patients with recurrent acute pancreatitis without an obvious cause actually have occult gallstone disease due to microlithiasis. Examination of duodenal aspirates in such cases often reveals cholesterol crystals, which confirm the diagnosis. Other diseases of the biliary tree and pancreatic ducts that can cause acute pancreatitis include choledochocele, ampullary tumors, pancreas divisum, and pancreatic duct stones, stricture, and tumor. Approximately 2% of patients with pancreatic carcinoma present with acute pancreatitis.

Pancreatitis in Patients with AIDS The incidence of acute pancreatitis is increased in patients with AIDS for two reasons: (1) the high incidence of infections involving the pancreas, such as infections with cytomegalovirus, *Cryptosporidium*, and the *Mycobacterium avium* complex; and (2) the frequent use by patients with AIDS of medications such as didanosine, pentamidine, and trimethoprim-sulfamethoxazole (Chap. 309).

℞ **TREATMENT** In most patients (approximately 85 to 90%) with acute pancreatitis, the disease is self-limited and subsides spontaneously, usually within 3 to 7 days after treatment is instituted. Conventional measures include (1) analgesics for pain, (2) intravenous fluids and colloids to maintain normal intravascular volume, (3) no oral alimentation, and (4) nasogastric suction to decrease gastrin release from the stomach and prevent gastric contents from entering the duodenum. Recent controlled trials, however, have shown that nasogastric suction offers no clear-cut advantages in the treatment of mild to moderately severe acute pancreatitis. Its use, therefore, must be considered elective rather than mandatory.

It has been demonstrated that CCK-stimulated pancreatic secretion is almost abolished in four different experimental models of acute pancreatitis. This finding probably explains why drugs to block pancreatic secretion in acute pancreatitis have failed to have any therapeutic benefit. For this and other reasons, anticholinergic drugs are not indicated in acute pancreatitis. In addition to nasogastric suction and anticholinergic drugs, other therapies designed to "rest the pancreas" by inhibiting pancreatic secretion have not changed the course of the disease. Although antibiotics have been used in the treatment of acute pancreatitis, randomized, prospective trials have shown no benefit from their use in acute pancreatitis of mild to moderate severity.

However, current experimental evidence favors the use of prophylactic antibiotics in severe acute pancreatitis. Results of four contemporary randomized clinical trials restricted to patients with prognostically severe acute pancreatitis have demonstrated an improved outcome, i.e., reduced rate of infection and/or mortality, associated with the antibiotic treatment. The carbapenem group of antibiotics, including imipenem, has a very broad spectrum including activity against *Pseudomonas*, *Staphylococcus*, and *Enterococcus*; and these agents penetrate well into pancreatic tissue. Furthermore, because secondary infection of necrotic pancreatic tissue (abscess, pseudocyst or obstructed biliary passages, ascending cholangitis complicating choledocholithiasis) contributes to many of the late deaths from pancreatitis, appropriate antibiotic therapy of established infections is quite important.

Several other drugs have been evaluated by prospective controlled trials and found ineffective in the treatment of acute pancreatitis. The list, by no means complete, includes glucagon, H_2 blockers, protease inhibitors such as aprotinin, glucocorticoids, calcitonin, nonsteroidal anti-inflammataory drugs (NSAIDs) and lexiplafant, a platelet-activating factor inhibitor. A recent meta-analysis of somatostatin, ocreotide, and the antiprotease gabexate methylate in therapy of acute pancreatitis suggested (1) a reduced mortality rate but no change in complications with octreotide, and (2) no effect on the mortality rate but reduced pancreatic damage with gabexate.

Intraabdominal *Candida* infection during acute necrotizing pancreatitis is increasing in frequency and is associated with an increased mortality rate. In one representatitve trial, intraabdominal *Candida* infection was found in 13 of 37 cases and was associated with a mortality rate fourfold greater than that associated with intraabdominal bacterial infection alone. Given the impact of *Candida* infection on the mortality rate in acute necrotizing pancreatitis and the apparent benefit of prophylactic chemotherapy, these data suggest earlier use of fungicides.

A CT scan, especially a contrast-enhanced dynamic CT (CECT) scan, provides valuable information on the severity and prognosis of acute pancreatitis (Fig. 304-1 and Table 304-4). In particular, a CECT scan allows estimation of the presence and extent of pancreatic necrosis. Recent studies suggest that the likelihood of prolonged pancreatitis or a serious complication is negligible when the CT severity index is 1 or 2 and low with scores of 3 to 6. However, patients with scores of 7 to 10 had a 92% morbidity rate and a 17% mortality rate. Necrosis is present in 20 to 30% of patients. Those with necrosis have a morbidity rate >20%, whereas those without necrosis have a morbidity rate <10% and a negligible mortality rate. A CECT scan is indicated in patients with three or more of Ranson's signs, in all seriously ill patients, and in patients who show evidence of clinical deterioration. The patient with mild to moderate pancreatitis usually requires treatment with intravenous fluids, fasting, and possibly nasogastric suction for 2 to 4 days. A clear liquid diet is frequently started on the third to sixth day, and a regular diet by the fifth to seventh day. The patient with unremitting *fulminant pancreatitis* usually requires inordinate amounts of fluid and close attention to complications such as cardiovascular collapse, respiratory insufficiency, and pancreatic infection. The latter should be managed by a combination of radiologic and surgical means (see below). While earlier uncontrolled studies suggested that *peritoneal lavage* through a percutaneous dialysis catheter was helpful in severe pancreatitis, subsequent studies indicate that this treatment does not influence the outcome of such attacks. Aggressive surgical pancreatic debridement (necrosectomy) should be undertaken soon after confirmation of the presence of infected necrosis, and multiple operations may be required. Since the mortality rate from sterile acute necrotizing pancreatitis is approximately 10%, laparotomy with adequate drainage and removal of necrotic tissue should be considered if conventional therapy does not halt the patient's deterioration. The use of parenteral nutrition makes it possible to give nutritional support to patients with severe, acute, or protracted pancreatitis who are unable to eat normally. Patients with severe gallstone-induced pancreatitis may improve dramatically if papillotomy is carried out within the first 36 to 72 h of the attack. Studies indicate that only those patients with gallstone pancreatitis who are in the very severe group should be considered for urgent endoscopic retrograde cholangiopancreatography (ERCP). Finally, the treatment for patients with hypertriglyceridemia-associated pancreatitis includes (1) weight loss to ideal weight, (2) a lipid-restricted diet, (3) exercise, (4) avoidance of alcohol and of drugs that can elevate serum triglycerides (i.e., estrogens, vitamin A, thiazides, and beta-blockers), and (5) control of diabetes.

Table 304-4 Severity Index in Acute Pancreatitis

	Points
Grade of acute pancreatitis	
A. Normal pancreas	0
B. Pancreatic enlargement alone	1
C. Inflammation compared with pancreas and peripancreatic fat	2
D. One peripancreatic fluid collection	3
E. Two or more fluid collections	4
Degree of pancreatic necrosis	
A. No necrosis	0
B. Necrosis of one-third of pancreas	2
C. Necrosis of one-half of pancreas	4
D. Necrosis of more than one-half of pancreas	6

INFECTED PANCREATIC NECROSIS, ABSCESS, AND PSEUDOCYST Infected pancreatic necrosis should be differentiated from pancreatic abscess. The former is a diffuse infection of an acutely inflamed, necrotic pancreas occurring in the first 1 to 2 weeks after the onset of pancreatitis. In contrast, a pancreatic abscess is an ill-defined, liquid collection of pus that evolves over a longer period, often 4 to 6 weeks. It tends to be less life-threatening and is associated with a lower rate of surgical mortality. Infected pancreatic necrosis should be treated by surgical debridement because the solid component of the infected pancreas is not amenable to effective radiologically guided percutaneous evacuation. Pancreatic abscess can be treated surgically or, in selected cases, by percutaneous drainage. The necrotic pancreas becomes secondarily infected in 40 to 60% of patients, most frequently with gram-negative bacteria of alimentary origin. Whether infection occurs depends on several factors, including the extent of pancreatic and peripancreatic necrosis, the degree of pancreatic ischemia and hypoperfusion, and the presence of organ or multiorgan failure.

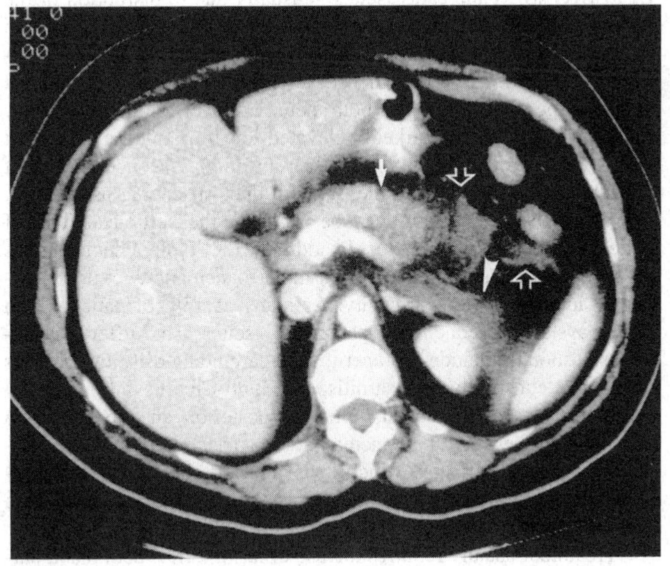

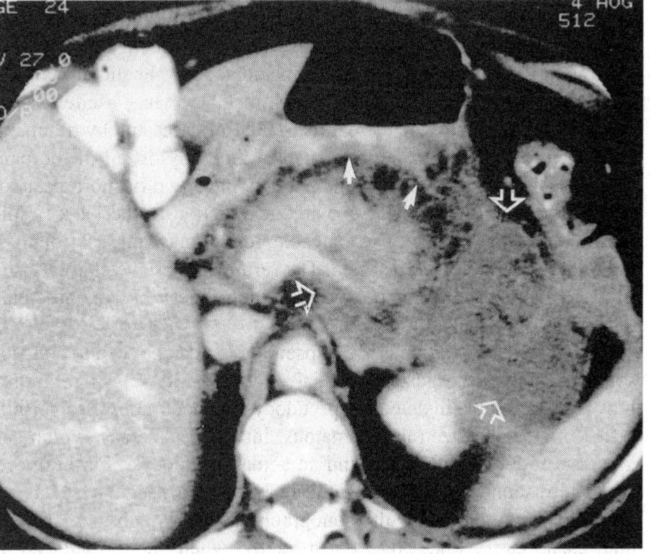

FIGURE 304-1 Acute pancreatitis: CT evolution. *A.* Contrast-enhanced CT scan of the abdomen performed on admission of a patient with clinical evidence of acute pancreatitis. Note the mildly decreased density of the body of the pancreas to the left of the midline (*arrow*). There are a few linear strands in the peripancreatic fat, suggesting inflammation (*open arrows*). A small amount of fluid is seen in the anterior pararenal space (*arrowhead*). *B.* Nine days after admission, there is a marked worsening with severe inflammation of the pancreas evidenced by anterior displacement of the posterior gastric wall (*arrows*), increased inflammation of the peripancreatic fat, and increased pancreatic effusion in the anterior perirenal space and around the splenic vein (*open arrows*). *(Courtesy of Dr. PR Ros, University of Florida College of Medicine.)*

The early diagnosis of pancreatic infection can be accomplished by CT-guided needle aspiration. In one study, 60 patients, representing 5% of all admissions for acute pancreatitis, were suspected of harboring a pancreatic infection on the basis of fever, leukocytosis, and an abnormal CT scan (pseudocyst or extrapancreatic fluid collection). Importantly, 60% of these patients had a pancreatic infection, and 55% of these infections developed in the first 2 weeks. These findings suggest that only guided aspiration can reliably distinguish sterile from infected pancreatic necrosis. The following are guidelines for patients meeting the above selection criteria: (1) Pseudocysts should be aspirated promptly, because more than half may be infected; (2) extrapancreatic fluid collections need not be aspirated promptly, because most are sterile; (3) if a necrotic pancreas is found initially to be sterile but fever and leukocytosis persist, several days of observation should be allowed to pass before reaspiration is considered, as clinical improvement frequently occurs; and (4) if fever and leukocytosis recur after an interval of well-being, reaspiration should be considered.

Severe pancreatitis with the presence of three or more risk factors, postoperative pancreatitis, early oral feeding, early laparotomy, and perhaps injudicious use of antibiotics predispose to the development of pancreatic abscess, which occurs in 3 to 4% of patients with acute pancreatitis. Pancreatic abscess also may develop because of a communication between a pseudocyst and the colon, inadequate surgical drainage of a pseudocyst, or needling of a pseudocyst. The characteristic signs of abscess are fever, leukocytosis, ileus, and rapid deterioration in a patient previously recovering from pancreatitis. Sometimes, however, the only manifestations are persistent fever and signs of continuing pancreatic inflammation. Drainage of pancreatic abscesses by percutaneous catheter techniques, using CT guidance, has been only moderately successful (resolution in 50 to 60% of patients). Accordingly, laparotomy with radical sump drainage and possibly resection of necrotic tissue is usually required, because the mortality rate for undrained pancreatic abscess approaches 100%. Multiple abscesses are common, and reoperation is frequently necessary.

Pseudocysts of the pancreas are collections of tissue, fluid, debris, pancreatic enzymes, and blood which develop over a period of 1 to 4 weeks after the onset of acute pancreatitis; they form in approximately 15% of patients with acute pancreatitis. In contrast to true cysts, pseudocysts do not have an epithelial lining; their walls consist of necrotic tissue, granulation tissue, and fibrous tissue. Disruption of the pancreatic ductal system is common. However, the subsequent course of this disruption varies widely, ranging from spontaneous healing to continuous leakage of pancreatic juice, which results in tense ascites. Pseudocysts are preceded by pancreatitis in 90% of cases and by trauma in 10%. Approximately 85% are located in the body or tail of the pancreas and 15% in the head. Some patients have two or more pseudocysts. Abdominal pain, with or without radiation to the back, is the usual presenting complaint. A palpable, tender mass may be found in the middle or left upper abdomen. The serum amylase level is elevated in 75% of patients at some point during their illness and may fluctuate markedly.

On x-ray examination, 75% of pseudocysts can be seen to displace some portion of the gastrointestinal tract (Fig. 304-2). Sonography, however, is reliable in detecting pseudocysts. Sonography also permits differentiation between an edematous, inflamed pancreas, which can give rise to a palpable mass, and an actual pseudocyst. Furthermore, serial ultrasound studies will indicate whether a pseudocyst has resolved. CT complements ultrasonography in the diagnosis of pancreatic pseudocyst (Fig. 304-2), especially when the pseudocyst is infected.

In studies with sonography, pseudocysts were seen to resolve in 25 to 40% of patients. Pseudocysts that are greater than 5 cm in diameter and that persist for longer than 6 weeks should be considered for drainage. Recent natural history studies have suggested that noninterventional, expectant management is the best course in selected patients with minimal symptoms and no evidence of active alcohol use in whom the pseudocyst appears mature by radiography and does not resemble a cystic neoplasm. A significant number of these pseudocysts resolve spontaneously more than 6 weeks after their formation. Also, these studies demonstrate that large pseudocyst size is not an absolute indication for interventional therapy and that many peripancreatic fluid collections detected on CT in cases of acute pancreatitis resolve spontaneously. A pseudocyst that does not resolve spontaneously may lead to serious complications, such as (1) pain caused by expansion of the lesion and pressure on other viscera, (2) rupture, (3) hemorrhage, and (4) abscess. Rupture of a pancreatic pseudocyst is a particularly serious complication. Shock almost always supervenes, and mortality rates range from 14% if the rupture is not associated with hemorrhage to over 60% if hemorrhage has occurred. Rupture and hemorrhage are the prime causes of death from pancreatic pseudocyst. A triad of findings—an increase in the size of the mass, a localized bruit over the mass, and a sudden decrease in hemoglobin level and hematocrit without obvious external blood loss—should alert one to the possibility of hemorrhage from a pseudocyst. Thus, in patients who are stable and free of complications and in whom serial ultrasound studies show that the pseudocyst is shrinking, conservative therapy is indicated. Conversely, if the pseudocyst is expanding and is complicated by rupture, hemorrhage, or abscess, the patient should be operated on. With ultrasound or CT guidance, sterile chronic pseudocysts can be treated safely with single or repeated needle aspiration or more prolonged catheter drainage with a success rate of 45 to 75%. The success rate of these techniques for infected pseudocysts is considerably less (40 to 50%). Patients who do not respond to drainage require surgical therapy for internal or external drainage of the cyst.

Pseudoaneurysms develop in up to 10% of patients with acute pancreatitis at sites reflecting the distribution of pseudocysts and fluid collections (Fig. 304-2*D*). The splenic artery is most frequently involved, followed by the inferior and superior pancreatic duodenal arteries. This diagnosis should be suspected in patients with pancreatitis who develop upper gastrointestinal bleeding without an obvious cause or in whom thin-cut CT scanning reveals a contrast-enhanced lesion within or adjacent to a suspected pseudocyst. Arteriography is necessary to confirm the diagnosis.

PANCREATIC ASCITES AND PANCREATIC PLEURAL EFFUSIONS Pancreatic ascites is usually due to disruption of the main pancreatic duct, often by an internal fistula between the duct and the peritoneal cavity or a leaking pseudocyst (Chap. 43). This diagnosis is suggested in a patient with an elevated serum amylase level in whom the ascites fluid has both increased levels of albumin [30 g/L (>3.0 g/dL)] and a markedly elevated level of amylase. The fluid in true pancreatic ascites usually has an amylase concentration of >20,000 U/L as a result of the ruptured duct or leaking pseudocyst. Lower amylase elevations may be found in the peritoneal fluid of patients with acute pancreatitis. In addition, ERCP often demonstrates passage of contrast material from a major pancreatic duct or a pseudocyst into the peritoneal cavity. As many as 15% of patients with pseudocysts have concurrent pancreatic ascites. The differential diagnosis should include intraperitoneal carcinomatosis, tuberculous peritonitis, constrictive pericarditis, and Budd-Chiari syndrome.

If the pancreatic duct disruption is posterior, an internal fistula may develop between the pancreatic duct and the pleural space, producing a pleural effusion, which is usually left-sided and often massive. This complication often requires thoracentesis or chest tube drainage.

Treatment usually requires the use of nasogastric suction and parenteral alimentation to decrease pancreatic secretion. In addition, paracentesis is performed to keep the peritoneal cavity free of fluid and, it is hoped, to effect sealing of the leak. The long-acting somatostatin analogue octreotide, which inhibits pancreatic secretion, is useful in cases of pancreatic ascites and pleural effusion. If ascites continues to recur after 2 to 3 weeks of medical management, the patient should

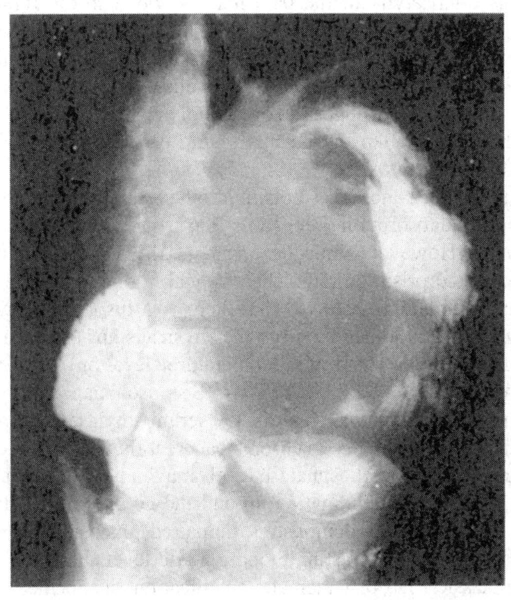

A

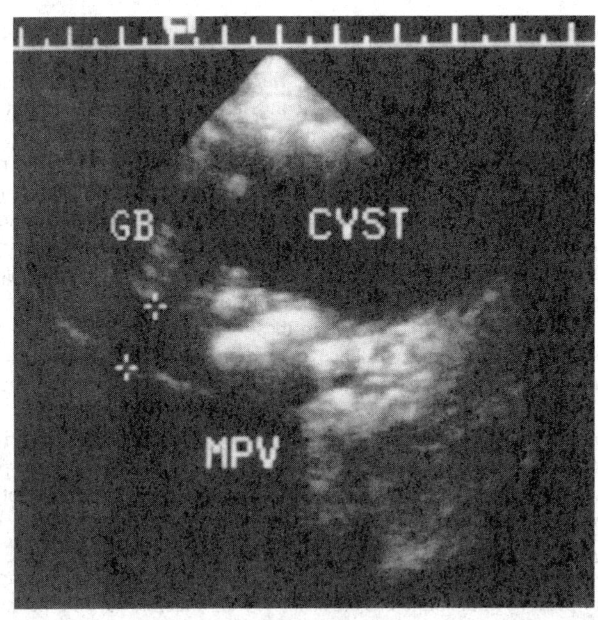

B

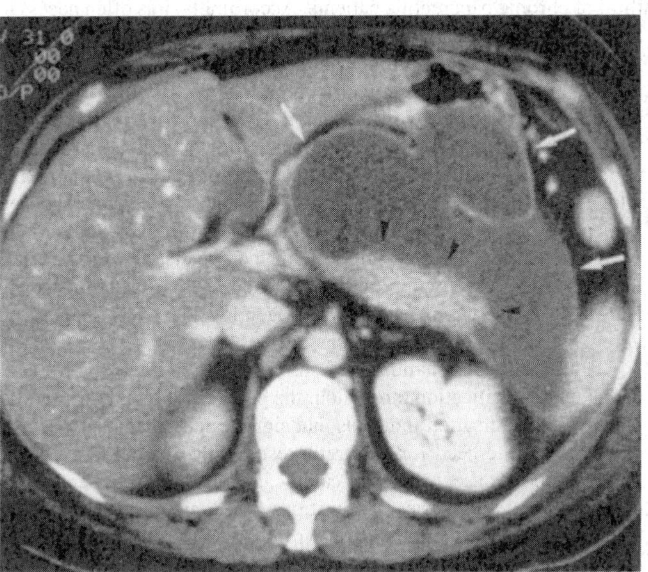

C

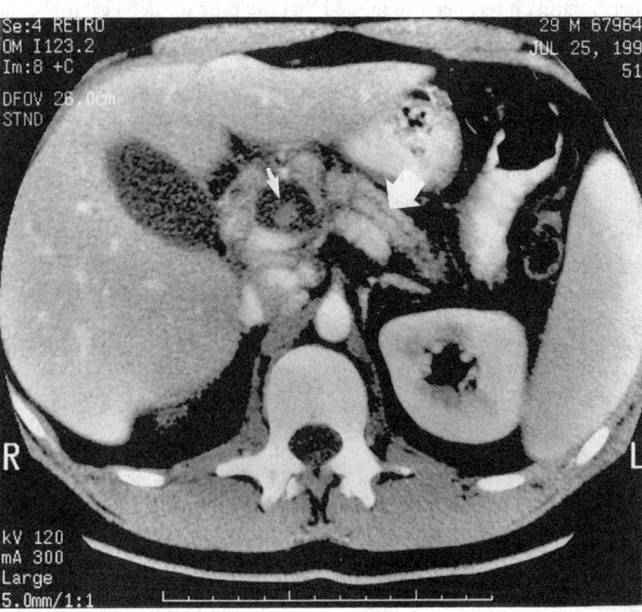

D

FIGURE 304-2 Pseudocyst of pancreas. *A*. Upper gastrointestinal x-ray showing displacement of stomach by pseudocyst. *B*. Sonogram showing pseudocyst (*cyst*). GB, gallbladder; MVP, portal vein. Behind the large pseudocyst is seen the calcified head of the pancreas. A dilated common bile duct (*asterisk*) is noted. *C*. CT scan showing pseudocyst. Note the large, lobulated fluid collection (*arrows*) surrounding the tail of the pancreas (*arrowheads*). Note also the dense, thin rim in the periphery representing the fibrous capsule of the pseudocyst. *D*. Spiral CT showing a pseudocyst (*small arrow*) with a pseudoaneurysm (light area in pseudocyst). Note the demonstration of the main pancreatic duct (*big arrow*), even though this duct is minimally dilated by ERCP. *(A, B courtesy of Dr. CE Forsmark, University of Florida College of Medicine; C, D courtesy of Dr. PR Ros, University of Florida College of Medicine.)*

be operated on after pancreatography to define the anatomy of the abnormal duct. A disrupted main pancreatic duct can also be treated effectively by stenting. Patients in whom ERCP identifies two or more sites of extravasation are unlikely to respond to conservative management and/or stenting.

CHRONIC PANCREATITIS AND PANCREATIC EXOCRINE INSUFFICIENCY

GENERAL AND ETIOLOGIC CONSIDERATIONS Chronic inflammatory disease of the pancreas may present as episodes of acute inflammation in a previously injured pancreas or as chronic damage with persistent pain or malabsorption. The causes of relapsing chronic pancreatitis are similar to those of acute pancreatitis (Table 304-1), except that there is an appreciable incidence of cases of undetermined origin. In addition, the pancreatitis associated with gallstones is predominantly acute or relapsing-acute in nature. A cholecystectomy is almost always performed in patients after the first or second attack of gallstone-associated pancreatitis. Patients with chronic pancreatitis may present with persistent abdominal pain, with or without steatorrhea; some (~15%) present with steatorrhea and no pain.

Patients with chronic pancreatitis in whom there is extensive destruction of the pancreas (less than 10% of exocrine function remaining) have steatorrhea and azotorrhea. Among American adults, alcoholism is the most common cause of clinically apparent pancreatic exocrine insufficiency, while cystic fibrosis is the most frequent cause in children. In up to 25% of American adults with chronic pancreatitis, the cause is not known; that is, they have idiopathic chronic pancreatitis. Mutations of the cystic fibrosis transmembrane conductance regulator (CFTR) gene have been documented in patients with idiopathic chronic pancreatitis. It has been estimated that in patients with idiopathic pancreatitis the frequency of a single CFTR mutation is 11 times the expected frequency and the frequency of two mutant alleles is 80 times the expected frequency. The results of sweat chloride testing are not diagnostic of cystic fibrosis in these patients. However, these patients have functional evidence of a defect in CFTR-mediated ion transport in nasal epithelium. It is suggested that up to 25% of patients with idiopathic chronic pancreatitis may have abnormalities of the CFTR gene. The therapeutic and prognostic implication of these findings remain to be determined. In other parts of the world, severe protein-calorie malnutrition is a common cause. Table 304-5 lists other causes of pancreatic exocrine insufficiency, but they are relatively uncommon.

PATHOPHYSIOLOGY The events that initiate an inflammatory process in the pancreas are still not well understood, and the many hypotheses will not be reviewed here. In the case of alcohol-induced pancreatitis, it has been suggested that the primary defect may be the precipitation of protein (inspissated enzymes) in the ducts. The resulting ductal obstruction could lead to duct dilation, diffuse atrophy of the acinar cells, fibrosis, and eventual calcification of some of the protein plugs. However, the fact that some alcoholic patients with recurrent acute pancreatitis show no evidence of chronic pancreatitis does not support this hypothesis. In fact, experimental and clinical observations have shown that alcohol has direct toxic effects on the pancreas. While patients with alcohol-induced pancreatitis generally consume large amounts of alcohol, some consume very little (50 g/d or less). Thus prolonged consumption of "socially acceptable" amounts of alcohol is compatible with the development of pancreatitis. In addition, the finding of extensive pancreatic fibrosis in patients who died during their first attack of clinical acute alcohol-induced pancreatitis supports the concept that such patients already have chronic pancreatitis.

CLINICAL FEATURES Patients with relapsing chronic pancreatitis may present with symptoms identical to those of acute pancreatitis, but pain may be continuous, intermittent, or absent. The pathogenesis of this pain is poorly understood. Although the classic description is of epigastric pain radiating through the back, the pain pattern is often atypical; the pain may be worst in the right or left upper quadrant of the back or may be diffuse throughout the upper abdomen; it may even be referred to the anterior chest or flank. Characteristically it is persistent, deep-seated, and unresponsive to antacids. It often is worsened by ingestion of alcohol or a heavy meal (especially one rich in fat). Often the pain is severe enough to necessitate the frequent use of narcotics.

Weight loss, abnormal stools, and other signs or symptoms suggestive of malabsorption (see Table 286-5) are common in chronic pancreatitis. However, clinically apparent deficiencies of fat-soluble vitamins are surprisingly rare. The physical findings in these patients are usually not impressive, so that there is a disparity between the severity of the abdominal pain and the physical signs (other than some abdominal tenderness and mild temperature elevation).

Table 304-5 Causes of Pancreatic Exocrine Insufficiency

- Alcohol, chronic alcoholism
- Idiopathic pancreatitis
- Cystic fibrosis
- Hypertriglyceridemia
- Severe protein-calorie malnutrition with hypoalbuminemia
  - Tropical pancreatitis (Africa, Asia)
- Pancreatic and duodenal neoplasms
- Pancreatic resection
- Gastric surgery
  - Subtotal gastrectomy with Billroth I anastomosis
  - Subtotal gastrectomy with Billroth II anastomosis
  - Truncal vagotomy and pyloroplasty
- Gastrinoma (Zollinger-Ellison syndrome)
- Hereditary pancreatitis
- Traumatic pancreatitis
- Abdominal radiotherapy
- Hemochromatosis
- Shwachman's syndrome (pancreatic insufficiency and bone marrow dysfunction)
- Trypsinogen deficiency
- Enterokinase deficiency
- Isolated deficiencies of amylase, lipase, or proteases
- α_1-Antitrypsin deficiency

DIAGNOSTIC EVALUATION (See also Chap. 303) In contrast to relapsing acute pancreatitis, the serum amylase and lipase levels are usually not elevated in chronic pancreatitis. Elevations of serum bilirubin and alkaline phosphatase levels may indicate cholestasis secondary to chronic inflammation around the common bile duct (Fig. 304-3). Many patients demonstrate impaired glucose tolerance, and some have an elevated fasting blood glucose level.

The classic triad of pancreatic calcification, steatorrhea, and diabetes mellitus usually establishes the diagnosis of chronic pancreatitis and exocrine pancreatic insufficiency but is found in less than one-third of chronic pancreatitis patients. Accordingly, it is often necessary to perform an intubation test such as the *secretin stimulation test*, which usually gives abnormal results when 60% or more of pancreatic exocrine function has been lost. Approximately 40% of patients with chronic pancreatitis have *cobalamin (vitamin B_{12})* malabsorption, which can be corrected by the administration of oral pancreatic enzymes. There is usually a marked excretion of fecal fat (Chap. 286), which can be reduced by the administration of oral pancreatic enzymes. The serum trypsinogen (Chap. 303) and the D-xylose urinary excretion test are useful in patients with "pancreatic steatorrhea," since the trypsinogen level will be abnormal, and D-xylose excretion usually is normal. A decreased serum trypsinogen level strongly suggests severe pancreatic exocrine insufficiency.

The radiographic hallmark of chronic pancreatitis is the presence of scattered calcification throughout the pancreas (Fig. 304-3). Diffuse pancreatic calcification indicates that significant damage has occurred and obviates the need for a secretin test. While alcohol is by far the most common cause, pancreatic calcification also may be seen in cases of severe protein-calorie malnutrition, hereditary pancreatitis, posttraumatic pancreatitis, hyperparathyroidism, islet cell tumors, and idiopathic chronic pancreatitis. A large prospective study has shown convincingly that pancreatic calcification decreases or even disappears spontaneously in one-third of patients with severe chronic pancreatitis; this outcome may also follow ductal decompression. Pancreatic calcification is a dynamic process that is incompletely understood.

Sonography, CT, and ERCP greatly aid the diagnosis of pancreatic disease. In addition to excluding pseudocysts and pancreatic cancer, sonography and CT may show calcification or dilated ducts associated with chronic pancreatitis (Fig. 304-4). ERCP is the only major technique that provides a direct view of the pancreatic duct. In patients with alcohol-induced pancreatitis, ERCP may reveal a pseudocyst missed by sonography or CT.

COMPLICATIONS OF CHRONIC PANCREATITIS The complications of chronic pancreatitis are protean. *Cobalamin (vitamin B_{12})* malabsorption occurs in 40% of patients with alcohol-induced chronic pancreatitis and in virtually all with cystic fibrosis. It is consistently corrected by the administration of pancreatic enzymes (containing proteases). It may be due to excessive binding of cobalamin by cobalamin-binding proteins other than intrinsic factor, which ordinarily are destroyed by pancreatic proteases and therefore do not compete with intrinsic factor for cobalamin binding. Although most patients show *impaired glucose tolerance*, diabetic ketoacidosis and coma are uncommon. Similarly, end-organ damage (retinopathy, neu-

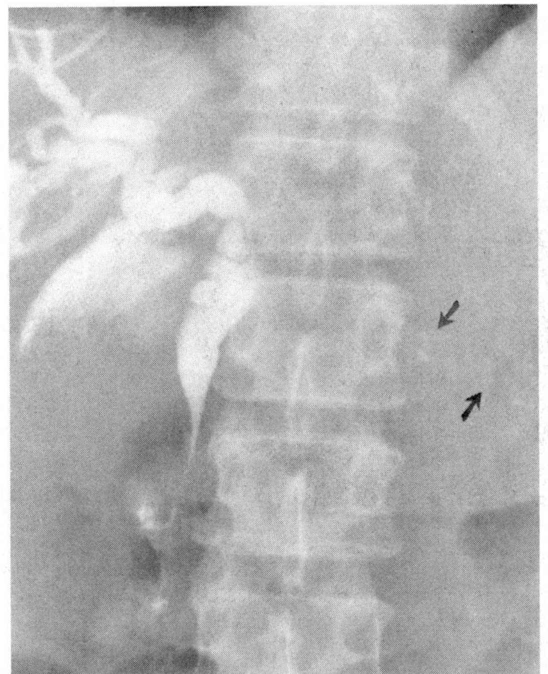

A

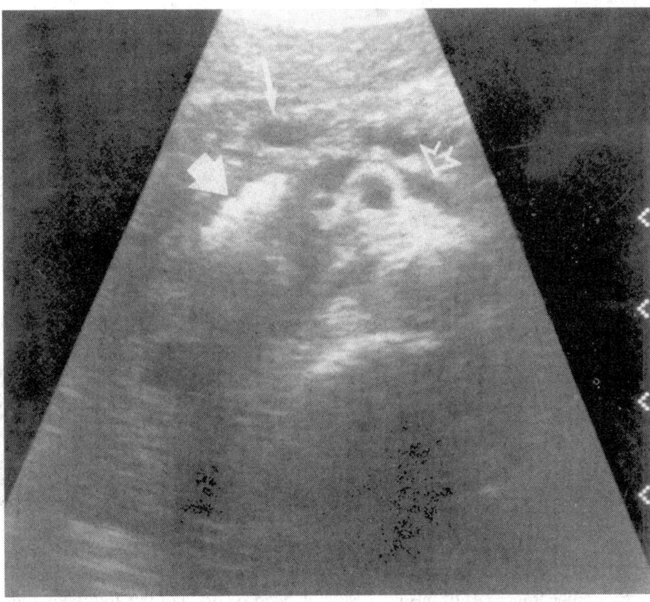

B

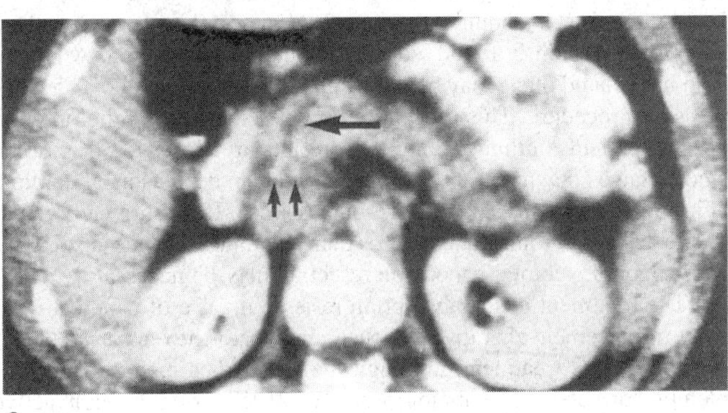

C

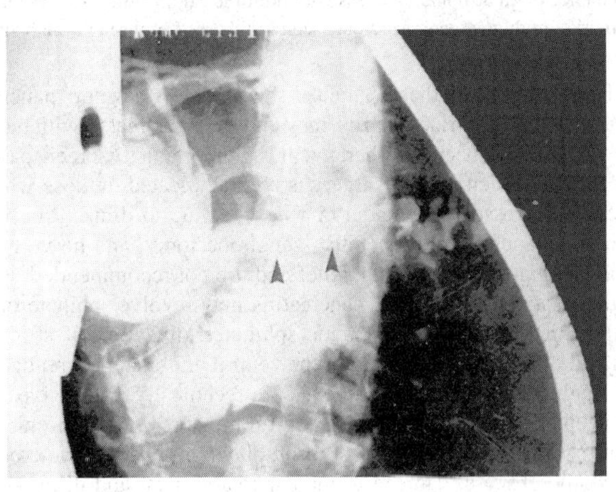

D

FIGURE 304-3 Radiologic abnormalities in chronic pancreatitis. *A*. Pancreatic calcification (*arrows*) and stenosis (tapering) of the intrahepatic portion of the common bile duct demonstrated by percutaneous transhepatic cholangiography. *B*. Pancreatic calcification (*large white arrow*) demonstrated by sonography. Note dilated pancreatic duct (*thin white arrow*) and splenic vein (*open arrow*). *C*. Pancreatic calcification (*vertical arrows*) and dilated pancreatic duct (*horizontal arrow*) demonstrated by CT scan. *D*. Endoscopic retrograde cholangiogram shows grossly dilated pancreatic ducts (*arrows*) in a patient with long-standing pancreatitis.

ropathy, nephropathy) is also uncommon, and the appearance of these complications should raise the question of concomitant genetic diabetes mellitus. A nondiabetic retinopathy, peripheral in location and secondary to vitamin A and/or zinc deficiency, is common in these patients. *Effusions* containing high concentrations of amylase may occur into the pleural, pericardial, or peritoneal space. *Gastrointestinal bleeding* may occur from peptic ulceration, gastritis, a pseudocyst eroding into the duodenum, or ruptured varices secondary to splenic vein thrombosis due to inflammation of the tail of the pancreas. *Icterus* may occur, caused either by edema of the head of the pancreas, which compresses the common bile duct, or by chronic cholestasis secondary to a chronic inflammatory reaction around the intrapancreatic portion of the common bile duct (Fig. 304-3). The chronic obstruction may lead to cholangitis and ultimately to biliary cirrhosis. *Subcutaneous fat necrosis* may appear as tender red nodules on the lower extremities. *Bone pain* may be secondary to intramedullary fat necrosis. Inflammation of the large and small joints of the upper and lower extremities may occur. The incidence of pancreatic carcinoma is increased in patients with chronic pancreatitis who have been followed for 2 or more years. Twenty years after the diagnosis of chronic pancreatitis, the cumulative risk of pancreatic carcinoma is 4%. Perhaps the most common and troublesome complication is addiction to narcotics.

℞ TREATMENT Therapy for patients with chronic pancreatitis is directed toward two major problems—pain and malabsorption. Patients with intermittent attacks of pain are treated essentially like those with acute pancreatitis (see above). Patients with severe and persistent pain should avoid alcohol completely and avoid large meals rich in fat. Since the pain is often severe enough to require frequent use of narcotics (and hence addiction), a number of surgical procedures have been developed for pain relief. ERCP allows the surgeon to plan the operative approach. If there is a stricture of the pancreatic duct, a *local resection* may ameliorate the pain. Unfortunately, isolated localized strictures are not common. In most patients with alcohol-induced disease, the pancreas is diffusely involved, and surgically correctible localized ductal disease is rare. When there is primary ductal obstruction and dilation, ductal decompression may provide effective pain palliation. Short-term pain relief may be achieved in up to 80% of patients, while long-term pain relief occurs in approximately 50%. In some of these patients, however, pain relief can be achieved only by resecting 50 to 95% of the gland. Although pain relief is achieved

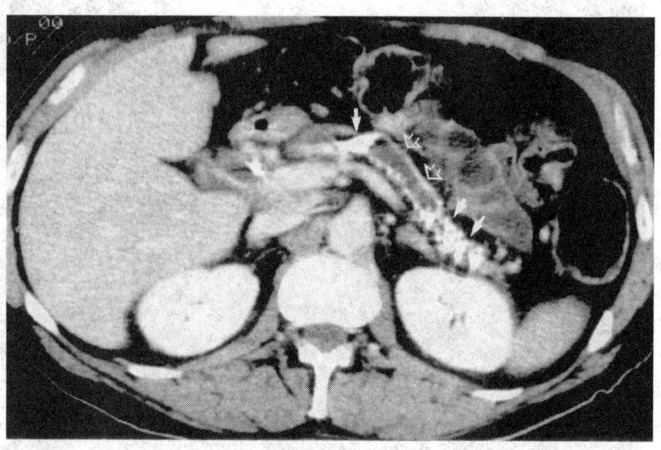

A

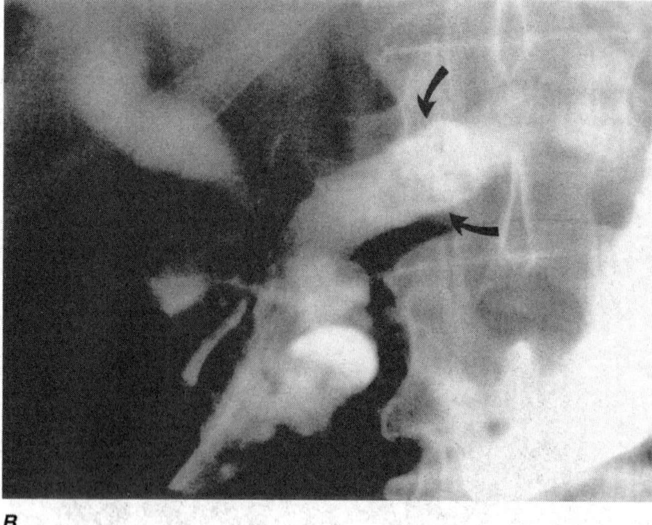

B

FIGURE 304-4 Chronic pancreatitis and pancreatic calculi: CT scan and ERCP appearance. *A.* In this contrast-enhanced CT scan of the abdomen, there is evidence of an atrophic pancreas with multiple calcifications (*arrows*). Note the markedly dilated pancreatic duct seen in this section through the body and tail (*open arrows*). *B.* ERCP in the same patient demonstrates the dilated pancreatic duct as well as an intrapancreatic duct calculus (*arrows*). These findings correlate nicely with the CT scan appearance.

in three-quarters of these patients, they tend to develop pancreatic endocrine and exocrine insufficiency and must be treated with pancreatic enzyme replacement therapy. It is important to screen patients carefully, for such radical surgery is contraindicated in those who are severely depressed or suicidal or who continue to drink. Procedures such as splanchnicectomy, celiac ganglionectomy, and nerve blocks usually bring only temporary relief and are not recommended. Endoscopic treatment of chronic pancreatitis may involve sphincterotomy of the minor or major pancreatic sphincter, dilatation of strictures, removal of calculi, or stenting of the ventral or dorsal pancreatic duct. Although many of these techniques are technically impressive, none has been subjected to a randomized trial in patients with chronic pancreatitis. In addition, significant complications—acute pancreatitis, pancreatic abscess, damage to the pancreatic duct, and death—have occurred in up to 36% of patients after stent placement.

Three double-blind trials have demonstrated that administration of pancreatic enzymes decreases abdominal pain in selected patients with chronic pancreatitis. In these trials, approximately 75% of the patients evaluated experienced pain relief. The patients most likely to respond are those with mild to moderate exocrine pancreatic dysfunction, as evidenced by an abnormal secretin test, normal fat absorption, and minimal abnormalities on ERCP examination. These clinical observations seem to fit with data from human beings and experimental animals demonstrating a negative feedback regulation for pancreatic exocrine secretion controlled by the amount of proteases within the lumen of the proximal small intestine. It seems reasonable to use the following approach for patients with severe, persistent, or continuous abdominal pain thought to be caused by chronic pancreatitis. After other causes of abdominal pain (peptic ulcer, gallstones, etc.) have been excluded, a pancreatic *sonogram* should be done. If no mass is found, a *secretin test* may be performed, because its results usually are abnormal in cases of chronic pancreatitis with pain. If the results are abnormal (i.e., decreased bicarbonate concentration or volume output), a 3- to 4-week *trial of pancreatic enzyme administration* is appropriate. Eight conventional tablets or capsules are taken at meals and at bedtime. There are a number of studies suggesting that patients may have small-duct chronic pancreatitis and chronic abdominal pain with a normal appearance on radiographic evaluations (ultrasound, CT, ERCP) but abnormal results on hormone stimulation tests (secretin test) and/or abnormal pancreatic histology. Such minimal-change chronic pancreatitis may respond well to pancreatic enzyme therapy (non-enteric-coated) for relief of abdominal pain. If no relief is obtained, and especially if the volume secreted during the secretin test is very low, ERCP should be performed. If a pseudocyst or a localized ductal obstruction is found, surgery should be considered. A patient who has dilated ducts may be a candidate for a surgical ductal decompression procedure. This procedure provides short-term relief in up to 80% of patients, although long-term results are closer to 50%. Some studies have shown octreotide to be effective in decreasing abdominal pain in patients with severe large-duct disease. If no surgically remediable lesion is found and severe pain continues despite abstinence from alcohol, subtotal pancreatic resection may be necessary.

The treatment of malabsorption rests on the use of pancreatic enzyme replacement therapy. Diarrhea and steatorrhea are usually improved by this treatment, although the steatorrhea may not be completely corrected. The major problem is delivering enough active enzyme into the duodenum. Steatorrhea could be abolished if 10% of the normal amount of lipase could be delivered to the duodenum at the proper time. This concentration of lipase cannot be achieved with the current preparations of pancreatic enzymes, even if the latter are given in large doses. The reason for these poor results may be that lipase is inactivated by gastric acid, that food empties from the stomach faster than do the pancreatic enzymes, and that batches of commercially available pancreatic extracts vary in enzyme activity.

For the usual patient, two or three enteric-coated capsules or eight conventional (non-enteric-coated) tablets of a potent enzyme preparation should be administered with meals. Some patients using conventional tablets require adjuvant therapy to improve enzyme replacement treatment. H_2 receptor antagonists, sodium bicarbonate, and proton pump inhibitors are effective adjuvants. Antacids containing calcium carbonate or magnesium hydroxide are not effective and may actually result in increased steatorrhea. Several publications have reported colonic strictures in patients with cystic fibrosis receiving extraordinarily high doses of high-potency pancreatic enzyme preparations. Such lesions have not been reported in adults with chronic pancreatitis.

Supportive measures include diet restriction and pain medications. The diet should be moderate in fat (30%), high in protein (24%), and low in carbohydrate (40%). Restriction of long-chain triglyceride intake can help patients who do not respond satisfactorily to pancreatic enzyme therapy. Use of foods containing mainly medium-chain fatty acids, which do not require lipase for digestion, may be beneficial. Nonnarcotic analgesics should be emphasized. Patients taking narcotic drugs for pain relief often become addicted and continue to have pain.

Table 304-6 Pancreatic Endocrine Tumors

Syndrome	Hormone(s) Produced	Primary Hormone Effects	Pathologic Features	Clinical Features
Zollinger-Ellison	Gastrin	Gastric acid hypersecretion with basal acid outputs usually >15 mmol/h (>15 mEq/h)	Delta cell islet tumors; 10% aberrant (duodenal); 60% malignant	Severe peptic ulcer disease often refractory to therapy; ectopic ulcers; diarrhea; multiple endocrine adenomas (parathyroid, pituitary, adrenal, thyroid)
Insulinoma	Insulin	Hypoglycemia with inappropriately increased serum insulin levels	Beta cell islet tumors; 80–90% benign	Hypoglycemic symptoms
Glucagonoma	Glucagon; pancreatic polypeptide	Hyperglucagonemia → glucose intolerance	Alpha cell islet tumors; 60% malignant	Slow-growing pancreatic tumor; hyperglycemia; ezcematoid dermatitis, or necrolytic erythema weight loss; anemia; gastric and intestinal motor abnormalities
Somatostatinoma	Somatostatin; pancreatic polypeptide	Somatostatin inhibits insulin, gastrin, and pancreatic enzyme secretion; decreased bile flow	Delta cell islet tumor	Pancreatic tumor; diarrhea; steatorrhea; gallstones; diabetes mellitus; anemia
Pancreatic cholera	Vasoactive intestinal peptide ? Gastric inhibitory polypeptide ? Prostaglandin E ? Pancreatic peptide	Net secretion of salt and water by gut	? Delta cell tumor; >50% malignant	Pancreatic tumor with severe watery diarrhea; flushing; weight loss; hypokalemia; hypercalcemia; hypochlorhydria; hyperglycemia; inordinate fecal water and electrolyte losses
Carcinoid	Serotonin; prostaglandins	Altered gut motility; diarrhea	Enterochromaffin cells; non-beta-cell islet tumors	Carcinoid syndrome with flushing; wheezing; diarrhea; alcohol intolerance; hepatomegaly

Patients with severe exocrine pancreatic insufficiency secondary to alcohol who continue to drink have a high mortality rate (in one series, 50% of patients who were followed for 5 to 12 years died during this period) and significant morbidity (weight loss, lassitude, vitamin deficiency, and narcotic addiction). Chronic pancreatitis carries significant medical and social costs. A recent study found that pancreatitis led to retirement in 11% of patients with the disease, accounting for 45% of all retirements. In 87% of patients with chronic pancreatitis unable to maintain gainful employment, alcoholism was a contributing factor. Patients with chronic pancreatitis also use substantial medical resources. In 1987 in the United States, this diagnosis accounted for 122,000 recorded outpatient visits and 56,000 hospital admissions. Pain may abate if progressive severe exocrine insufficiency continues. Patients who abstain from alcohol and use vigorous replacement therapy for maldigestion-malabsorption do reasonably well.

HEREDITARY PANCREATITIS Hereditary pancreatitis is a rare disease that is similar to chronic pancreatitis except for an early age of onset and evidence of hereditary factors (involving an autosomal dominant gene with incomplete penetrance). A genome-wide search using genetic linkage analysis identified the hereditary pancreatitis gene on chromosome 7. An R117H mutation in the cationic trypsinogen gene occurs in most of the families with hereditary pancreatitis that have been studied. Molecular modeling predicts the formation of hydrolysis-resistant trypsin that could lead to pancreatic autodigestion. These patients have recurring attacks of severe abdominal pain which may last from a few days to a few weeks. The serum amylase and lipase levels may be elevated during acute attacks but usually are normal. Patients frequently develop pancreatic calcification, diabetes mellitus, and steatorrhea, and, in addition, they have an increased incidence of pancreatic carcinoma. Such patients often require ductal decompression for pain relief. Abdominal complaints in relatives of patients with hereditary pancreatitis should raise the question of pancreatic disease.

PANCREATIC ENDOCRINE TUMORS

→*Pancreatic endocrine tumors are summarized in Table 304-6 and are discussed in Chap. 93.*

OTHER CONDITIONS

ANNULAR PANCREAS When the ventral pancreatic anlage fails to migrate correctly to make contact with the dorsal anlage, the result may be a ring of pancreatic tissue encircling the duodenum. Such an annular pancreas may cause intestinal obstruction in the neonate or the adult. Symptoms of postprandial fullness, epigastric pain, nausea, and vomiting may be present for years before the diagnosis is entertained. The radiographic findings are symmetric dilation of the proximal duodenum with bulging of the recesses on either side of the annular band, effacement but not destruction of the duodenal mucosa, accentuation of the findings in the right anterior oblique position, and lack of change on repeated examinations. The differential diagnosis should include duodenal webs, tumors of the pancreas or duodenum, postbulbar peptic ulcer, regional enteritis, and adhesions. Patients with annular pancreas have an increased incidence of pancreatitis and peptic ulcer. Because of these and other potential complications, the treatment is surgical even if the condition has been present for years. Retrocolic duodenojejunostomy is the procedure of choice, although some surgeons advocate Billroth II gastrectomy, gastroenterostomy, and vagotomy.

PANCREAS DIVISUM Pancreas divisum occurs when the embryologic ventral and dorsal pancreatic anlagen fail to fuse, so that pancreatic drainage is accomplished mainly through the accessory papilla. Pancreas divisum is the most common congenital anatomic variant of the human pancreas. Current evidence indicates that this anomaly does not predispose to the development of pancreatitis in the great majority of patients who harbor it. However, the combination of pancreas divisum and a small accessory orifice could result in dorsal duct obstruction. The challenge is to identify this subset of patients with dorsal duct pathology. Cannulation of the dorsal duct by ERCP is not as easily done as is cannulation of the ventral duct. Patients with pancreatitis and pancreas divisum demonstrated by ERCP should be treated with conservative measures. In many of these patients, pancreatitis is idiopathic and unrelated to the pancreas divisum. Endoscopic or surgical intervention is indicated only when the above methods fail. If marked dilation of the dorsal duct can be demonstrated, surgical ductal decompression should be performed. The appropriate therapy for patients without dilation of the dorsal duct is not yet defined. It should be stressed that the ERCP appearance of pancreas divisum—i.e., a small-caliber ventral duct with an arborizing pattern—may be mistaken as representing an obstructed main pancreatic duct secondary to a mass lesion.

MACROAMYLASEMIA In macroamylasemia, amylase circulates in the blood in a polymer form too large to be easily excreted by the kidney. Patients with this condition demonstrate an elevated serum amylase value, a low urinary amylase value, and a C_{am}/C_{cr} ratio of less than 1%. The presence of macroamylase can be documented by chromatography of the serum. The prevalence of macroamylasemia is 1.5% of the nonalcoholic general adult hospital population. Usually macroamylasemia is an incidental finding and is not related to disease of the pancreas or other organs.

Macrolipasemia has now been documented in a few patients with cirrhosis or non-Hodgkin's lymphoma. In these patients, the pancreas appeared normal on ultrasound and CT examination. Lipase was shown to be complexed with immunoglobulin A. Thus, the possibility of *both* macroamylasemia and macrolipasemia should be considered in patients with elevated blood levels of these enzymes.

ACKNOWLEDGMENT

This chapter represents a revised version of a chapter by Dr. Norton J. Greenberger, Dr. Phillip P. Toskes, and Dr. Kurt J. Isselbacher that was in the previous editions of this textbook.

BIBLIOGRAPHY

ADAMS DB et al: Outcome after lateral pancreaticojejunostomy for chronic pancreatitis. Ann Surg 219:481, 1994

ANDRIULLI A et al: Meta-analysis of somatostatin, octreotide, and gabexate mesilate in the therapy of acute pancreatitis. Aliment Pharmacol Ther 12:237, 1998

BALTHAZAR EJ et al: Acute pancreatitis: Value of CT in establishing prognosis. Radiology 174:331, 1990

BANKS PA et al: CT-guided aspiration of suspected pancreatic infection: Bacteriology and clinical outcome. Int J Pancreatol 18:265, 1995

BASSI C et al: Controlled clinical trial of perfloxicin versus imipenem in severe acute pancreatitis. Gastroenterology 115:1513, 1998

BOZKURT T et al: Comparison of pancreatic morphology and exocrine functional impairment in patients with chronic pancreatitis. Gut 35:1132, 1994

CAVALLINI G et al: Gabexate for the prevention of pancreatic damage related to endoscopic retrograde cholangiopancreatography. N Engl J Med 335:919, 1996

CHEY WY: Neurohormonal control of the exocrine pancreas. Curr Opin Gastroenterol 13: 375, 1997

COHN JA et al: Relation between mutations of the cystic fibrosis gene and idiopathic pancreatitis. N Engl J Med 339:653, 1998

FORSMARK CE, TOSKES PP: What does an abnormal pancreatogram mean? Gastrointest Endosc Clin North Am 5:105, 1995

GELTECK CJ et al: Severe hypertriglyceridemia and pancreatitis when estrogen replacement therapy is given to hypertriglyceridemic women. J Lab Clin Med 123:59, 1994

HOERAUF A et al: Intra-abdominal Candida infection during acute necrotizing pancreatitis has a high prevalence and is associated with increased mortality. Crit Care Med 26: 2010, 1998

JOSEPHSON S, TOSKES PP: Chronic pancreatitis: Medical management. Practical Gastroenterol 20:6, 1996

LEE SP et al: Biliary sludge as a cause of acute pancreatitis. N Engl J Med 326:589, 1992

LOWENFELS AB et al: Prognosis of chronic pancreatitis: An international multi-center study. Am J Gastroenterol 89:1467, 1994

MONTORSI M et al: Efficacy of octreotide in the prevention of pancreatic fistula after elective pancreatic resections: A prospective, controlled randomized clinical trial. Surgery 117:26, 1995

PETTI JJ et al: Pancolonic disease in cystic fibrosis and high dose pancreatic enzyme therapy. J Pediatr 125:587, 1994

POWELL JJ et al: Antibiotic prophylaxis in the initial management of severe acute pancreatitis. Br J Surg 85:582, 1998

SHARER N et al: Mutations of the cystic fibrosis gene in patients with chronic pancreatitis. N Engl J Med 339:645, 1998

SHERMAN S et al: Stent-induced pancreatic ductal and parenchymal changes: Correlation of endoscopic ultrasound with ERCP. Gastrointest Endosc 44:276, 1996

STEER ML et al: Chronic pancreatitis. N Engl J Med 332:1482, 1995

TODD HB, DESIREE EM: Acute necrotizing pancreatitis. N Engl J Med 340:1412, 1999

WALSH TN: Minimal change chronic pancreatitis. Gut 33:1566, 1992

WHITCOMB DC et al: Hereditary pancreatitis is caused by a mutation in the cationic trypsinogen gene. Nat Genet 13:141, 1996

PART TWELVE

DISORDERS OF THE IMMUNE SYSTEM, CONNECTIVE TISSUE, AND JOINTS

Section 1
DISORDERS OF THE IMMUNE SYSTEM

305 INTRODUCTION TO THE IMMUNE SYSTEM

Barton F. Haynes, Anthony S. Fauci

ADCC antibody-dependent cellular cytotoxicity	MHC major histocompatibility complex
APCs antigen-presenting cells	MIP macrophage inflammatory protein
ATG anti-thymocyte globulin	NK natural killer
BCR B cell receptors	NK-Rs NK receptors
CTLs cytotoxic T lymphocytes	PAMPs pathogen-associated molecular patterns
FDCs follicular dendritic cells	PRRs pattern recognition receptors
GM-CSF granulocyte-macrophage colony stimulating factor	PTKs protein tyrosine kinases
HEVs high endothelial venules	RAG recombinase activating gene
IDDM insulin-dependent diabetes mellitus	STAT signal transducers and activators of transcription
IFN interferon	TCR T cell receptor
IL interleukin	TGF transforming growth factor
IVIg intravenous immunoglobulin	TNF tumor necrosis factor
LAK lymphokine-activated killer	X-SCID x-linked form of severe combined immune deficiency syndrome
LGLs large granular lymphocytes	
LPS lipopolysacchride	
MAB monoclonal antibody	
MCP monocyte chemotactic protein	

DEFINITIONS

- *Adaptive immune system*—recently evolved system of immune responses mediated by T and B lymphocytes. Immune responses by these cells are based on specific antigen recognition by clonotypic receptors that are products of genes that rearrange during development and throughout the life of the organism. Additional cells of the adaptive immune system include various types of antigen-presenting cells.
- *Antibody*—B cell–produced molecules encoded by genes that rearrange during B cell development consisting of immunoglobulin heavy and light chains that together form the central component of the B cell receptor for antigen. Antibody can exist as B cell surface antigen-recognition molecules or as secreted molecules in plasma and other body fluids.
- *Antigens*—foreign or self molecules that are recognized by the adaptive and innate immune systems resulting in innate immune cell triggering, T cell activation, and/or B cell antibody production.
- *Antimicrobial peptides*—small peptides <100 amine acids in length that are produced by cells of the innate immune system and have anti-infectious agent activity.
- *B lymphocytes*—bone marrow–derived or bursal-equivalent lymphocytes that express surface immunoglobulin (the B cell receptor for antigen) and secrete specific antibody after interaction with antigen.
- *B cell receptor for antigen*—complex of surface molecules that rearrange during postnatal B cell development, made up of surface immunoglobulin (Ig) and associated Ig $\alpha\beta$ chain molecules that recognize nominal antigen via Ig heavy and light chain variable regions, and signal the B cell to terminally differentiate to make antigen-specific antibody.
- *Complement*—cascading series of plasma enzymes and effector proteins whose function is to lyse pathogens and/or target them to be phagocytized by neutrophils and monocyte/macrophage lineage cells of the reticuloendothelial system.
- *Co-stimulatory molecules*—molecules of antigen-presenting cells (such as B7-1 and B7-2 or CD40) that lead to T cell activation when ligated by ligands on activated T cells (such as CD28 or CD40 ligand).
- *Cytokines*—soluble proteins that interact with specific cellular receptors that are involved in the regulation of the growth and activation of immune cells and mediate normal and pathologic inflammatory and immune responses.
- *Dendritic cells*—myeloid and/or lymphoid lineage antigen-presenting cells of the adaptive immune system. Immature dendritic cells, or dendritic cell precursors, are key components of the innate immune system by responding to infections with production of high levels of cytokines. Dendritic cells are key initiators both of innate immune responses via cytokine production and of adaptive immune responses via presentation of antigen to T lymphocytes.
- *Innate immune system*—ancient immune recognition system of host cells bearing germline encoded pattern recognition receptors (PRRs) that recognize pathogens and trigger a variety of mechanisms of pathogen elimination. Cells of the innate immune system include natural killer (NK) cell lymphocytes, monocytes/macrophages, immature or dendritic cell precursors, neutrophils, basophils, eosinophils, tissue mast cells, and epithelial cells.
- *Large granular lymphocytes*—lymphocytes of the innate immune system with azurophilic cytotoxic granules that have NK cell activity capable of killing foreign and host cells with little or no self major histocompatibility complex (MHC) class I molecules.
- *Natural killer cells*—large granular lymphocytes that kill target cells that express little or no HLA class I molecules, such as malignantly transformed cells and virally infected cells. NK cells express receptors that inhibit killer cell function when self MHC class I is present.
- *Pathogen-associated molecular patterns*—Invariant molecular structures expressed by large groups of microorganisms that are recognized by host cellular PRRs in the mediation of innate immunity.
- *Pattern recognition receptors*—germline-encoded receptors expressed by cells of the innate immune system that recognize pathogen-associated molecular patterns (PAMPs).
- *T cells*—thymus-derived lymphocytes that mediate adaptive cellular immune responses including T helper and cytotoxic T lymphocyte effector cell functions.
- *T cell receptor for antigen*—complex of surface molecules that rearrange during postnatal T cell development made up of clonotypic T cell receptor (TCR) α and β chains that are associated with the CD3 complex composed of invariant γ, δ, ε, ζ, and η chains. The clonotypic TCR α and β chains recognize peptide fragments of protein antigen physically bound in antigen-presenting cell MHC class I or II molecules, leading to signaling via the CD3 complex to mediate effector functions.
- *Tolerance*—recognition of foreign or self antigens by B and T lymphocytes in the absence of expression of antigen-presenting cell co-stimulatory molecules that leads to B and T cell nonresponsiveness to antigens. Active T lymphocyte tolerance can be achieved through blockade of the B7/CD28 co-stimulatory pathway.

INTRODUCTION The human immune system has evolved over millions of years from both invertebrate and vertebrate organisms to develop sophisticated defense mechanisms highly specific for invading pathogens. Immune systems evolved to protect the host from microbes and their virulence factors. From invertebrates, humans have inherited the innate immune system, an ancient defense system that uses germ line–encoded proteins to recognize pathogens. Cells of the innate immune system, such as macrophages and NK lymphocytes, recognize pathogen molecular motifs that are highly conserved among many microbes (PAMPs) and use a diverse set of receptor molecules (PRRs). Important components of the recognition of microbes by the innate immune system are: (1) recognition by germ line–encoded host molecules, (2) recognition of key microbe virulence factors but not recognition of self molecules, and (3) nonrecognition of benign foreign molecules or microbes. It is particularly important for the innate immune system to not recognize foreign nonpathogenic molecules that are common in the environment, since reaction against them would cause continuous inflammatory disease. Upon contact with pathogens, macrophages and NK cells may kill pathogens directly or may activate a series of events that both slows the infection and recruits the more recently evolved arm of the human immune system, the adaptive immune system.

Adaptive immunity is found only in vertebrates and is based on the generation of antigen receptor T and B lymphocytes by germ-line gene rearrangements that occur during the development of each person. By a complex series of molecular mechanisms of gene rearrangement, individual T or B cells express unique antigen receptors on their surface, such that taken together the pools of adult human T and B lymphocytes contain cells capable of specifically recognizing the diverse antigens of the myriad of infectious agents in the environment. Coupled with finely tuned specific recognition mechanisms that maintain tolerance to self antigen, T and B lymphocytes of the adaptive immune system with their postnatally rearranged clonotypic antigen receptors bring both *specificity* and *immune memory* to vertebrate host defenses.

This chapter describes the cellular components, molecules, and mechanisms that make up the innate and adaptive immune systems and describes how adaptive immunity is recruited to the defense of the host by innate immune responses. An appreciation of the cellular and molecular bases of innate and adaptive immune responses is critical to understanding the pathogenesis of inflammatory, autoimmune, infectious, and immunodeficiency diseases.

THE CD CLASSIFICATION OF HUMAN LYMPHOCYTE DIFFERENTIATION ANTIGENS The development of monoclonal antibody technology led to the discovery of a large number of new leukocyte surface molecules. In 1982, the First International Workshop on Leukocyte Differentiation Antigens was held to establish a nomenclature for cell-surface molecules of human leukocytes. From this and subsequent leukocyte differentiation workshops has come the cluster of differentiation (CD) classification of leukocyte antigens (Table 305-1). The data presented in Table 305-1 establish a context to facilitate discussion and study of the complex series of events that transpire during normal and aberrant innate and adaptive human immune responses.

THE INNATE IMMUNE SYSTEM All multicellular organisms, including humans, have developed the use of a limited number of germ line–encoded molecules that recognize large groups of pathogens. Because of the myriad human pathogens, host molecules of the human innate immune system must recognize PAMPs, the common molecular structures shared by many pathogens. PAMPs must be conserved structures vital to pathogen virulence and survival, such as bacterial endotoxin, so that pathogens cannot mutate molecules of PAMPs to evade human innate immune responses. In addition, one major end product of innate immunity is the destruction of the invading pathogen, thus necessitating that PAMPs recognized by innate immune responses be completely distinct from self molecules. PPRs are host proteins of the innate immune system that recognize PAMPs and are human molecules whose ancestors are evolutionarily ancient (Tables 305-2, 305-3). Thus, recognition of pathogen molecules by hematopoietic and nonhematopoietic cell types leads to activation/production of the complement cascade, cytokines, and antimicrobial peptides as effector molecules.

PATTERN RECOGNITION Major PRR families of proteins include C-type lectins, leucine-rich proteins, macrophage scavenger receptor proteins, plasma pentraxins, lipid transferase, and integrins (Table 305-3). A major group of PRR collagenous glycoproteins with C-type lectin domains are termed *collectins* and include the serum protein, mannose-binding lectin. Mannose-binding lectin and other collectins, as well as two other protein families—the pentraxins (such as C-reactive protein and serum amyloid P) and macrophage scavenger receptors—all have the property of opsonizing (coating) bacteria for phagocytosis by macrophages and can also activate the complement cascade to lyse bacteria. Integrins are cell-surface adhesion molecules that signal cells after cells bind bacterial lipopolysacchride (LPS) and activate phagocytic cells to ingest pathogens.

A remarkable series of recent discoveries has revealed the mechanisms of connection between the innate and adaptive immune systems; these include (1) the plasma protein, LPS-binding protein, which binds and transfers LPS to the macrophage LPS receptor, CD14; and (2) a human family of proteins called *Toll proteins*, which are associated with CD14, bind LPS, and signal the macrophage to produce cytokines and upregulate cell-surface molecules that signal the initiation of adaptive immune responses (Fig. 305-1, Table 305-3, and Table 305-4). Proteins in the Toll family are expressed on macrophages (Toll 2 and Toll 4) and on dendritic cells and B cells (RP105). Upon ligation these receptors activate a series of intracellular events that lead to the killing of bacteria as well as to the recruitment and ultimate activation of antigen-specific T and B lymphocytes (Fig. 305-1). Importantly, signaling by massive amounts of LPS through Toll receptors leads to the release of large amounts of cytokines that mediate LPS-induced shock. Mutations in Toll proteins in mice protect from LPS shock, and mutations in Toll proteins in humans similarly protect from LPS-induced inflammatory diseases such as LPS-induced asthma.

Cells of invertebrates and vertebrates produce antimicrobial small peptides containing fewer than 100 amino acids that can act as endogenous antibodies (Table 305-2). Some of these peptides are produced by epithelia that line various organs, while others are found in macrophages or neutrophils that ingest pathogens. Antimicrobial peptides have been identified that kill bacteria such as *Pseudomonas* spp., *Escherichia coli*, and *Mycobacterium tuberculosis*.

EFFECTOR CELLS OF INNATE IMMUNITY Cells of the innate immune system and their roles in the first line of host defense are described in Table 305-4. Equally important as their roles in the mediation of innate immune responses are the roles that each cell type plays in recruiting T and B lymphocytes of the adaptive immune system to engage in specific antipathogen responses.

Monocytes-Macrophages Monocytes arise from precursor cells within bone marrow (Fig. 305-2) and circulate with a half-life ranging from 1 to 3 days. Monocytes leave the peripheral circulation by marginating in capillaries and migrating into a vast extravascular pool. Tissue macrophages arise from monocytes that have migrated out of the circulation and by in situ proliferation of macrophage precursors in tissue. Common locations where tissue macrophages (and certain of their specialized forms) are found are lymph node, spleen, bone marrow, perivascular connective tissue, serous cavities such as the peritoneum, pleura, skin connective tissue, lung (alveolar macrophage), liver (Kupffer cell), bone (osteoclast), central nervous system (microglia), and synovium (type A lining cell).

In general, monocytes-macrophages are on the first line of defense associated with innate immunity; however, they also play a major role in recruitment of adaptive immune responses by mediation of functions such as binding LPS, the presentation of antigen to T lymphocytes, and the secretion of factors such as interleukin (IL) 1, tumor necrosis factor (TNF), IL-12, and IL-6, which are central to antigen-

Table 305-1 Human Leukocyte Surface Antigens - the CD Classification of Leukocyte Differentiation Antigens

Surface Antigen (Other Names)	Family	Molecular Mass, kDa	Distribution	Ligand(s)	Function
CD1a (T6, HTA-1)	Ig	49	CD, cortical thymocytes	Not known	Possible role in T cell development
CD1b	Ig	45	CD, cortical thymocytes	Not known	Antigen presentation of lipids
CD1c	Ig	43	DC, cortical thymocytes, subset of B cells	Not known	Unknown
CD1d	Ig	?	Cortical thymocytes, intestinal epithelium	Not known	Presentation of peptide antigens
CD2 (T12, LFA-2)	Ig	50	T, NK	CD58, CD48, CD59, CD15	Alternative T cell activation, T cell anergy, T cell cytokine production, T- or NK-mediated cytolysis, T cell apoptosis, cell adhesion
CD3 (T3, Leu-4)	Ig	γ:25–28, δ:21–28, ε:20–25, η:21–22, ζ:16	T	Associates with the TCR	T cell activation and function; ζ is the signal transduction components of the CD3 complex
CD4 (T4, Leu-3)	Ig	55	T, myeloid	MHC-II, HIV, gp120, IL-16, SABP	T cell selection, T cell activation, signal transduction with p56*lck*, primary receptor for HIV
CD7 (3A1, Leu-9)	Ig	40	T, NK	K-12 (CD7L)	T and NK cell signal transduction and regulation of IFN-γ, TNF-α production
CD8 (T8, Leu-2)	Ig	34	T	MHC-I	T cell selection, T cell activation, signal transduction with p56*lck*
CD10 (CALLA,	Zn metalloprotease	100	Early T and B precursors, G,	Not known	Possible role in B cell development; Zn metalloprotease
CD11a (LFA-1α, αL integrin)	α Integrin	170–180	All leukocytes	CD54, CD102, CD50	Cell adhesion, co-stimulation
CD11b (αM integrin, Mac-1, CR3)	α Integrin	165–170	G, M, NK, subset of B and T	iC3b, fibrinogen, CD23	Cell adhesion, phagocytosis, absent in Leukocyte Adhesion Deficiency-1 patients
CD11c (αX integrin, CR4)	α Integrin	145–150	G, M, NK, subset of B and T	iC3b, fibrinogen, CD23	Cell adhesion, phagocytosis, absent in Leukocyte adhesion deficiency (LAD) 1 patients
CD14 (LPS-receptor)	LRG	53–55	M, G (weak), not by myeloid progenitors	Endotoxin (lipopolysaccharide), lipoteichoic acid, PI	Endotoxin (LPS) receptor
CD16a (FcγRIIIA, Leu-11)	Ig	50–65	NK, G, M, subset of T	IgG	Low affinity receptor for IgG, ADCC, activation of cytotoxicity, cytokine production
CD16b (FcγRIIIB)	Ig	50–65	G	IgG	Low-affinity IgG receptor, GPI-linked
CD18 (β2 integrin)	β Integrin	95	All leukocytes	See CD11a, CD11b, CD11c	Associates with CD11a, CD11b, and CD11c; defect in CD18 causes LAD-1
CD19 B4	Ig	95	B (except plasma cells), FDC	Not known	Associates with CD21 and CD81 to form a complex involved in signal transduction in B cell development, activation, and differentiation
CD20 (B1)	Unassigned	33–37	B (except plasma cells)	Not known	Cell signaling, may be important for B cell activation and proliferation
CD21 (B2, CR2, EBV-R, C3dR)	RCA	145	Mature B, FDC, subset of thymocytes	C3d, C3dg, iC3b, CD23, EBV	Associates with CD19 and CD81 to form a complex involved in signal transduction in B cell development, activation, and differentiation; Epstein-Barr virus receptor
CD22 (BL-CAM)	Ig	130–140	Mature B	CDw75	Cell adhesion, signaling through association with p72*sky*, p53/56*lyn*, PI3 kinase, SHP1, fLCγ
CD23 (FcεRII, B6, Leu-20, BLAST-2)	C-type lectin	45	B, M, FDC	IgE, CD21, CD11b, CD11c	Regulates IgE synthesis, cytokine release by monocytes
CD27	TNFR	55	T, B, mature thymocytes, subset NK	CD70	Co-stimulatory for T cell activation
CD28	Ig	44	T, plasma cells	CD80, CD86	Co-stimulatory for T cell activation; involved in the decision between T cell activation and anergy

(continued)

Table 305-1 Human Leukocyte Surface Antigens - the CD Classification of Leukocyte Differentiation Antigens—*(continued)*

Surface Antigen (Other Names)	Family	Molecular Mass, kDa	Distribution	Ligand(s)	Function
CD29 (β1 integrin)	β Integrin	130	Broad	See CD49a–f	Associates with CD49a–f to function in cell adhesion
CD30 (Ki-1 antigen)	TNFR	105–120	M; activated T, B, NK; Hodgkin's cells, certain non-hodgkin's lymphomas	CD153	TCR-mediated cell death, activates NfκB, thymocytes negative selection
CD32 (FcγRII)	Ig	40	M, MP, G, B, P, DC, subset EC	IgG	Low-affinity receptor for IgG mediates endocytosis, cytotoxicity, and immunomodulation
CD34	Sialomucin	90	Hematopoietic progenitor cells, endothelium	L-selectin	Cell adhesion
CD35 (CR1, C3bR, C4bR)	RCA	160–255	G, M, E, B, subset T, RBC, FDC, others	C3b, C4b, iC3b, C3dg, iC3, iC4	Binding of C4b/C3b coated particles, removing and processing immune complexes
CD38 (T10)	Unassigned	45	Early B and T, activated B and T, thymocytes, GC B cells, plasma cells	Not known	Co-stimulatory for T cell and B cell activation, ADP ribosyl cyclase activity
CD40	TNFR	48–50	B, DC, EC, thymic epithelium, MP, cancers	CD154	B cell activation, proliferation, and differentiation, formation of GCs, isotype switching, rescue from apoptosis
CD44 (H-CAM, Hermes, In(Lu)-related)	Hyaladherin	85	Broad	Hyaluronan, MIP-1β, osteopontin, ankyrin	Cell adhesion, signaling, activation
CD44R (CD44v)	Hyaladherin	85–250	Epithelia, M, activated leukocytes	Hyaluronan, MIP-1β, bFGF, ostopontin, ankyrin	Unclear, but possibly mediates cell movement through ECM and the metastasis of certain epithelial malignancies
CD45 (LCA, T200, B220)	PTP	180, 200, 210, 220	All leukocytes	Galectin-1, CD2, CD3, CD4	T and B activation, thymocyte development, signal transduction, apoptosis
CD45RA	PTP	210, 220	Subset T, medullary thymocytes, "naive" T	Galectin-1, CD2, CD3, CD4	Isoforms of CD45 containing exon 4 (A), restricted to a subset of T cells
CD45RB	PTP	200, 210, 220	All leukocytes	Galectin-1, CD2, CD3, CD4	Isoforms of CD45 containing exon 5 (B)
CD45RC	PTP	210, 220	Subset T, medullary thymocytes, "naive" T	Galectin-1, CD2, CD3, CD4	Isoforms of CD45 containing exon 6 (C), restricted to a subset of T cells
CD45RO	PTP	180	Subset T, cortical thymocytes, "memory" T	Galectin-1, CD2, CD3, CD4	Isoforms of CD45 containing no differentially spliced exons, restricted to a subset of T cells
CD49a (VLA-1, α1 integrin)	α Integrin	200–210	M, activated T, NK, subset EC, fibroblasts, neuronal cells	Laminin, collagen I, collagen IV	Cell adhesion, associates with β1 integrin (CD29)
CD49b (VLA-2, α2 integrin, GPIa)	α Integrin	155–165	T and B, P, EC, fibroblasts, subset epithelia	Collagen I, II, III, IV; laminin	Cell adhesion, rgulation of matrix metalloproteinase I and collagen I expression, associates with β1 integrin (CD29)
CD49c (VLA-3, α3 integrin)	α Integrin	145–150	B, subset epithelia, fibroblasts	Fibronectin, collagen, laminin	Cell adhesion, associates with β1 integrin (CD29)
CD49d (VLA-4, α4 integrin)	α Integrin	145–150	B, T, M, NK, DC, subset cancers	CD106, MadCAM-1, fibronectin, invasin, thrombospondin	Cell adhesion, lymphocyte migration, associates with β1 integrin (CD29)
CD49e (VLA-5, α5 integrin, FNR-α)	α Integrin	160	T, M, P, EC, fibroblasts, muscle cells, subset epithelia, progenitor cells	L1, fibronectin	Cell adhesion, migration, matrix assembly, associates with β1 integrin (CD29)
CD49f (VLA-6, α6 integrin)	α Integrin	150	T, M, eosinophils, P, epithelia	Laminin	Cell adhesion, spreading and migration, associates with β1 integrin (CD29)
CD54 (ICAM-1)	Ig	75–115	M, activated T and B, activated EC, activated fibroblasts, subset epithelia	CD11a/CD18, CD11b/CD18, rhinovirus	Cell adhesion, receptor for rhinovirus
CD58 (LFA-3)	Ig	40–70	Broad	CD2	Cell adhesion
CD64 (FCRI)	Ig	72	Myeloid cells	IgG	Binds IgG

(continued)

Table 305-1—*(continued)*

Surface Antigen (Other Names)	Family	Molecular Mass, kDa	Distribution	Ligand(s)	Function
CD70 (CD27L, Ki-24 antigen)	TNF	55–170	Activated T and B, Hodgkin's cells, anaplastic large cell lymphoma	CD27	Antibodies inhibit T cell proliferation in some systems; used for typing lymphomas
CD73 (ecto 5′ nucleotidase)	Unassigned	69–72	Subset of T and B, FDC, EC, epithelia	AMP	Co-stimulatory molecule, may be involved in B-FDC interactions
CD79a	Ig	47	B	Not known	Complexes with sIg to form the BCR
CD79b	Ig	37	B	Not known	Complexes with sIg to form the BCR
CD80 (B7-1, BB1)	Ig	60	Activated B and T, MP, DC	CD28, CD152	Co-regulator of T cell activation; signaling through CD28 stimulates and through CD152 inhibits T cell activation
CD83	Ig	43	DC	Not known	Unknown
CD86 (B7-2, B70)	Ig	80	Subset B, DC, EC, activated T, thymic epithelium	CD28, CD152	Co-regulator of T cell activation; signaling through CD28 stimulates and through CD152 inhibits T cell activation
CD95 (APO-1, Fas)	TNFR	135	Activated T and B	Fas ligand	Mediates apoptosis
CD132 (Common γ chain)	Class I CKR	64–70	T, B, MK, M, G	IL-2, -4, -7, -9, -15	Signal transduction component of the IL-2, -4, -7, -9, and -15 receptors
CD134 (OX40)	TNFR	50	Activated T	gp34	Cell adhesion and T cell co-stimulation
CD152 (CTLA-4)	Ig	30–33	Activated T	CD80, CD86	Inhibits T cell proliferation
CD153 (CD30L)	TNF	38–40	Activated T	CD30	T cell proliferation and cytokine production
CD154 (CD40L)	TNF	33	Activated CD4+ T, subset CD8+ T, NK, M, basophil	CD40	Co-stimulatory for T cell activation, B cell proliferation and differentiation

ABBREVIATIONS: ADCC, antibody-dependent cellular cytotoxicity; AMP, adenosine monophosphate; BL-CAM, B-lymphocyte cell adhesion molecule; BLAST, B cell–specific activation antigen; CALLA, common acute lymphoblasticleukemia antigen; CKR, cytokine receptor; CTLA, cytotoxic T lymphocyte–associated protein; DC, dendritic cells; EBV, Epstein-Barr virus; EC, endothelial cells; ECM, extracellular matrix; FcγRIIIA, low-affinity IgG receptor isoform A; FDC, follicular dendritic cells; G, granulocytes; GC, germinal center; GPI, glycosyl phosphotidylinositol; H-CAM, homing-associated cell adhesion molecule; HTA, human thymocyte antigen; ICAM, intercellular adhesion molecule; IgG, immunoglobulin G; In(Lu), inhibitor lutheran; LCA, leukocyte common antigen; LFA, lymphocyte function antigen; LPS, lipopolysaccharide; LRG, leucine rich repeats; M, monocytes; MAC, macrophage; MadCAM, mucosal addressin cell adhesion molecule; MHC-I, major histocompatibility complex class I; MP, macrophages; Mr, relative molecular mass; NK, natural killer cells; P, platelets; PBT, peripheral blood T cells; PI, phosphotidylinositol; PI3K, phosphotidylinositol 3-kinase; PLC, phospholipase C; PTP, protein tyrosine phosphatase; RBC, red blood cells; SABP, secretory actin binding protein; TCR, T cell receptor; TNF, tumor necrosis factor; TNFR, tumor necrosis factor receptor; VLA, very late activation antigen.

SOURCE: Compiled with permission from T Kishimoto et al (eds): *Leukocyte Typing VI*, New York, Garland Publishing 1997; R Brines et al: Immunology Today 18S:1, 1997; and S Shaw ed: *Protein Reviews on the Web* www.ncbi.nlm.nih.gov/prow.

specific activation of T and B lymphocytes (Fig. 305-1). Although monocytes-macrophages were originally thought to be the major antigen-presenting cells (APCs) of the immune system, it is now clear that dendritic/Langerhans cells are the most potent and effective APCs in the body (see below). Monocytes-macrophages mediate innate immune effector functions such as destruction of antibody-coated bacteria, tumor cells, or even normal hematopoietic cells in certain types of autoimmune cytopenias. Activated macrophages can also mediate antigen-nonspecific lytic activity and eliminate cell types such as tumor cells in the absence of antibody. This activity is largely mediated by cytokines (i.e., TNF-α and IL-1). Monocytes-macrophages express lineage-specific molecules (e.g., the cell-surface LPS receptor, CD14) as well as surface receptors for a number of molecules, including the Fc region of IgG (CD16, CD32, CD64), activated complement components (CD35) (Table 305-1), and various cytokines (Table 305-5). Finally, macrophage secretory products are more diverse than those of any other cell of the immune system. Among monocyte-macrophage-secreted products are hydrolytic enzymes, products of oxidative metabolism, TNF-α, IL-1, -6, -10, -12, -15, -18, and a number of chemoattractant cytokines (chemokines) involved in the orchestration of an immune response in tissues (Table 305-5).

Dendritic/Langerhans Cells Dendritic/Langerhans cells are bone marrow–derived APCs that are distinct from monocytes-macrophages and are derived from both lymphoid and myeloid lineages. They generally lack the standard T, B, NK, and monocyte cell markers but do express CD83 and other molecules that aid in their identification. They can be expanded in culture, and their function is enhanced by the cytokines granulocyte-macrophage colony stimulating factor (GM-CSF), IL-1, IL-4, and TNF-α. They are distinguished by an exceptional ability to present antigen, by expression of high levels of MHC class II and co-stimulatory molecules, and by dendritic morphology with multiple thin membrane projections (veils).

Dendritic cells are referred to as Langerhans cells when they are present in the skin and beneath the mucosal surface. They comprise the dendritic cells of the blood and the spleen and the veil cells of afferent lymphatics, and they form part of the interdigitating cell network of lymphoid organs. In responses involving the innate immune

Table 305-2 Major Components of the Innate Immune System

Pattern recognition receptors (PRR)	C type lectins, leucine-rich proteins, scavenger receptors, pentraxins, lipid transferases, integrins
Antimicrobial peptides	α-Defensins, β-defensins, cathelin, protegrin, granulsyin, histatin, secretory leukoprotease inhibitor, and probiotics
Cells	Macrophages, dendritic cells, NK cells, NK-T cells, neutrophils, eosinophils, mast cells, basophils, and epithelial cells
Complement components	Classic and alternative complement pathway, and proteins that bind complement components
Cytokines	Autocrine, paracrine, endocrine cytokines that mediate host defense and inflammation, as well as recruit, direct, and regulate adaptive immune responses

NOTE: NK cells, natural killer cells.

Table 305-3 Major Pattern Recognition Receptors (PRR) of the Innate Immune System

PRR Protein Family	Sites of Expression	Examples	Ligands (PAMPs)	Functions of PRR
C-type lectins				
Humoral	Plasma proteins	Collectins	Bacterial and viral carbohydrates	Opsonization of bacteria and virus, activation of complement
Cellular	Macrophages, dendritic cell	Macrophage mannose receptor	Terminal mannose	Phagocytosis of pathogens
	Natural killer (NK) cells	NKG2-A	Carbohydrate on HLA molecules	Inhibits killing of host cells expressing HLA+ self peptides
Leucine-rich proteins	Macrophage, epithelial cells	CD14	Lipopolysaccharide (LPS)	Binds LPS and Toll proteins
	Macrophage, many others	Toll proteins (Toll2, Toll4 on macrophages, RP105 on B cells and dendritic cells)	Lipopolysaccharide	Binds LPS and activates the cell to produce cytokines to activate adaptive immunity. Also LPS ligation of Toll or RR105 proteins on macrophages, dendritic cells, or B cell induces B7-1 (CD80) and B7-2 (CD86) co-stimulatory molecules that are required for T and B cell antigen presentation in adaptive immune responses
Scavenger receptors	Macrophage	Macrophage scavenger receptors	Bacterial cell walls	Phagocytosis of bacteria
Pentraxins	Plasma protein	C-creative proteins	Phosphotidyl choline	Opsonization of bacteria, activation of complement
	Plasma protein	Serum amyloid P	Bacterial cell walls	Opsonization of bacteria, activation of complement
Lipid transferases	Plasma protein	LPS binding protein	LPS	Binds LPS, transfers LPS to CD14
Integrins	Macrophages, dendritic cells, NK cells	CD11b,c; CD18	LPS	Signals cells, activates phagocytosis

NOTE: PAMPs, pathogen-associated molecular patterns.
SOURCE: Adapted with permission from Medzhitov and Janeway, 1997a.

system, bacterial LPS binds to dendritic cell RP105 Toll-like protein, upregulating dendritic cell molecules, such as MHC class II, B7-1 (CD80), and B7-2 (CD86), which enhance specific antigen presentation and induce dendritic cell cytokine production.

A critical cell type of the innate immune system is the dendritic cell precursor that, in response to viral infections, produces high levels of interferon (IFN) α. IFN-α in turn activates NK cells to kill virally infected cells and activates monocytes-macrophages and other APCs to recruit antigen-specific T and B cells to respond to viral infections. thus, immature dendritic cells are important components of innate immunity, while mature dendritic cells, as APCs, are important components of adaptive immunity.

Follicular Dendritic Cells Follicular dendritic cells (FDCs) are APCs for B cells and their lineage is distinct from that of dendritic/Langerhans cells, the major APCs for T cells. FDCs are located in the germinal centers of follicles of secondary lymphoid organs. Their main function is to trap and retain antigens in the germinal centers of lymphoid organs and to present these antigens to B cells. Antigen is retained on their membranes in the form of antigen-antibody complexes that bind to the cell via the cellular receptor for C3. FDCs have extensive, thin, finger-like projections that surround the B cells in the germinal centers, allowing for maximal exposure of trapped antigen. The retention of antigen on the surface of FDC membranes is critical for the selection and growth of high-affinity clones of B cells and for the maintenance of B cell memory. Of note, HIV is trapped in large quantities on the processes of FDCs in lymphoid organs, allowing the lymphoid tissue to serve as a reservoir of virus and a source of infection for CD4+ T cells migrating into the area to provide help to B cells in the initiation and propagation of an HIV-specific humoral response (Chap. 309).

Large Granular Lymphocytes/Natural Killer Cells Large granular lymphocytes (LGLs) account for approximately 5 to 10% of peripheral blood lymphocytes. LGLs are nonadherent, nonphagocytic cells with large azurophilic cytoplasmic granules. LGLs express surface receptors for the Fc portion of IgG (CD16) and for NCAM-I (CD56), and many LGLs express some T lineage markers, particularly CD8, and proliferate in response to IL-2. LGLs arise in both bone marrow and thymic microenvironments (Fig. 305-2).

Functionally, LGLs share features with both monocytes-macrophages and neutrophils in that LGLs mediate both antibody-dependent cellular cytotoxicity (ADCC) and NK activity. ADCC is the binding of an opsonized (antibody-coated) target cell to an Fc receptor–bearing effector cell via the Fc region of antibody, resulting in lysis of the target by the effector cell. NK cell activity is the nonimmune (i.e., effector cell never having had previous contact with the target), MHC-unrestricted, non-antibody-mediated killing of target cells, which are usually malignant cell types, transplanted foreign cells, or virus-infected cells. Thus, LGLs that mediate NK cell activity may play an important role in immune surveillance and destruction of cells that spontaneously undergo malignant transformation in vivo. Subsets of NK cells may play a role in hematopoietic cell engraftment; some subsets stimulate bone marrow stem cells, and others stimulate engraftment. Lymphokine-activated killer (LAK) cells are NK lymphocytes that proliferate in vitro to high concentrations of IL-2 and develop the ability to kill tumor cells more efficiently than unstimulated NK cells. Rare patients with complete absence of NK cells have been described who lack both NK cell activity and CD56+, CD16+ lymphocytes but have normal T and B cell function. NK cell hyporesponsiveness is also observed in patients with the *Chédiak-Higashi syndrome*, an autosomal recessive disease associated with fusion of cytoplasmic granules and defective degranulation of neutrophil lysosomes.

The ability of NK cells to kill target cells is inversely related to target cell expression of MHC class I molecules. Thus, NK cells kill target cells with low or no levels of MHC class I expression and are prevented from killing target cells with high levels of class I expression. Recent studies have demonstrated the presence of NK receptors (NK-Rs) or killer cell inhibitory receptors (KIRs) that bind to either classic MHC class I molecules in a polymorphic way or the MHC-class Ib molecule HLA-E (Fig. 305-3). In every person, NK cells express at least one NK-R that recognizes a self–MHC class I allele. NK-Rs of the Ig superfamily bind specific MHC class I molecules; for example, the NK-R p140 binds HLA-A3, and another NK-R, p70, binds HLA-B27 (Fig. 305-3). A second NK-R of the C-type lectin family of proteins is termed *CD94/NKG2A* and binds the MHC-related protein HLA-E (Fig. 305-3). HLA-E has an MHC class I structure but exclusively binds the leader sequence peptides of classic MHC class I molecules in the HLA-E MHC-like "notch" (see "Molecular Basis of T Cell Recognition of Antigen," below). In this manner, CD94/NKG2A NK cell molecules survey and monitor the total level of classic MHC class I molecules on the surface of host cells. When cell-surface levels of host MHC class I molecules decrease, such as occurs during malignant transformation or viral infection of host cells, the altered host cell with diminished MHC class I expression is recognized by NK-Rs, and the NK cell is activated to kill the host tumor or virally infected cells. The ability of NK-Rs to bind to self-MHC and inhibit NK killing of normal host cells is a key protective mechanism for prevention of NK cell–mediated autoimmune disease.

Some NK cells express CD3 and are termed *NK/T cells.* NK/T cells can also express oligoclonal forms of the TCR for antigen that can recognize lipid molecules of intracellular bacteria when presented in the context of CD1 molecules on APCs. This mode of recognition of intracellular bacteria such as *Listeria monocytogenese* and *M. tuberculosis* by NK/T cells is thought to be an important defense mechanism against these organisms that, via usage of a clonal form of TCRs for antigen, incorporates components of both the innate and adaptive immune systems.

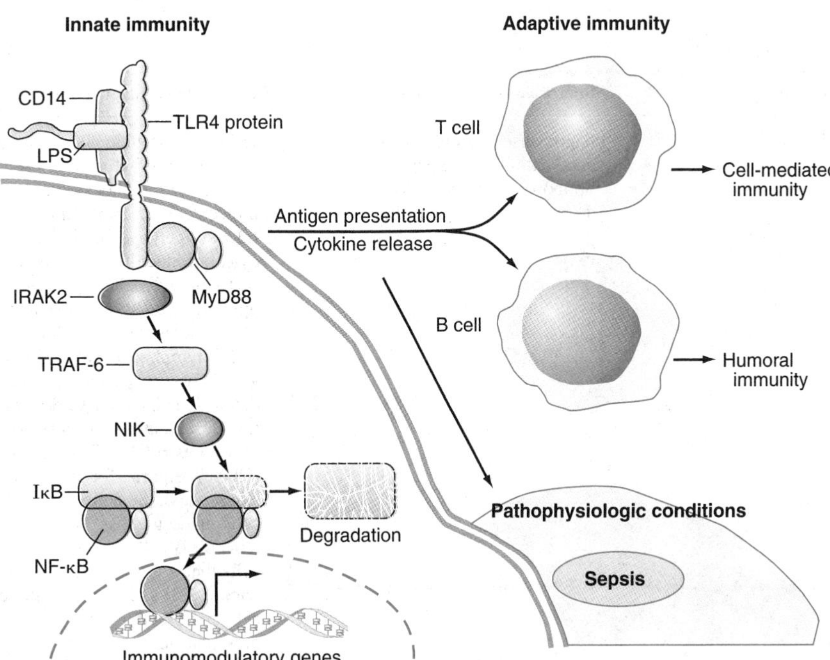

FIGURE 305-1 Role of Toll-like receptors (TLR) in the regulation of the response of macrophages to bacterial lipopolysaccharide (LPS). Lipopolysaccharide, a component of the cell wall of gram-negative bacteria, binds with high affinity to CD14, a glycosyl phosphatidylinositol-linked protein expressed on the surface of macrophages, and to TLR4 protein. This leads to activation of the transmembrane TLR4 protein, initiating an intracellular signaling cascade. Signaling by the TLR4 protein to the transcriptional regulatory complex of NF-κB and IκB occurs through the recruitment of MyD88 (a transcription factor) and the interleukin-1 receptor–associated kinase 2 (IRAK2) and involves the adapter tumor necrosis factor receptor–associated factor 6 (TRAF-6) and the NF-κB-inducing kinase (NIK). These kinases phosphorylate IκB, causing its rapid degradation and the release of NF-κB, which then passes into the nucleus. Once in the nucleus, NF-κB binds to specific sequences in the promoter regions of immunomodulatory genes. This leads to the expression of immunomodulatory genes, including cytokines and co-stimulatory molecules. These gene products act on T and B cells to initiate the adaptive immune response. Under pathophysiologic conditions, high levels of immune system activation by bacterial LPS may lead to septic shock. *(With permission from Modlin et al.)*

Neutrophils, Eosinophils, and Basophils Granulocytes are present in nearly all forms of inflammation and are amplifiers and effectors of innate immune responses. Unchecked accumulation and activation of granulocytes can lead to host tissue damage, as seen in neutrophil- and eosinophil-mediated *systemic necrotizing vasculitis.* Granulocytes are derived from stem cells in bone marrow (Fig. 305-2). Each type of granulocyte (neutrophil, eosinophil, or basophil) is derived from a different subclass of progenitor cell, which is stimulated to proliferate by colony stimulating factors (Table 305-5). During terminal maturation of granulocytes, class-specific nuclear morphology and cytoplasmic granules appear that allow for histologic identification of granulocyte type.

Neutrophils express Fc receptors for IgG (CD16) and receptors for activated complement components (C3b or CD35) (Table 305-1). Upon interaction of neutrophils with opsonized bacteria or immune complexes, azurophilic granules (containing myeloperoxidase, lysozyme, elastase, and other enzymes) and specific granules (containing lactoferrin, lysozyme, collagenase, and other enzymes) are released, and microbicidal superoxide radicals (O_2^-) are generated at the neutrophil surface. The generation of superoxide leads to inflammation by direct injury to tissue and by alteration of macromolecules such as collagen and DNA.

Eosinophils express Fc receptors for IgG (CD32) and are potent cytotoxic effector cells for various parasitic organisms. Intracytoplasmic contents of eosinophils, such as major basic protein, eosinophil cationic protein, and eosinophil-derived neurotoxin, are capable of directly damaging tissues and may be responsible in part for the organ system dysfunction in the *hypereosinophilic syndromes* (Chap. 64). Since the eosinophil granule contains anti-inflammatory types of enzymes (histaminase, arylsulfatase, phospholipase D), eosinophils may homeostatically downregulate or terminate ongoing inflammatory responses.

The normal functions of basophils and tissue mast cells are not completely understood; they are potent reservoirs of cytokines such as IL-4. The capacity of basophil cytokines and mediators to increase local delivery of antibodies and complement by increasing vascular permeability is hypothetical. Thus, the basophil is identified principally with allergic reactions and some delayed cutaneous hypersensitivity states. Certainly, the promotion of increased vascular permeability by basophils is important in the genesis of inflammatory lesions in some vasculitis syndromes (Chap. 317). Basophils express high-affinity surface receptors for IgE (FcRI) and, upon cross-linking of basophil-bound IgE by antigen, release histamine, eosinophil chemotactic factor of anaphylaxis, and neutral protease—all mediators of immediate (anaphylaxis) hypersensitivity responses (Table 305-6). In addition, basophils express surface receptors for activated complement components (C3a, C5a), through which mediator release can be directly effected. →*For further discussion of tissue mast cells, see Chap. 310.*

THE COMPLEMENT SYSTEM The complement system, an important soluble component of the innate immune system, is a series of plasma enzymes, regulatory proteins, and proteins that are activated in a cascading fashion, resulting in cell lysis. There are two arms of the complement system (Fig. 305-4). Activation of the classic complement pathway via C1, C4, and C2 and activation of the alter-

Table 305-4 Cells of the Innate Immune System and Their Major Roles in Triggering Adaptive Immunity

Cell Type	Major Role in Innate Immunity	Major Role in Adaptive Immunity
Macrophages	Phagocytose and kill bacteria; produce antimicrobial peptides; bind lipopolysaccharide (LPS); produce inflammatory cytokines	Produce interleukin (IL) 1 and tumor necrosis factor (TNF) α to upregulate lymphocyte adhesion molecules and chemokines to attract antigen-specific lymphocytes; produce IL-12 to recruit T_H1 helper T cell responses; upregulate co-stimulatory and MHC molecules to facilitate T and B lymphocyte recognition and activation; macrophages and dendritic cells, after LPS signaling, upregulate co-stimulatory molecules B7-1 (CD80) and B7-2 (CD86) required for activation of antigen-specific antipathogen T cells; there are also Toll-like proteins on B cells and dendritic cells that after LPS ligation induce CD80 and CD86 on these cells for T cell antigen presentation.
Precursors of dendritic cells or immature dendritic cells	Produce large amounts of interferon (IFN)α, which has antitumor and antiviral activity	IFN-α is a potent activator of macrophage and mature dendritic cells to phagocytose invading pathogens and present pathogen antigens to T and B cells
Natural killer (NK) cells	Kill foreign and host cells that have low levels of MHC+ self peptides. Express NK receptors that inhibit NK function in the presence of high expression of self-MHC.	Produce TNF-α and IFN-γ that recruit T_H1 helper T cell responses
NK-T cells	Lymphocytes with both T cell and NK surface markers that recognize lipid antigens of intracellular bacteria such as *M. tuberculosis* by CD1 molecules and kill host cells infected with intracellular bacteria.	Produce IL-4 to recruit T_H2 helper T cell responses, IgG1 and IgE production
Neutrophils	Phagocytose and kill bacteria, produce antimicrobial peptides	Produce nitric oxide synthase and nitric oxide that inhibit apoptosis in lymphocytes and can prolong adaptive immune responses
Eosinophils	Kill invading parasites	Produce IL-5 that recruits Ig-specific antibody responses
Mast cells and basophils	Release TNF-α, IL-6, IFN-γ in response to a variety of bacterial PAMPs	Produce IL-4 that recruits T_H2 helper T cell responses and recruit IgG1- and IgE-specific antibody responses
Epithelial cells	Produce anti-microbial peptides; tissue specific epithelia produce mediator of local innate immunity, e.g. lung epithelial cells produce surfactant proteins (proteins within the collectin family) that bind and promote clearance of lung invading microbes	Produce TGF-β that triggers IgA-specific antibody responses

NOTE: MHC, major histocompatibility complex; PAMP, pathogen-associated molecular patterns.
SOURCE: Adapted with permission from Medzhitov and Janeway, 1997a.

native complement pathway via factor D, C3, and factor B both lead to cleavage and activation of C3. C3 is a protein whose activation fragments, when bound to target surfaces such as bacteria and other foreign antigens, are critical for opsonization (coating by antibody and complement) in preparation for phagocytosis.

The protein fragment C3b, split from C3, is necessary for activation of the terminal complement components C5 through C9. These form the membrane attack complex, which, when inserted into cell membranes, brings about osmotic lysis of the cell.

C3b also joins with a cleavage product of factor B (called Bb) to form C3bBb, also known as the *alternative pathway C3 convertase*. Activation of the classic complement pathway results in cleavage of C4 and C2 with a resulting complex of fragments, C4b2a, also called the *classic pathway C3 convertase*. Both the classic pathway C3 convertase (C4b2a) and the alternative pathway C3 convertase (C3bBb) function to cleave C3 to form active C3b, thus driving activation of the C5–9 membrane attack complex. The fact that C3b can combine with Bb to form the alternative pathway C3 convertase gives rise to a potent positive-feedback loop for production of C3b and thus continued activation of terminal complement components.

The classic complement pathway is activated by interaction of antigen and antibody to form immune complexes that bind C1q, a subunit of C1. Immunoglobulin isotypes that bind C1q and activate the classic pathway are IgM, IgG1, IgG2, and IgG3. In contrast, IgA1, IgA2, and IgD activate complement via the alternative pathway. Activation of the complement cascade via the classic pathway by IgG- or IgM-containing immune complexes is a rapid and efficient pathway to activation of terminal complement components. In contrast, activation of the alternative complement pathway via IgA-containing immune complexes or by bacterial endotoxin is a slower and less efficient pathway to terminal component activation. Thus the immunoglobulin isotype composition of immune complexes is a critical factor in determining complement activation and the efficiency of clearance of immune complexes by C3 receptor–bearing cells.

In addition to the role of complement in opsonization of bacteria and cell lysis, several complement fragments are potent mediators of immune cell activation. C3a and C5a bind to receptors on mast cells and basophils, resulting in release of histamine and other mediators of anaphylaxis. C5a is also a potent chemoattractant for neutrophils and monocytes-macrophages (Table 305-7).

CYTOKINES Cytokines are soluble proteins produced by a wide variety of hematopoietic and nonhematopoietic cell types (Table 305-5). They are critical for both normal innate and adaptive immune responses, and their expression may be perturbed in most immune, inflammatory, and infectious disease states.

Cytokines are involved in the regulation of the growth, development, and activation of immune system cells and in the mediation of the inflammatory response. In general, cytokines are characterized by considerable redundancy in that different cytokines have similar functions. In addition, many cytokines are pleiotropic in that they are capable of acting on many different cell types. This pleiotropism results from the expression on multiple cell types of receptors for the same cytokine (see below), leading to the formation of "cytokine networks." The action of cytokines may be: (1) autocrine when the target cell is the same cell that secretes the cytokine, (2) paracrine when the target cell is nearby, and (3) endocrine when the cytokine is secreted into the circulation and acts distal to the source. A number of classifications have been proposed for the grouping of cytokines according to functions; however, these are all imperfect because of the fact that a number of cytokines overlap these groupings. One empirical classification divides the cytokines into the following three groups:

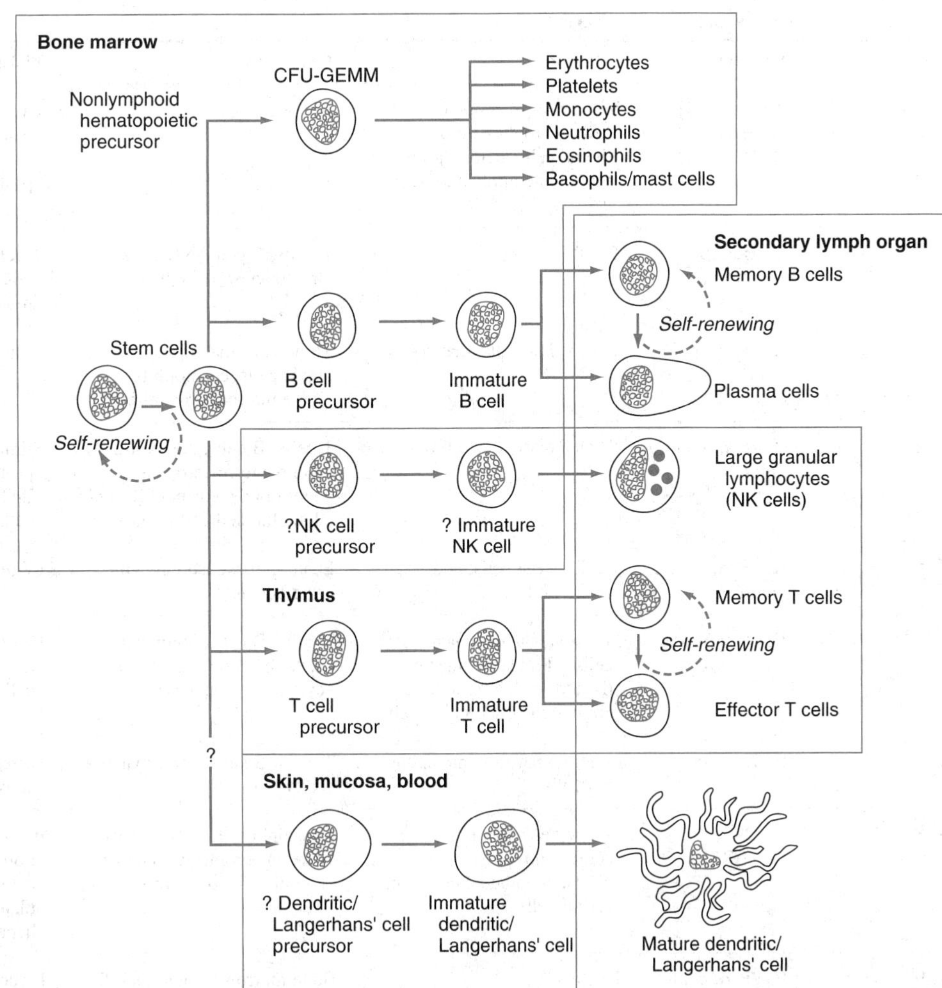

FIGURE 305-2 Hematopoietic stem cell differentiation in bone marrow, thymus, and secondary lymphoid organs. *[After BF Haynes, SM Denning, in G Stamatoyannopoulos et al (eds): The Molecular Basis of Blood Diseases, 2d ed. Philadelphia, Saunders, 1993, with permission].*

1. Immunoregulatory cytokines involved in the activation, growth, and differentiation of lymphocytes and monocytes, e.g., IL-2, IL-4, IL-10, IFN-γ, and transforming growth factor (TGF) β
2. Proinflammatory cytokines produced predominantly by mononuclear phagocytes in response to infectious agents (e.g., IL-1, TNF-α, and IL-6) and the chemokine family of inflammatory cytokines, within which are included IL-8, monocyte chemotactic protein (MCP)-1, MCP-2, MCP-3, macrophage inflammatory protein (MIP)-1α, MIP-1β, and regulation-upon-activation, normal T expressed and secreted (RANTES) (Chap. 64)
3. Cytokines that regulate immature leukocyte growth and differentiation, e.g., IL-3, IL-7, and GM-CSF.

In general, cytokines exert their effects by influencing gene activation that results in cellular activation, growth, differentiation, functional cell-surface molecule expression, and cellular effector function. In this regard, cytokines can have dramatic effects on the regulation of immune responses and the pathogenesis of a variety of diseases. Indeed, T cells have been categorized on the basis of the pattern of cytokines that they secrete that results in either humoral immune response (T_H2) or a cell-mediated immune response (T_H1).

Cytokine receptors can be grouped into five general families based on similarities in their extracellular amino acid sequences and conserved structural domains (Fig. 305-5). The *immunoglobulin (Ig) superfamily* represents a large number of cell-surface and secreted proteins. All members of the Ig superfamily must have at least one common domain in their protein structure. The IL-1 receptors (type 1, type 2) are examples of cytokine receptors with extracellular Ig domains.

The hallmark of the *hematopoietic growth factor (type 1) receptor* family is that the extracellular regions of each receptor contain two conserved motifs. One motif located at the N terminus is rich in cysteine residues. The other motif is located at the C terminus proximal to the transmembrane region and comprises five amino acid residues, tryptophan-serine-X-tryptophan-serine (WSXWS). Cytokine receptors expressing the WSXWS motif are also referred to as "type I family of cytokine receptors." This family can be further grouped on the basis of the number of receptor subunits they have and on the utilization of shared subunits. The shared common receptors often have a critical role in signal transduction. A number of cytokine receptors, i.e., IL-6, IL-11, IL-12, and leukemia inhibitory factor, are paired with gp130. There is also a common 150-kDa subunit shared by IL-3, IL-5, and GM-CSF receptors. The gamma chain (γ_c) of the IL-2 receptor is common to the IL-2, IL-4, IL-7, IL-9, and IL-15 receptors. Thus, the specific cytokine receptor is responsible for ligand-specific binding, while the subunits such as gp130, the 150-kDa subunit, and γ_c are important in signal transduction. The γ_c gene is on the X chromosome, and mutations in the γ_c protein result in the X-linked form of severe combined immune deficiency syndrome (X-SCID) (Chap. 308).

The members of the *interferon (type II) receptor* family include the receptors for IFN-γ, and -β, which share a similar 210-amino-acid binding domain with conserved cysteine pairs at both the amino and carboxy termini. The receptors for the interferons consist of at least two distinct subunits.

The members of the *TNF (type III) receptor family* share a common binding domain composed of repeated cysteine-rich regions. Members of this family include the p55 and p75 receptors for TNF (TNFR1 and TNFR2, respectively); CD40 antigen, which is an important B cell–surface marker involved in immunoglobulin isotype switching; fas/Apo-1, whose triggering induces apoptosis (programmed cell death); CD27 and CD30, which are found on activated T cells and B cells; and nerve growth factor receptor.

The common motif for the *seven transmembrane helix family* was originally found in receptors linked to GTP-binding proteins. This family includes receptors for chemokines, β-adrenergic receptors, and retinal rhodopsin. It is important to note that two members of the chemokine receptor family, CXC chemokine receptor type 4 (CXCR4)

Table 305-5 Cytokines and Cytokine Receptors

Cytokine	Receptor	Cell Source	Cell Target	Biologic Activity
IL-1α,β	Type 1 IL-1R, type 2 IL-1R	Monocytes/macrophages, B cells, fibroblasts, most epithelial cells including thymic epithelium, endothelial cells	All cells	Upregulates adhesion molecule expression, neutrophil and macrophage emigration; mimics shock, fever; upregulates hepatic acute-phase protein production; facilitates hematopoiesis
IL-2	IL-2R α,β, common γ	T cells	T cells, B cells, NK cells, monocytes/macrophages	T cell activation and proliferation, B cell growth, NK cell proliferation and activation, enhanced monocyte/macrophage cytolytic activity
IL-3	IL-3R, common β	T cells, NK cells, mast cells	Monocytes/macrophages, mast cells, eosinophils, bone marrow progenitors	Stimulation of hematopoietic progenitors
IL-4	IL-4R α, common γ	T cells, mast cells, basophils	T cells, B cells, NK cells, monocytes/macrophages, neutrophils, eosinophils, endothelial cells, fibroblasts	Stimulates T_H2 helper T cell differentiation and proliferation; stimulates B cell Ig class switch to IgG1 and IgE; anti-inflammatory action on T cells, monocytes
IL-5	IL-5R α, common β	T cells, mast cells, and eosinophils	Eosinophils, basophils, murine B cells	Regulates eosinophil migration and activation
IL-6	IL-6R, gp130	Monocytes/macrophages, B cells, fibroblasts, most epithelium including thymic epithelium, endothelial cells	T cells, B cells, epithelial cells, hepatocytes, monocytes/macrophages	Induction of acute-phase protein production, T and B cell differentiation and growth, myeloma cell growth, osteoclast growth and activation
IL-7	IL-7R α, common γ	Bone marrow, thymic epithelial cells	T cells, B cells, bone marrow cells	Differentiation of B, T, and NK cell precursors, activation of T and NK cells
IL-8	CXCR1, CXCR2	Monocytes/macrophages, T cells, neutrophils, fibroblasts, endothelial cells, epithelial cells	Neutrophils, T cells, monocytes/macrophages, endothelial cells, basophils	Induces neutrophil, monocyte, and T cell migration; induces neutrophil adherance to endothelial cells and histamine release from basophils; stimulates angiogenesis; suppresses proliferation of hepatic precursors
IL-9	IL-9R α, common γ	T cells	Bone marrow progenitors, B cells, T cells, mast cells	Induces mast cell proliferation and function, synergizes with IL-4 in IgG and IgE production, T cell growth, activation, and oncogenesis
IL-10	IL-10R	Monocytes/macrophages, T cells, B cells, keratinocytes, mast cells	Monocytes/macrophages, T cells, B cells, NK cells, mast cells	Inhibits macrophage proinflammatory cytokine production; downregulates cytokine class II antigen and B7-1 and B7-2 expression; inhibits differentiation of T_H1 helper T cells; inhibits NK cell function; stimulates mast cell proliferation and function and B cell activation and differentiation
IL-11	IL-11R, gp130	Bone marrow stromal cells	Megakaryocytes, B cells, hepatocytes	Induces megakaryocyte colony formation and maturation; enhances antibody responses; stimulates acute-phase protein production
IL-12 (35-kDa and 40-kDa subunits)	IL-12R	Activated macrophages, dendritic cells, neutrophils	T cells, NK cells	Induces T_H1 T helper cell formation and lymphokine-activated killer cell formation; increases CD8+ CTL activity
IL-13	IL-13/IL-4R	T cells (T_H2)	Monocytes/macrophages, B cells, endothelial cells, keratinocytes	Upregulation of VCAM-1 and C-C chemokine expression on endothelial cells; B cell activation and differentiation; inhibits macrophage proinflammatory cytokine production
IL-14	Unknown	T cells	Normal and malignant B cells	Induces B cell proliferation
IL-15	IL-15R α, common γ, IL-2R β	Monocytes/macrophages, epithelial cells, fibroblasts	T cells, NK cells	T cell activation and proliferation; promotes angiogenesis and NK cells
IL-16	CD4	Mast cells, eosinophils, CD8+ T cells, respiratory epithelium	CD4+ T cells, monocytes/macrophages, eosinophils	Chemoattraction of CD4+ T cells, monocytes, and eosinophils; inhibits HIV replication; inhibits T cell activation through CD3/T cell receptor

(continued)

Table 305-5—*(continued)*

Cytokine	Receptor	Cell Source	Cell Target	Biologic Activity
IL-17	IL17R	CD4+ T cells	Fibroblasts, endothelium, epithelium	Enhanced cytokine secretion
IL-18	IL-18R (IL-1R-related protein)	Keratinocytes, macrophages	T cells, B cells, NK cells	Upregulated IFN-γ production, enhanced NK cell cytotoxicity
IFN-α	Type I interferon receptor	All cells	All cells	Antiviral activity; stimulates T cell, macrophage, and NK cell activity; direct antitumor effects; upregulates MHC class I antigen expression; used therapeutically in viral and autoimmune conditions
IFN-β	Type I interferon receptor	All cells	All cells	Antiviral activity; stimulates T cell, macrophage, and NK cell activity; direct antitumor effects; upregulates MHC class I antigen expression; used therapeutically in viral and autoimmune conditions
IFN-γ	Type II interferon receptor	T cells, NK cells	All cells	Regulates macrophage and NK cell activation; stimulates immunoglobulin secretion by B cells; induction of class II histocompatibility antigens; T_H1 T cell differentiation
TNF-α	TNF-RI, TNF-RII	Monocytes/macrophages, mast cells, basophils, eosinophils, NK cells, B cells, T cells, keratinocytes, fibroblasts, thymic epithelial cells	All cells except erythrocytes	Fever, anorexia, shock, capillary leak syndrome, enhanced leukocyte cytotoxicity, enhanced NK cell function, acute-phase protein synthesis, proinflammatory cytokine induction
TNF-β	TNF-RI, TNF-RII	T cells, B cells	All cells except erythrocytes	Cell cytotoxicity, lymph node and spleen development
LTβ	LTβR	T cells	All cells except erythrocytes	Cell cytotoxicity, normal lymph node development
G-CSF	G-CSFR; gp130	Monocytes/macrophages, fibroblasts, endothelial cells, thymic epithelial cells, stromal cells	Myeloid cells, endothelial cells	Regulates myelopoiesis; enhances survival and function of neutrophils; clinical use in reversing neutropenia after cytotoxic chemotherapy
GM-CSF	GM-CSFR; common β	T cells, monocytes/macrophages, fibroblasts, endothelial cells, thymic epithelial cells	Monocytes/macrophages, neutrophils, eosinophils, fibroblasts, endothelial cells	Regulates myelopoiesis; enhances macrophage bactericidal and tumoricidal activity; mediator of dendritic cell maturation and function; upregulates NK cell function; clinical use in reversing neutropenia after cytotoxic chemotherapy
M-CSF	M-CSFR (c-*fms* proto-oncogene)	Fibroblasts, endothelial cells, monocytes/macrophages, T cells, B cells, epithelial cells including thymic epithelium	Monocytes/macrophages	Regulates monocyte/macrophage production and function
LIF	LIFR; gp130	Activated T cells, bone marrow stromal cells, thymic epithelium	Megakaryocytes, monocytes, hepatocytes, possibly lymphocyte subpopulations	Induces hepatic acute-phase protein production; stimulates macrophage differentiation; promotes growth of myeloma cells and hematopoietic progenitors; stimulates thromboiesis
OSM	OSMR; LIFR; gp130	Activated monocytes/macrophages and T cells, bone marrow stromal cells, some breast carcinoma cell lines, myeloma cells	Neurons, hepatocytes, monocytes/macrophages, adipocytes, alveolar epithelial cells, embryonic stem cells, melanocytes, endothelial cells, melanocytes, endothelial cells, fibroblasts, myeloma cells	Induces hepatic acute-phase protein production; stimulates macrophage differentiation; promotes growth of myeloma cells and hematopoietic progenitors; stimulates thrombopoiesis; stimulates growth of Kaposi's sarcoma cells.
SCF	SCFR (c-*kit*-proto-oncogene)	Bone marrow stromal cells and fibroblasts	Embryonic stem cells, myeloid and lymphoid precursors, mast cells	Stimulates hematopoietic progenitor cell growth, mast cell growth; promotes embryonic stem cell migration

(continued)

Table 305-5 Cytokines and Cytokine Receptors—*(continued)*

Cytokine	Receptor	Cell Source	Cell Target	Biologic Activity
TGF-β (3 isoforms)	Type I, II, III TGF-β receptor	Most cell types	Most cell types	Downregulates T cell, macrophage, and granulocyte responses; stimulates synthesis of matrix proteins; stimulates angiogenesis
Lymphotactin/ SCM-1	Unknown	NK cells, mast cells, double negative thymocytes, activated CD8+ T cells	T cells, NK cells	Chemoattractant for lymphocytes; only known chemokine of C class
MCP-1	CCR2	Fibroblasts, smooth-muscle cells, activated PBMCs	Monocytes/macrophages, NK cells, memory T cells, basophils	Chemoattractant for monocytes, activated memory T cells, and NK cells; induces granule release from CD8+ T cells and NK cells; potent histamine-releasing factor for basophils; suppresses proliferation of hematopoietic precursors; regulates monocyte protease production
MCP-2	CCR1, CCR2	Fibroblasts, activated PBMCs	Monocytes/macrophages, T cells, eosinophils, basophils, NK cells	Chemoattractant for monocytes, memory and naive T cells, eosinophils, ? NK cells; activates basophils and eosinophils; regulates monocyte protease production
MCP-3	CCR1, CCR2	Fibroblasts, activated PBMCs	Monocytes/macrophages, T cells, eosinophils, basophils, NK cells, dendritic cells	Chemoattractant for monocytes, memory and naive T cells, dendritic cells, eosinophils, ? NK cells; activates basophils and eosinophils; regulates monocyte protease production
MCP-4	CCR2, CCR3	Lung, colon, small intestinal epithelial cells, activated endothelial cells	Monocytes/macrophages, T cells, eosinophils, basophils	Chemoattractant for monocytes, T cells, eosinophils, and basophils
Eotaxin	CCR3	Pulmonary epithelial cells, heart	Eosinophils, basophils	Potent chemoattractant for eosinophils and basophils; induces allergic airways disease; acts in concert with IL-5 to activate eosinophils; antibodies to eotaxin inhibit airway inflammation
TARC	CCR4	Thymus, dendritic cells, activated T cells	T cells, NK cells	Chemoattractant for T and NK cells
MDC	CCR4	Monocytes/macrophages, dendritic cells, thymus	Activated T cells	Chemoattractant for activated T cells; inhibits infection with T cell tropic HIV
MIP-1α	CCR1, CCR5	Monocytes/macrophages, T cells	Monocytes/macrophages, T cells, dendritic cells, NK cells, eosinophils, basophils	Chemoattractant for monocytes, T cells, dendritic cells, NK cells; weak chemoattractant for eosinophils and basophils; activates NK cell function; suppresses proliferation of hematopoietic precursors; necessary for myocarditis associated with Coxsackie virus infection; inhibits infection with monocytotropic HIV
MIP-1β	CCR5	Monocytes/macrophages, T cells	Monocytes/macrophages, T cells, NK cells, dendritic cells	Chemoattractant for monocytes, T cells, and NK cells; activates NK cell function; inhibits infection with monocytotropic HIV
RANTES	CCR1, CCR2, CCR5	Monocytes/macrophages, T cells, fibroblasts, eosinophils	Monocytes/macrophages, T cells, NK cells, dendritic cells, eosinophils, basophils	Chemoattractant for monocytes/macrophages, CD4+ CD45RO+ T cells, CD8+ T cells, NK cells, eosinophils, and basophils, induces histamine release from basophils; inhibits infection with monocytotropic HIV
LARC/MIP-3α/Exodus-1	CCR6	Dendritic cells, fetal liver cells, activated T cells	T cells, B cells	Chemoattractant for lymphocytes
ELC/MIP-3β	CCR7	Thymus, lymph node, appendix	Activated T cells and B cells	Chemoattractant for B and T cells; receptor upregulated on EBV-infected B cells and HSV-infected T cells
I-309/TCA-3	CCR8	Activated T cells	Monocytes/macrophages, T cells	Chemoattractant for monocytes; prevents glucocorticoid-induced apoptosis in some T cell lines
SLC/TCA-4/Exodus-2	Unknown	Thymic epithelial cells, lymph node, appendix, and spleen	T cells	Chemoattractant for T lymphocytes; inhibits hematopoiesis

(continued)

Table 305-5—*(continued)*

Cytokine	Receptor	Cell Source	Cell Target	Biologic Activity
DC-CK1/ PARC	Unknown	Dendritic cells in secondary lymphoid tissues	Naive T cells	May have a role in the induction of immune responses
TECK	Unknown	Dendritic cells, thymus, liver, small intestine	T cells, monocytes/macrophages, dendritic cells	Thymic dendritic cell–derived cytokine, possibly involved in T cell development
GRO-α/MGSA	CXCR2	Activated granulocytes, monocytes/macrophages, and epithelial cells	Neutrophils, epithelial cells, ?endothelial cells	Neutrophil chemoattractant and activator; mitogenic for some melanoma cell lines; suppresses proliferation of hematopoietic precursors; angiogenic activity
GROβ/ MIP-2α	CXCR2	Activated granulocytes and monocytes/macrophages	Neutrophils and ?endothelial cells	Neutrophil chemoattractant and activator; angiogenic activity
NAP-2	CXCR2	Platelets	Neutrophils, basophils	Derived from platelet basic protein; neutrophil chemoattractant and activator
IP-10	CXCR3	Monocytes/macrophages, T cells, fibroblasts, endothelial cells, epithelial cells	Activated T cells, tumor-infiltrating lymphocytes, ?endothelial cells, ?NK cells	IFN-γ-inducible protein that is a chemoattractant for T cells; suppresses proliferation of hematopoietic precursors
MIG	CXCR3	Monocytes/macrophages, T cells, fibroblasts	Activated T cells, tumor-infiltrating lymphocytes	IFN-γ-inducible protein that is a chemoattractant for T cells; suppresses proliferation of hematopoietic precursors
SDF-1	CXCR4	Fibroblasts	T cells, dendritic cells, ? basophils, ? endothelial cells	Low-potency, high-efficacy T cell chemoattractant; required for B lymphocyte development; prevents infection of CD4+, CXCR4+ cells by T cell tropic HIV
Fractalkine	CX3CR1	Activated endothelial cells	NK cells, T cells, monocytes/ macrophages	Cell surface chemokine/mucin hybrid molecule that functions as a chemoattractant, leukocyte activator, and cell adhesion molecule
PF-4	Unknown	Platelets, megakaryocytes	Fibroblasts, endothelial cells	Chemoattractant for fibroblasts; suppresses proliferation of hematopoietic precursors; inhibits endothelial cell proliferation and angiogenesis

NOTE: CCR, CC-type chemokine receptor; CSF, colony stimulating factor; CXCR, CXC-type chemokine receptor; DC-CK, dendritic cell chemokine; EBV, Epstein-Barr virus; ELC, EBI1 ligand chemokine (MIP-1β); G-CSF, granulocyte CSF; GM-CSF, granulocyte-macrophage CSF; GRO, growth-related peptide; IFN, interferon; IL, interleukin; IP, IFN-γ-inducible protein; LARC, liver and activation-regulated chemokine; LIF, leukemia inhibitory factor; LT, lymphotoxin; MCP, monocyte chemotactic protein; M-CSF, macrophage CSF; MDC, macrophage-derived chemokine; MGSA, melanoma growth-stimulating activity; MHC, major histocompatibility complex; MIG, monoteine induced by IFN-γ; MIP, macrophage inflammatory protein; NAP, neutrophil-activating protein; NK, natural killer; OSM, oncostatin M; PARC, pulmonary and activation-regulated chemokine; PMBC, peripheral blood mononuclear cells; PF, platelet factor; RANTES, regulated on activation, normally T cell expressed and secreted; SCF, stem cell factor; SDF, stromal cell–derived factor; SLC, secondary lymphoid tissue chemokine; TARC, thymus and activation-regulated chemokine; TCA, T cell activation protein; TECK, thymus-express chemokine; TGF, transforming growth factor; TNF, tumor necrosis factor; VCAM, vascular cell adhesion molecule.

SOURCE: From JS Sundy et al, in J Gallin and R Snyderman (eds): *Inflammation, Basic Principles and Clinical Correlates*, 3d ed. Philadelphia, Lippincott Williams & Wilkins, 1999, with permission.

and β chemokine receptor type 5 (CCR5), have recently been found to serve as the two major coreceptors for binding and entry of HIV into CD4-expressing host cells (Chap. 309). Both cytokines and their receptors share similar structures and functions. For example, ligands for the TNF receptor family of receptors regulate and determine activation for programmed cell death (*apoptosis*) and all ligate molecules of the same structural family. Similarly IL-3, IL-5, and GM-CSF are all produced by T helper (T_H) 2 cells, and the receptors of these cytokines share common γ chains. Thus, cytokines and their receptors may have diversified together during evolution.

Significant advances have been made in defining the signaling pathways through which cytokines exert their effects intracellularly. This is particularly true with regard to the diverse family of hematopoietin receptors. The Janus family of protein tyrosine kinases (JAK) is a critical element involved in signaling via the hematopoietin receptors. There are four known JAK kinases, JAK1, JAK2, JAK3, and Tyk2, which preferentially bind different receptor subunits. Cytokine binding to its receptor brings the cytokine receptor subunits into apposition and allows a pair of JAKs to transphosphorylate and activate one another. The JAKs then phosphorylate the receptor on the tyrosine residues and allow signaling molecules to bind to the receptor, where these molecules in turn can become phosphorylated. These signaling molecules can bind the receptor because they have domains (SH2, or src homology 2 domains) that can bind phosphorylated tyrosine residues. There are a number of these important signaling molecules that bind the receptor, such as the adapter molecule SHC, which can couple the receptor to the activation of the mitogen-activated protein kinase pathway. In addition, a very important class of substrate of the JAKs is the signal transducers and activators of transcription (STAT) family of transcription factors. STATs have SH2 domains that enable them to bind to phosphorylated receptors, where they are then phosphorylated by the JAKs. It appears that different STATs have specificity for different receptor subunits. The STATs then dissociate from the receptor and translocate to the nucleus, bind to DNA motifs that they recognize, and regulate gene expression. The STATs preferentially bind DNA motifs that are slightly different from one another and thereby presumably control transcription of specific genes. The importance of this pathway is particularly relevant to lymphoid development. Mutations of JAK3 itself also result in a disorder identical to X-SCID; however, since JAK3 is found on chromosome 19 and not on the X chromosome, JAK3 deficiency occurs in boys and girls (Chap. 308). In this chapter the cytokines that affect various cell types are discussed in the context of each of the cell types.

THE ADAPTIVE IMMUNE SYSTEM Adaptive immunity is characterized by antigen-specific responses to a foreign antigen or pathogen and, compared to innate immunity which occurs immediately

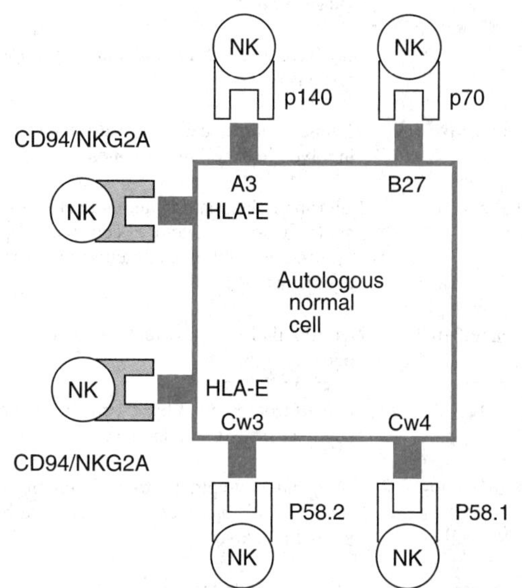

FIGURE 305-3 A schematic representation of the human natural killer (NK) receptor repertoire. The NK cells of a given individual express clonally distributed NK-Rs for self-HLA class I molecules. In this representative donor (HLA haplotype: HLA-A1, A3; HLA-B7, B27; HLA-Cw3, Cw4), NK cells express at least one inhibitory receptor that interacts with self-HLA alleles. The NK-Rs depicted in white are those belonging to the Ig superfamily that recognize allelic forms of HLA class I molecules. CD94/NKG2A receptors (stippled blue) bind to the MHC class I–like molecules, HLA-E, that present leader sequence peptides of classic MHC class I molecules to CD94/NKG2A molecules. The receptors belonging to the Ig superfamily do not cover the whole set of HLA class I alleles and are not expressed by 100% of NK cells. CD94/NKG2A receptors play important roles in monitoring the total level of MHC class I molecules on viral and malignantly transformed cells. *(Adapted from Moretta A et al, with permission.)*

(1 to 2 days), generally takes several days or longer to materialize. A key feature of adaptive immunity is memory for the antigen such that subsequent antigen exposures lead to more rapid and often more vigorous immune responses. The adaptive immune system consists of dual limbs of cellular and humoral immunity. The principal effectors of cellular immunity are T lymphocytes, while the principal effectors of humoral immunity are B lymphocytes (Table 305-8). Both B and T lymphocytes derive from a common stem cell (Fig. 305-2).

The proportion and distribution of immunocompetent cells in various tissues reflect cell traffic, homing patterns, and functional capabilities. Bone marrow is the major site of maturation of B cells, monocytes-macrophages, and granulocytes and contains pluripotent stem cells which, under the influence of various colony stimulating factors, are capable of giving rise to all hematopoietic cell types (Fig. 305-2). T cell precursors also arise from hematopoietic stem cells and home to the thymus for maturation. Mature T lymphocytes, B lymphocytes, monocytes, and dendritic/Langerhans cells enter the circulation and home to peripheral lymphoid organs (lymph nodes, spleen) and the gut-associated lymphoid tissue (tonsil, Peyer's patches, and appendix) as well as the skin and mucous membranes and await activation by foreign antigen.

T CELLS The pool of effector T cells is established in the thymus early in life and is maintained throughout life both by new T cell production in the thymus and by antigen-driven expansion of virgin peripheral T cells into "memory" T cells that reside in peripheral lymphoid organs. The thymus exports approximately 2% of the total number of thymocytes per day throughout life, with the total number of daily thymic emigrants decreasing by approximately 3% per year during the first four decades of life. Thymic emigrants can be identified

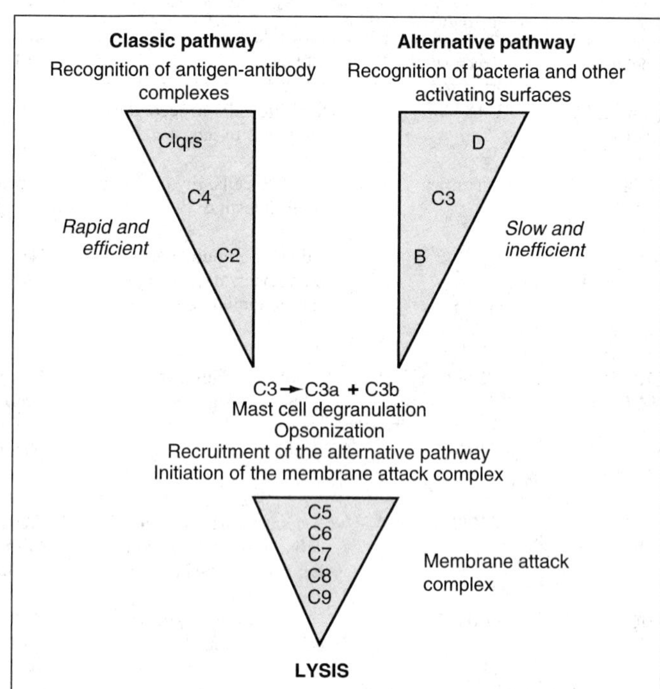

FIGURE 305-4 Components of the complement system. *(After Paul, with permission.)*

Table 305-6 Mediators Released from Human Mast Cells and Basophils

Mediator	Actions
Histamine	Smooth-muscle contraction, increased vascular permeability
Slow-reacting substance of anaphylaxis (SRSA) (leukotriene C4, D4, E4)	Smooth-muscle contraction
Eosinophil chemotactic factor of anaphylaxis (ECF-A)	Chemotactic attraction of eosinophils
Platelet-activating factor	Activates platelets to secrete serotonin and other mediators: smooth-muscle contraction; induces vascular permeability
Neutrophil chemotactic factor (NCF)	Chemotactic attraction of neutrophils
Leukotactic activity (leukotriene B4)	Chemotactic attraction of neutrophils
Heparin	Anticoagulant
Basophil kallikrein of anaphylaxis (BK-A)	Cleaves kininogen to form bradykinin

Table 305-7 Biologic Activities of Some Complement Components

Component	Activity
C4a weak anaphylatoxin	Evokes histamine release from basophils and mast cells
C3a	Anaphylatoxin; evokes histamine release from basophils and mast cells
C5a	Anaphylatoxin; evokes histamine release from basophils and mast cells; potent chemoattractant for monocytes and neutrophils
C3b, C3bi	Enhancement of phagocytosis by neutrophils and monocytes; promotes immune-complex binding to cells within monocyte-macrophage system, as well as neutrophils; C3b with Bb forms alternative pathway C3 convertase and amplifies alternative pathway; promotes solubilization of immune complexes
C5–9	Membrane attack complex; forms transmembrane channels leading to cell destruction

SOURCE: After S Ruddy, in WN Kelley et al (eds): *Textbook of Rheumatology*, 4th ed. Philadelphia, Saunders, 1993, with permission.

by the expression of certain combinations of T cell surface markers and by the presence in nuclei of excised (deleted) pieces of rearranged TCR DNA, called *T cell receptor excision circles*.

Mature T lymphocytes constitute 70 to 80% of normal peripheral blood lymphocytes (only 2% of the total-body lymphocytes are contained in peripheral blood), 90% of thoracic duct lymphocytes, 30 to 40% of lymph node cells, and 20 to 30% of spleen lymphoid cells. In lymph nodes, T cells occupy deep paracortical areas around B cell germinal centers, and in the spleen, they are located in periarteriolar areas of white pulp (Chap. 63). T cells are the primary effectors of cell-mediated immunity, with subsets of T cells maturing into CD8+ cytotoxic T cells capable of lysis of virus-infected or foreign cells. In general, CD4+ T cells are also the primary regulatory cells of T and B lymphocyte and monocyte function by the production of cytokines and by direct cell contact. In addition, T cells regulate erythroid cell maturation in bone marrow, and through cell contact (CD40 ligand) have an important role in activation of B cells and induction of Ig isotype switching.

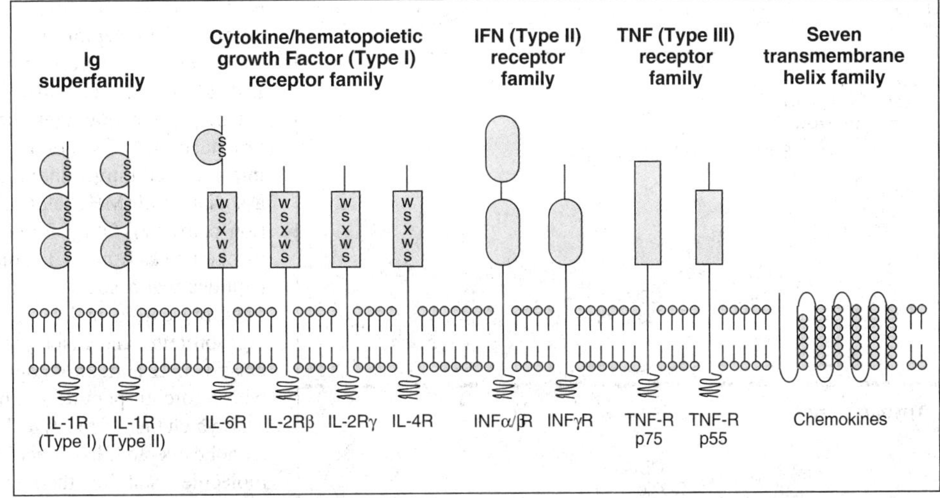

FIGURE 305-5 Cytokine family receptor members. Cytokine receptors have been segregated into several large families based on similarities in the extracellular amino acid sequences and conserved structural domains. There are five cytokine receptor family members. See text for details. *(After Abbas et al, with permission.)*

Human T cells express cell-surface proteins that mark stages of intrathymic T cell maturation or identify specific functional subpopulations of mature T cells. Many of these molecules mediate or participate in important T cell functions (Table 305-1; Fig. 305-6).

A number of cytokines regulate the process of T cell proliferation and differentiation (Table 305-5). The earliest identifiable T cell precursors in bone marrow are CD34+ pro-T cells (i.e., cells in which TCR genes are neither rearranged nor expressed). In the thymus, CD34+ T cell precursors begin cytoplasmic (c) synthesis of components of the CD3 complex of TCR-associated molecules (Fig. 305-6.) Within T cell precursors, TCR for antigen gene rearrangement begins under the influence of IL-7 and yields two T cell lineages, expressing either TCR$\alpha\beta$ chains or TCR$\gamma\delta$ chains. T cells expressing the TCR$\alpha\beta$ chains comprise the majority of peripheral T cells in blood, lymph node, and spleen and terminally differentiate into either CD4+ or CD8+ cells. Cells expressing TCR$\gamma\delta$ chains circulate as a minor population in blood; their functions, although not fully understood, have been postulated to be those of immune surveillance at epithelial surfaces and cellular defenses against mycobacterial organisms and other intracellular bacteria (see below). Immature cortical thymocytes express, in addition to CD1, both CD4 and CD8 (i.e., they are double positive); however, upon reaching functional maturity, T cell expression of CD1 ceases, and CD4 and CD8 are reciprocally expressed. (i.e., T cells become single positive for either CD4 or CD8).

In the thymus, the recognition of self-peptides on thymic epithelial cells, thymic macrophages, and dendritic cells plays an important role in shaping the T cell repertoire to recognize foreign antigen (*positive selection*) and in eliminating highly autoreactive T cells (*negative selection*). As immature cortical thymocytes begin to express surface TCR for antigen, autoreactive thymocytes are destroyed (negative selection), thymocytes with TCRs capable of interacting with foreign antigen peptides in the context of self–MHC antigens are activated and develop to maturity (positive selection), and thymocytes with TCR that are incapable of binding to self–MHC antigens die of attrition (*no selection*). Mature thymocytes that are positively selected are either CD4+ helper T cells or MHC class II–restricted cytotoxic (killer) T cells, or they are CD8+ T cells destined to become MHC class I–restricted cytotoxic T cells. For T cells to be *MHC class I–* or *class II–restricted* means that T cells recognize antigen peptide fragments only when they are presented in the antigen-recognition site of a class I or class II MHC molecule, respectively (see below).

After thymocyte maturation and selection, mature CD4 and CD8 thymocytes leave the thymus and migrate to all sites of the peripheral immune system. It is important to note that the adult thymus continues to function, albeit with decreasing output, well into adult life, with detectable function though age 50. Thus, the thymus continues to be a contributor to the peripheral immune system, both normally and when the peripheral T cell pool is damaged, such as occurs in AIDS and cancer chemotherapy.

MOLECULAR BASIS OF T CELL RECOGNITION OF ANTIGEN The TCR for antigen is a complex of molecules consisting of an antigen-binding heterodimer of either $\alpha\beta$ or $\gamma\delta$ chains noncovalently linked with five CD3 subunits (γ, δ, ϵ, ζ, and η) (Fig. 305-7). The CD3 ζ chains are either disulfide-linked homodimers (CD3-ζ_2) or disulfide-linked heterodimers composed of one ζ chain and one η chain. TCR$\alpha\beta$ or TCR$\gamma\delta$ molecules must be associated with CD3 molecules to be inserted into the T cell surface membrane, TCRα being paired with TCRβ and TCRγ being paired with TCRδ. Molecules of the CD3 complex mediate transduction of T cell activation signals via TCRs, while TCRα and β or γ and δ molecules combine to form the TCR antigen-binding site.

The α, β, γ, and δ TCR for antigen molecules have amino acid sequence homology and structural similarities to immunoglobulin heavy and light chains and are thus members, along with other important molecules of immune cells of the *immunoglobulin gene superfamily* of molecules (e.g., MHC class I or II, CD3, CD4, CD8). The genes encoding the TCR molecules are encoded as clusters of gene segments that rearrange during the course of T cell maturation.

Table 305-8 Components of the Adaptive Immune System

Cellular
Thymus-derived (T) lymphocytes—T cell precursors in the thymus; naive mature T lymphocytes before antigen exposure; memory T lymphocytes after antigen contact; helper T lymphocytes for B and T cell responses; cytotoxic T lymphocytes that kill pathogen-infected target cells

Humoral
Bone-marrow-derived (B) lymphocytes—B cell precursors in bone marrow; naive B cells prior to antigen recognition, memory B cells after antigen contact; plasma cells that secrete specific antibody

Cytokines
Soluble proteins that direct, focus, and regulate specific T versus B lymphocyte immune responses

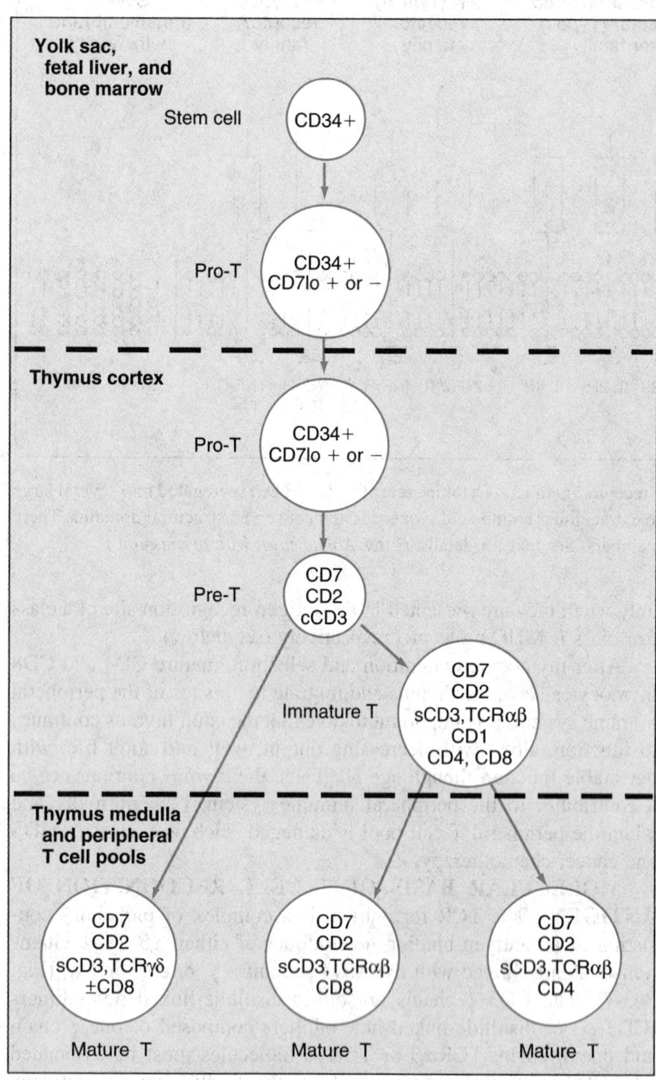

FIGURE 305-6 Human T cell maturation. sCD3, surface CD3 expression; cCD3, cytoplasmic CD3 expression; TCR, T cell receptor.

This creates an efficient and compact mechanism for housing the diversity requirements of antigen receptor molecules. The TCRα chain is on chromosome 14 and consists of a series of V (variable), J (joining), and C (constant) regions. The TCRβ chain is on chromosome 7 and consists of multiple V, D (diversity), J, and C TCRβ loci. The TCRγ chain is on chromosome 7, and the TCRδ chain is in the middle of the TCRα locus on chromosome 14. Thus, molecules of the TCR for antigen have constant (framework) and variable regions, and the gene segments encoding the α, β, γ, and δ chains of these molecules are recombined and selected in the thymus, culminating in synthesis of the completed molecule. In both T and B cell precursors (see below), DNA rearrangements of antigen receptor genes involves the same enzymes, recombinase activating gene (RAG)1 and RAG2, both DNA-dependent protein kinases.

TCR diversity is created by the different V, (D), and J segments that are possible for each receptor chain by the many permutations of V, D, and J segment combinations, by "N-region diversification" due to the addition of nucleotides at the junction of rearranged gene segments, and the pairing of individual chains to form a TCR dimer. As T cells mature in the thymus, the repertoire of antigen-reactive T cells is modified by selection processes that eliminate many autoreactive T cells, enhance the proliferation of cells that function appropriately with self-MHC molecules and antigen, and allow T cells with nonproductive TCR rearrangements to die. Like B cell antigen receptors (Ig molecules), TCRs may also undergo affinity maturation by somatic mutation of the receptor, once they leave the thymus.

T cells do not recognize native protein or carbohydrate antigens. Instead, T cells recognize only short (approximately 9 to 13 amino acids) peptide fragments derived from protein antigens taken up or produced in APCs. Foreign antigens may be taken up by endocytosis into acidified intracellar vesicles and degraded into small peptides that associate with MHC class II molecules (exogenous antigen-presentation pathway). Other foreign antigens arise endogenously in the cytosol (such as from replicating viruses) and are broken down into small peptides that associate with MHC class I molecules (endogenous antigen-presenting pathway). Thus, APCs proteolytically degrade foreign proteins and display peptide fragments embedded in the MHC class I or II antigen-recognition site on the MHC molecule surface, where foreign peptide fragments are available to bind to TCR$\alpha\beta$ or TCR$\gamma\delta$ chains of reactive T cells (Fig. 305-8). CD4 molecules act as an adhesive and, by direct binding to MHC class II (DR, DQ, or DP) molecules, stabilize the interaction of TCR with peptide antigen (Fig. 305-7). Similarly, CD8 molecules also act as adhesives to stabilize the TCR-antigen interaction by direct CD8 molecule binding to MHC class I (A, B, or C) molecules.

Antigens that arise in the cytosol and are processed via the endogenous antigen-presentation pathway are cleaved into small peptides by a 28-subunit complex of proteases called the *proteasome*. From the proteasome, antigen peptide fragments are transported from the cytosol into the lumen of the endoplasmic reticulum by a heterodimeric complex termed *transporters associated with antigen processing*, or TAP proteins. There, MHC class I molecules in the endoplasmic reticulum membrane physically associate with processed cytosolic peptides. Following peptide association with class I molecules, peptide–class I complexes are exported to the Golgi apparatus, and then to the cell surface, for recognition by CD8+ T cells.

Antigens taken up from the extracellular space via endocytosis into intracellular acidified vesicles are degraded by vesicle proteases into peptide fragments. Intracellular vesicles containing MHC class II molecules fuse with peptide-containing vesicles, thus allowing peptide fragments to physically bind to MHC class II molecules. Peptide–MHC class II complexes are then transported to the cell surface for recognition by CD4+ T cells.

Whereas it is generally agreed that the TCR$\alpha\beta$ receptor recognizes peptide antigens in the context of MHC class I or class II molecules, recent data suggest that lipids in the cell wall of intracellular bacteria such as *M. tuberculosis* can also be presented to a wide variety of T cells, including subsets of CD4−, CD8− TCR$\alpha\beta$ T cells, TCR$\gamma\delta$ T cells, and a subset of CD8+ TCR$\alpha\beta$ T cells. Importantly, bacterial lipid antigens are not presented in the context of MHC class I or II molecules, but rather are presented in the context of MHC-related CD1 molecules. Some $\gamma\delta$ T cells that recognize lipid antigens via CD1 molecules have very restricted TCR usage, do not need antigen priming to respond to bacterial lipids, and may actually be a form of innate rather than acquired immunity to intracellular bacteria.

Just as foreign antigens are degraded and their peptide fragments presented in the context of MHC class I or class II molecules on APCs, endogenous self-proteins are also degraded and self-peptide fragments are presented to T cells in the context of MHC class I or class II molecules on APCs. In peripheral lymphoid organs, T cells are present that are capable of recognizing self-protein fragments but normally are *anergic* or *tolerant*, i.e., nonresponsive to self-antigenic stimulation, due to lack of self-antigen upregulating APC *co-stimulatory molecules* such as B7-1 and B7-2 (see below).

Once engagement of mature T cell TCR by foreign peptide occurs in the context of self–MHC class I or class II molecules, binding of non-antigen-specific adhesion ligand pairs such as CD54-CD11/CD18 and CD58-CD2 stabilizes MHC peptide–TCR binding and the expression of these adhesion molecules is upregulated (Fig. 305-7). Once antigen ligation of the TCR occurs, the T cell membrane is partitioned into *lipid membrane microdomains*, or *lipid rafts*, that coalesce the key signaling molecules TCR/CD3 complex, CD28, CD2, LAT (linker for activation of T cells), intracellular activated (dephosphorylated) src family protein tyrosine kinases (PTKs), and the key CD3ζ-associated protein-70 (ZAP-70) PTK (Fig. 305-7). Importantly, during T cell activation, the dephosphorylating molecule, CD45, with protein tyrosine phosphatase activity is partitioned away from the TCR complex to allow activating phosphorylation events to occur. The coalescence of signaling molecules of activated T lymphocytes in *microdomains* has suggested that T cell–APC interactions can be considered *immunologic synapses*, analogous in function to neuronal synapses.

After TCR-MHC binding is stabilized, activation signals are transmitted through the cell to the nucleus that lead to the expression of gene products important in mediating the wide diversity of T cell functions such as the secretion of IL-2. The TCR does not have intrinsic signaling activity but is linked to a variety of signaling pathways via immunoreceptor tyrosine-based activation motifs (ITAMs) expressed on the various CD3 chains that bind to proteins that mediate signal transduction. Each of the pathways results in the activation of particular transcription factors that control the expression of cytokine and cytokine receptor genes. Thus, antigen-MHC binding to the TCR induces the activation of the src family of PTKs, fyn and lck (lck is associated with CD4 or CD8 co-stimulatory molecules); phosphorylation of CD3ζ chain; activation of the related tyrosine kinases ZAP-70 and syk; and downstream activation of the calcium-dependent calcineurin pathway, the ras pathway, and the protein kinase C pathway. Each of these pathways leads to activation of specific families of transcription factors (including NF-AT, fos and jun, and rel/NF-κB) that form heteromultimers capable of inducing expression of IL-2, IL-2 receptor, IL-4, TNF-α, and other T cell mediators. The src family kinases require dephosphorylation of an inactivation site by CD45 phosphatase before they can be phosphorylated on an activation site. Furthermore, the activity through the receptor is downregulated by the csk-PEP enzyme, a phosphatase that inactivates the src family kinases.

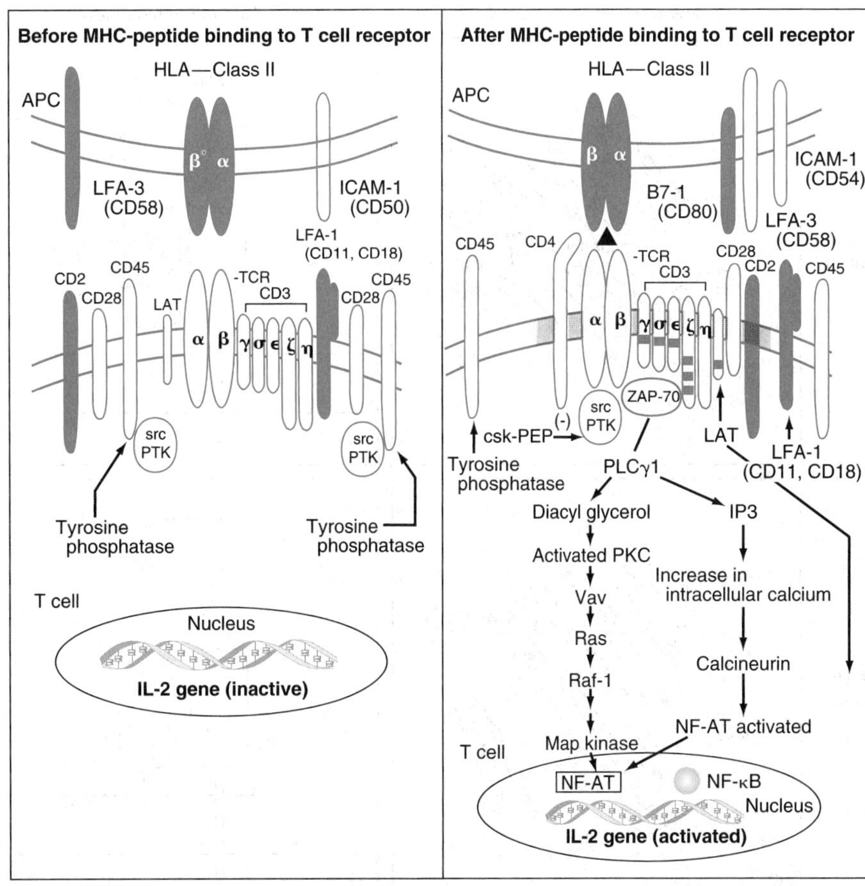

FIGURE 305-7 Molecules involved in human T cell recognition of antigen and in human T cell activation. *A*. Schematic arrangement of antigen-presenting cell (APC) molecules (top cell) and T cell molecules (bottom cell) before MHC-peptide binding to T cell receptor (TCR). *B*. The changes that occur in T cell and APC molecules after MHC-peptide binding to TCR. The black triangle at the tip of the αβ chains of MHC class II molecules represents a peptide fragment of "processed" protein antigen. After TCR ligation, src protein tyrosine kinase (PTK) is activated via dephosphorylation and the TCR complex is joined by CD4, CD2, and CD28 as well as the linker for activated T lymphocytes (LAT) in a lipid microdomain area (gray area). Activation signals are mediated via immunoreceptor tyrosine-based activation (ITAM) sequences in LAT and CD3 chains (blue bars) that bind to enzymes and transduce activation signals to the nucleus via the indicated intracellular activation pathways. See text for details of the activation and signal transduction process. *(Adapted from Thomas; from Robey and Allison; and from Weiss and Littman, with permission.)*

In addition to the signals delivered to the T cell from the TCR and CD4 and CD8 molecules, co-stimulatory receptors [such as CD28 activated by CD80 (B7-1) and/or CD86 (B7-2)] also deliver important signals that upregulate the function of the T cell. The CD28 signal transduction pathway appears particularly important. CD28 signals through phosphoinositide-3-phosphate kinase; its downstream effects are not completely clear. However, if signal transduction through CD28 does not occur in concert with TCR ligation, or if CD28 is blocked, the T cell becomes inactivated or anergic (nonresponsive or tolerant) rather than activated.

CTLA-4 (CD52) is an Ig superfamily molecule on T cells that, like CD28, is a ligand for B7-1 and B7-2 but has a higher affinity for B7-1 and B7-2 than does CD28. T cell CTLA-4 ligation sends a negative signal to the T cell to become tolerant or nonresponsive to antigen stimulation after TCR-MHC ligation. Blocking of CD28-mediated co-stimulation occurs when a second ligand for B7-1 and B7-2 ligates an APC while the TCR is bound to MHC. Thus, a convergence of molecular and biochemical events involving co-stimulatory molecules is required for normal T cell recognition of antigen and consequent T cell activation. In order to exploit this biology for therapeutic purposes, one clinical strategy currently being tested is administration of soluble recombinant CTLA-4 protein to patients at the time of organ transplantation in order to induce a cohort of organ transplant–specific tolerant T cells and thereby reduce the rejection of organ allografts. Alternatively, blocking CTLA-4/B7 interactions with soluble CD28 or CTLA-4 monoclonal antibodies might possibly be therapeutically useful to enhance immune responses to human cancers (see "Immunotherapy," below).

T CELL SUPERANTIGENS Conventional antigens bind to MHC class I or II molecules in the groove of the αβ heterodimer and bind to T cells via the V regions of the TCRα and -β chains (Fig. 305-7). In contrast, superantigens bind directly to the lateral portion of the TCRβ chain and MHC class II β chain and stimulate T cells based solely on the Vβ gene segment utilized independent of the D, J, and Vα sequences present. *Superantigens* are protein molecules capable of activating up to 20% of the peripheral T cell pool, whereas conventional antigens activate fewer than 1 in 10,000 T cells. T cell superantigens include staphylococcal enterotoxins, other bacterial products, and certain nonhuman retroviral proteins. Superantigen stimulation of human peripheral T cells occurs in the clinical setting of the *staphylococcal toxic shock syndrome*, leading to massive overproduction of T cell cytokines (Chap. 139).

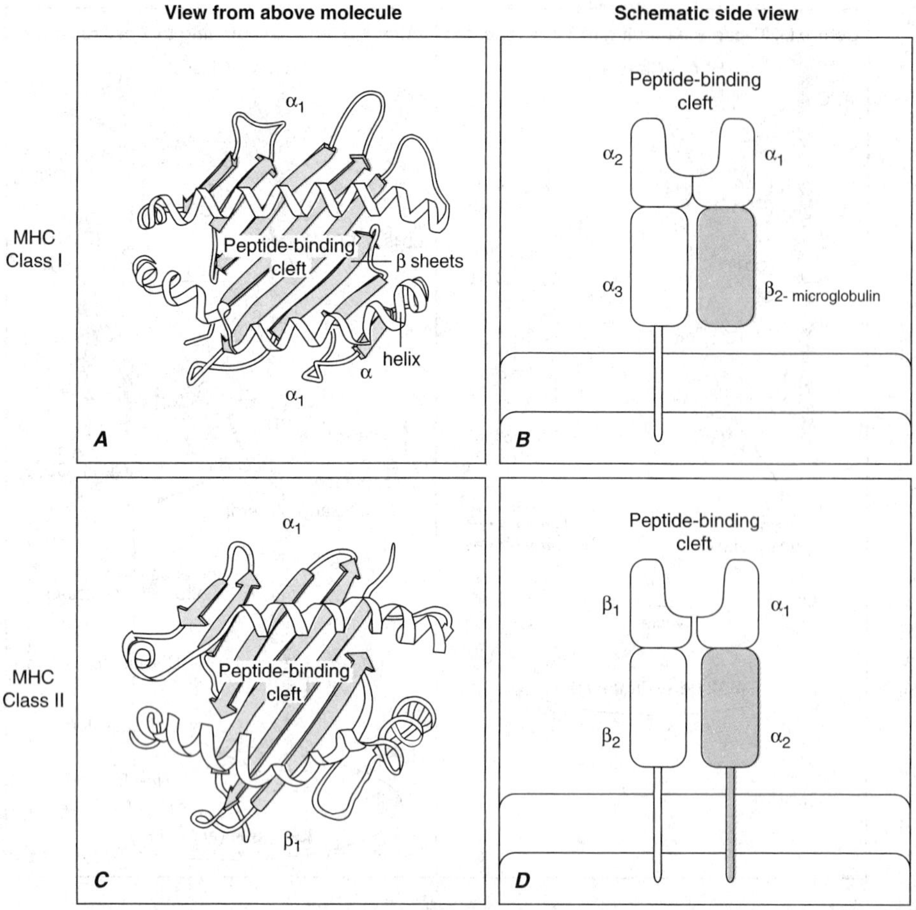

FIGURE 305-8 Structure of MHC class I and MHC class II molecules. *A* and *B*. Top and schematic side views of an MHC class I molecule. *C* and *D*. Top and schematic side views of an MHC class II molecule. Peptide-binding cleft is the location of short peptide fragments derived from proteolytic cleavage of either foreign or self-proteins. Whereas the peptide-binding cleft of class I comprises the α_1, α_2, and α_3 domains of the class I α chain, the peptide-binding cleft of class II comprises the β_1 and α_1 domains of the class II β and α chains, respectively. *(From Janeway et al, with permission.)*

B CELLS Mature B cells comprise 10 to 15% of human peripheral blood lymphocytes, 50% of splenic lymphocytes, and approximately 10% of bone marrow lymphocytes. B cells express on their surface intramembrane immunoglobulin (Ig) molecules that function as B cell receptors (BCR) for antigen in a complex of Ig-associated α and β signaling molecules with properties similar to those described in T cells (Fig. 305-9). Unlike T cells, which recognize only processed peptide fragments of conventional antigens embedded in the notches of MHC class I and class II antigens of APCs, B cells are capable of recognizing and proliferating to whole unprocessed native antigens via antigen binding to B cell surface Ig (sIg) receptors. B cells also express surface receptors for the Fc region of IgG molecules (CD32) as well as receptors for activated complement components (C3d or CD21, C3b or CD35). The primary function of B cells is to produce antibodies. B cells also serve as APCs and are highly efficient at antigen processing. Their antigen-presenting function is enhanced by a variety of cytokines. Mature B cells are derived from bone marrow precursor cells that arise continuously throughout life (Figs. 305-2, 305-10).

B lymphocyte development can be separated into antigen-independent and antigen-dependent phases. Antigen-independent B cell development occurs in primary lymphoid organs, including fetal liver and bone marrow, and includes all stages of B cell maturation up to the sIg+ mature B cell. Antigen-dependent B cell maturation is driven by the interaction of antigen with the mature B cell sIg, leading to memory B cell induction, Ig class switching, and plasma cell formation. Antigen-dependent stages of B cell maturation occur in secondary lymphoid organs, including lymph node, spleen, and gut Peyer's patches. In contrast to the T cell repertoire that is for the most part generated intrathymically before contact with foreign antigen, the repertoire of B cells expressing diverse antigen-reactive sites is modified by further alteration of Ig genes after stimulation by antigen—a process called *somatic mutation*—which occurs in lymph node germinal centers.

During B cell development, diversity of the antigen-binding variable region of Ig is generated by an ordered set of Ig gene rearrangements that are similar to the rearrangements undergone by TCR α, β, γ, and δ genes. Heavy chain rearrangements precede those for light chains. For the heavy chain, there is first a rearrangement of D segments to J segments, followed by a second rearrangement between a V gene segment and the newly formed D-J sequence; the C segment is aligned to the V-D-J complex to yield a functional Ig heavy chain gene (V-D-J-C). During later stages, a functional κ or λ light chain gene is generated by rearrangement of a V segment to a J segment, ultimately yielding an intact Ig molecule composed of heavy and light chains.

The process of Ig gene rearrangement is regulated to result in a single antibody specificity produced by each B cell, with each Ig molecule comprising one type of heavy chain and one type of light chain. Although each B cell contains two copies of Ig light and heavy chain genes, only one gene of each type is productively rearranged and expressed in each B cell, a process termed *allelic exclusion.*

There are approximately 300 V_κ genes and 5 J_κ genes, resulting in the pairing of V_κ and J_κ genes to create over 1500 different light chain combinations. The number of distinct κ light chains that can be generated is increased by

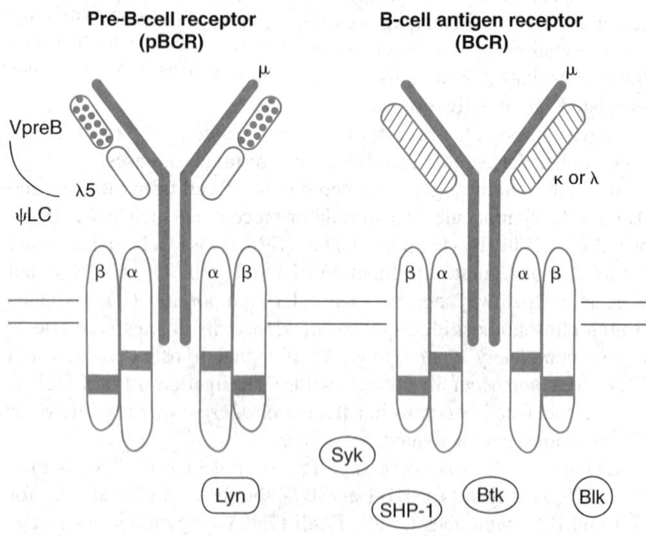

FIGURE 305-9 The pre-B cell receptor and B-cell antigen receptor associate with the signal-transducing heterodimer Igα/Igβ. Solid horizontal bars in α and β chains denote the immunoreceptor tyrosine-based activation motif (ITAM). Signals from the antigen receptors are further propagated downstream by other signaling molecules such as the syk and the src family of tyrosine kinases (fyn, lyn, blk, and btk), as well as by the phosphatase, SHP-1. *(Adapted from Lam and Rajewsky, with permission.)*

somatic mutations within the V_κ and J_κ genes, thus creating large numbers of possible specificities from a limited amount of germ-line genetic information. As noted above, in heavy chain Ig gene rearrangement, the VH domain is created by the joining of three types of germ-line genes called V_H, D_H, and J_H, thus allowing for even greater diversity in the variable region of heavy chains than of light chains.

The most immature B cell precursors (early pro-B cells) lack cytoplasmic Ig (cIg) and sIg (Fig. 305-10). The large pre-B cell is marked by the acquisition of the surface pre-BCR composed of μ heavy (H) chains and a pre-B light chain, termed ψLC (Fig. 305-9). ψLC is a surrogate light chain receptor encoded by the nonrearranged V pre-B and the λ5 light chain locus (the pre-BCR). Pro- and pre-B cells are driven to proliferate and mature by signals from bone marrow stroma, in particular, IL-7. Light chain rearrangement occurs in the small pre-B cell stage such that the full BCR is expressed at the immature B cell stage. Immature B cells have rearranged Ig light chain genes and express sIgM. As immature B cells develop into mature B cells, sIgD is expressed as well as sIgM. At this point, B lineage development in bone marrow is complete, and B cells exit into the peripheral circulation and migrate to secondary lymphoid organs to encounter specific antigens.

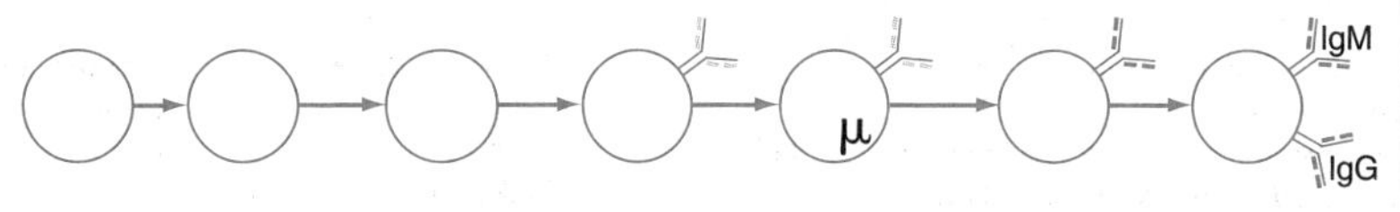

	Stem cell	Early pro-B cell	Late pro-B cell	Large pre-B cell	Small pre-B cell	Immature B cell	Mature B cell
					μ		IgM IgG
H-chain genes	Germline	DJ Rearranged	V-DJ Rearranged	VDJ Rearranged	VDJ Rearranged	VDJ Rearranged	VDJ Rearranged
L-chain genes	Germline	Germline	Germline	Germline	V-J Rearrangment	VJ Rearranged	VJ Rearranged
Surface Ig	Absent	Absent	Absent	μ H-chain at surface as part of pre-β receptor	μ H-chain in cytoplasm and at surface	IgM expressed on cell surface	IgD and IgM made from alternatively spliced H-chain transcripts
Surface Marker Proteins	CD34	CD34 CD10 CD19 CD38	CD10 CD19 CD20 CD38 CD40	CD19 CD20 CD38 CD40	CD19 CD20 CD38 CD40	CD19 CD20 CD40	CD19 CD20 CD21 CD40

FIGURE 305-10 Developmental stages of B cells. Elements of the developing B cell receptor for antigen (BCR) are shown schematically. The classification into the various stages of B cell development is primarily defined by rearrangement of the immunoglobulin (Ig), heavy (H), and light (L) chain genes and by the absence or presence of specific surface markers. *(Adapted from Janeway et al, with permission.)*

Random rearrangements of Ig genes occasionally generates self-reactive antibodies, and mechanisms must be in place to correct these mistakes. One such mechanism is BCR editing, whereby autoreactive BCRs are mutated to not react with self-antigens. If receptor editing is unsuccessful in eliminating autoreactive B cells, then autoreactive B cells undergo negative selection in the bone marrow through induction of apoptosis after BCR engagement of self-antigen.

After leaving the bone marrow, B cells populate peripheral B cell sites, such as lymph node and spleen, and await contact with foreign antigens that react with each B cell's clonotypic receptor. As antigen-driven B cell activation occurs through the BCR, a process known as *somatic hypermutation* takes place whereby point mutations in rearranged H- and L-genes give rise to mutant sIg molecules, some of which bind antigen better than the original sIg molecules. Somatic hypermutation, therefore, is a process whereby memory B cells in peripheral lymph organs have the best binding, or the highest affinity antibodies. This overall process of generating the best antibodies is called *affinity maturation of antibody*.

Lymphocytes that synthesize IgG, IgA, and IgE are derived from sIgM+, sIgD+ mature B cells. Ig class switching occurs in lymph node and other peripheral lymphoid tissue germinal centers. Pairs of CD40+ B cells and CD40 ligand+ T cells bind and drive B cell Ig switching via T cell–produced cytokines such as IL-4 and TGF-β. IL-1, -2, -4, -5, and -6 synergize to drive mature B cells to proliferate and differentiate into Ig-secreting cells.

Humoral Mediators of Adaptive Immunity: Immunoglobulins Immunoglobulins are the products of differentiated B cells and mediate the humoral arm of the immune response. The primary functions of antibodies are to bind specifically to antigen and bring about the inactivation or removal of the offending toxin, microbe, parasite, or other foreign substance from the body. The structural basis of Ig molecule function and Ig gene organization has provided insight into the role of antibodies in normal protective immunity, pathologic immune-mediated damage by immune complexes, and autoantibody formation against host determinants.

All immunoglobulins have the basic structure of two heavy and two light chains (Figs. 305-9 and 305-11). Immunoglobulin isotype (i.e., G, M, A, D, E) is determined by the type of Ig heavy chain present. IgG and IgA isotypes can be divided further into subclasses (G1, G2, G3, G4, and A1, A2) based on specific antigenic determinants on Ig heavy chains. The characteristics of human immunoglobulins are outlined in Table 305-9. The four chains are covalently linked by disulfide bonds. Each chain is made up of a V region and C regions (also called *domains*), themselves made up of units of approximately 110 amino acids. Light chains have one variable (V_L) and one constant (C_L) unit; heavy chains have one variable unit (V_H) and three or four constant (C_H) units, depending on isotype. As the name suggests, the constant, or C, regions of Ig molecules are made up of homologous sequences and share the same primary structure as all other Ig chains of the same isotype and subclass. Constant regions are involved in biologic functions of Ig molecules. The C_{H2} domain of IgG and the C_{H4} units of IgM are involved with the binding of the C1q portion of C1. The C_H region at the carboxy-terminal end of the IgG molecule, the Fc region (Fig. 305-11), binds to surface Fc receptors (CD16, CD32, CD64) of macrophages, LGLs, B cells, neutrophils, and eosinophils.

Variable regions (V_L and V_H) constitute the antibody-binding (Fab) region of the molecule. Within the V_L and V_H regions are hy-

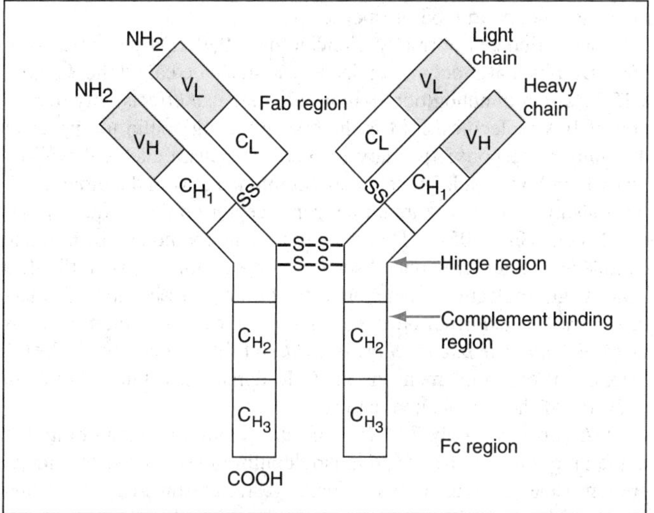

FIGURE 305-11 Schematic structure of the immunoglobulin G (IgG) molecule.

Table 305-9 Physical, Chemical, and Biologic Properties of Human Immunoglobulins

Property	IgG	IgA	IgM	IgD	IgE
Usual molecular form	Monomer	Monomer, dimer	Pentamer, hexamer	Monomer	Monomer
Other chains	None	J chain, SC	J chain	None	None
Subclasses	G1, G2, G3, G4	A1, A2	None	None	None
Heavy chain allotypes	Gm (=30)	No A1, A2m (2)	None	None	None
Molecular mass, kDa	150	160, 400	950, 1150	175	190
Sedimentation constant, Sw20	6.6S	7S, 11S	19S	7S	8S
Carbohydrate content, %	3	7	10	9	13
Serum level in average adult, mg/mL	9.5–12.5	1.5–2.6	0.7–1.7	0.04	0.0003
Percentage of total serum Ig	75–85	7–15	5–10	0.3	0.019
Serum half-life, days	23	6	5	3	2.5
Synthesis rate, mg/kg per day	33	65	7	0.4	0.016
Antibody valence	2	2,4	10,12	2	2
Classical complement activation	+(G1, 2?, 3)	–	++	–	–
Alternate complement activation	+(G4)	+	–	+	–
Binding cells via Fc	Macrophages, neutrophils, large granular lymphocytes	Lymphocytes	Lymphocytes	None	Mast cells, basophils, B cells
Biologic properties	Placental transfer, secondary Ab for most antipathogen responses	Secretory immunoglobulin	Primary Ab responses	Marker for mature B cells	Allergy, antiparasite responses

SOURCE: After L Carayannopoulos and JD Capra, in WE Paul (ed): *Fundamental Immunology*, 2d ed. New York, Raven, 1989, with permission.

pervariable regions (extreme sequence variability) that constitute the antigen-binding site unique to each Ig molecule. The idiotype is defined as the specific region of the Fab portion of the Ig molecule to which antigen binds. Antibodies against the idiotype portion of an antibody molecule are called *anti-idiotype antibodies*. The formation of such antibodies in vivo during a normal B cell antibody response may generate a negative (or "off") signal to B cells to terminate antibody production.

IgG comprises approximately 75 to 85% of total serum immunoglobulin. The four IgG subclasses are numbered in order of their level in serum, IgG1 being found in greatest amounts and IgG4 the least. IgG subclasses have clinical relevance in their varying ability to bind macrophage and neutrophil Fc receptors and to activate complement (Table 305-9). Moreover, selective deficiencies of certain IgG subclasses give rise to clinical syndromes in which the patient is inordinately susceptible to bacterial infections. IgG antibodies are frequently the predominant antibody made after rechallenge of the host with antigen (secondary antibody response).

IgM antibodies normally circulate as a 950-kDa pentamer with 160-kDa bivalent monomers joined by a molecule called the *J chain*, a 15-kDa nonimmunoglobulin molecule that also effects polymerization of IgA molecules. IgM is the first immunoglobulin to appear in the immune response (primary antibody response) and is the initial type of antibody made by neonates. Membrane IgM in the monomeric form also functions as a major antigen receptor on the surface of mature B cells (Fig. 305-9). IgM is an important component of immune complexes in autoimmune diseases. For example, IgM antibodies against IgG molecules (rheumatoid factors) are present in high titers in *rheumatoid arthritis*, other collagen diseases, and some infectious diseases (*subacute bacterial endocarditis*). IgM antibody binds the C1 component of complement via the CH4 domain and thus is a potent activator of the complement cascade.

IgA comprises only 7 to 15% of total serum immunoglobulin but is the predominant class of immunoglobulin in secretions. IgA in secretions (tears, saliva, nasal secretions, gastrointestinal tract fluid, and human milk) is in the form of secretory IgA (sIgA), a polymer consisting of two IgA monomers, a joining molecule, again called the J chain, and a glycoprotein called the *secretory protein*. Of the two IgA subclasses, IgA1 is primarily found in serum, whereas IgA2 is more prevalent in secretions. IgA fixes complement via the alternative complement pathway and has potent antiviral activity in humans by prevention of virus binding to respiratory and gastrointestinal epithelial cells.

IgD is found in minute quantities in serum and, together with IgM, is a major receptor for antigen on the B cell surface (Table 305-9). IgE, which is present in serum in very low concentrations, is the major class of immunoglobulin involved in arming mast cells and basophils by binding to these cells via the Fc region. Antigen cross-linking of IgE molecules on basophil and mast cell surfaces results in release of mediators of the immediate hypersensitivity response (Table 305-6).

CELLULAR INTERACTIONS IN REGULATION OF NORMAL IMMUNE RESPONSES The net result of activation of the humoral (B cell) and cellular (T cell) arms of the adaptive immune system by foreign antigen is the elimination of antigen directly by specific effector T cells or in concert with specific antibody. In addition, regulatory T cells are activated that modulate effector T cell activation and B cell antibody production. Figure 305-12 is a simplified schematic diagram of the T and B cell responses indicating some of these cellular interactions.

The expression of adaptive immune cell function is the result of a complex series of immunoregulatory events that occur in phases. Both T and B lymphocytes mediate immune functions, and each of these cell types, when given appropriate signals, passes through stages, from activation and induction through proliferation, differentiation, and ultimately effector functions. The effector function expressed may be at the end point of a response, such as secretion of antibody by a differentiated plasma cell, or it might serve a regulatory function that modulates other functions, such as is seen with CD4+ inducer or CD8+ regulatory T lymphocytes, which modulate both differentiation of B cells and activation of CD8+ or CD4+ cytotoxic T cells.

CD4 helper T cells can be subdivided on the basis of cytokines produced (Fig. 305-13). Activated T_H1-type helper T cells secrete IL-2, IFN-γ, IL-3, TNF-α, GM-CSF, and TNF-β, while activated T_H2-type helper T cells secrete IL-3, -4, -5, -6, -10, and -13. T_H1 CD4+ T cells, through elaboration of IFN-γ, have a central role in mediating intracellular killing by a variety of pathogens. T_H1 CD4+ T cells also provide T cell help for generation of cytotoxic T cells and some types of opsonizing antibody, and generally respond to antigens that lead to delayed hypersensitivity types of immune responses for many intracellular viruses and bacteria (such as HIV or *M. tuberculosis*). In contrast, T_H2 cells have a primary role in regulatory humoral immunity and isotype switching. In addition, T_H2 cells, through production of IL-4 and IL-10, have a regulatory role in limiting proinflammatory responses mediated by T_H1 cells (Table 305-5). In addition, T_H2 CD4+ T cells provide help to B cells for specific Ig production and respond to antigens that require high antibody levels for foreign antigen elimination (extracellular encapsulated bacteria such as *Streptococcus pneumoniae* and certain parasite infections). Different cytokines can drive the immune response preferentially towards a T_H1 or a T_H2 response. For example, APC-derived IL-12 induces CD4+ T cell differentiation towards a T_H1 type cell, whereas IL-4 drives differentiation towards a T_H2 type cell (Fig. 305-13).

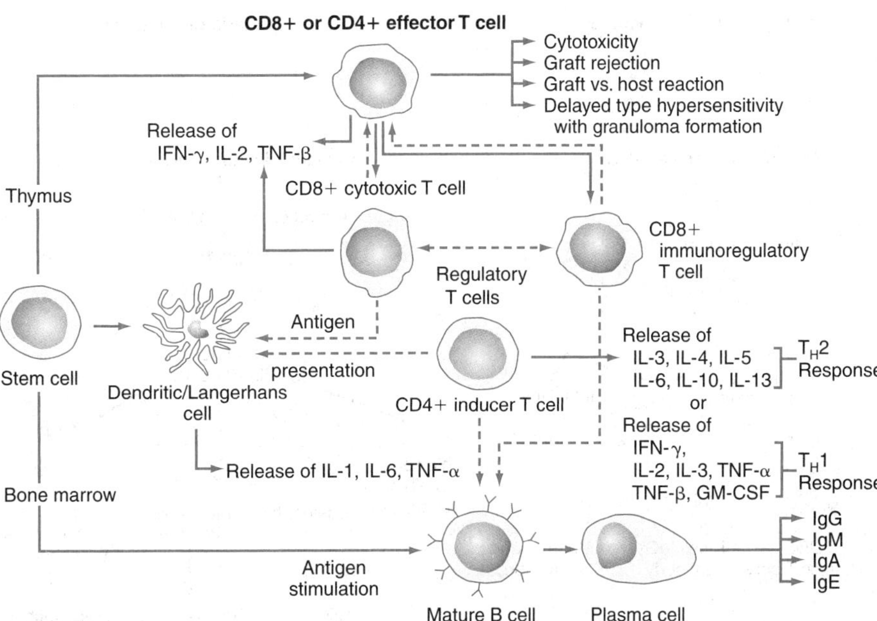

FIGURE 305-12 Schematic model of intercellular interactions of adaptive immune system cells. In this figure the solid arrows denote that cells develop from precursor cells or produce cytokines or antibodies; dotted lines indicate intercellular interactions. Stem cells differentiate into either T cells, antigen-presenting dendritic cells (also called Langerhans cells when located in skin or thymus), or B cells. Foreign antigen is processed by dendritic cells, and peptide fragments of foreign antigen are presented to CD4+ and/or CD8+ T cells. CD8+ T cell activation leads to induction of cytotoxic T lymphocyte (CTL) or killer T cell generation, as well as induction of cytokine-producing CD8+ immunoregulatory cells. For antibody production against the same antigen, active antigen is bound to sIg within the B cell receptor complex and drives B cell maturation into plasma cells that secrete Ig. Regulatory T_H1 or T_H2 CD4+ T cells producing interleukin (IL) 4, IL-5, or interferon (IFN)γ regulate the Ig class switching and determine the type of antibody produced. GM-CSF, granulocyte-macrophage colony stimulating factor; TNF, tumor necrosis factor.

As shown in Fig. 305-12, upon activation by APCs such as dendritic cells, regulatory T cell subsets that produce IL-2, IL-3, IFN-γ, and/or IL-4, -5, -6, -10, and -13 are generated that exert positive and negative influences on effector T and B cells. For B cells, trophic effects are mediated by a variety of cytokines, particularly T cell–derived IL-3, -4, -5, and -6, which act at sequential stages of B cell maturation, resulting in B cell proliferation, differentiation, and ultimately antibody secretion (Table 305-5). For cytotoxic T cells, trophic factors include inducer T cell secretion of IL-2, IFN-γ, and IL-12 (Table 305-5). In addition, B cells themselves are capable of serving as APCs, processing and presenting antigens to T cells, and secreting TNF-α and IL-6.

Although B cells recognize native antigen via B cell surface Ig receptors, B cells require T cell help to produce high-affinity antibody of multiple isotypes that are the most effective in eliminating foreign antigen. This T cell dependence likely functions in the regulation of B cell responses and in protection against excessive autoantibody production. T cell–B cell interactions that lead to high-affinity antibody production require: (1) processing of native antigen by B cells and expression of peptide fragments on the B cell surface for presentation to T_H cells, (2) the ligation of B cells both by the T cell receptor complex and the CD40 ligand, (3) induction of the process termed *antibody isotype switching* in antigen-specific B cell clones, and (4) induction of the process of *affinity maturation* of antibody in the germinal centers of B cell follicles of lymph node and spleen.

Naive B cells express cell-surface IgD and IgM, and initial contact of naive B cells with antigen is via binding of native antigen to B cell–surface IgM. T cell cytokines, released following T_H2 cell contact with B cells or by a "bystander" effect, induce changes in Ig gene conformation that promote recombination of Ig genes. These events then result in the "switching" of expression of heavy chain exons in a triggered B cell, leading to the secretion of IgG, IgA, or, in some cases, IgE antibody with the same V region antigen specificity as the original IgM antibody, for response to a wide variety of extracellular bacteria, protozoa, and helminths. CD40 ligand expression by activated T cells is critical for induction of B cell antibody isotype switching and for B cell responsiveness to cytokines. Patients with mutations in T cell CD40 ligand have B cells that are unable to undergo isotype switching, resulting in lack of memory B cell generation and the immunodeficiency syndrome of *X-linked hyper-IgM syndrome* (Chap. 308).

MECHANISMS OF IMMUNE-MEDIATED DAMAGE TO MICROBES OR HOST TISSUES Several responses by the host innate and adaptive immune systems to foreign microbes culminate in rapid and efficient elimination of microbes. In these scenarios, the classic weapons of the adaptive immune system (T cells, B cells) interface with cells (macrophages, dendritic cells, NK cells, neutrophils, eosinophils, basophils) and soluble products (microbial peptides, pentraxins, complement and coagulation systems) of the innate immune system (Chaps. 64 and 310).

There are five general phases of host defenses: (1) migration of leukocytes to sites of antigen localization; (2) antigen nonspecific recognition of pathogens by macrophages and other cells and systems of the innate immune system; (3) specific recognition of foreign antigens mediated by T and B lymphocytes; (4) amplification of the inflammatory response with recruitment of specific and nonspecific effector cells by complement components, cytokines, kinins, arachidonic acid metabolites, and mast cell–basophil products; and (5) macrophage, neutrophil, and lymphocyte participation in destruction of antigen with ultimate removal of antigen particles by phagocytosis (by macrophages or neutrophils) or by direct cytotoxic mechanisms (involving macrophages, neutrophils, and lymphocytes). Under normal circumstances, orderly progression of host defenses through these phases results in a well-controlled immune and inflammatory response that protects the host from the offending antigen. However, dysfunction of any of the host defense systems can damage host tissue and produce clinical disease. Furthermore, for certain pathogens or antigens, the normal immune response itself might contribute substantially to the tissue damage. For example, the immune and inflammatory response in the brain to certain pathogens such as *M. tuberculosis* may be responsible for much of the morbidity of this disease in that organ system (Chap. 169). In addition, the morbidity associated with certain pneumonias

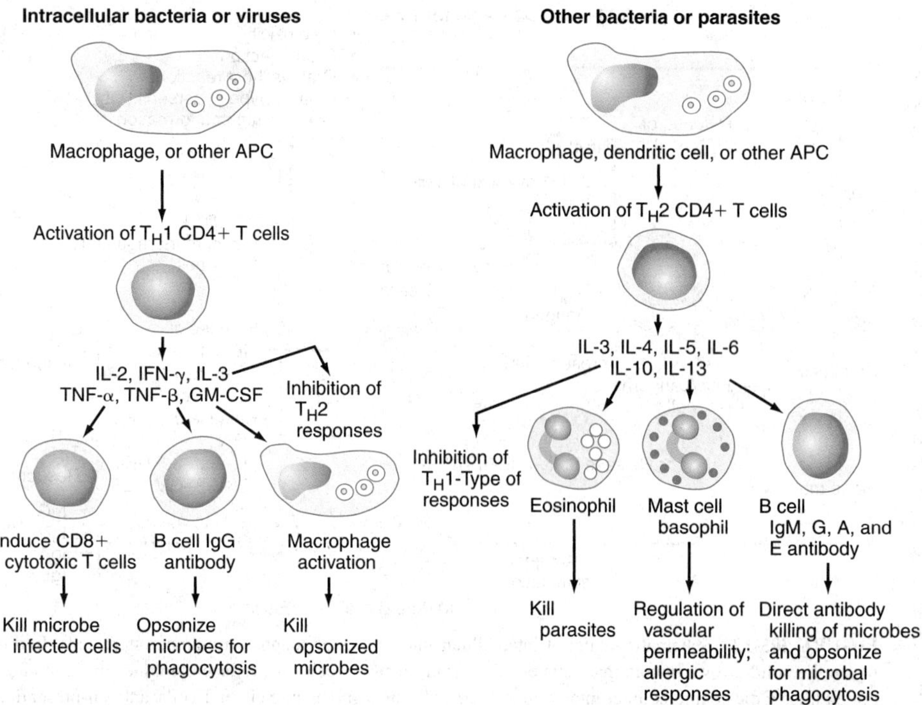

FIGURE 305-13 CD4+ helper T 1 (T_H1) cells and T_H2 T cells secrete distinct but overlapping sets of cytokines. T_H1 CD4+ cells are frequently activated in immune and inflammatory reactions against intracellular bacteria or viruses, while T_H2 CD4+ cells are frequently activated for certain types of antibody production against parasites and extracellular encapsulated bacteria; they are also activated in allergic diseases. APC, antigen-presenting cell; GM-CSF, granulocyte-macrophage colony stimulating factor; IFN, interferon; IL, interleukin; TNF, tumor necrosis factor. *(Adapted from Romagnani, with permission.)*

such as that caused by *Pneumocystis carinii* may be associated more with inflammatory infiltrates than with the tissue destructive effects of the microorganism itself (Chap. 209). Thus, it is important to appreciate how normally protective proinflammatory responses that mediate intracellular killing are regulated. What follows are brief discussions of mechanisms of leukocyte migration to sites of inflammation, immune complex formation, immediate-type hypersensitivity responses, cytotoxic reactions of antibody, delayed cellular types of hypersensitivity responses, and programmed cell death of immune competent cells.

The Molecular Basis of Lymphocyte–Endothelial Cell Interactions The control of lymphocyte circulatory patterns between the bloodstream and peripheral lymphoid organs operates at the level of lymphocyte–endothelial cell interactions to control the specificity of lymphocyte subset entry into organs. Similarly, lymphocyte–endothelial cell interactions regulate the entry of lymphocytes into inflamed tissue. Adhesion molecule expression on lymphocytes and endothelial cells regulates the retention and subsequent egress of lymphocytes within tissue sites of antigenic stimulation, delaying cell exit from tissue and preventing reentry into the circulating lymphocyte pool. All types of lymphocyte migration begin with lymphocyte attachment to specialized regions of vessels, termed *high endothelial venules* (HEVs). An important concept for many of the adhesion molecules listed in Table 305-10 is that the molecules do not generally bind their ligand until a conformational change (ligand activation) occurs in the adhesion molecule that allows ligand binding. Induction of a conformation-dependent determinant on an adhesion molecule can be accomplished by cytokines or via ligation of other adhesion molecules on the cell.

The first stage of lymphocyte–endothelial cell interactions, *attachment and rolling*, occurs when lymphocytes leave the stream of flowing blood cells in a postcapillary venule and roll along venule endothelial cells (Fig. 305-14). Lymphocyte rolling is mediated by the L-selectin molecule (LECAM-1, LAM-1) and slows cell transit time through venules, allowing time for activation of adherent cells.

The second stage of lymphocyte–endothelial cell interactions, *adhesion triggering*, requires stimulation of lymphocytes by chemoattractants or by endothelial cell–derived cytokines. Cytokines thought to participate in adherent cell triggering include members of the IL-8 family, platelet-activation factor, leukotriene B_4, and C5a. Following activation by chemoattractants, lymphocytes shed L-selectin from the cell surface and upregulate cell CD11b/18 (MAC-1) or CD11a/18 (LFA-1) molecules, resulting in firm attachment of lymphocytes to HEVs.

Lymphocyte homing to peripheral lymph nodes involves adhesion of L-selectin to carbohydrate of peripheral node HEVs, whereas homing of lymphocytes to intestine Peyer's patches primarily involves adhesion of the $\alpha4,\beta7$ integrin to MAdCAM-1 oligosaccharides on the Peyer's patch HEVs. However, for migration to mucosal Peyer's patch lymphoid aggregates, naive lymphocytes primarily use L-selectin, whereas memory lymphocytes use $\alpha4,\beta7$ integrin. $\alpha4,\beta1$ integrin (CD49d/CD29, VLA-4)–VCAM-1 interactions are important in the initial interaction of memory lymphocytes with HEVs of multiple organs in sites of inflammation.

The third stage of leukocyte emigration in HEVs, *sticking and arrest*, is sticking of the lymphocyte and arrest at the site of sticking, mediated predominantly by ligation of $\alpha L,\beta2$ integrin LFA-1 to the integrin ligands ICAM-1 and ICAM-2 on HEVs. While the first three stages of lymphocyte attachment to HEVs takes only a few seconds, the fourth stage of lymphocyte emigration, *transendothelial migration*, takes approximately 10 min. Although the molecular mechanisms that control lymphocyte transendothelial migration are not fully characterized, the HEV CD44 molecule and molecules of the HEV glycocalyx (extracellular matrix) are thought to play important regulatory roles in this process (Fig. 305-14). Finally, expression of matrix metalloproteases capable of di-

Table 305-10 Complement Deficiencies and Associated Diseases

Component	Associated Diseases
CLASSIC PATHWAY	
C1q, C1r, C1s, C4	Immune-complex syndromes,[a] pyogenic infections
C2	Immune-complex syndromes,[a] few with pyogenic infections
C1 inhibitor	Rare immune-complex disease, few with pyogenic infections
C3 AND ALTERNATIVE PATHWAY C3	
C3	Immune-complex syndromes,[a] pyogenic infections
D	Pyogenic infections
Properdin	*Neisseria* infections
I	Pyogenic infections
H	Hemolytic uremic syndrome
MEMBRANE ATTACK COMPLEX	
C5, C6, C7, C8	Recurrent *Neisseria* infections, immune-complex disease
C9	Rare *Neisseria* infections

[a] Immune-complex syndromes include systemic lupus erythematosus (SLE) and SLE-like syndromes, glomerulonephritis, and vasculitis syndromes.
SOURCE: After JA Schifferli and DK Peters, Lancet 88:957, 1983, with permission.

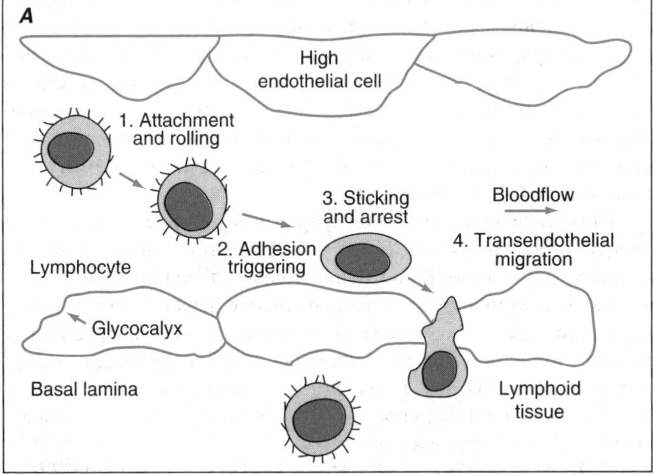

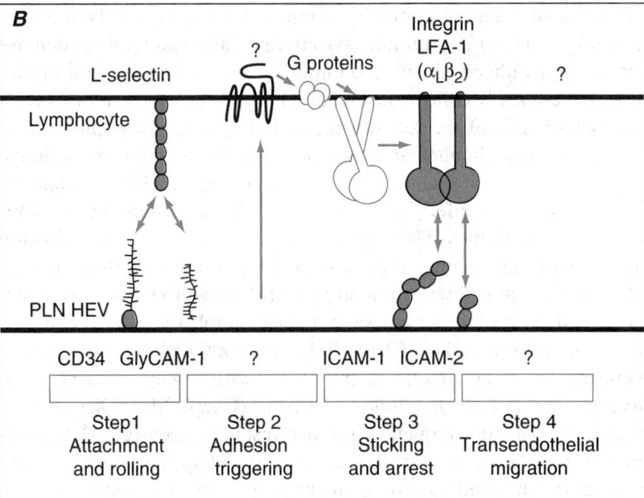

FIGURE 305-14 Lymphocyte emigration in high endothelial venules (HEV). *A.* Lymphocytes circulating in blood initiate contact with high endothelial cells via microvilli. This initial adhesion is transient and is often manifested in rolling of the interacting cells along the HEV endothelium (step 1: attachment and rolling). Activation of lymphocyte adhesiveness (step 2: adhesion triggering) results in firm attachment, which becomes stable to physiologic shear force (step 3: sticking and arrest). Lymphocytes then migrate through endothelial cell junctions and enter lymphoid tissue after crossing the HEV basal lamina (step 4: transendothelial migration). The luminal surface of HEV is coated by a prominent glycocalyx, and this may play an important role in lymphocyte emigration (see text for details). *B.* The initial interaction of lymphocytes with HEV in peripheral lymph nodes (PLNs) is mediated by L-selectin, which recognizes the following HEV mucin-like counter-receptors: CD34 and glycosylation-dependent cell adhesion molecule 1 (GlyCAM-1). Activation of lymphocyte adhesiveness occurs via G protein–coupled receptors, but the local factors involved in physiologic activation of lymphocytes in HEV are not yet characterized. The integrin leukocyte function–associated molecule 1 (LFA-1) (ab;CD11a/CD18) and its HEV counter-receptors intercellular adhesion molecule 1 (ICAM-1) and ICAM-2 play a major role in lymphocyte arrest in PLN HEV. The molecular mechanisms involved in lymphocyte transendothelial migration remain poorly characterized. *(After Girard and Springer, with permission.)*

gesting the subendothelial basement membrane, rich in nonfibrillar collagen, appears to be required for the penetration of lymphoid cells into the extravascular sites.

Abnormal induction of HEV formation and use of the molecules discussed above have been implicated in the induction and maintenance of inflammation in a number of chronic inflammatory diseases. In animal models of insulin-dependent diabetes mellitus (IDDM), MAdCAM-1 and GlyCAM-1 have been shown to be highly expressed on HEVs in inflamed pancreatic islets, and treatment of these animals with inhibitors of L-selectin and $\alpha 4$ integrin function blocked the development of IDDM (Chap. 333). A similar role for abnormal induction of the adhesion molecules of lymphocyte emigration has been suggested in rheumatoid arthritis (Chap. 312), Hashimoto's thyroiditis (Chap. 330), Graves' disease (Chap. 330), multiple sclerosis (Chap. 371), Crohn's disease (Chap. 287), and ulcerative colitis (Chap. 287).

Immune-Complex Formation Clearance of antigen by immune-complex formation between antigen and antibody is a highly effective mechanism of host defense. However, depending on the level of immune complexes formed and their physicochemical properties, immune complexes may or may not result in host and foreign cell damage. After antigen exposure, certain types of soluble antigen-antibody complexes freely circulate and, if not cleared by the reticuloendothelial system, can be deposited in blood vessel walls and in other tissues such as renal glomeruli (Chap. 317).

Immediate-Type Hypersensitivity Helper T cells that drive antiallergen IgE responses are usually T_H2-type inducer T cells that secrete IL-4, IL-5, IL-6, and IL-10. Mast cells and basophils have high-affinity receptors for the Fc portion of IgE (FcRI), and cell-bound antiallergen IgE effectively "arms" basophils and mast cells. Mediator release is triggered by antigen (allergen) interaction with Fc receptor–bound IgE; the mediators released are responsible for the pathophysiologic changes of allergic diseases (Table 305-6). Mediators released from mast cells and basophils can be divided into three broad functional types: (1) those that increase vascular permeability and contract smooth muscle (histamine, platelet-activating factor, SRS-A, BK-A), (2) those that are chemotactic for or activate other inflammatory cells (ECF-A, NCF, leukotriene B_4), and (3) those that modulate the release of other mediators (BK-A, platelet-activating factor) (Chap. 310).

Cytotoxic Reactions of Antibody In this type of immunologic injury, complement-fixing (C1-binding) antibodies against normal or foreign cells or tissues (IgM, IgG1, IgG2, IgG3) bind complement via the classic pathway and initiate a sequence of events similar to that initiated by immune-complex deposition, resulting in cell lysis or tissue injury. Examples of antibody-mediated cytotoxic reactions include red cell lysis in *transfusion reactions*, *Goodpasture's syndrome* with anti-glomerular basement membrane antibody formation, and *pemphigus vulgaris* with antiepidermal antibodies inducing blistering skin disease.

Classic Delayed-Type Hypersensitivity Reactions Inflammatory reactions initiated by mononuclear leukocytes and not by antibody alone have been termed *delayed-type hypersensitivity reactions*. The term *delayed* has been used to contrast a secondary cellular response that appears 48 to 72 h after antigen exposure with an *immediate* hypersensitivity response generally seen within 12 h of antigen challenge and initiated by basophil mediator release or preformed antibody. For example, in an individual previously infected with *M. tuberculosis* organisms, intradermal placement of tuberculin purified-protein derivative as a skin test challenge results in an indurated area of skin at 48 to 72 h, indicating previous exposure to tuberculosis.

The cellular events that result in classic delayed-type hypersensitivity responses are centered around T cells (predominantly, though not exclusively, IFN-γ, IL-2, and TNF-α-secreting T_H1-type helper T cells) and macrophages. First, local immune and inflammatory responses at the site of foreign antigen upregulate endothelial cell adhesion molecule expression, promoting the accumulation of lymphocytes at the tissue site. In the general scheme outlined in Fig. 305-12, antigen is processed by dendritic/Langerhans cells or monocytes-macrophages and presented to small numbers of CD4+ T cells expressing a TCR specific for the antigen. IL-12 produced by APCs induces T cells to produce IFN-γ (T_H-1 response). IL-1 and IL-6 secreted by APCs amplify the clonal expansion of antigen-specific T cells, and other cytokines (primarily IL-2, IFN-γ, and TNF-β) are secreted that promote recruitment of diverse populations of T cells and macrophages to the site of the cellular inflammatory response. In particular, CD8+ cytotoxic T cells are induced by IL-2 to become active killer cells. Once recruited, macrophages frequently undergo epithelioid cell transformation and fuse to form multinucleated giant cells. This type of mononuclear cell infiltrate is termed *granulomatous inflammation.* Examples of diseases in which delayed-type hypersensitivity plays a major role are fungal infections (*histoplasmosis*) (Chap. 201), mycobacterial infections (*tuberculosis, leprosy*) (Chaps. 169 and 170), chlamydial infections (*lymphogranuloma venereum*) (Chap. 179), helminth infections (*schistosomiasis*) (Chap. 224), reactions to toxins (*berylliosis*) (Chap. 254), and hypersensitivity reactions to organic dusts (*hypersensitivity pneumonitis*) (Chap. 253). In addition, delayed-type hypersensitivity responses play important roles in tissue damage in autoimmune diseases such as *rheumatoid arthritis, temporal arteritis,* and *Wegener's granulomatosis* (Chaps. 312 and 317).

The Cellular and Molecular Control of Programmed Cell Death (Apoptosis) The process of apoptosis plays a crucial role in regulating normal immune responses to antigen. In general, a wide variety of stimuli trigger cell surface receptors (e.g., TNF receptor family members or related proteins) or cytoplasmic receptors (e.g., ceramide, glucocorticoids) that activate groups of proteases such as FADD-like IL-1β-converting enzyme (FLICE) or Caspase 8 (Fig. 305-15). These proteases either cleave molecules that lead to cell death themselves or activate other enzymes to cleave molecules that eventuate in cell death (Fig. 305-15). The end stages of this sequence of events lead to cell death characterized by degradation of cytoplasmic (actin) and nuclear cytoskeletal proteins as well as cleavage of DNA at regular intervals (nucleosomes), leading to nuclear disintegration seen on electron microscopy and "laddering" of DNA when analysed by agarose gel electrophoresis. The level of expression of certain cytosolic proteins, such as Bcl-2 and Bcl-XL, negatively regulates the process of apoptosis by inhibiting activation of cytosolic proteases that induce cell death. For example, T cells that are negatively selected in the thymus are induced to undergo apoptosis and have low levels of proteins such as Bcl-2, whereas medullary thymocytes that have been triggered to proliferate and survive thymocyte selection (positive selection) have high levels of Bcl-2.

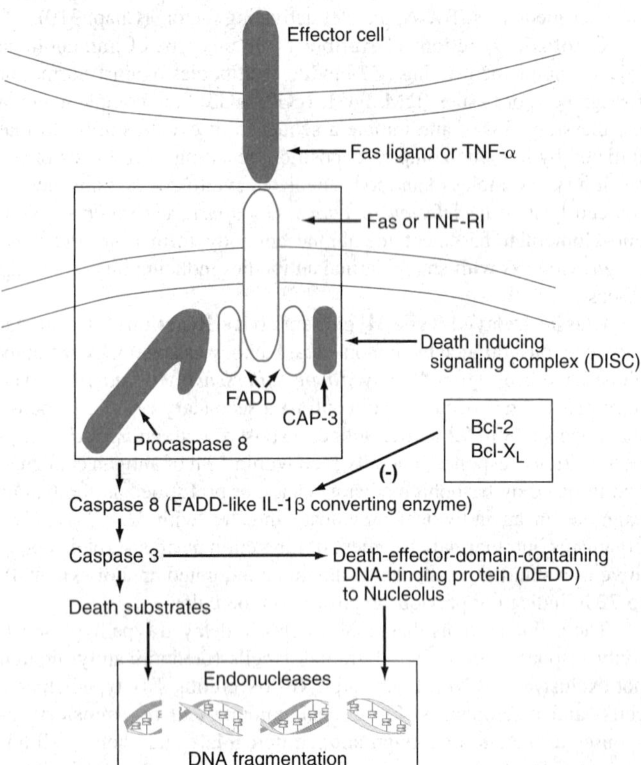

FIGURE 305-15 Intracellular signaling pathways that regulate programmed cell death. Bcl-2 and Bcl-XL are two proteins that inhibit programmed cell death. Caspase activation may result in the translocation of the death-effector domain containing DNA binding protein (DEDD) that inhibits DNA transcription in the nucleolus. Upon ligation of CD95 by Fas ligand or tumor necrosis factor receptor I (TNF-RI) by TNF-α, a death-inducing signaling complex (DISC) is formed from Procaspase 8, FADD, and Cap-3 proteins. Signaling caspases are activated, eventuating in endonucleases being produced that fragment DNA, leading to cell death. IL, interleukin. *(Adapted with permission from Scaffidi et al.)*

Thus, in the immune system, apoptosis is a mechanism induced to remove autoreactive T cells from the thymus during negative selection, to remove autoreactive B and T cells from peripheral lymphoid organs upon contact with antigen or antigen-reactive helper T cells in spleen and lymph node, and to remove virus-infected or malignant cells after contact with antigen-specific CD8+ cytotoxic T lymphocytes. Induction of apoptosis is one of two principal mechanisms of target cell lysis by cytotoxic T lymphocytes, the other consisting of the release of cytotoxic perforin molecules.

CLINICAL EVALUATION OF IMMUNE FUNCTION Clinical assessment of immunity requires investigation of the four major components of the immune system that participate in host defense and in the pathogenesis of autoimmune diseases: (1) humoral immunity (B cells); (2) cell-mediated immunity (T cells, monocytes); (3) phagocytic cells of the reticuloendothelial system (macrophages), as well as polymorphonuclear leukocytes; and (4) complement. Clinical problems that require an evaluation of immunity include chronic infections, recurrent infection, unusual infecting agents, and certain autoimmune syndromes. The type of clinical syndrome under evaluation can provide information regarding possible immune defects (Chap. 308). Defects in cellular immunity generally result in viral, mycobacterial, and fungal infections. An extreme example of deficiency in cellular immunity is AIDS (Chap. 309). Antibody deficiencies result in recurrent bacterial infections, frequently with organisms such as *S. pneumoniae* and *Haemophilus influenzae* (Chap. 308). Disorders of phagocyte function frequently are manifested by recurrent skin infections, often due to *Staphylococcus aureus* (Chap. 64). Finally, deficiencies of early and late complement components are associated with autoimmune phenomena and recurrent *Neisseria* infections (Table 305-10). →***For further discussion of useful initial screening tests of immune function, see Chap. 308.***

IMMUNOTHERAPY Most current therapies for autoimmune and inflammatory diseases involve the use of nonspecific immune-modulating or immunosuppressive agents such as glucocorticoids or cytotoxic drugs. The goal of development of new treatments for immune-mediated diseases is to design ways to specifically interrupt pathologic immune responses, leaving nonpathologic immune responses intact. Novel ways to interrupt pathologic immune responses that are under investigation include: the use of anti-inflammatory cytokines or specific cytokine inhibitors as anti-inflammatory agents; the use of monoclonal antibodies against T or B lymphocytes as therapeutic agents; the induction of anergy by administration of soluble CTLA-4 protein, the use of intravenous Ig for certain infections and immune complex–mediated diseases, and the use of specific cytokines to reconstitute components of the immune system (Table 305-11) (Chaps. 64, 308, and 309).

Cytokines and Cytokine Inhibitors Recently a humanized mouse anti-TNF-α monoclonal antibody (MAB) has been tested in both rheumatoid arthritis and ulcerative colitis. Use of anti-TNF-α antibody therapy has resulted in clinical improvement in patients with these diseases and has opened the way for targeting TNF-α to treat other severe forms of autoimmune and/or inflammatory disease. Anti-TNF-α MAB has been approved for treatment of patients with rheumatoid arthritis.

Other cytokine inhibitors under investigation are recombinant soluble TNF-α receptor (R) fused to human Ig and soluble IL-1 receptor (termed *IL-1 receptor antagonist,* or IL-1 ra). Soluble TNF-αR and IL-1 ra act to inhibit the activity of pathogenic cytokines in rheumatoid arthritis, i.e., TNF-α and IL-1 respectively. Similarly, anti-IL-6, IFN-β, and IL-11 act to inhibit pathogenic proinflammatory cytokines.

Table 305-11 Current Status of Development of Immunomodulatory Agents

Agents	Rationale	Status
CYTOKINES AND CYTOKINE INHIBITORS TO INHIBIT IMMUNE RESPONSES AND INFLAMMATION		
Anti-TNF-α monoclonal antibody	Inhibit TNF-α	FDA approved for rheumatoid arthritis; in trials for Crohn's colitis
Recombinant TNF-receptor-IG fusion protein	Inhibit TNF-α	In trials for rheumatoid arthritis
Recombinant IL-1 receptor antagonist (IL-1Ra)	Inhibit IL-1α and β	In trials for rheumatoid arthritis
Anti-IL-6 monoclonal antibody	Inhibit IL-6	Tested in phase I trial in rheumatoid arthritis
Inferferon-β	Inhibit IL-1, decrease synovial T cells	In trials for use in rheumatoid arthritis
Interferon-γ	Induce monocyte/macrophage activation	Effective in treating monocyte/macrophage phagocytic defects in chronic granulomatous disease
IL-11	Inhibit TNF-α and IL-1 production	In trials for Crohn's colitis
IL-12	Stimulate anti-tumor and anti-viral or bacterial cytotoxic T lymphocyte responses	Trials underway for use in cancer patients; trials planned in humans to prevent/treat severe infections
MONOCLONAL ANTIBODIES AGAINST T OR B CELLS		
Anti-CD3 anti-T cell monoclonal antibody	Inhibit T cell function; Induce T cell lymphopenia	FDA approved for treatment of cardiac and renal allograft rejection
Anti-CD4 monoclonal antibody	Inhibit CD4+ T cell function	In trials for rheumatoid arthritis
Anti-CD40 ligand (CD154) monoclonal antibody	Inhibit CD40-CD40 ligand interaction; induces T cell tolerance	In primate trials for prevention of renal allograft rejection
SOLUBLE T CELL MOLECULE		
Soluble CTLA-4 protein	Inhibit CD28-B7-1 and B7-2 interactions; induce tolerance to organ grafts; inhibit autoimmune T cell reactivity in autoimmune diseases	In trials for preventing GVHD in bone marrow transplantation and for treatment of psoriasis
INTRAVENOUS IMMUNOGLOBULIN		
IVIg	Reticuloendothelial cell blockage; complement inhibition; regulation of idiotype/anti-idiotype antibodies; modulation of cytokine production; modulation of lymphocyte production	FDA approved for Kawasaki's disease and immune thrombocytopenia purpura; treatment of graft versus host disease, multiple sclerosis, myasthenia gravis, Guillain-Barre Syndrome, and chronic inflammatory demylenating polyneuropathy supported by clinical trials
CYTOKINES FOR IMMUNE RECONSTITUTION		
IL-2	Induce proliferation of peripheral memory CD4+ and CD8+ T cells	In trial for treatment of HIV infection
IL-7	Induce renewed thymopoiesis	Under consideration for treatment of diseases associated with T cell deficiency

Anti-IL-6 inhibits IL-6 activity, while IFN-β and IL-11 decrease IL-1 and TNF-α production.

Recent studies have identified mutations in the IL-12 gene in patients susceptible to severe myobacterial infections. IL-12 is a critical cytokine for induction of IFN-γ and cytotoxic T lymphocytes (CTLs) against intracellular organisms; it is under study for treatment of severe infections such as that caused by *M. tuberculosis* and for treatment of various cancers. In this latter setting, IL-12 is being studied for its ability to enhance antitumor cellular immunity by enhancing the induction of antitumor CTL.

Of particular note has been the successful use of IFN-γ in the treatment of the phagocytic cell defect in *chronic granulomatous disease* (Chap. 64). Intermittent infusions of IL-2 in HIV-infected individuals in the early or intermediate stages of disease have resulted in substantial and sustained increases in CD4+ T cells.

Monoclonal Antibodies to T and B Cells The OKT3 MAB against human T cells has been used for several years as a T cell–specific immunosuppressive agent that can substitute for horse antithymocyte globulin (ATG) in the treatment of solid organ transplant rejection. OKT3 produces fewer allergic reactions than ATG but does induce human anti-mouse Ig antibody—thus limiting its use. Anti-CD4 MAB therapy has been used in trials to treat patients with rheumatoid arthritis. While inducing profound immunosuppression, anti-CD4 MAB treatment also induces considerable susceptibility to severe infections. Treatment of patients with a MAB against the T cell molecule CD40 ligand (CD154) is under investigation to induce tolerance to organ transplants, with promising results reported in animal studies.

Tolerance Induction Specific immunotherapy has moved into a new era with the introduction of soluble CTLA-4 protein into clinical trials. Use of this molecule to block T cell activation via TCR/CD28 ligation during organ or bone marrow transplantation has showed promising results in animals and in early human clinical trials. Specifically, treatment of bone marrow with CTLA-4 protein reduces rejection of the graft in HLA-mismatched bone marrow transplantation. In addition, promising results with soluble CTLA-4 have been reported in the downmodulation of autoimmune T cell responses in the treatment of psoriasis.

Intravenous Immunoglobulin (IVIg) IVIg has been successfully used to block reticuloendothelial cell function and immune complex clearance in various immune cytopenias such as immune thrombocytopenia (Chap. 116). In addition, IVIg is useful for prevention of tissue damage in certain inflammatory syndromes such as Kawasaki's disease (Chap. 317) and as Ig replacement therapy for certain types of immunoglobulin deficiencies (Chap. 308). In addition, controlled clinical trials support the use of IVIg in selected patients with graft-versus-host disease, multiple sclerosis, myasthenia gravis, Guillain-Barré syndrome, and chronic demyelinating polyneuropathy (Table 305-11).

Thus, a number of recent insights into immune system function have spawned a new field of interventional immunotherapy and have enhanced the prospect for development of specific and nontoxic therapies for immune and inflammatory diseases.

BIBLIOGRAPHY

ABBAS AK et al (eds): *Cellular and Molecular Immunology*, 2d ed. Philadelphia, Saunders, 1994

ARMITAGE RJ et al: CD40L: A multifunctional ligand. Semin Immunol 5:401, 1993

BENSCHOP RJ, CAMBIER JC: B cell development: Signal transduction by antigen receptors and their surrogates. Curr Opin Immunol 11:143, 1999

DURIE FH et al: The role of CD40 in the regulation of humoral and cell-mediated immunity. Immunol Today 15:406, 1994

FOXWELL BMJ et al: Interleukin-7 can induce the activation of Jak-1, Jak-3, and STAT5 proteins in immune T cells. Eur J Immunol 25:3041, 1995

GEORGE AJT et al: Disease susceptibility, transplantation and the MHC. Immunol Today 16:209, 1995

GIRARD JP, SPRINGER TA: High endothelial venules (HEVs): Specialized endothelium for lymphocyte migration. Immunol Today 16:449, 1995

GLEICH GJ: Eosinophils, basophils and mast cells. J Allergy Clin Immunol 84:1024, 1989

HAYNES BF et al: The role of the thymus in immune reconstitution in aging bone marrow transplantation and AIDS. Ann Rev Immunol, 18:529, 2000

HERMAN A et al: Superantigens: Mechanism of T-cell stimulation and the role in immune responses. Annu Rev Immunol 9:745, 1991

JANEWAY CA et al (eds): *Immunobiology. The Immune System in Health and Disease*, 4th ed. New York, Garland, 1999

JUNE CH et al: The B7 and CD28 receptor families. Immunol Today 15:321, 1994

KELLEY WN et al (eds): *Textbook of Rheumatology*, 4th ed. Philadelphia, Saunders, 1993, chaps. 6, 7, 10, 13, 15, 16

KOPP EB, MEDZHITOV R: The Toll-receptor family and control of innate immunity. Curr Opin Immunol 11:13, 1999

KROEMER G et al: The biochemistry of programmed cell death. FASEB J 9:1277, 1995

LAM K-P, RAJEWSKY K: B cell development, in *Inflammation: Basic Principles and Clinical Correlates*, 3d ed. J Gallin, R Snyderman (eds). Philadelphia, Lippincott Williams & Wilkins, 1999, pp 151–166

MEDZHITOV R, JANEWAY CA Jr.: Innate immunity: Impact on the adaptive immune response. Curr Opin Immunol 9:4, 1997a

———, ———: Innate immunity: The virtues of a nonclonal system of recognition. Cell 91:295, 1997b

MODLIN RL et al: The Toll of innate immunity on microbial pathogens. N Engl J Med 340:1834, 1999

MORETTA A et al: Major histocompatibility complex class I–specific receptors on human natural killer and T lymphocytes. Immunol Rev 155:105, 1997

PAUL WE (ed): *Fundamental Immunology*, 2d ed. New York, Raven, 1989

ROBEY E, ALLISON IP: T-cell activation: Integration of signals from the antigen receptor and costimulatory molecules. Immunol Today 16:306, 1995

ROMAGNANI S: CD4 effector cells, Chapter 12, in *Inflammation: Basic Principles and Clinical Correlates*, 3d ed, J Gallin, R Snyderman, eds. Philadelphia, Lippincott Williams & Wilkins, 1999, pp 177–184

SCAFFIDI C et al: Apoptosis signaling in lymphocytes. Curr Opin Immunol 11:277, 1999

SIEGAL FP et al: The nature of the principal type 1 interferon-producing cells in human blood. Science 284:1835, 1999

SPRINGER TA: Traffic signals for lymphocyte recirculation and leukocyte emigration: The multistep paradigm. Cell 76:301, 1994

SUGITA M et al: Molecule of the month: CD1—a new paradigm for antigen presentation and T cell activation. Clin Immunol Immunopathol 87:8, 1998

THOMAS ML: The regulation of antigen-receptor signaling by protein tyrosine phosphatases: A hole in the story. Curr Opin Immunol 11:270, 1997

WEISS A, LITTMAN DR: Signal transduction by lymphocyte antigen receptor. Cell 76: 263, 1995

VAN LEEUWEN JEM, SAMELSON LE: T cell antigen-receptor signal transduction. Curr Opin Immunol 11:242, 1999

306

Gerald T. Nepom, Joel D. Taurog

THE MAJOR HISTOCOMPATIBILITY GENE COMPLEX

AS	ankylosing spondylitis	RA	rheumatoid arthritis
CTL	cytolytic T lymphocytes	ReA	reactive arthritis
ER	endoplasmic reticulum	SLE	systemic lupus erythematosus
KIR	killer cell–inhibitory cell receptor	TCRs	T cell receptors
MHC	major histocompatibility complex	TNF	tumor necrosis factor
NK	natural killer		

THE HLA COMPLEX AND ITS PRODUCTS

The human major histocompatibility complex (MHC), commonly called the human leukocyte antigen (HLA) complex, is a 4-megabase (Mb) region on chromosome 6 (6p21.3) that is densely packed with expressed genes. The best known of these genes are the HLA class I and class II genes, whose products are critical for immunologic specificity and transplantation histocompatibility; they play a major role in susceptibility to a number of autoimmune diseases. Many other genes in the HLA region are also essential to the innate and antigen-specific functioning of the immune system. The HLA region shows extensive conservation with the MHC of other mammals in terms of genomic organization, gene sequence, and protein structure and function. Much of our understanding of the MHC has come from investigation of the MHC in mice, where it is termed the *H-2 complex*, and to a lesser degree from other species as well. Nonetheless, in this chapter the discussion will be confined to information applicable to the MHC in humans.

The *HLA class I genes* are located in a 2-Mb stretch of DNA at the telomeric end of the HLA region (Fig. 306-1). The classic (MHC class Ia) HLA-A, -B, and -C loci, the products of which are integral participants in the immune response to intracellular infections, tumors, and allografts, are expressed in all nucleated cells and are highly polymorphic in the population. *Polymorphism* refers to a high degree of allelic variation within a genetic locus that leads to extensive variation between different individuals expressing different alleles. Over 100 alleles at HLA-A, 200 at HLA-B, and 50 at HLA-C have been identified in different human populations. Each of the alleles at these loci encodes a *heavy chain* (also called an *α chain*) that associates noncovalently with the nonpolymorphic light chain *β_2-microglobulin*, encoded on chromosome 15.

The *nomenclature* of HLA genes and their products reflects the grafting of newer DNA sequence information on an older system based on serology. Among class I genes, alleles of the HLA-A, -B, and -C loci were originally identified in the 1950s, 1960s, and 1970s by alloantisera, derived primarily from multiparous women, who in the course of normal pregnancy produce antibodies against paternal antigens expressed on fetal cells. The serologic allotypes were designated by consecutive numbers, e.g., HLA-A1, HLA-B8. The HLA-C locus alleles were designated HLA-Cw, rather than HLA-C, partly to distinguish them from the HLA-encoded complement loci C2 and C4. With the application of DNA sequence analysis and other molecular techniques in the 1980s, and particularly polymerase chain reaction–based techniques since the late 1980s, most serologically defined specificities were found to include a number of closely related alleles differing by only a few amino acids. These are commonly termed *subtypes* of the parent specificity. Currently, under World Health Organization nomenclature, class I alleles are given a single designation that indicates locus, serologic specificity, and sequence-based subtype. For example, HLA-A*0201 indicates subtype 1 of the serologically defined allele HLA-A2. As new alleles are discovered, they are named and numbered based on sequence homology to known alleles or, in the absence of strong homology, designated as consecutively numbered separate alleles, irrespective of serologic reactivity. Subtypes that differ from each other at the nucleotide but not the amino acid sequence level are designated by an extra numeral; e.g., HLA-B*07021 and HLA-B*07022 are two variants of the HLA-B7 subtype of HLA-B*0702. The nomenclature of class II genes, discussed below, is made more complicated by the fact that both chains of a class II molecule are encoded by closely linked HLA-encoded loci, both of which may be polymorphic, and by the presence of differing numbers of isotypic DRB loci in different individuals. It has become clear that accurate HLA genotyping requires DNA sequence analysis, and the identification of alleles at the DNA sequence level has contributed greatly to the understanding of the role of HLA molecules as peptide-binding ligands, to the analysis of associations of HLA alleles with certain diseases, to the study of the population genetics of HLA, and to a clearer understanding of the contribution of HLA differences in allograft rejection and graft-vs.-host disease. Current databases of HLA class I and class II sequences can be accessed by internet (e.g., from the American Society for Histocompatibility and Immunogenetics, www.swmed.edu/home_pages/ASHI/sequences/seq3.htm), and frequent updates of HLA gene lists are published in several journals.

As shown in Fig. 306-2 and discussed below in detail, a characteristic structural feature of class I and class II HLA molecules is the *peptide-binding groove* that enables these molecules to form highly stable complexes with a wide array of peptide sequences that can be recognized as antigens by T cells. In the case of class I molecules, peptide binding provides a display on the cell surface of peptides derived from intracellular proteins, and this serves as a readout to CD8+ T cells of the proteins being produced within somatic cells. The polymorphism at the loci encoding these molecules predominantly affects the amino acid residues that make up the peptide-binding groove, further amplifying the array of peptides that can be bound by different HLA molecules and generating important functional immune differences and transplantation incompatibility among different individuals.

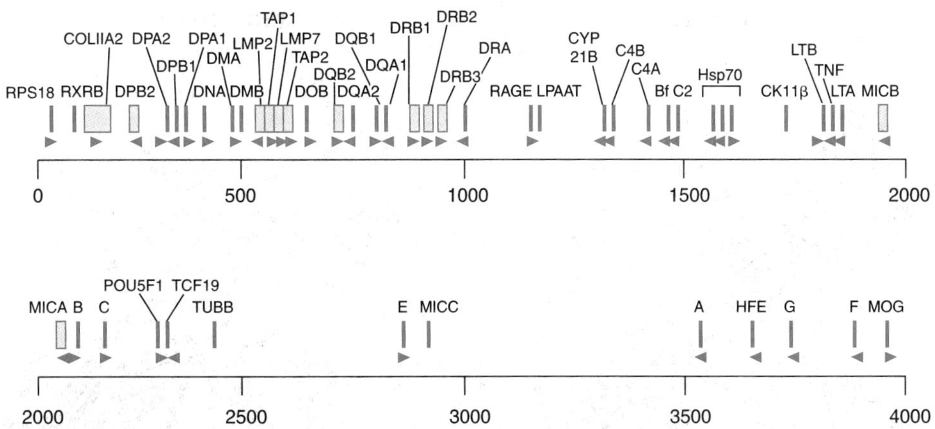

FIGURE 306-1 Physical map of the HLA region, showing the class I and class II loci, other immunologically important loci, and a sampling of other genes mapped to this region. Gene orientation is indicated by arrowheads. Scale is in kilobase (kb). The approximate genetic distance from DP to A is 3.2 cM. This includes 0.8 cM between A and B (including 0.2 cM between C and B), 0.4 to 0.8 cM between B and DR-DQ, and 1.6 to 2.0 cM between DR-DQ and DP.

The nonclassic, or class Ib, MHC molecules, HLA-E, -F, and -G, are much less polymorphic than MHC Ia and, except for HLA-E, have a more limited tissue distribution. The HLA-E molecule, which has a peptide repertoire restricted to signal peptides cleaved from classic MHC class I molecules, is the major self-recognition target for the natural killer (NK) cell inhibitory receptors NKG2A or NKG2C paired with CD94 (see below and Chap. 305). HLA-G is expressed selectively in extravillous trophoblasts, the fetal cell population directly in contact with maternal tissues. It binds a wide array of peptides, is expressed in six different alternatively spliced forms, and provides inhibitory signals to both NK cells and T cells, presumably in the service of maintaining maternofetal tolerance. The function of HLA-F remains largely unknown. Although HLA-C is considered a classic class I molecule, its degree of polymorphism and level of surface expression are significantly lower than those of HLA-A and HLA-B. Moreover, unlike HLA-A and -B molecules, which function primarily by presenting antigen to CD8+ T cells expressing $\alpha\beta$ T cell receptors (TCRs), the primary function of HLA-C molecules appears to be to serve as targets of NK cell recognition (see below).

Additional class I–like genes have been identified, some HLA-linked and some encoded on other chromosomes, that show only distant homology to the class Ia and Ib molecules but that share the three-dimensional class I structure. Those on chromosome 6p21 include MIC-A and MIC-B, which are encoded centromeric to HLA-B; and HLA-HFE, located 3 to 4 cM (centi-Morgan) telomeric of HLA-F. MIC-A and MIC-B do not bind peptide but are expressed on gut and other epithelium in a stress-inducible manner and serve as activation signals for certain $\gamma\delta$ T cells and NK cells, whereas HLA-HFE encodes the gene defective in hereditary hemochromatosis (Chap. 345). Among the non-HLA, class I–like genes, CD1 refers to a family of molecules that present glycolipids or other nonpeptide ligands to certain T cells, including T cells with NK activity; FcRn binds IgG within lysosomes and protects it from catabolism (Chap. 305); and Zn-α_2-glycoprotein 1 binds a nonpeptide ligand and promotes catabolism of triglycerides in adipose tissue. Like the HLA-A, -B, -C, -E, -F, and -G heavy chains, each of which forms a heterodimer with β_2-microglobulin (Fig. 306-2), the class I–like molecules HLA-HFE, FcRn, and CD1 also bind to β_2-microglobulin, but MIC-A, MIC-B, and Zn-α_2-glycoprotein 1 do not.

The *HLA class II region* is also illustrated in Fig. 306-1. Multiple class II genes are arrayed within the centromeric 1 Mb of the HLA region, forming distinct haplotypes. A *haplotype* refers to an array of alleles at polymorphic loci along a chromosomal segment. In the context of HLA, haplotype can refer either to a large segment of the HLA region encompassing many of the polymorphic HLA loci (also called an *extended haplotype* or to a more restricted segment such as the tightly linked DR and DQ loci. Multiple class II genes are present on a single haplotype, clustered into three major subregions: HLA-DR, -DQ, and -DP. Each of these subregions contains at least one functional alpha (A) locus and one functional beta (B) locus. Together these encode proteins that form the α and β polypeptide chains of a mature class II HLA molecule. Thus, the DRA and DRB genes encode an HLA-DR molecule; products of the DQA1 and DQB1 genes form an HLA-DQ molecule; and the DPA1 and DPB1 genes encode an HLA-DP molecule. There are several DRB genes (DRB1, DRB2, and DRB3, etc.), so that two expressed DR molecules are encoded on most haplotypes by combining the α-chain product of the DRA gene with separate β chains.

The class II region was originally termed the *D-region*. The allelic gene products were first detected by their ability to stimulate lymphocyte proliferation by *mixed lymphocyte reaction*, and were named Dw1, Dw2, etc. Subsequently, serology was used to identify gene products on peripheral blood B cells, and the antigens were termed *DR* (D-related). After additional class II loci were identified, these came to be known as DQ and DP.

The HLA class II DRB and DPB loci are extremely polymorphic, with over 200 DR alleles and over 75 DP alleles, respectively. In the DQ region, both DQA1 and DQB1 are polymorphic, with 20 DQA1 alleles and over 40 DQB1 alleles. The current nomenclature is largely analogous to that discussed above for class I, using the convention "locus*allele." Thus, for example, subtypes of the serologically defined specificity DR4, encoded by the DRB1 locus, are termed DRB1*0401, -0402, etc. In addition to allelic polymorphism, products of different DQA1 alleles can, with some limitations, pair with products of different DQB1 alleles through both *cis* and *trans* pairing to create combinatorial complexity and expand the number of expressed class II molecules. Because of the enormous allelic diversity in the general population, most individuals are heterozygous at all of the class I and class II loci. Thus, most individuals express six classic class I molecules (two each of HLA-A, -B, and -C) and approximately eight class II molecules—two DP, two DR (more in the case of haplotypes with additional functional DRB genes), and up to four DQ (two *cis* and two *trans*).

The localization of polymorphic residues in class II molecules is similar to that for class I, i.e., it is predominantly in sites that affect peptide binding (see below). In the case of class II molecules, the peptides displayed on the cell surface are primarily derived from proteins acquired from the extracellular environment, processed through the endosomal-lysosomal pathway, and presented to CD4+ T cells.

OTHER GENES IN THE MHC **Immunologically Relevant Genes** In addition to the class I and class II genes themselves,

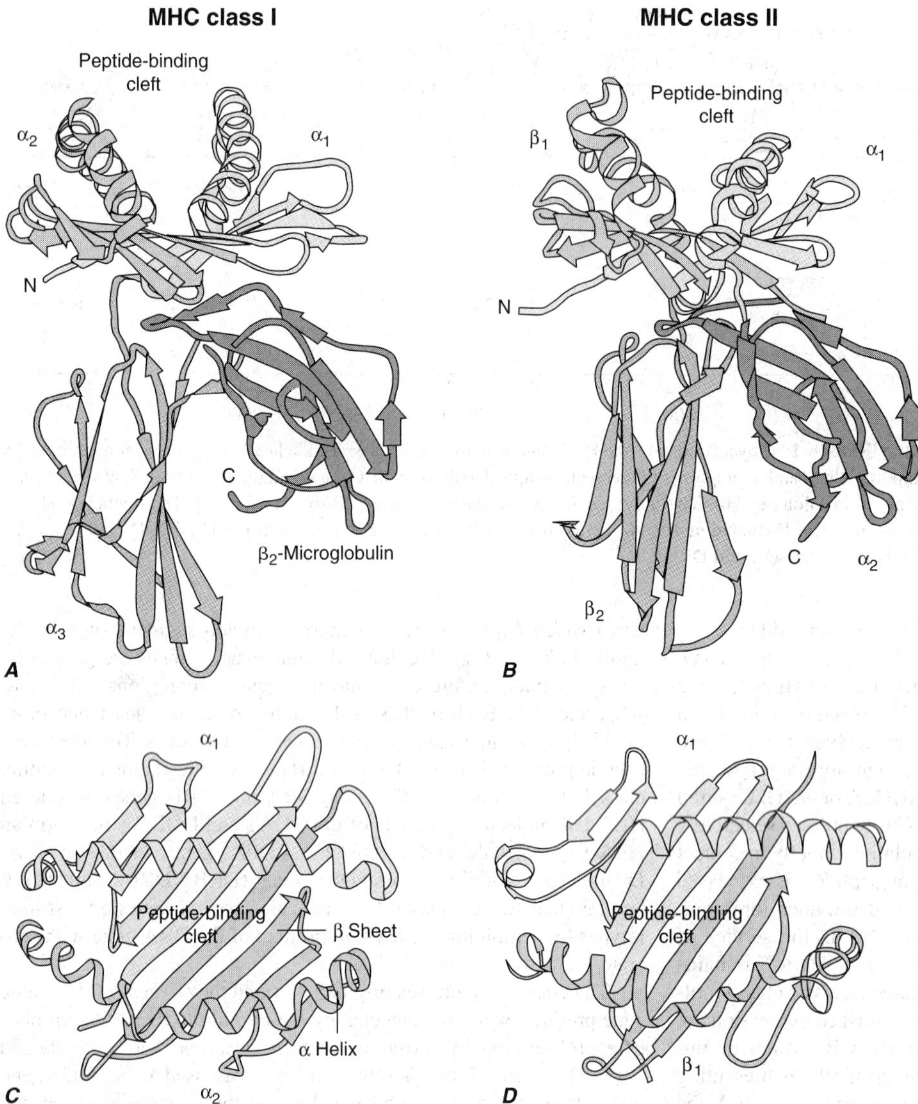

FIGURE 306-2 Side (*A, B*) and top (*C, D*) views of the MHC class I and class II molecules. The α_1 and α_2 domains of class I and the α_1 and β_1 domains of class II form a β-sheet platform that forms the floor of the peptide-binding groove, and α helices that form the sides of the groove. The α_3 (*A*) and β_2 domains (*B*) project from the cell surface and form the contact sites for CD8 and CD4, respectively. *(Adapted from C. Janeway et al, Immunobiology Bookshelf, 2d ed., Garland Publishing, New York, 1997, with permission.)*

there are numerous genes interspersed among the HLA loci that have interesting and important immunologic functions. The current concept of the function of MHC genes now encompasses many of these additional genes. As discussed in more detail below, TAP and LMP genes encode molecules that participate in intermediate steps in the HLA class I biosynthetic pathway, and deficiencies of the TAP or LMP genes can markedly alter class I–mediated immune recognition. Another set of HLA genes, DMA and DMB, performs an analogous function for the class II pathway. These genes encode an intracellular molecule that facilitates the proper complexing of HLA class II molecules with antigen (see below). The HLA class III region is a name given to a cluster of genes between the class I and class II complexes, which includes genes for the two closely related cytokines tumor necrosis factor (TNF) α and lymphotoxin (TNF-β); the complement components C2, C4, and Bf; heat shock protein (HSP)70; and the enzyme 21-hydroxylase.

The class I genes HLA-A, -B, and -C are expressed in all nucleated cells, although generally to a higher degree on leukocytes than on other cells. In contrast, the class II genes show a more restricted distribution: HLA-DR and HLA-DP genes are constitutively expressed on most cells of the myeloid cell lineage, whereas all three class II gene families (HLA-DR, -DQ, and -DP) are inducible by certain stimuli provided by inflammatory cytokines such as interferon γ. Within the lymphoid lineage, expression of these class II genes is constitutive on B cells and inducible on human T cells. Most endothelial and epithelial cells in the body, including the vascular endothelium and the intestinal epithelium, are also inducible for class II gene expression. Thus, while these somatic tissues normally express only class I and not class II genes, during times of local inflammation they are recruited by cytokine stimuli to express class II genes as well, thereby becoming active participants in ongoing immune responses. Other HLA genes involved in the immune response, such as TAP and LMP, are also susceptible to upregulation by signals such as interferon γ.

Other Genes and Genetic Elements Large-scale genomic sequencing projects have recently yielded sequence data for the entire HLA region, which can be accessed on the internet (e.g., www.sanger.ac.uk/HGP/Chr6/). As a result, many new genes have been discovered, the functions of which remain to be determined, as well as numerous microsatellite regions and other genetic elements. The gene density of the class II region is high, with approximately one protein encoded every 30 kb; that of the class I and class III regions is even higher, with approximately one protein encoded every 15 kb. It is also of interest that these regions also differ with respect to the GC (guanidine + cytosine) content. Vertebrate genomes have a long-range mosaic structure with regard to relative GC content that is related to chromosome banding. Regions of homogeneous GC content are termed *isochores*. The HLA class I and class III regions belong to the H3 (highest GC) isochore, with 53% GC, whereas the class II region belongs to the L or H1 isochores (low GC), with 40 to 45% GC. An abrupt demarcation between these two isochores occurs near the boundary separating the class II and class III regions.

LINKAGE DISEQUILIBRIUM In addition to extensive polymorphism at the class I and class II loci, another characteristic feature of the HLA complex is *linkage disequilibrium*. This is formally defined as a deviation from Hardy-Weinberg equilibrium for alleles at linked loci. This is reflected in the very low recombination rates between certain loci within the HLA. For example, recombination between DR and DQ loci is almost never observed in family studies, and characteristic haplotypes with particular arrays of DR and DQ alleles are found in every population. Similarly, the complement components C2, C4, and Bf are almost invariably inherited together, and the alleles at these loci are found in characteristic haplotypes. In contrast, there is a recombinational hotspot between DQ and DP, which are separated by 1 to 2 cM of genetic distance, despite their close physical proximity. Certain extended haplotypes encompassing the interval from DQ into the class I region are commonly found, the most notable being the haplotype DR3-B8-A1, which is found, in whole or in part, in 10 to 30% of northern European Caucasians. The genetic mechanisms that account for linkage disequilibrium in HLA have not been determined.

It has been hypothesized that selective pressures may maintain certain haplotypes, but this remains to be demonstrated. As discussed below under HLA and immunologic disease, one consequence of the phenomenon of linkage disequilibrium has been the difficulty it produces in assigning HLA disease associations to a single allele at a single locus.

MHC STRUCTURE AND FUNCTION

Class I and class II molecules display a distinctive structural architecture that contains specialized functional domains responsible for the unique genetic and immunologic properties of the HLA complex. The principal known function of both class I and class II HLA molecules is to bind antigenic peptides in order to present antigen to an appropriate T cell. The ability of a particular peptide to bind to an individual HLA molecule satisfactorily is a direct function of the molecular fit between the amino acid residues on the peptide with respect to the amino acid residues of the HLA molecule. The bound peptide forms a tertiary structure called the *MHC-peptide complex*, which communicates with T lymphocytes through binding to the TCR molecule. The first site of TCR-MHC-peptide interaction in the life of a T cell occurs in the thymus, where self-peptides are presented to developing thymocytes by MHC molecules expressed on thymic epithelium and hematopoietically derived antigen-presenting cells, which are primarily responsible for positive and negative selection, respectively (see Chap. 305 for details of thymic selection of the T cell repertoire). Mature T cells encounter MHC molecules in the periphery both in the maintenance of tolerance (Chap. 305) and in the initiation of immune responses. Because most antibody responses and all T cell responses are T cell dependent (Chap. 305), the MHC-peptide-TCR interaction is the central event in the initiation of most antigen-specific immune responses, since it is the event that actually confers the specificity. Thus, the population of MHC–T cell complexes expressed in the thymus shapes the TCR repertoire. For potentially immunogenic peptides, the ability of a given peptide to be generated and bound by an HLA molecule is a primary determinant of whether or not an immune response to that peptide can be generated; the repertoire of peptides that a particular individual's HLA molecules can bind exerts a major influence over the specificity of that individual's immune response.

When a TCR molecule binds to an HLA-peptide complex, it forms intermolecular contacts with both the antigenic peptide and with the HLA molecule itself. The outcome of this recognition event depends on the density and duration of the binding interaction, accounting for a dual specificity requirement for activation of the T cell. That is, the TCR must be specific both for the antigenic peptide and for the HLA molecule. The polymorphic nature of the presenting molecules, and the influence that this exerts on the peptide repertoire of each molecule, results in the phenomenon of *MHC restriction* of the T cell specificity for a given peptide. The binding of CD8 or CD4 molecules, respectively, to the class I or class II molecule also contributes to the interaction between T cell and the HLA-peptide complex, by providing for the selective activation of the appropriate T cell.

CLASS I STRUCTURE (Fig. 306-2*A*) As noted above, MHC class I molecules provide a cell-surface display of peptides derived from intracellular proteins; they also provide the signal for self-recognition by NK cells. Surface-expressed class I molecules consist of an MHC-encoded 44-kDa glycoprotein heavy chain, a non-MHC-encoded 12-kDa light chain β_2-microglobulin; and an antigenic peptide, typically 8 to 11 amino acids in length and derived from intracellularly produced protein. The heavy chain contains three domains, termed α_1, α_2, and α_3. The α_1 and α_2 domains form an "intrachain dimer," which together form a peptide-binding groove. In HLA-A and -B molecules, the groove is approximately 3 nm in length by 1-2 nm in maximum width (30 Å $\times$ 12 Å), whereas it is apparently somewhat wider in HLA-C. In cell surface–expressed class molecules, each domain contributes four of the eight strands of antiparallel β sheet, the membrane-distal side of which forms the floor of the groove, and one of the pair of α helices, the two coils of which form the walls of the groove (Fig. 306-2*A*). The membrane-anchored α_3 domain and noncovalently associated β_2-microglobulin chain reside on the membrane-proximal side of the β sheet, each folded in the conformation of an immunoglobulin domain. The peptide is noncovalently bound in an extended conformation within the peptide-binding groove, with both N– and C-terminal ends anchored in pockets within the groove (A and F pockets, respectively) and, in many cases, with a prominent kink, or arch, approximately one-third of the way from the N-terminus that elevates the peptide main chain off the floor of the groove.

A remarkable property of peptide binding by MHC molecules is the ability to form highly stable complexes with a wide array of peptide sequences. This is accomplished by a combination of peptide sequence–independent and –dependent bonding. The former consists of hydrogen bond and van der Waals interactions between conserved residues in the peptide-binding groove and charged or polar atoms along the peptide backbone. The latter are dependent upon the six side pockets that are formed by the irregular surface produced by protrusion of amino acid side chains from within the binding groove. The side chains lining the pockets interact with some of the peptide side chains. The sequence polymorphism among different class I alleles and isotypes predominantly affects the residues that line these pockets, and the interactions of these residues with peptide residues constitute the sequence-dependent bonding that confers a particular sequence "motif" on the range of peptides that can bind any given MHC molecule.

CLASS I BIOSYNTHESIS (Fig. 306-3*A*) The biosynthesis of the classical MHC class I molecules reflects their role in presenting endogenous peptides. The heavy chain is cotranslationally inserted into the membrane of the endoplasmic reticulum (ER), where it becomes glycosylated and associates sequentially with the chaperone proteins calnexin and ERp57. It then forms a complex with β_2-microglobulin, and this complex associates with the chaperone calreticulin and the MHC-encoded molecule tapasin. Meanwhile, peptides generated within the cytosol from intracellular proteins by the multisubunit, multicatalytic proteasome complex are actively transported into the ER by MHC-encoded TAP (transporter associated with antigen processing) heterodimer. Following association with chaperones and trimming by peptidases within the ER, peptides bind to nascent class I molecules for which they have requisite affinity, to form complete, folded heavy chain–β_2-microglobulin–peptide trimer complexes. These are transported rapidly from the ER, through the *cis*- and *trans*-Golgi, where the N-linked oligosaccharide is further processed, and thence to the cell surface. Other proteins have been implicated in MHC class I assembly, e.g., the chaperones BiP and HSP70, but their roles in the pathway are not clear. The pathways for surface MHC class I degradation are poorly understood. A small proportion of heavy chains within properly assembled MHC class I molecules apparently become unfolded and subsequently degraded in the lysosomal pathway.

Most of the peptides transported by TAP are produced in the cytosol by proteolytic cleavage of intracellular proteins by the multisubunit, multicatalytic proteasome. Inhibitors of the proteasome dramatically reduce expression of class I-presented antigenic peptides, but other proteolytic systems may also generate peptides bound to class I. The MHC-encoded proteasome subunits LMP2 and LMP7 may influence the spectrum of peptides produced, but they are not essential for proteasome function. Under certain circumstances, peptides derived from extracellular proteins in particulate form can become associated with class I molecules, but not necessarily by entering the class I pathway. Peptides are apparently bound to chaperones in the cytosol, including HSP90 and HSP70.

CLASS I FUNCTION **Peptide Antigen Presentation** It is estimated that on any given cell, a given class I allele binds several hundred to several thousand distinct peptide species. The vast majority of these peptides are self peptides to which the host immune system is tolerant by one or more of the mechanisms that maintain tolerance, e.g., clonal deletion in the thymus or clonal anergy or clonal ignorance

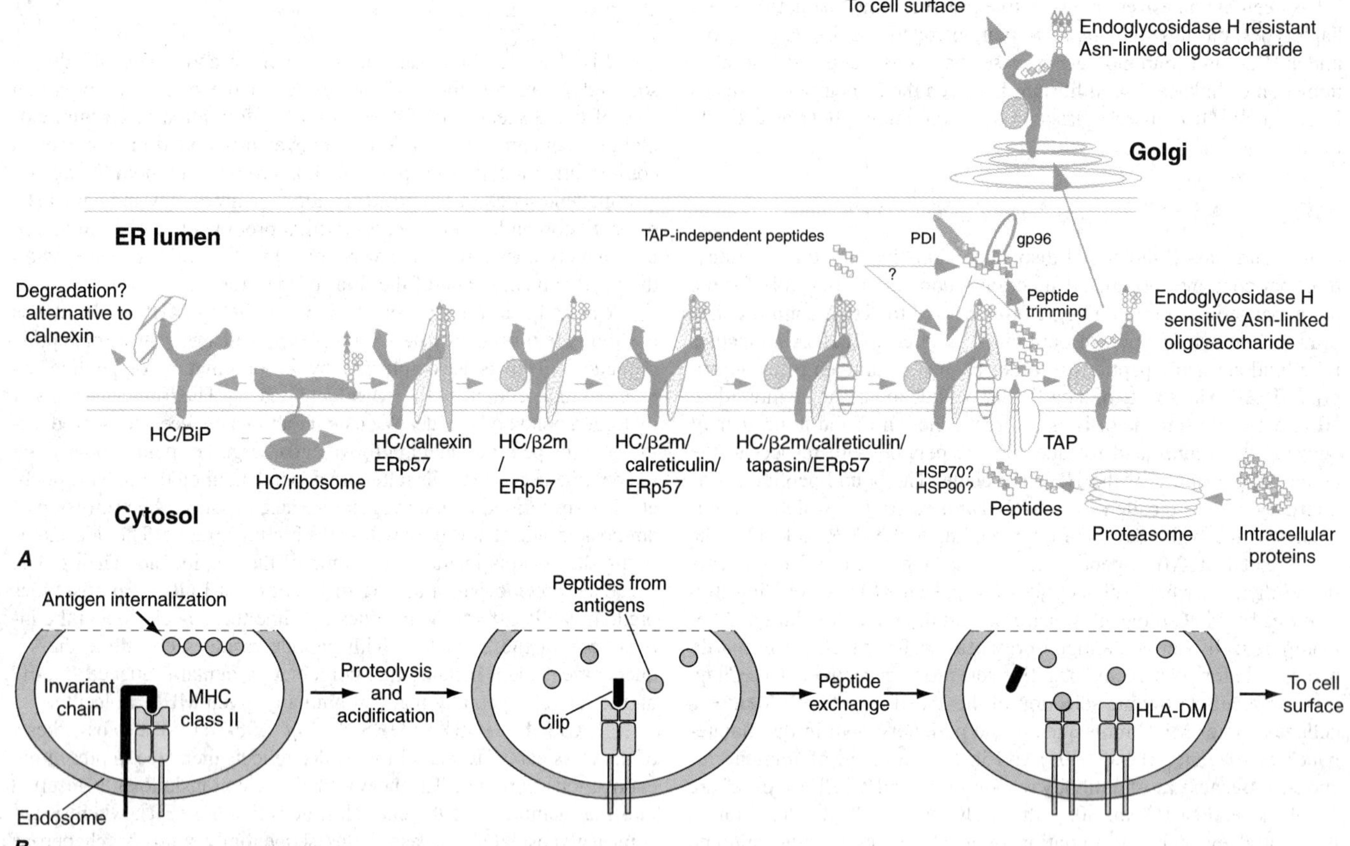

FIGURE 306-3 Biosynthesis of class I (*A*) and class II (*B*) molecules. *A.* Nascent heavy chain (HC) becomes associated with β_2-microglobulin (β2m) and peptide through interactions with a series of chaperones. Peptides generated by the proteasome are transported into the endoplasmic reticulum (ER) by TAP. Peptides undergo N-terminal trimming in the ER and become associated with chaperones, including gp96 and PDI. Once peptide binds to HC-β2m, the HC-β2m-peptide trimeric complex exits the ER and is transported by the secretory pathway to the cell surface. In the Golgi, the N-linked oligosaccharide undergoes maturation, with addition of sialic acid residues. Molecules are not necessarily drawn to scale. *B.* Pathway of HLA class II molecule assembly and antigen processing. After transport through the Golgi and post-Golgi compartment, the class II–invariant chain complex moves to an acidic endosome, where the invariant chain is proteolytically cleaved into fragments and displaced by antigenic peptides, facilitated by interactions with the DMA-DMB chaperone protein. This class II molecule–peptide complex is then transported to the cell surface.

in the periphery (Chaps. 305 and 307). However, class I molecules bearing foreign peptides expressed in a permissive immunologic context activate CD8 T cells, which, if naïve, will then differentiate into cytolytic T lymphocytes (CTL). These T cells and their progeny, through their $\alpha\beta$ T cell receptors, are then capable of Fas/CD95- and/or perforin-mediated cytotoxicity and/or cytokine secretion (Chap. 305) upon further encounter with the class I–peptide combination that originally activated it, and also with other combinations of class I molecules plus peptide that present a similar immunochemical stimulus to the TCR. As alluded to above, this phenomenon by which T cells recognize foreign antigens in the context of specific MHC alleles is termed *MHC restriction*, and the specific MHC molecule is termed the *restriction element*. The most common source of foreign peptides presented by class I molecules is viral infection, in the course of which peptides from viral proteins enter the class I pathway. The generation of a strong CTL response that destroys virally infected cells represents an important antigen-specific defense against many viral infections (Chap. 305). In the case of some viral infections—hepatitis B, for example—CTL-induced target cell apoptosis is thought to be a more important mechanism of tissue damage than any direct cytopathic effect of the virus itself. The importance of the class I pathway in the defense against viral infection is underscored by the identification of a number of viral products that interfere with the normal class I biosynthetic pathway and thus block the immunogenetic expression of viral antigens.

Other examples of intracellularly generated peptides that can be presented by class I molecules in an immunogenic manner include peptides derived from nonviral intracellular infectious agents (e.g., *Listeria*, *Plasmodium*), tumor antigens, minor histocompatibility antigens, and presumably certain autoantigens. There are also situations in which cell surface–expressed class I molecules are thought to acquire and present exogenously derived peptides.

The role of class I HLA molecules in transplantation and in infectious and autoimmune diseases is discussed below.

NK Cell Recognition (See also Chap. 305) NK cells, which play an important role in innate immune responses, are activated to cytotoxicity and cytokine secretion by contact with cells that lack MHC class I expression, and NK cell activation is inhibited by cells that express MHC class I. In humans, the recognition of class I molecules by NK cells is carried out by two classes of receptor families, the killer cell–inhibitory cell receptor (KIR) family and the CD94/NKG2 family. The KIR family, encoded on chromosome 19q13.4, comprises glycoproteins of the immunoglobulin (Ig) superfamily that bind HLA class I molecules and inhibit NK cell–mediated cytotoxicity. An estimated 40 genes are divided into two subfamilies, KIR2D and KIR3D, which contain either two or three Ig domains, respectively. The KIR2D molecules primarily recognize alleles of HLA-C. The latter all possess either asparagine at position 77 and lysine at position 80, or serine at 77 and asparagine at 80 in the α_1 domain of the heavy chain. Different members of the KIR2D family recognize the alternative forms of this polymorphism as well as other residues of the HLA-C heavy chain. The KIR3D molecules predominantly recognize HLA-B alleles. The latter carry a supertypic polymorphism defined serologically by two allotypes, HLA-Bw4 and -Bw6, that are determined by residues 77 to 83 in the α_1 domain of the heavy chain. It is primarily alleles of the Bw4 supertype that bind KIR3D molecules. Although there is KIR recognition of some HLA-A and -Bw6 alleles, many of these alleles appear not to have a corresponding KIR ligand.

The second family of inhibitory NK receptors for HLA is encoded in the NK complex on chromosome 12p12.3-13.1 and consists of CD94 and four NKG2 genes: A, C, E, and D/F. These molecules are C-type (calcium-binding) lectins and are thought to exist as disulfide-bonded heterodimers between CD94 and the various NKG2 glycoproteins. CD94/NKG2A apparently binds to HLA-E and -G and several alleles of HLA-A, -B, and -C. CD94/NKG2C binds primarily to HLA-E. The specificities of the other NKG2 molecules are not yet established. →*The function of NK cells in immune responses is discussed in Chap. 305.*

CLASS II STRUCTURE A specialized functional architecture similar to that of the class I molecules can be seen in the example of a class II molecule depicted in Fig. 306-2*B*, with an antigen-binding cleft arrayed above a supporting scaffold that extends the cleft toward the external cellular environment. However, in contrast to the HLA class I molecular structure, β_2-microglobulin is not associated with class II molecules. Rather, the class II molecule is a heterodimer, composed of a 29-kDa β chain and a 34-kDa α chain. The amino-terminal domains of each chain form the antigen-binding elements, which, like the class I molecule, cradle a bound peptide in a groove bounded by extended α-helical loops, one encoded by the A (α chain) gene and one by the B (β chain) gene. Like the class I groove, the class II antigen-binding groove is punctuated by pockets that contact the side chains of amino acid residues of the bound peptide; unlike the class I groove, it is open at both ends. Therefore, peptides bound by class II molecules vary greatly in length, since both the N- and C-terminal ends of the peptides can extend through the open ends of this groove. Approximately 11 amino acids within the bound peptide form intimate contacts with the class II molecule itself, with backbone hydrogen bonds and specific side chain interactions combining to provide stability and specificity, respectively, to the binding (Fig. 306-4).

The genetic polymorphisms that distinguish different class II genes correspond to changes in the amino acid composition of the class II molecule, and these variable sites are clustered predominantly around the pocket structures within the antigen-binding groove. As with class I, this is a critically important feature of the class II molecule, which explains how genetically different individuals have functionally different HLA molecules.

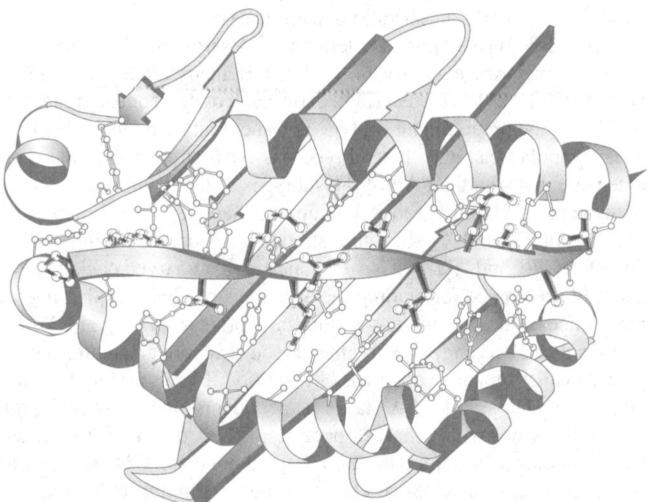

FIGURE 306-4 Top view of the HLA-DR1 molecule containing the peptide 306-318 from influenza hemagglutinin. The N terminus of the peptide is at left, and the peptide lies relatively flat within the peptide-binding groove in an extended conformation with a pronounced twist. Some 35% of the peptide surface is potentially available for interaction with the antigen receptor on T cells. Pockets in the peptide-binding site accommodate 5 of the 13 side chains of the bound peptide, manifesting the peptide specificity of HLA-DR1. Twelve hydrogen bonds between conserved HLA-DR1 residues and the main chain of the peptide provide a universal mode of peptide binding. The ends of the binding groove are open, and longer variants of the peptide can extend out from each end. In contrast, peptides bound to class I molecules are anchored into pockets at their N and C termini by conserved residues, and the middle portion of the peptide is typically kinked upwards out of the groove. *(Adapted from LJ Stern et al: Nature 368:215, 1994. Copyright 1994 Macmillan Magazines Ltd, with permission.)*

As noted above, the class I–peptide complex is preferentially recognized by CD8 T cells, and the class II–peptide complex is preferentially recognized by CD4 T cells. These interactions provide an important signal for activation of specific T cell lineages during antigen-recognition events. The CD8 recognition site is located on the α_3 domain of the MHC class I molecule, and the CD4 recognition site is located on the β_2 domain of the class II molecule, in both cases remote from the peptide-binding site.

BIOSYNTHESIS AND FUNCTION OF CLASS II MOLECULES The intracellular assembly of class II molecules occurs within a specialized compartmentalized pathway that differs dramatically from the class I pathway described above. As illustrated in Fig. 306-3*B*, the class II molecule assembles in the ER in association with a chaperone molecule, known as the *invariant chain*. The invariant chain performs at least two roles. First, it binds to the class II molecule and blocks the peptide-binding groove, thus preventing antigenic peptides from binding. This role of the invariant chain appears to account for one of the important differences between class I and class II MHC pathways, since it can explain why class I molecules present endogenous peptides from proteins newly synthesized in the ER, but class II molecules generally do not. Second, the invariant chain contains molecular localization signals that direct the class II molecule to traffic into post-Golgi compartments known as *endosomes*, which develop into specialized acidic compartments where proteases cleave the invariant chain, and antigenic peptides can now occupy the class II groove. It is at this stage in the intracellular pathway that the MHC-encoded DM molecule catalytically facilitates the exchange of peptides within the class II groove to help optimize the specificity and stability of the MHC-peptide complex.

Once this MHC-peptide complex is deposited in the outer cell membrane, it becomes the target for T cell recognition via a specific TCR expressed on lymphocytes. Because the endosome environment contains internalized proteins retrieved from the extracellular environment, the class II–peptide complex often contains bound antigens that were originally derived from extracellular proteins. In this way, the class II peptide loading pathway provides a mechanism for immune surveillance of the extracellular space. This appears to be an important feature that permits the class II molecule to bind foreign peptides, distinct from the endogenous pathway of class I–mediated presentation.

ROLE OF HLA IN TRANSPLANTATION The development of modern clinical transplantation in the decades since the 1950s provided a major impetus for elucidation of the HLA system, as allograft survival is highest when donor and recipient are HLA-identical. Although many molecular events participate in transplantation rejection, allogeneic differences at class I and class II loci play a major role. Class I molecules can promote T cell responses in several different ways. In the cases of allografts in which the host and donor are mismatched at one or more class I loci, host T cells can be activated by classical *direct alloreactivity*, in which the antigen receptors on the host T cells react with the foreign class I molecule expressed on the allograft. In this situation, the response of any given TCR may be dominated by the allogeneic MHC molecule, the peptide bound to it, or some combination of the two. Another type of host antigraft T cell response involves the uptake and processing of donor MHC antigens by host antigen-presenting cells and the subsequent presentation of the resulting peptides by host MHC molecules. This mechanism is termed *indirect alloreactivity*, or *cross-priming*. It appears to play a quantitatively significant role in allograft rejection, although the molecular and cellular basis for the antigen processing remain to be completely elucidated. In the case of class I molecules on allografts that are shared by the host and the donor, a host T cell response may still be triggered because of peptides that are presented by the class I molecules of the graft but not of the host. The most common basis for the existence of these endogenous antigenic peptides, called *minor histocompatibility antigens*, is a genetic difference between donor and host at a non-MHC locus encoding the structural gene for the protein from which the peptide is derived. These loci are termed *minor histocompatibility loci*, and nonidentical individuals typically differ at many such loci, although only a few provide peptides for any given HLA allele. In recent years, the peptides and parent proteins for a number of human and experimental rodent minor histocompatibility antigens have been identified. In many of these cases of allograft rejection, T cell help for the generation of class I–restricted CD8 cells is provided by CD4 T cells reacting to analogous II differences. Moreover, class II differences alone are sufficient to drive allograft rejection.

ASSOCIATION WITH INFECTIOUS DISEASE It has long been postulated that infectious agents provide the driving force for the allelic diversification seen in the HLA system. This has been difficult to confirm definitively, but one corollary of this hypothesis, namely, that it would be unusual to find HLA alleles strongly associated with susceptibility to any particular infectious disease, has generally been observed. Some modest associations of susceptibility to tuberculosis and leprosy have been found for several subtypes of HLA-DR2 (DRB1*15), and progression of HIV has been associated with several HLA haplotype including HLA-B35, HLA-CW*04, and HLA-A1-B8-DR3 in some studies (Chap. 309). With regard to resistance to infectious disease, the best documented example has been shown for malaria, in which B*5301, DRB1*1302, and DRB1*0101 have been shown to exert varying degrees of protection against severe disease. Slow progression of HIV has been associated with several HLA haplotypes (Chap. 309), and reduced persistence of hepatitis B and C viruses has been associated, respectively, with DRB1*1302 and with DR5.

A polymorphism in the promoter of the TNF-α gene in the HLA class III region, which is associated with quantitative variation in the production of TNF, has recently been shown to have an association with the manifestations of a number of infectious diseases, including cerebral malaria, mucocutaneous leishmaniasis, lepromatous leprosy, scarring trachoma, persistent hepatitis B infection, and fatal meningicoccal meningitis.

ASSOCIATION OF HLA ALLELES WITH SUSCEPTIBILITY TO IMMUNOLOGICALLY MEDIATED DISEASES Because of the immense polymorphism of HLA loci and strong linkage disequilibrium within the HLA region, it became possible, once a sufficient number of alleles had been defined by the early 1970s, to find associations of particular HLA alleles with certain disease states by comparing allele frequencies in patients with any particular disease and in control populations. A large number of such associations were identified during the 1970s. Most subsequent work in this field has been devoted to refining these associations to molecularly defined alleles and attempting to elucidate the contribution of HLA to disease pathogenesis. Table 306-1 lists the major diseases associated with HLA class I and class II genes. The strength of genetic association is reflected in the term *relative risk*, which is a statistical odds ratio representing the risk of disease in an individual carrying a particular genetic marker compared with the risk in individuals in that population without that marker. The nomenclature shown in Table 306-1 reflects both the HLA serotype (e.g., DR3, DR4) and the HLA genotype (e.g., DRB1*0301, DRB1*0401). Both because of the strong linkage disequilibrium within HLA and because the serologically identified loci represent only a small fraction of the total genes within the region, for many years it could not be established whether the associated alleles themselves participated in disease pathogenesis or were merely markers that were in linkage disequilibrium with the true disease allele. In recent years, it has become clear that it is very likely that the class I and class II alleles themselves are the true disease alleles for most of these associations. However, as discussed below, because of the extremely strong linkage disequilibrium between the DR and DQ loci, in some cases it has been difficult to determine the specific locus or combination of class II loci involved. At a minimum, different populations with different DR-DQ haplotypes need to be compared.

As might be predicted from the known function of the class I and class II gene products, almost all of the diseases associated with specific HLA alleles have an immunologic component to their pathogenesis. In some cases, as discussed below, specific protein and even peptide antigens have been implicated, but in no case is the molecular and cellular pathogenesis well understood. From a genetic point of view, strong HLA associations with disease (those associations with a relative risk of 10 or greater) are unusual because the implicated HLA alleles are normal, rather than defective, alleles. However, even in diseases with very strong HLA associations such as ankylosing spondylitis (AS) and type I diabetes mellitus, the non-HLA contribution exceeds 50% of the genetic predisposition, and the concordance of disease in monozygotic twins is considerably higher than in HLA-identical dizygotic twins or other sibling pairs. Genome-wide linkage analyses in these two diseases have found that the non-HLA genetic contribution comes from several other regions, although the linkage to HLA is by far the strongest.

Another group of diseases is genetically linked to HLA, not because of the immunologic function of HLA alleles, but rather because they are caused by autosomal dominant or recessive abnormal alleles at loci that happen to reside in or near the HLA region. Examples of these are 21-hydroxylase deficiency, hemochromatosis, and spinocerebellar ataxia (Chaps. 338, 345, and 364, respectively).

CLASS I DISEASE ASSOCIATIONS Although the associations of human disease with particular HLA alleles or haplotypes predominantly involve the class II region, there are also several prominent disease associations with class I alleles. These include the association of Behçet's disease (Chap. 316) with HLA-B51, psoriasis vulgaris (Chap. 56) with HLA-Cw6, and, most prominently, the spondyloarthropathies (Chap. 315) with HLA-B27. The latter is among the strongest of all HLA associations with disease.

HLA-B27 was originally defined as a serologic determinant. It currently includes a family of 15 HLA-B locus alleles, designated HLA-B*2701-2715, as determined by nucleotide sequencing. HLA-B*2705 is the predominant subtype in Caucasians and most other non-Asian populations, and this subtype has been subjected to the most extensive investigation. All of the subtypes share a common B pocket in the peptide-binding groove, containing characteristic residues His9, Thr24, Glu45, and Cys67, and almost all share adjacent residues Ala69, Lys70, and Ala71. This deep, negatively charged pocket shows a strong preference for binding the arginine side chain, explaining the preference of the B27 binding group for peptides with Arg at P2 (peptide residue 2), as suggested by the crystal structure and confirmed by peptide isolation and sequencing. In addition, B27 is among the most negatively charged of HLA class I heavy chains, and the overall preference is for positively charged peptides. B27 is distinguished among class I alleles as a dominant restricting element for CTL recognition of antigens from a wide variety of viruses, including HIV, and it is associated with prolonged survival in HIV infection (Chap. 309).

HLA-B27 and Disease HLA-B27 is very highly associated with AS (Chap. 315), both in its idiopathic form and in association with chronic inflammatory bowel disease or psoriasis vulgaris. It is also associated with reactive arthritis (ReA; Chap. 315), with other idiopathic forms of peripheral arthritis (undifferentiated spondyloarthropathy), and with recurrent acute anterior uveitis. B27 is found in 50 to 90% of individuals with these conditions, compared with a prevalence of ~7% in North American Caucasians. The prevalence of B27 in patients with idiopathic AS is 90%, and in AS complicated by iritis or aortic insufficiency is close to 100%. The absolute risk of spondyloarthropathy in unselected B27+ individuals has been variously estimated at 2 to 13% and >20% if a B27+ first-degree relative is affected. The concordance rate of AS in identical twins is very high, approximately 75%. It can be concluded that the B27 molecule itself is involved in disease pathogenesis, based on strong evidence from clinical epidemiology and on the occurrence of a spondyloarthropathy-like disease in HLA-B27 transgenic rats. A well-established association with both AS and ReA exists for subtypes B*2702, -04, and -05, and anecdotal association has been reported for subtypes B*2701, -03, -07, -08, -10, and -11. The propensity of the B27 molecule to induce disease thus presumably derives from one or more unique features of its structure that are shared by several B27 subtypes. It remains a central unanswered question whether the pathogenesis of B27-associated disease derives from the specificity of a particular peptide or family of peptides bound to B27 or whether another mechanism is involved that is independent of the peptide specificity of B27. The first alternative can be further subdivided into mechanisms that involve T cell recognition of B27-peptide complexes, and those that do not. A variety of other roles for B27 in disease pathogenesis have been postulated, including molecular or antigenic mimicry between B27 and certain bacteria and reduced killing of intracellular bacteria in cells expressing B27. However, the most straightforward possibility is the presentation of peptides to CD8 T cells in a way that somehow promotes joint inflammation, i.e., the "arthritogenic peptide" hypothesis. This concept has been supported in ReA by the finding of CD8-restricted antigen-specific T cells, particularly in *Yersinia*-induced ReA. It is of particular interest that the HSP60 molecule from *Y. enterocolitica* has been shown to give rise to dominant antigens recognized by both synovial B27-restricted CD8 and class II–restricted CD4 T cells. This suggests a T cell pathogenesis involving intramolecular help and/or epitope spreading in which a B27-restricted response could well be primary.

In contrast to ReA, there is little direct evidence regarding the molecular role of HLA-B27 in ankylosing spondylitis. However, correlations between disease susceptibility and the peptide-binding specificity of the B27 subtypes have been found that support the "arthritogenic peptide" hypothesis in AS. Specifically, a lack of disease susceptibility has been documented for the subtypes B*2706, found mainly amongst Southeast Asians, and B*2709, found mainly amongst Sardinians. B*2709 differs from B*2705 only at residue 116, carrying His instead of Asp. B*2706 differs from B*2704 at 114 and 116, carrying Asp and Tyr instead of His and Asp. These residues, which lie in the floor of the peptide-binding groove, interact with the C-terminal end of the bound peptide. Unlike the disease-associated subtypes, B*2706 and B*2709 have been found not to carry peptides with C-terminal Tyr. This has led to the hypothesis of a disease-prone B27-bound peptide with C-terminal Tyr.

Table 306-1 Significant HLA Class I and Class II Associations with Disease[a]

	Marker	Gene	Strength of Association
SPONDYLOARTHROPATHIES			
Ankylosing spondylitis	B27	B*2702, -04, -05	++++
Reiter's syndrome	B27		++++
Acute anterior uveitis	B27		+++
Reactive arthritis (*Yersinia, Salmonella, Shigella, Chlamydia*)	B27		+++
Psoriatic spondylitis	B27		+++
COLLAGEN-VASCULAR DISEASES			
Juvenile arthritis, pauciarticular	DR8		++
	DR5		++
Rheumatoid arthritis	DR4	DRB1*0401, -04, -05	+++
Sjögren's syndrome	DR3		++
Systemic lupus erythematosus			
Caucasian	DR3		+
Japanese	DR2		++
AUTOIMMUNE GUT AND SKIN			
Gluten-sensitive enteropathy (celiac disease)	DR3	DQA1*0501 DQB1*0201	+++
Chronic active hepatitis	DR3		++
Dermatitis herpetiformis	DR3		+++
Psoriasis vulgaris	Cw6		++
Pemphigus vulgaris	DR4	DRB1*0402	+++
	DR6	DQB1*0503	
AUTOIMMUNE ENDOCRINE			
Type 1 diabetes mellitus	DR4	DQB1*0302	+++
	DR3		++
	DR2	DQB1*0602	—[b]
Hyperthyroidism (Graves')	B8		+
	DR3		+
Hyperthyroidism (Japanese)	B35		+
Adrenal insufficiency	DR3		++
AUTOIMMUNE NEUROLOGIC			
Myasthenia gravis	B8		+
	DR3		+
Multiple sclerosis	DR2	DRB1*1501 DRB5*0101	++
OTHER			
Behçet's disease	B51		++
Congenital adrenal hyperplasia	B47	21-OH (Cyp21B)	+++
Narcolepsy	DR2		++++
Goodpasture's syndrome (anti-GBM)	DR2		++

[a] Various diseases associated with HLA genes are listed, with the HLA serotype or linked marker most frequently found related to disease. Genes are listed for cases where specific alleles have been identified as responsible for this association. The strength of association reflects the likelihood of disease in individuals with the marker compared to individuals who do not carry the marker; ++++, relative risk > 10; +++, relative risk > 5; ++, relative risk > 3; +, relative risk > 1.5.

[b] Strong negative association, i.e., genetic association with protection from diabetes.

CLASS II DISEASE ASSOCIATIONS The majority of associations between HLA and disease are with class II alleles (Table 306-1). Several diseases have complex HLA genetic associations.

Celiac Disease In the case of celiac disease (Chap. 286), it is probable that the HLA-DQ genes are the primary basis for the disease association. HLA-DQ genes present on both the celiac-associated DR3 and DR7 haplotypes include the DQB1*0201 gene, and further detailed studies have documented a specific class II $\alpha\beta$ dimer encoded by the DQA1*0501 and DQB1*0201 genes, which appears to account for the HLA genetic contribution to celiac disease susceptibility. This specific HLA association with celiac disease may have a straightforward explanation: peptides derived from the wheat gluten component gliaden are bound to the molecule encoded by DQA1*0501 and DQB1*0201 and presented to T cells. A gliaden-derived peptide that has been implicated in this immune activation binds the DQ class II dimer best when the peptide contains a glutamine to glutamic acid substitution. It has been proposed that tissue transglutaminase, an enzyme present at increased levels in the intestinal cells of celiac patients, converts glutamine to glutamic acid in gliadin, creating peptides that are capable of being bound by the DQ2 molecule and presented to T cells.

Pemphigus Vulgaris In the case of pemphigus vulgaris (Chap. 58), there are two HLA haplotypes associated with disease: DRB1*0402-DQB1*0302 and DRB1*1401-DQB1*0503. Peptides derived from epidermal autoantigens have been implicated that preferentially bind to the DRB1*0402-encoded molecule, suggesting that specific peptide binding by this disease-associated class II molecule is important in disease. However, there are no class II genes in common between the disease-associated DR4 and DR14 haplotypes, and there is no evidence for any interaction of the latter haplotype interacting with the epidermal peptides that bind the DRB1*0402-encoded molecule. Thus, the most likely interpretation is that each of these class II associations with pemphigus represents a different pathway to a comparable clinical outcome.

Juvenile Arthritis Pauciarticular juvenile arthritis (Chap. 312) is an autoimmune disease associated with genes at the DRB1 locus and also with genes at the DPB1 locus. Patients with both DPB1*0201 and a DRB1 susceptibility allele (usually DRB1*08 or -*05) have a higher relative risk than expected from the additive effect of those genes alone. In juvenile patients with rheumatoid factor–positive polyarticular disease, heterozygotes carrying both DRB1*0401 and -*0404 have a relative risk >100, reflecting an apparent synergy in individuals inheriting both of these susceptibility genes.

Type 1 Diabetes Mellitus There are several aspects of the genetics of type 1 diabetes (Chap. 333) that illustrate the complex nature of HLA associations with autoimmune diseases. First, type 1 (autoimmune) diabetes mellitus is associated with both DR3 and DR4 serotypes and their corresponding genes. The presence of both the DR3 and DR4 haplotypes in one individual confers the highest known genetic risk for type diabetes, and individuals carrying either of these haplotypes also carry some increased risk. Specific class II genes on each haplotype have been thoroughly studied, and the strongest association is with DQB1*0302, a specific gene on the diabetes-associated DR4 haplotypes. Thus, all DR4 haplotypes that carry a DQB1*0302 gene are associated with type 1 diabetes, whereas related DR4 haplotypes that carry a different DQB1 gene are not. The primary class II determinant of susceptibility, therefore, is HLA-DQB1*0302. However, the relative risk associated with inheritance of this gene can be modified, depending on other HLA genes present either on the same or a second haplotype. For example, just as the presence of a second haplotype containing DR3 is associated with an increased risk of diabetes, the presence of a DR2-positive haplotype containing a DQB1*0602 gene is associated with decreased risk. This gene, DQB1*0602, is considered "protective" for type 1 diabetes. Even some DRB1 genes that can occur on the same haplotype as DQB1*0302 may modulate risk, so that individuals with the DR4 haplotype that contains DRB1*0403 are less susceptible to type 1 diabetes than individuals with other DR4-DQB1*0302 haplotypes.

Although the presence of a DR3 haplotype in combination with the DR4-DQB1*0302 haplotype is a very high risk combination for diabetes susceptibility, the specific gene on the DR3 haplotype that is responsible for this synergy has not yet been identified. This is because the predominant HLA-DR3 haplotype in Caucasians has very tight linkage with other genes within the MHC, including HLA-A1, -B8, -Cw7, and -C4A, as discussed above. Thus, any of a large variety of genes within the HLA region on this DR3 haplotype may be the primary gene(s) responsible for contributing to diabetes susceptibility. An example that more directly implicates other genes linked to DR3 is the association between HLA genes and systemic lupus erythematosus (SLE; Chap. 311). The C4A null alleles that are present on the HLA-DR3 haplotypes in SLE are also often present in patients without DR3, notably those with HLA-DR2. This implies the presence of a C4A silent allele, which is a defective structural gene for the C4 complement component, rather than the expression of any particular class II gene, as a potential susceptibility gene within HLA associated with SLE.

HLA and Rheumatoid Arthritis The HLA genes most highly associated with rheumatoid arthritis (RA) are DRB1*0401 and DRB1*0404 (Chap. 312). These genes encode a distinctive sequence of amino acids from codons 67 to 74 of the DRβ molecule: RA-associated class II molecules carry the sequence LeuLeuGluGlnArgArgAlaAla or LeuLeuGluGlnLysArgAlaAla in this region, while non-RA-associated genes carry one or more differences in this region. These residues form a portion of the molecule that lies in the middle of the α-helical portion of the DRB1-encoded class II molecule, termed the *shared epitope*.

These DR4+ RA-associated alleles are most frequent among patients with more severe, erosive disease. The frequency of these DR4+ alleles is lower among patients with RA who are rheumatoid factor–negative and those with nonerosive forms of the disease. Although the frequency of these DRB1 susceptibility alleles in RA patients is high, the same genes are also prevalent in the unaffected population, and thus the absolute risk associated with these susceptibility alleles is low. The highest risk for susceptibility to RA comes in individuals who carry both a DRB1*0401 and DRB1*0404 gene. Some forms of RA are associated with other HLA genes, such as DRB1*01, -*1001, and -*1402, which also carry the shared epitope sequence, strongly suggesting that this part of the class II molecule contributes directly to disease pathogenesis.

MOLECULAR MECHANISMS FOR HLA DISEASE ASSOCIATIONS As noted above, HLA molecules play a key role in the selection and establishment of the antigen-specific T cell repertoire and a major role in the subsequent activation of those T cells during the initiation of an immune response. Precise genetic polymorphisms characteristic of individual alleles dictate the specificity of these interactions and thereby instruct and guide antigen-specific immune events. These same genetically determined pathways are therefore implicated in disease pathogenesis when specific HLA genes are responsible for autoimmune disease susceptibility.

The fate of developing T cells within the thymus is determined by the affinity of interaction between TCR and HLA molecules bearing self peptides; thus, the particular HLA types of each individual control the precise specificity of the T cell repertoire (Chap. 305). The primary basis for HLA-associated disease susceptibility may well lie within this thymic maturation pathway. The positive selection of potentially autoreactive T cells, based on the presence of specific HLA susceptibility genes, may establish the threshold for disease risk in a particular individual.

At the time of onset of a subsequent immune response, the primary role of the HLA molecule is to bind peptide and present it to antigen-specific T cells. The HLA complex can therefore be viewed as encoding genetic determinants of precise immunologic activation events. Antigenic peptides that bind particular HLA molecules are capable of stimulating T cell immune responses; peptides that do not bind are not presented to T cells and are not immunogenic. This genetic control of the immune response is mediated by the polymorphic sites within the HLA antigen-binding groove that interact with the bound peptides. In autoimmune and immune-mediated diseases, it is likely that specific tissue antigens that are targets for pathogenic lymphocytes are complexed with the HLA molecules encoded by specific susceptibility alleles. In autoimmune diseases with an infectious etiology, it is likely that immune responses to peptides derived from the initiating pathogen are bound and presented by particular HLA molecules to activate T lymphocytes that play a triggering or contributory role in disease pathogenesis. The concept that early events in disease initiation are triggered by specific HLA-peptide complexes offers some prospects for therapeutic intervention, since it may be possible to design compounds that interfere with the formation or function of specific HLA-peptide-TCR interactions.

When considering mechanisms of HLA associations with the immune response and with disease it is well to remember that just as HLA genetics are complex, so are the mechanisms likely to be heterogeneous. Immune-mediated disease is a multistep process in which one of the HLA-associated functions is to establish a repertoire of potentially reactive T cells, while another HLA-associated function is to provide the essential peptide-binding specificity for T cell recognition. For diseases with multiple HLA genetic associations, it is possible that both of these interactions occur and synergize to advance an accelerated pathway of disease.

BIBLIOGRAPHY

BRAUD VM et al: Functions of nonclassical MHC and non-MHC-encoded class I molecules. Curr Opin Immunol 11:100, 1999

BUSCH R, MELLINS ED: Developing and shedding inhibitions: How MHC class II molecules reach maturity. Curr Opin Immunol 8:51, 1996

GODKIN A, JEWELL D: The pathogenesis of celiac disease. Gastroenterology 115:206, 1998

HAMMER J et al: HLA class II peptide binding specificity and autoimmunity. Adv Immunol 66:67, 1997

HILL AV: The immunogenetics of human infectious diseases. Annu Rev Immunol 16:593, 1998

LOPEZ-LARREA C et al: The role of HLA-B27 polymorphism and molecular mimicry in spondyloarthropathy. Mol Med Today 4:540, 1998

NEPOM GT: Major histocompatibility complex–directed susceptibility to rheumatoid arthritis. Adv Immunol 68:315, 1998

———, KWOK WW: Molecular basis for HLA-DQ associations with IDDM. Diabetes 47:1177, 1998

PAMER E, CRESSWELL P: Mechanisms of MHC class I–restricted antigen processing. Annu Rev Immunol 16:323, 1998

STERN LJ, WILEY DC: Antigenic peptide binding by class I and class II histocompatibility proteins. Structure 2(4):245, 1994

TAUROG JD et al: Inflammatory disease in HLA-B27 transgenic rats. Immunol Rev 169: 209, 1999

307

Peter E. Lipsky, Betty Diamond

AUTOIMMUNITY AND AUTOIMMUNE DISEASES

One of the classically accepted features of the immune system is the capacity to distinguish self from non-self. Although they are able to recognize and generate reactions to a vast array of foreign materials, most animals do not mount immune responses to self-antigens under ordinary circumstances and thus are tolerant to self. Although recognition of self plays an important role in generating both the T cell and B cell repertoires of immune receptors and plays an essential role in the recognition of nominal antigen by T cells, the development of potentially harmful immune responses to self-antigens is, in general, precluded. Autoimmunity, therefore, represents the end result of the breakdown of one or more of the basic mechanisms regulating immune tolerance.

The presence or absence of pathologic consequences resulting from self-reactivity determines whether autoimmunity leads to the development of an autoimmune disease. The essential feature of an autoimmune disease is that tissue injury is caused by the immunologic reaction of the organism with its own tissues. Autoimmunity, on the other hand, refers merely to the presence of antibodies or T lymphocytes that react with self-antigens and does not necessarily imply that the development of self-reactivity has pathogenic consequences.

Autoimmunity may occur as an isolated event or in the setting of specific clinical syndromes. Autoimmunity may be seen in normal individuals and in higher frequency in normal older people. In addition, autoreactivity may develop during various infectious conditions. The expression of autoimmunity may be self-limited, as occurs with many infectious processes, or persistent. In both circumstances there is a tendency to develop autoreactivity directed against a variety of different tissues or organs. As mentioned above, autoimmunity does not necessarily lead to tissue damage, and even in the presence of organ pathology, it may be difficult to determine whether the damage is mediated by autoreactivity. Thus, the presence of self-reactivity may be either the cause or a consequence of an ongoing pathologic process. Furthermore, when autoreactivity is induced by an inciting event, such as infection or tissue damage from trauma or infarction, there may or may not be ensuing pathology.

MECHANISMS OF AUTOIMMUNITY Since Ehrlich first postulated the existence of mechanisms to prevent the generation of self-reactivity in 1900, ideas concerning the nature of this inhibition have developed in parallel with the progressive increase in understanding of the immune system. Burnet's clonal selection theory included the idea that interaction of lymphoid cells with their specific antigens during fetal or early postnatal life would lead to elimination of such "forbidden clones." This idea became untenable, however, when it was shown by a number of investigators that autoimmune diseases could be induced by simple immunization procedures, that autoantigen-binding cells could be demonstrated easily in the circulation of normal individuals, and that self-limited autoimmune phenomena frequently developed during infections. These observations indicated that clones of cells capable of responding to autoantigens were present in the repertoire of antigen-reactive cells in normal adults and suggested that mechanisms in addition to clonal deletion were responsible for preventing their activation.

Table 307-1 Mechanisms Preventing Autoimmunity

1. Sequestration of self-antigen
2. Generation and maintenance of tolerance
   a. Central deletion of autoreactive lymphocytes
   b. Peripheral anergy of autoreactive lymphocytes
   c. Receptor replacement by autoreactive lymphocytes
3. Regulatory mechanisms
   a. Anti-idiotype regulation
   b. Regulatory T cells

Currently, three general processes are thought to be involved in the maintenance of selective unresponsiveness to autoantigens (Table 307-1): (1) sequestration of self-antigens, rendering them inaccessible to the immune system; (2) specific unresponsiveness (tolerance or anergy) of relevant T or B cells; and (3) limitation of potential reactivity by regulatory mechanisms. These mechanisms permit the host to respond to the vast universe of foreign antigens but preclude responses to autoantigens that might have pathogenic consequences.

Derangements of these normal processes may predispose to the development of autoimmunity (Table 307-2). In general, these abnormal responses relate to stimulation by exogenous agents, usually bacterial or viral, or endogenous abnormalities in the cells of the immune system. Thus, autoreactivity can result from exogenous stimulation of the immune system in a manner that overcomes the regulated unresponsiveness to self-antigens. Microbial superantigens, such as staphylococcal protein A and staphylococcal enterotoxins, are substances that can stimulate a broad range of T and B cells based upon specific interactions with selected families of immune receptors irrespective of their antigen specificity. If autoantigen reactive T and/or B cells express these receptors, autoimmunity might develop. Alternatively, mo-

Table 307-2 Mechanisms of Autoimmunity

- I. Exogenous
  - A. Molecular mimicry
  - B. Superantigenic stimulation
  - C. Microbial adjuvanticity
- II. Endogenous
  - A. Altered antigen presentation
    1. Loss of immunologic privilege
    2. Presentation of novel or crytic epitopes (epitope spreading)
    3. Alteration of self-antigen
    4. Enhanced function of antigen-presenting cells
       a. Costimulatory molecule expression
       b. Cytokine production
  - B. Increased T cell help
    1. Cytokine production
    2. Costimulatory molecules
  - C. Increased B cell function
  - D. Apoptotic defects
  - E. Cytokine imbalance
  - F. Altered immunoregulation
    1. Anti-idiotype regulation
    2. Regulatory T cells

lecular mimicry or cross-reactivity between a microbial product and a self-antigen might lead to activation of autoreactive lymphocytes. One of the best examples of autoreactivity and autoimmune disease resulting from molecular mimicry is rheumatic fever, in which antibodies to the M protein of streptococci cross-react with myosin, laminin, and other matrix proteins. Deposition of these autoantibodies in the heart initiates an inflammatory response. Molecular mimicry between microbial proteins and host tissues has been reported in insulin-dependent diabetes mellitus (IDDM), rheumatoid arthritis, and multiple sclerosis. The capacity of nonspecific stimulation of the immune system to predispose to the development of autoimmunity has been explored in a number of models; one is provided by the effect of adjuvants on the production of autoimmunity. Autoantigens become much more immunogenic when administered with adjuvant. It is presumed that infectious agents may be able to overcome self-tolerance because they possess molecules, such as bacterial endotoxin, that have adjuvant-like effects on the immune system.

Endogenous derangements of the immune system may also contribute to the loss of immunologic tolerance, or anergy, to self-antigens and the development of autoimmunity (Table 307-2). Many autoantigens reside in immunologically privileged sites, such as the brain or the anterior chamber of the eye. These sites are characterized by the inability of engrafted tissue to elicit immune responses. Immunologic privilege results from a number of events, including the limited entry of proteins from those sites into lymphatics, the local production of immunosuppressive cytokines such as transforming growth factor (TGF) β, and the local expression of molecules such as Fas ligand that can induce apoptosis of activated T cells. Lymphoid cells remain in a state of immunologic ignorance (neither activated nor anergized) to proteins expressed uniquely in immunologically privileged sites. If the privileged site is damaged by trauma or inflammation, or if T cells are activated elsewhere, proteins expressed at this site can become the targets of immunologic assault. Such an event may occur in multiple sclerosis and sympathetic ophthalmia, in which antigens uniquely expressed in the brain and eye, respectively, become the target of activated T cells.

Alterations in antigen presentation may also contribute to autoimmunity. This may occur by epitope spreading, in which protein determinants (*epitopes*) not routinely seen by lymphocytes (*cryptic epitopes*) are recognized as a result of immunologic reactivity to associated molecules. For example, animals immunized with one protein component of the spliceosome may be induced to produce antibodies to multiple other spliceosome proteins. Finally, inflammation, drug exposure, or normal senescence may cause a primary chemical alteration in proteins, resulting in the generation of immune responses that cross-react with normal self-proteins. Alterations in the availability and presentation of autoantigens may be important components of immunoreactivity in certain models of organ-specific autoimmune diseases. In addition, these factors may be relevant in understanding the pathogenesis of various drug-induced autoimmune conditions. However, the diversity of autoreactivity manifest in non-organ-specific systemic autoimmune diseases suggests that these conditions might result from a more general activation of the immune system rather than from an alteration in individual self-antigens.

A number of experimental models have suggested that intense stimulation of T lymphocytes can produce nonspecific signals that bypass the need for antigen-specific helper T cells and lead to polyclonal B cell activation with the formation of multiple autoantibodies. For example, antinuclear, antierythrocyte, and antilymphocyte antibodies are produced during the chronic graft-versus-host reaction. In addition, true autoimmune diseases, including autoimmune hemolytic anemia and immune complex–mediated glomerulonephritis, can also be induced in this manner. While it is clear that such diffuse activation of helper T cell activity can cause autoimmunity, nonspecific stimulation of B lymphocytes can also lead to the production of autoantibodies. Thus, the administration of polyclonal B cell activators, such as bacterial endotoxin, to normal mice leads to the production of a number of autoantibodies, including those directed to DNA and IgG (rheumatoid factor).

Primary alterations in the activity of T and/or B cells, cytokine imbalances, or defective immunoregulatory circuits may also contribute to the emergence of autoimmunity. Although the biochemical bases of many of these abnormalities have not been documented, they may contribute to the emergence of autoimmunity either alone or in concert. For example, decreased apoptosis, as can be seen in animals with defects in Fas (CD95) or Fas ligand or in patients with related abnormalities, can be associated with the development of autoimmunity. Similarly, diminished production of tumor necrosis factor (TNF) α and interleukin (IL)10 has been reported to be associated with the development of autoimmunity.

An alternative explanation for the development of autoimmunity is that self-reactivity results not from overstimulation of the immune system but rather from an abnormality of immunoregulatory mechanisms. Observations made in both human autoimmune disease and animal models suggest that defects in the generation and expression of regulatory T cell activity may allow for the production of autoantibodies. The importance of defects in immunoregulatory cells is confirmed by the finding that administration of normal suppressor T cells or factors derived from them can prevent the development of autoimmune disease in rodent models of autoimmunity.

One of the mechanisms that regulates normal humoral immune responses is the production of anti-idiotype antibodies. These are immunoglobulin molecules directed against antigen-binding determinants of the specific antibodies originally elicited by the immunogen. Production of anti-idiotype antibodies may be dependent on helper T cell activity even when the initial immunogen is T cell independent. Therefore, it is possible that abnormalities in the generation of appropriate anti-idiotype antibodies, either at the B or T cell level, are responsible for the development of autoimmunity in certain circumstances.

It should be apparent that no single mechanism can explain all the varied manifestations of autoimmunity. Indeed, it appears likely, especially in systemic autoimmune diseases, that a number of abnormalities may converge to induce the complete syndrome. Moreover, one abnormality may cause a second, which, in concert with the first, facilitates the expression of autoimmunity. This possibility is consistent with recent findings in murine models of IDDM; systemic lupus erythematosus (SLE), rheumatoid arthritis, and multiple sclerosis in which multiple genetic regions, many of which are involved in controlling immune reactivity, appear to contribute to the development of autoimmune disease.

Despite the plethora of immunologic derangements identified in systemic autoimmune diseases such as SLE, the primary abnormality causing the disease remains unclear. In fact, detailed examination of a number of murine strains that spontaneously develop a lupus-like syndrome has failed to demonstrate a common immunologic abnormality. Additional factors that appear to be important determinants in the induction of autoimmunity include age, sex, genetic background, exposure to infectious agents, and environmental contacts. How all of these disparate factors affect the capacity to develop self-reactivity is currently being intensively investigated.

GENETIC CONSIDERATIONS Evidence in humans that there are susceptibility genes for autoimmunity comes from family studies and especially from studies of twins. Studies in IDDM, rheumatoid arthritis, multiple sclerosis, and SLE have shown that approximately 15 to 30% of pairs of monozygotic twins show disease concordance, compared with <5% of dizygotic twins. The occurrence of different autoimmune diseases within the same family has suggested that certain susceptibility genes may predispose to a variety of autoimmune diseases. In addition to this evidence from humans, certain inbred mouse strains reproducibly develop specific spontaneous or experimentally induced autoimmune diseases, whereas others do not. These findings have led to an extensive search for genes that determine susceptibility to autoimmune disease.

The most consistent association for susceptibility to autoimmune disease has been with the major histocompatibility complex (MHC). Many human autoimmune diseases are associated with particular HLA alleles (Chap. 306). It has been suggested that the association of MHC genotype with autoimmune disease relates to differences in the ability of different allelic variations of MHC molecules to present autoantigenic peptides to autoreactive T cells. An alternative hypothesis involves the role of MHC alleles in shaping the T cell receptor repertoire during T cell ontongeny in the thymus. Additionally, specific MHC gene products themselves may be the source of peptides that can be recognized by T cells. Cross-reactivity between such MHC peptides and peptides derived from proteins produced by common microbes may trigger autoimmunity by molecular mimicry. However, MHC genotype alone does not determine the development of autoimmunity. Identical twins are far more likely to develop the same autoimmune disease than MHC-identical nontwin siblings, suggesting that genetic factors other than the MHC also affect disease susceptibility. Recent studies of the genetics of IDDM, SLE, and multiple sclerosis in humans and mice have shown that there are several independently segregating disease susceptibility loci in addition to the MHC.

There is evidence that several other genes are important in increasing susceptibility to autoimmune disease. In humans, inherited homozygous deficiency of the early proteins of the classic pathway of complement (C1, C4, or C2) is very strongly associated with the development of SLE. In mice and humans, abnormalities in the genes encoding proteins involved in the regulation of apoptosis, including Fas (CD95) and Fas ligand (CD95 ligand), are strongly associated with the development of autoimmunity. There is also evidence that inherited variation in the level of expression of certain cytokines, such as TNF-α or IL-10, may also increase susceptibility to autoimmune disease.

A further important factor in disease susceptibility is the hormonal status of the patient. Many autoimmune diseases show a strong sex bias, which appears in most cases to relate to the hormonal status of women. ■

Table 307-3 Mechanisms of Tissue Damage in Autoimmune Disease

Effector	Mechanism	Target	Disease
Autoantibody	Blocking or inactivation	α Chain of the nicotinic acetylcholine receptor	Myasthenia gravis
		Phospholipid–β_2-glycoprotein 1 complex	Antiphospholipid syndrome
		Insulin receptor	Insulin-resistant diabetes mellitus
		Intrinsic factor	Pernicious anemia
	Stimulation	TSH receptor (LATS)	Graves' disease
		Proteinase-3 (ANCA)	Wegener's granulomatosis
		Epidermal cadherin$_1$ Desmoglein 3	Pemphigus vulgaris
	Complement activation	α_3 Chain of collagen IV	Goodpastures' syndrome
	Immune-complex formation	Double-stranded DNA	Systemic lupus erythematosus
		Ig	Rheumatoid arthritis
	Opsonization	Platelet GpIIb:IIIa	Autoimmune thrombocytopenic purpura
		Rh antigens, I antigen	Autoimmune hemolytic anemia
	Antibody-dependent cellular cytotoxicity	Thyroid peroxidase, thyroglobulin	Hashimoto's thyroiditis
T cells	Cytokine production	?	Rheumatoid arthritis, Multiple sclerosis, insulin-dependent diabetes mellitus
	Cellular cytotoxicity	?	Insulin-dependent diabetes mellitus

NOTE: ANCA, antineutrophil cytoplasmic antibody; LATS, long-acting thyroid stimulator; TSH, thyroid-stimulating hormone.

IMMUNOPATHOGENIC MECHANISMS IN AUTOIMMUNE DISEASES The mechanisms of tissue injury in autoimmune diseases can be divided into antibody-mediated and cell-mediated processes. Representative examples are listed in Table 307-3.

The pathogenicity of autoantibodies can be mediated through several mechanisms, including opsonization of soluble factors or cells, activation of an inflammatory cascade via the complement system, and interference with the physiologic function of soluble molecules or cells.

In autoimmune thrombocytopenic purpura, opsonization of platelets targets them for elimination by phagocytes. Likewise, in autoimmune hemolytic anemia, binding of immunoglobulin to red cell membranes leads to phagocytosis and lysis of the opsonized cell. Goodpastures' syndrome, a disease characterized by lung hemorrhage and severe glomerulonephritis, represents an example of antibody binding leading to local activation of complement and neutrophil accumulation and activation. The autoantibody in this disease binds to the α_3 chain of type IV collagen in the basement membrane. In SLE, activation of the complement cascade at sites of immunoglobulin deposition in renal glomeruli is considered to be a major mechanism of renal damage.

Autoantibodies can also interfere with normal physiologic functions of cells or soluble factors. Autoantibodies against hormone receptors can lead to stimulation of cells or to inhibition of cell function through interference with receptor signaling. For example, long-acting thyroid stimulators (LATS), which are autoantibodies that bind to the receptor for thyroid-stimulating hormone (TSH), are present in Graves' disease and function as agonists, causing the thyroid to respond as if there were an excess of TSH. Alternatively, antibodies to the insulin receptor can cause insulin-resistant diabetes mellitus through receptor blockade. In myasthenia gravis, autoantibodies to the acetylcholine receptor can be detected in 85 to 90% of patients and are responsible for muscle weakness. The exact location of the antigenic epitope, the valence and affinity of the antibody, and perhaps other characteristics determine whether activation or blockade results from antibody binding.

Antiphospholipid antibodies are associated with thromboembolic events in primary and secondary antiphospholipid syndrome and have also been associated with fetal wastage. The major antibody is directed to the phospholipid–β_2-glycoprotein I complex and appears to exert a procoagulant effect. In pemphigus vulgaris, autoantibodies bind to a component of the epidermal cell desmosome, desmoglein 3, and play a role in the induction of the disease. They exert their pathologic effect by disrupting cell-cell junctions through stimulation of the production of epithelial proteases, leading to blister formation. Cytoplasmic antineutrophil cytoplasmic antibody (c-ANCA), found in Wegener's granulomatosis, is an antibody to an intracellular antigen, the 29-kDa serine protease (proteinase-3). In vitro experiments have shown that IgG c-ANCA causes cellular activation and degranulation of primed neutrophils.

It is important to note that autoantibodies of a given specificity may cause disease only in genetically susceptible hosts, as has been shown in experimental models of myasthenia gravis. Finally, some autoantibodies seem to be markers for disease but have as yet no known pathogenic potential.

AUTOIMMUNE DISEASE Manifestations of autoimmunity are found in a large number of pathologic conditions. However, their presence does not necessarily imply that the pathologic process is an autoimmune disease. A number of attempts to establish formal criteria for the diagnosis of autoimmune diseases have been made, but none is universally accepted. One set of criteria is shown in Table 307-4; however, this should be viewed merely as a guide in consideration of the problem.

To classify a disease as autoimmune, it is necessary to demonstrate that the immune response to a self-antigen causes the observed pathology. Initially, the demonstration that antibodies against the affected tissue could be detected in the serum of patients suffering from various diseases was taken as evidence that these diseases had an autoimmune basis. However, such autoantibodies are also found when tissue damage is caused by trauma or infection, and the autoantibody is secondary to tissue damage. Thus, it is necessary to show that autoimmunity is pathogenic before classifying a disease as autoimmune.

If the autoantibodies are pathogenic, it may be possible to transfer disease to experimental animals by the administration of autoantibodies, with the subsequent development of pathology in the recipient similar to that seen in the patient from whom the antibodies were obtained. This has been shown, for example, in Graves' disease. Some autoimmune diseases can be transferred from mother to fetus and are observed in the newborn babies of diseased mothers. The symptoms of the disease in the newborn usually disappear as the levels of the maternal antibody decrease. An exception is congenital heart block, in which damage to the developing conducting system of the heart as a result of transfer of anti-Ro antibody from the mother results in permanent heart block.

In most situations, the critical factors that determine when the development of autoimmunity results in autoimmune disease have not been delineated. The relationship of autoimmunity to the development of autoimmune disease may relate to the fine specificity of the antibodies or T cells or their specific effector capabilities. In many circumstances a mechanistic understanding of the pathogenic potential of autoantibodies has not been established. In some autoimmune diseases, biased production of cytokines by helper T (T_H) cells may play a role in pathogenesis. In this regard, T cells can differentiate into specialized effector cells that predominantly produce interferon γ (T_H1) or IL-4 (T_H2) (Chap. 305). The former facilitate macrophage activation and classic cell-mediated immunity, whereas the latter are thought to have regulatory functions and are involved in the resolution of normal immune responses and also the development of responses to a variety of parasites. In a number of autoimmune diseases, such as rheumatoid arthritis, multiple sclerosis, IDDM, and Crohn's disease, there appears to be biased differentiation of T_H1 cells, with resultant organ damage.

Table 307-4 Human Autoimmune Disease: Presumptive Evidence for an Immunologic Pathogenesis

Major Criteria

1. Presence of autoantibodies or evidence of cellular reactivity to self
2. Documentation of relevant autoantibody or lymphocytic infiltrate in the pathologic lesion.
3. Demonstration that relevant autoantibody or T cells can cause tissue pathology
   a. Transplacental transmission
   b. Adaptive transfer into animals
   c. In vitro impact on cellular function

Supportive Evidence

1. Reasonable animal model
2. Beneficial effect from immunosuppressive agents
3. Association with other evidence of autoimmunity
4. No evidence of infection or other obvious cause

ORGAN-SPECIFIC VERSUS SYSTEMIC AUTOIMMUNE DISEASES Autoimmune diseases form a spectrum, from those specifically affecting a single organ to systemic disorders with involvement of many organs (Table 307-5). Hashimoto's autoimmune thyroiditis is probably the best studied example of an organ-specific autoimmune disease (Chap. 330). In this disorder, there is a specific lesion in the thyroid associated with infiltration of mononuclear cells and damage to follicular cells. Antibody to thyroid constituents can be demonstrated in nearly all cases. Other organ- or tissue-specific autoimmune disorders include pemphigus vulgaris, autoimmune hemolytic anemia, idiopathic thrombocytopenic purpura, Goodpasture's syndrome, myasthenia gravis, and sympathetic ophthalmia. One important feature of some organ-specific autoimmune diseases is the tendency for overlap, such that an individual with one specific syndrome is more likely to develop a second syndrome. For example, there is a high incidence of pernicious anemia in individuals with autoimmune thyroiditis. More striking is the tendency for individuals with an organ-specific autoimmune disease to develop multiple other manifestations of autoimmunity without the development of associated organ pathology. Thus, as many as 50% of individuals with pernicious anemia have non-cross-reacting antibodies to thyroid constituents, whereas patients with myasthenia gravis may develop antinuclear antibodies, antithyroid antibodies, rheumatoid factor, antilymphocyte antibodies, and polyclonal hypergammaglobulinemia. Part of the explanation for this may relate to the genetic elements shared by individuals with these different diseases.

SYSTEMIC AUTOIMMUNE DISEASE Systemic autoimmune diseases differ from organ-specific diseases in that pathologic lesions are found in multiple, diverse organs and tissues. The hallmark of these conditions is the demonstration of associated relevant autoimmune manifestations that are likely to be etiologic in the organ pathology. SLE is the best example of such a disorder. Although a number of other diseases such as Sjögren's syndrome possess certain of the features of a systemic autoimmune disease, SLE represents the prototype of these disorders because of its abundance of autoimmune manifestations.

SLE is a disease of protean manifestations that characteristically involves the kidneys, joints, skin, serosal surfaces, blood vessels, and central nervous system (Chap. 311). The disease is associated with a vast array of autoantibodies whose production appears to be a part of a generalized hyperreactivity of the humoral immune system. Other features of SLE include generalized B cell hyperresponsiveness, polyclonal hypergammaglobulinemia, and increased titers of antibodies to commonly encountered viral antigens.

A number of the autoantibodies found in SLE have clearly been implicated in certain of the pathologic features of the disease. Clas-

Table 307-5 Some Autoimmune Diseases

ORGAN SPECIFIC	
Graves' disease	Autoimmune hemolytic anemia
Hashimoto's thyroiditis	Autoimmune thrombocytopenic purpura
Autoimmune polyglandular syndrome	Pernicious anemia
Insulin-dependent diabetes mellitus	Myasthenia gravis
Insulin-resistant diabetes mellitus	Multiple sclerosis
Immune-mediated infertility	Guillain-Barré syndrome
Autoimmune Addison's disease	Stiff-man syndrome
Pemphigus vulgaris	Acute rheumatic fever
Pemphigus foliaceus	Sympathetic ophthalmia
Dermatitis herpetiformis	
Autoimmune alopecia	Goodpasture's syndrome
Vitiligo	
ORGAN NONSPECIFIC (SYSTEMIC)	
Systemic lupus erythematosus	Wegener's granulomatosis
Rheumatoid arthritis	Antiphospholipid syndrome
Systemic necrotizing vasculitis	Sjögren's syndrome

Table 307-6 Immunopathogenic Mechanisms in Systemic Lupus Erythematosus

Mechanism	Autoantibody	Pathologic Consequence
Inactivation or blocking	Antilymphocyte	Depressed T lymphocyte function Inhibition of suppressor T cell function
	Anticoagulants	Inhibition of clotting
	Antineuron	CNS dysfunction
	Antineutrophil	Depressed phagocytosis
	Anti-Ro	Congenital heat block
	Antiphospholipid	Thrombosis
Opsonization	Antierythrocyte	Hemolytic anemia
	Antiplatelet	Thrombocytopenia
	Antilymphocyte	Lymphopenia
	Antineutrophil	Neutropenia
Immune-complex deposition or in situ formation	Anti-DNA Antinucleoprotein, Anti-RNP, anti-IgG	Renal disease

NOTE: CNS, central nervous system.

sically, SLE has been considered a disorder in which immune complexes are the major pathogenic entity. While immune-complex deposition or in situ formation of complexes appears to be a major pathogenic mechanism in lupus renal disease, additional autoimmune processes may be implicated in the pathogenesis of other features of the disease (Table 307-6).

The etiology of SLE remains unknown, and the interplay of a number of factors appears to be involved in its pathogenesis. Race and gender play an important role as evidenced by the increased incidence in young black females. The role of environmental factors is suggested by the high incidence of autoantibodies, especially antilymphocyte antibodies, in nonconsanguineous household contacts of individuals with SLE. The importance of genetic influences is suggested by family studies indicating that first-degree relatives of SLE patients have an increased likelihood of developing autoimmunity and autoimmune disease. The very high concordance rate for SLE and even higher rate for autoimmunity in monozygotic twins supports this concept. Finally, the association of SLE with MHC genes confirms the importance of immunogenetic factors in its pathogenesis. Current hypotheses concerning the immunopathogenesis of SLE suggest that autoantibody formation may result from a combination of exaggerated B cell activation owing either to excessive exogenous stimulation or endogenous hyperactivity and inadequate regulatory T cell or anti-idiotype regulation. Genetic elements may contribute to each of these abnormalities.

BIBLIOGRAPHY

ANDRE I et al: Checkpoints in the progression of autoimmune disease: Lessons from diabetes models. Proc Natl Acad Sci USA 93:2260, 1996

BERNAL A et al: Superantigens in human disease. J Clin Immunol 19:149, 1999

GIANANI R, SARVETNICK N: Viruses, cytokines, antigens, and autoimmunity. Proc Natl Acad Sci USA 93:2257, 1996

MADAIO MP: The role of autoantibodies in the pathogenesis of lupus nephritis. Semin Nephrol 19:48, 1999

MCDEVITT HO: The role of MHC class II molecules in susceptibility and resistance to autoimmunity. Curr Opin Immunol 10:677, 1998

MOLLER E: Mechanisms for induction of autoimmunity in humans. Acta Paediatr Suppl 424:16, 1998

O'GARRA A et al: CD4+ T-cell subsets in autoimmunity. Curr Opin Immunol 9:872, 1997

PARISH CR, O'NEILL ER: Dependence of the adaptive immune response on innate immunity: Some questions answered but new paradoxes emerge. Immunol Cell Biol 75: 523, 1997

RAY S et al: Pathogenic autoantibodies are routinely generated during the response to foreign antigen: A paradigm for autoimmune disease. Proc Natl Acad Sci USA 93: 2019, 1996

RIDWAY WM, FATHMAN CG: The association of MHC with autoimmune disease: Understanding the pathogenesis of autoimmune diabetes. Clin Immunol Immunopathol 86:3, 1998

ROSE NR: The role of infection in the pathogenesis of autoimmune disease. Semin Immunol 10:5, 1998

STEINMAN L, CONLON P: Viral damage and the breakdown of self-tolerance. Nat Med 3:1085, 1997

VANDERLUGT C, MILLER SD: Epitope spreading. Curr Opin Immunol 8:831, 1996

VON HERRATH MG, OLDSTONE MBA: Virus-induced autoimmune disease. Curr Opin Immunol 8:878, 1996

VYSE TJ, TODD JA: Genetic analysis of autoimmune disease. Cell 85:311, 1996

308

Max D. Cooper, Harry W. Schroeder, Jr.

PRIMARY IMMUNE DEFICIENCY DISEASES

ADA adenosine deaminase
AT ataxia-telangiectasia
Btk Bruton's tyrosine kinase
EBV Epstein-Barr virus
IFNGR1 interferon γ receptor 1
IFNGR2 interferon γ receptor signal-transducing chain
MHC major histocompatibility complex
NK natural killer
PNP purine nucleoside phosphorylase
PPD purified protein derivative
SCID severe combined immunodeficiency
TCR T cell receptors
WHN winged-helix-nude

Immunologic functions are mediated by developmentally independent, but functionally interacting, families of lymphocytes. The activities of B and T lymphocytes and their products in host defense are closely integrated with the functions of other cells of the reticuloendothelial system. Dendritic cells, Langerhans' cells in the skin, and macrophages play an important role in the trapping and presentation of antigens to T and B cells to initiate the immune response. Macrophages also become effector cells, especially when activated by cytokine products of lymphocytes. The scavenger activity of macrophages and polymorphonuclear leukocytes is directed and made specific by antibodies in concert with cytokines and the complement system. Natural killer (NK) cells, a population of granular lymphocytes with receptors specific for MHC class I molecules, may spontaneously kill tumor and virus-infected cells, activities that are enhanced by the cytokine products of immune and inflammatory cells. Killing by NK cells can also be targeted by IgG antibodies for which NK cells have cell-surface receptors. The interaction of basophils and tissue mast cells with IgE antibodies in causation of immediate-type hypersensitivity is discussed in Chap. 310. Consideration of these interrelationships is an important part of the analysis of patients with suspected immune deficiency.

DIFFERENTIATION OF T AND B CELLS The functional deficits that occur in both congenital and acquired immunodeficiencies are usefully viewed as being caused by defects at various points along the differentiation pathways of immunocompetent cells. A subpopulation of hematopoietic stem cells become restricted to lymphoid differentiation prior to migration to the thymus, where T cells are generated, and in the fetal liver and adult bone marrow, where B cell development begins (Fig. 308-1). Immature T and B cells then migrate through the circulation to the spleen, lymph nodes, intestine and other peripheral lymphoid organs. In these sites, they may encounter antigens presented by dendritic cells or macrophages and respond with proliferation, differentiation and mediation of immune responses. Chap. 305 provides a general account of their roles in cellular and humoral immunity.

Differentiation of T or B cells may be arrested at either the primary or secondary stages. Reflecting the complex cellular interactions involved in immune responses and the pivotal role played by T lymphocytes, immune deficiencies primarily involving T cells are usually also associated with abnormal B cell function. Conversely, immuno-

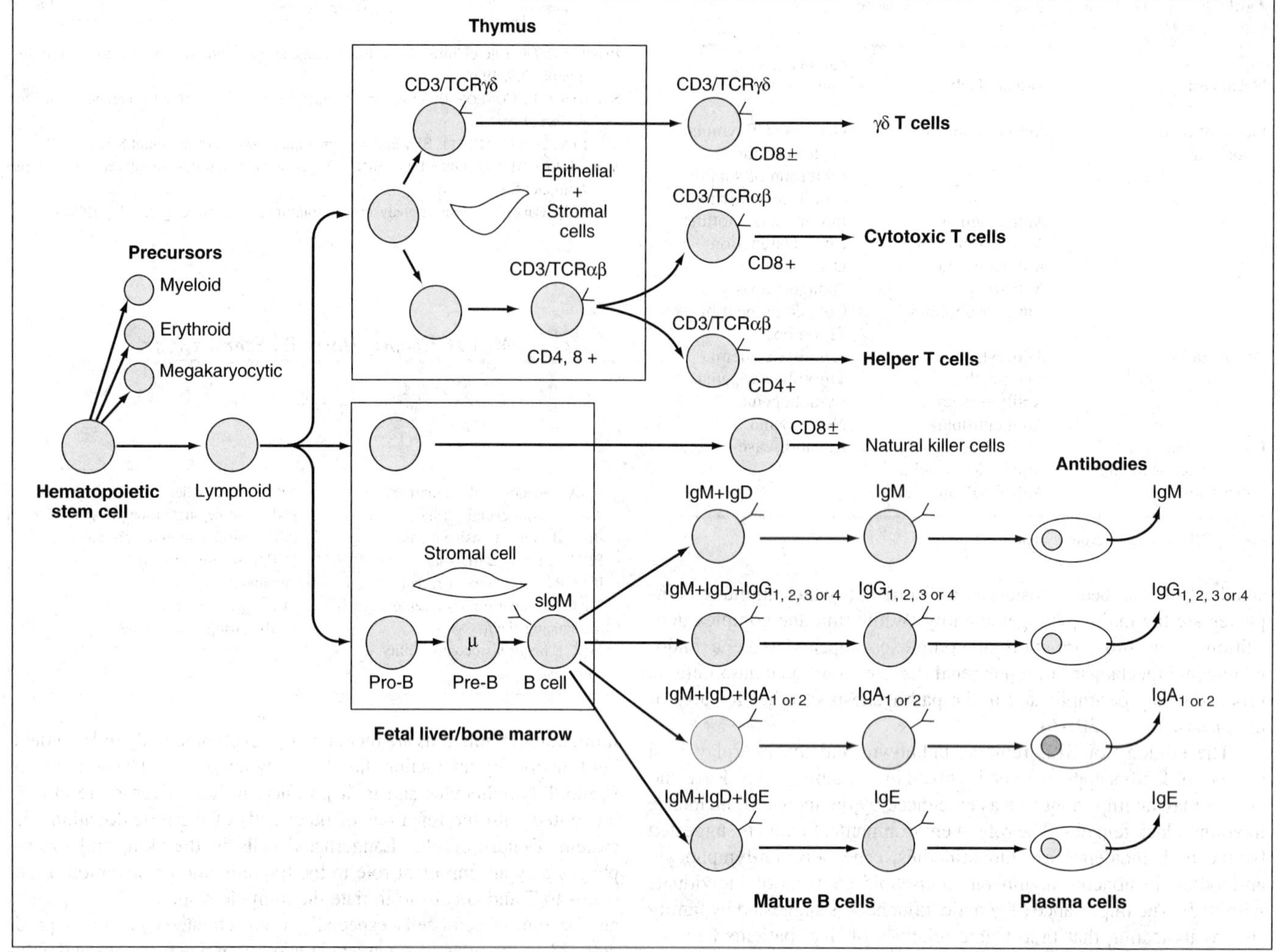

FIGURE 308-1 Hypothetical model outlining the differentiation of hematopoietic stem cells along T, B, and NK cell lineages. The antigen presenting dendritic cells, not shown here, are derived from both lymphoid and myeloid progenitors. Failure to develop T and B cells may result from defective stem cells or from inborn metabolic errors affecting both cell types. Rarely, other hematopoietic cell lines are also absent. Absence of either T or B cells suggests malfunction of central lymphoid tissues, including the thymus and the fetal liver–bone marrow complex. B cell deficiency may result from failure to generate pre-B cells from their stem cell precursors or from failure of pre-B cells to give rise to their B lymphocyte progeny. Similarly, differentiation may be arrested at several levels within the T cell lineage; arrests at the thymocyte level and failure to develop the helper subset have been observed in immunodeficient patients. Agammaglobulinemia and deficiencies of some T cell functions may occur despite the presence of normal numbers of B or T cells in the circulation. Failure of B lymphocytes to differentiate to plasma cells can be due to intrinsic cellular abnormalities or to faulty T cell regulation.

deficiencies manifested primarily by inability to produce antibodies may be caused by T cell defects not associated with abnormal cell-mediated immunity.

CLINICAL DISEASE FEATURES COMMON TO IMMUNE DEFICIENCY Immunodeficiency syndromes, whether congenital, spontaneously acquired, or iatrogenic, are characterized by unusual susceptibility to infection and not infrequently to autoimmune disease and lymphoreticular malignancies. The types of infection often provide the first clue to the nature of the immunologic defect.

Patients with *defects in humoral immunity* have recurrent or chronic sinopulmonary infection, meningitis, and bacteremia, most commonly caused by pyogenic bacteria such as *Haemophilus influenzae*, *Streptococcus pneumoniae*, and staphylococci. These and other pyogenic organisms also cause frequent infections in individuals who have either neutropenia or a deficiency of the pivotal third component of complement (C3). The tripartite collaboration of antibody, complement, and phagocytes in host defense against pyogenic organisms makes it important to assess all three systems in individuals with unusual susceptibility to bacterial infections.

Antibody-deficient patients in whom cell-mediated immunity is intact have an interesting response to viral infections. The clinical course of primary infection with viruses such as varicella zoster or rubeola, unless complicated by bacterial infection, does not differ significantly from that of the normal host. However, long-lasting immunity may not develop, and as a result, multiple bouts of chickenpox and measles may occur. Such observations suggest that intact T cells may be sufficient for control of established viral infections, while antibodies play an important role in limiting the initial dissemination of virus and in providing long-lasting protection. Exceptions to this generalization are becoming more widely recognized. Agammaglobulinemic patients fail to clear hepatitis B virus from their circulation and have a progressive, and often fatal, course. Poliomyelitis has occurred following live-virus vaccination in some patients. Chronic encephalitis, which may progress over a period of months to years, is a particular threat in congenitally agammaglobulinemic boys. Echoviruses and adenoviruses have been isolated from brain, spinal fluid, or other sites in such patients.

The occurrence of an unusually serious infection, for example, *H. influenzae* meningitis in an older child or adult, warrants consideration of humoral immune deficiency. Recurrent bacterial pneumonias also suggest this possibility. Chronic otitis media occurs frequently in patients with hypogammaglobulinemia and is significant because of its relative rarity in normal adults. Pansinusitis, although almost invariably present in immunoglobulin deficiency, is a less helpful finding because it is not rare in apparently normal people. Bacterial infections of the skin or urinary tract are less frequent problems in hypogammaglobulinemic patients.

Infestation with the intestinal parasite *Giardia lamblia* is a frequent cause of diarrhea in antibody-deficient patients.

Abnormalities of cell-mediated immunity predispose to disseminated virus infections, particularly with latent viruses such as herpes simplex (Chap. 182), varicella zoster (Chap. 183), and cytomegalovirus (Chap. 185). In addition, patients so affected almost invariably develop mucocutaneous candidiasis and frequently acquire systemic fungal infections. Pneumonia caused by *Pneumocystis carinii* is also common (Chap. 209). Severe enteritis caused by *Cryptosporidium* infection may extend to the biliary tract to result in sclerosing cholangitis.

T cell deficiency is always accompanied by some abnormality of antibody responses (Fig. 308-1), although this may not be reflected by hypogammaglobulinemia. This explains in part why patients with primary T cell defects are also subject to overwhelming bacterial infection.

The most severe form of immune deficiency occurs in individuals, often infants, who lack both cell-mediated and humoral immune functions. Individuals with severe combined immunodeficiency (SCID) are susceptible to the whole range of infectious agents including organisms not ordinarily considered pathogenic. Multiple infections with viruses, bacteria, and fungi occur, often simultaneously. Because donor lymphocytes cannot be rejected by these recipients, blood transfusions can produce fatal graft-versus-host disease.

EVALUATION OF IMMUNODEFICIENT PATIENTS A careful history and physical examination will usually indicate whether the major problem involves the antibody-complement-phagocyte system or cell-mediated immunity. A history of contact dermatitis due to poison ivy suggests intact cellular immunity. Persistent mucocutaneous candidiasis suggests deficient cell-mediated immunity. Lymphopenia and the absence of palpable lymph nodes may be important findings. However, patients with profound immunodeficiency may have diffuse lymphoid hyperplasia. Most immunodeficiencies may be diagnosed by thoughtful use of tests available in local or regional clinical laboratories. More precise evaluation of immunologic functions and treatment may require referral to specialized centers. Table 308-1 presents a résumé of widely available laboratory investigations.

Humoral Immunity With rare exceptions, deficiency of humoral immunity is accompanied by diminished serum concentration of one or more classes of immunoglobulin. Normal values vary with age, and adult concentrations of IgM (1.0 ± 0.4 g/L) are reached at about 1 year, of IgG (10.0 ± 3.0 g/L) at 5 to 6 years, and of IgA (2.5 ± 1.0 g/L) by puberty (Chap. 305). The wide range of values among normal adults creates difficulty in defining the lower limits of normal. Reasonable estimates for low values are below 0.4 g/L for IgM, 5 g/L for IgG, and 0.5 g/L for IgA. In the presence of borderline hypogammaglobulinemia, assessing the patient's capacity to produce specific antibodies becomes particularly important. Isohemagglutinins, anti-streptolysin O, and "febrile agglutinins" are valuable standard assays, and measurements of pre- and postimmunization titers to tetanus toxoid, diphtheria toxoid, *H. influenzae* capsular polysaccharide, and *S. pneumoniae* serotypes provide a comprehensive assessment of humoral responsiveness.

Estimation of numbers of circulating B and T lymphocytes is of value in determining the pathogenesis of certain types of immune deficiency. B lymphocytes are identified by the presence of membrane-bound immunoglobulins, their associated α- and β-chain units, and other lineage-specific molecules on the B cell surface (Table 308-1), which can be identified and enumerated by specific monoclonal antibodies.

Since antibody deficiency may be mimicked clinically by deficiency of complement components, measurement of total hemolytic complement (CH_{50}) should be a part of the evaluation of host defense. Measurement of C3 alone is inadequate for screening, since deficiencies of both early and late complement components may predispose to bacterial infection (Chap. 305).

Table 308-1 Laboratory Evaluation of Host Defense Status

Initial Screening Assays[a]

Complete blood count with differential smear

Serum immunoglobulin levels: IgM, IgG, IgA, IgD, IgE

Other Readily Available Assays

Quantification of blood mononuclear cell populations by immunofluorescence assays employing monoclonal antibody markers[b]

- T cells: CD3, CD4, CD8, TCR$\alpha\beta$, TCR$\gamma\delta$
- B cells: CD19, CD20, CD21, Ig(μ, δ, γ, α, κ, λ), Ig-associated molecules (α, β)
- NK cells: CD16/CD56
- Monocytes: CD15
- Activation markers: HLA-DR, CD25, CD80 (B cells), CD154 (T cells)

T cell functional evaluation

1. Delayed hypersensitivity skin tests (PPD, *Candida*, histoplasmin, tetanus toxoid)
2. Proliferative response to mitogens (anti-CD3 antibody, phytohemagglutinin, concanavalin A) and allogeneic cells (mixed lymphocyte response)
3. Cytokine production

B cell functional evaluation

1. Natural or commonly acquired antibodies: isohemagglutinins; antibodies to common viruses (influenza, rubella, rubeola) and bacterial toxins (diphtheria, tetanus)
2. Response to immunization with protein (tetanus toxoid) and carbohydrate (pneumococcal vaccine, *H. influenzae B* vaccine) antigens
3. Quantitative IgG subclass determinations

Complement

1. CH_{50} assays (classic and alternative pathways)
2. C3, C4, and other components

Phagocyte function

1. Reduction of nitroblue tetrazolium
2. Chemotaxis assays
3. Bactericidal activity

[a] Together with a history and physical examination, these tests will identify more than 95% of patients with primary immunodeficiencies.

[b] The menu of monoclonal antibody markers may be expanded or contracted to focus on particular clinical questions.

Cellular Immunity T lymphocytes may be enumerated by their expression of the TCR/CD3 complex of surface molecules. The CD4 molecule serves as a marker for helper T cells, although macrophages also express this molecule in relatively low levels. Conversely, CD8$\alpha\beta$ heterodimers are expressed by cytotoxic T cells. CD8 is also expressed by some $\gamma\delta$ T cells and by NK cells, although usually as CD8$\alpha\alpha$ homodimeric molecules.

Normal levels of serum immunoglobulins and antibody responsiveness are reliable indices of intact helper T cell function. T lymphocyte function can be measured directly by delayed hypersensitivity skin testing using a variety of antigens to which the majority of older children and adults have been sensitized. A generally useful skin test antigen is a 1:5 dilution of tetanus toxoid injected intradermally, since almost all individuals will have been sensitized. Purified protein derivative (PPD), histoplasmin, mumps antigen, and extracts of *Candida* or *Trichophyton* also may be used.

T lymphocyte function may be estimated in vitro by the capacity of cells to proliferate in response to antigens to which the patient has been sensitized, to lymphocytes from an unrelated donor, to antibodies that cross-link the CD3/TCR complex, or to the T cell mitogens, such as phytohemagglutinin and concanavalin A. The response is usually quantified by measurement of incorporation of radioactive thymidine into newly synthesized DNA. The production of cytokines (or interleukins) by activated T cells, can be measured as can the ability of T cells activated in mixed lymphocyte culture to lyse target cells. Finally, assays exist for detection of defects in T cell surface receptors and specific elements of their signal transduction pathways.

CLASSIFICATION *Primary immunodeficiencies* may be either congenital or manifested later in life and are currently classified according to mode of inheritance and whether the genetic defect affects T cells, B cells, or both (Table 308-2). The following discussion emphasizes three related concepts: (1) that immunodeficiencies are logically viewed as defects of cellular differentiation; (2) that these defects may involve either primary development of T or B cells or the antigen-dependent phase of their differentiation; and (3) that defects of B cell differentiation may in some instances reflect faulty T-B collaboration.

Secondary immunodeficiencies are those not caused by intrinsic abnormalities in development or function of T and B cells. The best known of these is AIDS, which may follow infection with the human immunodeficiency virus (Chap. 309). Other examples are immune deficiency associated with malnutrition, protein-losing enteropathy, and intestinal lymphangiectasia. Also considered secondary are immunodeficiencies resulting from hypercatabolic states such as occur in myotonic dystrophy, immunodeficiency associated with lymphoreticular malignancy, and immunodeficiency resulting from treatment with x-rays, antilymphocyte antibodies, or immunosuppressive drugs.

Incidence As a group, the primary immunodeficiencies are relatively common. The most frequent, isolated IgA deficiency, occurs in approximately 1 in 600 individuals in North America. Common variable immunodeficiency, a related disorder characterized by panhypogammaglobulinemia, is the next most common disorder. Both of these immunodeficiency states often become clinically evident in young adults.

The more severe forms of primary immunodeficiency are relatively rare, have their onset early in life, and all too frequently result in death during childhood. However, patients with congenital hypogammaglobulinemia may survive to middle age and beyond with replacement antibody therapy. In a referral center for patients with immunodeficiency diseases, approximately two-thirds of the immunodeficient patients will be adults.

Severe Combined Immunodeficiency The SCID syndrome is characterized by gross functional impairment of both humoral and cell-mediated immunity and by susceptibility to devastating fungal, bac-

Table 308-2 Classification of Primary Immunodeficiencies

COMBINED IMMUNODEFICIENCIES	
Severe combined immunodeficiency (SCID):	Primary T cell immunodeficiency:
Recombinase activating gene (RAG 1/2) deficiency	DiGeorge syndrome
Adenosine deaminase (ADA) deficiency	Nude syndrome
Interleukin receptor γ chain (γ_c) deficiency	T cell receptor deficiency
Janus-associated kinase 3 (JAK3) deficiency	MHC class II deficiency
Reticular dysgenesis	TAP-2 deficiency (MHC class I deficiency)
	ZAP70 tyrosine kinase deficiency
	Purine nucleotide phosphorylase (PNP) deficiency
PREDOMINANTLY ANTIBODY DEFICIENCIES	
X-linked agammaglobulinemia (Bruton's tyrosine kinase deficiency)	Ig heavy chain gene deletions
Autosomal recessive agammaglobulinemia:	IgA deficiency
Mu heavy chain deficiency	Selective deficiency of IgG subclasses (with or without IgA deficiency)
Surrogate light chain (γ5/14.1) deficiency)	Common variable immunodeficiency (CVID)
Hyper-IgM syndrome:	Antibody deficiency with normal immunoglobulins
X-linked (CD40 ligand deficiency)	Transient hypogammaglobulinemia of infancy
Other	
OTHER WELL-DEFINED IMMUNODEFICIENCY SYNDROMES	
Interferon γ receptor (IFNGR1, IFNGR2) deficiency	Ataxia telangiectasia (ATM deficiency)
Interleukin 12 and interleukin 12 receptor deficiency	X-linked lymphoproliferative syndrome (SH2D1A/SAP deficiency)
Immunodeficiency with thymoma	Hyper IgE syndrome
Wiskott-Aldrich syndrome (WAS protein deficiency)	
IMMUNODEFICIENCY ASSOCIATED WITH OR SECONDARY TO OTHER DISEASES	
Chromosomal Instability or defective repair:	Immunodeficiency with dermatologic defects:
Bloom syndrome	Ectrodactyly-ectodermal dysplasia-clefting syndrome
Xeroderma pigmentosum	Immunodeficiency with absent thumbs, anosmia and ichthyosis
Fanconi anemia	Partial albinism
ICF syndrome	Dyskeratosis congenita
Nijmegen breakage syndrome	Netherton syndrome
Seckel syndrome	Anhidrotic ectodermal dysplasia
Chromosomal defects:	Papillon-Lefevre syndrome
Down syndrome (Trisomy 21)	Congenital ichthyosis
Turner syndrome	Hereditary metabolic defects:
Deletions or rings of chromosome 18 (18p- and 18q-)	Acrodermatitis enteropathica
Skeletal abnormalities:	Transcobalamin 2 deficiency
Short-limbed skeletal dysplasia (short-limbed dwarfism)	Type 1 hereditary orotic aciduria
Cartilage-hair hypoplasia (metaphyseal chondroplasia)	Intractable diarrhea, abnormal facies, trichorrhexis and immunodeficiency
Immunodeficiency with generalized growth retardation:	Methylmalonic acidemia
Schimke immuno-osseous dysplasia	Biotin dependent carboxylase deficiency
Dubowitz syndrome	Mannosidosis
Kyphomelic dysplasia with SCID	Glycogen storage disease, type 1b
Mulibrey's nannism	Chediak-Higashi syndrome
Growth retardation, facial anomalies and immunodeficiency	Hypercatabolism of immunoglobulin:
Progeria (Hutchinson-Gilford syndrome)	Familial hypercatabolism
	Intestinal lymphangiectasia
	Other:
	Chronic muco-cutaneous candidiasis
	Hereditary or congenital hyposplenia or asplenia
	Ivermark syndrome

terial, and viral infections. It is usually congenital, may be inherited either as an X-linked or autosomal recessive defect, or may occur sporadically. Affected infants rarely survive beyond 1 year without treatment.

The syndrome has been associated with a diversity of defects in development of immunocompetent cells, which are caused by mutations in genes whose products are necessary for the normal differentiation of T, B, and, sometimes, NK cells.

In one autosomal recessive form of SCID characterized by severe lymphopenia, the failure in T and B cell development is due to *mutations in the* RAG-*1* or RAG-*2 genes*, the combined activities of which are needed for V(D)J recombination. A function-loss *mutation in the DNA-dependent tyrosine kinase gene* in SCID mice may prove to be a cause for SCID in humans as well, since this is another essential enzyme in the V(D)J gene rearrangement process. About half of patients with autosomal recessive SCID are deficient in an enzyme involved in purine metabolism, adenosine deaminase (ADA), due to *mutations in the* ADA *gene*. The abortive lymphoid differentiation associated with ADA deficiency is due to intracellular accumulation of adenosine and deoxyadenosine nucleotides that interferes with critical metabolic functions, including DNA synthesis.

SCID also may occur with an X-linked inheritance pattern. Aborted thymocyte differentiation and an absence of peripheral T cells and NK cells is seen in *X-linked* SCID. B lymphocytes are present in normal numbers but are functionally defective. The defective gene encodes a common γ chain of the receptors for IL-2, -4, -7, -9, and -15, thus disrupting the action of this important set of lymphokines.

The same $T^-NK^-B^+$ SCID phenotype seen in X-linked SCID can be inherited as an autosomal recessive disease due to mutations in the gene for *JAK3 protein kinase deficiency*. This enzyme associates with the common γ chain of the receptors for IL-2, -4, -7, -9, and -15 to serve as a key element in their signal transduction pathways.

℞ TREATMENT The cellular defects in SCID patients logically rest with the pluripotent hematopoietic stem cells or their lymphoid progenitor progeny. Accordingly, the immunological deficits in all of the different types of SCID patients have been repaired by transplantation of histocompatible bone marrow as a source of stem cells, thereby implying that the stromal microenvironments of these individuals are intact and capable of supporting T and B cell development. However, antibody deficiency requiring immunoglobulin replacement therapy may persist for years in the γc deficient and JAK3 deficient patients, unless the defective B cells are eliminated prior to bone marrow transplantation to allow their replacement with normal B cells of donor origin. In ADA-deficient patients without histocompatible bone marrow donors, the administration of exogenous ADA (conjugated to polyethylene glycol to prolong its half-life) may improve immunological function and clinical status. ADA gene therapy has also been used with limited success in these patients. Treatment of SCID patients should be performed in centers with a strong research interest in this problem. It is crucial that these patients be recognized early and not be given live viral vaccines or blood transfusions, which may cause fatal graft-versus-host disease.

Primary T Cell Immunodeficiency Reflecting the diversity of T cell functions, abnormalities of T cell development may be responsible for a wide spectrum of immune deficiencies, including combined immunodeficiency, selective defects in cell-mediated immunity, and syndromes presenting as antibody deficiency. These defects may be acquired (Chap. 309) as well as congenital.

DiGeorge's syndrome This classic example of isolated T cell deficiency results from maldevelopment of thymic epithelial elements derived from the third and fourth pharyngeal pouches. The gene defect has been mapped to chromosome 22q11 in most patients with DiGeorge's syndrome, and to chromosome 10p in others. Defective development of organs dependent on cells of embryonic neural crest origin includes: congenital cardiac defects, particularly those involving the great vessels; hypocalcemic tetany, due to failure of parathyroid development; and absence of a normal thymus. Facial abnormalities may include abnormal ears, shortened philtrum, micrognathia, and hypertelorism. Serum immunoglobulin concentrations are frequently normal, but antibody responses, particularly of IgG and IgA isotypes, are usually impaired. T cell levels are reduced, whereas B cell levels are normal. Affected individuals usually have a small, histologically normal thymus located near the base of the tongue or in the neck, allowing most patients to develop functional T cells in numbers that may or may not be adequate for host defense.

The nude syndrome The human disease counterpart to the *nude* mouse is also caused by mutations of the *whn (winged-helix-nude)* gene that result in impairment of hair follicle and epithelial thymic development. The human *nude* phenotype is characterized by congenital baldness, nail dystrophy and severe T cell immunodeficiency.

T cell receptor deficiency Since the expression and function of antigen-specific T cell receptors (TCR) is dependent on their companion CD3γ, δ, ϵ, and ζ-η chains, defective genes for any of these receptor components can impair T cell development and function. Immunodeficiencies due to inherited CD3γ and CD3ϵ mutations have been identified. CD3γ mutations result in a selective deficit in CD8 T cells, whereas CD3ϵ mutations lead to a preferential reduction in CD4 T cells, thus implying differences in the signal transduction roles for each CD3 component.

Major histocompatibility complex (MHC) class II deficiency Because T cells are required for B cell responses to most antigens, any gene defect (or acquired disorder) that interferes with T cell development and cell-mediated immunity will also compromise antibody production and humoral immunity. MHC class II deficiency results in one such immunodeficiency in that the TCR$\alpha\beta$ must see protein antigens as peptide fragments held within the α helical grooves of class II and class I molecules encoded by the MHC. Antigen-presenting cells in individuals with this relatively rare disorder fail to express the class II molecules DP, DQ, and DR on their surface. Limited numbers of helper CD4 T cells are therefore generated in the thymus, and they fail to see antigen in the periphery. Affected individuals experience recurrent bronchopulmonary infections, chronic diarrhea, and severe viral infections that usually prove fatal before 4 years of age. The defect is caused by mutations in genes that encode essential transcriptional factors that bind to promoter elements for the MHC class II genes. The class II transactivator gene is mutated in one subgroup of MHC class II deficient patients, whereas mutations in RFX genes encoding additional transcriptional factors for MHC class II genes are responsible for the defective development and function of CD4 T cells in other families: RFXANK in subgroup B, RFX5 in subgroup C, and RFXAP in subgroup D.

Zap70 tyrosine kinase deficiency Recurrent and opportunistic infections begin within the first year of life in individuals with a deficiency in ZAP70 tyrosine kinase, a pivotal component in the TCR/CD3 signal transduction cascade. The rare inheritance of mutations in both alleles of the ZAP70 gene results in a selective deficiency of CD8 T cells and dysfunction of CD4 T cells, which are present in normal numbers. Severe immunodeficiency is the inevitable consequence.

Purine nucleoside phosphorylation deficiency Function-loss mutations of the purine nucleoside phosphorylase (PNP) gene are associated with an often severe and selective deficiency of T lymphocyte function. This enzyme functions in the same purine salvage pathway as ADA; toxic effects of the PNP deficiency may result from the intracellular accumulation of deoxyguanosine triphosphate.

Ataxia-telangiectasia Ataxia-telangiectasia (AT) is an autosomal recessive genetic disorder characterized by cerebellar ataxia, oculocutaneous telangiectasia, and immunodeficiency. The mutant ATM gene has sequence similarity to the phosphatidyl-inositol-3 kinases that are involved in signal transduction. The ATM gene belongs to a conserved family of genes that monitor DNA repair and coordinate DNA synthesis with cell division. The deleterious effects of the ATM gene are widespread. Truncal ataxia may become evident when walking begins and is progressive. Telangiectasia, primarily represented by dilated blood vessels in the ocular sclera, a butterfly area of the face and on the ears, is an early diagnostic feature. Immunodeficiency may be clinically manifest by recurrent and chronic sinopulmonary infection leading to bronchiectasis, although not all patients have overt immunodeficiency. Ovarian agenesis is a frequent occurrence. Persistence of very high serum levels of oncofetal proteins, including α fetoprotein and carcinoembryonic antigen, may be of diagnostic value. Frequent causes of death are chronic pulmonary disease and malignancy. Lymphomas are most common, although carcinomas also have occurred.

The immunologic abnormalities seem to be related to maldevelopment of the thymus. The markedly hypoplastic thymus is similar in appearance to an embryonic thymus. The peripheral T cell pool is reduced in size, especially in lymphoid tissue compartments. Cutaneous anergy and delayed rejection of skin grafts are common. Although B lymphocyte development is normal, most patients are deficient in serum IgE and IgA, and a smaller number have reduced serum levels of IgG, particularly of the IgG2, IgG4 subclasses.

The defect in DNA repair mechanisms in these patients renders their cells highly susceptible to radiation-induced chromosomal damage and resultant tumor development. AT is a rare disorder, one in 10,000 to 100,000 incidence, but 1% of the population is heterozygous for an AT mutation. This is important because the heterozygous state also predisposes to enhanced cellular radiosensitivity and cancer, especially breast cancer in females (Chap. 364).

℞ TREATMENT Therapeutic options other than symptomatic treatment are limited for this group of patients. Live vaccines and blood transfusions containing viable T cells should be assiduously avoided. Exposure to X-irradiation should also be avoided in patients with AT. Therapeutic intervention in the form of an epithelial thymic transplant should repair the T cell deficiency in patients with the *nude* syndrome and in the most severe cases of DiGeorge's syndrome where T cells are absent. Preventive therapy for *P. carinii* in the form of trimethoprim-sulfamethoxazole should be considered. Immunoglobulin infusions are also recommended for those T cell deficient individuals with severe antibody deficiency reflected by low serum levels of IgG.

Immunoglobulin Deficiency Syndromes • *X-LINKED AGAMMAGLOBULINEMIA* Males with this syndrome often begin to have recurrent bacterial infections late in the first year of life, when maternally derived immunoglobulins have disappeared. Although B cell progenitors are found in the bone marrow, affected individuals have very few immunoglobulin-bearing B lymphocytes in their circulation and lack primary and secondary lymphoid follicles. The developmental block is evident at the pre-B cell level (Fig. 308-1). Mutations of Bruton's tyrosine kinase (Btk) gene are responsible for X-linked agammaglobulinemia. B cells in heterozygous female carriers exclusively utilize the X chromosome with the normal Btk gene, while T cells and myeloid cells express either X chromosome. *X-linked agammaglobulinemia with growth hormone deficiency* is a rare variant disorder caused by another gene defect that maps to the same region of the X chromosome.

Agammaglobulinemia is a misnomer, since most of these patients synthesize some immunoglobulins. Within the same family, some affected males may have substantial levels of IgM, IgG, and IgA, while others are nearly agammaglobulinemic. Btk-deficient patients typically are very deficient in circulating B lymphocytes. The few B lymphocytes that escape the block in pre-B cell differentiation are impaired in their responsiveness to antigenic stimulation, making antibody replacement therapy essential in these patients.

Sinopulmonary bacterial infections constitute the most frequent clinical problem. Mycoplasma infections also cause arthritis in some of these patients. Chronic encephalitis of viral etiology, sometimes associated wtih dermatomyositis, can be a fatal complication. These complications are reduced by treatment with intravenous immunoglobulin.

Autosomal recessive agammaglobulinemia This syndrome can result from mutations in a variety of genes whose products are required for B lineage differentiation. For example, signals induced via pre-B receptors are essential for pre-B cell development. Consequently, mutations in any of the genes coding pre-B receptor components—μ heavy chains, surrogate light chains (VpreB and λ5/14.1), Igα and Igβ—can block B lineage differentiation. Congenital absence of B cells, agammaglobulinemia and recurrent bacterial infections have been seen in children with function-loss mutations in both alleles of the μ heavy chain gene or the λ5/14.1 surrogate light chain gene. Disruption of B cell development may also occur as a consequence of mutations in genes coding transcription factors for pre-B receptor genes or for key elements in the pre-B receptor signaling pathway.

Transient hypogammaglobulinemia of infancy This diagnosis is reserved for those rare instances in which normal physiologic hypogammaglobulinemia of infancy is unusually prolonged and severe. IgG levels normally drop to 3.0 to 4.0 g/L between 3 and 6 months of age as maternally derived IgG is catabolized. The IgG levels subsequently rise, reflecting the infants' increased synthetic capacity. Periodic immunologic assessment is needed to differentiate transient hypogammaglobulinemia from other forms of antibody deficiency. Antibody replacement therapy is recommended only in the face of severe or recurrent infections.

IgA deficiency An inability to produce antibodies of the IgA1 and IgA2 subclasses occurs in approximately 1 in 600 individuals of European origin, a much higher incidence than is seen for other primary immunodeficiencies. IgA deficiency is much less common in people of Asian and African origin. In Japan, for example, the incidence is approximately 1 in 18,500. While the precise genetic basis for this difference in incidence is unknown, IgA deficiency is frequently associated with certain MHC haplotypes that are more common in Caucasians.

Individuals with isolated IgA deficiency may appear healthy or present with an increased number of respiratory infections of varying severity, and a few have progressive pulmonary disease leading to bronchiectasis. Chronic diarrheal diseases also occur. Reductions in the IgG2 and IgG4 subclasses are associated with the increased infections in some IgA-deficient individuals. The incidence of asthma and other atopic diseases among IgA-deficient patients is high. Conversely, the incidence of IgA deficiency among atopic children has been found to be more than 20 times that in the normal population. IgA deficiency is also significantly associated with arthritis (Chap. 312) and systemic lupus erythematosus (Chap. 311). IgA-deficient patients frequently produce autoantibodies. Some of them develop significant levels of antibodies to IgA, which may render them vulnerable to severe anaphylactic reactions when transfused with normal blood or blood products.

An accurate picture of the clinical consequences of IgA deficiency requires lifelong study of affected individuals. Among 204 healthy young adults whose IgA deficiency was identified when they served as blood donors, 80% were found to experience episodes of infections, drug allergy, autoimmune disorders, or atopic disease during the next 20 years of their life. They had an increased susceptibility to pneumonia, recurrent episodes of respiratory infections, and a higher incidence of autoimmune diseases, including vitiligo, autoimmune thyroiditis, and possibly rheumatoid arthritis.

IgA deficiency is often familial. It can also occur in association with congenital intrauterine infections, such as toxoplasmosis, rubella, and cytomegalovirus infection, or following treatment with phenytoin, penicillamine, or other medications in genetically susceptible individuals. The pathogenesis of IgA deficiency, whether genetic or triggered by environmental insult, involves a block in B cell differentiation that may reflect defective interaction between T and B cells.

Treatment of IgA deficiency is essentially symptomatic. IgA cannot be effectively replaced by exogenous immunoglobulin or plasma, and use of either can increase the risk of development of antibodies to IgA. IgA-deficient patients in need of transfusion should be screened for the presence of antibodies to IgA and ideally should be given blood only from IgA-deficient donors. Immunoglobulin infusions may benefit the exceptional IgA deficient person in whom IgG2 and IgG4 subclass deficiencies are associated with severe infections, but the risk of anaphylactic reactions to contaminating IgA must always be considered in treating these patients.

IgG subclass deficiencies Selective deficiencies in one or more of the four IgG subclasses are seen in some patients with repeated infections. The IgG subclass deficiency may easily go undetected when the total serum IgG level is measured, because IgG2, IgG3, and IgG4 together account for only 30 to 40% of the IgG antibodies. Even a deficiency in IgG1 may be masked by increases in the remaining IgG isotypes. However, the availability of subclass-specific monoclonal antibodies allows precise measurement of IgG subclass levels.

Homozygous deletions of genes encoding the constant region of the different γ chains is the basis for the IgG subclass deficiency in some individuals. For example, deletion of the $C_{\alpha 1}$, $C_{\gamma 2}$, $C_{\gamma 4}$, and C_{ϵ} genes in the heavy chain locus on both chromosomes 14 was responsible for one individual's inability to make IgA1, IgG2, IgG4, and IgE. Because other components of their immune system are intact, individuals with this and other patterns of C_H-gene deletions may not have unusual infections.

Most of the IgG subclass–deficient individuals with repeated infections appear to have regulatory defects that prevent normal B cell differentiation. The defect may extend to other isotypes. IgA deficiency may accompany IgG2 and IgG4 subclass deficiencies (see "IgA Deficiency" above); an inability to produce IgM antibodies to polysaccharide antigens often reflects a broader defect in antibody responsiveness. While patients with IgG subclass deficiency may benefit from administration of immunoglobulin, a thorough assessment of humoral immunity is needed to identify the relatively few who need this therapy.

Common variable immunodeficiency This diagnostic category includes a heterogeneous group of males and females, mostly adults, who have in common the clinical manifestations of deficient production of all the different classes of antibodies. The majority of these hypogammaglobulinemic patients have normal numbers of B lymphocytes that are clonally diverse but phenotypically immature. B lymphocytes in these patients are able to recognize antigens and can proliferate in response, but they largely fail to become mature plasma cells. This abortive differentiation pattern leads to the frequent occurrence of nodular B lymphocyte hyperplasia, resulting in splenomegaly and intestinal lymphoid hyperplasia, sometimes of massive proportion.

It is important to note that common variable immunodeficiency and IgA deficiency represent polar ends of a clinical spectrum due to the same underlying gene defect in a large subset of these patients. The two disorders feature similar B cell differentiation arrests, differing only in the numbers of immunoglobulin classes involved. Over a period of years, IgA deficient patients may progress to the pan-hypogammaglobulinemia phenotype characteristic of common variable immunodeficiency, and vice versa. Both disorders occur frequently within the same family, and the same MHC haplotypes are associated with both immunodeficiency patterns. Family studies suggest an underlying susceptibility gene in the MHC class III region for both disorders.

It is important to consider the diagnosis of common variable immunodeficiency in adults with chronic pulmonary infections, some of whom will present with bronchiectasis. Intestinal diseases—including chronic giardiasis, intestinal malabsorption, and atrophic gastritis with pernicious anemia—are common in this group of patients. Patients with common variable immunodeficiency also may present with signs and symptoms highly suggestive of lymphoid malignancy, including fever, weight loss, anemia, thrombocytopenia, splenomegaly, generalized lymphadenopathy, and lymphocytosis. Histologic examination of lymphoid tissues usually reveals germinal center hyperplasia which may be difficult to distinguish from nodular lymphoma (Chap. 112). Demonstration of a normal distribution of immunoglobulin isotypes and light chain classes for circulating and tissue B lymphocytes can serve to distinguish these patients from those having a monoclonal B cell malignancy with secondary hypogammaglobulinemia. The administration of intravenous immunoglobulin in adequate doses (see below) is an essential part of the prevention and treatment of all these complications.

X-linked immunodeficiency with hyper IgM In this syndrome, typically the IgG and IgA levels are very low, while IgM levels may be very high, normal, or even low. The development of B lymphocytes bearing IgM and IgD and the absence of IgG and IgA B lymphocytes indicate a defect in isotype switching. The defective gene in these patients encodes a transiently expressed molecule on activated T cells that is the ligand for the CD40 molecule on dendritic cells (DC) and B cells. Gene mutations that preclude normal CD40 ligand expression prevent normal T and B cell cooperation, germinal center formation, V-region diversification by somatic hypermutation, and isotype switching. T cell responses are also compromised in these CD40 ligand deficient patients because their T cells are deprived of an important feedback stimulus as a consequence of the defective T, DC, B cell interactions (Chap. 305). Consequently, these patients experience more severe infections than those occurring with other hypogammaglobulinemic states. In addition to recurrent bacterial infections, pneumonia may be caused by *P. carinii*, cytomegalovirus, *Aspergillus*, *Cryptosporidium*, and other unusual organisms. Enteritis due to cryptosporidial infection may extend into the biliary tract to result in a sclerosing cholangitis and hepatic cirrhosis. Neutropenia is frequent in affected males and increases their vulnerability to infections.

Immunodeficiency with hyper IgM is also seen in patients of both sexes who lack mutations in their CD40 ligand gene. While the phenotype in the non-X-linked form of immunodeficiency with hyper IgM is similar, the clinical course is usually milder than in CD40 ligand deficient patients. Candidate disease genes in this syndrome include the CD40 gene and genes coding signaling elements in the CD40 signaling pathway.

℞ TREATMENT Replacement therapy with human immunoglobulin is the therapeutic cornerstone for antibody-deficient patients who have recurrent infections and who are deficient in IgG. Maintenance of serum IgG levels above 5.0 g/L will prevent most systemic infections in the patients. These serum levels usually can be achieved by intravenous administration of immunoglobulin, 400 to 500 mg/kg, at 3- to 4-week intervals. In patients with mild to moderate IgG deficiency (3.0 to 5.0 g/L) or isolated IgG subclass deficiencies, the decision to treat should be based on evaluation of clinical symptoms and antibody responses to antigenic challenge. Since immunoglobulin preparations are comprised almost entirely of IgG antibodies, they are of no value for repairing deficiencies of immunoglobulins other than IgG. Infusions of immunoglobulin are also not benign. While HIV transmission has not been reported, previous epidemics of hepatitis C virus infections in hypogammaglobulinemic patients receiving contaminated immunoglobulin preparations have led to improved safety measures for current commercial preparations. Some antibody-deficient patients develop symptoms of diaphoresis, tachycardia, flank pain, and hypotension during immunoglobulin infusion. This reaction may be mediated by aggregates of IgG or other biologically active substances and often is resolved by slowing the rate of immunoglobulin infusion. More serious anaphylactic reactions may occur as a consequence of antibodies produced by the patient against donor immunoglobulins, particularly IgA (Chap. 114). The potential for severe adverse reactions merits administration of the initial immunoglobulin infusion under medical supervision in a hospital or clinic setting.

A heightened index of suspicion of infection is essential for antibody-deficient patients. Identification of infectious agents in order to select appropriate antibiotic, antiparasitic, or antiviral therapy is also very important. Immunoglobulin infusions usually do not suffice to eliminate chronic sinopulmonary infections with *H. influenzae* and other microorganisms, and a prolonged course of antibiotic therapy may be required to effectively treat these infections and prevent progression to pulmonary fibrosis and bronchiectasis. Maintenance of good pulmonary toilet with regular postural drainage can also be especially important in management of these patients. Infestation with *G. lamblia*, a common cause of chronic diarrhea in antibody deficient patients, usually responds to therapy with metronidazole.

Cryptosporidial infections in CD40 ligand deficient patients may respond to long-term treatment with amphotericin B and flucytosine. The neutropenia frequently associated with infections in these patients may or may not resolve with improvement of infections and antibody replacement therapy. Bone marrow transplantation following myeloablative pretransplantation therapy can be curative for boys with this devastating immunodeficiency. This treatment has a much greater chance of success when performed during childhood.

Miscellaneous Immunodeficiency Syndromes Infection with *Candida albicans* is the almost universal accompaniment of severe deficiencies in cell-mediated immunity. *Chronic mucocutaneous candidiasis* is different because superficial candidiasis is usually the only major manifestation of immunodeficiency in this syndrome. These patients rarely develop systemic infection with *Candida* or other fungal agents and are not unusually susceptible to virus or bacterial disease. No uniformity of immunologic defects has been identified in these patients, although defects of antibody formation have been detected occasionally. Humoral immunity, including ability to make specific anti-*Candida* antibodies, is usually normal. Many patients are anergic, some to a variety of antigens and some only to *Candida*. The syndrome is often congenital and may be associated with single or multiple endocrinopathies as well as iron deficiency. Treatment of associated conditions may lead to improvement or even cure of *Candida* infection. In other patients, intensive treatment with amphotericin B coupled with surgical removal of infected nails has led to sustained improvement. Oral antifungal agents, such as fluconazole and itraconazole, also may be effective.

Interferon γ receptor deficiency This immunodeficiency is characterized by serious infections caused by bacille Calmette-Guerin vaccine and environmental non-tuberculous mycobacteria. Associated salmonella infections occur in a minority of the cases. This syndrome can be caused by mutations in the interferon γ receptor signal-transducing chain (IFNGR2). Two additional forms of this syndrome are caused by different types of mutations in the interferon γ receptor 1 (IFNGR1) gene that encodes the ligand binding chain of the interferon γ receptor. Null mutations in both IFNGR1 alleles are responsible for a more severe autosomal recessive form. A less severe form, inherited in an autosomal dominant pattern, is caused by IFNGR1 mutations in a small deletional hotspot that result in a truncated receptor chain lacking the cytoplasmic tail. Accumulation of the truncated receptor on the surface of macrophages compromises their response to interferon γ and the killing of ingested mycobacterium.

Interleukin 12 receptor deficiency Mutations in the gene coding the β_1 subunit of the IL-12 receptor can cause this syndrome. Affected patients suffer from disseminated mycobacterial infections attributable to bacille Calmette-Guerin and nontuberculous mycobacteria, and in some cases non-typhi salmonella infections. Although the clinical manifestations are usually less severe than in patients with complete IFNGR1 deficiency, IL-12 receptor deficiency may predispose individuals to clinical tuberculosis as well. Deficient interferon γ production by the otherwise normal NK and T cells is seen in IL-12 receptor deficient patients, and therapeutic use of interferon γ may cure their mycobacterial infection.

Immunodeficiency with thymoma The association of hypogammaglobulinemia with spindle cell thymoma usually occurs relatively late in adult life. Bacterial infections and severe diarrhea often reflect the antibody deficiency, whereas fungal and viral infections are infrequent complications. T cell numbers and cell-mediated immunity are usually intact, but these patients are very deficient in circulating B lymphocytes and pre-B cells in the bone marrow. They also frequently have eosinopenia and may develop erythroid aplasia. Complete bone marrow failure sometimes occurs. The relationship between the thymoma and apparent abnormalities of hematopoietic stem cells remains conjectural, and treatment is limited to immunoglobulin administration and symptomatic therapy.

Wiskott-Aldrich syndrome This X-linked disease characterized by eczema, thrombocytopenia, and repeated infections, is caused by mutations in the WASP gene. The WASP protein is expressed in cells of all hematopoietic lineages. It may serve a cytoskeletal organizing role for signaling elements that are particularly important in platelets and T cells. The platelets are small and have a shortened half-life. Affected male infants often present with bleeding, and most do not survive childhood, dying of complications of bleeding, infection, or lymphoreticular malignancy. The immunologic defects include low serum concentrations of IgM, while IgA and IgG are normal and IgE is frequently increased. The number and class distribution of B lymphocytes are usually normal. Functionally, these patients are unable to make antibodies to polysaccharide antigens normally; responses to protein antigens may also be impaired late in the course of the disease. Most patients eventually acquire T cell deficiencies. Affected boys frequently become anergic, and their T cells do not respond normally to antigenic challenge. This results in vulnerability to overwhelming infections with herpes simplex virus and other infectious agents.

Transplantation of histocompatible bone marrow from a sibling donor following myeloablative therapy can correct both the hematologic and immunologic abnormalities. In patients lacking a suitable donor, intravenous immunoglobulin infusions or splenectomy may improve platelet counts and reduce the risk of serious hemorrhage. Because of the increased risk of pneumococcal bacteremia, splenectomized patients should receive prophylactic penicillin.

X-linked lymphoproliferative syndrome This disease involves a selective impairment in immune elimination of Epstein-Barr virus (EBV). A fulminant and fatal outcome is the consequence of EBV infection in approximately half of the affected males. Hypogammaglobulinemia is the outcome in 30%, and B cell malignancies are acquired in approximately 25% of EBV-infected patients. The disease may be manifested from early childhood onward, depending on the time of EBV infection. Carrier females handle EBV infections normally. Generation of cytotoxic T cells appears to be the primary mechanism of control of EBV infection in normal persons. In males with the X-linked lymphoproliferative syndrome, this process is impaired as a consequence of mutations in a gene coding for a T cell signaling element called SH2D1A or SAP. Intravenous immunoglobulins should be administered to affected males who develop hypogammaglobulinemia. Bone marrow transplantation from an HLA-matched donor may be curative, especially in younger children with this syndrome. However, myeloablative chemotherapy is a necessary prerequisite to successful bone marrow transplantation, thereby increasing the risk of this procedure.

Hyper-IgE syndrome The hyper IgE syndrome (Chap. 64) is characterized by recurrent abscesses involving skin, lungs, and other organs and very high IgE levels. IgE levels may decline with time to reach normal levels in approximately 20% of affected adults. Staphylococcal infection is common to all patients, but most have infections with other pyogenic organisms as well. Abnormal neutrophil chemotaxis is an inconsistent finding, and diminished antibody responses to secondary immunization have been noted. Non-immunologic features include impaired shedding of the primary teeth, recurrent bone fractures, hyperextensible joints and scoliosis. Males and females are affected in an inheritance pattern suggesting an autosomal dominant defect with variable penetrance, but the gene defect has not been identified. Prophylaxis with penicillinase-resistant penicillins or cephalosporins is highly recommended to prevent staphylococcal infections. Pneumatoceles, a frequent complication of pneumonias, may require surgical excision.

Metabolic Abnormalities Associated with Immunodeficiency The relation of deficiencies of the purine salvage enzymes adenosine deaminase and purine nucleoside phosphorylase to immunodeficiency was discussed earlier. The syndrome of *acrodermatitis enteropathica* includes severe desquamating skin lesions, intractable diarrhea, bizarre neurologic symptoms, variable combined immunodeficiency, and an often fatal outcome. This disease is apparently caused by an inborn error of metabolism resulting in malabsorption of dietary zinc and can be treated effectively by parenteral or large oral doses of zinc. Zinc deficiency might in part account for the immunodeficiency that accompanies severe malnutrition. Inherited *deficiency of transcobalamin II*, the serum carrier molecule responsible for transport of vitamin B_{12} to tissues, is associated with failure of immunoglobulin production as well as megaloblastic anemia, leukopenia, thrombocytopenia, and severe malabsorption. All abnormalities of this rare disorder are reversed by administration of vitamin B_{12}.

Table 308-3 Genes or Genetic Loci Associated with Primary Immunodeficiencies

Disorder	Gene or Locus	Chromosome
Severe combined immunodeficiency (SCID):		
Recombinase activating gene deficiency	RAG1, RAG2	11p13
Adenosine deaminase deficiency	ADA	20q13.11
Interleukin receptor γ chain deficiency	IL2RG	Xq13
Janus-associated kinase 3 deficiency	JAK3	19p13.1
DNA-dependent protein kinase deficiency	PRKDC	8q11
Primary T cell immunodeficiency:		
DiGeorge syndrome	DGCR1	22q11
	DGCR2	10q13
Nude syndrome	WHN	17q11-q12
T cell receptor deficiency:		
CD3γ	CD3G	7q35
CD3ϵ	CD3E	11q23
MHC class II deficiency:		
MHC class II transactivator (group A)	CIITA	16p13
Regulatory factor X, ankyrin-repeat containing (group B)	RFXANK	19p12
Regulatory factor X, 5 (group C)	RFX5	1q21.1-q21.3
Regulatory factor X-associated protein (group D)	RFXAP	13q14
Transporter, ATP-binding cassette, major histocompatibility complex, 2 deficiency	TAP2	6p21.3
Zeta-chain-associated protein kinase deficiency	ZAP70	2q12
Purine nucleotide phosphorylase deficiency	NP	14q13.1
Predominantly antibody deficiencies:		
X-linked agammaglobulinemia	BTK	Xq21.3-q22
Ig heavy chain deletions	IGHG1	14q32.33
Surrogate light chain deficiency	IGLL5	22q11.21
X-linked hyper-IgM syndrome	HIGM1	Xq26
IgA deficiency/common variable immunodeficiency	MHC class III	6p21.3
Other well-defined immunodeficiency syndromes:		
Interferon γ receptor deficiency	IFNGR1	6q23-q24
	IFNGR2	21q22.1-22.2
Interleukin 12 deficiency	IL12B	5q31-q33
Interleukin 12 receptor deficiency	IL12RB1	19p13.1
Wiskott-Aldrich syndrome	WAS	Xp11.23-p11.22
Ataxia telangiectasia	ATM	11q22.3
X-linked lymphoproliferative syndrome	SH2D1A/SAP	Xq25

CONCLUSION Defective genes have been identified for most of the primary immunodeficiency diseases that are currently recognized (Table 308-3). It can be anticipated that many different gene mutations will be identified in other individuals with increased susceptibility to infection. Identification of the mutant genes is the first step toward a better understanding of the pathogenesis of immunodeficiency disease and improved therapeutic strategies. Successful gene repair is the ultimate goal for these individuals.

ACKNOWLEDGMENT

This chapter represents a revised version of a chapter by Dr. Max D. Cooper and Dr. Alexander R. Lawton III that has appeared in previous editions of this textbook.

BIBLIOGRAPHY

BUCKLEY RH et al: Hematopoietic stem-cell transplantation for the treatment of severe combined immunodeficiency. N Engl J Med 340:508, 1999

BURROWS PD, COOPER MD: IgA deficiency. Adv Immunol 65:245, 1997

CANDOTTI F, BLAESE RM: Gene therapy of primary immunodeficiencies. Springer Semin Immunopathol 19:493, 1998

CHAPEL HM: Safety and availability of immunoglobulin replacement therapy in relation to potentially transmissable agents. Clin Exp Immunol 118(Suppl 1):29, 1999

DICKLER HB, GELFAND EW: Current perspectives on the use of intravenous immunoglobulin. Adv Int Med 41:641, 1996

FISCHER A, MALISSEN B: Natural and engineered disorders of lymphocyte development. Science 280:237, 1998

GREWAL IS, FLAVELL RA: CD40 and CD154 in cell-mediated immunity. Ann Rev Immunol 16:111, 1998

JOUANGUY E et al: A human IFNGR1 small deletion hotspot associated with dominant susceptibility to mycobacterial infection. Nat Genet 21:370, 1999

KOSKINEN S: Long-term follow-up of health in blood donors with primary selective IgA deficiency. J Clin Immunol 16:165, 1996

MASTERNAK K et al: A gene encoding a novel RFX-associated transactivator is mutated in the majority of MHC class II deficiency patients. Nat Genet 20:273, 1998

OCHS HD et al: *Primary Immunodeficiency Diseases*. New York, Oxford Univ Press, 1999

ROSEN FS et al: Primary immunodeficiency diseases. Report of a WHO Scientific Group. Clin Exp Immunol 109(Suppl 1):1, 1997

SAYOS J et al: The X-linked lymphoproliferative-disease gene product SAP regulated signals induced through the co-receptor SLAM. Nature 395:462, 1998

SCHROEDER HW JR et al: Susceptibility locus for IgA deficiency and Common Variable Immunodeficiency in the HLA-DR3, -B8, -A1 Haplotype. Mol Med 4:72, 1998

309

Anthony S. Fauci, H. Clifford Lane

HUMAN IMMUNODEFICIENCY VIRUS (HIV) DISEASE: AIDS AND RELATED DISORDERS

ADCC antibody-dependent cellular cytotoxicity
CDC Centers for Disease Control and Prevention
CIDP chronic inflammatory demyelinating polyneuropathy
CMV cytomegalovirus
CNS central nervous system
CRFs circulating recombinant forms
CSF cerebrospinal fluid
CT computed tomography
CTLs cytolytic T lymphocytes
EBV Epstein-Barr virus
EIA enzyme immunoassay
ELISA enzyme-linked immunosorbent assay
FDA Food & Drug Administration
FDCs follicular dendritic cells
GM-CSF granulocyte-macrophage colony stimulating factor
HAART highly active antiretroviral therapy
HBV hepatitis B virus
HCV hepatitis C virus
HHV human herpesvirus
HSV herpes simplex virus
HTLV human T lymphotropic viruses
ICL idiopathic CD4+ lymphocytopenia
IDUs injection drug users
IFN interferon
IL interleukin
KS Kaposi's sarcoma
KSHV Kaposi's sarcoma–associated herpesvirus
LIP lymphoid interstitial pneumonitis
MAC *M. avium* complex
MHC major histocompatibility complex
MIP macrophage inflammatory protein
MMSE Mini-Mental Status Examination
MRI magnetic resonance imaging
NK natural killer
NIP nonspecific interstitial pneumonitis
PCP *P. carinii* pneumonia
PCR polymerase chain reaction
PML progressive multifocal leukoencephalopathy
PPD purified protein derivative
RT-PCR reverse transcriptase PCR
SDF stromal cell–derived factor
SIADH syndrome of inappropriate antidiuretic hormone (vasopressin) secretion
SIV simian immunodeficiency virus
STD sexually transmitted disease
TAP transporter associated with antigen-presenting
TB tuberculosis
TGF transforming growth factor
TMP/SMZ trimethoprim/sulfamethoxazole
TNF tumor necrosis factor
VDRL Venereal Disease Research Laboratory
WBC white blood cell count

AIDS was first recognized in the United States in the summer of 1981, when the U.S. Centers for Disease Control and Prevention (CDC) reported the unexplained occurrence of *Pneumocystis carinii* pneumonia in five previously healthy homosexual men in Los Angeles and of Kaposi's sarcoma (KS) in 26 previously healthy homosexual men in New York and Los Angeles. Within months, the disease became recognized in male and female injection drug users (IDUs) and soon thereafter in recipients of blood transfusions and in hemophiliacs. As the epidemiologic pattern of the disease unfolded, it became clear that a microbe transmissible by sexual (homosexual and heterosexual) contact and blood or blood products was the most likely etiologic agent of the epidemic.

In 1983, HIV was isolated from a patient with lymphadenopathy, and by 1984 it was demonstrated clearly to be the causative agent of AIDS. In 1985, a sensitive enzyme-linked immunosorbent assay (ELISA) was developed, which led to an appreciation of the scope of HIV infection among cohorts of individuals in the United States who admitted to practicing high-risk behavior (see below) as well as among selected populations that had been screened, such as blood donors, military recruits and active-duty military personnel, Job Corps applicants, and patients in selected sentinel hospitals. In addition, seroprevalance studies revealed the enormity of the global pandemic, particularly in developing countries (see below).

Table 309-1 1993 Revised Classification System for HIV Infection and Expanded AIDS Surveillance Case Definition for Adolescents and Adults[a]

	Clinical Categories		
CD4+ T Cell Categories	A Asymptomatic, Acute (Primary) HIV or PGL[b]	B Symptomatic, Not A or C Conditions	C AIDS-Indicator Conditions
>500/μL	A1	B1	C1
200–499/μL	A2	B2	C2
<200/μL	A3	B3	C3

[a] The shaded areas indicate the expanded AIDS surveillance case definition.
[b] PGL, progressive generalized lymphadenopathy.
SOURCE: MMWR 42(No. RR-17), December 18, 1992.

The staggering worldwide growth of the HIV pandemic has been matched by an explosion of information in the areas of HIV virology, the pathogenesis (both immunologic and virologic) and treatment of HIV disease, the treatment and prophylaxis of the opportunistic diseases associated with HIV infection, and vaccine development. The information flow related to HIV disease is enormous, and it has become almost impossible for the health care generalist to stay abreast of the literature. The purpose of this chapter is to present the most current information available on the scope of the epidemic; on its pathogenesis, treatment, and prevention; and on prospects for vaccine development. Above all, the aim is to provide a solid scientific basis and practical guidelines for a state-of-the-art approach to the HIV-infected patient.

DEFINITION With the identification of HIV in 1983 and its proof as the etiologic agent of AIDS in 1984, and with the availability of sensitive and specific diagnostic tests for HIV infection, the case definition of AIDS has undergone several revisions over the years. The latest revision took place in 1993; this revised CDC classification system for HIV-infected adolescents and adults categorizes persons on the basis of clinical conditions associated with HIV infection and CD4+ T lymphocyte counts. The system is based on three ranges of CD4+ T lymphocyte counts and three clinical categories and is represented by a matrix of nine mutually exclusive categories (Tables 309-1 and 309-2). Using this system, any HIV-infected individual with a CD4+ T cell count of <200/μL has AIDS by definition, regardless of the presence of symptoms or opportunistic diseases (Table 309-1). The clinical conditions in clinical category C now include pulmonary tuberculosis (TB), recurrent pneumonia, and invasive cervical cancer (Table 309-2). Once individuals have had a clinical condition in category B, their disease cannot again be classified as category A, even if the condition resolves; the same holds true for category C in relation to category B.

While the definition of AIDS is complex and comprehensive, the clinician should not focus on whether AIDS is present but should view HIV disease as a spectrum ranging from primary infection, with or without the acute syndrome, to the asymptomatic stage, to advanced disease (see below). The definition of AIDS was established not for the practical care of patients but for surveillance purposes.

ETIOLOGIC AGENT

The etiologic agent of AIDS is HIV, which belongs to the family of human retroviruses (Retroviridae) and the subfamily of lentiviruses (Chap. 191). Nononcogenic lentiviruses cause disease in other animal species, including sheep, horses, goats, cattle, cats, and monkeys. The

Table 309-2 Clinical Categories of HIV Infection

Category A: Consists of one or more of the conditions listed below in an adolescent or adult (>13 years) with documented HIV infection. Conditions listed in categories B and C must not have occurred.
- Asymptomatic HIV infection
- Persistent generalized lymphadenopathy
- Acute (primary) HIV infection with accompanying illness or history of acute HIV infection

Category B: Consists of symptomatic conditions in an HIV-infected adolescent or adult that are not included among conditions listed in clinical category C and that meet at least one of the following criteria: (1) The conditions are attributed to HIV infection or are indicative of a defect in cell-mediated immunity; or (2) the conditions are considered by physicians to have a clinical course or to require management that is complicated by HIV infection. Examples include, but are not limited to, the following:
- Bacillary angiomatosis
- Candidiasis, oropharyngeal (thrush)
- Candidiasis, vulvovaginal; persistent, frequent, or poorly responsive to therapy
- Cervical dysplasia (moderate or severe)/cervical carcinoma in situ
- Constitutional symptoms, such as fever (38.5°C) or diarrhea lasting >1 month
- Hairy leukoplakia, oral
- Herpes zoster (shingles), involving at least two distinct episodes or more than one dermatome
- Idiopathic thrombocytopenic purpura
- Listeriosis
- Pelvic inflammatory disease, particularly if complicated by tuboovarian abscess
- Peripheral neuropathy

Category C: Conditions listed in the AIDS surveillance case definition.
- Candidiasis of bronchi, trachea, or lungs
- Candidiasis, esophageal
- Cervical cancer, invasive[a]
- Coccidioidomycosis, disseminated or extrapulmonary
- Cryptococcosis, extrapulmonary
- Cryptosporidiosis, chronic intestinal (>1 month's duration)
- Cytomegalovirus disease (other than liver, spleen, or nodes)
- Cytomegalovirus retinitis (with loss of vision)
- Encephalopathy, HIV-related
- Herpes simplex: chronic ulcer(s) (>1 month's duration); or bronchitis, pneumonia, or esophagitis
- Histoplasmosis, disseminated or extrapulmonary
- Isosporiasis, chronic intestinal (>1 month's duration)
- Kaposi's sarcoma
- Lymphoma, Burkitt's (or equivalent term)
- Lymphoma, primary, of brain
- *Mycobacterium avium* complex or *M. kansasii*, disseminated or extrapulmonary
- *Mycobacterium tuberculosis*, any site (pulmonary[a] or extrapulmonary)
- *Mycobacterium*, other species or unidentified species, disseminated or extrapulmonary
- *Pneumocystis carinii* pneumonia
- Pneumonia, recurrent[a]
- Progressive multifocal leukoencephalopathy
- *Salmonella* septicemia, recurrent
- Toxoplasmosis of brain
- Wasting syndrome due to HIV

[a] Added in the 1993 expansion of the AIDS surveillance case definition.
SOURCE: MMWR 42(No. RR-17), December 18, 1992.

four recognized human retroviruses belong to two distinct groups: the human T lymphotropic viruses (HTLV) I and HTLV-II, which are transforming retroviruses; and the human immunodeficiency viruses, HIV-1 and HIV-2, which are cytopathic viruses (Chap. 191). The most common cause of HIV disease throughout the world, and certainly in the United States, is HIV-1. HIV-1 comprises several subtypes with different geographic distributions (see below). HIV-2 was first identified in 1986 in West African patients and was originally confined to West Africa. However, a number of cases that can be traced to West Africa or to sexual contacts with West Africans have been identified throughout the world. HIV-2 is more closely related phylogenetically to the simian immunodeficiency virus (SIV) found in sooty mangabeys than it is to HIV-1. In 1999, it was demonstrated that HIV-1 infection in humans was zoonotic and had originated from the *Pan troglodytes troglodytes* species of chimpanzees in whom the virus had co-evolved over centuries. The taxonomic relationship among primate lentiviruses is shown in Fig. 309-1.

MORPHOLOGY OF HIV Electron microscopy shows that the HIV virion is an icosahedral structure (Fig. 309-2*A*) containing numerous external spikes formed by the two major envelope proteins, the external gp120 and the transmembrane gp41. The virion buds from the surface of the infected cell and incorporates a variety of host proteins, including major histocompatibility complex (MHC) class I and II antigens (Chap. 306), into its lipid bilayer. The structure of HIV-1 is schematically diagrammed in Fig. 309-2*B* (Chap. 191).

REPLICATION CYCLE OF HIV HIV is an RNA virus whose hallmark is the reverse transcription of its genomic RNA to DNA by the enzyme *reverse transcriptase*. The replication cycle of HIV begins with the high-affinity binding of the gp120 protein via a portion of its V1 region near the N terminus to its receptor on the host cell surface, the CD4 molecule (Fig. 309-3). The CD4 molecule is a 55-kDa protein found predominantly on a subset of T lymphocytes that are responsible for helper or inducer function in the immune system (Chap. 305). It is also expressed on the surface of monocytes/macrophages and dendritic/Langerhans cells. In order for HIV-1 to fuse to and enter its target cell, it must also bind to one of a group of co-receptors. The two major co-receptors for HIV-1 are CCR5 and CXCR4. Both receptors belong to the family of seven-transmembrane-domain G protein–coupled cellular receptors, and the use of one or the other or both receptors by the virus for entry into the cell is an important determinant of the cellular tropism of the virus (see below for details). Following binding, the conformation of the viral envelope changes dramatically, and fusion with the host cell membrane occurs in a coiled-spring fashion via the newly exposed gp41 molecule (Fig. 309-4); the HIV genomic RNA is uncoated and internalized into the target cell (Fig. 309-3). The reverse transcriptase enzyme, which is contained in the infecting virion, then catalyzes the reverse transcription of the genomic RNA into double-stranded DNA. The DNA translocates to the nucleus, where it is integrated randomly into the host cell chromosomes through the action of another virally encoded enzyme, *integrase*. This provirus may remain transcriptionally inactive (latent), or it may manifest varying levels of gene expression, up to active production of virus.

Cellular activation plays an important role in the life cycle of HIV and is critical to the pathogenesis of HIV disease (see below). Following initial binding and internalization of virions into the target cell, incompletely reverse-transcribed DNA intermediates are labile in quiescent cells and will not integrate efficiently into the host cell genome unless cellular activation occurs shortly after infection. Furthermore, some degree of activation of the host cell is required for the initiation of transcription of the integrated proviral DNA into either genomic RNA or mRNA. In this regard, activation of HIV expression from the latent state depends on the interaction of a number of cellular and viral factors. Following transcription, HIV mRNA is translated into proteins that undergo modification through glycosylation, myristylation, phosphorylation, and cleavage. The viral particle is formed by the assembly of HIV proteins, enzymes, and genomic RNA at the plasma membrane of the cells. Budding of the progeny virion occurs through the host cell membrane, where the core acquires its external envelope (Chap. 191). The virally encoded protease then catalyzes the cleavage of the gag-pol precursor to yield the mature virion. Each point in the life cycle of HIV is a real or potential target for therapeutic intervention (see below). Thus far, the reverse transcriptase and protease enzymes have proven to be susceptible to pharmacologic disruption (see below).

HIV GENOME Figure 309-5 illustrates the arrangement of the HIV genome schematically. Like other retroviruses, HIV-1 has genes that encode the structural proteins of the virus: *gag* encodes the proteins that form the core of the virion (including p24 antigen); *pol* encodes the enzymes responsible for reverse transcription and integra-

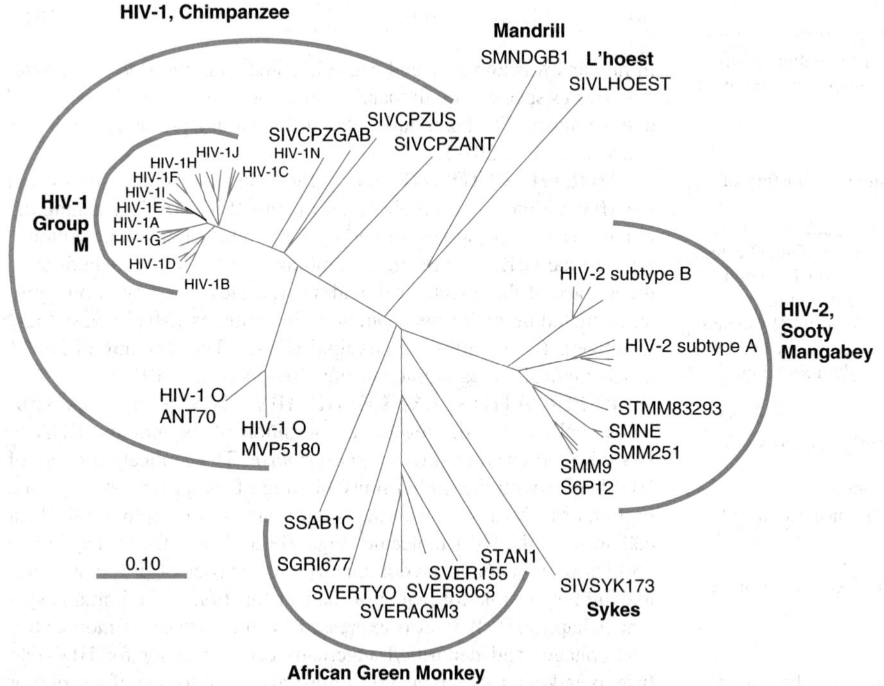

FIGURE 309-1 A phylogenetic tree, based on the complete genomes of primate immunodeficiency viruses. The scale at the bottom (0.10) indicates a 10% difference at the nucleotide level. *(Prepared by Brian Foley, PhD, of the HIV Sequence Database, Theoretical Biology and Biophysics Group, Los Alamos National Laboratory, from the complete genome alignment available at hiv-web.lanl.gov under the alignments section.)*

tion; and *env* encodes the envelope glycoproteins. However, HIV-1 is more complex than other retroviruses, particularly those of the nonprimate group, in that it also contains at least six other genes (*tat, rev, nef, vif, vpr,* and *vpu*), which code for proteins involved in the regulation of gene expression (Chap. 191). Several of these proteins are felt to play a role in the pathogenesis of HIV disease. For example, Tat, Nef, and Vpu have all been shown to downregulate MHC class I expression; this may be a strategy that the virus employs to evade immune-mediated elimination by CD8+ cytolytic T cells. Nef also downregulates cell surface expression of CD4 by inducing endocytosis and lysosomal degradation. Supernatants from Nef-expressing macrophages have been shown to induce chemotaxis and activation of resting T lymphocytes leading to productive HIV infection. In addition to its primary function as a transcriptional enhancer in infected cells, Tat may also be secreted and directly activate potential target cells. In addition, in its secreted form Tat has been shown to be immunosuppressive directly as well as indirectly by inducing secretion of interferon (IFN)α from monocytes/macrophages. Flanking these genes are the long terminal repeats (LTRs), which contain regulatory elements involved in gene expression (see below) such as the polyadenylation signal sequence; the TATA promotor sequence; the NF-κB and Sp1 enhancer binding sites; the transactivating response (TAR) sequences, where the Tat protein binds; and the negative regulatory element (NRE), whose deletion increases the level of gene expression (Fig. 309-5). The major difference between the genomes of HIV-1 and HIV-2 is the fact that HIV-2 lacks the *vpu* gene and has a *vpx* gene not contained in HIV-1.

MOLECULAR HETEROGENEITY OF HIV-1 Molecular analyses of various HIV isolates reveal sequence variations over many parts of the viral genome. For example, in different isolates, the degree of difference in the coding sequences of the viral envelope protein ranges from a few percent (very close) to 50%. These changes tend to cluster in hypervariable regions. One such region, called V3, is a target for neutralizing antibodies and contains recognition sites for T cell responses (see below). Variability in this region is likely due to selective pressure from the host immune system. The extraordinary variability of HIV-1 is in marked contrast to the relative genetic stability of HTLV-I and -II.

There are two groups of HIV-1: group M (major), which is responsible for most of the infections in the world; group O (outlier), a relatively rare viral form found originally in Cameroon, Gabon, and France; and a third group (group N) first identified in a Cameroonian woman with AIDS. The M group comprises eight subtypes, or *clades*, designated A, B, C, D, F, G, H, and J, as well as four major circulating recombinant forms (CRFs). These four CRFs are the AE virus, prevalent in southeast Asia and often referred to simply as E, despite the fact that the parental E virus has never been found; AG from west and central Africa; AGI from Cyprus and Greece; and AB from Russia. These 8 subtypes and 4 CRFs create the major branches in the phylogenetic tree that represents the lineage of the M group of HIV-1 (Fig. 309-6; also see hiv-web.lanl.gov/ALIGN_CURRENT/SUBTYPE-REF/Table1.html).

The global patterns of HIV-1 variation likely result from accidents of viral trafficking. Subtype B viruses, which now differ by up to 17% in their *env* coding sequences, are the overwhelmingly predominant viruses seen in the United States, Canada, certain countries in South America, western Europe, and Australia. Other subtypes are also present in these countries to varying degrees. It is thought that, purely by chance, subtype B was seeded into the United States in the late 1970s, thereby establishing an overwhelming founder effect. Subtype C viruses (of the M group) are the most common form worldwide; many countries have cocirculating viral subtypes

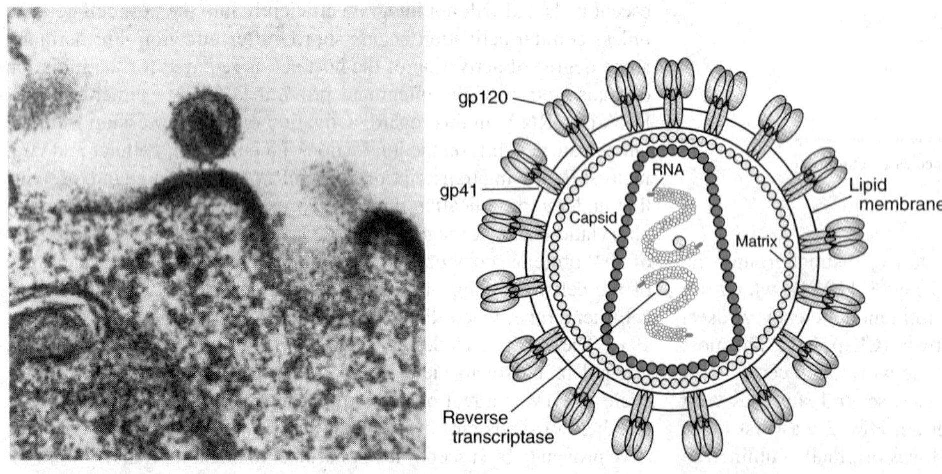

FIGURE 309-2 *A.* Electron micrograph of HIV. Figure illustrates a typical virion following budding from the surface of a CD4+ T lymphocyte, together with two additional incomplete virions in the process of budding from the cell membrane. *B.* Structure of HIV-1, including the gp120 outer membrane, gp41 transmembrane components of the envelope, genomic RNA, enzyme reverse transcriptase, p18(17) inner membrane (matrix), and p24 core protein (capsid) (copyright © by George V. Kelvin). *(Adapted from RC Gallo: Sci Am 256:46, 1987.)*

that are giving rise to CRFs. Figure 309-7 schematically diagrams the worldwide distribution of HIV-1 subtypes by region. The predominant subtype in Europe and the Americas is subtype B. In Africa, >75% of strains recovered to date have been of subtypes A, C, and D, with C being the most common. In Asia, HIV-1 isolates of subtypes E, C, and B predominate. Subtype E accounts for most infections in Southeast Asia, while subtype C is prevalent in India (see "HIV Infections and AIDS Worldwide," below). Sequence analyses of HIV-1 isolates from infected individuals indicate that recombination among viruses of different clades likely occurs as a result of infection of an individual with viruses of more than one clade, particularly in geographic areas where clades overlap.

TRANSMISSION

HIV is transmitted by both homosexual and heterosexual contact; by blood and blood products; and by infected mothers to infants either intrapartum, perinatally, or via breast milk. After approximately 20 years of scrutiny, there is no evidence that HIV is transmitted by casual contact or that the virus can be spread by insects, such as by a mosquito bite.

SEXUAL TRANSMISSION HIV infection is predominantly a sexually transmitted disease (STD) worldwide. Although approximately 42% of new HIV infections in the United States are among men who have sex with men, heterosexual transmission is clearly the most common mode of infection worldwide, particularly in developing countries. Furthermore, the yearly incidence of new cases of AIDS attributed to heterosexual transmission of HIV is steadily increasing in the United States, mainly among minorities, particularly women in minority groups (Fig. 309-8).

HIV has been demonstrated in seminal fluid both within infected mononuclear cells and in the cell-free state. The virus appears to concentrate in the seminal fluid, particularly in situations where there are increased numbers of lymphocytes and monocytes in the fluid, as in genital inflammatory states such as urethritis and epididymitis, conditions closely associated with other STDs (see below). The virus has also been demonstrated in cervical smears and vaginal fluid. There is a strong association of transmission of HIV with receptive anal intercourse, probably because only a thin, fragile rectal mucosal membrane separates the deposited semen from potentially susceptible cells in and beneath the mucosa and trauma may be associated with anal intercourse. Anal douching and sexual practices such as insertion of hard objects or a clenched fist into the rectum ("fisting") traumatize the rectal mucosa, thereby increasing the likelihood of infection during receptive anal intercourse. It is likely that anal intercourse provides at least two modalities of infection: (1) direct inoculation into blood in cases of traumatic tears in the mucosa; and (2) infection of susceptible target cells, such as Langerhans cells, in the mucosal layer in the absence of trauma (see below). Although the vaginal mucosa is several layers thicker than the rectal mucosa and less likely to be traumatized during intercourse, it is clear that the virus can be transmitted to either partner through vaginal intercourse. In a 10-year prospective study in the United States of heterosexual transmission of HIV, male-to-female transmission was approximately eight times more efficient than female-to-male transmission. This difference may be due in part to the prolonged exposure to infected seminal fluid of the vaginal and cervical mucosa, as well as the endometrium (when semen enters through the cervical os). By comparison, the penis and urethral orifice are exposed relatively briefly to infected vaginal fluid. Among various co-

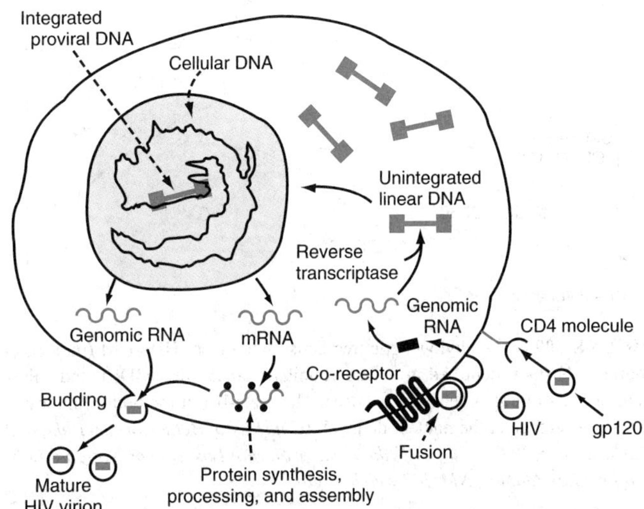

FIGURE 309-3 The replication cycle of HIV. See text for description. *(Adapted from AS Fauci, 1988.)*

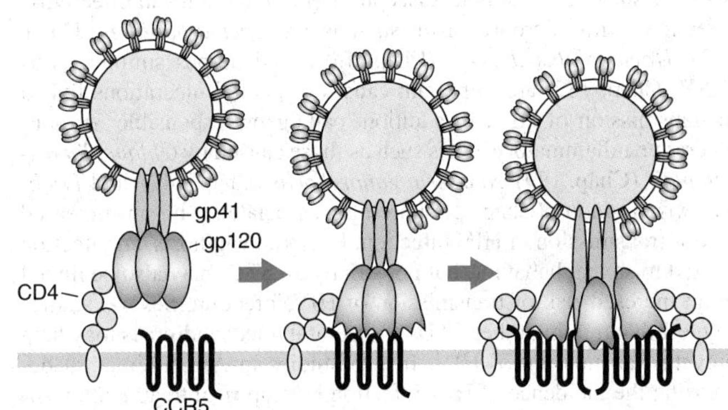

FIGURE 309-4 Binding and fusion of HIV-1 with its target cell. HIV 1 binds to its target cell via the CD4 molecule, leading to a conformational change in the gp120 molecule that allows it to bind to the co-receptor CCR5 (for R5-using viruses). The virus then fuses with the host cell membrane in a coiled-spring fashion via the newly exposed gp41 molecule (see text for details). *(Adapted from Doms and Peiper.)*

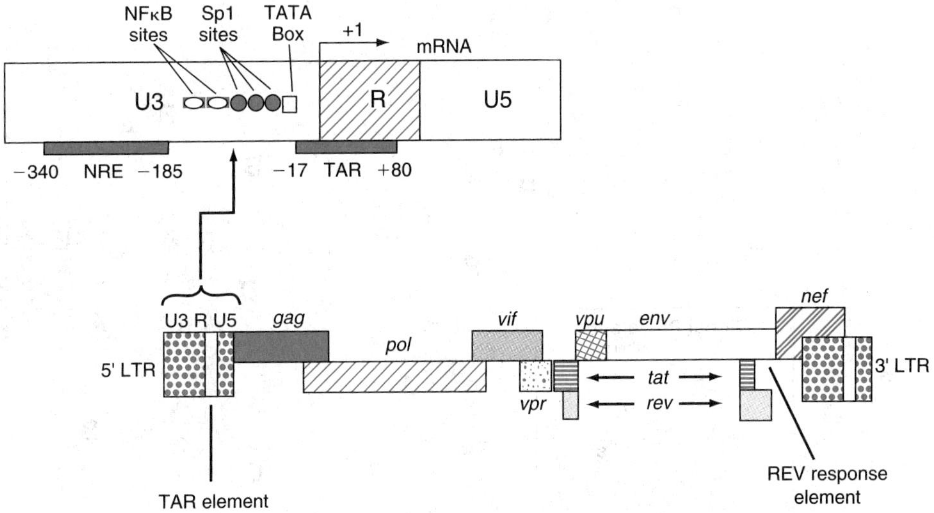

FIGURE 309-5 The genome of HIV. An expanded version of the 5′ long terminal repeat (LTR) is also shown. *(Adapted from WC Greene: N Engl J Med 324:308, 1991, and ZF Rosenberg, AS Fauci: Immunol Today 11: 176, 1990).*

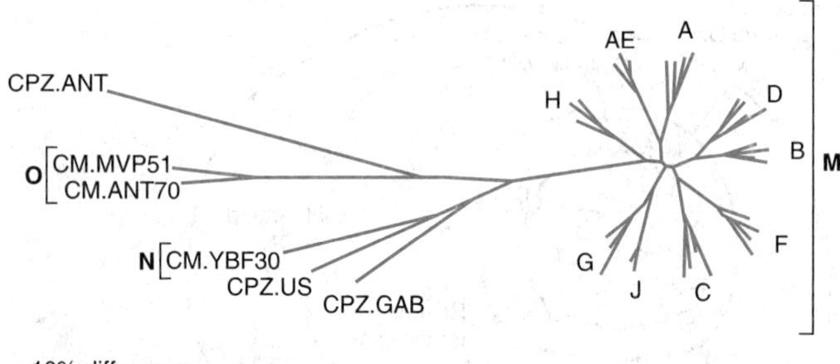

FIGURE 309-6 A phylogenetic tree constructed from HIV-1 M (major), O (outlier), N (first identified in a Cameroonian woman with AIDS), and chimpanzee (CPZ) viral envelope sequences. The scale-bar at the bottom indicates a 10% difference at the nucleotide level. *(Courtesy of Bette Korber, PhD, and Carla Kuiken, PhD, of the HIV database project at Los Alamos National Laboratory, Los Alamos, NM, hiv-web.lanl.gov.)*

factors examined in this study, a history of STDs (see below) was most strongly associated with HIV transmission. In this regard, there is a close association between genital ulcerations and transmission, from the standpoints of both susceptibility to infection and infectivity. Infections with microorganisms such as *Treponema pallidum* (Chap. 172), *Haemophilus ducreyi* (Chap. 149), and herpes simplex virus (HSV; Chap. 182) are important causes of genital ulcerations linked to transmission of HIV. In addition, pathogens responsible for nonulcerative inflammatory STDs such as those caused by *Chlamydia trachomatis* (Chap. 179), *Neisseria gonorrhoeae* (Chap. 147), and *Trichomonas vaginalis* (Chap. 218) are also associated with an increased risk of transmission of HIV infection. Bacterial vaginosis, an infection related to sexual behavior, but not strictly an STD, may also be linked to an incresed risk of transmission of HIV infection. Several studies suggest that treating other STDs and genital tract syndromes may help prevent transmission of HIV. In two studies in Africa aimed at decreasing the incidence of HIV infection by empirical treatment of village inhabitants for other STDs, there were divergent results. In Mwanza, Tanzania, empirical treatment for STDs resulted in a decrease in STDs, including HIV infection. In contrast, in the Rakai district of Uganda, empirical treatment of STDs resulted in a decrease in these diseases but not a decrease in HIV infections. The prevalance

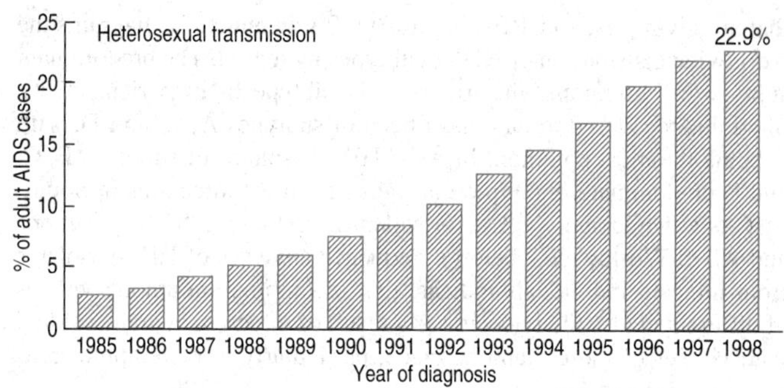

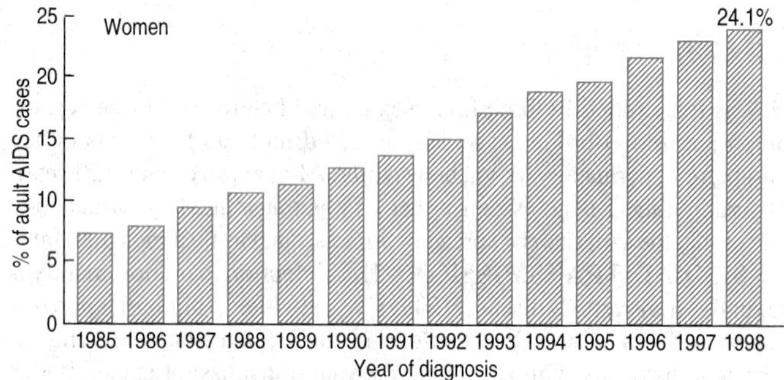

FIGURE 309-8 Adult AIDS cases in the United States among heterosexuals and women, 1985 through 1998. *Upper*. Estimated proportion of cases in which infection was acquired by heterosexual transmission; data adjusted for reporting delays and reclassification of cases in which no risk factor was reported or identified. *Lower*. Cases among women. *(Courtesy of the Centers for Disease Control and Prevention.)*

of HIV infection in Uganda was considerably greater than that in Tanzania at the time of the studies, and, according to a model of the dynamics of sexual spread of HIV, treatment of other STDs would be expected to have less of an effect on decreasing the transmission of HIV in a population with a higher prevalence than in a population with a lower prevalence of HIV infection. Subsequent studies in Uganda indicated that the chief predictor of heterosexual transmission of HIV was the level of plasma viremia. In some studies the use of oral contraceptives was associated with an increase in incidence of HIV infection over and above that which might be expected by not using a condom for birth control. Finally, lack of circumcision has been

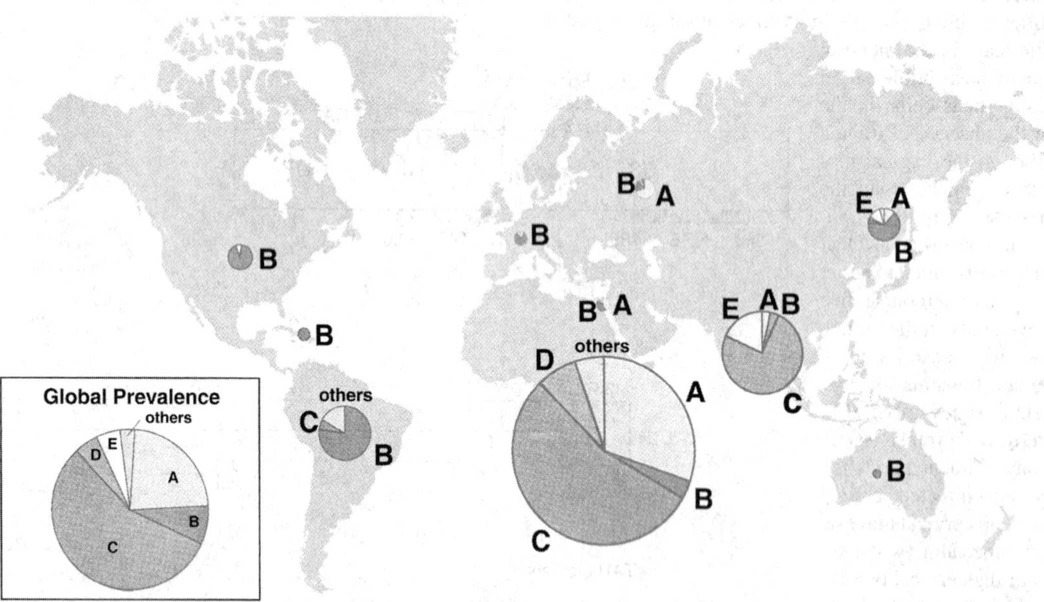

FIGURE 309-7 Geographic distribution of HIV-1 subtypes, 1999. The prevalence of HIV-1 genetic subtypes varies by geographic region. The proportions of subtypes in different regions are indicated by pie charts. *[From the Joint United Nations Programme on HIV/AIDS (UNAIDS).]*

strongly associated with a higher risk of HIV infection in certain cohorts. This difference may be due to increased susceptibility of uncircumcised men to ulcerative STDs, as well as other factors such as microtrauma. In addition, the moist environment under the foreskin may promote the presence or persistence of microbial flora which, via inflammatory changes, may lead to higher concentrations of target cells for HIV in the foreskin. Some studies suggest that only circumcision performed before age 20 is associated with a reduced risk of HIV infection. Thus, in certain cases, these phenomena can also be considered as cofactors for HIV transmission.

Oral sex is a much less efficient mode of transmission of HIV than is receptive anal intercourse. However, there is a misperception by some persons that oral sex, particularly among homosexual men, can be proposed as a form of "safe sex" and a substitute for receptive anal intercourse. This is a dangerous approach, as there have been several reports of documented HIV transmission resulting solely from receptive fellatio and insertive cunnilingus. For example, one study reported that in 12 subjects where the precise date of seroconversion could be identified, 4 individuals reported oral-genital contact as their sole risk factor. There are probably many more cases that go unreported because of the frequent practice of both oral sex and receptive anal intercourse by the same person. The association of alcohol consumption and illicit drug use with unsafe sexual behavior, both homosexual and heterosexual, leads to an increased risk of sexual transmission of HIV.

TRANSMISSION BY BLOOD AND BLOOD PRODUCTS HIV can be transmitted to individuals who receive HIV-tainted blood transfusions, blood products, or transplanted tissue, as well as to IDUs who are exposed to HIV while sharing injection paraphernalia such as needles, syringes, the water in which drugs are mixed, or the cotton through which drugs are filtered. Parenteral transmission of HIV during injection drug use does not require intravenous puncture; subcutaneous ("skin popping") or intramuscular ("muscling") injections can transit HIV as well, even though these behaviors are sometimes erroneously perceived as low-risk. Among IDUs, the risk of HIV infection increases with the duration of injection drug use; the frequency of needle sharing; the number of partners with whom paraphernalia are shared, particularly in the setting of "shooting galleries" where drugs are sold and large numbers of IDUs may share a limited number of "works"; comorbid psychiatric conditions such as antisocial personality disorder; the use of cocaine in injectable form or smoked as "crack"; and the use of injection drugs in a geographic location with a high prevalence of HIV infection, such as certain inner-city areas in the United States.

From the late 1970s until the spring of 1985, when mandatory testing of donated blood for HIV-1 was initiated, it has been estimated that over 10,000 individuals in the United States were infected through transfusions of blood or blood products (Chap. 114). Approximately 8900 individuals in the United States who survived the illness for which they received HIV-contaminated blood transfusions, blood components, or transplanted tissue have developed AIDS. It is estimated that 90 to 100% of individuals who were exposed to such HIV-contaminated products became infected. Transfusions of whole blood, packed red blood cells, platelets, leukocytes, and plasma are all capable of transmitting HIV infection. In contrast, hyperimmune gamma globulin, hepatitis B immune globulin, plasma-derived hepatitis B vaccine, and Rh_0 immune globulin have not been associated with transmission of HIV infection. The procedures involved in processing these products either inactivate or remove the virus.

In addition to the above, several thousand individuals in the United States with hemophilia or other clotting disorders were infected with HIV by receipt of HIV-contaminated fresh frozen plasma or concentrates of clotting factors; approximately 5310 of these individuals have developed AIDS. Currently, in the United States and in most developed countries, the following measures have made the risk of transmission of HIV infection by transfused blood or blood products extremely small: (1) the screening of all blood for p24 antigen and for HIV antibody by ELISA, with a confirmatory western blot where applicable; (2) the self-deferral of donors on the basis of risk behavior; (3) the screening out of HIV-negative individuals with positive surrogate laboratory parameters of HIV infection, such as hepatitis B and C; and (4) serologic testing for syphilis. It is currently estimated that the risk of infection with HIV in the United States via transfused screened blood is approximately 1 in 676,000 donations. Therefore, among the 12 million donations collected in the United States each year, an estimated 18 infectious donations are available for transfusion. The addition of nucleic acid testing to the blood screening protocol to capture some of these rare HIV antibody–negative units should decrease even further the chances of transmission by transfused blood or blood products. There have been several reports of sporadic breakdowns in routinely available screening procedures in certain countries, where contaminated blood was allowed to be transfused, resulting in small clusters of patients becoming infected. There have been no reported cases of transmission of HIV-2 in the United States via donated blood, and, currently, donated blood is screened for both HIV-1 and HIV-2 antibodies. The chance of infection of a hemophiliac via clotting factor concentrates has essentially been eliminated because of the added layer of safety resulting from heat treatment of the concentrates.

Prior to the screening of donors, a small number of cases of transmission of HIV via semen used in artificial insemination and tissues used in organ transplantation were well documented. At present, donors of such tissues are prescreened for HIV infection.

OCCUPATIONAL TRANSMISSION OF HIV: HEALTH CARE WORKERS AND LABORATORY WORKERS There is a small, but definite, occupational risk of HIV transmission in health care workers and laboratory personnel and potentially in others who work with HIV-infected specimens, particularly when sharp objects are used. An estimated 600,000 to 800,000 health care workers are stuck with needles or other sharp medical instruments in the United States each year. Large, multi-institutional studies have indicated that the risk of HIV transmission following skin puncture from a needle or a sharp object that was contaminated with blood from a person with documented HIV infection is approximately 0.3% (see "HIV and the Health Care Worker," p. 1909). The risk of hepatitis B infection following a similar type of exposure is 6 to 30% in nonimmune individuals; if a susceptible worker is exposed to HBV, postexposure prophylaxis with hepatitis B immune globulin and initiation of HBV vaccine is more than 90% effective in preventing HBV infection. The risk of HCV infection following percutaneous injury is approximately 1.8% (Chap. 295). An increased risk for HIV infection following percutaneous exposures to HIV-infected blood is associated with exposures involving a relatively large quantity of blood, as in the case of a device visibly contaminated with the patient's blood, a procedure that involves a needle placed directly in a vein or artery, or a deep injury. In addition, the risk increases for exposures to blood from patients with advanced-stage disease, probably owing to the higher titer of HIV in the blood as well as to other factors, such as the presence of more virulent strains of virus (see "HIV and the Health Care Worker," p. 1909).

There have been reports of health care workers who became infected through the exposure of mucous membranes or abraded skin to HIV-infected material; however, the risk associated with mucocutaneous exposure has been difficult to quantify, because transmission by this route is extremely rare. Factors that might be associated with mucocutaneous transmission of HIV include exposure to an unusually large volume of blood, prolonged contact, and a potential portal of entry. A prospective study has indicated that the use of antiretroviral drugs as postexposure prophylaxis decreases the risk of infection compared to historic controls in occupationally exposed health care workers. Transmission of HIV through intact skin has not been documented (see "HIV and the Health Care Worker," p. 1909).

Since the beginning of the HIV epidemic, there have been at least three reported instances in which transmission of infection from a health care worker to patients seemed highly probable. The first involved a dentist in Florida who apparently infected six of his patients, most likely through contaminated instruments. Another case involved an orthopedic surgeon in France who apparently infected a patient during placement of a total hip prosthesis. A third case involved the apparent transmission of HIV from a nurse to a surgical patient in France. An additional situation involved the apparent infection of four patients by an HIV-negative general surgeon in Australia during routine outpatient surgery. The cause of the transmission was felt to be a failure on the part of the surgeon to sterilize instruments properly between procedures following prior surgery on an infected patient. Despite these few cases, the risk of transmission from an infected health care worker to patients is extremely low; in fact, too low to be measured accurately. Indeed several epidemiologic studies have been performed tracing thousands of patients of HIV-infected dentists, physicians, surgeons, obstetricians, and gynecologists and no other cases of HIV infection that could be linked to the health care providers were identified. The very occurrence of transmission of HIV as well as hepatitis B and C to and from health care workers in the workplace underscores the importance of the use of universal precautions when caring for all patients (see below and Chap. 134).

MATERNAL-FETAL/INFANT TRANSMISSION HIV infection can be transmitted from an infected mother to her fetus during pregnancy or to her infant during delivery. This is an extremely important form of transmission of HIV infection in developing countries, where the proportion of infected women to infected men is approximately 1:1. Virologic analysis of aborted fetuses indicate that HIV can be transmitted to the fetus as early as the first and second trimester of pregnancy. However, maternal transmission to the fetus occurs most commonly in the perinatal period. This conclusion is based on a number of considerations, including the time frame of identification of infection by the sequential appearance of classes of antibodies to HIV (i.e., the appearance of HIV-specific IgA antibody within 3 to 6 months after birth); a positive viral culture; the appearance of p24 antigenemia weeks to months after delivery, but not at the time of delivery; a polymerase chain reaction (PCR) assay of infant blood following delivery that is negative at birth and positive several months later; the demonstration that the firstborn twin of an infected mother is more commonly infected than is the second twin; and the evidence that cesarean section results in decreased transmission to the infant.

In the absence of prophylactic antiretroviral therapy to the mother during pregnancy, labor, and delivery, and to the fetus following birth (see below), the probability of transmission of HIV from mother to infant/fetus ranges from 15 to 25% in industrialized countries and from 25 to 35% in developing countries. These differences may relate to the adequacy of prenatal care as well as to the stage of HIV disease and the general health of the mother during pregnancy. Higher rates of transmission have been associated with many factors, including high maternal levels of plasma viremia, low maternal CD4+ T cell counts and HIV p24 antibody levels, maternal vitamin A deficiency, a prolonged interval between membrane rupture and delivery, presence of chorioamnionitis at delivery, STDs during pregnancy, cigarette smoking and hard drug use during pregnancy, preterm labor, obstetric procedures such as amniocentesis and amnioscopy, and other factors that may increase the exposure of the infant to the mother's blood. With regard to levels of viremia, several studies indicate that the risk of transmission increases with the maternal plasma HIV RNA level. In one series of 552 singleton pregnancies in the United States, the rate of mother-to-baby transmission was 0% among women with <1000 copies of HIV RNA per milliliter of blood, 16.6% among women with 1000 to 10,000/mL, 21.3% among women with 10,001 to 50,000/mL, 30.9% among women with 50,001 to 100,000/mL, and 40.6% among women with >100,000/mL. However, there may be no lower "threshold" below which transmission never occurs, since other studies have reported transmission by women with viral RNA levels below the level of detectability of 50 copies per milliliter. Finally, it has been speculated that if the mother experiences acute primary infection during pregnancy, there is a higher rate of transmission to the fetus, owing to the high levels of viremia that occur during primary infection (see below). In the United States and other industrialized countries, zidovudine treatment of HIV-infected pregnant women from the beginning of the second trimester through delivery and of the infant for 6 weeks following birth has dramatically decreased the rate of intrapartum and perinatal transmission of HIV infection from 22.6% in the untreated group to <5%. It is expected that the rate of transmission will decrease even further as more potent combinations of drugs are used in HIV-infected pregnant women (see below).

In developed countries, current recommendations to reduce perinatal transmission of HIV include universal voluntary HIV testing and counseling of pregnant women, zidovudine prophylaxis, obstetric management that attempts to minimize exposure of the infant to maternal blood and genital secretions, and avoidance of breast feeding. It is also recommended that the choice of antiretroviral therapy for pregnant women should be based on the same considerations used for women who are not pregnant, with discussion of the recognized and unknown risks and benefits of such therapy during pregnancy. The cost and logistics of the above protocol are not feasible for developing countries, particularly those in sub-Saharan Africa where the per capita health care delivery allocation is often only a few dollars per year. Studies have demonstrated that truncated regimens of zidovudine alone or in combination with lamivudine given to the mother during the last few weeks of pregnancy or even only during labor and delivery, and to the infant for a week or less, reduced transmission to the infant by 50% compared to placebo. One important study in Uganda demonstrated that a single dose of nevirapine given to the mother at the onset of labor followed by a single dose to the newborn within 72 h of birth decreased transmission to 13% compared to 25% transmission at age 14 to 16 weeks when the mother received multiple doses of zidovudine throughout labor and delivery and the infant received zidovudine daily for a full week following birth. The cost of the nevirapine for the mother and infant was a mere $4.00, which would make this regimen affordable for many developing countries. Approximately 1800 babies are born infected each day throughout the world, and 90% of these are in sub-Saharan Africa; thus, implementation of such a regimen could potentially save 1000 babies per day from becoming infected.

Although most transmission of HIV occurs during pregnancy and at birth, breast feeding may account for 5 to 15% of infants becoming infected after delivery. This is an important modality of transmission of HIV infection in developing countries, particularly where mothers continue to breast feed for prolonged periods. The risk factors for mother-to-child transmission of HIV via breast feeding are not fully understood; factors that increase the likelihood of transmission include detectable levels of HIV in breast milk, the presence of mastitis, low maternal CD4+ T cell counts, and maternal vitamin A deficiency. The risk of HIV infection via breast feeding is highest in the early months of breast feeding. In addition, exclusive breast feeding has been reported to carry a lower risk of HIV transmission than mixed feeding. Certainly, in developed countries breast feeding by an infected mother should be avoided. However, there is disagreement regarding recommendations for breast feeding in certain developing countries, where breast milk is the only source of adequate nutrition as well as immunity against potentially serious infections for the infant. Studies are being conducted to determine whether intermittent administration of nevirapine, which has a relatively long half-life, to uninfected babies born of infected mothers decreases the incidence of infection via breast feeding.

TRANSMISSION BY OTHER BODY FLUIDS There is no convincing evidence that saliva can transmit HIV infection, either through kissing or through other exposures, such as occupationally to health care workers. HIV can be isolated from saliva of only a small proportion of infected individuals, typically in titers that are low compared to those in blood and genital secretions. In addition, saliva contains endogenous antiviral factors; among these factors, HIV-specific immunoglobulins of IgA, IgG, and IgM isotypes are detected readily in salivary secretions of infected individuals. It has been suggested that large glycoproteins such as mucins and thrombospondin-1 sequester HIV into aggregates for clearance by the host. In addition, a number of soluble salivary factors inhibit HIV to various degrees in vitro, probably by targeting host cell receptors rather than the virus itself. Perhaps the best-studied of these, secretory leukocyte protease inhibitor (SLPI), blocks HIV infection in several cell culture systems, and it is found in saliva at levels that approximate those required for inhibition of HIV in vitro. It has also been suggested that submandibular saliva reduces HIV infectivity by stripping gp120 from the surface of virions, and that saliva-mediated disruption and lysis of HIV-infected cells occurs because of the hypotonicity of oral secretions. There have been outlier cases of suspected transmission by saliva, but these have probably been blood-to-blood transmissions. One case was reported of a 91-year-old man who was bitten during a robbery attempt by an HIV-infected person. He seroconverted, and there was no question that the source of the infection was the human bite. However, the individual who bit him had bleeding gums, and it was thought that the infection was actually transmitted via blood. In addition, a most unusual form of HIV transmission from infected children to mothers in the former Soviet Union has been identified. In those cases, the children (infected through transfusion) were said to have bleeding sores in the mouth, and the mothers were said to have lacerations and abrasions on and around the nipples of the breast resulting from trauma from the children's teeth. Breast feeding had been continued until the children were older than is usual in other developed countries.

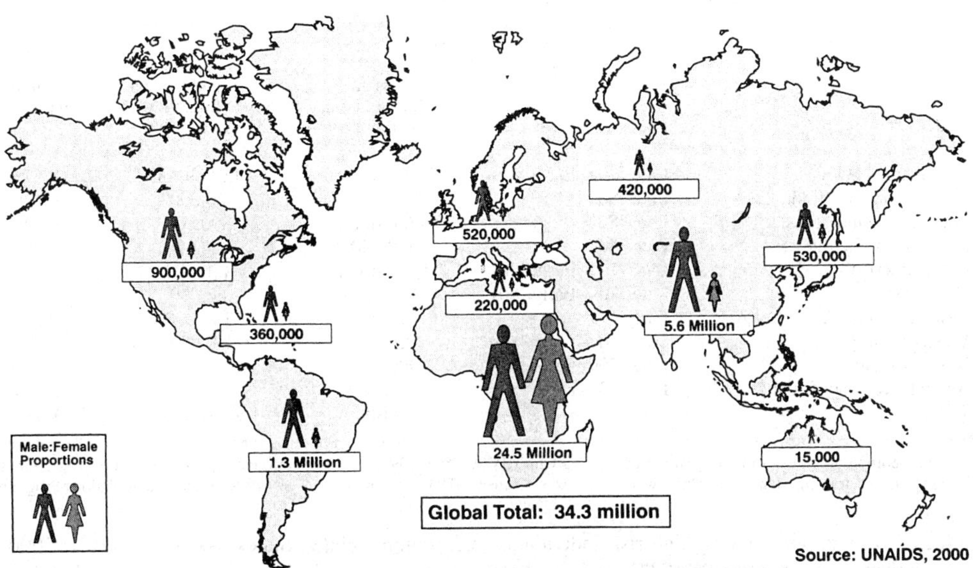

FIGURE 309-9 Estimated number of adults and children living with HIV infection as of January 1, 2000. *(From UNAIDS.)*

Although virus can be identified, if not isolated, from virtually any body fluid, there is no evidence that HIV transmission can occur as a result of exposure to tears, sweat, and urine. However, there have been isolated cases of transmission of HIV infection by body fluids that may or may not have been contaminated with blood. Most of these situations occurred in the setting of a close relative providing intensive nursing care for an HIV-infected person without observing universal precautions. These cases underscore the importance of observing universal precautions in the handling of body fluids and wastes from HIV-infected individuals (see below).

EPIDEMIOLOGY

HIV INFECTION AND AIDS WORLDWIDE HIV infection/AIDS is a global pandemic, with cases reported from virtually every country. The current estimate of the number of cases of HIV infection among adults worldwide is approximately 33 million, two-thirds of whom are in sub-Saharan Africa; 47% of cases are women. In addition, an estimated 1.3 million children under 15 are living with HIV/AIDS. The global distribution of these cases is illustrated in Fig. 309-9. According to the Joint United Nations Programme on HIV/AIDS (UNAIDS), in 1999 alone there were an estimated 5.4 million new cases of infection worldwide (more than 15,000 new infections each day) and 2.8 million death from AIDS, making it the fourth leading cause of mortality worldwide. The estimated number of AIDS-related deaths worldwide through the year 2000 is illustrated in Fig. 309-10. The HIV epidemic has occurred in "waves" in different regions of the world, each wave having somewhat different characteristics depending on the demographics of the country and region in question and the timing of the introduction of HIV into the population. As noted above, different subtypes, or clades, of HIV-1 are prevalent in different regions of the world (see above and Fig. 309-7), increasing the difficulty in the development of vaccines and perhaps accounting for different degrees of virulence. It is unlikely that a single vaccine will be applicable to all regions of the world. In this regard, in addition to HIV-1 subtype B, the predominant subtype in the United States, HIV-1 subtypes A, AE, AG, C, D, and O have been detected in individuals in the United States, as might be expected given the degree of international travel that occurs.

Table 309-3 provides the statistics and demographic features of HIV/AIDS in different regions of the world. Although the epidemic was first recognized in the United States and shortly thereafter in western Europe, it very likely began in sub-Saharan Africa (see above), which has been particularly devastated by the epidemic, with the prevalance of infection in many cities in the double digits. According to the United Nations Population Division, by the year 2015 life expectancy in the nine countries in Africa with the highest HIV prevalence rates will fall, on average, 17 years. In certain sub-Saharan African countries such as Zimbabwe and Botswana, available seroprevalence data indicate >25% of the adult population aged 15 to 49 is HIV-

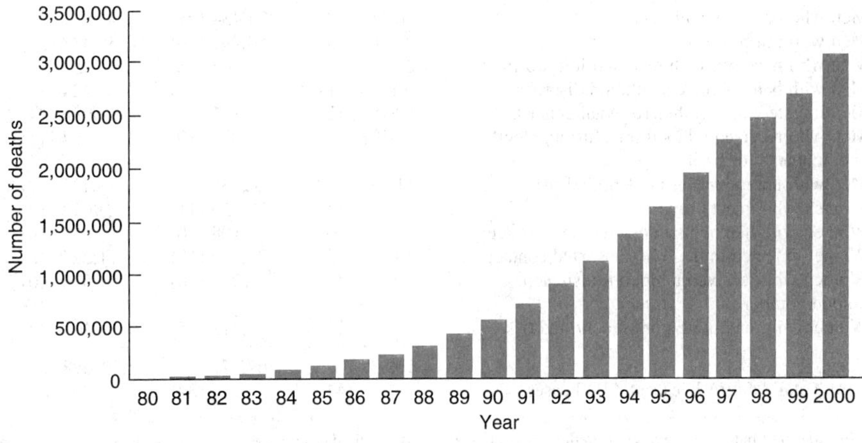

FIGURE 309-10 Estimated/projected annual number of deaths due to AIDS from 1980 through 2000. *(From UNAIDS.)*

Table 309-3 Regional HIV/AIDS Statistics and Features, 1 January 2000

Region	Epidemic Started	Adults and Children Living with HIV/AIDS	Adults and Children Newly Infected with HIV in 1999	Adult Prevalence Rate[a]	HIV-Positive Adult Women, %	Main Mode of Transmission[b] for Adults Living with HIV/AIDS
Sub-Saharan Africa	Late '70s–Early '80s	24.5 million	4.0 million	8.57%	55	Hetero
North Africa & Middle East	Late '80s	220,000	20,000	0.12%	20	IDU, Hetero
South & Southeast Asia	Late '80s	5.6 million	800,000	0.54%	35	Hetero
East Asia & Pacific	Late '80s	530,000	120,000	0.06%	13	IDU, Hetero, MSM
Latin America	Late '70s–Early '80s	1.3 million	150,000	0.49%	25	MSM, IDU, Hetero
Caribbean	Late '70s–Early '80s	360,000	60,000	2.11%	35	Hetero, MSM
Eastern Europe & Central Asia	Early '90s	420,000	130,000	0.21%	25	IDU, MSM
Western Europe	Late '70s–Early '80s	520,000	30,000	0.23%	25	MSM, IDU
North America	Late '70s–Early '80s	900,000	45,000	0.58%	20	MSM, IDU, Hetero
Australia & New Zealand	Late '70s–Early '80s	15,000	500	0.13%	10	MSM, IDU
Total		**34.3 million**	**5.4 million**	**1.07%**	**47**	

[a] The proportion of adults (15 to 49 years of age) living with HIV/AIDS in 1999.
[b] MSM (sexual transmission among men who have sex with men), IDU (transmission through injecting drug use), Hetero (heterosexual transmission).
SOURCE: Joint United Nations Programme on HIV/AIDS (UNAIDS).

infected. In addition, among high-risk individuals (e.g., commercial sex workers, patients attending STD clinics) who live in urban areas of sub-Saharan Africa, seroprevalence is now >50% in many countries. The epidemic in Asian countries, particularly India and Thailand, has lagged temporally behind that in Africa; however, the number of new cases in this region is accelerating rapidly, and the magnitude of the epidemic is projected to exceed that of sub-Saharan Africa in the early part of the twenty-first century. The estimated number of cases in China is still relatively small; however, the potential exists for a major expansion of the epidemic in that nation of over 1 billion people.

The major mode of transmission of HIV worldwide is unquestionably heterosexual sex; this is particularly true and has been so since the begining of the epidemic in developing countries, where the numbers of infected men and women are approximately equal. The epidemic in most developed countries was first introduced among homosexual men and, to a greater or lesser degree (depending on the individual country), among IDUs. In this regard, the total numbers of AIDS cases in those countries still reflect a high proportion of cases among these high-risk groups. However, in most developed countries, including the United States (see below), there has been a gradual shift such that among new cases of AIDS, there is a greater prevalence among heterosexuals and IDUs than among homosexual men.

AIDS IN THE UNITED STATES AIDS has had and will continue to have an extraordinary public health impact in the United States. As of January 1, 2000, >724,600 cumulative cases of AIDS had been reported in adults and adolescents in the United States (Table 309-4) and approximately 425,000 AIDS-related deaths had been reported. It is the fifth leading cause of death among Americans aged 25 to 44 (Fig. 309-11), having dropped from first within the past few years. The death rate from AIDS declined 42% from 1996 to 1997 and 18% from 1997 to 1998. This trend is due to several factors including the improved prophylaxis and treatment of opportunistic infections, the growing experience among health professions in caring for HIV-infected individuals, improved access to health care, and the decrease in infections due to saturational effects and prevention efforts. However, the most influential factor clearly has been the increased use of potent antiretroviral drugs, generally administered in a combination of three or four agents, usually including a protease inhibitor (see below). When one looks at the totality of data collected from the beginning of the epidemic, approximately one-half of cases are among men who have had sex with men. However, over the past few years, the numbers of newly reported cases of AIDS among other groups, including IDUs and heterosexuals, have surpassed the numbers of newly reported cases among men who have had sex with men. The proportion of new cases of AIDS per year attributed to heterosexual contact has increased dramatically over the past 15 years in the United States (Fig. 309-8). Women are increasingly affected; the proportion of AIDS cases in the United States reported among adult and adolescent females has increased from <5% to 24% from 1985 to 1998 (Fig. 309-8). Most cases

Table 309-4 AIDS Cases in Adults/Adolescents in the United States as of 1 January 2000

Exposure Category	White, Not Hispanic No. (%)	Black, Not Hispanic No. (%)	Hispanic No. (%)	Asian/Pacific Islander No. (%)	American Indian/Alaska Native No. (%)	Total[a] No. (%)
Men who have sex with men	216,564 (68)	74,434 (28)	45,867 (35)	3389 (64)	987 (47)	341,597 (47)
Men who inject drugs	26,856 (8)	68,491 (26)	38,338 (29)	244 (5)	273 (13)	134,356 (19)
Men who have sex with men and inject drugs	23,880 (7)	14,965 (6)	7253 (6)	172 (3)	295 (14)	46,582 (6)
Men with hemophilia/coagulation disorder	3725 (1)	551 (0)	424 (0)	67 (1)	30 (1)	4803 (1)
Men infected through heterosexual contact	5181 (2)	15,121 (6)	5986 (4)	165 (3)	47 (2)	26,530 (4)
Men who received a blood transfusion, blood components, or tissue	3133 (1)	1028 (0)	564 (1)	112 (2)	8 (0)	4863 (1)
Men with unreported or unidentified risk	11,198 (3)	24,658 (9)	9425 (7)	521 (10)	103 (5)	46,112 (6)
Women who inject drugs	11,074 (3)	29,059 (11)	9613 (7)	107 (2)	164 (8)	50,073 (7)
Women with hemophilia/coagulation disorder	102 (0)	108 (0)	53 (0)	5 (0)	2 (0)	272 (0)
Women infected through heterosexual contact	10,528 (3)	25,719 (10)	11,222 (8)	310 (6)	127 (6)	47,946 (7)
Women who received a blood transfusion, blood components, or tissue	1789 (1)	1230 (0)	536 (0)	96 (2)	14 (1)	3668 (1)
Women with unreported or unidentified risk	2805 (1)	12,413 (5)	2407 (2)	111 (2)	51 (2)	17,851 (2)
Total	316,835	267,777	131,698	5299	2101	724,656
% of Total Adult/Adolescent AIDS cases	(44)	(37)	(18)	(<1)	(<1)	(100)

[a] Includes 943 individuals whose race/ethnicity is unknown, and 3 individuals whose sex is unknown.
SOURCE: Centers for Disease Control and Prevention, 2000.

of transmission by injection drug use and heterosexual contact are reported from the northeast and southeast regions of the country, particularly among minorities. HIV infection and AIDS have disproportionately affected minority populations in the United States. The rates of AIDS cases per 100,000 population reported among adults and adolescents in 1999 were 84.2 for African Americans, 34.6 for Hispanics, 9.0 for whites, 11.3 for American Indians/Alaska Natives, and 4.3 for Asian/Pacific Islanders (Fig. 309-12).

As of January 1, 2000, 8718 cases of AIDS in children <13 years old had been reported, and approximately 60% of these children have died (Table 309-5). Approximately 90% of these children were born to mothers who were HIV-infected or who were at risk for HIV infection and, in approximately 60% of those cases, the mother was either an IDU or the heterosexual partner of an IDU. About 42% of women with AIDS have become infected through injection drug use, compared to 22% of men with AIDS; 40% of women have become infected by heterosexual contact, compared to 4% of men with AIDS. Only 1% of AIDS cases are among hemophiliacs, and 1% are among recipients of blood transfusions, blood products, or transplanted tissue. The relative contribution of the latter groups will gradually decrease, even though individuals infected previously through this mode of transmission will continue to develop AIDS. The risk of additional infections via this mode of transmission in the United States is extremely small (see above). In recent years, the incidence of AIDS has decreased considerably, with ~46,000 new cases in 1999 compared to ~60,000 in 1996. This trend likely reflects both reduced infection rates since the mid-1980s; more widespread use of prophylactic therapies, which delay the onset of AIDS; and the use of highly effective antiretroviral therapy early in the course of HIV infection (see below). Also, the demography of newly infected individuals has changed considerably since the mid-1980s (see below).

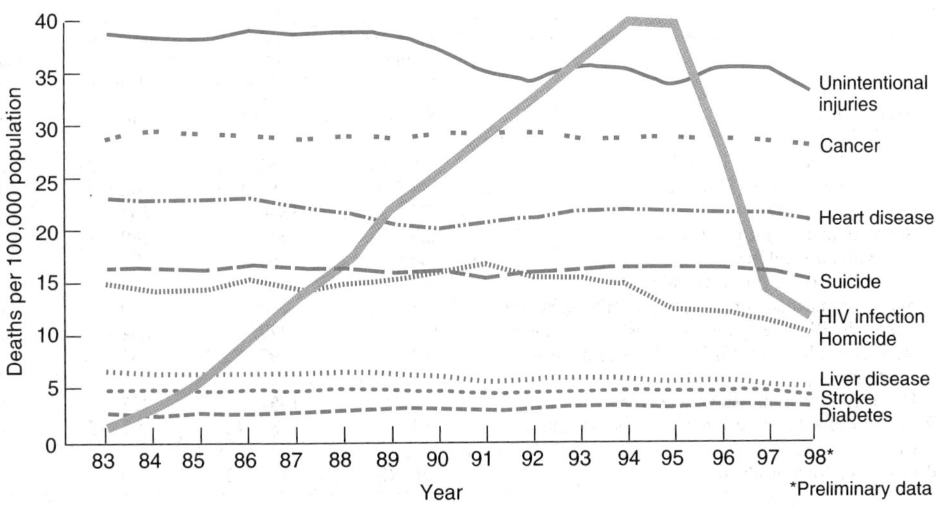

FIGURE 309-11 Death rates from leading causes of death in persons aged 25–44 years in the United States from 1983 through 1998. *(From National Center for Health Statistics.)*

HIV PREVALENCE AND INCIDENCE IN THE UNITED STATES It is estimated that between 650,000 and 900,000 adults and adolescents in the United States are living with HIV infection, including 120,000 to 160,000 women. This estimate results in an overall nationwide prevalence of HIV infection of approximately 0.3%. Prevalence is highest among young adults in their late twenties and thirties and among minorities. An estimated 3% of black men and 1% of black women in their thirties are living with HIV infection. The number of new infections per year is estimated to be approximately 40,000, and this number has remained stable for at least 9 years. The estimated proportion of HIV infections has declined among white males, especially those >30, while the proportion of new HIV infections appears to have increased among women and minorities. Among newly infected persons in the United States, ~70% are men and ~30% are women (Fig. 309-13). Of these newly infected individuals, half are <25 years. Of new infections among men, the CDC estimates that ~60% were infected through homosexual sex, 25% through injection drug use, and 15% through heterosexual sex. Of new infections among women, ~75% were infected through heterosexual sex and 25% through injection drug use.

HIV infection and AIDS are widespread in the United States; although the epidemic on the whole is plateauing, it is spreading rapidly among certain populations, stabilizing in others, and decreasing in others. Similar to other STDs, HIV infection will not spread homogeneously throughout the population of the United States. However, it is clear that anyone who practices high-risk behavior is at risk for HIV infection. In addition, the alarming increase in infections and AIDS cases among heterosexuals (particularly sexual partners of IDUs, women, and adolescents) as well as the spread in certain inner city areas (particularly among underserved minority populations with inadequate access to health care) testifies to the fact that the epidemic of HIV infection in the United States is a public health problem of major proportions.

PATHOPHYSIOLOGY AND PATHOGENESIS

The hallmark of HIV disease is a profound immunodeficiency resulting primarily from a progressive quantitative and qualitative deficiency of the subset of T lymphocytes referred to as *helper T cells*, or *inducer T cells*. This subset of T cells is defined phenotypically by the presence on its surface of the CD4 molecule (Chap. 305), which serves as the primary cellular receptor for HIV. A co-receptor must also be present together with CD4 for efficient fusion and entry of HIV-1 into its target cells (Figs. 309-3 and 309-4). HIV uses two major co-receptors for fusion and entry; these co-receptors are also the primary receptors for certain chemoattractive cytokines termed *chemokines* and belong to the seven-transmembrane-domain G protein–coupled family of receptors. CCR5 and CXCR4 are the major co-receptors used by HIV (see above and below). Although a number of mechanisms responsible for cytopathicity and immune dysfunction of CD4+ T cells have been demonstrated in vitro, particularly direct infection and destruction of these cells by HIV (see below), it remains unclear which mechanisms or combination of mechanisms are primarily responsible for their progressive depletion and functional impairment in vivo. When the number of CD4+ T cells declines below a certain level (see below), the patient is at high risk of developing a variety of opportunistic diseases,

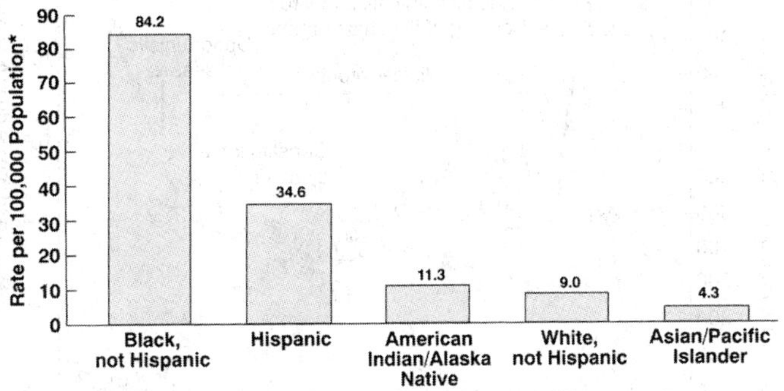

FIGURE 309-12 Rates of adult/adolescent AIDS cases per 100,000 population diagnosed in 1999 in various racial/ethnic groups in the United States. *(From Centers for Disease Control and Prevention, 2000.)*

Table 309-5 Pediatric (<13 Years) AIDS Cases in the United States as of 1 January, 2000

Exposure Category	White, Not Hispanic No. (%)	Black, Not Hispanic No. (%)	Hispanic No. (%)	Asian/Pacific Islander No. (%)	American Indian/ Alaska Native No. (%)	Total[a] No. (%)
Hemophilia/Coagulation Disorder	158 (10)	34 (1)	38 (2)	3 (6)	2 (7)	235 (3)
Mother with/at Risk for HIV infection	1144 (75)	4881 (96)	1846 (92)	31 (65)	27 (90)	7943 (91)
Injecting drug use	477	1880	737	4	13	3116
Sex with injecting drug user	223	718	489	5	7	1443
Sex with bisexual male	66	63	39	2	—	171
Sex with person with hemophilia	17	7	8	—	—	32
Sex with transfusion recipient with HIV infection	8	8	9	—	—	25
Sex with HIV-infected person, risk not specified	140	777	254	9	3	1185
Receipt of blood transfusion, blood components, or tissue	42	97	33	1	—	153
Has HIV infection, risk not specified	171	1351	277	10	4	1818
Receipt of blood transfusion, blood components, or tissue	189 (12)	89 (2)	91 (5)	10 (21)	— —	379 (4)
Risk not reported or identified	26 (2)	100 (2)	30 (1)	4 (8)	1 (3)	161 (2)
Total	1517	5104	2005	48	30	8718
% of Total Pediatric AIDS Cases	(17)	(58)	(23)	(<1)	(<1)	(100)

[a] Includes 14 children whose race/ethnicity is unknown.
SOURCE: Centers for Disease Control and Prevention, 2000.

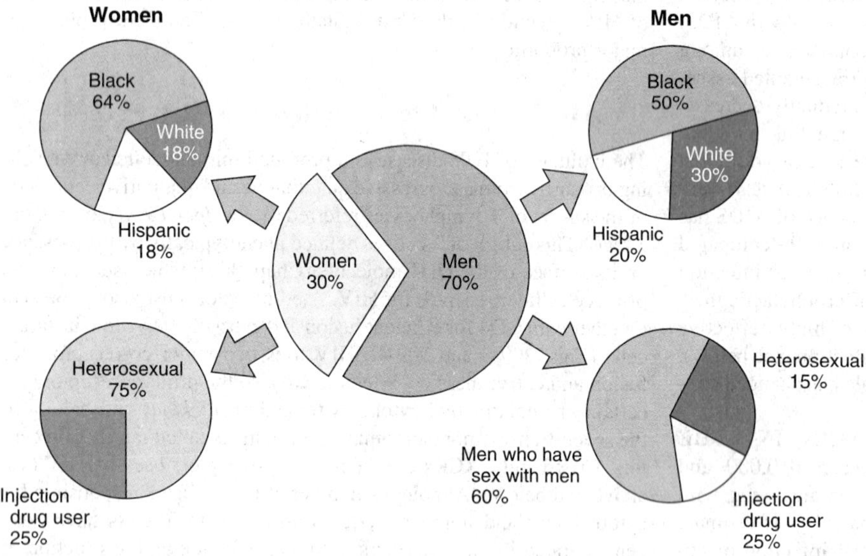

FIGURE 309-13 Estimated new HIV infections by race and risk in the United States in 1998. *(From Centers for Disease Control and Prevention, 1999 National HIV Prevention Conference.)*

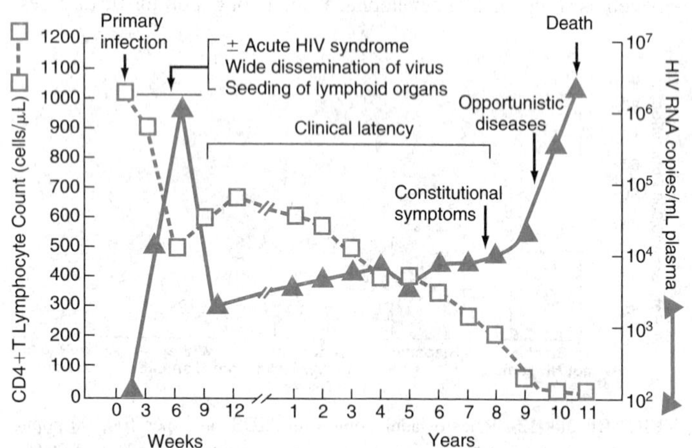

FIGURE 309-14 Typical course of an HIV-infected individual. See text for detailed description. *(From Fauci et al.)*

particularly the infections and neoplasms that are AIDS-defining illnesses. Some features of AIDS, such as KS and neurologic abnormalities (see below), cannot be explained completely by the immunosuppressive effects of HIV, since these complications may occur prior to the development of severe immunologic impairment.

The combination of viral pathogenic and immunopathogenic events that occurs during the course of HIV disease from the moment of initial (primary) infection through the development of advanced-stage disease is complex and varied. It is important to appreciate that the pathogenic mechanisms of HIV disease are multifactorial and multiphasic and are different at different stages of the disease. Therefore, it is essential to consider the typical clinical course of an untreated HIV-infected individual in order to more fully appreciate these pathogenic events (Fig. 309-14).

PRIMARY HIV INFECTION, INITIAL VIREMIA, AND DISSEMINATION OF VIRUS The events associated with primary HIV infection are likely critical determinants of the subsequent course of HIV disease. In particular, the dissemination of virus to lymphoid organs is a major factor in the establishment of a chronic and persisent infection (see below). The initial infection of susceptible cells may vary somewhat with the route of infection. Virus that enters directly into the bloodstream via infected blood or blood products (i.e., transfusions, use of contaminated needles for injecting drugs, sharp-object injuries, maternal-to-fetal transmission either intrapartum or perinatally, or sexual intercourse where there is enough trauma to cause bleeding) is likely cleared from the circulation to the spleen and other lymphoid organs, where it replicates to a critical level and then leads to a burst of viremia that disseminates virus throughout the body. It is uncertain which cell in the blood or lymphoid tissue is the first to actually become infected; however, studies in animal models suggest that dendritic lineage cells may be the initial cells infected. Depending on their stage of maturation, dendritic cells can either be directly infected with virus and pass virus on to CD4+ T cells or physically bring the virus into contact with CD4+ T cells without themselves becoming infected. Studies in the monkey model of mucosal exposure to SIV strongly suggest that the initial cell to become infected at the site of exposure is the Langerhans cell, which is a dendritic lineage cell, and that this cell passes the virus on to CD4+ T cells in the draining lymph nodes. This mechanism likely operates in humans when HIV enters "locally" (as opposed to directly into the blood), via the vagina, rectum, or urethra during intercourse or via the upper gastrointestinal tract from swallowed infected semen, vaginal fluid, or breast milk. Certainly, CD4+ T cells and to a lesser extent cells of monocyte lineage are the major ultimate targets of HIV infection. In primary HIV infection, virus replication in CD4+ T cells intensifies prior to the initiation of an HIV-specific immune response (see below), leading to a burst of viremia (Fig. 309-14) and then to a rapid dissemination of virus to other lymphoid organs, the brain, and other tissues. Individuals who experience the "acute HIV syndrome," which occurs to varying degrees in approximately 50% of individuals with primary infection, have high levels of viremia that last for several weeks (see below). The acute mononucleosis-like symptoms are well correlated with the presence of viremia. Virtually all patients appear to develop some degree of viremia during primary infection, which contributes to virus dissemination, even though they remain asymptomatic or do not recall experiencing symptoms. Careful examination of lymph nodes from more than one site in patients with established HIV infection who did not report symptoms of a primary infection strongly indicate that wide dissemination to lymphoid tissue occurs in most patients. A more detailed description of the role of lymphoid tissue in the immunopathogenesis of HIV disease is given below. It appears that the initial level of plasma viremia in primary HIV infection does not necessarily determine the rate of disease progression; however, the set point of the level of steady-state plasma viremia after approximately 1 year does seem to correlate with the rapidity of disease progression (see below).

ESTABLISHMENT OF CHRONIC AND PERSISTENT INFECTION **Persistent Virus Replication** HIV infection is relatively unique among human viral infections. Despite the robust cellular and humoral immune responses that are mounted following primary infection (see below), once infection has been established the virus is virtually never cleared completely from the body. Rather, a chronic infection develops that persists with varying degrees of virus replication for a median of approximately 10 years before the patient becomes clinically ill (see below). It is this establishment of a chronic, persistent infection that is the hallmark of HIV disease. Throughout the often protracted course of chronic infection, virus replication can almost invariably be detected in untreated patients, both by highly sensitive assays for plasma viremia as well as by demonstration of virus replication in lymphoid tissue. In human viral infections, with very few exceptions, if the host survives, the virus is completely cleared from the body and a state of immunity against subsequent infection develops. HIV infection very rarely kills the host during primary infection. Certain viruses, such as HSV (Chap. 182), are not completely cleared from the body after infection, but instead enter a latent state; in these cases, clinical latency is accompanied by microbiologic latency. This is not the case with HIV infection, in which some degree of virus replication invariably occurs during the period of clinical latency (see below). Chronicity associated with persistent virus replication can also be seen in certain cases of hepatitis B and C infections (Chap. 297); however, in these infections the immune system is not a target of the virus. As mentioned above, HIV usually does not abruptly kill the host; rather it generally succeeds in escaping from a rather vigorous immune response and establishing a state of chronic infection with varying degrees of persistently active virus replication.

Evasion of Immune System Control Clearly, HIV successfully evades elimination by the immune system in order to establish chronicity. The mechanisms whereby this occurs are not completely clear; however, several have been proposed as playing a role in this phenomenon. HIV has an extraordinary ability to mutate, but this mechanism probably acts mainly after the establishment of chronic infection and contributes to the maintenance of chronicity. Since the transmitted virus and the virus that initially becomes established as a chronic infection are relatively homogeneous, the initial escape from immune system control likely involves mechanisms other than viral mutation. Molecular analysis of clonotypes has demonstrated that clones of CD8+ cytolytic T lymphocytes (CTLs) that expand greatly during primary HIV infection and likely represent the high-affinity clones that would be expected to be most efficient in eliminating virus-infected cells are no longer detectable after their initial burst of expansion. The marked diminution of frequency or disappearance of these HIV-specific cells cannot be explained by mutations in the viral epitope to which they are directed, since virus-sequencing studies indicate that the initial viral epitope is still present when the clones are no longer detected. Furthermore, other, less expanded clones of CD8+ T cells that recognize the same viral epitope persist and likely account for the partial control of virus replication. It is thought that the initially expanded clones may have been deleted owing to the overwhelming exposure to viral antigens during the initial burst of viremia, similar to the exhaustion of CD8+ CTLs that has been reported in the murine model of lymphocytic choriomeningitis virus (LCMV) infection. To compound this phenomenon, virus replication and thus saturation of antigen-presenting cells with viral antigen take place in the lymphoid tissue (see below), which is also the site of generation of HIV-specific CTLs.

Another potential mechanism of HIV escape is related to the fact that, during primary HIV infection and the transition to established chronic infection, both activated HIV-specific CTLs and CTL precursors are preferentially and paradoxically segregated in the peripheral blood, where very little active virus replication takes place, rather than in the lymphoid tissue, which is the main site of virus replication and spread, and the major source of plasma viremia. Finally, the escape of HIV from elimination during primary infection allows the formation of a large pool of latently infected cells that cannot be eliminated by virus-specific CTLs (see below). Thus, despite a potent immune response and the marked downregulation of virus replication following primary HIV infection, HIV succeeds in establishing a state of chronic infection with a variable degree of persistent virus replication. In most cases, during this period the patient makes the clinical transition from acute primary infection to a relatively prolonged state of clinical latency (see below).

Reservoir of Latency Infected Cells It has been clearly demonstrated that there exists in virtually all HIV-infected individuals a pool of latently infected, resting CD4+ T cells, and that this pool of cells likely serves as at least one component of the persistent reservoir of virus. Such cells manifest postintegration latency in that the HIV provirus integrates into the genome of the cell and can remain in this state until an activation signal drives the expression of HIV transcripts and ultimately replication-competent virus. This form of latency is to be distinguished from preintegration latency, in which HIV enters a resting CD4+ T cell and, in the absence of an activation signal, only a limited degree of reverse transcription of the HIV genome occurs. This period of preintegration latency may last hours to days, and if no activation signal is delivered to the cell, the proviral DNA loses its capacity to initiate a productive infection. If these cells do become activated, reverse transcription proceeds to completion and the virus continues along its replication cycle (see above and Fig. 309-15). The pool of cells that are in the postintegration state of latency are established early during the course of primary HIV infection. Despite the suppression of plasma viremia to below detectable levels (<50 copies of HIV RNA per milliliter) by potent combinations of several antiretroviral drugs for as long as 3 years, this pool of latently infected cells persists and can give rise to replication-competent virus. This persistent pool of latently infected cells is a major obstacle to any goal of eradication of virus from infected individuals.

Viral Dynamics It was originally thought that very little virus replication occurred during clinical latency. However, studies of lymphoid tissue using PCR analysis for HIV RNA and in situ hybridization for individual virus-expressing cells clearly demonstrated that

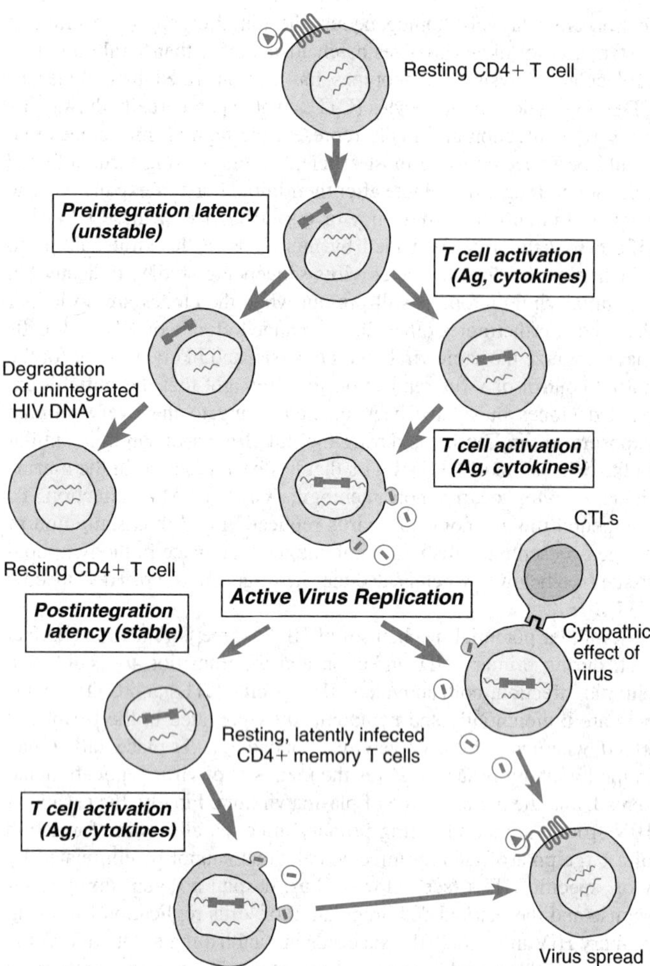

FIGURE 309-15 Generation of latently infected, resting CD4+ T cells in HIV-infected individuals. See text for details; Ag, antigen; CTLs, cytolytic T lymphocytes. *(Courtesy of TW Chun.)*

HIV replication occurs throughout the course of HIV infection, even during clinical latency when it is very difficult to culture virus from unfractionated peripheral blood mononuclear cells. The availability of sensitive PCR techniques led to the demonstration that some degree of plasma viremia is present in virtually all untreated patients at all stages of HIV disease. Subsequently, the dynamics of viral production and turnover were quantified using mathematical modeling in the setting of the administration of reverse transcriptase and protease inhibitors to HIV-infected individuals in clinical studies. Treatment with these drugs resulted in a precipitous decline in the level of plasma viremia, which typically fell by 99% within 2 weeks. The number of CD4+ T cells in the blood increased concurrently, which implies that the killing of CD4+ T cells is linked directly to the levels of replicating virus. However, it is generally agreed that a significant component of the early rise in CD4+ T cell numbers following the initiation of therapy is due to the redistribution of cells into the peripheral blood from other body compartments. It was determined on the basis of the emergence of resistant mutants during therapy that 93 to 99% of the circulating virus originated from recently infected, rapidly turning over CD4+ T cells and that approximately 1 to 7% of circulating virus originated from longer-lived cells, likely monocyte/macrophages. A negligible amount of circulating virus originated from the pool of latently infected cells (see above) (Fig. 309-16). It was also determined that the half-life of a circulating virion was approximately 30 min and that of productively infected cells was 1 day. Given the relatively steady level of plasma viremia and of infected cells, it appears that extremely large amounts of virus (approximately 10^{10} to 10^{11} virions)

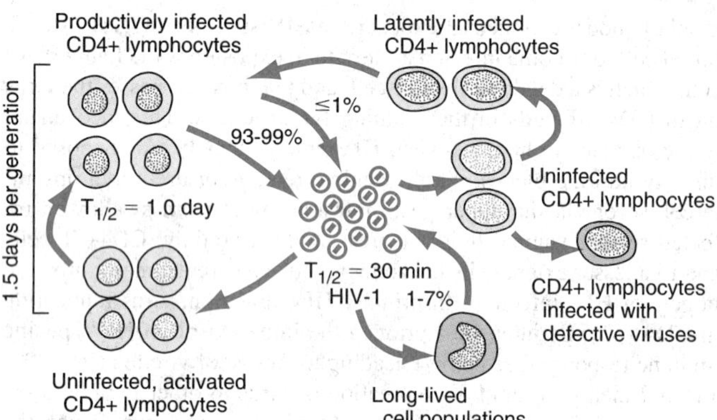

FIGURE 309-16 Dynamics of HIV infection in vivo. See text for detailed description. *(From Perelson et al, 1996.)*

are produced and cleared from the circulation each day. In addition, data suggest that the minimum duration of the HIV-1 replication cycle in vivo averages 1.5 days. Other studies have demonstrated that the decrease in plasma viremia that results from antiretroviral therapy correlates closely with a decrease in virus replication in lymph nodes, further confirming that lymphoid tissue is the main site of HIV replication and the main source of plasma viremia. Using a mathematical formula that assumed a two-phase decay of virus-infected cells, it was originally estimated that virus could be eradicated within 2.3 to 3.1 years from an HIV-infected individual who was receiving antiretroviral therapy that successfully suppressed all virus replication. However, recent data taking into account the pool of latently infected cells (see above) indicate that there is a third, much longer phase of decay that results in a projected time to viral eradication ranging from 10 to 60 years. Concomitant with this finding was the realization that even the most potent combinations of antiretroviral drugs did not completely suppress virus replication, as indicated by the detection of variable degress of cell-associated HIV RNA by sensitive PCR assays in most patients despite the absence of detectable plasma virema. Therefore, it is highly unlikely that virus will be eradicated from HIV-infected individuals with the currently available antiretoviral drugs despite the favorable clinical outcomes that have resulted from such therapy (see below).

The level of steady-state viremia, called the viral *set point*, at approximately 1 year has important prognostic implications for the progression of HIV disease. It has been demonstrated that HIV-infected individuals who have a low set point at 6 months to 1 year progress to AIDS much more slowly than individuals whose set point is very high at that time (Fig. 309-17). Levels of viremia generally increase

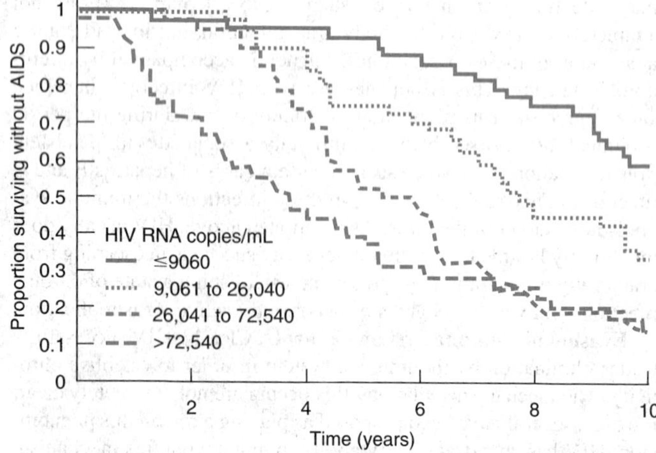

FIGURE 309-17 Relationship between levels of virus and rates of disease progression. Kaplan-Meier curves for AIDS-free survival stratified by baseline HIV-1 RNA categories (copies per milliliter). *(From Mellors et al.)*

as disease progresses. Measurement of the level of viremia is playing an increasingly important role in guiding therapeutic decisions in HIV-infected individuals (see below).

Immunopathogenic Events during Clinical Latency With few exceptions, the level of CD4+ T cells in the blood decreases gradually and progressively in HIV-infected individuals. The slope of this decline, together with the level of plasma viremia (see above), predict well the pattern of the clinical course and the development of advanced disease. Most patients are entirely asymptomatic while this progressive decline is taking place (see below) and are often described as being in a state of *clinical latency*. However, clinical latency does not mean disease latency, since progression is generally relentless during this period. Furthermore, clinical latency should not be confused with microbiologic latency. Although there are cells present in an infected individual that are latently infected and do not express detectable viral RNA, there is virtually always some degree of ongoing virus replication, even during the early stages of HIV disease.

ADVANCED HIV DISEASE In untreated patients or in patients in whom therapy has not adequately controlled virus replication (see below), after a variable period, usually measured in years, the CD4+ T cell count falls below a critical level (<200 cells per microliter), and the patient becomes highly susceptible to opportunistic disease (Fig. 309-14). For this reason, the CDC case definition of AIDS was modified to include all HIV-infected individuals with CD4+ T cell counts below this level (Table 309-1). Patients may experience constitutional signs and symptoms or may develop an opportunistic disease abruptly without any prior symptoms, although the latter scenario is unusual. The depletion of CD4+ T cells continues to be progressive and unrelenting in this phase. It is not uncommon for CD4+ T cell counts to drop as low as 10/μL or even to zero, yet the patients may survive for months or even for >1 year. This situation has become increasingly common as patients are treated more aggressively and are given prophylaxis against the common life-threatening opportunistic infections (see below). In addition, control of plasma viremia by antiretroviral therapy, even in individuals with extremely low CD4+ T cell counts, has increased survival in these patients despite the fact that their CD4+ T cell counts may not significantly increase as a result of therapy. Ultimately, patients who progress to this severest form of immunodeficiency usually succumb to opportunistic infections or neoplasms (see below).

LONG-TERM SURVIVORS AND LONG-TERM NONPROGRESSORS The median time from primary HIV infection to the development of AIDS in untreated individuals is approximately 10 years. Treatment with effective combinations of antiretroviral drugs has clearly extended this period; the full extent of this benefit has yet to be realized. The definitions of *long-term survivor* and *long-term nonprogressor* continue to evolve as more data are collected from prospective cohort studies. Predictions from one study that antedated the availability of effective antiretroviral therapy estimated that approximately 13% of homosexual/bisexual men who were infected at an early age may remain free of clinical AIDS for >20 years. Currently, individuals are considered to be long-term survivors if they remain alive for 10 to 15 years after initial infection. In most such individuals the disease has progressed, in that they have significant immunodeficiency, and many have experienced opportunistic diseases. Some of these individuals have CD4+ T cell counts that have decreased to ≤200/μL but have remained stable at that level for years. The mechanisms of this stabilization are not entirely clear but may relate to the beneficial effects of antiretroviral therapy and prophylaxis against opportunistic infections. In addition, a number of viral and/or host determinants likely contribute to the long-term survival of these individuals. In some individuals, the virus may either have been less virulent initially or may have mutated to a less virulent form under the influence of antiretroviral therapy. Quantitative and qualitative aspects of the HIV-specific immune response, as well as recognized and unrecognized genetic factors (see below), may also contribute to the long-term survival of these individuals.

Fewer than 5% of HIV-infected individuals are characterized as long-term nonprogressors. All long-term nonprogressors are long-term survivors; however, the reverse is not true. Individuals who have been infected with HIV for a long period (≳10 years), whose CD4+ T cell counts are in the normal range and have remained stable over years, and who have not received antiretroviral therapy are considered to be long-term nonprogressors. These patients are characterized by a low viral burden (low number of HIV-infected cells), low levels of plasma viremia, generally normal immune function according to commonly measured parameters (skin tests, in vitro lymphocyte responses to various mitogens and antigens), and normal-appearing lymphoid tissue architecture as determined on lymph node biopsy. In general, long-term nonprogressors manifest robust HIV-specific immune responses, both humoral (neutralizing antibodies) and cell-mediated (HIV-specific CTLs). However, this may also be true of some individuals early in the course of disease who ultimately progress to advanced disease. Although viremia is consistently very low in long-term nonprogressors, many have persistent viremia as determined by sensitive PCR assays. No qualitative abnormalities in the virus have been detected in most of these patients. However, a small subset of patients do have defective virus; in particular, in one cohort of five long-term nonprogressors, the virus had a defect in the *nef* gene. In another report, a blood donor in Australia who was HIV-infected and a group of seven individuals who were infected by blood or blood products from that donor remained free of HIV-related disease and maintained normal and stable CD4+ T cell counts for several years after infection. Sequence analysis of viruses isolated from the donor and recipients revealed similar deletions in the *nef* gene and the region of overlap of *nef* and the U3 region of the HIV long terminal repeat (Fig. 309-5). However, several of these individuals have now begun to show indications of progressive immunodeficiency, and thus they can no longer be considered nonprogressors. The precise role of host factors in long-term nonprogression remains unclear. There is no obvious and consistent genetic determinant for nonprogression. However, several genetic mutations have been demonstrated to result in a delay in the progression of HIV disease. These include heterozygosity for the *CCR5*-Δ32 deletion, heterozygosity for the *CCR2*-64I mutation, homozygosity for the *SDF1*-3′A mutation, and heterozygosity for the *RANTES-28G* mutation (see "Genetic Factors in HIV Pathogenesis," below). Since CCR5 is the major co-receptor for R5 or macrophage-tropic strains of HIV and since individuals who are homozygous for the *CCR5*-Δ32 deletion are, with rare exceptions, protected against HIV infection, the potential mechanism for slow progression in heterozygotes is clear. In addition, certain single nucleotide polymorphisms in the *CCR5* promoter have been shown to be associated with slower progression of disease. The reason for the slowing of progression of HIV disease in individuals who are heterozygous for the *CCR2*-64I mutation is less clear; however, it has been demonstrated that CXCR4 can dimerize with the CCR2V64I mutant but not with wild-type CCR2. This dimerization may reduce the amount of CXCR4 on the cell surface and as a result inhibit infection with X4 viruses. Homozygosity for the *SDF1*-3′A mutation may upregulate the *SDF1* gene enabling SDF-1, which is the natural ligand for CXCR4, to compete more effectively with X4 or T cell tropic virus for the CXCR4 coreceptor. The *RANTES-28G* mutation increases RANTES expression, which is the natural ligand for CCR5 and may thus inhibit infection with R5 viruses. Finally, maximal HLA heterozygosity of class I loci (A, B, and C) has been shown to be associated with delayed progression of HIV disease. Although long-term nonprogressors have robust HIV-specific immune responses as well as competent CD8+ T cell suppressors of HIV replication, it is unclear whether these factors are directly responsible for the state of nonprogression. A substantial proportion of HIV-infected individuals manifest comparable immune responses early in the course of their disease and still experience disease progression. Long-term nonprogressors likely represent a heterogeneous group. The lack of disease progression may be explained in some by a defect in the virus; in others by any of a variety of host factors, including recognized and as yet unrecognized genetic factors; and in others by a combination of both.

ROLE OF LYMPHOID ORGANS IN HIV PATHOGENESIS Lymphoid tissues are the major anatomic sites for the establishment and propagation of HIV infection (see above). For practical reasons, most studies on the pathogenesis of HIV infection have focused on peripheral blood mononuclear cells. However, lymphocytes in the peripheral blood represent only approximately 2% of the total body lymphocyte pool and so may not always accurately reflect the status of the entire immune system; most of the body's lymphocytes reside in lymphoid organs, such as the lymph nodes, spleen, and gut-associated lymphoid tissue. Furthermore, virus replication occurs mainly in lymphoid tissue and not in blood; the level of plasma viremia reflects virus production in lymphoid tissue. Finally, since HIV disease is an infectious disease of the immune system, it is critical to appreciate the pathogenic events that occur in the lymphoid tissue in HIV infection.

Some patients experience progressive generalized lymphadenopathy (see below) early in the course of the infection; others experience varying degrees of transient lymphadenopathy. Lymphadenopathy reflects the cellular activation and immune response to the virus in the lymphoid tissue, which is generally characterized by follicular or germinal-center hyperplasia. Lymph node involvement is a common denominator of virtually all patients with HIV infection, even those without easily detectable lymphadenopathy.

Simultaneous examination of lymph node and peripheral blood in the same patients during various stages of HIV disease, including the early asymptomatic stage (when CD4+ T cell counts generally are $>500/\mu L$), the intermediate stage (when counts are usually 200 to 500/μL) and the advanced stage (when counts are $<200/\mu L$) has led to substantial insight into the pathogenesis of HIV disease. Using a combination of PCR techniques for HIV DNA and RNA in tissue and RNA in plasma, in situ hybridization for HIV RNA, and light and electron microscopy, the following picture has emerged. In most untreated patients, early in the course of infection when the viral set point has been reached and prior to significant immunodeficiency (CD4+ T cell counts $>500/\mu L$), levels of plasma viremia are variable but generally low; the viral burden (number of infected cells) in the peripheral blood is usually extremely low, and expression of HIV in these cells is minimal or undetectable. Remarkably, at this time copious amounts of extracellular virions are trapped on the processes of the follicular dendritic cells (FDCs) in the germinal centers of the lymph nodes (Fig. 309-18*A*). In situ hybridization reveals expression of virus in individual cells of the paracortical area and, to a lesser extent, the germinal center (Fig. 309-18*B*). The number of cells expressing virus is low early in the course of disease and increases as disease progresses. Examination of lymph nodes during primary HIV infection in humans (see above) and SIV infection in macaques indicates that during the transition from primary infection to established chronic infection, germinal centers form and virus is trapped. This trapping, together with the generation of a vigorous HIV-specific immune response, likely contributes to the rapid decrease in plasma viremia seen in most patients following the initial burst of viremia associated with primary infection. A considerable amount of virus can be trapped during the period of high viremia associated with primary infection. The persistence of trapped virus after chronic infection likely reflects a steady state whereby trapped virus turns over and is replaced by fresh virions, which are produced persistently, albeit usually at low levels during the early, clinically latent stage of disease.

During early-stage HIV disease, the architecture of the germinal centers is generally preserved and may even be hyperplastic owing to in situ proliferation of cells (mostly B lymphocytes) and recruitment to the lymph nodes of a number of cell types (B cells, CD4+ and CD8+ T cells). Electron microscopy demonstrates a fine network of FDCs with many long, finger-like processes that envelop virtually every lymphocyte in the germinal center (Fig. 309-18*C*). Extracellular virions can be seen attached to the processes, yet the FDCs appear to be relatively healthy. The trapping of antigen is a physiologically normal function for the FDCs, which present antigen to B cells and contribute to the generation of B cell memory. However, in the case of HIV, the trapped virions serve as a persistent source of cellular activation, resulting in the secretion of proinflammatory cytokines such as interleukin (IL) 1β, tumor necrosis factor (TNF)α, and IL-6, which can upregulate virus replication in infected cells (see below). Furthermore, although trapped virus is coated by neutralizing antibodies, it has been demonstrated that these virions remain infectious for CD4+ T cells while attached to the processes of the FDCs. CD4+ T cells that migrate into the germinal center to provide help to B cells in the generation of an HIV-specific immune response thus are susceptible to infection by these trapped virions. Thus, in HIV infection, a normal physiologic function of the immune system, which contributes to the clearance of virus as well as to the generation of a specific immune response, can also have deleterious consequences. It is difficult to demonstrate infection of the FDCs at this point, or even in advanced disease; however, rare examples of virus budding off FDCs have been reported.

As the disease progresses, the architecture of the germinal centers begins to show disruption, and the trapping efficiency of the lymph node diminishes. Electron microscopy reveals swollen organelles, and the FDCs begin to undergo cell death. The mechanisms of FDC death remain unclear; there is no indication by electron microscopy of copious virus replication or budding of virions off the cell in great quantities. At this stage, the level of plasma viremia generally increases. In addition, both the relative number of infected cells in the blood and the expression of virus from these cells increases, approaching the levels in the lymph nodes. As the disease progresses to an advanced stage, there is complete disruption of the architecture of the germinal centers, accompanied by dissolution of the FDC network and massive dropout of FDCs (Fig. 309-18*D*). The trapping function of the lymph nodes is completely lost, and virus freely spills out into the circulation. Simultaneous PCR analysis of lymph node and peripheral blood mononuclear cells indicates that the relative number of infected cells in the blood and their expression of virus begin to equal the levels in the lymph nodes at this stage. Advanced disease is accompanied by high levels of plasma viremia, which represent a true increase in virus replication, due in part to a further diminution of immune control of virus replication (see below) as well as to the loss of the mechanical trapping function of the lymph nodes. At this point, the lymph nodes are "burnt out." This destruction of lymphoid tissue compounds the immunodeficiency of HIV disease and contributes to the inability to mount adequate immune responses against opportunistic pathogens. The events from primary infection to the ultimate destruction of the immune system are illustrated in Fig. 309-19.

ROLE OF CELLULAR ACTIVATION IN HIV PATHOGENESIS The immune system is normally in a state of homeostasis, awaiting perturbation by foreign antigenic stimuli. Activation of the immune system is an essential component of an appropriate immune response to a foreign antigen. Once the immune response deals with and clears the antigen, the system returns to relative quiescence (Chap. 305). In HIV infection, however, the immune system is chronically activated owing to the chronicity of infection and the persistence of virus replication (see above). This activated state is reflected by hyperactivation of B cells leading to hypergammaglobulinemia; spontaneous lymphocyte proliferation; activation of monocytes; expression of activation markers on CD4+ and CD8+ T cells; lymph node hyperplasia, particularly early in the course of disease (see above); increased secretion of proinflammatory cytokines (see below); elevated levels of neopterin, β_2-microglobulin, acid-labile interferon, and soluble IL-2 receptors; and autoimmune phenomena (see below). Even in the absence of direct infection of a target cell, HIV envelope proteins can interact with cellular receptors (CD4 molecules and chemokine receptors) to deliver potent activation signals resulting in calcium flux, the phosphorylation of certain proteins involved in signal transduction, co-localization of cytoplasmic proteins including those involved in cell trafficking, secretion of certain cytokines, immune dysfunction, and under certain circumstances, apoptosis (see below).

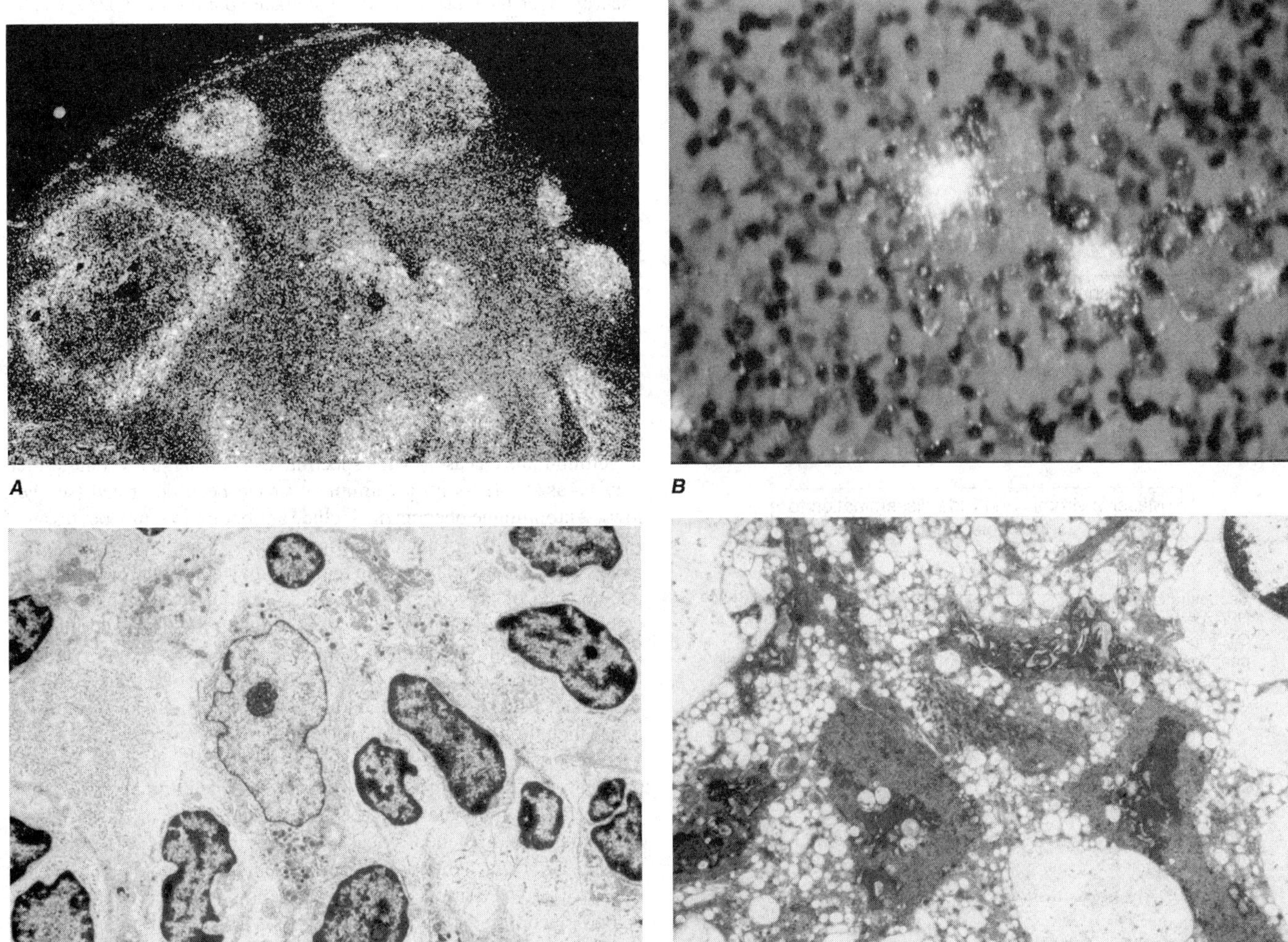

A B C D

FIGURE 309-18 HIV in the lymph nodes of HIV-infected individuals. *A.* Cervical lymph node from an asymptomatic individual with very low levels of plasma viremia. In situ hybridization using a molecular probe for HIV RNA reveals copious virus demarcating the numerous germinal centers (bright areas) of the node. The virus was extracellular and bound to the processes of the follicular dendritic cells (FDCs), which form a matrix within the confines of the germinal centers. Original ×25. *B.* Individual cells infected with HIV. Two cells in the paracortical area of the lymph node are shown expressing HIV RNA by in situ hybridization using a radiolabeled molecular probe. Original ×250. *C.* FDCs in cervical node of an asymptomatic HIV-infected individual. Electron microscopy reveals an FDC with a prominent nucleolus surrounded by several lymphocytes within the germinal center of the node. Higher magnification of several fields indicates that multiple processes of the FDCs are in contact with several lymphocytes. Original ×1920. *D.* Dissolution of FDCs in the germinal center of a cervical lymph node from a patient with advanced HIV disease. Widespread death of FDCs is associated with a loss of ability of the lymph node to trap virus late in the course of HIV disease. Original ×3744. *(A and B courtesy of Dr. Cecil Fox; C and D courtesy of Dr. Jan Orenstein. Adapted from G Pantaleo et al: N Engl J Med 328:327, 1993.)*

Persistent immune activation may have several deleterious consequences. From a virologic standpoint, although quiescent CD4+ T cells can be infected with HIV, reverse transcription, integration, and virus spread are much more efficient in activated cells. Furthermore, cellular activation induces expression of virus in cells latently infected with HIV (see above). From an immunologic standpoint, chronic exposure of the immune system to a particular antigen over an extended period may ultimately lead to an inability to sustain an adequate immune response to the antigen. Furthermore, the ability of the immune system to respond to a broad spectrum of antigens may be compromised if immune-competent cells are maintained in a state of chronic activation. In addition, activation of the immune system may favor the elimination of cells via programmed cell death (apoptosis) (see below) as well as the secretion of certain cytokines that can induce HIV expression (see below).

Role of Apoptosis *Apoptosis* is a form of programmed cell death that is a normal mechanism for the elimination of effete cells in organogenesis as well as in the cellular proliferation that occurs during a normal immune response (Chap. 305). Apoptosis is strictly dependent on cellular activation. It has been hypothesized that, in HIV infection, sequential activation signals delivered to CD4+ T cells induce apoptosis. Cross-linking of the CD4 molecule by gp120 or gp120/anti-gp120 complexes delivers the first of two signals required for apoptosis. The second signal supposedly leading to cell death is delivered via the T cell receptor by antigen. According to this hypothesis, direct infection of CD4+ T cells is not required for apoptosis to occur, although it has been demonstrated that alterations in tyrosine kinase activity of HIV-infected cells may induce the cell to undergo apoptosis. HIV can trigger both Fas-dependent and Fas-independent pathways of apoptosis. Mechanisms involved in this process include upregulation of Fas and Fas ligand, upregulation of caspase-1 and caspase-8, downregulation of the anti-apoptotic Bcl-2 protein, and activation of cyclin-dependent kinases. Certain viral gene products have been associated with enhanced susceptibility to apoptosis including envelope, Nef, and Vpu. A number of studies, including those examining lymphoid tissue, have demonstrated that the rate of apoptosis is elevated in HIV infection and that apoptosis is seen in "bystander" cells such as CD8+ T cells and B cells as well as in CD4+ T cells.

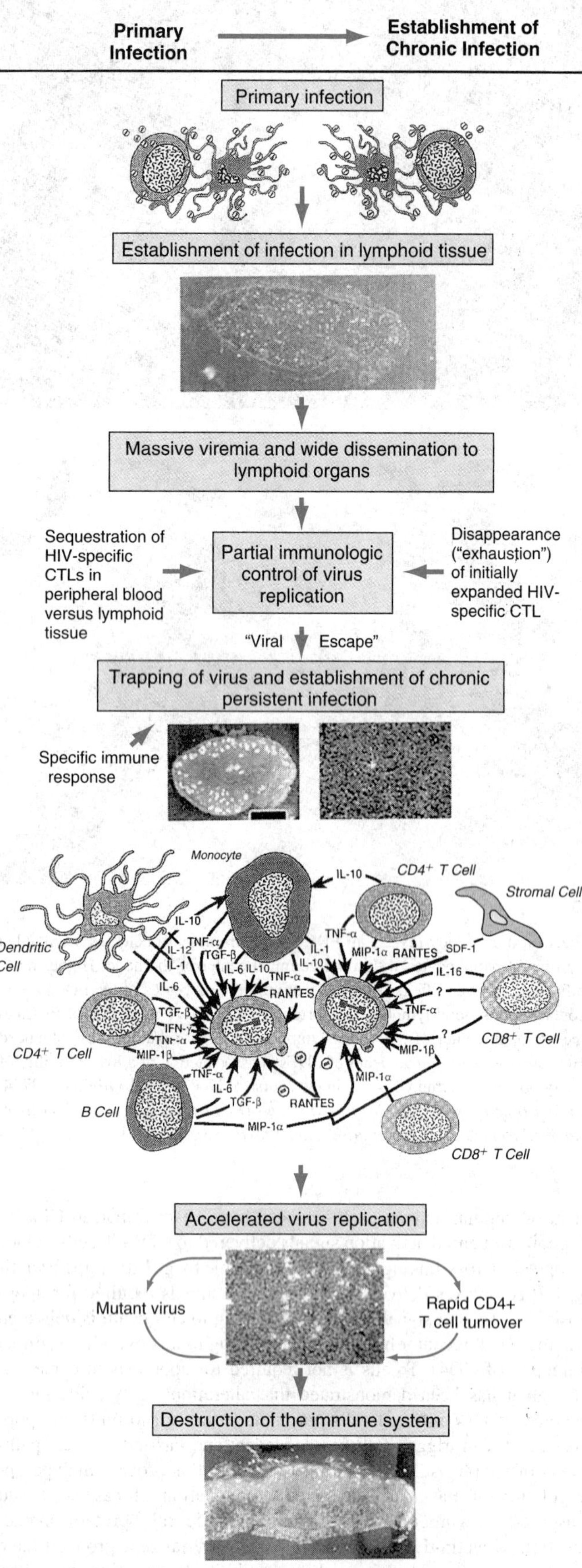

FIGURE 309-19 Events that transpire from primary HIV infection through the establishment of chronic persistent infection to the ultimate destruction of the immune system. See text for details; CTLs, cytolytic T lymphocytes.

Macrophages have been shown to mediate apoptosis of CD8+ T cells by a mechanism involving gp120-induced upregulation of Fas ligand expression on macrophages and enhanced secretion of macrophage-derived TNF-α. The intensity of apoptosis correlates with the general state of activation of the immune system and not with the stage of disease or with viral burden. The potential role of apoptosis in the pathogenesis of HIV disease is underscored by results from animal studies that show an increased frequency of apoptosis in CD4+ T cells in primates infected with pathogenic strains of SIV but not in primates infected with nonpathogenic strains of SIV. It is likely that apoptosis of immune-competent cells contributes to the immune abnormalities in HIV disease; however, this is probably a nonspecific mechanism that merely reflects the aberrant state of immune activation.

Autoimmune Phenomena The autoimmune phenomena that are common in HIV-infected individuals reflect, at least in part, chronic immune system activation as well as molecular mimickry by viral components. Although these phenomena usually occur in the absence of autoimmune disease, a wide spectrum of clinical manifestations that may be associated with autoimmunity have been described (see below). Autoimmune phenomena include antibodies to lymphocytes and, less commonly, to platelets and neutrophils. Antiplatelet antibodies have some clinical relevance, in that they may contribute to the thrombocytopenia of HIV disease (see below). Antibodies to nuclear and cytoplasmic components of cells have been reported, as have antibodies to cardiolipin; CD4 molecules; CD43 molecules, C1q-A; variable regions of the T cell receptor α, β, and γ chains; Fas; denatured collagen; and IL-2. In addition, autoantibodies to a range of serum proteins, including albumin, immunoglobulin, and thyroglobulin, have been reported. There is antigenic cross-reactivity between HIV viral proteins (gp120 and gp41) and MHC class II determinants, and anti-MHC class II antibodies have been reported in HIV infection. These antibodies could potentially lead to the elimination of MHC class II-bearing cells via antibody-dependent cellular cytotoxicity (ADCC) (Chap. 305). In addition, regions of homology exist between HIV envelope glycoproteins and IL-2 as well as MHC class I molecules.

Cofactors Contributing to HIV Pathogenesis Both endogenous and exogenous factors can contribute to HIV pathogenesis by a number of mechanisms; paramount among these is the upregulation of virus expression, a process intimately connected with cellular activation. The main endogenous factors that regulate HIV expression are cytokines (see below). Among exogenous factors, other microbes likely have important effects on HIV replication and HIV pathogenesis. They can thus be considered real or potential *cofactors* in the pathogenesis of HIV disease. Co-infection or simultaneous cotransfection of cells with HIV and other viruses or viral genes has demonstrated that certain viruses, such as HSV type 1, cytomegalovirus (CMV), human herpesvirus (HHV) 6, Epstein-Barr virus (EBV), hepatitis B virus (HBV), adenovirus, pseudorabies virus, and HTLV-I can upregulate HIV expression. Other microbes, such as *Mycoplasma* have been reported to contribute to the induction of HIV expression. *Mycobacterium tuberculosis* is a common opportunistic infection in HIV-infected individuals (see below and Chap. 169). In addition to the fact that HIV-infected individuals are more likely to develop active TB after exposure, it has been demonstrated that active TB can accelerate the course of HIV infection. It has also been shown that levels of plasma viremia are greatly elevated in HIV-infected individuals with active TB, compared to pre-TB levels and levels of viremia after successful treatment of the active TB. In vitro studies demonstrated that virus replication was markedly enhanced in lymphocytes of HIV-infected individuals who were skin test–positive for purified protein derivative (PPD) when PPD antigen was added to culture, resulting in cellular activation. Confirmatory evidence that antigen-induced activation was a major contributor to the accelerated viremia in HIV-infected individuals with active TB was provided by studies in which HIV-infected individuals were immunized with common recall antigens such as tetanus toxoid, influenza, or pneumococcal polysaccharide. Under these circumstances, a transient elevation of plasma viremia accompanied the cellular activation induced by the immunization. A greater degree of induction of virus was seen in those individuals with early stage as opposed to advanced stage HIV disease, and the degree of virus induction correlated with the level of immune system activation.

THE CYTOKINE NETWORK IN HIV PATHOGENESIS

Cytokine Regulation of HIV Expression The immune system is homeostatically regulated by a complex network of immunoregulatory cytokines, which are pleiotropic and redundant and operate in an autocrine and paracrine manner. They are expressed continuously, even during periods of apparent quiescence of the immune system. On perturbation of the immune system by antigenic challenge, the expression of cytokines increases to varying degrees (Chap. 305). Cytokines that are important components of this immunoregulatory network have been demonstrated to play a major role in the regulation of HIV expression in vitro. A number of in vitro model systems of chronically infected monocyte or T cell lines, primary cultures of peripheral blood or lymph node mononuclear cells from HIV-infected individuals, and acutely infected primary cell cultures have been used to demonstrate the role of cytokines in the regulation of HIV expression. Potent modulation of HIV expression has been demonstrated either by manipulating endogenous cytokines or by adding exogenous cytokines to culture. Cytokines that induce HIV expression in one or more of these systems include IL-1, IL-2, IL-3, IL-6, IL-12, TNF-α, and TNF-β, macrophage colony stimulating factor (M-CSF), and granulocyte-macrophage colony stimulating factor (GM-CSF). Among these cytokines, the most consistent and potent inducers of HIV expression are the *proinflammatory cytokines* TNF-α, IL-1β, and IL-6. IFN-α and -β suppress HIV replication, whereas transforming growth factor (TGF) β, IL-4, IL-10, and IFN-γ can either induce or suppress HIV expression, depending on the system involved. The *CC-chemokines* RANTES, macrophage inflammatory protein (MIP) 1α, and MIP-1β (Chap. 305) inhibit infection by and spread of R5 (macrophage-tropic) HIV-1 strains, while *stromal cell–derived factor* (SDF) 1 inhibits infection by and spread of X4 (T cell–tropic) strains (see below). Several of these cytokines act synergistically in regulating HIV infection and replication, and others function in an autocrine and paracrine manner, similar to their physiologic function in the regulation of the immune system. Blocking of endogenous HIV-inducing cytokines or addition of inhibitors of HIV suppressor cytokines in cultures of peripheral blood and lymph node mononuclear cells from HIV-infected individuals has demonstrated that HIV replication is controlled tightly by endogenous cytokines acting in an autocrine and paracrine manner. Indeed, the net level of virus replication in an HIV-infected individual at least in part reflects a balance between inductive and suppressive host factors, mediated mainly by cytokines. An example of this endogenous regulation is the case of IL-10, which inhibits HIV replication in acutely infected monocyte/macrophages by blocking the secretion of the HIV-inducing cytokines TNF-α and IL-6. In addition, IL-4, IL-13, and TGF-β inhibit HIV expression in chronically infected monocytic cell lines stimulated by lipopolysaccharide and GM-CSF by increasing the ratio of expression of endogenous IL-1 receptor antagonist to IL-1β.

The molecular mechanisms of HIV regulation are best understood for TNF-α, which activates NF-κB proteins that function as transcriptional activators of HIV expression. The HIV-inducing effect of IL-1β is thought to occur at the level of viral transcription in an NF-κB-independent manner. IL-6, GM-CSF, and IFN-γ regulate HIV expression mainly by posttranscriptional mechanisms. Elevated levels of TNF-α and IL-6 have been demonstrated in plasma and cerebrospinal fluid (CSF), and increased expression of TNF-α, IL-1β, IFN-γ, and IL-6 has been demonstrated in the lymph nodes of HIV-infected individuals. The mechanisms whereby the CC-chemokines RANTES, MIP-1α, and MIP-1β inhibit infection of R5 strains of HIV very likely involve blocking of the binding of the virus to its co-receptor, the CC-chemokine receptor CCR5 (see above and below). Of note is the fact that CC-chemokines that inhibit infection by R5 strains of virus actually enhance infection by X4 strains of virus by inducing intracellular signal transduction through the CCR5 and CD4 molecules. In addition, products of bacterial pathogens as well as of certain viruses including HIV-1 itself can induce the expression of CXCR4 and thus potentially favor infection with X4 strains of virus that utilize this co-receptor.

Dysregulation of Cytokines HIV-infected individuals show an imbalance in the T cell limbs of the immune response, which are defined by the patterns of cytokine secretion. T helper (T_H)1 cells are characterized by secretion of IL-2 and IFN-γ and favor cell-mediated immune responses, whereas T_H2 cells are characterized by secretion of IL-4, IL-5, and IL-10 and favor humoral immune responses (Chap. 305). Since several cell types in addition to CD4+ T cells secrete these cytokines, it is more accurate to refer to immune responses that reflect one or the other cytokine pattern as *T_H1 or T_H2 type responses.* HIV-infected individuals show a decrease in T_H1 type responses relative to T_H2 type cytokine patterns. They manifest a progressive loss in expression of the IL-2 receptor and in the ability to produce the immunoregulatory cytokines IL-2 and IL-12; these cytokines are critical for effective cell-mediated immune responses in that they stimulate proliferation and lytic activity of CTLs and natural killer (NK) cells. Furthermore, IL-12 is important for the stimulation of T_H1 type cytokines such as IL-2 and IFN-γ that favor the development of cell-mediated immune responses. T_H1 type cytokines such as IL-2, IL-12, TNF-α, and IFN-γ upregulate CCR5 expression, while T_H2 type cytokines such as IL-4 and IL-10 upregulate CXCR4 expression and downregulate CCR5 expression. It has also been demonstrated that in vitro apoptosis can be inhibited in T cells from HIV-infected donors by antibodies to IL-4 and IL-10 and enhanced by antibodies to IL-12. Although it has been proposed that a clear-cut switch from a T_H1 type to a T_H2 type of cytokine pattern is a critical step in the pathogenesis of HIV disease, no sharp dichotomy between these two types of cytokine patterns that is directly related to progression of disease has been corroborated. Cytokine dysregulation in HIV infection is complex and cannot be neatly classified in terms of the polarity of T_H1 and T_H2 responses.

CELLULAR TARGETS OF HIV Although the CD4+ T lymphocytes and CD4+ cells of monocyte lineage are the principal targets of HIV, virtually any cell that expresses the CD4 molecule together with co-receptor molecules (see above and below) can potentially be infected with HIV. Circulating dendritic cells have been reported to express low levels of CD4, and depending on their stage of maturation, these cells can be infected with HIV (see below). Epidermal Langerhans cells express CD4 and have been infected by HIV in vivo. In vitro, HIV has been reported also to infect a wide range of cells and cell lines that express low levels of CD4, no detectable CD4, or only CD4 mRNA; among these are FDCs; megakaryocytes; eosinophils; astrocytes; oligodendrocytes; microglial cells; CD8+ T cells; B cells; NK cells; renal epithelial cells; cervical cells; rectal and bowel mucosal cells such as enterochromaffin, goblet, and columnar epithelial cells; trophoblastic cells; and cells from a variety of organs, such as liver, lung, heart, salivary gland, eye, prostate, testis, and adrenal gland. Since the only cells that have been shown unequivocally to be infected with HIV and to support replication of the virus are CD4+ T lymphocytes and cells of monocyte/macrophage lineage, the relevance of the in vitro infection of these other cell types is questionable.

Of potentially important clinical relevance is the demonstration that thymic precursor cells, which were assumed to be negative for CD3, CD4, and CD8 molecules, actually do express low levels of CD4 and can be infected with HIV in vitro. In addition, human thymic epithelial cells transplanted into an immunodeficient mouse can be infected with HIV by direct inoculation of virus into the thymus. Since these cells may play a role in the normal regeneration of CD4+ T cells, it is possible that their infection and depletion contribute, at least in part, to the impaired ability of the CD4+ T cell pool to completely reconstitute itself in certain infected individuals in whom antiretroviral therapy has suppressed viral replication to below detectable levels (<50 copies of HIV RNA per milliliter; see below). In addition, CD34+ monocyte precursor cells have been shown to be infected in

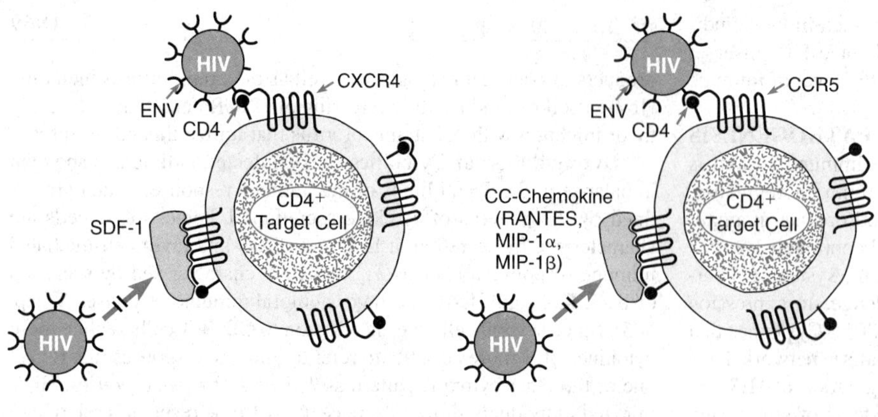

FIGURE 309-20 Model for the role of co-receptors CXCR4 and CCR5 in the efficient binding and entry of X4 (T cell–tropic) and R5 (macrophage-tropic) strains of HIV-1, respectively, into CD4+ target cells. Blocking of this initial event in the virus life cycle can be accomplished by inhibition of binding to the co-receptor by the normal ligand for the receptor in question. The ligand for CXCR4 is stromal cell–derived factor (SDF-1); the ligands for CCR5 are RANTES, MIP-1α, and MIP-1β.

vivo in patients with advanced HIV disease. It is likely that these cells express low levels of CD4, and therefore it is not essential to invoke CD4-independent mechanisms to explain the infection.

ROLE OF CO-RECEPTORS IN CELL TROPISM OF HIV Different strains of HIV-1 utilize two major co-receptors along with CD4 to bind to, fuse with, and enter target cells; these co-receptors are CCR5 and CXCR4, which are receptors for certain chemokines and belong to the seven-transmembrane-domain G protein–coupled family of receptors (see above). Strains of HIV that utilize CCR5 as a co-receptor are referred to as *R5 viruses*. These viruses were formerly classified as *macrophage tropic viruses* since they readily infect macrophages but not T cell lines. Strains of HIV that utilize CXCR4 are referred to as *X4 viruses*. These viruses are also referred to as *T cell–tropic viruses* since they readily infect T cell lines but not macrophages. In actuality, X4 viruses enter macrophages but do not proceed efficiently along the replication cycle unless an appropriate signal is delivered to the cell. Many virus strains are *dual tropic* in that they utilize both CCR5 and CXCR4; these are referred to as *R5X4 viruses*. Other terminology that has been associated with R5 versus X4 viruses is *non-syncytium-inducing viruses* versus *syncytium-inducing viruses*, respectively, based on the observation that R5 viruses generally do not form syncytia in culture with certain T cell lines, whereas X4 viruses readily form syncytia. In reality, under certain conditions both R5 and X4 viruses are capable of forming syncytia in culture.

The natural chemokine ligands for the major HIV co-receptors can readily block entry of HIV. For example, the CC-chemokines RANTES, MIP-1α, and MIP-1β, which are the natural ligands for CCR5, block entry of R5 viruses, whereas SDF-1, the natural ligand for CXCR4, blocks entry of X4 viruses. The mechanism of inhibition of viral entry is a steric inhibition of binding that is not dependent on signal transduction (Fig. 309-20).

The transmitting virus is almost invariably an R5 virus that predominates during the early stages of HIV disease. In approximately 40% of HIV-infected individuals, there is a transition to a predominantly X4 virus that is associated with a relatively rapid progression of disease. However, at least 60% of infected individuals progress in their disease while maintaining predominance of an R5 virus. Other chemokine receptor family members may function as coreceptors for HIV and SIV entry, but to a much lesser extent than do CCR5 and CXCR4; these include CCR3, BOB/GPR15, Bonzo/STRL33/TYMSTR, CCR2, CCR8, CX_3CR1(V28), and GPR1.

The basis for the tropism of different envelope glycoproteins for either CCR5 or CXCR4 relates to the ability of the HIV envelope, particularly the third variable region (V3 loop) of gp120, to interact with these co-receptors. In this regard, binding of gp120 to CD4 induces a conformational change in gp120 that increases its affinity for CCR5. It appears that the interaction of gp120 with CXCR4 is less dependent on the conformational change induced in gp120 by CD4. In fact, there are X4 strains of HIV that bind to CXCR4 in the absence of surface-bound or soluble CD4. Finally, R5 viruses are more efficient in infecting monocyte/macrophages and microglial cells of the brain (see "Neuropathogenesis," below).

ABNORMALITIES OF MONONUCLEAR CELLS CD4+ T Cells The range of T cell abnormalities in advanced HIV infection is broad. The defects are both quantitative and qualitative and involve virtually every limb of the immune system (see below), indicating the critical dependence of the integrity of the immune system on the inducer/helper function of CD4+ T cells. Virtually all of the immune defects in advanced HIV disease can ultimately be explained by the quantitative depletion of CD4+ T cells. However, T cell dysfunction (see below) can be demonstrated in patients early in the course of infection, even when the CD4+ T cell count is in the low-normal range. The degree and spectrum of dysfunctions increase as the disease progresses. One of the first abnormalities to be detected is a defect in response to remote recall antigens, such as tetanus toxoid and influenza, at a time when mononuclear cells can still respond normally to mitogenic stimulation. Defects in responses to soluble antigens are followed in time by the loss of T cell proliferative responses to alloantigens, and subsequently to mitogens. Essentially every T cell function has been reported to be abnormal at some stage of HIV infection. These abnormalities include defective T cell cloning and colony-forming efficiencies, impaired expression of IL-2 receptors, defective IL-2 production, and decreased IFN-γ production in response to antigens. The proportion of CD4+ T cells that express CD28, which is a major co-stimulatory molecule necessary for the normal activation of T cells, is reduced during HIV infection. Cells lacking expression of CD28 do not respond to activation signals and may express markers of terminal activation including HLA-DR, CD38, and CD45RO. CD4+ T cells from HIV-infected individuals express abnormally low levels of CD40 ligand, which may explain the dysregulation of B cell function observed in HIV disease.

It is difficult to explain completely the profound immunodeficiency noted in HIV-infected individuals solely on the basis of direct infection and quantitative depletion of CD4+ T cells. This is particularly apparent during the early stages of HIV disease, when CD4+ T cell numbers may be only marginally decreased. Certainly, at the stage of advanced disease when the CD4+ T cell count is in the range of 0 to 50/μL, quantitative depletion alone can explain the immune defects. However, it is likely that CD4+ T cell dysfunction results from a combination of depletion of cells due to direct infection and a number of virus-related but indirect effects on the cell (Table 309-6).

Single-cell killing and the formation of syncytia between infected and uninfected cells have been demonstrated clearly in vitro, although

Table 309-6 Mechanisms of CD4+ T Cell Dysfunction and Depletion

Direct Mechanisms	Indirect Mechanisms
Accumulation of unintegrated viral DNA	Aberrant intracellular signaling events
Interference with cellular RNA processing	Syncytium formation
	Autoimmunity
Intracellular gp120-CD4 autofusion events	Innocent bystander killing of viral antigen–coated cells
Loss of plasma membrane integrity due to viral budding	Apoptosis
	Inhibition of lymphopoiesis
Elimination of HIV-infected cells by virus-specific immune responses	

the precise mechanisms of cell death in vivo have not been determined. Cytopathicity in an infected cell in vitro may result from a number of mechanisms, including copious budding of virions from the cell surface with resulting disruption of the integrity of the cell membrane; interference with cellular RNA processing or the accumulation of high levels of heterodisperse RNA molecules; disruption of cellular protein synthesis owing to high levels of viral RNA; accumulation of high levels of unintegrated viral DNA in the cell cytoplasm; induction of aberrant patterns of protein tyrosine phosphorylation; and the interaction between HIV gp120 and CD4 intracellularly. Strain differences in single-cell killing are determined largely by gp120 sequences, which supports the importance of the viral envelope in this process. *Syncytia formation* involves fusion of the cell membrane of an infected cell with the cell membranes of variable numbers of uninfected CD4+ cells. Although cell fusion has not been shown to be an important pathogenic process in vivo, a direct relationship between the presence of syncytia and the degree of cytopathic effect has been demonstrated in vitro, and a correlation has been reported between the presence of virus isolates that readily induce syncytia in vitro and a more aggressive clinical course in the patient. Efficient syncytia formation depends on the leukocyte adhesion molecule LFA-1 (Chap. 305) on human CD4+ T cells acutely infected with HIV in vitro.

Humoral and cellular immune responses to HIV may contribute to protective immunity by eliminating virus and virus-infected cells (see below). However, since the main targets of HIV infection are immune-competent cells, these responses may contribute to immune-cell depletion and immunologic dysfunction by eliminating both infected cells and "innocent bystander" cells. Soluble viral proteins, particularly gp120, can bind with high affinity to the CD4 molecules on uninfected T cells and monocytes; in addition, virus and/or viral proteins can bind to dendritic cells or FDCs. HIV-specific antibody can recognize these bound molecules and potentially collaborate in the elimination of the cells by ADCC.

Nonpolymorphic determinants of MHC class I products share a degree of homology with gp120 and gp41 proteins of HIV. Such similarities may lead to the generation of autoantibodies to self-MHC determinants. In fact, anti-HLA-DR antibodies have been demonstrated in the sera of HIV-infected individuals (see "Autoimmune Phenomena," above). These antibodies could contribute to the elimination of HLA-DR–expressing cells by ADCC; in addition, it has been suggested that these antibodies may inhibit certain T cell functions that involve HLA-DR molecules.

HIV envelope glycoproteins gp120 and gp160 manifest high-affinity binding to CD4 as well as to various chemokine receptors (see above). Intracellular signals transduced by gp120 have been associated with a number of immunopathogenic processes including anergy, apoptosis, and abnormalities of cell trafficking. The molecular mechanisms responsible for these abnormalities include dysregulation of the T cell receptor–phosphoinositide pathway, p56lck activation, phosphorylation of focal adhesion kinase, activation of the MAP kinase and ras signaling pathways, and downregulation of the co-stimulatory molecules CD40 ligand and CD80.

Finally, the inexorable decline in CD4+ T cell counts that occurs in most HIV-infected individuals may result in part from the inability of the immune system to regenerate the CD4+ T cell pool rapidly enough to compensate for both HIV-mediated destruction of cells and natural attrition of cells. At least two major mechanisms may contribute to the failure of the CD4+ T cell pool to reconstitute itself adequately over the course of HIV infection. The first is the destruction of lymphoid precursor cells, including thymic and bone marrow progenitor cells (see above); the other is the gradual disruption of the lymphoid tissue microenvironment, which is essential for efficient regeneration of immune-competent cells (see above).

CD8+ T Cells The level of CD8+ T cells varies throughout the course of disease. Following the resolution of acute primary infection, CD8+ T cells generally rebound to higher than normal levels and may remain that way throughout the clinically latent stage of disease. This CD8+ T lymphocytosis may in part reflect the expansion of clones of HIV-specific CD8+ CTLs. During the late stages of HIV infection, there may be a significant reduction in the numbers of CD8+ T cells. HIV-specific CD8+ CTLs have been demonstrated in HIV-infected individuals early in the course of disease (see below). As the disease progresses, this functional capability decreases and may be lost entirely. The cause of this loss of cytolytic activity is unclear. However, it has been demonstrated that, as disease progresses, CD8+ T cells assume an abnormal phenotype characterized by expression of activation markers such as HLA-DR with an absence of expression of the IL-2 receptor (CD25) and a loss of clonogenic potential. It has been reported that the phenotype of CD8+ T cells in HIV-infected individuals may be of prognostic significance. Those individuals whose CD8+ T cells developed a phenotype of HLA-DR+/CD38− following seroconversion had stabilization of their CD4+ T cell counts, whereas those whose CD8+ T cells developed a phenotype of HLA-DR+/CD38+ had a more aggressive course and a poorer prognosis. In addition to the defects in HIV-specific CTLs, functional defects in other MHC-restricted CTLs, such as those directed against influenza and CMV, have been demonstrated. Since the integrity of CD8+ T cell function depends in part on adequate inductive signals from CD4+ T cells, the defect in CD8+ CTLs is likely compounded by the quantitative loss of CD4+ T cells.

B Cells B cells from HIV-infected individuals manifest abnormal activation, which is reflected by spontaneous proliferation and immunoglobulin secretion and by increased spontaneous secretion of TNF-α and IL-6. The enhanced spontaneous in vitro transformation of B cells with EBV is probably due to defective T cell immune surveillance and has as its in vivo counterpart an increase in the incidence of EBV-related B cell lymphomas. Untransformed B cells cannot be infected with HIV. However, HIV or its products can activate B cells directly; portions of the HIV gp41 envelope protein have been reported to induce polyclonal B cell activation. In addition, it has been reported that products of the VH_3 genes on the surface of B cells can serve as a receptor for HIV. It is likely that in vivo activation of B cells by virus products accounts at least in part for the spontaneous activation of these cells noted ex vivo. B cells from HIV-infected individuals express abnormally low levels of HLA-DR on their surface and fail to upregulate CD70 normally following stimulation with activated T cells; this latter defect is associated with impaired CD70-dependent immunoglobulin synthesis. In advanced HIV disease, B cells fail to proliferate and differentiate in response to ligation of the B cell antigen receptor and CD40, suggesting a defect in signal transduction. In vivo, this activated state manifests itself by hypergammaglobulinemia and by the presence of circulating immune complexes and autoantibodies (see above). HIV-infected individuals respond poorly to primary and secondary immunizations with protein and polysaccharide antigens. These B cell defects are likely responsible in part for the increase in certain bacterial infections seen in advanced HIV disease in adults, as well as for the important role of bacterial infections in the morbidity and mortality of HIV-infected children, who cannot mount an adequate humoral response to common bacterial pathogens. The absolute number of circulating B cells may be depressed in primary HIV infection; however, this phenomenon is usually transient and likely reflects in part a redistribution of cells out of the circulation and into the lymphoid tissue. In certain patients, the number of circulating B cells decreases in advanced-stage disease.

Monocyte/Macrophages Circulating monocytes are generally normal in number in HIV-infected individuals. Monocytes express the CD4 molecule and several co-receptors for HIV on their surface, including CCR5, CXCR4, and CCR3, and thus are targets of HIV infection. Of note is the fact that the degree of cytopathicity of HIV for cells of the monocyte lineage is low, and HIV can replicate extensively in cells of the monocyte lineage with little cytopathic effect. Hence, monocyte-lineage cells may play a role in the dissemination of HIV in the body and can serve as reservoirs of HIV infection, thus representing an obstacle to the eradication of HIV by antiretroviral drugs.

In vivo infection of circulating monocytes is difficult to demonstrate; however, infection of tissue macrophages and macrophage-lineage cells in the brain (infiltrating macrophages or resident microglial cells) and lung (pulmonary alveolar macrophages) can be demonstrated easily. Infection of monocyte precursors in the bone marrow may directly or indirectly be responsible for certain of the hematologic abnormalities in HIV-infected individuals. A number of abnormalities of circulating monocytes have been reported in HIV-infected individuals, including decreased secretion of IL-1 and IL-12; increased secretion of IL-10; defects in antigen presentation and induction of T cell responses due to decreased MHC class II expression; and abnormalities of Fc receptor function, C3 receptor–mediated clearance, oxidative burst responses, and certain cytotoxic functions such as ADCC, possibly related to low levels of expression of Fc and complement receptors. The mechanisms of the monocyte defects are uncertain but almost certainly cannot be even partly explained by direct infection with HIV. Exposure of monocytes to viral proteins such as gp120 and Tat, as well as to certain cytokines, can cause abnormal activation, and this may play a role in cellular dysfunction (see above).

Dendritic and Langerhans Cells There has been considerable disagreement regarding the HIV infectibility and hence the depletion as well as the dysfunction of circulating dendritic cells. Depending on their state of maturation, dendritic cells express varying levels of CD4 as well as several chemokine receptors. In this regard, it appears that the ability of a dendritic cell to become infected depends in part on its state of maturation. Mature dendritic cells have been demonstrated to be infectable by both R5 and X4 isolates of HIV-1. Immature tissue dendritic cells have been less well studied in their native state. Certain groups have reported infection and dysfunction of dendritic cells from HIV-infected individuals, particularly a decreased ability to present antigen to T cells, and other groups have found little if any HIV infection or functional abnormalities. In this regard, there is general agreement regarding the ability of skin and mucous membrane Langerhans cells to be infected (see above). These latter cells likely play an important role in the initiation and propagation of HIV infection (see above). Even in those dendritic cells in which infection occurs, the efficiency of infection and level of productivity of infection is quite low compared to CD4+ T cells.

Natural Killer Cells The role of NK cells is to provide immunosurveillance against virus-infected cells, certain tumor cells, and allogeneic cells (Chap. 305). Functional abnormalities in NK cells have been observed throughout the course of HIV disease, and the severity of these abnormalities increases as disease progresses. Most studies report that NK cells are normal in number and phenotype in HIV-infected individuals; however, a numerical decrease in the CD16+/CD56+ subpopulation of NK cells has been reported together with an increase in activation markers. The abnormality in NK cell function is thought to result from a defect in postbinding lysis. However, the lytic machinery does not appear to be impaired, since NK cells from HIV-infected individuals mediate ADCC normally. The addition of either IL-2, IL-12, IL-15, or IFN-α to cultures improves the defective in vitro NK cell function of HIV-infected individuals. Enhanced expression of cytolytic inhibitory receptors in HIV-infected individuals may contribute to the abnormalities in NK function. Furthermore, selective HIV-mediated downregulation of HLA-A and -B, but not HLA-C and -D molecules may inhibit NK-mediated killing of HIV-infected target cells. Finally, NK cells serve as important sources of HIV-inhibitory CC-chemokines. NK cells isolated from HIV-infected individuals constitutively produce high levels of MIP-1α, MIP-1β, and RANTES. In addition, high levels of these chemokines are seen when NK cells are stimulated with IL-2 or IL-15 or when CD16 is cross-linked or during the process of lytic killing of target cells.

GENETIC FACTORS IN HIV PATHOGENESIS Several reports have described MHC alleles and other host factors that may influence the pathogenesis and course of HIV disease. These include associations with certain HIV-related manifestations, such as KS and diffuse lymphadenopathy, or with the type of clinical course, such as long-term survival or rapid progression (Table 309-7). A number of mechanisms have been proposed whereby MHC-encoded molecules might predispose an individual either to rapid progression or to nonprogression to AIDS. These proposed mechanisms include the ability to present certain immunodominant HIV T helper or CTL epitopes, leading to a relatively protective immune response against HIV and hence to slow progression of disease. In contrast, certain MHC class I or class II alleles might predispose an individual to an immunopathogenic response against viral epitopes in certain tissues, such as the central nervous system (CNS) or lungs, or against certain HIV-infected cell types, such as macrophages or dendritic cells/Langerhans cells. In addition, certain rare MHC class I and class II alleles might facilitate rapid recognition of HIV-infected cells from the infecting partner in primary HIV infection and promote rejection of these cells by alloreactive responses. Similarly, common MHC alleles could lead to less effective removal of HIV-infected allogeneic cells. It has been clearly demonstrated that maximal *HLA* heterozygosity for class I loci (A, B, and C) is associated with a delayed onset of AIDS among HIV-infected individuals, whereas homozygosity for these loci was associated with a more rapid progression to AIDS and death. This observation is likely due to the fact that individuals heterozygous at *HLA* loci are able to present a greater variety of antigenic peptides to cytotoxic T lymphocytes than are homozygotes resulting in a more effective immune response against a number of pathogens including HIV. Of particular note is the fact that the HLA class I alleles B*35 and Cw*04 were consistently associated with rapid development of AIDS. Other data have indicated that transporter associated with antigen-presenting (TAP) genes play a role in determining the outcome of HIV infection. HLA profiles that reflect certain combinations of MHC-encoded TAP and class I and class II genes are strongly associated with different rates of progression to AIDS.

Rare individuals have been reported who had had repetitive sexual exposure to HIV in high-risk situations but remained uninfected. The peripheral blood mononuclear cells of two such individuals were found to be highly resistant to infection in vitro with R5 strains of HIV-1, but they were readily infected with X4 strains. Genetic analysis revealed that these two individuals inherited a homozygous defect in the gene that codes for CCR5, the cellular co-receptor for R5 strains of HIV-1. The defective *CCR5* allele contained a 32-bp deletion corresponding to the second extracellular loop of the receptor. The encoded protein was severely truncated, and the receptor was nonfunctional, explaining the refractoriness to infection with R5 strains of HIV-1. Population studies revealed that approximately 1% of the Caucasian population of western European ancestry possessed the homozygous defect. Up to 20% of this group had the heterozygous defect. Of note, cohort studies of hundreds of DNA samples originating from western and central Africa and Japan did not reveal a single mutant allele, suggesting that the allele is either absent or extremely rare in Africa and Japan. In a cohort of 1400 HIV-1–infected Caucasian individuals, no subject homozygous for the mutation was found, strongly supporting the concept that the homozygous defect confers protection against infection. This finding is particularly compelling in light of the fact that transmitting viruses are strongly biased towards R5 strains of HIV-1 (see above). Furthermore, there was a higher frequency of individuals heterozygous for the genetic defect among HIV-infected patients who were long-term nonprogressors compared to HIV-infected individuals who progressed more rapidly (see above). Of note, several individuals have been identified who were homozygous for the *CCR5* Δ32 defect who in fact did become infected with HIV. These individuals were found to have an X4 strain of HIV that was associated in some cases with an accelerated course of disease. Slow progression of HIV disease is also seen in individuals who are heterozygous for the *CCR2V64I* mutation; this is felt to be due to dimerization of CXCR4 with the mutated CCR2V64I resulting in a decreased expression of CXCR4 on the cell surface. Individuals who are homozygous for the *SDF1-3′*A mutation manifest slow progression, likely due to the upregulation of SDF-1 and resulting inhibition of binding of X4 viruses

Table 309-7 Genetic Factors Implicated in the Pathogenesis of HIV Disease

Factor	Association
MAJOR HISTOCOMPATIBILITY LOCI-ENCODED GENES	
B35, C4, DR1, DQ1	Kaposi's sarcoma
DR1	Kaposi's sarcoma
DR2, DR5	Kaposi's sarcoma
DR5	Kaposi's sarcoma
Aw23, Bw49	Kaposi's sarcoma
B62	Fever, skin rash in primary HIV infection
Aw19	HIV seropositivity in individuals multiply exposed to HIV
A1, A24, C7, B8, DR3	Rapid progression to AIDS
DR4, DQB1*0302	Rapid progression to AIDS
DR3, DQ1	Rapid progression to AIDS
B*35	Rapid progression to AIDS
Cw*04	Rapid progression to AIDS
TAP2.1	Promotes HIV progression to AIDS
DR5	Thrombocytopenia and lymphadenopathy in HIV infection
DR5, DR6	Diffuse infiltrative CD8+ lymphocytosis with Sjögren-like syndrome in HIV infection
Bw4	Slow decline in CD4+T cell count
B13, B27, B51, B57, DQB1*0302,0303	Protects from progression to AIDS
B*5701	Strong protection from progression to AIDS
A26, B38, TAP1.4, TAP2.3	Ability to clear HIV infection in transiently infected seronegative individuals
A28, Bw70, Aw69, B18	Protection from HIV infection
A32, B4, C2	Long-term survival in HIV infection
A11, A32, B13, C2, DQA1*0301, DQB1*0302, DRB1*0400, DRB4*0101	Long-term survival in HIV infection
Heterozygosity for Class I loci (A, B, and C)	Delayed onset to AIDS
Homozygosity for Class I loci (A, B, and C)	Rapid onset to AIDS and death
OTHER GENES	
p53 tumor suppressor gene	Controls HIV replicative patterns and determinant of viral latency
CCR5 gene	Homozygous defect involving a 32-bp deletion corresponding to the second extracellular loop of the receptor results in resistance to infection; heterozygous defect appears to result in partial protection against disease progression. Also, several single nucleotide polymorphisms in the CCR5 promoter have been shown to be associated with variable rates of progression in AIDS.
CCR2 gene	Heterozygosity for CCRV641 mutation is associated with delay in progression of HIV disease
CX_3CR1 gene	Mutations in I249 and M280 associated with rapid progression to AIDS
RANTES gene	A mutation of the RANTES gene (RANTES-28G) results in increased transcription and expression of RANTES on mononuclear cells with resulting inhibition of infection with R5 strains of HIV and delay of disease progression
SDF1 gene	Homozygosity for SDF1-3′A mutation is associated with a delay in progression of HIV disease
IL-10 gene	Individuals carrying the IL10-5′592A promoter allele were at increased risk for HIV infection and, once infected, progressed more rapidly than homozygotes for the alternative IL10-5′-592 C/C genotype

SOURCES: Adapted from Haynes et al; R Liu et al; Samson et al; Carrington et al; also see Bibliography.

to mononuclear cells. Delayed progression of disease is also seen in those individuals who have any of a number of single nucleotide polymorphisms in the *CCR5* promoter. In addition, individuals who carry a certain allele (IL-10-5′592A) of the IL-10 promoter are at increased risk of infection and, once infected, progress more rapidly than homozygotes for the alternative genotype. The mechanism of this effect is felt to be a downregulation of the inhibitory cytokine IL-10 resulting in facilitation of HIV replication. Finally, individuals with a mutation of the *RANTES* gene (*RANTES-28G*) manifest a delay in disease progression due likely to the increased expression of RANTES and resulting inhibition of infection with R5 viruses (Table 309-7).

NEUROPATHOGENESIS HIV-infected individuals can experience a variety of neurologic abnormalities due either to opportunistic infections and neoplasms (see below) or to direct effects of HIV or its products. With regard to the latter, HIV has been demonstrated in the brain and CSF of infected individuals with and without neuropsychiatric abnormalities. The main cell types that are infected in the brain in vivo are those of the monocyte/macrophage lineage, including monocytes that have migrated to the brain from the peripheral blood as well as resident microglial cells. HIV entry into brain is felt to be due, at least in part, to the ability of virus-infected and immune-activated macrophages to induce adhesion molecules such as E-selectin and vascular cell adhesion molecule-1 (VCAM-1) on brain endothelium. Other studies have demonstrated that HIV gp120 enhances the expression of intercellular adhesion molecule-1 (ICAM-1) in glial cells; this effect may facilitate entry of HIV-infected cells into the CNS and may promote syncytia formation. Virus isolates from the brain are preferentially R5 strains as opposed to X4 strains (see above); in this regard, HIV-infected individuals who are heterozygous for *CCR5Δ32* appear to be relatively protected against the development of HIV encephalopathy compared to wild-type individuals. Distinct HIV envelope sequences are associated with the clinical expression of the AIDS dementia complex (see below). Although there have been reports of infrequent HIV infection of neuronal cells and astrocytes, there is no convincing evidence that brain cells other than those of monocyte/macrophage lineage can be productively infected in vivo. Nonetheless, it has been demonstrated that galactosyl ceramide may be an essential component of the HIV gp120 receptor on neural cells, and antibodies to galactosyl ceramide inhibit entry of HIV into neural cell lines in vitro.

HIV-infected individuals may manifest white matter lesions as well as neuronal loss. Given the relative absence of evidence of HIV infection of neurons either in vivo or in vitro, it is unlikely that direct infection of these cells accounts for their loss. Rather, the HIV-mediated effects on brain tissue are thought to be due to a combination of direct effects, either toxic or function-inhibitory, of gp120 on neuronal cells and effects of a variety of neurotoxins released from infiltrating monocytes, resident microglial cells, and astrocytes. In this regard, it has been demonstrated that both HIV-1 Nef and Tat can induce chemotaxis of leukocytes, including monocytes, into the CNS. Neurotoxins can be released from monocytes as a consequence of infection and/or immune activation. Monocyte-derived neurotoxic factors have been reported to kill neurons via the *N*-methyl-D-aspartate (NMDA) receptor. In addition, HIV gp120 shed by virus-infected monocytes could cause neurotoxicity by antagonizing the function of vasoactive intestinal peptide (VIP), by elevating intracellular calcium levels, and by decreasing nerve growth factor levels in the cerebral cortex. A variety of monocyte-derived cytokines can contribute directly or indirectly to the neurotoxic effects in HIV infection; these include TNF-α, IL-1, IL-6, TGF-β, IFN-γ, platelet-activating factor, and endothelin. Certain studies have correlated levels of CC-chemokines MIP-1α, MIP-1β, and RANTES in CSF with HIV-related encephalopathy. In addition, infection and/or activation of monocyte-lineage cells can result in increased production of eicosanoids, nitric oxide, and quinolinic acid, which may contribute to neurotoxicity. Astrocytes may play diverse roles in HIV neuropathogenesis. Reactive gliosis or astrocytosis has been demonstrated in the brains of HIV-infected individuals, and TNF-α and IL-6 have been shown to induce astrocyte proliferation. In addition, astrocyte-derived IL-6 can induce HIV expression in infected cells in vitro. Furthermore, it has been suggested that astrocytes may downregulate macrophage-produced neurotoxins. It has been reported that HIV-infected individuals with the E4 allele for apolipoprotein E (apo E) are at increased risk for AIDS encephalopathy and peripheral neuropathy. The likelihood that HIV or its products are involved in neuropathogenesis is supported by the observation that neuropsychiatric abnormalities may undergo remarkable and rapid improvement upon the initiation of antiretroviral therapy, particularly in HIV-infected children.

PATHOGENESIS OF KAPOSI'S SARCOMA KS is an opportunistic disease in HIV-infected individuals. Unlike opportunistic infections, its occurrence is not strictly related to the level of depression of CD4+ T cell counts (see below). There are at least four distinct epidemiologic forms of Kaposi's sarcoma: (1) the classic form that occurs in older men of predominantly Mediterranean or eastern European Jewish backgrounds with no recognized contributing factors; (2) the equatorial African form that occurs in all ages, also without any recognized precipitating factors; (3) the form associated with organ transplantation and its attendent iatrogenic immunosuppressed state; and (4) the form associated with HIV-1 infection. The pathogenesis of KS is complex and has not been fully delineated. KS does not result from a neoplastic transformation of cells in the classic sense and so is not truly a sarcoma. It is a manifestation of excessive proliferation of spindle cells that are believed to be of vascular origin and have features in common with endothelial and smooth-muscle cells. In HIV disease the development of KS is dependent on the interplay of a variety of factors including HIV-1 itself, HHV-8, immune activation, and cytokine secretion. A number of epidemiologic and virologic studies have clearly linked HHV-8, which is also referred to as *Kaposi's sarcoma–associated herpesvirus* (KSHV), to KS not only in HIV-infected individuals but also in individuals with the other forms of KS. KSHV is a γ-herpesvirus related to EBV and herpesvirus saimiri. It encodes a homologue to human IL-6 and in addition to KS has been implicated in the pathogenesis of body cavity lymphoma, multiple myeloma, and monoclonal gammopathy of undetermined significance. Sequences of HHV-8 are found universally in the lesions of KS, and patients with KS are virtually all seropositive for HHV-8. HHV-8 DNA sequences can be found in the B cells of 30 to 50% of patients with KS and 7% of patients with AIDS without clinically apparent KS.

Between 1 and 2% of eligible blood donors are positive for antibodies to HHV-8, while the prevalence of HHV-8 seropositivity in HIV-infected men is 30 to 35%. The prevalence in HIV-infected women is approximately 4%. This finding is reflective of the lower incidence of KS in women. It has been debated whether HHV-8 is actually the transforming agent in KS; the bulk of the cells in the tumor lesions of KS are not neoplastic cells. However, a recent study has demonstrated that endothelial cells can be transformed in vitro by HHV-8. Despite the complexity of the pathogenic events associated with the development of KS in HIV-infected individuals, it is generally felt that HHV-8 is indeed the etiologic agent of this disease. The initiation and/or propagation of KS requires an activated state and is mediated, at least in part, by cytokines. A number of factors, including TNF-α, IL-1β, IL-6, GM-CSF, basic fibroblast growth factor, and oncostatin M, function in an autocrine and paracrine manner to sustain the growth and chemotaxis of the KS spindle cells. It has been suggested that the HIV Tat protein plays a major role in the pathogenesis of KS. In this regard, it has been demonstrated that IFN-γ can induce endothelial cells to proliferate and to invade the extracellular matrix in response to HIV Tat. This occurs as a result of the upregulation by IFN-γ of the expression and activity of the receptors for Tat, which are the integrins $\alpha_5\beta_1$ and $\alpha_v\beta_3$. In addition, the HIV-1 Tat protein has been shown to act synergistically with basic fibroblast growth factor in the induction of lesions resembling KS lesions in mice. Glucocorticoids have been shown to have a stimulatory effect, and human chorionic gonadotrophin an inhibitory effect, on KS spindle cells, suggesting that modulation of the balance of autocrine factors may have therapeutic potential in KS.

IMMUNE RESPONSE TO HIV

As detailed above and below, following the initial burst of viremia during primary infection, HIV-infected individuals mount a robust immune response that usually substantially curtails the levels of plasma viremia and likely contributes to delaying the ultimate development of clinically apparent disease for a median of 10 years. This immune response contains elements of both humoral and cell-mediated immunity (Table 309-8; Fig. 309-21). It is directed against multiple antigenic determinants of the HIV virion as well as against viral proteins expressed on the surface of infected cells. Ironically, those CD4+ T cells with T cell receptors specific for HIV are theoretically those CD4+ T cells most likely to bind to infected cells and themselves be infected and destroyed. Thus, an early consequence of HIV infection may be interference with the generation of an effective immune response through the elimination of HIV-specific CD4+ T lymphocytes.

Although a great deal of investigation has been directed toward delineating and better understanding the components of this immune response, it remains unclear which of these phenomena are most important in delaying progression of infection and which, if any, play a role in the pathogenesis of HIV disease.

HUMORAL IMMUNE RESPONSE Antibodies to HIV usually appear within 6 weeks and almost invariably within 12 weeks of primary infection (Fig. 309-22); rare exceptions are individuals who have defects in the ability to produce HIV-specific antibodies. Detection of these antibodies forms the basis of most diagnostic screening tests for HIV infection. The appearance of HIV-binding antibodies detected by ELISA and western blot assays occurs prior to the appearance of neutralizing antibodies; the latter generally appear following the initial decreases in plasma viremia, which is more closely related to the appearance of HIV-specific CD8+ T lymphocytes. The first antibodies detected are those directed against the structural or gag proteins of HIV, p24 and p17, and the gag precursor p55. The development of antibodies to p24 is associated with a decrease in the serum levels of free p24 antigen. Antibodies to the gag proteins are followed by the appearance of antibodies to the envelope proteins (gp160, gp120, p88, and gp41) and to the products of the *pol* gene (p31, p51, and p66). In addition, one may see antibodies to the low-molecular-weight regulatory proteins encoded by the HIV genes *vpr*, *vpu*, *vif*, *rev*, *tat*, and *nef*.

While antibodies to multiple antigens of HIV are produced, the precise functional significance of these different antibodies is unclear. The best studied have been the antibodies directed towards the envelope proteins of the virus. As noted above, the envelope of HIV con-

Table 309-8 Elements of the Immune Response to HIV

- Humoral immunity
  - Binding antibodies
  - Neutralizing antibodies
    - Type specific
    - Group specific
  - Antibodies participating in antibody-dependent cellular cytotoxicity (ADCC)
    - Protective
    - Pathogenic (bystander killing)
  - Enhancing antibodies
- Cell-mediated immunity
  - Helper CD4+ T lymphocytes
  - Class I MHC–restricted cytotoxic CD8+ T lymphocytes
  - CD8+ T cell–mediated inhibition (noncytolytic)
  - ADCC
  - Natural killer cells

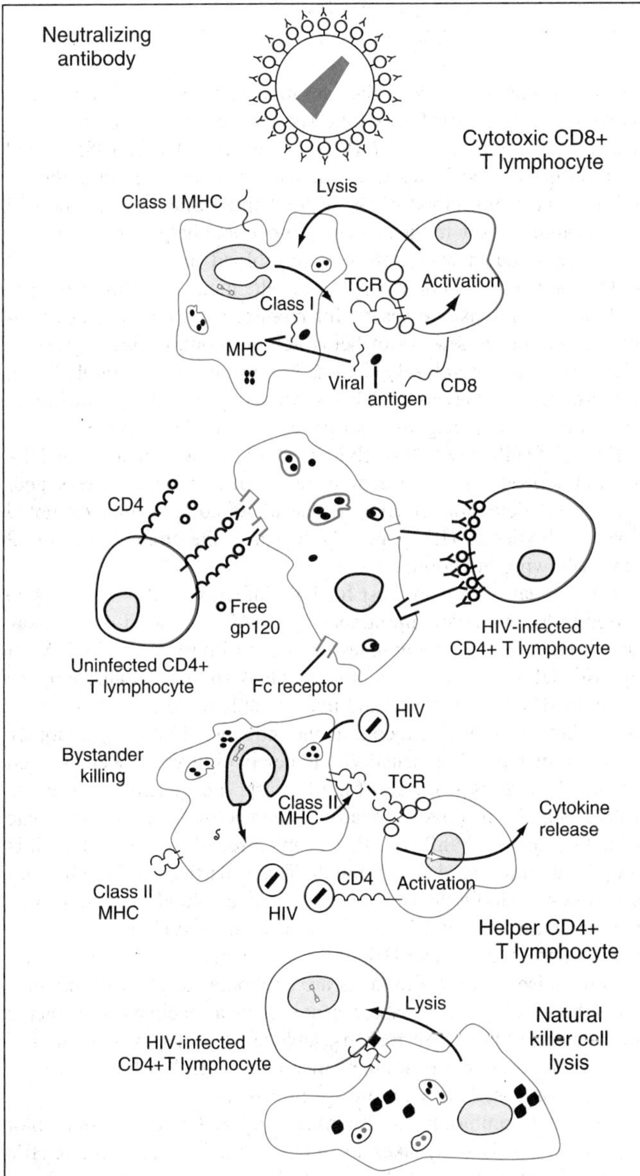

FIGURE 309-21 Schematic representation of the different immunologic effector mechanisms felt to be active in the setting of HIV infection. Detailed descriptions are given in the text. TCR, T cell receptor.

sists of an outer envelope glycoprotein with a molecular mass of 120 kDa and a transmembrane glycoprotein with a molecular mass of 41 kDa. These are initially synthesized as a 160-kDa precursor that is cleaved by cellular proteases. Most of the antienvelope antibodies are directed either toward an epitope in the gp41 region comprising amino acids 579 to 613 or toward a hypervariable region in the gp120 molecule, known as the *V3 loop region*, comprising amino acids 303 through 338. This V3 region is a major site for the development of mutations that lead to variants of HIV that are not well recognized by the immune system.

Antibodies directed toward the envelope proteins of HIV have been characterized both as being protective and as possibly contributing to the pathogenesis of HIV disease. Among the protective antibodies are those that function to neutralize HIV directly and prevent the spread of infection to additional cells, as well as those that participate in ADCC. *Neutralizing antibodies* may be a component of primary HIV infection, and some long-term nonprogressors have been reported to have increased titers of neutralizing antibodies. Neutralizing antibodies appear to be of two forms, type-specific and group-specific. *Type-specific neutralizing antibodies* are generally directed to the V3 loop region. These antibodies neutralize only viruses of a given strain and are present in low titer in most infected individuals. *Group-specific neutralizing antibodies* are capable of neutralizing a wide variety of HIV isolates. At least two forms of group specific antibodies have been identified: those binding to amino acids 423 to 437 of gp120 and those binding to amino acids 728 to 745 of gp41. The other major class of protective antibodies are those that participate in ADCC, which is actually a form of cell-mediated immunity (Chap. 305) in which NK cells that bear Fc receptors are armed with specific anti-HIV antibodies that bind to the NK cells via their Fc portion. These armed NK cells then bind to and destroy cells expressing HIV antigens. Antibodies to both gp120 and gp41 have been shown to participate in ADCC-mediated killing of HIV-infected cells. The levels of antienvelope antibodies capable of mediating ADCC are highest in the earlier stages of HIV infection. In vitro, IL-2 can augment ADCC-mediated killing.

In addition to playing a role in host defense, HIV-specific antibodies have also been implicated in disease pathogenesis. Antibodies directed to gp41, when present in low titer, have been shown in vitro to be capable of facilitating infection of cells through an Fc receptor–mediated mechanism known as *antibody enhancement*. Thus, the same regions of the envelope protein of HIV that give rise to antibodies capable of mediating ADCC also elicit the production of antibodies that can facilitate infection of cells in vitro. In addition, it has been postulated that anti-gp120 antibodies that participate in the ADCC killing of HIV-infected cells might also kill uninfected CD4+ T cells if the uninfected cells had bound free gp120, a phenomenon referred to as *bystander killing*.

CELLULAR IMMUNE RESPONSE Given the fact that T cell–mediated immunity is known to play a major role in host defense against most viral infections (Chap. 305), it is generally thought to be an important component of the host immune response to HIV. T cell immunity can be divided into two major categories, mediated respectively by the *helper/inducer CD4+ T cells* and the *cytotoxic/immunoregulatory CD8+ T cells*.

It has been difficult to demonstrate the presence of HIV-specific CD4+ T cells in HIV-infected patients directly, particularly in those with advanced disease. This difficulty may be related to the fact that these cells, with their high affinity for binding to HIV-infected cells, may be among the first to be infected and destroyed during HIV infection. CD4+ T lymphocytes with reactivity to the p24 antigen of HIV have been reported to be present in a subset of long-term nonprogressors and in a subset of patients in whom therapy was initiated shortly following infection. While a reverse correlation exists between the presence of these cells and levels of plasma HIV viremia, it is

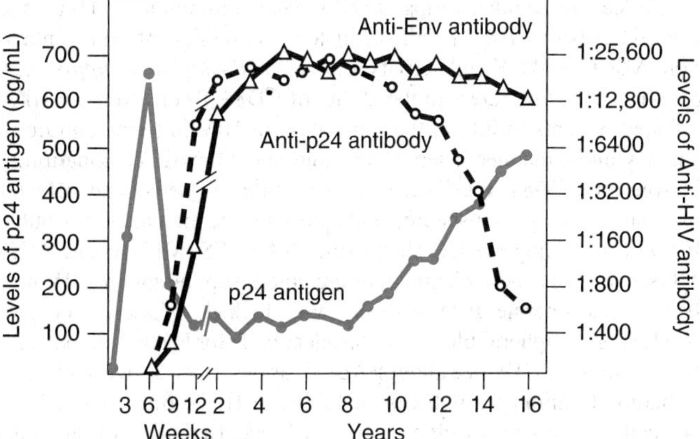

FIGURE 309-22 Relationship between antigenemia and the development of antibodies to HIV. Antibodies to HIV proteins are generally seen 6 to 12 weeks following infection and 3 to 6 weeks after the development of plasma viremia. Late in the course of illness, antibody levels to p24 decline, generally in association with a rising titer of p24 antigen.

unclear whether or not there is a causal relationship between these parameters. Through the use of computer modeling, several regions of the HIV-1 envelope molecule have been identified that are structurally analogous to other known T cell epitopes by virtue of having structures known as *amphipathic helices*. Peptides from these envelope regions have been used to identify the presence of CD4+ T cells specific for these regions in the peripheral blood of HIV-infected individuals. Other studies have demonstrated that peripheral blood T cells of some healthy, HIV-negative individuals also react to the envelope proteins of HIV. It is unclear whether or not this represents the presence of a degree of protective immunity in these individuals.

MHC class I–restricted, HIV-specific CD8+ T cells have been identified in the peripheral blood of patients with HIV-1 infection. These cells include cytotoxic T cells (CTLs) and T cells that can be induced by HIV antigens to express cytokines such as IFN-γ. CTLs have been identified in the peripheral blood of patients within weeks of HIV infection. These CD8+ T lymphocytes, through their HIV-specific antigen receptors, bind to and cause the lytic destruction of target cells bearing identical MHC class I molecules associated with HIV antigens. Two types of CTL activity can be demonstrated in the peripheral blood or lymph node mononuclear cells of HIV-infected individuals. The first type directly lyses appropriate target cells in culture without prior in vitro stimulation (*spontaneous CTL activity*). The other type of CTL activity reflects the *precursor frequency of CTLs* (CTLp); this type of CTL activity can be demonstrated by stimulation of CD8+ T cells in vitro with a mitogen such as phytohemagglutinin or anti-CD3 antibody. Following primary HIV infection, the qualitative nature of the HIV-specific CTL response is an important predictor of eventual clinical outcome. Patients who mount a broad CD8+ CTL response generally have a more favorable clinical course than do patients who mount a more restricted CTL response. These data are consistent with studies in the SIV model where deletion of CD8+ T cells leads to a more accelerated clinical course.

In addition to CTLs, CD8+ T cells capable of being induced by HIV antigens to express cytokines such as IFN-γ also appear in the setting of HIV-1 infection. It is not clear whether these are the same or different effector pools compared to those cells mediating cytotoxicity; in addition, the relative roles of each in host defense against HIV are not fully understood. It does appear that these CD8+ T cells are driven to in vivo expansion by HIV antigen. There is a direct correlation between levels of CD8+ T cells capable of producing IFN-γ in response to HIV antigens and plasma levels of HIV-1 RNA. Thus, while these cells are clearly induced by HIV-1 infection, their overall ability to control infection remains unclear. Multiple HIV antigens, including Gag, Env, Pol, Tat, Rev, and Nef, can elicit CD8+ T cell responses.

At least three other forms of cell-mediated immunity to HIV have been described: CD8+ T cell–mediated suppression of HIV replication, ADCC, and NK cell activity. *CD8+ T cell–mediated suppression of HIV replication* refers to the ability of CD8+ T cells from an HIV-infected patients to inhibit the replication of HIV in tissue culture in a noncytolytic manner. There is no requirement for HLA compatibility between the CD8+ T cells and the HIV-infected cells. This effector mechanism is thus nonspecific and appears to be mediated by soluble factor(s) including the CC-chemokines RANTES, MIP-1α and MIP-1β (see above). These chemokines are potent suppressors of HIV replication and operate at least in part via blockade of the co-receptor (CCR5) on peripheral blood mononuclear cells for R5 or macrophage-tropic strains of HIV (see above). *ADCC*, as described above in relation to humoral immunity, involves the killing of HIV-expressing cells by NK cells armed with specific antibodies directed against HIV antigens. Finally, *NK cells* alone have been shown to be capable of killing HIV-infected target cells in tissue culture. This primitive cytotoxic mechanism of host defense is directed toward nonspecific surveillance for neoplastic transformation and viral infection through recognition of altered class I MHC molecules.

DIAGNOSIS AND LABORATORY MONITORING OF HIV INFECTION

The establishment of HIV as the causative agent of AIDS and related syndromes early in 1984 was followed by the rapid development of sensitive screening tests for HIV infection. By March, 1985, blood donors in the United States were routinely screened for antibodies to HIV. In June 1996, blood banks in the United States added the p24 antigen capture assay to the screening process to help identify the rare infected individuals who were donating blood in the time (up to 3 months) between infection and the development of antibodies. The development of sensitive assays for monitoring levels of plasma viremia ushered in a new era of being able to monitor the progression of HIV disease more closely. Utilization of these tests, coupled with the measurement of levels of CD4+ T lymphocytes in peripheral blood, is essential in the management of patients with HIV infection.

DIAGNOSIS OF HIV INFECTION The diagnosis of HIV infection depends upon the demonstration of antibodies to HIV and/or the direct detection of HIV or one of its components. As noted above, antibodies to HIV generally appear in the circulation 2 to 12 weeks following infection.

The standard screening test for HIV infection is the ELISA, also referred to as an enzyme immunoassay (EIA). This solid-phase assay is an extremely good screening test with a sensitivity of >99.5%. Most diagnostic laboratories use a commercial EIA kit that contains antigens from both HIV-1 and HIV-2 and thus are able to detect either. These kits use both natural and recombinant antigens and are continuously updated to increase their sensitivity to newly discovered species, such as group O viruses (Fig. 309-6). EIA tests are generally scored as positive (highly reactive), negative (nonreactive), or indeterminate (partially reactive). While the EIA is an extremely sensitive test, it is not optimal with regard to specificity. This is particularly true in studies of low-risk individuals, such as volunteer blood donors. In this latter population, only 10% of EIA-positive individuals are subsequently confirmed to have HIV infection. Among the factors associated with false-positive EIA tests are antibodies to class II antigens, autoantibodies, hepatic disease, recent influenza vaccination, and acute viral infections. For these reasons, anyone suspected of having HIV infection based upon a positive or inconclusive EIA result must have the result confirmed with a more specific assay.

The most commonly used confirmatory test is the western blot (Fig. 309-23). This assay takes advantage of the fact that multiple HIV antigens of different, well-characterized molecular weights elicit the production of specific antibodies. These antigens can be separated on the basis of molecular weight, and antibodies to each component can be detected as discrete bands on the western blot. A negative western blot is one in which no bands are present at molecular weights corresponding to HIV gene products. In a patient with a positive or indeterminate EIA and a negative western blot, one can conclude with certainty that the EIA reactivity was a false positive. On the other hand, a western blot demonstrating antibodies to products of all three of the major genes of HIV (*gag*, *pol*, and *env*) is conclusive evidence of infection with HIV. Criteria established by the U.S. Food & Drug Administration (FDA) in 1993 for a positive western blot state that a result is considered positive if antibodies exist to two of the three HIV proteins: p24, gp41, and gp120/160. Using these criteria, approximately 10% of all blood donors deemed positive for HIV-1 infection lacked an antibody band to the *pol* gene product p31. Some 50% of these blood donors were subsequently found to be false positives. Thus, the absence of the p31 band should increase the suspicion that one may be dealing with a false-positive test result. In this setting it is prudent to obtain additional confirmation with an RNA-based test and/or a follow-up western blot. By definition, western blot patterns of reactivity that do not fall into the positive or negative categories are considered "indeterminate." There are two possible explanations for an indeterminate western blot result. The most likely explanation in a low-risk individual is that the patient being tested has antibodies that cross-react with one of the proteins of HIV. The most common patterns of cross-reactivity are antibodies that react with p24 and/or p55. The least likely explanation in this setting is that the individual is infected with HIV and is in the process of mounting a classic antibody response. In either instance, the western blot should be repeated in 1 month to determine whether or not the indeterminate pattern is a pattern in evolution. In addition, one may attempt to confirm a diagnosis of HIV infection with the p24 antigen capture assay or one of the tests for HIV RNA (discussed below). While the western blot is an excellent confirmatory test for HIV infection in patients with a positive or indeterminate EIA, it is a poor screening test. Among individuals with a negative EIA and PCR for HIV, 20 to 30% may show one or more bands on western blot. While these bands are usually faint and represent cross-reactivity, their presence creates a situation in which other diagnostic modalities [such as DNA PCR, RNA PCR, the (b)DNA assay, or p24 antigen capture] must be employed to ensure that the bands do not indicate early HIV infection.

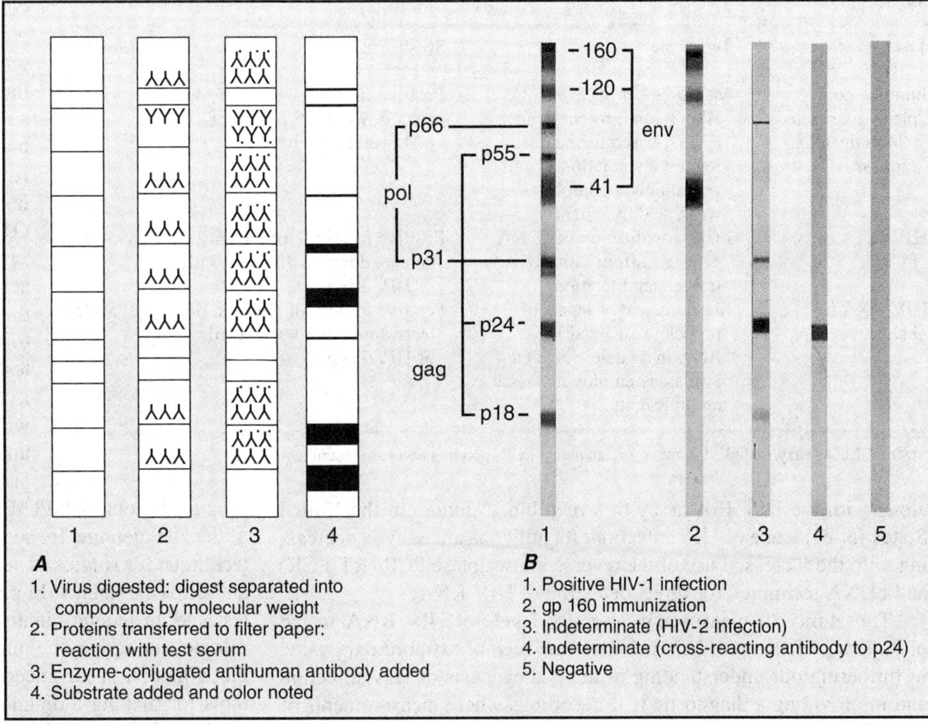

FIGURE 309-23 *A.* Schematic representation of how a western blot is performed. *B.* Examples of patterns of western blot reactivity. In each instance the western blot strip contains antigens to HIV-1. The sera from the patient immunized to the HIV-1 envelope only contains antibodies to the HIV-1 envelope proteins. The sera from the patient with HIV-2 infection cross-reacts with both *reverse transcriptase* and *gag* gene products of HIV-1.

A guideline for the use of these serologic tests in attempting to make a diagnosis of HIV infection is depicted in Fig. 309-24. In patients in whom HIV infection is suspected, the appropriate initial test is the EIA. If the result is negative, unless there is strong reason to suspect early HIV infection (as in a patient exposed within the previous 3 months), the diagnosis is ruled out and retesting should be performed only as clinically indicated. If the EIA is indeterminate or positive, the test should be repeated. If the repeat is negative on two occasions, one can assume that the initial positive reading was due to a technical error in the performance of the assay and that the patient is negative. If the repeat is indeterminate or positive, one should proceed to the HIV-1 western blot. If the western blot is positive, the diagnosis is HIV-1 infection. If the western blot is negative, the EIA can be assumed to have been a false positive for HIV-1 and the diagnosis of HIV-1 infection is ruled out. It would be prudent at this point to perform specific serologic testing for HIV-2 following the same type of algorithm. If the western blot for HIV-1 is indeterminate, it should be repeated in 4–6 weeks; in addition, one may proceed to a p24 antigen capture assay, HIV-1 RNA assay, or HIV-1 DNA PCR and specific serologic testing for HIV-2. If the p24 and HIV RNA assays are negative and there is no progression in the western blot, a diagnosis of HIV-1 is ruled out. If either the p24 or HIV-1 RNA assay is positive and/or the HIV-1 western blot shows progression, a tentative diagnosis of HIV-1 infection can be made and later confirmed with a follow-up western blot demonstrating a positive pattern.

As mentioned above, a variety of laboratory tests are available for the direct detection of HIV or its components (Table 309-9; Fig. 309-25). These tests may be of considerable help in making a diagnosis of HIV infection when the western blot results are indeterminate. In addition, the tests detecting levels of HIV RNA can be used to determine prognosis and to assess the response to antiretroviral therapies. The simplest of the direct detection tests is the *p24 antigen capture assay*. This is an EIA-type assay in which the solid phase consists of antibodies to the p24 antigen of HIV. It detects the viral protein p24 in the blood of HIV-infected individuals where it exists either as free antigen or complexed to anti-p24 antibodies. Overall, approximately 30% of individuals with untreated HIV infection have detectable levels of free p24 antigen. This increases to about 50% when samples are treated with a weak acid to dissociate antigen-antibody complexes. Throughout the course of HIV infection, an equilibrium exists between p24 antigen and anti-p24 antibodies. During the first few weeks of infection, before an immune response develops, there is a brisk rise in p24 antigen levels (Fig. 309-22). After the development of anti-p24 antibodies, these levels decline. Late in the course of infection, when circulating levels of virus are high, p24 antigen levels also increase, particularly when detected by techniques involving dissociation of antigen-antibody complexes. This assay has its greatest use as a screening test for HIV infection in patients suspected of having the acute HIV syndrome, as high levels of p24 antigen are present prior to the development of antibodies. In addition, it is currently routinely used

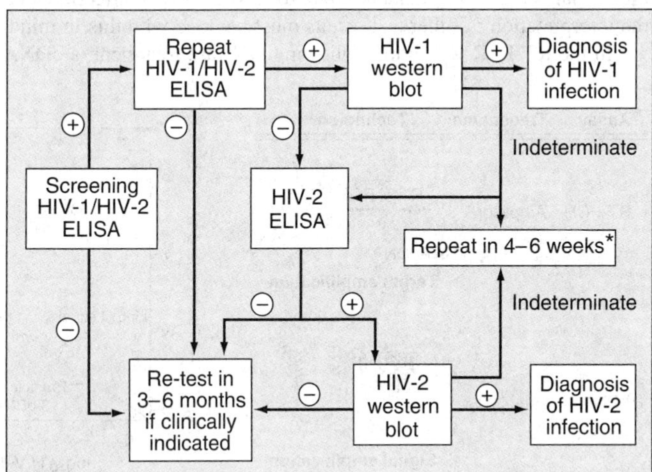

FIGURE 309-24 Algorithm for the use of serologic tests in the diagnosis of HIV-1 or HIV-2 infection. * Stable indeterminate western blot 4 to 6 weeks later makes HIV infection unlikely. However, it should be repeated twice at 3-month intervals to rule out HIV infection. Alternatively, one may test for HIV-1 p24 antigen on HIV RNA.

Table 309-9 Characteristics of Tests for Direct Detection of HIV

Test	Technique	Sensitivity	Cost/Test
Immune complex–dissociated p24 antigen capture assay	Measurement of levels of HIV-1 core protein in an ELISA-based format following dissociation of antigen-antibody complexes by weak acid treatment	Positive in 50% of patients; detects down to 15 pg/mL of p24 protein	\$1–2
HIV RNA by PCR	PCR amplification of cDNA generated from viral RNA (target amplification)	Positive in >98% of patients; detects down to 40 copies/mL of HIV RNA	\$75–150
HIV RNA by bDNA	Measurement of levels of particle-associated HIV RNA in a nucleic acid capture assay employing signal amplification	Positive in 90% of patients; detects down to 50 copies/mL of HIV RNA	\$75–150

NOTE: ELISA, enzyme-linked immunosorbent assay; PCR, polymerase chain reaction.

along with the HIV EIA assay to screen blood donors in the United States for evidence of HIV infection. Its utility as an assay is decreasing with the increased use of the reverse transcriptase PCR (RT-PCR) and bDNA technique for direct detection of HIV RNA.

The ability to measure and monitor levels of HIV RNA in the plasma of patients with HIV infection has been of extraordinary value in furthering our understanding of the pathogenesis of HIV infection and in providing a diagnostic tool in settings where measurements of anti-HIV antibodies may be misleading, such as in acute infection and neonatal infection. Two assays are predominantly used for this purpose. They are the *RT-PCR* (Amplicor) and the *bDNA* (Quantiplex). It should be pointed out that the only test approved by the FDA at this time for the measurement of HIV RNA levels is the RT-PCR test. While this approval is limited to the use of the test for determining prognosis, it is the general consensus that this test as well as the bDNA test are also of value for monitoring the effects of therapy and in making a diagnosis of HIV infection. In addition to these two commercially available tests, the *DNA PCR* is also employed by research laboratories for making a diagnosis of HIV infection by amplifying HIV proviral DNA from peripheral blood mononuclear cells. The commercially available RNA detection tests have a sensitivity of 40 to 50 copies of HIV RNA per milliliter of plasma, while the DNA PCR tests can detect proviral DNA at a frequency of one copy per 10,000 to 100,000 cells. Thus, these tests are extremely sensitive. One frequent consequence of a high degree of sensitivity is some loss of specificity, and false-positive results have been reported with each of these techniques. For this reason, a positive EIA with a confirmatory western blot remains the "gold standard" for a diagnosis of HIV infection, and the interpretation of other test results must be done with this in mind.

In the RT-PCR technique, following DNAase treatment, a cDNA copy is made of all RNA species present in plasma. Insofar as HIV is an RNA virus, this will result in the production of DNA copies of the HIV genome in amounts proportional to the amount of HIV RNA present in plasma. This proviral DNA is then amplified and characterized using standard PCR techniques, employing primer pairs that can distinguish genomic cDNA from messenger cDNA. The bDNA assay involves the use of a solid-phase nucleic acid capture system and signal amplification through successive nucleic acid hybridizations to detect small quantities of HIV RNA. Both tests can achieve a tenfold increase in sensitivity to 40 to 50 copies of HIV RNA per milliliter with a preconcentration step in which plasma undergoes ultracentrifugation to pellet the viral particles. In addition to being a diagnostic and prognostic tool, RT-PCR is also useful for amplifying defined areas of the HIV genome for sequence analysis and has become an important technique for studies of sequence diversity and microbial resistance to antiretroviral agents. In patients with a positive or indeterminate EIA test and an indeterminate western blot, and in patients in whom serologic testing may be unreliable (such as patients with hypogammaglobulinemia or advanced HIV disease), these tests provide valuable tools for making a diagnosis of HIV infection. They should only be used for diagnosis when standard serologic testing has failed to provide a definitive result.

LABORATORY MONITORING OF PATIENTS WITH HIV INFECTION The epidemic of HIV infection and AIDS has provided the clinician with new challenges for integrating clinical and laboratory data to effect optimal patient management. The close relationship between clinical manifestations of HIV infection and CD4+ T cell count has made measurement of the latter a routine part of the evaluation of HIV-infected individuals. Determinations of CD4+ T cell counts and measurements of the levels of HIV RNA in serum or plasma provide a powerful set of tools for determining prognosis and monitoring response to therapy. While the CD4+ T cell count provides information on the current immunologic status of the patient, the HIV RNA level predicts what will happen to the CD4+ T cell count in the near future, and hence provides an important piece of prognostic information.

CD4+ T Cell Counts The CD4+ T cell count is the laboratory test generally accepted as the best indicator of the immediate state of immunologic competence of the patient with HIV infection. This measurement, which is the product of the percent of CD4+ T cells (determined by flow cytometry) and the total lymphocyte count [determined by the white blood cell count (WBC) and the differential count] has been shown to correlate very well with the level of immunologic competence. Patients with CD4+ T cell counts <200/μL are at high risk of infection with *P. carinii*, while patients with CD4+ T cell counts <50/μL are at high risk of infection with CMV and mycobacteria of the *M. avium complex* (MAC) (Fig. 309-26). Patients with HIV infection should have CD4+ T cell measurements performed at the time of diagnosis and every 3 to 6 months thereafter. More frequent measurements should be made if a declining trend is noted. According to most guidelines, a CD4 T cell count <500/μL is an indication for consideration of initiating antiretroviral therapy, and a decline in CD4+ T cell count of >25% is an indication for considering a change in

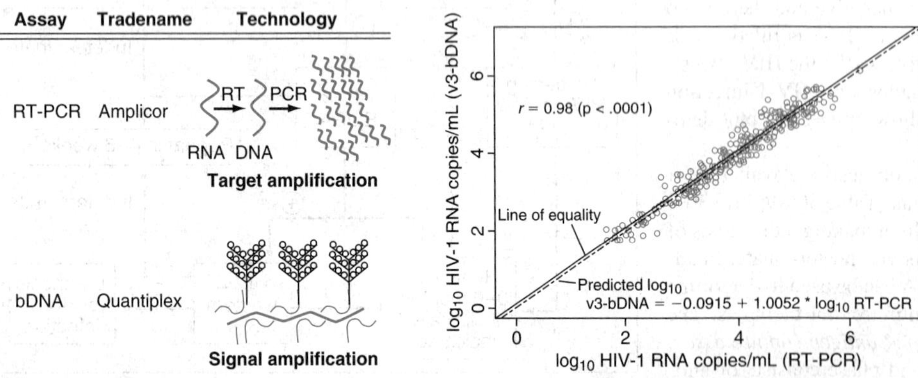

FIGURE 309-25 Comparison of RT-PCR and bDNA assays. *A*. Schematic representation of RT-PCR and bDNA assays. See text for detailed description. *B*. Scatter plot of $\log_{10}$v3 bDNA versus $\log_{10}$ RT-PCR with the line of equity (solid) and the fitted regression line (hatched). The equation for the fitted regression line is given in the lower-right-hand corner. There is good agreement between the two assays. v3, version 3 of the bDNA assay. *(From Highbarger et al.)*

therapy. Once the CD4+ T cell count is <200/μL, patients should be placed on a regimen for *P. carinii* prophylaxis, and once the count is <50/μL, primary prophylaxis for MAC infection is indicated. As with any laboratory measurement, one may wish to obtain two determinations prior to any significant changes in patient management based upon CD4+ T cell count alone.

HIV RNA Determinations Facilitated by highly sensitive techniques for the precise quantitation of small amounts of nucleic acids, the measurement of serum or plasma levels of HIV RNA has become an essential component in the monitoring of patients with HIV infection. As discussed under diagnosis of HIV infection, the two most commonly used techniques are the RT-PCR assay and the bDNA assay. Both assays generate data in the form of number of copies of HIV RNA per milliliter of serum or plasma and, by employing a 1:10 concentration step with ultracentrifugation, can detect as few as 40 to 50 copies of HIV RNA per milliliter of plasma. Although earlier versions of the bDNA assay generated values that were approximately 50% of those of the RT-PCR assay, the more recent versions (version 3 or higher) provide numbers essentially identical to those of the RT-PCR test (Fig. 309-25). While it is common practice to describe levels of HIV RNA below these cut-offs as "undetectable," this is a term that should be avoided as it is imprecise and leaves the false impression that the level of virus is 0. By utilizing more sensitive, nested PCR techniques and by studying tissue levels of virus as well as plasma levels, HIV RNA can be detected in virtually every patient with HIV infection. Measurements of changes in HIV RNA levels over time have been of great value in delineating the relationship between levels of virus and rates of disease progression (Fig. 309-17), the rates of viral turnover, the relationship between immune system activation and viral replication, and the time to development of drug resistance. HIV RNA measurements are greatly influenced by the state of activation of the immune system and may fluctuate greatly in the setting of secondary infections or immunization. For these reasons, decisions based upon HIV RNA levels should never be made on a single determination. Measurements of plasma HIV RNA levels should be made at the time of HIV diagnosis and every 3 to 4 months thereafter in the untreated patient. In general, most guidelines suggest that therapy be initiated in patients with >20,000 copies of HIV RNA per milliliter (see below). Following the initiation of therapy or any change in therapy, plasma HIV RNA levels should be monitored approximately every 4 weeks until the effectiveness of the therapeutic regimen is determined by the development of a new steady-state level of HIV RNA. In most instances of effective therapy this will be <50 copies per milliliter. This level of virus is generally achieved within 6 months of the initiation of effective treatment. During therapy, levels of HIV RNA should be monitored every 3 to 4 months to evaluate the continuing effectiveness of therapy.

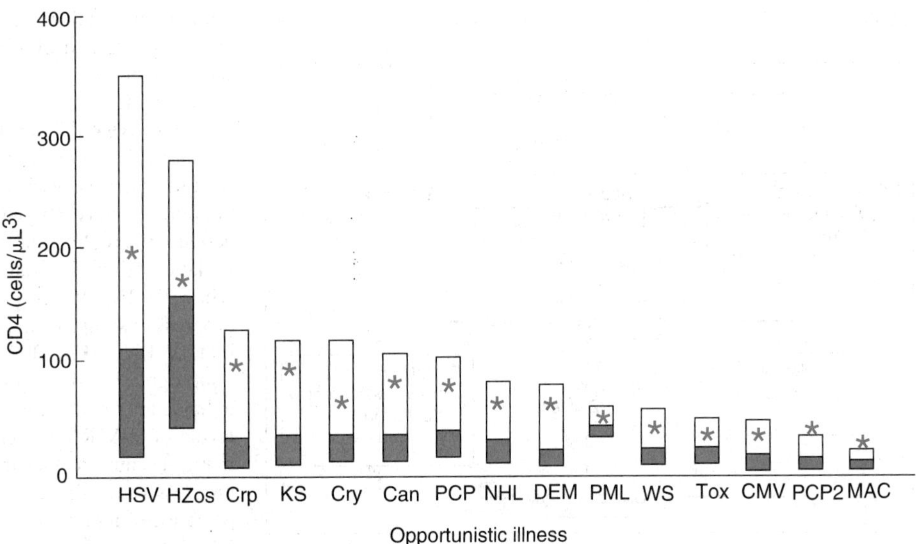

FIGURE 309-26 Relationship between CD4+ T cell counts and the development of opportunistic diseases. Boxplot of the median (line inside the box), first quartile (bottom of the box), third quartile (top of the box), and mean (asterisk) CD4+ lymphocyte count at the time of the development of opportunistic disease. Can, candidal esophagitis; CMV, cytomegalovirus infection; Crp, cryptosporidiosis; Cry, cryptococcal meningitis; DEM, AIDS dementia complex; HSV, herpes simplex virus infection; HZos, herpes zoster; KS, Kaposi's sarcoma; MAC, *Mycobacterium avium* complex bacteremia; NHL, non-Hodgkin's lymphoma; PCP, primary *Pneumocystis carinii* pneumonia; PCP2, secondary *Pneumocystis carinii* pneumonia; PML, progressive multifocal leukoencephalopathy; Tox, *Toxoplasma gondii* encephalitis; WS, wasting syndrome. *(From Moore and Chaisson.)*

HIV Resistance Testing The availability of multiple antiretroviral drugs as treatment options has generated a great deal of interest in the potential for measuring the sensitivity of an individual's HIV virus(es) to different antiretroviral agents. HIV resistance testing can be done through either genotypic or phenotypic measurements. In the genotypic assays, sequence analyses of the HIV genomes obtained from patients are compared to sequences of viruses with known antiretroviral resistance profiles. In the phenotypic assays, the in vivo growth of viral isolates obtained from the patient are compared to the growth of reference strains of the virus in the presence or absence of different antiretroviral drugs. A modification of this phenotypic approach utilizes a comparison of the enzymatic activities of the reverse transcriptase or protease genes obtained by molecular cloning of patients' isolates to the enzymatic activities of genes obtained from reference strains of HIV in the presence or absence of different drugs targeted to these genes. These tests are quite good in identifying those antiretroviral agents that have been utilized in the past in a given patient. Their clinical value in identifying which antiretroviral regimen is best for an individual patient is still under investigation.

Other Tests A variety of other laboratory tests have been studied as potential markers of HIV disease activity. Among these are quantitative culture of replication-competent HIV from plasma, peripheral blood mononuclear cells, or resting CD4+ T cells; circulating levels of β_2-microglobulin, soluble IL-2 receptor, IgA, acid-labile endogenous interferon, or TNF-α; and the presence or absence of activation markers such as CD38 or HLA-DR on CD8+ T cells. While these measurements have value as markers of disease activity and help to increase our understanding of the pathogenesis of HIV disease, they do not currently play a major role in the monitoring of patients with HIV infection.

CLINICAL MANIFESTATIONS

The clinical consequences of HIV infection encompass a spectrum ranging from an acute syndrome associated with primary infection to a prolonged asymptomatic state to advanced disease. It is best to regard HIV disease as beginning at the time of primary infection and progressing through various stages. As mentioned above, active virus replication and progressive immunologic impairment occur throughout the course of HIV infection in most patients. With the exception of long-term nonprogressors (see above), HIV disease in untreated patients inexorably progresses even during the clinically latent stage.

THE ACUTE HIV SYNDROME It is estimated that 50 to 70% of individuals with HIV infection experience an acute clinical syndrome approximately 3 to 6 weeks after primary infection (Fig. 309-27). Varying degrees of clinical severity have been reported, and although it has been suggested that symptomatic seroconversion lead-

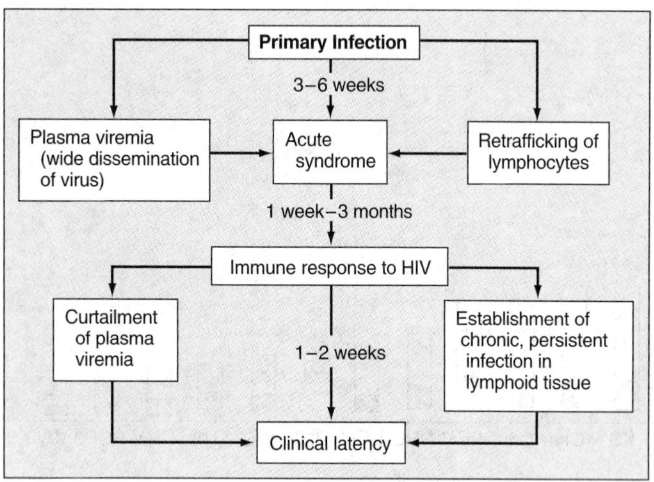

FIGURE 309-27 The acute HIV syndrome. See text for detailed description. *(Adapted from G Pantaleo et al: N Engl J Med 328:327, 1993.)*

ing to the seeking of medical attention indicates an increased risk for an accelerated course of disease, this has not been shown definitively. In fact, there does not appear to be a correlation between the level of the initial burst of viremia in acute HIV infection and the subsequent course of disease. The typical clinical findings are listed in Table 309-10; they occur along with a burst of plasma viremia. The syndrome is typical of an acute viral syndrome and has been likened to acute infectious mononucleosis. Symptoms usually persist for 1 to several weeks and gradually subside as an immune response to HIV develops and the levels of plasma viremia decrease. Opportunistic infections have been reported during this stage of infection, reflecting the immunodeficiency that results from reduced numbers of CD4+ T cells and likely also from the dysfunction of CD4+ T cells owing to cross-linking of the CD4 molecule on the cell surface by viral envelope proteins (see "Mechanisms of CD4+ T Lymphocyte Depletion and Dysfunction," above) associated with the extremely high levels of plasma viremia. A number of immunologic abnormalities accompany the acute HIV syndrome, including multiphasic perturbations of the numbers of circulating lymphocyte subsets. The number of total lymphocytes and T cell subsets (CD4+ and CD8+) are initially reduced. An inversion of the CD4+/CD8+ T cell ratio occurs later because of a rise in the number of CD8+ T cells. In fact, there may be a selective and transient expansion of CD8+ T cell subsets, as determined by T cell receptor analysis (see above). The total circulating CD8+ T cell count may remain elevated or return to normal; however, CD4+ T cell levels usually remain somewhat depressed, although there may be a slight rebound towards normal. Lymphadenopathy occurs in approximately 70% of individuals with primary HIV infection. Most patients recover spontaneously from this syndrome and many are left with only a mildly depressed CD4+ T cell count that remains stable for a variable period before beginning its progressive decline (see below); in some individuals, the CD4+ T cell count returns to the normal range. Approximately 10% of patients manifest a fulminant course of immunologic and clinical deterioration after primary infection, even after the disappearance of symptoms. In most patients, primary infection with or without the acute syndrome is followed by a prolonged period of clinical latency.

Table 309-10 Clinical Findings in the Acute HIV Syndrome

General	Neurologic
Fever	Meningitis
Pharyngitis	Encephalitis
Lymphadenopathy	Peripheral neuropathy
Headache/retroorbital pain	Myelopathy
Arthralgias/myalgias	Dermatologic
Lethargy/malaise	Erythematous maculopapular rash
Anorexia/weight loss	Mucocutaneous ulceration
Nausea/vomiting/diarrhea	

SOURCE: From Tindall and Cooper.

THE ASYMPTOMATIC STAGE—CLINICAL LATENCY Although the length of time from initial infection to the development of clinical disease varies greatly, the median time for untreated patients is approximately 10 years. As emphasized above, HIV disease with active virus replication is ongoing and progressive during this asymptomatic period. The rate of disease progression is directly correlated with HIV RNA levels. Patients with high levels of HIV RNA in plasma progress to symptomatic disease faster than do patients with low levels of HIV RNA (Fig. 309-17). Some patients referred to as long-term nonprogressors show little if any decline in CD4+ T cell counts over extended periods of time. These patients generally have extremely low levels of HIV RNA. Certain other patients remain entirely asymptomatic despite the fact that their CD4+ T cell counts show a steady progressive decline to extremely low levels. In these patients, the appearance of an opportunistic disease may be the first manifestation of HIV infection. During the asymptomatic period of HIV infection, the average rate of CD4+ T cell decline is approximately 50/μL per year. When the CD4+ T cell count falls to <200/μL, the resulting state of immunodeficiency is severe enough to place the patient at high risk for opportunistic infection and neoplasms, and hence for clinically apparent disease.

SYMPTOMATIC DISEASE Symptoms of HIV disease can appear at any time during the course of HIV infection. Generally speaking, the spectrum of illness that one observes changes as the CD4+ T cell count declines. The more severe and life-threatening complications of HIV infection occur in patients with CD4+ T cells counts <200/μL. A diagnosis of AIDS is made in anyone with HIV infection and a CD4+ T cell count <200/μL and in anyone with HIV infection who develops one of the HIV-associated diseases considered to be indicative of a severe defect in cell-mediated immunity (category C, Table 309-2). While the causative agents of the secondary infections are characteristically opportunistic organisms such as *P. carinii*, atypical mycobacteria, CMV, and other organisms that do not ordinarily cause disease in the absence of a compromised immune system, they also include common bacterial and mycobacterial pathogens. Approximately 80% of deaths among AIDS patients are as a direct result of an infection other than HIV, with bacterial infections heading the list. Following the widespread use of combination antiretroviral therapy and implementation of guidelines for the prevention of opportunistic infections (Table 309-11), the incidence of secondary infections has decreased dramatically (Fig. 309-28). Overall, the clinical spectrum of HIV disease is constantly changing as patients live longer and new and better approaches to treatment and prophylaxis are developed. In general, it should be stressed that a key element of treatment of symptomatic complications of HIV disease, whether they are primary or secondary, is achieving good control of HIV replication through the use of combination antiretroviral therapy and instituting primary and secondary prophylaxis as indicated.

Disease of the Respiratory System Acute bronchitis and sinusitis are prevalent during all stages of HIV infection. The most severe cases tend to occur in patients with lower CD4+ T cell counts. Sinusitis presents as fever, nasal congestion, and headache. The diagnosis is made by computed tomography (CT) or magnetic resonance imaging (MRI). The maxillary sinuses are most commonly involved; however, disease is also frequently seen in the ethmoid, sphenoid, and frontal sinuses. While some patients may improve without antibiotic therapy, radiographic improvement is quicker and more pronounced in patients who have received antimicrobial therapy. It is postulated that this high incidence of sinusitis results from an increased frequency of infection with encapsulated organisms such as *H. influenzae* and *Streptococcus pneumoniae*. In patients with low CD4+ T cell counts one may see mucormycosis infections of the sinuses. In contrast to the course of this infection in other patient populations, mucormycosis of the sinuses in patients with HIV infection may progress more slowly. In this set-

Table 309-11 1999 USPHS/IDSA Guidelines for the Prevention of Opportunistic Infections in Persons Infected with HIV

Pathogen	Indications	First Choice(s)	Alternatives
STRONGLY RECOMMENDED AS STANDARD OF CARE FOR PRIMARY AND SECONDARY PROPHYLAXIS			
Pneumocystis carinii	CD4 count <200/μl or Oropharyngeal candidiasis or Unexplained fever >2 weeks Prior bout of PCP	Trimethoprim/sulfamethoxazole (TMP/SMZ), 1 DS tablet qd	Dapsone 50 mg bid PO or 100 mg/d PO Dapsone 50 mg/d PO+ Pyrimethamine 50 mg/wk PO+ Leucovorin 25 mg/wk PO TMP/SMZ, 1 SS tablet qd Dapsone 200 mg PO+ Pyrimethamine 50 mg + Leucovorin 25 mg PO weekly Aerosolized pentamidine, 300 mg qm via Respirgard II nebulizer Atovoquone 1500 mg/d PO TMP/SMZ 1 DS tablet PO 3×/wk
Mycobacterium tuberculosis			
Isoniazid sensitive	Skin test >5 mm or Prior positive test without treatment or Contact with case of active TB	Isoniazid 300 mg PO+ Pyridoxine 500 mg/d PO ×9 mo	Rifabutin 300 mg PO+ Pyrazinamide 20 (mg/kg)/d PO ×2 mo
		Isoniazid 900 mg PO+ Pyridoxine 100 mg PO 2 ×/wk ×9 mo	Rifampin 600 mg/d PO ×4 mo
Isoniazid resistant	Same with high probability of exposure to isoniazid-resistant TB	Rifampin 600 mg PO+ Pyrazinamide 20 (mg/kg)/d PO q ×2 mo	Rifabutin 300 mg PO+ daily Pyrazinamide 20 (mg/kg)/d PO ×2 mo Rifampin 600 mg/d PO ×4 mo Rifabutin 300 mg/d PO ×4 mo
Multidrug resistant	Same with high probability of exposure to multidrug resistant TB	Consult local public health authorities	
Mycobacterium-avium complex	CD4 count <50/μl	Azithromycin 1200 mg weekly PO Clarithromycin 500 mg bid PO	Rifibutin 300 mg/d PO Azithromycin 1200 mg weekly PO+ Rifabutin 300 mg/d PO
	Prior documented disseminated disease	Clarithromycin 500 mg bid PO + Ethambutol 15 (mg/kg)/d PO+/− Rifabutin 300 mg/d PO	Azithromycin 500 mg/d PO+ Ethambutol 15 (mg/kg)/d PO+/− Rifabutin 300 mg/d PO
Toxoplasma gondii	IgG antibody and CD4 count <100/μl	TMP/SMZ 1 DS tablet qd	TMP/SMZ 1 SS tablet qd Dapsone 50 mg/d PO+ Pyrimethamine 50 mg weekly PO+ Leucovorin 25 mg weekly PO Atovoquone 1500 mg/d PO
	Prior toxoplasmic encephalitis	Sulfadiazine 500–1000 mg qid PO+ Pyrimethamine 25–75 mg/d PO+ Leucovorin 10 mg/d PO	Clindamycin 300–450 mg 16–8h PO+ Pyrimethamine 25–75 mg/d PO+ Leucovorin 10–25 mg/d PO
Varicella zoster virus	Significant exposure to chickenpox or shingles in a patient with no history of immunization or prior exposure to either	Varicella zoster immune globulin 6.25 mL within 96 h	
Cryptococcus neoformans	Prior documented disease	Fluconazole 200 mg/d PO	Amphotericin B 0.6–1.0 mg/kg 3 ×/wk IV Itraconazole 200 mg/d PO
Histoplasma capsulatum	Prior documented disease	Itraconazole 200 mg bid PO	Amphotericin B 1.0 (mg/kg)/wk IV
Coccidioides immitis	Prior documented disease	Fluconazole 400 mg/d PO	Amphotericin B 1.0 (mg/kg)/wk IV Itraconazole 200 mg/d PO
Salmonella species	Prior bacteremia	Ciprofloxacin 500 mg bid PO for several months	
Cytomegalovirus	Prior end-organ disease (any)	Ganciclovir, 5–6 mg/kg 5–7 days/wk IV Ganciclovir 1000 mg tid PO Foscarnet 90–120 (mg/kg)/d IV	Cidofovir 5 mg/kg every other week IV
	Prior retinitis	Ganciclovir sustained-release implant q6–9mo + ganciclovir 1–1.5 g tid PO	Fomivirsen, 1 vial injected into the vitreous q2–4wk
IMMUNIZATIONS GENERALLY RECOMMENDED			
Hepatitis B virus	All susceptible (anti-HBc and anti-HBs negative) patients	Hepatitis B vaccine: 3 doses	
Hepatitis A virus	All susceptible (anti-HAV negative) patients with chronic hepatitis C	Hepatitis A vaccine: 2 doses	
Influenza virus	All patients annually	Whole or split virus 1 dose yearly	

(continued)

Table 309-11 1999 USPHS/IDSA Guidelines for the Prevention of Opportunistic Infections in Persons Infected with HIV—*(continued)*

Pathogen	Indications	First Choice(s)	Alternatives
Streptococcus pneumoniae	All patients	Pneumoccal vaccine 0.5 mL IM ×1 if CD4 count >200/μl Reimmunize patients initially immunized at a CD4 count <200/μl whose CD4 count then increases to >200/μl	
RECOMMENDED FOR PREVENTION OF SEVERE OR FREQUENT RECURRENCES			
Herpes simplex	Frequent/severe recurrences	Acyclovir 200 mg tid PO Acyclovir 40 mg bid PO Famciclovir 500 mg bid PO	
Candida	Frequent/severe recurrences	Fluconazole 100–200 mg/d PO Itraconazole solution 200 mg/d PO Ketoconazole 200 mg/d PO	

NOTE: DS, double strength; SS, single strength; PCP, *Pneumocystis carinii* pneumonia; TB, tuberculosis

ting aggressive, frequent local debridement in addition to local and systemic amphotericin B may be needed for effective treatment.

Pulmonary disease is one of the most frequent complications of HIV infection. The most common manifestation of pulmonary disease is pneumonia. The two most common causes of pneumonia are bacteria infections and *P. carinii* infection. Other major causes of pulmonary infiltrates include mycobacterial infections, fungal infections, nonspecific interstitial pneumonitis, KS, and lymphoma.

Pneumonia is seen with an increased frequency in patients with HIV infection. Patients with HIV infection appear to be particularly prone to infections with encapsulated organisms. *S. pneumoniae* (Chap. 138) and *H. influenzae* (Chap. 149) are responsible for most cases of bacterial pneumonia in patients with AIDS. This may be a consequence of altered B cell function and/or defects in neutrophil function that may be secondary to HIV disease (see above). Pneumococcal infection may be the earliest serious infection to occur in patients with HIV disease. This can present as pneumonia, sinusitis, and/or bacteremia. Patients with HIV infection have a sixfold increase in the incidence of pneumococcal pneumonia and a 100-fold increase in the incidence of pneumococcal bacteremia. Pneumococcal disease may be seen in patients with relatively intact immune systems. In one study, the baseline CD4+ T cell count at the time of a first episode of pneumococcal pneumonia was ~300/μL. Of interest is the fact that the inflammatory response to pneumococcal infection appears proportional to the CD4+ T cell count. Due to this high risk of pneumococcal disease, immunization with pneumococcal polysaccharide is one of the generally recommended prophylactic measures for patients with HIV infection and CD4+ T cell counts >200/μL. It is less clear if this intervention is of benefit in patients with more advanced disease and high viral loads.

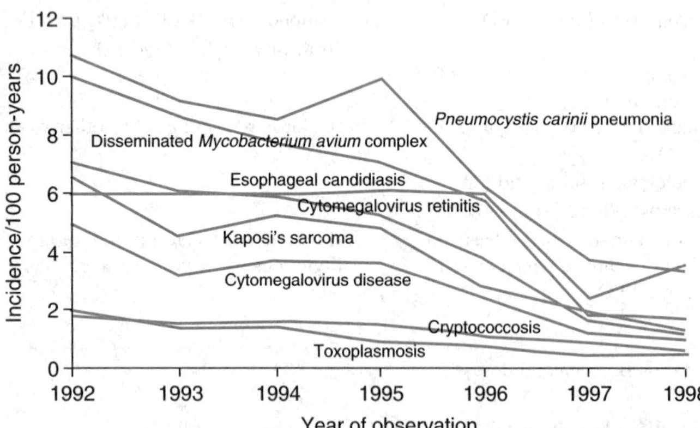

FIGURE 309-28 Decrease in the incidence of opportunistic infections and Kaposi's sarcoma in HIV-infected individuals with CD4+ T cell counts <100/μL from 1992 through 1998. *[Adapted and updated from Palella et al, and JE Kaplan et al: Clin Infect Dis 30(S1):S5, 2000, with permission.]*

P. carinii pneumonia (PCP), once the hallmark of AIDS, has dramatically declined in incidence following the development of effective prophylactic regimens and the widespread use of combination antiretroviral therapy. The risk of PCP is most common among those who have experienced a previous bout of PCP and those who have CD4+ T cell counts of <200/μL. Overall, 79% of patients with PCP have CD4+ T cell counts <100/μL and 95% of patients have CD4+ T cell counts <200/μL. Recurrent fever, night sweats, thrush, and unexplained weight loss are also associated with an increased incidence of PCP. For these reasons, it is strongly recommended that all patients with CD4+ T cell counts <200/μL (or a CD4 percentage <15) receive some form of PCP prophylaxis. At present the incidence of PCP is approaching zero in patients with known HIV infection receiving appropriate antiretroviral therapy and prophylaxis. Primary PCP is now occurring at a median CD4+ T cell count of 36/μL, while secondary PCP is occurring at a median CD4+ T cell count of 10/μL. Patients with PCP generally present with fever and a cough that is usually nonproductive or productive of only scant amounts of white sputum. They may complain of a characteristic retrosternal chest pain that is worse on inspiration and is described as sharp or burning. HIV-associated PCP may have an indolent course characterized by weeks of vague symptoms and should be included in the differential diagnosis of fever, pulmonary complaints, or unexplained weight loss in any patient with HIV infection and <200 CD4+ T cells/μL. The most common finding on chest x-ray is either a normal film, if the disease is suspected early, or a faint bilateral interstitial infiltrate. The classic finding of a dense perihilar infiltrate is unusual in patients with AIDS. In patients with PCP who have been receiving aerosolized pentamidine for prophylaxis, one may see an x-ray picture of upper lobe cavitary disease, reminiscent of TB. Other less common findings on chest x-ray include lobar infiltrates and pleural effusions. Routine laboratory evaluation is usually of little help in the differential diagnosis of PCP. A mild leukocytosis is common, although this may not be obvious in patients with prior neutropenia. Arterial blood gases may indicate hypoxemia with a decline in Pa_{O_2} and an increase in the arterial-alveolar (a − A) gradient. Arterial blood gas measurements not only aid in making the diagnosis of PCP but also provide important information for staging the severity of the disease and directing treatment. A definitive diagnosis of PCP requires demonstration of the trophozoite or cyst form of the organism in samples obtained from induced sputum, bronchoalveolar lavage, transbronchial biopsy, or open lung biopsy. PCR has been used to detect specific DNA sequences for *P. carinii* in clinical specimens where histologic examinations have failed to make a diagnosis.

In addition to pneumonia, a number of other clinical problems have been reported in HIV-infected patients as a result of infection with *P. carinii*. Otic involvement may be seen as a primary infection, presenting as a polypoid mass involving the external auditory canal. In patients receiving aerosolized penamidine for prophylaxis against PCP one may see a variety of extrapulmonary manifestations of *P. carinii*.

These include ophthalmic lesions of the choroid, a necrotizing vasculitis that resembles Burger's disease, bone marrow hypoplasia, and intestinal obstruction. Other organs that have been involved include lymph nodes, spleen, liver, kidney, pancreas, pericardium, heart, thyroid, and adrenals. Organ infection may be associated with cystic lesions that may appear calcified on CT or ultrasound. The standard treatment for PCP or disseminated pneumocystosis is trimethoprim/sulfamethoxazole (TMP/SMZ). A high incidence of side effects, particularly skin rash and bone marrow suppression, is seen with TMP/SMZ in patients with HIV infection. Alternative treatments for mild to moderate PCP include dapsone/trimethoprim and clindamycin/primaquine. Intravenous pentamidine is the treatment of choice for severe disease in the patient unable to tolerate TMP/SMZ. For patients with a Pa_{O_2} <70 mmHg or with an a − A gradient >35 mmHg, adjunct glucocorticoid therapy should be used in addition to specific antimicrobials. Overall, treatment should be for 21 days and followed by secondary prophylaxis. Prophylaxis for PCP is indicated for any HIV-infected individual who has experienced a prior bout of PCP, any patient with a CD4+ T cell count of <200/μL or a CD4 percentage <15, any patient with unexplained fever for >2 weeks, and any patient with a history of oropharyngeal candidiasis. The preferred regimen for prophylaxis is TMP/SMZ, one double-strength tablet daily. This regimen also provides protection against toxoplasmosis and some bacterial respiratory pathogens. For patients who cannot tolerate TMP/SMZ, alternatives include dapsone plus pyrimethamine plus leucovorin, aerosolized pentamidine administered by the Respirgard II nebulizer, and atovaquone. Primary prophylaxis for PCP can be discontinued in those patients treated with combination antiretroviral therapy who maintain good suppression of HIV (<500 copies per milliliter) and CD4+ T cell counts >200/μL for at least 3 to 6 months. There is as yet insufficient information to know if the same recommendation will hold for discontinuation of secondary prophylaxis.

M. tuberculosis, once thought to be on its way to extinction in the United States, experienced a resurgence associated with the HIV epidemic (Chap. 169). Worldwide, approximately one-third of all AIDS-related deaths are associated with TB. In the United States approximately 5% of AIDS patients have active TB. HIV infection increases the risk of developing active tuberculosis by a factor of 15 to 30. For the patient with untreated HIV infection and a positive PPD skin test, the rate of reactivation TB is 7 to 10% per year. Untreated TB can accelerate the course of HIV infection. Levels of plasma HIV RNA increase in the setting of active TB and decline in the setting of successful TB treatment. Active TB is most common in patients 25 to 44 years of age, in African-Americans and Hispanics, in patients in New York City and Miami, and in patients in developing countries. In these demographic groups, 20 to 70% of the new cases of active TB are in patients with HIV infection. The epidemic of TB embedded in the epidemic of HIV infection probably represents the greatest health risk to the general public and the health care profession associated with the HIV epidemic. In contrast to infection with atypical mycobacteria such as MAC, active TB often develops relatively early in the course of HIV infection and may be an early clinical sign of HIV disease. In one study, the median CD4+ T cell count at presentation of TB was 326/μL. The clinical manifestations of TB in HIV-infected patients are quite varied and generally show different patterns as a function of the CD4+ T cell count. In patients with relatively high CD4+ T cell counts, the typical pattern of pulmonary reactivation occurs in which patients present with fever, cough, dyspnea on exertion, weight loss, night sweats, and a chest x-ray revealing cavitary apical disease of the upper lobes. In patients with lower CD4+ T cell counts, disseminated disease is more common. In these patients the chest x-ray may reveal diffuse or lower lobe bilateral reticulonodular infiltrates consistent with miliary spread, pleural effusions, and hilar and/or mediastinal adenopathy. Infection may be present in bone, brain, meninges, gastrointestinal tract, lymph nodes (particularly cervical lymph nodes), and viscera. Approximately 60 to 80% of patients have pulmonary disease, and 30 to 40% have extrapulmonary disease. Respiratory isolation and a negative-pressure room should be used for patients in whom a diagnosis of pulmonary TB is being considered. This approach is critical to limit nosocomial and community spread of infection. Culture of the organism from an involved site provides a definitive diagnosis. Blood cultures are positive in 15% of patients. In the setting of fulminant disease one cannot rely upon the accuracy of a negative PPD skin test to rule out a diagnosis of TB. TB is one of the conditions associated with HIV infection for which cure is possible. Therapy for TB is generally the same in the HIV-infected patient as in the HIV-negative patient (Chap. 169). Due to pharmacokinetic interactions, rifabutin should be substituted for rifampin in patients receiving the HIV protease inhibitors or nonnucleoside reverse transcriptase inhibitors; both drugs should be avoided in patients receiving ritonavir. Treatment is most effective in programs that involve directly observed therapy. Effective prevention of active TB can be a reality if the health care professional is aggressive in looking for evidence of latent TB by making sure that all patients with HIV infection receive a PPD skin test. Anergy testing is not of value in this setting. HIV-infected individuals with a skin test reaction of >5 mm or those who are close household contacts of persons with active TB should receive treatment with 9 months of isoniazid, or 2 months of therapy with rifampin and pyrazinamide, or 2 months of therapy with rifabutin and pyrazinamide.

Atypical mycobacterial infections are also seen with an increased frequency in patients with HIV infection. Infections with at least 12 different mycobacteria have been reported, including *M. bovis* and representatives of all four Runyon groups. The most common atypical mycobacterial infection is with *M. avium* or *M. intracellulare* species, the *M. avium* complex (MAC). Infections with MAC are seen mainly in patients in the United States and are rare in Africa. It has been suggested that prior infection with *M. tuberculosis* decreases the risk of MAC infection. MAC infections probably arise from organisms that are ubiquitous in the environment, including both soil and water. The presumed portals of entry are the respiratory and gastrointestinal tract. MAC infection is a late complication of HIV infection, occurring in patients with CD4+ T cell counts of <50/μL. The average CD4+ T cell count at the time of diagnosis is 10/μL. The most common presentation is disseminated disease with fever, weight loss, and night sweats. At least 85% of patients with MAC infection are mycobacteremic, and large numbers of organisms can often be demonstrated on bone marrow biopsy. The chest x-ray is abnormal in approximately 25% of patients, with the most common pattern being that of a bilateral, lower lobe infiltrate suggestive of miliary spread. Alveolar or nodular infiltrates and hilar and/or mediastinal adenopathy can also occur. Other clinical findings include endobronchial lesions, abdominal pain, diarrhea, and lymphadenopathy. The diagnosis is made by the culture of blood or involved tissue. The finding of two consecutive sputum samples positive for MAC is highly suggestive of pulmonary infection. Cultures may take 2 weeks to turn positive. Therapy consists of a macrolide, usually clarithromycin, with ethambutol. Some physicians elect to add a third drug from among rifabutin, ciprofloxacin, or amikacin in patients with extensive disease. Therapy is generally for life; however, with the advent of highly active antiretroviral therapy (HAART), it may be possible to discontinue therapy in patients with sustained suppression of HIV replication and CD4+ T cell counts >100/μL for >6 months. Primary prophylaxis for MAC is indicated in patients with HIV infection and CD4+ T cell counts <50/μL. This may be discontinued in patients in whom HAART induces a sustained suppression of viral replication and increases in CD4+ T cell counts to >100/μL for 3 to 6 months.

Rhodococcus equi is a gram-positive pleomorphic acid-fast non-spore-forming bacillus that can cause pulmonary and/or disseminated infection in patients with HIV infection. Fever and cough are the most common presenting signs. Radiographically one may see cavitary lesions and consolidation. Blood cultures are often positive. Treatment is based upon antimicrobial sensitivity testing.

Fungal infections of the lung can be seen in patients with AIDS. Patients with pulmonary cryptococcal disease present with fever, cough, dyspnea, and in some cases, hemoptysis. A focal or diffuse interstitial infiltrate is seen on chest x-ray in >90% of patients. In addition, one may see lobar disease, cavitary disease, pleural effusions, and hilar or mediastinal adenopathy. Over half of patients are fungemic, and 90% of patients have concomitant CNS infection. *Coccidioides immitis* is a mold that is endemic in the southwest United States. It can cause a reactivation pulmonary syndrome in patients with HIV infection. Most patients with this condition will have CD4+ T cell counts <250/μL. Patients present with fever, weight loss, cough, and extensive, diffuse reticulonodular infiltrates on chest x-ray. One may also see nodules, cavities, pleural effusions, and hilar adenopathy. While serologic testing is of value in the immunocompetent host, serologies are negative in 25% of HIV-infected patients with coccidioidal infection. Invasive aspergillosis is not an AIDS-defining illness and is generally not seen in patients with AIDS in the absence of neutropenia or administration of glucocorticoids. *Aspergillus* infection may have an unusual presentation in the respiratory tract of patients with AIDS where it gives the appearance of a pseudomembranous tracheobronchitis. Primary pulmonary infection of the lung may be seen with *histoplasmosis*. The most common pulmonary manifestation of histoplasmosis, however, is in the setting of disseminated disease, presumably due to reactivation. In this setting respiratory symptoms are usually minimal, with cough and dyspnea occurring in 10 to 30% of patients. The chest x-ray is abnormal in about 50% of patients, showing either a diffuse interstitial infiltrate or diffuse small nodules.

Two forms of *idiopathic interstitial pneumonia* have been identified in patients with HIV infection: lymphoid interstitial pneumonitis (LIP) and nonspecific interstitial pneumonitis (NIP). LIP, a common finding in children, is seen in about 1% of adult patients with HIV infection. This disorder is characterized by a benign infiltrate of the lung and is felt to be part of the polyclonal activation of lymphocytes seen in the context of HIV and EBV infections. Transbronchial biopsy is diagnostic in 50% of the cases, with an open-lung biopsy required for diagnosis in the remainder of cases. This condition is generally self-limited and no specific treatment is necessary. Severe cases have been managed with brief courses of glucocorticoids. Although rarely a clinical problem since the use of HAART, evidence of NIP may be seen in up to half of all patients with untreated HIV infection. Histologically, interstitial infiltrates of lymphocytes and plasma cells in a perivascular and peribronchial distribution are present. When symptomatic, patients present with fever and nonproductive cough occasionally accompanied by mild chest discomfort. Chest x-ray is usually normal or may reveal a faint interstitial pattern. Similar to LIP, this is a self-limited process for which no therapy is indicated.

Neoplastic diseases of the lung including KS and lymphoma are discussed below in the section on malignancies.

Diseases of the Cardiovascular System While heart disease is a relatively common postmortem finding in HIV-infected patients (25 to 75% in autopsy series), it is less of a problem clinically. The most common clinically significant finding is a dilated cardiomyopathy associated with congestive heart failure referred to as *HIV-associated cardiomyopathy*. This generally occurs as a late complication of HIV infection and, histologically, displays elements of myocarditis. For this reason some have advocated treatment with intravenous Ig. HIV can be directly demonstrated in cardiac tissue in this setting, and there is debate over whether or not it plays a direct role in this condition. Patients present with typical findings of congestive heart failure, namely edema and shortness of breath. Patients with HIV infection may also develop cardiomyopathy as a side effect of IFN-α or nucleoside analogue therapy, which is reversible once therapy is stopped. KS, cryptococcosis, Chagas disease, and toxoplasmosis can involve the myocardium, leading to cardiomyopathy. In one series, most patients with HIV infection and a treatable myocarditis were found to have myocarditis associated with toxoplasmosis. Most of these patients also had evidence of CNS toxoplasmosis. Thus, MRI or double-dose contrast CT scan of the brain should be included in the workup of any patient with advanced HIV infection and cardiomyopathy.

A variety of other cardiovascular problems are found in patients with HIV infection. Pericardial effusions may be seen in the setting of advanced HIV infection. Predisposing factors include TB, congestive heart failure, mycobacterial infection, cryptococcal infection, pulmonary infection, lymphoma, and KS. While pericarditis is quite rare, in one series 5% of patients with HIV disease had pericardial effusions that were considered to be moderate or severe. Tamponade and death have occurred in association with pericardial KS, presumably owing to acute hemorrhage. A high percentage of patients have hypertriglyceridemia and elevations in serum cholesterol, and coronary artery disease has been a relatively frequent finding at autopsy. This problem appears to becoming even more prevalent as a side effect of HAART. While clinically significant ischemic heart disease has not been reported to be occurring with an increased frequency in this patient population, many are concerned that it is just a matter of time before this is the case. Nonbacterial thrombotic endocarditis has been reported and should be considered in patients with unexplained embolic phenomena. Intravenous pentamidine, when given rapidly, can result in hypotension as a consequence of cardiovascular collapse.

Diseases of the Oropharynx and Gastrointestinal System Oropharyngeal and gastrointestinal diseases are common features of HIV infection. They are most frequently due to secondary infections. In addition, oral and gastrointestinal lesions may occur with KS and lymphoma.

Oral lesions, including *thrush*, *hairy leukoplakia*, and *aphthous ulcers*, are particularly common in patients with untreated HIV infection. Thrush, due to *Candida* infection, and oral hairy leukoplakia, presumed due to EBV, are usually indicative of fairly advanced immunologic decline; they generally occur in patients with CD4+ T cell counts of <300/μL. In one study, 59% of patients with oral candidiasis went on to develop AIDS in the next year. Thrush appears as a white, cheesy exudate, often on an erythematous mucosa in the posterior oropharynx (**see Plate IID-43**). While most commonly seen on the soft palate, early lesions are often found along the gingival border. The diagnosis is made by direct examination of a scraping for pseudohyphal elements. Culturing is of no diagnostic value, as most patients with HIV infection will have a positive throat culture for *Candida* even in the absence of thrush. Oral hairy leukoplakia presents as white, frondlike lesions, generally along the lateral borders of the tongue and sometimes on the adjacent buccal mucosa (**see Plate IID-42**). Despite its name, oral hairy leukoplakia is not considered a premalignant condition. Lesions are associated with florid replication of EBV. While usually more disconcerting as a sign of HIV-associated immunodeficiency than a clinical problem in need of treatment, severe cases have been reported to respond to topical podophyllin or systemic therapy with acyclovir. Aphthous ulcers of the posterior oropharynx are also seen with regularity in patients with HIV infection. These lesions are of unknown etiology and can be quite painful and interfere with swallowing. Topical anesthetics provide immediate symptomatic relief of short duration. The fact that thalidomide is an effective treatment for this condition suggests that the pathogenesis may involve the action of tissue-destructive cytokines. Palatal, glossal, or gingival ulcers may also result from cryptococcal disease or histoplasmosis.

Esophagitis (Fig. 309-29) may present with odynophagia and retrosternal pain. Upper endoscopy is generally required to make an accurate diagnosis. Esophagitis may be due to *Candida*, CMV, or HSV. While CMV tends to be associated with a single large ulcer, HSV infection is more often associated with multiple small ulcers. The esophagus may also be the site of KS and lymphoma. Like the oral mucosa, the esophageal mucosa may have large, painful ulcers of unclear etiology that may respond to thalidomide. While achlorhydria is a common problem in patients with HIV infection, other gastric problems are generally rare. Among the conditions involving the stomach are KS and lymphoma. Infections of the small and large intestine leading to diarrhea, abdominal pain, and occasionally fever are among the most significant gastrointestinal problems in the HIV-infected patients. They include infections with bacteria, protozoa, and viruses.

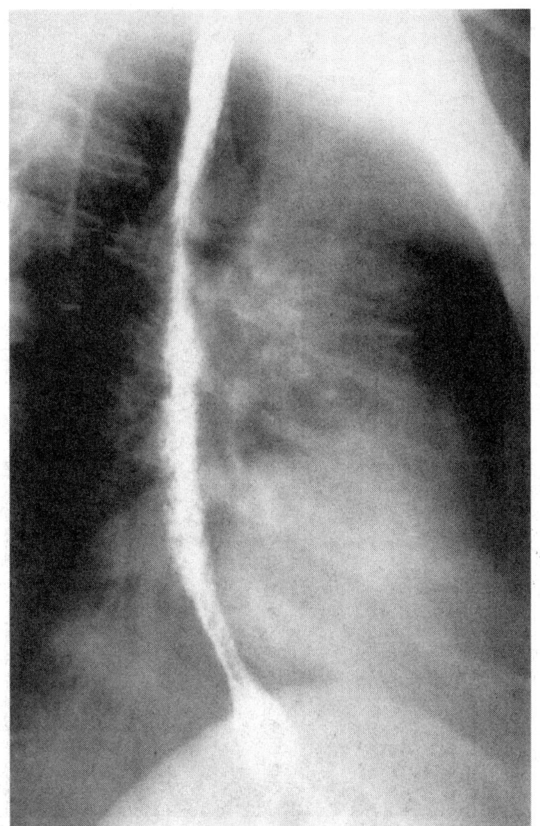

FIGURE 309-29 Barium swallow of a patient with *Candida* esophagitis. The flow of barium along the mucosal surface is grossly irregular.

Bacteria and fungi may be responsible for secondary infections of the gastrointestinal tract. Infections with enteric pathogens such as *Salmonella*, *Shigella*, and *Campylobacter* are more common in homosexual men and are often more severe and more apt to relapse in patients with HIV infection. Patients with untreated HIV have approximately a 20-fold increased risk of infection with *S. typhimurium*. They may present with a variety of nonspecific symptoms including fever, anorexia, fatigue, and malaise of several weeks' duration. Diarrhea is common but may be absent. Diagnosis is made by culture of blood and stool. Long-term therapy with ciprofloxacin is the recommended treatment. HIV-infected patients also have an increased incidence of *S. typhi* infection in areas of the world where typhoid is a problem. *Shigella* spp., particularly *S. flexneri*, can cause severe intestinal disease in HIV-infected individuals. Up to 50% of patients will develop bacteremia. *Campylobacter* infections occur with an increased frequency in patients with HIV infection. While *C. jejuni* is the strain most frequently isolated, infections with many other strains have been reported. Patients usually present with crampy abdominal pain, fever, and bloody diarrhea. Infection may present as proctitis. Stool examination reveals the presence of fecal leukocytes. Systemic infection can occur, with up to 10% of infected patients exhibiting bacteremia. Most strains are sensitive to erythromycin. Abdominal pain and diarrhea may be seen with MAC infection.

Fungal infections may also be a cause of diarrhea in patients with HIV infection. Histoplasmosis, coccidioidomycosis, and penicilliosis have all been identified as a cause of fever and diarrhea in patients with HIV infection. Peritonitis has been seen with *C. immitis*.

Cryptosporidia, microsporidia, and *Isospora belli* (Chap. 218) are the most common opportunistic protozoa that infect the gastrointestinal tract and cause diarrhea in HIV-infected patients. Cryptosporidial infection may present in a variety of ways, ranging from a self-limited or intermittent diarrheal illness in patients in the early stages of HIV infection to a severe, life-threatening diarrhea in severely immunodeficient individuals. In patients with untreated HIV infection and CD4+ T cell counts of $<300/\mu L$, the incidence of cryptosporidiosis is approximately 1% per year. In 75% of cases the diarrhea is accompanied by crampy abdominal pain, and 25% of patients have nausea and/or vomiting. Cryptosporidia may also cause biliary tract disease in the HIV-infected patient, leading to cholecystitis with or without accompanying cholangitis. The diagnosis of cryptosporidial diarrhea is made by stool examination. The diarrhea is noninflammatory, and the characteristic finding is the presence of oocysts that stain with acid-fast dyes. Therapy is predominantly supportive, and marked improvements have been reported in the setting of effective antiretroviral therapy. Treatment with up to 2000 mg/d of nitazoxanide (NTZ) is associated with improvement in symptoms or a decrease in shedding of organisms in about half of patients. Its overall role in the management of this condition remains unclear. Patients can minimize their risk of developing cryptosporidiosis by avoiding contact with human and animal feces and by not drinking untreated water from lakes or rivers.

Microsporidia are small, unicellular, obligate intracellular parasites that reside in the cytoplasm of enteric cells (Chap. 218). The main species causing disease in humans is *Enterocytozoon bieneusi*. The clinical manifestations are similar to those described for Cryptosporidia and include abdominal pain and diarrhea. The small size of the organism may make it difficult to detect; however, with the use of chromotrope-based stains, organisms can be identified in stool samples by light microscopy. Definitive diagnosis generally depends on electron microscopic examination of a stool specimen, intestinal aspirate, or intestinal biopsy specimen. In contrast to cryptosporidia, microsporidia have been noted in a variety of extraintestinal locations, including the eye, muscle, and liver, and have been associated with conjunctivitis and hepatitis. Albendazole, 400 mg bid, has been reported to be of benefit in some patients.

I. belli is a coccidian parasite (Chap. 218) most commonly found as a cause of diarrhea in patients from the Caribbean and Africa. Its cysts appear in the stool as large, acid-fast structures that can be differentiated from those of cryptosporidia on the basis of size, shape, and number of sporocysts. The clinical syndromes of *Isospora* infection are identical to those caused by cryptosporidia. The important distinction is that infection with *Isospora* is generally relatively easy to treat with TMP/SMZ. While relapses are common, a thrice-weekly regimen, similar to that used to provide prophylaxis against PCP, appears adequate to prevent recurrence.

CMV colitis was once seen in 5 to 10% of patients with AIDS. It is much less common with the advent of HAART. CMV colitis presents as diarrhea, abdominal pain, weight loss, and anorexia. The diarrhea is usually nonbloody, and the diagnosis is achieved through endoscopy and biopsy. Multiple mucosal ulcerations are seen at endoscopy, and biopsies reveal characteristic intranuclear inclusion bodies. Bacteremia may result as a consequence of thinning of the bowel wall. Treatment is with either ganciclovir or foscarnet for 3 to 6 weeks. Relapses are common, and maintenance therapy is typically necessary in patients whose HIV infection is poorly controlled. Patients with CMV disease of the gastrointestinal tract should be carefully monitored for evidence of retinitis.

In addition to disease caused by specific secondary infections, patients with HIV infection may also experience a chronic diarrheal syndrome for which no etiologic agent other than HIV can be identified. This entity is referred to as *AIDS enteropathy* or *HIV enteropathy*. It is most likely a direct result of HIV infection in the gastrointestinal tract. Histologic examination of the small bowel in these patients reveals low-grade mucosal atrophy with a decrease in mitotic figures, suggesting a hyporegenerative state. Patients often have decreased or absent small-bowel lactase and malabsorption with accompanying weight loss.

The initial evaluation of a patient with HIV infection and diarrhea should include a set of stool examinations, including culture, examination for ova and parasites, and examination for *Clostridium difficile* toxin. Approximately 50% of the time this workup will demonstrate infection with pathogenic bacteria, mycobacteria, or protozoa. If the initial stool examinations are negative, additional evaluation, including upper and/or lower endoscopy with biopsy, will yield a diagnosis of microsporidial or mycobacterial infection of the small intestine ~30% of the time. In patients for whom this diagnostic evaluation is nonrevealing, a presumptive diagnosis of HIV enteropathy can be made if the diarrhea has persisted for >1 month. An algorithm for the evaluation of diarrhea in patients with HIV infection is given in Fig. 309-30.

Rectal lesions are common in HIV-infected patients, particularly the perirectal ulcers and erosions due to the reactivation of HSV (Fig. 309-31). These may appear quite atypical, as denuded skin without vesicles, and they respond well to treatment with acyclovir, famciclovir, or foscarnet. Other rectal lesions encountered in the patients with HIV infection include condylomata acuminata, KS, and intraepithelial neoplasia.

Hepatobiliary Disease Diseases of the hepatobiliary system are a major problem in patients with HIV infection. It has been estimated that approximately one-third of the deaths of patients with HIV infection are in some way related to liver disease. While this is predominantly a reflection of the problems encountered in the setting of co-infection with hepatitis B or C, it is also a reflection of the hepatic injury, predominantly in the form of hepatic steatosis, that can be seen in the context of nucleoside analogue antiretroviral therapy.

Over 95% of HIV-infected individuals have evidence of infection with HBV; 5–40% of patients are co-infected with hepatitis C virus (HCV); and co-infection with hepatitis D, E, and/or G viruses is common. HIV infection has a significant impact on the course of hepatitis virus infection. It is associated with approximately a threefold increase in the development of persistent hepatitis B surface antigenemia. Patients infected with both HBV and HIV have decreased evidence of inflammatory liver disease. The presumption that this is due to the immunosuppressive effects of HIV infection is supported by the observations that this situation can be reversed, and one may see the development of more severe hepatitis following the initiation of effective antiretroviral therapy. IFN-α is less successful as a treatment of HBV in patients with HIV co-infection, and lamivudine is the treatment of choice. It is important to remember that lamivudine is also a

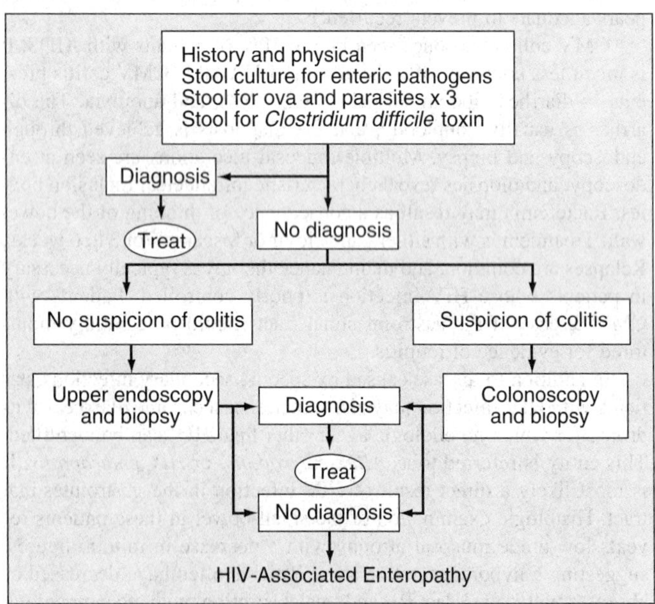

FIGURE 309-30 Algorithm for the evaluation of diarrhea in a patient with HIV infection. HIV-associated enteropathy is a diagnosis of exclusion and can be made only after other, generally treatable, forms of diarrheal illness have been ruled out.

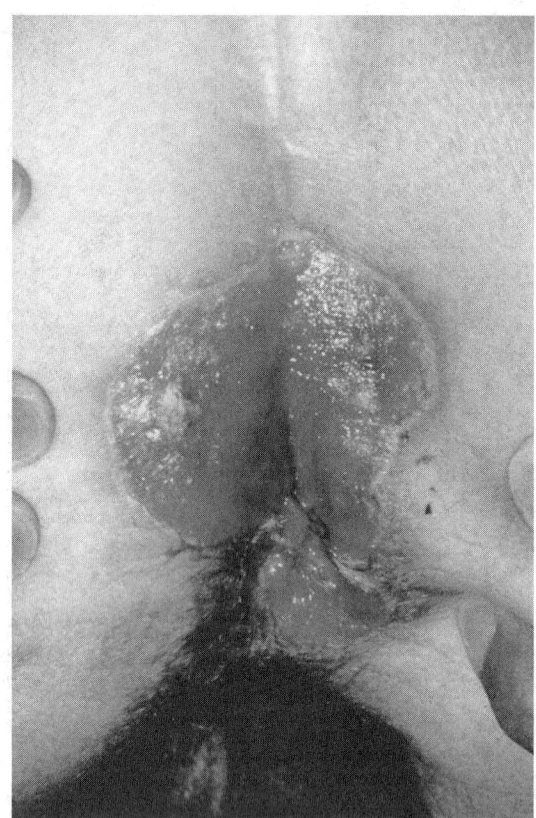

FIGURE 309-31 Severe, erosive perirectal herpes simplex in a patient with AIDS.

potent antiretroviral agent in the setting of combination antiretroviral therapy. It should not be used as a single agent in patients with HIV infection, even if it is only being used to treat HBV, in order to avoid the rapid development of lamivudine-resistant quasispecies of HIV. In contrast to the situation with HBV, HCV infection is more severe in the patient with HIV infection. In the setting of HIV and HCV co-infection, levels of HCV are approximately tenfold higher than in the HIV-negative patient with HCV infection. The incidence of HCV-associated liver failure appears to be higher by a similar factor in patients with HIV infection. Hepatitis A virus infection is not seen with an increased frequency in patients with HIV infection. It is recommended that all patients with HIV infection who have not experienced natural infection be immunized with hepatitis A and/or hepatitis B vaccines.

A variety of other infections may also involve the liver. Granulomatous hepatitis may be seen as a consequence of mycobacterial or fungal infections, particularly MAC infection. Hepatic masses may be seen in the context of TB, peliosis hepatis, or fungal infection. Among the fungal opportunistic infection *C. immitis* and *Histoplasma capsulatum* are those most likely to involve the liver. Biliary tract disease in the form of papillary stenosis or sclerosing cholangitis has been reported in the context of cryptosporidiosis, CMV infection, and KS.

Many of the drugs used to treat HIV infection are metabolized by the liver and can cause liver injury. Nucleoside analogues work by inhibiting DNA synthesis. This can result in toxicity to mitochondria, which can lead to disturbances in oxidative metabolism. This may be manifest as hepatic steatosis and, in severe cases, lactic acidosis and fulminant liver failure. It is important to be aware of this condition and to watch for it in patients with HIV infection receiving nucleoside analogues. It is reversible if diagnosed early and the offending agent(s) discontinued. Indinavir may cause mild to moderate elevations in serum bilirubin in 10 to 15% of patients in a syndrome similar to Gilbert's syndrome.

Pancreatic injury is most commonly a consequence of drug toxicity, notably that secondary to pentamidine or dideoxynucleosides.

While up to half of patients in some series have biochemical evidence of pancreatic injury, <5% of patients show any clinical evidence of pancreatitis that is not linked to a drug toxicity.

Diseases of the Kidney and Genitourinary Tract Diseases of the kidney or genitourinary tract may be a direct consequence of HIV infection, due to an opportunistic infection or neoplasm, or related to drug toxicity. *HIV-associated nephropathy* was first described in IDUs and was initially thought to be IDU nephropathy in patients with HIV infection; it is now recognized as a true direct complication of HIV infection. HIV-associated nephropathy can be an early manifestation of HIV infection and is also seen in children. Over 90% of reported cases have been in African-American or Hispanic individuals; the disease is not only more prevalent in these populations but also more severe. Proteinuria is the hallmark of this disorder. Overall, microalbuminuria is seen in ~20% of untreated HIV-infected patients; significant proteinuria is seen in closer to 2%. Edema and hypertension are rare. Ultrasound examination reveals enlarged, hyperechogenic kidneys. A definitive diagnosis is obtained through renal biopsy. Histologically, focal segmental glomerulosclerosis is present in 80%, and mesangial proliferation in 10 to 15% of cases. Prior to effective antiretroviral therapy, this disease was characterized by relatively rapid progression to end-stage renal disease. Treatment with prednisone, 60 mg/d, has been reported to be of benefit in some cases. The incidence of this disease in patients receiving adequate antiretroviral therapy has not been well defined; however, the impression is that it has decreased in frequency. It is the leading cause of end-stage renal disease in patients with HIV infection.

Among the drugs commonly associated with renal damage in patients with HIV disease are pentamidine, amphotericin, adefovir, cidofovir, and foscarnet. TMP/SMZ may compete for tubular secretion with creatinine and cause an increase in the serum creatinine level. Sulfadiazine may crystallize in the kidney and result in an easily reversible form of renal shutdown. One of the most common drug-induced renal complications is indinavir-associated renal calculi. This condition is seen in ~10% of patients receiving this HIV protease inhibitor. It may present with a variety of manifestations, ranging from asymptomatic hematuria to renal colic. Adequate hydration is the mainstay of treatment and prevention for this condition.

Genitourinary tract infections are seen with a high frequency in patients with HIV infection; they present with dysuria, hematuria, and/or pyuria and are managed in the same fashion as in patients with HIV infection. Infections with *T. pallidum*, the etiologic agent of *syphilis*, play an important role in the HIV epidemic (Chap. 172). In HIV-negative individuals, genital syphilitic ulcers as well as the ulcers of chancroid are major predisposing factors for heterosexual transmission of HIV infection. While most HIV-infected individuals with syphilis have a typical presentation, a variety of formerly rare clinical problems may be encountered in the setting of dual infection. Among them are *lues maligna*, an ulcerating lesion of the skin due to a necrotizing vasculitis; unexplained fever; nephrotic syndrome; and neurosyphilis. The most common presentation of syphilis in the HIV-infected patient is that of *condylomata lata*, a form of secondary syphilis. Neurosyphilis may be asymptomatic or may present as acute meningitis, neuroretinitis, deafness, or stroke. The rate of neurosyphilis may be as high as 1% in patients with HIV infection. As a consequence of the immunologic abnormalities seen in the setting of HIV infection, diagnosis of syphilis through standard serologic testing may be challenging. On the one hand, a significant number of patients have false-positive Venereal Disease Research Laboratory (VDRL) tests due to polyclonal B cell activation. On the other hand, the development of a new positive VDRL may be delayed in patients with new infections, and the anti-fluorescent treponema antibody (anti-FTA) test may be negative due to immunodeficiency. Thus, dark-field examination of appropriate specimens should be performed in any patient in whom syphilis is suspected, even if the patient has a negative VDRL. Similarly, any patient with a positive serum VDRL test, neurologic findings, and an abnormal spinal fluid examination should be considered to have neurosyphilis, regardless of the CSF VDRL result. In any setting, patients treated for syphilis need to be carefully monitored to ensure adequate therapy.

Vulvovaginal candidiasis is a common problem in women with HIV infection. Symptoms include pruritus, discomfort, dyspareunia, and dysuria. Vulvar infection may present as a moribilliform rash that may extend to the thighs. Vaginal infection is usually associated with a white discharge, and plaques may be seen along an erythematous vaginal wall. Diagnosis is made by microscopic examination of the discharge for pseudohyphal elements in a 10% potassium hydroxide solution. Mild disease can be treated with topical therapy. More serious disease can be treated with fluconazole. Other causes of vaginitis include *Trichomonas* and mixed bacteria.

Diseases of the Endocrine System and Metabolic Disorders A variety of endocrine and metabolic disorders are seen in the context of HIV infection. Between 33 and 75% of patients with HIV infection receiving HAART develop a syndrome often referred to as *lipodystrophy*, consisting of elevations in plasma triglycerides, total cholesterol, apolipoprotein B, and high-density lipoprotein cholesterol as well as hyperinsulinemia. Many of these patients have been noted to have a characteristic set of body habitus changes associated with fat redistribution, consisting of truncal obesity coupled with peripheral wasting (Fig. 309-32). Truncal obesity is apparent as an increase in abdominal girth related to increases in mesenteric fat, a dorsocervical fat pad ("buffalo hump") reminiscent of patients with Cushing's syndrome, and enlargement of the breasts. The peripheral wasting is particularly noticeable in the face and buttocks and by the prominence of the veins in the legs. Other related problems include insulin-requiring diabetes mellitus and avascular necrosis of the femoral head. These changes may develop at any time ranging from approximately 6 weeks to several years following the initiation of HAART. The syndrome has been reported in association with regimens containing a variety of different drugs, and while initially reported in the setting of protease inhibitor therapy, it appears similar changes can be induced by potent protease-sparing regimens. National Cholesterol Education Program (NCEP) guidelines should be followed in the management of these lipid abnormalities (Chap. 242). Due to concerns regarding drug interactions, the most commonly utilized agents in this setting are gemfibrozil and atorvostatin.

Patients with advanced HIV disease may develop hyponatremia due to the syndrome of inappropriate antidiuretic hormone (vasopressin) secretion (SIADH) as a consequence of increased free water intake and decreased free water excretion. SIADH is usually seen in conjunction with pulmonary or CNS disease. Low serum sodium may also be due to adrenal insufficiency; concomitant high serum potassium should alert one to this possibility. Adrenal gland disease may be due to mycobacterial infections, CMV disease, cryptococcal disease, histoplasmosis, or ketoconazole toxicity.

Thyroid function is generally normal in patients with HIV infection although approximately 2 to 3% of patients may have elevations in thyroid stimulating hormone (TSH). In advanced HIV disease, infection of the thyroid gland may occur with opportunistic pathogens, including *P. carinii*, CMV, mycobacteria, *Toxoplasma gondii*, and *Cryptococcus neoformans*. These infections are generally associated with a nontender, diffuse enlargement of the thyroid gland. Thyroid function is usually normal. Diagnosis is made by fine-needle aspirate or open biopsy.

Advanced HIV disease is associated with *hypogonadism* in approximately 50% of men. While this is generally a complication of underlying illness, testicular dysfunction may also be a side effect of ganciclovir therapy. In some surveys, up to two-thirds of patients report decreased libido and one-third complain of impotence. Androgen replacement therapy should be considered in patients with symptomatic hypogonadism. HIV infection does not seem to have a significant effect on the menstrual cycle outside the setting of advanced disease.

Rheumatologic Diseases Immunologic and rheumatologic disorders are common in patients with HIV infection and range from

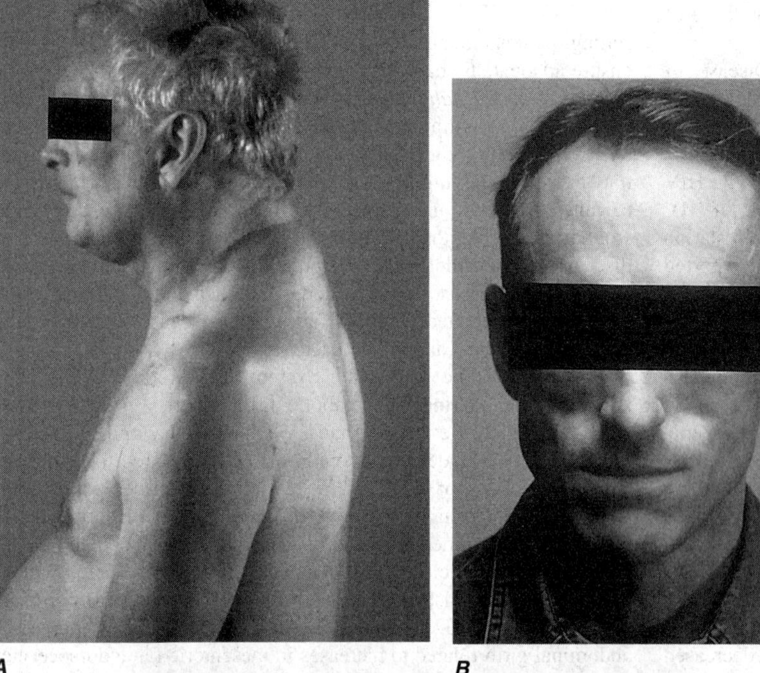

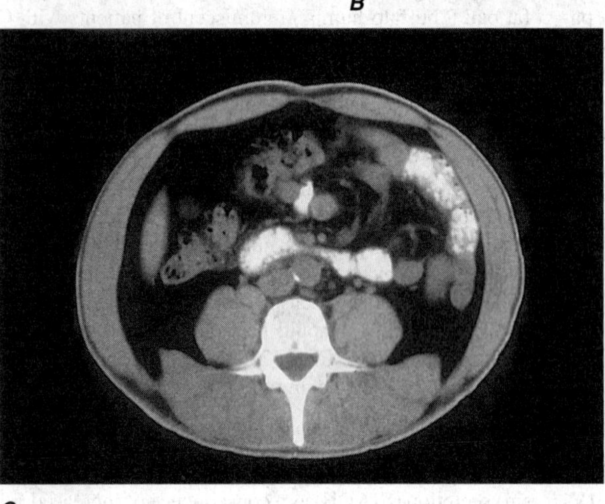

FIGURE 309-32 Characteristics of lipodystrophy. *A*. Truncal obesity and buffalo hump. *B*. Facial wasting. *C*. Accumulation of intraabdominal fat on CT scan.

excessive immediate-type hypersensitivity reactions (Chap. 310) to an increase in the incidence of reactive arthritis (Chap. 315) to conditions characterized by a diffuse infiltrative lymphocytosis. These phenomena occur in an apparent paradox to the profound immunodeficiency and immunosuppression that characterizes HIV infection. In addition, following the initiation of antiretroviral therapy, one may see a variety of exaggerated immune responses to existing opportunistic infections referred to as *immune reactivation syndromes*.

Drug allergies are the most significant allergic reactions occurring in HIV-infected patients and appear to become more common as the disease progresses. They occur in 65% of patients who receive therapy with TMP/SMZ for PCP. In general, these drug reactions are characterized by erythematous, morbilliform eruption that are pruritic, tend to coalesce, and are often associated with fever. Nonetheless, ~33% of patients can be maintained on the offending therapy, and thus these reactions are not an immediate indication to stop the drug. Anaphylaxis is extremely rare in patients with HIV infection, and patients who have a cutaneous reaction during a single course of therapy can still be considered candidates for future treatment or prophylaxis with the same agent. The one exception to this is the nucleoside analogue abacavir, where fatal hypersensitivity reactions have been reported with rechallenge. A hypersensitivity reaction to abacavir is an absolute contraindication to future therapy. For other agents, including TMP/SMZ, desensitization regimens are moderatively successful. While the mechanisms underlying these allergic-type reactions remain unknown, patients with HIV infection have been noted to have elevated IgE levels that increase as the CD4+ T cell count declines. The numerous examples of patients with multiple drug reactions suggest that a common pathway is involved.

HIV infection shares many similarities with a variety of autoimmune diseases, including a substantial polyclonal B cell activation that is associated with a high incidence of antiphospholipid antibodies, such as anticardiolipin antibodies, VDRL antibodies, and lupus-like anticoagulants. In addition, HIV-infected individuals have an increased incidence of antinuclear antibodies. Despite these serologic findings, there is no evidence that HIV-infected individuals have an increase in two of the more common autoimmune diseases, i.e., systemic lupus erythematosus and rheumatoid arthritis. In fact, it has been observed that these diseases may be somewhat ameliorated by the concomitant presence of HIV infection, suggesting that an intact CD4+ T cell limb of the immune response plays an integral role in the pathogenesis of these conditions. Similarly, there are anecdotal reports of patients with common variable immunodeficiency (Chap. 308), characterized by hypogammaglobulinemia who have had a normalization of Ig levels following the development of HIV infection, suggesting a possible role for overactive CD4+ T cell immunity in certain forms of that syndrome. The one autoimmune disease that may occur with an increased frequency in patients with HIV infection is a variant of primary Sjögren's syndrome (Chap. 314). Patients with HIV infection may develop a syndrome consisting of parotid gland enlargement, dry eyes, and dry mouth that is associated with lymphocytic infiltrates of the salivary gland and lung. In contrast to Sjögren's syndrome, in which these infiltrates are composed predominantly of CD4+ T cells, in patients with HIV infection the infiltrates are composed predominantly of CD8+ T cells. In addition, while patients with Sjögren's syndrome are mainly women who have autoantibodies to Ro and La and who frequently have HLA-DR3 or -B8, MHC haplotypes, HIV-infected individuals with this syndrome are usually African-American men who do not have anti-Ro or anti-La and who most often are HLA-DR5. This syndrome appears to be less common with the increased use of effective antiretroviral therapy. The term *diffuse infiltrative lymphocytosis syndrome* (DILS) has been proposed to describe this entity and to distinguish it from Sjögren's syndrome.

Approximately one-third of HIV-infected individuals experience arthralgias; furthermore, 5 to 10% are diagnosed as having some form of reactive arthritis, such as Reiter's syndrome or psoriatic arthritis (Chaps. 315 and 324). These syndromes occur with increasing frequency as the competency of the immune system declines. This association may be related to an increase in the number of infections with organisms that may trigger a reactive arthritis with progressive immunodeficiency. Reactive arthritides in HIV-infected individuals generally respond well to standard treatment; however, therapy with methotrexate has been associated with an increase in the incidence of opportunistic infections and should be used with caution and only in severe cases.

HIV-infected individuals also experience a variety of joint problems without obvious cause that are referred to generically as *HIV- or AIDS-associated arthropathy*. This syndrome is characterized by subacute oligoarticular arthritis developing over a period of 1 to 6 weeks and lasting 6 weeks to 6 months. It generally involves the large joints, predominantly the knees and ankles, and is nonerosive with only a mild inflammatory response. X-rays of the joint are nonrevealing. Nonsteroidal anti-inflammatory drugs are only marginally helpful; however, relief has been noted with the use of intraarticular glucocorticoids. A second form of arthritis also thought to be secondary to HIV infection is called *painful articular syndrome*. This condition, found in as many as 10% of AIDS patients, presents as an acute, severe, sharp pain in the affected joint. It affects primarily the knees, elbows, and shoulders; lasts 2 to 24 h; and may be severe enough to require narcotic analgesics. The cause of this arthropathy is unclear; however, it is thought to result from a direct effect of HIV on the joint. This condition is reminiscent of the fact that other lentiviruses, in particular the caprine arthritis-encephalitis virus, are capable of directly causing arthritis.

A variety of other immunologic or rheumatologic diseases have been reported in HIV-infected individuals, either de novo or in association with opportunistic infections or drugs. Using the criteria of widespread musculoskeletal pain of at least 3 months' duration and the presence of at least 11 of 18 possible tender points by digital palpation, 11% of an HIV-infected cohort containing 55% IDUs were diagnosed as having *fibromyalgia* (Chap. 325). While the incidence of frank arthritis was less in this population than in other studied populations that consisted predominantly of homosexual men, these data support the concept that there are musculoskeletal problems that occur as a direct result of HIV infection. In addition there have been reports of leukocytoclastic vasculitis in the setting of zidovudine therapy. CNS angiitis and polymyositis have also been reported in HIV-infected individuals. Septic arthritis is surprisingly rare, especially given the increased incidence of staphylococcal bacteremias seen in this population. When septic arthritis has been reported, it has usually been due to systemic fungal infections with *C. neoformans*, *Sporothrix schenckii*, or *H. capsulatum*, or systemic mycobacterial infection with *M. haemophilum*.

Following the initiation of effective antiretroviral therapy, a paradoxical worsening of preexisting, untreated opportunistic infections may be noted. These *immune reactivation syndromes* are particularly common in patients with underlying untreated mycobacterial infections. They appear to be related to a phenomenon similar to type IV hypersensitivity reactions and reflect the immediate improvements in immune function that occur as levels of HIV RNA drop and the immunosuppressive effects of HIV infection are controlled. In severe cases the use of immunosuppressive drugs such as glucocorticoids may be required to blunt the inflammatory component of these reactions while specific antimicrobial therapy takes effect.

Diseases of the Hematopoietic System Disorders of the hematopoietic system including lymphadenopathy, anemia, leukopenia, and/or thrombocytopenia are common throughout the course of HIV infection and may be the direct result of HIV, manifestations of secondary infections and neoplasms, or side effects of therapy (Table 309-12). Direct histologic examination and culture of lymph node or bone marrow tissue are often diagnostic. A significant percentage of bone marrow aspirates from patients with HIV infection have been reported to contain lymphoid aggregates, the precise significance of which is unknown.

Table 309-12 Causes of Bone Marrow Suppression in Patients with HIV Infection

HIV infection	Medications:
Mycobacterial infections	Zidovudine
Fungal infections	Dapsone
B19 parvovirus infection	Trimethoprim/sulfamethoxazole
Lymphoma	Pyrimethamine
	5-Flucytosine
	Ganciclovir
	Interferon-α
	Trimetrexate
	Foscarnet

Some patients, otherwise asymptomatic, may develop *persistent generalized lymphadenopathy* as an early clinical manifestation of HIV infection. This condition is defined as the presence of enlarged lymph nodes (>1 cm) in two or more extrainguinal sites for >3 months without an obvious cause. The lymphadenopathy is due to marked follicular hyperplasia in the node in response to HIV infection. The nodes are generally discrete and freely movable. This feature of HIV disease may be seen at any point in the spectrum of immune dysfunction and is not associated with an increased likelihood of developing AIDS. Paradoxically, a loss in lymphadenopathy or a decrease in lymph node size outside the setting of antiretroviral therapy may be a prognostic marker of disease progression. In patients with CD4+ T cell counts >200/μL, the differential diagnosis of lymphadenopathy includes KS and TB. In patients with more advanced disease, lymphadenopathy may also be due to lymphoma, atypical mycobacterial infection, toxoplasmosis, systemic fungal infection, or bacillary angiomatosis. While indicated in patients with CD4+ T cell counts <200/μL, lymph node biopsy is not indicated in patients with early-stage disease unless there are signs and symptoms of systemic illness, such as fever and weight loss, or unless the nodes begin to enlarge, become fixed, or coalesce.

Anemia is the most common hematologic abnormality in HIV-infected patients. While generally mild, anemia can be quite severe and require chronic blood transfusions. Among the specific reversible causes of anemia in the setting of HIV infection are drug toxicity, systemic fungal and mycobacterial infections, nutritional deficiencies, and parvovirus B19 infections. Zidovudine has a somewhat selective ability to block erythroid maturation, an effect that precedes effects on other marrow elements. A characteristic feature of zidovudine therapy is an elevated mean corpuscular volume (MCV). Another drug used in patients with HIV infection that has a selective effect on the erythroid series is dapsone. This drug can cause a serious hemolytic anemia in patients who are deficient in glucose-6-phosphate dehydrogenase and can create a functional anemia in others through induction of methemoglobinemia. Folate levels are usually normal in HIV-infected individuals; however, vitamin B_{12} levels may be depressed as a consequence of achlorhydria or malabsorption. True autoimmune hemolytic anemia is rare, although ~20% of patients with HIV infection may have a positive direct antiglobulin test as a consequence of polyclonal B cell activation. Infection with parvovirus B19 may also cause anemia. It is important to recognize this possibility given the fact that it responds well to treatment with intravenous immunoglobulin. Erythropoietin levels in patients with HIV infection and anemia are generally less than expected given the degree of anemia. Treatment with erythropoietin at doses of 100 μg/kg three times a week may result in an increase in hemoglobulin levels. An exception to this is a subset of patients with zidovudine-associated anemia in whom erythropoietin levels may be quite high.

During the course of HIV infection, neutropenia may be seen in approximately half of patients. In most instances it is mild; however, it can be severe and can put patients at risk of spontaneous bacterial infections. This is most frequently seen in patients with severely advanced HIV disease and in patients receiving any of a number of potentially myelosuppressive therapies. In the setting of neutropenia, diseases that are not commonly seen in HIV-infected patients, such as aspergillosis or mucormycosis, may occur. The potential role of colony-stimulating factors in the management of patients with HIV infection has undergone extensive evaluation. Both granulocyte colony stimulating factor (G-CSF) and GM-CSF increase neutrophil counts in patients with HIV infection regardless of the cause of the neutropenia. Earlier concerns about the potential of these agents to also increase levels of HIV were not confirmed in controlled clinical trials.

Thrombocytopenia may be an early consequence of HIV infection. Approximately 3% of patients with untreated HIV infection and CD4+ T cell counts ≥400/μL have platelet counts <150,000/μL. For untreated patients with CD4+ T cell counts <400/μL, this incidence increases to 10%. Thrombocytopenia is rarely a serious clinical problem in patients with HIV infection and generally responds well to antiretroviral therapy. Clinically, it resembles the thrombocytopenia seen in patients with idiopathic thrombocytopenic purpura (Chap. 116). Immune complexes containing anti-gp120 antibodies and anti-anti gp120 antibodies have been noted in the circulation and on the surface of platelets in patients with HIV infection. Patients with HIV infection have also been noted to have a platelet-specific antibody directed towards a 25-kDa component of the surface of the platelet. Other data suggest that the thrombocytopenia in patients with HIV infection may be due to a direct effect of HIV on megakaryocytes. Whatever the cause, it is very clear that the most effective medical approach to this problem has been the use of combination antiretroviral therapy. For patients with platelet counts <20,000/μL a more aggressive approach combining intravenous Ig or anti-Rh Ig for an immediate response with antiretroviral therapy for a more lasting response is appropriate. Splenectomy is a rarely needed option and is reserved for patients refractory to medical management. Because of the risk of serious infection with encapsulated organisms, all patients with HIV infection about to undergo splenectomy should be immunized with pneumococcal polysaccharide. It should be noted that, in addition to causing an increase in the platelet count, removal of the spleen will result in an increase in the peripheral blood lymphocyte count, making CD4+ T cell counts unreliable. In this setting, the clinician should rely on the CD4+ T cell percent for making diagnostic decisions with respect to the likelihood of opportunistic infections. A CD4+ T cell percent of 15 is approximately equivalent to a CD4+ T cell count of 200/μL. In patients with early HIV infection, thrombocytopenia has also been reported as a consequence of classic thrombotic thrombocytopenic purpura (Chap. 116). This clinical syndrome, consisting of fever, thrombocytopenia, hemolytic anemia, and neurologic and renal dysfunction, is a rare complication of early HIV infection. As in other settings, the appropriate management is the use of salicylates and plasma exchange. Other causes of thrombocytopenia include lymphoma, mycobacterial infections, and fungal infections.

Dermatologic Diseases Dermatologic problems occur in >90% of patients with HIV infection. From the macular, roseola-like rash seen with the acute seroconversion syndrome to extensive end-stage KS, cutaneous manifestations of HIV disease can be seen throughout the course of HIV infection. Among the more common nonneoplastic problems are seborrheic dermatitis, eosinophilic pustular folliculitus, and opportunistic infections. Extrapulmonary pneumocystosis may cause a necrotizing vasculitis. Neoplastic conditions are covered below in the section on malignant diseases.

Seborrheic dermatitis occurs in 3% of the general population and in up to 50% of patients with HIV infection. Seborrheic dermatitis increases in prevalence and severity as the CD4+ T cell count declines. In HIV-infected patients, seborrheic dermatitis may be aggravated by concomitant infection with *Pityrosporum*, a yeastlike fungus; use of topical antifungal agents has been recommended in cases refractory to standard topical treatment.

Eosinophilic pustular folliculitis is a rare dermatologic condition that is seen with increased frequency in patients with HIV infection. It presents as multiple, urticarial perifollicular papules that may coalesce into plaquelike lesions. Skin biopsy reveals an eosinophilic infiltrate of the hair follicle, which in certain cases has been associated with the presence of a mite. Patients typically have an elevated serum IgE level and may respond to treatment with topical anthelminthics. Patients with HIV infection have also been reported to develop a severe form of *Norwegian scabies* with hyperkeratotic psoriasiform lesions.

Both *psoriasis* and *ichthyosis*, although they are not reported to be increased in frequency, may be particularly severe when they occur in patients with HIV infection. Preexisting psoriasis may become guttate in appearance and more refractory to treatment in the setting of HIV infection.

Reactivation herpes zoster (*shingles*) is seen in 10 to 20% of patients with HIV infection. This reactivation syndrome of varicella-zoster virus indicates a modest decline in immune function and may be the first indication of clinical immunodeficiency. In one series, patients who developed shingles did so an average of 5 years after HIV infection. In a cohort of patients with HIV infection and localized zoster, the subsequent rate of the development of AIDS was 1% per month. In that study, AIDS was more likely to develop if the outbreak of zoster was associated with severe pain, extensive skin involvement, or involvement of cranial or cervical dermatomes. The clinical manifestations of reactivation zoster in HIV-infected patients, although indicative of immunologic compromise, are not as severe as those seen in other immunodeficient conditions. Thus, while lesions may extend over several dermatomes **(see Plate IID-37)** and frank cutaneous dissemination may be seen, visceral involvement has not been reported. In contrast to patients without a known underlying immunodeficiency state, patients with HIV infection tend to have recurrences of zoster with a relapse rate of approximately 20%. Acyclovir or famciclovir is the treatment of choice. Foscarnet is of value in patients with acyclovir-resistant virus.

Infection with *herpes simplex virus* in HIV-infected individuals is associated with recurrent orolabial, genital, and perianal lesions as part of recurrent reactivation syndromes (Chap. 182). As HIV disease progresses and the CD4+ T cell count declines, these infections become more frequent and severe. Lesions often appear as beefy red, are exquisitely painful, and have a tendency to occur high in the gluteal cleft (Fig. 309-31). Perirectal HSV may be associated with proctitis and anal fissures. HSV should be high in the differential diagnosis of any HIV-infected patient with a poorly healing, painful perirectal lesion. In addition to recurrent mucosal ulcers, recurrent HSV infection in the form of *herpetic whitlow* can be a problem in patients with HIV infection, presenting with painful vesicles or extensive cutaneous erosion. Acyclovir or famciclovir is the treatment of choice in these settings.

Diffuse skin eruptions due to *Molluscum contagiosum* may be seen in patients with advanced HIV infection. These flesh-colored, umbilicated lesions may be treated with local therapy. They tend to regress with effective antiretroviral therapy. Similarly, *condyloma acuminatum* lesions may be more severe and more widely distributed in patients with low CD4+ T cell counts. Atypical mycobacterial infections may present as erythematous cutaneous nodules as may fungal infections, *Bartonella*, *Acanthamoeba*, and KS.

The skin of patients with HIV infection is often a target organ for drug reactions (Chap. 59). Although most skin reactions are mild and not necessarily an indication to discontinue therapy, patients may have particularly severe cutaneous reactions, including erythroderma and *Stevens-Johnson syndrome*, as a reaction to drugs, particularly sulfa drugs, the nonnucleoside reverse transcriptase inhibitors, abacavir, and amprenavir. Similarly, patients with HIV infection are often quite photosensitive and burn easily following exposure to sunlight or as a side effect of radiation therapy (see Chap. 60).

HIV infection and its treatment may be accompanied by cosmetic changes of the skin that are not of great clinical importance but may be troubling to patients. Yellowing of the nails and straightening of the hair, particularly in African-American patients, have been reported as a consequence of HIV infection. Zidovudine therapy has been associated with elongation of the eyelashes and the development of a bluish discoloration to the nails, again more common in African-American patients. Therapy with clofazimine may cause a yellow-orange discoloration of the skin.

Neurologic Diseases Clinical disease of the nervous system accounts for a significant degree of morbidity in a high percentage of patients with HIV infection (Table 309-13). The neurologic problems that occur in HIV-infected individuals may be either primary to the pathogenic processes of HIV infection or secondary to opportunistic infections or neoplasms (see above). Among the more frequent opportunistic diseases that involve the CNS are toxoplasmosis, cryptococcosis, progressive multifocal leukoencephalopathy, and primary

Table 309-13 Neurologic Diseases in Patients with HIV Infection

Opportunistic infections
- Toxoplasmosis
- Cryptococcosis
- Progressive multifocal leukoencephalopathy
- Cytomegalovirus
- Syphilis
- Mycobacterium tuberculosis
- HTLV-I infection

Neoplasms
- Primary CNS lymphoma
- Kaposi's sarcoma

Result of HIV-1 infection
- Aseptic meningitis
- HIV encephalopathy (AIDS dementia complex)
- Myelopathy
  - Vacuolar myelopathy
  - Pure sensory ataxia
  - Paresthesia/dysesthesia
- Peripheral neuropathy
  - Acute inflammatory demyelinating polyneuropathy (Guillain-Barré syndrome)
  - Chronic inflammatory demyelinating polyneuropathy (CIDP)
  - Mononeuritis multiplex
  - Distal symmetric polyneuropathy
- Myopathy

CNS lymphoma. Other less common problems include mycobacterial infections; syphilis; and infection with CMV, HTLV-I, or *Acanthamoeba*. Overall, secondary diseases of the CNS occur in approximately one-third of patients with AIDS. These data antedate the widespread use of combination antiretroviral therapy, and this frequency is considerably less in patients receiving effective antiretroviral drugs. Primary processes related to HIV infection of the nervous system are reminiscent of those seen with other lentiviruses, such as the Visna-Maedi virus of sheep. Neurologic problems occur throughout the course of disease and may be inflammatory, demyelinating, or degenerative in nature. While only one of these, the *AIDS dementia complex*, or *HIV encephalopathy*, is considered an AIDS-defining illness, most HIV-infected patients have some neurologic problem during the course of their disease. As noted in the section on pathogenesis, damage to the CNS may be a direct result of viral infection of the CNS macrophages or glial cells or may be secondary to the release of neurotoxins and potentially toxic cytokines such as IL-1β, TNF-α, IL-6, and TGF-β. Virtually all patients with HIV infection have some degree of nervous system involvement with the virus. This is evidenced by the fact that CSF findings are abnormal in approximately 90% of patients, even during the asymptomatic phase of HIV infection. CSF abnormalities include pleocytosis (50 to 65% of patients), detection of viral RNA (~75%), elevated CSF protein (35%), and evidence of intrathecal synthesis of anti-HIV antibodies (90%). It is important to point out that evidence of infection of the CNS with HIV does not imply impairment of cognitive function. The neurologic function of an HIV-infected individual should be considered normal unless clinical signs and symptoms suggest otherwise.

Aseptic meningitis may be seen in any but the very late stages of HIV infection. In the setting of acute primary infection patients may experience a syndrome of headache, photophobia, and meningismus. Rarely, an acute encephalopathy due to encephalitis may occur. Cranial nerve involvement may be seen, predominantly cranial nerve VII but occasionally V and/or VIII. CSF findings include a lymphocytic pleocytosis, elevated protein level, and normal glucose level. This syndrome, which cannot be clinically differentiated from other viral meningitides (Chap. 373), usually resolves spontaneously within 2 to 4 weeks; however, in some patients, signs and symptoms may become chronic. Aseptic meningitis may occur any time in the course of HIV infection; however, it is rare following the development of AIDS. This fact suggests that clinical aseptic meningitis in the context of HIV infection is an immune-mediated disease.

C. neoformans is the leading infectious cause of meningitis in patients with AIDS (Chap. 204). It is the initial AIDS-defining illness in approximately 2% of patients and generally occurs in patients with CD4+ T cell counts <100/μL. Cryptococcal meningitis is particularly common in patients with AIDS in Africa, occurring in ~20% of patients. Most patients resent with a picture of subacute meningoencephalitis with fever, nausea, vomiting, altered mental status, headache, and meningeal signs. The incidence of seizures and focal neurologic deficits is low. The CSF profile may be normal or may show only modest elevations in WBC or protein levels. In addition to meningitis, patients may develop cryptococcomas. Approximately one-third of patients also have pulmonary disease. Uncommon manifestations of cryptococcal infection include skin lesions that resemble *molluscum contagiosum*, lymphadenopathy, palatal and glossal ulcers, arthritis, gastroenteritis, myocarditis, and prostatitis. The prostate gland may serve as a reservoir for smoldering cryptococcal infection. The diagnosis of cryptococcal meningitis is made by identification of organisms in spinal fluid with India ink examination or by the detection of cryptococcal antigen. A biopsy may be needed to make a diagnosis of CNS cryptococcoma. Treatment is with intravenous amphotericin B, at a dose of 0.7 mg/kg daily, with flucytosine, 25 mg/kg qid for 2 weeks, followed by fluconazole, 400 mg/d orally for 8 weeks, and then fluconazole, 200 mg/d for life. Other fungi that may cause meningitis in patients with HIV infection are *C. immitis* and *H. capsulatum*. Meningoencephalitis has also been reported due to *Acanthamoeba* or *Naegleria*.

HIV encephalopathy, also called HIV-associated dementia or AIDS dementia complex, consists of a constellation of signs and symptoms of CNS disease that generally occurs late in the course of HIV infection and progresses slowly over months. A major feature of this entity is the development of dementia, defined as a decline in cognitive ability from a previous level. It may present as impaired ability to concentrate, increased forgetfulness, difficulty reading, or increased difficulty performing complex tasks. Initially these symptoms may be indistinguishable from findings of situational depression or fatigue. In contrast to "cortical" dementia (such as Alzheimer's disease), aphasia, apraxia, and agnosia are uncommon, leading some investigators to classify HIV encephalopathy as a "subcortical dementia" (see below). In addition to dementia, patients with HIV encephalopathy may also have motor and behavioral abnormalities. Among the motor problems are unsteady gait, poor balance, tremor, and difficulty with rapid alternating movements. Increased tone and deep tendon reflexes may be found in patients with spinal cord involvement. Late stages may be complicated by bowel and/or bladder incontinence. Behavioral problems include apathy and lack of initiative, with progression to a vegetative state in some instances. Some patients develop a state of agitation or mild mania. These changes usually occur without significant changes in level of alertness. This is in contrast to the finding of somnolence in patients with dementia due to toxic/metabolic encephalopathies.

HIV encephalopathy is the initial AIDS-defining illness in approximately 3% of patients with HIV infection and thus only rarely precedes clinical evidence of immunodeficiency. Clinically significant encephalopathy eventually develops in approximately one-fourth of patients with AIDS. As immunologic function declines, the risk and severity of HIV encephalopathy increases. Autopsy series suggest that 80 to 90% of patients with HIV infection have histologic evidence of CNS involvement. Several classification schemes have been developed for grading HIV encephalopathy; a commonly used clinical staging system is outlined in Table 309-14.

The precise cause of HIV encephalopathy remains unclear, although the condition is thought to be a result of direct effects of HIV on the CNS. HIV has been found in the brains of patients with HIV encephalopathy by Southern blot, in situ hybridization, PCR, and electron microscopy. Multinucleated giant cells, macrophages, and microglial cells appear to be the main cell types harboring virus in the CNS. Histologically, the major changes are seen in the subcortical

Table 309-14 Clinical Staging of HIV Encephalopathy (AIDS Dementia Complex)

Stage	Definition
Stage 0 (normal)	Normal mental and motor function
Stage 0.5 (equivocal/ subclinical)	Absent, minimal, or equivocal symptoms without impairment of work or capacity to perform activities of daily living. Mild signs (snout response, slowed ocular or extremity movements) may be present. Gait and strength are normal.
Stage 1 (mild)	Able to perform all but the more demanding aspects of work or activities of daily living but with unequivocal evidence (signs or symptoms that may include performance on neuropsychological testing) of functional, intellectual, or motor impairment. Can walk without assistance.
Stage 2 (moderate)	Able to perform basic activities of self-care but cannot work or maintain the more demanding aspects of daily life. Ambulatory, but may require a single prop.
Stage 3 (severe)	Major intellectual incapacity (cannot follow news or personal events, cannot sustain complex conversation, considerable slowing of all output) or motor disability (cannot walk unassisted, usually with slowing and clumsiness of arms as well).
Stage 4 (end-stage)	Nearly vegetative. Intellectual and social comprehension and output are at a rudimentary level. Nearly or absolutely mute. Paraparetic or paraplegic with urinary and fecal incontinence.

SOURCE: Adapted from JJ Sidtis, RW Price, Neurology 40:197, 1990.

Table 309-15 Mini-Mental Status Examination

Question	Scoring	Maximum Score
1. Where are you (state, county, city, hospital, clinic)?	1 point for each	5
2. What are the (day, date, month, season, year, time)?	1 point for each	5
3. "Say these three words after me: (yellow, apple, Ohio)"	1 point for each	3
4. Ask patient to begin with 100 and count backwards by 7's. Or, if patient refuses, ask to spell "world" backwards.	Stop after 5, score no. correct Or 1 point for each correct letter	5
5. Recall the three words given in question no. 3.	1 point for each	3
6. Ask the patient to name "watch" then "pencil."	1 point for each	2
7. Ask the patient to repeat "No ifs, ands, or buts."	1 point if correct	1
8. Three-stage command: Take this paper in your right hand, fold it in half, and put it on the floor.	1 point for each correct	3
9. Ask the patient to read silently and obey the command (print in block letters): CLOSE YOUR EYES.	1 point if correct	1
10. Ask the patient to write a sentence.	1 point if it contains a subject and verb and makes sense (ignore spelling and grammar)	1
11. "Draw a clock with numbers and hands showing the time to be 8: 20	2 points if correct	2
12. Have the patient copy this design:	1 point if all sides and angles are preserved and if intersecting sides form a quadrangle	1

areas of the brain and include pallor and gliosis, multinucleated giant cell encephalitis, and vacuolar myelopathy. Less commonly, diffuse or focal spongiform changes occur in the white matter.

There are no specific criteria for a diagnosis of HIV encephalopathy, and this syndrome must be differentiated from a number of other diseases that affect the CNS of HIV-infected patients (Table 309-13). The diagnosis of dementia depends upon demonstrating a decline in cognitive function. This can be accomplished objectively with the use of a Mini-Mental Status Examination (MMSE) (Table 309-15) in patients for whom prior scores are available. For this reason, it is advisable for all patients with a diagnosis of HIV infection to have a baseline MMSE. However, changes in MMSE scores may be absent in patients with mild HIV encephalopathy. Imaging studies of the CNS, by either MRI or CT, often demonstrate evidence of cerebral atrophy (Fig. 309-33). MRI may also reveal small areas of increased density on T2-weighted images. Lumbar puncture is an important element of the evaluation of patients with HIV infection and neurologic abnormalities. It is generally most helpful in ruling out or making a diagnosis of opportunistic infections. In HIV encephalopathy, patients may have the nonspecific findings of an increase in CSF cells and protein level. While HIV RNA can often be detected in the spinal fluid and HIV can be cultured from the CSF, this finding is not specific for HIV encephalopathy. There appears to be no correlation between the presence of HIV in the CSF and the presence of HIV encephalopathy. Elevated levels of β_2-microglobulin, neopterin, and quinolinic acid (a metabolite of tryptophan reported to cause CNS injury) have been noted in the CSF of patients with HIV encephalopathy. These findings suggest that these factors as well as inflammatory cytokines may be involved in the pathogenesis of this syndrome.

Combination antiretroviral therapy is of benefit in patients with HIV encephalopathy. Improvement in neuropsychiatric test scores has been noted for both adult and pediatric patients treated with antiretrovirals. The rapid improvement in cognitive function noted with the initiation of antiretroviral therapy suggests that at least some component of this problem is quickly reversible, again supporting at least a partial role of soluble mediators in the pathogenesis. It should also be noted that these patients have an increased sensitivity to the side effects of neuroleptic drugs. The use of these drugs for symptomatic treatment is associated with an increased risk of extrapyramidal side effects; therefore, patients with HIV encephalopathy who receive these agents must be monitored carefully.

Seizures may be a consequence of opportunistic infections, neoplasms, or HIV encephalopathy (Table 309-16). The seizure threshold is often lower than normal in these patients owing to the frequent presence of electrolyte abnormalities. Seizures are seen in 15 to 40% of patients with cerebral toxoplasmosis, 15 to 35% of patients with primary CNS lymphoma, 8% of patients with cryptococcal meningitis, and 7 to 50% of patients with HIV encephalopathy. Seizures may also be seen in patients with CNS tuberculosis, aseptic meningitis, and progressive multifocal leukoencephalopathy. Seizures may be the presenting clinical symptom of HIV disease. In one study of 100 patients with HIV infection presenting with a first seizure, cerebral mass lesions were the most common cause, responsible for 32 of the 100 new-onset seizures. Of these 32 cases, 28 were due to toxoplasmosis and 4 to lymphoma. HIV encephalopathy accounted for an additional 24 new-onset seizures. Cryptococcal meningitis

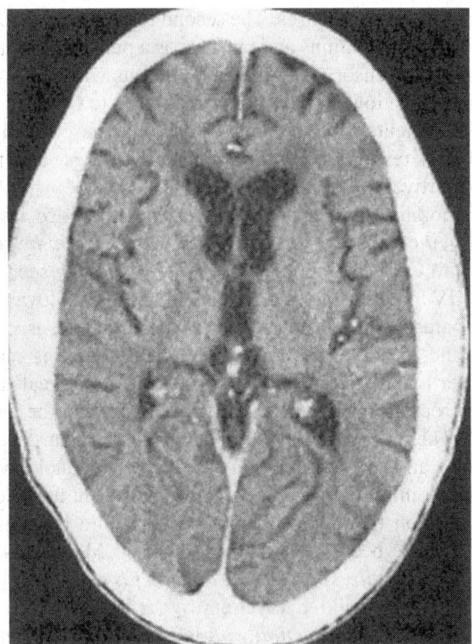

FIGURE 309-33 AIDS dementia complex. Postcontrast CT scan through the lateral ventricles of a 47-year old man with AIDS, altered mental status, and dementia. The lateral and third ventricles and the cerebral sulci are abnormally prominent. Mild white matter hypodensity is also seen adjacent to the frontal horns of the lateral ventricles.

was the third most common diagnosis, responsible for 13 of the 100 seizures. In 23 cases, no cause could be found, and it is possible that these cases represent a subcategory of HIV encephalopathy. Of these 23 cases, 16 (70%) had two or more seizures, suggesting that anticonvulsant therapy is indicated in all patients with HIV infection and seizures unless a rapidly correctable cause is found. While phenytoin remains the initial treatment of choice, hypersensitivity reactions to this drug have been reported in >10% of patients with AIDS, and therefore the use of phenobarbital or valproic acid must be considered as alternatives.

Patients with HIV infection may present with *focal neurologic deficits* from a variety of causes. The most common cause are toxoplasmosis, progressive multifocal leukoencephalopathy, and CNS lymphoma. Other causes include cryptococcal infections (discussed above; also Chap. 204), stroke, and reactivation Chagas' disease.

Toxoplasmosis has been one of the most common causes of secondary CNS infections in patients with AIDS, but its incidence is decreasing in the era of HAART. It is most common in patients from the Caribbean and from France. Toxoplasmosis is generally a late complication of HIV infection and usually occurs in patients with CD4+ T cell counts <200/μL. Cerebral toxoplasmosis is thought to represent a reactivation syndrome. It is 10 times more common in patients with antibodies to the organism than in patients who are seronegative. Patients diagnosed with HIV infection should be screened for IgG antibodies to *T. gondii* during the time of their initial workup. Those who are seronegative should be counseled about ways to minimize the risk

Table 309-16 Causes of Seizures in Patients with HIV Infection

Disease	Overall Contribution to First Seizure, %	Fraction of Patients Who Have Seizures, %
HIV encephalopathy	24–47	7–50
Cerebral toxoplasmosis	28	15–40
Cryptococcal meningitis	13	8
Primary central nervous system lymphoma	4	15–30
Progressive multifocal leukoencephalopathy	1	

SOURCE: From Holtzman et al.

of primary infection including avoiding the consumption of undercooked meat and careful hand washing after contact with soil or changing the cat litter box. The most common clinical presentation in patients with HIV infection is fever, headache, and focal neurologic deficits. Patients may present with seizure, hemiparesis, or aphasia as a manifestation of these focal deficits or with a picture more influenced by the accompanying cerebral edema and characterized by confusion, dementia, and lethargy, which can progress to coma. The diagnosis is usually suspected on the basis of MRI findings of multiple lesions in multiple locations, although in come cases only a single lesion is seen. Pathologically, these lesions generally exhibit inflammation and central necrosis and, as a result, demonstrate ring enhancement on contrast MRI (Fig. 309-34) or, if MRI is unavailable or contraindicated, on double-dose contrast CT. There is usually evidence of surrounding edema. In addition to toxoplasmosis, the differential diagnosis of single or multiple enhancing mass lesions in the HIV-infected patient includes primary CNS lymphoma (see below) and, less commonly, TB or fungal or bacterial abscesses. The definitive diagnostic procedure is brain biopsy. However, given the morbidity than can accompany this procedure, it is usually reserved for the patient who has failed 2 to 4 weeks of empirical therapy. If the patient is seronegative for *T. gondii*, the likelihood that a mass lesion is due to toxoplasmosis is <10%. In that setting, one may choose to be more aggressive and perform a brain biopsy sooner. Standard treatment is sulfadiazine and pyrimethamine with leucovorin as needed for a minimum of 4 to 6 weeks. Alternative therapeutic regimens include clindamycin in combination with pyrimethamine; atovaquone plus pyrimethamine; and azithromycin plus pyrimethamine plus rifabutin. Relapses are common, and it is recommended that patients with a history of prior toxoplasmic encephalitis receive maintenance therapy with sulfadiazine, pyrimethamine, and leucovorin. Patients with CD4+ T cell counts <100/μL and IgG antibody to *Toxoplasma* should receive primary prophylaxis for toxoplasmosis. Fortunately, the same daily regimen of a single double-strength tablet of TMP/SMZ used for *P. carinii* prophylaxis provides adequate primary protection against toxoplasmosis. It is likely that future recommendations will allow for discontinuation of prophylaxis for toxoplasmosis in the setting of effective antiretroviral therapy and increases in CD4+ T cell counts to >100/μL for 3 to 6 months.

JC virus, a human papilloma virus that is the etiologic agent of *progressive multifocal leukoencephalopathy* (PML), is an important opportunistic pathogen in patients with AIDS (Chap. 373). While approximately 70% of the general adult population have antibodies to

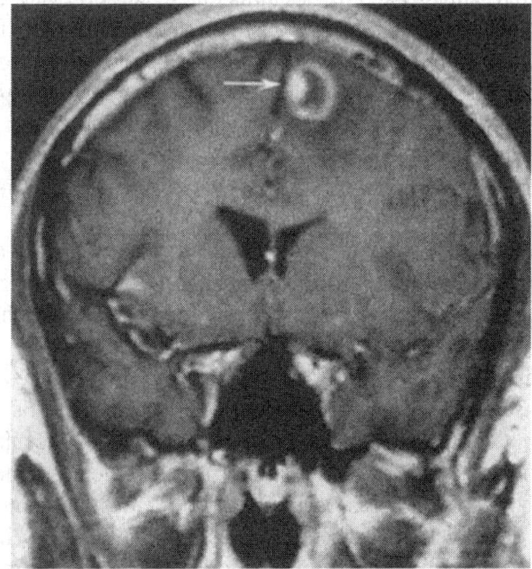

FIGURE 309-34 CNS toxoplasmosis. A coronal postcontrast T1 weighted MR scan demonstrates a peripheral enhancing lesion in the left frontal lobe, associated with an eccentric nodular area of enhancement (*arrow*); this so-called "eccentric target sign" is typical of toxoplasmosis.

JC virus, indicative of prior infection, <10% of healthy adults show any evidence of ongoing viral replication. PML is the only known clinical manifestation of JC virus infection. It is a late manifestation of AIDS and is seen in ~4% of patients with AIDS. The lesions of PML begin as small foci of demyelination in subcortical white matter that eventually coalesce. The cerebral hemispheres, cerebellum, and brainstem may all be involved. Patients typically have a protracted course with multifocal neurologic deficits, with or without changes in mental status. Ataxia, hemiparesis, visual field defects, aphasia, and sensory defects may occur. MRI typically reveals multiple, nonenhancing white matter lesions that may coalesce and have a predeliction for the occipital and parietal lobes. The lesions show signal hyperintensity on T2-weighted images and diminished signal on T1-weighted images. Prior to the availability of potent antiretroviral combination therapy, the majority of patients with PML died within 3 to 6 months of the onset of symptoms. There is no specific treatment for PML; however, regressions of more than 2.5 years in duration have been reported in patients with PML treated with HAART for their HIV disease. Factors influencing a favorable prognosis include a CD4+ T cell count >100/μL at baseline and the ability to maintain an HIV viral load of <500 copies per milliliter. Baseline viral load does not have independent predictive value of survival. Of note, PML is one of the few opportunistic infections that continue to occur with some frequency despite the widespread use of HAART.

Reactivation American trypanosomiasis may present as acute meningoencephalitis with focal neurologic signs, fever, headache, vomiting, and seizures. In South America, reactivation of *Chagas' disease* is considered to be an AIDS-defining condition and may be the initial AIDS-defining condition. Lesions appear radiographically as single or multiple hypodense areas, typically with ring enhancement and edema. They are found predominantly in the subcortical areas, a feature that differentiates them from the deeper lesions of toxoplasmosis. *Trypanosoma cruzi* amastigotes, or trypanosomes, can be identified from biopsy specimens or CSF. Other CSF findings include elevated protein and a mild (<100 cells/μL) lymphocytic pleocytosis. Organisms can also be identified by direct examination of the blood. Treatment consists of benzimidazole (2.5 mg/kg bid) or nifurtimox (1 mg/kg tid) for at least 60 days, followed by maintenance therapy for life with either drug at a dose of 5 mg/kg three times a week.

Stroke may occur in patients with HIV infection. In contrast to the other causes of focal neurologic deficits in patients with HIV infection, the symptoms of a stroke are sudden in onset. Among the secondary infectious diseases in patients with HIV infection that may be associated with stroke are vasculitis due to cerebral varicella zoster or neurosyphilis and septic embolism in association with fungal infection. Other elements of the differential diagnosis of stroke in the patient with HIV infection include atherosclerotic cerebral vascular disease, thrombotic thrombocytopenic purpura, and cocaine or amphetamine use.

Primary CNS lymphoma is discussed below in the section on neoplastic diseases.

Spinal cord disease, or myelopathy, is present in approximately 20% of patients with AIDS, often as part of HIV encephalopathy. In fact, 90% of the patients with HIV-associated myelopathy have some evidence of dementia, suggesting that similar pathologic processes may be responsible for both conditions. Three main types of spinal cord disease are seen in patients with AIDS. The first of these is a vacuolar myelopathy, as discussed above under HIV encephalopathy. This condition is pathologically similar to subacute combined degeneration of the cord such as occurs with pernicious anemia. Although vitamin B_{12} deficiency can be seen in patients with AIDS, it does not appear to be responsible for the myelopathy seen in the majority of patients. Vacuolar myelopathy is characterized by a subacute onset and often presents with gait disturbances, predominantly ataxia and spasticity; it may progress to include bladder and bowel dysfunction. Physical findings include evidence of increased deep tendon reflexes and extensor plantar responses. The second form of spinal cord disease involves the dorsal columns and presents as a pure sensory ataxia. The third form is also sensory in nature and presents with paresthesias and dysesthesias of the lower extremities. In contrast to the cognitive problems seen in patients with HIV encephalopathy, these spinal cord syndromes do not respond well to antiretroviral drugs, and therapy is mainly supportive.

One important disease of the spinal cord that also involves the peripheral nerves is a *myelopathy* and *polyradiculopathy* seen in association with CMV infection. This entity is generally seen late in the course of HIV infection and is fulminant in onset, with lower extremity and sacral paresthesias, difficulty in walking, areflexia, ascending sensory loss, and urinary retention. The clinical course is rapidly progressive over a period of weeks. CSF examination reveals a predominantly neutrophilic pleocytosis, and CMV DNA can be detected by CSF PCR. Therapy with ganciclovir or foscarnet can lead to rapid improvement, and prompt initiation of foscarnet or ganciclovir therapy is important in minimizing the degree of permanent neurologic damage. Combination therapy with both drugs should be considered in patients who have been previously treated for CMV disease.→*Other diseases involving the spinal cord in patients with HIV infection include* **HTLV-I-associated myelopathy** *(HAM) (Chap. 191), neurosyphilis (Chap. 172), infection with herpes simplex (Chap. 182) or varicella-zoster (Chap. 183), TB (Chap. 169), and lymphoma (Chap. 112).*

Peripheral neuropathies are common in patients with HIV infection. They occur at all stages of illness and take a variety of forms. Early in the course of HIV infection, an acute inflammatory demyelinating polyneuropathy resembling Guillain-Barré syndrome may occur (Chap. 378). In other patients, a progressive or relapsing-remitting inflammatory neuropathy resembling chronic inflammatory demyelinating polyneuropathy (CIDP) has been noted. Patients commonly present with progressive weakness, areflexia, and minimal sensory changes. CSF examination often reveals a mononuclear pleocytosis, and peripheral nerve biopsy demonstrates a perivascular infiltrate suggesting an autoimmune etiology. Plasma exchange or intravenous immunoglobulin has been tried with variable success. Because of the immunosuppressive effects of glucocorticoids, they should be reserved for severe cases of CIDP refractory to other measures. Another autoimmune peripheral neuropathy seen in patients with AIDS is mononeuritis multiplex (Chaps. 378 and 317) due to a necrotizing arteritis of peripheral nerves. The most common peripheral neuropathy in patients with HIV infection is a *distal sensory polyneuropathy* that may be a direct consequence of HIV infection or a side effect of dideoxynucleoside therapy. Two-thirds of patients with AIDS may be shown by electrophysiologic studies to have some evidence of peripheral nerve disease. Presenting symptoms are usually painful burning sensations in the feet and lower extremities. Findings on examination include a stocking-type sensory loss to pinprick, temperature, and touch sensation and a loss of ankle reflexes. Motor changes are mild and are usually limited to weakness of the intrinsic foot muscles. Response of this condition to antiretrovirals has been variable, perhaps because antiretrovirals are responsible for the problem in some instances. When due to dideoxynucleoside therapy, patients with lower extremity peripheral neuropathy may complain of a sensation that they are walking on ice. Other entities in the differential diagnosis of peripheral neuropathy include diabetes mellitus, vitamin B_{12} deficiency, and side effects from metronidazole or dapsone. For distal symmetric polyneuropathy that fails to resolve following the discontinuation of dideoxynucleosides, therapy is symptomatic; gabapentin, carbamazepine, tricyclics, or analgesics may be effective for dysesthesias. Some patients may respond to combination antiretroviral therapy, and preliminary data suggest that nerve growth factor may benefit some cases.

Myopathy may complicate the course of HIV infection; causes include HIV infection itself, zidovudine, and the generalized wasting syndrome. HIV-associated myopathy may range in severity from an asymptomatic elevation in creatine kinase levels to a subacute syndrome characterized by proximal muscle weakness and myalgias.

Quite pronounced elevations in creatine kinase may occur in asymptomatic patients, particularly after exercise. The clinical significance of this as an isolated laboratory finding is unclear. A variety of both inflammatory and noninflammatory pathologic processes have been noted in patients with more severe myopathy, including myofiber necrosis with inflammatory cells, nemaline rod bodies, cytoplasmic bodies, and mitochondrial abnormalities. Profound muscle wasting, often with muscle pain, may be seen after prolonged zidovudine therapy. This toxic side effect of the drug is dose-dependent and is related to its ability to interfere with the function of mitochondrial polymerases. It is reversible following discontinuation of the drug. Red ragged fibers are a histologic hallmark of zidovudine-induced myopathy.

Ophthalmologic Disease Ophthalmologic problems occur in approximately half of patients with advanced HIV infection. The most common abnormal findings on funduscopic examination are cotton-wool spots. These are hard white spots that appear on the surface of the retina and often have an irregular edge. They represent areas of retinal ischemia secondary to microvascular disease. At times they are associated with small areas of hemorrhage and thus can be difficult to distinguish from CMV retinitis. In contrast to CMV retinitis, however, these lesions are not associated with visual loss and tend to remain stable or improve over time.

One of the most devastating consequences of HIV infection is CMV retinitis. Patients at high risk of CMV retinitis (CD4+ T cell count $<100/\mu L$) should undergo an ophthalmologic examination every 3 to 6 months. The majority of cases of CMV retinitis occur in patients with a CD4+ T cell count $<50/\mu L$. Prior to the availability of HAART, this CMV reactivation syndrome was seen in 25 to 30% of patients with AIDS. CMV retinitis usualy presents as a painless, progressive loss of vision. Patients may also complain of blurred vision, "floaters," and scintillations. The disease is usually bilateral, affecting one eye more than the other. The diagnosis is made on clinical grounds by an experienced ophthalmologist. The characteristic retinal appearance is that of perivascular hemorrhage and exudate **(see Plate III-1)**. In situations where the diagnosis is in doubt due to an atypical presentation or an unexpected lack of response to therapy, vitreous or aqueous humor sampling with molecular diagnostic techniques may be of value. CMV infection of the retina results in a necrotic inflammatory process, and the visual loss that develops is irreversible. As a consequence of retinal atrophy in areas or prior inflammation, CMV retinitis may be complicated by rhegmatogenous retinal detachment. Therapy for CMV retinitis consists of intravenous ganciclovir or foscarnet, with cidofovir as an alternative. Combination therapy with ganciclovir and foscarnet has been shown to be slightly more effective than either ganciclovir or foscarnet alone in the patient with relapsed CMV retinitis. A 3-week induction course is followed by maintenance therapy with one of these drugs systemically. While the majority of patients will require intravenous maintenance therapy, a ganciclovir prodrug with better oral bioavailability has shown promise in clinical trials. If CMV disease is limited to the eye, a ganciclovir-releasing intraocular implant, periodic injections of the antisense nucleic acid preparation formivirsen, or intravitreal injections of ganciclovir or foscarnet may be considered; some choose to combine intraocular implants with oral ganciclovir. Intravitreal injections of cidofovir are generally avoided due to the increased risk of uveitis and hypotony. Maintenance therapy is continued until the CD4+ T cell count remains >100 to $150/\mu L$ for >6 months. The majority of patients with HIV infection and CMV disease develop some degree of uveitis with the initiation of antiretroviral therapy. The etiology of this is unknown; however, it has been suggested that this may be due to the generation of an enhanced immune response to CMV. In some instances this has required the use of topical glucocorticoids.

Both HSV and varicella zoster virus can cause a rapidly progressing, bilateral necrotizing retinitis referred to as the *acute retinal necrosis syndrome*. This syndrome, in contrast to CMV retinitis, is associated with pain, keratitis, and iritis. It is often associated with orolabial HSV or trigeminal zoster. Ophthalmologic examination reveals widespread pale gray peripheral lesions. This condition is often complicated by retinal detachment. It is important to recognize and treat this condition with intravenous acyclovir as quickly as possible to minimize the loss of vision.

Several other secondary infections may cause ocular problems in HIV-infected patients. *P. carinii* can cause a lesion of the choroid that may be detected as an incidental finding on ophthalmologic examination. These lesions are typically bilateral, are from half to twice the disc diameter in size, and appear as slightly elevated yellow-white plaques. They are usually asymptomatic and may be confused with cotton-wool spots. Chorioretinitis due to toxoplasmosis can be seen alone or, more commonly, in association with CNS toxoplasmosis.

Additional Disseminated Infections and Wasting Syndrome Infections with species of the small, gram-negative rickettsia-like organism *Bartonella* (Chap. 163) are seen with increased frequency in patients with HIV infection. While not considered an AIDS-defining illness by the CDC, many experts view infection with *Bartonella* as indicative of a severe defect in cell-mediated immunity. It is usually seen in patients with CD4+ T cell counts $<100/\mu L$. Among the clinical manifestations of *Bartonella* infection are bacillary angiomatosis, cat-scratch disease, and trench fever. *Bacillary angiomatosis* is usually due to infection with *B. henselae*. It is characterized by a vascular proliferation that leads to a variety of skin lesions that have been confused with the skin lesions of KS. In contrast to the lesions of KS, the lesions of bacillary angiomatosis generally blanch, are painful, and typically occur in the setting of systemic symptoms. Infection can extend to the lymph nodes, liver (peliosis hepatis), spleen, bone, heart, CNS, respiratory tract, and gastrointestinal tract. *Cat-scratch disease* generally begins with a papule at the site of inoculation. This is followed several weeks later by the development of regional adenopathy and malaise. Infection with *B. quintana* is transmitted by lice and has been associated with case reports of trench fever, endocarditis, adenopathy, and bacillary angiomatosis. The organism is quite difficult to culture, and diagnosis often relies upon identifying the organism in biopsy specimens using the Warthin-Starry or similar stains. Treatment is with either erythromycin or doxycyline for at least 3 months.

Histoplasmosis is an opportunistic infection that is seen most frequently in patients in the Mississippi and Ohio River valleys, Puerto Rico, the Dominican Republic, and South America. These are all areas in which infection with *H. capsulatum* is endemic (Chap. 201). Because of this limited geographic distribution, the percentage of AIDS cases in the United States with histoplasmosis is only approximately 0.5. Histoplasmosis is generally a late manifestation of HIV infection; however, it may be the initial AIDS-defining condition. In one study, the median CD4+ T cell count for patients with histoplasmosis and AIDS was $33/\mu L$. While disease due to *H. capsulatum* may present as a primary infection of the lung, disseminated disease, presumably due to reactivation, is the most common presentation in HIV-infected patients. Patients usually present with a 4- to 8-week history of fever and weight loss. Hepatosplenomegaly and lymphadenopathy are each seen in about 25% of patients. CNS disease, either meningitis or a mass lesion, is seen in 15% of patients. Bone marrow involvement is common, with thrombocytopenia, neutropenia, and anemia occurring in 33% of patients. Approximately 7% of patients have mucocutaneous lesions consisting of a maculopapular rash and skin or oral ulcers. Respiratory symptoms are usually mild, with chest x-ray showing a diffuse infiltrate or diffuse small nodules in approximately half of cases. Diagnosis is made by culturing the organisms from blood, bone marrow, or tissue. Treatment is typically with amphotericin B, 0.7 to 1.0 mg/kg daily to a total dose of 1 g followed by maintenance therapy with itraconazole. In the setting of mild infection, it may be appropriate to treat with itraconazole alone.

Following the spread of HIV infection to southeast Asia, disseminated infection with *Penicillium marneffei* was recognized as a complication of HIV infection and is considered an AIDS-defining condition in those parts of the world where it occurs. *P. marneffei* is the third most common AIDS-defining illness in Thailand, following TB and cryptococcosis. It is more frequently diagnosed in the rainy than the dry season. Clinical features include fever, generalized lymphadenopathy, hepatosplenomegaly, anemia, thrombocytopenia, and papular skin lesions with central umbilication. Treatment is with amphotericin B followed by itraconazole.

Visceral leishmaniasis (Chap. 215) is recognized with increasing frequency in patients with HIV infection who live in or travel to areas endemic for this protozoal infection transmitted by sandflies. The clinical presentation is one of hepatosplenomegaly, fever, and hematologic abnormalities. Lymphadenopathy and other constitutional symptoms may be present. Organisms can be isolated from cultures of bone marrow aspirates. Histologic stains may be negative, and antibody titers are of little help. Patients with HIV infection usually respond well initially to standard therapy with pentavalent antimony compounds. Eradication of the organism is difficult, however, and relapses are common.

Generalized wasting is an AIDS-defining condition; it is defined as involuntary weight loss of >10% associated with intermittent or constant fever and chronic diarrhea or fatigue lasting >30 days in the absence of a defined cause other than HIV infection. It is the initial AIDS-defining condition in approximately 10% of patients with AIDS in the United States. A constant feature of this syndrome is severe muscle wasting with scattered myofiber degeneration and occasional evidence of myositis. Glucocorticoids may be of some benefit; however, this approach must be carefully weighed against the risk of compounding the immunodeficiency of HIV infection. Androgenic steroids, growth hormone, and total parenteral nutrition have been used as therapeutic interventions with variable success.

Neoplastic Diseases The neoplastic diseases clearly seen with an increased frequency in patients with HIV infection are KS and non-Hodgkin's lymphoma. In addition, there also appears to be an increased incidence of Hodgkin's disease; multiple myeloma; leukemia; melanoma; and cervical, brain, testicular, oral, and anal cancers. Recent years have witnessed a marked reduction in the incidence of KS (Fig. 309-28), felt to be primarily due to the use of potent antiretroviral therapy. Rates of non-Hodgkin's lymphoma have declined as well; however, this decline has not been as dramatic as the decline in rates of KS.

Kaposi's sarcoma is a multicentric neoplasm consisting of multiple vascular nodules appearing in the skin, mucous membranes, and viscera. The course ranges from indolent, with only minor skin or lymph node involvement, to fulminant, with extensive cutaneous and visceral involvement. In the initial period of the AIDS epidemic, KS was a prominent clinical feature of the first cases of AIDS, occurring in 79% of the patients diagnosed in 1981. By 1989 it was seen in only 25% of cases, by 1992 the number had decreased to 9%, and by 1997 the number was <1%. HHV-8 or KSHV has been strongly implicated as a viral cofactor in the pathogenesis of KS (see above).

Clinically, KS has varied presentations and may be seen at any stage of HIV infection, even in the presence of a normal CD4+ T cell count. The initial lesion may be a small, raised reddish-purple nodule on the skin, a discoloration on the oral mucosa, or a swollen lymph node **(see Plate IIB-20)**. Lesions often appear in sun-exposed areas, particularly the tip of the nose, and have a propensity to occur in areas of trauma (Koebner phenomenon). Because of the vascular nature of the tumors and the presence of extravasated red blood cells in the lesions, their color ranges from reddish to purple to brown and often take the appearance of a bruise, with yellowish discoloration and tattooing. Lesions range in size from a few millimeters to several centimeters in diameter and may be either discrete or confluent. KS lesions most commonly appear as raised macules; however, they also can be papular, particularly in patients with higher CD4+ T cell counts. Confluent lesions may give rise to surrounding lymphedema and may be disfiguring when they involve the face and disabling when they involve the lower extremities or the surfaces of joints. Apart from skin, lymph nodes, gastrointestinal tract, and lung are the organ systems most commonly affected by KS. Lesions have been reported in virtually every organ, including the heart and the CNS. In contrast to most malignancies, in which lymph node involvement implies metastatic spread and a poor prognosis, lymph node involvement may be seen very early in Kaposi's sarcoma and is of no special clinical significance. In fact, some patients may present with disease limited to the lymph nodes. These are generally patients with relatively intact immune function and thus the patients with the best prognosis. Pulmonary involvement with KS generally presents with shortness of breath. Some 80% of patients with pulmonary KS also have cutaneous lesions. The chest x-ray characteristically shows bilateral lower lobe infiltrates that obscure the margins of the mediastinum and diaphragm (Fig. 309-35). Pleural effusions are seen in 70% of cases of pulmonary KS, a fact that is often helpful in the differential diagnosis. Gastrointestinal involvement is seen in 50% of patients and usually takes one of two forms. The first is mucosal involvement, which may lead to bleeding that can be severe. These patients sometimes also develop symptoms of gastrointestinal obstruction if lesions become large. The second gastrointestinal manifestation is due to biliary tract involvement. KS lesions may infiltrate the gallbladder and biliary tree, leading to a clinical picture of obstructive jaundice similar to that seen with sclerosing cholangitis. Several staging systems have been proposed for KS. One in common use was developed by the National Institute of Allergy and Infectious Diseases AIDS Clinical Trials Group; it distinguishes patients on the basis of tumor extent, immunologic function, and presence or absence of systemic disease (Table 309-17).

A diagnosis of KS is based upon biopsy of a suspicious lesion. Histologically one sees a proliferation of spindle cells and endothelial cells, extravasation of red blood cells, hemosiderin-laden macrophages, and, in early cases, an inflammatory cell infiltrate. Included in the differential diagnosis are lymphoma (particularly for oral lesions), bacillary angiomatosis, and cutaneous mycobacterial infections.

Management of KS (Table 309-18) should be carried out in consultation with an expert since definitive treatment guidelines do not exist. In the majority of cases effective antiretroviral therapy will go a long way in achieving control. Indeed, spontaneous regressions have been reported in the setting of HAART. For patients in whom tumor persists or in whom control of HIV replication is not possible, a variety of options exist. In some cases, lesions remain quite indolent, and many of these patients can be managed with no specific treatment. Fewer than 10% of AIDS patients with KS die as a consequence of their malignancy, and death from secondary infections is considerably more common. Thus, whenever possible one should avoid treatment regimens that may further suppress the immune system and increase susceptibility to opportunistic infections. Treatment is indicated under two main circumstances. The first is when a single lesion or a limited

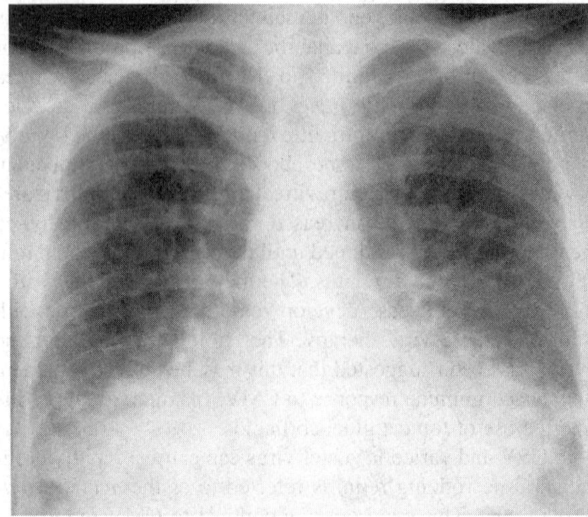

FIGURE 309-35 Chest x-ray of a patient with AIDS and pulmonary Kaposi's sarcoma. The characteristic findings include dense bilateral lower lobe infiltrates obscuring the heart borders and a pleural effusion.

number of lesions are causing significant discomfort or cosmetic problems, such as with prominent facial lesions, lesions overlying a joint, or lesions in the oropharynx that interfere with swallowing or breathing. Under these circumstances, treatment with localized radiation, intralesional vinblastine, or cryotherapy may be indicated. It should be noted that patients with HIV infection are particularly sensitive to the side effects of radiation therapy. This is especially true with respect to the development of radiation-induced mucositis; doses of radiation directed at mucosal surfaces, particularly in the head and neck region, should be adjusted accordingly. The use of systemic therapy, either IFN-α or chemotherapy, should be considered in patients with a large number of lesions or in patients with visceral involvement. The single most important determinant of response appears to be the CD4+ T cell count. This relationship between response rate and baseline CD4+ T cell count is particularly true for IFN-α. The response rate for patients with CD4+ T cell counts >600/μL is approximately 80%, while the response rate for patients with counts <150/μL is <10%. In contrast to the other systemic therapies, IFN-α provides an added advantage of having antiretroviral activity; thus, it may be the appropriate first choice for single-agent systemic therapy for early patients with disseminated disease. A variety of chemotherapeutic agents have also been shown to have activity against KS. Three of them, liposomal daunorubicin, liposomal doxorubicin, and paclitaxel have been approved by the FDA for this indication. Liposomal daunorubicin is approved as first-line therapy for patients with advanced KS. It has fewer side effects than conventional chemotherapy. In contrast, liposomal doxorubicin and paclitaxel are only approved for KS patients who have failed standard chemotherapy. Response rates vary from 23 to 88%, appear to be comparable to what had been achieved earlier with combination chemotherapy regimens, and are greatly influenced by CD4+ T cell count.

Table 309-17 National Institute of Allergy and Infectious Diseases AIDS Clinical Trials Group TIS Staging System for Kaposi's Sarcoma

Parameter	Good Risk (stage 0): All of the Following	Poor Risk (stage 1): Any of the Following
Tumor (T)	Confined to skin and/or lymph nodes and/or minimal oral disease	Tumor-associated edema or ulceration Extensive oral lesions Gastrointestinal lesions Nonnodal visceral lesions
Immune system (I)	CD4+ T cell count ≥200/μL	CD4+ T cell count <200/μL
Systemic illness (S)	No B symptoms[a] Karnofsky performance status >70 No history of opportunistic infection, neurologic disease, lymphoma, or thrush	B symptoms[a] present Karnofsky performance status <70 History of opportunistic infection, neurologic disease, lymphoma, or thrush

[a] Defined as unexplained fever, night sweats, >10% involuntary weight loss, or diarrhea persisting for more than 2 weeks.

Lymphomas occur with an increased frequency in patients with congenital or acquired T cell immunodeficiencies (Chap. 308). AIDS is no exception; at least 6% of all patients with AIDS develop lymphoma at some time during the course of their illness. This is a 120-fold increase in incidence compared to the general population. In contrast to the situation with KS and most opportunistic infections, the incidence of AIDS-associated lymphomas has not experienced as dramatic a decrease as a consequence of the widespread use of effective antiretroviral therapy. Lymphoma occurs in all risk groups, with the highest incidence in patients with hemophilia and the lowest incidence in patients from the Caribbean or Africa with heterosexually acquired infection. Lymphoma is a late manifestation of HIV infection, generally occurring in patients with CD4+ T cell counts of <200/μL. As HIV disease progresses, the risk of lymphoma increases. In contrast to KS, which occurs at a relatively constant rate throughout the course of HIV disease, the attack rate for lymphoma increases exponentially with increasing duration of HIV infection and decreasing level of immunologic function. At 3 years following a diagnosis of HIV infection, the risk of lymphoma is 0.8% per year; by 8 years after infection, it is 2.6% per year. As people with HIV infection live longer as a consequence of improved antiretroviral therapy and better treatment and prophylaxis of opportunistic infections, it is anticipated that the incidence of lymphomas will increase.

Three main categories of lymphoma are seen in patients with HIV infection: grade III or IV immunoblastic lymphoma, Burkitt's lymphoma, and primary CNS lymphoma. Approximately 90% of these lymphomas are B cell in phenotype, and half contain EBV DNA. These tumors may be either monoclonal or oligoclonal in nature and are probably in some way related to the pronounced polyclonal B cell activation seen in patients with AIDS.

Immunoblastic lymphomas account for ~60% of the cases of lymphoma in patients with AIDS. These are generally high grade and would have been classified as diffuse histiocytic lymphomas in earlier classification schemes. This tumor is more common in older patients, increasing in incidence from 0% in HIV-infected individuals <1 year old to >3% in those >50. One variant of immunoblastic lymphoma is body cavity lymphoma. This malignancy presents with lymphomatous pleural, pericardial, and/or peritoneal effusions in the absence of discrete nodal or extranodal masses. The tumor cells do not express surface markers for B cells or T cells. HHV-8 DNA sequences have been found in the genome of the malignant cells (see above).

Small non-cleaved cell lymphoma (*Burkitt's lymphoma*) accounts for ~20% of the cases of lymphoma in patients with AIDS. It is most frequent in patients 10 to 19 years old and usually demonstrates characteristic c-*myc* translocations from chromosome 8 to chromosomes 14 or 22. Burkitt's lymphoma is not commonly seen in the setting of immunodeficiency other than HIV-associated immunodeficiency, and the incidence of this particular tumor is over 1000-fold higher in the setting of HIV infection than in the general population. In contrast to African Burkitt's lymphoma, where 97% of the cases contain EBV genome, only 50% of HIV-associated Burkitt's lymphomas are EBV-positive.

Primary CNS lymphoma accounts for approximately 20% of the cases of lymphoma in patients with HIV infection. In contrast to HIV-associated Burkitt's lymphoma, primary CNS lymphomas are usually positive for EBV. In one study, the incidence of Epstein-Barr positivity was 100%. This malignancy does not have a predilection for any particular age group. The median CD4+ T cell count at the time of diagnosis is approximately 50/μL. Thus, CNS lymphoma generally presents at a later stage of HIV infection than systemic lymphoma. This fact may at least in part explain the poorer prognosis for this subset of patients.

The clinical presentation of lymphoma in patients with HIV infection is quite varied, ranging from focal seizures to rapidly growing

Table 309-18 Management of AIDS-Associated Kaposi's Sarcoma

Observation and optimization of antiretroviral therapy
Single or limited number of lesions
- Radiation
- Intralesional vinblastine
- Cryotherapy

Extensive disease
- Initial therapy
  - Interferon-α (if CD4+ T cells >150/μL)
  - Liposomal danorubicin
- Subsequent therapy
  - Liposomal doxorubicin
  - Paclitaxel
- Combination chemotherapy with low-dose doxorubicin, bleomycin, and vinblastine (ABV)
- Radiation treatment

mass lesions in the oral mucosa (Fig. 309-36) to persistent unexplained fever. At least 80% of patients present with extranodal disease, and a similar percentage have B-type symptoms of fever, night sweats, or weight loss. Virtually any site in the body may be involved. The most common extranodal site is the CNS, which is involved in approximately one-third of all patients with lymphoma. Approximately 60% of these cases are primary CNS lymphoma. Primary CNS lymphoma generally presents with focal neurologic deficits, including cranial nerve findings, headaches, and/or seizures. MRI or CT generally reveals a limited number (one to three) of 3- to 5-cm lesions (Fig. 309-37). The lesions often show ring enhancement on contrast administration and may occur in any location. Locations that are most commonly involved with CNS lymphoma are deep in the white matter. Contrast enhancement is usually less pronounced than that seen with toxoplasmosis. The main diseases in the differential diagnosis are cerebral toxoplasmosis and cerebral Chagas' disease. In addition to the 20% of lymphomas in HIV-infected individuals that are primary CNS lymphomas, CNS disease is also seen in HIV-infected patients with systemic lymphoma. Approximately 20% of patients with systemic lymphoma have CNS disease in the form of leptomeningeal involvement. This fact underscores the importance of lumbar puncture in the staging evaluation of patients with systemic lymphoma.

Systemic lymphoma is seen at earlier stages of HIV infection than primary CNS lymphoma. In one series the mean CD4+ T cell count was 189/μL. In addition to lymph node involvement, systemic lymphoma may commonly involve the gastrointestinal tract, bone marrow, liver, and lung. Gastrointestinal tract involvement is seen in ~25% of patients. Any site in the gastrointestinal tract may be involved, and patients may complain of difficulty swallowing or abdominal pain. The diagnosis is usually suspected on the basis of CT or MRI of the abdomen. Bone marrow involvement is seen in ~20% of patients and may lead to pancytopenia. Liver and lung involvement are each seen in ~10% of patients. Pulmonary disease may present as either a mass lesion, multiple nodules, or an interstitial infiltrate.

Both conventional and unconventional approaches have been employed in an attempt to treat HIV-related lymphomas. Systemic lymphoma is generally treated by the oncologist with combination chemotherapy. Earlier disappointing figures are being replaced with more optimistic results for the treatment of systemic lymphoma following the availability of more effective combination antiretroviral therapy. As in most situations in patients with HIV disease, those with the higher CD4+ T cell counts tend to do better. Response rates as high as 72% and disease-free intervals >15 months have been reported. Treatment of primary CNS lymphoma remains a significant challenge. Treatment is complicated by the fact that this illness usually occurs in patients with advanced HIV disease. Palliative measures such as radiation therapy provide some relief. The prognosis remains poor in this group, with median survival <1 year.

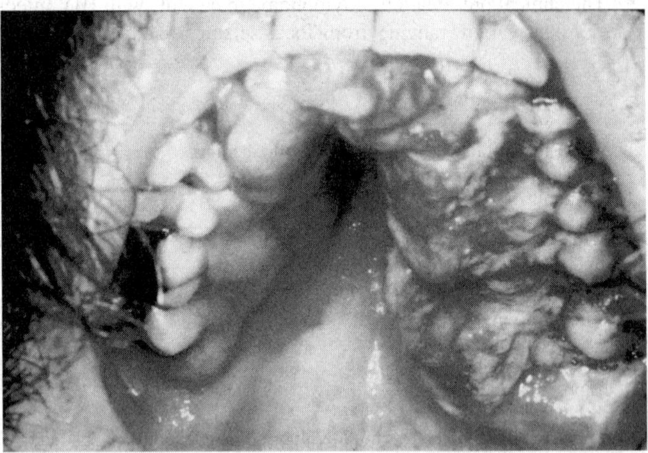

FIGURE 309-36 Diffuse histiocytic lymphoma involving the hard palate of a patient with AIDS.

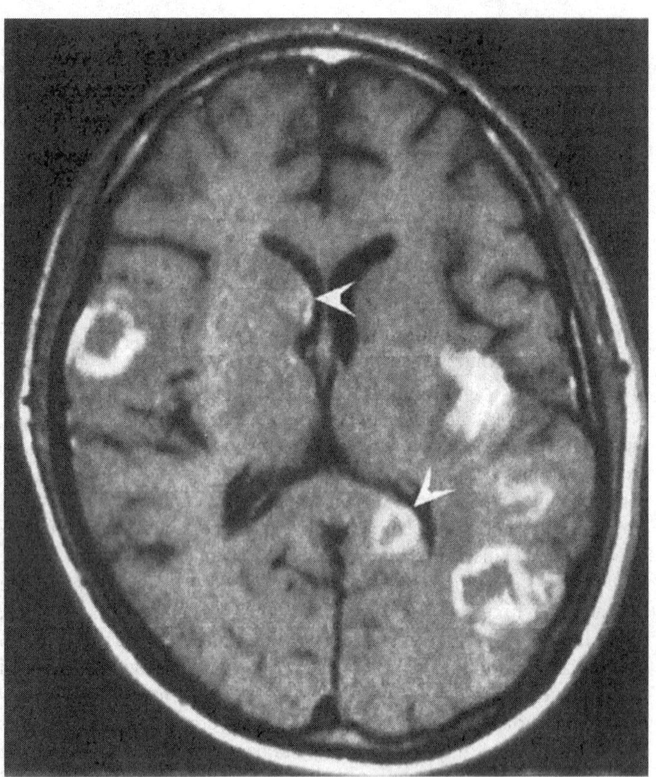

FIGURE 309-37 CNS lymphoma. Postcontrast T1 weighted MR scan with AIDS, an altered mental status, and hemiparesis. Multiple enhancing lesions, some ring-enhancing are present. The left Sylvian lesion shows gyral and subcortical enhancement, and the lesions in the caudate and splenium (*arrowheads*) show enhancement of adjacent ependymal surfaces.

Evidence of infection with *human papilloma virus*, associated with *intraepithelial dysplasia of the cervix or anus*, is approximately twice as common in HIV-infected individuals as in the general population and can lead to intraepithelial neoplasia and eventually invasive cancer. It is anticipated that both anal and cervical carcinomas will be seen with increased frequency in the HIV-infected population as survival is prolonged with combination antiretroviral therapy. In two separate studies, HIV-infected men without anorectal symptoms were studied for evidence of dysplasia, and Papanicolauo (Pap) smears were found to be abnormal in 40%. These changes were persistent at 1 year follow-up, raising the possibility of a subsequent transition to a more malignant condition. While the incidence of an abnormal Pap smear of the cervix is ~5% in otherwise healthy women, the incidence of abnormal cervical smears in women with HIV infection is 60%. Based on this finding, *invasive cervical cancer* was added to the list of AIDS-defining conditions. Thus far, however, only small increases in the incidence of cervical or anal cancer have been seen as a consequence of HIV infection. However, given this high rate of dysplasia, a comprehensive gynecologic and rectal examination, including Pap smear, is indicated at the initial evaluation and 6 months later for all patients with HIV infection. If these examinations are negative at both time points, the patient should be followed with yearly evaluations. If an initial or repeat Pap smear shows evidence of severe inflammation with reactive squamous changes, the next Pap smear should be performed at 3 months. If, at any time, a Pap smear shows evidence of squamous intraepithelial lesions, colposcopic examination with biopsies as indicated should be performed.

IDIOPATHIC CD4+ T LYMPHOCYTOPENIA

A syndrome was recognized in 1992 that was characterized by an absolute CD4+ T cell count of <300/μL or <20% of total T cells on more than one occasion; no evidence of HIV-1, HIV-2, HTLV-I, or HTLV-II on testing; and the absence of any defined immunodeficiency or therapy associated with decreased levels of CD4+ T cells. By mid-1993, approximately 100 patients had been described. After extensive multicenter investigations, a series of reports were published in early 1993, which together allowed a number of conclusions. Idiopathic CD4+ lymphocytopenia (ICL) is a very rare syndrome, as determined by studies of blood donors and cohorts of HIV-seronegative homosexual men. Cases were clearly identified as early as 1983, and cases remarkably similar to ICL had been identified decades ago. The definition of ICL based on CD4+ T cell counts coincided with the ready availability of testing for CD4+ T cells in patients suspected of being immunosuppressed. Although, as a result of immune deficiency, certain patients with ICL develop some of the opportunistic diseases (particularly cryptococcosis) seen in HIV-infected patients, the syndrome is demographically, clinically, and immunologically unlike HIV infection and AIDS. Fewer than half of the reported ICL patients had risk factors for HIV infection, and there were wide geographic and age distributions. The fact that a significant proportion of patients did have risk factors probably reflects a selection bias, in that physicians who take care of HIV-infected patients are more likely to monitor CD4+ T cells. Approximately one-third of the patients are women, compared to 16% of women among HIV-infected individuals in the United States. Many patients with ICL remained clinically stable, and their condition did not deteriorate progressively as is common with seriously immunodeficient HIV-infected patients. Certain patients with ICL even experienced spontaneous reversal of the CD4+ T lymphocytopenia. Immunologic abnormalities in ICL are somewhat different from those of HIV infection. ICL patients often also have decreases in CD8+ T cells and in B cells. Furthermore, immunoglobulin levels were either normal or, more commonly, decreased in patients with ICL, compared to the usual hypergammaglobulinemia of HIV-infected individuals. Finally, virologic studies revealed no evidence of HIV-1, HIV-2, HTLV-I, or HTLV-II or of any other mononuclear cell–tropic virus. Furthermore, there was no epidemiologic evidence to suggest that a transmissible microbe was involved. The cases of ICL were widely dispersed, with no clustering. Close contacts and sexual partners who were studied were clinically well and were serologically, immunologically, and virologically negative for HIV. ICL is a heterogeneous syndrome, and it is highly likely that there is no common cause; however, there may be common causes among subgroups of patients that are currently unrecognized.

Patients who present with laboratory data consistent with ICL should be worked up for underlying diseases that could be responsible for the immune deficiency. If no underlying cause is detected, no specific therapy should be initiated. However, if opportunistic diseases occur, they should be treated appropriately (see above). Depending on the level of the CD4+ T cell count, patients should receive prophylaxis for the commonly encountered opportunistic infections.

℞ TREATMENT **General Principles of Patient Management** The treatment of patients with HIV infection requires not only a comprehensive knowledge of the possible disease processes that may occur but also the ability to deal with the problems of a chronic, potentially life-threatening illness. Great advances have been made in the treatment of patients with HIV infection. The appropriate use of potent combination antiretroviral therapy and other treatment and prophylactic interventions is of critical importance in providing each patient with the best opportunity to live a long and healthy life despite the presence of HIV infection. In contrast to the earlier days of this epidemic, a diagnosis of HIV infection need no longer be equated with an inevitably fatal disease. In addition to medical interventions, the health care provider has a responsibility to provide each patient with appropriate counseling and education concerning their disease as part of a comprehensive care plan. Patients must be educated about the potential transmissibility of their infection and about the fact that while health care providers may refer to levels of the virus as "undetectable" this is more a reflection of the sensitivity of the assay being used to measure the virus than a comment on the presence or absence of the virus. It is important for patients to be aware and that the virus is still present and capable of being transmitted at all stages of HIV disease. Thus, there needs to be frank discussions concerning sexual practices and the sharing of needles. The treating physician must not only be aware of the latest medications available for patients with HIV infection but must also educate patients concerning the natural history of their illness and listen and be sensitive to their fears and concerns. As with other diseases, therapeutic decisions should be made in consultation with the patient, when possible, and with the patient's proxy if the patient is incapable of making decisions. In this regard, it is recommended that all patients with HIV infection, and in particular those with CD4+ T cell counts $<200/\mu L$, designate a trusted individual with durable power of attorney to make medical decisions on their behalf, if necessary.

No matter how well prepared a patient is for adversity, the discovery of a diagnosis of HIV infection is a devastating event. For this reason, it is recommended that anyone about to undergo testing have "pretest counseling" to prepare him or her at least partially should the results demonstrate the presence of HIV infection. Following a diagnosis of HIV infection, the health care provider should be prepared to activate support systems immediately for the newly diagnosed patient. These should include an experienced social worker or nurse who can spend time talking to the person and ensuring that he or she is emotionally stable. Most communities have HIV crisis centers that can be of great help in these difficult situations.

Following a diagnosis of HIV infection, there are several examinations and laboratory studies that should be performed to help determine the extent of disease and provide baseline standards for future reference (Table 309-19). In addition to routine chemistry and hematology screening panels and chest x-ray, one should also obtain a CD4+ T cell count, two separate plasma HIV RNA levels, a VDRL test, and an anti-*Toxoplasma* antibody titer. A PPD test should be done, and a MMSE performed and recorded. Patients should be immunized with pneumococcal polysaccharide and, if seronegative for these viruses, with hepatitis A and hepatitis B vaccines. In addition, patients should be counseled with regard to sexual practices and needle sharing, and counseling should be offered to those whom the patient knows or suspects may also be infected. Once these baseline activities are performed, short- and long-term medical management strategies should be developed based uoon the most recent information available and modified as new information becomes available. The field of HIV medicine is changing rapidly, and it is difficult to remain fully up to date. Fortunately there are a series of excellent sites on the World Wide Web that are frequently updated, and they provide the most recent information on a variety of topics, including consensus panel reports on treatment (Table 309-20).

Antiretroviral Therapy Combination antiretroviral therapy, or HAART, is the cornerstone of management of patients with HIV infection. Following the initiation of widespread use of HAART in the

Table 309-19 Initial Evaluation of the Patient with HIV Infection

History and physical examination
Routine chemistry and hematology
CD4+ T lymphocyte count
Two plasma HIV RNA levels
VDRL test
Anti-*Toxoplasma* antibody titer
PPD skin test
Mini-mental status examination
Serologies for hepatitis A and hepatitis B
Immunization with pneumococcal polysaccharide
Immunization with hepatitis A and hepatitis B if seronegative
Counseling regarding natural history and transmission
Help contacting others who might be infected

NOTE: VDRL, Venereal Disease Research Laboratory; PPD, purified protein derivative.

Table 309-20 Resources Available on the World Wide Web Regarding HIV Disease

www.hivatis.org	HIV AIDS Treatment Information Services; posts federally approved treatment guidelines for HIV and AIDS
www.actis.org	AIDS Clinical Trials Information Service (ACTIS); information on federally funded and privately funded clinical trials; CDC information services.
www.cdcnpin.org	Updates on epidemiologic data from the CDC
www.cc.nih.gov/phar/hiv-mgt	Online images of HIV drugs and information regarding dosing

NOTE: CDC, Centers for Disease Control and Prevention.

United States in 1995 to 1996, marked declines have been noted in the incidence of most AIDS-defining conditions (Fig. 309-28). Suppression of HIV replication is an important component in prolonging life as well as improving the quality of life in patients with HIV infection. Unfortunately, many of the most important questions related to the treatment of HIV disease currently lack definitive answers. Among them are the questions of when should therapy be started, what is the best initial regimen, when should a given regimen be changed, and what should it be changed to when a change is made. Notwithstanding these uncertainties, the physician and patient must come to a mutually agreeable plan based upon the best available data. In an effort to facilitate this process, the United States Department of Health and Human Services has published a series of frequently updated guidelines including the "*Principles of Therapy of HIV Infection*," "*Guidelines for the Use of Antiretroviral Agents in HIV-Infected Adults and Adolescents*," and "*Guidelines for the Prevention of Opportunistic Infections in Persons Infected with Human Immunodeficiency Virus*." At present, an extensive clinical trials network, involving both clinical investigators and patient advocates, is in place attempting to develop improved approaches to therapy. Consortia comprising representatives of academia, industry, and the federal government are involved in the process of drug development, including clinical trials. As a result, new therapies and new therapeutic strategies are continually emerging. New drugs are often available through expanded access programs prior to official licensure. Given the complexity of this field, decisions regarding antiretroviral therapy are best made in consultation with experts. Currently licensed drugs for the treatment of HIV infection fall into two main categories: those that inhibit the viral reverse transcriptase enzyme (Table 309-21, Fig. 309-3*B*) and those that inhibit the viral protease enzyme. There are numerous drug-drug interactions that one must take into consideration when using these agents (Table 309-22).

The FDA-approved reverse transcriptase inhibitors include the *nucleoside analogues* zidovudine, didanosine, zalcitabine, stavudine, lamivudine, and abacavir and the *nonnucleoside reverse transcriptase inhibitors* nevirapine, delavirdine, and efavirenz (Fig. 309-38; Table 309-21). These were the first class of drugs that were licensed for the treatment of HIV infection. They are indicated for this use as part of combination regimens. It should be stressed that none of these drugs should be used as monotherapy for HIV infection. Thus, when lamivudine is used to treat hepatitis B infection in the setting of HIV infection, one should ensure that the patient is also on additional antiretroviral medication. The reverse transcriptase inhibitors block the HIV replication cycle at the point of RNA-dependent DNA synthesis, the reverse transcription step. While the nonnucleoside reverse transcriptase inhibitors are quite selective for the HIV-1 reverse transcriptase, the nucleoside analogues inhibit a variety of DNA polymerization reactions in addition to those of the HIV-1 reverse transcriptase. For this reason, serious side effects are more common with the nucleoside analogues and include mitochondrial damage that can lead to hepatic steatosis and lactic acidosis as well as peripheral neuropathy and pancreatitis.

Zidovudine (AZT; 3′-azido-2′,3′-dideoxythymidine) was the first drug approved for the treatment of HIV infection and is the prototype nucleoside analogue. These compounds, in which the hydroxyl group in the 3′ position of the ribose moiety is substituted with a hydrogen or other chemical group, act as DNA chain terminators owing to their inability to form a 3′-5′ phosphodiester linkage with another nucleoside. They bind much more avidly to the active site of the RNA-dependent DNA polymerase of HIV (reverse transcriptase) than to the active site of mammalian cell DNA polymerases; this explains their selective effect on HIV replication. Zidovudine also has a relatively high avidity for the DNA polymerase-γ of human mitochondria. This may contribute to the development of the fatty liver and the myopathy sometimes observed in patients taking zidovudine. As with all the nucleoside analogues, the active form of zidovudine is the triphosphate, and the rate of phosphorylation, a thymidine kinase–dependent pathway, may be different in different cells. This may explain why zidovudine is more effective at inhibiting HIV replication in some cells than others. The clinical efficacy of zidovudine was clearly established in 1986 in a phase II, randomized, placebo-controlled trial in patients with advanced HIV disease. However, while treatment of patients with early stages of HIV infection was associated with increases in CD4+ T cell count, it was not associated with a better overall outcome than later intervention. Subsequent trials established the ability of this drug to dramatically decrease the incidence of perinatal transmission of HIV from infected mother to infant. Eventually a series of studies demonstrated the superiority of combination antiretroviral regimens over zidovudine alone, and combination therapy (discussed below) remains the standard of treatment today. Among the side effects of zidovudine at the initiation of therapy are fatigue, malaise, nausea, and headache. These side effects often subside over time. Patients on zidovudine may develop a macrocytic anemia, myopathy, cardiomyopathy, and lactic acidosis associated with fatty infiltration of the liver. As with every antiretroviral drug, HIV has the ability to develop resistance to zidovudine. Zidovudine resistance has been reported to occur ~6 months following the initiation of zidovudine monotherapy. More recently, zidovudine-resistant viruses have been noted in patients with acute infection prior to the initiation of therapy, implying that zidovudine-resistant viruses can be transmitted from person to person. Resistance emerges more rapidly in late-stage patients, presumably as a consequence of a greater degree of viral replication and thus a greater opportunity for mutation. A variety of amino acid changes including substitutions, insertions, and deletions have been reported to confer zidovudine resistance (Fig. 309-39). A combination preparation, Combivir, consists of zidovudine and lamivudine.

Didanosine (ddI; 2′,3′-dideoxyinosine) was the second drug licensed for the treatment of HIV infection, followed shortly thereafter by zalcitabine. Didanosine is metabolized to dideoxyadenosine in vivo. It is best absorbed on an empty stomach at a high pH. For this reason, the current formulations of didanosine contain a buffer, and each dose must be administered in no fewer than two tablets to ensure adequate buffering of stomach acid. The toxicity profile of didanosine is quite different from that of zidovudine. The most common toxicity is a painful sensory peripheral neuropathy that occurs in ~30% of patients receiving >400 mg/d. It generally resolves with discontinuation of the drug and may not recur if the drug is resumed at a reduced dose. At higher doses than are currently used one may see pancreatitis in ~10% of patients. Pancreatitis associated with didanosine therapy can be fatal. Didanosine should be discontinued if a patient experiences abdominal pain consistent with pancreatitis or if an elevated serum amylase or lipase is found in association with an edematous pancreas on ultrasound. Didanosine is contraindicated in patients with a prior history of pancreatitis, regardless of etiology.

Zalcitabine (ddC; 2′,3′-dideoxycytidine) is rarely used today in the management of patients with HIV infection. Among the nucleoside analogues licensed for the treatment of HIV infection, it is probably the weakest. The main toxicity of ddC is pancreatitis.

Stavudine (d4T; 2′,3′-didehydro-3′-deoxythymidine) was the fourth drug licensed for the treatment of HIV infection. Like zidovudine, stavudine is a thymidine analogue. These two drugs are antagonistic in vitro and in vivo and should not be given together. Peripheral neuropathy and hepatic steatosis are the main toxicities of stavudine. It is commonly used with lamivudine as part of an initial treatment regimen.

Lamivudine (3TC; 2′,3′-dideoxy-3′-thiacytidine) is the fifth of the nucleoside analogues to be licensed in the United States. It is licensed for use in combination with zidovudine in situations where zidovudine is indicated. In actual practice, lamivudine, is a frequent element of many different combination regimens currently in use. It is available either alone or in combination with zidovudine (Combivir). One reason behind the excellent synergy seen between lamivudine and the other nucleoside analogues may be that strains of HIV resistant to lamivudine (M184V substitution) appear to have enhanced sensitivity to other nucleosides, and thus development of dual resistance is quite difficult. In addition, there is a suggestion that 3TC-resistant strains of HIV may

Table 309-21 Antiretroviral Drugs Used in the Treatment of HIV Infection

Drug	Status	Indication	Dose as Monotherapy	Dose in Combination	Supporting Data	Toxicity
REVERSE TRANSCRIPTASE INHIBITORS						
Zidovudine (AZT, azidothymidine, Retrovir, 3′azido-3′-deoxythymidine)	Licensed	Treatment of HIV infection when antiretroviral therapy is indicated	Not indicated	200 mg q8h or 300 mg bid	19 vs 1 death in original placebo-controlled trial in 281 patients with AIDS or ARC. Decreased progression to AIDS in patients with CD4+ T cell counts <500/μL, *n* = 2051	Anemia, granulocytopenia, myopathy, lactic acidosis, hepatomegaly with steatosis, headache, nausea
		Prevention of maternal-fetal HIV transmission	*Mother:* 100 mg 5 ×/d until the start of labor, then 2 mg/kg over 1 h IV, followed by 1 mg/kg per h IV until clamping of umbilical cord; *Infant:* 2 mg/kg q6h PO beginning within 12 h birth, or 1.5 mg/kg q6h IV over 30 min		In pregnant women with CD4+ T cell count ≥200/μL, AZT PO beginning at weeks 14–34 of gestation plus IV drug during labor and delivery plus PO AZT to infant for 6 wk decreased transmission of HIV by 67.5% (from 25.5% to 8.3%), *n* = 363	
Didanosine (Videx, ddI, dideoxyinosine, 2′,3′-dideoxyinosine)	Licensed	For treatment of HIV infection when antiretroviral therapy is warranted	Not indicated	Requires 2 tablets to achieve adequate buffering of stomach acid; should be administered on an empty stomach ≥60 kg: 200 mg bid <60 kg: 125 mg bid 200 mg bid 125 mg bid	Clinically superior to AZT as monotherapy in 913 patients with prior AZT therapy. Clinically superior to AZT and comparable to AZT + ddI and AZT + ddC in 1067 AZT-naive patients with CD4+ T cell counts of 200–500/μL	Pancreatitis, peripheral neuropathy, abnormalities on liver function tests
Zalcitabine (ddC, HIVID, 2′3′-dideoxycytidine)	Licensed	In combination with other antiretroviral agents for the treatment of HIV infection	Not indicated	0.75 mg tid	Clinically inferior to AZT monotherapy as initial treatment. Clinically as good as ddI in advanced patients intolerant to AZT. In combination with AZT, was clinically superior to AZT alone in patients with AIDS or CD4+ T cell count <350/μL	Peripheral neuropathy, pancreatitis, lactic acidosis, hepatomegaly with steatosis, oral ulcers
Stavudine (d4T, Zerit, 2′3′-didehydro-3′-dideoxythymidine)	Licensed	Treatment of HIV-infected patients who have received prolonged prior zidovudine therapy	Not indicated	≥60 kg: 40 mg bid <60 kg: 30 mg bid	Superior to AZT with respect to changes in CD4+ T cell counts in 359 patients who had received ≥24 wk of AZT. Following 12 wk of randomization, the CD4+ T cell count had decreased in AZT-treated controls by a mean of 22/μL, while in stavudine-treated patients, it had increased by a mean of 22/μL	Peripheral neuropathy, pancreatitis

(continued)

Table 309-21 Antiretroviral Drugs Used in the Treatment of HIV Infection—*(continued)*

Drug	Status	Indication	Dose as Monotherapy	Dose in Combination	Supporting Data	Toxicity
Lamivudine (Epivir, 2′3′-dideoxy-3′-thiacytidine, 3TC)	Licensed	In combination with other antiretroviral agents for the treatment of HIV infection	Not indicated	150 mg bid	Superior to AZT alone with respect to changes in CD4 counts in 495 patients who were zidovudine-naive and 477 patients who were zidovudine-experienced. Overall CD4+ T cell counts for the zidovudine group were at baseline by 24 wk, while in the group treated with zidovudine plus lamivudine, they were 10–50 cells/μL above baseline. 54% decrease in progression to AIDS/death compared to AZT alone	
Abacavir (Ziagen)	Licensed	For treatment of HIV infection in combination with other antiretroviral agents	Not indicated	300 mg bid	Abacavir + AZT + 3TC equivalent to indinavir + AZT + 3TC with regard to viral load suppression (~60% in each group with <400 HIV RNA copies/mL plasma) and CD4 cell increase (~100/μL in each group) at 24 weeks	Hypersensitivity reaction (can be fatal); fever, rash, nausea, vomiting, malaise or fatigue, and loss of appetite
Delavirdine (Rescriptor)	Licensed	For use in combination with appropriate antiretrovirals when treatment is warranted	Not indicated	400 mg tid	Delavirdine + AZT superior to AZT alone with regard to viral load suppression at 52 weeks	Skin rash, abnormalities in liver function tests
Nevirapine (Viramune)	Licensed	In combination with nucleoside analogues for treatment of progressive HIV infection	Not indicated	200 mg/d × 14 days then 200 mg bid	Increases in CD4+ T cell count, decrease in HIV RNA when used in combination with nucleosides	Skin rash, abnormalities in liver function tests
Efavirenz (Sustiva)	Licensed	For treatment of HIV infection in combination with other antiretroviral agents	Not indicated	600 mg qhs	Efavirenz + AZT + 3TC comparable to indinavir + AZT + 3TC with regard to viral load suppression (a higher percentage of the efavirenz group achieved viral load <50 copies/mL; however, the discontinuation rate in the indinavir group was unexpectedly high, accounting for most treatment "failures") and CD4 cell increase (~140/μL in each group) at 24 weeks	Rash, dysphoria, elevated liver function tests
PROTEASE INHIBITORS						
Saquinavir mesylate (Invirase—hard gel capsule)	Licensed	In combination with other antiretroviral agents when therapy is warranted	Not indicated	600 mg q8h	Increases in CD4+ T cell counts, reduction in HIV RNA most pronounced in combination therapy with ddC. 50% reduction in first AIDS-defining event or death in combination with ddC compared to either agent alone	Diarrhea, nausea, headaches, hyperglycemia, fat redistribution, lipid abnormalities
(Fortovase—soft gel capsule)	Licensed	For use in combination with other antiretroviral agents when treatment is warranted	Not indicated	1200 mg tid	Reduction in the mortality rate and AIDS-defining events for patients who received hard-gel formulation in combination with ddC	Diarrhea, nausea, abdominal pain, headaches, hyperglycemia, fat redistribution, lipid abnormalities

(continued)

Table 309-21—*(continued)*

Drug	Status	Indication	Dose as Monotherapy	Dose in Combination	Supporting Data	Toxicity
Ritonavir (Norvir)	Licensed	In combination with nucleoside analogues for treatment of HIV infection when treatment is warranted	Not indicated	600 mg bid	Reduction in the cumulative incidence of clinical progression or death from 34 to 17% in patients with CD4+ T cell count <100/μL treated for a median of 6 months	Nausea, abdominal pain, hyperglycemia, fat redistribution, lipid abnormalities, may alter levels of many other drugs, including saquinavir
Indinavir sulfate (Crixivan)	Licensed	For treatment of HIV infection when antiretroviral treatment is warranted	Not indicated	800 mg q8h	Increase in CD4+ T cell count by 100/μL and 2-log decrease in HIV RNA levels when given in combination with zidovudine and lamivudine. Decrease of 50% in risk of progression to AIDS or death when given with zidovudine and lamivudine compared with zidovudine and lamivudine alone	Nephrolithiasis, indirect hyperbilirubinemia, hyperglycemia, fat redistribution, lipid abnormalities
Nelfinavir mesylate (Viracept)	Licensed	For treatment of HIV infection when antiretroviral therapy is warranted	Not indicated	750 mg tid or 1250 mg bid	2.0-log decline in HIV RNA when given in combination with stavudine	Diarrhea, loose stools, hyperglycemia, fat redistribution, lipid abnormalities
Amprenavir (Agenerase)	Licensed	In combination with other antiretroviral agents for treatment of HIV infection	Not indicated	1200 mg bid	In treatment-naïve patients, amprenavir + AZT + 3TC superior to AZT + 3TC with regard to viral load suppression (53% vs 11% with <400 HIV RNA copies/mL plasma at 24 weeks). CD4+ T cell responses similar between treatment groups. In treatment-experienced patients, amprenavir + NRTIs similar to indinavir + NRTIs with regard to viral load suppression (43% vs 53% with <400 HIV RNA copies/mL plasma at 24 weeks). CD4+ T cell responses superior in the indinavir + NRTIs group	Nausea, vomiting, diarrhea, rash, oral paresthesias, elevated liver function tests, hyperglycemia, fat redistribution, lipid abnormalities
Lopinavir/ritonavir (Kaletra)	Licensed	For treatment of HIV infection	Not indicated	400 mg/100 mg bid	In treatment of naïve patients, lopinavir/ritonavir + d4T + 3TC superior to nelfinavir + d4T + 3TC with regard to viral load suppression (79% vs 64% with <400 HIV RNA copies/mL at 40 weeks). CD4+ T cell increases similar in both groups.	Diarrhea, hyperglycemia, fat redistribution, lipid abnormalities

NOTE: ARC, AIDS-related complex; NRTIs, nonnucleoside reverse transcriptase inhibitors.

be less virulent and are less able to generate new mutants than are strains of HIV that are 3TC-sensitive. Lamivudine is among the best tolerated and least toxic nucleoside analogues.

Abacavir {(1S,cis)-4-[2-amino-6-(cyclopropylamino)-9H-purin-9-yl]-2-cyclopentene-1-methanol sulfate (salt)(2:1)} is a synthetic carbocyclic analogue of the nucleoside guanosine. It is licensed to be used in combination with other antiretroviral agents for the treatment of HIV-1 infection. Hypersensitivity reactions have been reported in ~5% of patients treated with this drug, and patients developing signs or symptoms of hypersensitivity such as fever, skin rash, fatigue, and gastrointestinal symptoms should discontinue the drug and not restart it. Fatal hypersensitivity reactions have been reported with rechallenge. Abacavir-resistant strains of HIV are typically also resistant to lamivudine, didanosine, and zalcitabine.

Nevirapine, *delavirdine*, and *efavirenz* are nonnucleoside inhibitors of the HIV-1 reverse transcriptase. They are licensed for use in combination with nucleoside analogues for the treatment of HIV-infected adults. These agents inhibit reverse transcriptase by binding to regions of the enzyme outside the active site and causing conformational changes in the enzyme that render it inactive. Although these agents are active in the nanomolar range, they are also very selective for the reverse transcriptase of HIV-1, have no activity against HIV-2, and, when used as monotherapy, are associated with the rapid emergence of drug-resistant mutants (Table 309-21; Fig. 309-39). Efavirenz is administered once a day, nevirapine twice a day, and delavirdine three times a day. All three drugs are associated with the development of a maculopapular rash, generally seen within the first few weeks of therapy. While it is possible to treat through this rash, it is important

Table 309-22 Drug-Drug Interactions Involving Antiretroviral Agents

Index Drug	Interacting Drug(s)	Mechanism/Effect	Recommendation
Amprenavir	Efavirenz	Induction of metabolism, decreased amprenavir AUC	Consider dosage increase to 1200 mg tid or add ritonavir 200 mg bid
	Indinavir	Inhibition of metabolism—drug levels increased 64%	Combination under investigation
	Ketoconazole	Inhibition of metabolism—drug levels increased 32%	Combination under investigation
	Ritonavir	Inhibition of metabolism—amprenavir AUC increased 2.5-fold	Combination under investigation to optimize amprenavir levels
Amprenavir, indinavir, saquinavir, ritonavir, nelfinavir	Rifampin	Induction of metabolism—marked decrease in protease inhibitor drug levels	Avoid concomitant use
Antiarrhythmics (flecainaide, quinidine, propafenone, amiodarone)	Ritonavir	Inhibition of metabolism—potential for increased levels and toxicity	Use with caution or avoid concomitant use
Atovaquone	Rifampin	Induction of metabolism—decreased drug levels	Concentrations may not be therapeutic—avoid or increase dose
Benzodiazepines (flurazepam, diazepam, midazolam, triazolam)	Protease inhibitors, delavirdine	Inhibition of metabolism—increased drug levels	Monitor for toxicity such as increased sedation, decrease dose, or use temazepam, lorazepam
Cidofovir	Nephrotoxic drugs (aminoglycosides, amphotericin, foscarnet)	Potential for increased side effects	Monitor renal function
Cisapride	Protease inhibitors, azole antifungals, macrolides, delavirdine	Inhibition of metabolism	Cardiotoxic life-threatening effects possible—avoid concomitant use
Clarithromycin	Efavirenz	Induction of metabolism—40% decrease in clarithromycin AUC	Clinical significance unknown, but clarithromycin effectiveness may be altered
	Nevirapine	Induction of metabolism—decrease in clarithromycin AUC by 30%, increase in 14-OH clarithromycin by 58%	No dosage adjustments necessary
	Ritonavir	Inhibition of metabolism—drug levels increased 77%	No adjustment needed in normal renal function
Delavirdine	Adefovir	Decrease in delavirdine AUC by 35–44%	No clinical data, but potential for decreased DLV efficacy
	Agents that increase gastric pH—antacids, H_2 blockers, proton pump inhibitors, didanosine	Delavirdine absorption decreased with increased pH	Avoid concomitant use with H_2 blockers and proton pump inhibitors; separate from antacids by at least 2 h
	Rifabutin	Induction of metabolism—50–60% decrease in delavirdine levels	Clinical significance unknown; may require increased delavirdine dose
	Rifampin	Induction of metabolism—marked decrease in drug levels	Avoid concomitant use
Didanosine (ddl)	Allopurinol	Increased ddl AUC by 2-fold	Clinical significance unknown
	Methadone	Decrease in ddl AUC by 52%	No clinical data, but potential for decreased ddl efficacy
Efavirenz	Fluconazole	Inhibition of metabolism—efavirenz AUC increased 15%	No dosage adjustment necessary
	Indinavir	Induction of hepatic metabolism—indinavir AUC decreased 35%	Consider increasing indinavir dose to 1000 mg q8h
	Nelfinavir	Nelfinavir AUC increased 21%	No dosage adjustment necessary
	Rifampin	Induction of metabolism—significant reduction in efavirenz AUC	Clinical significance unknown; increase in efavirenz dose may be required
	Rifampin	Induction of metabolism—efavirenz AUC decreased 26%	Clinical significance unknown
	Ritonavir	Inhibition of metabolism—efavirenz AUC increased 21%	No dosage adjustment necessary
Ergot alkaloids (ergotamine, dihydroergotamine, ergoloid mesylates)	Protease inhibitors, azole antifungals, macrolides, delavirdine	Inhibition of metabolism—potential for acute toxicity	Use with caution or avoid concomitant use; monitor for toxicity such as peripheral vasoconstriction, nausea and vomiting, and impaired mental status
Ethinyl estradiol	Efavirenz	Inhibition of metabolism—37% increase in estradiol AUC	No dosage adjustment necessary
	Ritonavir, nelfinavir	Induction of metabolism—decreased levels of oral contraceptive	Use alternative methods of contraception
Fluvastatin, lovastatin, simvastatin	Protease inhibitors, azole antifungals, macrolides, delavirdine	Inhibition of metabolism—potential for increased levels and toxicity	Potential for hypolipidemic toxicity (dizziness, headache, GI side effects); monitor patient closely and consider dose reduction or use pravastatin or atorvastatin
Foscarnet	Nephrotoxic drugs (aminoglycosides, amphotericin, cidofovir)	Potential for increased toxicity	Monitor renal function

(continued)

Table 309-21—*(continued)*

Index Drug	Interacting Drug(s)	Mechanism/Effect	Recommendation
Ganciclovir	Drugs causing bone marrow suppression (i.e., TMP/SMZ, zidovudine)	Potential for increased hematologic toxicity	Monitor for anemia and neutropenia—adjust/change doses and drugs if required; consider supportive therapy with G-CSF
Indinavir, saquinavir, ritonavir, nelfinavir, amprenavir	Anticonvulsants (carbamazepine, phenytoin, phenobarbital)	Induction of metabolism—potential decrease in drug levels	Clinical effects unknown; monitor blood levels, consider dosage increase, or avoid concomitant use
Indinavir	Delavirdine	Increased indinavir levels	Consider reducing indinavir dose to 600 mg q8h
	St. John's wort	Decreased indinavir levels	Avoid use of St. John's wort
	Didanosine, antacids	ddl buffer decreases absorption of indinavir	Separate doses by at least 1 h
	Methadone	Indinavir C_{max} decreased 16–36%; indinavir C_{min} increased by 50–100%	No dosage adjustments necessary
	Nelfinavir	Inhibition of metabolism—indinavir drug levels increased by 51%, nelfinavir drug levels by 83%	Combination currently under evaluation
	Nevirapine	Induction of metabolism—decreased drug levels of indinavir by 30%	Consider increasing indinavir dose to 1000 mg q8h
	Ritonavir	Inhibition of metabolism—indinavir AUC increased 3-7-fold	bid regimens under investigation to optimize indinavir levels—various doses under study including 800 mg indinavir/200 mg ritonavir bid
Meperidine	Ritonavir	Likely induction of metabolism—Decrease in meperidine AUC 67%, increase in normeperidine 47%	Potential for decreased meperidine effectiveness—may require increased dose; caution with chronic dosing
Methadone	Abacavir	Methadone clearance decreased 22%	Low potential for opiate withdrawal; monitor closely and increase methadone dose as required to control symptoms
	Fluconazole	Inhibition of metabolism—drug levels increased 30%	Monitor for methadone toxicity such as respiratory depression, drop in blood pressure, and mental status changes; consider dosage adjustment
	Nevirapine	Induction of metabolism—substantial decrease in methadone levels	Potential for opiate withdrawal; monitor closely and increase methadone dose as required to control symptoms
Nelfinavir	Ritonavir	Inhibition of metabolism—increased drug levels of nelfinavir by 152%	Currently under investigation
Pentamidine	Drugs that cause pancreatitis (didanosine, zalcitabine)	Increased risk of pancreatitis	Monitor amylase, lipase
Quinolone antibiotics (ciprofloxacin, levofloxacin, ofloxaxin, etc)	Didanosine, antacids, iron products, calcium products, sucralfate	Chelation resulting in marked decrease in quinolone drug levels	Administer cation preparations at least 2 h after quinolone
Rifabutin	Amprenavir, ritonavir, indinavir, nelfinavir	Inhibition of metabolism—marked increase in rifabutin drug levels	Use 150 mg qd with indinavir, nelfinavir, emprenavir, Use 150 mg every other day with ritonavir
	Fluconazole	Inhibition of metabolism—marked increase in rifabutin drug levels	Monitor for rifabutin toxicity such as uveitis, nausea, neutropenia
Saquinavir	Nevirapine	Induction of metabolism—drug levels decreased 27%	Clinical significance unknown—consider dosage increase of saquinavir or add ritonavir
	Ritonavir	Inhibition of metabolism—3-fold or higher increase in saquinavir drug levels	Various combinations used to optimize saquinavir therapy including 400 mg saquinavir/400 mg ritonavir
	Efavirenz	Induction of metabolism—saquinavir AUC decreased 62%	Avoid concomitant use unless saquinavir is administered with ritonavir
Sildenafil	Ritonavir	Inhibition of metabolism—sildenafil AUC increased 11-fold	Use 25-mg sildenafil dose and do not repeat for 48 h
	Saquinavir, indinavir	Inhibition of metabolism—sildenafil AUC increased 3–4-fold	Use 25-mg sildenafil dose
Terfenadine, astemizole	Protease inhibitors, azole antifungals, macrolides, delavirdine	Inhibition of metabolism	Cardiotoxic life-threatening effects possible—avoid concomitant use
Theophylline	Ritonavir	Induction of metabolism—decreased blood levels	Monitor theophylline levels
Tipranavir	Ritonavir	Inhibition of metabolism—tipranavir AUC increased 7–45-fold	Combination under investigation to optimize tipranavir levels
TMP/SMZ	Rifampin	TMP AUC decreased 63%, SMZ AUC decreased 23%	Clinical significance unknown
Zalcitabine, stavudine, didanosine	Drugs that cause peripheral neuropathy—INH, d4T, ddI, ddC	Potential for increased risk of peripheral neuropathy	Monitor for signs and symptoms such as numbness and tingling in extremities
Zidovudine	Drugs causing bone marrow suppression (i.e., TMP/SMZ, ganciclovir, sulfadiazine)	Increased bone marrow suppression	Monitor for anemia, neutropenia—may require supportive therapy (EPO, G-CSF)

NOTE: AUC, area under the curve; *C*, concentration; EPO, erythropoietin; G-CSF, granulocyte colony stimulating factor; TMP/SMZ, trimethoprim/sulfamethoxazole.

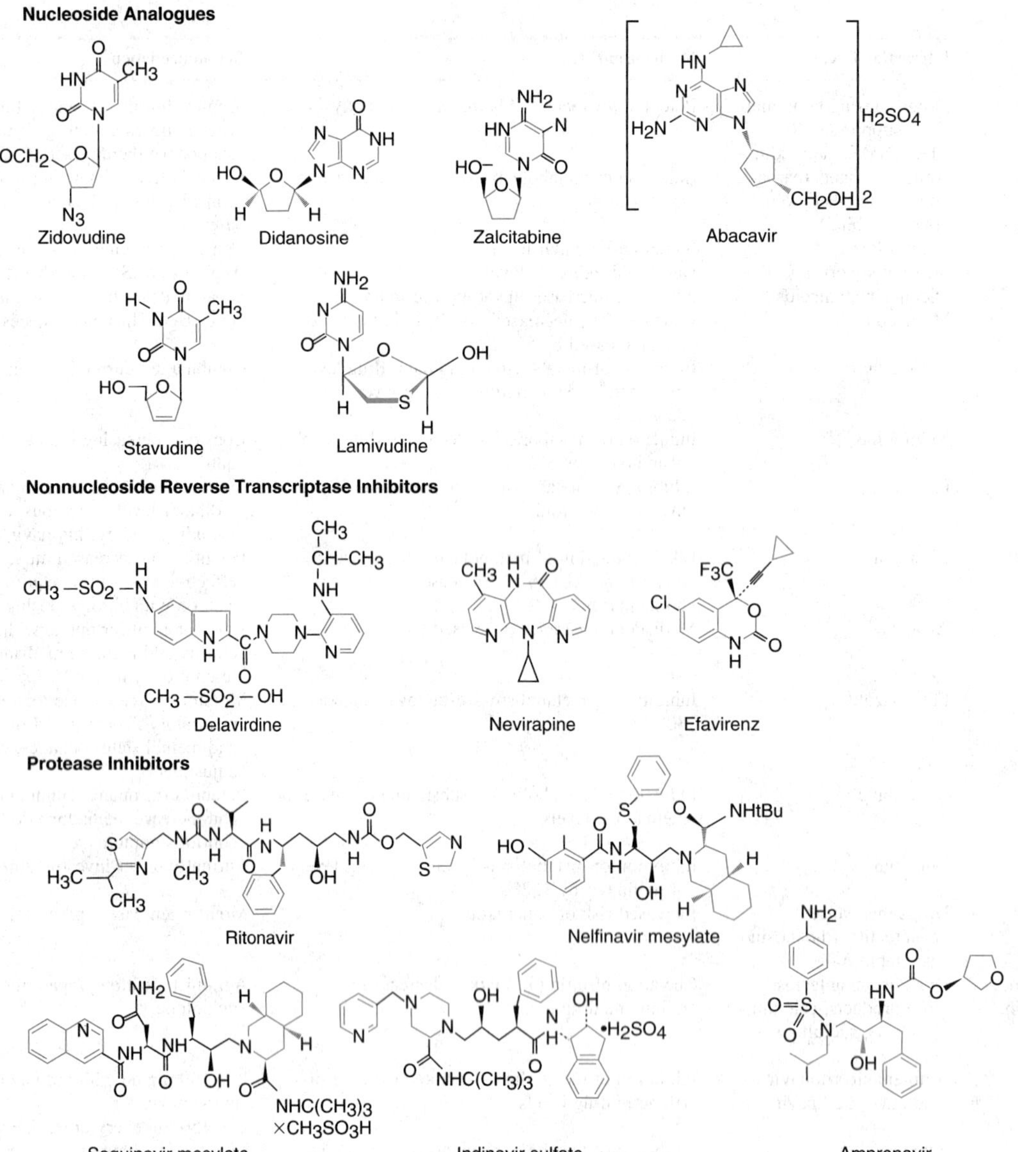

FIGURE 309-38 Molecular structures of antiretroviral agents.

to be sure that one is not dealing with a more severe eruption such as Stevens-Johnson syndrome by looking carefully for signs of mucosal involvement, significant fever, or painful lesions with desquamation. In addition to skin rash, many patients treated with efavirenz note a feeling of light-headedness, dizziness, or out of sorts following the initiation of therapy. Some complain of vivid dreams. These symptoms tend to disappear after several weeks of therapy. Aside from difficulties with dreams, taking efavirenz at bedtime may minimize the side effects. Nevirapine and efavirenz are both commonly used as part of initial treatment regimens in combination with two nucleoside analogues. Another common use of these drugs is as part of salvage regimens in patients whose current regimen is inadequate.

The introduction of the HIV-1 protease inhibitors (saquinavir, indinavir, ritonavir, nelfinavir, and amprenavir) to the therapeutic armamentarium of antiretrovirals has had a profound impact on the efficacy of antiretroviral therapy. When used as part of initial regimens in combination with reverse transcriptase inhibitors, these agents have been shown to be capable of suppressing levels of HIV replication to under 50 copies per milliliter in the majority of patients for a minimum of 3 years. As in the case of reverse transcriptase inhibitors, resistance to protease inhibitors can develop rapidly in the setting of monotherapy, and thus these agents should be used as part of combination therapeutic regimens. A summary of known resistance mutations for reverse transcriptase and protease inhibitors is shown in Fig. 309-39.

Saquinavir was the first of the HIV-1 protease inhibitors to be licensed. Initially provided as a hard gel (Invirase) with poor bioavailability, the current soft-get formulation (Fortavase) provides good plasma levels of drug, particularly when administered in conjunction with ritonavir. Saquinavir is metabolized by the cytochrome P450 system, and ritonavir therapy results in inhibition of cytochrome P450 action. Thus, when both drugs are administered together there is the potential for increases in saquinavir levels. The use of low doses of ritonavir to provide pharmacodynamic boosting of other agents has become a fairly common strategy in HIV therapy. Saquinavir is perhaps the best-tolerated protease inhibitor and the one with the fewest side effects.

Ritonavir was the first protease inhibitor for which clinical efficacy was demonstrated. In a study of 1090 patients with CD4+ T cell counts $<100/\mu L$ who were randomized to receive either placebo or ritonavir in addition to any other licensed medications, patients receiving ritonavir had a reduction in the cumulative incidence of clinical progression or death from 34% to 17%. Mortality decreased from 10.1% to 5.8%. At full doses, ritonavir is poorly tolerated. Among the main side effects are nausea, diarrhea, abdominal pain, and circumoral paresthesia. Ritonavir has a high affinity for several isoforms of cytochrome

P450, and its use can result in large increases in the plasma concentrations of drugs metabolized by this pathway. Among the agents affected in this manner are saquinavir, indinavir, macrolide antibiotics, R-warfarin, ondansetron, rifampin, most calcium channel blockers, glucocorticoids, and some of the chemotherapeutic agents used to treat KS. In addition, ritonavir may increase the activity of glucuronyltransferases, thus decreasing the levels of drugs metabolized by this pathway. Overall, great care must be taken when prescribing additional drugs to patients taking ritonavir. As mentioned above, the pharmacodynamic boosting property of ritonavir, seen with doses as low as 100 to 200 mg twice a day, is often used in the setting of HIV infection to derive more convenient regimens. For example, when given with low-dose ritonavir, saquinavir and indinavir can both be given on twice-a-day schedules and taken with food.

Indinavir is among the best studied of the HIV-1 protease inhibitors. It was the first protease inhibitor used in combination with dual nucleoside therapy. The combination of zidovudine, lamivudine, and indinavir was the first "triple combination" shown to have a profound effect on HIV replication. The main side effects of indinavir are nephrolithiasis (seen in 4% of patients) and asymptomatic indirect hyperbilirubinemia (seen in 10%). Indinavir is predominantly metabolized by the liver. The dose should be lowered in patients with cirrhosis. Indinavir shares metabolic pathways with terfenadine, astemizole, cisapride, triazolam, and midazolam. To avoid the potential for cardiac arrhythmias or prolonged sedation, these drugs should not be administered to patients taking indinavir. Levels of indinavir are decreased during concurrent therapy with rifabutin or nevirapine and increased during concurrent therapy with ketoconazole, delavirdine, efavirenz, or ritonavir. Dosages should be modified appropriately in these circumstances (Table 309-22).

A. Mutations in the Protease Gene Selected by Protease Inhibitors
Protease Inhibitors

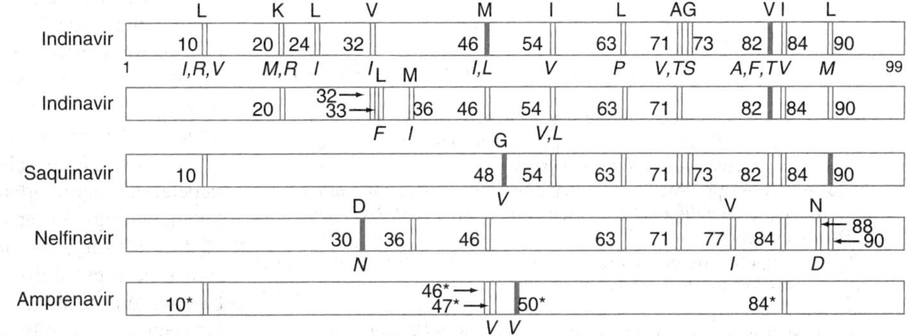

B. Mutations in the Reverse Transcriptase (RT) Gene Selected by RT Inhibitors
Nucleoside RT Inhibitors

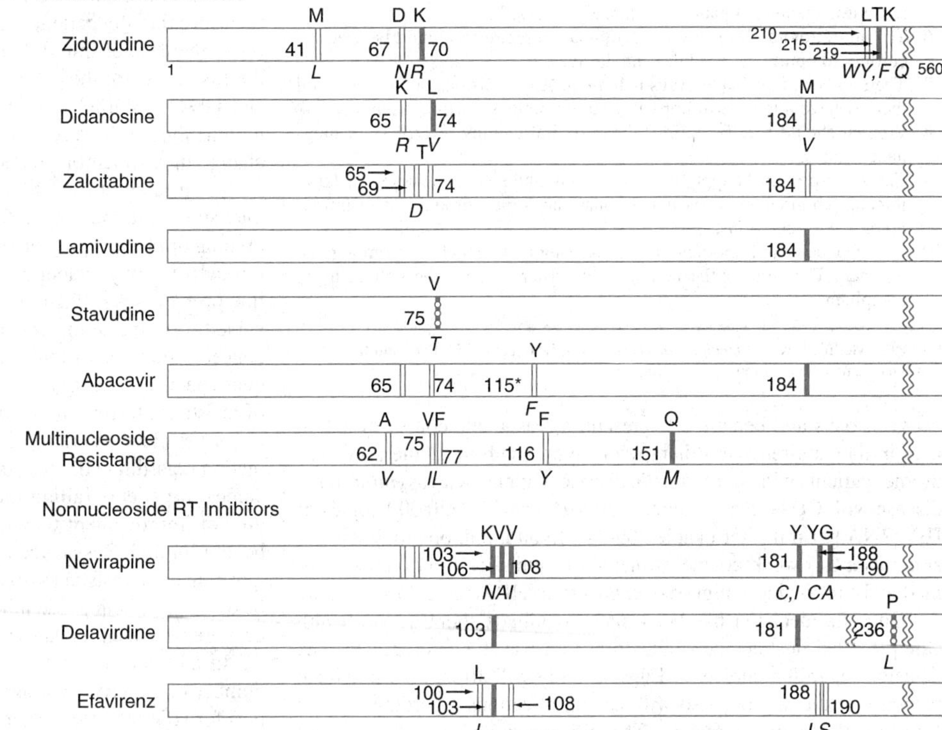

FIGURE 309-39 Amino acid substitutions conferring resistance to antiretroviral drugs. The most common HIV-1 mutations selected by protease inhibitors *(A)*, and nucleoside and nonnucleoside reverse transcriptase inhibitors *(B)*. For each amino acid residue listed, the letter above the listing indicates the amino acid associated with the wild-type virus. The italicized letter below the residue indicates the substitution that confers drug resistance. *(From Hirsch et al.)*

Nelfinavir was approved in 1997 and *amprenavir* was approved in 1999 for the treatment of adult or pediatric HIV infection when antiretroviral therapy is warranted. As with most of the newer antiretroviral agents, these approvals were based on randomized, controlled trials that demonstrated decreases in plasma HIV RNA levels and increases in CD4+ T cell counts. Both agents have unique resistance profiles. Nelfinavir resistance is associated with a D30N substitution in the protease gene. Viruses harboring this single mutation retain sensitivity to other protease inhibitors, and it has been suggested that for this reason nelfinavir is a good initial protease inhibitor. It is not clear, however, whether this theoretical consideration will be borne out in the results of clinical trials. Protease inhibitor resistance typically involves multiple amino acid substitutions and reduced susceptibility across the class. Amprenavir resistance is associated with a unique substitution at amino acid 50 (I50V), and it has been suggested that amprenavir may be of particular value in salvage regimens. This assumption also awaits verification in controlled clinical trials. Nelfinavir and amprenavir are both associated with gastrointestinal side effects. About 1% of patients receiving amprenavir have experienced severe and life-threatening skin reactions. An additional disadvantage of amprenavir is that the current formulation requires the patient to take 8 large capsules twice a day.

One of the main problems that has been encountered with the widespread use of HAART therapy has been a syndrome of hyperlipidemia and fat distribution often referred to as *lipodystrophy syndrome* (discussed above under metabolic abnormalities).

The principles of therapy for HIV infection have been articulated by a panel sponsored by the U.S. Department of Health and Human Services and the Henry J. Kaiser Family Foundation. These principles are summarized in Table 309-23. However, *one element of HIV disease not currently covered by these principles is that eradication of HIV infection has not yet been possible*. Treatment decisions must take into account the fact that one is dealing with a chronic infection. While early therapy is generally the rule in infectious diseases, immediate treatment of every HIV-infected individual upon diagnosis may not be prudent, and therapeutic decisions must take into account the balance

Table 309-23 Principles of Therapy of HIV Infection

1. Ongoing HIV replication leads to immune system damage and progression to AIDS.
2. Plasma HIV RNA levels indicate the magnitude of HIV replication and the rate of CD4+ T cell destruction. CD4+ T cell counts indicate the current level of competence of the immune system.
3. Rates of disease progression differ among individuals, and treatment decisions should be individualized based upon plasma HIV RNA levels and CD4+ T cell counts.
4. Maximal suppression of viral replication is a goal of therapy; the greater the suppression the less likely the appearance of drug-resistance quasispecies.
5. The most effective therapeutic strategies involve the simultaneous initiation of combinations of effective anti-HIV drugs with which the patient has not been previously treated and that are not cross-resistant with antiretroviral agents that patient has already received.
6. The antiretroviral drugs used in combination regimens should be used according to optimum schedules and dosages.
7. The number of available drugs is limited. Any decisions on antiretroviral therapy have a long-term impact on future options for the patient.
8. Women should receive optimal antiretroviral therapy regardless of pregnancy status.
9. The same principals apply to children and adults. The treatment of HIV-infected children involves unique pharmacologic, virologic, and immunologic considerations.
10. Compliance is an important part of ensuring maximal effect from a given regimen. The simpler the regimen, the easier it is for the patient to be compliant.

SOURCE: Modified from, *Principles of Therapy of HIV Infection*, USPHS and the Henry J. Kaiser Family Foundation.

between risks and benefits. At present, a reasonable course of action is to initiate antiretroviral therapy in anyone with the acute HIV syndrome; patients with symptomatic disease; patients with asymptomatic disease with CD4+ T cell counts $<500/\mu L$ or with $>20,000$ copies of HIV RNA per milliliter (Table 309-24). In addition, one may wish to administer a 6-week course of therapy to uninfected individuals immediately following a high-risk exposure to HIV (see below).

Once the decision has been made to initiate therapy, the health care provider must decide which drugs to use as the first regimen. The decision regarding choice of drugs not only will affect the immediate response to therapy but also will have implications regarding options for future therapeutic regimens. The initial regimen is usually the most effective insofar as the virus has yet to develop significant resistance. The two options for initial therapy most commonly in use today are two different three-drug regimens. The first regimen utilizes two nucleoside analogues (one of which is usually lamivudine) and a protease inhibitor. The second regimen utilizes two nucleoside analogues and a nonnucleoside reverse transcriptase inhibitor. Unfortunately there are no clear data at present on which to base distinctions between these two approaches. Following the initiation of therapy one should expect a 1 log (tenfold) reduction in plasma HIV RNA levels within 1 to 2 months and eventually a decline in plasma HIV RNA levels to <50 copies per milliliter. During this same time there should be a rise in the CD4+ T cell count of 100 to $150/\mu L$ that is particularly brisk during the first month of therapy. Many clinicians feel that failure to achieve this endpoint is an indication for a change in therapy. Other reasons for a change in therapy include a persistently declining CD4+ T cell count, clinical deterioration, or drug toxicity (Table 309-25). As in the case of initiating therapy, changing therapy may have a lasting impact on future therapeutic options. When changing therapy because of treatment failure (clinical progression or worsening laboratory parameters), it is important to attempt to provide a regimen with at least two new drugs. In the patient in whom a change is made for reasons of drug toxicity, a simple replacement of one drug is reasonable. It should be stressed that in attempting to sort out a drug toxicity it may be advisable to hold all therapy for a period of time to distinguish between drug toxicity and disease progression. Drug toxicity will usually begin to show signs of reversal within 1 to 2 weeks. Prior to changing a treatment regimen because of drug failure, it is important to ensure that the patient has been adherent to the prescribed regimen. As in the case of initial therapy, the simpler the therapeutic regimen, the easier it is for the patient to be compliant. Plasma HIV RNA levels and CD4+ T lymphocyte counts should be monitored every 3 to 4 months during therapy and more frequently if one is contemplating a change in regimen or immediately following a change in regimen.

In an attempt to determine an optimal therapeutic regimen, one may attempt to measure antiretroviral drug susceptibility through genotyping or phenotyping of HIV quasispecies. Genotyping may be done through dideoxynucleotide sequencing, DNA chip hybridization, or line probe assays. Phenotypic assays measure the performance of reverse transcriptase or protease in the presence or absence of different concentrations of different drugs. These assays will generally detect quasispecies present at a frequency of at least 10%. The precise role of resistance testing in the management of patients with HIV infection is not yet clear. While randomized studies have suggested that information regarding HIV resistance profiles may improve therapeutic outcomes in patients failing their current antiretroviral regimen, the degree of improvement thus far has been small and the duration of the benefit limited. Resistance testing may be of particular value in distinguishing drug-resistant virus from poor patient compliance; it may also be of value to help guide initial therapy in a setting where transmission of a drug-resistant isolate is felt to be likely.

In addition to the licensed medications discussed above, a large number of experimental agents are being evaluated as possible therapies for HIV infection. Therapeutic strategies are being developed that interfere with virtually every step of the replication cycle of the virus (Fig. 309-3). In addition, as more is discovered about the role of the immune system in controlling viral replication, additional strategies, generically referred to as "immune-based therapies," are being developed as a complement to antiviral therapy. Among the antiviral agents in early clinical trials are additional nucleoside analogues, nucleotide analogues, additional protease inhibitors including nonpeptidomimetic compounds, integrase inhibitors, antisense nucleic acids, and fusion inhibitors. Among the immune-based therapies being evaluated are IFN-α, bone marrow transplantation, adoptive transfer of lymphocytes

Table 309-24 Indications for the Initiation of Antiretroviral Therapy in Patients with HIV Infection

I. Acute infection syndrome
II. Chronic infection
  A. Symptomatic disease
  B. Asymptomatic diseases[a]
    1. CD4+ T cell count $<500/\mu L$ or decreasing
    2. HIV RNA $>20,000$ copies per milliliter or increasing
III. Postexposure prophylaxis

[a] This is the area of greatest controversy. Some experts would wait until the CD4 cell count declines to $200/\mu l$, whereas others would treat everyone regardless of CD4+ T cell count.

SOURCE: *Guidelines for the Use of Antiretroviral Agents in HIV-Infected Adults and Adolescents*. USPHS.

Table 309-25 Indications for Changing Antiretroviral Therapy in Patients with HIV Infection[a]

Less than a 1-log drop in plasma HIV RNA by 4 weeks following the initiation of therapy
A reproducible significant increase (defined as 3-fold or greater) from the nadir of plasma HIV RNA level not attributable to intercurrent infection, vaccination, or test methodology
Persistently declining CD4+ T cell numbers
Clinical deterioration
Side effects

[a] Generally speaking, a change should involve the initiation of at least 2 drugs felt to be effective in the given patient. The exception to this is when change is being made to manage toxicity, in which case a single substitution is reasonable.

SOURCE: *Guidelines for the Use of Antiretroviral Agents in HIV-Infected Adults and Adolescents*. USPHS.

genetically modified to resist infection or enhance HIV-specific immunity, active immunotherapy with inactivated HIV, and IL-2.

HIV AND THE HEALTH CARE WORKER

Health care workers, especially those who deal with large numbers of HIV-infected patients, have a small but definite risk of becoming infected with HIV as a result of professional activities. As of January 1, 2000, 56 health care workers in the United States had been documented as having seroconverted to HIV following occupational exposure; 25 have developed AIDS. The individuals who seroconverted include 19 laboratory workers (16 of whom were clinical laboratory workers), 23 nurses, 6 physicians, 2 surgical technicians, 1 dialysis technician, 1 respiratory therapist, 1 health aide, 1 embalmer/morgue technician, and 2 housekeeper/maintenance workers. The exposures included 48 percutaneous (puncture/cut injury), 5 mucocutaneous (mucous membrane and/or skin), 2 both percutaneous and mucocutaneous, and 1 unknown route of exposure. Fifty exposures were to HIV-infected blood, three to concentrated virus in a laboratory, one to visibly bloody fluid, and one to unspecified fluid. As of January 1, 2000, there had been 136 other cases of HIV infection or AIDS among health care workers who have not reported other risk factors for HIV infection and who report a history of exposure to blood, body fluids, or HIV-infected laboratory material, but for whom seroconversion after exposure was not documented. The number of these workers who actually acquired their infection through occupational exposures is not known. Taken together, the data from several large studies suggest that the risk of HIV infection following a percutaneous injury with an HIV-contaminated hollow-bore needle (in contrast to a solid-bore needle, i.e., a suture needle) is approximately 0.3%. A seroprevalence survey of 3420 orthopedic surgeons, 75% of whom practiced in an area with a relatively high prevalence of HIV infection and 39% of whom reported percutaneous exposure to patient blood, usually through an accident involving a suture needle, failed to reveal any cases of possible occupational infection, suggesting that the risk of infection with a suture needle may be considerably less than that with a blood-drawing needle.

Most cases of health care worker seroconversion occur as a result of needle-stick injuries. When one considers the circumstances that result in needle-stick injuries, it is immediately obvious that adhering to the standard guidelines for dealing with sharp objects would result in a significant decrease in this type of accident. In one study, 27% of needle-stick injuries resulted from improper disposal of the needle (over half of these were due to recapping the needle), 23% occurred during attempts to start an intravenous line, 22% occurred during blood drawing, 16% were associated with an intramuscular or subcutaneous injection, and 12% were associated with giving an intravenous infusion.

Recommendations regarding postexposure prophylaxis must take into account that several circumstances determine the risk of transmission of HIV following occupational exposure. In this regard, five factors have been associated with an increased risk for occupational transmission of HIV infection: deep injury, the presence of visible blood on the instrument causing the exposure, injury with a device that had been placed in the vein or artery of the source patient, terminal illness in the source patient, and lack of postexposure antiretroviral therapy in the exposed health care worker. Other important considerations include pregnancy in the health care worker and the possibility of exposure to drug-resistant virus. Regardless of the decision to use postexposure prophylaxis, the wound should be cleansed immediately and antiseptic applied. If a decision is made to offer postexposure prophylaxis, U.S. Public Health Service guidelines recommend (1) a combination of two nucleoside analogue reverse transcriptase inhibitors given for 4 weeks for routine exposures, or (2) a combination of two nucleoside analogue reverse transcriptase inhibitors plus a protease inhibitor given for 4 weeks for high-risk or otherwise complicated exposures, although most clinicians administer the latter regimen in all cases in which a decision is made to treat. Further details are available from the U.S. Public Health Service *Guidelines for the Management of Health-Care Worker Exposures to HIV and Recommendations for Postexposure Prophylaxis* (CDC, 1998).

Health care workers can minimize their risk of occupational HIV infection by following the CDC guidelines of July 1991, which include adherence to universal precautions, refraining from direct patient care if one has exudative lesions or weeping dermatitis, and disinfecting and sterilizing reusable devices employed in invasive procedures. The premise of universal precautions is that every specimen should be handled as if it came from someone infected with a bloodborne pathogen. All samples should be double-bagged, gloves should be worn when drawing blood, and spills should be immediately disinfected with bleach.

In attempting to put this small but definite risk to the health care worker in perspective, it is important to point out that approximately 200 health care workers die each year as a result of occupationally acquired hepatitis B infection. The tragedy in this instance is that these infections and deaths due to HBV could be greatly decreased by more extended use of the HBV vaccine. The risk of HBV infection following a needle-stick injury from a hepatitis antigen–positive patient is much higher than the risk of HIV infection (see "Transmission," above). There are multiple examples of needle-stick injuries where the patient was positive for both HBV and HIV and the health care worker became infected only with HBV. For these reasons, it is advisable, given the high prevalence of HBV infection in HIV-infected individuals, that all health care workers dealing with HIV-infected patients be immunized with the HBV vaccine.

TB is another infection common to HIV-infected patients that can be transmitted to the health care worker. For this reason, all health care workers should know their PPD status, have it checked yearly, and receive one year of isoniazid treatment if their skin test converts to positive. In addition, all patients in whom a diagnosis of TB is being entertained should be placed immediately in respiratory isolation, pending results of the diagnostic evaluation. The emergence of drug-resistant organisms has made TB an increasing problem for health care workers. This is particularly true for the health care worker with preexisting HIV infection.

One of the most charged issues ever to come between health care workers and patients is that of transmission of infection from HIV-infected health care workers to their patients. This is discussed under "Occupational Transmission of HIV: Health Care Workers and Laboratory Workers," p. 1857. Theoretically, the same universal precautions that are used to protect the health care worker from the HIV-infected patient will also protect the patient from the HIV-infected health care worker.

VACCINES

Historically, vaccines have provided a safe, cost-effective, and efficient means of preventing illness, disability, and death from infectious diseases. Given the fact that human behavior, especially human sexual behavior, is extremely difficult to change, the best hope for preventing the spread of HIV infection rests with the development of a safe and effective vaccine. This task is problematic for a number of reasons, including the high mutability of the virus, the fact that the infection can be transmitted by cell-free or cell-associated virus, the likely need for the development of effective mucosal immunity, and the fact that it has been difficult to establish the precise correlates of protective immunity to HIV infection. Some HIV-infected individuals are long-term nonprogressors (see above), and a number of individuals have been exposed to HIV multiple times but remain uninfected; these facts suggest that there are protective elements of an HIV-specific immune response. In addition, studies using animal models, specifically SIV in the monkey and HIV-1 in the chimpanzee, have been encouraging and suggest that an HIV vaccine is possible. It should be pointed out that while the ideal goal of an HIV vaccine is to prevent infection, a vaccine given to an uninfected individual that significantly alters the

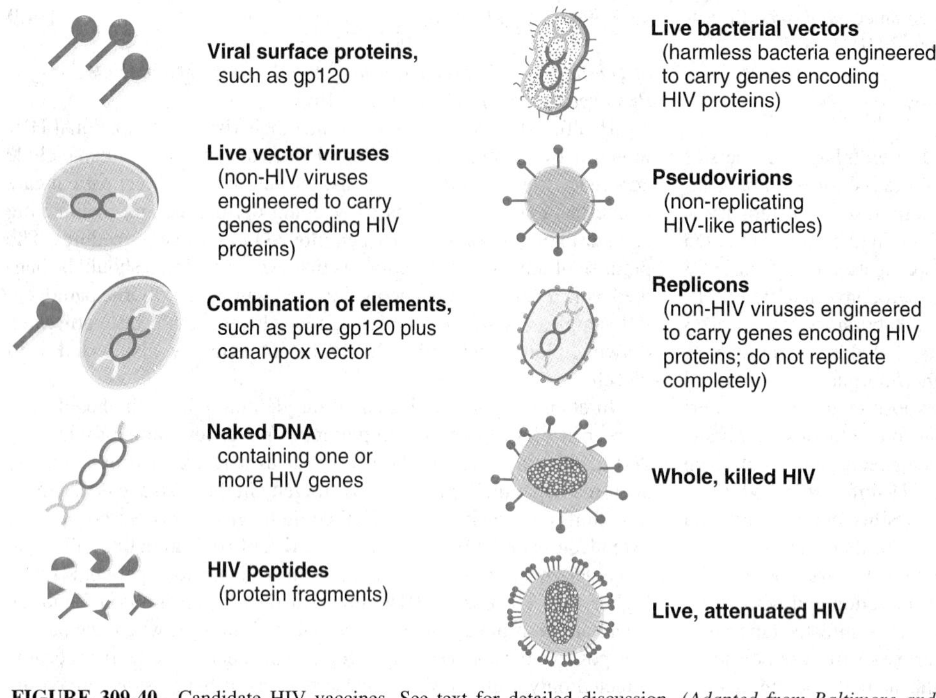

FIGURE 309-40 Candidate HIV vaccines. See text for detailed discussion. *(Adapted from Baltimore and Heilman, 1998. Copyright © Slim Films.)*

course of disease or the infectivity of the individual, should that person become infected, could have an impact not only on the individual in question but also on the spread of infection in the community.

A number of clinical trials ranging from several small phase I trials to determine safety, to fewer intermediate-sized phase II trials to determine safety and immunogenicity, to a single phase III trial to determine efficacy have been or are currently being conducted in humans. The single phase III trial is testing a bivalent gp 120 protein; this product has been shown to induce antibodies but not cytolytic T cells responses in phase I and II trials. The furthest advanced among phase II trials involves a combination approach using a live canarypox vector expressing one or multiple HIV epitopes given together with gp120 or using the gp120 as a boost. This approach has resulted in neutralizing antibodies in virtually all recipients and HIV-specific cytolytic T cells in approximately 30% of individuals at any given time during the course of the trial.

Other approaches currently being tested in phase I and/or phase II trials in humans include naked DNA; vaccines employing vectors such as modified vaccinia Ankara (MVA), salmonella, Venezuela equine encephalitis (VEE) virus, among others; peptide and subunit vaccines; and pseudovirions (Fig. 309-40). Live attenuated HIV vaccines have not proceeded into human trials at this time because of safety concerns. It is clear that it will take several years of clinical trials to establish the efficacy or lack thereof of a candidate vaccine for HIV.

PREVENTION

Education, counseling, and behavior modification are the cornerstones of an HIV prevention strategy. Widespread voluntary testing of individuals who have practiced or are practicing high-risk behavior, together with counseling of infected individuals, is recommended. Information gathered from such an approach should serve as the basis for behavior-modification programs, both for infected individuals who may be unaware of their HIV status and who could infect others and for uninfected individuals practicing high-risk behavior. The practice of "safer sex" is the most effective way for sexually active uninfected individuals to avoid contracting HIV infection and for infected individuals to avoid spreading infection. Abstinence from sexual relations is the only absolute way to prevent sexual transmission of HIV infection. However, this may not be feasible, and there are a number of relatively safe practices that can markedly decrease the chances of transmission of HIV infection. Partners engaged in monogamous sexual relationships who wish to be assured of safety should both be tested for HIV antibody. If both are negative, it must be understood that any divergence from monogamy puts both partners at risk; open discussion of the importance of honesty in such relationships should be encouraged. When the HIV status of either partner is not known, or when one partner is positive, there are a number of options. Use of condoms can markedly decrease the chance of HIV transmission. It should be remembered that condoms are not 100% effective in preventing transmission of HIV infection, and there is an ~10% failure rate of condoms used for contraceptive purposes. Most condom failures result from breakage or improper usage, such as not wearing the condom for the entire period of intercourse. Latex condoms are preferable, since virus has been shown to leak through natural skin condoms. Petroleum-based gels should never be used for lubrication of the condom, since they increase the likelihood of condom rupture. There has been a tendency among homosexual men to practice fellatio as a "minimal risk" activity compared to receptive anal intercourse. It should be emphasized that receptive oral fellatio is definitely not safe sex, and there has been clear-cut documentation of transmission of HIV where receptive fellatio was the only sexual act performed (see "Transmission," above). Topical microbicides for vaginal and anal use are being pursued actively as a means by which individuals could avoid infection when the insertive partner cannot be relied on to use a condom. Kissing is considered safe, although there is a theoretical possibility of transmission via virus in saliva. The low concentration of virus in saliva of infected individuals, as well as the presence in saliva of HIV-inhibitory proteins (see above), lessens any risk of transmission by kissing.

The most effective way to prevent transmission of HIV infection among IDUs is to stop the use of injectable drugs. Unfortunately, that is extremely difficult to accomplish unless the individual enters a treatment program. For those who will not or cannot participate in a drug treatment program and who will continue to inject drugs, the avoidance of sharing of needles and other paraphernalia ("works") is the next best way to avoid transmission of infection. The cultural and social factors that contribute to the sharing of paraphernalia are complex and difficult to overcome. In addition, needles and syringes may be in short supply. Under these circumstances, paraphernalia should be cleaned after each usage with a virucidal solution, such as undiluted sodium hypochlorite (household bleach). Data from a number of studies have indicated that programs that provide sterile needles to addicts in exchange for used needles have resulted in a decrease in HIV transmission without increasing the use of injection drugs. It is important for IDUs to be tested for HIV infection and counseled, to avoid transmission to their sexual partners. Secondary and tertiary spread of HIV infection by the heterosexual route within settings of a high level of injection drug use has increased greatly in the United States (see above).

Transmission of HIV via transfused blood or blood products has been decreased dramatically by a combination of screening of all blood donors for HIV infection by assays for both HIV antibody and p24 antigen and self-deferral of individuals at risk for HIV infection. In addition, clotting factor concentrates are heat-treated, essentially eliminating the risk to hemophiliacs who require these products. Autologous transfusions are preferable to transfusions from another individual. However, logistic constraints as well as the unpredictability of the need for most transfusions limit the feasibility of this approach. At present the risk of becoming HIV-infected from a contaminated blood transfusion is approximately 1 in 676,000 donations.

HIV can be transmitted via breast milk and colostrum. The avoidance of breast feeding may not be practical in developing countries, where nutritional concerns override the risk of HIV transmission. However, it is becoming appreciated that from 5 to 15% of infants who were born of HIV-infected mothers and who were fortunate enough not to have been infected intrapartum or peripartum become infected via breast feeding. Therefore, even in developing countries, breast feeding from an infected mother should be avoided if at all possible. Unfortunately, this is rarely the case, and given the disadvantages of withholding breast feeding in developing countries (see above), health authorities in most developing countries continue to recommend breast feeding despite the potential for HIV transmission. In developed countries such as the United States, where bottled formula and milk are readily accessible, breast feeding is absolutely contraindicated when a mother is HIV positive.

BIBLIOGRAPHY

ALKHATIB G et al: CC CKR5: A RANTES, MIP-1α, MIP-1β receptor as a fusion cofactor for macrophage-tropic HIV-1. Science 272:1955, 1996

ANTMAN K, CHANG Y: Kaposi's sarcoma. N Engl J Med 342:1027, 2000

BALOTTA C et al: Identification of two distinct subsets of long-term nonprogressors with divergent viral activity by stromal-derived factor 1 chemokine gene polymorphism analysis. J Infect Dis 180:285, 1999

BALTIMORE D, HEILMAN C: HIV vaccines: Prospects and challenges. Sci Am 279:98, 1998

BERGER JR, MAJOR EO: Progressive multifocal leukoencephalopathy. Semin Neurol 19: 193, 1999

BLEUL CC et al: The lymphocyte chemoattractant SDF-1 is a ligand for LESTR/fusin and blocks HIV-1 entry. Nature 382:829, 1996

BREAM JH et al: CCR5 promoter alleles and specific DNA binding factors. Science 284: 223a, 1999

CAMERON DW et al: Randomised placebo-controlled trial of ritonavir in advanced HIV-1 disease. Lancet 351:543, 1998

CAO Y et al: Virologic and immunologic characterization of long-term survivors of human immunodeficiency virus type-1 infection. N Engl J Med 332:201, 1995

CARDO DM et al: A case-control study of HIV seroconversion in health care workers after percutaneous exposure. N Engl J Med 337:1485, 1997

CARR A et al: Pathogenesis of HIV-1 protease inhibitor–associated peripheral lipodystrophy, hyperlipidemia and insulin resistance. Lancet 351:1881, 1998

CARRINGTON M et al: HLA and HIV-1: Heterozygote advantage and B*35-cw*04 disadvantage. Science 283:1, 1999

CENTERS FOR DISEASE CONTROL AND PREVENTION: Human immunodeficiency virus transmission in household settings—United States. MMWR 347:353, 1994

———: Public Health Service guidelines for the management of health-care worker exposures to HIV and recommendations for postexposure prophylaxis. MMWR 47(RR-7):1, 1998

———: Diagnosis and reporting of HIV and AIDS in states with integrated HIV and AIDS surveillance—United States, January 1994–June 1997. MMWR 47:309, 1998

———: Guidelines for the use of antiretroviral agents in HIV-infected adults and adolescents. MMWR 47(RR-5):43, 1998 (See updates at www.hivatis.org)

———: Public Health Service Task Force recommendations for the use of antiretroviral drugs in pregnant women infected with HIV-1 for maternal health and for reducing perinatal HIV-1 transmission in the United States. MMWR 47(RR-2):1, 1998 (See updates at www.hivatis.org)

———: HIV/AIDS surveillance report, 1999; 11(No. 2):1, 2000

———: 1999 USPHS/IDSA guidelines for the prevention of opportunistic infections in persons infected with human immunodeficiency virus. U.S. Public Health Service (USPHS) and Infectious Diseases Society of America (IDSA). MMWR 48(RR-10): 1, 1999

CHOE H et al: The β-chemokine receptors CCR3 and CCR5 facilitate infection by primary HIV-1 isolates. Cell 85:1135, 1996

CHUN TW, FAUCI AS: Latent reservoirs of HIV: Obstacles to the eradication of virus. Proc Natl Acad Sci USA 96:10958, 1999

——— et al: Presence of an inducible HIV-1 latent reservoir during highly active antiretroviral therapy. Proc Natl Acad Sci USA 94:13193, 1997

——— et al: Re-emergence of HIV after stopping therapy. Nature 401:874, 1999

———: Relationship between preexisting viral reservoirs and the reemergence of plasma viremia after discontinuation of highly active anti-retroviral therapy. Nat Med 6:757, 2000

CLIFFORD DB et al: HAART improves prognosis in HIV-associated progressive multifocal leukoencephalopathy. Neurology 52:623, 1999

COCCHI F et al: Identification of RANTES, MIP-1α, and MIP-1β as the major HIV-suppressive factors produced by CD8+ T cells. Science 270:1811, 1995

COHEN GB et al: The selective downregulation of class 1 major histocompatibility complex proteins by HIV-1 protects HIV-infected cells from NK cells. Immunity 10:661, 1999

COHEN OJ et al: The immunology of human immunodeficiency virus infection, in: *Principles and Practice of Infectious Diseases*, 5th ed, GL Mandell, JE Bennett, and R Dolin (eds.). Philadelphia, Churchill Livingstone, pp 1374–1397, 2000

———, FAUCI AS: Benchmarks for antiretroviral therapy [comment]. J Clin Invest 105: 709, 2000

CONNORS M et al: HIV infection induces changes in CD4+ T cell phenotype and depletions within the CD4+ T cell repertoire that are not immediately restored by antiviral or immune-based therapies. Nature Med 3:533, 1997

CORDER EH et al: HIV-infected subjects with the E4 allele for APOE have excess dementia and peripheral neuropathy. Nat Med 4:1182, 1998

COUTSOUDIS A et al: Influence of infant-feeding patterns on early mother-to-child transmission of HIV-1 in Durban, South Africa: A prospective cohort study. Lancet 354: 471, 1999

DAVEY RT JR et al: HIV-1 and T cell dynamics after interruption of highly active antiretroviral therapy (HAART) in patients with a history of sustained viral suppression. Proc Natl Acad Sci USA 21:96,15109, 1999

——— et al: Immunologic and virologic effects of subcutaneous interleukin 2 in combination with antiretroviral therapy: A randomized controlled trial. JAMA 284:183, 2000

DENG HK et al: Identification of a major co-receptor for primary isolates of HIV-1. Nature 381:661, 1996

DEPARTMENT OF ECONOMIC AND SOCIAL AFFAIRS OF THE UNITED NATIONS SECRETARIAT: The Demographic Impact of HIV/AIDS. New York, 1999

DOMS RW, PEIPER SC: Unwelcomed guests with master keys: How HIV uses chemokine receptors for cellular entry. Virology 235:179, 1997

DONOVAN B, ROSS MW: Preventing HIV: Determinants of sexual behaviour. Lancet 355: 1897, 2000

DONG KL et al: Changes in body habitus and serum lipid abnormalities in HIV-positive women on highly active antiretroviral therapy. J Acquir Immune Defic Syndr 21:107, 1999

DORANZ BJ et al: A dual-tropic primary HIV-1 isolate that uses fusin and the β-chemokine receptors CKR-5, CKR-3, and CKR-2b as fusion cofactors. Cell 85:1149, 1996

DOUEK D et al: Changes in thymic function with age and during treatment of HIV infection. Nature 396:690, 1999

DRAGIC T et al: HIV-1 entry into CD4+ cells is mediated by the chemokine receptor CC-CKR-5. Nature 381:667, 1996

EMERY S, LANE HC: Immune reconstitution in HIV infection. Curr Opin Immunol 9:568, 1997

FAUCI AS: The AIDS epidemic—considerations for the 21st century. N Engl J Med 341: 1046, 1999

———: The human immunodeficiency virus: Infectivity and mechanisms of pathogenesis. Science 239:617, 1988

———: CD4+ T lymphocytopenia without HIV infection—no lights, no camera, just facts. N Engl J Med 328:429, 1993

———: Multifactorial nature of human immunodeficiency virus disease: Implications for therapy. Science 262:1011, 1993

———: An HIV vaccine: Breaking the paradigms. Proc Assoc Am Physicians 108:6, 1996

———: Host factors and the pathogenesis of HIV-induced disease. Nature 384:529, 1996

———: The AIDS epidemic—considerations for the 21st century. N Engl J Med 341: 1046, 1999

——— et al: Immunopathogenic mechanisms of HIV infection. Ann Intern Med 124:654, 1996

FAUKE S et al: Rapid progression to AIDS in HIV+ individuals with a structural variant of the chemokine receptor CX_3CR1. Science 287:2274, 2000

FIORELLI V et al: IFN-γ induces endothelial cells to proliferate and to invade the extracellular matrix in response to the HIV-1 tat protein: Implications for AIDS–Kaposi's sarcoma pathogenesis. J Immunol 162:1165, 1999

FLEXNER C: HIV-protease inhibitors. N Engl J Med 338:1281, 1998

FLORE O et al: Transformation of primary human endothelial cells by Kaposi's sarcoma–associated herpesvirus. Nature 394:588, 1998

GALLO R: The enigmas of Kaposi's sarcoma. Science 282:1837, 1998

GAO F et al: Origin of HIV-1 in the chimpanzee *Pan troglodytes troglodytes*. Nature 397: 436, 1999

GARCIA P et al: Maternal level of plasma human immunodeficiency virus type 1 RNA and the risk of perinatal transmission. N Engl J Med 341:394, 1999

GERBERDING J: Provider-to-patient HIV transmission: How to keep it exceedingly rare. Ann Intern Med 130:64, 1999

GILKS CF et al: Invasive pneumococcal disease in a cohort of predominantly HIV-1 infected female sex-workers in Nairobi, Kenya. Lancet 347:718, 1996

GOEDERT JJ et al: Spectrum of AIDS-associated malignant disorders. Lancet 351:1833, 1998

GUAY LA et al: Intrapartum and neonatal single-dose nevirapine compared with zidovudine for prevention of mother-to-child transmission of HIV-1 in Kampala, Uganda: HIVNET 012 randomised trial. Lancet 354:795, 1999

Gulick RM et al: Treatment with indinavir, zidovudine and lamivudine in adults with human immunodeficiency virus infection and prior antiretroviral therapy. N Engl J Med 337:734, 1997

Halperin DT, Bailey RC: Male circumcision and HIV infection: 10 years and counting. Lancet 354:1813, 1999

Haynes BF et al: Toward an understanding of the correlates of protective immunity to HIV infection. Science 271:324, 1996

Highbarger HC et al: Comparison of the quantiplex version 3.0 assay and a sensitized amplicor monitor assay for measurement of human immunodeficiency virus type 1 RNA levels in plasma samples. J Clin Microbiol 37:3612, 1999

Hirsch MS et al: Antiretroviral drug resistance testing in adults with HIV infection: Implications for clinical management. International AIDS Society—USA Panel. JAMA 279:1984, 1998

Hitchcock P, Fransen L: Preventing HIV infection: Lessons from Mwanza and Rakai. Lancet 353:513, 1999

Ho DD et al: Rapid turnover of plasma virions and CD4 lymphocytes in HIV infection. Nature 373:123, 1995

Holtzman DM et al: New-onset seizures associated with human immunodeficiency virus infection: Causation and clinical features in 100 cases. Am J Med 87:173, 1989

Jacobsen H et al: In vivo resistance to human immunodeficiency virus type 1 proteinase inhibitor: Mutations, kinetics and frequencies. J Infect Dis 173:1379, 1996

Jacobson JM et al: Thalidomide for the treatment of oral aphthous ulcers in patients with human immunodeficiency virus infection. N Engl J Med 336:1487, 1997

Joint United Nations Programme on HIV/AIDS (UNAIDS): Report on the Global HIV/AIDS Epidemic, June 2000. Geneva, 2000

Kahn JO, Walker BD: Acute human immunodeficiency virus type 1 infection. N Engl J Med 339:33, 1998

Kaplan JE et al: 14-year followup of HIV-infected homosexual men with lymphadenopathy syndrome. J Acquired Immune Defic Syndr Hum Retrovirol 11:206, 1996

Kaslow RA et al: Influence of combinations of human major histocompatibility complex genes on the course of HIV-1 infection. Nat Med 2:405, 1996

Kedes D et al: The seroepidemiology of human herpesvirus 8 (Kaposi's sarcoma–associated herpesvirus): Distribution of infection in KS risk groups and evidence for sexual transmission. Nat Med 2:918, 1996

Keet I et al: Consistent associations of HLA class I and II and transporter gene products with progression of human immunodeficiency virus type 1 infection in homosexual men. J Infect Dis 180:299, 1999

Kirchhoff F et al: Brief report: Absence of intact *nef* sequences in a long-term survivor with nonprogressive HIV-1 infection. N Engl J Med 332:228, 1995

Klein RS et al: Chemokine receptor expression and signaling in macaque and human fetal neurons and astrocytes: Implications for the neuropathogenesis of AIDS. J Immunol 163:1636, 1999

Kleinman S et al: False-positive HIV-1 test results in a low-risk screening setting of voluntary blood donation. JAMA 280:1080, 1998

Kodel U et al: HIV type 1 nef protein is a viral factor for leukocyte recruitment into the central nervous system. J Immunol 163:1245, 1999

Kovacs JA, Masur H: Prophylaxis against opportunistic infections in patients with human immunodeficiency virus infection. N Engl J Med 342:1416, 2000

Lackritz EM et al: Estimated risk of HIV transmission by screened blood in the United States. N Engl J Med 333:1721, 1995

Landesman SH et al: Obstetrical factors and the transmission of human immunodeficiency virus type 1 from mother to child. N Engl J Med 334:1617, 1997

Learmont JC et al: Immunologic and virologic status after 14 to 18 years of infection with an attenuated strain of HIV-1. A report from the Sydney Blood Bank Cohort. N Engl J Med 340:1715, 1999

Letendre S et al: Cerebrospinal fluid β chemokine concentrations in neurocognitively impaired individuals infected with human immunodeficiency virus type 1. J Infect Dis 180:310, 1999

Littman D: Chemokine receptors: Keys to AIDS pathogenesis? Cell 93:677, 1998

Liu H et al: Polymorphism in RANTES chemokine promoter affects HIV-1 disease progression. Proc Nat Acad Sci USA 96:4581, 1999

Liu R et al: Homozygous defect in HIV-1 coreceptor accounts for resistance of some multiply exposed individuals to HIV-1 infection. Cell 86:367, 1996

Lot F et al: Probable transmission of HIV from an orthopedic surgeon to a patient in France. Ann Intern Med 130:1, 1999

Maiman M et al: Cervical cancer as an AIDS-defining illness. Obstet Gynecol 89:76, 1997

Mannheimer SB, Soave R: Protozoal infections in patients with AIDS. Cryptosporidiosis, isosporiasis, cyclosporiasis, and microsporidiosis. Infect Dis Clin North Am 8: 483, 1994

Martin JA et al: *Births and Deaths: Preliminary Data for 1998*. National Vital Statistics Reports, vol 27, no. 25. Hyattsville, MD, National Center for Health Statistics, 1999

Mellado M et al: Chemokine control of HIV-1 infection. Nature 400:723, 1999

Mellors JW et al: Prognosis in HIV-1 infection predicted by the quantity of virus in plasma. Science 272:1167, 1996

Migueles SA et al: HLAB*5701 is highly associated with restriction of virus replication in a subgroup of HIV-infected long term nonprogressors. Proc Nat Acad Sci USA 97:2709, 2000

Miller KD et al: Visceral abdominal fat accumulation associated with the use of indinavir. Lancet 351:871, 1998

Miotti P et al: HIV transmission through breastfeeding: A study in Malawi. JAMA 282: 744, 1999

Mofenson LM et al: Risk factors for perinatal transmission of human immunodeficiency virus type 1 in women treated with zidovudine. N Engl J Med 334:385, 1999

———, McIntyre JA: Advances and research directions in the prevention of mother-to-child HIV-1 transmission. Lancet 355:2237, 2000

Moore PS, Chang Y: Detection of herpesvirus-like DNA sequences in Kaposi's sarcoma in patients with and those without HIV infection. N Engl J Med 332:1181, 1995

Moore RD, Chaisson RE: Natural history of opportunistic diseases in an HIV-infected urban clinical cohort. Ann Intern Med 124:633, 1996

National Institute for Occupational Safety and Health, Centers for Disease Control and Prevention: *Preventing Needlestick Injuries in Health Care Settings*, 1999

Oberlin E et al: The CXC chemokine receptor SDF-1 is the ligand for LESTR/fusin and prevents infection by T-cell-line-adapted HIV-1. Nature 382:833, 1996

O'Brien SJ: AIDS: A role for host genes. Hosp Pract (Off Ed) 33:53, 1998

———, Dean M: In search of AIDS-resistance genes. Sci Am 277:44, 1997

O'Brien WA et al: Changes in plasma HIV-1 RNA and CD4+ lymphocyte count and the risk of progression to AIDS. N Engl J Med 334:426, 1996

——— et al: Changes in plasma HIV RNA levels and CD4+ T lymphocyte counts predict both response to antiretroviral therapy and therapeutic failure. Ann Intern Med 126: 939, 1997

Ogg GS et al: Quantitation of HIV-1 specific cytotoxic T-lymphocytes and plasma load of viral RNA. Science 279:2103, 1998

Padian NS et al: Heterosexual transmission of human immunodeficiency virus (HIV) in northern California: Results from a ten-year study. Am J Epidemiol 146:350, 1997

Pagano MA et al: Cerebral tumor-like American trypanosomiasis in acquired immunodeficiency syndrome. Ann Neurol 45:403, 1999

Palella FJ et al: Declining morbidity and mortality among patients with advanced human immunodeficiency virus infection. N Engl J Med 338:853, 1998

Pantaleo G, Fauci AS: HIV infection is active and progressive in lymphoid tissue during the clinically latent stage of disease. Nature 362:355, 1993

———, ———: New concepts in the pathogenesis of HIV infection. Annu Rev Immunol 13:487, 1995

——— et al: Studies in subjects with long-term nonprogressive human immunodeficiency virus infection. N Engl J Med 332:209, 1995

Peckham C, Gibb D: Mother-to-child transmission of the human immunodeficiency virus. N Engl J Med 333:298, 1995

Perelson AS et al: HIV-1 dynamics in vivo: Virion clearance rate, infected cell lifespan, and viral generation time. Science 271:1582, 1996

——— et al: Decay characteristics of HIV-1 infected compartments during combination therapy. Nature 386:188, 1997

Price RW: Neurological complications of HIV infection. Lancet 348:445, 1996

Quinn TC et al: Viral load and heterosexual transmission of human immunodeficiency virus type 1. Rakai Project Study Group. N Engl J Med 342:921, 2000

Rettig MB et al: Kaposi's sarcoma–associated herpesvirus infection of bone marrow dendritic cells from multiple myeloma patients. Science 276:1851, 1997

Rich JD et al: Misdiagnosis of HIV infection by HIV-1 plasma viral load testing: A case series. Ann Intern Med 130:37, 1999

Richman DD: Normal physiology and HIV pathophysiology of human T-cell dynamics [In Process Citation]. J Clin Invest 105:565, 2000

Robertson DL et al: Recombination in HIV-1. Nature 374:124, 1995

Rosenberg ES: Vigorous HIV-1 specific CD4+ T cell responses associated with control of viremia. Science 278:1447, 1997

Samson M et al: Resistance to HIV-1 infection in Caucasian individuals bearing mutant alleles of the CCR-5 chemokine receptor gene. Nature 382:722, 1996

Schmitz JE et al: Control of viremia in simian immunodeficiency virus infection by CD8 lymphocytes. Science 283:852, 1999

Sewankambo N et al: HIV-1 infection associated with abnormal vaginal flora morphology and bacterial vaginosis. Lancet 350:546, 1997

Silva-Cardoso J et al: Pericardial involvement in human immunodeficiency virus infection. Chest 115:418, 1999

Simon F et al: Identification of a new human immunodeficiency virus type distinct from group M and group O. Nat Med 4:1032, 1998

Smith KJ et al: Cutaneous findings in HIV-1 positive patients: A 42-month prospective study. J Am Acad Dermatol 31:746, 1994

Soto-Ramirez LE et al: HIV-1 Langerhans' cell tropism associated with heterosexual transmission of HIV. Science 271:1291, 1996

Sparano JA: Treatment of AIDS-related lymphomas. Curr Opin Oncol 7:442, 1995

Spira AI et al: Cellular targets of infection and route of viral dissemination after an intravaginal inoculation of simian immunodeficiency virus into rhesus macaques. J Exp Med 183:215, 1996

Stansell JD et al: Predictors of *Pneumocystis carinii* pneumonia in HIV-infected persons. Am J Respir Crit Care Med 155:60, 1997

Sullivan PS et al: Persistently negative HIV-1 antibody enzyme immunoassay screening results for patients with HIV-1 infection and AIDS: Serologic, clinical, and virologic results. AIDS 13:89, 1999

SWINGLER S et al: HIV-1 nef mediates lymphocyte chemotaxis and activation by infected macrophages. Nat Med 5:997, 1999

TAVEL JA et al: Guide to major clinical trials of antiretroviral therapy in human immunodeficiency virus-infected patients: Protease inhibitors, non-nucleoside reverse transcriptase inhibitors, and nucleotide reverse transcriptase inhibitors. Clin Infect Dis 28:643, 1999

TINDALL B, COOPER DA: Primary HIV infection. Host responses and intervention strategies. AIDS 5:1, 1991

VANHEMS P et al: Comprehensive classification of symptoms and signs reported among 218 patients with acute HIV-1 infection. J Acquir Immune Defic Syndr 21:99, 1999

VITTINGHOFF E et al: Per-contact risk of human immunodeficiency virus transmission between male sexual partners. Am J Epidemiol 150:306, 1999

WALKER CM et al: CD8+ lymphocytes can control HIV infection in vitro by suppressing virus replication. Science 234:1563, 1986

WEI X et al: Viral dynamics in human immunodeficiency virus type 1 infection. Nature 373:117, 1995

WEISS JM et al: HIV-1 tat induces monocyte chemoattractant protein-1 mediated monocyte transmigration across a model of the human blood-brain barrier and up-regulates CCR5 expression on human monocytes. J Immunol 163:2953, 1999

WHALEN C et al: Accelerated course of human immunodeficiency virus infection after tuberculosis. Am J Respir Crit Care Med 151:129, 1995

WORLD HEALTH ORGANIZATION: *The World Health Report 1999: Making a Difference.* Geneva, 1999

Section 2
DISORDERS OF IMMUNE-MEDIATED INJURY

310

K. Frank Austen

ALLERGIES, ANAPHYLAXIS, AND SYSTEMIC MASTOCYTOSIS

BPL benzylpenicilloyl-polylysine	IP_3 inositol-1,4,5-triphosphate
C1INH C1 inhibitor	ITAMs immunoreceptor tyrosine-based activation motifs
CPA carboxypeptidase A	LT leukotriene
1,2-DAGs 1,2-diacylglycerols	MDM minor determinant mixture
ELISA enzyme-linked immunosorbent assays	MHC major histocompatibility complex
FLAP 5-lipoxygenase activating protein	PAF platelet-activating factor
GM-CSF granulocyte-macrophage colony-stimulating factor	PG prostaglandin
IFN interferon	SCF stem cell factor
IL interleukin	TCR T cell receptor
	TNF-α tumor necrosis factor α

The term *atopic allergy* implies a familial tendency to manifest such conditions as asthma, rhinitis, urticaria, and eczematous dermatitis (atopic dermatitis) alone or in combination. However, individuals without an atopic background may also develop hypersensitivity reactions, particularly urticaria and anaphylaxis, associated with the same class of antibody, IgE, found in atopic individuals. Inasmuch as the mast cell is the key effector cell of the biologic response in allergic rhinitis, urticaria, anaphylaxis, and systemic mastocytosis, the introduction to these clinical problems will consider the developmental biology, activation pathway, product profile, and target tissues for this cell type.

The fixation of IgE to human mast cells and basophils, a process termed *sensitization*, prepares these cells for subsequent antigen-specific activation. The interaction of the high-affinity Fc receptor for IgE, designated FcϵRI, upregulates the cellular expression of the receptor, possibly by ligand-mediated stabilization. FcϵRI is composed of one α, one β, and two disulfide-linked γ chains, which together cross the plasma membrane seven times. The α chain is solely responsible for IgE binding, and the β and γ chains are responsible for signal transduction that results from the aggregation of the tetrameric receptors by polymeric antigen.

The interaction of specific multivalent antigen with receptor-bound IgE results in clustering of the receptors to initiate signal transduction through the action of a *src* family–related tyrosine kinase, termed *Lyn*, that is constitutively associated with the β chain. Lyn transphosphorylates the canonical immunoreceptor tyrosine-based activation motifs (ITAMs) of the β and γ chains of the receptor, resulting in recruitment of more active Lyn to the β chain and of the Syk/zap-70 family tyrosine kinases. The two phosphorylated tyrosines in the ITAMs function as binding sites for the tandem *src* homology two (SH2) domains within these kinases. It appears that Syk activates not only phospholipase Cγ but also phosphatidylinositol-3-kinase to provide phosphatidyl-3,4,5-triphosphate, which allows membrane targeting of the Tec family kinases (Btk and Itk) and their activation by Lyn. The resulting Tec kinase–dependent phosphorylation of phospholipase Cγ with cleavage of its phospholipid membrane substrate provides inositol-1,4,5-triphosphate (IP_3) and 1,2-diacylglycerols (1,2-DAGs) so as to mobilize intracellular calcium and activate protein kinase C. The subsequent opening of calcium-regulated activated channels provides the sustained elevations of intracellular calcium required to recruit the mitogen-activated protein kinases, JNK and p38 (serine/threonine kinases), which provide cascades to augment arachidonic acid release and to mediate nuclear translocation of transcription factors for various cytokines. The calcium ion–dependent activation of phospholipases cleaves membrane phospholipids to generate lysophospholipids, which, like 1,2-DAG, are fusogenic and may facilitate the fusion of the secretory granule perigranular membrane with the cell membrane, a step that releases the membrane-free granule containing the preformed or primary mediators of mast cell effects.

The secretory granule of the human mast cell has a crystalline structure, unlike mast cells of lower species, and IgE-dependent cell activation can be characterized morphologically by solubilization and swelling of the granule contents within the first minute of receptor perturbation; this reaction is followed by the ordering of intermediate filaments about the swollen granule, movement toward the cell surface, and fusion of the perigranular membrane with that of other granules and with the plasmalemma to form extracellular channels for mediator release while maintaining cell viability.

In addition to exocytosis, aggregation of FcϵRI initiates two other pathways for generation of bioactive products, namely, lipid mediators and cytokines. The biochemical steps involved in expression of such cytokines as tumor necrosis factor α (TNF-α), interleukin (IL) 6, IL-4, IL-5, granulocyte-macrophage colony-stimulating factor (GM-CSF), and others have not been specifically defined for mast cells. Nonetheless, inhibition studies of cytokine production (IL-1β, TNF-α, and IL-6) in mouse mast cells with cyclosporine or FK506 reveal binding to the ligand-specific immunophilin and attenuation of the calcium ion- and calmodulin-dependent serine/threonine phosphatase, calcineurin.

Lipid mediator generation (Fig. 310-1) involves translocation of calcium ion–dependent cytosolic phospholipase A_2 to the perinuclear membrane, with subsequent release of arachidonic acid for metabolic processing by the distinct prostanoid and leukotriene pathways. The constitutive prostaglandin endoperoxide synthase (PGHS-1/cyclooxygenase-1) and the de novo inducible PGHS-2 (cyclooxygenase-2)

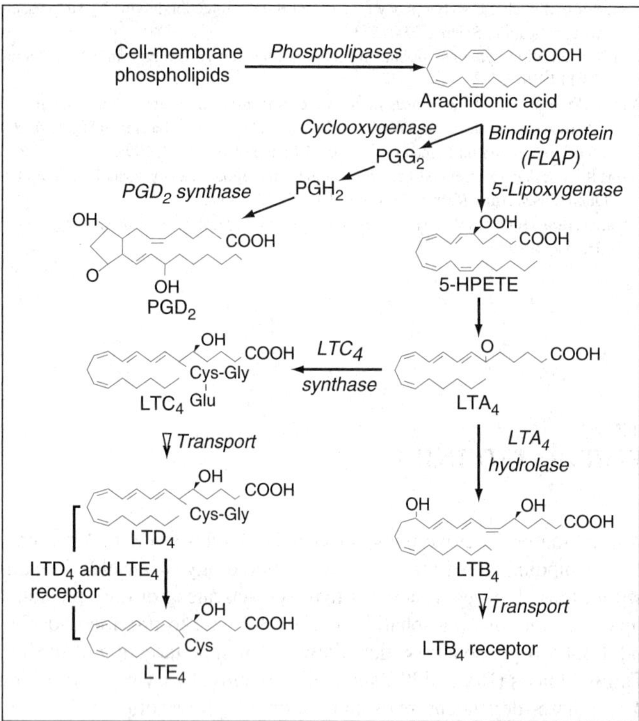

FIGURE 310-1 Pathways for biosynthesis and release of membrane-derived lipid mediators from mast cells. In the 5-lipoxygenase pathway leukotriene A_4 (LTA_4) is the intermediate from which the terminal-pathway enzymes generate the distinct final products, leukotriene C_4 (LTC_4) and leukotriene B_4 (LTB_4), which leave the cell by separate saturable transport systems. Gamma glutamyl transpeptidase and a dipeptidase then cleave glutamic acid and glycine from LTC_4 to form LTD_4 and LTE_4, respectively, for which there appears to be a common receptor. The only mast cell product of the cyclooxygenase system is PGD_2.

convert released arachidonic acid to the sequential intermediates prostaglandin (PG) G_2 and PGH_2. The glutathione-dependent hematopoietic PGD_2 synthase then converts PGH_2 to PGD_2, the predominant mast cell prostanoid.

For processing by the leukotriene pathway, the released arachidonic acid is translocated to an integral perinuclear membrane protein, the 5-lipoxygenase activating protein (FLAP). The calcium ion–dependent activation of 5-lipoxygenase involves translocation to the perinuclear membrane, which allows conversion of the arachidonic acid to the sequential intermediates, 5-hydroperoxyeicosatetraenoic acid and leukotriene (LT) A_4. LTA_4 is conjugated with reduced glutathione by LTC_4 synthase, an integral membrane protein with significant homology to FLAP. Intracellular LTC_4 is released by a carrier-specific export step for extracellular conversion to the receptor-active cysteinyl leukotrienes LTD_4 and LTE_4 by sequential removal of glumatic acid and glycine. A cytosolic LTA_4 hydrolase converts some LTA_4 to the dihydroxy leukotriene LTB_4, which then undergoes specific export for extracellular receptor–mediated actions. The lysophospholipid formed during release of arachidonic acid from 1-*O*-alkyl-2-acyl-*sn*-glyceryl-3-phosphorylcholine can be acetylated in the second position to form platelet-activating factor (PAF).

Unlike other cells of bone marrow origin, mast cells leave the marrow and circulate as committed progenitors lacking their definitive secretory granules. These committed progenitors express the receptor, c-*kit*, for stem cell factor (SCF) before the expression of FcεRI. Whereas c-*kit* is lost or markedly diminished in expression by other cell types, it is retained by mature, differentiated mast cells and is an absolute requirement for the development of constitutive tissue mast cells residing in skin and connective tissue sites and for the T cell–dependent mast cells residing in mucosal surfaces or undergoing reactive hyperplasia. Indeed, in clinical T cell deficiencies, mast cells are absent from the intestinal mucosa but are present in the submucosa. It is thus assumed that unrecognized mast cell progenitors enter the tissue and undergo regulated proliferation, differentiation, and maturation. Based on the immunodetection of secretory granule neutral proteases, mast cells in the lung parenchyma and intestinal mucosa selectively express tryptase; those in the intestinal and airway submucosa, skin, lymph nodes, and breast parenchyma express tryptase, chymase, and carboxypeptidase A (CPA); and occasional mast cells in intestinal submucosa express chymase and CPA but not tryptase. The secretory granules of mast cells selectively positive for tryptase in lung and intestinal mucosa exhibit closed scrolls with a periodicity suggestive of a crystalline structure by electron microscopy; whereas the secretory granules of mast cells with mutiple proteases residing in skin, lymph nodes, breast parenchyma, and submucosa of airways and intestine are scroll-poor, with an amorphous or latticelike appearance.

Mast cells are distributed at cutaneous and mucosal surfaces and in deeper tissues about venules and could regulate the entry of foreign substances by their rapid response capability (Fig. 310-2). Upon stimulus-specific activation in vitro, histamine and secretory granule–associated acid hydrolases are solubilized, whereas the neutral proteases, which are cationic, remain largely complexed to the anionic proteoglycans, heparin and chrondroitin sulfate E. The macromolecular complex serves to deliver the neutral proteases so that the endo- and exoproteases can function in concert at the substrate site to clear damaged tissue and facilitate repair. Histamine and the various lipid mediators (PGD_2, LTD_4/E_4, PAF) alter venular permeability, thereby allowing influx of plasma proteins such as complement and immunoglobulins, whereas LTB_4 mediates leukocyte–endothelial cell adhesion with subsequent directed migration (chemotaxis). The accumulation of leukocytes and opsonins would facilitate defense of the microenvironment. The cysteinyl leukotrienes constrict both vascular and nonvascular smooth muscle and are much more potent than histamine in constricting human airway smooth muscle when administered by aerosol.

The cellular component of the inflammatory response elicited by preformed secretory granule–associated and membrane-

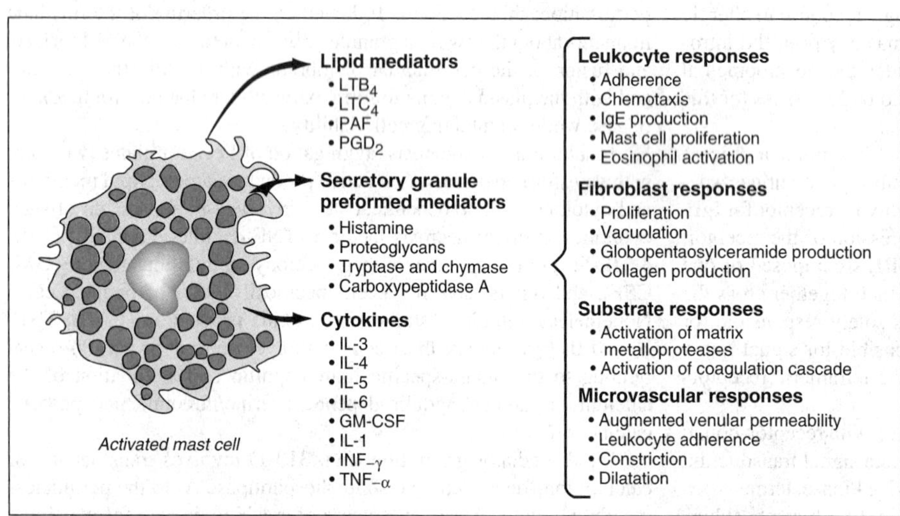

FIGURE 310-2 Bioactive mediators of three categories generated by IgE-dependent activation of murine mast cells can elicit common but sequential target cell effects leading to acute and sustained inflammatory responses.

derived lipid mediators would be augmented and sustained by the addition of cytokines of mast cell or T cell origin to the microenvironment. Activation of human skin mast cells in situ elicits TNF-α production and release, which in turn induces endothelial cell responses favoring leukocyte adhesion. Activation of purified human lung mast cells in vitro results in substantial production of IL-5 and lesser quantities of IL-4. Bronchial biopsies of patients with bronchial asthma reveal that mast cells are immunohistochemically positive for IL-4 and IL-5, but that the predominant localization of IL-4, IL-5, and GM-CSF is to T cells, defined as T_H2 by this profile. It is speculated that IL-4 modulates the T cell phenotype to the T_H2 subtype, and that IL-5 or GM-CSF converts infiltrating eosinophils to an activated, autoaggressive phenotype with augmented capacity for cytotoxicity and generation of O_2^- and the cysteinyl leukotrienes.

The view of immediate and late cellular phase of allergic inflammation is supported by the response of the skin, nose, or lung of allergic humans to local allergen challenge; greater quantities of allergen are needed to elicit the cellular phase. In the immediate phase of a local challenge, there is pruritus and watery discharge from the nose, bronchospasm and mucous secretion in the lungs, and a wheal-and-flare response with pruritus in the skin. The reduced nasal patency, reduced pulmonary function, or evident erythema with swelling at the skin site in a late-phase response at 6 to 8 h are associated with biopsy findings of infiltrating and activated T_H2 type T cells, eosinophils, basophils, and even some neutrophils. This allergic inflammation proceeding from early mast cell activation to late cellular infiltration is believed to promote end-organ hyperresponsivity, as would be characteristic of perennial rhinitis or bronchial asthma; for attenuation, it requires introduction of an anti-inflammatory agent such as a glucocorticoid. The particular chemokines responsible for directed migration of eosinophils and T cells after their integrin-dependent endothelial cell adhesion are not yet defined, although eotaxin is a likely contributor since both cell types, as well as basophils, express the selective receptor CCR-3.

Consideration of the mechanism of immediate type hypersensitivity diseases in the human has focused largely on the IgE-dependent recognition of otherwise nontoxic substances. A region of chromosome 5 (5q23-31) contains genes implicated in the control of IgE levels including IL-4 and IL-13, as well as IL-3 and IL-9 involved in reactive mast cell hyperplasia and IL-5 and GM-CSF central to eosinophil development and their enhanced tissue viability. Genes with linkage to the specific IgE response to particular allergens include those encoding the major histocompatibility complex (MHC) and certain chains of the T cell receptor (TCR-$\alpha\delta$). The complexity of atopy and the associated diseases is such that susceptibility, severity, and therapeutic responses most likely relate not only to specific IgE but also to constitutive target tissue reactivity and the superimposed effects of the local inflammatory response mediated by T_H2 cells, mast cells, basophils, and eosinophils.

The induction of allergic disease requires sensitization of a predisposed individual to specific allergen. This sensitization can occur anytime in life, although the greatest propensity for the development of allergic disease appears to occur in childhood and early adolescence. Exposure of a susceptible individual to an allergen results in processing of the allergen by antigen-presenting cells, including macrophage-like cells located throughout the body at surfaces that contact the outside environment, such as the nose, lungs, eyes, skin, and intestine. These antigen-presenting cells process the allergen protein and present the epitope-bearing peptides via their MHC to particular T cell subsets. The T cell response depends both on cognate recognition through various ligand/receptor interactions and on the cytokine microenvironment, with IL-4 directing a T_H2 response and interferon (IFN)γ a T_H1 profile. T cells can potentially induce several responses to an allergen, including those typical of contact dermatitis, known as the T_H1 type response, and those mediated by IgE, known as the T_H2 allergic response. The T_H2 response is associated with activation of specific B cells that transform into plasma cells. Synthesis and release into the serum of allergen-specific IgE by plasma cells result in sensitization of IgE Fc receptor–bearing cells including mast cells and basophils, which subsequently are capable of becoming activated upon exposure to the specific allergen. In certain diseases, including those associated with atopy, the monocyte and eosinophil populations can express a trimeric high-affinity receptor, FcϵRI, which lacks the β chain, and yet respond to its aggregation.

ANAPHYLAXIS

DEFINITION The life-threatening anaphylactic response of a sensitized human appears within minutes after administration of specific antigen and is manifested by respiratory distress often followed by vascular collapse or by shock without antecedent respiratory difficulty. Cutaneous manifestations exemplified by pruritus and urticaria with or without angioedema are characteristic of such systemic anaphylactic reactions. Gastrointestinal manifestations include nausea, vomiting, crampy abdominal pain, and diarrhea.

PREDISPOSING FACTORS AND ETIOLOGY There is no convincing evidence that age, sex, race, occupation, or geographic location predisposes a human to anaphylaxis except through exposure to some immunogen. According to most studies, atopy does not predispose individuals to anaphylaxis from penicillin therapy or venom of a stinging insect but is a risk factor for allergens in food or latex.

The materials capable of eliciting the systemic anaphylactic reaction in humans include the following: heterologous proteins in the form of hormones (insulin, vasopressin, parathormone), enzymes (trypsin, chymotrypsin, penicillinase, streptokinase), pollen extracts (ragweed, grass, trees), nonpollen extracts (dust mites, dander of cats, dogs, horses, and laboratory animals), food (milk, eggs, seafood, nuts, grains, beans, gelatin in capsules), antiserum (antilymphocyte gamma globulin), occupation-related proteins (latex rubber products), and Hymenoptera venom (yellow jacket, yellow and baldfaced hornets, paper wasp, honey bee, imported fire ants); polysaccharides such as dextran and thiomerosal as a vaccine preservative; and most commonly drugs such as protamine and antibiotics (penicillins, cephalosporins, amphotericin B, nitrofurantoin, quinolones), local anesthetics (procaine, lidocaine), muscle relaxants (suxamethonium, gallamine, pancuronium), vitamins (thiamine, folic acid), diagnostic agents (sodium dehydrocholate, sulfobromophthalein), and occupation-related chemicals (ethylene oxide), which are considered to function as haptens that form immunogenic conjugates with host proteins. The conjugating hapten may be the parent compound, a nonenzymatically derived storage product, or a metabolite formed in the host.

PATHOPHYSIOLOGY AND MANIFESTATIONS Individuals differ in the time of appearance of symptoms and signs, but the hallmark of the anaphylactic reaction is the onset of some manifestation within seconds to minutes after introduction of the antigen, generally by injection or less commonly by ingestion. There may be upper or lower airway obstruction or both. Laryngeal edema may be experienced as a "lump" in the throat, hoarseness, or stridor, while bronchial obstruction is associated with a feeling of tightness in the chest and/or audible wheezing. Patients with bronchial asthma are predisposed to severe involvement of the lower airways. A characteristic feature is the eruption of well-circumscribed, discrete cutaneous wheals with erythematous, raised, serpiginous borders and blanched centers. These urticarial eruptions are intensely pruritic and may be localized or disseminated. They may coalesce to form giant hives, and they seldom persist beyond 48 h. A localized, nonpitting, deeper edematous cutaneous process, angioedema, may also be present. It may be asymptomatic or cause a burning or stinging sensation.

In fatal cases with clinical bronchial obstruction, the lungs show marked hyperinflation on gross and microscopic examination. The microscopic findings in the bronchi, however, are limited to luminal secretions, peribronchial congestion, submucosal edema, and eosinophilic infiltration, and the acute emphysema is attributed to intractable bronchospasm that subsides with death. The angioedema resulting in death by mechanical obstruction occurs in the epiglottis and larynx, but the process is also evident in the hypopharynx and to some extent in the trachea; on microscopic examination there is wide separation of the collagen fibers and the glandular elements; vascular congestion and eosinophilic infiltration are also present. Patients dying of vascular collapse without antecedent hypoxia from respiratory insufficiency have visceral congestion with a presumptive loss of intravascular blood volume. The associated electrocardiographic abnormalities, with or without infarction, noted in some patients may reflect a primary cardiac event or be secondary to a critical reduction in blood volume.

The angioedematous and urticarial manifestations of the anaphylactic syndrome have been attributed to release of endogenous histamine. A role for the cysteinyl leukotrienes in altering pulmonary mechanics by causing marked bronchiolar constriction seems likely. Vascular collapse without respiratory distress in response to experimental challenge with the sting of a hymenopteran was associated not only with marked and prolonged elevations in blood histamine but also with evidence of intravascular coagulation and kinin generation. The findings that patients with systemic mastocytosis and episodic hypotension proceeding to vascular collapse excrete large amounts of PGD_2 metabolites in addition to histamine and that these events are controlled by administration of a nonsteroidal agent but not by antihistamines alone suggest that PGD_2 is also of importance in the hypotensive anaphylactic reactions. The cysteinyl leukotrienes may be involved in the pathobiologic process in patients with myocardial ischemia without or with infarction.

DIAGNOSIS The diagnosis of an anaphylactic reaction depends largely on an accurate history revealing the onset of the appropriate symptoms and signs within minutes after the responsible material is encountered. When only a portion of the full syndrome is present, such as isolated urticaria, sudden bronchospasm in a patient with asthma, or vascular collapse after intravenous administration of an agent, it may be appropriate to consider a complement-mediated immune complex reaction, an idiosyncratic response to any of the nonsteroidal anti-inflammatory agents, or the direct effect of certain drugs or diagnostic agents on mast cells. Intravenous administration of a chemical mast cell–degranulating agent, including opiate derivatives and radiographic contrast media, may elicit generalized urticaria, angioedema, and a sensation of retrosternal oppression with or without clinically detectable bronchoconstriction or hypotension. Aspirin and other nonsteroidal anti-inflammatory agents such as indomethacin, aminopyrine, and mefenamic acid may precipitate a life-threatening episode of obstruction of upper or lower airways, especially in patients with asthma, that is clinically reminiscent of anaphylaxis but is not associated with a detectable IgE response. This syndrome, which is commonly associated with nasal polyposis, is due to inhibition of PGHS-1 with corresponding unregulated, amplified generation of the cysteinyl leukotrienes via the 5-lipoxygenase/LTC_4 synthase pathway. In the transfusion anaphylactic reaction that occurs in patients with IgA deficiency, the responsible specificity resides in IgG or IgE anti-IgA; the mechanism of the reaction mediated by IgG anti-IgA is presumed to be complement activation with secondary mast cell participation.

The presence of specific IgE in the heart blood of patients dying of systemic anaphylaxis has been demonstrated at postmortem by passive transfer of the serum intradermally into a normal recipient, followed in 24 h by antigen challenge into the same site, with subsequent development of a wheal and flare, the Prausnitz-Küstner reaction. To avoid the hazards of transferring hepatitis or other infections to a recipient, it is preferable to use the serum to seek passive sensitization of a human leukocyte suspension enriched with basophils for subsequent antigen-induced histamine release. Furthermore, radioimmunoassays have demonstrated specific IgE antibodies in patients with anaphylactic reactions, but such approaches require purified antigens. Elevations of β-tryptase levels in serum implicate mast cell activation in an adverse systemic reaction and are particularly informative with episodes of hypotension during general anesthesia or when there has been a fatal outcome.

℞ **TREATMENT** Early recognition of an anaphylactic reaction is mandatory, since death occurs within minutes to hours after the first symptoms. Mild symptoms such as pruritus and urticaria can be controlled by administration of 0.2 to 0.5 mL of 1:1000 epinephrine subcutaneously, with repeated doses as required at 20-min intervals for a severe reaction. If the antigenic material was injected into an extremity, the rate of absorption may be reduced by prompt application of a tourniquet proximal to the reaction site, administration of 0.2 mL of 1:1000 epinephrine into the site, and removal without compression of an insect stinger, if present. An intravenous infusion should be initiated to provide a route for administration of 2.5 mL epinephrine, diluted 1:10,000, at 5- to 10-min intervals, volume expanders such as normal saline, and vasopressor agents such as dopamine if intractable hypotension occurs. Replacement of intravascular volume due to postcapillary venular leakage may require several liters of saline. Epinephrine provides both α- and β-adrenergic effects, resulting in vasoconstriction, bronchial smooth-muscle relaxation, and attenuation of enhanced venular permeability. Beta blockers are relatively contraindicated in persons at risk for anaphylactic reactions, especially those sensitive to Hymenoptera venom or those undergoing immunotherapy for respiratory system allergy. When epinephrine fails to control the anaphylactic reaction, hypoxia due to airway obstruction or related to a cardiac arrhythmia, or both, must be considered. Oxygen via a nasal catheter or intermittent positive-pressure breathing of oxygen with 0.5 mL isoproterenol diluted 1:200 in saline may be helpful, but either endotracheal intubation or a tracheostomy is mandatory for oxygen delivery if progressive hypoxia develops. Ancillary agents such as the antihistamine diphenhydramine, 50 to 100 mg intramuscularly or intravenously, and aminophylline, 0.25 to 0.5 g intravenously, are appropriate for urticaria-angioedema and bronchospasm, respectively. Intravenous glucocorticoids are not effective for the acute event but may alleviate later recurrence of bronchospasm, hypotension, or urticaria. Furthermore, in a syndrome termed *idiopathic anaphylaxis* with recurrent angioedema of the upper airways, glucocorticoid administration may be beneficial by reducing the frequency of attacks and/or the severity of episodes.

PREVENTION Prevention of anaphylaxis must take into account the sensitivity of the recipient, the dose and character of the diagnostic or therapeutic agent, and the effect of the route of administration on the rate of absorption. If there is a definite history of a past anaphylactic reaction, even though mild, it is advisable to select another agent or procedure. A knowledge of cross-reactivity among agents is critical since, for example, cephalosporins share a common β-lactam ring with the penicillins. A skin test should be performed before the administration of certain materials that are likely to elicit anaphylactic reactions, such as allergenic extracts, or when the nature of the past adverse reaction is unknown. A scratch test should precede an intradermal test in very sensitive patients. With regard to penicillin, two-thirds of patients with a positive reaction history and positive skin tests to benzylpenicilloyl-polylysine (BPL) and/or the minor determinant mixture (MDM) of benzylpenicillin products experience allergic reactions with treatment, and these are almost uniformly of the anaphylactic type in those patients with minor determinant reactivity. Even patients without a history of previous clinical reactions have a 2 to 6 percent incidence of positive skin tests to the two test materials, and about 3 per 1000 with a negative history experience anaphylaxis with therapy, with a mortality of about 1 per 100,000. Skin testing for antibiotics should be performed only on patients with a positive clinical history consistent with an IgE-mediated reaction and in imminent need of the antibiotic in question; skin testing is of no value for non-IgE-mediated eruptions. Desensitization with most antibiotics can proceed by the intravenous, subcutaneous, or oral route. Typically, graded quantities of the antibiotic are given by the selected route using double doses until a therapeutic dosage is achieved. Due to the risk of systemic anaphylaxis during the course of desensitization, such a procedure should be performed only in a setting in which resuscitation equipment is at hand and an intravenous line is in place. It is critical to give the therapeutic agent at regular intervals to prevent the reestablishment of a sensitized cell pool of large size.

A different form of protection involves the development of blocking antibody of the IgG class, which is protective against Hymenoptera venom–induced anaphylaxis by interacting with antigen so that less reaches the sensitized tissue mast cells; to be effective, this immunotherapy requires the use of specific or cross-reacting Hymenoptera venom. Because sensitization can be transient, the maximal risk for systemic anaphylactic reactions in persons with Hymenoptera sensitivity occurs in association with a currently positive skin test. Although there is only low-grade cross-reactivity between honey bee and yellow jacket venoms, there is a high degree of cross-reactivity between yellow jacket venom and the rest of the vespid venoms (yellow or bald-faced hornets and wasps). Prevention involves modification of outdoor activities to exclude bare feet, wearing perfumed toiletries, eating in areas attractive to insects, clipping hedges or grass, and hauling away trash or fallen fruit. As with each anaphylactic sensitivity, the individual should wear an informational bracelet and have immediate access to an unexpired epinephrine kit. The limitations of lifestyle and the psychological duress can be addressed by venom immunotherapy to achieve a venom-specific IgG titer. Although it has been recommended that venom therapy be continued indefinitely or until the skin and specific serum IgE tests are unremarkable, there is evidence that 5 years of treatment induces a state of resistance to sting reactions that is independent of serum levels of specific IgG or IgE. This contrasts with the definite relation of sting immunity to specific IgG earlier in the treatment regime. For children with a systemic reaction limited to skin, the likelihood of progression to more serious respiratory or vascular manifestations is low, and thus immunotherapy is not recommended.

URTICARIA AND ANGIOEDEMA

DEFINITION Urticaria and angioedema may appear separately or together as cutaneous manifestations of localized nonpitting edema; a similar process may occur at mucosal surfaces of the upper respiratory or gastrointestinal tract. *Urticaria* involves only the superficial portion of the dermis, presenting as well-circumscribed wheals with erythematous raised serpiginous borders with blanched centers that may coalesce to become giant wheals. *Angioedema* is a well-demarcated localized edema involving the deeper layers of the skin, including the subcutaneous tissue. Recurrent episodes of urticaria and/or angioedema of less than 6 weeks' duration are considered acute, whereas attacks persisting beyond this period are designated chronic.

PREDISPOSING FACTORS AND ETIOLOGY The occurrence of urticaria and angioedema is probably more frequent than usually described because of the evanescent, self-limited nature of such eruptions, which seldom require medical attention when limited to the skin. Although persons in any age group may experience acute or chronic urticaria and/or angioedema, these lesions increase in frequency after adolescence, with the highest incidence occurring in persons in the third decade of life; indeed, one survey of college students indicated that 15 to 20% had experienced a pruritic wheal reaction.

The classification of urticaria-angioedema presented in Table 310-1 focuses on the different mechanisms for eliciting clinical disease and can be useful for differential diagnosis; nonetheless, most cases of chronic urticaria are idiopathic. Urticaria and/or angioedema occurring during the appropriate season in patients with seasonal respiratory allergy or as a result of exposure to animals or molds is attributed to inhalation or physical contact with pollens, animal dander, and mold spores, respectively. However, urticaria and angioedema secondary to inhalation are relatively uncommon compared to urticaria and angioedema elicited by ingestion of fresh fruits, shellfish, fish, milk products, chocolate, legumes including peanuts, and various drugs that may elicit not only the anaphylactic syndrome with prominent gastrointestinal complaints but also chronic urticaria.

Table 310-1 Classification of Urticaria and/or Angioedema

1. IgE-dependent
   a. Specific antigen sensitivity (pollens, foods, drugs, fungi, molds, Hymenoptera venom, helminths)
   b. Physical: dermographism, cold, solar, cholinergic, vibratory, exercise-related
2. Complement-mediated
   a. Hereditary angioedema: type 1, type 2
   b. Acquired angioedema: type 1, type 2
   c. Necrotizing vasculitis
   d. Serum sickness
   e. Reactions to blood products
3. Nonimmunologic
   a. Direct mast cell–releasing agents: opiates, antibiotics, curare, D-tubocurarine, radiocontrast media
   b. Agents that alter arachidonic acid metabolism: aspirin and nonsteroidal anti-inflammatory agents, azo dyes, and benzoates
4. Idiopathic

Additional etiologies include physical stimuli such as cold, heat, solar rays, exercise, and mechanical irritation. The physical urticarias can be distinguished by the precipitating event and other aspects of the clinical presentation. *Dermographism*, which occurs in 1 to 4% of the population, is defined by the appearance of a linear wheal at the site of a brisk stroke with a firm object or by any configuration appropriate to the eliciting event. Dermographism has a prevalence that peaks in the second to third decades. It is not influenced by an atopic diathesis and has a duration generally of less than 5 years. *Pressure urticaria*, which often accompanies dermographism or chronic idiopathic urticaria, presents in response to a sustained stimulus such as a shoulder strap or belt, running (feet), or manual labor (hands). *Cholinergic urticaria* is distinctive in that the pruritic wheals are of small size (1 to 2 mm) and are surrounded by a large area of erythema; attacks are precipitated by fever, a hot bath or shower, or exercise and are presumptively attributed to a rise in core body temperature. *Exercise-related anaphylaxis* can be limited to erythema and pruritic urticaria but may progress to angioedema of the face, oropharynx, larynx, or intestine or to vascular collapse; it is distinguished from cholinergic urticaria by presenting with wheals of conventional size and by not occurring with fever or a hot bath. *Cold urticaria*, either acquired or hereditary, is local at body areas exposed to low ambient temperature or cold objects (ice cube) but can progress to vascular collapse with immersion in cold water (swimming). *Solar urticaria* is subdivided into three groups by the response to specific portions of the light spectrum. *Vibratory angioedema* may occur after years of occupational exposure or can be idiopathic; it may be accompanied by cholinergic urticaria. Other rare forms of physical allergy, always defined by stimulus-specific elicitation, include *local heat urticaria*, *aquagenic urticaria* from contact with water of any temperature (sometimes associated with polycythemia vera), and *contact urticaria* from direct interaction with some chemical substance.

Angioedema without urticaria occurs with C1 inhibitor (C1INH) deficiency that may be inborn as an autosomal dominant characteristic or may be acquired. The urticaria and angioedema associated with classic serum sickness or with hypocomplementemic cutaneous necrotizing angiitis are believed to be immune-complex diseases. The drug reactions to mast cell granule–releasing agents and to nonsteroidal anti-inflammatory drugs may be systemic, resembling anaphylaxis, or limited to cutaneous sites.

PATHOPHYSIOLOGY AND MANIFESTATIONS Uricarial eruptions are distinctly pruritic, involve any area of the body from the scalp to the soles of the feet, and appear in crops of 24- to 72-h duration, with old lesions fading as new ones appear. The most common sites for urticaria are the extremities and face, with angioedema often being periorbital and in the lips. Although self-limited in duration, angioedema of the upper respiratory tract may be life-threatening due to laryngeal obstruction, while gastrointestinal involvement may present with abdominal colic, with or without nausea and vomiting, and may precipitate unnecessary surgical intervention. No residual discoloration occurs with either urticaria or angioedema unless there is an underlying process leading to superimposed extravasation of erythrocytes.

The pathology of urticaria and angioedema is usually characterized by edema of the dermis in urticaria and of the subcutaneous tissue as well as the dermis in angioedema. Collagen bundles in affected areas are widely separated, and the venules are sometimes dilated. The perivenular infiltrate may consist of lymphocytes, eosinophils, and neutrophils that are present in varying combination and number throughout the dermis.

Perhaps the best-studied example of IgE- and mast cell–mediated urticaria and angioedema is *cold urticaria*. Cryoglobulins may be recognized, but not in the majority of patients. Immersion of an extremity in an ice bath precipitates angioedema of the distal portion with urticaria at the air interface within minutes of the challenge. Histologic studies reveal marked mast cell degranulation with associated edema of the dermis and subcutaneous tissues. The venous effluent of the cold-challenged and angioedematous extremity reveals a marked rise in plasma content of histamine, whereas the venous effluent of the contralateral normal extremity contains none of this mediator. Elevated levels of histamine have been found in the plasma of venous effluent and in the fluid of suction blisters at experimentally induced lesional sites in patients with dermographism, pressure urticaria, vibratory angioedema, light urticaria, and heat urticaria. By ultrastructural analysis, the pattern of mast cell degranulation in cold urticaria resembles an IgE-mediated response with solubilization of granule contents, fusion of the perigranular and cell membranes, and discharge of granule contents, whereas in a dermographic lesion there is an additional superimposed zonal (piecemeal) degranulation. Elevations of plasma histamine levels with biopsy-proven mast cell degranulation have also been demonstrated with systemic attacks of *cholinergic urticaria* and *exercise-related anaphylaxis* precipitated experimentally in subjects exercising on a treadmill while wearing a wet suit; however, only in cholinergic urticaria is there a concomitant decrease in pulmonary function.

DIAGNOSIS The rapid onset and self-limited nature of urticarial and angioedematous eruptions are distinguishing features. Additional characteristics are the occurrence of the urticarial crops in various stages of evolution and the asymmetric distribution of the angioedema. Urticaria and/or angioedema involving IgE-dependent mechanisms are often appreciated by historic considerations implicating specific allergens or physical stimuli, by seasonal incidence, and by exposure to certain environments. Direct reproduction of the lesion with physical stimuli is particularly valuable because it so often establishes the cause of the lesion. The diagnosis of an environmental allergen based on the clinical history can be confirmed by skin testing or assay for allergen-specific IgE in serum. IgE-mediated urticaria and/or angioedema may or may not be associated with an elevation of total IgE or with peripheral eosinophilia. Fever, leukocytosis, and an elevated sedimentation rate are absent.

The classification of urticarial and angioedematous states noted in Table 310-1 in terms of possible mechanisms necessarily includes some differential diagnostic points. Hypocomplementemia is not observed in IgE-mediated mast cell disease and may reflect either an acquired abnormality generally attributed to the formation of immune complexes or a genetic deficiency of C1INH. Chronic recurrent urticaria, generally in females, associated with arthralgias, an elevated sedimentation rate, and normo- or hypocomplementemia suggests an underlying cutaneous necrotizing angiitis. Vasculitic urticaria typically persists longer than 72 h, whereas conventional urticaria often has a duration of less than 24 to 48 h. Confirmation depends on a biopsy that reveals cellular infiltration, nuclear debris, and fibrinoid necrosis of the venules. The same pathobiologic process accounts for the urticaria in association with such diseases as systemic lupus erythematosus or viral hepatitis with or without an associated arteritis. Serum sickness per se or a similar clinical entity due to drugs includes not only urticaria but also pyrexia, lymphadenopathy, myalgia, and arthralgia or arthritis. Urticarial reactions to blood products or intravenous administration of immunoglobulin are defined by the event and generally are not progressive unless the recipient is IgA-deficient in the former case or the reagent is aggregated in the latter.

Hereditary angioedema is an autosomal dominant disease due to a deficiency of antigenic and/or functional C1INH. The diagnosis is suggested not only by family history but also by the lack of pruritus and of urticarial lesions, the prominence of recurrent gastrointestinal attacks of colic, and episodes of laryngeal edema. Laboratory diagnosis depends on demonstrating a deficiency of C1INH antigen (type 1) in most kindreds, but some kindreds have an antigenically intact nonfunctional protein (type 2) and require a functional assay to establish the diagnosis. The natural substrates of uninhibited C1 protease, C4 and C2, are chronically depleted but fall further during attacks due to the activation of additional C1. Because the C1INH protein also regulates the Hageman factor–initiated activation of kallikrein and of plasmin, the vasoactive peptides responsible for the angioedema are likely some combination of bradykinin and a plasmin-derived fragment of C1-cleaved C2. An acquired form of C1INH deficiency, associated with lymphoproliferative disorders, has the same clinical manifestations but differs in the lack of a familial element; in the reduction of C1 function and C1q protein as well as C1INH, C4, and C2; and in the presence of an anti-idiotypic antibody to the monoclonal immunoglobulin expressed on the B cells. A second acquired form of C1INH deficiency with angioedema due to the appearance of IgG anti-C1INH may be associated with systemic lupus erythematosus.

Urticaria and angioedema must be differentiated from contact sensitivity, a vesicular eruption that progresses to chronic thickening of the skin with continued allergenic exposure. They must also be differentiated from atopic dermatitis, a condition that may present as erythema, edema, papules, vesiculation, and oozing proceeding to a subacute and chronic stage in which vesiculation is less marked or absent and scaling, fissuring, and lichenification predominate in a distribution that characteristically involves the flexor surfaces. In cutaneous mastocytosis, the reddish brown macules and papules, characteristic of urticaria pigmentosa, urticate with pruritus upon trauma; and in systemic mastocytosis, without or with urticaria pigmentosa, there is an episodic systemic flushing with or without urticaria but no angioedema.

Rx **TREATMENT** Identification of the etiologic factor(s) and their elimination provide the most satisfactory therapeutic program; this approach is feasible to varying degrees with IgE-mediated reactions to allergens or physical stimuli. For most forms of urticaria, H_1 antihistamines such as chlorpheniramine or diphenhydramine, and including the nonsedating class such as loratadine or cetirizine, are effective in attenuating both urtication and pruritus. Cyproheptadine and especially hydroxyzine have proven effective when H_1 antihistamines have been inadequate. Doxepin, a dibenzoxepin tricyclic compound with both H_1 and H_2 receptor antagonist activity, is yet another alternative. Topical glucocorticoids are of no value in the management of urticaria and/or angioedema. Systemic glucocorticoids are generally avoided in idiopathic, allergen-induced, or physical urticarias due to their long-term toxicity. However, systemic glucocorticoids are useful in the management of patients with pressure urticaria, with vasculitic urticaria (especially with eosinophil prominence), with idiopathic angioedema with or without urticaria, or with chronic urticaria that responds poorly to conventional treatment. With persistent vasculitic urticaria, hydroxychloroquine or colchicine may be added to the regimen after hydroxyzine and before or along with systemic glucocorticoids.

The therapy of inborn C1INH deficiency has been simplified by the finding that attenuated androgens correct the biochemical defect and afford prophylactic protection. Since the affected individuals are heterozygous, with the depletion of C1INH being due to deficient synthesis and consequent excessive utilization of the limited amount available, the efficacy of the attenuated androgens is attributed to production by the normal gene of an amount of functional C1INH sufficient to control the spontaneous activation of C1 to C1 protease. Since the use of such agents for children and pregnant women is not yet accepted, the antifibrinolytic agent ϵ-aminocaproic acid may be used occasionally to control spontaneous attacks or for preoperative prophylaxis in some patients. This agent should not be used in patients with thrombotic tendencies or ischemia due to arterial athrosclerosis. Infusion of isolated C1INH protein appears useful in prophylaxis and to ameliorate an attack but is not yet widely available.

SYSTEMIC MASTOCYTOSIS

DEFINITION *Systemic mastocytosis* is defined by mast cell hyperplasia that in most instances is indolent and nonneoplastic. Since human mast cells originate from pluripotent bone marrow cells (CD34+), circulate as nonmetachromatically staining, c-*kit*-positive mononuclear cells, and undergo tissue-specific proliferation and maturation, the hyperplasia is generally recognized only in bone marrow and in the normal peripheral distribution sites of the cells, such as skin, gastrointestinal mucosa, liver, and spleen. Mastocytosis occurs at any age and has a slight preponderance in males. The prevalence of systemic mastocytosis is not known, a familial occurrence has not been established, and atopy is not increased.

CLASSIFICATION, PATHOPHYSIOLOGY, AND CLINICAL MANIFESTATIONS A recent consensus classification for systemic mastocytosis recognizes four forms (Table 310-2). The form designated as *indolent* accounts for the majority of patients and is not known to alter life expectancy. When a patient is classified as having indolent systemic mastocytosis, the concomitant clinical findings must be carefully noted, since they define the complications and directions for management. In systemic mastocytosis *associated with hematologic disorders*, the prognosis is determined by the nature of that disorder, which can range from dysmyelopoiesis to leukemia. In *aggressive* systemic mastocytosis, mast cell proliferation in parenchymal organs such as liver, spleen, and lymph nodes is marked and in a subset of patients is associated with prominent eosinophilia in affected organs or peripheral blood; the prognosis is poor due to widespread tissue infiltration. *Mast cell leukemia* is the rarest form of the disease and is invariably fatal at present; in contrast to the other forms, the peripheral blood contains circulating, metachromatically staining, atypical mast cells. In types II and IV systemic mastocytosis there is a point mutation of the c-*kit* tyrosine kinase in the leukocytes and mast cells, respectively; this mutation can also be detected in lesional tissue such as the small, reddish brown macules or papules, termed *urticaria pigmentosa*, at skin sites of patients with type I. The most common mutation, a substitution of valine for aspartate in codon 816 (V816D), leads to constitutively activated c-*kit*, which then drives proliferation independently of SCF. More than half of the cases of type II systemic mastocytosis with a V816D mutation exhibit cytogenetic abnormalities on routine karyotyping. In types I and III there is excessive production of the c-*kit* ligand (SCF) in the microenvironment of the mast cells, and this may be autocrine in type III. In infants and children (type I) with

Table 310-2 Classification of Systemic Mastocytosis

Type	Description
I	*Indolent* with cutaneous manifestations, vascular collapse, ulcer disease, malabsorption, skeletal disease, hepatosplenomegaly, or lymphadenopathy
II	*Concomitant hematologic disorder*, either myelodysplastic or myeloproliferative
III	*Aggressive* per se or lymphadenopathic mastocytosis with eosinophilia
IV	*Mastocytic leukemia*

cutaneous manifestations, namely, urticaria pigmentosa or bullous lesions, visceral involvement is usually lacking, and resolution is common because there are no mutations to activate the tyrosine kinase. The clinical manifestations of systemic mastocytosis, particularly types I and II, distinct from a leukemic complication, are due to tissue occupancy by the mast cell mass, the tissue response to that mass, and the release of bioactive substances acting at both local and distal sites. The pharmacologically induced manifestations are pruritus, flushing, palpitations and vascular collapse, gastric distress, lower abdominal crampy pain, and recurrent headache. The increase in cell burden is evidenced by the lesions of urticaria pigmentosa at skin sites, but it also contributes to bone pain and malabsorption. The mast cell–mediated fibrotic changes are limited to liver, spleen, and bone marrow and presumably relate to the functional characteristics of mast cells developing at those sites, as opposed to those at sites without fibrosis, such as the gastrointestinal tissue or skin. Immunofluorescent analysis of bone marrow and skin lesions in indolent mastocytosis and of spleen, lymph node, and skin in aggressive systemic mastocytosis has revealed only one mast cell phenotype, namely, scroll-poor cells expressing tryptase, chymase, and CPA.

The cutaneous lesions of urticaria pigmentosa respond to trauma with urtication and erythema (Darier's sign). The apparent incidence of these lesions is 90 percent or greater in patients with indolent systemic mastocytosis. Approximately 1 percent of patients with indolent mastocytosis have skin lesions that appear as tan-brown macules with striking patchy erythema and associated telangiectasia (telangiectasia macularis eruptiva perstans). In the upper gastrointestinal tract, histamine-mediated hypersecretion is the most common problem, with resultant gastritis and peptic ulcer. In the lower intestinal tract, the occurrence of diarrhea and abdominal pain is attributed to increased motility due to mast cell mediators, and this can be aggravated by malabsorption with secondary nutritional insufficiency and osteomalacia. The periportal fibrosis associated with mast cell infiltration and a prominence of eosinophils may lead to portal hypertension and ascites. In some patients, flushing and recurrent vascular collapse are markedly aggravated by an idiosyncratic response to a minimal dosage of nonsteroidal anti-inflammatory agents. The neuropsychiatric disturbances are clinically most evident as impaired recent memory, decreased attention span, and "migraine-like" headaches. Patients in every category of systemic mastocytosis may experience exacerbation of a specific clinical sign or symptom with alcohol ingestion, use of mast cell–interactive narcotics, or ingestion of nonsteroidal anti-inflammatory agents.

DIAGNOSIS Although the diagnosis is generally suspected on the basis of the clinical history and physical findings, the contention can be strengthened by certain laboratory procedures and established only by a tissue diagnosis. A 24-h urine collection for measurement of histamine, histamine metabolites, or metabolites of PGD_2 is currently the most common noninvasive approach. A convenient alternative is to measure blood levels of the mast cell–derived neutral protease tryptase. The α form of tryptase is elevated in more than one-half of patients with type I systemic mastocytosis and in virtually all those with types II and III, whereas the β form is increased in patients undergoing an anaphylactic reaction. Additional studies directed by the presentation include a bone scan or skeletal survey; contrast studies of the upper gastrointestinal tract with small-bowel follow-through, computed tomography scan, or endoscopy; and a neuropsychiatric evaluation, including an electroencephalogram. The tissue diagnosis is straightforward if there are lesions of urticaria pigmentosa, but the diagnosis of systemic mastocytosis requires involvement of other organs and is most frequently established by bone marrow biopsy and aspiration. The bone marrow lesions consist of focal and paratrabecular aggregates of spindle-shaped mast cells, often mixed with eosinophils, lymphocytes, and, on occasion, plasma cells, histiocytes, and fibroblasts.

The differential diagnosis requires the exclusion of other flushing disorders. The 24-h urine assessment of 5-hydroxy-indoleacetic acid and metanephrines should exclude a carcinoid tumor or a pheochromocytoma. Most patients with recurrent anaphylaxis, including the idiopathic group, present with angioedema and/or wheezing, which are not manifestations of systemic mastocytosis.

℞ **TREATMENT** The management of systemic mastocytosis uses a stepwise and symptom/sign–directed approach that includes an H_1 antihistamine for flushing and pruritus, an H_2 antihistamine or proton pump inhibitor for gastric acid hypersecretion, oral cromolyn sodium for diarrhea and abdominal pain, and a nonsteroidal anti-inflammatory agent for severe flushing associated with vascular collapse despite use of H_1 and H_2 antihistamines to block biosynthesis of PGD_2. Systemic glucocorticoids appear to alleviate the malabsorption. Headaches are generally managed with tricyclic antidepressants and other neurotransmitter-modifying agents. Ketotifen has been used to alleviate flushing in patients with gastric intolerance to nonsteroidal anti-inflammatory agents and in patients with bone pain or intractable headaches. The efficacy of IFN-α in aggressive systemic mastocytosis is controversial, and this may relate to the difficulty in achieving the necessary dosage in some patients due to the attendant side effects. Treatment with hydroxyurea to reduce the mast cell lineage progenitors may have merit in type III systemic mastocytosis. Chemotherapy is appropriate for the frank leukemias in types II and IV.

ALLERGIC RHINITIS

DEFINITION Allergic rhinitis is characterized by sneezing; rhinorrhea; obstruction of the nasal passages; conjunctival, nasal, and pharyngeal itching; and lacrimation, all occurring in a temporal relationship to allergen exposure. Although commonly seasonal due to elicitation by airborne pollens, it can be perennial in an environment of chronic exposure. The incidence of allergic rhinitis in North America is about 7%, with the peak occurring in childhood and adolescence.

PREDISPOSING FACTORS AND ETIOLOGY Allergic rhinitis generally presents in atopic individuals, i.e., in persons with a family history of a similar or related symptom complex and a personal history of collateral allergy expressed as eczematous dermatitis, urticaria, and/or asthma (Chap. 252). Symptoms generally appear before the fourth decade of life and tend to diminish gradually with aging, although complete spontaneous remissions are uncommon. A relatively small number of weeds that depend on wind rather than insects for cross-pollination, as well as certain grasses and trees, produce sufficient quantities of pollen suitable for wide distribution by air currents to elicit seasonal allergic rhinitis. The dates of pollination of these species generally vary little from year to year in a particular locale but may be quite different in another climate. In the temperate areas of North America, trees typically pollinate from March through May, grasses in June and early July, and ragweed from mid-August to early October. Molds, which are widespread in nature because they occur in soil or decaying organic matter, may propagate spores in a pattern dependent on climatic conditions. Perennial allergic rhinitis occurs in response to allergens that are present throughout the year such as in desquamating epithelium in animal dander or cockroach-derived proteins, the processed materials or chemicals utilized in an industrial setting, or the dust accumulating at work or at home. Dust has a diverse allergen content including *Dermatophagoides farinae* and *D. pteronyssinus*, which may be present alone or together in house dust. Dust mites are scavengers of flecks of human skin and coat the digestate with mite-specific protein for subsequent excretion as part of a fecal ball. In up to two-thirds of patients with perennial rhinitis, no clear-cut allergen can be demonstrated. The ability of allergens to cause rhinitis rather than lower respiratory symptoms may be attributed to their size, 10 to 100 μm, and retention within the nose.

PATHOPHYSIOLOGY AND MANIFESTATIONS Episodic rhinorrhea, sneezing, obstruction of the nasal passages with lacrimation, and pruritus of the conjunctiva, nasal mucosa, and oropharynx are the hallmarks of allergic rhinitis. The nasal mucosa is pale and boggy, the conjunctiva congested and edematous, and the pharynx is generally unremarkable. Swelling of the turbinates and mucous membranes with obstruction of the sinus ostia and eustachian tubes precipitates secondary infections of the sinuses and middle ear, respectively, commonly in perennial but rarely in seasonal disease. Nasal polyps, representing mucosal protrusions containing edema fluid with variable numbers of eosinophils, arise concurrently with edema and/or infection within the sinuses and increase obstructive symptoms.

The nose presents a large mucosal surface area through the folds of the turbinates and serves to adjust the temperature and moisture content of inhaled air and to filter out particulate materials above 10 μm in size by impingement in a mucous blanket; ciliary action moves the entrapped particles toward the pharynx. Entrapment of pollen and digestion of the outer coat by mucosal enzymes such as lysozymes release protein allergens generally of 10,000 to 40,000 molecular weight. The initial interaction occurs between the allergen and intraepithelial mast cells and then proceeds to involve deeper perivenular mast cells, both of which are sensitized with specific IgE. During the symptomatic season when the mucosae are already swollen and hyperemic, there is enhanced adverse reactivity to the seasonal pollen as well as to antigenically unrelated pollens for which there is underlying hypersensitivity due to improved penetration of the allergens. Biopsy specimens of nasal mucosa during seasonal rhinitis show submucosal edema with infiltration by eosinophils, along with some basophils and neutrophils.

The mucosal surface fluid contains IgA that is present because of its secretory piece and also IgE, which apparently arrives by diffusion from plasma cells in proximity to mucosal surfaces. IgE fixes to mucosal and submucosal mast cells, and the intensity of the clinical response to inhaled allergens is quantitatively related to the naturally occurring pollen dose. Specific IgE is distributed also to circulating basophilic leukocytes; patients with more severe clinical disease have basophils that release histamine in response to lesser concentrations of allergen in vitro than do cells from patients with milder disease. In sensitive individuals, the introduction of allergen into the nose is associated with sneezing, "stuffiness," and discharge, and the fluid contains histamine, PGD_2, and leukotrienes. Thus the mast cells of the nasal mucosa and submucosa generate and release mediators through IgE-dependent reactions that are capable of producing tissue edema and eosinophilic infiltration.

DIAGNOSIS The diagnosis of seasonal allergic rhinitis depends largely on an accurate history of occurrence coincident with the pollination of the offending weeds, grasses, or trees. The continuous character of perennial allergic rhinitis due to contamination of the home or place of work makes historic analysis difficult, but there may be a variability in symptoms that can be related to exposure to animal dander, dust mite and/or cockroach allergens, or work-related allergens such as latex. Patients with perennial rhinitis commonly develop the problem in adult life, are more often women than men, and manifest nasal polyps and thickening of the sinus membranes demonstrated by radiography. The term *vasomotor rhinitis* designates a condition of enhanced reactivity of the nasopharynx in which a symptom complex resembling perennial allergic rhinitis occurs with nonspecific stimuli. Other entities to be excluded are structural abnormalities of the nasopharynx; exposure to irritants; upper respiratory infection; pregnancy with prominent nasal mucosal edema; prolonged topical use of α-adrenergic agents in the form of nose drops (rhinitis medicamentosa); and the use of certain therapeutic agents such as rauwolfia, β-adrenergic antagonists, or estrogens.

The nasal secretions of allergic patients are rich in eosinophils, and peripheral eosinophilia is a common feature. Local or systemic neutrophilia implies infection. Total serum IgE is frequently elevated, but the demonstration of immunologic specificity for IgE is critical to an etiologic diagnosis. A skin test by the epicutaneous route (scratch or prick) with the allergens of interest provides a rapid and reliable approach to identifying allergen-specific IgE that has sensitized cutaneous mast cells. An intradermal test may follow if indicated by history when the epicutaneous test is negative, but it is less reliable due to the reactivity of some asymptomatic individuals at the test dose. Skin testing by scratch or prick for food allergens is controversial but does seem to have predictive value for the absence of specific IgE sensitivity. A double-blind, placebo-controlled challenge may document a food allergy, but such a procedure does bear the risk of an anaphylactic reaction. An elimination diet is safer but is tedious and less definitive. Food allergy is uncommon as a cause of allergic rhinitis.

Newer methodology for detecting total IgE, including the development of enzyme-linked immunosorbent assays (ELISA) employing anti-IgE bound to either a solid-phase or a liquid-phase paramagnetic particle, provides rapid and cost effective determinations. Measurements of specific anti-IgE in serum are obtained by its binding to a solid-phase allergen and quantitation by subsequent uptake of radiolabeled anti-IgE. This radioallergosorbent technique correlates with the bioassay of specific IgE by skin test, which is mast cell–dependent, and by histamine release from peripheral blood leukocytes, which is basophil-dependent. As compared to the skin test, the assay of specific IgE in serum is less sensitive but has high specificity. Furthermore, ELISA utilizing reactions that generate visible light or fluorescence have replaced the radioimmunoassays, and newer chemiluminescent tracers provide additional sensitivity for detection of minute quantities of allergen-specific IgE.

PREVENTION Avoidance of exposure to the offending allergen is the most effective means of controlling allergic diseases; removal of pets from the home to avoid animal danders, utilization of air filtration devices to minimize the concentrations of airborne pollens, elimination of cockroach-derived proteins by chemical destruction of the pest and careful food storage, travel to nonpollinating areas during the critical periods, and even a change of domicile to eliminate a mold spore problem may be necessary. Control of dust mites by allergen avoidance includes use of plastic-lined covers for mattresses, pillows, and comforters, and elimination of carpets and drapes.

℞ **TREATMENT** Management with pharmacologic agents represents the standard approach to seasonal or perennial allergic rhinitis. Antihistamines of the H_1 class are effective for nasopharyngeal itching, sneezing, and watery rhinorrhea and for such ocular manifestations as itching, tearing, and erythema, but they are not efficacious for the nasal congestion. The older antihistamines are sedating, and their anticholinergic (muscarinic) effects include visual disturbance, urinary retention, and even arrhythmias. Because the newer H_1 antihistaminics such as loratadine and cetirizine are less lipophilic, their ability to cross the blood-brain barrier is reduced, and thus their sedating and anticholinergic side effects are minimized. Because life-threatening ventricular arrhythmias with some fatalities have been caused by prolongation of the QT interval resulting from inhibition of the metabolism of terfenadine and astemizole by their interactions with macrolide antibiotics, these agents have been subtantially replaced by loratadine, fexofenadine, and cetirizine. α-Adrenergic agents such as phenylephrine or oximetazoline are generally used topically to alleviate nasal congestion and obstruction, but the duration of efficacy is limited because of rebound rhinitis and such systemic responses as insomnia, irritability, and hypertension. The latter are more frequent with use of oral α-adrenergic agonists, which nonetheless are useful in relieving nasal congestion and diminishing the sedating effects of conventional antihistamines. Cromolyn sodium, a nasal spray, is essentially without side effects and is used prophylactically on a continuous basis during the season to attenuate allergen activation of nasal mast cells. The clinical efficacy of cromolyn sodium and that of nonsedating antihistamines are roughly equivalent. Intranasal high-potency glucocorticoids are the most potent drugs available for the relief of established rhinitis, seasonal or perennial, and even vasomotor rhinitis; they provide efficacy with substantially reduced side effects as compared with this same class of agent administered orally. Their most frequent side effect is local irritation, with *Candida* overgrowth being a rare occurrence. The topical-to-systemic activity of flunisolide or budesonide is significantly greater than for beclomethasone or triamcinolone with much less systemic absorption. For patients who do not benefit adequately from a full dosage of a nonsedating H_1 antihistamine and a maintenance dosage of cromolyn sodium, an α-adrenergic agent for short-term relief should be replaced by high-potency topical glucocorticoids. For systemic symptoms not related to the nasopharynx, such as allergic conjunctivitis, treatment may be local.

Immunotherapy, often termed *hyposensitization*, consists of repeated subcutaneous injections of gradually increasing concentrations of the allergen(s) considered to be specifically responsible for the symptom complex. Controlled studies of ragweed, grass, dust mite, and cat dander allergens administered for treatment of allergic rhinitis have demonstrated at least partial relief of symptoms and signs. The duration of such immunotherapy is 3 to 5 years, with discontinuation being based on minimal symptoms over two consecutive seasons of exposure. Clinical benefit appears related to the administration of a high dose of allergen at weekly or biweekly intervals. Patients should remain at the treatment site for at least 20 min after allergen administration so that any anaphylactic consequence can be managed. Local reactions with erythema and induration are not uncommon and may persist for 1 to 3 days. Immunotherapy is contraindicated in patients with significant cardiovascular disease or unstable asthma and should be conducted with particular caution in any patient requiring β-adrenergic blocking therapy because of the difficulty in managing an anaphylactic complication. The immunologic characteristics of a response include a rise in antibodies of the IgG class, a small increase in specific IgE early in the treatment course followed by a plateau or decline, and a decline in the percentage of histamine released from peripheral blood basophilic leukocytes challenged with a fixed concentration of the allergen. The antibodies of the IgG class might well reduce or neutralize the quantity of allergen available for interaction with the tissue mast cells but, more important, could modify the seasonal booster response in specific IgE synthesis. None of the individual parameters of the response to immunotherapy correlates well with the assessments of clinical efficacy, suggesting that benefit is derived from a complex of effects that likely includes a reduction in T cell cytokine production. Immunotherapy should be reserved for clearly documented seasonal or perennial rhinitis, clinically related to defined allergen exposure with confirmation by the presence of allergen-specific IgE, which has failed management by allergen avoidance and pharmacotherapy due to lack of efficacy or side effects. A sequence for the management of allergic or perennial rhinitis based on an allergen-specific diagnosis and stepwise management as required for symptom control would include the following: (1) identification of the offending allergen(s) by history with confirmation of the presence of allergen-specific IgE by skin test (epicutaneous) and/or serum assay; (2) avoidance of the offending allergen; (3) for mild symptoms, prophylactic management with topical cromolyn sodium or treatment with a single bedtime dose of chlorpheniramine (if the latter is associated with undue side effects, substitute a second-generation nonsedating antihistimine); combination with an oral decongestant such as pseudoephedrine can be beneficial; (4) for prominent symptoms, utilization of topical beclomethasone, budesonide, fluticasone, momestasone, or triamcinalone may be needed for a satisfactory clinical outcome; and (5) for management failures despite avoidance and pharmacotherapy, progression to immunotherapy.

BIBLIOGRAPHY

AUSTEN KF, METCALFE DD: Anaphylactic syndrome, in *Immunological Diseases*, 5th ed, M Frank et al (eds). Boston, Little, Brown, 1995

BINGHAM CO, AUSTEN KF: The molecular and cellular biology of the mast cell, in *Fitzpatrick's Dermatology in General Medicine*, 5th ed, IM Freedberg et al (eds). New York, McGraw-Hill, 1999, pp 414–423

EWAN PW: Anaphylaxis. BMJ 316:1442, 1997

METCALFE DD: The mastocytosis syndrome, in *Fitzpatrick's Dermatology in General Medicine*, 5th ed, IM Freedberg et al (eds). New York, McGraw-Hill, 1999, pp 1902–1908

O'HOLLAREN MT: Update in allergy and immunology. Ann Intern Med 129:1036, 1998

PENROSE JF et al: Leukotrienes: Biosynthetic pathways, release, and receptor-mediated actions with relevance to disease states, in *Inflammation: Basic Principles and Clinical Correlates*, 3rd ed, JI Gallin and R Snyderman (eds). Philadelphia, Lippincott Williams & Wilkins, 1999

SOTER NA: Urticaria and angioedema, in *Fitzpatrick's Dermatology in General Medicine*, 5th ed, IM Freedberg et al (eds). New York, McGraw-Hill, 1999, pp 1409–1419

VALENTINE MD: Insect venom allergy, in *Immunological Diseases*, 5th ed, M Frank et al (eds). Boston, Little, Brown, 1995

311 SYSTEMIC LUPUS ERYTHEMATOSUS

Bevra Hannahs Hahn

aCL anticardiolipin	LA lupus anticoagulant
ANA antinuclear antibody	MCP metacarpophalangeal
CNS central nervous system	MRI magnetic resonance imaging
CSF cerebrospinal fluid	NSAIDs nonsteroidal anti-inflammatory drugs
CT computed tomography	PIP proximal interphalangeal
DEJ dermal-epidermal junction	SCLE subacute cutaneous lupus erythematosus
DLE discoid lupus erythematosus	SLE systemic lupus erythematosus
ERT estrogen replacement therapy	UV ultraviolet
GI gastrointestinal	
GN glomerulonephritis	

DEFINITION AND PREVALENCE Systemic lupus erythematosus (SLE) is a disease of unknown etiology in which tissues and cells are damaged by pathogenic autoantibodies and immune complexes. Ninety percent of cases are in women, usually of child-bearing age, but children, men, and the elderly can be affected. In the United States, the prevalence of SLE in urban areas varies from 15 to 50 per 100,000 population; it is more common in blacks than in whites. Hispanic and Asian populations are also susceptible.

PATHOGENESIS AND ETIOLOGY SLE results from tissue damage caused by pathogenic subsets of autoantibodies and immune complexes. The abnormal immune responses include (1) polyclonal and antigen-specific T and B lymphocyte hyperactivity, and (2) inadequate regulation of that hyperactivity. These abnormal immune responses probably depend upon interactions between susceptibility genes and environment. Evidence for genetic predisposition includes increased concordance for disease in monozygotic (24 to 58%) compared with dizygotic (0 to 6%) twins, a $\lambda_s > 10$, and a 10 to 15% frequency of patients with more than one affected family member. Studies of association, linkage, and genome scanning show complex genetic susceptibility. Most people with homozygous deficiencies of early components of complement (C1q, C2, C4) have SLE or similar disease (accounting for <5% of SLE patients), suggesting that these genes are major predisposing factors. Most patients must inherit multiple susceptibility genes, and probably experience environmental stimuli as well, to develop clinical disease. A defective or deleted class III allele, C4AQO, is the most common genetic marker associated with SLE in many ethnic groups (40 to 50% of patients compared with 15% of healthy controls). One extended haplotype, B8.DR3.DQw2.C4AQO, predisposes to SLE in populations with Northern European heritage. SLE is associated with HLA-DR2 or -DR3 in many groups, and single-gene associations occur between HLA class II (especially DQ_β) and autoantibodies that associate with clinical subsets of lupus. For example, antibodies to Ro/La (SS-A/SS-B) are associated with subacute cutaneous lupus and certain DQA and DQB genes that are usually inherited with DR3. Normal alleles of FcγRIIA or of FcγRIIIA that bind IgG2 or IgG1 and IgG3, respectively, less efficiently than other alleles are associated with SLE, particularly with nephritis. FcγRIIA predisposes to SLE in African Americans and South Koreans; FcγRIIIA predisposes across different ethnic groups. Such alleles might account for impaired clearing of autoantibodies and immune complexes, thus predisposing to their deposition in tissues. Genome scanning from several laboratories has shown two regions of chromosome 1 that link to disease in sibpairs or multiplex families. One region, 1q23, contains the FcγRIIA gene; the other, 1q41-42, contains poly (ADP-ribosyl) polymerase (PARP), which may be another predisposing gene that plays a role in DNA repair and apoptosis. Other results of genome scanning suggest that at least 10 other regions on various chromosomes, in addition to HLA and the two regions on chromosome 1 discussed above, participate in susceptibility. Some genes may be "autoimmunity" genes common to different autoimmune diseases across different ethnic groups; others are likely to be restricted to a single disease and/or a single ethnic group. Family studies suggest that females are more likely than males to express the autoimmune manifestations of their genotypes.

Environmental factors that cause flares of SLE are largely unknown, with the exception of ultraviolet (UV)-B (and sometimes UV-A) light. As many as 70% of patients are photosensitive. Other factors, such as ingested alfalfa sprouts, and chemicals, such as hydrazines, have been implicated. Searches for viral/retroviral disease inducers have been inconclusive. Although some drugs can induce lupus-like disease, there are notable clinical and autoantibody differences between drug-induced and spontaneous lupus. Femaleness is clearly a susceptibility factor, since the prevalence in women of child-bearing years is seven to nine times higher than in men, whereas the female: male ratio is 3:1 in pre- and postmenopausal years. Metabolism of estrogenic and androgenic hormones may be abnormal in lupus patients. Sex hormones also influence immune tolerance.

Abnormal immune responses permit sustained production of pathogenic subsets of autoantibodies and immune complexes. Some autoantibodies, such as anti-DNA, can bind to tissue via charge or cross-reactivity, or in immune complexes, and cause complement-mediated damage. Some subsets of anti-DNA and anti-RNP can bind and enter living cells, altering their function. Other autoantibodies cause damage by direct binding to cell membranes (erythrocytes, platelets) that cause those cells to be phagocytized and destroyed. T cell help is critical to development of full-blown disease; cells of CD4+CD8−, CD4−CD8+, and CD4− CD8− phenotypes all help autoantibody production in SLE. The abnormalities that permit hyperactivated self-reactive B and T cells to dominate immune repertoires in murine and human SLE are multiple and include defects in cell activation, tolerance, apoptosis, idiotypic networks, immune complex clearance, and generation of regulatory cells. The structure of antigens that stimulate autoantibodies is under investigation. Some are clearly derived from self (nucleosomes, ribonucleoprotein, erythrocyte and lymphocyte surface antigens); others may be from the external environment and mimic self (e.g., components of vesicular stomatitis virus mimic peptides in Sm antigen). Many DNA/protein and RNA/protein antigens may be presented to the immune system in surface blebs of apoptotic cells. Since UV light induces apoptosis in skin cells, this might be a mechanism for flaring disease. Autoantibodies characteristic of SLE are listed in Table 311-1.

In summary, some individuals are genetically predisposed to SLE. Under the influence of multiple genes, possibly triggered by environmental challenges and highly influenced by sex, they may develop a number of different clinical syndromes that fulfill diagnostic criteria for SLE. The etiology of these syndromes is complex and probably differs between patients.

CLINICAL MANIFESTATIONS At onset, SLE may involve only one organ system (additional manifestations occur later) or may be multisystemic. Clinical manifestations are listed in Table 311-2; those that fulfill American Rheumatism Association (currently the American College of Rheumatology) updated criteria for a diagnosis of SLE are listed in Table 311-3. Autoantibodies are detectable at disease onset. Severity varies from mild and intermittent to persistent and fulminant. Most patients experience exacerbations interspersed with periods of relative quiescence. True remissions with no symptoms and requiring no therapy occur in up to 20% but are usually not permanent. Systemic symptoms are usually prominent and include fatigue, malaise, fever, anorexia, and weight loss.

Musculoskeletal Manifestations Almost all patients experience arthralgias and myalgias; most develop intermittent arthritis. Pain is often out of proportion to physical findings. Symmetric fusiform swelling in joints [most frequently proximal interphalangeal (PIP) and metacarpophalangeal (MCP) joints of the hands, wrists, and knees], diffuse puffiness of hands and feet, and tenosynovitis can be seen. Joint deformities are unusual, with 10% of patients developing swan-neck deformities of fingers and ulnar drift at MCP joints. Erosions are rare; subcutaneous nodules occur. Myopathy can be inflammatory (during periods of active disease), or secondary to treatment (hypokalemia, glucocorticoid myopathy, hydroxychloroquine myopathy). Ischemic necrosis of bone is a common cause of hip, knee, or shoulder pain in patients receiving glucocorticoids.

Cutaneous Manifestations The malar ("butterfly") rash is a photosensitive, fixed erythematous rash, flat or raised, over the cheeks and bridge of the nose, often involving the chin and ears. Scarring is absent; telangiectases may develop. A more diffuse maculopapular rash, predominant in sun-exposed areas, is also common and usually indicates disease flare. Loss of scalp hair is usually patchy but can be extensive; hair often regrows in SLE lesions but not in lesions of discoid lupus erythematosus (DLE). DLE occurs in about 20% of patients with SLE and can be disfiguring, since the lesions have central atrophy and scarring, with permanent loss of appendages. DLE lesions are circular with an erythematous raised rim, scaliness, follicular plugging, and telangiectasia. They occur over the scalp, ears, face, and sun-exposed areas of the arms, back, and chest. Only 5% of patients with DLE subsequently develop SLE. Less frequent SLE skin lesions include urticaria, bullae, erythema multiforme, lichen planus–like lesions, and panniculitis ("lupus profundus").

Table 311-1 Autoantibodies in Patients with SLE

	Incidence, %	Antigen Detected	Clinical Importance
Antinuclear antibodies	98	Multiple nuclear	Human cell substrates are more sensitive than murine. Repeatedly negative tests make SLE unlikely.
Anti-DNA	70	DNA (ds)	Anti-dsDNA is relatively disease-specific; anti-ssDNA is not. High titers are associated with nephritis and clinical activity in some patients.
Anti-Sm	30	Protein complexed to 6 species of small nuclear RNA	Specific for SLE.
Anti-RNP	40	Protein complexed to U1RNA	High titer in syndromes with features of polymyositis, lupus, scleroderma, and mixed connective tissue disease. If present in SLE without anti-DNA, risk for nephritis is low.
Anti-Ro (SS-A)	30	Protein complexed to y_1-y_5 RNA	Associated with Sjögren's syndrome, subacute cutaneous lupus, inherited C′ deficiencies, ANA-negative lupus, lupus in the elderly, neonatal lupus, congenital heart block. Can cause nephritis.
Anti-La (SS-B)	10	Phosphoprotein	Always associated with anti-Ro. Risk for nephritis is low if present. Associated with Sjögren's syndrome.
Antihistone	70	Histones	More frequent in drug-induced LE (95%) than in spontaneous SLE.
Antiphospholipid	50	Phospholipids	Three types—lupus anticoagulant (LA), anticardiolipin (aCL), and false-positive test for syphilis (BFP). The LA and aCL (particular high-titer IgG) are associated with clotting, fetal loss, thrombocytopenia, and valvular heart disease. Antibodies to β_2-glycoprotein I are part of this group.
Antierythrocyte	60	Erythrocyte	A small proportion of these patients develop overt hemolysis.
Antiplatelet	30	Platelet surface + cytoplasm	Associated with thrombocytopenia in 15% of patients.
Antilymphocyte	70	Lymphocyte surface	Probably associated with leukopenia and abnormal T cell function.
Antineuronal	60	Neuronal and lymphocyte surface	In some series, high titers of IgG correlate with diffuse CNS lupus.
Antiribosomal P	20	Ribosomal P protein	In some series, antibody in serum correlates with psychosis or depression due to CNS SLE.

Patients with subacute cutaneous lupus erythematosus (SCLE) are a distinct subset with recurring extensive dermatitis. Arthritis and fatigue are frequent; central nervous system and renal involvement are not. Some patients are antinuclear antibody (ANA)–negative. Most have antibodies to Ro (SS-A) or to single-stranded (ss) DNA. Skin lesions are photosensitive and either annular or papulosquamous psoriasiform; they occur over the arms, trunk, and face but do not scar.

Patients with SLE, DLE, or SCLE can develop vasculitic skin lesions. These include purpura, subcutaneous nodules, nail fold infarcts, ulcers, vasculitic urticaria, panniculitis, and gangrene of digits. Shallow, slightly painful ulcers in the mouth and nose are frequent in patients with SLE.

Renal Manifestations Most patients with SLE have immunoglobulins deposited in glomeruli, but only one-half have clinical nephritis, defined by proteinuria. Early in the disease most are asymptomatic, although some develop the edema of nephrotic syndrome. Urinalysis shows hematuria, cylindruria, and proteinuria. Most patients with mesangial or mild focal proliferative nephritis (see discussion under "Pathology," below) maintain good renal function. Patients with diffuse proliferative nephritis develop renal failure if untreated. Because severe nephritis requires aggressive immunosuppression with high-dose glucocorticoids and cytotoxic drugs and mild lesions do not, renal biopsy may provide information that affects therapy. Patients with rapidly deteriorating renal function and active urine sediment require prompt, aggressive therapy; biopsy is not necessary unless they fail to respond. However, patients with a slow rise in serum creatinine to levels >265 μmol/L (3 mg/dL) should be biopsied; a high proportion of sclerotic glomeruli on biopsy suggests that these patients are unlikely to respond to immunosuppressive therapies and are candidates for dialysis or transplantation. Patients with persistently abnormal urinalyses, high titers of anti-dsDNA, and/or hypocomplementemia are at risk for severe nephritis; kidney biopsy may guide therapy.

Nervous System Any region of the brain can be involved in SLE, as can the meninges, spinal cord, and cranial and peripheral nerves. Central nervous system (CNS) events may be single or multiple and often occur when SLE is active in other organ systems. Mild cognitive dysfunction is the most frequent manifestation. Headaches are common and may be migraine-like or nonspecific. Seizures of any type may occur. Less frequent manifestations include psychosis, acute confusional states, demyelinating disorders, cerebrovascular disease, movement disorders, aseptic meningitis, myelopathy, mononeuropathy or polyneuropathy of cranial or peripheral nerves, autonomic dysfunction, acute demyelinating polyneuropathy (Guillain-Barré), mood disorders, optic neuritis, subarachnoid hemorrhage, pseudotumor cer-

Table 311-2 Clinical Manifestations of SLE

Manifestation	Percent of Patients Positive during Course of Disease	
Systemic		95
Fatigue, malaise, fever, anorexia, nausea, weight loss		
Musculoskeletal		95
Arthralgias/myalgias	95	
Nonerosive polyarthritis	60	
Hand deformities	10	
Myopathy/myositis	40/5	
Ischemic necrosis of bone	15	
Cutaneous		80
Malar rash	50	
Discoid rash	15	
Photosensitivity	70	
Oral ulcers	40	
Other rashes—maculopapular, urticarial, bullous, subacute cutaneous lupus	40	
Alopecia	40	
Vasculitis	20	
Panniculitis	5	
Hematologic		85
Anemia (of chronic disease)	70	
Hemolytic anemia	10	
Leukopenia ($<4000/mm^3$)	65	
Lymphopenia ($<1500/mm^3$)	50	
Thrombocytopenia ($<100,000/mm^3$)	15	
Circulating anticoagulant	10–20	
Splenomegaly	15	
Lymphadenopathy	20	
Neurologic		60
Cognitive dysfunction	50	
Mood disorder	40	
Headache	25	
Seizures	20	
Mono- or polyneuropathy	15	
Cerebrovascular disease	10	
Demyelinating syndrome	8	
Acute confusional state	5	
Movement disorder	2	
Neurologic *(Continued)*		
Aseptic meningitis	<1	
Myelopathy	<1	
Other (see text)	5	
Cardiopulmonary		60
Pleurisy	50	
Pericarditis	30	
Myocarditis	10	
Endocarditis (Libman-Sacks)	10	
Valvular insufficiency	2	
Coronary artery disease	8	
Pleural effusions	30	
Lupus pneumonitis	10	
Interstitial fibrosis	5	
Pulmonary hypertension	<5	
ARDS/hemorrhage	<5	
Renal		50
Proteinuria >500 mg/24 h	50	
Cellular casts	50	
Nephrotic syndrome	25	
Renal failure	5–10	
Gastrointestinal		45
Nonspecific (anorexia, nausea, mild pain, diarrhea)	30	
Vasculitis with bleeding or perforation	5	
Ascites	<5	
Abnormal liver enzymes	40	
Thrombosis		15
Venous	10	
Arterial	5	
Fetal loss		30 (of pregnancies)
Ocular		15
Retinal vasculitis	5	
Conjunctivitis/episcleritis	10	
Sicca syndrome	15	

ebri, and hypothalamic dysfunction with inappropriate secretion of vasopressin. Depression and anxiety are frequent.

Laboratory diagnosis of CNS lupus can be difficult. Abnormal electroencephalograms occur in about 70% of patients with neurologic complaints and usually show diffuse slowing or focal abnormalities. Cerebrospinal fluid (CSF) shows elevated protein levels in 50% and increased mononuclear cells in 30% of patients; oligoclonal bands and increased Ig synthesis may be found. Lumbar puncture is recommended when the diagnosis of CNS lupus is in doubt or when infection is a possible cause of symptoms. Magnetic resonance imaging (MRI) with contrast is the most sensitive radiographic technique to detect acute and chronic lesions of SLE; changes are often nonspecific. Patients with focal neurologic lesions are more likely to have positive MRI scans than those with diffuse manifestations. Computed tomography (CT) scans are useful to rule out bleeding or mass lesions, if indicated. Angiograms can detect vasculitis and vascular occlusions or emboli; they cannot visualize vessels smaller than 50 μm; lupus vasculitis usually involves smaller vessels. Laboratory measures of disease activity often do not correlate with neurologic manifestations. Neurologic problems (with the exception of deficits resulting from large infarcts) usually improve with immunosuppressive therapy and/or time; recurrences are seen in approximately one-third of patients.

Vascular System Thrombosis in vessels of any size can be a major problem. Although vasculitis may underly thrombosis, there is increasing evidence that antibodies against phospholipids [lupus anticoagulant (LA), anticardiolipin (aCL)] are associated with clotting without inflammation. The source of cerebral emboli may be the lesions of Libman-Sacks endocarditis. In addition, degenerative vascular changes after years of exposure of blood vessels to circulating immune complexes and hyperlipidemia from glucocorticoid therapy predispose to degenerative cerebral and coronary artery disease in lupus patients. Therefore, anticoagulation is more appropriate than immunosuppression in some patients.

Hematologic Manifestation Anemia of chronic disease occurs in most patients when lupus is active. Hemolysis occurs in a small proportion of those with positive Coombs' tests; it is usually responsive to high-dose glucocorticoids; resistant cases may respond to splenectomy. Leukopenia (usually lymphopenia) is common but is rarely associated with recurrent infections and does not require treatment. Mild thrombocytopenia is common; severe thrombocytopenia with bleeding and purpura occurs in 5% of patients and should be treated with high-dose glucocorticoids. Short-term improvement can be achieved by administration of intravenous gamma globulin. If the platelet count fails to reach acceptable levels in 2 weeks, addition of cytotoxic drugs, cyclosporine, danazole, and/or splenectomy should be considered.

The LA belongs to a family of antiphospholipid antibodies. It is recognized by prolongation of the partial thromboplastin time and failure of added normal plasma to correct the prolongation. More sensitive tests include the Russell viper venom time. aCL are detected in enzyme-linked immunosorbent assays. Clinical manifestations of LA and aCL include thrombocytopenia, recurrent venous or arterial clotting, recurrent fetal loss, and valvular heart disease. If the LA is associated with hypoprothrombinemia or thrombocytopenia, bleeding may occur. Less commonly, antibodies to clotting factors (VIII, IX) arise; they cause bleeding. Bleeding syndromes usually respond to glucocorticoids; clotting syndromes do not.

Cardiopulmonary System Pericarditis is the most frequent manifestation of cardiac lupus; effusions can occur and occasionally lead to tamponade; constrictive pericarditis is rare. Myocarditis can cause arrhythmias, sudden death, and/or heart failure. Valvular insufficiency (usually aortic or mitral) can occur, with or without Libman-Sacks endocarditis. Lesions on valves are best detected by transesophageal echocardiography. Myocardial infarcts usually result from degenerative disease, although they can result from vasculitis.

Pleurisy and pleural effusions are common manifestations of SLE. Lupus pneumonitis causes fever, dyspnea, and cough; x-rays show

Table 311-3 The 1982 Criteria for Classification of Systemic Lupus Erythematosus, Updated 1997

1. Malar rash	Fixed erythema, flat or raised, over the malar eminences
2. Discoid rash	Erythematous raised patches with adherent keratotic scaling and follicular plugging; atrophic scarring may occur
3. Photosensitivity	Exposure to UV light causes rash
4. Oral ulcers	Includes oral and nasopharyngeal, observed by physician
5. Arthritis	Nonerosive arthritis involving two or more peripheral joints, characterized by tenderness, swelling, or effusion
6. Serositis	Pleuritis or pericarditis documented by ECG or rub or evidence of pericardial effusion
7. Renal disorder	Proteinuria > 0.5 g/d or > 3+, or cellular casts
8. Neurologic disorder	Seizures without other cause or psychosis without other cause
9. Hematologic disorder	Hemolytic anemia or leukopenia (< 4000/μL) or lymphopenia (< 1500/μL) or thrombocytopenia (< 100,000/μL) in the absence of offending drugs
10. Immunologic disorder	Anti-dsDNA, anti-Sm, and/or anti-phospholipid
11. Antinuclear antibodies	An abnormal titer of ANAs by immunofluorescence or an equivalent assay at any point in time in the absence of drugs known to induce ANAs

If four of these criteria are present at any time during the course of disease, a diagnosis of systemic lupus can be made with 98% specificity and 97% sensitivity.

SOURCE: Criteria published by EM Tan et al, Arthritis Rheum 25:1271, 1982; updated by MC Hochberg, Arthritis Rheum 40:1725, 1997.

fleeting infiltrates and/or areas of platelike atelectasis; this syndrome responds to glucocorticoids. However, *the most common cause of pulmonary infiltrates in patients with SLE is infection.* Interstitial pneumonitis leading to fibrosis occurs occasionally; the inflammatory phase may respond to treatment; the fibrosis does not. Pulmonary hypertension is an uncommon, grave manifestation of SLE. Infrequent pulmonary manifestations with high mortality rates include adult respiratory distress syndrome and massive intraalveolar hemorrhage.

Gastrointestinal System Common gastrointestinal (GI) symptoms include nausea, diarrhea, and vague discomfort. Symptoms may result from lupus peritonitis and may herald a flare of SLE. Vasculitis of the intestine is the most dangerous manifestation, presenting with acute crampy abdominal pain, vomiting, and diarrhea. Intestinal perforation can occur and usually requires immediate surgery. Patients with pseudoobstruction have abdominal pain; x-rays show dilated loops of small bowel which may be edematous; surgery should be avoided unless frank obstruction is present. Glucocorticoid therapy is useful for all these GI syndromes. Some patients have GI motility disorders similar to those in scleroderma; they are not benefited by steroids. Acute pancreatitis occurs and can be severe, resulting from active SLE or from therapy with glucocorticoids or azathioprine. Elevated amylase levels may reflect pancreatitis, salivary gland inflammation, or macroamylasemia. Elevated serum transaminase levels are common in patients with active SLE but are not associated with significant hepatic damage; they return to normal as the disease is treated.

Ocular Manifestation Retinal vasculitis is a serious manifestation; blindness can develop over a few days, and aggressive immunosuppression should be instituted. Examination shows areas of sheathed, narrow retinal arterioles and cytoid bodies (white exudates) adjacent to vessels. Other ocular abnormalities include conjunctivitis, episcleritis, optic neuritis, and the sicca syndrome.

PATHOLOGY **Cutaneous Lesions** Lesions of acute SLE, DLE, and SCLE show similar histopathology, with degeneration of the basal layer of the epidermis, disruption of the dermal-epidermal junction (DEJ), and mononuclear infiltrates around vessels and appendages in the upper dermis. In DLE, follicular plugging and hyperkeratosis are prominent. Deposits of Ig and C′ are seen in the DEJ in 80 to 100% of lesional and 50% of nonlesional skin in active SLE; the proportions are lower during remissions. Only 50% of SCLE lesions are positive for Ig and C′ deposits. Ig deposition in the DEJ is not specific for SLE. Vasculitic skin lesions usually show leukocytoclastic angiitis.

Renal Lesions Glomerulonephritis (GN) is caused by deposition of circulating immune complexes or in situ complex formation in mesangium and glomerular basement membrane. Renal biopsy should be considered when results would affect therapy. Information regarding location of immune deposits, histologic pattern of renal damage, and activity and chronicity of lesions are all useful in predicting prognosis and selecting appropriate treatment. In mild GN unlikely to lead to renal failure, Ig deposits are confined to the mesangium, and histology shows no changes or mesangial proliferation. If Ig and C′ are deposited outside the mesangium in capillary glomerular basement membrane, prognosis worsens. Histologic changes that should be treated with aggressive immunosuppression include focal proliferative, membranoproliferative, and diffuse proliferative GN (Chap. 275). Progression from focal to diffuse lesions can occur. Membranous changes without proliferation are uncommon but have a better prognosis than proliferative GN. Activity and chronicity scores indicate severity and reversibility of lesions. *Reversible "active" lesions* associated with high risk of progression to renal failure are glomerular necrosis, cellular epithelial crescents, hyaline thrombi, interstitial inflammatory infiltrates, and necrotizing vasculitis. *Irreversible changes unlikely to respond to immunosuppression* and highly associated with renal failure include glomerular sclerosis, fibrous crescents, interstitial fibrosis, and tubular atrophy. In patients with high chronicity scores, treatment of lupus should be determined by extrarenal disease.

LABORATORY MANIFESTATIONS The presence of characteristic antibodies (Table 311-1) confirms the diagnosis of SLE. ANAs are the best screening test. If the test substrate contains human nuclei (WIL-2 or HEP-2 cells), more than 95% of lupus patients will be positive. A positive ANA test is not specific for SLE; ANAs occur in some normal individuals (usually in low titer); the frequency increases with aging. Other autoimmune diseases, viral infections, chronic inflammatory processes, and several drugs induce ANAs. Therefore, a positive ANA test supports the diagnosis of SLE but is not specific; a negative ANA test makes the diagnosis unlikely but not impossible. Antibodies to double-stranded DNA (dsDNA) and to Sm are relatively specific for SLE; other autoantibodies listed in Table 311-1 are not. However, determining the complete autoantibody profile of each patient helps predict clinical subsets. High serum levels of ANAs and anti-dsDNA and low levels of complement usually reflect disease activity, especially in patients with nephritis. Total functional hemolytic complement (CH_{50}) levels are the most sensitive measure of complement activation but are also most subject to laboratory error. Quantitative levels of C3 and C4 are widely available. Very low levels of CH_{50} with normal levels of C3 suggest inherited deficiency of a complement component, which is highly associated with SLE and with ANA negativity.

Hematologic abnormalities include anemia (usually normochromic normocytic but occasionally hemolytic), leukopenia, lymphopenia, and thrombocytopenia. The Westergren erythrocyte sedimentation rate correlates with disease activity in some patients.

Urinalysis should be performed and serum creatinine levels should be measured periodically in patients with SLE. With active nephritis, the urinalysis usually shows proteinuria, hematuria, and cellular or granular casts. Urinary protein excretion measured over 24 h increases during periods of activity. (See the discussion under "Pathology" for a description of renal biopsy.)

PREGNANCY Fertility rates are normal in patients with SLE, but spontaneous abortion and stillbirths are frequent (10 to 30%), especially in women with LA and/or aCL. The treatment of choice for pregnant women with prior fetal loss and antiphospholipid antibodies

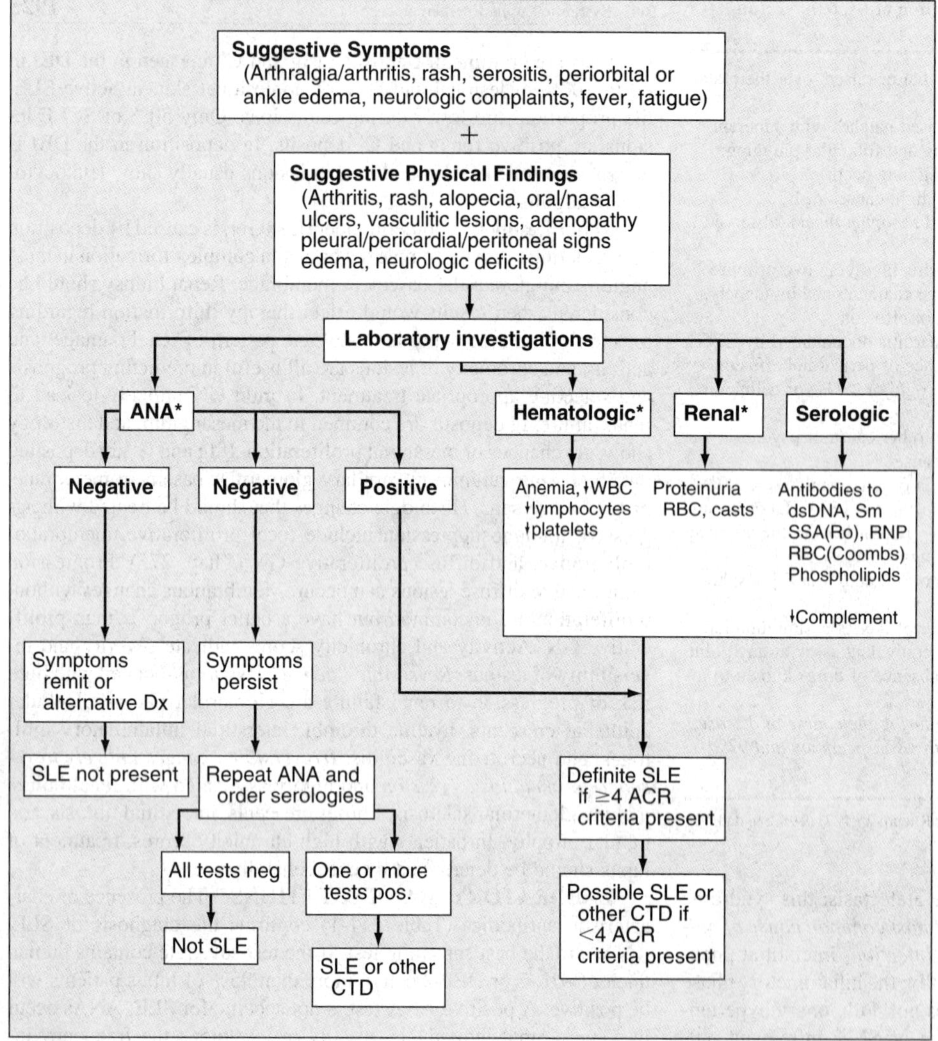

FIGURE 311-1 Algorithm for the diagnosis of SLE. ANA, antinuclear antibody; ACR, American College of Rheumatology; CTD, connective tissue disease; WBC, white blood cell count; RBC, red blood cell count, *, recommended in initial evaluation.

is low-dose heparin, e.g., 5000 units subcutaneously twice a day. This may be associated with maternal bone loss. If there are contraindications to heparin therapy, low-dose aspirin or low- to moderate-dose glucocorticoids may be used.

Pregnancy has varied effects on SLE activity. Disease flares in a small proportion, especially during the 6 weeks postpartum. If severe renal or cardiac disease is absent and SLE activity is controlled, most patients complete pregnancy safely and deliver normal infants. Glucocorticoids (except dexamethasone and betamethasone) are inactivated by placental enzymes and do not cause fetal abnormalities in humans; they should be used to suppress disease activity. Neonatal lupus, caused by transmission of maternal anti-Ro across the placenta, consists of transient skin rash and (rarely) permanent heart block. Transient thrombocytopenia from maternal antiplatelet antibodies also occurs.

DIFFERENTIAL DIAGNOSIS The American Rheumatism Association published diagnostic criteria for SLE (Table 311-3) which were updated in 1997. Any four of the manifestations listed establish a diagnosis of SLE. Early disease confined to a few systems is more difficult to classify; it may take several years for a patient to fulfill criteria. Disorders with which SLE can be confused include rheumatoid arthritis; various forms of dermatitis; neurologic disorders such as epilepsy, multiple sclerosis, and psychiatric disorders; and hematologic diseases such as idiopathic thrombocytopenic purpura. Many autoimmune disorders have overlapping features so that exact classification may be difficult. Mixed connective tissue disease has features of SLE, rheumatoid arthritis, polymyositis, and scleroderma, accompanied by high titers of anti-ribonucleoprotein antibodies (Chap. 313); patients have a low incidence of nephritis and CNS disease and a high incidence of pulmonary manifestations and evolution into scleroderma. The possibility of drug-induced lupus should always be considered. Figure 311-1 presents an algorithm for diagnosis of SLE.

DRUG-INDUCED LUPUS Several drugs can cause a syndrome resembling SLE, including procainamide, hydralazine, isoniazid, chlorpromazine, D-penicillamine, practolol, methyldopa, quinidine, interferon α, and possibly hydantoin, ethosuximide, and oral contraceptives. The syndrome is rare with all but procainamide, the most frequent offender, and hydralazine. There is genetic predisposition to drug-induced lupus, partly determined by drug acetylation rates. Procainamide induces ANA in 50 to 75% of individuals within a few months; hydralazine induces ANA in 25 to 30%. Between 10 and 20% of ANA-positive individuals develop lupus-like symptoms. Most common are systemic complaints and arthralgias; polyarthritis and pleuropericarditis occur in 25 to 50%. Renal and CNS involvement are rare. All patients have ANA and most have antibodies to histones. Antibodies to dsDNA and hypocomplementemia are rare—a helpful point in distinguishing drug-induced from idiopathic lupus. Anemia, leukopenia, LA, aCL, thrombocytopenia, cryoglobulins, rheumatoid factors, false-positive VDRL, and positive direct Coombs' tests can occur. The initial therapeutic approach is withdrawal of the offending drug; most patients improve in a few weeks. If symptoms are severe, a short course (2 to 10 weeks) of glucocorticoids is indicated. Symptoms rarely persist more than 6 months; ANA may persist for years. Most lupus-inducing drugs can be used safely in patients with idiopathic SLE.

PROGNOSIS Survival in patients with SLE is 90 to 95% at 2 years, 82 to 90% at 5 years, 71 to 80% at 10 years, and 63 to 75% at 20 years. The following factors have been associated with poor prognosis (approximately 50% mortality in 10 years): high serum creatinine levels [$>$124 μmol/L($>$1.4 mg/dL)], hypertension, nephrotic syndrome (24-h urine protein excretion $>$2.6 g), anemia [hemoglobin $<$ 124 g/L($<$12.4g/dL)], hypoalbuminemia and hypocomplementemia at the time of diagnosis, and low socioeconomic status. Other factors associated with a poor prognosis in most studies include thrombocytopenia, serious CNS involvement, antibodies to phospholipids, and African American race. Disability in SLE patients is common. However, approximately 20% of patients experience disease remissions (usually transient), and the likelihood of remission increases with each decade after diagnosis. Infections and active SLE, especially renal failure, are the leading causes of death in the first decade of disease. Thromboembolic events are frequent causes of death in the second decade.

℞ **TREATMENT** There is no cure for SLE. Complete sustained remissions are rare. Therefore, patient and physician should plan to control acute, severe flares and to develop maintenance strategies in which symptoms are suppressed to an acceptable level, usually at the cost of some drug side effects. Approximately 25% of SLE patients have mild disease with no life-threatening manifestations, although pain and fatigue may be disabling. These patients should be managed without glucocorticoids. Arthralgias, arthritis, myalgias, fever, and mild serositis may improve on nonsteroidal anti-inflammatory drugs (NSAIDs) including salicylates. However, NSAID toxicities such as elevated serum transaminases, aseptic meningitis, and renal impairment are especially frequent in SLE. The role of NSAIDs, which are primarily COX-2 inhibitors, in treatment of SLE has not been studied; they are likely to be useful. The dermatitides of SLE, fatigue, and lupus arthritis may respond to antimalarials. Doses of 400 mg hydroxychloroquine daily may improve skin lesions in a few weeks. Side effects are uncommon and include retinal toxicity, rash, myopathy, and neuropathy. Regular ophthalmologic examinations should be performed at least annually, since retinal toxicity is related to cumulative dose. Other therapies include sunscreens (an SPF rating $\geq$ 15 is recommended), topical or intralesional glucocorticoids, quinacrine, retinoids, and dapsone. Recent studies suggest that daily oral doses of dihydroepiandrosterone may lower disease activity in patients with mild SLE. Systemic glucocorticoids should be reserved for patients with disabling disease unresponsive to these conservative measures.

Life-threatening, severely disabling manifestations of SLE that are responsive to immunosuppression should be treated with high doses of *glucocorticoids* (1 to 2 mg/kg per day). When disease is active, glucocorticoids should be given in divided doses every 8 to 12 h. After the disease is controlled, therapy should be consolidated to one morning dose; thereafter the daily dose should be tapered as rapidly as clinical disease permits. Ideally, patients should be slowly converted to alternate-day therapy with a single morning dose of short-acting glucocorticoid (prednisone, prednisolone, methylprednisolone) to minimize side effects. However, the disease may flare on the day off steroids, in which case the lowest single daily dose that suppresses disease should be used. Acutely ill lupus patients, including those with proliferative GN, can be treated with 3 to 5 days of 1000 mg intravenous "pulses" of methylprednisolone, followed by maintenance daily or alternate-day glucocorticoids. Disease flares are probably controlled more rapidly by this approach, but it is unclear whether long-term outcome is changed.

Undesirable effects of chronic glucocorticoid therapy include cushingoid habitus, weight gain, hypertension, infection, capillary fragility, acne, hirsutism, accelerated osteoporosis, ischemic necrosis of bone, cataracts, glaucoma, diabetes mellitus, myopathy, hypokalemia, irregular menses, irritability, insomnia, and psychosis. Prednisone doses of 15 mg daily (or less) given before noon usually do not suppress the hypothalamic-pituitary axis. Some side effects can be minimized; sustained hyperglycemia, hypertension, edema, and hypokalemia should be treated; infections should be identified and treated early; immunizations with influenza and pneumococcal vaccines are safe if disease is stable. To minimize osteoporosis, supplemental calcium (1000 mg daily) should be added in most patients; in those with 24-h urinary calcium excretion <120 mg, vitamin D, 50,000 units one to three times weekly, can be added (monitor for hypercalcemia). Estrogen replacement therapy (ERT) should be considered at menopause. There is debate regarding the ability of oral contraceptives or ERT to cause flares of SLE in some patients; these therapies should be withheld from patients with a history of thrombosis. Calcitonin and bisphosphonates (alendronate, didronel, or acetonel) are also useful in preventing and treating osteoporosis.

The use of *cytotoxic agents* (azathioprine, chlorambucil, cyclophosphamide, methotrexate, mycophenolate mofetil) in SLE is probably beneficial in controlling active disease, reducing the rate of disease flares, and reducing steroid requirements. Patients with lupus nephritis have significantly less renal failure and better survival if treated with combinations of glucocorticoids plus intravenous cyclophosphamide; azathioprine as the second drug is less beneficial but is also effective in preventing renal failure. Open trials suggest that mycophenolate, and possibly methotrexate, are also effective second

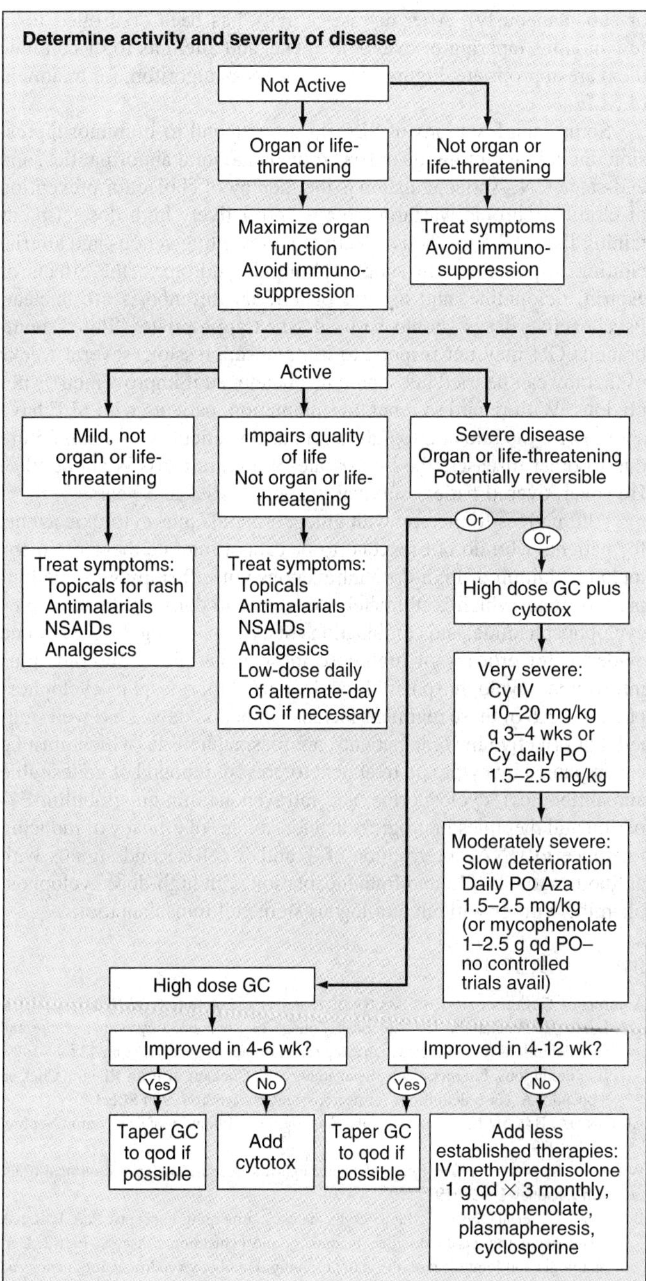

FIGURE 311-2 Algorithm for the treatment of SLE. GC, glucocorticoids; high-dose GC, methylprednisolone 1000 mg, IV, qd × 3, then 1 to 2 mg/kg prednisone per day orally, or 1 to 2 mg/kg prednisone per day orally; cytotox, cytotoxic drugs such as cyclophosphamide (Cy) and azathioprine (Aza); qod, alternate day therapy; NSAIDs, nonsteroidal anti-inflammatory agents.

drugs and sometimes benefit patients who fail to respond to cyclophosphamide plus glucocorticoids. Undesirable side effects of cytotoxic drugs include bone marrow suppression, increased infection with opportunistic organisms such as herpes zoster, irreversible ovarian failure, hepatotoxicity (azathioprine, methotrexate, and mycophenolate), bladder toxicity (cyclophosphamide), alopecia, and increased risk for malignancy. Azathioprine is the least toxic; recommended doses are 2 to 3 mg/kg per day orally. Cyclophosphamide is the most effective and the most toxic. Intravenous pulse doses (10 to 15 mg/kg) once every 4 weeks have less urinary bladder toxicity than daily oral doses. Cyclophosphamide can also be used in daily oral doses (1.5 to 2.5 mg/kg per day of each). Mycophenolate can be given orally (1 to 2.5 g a day in divided doses) or methotrexate (5 to 20 mg once a week, orally or subcutaneously). After disease activity has been controlled for a few months, tapering of cytotoxic agents and attempts to discontinue them are appropriate. Figure 311-2 presents an algorithm for treatment of SLE.

Some manifestations of SLE do not respond to immunosuppression, including clotting disorders, some behavioral abnormalities, and end-stage GN. Anticoagulation is the therapy of choice for prevention of clotting; chronic warfarin therapy in relatively high doses (maintaining INR at 2.5 to 3.0) is effective in preventing venous and arterial clotting in patients with antiphospholipid syndromes; the effects of aspirin, ticlopidine, and heparin on arterial thrombosis are unclear. Psychoactive drugs should be used when appropriate. "Pure" membranous GN may not respond to immunosuppression; several weeks of therapy can be tried but should be abandoned if improvement is not obvious. With regard to renal transplantation, patients with SLE have about twice the rate of allograft failure as do patients with renal failure due to other diseases; the 5-year rate of allograft loss is about 50%. However, overall patient survival is good, >90% at 5 years.

Alternatives to therapy with glucocorticoids plus cytotoxic agents for patients who do not respond to or cannot tolerate these regimens include addition of high-dose intravenous pulse therapy with methylprednisolone, which is ultimately converted to daily prednisone, plus cyclophosphamide, and combinations of cytotoxic drugs; there is some evidence for efficacy of high-dose intravenous glucocorticoids plus intravenous cyclophosphamide and of azathioprine plus cyclophosphamide. All of these regimens increase infection rates. Less well studied, but effective in some patients, are plasmapheresis (which must be accompanied by cytotoxic treatment to prevent rebound of undesirable autoantibodies), cyclosporine, and intravenous immunoglobulin. Experimental therapies in progress include studies of efficacy of inducing tolerance to DNA, interruption of T and B cell second signals with antibodies to CD40L, and immunoablation with high-dose cyclophosphamide with or without autologous stem cell transplantation.

BIBLIOGRAPHY

American College of Rheumatology: Ad Hoc Committee on Neuropsychiatric Lupus Nomenclature: The American College of Rheumatology nomenclature and case definitions for neuropsychiatric lupus syndromes. Arthritis Rheum 42:599, 1999. [For definitions: Internet: www.rheumatology.org Click on Arthritis Rheum. Click on Appendix A: Case definitions for neuropsychiatric syndromes in SLE.]

Austin HA, Balow JE: Natural history and treatment of lupus nephritis. Semin Nephrol 19:2, 1999

Bansal VK, Beto JA: Treatment of lupus nephritis: A meta-analysis of clinical trials. Am J Kidney Dis 29:193, 1997

Boumpas DT et al: Systemic lupus erythematosus: Emerging concepts. Part 1: Renal, neuropsychiatric, cardiovascular, pulmonary and hematologic disease. Part 2: Dermatologic and joint disease, the antiphospholipid antibody syndrome, pregnancy and hormonal therapy, morbidity and mortality, and pathogenesis. Ann Intern Med 123: 42, 940, 1995

Cowchock S: Treatment of antiphospholipid syndrome in pregnancy. Lupus 7(Suppl 2): S95, 1998

Hahn BH: Mechanisms of disease: Antibodies to DNA. N Engl J Med 338:1359, 1998

Harley JB et al: The genetics of human systemic lupus erythematosus. Curr Opin Immunol 10:690, 1998

Kimberly RP: Glucocorticoids. Curr Opin Rheumatol 6:273, 1994

Quismorio FP Jr: Clinical application of serologic abnormalities in systemic lupus erythematosus, in *Dubois' Lupus Erythematosus*, 5th ed, DJ Wallace, BH Hahn (eds). Baltimore, Williams & Wilkins, 1997, pp. 925–942

Stone JH et al: Outcome of renal transplantation in ninety-seven cyclosporine-era patients with systemic lupus erythematosus and matched controls. Arthritis Rheum 41:1438, 1998

Tumlin JA: Lupus nephritis: Novel immunosuppressive modalities and future directions. Semin Nephrol 19:67, 1999

Ward MM et al: Long-term survival in systemic lupus erythematosus: Patient characteristics associated with poorer outcomes. Arthritis Rheum 38:274, 1995

Werth VP et al: Pathogenetic mechanisms and treatment of cutaneous lupus erythematosus. Curr Opin Rheumatol 9:400, 1997

312

Peter E. Lipsky

RHEUMATOID ARTHRITIS

Cox	cyclooxygenase	IFN	interferon
CSIs	Cox-2-specific inhibitors	IL	interleukin
DMARDs	disease-modifying antirheumatic drugs	NSAIDs	nonsteroidal anti-inflammatory drugs
EBV	Epstein-Barr virus	RA	rheumatoid arthritis
GM-CSF	granulocyte-macrophage colony stimulating factor	TGF-β	transforming growth factor β
		TNF	tumor necrosis factor

Rheumatoid arthritis (RA) is a chronic multisystem disease of unknown cause. Although there are a variety of systemic manifestations, the characteristic feature of RA is persistent inflammatory synovitis, usually involving peripheral joints in a symmetric distribution. The potential of the synovial inflammation to cause cartilage destruction and bone erosions and subsequent changes in joint integrity is the hallmark of the disease. Despite its destructive potential, the course of RA can be quite variable. Some patients may experience only a mild oligoarticular illness of brief duration with minimal joint damage, whereas others will have a relentless progressive polyarthritis with marked functional impairment.

EPIDEMIOLOGY AND GENETICS The prevalence of RA is approximately 0.8% of the population (range 0.3 to 2.1%); women are affected approximately three times more often than men. The prevalence increases with age, and sex differences diminish in the older age group. RA is seen throughout the world and affects all races. However, the incidence and severity seem to be less in rural sub-Saharan Africa and in Caribbean blacks. The onset is most frequent during the fourth and fifth decades of life, with 80% of all patients developing the disease between the ages of 35 and 50. The incidence of RA is more than six times as great in 60- to 64-year-old women compared to 18- to 29-year-old women.

Family studies indicate a genetic predisposition. For example, severe RA is found at approximately four times the expected rate in first-degree relatives of individuals with disease associated with the presence of the autoantibody, rheumatoid factor; approximately 10% of patients with RA will have an affected first-degree relative. Moreover, monozygotic twins are at least four times more likely to be concordant for RA than dizygotic twins, who have a similar risk of developing RA as nontwin siblings. Only 15 to 20% of monozygotic twins are concordant for RA, however, implying that factors other than genetics play an important etiopathogenic role. Of note, the highest risk for concordance of RA is noted in twins who have two HLA-DRB1 alleles known to be associated with RA. The class II major histocompatibility complex allele HLA-DR4. (DRB1*0401) and related alleles are known to be major genetic risk factors for RA. Early studies showed that as many as 70% of patients with classic or definite RA express HLA-DR4 compared with 28% of control individuals. An association with HLA-DR4 has been noted in many populations, including North American and European whites, Chippewa Indians, Japanese, and native populations in India, Mexico, South America, and southern China. In a number of groups, including Israeli Jews, Asian Indians, and Yakima Indians of North America, however, there is no association between the development of RA and HLA-DR4. In these individuals, there is an association between RA and HLA-DR1 in the former two groups and HLA-Dw16 in the latter. Molecular analysis of HLA-DR antigens has provided insight into these apparently disparate findings. The HLA-DR molecule is composed of two chains, a nonpolymorphic α chain and a highly polymorphic β chain. Allelic variations in the HLA-DR molecule reflect differences in the amino acids of the β chain, with the major amino acid changes occurring in the three hypervariable regions of the molecule. Each of the HLA-DR molecules that is associated with RA has the same or a very similar sequence of amino acids in the third hypervariable region of the β chain of the molecule. Thus the β chains of the HLA-DR molecules associated with RA, including HLA-Dw4 (DRβ1*0401), HLA-Dw14 (DRβ1*0404), HLA-Dw15 (DRβ1*0405), HLA-DR1 (DRβ1*0101), and HLA-Dw16 (DRβ1*1402), contain the same amino acids at positions 67 through 74, with the exception of a single change of one basic amino acid for another (arginine → lysine) in position 71 of HLA-Dw4. All other HLA-DR β chains have amino acid changes in this region that alter either their charge or hydrophobicity. These results indicate that a particular amino acid sequence in the third hypervariable region of the HLA-DR molecule is a major genetic element conveying susceptibility to RA, regardless of whether it occurs in HLA-DR4, HLA-Dw16, or HLA-DR1. It has been estimated that the risk of developing RA in a person with HLA-Dw4 (DRβ1*0401) or HLA-Dw14 (DRβ1*0404) is 1 in 35 and 1 in 20, respectively, whereas the presence of both alleles puts persons at an even greater risk. The lack of association of HLA-DR4 and RA in certain populations is explained by the major member of the DR4 family found in that population. HLA-DR4 is a family of closely related, serologically defined molecules, including HLA-Dw4, -Dw10, -Dw13, and -Dw15. Different members of the HLA-DR family of molecules are found to predominate in different ethnic groups. Thus, in HLA-DR4–positive North American whites, HLA-Dw4 and -Dw14 are the most frequent, whereas HLA-Dw15 is most frequent in Japanese and southern Chinese. Each of these is associated with RA. By contrast, HLA-Dw10, which is not associated with RA and contains nonconservative amino acid changes in positions 70 and 71 of the β chain, is most common in Israeli Jews. Therefore, HLA-DR4 is not associated with RA in this population. In certain groups of patients, there does not appear to be a clear association between HLA-DR4–related epitopes and RA. Thus, nearly 75% of African American RA patients do not have this genetic element. Moreover, there is an association with HLA-DR10 (DRB1*1001) in Spanish and Italian patients, with HLA-DR9 (DRB1*0901) in Chileans, and with HLA-DR3 (DRB1*0301) in Arab populations.

Additional genes in the HLA-D complex may also convey altered susceptibility to RA. Certain HLA-DR alleles, including HLA-DR5 (DRB1*1101), HLA-DR2 (DRB1*1501), HLA-DR3 (DRB1*0301), and HLA-DR7 (DRB1*0701), may protect against the development of RA in that they tend to be found at lower frequency in RA patients than in controls. Moreover, the HLA-DQ alleles, DQB1*0301 and DQB1*0302, that are in linkage disequilibrium with HLA-DR4 and DQB1*0501, have also been associated with RA. This has raised the possibility that HLA-DQ alleles may represent the actual RA susceptibility genes, whereas specific HLA-DR alleles may convey protection. In this model, the complement of HLA-DR and DQ alleles determines RA susceptibility. Disease manifestations have also been associated with HLA phenotype. Thus, early aggressive disease and extraarticular manifestations are more frequent in patients with DRB1*0401 or DRB1*0404, and more slowly progressive disease in those with DRB1*0101. The presence of both DRB1*0401 and DRB1*0404 appears to increase the risk for both aggressive articular and extraarticular disease. It has been estimated that HLA genes contribute only a portion of the genetic susceptibility to RA. Thus genes outside the HLA complex also contribute. These include genes controlling the expression of the antigen receptor on T cells and both immunoglobulin heavy and light chains. Moreover, polymorphisms in the tumor necrosis factor (TNF) α and the interleukin (IL) 10 genes are also associated with RA, as is a region on chromosome 3 (3q13).

Genetic risk factors do not fully account for the incidence of RA, suggesting that environmental factors also play a role in the etiology of the disease. This is emphasized by epidemiologic studies in Africa that have indicated that climate and urbanization have a major impact on the incidence and severity of RA in groups of similar genetic background.

ETIOLOGY The cause of RA remains unknown. It has been suggested that RA might be a manifestation of the response to an infectious agent in a genetically susceptible host. Because of the worldwide distribution of RA, it has been hypothesized that if an infectious agent is involved, the organism must be ubiquitous. A number of possible causative agents have been suggested, including *Mycoplasma*, Epstein-Barr virus (EBV), cytomegalovirus, parvovirus, and rubella virus, but convincing evidence that these or other infectious agents cause RA has not emerged. The process by which an infectious agent might cause chronic inflammatory arthritis with a characteristic distribution also remains a matter of controversy. One possibility is that there is persistent infection of articular structures or retention of microbial products in the synovial tissues which generates a chronic inflammatory response. Alternatively, the microorganism or response to the microorganism might induce an immune response to components of the joint by altering its integrity and revealing antigenic peptides. In this regard, reactivity to type II collagen and heat shock proteins has been demonstrated. Another possibility is that the infecting microorganism might prime the host to cross-reactive determinants expressed within the joint as a result of "molecular mimicry." Recent evidence of similarity between products of certain gram-negative bacteria and EBV and the HLA-DR4 molecule itself has supported this possibility. Finally, products of infecting microorganisms might induce the disease. Recent work has focused on the possible role of "superantigens" produced by a number of microorganisms, including staphylococci, streptococci and *M. arthritidis*. Superantigens are proteins with the capacity to bind to HLA-DR molecules and particular V_β segments of the heterodimeric T cell receptor and stimulate specific T cells expressing the V_β gene products (Chap. 305). The role of superantigens in the etiology of RA remains speculative. Of all the potential environmental triggers, the only one clearly associated with the development of RA is cigarette smoking.

PATHOLOGY AND PATHOGENESIS Microvascular injury and an increase in the number of synovial lining cells appear to be the earliest lesions in rheumatoid synovitis. The nature of the insult causing this response is not known. Subsequently, an increased number of synovial lining cells is seen along with perivascular infiltration with mononuclear cells. Before the onset of clinical symptoms, the perivascular infiltrate is predominantly composed of myeloid cells, whereas in symptomatic arthritis, T cells can also be found, although their number does not appear to correlate with symptoms. As the process continues, the synovium becomes edematous and protrudes into the joint cavity as villous projections.

Light-microscopic examination discloses a characteristic constellation of features, which include hyperplasia and hypertrophy of the synovial lining cells; focal or segmental vascular changes, including microvascular injury, thrombosis, and neovascularization; edema; and infiltration with mononuclear cells, often collected into aggregates around small blood vessels (Fig. 312-1). The endothelial cells of the rheumatoid synovium have the appearance of high endothelial venules of lymphoid organs and have been altered by cytokine exposure to facilitate entry of cells into tissue. Rheumatoid synovial endothelial cells express increased amounts of various adhesion molecules involved in this process. Although this pathologic picture is typical of RA, it can also be seen in a variety of other chronic inflammatory arthritides. The mononuclear cell collections are variable in composition and size. The predominant infiltrating cell is the T lymphocyte. CD4+ T cells predominate over CD8+ T cells and are frequently found in close proximity to HLA-DR+ macrophages and dendritic cells. Increased numbers of a separate population of T cells expressing the $\gamma\delta$ form of the T cell receptor have also been found in the synovium, although they remain a minor population there and their role in RA has not been delineated. The major population of T cells in the rheumatoid synovium is composed of CD4+ memory T cells that form the majority of cells aggregated around postcapillary venules. Scattered throughout the tissue are CD8+ T cells. Both populations express the early activation antigen, CD69. Besides the accumulation of T cells, rheumatoid synovitis is also characterized by the infiltration of variable numbers of B cells and antibody-producing plasma cells. In advanced disease, structures similar to germinal centers of secondary lymphoid organs may be observed in the synovium. Both polyclonal immuno-

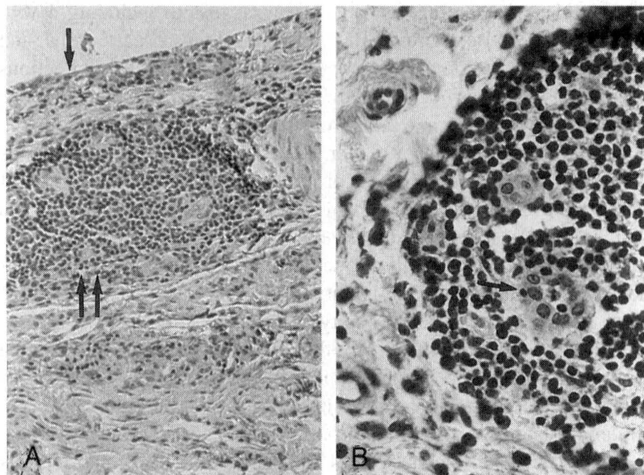

FIGURE 312-1 Histology of rheumatoid synovitis. *A*. The characteristic features of rheumatoid inflammation with hyperplasia of the lining layer *(arrow)* and mononuclear infiltrates in the sublining layer *(double arrow)*. *B*. A higher magnification of the largely CD4+ T cell infiltrate around postcapillary venules *(arrow)*.

globulin and the autoantibody rheumatoid factor are produced within the synovial tissue, which leads to the local formation of immune complexes. Finally, the synovial fibroblasts in RA manifest evidence of activation in that they produce a number of enzymes such as collagenase and cathepsins that can degrade components of the articular matrix. These activated fibroblasts are particularly prominent in the lining layer and at the interface with bone and cartilage. Osteoclasts are also prominent at sites of bone erosion.

The rheumatoid synovium is characterized by the presence of a number of secreted products of activated lymphocytes, macrophages, and fibroblasts. The local production of these cytokines and chemokines appears to account for many of the pathologic and clinical manifestations of RA. These effector molecules include those that are derived from T lymphocytes such as interleukin IL-2, interferon (IFN) γ, IL-6, IL-10, granulocyte-macrophage colony stimulating factor (GM-CSF), TNF-α, transforming growth factor β (TGF-β); IL-13, IL-16, and IL-17; those originating from activated myeloid cells, including IL-1, TNF-α, IL-6, IL-8, IL-10, IL-12, GM-CSF, macrophage CSF, platelet-derived growth factor, insulin-like growth factor, and TGF-β; as well as those secreted by other cell types in the synovium, such as fibroblasts and endothelial cells, including IL-1, IL-6, IL-8, GM-CSF, IL-15, IL-16, IL-18, and macrophage CSF. The activity of these chemokines and cytokines appears to account for many of the features of rheumatoid synovitis, including the synovial tissue inflammation, synovial fluid inflammation, synovial proliferation, and cartilage and bone damage, as well as the systemic manifestations of RA. In addition to the production of effector molecules that propagate the inflammatory process, local factors are produced that tend to slow the inflammation, including specific inhibitors of cytokine action and additional cytokines, such as TGF-β, which inhibits many of the features of rheumatoid synovitis including T cell activation and proliferation, B cell differentiation, and migration of cells into the inflammatory site.

These findings have suggested that the propagation of RA is an immunologically mediated event, although the original initiating stimulus has not been characterized. One view is that the inflammatory process in the tissue is driven by the CD4+ T cells infiltrating the synovium. Evidence for this includes (1) the predominance of CD4+ T cells in the synovium; (2) the increase in soluble IL-2 receptors, a product of activated T cells, in blood and synovial fluid of patients with active RA; and (3) amelioration of the disease by removal of T cells by thoracic duct drainage or peripheral lymphapheresis or suppression of their function by drugs, such as cyclosporine or nondepleting monoclonal antibodies to CD4. In addition, the association of RA with certain HLA-DR or -DQ alleles, whose only known functions are to shape the repertoire of CD4+ T cells during ontogeny in the thymus and bind and present antigenic peptides to CD4+ T cells in the periphery, strongly implies a role for CD4+ T cells in the pathogenesis of the disease. Finally, patients with established RA who become infected with HIV also have been noted to improve, although this has not been a uniform finding. Within the rheumatoid synovium, the CD4+ T cells differentiate predominantly into Th1-like effector cells producing the proinflammatory cytokine IFN-γ and appear to be deficient in differentiation into Th2-like effector cells capable of producing the anti-inflammatory cytokine IL-4. As a result of the ongoing secretion of IFN-γ without the regulatory influences of IL-4, macrophages are activated to produce the proinflammatory cytokines IL-1 and TNF-α and also increase expression of HLA molecules. Moreover, T lymphocytes express surface molecules such as CD154 (CD40 ligand) and also produce a variety of cytokines that promote B cell proliferation and differentiation into antibody-forming cells and therefore also may promote local B cell stimulation. The resultant production of immunoglobulin and rheumatoid factor can lead to immune-complex formation with consequent complement activation and exacerbation of the inflammatory process by the production of the anaphylatoxins, C3a and C5a, and the chemotactic factor C5a. The tissue inflammation is reminiscent of delayed type hypersensitivity reactions occurring in response to soluble antigens or microorganisms, although it has become clear that the number of T cells producing cytokines such as IFN-γ is less than is found in typical delayed type hypersensitivity reactions, perhaps owing to the large amount of reactive oxygen species produced locally in the synovium that can dampen T cell function. It remains unclear whether the persistent T cell activity represents a response to a persistent exogenous antigen or to altered autoantigens such as collagen, immunoglobulin, or one of the heat shock proteins, or perhaps both. Alternatively, it could represent persistent responsiveness to activated autologous cells such as might occur as a result of EBV infection or persistent response to a foreign antigen or superantigen in the synovial tissue. Finally, rheumatoid inflammation could reflect persistent stimulation of T cells by synovial-derived antigens that cross-react with determinants introduced during antecedent exposure to foreign antigens or infectious microorganisms.

Overriding the chronic inflammation in the synovial tissue is an acute inflammatory process in the synovial fluid. The exudative synovial fluid contains more polymorphonuclear leukocytes than mononuclear cells. A number of mechanisms play a role in stimulating the exudation of synovial fluid. Locally produced immune complexes can activate complement and generate anaphylatoxins and chemotactic factors. Local production, by a variety of cells, of chemokines and cytokines with chemotactic activity as well as inflammatory mediators such as leukotriene B_4 and products of complement activation can attract neutrophils. Moreover, many of these same agents can also stimulate the endothelial cells of postcapillary venules to become more efficient at binding circulating cells. The net result is the enhanced migration of polymorphonuclear leukocytes into the synovial site. In addition, vasoactive mediators such as histamine produced by the mast cells that infiltrate the rheumatoid synovium may also facilitate the exudation of inflammatory cells into the synovial fluid. Finally, the vasodilatory effects of locally produced prostaglandin E_2 may also facilitate entry of inflammatory cells into the inflammatory site. Once in the synovial fluid, the polymorphonuclear leukocytes can ingest immune complexes, with the resultant production of reactive oxygen metabolites and other inflammatory mediators, further adding to the inflammatory milieu. Locally produced cytokines and chemokines can additionally stimulate polymorphonuclear leukocytes. The production of large amounts of cyclooxygenase and lipoxygenase pathway products of arachidonic acid metabolism by cells in the synovial fluid and tissue further accentuates the signs and symptoms of inflammation.

The precise mechanism by which bone and cartilage destruction occurs has not been completely resolved. Although the synovial fluid contains a number of enzymes potentially able to degrade cartilage, the majority of destruction occurs in juxtaposition to the inflamed synovium, or pannus, that spreads to cover the articular cartilage. This vascular granulation tissue is composed of proliferating fibroblasts, small blood vessels, and a variable number of mononuclear cells and produces a large amount of degradative enzymes, including collagenase and stromelysin, that may facilitate tissue damage. The cytokines IL-1 and TNF-α play an important role by stimulating the cells of the pannus to produce collagenase and other neutral proteases. These same two cytokines also activate chondrocytes in situ, stimulating them to produce proteolytic enzymes that can degrade cartilage locally and also inhibiting synthesis of new matrix molecules. Finally, these two cytokines may contribute to the local demineralization of bone by activating osteoclasts that accumulate at the site of local bone resorption. Prostaglandin E_2 produced by fibroblasts and macrophages may also contribute to bone demineralization. The common final pathway of bone erosion is likely to involve the activation of osteoclasts that are present in large numbers at these sites. Systemic manifestations of RA can be accounted for by release of inflammatory effector molecules from the synovium. These include IL-1, TNF-α, and IL-6, which account for many of the manifestations of active RA, including malaise, fatigue, and elevated levels of serum acute-phase reactants. The importance of TNF-α in producing these manifestations is emphasized by the prompt amelioration of symptoms following administration of a monoclonal antibody to TNF-α or a soluble TNF-α receptor Ig construct to patients with RA. In addition, immune complexes produced within the synovium and entering the circulation may account for other features of the disease, such as systemic vasculitis.

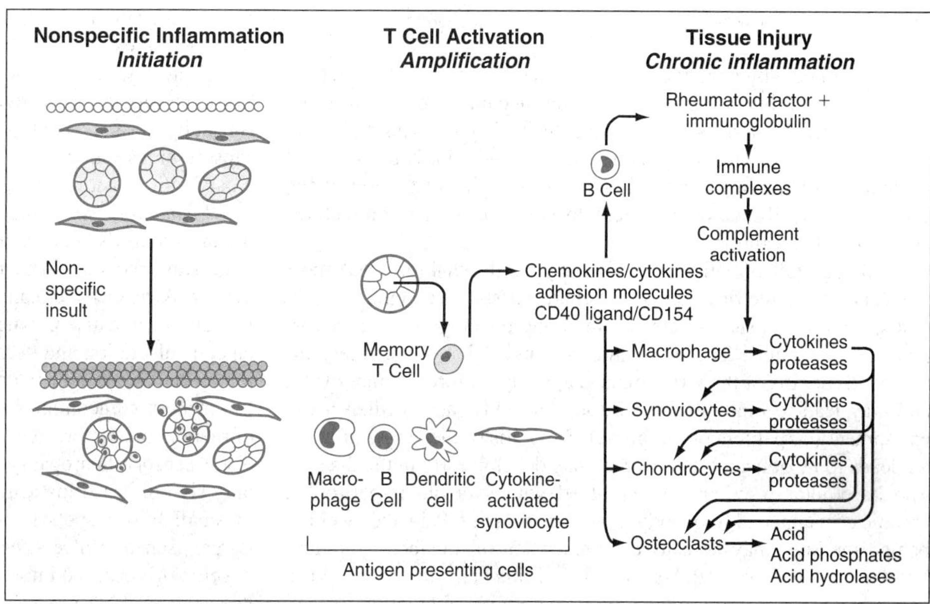

FIGURE 312-2 The progression of rheumatoid synovitis. This figure depicts the evolution of the pathogenic mechanisms and ultimate pathologic changes involved in the development of rheumatoid synovitis. The stages of rheumatoid arthritis are proposed to be an initiation phase of nonspecific inflammation, followed by an amplification phase resulting from T cell activation, and finally a stage of chronic inflammation with tissue injury. A variety of stimuli may initiate the initial phase of nonspecific inflammation, which may last for a protracted period of time with no or moderate symptoms. When activation of memory T cells in response to a variety of peptides presented by antigen-presenting cells occurs in genetically susceptible individuals, amplification of inflammation occurs with the promotion of local rheumatoid factor production and enhanced capacity to mediate tissue damage.

As shown in Fig. 312-2, the pathology of RA evolves over the duration of this chronic disease. The earliest event appears to be a nonspecific inflammatory response initiated by an unknown stimulus and characterized by accumulation of macrophages and other mononuclear cells within the sublining layer of the synovium. The activity of these cells is demonstrated by the increased appearance of macrophage-derived cytokines, including TNF-α, IL-1β, and IL-6. Subsequently, activation of CD4+ T cells is induced, presumably in response to antigenic peptides displayed by a variety of antigen-presenting cells in the synovial tissue. The activated T cells are capable of producing cytokines, especially IFN-γ, which amplify and perpetuate the inflammation. The presence of activated T cells expressing CD154 (CD40 ligand) can induce polyclonal B cell stimulation and the local production of rheumatoid factor. The cascade of cytokines produced in the synovium activates a variety of cells in the synovium, bone, and cartilage to produce effector molecules that can cause tissue damage characteristic of chronic inflammation. It is important to emphasize that there is no current way to predict the progress from one stage of inflammation to the next, and once established, each can influence the other. Important features of this model include the following: (1) the major pathologic events vary with time in this chronic disease; (2) the time required to progress from one step to the next may vary in different patients and the events, once established, may persist simultaneously; (3) once established, the major pathogenic events operative in an individual patient may vary at different times; and (4) the process is chronic and reiterative, with successive events stimulating progressive amplification of inflammation. These considerations have important implications with regard to appropriate treatment.

CLINICAL MANIFESTATIONS **Onset** Characteristically, RA is a chronic polyarthritis. In approximately two-thirds of patients, it begins insidiously with fatigue, anorexia, generalized weakness, and vague musculoskeletal symptoms until the appearance of synovitis becomes apparent. This prodrome may persist for weeks or months and defy diagnosis. Specific symptoms usually appear gradually as several joints, especially those of the hands, wrists, knees, and feet, become affected in a symmetric fashion. In approximately 10% of individuals, the onset is more acute, with a rapid development of polyarthritis, often accompanied by constitutional symptoms, including fever, lymphadenopathy, and splenomegaly. In approximately one-third of patients, symptoms may initially be confined to one or a few joints. Although the pattern of joint involvement may remain asymmetric in a few patients, a symmetric pattern is more typical.

Signs and Symptoms of Articular Disease Pain, swelling, and tenderness may initially be poorly localized to the joints. Pain in affected joints, aggravated by movement, is the most common manifestation of established RA. It corresponds in pattern to the joint involvement but does not always correlate with the degree of apparent inflammation. Generalized stiffness is frequent and is usually greatest after periods of inactivity. Morning stiffness of greater than 1-h duration is an almost invariable feature of inflammatory arthritis and may serve to distinguish it from various noninflammatory joint disorders. Notably, however, the presence of morning stiffness may not reliably distinguish between chronic inflammatory and noninflammatory arthritides, as it is also found frequently in the latter. The majority of patients will experience constitutional symptoms such as weakness, easy fatigability, anorexia, and weight loss. Although fever to 40°C occurs on occasion, temperature elevation in excess of 38°C is unusual and suggests the presence of an intercurrent problem such as infection.

Clinically, synovial inflammation causes swelling, tenderness, and limitation of motion. Warmth is usually evident on examination, especially of large joints such as the knee, but erythema is infrequent. Pain originates predominantly from the joint capsule, which is abundantly supplied with pain fibers and is markedly sensitive to stretching or distention. Joint swelling results from accumulation of synovial fluid, hypertrophy of the synovium, and thickening of the joint capsule. Initially, motion is limited by pain. The inflamed joint is usually held in flexion to maximize joint volume and minimize distention of the capsule. Later, fibrous or bony ankylosis or soft tissue contractures lead to fixed deformities.

Although inflammation can affect any diarthrodial joint, RA most often causes symmetric arthritis with characteristic involvement of certain specific joints such as the proximal interphalangeal and metacarpophalangeal joints. The distal interphalangeal joints are rarely involved. Synovitis of the wrist joints is a nearly uniform feature of RA and may lead to limitation of motion, deformity, and median nerve entrapment (carpal tunnel syndrome). Synovitis of the elbow joint often leads to flexion contractures that may develop early in the disease. The knee joint is commonly involved with synovial hypertrophy, chronic effusion, and frequently ligamentous laxity. Pain and swelling behind the knee may be caused by extension of inflamed synovium into the popliteal space (Baker's cyst). Arthritis in the forefoot, ankles, and subtalar joints can produce severe pain with ambulation as well as a number of deformities. Axial involvement is usually limited to the upper cervical spine. Involvement of the lumbar spine is not seen, and lower back pain cannot be ascribed to rheumatoid inflammation. On occasion, inflammation from the synovial joints and bursae of the upper cervical spine leads to atlantoaxial subluxation. This usually presents as pain in the occiput but on rare occasions may lead to compression of the spinal cord.

With persistent inflammation, a variety of characteristic joint changes develop. These can be attributed to a number of pathologic events, including laxity of supporting soft tissue structures; damage or weakening of ligaments, tendons, and the joint capsule; cartilage degradation; muscle imbalance; and unopposed physical forces associated with the use of affected joints. Characteristic changes of the hand include (1) radial deviation at the wrist with ulnar deviation of the digits, often with palmar subluxation of the proximal phalanges ("Z" deformity); (2) hyperextension of the proximal interphalangeal joints, with compensatory flexion of the distal interphalangeal joints (swan-neck deformity); (3) flexion contracture of the proximal interphalangeal joints and extension of the distal interphalangeal joints (boutonnière deformity); and (4) hyperextension of the first interphalangeal joint and flexion of the first metacarpophalangeal joint with a consequent loss of thumb mobility and pinch. Typical joint changes may also develop in the feet, including eversion at the hindfoot (subtalar joint), plantar subluxation of the metatarsal heads, widening of the forefoot, hallux valgus, and lateral deviation and dorsal subluxation of the toes.

Extraarticular Manifestations RA is a systemic disease with a variety of extraarticular manifestations. Although these occur frequently, not all of them have clinical significance. However, on occasion, they may be the major evidence of disease activity and source of morbidity and require management per se. As a rule, these manifestations occur in individuals with high titers of autoantibodies to the Fc component of immunoglobulin G (rheumatoid factors).

Rheumatoid nodules develop in 20 to 30% of persons with RA. They are usually found on periarticular structures, extensor surfaces, or other areas subjected to mechanical pressure, but they can develop elsewhere, including the pleura and meninges. Common locations include the olecranon bursa, the proximal ulna, the Achilles tendon, and the occiput. Nodules vary in size and consistency and are rarely symptomatic, but on occasion they break down as a result of trauma or become infected. They are found almost invariably in individuals with circulating rheumatoid factor. Histologically, rheumatoid nodules consist of a central zone of necrotic material including collagen fibrils, noncollagenous filaments, and cellular debris; a midzone of palisading macrophages that express HLA-DR antigens; and an outer zone of granulation tissue. Examination of early nodules has suggested that the initial event may be a focal vasculitis. In some patients, treatment with methotrexate can increase the number of nodules dramatically.

Clinical weakness and atrophy of skeletal muscle are common. Muscle atrophy may be evident within weeks of the onset of RA and is usually most apparent in musculature approximating affected joints. Muscle biopsy may show type II fiber atrophy and muscle fiber necrosis with or without a mononuclear cell infiltrate.

Rheumatoid vasculitis (Chap. 317), which can affect nearly any organ system, is seen in patients with severe RA and high titers of circulating rheumatoid factor. Rheumatoid vasculitis is very uncommon in African Americans. In its most aggressive form, rheumatoid vasculitis can cause polyneuropathy and mononeuritis multiplex, cutaneous ulceration and dermal necrosis, digital gangrene, and visceral infarction. While such widespread vasculitis is very rare, more limited forms are not uncommon, especially in white patients with high titers of rheumatoid factor. Neurovascular disease presenting either as a mild distal sensory neuropathy or as mononeuritis multiplex may be the only sign of vasculitis. Cutaneous vasculitis usually presents as crops of small brown spots in the nail beds, nail folds, and digital pulp. Larger ischemic ulcers, especially in the lower extremity, may also develop. Myocardial infarction secondary to rheumatoid vasculitis has been reported, as has vasculitic involvement of lungs, bowel, liver, spleen, pancreas, lymph nodes, and testes. Renal vasculitis is rare.

Pleuropulmonary manifestations, which are more commonly observed in men, include pleural disease, interstitial fibrosis, pleuropulmonary nodules, pneumonitis, and arteritis. Evidence of pleuritis is found commonly at autopsy, but symptomatic disease during life is infrequent. Typically, the pleural fluid contains very low levels of glucose in the absence of infection. Pleural fluid complement is also low compared with the serum level when these are related to the total protein concentration. Pulmonary fibrosis can produce impairment of the diffusing capacity of the lung. Pulmonary nodules may appear singly or in clusters. When they appear in individuals with pneumoconiosis, a diffuse nodular fibrotic process (Caplan's syndrome) may develop. On occasion, pulmonary nodules may cavitate and produce a pneumothorax or bronchopleural fistula. Rarely, pulmonary hypertension secondary to obliteration of the pulmonary vasculature occurs. In addition to pleuropulmonary disease, upper airway obstruction from cricoarytenoid arthritis or laryngeal nodules may develop.

Clinically apparent heart disease attributed to the rheumatoid process is rare, but evidence of asymptomatic pericarditis is found at autopsy in 50% of cases. Pericardial fluid has a low glucose level and is frequently associated with the occurrence of pleural effusion. Although pericarditis is usually asymptomatic, on rare occasions death has occurred from tamponade. Chronic constrictive pericarditis may also occur.

RA tends to spare the central nervous system directly, although vasculitis can cause peripheral neuropathy. *Neurologic manifestations* may also result from atlantoaxial or midcervical spine subluxations. Nerve entrapment secondary to proliferative synovitis or joint deformities may produce neuropathies of median, ulnar, radial (interosseous branch), or anterior tibial nerves.

The rheumatoid process involves the *eye* in fewer than 1% of patients. Affected individuals usually have long-standing disease and nodules. The two principal manifestations are episcleritis, which is usually mild and transient, and scleritis, which involves the deeper layers of the eye and is a more serious inflammatory condition. Histologically, the lesion is similar to a rheumatoid nodule and may result in thinning and perforation of the globe (scleromalacia perforans). From 15 to 20% of persons with RA may develop Sjögren's syndrome with attendant keratoconjunctivitis sicca.

Felty's syndrome consists of chronic RA, splenomegaly, neutropenia, and, on occasion, anemia and thrombocytopenia. It is most common in individuals with long-standing disease. These patients frequently have high titers of rheumatoid factor, subcutaneous nodules, and other manifestations of systemic rheumatoid disease. Felty's syndrome is very uncommon in African Americans. It may develop after joint inflammation has regressed. Circulating immune complexes are often present, and evidence of complement consumption may be seen. The leukopenia is a selective neutropenia with polymorphonuclear leukocyte counts of <1500 cells per microliter and sometimes <1000 cells per microliter. Bone marrow examination usually reveals moderate hypercellularity with a paucity of mature neutrophils. However, the bone marrow may be normal, hyperactive, or hypoactive; maturation arrest may be seen. Hypersplenism has been proposed as one of the causes of leukopenia, but splenomegaly is not invariably found and splenectomy does not always correct the abnormality. Excessive margination of granulocytes caused by antibodies to these cells, complement activation, or binding of immune complexes may contribute to granulocytopenia. Patients with Felty's syndrome have increased frequency of infections usually associated with neutropenia. The cause of the increased susceptibility to infection is related to the defective function of polymorphonuclear leukocytes as well as the decreased number of cells.

Osteoporosis secondary to rheumatoid involvement is common and may be aggravated by glucocorticoid therapy. Glucocorticoid treatment may cause significant loss of bone mass, especially early in the course of therapy, even when low doses are employed. Osteopenia in RA involves both juxtaarticular bone and long bones distant from involved joints. RA is associated with a modest decrease in mean bone mass and a moderate increase in the risk of fracture. Bone mass appears to be adversely affected by functional impairment and active inflammation, especially early in the course of the disease.

RA in the Elderly The incidence of RA continues to increase past age 60. It has been suggested that elderly-onset RA might have a poorer prognosis, as manifested by more persistent disease activity, more frequent radiographically evident deterioration, more frequent systemic involvement, and more rapid functional decline. Aggressive disease is largely restricted to those patients with high titers of rheumatoid factor. By contrast, elderly patients who develop RA without elevated titers of rheumatoid factor (seronegative disease) generally have less severe, often self-limited disease.

LABORATORY FINDINGS No tests are specific for diagnosing RA. However, rheumatoid factors, which are autoantibodies reactive with the Fc portion of IgG, are found in more than two-thirds of adults with the disease. Widely utilized tests largely detect IgM rheumatoid factors. The presence of rheumatoid factor is not specific for RA. Rheumatoid factor is found in 5% of healthy persons. The frequency of rheumatoid factor in the general population increases with age, and 10 to 20% of individuals over 65 years old have a positive test. In addition, a number of conditions besides RA are associated with the presence of rheumatoid factor. These include systemic lupus erythematosus, Sjögren's syndrome, chronic liver disease, sarcoidosis, interstitial pulmonary fibrosis, infectious mononucleosis, hepatitis B, tuberculosis, leprosy, syphilis, subacute bacterial endocarditis, visceral leishmaniasis, schistosomiasis, and malaria. In addition, rheumatoid factor may appear transiently in normal individuals after vaccination or transfusion and may also be found in relatives of individuals with RA.

The presence of rheumatoid factor does not establish the diagnosis of RA as the predictive value of the presence of rheumatoid factor in determining a diagnosis of RA is poor. Thus fewer than one-third of unselected patients with a positive test for rheumatoid factor will be found to have RA. Therefore, the rheumatoid factor test is not useful as a screening procedure. However, the presence of rheumatoid factor can be of prognostic significance because patients with high titers tend to have more severe and progressive disease with extraarticular manifestations. Rheumatoid factor is uniformly found in patients with nodules or vasculitis. In summary, a test for the presence of rheumatoid factor can be employed to confirm a diagnosis in individuals with a suggestive clinical presentation and, if present in high titer, to designate patients at risk for severe systemic disease. A number of additional autoantibodies may be found in patients with RA, including antibodies to filaggrin, citrulline, calpastatin, components of the spliceosome (RA-33), and an unknown antigen, Sa. Some of these may be useful in diagnosis in that they may occur early in the disease before

rheumatoid factor is present or may be associated with aggressive disease.

Normochromic, normocytic anemia is frequently present in active RA. It is thought to reflect ineffective erythropoiesis; large stores of iron are found in the bone marrow. In general, anemia and thrombocytosis correlate with disease activity. The white blood cell count is usually normal, but a mild leukocytosis may be present. Leukopenia may also exist without the full-blown picture of Felty's syndrome. Eosinophilia, when present, usually reflects severe systemic disease.

The erythrocyte sedimentation rate is increased in nearly all patients with active RA. The levels of a variety of other acute-phase reactants including ceruloplasmin and C-reactive protein are also elevated, and generally such elevations correlate with disease activity and the likelihood of progressive joint damage.

Synovial fluid analysis confirms the presence of inflammatory arthritis, although none of the findings is specific. The fluid is usually turbid, with reduced viscosity, increased protein content, and a slightly decreased or normal glucose concentration. The white cell count varies between 5 and 50,000/μL; polymorphonuclear leukocytes predominate. A synovial fluid white blood cell count >2000/μL with more than 75% polymorphonuclear leukocytes is highly characteristic of inflammatory arthritis, although not diagnostic of RA. Total hemolytic complement, C3, and C4 are markedly diminished in synovial fluid relative to total protein concentration as a result of activation of the classic complement pathway by locally produced immune complexes.

RADIOGRAPHIC EVALUATION Early in the disease, roentgenograms of the affected joints are usually not helpful in establishing a diagnosis. They reveal only that which is apparent from physical examination, namely, evidence of soft tissue swelling and joint effusion. As the disease progresses, abnormalities become more pronounced, but none of the radiographic findings is diagnostic of RA. The diagnosis, however, is supported by a characteristic pattern of abnormalities, including the tendency toward symmetric involvement. Juxtaarticular osteopenia may become apparent within weeks of onset. Loss of articular cartilage and bone erosions develop after months of sustained activity. The primary value of radiography is to determine the extent of cartilage destruction and bone erosion produced by the disease, particularly when one is monitoring the impact of therapy with disease-modifying drugs or surgical intervention. Other means of imaging bones and joints, including ^{99m}Tc bisphosphonate bone scanning and magnetic resonance imaging, may be capable of detecting early inflammatory changes that are not apparent from standard radiography but are rarely necessary in the routine evaluation of patients with RA.

CLINICAL COURSE AND PROGNOSIS The course of RA is quite variable and difficult to predict in an individual patient. Most patients experience persistent but fluctuating disease activity, accompanied by a variable degree of joint abnormalities and functional impairment. After 10 to 12 years, fewer than 20% of patients will have no evidence of disability or joint abnormalities. Within 10 years, approximately 50% of patients will have work disability. A number of features are correlated with a greater likelihood of developing joint abnormalities or disabilities. These include the presence of more than 20 inflamed joints, a markedly elevated erythrocyte sedimentation rate, radiographic evidence of bone erosions, the presence of rheumatoid nodules, high titers of serum rheumatoid factor, the presence of functional disability, persistent inflammation, advanced age at onset, the presence of comorbid conditions, low socioeconomic status or educational level, or the presence of HLA-DRB1*0401 or -DRB*0404. The presence of one or more of these implies the presence of more aggressive disease with a greater likelihood of developing progressive joint abnormalities and disability. Persistent elevation of the erythrocyte sedimentation rate, disability, and pain on longitudinal follow-up are good predictors of work disability. Patients who lack these features have more indolent disease with a slower progression to joint abnormalities and disability. The pattern of disease onset does not appear to predict the development of disabilities. Approximately 15% of patients with RA will have a short-lived inflammatory process that remits without major disability. These individuals tend to lack the aforementioned features associated with more aggressive disease.

Several features of patients with RA appear to have prognostic significance. Remissions of disease activity are most likely to occur during the first year. White females tend to have more persistent synovitis and more progressively erosive disease than males. Persons who present with high titers of rheumatoid factor, C-reactive protein, and haptoglobin also have a worse prognosis, as do individuals with subcutaneous nodules or radiographic evidence of erosions at the time of initial evaluation. Sustained disease activity of more than 1 year's duration portends a poor outcome, and persistent elevation of acute-phase reactants appears to correlate strongly with radiographic progression. A large proportion of inflamed joints manifest erosions within 2 years, whereas the subsequent course of erosions is highly variable; however, in general, radiographic damage appears to progress at a constant rate in patients with RA. Foot joints are affected more frequently than hand joints. Despite the decrease in the rate of progressive joint damage with time, functional disability, which develops early in the course of the disease, continues to worsen at the same rate, although the most rapid rate of functional loss occurs within the first 2 years of disease.

The median life expectancy of persons with RA is shortened by 3 to 7 years. Of the 2.5-fold increase in mortality rate, RA itself is a contributing feature in 15 to 30%. The increased mortality rate seems to be limited to patients with more severe articular disease and can be attributed largely to infection and gastrointestinal bleeding. Drug therapy may also play a role in the increased mortality rate seen in these individuals. Factors correlated with early death include disability, disease duration or severity, glucocorticoid use, age at onset, and low socioeconomic or educational status.

DIAGNOSIS The mean delay from disease onset to diagnosis is 9 months. This is often related to the nonspecific nature of initial symptoms. The diagnosis of RA is easily made in persons with typical established disease. In a majority of patients, the disease assumes its characteristic clinical features within 1 to 2 years of onset. The typical picture of bilateral symmetric inflammatory polyarthritis involving small and large joints in both the upper and lower extremities with sparing of the axial skeleton except the cervical spine suggests the diagnosis. Constitutional features indicative of the inflammatory nature of the disease, such as morning stiffness, support the diagnosis. Demonstration of subcutaneous nodules is a helpful diagnostic feature. Additionally, the presence of rheumatoid factor, inflammatory synovial fluid with increased numbers of polymorphonuclear leukocytes, and radiographic findings of juxtaarticular bone demineralization and erosions of the affected joints substantiate the diagnosis.

The diagnosis is somewhat more difficult early in the course when only constitutional symptoms or intermittent arthralgias or arthritis in an asymmetric distribution may be present. A period of observation may be necessary before the diagnosis can be established. A definitive diagnosis of RA depends predominantly on characteristic clinical features and the exclusion of other inflammatory processes. The isolated finding of a positive test for rheumatoid factor or an elevated erythrocyte sedimentation rate, especially in an older person with joint pains, should not itself be used as evidence of RA.

In 1987, the American College of Rheumatology developed revised criteria for the classification of RA (Table 312-1). These criteria demonstrate a sensitivity of 91 to 94% and a specificity of 89% when used to classify patients with RA compared with control subjects with rheumatic diseases other than RA. Although these criteria were developed as a means of disease classification for epidemiologic purposes, they can be useful as guidelines for establishing the diagnosis. Failure to meet these criteria, however, especially during the early stages of the disease, does not exclude the diagnosis. Moreover, in patients with early arthritis, the criteria do not discriminate effectively between patients who subsequently develop persistent, disabling, or erosive disease and those who do not.

Table 312-1 The 1987 Revised Criteria for the Classification of Rheumatoid Arthritis

1. Guidelines for classification
   a. Four of seven criteria are required to classify a patient as having rheumatoid arthritis (RA).
   b. Patients with two or more clinical diagnoses are not excluded.
2. Criteria[a]
   a. Morning stiffness: Stiffness in and around the joints lasting 1 h before maximal improvement.
   b. Arthritis of three or more joint areas: At least three joint areas, observed by a physician simultaneously, have soft tissue swelling or joint effusions, not just bony overgrowth. The 14 possible joint areas involved are right or left proximal interphalangeal, metacarpophalangeal, wrist, elbow, knee, ankle, and metatarsophalangeal joints.
   c. Arthritis of hand joints: Arthritis of wrist, metacarpophalangeal joint, or proximal interphalangeal joint.
   d. Symmetric arthritis: Simultaneous involvement of the same joint areas on both sides of the body.
   e. Rheumatoid nodules: Subcutaneous nodules over bony prominences, extensor surfaces, or juxtaarticular regions observed by a physician.
   f. Serum rheumatoid factor: Demonstration of abnormal amounts of serum rheumatoid factor by any method for which the result has been positive in less than 5% of normal control subjects.
   g. Radiographic changes: Typical changes of RA on posteroanterior hand and wrist radiographs that must include erosions or unequivocal bony decalcification localized in or most marked adjacent to the involved joints.

[a] Criteria a–d must be present for at least 6 weeks. Criteria b–e must be observed by a physician.

SOURCE: From FC Arnett et al: Arthritis Rheum 31:315, 1988.

℞ **TREATMENT General Principles** The goals of therapy of RA are (1) relief of pain, (2) reduction of inflammation, (3) protection of articular structures, (4) maintenance of function, and (5) control of systemic involvement. Since the etiology of RA is unknown, the pathogenesis is not completely delineated, and the mechanisms of action of many of the therapeutic agents employed are uncertain, therapy remains largely empirical. None of the therapeutic interventions is curative, and therefore all must be viewed as palliative, aimed at relieving the signs and symptoms of the disease. The various therapies employed are directed at nonspecific suppression of the inflammatory or immunologic process in the hope of ameliorating symptoms and preventing progressive damage to articular structures.

Management of patients with RA involves an interdisciplinary approach, which attempts to deal with the various problems that these individuals encounter with functional as well as psychosocial interactions. A variety of physical therapy modalities may be useful in decreasing the symptoms of RA. Rest ameliorates symptoms and can be an important component of the total therapeutic program. In addition, splinting to reduce unwanted motion of inflamed joints may be useful. Exercise directed at maintaining muscle strength and joint mobility without exacerbating joint inflammation is also an important aspect of the therapeutic regimen. A variety of orthotic and assistive devices can be helpful in supporting and aligning deformed joints to reduce pain and improve function. Education of the patient and family is an important component of the therapeutic plan to help those involved become aware of the potential impact of the disease and make appropriate accommodations in life-style to maximize satisfaction and minimize stress on joints.

Medical management of RA involves five general approaches. The first is the use of aspirin and other nonsteroidal anti-inflammatory drugs (NSAIDs) and simple analgesics to control the symptoms and signs of the local inflammatory process. These agents are rapidly effective at mitigating signs and symptoms, but they appear to exert minimal effect on the progression of the disease. Recently, specific inhibitors of the isoform of cyclooxygenase (Cox) that is upregulated at inflammatory sites (Cox-2) have been developed. Cox-2-specific inhibitors (CSIs) have been shown to be as effective as classic NSAIDs, which inhibit both isoforms of Cox, but to cause significantly less gastroduodenal ulceration. The second line of therapy involves use of low-dose oral glucocorticoids. Although low-dose glucocorticoids have been widely used to suppress signs and symptoms of inflammation, recent evidence suggests that they may also retard the development and progression of bone erosions. Intraarticular glucocorticoids can often provide transient symptomatic relief when systemic medical therapy has failed to resolve inflammation. The third line of agents includes a variety of agents that have been classified as the disease-modifying or slow-acting antirheumatic drugs. These agents appear to have the capacity to decrease elevated levels of acute-phase reactants in treated patients and, therefore, are thought to modify the inflammatory component of RA and thus its destructive capacity. Recently, combinations of disease-modifying antirheumatic drugs (DMARDs) have shown promise in controlling the signs and symptoms of RA. A fourth group of agents are the TNF-α neutralizing agents, which have been shown to have a major impact on the signs and symptoms of RA. A fifth group of agents are the immunosuppressive and cytotoxic drugs that have been shown to ameliorate the disease process in some patients. Additional approaches have been employed in an attempt to control the signs and symptoms of RA. Substituting omega-3 fatty acids such as eicosapentaenoic acid found in certain fish oils for dietary omega-6 essential fatty acids found in meat has also been shown to provide symptomatic improvement in patients with RA. A variety of nontraditional approaches have also been claimed to be effective in treating RA, including diets, plant and animal extracts, vaccines, hormones, and topical preparations of various sorts. Many of these are costly, and none has been shown to be effective. However, belief in their efficacy ensures their continued use by some patients.

Drugs • ***Nonsteroidal anti-inflammatory drugs*** Besides aspirin, many NSAIDs are available to treat RA. As a result of the capacity of these agents to block the activity of the Cox enzymes and therefore the production of prostaglandins, prostacyclin, and thromboxanes, they have analgesic, anti-inflammatory, and antipyretic properties. In addition, the agents may exert other anti-inflammatory effects. These agents are all associated with a wide spectrum of toxic side effects. Some, such as gastric irritation, azotemia, platelet dysfunction, and exacerbation of allergic rhinitis and asthma, are related to the inhibition of cyclooxygenase activity, whereas a variety of others, such as rash, liver function abnormalities, and bone marrow depression, may not be. None of the NSAIDs has been shown to be more effective than aspirin in the treatment of RA. However, these nonaspirin drugs are associated with a lower incidence of gastrointestinal intolerance. None of the newer NSAIDs appears to show significant therapeutic advantages over the other available agents. In addition, there is no consistent advantage of any of these newer agents over the others with respect to the incidence or severity of toxic manifestations. Recent evidence indicates that two separate enzymes, Cox-1 and -2, are responsible for the initial metabolism of arachidonic acid into various inflammatory mediators. The former is constitutively present in many cells and tissues, including the stomach and the platelet, whereas the latter is specifically induced in response to inflammatory stimuli. Inhibition of Cox-2 accounts for the anti-inflammatory effects of NSAIDs, whereas inhibition of Cox-1 induces much of the mechanism-based toxicity. As the currently available NSAIDs inhibit both enzymes, therapeutic benefit and toxicity are intertwined. CSIs have now been approved for the treatment of RA. Clinical trials have shown that CSIs suppress the signs and symptoms of RA as effectively as classic Cox-nonspecific NSAIDs but are associated with a significantly reduced incidence of gastroduodenal ulceration. This suggests that CSIs might be considered instead of classic Cox-nonspecific NSAIDs, especially in persons with increased risk of NSAID-induced major upper gastrointestinal side effects, including persons over 65, those with a history of peptic ulcer disease, persons receiving glucocorticoids or anticoagulants, or those requiring high doses of NSAIDs.

Disease-modifying antirheumatic drugs Clinical experience has delineated a number of agents that appear to have the capacity to alter the course of RA. This group of agents includes methotrexate, gold compounds, D-penicillamine, the antimalarials, and sulfasalazine. Despite having no chemical or pharmacologic similarities, in practice these agents share a number of characteristics. They exert minimal direct nonspecific anti-inflammatory or analgesic effects, and therefore NSAIDs must be continued during their administration, except in a few cases when true remissions are induced with them. The appearance of benefit from DMARD therapy is usually delayed for weeks or months. As many as two-thirds of patients develop some clinical improvement as a result of therapy with any of these agents, although the induction of true remissions is unusual. In addition to clinical improvement, there is frequently an improvement in serologic evidence of disease activity, and titers of rheumatoid factor and C-reactive protein and the erythrocyte sedimentation rate frequently decline. Moreover, emerging evidence suggests that DMARDs actually retard the development of bone erosions or facilitate their healing. Furthermore, developing evidence suggests that early aggressive treatment with DMARDs may be effective at slowing the appearance of bone erosions.

Which DMARD should be the drug of first choice remains controversial, and trials have failed to demonstrate a consistent advantage of one over the other. Despite this, methotrexate has emerged as the DMARD of choice because of its relatively rapid onset of action, its capacity to effect sustained improvement with ongoing therapy, and the high level of patient retention on therapy. Each of the DMARDs is associated with considerable toxicity, and therefore careful patient monitoring is necessary. Toxicity of the various agents also becomes important in determining the drug of first choice. Of note, failure to respond or development of toxicity to one DMARD does not preclude responsiveness to another. Thus, a similar percentage of RA patients who have failed to respond to one DMARD will respond to another when it is given as the second disease-modifying drug.

No characteristic features of patients have emerged that predict responsiveness to a DMARD. Moreover, the indications for the initiation of therapy with one of these agents are not well defined, although recently the trend has been to begin DMARD therapy early in the course of the disease, and data have begun to emerge to support the conclusion that this approach may slow the development of bone erosions, although this remains controversial.

The folic acid antagonist methotrexate, given in an intermittent low dose (7.5 to 30 mg once weekly), is currently a frequently utilized DMARD. Most rheumatologists recommend use of methotrexate as the initial DMARD, especially in individuals with evidence of aggressive RA. Recent trials have documented the efficacy of methotrexate and have indicated that its onset of action is more rapid than other DMARDs, and patients tend to remain on therapy with methotrexate longer than they remain on other DMARDs because of better clinical responses and less toxicity. Long-term trials have indicated that methotrexate does not induce remission but rather suppresses symptoms while it is being administered. Maximal improvement is observed after 6 months of therapy, with little additional improvement thereafter. Major toxicity includes gastrointestinal upset, oral ulceration, and liver function abnormalities that appear to be dose-related and reversible and hepatic fibrosis that can be quite insidious, requiring liver biopsy for detection in its early stages. Drug-induced pneumonitis has also been reported. Liver biopsy is recommended for individuals with persistent or repetitive liver function abnormalities. Concurrent administration of folic acid or folinic acid may diminish the frequency of some side effects without diminishing effectiveness.

Glucocorticoid Therapy Systemic glucocorticoid therapy can provide effective symptomatic therapy in patients with RA. Low-dose (<7.5 mg/d) prednisone has been advocated as useful additive therapy to control symptoms. Moreover, recent evidence suggests that low-dose glucocorticoid therapy may retard the progression of bone erosions. Monthly pulses with high-dose glucocorticoids may be useful-

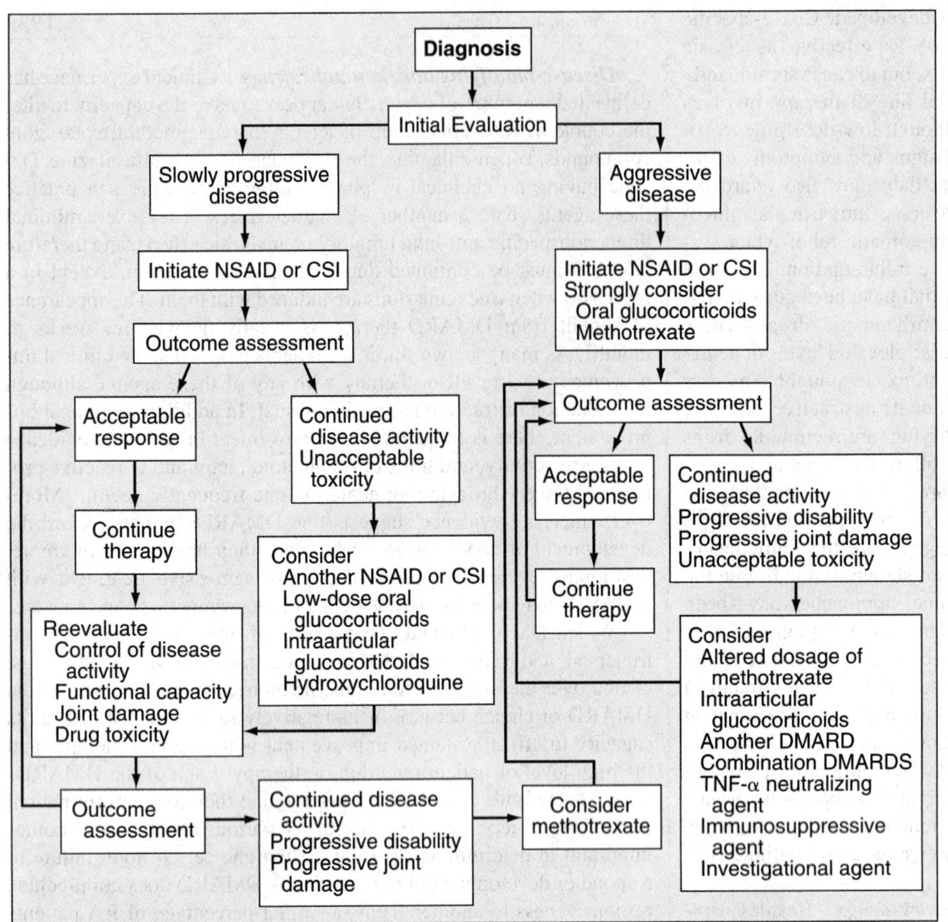

FIGURE 312-3 Algorithm for the medical management of rheumatoid arthritis. NSAID, nonsteroidal anti-inflammatory drug; CSI, Cox-2 specific inhibitor; DMARD, disease-modifying antirheumatic drug; TNF-α, tumor necrosis factor α.

Surgery Surgery plays a role in the management of patients with severely damaged joints. Although arthroplasties and total joint replacements can be done on a number of joints, the most successful procedures are carried out on hips, knees, and shoulders. Realistic goals of these procedures are relief of pain and reduction of disability. Reconstructive hand surgery may lead to cosmetic improvement and some functional benefit. Open or arthroscopic synovectomy may be useful in some patients with persistent monarthritis, especially of the knee. Although synovectomy may offer short-term relief of symptoms, it does not appear to retard bone destruction or alter the natural history of the disease. In addition, early tenosynovectomy of the wrist may prevent tendon rupture.

in some patients and may hasten the response when therapy with a DMARD is initiated.

TNF-α neutralizing agents Recently, biologic agents that bind and neutralize TNF-α have become available. One of these is a TNF-α type II receptor fused to IgG1 (etanercept), and the second is a chimeric mouse/human monoclonal antibody to TNF-α (infliximab). Clinical trials have shown that parenteral administration of either TNF-α neutralizing agent is remarkably effective at controlling signs and symptoms of RA in patients who have failed DMARD therapy. Repetitive therapy with these agents is effective with or without concomitant methotrexate. Although these agents are notably effective in persistently controlling signs and symptoms of RA in a majority of patients, their impact on the progression of bone erosions has not been proven. Side effects include the potential for an increased risk of serious infections and the development of anti-DNA antibodies, but with no associated evidence of signs and symptoms of systemic lupus erythematosus. Although these side effects are uncommon, their occurrence mandates that TNF-α neutralizing therapy be supervised by physicians with experience in their use.

Immunosuppressive Therapy The immunosuppressive drugs azathioprine, leflunomide, cyclosporine, and cyclophosphamide have been shown to be effective in the treatment of RA and to exert therapeutic effects similar to those of the DMARDs. However, these agents appear to be no more effective than the DMARDs. Moreover, they cause a variety of toxic side effects, and cyclophosphamide appears to predispose the patient to the development of malignant neoplasms. Therefore, these drugs have been reserved for patients who have clearly failed therapy with DMARDs. On occasion, extraarticular disease such as rheumatoid vasculitis may require cytotoxic immunosuppressive therapy.

Approach to the Patient

An approach to the medical management of patients with RA is depicted in Fig. 312-3. The principles underlying care of these patients reflect the variability of the disease, the frequent persistent nature of the inflammation and its potential to cause disability, the relationship between sustained inflammation and bone erosions, and the need to reevaluate the patient frequently for symptomatic response to therapy, progression of disability and joint damage, and side effects of treatment. At the onset of disease it is difficult to predict the natural history of an individual patient's illness. Therefore, the usual approach is to attempt to alleviate the patient's symptoms with NSAIDs or CSIs. Some patients may have mild disease that requires no additional therapy.

At some time during most patients' course, the possibility of initiating DMARD therapy and/or low-dose oral glucocorticoids is entertained. With aggressive disease this might occur sooner, often within 1 to 3 months of diagnosis, whereas in patients with more indolent disease, smoldering activity may not require such therapy for many years. The development of bone erosions or radiographic evidence of cartilage loss is clear-cut evidence of the destructive potential of the inflammatory process and indicates the need for DMARD therapy. The other indications as outlined above, including persistent pain, joint swelling, or functional impairment, are much more subjective, however. As persistent inflammation, involvement of multiple joints, elevated levels of acute-phase reactants, and rheumatoid factor titers correlate with the development of disability and/or bony erosions, some have advocated the use of these prognostic indicators of aggressive disease in the decision to employ DMARDs early in the course of RA. The decision to begin use of a DMARD and/or low-dose oral glucocorticoids requires experience and clinical judgment as well as the ability to assess joint swelling and functional activity and the patient's pain tolerance and expectation of therapy accurately. In this setting, the fully informed patient must play an active role in the decision to begin DMARD and/or low-dose oral glucocorticoid therapy, after careful review of the therapeutic and toxic potential of the various drugs.

If a patient responds to a DMARD, therapy is continued with careful monitoring to avoid toxicity. All DMARDs provide a suppressive effect and therefore require prolonged administration. Even with successful therapy, local injection of glucocorticoids may be necessary to diminish inflammation that may persist in a limited number of joints. In addition, NSAIDs or CSIs may be necessary to mitigate symptoms. Even after inflammation has totally resolved, symptoms from loss of cartilage and supervening degenerative joint disease or altered joint function may require additional treatment. Surgery may also be necessary to relieve pain or diminish the functional impairment secondary to alterations in joint function. Recently an alternative approach to treat patients with RA has been suggested. This involves the initiation of therapy with multiple agents early in the course of disease in an attempt to control inflammation, followed by maintenance on one or more agents as necessary to control disease activity. The effectiveness of this therapeutic alternative has not been proved.

BIBLIOGRAPHY

ABU-SHAKRA M et al: Clinical and radiographic outcomes of rheumatoid arthritis patients not treated with disease-modifying drugs. Arthritis Rheum 41:1190, 1998

BUCHT A et al: Expression of interferon-gamma (IFN-γ), IL-10, IL-12 and transforming growth factor-beta (TGF-β) mRNA in synovial fluid cells from patients in the early and late phases of Rheumatoid arthritis (RA). Clin Exp Immunol 103:357, 1996

GOUGH A et al: Osteoclastic activation is the principal mechanism leading to secondary osteoporosis in rheumatoid arthritis. J Rheumatol 25:1282, 1998

GRAUDAL NA et al: Radiographic progression in rheumatoid arthritis. Arthritis Rheum 41:1470, 1998

HARRISON BJ et al: The performance of the 1987 ARA classification criteria for rheumatoid arthritis in a population-based cohort of patients with early inflammatory polyarthritis. J Rheumatol 25:2324, 1998

KAARELA K, KAUTIAINEN H: Continuous progression of radiological destruction in seropositive rheumatoid arthritis. J Rheumatol 24:1285, 1997

KANIK KS et al: Distinct patterns of cytokine secretion characterize new onset synovitis versus chronic rheumatoid arthritis. J Rheumatol 25:16, 1998

KIM H-J et al: Plasma cell development in synovial germinal centers in patients with rheumatoid and reactive arthritis. J Immunol 162:3053, 1999

KOTAKE S et al: IL-17 in synovial fluids from patients with rheumatoid arthritis is a potent stimulator of osteoclastogenesis. J Clin Invest 103:1345, 1999

KRAAN MC et al: Asymptomatic synovitis precedes clinically manifest arthritis. Arthritis Rheum 41:1481, 1998

KWOH CK et al: American College of Rheumatology Guidelines for the Management of Rheumatoid Arthritis. Arthritis Rheum 39:713, 1996

LAWRENCE RC et al: Estimates of the prevalence of arthritis and selected musculoskeletal disorders in the United States. Arthritis Rheum 41:778, 1998

LIPSKY PE, DAVIS LS: The central involvement of T cells in rheumatoid arthritis. Immunologist 6:121, 1998

MACDONALD KPA et al: Functional CD40 ligand is expressed by T cells in rheumatoid arthritis. J Clin Invest 100:2404, 1997

MAINI RN et al: Therapeutic efficacy of multiple intravenous infusions of anti-tumor necrosis factor α monoclonal antibody combined with low-dose weekly methotrexate in rheumatoid arthritis. Arthritis Rheum 41:1552, 1998

MORELAND LW et al: Treatment of rheumatoid arthritis with a recombinant human necrosis factor receptor (p75)-Fc fusion protein. N Engl J Med 337:141, 1997

MORITA Y et al: Expression of interleukin-12 in synovial tissue from patients with rheumatoid arthritis. Arthritis Rheum 41:306, 1998

MU H et al: Tumor necrosis factor α microsatellite polymorphism is associated with rheumatoid arthritis severity through an interaction with the HLA-DRB1 shared epitope. Arthritis Rheum 42:438, 1999

PLANT MJ et al: Patterns of radiological progression in early rheumatoid arthritis: Results of an 8-year prospective study. J Rheumatol 25:417, 1998

RAU R et al: Long-term combination therapy of refractory and destructive rheumatoid arthritis with methotrexate (MTX) and intramuscular gold or other disease-modifying antirheumatic drugs compared to MTX monotherapy. J Rheumatol 25:1485, 1998

SCHULZE-KOOPS H et al: Reduction of Th1 cell activity in the peripheral circulation of patients with rheumatoid arthritis after treatment with a non-depleting humanized monoclonal antibody to CD4. J Rheumatol 25:2065, 1998

SHARIF M et al: Changes in biochemical markers of joint tissue metabolism in a randomized controlled trial of glucocorticoid in early rheumatoid arthritis. Arthritis Rheum 41:1203, 1998

SIMMS RW et al: American College of Rheumatology Guidelines for Monitoring Drug Therapy in Rheumatoid Arthritis. Arthritis Rheum 39:723, 1996

SIMON LS et al: Preliminary study of the safety and efficacy of SC-58635, a novel cyclooxygenase 2 inhibitor. Arthritis Rheum 41:1591, 1998

SMOLEN JS et al: Efficacy and safety of leflunomide compared with placebo and sulphasalazine in active rheumatoid arthritis: A double-blind, randomised, multicentre trial. Lancet 353:259, 1999

STEIN CM et al: Combination treatment of severe rheumatoid arthritis with cyclosporine and methotrexate for forty-eight weeks. Arthritis Rheum 40:1843, 1997

SYMMONS DPM et al: Long-term mortality outcome in patients with rheumatoid arthritis: Early presenters continue to do well. J Rheumatol 25:1072, 1998

THOMAS R, LIPSKY PE: Could endogenous self-peptides presented by dendritic cells initiate rheumatoid arthritis? Immunol Today 17:559, 1996

VINCENT C et al: Immunoblotting detection of autoantibodies to human epidermis filaggrein: A new diagnostic test for rheumatoid arthritis. J Rheumatol 25:838, 1998

WAGNER U et al: HLA markers and prediction of clinical course and outcome in rheumatoid arthritis. Arthritis Rheum 40:341, 1997

WEINBLATT WE et al: Long-term prospective study of methotrexate in rheumatoid arthritis: Conclusion after 132 months of therapy. J Rheumatol 25:238, 1998

——— et al: A trial of etanercept, a recombinant tumor necrosis factor receptor: Fc fusion protein, in patients with rheumatoid arthritis receiving methotrexate. N Engl J Med 340:253, 1999

WEYAND DM et al: The influence of sex on the phenotype of rheumatoid arthritis. Arthritis Rheum 41:817, 1998

WOLFE F, HAWLEY D: The long-term outcomes of rheumatoid arthritis: Work disability: A prospective 18-year study of 823 patients. J Rheumatol 25:2108, 1998

———, SHARP JT: Radiographic outcome of recent-onset rheumatoid arthritis. Arthritis Rheum 41:1571, 1998

313

Bruce C. Gilliland

SYSTEMIC SCLEROSIS (SCLERODERMA)

EMS eosinophilia-myalgia syndrome	PDGF platelet-derived growth factor
GVHD graft-versus-host disease	RNP ribonucleoprotein
ICAM-1 intercellular adhesion molecule-1	SLE systemic lupus erythematosus
IL interleukin	SSc systemic sclerosis
MCTD mixed connective tissue disease	TGF transforming growth factor

DEFINITION Systemic sclerosis (SSc) is a chronic multisystem disorder of unknown etiology characterized clinically by thickening of the skin caused by accumulation of connective tissue and by involvement of visceral organs, including the gastrointestinal tract, lungs, heart, and kidneys. Classification of SSc and sclerodermal-like disorders is shown in (Table 313-1). Vascular abnormalities, especially of the microvasculature are a prominent feature of SSc. The degree and rate of skin and internal organ involvement vary among patients.

Table 313-1 Classification of Scleroderma/Systemic Sclerosis and Scleroderma-Like Disorders

Systemic sclerosis
- Limited cutaneous disease
- Diffuse cutaneous disease
- Sine scleroderma
- Undifferentiated connective tissue disease
- Overlap syndromes

Localized scleroderma
- Morphea
- Linear scleroderma
- *En coup de sabre*

Chemically induced scleroderma-like disorders
- Toxic-oil syndrome
- Vinyl chloride–induced disease
- Bleomycin-induced fibrosis
- Pentazocine-induced fibrosis
- Epoxy- and aromatic hydrocarbons–induced fibrosis
- Eosinophilia-myalgia syndrome

Other scleroderma-like disorders
- Scleredema adultorum of Buschke
- Scleromyxedema
- Chronic graft-vs.-host disease
- Eosinophilic fasciitis
- Digital sclerosis in diabetes
- Primary amyloidosis and amyloidosis associated with multiple myeloma

Two subsets, however, can be identified, even though there is some overlap (Table 313-2). One subset is referred to as *diffuse cutaneous scleroderma* and is characterized by the rapid development of symmetric skin thickening of proximal and distal extremities, face, and trunk. These patients are at greater risk for developing kidney and other visceral disease early in their course. The other subset is *limited cutaneous scleroderma*, which is defined by symmetric skin thickening limited to distal extremities and face. This subset frequently has features of the *CREST syndrome*, standing for *c*alcinosis, *R*aynaud's phenomenon, *e*sophageal dysmotility, *s*clerodactyly, and *t*elangiectasia. The prognosis in limited cutaneous scleroderma is better except for those patients who, after many years, develop pulmonary arterial hypertension or biliary cirrhosis. Involvement of visceral organs may also occur in the absence of any skin involvement, which is referred to as *systemic sclerosis sine scleroderma*. Survival is determined by the severity of visceral disease, especially involving the lungs, heart, and/or kidneys.

Preliminary criteria for the classification of systemic sclerosis were developed by the American Rheumatism Association (now called the American College of Rheumatology) for the purpose of uniformity in clinical studies. A major criterion was the presence of sclerodermatous skin changes of the fingers of both hands plus involvement at any location proximal to the metacarpal phalangeal joints, entire extremity, face, neck, chest, and abdomen. Minor criteria were sclerodactyly, digital pitting scars or tissue loss of the volar pads of the fingertips, and bibasilar pulmonary fibrosis. The diagnosis of SSc was based on the presence of the major criterion or two or more minor criteria. The sensitivity of these criteria was 97%, and the specificity 98%. These criteria are not, however, applicable to clinical practice as many patients have SSc who do not meet these criteria. Scleroderma can also occur in a localized form limited to the skin, subcutaneous tissue, and muscle and without systemic involvement. Localized scleroderma occurs most often in children and young women but can affect any age group. The two localized forms are *morphea*, which occurs as single or multiple plaques of skin induration, and *linear scleroderma*, which involves an extremity or face. Linear scleroderma of one side of the forehead and scalp produces a disfiguration referred to as *en coup de sabre* because it resembles a wound from a sword. It may be associated with hemiatrophy of the same side of the face.

SSc also occurs in association with features of other connective tissue diseases. The term *overlap syndrome* has been used to describe such patients. Undifferentiated connective tissue disease has been suggested as a designation for patients who do not have diagnostic criteria for any one connective tissue disease. *Mixed connective tissue disease* (MCTD), a syndrome involving features of systemic lupus erythematosus (SLE), SSc, polymyositis, and rheumatoid arthritis and very high titers of circulating antibody to nuclear ribonucleoprotein (RNP) antigen, will be discussed later in the chapter. *Eosinophilic fasciitis*

Table 313-2 Subsets of Systemic Sclerosis

	Diffuse	Limited[a]
Skin involvement	Distal and proximal extremities, face, trunk	Distal to elbows, face
Raynaud's phenomenon	Onset within 1 year or at time of skin changes	May precede skin disease by years
Organ involvement	Pulmonary (interstitial fibrosis); renal (renovascular hypertensive crisis); gastrointestinal; cardiac	Gastrointestinal; pulmonary arterial hypertension after 10–15 years of disease in <10% of patients; biliary cirrhosis
Nail fold capillaries	Dilatation and dropout	Dilatation without significant dropout
Antinuclear antibodies	Antitopoisomerase 1	Anticentromere

[a] Also referred to as CREST (*c*alcinosis, *R*aynaud's, *e*sophageal dysmotility, *s*clerodactyly, *t*elangiectasia).

and the *eosinophilia-myalgia syndrome* (EMS) associated with contaminated L-tryptophan ingestion (Chap. 382) are scleroderma-like illnesses and will also be discussed in this chapter.

EPIDEMIOLOGY SSc has a worldwide distribution and affects all races. The onset of disease is unusual in childhood and young men. The incidence increases with age, peaking in the third to fifth decade. Women overall are affected approximately three times as often as men and even more often during the late childbearing years (≥8:1). SSc is more frequent and severe in young black women. The annual incidence has been estimated to be 19 cases per million population. The reported prevalence of SSc is between 19 and 75 per 100,000 persons. An exceptionally high prevalence of SSc (472 per 100,000 persons) has been noted in the Choctaw Native Americans in Oklahoma—the highest found to date in any ethnic group. Both incidence and prevalence may be underestimated because patients with early and atypical disease may be overlooked in surveys. The role of heredity has not been clarified. Several examples of familial SSc have been reported, and the finding of other connective tissue diseases and antinuclear antibodies in relatives of involved patients suggests a hereditary predisposition. However, spouses of SSc patients also have an increased incidence of antinuclear antibodies, suggesting environmental factors. Discordance of SSc in identical twins speaks against a significant genetic predisposition to disease. Immunogenetic studies have not shown strong associations between the major histocompatibility complex and susceptibility to SSc. Some studies have shown an association of SSc with HLA-A1, -B8, -DR3, or with DR3/DR52. C4A null alleles (C4AQ0) and HLA-DQA2 have been reported by some investigators to be markers for disease susceptibility. A more consistent relationship has been found between certain HLA types and the occurrence of specific autoantibodies in SSc patients. Anticentromere antibodies have been shown to be associated with HLA-DQB1*05 allele and, less often, with -DQB1*0301, -*0401, or -*0402. Antitopoisomerase 1 antibodies, on the other hand, are associated most frequently with HLA-DQB1*0301 in several populations, including Caucasians and African Americans.

Several environmental factors have been associated with the development of SSc and scleroderma-like illnesses. SSc appears to be more common in coal and gold miners, especially in those with more extensive exposure, suggesting that silica dust may be a predisposing factor. Workers exposed to polyvinyl chloride may develop Raynaud's phenomenon, acroosteolysis, scleroderma-like skin lesions, pulmonary fibrosis, and nail fold capillary abnormalities similar to those observed in SSc. These workers may also develop hepatic fibrosis and angiosarcoma. The observation that individuals exposed to similar amounts of vinyl chloride do not develop the same degree of disease suggests that a genetic factor may determine susceptibility and disease severity. The development of scleroderma has also been associated with exposure to epoxy resins and aromatic hydrocarbons such as benzine, toluene, and trichloroethylene. In 1981, in Spain, a multisystem disease resembling scleroderma occurred following the ingestion of aniline-adulterated cooking oil (rapeseed oil). Approximately 20,000 people were affected. The patients initially developed interstitial pneumonitis, eosinophilia, arthralgias, arthritis, and myositis, followed subsequently by joint contractures, skin thickening, Raynaud's phenomenon, pulmonary hypertension, sicca syndrome, and resorption of the distal fingertips. Extensive sclerosis of the dermis and subcutaneous tissue has been noted in patients receiving pentazocine, a nonnarcotic analgesic agent. Bleomycin, an anticancer agent, produces fibrotic skin nodules, linear hyperpigmentation, alopecia, Raynaud's phenomenon, gangrene of fingers, and pulmonary fibrosis affecting mainly the lower lobes. Scleroderma and other connective tissue diseases have been reported in women who have had silicone breast implants. Recent studies have not shown that women with these implants carry an increased risk for developing scleroderma or other connective tissue diseases. Localized fibrosis, however, can occur around the implant. While environmental factors or undefined infectious agents may be of etiologic significance, the cause of SSc remains unknown.

PATHOGENESIS The outstanding feature of SSc is overproduction and accumulation of collagen and other extracellular matrix proteins, including fibronectin, tenascin, and glycosaminoglycans, in skin and other organs. The disease process involves immunologic mechanisms, vascular endothelial cell activation and/or injury, and activation of fibroblasts resulting in production of excessive collagen.

An early event in SSc that precedes fibrosis is vascular injury involving small arteries, arterioles, and capillaries in the skin, gastrointestinal tract, kidneys, heart, and lungs. Raynaud's phenomenon, the initial symptom of SSc in the majority of patients, is a clinical expression of the abnormal regulation of blood flow resulting from vascular injury. Injury to endothelial cells and basal lamina occurs early and is followed by thickening of the intima, narrowing of the lumen, and eventual obliteration of the vessel. As vascular damage progresses, the microvascular bed in the skin and other sites is diminished, producing a state of chronic ischemia. Vascular abnormalities can be observed in the nail folds by wide-field microscopy, which shows dropout of capillaries with dilatation and tortuosity of remaining ones. In the skin, remaining capillaries may proliferate and dilate to become visible telangiectasia. Endothelial cell damage is reflected in elevated levels of factor VIII/von Willebrand factor in the sera of some patients with SSc.

Several mechanisms for endothelial injury or activation have been proposed in SSc. Any or all of these mechanisms may be involved in a given patient; some evidence for each exists. A cytotoxic factor for endothelium has been identified in some patients that degrades the basal lamina, releasing fragments of type IV collagen and laminin. This factor, a type IV collagenase, is secreted by activated T cells and is referred to as *granzyme 1* because of its location in cytolytic T cells. Type IV collagen and laminin fragments may stimulate an immune response to the basal lamina. Both antibodies and cell-mediated immunity to type IV collagen and laminin have been observed in some SSc patients and may be involved in endothelial injury or may be an epiphenomenon. Anti-endothelial cell antibodies (AECA) may be another mechanism for microvascular damage. In 25% of SSc patients, AECA have been shown to mediate antibody-dependent cell cytotoxicity against human endothelial cells. Circulating AECA in general have been reported in the sera of SSc patients in amounts ranging from 21 to 85%. This wide variation reflects patient selection, type of assay, and the source of endothelium. These antibodies are not specific for SSc and are found in other connective tissue diseases. The frequency of AECA is higher in patients with diffuse cutaneous SSc. They have also been shown to be associated with digital infarcts, pulmonary hypertension, and impaired alveolocapillary diffusion. Studies have show that AECA initiate programmed cell death (apoptosis), which may be an important event in the pathogenesis of SSc. These antibodies also induce expression of vascular cell adhesion molecule-1 (VCAM-1), intercellular adhesion molecule-1 (ICAM-1), E-selectin, and P-selectin on endothelial cells in SSc and stimulate the production of chemoattractants [interleukin (IL) 1, IL-8, monocyte chemotactic protein], leading to the binding of lymphocytes to the endothelium and their migration into the perivascular tissue. Elevated serum levels of VCAM-1, ICAM-1, and P-selectin are observed in early stages of SSc.

The injury to the endothelium leads to a state favoring vasoconstriction and ischemia. The damaged endothelium produces decreased amounts of prostacylin, which is an important vasodilator and inhibitor of platelet aggregation. Platelets are activated on binding to the damaged endothelium and release thromboxane, a potent vasoconstrictor. Activated platelets also release platelet-derived growth factor (PDGF), which is chemotactic and mitogenic for both smooth-muscle cells and fibroblasts, and transforming growth factor (TGF)β, which stimulates fibroblast collagen synthesis. These and other cytokines stimulate intimal fibrosis and, with their passage through the injured endothelium, may produce adventitial and perivascular fibrosis. Endothelin-1, a vasoconstricting factor released from endothelial cells on cold exposure, is also increased in SSc patients. In addition, it stimulates fibroblasts and smooth-muscle cells. The vasoconstriction action of endothelin-1 is normally opposed by endothelium-derived relaxation factor (EDRF, nitric oxide), also secreted by endothelial cells. The normal compensatory increase in EDRF is not seen in some patients with SSc, suggesting impairment of its synthesis. A deficiency of vasodilatory neuropeptides resulting from sensory system nerve damage may also produce a condition favoring vasoconstriction. Vasoconstriction itself also contributes to endothelial damage through a mechanism of reperfusion injury, resulting in vascular occlusion and fibrosis.

Existing evidence indicates that cell-mediated immunity plays a central role in the development of fibrosis in SSc. T cells, macrophages, endothelial cells, and other cells along with cytokines and growth factors interact in a complex manner to stimulate fibrosis. The vascular endothelium has been proposed as a target for cell-mediated immunity. Laminin and type IV collagen, components of the subendothelial basement membrane, induce in vitro transformation of lymphocytes from SSc patients. In the early stages of SSc, a mononuclear cell infiltrate consisting predominantly of activated helper-inducer T cells surrounds small blood vessels in the dermis. Subsequently, mononuclear cell infiltrates are found in macroscopically normal-appearing skin adjacent to areas of fibrosis. T cell hyperactivity is reflected by increased serum levels of CD4+ T cells. The ratio of CD4+ to CD8+ T cells is also increased. Elevated circulating levels of IL-2, a product of activated T cells, and IL-2 receptors have been shown to be associated with active fibrosis. In addition, serum levels of IL-4 are increased in SSc patients. IL-4, a product of activated T cells, stimulates fibroblast chemotaxis and proliferation and collagen production. In a recent study, CD8+ T cells isolated from bronchoalveolar lavage fluid from SSc patients made IL-4 and/or IL-5 mRNA. SSc patients with these type 2 cytokines were more likely to have alveolitis and a lower forced vital capacity. Although larger studies are needed, the findings suggest that these cytokines are involved in the pathogenesis of interstitial pulmonary fibrosis. Another cytokine, interferon γ, is produced by activated T cells and stimulates macrophages but inhibits collagen synthesis by fibroblasts. Reduced serum levels of interferon γ are found in some SSc patients. In vitro stimulation of T cells from SSc patients did not show an increased production of interferon γ compared to normal individuals, suggesting an inability in SSc patients to suppress fibrosis normally.

Macrophages are present in increased numbers in the infiltrates of SSc lesions, including the pulmonary alveoli. Activated macrophages secrete several important products involved in the pathogenesis of SSc including IL-1, IL-6, tumor necrosis factor (TNF) α, TGF-β, and PDGF. IL-1 has been shown to stimulate fibroblast proliferation and collagen synthesis. The important role for IL-6 may be in stimulating the local release of tissue inhibitor of metalloproteinase (TIMP) by fibroblasts and thereby limiting the breakdown of collagen. TNF-α, in conjunction with interferon γ, can cause endothelial cell cytolysis and also induces the expression of endothelial cell adhesion molecules (see above), which are responsible for the binding of T cells and subsequent vascular injury. The role of TGF-β and PDGF secreted by macrophages and other cells is discussed below. In addition to the above cytokines, macrophages secrete *fibronectin*, a large matrix protein that is increased in SSc lesions. Fibronectin is also secreted by fibroblasts. Fibronectin interacts with collagen in the SSc lesions where it binds fibroblasts and mononuclear cells through receptors called *integrins*. Fibronectin functions as a chemoattractant and mitogen for fibroblasts.

Additional support for involvement of cell-mediated immunity in the pathogenesis of SSc is the appearance of scleroderma-like lesions in patients with graft-versus-host disease (GVHD) after bone marrow transplantation and in a murine model of chronic GVHD, conditions known to be associated with activated T cells. GVHD and SSc are both associated with progressive skin induration, joint contractures, and gastrointestinal and pulmonary involvement and are frequently accompanied by Sjögren's syndrome. Antinuclear antibodies are present in both diseases. Raynaud's phenomenon and kidney involvement are infrequent in GVHD.

Mast cells may also be involved in the development of fibrosis.

Increased numbers of mast cells are found in the dermis in both involved and uninvolved skin. Mast cell degranulation has been noted in skin that subsequently became fibrosed. Interaction with T cells may be one mechanism for mast cell degranulation resulting in release of products that stimulate fibroblast collagen synthesis. Release of histamine from mast cells may also contribute to edema observed in early disease.

Fibroblast growth and synthesis of collagen, fibronectin, and glycosaminoglycans are increased in SSc. Fibroblasts from SSc appear to have aberrant regulation of growth compared with fibroblasts from normal persons. When fibroblasts from affected SSc skin are removed and cultured in vitro, they continue to produce excessive quantities of collagen. The collagen is biochemically normal, and the proportion of type I to type III is the same as in normal skin. Fibroblasts from SSc patients appear to be in a state of permanent activation, most likely as a result of stimulation by cytokines. These activated cells are thought to represent an expanded subpopulation of fibroblasts that inherently express increased matrix genes. Studies have revealed a subpopulation of SSc fibroblasts that produces two to three times more collagen than other cells from the same tissue. Fibroblasts expressing elevated levels of mRNA for types I and III collagen have been demonstrated by in situ hybridization, particularly around dermal blood vessels in affected SSc skin. Collagen deposition is also initially perivascular in other organs including myocardium, muscle, and kidney. A small number of fibroblasts express increased levels of mRNA for types VI and VII collagen. Type VII collagen is normally found at the dermal-epidermal basement membrane zone and is the major component of anchoring fibrils that act to stabilize the attachment of the basement membrane to the underlying dermis. In SSc patients, type VII collagen is found throughout the dermis and may account for the indurated, tightly bound skin in this disease. PDGF receptors are expressed on SSc fibroblasts not only from affected areas but also from macroscopically normal-appearing skin. Fibroblasts from normal persons lack expression of these receptors. TGF-β has been shown to upregulate the expression of these receptors in SSc fibroblasts but not in normal cells and, in conjunction with PDGF, stimulates SSc fibroblast proliferation. Macrophages and fibroblasts are capable of secreting PDGF and TGF-β, and activated T cells release TGF-β. TGF-β also induces the autocrine production of PDGF-related peptides, referred to as connective tissue growth factor (CTGF), by fibroblasts. TGF-β interacts with CTGF on fibroblasts to stimulate fibroblast proliferation and collagen synthesis. Serum levels of CTGF have been found to be elevated in SSc and correlate with the degree of dermal and pulmonary fibrosis.

Fibroblasts may activate T cells to release cytokines that stimulate fibrosis. Fibroblasts in SSc patients have been shown to have increased expression of an adhesion molecule, ICAM-1, which binds to specific integrins on T cells. This binding allows interaction between T cell antigen receptor and class II molecules and antigen on fibroblasts, resulting in T cell activation and cytokine release. T cells may also be activated by their interaction with extracellular matrix molecules including collagen, fibronectin, and laminin.

Recent studies have suggested that microchimerism may be involved in the pathogenesis of SSc. Microchimerism in SSc is of interest because of the clinical similarities between SSc and GVHD after allogeneic bone marrow transplantation. Also relevant are the predilection for women in SSc and the increased incidence of SSc in women after the childbearing years. Fetal progenitor cells can persist in the serum of normal women for many years after childbirth. Compared to normal controls, both the quantity and frequency of fetal cells have been found to be increased in the serum of SSc patients. Microchimerism can also occur in nulligravid women and in men with SSc as non-host cells may come from blood transfusion, engraftment of cells from a twin, or from maternal cells in utero. Two-directional traffic of cells occurs during pregnancy. The mechanism by which microchimerism is involved in the pathogenesis is not known, but it is conceivable that these small numbers of non-host cells interfere with immune regulation, leading to autoimmunity.

Chromosomal abnormalities have been noted in >90% of SSc patients. These acquired abnormalities include chromatid breaks, acentric fragments, and ring chromosomes and are found in ~30% of mitotic cells. A chromosomal breakage factor has been found in the serum of SSc patients and their first-degree relatives. The significance of these chromosomal abnormalities is unknown.

PATHOLOGY **Skin** In the skin, a thin epidermis overlies compact bundles of collagen that lie parallel to the epidermis. Fingerlike projections of collagen extend from the dermis into the subcutaneous tissue and bind the skin to the underlying tissue. Dermal appendages are atrophied, and rete pegs are lost. In early stages of disease, a mononuclear cell infiltrate of predominantly T cells surrounds small dermal blood vessels. Increased numbers of T cells, monocytes, plasma cells, and mast cells are found, particularly in the lower dermis of involved skin.

Gastrointestinal Tract In the lower two-thirds of the esophagus, the histologic findings consist of a thin mucosa and increased collagen in the lamina propria, submucosa, and serosa. The degree of fibrosis is less than in the skin. Atrophy of the muscularis in the esophagus and throughout the involved portions of the gastrointestinal tract is more prominent than the amount of fibrotic replacement of muscle. Ulceration of the mucosa is often present and may be due to either SSc or superimposed peptic esophagitis. Chronic esophageal reflux can lead to metaplasia of the lower esophagus (Barrett's esophagus), which is a premalignant lesion. Striated muscles in the upper third of the esophagus are relatively spared. Similar changes may be found throughout the gastrointestinal tract, especially in the second and third portions of the duodenum, in the jejunum, and in the large intestine. Atrophy of the muscularis of the large intestine may lead to the development of large-mouth diverticula. In the later stages of the disease, the involved portions of the gastrointestinal tract become dilated. Infiltration of lymphocytes and plasma cells in the lamina propria is also present.

Lung With pulmonary involvement, diffuse interstitial fibrosis, thickening of the alveolar membrane, and peribronchial and pleural fibrosis are observed. Bronchiolar epithelial proliferation accompanies the pulmonary fibrosis. Rupture of septa produces small cysts and areas of bullous emphysema. Small pulmonary arteries and arterioles show intimal thickening, fragmentation of the elastica, and muscular hypertrophy; this may occur without interstitial pulmonary fibrosis and produce pulmonary hypertension, particularly in a subset of patients with limited cutaneous SSc.

Musculoskeletal System The synovium in patients with arthritis is similar to that seen in early rheumatoid arthritis and shows edema with infiltration of lymphocytes and plasma cells. A characteristic finding is a thick layer of fibrin overlying and within the synovium. Later in the disease the synovium may become fibrotic. Fibrinous deposits appear on the surfaces of tendon sheaths and in the overlying fascia and may lead to audible creaking over moving tendons.

Histologic features of primary myopathy consist of interstitial and perivascular lymphocytic infiltrations, degeneration of muscle fibers, and interstitial fibrosis. Arterioles may be thickened, and capillaries may be decreased in number. Pathologic and electrophysiologic findings of polymyositis in proximal muscles are present in the few patients who are considered to have the overlap syndrome of SSc and polymyositis.

Heart Cardiac involvement consists of degeneration of myocardial fibers and irregular areas of interstitial fibrosis that are most prominent around blood vessels. Intermittent spasm of blood vessels may result in contraction band necrosis, similar to change observed in myocardial infarction in patients with atherosclerotic coronary artery disease. Fibrosis also involves the conduction system, leading to atrioventricular conduction defects and arrhythmias. The wall of smaller coronary arteries may be thickened. Fibrinous pericarditis and pericardial effusions are found in some patients.

Kidney Renal involvement is found in over half the patients and consists of intimal hyperplasia of the interlobular arteries; fibrinoid necrosis of the afferent arterioles, including the glomerular tuft; and thickening of the glomerular basement membrane. Small cortical infarctions and glomerulosclerosis may be present. The renal pathologic change is often indistinguishable from that observed in malignant hypertension. Renal vascular lesions, however, may be present in the absence of hypertension. Immunofluorescence studies of kidney have shown IgM, complement components, and fibrinogen in the walls of affected vessels. Angiographic renal studies in patients with SSc may show constriction of the intralobular arteries, a finding that simulates the vasospasm of the digital arteries observed in Raynaud's phenomenon. Cold-induced Raynaud's phenomenon has been shown to decrease renal blood flow.

Other Organs Primary liver involvement is not common. Primary biliary cirrhosis occurs in some patients, particularly in those with the limited cutaneous form of SSc. Fibrosis of the thyroid gland may develop in the presence or absence of autoimmune thyroiditis.

Thickening of the periodontal membrane with replacement of the lamina dura is demonstrated radiographically as widening of the periodontal space and may cause gingivitis and loosening of the teeth. The decreased oral aperture and mucosal dryness make eating and oral hygiene difficult.

CLINICAL MANIFESTATIONS (See Table 313-3) **Raynaud's Phenomenon** SSc usually begins insidiously; the first symptoms are frequently Raynaud's phenomenon and puffy fingers. Some 95% of patients will experience Raynaud's phenomenon, which is defined as episodic vasoconstriction of small arteries and arterioles of fingers, toes, and sometimes the tip of the nose and earlobes. Episodes are brought on by cold exposure, vibration, or emotional stress. Patients experience pallor and/or cyanosis followed by rubor on rewarming. Pallor and/or cyanosis are usually associated with coldness and numbness of fingers and/or toes, and rubor with pain and tingling. Not all patients appreciate the three color phases. A history of digit pallor appears to be the most reliable symptom for the presence of Raynaud's phenomenon. Raynaud's phenomenon may precede skin changes by several months or even years in those patients who subsequently develop the limited cutaneous form of SSc. In diffuse cutaneous SSc, skin changes are seen typically within a year of the onset of Raynaud's phenomenon. After 2 or more years of Raynaud's phenomenon, few patients who have this as their only symptom will subsequently develop SSc.

Skin Features In early disease, fingers and hands are swollen. Swelling may also involve forearms, feet, lower legs, and face. However, lower extremities are relatively spared. This edematous phase may last for a few weeks, months, or even longer. The edema may be pitting or nonpitting and accompanied by erythema. The skin changes begin distally in the extremities and advance proximally. The skin gradually becomes firm, thickened, and eventually tightly bound to underlying subcutaneous tissue (indurative phase). In patients with diffuse cutaneous scleroderma, skin changes will become generalized, involving initially the extremities, followed by the face and trunk over a period of time, varying from months to a few years. In some patients, the skin changes may develop gradually over several years. Rapid progression of these changes over a 1- to 3-year period is associated with a greater risk of visceral disease, particularly of the lungs, heart, or kidneys. Also in diffuse cutaneous SSc, the skin changes usually peak in 3 to 5 years and then slowly improve. On the other hand, patients with limited cutaneous scleroderma will usually have a more gradual progression of skin changes, which are restricted to fingers or distal extremity and face and may continue to worsen. In both subsets of SSc, skin thickening is usually greater in the distal extremity. After many years of disease, the skin may soften and return to normal thickness or become thin and atrophic.

Table 313-3 Clinical Features of Systemic Sclerosis

Clinical Feature	Percent of Patients with Clinical Feature during Course of Disease: Limited[a]	Diffuse[a]
Raynaud's phenomenon	95–100	90–95
Skin thickening	98[b]	100
Subcutaneous calcinosis	50	10
Telangiectasia	85	40
Arthralgias/arthritis	40	70
Myopathy	5	50
Esophageal dysmotility	80	80
Pulmonary fibrosis	35	40
Isolated pulmonary arterial hypertension	<10	<1
Congestive heart failure	<1	30
Renal crisis	<1	15

[a] Limited cutaneous and diffuse cutaneous subsets of SSc.
[b] 2% or fewer of patients have SSc sine scleroderma.

In the extremities, the taut skin over fingers gradually limits full extension, and flexion contractures develop. Ulcers may appear on the volar pads of the fingertips and over bony prominences such as elbows, malleoli, and the extensor surface of the proximal interphalangeal joints of the hands. These ulcers may become secondarily infected. The volar pads of the fingertips develop pitting scars and lose soft tissue. In some instances, resorption of the terminal phalanges occurs. Skin over the extremities, face, and trunk may become darkly pigmented, even without exposure to the sun. Hyperpigmentation of the skin may occur over superficial blood vessels and tendons. Areas of hypopigmentation may also develop, similar to vitiligo, involving the eyebrows, scalp, and trunk. The sparing of pigment around hair follicles gives the skin a "salt-and-pepper" appearance. Other patients may develop a diffuse tanning of the skin. The skin loses hair, oil, and sweat glands and so becomes dry and coarse. Vaginal dryness occurs and may cause dyspareunia.

In some patients, particularly those with the limited cutaneous form of disease, calcific deposits develop in intracutaneous and subcutaneous tissue. The sites commonly involved are periarticular tissue, digital pads, olecranon and prepatellar bursae, and skin along the extensor surface of the forearms. The overlying skin may break down, with drainage of calcific material. Involvement of the face results in thinning of the lips, loss of skin wrinkles and facial expression, as well as microstomia, which may make eating and dental hygiene difficult. The nose takes on a pinched or beaklike appearance. Wrinkles appear around the mouth perpendicular to the lips. Small telangiectatic mats may appear on the fingers, face, lips, tongue, and buccal mucosa after several years. They are seen more frequently in patients with limited cutaneous SSc but are also observed in patients with long-standing diffuse cutaneous SSc. The capillary beds of nail folds of the fingers may show enlargement of capillaries with little or no capillary loss, usually indicative of limited cutaneous scleroderma. In diffuse cutaneous scleroderma, there is disorganization of the capillary beds with dilated capillaries interspersed with areas where capillaries have disappeared. These capillary changes, which are observed by wide-angle microscopy or with an ophthalmoscope used as a magnifier, are not found in patients who have only Raynaud's phenomenon.

Musculoskeletal Features More than half the patients with SSc complain of pain, swelling, and stiffness of the fingers and knees. A symmetric polyarthritis resembling rheumatoid arthritis may be seen. In more advanced stages of the disease, leathery crepitation can be palpated over moving joints, especially the knee. Extensive fibrotic thickening of the tendon sheaths in the wrist can produce a carpal tunnel syndrome. Muscle weakness is usually present in patients with severe skin involvement and, in most cases, is due to disuse atrophy. There is a distinctive histologic myopathy that accompanies SSc that is not associated with muscle enzyme abnormalities. A few patients develop a myositis characterized by proximal muscle weakness and muscle enzyme elevations that are identical to polymyositis (overlap syndrome). In addition to terminal phalanges, resorption of bone may involve ribs, clavicle, and angle of mandible.

Gastrointestinal Features The majority of patients from both subsets of SSc have gastrointestinal involvement. Symptoms attributable to esophageal involvement are present in >50% of patients and include epigastric fullness, burning pain in the epigastric or retrosternal regions, and regurgitation of gastric contents. These symptoms, most noticeable when the patient is lying flat or bending over, are due to the reduced tone of the gastroesophageal sphincter and to dilatation of the distal esophagus. Peptic esophagitis frequently occurs and may lead to strictures and narrowing of the lower esophagus. However, it seldom results in bleeding. Barrett's metaplasia may develop, but transition to adenocarcinoma is uncommon. Dysphagia, particularly of solid foods, may occur independent of other esophageal symptoms and is caused by loss of esophageal motility due to neuromuscular dysfunction. Manometry or cineradiography reveals decreased amplitude or disappearance of peristaltic waves in the lower two-thirds of the esophagus. Raynaud's phenomenon in the absence of a connective tissue disease is also associated with esophageal dysmotility. Later in the course of the illness, dilatation and atony of the lower portion of the esophagus as well as reflux are seen. With gastric involvement, barium studies show dilatation, atony, and delayed gastric emptying. Patients may complain of early satiety. Gastric outlet obstruction can also occur.

Hypomotility of the small intestine produces symptoms of bloating and abdominal pain and may suggest an intestinal obstruction or paralytic ileus (pseudoobstruction). Malabsorption syndrome with weight loss, diarrhea, and anemia is due to bacterial overgrowth in the atonic intestine or possibly to obliteration of lymphatics by fibrosis. Roentgenographic features of the second and third portions of the duodenum and of the jejunum include dilatation, loss of the usual feathery pattern, and delayed disappearance of barium. Pneumatosis intestinalis occasionally occurs and appears as radiolucent cysts or linear streaks within the wall of the small intestine. Benign pneumoperitoneum may result from the rupture of these cysts. Involvement of the large intestine may cause chronic constipation and fecal impaction with episodes of bowel obstruction. A segment of atonic bowel may act as a fulcrum for intussuception to occur. Barium studies of the large intestine may show dilatation, atony, and large-mouth diverticula. Laxity of the anal sphincter may cause incontinence or rarely anal prolapse. Some patients may have gastrointestinal features of SSc with little or no cutaneous or other organ involvement, referred to as *SSc sine scleroderma.* Vascular ectasia may develop in the stomach and intestine and can be the source of gastrointestinal bleeding. These dilated submucosal capillaries in the stomach appear on endoscopy as broad stripes—hence the term "watermelon stomach."

Pulmonary Features Pulmonary involvement occurs in at least two-thirds of SSc patients and is now the leading cause of death in SSc, replacing renal disease, which can usually be treated effectively. The most common symptom is exertional dyspnea, often accompanied by a dry, nonproductive cough. Bilateral basilar rales may be present. In the majority of patients, symptoms usually correlate with radiologic evidence of pulmonary fibrosis and with restrictive lung disease on pulmonary function tests.

Pulmonary function tests are frequently abnormal and show a reduction in vital capacity and decreased lung compliance. Impairment of gas exchange is reflected by a low diffusing capacity and low P_{O_2} with exercise. These abnormalities may be present even when the chest radiograph is normal. Chest film may show a pattern of linear densities, mottling, and honeycombing involving most prominently the lower two-thirds of the lung. Early interstitial pulmonary disease can be detected by high-resolution computed tomography (HRCT) and bronchoalveolar lavage (BAL). Active inflammatory alveolitis gives a "ground glass" appearance on HRCT. The recovery by BAL of increased numbers of cells, mostly alveolar macrophages accompanied by neutrophils or eosinophils, is evidence for alveolitis.

Both interstitial fibrosis and vascular lesions are found in the lungs of patients with SSc. Interstitial pulmonary fibrosis may be the predominant lesion in patients with diffuse or limited cutaneous SSc. Patients with diffuse cutaneous involvement who have antitopoisomerase 1 antibodies are particularly at risk of developing severe pulmonary fibrosis. In the absence of significant interstitial fibrosis, a severe form of pulmonary arterial hypertension may develop after many years of disease in a subset of patients with limited cutaneous SSc. Fewer than 10% of patients will develop this complication, which is caused by narrowing and obliteration of pulmonary arteries and arterioles by intimal fibrosis and medial hypertrophy. Pulmonary hypertension is manifested initially by exertional dyspnea and eventually by the appearance of right-sided heart failure. Pulmonary artery pressure can be measured noninvasively by two-dimensional echocardiography. The prognosis is extremely poor with the development of pulmonary hypertension; the mean duration of survival is approximately 2 years.

A less common pulmonary problem is aspiration pneumonia resulting from gastric reflux due to lower esophageal atony. Restriction of chest movement caused by extensive fibrotic skin involvement of the thorax rarely occurs. Superimposed bacterial or viral infection can be a serious complication in patients with pulmonary fibrosis. An increased frequency of alveolar cell and bronchogenic carcinoma is seen in patients with pulmonary fibrosis.

Cardiac Features Primary cardiac involvement in SSc includes pericarditis with or without effusions, heart failure, and varying degrees of heart block or arrhythmias. The majority of patients with diffuse cutaneous SSc have cardiac abnormalities. Cardiomyopathy attributable to myocardial fibrosis appears in $<10\%$ of patients and involves primarily those patients with diffuse cutaneous scleroderma. Radionuclide studies have shown abnormalities of left ventricular function due to myocardial fibrosis. Cold-induced vasospasm of the hands produces defects in myocardial thallium perfusion. The characteristic pathologic feature of contraction band necrosis results from cardiac muscle damage caused by intermittent vasospasm of coronary vessels. Patients may experience angina pectoris even though coronary angiograms are normal. Patients can also develop left ventricular failure secondary to systemic hypertension or cor pulmonale secondary to pulmonary arterial hypertension.

Renal Features Renal failure was the leading cause of death in SSc until the advent of effective treatment. Significant renal disease occurs mostly in those patients with diffuse cutaneous scleroderma. A high risk of renal crisis is present in those patients who have rapidly progressive widespread skin thickening in their first 2 to 3 years of disease. Renal crisis is characterized by malignant hypertension, which can progress rapidly to renal failure. These patients manifest hypertensive encephalopathy, severe headache, retinopathy, seizures, and left ventricular failure. Hematuria and proteinuria are followed by oliguria and renal failure. The mechanism for the hypertensive crisis is activation of the renin-angiotensin system. Before the advent of effective antihypertensive drugs, the majority of these patients died within 6 months. A small number of patients may develop renal crises in the absence of hypertension. Renal failure can also develop insidiously later in the course of disease in the setting of mild to moderate hypertension and proteinuria. In these patients or those with clinically unrecognized renal disease, reduction of renal plasma flow secondary to heart failure or volume depletion resulting from overdiuresis may precipitate renal crisis. An indicator of impending renal failure is microangiopathic anemia, which may occur in a normotensive patient. The presence of a large chronic pericardial effusion may also herald subsequent renal failure.

Other Features Symptoms of dry eyes and/or dry mouth are frequently present in patients with SSc. Lip biopsy may show lymphocytic infiltration of minor salivary glands characteristic of Sjögren's syndrome or intraglandular or periglandular fibrosis secondary to SSc. Antibodies to SS-A (Ro) and/or SS-B (La) are found in those patients with lip biopsies consistent with Sjögren's syndrome (overlap syndrome-SSc and Sjögren's syndrome) and not in those with salivary gland fibrosis.

Hypothyroidism occurs in a significant number of patients and may be associated with high levels of antithyroid antibodies. Fibrosis of the thyroid gland may be present but also occurs in the absence of autoimmune thyroiditis. Other manifestations of SSc include trigeminal neuralgia and male impotence secondary to decreased penile tumescence. These men have normal serum levels of testosterone and gonadotropins. Pathogenesis of this abnormality has been considered to be caused by vascular and/or autonomic nervous system abnormalities. Biliary cirrhosis is occasionally observed in patients with limited cutaneous SSc.

LABORATORY FINDINGS The erythrocyte sedimentation rate may be elevated. Hypoproliferative anemia related to chronic inflammation is the most common cause of anemia in SSc. Anemia may also be caused by iron deficiency secondary to gastrointestinal bleeding. Bacterial overgrowth due to atony of the small bowel may lead to vitamin B_{12} and/or folic acid–deficiency anemia. Microangiopathic hemolytic anemia is most often associated with renal involvement and is caused by the presence of intravascular fibrin in renal arterioles. Polyclonal hypergammaglobulinemia, consisting mostly of IgG, is found in approximately half the patients. Rheumatoid factor, in low titer, is present in 25% of patients. Cryoglobulins may be present in the serum. Antinuclear antibodies detected by using a cultured human laryngeal carcinoma cell line (HEp-2) substrate are present in 95% of patients (Table 313-4). Antinuclear antibodies that have a high specificity for SSc are antitopoisomerase 1 (Scl-70), antinucleolar, and anticentromere. Antitopoisomerase 1, originally called anti-Scl-70, recognizes the nuclear enzyme DNA topoisomerase 1, a nuclear enzyme involved in the unwinding of DNA for replication and RNA transcription. These antibodies are found in ~20% of all SSc patients and in ~40% of those with diffuse cutaneous SSc. They are associated with diffuse cutaneous involvement, interstitial pulmonary disease, and renal and other visceral organ involvement. A very high frequency of these antibodies has been reported in Choctaw Native Americans in association with diffuse cutaneous SSc. They are seldom present in other disorders or in conjunction with anticentromere antibodies. Anticentromere antibodies react with protein antigens located in the kinetochore region of chromosomes and are present in 40 to 80% of patients with limited cutaneous scleroderma or CREST syndrome. Anticentromere antibodies are found in only about 2 to 5% of patients with diffuse cutaneous scleroderma and rarely in other connective tissue diseases. They are found occasionally in patients with only Raynaud's phenomenon and may indicate subsequent development of limited cutaneous disease. Antinucleolar antibodies are relatively specific for SSc and are present in ~20 to 30% of patients. Several antinucleolar antibodies have been associated with SSc: Anti-RNA polymerases I, II, and III are found in patients with diffuse cutaneous SSc who have a higher prevalence of renal and cardiac involvement. Anti-Th RNP has been found in patients with limited cutaneous SSc, and anti-PM-Scl, formerly referred to as anti-PM1, along with anti-Ku, may be found in a subset of patients with overlapping features of limited cutaneous SSc and polymyositis. Anti-U_3 RNP (anti-fibrillarin) is also highly specific for SSc and may be associated with skeletal muscle disease, bowel involvement, and pulmonary arterial hypertension. Anti-U_1 RNP is found in ~5 to 10% of SSc patients and in 95 to 100% of those patients with the overlap syndrome of MCTD. The titers in MCTD are usually high (see below). Anti-SS-A (Ro) and/or anti-SS-B (La) are present in those patients with overlap syndrome of SSc and Sjögren's syndrome.

Table 313-4 Autoantibodies in Systemic Sclerosis

Autoantibody	Clinical Association	Percent[a]
Antitopoisomerase 1	Diffuse cutaneous SSc	40
Anticentromere	Limited cutaneous SSc	60–80
Anti-RNA polymerase I, II, III	Diffuse cutaneous SSc	5–40
Anti-Th RNP	Limited cutaneous SSc	14
Anti-U_1 RNP	Limited cutaneous SSc	5–10
	Mixed connective tissue disease	95–100
Anti-PM/Scl	Overlap (SSc, polymyositis)	25

[a] Approximate percentages for the predominant clinical association.

DIAGNOSIS The diagnosis of SSc presents no difficulty in the presence of Raynaud's phenomenon, with typical skin lesions and visceral involvement. Although Raynaud's phenomenon may be the first symptom of SSc, most patients with Raynaud's phenomenon alone do not develop a connective tissue disease. Other causes of Raynaud's phenomenon include thoracic outlet (scalenus anticus and cervical rib) syndromes, shoulder-hand syndrome, trauma (jackhammer or vibratory machine operators), previous cold injury, vinyl chloride exposure, and circulating cryoglobulins or cold agglutinins. Linear scleroderma and morphea are localized forms of scleroderma that can usually be distinguished clinically. In early disease, SSc may initially be confused with rheumatoid arthritis, SLE, or polymyositis when articular or muscle involvement is prominent. SSc without cutaneous involvement should be considered in patients with unexplained pulmonary fibrosis, pulmonary hypertension, cardiomyopathies, heart block, dysphagia, or malabsorption syndrome. Several conditions have scleroderma-like features but lack the visceral involvement. Scleredema (scleredema adultorum of Buschke) occurs predominantly in children and is characterized by painless edematous induration involving the face, scalp, neck, trunk, and proximal portions of the extremities. Involvement of the hands and feet usually does not occur. Scleredema may be associated with previous streptococcal infection and is usually self-limited, resolving in 6 to 12 months. Histology reveals accumulation of mucopolysaccharides in the dermis and skeletal muscle. A rare entity, scleromyxedema is manifested by yellowish or pale red papules in association with diffuse skin thickening that may involve the face and hands. Acid mucopolysaccharide deposits are found in the dermis. Monoclonal IgG may be detected in some of these patients. Patients with insulin-dependent diabetes mellitus may develop digital sclerosis and contractures (prayer hand deformity). Primary amyloidosis and amyloidosis associated with multiple myeloma may involve the skin of the extremities and face diffusely to give the appearance of scleroderma. Biopsy will clearly differentiate these entities.

COURSE AND PROGNOSIS The course of SSc is quite variable. Until the disease differentiates into recognizable subsets, prognosis in early disease is difficult to predict. Patients with limited cutaneous scleroderma, especially those with anticentromere antibodies, have a good prognosis, with the notable exception of those few patients, <10%, who after ≥10 to 20 years develop pulmonary arterial hypertension. Malabsorption syndrome and primary biliary cirrhosis are the causes of morbidity and mortality in some patients with limited cutaneous disease. On the other hand, the prognosis is generally worse in patients with diffuse cutaneous disease, particularly when the onset occurs at an older age. In addition, males have a worse prognosis. Renal and other visceral organ disease may develop early in the course of those patients with rapidly progressive generalized skin thickening. Death occurs most often from pulmonary, cardiac, and renal involvement. With the advent of effective therapy for renal crisis along with renal dialysis for those patients with renal failure, survival has greatly improved. In patients with diffuse cutaneous disease, the 5-year cumulative survival rate is ~70% and the 10-year is ~55%. In limited cutaneous disease the 5-year is ~90% and the 10-year is ~75%.

Skin may spontaneously soften after years of disease. Softening occurs in the reverse order of original skin involvement, beginning with the trunk and followed by the proximal and then the distal extremities. Sclerodactyly and flexion contractures may persist. Skin thickness may eventually approach normal; however, the skin may be atrophic.

℞ **TREATMENT** Even though SSc cannot be cured, treatment of involved organ systems can relieve symptoms and improve function. The doctor-patient relationship is extremely important in caring for patients with this chronic debilitating illness. Once the diagnosis of SSc has been made, the patient and family should be instructed about this disorder. The patient will need repeated explanations and reassurances throughout his or her illness. Depending on the severity of illness, the patient will require monitoring of blood pressure, blood counts, urinalysis, and monitoring of renal and pulmonary function on a regular basis.

Effectiveness of drug therapy in SSc is difficult to evaluate because of the variable course and severity of the disease. Many drugs have been used in the treatment of SSc without any consistent or prolonged benefit. In uncontrolled studies, D-penicillamine has been reported to reduce skin thickening and prevent development of significant organ involvement when compared to similar historic controls. Five-year cumulative survival rates of 80% have been reported in D-penicillamine-treated patients. This drug interferes with inter- and intramolecular cross-linking of collagen and is also immunosuppressive. Its immunosuppressive activity may also lead to decreased collagen production. Penicillamine is better tolerated when started at a low dose, usually 250 mg/d, and then increased at 1- to 3-month intervals up to 1.5 g/d as tolerated. Although a few patients can tolerate higher doses, most patients are maintained on a dose between 0.5 and 1 g/d. For optimal absorption, it is important to give this drug 1 h before or 2 h after a meal. This drug can be quite toxic; its more serious complications include glomerulonephritis with nephrotic syndrome, aplastic anemia, leukopenia, thrombocytopenia, and myasthenia gravis. Other side effects are fever, rash, anorexia, nausea, and loss of taste. Patients should have monthly complete blood counts (including platelet count) and urinalyses. The results of a 2-year double-blind randomized study comparing high-dose D-penicillamine (750 to 1000 mg/d) with low-dose D-penicillamine (125 mg every other day) in patients with early diffuse cutaneous SSc were recently reported. The degree of skin thickening and the occurrence of renal crises and other organ involvement as well as mortality were not significantly different between the high- and low-dose treated groups. This study suggested that there was no advantage in using doses >125 mg every other day. Azathioprine, methotrexate, cyclophosphamide, and other immunosuppressives have also been used in SSc and should be reserved for those patients with rapidly progressive disease. Control studies are lacking. Trials of treatment with recombinant interferon γ, 5-fluorouracil, and extracorporeal photochemotherapy have shown improvement in some disease parameters. No therapy, however, has been clearly demonstrated in a controlled, prospective study to suppress or reverse the disease process of SSc. Because of the poor prognosis in SSc patients who have a rapid onset of diffuse cutaneous disease and early visceral organ involvement (pulmonary, cardiac, or renal), clinical trials are under way using high-dose immunosuppressive therapy followed by autologous stem cell transplantation. The rationale is that high doses of an immunosuppressive drug such as cyclophosphamide may reverse or modify the disease course. The autologous stem cell transplantation permits the rapid reconstitution of hematopoiesis.

Antiplatelet therapy may play a role in the treatment of SSc, since the biologic products of platelets affect blood vessels. Low doses of aspirin block the formation of thromboxane A_2, a powerful vasoconstrictor and platelet aggregator. In addition, dipyridamole, 200 to 400 mg in divided daily doses, also decreases platelet adhesion to damaged vessel walls. While these drugs have a reasonable therapeutic rationale, a 2-year double-blind study did not show any benefit from their use. Reports of beneficial effects of colchicine or chlorambucil have not been documented in controlled studies.

Glucocorticoids are indicated in those patients with inflammatory myositis or pericarditis. The initial dose is 40 to 60 mg/d and is tapered based on clinical improvement (see below). They should not be used for the indolent primary form of muscle disease of SSc. Prednisone in the range of 20 to 40 mg/d may decrease edema associated with the edematous phase of early skin involvement. Glucocorticoids are not otherwise indicated in the long-term treatment of SSc. High doses of glucocorticoids may play a role in precipitating acute renal failure. A retrospective case-control study in patients with early diffuse cutaneous SSc showed a significant association between prior high-dose glucocorticoids (prednisone $\geq$ 15 mg/d) and the development of scleroderma renal crisis. Based on these observations, immunosuppressive drugs (e.g. methotrexate, azathioprine, or cyclophosphamide) should be considered in treating the inflammatory myositis, pericarditis, or early inflammatory skin disease.

The management of Raynaud's phenomenon is directed at control of vasospasm. Patients should be advised to dress warmly and wear mittens and socks, not to smoke, to remove causes of external stress, and to avoid drugs such as amphetamine and ergotamine. Cold drafts should be avoided. Air-conditioned rooms in warm climates can also be a problem for patients with Raynaud's phenomenon. Beta-blocking drugs may make Raynaud's phenomenon worse. Warmth of the central body induces peripheral vasodilatation. Drugs that block sympathetic vasoconstriction, such as reserpine, α-methyldopa, phenoxybenzamine, and prazosin, may be useful in the treatment of Raynaud's phenomenon, but their side effects often curtail extended use. The calcium channel blockers nifedipine, diltiazem, and the longer acting amlodipine can be effective in alleviating Raynaud's phenomenon, but side effects of light-headedness and palpitations may limit their use. The sustained-release form of nifedipine is better tolerated; the dose is 30 mg/d up to 60 or 90 mg/d as required to control symptoms. Nitroglycerine paste, applied to an affected digit, may improve local blood flow. In a 12-week pilot study, losartan, a specific nonpeptide angiotensen II type 1 receptor antagonist, reduced the severity and frequency of Raynaud's phenomenon episodes. Ketanserin, an oral serotonin antagonist, also has been shown to be effective. Selective serotonin reuptake inhibitors (e.g., fluoxetine) may be beneficial in some patients. These drugs decrease platelet 5-hydroxytryptamine, which is thought to play a role in the pathogenesis of Raynaud's phenomenon. Studies with intravenous iloprost, a prostacyclin analogue, have shown a decrease in frequency and severity of Raynaud's phenomenon and healing of digital ulcers in some patients. Iloprost is still not available in the United States for general use. Intravenous alprostadil, a prostaglandin, can be effective in treating severe Raynaud's phenomenon with digital ulcers. Epoprostenol (prostacyclin), used in the treatment of pulmonary hypertension, also improves Raynaud's phenomenon. Pentoxifylline may also improve perfusion by increasing the deformability of the red cell plasma membranes. Techniques of biofeedback have also been used with variable success for teaching patients to control the temperature of their hands. Stellate ganglion blockage may be useful in temporarily alleviating severe ischemic pain in the fingers. Surgical sympathectomy usually provides only temporary improvement, and it, along with other forms of therapy, does not prevent progression of the vascular lesion. Digital sympathectomy can be effective in some patients. The response to any therapy for Raynaud's phenomenon is limited by the degree of existing structural narrowing of digital arteries. In patients with severe Raynaud's phenomenon and refractory digital ulcers, distal ulnar artery occlusion should be considered. A positive Allen test is suggestive, and the diagnosis is confirmed by angiography. When ulnar artery occlusion is present, revascularization and a digital sympathectomy may be beneficial. Gangrene of distal digits may occur and require surgical amputation.

Numerous drugs have been claimed to soften the hidebound skin, but documentation in controlled studies is lacking. These drugs include D-penicillamine, colchicine, *p*-aminobenzoic acid, and vitamin E. In a recent randomized, double-blind, placebo-controlled trial, recombinant human relaxin given by continuous subcutaneous infusion for 24 weeks was associated with reduced skin thickening and improved mobility in patients with moderate to severe diffuse cutaneous scleroderma. Relaxin, a hormone associated with pregnancy, has been shown to have antifibrotic properties. Dryness of the skin may be reduced by avoiding frequent use of detergent soaps and by regularly applying hydrophilic ointments and bath oils. Regular exercise helps to maintain flexibility of extremities and pliability of skin. Massaging the skin several times a day may also be beneficial. Fingertip ulcerations can be protected by applying a guard or cage over the end of the finger. The use of an occlusive dressing, such as the hydrocolloid duo-DERM or other membranes, over a noninfected ulcer may promote healing and protect the finger. Skin ulcers should be kept clean by soaking or by surgical or chemical debridement. Sympatholytic drugs or local nitroglycerine paste applied to or adjacent to the ulcer may be beneficial in promoting healing. Infected ulcers can usually be treated with topical antibiotics but may require systemic antibiotics, especially when there is a question of underlying osteomyelitis. The development of calcinosis cannot be prevented, nor can deposits be dissolved. Warfarin has been reported to reduce calcinosis in a few patients.

In patients experiencing dry mouth, frequent sips of water help to relieve symptoms. Pilocarpine hydrochloride tablets may increase salivary secretions in some patients. Patients with dry eyes should use artificial tears regularly.

Patients with reflux esophagitis are treated with small, frequent meals, antacids between meals, and elevation of the head of the bed. Patients should be advised not to lie down for a few hours after a meal and to avoid coffee, tea, alcohol, peppermint, and chocolate, which reduce the pressure of the lower esophageal sphincter. Fatty foods and late-evening snacks should be avoided. Cimetidine, ranitidine or other newer H_2 blockers may be beneficial. Gastric acid (proton) pump inhibitors are more effective in treating erosive esophagitis than are H_2 blockers. Metoclopramide and cisapride increase gastrointestinal motility but do not significantly improve esophageal motility. They both increase lower esophageal sphincter tone and can be of help in some patients. Cisapride is no longer available (as of July 2000) because it caused life-threatening arrhythmias. Nifedipine and, to a lesser extent, diltiazem reduce lower esophageal sphincter tone resulting in esophageal reflux. Patients with dysphagia should be instructed to chew their food thoroughly and wash it down with fluids. Malabsorption syndrome due to duodenal hypomotility and bacterial overgrowth causes bloating and diarrhea, which may improve with intermittent use of appropriate antibiotics. Antibiotics are rotated every 2 weeks. Commonly used antibiotics are metronidazole, vancomycin, erythromycin, ciprofloxacin, neomycin, and tetracycline. Patients with severe debilitating malabsorption may benefit from parenteral hyperalimentation. Patients with chronic intestinal pseudoobstruction might respond to octreotide. Stool softeners and mild laxatives are usually adequate for treating constipation caused by hypomotility of the colon.

Articular symptoms are treated with nonsteroidal anti-inflammatory agents. Low-dose prednisone ($\leq$10 mg/d) may improve symptoms in those not responding to these agents. Physical therapy may help to reduce the loss of joint mobility that occurs in SSc.

In patients with diffuse cutaneous SSc, the early recognition of alveolitis as previously described (see "Pulmonary Features") may allow treatment that might slow or prevent the development of pulmonary fibrosis. Cyclophosphamide has been reported in uncontrolled studies to be beneficial, and a controlled study is presently being done. The role of glucocorticoids in preventing progression of interstitial lung disease is not clear but may be of benefit in early disease. Pulmonary fibrosis is not reversible, and therefore treatment is directed at symptoms or complications. Pulmonary infection requires prompt treatment with antibiotics. Hypoxia necessitates giving low concentrations of oxygen. Patients should receive polyvalent pneumoccal vaccine (Pneumovax) and yearly influenza immunizations.

For patients with limited cutaneous SSc who develop isolated pulmonary arterial hypertension, treatment is limited. The usual treatment is supplemental oxygen, anticoagulation, and the administration of a vasodilator. A calcium channel blocker such as nifedipine lowers pulmonary arterial resistance and improves cardiac function, but in most patients this is only for a short period of time. Few patients survive more than 5 years. Heart-lung or single-lung transplantation may be a therapeutic option only in those patients without other significant systemic involvement. Current reports of intravenous epoprostenol (prostacyclin) in the treatment of SSc-associated pulmonary hypertension have been encouraging. Epoprostenol is infused continuously via a central line with a portable pump. Improvement in symptoms of right heart failure and exercise tolerance occurred. Also hemodynamic tests showed a decrease in the pulmonary vascular resistance and pulmonary artery pressure both in the short term and in a few patients after 1 or 2 years.

Recognition of early signs of renal hypertensive crisis is important in order to preserve renal function and prevent hypertensive encephalopathy. Renal involvement is often accompanied by hypertension and mild to moderate proteinuria. An occasional patient may be normotensive. Antihypertensive agents are often effective in lowering blood pressure and stabilizing or reversing renal failure. These drugs include propranolol, clonidine, and minoxidil. Particularly effective are the angiotensin-converting enzyme inhibitors, which include captopril, enalapril, and lisinopril. Dialysis may be required in patients with progressive renal failure. Some patients, however, have a slow return of renal function after several months and may no longer require dialysis. Patients are usually not candidates for kidney transplantation because of the other systemic manifestations of SSc.

Patients with cardiac failure require careful monitoring of digitalis and diuretic administration. Noninflammatory pericardial effusions may also improve with diuretics. Care should be taken to avoid overdiuresis, which may lead to decreased renal blood flow, decreased cardiac output, and renal failure.

MIXED CONNECTIVE TISSUE DISEASE MCTD is an overlap syndrome characterized by combinations of clinical features of SLE (Chap. 311), SSc, polymyositis (Chap. 382), and rheumatoid arthritis (Chap. 312) and the presence of very high titers of circulating autoantibodies to nuclear RNP antigen. This antibody in high titer, now referred to as *anti-U_1 RNP*, has been a justification for considering MCTD as a distinct clinical entity. MCTD has been challenged as a distinct disorder by those who consider it as a subset of SLE or scleroderma. Others prefer to classify MCTD as an undifferentiated connective tissue disease. MCTD occurs worldwide and in all races. The peak onset of disease is in the second and third decades, but MCTD is seen in children and the elderly. Women are predominantly affected. The pathogenic mechanisms in MCTD reflect the disorders making up this syndrome.

Clinical Features The presenting symptoms of MCTD are most often Raynaud's phenomenon, puffy hands, arthralgias, myalgias, and fatigue. Occasionally, patients may present with the acute onset of high fever, polymyositis, arthritis, and neurologic features such as trigeminal neuralgia and aseptic meningitis. The various features of the connective tissue disorders making up MCTD develop over months and years.

The fingers as well as the entire hand may be puffy, followed later by sclerodactyly. Sclerodermal changes are usually limited to the distal extremities and sometimes the face but spare the trunk. Telangiectasia and calcinosis may develop. Some patients have mucocutaneous features of SLE including a classic malar rash, photosensitivity, discoid lesions, alopecia, and painful oral ulcerations. An erythematous rash over the knuckles, elbows, and knees and heliotropic eyelids, typical of dermatomyositis, are uncommon.

Joint pain, stiffness, and swelling involving the peripheral joints occur frequently. Deformities of the hands similar to those of rheumatoid arthritis may develop but usually without bony erosions. A destructive polyarthritis is occasionally observed. Myalgias are a frequent symptom. Some patients develop typical symptoms of polymyositis with proximal muscle weakness, abnormal electromyographic findings, elevated levels of muscle enzymes, and inflammatory changes on muscle biopsy.

Approximately 85% of patients have pulmonary involvement, which is often asymptomatic. Diffusing capacity for carbon monoxide may be the only abnormality. Pleurisy commonly occurs but is seldom associated with large pleural effusions. Some patients develop interstitial lung disease. Pulmonary arterial hypertension is the most common cause of death in MCTD.

Approximately 25% of patients develop renal disease. Membranous glomerulonephritis is most common and usually mild but can cause nephrotic syndrome. Diffuse proliferative glomerulonephritis is unusual in MCTD, perhaps because of the protective role believed to be played by the high titers of anti-U_1 RNP. Renal crisis secondary to malignant renovasculature hypertension, as occurs in scleroderma, is seen in a few patients.

Gastrointestinal involvement is seen in ~70% of patients. The most common manifestations are esophageal dysmotility, lower esophageal sphincter laxity, and gastroesophageal reflux. Bowel manifestations mimic those of scleroderma bowel disease.

Pericarditis occurs in 30% of patients. Other cardiac features include myocarditis, arrhythmia, conduction disturbances, and mitral valve prolapse. Other clinical features of MCTD include trigeminal neuropathy, peripheral neuropathy, aseptic meningitis, lymphadenopathy, and Sjögren's syndrome. The majority of patients have developed, or will develop within 5 years of presentation, diagnostic clinical criteria for one of the overlapping connective tissue diseases, most often SLE or SSc.

Laboratory Findings Anemia of chronic inflammation is seen in the majority of patients. A positive direct Coombs' test is found in many patients, but hemolytic anemia is unusual. Leukopenia, thrombocytopenia, or both are present in some patients. Hypergammaglobulinemia is common, and rheumatoid factor is present in 50% of patients.

All patients, by definition of MCTD, have antibodies to U_1 RNP. The specificity of this antibody is to the 70-kDa protein complexed to small nuclear RNA. The anti-U_1 RNP antibodies are associated with HLA-DR4 but not with -DR2 and -DR3 as found in SLE. Molecular mimicry has been demonstrated between U_1 RNP and retroviral antigens by some laboratories.

℞ **TREATMENT** The treatment of MCTD is essentially the same as would be indicated for the respective connective tissue diseases defining this syndrome. More than half the patients have a favorable course. The 10-year survival rate overall is approximately 80% but varies depending on the connective tissue disease that may eventually develop.

EOSINOPHILIC FASCIITIS Eosinophilic fasciitis is a scleroderma-like syndrome of unknown cause characterized by inflammation followed later by sclerosis of the dermis, subcutis, and deep fascia. The disease affects adults and often occurs after strenuous physical activity. Patients do not have Raynaud's phenomenon or internal organ involvement. Several immunologic abnormalities have been associated with eosinophilic fasciitis and include aplastic anemia, myelodysplastic syndrome, and thrombocytopenia. Patients usually have the abrupt onset of symmetric tenderness and swelling of the extremities, rapidly followed by induration of the skin and subcutaneous tissue. The skin takes on a cobblestone or puckered appearance. Carpal tunnel syndrome appears early in the course, and flexion contractures develop later. A low-grade myositis is often present, but creatinine kinase levels are usually normal. A marked eosinophilia is found in the early stage of disease and subsequently decreases. Increased levels of polyclonal IgG and immune complexes are often present in the serum. A full-thickness biopsy consisting of skin, fascia, and superficial muscle shows perivascular infiltration of histiocytes, eosinophils, lymphocytes, and plasma cells. Biopsies later in the course show sclerosis. Spontaneous improvement and occasionally complete remission may occur after 2 to 5 years of disease. Some patients have persistent disease, while others are left with flexion contractures. Administration of glucocorticoids may provide symptomatic improvement and will decrease the eosinophilia. Improvement has been reported with the use of the H_2 blocker cimetidine.

EOSINOPHILIA-MYALGIA SYNDROME In 1989, reports of patients with scleroderma-like skin changes, myalgias, and eosinophilia dramatically increased. Most, but not all, of these cases were associated with ingestion of L-tryptophan manufactured by a single Japanese company. Batches of L-tryptophan implicated in EMS were found to contain trace amounts of a contaminant identified as a dimer of L-tryptophan that appeared in 1988 after changes were made in the method of manufacturing this drug. It is not clear whether this chemical contaminant is the etiologic agent or whether another unidentified substance is responsible. *L-Tryptophan products were taken off the market in 1990.* The onset of EMS can be either abrupt or insidious. In the early phases of the disease, clinical manifestations include low-grade fever, fatigue, dyspnea, cough, arthralgias/arthritis, evanescent erythematous rashes, muscle cramping, and severe myalgias. Pulmonary infiltrates may be present. Over the next 2 to 3 months, scleroderma-like skin changes appear. Some patients develop a peripheral neuropathy, which may persist. An ascending polyneuropathy may lead to paralysis and respiratory failure requiring ventilatory assistance. Cognitive dysfunction with impairment of memory and concentration has been recognized in this syndrome. Myocarditis and cardiac arrhythmias occur in some patients, and a few patients develop pulmonary hypertension. Approximately a third of patients have features of eosinophilic fasciitis. EMS most closely resembles toxic oil syndrome; however, Raynaud's phenomenon does not occur, and there is a lower prevalence of pulmonary hypertension and thromboembolic disease. The peripheral eosinophil count is $>1000/\mu L$ in most patients. The histologic findings on biopsy of skin, fascia, and superficial muscle are similar to those found in eosinophilic fasciitis. The clinical features of EMS may persist after L-tryptophan has been discontinued. EMS may run a chronic course, and response to therapy has been variable. Treatment has included glucocorticoids, antimalarial drugs, immunosuppressive drugs, and plasmapheresis. Prednisone was beneficial during the acute inflammatory phase of the disease in the majority of patients and resulted in resolution of pulmonary infiltrates, peripheral edema, and eosinophilia. In the later phase of the illness, no treatment was found to be of particular value. The pathogenesis of this disease is not known. A follow-up of patients 2 years after their onset of illness showed that most symptoms and physical findings had resolved or improved except for cognitive dysfunction, which became worse in approximately one-third of the patients, and peripheral neuropathy, which remained unchanged (Chap. 382).

BIBLIOGRAPHY

ARNETT FC: HLA and autoimmunity in scleroderma (systemic sclerosis). Int Rev Immunol 12:107, 1995

BENNETT RM: Mixed connective tissue disease and other overlap syndromes, in *Textbook of Rheumatology*, 5th ed, WN Kelley et al (eds). Philadelphia, Saunders, 1997, p 1065

BLACK CM: Systemic sclerosis: Management, in *Rheumatology*, 2 ed, JH Klippel, PA Dieppe (eds). London, Mosby International, 1998, 7:11.1

BOLSTER MB, SILVER RM: Assessment and management of scleroderma lung disease. Curr Opin Rheumatol 11:508, 1999

BORDRON A et al: The binding of some human antiendothelial cell antibodies induces endothelial cell apoptosis. J Clin Invest 101:2029, 1998

CARPENTIER PH, MARICQ HR: Microvasculature in systemic sclerosis. Rheum Dis Clin North Am 16:75, 1990

CLEMENTS PJ, FURST DE: Choosing appropriate patients with systemic sclerosis for treatment by autologous stem cell transplantation. J Rheumatol 24(Suppl 48):85, 1997

——— et al: High-dose versus low-dose D-penicillamine in early diffuse systemic sclerosis: Analysis of a two-year, double-blind, randomized, controlled clinical trial. Arthritis Rheum 42:1194, 1999

EVANS PC et al: Long-term fetal microchimerism in peripheral blood mononuclear cell subsets in healthy women and women with scleroderma. Blood 93:2033, 1999

HARVEY GR, MCHUGH NJ: Serologic abnormalities in systemic sclerosis. Curr Opin Rheumatol 11:495, 1999

HERTZMAN PA et al: The eosinophilia-myalgia syndrome: Status of 205 patients and results of treatment 2 years after onset. Ann Intern Med 122:851, 1995

KAHALEH B, MATUCCI-CERINIC M: Raynaud's phenomenon and scleroderma: Dysregulated neuroendothelial control of vascular tone. Arthritis Rheum 38:1, 1995

KLINGS ES et al: Systemic sclerosis–associated pulmonary hypertension: Short- and long-term effects of epoprostenol (prostacyclin). Arthritis Rheum 42:2638, 1999

LAKHANPAL S et al: Eosinophilic fasciitis: Clinical spectrum and therapeutic response in 52 cases. Semin Arthritis Rheum 17:221, 1988

LEROY EC: Pathogenesis of systemic sclerosis (scleroderma), in *Arthritis and Allied Conditions*, 13th ed, WJ Koopman (ed). Baltimore, Williams & Wilkins, 1997, p 1481

——— et al: Systemic sclerosis (scleroderma): Classification, subsets and pathogenesis. J Rheumatol 15:202, 1988

MCSWEENEY PA: High-dose immunosuppressive therapy for rheumatoid arthritis: Some answers, more questions. Arthritis Rheum 42:2269, 1999

MEDSGER TA JR: Systemic sclerosis (scleroderma), Clinical aspects, in *Arthritis and Allied Conditions*, 13th ed, WJ Koopman (ed). Baltimore, Williams & Wilkins, 1997, p 1433

NELSON JL: Microchimerism and the pathogenesis of systemic sclerosis. Curr Opin Rheumatol 10:564, 1998

POSTLETHWAITE AE: Role of T cells and cytokines in effecting fibrosis. Int Rev Immunol 12:247, 1995

REICHLIN M: Undifferentiated connective tissue diseases, overlap syndromes, and mixed connective tissue disease, in *Arthritis and Allied Conditions*, 13th ed, WJ Koopman (ed). Baltimore, Williams & Wilkins, 1997, p 1309

RENAUDINEAU Y et al: Anti-endothelial cell antibodies in systemic sclerosis. Clin Diagn Lab Immunol 6:156, 1999

ROSE S et al: Gastrointestinal manifestations of scleroderma. Gastroenterol Clin North Am 27:563, 1998

SATO S et al: Serum levels of connective tissue growth factor are elevated in patients with SSc: Association with extent of skin sclerosis and severity of pulmonary fibrosis. J Rheumatol 27:149, 2000

SEIBOLD JR: Scleroderma, in *Textbook of Rheumatology*, 5th ed, WN Kelley et al (eds). Philadelphia, Saunders, 1997, p 1133

SEIBOLD JR et al: Recombinant human relaxin in the treatment of scleroderma, a randomized, double-blind, placebo-controlled trial. Ann Intern Med 132:871, 2000

SILVER RM: Variant forms of scleroderma, in *Arthritis and Allied Conditions*, 13th ed, WJ Koopman (ed). Baltimore, Williams & Wilkins, 1997, p 1465

——— et al: Trytophan metabolism via the kyurenine pathway in patients with the esoinophilia myalgia syndrome. Arthritis Rheum 35:1097, 1992

STEEN VD: Renal involvement in systemic sclerosis. Clin Dermatol 12:253, 1994

———, MEDSGER TA: Case-control study of corticosteroids and other drugs that either precipitate or protect from the development of scleroderma renal crisis. Arthritis Rheum 41:1613, 1998

——— et al: Therapy for severe interstitial lung disease in systemic sclerosis. A retrospective study. Arthritis Rheum 37:1290, 1994

SUBCOMMITTEE FOR SCLERODERMA CRITERIA OF THE AMERICAN RHEUMATISM ASSOCIATION DIAGNOSTIC AND THERAPEUTIC CRITERIA COMMITTEE: Preliminary criteria for the classification of systemic sclerosis (scleroderma). Arthritis Rheum 23: 581, 1980

TAN FK et al: Association of microsatellite markers near the fibrillin 1 gene on human chromosome 15q with scleroderma in a Native American population. Arthritis Rheum 41:1729, 1998

VARGA J, BASHEY RI: Regulation of connective tissue synthesis in systemic sclerosis. Int Rev Immunol 12:187, 1995

V'AZQUEZ AD, ROTHFIELD NF: Autoantibodies in systemic sclerosis. Int Rev Immunol 12:145, 1995

314 SJÖGREN'S SYNDROME

Haralampos M. Moutsopoulos

DEFINITION Sjögren's syndrome is a chronic, slowly progressive autoimmune disease characterized by lymphocytic infiltration of the exocrine glands resulting in xerostomia and dry eyes. Approximately one-third of patients present with systemic manifestations. A small but significant number of the patients may develop malignant lymphoma. The disease can be seen alone (primary Sjögren's syndrome) or in association with other autoimmune rheumatic diseases (secondary Sjögren's syndrome) (Table 314-1).

INCIDENCE AND PREVALENCE The disease affects predominantly middle-aged women (female-to-male ratio 9:1), although it occurs in all ages, including childhood. The prevalence of primary Sjögren's syndrome is approximately 0.5 to 1.0%. In addition, 30% of patients with autoimmune rheumatic diseases suffer from secondary Sjögren's syndrome.

PATHOGENESIS Sjögren's syndrome is characterized by lymphocytic infiltration of the exocrine glands and B lymphocyte hyperreactivity, as illustrated by circulating autoantibodies. The latter is accompanied by an oligomonoclonal B cell process, which is characterized by serum and urine monoclonal light chains and cryoprecipitable monoclonal immunoglobulins.

Sera of patients with Sjögren's syndrome often contain a number of autoantibodies directed against non-organ-specific antigens such as immunoglobulins (rheumatoid factors) and extractable nuclear and cy-

Table 314-1 Association of Sjögren's Syndrome with Other Autoimmune Diseases

Rheumatoid arthritis	Primary biliary cirrhosis
Systemic lupus erythematosus	Vasculitis
Scleroderma	Chronic active hepatitis
Mixed connective tissue disease	

toplasmic antigens (Ro/SS-A, La/SS-B). Ro/SS-A autoantigen consists of three polypeptide chains (52, 54, and 60 kDa) in conjunction with RNAs, whereas the 48-kDa La/SS-B protein is bound to RNA III polymerase transcripts. The presence of autoantibodies to Ro/SS-A and La/SS-B antigens in Sjögren's syndrome is associated with earlier disease onset, longer disease duration, salivary gland enlargement, severity of lymphocytic infiltration of minor salivary glands, and certain extraglandular manifestations such as lymphadenopathy, purpura, and vasculitis. Antibodies to α-fordin (120 kDa), a salivary gland–specific protein, have recently been found in sera of patients with Sjögren's syndrome but not in sera of patients with other connective tissue diseases.

Phenotypic and functional studies have shown that the predominant cell infiltrating the affected exocrine glands is the helper/inducer T cell with characteristics of memory cells. Both B and T infiltrating lymphocytes are activated, as illustrated by production of immunoglobulins with autoantibody activity, spontaneous release of interleukin 2, and expression on the T cell surface of activation markers such as class II HLA as well as costimulatory molecules and lymphocyte function–associated antigen 1. Macrophages and natural killer cells are rarely detected in infiltrates, while epithelial cells of the affected glands inappropriately express class II molecules and possess messages for c-*myc* protooncogene and proinflammatory cytokines. All these phenomena suggest that the epithelial cell of the exocrine glands in Sjögren's syndrome may act as an antigen-presenting cell. In contrast to infiltrating lymphocytes, these cells undergo apoptotic death, resulting in exocrine gland dysfunction.

Immunogenetic studies have demonstrated that HLA-B8, -DR3, and -DRw52 are prevalent in patients with primary Sjögren's syndrome as compared with the normal control population. Molecular analysis of HLA class II genes has revealed that patients with Sjögren's syndrome, regardless of their ethnic origin, are highly associated with the HLA DQA1*0501 allele.

CLINICAL MANIFESTATIONS The majority of the patients with Sjögren's syndrome have symptoms related to diminished lacrimal and salivary gland function. In most patients, the primary syndrome runs a slow and benign course. The initial manifestations can be mucosal dryness or nonspecific, and 8 to 10 years elapse from the initial symptoms to full-blown development of the disease.

The principal oral symptom of Sjögren's syndrome is dryness (xerostomia). Patients complain of difficulty in swallowing dry food, inability to speak continuously, a burning sensation, increase in dental caries, and problems in wearing complete dentures. Physical examination shows a dry, erythematous, sticky oral mucosa. There is atrophy of the filiform papillae on the dorsum of the tongue, and saliva from the major glands is either not expressible or is cloudy. Enlargement of the parotid or other major salivary glands occurs in two-thirds of patients with primary Sjögren's syndrome but is uncommon in those with the secondary syndrome. Diagnostic tests include sialometry, sialography, and scintigraphy. The labial minor salivary gland biopsy permits histopathologic confirmation of the focal lymphocytic infiltrates.

Ocular involvement is the other major manifestation of Sjögren's syndrome. Patients usually complain of dry eyes, with a sandy or gritty feeling under the eyelids. Other symptoms include burning, accumulation of thick strands at the inner canthi, decreased tearing, redness, itching, eye fatigue, and increased photosensitivity. These symptoms are attributed to the destruction of corneal and bulbar conjunctival epithelium, defined as keratoconjunctivitis sicca. Diagnostic evaluation of keratoconjunctivitis sicca includes measurement of tear flow by Schirmer's I test and tear composition as assessed by the tear breakup time or tear lysozyme content. Slit-lamp examination of the cornea and conjunctiva after rose Bengal staining reveals punctate corneal ulcerations and attached filaments of corneal epithelium.

Involvement of other exocrine glands occurs less frequently and includes a decrease in mucous gland secretions of the upper and lower respiratory tree, resulting in dry nose, throat, and trachea (xerotrachea), and diminished secretion of the exocrine glands of the gastrointestinal tract, leading to esophageal mucosal atrophy, atrophic gastritis, and subclinical pancreatitis. Dyspareunia due to dryness of the external genitalia and dry skin also may occur.

Extraglandular (systemic) manifestations are seen in one-third of patients with Sjögren's syndrome (Table 314-2), while they are very rare in patients with Sjögren's syndrome associated with rheumatoid arthritis. These patients complain more often of easy fatigability, low-grade fever, Raynaud's phenomenon, myalgias, and arthralgias. Most patients with primary Sjögren's syndrome experience at least one episode of nonerosive arthritis during the course of their disease. Manifestations of pulmonary involvement are frequent but rarely important clinically. Dry cough is the major manifestation that is attributed to small airway disease. Renal involvement includes interstitial nephritis, clinically manifested by hypostenuria and renal tubular dysfunction with or without acidosis. Untreated acidosis may lead to nephrocalcinosis. Glomerulonephritis is a rare finding that occurs in patients with systemic vasculitis, cryoglobulinemia, or systemic lupus erythematosus overlapping with Sjögren's syndrome. Vasculitis affects small and medium-sized vessels. The most common clinical features are purpura, recurrent urticaria, skin ulcerations, glomerulonephritis, and mononeuritis multiplex. Sensorineural hearing loss was found in one-half of patients with Sjögren's syndrome and correlated with the presence of anticardiolipin antibodies.

It has been suggested that primary Sjögren's syndrome with vasculitis also may present with multifocal, recurrent, and progressive nervous system disease, such as hemiparesis, transverse myelopathy, hemisensory deficits, seizures, and movement disorders. Aseptic meningitis and multiple sclerosis also have been reported in these patients.

Lymphoma is a well-known manifestation of Sjögren's syndrome that usually presents later in the illness. Persistent parotid gland enlargement, lymphadenopathy, cutaneous vasculitis, peripheral neuropathy, lymphopenia, and cryoglobulinemia are manifestations suggesting the development of lymphoma. Most lymphomas are extranodal, marginal zone B cell, and low grade. Salivary glands are the most common site of involvement.

Routine laboratory tests reveal mild normochromic, normocytic anemia. An elevated erythrocyte sedimentation rate is found in approximately 70% of patients.

DIAGNOSIS AND DIFFERENTIAL DIAGNOSIS A European multicenter study has developed diagnostic criteria of Sjögren's syndrome (Table 314-3), which have been validated and present high specificity and sensitivity. A diagnostic algorithm is depicted in Fig. 314-1.

Table 314-2 Incidence of Extraglandular Manifestations in Primary Sjögren's Syndrome

Clinical Manifestation	Percent
Arthralgias/arthritis	60
Raynaud's phenomenon	37
Lymphadenopathy	14
Lung involvement	14
Vasculitis	11
Kidney involvement	9
Liver involvement	6
Lymphoma	6
Splenomegaly	3
Peripheral neuropathy	2
Myositis	1

Table 314-3 Diagnostic Criteria for Sjögren's Syndrome[a]

Criteria	Definitions
1. Ocular symptoms	Dry eyes every day for more than 3 months, recurrent sensation of sand or gravel in the eyes, or use of tear substitutes more than three times a day
2. Oral symptoms	Daily feeling of dry mouth for more than 3 months, recurrent or persistently swollen salivary glands, or use of liquids to aid in swallowing dry food
3. Ocular signs	Positive Schirmer's I test (<5 mm in 5 min), or a rose Bengal score of ≥4 according to van Bijsterveld's scoring system
4. Histopathology	Focus score 1 in a minor salivary gland biopsy
5. Salivary gland involvement	Positive result in one of the following tests: salivary scintigraphy, parotid sialography, salivary flow (≤1.5 mL in 15 min)
6. Autoantibodies	Antibodies to Ro(SS-A) or La(SS-B), antinuclear antibodies, or rheumatoid factor

[a] Probable Sjögren's syndrome: three items are present.
Definite Sjögren's syndrome: four or more items are present.

The differential diagnosis of Sjögren's syndrome includes other conditions that may cause dry mouth or eyes or parotid salivary gland enlargement (Table 314-4). Infections with HIV and hepatitis C virus (Chap. 309) and sarcoidosis (Chap. 318) appear to produce a clinical picture indistinguishable from that of Sjögren's syndrome (Table 314-5).

Rx **TREATMENT** Sjögren's syndrome remains fundamentally an incurable disease. Hence treatment is aimed at symptomatic relief and limiting the damaging local effects of chronic xerostomia and keratoconjunctivitis sicca by substitution of the missing secretions.

The sicca complex is treated with fluid replacement supplied as often as necessary. To replace deficient tears, there are several readily available ophthalmic preparations (Tearisol; Liquifilm; 0.5% methylcellulose; Hypo Tears). It may be necessary for severely affected patients to use these preparations as often as every 30 min. If corneal ulceration is present, eye patching and boric acid ointments are recommended. Certain drugs that may increase lacrimal and salivary hy-

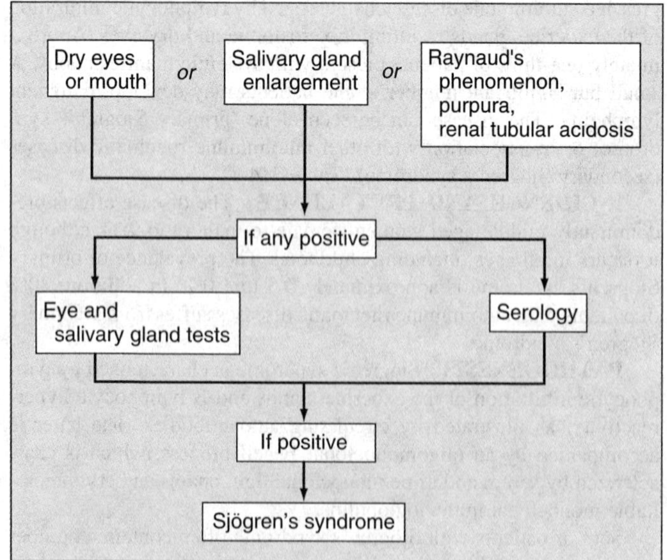

FIGURE 314-1 Algorithm for the diagnosis of Sjögren's syndrome.

Table 314-4 Differential Diagnosis of Sicca Symptoms

Xerostomia	Dry Eye	Bilateral Parotid Gland Enlargement
Viral infections	Inflammation	Viral infections
Drugs	Stevens-Johnson syndrome	Mumps
Psychotherapeutic	Pemphigoid	Influenza
Parasympatholytic	Chronic conjunctivitis	Epstein-Barr
Antihypertensives	Chronic blepharitis	Coxsackievirus A
Psychogenic	Sjögren's syndrome	Cytomegalovirus
Irradiation	Toxicity	HIV
Diabetes mellitus	Burns	Sarcoidosis
Trauma	Drugs	Amyloidosis
Sjögren's syndrome	Neurologic conditions	Sjögren's syndrome
	Impaired lacrimal gland function	Metabolic
	Impaired eyelid function	Diabetes mellitus
	Miscellaneous	Hyperlipoproteinemias
	Trauma	Chronic pancreatitis
	Hypovitaminosis A	Hepatic cirrhosis
	Blink abnormality	Endocrine
	Lid scarring	Acromegaly
	Anesthetic cornea	Gonadal hypofunction
	Epithelial irregularity	

Table 314-5 Differential Diagnosis of Sjögren's Syndrome with HIV Infection

HIV Infection and Sicca Syndrome	Sjögren's Syndrome	Sarcoidosis
Predominant in young males	Predominant in middle-aged women	Invariable
Lack of autoantibodies to Ro/SS-A and/or La/SS-B	Presence of autoantibodies	Lack of autoantibodies to Ro/SS-A and/or La/SS-B
Lymphoid infiltrates of salivary glands by CD8+ lymphocytes	Lymphoid infiltrates of salivary glands by CD4+ lymphocytes	Granulomas in salivary glands
Association with HLA-DR5	Association with HLA-DR3 and -DRw52	Unknown
Positive serologic tests for HIV	Negative serologic tests for HIV	Negative serologic tests for HIV

pofunction such as diuretics, antihypertensive drugs, and antidepressants should be avoided. Propionic acid gels may be used to treat vaginal dryness.

Pilocarpine (5 mg thrice daily) given orally appears to improve sicca manifestations. Hydroxychloroquine (200 mg/day) is helpful for arthralgias. Glucocorticoids (1 mg/kg per day) or other immunosuppressive agents (i.e., cyclophosphamide) are indicated for the treatment of extraglandular manifestations, particularly when renal or severe pulmonary involvement and systemic vasculitis have been documented.

BIBLIOGRAPHY

DAFNI UG et al: Prevalence of Sjögren's syndrome in a closed rural community. Ann Rheum Dis 56:521, 1997

HANEJI N et al: Identification of alpha-fodrin as a candidate autoantigen in primary Sjögren's syndrome. Science 276:604, 1997

MANOUSSAKIS MN et al: Expression of B7 costimulatory molecules by salivary gland epithelial cells in patients with Sjögren's syndrome. Arthritis Rheum 42:229, 1999

PAPIRIS SA et al: Lung involvement in Sjögren's syndrome. Semin Respir Crit Care Med 20, 179, 1999

POLIHRONIS M et al: Modes of epithelial cell death and repair in Sjögren's syndrome. Clin Exp Immunol 114:485, 1998

TUMIATI B et al: Hearing loss in the Sjögren syndrome. Ann Intern Med 126:450, 1997

TZIOUFAS AG, MOUTSOPOULOS HM: Sjögren's syndrome, in *Rheumatology*, JH Klippel, PA Dieppe (eds). London, Mosby, 1998

315

Joel D. Taurog, Peter E. Lipsky

ANKYLOSING SPONDYLITIS, REACTIVE ARTHRITIS, AND UNDIFFERENTIATED SPONDYLOARTHROPATHY

The spondyloarthropathies are a group of disorders that share certain clinical features and an association with the HLA-B27 allele. These disorders include ankylosing spondylitis, Reiter's syndrome, reactive arthritis, psoriatic arthritis and spondylitis, enteropathic arthritis and spondylitis, juvenile-onset spondyloarthropathy, and undifferentiated spondyloarthropathy. The similarities in clinical manifestations and genetic predisposition suggest that these disorders share pathogenic mechanisms. Specific definitions and diagnostic criteria for the individual conditions will be provided in subsequent sections of this chapter.

ANKYLOSING SPONDYLITIS

Ankylosing spondylitis (AS) is an inflammatory disorder of unknown cause that primarily affects the axial skeleton; peripheral joints and extraarticular structures may also be involved. The disease usually begins in the second or third decade; the prevalence in men is approximately three times that in women. It is considered the prototype of the spondyloarthropathies. Older names include *Marie-Strümpell disease* or *Bechterew's disease*.

EPIDEMIOLOGY AS shows a striking correlation with the histocompatibility antigen HLA-B27 and occurs worldwide roughly in proportion to the prevalence of this antigen (Chap. 306). In North American Caucasians, the general prevalence of B27 is 7%, whereas over 90% of patients with AS have inherited this antigen. The association with B27 is independent of disease severity.

In population surveys, 1 to 6% of adults inheriting B27 have been found to have AS. In contrast, in families of patients with AS, the prevalence is 10 to 30% among adult first-degree relatives inheriting B27. The concordance rate in identical twins is estimated to exceed 65%. It is currently believed that susceptibility to AS is determined almost entirely by genetic factors, with as yet unidentified allelic genes in addition to B27 comprising about two-thirds of the genetic component and B27 itself comprising about one-third. AS is strongly associated with inflammatory bowel disease (IBD), including both ulcerative colitis and Crohn's disease. IBD is a risk factor for AS independent of HLA-B27, although 50 to 75% of patients with both AS and IBD are B27 positive. →*See also Chap. 287.*

PATHOLOGY The *enthesis*, the site of ligamentous attachment to bone, is thought to be the primary site of pathology in AS, particularly in the lesions around the pelvis and spine. Enthesitis is associated with prominent edema of the adjacent bone marrow and is often characterized by erosive lesions that eventually undergo ossification.

Sacroiliitis is usually one of the earliest manifestations of AS, with features of both enthesitis and synovitis. The early lesions consist of subchondral granulation tissue containing lymphocytes, plasma cells, mast cells, macrophages, and chondrocytes; infiltrates of lymphocytes and macrophages in ligamentous and periosteal zones; and subchondral bone marrow edema. Synovitis follows and may progress to pannus formation. Islands of new bone formation can be found within the inflammatory infiltrates. Usually, the thinner iliac cartilage is eroded before the thicker sacral cartilage. The irregularly eroded, sclerotic margins of the joint are gradually replaced by fibrocartilage regeneration and then by ossification. Ultimately, the joint may be totally obliterated. This progression is evident by imaging techniques (see below).

In the spine, early in the process there is inflammatory granulation tissue at the junction of the annulus fibrosus of the disk cartilage and the margin of vertebral bone. The outer annular fibers are eroded and eventually replaced by bone, forming the beginning of a bony excrescence called a *syndesmophyte*, which then grows by continued enchondral ossification, ultimately bridging the adjacent vertebral bodies. Ascending progression of this process leads to the "bamboo spine" observed radiographically. Other lesions in the spine include diffuse osteoporosis, erosion of vertebral bodies at the disk margin, "squaring" of vertebrae, and inflammation and destruction of the disk-bone border. Inflammatory arthritis of the apophyseal joints is common, with erosion of cartilage by pannus, often followed by bony ankylosis.

Bone mineral density is significantly diminished in the spine and proximal femur early in the course of the disease, before the advent of significant immobilization. The mechanism for this is not known.

Peripheral arthritis in AS can show synovial hyperplasia, lymphoid infiltration, and pannus formation, but the process lacks the exuberant synovial villi, fibrin deposits, ulcers, and accumulations of plasma cells seen in rheumatoid arthritis (Chap. 312). Central cartilaginous erosions caused by proliferation of subchondral granulation tissue are common in AS but rare in rheumatoid arthritis.

Acute anterior uveitis (iritis) occurs in at least 20% of patients with AS. Few cases have been studied histologically, none at an early stage. After recurrent attacks, the iris shows nonspecific inflammatory changes, scarring, increased vascularity, and pigment-laden macrophages. Pupillary synechiae and cataract formation are common sequelae.

Aortic insufficiency develops in a small percentage of cases. There is thickening of the aortic valve cusps and the aorta near the sinuses of Valsalva, with dense adventitial scar tissue and intimal fibrous proliferation. The scar tissue can extend into the ventricular septum with resultant heart block.

Microscopic inflammatory lesions of the colon and ileocecal valve have been found in 25 to 50% of patients with AS, even in those lacking any clinical evidence of IBD. IgA nephropathy has been reported with increased frequency.

PATHOGENESIS The pathogenesis of AS is incompletely understood. A number of features of the disease implicate immune-mediated mechanisms, including elevated serum levels of IgA and acute-phase reactants, inflammatory histology, and close association with HLA-B27. The inflamed sacroiliac joint is infiltrated with CD4+ and CD8+ T cells and macrophages and shows high levels of tumor necrosis factor α. Transforming growth factor β is detectable near the sites of new bone formation. No specific event or exogenous agent that triggers the onset of disease has been identified, although overlapping features with reactive arthritis and IBD suggest that enteric bacteria may play a role. Elevated serum titers of antibodies to certain enteric bacteria, particularly *Klebsiella pneumoniae*, are common in AS patients, but no role for these antibodies in the pathogenesis of AS has been identified. Evidence that B27 plays a direct role is provided by the finding that rats transgenic for B27 spontaneously develop spondylitis, along with colitis, peripheral arthritis, and other lesions characteristic of the spondyloarthropathies (see below).

Some evidence has accumulated for autoimmunity to the cartilage proteoglycan aggrecan, and particularly its G1 globulin domain and link protein. AS patients have been found to have cellular immunity to these molecules, and mice immunized with the G1 domain develop spondylitis and discitis. Sharing of proteoglycan antigenic epitopes among the pathologic sites in the skeleton, uveal tract, and aorta in AS suggests a possible explanation for the distribution of pathologic sites in AS.

CLINICAL MANIFESTATIONS The symptoms of the disease are usually first noticed in late adolescence or early adulthood; the median age in western countries is 23 in both genders. In 5% of patients, symptoms begin after age 40. The initial symptom is usually dull pain, insidious in onset, felt deep in the lower lumbar or gluteal region, accompanied by low-back morning stiffness of up to a few hours' duration that improves with activity and returns following periods of inactivity. Within a few months of onset, the pain has usually become persistent and bilateral. Nocturnal exacerbation of pain that forces the patient to rise and move around may be frequent.

In some patients bony tenderness may accompany back pain or stiffness, while in others it may be the predominant complaint. Common sites include the costosternal junctions, spinous processes, iliac crests, greater trochanters, ischial tuberosities, tibial tubercles, and heels. Occasionally, bony chest pain is the presenting complaint. Arthritis in the hips and shoulders ("root" joints) occurs in 25 to 35% of patients, in many cases early in the disease course. Arthritis of peripheral joints other than the hips and shoulders, usually asymmetric, occurs in up to 30% of patients and can occur at any stage of the disease. Neck pain and stiffness from involvement of the cervical spine are usually relatively late manifestations. Occasional patients, particularly in the older age group, present with predominantly constitutional symptoms such as fatigue, anorexia, fever, weight loss, or night sweats.

AS often has a juvenile onset in developing countries. In these individuals, peripheral arthritis and enthesitis usually predominate, with axial symptoms supervening in late adolescence.

The most common extraarticular manifestation is acute anterior uveitis, which can antedate the spondylitis. Attacks are typically unilateral, causing pain, photophobia, and increased lacrimation. These tend to recur, often in the opposite eye. Cataracts and secondary glaucoma are not uncommon sequelae. Aortic insufficiency, sometimes producing symptoms of congestive heart failure, occurs in a few percent of patients, occasionally early in the course of the spinal disease. Third-degree heart block may occur alone or together with aortic insufficiency. The block is in the atrioventricular node in 95% of cases. Up to half the patients have inflammation in the colon or ileum. This is usually asymptomatic, but in 5 to 10% of patients with AS, frank IBD will develop.

Initially, physical findings mirror the inflammatory process. The most specific findings involve loss of spinal mobility, with limitation of anterior and lateral flexion and extension of the lumbar spine and of chest expansion. Limitation of motion is usually out of proportion to the degree of bony ankylosis, reflecting muscle spasm secondary to pain and inflammation. Pain in the sacroiliac joints may be elicited either with direct pressure or with maneuvers that stress the joints, but these techniques are unreliable in discriminating inflammatory sacroiliitis. In addition, there is commonly tenderness upon palpation at the sites of symptomatic bony tenderness and paraspinous muscle spasm.

The Schober test is a useful measure of flexion of the lumbar spine. The patient stands erect, with heels together, and marks are made directly over the spine 5 cm below and 10 cm above the lumbosacral junction (identified by a horizontal line between the posterosuperior iliac spines.) The patient then bends forward maximally, and the distance between the two marks is measured. The distance between the two marks increases 5 cm or more in the case of normal mobility and less than 4 cm in the case of decreased mobility. Chest expansion is measured as the difference between maximal inspiration and maximal forced expiration in the fourth intercostal space in males or just below the breasts in females. Normal chest expansion is 5 cm or greater.

Limitation or pain with motion of the hips or shoulders is usually present if either of these joints is involved. Careful examination is also necessary to detect inflammatory disease of peripheral joints. It should be emphasized that early in the course of mild cases, symptoms may be subtle and nonspecific, and the physical examination may be completely normal.

The course of the disease is extremely variable, ranging from the individual with mild stiffness and radiographically equivocal sacroiliitis to the patient with a totally fused spine and severe bilateral hip arthritis, possibly accompanied by severe peripheral arthritis and extraarticular manifestations. Pain tends to be persistent early in the disease and then to become intermittent, with alternating exacerbations and quiescent periods. In a typical severe untreated case with progression of the spondylitis to syndesmophyte formation, the patient's posture undergoes characteristic changes. The lumbar lordosis is obliterated with accompanying atrophy of the buttocks. The thoracic kyphosis is accentuated. If the cervical spine is involved, there may be a forward stoop of the neck. Hip involvement with ankylosis may lead to flexion contractures, compensated by flexion at the knees. The progression of the disease may be followed by measuring the patient's height, chest expansion, Schober test, and occiput-to-wall distance when the patient stands erect with the heels and back flat against the wall. Occasional individuals are encountered with advanced physical findings suggestive of long-standing AS who report having never had significant symptoms.

In some but not all studies, onset of the disease in adolescence correlates with a worse prognosis, but there is general agreement that early severe hip involvement is an indication of progressive disease. The disease in women tends to progress less frequently to total spinal ankylosis, although there is some evidence for an increased prevalence of isolated cervical ankylosis and peripheral arthritis in women. In industrialized countries, peripheral arthritis (distal to hips and shoulders) occurs overall in about 25% of patients, usually as a late manifestation, whereas in developing countries, the prevalence is much higher, with onset typically early in the disease course. Pregnancy has no consistent effect on AS, with symptoms improving, remaining the same, or deteriorating in about one-third of pregnant patients, respectively.

The most serious complication of the spinal disease is spinal fracture, which can occur with even minor trauma to the rigid, osteoporotic spine. The cervical spine is most commonly involved. These fractures are often displaced and cause spinal cord injury. Cauda equina syndrome and slowly progressive upper pulmonary lobe fibrosis are rare complications of long-standing AS. The prevalence of aortic insufficiency and of cardiac conduction disturbances, including third-degree heart block, increases with prolonged disease. Subclinical pulmonary lesions and cardiac dysfunction may be relatively common. Prostatitis has been reported to have an increased prevalence in men with AS. Amyloidosis is only rarely associated (Chap. 319).

Several validated measures of disease activity and functional outcome have recently been developed for AS. Despite the persistence of the disease, most patients remain gainfully employed. The effect of AS on survival is controversial. Some, but not all, studies have suggested that AS shortens life span, compared with the general population. Mortality attributable to AS is largely the result of spinal trauma, aortic insufficiency, respiratory failure, amyloid nephropathy, or complications of therapy such as upper gastrointestinal hemorrhage.

LABORATORY FINDINGS No laboratory test is diagnostic of AS. In most ethnic groups, the HLA-B27 gene is present in approximately 90% of patients with AS. Most, but not all, patients with active disease have an elevated erythrocyte sedimentation rate and an elevated level of C-reactive protein. A mild normochromic, normocytic anemia may be present. Patients with severe disease may show an elevated alkaline phosphatase level. Elevated serum IgA levels are common. Rheumatoid factor and antinuclear antibodies are largely absent unless caused by a coexistent disease. Synovial fluid from inflamed peripheral joints in AS is not distinctly different from that of other inflammatory joint diseases. In cases with restriction of chest wall motion, decreased vital capacity and increased functional residual capacity are common, but airflow measurements are normal and ventilatory function is usually well maintained.

RADIOGRAPHIC FINDINGS Radiographically demonstrable sacroiliitis is usually present in AS. The earliest changes in the sacroiliac joints demonstrable by standard radiography are blurring of the cortical margins of the subchondral bone, followed by erosions and sclerosis. Progression of the erosions leads to "pseudowidening" of the joint space; as fibrous and then bony ankylosis supervene, the joints may become obliterated radiographically. The changes and progression of the lesions are usually symmetric.

Roentgenographic abnormalities generally appear in the sacroiliac joints before appearing elsewhere in the spine. In the lumbar spine, progression of the disease leads to straightening, caused by loss of lordosis, and reactive sclerosis, caused by osteitis of the anterior corners of the vertebral bodies with subsequent erosion, leading to "squaring" of the vertebral bodies. Progressive ossification of the superficial layers of the annulus fibrosus leads to eventual formation of marginal syndesmophytes, visible on plain films as bony bridges connecting successive vertebral bodies anteriorly and laterally.

In mild cases, years may elapse before unequivocal sacroiliac abnormalities are evident on plain radiographs. Computed tomography (CT) and magnetic resonance imaging (MRI) can detect abnormalities reliably at an earlier stage than plain radiography. MRI has emerged as a highly sensitive and specific technique for identifying early intra-articular inflammation, cartilage changes, and underlying bone marrow edema in sacroiliitis (Fig. 315-1). In suspected cases in which conventional radiography does not reveal definite sacroiliac abnormalities or is undesirable (e.g., in young women or children), dynamic MRI is the procedure of choice for establishing a diagnosis of sacroiliitis.

Reduced bone mineral density can be detected by dual-energy x-ray absorptiometry of the femoral neck and the lumbar spine. Falsely elevated readings related to spinal ossification can be avoided by using a lateral projection of the L3 vertebral body.

DIAGNOSIS The diagnosis of early AS before the development of irreversible deformity can be difficult to establish. Currently, modified New York criteria (1984) are widely used for diagnosis. These consist of the following: (1) a history of inflammatory back pain (see below); (2) limitation of motion of the lumbar spine in both the sagittal and frontal planes; (3) limited chest expansion, relative to standard values for age and sex; and (4) definite radiographic sacroiliitis. Using these criteria, the presence of radiographic sacroiliitis plus any one of the other three criteria is sufficient for a diagnosis of definite AS. These

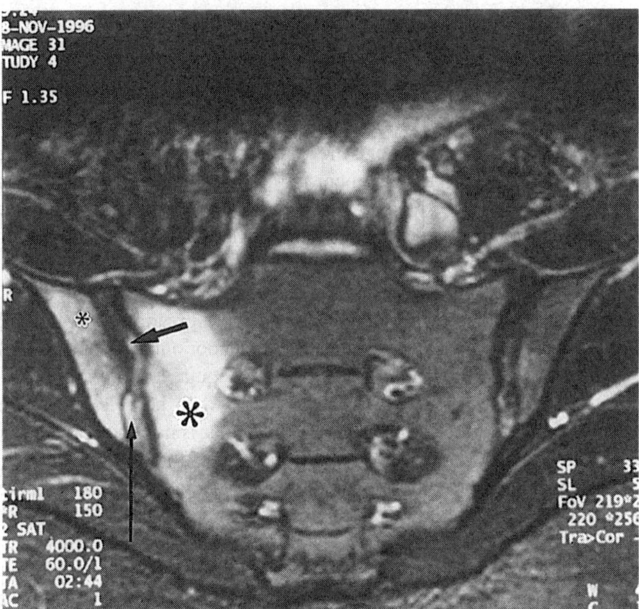

FIGURE 315-1 Early sacroiliitis of ankylosing spondylitis. Magnetic resonance imaging of the sacroiliac joints of a 23-year-old woman with progressive right-sided inflammatory back pain of 6 months' duration. Conventional radiographs were normal. A fat-suppressed image employing a short tau inversion recovery (STIR) sequence shows acute sarcoiliitis on the right side, with edema in the juxtaarticular bone marrow (*asterisks*), in the region of the synovium and joint capsule (*thin arrow*), and in the region of the interosseous ligaments (*thick arrow*). Early chronic changes, including cortical erosions and joint space widening, were evident in the right sacroiliac joint in T1-, contrast-enhanced T1-, and T2*-weighted images (not shown). The patient subsequently developed radiographically evident bilateral sacroiliitis fulfilling the criteria for ankylosing spondylitis. *(Photo provided by Dr. Jürgen Braun, Freie Universität Berlin; previously published in Zeitschrift für Rheumatologie 58:61, 1999. Reproduced with permission.)*

criteria may need to be further modified to include sacroiliitis demonstrated by MRI to increase their sensitivity.

The presence of B27 is neither necessary nor sufficient for the diagnosis, but the B27 test can be helpful in patients with suggestive clinical findings who have not yet developed radiographic sacroiliitis. Moreover, the absence of B27 in a typical case of AS significantly increases the probability of coexistent IBD.

AS must be differentiated from numerous other causes of low-back pain, some of which are far more common than AS. The inflammatory back pain of AS is usually distinguished by the following five features: (1) age of onset below 40, (2) insidious onset, (3) duration greater than 3 months before medical attention is sought, (4) morning stiffness, and (5) improvement with exercise or activity. The most common causes of back pain other than AS are primarily mechanical or degenerative rather than inflammatory and do not show these features. Less common metabolic, infectious, and malignant causes of back pain also must be differentiated from AS. Ochronosis can produce a phenotype that is clinically and radiographically similar to AS.

Marked calcification and ossification of paraspinous ligaments occur in *diffuse idiopathic skeletal hyperostosis* (DISH). Although DISH is often categorized as a variant of osteoarthritis, diarthrodial joints are not involved. Ligamentous calcification and ossification are usually most prominent in the anterior spinal ligament and give the appearance of "flowing wax" on the anterior bodies of the vertebrae. However, a radiolucency may be seen between the newly deposited bone and the vertebral body, differentiating DISH from the marginal osteophytes in spondylosis. Intervertebral disk spaces are preserved, and sacroiliac and apophyseal joints appear normal, helping to differentiate DISH from spondylosis and from AS, respectively.

DISH occurs in the middle-aged and the elderly and is more common in men than in women. Patients are frequently asymptomatic but may have stiffness. Radiographic changes are generally much more severe than might be predicted from the mild symptoms caused by DISH.

℞ **TREATMENT** There is no definitive treatment for AS. The principal goal of management is the conscientious participation by the patient in an exercise program designed to maintain functional posture and to preserve range of motion. There is evidence that exercise increases mobility and improves function. The proportion of patients wtih severe deformity has decreased markedly in recent decades, probably because of earlier diagnosis and widespread use of physical therapy. Smoking has been associated with a poor outcome and should be emphatically discouraged. Most patients require anti-inflammatory agents to achieve sufficient symptomatic relief to be able to remain functional and carry out the exercise program. It is not known whether drug treatment alone can alter the progression of the disease.

Several nonsteroidal anti-inflammatory drugs (NSAIDs) have proved effective in reducing the pain and stiffness of AS and are commonly used. Indomethacin is particularly effective as a 75-mg slow-release preparation taken once or twice daily. Although phenylbutazone, at doses of 200 to 400 mg/d, has been considered the most effective anti-inflammatory agent in AS, because of its greater potential for serious side effects such as aplastic anemia and agranulocytosis, its use in the United States is confined to patients with very severe disease whose symptoms do not respond at all to other agents. Recent controlled trials suggest that sulfasalazine,[1] in doses of 2 to 3 g/d, is useful in reducing peripheral joint symptoms as well as reversing laboratory evidence of inflammation. Some studies have not shown it to benefit axial arthritis, and its effect on natural progression of the disease is unproven. The peripheral arthritis may also respond to the folic acid antagonist methotrexate.[1] No therapeutic role for gold, penicillamine, immunosuppressive drugs, or oral glucocorticoids has been documented in AS. Occasionally, intralesional or intraarticular glucocorticoid injections may be beneficial in patients with persistent enthesopathy or synovitis unresponsive to anti-inflammatory agents. Recent studies have suggested that symptomatic benefit can be achieved from CT-guided glucocorticoid injections into the sacroiliac joints, but the effects are not sustained. Anecdotal benefit has been reported for diverse agents such as pamidronate, thalidomide, pulse intravenous methylprednisolone, and tumor necrosis factor α antagonists. Controlled trials of these and other agents are needed, since for many patients current therapy is inadequate even for control of pain and stiffness.

The most common indication for surgery in patients with AS is severe hip joint arthritis, the pain and stiffness of which are usually dramatically relieved by total hip arthroplasty. A small number of patients may benefit from surgical correction of extreme flexion deformities of the spine or of atlantoaxial subluxation.

Attacks of iritis are usually effectively managed with local glucocorticoid administration in conjunction with mydriatic agents, although systemic glucocorticoids or even immunosuppressive drugs may be required in some cases. Coexistent cardiac disease may require pacemaker implantation and/or aortic valve replacement.

REACTIVE ARTHRITIS AND UNDIFFERENTIATED SPONDYLOARTHROPATHY

Reactive arthritis (ReA) refers to acute nonpurulent arthritis complicating an infection elsewhere in the body. In recent years, the term has been used primarily to refer to spondyloarthropathies following enteric or urogenital infections and occurring predominantly in individuals with the histocompatibility antigen HLA-B27. Included in this category is the constellation of clinical findings formerly commonly called *Reiter's syndrome*. →***Other forms of reactive and infection-related arthritis not associated with B27 and showing a different spectrum of clinical features, such as rheumatic fever or Lyme disease, are discussed in Chaps. 235 and 176.***

HISTORIC BACKGROUND The association of acute arthritis with episodes of diarrhea or urethritis has been recognized for centuries. A large number of cases during World Wars I and II focused attention on the triad of arthritis, urethritis, and conjunctivitis, which became known as Reiter's syndrome, often occurring with additional mucocutaneous lesions.

The identification of bacterial species capable of triggering the clinical syndrome and the finding that up to 85% of the patients possess the B27 antigen have led to the unifying concept of ReA as a clinical syndrome triggered by specific etiologic agents in a genetically susceptible host. A similar spectrum of clinical manifestations can be triggered by enteric infection with any of several *Shigella*, *Salmonella*, *Yersinia*, and *Campylobacter* species, by genital infection with *Chlamydia trachomatis*; and possibly by other agents as well. Although Reiter's syndrome can be said to represent one part of the spectrum of the clinical manifestations of ReA, particularly that induced by *Shigella* or *Chlamydia*, the term is now largely of historic interest only. Since most patients with spondyloarthropathy do not have the classic features of Reiter's syndrome, it has become customary to employ the term *reactive arthritis*, regardless of whether or not there is evidence for a triggering infection. For the purposes of this chapter, the use of ReA will be restricted to those cases of spondyloarthropathy in which there is at least presumptive evidence for a related antecedent infection. Patients with clinical features of ReA who lack both evidence of an antecedent infection and the classic findings of Reiter's syndrome (urethritis, arthritis, conjunctivitis) will be considered to have *undifferentiated spondyloarthropathy*, which is discussed at the end of this chapter.

EPIDEMIOLOGY Like AS, ReA occurs predominantly in individuals who have inherited the B27 gene; in most series, 60 to 85% of patients are B27 positive. In epidemics of arthritogenic bacterial

[1]Azathioprine, methotrexate, and sulfasalazine have not been approved for this purpose by the U.S. Food and Drug Administration at the time of publication.

infection, e.g., *S. flexneri*, it has been estimated that ReA develops in ~20% of exposed B27-positive individuals. In families with multiple cases of AS or ReA, the two conditions have been said to "breed true," i.e., to be uncommonly found together within an individual family. Whether this is caused by genetic or environmental factors is not known. The disease is most common in individuals 18 to 40 years of age, but it can occur both in children over 5 years of age and in older adults.

The sex ratio in ReA following enteric infection is nearly 1:1, whereas venereally acquired ReA is predominantly confined to men. The overall prevalence and incidence of ReA are difficult to assess because of the variable prevalence of the triggering infections and genetic susceptibility factors in different populations. For example, in Olmsted County, MN, the incidence was estimated as 3.5 cases per 100,000 population per year. In contrast, in a population with a high rate of genitourinary and/or gastrointestinal infections such as urban homosexual and bisexual men, the prevalence may approach 1 per 1000.

A particularly severe form of peripheral spondyloarthropathy has been described in patients with AIDS (Chap. 309). Most of these patients are HLA-B27 positive, but HIV infection per se is not an independent risk factor for spondyloarthropathy.

PATHOLOGY Synovial histology is similar to that of other inflammatory arthropathies. Enthesitis is a common clinical finding in ReA; the histology of this lesion resembles that of AS. Microscopic histopathologic evidence of inflammation has occasionally been noted in the colon and ileum of patients with postvenereal ReA, but much less commonly than in postenteric ReA. The skin lesions of keratoderma blenorrhagica, which is associated mainly with venereally acquired ReA, are histologically indistinguishable from psoriatic lesions.

ETIOLOGY AND PATHOGENESIS The first bacterial infection noted to be causally related to ReA was *S. flexneri*. An outbreak of shigellosis among Finnish troops in 1944 resulted in numerous cases of ReA. Of the four species *S. sonnei*, *S. boydii*, *S. flexneri*, and *S. dysenteriae*, *S. flexneri* has most often been implicated in cases of ReA, both sporadic and epidemic. *S. sonnei*, although responsible for the majority of cases of shigellosis in the United States, has only rarely been implicated in cases of ReA.

Other bacteria that have been definitively identified as triggers of ReA include several *Salmonella* spp., *Y. enterocolitica*, *C. jejuni*, and *C. trachomatis*. There is suggestive evidence implicating several other microorganisms, including *Y. pseudotuberculosis*, *Clostridium difficile*, and *Ureaplasma urealyticum*. *Chlamydia pneumoniae*, a respiratory pathogen, has also recently been implicated in triggering ReA. There are also numerous isolated reports of acute arthritis preceded by other bacterial, viral, or parasitic infections, but whether the microorganisms involved are actual triggers of ReA remains to be determined.

It has not been determined whether ReA occurs by the same pathogenic mechanism following infection with each of these microorganisms, nor has the mechanism been fully elucidated in the case of any one of the known bacterial triggers. Most, if not all, of the triggering organisms produce lipopolysaccharide (LPS) and share a capacity to attack mucosal surfaces, to invade host cells, and survive intracellularly. Antigens from *Chlamydia*, *Yersinia*, *Salmonella*, and *Shigella* have been shown to be present in the synovium and/or synovial fluid leukocytes of patients with ReA for long periods following the acute attack. In ReA triggered by *Y. enterocolitica*, bacterial LPS and heat shock protein antigens have been found in peripheral blood cells years after the triggering infection. In the case of *C. trachomatis*, synovial persistence of microbial DNA and RNA suggests the presence of viable organisms, despite uniform failure to culture the organism from these specimens. There is thus evidence that ReA, at least in some cases, may be a form of chronic infection, rather than solely "reactive." T cells that specifically respond to antigens of the inciting organism are typically found in inflamed synovium but not in peripheral blood of patients with ReA. These T cells are predominantly CD4+, but CD8+ B27-restricted bacteria-specific cytolytic T cells have also been isolated in *Yersinia*- and *C. trachomatis*-induced ReA. Specific peptide antigens from these organisms have been identified as dominant T cells epitopes. Unlike the synovial CD4 T cells in rheumatoid arthritis, which are predominantly of the T_H1 phenotype, those in ReA also show a T_H2 phenotype. It is likely that antigen-specific T cells play an important role in the pathogenesis of ReA, but the precise mechanisms remain to be determined.

The role of HLA-B27 in ReA also remains to be determined. Transgenic rats with high expression of B27 spontaneously develop a multiple organ system inflammatory disease affecting the gut, peripheral and axial joints, male genital tract, and skin that resembles these human conditions clinically and histologically. When raised in a germ-free environment, the B27 rats do not develop gut or joint inflammation, but the skin and genital lesions are not prevented. These findings suggest that bacteria are necessary, and normal gut bacteria are sufficient, to induce B27-related joint inflammation. In both the rat and human diseases, it remains to be determined whether the primary process is an autoimmune response against host tissues or an immune response against antigens of the triggering organism that have disseminated to the target tissues, and the specific role of B27 itself remains to be determined. A potentially very informative converse observation, in which humans develop a disease process resembling one first described in rats, is the recent finding that 0.4 to 0.8% of individuals treated with intravesicular bacillus Calmette-Guérin for bladder cancer develop reactive arthritis, and 60% of these patients are B27 positive. The process closely mimics adjuvant-induced arthritis in rats given complete Freund's adjuvant, first described over 40 years ago, which is currently thought to be mediated by CD4+ T cells specific for mycobacterial heat shock protein.

An intriguing in vitro finding indicates that the presence of HLA-B27 significantly prolongs the intracellular survival of *Y. enterocolitica*, and *S. enteritides* in human and mouse cell lines. A unifying hypothesis suggests that prolonged intracellular bacterial survival, promoted by B27, other factors, or both, permits trafficking of infected leukocytes from the site of primary infection to joints, where a T cell response to persistent bacterial antigens promotes arthritis. Evidence exists supporting each step of this scheme.

CLINICAL FEATURES The clinical manifestations of ReA constitute a spectrum that ranges from an isolated, transient monarthritis to severe multisystem disease. In the majority of cases, a careful history will elicit some evidence of an antecedent infection 1 to 4 weeks before the onset of symptoms of the reactive disease. However, in a sizable minority, no clinical or laboratory evidence of an antecedent infection can be found. In many cases of presumed venereally acquired reactive disease, there is a history of a recent new sexual partner, even in the absence of laboratory evidence of infection.

Constitutional symptoms are common, including fatigue, malaise, fever, and weight loss. The musculoskeletal symptoms are usually acute in onset. Arthritis is usually asymmetric and additive, with involvement of new joints occurring over a period of a few days to 1 to 2 weeks. The joints of the lower extremities, especially the knee, ankle, and subtalar, metatarsophalangeal, and toe interphalangeal joints, are the most common sites of involvement, but the wrist and fingers can be involved as well. The arthritis is usually quite painful, and tense joint effusions are not uncommon, especially in the knee. Dactylitis, or "sausage digit," a diffuse swelling of a solitary finger or toe, is a distinctive feature of both ReA and psoriatic arthritis (Chap. 324). It is not specific, however, in that it is also seen in polyarticular gout and sarcoidosis. Tendinitis and fasciitis are particularly characteristic lesions, producing pain at multiple insertion sites, especially the Achilles insertion, the plantar fascia, and sites along the axial skeleton. Spinal and low-back pain are quite common and may be caused by insertional inflammation, muscle spasm, acute sacroiliitis, or, presumably, arthritis in intervertebral articulations.

Urogenital lesions may occur throughout the course of the disease. In males, urethritis may be marked or relatively asymptomatic and may be either an accompaniment of the triggering infection or a result of the reactive phase of the disease. Prostatitis is also common. Similarly, in females, cervicitis or salpingitis may be caused either by the infectious trigger or by the sterile reactive process.

Ocular disease is common, ranging from transient, asymptomatic conjunctivitis to an aggressive anterior uveitis that occasionally proves refractory to treatment and may result in blindness.

Mucocutaneous lesions are frequent. Oral ulcers tend to be superficial, transient, and often asymptomatic. The characteristic skin lesions, *keratoderma blenorrhagica*, consist of vesicles that become hyperkeratotic, ultimately forming a crust before disappearing. They are most common on the palms and soles but may occur elsewhere as well. In patients with HIV infection, these lesions are often extremely severe and extensive, to the point of dominating the clinical picture (Chap. 309). Lesions on the glans penis, termed *circinate balanitis*, are common; these consist of vesicles that quickly rupture to form painless superficial erosions, which in circumcised individuals can form crusts similar to those of keratoderma blenorrhagica. Nail changes are common and consist of onycholysis, distal yellowish discoloration, and/or heaped-up hyperkeratosis.

Less frequent or rare manifestations of ReA include cardiac conduction defects, aortic insufficiency, central or peripheral nervous system lesions, and pleuropulmonary infiltrates.

Long-term follow-up studies suggest that some joint symptoms persist in 30 to 60% of patients with ReA. Recurrences of the acute syndrome are common, and as many as 25% of patients either become unable to work or are forced to change occupations because of persistent joint symptoms. Chronic heel pain is often a particularly distressing symptom. Some aspects of ankylosing spondylitis are also common sequelae (see below). In some but not all studies, HLA-B27-positive patients have shown a worse outcome than B27-negative patients. The extent to which the long-term prognosis varies with different inciting agents is not known. However, patients with *Yersinia*-induced arthritis appear to have less chronic disease than those whose initial episode follows epidemic shigellosis.

LABORATORY AND RADIOGRAPHIC FINDINGS The erythrocyte sedimentation rate is usually elevated during the acute phase of the disease. Mild anemia may be present, and acute-phase reactants tend to be increased. Synovial fluid is nonspecifically inflammatory, showing an elevated white cell count with a predominance of neutrophils. In most ethnic groups, 50 to 75% of the patients are B27 positive. It is unusual for the triggering infection to persist at the site of primary mucosal infection through the time of onset of the reactive disease, but it may occasionally be possible to culture the organism, e.g., in the case of *Yersinia*- or *Chlamydia*-induced disease. Serologic evidence of a recent infection may be present, such as a marked elevation of antibodies to *Yersinia, Salmonella*, or *Chlamydia*.

In early or mild disease, radiographic changes may be absent or confined to juxtaarticular osteoporosis. With long-standing persistent disease, marginal erosions and loss of joint space can be seen in affected joints. Periostitis with reactive new bone formation is characteristic of the disease, as it is with all the spondyloarthropathies. Spurs at the insertion of the plantar fascia are common.

Sacroiliitis and spondylitis may be seen as late sequelae. The sacroiliitis is more commonly asymmetric than in AS, and the spondylitis, rather than ascending symmetrically from the lower lumbar segments, can begin anywhere along the lumbar spine. The syndesmophytes may be coarse and nonmarginal, arising from the middle of a vertebral body, a pattern rarely seen in primary AS. Progression to spinal fusion as a sequela of ReA is uncommon.

DIAGNOSIS ReA is a clinical diagnosis, there being no definitively diagnostic laboratory test or radiographic finding. The diagnosis should be entertained in any patient with an acute inflammatory, asymmetric, additive arthritis or tendinitis. The evaluation of such a patient should include careful questioning regarding possible antecedent triggering events such as an episode of diarrhea or dysuria. On physical examination, careful attention must be paid to the distribution of the joint and tendon involvement and to possible sites of extraarticular involvement, such as the eyes, mucous membranes, skin, nails, and genitalia. Synovial fluid aspiration and analysis may be helpful in excluding septic or crystal-induced arthritis. Culture or serology may help to identify a triggering infection. The role of molecular methods of microbial detection has not been established (see below).

Although typing for B27 is not needed to secure the diagnosis in clear-cut cases, it may have prognostic significance in terms of severity, chronicity, and the propensity for spondylitis and uveitis. Furthermore, it can be helpful diagnostically in atypical cases, a positive test increasing and a negative test decreasing the probability of ReA.

It is particularly important to differentiate ReA from disseminated gonococcal disease, both of which can be venereally acquired and associated with urethritis (Chap. 147). Gonococcal arthritis and tenosynovitis tend to involve both upper and lower extremities equally, whereas in ReA lower extremity symptoms usually predominate. Back pain is common in ReA but is not a feature of gonococcal disease, whereas the vesicular skin lesions characteristic of disseminated gonococcal disease are not found in ReA. A positive gonococcal culture from the urethra or cervix does not exclude a diagnosis of ReA; however, culturing gonococci from blood, skin lesion, or synovium establishes the diagnosis of disseminated gonococcal disease. Polymerase chain reaction (PCR) technology has recently been used in the diagnosis of infections with *Neisseria gonorrheae* and with *C. trachomatis*. Occasionally, the only definitive way to distinguish the two is through a therapeutic trial of antibiotics.

ReA shares many features in common with psoriatic arthropathy, including the asymmetry of the arthritis, a propensity for "sausage digits" and nail involvement, an association with uveitis, and skin lesions of similar histology (Chap. 324). However, psoriatic arthritis is usually gradual in onset, the arthritis tends to affect primarily the upper extremities, and there is less associated periarthritis. Psoriatic arthritis is not associated with mouth ulcers or urethritis, or, usually, with bowel symptoms. Although psoriatic arthropathy shows some distinctive radiographic features that are not found in ReA, these occur only late in the disease and are of little help diagnostically. Only psoriatic spondylitis, not the peripheral arthritis, is associated with B27, about 50% of patients being positive. Occasional patients, usually B27 positive, following what appears to be a typical episode of ReA, will develop typical psoriasis and persistent arthritis such that the two entities become indistinguishable.

Undifferentiated spondyloarthropathy, or simply "spondyloarthropathy," is diagnosed in patients who lack evidence of an antecedent infection that might trigger ReA and who do not meet criteria for AS but who show clinical features of these disorders.

℞ **TREATMENT** Most patients with ReA are benefitted to some degree by NSAIDs, although rarely are symptoms of the acute arthritis completely ameliorated, and some patients fail to respond at all. Indomethacin, 75 to 150 mg/d in divided doses, is the initial treatment of choice. Other NSAIDs may be tried, with phenylbutazone, 100 mg tid or qid, being the NSAID of last resort, to be used only in severe, refractory cases because of its potentially serious side effects.

It is unclear whether antibiotics have a role in the therapy of ReA. One controlled study suggested that prolonged administration of a long-acting tetracycline may accelerate recovery from *Chlamydia*-induced ReA, but subsequent results have been less encouraging, and therapy for other bacterial triggers of ReA has shown little or no benefit. However, there is evidence that prompt, appropriate antibiotic treatment of acute chlamydial urethritis may prevent subsequent ReA. Currently, expert opinion supports the use of antibiotic therapy in established urogenital ReA but not in gastrointestinal ReA.

Two recent multicenter trials have suggested that sulfasalazine, up to 3 g/d in divided doses, may be beneficial to patients with persistent ReA.[1] Patients with debilitating symptoms refractory to NSAID and sulfasalazine therapy may respond to immunosuppressive agents such as azathioprine, 1 to 2 mg/kg per day, or to methotrexate, 7.5 to

15 mg per week. Systemic glucocorticoids are not generally recommended but in rare instances may be helpful in mobilizing a severely affected bedridden patient. Antimalarials, gold, and penicillamine are not useful in the treatment of ReA. Trials of new agents proven useful in rheumatoid arthritis, such as COX-2 inhibitors, leflunomide, and tumor necrosis factor α inhibitors, remain to be implemented.

Tendinitis and other enthesitic lesions occasionally may benefit from intralesional glucocorticoids. Uveitis may require aggressive treatment with glucocorticoids to prevent serious sequelae. Skin lesions ordinarily require only symptomatic treatment. In patients with HIV infection and ReA, many of whom have severe skin lesions, the skin lesions in particular appear to respond to systemic treatment with anti-retroviral agents (Chap. 309). Cardiac complications are managed conventionally; management of neurologic complications is symptomatic.

Patients need to be educated about the nature of the disease and the factors that predispose to its recurrence. Comprehensive management includes counseling of patients in the avoidance of sexually transmitted disease and exposure to enteropathogens, as well as appropriate use of physical therapy, vocational counseling, and continued surveillance for long-term complications such as ankylosing spondylitis.

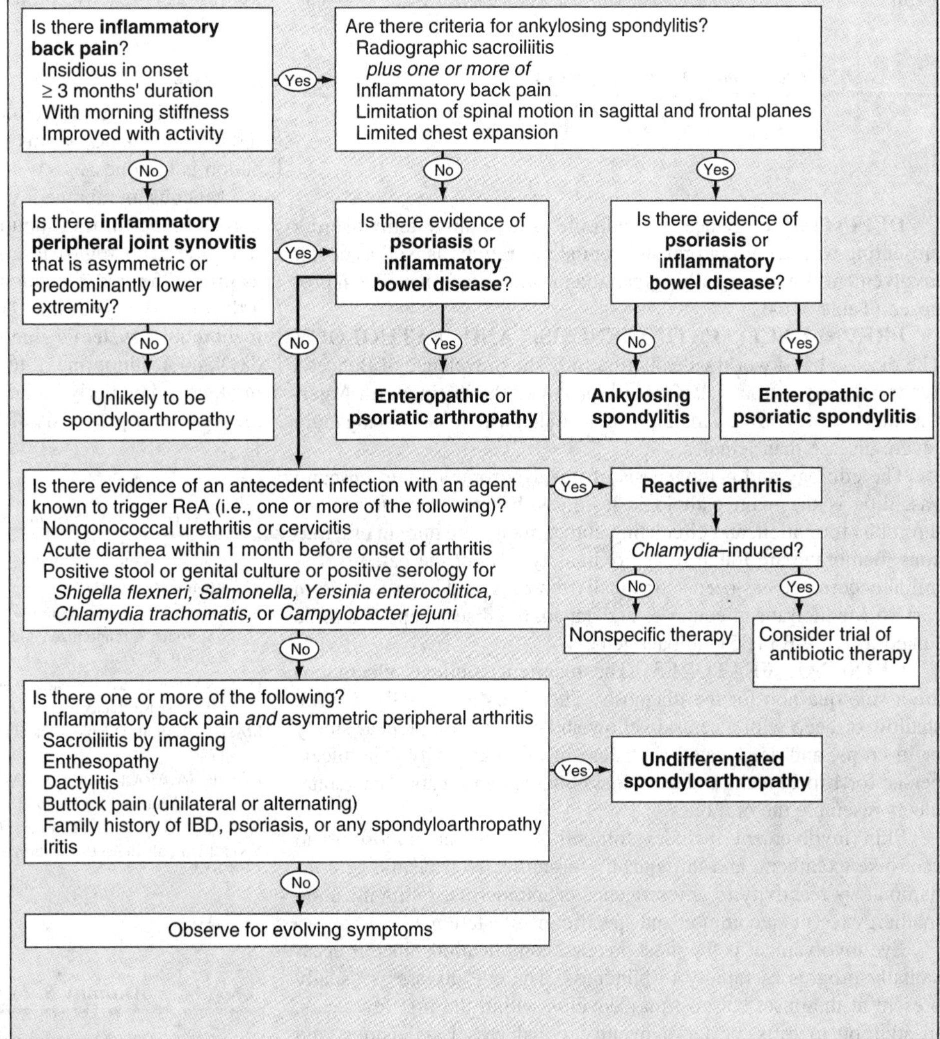

FIGURE 315-2 Algorithm for diagnosis of the spondyloarthropathies.

UNDIFFERENTIATED AND JUVENILE-ONSET SPONDYLOARTHROPATHY

It is not uncommon for clinicians to encounter patients, usually young adults, who do not have IBD or psoriasis, lack evidence of an antecedent triggering infection, and do not have the classic triad of Reiter's syndrome or meet criteria for ankylosing spondylitis, who nonetheless present with some features of one or more of the spondyloarthropathies discussed above. For example, a patient may present with inflammatory synovitis of one knee, Achilles tendinitis, and dactylitis of one digit ("sausage digit"), or sacroiliitis in the absence of other criteria for AS. It is now common to consider such patients as having *undifferentiated spondyloarthropathy*, or simply *spondyloarthropathy*. Other terms for this condition have included *seronegative oligoarthritis*, *undifferentiated oligoarthritis*, and the now-outmoded *incomplete Reiter's syndrome*. There is strong evidence that some, perhaps most, of these patients have ReA in which the triggering infection remains clinically silent. In some other cases, the patient subsequently develops IBD or psoriasis or the process eventually meets criteria for ankylosing spondylitis. Approximately half the patients with undifferentiated spondyloarthropathy are HLA-B27 positive, and thus the absence of B27 is not useful in establishing or excluding the diagnosis.

In *juvenile-onset spondyloarthropathy*, which begins most commonly in boys (60 to 80%) between ages 7 and 16, an asymmetric, predominantly lower extremity oligoarthritis and enthesitis without extraarticular features is the typical mode of presentation. The prevalence of B27 in this condition, which has been termed the *SEA syndrome* (*s*eronegative, *e*nthesopathy, *a*rthropathy), is approximately 80%. Many, but not all, of these patients go on to develop typical ankylosing spondylitis in late adolescence or adulthood.

Management of undifferentiated spondyloarthropathy is similar to that of the other spondyloarthropathies, with NSAIDs and physical therapy forming the mainstays of treatment. Textbooks of pediatrics should be consulted for information on management of juvenile-onset spondyloarthropathy. An algorithm for the diagnosis of the spondyloarthropathies in adults is presented in Fig. 315-2.

BIBLIOGRAPHY

Bergfeldt L: HLA-B27-associated cardiac disease. Ann Intern Med 127:621, 1997

Braun J et al: Prevalence of spondylarthropathies in HLA-B27 positive and negative blood donors. Arthritis Rheum 41:58, 1998

——— et al: Radiologic diagnosis and pathology of spondyloarthropathies. Rheum Dis Clin North Am 24:697, 1998

Brown MA et al: Susceptiblity to ankylosing spondylitis in twins: The role of genes, HLA, and the environment. Arthritis Rheum 40:1823, 1997

Calin A, Taurog JD (eds): *The Spondyloarthritides*. Oxford, Oxford Univ Press, 1998

Dougados M et al: Spondylarthropathy treatment: Progress in medical treatment, physical therapy and rehabilitation. Baillieres Clin Rheumatol 12:717, 1998

Gladman DD: Psoriatic arthritis. Rheum Dis Clin North Am 24:829, 1998

Lee YS et al: Skeletal status of men with early and late ankylosing spondylitis. Am J Med 103:233, 1997

Power WJ et al: Outcomes in anterior uveitis associated with the HLA-B27 haplotype. Ophthalmology 105:1646, 1998

316

Haralampos M. Moutsopoulos

BEHÇET'S SYNDROME

DEFINITION Behçet's syndrome is a multisystem disorder presenting with recurrent oral and genital ulcerations as well as ocular involvement. Internationally agreed diagnostic criteria have been proposed (Table 316-1).

PREVALENCE, PATHOGENESIS, AND PATHOLOGY The disease has a worldwide distribution. The prevalence of Behçet's syndrome ranges from 1:10,000 in Japan to 1:500,000 in North America and Europe. It affects mainly young adults, with males having more severe disease than females.

The etiology and pathogenesis of this syndrome remain obscure; vasculitis is the main pathologic lesion with a tendency to venous thrombus formation, and circulating autoantibodies to human oral mucous membrane are found in approximately 50% of the patients. Familial occurrence has been sporadically reported; and in patients from eastern Mediterranean countries and Japan, the disease appears to be linked to HLA-B5 (B51) alloantigens.

CLINICAL FEATURES The recurrent aphthous ulcerations are a sine qua non for the diagnosis. The ulcers are usually painful, shallow or deep with a central yellowish necrotic base, appear singly or in crops, and are located anywhere in the oral cavity. The ulcers persist for 1 to 2 weeks and subside without leaving scars. The genital ulcers resemble the oral ones.

Skin involvement includes folliculitis, erythema nodosum, an acne-like exanthem, and infrequently vasculitis. Nonspecific skin inflammatory reactivity to any scratches or intradermal saline injection (pathergy test) is a common and specific manifestation.

Eye involvement is the most dreaded complication, since it occasionally progresses rapidly to blindness. The eye disease is usually present at the onset but also may develop within the first few years. In addition to iritis, posterior uveitis, retinal vessel occlusions, and optic neuritis can be seen in some patients with the syndrome. Hypopyon uveitis, which is considered the hallmark of Behçet's syndrome, is in fact a rare manifestation.

The arthritis of Behçet's syndrome is not deforming and affects the knees and ankles.

Superficial or deep peripheral vein thrombosis is seen in one-fourth of the patients. Pulmonary emboli are a rare complication. The superior vena cava is obstructed occasionally, producing a dramatic clinical picture. Arterial involvement occurs infrequently and presents with aortitis or peripheral arterial aneurysm and arterial thrombosis. Pulmonary artery vasculitis presenting with dyspnea, cough, chest pain, hemoptysis, and infiltrates on chest roentgenograms has been reported recently in 5% of patients.

Central nervous system involvement is found more frequently in patients from northern Europe and the United States. The most common lesions are benign intracranial hypertension, a multiple sclerosis–like picture, pyramidal involvement, and psychiatric disturbances.

Gastrointestinal involvement is reported in patients from Japan and includes mucosal ulcerations of the gut.

Laboratory findings are mainly nonspecific indices of inflammation such as leukocytosis and elevated erythrocyte sedimentation rate as well as C-reactive protein levels; antibodies to human oral mucosa are also found.

Table 316-1 Diagnostic Criteria of Behçet's Disease

Recurrent oral ulceration plus two of the following:
- Recurrent genital ulceration
- Eye lesions
- Skin lesions
- Pathergy test

℞ **TREATMENT** The severity of the syndrome usually abates with time. Apart from the patients with neurologic complications, the life expectancy seems to be normal, and the only serious complication is blindness.

Mucous membrane involvement may respond to topical glucocorticoids in the form of mouthwash or paste. In more serious cases thalidomide (100 mg/d) is effective. Thrombophlebitis is treated with aspirin, 325 mg/d. Colchicine or interferon α can be beneficial for the arthritis of the syndrome. Uveitis and central nervous system involvement require systemic glucocorticoid therapy (prednisone, 1 mg/kg per day) and azathioprine, 2 to 3 mg/kg per day, or cyclosporine, 5 to 10 mg/kg per day. Early initiation of azathioprine tends to favorably affect the long-term prognosis of Behçet's syndrome.

BIBLIOGRAPHY

HAMURYUDAN V et al: Systemic interferon α2b treatment in Behçet's syndrome. J Rheumatol 21:1098, 1994

——— et al: Azathioprine in Behçet's syndrome: Effects on long-term prognosis. Arthritis Rheum 40:769, 1997

——— et al: Thalidomide in the treatment of the mucocutaneous lesions of the Behçet syndrome. A randomized double-blind, placebo-controlled trial. Ann Intern Med 128: 443, 1998

INTERNATIONAL STUDY GROUP FOR BEHÇET'S DISEASE: Criteria of diagnosis of Behçet's disease. Lancet 335:1078, 1990

MASUDA K et al: Double masked trial of cyclosporin in Behçet's disease. Lancet 1:1093, 1989

PAPIRIS SA, MOUTSOPOULOS HM: Rare rheumatic disorders: Behçet's disease. Baillieres Clin Rheumatol 7:173, 1993

SAKANE T et al: Behçet's disease. N Engl J Med 341:1284, 1999

YAZICI H et al: Behçet's syndrome. Curr Opin Rheumatol 11:53, 1999

317

Anthony S. Fauci

THE VASCULITIS SYNDROMES

AIL angiocentric immunoproliferative lesions	IFN interferon
	IL interleukin
ANCA antineutrophil cytoplasmic antibodies	PAN classic polyarteritis nodosa
	TNF tumor necrosis factor
ELAM-1 endothelial-leukocyte adhesion molecule 1	VCAM-1 vascular cell adhesion molecule 1
ESR erythrocyte sedimentation rate	WBC white blood count

DEFINITION *Vasculitis* is a clinicopathologic process characterized by inflammation of and damage to blood vessels. The vessel lumen is usually compromised, and this is associated with ischemia of the tissues supplied by the involved vessel. A broad and heterogeneous group of syndromes may result from this process, since any type, size, and location of blood vessel may be involved. Vasculitis and its consequences may be the primary or sole manifestation of a disease; alternatively, vasculitis may be a secondary component of another primary disease. Vasculitis may be confined to a single organ such as the skin, or it may simultaneously involve several organ systems.

CLASSIFICATION OF VASCULITIC SYNDROMES A major feature of the vasculitic syndromes as a group is the fact that there is a great deal of heterogeneity at the same time as there is considerable overlap among them. This has led to both difficulty and confusion with regard to the categorization of these diseases. The classification scheme listed in Table 317-1 takes into account this heterogeneity and overlap and will serve as a matrix to emphasize the fact that certain syndromes are predominantly systemic in nature and almost invariably lead to irreversible organ system dysfunction and even

Table 317-1 Classification of the Vasculitis Syndromes

I. Systemic necrotizing vasculitis
  A. Polyarteritis nodosa (PAN)
    1. Classic PAN
    2. Microscopic polyangiitis
  B. Allergic angiitis and granulomatosis of Churg-Strauss
  C. Polyangiitis overlap syndrome
II. Wegener's granulomatosis
III. Temporal arteritis
IV. Takayasu's arteritis
V. Henoch-Schönlein purpura
VI. Predominantly cutaneous vasculitis (hypersensitivity vasculitis)
  A. Exogenous stimuli proven or suspected
    1. Drug-induced vasculitis
    2. Serum sickness and serum sickness–like reactions
    3. Vasculitis associated with infectious diseases
  B. Endogenous antigens likely involved
    1. Vasculitis associated with neoplasms (particularly lymphoid malignancies)
    2. Vasculitis associated with connective tissue diseases
    3. Vasculitis associated with other underlying diseases
    4. Vasculitis associated with congenital deficiencies of the complement system
VII. Other vasculitic syndromes
  A. Kawasaki disease
  B. Isolated central nervous system vasculitis
  C. Thromboangiitis obliterans (Buerger's disease)
  D. Behçet's syndrome
  E. Miscellaneous vasculitides

death if untreated, while others are usually localized to the skin and rarely result in irreversible dysfunction of vital organs. The distinguishing and overlapping features of the diseases listed in Table 317-1, which justify this classification scheme, will be discussed below.

PATHOPHYSIOLOGY AND PATHOGENESIS Generally, most of the vasculitic syndromes are assumed to be mediated at least in part by immunopathogenic mechanisms (Table 317-2). However, evidence to this effect is for the most part indirect and may reflect epiphenomena as opposed to true causality.

Pathogenic Immune-Complex Formation Vasculitis is generally considered within the broader category of *immune-complex diseases* that include serum sickness and certain of the connective tissue diseases of which systemic lupus erythematosus (Chap. 311) is the prototype. Although deposition of immune complexes in vessel walls is the most widely accepted pathogenic mechanism of vasculitis, the causal role of immune complexes has not been clearly established in most of the vasculitic syndromes. Circulating immune complexes need not result in deposition of the complexes in blood vessels with ensuing vasculitis, and many patients with active vasculitis do not have demonstrable circulating or deposited immune complexes. The actual antigen contained in the immune complex has only rarely been identified in vasculitic syndromes. In this regard, hepatitis B antigen has been identified in both the circulating and deposited immune complexes in a subset of patients with systemic vasculitis, most notably within the polyarteritis nodosa group (see below). Essential mixed cryoglobulinemia has been associated with hepatitis C virus infection; hepatitis C virions and hepatitis C virus antigen-antibody complexes have been identified in the cryoprecipitates of these patients. An association between persistent parvovirus B19 infection and certain vasculitides has been reported; however, the pathogenic mechanisms related to this association are unclear.

Table 317-2 Potential Mechanisms of Vessel Damage in Vasculitis Syndromes

Pathogenic immune complex formation and/or deposition
  Henoch-Schönlein purpura
  Vasculitis associated with collagen vascular diseases
  Serum sickness and cutaneous vasculitis syndromes
  Hepatitis C–associated essential mixed cryoglobulinemia
  Hepatitis B–associated polyarteritis nodosa
Production of antineutrophilic cytoplasmic autoantibodies
  Wegener's granulomatosis
  Churg-Strauss syndrome
  Microscopic polyangiitis
Pathogenic T lymphocye responses and granuloma formation
  Temporal arteritis
  Takayasu's arteritis
  Wegener's granulomatosis
  Churg-Strauss syndrome
  Kawasaki disease

SOURCE: Adapted from MC Sneller, AS Fauci: Med Clin North Am 81:221, 1997.

The mechanisms of tissue damage in immune complex–mediated vasculitis resemble those described for serum sickness. In this model, antigen-antibody complexes are formed in antigen excess and are deposited in vessel walls whose permeability has been increased by vasoactive amines such as histamine, bradykinin, and leukotrienes released from platelets or from mast cells as a result of IgE-triggered mechanisms. The deposition of complexes results in activation of complement components, particularly C5a, which is strongly chemotactic for neutrophils. These cells then infiltrate the vessel wall, phagocytose the immune complexes, and release their intracytoplasmic enzymes, which damage the vessel wall. As the process becomes subacute or chronic, mononuclear cells infiltrate the vessel wall. The common denominator of the resulting syndrome is compromise of the vessel lumen with ischemic changes in the tissues supplied by the involved vessel.

Antineutrophil Cytoplasmic Antibodies (ANCA) ANCA are antibodies directed against certain proteins in the cytoplasm of neutrophils. They are present in a high percentage of patients with systemic vasculitis, particularly Wegener's granulomatosis, as well as in patients with microscopic polyangiitis and in patients with necrotizing and crescentic glomerulonephritis. There are two major categories of ANCA based on different targets for the antibodies. The terminology of *cytoplasmic* (c) *ANCA* refers to the diffuse, granular cytoplasmic staining pattern observed by immunofluorescence microscopy when serum antibodies bind to indicator neutrophils. Proteinase-3, the 29-kDa neutral serine proteinase present in neutrophil azurophilic granules is the major c-ANCA antigen. More than 90% of patients with typical Wegener's granulomatosis and active glomerulonephritis have a positive c-ANCA titer. The terminology of *perinuclear* (p) *ANCA* refers to the more localized perinuclear or nuclear staining pattern of the indicator neutrophils. The major target for p-ANCA is the enzyme myeloperoxidase; other targets of p-ANCA include elastase, cathepsin G, lactoferrin, lysozyme, and bactericidal/permeability-increasing protein. p-ANCA have been reported to occur in variable percentages of patients with microscopic polyangiitis, polyarteritis nodosa, Churg-Strauss syndrome, crescentic glomerulonephritis, and Goodpasture's syndrome as well as in association with nonvasculitic entities such as certain rheumatic and nonrheumatic autoimmune diseases, inflammatory bowel disease, certain drugs, and infections such as endocarditis and bacterial airway infections in patients with cystic fibrosis.

It is unclear why patients with these vasculitis syndromes develop ANCA, whereas ANCA are rare in other inflammatory diseases. However, once ANCA are present, there are a number of in vitro observations that suggest feasible mechanisms whereby these antibodies can contribute to the pathogenesis of the vasculitis syndromes. When neutrophils are in the resting state, proteinase-3 exists in the azurophilic granules of the cytoplasm, apparently inaccessible to serum antibodies. However, when neutrophils are primed by tumor necrosis factor (TNF)α or interleukin (IL)1, proteinase-3 translocates to the cell membrane where it can interact with extracellular ANCA. The neutrophils then degranulate and produce reactive oxygen species that can cause tissue damage. Endothelial cells also translocate their cytoplasmic proteinase-3 to the cell membrane upon priming with TNF-α, IL-1, or interferon (IFN)γ, thus rendering them susceptible to interaction with ANCA and leading possibly to tissue damage due to complement-mediated cytotoxicity or antibody-dependent cellular cytotoxicity. Despite the attractiveness of these in vitro data, there is no conclusive evidence that ANCA are directly involved in the pathogenesis of the vasculitis syndromes, and they may represent merely an epiphenomenon; in fact, a number of clinical and laboratory observations argue against a primary pathogenic linkage. Patients may have vasculitis in the absence of ANCA; the absolute height of the antibody titers does not correlate well with disease activity; and patients with vasculitis, particularly Wegener's granulomatosis, in remission may continue to have high c-ANCA titers for years. Thus, their role in the pathogenesis of systemic vasculitis remains an open question.

Pathogenic T Lymphocyte Responses and Granuloma Formation In addition to the classic immune complex–mediated mechanisms of vasculitis as well as ANCA, other immunopathogenic mechanisms may be involved in damage to vessels. The most prominent of these are delayed hypersensitivity and cell-mediated immune injury as reflected in the histopathologic feature of granulomatous vasculitis. However, immune complexes themselves may induce granulomatous responses. Vascular endothelial cells can express HLA class II molecules following activation by cytokines such as IFN-γ. This allows these cells to participate in immunologic reactions such as interaction with CD4+ T lymphocytes in a manner similar to antigen-presenting macrophages. Endothelial cells can secrete IL-1 which may activate T lymphocytes and initiate or propagate in situ immunologic processes within the blood vessel. In addition, IL-1 and TNF-α are potent inducers of endothelial-leukocyte adhesion molecule 1 (ELAM-1) and vascular cell adhesion molecule 1 (VCAM-1), which may enhance the adhesion of leukocytes to endothelial cells in the blood vessel wall. Other mechanisms such as direct cellular cytotoxicity or antibody directed against vessel components or antibody-dependent cellular cytotoxicity have been suggested in certain types of vessel damage. However, there is no convincing evidence to support their causal contribution to the pathogenesis of any of the recognized vasculitic syndromes.

It is unknown why certain individuals develop vasculitis in response to certain antigenic stimuli, whereas others do not. However, it is likely that a number of factors are involved in the ultimate expression of a vasculitic syndrome. These include the genetic predisposition and the regulatory mechanisms associated with immune response to certain antigens. When immune complexes are involved in the pathogenic process, the ability of the reticuloendothelial system to clear circulating complexes from the blood, the size and physicochemical properties of immune complexes, the relative degree of turbulence of blood flow, the intravascular hydrostatic pressure in different vessels, and the preexisting integrity of the vessel endothelium likely explain why only certain types of immune complexes cause vasculitis and why the vasculitic process is selective for only certain vessels in individual patients.

Approach to the Patient

Given the heterogeneous nature of the vasculitis syndromes, workup of a patient with suspected vasculitis should follow a series of progressive steps that establish the diagnosis of vasculitis, determine where possible the category of the vasculitis syndrome (Table 317-1), and determine the pattern and extent of disease activity. This information should then be utilized to determine the choice of therapeutic options (Fig. 317-1). This approach is of considerable importance since several of the vasculitis syndromes require aggressive therapy with glucocorticoids and immunosuppressive agents, while other syndromes usually resolve spontaneously and require symptomatic treatment only. Vasculitis is often suspected on clinical and laboratory grounds (see individual syndromes below). Depending on the individual category of vasculitis, measurement of ANCA titers may be helpful in this regard. However, a diagnosis of a vasculitis syndrome should not be made nor should treatment be initiated on the basis of a positive ANCA titer alone. The definitive diagnosis of vasculitis is made upon biopsy of involved tissue. The yield of "blind" biopsies of organs with

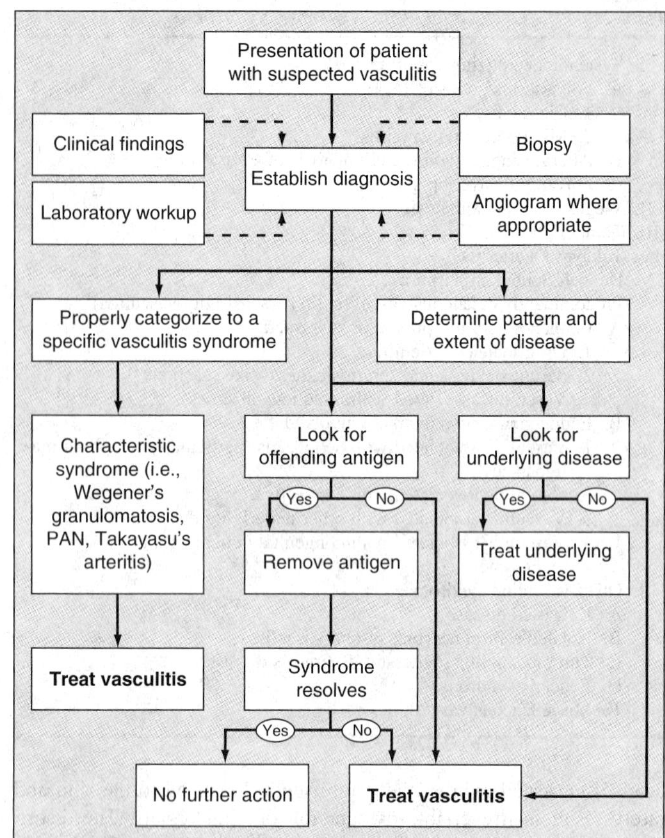

FIGURE 317-1 Algorithm for the approach to a patient with suspected diagnosis of vasculitis.

no subjective or objective evidence of involvement is very low and should be avoided. When syndromes such as classic polyarteritis nodosa, Takayasu's arteritis, or the polyangiitis overlap syndrome are suspected, angiogram of organs with suspected involvement should be performed. However, angiograms should not be performed routinely when patients present with localized cutaneous vasculitis with no clinical indication of visceral involvement.

The constellation of clinical, laboratory, biopsy, and radiographic findings usually allows proper categorization to a specific syndrome, and therapy where appropriate should be initiated according to this information (see individual syndromes below). If an offending antigen that precipitates the vasculitis is recognized, the antigen should be removed where possible. If the syndrome resolves, no further action should be taken. If disease activity continues, treatment should be initiated. If the vasculitis is associated with an underlying disease such as an infection, neoplasm, or connective tissue disease, the underlying disease should be treated. If the syndrome resolves, no further action should be taken. If the syndrome does not resolve or if there is no recognizable underlying disease and the vasculitis persists, treatment should be initiated according to the category of the vasculitis syndrome. Treatment options will be considered under the individual syndromes, and general principles of therapy will be considered at the end of the chapter.

SYSTEMIC NECROTIZING VASCULITIS

POLYARTERITIS NODOSA AND MICROSCOPIC POLYANGIITIS Definition *Classic polyarteritis nodosa* (PAN) was described in 1866 by Kussmaul and Maier. It is a multisystem, necrotizing vasculitis of small and medium-sized muscular arteries in which involvement of the renal and visceral arteries is characteristic. Classic PAN does not involve pulmonary arteries, although bronchial vessels may be involved; granulomas, significant eosinophilia, and an allergic diathesis are not part of the classic syndrome. The term *mi-*

croscopic polyangiitis (microscopic polyarteritis) was introduced into the literature by Davson in 1948. The Chapel Hill Consensus Conference on the Nomenclature of Systemic Vasculitis held in 1992 officially adopted the term to connote a necrotizing vasculitis with few or no immune complexes (pauci-immune) affecting small vessels (capillaries, venules, or arterioles). Since necrotizing arteritis involving small and medium-sized arteries may also be present, it shares features with classic PAN except that glomerulonephritis is very common in microscopic polyangiitis, and pulmonary capillaritis often occurs.

Incidence and Prevalence It is difficult to establish an accurate incidence of these diseases because of the fact that many reports of PAN actually have included both classic PAN and microscopic polyangiitis as well as other related vasculitides. Both diseases are uncommon, but classic PAN is felt to be more uncommon than microscopic polyangiitis. The mean age of onset of both PAN and microscopic polyangiitis is approximately 50 years of age, and males are slightly more frequently affected than females in both diseases.

Pathophysiology and Pathogenesis The vascular lesion in classic PAN is a necrotizing inflammation of small and medium-sized muscular arteries. The lesions are segmental and tend to involve bifurcations and branchings of arteries. They may spread circumferentially to involve adjacent veins. However, involvement of venules is not seen in classic PAN and, if present, suggests microscopic polyangiitis or the polyangiitis overlap syndrome (see below). In the acute stages of disease, polymorphonuclear neutrophils infiltrate all layers of the vessel wall and perivascular areas, which results in intimal proliferation and degeneration of the vessel wall. Mononuclear cells infiltrate the area as the lesions progress to the subacute and chronic stages. Fibrinoid necrosis of the vessels ensues with compromise of the lumen, thrombosis, infarction of the tissues supplied by the involved vessel, and, in some cases, hemorrhage. As the lesions heal, there is collagen deposition, which may lead to further occlusion of the vessel lumen. Aneurysmal dilatations up to 1 cm in size along the involved arteries are characteristic of classic PAN. Granulomas and substantial eosinophilia with eosinophilic tissue infiltrations are not characteristically found and suggest allergic angiitis and granulomatosis (see below).

Multiple organ systems are involved, and the clinicopathologic findings reflect the degree and location of vessel involvement and the resulting ischemic changes. As mentioned above, pulmonary arteries are not involved in classic PAN, and bronchial artery involvement is uncommon, whereas pulmonary capillaritis occurs frequently in microscopic polyangiitis. The pathology in the kidney in classic PAN is predominantly that of arteritis without glomerulonephritis. In contrast, glomerulonephritis is very common in microscopic polyangiitis. In patients with significant hypertension, typical pathologic features of glomerulosclerosis may be seen alone or superimposed on lesions of glomerulonephritis. In addition, pathologic sequelae of hypertension may be found elsewhere in the body.

The presence of hepatitis B antigenemia in approximately 20 to 30% of patients with systemic vasculitis, particularly of the classic PAN type, together with the isolation of circulating immune complexes composed of hepatitis B antigen and immunoglobulin, and the demonstration by immunofluorescence of hepatitis B antigen, IgM, and complement in the blood vessel walls, strongly suggest the role of immunologic phenomena in the pathogenesis of this disease. Hepatitis C infection has been reported in approximately 5% of patients with PAN; however, its pathogenic role in the vasculitis is unclear at present. Hairy cell leukemia can be associated with classic PAN; the pathogenic mechanisms of this association are unclear.

Clinical and Laboratory Manifestations Nonspecific signs and symptoms are the hallmarks of classic PAN. Fever, weight loss, and malaise are present in over one-half of cases. Patients usually present with vague symptoms such as weakness, malaise, headache, abdominal pain, and myalgias. Specific complaints related to the vascular involvement within a particular organ system may also dominate the presenting clinical picture as well as the entire course of the illness (Table 317-3). In classic PAN, renal involvement most commonly manifests as hypertension, renal insufficiency, or hemorrhage due to microaneurysms. In microscopic polyangiitis acute glomerulonephritis is the characteristic renal lesion.

Table 317-3 Clinical Manifestations Related to Organ System Involvement in Classic Polyarteritis Nodosa

Organ System	Percent Incidence	Clinical Manifestations
Renal	60	Renal failure, hypertension
Musculoskeletal	64	Arthritis, arthralgia, myalgia
Peripheral nervous system	51	Peripheral neuropathy, mononeuritis multiplex
Gastrointestinal tract	44	Abdominal pain, nausea and vomiting, bleeding, bowel infarction and perforation, cholecystitis, hepatic infarction, pancreatic infarction
Skin	43	Rash, purpura, nodules, cutaneous infarcts, livedo reticularis, Raynaud's phenomenon
Cardiac	36	Congestive heart failure, myocardial infarction, pericarditis
Genitourinary	25	Testicular, ovarian, or epididymal pain
Central nervous system	23	Cerebral vascular accident, altered mental status, seizure

SOURCE: From TR Cupps, AS Fauci: *The Vasculitides*. Philadelphia, Saunders, 1981.

There are no diagnostic serologic tests for classic PAN. In over 75% of patients, the leukocyte count is elevated with a predominance of neutrophils. Eosinophilia is seen only rarely and, when present at high levels, suggests the diagnosis of allergic angiitis and granulomatosis. The anemia of chronic disease may be seen, and an elevated erythrocyte sedimentation rate (ESR) is almost always present. Other common laboratory findings reflect the particular organ involved. Hypergammaglobulinemia may be present, and up to 30% of patients have a positive test for hepatitis B surface antigen. Positive ANCA titers (usually of the p-ANCA type) are found in a low percentage (<20%) of patients with classic PAN. Microscopic polyangiitis is strongly associated with ANCA that are usually of the p-ANCA type, but c-ANCA have also been reported. In contrast, the ANCA in Wegener's granulomatosis (see below) are almost always of the c-ANCA type. Arteriograms may demonstrate characteristic abnormalities such as aneurysms in the small and medium-sized muscular arteries of the kidneys and abdominal viscera in classic PAN.

Diagnosis The diagnosis of classic PAN is based on the demonstration of characteristic findings of vasculitis on biopsy material of involved organs. In the absence of easily accessible tissue for biopsy, the angiographic demonstration of involved vessels, particularly in the form of aneurysms of small and medium-sized arteries in the renal, hepatic, and visceral vasculature, is sufficient to make the diagnosis. Aneurysms of vessels are not pathognomonic of classic PAN; furthermore, aneurysms need not always be present, and angiographic findings may be limited to stenotic segments and obliteration of vessels. Biopsy of symptomatic organs such as nodular skin lesions, painful testes, and muscle groups provides the highest diagnostic yields, while blind biopsy of asymptomatic organs is frequently negative. The presence of small vessel vasculitis, particularly in the setting of glomerulonephritis and pulmonary capillaritis distinguishes microscopic polyangiitis from classic PAN. In this regard, biopsy of the kidney or lung may establish the diagnosis of microscopic polyangiitis.

Prognosis The prognosis of untreated classic PAN as well as that of microscopic polyangiitis is extremely poor. The usual clinical course is characterized either by fulminant deterioration or by relentless progression associated with intermittent acute flare-ups. In classic PAN, death usually results from renal failure; from gastrointestinal complications, particularly bowel infarcts and perforation; and from cardiovascular causes. In microscopic polyangiitis, death usually results from renal failure or pulmonary hemorrhage. Intractable hypertension often compounds dysfunction in other organ systems, such as the kidneys, heart, and central nervous system, leading to additional late morbidity and mortality in classic PAN. The 5-year survival rate of untreated patients has been reported to be between 10 and 20% for both diseases; this rate has increased substantially as a result of treatment (see below).

℞ TREATMENT Extremely favorable therapeutic results have been reported in classic PAN with the combination of prednisone, 1 mg/kg per day, and cyclophosphamide, 2 mg/kg per day (see "Wegener's Granulomatosis" for a detailed description of this therapeutic regimen). This regimen has been reported to result in up to a 90% long-term remission rate even following the discontinuation of therapy. In less severe cases of classic PAN, glucocorticoids alone have resulted in disease remission. In addition, long-term remissions have been reported in PAN associated with hepatitis B virus antigenemia using the antiviral agent vidarabine in combination with plasma exchange with and without glucocorticoids. Favorable results have also been reported in the treatment of PAN related to hepatitis B virus with IFN-α and plasma exchange. Careful attention to the treatment of hypertension can lessen the acute and late morbidity and mortality associated with renal, cardiac, and central nervous system complications of PAN. The treatment regimen for microscopic polyangiitis is similar to that for Wegener's granulomatosis (see below), particularly if glomerulonephritis is present.

ALLERGIC ANGIITIS AND GRANULOMATOSIS (CHURG-STRAUSS DISEASE) Definition *Allergic angiitis and granulomatosis* was described in 1951 by Churg and Strauss and is a disease characterized by granulomatous vasculitis of multiple organ systems, particularly the lung. It is characterized by vasculitis of blood vessels of various types or sizes (including veins and venules), intra- and extravascular granuloma formation together with eosinophilic tissue infiltration, and a strong association with severe asthma and peripheral eosinophilia.

Incidence and Prevalence Allergic angiitis and granulomatosis is an uncommon disease whose exact incidence, similar to classic PAN, is difficult to determine due to the grouping of multiple types of vasculitic syndromes in many reported series. The disease can occur at any age with the possible exception of infants. The mean age of onset is 44 years, with a male-to-female ratio of 1.3:1.

Pathophysiology and Pathogenesis The vasculitis of allergic angiitis and granulomatosis involves small and medium-sized muscular arteries, capillaries, veins, and venules. The characteristic histopathologic features of allergic angiitis and granulomatosis are granulomatous reactions that may be present in the tissues or even within the walls of the vessels themselves. These are usually associated with infiltration of the tissues with eosinophils. This process can occur in any organ in the body; lung involvement is predominant, with skin, cardiovascular system, kidney, peripheral nervous system, and gastrointestinal tract also commonly involved. Although the precise pathogenesis of this disease is uncertain, its strong association with asthma and its clinicopathologic manifestations including eosinophilia, granulomata, and vasculitis, which strongly suggest hypersensitivity phenomena, point to aberrant immunologic phenomena.

Clinical and Laboratory Manifestations Patients with allergic angiitis and granulomatosis exhibit nonspecific manifestations such as fever, malaise, anorexia, and weight loss, which are characteristic of a multisystem disease. The pulmonary findings in allergic angiitis and granulomatosis clearly dominate the clinical picture with severe asthmatic attacks and the presence of pulmonary infiltrates. Clinically recognizable heart disease occurs in approximately one-third of patients. Heart involvement is seen at autopsy in 62% of cases and is the cause of death in 23% of patients. Skin lesions occur in approximately 70% of patients and include purpura in addition to cutaneous and subcutaneous nodules. The renal disease in allergic angiitis and granulomatosis is less common and generally less severe than that of classic PAN and microscopic polyangiitis.

The characteristic laboratory finding in virtually all patients with allergic angiitis and granulomatosis is a striking eosinophilia, which reaches levels greater than 1000 cells/μL in more than 80% of patients. The other laboratory findings are similar to those of classic PAN and microscopic polyangiitis and reflect the organ systems involved. Allergic angiitis and granulomatosis is associated with p-ANCA.

Diagnosis The diagnosis of allergic angiitis and granulomatosis is made by biopsy in a patient with the characteristic clinical manifestations (see above). Granulomatous vasculitis with eosinophilic tissue involvement together with peripheral eosinophilia are typical.

Prognosis The prognosis of untreated allergic angiitis and granulomatosis is poor, with a reported 5-year survival of 25%. The cause of death is likely to be related to pulmonary and cardiac disease.

℞ TREATMENT Glucocorticoid therapy has been reported to increase the 5-year survival to more than 50%. In certain patients, the disease may be quite mild and may remit spontaneously or with short courses of glucocorticoids. In glucocorticoid failures or in patients who present with fulminant multisystem disease, the treatment of choice is a combined regimen of cyclophosphamide and alternate-day prednisone, which has resulted in a high rate of complete remission (see "Wegener's Granulomatosis" for a detailed description of this therapeutic regimen).

POLYANGIITIS OVERLAP SYNDROME Many patients with systemic vasculitis manifest clinicopathologic characteristics that do not fit precisely into any classification but have overlapping features of classic PAN, allergic angiitis and granulomatosis, Wegener's granulomatosis, Takayasu's arteritis, and the hypersensitivity group of vasculitides. This subgroup has been referred to as the *polyangiitis overlap syndrome* and is part of the major grouping of systemic necrotizing vasculitis. This entity has been designated with a distinct classification in order to avoid confusion in attempting to fit such overlap syndromes into one or other of the more classic vasculitic syndromes. This subgroup is truly a systemic vasculitis with the same potential for resulting in irreversible organ system dysfunction as the other systemic necrotizing vasculitides. The diagnostic and therapeutic considerations as well as the prognosis for this subgroup are the same as those for classic PAN, microscopic polyangiitis, and allergic angiitis and granulomatosis.

WEGENER'S GRANULOMATOSIS

DEFINITION *Wegener's granulomatosis* is a distinct clinicopathologic entity characterized by granulomatous vasculitis of the upper and lower respiratory tracts together with glomerulonephritis. In addition, variable degrees of disseminated vasculitis involving both small arteries and veins may occur.

INCIDENCE AND PREVALENCE Wegener's granulomatosis is an uncommon disease whose true incidence is difficult to determine. It is extremely rare in blacks compared with whites; the male-to-female ratio is 1:1. The disease can be seen at any age; approximately 15% of patients are less than 19 years of age, but only rarely does the disease occur before adolescence; the mean age of onset is approximately 40 years.

PATHOPHYSIOLOGY AND PATHOGENESIS The histopathologic hallmarks of Wegener's granulomatosis are necrotizing vasculitis of small arteries and veins together with granuloma formation, which may be either intravascular or extravascular (Fig. 317-2). Lung involvement typically appears as multiple, bilateral, nodular cavitary infiltrates (Fig. 317-3), which on biopsy almost invariably reveal the typical necrotizing granulomatous vasculitis. Endobronchial disease, either in its active form or as a result of fibrous scarring, may lead to obstruction with atelectasis. Upper airway lesions, particularly

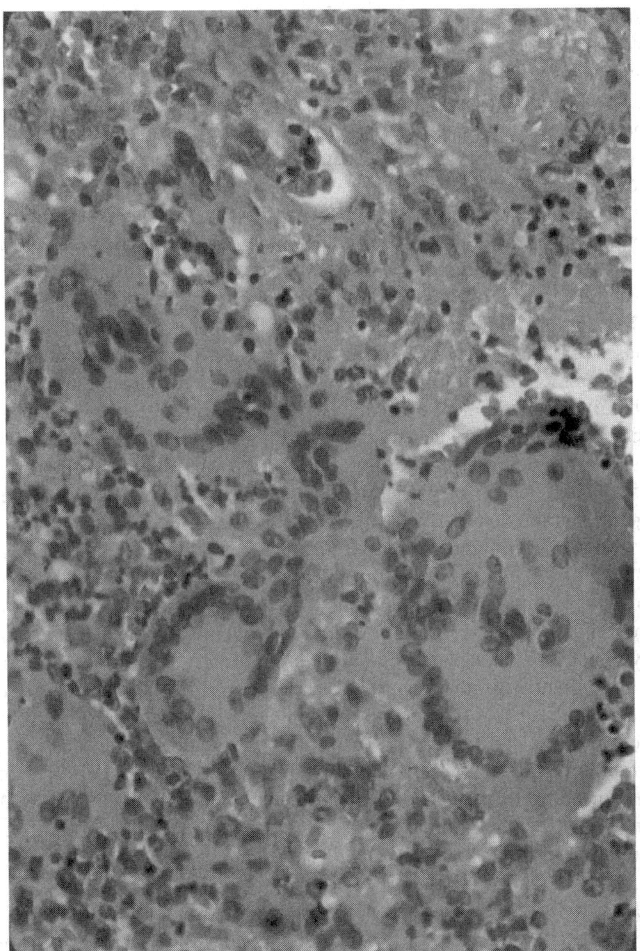

FIGURE 317-2 Lung biopsy in a patient with Wegener's granulomatosis. Biopsy revealed necrotizing vasculitis with granuloma formation. This section demonstrates several well-formed multinucleated giant cells in an area of granulomatous inflammation.

those in the sinuses and nasopharynx, typically reveal inflammation, necrosis, and granuloma formation with or without vasculitis.

In its earliest form, renal involvement is characterized by a focal and segmental glomerulitis that may evolve into a rapidly progressive crescentic glomerulonephritis. Granuloma formation is only rarely seen on renal biopsy. In addition to the classic triad of upper and lower

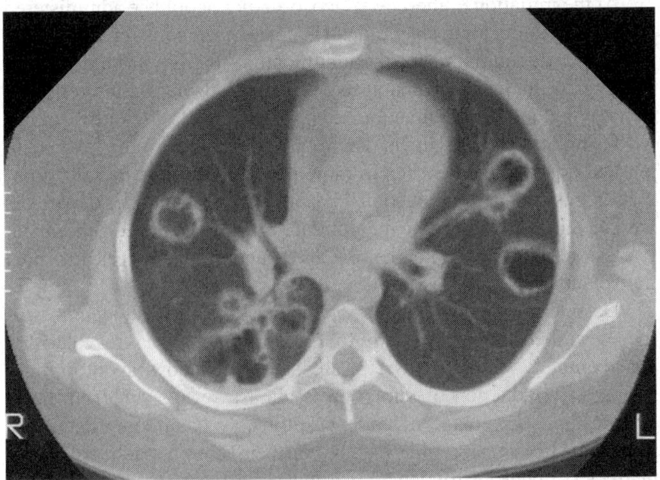

FIGURE 317-3 Computed tomography scan of a patient with Wegener's granulomatosis. The patient developed multiple, bilateral, and cavitary infiltrates.

respiratory tracts and kidney disease, virtually any organ can be involved with vasculitis, granuloma, or both.

The immunopathogenesis of this disease is unclear, although the involvement of upper airways and lungs with granulomatous vasculitis suggests an aberrant hypersensitivity response to an exogenous or even endogenous antigen that enters through or resides in the upper airway. Chronic nasal carriage of *Staphylococcus aureus* has been reported to be associated with a higher relapse rate of Wegener's granulomatosis; however, there is no evidence for a role of this organism in the pathogenesis of the disease.

Peripheral blood mononuclear cells obtained from patients with Wegener's granulomatosis manifest increased secretion of IFN-γ but not of IL-4, IL-5, or IL-10 compared to normal controls. The increased IFN-γ production is inhibited by exogenous IL-10. In addition, TNF-α production from peripheral blood mononuclear cells and CD4+ T is elevated. Furthermore, monocytes from patients with Wegener's granulomatosis produce increased amounts of IL-12. These findings indicate an unbalanced Th1-type T cell cytokine pattern in this disease that may have pathogenic and perhaps ultimately therapeutic implications.

A high percentage of patients with Wegener's granulomatosis develop ANCA; c-ANCA are the predominant ANCA in this disease. As with the other categories of vasculitis, there is no clear evidence that ANCA play a primary role in the pathogenesis of Wegener's granulomatosis.

CLINICAL AND LABORATORY MANIFESTATIONS

A typical patient presents with severe upper respiratory tract findings such as paranasal sinus pain and drainage and purulent or bloody nasal discharge with or without nasal mucosal ulceration (Table 317-4). Nasal septal perforation may follow, leading to saddle nose deformity. Serous otitis media may occur as a result of eustachian tube blockage.

Pulmonary involvement may be manifested as asymptomatic infiltrates or may be clinically expressed as cough, hemoptysis, dyspnea, and chest discomfort. It is present in 85 to 90% of patients. Subglottic stenosis resulting from active disease or scarring occurs in approximately 16% of patients and may result in severe airway obstruction.

Eye involvement (52% of patients) may range from a mild conjunctivitis to dacryocystitis, episcleritis, scleritis, granulomatous sclerouveitis, ciliary vessel vasculitis, and retroorbital mass lesions leading to proptosis.

Skin lesions (46% of patients) appear as papules, vesicles, palpable purpura, ulcers, or subcutaneous nodules; biopsy reveals vasculitis, granuloma, or both. Cardiac involvement (8% of patients) manifests as pericarditis, coronary vasculitis, or, rarely, cardiomyopathy. Nervous system manifestations (23% of patients) include cranial neuritis, mononeuritis multiplex, or, rarely, cerebral vasculitis and/or granuloma.

Renal disease (77% of patients) generally dominates the clinical picture and, if left untreated, accounts directly or indirectly for most of the mortality in this disease. Although it may smolder in some cases as a mild glomerulitis with proteinuria, hematuria, and red blood cell casts, it is clear that once clinically detectable renal functional impairment occurs, rapidly progressive renal failure usually ensues unless appropriate treatment is instituted.

While the disease is active, most patients have nonspecific symptoms and signs such as malaise, weakness, arthralgias, anorexia, and weight loss. Fever may indicate activity of the underlying disease but more often reflects secondary infection, usually of the upper airway.

Characteristic laboratory findings include a markedly elevated ESR, mild anemia and leukocytosis, mild hypergammaglobulinemia (particularly of the IgA class), and mildly elevated rheumatoid factor. Thrombocytosis may be seen as an acute-phase reactant. In typical Wegener's granulomatosis with granulomatous vasculitis of the respiratory tract and glomerulonephritis, approximately 90% of patients have a positive c-ANCA. However, in the absence of renal disease, the sensitivity drops to approximately 70%.

Table 317-4 Wegener's Granulomatosis: Frequency of Clinical Manifestations in 158 Patients Studied at the National Institutes of Health

Manifestation	Percent at Disease Onset	Percent Throughout Course of Disease
Kidney		
Glomerulonephritis	18	77
Ear/nose/throat	73	92
Sinusitis	51	85
Nasal disease	36	68
Otitis media	25	44
Hearing loss	14	42
Subglottic stenosis	1	16
Ear pain	9	14
Oral lesions	3	10
Lung	45	85
Pulmonary infiltrates	25	66
Pulmonary nodules	24	58
Hemoptysis	12	30
Pleuritis	10	28
Eyes		
Conjunctivitis	5	18
Dacryocystitis	1	18
Scleritis	6	16
Proptosis	2	15
Eye pain	3	11
Visual loss	0	8
Retinal lesions	0	4
Corneal lesions	0	1
Iritis	0	2
Other[a]		
Arthralgias/arthritis	32	67
Fever	23	50
Cough	19	46
Skin abnormalities	13	46
Weight loss (greater than 10% body weight)	15	35
Peripheral neuropathy	1	15
Central nervous system disease	1	8
Pericarditis	2	6
Hyperthyroidism	1	3

[a] Fewer than 1% had parotid, pulmonary artery, breast, or lower genitourinary (urethra, cervix, vagina, testicular) involvement.

SOURCE: Hoffman et al.

DIAGNOSIS The diagnosis of Wegener's granulomatosis is a clinicopathologic one made by the demonstration of necrotizing granulomatous vasculitis on biopsy of appropriate tissue in a patient with the clinical findings of upper and lower respiratory tract disease together with evidence of glomerulonephritis. Pulmonary tissue, preferably obtained by open thoracotomy, offers the highest diagnostic yield, almost invariably revealing granulomatous vasculitis. Biopsy of upper airway tissue usually reveals granulomatous inflammation with necrosis but may not show vasculitis. Renal biopsy confirms the presence of glomerulonephritis.

The specificity of a positive c-ANCA titer for Wegener's granulomatosis is very high, especially if active glomerulonephritis is present. However, the presence of c-ANCA should be adjunctive and, with very rare exceptions, should not substitute for a tissue diagnosis. False-positive ANCA titers have been reported in certain infectious and neoplastic diseases.

In its typical presentation, the classic clinicopathologic complex of Wegener's granulomatosis usually provides ready differentiation from other disorders. However, if all the typical features are not present at once, it needs to be differentiated from the other vasculitides, particularly allergic angiitis and granulomatosis, Goodpasture's syndrome (Chap. 275), tumors of the upper airway or lung, and infectious diseases such as histoplasmosis (Chap. 201), mucocutaneous leishmaniasis (Chap. 215), and rhinoscleroma (Chap. 30) as well as noninfectious granulomatous diseases.

Of particular note is the differentiation from *midline granuloma* and *upper airway neoplasms*, which are part of the spectrum of *midline destructive diseases*. These diseases lead to extreme tissue destruction and mutilation localized to the midline upper airway structures including the sinuses; erosion through the skin of the face commonly occurs, a feature that is extremely rare in Wegener's granulomatosis. Although blood vessels may be involved in the intense inflammatory reaction and necrosis, primary vasculitis is seen rarely. When systemic involvement occurs, it usually declares itself as a neoplastic process. In this regard, it is likely that midline granuloma is part of the spectrum of *angiocentric immunoproliferative lesions* (AIL). The latter are considered to represent a spectrum of postthymic T cell proliferative lesions and should be treated as such (Chap. 112). The term *idiopathic* has been applied to midline granuloma when extensive diagnostic workup including multiple biopsies has failed to reveal anything other than inflammation and necrosis. Under these circumstances, it is possible that the tumor cells were masked by the intensive inflammatory response. Such cases have responded to local irradiation with 50 Gy (5000 rad). Upper airway lesions should never be irradiated in Wegener's granulomatosis.

Wegener's granulomatosis must also be differentiated from *lymphomatoid granulomatosis*, the latter also being a part of the spectrum of AIL. Lymphomatoid granulomatosis is characterized by lung, skin, central nervous system, and kidney involvement in which atypical lymphocytoid and plasmacytoid cells infiltrate tissue in an angioinvasive manner. In this regard, it clearly differs from Wegener's granulomatosis in that it is not an inflammatory vasculitis in the classic sense but an infiltration of vessels with atypical mononuclear cells; granuloma may be present in involved tissues. Approximately 50% of patients develop a true malignant lymphoma. The presence of c-ANCA in Wegener's granulomatosis proves extremely helpful in the differentiation from all the preceding diseases.

℞ **TREATMENT** Wegener's granulomatosis was formerly universally fatal, usually within a few months after the onset of clinically apparent renal disease. Glucocorticoids alone led to some symptomatic improvement, with little effect on the ultimate course of the disease. It has been well established that the most effective therapy in this disease is cyclophosphamide given in doses of 2 mg/kg per day orally together with glucocorticoids. The leukocyte count should be monitored closely during therapy, and the dosage of cyclophosphamide should be adjusted in order to maintain the count above 3000/μL, which generally maintains the neutrophil count at approximately 1500/μL. With this approach, clinical remission can usually be induced and maintained without causing severe leukopenia with its associated risk of infection. Cyclophosphamide should be continued for 1 year following the induction of complete remission and gradually tapered and discontinued thereafter.

At the initiation of therapy, glucocorticoids should be administered together with cyclophosphamide. This can be given as prednisone, 1 mg/kg per day initially (for the first month of therapy) as a daily regimen, with gradual conversion to an alternate-day schedule followed by tapering and discontinuation after approximately 6 months.

Using the above regimen, the prognosis of this disease is excellent; marked improvement is seen in more than 90% of patients, and complete remissions are achieved in 75% of patients. A number of patients who developed irreversible renal failure but who achieved subsequent remission on appropriate therapy have undergone successful renal transplantation.

Despite the dramatic remissions induced by the therapeutic regimen described above, long-term follow-up of patients has revealed that approximately 50% of remissions are later associated with one or more relapses. Reinduction of remission is almost always achieved; however, a high percentage of patients ultimately have some degree of morbidity from irreversible features of their disease, such as varying degrees of renal insufficiency, hearing loss, tracheal stenosis, saddle nose deformity, and chronically impaired sinus function. In evaluating patients for relapse, the ANCA titer can be misleading. Many patients who achieve remission continue to have elevated titers for years. In addition, over 40% of patients who were in remission and had a fourfold increase in c-ANCA titer did not have a relapse in disease. In this regard, therapy should not be reinstituted or increased on the basis of a rise in the ANCA titer alone; however, such a finding should prompt the clinician to examine the patient carefully for any objective evidence of active disease and to monitor that patient more closely.

Certain types of morbidity are related to toxic side effects of treatment. Since the preceding therapeutic regimen calls for conversion to alternate-day glucocorticoid therapy within 3 months and ultimate discontinuation within 6 to 12 months, glucocorticoid-related side effects such as diabetes mellitus, cataracts, life-threatening infectious disease complications, serious osteoporosis, and severe cushingoid features are infrequently encountered except in those patients requiring prolonged courses of daily glucocorticoids. However, cyclophosphamide-related toxicities are more frequent and severe. Cystitis to varying degrees occurs in 50% of patients, bladder cancer in 6%, and myelodysplasia in 2%.

Some reports have indicated therapeutic success with less frequent and severe toxic side effects using intermittent boluses of intravenous cyclophosphamide (1 g/m^2 per month) in place of daily drug administered orally. However, we and others have found an increased rate of relapse with bolus intravenous cyclophosphamide. We therefore strongly recommend that the drug be given as daily oral therapy.

Despite concerns regarding toxicity, a regimen of daily cyclophosphamide and glucocorticoids is clearly the treatment of choice in patients with immediately life-threatening disease such as rapidly progressive glomerulonephritis. However, methotrexate together with glucocorticoids may be considered as an alternative for initial therapy for certain patients whose disease is not immediately life-threatening or as a switch regimen in those patients who have experienced significant cyclophosphamide toxicity. In one study, patients in this category were given oral prednisone as described above, and methotrexate was administered orally starting at a dosage of 0.3 mg/kg, with a maximum of 15 mg/week. If the treatment was well tolerated after 1 to 2 weeks, the dosage was increased by 2.5 mg weekly up to a dosage of 20 to 25 mg/week and maintained at that level. Remissions were achieved in 33 of 42 patients (79%). Nineteen patients relapsed; 15 of these 19 relapses occurred when patients were receiving 15 mg or less of methotrexate per week; 13 of these 19 were treated with a second course of methotrexate and prednisone and 10 of 13 achieved a second remission. Toxicities of methotrexate included elevated transaminase levels (24%), leukopenia (7%), opportunistic infection (9.5%), methotrexate pneumonitis (7%), and stomatitis (2%).

Azathioprine, in doses of 1 to 2 mg/kg per day, has proven effective in some patients, particularly in maintaining remission in those in whom remission was induced by cyclophosphamide. The drug should be administered together with the glucocorticoid regimen described above. Although certain reports have indicated that trimethoprim-sulfamethoxazole may be of benefit in the treatment of Wegener's granulomatosis, there are no firm data to substantiate this, particularly in patients with serious renal and pulmonary disease. In a study examining the effect of trimethoprim-sulfamethoxazole on relapse, decreased relapses were shown only with regard to upper airway disease, and no differences in major organ relapses were observed. Trimethoprim-sulfamethoxazole alone should never be used to treat active Wegener's granulomatosis outside of the upper airway.

TEMPORAL ARTERITIS

DEFINITION *Temporal arteritis*, also referred to as *cranial arteritis* or *giant cell arteritis*, is an inflammation of medium- and large-sized arteries. It characteristically involves one or more branches of the carotid artery, particularly the temporal artery; hence the name. However, it is a systemic disease that can involve arteries in multiple locations.

INCIDENCE AND PREVALENCE The incidence of temporal arteritis varies widely in different studies and in different geographic regions. A high incidence has been found in Scandanavia and in regions of the United States with large Scandanavian populations, compared to a lower incidence in southern Europe. The annual incidence rates in individuals 50 years of age and older range from 0.49 to 23.3 per 100,000 population. It occurs almost exclusively in individuals older than 55 years; however, well-documented cases have occurred in patients 40 years old or younger. It is more common in women than in men and is rare in blacks. Familial aggregation has been reported, as has an association with HLA-DR4. In addition, genetic linkage studies have demonstrated an association of temporal arteritis with alleles at the HLA-DRB1 locus, particularly HLA-DRB1*04 variants. The disease is closely associated with *polymyalgia rheumatica*, which is more common than temporal arteritis. In Olmsted County, Minnesota, the annual incidence of polymyalgia rheumatica in individuals 50 years of age and older is 52.5 per 100,000 population.

PATHOPHYSIOLOGY AND PATHOGENESIS Although the temporal artery is most frequently involved in this disease, patients often have a systemic vasculitis of multiple medium- and large-sized arteries, which may go undetected. Histopathologically, the disease is a panarteritis with inflammatory mononuclear cell infiltrates within the vessel wall with frequent giant cell formation. There is proliferation of the intima and fragmentation of the internal elastic lamina. Pathophysiologic findings in organs result from the ischemia related to the involved vessels. Distinct cytokine patterns as well as T lymphocytes expressing specific antigen receptors have been described suggesting the involvement of immunopathogenic mechanisms in temporal arteritis. IL-6 and IL-1β expression has been detected in a majority of circulating monocytes of patients with temporal arteritis and polymyalgia rheumatica. T cells recruited to vasculitic lesions in patients with temporal arteritis produce predominantly IL-2 and IFN-γ, and the latter has been suggested to be involved in the progression to overt arteritis. Sequence analysis of the T cell receptor of tissue-infiltrating T cells in lesions of temporal arteritis indicates restricted clonal expansion, suggesting that an antigen residing in the arterial wall is recognized by a small fraction of T cells.

CLINICAL AND LABORATORY MANIFESTATIONS The disease is characterized clinically by the classic complex of fever, anemia, high ESR, and headaches in an elderly patient. Other manifestations include malaise, fatigue, anorexia, weight loss, sweats, and arthralgias. The polymyalgia rheumatica syndrome is characterized by stiffness, aching, and pain in the muscles of the neck, shoulders, lower back, hips, and thighs.

In patients with involvement of the temporal artery, headache is the predominant symptom and may be associated with a tender, thickened, or nodular artery, which may pulsate early in the disease but become occluded later. Scalp pain and claudication of the jaw and tongue may occur. A well-recognized and dreaded complication of temporal arteritis, particularly in untreated patients, is ocular involvement due primarily to ischemic optic neuropathy, which may lead to serious visual symptoms, even sudden blindness in some patients. However, most patients have complaints relating to the head or eyes for months before objective eye involvement. Attention to such symptoms with institution of appropriate therapy (see below) will usually avoid this complication. Claudication of the extremities, strokes, myocardial infarctions, and infarctions of visceral organs have been reported. Of note, temporal arteritis is associated with a markedly increased risk of aortic aneurysm, which is usually a late complication and may lead to dissection and death.

Characteristic laboratory findings in addition to the elevated ESR include a normochromic or slightly hypochromic anemia. Liver function abnormalities are common, particularly increased alkaline phosphatase levels. Increased levels of IgG and complement have been reported. Levels of enzymes indicative of muscle damage such as serum creatine kinase are not elevated.

DIAGNOSIS The diagnosis of temporal arteritis and its associated clinicopathologic syndrome can often be made clinically by the demonstration of the classic picture of fever, anemia, and high ESR with or without symptoms of polymyalgia rheumatica in an elderly patient. The diagnosis is confirmed by biopsy of the temporal artery. Since involvement of the vessel may be segmental, the diagnosis may be missed on routine biopsy; serial sectioning of biopsy specimens is recommended. When the temporal arteries appear clinically normal, but temporal arteritis is strongly suspected, a biopsy segment of a few centimeters may be required to establish the diagnosis. Ultrasonography of the temporal artery has been reported to be helpful in diagnosis. A temporal artery biopsy should be obtained as quickly as possible in the setting of ocular signs and symptoms, and under these circumstances therapy should not be delayed pending a biopsy. In this regard, it has been reported that temporal artery biopsies may show vasculitis even after more than 14 days of glucocorticoid therapy. A dramatic clinical response to a trial of glucocorticoid therapy can confirm the diagnosis.

℞ **TREATMENT** Temporal arteritis and its associated symptoms are exquisitely sensitive to glucocorticoid therapy. Treatment should begin with prednisone, 40 to 60 mg per day for approximately 1 month, followed by a gradual tapering to a maintenance dose of 7.5 to 10 mg per day. In order to lessen glucocorticoid side effects in elderly individuals, conversion to alternate-day therapy may be attempted, but only after the disease has been put into remission with daily therapy. When ocular signs and symptoms occur, it is important that therapy be initiated or adjusted to control them. Because of the possibility of relapse, therapy should be continued for at least 1 to 2 years. The ESR can serve as a useful indicator of inflammatory disease activity in monitoring and tapering therapy and can be used to judge the pace of the tapering schedule. However, minor increases in the ESR can occur as glucocorticoids are being tapered and do not necessarily reflect an exacerbation of arteritis, particularly if the patient remains symptom free. Under these circumstances, the tapering should continue with caution. If one attempts to maintain a normal ESR throughout the tapering period, glucocorticoid toxicity will almost surely occur. The prognosis is generally good, and most patients achieve complete remission that is often maintained after withdrawal of therapy.

TAKAYASU'S ARTERITIS

DEFINITION *Takayasu's arteritis* is an inflammatory and stenotic disease of medium- and large-sized arteries characterized by a strong predilection for the aortic arch and its branches. For this reason, it is often referred to as the *aortic arch syndrome*.

INCIDENCE AND PREVALENCE Takayasu's arteritis is an uncommon disease, much less common than temporal arteritis. It is most prevalent in adolescent girls and young women. Although it is more common in the Orient, it is neither racially nor geographically restricted.

PATHOPHYSIOLOGY AND PATHOGENESIS The disease involves medium- and large-sized arteries, with a strong predilection for the aortic arch and its branches; the pulmonary artery may also be involved. The most commonly affected arteries seen by angiography are listed in Table 317-5. The involvement of the major branches of the aorta is much more marked at their origin than distally. The disease is a panarteritis with inflammatory mononuclear cell infiltrates and occasionally giant cells. There are marked intimal proliferation and fibrosis, scarring and vascularization of the media, and disruption and degeneration of the elastic lamina. Narrowing of the lumen occurs with or without thrombosis. The vasa vasorum are frequently involved. Pathologic changes in various organs reflect the compromise of blood flow through the involved vessels.

Immunopathogenic mechanisms, the precise nature of which is uncertain, are suspected in this disease. As with several of the vasculitis syndromes, circulating immune complexes have been demonstrated, but their pathogenic significance is unclear.

Table 317-5 Frequency of Arteriographic Abnormalities and Potential Clinical Manifestations of Arterial Involvement in Takayasu's Arteritis

Artery	Percent of Arteriographic Abnormalities	Potential Clinical Manifestations
Subclavian	93	Arm claudication, Raynaud's phenomenon
Common carotid	58	Visual changes, syncope, transient ischemic attacks, stroke
Abdominal aorta[a]	47	Abdominal pain, nausea, vomiting
Renal	38	Hypertension, renal failure
Aortic arch or root	35	Aortic insufficiency, congestive heart failure
Vertebral	35	Visual changes, dizziness
Coeliac axis[a]	18	Abdominal pain, nausea, vomiting
Superior mesenteric[a]	18	Abdominal pain, nausea, vomiting
Iliac	17	Leg claudication
Pulmonary	10–40	Atypical chest pain, dyspnea
Coronary	<10	Chest pain, myocardial infarction

[a] Arteriographic lesions at these locations are usually asymptomatic but may potentially cause these symptoms.

SOURCE: Kerr et al.

CLINICAL AND LABORATORY MANIFESTATIONS Takayasu's arteritis is a systemic disease with generalized as well as local symptoms. The generalized symptoms include malaise, fever, night sweats, arthralgias, anorexia, and weight loss, which may occur months before vessel involvement is apparent. These symptoms may merge into those related to pain over the involved vessels, followed by symptoms of ischemia in organs supplied by the compromised vessels. Pulses are commonly absent in the involved vessels, particularly the subclavian artery. The frequency of arteriographic abnormalities and the potentially associated clinical manifestations are listed in Table 317-5.

The clinical course may be fulminant, may progress gradually, or may stabilize. Complications are related to the distribution of the involved vessels. Death usually occurs from congestive heart failure or cerebrovascular accidents.

Characteristic laboratory findings include an elevated ESR, mild anemia, and elevated immunoglobulin levels.

DIAGNOSIS The diagnosis of Takayasu's arteritis should be suspected strongly in a young woman who develops a decrease or absence of peripheral pulses, discrepancies in blood pressure, and arterial bruits. The diagnosis is confirmed by the characteristic pattern on arteriography, which includes irregular vessel walls, stenosis, poststenotic dilatation, aneurysm formation, occlusion, and evidence of increased collateral circulation. Complete aortic arteriography should be obtained, unless this is renally contraindicated, in order to fully delineate the distribution and degree of arterial disease. Histopathologic demonstration of inflamed vessels adds confirmatory data; however, tissue is rarely readily available for examination.

℞ **TREATMENT** The course of the disease is variable, and spontaneous remissions may occur. Reported mortality statistics range from less than 10 to 75%. Although glucocorticoid therapy in doses of 40 to 60 mg prednisone per day alleviates symptoms, there are no convincing studies that indicate that they alone increase survival. The combination of glucocorticoid therapy for acute signs and symptoms and an aggressive surgical and/or angioplastic approach to stenosed vessels has markedly improved survival and decreased morbidity by lessening the risk of stroke, correcting hypertension due to renal artery stenosis, and improving blood flow to ischemic viscera and limbs. Unless it is urgently required, surgical correction of stenosed arteries should be undertaken only when the vascular inflammatory process is well controlled with medical therapy. Most recent mortality figures using this therapeutic approach are less than 10%. In individuals who are refractory to glucocorticoids, methotrexate in doses up to 25 mg per week has yielded encouraging results; however, long-term studies will be needed to confirm this.

HENOCH-SCHÖNLEIN PURPURA

DEFINITION *Henoch-Schönlein purpura*, also referred to as *anaphylactoid purpura*, is a distinct systemic vasculitis syndrome that is characterized by palpable purpura (most commonly distributed over the buttocks and lower extremities), arthralgias, gastrointestinal signs and symptoms, and glomerulonephritis. It is a small vessel vasculitis.

INCIDENCE AND PREVALENCE Henoch-Schönlein purpura is usually seen in children; most patients range in age from 4 to 7 years; however, the disease may also be seen in infants and adults. It is not a rare disease; in one series it accounted for between 5 and 24 admissions per year at a pediatric hospital. The male-to-female ratio is 1.5:1. A seasonal variation with a peak incidence in spring has been noted.

PATHOPHYSIOLOGY AND PATHOGENESIS The presumptive pathogenic mechanism for Henoch-Schönlein purpura is immune-complex deposition. A number of inciting antigens have been suggested including upper respiratory tract infections, various drugs, foods, insect bites, and immunizations. IgA is the antibody class most often seen in the immune complexes and has been demonstrated in the renal biopsies of these patients.

CLINICAL AND LABORATORY MANIFESTATIONS In pediatric patients, presenting symptoms related to the skin, gut, and joints are present in 50% of cases. In adults, presenting symptoms related to the skin are seen in over 70% of patients, while initial complaints related to the gut or the joints are noted in fewer than 20% of cases. The typical palpable purpura is seen in virtually all patients; most patients develop polyarthralgias in the absence of frank arthritis. Gastrointestinal involvement, which is seen in almost 70% of pediatric patients, is characterized by colicky abdominal pain usually associated with nausea, vomiting, diarrhea, or constipation and is frequently accompanied by the passage of blood and mucus per rectum; bowel intussusception may occur rarely. The renal involvement is usually characterized by mild glomerulonephritis leading to proteinuria and microscopic hematuria, with red blood cell casts in the majority of patients (Chap. 275); it usually resolves spontaneously without therapy. Rarely, a progressive glomerulonephritis will develop. Renal failure is the most common cause of death in the rare patient who dies of Henoch-Schönlein purpura. Although certain studies have found that renal disease is more severe in adults, this has not been a consistent finding. However, the course of renal disease in adults may be more insidious and thus requires close follow-up. Myocardial involvement can occur in adults but is rare in children.

Routine laboratory studies generally show a mild leukocytosis, a normal platelet count, and occasionally eosinophilia. Serum complement components are normal, and IgA levels are elevated in about one-half of patients.

℞ **TREATMENT** The prognosis of Henoch-Schönlein purpura is excellent. Most patients recover completely, and some do not require therapy. Treatment is similar for adults and children. When glucocorticoid therapy is required, prednisone in doses of 1 mg/kg per day and tapered according to clinical response has been shown to be useful in decreasing tissue edema, arthralgias, and abdominal discomfort; however, it has not proven beneficial in the treatment of skin or renal disease and does not appear to shorten the duration of active disease or lessen the chance of recurrence. Patients with rapidly progressive glomerulonephritis have been anecdotally reported to benefit from intensive plasma exchange combined with immunosuppressive drugs.

PREDOMINANTLY CUTANEOUS VASCULITIS

DEFINITION The term *predominantly cutaneous vasculitis* has been used interchangeably with the terms *hypersensitivity vasculitis* and *cutaneous leukocytoclastic vasculitis*. Due to the heterogeneity of this group of disorders, none of these terms is totally adequate. The common denominator of this group of diseases is the involvement of small vessels of the skin. The syndrome is presumed to be associated with an aberrant hypersensitivity reaction to an antigen such as an infectious agent, a drug, or other foreign or endogenous substances. In most instances, however, an antigen is never identified and the disease remains idiopathic. The term *hypersensitivity vasculitis* is a misleading term since most of the other groups of vasculitis syndromes are probably also associated with some form of hypersensitivity or aberrant immunologic reaction to as yet unidentified antigens. The term *cutaneous leukocytoclastic vasculitis* is a better term; however, not all of these vasculitides are truly leukocytoclastic in nature. We have elected to use the term *"predominantly" cutaneous vasculitis* since skin involvement generally dominates the clinical picture, but the skin is not always the exclusive organ involved. Indeed, any organ system can be involved with this type of vasculitis; however, the extracutaneous involvement is usually much less severe than that of the systemic necrotizing vasculitides.

INCIDENCE AND PREVALENCE Although the exact incidence of this group of vasculitis syndromes is uncertain, it is clearly more common than the systemic necrotizing vasculitis group. The disease can occur at any age and in both sexes; however, different subgroups have a higher incidence in certain age groups, and some are more common in males than females, or vice versa.

PATHOPHYSIOLOGY AND PATHOGENESIS The typical histopathologic feature of the predominantly cutaneous vasculitides is the presence of vasculitis of small vessels. Postcapillary venules are the most commonly involved vessels; capillaries and arterioles may be involved less frequently. This vasculitis is characterized by a *leukocytoclasis*, a term that refers to the nuclear debris remaining from the neutrophils that have infiltrated in and around the vessels during the acute stages. In the subacute or chronic stages, mononuclear cells predominate; in certain subgroups, eosinophilic infiltration is seen. Erythrocytes often extravasate from the involved vessels, leading to palpable purpura.

Immune-complex deposition is generally considered to be the immunopathogenic mechanism of this type of vasculitis; however, formal proof that this is the case has not been established for all subgroups (see above). The predominantly cutaneous vasculitides can be broken down empirically into two major categories depending on the type of putative antigen involved in the hypersensitivity reaction. In the originally described group, the antigen was foreign to the host, i.e., a drug, microbe, or foreign protein. In this regard, essential mixed cryoglobulinemia has been associated with hepatitis C virus infection. In the second category, the antigen is felt to be endogenous to the host. Examples of these are the "self" proteins such as DNA or immunoglobulin, which form immune complexes with their respective antibodies and lead to vasculitic complications in systemic lupus erythematosus and rheumatoid arthritis, respectively; other examples are the recognized and putative tumor antigens that form immune complexes with antibody and lead to vasculitis associated with certain neoplasms. Certain lymphoid malignancies may also secrete cytokines that contribute to the pathogenic process.

CLINICAL AND LABORATORY MANIFESTATIONS The hallmark of this broad group of vasculitides is the predominance of skin involvement. Skin lesions may appear typically as palpable purpura; however, other cutaneous manifestations of the vasculitis may occur, including macules, papules, vesicles, bullae, subcutaneous nodules, ulcers, and recurrent or chronic urticaria. Despite the fact that skin lesions predominate, other organ systems may be involved to varying degrees, and the extent to which this occurs may define a relatively distinct subgroup. Even in patients with isolated cutaneous involvement, the disease may be characterized by systemic signs and symptoms such as fever, malaise, myalgia, and anorexia. The skin lesions may be pruritic or even quite painful, with a burning or stinging sensation. Lesions most commonly occur in the lower extremities in ambulatory patients or in the sacral area in bedridden patients due to the effects of hydrostatic forces on the postcapillary venules. Edema may accompany certain lesions, and hyperpigmentation often occurs in areas of recurrent or chronic lesions.

There are no specific laboratory tests diagnostic of this category of vasculitis. A mild leukocytosis with or without eosinophilia is characteristic, as is an elevated ESR. Cryoglobulins and rheumatoid factor may be seen in certain cases, and serum complement levels follow no definite pattern. Laboratory abnormalities related to specific organ dysfunction reflect the involvement of these organs in the particular syndrome in question.

Drug-Induced Vasculitis Cutaneous drug reactions take a number of forms, and vasculitis is only one of these (Chaps. 57 and 59). Vasculitis associated with drug reactions usually presents as palpable purpura that may be generalized or limited to the lower extremities or other dependent areas; however, urticarial lesions, ulcers, and hemorrhagic blisters may also occur (Chap. 59). Signs and symptoms may be limited to the skin, although systemic manifestations such as fever, malaise, and polyarthralgias may occur. Although the skin is the predominant organ involved, systemic vasculitis may result from drug reactions. Drugs that have been implicated in vasculitis include allopurinol, thiazides, gold, sulfonamides, phenytoin, and penicillin (Chap. 59).

Serum Sickness and Serum Sickness–Like Reactions These reactions are characterized by the occurrence of fever, urticaria, polyarthralgias, and lymphadenopathy 7 to 10 days after primary exposure and 2 to 4 days after secondary exposure to a heterologous protein (classic serum sickness) or a nonprotein drug such as penicillin or sulfa (serum sickness–like reaction). Most of the manifestations are not due to a vasculitis; however, occasional patients will have typical cutaneous venulitis that may progress rarely to a systemic vasculitis.

Vasculitis Associated with Other Underlying Primary Diseases A number of diseases have vasculitis as a secondary manifestation of the underlying primary process. Foremost among these are the connective tissue diseases, particularly *systemic lupus erythematosus* (Chap. 311), *rheumatoid arthritis* (Chap. 312), and *Sjögren's syndrome* (Chap. 314). The most common form of vasculitis in these conditions is the small vessel venulitis isolated to the skin and clinically indistinguishable from the predominantly cutaneous vasculitides noted in response to an exogenous antigen. However, certain patients may develop a fulminant systemic necrotizing vasculitis indistinguishable from the PAN group.

Cryoglobulinemia may be seen in a number of the diverse vasculitic syndromes. *Essential mixed cryoglobulinemia* (Chap. 275) may present as a predominantly cutaneous vasculitis. However, typically, it is associated with glomerulonephritis, arthralgias, hepatosplenomegaly, and lymphadenopathy in addition to skin involvement.

Vasculitis can be associated with certain *malignancies*, particularly lymphoid or reticuloendothelial neoplasms. Leukocytoclastic venulitis confined to the skin is the most common finding; however, widespread systemic vasculitis may occur. Of particular note is the association of *hairy cell leukemia* (Chap. 112) with classic PAN.

A leukocytoclastic vasculitis predominantly involving the skin with occasional involvement of other organ systems may be a minor component of many other diseases. These include *subacute bacterial endocarditis, Epstein-Barr virus infection, HIV infection, chronic active hepatitis*, as well as a number of other infections; *ulcerative colitis, congenital deficiencies of various complement components, retroperitoneal fibrosis*, and *primary biliary cirrhosis*. Association of predominantly cutaneous vasculitis with *α_1-antitrypsin deficiency, intestinal bypass surgery*, and *relapsing polychondritis* has been reported.

DIAGNOSIS The diagnosis of this category of vasculitis is made by the demonstration of vasculitis on biopsy. Given the predominance of cutaneous involvement, biopsy material is generally readily available. An important principle in the diagnostic approach to patients with presumed isolated cutaneous vasculitis is to search for an etiology of the vasculitis—be it an exogenous agent such as a drug or an infection or an endogenous condition such as an underlying disease (Fig. 317-1). In addition, a careful physical and laboratory examination should be performed to rule out the possibility of systemic disease. This should start with the least invasive diagnostic approach and proceed to the more invasive only if clinically indicated.

℞ TREATMENT Most cases of predominantly cutaneous vasculitis resolve spontaneously, and others remit and relapse before finally remitting completely. In those patients in whom persistent cutaneous disease evolves or in whom extracutaneous organ system involvement occurs, a variety of therapeutic regimens have been tried with variable results. In general, the treatment of this type of vasculitis has not been satisfactory. Fortunately, since the disease is generally limited to the skin, this lack of consistent response to therapy usually does not lead to a life-threatening situation. When an antigenic stimulus is recognized as the precipitating factor in the vasculitis, it should be removed; if this is a microbe, appropriate antimicrobial therapy should be instituted. If the vasculitis is associated with another underlying disease, treatment of the latter often results in resolution of the former. In situations where disease is apparently self-limited, no therapy, except possibly symptomatic therapy, is indicated. When disease persists and when there is no evidence of an inciting agent, an associated disease, or an underlying systemic vasculitis, the decision to treat should be based on weighing the balance between the degree of symptoms and the risk of treatment. If the decision is made to treat, glucocorticoid therapy should be instituted, usually as prednisone, 1 mg/kg per day, in a regimen aimed at rapid tapering where possible, either directly to discontinuation or by conversion to an alternate-day regimen followed by ultimate discontinuation. In cases that prove refractory to glucocorticoids, a trial of an immunosuppressive agent may be indicated. Patients with chronic vasculitis isolated to cutaneous venules rarely respond dramatically to any therapeutic regimen, and immunosuppressive agents should be used only as a last resort in these patients. Methotrexate and azathioprine have been used in such situations in anecdotal reports (see above for specific regimens). Although cyclophosphamide is the most effective therapy for the systemic vasculitides, it should almost never be used for predominantly cutaneous vasculitis because of the potential toxicity. Plasmapheresis has been used with some success in fulminant cases. Dapsone has been tried in a number of patients with isolated cutaneous vasculitis with rare anecdotal reports of success. However, this drug has been consistently beneficial as therapy for cutaneous vasculitis only in patients with erythema elevatum diutinum (see below).

KAWASAKI DISEASE

Kawasaki disease (mucocutaneous lymph node syndrome) is an acute, febrile, multisystem disease of children. It is characterized by unresponsiveness to antibiotics, nonsuppurative cervical adenitis, and changes in the skin and mucous membranes such as edema; congested conjunctivae; erythema of the oral cavity, lips, and palms; and desquamation of the skin of the fingertips. Although the disease is generally benign and self-limited, it is associated with coronary artery aneurysms in approximately 25% of cases, with an overall case fatality rate of 0.5 to 2.8%. These complications usually occur between the third and fourth weeks of illness during the convalescent stage. Vasculitis of the coronary arteries is seen in almost all the fatal cases that have been autopsied. There is typical intimal proliferation and infiltration of the vessel wall with mononuclear cells. Beadlike aneurysms and thromboses may be seen along the artery. Most investigators agree that many of the cases of PAN formerly reported in children were actually arteritic complications of unrecognized Kawasaki disease. Other manifestations include pericarditis, myocarditis, myocardial ischemia and infarction, and cardiomegaly.

It is likely that immune-mediated injury to blood vessel endothelium is involved in the pathogenesis of this disease. Patients with Kawasaki disease have been demonstrated to have evidence of increased immune activation characterized by increased activated helper T cells and monocytes, elevated serum-soluble IL-2 receptor levels, elevated levels of spontaneous IL-1 production by peripheral blood mononuclear cells, anti-endothelial cell antibodies, and increased cytokine-inducible activation antigens on their vascular endothelium. A strong association has been reported between a novel form of *S. aureus* that releases toxic shock syndrome toxin 1 and Kawasaki disease, suggesting that this was the causative organism and was acting as a superantigen similar to the superantigen effect in toxic shock syndrome. However, analysis of the T cell receptor repertoire of patients with Kawasaki disease has yielded conflicting data as to whether the T cell response is driven by a superantigen or by a conventional antigen.

Apart from the up to 2.8% of patients who develop fatal complications, the prognosis of this disease for uneventful recovery is excellent. High-dose intravenous γ globulin (2 g/kg as a single infusion over 10 h) together with aspirin (100 mg/kg per day for 14 days followed by 3 to 5 mg/kg per day for several weeks) have been shown to be effective in reducing the prevalence of coronary artery abnormalities when administered early in the course of the disease.

ISOLATED VASCULITIS OF THE CENTRAL NERVOUS SYSTEM

Isolated vasculitis of the central nervous system is an uncommon clinicopathologic entity characterized by vasculitis restricted to the vessels of the central nervous system without other apparent systemic vasculitis. Although the arteriole is most commonly affected, vessels of any size can be involved. The inflammatory process is usually composed of mononuclear cell infiltrates with or without granuloma formation. Cases have been associated with cytomegalovirus, syphilis, pyogenic bacterial, and varicella-zoster infections, as well as with Hodgkin's disease and amphetamine abuse; however, in most cases no underlying disease process has been identified.

Patients may present with severe headaches, altered mental function, and focal neurologic defects. Systemic symptoms are generally absent. Devastating neurologic abnormalities may occur depending on the extent of vessel involvement. The diagnosis is generally made by demonstration of characteristic vessel abnormalities on arteriography and confirmed by biopsy of the brain parenchyma and leptomeninges. In the absence of a brain biopsy, care should be taken not to misinterpret as true primary vasculitis angiographic abnormalities that might actually be vessel spasm related to another cause. The prognosis of this disease is poor; however, in certain patients the disease may remit spontaneously, and some reports indicate that glucocorticoid therapy alone or together with cyclophosphamide in steroid-resistant patients administered as described above for the systemic vasculitides has induced sustained clinical remissions in a small number of patients.

THROMBOANGIITIS OBLITERANS (BUERGER'S DISEASE)

Thromboangiitis obliterans is an inflammatory occlusive peripheral vascular disease of unknown etiology that affects arteries and veins. Thrombosis of the vessels is likely the primary event, and so this disease is not a classic vasculitis. However, it is considered among the vasculitides because of the intense inflammatory response within the thrombus and the fact that there is often a vasculitis of the vasa vasorum in the arterial wall. →*The disease is discussed in detail in Chap. 248.*

BEHÇET'S SYNDROME

Behçet's syndrome is a clinicopathologic entity characterized by recurrent episodes of oral and genital ulcers, iritis, and cutaneous lesions. The underlying pathologic process is a leukocytoclastic venulitis, although vessels of any size and in any organ can be involved. →*This disorder is described in detail in Chap. 316.*

MISCELLANEOUS VASCULITIDES

A variety of disorders, many of which are uncommon, are characterized by varying degrees of inflammatory responses involving blood vessels. *Cogan's syndrome* is a disease characterized by nonsyphilitic interstitial keratitis together with vestibuloauditory symptoms. It may be associated with a systemic vasculitis involving vessels of different sizes as well as the aortic valve.

Erythema elevatum diutinum is a rare chronic skin disorder of unknown etiology characterized by persistent red, purple, and yellowish papules, plaques, and nodules usually distributed symmetrically over the extensor surface of the limbs; on biopsy, they demonstrate a leukocytoclastic venulitis together with a marked dermal inflammatory infiltrate. An association with streptococcal infections has been reported. The disease responds dramatically to dapsone therapy.

Certain *infections* may directly trigger an inflammatory vasculitic process. For example, rickettsias can invade and proliferate in the endothelial cells of small blood vessels causing a vasculitis (Chap. 177). In addition, the inflammatory response around blood vessels associated with certain systemic fungal diseases such as histoplasmosis (Chap. 201) may mimic a primary vasculitic process.

PRINCIPLES OF TREATMENT

Once a diagnosis of vasculitis has been established, a decision regarding therapeutic strategy must be made (Fig. 317-1). The vasculitis syndromes represent a wide spectrum of diseases with varying degrees of severity. Some require immediate and aggressive therapy with glucocorticoids and immunosuppressive agents, while others should be treated conservatively and symptomatically, usually with nonsteroidal anti-inflammatory drugs. Since the potential toxic side effects of certain therapeutic regimens may be substantial, the risk-versus-benefit ratio of any therapeutic approach should be weighed carefully. Specific therapeutic regimens are discussed above for the individual vasculitis syndromes; however, certain general principles regarding therapy should be considered. On the one hand, glucocorticoids and/or immunosuppressive therapy should be instituted immediately in diseases where irreversible organ system dysfunction and high morbidity and mortality have been clearly established. Wegener's granulomatosis is the prototype of a severe systemic vasculitis requiring such a therapeutic approach (see above). On the other hand, when feasible, aggressive therapy should be avoided for vasculitic manifestations that rarely result in irreversible organ system dysfunction and that usually do not respond to such therapy. For example, isolated cutaneous vasculitis usually resolves with symptomatic treatment, and prolonged courses of glucocorticoids uncommonly result in clinical benefit. Immunosuppressive agents have not proven to be beneficial in isolated cutaneous vasculitis, and their toxic side effects generally outweigh any potential beneficial effects. Glucocorticoids should be initiated in those systemic vasculitides that cannot be specifically categorized or for which there is no established standard therapy; immunosuppressive therapy should be added in these diseases only if an adequate response does not result or if remission can only be achieved and maintained with an unacceptably toxic regimen of glucocorticoids. When remission is achieved, one should continually attempt to taper glucocorticoids to an alternate-day regimen and discontinue when possible. When using immunosuppressive regimens, one should taper and discontinue the drug as soon as is feasible upon induction of remission (see below).

When glucocorticoids are used, prednisone is generally the formulation of choice and is administered as 1 mg/kg per day orally, first in divided doses and then converted to a single daily dose. After clinical improvement is noted (usually within a month), the regimen is gradually converted to an alternate-day schedule, followed by tapering and discontinuation after approximately 6 months or as the clinical response dictates. When an immunosuppressive agent is required, cyclophosphamide is the drug of choice and its efficacy has been clearly established in Wegener's granulomatosis and the severe systemic vasculitides (see above). It should be given in doses of 2 mg/kg per day orally. It is recommended that the drug be taken as a single dose in the morning together with large amounts of fluid. Dose adjustments should be based on the leukocyte count, which should be maintained above 3000/μL. Leukocyte counts at any given time will reflect the dosage of cyclophosphamide taken the previous week. Of note, neutropenia may become more pronounced as glucocorticoids are tapered. The regimen that has proven successful in Wegener's granulomatosis (see above) and that should be followed for the other severe systemic vasculitides has called for continuation of cyclophosphamide for approximately 1 year following the induction of complete remission, with gradual tapering (by 25-mg decrements of the daily dose) over several months until discontinuation. No other drug has proven to be as effective as cyclophosphamide for severe life-threatening vasculitis. However, immediate and long-range toxic side effects may be severe. Alternative immunosuppressive regimens may be instituted where indicated in those patients who cannot tolerate cyclophosphamide due to unacceptable side effects or who do not wish to take cyclophosphamide because of the potential side effects, particularly infertility or sterility in individuals of child-bearing age. Methotrexate has been shown to be an acceptable alternative to cyclophosphamide when the latter drug cannot be used. Methotrexate is administered as a single weekly dose initially at a dosage of 0.3 mg/kg, not to exceed 15 mg/week. If the treatment is well tolerated after 1 to 2 weeks, the dosage should be increased by 2.5 mg weekly up to a dosage of 20 to 25 mg/week and maintained at that level. Azathioprine at a dosage of 2 mg/kg per day orally has also been employed as an alternative to cyclophosphamide in severe systemic vasculitis with less favorable results. In unusual cases in which none of the above regimens have resulted in remission of the vasculitis, certain experimental approaches have been used, such as plasmapheresis together with immunosuppressive drugs, with anecdotal reports of limited success. In addition, other immunosuppressive agents such as cyclosporine have been employed with minimal success.

Physicians should be thoroughly aware of the toxic side effects of therapeutic agents employed (Table 317-6). Side effects of glucocorticoid therapy are markedly decreased in frequency and duration in patients on alternate-day regimens compared to daily regimens. When cyclophosphamide is administered chronically in doses of 2 mg/kg per day for substantial periods of time (one to several years), the incidence of cystitis as defined by nonglomerular hematuria is approximately 50% and the incidence of bladder cancer is 6%. Bladder cancer can occur several years after discontinuation of cyclophosphamide therapy; therefore, monitoring for bladder cancer should continue indefinitely in patients who have received prolonged courses of daily cyclophosphamide. Significant alopecia is unusual in the chronically administered, low-dose regimen. When patients are receiving low-dose cyclophosphamide, the white blood count (WBC) is maintained above 3000/μL, and the patient is not receiving daily glucocorticoids, the incidence of life-threatening opportunistic infections is very low. However, the WBC is not an accurate predictor of risk of opportunistic infections in patients receiving methotrexate; infections with *Pneumocystis carinii* and certain fungi can be seen in the face of WBC that are within normal limits. All vasculitis patients who are not allergic to sulfa and who are receiving daily glucocorticoids in combination with an immunosuppressive drug should receive trimethoprim-sulfamethoxazole as prophylaxis against *P. carinii* infection.

Finally, it should be emphasized that each patient is unique and requires individual decision-making. The above outline should serve as a framework to guide therapeutic approaches; however, flexibility should be practiced in order to provide maximal therapeutic efficacy with minimal toxic side effects in each patient.

Table 317-6 Major Toxic Side Effects of Drugs Commonly Used in the Treatment of Systemic Vasculitis

GLUCOCORTICOIDS	
Osteoporosis	Growth suppression in children
Cataracts	Hypertension
Glaucoma	Avascular necrosis of bone
Diabetes mellitus	Myopathy
Electrolyte abnormalities	Alterations in mood
Metabolic abnormalities	Psychosis
Suppression of inflammatory and immune responses leading to opportunistic infections	Pseudotumor cerebri
Cushingoid features	Peptic ulcer diathesis
	Pancreatitis
CYCLOPHOSPHAMIDE	
Bone marrow suppression	Hypogammaglobulinemia
Cystitis	Pulmonary fibrosis
Bladder carcinoma	Myelodysplasia
Gonadal suppression	Oncogenesis
Gastrointestinal intolerance	
METHOTREXATE	
Gastrointestinal intolerance	Pneumonitis
Stomatitis	Teratogenicity
Neutropenia	Opportunistic infections
Hepatotoxicity (may lead to fibrosis or cirrhosis)	

BIBLIOGRAPHY

FAUCI AS et al: Wegener's granulomatosis: Prospective clinical and therapeutic experience with 85 patients for 21 years. Ann Intern Med 98:76, 1983

GUILLEVIN L et al: Treatment of polyarteritis nodosa related to hepatitis B virus with interferon-alpha and plasma exchanges. Ann Rheum Dis 53:334, 1994

——— et al: Microscopic polyangiitis. Clinical and laboratory findings in eighty-five patients. Arthritis Rheum 42:421, 1999

HOFFMAN GS, SPECKS U: Antineutrophil cytoplasmic antibodies. Arthritis Rheum 41:1521, 1998

——— et al: Wegener's granulomatosis: An analysis of 158 patients. Ann Intern Med 116:488, 1992

HUNDER GG: Giant cell arteritis and polymyalgia rheumatica. Med Clin North Am 81:195, 1997

JENNETTE JC et al: Nomenclature of systemic vasculitis. Proposal of an international consensus conference. Arthritis Rheum 37:187, 1994

KERR G et al: Takayasu arteritis. Ann Intern Med 120:919, 1994

LANGFORD CA et al: Use of cytotoxic agents and cyclosporine in the treatment of autoimmune disease. Part 2: Inflammatory bowel disease, systemic vasculitis, and therapeutic toxicity. Ann Intern Med 129:49, 1998

LEUNG DYM et al: The immunopathogenesis and management of Kawasaki syndrome. Arthritis Rheum 41:1538, 1998

LUDVIKSSON BR et al: Active Wegener's granulomatosis is associated with HLA-DR+ CD4+ T cells exhibiting an unbalanced Th-1 type T cell cytokine pattern: Reversal with IL-10. J Immunol 160:3602, 1998

SNELLER MC, FAUCI AS: Pathogenesis of vasculitis syndromes. Adv Rheumatol 81:221, 1997

——— et al: An analysis of forty-two Wegener's granulomatosis patients treated with methotrexate and prednisone. Arthritis Rheum 38:608, 1995

SOMER T, FINEGOLD SM: Vasculitis associated with infections, immunization, and antimicrobial drugs. Clin Infect Dis 20:1010, 1995

TALAR-WILLIAMS C et al: Cyclophosphamide-induced cystitis and bladder cancer in patients with Wegener's granulomatosis. Ann Intern Med 124:477, 1996

WEYLAND CM et al: Distinct vascular lesions in giant cell arteritis share identical T cell clonotypes. J Exp Med 179:951, 1994

——— et al: Tissue cytokine patterns in patients with polymyalgia rheumatica and giant cell arteritis. Ann Intern Med 121:484, 1994

318 SARCOIDOSIS

Ronald G. Crystal

DEFINITION Sarcoidosis is a chronic, multisystem disorder of unknown cause characterized in affected organs by an accumulation of T lymphocytes and mononuclear phagocytes, noncaseating epithelioid granulomas, and derangements of the normal tissue architecture. Although there are usually skin anergy and depressed cellular immune processes in the blood, sarcoidosis is characterized at the sites of disease by exaggerated T helper 1 (T_H1) lymphocyte immune processes. All parts of the body can be affected, but the organ most frequently affected is the lung. Involvement of the skin, eye, liver, and lymph nodes is also common. The disease is often acute or subacute and self-limiting, but in many individuals it is chronic, waxing and waning over many years.

ETIOLOGY The cause of sarcoidosis is unknown. Various infectious and noninfectious agents have been implicated, but there is no proof that any specific agent is responsible. However, all available evidence is consistent with the concept that the disease results from an exaggerated cellular immune response (acquired, inherited, or both) to a limited class of persistent antigens or self-antigens.

INCIDENCE AND PREVALENCE Sarcoidosis is a relatively common disease affecting individuals of both sexes and almost all ages, races, and geographic locations. Females appear to be slightly more susceptible than males. Cases of sarcoidosis have been described in all of the major races, and the disease is found throughout the world. It has been suggested that sarcoidosis is more common in certain geographic areas such as the southeastern part of the United States, but when case-matched controls have been used, these geographic differences are less convincing. There is a remarkable diversity of the prevalence of sarcoidosis among certain ethnic and racial groups, with a range of <1 to 64 per 100,000 worldwide. The prevalence of sarcoidosis is from 10 to 40 per 100,000 in the United States and Europe. In the United States, most patients are black, with a ratio of blacks to whites ranging from 10:1 to 17:1. In Europe, however, the disease affects mostly whites. Furthermore, while the prevalence per 100,000 in Sweden is 64, in France it is 10, in Poland 3, yet for Irish females living in London it is 200. In contrast, the disease is very rare among Inuit, Canadian Indians, New Zealand Maoris, and Southeast Asians.

Most patients present with sarcoidosis between the ages of 20 and 40, but the disease can occur in children and in the elderly. Several hundred kindred groups with familial sarcoidosis have been described, and the disease has been observed in twins, more commonly in monozygotic than in dizygotic pairs. There also have been several instances of husband-wife pairs identified, and geographic foci of sarcoidosis among unrelated individuals living closely within a community, arguing for some environmental factors in the pathogenesis of the disease. Although the disease is believed to result from exaggerated cellular immune responses to a limited class of antigens, no clear patterns in any HLA locus have emerged. Unlike many diseases in which the lung is involved, sarcoidosis favors nonsmokers.

PATHOPHYSIOLOGY AND IMMUNOPATHOGENESIS The first manifestation of the disease is an accumulation of mononuclear inflammatory cells, mostly CD4+ T_H1 lymphocytes and mononuclear phagocytes, in affected organs. This inflammatory process is followed by the formation of granulomas, aggregates of macrophages and their progeny, epithelioid cells, and multinucleated giant cells. The typical sarcoid granuloma is a compact structure composed of an aggregate of mononuclear phagocytes surrounded by a rim of CD4+ T lymphocytes and, to a far lesser extent, B lymphocytes. The overall structure is relatively discrete and is interspersed with fine collagen fibrils, presumably remnants of the underlying connective tissue matrix. The giant cells within the granuloma can be of the Langhans' or foreign-body variety and often contain inclusions such as Schaumann bodies (conchlike structures), asteroid bodies (stellate-like structures), and residual bodies (refractile calcium-containing inclusions).

Together the accumulated T cells, mononuclear phagocytes, and granulomas represent the active disease. Other than the fact that they take up space and thus their bulk modifies the local architecture, for all except late stage cases, there is no evidence that the mononuclear inflammatory cells dispersed in the tissue or in the granuloma injure the affected organ by releasing mediators that damage the normal parenchymal cells or the extracellular matrix. Rather, organ dysfunction in sarcoidosis results mostly from the accumulated inflammatory cells distorting the architecture of the affected tissue; if a sufficient number of structures vital to the function of the tissue are involved, the disease becomes clinically apparent in that organ. Thus, while autopsy series show that, to some extent, sarcoidosis involves most organs in the majority of patients, the disease manifests clinically only in organs where it affects function (such as the lung and eye) or in organs where it is readily observed (such as the skin or, by x-ray, the hilar nodes). For example, in the lung, the inflammatory cells and granulomas distort the walls of the alveoli, bronchi, and blood vessels (Fig. 318-1*A*), thus altering the intimate relationships between air and blood necessary for normal gas exchange. When a sufficient amount of pulmonary tissue is involved, it is sensed by the individual as dyspnea. In contrast, most individuals with sarcoidosis have granulomatous mononuclear cell inflammation in the liver but usually do not have symptoms or significant functional derangements referable to that organ, likely because the disease process does not modify the local structures sufficiently to affect function.

If the disease is suppressed, either spontaneously or with therapy, the mononuclear inflammation is reduced in intensity and the number of granulomas is reduced. The granulomas resolve either by dispersion of the cells or by centripetal proliferation of fibroblasts from the periphery of the granuloma inward, to form a small scar. In chronic cases, the mononuclear cell inflammation persists for years. If the intensity of the inflammation is sufficiently high for a sufficiently long period, the derangements to the affected tissues result in extensive damage, the development of fibrosis, and permanent loss of organ function.

All available evidence suggests that active sarcoidosis results from an exaggerated cellular immune response to a variety of antigens or self-antigens, in which the process of T lymphocyte triggering, proliferation, and activation is skewed in the direction of CD4+ T_H1 lymphocyte processes (Fig. 318-1*B*). The result is an exaggerated T_H1 T lymphocyte response and thus the accumulation of large numbers of activated T_H1 cells in the affected organs. Since the activated T_H1 lymphocyte releases mediators that attract and activate mononuclear phagocytes, it is likely that the process of granuloma formation is a secondary phenomenon that is a consequence of the exaggerated T_H1 cell process. In this context, the current hypotheses of the cause of sarcoidosis, not mutually exclusive, include the following: (1) The disease is caused by a class of persistent antigens, nonself or self, that trigger only the T_H1 cell arm of the immune response; (2) the disease results from an inadequate suppressor arm of the immune response, such that T_H1 cell processes cannot be shut down in a normal fashion; or (3) the disease results from inherited (and/or acquired) differences in immune response genes, such that the response to a variety of antigens is an exaggerated, T_H1 cell process.

Independent of the inciting agent(s) or the reason why there is an exaggerated T_H1 cell response, there is a general understanding of the processes responsible for the maintenance of the inflammation and the development of the granuloma. The T_H1 lymphocytes accumulate at the sites of disease, at least in part, because they proliferate in these sites at an exaggerated rate. This T cell proliferation is maintained by the spontaneous release of interleukin (IL) 2, the T cell growth factor, by activated T_H1 cells in the local milieu. In this regard, sarcoidosis is a remarkable example of compartmentalization of the immune system and a dramatic illustration of why disease activity of sarcoidosis cannot be assessed by evaluating the immune system only in the blood.

Whereas the T_H1 cells in the involved organs are releasing IL-2 and proliferating at an enhanced rate, the T cells in other sites, such as blood, are quiescent. Furthermore, while there is a marked enhancement of the number of T_H1 cells at the sites of disease, the numbers of T_H1 cells in the blood are normal or slightly reduced. In the involved organs, the ratio of CD4+ to CD8+ T cells may be as high as 10:1 compared to the ratio of 2:1 found in normal tissues or in the blood of affected individuals.

In addition to driving other T_H1 cells in the affected organs to proliferate, the T_H1 cells at the sites of disease are activated and release mediators that both recruit and activate mononuclear phagocytes. The activated T_H1 cells accomplish this by releasing a variety of mediators (lymphokines) including proteins capable of recruiting blood monocytes to the local milieu of the activated T cells and interferon γ, a protein that, among its many actions, activates mononuclear phagocytes. Together with cytokines such as interleukin (IL)-12 and others released locally, these mediators recruit blood monocytes to the affected organs and activate them, providing the building blocks for the formation of the granuloma.

In addition to these exaggerated cellular immune processes, active sarcoidosis is also characterized by hyperglobulinemia. Included among the immunoglobulins are antibodies against a variety of infectious agents as well as IgM anti-T cell antibodies. However, there is no evidence that any of these antibodies plays a role in the pathogenesis of the disease, and they are thought to result from the nonspecific polyclonal stimulation of B cells by the activated T cells at the site of disease.

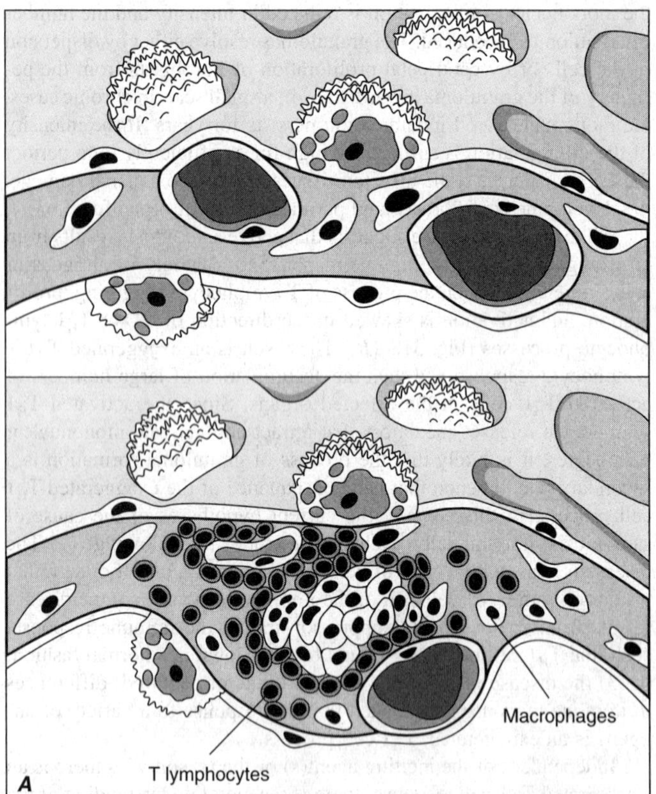

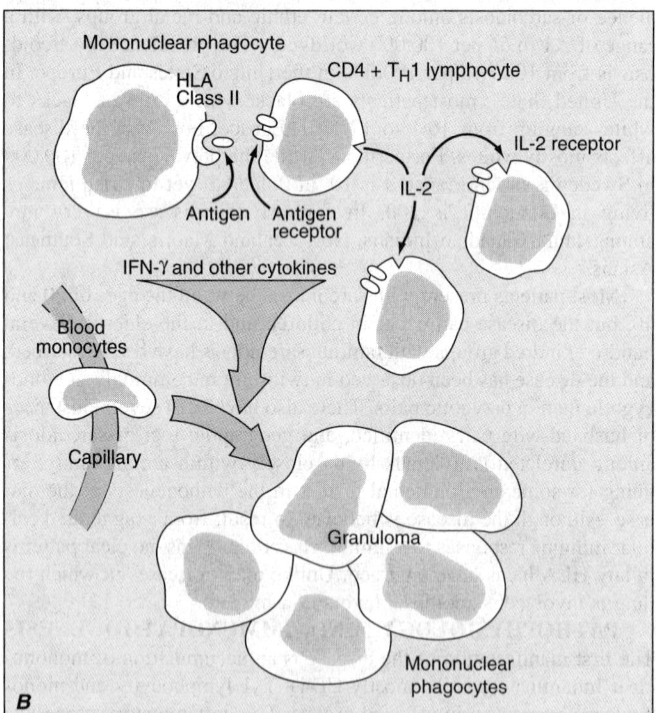

FIGURE 318-1 Pathogenesis of sarcoidosis. *A.* Histologic abnormalities. Normal alveoli (*top*) and alveoli in active sarcoidosis (*bottom*). The latter are distorted by the accumulated CD4+ T_H1 lymphocytes, alveolar macrophages, and macrophages aggregated into granulomas. There is mild damage to alveolar epithelial and endothelial cells. *B.* The exaggerated processes of T_H1 lymphocytes in affected organs result in the accumulation of these cells along with macrophages and macrophages aggregated into granulomas. The trigger for the T_H1 lymphocytes is unknown. It may be a limited class of antigens or self-antigens presented in the context of class II HLA surface molecules by mononuclear phagocytes to the T_H1 lymphocyte. The antigen class II HLA complex is identified by the T cell antigen receptor, and the T cell is activated. Consequent to this process the immune response is exaggerated and skewed to produce activated T_H1 lymphocytes that release IL-2, which drives the accumulation of more T lymphocytes. The activated T_H1 lymphocytes also release interferon γ (INF-γ). Together with cytokines such as IL-12, macrophage inflammatory protein 1α and granulocyte-macrophage colony stimulating factor released in the local milieu, there is recruitment and activation of blood monocytes and subsequent granuloma formation.

If the damage in the affected organs is sufficiently extensive that the remaining parenchymal cells cannot reestablish the normal tissue architecture, the usual result is fibrosis, the proliferation of mesenchymal cells, and deposition of their connective tissue products. There is convincing evidence that the fibroblast proliferation is directed by tissue macrophages spontaneously releasing growth signals for fibroblasts, including platelet-derived growth factor, fibronectin, and insulin-like growth factor 1. It is not known, however, why this fibrotic process occurs only in a relatively small proportion of individuals with sarcoidosis.

CLINICAL MANIFESTATIONS Sarcoidosis is a systemic disease, and thus the clinical manifestations may be generalized or focused on one or more organs. However, because the lung is almost always involved, most patients have symptoms referable to the respiratory system. Independent of the site, the clinical manifestations of the disease relate directly to the exaggerated T_H1 lymphocyte–mononuclear phagocyte granulomatous inflammatory process itself or to the sequelae resulting from the permanent damage caused by this process.

Sarcoidosis is occasionally discovered in a completely asymptomatic individual, but more commonly it presents abruptly over 1 to 2 weeks or the affected individual develops symptoms insidiously over several months. Independent of the mode of presentation, ~75% of all cases present in individuals younger than 40 years.

The asymptomatic form is usually detected by a routine examination, such as a chest film. In the United States, this form represents about 10 to 20% of all cases, but in countries where chest films are mandatory in preemployment screening programs, the proportion of asymptomatic patients is higher.

So-called acute or subacute sarcoidosis develops abruptly over a period of a few weeks and represents 20 to 40% of all cases. These individuals usually have constitutional symptoms such as fever, fatigue, malaise, anorexia, or weight loss. These symptoms are usually mild, but in approximately 25% of the acute cases the constitutional complaints are extensive. Many patients have respiratory symptoms, including cough, dyspnea, a vague retrosternal chest discomfort and/or polyarthritis. Two syndromes have been identified in the acute group. Löfgren's syndrome, frequent in Scandinavian, Irish, and Puerto Rican females, includes the complex of erythema nodosum **(Plate IIE-70)** and x-ray findings of bilateral hilar adenopathy, often accompanied by joint symptoms, including arthritis at the ankles, knees, wrists, or elbows. The Heerfordt-Waldenström syndrome describes individuals with fever, parotid enlargement, anterior uveitis, and facial nerve palsy.

The insidious form of sarcoidosis develops over months and is associated usually with respiratory complaints without constitutional symptoms. In the United States, 40 to 70% of all patients with sarcoidosis patients are in this category. About 10% of these individuals have symptoms referable to organs other than the lung. It is the individuals who present with the insidious form of sarcoidosis who most commonly go on to develop chronic sarcoidosis, with permanent damage to the lung and other organs.

Despite the fact that sarcoidosis is a systemic disease and some evidence of inflammation can be detected in most organs in the majority of patients, sarcoidosis is important clinically because of the pulmonary abnormalities and, to a lesser extent, lymph node, skin, liver, and eye involvement. Far less commonly, other organs are involved significantly.

Lung Of individuals with sarcoidosis, 90% have abnormal findings on chest x-ray at some time during their course (Fig. 318-2*A*). Overall, ~50% develop permanent pulmonary abnormalities, and 5 to 15% have progressive fibrosis of the lung parenchyma. Sarcoidosis of the lung is primarily an interstitial lung disease (Chap. 259) in which the inflammatory process involves the alveoli, small bronchi, and small blood vessels. These individuals typically have symptoms of dyspnea, particularly with exercise, and a dry cough. In acute and subacute cases, physical examination usually reveals dry rales. Hemoptysis is rare, as is production of sputum. Occasionally, the large airways are involved to a degree sufficient to cause dysfunction. Distal atelectasis can result from endobronchial sarcoidosis or from external compression from enlarged intrathoracic nodes. Rarely, wheezing is heard, incorrectly suggesting asthma. Large-vessel pulmonary granulomatous arteritis is common, but it rarely causes major problems. If it dominates the pulmonary lesions, it is sometimes called *necrotizing sarcoidal granulomatosis*. The pleura is involved in 1 to 5% of cases, almost always manifesting as a unilateral pleural effusion with characteristics of an exudate containing lymphocytes. The effusions usually clear within a few weeks, but chronic pleural thickening can result. Pneumothorax is very rare.

Lymph Nodes Lymphadenopathy is very common in sarcoidosis. Intrathoracic nodes are enlarged in 75 to 90% of all patients; usually this involves the hilar nodes, but the paratracheal nodes are commonly involved (Fig. 318-2*A*). Less frequently, there is enlargement of subcarinal, anterior mediastinal, or posterior mediastinal nodes. Peripheral lymphadenopathy is very common, particularly involving the cervical, axillary, epitrochlear, and inguinal nodes. The nodes in the retroperitoneal area and in the mesenteric chain also can enlarge. All these nodes are nonadherent, with a firm, rubbery texture. Palpation causes no pain. Unlike nodes in tuberculosis, the nodes do not ulcerate. The lymphadenopathy rarely causes a problem for the affected individual; however, if it is massive, it can be disfiguring and can impinge on other organs and lead to functional impairment.

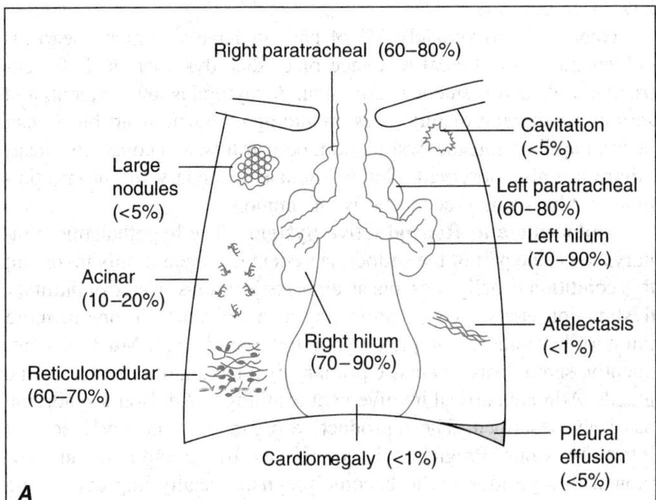

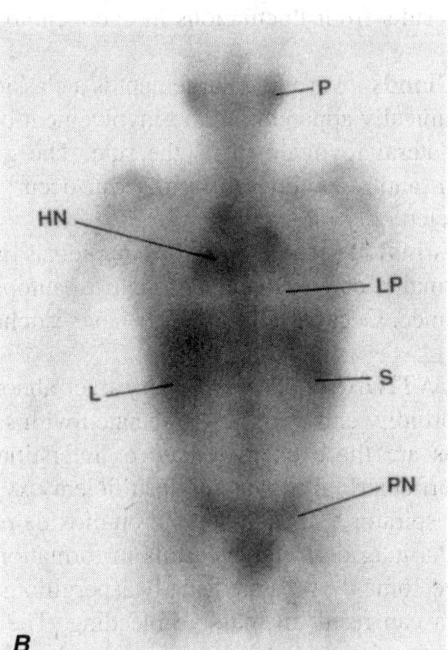

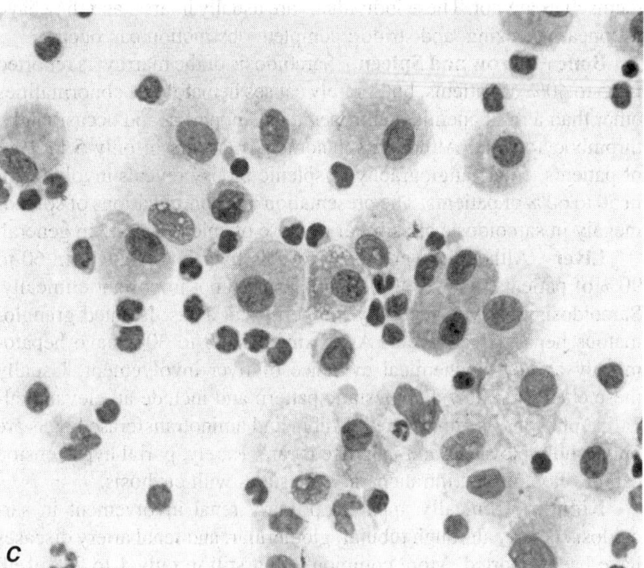

FIGURE 318-2 Common laboratory findings of sarcoidosis. *A.* Schematic view of the abnormal findings on the chest x-ray. Shown are changes observed with the average frequency of occurrence. *B.* Typical gallium-67 scan of an individual with active sarcoidosis. The isotope has accumulated in the lung parenchyma (LP), liver (L), spleen (S), parotid (P), hilar nodes (HN), and pelvic nodes (PN). *C.* Cells recovered by bronchoalveolar lavage of an individual with active pulmonary sarcoidosis. The lavage analysis reflects the inflammation in the tissue. Shown are alveolar macrophages (*large cells*) and lymphocytes (*small cells*). The cell population is dominated by the T_H1 subset of CD4+ lymphocytes, in contrast to normal individuals, in whom lymphocytes represent <20% of the cell population.

Skin Sarcoidosis involves the skin in ~25% of patients. The most common lesions are erythema nodosum **(Plate IIE-70)**, plaques, maculopapular eruptions, subcutaneous nodules, and lupus pernio. Erythema nodosum, comprising bilateral, tender red nodules on the anterior surface of the legs, is not specific for sarcoidosis but is common, particularly in acute sarcoidosis, in combination with systemic symptoms and polyarthralgias. Treatment is not required, since the lesions resolve spontaneously in 2 to 4 weeks. Erythema nodosum is much more common among patients with sarcoidosis in Europe than in the United States. Skin plaques associated with sarcoidosis are purple, indolent lesions, often raised, and usually occur on the face, buttocks, and extremities. The maculopapular eruptions occur on the face around the eyes and nose, on the back, and on the extremities. These are elevated lesions <1 cm in diameter with a flat, waxy top. Subcutaneous nodules are most common on the trunk and extremities. Lupus pernio is characterized by indurated blue-purple, swollen, shiny lesions on the nose, cheeks, lips, ears, fingers, and knees. The lesions on the tip of the nose cause a bulbous appearance, sometimes associated with varicosities. The nasal mucosa is usually involved, and underlying bone can be destroyed. Sarcoidosis also can involve old surgical scars and tattoos. Although it may be disfiguring, cutaneous sarcoidosis rarely causes major problems. Clubbing of the fingers is occasionally observed in sarcoidosis, usually in association with extensive pulmonary fibrosis.

Eye Eye involvement occurs in ~25% of patients with sarcoidosis, and it can cause blindness. The usual lesions involve the uveal tract, iris, ciliary body, and choroid. Of those patients with eye involvement, ~75% have anterior uveitis and 25 to 35% have posterior uveitis. There is blurred vision, tearing, and photophobia. The uveitis can develop rapidly and may clear spontaneously over a 6- to 12-month period. It also can develop insidiously and be chronic. Conjunctival involvement is also common, usually with small, yellow nodules. When the lacrimal gland is involved, a keratoconjunctivitis sicca syndrome, with dry, sore eyes, can result.

Upper Respiratory Tract The nasal mucosa is involved in up to 20% of patients, usually presenting with nasal stuffiness. Any of the structures of the mouth can be involved, particularly the tonsils. Sarcoidosis involves the larynx in ~5% of patients. The epiglottis and areas around the true vocal cords are usually involved, but the cords themselves are not. These individuals are usually hoarse, and they have dyspnea, wheezing, and stridor; complete obstruction can occur.

Bone Marrow and Spleen Sarcoidosis of the marrow is reported in 15 to 40% of patients, but it rarely causes hematologic abnormalities other than a mild anemia, neutropenia, eosinophilia, and occasionally, thrombocytopenia. Although splenomegaly occurs in only 5 to 10% of patients, celiac angiography or splenic biopsy reveals involvement in 50 to 60% of patients. The presentation and complications of splenomegaly in sarcoidosis are similar to those of splenomegaly in general.

Liver Although liver biopsy reveals liver involvement in 60 to 90% of patients, liver dysfunction is usually not important clinically. Sarcoidosis involves generally the periportal areas. Isolated granulomatous hepatitis can occur. Approximately 20 to 30% have hepatomegaly and/or biochemical evidence of liver involvement. Usually these changes reflect a cholestatic pattern and include an elevated alkaline phosphatase level; the bilirubin and aminotransferase levels are only mildly elevated, and jaundice is rare. Rarely, portal hypertension can develop, as can intrahepatic cholestasis with cirrhosis.

Kidney Clinically apparent primary renal involvement in sarcoidosis is rare, although tubular, glomerular, and renal artery diseases have been reported. More commonly, but still in only 1 to 2% of all patients, there is a disorder of calcium metabolism with hypercalciuria, with or without hypercalcemia. If chronic, nephrocalcinosis and nephrolithiasis can result. It is believed that the calcium abnormalities are associated with enhanced calcium absorption in the gut, which is related to an abnormally high level of circulating 1,25-dihydroxyvitamin D produced by mononuclear phagocytes in the granulomas.

Nervous System All components of the nervous system can be involved in sarcoidosis. Neurologic findings are observed in about 5% of patients. Seventh nerve involvement with unilateral facial paralysis is most common. It occurs suddenly and is usually transient. Other common manifestations of neurosarcoid include optic nerve dysfunction, papilledema, palate dysfunction, hearing abnormalities, hypothalamic and pituitary abnormalities, chronic meningitis, and, occasionally, space-occupying lesions. Psychiatric disturbances have been described, and seizures can occur. Rarely, multiple lesions occur that mimic multiple sclerosis, spinal cord abnormalities, and peripheral neuropathy.

Musculoskeletal System The bones, joints, and/or muscles can be involved in sarcoidosis. Bone lesions are observed in 5% of patients and include variable-sized cysts in areas of expanded bone; well-defined, round, punched-out lesions; or lattice-like changes. Hand and foot bones are the common sites, but most bones can be involved. Occasionally, the bone lesions are tender and painful. Joint involvement is more common, with an incidence of 25 to 50% in known cases of sarcoidosis. Arthralgias and frank arthritis occur mostly in large joints; they can be migratory and are usually transient, but they can be chronic and result in deformities. Although muscle biopsy frequently demonstrates granulomatous inflammation, muscle dysfunction is rare. However, nodules, polymyositis, and chronic myopathy have been described.

Heart Approximately 5% of patients have significant heart involvement, with clinical evidence of cardiac dysfunction. Left ventricular wall involvement is common. Arrhythmias are frequent, and serious conduction disturbances, including complete heart block, can occur. Papillary muscle dysfunction, pericarditis, and congestive heart failure are also observed. Cor pulmonale secondary to chronic pulmonary fibrosis may occur but is uncommon.

Endocrine and Reproductive System The hypothalamic-pituitary axis is the part of the endocrine system most commonly involved; this condition usually presents as diabetes insipidus. Anterior pituitary dysfunction is also seen, manifesting as a deficiency in one or more pituitary hormones. Complete hypopituitarism is rare. Much less frequently, sarcoidosis can cause primary dysfunction of other endocrine glands. Adrenal cortical involvement resulting in Addison's syndrome has been described. The reproductive organs may be involved, but infertility is rare. Pregnancy is not affected by sarcoidosis, and common with sarcoidosis who become pregnant usually improve during pregnancy. However, the disease may flare post partum; presumably this variation results from fluctuations in endogenous glucocorticoid production.

Exocrine Glands Parotid enlargement is a classic feature of sarcoidosis, but clinically apparent parotid involvement occurs in <10% of patients. Bilateral involvement is the rule. The gland is usually nontender, firm, and smooth. Xerostomia can occur; other exocrine glands are affected only rarely.

Gastrointestinal Tract Although sarcoidosis involvement of the gastrointestinal tract is found occasionally at autopsy, it rarely has clinical importance. Occasionally, patients have esophageal or gastric symptoms.

COMPLICATIONS The respiratory tract abnormalities cause most of the morbidity and mortality associated with sarcoidosis. The major problems are those characteristic of interstitial lung disease (Chap. 259), particularly dyspnea and insufficient oxygen delivery to vital organs. Respiratory failure with carbon dioxide retention is rare. In some patients, lung destruction results in formation of bullae that may harbor mycetomas, which are usually aspergillomas; erosion into the parenchyma can result in massive bleeding. The most common complications apart from the lung are associated with the eye; however, with therapy, blindness is rare. Complications of other organs include a gamut of abnormalities. The most serious are central nervous system (CNS) lesions or cardiac involvement leading to congestive heart failure or sudden death.

LABORATORY ABNORMALITIES Common abnormalities in the blood include lymphocytopenia, an occasional mild eosinophilia, an increased erythrocyte sedimentation rate, hyperglobulinemia, and an elevated level of angiotensin-converting enzyme (ACE). False-positive tests for rheumatoid factor or antinuclear antibodies can be observed. Hypercalcemia is rare. Other serum abnormalities relate to involvement of specific organs such as liver, kidney, or endocrine glands.

Because the lung is involved so commonly, the routine chest film is almost always abnormal (Fig. 318-2*A*). The three classic x-ray patterns of pulmonary sarcoidosis are type I—bilateral hilar adenopathy with no parenchymal abnormalities; type II—bilateral hilar adenopathy with diffuse parenchymal changes; and type III—diffuse parenchymal changes without hilar adenopathy. The type III pattern is sometimes split into two categories, with films that show fibrosis and upper lobe retraction classified separately. Although patients with type I x-ray patterns tend to have the acute or subacute, reversible form of the disease while those with types II and III often have the chronic, progressive disease, these patterns do not represent consecutive "stages" of sarcoidosis. Thus, except for epidemiologic purposes, this x-ray categorization is mostly of historic interest. The hilar adenopathy is almost always bilateral, but unilateral node enlargement can be seen. Nodes are also common in the paratracheal region. The diffuse parenchymal changes are typically reticulonodular infiltrates, but an acinar pattern is observed occasionally. Large nodules, similar to those of metastatic disease, are unusual but can occur. When there is massive fibrosis, the hila are pulled upward and there are conglomerate masses in the midlung zones. Some of the unusual chest x-ray findings in sarcoidosis include "egg shell" calcification of hilar nodes, pleural effusions, cavitation, atelectasis, pulmonary hypertension, pneumothorax, and cardiomegaly. Computed tomography of the chest is rarely helpful for either diagnosis or prognosis but can identify early fibrosis, and a "ground-glass" appearance is thought to be consistent with an active alveolitis.

A

History, physical examination

Sarcoidosis?

Rule out other disorders	Major diagnostic tests	Ancillary diagnostic
HIV	Routine blood	Skin test for anergy
Neoplastic	Chest x-ray	Angiotensin-converting enzyme
Mycobacterial	Organ function	Gallium-67 scan
Fungal	Biopsy	Bronchoalveolar lavage
Other interstitial lung disorders		24-h urine calcium

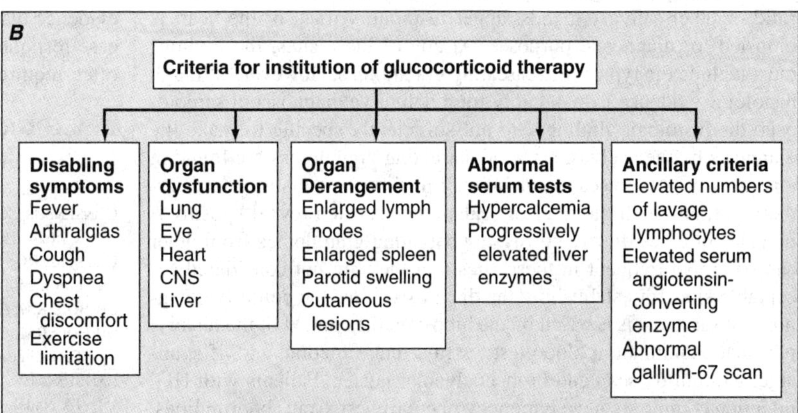

FIGURE 318-3 Diagnostic and therapeutic algorithms relevant to sarcoidosis. *A*. Diagnosis of sarcoidosis. If the history and physical examination suggest sarcoidosis, the diagnosis is made by a combination of history, physical examination, and diagnostic test. No tests are definitive for sarcoidosis; the diagnosis is made by a combination of findings. The major diagnostic tests carry the most weight, with biopsy and histologic assessment of the relevant organ the most important. Assessment of function of the organ systems that appear to be affected help with diagnosis and decisions about therapy. *B*. Therapy of sarcoidosis. Once the definitive diagnosis is made, the decision to not treat or to institute treatment with glucocorticoids is based on the presence or absence of disabling symptoms, organ dysfunction, organ derangement, and results of various tests of disease activity. Any organ can be threatened by sarcoidosis, but lung, eye, heart, liver, and central nervous system are at greatest risk. The disease can wax and wane, and periodic assessments at 3- to 6-month intervals are used to reevaluate decisions regarding therapy.

The lung function abnormalities of sarcoidosis are typical for interstitial lung disease (Chap. 259) and include decreased lung volumes and diffusing capacity with a normal or supernormal ratio of the forced expiratory volume in 1 s to the forced vital capacity. Occasionally there is evidence of airflow limitation. There is usually mild hypoxemia and a mild, compensated hypocarbia.

The gallium-67 lung scan is usually abnormal, showing a pattern of diffuse uptake. If present, enlarged nodes are detected in these scans, as is inflammation in a variety of extrathoracic sites that usually have no clinical importance (Fig. 318-2*B*). Bronchoalveolar lavage typically demonstrates an increased proportion of lymphocytes, most of which are members of the activated T_H1 subset of CD4+ T lymphocytes (Fig. 318-2*C*). The remaining cells are mostly alveolar macrophages. In patients with significant fibrosis, a few neutrophils are also found. Eosinophils are rare.

The other laboratory features of sarcoidosis depend on the specific organ involved.

DIAGNOSIS For a typical case, the diagnosis of sarcoidosis is made by a combination of clinical, radiographic, and histologic findings (Fig. 318-3*A*). In a young adult with constitutional complaints, respiratory symptoms, erythema nodosum, blurred vision, and bilateral hilar adenopathy, the diagnosis is almost always sarcoidosis. Commonly, however, the findings are more subtle. Furthermore, because sarcoidosis can occur in almost any place in the body, like tuberculosis or syphilis, it can be confused with many other disorders. In this context, the differential diagnosis of sarcoidosis must cover a wide range. However, it is confused most commonly with neoplastic diseases such as lymphoma or with disorders characterized also by a mononuclear cell granulomatous inflammatory process, such as the mycobacterial and fungal disorders.

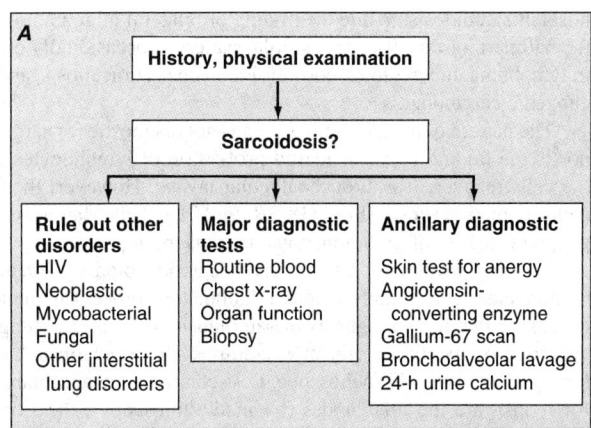

The presence of skin anergy is typical but not diagnostic of sarcoidosis. Individuals with sarcoidosis who develop active tuberculosis react strongly to skin tests with purified protein derivative. The Kveim-Siltzbach skin test, the intradermal injection of a heat-treated suspension of a sarcoidosis spleen extract which is biopsied 4 to 6 weeks later, yields sarcoidosis-like lesions in 70 to 80% of individuals with sarcoidosis, with <5% false-positive results. However, the material is not widely available, and with the use of the transbronchial biopsy to obtain lung parenchyma for diagnostic purposes, the Kveim-Siltzbach test is not in general use.

No blood findings are diagnostic of the disease. Serum levels of ACE are elevated in approximately two-thirds of patients with sarcoidosis. Approximately 5% of all positive tests are not sarcoidosis and are seen in a variety of disorders, including asbestosis, silicosis, berylliosis, fungal infection, granulomatous hepatitis, hypersensitivity pneumonitis, leprosy, lymphoma, and tuberculosis. Hypercalcemia or an elevated 24-h urine calcium level is consistent with the diagnosis but is not specific.

The chest x-ray cannot be used as the sole criterion for the diagnosis of sarcoidosis. While the finding of bilateral hilar adenopathy is the hallmark of this disease, a similar pattern is occasionally observed in lymphoma, tuberculosis, coccidioidomycosis, brucellosis, and bronchogenic carcinoma.

The pattern of the gallium-67 scan is not diagnostic for sarcoidosis, nor is the finding of an increased proportion of lymphocytes among the cells recovered by bronchoalveolar lavage. However, the typical patterns of these tests (Fig. 318-2*B* and *C*) put the diagnosis in the general category of granulomatous lung disorders.

Whether or not the presentation is "classic," biopsy evidence of a mononuclear cell granulomatous inflammatory process is mandatory to make a definitive diagnosis of sarcoidosis. Because the lung is involved so frequently, it is the most common site to be biopsied, usually through a fiberoptic bronchoscope. Less common, but acceptable, sites for biopsy are the hilar nodes (by mediastinoscopy), the skin, conjunctiva, or lip. Rarely, the spleen, intraabdominal nodes, muscle, parotid or other salivary glands, upper respiratory tract, or the heart is biopsied for diagnostic purposes. At any of these sites, the findings must include the typical noncaseating granulomas. However, although histologic evidence is mandatory for a definitive diagnosis of sarcoidosis, the histologic findings are not sufficiently specific to make the diagnosis by themselves, since noncaseating granulomas are found in a number of other diseases, including infections and malignancy. Furthermore, although the liver or scalene nodes often reveal "positive" biopsies in cases of sarcoidosis, noncaseating granulomas from other causes are so frequent in these sites that they are not considered acceptable sites for establishing the diagnosis. Thus the definitive diagnosis of sarcoidosis is based on the biopsy in the context of the history, physical examination, blood tests, x-ray, lung function, and, if available, gallium-67 scan and bronchoalveolar lavage. Patients with HIV infection commonly have lymphocytopenia, chest x-ray abnormalities, positive gallium-67 chest scans, and increased proportions of lavage lymphocytes (early in the course of the disease), and they can have lung granulomas; thus, serologic testing for HIV infection should always be done in individuals suspected of having sarcoidosis.

PROGNOSIS Overall, the prognosis in sarcoidosis is good. Most individuals who present with the acute disease are left with no significant sequelae. Approximately half of all patients have some permanent organ dysfunction, but for most this is mild, stable, and progresses rarely. In ~15 to 20% of patients, the disease remains active or recurs intermittently. Death is attributable directly to the disease in ~10% of all those affected.

℞ **TREATMENT** The therapy of choice for sarcoidosis is glucocorticoids (Fig. 318-3*B*), Various other drugs have been tried, including indomethacin, oxyphenbutazone, chloroquine, hydroxychloroquine, methotrexate, *p*-aminobenzoate, allopurinol, levamisole, azothioprine, and cyclophosphamide; but there is no evidence, apart from anecdotal, uncontrolled reports, to support their efficacy. Cyclosporine is ineffective for the pulmonary manifestations of the disease; anecdotal reports suggest that it may be useful in extrathoracic sarcoid not responding to glucocorticoids.

The major problem in treating sarcoidosis is in deciding when to treat. Because the disease clears spontaneously in ~50% of patients, and because the permanent organ derangements often do not improve with glucocorticoid treatment, there is controversy among clinicians as to the criteria for treatment. However, there is no question that glucocorticoids suppress effectively the activated T_H1 lymphocyte processes occurring at the sites of disease. Thus, the major problem in making decisions concerning therapy in sarcoidosis is to determine the extent and activity of the inflammatory process in the organs at greatest risk, such as the lung, eye, heart, and CNS.

For the lung, this is based on a combination of history, physical findings, chest x-ray, and pulmonary function tests. Centers that see large numbers of these individuals sometimes use criteria based on gallium-67 lung scans and bronchoalveolar lavage findings. The serum level of ACE has been suggested as a criterion for disease activity, but it is not specific for the lung. Unless the respiratory impairment is devastating, active pulmonary sarcoidosis is observed usually without therapy for 2 to 3 months; if the inflammation does not subside spontaneously, therapy is instituted. For the eye, decisions concerning therapy are based on slit-lamp examination and tests for visual acuity. For the heart and CNS, decisions are based on an estimate of the severity of the involvement; patients with minor dysfunction are usually observed, while patients with significant cardiac or neurologic abnormalities are treated. Usually, it is not necessary to treat the systemic symptoms, but occasionally the extent of the fevers, fatigue, and/or weight loss necessitate therapy.

The usual therapy for sarcoidosis is prednisone, 1 mg/kg, for 4 to 6 weeks, followed by a slow taper over 2 to 3 months. This regimen is repeated if the disease again becomes active. Alternate-day therapy is used by some clinicians, but there is no evidence that it is as effective. High-dose bolus intravenous glucocorticoids are used occasionally but are probably not as effective as oral therapy. There is no evidence that inhaled glucocorticoids are efficacious. Mild ocular disease responds usually to local therapy, but suppression of the uveitis often requires systemic glucocorticoids.

BIBLIOGRAPHY

BAUGHMAN RP, LOWER EE: Alternatives to corticosteroids in the treatment of sarcoidosis. Sarcoidosis Vasc Diffuse Lung Dis 14:121, 1997

CONSENSUS CONFERENCE: Activity of sarcoidosis. Third WASOG Meeting. Eur Respir J 7:624, 1994

CRYSTAL RG: Interstitial lung disease of unknown etiology: Disorders characterized by chronic inflammation of the lower respiratory tract. N Engl J Med 310:154, 235, 1984

DU BOIS RM: Corticosteroids in sarcoidosis: Friend or foe? Eur Respir J 7:1203, 1994

DU BOIS RM: Granulomatous processes, in *The Lung: Scientific Foundations*, 2d ed, RG Crystal et al (eds). Philadelphia, Lippincott-Raven, 1996, pp 2395–2409

FANBURG BL, PITT EA: Sarcoidosis, in *Textbook of Respiratory Medicine*, JF Murray, JA Nadel (eds). Philadelphia, Saunders, 1988, pp 1486–1500

JAMES DG (ed): *Sarcoidosis and Other Granulomatous Disorders*. New York, Marcel Dekker, 1994

JOHNS CJ, MICHELE TM: The clinical management of sarcoidosis. A 50-year experience at the Johns Hopkins Hospital. Medicine 78:65, 1999

JUDSON MA et al: Defining organ involvement in sarcoidosis: The ACCESS proposed instrument. Sarcoidosis Vasc Diffuse Lung Dis 16:75, 1999

MOLLER DR: T-cell receptor genes in sarcoidosis. Sarcoidosis Vasc Diffuse Lung Dis 15: 158, 1998

———: Cells and cytokines involved in the pathogenesis of sarcoidosis. Sarcoidosis Vasc Diffuse Lung Dis 16:24, 1999

NAGAI S, IZUMI T: Pulmonary sarcoidosis: Population differences and pathophysiology. South Med J 88:1001, 1995

PINKSTON P et al: Spontaneous release of interleukin-2 by lung T-lymphocytes in active pulmonary sarcoidosis. N Engl J Med 208:793, 1983

ROBINSON BWS et al: Gamma interferon is spontaneously released by alveolar macrophages and lung T-lymphocytes in patients with pulmonary sarcoidosis. J Clin Invest 75:1488, 1985

ROBINSON DS et al: Granulomatous processes, in *The Lung: Scientific Foundations*, 2d ed, RG Crystal et al (eds). Philadelphia, Lippincott-Raven, 1996, pp 2395–2410

SHARMA OP: Pulmonary sarcoidosis and corticosteroids. Am Rev Resp Dis 147:1598, 1993

319

Jean D. Sipe, Alan S. Cohen

AMYLOIDOSIS

AD	Alzheimer's disease	IDOX	iododoxorubicin
AβPP	amyloid β-precursor protein	IL	interleukin
FAP	familial amyloid polyneuropathies	SAP	serum amyloid P
FHF	familial Hibernian fever	TNF	tumor necrosis factor
FMF	familial Mediterranean fever	TTR	transthyretin

DEFINITION AND CLASSIFICATION *Amyloidosis* results from the deposition of insoluble, fibrous amyloid proteins, mainly in the extracellular spaces of organs and tissues. Named by Virchow in 1854 on the basis of color after staining with iodine and sulfuric acid, all amyloid fibrils share an identical secondary structure, the β-pleated sheet conformation, and a unique ultrastructure. All amyloid deposits contain an identical nonfibrillar component, the pentraxin serum amyloid P (SAP), and are associated with glycosaminoglycans. Abnormal protein folding and assembly can also result in protein deposition (e.g., in brain or kidney) that lacks the classic fibrillar morphology of amyloid and the presence of SAP. Depending upon the biochemical nature of the amyloid precursor protein, amyloid fibrils can be deposited locally or may involve virtually every organ system of the body. Amyloid fibril deposition may have no apparent clinical consequences or may lead to severe pathophysiologic changes. Often the disease falls between these two extremes. Regardless of etiology, the clinical diagnosis of amyloidosis is usually not made until the disease is far advanced.

Although the fibril precursors differ in their amino acid sequences, the polypeptide backbones of these protein precursors assume similar fibrillar morphologies that render them resistant to proteolysis.

Table 319-1 Amyloid Fibril Proteins and Their Precursors in Humans

Amyloid Protein	Precursor	Systemic (S) or Localized (L)	Syndrome or Involved Tissues
AL	Immunoglobulin light chain	S, L	Primary Myeloma-associated
AH	Immunoglobulin heavy chain	S, L	Primary Myeloma-associated
ATTR	Transthyretin	S	Familial (prototype Portuguese, Japanese, Swedish) Senile systemic
		L?	Tenosynovium
AA	(Apo)serum AA	S	Secondary, reactive
$A\beta_2M$	β_2-microglobulin	S	Chronic hemodialysis
		L?	Joints
AApoAI	Apolipoprotein AI	S	Familial
		L	Aortic
AGel	Gelsolin	S	Familial (prototype Finnish)
ALys	Lysozyme	S	Familial
AFib	Fibrinogen α-chain	S	Familial
ACys	Cystatin C	S	Familial (protype Icelandic)
$A\beta$	$A\beta$ protein precursor ($A\beta PP$)	L	Alzheimer's disease, aging Familial (prototype Dutch)
$APrP^{sc}$	Prion protein	L	Spongiform encephalopathies
ACal	(Pro)calcitonin	L	C cell thyroid tumors
AIAPP	Islet amyloid polypeptide	L	Islets of Langerhans Insulinomas
AANF	Atrial natriuretic factor	L	Cardiac atria
APro	Prolactin	L	Aging pituitary Prolactinomas
AIns	Insulin	L	Iatrogenic
ALac[a]	Lactoferrin	L	Cornea

[a] Preliminary, awaiting for confirmation.
SOURCE: From P Westermark et al: Amyloid Int J Exp Clin Invest 6:63, 1999, reprinted with permission.

The amyloidoses are classified according to the biochemical nature of the fibril-forming protein (Table 319-1). *Systemic amyloidoses* include biochemically distinct forms that are neoplastic, inflammatory, genetic, or iatrogenic in origin, while *localized* or *organ-limited amyloidoses* are associated with aging and diabetes and occur in isolated organs, often endocrine, without evidence of systemic involvement.

Despite their biochemical and clinical differences, the various amyloidoses share common pathophysiologic features: (1) an amyloidogenic precursor in appropriate concentration; (2) appropriate host genetic background; (3) abnormalities in proteolysis of fibril precursors and nascent amyloid fibrils; and (4) alterations in extracellular matrix constituents such as glycosaminoglycans, including the presence of amyloid-enhancing factor and Apo E. The guidelines for nomenclature and classification of amyloid and amyloidosis were updated in 1998 by the Nomenclature Committee of the International Society for Amyloidosis (Table 319-1). Amyloid deposits should be classified using the capital letter A as the first letter of designation followed by the protein designation without any open space; for example, AL for amyloidosis involving immunoglobulin light chains.

ETIOLOGY AND PATHOGENESIS Light Chain Amyloidosis (AL) The most common form of systemic amyloidosis seen in current clinical practice is AL (primary idiopathic amyloidosis, or that associated with multiple myeloma) resulting from fibril formation by monoclonal antibody light chains in primary amyloidosis and in some cases of multiple myeloma (Chap. 113). Fewer than 20% of patients with AL have myeloma. The rest have other monoclonal gammopathies, light chain disease, or even agammaglobulinemia (producing light chains, but not intact immunoglobulin). About 15 to 20% of patients with myeloma have amyloidosis. A monoclonal population of bone marrow plasma cells is present and consistently produces either small lambda or kappa fragments or immunoglobulins that are processed (cleaved) in an abnormal fashion by macrophage enzymes to produce the partially degraded light chains responsible for AL amyloidosis. Lambda chain class predominates over kappa in AL by a 2:1 ratio, whereas in multiple myeloma and normal immunoglobulin synthesis, the reverse is true. Indeed, almost all lambda VI family chains have been associated with amyloid. The primary structure of each amyloid-forming light chain is unique, reflecting the features of the B cell clone that produced it. In patients with multiple myeloma, light chains can be deposited as casts in kidney tubules or as punctate deposits on basement membranes. Also, nonfibrillar deposition diseases have been described; thus there are three forms of human light chain–associated renal and systemic diseases: AL amyloidosis, cast nephropathy, and light chain deposition disease. Rarely, heavy chain amyloid deposition has been reported.

Amyloid A Amyloidosis (AA) AA amyloidosis (secondary, reactive, or acquired amyloidosis) occurs most frequently as a complication of chronic inflammatory disease. Effective treatment of the underlying inflammatory condition has reduced incidence in developed countries. In the past in the United States, tuberculosis (Chap. 169), osteomyelitis (Chap. 129), and leprosy (Chap. 170) were the most common precipitating diseases, and they remain so in developing countries. During inflammation, proinflammatory cytokines such as interleukin (IL) 1, IL-6, and tumor necrosis factor (TNF) stimulate the synthesis in liver of serum amyloid A, an injury-specific component of high-density lipoprotein. Thus, effective treatment of the underlying inflammatory disorder blocks the stimulus for precursor synthesis. Familial deposition of the AA protein occurs in some groups of patients with familial Mediterranean fever (FMF) and Familial Hibernian Fever (FHF) (Chap. 289). Colchicine treatment has been very effective both in blocking attacks of FMF and in reducing the incidence of AA amyloidosis in association with FMF. FMF is an autosomal recessive disorder subdivided into phenotype I, with irregularly occurring fever and abdominal, chest, or joint pain, preceding or accompanying renal amyloid; and phenotype II, in which renal amyloidosis is the first or only manifestation of the disease (Chap. 289). FMF is caused by mutations (16 identified to date) in the gene designated *MEFV* that encodes a 781-amino-acid protein named *pyrin* that appears to be a transcription factor. There is a strong correlation between the M694V mutation in MEFV and development of amyloidosis. FHF is an autosomal dominant disorder characterized by missense mutations in the TNF receptor.

Heredofamilial Amyloidoses Heredofamilial amyloidoses other than the AA form associated with FMF and FHF primarily involve the nervous system, and their mode of inheritance is autosomal dominant. Familial amyloid polyneuropathies (FAP) are dominant hereditary diseases affecting kinships originating in Portugal, Japan, Sweden, Finland, Greece, Italy, and elsewhere. FAP can be subclassified based on clinical symptoms and the biochemical nature of the fibrils; in nearly all cases the fibrils are variants of transthyretin (TTR), apolipoprotein AI, gelsolin, cystatin C, and rarely the α chain of fibrinogen A or lysozyme. The mutant proteins, although present from birth, are associated with a delayed onset of disease symptoms, usually after three to seven decades of life. The FAP transthyretin prototype is the lower limb neuropathy first described in Portugal. It has a poor prognosis and is characterized by progressively severe neuropathy, including marked autonomic nervous system involvement. In some of these individuals, bilateral "scalloped" pupils are pathognomonic of the disease.

ATTR The most frequently occurring form of FAP involves TTR, a 14-kDa protein originally described as prealbumin, that transports thyroxine and retinol-binding protein in the blood. The first mutation to be identified in Portuguese families and in families of Swedish origin was a single amino acid substitution, methionine for valine at position 30. To date, more than 60 TTR variants have been defined, several of which are nonamyloidogenic. Variant TTR gene carriers exhibit clinically heterogeneous amyloidoses according to the position and nature of the amino acid substitution. Substitution of proline for leucine at position 55 results in an early onset and rapidly progressing disease, whereas substitution of methionine for threonine at position 119 appears to protect against amyloid fibril formation. In Denmark, patients with a methionine substitution for leucine at position 111 have a severe cardiopathy. Nonpathogenic TTR mutants such as the substitution of serine for glycine at position 6 also exist, and several are associated with changes in association with retinol-binding protein.

AApoAI Deposition of one of five apolipoprotein AI variants (G26R, W50R, L60R, L90P, and deletion of residues 61-7 with VT inserts) can be associated with peripheral neuropathy that is clinically similar to the type of familial amyloidosis that is caused by variants of TTR. In some kindreds, the clinical presentation is renal failure without neurologic symptoms.

AGel A unique form of hereditary systemic amyloidosis has been reported primarily in Finland but also in patients of Japanese and Dutch backgrounds. Fibrils of gelsolin fragments, a calcium-binding protein that binds to and fragments actin filaments, are deposited in blood vessels and basement membranes, leading to clinical manifestations of lattice corneal dystrophy and cranial neuropathy, followed by peripheral neuropathy, dystrophic skin changes, and involvement of other organs. Two mutations at position 187, within the actin-binding domain of gelsolin, are associated with the disease.

ALys Hereditary nonneuropathic systemic amyloidosis has been described in English families in which lysozyme is the major fibril protein. Two mutations have been described—I56T and D67H.

AFib Hereditary nonneuropathic renal amyloidosis has been described in families with one of three mutations in the fibrinogen A α chains, R524L, E526V, or R554L.

Aβ_2M In long-term hemodialysis, amyloidosis is now well recognized as a serious bone and joint complication. β_2-microglobulin is the major constituent of the amyloid fibrils, and formation of advanced glycation end products of β_2-microglobulin has been implicated in the pathogenesis of Aβ_2M.

Localized or Organ-Limited Amyloidoses Depending upon the biochemical nature of the amyloid fibril protein, instead of systemic deposition involving the cardiovascular and gastrointestinal systems along with lymph nodes, spleen, liver, kidneys, and adrenals, amyloid deposition may be limited to a single organ such as the pancreas, brain, or heart. Recently, lactoferrin has been found to occur as amyloid fibrils in a rare form of corneal amyloidosis, and amyloid fibrils of prolactin have been identified in the pituitary gland and in a prolactin-producing tumor.

Polypeptide hormone–derived amyloidosis Amyloid deposits are common in polypeptide hormone–producing tissues and tumors. Calcitonin is deposited in the hereditary amyloid syndrome, medullary carcinoma of the thyroid (ACal) (Chap. 330). Also AANF (atrial natriuretic factor–derived) amyloid deposits are found in the sarcolemma of ~80% of persons over 80 years of age. AIAPP (islet amyloid polypeptide–derived, or amylin) is deposited as amyloid fibrils in 90% of individuals with type 2 diabetes (Chap. 333), in endocrine tumors (Chap. 93), and in insulinoma (Chap. 93). It is produced in β cells of the pancreas and stored and released together with insulin. Human insulin does not naturally form amyloid fibrils, although fibrils of porcine insulin, AIns, are sometimes found as subcutaneous nodules at sites of insulin injection in diabetic individuals.

Amyloidosis associated with Alzheimer's disease A novel protein, β-amyloid protein (Aβ), is the major fibril protein in the amyloid deposits of the cerebrovascular walls and the cores of the neuritic plaques of Alzheimer's disease (AD) patients and also in individuals with Down's syndrome (Chap. 66). The intracellular neurofibrillary tangles are composed of paired helical filaments arranged in a twisted conformation and have as their major component an abnormally phosphorylated τ-protein, a microtubule-associated protein whose semantic relation to the Aβ of AD is arguable. Aβ varies in length from 39 to 43 amino acids and is derived from a large transmembrane glycoprotein called amyloid β-precursor protein (AβPP). Mutations in AβPP are associated with familial AD and also with a different type of amyloidosis, hereditary cerebral hemorrhage with amyloidosis (Dutch type). Other forms of familial AD are associated with mutations in genes that encode presenilin proteins.

Prion diseases Prions are a unique class of infectious proteins associated with a group of neurodegenerative diseases, the transmissible spongiform encephalopathies. In humans, these diseases include kuru, Creutzfeldt-Jakob disease, Gerstmann-Straussler-Scheinker syndrome, and fatal familial insomnia (Chap. 373); in animals, scrapie and bovine spongiform encephalopathy (mad cow disease). PrP^{Sc} is a pathogenic, transmissible spongiform encephalopathy–specific form of the host-encoded prion protein (PrP); PrP^{Sc} differs from PrP in that it contains a high amount of β-pleated sheet structure and is insoluble and resistant to proteolytic enzymes. PrP^{Sc} deposits either consist of or can be readily converted to amyloid fibrils. APrP is similar to Aβ and ATTR in that both familial and sporadic forms occur. In addition, infectious prior diseases have resulted from the transmission of PrP^{Sc} by ritualistic cannibalism, corneal transplantation, treatment with cadaveric human growth hormone, and a variety of neurosurgical procedures. It has been suggested that the earlier onset familial forms of amyloidosis are due to accelerated fibril formation from mutant precursors, whereas in sporadic cases, amyloid fibrils are formed more slowly from normal precursor molecules. The mutant PrP molecules are nearer the threshold for transition to the amyloidogenic PrP^{Sc} than are the normal. The transition from normal to amyloidogenic PrP^{Sc} is irreversible but very slow. The disease progresses because, once formed, amyloidogenic PrP^{Sc} can seed the conversion of normal molecules into an amyloidogenic form.

CLINICAL MANIFESTATIONS The clinical manifestations of amyloidosis are varied and depend entirely on the biochemical nature of the fibril protein and thus the area of the body that is involved (Table 319-2). The diagnosis of amyloidosis is usually not made until after the point of irreversible organ damage. Proteinuria is often the first symptom associated with systemic amyloidosis, particularly of the AA and AL type; peripheral neuropathies are associated with FAP, and dementia and cognitive dysfunction with amyloid deposits in brain. Organ enlargement, especially of the liver, kidney, spleen, and heart, may be prominent; however, this does not occur in FAP, AD, or PrP diseases.

Table 319-2 Clinical Presentation of Systemic Amyloidosis

Disease	Symptoms
AL (primary)	Monoclonal immunoglobulin in urine or serum plus any of the following: Unexplained nephrotic syndrome Hepatomegaly Carpal tunnel syndrome Macroglossia Malabsorption or unexplained diarrhea or constipation Peripheral neuropathy Cardiomyopathy
AA (secondary)	Chronic infection (osteomyelitis, tuberculosis) or chronic inflammation (rheumatoid arthritis, granulomatous ileitis) plus development of any of the following: Proteinuria Hepatomegaly Unexplained gastrointestinal disease
Hereditary amyloidosis	Family history of neuropathy plus any of the following: Early sensorimotor disassociation Vitreous opacities Renal disease Autonomic nervous system symptoms Cardiovascular disease Gastrointestinal disease

Kidney Renal involvement may consist of mild proteinuria or frank nephrosis. In some cases, the urinary sediment may show a few red blood cells. The renal lesion is usually not reversible and in time leads to progressive azotemia and death. The prognosis does not appear to be related to the degree of the proteinuria; when azotemia finally develops, the prognosis is grave. Treatment by peritoneal or hemodialysis or kidney transplantation improves the prognosis considerably. Hypertension is rare, except in long-standing amyloidosis. Renal tubular acidosis or renal vein thrombosis may occur. Localized accumulation of amyloid may be noted in the ureter, bladder, or other parts of the genitourinary tract.

Heart Cardiac amyloidosis can present as intractable heart failure. Electrocardiographic abnormalities include a low-voltage QRS complex and abnormalities in atrioventricular and intraventricular conduction, often resulting in varying degrees of heart block. Owing to their propensity to develop conduction defects and arrhythmias, patients with cardiac amyloidosis appear to be especially sensitive to digitalis, and this drug should be used with caution.

With respect to systemic amyloidoses, cardiac amyloidosis is common in primary (AL) and heredofamilial amyloidosis and very rare in the secondary (AA) form. With respect to localized amyloidosis, cardiac amyloidosis of the wild type or nonvariant TTR type is common after 80 years of age; also atrial natriuretic factor may be present in the atria. In systemic amyloidosis, cardiac manifestations consist primarily of congestive failure and cardiomegaly (with or without murmurs) and a variety of arrhythmias and are comparable in AL and FAP, the predominant forms with cardiomyopathy (Chap. 238). Although these manifestations predominantly reflect diffuse myocardial amyloid, the endocardium, valves, and pericardium may also be involved. Pericarditis with effusion is rare, although the differential diagnosis of constrictive pericarditis versus restrictive cardiomyopathy frequently arises. Echocardiography has demonstrated symmetric thickening of the left ventricular wall, hypokinesia and decreased systolic contraction and thickening of the interventricular septum and left ventricular posterior wall, and left ventricular cavities of small to normal size. Two-dimensional echocardiography produces the characteristic findings of thickened right and left ventricles, a normal left ventricular cavity, and, especially, a diffuse hyperrefractile "granular sparkling" appearance. Hearts that are heavily infiltrated with amyloid may or may not show an enlarged silhouette. Fluoroscopy usually shows decreased mobility of the ventricular wall; angiographic studies usually demonstrate thickened ventricular wall, decreased ventricular mobility, and absence of rapid ventricular filling in early diastole.

Liver While hepatic involvement is common except in heredofamilial amyloidosis of the TTR type, liver function abnormalities are minimal and occur late in the disease. Portal hypertension occurs but is uncommon. Intrahepatic cholestasis has been noted in about 5% of patients with AL (primary) amyloidosis. Hepatomegaly is common, and AL hepatic amyloid is usually accompanied by the nephrotic syndrome and congestive heart failure with poor prognosis. Amyloidosis of the spleen characteristically is not associated with leukopenia and anemia.

Skin Involvement of the skin is one of the most characteristic manifestations of primary (AL) amyloidosis (Chap. 57). Other forms of amyloidosis such as lichen amyloidosis are thought to involve forms of keratin. In AL amyloidosis, the usually nonpruritic lesions may consist of slightly raised, waxy papules or plaques that are usually clustered in the folds of the axillae, anal, or inguinal regions; the face and neck; or mucosal areas such as ear or tongue. Periorbital ecchymoses ("black eye" or "raccoon syndrome") have been reported.

Gastrointestinal Tract Gastrointestinal symptoms are common in all systemic types of amyloidosis either from direct involvement of the gastrointestinal tract at any level or from infiltration of the autonomic nervous system with amyloid. Symptoms include obstruction, ulceration, malabsorption, hemorrhage, protein loss, and diarrhea (Chap. 286). Infiltration of the tongue is characteristic of primary amyloidosis (AL) or amyloidosis accompanying multiple myeloma and occasionally leads to macroglossia. When not enlarged, the tongue may become stiffened and firm to palpation. Gastrointestinal bleeding may occur from any of a number of sites, notably the esophagus, stomach, or large intestine, and may be severe. Amyloid infiltration of the esophagus may lead to an incompetent or nonrelaxing lower esophageal sphincter, nonspecific motility disorders of the esophageal body, or rarely achalasia. Small-bowel lesions may lead to clinical and x-ray changes of obstruction. A malabsorption syndrome is common. Amyloidosis (AA or secondary) may also develop in association with other entities involving the gastrointestinal tract, especially tuberculosis (Chap. 169), granulomatous enteritis (Chap. 287), lymphoma (Chap. 112), and Whipple's disease (Chap. 286); differentiation of these conditions, which give rise to secondary amyloidosis, from diffuse primary amyloidosis of the small bowel may be difficult. Similarly, amyloidosis of the stomach may closely mimic gastric carcinoma, with obstruction, achlorhydria, and the radiologic appearance of tumor masses.

Nervous System Neurologic manifestations, especially prominent in the heredofamilial amyloidoses may include peripheral neuropathy, postural hypotension, inability to sweat, Adies's pupil, hoarseness, and sphincter incompetence. The cranial nerves are generally spared, except in the Finnish hereditary amyloidosis. Carpal tunnel syndrome may be caused by several amyloidoses, especially primary (AL) and chronic hemodialysis ($A\beta_2M$) amyloid. Peripheral neuropathy is frequent in the former type. $A\beta$ amyloid occurs in the central nervous system as a component of senile plaques and in blood vessels ("congophilic angiopathy"). The protein concentration in the cerebrospinal fluid may be increased. Infiltrates of the cornea or vitreous body may be present in hereditary amyloid syndromes. Certain of these syndromes (advanced FAP) are characterized by a bilateral scalloping appearance of the pupil.

Endocrine Amyloid may infiltrate the thyroid or other endocrine glands but rarely causes endocrine dysfunction. Local amyloid deposits almost invariably accompany medullary carcinoma of the thyroid. Amyloid is often found in the adrenal gland, pituitary gland, and pancreas. Pancreatic islet amyloid as a complication of type 2 diabetes is especially prominent and is caused by the β cell peptide islet amyloid polypeptide. Little if any clinical dysfunction is present unless there is massive replacement of the gland by amyloid.

Joints and Muscles Amyloid can directly, although rarely, involve articular structures by its presence in the synovial membrane and synovial fluid or in the articular cartilage. In these cases it is almost always of the AL type and associated with multiple myeloma. Amyloid arthritis can mimic a number of the rheumatic diseases because it can present as a symmetric arthritis of small joints with nodules, morning stiffness, and fatigue (Chap. 320). The synovial fluid usually has a low white blood cell count, a good to fair mucin clot, a predominance of mononuclear cells, and no crystals. Studies of surgical specimens suggest a significant incidence of amyloid in cartilage, capsule, and synovium in osteoarthritis (Chap. 321). Amyloid infiltration of muscle may lead to a pseudomyopathy. Shoulder muscle infiltration can produce the "shoulder pad" sign. Amyloid is found in muscle inclusion body disease, where Aβ and/or PrP have been identified.

Deposition of β_2-microglobulin as amyloid fibrils in the musculoskeletal systems is a serious complication of long-term hemodialysis. Aβ_2M presents as the carpal tunnel syndrome, cystic bone lesions, and even destructive spondyloarthropathy.

Table 319-3 Diagnosis of Amyloidosis

BIOPSY	APPROPRIATE STAIN
Common sites	Congo red, viewed by polarization microscopy
Subcutaneous abdominal fat aspirate	Thioflavin (less specific)
Rectum	Potassium permanganate pretreatment, then Congo red stain
Skin	Other:
Gingiva	Cotton dyes (comparable with Congo red)
Occasional sites	Crystal violet (less sensitive)
Small intestine	**PROTEIN OR DNA STUDIES**
Muscle	Mutant protein identification
Nerve	Immunocytochemistry: immunofluorescent or immunoperoxidase stains with specific antisera
Rare sites	
Kidney	
Liver	
Bone marrow	
Synovium	
Spleen	

Respiratory System The nasal sinuses, larynx, and trachea may be involved by accumulation of AL amyloid, which blocks the ducts, in the case of the sinuses, or the air passages. Amyloidosis of the lung involves the bronchi and alveolar septa diffusely. The lower respiratory tract is affected most frequently in primary (AL) amyloidosis and in the disease associated with dysproteinemia. Pulmonary symptoms attributable to amyloid are present in about 30% of cases. Amyloid may be localized in the bronchi or pulmonary parenchyma and may resemble a neoplasm. In these cases, local excision should be attempted and, when successful, may be followed by prolonged remissions.

Hematopoietic System Hematologic changes may include fibrinogenopenia, increased fibrinolysis, and selective deficiency of clotting factors. Deficient factor X seems to be due to nonspecific calcium-dependent binding to the polyanionic amyloid fibrils. Splenectomy in the patient with such a factor X deficiency can relieve the deficiency and the associated bleeding disorder, since factor X has been shown to bind to the large masses of splenic amyloid. Endothelial damage together with the clotting abnormalities lead to a propensity toward abnormal bleeding.

DIAGNOSIS Amyloid fibrils are identified in biopsy or necropsy tissue sections (Table 319-3). The systemic amyloidoses offer a choice of biopsy sites; abdominal fat aspirates or renal or rectal biopsies are often performed. Microscopically, amyloid deposits stain pink with the hematoxylin-eosin stain and show metachromasia with crystal violet. The widely used and useful Congo red stain imparts a unique green birefringence when stained tissue sections are viewed using the polarizing microscope (Fig. 319-1). Fluorescent dyes such as thioflavin are sensitive screening stains for amyloid deposits in brain and other tissues; however, specificity should be confirmed. After amyloid has been identified by staining, it can be chemically classified by genomic DNA and protein studies and by immunohistochemistry. In the case of FAP, the presence of mutant TTR (or gelsolin, Apo AI, etc.) establishes the specific diagnosis of the disease. Isoelectric focusing is used as a simple screening test for variant transthyretins associated with familial TTR amyloidosis. In order to establish the relationship of immunoglobulin-related amyloid to multiple myeloma, electrophoretic and immunoelectrophoretic studies on serum and urine should be performed when the biopsy reveals amyloid deposition. Most of these patients will have only relatively small paraprotein components, and only a few will have frank multiple myeloma.

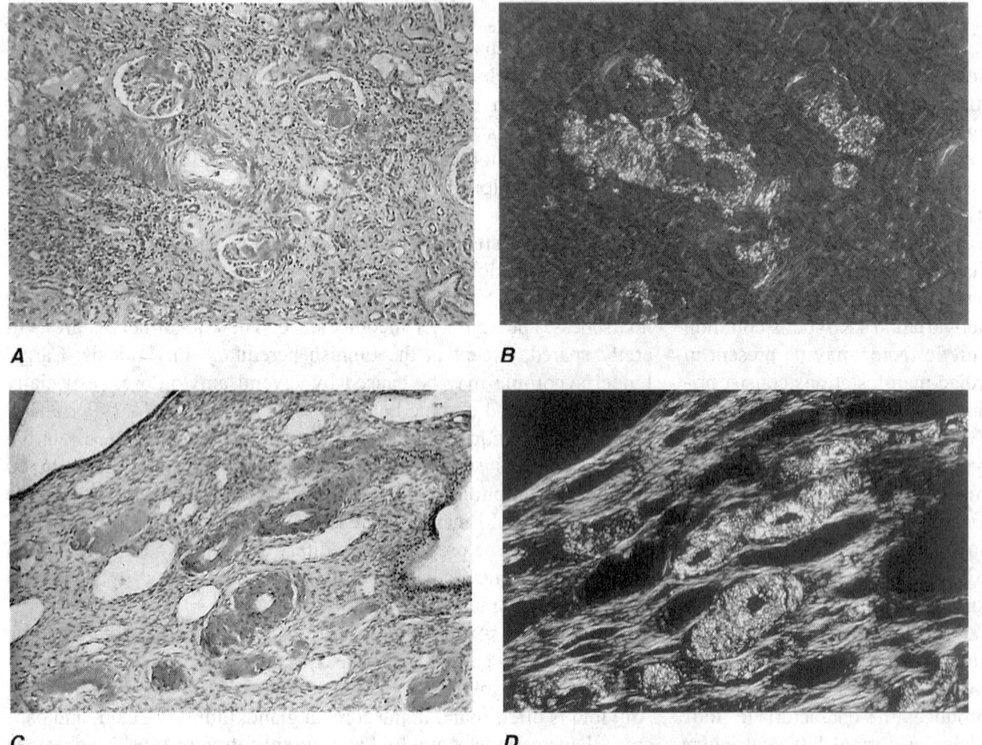

FIGURE 319-1 Microscopic tissue appearance of amyloid. *A.* Congo red stained section of amyloidotic kidney. *B.* Polarization microscopy of section *A* showing green birefringence of glomeruli and blood vessels. *C.* Congo red–stained section of uterus. *D.* Polarization microscopy of section *C* showing the vascular amyloid as well as amyloid in the muscle wall.

PROGNOSIS Generalized amyloidosis is usually a slowly progressive disease that leads to death in several years, but in some instances, prognosis is improving. The average survival in most large series of AL amyloid is ~12 months and in FAP is ~7 to 15 years. A number of individuals with amyloid have been followed 5 to 10 years and longer. The course of amyloidosis is difficult to document, because dating the time of origin of the disease is rarely possible. When amyloidosis develops in patients with rheumatoid arthritis, it seldom becomes evident when the arthritis is of less than 2 years' duration. When amyloidosis develops in patients with multiple myeloma, manifestations leading to initial hospitalization are more apt to be related to amyloid disease than to myeloma. In these cases, prognosis is very poor, and life expectancy is usually less than 6 months.

℞ TREATMENT Rational therapy should be directed at (1) reducing precursor production, (2) inhibiting the synthesis and extracellular deposition of amyloid fibrils, and (3) promoting lysis or mobilization of existing amyloid deposits. There are new specific therapies for the various amyloidoses. In certain of the heredofamilial amyloidoses, genetic counseling is an important aspect of treatment, and the removal of the site of synthesis of the mutant protein by liver transplantation has proven remarkably successful. Liver transplantation has been carried out since 1990 for FAP patients in Sweden, the United States, Portugal, Spain, and other countries. It appears that disease progression is halted and that there is some improvement in autonomic nervous system function. The utilization of chronic hemodialysis and of kidney transplantation has clearly improved the prognosis of renal amyloid.

In the case of AL amyloid, the fact that immunoglobulin light chain is made by plasma cells has led to the use of alkylating agents. However, these agents are toxic and not very effective. The most effective form of treatment currently is stem cell transplantation and immunosuppressive drugs (melphalan). Several long-term remissions have been reported, but serious complications, even death, can occur. A novel anthracycline, iododoxorubicin (IDOX), has been shown to bind to AL amyloid (similar to Congo red) in vivo and promote amyloid resorption. A subset of AL patients responds transiently to this experimental agent; and it is thought that IDOX may prove useful in combination with other forms of treatment. Cardiac tranplantation in

selected cases of AL or FAP amyloidosis has its advocates and has been successful.

Colchicine has been shown to be effective in preventing acute attacks and amyloidosis in patients with FMF (Chap. 289).

The major causes of death are heart disease and renal failure. Sudden death, presumably due to arrhythmias, is common. Occasionally, gastrointestinal hemorrhage, respiratory failure, intractable heart failure, and superimposed infections are the terminal events.

BIBLIOGRAPHY

BENSON MD, UEMICHI T: Transthyretin amyloidosis. Amyloid Int J Exp Clin Invest 3:44, 1996

COHEN AS: Amyloidosis. Bull Rheum Dis 40:1, 1991

———, JONES LA: Advances in amyloidosis. Curr Opin Rheumatol 5:62, 1993

———, SIPE JD: Amyloidosis, in *Clinical Immunology*, RR Rich et al (eds). St. Louis, Mosby Year Book, 1995, pp 1264–1272

FALK RH et al: The systemic amyloidoses. N Engl J Med 337:898, 1997

GLENNER GG, MURPHY MA: Amyloidosis of the nervous system. J Neurol Soc 94:1, 1989

HUSBY G et al: Serum amyloid A (SAA): Biochemistry, genetics and the pathogenesis of AA amyloidosis. Amyloid Int J Exp Clin Invest 1:119, 1994

LEWIS WD, SKINNER M: Liver transplantation for familial amyloidotic polyneuropathy: A potentially curative treatment. Amyloid Int J Exp Clin Invest 1:143, 1994

PRUSINER SB, DEARMOND SJ: Prion protein amyloid and neurodegeneration. Amyloid Int J Exp Clin Invest 2:39, 1995

SIPE JD: Amyloidosis. Crit Rev Clin Lab Sci 31:325, 1994

ZEMER D et al: Colchicine in the prevention and treatment of the amyloidosis of familial Mediterranean fever. N Engl J Med 314:1001, 1986

Section 3
DISORDERS OF THE JOINTS

320

John J. Cush, Peter E. Lipsky

APPROACH TO ARTICULAR AND MUSCULOSKELETAL DISORDERS

Musculoskeletal complaints account for more than 315,000,000 outpatient visits per year. Many of the musculoskeletal complaints that cause patients to seek medical attention are related to self-limited conditions requiring minimal evaluation and only symptomatic therapy and reassurance. However, some patients with similar symptoms have a more serious condition that requires further evaluation or additional laboratory testing to confirm the suspected diagnosis or determine the extent and nature of the pathologic process. A primary objective is to determine if a "red flag" or urgent rheumatologic condition is present and, if not, to formulate a differential diagnosis that leads to accurate diagnosis and timely therapy while avoiding excessive diagnostic testing and unnecessary treatment (Table 320-1) There are several urgent conditions that must be diagnosed promptly to avoid significant morbid or mortal sequelae. These red flag diagnoses include septic arthritis, acute crystal-induced arthritis (e.g., gout), and fracture. Each of these may be suspected by an acute onset with a monoarticular or focal presenting complaint (see below).

Individuals with musculoskeletal complaints should be evaluated in a uniform, logical manner by means of a thorough history, a comprehensive physical examination, and, if appropriate, laboratory testing. The goals of the initial encounter are to determine whether the musculoskeletal complaint is (1) *articular* or *nonarticular* in origin, (2) *inflammatory* or *noninflammatory* in nature, (3) *acute* or *chronic* in duration, and (4) *localized* or *widespread* (*systemic*) in distribution.

With such an approach and an understanding of the pathophysiologic processes that underlie musculoskeletal complaints, an adequate diagnosis can be made in the vast majority of individuals. However, some patients will not fit immediately into an established diagnostic category. Many musculoskeletal disorders resemble each other at the outset, and some take weeks or months to evolve into a readily recognizable diagnostic entity. This consideration should temper the desire always to establish a definitive diagnosis at the first encounter.

ARTICULAR VERSUS NONARTICULAR The musculoskeletal evaluation must discriminate the anatomic site(s) of origin of the patient's complaint. For example, ankle pain can result from a variety of pathologic conditions involving disparate anatomic structures, including gonococcal arthritis, calcaneal fracture, Achilles tendinitis, cellulitis, and peripheral neuropathy. Articular structures include the synovium, synovial fluid, articular cartilage, intraarticular ligaments, joint capsule, and juxtaarticular bone. Nonarticular (or periarticular) structures, such as supportive extraarticular ligaments, tendons, bursae, muscle, fascia, bone, nerve, and overlying skin, may be

Table 320-1 Evaluation of Patients with Musculoskeletal Complaints

Goals
- Accurate diagnosis
- Timely provision of therapy
- Avoidance of unnecessary diagnostic testing

Approach
- Anatomic localization of complaint (articular vs. nonarticular)
- Determination of the nature of the pathologic process (inflammatory vs. noninflammatory)
- Determination of the extent of involvement (monarticular, polyarticular, focal, widespread)
- Determination of chronology (acute vs. chronic)
- Formulation of a differential diagnosis

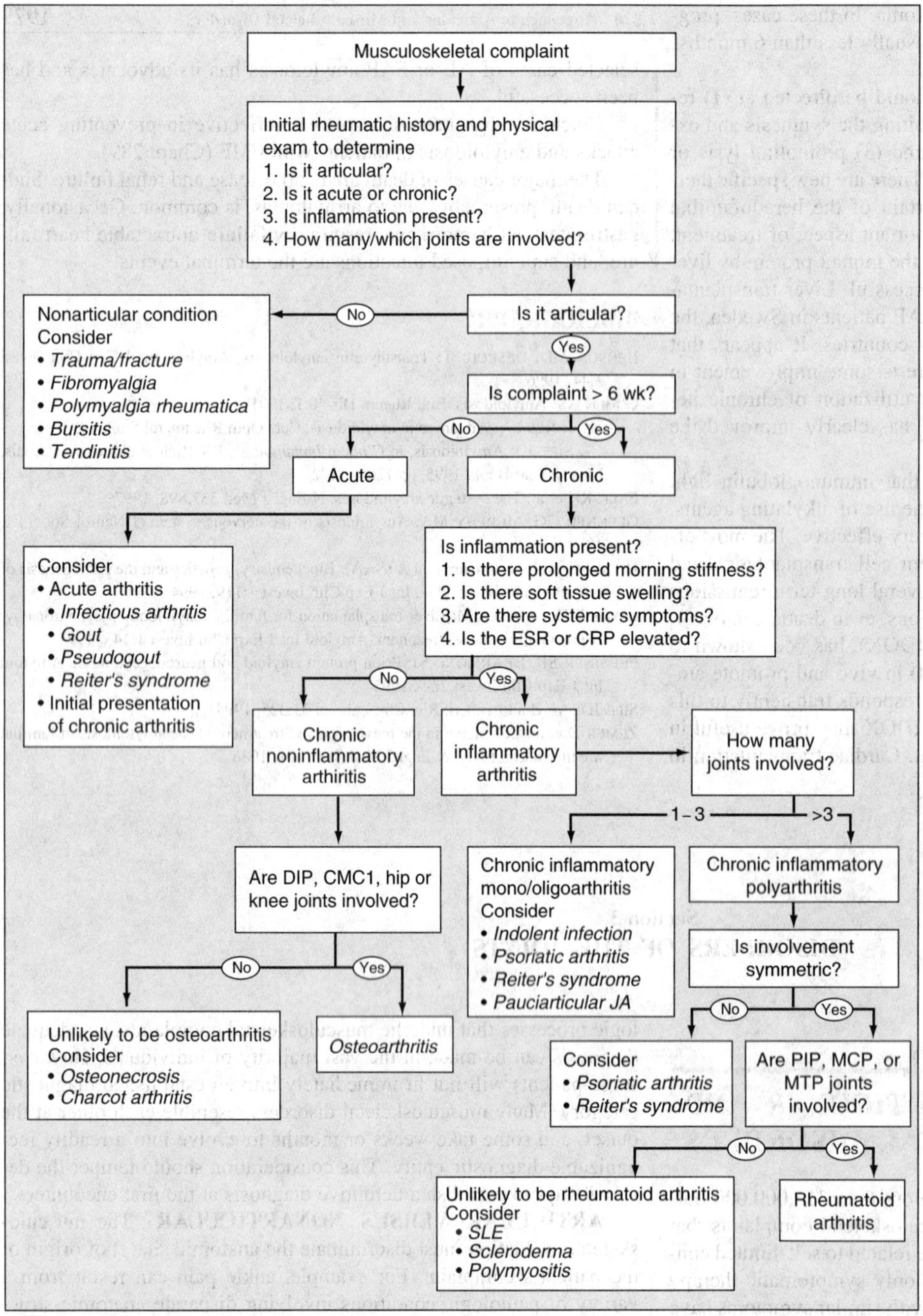

FIGURE 320-1 Algorithm for the diagnosis of musculoskeletal complaints. An approach to formulating a differential diagnosis (shown in italics). (ESR, erythrocyte sedimentation rate; CRP, C-reactive protein; DIP, distal interphalangeal; CMC, carpometacarpal; PIP, proximal interphalangeal; MCP, metacarpophalangeal; MTP, metatarsophalangeal; PMR, polymyalgia rheumatica; SLE, systemic lupus erythematosus; JA, juvenile arthritis.)

involved in the pathologic process. Pain from nonarticular structures may mimic true articular pain because of their proximity to the joint. Distinguishing between articular and nonarticular disease requires a careful and detailed examination. Articular disorders may be characterized by deep or diffuse joint pain, limited range of motion on active and passive movement, swelling caused by synovial proliferation or effusion or bony enlargement, crepitation, instability, locking, or deformity. By contrast, nonarticular disorders tend to be painful on active but not passive range of motion, demonstrate point or focal tenderness in regions distinct from articular structures, and have physical findings remote from the joint capsule. Moreover, nonarticular disorders seldom demonstrate crepitus, instability, deformity, or swelling.

INFLAMMATORY VERSUS NONINFLAMMATORY In the course of a musculoskeletal evaluation, the examiner should elicit symptoms and signs that will narrow or establish the diagnosis. A primary objective is to identify the nature of the underlying pathologic process. Musculoskeletal disorders are generally classified as inflammatory or noninflammatory. Inflammatory disorders may be infectious (infection with *Neisseria gonorrhoea* or *Mycobacterium tuberculosis*), crystal-induced (gout, pseudogout), immune-related [rheumatoid arthritis (RA), systemic lupus erythematosus (SLE)], reactive (rheumatic fever, Reiter's syndrome), or idiopathic. Inflammatory disorders may be identified by the presence of some or all of the four cardinal signs of inflammation (erythema, warmth, pain, and swelling), by systemic symptoms (prolonged morning stiffness, fatigue, fever, weight loss), or by laboratory evidence of inflammation (elevated erythrocyte sedimentation rate or C-reactive protein level, thrombocytosis, anemia of chronic disease, or hypoalbuminemia). Articular stiffness is common in chronic musculoskeletal disorders. However, the chronology and magnitude of stiffness may be diagnostically important. Morning stiffness related to inflammatory disorders (such as RA) is precipitated by prolonged rest, often lasts several hours, and may improve with activity and anti-inflammatory medications. By contrast, intermittent stiffness associated with noninflammatory conditions, such as osteoarthritis, is precipitated by brief periods of rest, usually lasts less than 60 min, and is exacerbated by activity. Noninflammatory disorders may be related to trauma (rotator cuff tear), ineffective repair (osteoarthritis), cellular overgrowth (pigmented villonodular synovitis), or pain amplification (fibromyalgia). They are often characterized by pain without swelling or warmth, the absence of inflammatory or systemic features, little or no morning stiffness, and normal laboratory findings.

Identification of the nature of the underlying process and the site of the complaint will enable the examiner to narrow the diagnostic considerations and to assess the need for immediate diagnostic or therapeutic intervention or for continued observation. Figure 320-1 presents a logical approach to the evaluation of patients with musculoskeletal complaints.

CLINICAL HISTORY Additional historic features may be helpful in establishing the nature and extent of the pathologic process and may provide important clues to the diagnosis. When evaluating patients with musculoskeletal complaints, the clinician should always consider the most common conditions (e.g., low back pain, osteoarthritis) seen in the general population (Fig. 320-2). Aspects of the patient profile, including age, sex, race, and family history, can provide important information. Certain diagnoses are more frequent in specific age groups. SLE, rheumatic fever, and Reiter's syndrome are more common in the young, whereas fibromyalgia and RA are most common in middle age, and osteoarthritis and polymyalgia rheumatica in the elderly. Some diseases are more common in a particular gender or race. Gout and the spondyloarthropathies (e.g., ankylosing spondylitis,

Reiter's syndrome) are more common in men, whereas SLE, RA, and fibromyalgia are more common in women. Polymyalgia rheumatica, giant cell arteritis, and Wegener's granulomatosis preferentially affect whites, whereas sarcoidosis and SLE are more common in blacks. *Familial aggregation* occurs in some disorders, such as ankylosing spondylitis, gout, RA, and Heberden's nodes of osteoarthritis.

The chronology of the complaint (*onset, evolution*, and *duration*) is an important diagnostic feature. The onset of disorders such as septic arthritis and gout tends to be abrupt, whereas osteoarthritis, RA, and fibromyalgia may develop more indolently. In terms of evolution, disorders are classified as acute (e.g., septic arthritis), chronic (e.g., osteoarthritis), intermittent (e.g., gout), migratory (e.g., rheumatic fever, gonococcal or viral arthritis), or additive (e.g., RA, Reiter's syndrome). Musculoskeletal disorders typically are called *acute* if they last less than 6 weeks and *chronic* if they last longer. Acute and intermittent arthropathies tend to be infectious, crystal-induced, or reactive. Noninflammatory and immune-related arthritides, such as osteoarthritis and RA, respectively, are often chronic. The duration of the patient's complaints may alter the diagnostic considerations. For example, the musculoskeletal signs and symptoms of hepatitis B virus infection may be identical with those of early RA at the onset but rarely persist beyond 3 weeks.

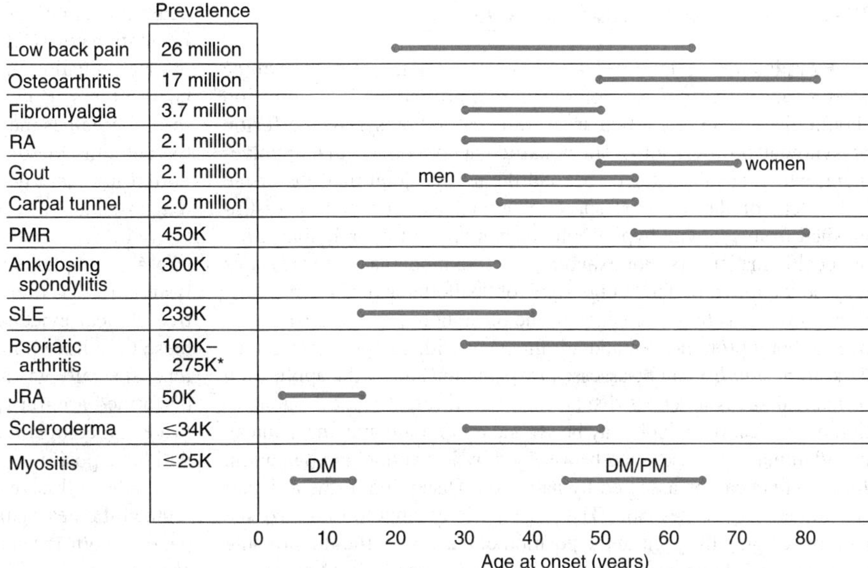

FIGURE 320-2 Age at onset for common rheumatic conditions; ranked by prevalance estimates in the United States in 1998. *Estimates vary.

The *number and distribution* of involved articulations should be noted. Articular disorders are classified as *monarticular* (one joint involved), *oligoarticular* or *pauciarticular* (two to three joints involved), or *polyarticular* (more than three joints involved). Nonarticular disorders can be classified as either *focal* or *widespread*. Complaints secondary to trauma and gout are typically focal or monarticular, whereas polymyositis, RA, and fibromyalgia are more diffuse or polyarticular. Joint involvement tends to be symmetric in RA but is often asymmetric in the spondyloarthropathies and in gout. The upper extremities are frequently involved in RA, whereas lower extremity arthritis is characteristic of Reiter's syndrome and gout at their onset. Involvement of the axial skeleton is common in osteoarthritis and ankylosing spondylitis but infrequent in RA, with the notable exception of the cervical spine.

The clinical history should also identify *precipitating events*, such as trauma, drug administration (Table 320-2), or antecedent or intercurrent illnesses, that may have contributed to the patient's complaint. Last, a thorough *rheumatic review of systems* may disclose associated features outside the musculoskeletal system and provide useful diagnostic information. A variety of musculoskeletal disorders may be associated with systemic features such as fever (SLE, infection), rash (SLE, Reiter's syndrome, dermatomyositis), myalgias, weakness (polymyositis, polymyalgia rheumatica), and morning stiffness (inflammatory arthritis). In addition, some conditions are associated with involvement of other organ systems, including the eyes (Behçet's disease, sarcoidosis, Reiter's syndrome), gastrointestinal tract (scleroderma, inflammatory bowel disease), genitourinary tract (Reiter's syndrome, gonococcemia, Behçet's disease), and nervous system (Lyme disease, SLE, vasculitis).

PHYSICAL EXAMINATION The goal of the physical examination is to ascertain the structures involved, the nature of the underlying pathology, the extent and functional consequences of the process, and the presence of systemic or extraarticular manifestations. A knowledge of topographic anatomy is necessary to identify the primary site(s) of involvement and differentiate articular from nonarticular disorders. The musculoskeletal examination depends largely on careful inspection, palpation, and a variety of specific physical maneuvers to elicit diagnostic signs (Table 320-3). Although most articulations of the appendicular skeleton can be examined in this manner, adequate inspection and palpation are not possible for many axial (e.g., zygapophyseal) and inaccessible (e.g., sacroiliac or hip) joints. For such joints, there is a greater reliance on specific maneuvers and imaging for assessment.

Table 320-2 Drug-Induced Musculoskeletal Conditions

Condition	Drugs
Arthralgias	Quinidine, amphotericin B, cimetidine, quinolones, chronic acyclovir, interferon, IL-2, nicardipine, vaccines, rifabutin
Myalgias/myopathy	Glucocorticoids, penicillamine, hydroxychloroquine, AZT, lovastatin, simvastatin, pravastatin, clofibrate, interferon, IL-2, alcohol, cocaine, taxol, docetaxel, colchicine, quinolones
Gout	Diuretics, aspirin, cytotoxics, cyclosporine, alcohol, moonshine, ethambutol
Drug-induced lupus	Hydralazine, procainamide, quinidine, phenytoin, methyldopa, isoniazid, chlorpromazine, lithium, penicillamine, tetracycline, infliximab
Osteonecrosis	Glucocorticoids, alcohol, radiation
Osteopenia	Glucocorticoids, chronic heparin, phenytoin, methotrexate
Scleroderma	Vinyl chloride, bleomycin, pentazocine, organic solvents, carbidopa, tryptophan, rapeseed oil
Vasculitis	Allopurinol, amphetamines, cocaine, thiazides, penicillamine, propylthiouracil

NOTE: IL-2, interleukin 2.

Table 320-3 Glossary of Musculoskeletal Terms

Crepitus A palpable (less commonly audible) vibratory or crackling sensation elicited with joint motion; fine joint crepitus is common and often insignificant in large joints; coarse joint crepitus indicates advanced cartilaginous and degenerative changes (as in osteoarthritis).
Subluxation Alteration of joint alignment such that articulating surfaces incompletely approximate each other
Dislocation Abnormal displacement of articulating surfaces such that the surfaces are not in contact
Range of motion For diarthrodial joints, the arc of measurable movement through which the joint moves in a single plane
Contracture Loss of full movement resulting from a fixed resistance due either to tonic spasm of muscle (reversible) or to fibrosis of periarticular structures (permanent)
Deformity Abnormal shape or size of a structure; may result from bony hypertrophy, malalignment of articulating structures, or damage to periarticular supportive structures
Enthesitis Inflammation of the entheses (tendinous or ligamentous insertions on bone)
Epicondylitis Infection or inflammation involving an epicondyle

Examination of involved and uninvolved joints will determine whether *warmth*, *erythema*, or *swelling* is present. The examination should distinguish true articular swelling caused by synovial effusion or synovial proliferation from nonarticular or periarticular involvement, which usually extends beyond the normal joint margins or the full extent of the synovial space. Synovial effusion can be distinguished from synovial hypertrophy or bony hypertrophy by palpation or specific maneuvers. For example, small to moderate knee effusions may be identified by the "bulge sign" or "ballottement of the patella." Bursal effusions (e.g., effusions of the olecranon or prepatellar bursa) overlie bony prominences and are fluctuant with sharply defined borders. Joint *stability* can be assessed by palpation and by the application of manual stress to assess displacement in different planes. Subluxation or dislocation, which may be secondary to traumatic, mechanical, or inflammatory causes, can be assessed by inspection and palpation. Joint *volume* can be assessed by palpation. Distention of the articular capsule usually causes pain. The patient will attempt to minimize the pain by keeping the joint in the position of least intraarticular pressure and greatest volume, usually partial flexion. Clinically, joint distention may be detected as obvious swelling, voluntary or fixed flexion deformities, or diminished range of motion—especially on extension, which decreases joint volume. Active and passive *range of motion* should be assessed in all planes, with contralateral comparison. Serial evaluations of joint motion may be made using a goniometer to quantify the arc of movement. Each joint should be passively manipulated through its full range of motion (including, as appropriate, flexion, extension, rotation, abduction, adduction, inversion, eversion, supination, pronation, and medial or lateral deviation or bending). Limitation of motion is frequently caused by effusion, pain, deformity, or contracture. *Contractures* may reflect antecedent synovial inflammation or trauma. Joint *crepitus* may be felt during palpation or maneuvers and may be prominent or coarse in osteoarthritis. Joint *deformity* usually indicates a long-standing or aggressive pathologic process. Deformities may result from ligamentous destruction, soft tissue contracture, bony enlargement, ankylosis, erosive disease, or subluxation. Examination of the musculature will permit assessment of strength and reveal atrophy, pain, or spasm. The examiner should look carefully for nonarticular or periarticular involvement, especially when articular complaints are not supported by objective findings referable to the joint capsule. The identification of musculoskeletal pain of soft tissue origin (nonarticular pain) will prevent unwarranted and often expensive additional evaluations. Specific maneuvers may reveal nonarticular abnormalities, such as a carpal tunnel syndrome (which can be identified by Tinel's or Phalen's sign). Other examples of soft tissue abnormalities include olecranon bursitis, epicondylitis (tennis elbow), enthesitis (e.g., Achilles tendinitis), and trigger points associated with fibromyalgia.

LABORATORY INVESTIGATIONS The vast majority of musculoskeletal disorders can be diagnosed easily by a complete history and physical examination. An additional objective of the initial encounter is to determine whether additional investigations or immediate therapy are required. A number of features indicate the need for additional evaluation. *Monarticular* conditions require additional evaluation, as do *traumatic* or *inflammatory* conditions and conditions accompanied by *neurologic changes* or *systemic manifestations* of serious disease. Finally, individuals with *chronic* symptoms (lasting more than 6 weeks), especially when there has been a lack of response to symptomatic measures, are candidates for additional evaluation. The extent and nature of the additional investigation should be dictated by the clinical features and suspected pathologic process. Laboratory tests should be used to confirm a specific clinical diagnosis and not be used as a tool to screen or evaluate patients with vague rheumatic complaints. Indiscriminate use of broad batteries of diagnostic tests and radiographic procedures are rarely useful or cost-effective.

Besides a complete blood count, including a white blood cell (WBC) and differential count, the routine evaluation should include determination of an acute-phase indicator, such as the erythrocyte sedimentation rate (ESR) or C-reactive protein (CRP), which can be useful in discriminating inflammatory from noninflammatory musculoskeletal disorders. Both tests are inexpensive and easily performed; the resulting values may be elevated with infections, inflammatory arthritis, autoimmune disorders, neoplasia, pregnancy, and advanced age. Serum uric acid determinations are only useful when gout has been diagnosed and therapy contemplated.

Serologic tests for rheumatoid factor, antinuclear antibodies (ANA), complement levels, Lyme disease antibodies, or antistreptolysin O (ASO) titer should be carried out only when there is substantive clinical evidence suggesting a relevant associated diagnosis, as these tests have poor predictive value when used in a screening fashion, especially when the pretest probability is low. They should not be performed arbitrarily in patients with minimal or nonspecific musculoskeletal complaints. For example, 4 to 5% of the general population will have positive tests for rheumatoid factor and ANAs, yet only 1% or 0.04% will have RA or SLE, respectively. IgM rheumatoid factor (autoantibodies against the Fc portion of IgG) is found in 80% of patients with RA and may also be seen in low titers in patients with chronic infections (tuberculosis, leprosy); other autoimmune diseases (SLE, Sjögren's syndrome); or chronic pulmonary, hepatic, or renal diseases. ANAs are found in nearly all patients with SLE and may also be seen in patients with other autoimmune diseases (polymyositis, scleroderma, antiphospholipid syndrome), drug-induced lupus (resulting from hydralazine, procainamide, or quinidine administration), or chronic hepatitic or renal disorders. The interpretation of a positive ANA determination may depend on the titer and on the pattern observed by immunofluorescence microscopy. Diffuse and speckled patterns are most common but least specific, whereas a peripheral, or rim, pattern is highly specific and is suggestive of autoantibodies against double-stranded (native) DNA. This pattern is seen only in patients with SLE.

Aspiration and analysis of synovial fluid are always indicated in acute monarthritis or when an infectious or crystal-induced arthropathy is suspected. Synovial fluid analysis may be crucial in distinguishing between noninflammatory and inflammatory processes. This distinction can be made on the basis of the appearance, viscosity, and cell count of the synovial fluid. Tests for synovial fluid glucose, protein, lactate dehydrogenase, lactic acid, or autoantibodies are not recommended, as they are insensitive or have little discriminatory value. Normal synovial fluid is clear or a pale straw color and is viscous, primarily because of the high levels of hyaluronate. Noninflammatory synovial fluid is clear, viscous, and amber-colored, with a WBC count of $<2000/\mu L$ and a predominance of mononuclear cells. The viscosity of synovial fluid is assessed by expressing fluid from the syringe one drop at a time. Normally there is a stringing effect, with a long tail behind each drop. Effusions due to osteoarthritis or trauma usually have normal viscosity. Inflammatory fluid is turbid and yellow, with an increased WBC (2000 to $50{,}000/\mu L$) and a predominance of polymorphonuclear leukocytes. Inflammatory fluid has a reduced viscosity, diminished hyaluronate, and little or no tail following each drop of synovial fluid. Such effusions are found in RA, gout, other inflammatory arthritides, and septic arthritis. Infectious fluid is turbid and opaque, with a WBC count usually $>50{,}000/\mu L$, a predominance of polymorphonuclear leukocytes ($>75\%$), and low viscosity. Such effusions are typical of septic arthritis, but they occur rarely with sterile inflammatory arthritides such as RA or gout. In addition, hemorrhagic synovial fluid may be seen with trauma, hemarthrosis, or neuropathic arthritis. An algorithm for synovial fluid aspiration and analysis is shown in Fig. 320-3. Synovial fluid should be analyzed immediately for appearance, viscosity, and cell count. Cellularity and the presence of crystals may be assessed by light or polarizing microscopy, respectively. Monosodium urate crystals, seen in gouty effusions, are long, needle-shaped, negatively birefringent, and usually intracellular, whereas calcium pyrophosphate dihydrate crystals, found in chondrocalcinosis and pseudogout, are usually short, rhomboid-shaped, and positively birefringent. Whenever infection is suspected, synovial fluid

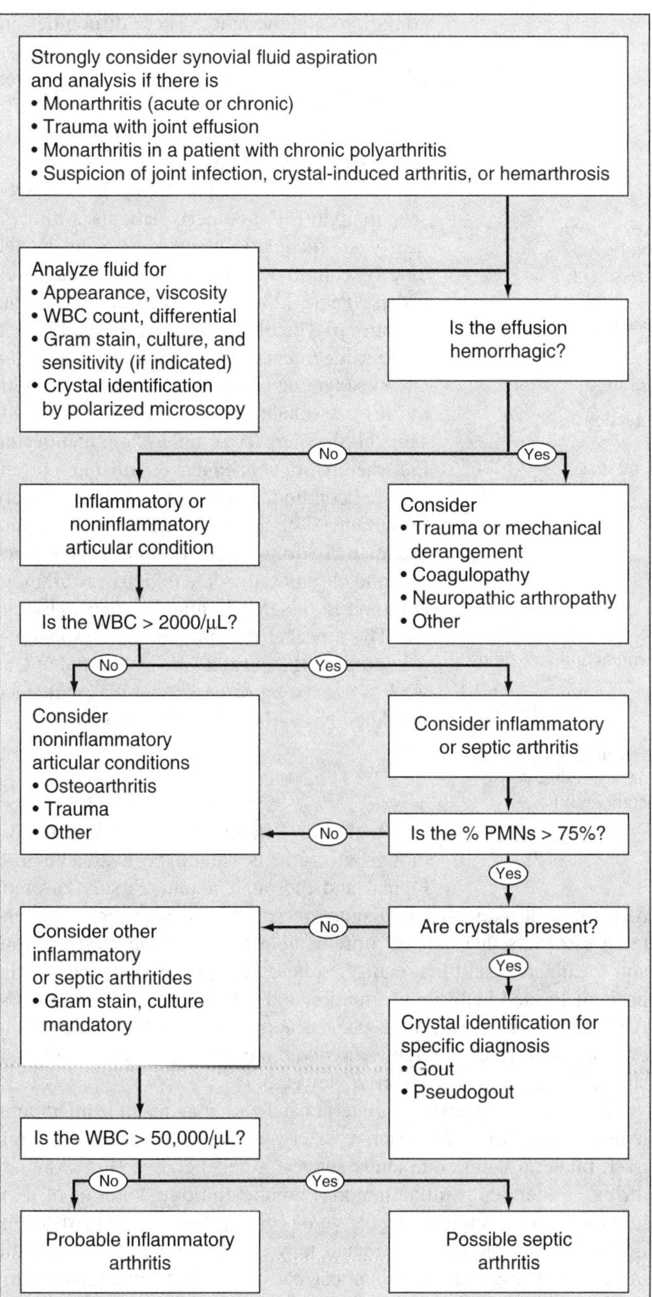

FIGURE 320-3 Algorithmic approach to the use and interpretation of synovial fluid aspiration and analysis.

should be Gram-stained and cultured appropriately. If gonococcal arthritis is suspected, immediate plating of the fluid on appropriate culture medium is indicated. Synovial fluid from chronic monarthritis patients should also be cultured for *M. tuberculosis* and fungi. Last, it should be noted that crystal-induced arthritis and infection occasionally occur together in the same joint.

DIAGNOSTIC IMAGING IN JOINT DISEASES Conventional radiography has been a valuable tool in the diagnosis and staging of articular disorders. Plain x-rays are most appropriate when there is a history of trauma, suspected chronic infection, progressive disability, or monarticular involvement; when therapeutic alterations are considered; or when a baseline assessment is desired for what appears to be a chronic process. However, in most inflammatory disorders, early radiography is rarely helpful in establishing a diagnosis and may only reveal soft tissue swelling or juxtaarticular demineralization. As the disease progresses, calcification (of soft tissues, cartilage, or bone), joint space narrowing, erosions, bony ankylosis, new bone formation (sclerosis, osteophyte formation, or periostitis), or subchondral cysts may develop and suggest specific clinical entities. Consultation with a radiologist will help define proper technique and positioning and prevent the need for further studies.

Additional imaging techniques may possess greater diagnostic sensitivity and facilitate early diagnosis in a limited number of articular disorders and are indicated in selected circumstances when conventional radiography is not adequate (Table 320-4). *Ultrasonography* is useful in the detection of soft tissue abnormalities that cannot be appreciated fully by clinical examination. Although ultrasonography is inexpensive and easily performed, only in a limited number of circumstances is it the preferred method of evaluation. The foremost application of ultrasound is in the diagnosis of synovial (Baker's) cysts, although rotator cuff tears and various tendon injuries may be evaluated with ultrasound by an experienced operator. *Radionuclide scintigraphy* provides useful information regarding the metabolic status of bone and, along with radiography, is well suited for total-body assessment of the extent and distribution of musculoskeletal involvement. It is a very sensitive but poorly specific means of detecting inflammatory or metabolic alterations in bone or periarticular soft tissue structures. The limited tissue resolution of scintigraphy may obscure the distinction between bony and periarticular processes and may necessitate the use of additional imaging modalities. Scintigraphy, using ^{99m}Tc, ^{67}Ga, or WBCs labeled with ^{111}In, has been applied to a variety of articular disorders with variable success (Table 320-4). [^{99m}Tc]pertechnetate or [^{99m}Tc]diphosphonate scintigraphy may be useful in identifying infection, neoplasia, inflammation, increased blood flow, bone remodeling, heterotopic bone formation, or avascular necrosis (Fig. 320-4). However, the poor specificity of ^{99m}Tc scanning has limited its use to investigational and serial assessments of joint or bone involvement, assessment of inflammatory or infectious processes, and surveys for bone metastases. ^{67}Ga binds to serum and cellular transferrin and lactoferrin and is preferentially taken up by neutrophils, macrophages, bacteria, and tumor tissue (e.g., lymphoma) and is useful in the identification of infection and malignancies. Scanning with ^{111}In-labeled WBCs has been used to detect both infectious and inflammatory arthritis. Although both have been used with success, ^{111}In-labeled WBC scanning is superior to ^{67}Ga in the early diagnosis of osteomyelitis and infected prosthetic joints. Prior treatment with antibiotics may reduce the diagnostic sensitivity of both ^{67}Ga and ^{111}In-labeled WBC scintigraphy.

Computed tomography (CT) provides rapid reconstruction of sagittal, coronal, and axial images and thus of the spatial relationships among anatomic structures. It has proved most useful in the assessment of the axial skeleton because of its ability to visualize in the axial plane. Articulations that are difficult to visualize by conventional radiography, such as the zygapophyseal, sacroiliac, sternoclavicular, and hip joints, can be evaluated effectively using CT. CT has been demonstrated to be useful in the diagnosis of low back pain syndromes, sacroiliitis, osteoid osteoma, tarsal coalition, osteomyelitis, intraarticular osteochondral fragments, and advanced osteonecrosis.

Magnetic resonance imaging (MRI) has significantly advanced the ability to image musculoskeletal structures. MRI can provide multiplanar images with fine anatomic detail and contrast resolution (Fig. 320-5). Other advantages are the absence of ionizing radiation and adverse effects and the superior ability to visualize bone marrow and soft tissue periarticular structures. However, the high cost and long procedural time of MRI limit its use in the evaluation of musculoskeletal disorders. MRI should be used only when it will provide necessary information that cannot be obtained by less expensive and noninvasive means.

MRI can image fascia, vessels, nerve, muscle, cartilage, ligaments, tendons, pannus, synovial effusions, cortical bone, and bone marrow. Visualization of particular structures can be enhanced by altering the pulse sequence to produce either T1-weighted or T2-weighted spin echo, gradient echo, or inversion recovery [including short tau inver-

Table 320-4 Diagnostic Imaging Techniques for Musculoskeletal Disorders

Method	Imaging Time, h	Cost[a]	Current Indications
Ultrasound[b]	<1	+	Synovial cysts Rotator cuff tears Tendon injury
Radionuclide scintigraphy			
^{99m}Tc	1–4	++	Metastatic bone survey Evaluation of Paget's disease Quantitative joint assessment Acute infection Acute and chronic osteomyelitis
^{111}In-WBC	24	+++	Acute infection Prosthetic infection Acute osteomyelitis
^{67}Ga	24–48	++++	Acute and chronic infection Acute osteomyelitis
Computed tomography	<1	+++	Herniated intervertebral disk Sacroiliitis Spinal stenosis Spinal trauma Osteoid osteoma Tarsal coalition
Magnetic resonance imaging	1/2–2	+++++	Avascular necrosis Osteomyelitis Intraarticular derangement and soft tissue injury Derangements of axial skeleton and spinal cord Herniated intervertebral disk Pigmented villonodular synovitis Inflammatory and metabolic muscle pathology

[a] Relative cost for imaging study.
[b] Results depend on operator.

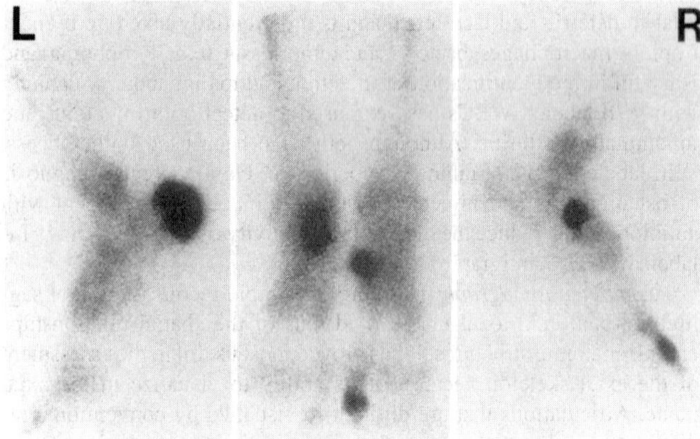

FIGURE 320-4 [^{99m}Tc]diphosphonate scintigraphy of the feet of a 33-year-old black male with Reiter's syndrome, manifested by sacroiliitis, urethritis, uveitis, asymmetric oligoarthritis, and enthesitis. This bone scan demonstrates increased uptake indicative of enthesitis involving the insertions of the left Achilles tendon, plantar aponeurosis, and right tibialis posterior tendon as well as arthritis of the right first interphalangeal joint.

sion recovery (STIR) images. Because of its sensitivity to changes in marrow fat, MRI is a sensitive although nonspecific means of detecting osteonecrosis and osteomyelitis (Fig. 320-5). Because of its enhanced soft tissue resolution, MRI is more sensitive than arthrography or CT for the diagnosis of soft tissue injuries (e.g., meniscal and rotator cuff tears), intraarticular derangements, and spinal cord damage following injury, subluxation, or synovitis of the vertebral facet joints.

RHEUMATOLOGIC EVALUATION OF THE ELDERLY Musculoskeletal disorders in elderly patients are often not diagnosed because the signs and symptoms may be insidious or chronic in these patients. In addition, the nature of the problem is often obscured by the presence of multiple interacting factors, including other medical conditions and therapies. These difficulties are compounded by the diminished reliability of laboratory testing in the elderly, who often manifest nonpathologic abnormal results. For example, erythrocyte sedimentation rates may be misleadingly elevated and low titer positive tests for rheumatoid factor and ANAs may be seen in up to 15% of elderly patients. Although nearly all rheumatic disorders can afflict the elderly, certain diseases and drug-induced disorders (Table 320-2) are more common in this age group. The elderly should be approached in the same manner as other patients with musculoskeletal complaints but with additional inquiries to exclude common geriatric musculoskeletal disorders. An emphasis on identifying the rheumatic consequences of intercurrent medical conditions and therapies is extremely important. Osteoarthritis, gout, polymyalgia rheumatica, drug-induced lupus erythematosus, and chronic salicylate toxicity are all more common in the elderly than in other individuals. The physical examination should identify the nature of the musculoskeletal complaint, as well as coexisting diseases that may influence the diagnosis and choice of treatment.

Approach to the Patient

Regional Rheumatic Complaints Although all patients should be evaluated in a logical and thorough manner, many cases of focal musculoskeletal complaints are caused by commonly encountered disorders that exhibit a predictable pattern of onset, evolution, and localization and that can often be diagnosed immediately on the basis of limited historic information and selected maneuvers or tests. Although nearly every joint can be approached in this manner, the evaluation of four commonly involved anatomic regions—the hand, shoulder, hip, and knee—are reviewed here.

Hand pain Focal or unilateral hand pain may result from trauma, overuse, infection, or a reactive or crystal-induced arthritis. By contrast, bilateral hand complaints suggest a degenerative (e.g., osteoarthritis), systemic, or inflammatory/immune etiology. Patterns of joint involvement are highly suggestive of certain disorders. The distribution of affected joints in the hand may provide important diagnostic information (Fig. 320-6). Thus, osteoarthritis (or degenerative arthritis) may manifest as distal interphalangeal (DIP) and proximal interphalangeal (PIP) joint pain with bony hypertrophy sufficient to produce Heberden's and Bouchard's nodes, respectively. Pain, with or without bony swelling, involving the base of the thumb (first carpometacarpal joint) is also highly suggestive of osteoarthritis. By contrast, RA tends to involve the PIP, metacarpophalangeal, intercarpal, and carpometacarpal joints (wrist) with pain, prolonged stiffness, and palpable synovial tissue hypertrophy. Psoriatic arthritis may also involve the DIP and PIP joints and the carpus with inflammatory pain, stiffness, and synovitis. Moreover, the diagnosis of psoriatic arthritis can be suggested by nail pitting or onycholysis. Soft tissue swelling may also be noted over the dorsum of the hand and wrist and may suggest an inflammatory extensor tendon tenosynovitis, possibly caused by gonococcal infection, gout, or inflammatory arthritis. The diagnosis of tenosynovitis may be suggested by local warmth and edema and is confirmed when pain is induced by maintaining the wrist in a fixed, neutral position and flexing the digits distal to the metacarpophalangeal joints to stretch the extensor tendon sheaths.

Focal wrist pain localized to the radial aspect may be caused by DeQuervain's tenosynovitis resulting from inflammation of the tendon sheath(s) involving the abductor pollicis longus or extensor pollicis brevis (Fig. 320-6). This condition commonly results from overuse or

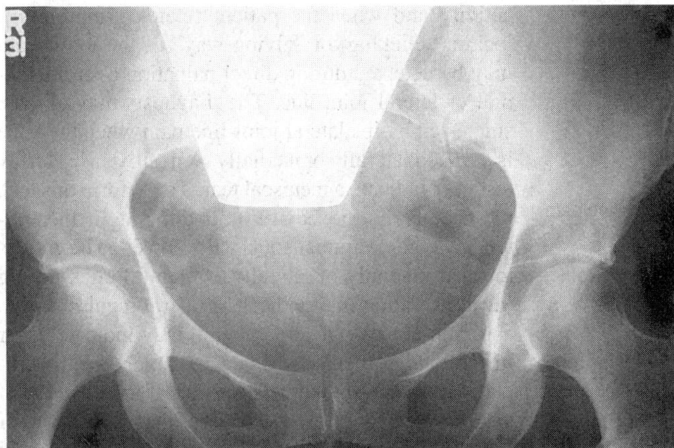

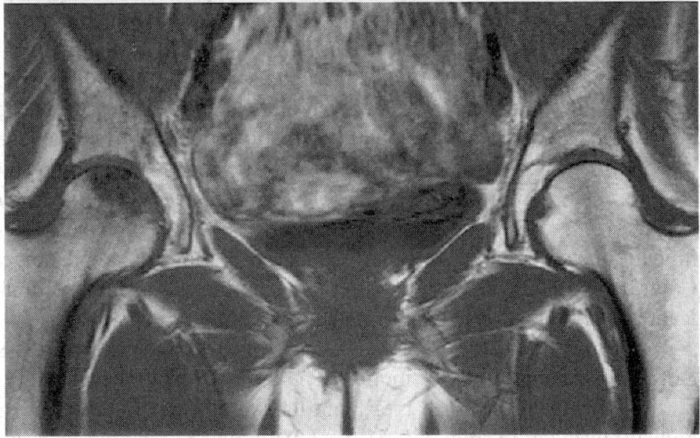

FIGURE 320-5 Superior sensitivity of magnetic resonance imaging in the diagnosis of osteonecrosis of the femoral head. A 45-year-old woman receiving high-dose glucocorticoids developed right hip pain. Conventional x-rays (*top*) demonstrated only mild sclerosis of the right femoral head. T1-weighted MRI (*bottom*) demonstrated low-density signal in the right femoral head, diagnostic of osteonecrosis.

develops after pregnancy and may be diagnosed with Finkelstein's test. A positive result in Finkelstein's test is present when local wrist pain is induced after the thumb is flexed across the palm and placed inside a clenched fist and the patient actively moves the hand downward with ulnar deviation at the wrist. Carpal tunnel syndrome is another common disorder of the upper extremity and results from compression of the median nerve within the carpal tunnel. Manifestations include paresthesias in the thumb and the second, third, and radial half of the fourth fingers, and sometimes, atrophy of thenar musculature. Carpal tunnel syndrome is commonly associated with pregnancy, edema, trauma, osteoarthritis, inflammatory arthritis, and infiltrative disorders (e.g., amyloidosis). The diagnosis is suggested by a positive Tinel's or Phalen's sign. With each test, paresthesia in a median nerve distribution is induced or increased by either "thumping" the volar aspect of the wrist (Tinel's sign) or pressing the extensor surfaces of the two flexed wrists against each another (Phalen's sign).

Shoulder pain During the evaluation of shoulder disorders, the examiner should carefully note any history of trauma, infection, inflammatory disease, occupational hazards, or previous cervical disease. In addition, the patient should be questioned as to the activities or movement(s) that elicit shoulder pain. Shoulder pain is frequently referred from the cervical spine, but it may also be referred from intrathoracic lesions (e.g., a Pancoast tumor) or from gallbladder, hepatic, or diaphragmatic disease. The shoulder should be put through its full range of motion both actively and passively (with examiner assistance): forward flexion, extension, abduction, adduction, and rotation. Manual inspection of the periarticular structures will often provide important diagnostic information. The examiner should apply direct manual pressure over the subacromial bursa, which lies lateral to and immediately beneath the acromion. Subacromial bursitis is a frequent cause of shoulder pain. Anterior to the subacromial bursa, the bicipital tendon traverses the bicipital groove. This tendon is best identified by palpating it in its groove as the patient rotates the humerus internally and externally. Direct pressure over the tendon may reveal pain indicative of bicipital tendinitis. Palpation of the acromioclavicular joint may disclose local pain, bony hypertrophy, or synovial swelling. Whereas osteoarthritis and RA commonly affect the acromioclavicular joint, osteoarthritis seldom involves the glenohumeral joint, unless there is a traumatic or occupational cause. The glenohumeral joint is best palpated anteriorly by placing the thumb over the humeral head (just medial and inferior to the coracoid process) and having the patient rotate the humerus internally and externally. Pain localized to this region is indicative of glenohumeral pathology. Synovial effusion or tissue is seldom palpable but, if present, may suggest infection, RA, or an acute tear of the rotator cuff.

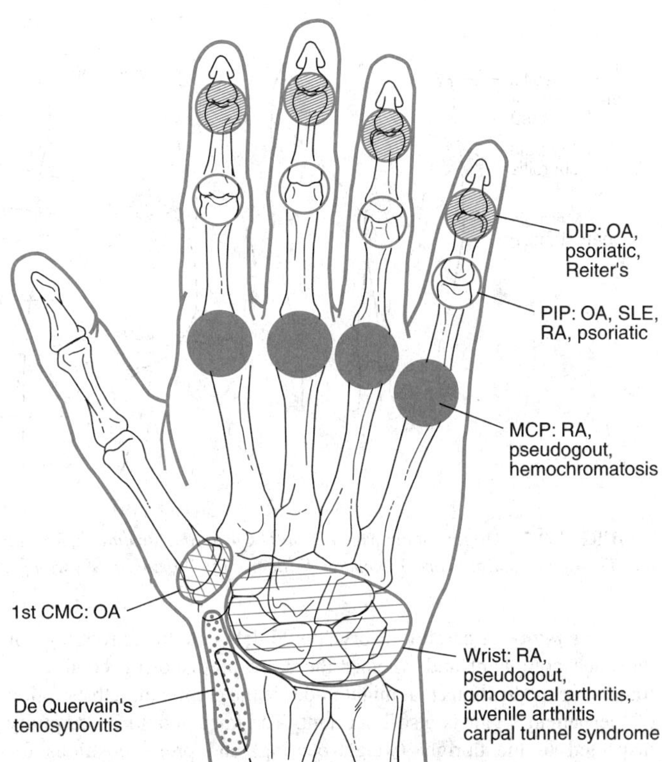

FIGURE 320-6 Sites of hand or wrist involvement and their potential disease associations. (DIP, distal interphalangeal; OA, osteoarthritis; PIP, proximal interphalangeal; SLE, systemic lupus erythematosus; RA, rheumatoid arthritis; MCP, metacarpophalangeal; CMC, carpometacarpal.) *(From JJ Cush, AF Kavanaugh, Rheumatology: Diagnosis and Therapeutics, Baltimore, Lippincott, Williams and Wilkins, 1999, with permission.)*

Rotator cuff tendinitis or tear is a very common cause of shoulder pain. The rotator cuff is formed by the tendons of the supraspinatus, infraspinatus, teres minor, and subscapularis muscles. Rotator cuff tendinitis is suggested by pain on active abduction (but not passive abduction), pain over the lateral deltoid muscle, night pain, and evidence of the impingement sign. This maneuver is performed by the examiner raising the patient's arm into forced flexion while stabilizing the scapula and preventing it from rotating. A positive sign is present if pain develops before 180° of forward flexion. A complete tear of the rotator cuff, which often results from trauma, may manifest in the same manner but is less common than tendinitis. The diagnosis is suggested by the drop arm test, in which the patient is asked to maintain the arm outstretched after it has been passively abducted. If the patient is unable to hold the arm up once 90° of abduction is reached, the test is positive. Tendinitis or tear of the rotator cuff can be confirmed by MRI or ultrasonography.

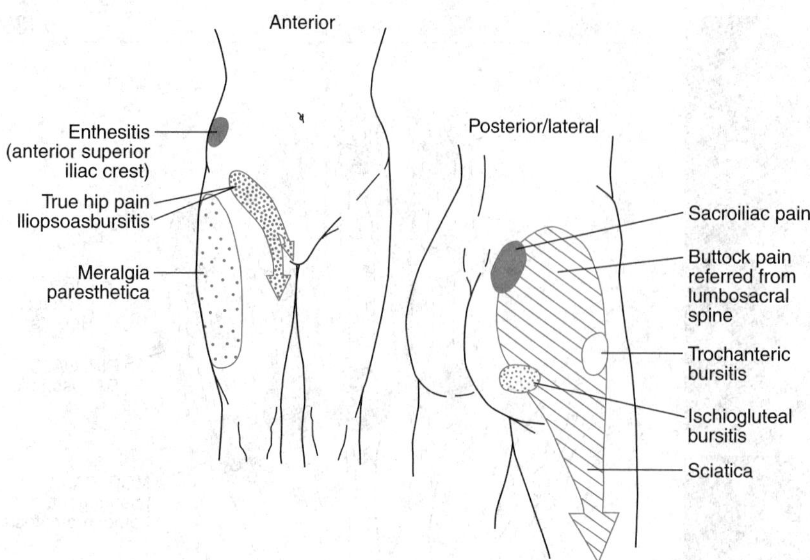

FIGURE 320-7 Origins of hip pain. *(From JJ Cush, AF Kavanaugh, Rheumatology: Diagnosis and Therapeutics, Baltimore, Lippincott, Williams and Wilkins, 1999, with permission.)*

Knee pain A careful history should delineate the chronology of the knee complaint and whether there are predisposing conditions, trauma, or medications that might underlie the complaint. Observation of the patient's gait is also important. The knee should be carefully inspected in the upright (weight-bearing) and prone positions for swelling, erythema, contusion, laceration, and malalignment. The most common form of malalignment in the knee is genu varum (bow-legs) and genu valgum (knock-knees). Bony swelling of the knee joint commonly results from hypertrophic osseous changes seen with disorders such as osteoarthritis and neuropathic arthropathy. Swelling caused by hypertrophy of intrasynovial structures (synovial enlargement or effusion) may manifest as a fluctuant, ballotable, or soft tissue enlargement in the suprapatellar pouch (superior reflection of the synovial cavity) or lateral and medial to the patella. Synovial effusions may also be detected by balloting the patella downward toward the femoral groove or by eliciting a bulge sign. To elicit this sign, the examiner positions the knee in extension and manually compresses or milks synovial fluid down from the suprapatellar pouch and lateral to the patellae. Manual pressure lateral to the patella may cause an observable shift in synovial fluid (bulge) to the medial aspect. This maneuver is only effective for detecting small to moderate effusions (<100 mL). Inflammatory disorders such as RA, gout, and Reiter's syndrome may involve the knee joint and produce significant pain, stiffness, swelling, or warmth. A popliteal or *Baker's cyst* is best palpated with the knee partially flexed and is best seen with the patient standing with knees fully extended to visualize popliteal swelling or fullness from a posterior view.

Anserine bursitis is an often missed cause of knee pain in adults. The pes anserine bursa underlies the semimembranosus tendon and may become inflamed or painful owing to trauma, overuse, or inflammation. Anserine bursitis manifests primarily as point tenderness inferior and medial to the patella and overlying the medial tibial plateau. Swelling and erythema may not be present. Other forms of bursitis may also present as knee pain. The prepatellar bursa is superficial and is located over the inferior portion of the patella. The infrapatellar bursa is deeper and lies beneath the patellar ligament before its insertion on the tibial tubercle.

Internal derangement of the knee may result from trauma or degenerative processes. Damage to the meniscal cartilage (medial or lateral) frequently presents as chronic or intermittent knee pain. Such an injury should be suspected when there is a history of trauma or athletic activity and when the patient relates symptoms of locking, clicking, or "giving way" of the joint. Pain may be detected during direct palpation over the medial or lateral joint line. The diagnosis may also be suggested by ipsilateral joint-line pain when the knee is stressed laterally or medially. A positive McMurray test may indicate a meniscal tear. To perform this test, the knee is first flexed at 90°, and the leg is then extended while simultaneously the lower extremity is torqued medially or laterally. A painful click during inward rotation may indicate a lateral meniscus tear, and pain during outward rotation may indicate a tear in the medial meniscus. Finally, damage to the cruciate ligaments should be suspected if there is pain of acute onset, possibly with swelling, a history of trauma, or a synovial fluid aspirate that is grossly bloody. Examination of the cruciate ligaments is best accomplished by eliciting a drawer sign. With the patient recumbent, the knee should be partially flexed and the foot stabilized on the examining surface. The examiner should manually attempt to displace the tibia anteriorly or posteriorly with respect to the femur. If anterior movement is detected, then anterior cruciate ligament damage is likely. Conversely, significant posterior movement may indicate posterior cruciate damage. Contralateral comparison will assist the examiner in detecting significant anterior or posterior movement.

Hip pain The hip is best evaluated by observing the patient's gait and assessing range of motion. The vast majority of patients reporting "hip pain" localize their pain unilaterally to the posterior or gluteal musculature (Fig. 320-7). Such pain may or may not be associated with low back pain and tends to radiate down the posterolateral aspect of the thigh. This presentation frequently results from degenerative arthritis of the lumbosacral spine and commonly follows a dermatomal distribution with involvement of nerve roots between L5 and S1. Some individuals instead localize their "hip pain" laterally to the area overlying the trochanteric bursa. Because of the depth of this bursa, swelling and warmth are usually absent. Diagnosis of trochanteric bursitis can be confirmed by inducing point tenderness over the trochanteric bursa. Range of movement may be limited by pain. Pain in the hip joint is less common and tends to be located anteriorly, over the inguinal ligament; it may radiate medially to the groin or along the anteromedial thigh. Uncommonly, iliopsoas bursitis may mimic true hip joint pain. Diagnosis of iliopsoas bursitis may be suggested by a history of trauma or inflammatory arthritis. Pain associated with an iliopsoas bursitis is localized to the groin or anterior thigh and tends to worsen with hyperextension of the hip; many patients prefer to flex and externally rotate the hip to reduce the pain from a distended bursa.

BIBLIOGRAPHY

BEESON PB: Age and sex associations of 40 autoimmune diseases. Am J Med 96:457, 1994

BROWER AC: Imaging techniques and modalities, in *Arthritis in Black and White*, 2d ed., AC Brower (ed). Philadelphia, Saunders, 1996, p 1

CUSH JJ et al: Evaluation of musculoskeletal complaints, in *Rheumatology: Diagnosis and Therapeutics*. JJ Cush, AF Kavanaugh (eds). Williams & Wilkins, Baltimore, 1998, pp 1–15

LAWRENCE RC et al: Estimates of the prevalence of arthritis and selected musculoskeletal disorders in the United States. Arthritis Rheum 41:778, 1998

LIPSKY PE et al: Algorithms for the diagnosis and management of musculoskeletal complaints. Am J Med 103:49S, 1997

SHMERLING RH et al: Synovial fluid tests: What should be ordered? JAMA 264:1009, 1990

WARD MW: Laboratory testing for systemic rheumatic diseases. Postgrad Med 103:93, 1998

WERNICK R: Avoiding laboratory test misinterpretation. Geriatrics 44:61, 1989

321 OSTEOARTHRITIS

Kenneth D. Brandt

Cox cyclooxygenase	NSAID nonsteroidal anti-inflammatory drug
CSIs Cox-2-specific inhibitors	OA osteoarthritis
DISH diffuse idiopathic skeletal hyperostosis	PAI-1 plasminogen activator inhibitor-1
GI gastrointestinal	PGs proteoglycans
IGF-1 insulin-like growth factor-1	TGF-β transforming growth factor β
IL interleukin	TIMP tissue inhibitor of metalloproteinase
MMPs matrix metalloproteinases	

Osteoarthritis (OA), also erroneously called degenerative joint disease, represents failure of the diarthrodial (movable, synovial-lined) joint. In idiopathic (primary) OA, the most common form of the disease, no predisposing factor is apparent. Secondary OA is pathologically indistinguishable from idiopathic OA but is attributable to an underlying cause (Table 321-1).

EPIDEMIOLOGY AND RISK FACTORS OA is the most common joint disease of humans. Among the elderly, knee OA is the leading cause of chronic disability in developed countries; some 100,000 people in the United States are unable to walk independently from bed to bathroom because of OA of the knee or hip.

Under the age of 55 years the joint distribution of OA in men and women is similar; in older individuals, hip OA is more common in men, while OA of interphalangeal joints and the thumb base is more common in women. Similarly, radiographic evidence of knee OA and, especially *symptomatic* knee OA, is more common in women than in men (Table 321-2).

Racial differences exist in both the prevalence of OA and the pattern of joint involvement. The Chinese in Hong Kong have a lower incidence of hip OA than whites; OA is more frequent in native Americans than in whites. Interphalangeal joint OA and, especially, hip OA are much less common in South African blacks than in whites in the same population. Whether these differences are genetic or are due to differences in joint usage related to life-style or occupation is unknown.

In some cases, the relation of heredity to OA is less ambiguous. Thus, the mother and sister of a woman with distal interphalangeal joint OA (Heberden's nodes) are, respectively, twice and thrice as likely to exhibit OA in these joints as the mother and sister of an unaffected woman. Point mutations in the cDNA coding for articular cartilage collagen have been identified in families with chondrodysplasia and polyarticular secondary OA.

Age is the most powerful risk factor for OA. In a radiographic survey of women less than 45 years old, only 2% had OA; between the ages of 45 to 64 years, however, the prevalence was 30%, and for those older than 65 years it was 68%. In males, the figures were similar but somewhat lower in the older age groups.

Major trauma and repetitive joint use are also important risk factors for OA. Anterior cruciate ligament insufficiency or meniscus damage (and meniscectomy) may lead to knee OA. Although damage to the articular cartilage may occur at the time of injury or subsequently, with use of the affected joint, even normal cartilage will degenerate if the joint is unstable. A person with a trimalleolar fracture will almost certainly develop ankle OA.

The pattern of joint involvement in OA is influenced by prior vocational or avocational overload. Thus, while ankle OA is common in ballet dancers, elbow OA in baseball pitchers, and metacarpophalangeal joint OA in prize fighters, OA is not very common at any of these sites in the general population.

Table 321-1 Classification of OA

I. Idiopathic
  A. Localized OA
    1. Hands: Heberden's and Bouchard's nodes (nodal), erosive interphalangeal arthritis (nonnodal), 1st carpometacarpal joint
    2. Feet: hallux valgus, hallux rigidus, contracted toes (hammer/cock-up toes), talonavicular
    3. Knee:
      a. Medial compartment
      b. Lateral compartment
      c. Patellofemoral compartment
    4. Hip:
      a. Eccentric (superior)
      b. Concentric (axial, medial)
      c. Diffuse (coxae senilis)
    5. Spine:
      a. Apophyseal joints
      b. Intervertebral joints (disks)
      c. Spondylosis (osteophytes)
      d. Ligamentous (hyperostosis, Forestier's disease, diffuse idiopathic skeletal hyperostosis
    6. Other single sites, e.g., glenohumoral, acromioclavicular, tibiotalar, sacroiliac, temporomandibular
  B. Generalized OA includes 3 or more of the areas listed above (Kellgren-Moore)
II. Secondary
  A. Trauma
    1. Acute
    2. Chronic (occupational, sports)
  B. Congenital or developmental
    1. Localized diseases: Legg-Calvé-Perthes, congenital hip dislocation, slipped epiphysis
    2. Mechanical factors: unequal lower extremity length, valgus/varus deformity, hypermobility syndromes
    3. Bone dysplasias: epiphyseal dysplasia, spondyloepiphyseal dysplasia, osteonychondystrophy
  C. Metabolic
    1. Ochronosis (alkaptonuria)
    2. Hemochromatosis
    3. Wilson's disease
    4. Gaucher's disease
  D. Endocrine
    1. Acromegaly
    2. Hyperparathyroidism
    3. Diabetes mellitus
    4. Obesity
    5. Hypothyroidism
  E. Calcium deposition diseases
    1. Calcium pyrophosphate dihydrate deposition
    2. Apatite arthropathy
  F. Other bone and joint diseases
    1. Localized: fracture, avascular necrosis, infection, gout
    2. Diffuse: rheumatoid (inflammatory) arthritis, Paget's disease, osteopetrosis, osteochondritis
  G. Neuropathic (Charcot joints)
  H. Endemic
    1. Kashin-Beck
    2. Mseleni
  I. Miscellaneous
    1. Frostbite
    2. Caisson's disease
    3. Hemoglobinopathies

SOURCE: From Mankin et al.

Table 321-2 Risk Factors for OA

Age	Repetitive stress, e.g., vocational[a]
Female sex	Obesity[a]
Race	Congenital/developmental defects[a]
Genetic factors	Prior inflammatory joint disease
Major joint trauma[a]	Metabolic/endocrine disorders

[a] Potentially modifiable

SOURCE: Adapted from M Hochberg: J Rheumatol 18: 1438, 1991.

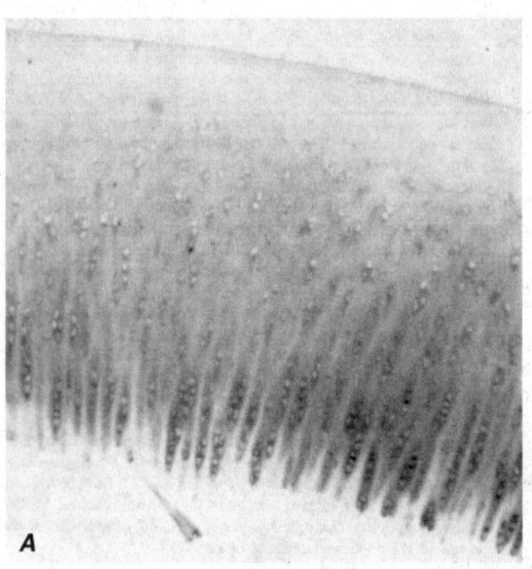

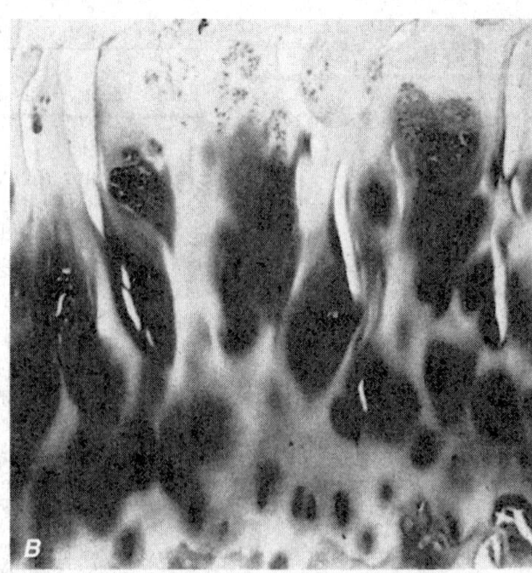

FIGURE 321-1 *A.* Normal articular cartilage. Note the intact surface and even distribution of chondrocytes. Mitotic figures are not present in normal adult articular cartilage. *B.* Osteoarthritic cartilage. Note the disruption of surface integrity, with vertical fissures (fibrillation) and irregular distribution of cells. Many of the chondrocytes have replicated and exist in clusters. Stained with safranin-O, which binds to the sulfated glycosaminoglycan chains of proteoglycans. Note patchy areas of diminished staining (pale extracellular matrix) due to proteoglycan depletion.

Given the growing participation of the population of this country in cardiovascular fitness programs, it is important to note that there are no convincing data to support an association between specific athletic activities and arthritis if major trauma is excluded. Neither long-distance running nor jogging has been shown to cause OA. This apparent lack of association may, however, be due to the lack of good long-term studies, the difficulty of retrospective assessment of activities, and selection bias, i.e., early discontinuation of the activity by those incurring joint damage. In contrast, vocational activities, such as those performed by jackhammer operators, cotton mill and shipyard workers, and coal miners, may lead to OA in the joints exposed to repetitive occupational use. Men whose jobs required knee bending and at least medium physical demands had a higher rate of radiographic evidence of knee OA, and more severe radiographic changes, than men whose jobs required neither.

Obesity is a risk factor for knee OA and hand OA. For those in the highest quintile for body mass index at baseline examination, the relative risk for developing knee OA in the ensuing 36 years was 1.5 for men and 2.1 for women. For *severe* knee OA, the relative risk rose to 1.9 for men and 3.2 for women, suggesting that obesity plays an even larger role in the etiology of the most serious cases of knee OA. Furthermore, obese individuals who have not yet developed OA can reduce their risk: A weight loss of only 5 kg was found to be associated with a 50% reduction in the odds of developing symptomatic knee OA.

The correlation between the pathologic severity of OA and symptoms is poor. Many individuals with radiographic changes of advanced OA have no symptoms. The risk factors for *pain* and *disability* in affected individuals are poorly understood. Disability in those with knee OA is more strongly associated with quadriceps muscle weakness than with either joint pain or radiographic severity of the disease. For the same degree of pathologic severity, women are more likely to be symptomatic than men, those on welfare more likely than those who are working, and those who are divorced more likely than those who are married. For individuals with OA who had poor social support, periodic telephone calls from a trained lay interviewer were as effective as a nonsteroidal anti-inflammatory drug (NSAID) in reducing joint pain, emphasizing the importance of psychosocial factors as determinants of pain.

PATHOLOGY Although the cardinal pathologic feature of OA is a progressive loss of articular cartilage, OA is not a disease of any single tissue but a disease of an *organ*, the synovial joint, in which all of the tissues are affected: the subchondral bone, synovium, meniscus, ligaments, and supporting neuromuscular apparatus as well as the cartilage.

The most striking morphologic changes in OA are usually seen in load-bearing areas of the articular cartilage. In the early stages the cartilage is thicker than normal, but with progression of OA the joint surface thins, the cartilage softens, the integrity of the surface is breached, and vertical clefts develop (fibrillation) (Fig. 321-1). Deep cartilage ulcers, extending to bone, may appear. Areas of fibrocartilaginous repair may develop, but the repair tissue is inferior to pristine hyaline articular cartilage in its ability to withstand mechanical stress. All of the cartilage is metabolically active, and the chondrocytes replicate, forming clusters (clones). Later, however, the cartilage becomes hypocellular.

Remodeling and hypertrophy of bone are also major features of OA. Appositional bone growth occurs in the subchondral region, leading to the bony "sclerosis" seen radiographically. The abraded bone under a cartilage ulcer may take on the appearance of ivory (eburnation). Growth of cartilage and bone at the joint margins leads to osteophytes (spurs), which alter the contour of the joint and may restrict movement. A patchy chronic synovitis and thickening of the joint capsule may further restrict movement. Periarticular muscle wasting is common and may play a major role in symptoms and, as indicated above, in disability.

PATHOGENESIS The main load on articular cartilage—the major target tissue in OA—is produced by contraction of the muscles that stabilize or move the joint. Although cartilage is an excellent shock absorber in terms of its bulk properties, at most sites it is only 1 to 2 mm thick—too thin to serve as the sole shock-absorbing structure in the joint. Additional protective mechanisms are provided by subchondral bone and periarticular muscles.

Articular cartilage serves two essential functions within the joint, both of which are mechanical. First, it provides a remarkably smooth bearing surface, so that, with joint movement, the bones glide effortlessly over each other. With synovial fluid as lubricant, the coefficient of friction for cartilage rubbed against cartilage, even under physiologic loading, is 15 times lower than that of two ice cubes passed across each other! Second, articular cartilage prevents the concentration of stresses, so the bones do not shatter when the joint is loaded.

OA develops in either of two settings: (1) the biomaterial properties of the articular cartilage and subchondral bone are normal, but excessive loading of the joint causes the tissues to fail, or (2) the applied load is reasonable, but the material properties of the cartilage or bone are inferior.

Although articular cartilage is highly resistant to wear under conditions of repeated oscillation, repetitive impact loading soon leads to joint failure. This fact accounts for the high prevalence of OA at specific sites related to vocational or avocational overloading. In general, the earliest changes occur at the sites in the joint that are subject to the greatest compressive loads. Some cases of "idiopathic" OA of the hip may be due to subtle congenital or developmental defects, such as congenital subluxation/dislocation, acetabular dysplasia, Legg-Calvé-Perthes disease, or slipped capital femoral epiphysis, which increase joint congruity and concentrate the dynamic load.

Clinical conditions that reduce the ability of the cartilage or subchondral bone to deform are associated with development of OA. In ochronosis, for example, accumulation of homogentisic acid polymers leads to stiffening of the cartilage; in osteopetrosis, stiffness of the subchondral trabeculae occurs. In both conditions, severe generalized

OA is usually apparent by the age of 40. If the subchondral bone is stiffened experimentally, repetitive impact loading soon leads to breakdown of the overlying cartilage. Conversely, osteoporosis, in which the bone is abnormally soft, may protect against OA.

The Extracellular Matrix of Normal Articular Cartilage Articular cartilage is composed of two major macromolecular species: proteoglycans (PGs), which are responsible for the compressive stiffness of the tissue and its ability to withstand load, and collagen, which provides tensile strength and resistance to shear. Although lysosomal proteases (cathepsins) have been demonstrated within the cells and matrix of normal articular cartilage, their low pH optimum makes it likely that the proteoglycanase activity of these enzymes will be confined to intracellular sites or the immediate pericellular area. However, cartilage also contains a family of matrix metalloproteinases (MMPs), including stromelysin, collagenase, and gelatinase, which can degrade all the components of the extracellular matrix at neutral pH. Each is secreted by the chondrocyte as a latent proenzyme that must be activated by proteolytic cleavage of its N-terminal sequence. The level of MMP activity in the cartilage at any given time represents the balance between activation of the proenzyme and inhibition of the active enzyme by tissue inhibitors. It has recently become apparent that much of the total tissue pool of aggrecan, the major PG in articular cartilage, is degraded by a proteinase that cleaves the protein core of the molecule at a site distinct from that at which the MMPs are active. The enzyme responsible for this cleavage is referred to as "aggrecanase" but has not been clearly identified.

The turnover of normal cartilage is effected through a degradative cascade, for which many investigators consider the driving force to be interleukin (IL) 1, a cytokine produced by mononuclear cells (including synovial lining cells) and synthesized by chondrocytes. IL-1 stimulates the synthesis and secretion of the latent MMPs and of tissue plasminogen activator. Plasminogen, the substrate for the latter enzyme, may be synthesized by the chondrocyte or may enter the cartilage from the synovial fluid. Both plasminogen and stromelysin may play a role in activation of the latent MMPs. In addition to its catabolic effect on cartilage, IL-1, at concentrations even lower than those needed to stimulate cartilage degradation, suppresses PG synthesis by the chondrocyte, inhibiting matrix repair (see below).

The balance of the system lies with at least two inhibitors, tissue inhibitor of metalloproteinase (TIMP) and plasminogen activator inhibitor-1 (PAI-1), which are synthesized by the chondrocyte and limit the degradative activity of MMPs and plasminogen activator, respectively. If TIMP or PAI-1 is destroyed or is present in concentrations that are insufficient relative to those of active enzymes, stromelysin and plasmin are free to act on matrix substrates. Stromelysin can degrade the protein core of the PG and activate latent collagenase. Conversion of latent stromelysin to an active, highly destructive protease by plasmin provides a second mechanism for matrix degradation.

Polypeptide mediators, e.g., insulin-like growth factor-1 (IGF-1) and transforming growth factor β (TGF-β), stimulate biosynthesis of PGs. They regulate matrix metabolism in normal cartilage and may play a role in matrix repair in OA. Notably, these growth factors modulate catabolic as well as anabolic pathways of chondrocyte metabolism; by down-regulating chondrocyte receptors for IL-1, they may decrease PG degradation.

In addition to its responsiveness to cytokines and a variety of other biologic mediators, chondrocyte metabolism in normal cartilage can be modulated directly by mechanical loading. Whereas static loading and prolonged cyclic loading inhibit synthesis of PGs and protein, loads of relatively brief duration may stimulate matrix biosynthesis.

Pathophysiology of Cartilage Changes in OA Most investigators feel that the primary changes in OA begin in the cartilage. A change in the arrangement and size of the collagen fibers is apparent. Biochemical data are consistent with the presence of a defect in the collagen network of the matrix, perhaps due to disruption of the "glue" that binds adjacent fibers. This is among the earliest matrix changes observed and appears to be irreversible.

Although "wear" may be a factor in the loss of cartilage, strong evidence supports the concept that lysosomal enzymes and MMPs account for much of the loss of cartilage matrix in OA. Whether their synthesis and secretion are stimulated by IL-1 or by other factors (e.g., mechanical stimuli), MMPs, plasmin, and cathepsins all appear to be involved in the breakdown of articular cartilage in OA. TIMP and PAI-1 may work to stabilize the system, at least temporarily, while growth factors, such as IGF-1, TGF-β, and basic fibroblast growth factor, are implicated in repair processes that may heal the lesion or, at least, stabilize the process. A stoichiometric imbalance exists between the levels of active enzyme and the level of TIMP, which may be only modestly increased.

Of current interest is the possible role of nitric oxide (NO) in articular cartilage damage in OA, since NO has been shown to stimulate synthesis of MMPs by chrondrocytes. Chondrocytes are a major source of NO, the synthesis of which is stimulated by IL-1 and tumor necrosis factor and by shear stresses on the tissue. In an experimental model of OA, treatment with a selective inhibitor of inducible NO synthase reduced the severity of cartilage damage.

The chondrocytes in OA cartilage undergo active cell division and are very active metabolically, producing increased quantities of DNA, RNA collagen, PG, and noncollagenous proteins. (For this reason, it is inaccurate to call OA a *degenerative* joint disease). Prior to cartilage loss and PG depletion, this marked biosynthetic activity may lead to an increase in PG concentration, which may be associated with thickening of the cartilage and a stage of homeostasis referred to as "compensated" OA. These mechanisms may maintain the joint in a reasonably functional state for years. The repair tissue, however, often does not hold up as well under mechanical stresses as normal hyaline cartilage and eventually, at least in some cases, the rate of PG synthesis falls off and "end-stage" OA develops, with full-thickness loss of cartilage.

CLINICAL FEATURES The joint pain of OA is often described as a deep ache and is localized to the involved joint. Typically, the pain of OA is aggravated by joint use and relieved by rest, but, as the disease progresses, it may become persistent. Nocturnal pain, interfering with sleep, is seen particularly in advanced OA of the hip and may be enervating. Stiffness of the involved joint upon arising in the morning or after a period of inactivity (e.g., an automobile ride) may be prominent but usually lasts less than 20 min. Systemic manifestations are not a feature of primary OA.

Because articular cartilage is aneural, the joint pain in OA must arise from other structures (Table 321-3). In some cases it may be due to stretching of nerve endings in the periosteum covering osteophytes; in others, to microfractures in subchondral bone or from medullary hypertension caused by distortion of blood flow by thickened subchondral trabeculae. Joint instability, leading to stretching of the joint capsule, and muscle spasm may also be sources of pain.

In some patients with OA, joint pain may be due to synovitis. In advanced OA, histologic evidence of synovial inflammation may be as marked as that in the synovium of a patient with rheumatoid arthritis. Synovitis in OA may be due to phagocytosis of shards of cartilage and bone from the abraded joint surface (wear particles), to release from the cartilage of soluble matrix macromolecules, or to crystals of calcium pyrophosphate or hydroxyapatite. In other cases, immune complexes, containing antigens derived from cartilage matrix, may be sequestered in collagenous tissue of the joint, leading to low-

Table 321-3 Causes of Joint Pain in Patients with OA

Source	Mechanism
Synovium	Inflammation
Subchondral bone	Medullary hypertension, microfractures
Osteophyte	Stretching of periosteal nerve endings
Ligaments	Stretch
Capsule	Inflammation, distention
Muscle	Spasm

grade chronic synovitis. In contrast, in the earlier stages of OA, even in the patient with chronic joint pain, synovial inflammation may be absent, suggesting that the joint pain is due to one of the other factors mentioned above.

Physical examination of the OA joint may reveal localized tenderness and bony or soft tissue swelling. Bony crepitus (the sensation of bone rubbing against bone, evoked by joint movement) is characteristic. Synovial effusions, if present, are usually not large. Palpation may reveal some warmth over the joint. Periarticular muscle atrophy may be due to disuse or to reflex inhibition of muscle contraction. In the advanced stages of OA, there may be gross deformity, bony hypertrophy, subluxation, and marked loss of joint motion. The notion that OA is inexorably progressive, however, is incorrect. In many patients the disease stabilizes; in some, regression of joint pain and even of radiographic changes occurs.

Although the diagnosis of OA is often straightforward because of the high prevalence of radiographic changes of OA in asymptomatic individuals, it is important to ensure that joint pain in a patient with radiographic evidence of OA is not due to some other cause, such as soft tissue rheumatism (e.g., anserine bursitis at the knee, trochanteric bursitis at the hip), radiculopathy, referral of pain from another joint (e.g., 25% of patients with hip disease have pain referred to the knee), entrapment neuropathy, vascular disease (claudication), or some other type of arthritis (e.g., crystal-induced synovitis, septic arthritis). These are all common pitfalls in the diagnosis of OA. It is usually not difficult to differentiate OA from a systemic rheumatic disease, such as rheumatoid arthritis, because, in the latter diseases, joint involvement is usually symmetric and polyarticular, with arthritis in wrists and metacarpophalangeal joints (which are generally not involved in OA), and there are also constitutional features such as prolonged morning stiffness, fatigue, weight loss, or fever.

LABORATORY AND RADIOGRAPHIC FINDINGS The diagnosis of OA is usually based on clinical and radiographic features. In the early stages, the radiograph may be normal, but joint space narrowing becomes evident as articular cartilage is lost. Other characteristic radiographic findings include subchondral bone sclerosis, subchondral cysts, and osteophytosis. A change in the contour of the joint, due to bony remodeling, and subluxation may be seen. Although tibiofemoral joint space narrowing has been considered to be a radiographic surrogate for articular cartilage thinning, in patients with early OA who do not have radiographic evidence of bony changes (e.g., subchondral sclerosis or cysts, osteophytes), joint space narrowing alone does not accurately indicate the status of the articular cartilage. Similarly, osteophytosis alone, in the absence of other radiographic features of OA, may be due to aging rather than to OA.

As indicated above, there is often great disparity between the severity of radiographic findings, the severity of symptoms, and functional ability in OA. Thus, while more than 90% of persons over the age of 40 have some radiographic changes of OA in weight-bearing joints, only 30% of these persons are symptomatic.

No laboratory studies are diagnostic for OA, but specific laboratory testing may help in identifying one of the underlying causes of secondary OA (Table 321-1). Because primary OA is not systemic, the erythrocyte sedimentation rate, serum chemistry determinations, blood counts, and urinalysis are normal. Analysis of synovial fluid reveals mild leukocytosis (<2000 white blood cells per microliter), with a predominance of mononuclear cells. Synovial fluid analysis is of particular value in excluding other conditions, such as calcium pyrophosphate dihydrate deposition disease (Chap. 322), gout (Chap. 322), or septic arthritis (Chap. 323).

Prior to the appearance of radiographic changes, the ability to diagnose OA clinically without an invasive procedure (e.g., arthroscopy) is limited. Approaches such as magnetic resonance imaging (MRI) and ultrasonography have not been sufficiently validated to justify their routine clinical use for diagnosis of OA or monitoring of disease progression.

OA AT SPECIFIC JOINT SITES **Interphalangeal Joints** Heberden's nodes, bony enlargements of the distal interphalangeal joints, are the most common form of idiopathic OA (Fig. 321-2). A similar process at the proximal interphalangeal joints leads to Bouchard's nodes. Often, these nodes develop gradually, with little or no discomfort. However, they may present acutely with pain, redness, and swelling, sometimes triggered by minor trauma. Gelatinous dorsal cysts filled with hyaluronic acid may develop at the insertion of the digital extensor tendon into the base of the distal phalanx.

Erosive OA In erosive OA distal and/or proximal interphalangeal joints of the hands are most prominently affected. Erosive OA is more destructive than typical nodal OA; x-ray evidence of collapse of the subchondral plate is characteristic, and bony ankylosis may occur. Joint deformity and functional impairment may be severe. Pain and tenderness are commonly episodic. The synovium is much more extensively infiltrated with mononuclear cells than in other forms of OA.

Generalized OA Generalized OA is characterized by involvement of three or more joints or groups of joints (distal interphalangeal and proximal interphalangeal joints are counted as one group each). Heberden's and Bouchard's nodes are prominent. Symptoms may be episodic, with "flare-ups" of inflammation marked by soft tissue swelling, redness, and warmth. The erythrocyte sedimentation rate may be elevated, but serum rheumatoid factor tests are negative.

Thumb Base The second most frequent area of involvement in OA is the thumb base. Swelling, tenderness, and crepitus on movement of the joint are typical. Osteophytes may lead to a "squared" appearance of the thumb base (Fig. 321-3). In contrast to Heberden's nodes, which usually do not interfere significantly with function, thumb base OA frequently causes loss of motion and strength. Pain with pinch leads to adduction of the thumb and contracture of the first web space, often resulting in compensatory hyperextension of the first metacarpophalangeal joint and swan-neck deformity of the thumb.

The Hip Congenital or developmental defects (e.g., acetabular dysplasia, Legg-Calvé-Perthes disease, slipped capital epiphysis) can lead to cases of hip OA. Some 20% of patients will develop bilateral involvement. Pain from hip OA is generally referred to the inguinal area but may be referred to the buttock or proximal thigh. Less commonly, hip OA presents as knee pain. Pain can be evoked by putting the involved hip through its range of motion. Flexion may be painless initially, but internal rotation will exacerbate pain. Loss of internal rotation occurs early, followed by loss of extension, adduction, and flexion due to capsular fibrosis and/or buttressing osteophytes.

The Knee OA of the knee may involve the medial or lateral femorotibial compartment and/or the patellofemoral compartment. Palpation may reveal bony hypertrophy (osteophytes) and tenderness.

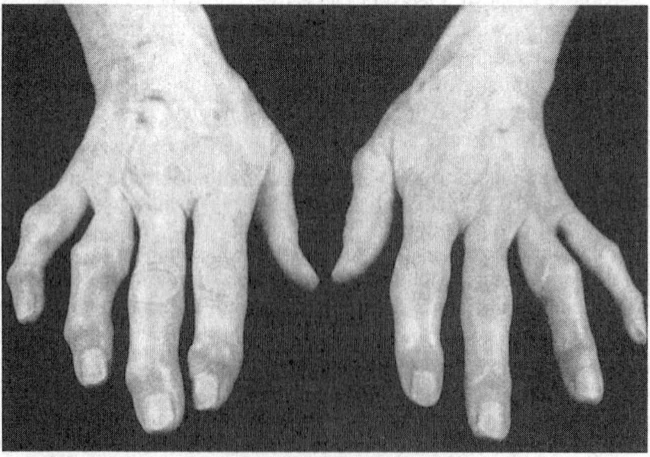

FIGURE 321-2 Nodal osteoarthritis. Note bony enlargement of distal and proximal interphalangeal joints (Heberden's nodes and Bouchard's nodes, respectively). *(Reprinted from the Clinical Slide Collection on the Rheumatic Diseases, © 1991, 1995. Reproduced with permission of the American College of Rheumatology.)*

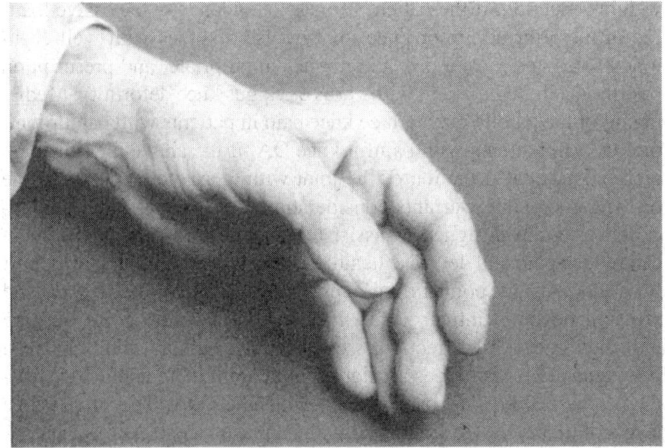

FIGURE 321-3 Osteoarthritis of the first carpometacarpal joint. Note the squared appearance of the thumb base, due to bony enlargement and remodeling of the joint.

Effusions, if present, are generally small. Joint movement commonly elicits bony crepitus. OA in the medial compartment may result in a varus (bow-leg) deformity; in the lateral compartment it may produce a valgus (knock-knee) deformity. A positive "shrug" sign (pain when the patella is compressed manually against the femur during quadriceps contraction) may be a sign of patellofemoral OA.

Chondromalacia patellae, which also is characterized by anterior knee pain and a positive shrug sign, is a syndrome of patellofemoral pain, often bilateral, in teenagers and young adults. It is more common in females than in males. It may be caused by a variety of factors (e.g., abnormal quadriceps angle, patella alta, trauma). Although exploration of the knee may reveal softening and fibrillation of cartilage on the posterior aspect of the patella, this change is usually not progressive; chondromalacia patellae is usually not a precursor of OA. In most cases, analgesics or NSAIDs and physical therapy are effective; in some, pain may be relieved by surgical correction of patellar malalignment.

The Spine Degenerative disease of the spine can involve the apophyseal joint, intervertebral disks, and paraspinous ligaments. *Spondylosis* refers to degenerative *disk* disease. The diagnosis of spinal OA should be reserved for patients with involvement of the apophyseal joints and not only disk degeneration. Symptoms of spinal OA include localized pain and stiffness. Nerve root compression by an osteophyte blocking a neural foramen, prolapse of a degenerated disk, or subluxation of an apophyseal joint may cause radicular pain and motor weakness.

Marked calcification and ossification of paraspinous ligaments occur in *diffuse idiopathic skeletal hyperostosis* (DISH). Although DISH is often categorized as a variant of OA, diarthrodial joints are not involved. Ligamentous calcification and ossification in the anterior spinal ligaments give the appearance of "flowing wax" on the anterior vertebral bodies. However, a radiolucency may be seen between the newly deposited bone and the vertebral body, differentiating DISH from the marginal osteophytes in spondylosis. Intervertebral disk spaces are preserved, and sacroiliac and apophyseal joints appear normal, helping to differentiate DISH from spondylosis and from ankylosing spondylitis, respectively. DISH occurs in the middle-aged and elderly and is more common in men than in women. Patients are frequently asymptomatic but may have musculoskeletal stiffness. The radiographic changes are generally much more severe than might be predicted from the mild symptoms.

℞ **TREATMENT** Treatment of OA is aimed at reducing pain, maintaining mobility, and minimizing disability. The vigor of the therapeutic intervention should be dictated by the severity of the condition in the individual patient. For those with only mild disease, reassurance, instruction in joint protection, and an occasional analgesic may be all that is required; for those with more severe OA, especially of the knee or hip, a comprehensive program comprising a spectrum of nonpharmacologic measures supplemented by an analgesic and/or NSAID is appropriate.

Nonpharmacologic Measures • ***Reduction of joint loading*** OA may be caused or aggravated by poor body mechanics. Correction of poor posture and a support for excessive lumbar lordosis can be helpful. Excessive loading of the involved joint should be avoided. Patients with OA of the knee or hip should avoid prolonged standing, kneeling, and squatting. Obese patients should be counseled to lose weight. In patients with medial-compartment knee OA, a wedged insole may decrease joint pain.

Rest periods during the day may be of benefit, but complete immobilization of the painful joint is rarely indicated. In patients with unilateral OA of the hip or knee, a cane, held in the contralateral hand, may reduce joint pain by reducing the joint contact force. Bilateral disease may necessitate use of crutches or a walker.

Physical therapy Application of heat to the OA joint may reduce pain and stiffness. A variety of modalities are available; often, the least expensive and most convenient is a hot shower or bath. Occasionally, better analgesia may be obtained with ice than with heat.

It is important to note that patients with OA of weight-bearing joints are less active and tend to be less fit with regard to musculoskeletal and cardiovascular status than normal controls. An exercise program should be designed to maintain range of motion, strengthen periarticular muscles, and improve physical fitness. The benefits of aerobic exercise include increases in aerobic capacity, muscle strength, and endurance; less exertion with a given workload; and weight loss. Those who exercise regularly live longer and are healthier than those who are sedentary. Patients with hip or knee OA can participate safely in conditioning exercises to improve fitness and health without increasing their joint pain or need for analgesics or NSAIDs.

Disuse of the OA joint because of pain will lead to muscle atrophy. Because periarticular muscles play a major role in protecting the articular cartilage from stress, strengthening exercises are important. In individuals with knee OA, strengthening of the periarticular muscles may result, within weeks, in a decrease in joint pain as great as that seen with NSAIDs.

Drug Therapy of OA Therapy for OA today is palliative; no pharmacologic agent has been shown to prevent, delay the progression of, or reverse the pathologic changes of OA in humans. Although claims have been made that some NSAIDs have a "chondroprotective effect," adequately controlled clinical trials in humans with OA to support this view are lacking. In management of OA pain, pharmacologic agents should be used as adjuncts to nonpharmacologic measures, such as those described above, which are the keystone of OA treatment.

Although NSAIDs often decrease joint pain and improve mobility in OA, the magnitude of this improvement is generally modest—on average, about 30% reduction in pain and 15% improvement in function. In a double-blinded, controlled trial in patients with symptomatic knee OA, an anti-inflammatory dose of ibuprofen (2400 mg/d) was no more effective than a low (i.e., essentially analgesic) dose of ibuprofen (1200 mg/d) or than acetaminophen (4000 mg/d), a drug with essentially no anti-inflammatory effect. Other studies confirm that an analgesic dose of ibuprofen may be as effective as anti-inflammatory doses of other NSAIDs, including the potent agent, phenylbutazone (400 mg/d), in symptomatic treatment of OA. Even in the presence of clinical signs of inflammation (e.g., synovial effusion, tenderness), relief of joint pain by acetaminophen may be as effective as that achieved with an NSAID. Nonetheless, if simple analgesics are inadequate, it is reasonable to cautiously prescribe an NSAID for a patient with OA.

It should be recognized that concern over the use of NSAIDs in OA has grown in recent years because of side effects of these agents, especially those related to the gastrointestinal (GI) tract. Those at greatest risk for OA, i.e., the elderly, appear also to be at greater risk than younger individuals for GI symptoms, ulceration, hemorrhage, and death as a result of NSAID use. The annual rate of hospitalization for peptic ulcer disease among elderly current NSAID users was 16 per 1000—four times greater than that for persons not taking an NSAID. Among those age 65 and older, as many as 30% of all hospitalizations and deaths related to peptic ulcer disease have been attributed to NSAID use. In addition to age, risk factors for hemorrhage and other ulcer complications associated with NSAID use include a history of peptic ulcer disease or of upper GI bleeding, concomitant use of glucocorticoids or anticoagulants, and, possibly, smoking and alcohol consumption (Table 321-4).

In patients who carry risk factors for an NSAID-associated GI catastrophe, a cyclooxygenase (Cox)-2–specific NSAID may be preferable to even a low dose of a nonselective Cox inhibitor. In contrast to the NSAIDs available to date—all of which inhibit Cox-1 as well as Cox-2—two Cox-2-specific inhibitors (CSIs), celecoxib and rofecoxib, are now available. Both appear to be comparable in efficacy to the nonselective NSAIDs. Endoscopic studies have shown that both agents are associated with an incidence of gastroduodenal ulcer lower than that of comparator NSAIDs and comparable to that of placebo. Of additional advantage with respect to the issue of upper GI bleeding, CSIs do not have a clinically significant effect on platelet aggregation or bleeding time, suggesting that CSIs may be especially advantageous in patients at high risk for incurring an NSAID-associated GI catastrophe. Long-term studies are now in progress that are designed to ascertain whether clinically important differences exist between CSIs and nonselective NSAIDs with respect to major GI clinical outcomes.

Systemic glucocorticoids have no place in the treatment of OA. However, intra- or periarticular injection of a depot glucocorticoid preparation may provide marked symptomatic relief for weeks to months. Because studies in animal models have suggested that glucocorticoids may produce cartilage damage, and frequent injections of large amounts of steroids have been associated with joint breakdown in humans, the injection should generally not be repeated in a given joint more often than every 4 to 6 months.

Intraarticular injection of hyaluronic acid has been approved recently for treatment of patients with knee OA who have failed a program of nonpharmacologic therapy and simple analgesics. Because the duration of benefit following treatment may exceed by months the synovial half-life of exogenous hyaluronic acid, the mechanism of action is unclear. The placebo response to intraarticular injection of hyaluronic acid is often large and sustained. Although relief of knee pain is achieved more slowly after hyaluronic acid injection than after intraarticular glucocorticoid injection, the effect may last much longer after hyaluronic acid injection than after glucocorticoid injection.

Capsaicin cream, which depletes local sensory nerve endings of substance P, a neuropeptide mediator of pain, may reduce joint pain and tenderness when applied topically by patients with hand or knee OA, even when used as monotherapy, i.e., without NSAIDs or systemic analgesics.

A Rational Approach to the Nonsurgical Management of OA Nonpharmacologic management is the foundation of treatment of OA pain and is as important as—and often more important than—drug treatment, which should play an adjunctive or complementary role in the management of this disease. Nonpharmacologic measures may comprise instruction of the patient in principles of joint protection; thermal modalities; exercises to strengthen periarticular muscles; weight reduction, if the patient is obese; avoidance of excessive loading of the arthritic hip or knee joint by use of shoes with well-cushioned soles and a cane or walker, when appropriate; and prescription of orthotics for the patient with varus or valgus knee deformity. Medial taping of the patella may reduce knee pain in patients with patellofemoral OA. In patients with painful knee OA, if the above measures are ineffective, tidal irrigation of the joint with a large quantity of saline or Ringer's lactate warrants consideration (see below). A health education program designed to assist the patient with self-management can reduce pain and decrease health care costs; the benefits may persist for years. At any point in the course of OA, if acute joint pain and effusion develop, intraarticular injection of glucocorticoids may be indicated once joint infection is excluded by synovial fluid analysis.

Table 321-4 Risk Factors for Upper Gastrointestinal Adverse Events in Patients Taking NSAIDs

Increasing age	History of upper gastrointestinal bleeding
Comorbidity (poor or fair general health)	Anticoagulation
Oral glucocorticoids	Combination NSAID therapy
History of peptic ulcer disease	Increasing NSAID dose

Figure 321-4 provides an algorithm that might be applied to treatment of a newly diagnosed patient with knee OA. The progressive levels of treatment are associated with increasing cost, decreasing convenience for the patient, and increasing risk of side effects. The scheme should not be interpreted dogmatically as a fixed progression of steps; rather, treatment of OA must be individualized. The treatment program should be flexible. For example, in some patients it may be reasonable to institute patellar taping or prescribe a wedged insole on the initial visit, or an intraarticular glucocorticoid injection on a later visit. As indicated above, maintaining regular contact with the patient, e.g., via periodic telephone calls, may reduce joint pain to a level beyond what can be achieved with an NSAID alone, and this, or some surrogate measure, warrants incorporation into the treatment program (Fig. 321-4).

Because of its low cost, excellent safety profile, and an efficacy in many patients comparable to that of NSAIDs, when an analgesic is required for treatment of OA pain it is reasonable to prescribe acetaminophen initially, in a dose up to 4000 mg/d. If this does not control joint symptoms within a reasonable period of time, a *low dose* of NSAID (e.g., ibuprofen, 1200 mg/d; naproxen, 500 mg/d) may be substituted for, or added to, the acetaminophen. If a nonselective NSAID is used, even in a low dose, it is reasonable to recommend coadministration of a gastroprotective agent, such as misoprostol, or a proton pump inhibitor, such as famotidine or omeprazole, which have been shown by endoscopy to be effective in treating and preventing NSAID gastropathy. Because the risk of an NSAID-associated GI catastrophe is dose-dependent, the lowest effective dose of NSAID should be employed. Salsalate and other nonacetylated salicylates, which have only a minimal effect on prostaglandin synthase, are as effective as other NSAIDs and have a lower rate of serious GI side effects. However, phototoxicity and central nervous system toxicity may limit their use.

If the above approach does not provide adequate symptomatic relief, tramadol, a weak opioid, for which the risks of tolerance and addiction appear to be minimal, may be prescribed. Mean daily doses have typically been in the range of 200 to 300 mg. Side effects (e.g., nausea and vomiting, constipation, and drowsiness) are common, but their frequency may be reduced by initiating treatment with a dose of only 25 mg/d, which is then gradually increased over the next several days. If this is not effective or opioids are contraindicated, an antiinflammatory dose of a CSI or of a nonselective NSAID may be prescribed, with coadministration of a gastroprotective agent in the latter instance.

When NSAIDs are required, they may be prescribed on an "as needed" basis, rather than in a fixed daily dose; pain control has been shown to be comparable and the risk of toxicity will be reduced. Once treatment with an NSAID or simple analgesic is initiated, the need for continuation of that treatment requires ongoing assessment. For many patients with OA, it will be possible eventually to reduce the dose of drug or to use the agent only intermittently, during exacerbations of joint pain.

Tidal Irrigation Copious irrigation of the OA knee to flush out fibrin, cartilage shards, and other debris may provide months of comfort for the patient whose joint pain has been refractory to analgesics, NSAIDs, and intraarticular glucocorticoid injections. It should be rec-

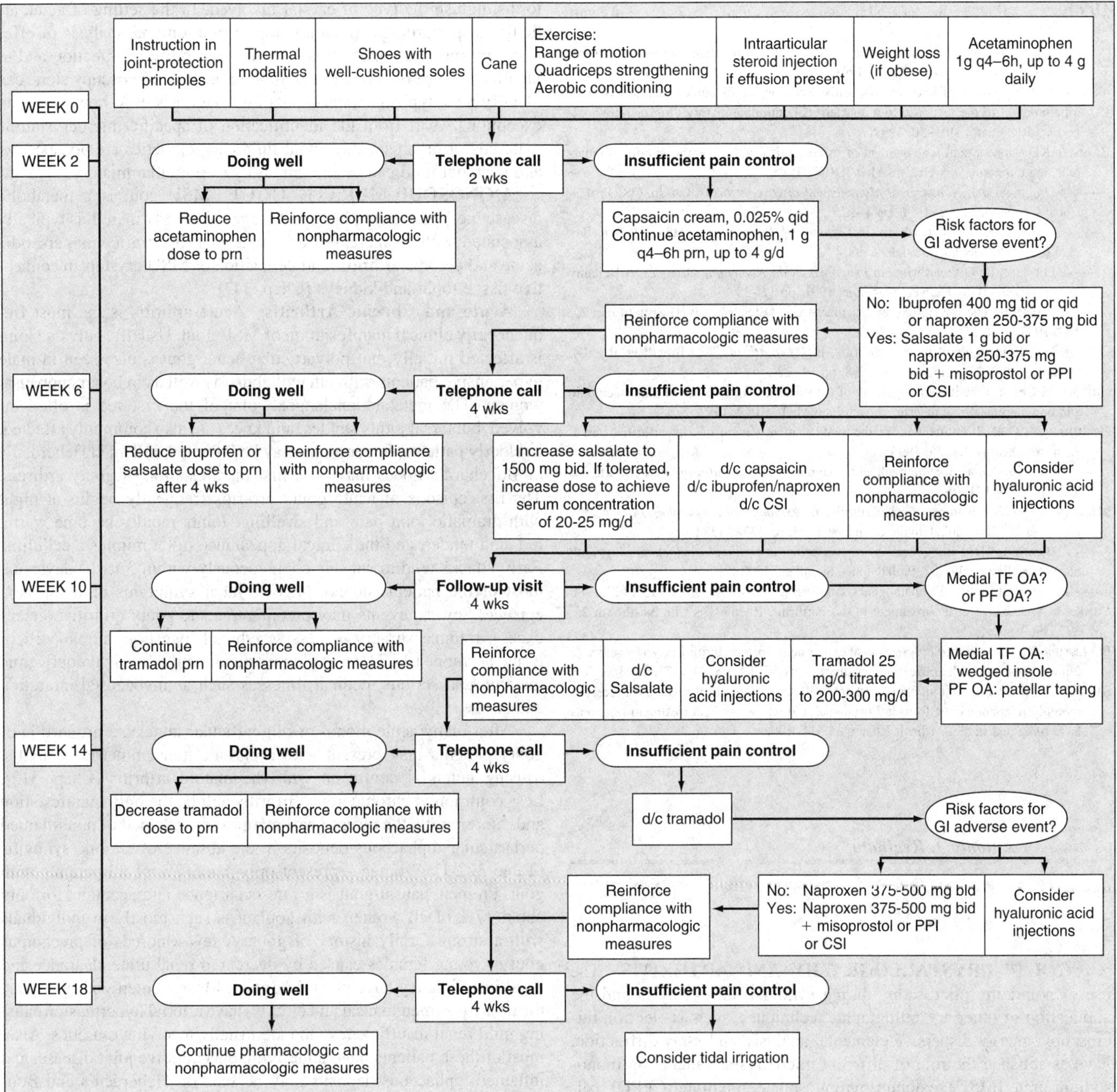

FIGURE 321-4 Algorithm for management of a newly diagnosed patient with knee OA. CSI, Cox-2-specific inhibitor; TF, tibiofemoral; PF, patellofemoral; PPI, proton pump inhibitor; d/c, discontinue *(Modified from Brandt, 1996, with permission.)*

ognized, however, that invasive procedures such as this are accompanied by a large placebo effect, and studies that include a sham lavage control group have not yet been reported.

Orthopedic Surgery Joint replacement surgery should be reserved for patients with advanced OA in whom aggressive medical management has failed. In such cases total joint arthroplasty may be remarkably effective in relieving pain and increasing mobility. Osteotomy, which is surgically more conservative, can eliminate concentrations of peak dynamic loading and may provide effective pain relief in patients with hip or knee OA. It is of greatest benefit when the disease is only moderately advanced. Arthroscopic removal of loose cartilage fragments can prevent locking and relieve pain. Chondroplasty (abrasion arthroplasty) has also had some popularity as treatment for OA, but well-controlled studies of its efficacy are lacking, and the fibrocartilage that resurfaces the abraded bone is inferior to normal hyaline cartilage in its ability to withstand mechanical loads. In patients who had undergone tibial osteotomy for medial compartment knee OA, knee pain and function were not related to the extent of cartilage regeneration 2 years later.

Autologous chondrocyte transplantation and attempts at cartilage repair using mesenchymal stem cells and autologous osteochondral plugs are currently being used experimentally for repair of focal chondral defects, but have not proved to be effective in treatment of OA.

ACKNOWLEDGMENT

Kathie Lane provided exemplary secretarial assistance during the preparation of this manuscript.

BIBLIOGRAPHY

ANDERSON JJ, FELSON DT: Factors associated with osteoarthritis of the knee in the first national health and nutrition examination survey (HANES I). Evidence for an association with overweight, race, and physical demands of work. Am J Epidemiol 128: 179, 1988

BRADLEY JD et al: Comparison of an anti-inflammatory dose of ibuprofen, an analgesic dose of ibuprofen, and acetaminophen in the treatment of patients with osteoarthritis of the knee. N Engl J Med 325:87, 1991

——— et al: Treatment of knee osteoarthritis: Relationship of clinical features of joint inflammation to the response to a nonsteroidal antiinflammatory drug or pure analgesic. J Rheumatol 19:1950, 1992

BRANDT KD: Nonsurgical management of osteoarthritis with an emphasis on nonpharmacologic measures. Arch Fam Med 4:1057, 1995

———: *Diagnosis and Nonsurgical Management of Osteoarthritis*. Caddo, OK, Professional Communications, 1996, pp 1–225

———: Management of osteoarthritis, in *Textbook of Rheumatology*, 6th ed, WN Kelley et al (eds). Philadelphia, Saunders, 2000

———, FLUSSER D: Osteoarthritis, in *Prognosis in the Rheumatic Diseases*, N Bellamy (ed). Lancaster, UK, Kluwer Academic, 1991, pp 11–35

———, RADIN E: The physiology of articular stress: Osteoarthrosis. Hospital Pract 22: 103, 1987

FELSON DT: Epidemiology of osteoarthritis, in *Osteoarthritis*, KD Brandt et al (eds). Oxford, Oxford University Press, 1998, pp 13–22

GRIFFIN MR et al: Practical management of osteoarthritis: Integration of pharmacologic and nonpharmacologic measures. Arch Fam Med 4:1049, 1995

HOCHBERG MC et al: Guidelines for the medical management of osteoarthritis: Part I. Arthritis Rheum 38:1535, 1995

——— et al: Guidelines for the medical management of osteoarthritis: Part II. Arthritis Rheum 38:1541, 1995

MANKIN HJ: Clinical features of osteoarthritis, in *Textbook of Rheumatology*, 4th ed, WN Kelley et al (eds). Philadelphia, Saunders, 1993, pp 1374–1384

———, BRANDT KD: Pathogenesis of osteoarthritis, in *Textbook of Rheumatology*, 6th ed, WN Kelley et al (eds). Philadelphia, Saunders, 2000

——— et al: Workshop on Etiopathogenesis of Osteoarthritis. J Rheumatol 13:1127, 1986

MINOR MA: Exercise in the treatment of osteoarthritis. Rheum Dis Clin North Am 25: 397, 1999

PELLETIER JP et al: Reduced progression of experimental osteoarthritis in vivo by selective inhibition of inducible nitric oxide synthase. Arthritis Rheum 41:1275, 1998

RENÉ J et al: Reduction of joint pain in patients with knee osteoarthritis who have received monthly telephone calls from lay personnel and whose medical treatment regimens have remained stable. Arthritis Rheum 35:511, 1992

322

Antonio J. Reginato

GOUT AND OTHER CRYSTAL ARTHROPATHIES

"GOUT" CRYSTALLOGRAPHY AND ARTHRITIS The use of polarizing microscopy during synovial fluid analysis and the application of other crystallographic techniques, such as electron microscopy, energy-dispersive elemental analysis, and x-ray diffraction, have established the role of different microcrystals, including monosodium urate (MSU), calcium pyrophosphate dihydrate (CPPD), calcium hydroxyapatite (HA), and calcium oxalate (CaOx), in inducing acute or chronic arthritis or periarthritis. In spite of differences in crystal morphology, chemistry, and physical properties, the clinical events that result from deposition of MSU, CPPD, HA, and CaOx may be indistinguishable (Table 322-1). Prior to the use of crystallographic techniques in rheumatology, much of what was considered to be MSU gouty arthritis in fact was not. Simkin has suggested that the generic term *gout* be used to describe the whole group of crystal-induced arthritides (MSU gout, CPPD gout, HA gout, and CaOx gout). This concept further emphasizes the identical clinical presentations of these entities (Table 322-1) and the need to perform synovial fluid analysis to distinguish the type of crystal involved. In the setting of acute articular or periarticular inflammation, aspiration and analysis of effusions are most important to assess the possibility of infection and to identify the type of crystals present. Polarization microscopy alone can identify most typical crystals and allow diagnosis. HA, however, is an exception. Apart from the identification of specific microcrystalline materials or organisms, synovial fluid characteristics are nonspecific, and synovial fluid can be inflammatory or noninflammatory.

Table 322-1 Musculoskeletal Manifestations of Crystal-Induced Arthritis

Acute mono- or polyarthritis	Destructive arthropathies
Bursitis	Pseudo-rheumatoid arthritis
Tendinitis	Pseudo-ankylosing spondylitis
Enthesitis	Spinal stenosis
Tophaceous deposits	Carpal tunnel syndrome
Peculiar type of osteoarthritis	Tendon rupture
Synovial osteochondromatosis	

MONOSODIUMURATE GOUT MSU gout is a metabolic disease most often affecting middle-aged to elderly men. It is typically associated with an increased uric acid pool, hyperuricemia, episodic acute and chronic arthritis, and deposition of MSU crystals in connective tissue tophi and kidneys (Chap. 347).

Acute and Chronic Arthritis Acute arthritis is the most frequent early clinical manifestation of MSU gout. Usually, only one joint is affected initially, but polyarticular acute gout is also seen in male hypertensive patients with ethanol abuse as well as in postmenopausal women. The metatarsophalangeal joint of the first toe is often involved, but tarsal joints, ankles, and knees are also commonly affected. In elderly patients, finger joints may be inflamed. Inflamed Heberden's or Bouchard's nodes may be a first manifestation of gouty arthritis. The first episode of acute gouty arthritis frequently begins at night with dramatic joint pain and swelling. Joints rapidly become warm, red, and tender, and the clinical appearance often mimics a cellulitis. Early attacks tend to subside spontaneously within 3 to 10 days, and most of the patients do not have residual symptoms until the next episode. Several events may precipitate acute gouty arthritis: dietary excess, trauma, surgery, excessive ethanol ingestion, adrenocorticotropic hormone (ACTH) and glucocorticoid withdrawal, hypouricemic therapy, and serious medical illnesses such as myocardial infarction and stroke.

After many acute mono- or oligoarticular attacks, a proportion of gouty patients may present with a chronic nonsymmetric synovitis, causing potential confusion with rheumatoid arthritis (Chap. 312). Less commonly, chronic gouty arthritis will be the only manifestation and, more rarely, the disease will manifest as inflamed or noninflamed periarticular tophaceous deposits in the absence of chronic synovitis (Table 322-1). Women represent only 5 to 17% of all patients with gout. Premenopausal gout is a rare occurrence and accounts for only about 17% of all women with gout; it is seen mostly in individuals with a strong family history of gout. A few kindreds of precocious gout in young females caused by decreased renal urate clearance and renal insufficiency have been described. Most women with gouty arthritis are postmenopausal and elderly, have arterial hypertension causing mild renal insufficiency, and are usually receiving diuretics. Also, most of these patients have underlying degenerative joint disease, and inflamed tophaceous deposits may be seen on Heberden's and Bouchard's nodes.

Laboratory diagnosis Even if the clinical appearance strongly suggests gout, the diagnosis should be confirmed by needle aspiration of acutely or chronically inflamed joints or tophaceous deposits. Acute septic arthritis, several of the other crystalline-associated arthropathies, palindromic rheumatism, and psoriatic arthritis may present with similar clinical features. During acute gouty attacks, strongly birefringent needle-shaped MSU crystals with negative elongation are largely intracellular (Fig. 322-1). Synovial fluid cell counts are elevated from 2000 to 60,000/μL. Effusions appear cloudy due to leukocytes, and large amounts crystals occasionally produce a thick pasty or chalky joint fluid. Bacterial infection can coexist with urate crystals in synovial fluid; if there is any suspicion of septic arthritis, joint fluid must also be cultured. MSU crystals can often be demonstrated in the first metatarsophalangeal (MTP) joint and in knees not acutely involved with gout. Arthrocentesis of these joints is a useful technique to establish the diagnosis of gout between attacks. Serum uric acid levels can be normal or low at the time of the acute attack, since lowering of uric acid with hypouricemic therapy or other medications limits the value of serum uric acid determinations for the diagnosis of gout. Despite these limitations, serum uric acid is almost always elevated at some time and can be used to follow the course of hypouricemic therapy. A 24-h urine collection for uric acid is valuable in assessing the risk of stones, in elucidating overproduction or underexcretion of uric acid, and in deciding which hypouricemic regimen to use (Chap. 347). Excretion of more than 800 mg of uric acid per 24 h on a regular diet suggests that causes of overproduction of purine should be considered. Urinalysis, blood urea nitrogen, serum creatinine, white blood cell (WBC) count, and serum lipids should be monitored because of possible pathologic sequelae of gout and other associated diseases requiring treatment.

Radiographic features Cystic changes, well-defined erosions described as punched-out lytic lesions with overhanging bony edges (Martel's sign), associated with soft tissue calcified masses are characteristic radiographic features of chronic tophaceous gout. However, similar radiographic signs can also be observed in erosive osteoarthritis, destructive apatite arthropathies, and rheumatoid arthritis.

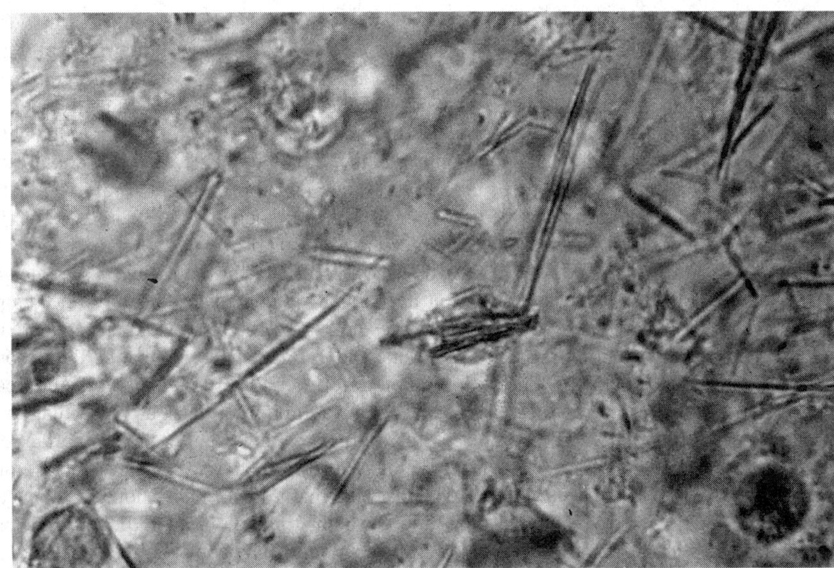

FIGURE 322-1 Extracellular and intracellular monosodiun urate crystals, as seen in a fresh preparation of synovial fluid, illustrate needle- and rod-shaped strongly negative birefringent crystals (compensated polarized light microscopy; 400×).

℞ TREATMENT **Acute Gouty Arthritis**

The mainstay of treatment during an acute attack is the administration of an anti-inflammatory drug such as colchicine, nonsteroidal anti-inflammatory drugs (NSAIDs), or glucocorticoids depending on the age of the patient and comorbid conditions. Both colchicine and NSAIDs may be quite toxic in the elderly, particularly in the presence of renal insufficiency and gastrointestinal disorders. In elderly patients, one may favor the use of intraarticular glucocorticoid injections for attacks involving one or two larger joints or cool applications along with lower oral doses of colchicine for gouty synovitis affecting small joints. Colchicine given orally is a traditional and effective treatment, if used early in the attack, in at least 85% of patients. One tablet (0.6 mg) is given every hour until relief of symptoms or gastrointestinal toxicity occurs, or a total of four to eight tablets have been taken in accordance with the age of the patient. The drug must be stopped promptly at the first sign of loose stools, and symptomatic treatment must be given for the diarrhea. Intravenous colchicine is sometimes used and can reduce, though not eliminate, the gastrointestinal side effects. Intravenous colchicine is most reliable for pre- or postoperative prophylaxis in 1- to 2-mg doses when patients cannot take medications orally. Life-threatening colchicine toxicity and sudden death have been described with the administration of more than 4 mg/d intravenously. The intravenous dose for acute gouty arthritis is 1 to 2 mg given slowly through an established venous line over 10 min in a soluset, and two additional doses of 1 mg each may be given at 6-h intervals, but the total dose should never exceed 4 mg. NSAIDs are affective in about 90% of patients, and the resolution of signs and symptoms usually occurs in 5 to 7 days. The most effective drugs are those with a short half-life and include indomethacin, 25 to 50 mg tid, ibuprofen, 800 mg tid, or diclofenac, 50 mg tid. Cyclooxigenase-2-specific inhibitors are probably equally effective but with less short-term gastrointestinal toxicity. Oral glucocorticoids such as prednisone, 30 to 50 mg/d as the initial dose and tapered over 5 to 7 days, a single intravenous dose of methylprednisolone, 7 mg of betametasone, or 60 mg of triamcinolone acetonide have been equally effective. ACTH as an intramuscular injection of 40 to 80 IU in a single dose or every 12 h for 1 to 2 days is effective in patients with acute polyarticular refractory gout or with a contraindication for using colchicine or NSAIDs.

Hypouricemic Therapy Attempts to normalize serum uric acid to <300 μmol/L (5.0 mg/dL) to prevent recurrent gouty attacks and eliminate tophaceous deposits entail a commitment to long-term hypouricemic regimens and medications that generally are required for life. Hypouricemic therapy should be considered when the hyperuricemia cannot be corrected by simple means (control of body weight, low-purine diet, increase in liquid ingestion, limitation of ethanol intake, and avoidance of diuretic use). The decision to initiate hypouricemic therapy is usually made taking into consideration the number of acute attacks, family history of gout, presence of MSU tophaceous deposits, uric acid excretion >800 mg per 24 hours, presence of uric acid stones, and risk for acute uric acid nephropathy during chemotherapy for myeloproliferative disorders. Uricosuric agents, such as probenecid, can be used in patients with good renal function who underexcrete uric acid, with <600 mg in a 24-hour urine sample. Urine volume must be maintained by ingestion of 1500 mL of water every day. Probenecid can be started at a dosage of 200 mg twice daily and increased gradually as needed up to 2 g in order to maintain a serum uric acid level <300 μmol/L (5 mg/dL). Probenecid is the drug of choice to treat elderly patients with hypertension and thiazide dependence; however, probenecid is not effective with a renal creatinine clearance <1 mL/s. These patients may require allopurinol or benzbromarone (not available in the United States), which is another uricosuric drug that is effective in patients with renal failure and who are receiving diuretics. Allopurinol is the best drug to lower serum urate in overproducers, stone formers, and patients with advanced renal failure. It can be given in a single morning dose, 300 mg initially and increasing up to 800 mg if needed. In most patients, it is not necessary to start at a lower dose; however, in patients with renal failure, the dosage should be adjusted depending on the serum creatinine concentration in order to minimize side effects. Patients with frequent acute attacks may require lower initial doses to prevent exacerbations. Toxicity of allopurinol has been recognized increasingly in patients with renal failure who use thiazide diuretics and in those patients allergic to penicillin and ampicillin. The most serious side effects include skin rash with progression to life-threatening toxic epidermal necrolysis, systemic vasculitis, bone marrow suppression, granulomatous hepatitis, and renal failure. Urate-lowering drugs should not be initiated during acute attacks. This is especially important in patients who have refractory acute arthritis or who had a flare-up previously with hypouricemic drugs. Colchicine prophylaxis in doses of 0.6 mg one to two times daily is usually continued, along with hypouricemic therapy, until the patient is normouricemic and without gouty attacks for 3 months. However, prophylactic colchicine treatment may be necessary as long as tophi are present.

CPPD DEPOSITION DISEASE **Pathogenesis** The deposition of CPPD crystals in articular tissues is most common in the elderly, affecting 10 to 15% of persons 65 to 75 years old and 30 to

60% of those more than 85 years old. In most cases this process is asymptomatic, and the cause of CPPD deposition is uncertain. Because over 80% of patients are more than 60 years old and 70% have preexisting joint damage from other conditions, it is likely that biochemical changes in aging cartilage favor crystal nucleation. Examples of such chemical alterations include the following. There is an increased production of inorganic pyrophosphate and decreased levels of pyrophosphatases in cartilage extracts from patients with CPPD arthritis. The increase in pyrophosphate production appears to be related to enhanced activity of ATP pyrophosphohydrolase and 5′-nucleotidase, which catalyze the reaction of ATP to adenosine and pyrophosphate. This pyrophosphate could combine with calcium to form CPPD crystals in matrix vesicles or on collagen fibers. There is a diminution in the levels of cartilage glycosaminoglycans that normally inhibit and regulate crystal nucleation. These deficiencies may lead to increased crystal deposition. In vitro studies have demonstrated that transforming growth factor $\beta 1$ and epidermal growth factor both stimulate the production of pyrophosphate by articular cartilage and thus may contribute to the deposition of CPPD crystals. The release of CPPD crystals into the joint space is followed by the phagocytosis of these crystals by neutrophils, which respond by releasing inflammatory substances. In addition, neutrophils release a glycopeptide that is chemotactic for other neutrophils, thus augmenting the inflammatory events. The same substance is present in MSU gout.

A minority of patients with CPPD arthropathy have metabolic abnormalities or hereditary CPPD disease (Table 322-2). These associations suggest that a variety of different metabolic products may enhance CPPD deposition. Included among these conditions are the "four H's" of hyperparathyroidism, hemochromatosis, hypophosphatasia, and hypomagnesemia. Hemochromatosis and hyperparathyroidism are good examples. Ferrous ions and hypercalcemia may either directly alter cartilage or inhibit inorganic pyrophosphatases, leading to enhanced susceptibility to CPPD deposition. The presence of CPPD arthritis in individuals less than 50 years old should lead to consideration of these metabolic disorders and inherited forms of disease, including those identified in a variety of ethnic groups (Table 322-2). Genomic DNA studies performed on four different kindreds have shown a possible location of the genetic defects on chromosome 8q in one, and on chromosome 5p in the other three. Identification of these genes will help elucidate the pathogenesis of both the familial and the more common sporadic form of the disease. Investigation should include inquiry for evidence of familial aggregation and evaluation of serum calcium, phosphorus, alkaline phosphatase, magnesium, serum ferritin, and transferritin saturation.

Clinical Manifestations CPPD arthropathy may be asymptomatic, acute, subacute, or chronic or cause acute synovitis superimposed on chronically involved joints. Acute CPPD arthritis was originally termed *pseudogout* by McCarty and coworkers because of its striking similarity to MSU gout. Other clinical manifestations of CPPD deposition include (1) induction or enhancement of peculiar forms of osteoarthritis; (2) induction of severe destructive disease that may radiographically mimic neuropathic arthritis; (3) production of symmetric proliferative synovitis, clinically similar to rheumatoid arthritis and frequently seen in familial forms with early onset; (4) intervertebral disk and ligament calcification with restriction of spine mobility, mimicking ankylosing spondylitis (also seen in hereditary forms); and (5) rarely spinal stenosis (most commonly seen in the elderly (Table 322-1).

Table 322-2 Conditions Associated with Calcium Pyrophosphate Dihydrate Disease

Aging
Disease-associated
- Primary hyperparathyroidism
- Hemochromatosis
- Hypophosphatasia
- Hypomagnesemia
- Chronic tophaceous gout
- Post-meniscectomy

Epiphyseal dysplasias
Hereditary: Slovakian-Hungarian, Spanish, Spanish-American (Argentian, Colombian, and Chilean), French, Swedish, Dutch, Canadian, Mexican-American, Italian-American, German-American, Japanese, Tunisian, Jewish, English

The knee is the joint most frequently affected in CPPD arthropathy. Other sites include the wrist, shoulder, ankle, elbow, and hands. Rarely, the temporomandibular joint and ligamentum flavum of the spinal canal are involved. Clinical and radiographic evidence indicates that CPPD deposition is polyarticular in at least two-thirds of patients. When the clinical picture resembles that of slowly progressive osteoarthritis, diagnosis may be more difficult. Joint distribution may provide important clues suggesting CPPD disease. For example, primary osteoarthritis rarely involves a metacarpophalangeal, wrist, elbow, shoulder, or ankle joint. If radiographs reveal punctate and/or linear radiodense deposits in fibrocartilaginous joint menisci or articular hyaline cartilage (chondrocalcinosis), the diagnostic certainty of CPPD is further enhanced. *Definitive diagnosis* requires demonstration of typical crystals in synovial fluid or articular tissue (Fig. 322-2). In the absence of joint effusion or indications to obtain a synovial biopsy, chondrocalcinosis is presumptive of CPPD deposition. One exception is chondrocalcinosis due to CaOx in some patients with chronic renal failure.

Acute attacks of CPPD arthritis may be precipitated by trauma, arthroscopy, or hyaluronate injections. Rapid diminution of serum calcium concentration, as may occur in severe medical illness or after surgery (especially parathyroidectomy), can also lead to pseudogout attacks.

In as many as 50% of cases, CPPD gout is associated with low-grade fever and, on occasion, temperatures as high as 40°C. Whether or not radiographic proof of chondrocalcinosis is evident in the involved joint(s), synovial analysis with microbial cultures is essential to rule out the possibility of infection. In fact, infection in a joint with any microcrystalline deposition process can lead to crystal shedding and subsequent synovitis from both crystals and microorganisms. Synovial fluid in acute CPPD gout has inflammatory qualities. The WBC count can range from several thousand cells to 100,000 cells/μL, the

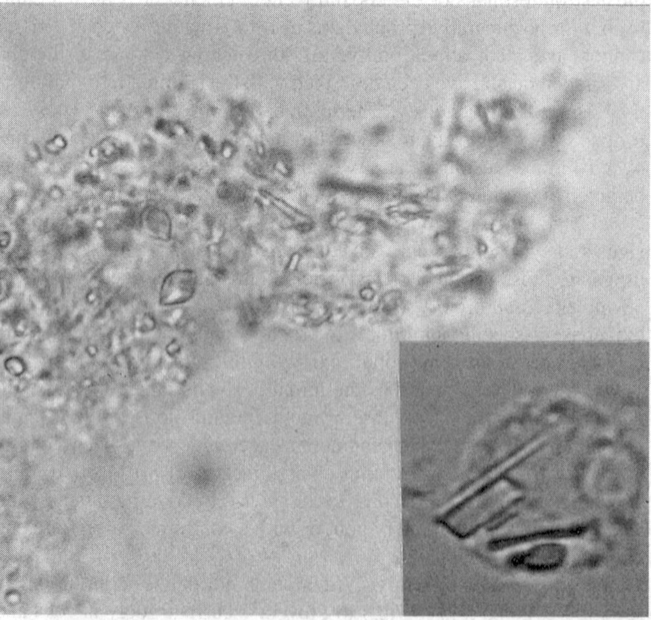

FIGURE 322-2 Intracellular and extracellular calcium pyrophosphate dihydrate crystals, as seen in a fresh preparation of synovial fluid, illustrate rectangular, rod-shaped, and rhomboid weakly positive birefringent crystals (compensated polarized light microscopy; 400×).

mean being about 24,000 cells/μL and the predominant cell being the neutrophil. Polarization microscopy usually reveals rhomboid crystals with weak positive birefringence inside fibrim and in neutrophils (Fig. 322-2).

TREATMENT Untreated acute attacks may last a few days to as long as a month. Treatment by joint aspiration and NSAIDs, or colchicine, or intraarticular glucocorticoid injection may result in return to prior status in 10 days or less. For patients with frequent recurrent attacks of CPPD gout, daily prophylactic treatment with low doses of colchicine may be helpful in decreasing the frequency of the attacks. Severe polyarticular attacks usually require short courses of glucocorticoids. Unfortunately, there is no effective way to remove CPPD deposits from cartilage and synovium. Uncontrolled studies suggest that radioactive synovectomy (with yttrium 90) or the administration of antimalarial agents may be helpful in controlling persistent synovitis. Patients with progressive destructive large-joint arthropathy usually require joint replacement.

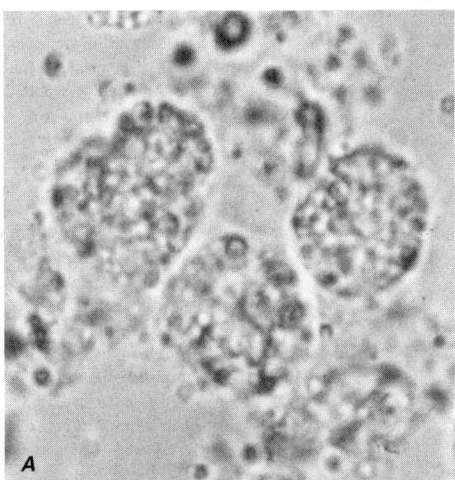

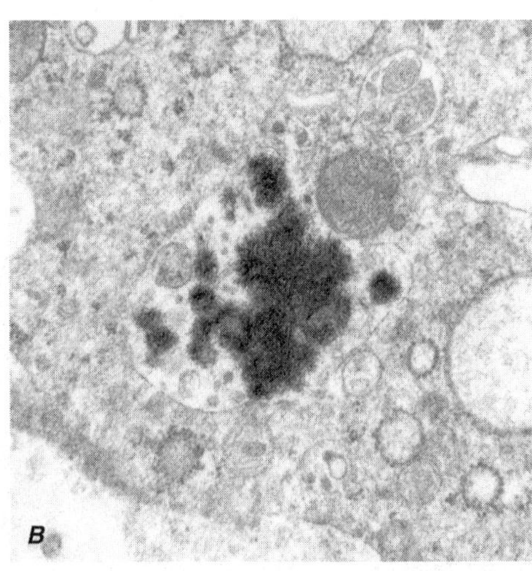

FIGURE 322-3 *A.* Cytoplasmic round inclusions inside synovial fluid cells represent aggregates of apatite crystals (fresh preparation, ordinary light microscopy; 288×). *B.* An electron micrograph demonstrates a cluster of dark apatite crystals within a synovial fluid mononuclear cell (21,600×).

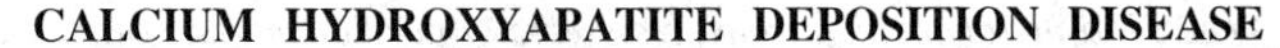

CALCIUM HYDROXYAPATITE DEPOSITION DISEASE

Pathogenesis HA is the primary mineral of bone and teeth. Abnormal accumulation can occur in areas of tissue damage (dystrophic calcification), in hypercalcemic or hyperparathyroid states (metastatic calcification), and in certain conditions of unknown cause (Table 322-3). In chronic renal failure, hyperphosphatemia enhances HA deposition both in and around joints.

HA may be released from exposed bone and cause the acute synovitis occasionally seen in chronic stable osteoarthritis (e.g., "hot" Heberden's nodes). HA deposition is also an important factor in an extremely destructive chronic arthropathy of the elderly that occurs most often in knees and shoulders (Milwaukee shoulder). Joint destruction is associated with attenuation or rupture of supporting structures, leading to instability and deformity. Progression tends to be indolent, and synovial fluid WBC counts are usually less than 1000/μL. Symptoms range from minimal to severe pain and disability that may lead to joint replacement surgery. Whether severely affected patients merely represent an extreme synovial tissue response to the HA crystals that are so common in osteoarthritis is uncertain. Synovial membrane tissue cultures exposed to HA (or CPPD) crystals markedly increased the release of collagenases and neutral proteases, underscoring the destructive potential of abnormally stimulated synovial lining cells.

Table 322-3 Conditions Associated with Hydroxyapatite Deposition Disease

Aging
Osteoarthritis
Hemorrhagic shoulder effusions in the elderly (Milwaukee shoulder)
Destructive arthropathy
Tendinitis, bursitis
Tumoral calcinosis (sporadic cases)
Disease-associated
Hyperparathyroidism
Milk alkali syndrome
Renal failure/long-term dialysis
Connective tissue diseases (e.g., progressive systemic sclerosis, CREST syndrome, idiopathic myositis, SLE)
Heterotopic calcification following neurologic catastrophes (e.g., stroke, spinal cord injury)
Hereditary
Bursitis, arthritis
Tumoral calcinosis
Fibrodysplasia ossificans progressiva

NOTE: CREST, calcinosis cutis, Raynaud's phenomenon, esophageal dysmotility, sclerodactyly, telangiectasia; SLE, systemic lupus erythematosus.

Clinical Manifestations Periarticular and articular deposits may coexist and be associated with acute and/or chronic damage to the joint capsule, tendons, bursa, or articular surfaces. The most common sites of HA deposition include bursae and tendons in and/or around the knees, shoulders, hips, and fingers. Clinical manifestations include asymptomatic radiographic abnormalities, acute synovitis, bursitis, tendinitis, and chronic destructive arthropathy. Most patients with HA arthropathy are elderly. Although the true incidence of HA arthritis is not known, 30 to 50% of patients with osteoarthritis have HA microcrystals in their synovial fluid. Such crystals can frequently be identified in clinically stable osteoarthritic joints, but they are more likely to come to attention in persons experiencing acute or subacute worsening of joint pain and swelling. The synovial fluid WBC count in HA arthritis is usually low (<2000/μL) but may at times have as many as 50,000/μL. Most synovial fluid analyses reveal a predominance of mononuclear cells. Occasionally, neutrophils may dominate.

Diagnosis Radiographic findings in HA arthropathy are not diagnostic. Intra- and/or periarticular calcifications with or without erosive, destructive, or hypertrophic changes may be present.

Definitive diagnosis of HA arthropathy depends on identification of crystals from synovial fluid or tissue (Fig. 322-3). Individual crystals are very small, nonbirefringent, and can only be seen by electron microscopy. Clumps of crystals may appear as 1- to 20-μm shiny intra- or extracellular globules that stain purplish with Wright's stain and bright red with alizarin red S. Absolute identification depends on electron microscopy with energy-dispersive elemental analysis, x-ray diffraction, or infrared spectroscopy.

TREATMENT Treatment of HA arthritis is nonspecific. Acute attacks of bursitis or synovitis may be self-limiting, resolving in from days to several weeks. Aspiration of effusions and the use of either NSAIDs or oral colchicine for 2 weeks or intra- or periarticular injection of glucocorticoid salts appear to shorten the duration and intensity of symptoms. In patients with underlying severe destructive articular changes, response to medical therapy is usually less rewarding.

CaOx DEPOSITION DISEASE

Pathogenesis *Primary oxalosis* is a rare hereditary metabolic disorder (Chap. 352). Enhanced production of oxalic acid may result from at least two different enzyme defects, leading to hyperoxalemia and deposition of calcium oxalate crystals in tissues. Nephrocalcinosis, renal failure, and death usually

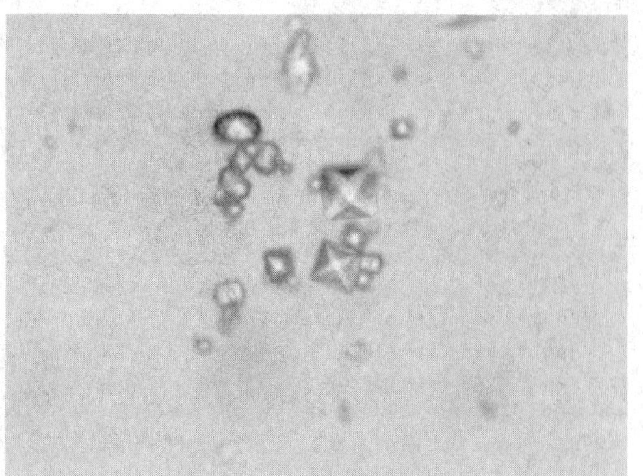

FIGURE 322-4 Bipyramidal and small polymorphic calcium oxalate crystals (ordinary light microscopy; 400×).

occur before age 20. Acute and/or chronic CaOx arthritis and periarthritis may complicate primary oxalosis during later years of illness.

Secondary oxalosis is more common than the primary disorder. It is one of the many metabolic abnormalities that complicate end-stage renal disease (ESRD). In ESRD, calcium oxalate deposits have long been recognized in visceral organs, blood vessels, bones, and even cartilage. However, it was not until 1982 that such deposits were demonstrated to be one of the causes of arthritis in chronic renal failure. Thus far, reported patients have been dependent on long-term hemodialysis or peritoneal dialysis (Chap. 272), and many had received ascorbic acid supplements. Ascorbic acid is metabolized to oxalate, which is inadequately cleared in uremia and by dialysis. Such supplements are now usually avoided in dialysis programs because of the risk of enhancing hyperoxalosis and its sequelae.

Clinical Manifestations and Diagnosis As was noted for the other calcium salts, CaOx aggregates can be found in bone, articular cartilage, synovium, and periarticular tissues. From these sites, crystals may be shed, causing acute synovitis. Persistent aggregates of CaOx may, like HA and CPPD, stimulate synovial proliferation and enzyme release, resulting in progressive articular destruction. Deposits have been documented in fingers, wrists, elbows, knees, ankles, and feet.

Each of the known microcrystalline arthropathies may be a complication of ESRD, and rare patients have more than one type of crystal present in a joint effusion. The advent of crystallographic techniques has made it clear that most arthritic problems in ESRD are not, as was once believed, due to MSU gout. Clinical features of acute CaOx arthritis may not be distinguishable from those due to sodium urate, CPPD, or HA. Radiographs may reveal chondrocalcinosis, a feature of either CPPD or CaOx deposition. CaOx-induced synovial effusions are usually noninflammatory, with fewer than 2000 leukocytes/μL. Neutrophils or mononuclear cells have predominated. CaOx crystals have a variable shape and variable birefringence to polarized light. The most easily recognized forms are bipyramidal and have strong positive birefringence (Fig. 322-4).

℞ **TREATMENT** Treatment of CaOx arthropathy with NSAIDs, colchicine, intraarticular glucocorticoids, and/or an increased frequency of dialysis has produced only slight improvement. In primary oxalosis, liver transplantation has induced a significant reduction in crystal deposits (Chap. 352).

BIBLIOGRAPHY

ANDREW LJ et al: Refinement of the chromosome 5p locus for familial calcium pyrophosphate dihydrate deposition disease. Am J Med Genet 64:136, 1999

BENHAMOU CL et al: Bone involvement in primary oxalosis (study of 20 cases). Rev Rhum Mal Osteoartic 58:763, 1991

DIEPPE PA et al: Apatite deposition disease: A new arthropathy. Lancet 1:266, 1976

DOHERTY M et al: Inorganic pyrophosphate in metabolic diseases predisposing to calcium pyrophosphate dihydrate crystal deposition. Arthritis Rheum 34:1297, 1991

EMERSON BE: The management of gout. N Engl J Med 334:445, 1996

GEORGE T, MANDEL B: Gout in the transplant patients. J Clin Rheumatol 1:328, 1995

MASUDA I et al: Inorganic pyrophosphate metabolism, in *Gout, Hyperuricemia and Other Crystal-Associated Arthropathies*, Ch J Smyth, VM Holers (eds). New York, Marcel Dekker, 1999, pp 359–367

PEREZ RUIZ F et al: Treatment of chronic gout in patients with renal function impairment. An open, randomized, actively controlled study. J Clin Rheumatol 5:49, 1999

REGINATO AJ, FALASCA GF: Calcium oxalate and other miscellaneous crystal-related arthropathies, in *Gout, Hyperuricemia and Other Crystal-Associated Arthropathies*, ChJ Smyth, VM Holers (eds). New York, Marcel Dekker, 1999, pp 370–393

———, SCHUMACHER HR: Apatite crystals in joint fluid: Clinical relevance and search for a simple and accurate diagnostic test. Rheumatol Rev 3:9, 1994

——— et al: Familial calcium pyrophosphate crystal deposition disease or calcium pyrophosphate gout. Rev Rheum [Engl Ed] 62:376, 1995

ROSENTHAL AK, RYAN LM: Treatment of refractory crystal-associated arthritis. Rheum Dis Clin North Am 21:151, 1995

SIMKIN PA: Oxalate crystals and the taxonomy of gout. JAMA 260:1285, 1988

323 INFECTIOUS ARTHRITIS

Scott J. Thaler, James H. Maguire

INTRODUCTION AND APPROACH TO THE PATIENT

While *Staphylococcus aureus*, *Neisseria gonorrhoeae*, and other bacteria are the most common causes of infectious arthritis, various mycobacteria, spirochetes, fungi, and viruses also infect joints. Since acute bacterial infection can rapidly destroy articular cartilage, all inflamed joints must be evaluated without delay to exclude noninfectious processes and to determine appropriate antimicrobial therapy and drainage procedures. For more detailed information on infectious arthritis due to specific organisms, the reader is referred to the chapters on those organisms.

Acute bacterial infection typically involves a single joint or a few joints. Subacute or chronic monarthritis or oligoarthritis suggests mycobacterial or fungal infection; episodic inflammation is seen in syphilis, Lyme disease, and the reactive arthritis that follows enteric infections and chlamydial urethritis (Table 323-1). Acute polyarticular inflammation occurs as an immunologic reaction during the course of endocarditis, rheumatic fever, disseminated neisserial infection, and acute hepatitis B. Bacteria and viruses occasionally infect multiple joints, the former most commonly in persons with rheumatoid arthritis.

Aspiration of synovial fluid, an essential element in the evaluation of potentially infected joints, can be performed without difficulty in most cases by the insertion of a large-bore needle into the site of maximal fluctuation or tenderness or by the route of easiest access. Ultrasonography or fluoroscopy may be used to guide aspiration of difficult-to-localize effusions of the hip and, occasionally, the shoulder and other joints. Normal synovial fluid contains <180 cells (predominantly mononuclear cells) per microliter. Synovial cell counts averaging 100,000/μL (range, 25,000 to 250,000/μL), with >90% neutrophils, are characteristic of acute bacterial infections. Crystal-induced, rheumatoid, and other noninfectious inflammatory arthritides are usually associated with <30,000 to 50,000 cells/μL; cell counts of 10,000 to 30,000/μL, with 50 to 70% neutrophils and the remainder lymphocytes, are common in mycobacterial and fungal infections. Definitive diagnosis of an infectious process relies on identification of the pathogen in stained smears of synovial fluid, isolation of the pathogen from cultures of synovial fluid and blood, or detection of microbial nucleic acids and proteins by polymerase chain reaction (PCR)–based assays and immunologic techniques.

ACUTE BACTERIAL ARTHRITIS Pathogenesis Bacteria enter the joint from the bloodstream, from a contiguous site of infection in bone or soft tissue, or by direct inoculation during surgery, injection, or trauma. In hematogenous infection, bacteria escape from synovial capillaries, which have no limiting basement membrane, and within hours provoke neutrophilic infiltration of the synovium. Neutrophils and bacteria enter the joint space; later, bacteria adhere to articular cartilage. Degradation of cartilage begins within 48 h as a result of increased intraarticular pressure, release of proteases and cytokines from chondrocytes and synovial macrophages, and invasion of the cartilage by bacteria and inflammatory cells. Histologic studies reveal bacteria lining the synovium and cartilage as well as abscesses extending into the synovium, cartilage, and—in severe cases—subchondral bone. Synovial proliferation results in the formation of a pannus over the cartilage, and thrombosis of inflamed synovial vessels develops. Bacterial factors that appear important in the pathogenesis of infective arthritis include various surface-associated adhesins in *S. aureus* that permit adherence to cartilage and endotoxins that promote chondrocyte-mediated breakdown of cartilage.

Table 323-1 Differential Diagnosis of Arthritis Syndromes

Acute Monarticular Arthritis	Chronic Monarticular Arthritis	Polyarticular Arthritis
Staphylococcus aureus	*Mycobacterium tuberculosis*	*Neisseria meningitidis*
Streptococcus pneumoniae	Nontuberculous mycobacteria	*N. gonorrhoeae*
β-Hemolytic streptococci	*Borrelia burgdorferi*	Nongonococcal bacterial arthritis
Gram-negative bacilli	*Treponema pallidum*	Bacterial endocarditis
Neisseria gonorrhoeae	*Candida* species	*Candida* species
Candida species	*Sporothrix schenckii*	Poncet's disease (tuberculous rheumatism)
Crystal-induced arthritis	*Coccidioides immitis*	
Fracture	*Blastomyces dermatitidis*	Hepatitis B virus
Hemarthrosis	*Aspergillus* species	Parvovirus B19
Foreign body	*Cryptococcus neoformans*	HIV
Osteoarthritis	*Nocardia* species	Human T lymphotropic virus type I
Ischemic necrosis	*Brucella* species	Rubella virus
Monarticular rheumatoid arthritis	Legg-Calvé-Perthes disease	Arthropod-borne viruses
	Osteoarthritis	Sickle cell disease flare
		Reactive arthritis
		Serum sickness
		Acute rheumatic fever
		Inflammatory bowel disease
		Systemic lupus erythematosus
		Rheumatoid arthritis/Still's disease
		Other vasculitides
		Sarcoidosis

Microbiology The hematogenous route of infection is the most common route in all age groups. In infants, group B streptococci, gram-negative enteric bacilli, and *S. aureus* are the usual pathogens. Since the advent of the *Haemophilus influenzae* vaccine, *S. aureus*, *Streptococcus pyogenes* (group A *Streptococcus*), and (in some centers) *Kingella kingae* have predominated among children <5 years of age. Among young adults and adolescents, *N. gonorrhoeae* is the most commonly implicated organism. *S. aureus* accounts for most nongonococcal isolates in adults of all ages; gram-negative bacilli, pneumococci, and β-hemolytic streptococci—particularly groups A and B, but also groups C, G, and F—are involved in up to one-third of cases in older adults, especially those with underlying comorbid illnesses.

Infections following surgical procedures or penetrating injuries are due most often to *S. aureus* and occasionally to other gram-positive bacteria or gram-negative bacilli. Infections with coagulase-negative staphylococci are unusual except after the implantation of prosthetic joints or arthroscopy. Anaerobic organisms, often in association with aerobic or facultative bacteria, are found after human bites and when decubitus ulcers or intraabdominal abscesses spread into adjacent joints. Polymicrobial infections complicate traumatic injuries with extensive contamination. Cat bites or scratches may introduce *Pasteurella multocida* into joints.

Nongonococcal Bacterial Arthritis • ***Epidemiology*** Although hematogenous infections with virulent organisms such as *S. aureus*, *H. influenzae*, and pyogenic streptococci occur in healthy persons, there is an underlying host predisposition in many cases of septic arthritis. Patients with rheumatoid arthritis have the highest incidence of infective arthritis, most often secondary to *S. aureus*, because of chronically inflamed joints, glucocorticoid therapy, and frequent breakdown of rheumatoid nodules, vasculitic ulcers, and skin overlying deformed joints. Diabetes mellitus, glucocorticoid therapy, hemodialysis, and malignancy all carry an increased risk of infection with *S. aureus* and gram-negative bacilli. Pneumococcal infections complicate alcoholism, deficiencies of humoral immunity, and hemoglobinopathies. Pneumococci, *Salmonella*, and *H. influenzae* cause septic arthritis in persons infected with HIV. Persons with primary immunoglobulin deficiency are at risk for mycoplasmal arthritis, which results in permanent joint damage if treatment with tetracycline and intravenous immunoglobulin replacement is not administered promptly. Intravenous drug users acquire staphylococcal and streptococcal infections from their own flora and acquire pseudomonal and other gram-negative infections from drugs and injection paraphernalia.

Clinical manifestations Some 90% of patients present with involvement of a single joint: most commonly the knee, less frequently the hip, and still less often the shoulder, wrist, or elbow. Small joints of the hands and feet are more likely to be affected after direct inoculation or a bite. Among intravenous drug users, infections of the spine, sacroiliac joints, or sternoclavicular joints are more common than infections of the appendicular skeleton. Polyarticular infection is most common among patients with rheumatoid arthritis and may resemble a flare of the underlying disease.

The usual presentation consists of moderate to severe pain that is uniform around the joint, effusion, muscle spasm, and decreased range of motion. Fever in the range of 38.3 to 38.9°C (101 to 102°F) and sometimes higher is common but may be lacking, especially in persons with rheumatoid arthritis, renal or hepatic insufficiency, or conditions requiring immunosuppressive therapy. The inflamed, swollen joint is usually evident on examination except in the case of a deeply situated joint, such as the hip, shoulder, or sacroiliac joint. Cellulitis, bursitis, and acute osteomyelitis, which may produce a similar clinical picture, should be distinguished from septic arthritis by their greater range of motion and less-than-circumferential swelling. A focus of extraarticular infection, such as a boil or pneumonia, should be sought. Peripheral-blood leukocytosis with a left shift and elevation of the erythrocyte sedimentation rate or C-reactive protein are common findings.

Plain radiographs show evidence of soft tissue swelling, joint-space widening, and displacement of tissue planes by the distended capsule. Narrowing of the joint space and bony erosions indicate advanced infection and a poor prognosis. Ultrasound is useful for detecting effusions in the hip, and computed tomography or magnetic resonance imaging can demonstrate infections of the sacroiliac joint, sternoclavicular joint, and the spine very well.

Laboratory findings Specimens of peripheral blood and synovial fluid should be obtained before antibiotics are administered. Blood cultures are positive in up to 50% of *S. aureus* infections but are less frequently positive in infections due to other organisms. The synovial fluid is turbid, serosanguineous, or frankly purulent. Gram-stained smears confirm the presence of large numbers of neutrophils. Levels of total protein and lactate dehydrogenase in synovial fluid are elevated, and the glucose level is depressed; however, these findings are not specific for infection, and measurement of these levels is not necessary to make the diagnosis. The synovial fluid should be examined for crystals, because gout and pseudogout can resemble septic arthritis clinically, and infection and crystal-induced disease occasionally occur together. Organisms are seen on synovial fluid smears in nearly three-quarters of infections with *S. aureus* and streptococci and in 30 to 50% of infections due to gram-negative and other bacteria. Cultures of synovial fluid are positive in >90% of cases. Inoculation of synovial fluid into bottles containing liquid media for blood cultures increases the yield of culture, especially if the pathogen is a fastidious organism or the patient is taking an antibiotic. Although not yet widely available, PCR-based assays for bacterial DNA will also be useful for the diagnosis of partially treated or culture-negative bacterial arthritis.

℞ TREATMENT Prompt administration of systemic antibiotics and drainage of the involved joint can prevent destruction of cartilage, postinfectious degenerative arthritis, joint instability, or deformity. Once samples of blood and synovial fluid have been obtained for culture, empirical antibiotics should be given that are directed against bacteria visualized on smears or against the pathogens that are likely, given the patient's age and risk factors. Initial therapy should consist of the intravenous administration of bactericidal agents; direct instillation of antibiotics into the joint is not necessary to achieve adequate levels in synovial fluid and tissue. An intravenous third-generation cephalosporin such as cefotaxime (1 g every 8 h) or ceftriaxone (1 to 2 g every 24 h) will provide adequate empirical coverage for most community-acquired infections in adults when smears show no organisms. Either oxacillin or nafcillin (2 g every 4 h) is used if there are gram-positive cocci on the smear. If methicillin-resistant *S. aureus* is a possible pathogen, as in hospitalized patients, intravenous vancomycin (1 g every 12 h) should be given. In addition, an aminoglycoside should be given to intravenous drug users or other patients in whom *Pseudomonas aeruginosa* may be the responsible agent.

Definitive therapy is based on the identity and antibiotic susceptibility of the bacteria isolated in culture. Infections due to staphylococci are treated with oxacillin, nafcillin, or vancomycin for 4 weeks. Pneumococcal and streptococcal infections due to penicillin-susceptible organisms respond to 2 weeks of therapy with penicillin G (2 million units intravenously every 4 h); infections caused by *H. influenzae* and by strains of *S. pneumoniae* that are resistant to penicillin are treated with cefotaxime or ceftriaxone for 2 weeks. Most enteric gram-negative infections can be cured in 3 to 4 weeks by a second- or third-generation cephalosporin given intravenously or by a fluoroquinolone, such as levofloxacin (500 mg intravenously or orally every 24 h). *P. aeruginosa* infection should be treated for at least 2 weeks with a combination regimen of an aminoglycoside plus either an extended-spectrum penicillin, such as mezlocillin (3 g intravenously every 4 h), or an antipseudomonal cephalosporin, such as ceftazidime (1 g intravenously every 8 h). If tolerated, this regimen is continued for an additional 2 weeks; alternatively, a fluoroquinolone, such as ciprofloxacin (750 mg orally bid), is given by itself or with the penicillin or cephalosporin in place of the aminoglycoside.

Timely drainage of pus and necrotic debris from the infected joint is required for a favorable outcome. Needle aspiration of readily accessible joints such as the knee may be adequate if loculations or particulate matter in the joint does not prevent its thorough decompression. Arthroscopic drainage and lavage may be employed initially or within several days if repeated needle aspiration fails to relieve symptoms, decrease the volume of the effusion and the synovial white cell count, and clear bacteria from smears and cultures. In some cases, arthrotomy is necessary to remove loculations and debride infected synovium, cartilage, or bone. Septic arthritis of the hip is best managed with arthrotomy, particularly in young children, in whom infection threatens the viability of the femoral head. Septic joints do not require immobilization except for pain control before symptoms are alleviated by treatment. Weight bearing should be avoided until signs of inflammation have subsided, but frequent passive motion of the joint is indicated to maintain full mobility. While addition of glucocorticoids to antibiotic treatment improves the outcome of *S. aureus* arthritis in experimental animals, no clinical trials have yet evaluated this approach in humans.

Gonococcal Arthritis • ***Epidemiology*** Gonococcal arthritis, accounting for 70% of episodes of infectious arthritis in persons <40 years of age, results from bacteremia arising from gonococcal infection or, more frequently, from asymptomatic gonococcal mucosal colonization of the urethra, cervix, or pharynx. Women are at greatest risk during menses or during pregnancy and overall are two to three times more likely than men to develop disseminated gonococcal infection and arthritis. Persons with complement deficiencies, especially of the terminal components, are prone to recurrent episodes of gonococcemia. Strains of gonococci that are most likely to cause disseminated infection include those that produce transparent colonies in culture, have the type IA outer-membrane protein, or are of the AUH-auxotroph type.

Clinical manifestations and laboratory findings The most common manifestation of disseminated gonococcal infection is a syndrome of fever, chills, rash, and articular symptoms. Small numbers of papules that progress to hemorrhagic pustules develop on the trunk and the extensor surfaces of the distal extremities. Migratory arthritis and tenosynovitis of the knees, hands, wrists, feet, and ankles are prominent. The cutaneous lesions and articular findings are believed to be the consequence of an immune reaction to circulating gonococci and immune-complex deposition in tissues. Thus, cultures of synovial fluid are consistently negative, and blood cultures are positive in <45% of patients. Synovial fluid may be difficult to obtain from inflamed joints and usually contains only 10,000 to 20,000 leukocytes/μL.

True gonococcal septic arthritis is less common than the disseminated gonococcal infection syndrome and always follows disseminated infection, which is unrecognized in one-third of patients. A single joint, such as the hip, knee, ankle, or wrist, is usually involved. Synovial fluid, which contains >50,000 leukocytes/μL, can be obtained with ease; the gonococcus is only occasionally evident in gram-stained smears, and cultures of synovial fluid are positive in <40% of cases. Blood cultures are almost always negative.

Because it is difficult to isolate gonococci from synovial fluid and blood, specimens for culture should be obtained from potentially infected mucosal sites. Cultures and gram-stained smears of skin lesions occasionally are positive. All specimens for culture should be plated onto Thayer-Martin agar directly or in special transport media at the bedside and transferred promptly to the microbiology laboratory in an atmosphere of 5% CO_2, as generated in a candle jar. PCR-based assays are extremely sensitive in detecting gonococcal DNA in synovial fluid. A dramatic alleviation of symptoms within 12 to 24 h after the initiation of appropriate antibiotic therapy supports a clinical diagnosis of the disseminated gonococcal infection syndrome if cultures are negative.

℞ TREATMENT Initial treatment consists of ceftriaxone (1 g intravenously or intramuscularly every 24 h) to cover possible penicillin-resistant organisms. Once local and systemic signs are clearly resolving, the 7-day course of therapy can be completed with an oral agent such as cefixime (400 mg bid) or ciprofloxacin (500 mg bid) or, if penicillin-susceptible organisms are isolated, amoxicillin (500 mg tid). Suppurative arthritis usually responds to needle aspiration of involved joints and 7 to 14 days of antibiotic treatment. Arthroscopic lavage or arthrotomy is rarely required.

It is noteworthy that arthritis symptoms similar to those seen in disseminated gonococcal infections occur in meningococcemia. A dermatitis-arthritis syndrome, purulent monarthritis, and reactive polyarthritis have been described. All respond to treatment with intravenous penicillin.

SPIROCHETAL ARTHRITIS Lyme Disease Lyme disease due to infection with the spirochete *Borrelia burgdorferi* causes arthritis in up to 70% of persons who are not treated. Intermittent arthralgias and myalgias, but not arthritis, occur within days or weeks of inoculation of the spirochete by the *Ixodes* tick. Later, there are three patterns of joint disease: (1) Fifty percent of untreated persons experience intermittent episodes of monarthritis or oligoarthritis involving the knee and/or other large joints. The symptoms wax and wane without treatment over months, and each year 10 to 20% of patients report loss of joint symptoms. (2) Twenty percent of untreated persons develop a pattern of waxing and waning arthralgias. (3) Ten percent of patients develop chronic inflammatory synovitis resulting in erosive lesions and destruction of the joint. Serologic tests for IgG antibodies to *B. burgdorferi* are positive in >90% of persons with Lyme arthritis, and a PCR-based assay detects *Borrelia* DNA in 85%.

℞ TREATMENT Lyme arthritis generally responds well to therapy. A regimen of oral doxycycline (100 mg bid for 30 days), oral amoxicillin (500 mg qid for 30 days), or parenteral ceftriaxone (2 g/d for 2 to 4 weeks) is recommended. Patients who do not respond to a total of 2 months of oral therapy or 1 month of parenteral therapy are unlikely to benefit from additional antibiotic therapy and are treated with anti-inflammatory agents or synovectomy. Failure of therapy is associated with host features such as the HLA-DR4 genotype, persistent reactivity to OspA (outer-surface protein A), and the presence of hLFA-1 (human leukocyte function–associated antigen-1), which cross-reacts with OspA.

Syphilitic Arthritis Articular manifestations occur in different stages of syphilis. In early congenital syphilis, periarticular swelling and immobilization of the involved limbs (Parrot's pseudoparalysis) complicate osteochondritis of long bones. Clutton's joint, a late manifestation of congenital syphilis that typically develops between the ages of 8 and 15 years, is caused by chronic painless synovitis with effusions of large joints, particularly the knees and elbows. Secondary syphilis may be associated with arthralgias; symmetric arthritis of the knees and ankles and occasionally of the shoulders and wrists; and sacroiliitis. The arthritis follows a subacute to chronic course with a mixed mononuclear and neutrophilic synovial-fluid pleocytosis (typical cell counts, 5000 to 15,000/μL). Immunologic mechanisms may contribute to the arthritis, and symptoms usually improve rapidly with penicillin therapy. In tertiary syphilis, Charcot's joint is a result of sensory loss due to tabes dorsalis. Penicillin is not helpful in this setting.

MYCOBACTERIAL ARTHRITIS Tuberculous arthritis accounts for ~1% of all cases of tuberculosis and for 10% of extrapulmonary cases. The most common presentation is chronic granulomatous monarthritis. An unusual syndrome, Poncet's disease, is a reactive symmetric form of polyarthritis that affects persons with visceral or disseminated tuberculosis. No mycobacteria are found in the joints, and symptoms resolve with antituberculous therapy.

Unlike tuberculous osteomyelitis, which typically involves the thoracic and lumbar spine (50% of cases), tuberculous arthritis primarily involves the large weight-bearing joints, in particular the hips, knees, and ankles, and only occasionally involves smaller non-weight-bearing joints. Progressive monarticular swelling and pain develop over months to years, and systemic symptoms are seen in only half of all cases. Tuberculous arthritis occurs as part of a disseminated primary infection or through late reactivation, often in persons with HIV infection or other immunocompromised hosts. Coexistent active pulmonary tuberculosis is unusual.

Aspiration of the involved joint yields fluid with an average cell count of 20,000/μL, with ~50% neutrophils. Acid-fast staining of the fluid yields positive results in fewer than one-third of cases, and cultures are positive in 80%. Culture of synovial tissue taken at biopsy is positive in ~ 90% of cases and shows granulomatous inflammation in most. DNA amplification methods such as PCR can shorten the time to diagnosis to 1 or 2 days. Radiographs reveal peripheral erosions at the points of synovial attachment, periarticular osteopenia, and eventually joint-space narrowing. Therapy for tuberculous arthritis is the same as that for tuberculous pulmonary disease, requiring the administration of multiple agents for 6 to 9 months. Therapy is more prolonged in immunosuppressed individuals, such as those infected with HIV.

Various atypical mycobacteria found in water and soil may cause chronic indolent arthritis. Such disease results from trauma and direct inoculation associated with farming, gardening, or aquatic activities. Smaller joints, such as the digits, wrists, and knees, are usually involved. Involvement of tendon sheaths and bursae is typical. The mycobacterial species involved include *Mycobacterium marinum*, *M. avium-intracellulare*, *M. terrae*, *M. kansasii*, *M. fortuitum*, and *M. chelonae*. In persons who have HIV infection or are receiving immunosuppressive therapy, hematogenous spread to the joints has been reported for *M. kansasii*, *M. avium-intracellulare*, and *M. haemophilum*. Diagnosis usually requires biopsy and culture, and therapy is based on antimicrobial susceptibility patterns.

FUNGAL ARTHRITIS Fungi are an unusual cause of chronic monarticular arthritis. Granulomatous articular infection with the endemic dimorphic fungi *Coccidioides immitis*, *Blastomyces dermatitidis*, and (less commonly) *Histoplasma capsulatum* results from hematogenous seeding or direct extension from bony lesions in persons with disseminated disease. Joint involvement is an unusual complication of sporotrichosis (infection with *Sporothrix schenckii*) among gardeners and other persons who work with soil or sphagnum moss. Articular sporotrichosis is six times more common among men than among women, and alcoholics and other debilitated hosts are at risk for polyarticular infection.

Candida infection involving a single joint, usually the knee, hip, or shoulder, results from surgical procedures, intraarticular injections, or (among critically ill patients with debilitating illnesses such as diabetes mellitus or hepatic or renal insufficiency and patients receiving immunosuppressive therapy) hematogenous spread. *Candida* infections in intravenous drug users typically involve the spine, sacroiliac joints, or other fibrocartilaginous joints. Unusual cases of arthritis due to *Aspergillus* species, *Cryptococcus neoformans*, *Pseudallescheria boydii*, and the dematiaceous fungi have also resulted from direct inoculation or disseminated hematogenous infection in immunocompromised persons.

The synovial fluid in fungal arthritis usually contains 10,000 to 40,000 cells/μL, with ~70% neutrophils. Stained specimens and cultures of synovial tissue often confirm the diagnosis of fungal arthritis when studies of synovial fluid give negative results. Treatment consists of drainage and lavage of the joint and systemic administration of amphotericin B, fluconazole, or itraconazole (the exact drug depending on the species involved). The doses and duration of therapy are the same as for disseminated disease (see Part Seven, Section 15). Intraarticular instillation of amphotericin B has been used in addition to intravenous therapy.

VIRAL ARTHRITIS Viruses produce arthritis by infecting synovial tissue during systemic infection or by provoking an immunologic reaction that involves joints. As many as 50% of women report persistent arthralgias and 10% frank arthritis within 3 days of the rash that follows natural infection with *rubella virus* and within 2 to 6 weeks after receipt of live virus vaccine. Episodes of symmetric inflammation of fingers, wrists, and knees uncommonly recur for longer than a year, but a syndrome of chronic fatigue, low-grade fever, headaches, and myalgias can persist for months or years. Intravenous immunoglobulin has been helpful in selected cases. Self-limited monarticular or migratory polyarthritis may develop within 2 weeks of the parotitis of *mumps*; this sequela is more common in men than in women. Approximately 10% of children and 60% of women develop arthritis after infection with *parvovirus B19*. In adults, arthropathy sometimes occurs without fever or rash. Pain and stiffness, with less prominent swelling (primarily of the hands but also of the knees, wrists, and ankles), usually resolve within weeks, although a small proportion of patients develop chronic arthropathy.

About 2 weeks before the onset of jaundice, up to 10% of persons with acute *hepatitis B* develop an immune complex–mediated, serum sickness–like reaction with maculopapular rash, urticaria, fever, and arthralgias. Less common developments include symmetric arthritis involving the hands, wrists, elbows, or ankles and morning stiffness that resembles a flare of rheumatoid arthritis. Symptoms resolve at the time jaundice develops. Approximately one-third of persons with chronic hepatitis C infection report persistent arthralgia or arthritis, both in the presence and in the absence of cryoglobulinemia. Painful arthritis involving larger joints often accompanies the fever and rash of several arthropod-borne viral infections, including those caused by *chikungunya, O'nyong-nyong, Ross River, Mayaro*, and *Barmah Forest* viruses. Symmetric arthritis involving the hands and wrists may occur during the convalescent phase of infection with *lymphocytic choriomeningitis virus*. Patients infected with an *enterovirus* frequently report arthralgias, and *echovirus* has been isolated from patients with acute polyarthritis.

Several arthritis syndromes are associated with *HIV* infection. Reiter's syndrome with painful lower-extremity oligoarthritis often follows an episode of urethritis in HIV-infected persons. HIV-associated Reiter's syndrome appears to be extremely common among persons with the HLA-B27 haplotype, but sacroiliac joint disease is unusual and is seen mostly in the absence of HLA-B27. Up to one-third of HIV-infected persons with psoriasis develop psoriatic arthritis. Painless monarthropathy and persistent symmetric polyarthropathy occasionally complicate HIV infection. Chronic persistent oligoarthritis of the shoulders, wrists, hands, and knees occurs in women infected with human T lymphotropic virus type I. Synovial thickening, destruction of articular cartilage, and leukemic-appearing atypical lymphocytes in synovial fluid are characteristic, but progression to T cell leukemia is unusual.

PARASITIC ARTHRITIS Arthritis due to parasitic infection is rare. The guinea worm *Dracunculus medinensis* may cause destructive joint lesions in the lower extremities as migrating gravid female worms invade joints or cause ulcers in adjacent soft tissues that become secondarily infected. Hydatid cysts infect bones in 1 to 2% of cases of infection with *Echinococcus granulosus*. The expanding destructive cystic lesions may spread to and destroy adjacent joints, particularly the hip and pelvis. In rare cases, chronic synovitis has been associated with the presence of schistosomal eggs in synovial biopsies. Monarticular arthritis in children with lymphatic *filariasis* appears to respond to therapy with diethylcarbamazine even in the absence of microfilariae in synovial fluid. Reactive arthritis has been attributed to *hookworm, Strongyloides, Cryptosporidium*, and *Giardia* infection in case reports, but confirmation is required.

POSTINFECTIOUS OR REACTIVE ARTHRITIS Reiter's syndrome, a reactive polyarthritis, develops several weeks after ~1% of cases of nongonococcal urethritis and 2% of enteric infections, particularly those due to *Yersinia enterocolitica, Shigella flexneri, Campylobacter jejuni*, and *Salmonella* species. Only a minority of these patients have the other findings of classic Reiter's syndrome, including urethritis, conjunctivitis, uveitis, oral ulcers, and rash. Studies have identified microbial DNA or antigen in synovial fluid or blood, but the pathogenesis of this condition is poorly understood.

Reiter's syndrome is most common among young men (except after *Yersinia* infection) and has been linked to the HLA-B27 locus as a potential genetic predisposing factor. Patients report painful, asymmetric oligoarthritis affecting mainly the knees, ankles, and feet. Low-back pain is common, and radiographic evidence of sacroiliitis is found in patients with long-standing disease. Most patients recover within 6 months, but prolonged recurrent disease is more common in cases following chlamydial urethritis. Anti-inflammatory agents help to relieve symptoms, but the role of prolonged antibiotic therapy in eliminating microbial antigen from the synovium is controversial.

Migratory polyarthritis and fever constitute the usual presentation of acute rheumatic fever in adults. This presentation is distinct from that of poststreptococcal reactive arthritis, which also follows infections with group A β-hemolytic *Streptococcus* but is not migratory, lasts beyond the typical 3-week maximum of acute rheumatic fever, and responds poorly to aspirin.

INFECTIONS IN PROSTHETIC JOINTS Infection complicates 1 to 4% of total joint replacements. The majority of infections are acquired intraoperatively or immediately postoperatively as a result of wound breakdown or infection; less commonly, these joint infections develop later after joint replacement and are the result of hematogenous spread or direct inoculation. The presentation may be acute, with fever, pain, and local signs of inflammation, especially in infections due to *S. aureus*, pyogenic streptococci, and enteric bacilli. Alternatively, infection may persist for months or years without causing constitutional symptoms when less virulent organisms, such as coagulase-negative staphylococci or diphtheroids, are involved. Such indolent infections are usually acquired during joint implantation and are discovered during evaluation of chronic unexplained pain or after a radiograph shows loosening of the prosthesis; the erythrocyte sedimentation rate and C-reactive protein are usually elevated in such cases.

The diagnosis is best made by needle aspiration of the joint; accidental introduction of organisms during aspiration must be meticulously avoided. Synovial fluid pleocytosis with a predominance of polymorphonuclear leukocytes is highly suggestive of infection, since other inflammatory processes uncommonly affect prosthetic joints. Culture and Gram's stain usually yield the responsible pathogen. Use of special media for unusual pathogens such as fungi, atypical mycobacteria, and *Mycoplasma* may be necessary if routine and anaerobic cultures are negative.

℞ **TREATMENT** Treatment includes surgery and high doses of parenteral antibiotics, which are given for 4 to 6 weeks because bone is usually involved. In most cases, the prosthesis must be replaced to cure the infection. Implantation of a new prosthesis is best delayed for several weeks or months because relapses of infection occur most commonly within this time frame. In some cases, reimplantation is not possible, and the patient must manage without a joint, with a fused joint, or even with amputation. Cure of infection without removal of the prosthesis is occasionally possible in cases that are due to streptococci or pneumococci and that lack radiologic evidence of loosening of the prosthesis. In these cases, antibiotic therapy must be initiated within several days of the onset of infection, and the joint should be drained vigorously either by open arthrotomy or arthroscopically. A high cure rate with retention of the prosthesis has been reported when the combination of oral rifampin and ciprofloxacin is given for 3 to 6 months to persons with staphylococcal prosthetic joint infection of short duration. This approach, which is based on the ability of rifampin to kill organisms adherent to foreign material and in the stationary growth phase, requires confirmation in prospective trials.

Prevention To avoid the disastrous consequences of infection, candidates for joint replacement should be selected with care. Rates of infection are particularly high among patients with rheumatoid arthritis, persons who have undergone previous surgery on the joint, and persons with medical conditions requiring immunosuppressive therapy. Perioperative antibiotic prophylaxis, usually with cefazolin, and measures to decrease intraoperative contamination, such as laminar flow, have lowered the rates of perioperative infection to <1% in many centers. After implantation, measures should be taken to prevent or rapidly treat extraarticular infections that might give rise to hematogenous spread to the prosthesis. The effectiveness of prophylactic antibiotics for the prevention of hematogenous infection following dental procedures has not been demonstrated; in fact, viridans streptococci and other components of the oral flora are extremely unusual causes of prosthetic joint infection. Accordingly, the American Dental Association and the American Academy of Orthopaedic Surgeons do not recommend antibiotic prophylaxis for most dental patients with total joint replacements. They do, however, recommend prophylaxis for patients who may be at high risk of hematogenous infection, including those with inflammatory arthropathies, immunosuppression, type 1 diabetes mellitus, joint replacement within 2 years, previous prosthetic joint infection, malnourishment, or hemophilia. The recommended regimen is amoxicillin (2 g orally) 1 h before dental procedures associated with a high incidence of bacteremia. Clindamycin (600 mg orally) is suggested for patients allergic to penicillin.

BIBLIOGRAPHY

BERMAN A et al: Human immunodeficiency virus infection associated arthritis: Clinical characteristics. J Rheumatol 26:1158, 1999

CUCURULL E, ESPINOZA LR: Gonococcal arthritis. Rheum Dis Clin North Am 24:305, 1998

CUNNINGHAM R et al: Clinical and molecular aspects of the pathogenesis of *Staphylococcus aureus* bone and joint infections. J Med Microbiol 44:157, 1996

DONATTO KC: Orthopedic management of septic arthritis. Rheum Dis Clin North Am 24: 275, 1998

GILLESPIE WJ: Prevention and management of infection after total joint replacement. Clin Infect Dis 25:1310, 1997

GOLDENBERG DL: Septic arthritis. Lancet 351:197, 1998

HARRINGTON JT: Mycobacterial and fungal arthritis. Curr Opin Rheumatol 10:335, 1998

WUORELA M, GRANFORS K: Infectious agents as triggers of reactive arthritis. Am J Med Sci 316:264, 1998

YTTERBERG SR: Viral arthritis. Curr Opin Rheumatol 11:275, 1999

ZIMMERLI W et al: Role of rifampin for treatment of orthopedic implant–related staphylococcal infections: A randomized controlled trial. Foreign-Body Infection (FBI) Study Group. JAMA 279:1537, 1998

324 *Peter H. Schur*

PSORIATIC ARTHRITIS AND ARTHRITIS ASSOCIATED WITH GASTROINTESTINAL DISEASE

PSORIATIC ARTHRITIS

Psoriatic arthritis (PsA) is a chronic inflammatory arthritis that affects 5 to 42% of people with psoriasis.

ETIOLOGY AND PATHOGENESIS To date, the cause and pathogenesis of PsA are unknown. Indirect evidence has suggested that interactions of infections, trauma, increased humoral and cellular immunity (e.g., to streptococci), cytokines (including TH1 and TH2), adhesion molecules, and abnormal fibroblast, dendritic cell, keratinocyte, and polymorphonuclear leukocyte (PMN) function are involved. Polyarthritis has developed in patients with psoriasis and hepatitis treated with interferon α. Most studies have observed an increased frequency of HLA-B17, CW6, and/or B27 in patients with psoriatic spondylitis, while B27, B38, B39, and DR7 have been noted in association with peripheral arthritis in different studies. Fulminant disease should make one suspect HIV disease (Chap. 309).

CLINICAL MANIFESTATIONS Three major types of PsA are generally recognized: asymmetric inflammatory arthritis, symmetric arthritis, and psoriatic spondylitis. A mean of 47% of patients (range, 16 to 70%) have an asymmetric inflammatory arthritis. Disease appears equally in men and women. Psoriasis tends to precede the arthritis by years. Many patients complain of morning stiffness. The proximal interphalangeal (PIP) and distal interphalangeal (DIP) joints are commonly involved [with characteristic sausage-shaped digits (dactylitis)], while knees, hips, ankles, temporomandibular joints, and wrists are less frequently involved. Most patients have onychodystrophy (onycholysis, ridging and pitting of nails), the course of which does not parallel that of the synovitis. The prognosis is good, with only one-fourth of the patients developing progressive destructive disease; one-third develop inflammatory ocular complications (conjunctivitis, iritis, episcleritis).

A mean of 25% of patients (range, 15 to 39%) develop symmetric arthritis resembling rheumatoid arthritis (Chap. 312). This disease occurs twice as frequently in women. Psoriasis and inflammatory arthritis usually develop simultaneously; most patients experience morning stiffness. The DIP, PIP, metacarpophalangeal (MCP), metatarsophalangeal (MTP), sternoclavicular, and, in particular, large peripheral joints are involved. Practically all patients have onychodystrophy, which helps distinguish them from patients with rheumatoid arthritis. Over half of the patients in this group go on to develop destructive arthritis, including arthritis mutilans. Eye complications are uncommon. Subcutaneous nodules are not present, but one-fourth of patients have rheumatoid factors. Unilateral upper limb edema has been described.

A mean of 23% of the patients (range 5 to 40%) have psoriatic "spondylitis," with or without peripheral joint involvement. Psoriasis tends to precede the arthritis by a few years, and low back pain with morning stiffness is common. Psoriatic spondylitis is more common in men. About half the patients in this group have spondylitis and the other half have sacroiliitis. The back disease is usually slowly progressive, with little clinical deterioration as compared with ankylosing spondylitis; the peripheral disease also tends not to be destructive except for the occasional patient with arthritis mutilans. Enthesopathy, i.e., inflammation of tendons and ligamentous attachments to bone, is characteristic, for example, of the Achilles tendon or of the plantar fascia causing heel pain. Many patients have onychodystrophy, but few have inflammatory ocular complications. Gut inflammation occurs in 30% (no gut inflammation was noted in patients with only peripheral arthritis).

Some authors have described additional subsets of psoriatic arthritis: predominant DIP joint involvement, arthritis mutilans, peripheral enthesitis, juvenile PsA, and SAPHO (synovitis, acne, pustulosis, hyperostosis, osteomyelitis).

The pathology of PsA is similar to that seen in rheumatoid arthritis: synoviocytic hyperplasia, early PMN infiltration and later mononuclear cell infiltration, cartilage erosion, and pannus formation. However, in PsA, the synovium is more vascular and there are fewer macrophages and less expression of endothelial cell leukocyte adhesion molecule-1 (ELAM-1). Fibrosis of the joint capsule and marrow is prominent in many patients.

LABORATORY FINDINGS There are few laboratory abnormalities. Elevated erythrocyte sedimentation rates, C-reactive proteins, and complement levels reflect inflammation. Rheumatoid factors are uncommon and are more likely to be observed in those with symmetric arthritis. Immunoglobulin levels, especially IgA levels, may be elevated (IgA antibodies to cytokeratins and antienterobacteria antibodies are elevated). Uric acid levels may be elevated; sodium urate crystals in joint fluids suggest gout.

Radiologic investigation reveals findings similar to those of rheumatoid arthritis: soft tissue swelling, loss of the cartilage space, erosions, bony ankylosis of fingers, subluxations, and subchondral cysts; of note, there is less demineralization. However, more unique and suggestive of psoriatic arthritis are erosions at DIP joints, expansion of the base of the terminal phalanx, tapering of the proximal phalanx and cuplike erosions and bony proliferation of the distal terminal phalanx ("pencil-in-cup" appearance), proliferation of bone near osseous erosions, terminal phalangeal osteolysis, bone proliferation and periostitis (especially of phalanges), and telescoping of one bone into its neighbor, leading to the "opera-glass" deformity (Fig. 324-1). The axial skeleton shows asymmetric or unilateral sacroiliitis, often asymptomatic paravertebral ossification, including cervical involvement, and large asymmetric nonmarginal syndesmophytes. Echocardiographic abnormalities resemble those of ankylosing spondilitis.

DIAGNOSIS The diagnosis of PsA should be considered in individuals with arthritis and psoriasis. Psoriasis should be distinguished from seborrheic dermatitis and eczema. Psoriatic lesions may be quite small peripherally and are often hidden in the scalp, umbilicus, and gluteal folds. Fungal infection of nails can be distinguished from psoriasis, for the latter will demonstrate pitting and onycholysis. Furthermore, onychodystrophy is uncommon (20% of cases) in uncomplicated psoriasis. It is often difficult to distinguish Reiter's syndrome (Chap. 315) from PsA, since both manifest dactylitis. Reiter's syndrome usually presents in younger individuals, especially males; is less frequently progressive or destructive; and is more likely to be associated with characteristic skin lesions (keratoderma blenorrhagica—which may, however, resemble pustular psoriasis), urethritis, and conjunctivitis. Gout can be distinguished by the presence of intraar-

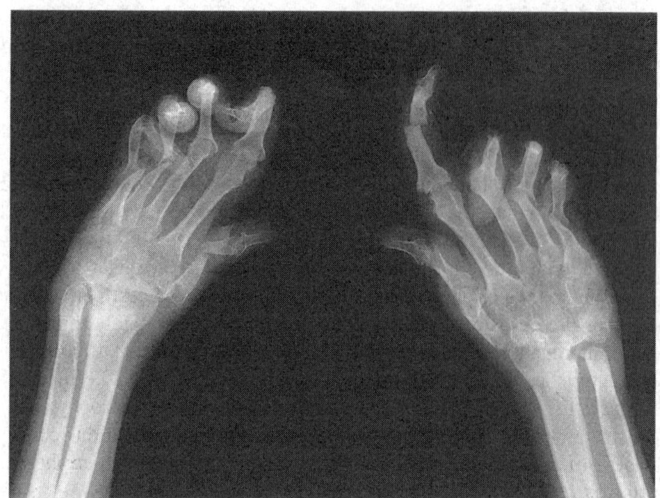

FIGURE 324-1 X-ray of hands of a patient with severe psoriatic arthritis characterized by destructive phalangeal changes (see text).

ticular sodium urate crystals (Chap. 322). Psoriasis in association with Heberden's nodes or Bouchard's nodes of the DIP and PIP joints, respectively, rather suggests osteoarthritis (Chap. 321). PsA differs from rheumatoid arthritis by the relative lack of rheumatoid factors; the tendency to asymmetry, dactylitis, iritis, enthesopathy, and onychodystrophy; the high frequency of HLA-B27, especially in patients with axial skeletal involvement; and characteristic radiologic features.

℞ **TREATMENT** The treatment of PsA begins with patient education and physical and occupational therapy to maintain muscle strength and joint and muscle function. Orthotics and occasional intraarticular glucocorticoids for isolated acutely and severely inflamed joints may be added as needed (Fig. 324-2). The mainstay, however, is the use of nonsteroidal anti-inflammatory drugs (NSAIDs), which reduce inflammation and alleviate pain for most patients. For patients with more severe involvement, a disease-modifying antirheumatic drug should be used. While hydroxychloroquine is often successful in

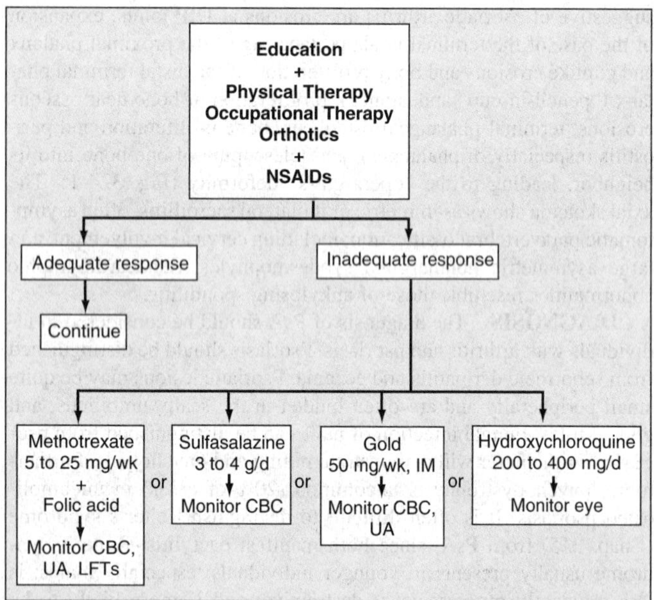

FIGURE 324-2 Algorithm for the treatment of psoriatic arthritis. See text for detailed description. NSAID, nonsteroidal anti-inflammatory drugs; CBC, complete blood count; UA, urinalysis; LFTs, liver function tests.

producing either amelioration or remission, it carries a significant risk of exacerbation of psoriasis and exfoliation. Sulfasalizine (2 to 4 g/d) has well-demonstrated efficacy for PsA. For more severe cases, especially with extensive skin involvement, 5 to 25 mg methotrexate per week is recommended. Most patients respond well with respect to both skin lesions and arthritis. Patients who are resistant to oral therapy may respond to parenteral therapy. Folic acid (1 mg/d) is recommended to prevent hematologic complications. Renal and liver function tests and a complete blood count should be performed every 6 to 8 weeks, and any abnormalities should suggest modification of the dosage. Liver biopsies are recommended after a total of 1.5 g methotrexate have been given and then every 2 years to identify the rare patient with fibrosis and cirrhosis, which necessitate withdrawal of the drug. Patients are advised to avoid nephrotoxic and hepatotoxic (e.g., ethanol) drugs. Patients with HIV infection may have worsening of their disease when treated with methotrexate. Intramuscular gold, cyclosporine (2 to 5 mg/kg per day), etretinate (0.5 mg/kg per day), and azathioprine have also proved successful. The arthritis may also respond to heliotherapy.

ARTHRITIS ASSOCIATED WITH GASTROINTESTINAL DISEASE

INFLAMMATORY BOWEL DISEASE Peripheral arthritis occurs in 9 to 30% of patients with inflammatory bowel disease (IBD) (e.g., ulcerative colitis or Crohn's disease; Chap. 287), and arthralgia is more common. Arthritis is somewhat more likely to occur in patients with large-bowel disease and in those patients with complications such as abscesses, pseudomembranous polyposis, perianal disease, massive hemorrhage, erythema nodosum, stomatitis, uveitis, and pyoderma gangrenosum. Males and females are affected equally. The arthritis tends to be acute, is associated with a flare-up of the bowel disease, occurs early in the course of the bowel disease, is self-limiting (90% of cases resolve within 6 months), and does not result in destruction. Most patients have a symmetric, migratory polyarthritis affecting primarily large joints of the lower extremity. Rheumatoid factors are not present. There is some association with HLA-BW62. Synovial fluids have 5000 to 12,000 white blood cells per microliter, mostly PMNs. Radiographs demonstrate soft tissue swelling and effusions without erosions or destruction. Pathologic examination of synovial biopsy specimens reveals only nonspecific inflammation. The peripheral arthritis responds to successful treatment of the bowel disease, such as colectomy (for ulcerative colitis), or administration of glucocorticoids, anti-tumor necrosis factor α therapy, or sulfasalazine. NSAIDs relieve pain and inflammation but should be used with caution because of possible gastrointestinal side effects.

Spondylitis occurs in 1.1 to 43% of patients with IBD (while gut inflammation develops in 68% of patients with spondyloarthropathies). Spondylitis often precedes IBD; their clinical courses are often strongly related. Males are affected more frequently. Patients typically complain of stiffness in the back and/or buttocks in the morning or after rest. The stiffness and associated pain are often relieved by exercise. Gastrointestinal infection/inflammation is thought to play a role in exacerbation of spondylitis. Physical examination reveals limitation of spinal flexion and reduced chest expansion. Some patients may have peripheral arthritis, especially of the hips and/or shoulders. Uveitis is a frequent complication. Radiographs of the back show the typical findings of ankylosing spondylitis and bilateral sacroiliitis. HLA-B27 is found in 53 to 75% of these patients. Treatment includes physical therapy, NSAIDs, glucocorticoids, and sulfasalazine. NSAIDs should be used with caution lest they exacerbate the IBD. The axial disease progresses slowly in a manner akin to that of ankylosing spondylitis.

Asymptomatic sacroiliitis detected by radiography occurs in 4 to 32% of patients with IBD. By contrast, 52% of patients with IBD have abnormalities on technetium pyrophosphate bone scans of the sacroiliac joint. There is no increased frequency of HLA-B27 in these patients. This "disease" does not necessarily progress to spondylitis.

Other complications of chronic IBD include (1) finger clubbing (observed in 4 to 13% of patients with Crohn's disease, especially those with small-bowel involvement), which may regress after surgery; (2) development of amyloid, especially in association with Crohn's disease; and (3) osteoporosis resulting from inactivity, malabsorption, and/or treatment with glucocorticoids. Osteomalacia can result from malabsorption. In this setting, with acutely increased back pain, one should suspect compression fracture.

INTESTINAL BYPASS ARTHRITIS Intestinal bypass surgery was developed for the treatment of obesity in 1952; 11 years later arthritis was recognized as a postoperative complication. Polyarthralgia, tenosynovitis, and sometimes arthritis occur weeks, even years, after surgery in 8 to 36% of patients. There is often an associated urticarial, vesicular, pustular, macular, or nodular eruption. X-rays generally show no joint damage. Tests for rheumatoid factors, antinuclear antibodies, and HLA-B27 are usually negative, while immune complexes (and cryoglobulins) are often present. They contain bacterial antigens, the corresponding antibodies, IgA secretory component, and complement components. These observations suggest that the syndrome has the following pathogenesis: Bacteria proliferate in intestinal blind loops; bacterial antigens are absorbed; and antibodies to these antigens develop and combine with them to form immune complexes, which deposit in synovial tissue to cause arthritis. NSAIDs and glucocorticoids can relieve the joint symptoms, but more lasting results can be achieved by tetracycline therapy to decrease the bacterial load; even better is reanastomosis of the bowel or resection of the blind loop.

WHIPPLE'S DISEASE (INTESTINAL LIPODYSTROPHY) Whipple's disease is rare and occurs mostly in middle-aged Caucasian males, who develop arthritis, prolonged diarrhea, malabsorption, and weight loss as a result of infection with the actinomyocete, *Tropheryma whippelii*. The organism has been found in waste water. Up to 90% of patients with the disease develop arthritis, usually prior to other symptoms. Knees and ankles and, to a lesser extent, fingers, hips, shoulders, elbows, and wrists are involved. The arthritis is acute in onset, migratory, usually lasts just a few days, and is rarely chronic or a cause of permanent joint damage. Associated symptoms may include fever (54%), edema, serositis (pleurisy, pericarditis, endocarditis), pneumonia, hypotension, lymphadenopathy (54%), hyperpigmentation (54%), subcutaneous nodules, clubbing, and uveitis. Central nervous system involvement may develop (80%), with cognitive changes, headache, diplopia, and papilledema, and may be appreciated by abnormalities in magnetic resonance images of the brain. Oculomasticatory myorhythmia and oculo-facial-skeletal myorhythmia are felt to be pathognomonic and are found in 20% of patients; they are always accompanied by supranuclear vertical gaze palsy. Laboratory abnormalities include anemia (75%), low serum levels of carotene (95%), and albumin (93%). The presence of HLA-B27 (8 to 30%) occurs in those patients with axial arthritis. Synovial fluids have been reported to contain 450 to 36,000 white blood cells per microliter (30 to 95% neutrophils) or a mild monocytosis. Joint x-rays rarely show erosions but may show a sacroiliitis in the occasional patients who have axial skeletal symptoms; abdominal computed tomographic scans may reveal lymphadenopathy. The lamina propria and/or foamy macrophages in small intestine contain PAS-staining bacterial remnants, presumably of *T. whippelii*. These inclusion-containing foamy macrophages have also been detected in the synovium, lymph nodes, and other tissues. Diagnosis is often established by polymerase chain reaction of the 165 ribosomal gene sequences of these bacteria in biopsied tissue, usually the duodenum. The syndrome responds best to therapy with penicillin (or ceftriaxone) and streptomycin for 2 weeks followed by trimethoprim-sulfamethoxazole for 1 to 2 years. However, central nervous system relapse may develop, which has been treated with cefixime.

REACTIVE ARTHRITIS A Reiter's-like syndrome of arthritis can develop 2 to 3 weeks following diarrhea caused by *Shigella, Salmonella, Yersinia, Chlamydia trachomatis*, or *Campylobacter* organisms. →*This condition is described in Chap. 315.*

BIBLIOGRAPHY

BOS JD, DE RIE MA: The pathogenesis of psoriasis: Immunological facts and speculations. Immunol Today 20:40, 1999

BRUCKLE W et al: Treatment of psoriatic arthritis with auranofin and gold sodium thiomalate. Clin Rheumatol 13:209, 1994

CLEGG DO et al: Comparison of sulfasalazine and placebo in the treatment of psoriatic arthritis. A Department of Veterans Affairs Cooperative Study. Arthritis Rheum 39: 2013, 1996

CUELLAR ML, ESPINOZA LR: Methotrexate use in psoriasis and psoriatic arthritis. Rheum Dis Clin North Am 23:797, 1997

DE KEYSER F et al: Bowel inflammation and the spondyloarthropathies. Rheum Dis Clin North Am 24:785, 1998

DURAND F et al: Whipple disease. Clinical review of 52 cases. The SNFMI Research Group on Whipple Disease. Societé Nationale Francaise de Medecine Interne. Medicine 76:170, 1997

ESPINOZA LR et al: Insights into the pathogenesis of psoriasis and psoriatic arthritis. Am J Med Sci 316:271, 1998

GLADMAN DD: Psoriatic arthritis. Rheum Dis Clin North Am 24:829, 1998

JONES G et al: Psoriatic arthritis: A quantitative overview of therapeutic options. The Psoriatic Arthritis Meta-Analysis Study Group. Br J Rheumatol 36:95, 1997

KAHN MF, CHAMOT AM: Sapho syndrome. Rheum Dis Clin North Am 18:225, 1992

KATZ JP, LICHTENSTEIN GR: Rheumatologic manifestations of gastrointestinal diseases. Gastroenterol Clin North Am 27:533, 1998

LOUIS ED et al: Diagnostic guidelines in central nervous system Whipple's disease. Ann Neurol 40:561, 1996

MAHRLE G et al: Low-dose short-term cyclosporine versus etretinate in psoriasis: Improvement of skin, nail, and joint involvement. J Am Acad Dermatol 32:78, 1995

MCGONAGLE D et al: Psoriatic arthritis. A unified concept twenty years on. Arthritis Rheum 42:1080, 1999

PORTER GG: Psoriatic arthritis. Plain radiology and other imaging techniques. Baillieres Clin Rheumatol 8:465, 1994

RAMZAN NN et al: Diagnosis and monitoring of Whipple disease by polymerase chain reaction. Ann Intern Med 126:520, 1997

325

Bruce C. Gilliland

RELAPSING POLYCHONDRITIS AND OTHER ARTHRITIDES

RELAPSING POLYCHONDRITIS

Relapsing polychondritis is an uncommon inflammatory disorder of unknown cause characterized by an episodic and generally progressive course affecting predominantly the cartilage of the ears, nose, and laryngotracheobronchial tree. Other manifestations include scleritis, neurosensory hearing loss, polyarthritis, vasculitis, cardiac abnormalities, skin lesions, and glomerulonephritis. The peak age of onset is between the ages of 40 to 50 years but relapsing polychondritis may affect children and the elderly. It is found in all races, and both sexes are equally affected. No familial tendency is apparent. A significantly higher frequency of HLA-DR4 has been found in patients with relapsing polychondritis than in normal individuals. A predominant subtype allele(s) of HLA-DR4 was not found. Approximately 30% of patients with relapsing polychondritis will have another rheumatologic disorder, the most frequent being systemic vasculitis, followed by rheumatoid arthritis, systemic lupus erythematosus (SLE), or Sjögren's syndrome. Nonrheumatic disorders associated with relapsing polychondritis include inflammatory bowel disease, primary biliary cirrhosis, and myelodysplastic syndrome.

Diagnostic criteria were suggested several years ago by McAdam et al. and modified by Damiani and Levine a few years later. These criteria continue to be generally used in clinical practice. McAdam et al. proposed the following: (1) recurrent chondritis of both auricles; (2) nonerosive inflammatory arthritis; (3) chondritis of nasal cartilage; (4) inflammation of ocular structures including conjunctivitis, keratitis, scleritis/episcleritis, and/or uveitis; (5) chondritis of the laryngeal and/or tracheal cartilages; and (6) cochlear and/or vestibular damage manifested by neurosensory hearing loss, tinnitus, and/or vertigo. The diagnosis is certain when three or more of these features were present with biopsy confirmation. Damiana and Levine later suggested that the diagnosis could be made when one or more of the above features and a positive biopsy were present, when two or more separate sites of cartilage inflammation were present that responded to glucocorticoids or dapsone, or when three or more of the above features were present. A biopsy is not necessary in most patients with clinically evident disease.

PATHOLOGY AND PATHOPHYSIOLOGY The earliest abnormality of cartilage noted histologically is a focal or diffuse loss of basophilic staining indicating depletion of proteoglycan from the cartilage matrix. Inflammatory infiltrates are found adjacent to involved cartilage and consist predominantly of mononuclear cells and occasional plasma cells. In acute disease, polymorphonuclear white cells may also be present. Destruction of cartilage begins at the outer edges and advances centrally. There is lacunar breakdown and loss of chondrocytes. Degenerating cartilage is replaced by granulation tissue and later by fibrosis and focal areas of calcification. Small loci of cartilage regeneration may be present. Immunofluorescence studies have shown immunoglobulins and complement at sites of involvement. Fine granular material observed in the degenerating cartilage matrix by electron microscopy has been interpreted to be enzymes or immunoglobulins.

Immunologic mechanisms play a role in the pathogenesis of relapsing polychondritis. Immunoglobulin and complement deposits are found at sites of inflammation. In addition, antibodies to type II collagen and to matrilin-1 and immune complexes are detected in the sera of some patients. The possibility that an immune response to type II collagen may be important in the pathogenesis is supported experimentally by the occurrence of auricular chondritis in rats immunized with type II collagen. Antibodies to type II collagen are found in the sera of these animals, and immune deposits are detected at sites of ear inflammation. Cell-mediated immunity may also be operative in causing tissue injury, since lymphocyte transformation can be demonstrated when lymphocytes of patients are exposed to cartilage extracts. Humoral and cellular immune responses to type IX and type XI collagen have been demonstrated in some patients. In a recent study, rats immunized with cartilage matrix protein (matrilin-1) were found to develop severe inspiratory stridor and swelling of the nasal septum. Cartilage matrix protein is a noncollagenous protein present in the extracellular matrix in cartilage. It is present in high concentrations in the trachea and is also present in the nasal septum but not in articular cartilage. The immunized rats had severe inflammation in the larynx close to the epiglottis, which was characterized by increased numbers of CD 4+ and CD 8+ T cells. All had IgG antibodies to cartilage matrix protein. The inflammation was believed to have been largely mediated by T cells. The results of the study suggest that immune responses to various cartilage proteins play a role in the pathogenesis of relapsing polychondritis.

Dissolution of cartilage matrix can be induced by the intravenous injection of crude papain, a proteolytic enzyme, into young rabbits, which results in collapse of their normally rigid ears within 4 h. Reconstitution of the matrix occurs in about 7 days. In relapsing polychondritis, loss of cartilage matrix also most likely results from action of proteolytic enzymes released from chondrocytes, polymorphonuclear white cells, and monocytes that have been activated by inflammatory mediators.

CLINICAL MANIFESTATIONS The onset of relapsing polychondritis is frequently abrupt with the appearance of one or two sites of cartilagenous inflammation. Fever, fatigue, and weight loss occur and may precede the clinical signs of relapsing polychondritis by several weeks. Relapsing polychondritis may go unrecognized for several months or even years in patients who only initially manifest intermittent joint pain and/or swelling, or who have unexplained eye inflammation, hearing loss, valvular heart disease, or pulmonary symptoms. The pattern of cartilagenous involvement and the frequency of episodes vary widely among patients.

Auricular chondritis is the most frequent presenting manifestation of relapsing polychondritis in 40% of patients and eventually affects about 85% of patients (Table 325-1). One or both ears are involved, either sequentially or simultaneously. Patients experience the sudden onset of pain, tenderness, and swelling of the cartilaginous portion of the ear. Earlobes are spared because they do not contain cartilage. The overlying skin has a beefy red or violaceous color. Prolonged or recurrent episodes result in a flabby or droopy ear as a sequela of cartilage destruction. Swelling may close off the eustachian tube (causing otitis media) or the external auditory meatus, either of which can impair hearing. Inflammation of the internal auditory artery or its cochlear branch produces hearing loss, vertigo, ataxia, nausea, and vomiting. The cartilage of the nose becomes inflamed during the first or subsequent attacks. Approximately 50% of patients will eventually have nose involvement. Patients may experience nasal stuffiness, rhinorrhea, and epistaxis. The bridge of the nose becomes red, swollen, and tender and may collapse, producing a saddle deformity. In some patients, the saddle deformity develops insidiously without overt inflammation. Saddle nose is observed more frequently in younger patients, especially in women.

Arthritis is the presenting manifestation in relapsing polychondritis in approximately one-third of patients and may be present for several months before other features appear. Eventually, more than half the patients will have arthritis. The arthritis is usually asymmetric and oligo- or polyarticular, and involves both large and small peripheral joints. An episode of arthritis lasts from a few days to several weeks and resolves spontaneously without residual joint deformity. Attacks of arthritis may not be temporally related to other manifestations of relapsing polychondritis. The joints are warm, tender, and swollen. Joint fluid has been reported to be noninflammatory. In addition to peripheral joints, inflammation may involve the costochondral, sternomanubrial, and sternoclavicular cartilages. Destruction of these cartilages may result in a pectus excavatum deformity or even a flail anterior chest wall. Relapsing polychondritis may occur in patients with preexisting rheumatoid arthritis, Reiter's syndrome, psoriatic arthritis, or ankylosing spondylitis.

Eye manifestations occur in more than half of patients and include conjunctivitis, episcleritis, scleritis, iritis, and keratitis. Ulceration and perforation of the cornea may occur and cause blindness. Other manifestations include eyelid and periorbital edema, proptosis, cataracts, optic neuritis, extraocular muscle palsies, retinal vasculitis, and renal vein occlusion.

Laryngotracheobronchial involvement occurs in ~50% of patients. Symptoms include hoarseness, a nonproductive cough, and tenderness over the larynx and proximal trachea. Mucosal edema, strictures, and/or collapse of laryngeal or tracheal cartilage may cause stridor and life-threatening airway obstruction necessitating tracheostomy. Collapse of cartilage in bronchi leads to pneumonia and, when extensive, to respiratory insufficiency.

Aortic regurgitation occurs in about 5% of patients and is due to progressive dilation of the aortic ring or to destruction of the valve

Table 325-1 Clinical Manifestations of Relapsing Polychondritis

	Frequency, %	
Clinical Feature	Presenting	Cumulative
Auricular chondritis	40	85
Hearing loss	10	30
Nasal chondritis	25	55
Saddle nose deformity	20	30
Ocular deformities	20	50
Respiratory disease	25	50
Arthritis	35	50
Aortic regurgitation	—	5
Vasculitis	3	10

SOURCE: Modified from Isaak et al: Ophthalmology 93:681, 1986.

cusps. Mitral and other heart valves are less often affected. Other cardiac manifestations include pericarditis, myocarditis, and conduction abnormalities. Aneurysms of the proximal, thoracic, or abdominal aorta may occur and occasionally rupture.

Systemic vasculitis may occur in association with relapsing polychondritis. Vasculitides include leukocytoclastic vasculitis, polyarteritis, temporal arteritis, and Takayasu's arteritis (Chap. 317). Neurologic abnormalities usually occur as a result of underlying vasculitis, manifesting as seizures, strokes, ataxia, and peripheral and cranial nerve neuropathies. Cranial nerves VI and VII are most often involved. Approximately 25% of patients have skin lesions, none of which is characteristic for relapsing polychondritis. These include purpura, erythema nodosum, erythema multiforme, angioedema/urticaria, livedo reticularis, and panniculitis. Segmental necrotizing glomerulonephritis with crescent formation has been noted in some patients in the absence of systemic vasculitis.

The course of disease is highly variable, with episodes lasting from a few days to several weeks and then subsiding spontaneously. Attacks may recur at intervals varying from weeks to months. In other patients, the disease has a chronic, smoldering course. In a few patients, the disease may be limited to one or two episodes of cartilage inflammation. In one study, the 5-year estimated survival rate was 74% and the 10-year survival rate 55%. In contrast to earlier series, only about half the deaths could be attributed to relapsing polychondritis or complications of treatment. Pulmonary complications accounted for only 10% of all fatalities. In general, patients with more widespread disease have a worse prognosis.

LABORATORY FINDINGS Mild leukocytosis and normocytic, normochromic anemia are often present. The erythrocyte sedimentation rate is usually elevated. Rheumatoid factor and antinuclear antibody tests are occasionally positive in low titers. Antibodies to type II collagen are present in most patients, but they are not specific. Circulating immune complexes may be detected, especially in patients with early active disease. Elevated levels of γ globulin may be present. Antineutrophil cytoplasmic antibodies (ANCA), either cytoplasmic (C-ANCA) or perinuclear (P-ANCA), are found in some patients with active disease. The upper and lower airways can be evaluated by imaging techniques such as linear tomography, laryngotracheography, and computed tomography, and by bronchoscopy. Bronchography is performed to demonstrate bronchial narrowing. Intrathoracic airway obstruction can also be evaluated by inspiratory-expiratory flow studies. The chest film may show narrowing of the trachea and/or the main bronchi, widening of the ascending or descending aorta due to an aneurysm, and cardiomegaly when aortic insufficiency is present. Radiographs may show calcification at previous sites of cartilage damage involving ear, nose, larynx, or trachea.

DIAGNOSIS Diagnosis is based on recognition of the typical clinical features. Biopsies of the involved cartilage from the ear, nose, or respiratory tract will confirm the diagnosis but are only necessary when clinical features are not typical. Patients with Wegener's granulomatosis may have a saddle nose and pulmonary involvement but can be distinguished by the absence of auricular involvement and the presence of granulomatous lesions in the tracheobronchial tree. Patients with Cogan's syndrome have interstitial keratitis and vestibular and auditory abnormalities, but this syndrome does not involve the respiratory tract or ears. Reiter's syndrome may initially resemble relapsing polychondritis because of oligoarticular arthritis and eye involvement, but it is distinguished in time by the appearance of urethritis and typical mucocutaneous lesions and the absence of nose or ear cartilage involvement. Rheumatoid arthritis may initially suggest relapsing polychondritis because of arthritis and eye inflammation. The arthritis in rheumatoid arthritis, however, is erosive and symmetric. In addition, rheumatoid factor titers are usually high compared with those in relapsing polychondritis. Bacterial infection of the pinna may be mistaken for relapsing polychondritis but differs by usually involving only one ear, including the earlobe. Auricular cartilage may also be damaged by trauma or frostbite.

Relapsing polychondritis may develop in patients with a variety

of autoimmune disorders, including SLE, rheumatoid arthritis, Sjögren's syndrome, and vasculitis. In most cases, these disorders antedate the appearance of polychondritis, usually by months or years. It is likely that these patients have an immunologic abnormality that predisposes them to development of this group of autoimmune disorders.

℞ **TREATMENT** In patients with active chondritis or associated vasculitis, prednisone, 40 to 60 mg/d, is often effective in suppressing disease activity; it is tapered gradually once disease is controlled. In some patients, prednisone can be stopped, while in others low doses in the range of 10 to 15 mg/d are required for continued suppression of disease. Immunosuppressive drugs such as methotrexate, cyclophosphamide, or azathioprine should be reserved for patients who fail to respond to prednisone or who require high doses for control of disease activity. Methotrexate has been found by some investigators to be very effective in treating relapsing polychondritis. Dapsone and cyclosporine have been reported to be beneficial in a few patients. Patients with significant ocular inflammation often require intraocular steroids as well as high doses of prednisone. Heart valve replacement or repair of an aortic aneurysm may be necessary. In patients with early subglottic disease, intralesional injection of glutocorticoids may be beneficial. When obstruction is severe, tracheostomy is required. Stents may be necessary in patients with tracheobronchial collapse.

OTHER ARTHRITIDES

NEUROPATHIC JOINT DISEASE Neuropathic joint disease (Charcot's joint) is a progressive destructive arthritis associated with loss of pain sensation, proprioception, or both. In addition, normal muscular reflexes that modulate joint movement are decreased. Without these protective mechanisms, joints are subjected to repeated trauma, resulting in progressive cartilage and bone damage. Neuropathic arthropathy was first described by Jean-Martin Charcot in 1868 in patients with tabes dorsalis. The term *Charcot joint* is commonly used interchangeably with *neuropathic joint*. Today, diabetes mellitus is the most frequent cause of neuropathic joint disease. A variety of other disorders are associated with neuropathic arthritis including leprosy, yaws, syringomyelia, meningomyelocoele, congenital indifference to pain, peroneal muscular atrophy (Charcot-Marie-Tooth disease), and amyloidosis. An arthritis resembling neuropathic joint disease is seen in patients who have received frequent intraarticular glucocorticoid injections into a weight-bearing joint and in patients with calcium pyrophosphate dihydrate crystal deposition disease. The distribution of joint involvement depends on the underlying neurologic disorder (Table 325-2). In tabes dorsalis, knees, hips, and ankles are most commonly affected; in syringomyelia, the glenohumeral joint, elbow, and wrist; and in diabetes mellitus, the tarsal and tarsometatarsal joints.

Pathology and Pathophysiology The pathologic changes in the neuropathic joint are similar to those found in the severe osteoarthritic joint. There is fragmentation and eventual loss of articular cartilage with eburnation of the underlying bone. Osteophytes are found at the joint margins. With more advanced disease, erosions are present on the joint surface. Fractures, devitalized bone, and intraarticular loose bodies may be present. Microscopic fragments of cartilage and bone are seen in the synovial tissue.

At least two underlying mechanisms are believed to be involved in the pathogenesis of neuropathic arthritis. An abnormal autonomic

Table 325-2 Disorders Associated with Neuropathic Joint Disease

Diabetes mellitus	Amyloidosis
Tabes dorsalis	Leprosy
Meningomyelocele	Congenital indifference to pain
Syringomyelia	Peroneal muscular atrophy

nervous system is thought to be responsible for the increased blood flow to the joint and subsequent resorption of bone. Loss of bone, particularly in the diabetic foot, may be the initial manifestation. With the loss of deep pain, proprioception, and protective neuromuscular reflexes, the joint is subjected to repeated injuries including ligamental tears and bone fractures. The mechanism of injury that occurs following frequent intraarticular glucocorticoid injections is thought to be due to the analgesic effect of glucocorticoids leading to overuse of an already damaged joint, which results in accelerated cartilage damage. It is not understood why only a few patients with neuropathies develop neuropathic arthritis.

Clinical Manifestations Neuropathic joint disease usually begins in a single joint and then progresses to involve other joints, depending on the underlying neurologic disorder. The involved joint progressively becomes enlarged from bony overgrowth and synovial effusion. Loose bodies may be palpated in the joint cavity. Joint instability, subluxation, and crepitus occur as the disease progresses. Neuropathic joints may develop rapidly, and a totally disorganized joint with multiple bony fragments may evolve in a patient within weeks or months. The amount of pain experienced by the patient is less than would be anticipated based on the degree of joint involvement. Patients may experience sudden joint pain from intraarticular fractures of osteophytes or condyles.

Neuropathic arthritis is encountered most often in patients with diabetes mellitus, with the incidence estimated in the range of 0.5%. The usual age of onset is ≥50 years following several years of diabetes, but exceptions occur. The tarsal and tarsometatarsal joints are most often affected, followed by the metatarsophalangeal and talotibial joints. The knees and spine are occasionally involved. In about 20%, neuropathic arthritis may be present in both feet. Patients often attribute the onset of foot pain to antecedent trauma such as twisting their foot. Neuropathic changes may develop rapidly following a foot fracture or dislocation. Swelling of the foot and ankle are often present. Downward collapse of the tarsal bones leads to convexity of the sole, referred to as a "rocker foot." Large osteophytes may protrude from the top of the foot. Calluses frequently form over the metatarsal heads and may lead to infected ulcers and osteomyelitis. Radiographs may show resorption and tapering of the distal metatarsal bones. The term *Lisfranc fracture-dislocation* is sometimes used to describe the destructive changes at the tarsometatarsal joints.

Diagnosis The diagnosis of neuropathic arthritis is based on the clinical features and characteristic radiographic findings in a patient with an underlying sensory neuropathy. The differential diagnosis of neuropathic arthritis includes osteomyelitis, osteonecrosis, advanced osteoarthritis, stress fractures, and calcium pyrophosphate dihydrate (CPPD) deposition disease. Radiographs in neuropathic arthritis initially show changes of osteoarthritis with joint space narrowing, subchondral bone sclerosis, osteophytes, and joint effusions followed later by marked destructive and hypertrophic changes. Soft tissue swelling, bone resorption, fractures, large osteophytes, extraarticular bone fragments, and subluxation are present with advanced arthropathy. The radiographic findings of neuropathic arthritis may be difficult to differentiate from those of osteomyelitis, especially in the diabetic foot. The joint margins in a neuropathic joint tend to be distinct, while in osteomyelitis, they are blurred. Imaging studies and cultures of fluid and tissue from the joint are often required to exclude osteomyelitis. Magnetic resonance imaging is helpful in differentiating these disorders. Another useful study is a bone scan using indium 111–labeled white blood cells or indium 111–labeled immunoglobulin G, which will show an increased uptake in osteomyelitis but not in a neuropathic joint. A technetium bone scan will not distinguish osteomyelitis from neuropathic arthritis as increased uptake is observed in both. The joint fluid in neuropathic arthritis is noninflammatory; may be xanthochromic or even bloody; and may contain fragments of synovium, cartilage, and bone. The finding of CPPD crystals suggests the diagnosis of a crystal associated neuropathic-like arthropathy. In the absence of CPPD crystals, the presence of increased number of leukocytes may indicate osteomyelitis.

℞ TREATMENT The primary focus of treatment is to provide stabilization of the joint. Treatment of the underlying disorder, even if successful, does not usually alter the joint disease. Braces and splints are helpful. Their use requires close surveillance, since patients may be unable to appreciate pressure from a poorly adjusted brace. In the diabetic patient, early recognition and treatment of a Charcot's foot by prohibiting weight bearing of the foot for at least 8 weeks may possibly prevent severe disease from developing. Fusion of a very unstable joint may improve function, but nonunion is frequent, especially when immobilization of the joint is inadequate.

HYPERTROPHIC OSTEOARTHROPATHY AND CLUBBING Hypertrophic osteoarthropathy (HOA) is characterized by clubbing of digits and, in more advanced stages, by periosteal new bone formation and synovial effusions. HOA occurs in primary and familial forms and usually begins in childhood. The secondary form of HOA is associated with intrathoracic malignancies, suppurative lung disease, congenital heart disease, and a variety of other disorders and is more common in adults. Clubbing is almost always a feature of HOA but can occur as an isolated manifestation (Fig. 325-1). The presence of clubbing in isolation is generally considered to represent either an early stage or an element in the spectrum of HOA. The presence of only clubbing in a patient usually has the same clinical significance as HOA.

Pathology and Pathophysiology In HOA, the bone changes in the distal extremities begin as periostitis followed by new bone formation. At this stage, a radiolucent area may be observed between the new periosteal bone and subjacent cortex. As the process progresses, multiple layers of new bone are deposited, which become contiguous with the cortex and result in cortical thickening. The outer portion of bone is laminated in appearance, with an irregular surface. Initially, the process of periosteal new bone formation involves the proximal and distal diaphyses of the tibia, fibula, radius, and ulna and, less frequently, the femur, humerus, metacarpals, metatarsals, and phalanges. Occasionally, scapulae, clavicles, ribs, and pelvic bones are also affected. In long-standing disease, these changes extend to involve metaphyses and musculotendinous insertions. The adjacent interosseous membranes may become ossified. The distribution of the bone manifestations is usually bilateral and symmetric. The soft tissue overlying the distal third of the arms and legs may be thickened. Mononuclear cell infiltration may be present in the adjacent soft tissue. Proliferation of connective tissue occurs in the nail bed and volar pad of digits, giving the distal phalanges a clubbed appearance. Small blood vessels in the clubbed digits are dilated and have thickened walls. In addition, the number of arteriovenous anastomoses is increased. The synovium of involved joints shows edema, varying degrees of synovial

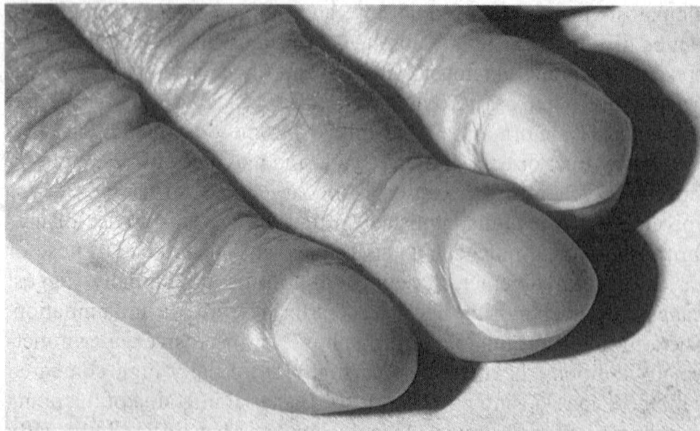

FIGURE 325-1 Clubbing of fingers. *(Reprinted from the Clinical Slide Collection on the Rheumatic Diseases, Copyright 1991, 1995. Used by permission of the American College of Rheumatology.)*

cell proliferation, thickening of the subsynovium, vascular congestion, vascular obliteration with thrombi, and small numbers of lymphocyte infiltrates.

Several theories have been suggested for the pathogenesis of HOA. Most have either been disproved or have not explained the development in all clinical disorders associated with HOA. Previously proposed neurogenic and humoral theories are no longer considered likely explanations for HOA. The neurogenic theory was based on the observation that vagotomy resulted in symptomatic improvement in a small number of patients with lung tumors and HOA. It was postulated that vagal stimuli from the tumor site led via a neural reflex to efferent nerve impulses to the distal extremities, resulting in HOA. This theory, however, did not explain HOA in conditions where vagal stimulation did not occur, as in cyanotic congenital heart disease or arterial aneurysms. The humoral theory postulated that soluble substances that are normally inactivated or removed during passage through the lung reached the systemic circulation in an active form and stimulated the changes of HOA. Substances proposed included prostaglandins, ferritin, bradykinin, estrogen, and growth hormone. These substances seemed unlikely candidates, since their blood levels in HOA patients overlapped those in individuals without HOA. Furthermore, these substances did not explain the development of localized HOA associated with arterial aneurysms or infected arterial grafts.

Recent studies have suggested a role for platelets in the development of HOA. It has been observed that megakaryocytes and large platelet particles, present in venous circulation, were fragmented in their passage through normal lung. In patients with cyanotic congenital heart disease and in other disorders associated with right-to-left shunts, these large platelet particles may bypass the lung and reach the distal extremities, where they can interact with endothelial cells. Platelet clumps have been demonstrated to form on an infected heart valve in bacterial endocarditis, in the wall of arterial aneurysms, and on infected arterial grafts. These platelet particles may also reach the distal extremities and interact with endothelial cells. Platelet-endothelial activation in the distal portion of extremities would then result in the release of platelet-derived growth factor (PDGF) and other factors leading to the proliferation of connective tissue and periosteum. Stimulation of fibroblasts by PDGF and transforming growth factor β (TGF-β) results in cell growth and collagen synthesis. Elevated plasma levels of von Willebrand factor antigen have been found in patients with both primary and secondary forms of HOA, indicating endothelial activation or damage. Abnormalities of collagen synthesis have been demonstrated in the involved skin of patients with primary HOA. Fibroblasts from affected skin were shown to have increased collagen synthesis, increased $\alpha1$(I) procollagen mRNA, and evidence for upregulation of collagen transcription. Other factors are undoubtedly involved in the pathogenesis of HOA, and further studies are needed to better understand this disorder.

Clinical Manifestations Primary HOA, also referred to as *pachydermoperiostitis* or *Touraine-Solente-Golé syndrome*, usually begins insidiously at puberty. In a smaller number of patients, the onset is in the first year of life. The disorder is inherited as an autosomal dominant trait with variable expression and is nine times more common in boys than in girls. Approximately one-third of patients have a family history of primary HOA.

Primary HOA is characterized by clubbing, periostitis, and unusual skin features. A small number of patients with this syndrome do not express clubbing. The skin changes and periostitis are prominent features of this syndrome. The skin becomes thickened and coarse. Deep nasolabial folds develop, and the forehead may become furrowed. Patients may have heavy-appearing eyelids and ptosis. The skin is often greasy, and there may be excessive sweating of the hands and feet. Patients may also experience acne vulgaris, seborrhea, and folliculitis. In a few patients, the skin over the scalp becomes very thick and corrugated, a feature that has been descriptively termed *cutis verticis gyrata*. The distal extremities, particularly the legs, become thickened owing to proliferation of new bone and soft tissue; when the process is extensive, the distal lower extremities resemble those of an elephant. The periostitis is usually not painful, as it may be in secondary HOA. Clubbing of the fingers may be extensive, producing large, bulbous deformities and clumsiness. Clubbing also affects the toes. Patients may experience articular and periarticular pain, especially in the ankles and knees, and joint motion may be mildly restricted owing to periarticular bone overgrowth. Noninflammatory effusions occur in the wrists, knees, and ankles. Synovial hypertrophy is not found. Associated abnormalities observed in patients with primary HOA include hypertrophic gastropathy, bone marrow failure, female escutcheon, gynecomastia, and cranial suture defects. In patients with primary HOA, the symptoms disappear when adulthood is reached.

HOA secondary to an underlying disease occurs more frequently than primary HOA. It accompanies a variety of disorders and may precede clinical features of the associated disorder by months. Clubbing is more frequent than the full syndrome of HOA in patients with associated illnesses. Because clubbing evolves over months and is usually asymptomatic, it is often recognized first by the physician and not the patient. Patients may experience a burning sensation in their fingertips. Clubbing is characterized by widening of the fingertips, enlargement of the distal volar pad, convexity of the nail contour, and the loss of the normal 15° angle between the proximal nail and cuticle. The thickness of the digit at the base of the nail is greater than the thickness at the distal interphalangeal joint. An objective measurement of finger clubbing can be made by determining the diameter at the base of the nail and at the distal interphalangeal joint of all 10 digits. Clubbing is present when the sum of the individual digit ratios is >10. At the bedside, clubbing can be appreciated by having the patient place the dorsal surface of the fourth fingers together. Normally, an open area is visible between the opposing fingers; when clubbing is present, this open space is no longer visible. The base of the nail feels spongy when compressed, and the nail can be easily rocked on its bed. Marked periungual erythema is usually present. When clubbing is advanced, the finger may have a drumstick appearance, and the distal interphalangeal joint can be hyperextended. Periosteal involvement in the distal extremities may produce a burning or deep-seated aching pain. The pain can be quite incapacitating and is aggravated by dependency and relieved by elevation of the affected limbs. The overlying soft tissue may be swollen, and the skin slightly erythematous. Pressure applied over the distal forearms and legs may be quite painful.

Patients may also experience joint pain, most often in the ankles, wrists, and knees. Joint effusions may be present; usually they are small and noninflammatory. The small joints of the hands are rarely affected. Severe joint or bone pain may be the presenting symptom of an underlying lung malignancy and may precede the appearance of clubbing. In addition, the progression of HOA tends to be more rapid when associated with malignancies, most notably bronchogenic carcinoma. Unlike primary HOA, excessive sweating and oiliness of the skin and thickening of the facial skin are uncommon in secondary HOA.

HOA occurs in 5 to 10% of patients with intrathoracic malignancies, the most common being bronchogenic carcinoma and pleural tumors (Table 325-3). Lung metastases infrequently cause HOA. HOA is also seen in patients with intrathoracic infections, including lung abscesses, empyema, bronchiectasis, chronic obstructive lung disease, and, uncommonly, pulmonary tuberculosis. HOA may also accompany chronic interstitial pneumonitis, sarcoidosis, and cystic fibrosis. In the latter, clubbing is more common than the full syndrome of HOA. Other causes of clubbing include congenital heart disease with right-to-left shunts, bacterial endocarditis, Crohn's disease, ulcerative colitis, sprue, and neoplasms of the esophagus, liver, and small and large bowel. In patients with congenital heart disease with right-to-left shunts, clubbing alone occurs more often than the full syndrome of HOA.

Unilateral clubbing has been found in association with aneurysms of major extremity arteries, infected arterial grafts, and with arteriovenous fistulas of brachial vessels. Clubbing of the toes but not fingers

Table 325-3 Disorders Associated with Hypertrophic Osteoarthropathy

Pulmonary	Cardiovascular
Bronchogenic carcinoma and other neoplasms	Cyanotic congenital heart disease
Lung abscesses, empyema, bronchiectasis	Subacute bacterial endocarditis
Chronic interstitial pneumonitis	Infected arterial grafts[a]
Cystic fibrosis	Aortic aneurysm[b]
Chronic obstructive lung disease	Aneurysm of major extremity artery[a]
Sarcoidosis	Patent ductus arteriosus[b]
Gastrointestinal	Arteriovenous fistula of major extremity vessel[a]
Inflammatory bowel disease	Thyroid (thyroid acropachy)
Sprue	Hyperthyroidism (Graves' disease)
Neoplasms: esophagus, liver, bowel	

[a] Unilateral involvement.
[b] Bilateral lower extremity involvement.

has been associated with an infected abdominal aortic aneurysm and patent ductus arteriosus. Clubbing of a single digit may follow trauma and has been reported in tophaceous gout and sarcoidosis. While clubbing occurs more commonly than the full syndrome in most diseases, periostitis in the absence of clubbing has been observed in the affected limb of patients with infected arterial grafts.

Hyperthyroidism (Graves' disease), treated or untreated, is occasionally associated with clubbing and periostitis of the bones of the hands and feet. This condition is referred to as *thyroid acropachy*. Periostitis is asymptomatic and occurs in the midshaft and diaphyseal portion of the metacarpal and phalangeal bones. The long bones of the extremities are seldom affected. Elevated levels of long-acting thyroid stimulator (LATS) are found in the serum of these patients.

Laboratory Findings The laboratory abnormalities reflect the underlying disorder. The synovial fluid of involved joints has <500 white cells per microliter, and the cells are predominantly mononuclear. Radiographs show a faint radiolucent line beneath the new periosteal bone along the shaft of long bones at their distal end. These changes are observed most frequently at the ankles, wrists, and knees. The ends of the distal phalanges may show osseous resorption. Radionuclide studies show pericortical linear uptake along the cortical margins of long bones that may be present before any radiographic changes.

℞ TREATMENT The treatment of HOA is to identify the associated disorder and treat it appropriately. The symptoms and signs of HOA may disappear completely with removal or effective chemotherapy of a tumor or with antibiotic therapy and drainage of a chronic pulmonary infection. Vagotomy or percutaneous block of the vagus nerve leads to symptomatic relief in some patients. Aspirin, other nonsteroidal anti-inflammatory drugs (NSAIDs), or analgesics may help control symptoms of HOA.

FIBROMYALGIA Fibromyalgia is a commonly encountered disorder characterized by widespread musculoskeletal pain, stiffness, paresthesia, nonrestorative sleep, and easy fatigability along with multiple tender points which are widely and symmetrically distributed. Fibromyalgia affects predominantly women in a ratio of 8 or 9 to 1 compared to men. This disorder is found in most countries, in most ethnic groups, and in all types of climates. The prevalence of fibromyalgia in the general population of a community in the United States using the 1990 American College of Rheumatology (ACR) classification criteria was reported to be 3.4% in women and 0.5% in men. Contrary to some previous reports, fibromyalgia was not found to be present mainly in young women but, rather, to be most prevalent in women ≥50 years. The prevalence increased with age, being 7.4% in women between the ages of 70 and 79. Although not common, fibromyalgia also occurs in children. The reported prevalence of fibromyalgia in some rheumatology clinics has been as high as 20%.

Pathogenesis Several causative mechanisms for fibromyalgia have been postulated. Disturbed sleep has been implicated as a factor in the pathogenesis. Nonrestorative sleep or awakening unrefreshed has been observed in most patients with fibromyalgia. Sleep electroencephalographic studies in patients with fibromyalgia have shown disruption of normal stage 4 sleep [non–rapid eye movement (NREM) sleep] by many repeated α-wave intrusions. The idea that stage 4 sleep deprivation has a role in causing this disorder was supported by the observation that symptoms of fibromyalgia developed in normal subjects whose stage 4 sleep was disrupted artificially by induced α-wave intrusions. This sleep disturbance, however, has been demonstrated in healthy individuals; in emotionally distressed individuals; and in patients with sleep apnea, fever, osteoarthritis, or rheumatoid arthritis. Low levels of serotonin metabolites have been reported in the cerebrospinal fluid of patients with fibromyalgia, suggesting that a deficiency of serotonin, a neurotransmitter that regulates pain and NREM sleep, might also be involved in the pathogenesis of fibromyalgia. Drugs that affect serotonin metabolism have not had a dramatic effect on fibromyalgia, however. Since patients experience pain from muscle and musculotendinous sites, many studies have been done to examine muscle, both structurally and physiologically. Inflammation or diagnostic muscle abnormalities have not been found. Evidence indicates deconditioning of muscles, and patients experience a greater degree of postexertional pain than do unaffected persons. Fibromyalgia patients as a group have been reported by some investigators to have reduced levels of growth hormone, which is important for muscle repair and strength. Growth hormone is secreted normally during stage 4 sleep, which is disturbed in patients with fibromyalgia. The reduction of growth hormone may explain the extended periods of muscle pain following exertion in these patients. The level of the neurotransmitter substance P has been reported to be increased in the cerebrospinal fluid of fibromyalgia patients and may play a role in spreading muscle pain. Patients with fibromyalgia have a decreased cortisol response to stress. Low urinary free cortisol and a diminished cortisol response to corticotropin-releasing hormone suggest an abnormal hypothalamic-pituitary-adrenal axis. Disturbances of the autonomic and peripheral nervous systems may account for the cold sensitivity and Raynaud's-like symptoms seen in patients with fibromyalgia.

Many patients with fibromyalgia have psychological abnormalities; there has been disagreement as to whether some of these abnormalities represent reactions to the chronic pain or whether the symptoms of fibromyalgia are a reflection of psychiatric disturbance. Many patients fit a psychiatric diagnosis, the most common being depression, anxiety, somatization, and hypochondriases. Studies have also shown a high prevalence of sexual and physical abuse and eating disorders. However, fibromyalgia also occurs in patients without significant psychiatric problems. Patients with fibromyalgia may have a lower pain threshold than usual, although not all investigators in the field agree on this point. A better understanding of fibromyalgia awaits further studies.

Clinical Manifestations Symptoms are generalized aching and stiffness of the trunk, hip, and shoulder girdles. Other patients complain of generalized muscle aching and weakness. Patients may complain of low back pain, which may radiate into the buttocks and legs. Others complain of pain and tightness in the neck and across the upper posterior shoulders. Patients complain of muscle pain after even mild exertion. Some degree of pain is always present. The pain has been described as a burning or gnawing pain or as soreness, stiffness, or aching. While pain may begin in one region, such as the shoulders, neck, or lower back, it eventually becomes widespread. Patients may complain of joint pain and perceive that their joints are swollen; however, joint examination yields normal findings. Stiffness is usually present on arising in the morning; usually it improves during the day, but in some patients it lasts all day. Patients may complain of numbness of their hands and feet. They may also feel colder overall than others in the home, and some may experience Raynaud's-like phenomena or actual Raynaud's phenomenon. Patients complain of feeling fatigued and exhausted and wake up tired. They also awaken frequently at night and have trouble falling back to sleep. Symptoms are made worse by stress or anxiety, cold, damp weather, and overexertion. Patients often feel better during warmer weather and vacations.

The characteristic feature on physical examination is the demonstration of specific tender points, which are exclusively more tender or painful than adjacent areas. The ACR Criteria for Fibromyalgia defines 18 tender points (Fig. 325-2). These points of tenderness are remarkably constant in location. A moderate degree of pressure should be used in digital palpation of these tender points. Some workers recommend that the tender site be palpated using a rolling motion, which may be more effective in eliciting the tenderness. The tender sites can also be examined using a dolorimeter, which is a spring-loaded pressure gauge. Digital palpation appears to be as effective and accurate for the diagnosis of fibromyalgia as dolorimetry. The amount of pressure applied by the examiner introduces variability in the interpretation, however. If too much pressure is applied, the pain will be produced even in normal subjects. Likewise, tenderness will not be appreciated if too little pressure is applied or the site is missed on palpation. Some investigators have quantitated their response, but the number of tender point sites is more diagnostic. Some patients are tender all over and not just at the specific tender point sites. These patients are still more tender over the specific tender point sites, however. Sites where there is usually no tenderness and which can be used as controls are the dorsum of the third digit between the proximal interphalangeal and distal interphalangeal joints, the medial third of the clavicle, the medial malleolus, and the forehead. If tenderness at these sites is also present, the diagnosis of fibromyalgia should be questioned and possible psychiatric disorders investigated. Whether such patients can be diagnosed as also having fibromyalgia is debatable.

Skinfold tenderness may be present, particularly over the upper

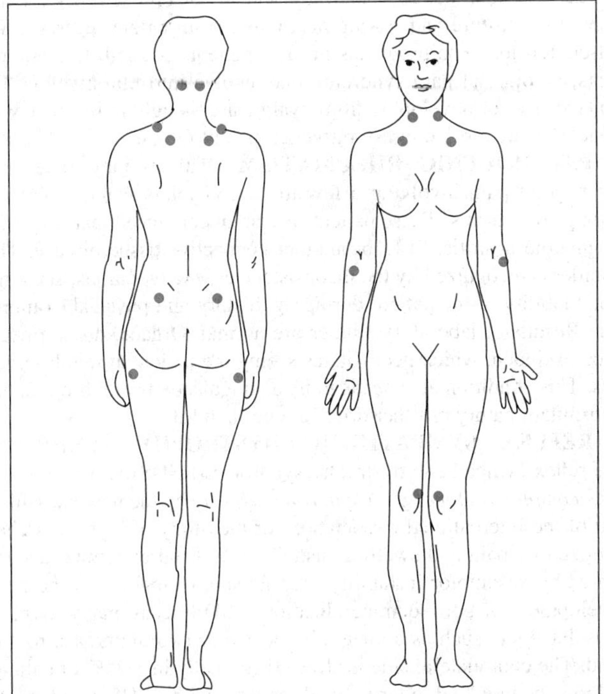

FIGURE 325-2 Tender points in fibromyalgia. Suboccipital muscle insertion at base of skull; anterior aspect of intertransverse process spaces at C5–7; midpoint of upper border of trapezius muscle; above scapular spine near medial border of scapula; second costochondral junction; lateral epicondyle; upper outer quadrant of buttocks; posterior aspect of trochanteric prominence; medial fat pad of knee (all bilateral). *(From the brochure "Fibromyalgia," Arthritis Information, Advise and Guidance, Disease Series. Used by permission of the Arthritis Foundation.)*

scapular region. Subcutaneous nodules may be felt at sites of tenderness. Nodules in similar locations are present in normal persons but are not tender.

Fibromyalgia may be triggered by emotional stress, medical illness, surgery, hypothyroidism, and trauma. It has appeared in some patients with human immunodeficiency virus (HIV) infection, parvovirus B19 infection, or Lyme disease. In the latter situation, fibromyalgia persisted despite adequate antibiotic treatment for Lyme disease. Disorders commonly associated with fibromyalgia include irritable bowel syndrome, irritable bladder, headaches (including migraine headaches), dysmenorrhea, premenstrual syndrome, restless legs syndrome, temporomandibular joint pain, and sicca syndrome.

The course of fibromyalgia is variable. Symptoms wax and wane in some patients, while in others pain and fatigue are persistent regardless of therapy. Studies from tertiary medical centers indicate a poor prognosis for most patients. The prognosis may be better in community-treated patients. In a community-based study reported after 2 years of treatment, 24% of patients were in remission, and 47% no longer fulfilled the ACR criteria for fibromyalgia.

Diagnosis Fibromyalgia is diagnosed by a history of widespread pain and the demonstration of at least 11 of the 18 tender point sites on digital palpation (Fig. 325-2). The ACR criteria are useful for standardizing the diagnosis; however, not all patients with fibromyalgia meet these criteria (Table 325-4). Some patients have fewer tender sites and more regional pain and may be considered to have probable fibromyalgia.

Results of joint and muscle examinations are normal in fibromyalgia patients, and there are no laboratory abnormalities. Fibromyalgia may occur in patients with rheumatoid arthritis, other connective tissue diseases, or other medical illness. A distinction is no longer made between primary and secondary fibromyalgia (concomitant with other disease), as the signs and symptoms are similar. Fibromyalgia and chronic fatigue syndrome have many similarities (Chap. 384). Both are associated with fatigue, abnormal sleep, musculoskeletal pain, and psychiatric conditions such as less severe forms of de-

Table 325-4 The American College of Rheumatology 1990 Criteria for the Classification of Fibromyalgia[a]

1. History of widespread pain. Pain is considered widespread when all of the following are present:
   a. Pain in the left side of the body
   b. Pain in the right side of the body
   c. Pain above the waist
   d. Pain below the waist
   e. Axial skeletal pain (cervical spine or anterior chest or thoracic spine or low back)
2. Pain on digital palpation in at least 11 of the following 18 tender point sites (see Fig. 325-2):
   a. Occiput: bilateral, at the suboccipital muscle insertion
   b. Low cervical: bilateral, at the anterior aspect of the intertransverse spaces at C5–7
   c. Trapezius: bilateral, at the midpoint of the upper border
   d. Supraspinatus: bilateral, at the origin, above the scapular spine near the medial border
   e. Second rib: bilateral, at the second costochondral junction, just lateral to the junction on the upper surface
   f. Lateral epicondyle: bilateral, 2 cm distal to the epicondyle
   g. Gluteal: bilateral, in the upper outer quadrant of the buttock
   h. Greater trochanter: bilateral, posterior to the trochanteric prominence
   i. Knee: bilateral, at the medial fat pad proximal to the joint line

Digital palpation should be performed with a moderate degree of pressure. For a tender point to be considered positive, the subject must state that the palpation was painful. "Tender" is not to be considered painful.

[a] For purposes of classification, patients will be said to have fibromyalgia if both criteria are satisfied. Widespread pain must have been present for at least 3 months. The presence of a second clinical disorder does not exclude the diagnosis of fibromyalgia.

SOURCE: Modified from F Wolfe et al: Arthritis Rheum 33:171, 1990.

pression and anxiety. Patients with chronic fatigue syndrome, however, are more likely to have symptoms suggesting a viral illness. These include mild fever, sore throat, and pain in the axillary and anterior and posterior cervical lymph nodes. The onset of chronic fatigue syndrome is usually sudden; patients are usually able to date the onset. Patients also have impaired memory and concentration. While many patients with chronic fatigue syndrome have tender points, the diagnosis does not require their presence. Polymyalgia rheumatica is distinguished from fibromyalgia in an elderly patient by the presence of more proximal muscle stiffness and pain and an elevated erythrocyte sedimentation rate. Patients should be evaluated for hypothyroidism, which may have symptoms similar to fibromyalgia or may accompany fibromyalgia.

The diagnosis of fibromyalgia has taken on a more complex significance in regard to labor and industry issues. This has become a significant issue since it has been reported that 10 to 25% of patients are not able to work in any capacity, while others require modification of their work. Disability evaluation in fibromyalgia is controversial. The diagnosis of fibromyalgia is not accepted by all. It is hard to evaluate patients' perceptions of their inability to function. The determination of tender points can also be subjective, on the part of both the physician and the patient, particularly when issues of compensation are pending. Patients also encounter difficulty in having their illness recognized as a disability. Physicians have been placed in the inappropriate role of assessing the patient's disability. Physicians are not in a position to quantitate disability at the workplace; that is better done by a work evaluation specialist. Better instruments are clearly needed for measuring disability, particularly in patients with fibromyalgia.

℞ **TREATMENT** Patients should be informed that they have a condition that is not crippling, deforming, or degenerative, and that treatment is available. Salicylates or other NSAIDs only partially improve symptoms. Glucocorticoids have been of little benefit and should not be used in these patients. Opiate analgesics should be avoided. Local measures such as heat, massage, injection of tender sites with steroids or lidocaine, and acupuncture provide only temporary relief of symptoms. Other therapies that may help to varying degrees including biofeedback, behavioral modification, hypnotherapy, and stress management and relaxation response training. The use of tricyclics such as amitriptyline (10 to 50 mg) and doxepin (10 to 25 mg) or a pharmacologically similar drug, cyclobenzaprine (10 to 40 mg), 1 to 2 h before bedtime will give the patient restorative sleep (stage 4 sleep), resulting in clinical improvement. Patients should be started on a low dose, which is increased gradually as needed. Side effects of these tricyclics and cyclobenzoprine limit their use; these include constipation, dry mouth, weight gain, drowsiness, and difficulty thinking. Depression and anxiety should be treated with appropriate drugs and, when indicated, with psychiatric counseling. Alprazolam and lorazepam can be used for anxiety, while trazodone, sertraline, fluoxetine, paroxetine or other newer selective serotonin reuptake inhibitors can be used as antidepressants. Patients may also benefit by regular aerobic exercises. Exercise should be of a low-impact type and begun at a low level. Eventually, the patient should be exercising 20 to 30 min 3 to 4 days a week. Regular stretching exercises are also very important. Life stresses should be identified and discussed with the patient, and the patient should be provided with help on how to cope with these stresses. Patients may benefit from a multidisciplinary team approach involving a mental health professional, a physical therapist, and a physical medicine and rehabilitation specialist. Group therapy may be beneficial. Patients should be well educated about their disorder and taught the importance of self help. There are patient support groups in many communities. While treatment of fibromyalgia is effective in some patients, others continue to have chronic disease, which is relieved only partially if at all.

MYOFASCIAL PAIN SYNDROME Myofascial pain syndrome is characterized by localized musculoskeletal pain and tenderness in association with trigger points. The pain is deep and aching and may be accompanied by a burning sensation. Myofascial pain may follow trauma, overuse, or prolonged static contraction of a muscle or muscle group, which may occur when reading or writing at a desk or working at a computer. In addition, this syndrome may be associated with underlying osteoarthritis of the neck or low back. Trigger points are a diagnostic feature of this syndrome. Pain is referred from trigger points to defined areas distant from the original tender points. Palpation of the trigger point reproduces or accentuates the pain. The trigger points are usually located in the center of a muscle belly, but they can occur at other sites, such as costosternal junctions, the xyphoid process, ligamentous and tendinous insertions, fascia, and fatty areas. Trigger point sites in muscle have been described as feeling indurated and taut, and palpation may cause the muscle to twitch. These findings, however, have been shown not to be unique for myofascial pain syndrome, since in a controlled study they were also present in fibromyalgia patients and normal subjects. Myofascial pain most often involves the posterior neck, low back, shoulders, and chest. Chronic pain in the muscles of the posterior neck may involve referral of pain from the trigger point in the erector neck muscle or upper trapezius to the head, leading to persistent headaches which may last for days. Trigger points in the paraspinal muscles of the low back may refer pain to the buttock. Pain may be referred down the leg from a trigger point in the gluteus medius and can mimic sciatica. A trigger point in the infraspinatus muscle may produce local and referred pain over the lateral deltoid and down the outside of the arm into the hand. Injection of a local anesthetic such as 1% lidocaine into the trigger point site often results in pain relief. Another useful technique is first to spray from the trigger point toward the area of referred pain with an agent such as ethyl chloride and then to stretch the muscle. This maneuver may need to be repeated several times. Massage and application of ultrasound to the affected area may also be beneficial. Patients should be instructed in methods to prevent muscle stresses related to work and recreation. Posture and resting positions are important in preventing muscle tension. The prognosis in most patients is good. In some patients, myofascial pain syndrome may evolve into fibromyalgia. Patients at risk for developing fibromyalgia are thought to be those with anxiety, depression, nonrestorative sleep, and fatigue.

PSYCHOGENIC RHEUMATISM Patients may experience severe joint pain involving a few to several joints without physical findings of arthritis. These patients are often convinced that they have rheumatoid arthritis, SLE, or another connective tissue disease. This disorder is recognized by the inconsistencies, exaggerations, and emotional lability of the patient during the history and physical examination. Results of laboratory studies are normal. Organic disease needs to be excluded, which necessitates seeing the patient at regular intervals. This condition also needs to be distinguished from fibromyalgia. Anti-inflammatory or other drugs are not helpful.

REFLEX SYMPATHETIC DYSTROPHY SYNDROME The reflex sympathetic dystrophy syndrome (RSDS) is now referred to as *complex regional pain syndrome, type 1*, by the new Classification of the International Association for the Study of Pain. It is characterized by pain and swelling, usually of a distal extremity, accompanied by vasomotor instability, trophic skin changes, and the rapid development of bony demineralization. RSDS occasionally involves an isolated site such as a knee, hip, or one or two digits of a foot or hand. The contralateral side is affected clinically in ~25% of patients and may be involved in virtually all patients with RSDS, as shown by scintigraphic studies. A precipitating event can be identified in at least two-thirds of cases. These events include trauma, such as fractures and crush injuries; myocardial infarction; strokes; peripheral nerve injury; and use of certain drugs, including barbiturates, anti-tuberculous drugs, and, more recently, cyclosporine administered to patients undergoing renal transplantation. The pathogenesis of RSDS is poorly understood and is thought to involve abnormal activity of the sympathetic nervous system following a precipitating event.

RSDS evolves through three clinical phases. The first phase is characterized by an intense burning pain and swelling of a distal extremity. The involved extremity is warm, edematous, and very tender, especially around joints. Sweating and hair growth are increased. Light touch causes pain, which may continue after the stimulus is removed. Passive or active motion of joints is very painful, and the joints are stiff. In the first phase, especially when both sides are involved, the clinical findings may suggest early rheumatoid arthritis. Redness and swelling over a distal extremity such as an ankle or wrist may also mimic inflammatory arthritis, or even an infectious arthritis. In 3 to 6 months, the skin gradually becomes thin, shiny, and cool. This is the second phase of the disease. The clinical features of the first and second phases often overlap. In another 3 to 6 months (third phase), the skin becomes atrophic and dry, and irreversible flexion contractures, palmar fibromatosis, and Dupuytren's contractures develop, resulting in a clawlike hand deformity. Similar changes occur in the feet. When RSDS occurs in the upper extremity, motion of the shoulder on the affected side may be painful and restricted, a condition referred to as *shoulder-hand syndrome* (see "Adhesive Capsulitis," below). →***Reflex sympathetic dystrophy syndrome, including its treatment, is covered in greater detail in Chap. 366.***

TIETZE'S SYNDROME AND COSTOCHONDRITIS Tietze's syndrome is manifested by painful swelling of one or more costochondral articulations. The age of onset is usually before 40, and both sexes are affected equally. In most patients only one joint is involved, usually the second or third costochondral joint. The onset of anterior chest pain may be sudden or gradual. The pain may radiate to the arms or shoulder and is aggravated by sneezing, coughing, deep inspirations, or twisting motions of the chest. The term *costochondritis* is often used interchangeably with *Tietze's syndrome*, but some workers restrict the former term to pain of the costochondral articulations without swelling. Costochondritis is observed in patients over age 40; tends to affect the third, fourth, and fifth costochondral joints; and occurs more often in women. Both syndromes may mimic cardiac or upper abdominal causes of pain. Rheumatoid arthritis, ankylosing spondylitis, and Reiter's syndrome may involve costochondral joints but are distinguished easily by their other clinical features. Other skeletal causes of anterior chest wall pain are xiphoidalgia and the slipping rib syndrome, which usually involves the tenth rib. Malignancies such as breast cancer, prostate cancer, plasma cell cytoma, and sarcoma can invade the ribs, thoracic spine, or chest wall and produce symptoms suggesting Tietze's syndrome. They should be easily distinguishable by radiographs and biopsy. Analgesics, anti-inflammatory drugs, and local glucocorticoid injections usually relieve symptoms.

MUSCULOSKELETAL DISORDERS ASSOCIATED WITH HYPERLIPIDEMIA (See also Chap. 344) Musculoskeletal manifestations may be the first indication of a hereditary disorder of lipoprotein metabolism. Patients with familial hypercholesterolemia (previously referred to as type II hyperlipoproteinemia) may have recurrent migratory polyarthritis involving knees and other large peripheral joints and, to a lesser degree, peripheral small joints. In a few patients, the arthritis is monarticular. Fever may accompany the arthritis. Pain ranges from moderate to very severe to incapacitating. The involved joints can be warm, erythematous, swollen, and tender. Arthritis usually has a sudden onset, lasts from a few days to 2 weeks, and does not cause joint damage. Episodes may suggest acute gout attacks. Several attacks occur a year. Synovial fluid from involved joints is not inflammatory and contains few white cells and no crystals. Joint involvement may actually represent inflammatory periarthritis or peritendinitis and not intraarticular disease. The recurrent, transient nature of the arthritis may suggest rheumatic fever, especially since patients with lipoproteinemia have an elevated erythrocyte sedimentation rate, and a falsely elevated antistreptolysin O titer. Patients may also experience Achilles tendinitis, which can be very painful. Attacks of tendinitis come on gradually and last only a few days. Fever is not present. Patients may be asymptomatic between attacks. During an attack the Achilles tendon is warm, erythematous, swollen, and tender to palpation. Achilles tendinitis and other joint manifestations often precede the appearance of xanthomas and may be the first clinical indication of hyperlipoproteinemia. Attacks of tendinitis may occur following treatment with a lipid-lowering drug. Patients also have tendinous xanthomas in the Achilles, patellar, and extensor tendons of the hands over the knuckles and feet. Xanthomas have also been reported in the peroneal tendon, the plantar aponeurosis, and the periosteum overlying the distal tibia. These xanthomas are located within tendon fibers. Tuberous xanthomas are soft subcutaneous masses located over the extensor surfaces of the elbows, knees, and hands, as well as on the buttocks. They appear in childhood in homozygous patients and after the age of 30 in heterozygous patients. Patients with elevated plasma levels of very low density lipoprotein (VLDL) and triglyceride (previously referred to as type IV hyperlipoproteinemia) may also have a mild inflammatory arthritis affecting large and small peripheral joints, usually in an asymmetric pattern with only a few joints involved at a time. The onset of arthritis is usually in middle age. Arthritis may be persistent or recurrent, with episodes lasting a few days to weeks. Joint pain is severe in some patients. Patients may experience morning stiffness. Joint tenderness and periarticular hyperesthesia may also be present, as may synovial thickening. Joint fluid is usually noninflammatory and without crystals, but may have increased white blood cell counts with predominantly mononuclear cells. The fluid is occasionally lactescent. Radiographs may show juxtaarticular osteopenia and cystic lesions. Large bone cysts have been noted in a few patients. Xanthoma and bone cysts are also observed in other lipoprotein disorders. The pathogenesis of arthritis in patients with familial hypercholesterolemia or with elevated levels of VLDL and triglyceride is not well understood. Salicylates, other NSAIDs, or analgesics usually provide relief of symptoms. Clinical improvement also may occur in patients treated with lipid lowering agents. Patients, however, treated with a HMG CoA reductase agent may experience myalgias and a few patients may develop polymysitis or even rhabdomyolysis (Chap. 382).

ARTHROPATHY OF ACROMEGALY Acromegaly is the result of excessive production of growth hormone by an adenoma in the anterior pituitary gland (Chap. 328). Middle-aged persons are most often affected. The excessive secretion of growth hormone along with insulin-like growth factor I stimulates proliferation of cartilage, periarticular connective tissue, and bone, resulting in several musculoskeletal abnormalities, including osteoarthritis, back pain, muscle weakness, and carpal tunnel syndrome.

An arthropathy resembling osteoarthritis is a common feature, affecting most often the knees, shoulders, hips, and hands. Single or multiple joints may be affected. The overgrowth of cartilage initially produces widening of the joint space. The newly synthesized cartilage is not developed in an organized manner, making it susceptible to fissuring, ulceration, and destruction. Ligamental laxity of the joint resulting from the growth of connective tissue also contributes to the development of osteoarthritis. With breakdown and loss of cartilage, the joint space narrows, and subchondral sclerosis and osteophytes appear on radiographs. Joint examination reveals marked crepitus and hypermobility. Joint fluid is noninflammatory. Calcium pyrophosphate dihydrate crystals are found in the cartilage in some cases of acromegaly arthropathy and, when shed into the joint, can produce attacks of pseudogout. Chondrocalcinosis may also be observed radiographically. Approximately half of the patients with acromegaly experience back pain, which is predominantly lumbosacral. Hypermobility of the spine may be a contributing factor in back pain. Radiograph of the spine shows normal or increased intervertebral disk spaces, hypertrophic anterior osteophytes, and ligamental calcification. These changes are similar to those observed in patients with diffuse idiopathic skeletal hyperostosis. Dorsal kyphosis in conjunction with elongation of the ribs contributes to the development of the barrel chest seen in acromegalic patients. The hands and feet become enlarged owing to soft tissue proliferation. The fingers are thickened and have spadelike distal tufts. One-third of patients have a thickened heel pad. Approximately 25% of patients have Raynaud's phenomenon.

Carpal tunnel syndrome occurs in about half of patients. The median nerve is compressed by the excessive growth of connective tissue in the carpal tunnel. The median nerve also becomes enlarged. Patients with acromegaly also develop proximal muscle weakness, which is thought to be caused by the effect of growth hormone on muscle. Results of muscle enzyme assays and electromyography are normal. Muscle biopsy specimens show muscle fibers of varying size and no inflammatory changes.

ARTHROPATHY OF HEMOCHROMATOSIS Hemochromatosis is a disorder of iron storage. Excessive amounts of iron are absorbed from the intestine, leading to iron deposition in parenchymal cells, which results in tissue damage and impairment of organ function (Chap. 345). Symptoms of hemochromatosis usually begin between the ages of 40 and 60 but can occur earlier. Arthritis, which occurs in 20 to 40% of patients, usually begins after the age of 50 and may be the first clinical feature of hemochromatosis. The arthropathy is an inflammatory osteoarthritis-like disorder affecting the small joints of the hands, followed later by larger joints such as knees, ankles, shoulders, and hips. The second and third metacarpophalangeal joints of both hands are often the first joints affected; they can provide an important clue to the possibility of hemochromatosis. Patients experience stiffness and pain. Morning stiffness usually lasts less than half an hour. The affected joints are enlarged and mildly tender. Synovial tissue is not appreciatively increased. Radiographs show irregular narrowing of the joint space, subchondral sclerosis, and subchondral cysts. There is juxtaarticular proliferation of bone, with frequent hooklike osteophytes. The synovial fluid is noninflammatory. The synovium shows mild to moderate proliferation of lining cells, fibrosis, and a low number of inflammatory cells, which are mononuclear. In approximately half of patients, there is evidence of calcium pyrophosphate deposition disease. Iron can be demonstrated in the lining cells of the synovium and also in chondrocytes.

Iron may damage the articular cartilage in several ways. Promotion by iron of superoxide-dependent lipid peroxidation may play a role in joint damage. In animal models, ferric iron has been shown to interfere with collagen formation. Iron has also been shown to increase the release of lysosomal enzymes from cells in the synovial membrane. Iron may also play a role in the development of chondrocalcinosis. Iron inhibits synovial tissue pyrophosphatase in vitro and, therefore, may inhibit pyrophosphatase in vivo, resulting in chondrocalcinosis. Iron in synovial cells may also inhibit the clearance of calcium pyrophosphate from the joint.

℞ TREATMENT The treatment of hemochromatosis is repeated phlebotomy. Unfortunately, this treatment has little effect on the arthritis, which, along with chondrocalcinosis, usually continues to progress. Treatment of the arthritis consists of administration of acetaminophen and NSAIDs. Placement of a hip or knee prosthesis has been successful in advanced disease.

HEMOPHILIC ARTHROPATHY Hemophilia is a sex-linked recessive genetic disorder characterized by the absence or deficiency of factor VIII (hemophilia A, or classic hemophilia) or factor IX (hemophilia B, or Christmas disease) (Chap. 117). Hemophilia A is by far the more common type, constituting 85% of cases. Spontaneous hemarthrosis is a common problem with both types of hemophilia and can lead to a chronic deforming arthritis. The frequency and severity of hemarthrosis are related to the degree of clotting factor deficiency. Hemarthrosis is not common in other inherited disorders of coagulation, such as von Willebrand's disease or factor V deficiency.

Hemarthrosis becomes evident after 1 year of age, when the child begins to walk and run. In order of frequency, the joints most commonly affected are the knees, ankles, elbows, shoulders, and hips. Small joints of the hands and feet are occasionally involved.

In the initial stage of arthropathy, hemarthrosis produces a warm, tensely swollen, and painful joint. The patient holds the affected joint in flexion and guards against any movement. Blood in the joint remains liquid because of the absence of intrinsic clotting factors and the absence of tissue thromboplastin in the synovium. The blood in the joint space is resorbed over a period of a week or longer, depending on the size of the hemarthrosis. Joint function usually returns to normal or baseline in about 2 weeks.

Recurrent hemarthrosis leads to the development of a chronic arthritis. The involved joints remain swollen, and flexion deformities develop. In the later stages of arthropathy, joint motion is restricted and function is severely limited. Joint ankylosis, subluxation, or laxity are features of end-stage disease.

Bleeding into muscle and soft tissue also causes musculoskeletal disorders. When bleeding into the iliopsoas muscle occurs, the hip is held in flexion because of the pain, resulting in a hip flexion contracture. Rotation of the hip is preserved, which distinguishes this problem from intraarticular hemorrhage. Expansion of the hematoma may place pressure on the femoral nerve, resulting in a femoral neuropathy. Another problem is shortening of the heel cord secondary to bleeding into the gastrocnemius. Hemorrhage into a closed compartment space, such as the volar compartment in the forearm, can result in muscle necrosis and flexion deformities of the wrist and fingers. When bleeding involves periosteum or bone, a pseudotumor forms. These occur distal to the elbows or knees in children and improve with treatment of the hemophilia. Surgical removal is indicated if the pseudotumor continues to enlarge. In adults, they occur in the femur and pelvis and are usually refractory to treatment. When bleeding occurs in muscle, cysts may develop within the muscle. Needle aspiration of a cyst is contraindicated because it can induce bleeding.

Septic arthritis can occur in hemophilia and is difficult at times to distinguish from acute hemarthrosis. Whenever there is suspicion of an infected joint, the joint should be aspirated immediately, the fluid cultured, and the patient started on a broad-spectrum antibiotic. The patient should be infused with the deficient clotting factor before the joint is tapped to decrease the risk of further bleeding.

Radiographs of joints reflect the stage of disease. In early stages there is only capsule distention; later, juxtaarticular osteopenia, marginal erosions, and subchondral cysts develop. In late disease, the joint space is narrowed and there is bony overgrowth. The changes are similar to those observed in osteoarthritis. Unique features of hemophilic arthropathy are widening of the femoral intercondylar notch, enlargement of the proximal radius, and squaring of the distal end of the patella.

Recurrent hemarthrosis produces synovial hyperplasia and hypertrophy. A pannus covers the cartilage. Cartilage is damaged by collagenase and other degradative enzymes released by mononuclear cells in the overlying synovium. Hemosiderin is found in synovial lining cells, the subsynovium, and chondrocytes and may also play a role in cartilage destruction.

℞ TREATMENT The treatment of hemarthrosis is initiated with the immediate infusion of factor VIII or IX at the first sign of joint or muscle hemorrhage. The patient is placed at bed rest, with the involved joint in as much extension as the patient can tolerate. Analgesic NSAIDs and local icing may help with the pain. NSAIDs can be given safely for short periods even though they have a stabilizing effect on platelets. Studies have shown no significant abnormalities in platelet function or bleeding time in hemophiliacs receiving ibuprofen. The new cyclooxygenase-2 inhibitors celecoxib and rofecoxib do not interfere with platelet function and can be safely given for pain. Synovectomy, open or arthroscopic, may be indicated in patients with chronic synovial proliferation and recurrent hemarthrosis. Hypertrophied synovium is very vascular and subject to bleeding. Both types of synovectomy reduce the number of hemarthroses and slow the roentgenographic progression of hemophilic arthropathy. Open surgical synovectomy, however, is associated with some loss of range of motion. Radiosynovectomy with either yttrium 90 silicate or phosphorus 31 colloid has also been effective and may be a useful alternative when surgical synovectomy is not practical. Total joint replacement is indicated for severe joint destruction and incapacitating pain. Because of the young age of hemophilic patients, total-joint prostheses may need to be replaced more than once during their lives.

ARTHROPATHIES ASSOCIATED WITH HEMOGLOBINOPATHIES **Sickle Cell Disease** Sickle cell disease (Chap. 106) is associated with several musculoskeletal abnormalities (Table 325-5). Children under the age of 5 may develop diffuse swelling, tenderness, and warmth of the hands and feet lasting from 1 to 3 weeks. The condition, referred to as *sickle cell dactylitis* or *hand-foot syndrome* has also been observed in sickle cell disease and sickle cell thalassemia. Dactylitis is believed to result from infarction of the bone marrow and cortical bone leading to periostitis and soft tissue swelling. Radiographs show periosteal elevation, subperiosteal new bone formation, and areas of radiolucency and increased density involving the metacarpals, metatarsals, and proximal phalanges. These bone changes disappear after several months. The syndrome leaves little or no residual damage. Because hematopoiesis ceases in the small bones of hands and feet with age, the syndrome is rarely seen after age 4 or 5 and does not occur in adults.

Sickle cell crisis is often associated with periarticular pain and joint effusions. The joint and periarticular area are warm and tender. Knees and elbows are most often affected, but other joints can be involved. Joint effusions are noninflammatory, with white cell counts <1000/μL; mononuclear cells predominate. There have been a few reports of sterile inflammatory effusion with high cell counts consisting of mostly polymorphonuclear white cells. Synovial biopsies have shown mild lining cell proliferation and microvascular thrombosis. Scintigraphic studies have shown decreased marrow uptake adjacent to the involved joint. The joint effusion and periarticular pain are considered to be the result of ischemia and infarction of the synovium and adjacent bone and bone marrow. The treatment is that for sickle cell crisis (Chap. 106).

Patients with sickle cell disease may also develop osteomyelitis, which commonly involves the long tubular bones (Chap. 129). These patients are particularly susceptible to bacterial infections, especially *Salmonella* infections, which are found in more than half of cases (Chap. 156). Radiographs of the involved site show periosteal elevation initially, followed by disruption of the cortex. Treatment of the infection results in healing of the bone lesion. Sickle cell disease is also associated with bone infarction resulting from thrombosis secondary to the sickling of red cells. Bone infarction also occurs in hemoglobin S-C disease and sickle cell thalassemia (Chap. 106). The bone pain in sickle cell crisis is due to bone and bone marrow infarction. In children, infarction of the epiphyseal growth plate interferes with normal growth of the affected extremity. Radiographically, infarction of the bone cortex results in periosteal elevation and irregular thickening of the bone cortex. Infarction in the bone marrow leads to lysis, fibrosis, and new bone formation.

Avascular necrosis of the head of the femur is seen in ~5% of patients. It also occurs in the humeral head and less commonly in the distal femur, tibial condyles, distal radius, vertebral bodies, and other juxtaarticular sites. The mechanism for avascular necrosis is most likely the same as for bone infarction. Subchondral hemorrhage may play a role in the deterioration of articular cartilage. Irregularity of the femoral head or of other bone surfaces affected by avascular necrosis eventually results in degenerative joint disease. Radiograph of the affected joint may show patchy radiolucency and density followed by

Table 325-5 Musculoskeletal Abnormalities in Sickle Cell Disease

Sickle cell dactylitis	Avascular necrosis
Joint effusions in sickle cell crises	Bone changes secondary to marrow hyperplasia
Osteomyelitis	Septic arthritis
Infarction of bone	Gouty arthritis
Infarction of bone marrow	

flattening of the bone. Magnetic resonance imaging is a sensitive technique for detecting early avascular necrosis as well as bone infarction elsewhere. Total hip replacement and placement of prostheses in other joints may improve function and relieve pain in those patients with severe joint destruction.

Septic arthritis is occasionally encountered in sickle cell disease (Chap. 323). Multiple joints may be infected. Joint infection may result from hematogenous spread or from spread of contiguous osteomyelitis. Microorganisms identified include staphylococcus, *Streptococcus*, *Escherichia coli*, and *Salmonella*. The latter is not seen as frequently in septic arthritis as it is in osteomyelitis. Acute gouty arthritis is uncommon in sickle cell disease, even though 40% of patients are hyperuremic. Hyperuricemia is due to overproduction of uric acid secondary to increased red cell turnover. Attacks may be polyarticular.

The bone marrow hyperplasia in sickle cell disease results in widening of the medullary cavities, thinning of the cortices, and coarse trabeculations and central cupping of the vertebral bodies. These changes are also seen to a lesser degree in hemoglobin S-C disease and sickle cell thalassemia. In normal individuals, red marrow is located mostly in the axial skeletal, but in sickle cell disease, red marrow is found in the bones of the extremities and even in the tarsal and carpal bones. Vertebral compression may lead to dorsal kyphosis, and softening of the bone in the acetabulum may result in protrusio acetabuli.

Thalassemia β-Thalassemia is a congenital disorder of hemoglobin synthesis characterized by impaired production of β chains (Chap. 106). Bone and joint abnormalities occur in β-thalassemia, being most common in the major and intermedia groups. In one study, approximately 50% of patients with β-thalassemia had evidence of symmetric ankle arthropathy, characterized by a dull aching pain aggravated by weight bearing. The onset was most often in the second or third decade of life. The degree of ankle pain in these patients varied. Some patients experienced self-limited ankle pain, which occurred only after strenuous physical activity and lasted several days to weeks. Other patients had chronic ankle pain, which became worse with walking. Symptoms eventually abated in a few patients. Compression of the ankle, calcaneus, or forefoot was painful in some patients. Synovial fluid from two patients was noninflammatory. Radiographs of ankle showed osteopenia, widened medullary spaces, thin cortices, and coarse trabeculations. These findings were largely the result of bone marrow expansion. The joint space was preserved. Specimens of bone from three patients revealed osteomalacia, osteopenia, and microfractures. Increased osteoblasts as well as increased foci of bone resorption were present on the bone surface. Iron staining was found in the bone trabeculae, in osteoid, and in the cement line. Synovium showed hyperplasia of lining cells which contained deposits of hemosiderin. This arthropathy was considered to be related to the underlying bone pathology. The role of iron overload or abnormal bone metabolism in the pathogenesis of this arthropathy is not known. The arthropathy was treated with analgesics and splints. Patients were also transfused to decrease hematopoiesis and bone marrow expansion.

Patients with β-thalassemia major and intermedia also have involvement of other joints, including the knees, hips, and shoulders. Acquired hemochromatosis with arthropathy has been described in a patient with thalassemia. Gouty arthritis and septic arthritis can occur. Avascular necrosis is not a feature of thalassemia because there is no sickling of red cells leading to thrombosis and infarction.

β-Thalassemia minor (trait) is also associated with joint manifestations. Chronic seronegative oligoarthritis affecting predominantly ankles, wrists, and elbows has been described. These patients had mild persistent synovitis without large effusions. Joint erosions were not seen. Recurrent episodes of an acute asymmetric arthritis also have been reported; episodes last less than a week and may affect knees, ankles, shoulders, elbows, wrists, and metacarpal phalangeal joints. The mechanism for this arthropathy is unknown. Treatment with nonsteroidal drugs was not particularly effective.

TUMORS OF JOINTS Primary tumors and tumor-like disorders of synovium are uncommon but should be considered in the differential diagnosis of monarticular joint disease. In addition, metastases to bone and primary bone tumors adjacent to a joint may produce joint symptoms. →*For further discussion, see Chap. 98.*

Pigmented villonodular synovitis is characterized by the slowly progressive, exuberant, benign proliferation of synovial tissue, usually involving a single joint. The most common age of onset is in the third decade, and women are affected slightly more often than men. The cause of this disorder is unknown.

The synovium has a brownish color and numerous large, finger-like villi that fuse to form pedunculated nodules. There is marked hyperplasia of synovial cells in the stroma of the villi. Hemosiderin granules and lipids are found in the cytoplasm of macrophages and in the interstitial tissue. Multinucleated giant cells may be present. The proliferative synovium grows into the subsynovial tissue and invades adjacent cartilage and bone.

The clinical picture of pigmented villonodular synovitis is characterized by the insidious onset of swelling and pain in one joint, most commonly the knee. Other joints affected include the hips, ankles, calcaneocuboid joints, elbows, and small joints of the fingers or toes. The disease may also involve the common flexor sheath of the hand or fingers. Less commonly, tendon sheaths in the wrist, ankle, or foot may be involved. Symptoms may be mild and intermittent and may be present for years before the patient seeks medical attention. Radiographs may show joint space narrowing, erosions, and subchondral cysts. The joint fluid contains blood and is dark red or almost black in color. Lipid-containing macrophages may be present in the fluid. The joint fluid may be clear if hemorrhages have not occurred.

The treatment of pigmented villonodular synovitis is complete synovectomy. With incomplete synovectomy, the villonodular synovitis recurs, and the rate of tissue growth may be faster than originally. Irradiation of the involved joint has been successful in some patients.

Synovial chondromatosis is a disorder characterized by multiple focal metaplastic growths of normal-appearing cartilage in the synovium or tendon sheath. Segments of cartilage break loose and continue to grow as loose bodies. When calcification and ossification of loose bodies occur, the disorder is referred to as *synovial osteochondromatosis*. The disorder is usually monarticular and affects young to middle-aged individuals. The knee is most often involved, followed by hip, elbow, and shoulder. Symptoms are pain, swelling, and decreased motion of the joint. Radiographs may show several rounded calcifications within the joint cavity. Treatment is synovectomy; however, the tumor may recur.

Hemangiomas occur in synovium and in tendon sheaths. The knee is affected most commonly. Recurrent episodes of joint swelling and pain usually begin in childhood. The joint fluid is bloody. Treatment is excision of the lesion. *Lipomas* occur most often in the knee, originating in the subsynovial fat on either side of the patellar tendon. Lipomas also appear in tendon sheaths of the hands, wrists, feet, and ankles. In some instances, surgical removal is necessary.

Synovial sarcoma is a malignant neoplasm often found near a large joint of both upper and lower extremities, being more common in the lower extremity. It seldom arises within the joint itself. Synovial sarcomas comprise 10% of sarcomas. The tumor is believed to arise from primitive mesenchymal tissue which differentiates into epithelial cells and/or spindle cells. Small foci of calcification may be present in the tumor mass. It occurs most often in young adults and is more common in men. The tumor presents as a slowly growing deep seated mass near a joint, without much pain. The area of the knee is the most common site, followed by the foot, ankle, elbow, and shoulder. Other primary sites include the buttocks, abdominal wall, retioperitoneum and mediastinum. The tumor spreads along tissue planes. The most common site of visceral metastasis is lung. The diagnosis is made by biopsy. Treatment is wide resection of the tumor including adjacent muscle and regional lymph nodes, followed by chemotherapy and radiation therapy. Currently used chemotherapeutic agents are doxorubicin, ifosfamide, and cisplatin. Amputation of the involved distal extremity may be required. Chemotherapy may be beneficial in some patients with metastatic disease. Isolated pulmonary mitostasis can be surgically removed. The 5-year survival with treatment has been reported as high as 88%.

BIBLIOGRAPHY

ALTMAN RD, TENENBAUM J: Hypertrophic osteoarthropathy, in *Textbook of Rheumatology*, 5th ed, WN Kelley et al (eds). Philadelphia, Saunders, 1997, pp 1514–1520

ARMAN MI et al: Brief report. Frequency and features of rheumatic findings in thalassaemia minor: A blind controlled study. Br J Rheumatol 31:197, 1992

BENNETT RM: The fibromyalgia syndrome, in *Textbook of Rheumatology*, 5th ed, WN Kelley et al (eds). Philadelphia, Saunders, 1997, pp 511–519

———: Emerging concepts in the neurobiology of chronic pain: Evidence of abnormal sensory processing in fibromyalgia. May Clin Proc 74:385, 1999

CANOSO JJ: Tumors of joints and related structures, in *Arthritis and Allied Conditions*, 13th ed, WJ Koopman (ed.). Baltimore, Williams & Wilkins, 1997, pp 1867–1886

CARELESS DJ, COHEN MG: Rheumatic manifestations of hyperlipidemia and antihyperlipidemia drug therapy. Semin Arthritis Rheum 23:90, 1993

CRONIN ME: Rheumatic aspects of endocrinopathies, in *Arthritis and Allied Conditions*, 13th ed, WJ Koopman (ed). Baltimore, Williams & Wilkins, 1997, pp 2233–2249

ELLMAN MH: Neuropathic joint disease (Charcot joints), in *Arthritis and Allied Conditions*, 13th ed, WJ Koopman (ed). Baltimore, Williams & Wilkins, 1997, pp 1641–1659

GOLDENBERG DL: Fibromyalgia syndrome a decade later: What have we learned? Arch Intern Med 159:777, 1999

HECK LW JR: Arthritis associated with hematologic disorders, storage diseases, disorders of lipid metabolism, and dysproteinemias, in *Arthritis and Allied Conditions*, 13th ed, WJ Koopman (ed). Baltimore, Williams & Wilkins, 1997, pp 1697–1717

LAMBERT RE, MCGUIRE JL: Iron storage disease, in *Textbook of Rheumatology*, 5th ed, WN Kelley et al (eds). Philadelphia, Saunders, 1997, pp 1423–1429

MARTINEZ-LAVIN M: Hypertrophic osteoarthropathy, in *Rheumatology*, JF Klippel, PA Dieppe (eds). St. Louis, Mosby, 1998, section 8, chap 46, pp 1–4

ROSENBERG EA, SCHILLER AC: Tumors and tumor-like lesions of joints and related structures, in *Textbook of Rheumatology*, 5th ed, WN Kelley et al (eds). Philadelphia, Saunders, 1997, pp 1593–1617

SCHUMACHER RH JR: Hemoglobinopathies and arthritis, in *Textbook of Rheumatology*, 5th ed, WN Kelley et al (eds). Philadelphia, Saunders, 1997, pp 1493–1498

UPCHURCH KS, BRETTLER DB: Hemophilic arthropathy, in *Textbook of Rheumatology*, 5th ed, WN Kelley et al (eds). Philadelphia, Saunders, 1997, pp 1485–1492

WOLFE F et al: The prevalence and characteristics of fibromyalgia in the general population. Arthritis Rheum 38:19, 1995

326

Bruce Gilliland

PERIARTICULAR DISORDERS OF THE EXTREMITIES

A number of periarticular disorders have become increasingly common over the past two to three decades, due in part to greater participation in recreational sports by individuals of a wide range of ages. This chapter discusses some of the more common periarticular disorders of the extremities.

BURSITIS Bursitis is inflammation of a bursa, which is a thin-walled sac lined with synovial tissue. The function of the bursa is to facilitate movement of tendons and muscles over bony prominences. Excessive frictional forces, trauma, systemic disease (e.g., rheumatoid arthritis, gout), or infection may cause bursitis. *Subacromial bursitis* (subdeltoid bursitis) is the most common form of bursitis. The subacromial bursa, which is contiguous with the subdeltoid bursa, is located between the undersurface of the acromion and the humeral head, and is covered by the deltoid muscle. Bursitis is caused by repetitive overhead motion and often accompanies rotator cuff tendinitis. Another frequently encountered form is *trochanteric bursitis*, which involves the bursa around the insertion of the gluteus medius onto the greater trochanter of the femur. Patients experience pain over the lateral aspect of the hip and upper thigh and have tenderness over the posterior aspect of the greater trochanter. External rotation and resisted abduction of the hip elicit pain. *Olecranon bursitis* occurs over the posterior elbow, and when the area is acutely inflamed, infection should be excluded by aspirating and culturing fluid from the bursa. *Achilles bursitis* involves the bursa located above the insertion of the tendon to the calcaneus and results from overuse and wearing tight shoes. *Retrocalcaneal bursitis* involves the bursa that is located between the calcaneus and posterior surface of the Achilles tendon. The pain is experienced at the back of the heel, and swelling appears on the medial and/or lateral side of the tendon. It occurs in association with spondyloarthropathies, rheumatoid arthritis, gout, or trauma. *Ischial bursitis* (weaver's bottom) affects the bursa separating the gluteus medius from the ischial tuberosity and develops from prolonged sitting and pivoting on hard surfaces. *Iliopsoas bursitis* affects the bursa that lies between the iliopsoas muscle and hip joint and is lateral to the femoral vessels. Pain is experienced over this area and is made worse by hip extension and flexion. Bursitis results from trauma or overuse but can also be seen in patients with rheumatoid arthritis. *Anserine bursitis* is an inflammation of the sartorius bursa located over the medial side of the tibia just below the knee and under the conjoint tendon and is manifested by pain on climbing stairs. Tenderness is present over the insertion of the conjoint tendon of the sartorius, gracilis, and semitendinosus. *Prepatellar bursitis* (housemaid's knee) occurs in the bursa situated between the patella and overlying skin and is caused by kneeling on hard surfaces. Treatment of bursitis consists of prevention of the aggravating situation, rest of the involved part, administration of a nonsteroidal anti-inflammatory drug (NSAID), or local glucocorticoid injection.

ROTATOR CUFF TENDINITIS AND IMPINGEMENT SYNDROME Tendinitis of the rotator cuff is the major cause of a painful shoulder and is currently thought to be caused by inflammation of the tendon(s). The rotator cuff consists of the tendons of the supraspinatus, infraspinatus, subscapularis, and teres minor muscles, and inserts on the humeral tuberosities. Of the tendons forming the rotator cuff, the supraspinatus tendon is the most often affected, probably because of its repeated impingement (impingement syndrome) between the humeral head and the undersurface of the anterior third of the acromion and coracoacromial ligament above as well as the reduction in its blood supply that occurs with abduction of the arm (Fig. 326-1). The tendon of the infraspinatus or the long head of the biceps is less commonly involved. The process begins with edema and hemorrhage of the rotator cuff, which evolves to fibrotic thickening and eventually to rotator cuff degeneration with tendon tears and bone spurs. Subacromial bursitis also accompanies this syndrome. Symptoms usually appear after injury or overuse, especially with activities involving elevation of the arm with some degree of forward flexion. Impingement syndrome occurs in persons participating in baseball, tennis, swimming, or occupations that require repeated elevation of the arm. Those over age 40 are particularly susceptible. Patients complain of a dull aching in the shoulder, which may interfere with sleep. Severe pain is experienced when the arm is actively abducted into an overhead position. The arc between 60 and 120° is especially painful. Tenderness is present over the lateral aspect of the humeral head just below the acromion. NSAIDs, local glucocorticoid injection, and physical therapy may relieve symptoms.

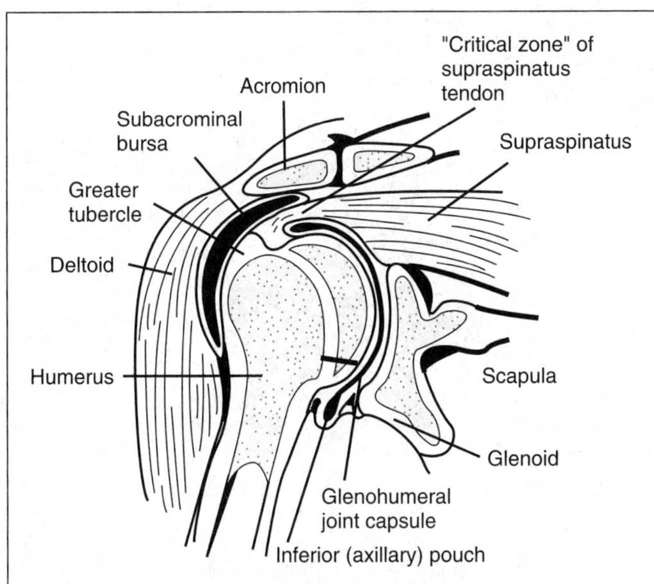

FIGURE 326-1 Coronal section of the shoulder illustrating the relationships of the glenohumeral joint, the joint capsule, the subacromial bursa, and the rotator cuff (supraspinatus tendon). *(From Kozin, with permission.)*

Patients may tear the supraspinatus tendon acutely by falling on an outstretched arm or lifting a heavy object. Symptoms are pain, along with weakness of abduction and external rotation of the shoulder. Atrophy of the supraspinatus muscles develops. The diagnosis is established by arthrogram or ultrasound. Surgical repair may be necessary in patients who fail to respond to conservative measures. In patients with moderate to severe tears and functional loss, surgery is indicated.

CALCIFIC TENDINITIS This condition is characterized by deposition of calcium salts, primarily hydroxyapatite, within a tendon. The exact mechanism of calcification is not known but may be initiated by ischemia or degeneration of the tendon. The supraspinatus tendon is most often affected because it is frequently impinged on and has a reduced blood supply when the arm is abducted. The condition usually develops after age 40. Calcification within the tendon may evoke acute inflammation, producing sudden and severe pain in the shoulder. However, it may be asymptomatic or not related to the patient's symptoms.

BICIPITAL TENDINITIS AND RUPTURE Bicipital tendinitis, or tenosynovitis, is produced by friction on the tendon of the long head of the biceps as it passes through the bicipital groove. When the inflammation is acute, patients experience anterior shoulder pain that radiates down the biceps into the forearm. Abduction and external rotation of the arm are painful and limited. The bicipital groove is very tender to palpation. Pain may be elicited along the course of the tendon by resisting supination of the forearm with the elbow at 90° (Yergason's supination sign). Acute rupture of the tendon may occur with vigorous exercise of the arm and is often painful. In a young patient, it should be repaired surgically. Rupture of the tendon in an older person may be associated with little or no pain and is recognized by the presence of persistent swelling of the biceps ("Popeye" muscle) produced by the retraction of the long head of the biceps. Surgery is usually not necessary in this setting.

ADHESIVE CAPSULITIS Often referred to as "frozen shoulder," adhesive capsulitis is characterized by pain and restricted movement of the shoulder, usually in the absence of intrinsic shoulder disease. Adhesive capsulitis, however, may follow bursitis or tendinitis of the shoulder or be associated with systemic disorders such as chronic pulmonary disease, myocardial infarction, and diabetes mellitus. Prolonged immobility of the arm contributes to the development of adhesive capsulitis, and reflex sympathetic dystrophy is thought to be a pathogenic factor. The capsule of the shoulder is thickened, and a mild chronic inflammatory infiltrate and fibrosis may be present.

Adhesive capsulitis occurs more commonly in women after age 50. Pain and stiffness usually develop gradually over several months to a year but progress rapidly in some patients. Pain may interfere with sleep. The shoulder is tender to palpation, and both active and passive movement are restricted. Radiographs of the shoulder show osteopenia. The diagnosis is confirmed by arthrography, in that only a limited amount of contrast material, usually <15 mL, can be injected under pressure into the shoulder joint.

In most patients, the condition improves spontaneously 1 to 3 years after onset, but some have permanent restriction of movement. Early mobilization of the arm following an injury to the shoulder may prevent the development of this disease. Slow but forceful injection of contrast material into the joint may lyse adhesions and stretch the capsule, resulting in improvement of shoulder motion. Manipulation under anesthesia may be helpful in some patients. Once the disease is established, therapy may have little effect on its natural course. Local injections of glucocorticoids, NSAIDs, and physical therapy may provide relief of symptoms.

LATERAL EPICONDYLITIS (TENNIS ELBOW) Lateral epicondylitis, or tennis elbow, is a painful condition involving the soft tissue over the lateral aspect of the elbow. The pain originates at or near the site of attachment of the common extensors to the lateral epicondyle and may radiate into the forearm and dorsum of the wrist. This painful condition is thought to be caused by small tears of the extensor aponeurosis resulting from repeated resisted contractions of the extensor muscles. The pain usually appears after work or recreational activities involving repeated motions of wrist extension and supination against resistance. Most patients with this disorder injure themselves in activities other than tennis, such as pulling weeds, carrying suitcases or briefcases, or using a screwdriver. The injury in tennis usually occurs when hitting a backhand with the elbow flexed. Shaking hands and opening doors can reproduce the pain. Striking the lateral elbow against a solid object may also induce pain.

The treatment is usually rest along with administration of an NSAID. Ultrasound, icing, and friction massage may also help relieve pain. When pain is severe, the elbow is placed in a sling or splinted at 90° of flexion. When the pain is acute and well localized, injection of a glucocorticoid using a small-gauge needle may be effective. Following injection, the patient should be advised to rest the arm for at least 1 month and avoid activities that would aggravate the elbow. Once symptoms have subsided, the patient should begin rehabilitation to strengthen and increase flexibility of the extensor muscles before resuming physical activity involving the arm. A forearm band placed 2.5 to 5.0 cm (1 to 2 in) below the elbow may help to reduce tension on the extensor muscles at their attachment to the lateral epicondyle. The patient should be advised to restrict activities requiring forcible extension and supination of the wrist. Improvement may take several months. The patient may continue to experience mild pain but, with care, can usually avoid the return of debilitating pain. In an occasional patient, surgical release of the extensor aponeurosis may be necessary.

MEDIAL EPICONDYLITIS Medial epicondylitis is an overuse syndrome resulting in pain over the medial side of the elbow with radiation into the forearm. The cause of this syndrome is considered to be repetitive resisted motions of wrist flexion and pronation, which lead to microtears and granulation tissue at the origin of the pronator teres and forearm flexors, particularly the flexor carpi radialis. This overuse syndrome is usually seen in patients >35 years and is much less common than lateral epicondylitis. It occurs most often in work-related repetitive activities but also occurs with recreational activities such as swinging a golf club (golfer's elbow) or throwing a baseball. On physical examination, there is tenderness just distal to the medial epicondyle over the origin of the forearm flexors. Pain can be reproduced by resisting wrist flexion and pronation with the elbow extended. Radiographs are usually normal. The differential diagnosis of patients with medial elbow symptoms include tears of the pronator teres, acute medial collateral ligament tear, and medial collateral ligament instability. Ulnar neuritis has been found in 25 to 50% of patients with medial epicondylitis and is associated with tenderness over the ulnar nerve at the elbow as well as hypesthesia and paresthesia on the ulnar side of the hand.

The initial treatment of medial epicondylitis is conservative, involving rest, NSAIDs, friction massage, ultrasound, and icing. Some patients may require splinting. Injections of glucocorticoids at the painful site may also be effective. Patients should be instructed to rest at least 1 month. Also, patients should be started on physical therapy once the pain has subsided. In patients with chronic debilitating medial epicondylitis that remains unresponsive after at least a year of treatment, surgical release of the flexor muscle at its origin may be necessary and is often successful.

BIBLIOGRAPHY

KOZIN F: Painful shoulder and the reflex sympathetic dystrophy syndrome, in *Arthritis and Allied Conditions*, 13th ed, WJ Koopman (ed). Baltimore, Williams & Wilkins, 1997, pp 1887–1922

LINTNER SA et al: Sports medicine, in *Textbook of Rheumatology*, 5th ed, WN Kelley et al (eds). Philadelphia, Saunders, 1997, pp 546–563

MATSEN FA III, ARNTZ CT: Subacromial impingement, in *The Shoulder*, L Reines (ed). Philadelphia, Saunders, 1990, pp 623–646

NEER CS II: Impingement lesions. Clin Orthop 173:70, 1983

PART THIRTEEN

ENDOCRINOLOGY AND METABOLISM

Section 1
ENDOCRINOLOGY

327 J. Larry Jameson

PRINCIPLES OF ENDOCRINOLOGY

CRH corticotropin-releasing hormone	POMC proopiomelanocortin
EGF epidermal growth factor	PTHrP parathyroid hormone–related peptide
GHRH growth hormone–releasing hormone	SERMs selective estrogen response modulators
GnRH gonadotropin-releasing hormone	SHBG sex hormone–binding globulin
GPCRs G protein–coupled receptors	STAT signal transduction and activators of transcription
hCG human chorionic gonadotropin	TBG thyroxine-binding globulin
HPA hypothalamic-pituitary-adrenal	TRH thyrotropin-releasing hormone
IGF insulin-like growth factor	
MEN multiple endocrine neoplasia	

The management of endocrine disorders requires an understanding of such disparate areas as intermediary metabolism, reproductive physiology, bone metabolism, and growth. Accordingly, the practice of endocrinology is intimately linked to a conceptual framework for understanding hormone secretion, hormone action, and principles of feedback control systems. The endocrine system is investigated primarily by measuring hormone concentrations, thereby arming the clinician with valuable diagnostic information. Most disorders of the endocrine system are amenable to effective treatment, once the correct diagnosis is determined. Endocrine deficiency disorders are treated with physiologic hormone replacement; hormone excess conditions, usually due to benign glandular adenomas, are managed by removing tumors surgically or by reducing hormone levels medically.

SCOPE OF ENDOCRINOLOGY

The specialty of endocrinology encompasses the study of glands and the hormones they produce. The term *endocrine* was coined by Starling to contrast the actions of hormones secreted internally (endocrine) with those secreted externally (*exocrine*) or into a lumen, such as the gastrointestinal tract. The term *hormone*, derived from a Greek phrase meaning "to set in motion," aptly describes the dynamic actions of these circulating substances as they elicit cellular responses and regulate physiologic processes through feedback mechanisms.

Unlike certain other specialties in medicine, it is not possible to define endocrinology strictly along anatomic lines. The classic endocrine glands—pituitary, thyroid, parathyroid, pancreatic islets, adrenal, and gonads—communicate broadly with other organs through the nervous system, hormones, cytokines, and growth factors. In addition to its traditional synaptic functions, the brain produces a vast array of peptide hormones, spawning the discipline of neuroendocrinology. Through the production of hypothalamic releasing factors, the central nervous system exerts a major regulatory influence over pituitary hormone secretion (Chap. 328). The peripheral nervous system modulates adrenal medulla and pancreatic islet hormone production. The immune and endocrine systems are also intimately intertwined. The adrenal glucocorticoid, cortisol, is a powerful immunosuppressant. Cytokines and interleukins (ILs) have profound effects on the functions of the pituitary, adrenal, thyroid, and gonads. Common endocrine diseases, such as autoimmune thyroid disease and type 1 diabetes mellitus, are caused by dysregulation of immune surveillance and tolerance. Less common diseases such as polyglandular failure, Addison's disease, and lymphocytic hypophysitis also have an immunologic basis.

The interdigitation of endocrinology with physiologic processes in other specialties sometimes blurs the role of hormones. For example, hormones play an important role in maintenance of blood pressure, intravascular volume, and peripheral resistance in the cardiovascular system. The heart is the principal source of atrial natriuretic peptide, which acts in classic endocrine fashion to induce natriuresis at a distant target organ (the kidney). Vasoactive substances such as catecholamines, angiotensin II, endothelin, and nitric oxide are involved in dynamic changes of vascular tone, in addition to their multiple roles in other tissues. Erythropoietin, a traditional circulating hormone, is made in the kidney and stimulates erythropoiesis in the bone marrow (Chap. 104). The kidney is also integrally involved in the renin-angiotensin axis (Chap. 331) and is a primary target of several hormones including parathyroid hormone (PTH), mineralocorticoids, and vasopressin. The gastrointestinal tract produces a surprising number of peptide hormones such as cholecystokinin, gastrin, secretin, and vasoactive intestinal peptide, among many others. Carcinoid and islet tumors can secrete excessive amounts of these hormones, leading to specific clinical syndromes (Chap. 93). Many of these gastrointestinal hormones are also produced in the central nervous system, where their functions remain poorly understood. As new hormones such as inhibin, ghrelin, and leptin are discovered, they become integrated into the science and practice of medicine on the basis of their functional roles rather than through their structures or mechanisms of action.

Characterization of hormone receptors frequently reveals unexpected relationships to factors in nonendocrine disciplines. The growth hormone (GH) receptor, for example, is a member of the cytokine receptor family. The G protein–coupled receptors (GPCRs), which mediate the actions of many peptide hormones, are used in numerous physiologic processes including vision, smell, and neurotransmission.

It is apparent that hormones and growth factors play an important functional role in all organ systems. Though endocrinologists are not usually involved in the administration of the hormones or growth factors used to treat diseases in other specialties (e.g., cardiology, hematology), the principles of endocrinology can be applied in these cases, thus emphasizing the impact of endocrinology across multiple disciplines.

NATURE OF HORMONES

Hormones can be divided into five major classes: (1) *amino acid derivatives* such as dopamine, catecholamines, and thyroid hormone; (2) *small neuropeptides* such as gonadotropin-releasing hormone (GnRH), thyrotropin-releasing hormone (TRH), somatostatin, and vasopressin; (3) *large proteins* such as insulin, luteinizing hormone (LH), and PTH produced by classic endocrine glands; (4) *steroid hormones* such as cortisol and estrogen that are synthesized from cholesterol-based precursors; and (5) *vitamin derivatives* such as retinoids (vitamin A) and vitamin D. A variety of *peptide growth factors*, most of which act locally, share actions with hormones. As a rule, amino acid derivatives and peptide hormone interact with cell-surface membrane receptors. Steroids, thyroid hormones, vitamin D, and retinoids are lipid-soluble and interact with intracellular nuclear receptors.

HORMONE AND RECEPTOR FAMILIES Many hormones and receptors can be grouped into families, reflecting their

Table 327-1 Membrane Receptor Families and Signaling Pathways

Receptors	Effectors	Signaling Pathways
G protein–coupled seven-transmembrane (GPCR)		
β-Adrenergic LH, FSH, TSH Glucagon PTH, PTHrP ACTH, MSH GHRH, CRH	$G_s\alpha$, adenylate cyclase Ca^{2+} channels	Stimulation of cyclic AMP production, protein kinase A Calmodulin, Ca^{2+}-dependent kinases
α-Adrenergic	$G_i\alpha$	Inhibition of cyclic AMP production
Somatostatin		Activation of K^+, Ca^{2+} channels
TRH, GnRH	G_q, G_{11}	Phospholipase C, diacylglycerol, IP_3, protein kinase C, Voltage-dependent Ca^{2+} channels
Receptor tyrosine kinase		
Insulin, IGF-I	Tyrosine kinases, IRS-1 to IRS-4	MAP kinases, PI 3-kinase, RSK
EGF, NGF	Tyrosine kinases, ras	Raf, MAP kinases, RSK
Cytokine receptor–linked kinase		
GH, PRL	JAK, tyrosine kinases	STAT, MAP kinase, PI 3-kinase, IRS-1, IRS-2
Serine Kinase		
Activin, TGF-β, MIS	Serine kinase	Smads

NOTE: IP_3, inositol triphosphate; IRS, insulin receptor substrates; MAP, mitogen-activated protein; MIS, müllerian-inhibiting substance; MSH, melanocyte-stimulating hormone; NGF, nerve growth factor; PI, phosphatylinositol; RSK, ribosomal S6 kinase; TGF-β, transforming growth factor β. For all other abbreviations, see text.

structural similarities (Table 327-1). The evolution of these families generates diverse but highly selective pathways of hormone action. Recognizing these relationships allows extrapolation of information gleaned from one hormone or receptor to other family members.

The glycoprotein hormone family, consisting of thyroid-stimulating hormone (TSH), follicle-stimulating hormone (FSH), LH, and human chorionic gonadotropin (hCG), illustrates many features of related hormones. The glycoprotein hormones are heterodimers that share the α subunit in common; the β subunits are distinct and confer specific biologic actions. The overall three-dimensional architecture of the β subunits is similar, reflecting the locations of conserved disulfide bonds that restrain protein conformation. The cloning of the β-subunit genes from multiple species suggests that this family arose from a common ancestral gene, probably by gene duplication and subsequent divergence to evolve new biologic functions.

As the hormone families enlarge and diverge, their receptors must co-evolve, if new biologic functions are to be derived. Related GPCRs, for example, have evolved for each of the glycoprotein hormones. These receptors are structurally similar, and each is coupled to the $G_s\alpha$ signaling pathway. However, there is minimal overlap of hormone binding. For example, TSH binds with high specificity to the TSH receptor but interacts weakly with the LH or the FSH receptor. Nonetheless, there can be subtle physiologic consequences of hormone cross-reactivity with other receptors. Very high levels of hCG during pregnancy stimulate the TSH receptor and increase thyroid hormone levels.

Insulin, insulin-like growth factor (IGF) I, and IGF-II share structural similarities that are most apparent when precursor forms of the proteins are compared. In contrast to the high degree of specificity seen with the glycoprotein hormones, there is moderate cross-talk among the members of the insulin/IGF family. High concentrations of an IGF-II precursor produced by certain tumors (e.g., sarcomas) can cause hypoglycemia, partly because of binding to insulin and IGF-I receptors (Chap. 334). High concentrations of insulin also bind to the IGF-I receptor, perhaps accounting for some of the clinical manifestations seen in severe insulin resistance.

Another important example of receptor cross-talk is seen with PTH and parathyroid hormone–related peptide (PTHrP) (Chap. 341). PTH is produced by the parathyroid glands, whereas PTHrP is expressed at high levels during development and by a variety of tumors. These hormones share amino acid sequence similarity, particularly in their amino-terminal regions. Both hormones bind to a single PTH receptor that is expressed in bone and kidney. Hypercalcemia and hypophosphatemia may therefore result from excessive production of either hormone, making it difficult to distinguish hyperparathyroidism from hypercalcemia of malignancy solely on the basis of serum chemistries. However, sensitive and specific assays for PTH now allow these disorders to be separated more readily.

Based on their specificities for DNA binding sites, the nuclear receptor family can be subdivided into type 1 receptors (GR, MR, AR, ER, PR) that bind steroids and type 2 receptors (TR, VDR, RAR, PPAR) that bind thyroid hormone, vitamin D, retinoic acid, or lipid derivatives. Certain functional domains in nuclear receptors, such as the zinc finger DNA-binding domains, are highly conserved. However, selective amino acid differences within this domain confer DNA sequence specificity. The hormone-binding domains are more variable, providing great diversity in the array of small molecules that can bind to different nuclear receptors. With few exceptions, hormone binding is highly specific for a single type of nuclear receptor. One exception involves the highly related glucocorticoid and mineralocorticoid receptors. Because the mineralocorticoid receptor also binds glucocorticoids with high affinity, an enzyme (11β-hydroxysteroid dehydrogenase) located in renal tubular cells inactivates glucocorticoids, allowing selective responses to mineralocorticoids such as aldosterone. However, when very high glucocorticoid concentrations occur, as in Cushing's syndrome, the glucocorticoid degradation pathway becomes saturated, allowing excessive cortisol levels to exert mineralocorticoid effects (sodium retention, potassium wasting). This phenomenon is particularly pronounced in ectopic adrenocorticotropic hormone (ACTH) syndromes (Chap. 331). Another example of relaxed nuclear receptor specificity involves the estrogen receptor, which can bind an array of compounds, some of which share little structural similarity to the high-affinity ligand estradiol. This feature of the estrogen receptor makes it susceptible to activation by "environmental estrogens" such as resveratrol, octylphenol, and many other aromatic hydrocarbons. On the other hand, this lack of specificity provides an opportunity to synthesize a remarkable series of clinically useful antagonists (e.g., tamoxifen) and selective estrogen response modulators (SERMs), such as raloxifene. These compounds generate distinct conformations that alter receptor interactions with components of the transcription machinery (see below), thereby conferring their unique actions.

HORMONE SYNTHESIS AND PROCESSING The synthesis of peptide hormones and their receptors occurs through a classic pathway of gene expression: transcription → mRNA → protein → posttranslational protein processing → intracellular sorting, membrane integration, or secretion (Chap. 65). Though endocrine genes contain regulatory DNA elements similar to those found in many other genes, their exquisite control by other hormones also necessitates the presence of specific hormone response elements. For example, the TSH genes are repressed directly by thyroid hormones acting through the thyroid hormone receptor, a member of the nuclear receptor family. Steroidogenic enzyme gene expression requires specific transcription factors such as steroidogenic factor-1 (SF-1), acting in conjunction with signals transmitted by trophic hormones (e.g., ACTH or LH). For some hormones, substantial regulation occurs at the level of translational efficiency. Insulin biosynthesis, while requiring ongoing gene transcription, is regulated primarily at the translational level in response to elevated levels of glucose or amino acids.

Many hormones are embedded within larger precursor polypeptides that are proteolytically processed to yield the biologically active hormone. Examples include: proopiomelanocortin (POMC) → ACTH; proglucagon → glucagon; proinsulin → insulin; pro-PTH → PTH, among others. In many cases, such as POMC and proglucagon, these precursors generate multiple biologically active peptides. It is provocative that hormone precursors are typically inactive, presumably adding an additional level of regulatory control. This is true not only for peptide hormones but also for certain steroids (testosterone → dihydrotestosterone) and thyroid hormone ($T_4 \rightarrow T_3$).

Hormone precursor processing is intimately linked to intracellular sorting pathways that transport proteins to appropriate vesicles and enzymes, resulting in specific cleavage steps, followed by protein folding and translocation to secretory vesicles. Hormones destined for secretion are translocated across the endoplasmic reticulum under the guidance of an amino-terminal signal sequence that is subsequently cleaved. Cell-surface receptors are inserted into the membrane via short segments of hydrophobic amino acids that remain embedded within the lipid bilayer. During translocation through the Golgi and endoplasmic reticulum, hormones and receptors are also subject to a variety of posttranslational modifications, such as glycosylation and phosphorylation, which can alter protein conformation, modify circulating half-life, and alter biologic activity.

Synthesis of most steroid hormones is based on modifications of the precursor, cholesterol. Multiple regulated enzymatic steps are required for the synthesis of testosterone (Chap. 335), estradiol (Chap. 336), cortisol (Chap. 331), and vitamin D (Chap. 340). This large number of synthetic steps predisposes to multiple genetic and acquired disorders of steroidogenesis (see below).

HORMONE SECRETION, TRANSPORT, AND DEGRADATION The circulating level of a hormone is determined by its rate of secretion and its circulating half-life. After protein processing, peptide hormones (GnRH, insulin, GH) are stored in secretory granules. As these granules mature, they are poised beneath the plasma membrane for imminent release into the circulation. In most instances, the stimulus for hormone secretion is a releasing factor or neural signal that induces rapid changes in intracellular calcium concentrations, leading to secretory granule fusion with the plasma membrane and release of its contents into the extracellular environment and blood stream. Steroid hormones, in contrast, diffuse into the circulation as they are synthesized. Thus, their secretory rates are closely aligned with rates of synthesis. For example, ACTH and LH induce steroidogenesis by stimulating the activity of *st*eroidogenic *a*cute *r*egulatory (StAR) protein (transports cholesterol into the mitochondrion) along with other rate-limiting steps (e.g., cholesterol side-chain cleavage enzyme, CYP11A1) in the steroidogenic pathway.

Hormone transport and degradation dictate the rapidity with which a hormonal signal decays. Some hormonal signals are evanescent (e.g., somatostatin), whereas others are longer lived (e.g., TSH). Because somatostatin exerts effects in virtually every tissue, a short half-life allows it concentrations and actions to be controlled locally. Structural modifications that impair somatostatin degradation have been useful for generating long-acting therapeutic analogues, such as octreotide (Chap. 328). On the other hand, the actions of TSH are highly specific for the thyroid gland. Its prolonged half-life accounts for relatively constant serum levels, even though TSH is secreted in discrete pulses.

An understanding of circulating hormone half-life is important for achieving physiologic hormone replacement, as the frequency of dosing and the time required to reach steady state are intimately linked to rates of hormone decay. T_4, for example, has a plasma half-life of 7 days. Consequently, >1 month is required to reach a new steady state, but single daily doses are sufficient to achieve constant hormone levels. T_3, in contrast, has a half-life of 1 day. Its administration is associated with more dynamic serum levels and it must be administered two to three times per day. Similarly, synthetic glucocorticoids vary widely in their half-lives; those with longer half-lives (e.g., dexamethasone) are associated with greater suppression of the hypothalamic-pituitary-adrenal (HPA) axis. Most protein hormones [e.g., ACTH, GH, prolactin (PRL); PTH, LH] have relatively short half-lives (<20 min), leading to sharp peaks of secretion and decay. The only accurate way to profile the pulse frequency and amplitude of these hormones is to measure levels in frequently sampled blood (every 10 min) over long durations (8 to 24 h). Because this is not practical in a clinical setting, an alternative strategy is to pool three to four samples drawn at about 30-min intervals, recognizing that pulsatile secretion makes it difficult to establish a narrow normal range. Rapid hormone decay is useful in certain clinical settings. For example, the short half-life of PTH allows the use of intraoperative PTH determinations to confirm successful removal of an adenoma. This is particularly valuable diagnostically when there is a possibility of multicentric disease or parathyroid hyperplasia, as occurs with multiple endocrine neoplasia (MEN) or renal insufficiency.

Many hormones circulate in association with serum-binding proteins. Examples include: (1) T_4 and T_3 binding to thyroxine-binding globulin (TBG), albumin, and thyroxine-binding prealbumin (TBPA); (2) cortisol binding to cortisol-binding globulin (CBG); (3) androgen and estrogen binding to sex hormone–binding globulin (SHBG) (also called testosterone-binding globulin, TeBG); (4) IGF-I and -II binding to multiple IGF-binding proteins (IGFBPs); (5) GH interactions with GH-binding protein (GHBP), a circulating fragment of the GH receptor extracellular domain; and (6) activin binding to follistatin. These interactions provide a hormonal reservoir, prevent otherwise rapid degradation of unbound hormones, restrict hormone access to certain sites (e.g., IGFBPs), and modulate the unbound, or "free," hormone concentrations. Although a variety of binding protein abnormalities have been identified, most have little clinical consequence, aside from creating diagnostic problems. For example, TBG deficiency can greatly reduce total thyroid hormone levels, but the free concentrations of T_4 and T_3 remain normal. Liver disease and certain medications can also influence binding protein levels (e.g., estrogen increases TBG) or cause displacement of hormones from binding proteins (e.g., salsalate displaces T_4 from TBG). Only free hormone is available to bind receptors and thereby elicit a biologic response. Short-term perturbations in binding proteins change the free hormone concentration, which in turn induces compensatory adaptations through feedback loops. SHBG changes in women are an exception to this self-correcting mechanism. When SHBG decreases because of insulin resistance or androgen excess, the free testosterone concentration is increased, potentially leading to hirsutism (Chap. 53). The increased free testosterone levels does not result in an adequate compensatory feedback correction because estrogen, and not testosterone, is the primary regulator of the reproductive axis.

HORMONE ACTION THROUGH RECEPTORS

Receptors for hormones are divided into two major classes—membrane and nuclear. *Membrane receptors* primarily bind peptide hormones and catecholamines. *Nuclear receptors* bind small molecules that can diffuse across the cell membrane, such as thyroid hormone, steroids, and vitamin D. Certain general principles apply to hormone-receptor interactions, regardless of the class of receptor. Hormones bind to receptors with specificity and a high affinity that generally coincides with the dynamic range of circulating hormone concentrations. Low concentrations of free hormone (usually 10^{-12} to 10^{-9} *M*) rapidly associate and dissociate from receptors in a bimolecular reaction, such that the occupancy of the receptor at any given moment is a function of hormone concentration and the receptor's affinity for the hormone. Receptor numbers vary greatly in different target tissues, providing one of the major determinants of specific cellular responses to circulating hormones. For example, ACTH receptors are located almost exclusively in the adrenal cortex, and FSH receptors are found only in the gonads. In contrast, insulin and thyroid hormone receptors are widely distributed, reflecting the need for metabolic responses in all tissues.

MEMBRANE RECEPTORS Membrane receptors for hormones can be divided into several major groups: (1) seven transmembrane GPCRs, (2) tyrosine kinase receptors, (3) cytokine receptors, and (4) serine kinase receptors (Fig. 327-1). The *seven transmembrane GPCR* family binds a remarkable array of hormones including large proteins (e.g., LH, PTH), small peptides (e.g., TRH, somatostatin), catecholamines (epinephrine, dopamine), and even minerals (e.g., calcium). The extracellular domains of GPCRs vary widely in size and are the major binding site for large hormones. The transmembrane-spanning regions are composed of hydrophobic α-helical domains that traverse the lipid bilayer. Like some channels, these domains are thought to circularize and form a hydrophobic pocket into which certain small ligands fit. Hormone binding induces conformational changes in these domains, transducing structural changes to the intracellular domain, which is a docking site for G proteins.

The large family of *G proteins,* so named because they bind guanine nucleotides (GTP, GDP), provides great diversity for coupling to different receptors. G proteins form a heterotrimeric complex that is composed of various α and $\beta\gamma$ subunits. The α subunit contains the guanine nucleotide–binding site and hydrolyzes GTP $\rightarrow$ GDP. The $\beta\gamma$ subunits are tightly associated and modulate the activity of the α subunit, as well as mediating their own effector signaling pathways. G protein activity is regulated by a cycle that involves GTP hydrolysis and dynamic interactions between the α and $\beta\gamma$ subunits. Hormone binding to the receptor induces GDP dissociation, allowing Gα to bind GTP and dissociate from the $\beta\gamma$ complex. Under these conditions, the Gα subunit is activated and mediates signal transduction through various enzymes such as adenylate cyclase or phospholipase C. GTP hydrolysis to GDP allows reassociation with the $\beta\gamma$ subunits and restores the inactive state. As described below, a variety of endocrinopathies result from G protein mutations or from mutations in receptors that modify their interactions with G proteins.

There are more than a dozen isoforms of the Gα subunit. $G_s\alpha$ stimulates, whereas $G_i\alpha$ inhibits adenylate cyclase, an enzyme that generates the second messenger, cyclic AMP, leading to activation of protein kinase A (Table 327-1). G_q subunits couple to phospholipase C, generating diacylglycerol and inositol triphosphate, leading to activation of protein kinase C and the release of intracellular calcium.

The *tyrosine kinase receptors* transduce signals for insulin and a variety of growth factors, such as IGF-I, epidermal growth factor (EGF), nerve growth factor, platelet-derived growth factor, and fibroblast growth factor. The cysteine-rich extracellular ligand-binding domains contain growth factor binding sites. After ligand binding, this class of receptors undergoes autophosphorylation, inducing interactions with intracellular adaptor proteins such as Shc and insulin receptor substrates 1 to 4. In the case of the insulin receptor, multiple kinases are activated including the Raf-Ras-MAPK and the Akt/protein kinase B pathways. The tyrosine kinase receptors play a prominent role in cell growth and differentiation as well as in intermediary metabolism.

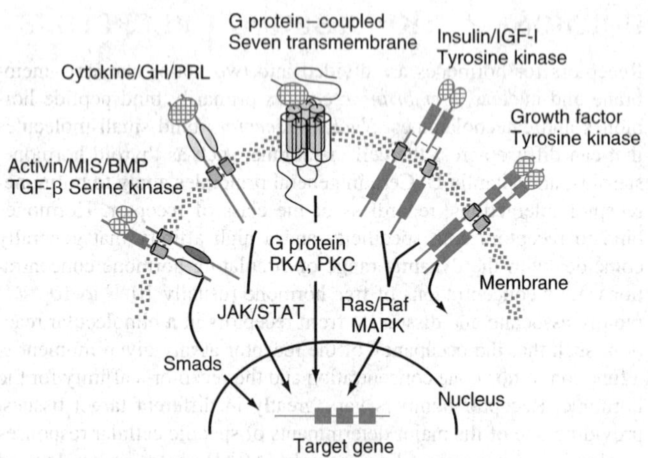

FIGURE 327-1 Membrane receptor signaling. For abbreviations, see text.

The GH and PRL receptors belong to the *cytokine receptor* family (Chap. 305). Analogous to the tyrosine kinase receptors, ligand binding induces receptor binding to intracellular kinases—the Janus kinases (JAKs), which phosphorylate members of the signal transduction and activators of transcription (STAT) family—as well as other signaling pathways (Ras, PI3-K, MAPK). The activated STAT proteins translocate to the nucleus and stimulate expression of target genes (Chap. 328).

The *serine kinase receptors* mediate the actions of activins, transforming growth factor β, müllerian-inhibiting substance (MIS, also known as anti-müllerian hormone, AMH), and bone morphogenic proteins (BMPs). This family of receptors (consisting of type I and II subunits) signal through proteins termed *smads* (fusion of terms for *Caenorhabditis elegans* sma + mammalian mad). Like the STAT proteins, the smads serve a dual role of transducing the receptor signal and acting as transcription factors. The pleomorphic actions of these growth factors dictate that they act primarily in a local (paracrine or autocrine) manner. Binding proteins, such as follistatin (which binds activin and other members of this family), function to inactivate the growth factors and restrict their distribution.

NUCLEAR RECEPTORS The family of nuclear receptors has grown to nearly 100 members, many of which are still classified as orphan receptors because their ligands, if they exist, remain to be identified (Fig. 327-2). Otherwise, most nuclear receptors are classified based on the nature of their ligands. Though all nuclear receptors ultimately act to increase or decrease gene transcription, some (e.g., glucocorticoid receptor) reside primarily in the cytoplasm, whereas others (e.g., thyroid hormone receptor) are always located in the nucleus. After ligand binding, the cytoplasmically localized receptors translocate to the nucleus.

The structures of nuclear receptors have been extensively studied, including by x-ray crystallography. The DNA binding domain, consisting of two zinc fingers, contacts specific DNA recognition sequences in target genes. Most nuclear receptors bind to DNA as dimers. Consequently, each monomer recognizes an individual DNA motif, referred to as a "half-site." The steroid receptors, including the glucocorticoid, estrogen, progesterone, and androgen receptors, bind to DNA as homodimers. Consistent with this twofold symmetry, their DNA recognition half-sites are palindromic. The thyroid, retinoid, PPAR, and vitamin D receptors bind to DNA preferentially as heterodimers in combination with retinoid X receptors (RXRs). Their DNA half-sites are arranged as direct repeats. Receptor specificity for DNA sequences is determined by (1) the sequence of the half-site, (2) the orientation of the half-sites (palindromic, direct repeat), and (3) the spacing between the half-sites. For example, vitamin D, thyroid and retinoid receptors recognize similar tandemly repeated half-sites (TAAGTCA), but these DNA repeats are spaced by three, four, and five nucleotides, respectively.

The carboxy-terminal hormone-binding domain mediates transcriptional control. For type II receptors, such as TR and RAR, co-repressor proteins bind to the receptor in the absence of ligand and silence gene transcription. Hormone binding induces conformational changes, triggering the release of co-repressors and inducing the recruitment of coactivators that stimulate transcription. Thus, these receptors are capable of mediating dramatic changes in the level of gene activity. Certain disease states are associated with defective regulation of these events. For example, mutations in the thyroid hormone receptor prevent co-repressor dissociation, resulting in a dominant form of hormone resistance (Chap. 330). In promyelocytic leukemia, fusion of RARα to other nuclear proteins causes aberrant gene silencing and prevents normal cellular differentiation. Treatment with retinoic acid reverses this repression and allows cellular differentiation and apoptosis to occur (Chap. 111). Type 1 steroid receptors do not interact with co-repressors, but ligand binding still mediates interactions with an array of coactivators. X-ray crystallography shows that various SERMs induce distinct receptor conformations. The tissue-specific responses caused by these agents in breast, bone, and uterus appear to reflect distinct interactions with coactivators. The receptor-coactivator complex stimulates gene transcription by several pathways including (1) recruitment of enzymes (histone acetyl transferases) that modify chromatin structure, (2) interactions with additional transcription factors on the target gene, and (3) direct interactions with components of the general transcription apparatus to enhance the rate of RNA polymerase II–mediated transcription.

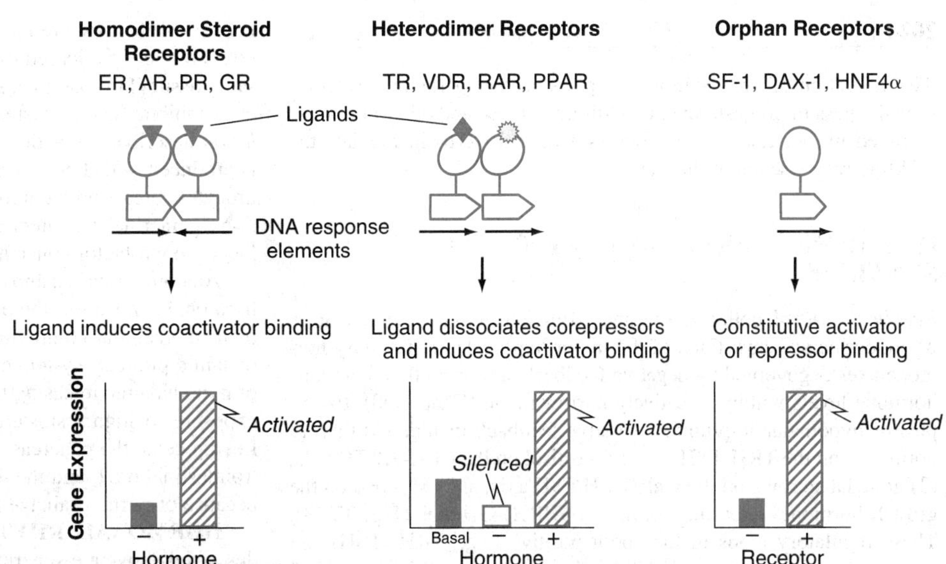

FIGURE 327-2 Nuclear receptor signaling. ER, estrogen receptor; AR, androgen receptor; PR, progesterone receptor; GR, glucocorticoid receptor; TR, thyroid hormone receptor; VDR, vitamin D receptor; RAR, retinoic acid receptor; PPAR, peroxisome proliferator activated receptor; SF-1, steroidogenic factor-1; DAX, *d*osage sensitive sex-reversal; *a*drenal hypoplasia congenita, *X*-chromosome; HNF4α, hepatic nuclear factor 4α

FUNCTIONS OF HORMONES

The functions of individual hormones are described in detail in subsequent chapters. Nonetheless, it is useful to illustrate how most biologic responses require integration of several different hormonal pathways. The physiologic functions of hormones can be divided into three general areas: (1) growth and differentiation, (2) maintenance of homeostasis, and (3) reproduction.

GROWTH Multiple hormones and nutritional factors mediate the complex phenomenon of growth (Chap. 328). Short stature may be caused by GH deficiency, hypothyroidism, Cushing's syndrome, precocious puberty, malnutrition or chronic illness, or genetic abnormalities that affect the epiphyseal growth plates (e.g., *FGFR3* or *SHOX* mutations). Many factors (GH, IGF-I, thyroid hormone) stimulate growth, whereas others (sex steroids) lead to epiphyseal closure. Understanding these hormonal interactions is important in the diagnosis and management of growth disorders. For example, delaying exposure to high levels of sex steroids may enhance the efficacy of GH treatment.

MAINTENANCE OF HOMEOSTASIS Though virtually all hormones affect homeostasis, the most important among these are the following:

1. Thyroid hormone—controls about 25% of basal metabolism in most tissues (Chap. 330)
2. Cortisol—exerts a permissive action for many hormones in addition to its own direct effects (Chap. 331)
3. PTH—regulates calcium and phosphorus levels (Chap. 341)
4. Vasopressin—regulates serum osmolality by controlling renal free water clearance (Chap. 329)
5. Mineralocorticoids—control vascular volume and serum electrolyte (Na^+, K^+) concentrations (Chap. 331)
6. Insulin—maintains euglycemia in the fed and fasted states (Chap. 333)

The defense against hypoglycemia is an impressive example of integrated hormone action (Chap. 334). In response to the fasted state and falling blood glucose, insulin secretion is suppressed, resulting in decreased glucose uptake and enhanced glycogenolysis, lipolysis, proteolysis, and gluconeogenesis to mobilize fuel sources. If hypoglycemia develops (usually from insulin administration or sulfonylureas), an orchestrated counterregulatory response occurs—glucagon and epinephrine rapidly stimulate glycogenolysis and gluconeogenesis, whereas GH and cortisol act over several hours to raise glucose levels and antagonize insulin action.

Although free water clearance is primarily controlled by vasopressin, cortisol and thyroid hormone are also important for facilitating renal tubular responses to vasopressin effects (Chap. 329). PTH and vitamin D function in an interdependent manner to control calcium metabolism (Chap. 340). PTH stimulates renal synthesis of 1,25 dihydroxyvitamin D, which increases calcium absorption in the gastrointestinal tract and enhances PTH action in bone. Increased calcium, along with vitamin D, feeds back to suppress PTH, thereby maintaining calcium balance.

Depending on the severity of a given stress and whether it is acute or chronic, multiple endocrine and cytokine pathways are activated to mount an appropriate physiologic response (Chap. 328). In severe acute stress such as trauma or shock, the sympathetic nervous system is activated and catecholamines are released, leading to increased cardiac output and a primed musculoskeletal system. Catecholamines also increase mean blood pressure and stimulate glucose production (Chap. 72). Multiple stress-induced pathways converge on the hypothalamus, stimulating several hormones including vasopressin and corticotropin-releasing hormone (CRH). These hormones, in addition to cytokines (tumor necrosis factor α, IL-2, IL-6), increase ACTH and GH production. ACTH stimulates the adrenal gland, increasing cortisol, which in turn helps to sustain blood pressure and dampen the inflammatory response. Increased vasopressin acts to conserve free water.

REPRODUCTION The stages of reproduction include: (1) sex determination during fetal development (Chap. 338); (2) sexual maturation during puberty (Chap. 8); (3) conception, pregnancy, lactation, and child-rearing (Chap. 336), and (4) cessation of reproductive capability at menopause. Each of these stages involves an orchestrated interplay of multiple hormones, a phenomenon well illustrated by the dynamic hormonal changes that occur during each 28-day menstrual cycle. In the early follicular phase, pulsatile secretion of LH and FSH stimulate the progressive maturation of the ovarian follicle. This results in a gradual increase of estrogen and progesterone leading to enhanced pituitary sensitivity to GnRH, which, when combined with accelerated GnRH secretion, triggers the LH surge and rupture of the mature follicle. Inhibin, a protein produced by the granulosa cells, enhances follicular growth and feeds back to the pituitary to selectively suppress FSH, without affecting LH. Growth factors, such as EGF and IGF-I modulate follicular responsiveness to gonadotropins. Vascular endothelial growth factor and prostaglandins play a role in follicle vascularization and rupture.

During pregnancy, the increased production of prolactin, in combination with placentally derived steroids (e.g., estrogen and progesterone), prepares the breast for lactation (Chap. 337). Estrogens induce the production of progesterone receptors, allowing for increased responsiveness to progesterone. In addition to these and other hormones involved in lactation, the nervous system and oxytocin mediate the suckling response and milk release.

HORMONAL FEEDBACK REGULATORY SYSTEMS

Feedback control, both negative and positive, is a fundamental feature of endocrine systems. Each of the major hypothalamic-pituitary-hormone axes is governed by negative feedback, a process that maintains hormone levels within a relatively narrow range (Chap. 328). Examples of hypothalamic-pituitary negative feedback include (1) thyroid hormones on the TRH-TSH axis, (2) cortisol on the CRH-ACTH axis, (3) gonadal steroids on the GnRH-LH/FSH axis, and (4) IGF-I on the growth hormone–releasing hormone (GHRH)-GH axis (Fig. 327-3). These regulatory loops include both positive (e.g., TRH, TSH) and negative components (e.g., T_4, T_3), allowing for exquisite control of hormone levels. As an example, a small reduction of thyroid hormone triggers a rapid increase of TRH and TSH secretion, resulting in thyroid gland stimulation and increased thyroid hormone production. When the thyroid hormone reaches a normal level, it feeds back to suppress TRH and TSH, and a new steady state is attained. Feedback regulation also occurs for endocrine systems that do not involve the pituitary gland, such as calcium feedback on PTH, glucose inhibition of insulin secretion, and leptin feedback on the hypothalamus. An understanding of feedback regulation provides important insights into endocrine testing paradigms (see below).

Positive feedback control also occurs but is not well understood. The primary example is estrogen-mediated stimulation of the midcycle LH surge. Though chronic low levels of estrogen are inhibitory, gradually rising estrogen levels stimulate LH secretion. This effect, which is illustrative of an endocrine rhythm (see below), involves activation of the hypothalamic GnRH pulse generator. In addition, estrogen-primed gonadotropes are extroardinarily sensitive to GnRH, leading to a 10- to 20-fold amplification of LH release.

PARACRINE AND AUTOCRINE CONTROL The aforementioned examples of feedback control involve classic endocrine pathways in which hormones are released by one gland and act on a distant target gland. However, local regulatory systems, often involving growth factors, are increasingly recognized. *Paracrine regulation* refers to factors released by one cell that act on an adjacent cell in the same tissue. For example, somatostatin secretion by pancreatic islet δ cells inhibits insulin secretion from nearby β cells. *Autocrine regulation* describes the action of a factor on the same cell from which it is produced. IGF-I acts on many cells that produce it, including chondrocytes, breast epithelium, and gonadal cells. Unlike endocrine actions, paracrine and autocrine control are difficult to document because local growth factor concentrations cannot be readily measured.

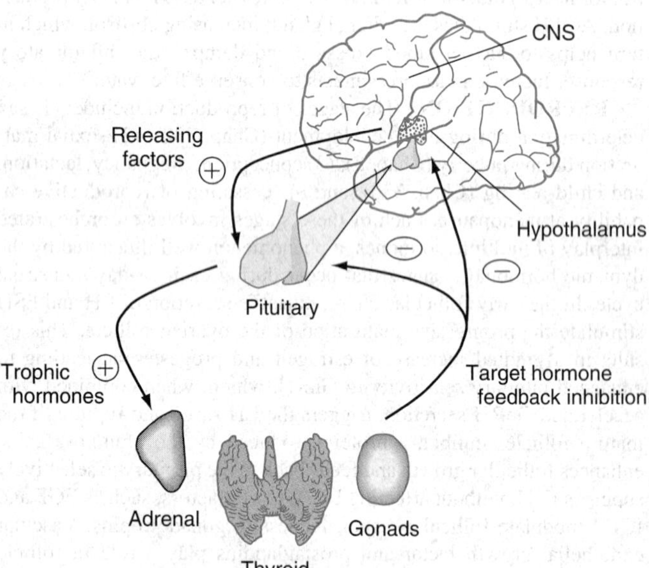

FIGURE 327-3 Feedback regulation of endocrine axes. CNS, central nervous system.

Anatomic relationships of glandular systems also greatly influence hormonal exposure—the physical organization of islet cells enhances their intercellular communication; the portal vasculature of the hypothalamic-pituitary system exposes the pituitary to high concentrations of hypothalamic releasing factors; testicular seminiferous tubules gain exposure to high testosterone levels produced by the interdigitated Leydig cells; the pancreas receives nutrient information from the gastrointestinal tract; and the liver is the proximal target of insulin action because of portal drainage from the pancreas.

HORMONAL RHYTHMS The feedback regulatory systems described above are superimposed on hormonal rhythms that are used for adaptation to the environment. Seasonal changes, the daily occurrence of the light-dark cycle, sleep, meals, and stress are examples of the many environmental events that affect hormonal rhythms. The *menstrual cycle* is repeated on average every 28 days, reflecting the time required to follicular maturation and ovulation (Chap. 336). Essentially all pituitary hormone rhythms are entrained to sleep and the *circadian cycle*, generating reproducible patterns that are repeated approximately every 24 h. The HPA axis, for example, exhibits characteristic peaks of ACTH and cortisol production in the early morning, with a nadir in the afternoon and evening. Recognition of these rhythms is important for endocrine testing and treatment. Patients with Cushing's syndrome characteristically exhibit increased midnight cortisol levels when compared to normal individuals (Chap. 331). In contrast, morning cortisol levels are similar in these groups, as cortisol is normally high at this time of day in normal individuals. The HPA axis is more susceptible to suppression by glucocorticoids administered at night as they blunt the early morning rise of ACTH. Understanding these rhythms allows glucocorticoid replacement that mimics diurnal production by administering larger doses in the morning than in the afternoon (Chap. 331).

Other endocrine rhythms occur on a more rapid time scale. Many peptide hormones are secreted in discrete bursts every few hours. LH and FSH secretion are exquisitely sensitive to GnRH pulse frequency. Intermittent pulses of GnRH are required to maintain pituitary sensitivity, whereas continuous exposure to GnRH causes pituitary gonadotrope desensitization. This feature of the hypothalamic-pituitary-gonadotrope (HPG) axis forms the basis for using long-acting GnRH agonists to treat central precocious puberty or to decrease testosterone levels in the management of prostate cancer.

It is important to be aware of the pulsatile nature of hormone secretion and the rhythmic patterns of hormone production when relating serum hormone measurements to normal values. For some hormones, integrated markers have been developed to circumvent hormonal fluctuations. Examples include 24-h urine collections for cortisol, IGF-I as a biologic marker of GH action, and HbA1c as an index of long-term (weeks to months) blood glucose control.

Often, one must interpret endocrine data only in the context of other hormonal results. For example, parathyroid hormone levels are typically assessed in combination with serum calcium concentrations. A high serum calcium level in association with elevated PTH is suggestive of hyperparathyroidism, whereas a suppressed PTH in this situation is more likely to be caused by hypercalcemia of malignancy or other causes of hypercalcemia. Similarly, TSH should be elevated when T_4 and T_3 concentrations are low, reflecting reduced feedback inhibition. When this is not the case, it is important to consider other abnormalities in the hormonal axis, such as secondary hypothyroidism, which is caused by a defect at the level of the pituitary.

PATHOLOGIC MECHANISMS OF ENDOCRINE DISEASE

Endocrine diseases can be divided into three major types of conditions: (1) hormone excess, (2) hormone deficiency, and (3) hormone resistance (Table 327-2).

CAUSES OF HORMONE EXCESS Syndromes of hormone excess can be caused by neoplastic growth of endocrine cells, autoimmune disorders, and excess hormone administration. Benign endocrine tumors, including parathyroid, pituitary, and adrenal adenomas, often retain the capacity to produce hormones, perhaps reflecting the fact that they are relatively well differentiated. Many endocrine tumors exhibit relatively subtle defects in their "set points" for feedback regulation. For example, in Cushing's disease, impaired feedback inhibition of ACTH secretion is associated with autonomous function. However, the tumor cells are not completely resistant to feedback, as revealed by the fact that ACTH is ultimately suppressed by higher doses of dexamethasone (e.g., high-dose dexamethasone test) (Chap. 331). Similar set point defects are also typical of parathyroid adenomas and autonomously functioning thyroid nodules.

The molecular basis of some endocrine tumors, such as the MEN syndromes (MEN-1, -2A, -2B), have provided important insights into tumorigenesis (Chap. 339). MEN-1 is characterized primarily by the triad of parathyroid, pancreatic islet, and pituitary tumors. MEN-2 predisposes to medullary thyroid carcinoma, pheochromocytoma, and hyperparathyroidism. The *MEN1* gene, located on chromosome 11q13, encodes a putative tumor-suppressor gene. Analogous to the paradigm first described for retinoblastoma, the affected individual inherits a mutant copy of the *MEN1* gene, and tumorigenesis ensues after a somatic "second hit" leads to loss of function of the normal *MEN1* gene (through deletion or point mutations).

Table 327-2 Causes of Endocrine Dysfunction

Type of Endocrine Disorder	Examples
Hyperfunction	
Neoplastic	
Benign	Pituitary adenomas, hyperparathyroidism, autonomous thyroid or adrenal nodules, pheochromocytoma
Malignant	Adrenal cancer, medullary thyroid cancer, carcinoid
Ectopic	Ectopic ACTH, SIADH secretion
Multiple endocrine neoplasia	MEN-1, MEN-2
Autoimmune	Graves' disease
Iatrogenic	Cushing's syndrome, hypoglycemia
Infectious/Inflammatory	Subacute thyroiditis
Activating receptor mutations	LH, TSH, Ca^{2+} and PTH receptors, $G_s\alpha$ (see Table 327-3)
Hypofunction	
Autoimmune	Hashimoto's thyroiditis, type 1 diabetes mellitus, Addison's disease, polyglandular failure
Iatrogenic	Radiation-induced hypopituitarism, hypothyroidism, surgical
Infectious/inflammatory	Adrenal insufficiency, hypothalamic sarcoidosis
Hormone mutations	GH, LHβ, FSHβ, vasopressin (see Table 327-3)
Enzyme defects	21-Hydroxylase deficiency (see Table 327-3)
Developmental defects	Kallmann syndrome, Turner syndrome, transcription factors (see Table 327-3)
Nutritional/vitamin deficiency	Vitamin D deficiency, iodine deficiency
Hemorrhage/infarction	Sheehan's syndrome, adrenal insufficiency
Hormone Resistance	
Receptor mutations	
Membrane	GH, vasopressin, LH, FSH, ACTH, GnRH, GHRH, PTH, leptin, Ca^{2+} (see Table 327-3)
Nuclear	AR, TR, VDR, ER,GR, $PPAR_\gamma$ (see Table 327-3)
Signaling pathway mutations	Albright's hereditary osteodystrophy
Postreceptor	Type 2 diabetes mellitus, leptin resistance

NOTE: AR, androgen receptor; ER, estrogen receptor; GR, glucocorticoid receptor; SIADH, syndrome of inappropriate antidiuretic hormone; TR, thyroid hormone receptor; VDR, vitamin D receptor. For all other abbreviations, see text.

In contrast to inactivation of a tumor-suppressor gene, as occurs in MEN-1 and most other inherited cancer syndromes, MEN-2 is caused by activating mutations in a single allele. In this case, activating mutations of the *RET* proto-oncogene, which encodes a receptor tyrosine kinase, leads to thyroid C-cell hyperplasia in childhood before the development of medullary thyroid carcinoma. Elucidation of the pathogenic mechanism has allowed early genetic screening for *RET* mutations in individuals at risk for MEN-2, permitting identification of those who may benefit from prophylactic thyroidectomy and biochemical screening for pheochromocytoma and hyperparathyroidism.

Mutations that activate hormone receptor signaling have been identified in several GPCRs (Table 327-3). For example, activating mutations of the LH receptor causes a dominantly transmitted form of male-limited precocious puberty, reflecting premature stimulation of testosterone synthesis in Leydig cells (Chap. 335). Activating mutations in these GPCRs are located primarily in the transmembrane domains and induce receptor coupling to $G_s\alpha$, even in the absence of hormone. Consequently, adenylate cyclase is activated and cyclic AMP levels increase in a manner that mimics hormone action. A similar phenomenon results from activating mutations in $G_s\alpha$. When these occur early in development, they cause McCune-Albright syndrome. When they occur only in somatotropes, the activating $G_s\alpha$ mutations cause GH-secreting tumors and acromegaly (Chap. 328).

In autoimmune Graves' disease, antibody interactions with the TSH receptor mimic TSH action, leading to hormone overproduction (Chap. 330). Analogous to the effects of activating mutations of the TSH receptor, these stimulating autoantibodies induce conformational changes that release the receptor from a constrained state, thereby triggering receptor coupling to G proteins.

CAUSES OF HORMONE DEFICIENCY Most examples of hormone deficiency states can be attributed to glandular destruction caused by autoimmunity, surgery, infection, inflammation, infarction, hemorrhage, or tumor infiltration (Table 327-2). Autoimmune damage to the thyroid gland (Hashimoto's thyroiditis) and pancreatic islet β cells (type 1 diabetes mellitus) are prevalent causes of endocrine disease. Mutations in a number of hormones, hormone receptors, transcription factors, enzymes, and channels can also lead to hormone deficiencies (Table 327-3).

HORMONE RESISTANCE Most severe hormone resistance syndromes are due to inherited defects in membrane receptors, nuclear receptors, or in the pathways that transduce receptor signals (Table 327-3). These disorders are characterized by defective hormone action, despite the presence of increased hormone levels. In complete androgen resistance, for example, mutations in the androgen receptor cause genetic (XY) males to have a female phenotypic appearance, even though LH and testosterone levels are increased (Chap. 338). In addition to these relatively rare genetic disorders, more common acquired forms of functional hormone resistance include insulin resistance in type 2 diabetes mellitus, leptin resistance in obesity, and GH resistance in catabolic states. The pathogenesis of functional resistance involves receptor downregulation and postreceptor desensitization of signaling pathways; functional forms of resistance are generally reversible.

Approach to the Patient

Because endocrinology interfaces with numerous physiologic systems, there is no standard endocrine history and examination. Moveover,

Table 327-3 Examples of Genetic Endocrine Diseases

Endocrine Mutation	Disorder[a]	Mode of Inheritance	Chromosome Location	Types of Mutation
Hormone Mutations				
Insulin	Hyperproinsulinemia	AR	11p15.5	P
Growth hormone	GH deficiency; dwarfism	AR,AD	17q22-q24	D,P
POMC	Adrenal insufficiency; obesity	AR	2p23.3	P
Parathyroid hormone	Hypoparathyroidism	AD	11p15.3-15.1	P
Thyroid-stimulating hormone	TSH deficiency; hypothyroidism	AR	1p22	D,P
Thyroglobulin	Hypothyroidism; goiter	AR	8q24.2-q24.3	P
Luteinizing hormone	LH deficiency; hypogonadism	AR	19q13.32	P
Follicle-stimulating hormone	FSH deficiency; hypogonadism	AR	11p13	P
Vasopressin/neurophysin II	Neurohypophyseal diabetes insipidus (DI)	AD	20p12.21	P
Anti-müllerian hormone	Retained müllerian ducts	AR	19p13.3-p13.2	P
Leptin	Obesity	AR	7q31.3	P
Binding Protein Mutations				
Thyroxine-binding globulin	Euthyroid hypothyroxinemia	XL	Xq21-22	D,P
Transthyretin	Euthyroid hyperthyroximemia	AD	18q11.2-12.1	P
Albumin	Euthyroid hyperthyroximemia	AD	4q11-q13	P
Membrane Receptor Mutations				
Insulin receptor	Insulin resistance	AR, AD	19p13.3-13	P
GnRH receptor	Hypogonadotropic hypogonadism	AR	4q21.2	P
GHRH receptor	GH deficiency; dwarfism	AR	7p15-p14	P
TRH receptor	Hypothalamic hypothyroidism	AR	8q23	P
Growth hormone receptor	Laron dwarfism	AR	5p13-p12	P
TSH receptor (inactive)	TSH resistance	AR	14q31	P
TSH receptor (activating)	Hyperthyroidism	AD, S	14q31	P
LH receptor (inactive)	Hypogonadism	AR	2p21	P
LH receptor (activating)	Male precocious puberty	AD,S	2p21	P
FSH receptor (inactivating)	Ovarian failure; ↓ spermatogenesis	AR	2p21-p16	P
PTH receptor (inactivating)	Blomstrand chondrodysplasia	AR	3p22-p21.1	P
PTH receptor (activating)	Jansen chondrodysplasia	AD	3p22-p21.1	P
ACTH receptor	Adrenal insufficiency	AR	18p11.2	P
Vasopressin V_2 receptor	Nephrogenic DI	XL	Xq27-q28	P
Calcium receptor (inactive)	Hypocalciuric hypercalcemia	AD,AR	3q21-q24	P
Calcium receptor (activating)	Hypoparathyroidism	AD	3q21-q24	P
MIS receptor	Retained müllerian ducts	AR	12q13	P
Leptin receptor	Obesity	AR	1p31	P
Melanocortin 4 receptor	Obesity	AD	18q22	P
$G_s\alpha$	Acromegaly	S	20q13.2-13.3	P
$G_s\alpha$	Albright osteodystrophy	AD; imprinting	20q13.2-13.3	P
$G_s\alpha$	McCune-Albright	Mosaic	20q13.2-13.3	P
Nuclear Receptor Mutations				
Vitamin D	Type II vitamin D–resistant rickets (VDRR)	AR	12q12-q14	P
Thyroid hormone	Thyroid hormone resistance	AD	3p24.3	P,D
Glucocorticoid	Glucocorticoid resistance	AR	5q31	P
Mineralocorticoid	Pseudohypoaldosteronism type 1	AD	4q31.1	P
Androgen	Androgen resistance	XL,S	Xcen-q13	P,D
Estrogen	Estrogen resistance	AR,S	6p25.1	P
PPAR $\gamma 2$	Obesity; insulin resistance	AD	3p25	P
Steroidogenic factor 1	XY sex-reversal; adrenal insufficiency	AD	9q33	P
DAX1	Adrenal hypoplasia congenita	XL	Xp21.3-p21.2	P,D
HNF 4α	MODY 1	AD	20q12-q13.1	P
Transcription Factor Mutations				
HNF 1α	MODY 3	AD	12q24.2	P
HNF 1β	MODY 5	AD	17cen-q21.3	P
Insulin promoter factor 1	MODY 4	AD	13q12.1	P
Pit1	GH, PRL, TSH deficiency	AR, AD	3p11	D,P
Prop1	GH, PRL, TSH, LH, FSH deficiency	AR	5q	P
Thyroid transcription factor 1	Congenital hypothyroidism	Unknown	14q13	Low expression
Thyroid transcription factor 2	Congenital hypothyroidism	AR	9q22	P
PAX-8	Congenital hypothyroidism	AR	2q12-q14	P
SRY translocation	XX male	XL	Ypter	Translocation
SRY mutation	XY female	YL	Ypter	P
SOX-9	XY female; campomelic dysplasia	AD	17q24.3-q25.1	P
Wilms' tumor	Frasier syndrome; Denys-Drash	AD	11p13	P
DAZ (RNA-binding protein)	Azoospermia	YL	Yq11	D
Endocrine Syndromes				
Kallmann	Hypogonadotropic hypogonadism	XL, AR, AD	Xp22.3	D,P,translocation
Prader-Willi	Hypogonadism, obesity, short stature	AD; imprint	15q11	D
Von Hippel–Lindau	Pheochromocytoma; renal Ca	AD	3p26-p25	D,P

(continued)

Table 327-3—*(continued)*

Endocrine Mutation	Disorder[a]	Mode of Inheritance	Chromosome Location	Types of Mutation
MEN-1	Neoplasia: Pit, pancreas, parathyroid	AD	11q13	P
MEN-2 (activating *ret* mutations)	Neoplasia: Parathyroid, pheo, MTC	AD	10q11.2	P
MEN-2b	MEN-2 and neurofibromas	AD	10q11.2	P
Carney complex	Cushing's; acromegaly, myxomas	AD	2p16	Unknown
Pendred syndrome	Goiter; deafness	AR	7q31	P,D
DiGeorge syndrome	Hypoparathyroidism; cardiac abn.	AD	22q11	D
Prohormone convertase 1	ACTH, GnRH, insulin deficiency	AR	5q15-q21	P
Polyglandular failure type 1	Polyglandular failure	AR	21q22.3	P
Enzyme and Channel Mutations				
Glucokinase	MODY 2	AD	7p15-p13	P
Sulfonylurea receptor	Nesidioblastosis	AR	11p15.1-p14	P
Potassium channel KCNJ11	Nesidioblastosis	AR	11p15.1	P
Sodium iodide symporter	Goiter, hypothyroidism	AR	19p12-13.2	P
Thyroid peroxidase	Goiter, hypothyroidism	AR	2pter-12	P
21-hydroxylase	CAH, androgen excess	AR	6p21	P,D
17α-Hydroxylase	Androgen deficiency, HTN	AR	10q24.3	P
17,20-Lyase activity	XY ambiguous genitalia	AR	10q24.3	P
11β-Hydroxylase	Androgen excess, HTN	AR	8q21	P
3β-Hydroxysteroid dehydrog.	CAH; Androgen deficiency	AR	1p13.1	P
Steroidogenic acute regulatory	Lipoid CAH	AR	8p11.2	P
5α-Reductase type 2	Male pseudohermaphroditism	AR	2p23	D,P
Aldosterone synthase	Glucocorticoid remediable HTN	AD	8q21	D, translocation
Amiloride sensitive Na channel	Liddle syndrome; HTN	AD	16p13-p12	P
Aquaporin 2	Nephrogenic DI	AR	12q13	P
PEX	Hypophosphatemic VDRR	XL	Xp22.2-pp22.1	P
1α Hydroxylase	Type 1 VDRR	AR	12q14	P

NOTE: AD, autosomal dominant; AR, autosomal recessive; CAH, congenital adrenal hyperplasia; D, deletion, HNF, hepatic nuclear factor; HTN, hypertension; MODY, maturity onset diabetes of the young; MTC, medullary thyroid carcinoma; P, point mutation; S, somatic cell mutation; XL, X-linked; YL, Y-linked. For other abbreviations, see text.
SOURCE: Adapted from DeGroot and Jameson, with permission.

because most glands are relatively inaccessible, the examination usually focuses on the manifestations of hormone excess or deficiency, as well as direct examination of palpable glands, such as the thyroid and gonads. For these reasons, it is important to evaluate patients in the context of their presenting symptoms, review of systems, family and social history, and exposure to medications that may affect the endocrine system. Astute clinical skills are required to detect subtle symptoms and signs suggestive of underlying endocrine disease. For example, a patient with Cushing's syndrome may manifest specific findings, such as central fat redistribution, striae, and proximal muscle weakness, in addition to features seen commonly in the general population, such as obesity, plethora, hypertension, and glucose intolerance. Similarly, the insidious onset of hypothyroidism—with mental slowing, fatigue, dry skin, and other features—can be difficult to distinguish from similar, nonspecific findings in the general population. Clinical judgment, based on knowledge of pathophysiology and experience, is required to decide when to embark on more extensive evaluation of these disorders. As described below, laboratory testing plays an essential role in endocrinology by allowing quantitative assessment of hormone levels and dynamics. Radiologic imaging tests, such as CT scan, MRI, thyroid scan, and ultrasound, are also used for the diagnosis of endocrine disorders. However, these tests are generally employed only after a hormonal abnormality has been established by biochemical testing.

Hormone Measurements and Endocrine Testing Radioimmunoassays are the most important diagnostic tool in endocrinology, as they allow sensitive, specific, and quantitative determination of steady-state and dynamic changes in hormone concentrations. Radioimmunoassays use antibodies to detect specific hormones. For many peptide hormones, these measurements are now configured as immunoradiometric assays (IRMAs), which use two different antibodies to increase binding affinity and specificity. There are many variations of these assays—a common format involves using one antibody to capture the antigen (hormone) onto an immobilized surface and a second antibody, labeled with a fluorescent or radioactive tag, to detect the antigen. These assays are sensitive enough to detect plasma hormone concentrations in the picomolar to nanomolar range, and they can readily distinguish structurally related proteins, such as PTH from PTHrP. A variety of other techniques are used to measure specific hormones, including mass spectroscopy, various forms of chromatography, and enzymatic methods; bioassays are now used rarely.

Most hormone measurements are based on plasma or serum samples. However, urinary hormone determinations remain useful for the evaluation of some conditions. Urinary collections over 24 h provide an integrated assessment of the production of a hormone or metabolite, many of which vary during the day. It is important to assure complete collections of 24-h urine samples; simultaneous measurement of creatinine provides an internal control for the adequacy of collection and can be used to normalize some hormone measurements. A 24-h urine free cortisol measurement largely reflects the amount of unbound cortisol, thus providing a reasonable index of biologically available hormone. Other commonly used urine determinations include: 17-hydroxycorticosteroids, 17-ketosteroids, vanillylmandelic acid (VMA), metanephrine, catecholamines, 5-hydroxyindoleacetic acid (5-HIAA), and calcium.

The value of quantitative hormone measurements lies in their correct interpretation in a clinical context. The normal range for most hormones is relatively broad, often varying by a factor of two- to tenfold. The normal ranges for many hormones are gender- and age-specific. Thus, using the correct normative database is an essential part of interpreting hormone tests. The pulsatile nature of hormones and factors that can affect their secretion, such as sleep, meals, and medications, must also be considered. Cortisol values increase fivefold between midnight and dawn; reproductive hormone levels vary dramatically during the female menstrual cycle.

For many endocrine systems, much information can be gained from basal hormone testing, particularly when different components of an endocrine axis are assessed simultaneously. For example, low testosterone and elevated LH levels suggest a primarily gonadal problem, whereas a hypothalamic-pituitary disorder is likely if both LH and testosterone are low. Because TSH is a sensitive indicator of thyroid function, it is generally recommended as a first-line test for thyroid disorders. An elevated TSH level is almost always the result of primary hypothyroidism, whereas a low TSH is most often caused by thyro-

Table 327-4 Examples of Prevalent Endocrine and Metabolic Disorders in the Adult

Disorder	Approx. Prevalence in Adults[a]	Screening/Testing Recommendations[b]	Specific Guidelines	Chapter
Obesity	23% BMI > 30 50% BMI > 25	Calculate BMI Measure waist circumference Exclude secondary causes Consider comorbid complications	NHLBI Clinical Guidelines on the Identification, Evaluation, and Treatment of Overweight and Obesity	77
Type 2 diabetes mellitus	>6%	Test every 3 years or more often in high-risk groups: Fasting plasma glucose (FPG) > 126 mg/dL Random plasma glucose > 200 mg/dL An elevated HbA1c Consider comorbid complications	Expert Committee on the Diagnosis and Classification of Diabetes Mellitus	333
Hyperlipidemia	5–10%	Cholesterol screening at least every 5 years; more often in high-risk groups Lipoprotein analysis (LDL, HDL) for increased cholesterol, CAD, diabetes Consider secondary causes	Expert Panel of the National Cholesterol Education Program (NCEP)	344
Hypothyroidism	5–10%, women 0.5–2%, men	TSH; confirm with free T_4		330
Graves' disease	1–3%, women 0.1%, men	TSH, free T_4		330
Thyroid nodules and neoplasia	5%	Physical examination of thyroid Fine-needle aspiration biopsy	American Thyroid Association	330
Osteoporosis	5%, women 1%, men	Bone mineral density measurements in individuals at risk Exclude secondary causes	World Health Organization	342
Hyperparathyroidism	0.1–0.5%, women > men	Serum calcium PTH, if calcium is elevated Assess comorbid conditions	NIH Consensus Conference on Diagnosis and Management of Asymptomatic Primary Hyperparathyroidism	341
Infertility	10%, couples	Investigate male and female member of couple Semen analysis in male Assess ovulatory cycles in female Specific tests as indicated		54
Polycystic ovarian syndrome	4–7% women	Free testosterone, DHEAS Consider comorbid conditions		336
Hirsutism	Variable	Free testosterone, DHEAS Exclude secondary causes Additional tests as indicated		53
Menopause	Median age, 51	FSH		336
Hyperprolactinemia	Common in women with amenorrhea or galactorrhea	PRL level MRI, if not medication-related		328
Erectile dysfunction	10–15%	PRL, testosterone Consider secondary causes (e.g., diabetes)		51
Gynecomastia	Common in older men	Often, no tests are indicated Consider Klinefelter syndrome Consider medications, hypogonadism, liver disease		337
Klinefelter syndrome	0.2%, men	Karyotype Testosterone		338
Turner syndrome	0.03%, women	Karyotype Consider comorbid conditions		338

[a] The prevalence of most disorders varies among ethnic groups and with aging.

[b] See individual chapters for additional information on evaluation and treatment. Early testing is indicated in patients with signs and symptoms of disease or in those at increased risk.

NOTE: BMI, body mass index; CAD, coronary artery disease; DHEAS, dehydroepiandrosterone; HDL, high-density lipoprotein; LDL, low-density lipoprotein; MRI, magnetic resonance imaging. For other abbreviations, see text.

toxicosis. These predictions can be confirmed by determining the free thyroxine level. Elevated calcium and PTH levels suggest hyperparathyroidism, whereas PTH is suppressed in hypercalcemia caused by malignancy or granulomatous diseases. A suppressed ACTH in the setting of hypercortisolemia, or increased urine free cortisol, is seen with hyperfunctioning adrenal adenomas.

It is not uncommon, however, for baseline hormone levels associated with pathologic endocrine conditions to overlap with the normal range. In this circumstance, dynamic testing is useful to further separate the two groups. There are a multitude of dynamic endocrine tests, but all are based on principles of feedback regulation, and most responses can be remembered based on the pathways that govern endocrine axes. *Suppression tests* are used in the setting of suspected endocrine hyperfunction. An example is the dexamethasone suppression test used to evaluate Cushing's syndrome (Chaps. 328 and 331). *Stimulation tests* are generally used to assess endocrine hypofunction. The ACTH stimulation test, for example, is used to assess the adrenal gland response in patients with suspected adrenal insufficiency. Other stimulation tests use hypothalamic-releasing factors such as TRH, GnRH, CRH, and GHRH to evaluate pituitary hormone reserve (Chap. 328). Insulin-induced hypoglycemia evokes pituitary ACTH and GH responses. Stimulation tests based on reduction or inhibition of endogenous hormones are less commonly used. Examples include metyrapone inhibition of cortisol synthesis and clomiphene inhibition of estrogen feedback.

Screening and Assessment of Common Endocrine Disorders Because many endocrine disorders are prevalent in the adult population (Table 327-4), most are diagnosed and managed by general internists, family practitioners, or other primary health care providers. The high prevalence and clinical impact of certain endocrine diseases justifies vigilance for features of these disorders during routine physical examinations; laboratory screening is indicated in selected high-risk populations.

BIBLIOGRAPHY

CANAFF L et al: Peptide hormone precursor processing: Getting sorted? Mol Cell Endocrinol 156:1, 1999

CARTER-SU C, SMIT LS: Signaling via JAK tyrosine kinases: Growth hormone receptor as a model system. Recent Prog Horm Res 53:61, 1998

CZEISLER CA, KLERMAN EB: Circadian and sleep-dependent regulation of hormone release in humans. Recent Prog Horm Res 54:97, 1999

DEGROOT LJ, JAMESON JL: *Endocrinology*, 4th ed. Philadelphia, Saunders, 2001 (in press)

GETHER U: Uncovering molecular mechanisms involved in activation of G protein–coupled receptors. Endocr Rev 21:90, 2000

GIGUERE V: Orphan nuclear receptors: From gene to function. Endocr Rev 20:689, 1999

JAMESON JL: *Hormone Resistance Syndromes*. Totowa, NJ, Humana, 1999

MARX SJ et al: Multiple endocrine neoplasia type 1: Clinical and genetic features of the hereditary endocrine neoplasias. Recent Prog Horm Res 54:397, 1999

MCKENNA NJ et al: Nuclear receptor coregulators: Cellular and molecular biology. Endocr Rev 20:321, 1999

VIRKAMAKI A et al: Protein-protein interaction in insulin signaling and the molecular mechanisms of insulin resistance. J Clin Invest 103:931, 1999

WILSON JD et al: *William's Textbook of Endocrinology*, 9th ed. Philadelphia, Saunders, 1998

328

Shlomo Melmed

DISORDERS OF THE ANTERIOR PITUITARY AND HYPOTHALAMUS

ACTH adrenocorticotropin hormone
AGHD adult GH deficiency
AVP arginine vasopressin
CNS central nervous system
CRH corticotropin-releasing hormone
CSF cerebrospinal fluid
CT computed tomography
FSH follicle-stimulating hormone
GH growth hormone
GHBP GH binding protein
GHRH growth hormone–releasing hormone
GHRPs growth hormone–releasing peptides
GnRH gonadotropin-releasing hormone
GPCR G protein–coupled receptor
hCG human chorionic gonadotropin
hMG human menopausal gonadotropin
HPA hypothalamo-pituitary-adrenal
IGFBPs IGF-binding proteins
IGF insulin-like growth factor
IL interleukin
JAK Janus kinase
LH luteinizing hormone
LOH loss of heterozygosity
MAP mitogen activated protein
MRI magnetic resonance imaging
POMC proopiomelanocortin
PRL prolactin
STAT signal transduction and activators of transcription
TNF tumor necrosis factor
TRH thyrotropin-releasing hormone
TSH thyroid-stimulating hormone

The anterior pituitary is often referred to as the "master gland" because, together with the hypothalamus, it orchestrates the complex regulatory functions of multiple other endocrine glands. The anterior pituitary gland produces six major hormones: (1) prolactin (PRL), (2) growth hormone (GH), (3) adrenocorticotropin hormone (ACTH), (4) luteinizing hormone (LH), (5) follicle-stimulating hormone (FSH), and (6) thyroid-stimulating hormone (TSH) (Table 328-1). Pituitary hormones are secreted in a pulsatile manner, reflecting stimulation by an array of specific hypothalamic releasing factors. Each of these pituitary hormones elicits specific responses in peripheral target tissues. The hormonal products of these peripheral glands, in turn, exert feedback control at the level of the hypothalamus and pituitary to modulate pituitary function (Fig. 328-1). Pituitary tumors cause characteristic hormone excess syndromes. Hormone deficiency may be inherited or acquired. Fortunately, efficacious treatments exist for the various pituitary hormone excess and deficiency syndromes. Nonetheless, these diagnoses are often elusive, emphasizing the importance of recognizing subtle clinical manifestations and performing the correct laboratory diagnostic tests. →*For discussion of disorders of the posterior pituitary, or neurohypophysis, see Chap. 329.*

ANATOMY AND DEVELOPMENT **Anatomy** The pituitary gland weighs ~600 mg and is located within the sella turcica ventral to the diaphragma sella; it comprises anatomically and functionally distinct anterior and posterior lobes. The sella is contiguous to vascular and neurologic structures, including the cavernous sinuses, cranial nerves, and optic chiasm. Thus, expanding intrasellar pathologic processes may have significant central mass effects in addition to their endocrinologic impact.

Hypothalamic neural cells synthesize specific releasing and inhibiting hormones that are secreted directly into the portal vessels of the pituitary stalk. Blood supply of the pituitary gland is derived from the superior and inferior hypophyseal arteries (Fig. 328-2). The hypothalamic-pituitary portal plexus provides the major blood source for the anterior pituitary, allowing reliable transmission of hypothalamic peptide pulses without significant systemic dilution; consequently, pituitary cells are exposed to sharp spikes of releasing factors and in turn release their hormones as discrete pulses (Fig. 328-3).

The posterior pituitary is supplied by the inferior hypophyseal arteries. In contrast to the anterior pituitary, the posterior lobe is directly innervated by hypothalamic neurons (supraopticohypophyseal and tuberohypophyseal nerve tracts) via the pituitary stalk (Chap. 329).

Table 328-1 Anterior Pituitary Hormone Expression and Regulation

Cell	Corticotrope	Somatotrope	Lactotrope	Thyrotrope	Gonadotrope
Tissue-specific transcription factor	PTX-1, CUTE	Prop I, Pit-I	Prop I, Pit I	Prop I, Pit 1, TEF	SF-1, DAX-1
Fetal appearance	6 weeks	8 weeks	12 weeks	12 weeks	12 weeks
Hormone	POMC	GH	PRL	TSH	FSH LH
Chromosomal locus	2 p	17q	6	α −6q; β-1p	β-11p; β-19q
Protein	Polypeptide	Polypeptide	Polypeptide	Glycoprotein α, β subunits	Glycoprotein α, β subunits
Amino acids	266 (ACTH 1–39)	191	199	211	210 204
Stimulators	CRH, AVP, gp-130 cytokines	GHRH, GHRP	Estrogen, TRH, VIP	TRH	GnRH, activins, estrogen
Inhibitors	Glucocorticoids	Somatostatin, IGF-I	Dopamine	T_3, T_4, dopamine, somatostatin, glucocorticoids	Sex steroids, inhibin
Target gland	Adrenal	Liver, other tissues	Breast, other tissues	Thyroid	Ovary, testis
Trophic effect	Steroid production	IGF-I production, growth induction, insulin antagonism	Milk production	T_4 synthesis and secretion	Sex steroid production, follicle growth germ cell maturation
Normal range	ACTH, 4–22 pg/L	<0.5 μg/L[a]	M < 15; F <20 μg/L	0.1–5 mU/L	M, 5–20 IU/L, F (basal), 5–20 IU/L

[a] Hormone secretion integrated over 24 h.

NOTE: M, male; F, female. For other abbreviations, see text.

SOURCE: Adapted from I Shimon, S Melmed, in P Conn, S Melmed (eds): *Endocrinology: Basic and Clinical Principles*. Totowa, NJ, Humana, 1996.

Thus, posterior pituitary production of vasopressin (antidiuretic hormone; ADH) and oxytocin is particularly sensitive to neuronal damage by lesions that affect the pituitary stalk or hypothalamus.

Pituitary Development The embryonic differentiation and maturation of anterior pituitary cells have been elucidated in considerable detail. Pituitary development from Rathke's pouch involves a complex interplay of lineage-specific transcription factors expressed in pluripotential stem cells and gradients of locally produced growth factors (Table 328-1). The transcription factor Pit-1 determines cell-specific expression of GH, PRL, and TSH in somatotropes, lactotropes, and thyrotropes. Expression of high levels of estrogen receptors in cells that contain Pit-1 favors PRL expression, whereas thyrotrope embronic factor (TEF) induces TSH expression. Pit-1 binds to GH, PRL, and TSH gene regulatory elements, as well as to recognition sites on its own promoter, providing a mechanism for perpetuating selective pituitary phenotypic stability. The transcription factor Prop-1 induces the pituitary development of Pit-1-specific lineages, as well as gonadotropes. Gonadotrope cell development is further defined by the cell-specific expression of the nuclear receptors, steroidogenic factor (SF-1) and DAX-1. Development of corticotrope cells, which express the proopiomelanocortin (POMC) gene, requires corticotropin upstream transcription element (CUTE) and the PTX-1 transcription factor. Abnormalities of pituitary development caused by mutations of Pit-1, Prop-1, SF-1, and DAX-1 result in a series of rare, selective or combined, pituitary hormone deficits.

HYPOTHALAMIC AND ANTERIOR PITUITARY INSUFFICIENCY

Hypopituitarism results from impaired production of one or more of the anterior pituitary trophic hormones. Reduced pituitary function can result from inherited disorders; more commonly, it is acquired and reflects the mass effects of tumors or the consequences of inflammation or vascular damage. These processes may also impair synthesis or secretion of hypothalamic hormones, with resultant pituitary failure (Table 328-2).

DEVELOPMENTAL AND GENETIC CAUSES OF HYPOPITUITARISM **Pituitary Dysplasia** Pituitary dysplasia may result in aplastic, hypoplastic, or ectopic pituitary gland development. Because pituitary development requires midline cell migration from the nasopharyngeal Rathke's pouch, midline craniofacial disorders, such as cleft lip and palate, basal encephalocele, hypertelorism, and optic nerve hypoplasia, may be associated with pituitary dysplasia. Acquired pituitary failure in the newborn can also be caused by birth trauma, including cranial hemorrhage, asphyxia, and breech delivery.

Septo-optic dysplasia Hypothalamic dysfunction and hypopituitarism may result from dysgenesis of the septum pellucidum or corpus callosum. Affected children have mutations in the *HESX1* gene, which is involved in early development of the ventral prosencephalon. These children exhibit cleft palate, syndactyly, ear deformities, hypertelorism, optic atrophy, micropenis, and anosmia. Pituitary dysfunction leads to diabetes insipidus, GH deficiency and short stature, and, occasionally, TSH deficiency.

Tissue-Specific Factor Mutations Several pituitary cell–specific transcription factors, such as Pit-1 and Prop-1, are critical for determining the development and function of specific anterior pituitary

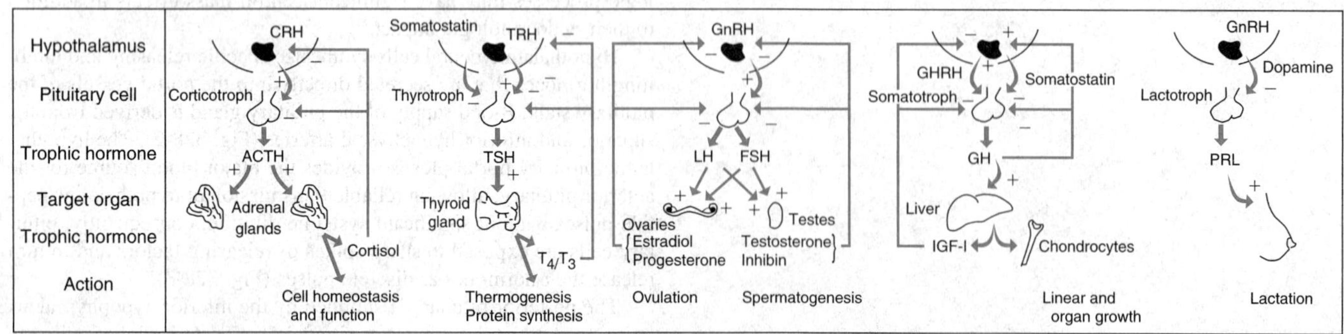

FIGURE 328-1 Diagram of pituitary axes. Hypothalamic hormones regulate anterior pituitary trophic hormones that, in turn, determine target gland secretion. Peripheral hormones feedback to regulate hypothalamic and pituitary hormones. For abbreviations, see text.

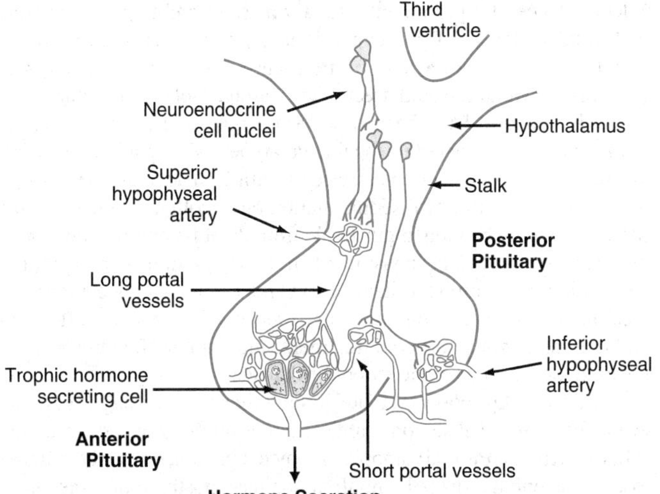

FIGURE 328-2 Diagram of hypothalamic-pituitary vasculature: The hypothalamic nuclei produce hormones that traverse the portal system and impinge on anterior pituitary cells to regulate pituitary hormone secretion. Posterior pituitary hormones are derived from direct neural extensions.

cell lineages. Autosomal dominant or recessive Pit-1 mutations cause combined GH, PRL, and TSH deficiencies. These patients present with growth failure and varying degrees of hypothyroidism. The pituitary may appear hypoplastic on magnetic resonance imaging (MRI).

Prop-1 is expressed early in pituitary development and appears to be required for Pit-1 function. Familial and sporadic *PROP1* mutations result in combined GH, PRL, TSH, and gonadotropin deficiency, with preservation of ACTH. Over 80% of these patients have growth retardation and, by adulthood, all are deficient in TSH and gonadotropins. Because of gonadotropin deficiency, they do not enter puberty spontaneously (Fig. 328-4).

Developmental Hypothalamic Dysfunction • ***Kallmann syndrome*** This syndrome results from defective hypothalamic gonadotropin-releasing hormone (GnRH) synthesis and is associated with anosmia or hyposmia due to olfactory bulb agenesis or hypoplasia (Chap. 335). The syndrome may also be associated with color blindness, optic atrophy, nerve deafness, cleft palate, renal abnormalities, cryptorchidism, and neurologic abnormalities such as mirror movements. Defects in the *KAL* gene, which maps to chromosome Xp22.3, prevent embryonic migration of GnRH neurons from the hypothalamic olfactory placode to the hypothalamus. Genetic abnormalities, in addition to *KAL* mutations, can also cause isolated GnRH deficiency, as autosomal recessive and dominant modes of transmission have been described. GnRH deficiency prevents progression through puberty. Males present with delayed puberty and pronounced hypogonadal features, including micropenis, probably the result of low testosterone levels during infancy (Chap. 335). Female patients present with primary amenorrhea and failure of secondary sexual development.

Kallmann syndrome and other causes of congenital GnRH deficiency are characterized by low LH and FSH levels and low concentrations of sex steroids (testosterone or estradiol). In sporadic cases of isolated gonadotropin deficiency, the diagnosis is often one of exclusion after eliminating other causes of hypothalamic-pituitary dysfunction. Repetitive GnRH administration restores normal pituitary gonadotropin responses, pointing to a hypothalamic defect.

Long-term treatment of males with human chorionic gonadotropin

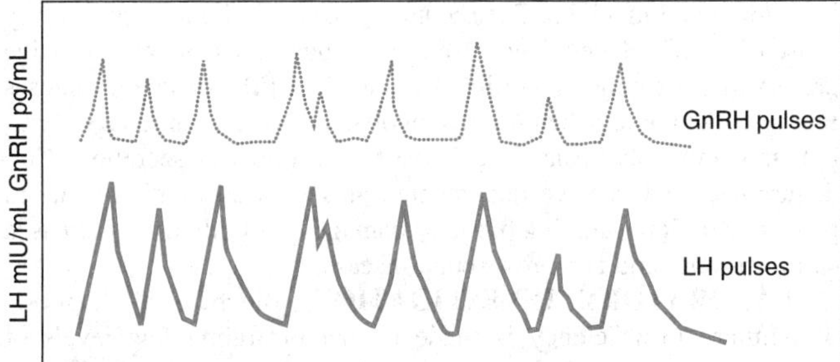

FIGURE 328-3 Hypothalamic gonadotropin-releasing hormone (GnRH) pulses induce secretory pulses of luteinizing hormone (LH).

Table 328-2 Etiology of Hypopituitarism[a]

Development/structural
- Transcription factor defect
- Pituitary dysplasia/aplasia
- Congenital CNS mass, encephalocele
- Primary empty sella
- Congenital hypothalamic disorders (septo-optic dysplasia, Prader-Willi syndrome, Laurence-Moon-Biedl syndrome, Kallmann syndrome)

Traumatic
- Surgical resection
- Radiation damage
- Head injuries

Neoplastic
- Pituitary adenoma
- Parasellar mass (meningioma, germinoma, ependymoma, glioma)
- Rathke's cyst
- Craniopharyngioma
- Hypothalamic hamartoma, gangliocytoma
- Pituitary metastases (breast, lung, colon carcinoma)
- Lymphoma and leukemia
- Meningioma

Infiltrative/inflammatory
- Hemochromatosis
- Lymphocytic hypophysitis
- Sarcoidosis
- Histiocytosis X
- Granulomatous hypophysitis

Vascular
- Pituitary apoplexy
- Pregnancy-related (infarction with diabetes; postpartum necrosis)
- Sickle cell disease
- Arteritis

Infections
- Fungal (histoplasmosis)
- Parasitic (toxoplasmosis)
- Tuberculosis
- *Pneumocystis carinii*

[a] Trophic hormone failure associated with pituitary compression or destruction usually occurs sequentially GH > FSH > LH > TSH > ACTH. During childhood, growth retardation is often the presenting feature, and in adults hypogonadism is the earliest symptom.

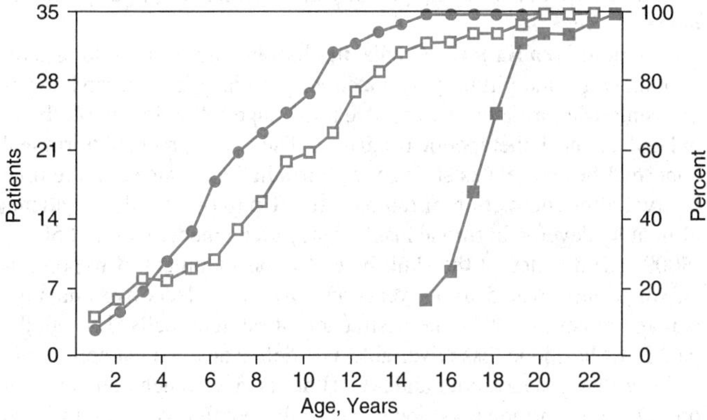

FIGURE 328-4 Gradual development of anterior pituitary hormone deficiencies in 35 patients with *PROP1* gene mutations. Combined pituitary hormone deficiency develops gradually. By adulthood, all patients have growth hormone (GH, ●), thyroid-stimulating hormone (TSH, □), and gonadotropin (LH, luteinizing hormone; FSH, follicle-stimulating hormone, ■) deficiency. *(Adapted from Deladoey et al, 1999.)*

(hCG) or testosterone restores pubertal development and secondary sex characteristics; females can be treated with cyclic estrogen and progestin. Fertility may also be restored by the administration of subcutaneous, pulsatile GnRH using a portable infusion pump.

Laurence-Moon-Bardet-Biedl syndrome This rare autosomal recessive disorder is characterized by mental retardation; obesity; and hexadactyly, brachydactyly, or syndactyly. Central diabetes insipidus may or may not be associated. GnRH deficiency occurs in 75% of males and half of affected females. Retinal degeneration begins in early childhood, and most patients are blind by age 30.

Fröhlich syndrome (adipose genital dystrophy) A broad spectrum of hypothalamic lesions may be associated with hyperphagia, obesity, and central hypogonadism. Decreased GnRH production in these patients results in attenuated pituitary FSH and LH synthesis and release.

Prader-Willi syndrome Chromosome 15q deletions are associated with hypogonadotropic hypogonadism, hyperphagia-obesity, chronic muscle hypotonia, mental retardation, and adult-onset diabetes mellitus (Chap. 66). Multiple somatic defects also involve the skull, eyes, ears, hands, and feet. Diminished hypothalamic oxytocin- and vasopressin-producing nuclei have been reported. Deficient GnRH synthesis is suggested by the observation that chronic GnRH treatment restores pituitary LH and FSH release.

ACQUIRED HYPOPITUITARISM Hypopituitarism may be caused by accidental or neurosurgical trauma; vascular events such as apoplexy; pituitary or hypothalamic neoplasms such as pituitary adenomas, craniopharyngiomas, or metastatic deposits; inflammatory disease such as lymphocytic hypophysitis; infiltrative disorders such as sarcoidosis, hemochromatosis (Chap. 345), and tuberculosis; or irradiation. It is often difficult to localize the site of hormonal dysfunction as many processes, including hemochromatosis and radiation, may affect both hypothalamic and pituitary function.

Hypothalamic Infiltration Disorders These disorders—including those associated with sarcoidosis, histiocytosis X, amyloidosis, and hemochromatosis—frequently involve both hypothalamic and pituitary neuronal and neurochemical tracts. Consequently, diabetes insipidus occurs in half of patients with these disorders. Growth retardation is seen if attenuated GH secretion occurs before pubertal epiphyseal closure. Hypogonadotropic hypogonadism and hyperprolactinemia are also common.

Inflammatory Lesions Pituitary damage and subsequent dysfunction can be seen with chronic infections such as tuberculosis, opportunistic fungal infections associated with AIDS, and in tertiary syphilis. Other inflammatory processes, such as granulomas or sarcoidosis, may mimic a pituitary adenoma. These lesions may cause extensive hypothalamic and pituitary damage, leading to trophic hormone failure.

Cranial Irradiation Cranial irradiation may result in long-term hypothalamic and pituitary dysfunction, especially in children and adolescents who are more susceptible to damage following whole-brain or head and neck therapeutic irradiation. The development of hormonal abnormalities correlates strongly with irradiation dosage and the time interval after completion of radiotherapy. Up to two-thirds of patients ultimately develop hormone insufficiency afer a median dose of 50 Gy (5000 rad) directed at the skull base. The development of hypopituitarism occurs over 5 to 15 years and usually reflects hypothalamic damage rather than absolute destruction of pituitary cells. Though the pattern of hormone loss is variable, GH deficiency is most commonly followed by gonadotropin and ACTH deficiency. When deficiency of one or more hormones is documented, the possibility of diminished reserve of other hormones is likely. Accordingly, anterior pituitary function should be evaluated over the long term in previously irradiated patients, and replacement therapy instituted when appropriate (see below).

Lymphocytic Hypophysitis This occurs mainly in pregnant or post-partum women; it usually presents with hyperprolactinemia and MRI evidence of a prominent pituitary mass resembling an adenoma, with mildly elevated PRL levels. Pituitary failure caused by diffuse lymphocytic infiltration may be transient or permanent but requires immediate evaluation and treatment. Rarely, isolated pituitary hormone deficiencies have been described, suggesting a selective autoimmune process targeted to specific cell types. Most patients manifest symptoms of progressive mass effects with headache and visual disturbance. The erythrocyte sedimentation rate is often elevated. As the MRI image may be indistinguishable from that of a pituitary adenoma, hypophysitis should be considered in a post-partum woman with a newly diagnosed pituitary mass before embarking on unnecessary surgical intervention. The inflammatory process often resolves after several months of glucocorticoid treatment, and pituitary function may be restored, depending on the extent of damage.

Pituitary Apoplexy Acute intrapituitary hemorrhagic vascular events can cause substantial damage to the pituitary and surrounding sellar structures. Pituitary apoplexy may occur spontaneously in a preexisting adenoma (usually nonfunctioning); postpartum (Sheehan's syndrome); or in association with diabetes, hypertension, sickle cell anemia, or acute shock. The hyperplastic enlargement of the pituitary during pregnancy increases the risk for hemorrhage and infarction. Apoplexy is an endocrine emergency that may result in severe hypoglycemia, hypotension, central nervous system (CNS) hemorrhage, and death. Acute symptoms include severe headache with signs of meningeal irritation, bilateral visual changes, ophthalmoplegia that varies, and, in severe cases, cardiovascular collapse and loss of consciousness. Pituitary computed tomography (CT) or MRI may reveal signs of intratumoral or sellar hemorrhage, with deviation of the pituitary stalk and compression of pituitary tissue.

Patients with no evident visual loss or impaired consciousness can be observed and managed conservatively with high-dose glucocorticoids. Those with significant or progressive visual loss or loss of consciousness require urgent surgical decompression. Visual recovery after surgery is inversely correlated with the length of time after the acute event. Therefore, severe ophthalmoplegia or visual deficits are indications for early surgery. Hypopituitarism is very common after apoplexy.

Empty Sella A partial or apparently totally empty sella is usually an incidental MRI finding. These patients usually exhibit normal pituitary function, implying that the surrounding rim of pituitary tissue is fully functional. Hypopituitarism, however, may develop insidiously. Pituitary masses may undergo clinically silent infarction with development of a partial or totally empty sella by cerebrospinal fluid (CSF) filling the dural herniation. Rarely, functional pituitary adenomas may arise within the rim of pituitary tissue, and these are not always visible on MRI.

PRESENTATION AND DIAGNOSIS The clinical manifestations of hypopituitarism depend on which hormones are lost and the extent of the hormone deficiency. GH deficiency causes growth disorders in children and leads to abnormal body composition in adults (see below). Gonadotropin deficiency causes menstrual disorders and infertility in women and decreased sexual function, infertility, and loss of secondary sexual characteristics in men. TSH and ACTH deficiency usually develop later in the course of pituitary failure. TSH deficiency leads to growth retardation in children and features of hypothyroidism in children and in adults. The secondary form of adrenal insufficiency caused by ACTH deficiency leads to hypocortisolism with relative preservation of mineralocorticoid production. PRL deficiency causes failure of lactation. When lesions involve the posterior pituitary tracts, polyuria and polydipsia reflect loss of vasopressin secretion. Epidemiologic studies have documented an increased mortality rate in patients with longstanding pituitary damage, primarily from increased cardiovascular and cerebrovascular disease.

LABORATORY INVESTIGATION Biochemical diagnosis of pituitary insufficiency is made by demonstrating low levels of trophic hormones in the setting of low target hormone levels. For example, low free thyroxine in the setting of a low or inappropriately normal TSH level suggests secondary hypothyroidism. Similarly, a

Table 328-3 Tests of Pituitary Insufficiency

Hormone	Test	Blood Samples	Interpretation
Growth hormone	Insulin tolerance test: Regular insulin (0.05–0.15 U/kg IV)	−30, 0, 30, 60, 120 min for glucose and GH	Glucose < 40 mg/dL; GH should be >3 μg/L
	GHRH test: 1 μg/kg IV	0, 15, 30, 45, 60, 120 min for GH	Normal response is GH >3 μg/L
	L-Arginine test: 30 g IV over 30 min	0, 30, 60, 120 min for GH	Normal response is GH >3 μg/L
	L-dopa test: 500 mg PO	0, 30, 60, 120 min for GH	Normal response is GH >3 μg/L
Prolactin	TRH test: 200–500 μg IV	0, 20, and 60 min for TSH and PRL	Normal prolactin is >2 μg/L and increase >200% of baseline
ACTH	Insulin tolerance test: Regular insulin (0.05–0.15 U/kg IV)	−30, 0, 30, 60, 90 min for glucose and cortisol	Glucose <40 mg/dL Cortisol should increase by >7 μg/dL or to >20 μg/dL
	CRH test: 1 μg/kg ovine CRH IV at 0800 h	0, 15, 30, 60, 90, 120 min for ACTH and cortisol	Basal ACTH increases 2- to 4-fold and peaks at 20–100 pg/mL Cortisol levels >20–25 μg/dL
	Metyrapone test: Metyrapone (30 mg/kg) at midnight	Plasma 11-deoxycortisol and cortisol at 8 A.M.; ACTH can also be measured	Plasma cortisol should be <4 μg/dL to assure an adequate response Normal response is 11-deoxycortisol >7.5 μg/dL or ACTH >75 pg/mL
	Standard ACTH stimulation test: ACTH 1-24 (Cosyntropin), 0.25 mg IM or IV	0, 30, 60 min for cortisol and aldosterone	Normal response is cortisol >21 μg/dL and aldosterone response of >4 ng/dL above baseline
	Low-dose ACTH test: ACTH 1-24 (Cosyntropin), 1 μg IV	0, 30, 60 min for cortisol	Cortisol should be >21 μg/dL
	3-day ACTH stimulation test consists of 0.25 mg ACTH 1-24 given IV over 8 h each day		Cortisol >21 μg/dL
TSH	Basal thyroid function tests: T_4, T_3, TSH	Basal tests	Low free thyroid hormone levels in the setting of TSH levels that are not appropriately increased
	TRH test: 200–500 μg IV	0, 20, 60 min for TSH and PRL	TSH should increase by >5 mU/L unless thyroid hormone levels are increased
LH, FSH	LH, FSH, testosterone, estrogen	Basal tests	Basal LH and FSH should be increased in postmenopausal women Low testosterone levels in the setting of low LH and FSH
	GnRH test: GnRH (100 μg) IV	0, 30, 60 min for LH and FSH	In most adults, LH should increase by 10 IU/L and FSH by 2 IU/L Normal responses are variable
Multiple hormones	Combined anterior pituitary test: GHRH (1 μg/kg), CRH (1 μg/kg), GnRH (100 μg), TRH (200 μg) are given IV	−30, 0, 15, 30, 60, 90, 120 min for GH, ACTH, cortisol, LH, FSH, and TSH	Combined or individual releasing hormone responses must be elevated in the context of basal target gland hormone values and may not be diagnostic (see text)

low testosterone level without elevation of gonadotropins suggests hypogonadotropic hypogonadism. Provocative tests may be required to assess pituitary reserve (Table 328-3). GH responses to insulin-induced hypoglycemia, arginine, L-dopa, growth hormone–releasing hormone (GHRH), or growth hormone–releasing peptides (GHRPs) can be used to assess GH reserve. PRL and TSH responses to thyrotropin-releasing hormone (TRH) reflect lactotrope and thyrotrope function. Corticotropin-releasing hormone (CRH) administration induces ACTH release, and administration of synthetic ACTH (cortrosyn) evokes adrenal cortisol release as an indirect indicator of pituitary ACTH reserve (Chap. 331). ACTH reserve is most reliably assessed during insulin-induced hypoglycemia. However, this test should be performed cautiously in patients with suspected adrenal insufficiency because of increased risk of hypoglycemia and hypotension.

Rx TREATMENT Hormone replacement therapy, including glucocorticoids, thyroid hormone, sex steroids, growth hormone, and vasopressin, is usually free of complications. Treatment regimens that mimic physiologic hormone production allow for maintenance of satisfactory clinical homeostasis. Effective dosage schedules are outlined in Table 328-4. Patients in need of glucocorticoid replacement require careful dose adjustments during stressful events such as acute illness, dental procedures, trauma, and acute hospitalization (Chap. 331).

HYPOTHALAMIC, PITUITARY, AND OTHER SELLAR MASSES

PITUITARY TUMORS Pituitary adenomas are the most common cause of pituitary hormone hypersecretion and hyposecretion syndromes in adults. They account for ~10% of all intracranial neoplasms. At autopsy, up to a quarter of all pituitary glands harbor an unsuspected microadenoma (<10 mm diameter). Similarly, pituitary imaging detects small pituitary lesions in at least 10% of normal individuals.

Pathogenesis Pituitary adenomas are benign neoplasms that arise from one of the five anterior pituitary cell types. The clinical and biochemical phenotype of pituitary adenomas depend on the cell type from which they are derived and are described in detail below. Thus, tumors arising from lactotrope (PRL), somatotrope (GH), corticotrope (ACTH), thyrotrope (TSH), or gonadotrope (LH, FSH) cells hypersecrete their respective hormones (Table 328-5). Plurihormonal tumors that express combinations of GH, PRL, TSH, ACTH, and the glycoprotein hormone α subunit may be diagnosed by careful immunocytochemistry or may, in fact, present with mixed clinical features of these hormonal hypersecretory syndromes. Morphologically, these tumors may arise from a single polysecreting cell type or consist of cells with mixed function within the same tumor.

Hormonally active tumors are characterized by autonomous hor-

Table 328-4 Hormone Replacement Therapy for Adult Hypopituitarism[a]

Trophic Hormone Deficit	Hormone Replacement
ACTH	Hydrocortisone (10–20 mg A.M.; 10 mg P.M.)
	Cortisone acetate (25 mg A.M.; 12.5 mg P.M.)
	Prednisone (5 mg A.M.; 2.5 mg P.M.)
TSH	L-Thyroxine (0.075–0.15 mg daily)
FSH/LH	Males
	Testosterone enanthate (200 mg IM every 2 weeks)
	Testosterone skin patch (5 mg/d)
	Females
	Conjugated estrogen (0.65–1.25 mg qd for 25 days)
	Progesterone (5–10 mg qd) on days 16–25
	Estradiol skin patch (0.5 mg, every other day)
	For fertility: Menopausal gonadotropins, human chorionic gonadotropins
GH	Adults: Somatotropin (0.3–1.0 mg SC qd)
	Children: Somatotropin [0.02–0.05 (mg/kg/day)]
Vasopressin	Intranasal desmopressin (5–20 μg twice daily)
	Oral 300–600 μg qd

[a] All doses shown should be individualized for specific patients and should be reassessed during stress, surgery, or pregnancy. Male and female fertility requirements should be managed as discussed in Chap. 54.

mone secretion with diminished responsiveness to the normal physiologic pathways of inhibition. Hormone production does not always correlate with tumor size. Small hormone-secreting adenomas may cause significant clinical perturbations, whereas larger adenomas that produce less hormone may be clinically silent and remain undiagnosed (if no central compressive effects occur). About one-third of all adenomas are clinically nonfunctioning and produce no distinct clinical hypersecretory syndrome. Most arise from gonadotrope cells and may secrete α- and β-glycoprotein hormone subunits or, very rarely, intact circulating gonadotropins. True pituitary carcinomas with documented extracranial metastases are exceedingly rare.

Almost all pituitary adenomas are monoclonal in origin, implying the acquisition of one or more somatic mutations that confer a selective growth advantage. In addition to direct studies of oncogene mutations, this idea is supported by X-chromosomal inactivation analyses of tumors in female patients heterozygous for X-linked genes. Consistent with their clonal origin, complete surgical resection of small pituitary adenomas usually cures hormone hypersecretion. Nevertheless, hypothalamic hormones, such as GHRH or CRH, also enhance the mitotic activity of their respective pituitary target cells, in addition to their role in pituitary hormone regulation. Thus, patients harboring rare abdominal or chest tumors elaborating ectopic GHRH or CRH may present with somatotrope or corticotrope hyperplasia.

Table 328-5 Classification of Pituitary Adenomas[a]

Adenoma Cell Origin	Hormone Product	Clinical Syndrome
Lactotrope	PRL	Hypogonadism, galactorrhea
Gonadotrope	FSH, LH, subunits	Silent or hypogonadism
Somatotrope	GH	Acromegaly/gigantism
Corticotrope	ACTH	Cushing's disease
Mixed growth hormone and prolactin cell	GH, PRL	Acromegaly, hypogonadism, galactorrhea
Other plurihormonal cell	Any	Mixed
Acidophil stem cell	PRL, GH	Hypogonadism, galactorrhea acromegaly
Mammosomatotrope	PRL, GH	Hypogonadism, galactorrhea acromegaly
Thyrotrope	TSH	Thyrotoxicosis
Null cell	None	Pituitary failure
Oncocytoma	None	Pituitary failure

[a] Hormone-secreting tumors are listed in decreasing order of frequency. All tumors may cause local pressure effects, including visual disturbances, cranial nerve palsy, and headache.

SOURCE: Adapted from S Melmed, in JL Jameson (ed): *Principles of Molecular Medicine*, Totowa, Humana Press, 1998.

Several etiologic genetic events have been implicated in the development of pituitary tumors. The pathogenesis of sporadic forms of acromegaly has been particularly informative as a model of tumorigenesis. GHRH, after binding to its G protein–coupled somatotrope receptor, utilizes cyclic AMP as a second messenger to stimulate GH secretion and somatotrope proliferation. A subset (~35%) of GH-secreting pituitary tumors contain mutations in Gsα (Arg 201 → Cys or His; Gln 227 → Arg). These mutations inhibit intrinsic GTPase activity, resulting in constitutive elevation of cyclic AMP, Pit-1 induction, and activation of cyclic AMP response element binding protein (CREB), thereby promoting somatotrope cell proliferation.

Characteristic loss of heterozygosity (LOH) in various chromosomes has been documented in large or invasive macroadenomas, suggesting the presence of putative tumor suppressor genes at these loci. LOH of chromosome region on 11q13, 13, and 9 is present in up to 20% of sporadic pituitary tumors including GH-, PRL-, and ACTH-producing adenomas and in some nonfunctioning tumors.

Compelling evidence also favors growth factor promotion of pituitary tumor proliferation. Basic fibroblast growth factor (bFGF) is abundant in the pituitary and has been shown to stimulate pituitary cell mitogenesis. Other factors involved in initiation and promotion of pituitary tumors include loss of negative-feedback inhibition (as seen with primary hypothyroidism or hypogonadism) and estrogen-mediated or paracrine angiogenesis. Growth characteristics and neoplastic behavior may also be influenced by several activated oncogenes, including *RAS* and pituitary tumor transforming gene (*PTTG*).

Genetic Syndromes Associated with Pituitary Tumors Several familial syndromes are associated with pituitary tumors, and the genetic mechanisms for some of these have been unraveled (Table 328-6).

Multiple endocrine neoplasia (MEN) 1 is an autosomal dominant syndrome characterized primarily by a genetic predisposition to parathyroid, pancreatic islet, and pituitary adenomas (Chap. 339). MEN-1 is caused by inactivating germline mutations in *MENIN*, a constitutively expressed tumor-suppressor gene located on chromosome 11q13. Loss of heterozygosity, or a somatic mutation of the remaining normal *MENIN* allele, leads to tumorigenesis. About half of affected patients develop prolactinomas; acromegaly and Cushing's syndrome are less commonly encountered.

Carney syndrome is characterized by spotty skin pigmentation, myxomas, and endocrine tumors including testicular, adrenal, and pituitary adenomas. Acromegaly occurs in about 20% of patients. This autosomal dominant syndrome is associated with microsatellite alterations on chromosome 2p16.

McCune-Albright syndrome consists of polyostotic fibrous dysplasia, pigmented skin patches, and a variety of endocrine disorders, including GH-secreting pituitary tumors, adrenal adenomas, and autonomous ovarian function (Chap. 343). Hormonal hypersecretion is due to constitutive cyclic AMP production caused by inactivation of the GTPase activity of Gsα. The Gsα mutations occur postzygotically, leading to a mosaic pattern of mutant expression.

Familial acromegaly is a rare disorder in which family members may manifest either acromegaly or gigantism. The disorder is associated with LOH at a chromosome 11q13 locus distinct from that of *MENIN*.

OTHER SELLAR MASSES *Craniopharyngiomas* are derived from Rathke's pouch. They arise near the pituitary stalk and commonly extend into the suprasellar cistern. These tumors are often large, cystic, and locally invasive. Many are partially calcified, providing a characteristic appearance on skull x-ray and CT images. More than half of all patients present before age 20, usually with signs of increased intracranial pressure, including headache, vomiting, papilledema, and hydrocephalus. Associated symptoms include visual field abnormalities, personality changes and cognitive deterioration, cranial nerve damage, sleep difficulties, and weight gain. Anterior pituitary dysfunction and diabetes insipidus are common. About half of affected children present with growth retardation.

Treatment usually involves transcranial or transsphenoidal surgical resection followed by postoperative radiation of residual tumor. This approach can result in long-term survival and ultimate cure, but most patients require lifelong pituitary hormone replacement. If the pituitary stalk is uninvolved and can be preserved at the time of surgery, the incidence of subsequent anterior pituitary dysfunction is significantly diminished.

Developmental failure of Rathke's pouch obliteration may lead to *Rathke's cysts*, which are small (<5 mm) cysts entrapped by squamous epithelium; these cysts are found in about 20% of individuals at autopsy. Although Rathke's cleft cysts do not usually grow and are often diagnosed incidentally, about a third present in adulthood with compressive symptoms, diabetes insipidus, and hyperprolactinemia due to stalk compression. Rarely, internal hydrocephalus develops. The diagnosis is suggested preoperatively by visualizing the cyst wall on MRI, which distinguishes these lesions from craniopharyngiomas. Cyst contents range from CSF-like fluid to mucoid material. *Arachnoid cysts* are rare and generate an MRI image isointense with cerebrospinal fluid.

Table 328-6 Genetic Syndromes Associated with Pituitary Tumors

Syndrome	Clinical Features	Chromosomal Location	Gene	Protein	Proposed Function/Defect
Multiple endocrine neoplasia type I (MEN-I)	Parathyroid, endocrine pancreas, anterior pituitary (mostly prolactinomas) tumors	11q13	*MEN1*	Menin	Nuclear, unknown
Familial acromegaly	GH-cell adenomas, acromegaly/gigantism	11q13 and other loci	Not *MEN1*	—	—
McCune-Albright syndrome	Polyostic fibrous dysplasia, pigmented skin patches; Endocrine abnormalities: precocious puberty, GH-cell adenomas, acromegaly/gigantism	20q13.2 (mosaic)	*GNAS1* (*gsp*)	Gsα	Signal transduction/inactive Inactive GTPase results in constitutive cyclic AMP elevation, independent of GHRH
Carney syndrome	Skin and cardiac myxomas, Cushing's syndrome, acromegaly	2p16	—	—	Telomere alteration?

SOURCE: Adapted from T Prezant, S Melmed, in S Webb (ed): *Pituitary Tumours*: Epidemiology, Pathogenesis, and Management. BioScientifica, Bristol, UK 1998.

Sella chordomas usually present with bony clival erosion, local invasiveness, and, on occasion, calcification. Normal pituitary tissue may be visible on MRI, distinguishing chordomas from aggressive pituitary adenomas. Mucinous material may be obtained by fine-needle aspiration.

Meningiomas arising in the sellar region may be difficult to distinguish from nonfunctioning pituitary adenomas. On MRI they may be asymmetric, and on CT they may show evidence of bony erosion. Meningiomas may cause compressive symptoms.

Histiocytosis X comprises a variety of syndromes associated with foci of eosinophilic granulomas. Diabetes insipidus, exophthalmos, and punched-out lytic bone lesions (*Hand-Schüller-Christian disease*) are associated with granulomatous lesions visible on MRI, as well as a characteristic axillary skin rash. Rarely, the pituitary stalk may be involved.

Pituitary metastases occur in ~3% of cancer patients. Blood-borne metastatic deposits are found almost exclusively in the posterior pituitary. Accordingly, diabetes insipidus can be a presenting feature of lung, gastrointestinal, breast, and other pituitary metastases. About half of pituitary metastases originate from breast cancer; about 25% of patients with breast cancer have such deposits. Rarely, pituitary stalk involvement results in anterior pituitary insufficiency. The MRI diagnosis of a metastatic lesion may be difficult to distinguish from an aggressive pituitary adenoma; the diagnosis may require histologic examination of excised tumor tissue. Primary or metastatic lymphoma, leukemias, and plasmacytomas also occur within the sella.

Hypothalamic hamartomas and *gangliocytomas* may arise from astrocytes, oligodendrocytes, and neurons with varying degrees of differentiation. These tumors may overexpress hypothalamic neuropeptides including GnRH, GHRH, or CRH. In GnRH-producing tumors, children present with precocious puberty, psychomotor delay, and laughing-associated seizures. Medical treatment of GnRH-producing hamartomas with long-acting GnRH analogues effectively suppresses gonadotropin secretion and controls pubertal development. Rarely, hamartomas are also associated with craniofacial abnormalities; imperforate anus; cardiac, renal, and lung disorders; and pituitary failure (*Pallister-Hall syndrome*). Hypothalamic hamartomas are often contiguous with the pituitary, and preoperative MRI diagnosis may not be possible. Histologic evidence of hypothalamic neurons in tissue resected at transsphenoidal surgery may be the first indication of a primary hypothalamic lesion.

Hypothalamic gliomas and *optic gliomas* occur mainly in childhood and usually present with visual loss. Adults have more aggressive tumors; about a third are associated with neurofibromatosis.

Brain germ-cell tumors may arise within the sellar region. These include *dysgerminomas*, which are associated with diabetes insipidus and visual loss and rarely metastasize. *Germinomas*, *embryonal carcinomas*, *teratomas*, and *choriocarcinomas* may arise in the parasellar region and produce hCG. These germ-cell tumors present with precocious puberty, diabetes insipidus, visual field defects, and thirst disorders. Many patients are GH-deficient with short stature.

METABOLIC EFFECTS OF HYPOTHALAMIC LESIONS The hypothalamus is subject to injury from mass lesions, granulomatous disorders, infections, and hemorrhage. Lesions involving the anterior and preoptic hypothalamic regions cause paradoxical vasoconstriction, tachycardia, and hyperthermia. Acute hyperthermia is usually due to a hemorrhagic insult, but poikilothermia may also occur. Central disorders of thermoregulation result from posterior hypothalamic damage. The *periodic hypothermia syndrome* comprises episodic attacks of rectal temperatures <30°C, sweating, vasodilation, vomiting, and bradycardia (Chap. 20). Damage to the ventromedial nuclei by craniopharyngiomas, hypothalamic trauma, or inflammatory disorders may be associated with *hyperphagia* and *obesity*. This region appears to contain an energy-satiety center where melanocortin receptors are influenced by leptin, insulin, POMC products, and gastrointestinal peptides (Chap. 77). Median eminence involvement results in diabetes insipidus in about 50% of patients. Hypothalamic gliomas in early childhood may be associated with a diencephalic syndrome characterized by progressive severe emaciation and growth failure. Polydipsia or hypodipsia are associated with damage to central osmoreceptors located in preoptic nuclei (Chap. 329). Slow-growing hypothalamic lesions can cause increased somnolence and disturbed sleep cycles as well as obesity, hypothermia, and emotional outbursts. Lesions of the central hypothalamus may stimulate sympathetic neurons, leading to elevated serum catecholamine and cortisol levels.

These patients are predisposed to cardiac arrhythmias, hypertension, and gastric erosions.

EVALUATION **Local Mass Effects** Clinical manifestations of sellar lesions vary, depending on the anatomic location of the mass and direction of its extension (Table 328-7). The dorsal roof of the sella presents the least resistance to soft tissue expansion from within the confines of the sella; consequently, pituitary adenomas frequently extend in a suprasellar direction. Bony invasion may ultimately occur as well.

Headaches are common features of small intrasellar tumors, even with no demonstrable suprasellar extension. Because of the confined nature of the pituitary, small changes in intrasellar pressure stretch the dural plate; however, the severity of the headache correlates poorly with adenoma size or extension.

Suprasellar extension can lead to visual loss by several mechanisms, the most common being compression of the optic chiasm, but direct invasion of the optic nerves or obstruction of CSF flow leading to secondary visual disturbances also occur. Pituitary stalk compression by a hormonally active or inactive intrasellar mass may compress the portal vessels, disrupting pituitary access to the hypothalamic hormones and dopamine; this results in hyperprolactinemia and concurrent loss of other pituitary hormones. This "stalk section" phenomenon may also be caused by trauma, whiplash injury with posterior clinoid stalk compression, or skull base fractures. Lateral mass invasion may impinge on the cavernous sinus and compress its neural contents, leading to cranial nerve III, IV, and VI palsies as well as effects on the ophthalmic and maxillary branches of the fifth cranial nerve (Chap. 367). Patients may present with diplopia, ptosis, ophthalmoplegia, and decreased facial sensation, depending on the extent of neural damage. Extension into the sphenoid sinus indicates that the pituitary mass has eroded through the sellar floor. Aggressive tumors may also invade the palate roof and cause nasopharyngeal obstruction, infection, and, rarely, CSF leakage. Both temporal and frontal lobes may be invaded, leading to uncinate seizures, personality disorders, and anosmia. Direct hypothalamic encroachment by an invasive pituitary mass may cause important metabolic sequelae, precocious puberty or hypogonadism, diabetes insipidus, sleep disturbances, dysthermia, and appetite disorders.

Table 328-7 Features of Sellar Mass Lesions[a]

Impacted Structure	Clinical Impact
Pituitary	Hypogonadism
	Hypothyroidism
	Growth failure and adult hyposomatotropism
	Hypoadrenalism
Optic tract	Loss of red perception
	Bitemporal hemianopia
	Superior or bitemporal field defect
	Scotoma
	Blindness
Hypothalamus	Temperature dysregulation
	Appetite and thirst disorders
	Obesity
	Diabetes insipidus
	Sleep disorders
	Behavioral dysfunction
	Autonomic dysfunction
Cavernous sinus	Opthalmoplegia ± ptosis or diplopia
	Facial numbness
Frontal lobe	Personality disorder
	Anosmia
Brain	Headache
	Hydrocephalus
	Psychosis
	Dementia
	Laughing seizures

[a] As the intrasellar mass expands, it first compresses intrasellar pituitary tissue, then usually invades dorsally through the dura to lift the optic chiasm or laterally to the cavernous sinuses. Bony erosion is rare, as is direct brain compression. Microadenomas may present with headache.

MRI Sagittal and coronal T1-weighted spin-echo MRI imaging, before and after administration of gadolinium, allow precise visualization of the pituitary gland with clear delineation of the hypothalamus, pituitary stalk, pituitary tissue and surrounding suprasellar cisterns, cavernous sinuses, sphenoid sinus, and optic chiasm. Pituitary gland height ranges from 6 mm in children to 8 mm in adults; during pregnancy and puberty, the height may reach 10 to 12 mm. The upper aspect of the adult pituitary is flat or slightly concave, but in adolescent and pregnant individuals, this surface may be convex, reflecting physiologic pituitary enlargement. The stalk should be vertical. CT scan is indicated to define the extent of bony erosion or the presence of calcification.

The soft tissue consistency of the pituitary gland is slightly heterogeneous on MRI. Anterior pituitary signal intensity resembles that of brain matter on T1-imaging (Fig. 328-5). Adenoma density is usually lower than that of surrounding normal tissue on T1-weighted imaging, and the signal intensity increases with T2-weighted images. The high phospholipid content of the posterior pituitary results in a bright enhancing signal.

Sellar masses are commonly encountered as incidental findings on MRI, and most of these are pituitary adenomas (incidentalomas). This finding is consistent with the observation that clinically silent pituitary microadenomas can be identified in up to 25% of pituitaries in autopsy series. In the absence of hormone hypersecretion, these small lesions can be safely monitored by MRI, which is performed annually and then less often if there is no evidence of growth. Resection should be considered for incidentally discovered macroadenomas, as about one-third become invasive or cause local pressure effects. If hormone hypersecretion is evident, specific therapies are indicated. When larger masses (>1 cm) are encountered, they should also be distinguished from nonadenomatous lesions. Meningiomas are often associated with bony hyperostosis; craniopharyngiomas may be calcified and are usually hypodense, whereas gliomas are hyperdense on T2-weighted images.

Ophthalmologic Evaluation Because optic tracts may be contiguous to an expanding pituitary mass, reproducible visual field assessment that uses perimetry techniques should be performed on all patients with sellar mass lesions that abut the optic chiasm. Loss of red perception is an early sign of optic tract pressure. Bitemporal hemianopia or superior bitemporal defects are classically observed, reflecting the location of these tracts within the inferior and posterior part of the chiasm. Early diagnosis reduces the risk of blindness, scotomas, or other visual disturbances.

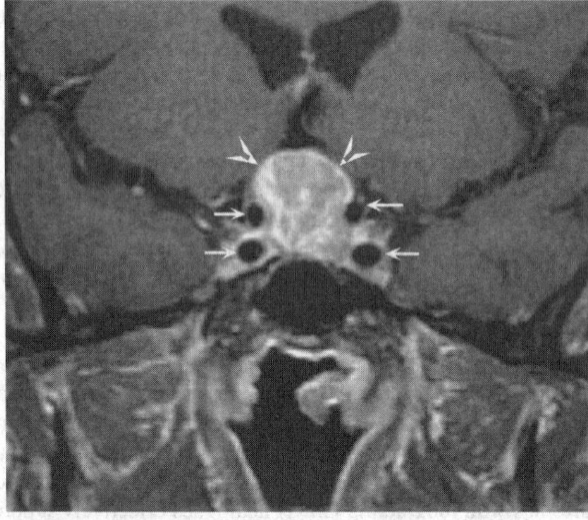

FIGURE 328-5 Pituitary adenoma. Coronal T1-weighted postcontrast MR image shows a homogeneously enhancing mass (arrowheads) in the sella turcica and suprasellar region compatible with a pituitary adenoma; the small arrows outline the carotid arteries.

Laboratory Investigation The presenting clinical features of functional pituitary adenomas (e.g., acromegaly, prolactinomas, or Cushing's disease) should guide the laboratory studies (see below). However, for a sellar mass with no obvious clinical features of hormone excess, laboratory studies are geared towards determining the nature of the tumor and assessing the possible presence of hypopituitarism. When a pituitary adenoma is suspected based on MRI, initial hormonal evaluation usually includes: (1) basal PRL; (2) insulin-like growth factor (IGF) I; (3) 24-h urinary free cortisol (UFC) and/or overnight oral dexamethasone (1 mg) suppression test; (4) α-subunit, FSH, and LH levels; and (5) thyroid function tests. Additional hormonal evaluation may be indicated based on the results of these tests. Pending more detailed assessment of hypopituitarism, a menstrual history, testosterone level, 8 A.M. cortisol, and thyroid function tests usually identify patients with pituitary hormone deficiencies that require hormone replacement before further testing or surgery.

Histologic Evaluation Immunohistochemical staining of pituitary tumor specimens obtained at transsphenoidal surgery confirm clinical and laboratory studies and provide a histologic diagnosis when hormone studies are equivocal and in cases of clinically nonfunctioning tumors. Occasionally, ultrastructural assessment by electron microscopy is required for diagnosis.

℞ TREATMENT **Overview** Successful management of sellar masses requires accurate diagnosis as well as selection of optimal therapeutic modalities. Most pituitary tumors are benign and slow-growing. Clinical features result from local mass effects and hormonal hypo- or hypersecretion syndromes caused directly by the adenoma or as a consequence of treatment. Thus, lifelong management and follow-up are necessary for these patients.

Improved MRI technology with gadolinium enhancement for pituitary visualization, new advances in transsphenoidal surgery and in stereotactic radiotherapy (including gamma-knife radiotherapy), and novel therapeutic agents have improved pituitary tumor management. The goals of pituitary tumor treatment include normalization of excess pituitary secretion, amelioration of symptoms and signs of hormonal hypersecretion syndromes, and shrinkage or ablation of large tumor masses with relief of adjacent structure compression. Residual anterior pituitary function should be preserved and can sometimes be restored by removing tumor mass. Ideally, adenoma recurrence should be prevented.

Transsphenoidal Surgery Transsphenoidal rather than transfrontal resection is the desired surgical approach for pituitary tumors, except for the rare invasive suprasellar mass surrounding the frontal or middle fossa, the optic nerves, or invading posteriorly behind the clivus. Intraoperative microscopy facilitates visual distinction between adenomatous and normal pituitary tissue, as well as microdissection of small tumors that may not be visible by MRI (Fig. 328-6). Transsphenoidal surgery also avoids the cranial invasion and manipulation of brain tissue required by subfrontal surgical approaches. Endoscopic techniques with three-dimensional intraoperative localization have improved visualization and access to tumor tissue. The endoscopic approach is also less traumatic, as the technique is endonasal and does not require a transsphenoidal retractor.

In addition to correction of hormonal hypersecretion, pituitary surgery is indicated for mass lesions that impinge on surrounding structures. Surgical decompression and resection are required for an expanding pituitary mass accompanied by pesistent headache, progressive visual field defects, cranial nerve palsies, internal hydrocephalus, and, occasionally, intrapituitary hemorrhage and apoplexy. Repeat surgery may be required for persistent postoperative CSF leakage. Transsphenoidal surgery is sometimes used for pituitary tissue biopsy and histologic diagnosis.

Whenever possible, the pituitary mass lesion should be selectively excised; normal tissue should be manipulated or resected only when critical for effective dissection. Nonselective hemihypophysectomy or total hypophysectomy may be indicated if no mass lesion is clearly discernible, multifocal lesions are present, or the remaining nontumorous pituitary tissue is obviously necrotic. This strategy increases the likelihood of hypopituitarism and the need for lifelong hormonal replacement.

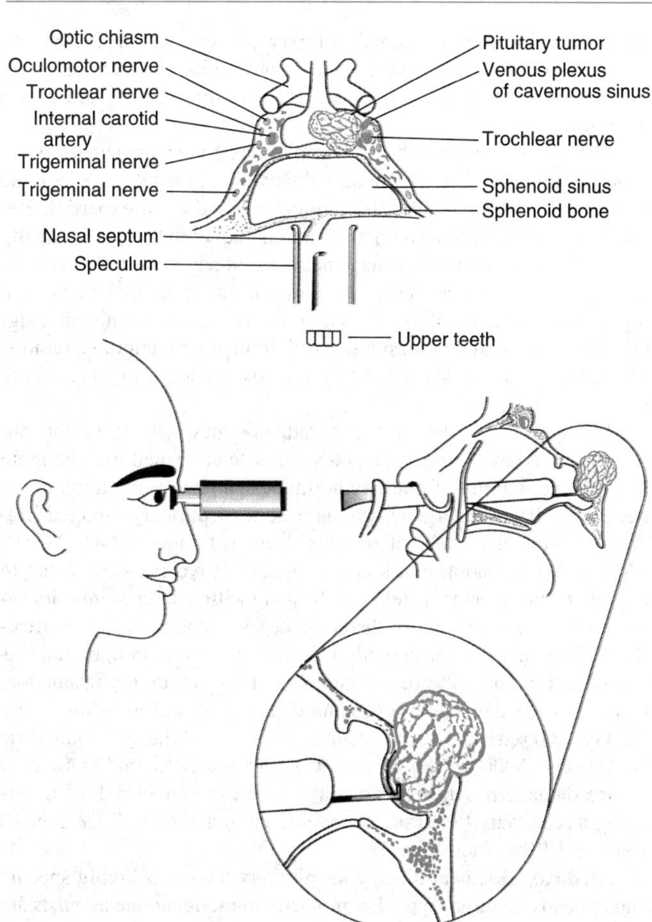

FIGURE 328-6 Transsphenoidal resection of pituitary mass via the endonasal approach. *(Adapted from Fahlbusch R: Endocrinol Metab Clin 21:669, 1992.)*

Preoperative local compression signs, including visual field defects or compromised pituitary function, may be reversed by surgery, particularly when these deficits are not long-standing. For large and invasive tumors, it is necessary to determine the optimal balance between maximal tumor resection and preservation of anterior pituitary function, especially for preserving growth and reproductive function in younger patients. Similarly, tumor invasion outside of the sella is rarely amenable to surgical cure; the surgeon must judge the risk:benefit ratio of extensive tumor resection.

Side effects Tumor size and the degree of invasiveness largely determine the incidence of surgical complications. Operative mortality is about 1%. Transient diabetes insipidus and hypopituitarism occur in up to 20% of patients. Permanent diabetes insipidus, cranial nerve damage, nasal septal perforation, or visual disturbances may be encountered in up to 10% of patients. CSF leaks occur in 4% of patients. Less common complications include carotid artery injury, loss of vision, hypothalamic damage, and meningitis. Permanent side effects are rarely encountered after surgery for microadenomas.

Radiation Radiation is used either as a primary therapy for pituitary or parasellar masses or, more commonly, as an adjunct to surgery or medical therapy. Focused megavoltage irradiation is achieved by precise MRI localization, using a high-voltage linear accelerator and accurate isocentric rotational arcing. A major determinant of accurate irradiation is to reproduce the patient's head position during multiple visits and to maintain absolute head immobility. A total of <50 Gy (5000 rad) is given as 180-cGy (180 rad) fractions split over about 6 weeks. Stereotactic radiosurgery delivers a large single high-energy dose from a cobalt 60 source (gamma knife), linear accelerator, or cyclotron. Long-term effects of gamma-knife surgery are as yet unknown.

The role of radiation therapy in pituitary tumor management depends on multiple factors including the nature of the tumor, age of the patient, and the availability of surgical and radiation expertise. Because of its relatively slow onset of action, radiation therapy is usually reserved for postsurgical management. As an adjuvant to surgery, radiation is used to treat residual tumor and in an attempt to prevent regrowth. Irradiation offers the only effective means for ablating significant residual tumor tissue derived from nonfunctioning tumors. PRL-, GH-, and ACTH-secreting tumor tissues are also amenable to medical therapy.

Side effects In the short term, radiation may cause transient nausea and weakness. Alopecia and loss of taste and smell may be more long-lasting. Failure of pituitary hormone synthesis is common in patients who have undergone head and neck or pituitary-directed irradiation. More than 50% of patients develop failure of GH, ACTH, TSH, and/or gonadotropin secretion within 10 years, usually due to hypothalamic damage. Lifelong follow-up with testing of anterior pituitary hormone reserve is therefore necessary after radiation treatment. Optic nerve damage with impaired vision due to optic neuritis is reported in about 2% of patients who undergo pituitary irradiation. Cranial nerve damage is uncommon now that radiation doses are ≤2 Gy (200 rad) at any one treatment session and the maximum dose is <50 Gy (5000 rad). The advent of stereotactic radiotherapy may reduce damage to adjacent structures. The cumulative risk of developing a secondary tumor after conventional radiation is 1.3% after 10 years and 1.9% after 20 years.

Medical Medical therapy for pituitary tumors is highly specific and depends on tumor type. For prolactinomas, dopamine agonists are the treatment of choice. For acromegaly and TSH-secreting tumors, somatostatin analogues and, occasionally, dopamine agonists are indicated. ACTH-secreting tumors and nonfunctioning tumors are generally not responsive to medication and require surgery and/or irradiation.

PROLACTIN

SYNTHESIS PRL consists of 198 amino acids and has a molecular mass of 21,500 kDa; it is weakly homologous to GH and human placental lactogen (hPL), reflecting the duplication and divergence of a common GH-PRL-hPL precursor gene on chromosome 6. PRL is synthesized in lactotropes, which comprise about 20% of anterior pituitary cells. Lactotropes and somatotropes are derived from a common precursor cell that may give rise to a tumor secreting both PRL and GH. Marked lactotrope cell hyperplasia develops during the last two trimesters of pregnancy and the first few months of lactation. These transient adaptive changes in the lactotrope population are induced by estrogen.

SECRETION Fetal PRL synthesis begins at 12 weeks' gestation (about 4 weeks after GH). Normal adult serum PRL levels are about 10 to 25 μg/L in women and 10 to 20 μg/L in men. PRL secretion is pulsatile, with the highest secretory peaks occurring during rapid eye movement sleep. Peak serum PRL levels (up to 30 μg/L) occur between 4:00 and 6:00 A.M. The circulating half-life of PRL is about 50 min.

PRL is unique among the pituitary hormones in that the predominant central control mechanism is inhibitory, reflecting dopamine-mediated suppression of PRL release. This regulatory pathway is exemplified by the spontaneous PRL hypersecretion that occurs after pituitary stalk section, often a consequence of mass lesions at the skull base.

Dopamine action is mediated by multiple receptor subtypes, each a member of the seven-transmembrane G protein–coupled receptor (GPCR) superfamily. In the pituitary, dopamine type 2 (D_2) receptors are predominant and mediate PRL inhibition. Targeted disruption (gene knockout) of the murine D_2 receptor results in hyperprolactinemia and lactotrope proliferation. Activation of D_2 receptors inhibits the cyclic AMP pathway, causing membrane hyperpolarization and closing of voltage-gated calcium channels; these events block secretory granule exocytosis by reducing intracellular free calcium. Because of the potent PRL inhibitory effects of dopamine, physiologic, pharmacologic, or pathologic alterations in dopamine action increase PRL levels. As discussed below, dopamine agonists play a central role in the management of hyperprolacinemic disorders.

TRH (pyro Glu-His-Pro-NH2) is a hypothalamic tripeptide that releases prolactin within 15 to 30 min after intravenous injection. The physiologic relevance of TRH for PRL regulation is unclear, as it appears to primarily regulate TSH (Chap. 330). *Vasoactive intestinal peptide* (VIP) also induces PRL release, whereas glucocorticoids and thyroid hormone suppress PRL secretion.

Serum PRL levels rise after exercise, meals, sexual intercourse, minor surgical procedures, general anesthesia, acute myocardial infarction, and other forms of acute stress. PRL levels also increase significantly (~tenfold) during pregnancy and decline rapidly within 2 weeks of parturition. If breastfeeding is initiated, basal PRL levels remain elevated; suckling stimulates reflex increases in PRL levels that last for about 30 to 45 min. Breast suckling activates neural afferent pathways in the hypothalamus that induce PRL release. With time, the suckling-induced responses diminish and interfeeding PRL levels return to normal.

ACTION The PRL receptor is a member of the type I cytokine receptor family that also includes GH and interleukin (IL) 6 receptors. Ligand binding leads to receptor dimerization followed by intracellular signaling mediated by the Janus kinase (JAK) pathway, which phosphorylates components of the signal transduction and activators of transcription (STAT) family. The STAT proteins translocate to the nucleus, where they act as transcription factors on target genes. In the breast, the lobuloalveolar epithelium proliferates in response to PRL, placental lactogens, elevated progesterone, and local paracrine growth factors; lactogenesis occurs as a result of complex multihormonal interactions (Chap. 337).

PRL acts to induce and maintain lactation, decrease reproductive function, and suppress sexual drive. These functions are geared towards ensuring that maternal lactation is sustained and not interrupted by pregnancy. PRL inhibits reproductive function at multiple levels, including suppression of hypothalamic GnRH and pituitary gonadotropin secretion, as well as impairing gonadal steroidogenesis in both female and male subjects. In the hypothalamus, PRL-mediated suppression of GnRH leads to loss of pulsatile LH secretion and abrogation of the preovulatory LH surge. In the ovary, PRL blocks folliculogenesis and inhibits granulosa cell aromatase activity, leading to hypoestrogenism and anovulation. PRL also has a luteolytic effect, generating a shortened, or inadequate, luteal phase of the menstrual cycle. In males, attenuated LH secretion leads to low testosterone levels and decreased spermatogenesis. These hormonal changes decrease libido and reduce fertility in patients with hyperprolactinemia (Chap. 54).

PRL exerts widespread metabolic effects to ensure maintenance of sustained lactation. Gastrointestinal calcium absorption is increased, bone calcium is mobilized, bile acids are elevated, and pancreatic β cell growth is induced by PRL. Centrally, PRL acts on brain centers involved in parenting behavior, appetite stimulation, and analgesia. Concomitant with these effects, maintenance of bone mineral density is abrogated; hyperprolactinemia is associated with enhanced risk for bone loss and the long-term development of osteoporosis. PRL receptors are abundant in the osteoblasts of developing bone, and the accompanying hypoestrogenemia contributes to accelerated bone loss in hyperprolactinemic women.

HYPERPROLACTINEMIA **Etiology** Hyperprolactinemia is the most common pituitary hormone hypersecretion syndrome in both males and females. PRL-secreting pituitary adenomas (prolactinomas) are the most common cause of PRL levels >100 μg/L (see below). Less pronounced PRL elevation can also be caused by microprolactinomas but is more commonly caused by drugs, pituitary stalk compression, hypothyroidism, or renal failure (Table 328-8).

Pregnancy and lactation are the important physiologic causes of hyperprolactinemia. Sleep-associated hyperprolactinemia reverts to normal within an hour of awakening. Nipple stimulation and sexual orgasm may also cause acute PRL increases. Chest wall stimulation or trauma (including chest surgery and herpes zoster) invoke the reflex suckling arc with resultant hyperprolactinemia. Chronic renal failure elevates PRL by decreasing peripheral PRL clearance. Primary hypothyroidism is associated with mild hyperprolactinemia, probably because of enhanced TRH secretion.

Lesions of the hypothalamic-pituitary region that disrupt hypothalamic dopamine synthesis, portal vessel delivery, or lactotrope responses are associated with hyperprolactinemia. Thus, hypothalamic tumors, cysts, infiltrative disorders, and radiation-induced damage cause elevated PRL levels, usually in the range of 30 to 100 μg/L. Plurihormonal adenomas (including GH and ACTH tumors) may directly hypersecrete PRL. Clinically nonfunctioning pituitary tumors commonly cause stalk pressure and hyperprolactinemia.

Drug-induced inhibition or disruption of dopaminergic receptor function results in hyperprolactinemia (Table 328-8). Thus, many antipsychotics and antidepressants cause hyperprolactinemia. Methyldopa inhibits dopamine synthesis and verapamil blocks dopamine release, also leading to hyperprolactinemia. Hormonal agents that induce PRL include estrogens, antiandrogens, and TRH.

Presentation and Diagnosis Amenorrhea, galactorrhea, and infertility are the hallmarks of hyperprolactinemia in women. If hyperprolactinemia develops prior to the menarche, primary amenorrhea results. More commonly, hyperprolactinemia develops later in life and leads to oligomenorrhea and, ultimately, to amenorrhea. Patients present with infertility, vaginal dryness, dyspareunia, and loss of libido. If hyperprolactinemia is sustained, vertebral bone mineral density can be reduced compared to age-matched controls, particularly when associated with pronounced hypoestrogenemia. Galactorrhea is present in up to 80% of hyperprolactinemic women. Though usually bilateral and spontaneous, it may be unilateral or only expressed manually. Patients may also complain of weight gain and mild hirsutism.

In men with hyperprolactinemia, diminished libido or visual loss (from optic nerve compression) are the usual presenting symptoms. Gonadotropin suppression leads to reduced testosterone, impotence, and oligospermia. True galactorrhea is uncommon in men with hyperprolactinemia. If the disorder is longstanding, secondary effects of hypogonadism are evident, including osteopenia, reduced muscle mass, and decreased beard growth.

The diagnosis of idiopathic hyperprolactinemia is made by exclusion of known causes of hyperprolactinemia in the setting of a normal pituitary MRI. Some of these patients may have small microadenomas below MRI sensitivity (~2 mm).

Laboratory Investigation Basal, fasting morning PRL levels (normally <20 μg/L) should be measured to assess hypersecretion. Because hormone secretion is pulsatile and levels vary widely in some individuals with hyperprolactinemia, it may be necessary to measure levels on several different occasions when clinical suspicion is high. Both false-positive and false-negative results may be encountered. In patients with markedly elevated PRL levels (>1000 μg/L), results may be falsely lowered because of assay artifacts; sample dilution is required to assess these high values accurately. Falsely elevated values may be caused by aggregated forms of circulating PRL, which are biologically inactive (macroprolactinemia). Hypothyroidism should be excluded by measuring TSH and T_4 levels.

Table 328-8 Etiology of Hyperprolactinemia[a]

I. Physiologic hypersecretion
   A. Pregnancy
   B. Lactation
   C. Chest wall stimulation
   D. Sleep
   E. Stress
II. Hypothalamic–pituitary stalk damage
   A. Tumors
      1. Craniopharyngioma
      2. Suprasellar pituitary mass extension
      3. Meningioma
      4. Dysgerminoma
      5. Metastases
   B. Empty sella
   C. Lymphocytic hypophysitis
   D. Adenoma with stalk compression
   E. Granulomas
   F. Rathke's cyst
   G. Irradiation
   H. Trauma
      1. Pituitary stalk section
      2. Suprasellar surgery
III. Pituitary hypersecretion
   A. Prolactinoma
   B. Acromegaly
IV. Systemic disorders
   A. Chronic renal failure
   B. Hypothyroidism
   C. Cirrhosis
   D. Pseudocyesis
   E. Epileptic seizures
V. Drug-induced hypersecretion
   A. Dopamine receptor blockers
      1. Phenothiazines: chlorpromazine, perphenazine
      2. Butyrophenones: haloperidol
      3. Thioxanthenes
      4. Metoclopramide
   B. Dopamine synthesis inhibitors
      1. α-methyldopa
   C. Catecholamine depletors
      1. Reserpine
   D. Opiates
   E. H_2 antagonists
      1. Cimetidine, ranitidine
   F. Imipramines
      1. Amitriptyline, amoxapine
   G. Serotonin-reuptake inhibitors
      1. Fluoxetine
   H. Calcium channel blockers
      1. Verapamil
   I. Hormones
      1. Estrogens
      2. Antiandrogens

NOTE: Hyperprolactinemia >100 μg/L almost invariably is indicative of a prolactin-secreting pituitary adenoma. Physiologic causes, hypothyroidism, and drug-induced hyperprolactinemia should be excluded before extensive evaluation.

℞ TREATMENT Treatment of hyperprolactinemia depends on the cause of elevated PRL levels. Regardless of the etiology, however, treatment should be aimed at normalizing PRL levels to alleviate suppressive effects on gonadal function, halt the galactorrhea, and preserve bone mineral density. Dopamine agonists are effective for many different causes of hyperprolactinemia (see "Treatment" for "Prolactinoma," below).

If the patient is taking a medication known to cause hyperprolactinemia, the drug should be withdrawn, if possible. For psychiatric patients who require neuroleptic agents, dose titration or the addition of a dopamine agonist can help restore normoprolactinemia and alleviate reproductive symptoms. However, dopamine agonists sometimes worsen the underlying psychiatric condition, especially at high doses. Hyperprolactinemia usually resolves after adequate thyroid hormone replacement in hypothyroid patients or after renal transplantation in patients or dialysis. Resection of hypothalamic or sellar mass lesions can reverse hyperprolactinemia caused by reduced dopamine tone. Granulomatous infiltrates rarely respond to glucocorticoid administration. In patients with irreversible hypothalamic damage, no treatment may be warranted. In up to 30% of patients with hyperprolactinemia—with or without a visible pituitary microadenoma—the condition resolves spontaneously.

PROLACTINOMA **Etiology and Prevalence** Tumors arising from lactotrope cells account for about half of all functioning pituitary tumors, with an annual incidence of ~3/100,000 population. Mixed tumors secreting combinations of GH and PRL, ACTH and PRL, and rarely TSH and PRL, are also seen. These plurihormonal tumors are usually recognized by immunohistochemistry, without apparent clinical manifestations from the production of additional hormones. Microadenomas are classified as <1 cm in diameter and do not usually invade the parasellar region. Macroadenomas are >1 cm in diameter, are locally invasive, and may impinge on adjacent structures. The female:male ratio for microprolactinomas is 20:1, whereas the gender ratio is near 1:1 for macroadenomas. Tumor size generally correlates directly with PRL concentrations; values >100 μg/L are usually associated with macroadenomas. Males tend to present with larger tumors than females, possibly because the features of hypogonadism are less readily evident. PRL levels remain stable in most patients, reflecting the slow growth of these tumors. About 5% of

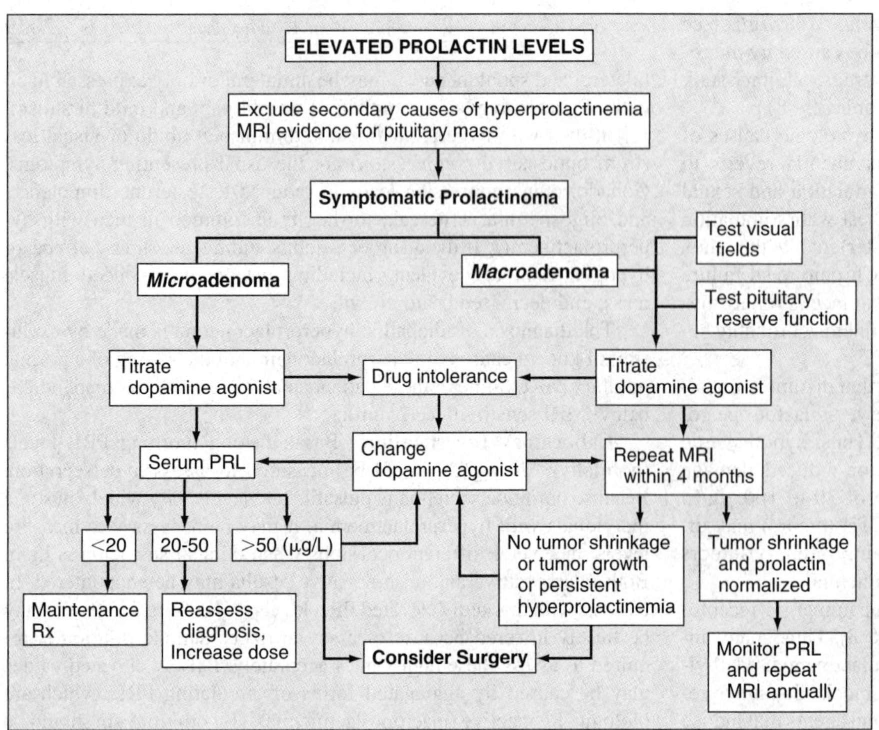

FIGURE 328-7 Management of prolactinoma. (MRI, magnetic resonance imaging; PRL, prolactin.)

microadenomas progress in the long term to macroadenomas. Hyperprolactinemia resolves spontaneously in about 30% of microadenomas.

Presentation and Diagnosis Women usually present with amenorrhea, infertility, and galactorrhea. If the tumor extends outside of the sella, visual field defects or other mass effects may be seen. Men often present with impotence, loss of libido, infertility, or signs of central CNS compression including headaches and visual defects. Assuming that known physiologic and medication-induced causes of hyperprolactinemia are excluded (Table 328-8), the diagnosis of prolactinoma is likely with a PRL level >100 μg/L. PRL levels <100μg/L may be caused by microadenomas, other sellar lesions that decrease dopamine inhibition, or nonneoplastic causes of hyperprolactinemia. For this reason, an MRI should be performed in all patients with hyperprolactinemia. It is important to remember that hyperprolactinemia caused by the mass effects of nonlactotrope lesions is also corrected by treatment with dopamine agonists. Consequently, PRL suppression by dopamine agonists does not necessarily indicate that the lesion is a prolactinoma.

Rx TREATMENT As microadenomas rarely progress to become macroadenomas, no treatment may be needed if fertility is not desired. Estrogen replacement is indicated to prevent bone loss and other consequences of hypoestrogenemia and does not appear to increase the risk of tumor enlargement. These patients should be monitored by regular serial PRL and MRI measurements.

For symptomatic microadenomas, therapeutic goals include control of hyperprolactinemia, reduction of tumor size, restoration of menses and fertility, and improvement of galactorrhea. Dopamine agonists should be titrated to achieve maximal PRL suppression and restoration of reproductive function (Fig. 328-7). A normalized PRL level does not assure reduced tumor size. However, tumor shrinkage is not usually seen in those who do not respond with lowered PRL levels. For macroadenomas, formal visual field testing should be performed before initiating dopamine agonists. MRI and visual fields should be assessed at 6- to 12-month intervals until the mass shrinks and annually thereafter until maximum size reduction has occurred.

Medical Oral dopamine agonists (cabergoline or bromocriptine) are the mainstay of therapy for patients with micro- or macroprolactinomas. Dopamine agonists suppress PRL secretion and synthesis as well as lactotrope cell proliferation.

Bromocriptine The ergot alkaloid bromocriptine mesylate is a dopamine receptor agonist that suppresses prolactin secretion by binding directly to lactotrope D_2 dopamine receptors. Bromocriptine is used as initial therapy for both micro- and macroprolactinomas. In microadenomas the drug rapidly lowers serum prolactin levels to normal in up to 70% of patients, decreases tumor size, and restores gonadal function. In patients with macroadenomas, prolactin levels are also normalized in 70% of patients and tumor mass shrinkage (≥50%) is achieved in up to 40% of patients. Mass effect symptoms, including headaches and visual disorders, usually improve dramatically within days after bromocriptine initiation; improvement of sexual function requires several weeks of treatment but may occur before complete normalization of prolactin levels. Drug withdrawal usually results in recurrent hyperprolactinemia and tumor reexpansion, with the risk of visual compromise. After initial control of PRL levels has been achieved, bromocriptine should be reduced to the lowest effective maintenance dose. In ~5% of treated patients, hyperprolactinemia may resolve and not recur when bromocriptine is discontinued after long-term treatment.

Therapy is initiated by administering a low bromocriptine dose (0.625 to 1.25 mg) at bedtime with a snack, followed by gradually increasing the dose. Most patients are successfully controlled with a daily dose of ≤7.5 mg (2.5 mg tid). About 20% of patients are resistant to dopaminergic treatment; they may have decreased D_2 dopamine receptor numbers or a postreceptor defect. D_2 receptor gene mutations in the pituitary have not been reported.

Nausea, vomiting, and postural hypotension with faintness may occur in ~25% of patients after the initial dose. These symptoms may persist in some patients. Other side effects include constipation, nasal stuffiness, dry mouth, nightmares, insomnia, and vertigo; decreasing the dose usually alleviates these problems. For the approximately 15% of patients who cannot tolerate oral bromocriptine, intravaginal administration of tablets is often efficacious.

Auditory hallucinations, delusions, and mood swings have been reported in up to 5% of patients and may be due to the dopamine agonist properties or to the lysergic acid derivative of the compound. Rare reports of leukopenia, thrombocytopenia, pleural fibrosis, cardiac arrhythmias, and hepatitis have been described.

Cabergoline An ergoline derivative, cabergoline is a long-acting dopamine agonist with high D_2 receptor affinity. The drug effectively suppresses PRL for >14 days after a single oral dose and induces prolactinoma shrinkage in most patients. Cabergoline (0.5 to 1.0 mg twice weekly) achieves normoprolactinemia and resumption of normal gonadal function in ~80% of patients with microadenomas; galactorrhea improves or resolves in 90% of patients. Cabergoline normalizes PRL and shrinks ~70% of macroprolactinomas. It may also be effective in patients resistant to bromocriptine. Adverse effects and drug intolerance are encountered less commonly than with bromocriptine.

Other dopamine agonists These include *pergolide mesylate*, an ergot derivative with dopaminergic properties; *lisuride*, an ergot derivative; and *quinagolide* (CV 205-502, Norprolac), a nonergot oral dopamine agonist with specific D_2 receptor activity.

Surgery Indications for surgical debulking include dopamine resistance or intolerance and the presence of an invasive macroadenoma with compromised vision that fails to improve rapidly after drug treatment. Initial PRL normalization is achieved in about 70% of microprolactinomas after surgical resection, but only 30% of macroadenomas can be successfully resected. However, follow-up studies have shown that recurrence of hyperprolactinemia occurs in up to 20% of patients within the first year after surgery; long-term recurrence rates exceed 50% for macroadenomas. Radiotherapy for prolactinomas is reserved for patients with aggressive tumors that do not respond to maximally tolerated dopamine agonists and/or surgery.

Pregnancy The pituitary increases in size during pregnancy, reflecting the stimulatory effects of estrogen and perhaps other growth factors. About 5% of microadenomas significantly increase in size, but 15 to 30% of macroadenomas may grow during pregnancy. Bromocriptine has been used for over 25 years to restore fertility in women with hyperprolactinemia, without evidence of untoward teratogenic effects. Nonetheless, most authorities recommend strategies to minimize fetal exposure to the drug. For women taking bromocriptine who desire pregnancy, mechanical contraception should be used through three regular menstrual cycles to allow for conception timing. When pregnancy is confirmed, bromocriptine should be discontinued and PRL levels followed serially, especially if headaches or visual symptoms occur. For women harboring macroadenomas, regular visual field testing is recommended, and the drug should be reinstituted if tumor growth is apparent. Although pituitary MRI may be safe during pregnancy, this procedure should be reserved for symptomatic patients with severe headache and/or visual field defects. Alternatively, surgical decompression may be indicated if vision is threatened. Though comprehensive data support the efficacy and relative safety of bromocriptine-facilitated fertility, patients should be advised of potential unknown deleterious effects and the risk of tumor growth during pregnancy. At present, the experience with cabergoline is too limited to recommend its routine use when fertility is desired.

GROWTH HORMONE

SYNTHESIS GH is the most abundant anterior pituitary hormone and is expressed early in fetal life (at 8 weeks' gestation). GH-secreting somatotrope cells constitute up to 50% of the total anterior pituitary cell population. Mammosomatotrope cells, which coexpress PRL with GH, can be identified using double immunostaining techniques. Somatotrope development is determined by expression of the cell-specific Pit-1 nuclear transcription factor. In addition to controlling cell differentiation, it also enhances GH gene expression. Five distinct genes on chromosome 17q22 encode GH and related proteins. The pituitary GH gene (*hGH-N*) produces two alternatively spliced products that give rise to 22-kDa GH (191 amino acids) and a less abundant, 20-kDa GH molecule, with similar biologic activity. Placental syncytiotrophoblast cells express a GH variant (*hGH-V*) gene; the related hormone human chorionic somatotropin (HCS) is expressed by distinct members of the gene cluster. HCS shares high homology with GH yet exhibits minimal growth-promoting properties.

SECRETION GH secretion is controlled by complex hypothalamic and peripheral factors. *GHRH* is a 44 amino acid hypothalamic peptide that stimulates GH synthesis and release. Synthetic agonists of the *GHRP* receptor stimulate GHRH and also directly stimulate GH release, but putative endogenous agonists remain incompletely characterized. *Somatostatin* (SRIF) is synthesized in the medial preoptic area of the hypothalamus and inhibits GH secretion. GHRH is secreted as discrete spikes that elicit GH pulses, whereas SRIF sets basal GH tone. SRIF is also expressed in many extrahypothalamic tissues, including the CNS, gastrointestinal system, and pancreas, where it also acts to inhibit the hormone secretion. *IGF-I*, the peripheral target hormone for GH, feeds back to inhibit GH; estrogens induce GH (Chap. 8), whereas glucocorticoid excess suppresses GH release.

Two distinct surface receptors on the somatotrope regulate GH synthesis and secretion. The GHRH receptor is a GPCR that signals through the intracellular cyclic AMP pathway. Activation of this receptor stimulates somatotrope cell proliferation as well as hormone production. Inactivating mutations of the GHRH receptor cause profound dwarfism (see below). A distinct surface receptor for GHRP has also been identified. This receptor is expressed in the hypothalamus and pituitary. A natural ligand, termed *ghrelin*, binds to the GHRP receptor; it is produced in large amounts in the stomach, though its physiologic role remains unknown. Hypothalamic somatostatin binds to five distinct receptor subtypes (SSTR1 to SSTR5) that are widely expressed in different tissues, including in the pituitary. SSTR2 and SSTR5 subtypes preferentially suppress GH (and TSH) secretion.

GH secretion is pulsatile, with greater levels at night generally correlating with the onset of sleep. GH secretory rates decline markedly with age so that hormone production in middle age is about 15% of production during puberty. These changes are paralleled by an age-related decline in lean muscle mass. GH secretion is also reduced in obese individuals, though IGF-I levels are preserved, suggesting a change in the setpoint for feedback control. Elevated GH levels occur within an hour of deep sleep onset as well as after exercise, physical stress, trauma, and during sepsis. Integrated 24-h GH secretion is higher in women and is also enhanced by estrogen replacement. Using assays in common clinical use, random GH measurements are undetectable in ~50% of daytime samples obtained from healthy subjects and are undetectable in most obese and elderly subjects. Thus, single random GH measurements do not distinguish patients with adult GH deficiency from normal persons.

GH secretion is profoundly influenced by nutritional factors. Using newer ultrasensitive chemiluminescence-based GH assays with a sensitivity of 0.002 μg/L, a glucose load can be shown to suppress GH to <0.7 μg/L in female and to <0.07 μg/L in male subjects. Increased GH pulse frequency and peak amplitudes occur with chronic malnutrition or prolonged fasting. GH is stimulated by high-protein meals and by L-arginine. GH secretion is induced by dopamine and apomorphine (a dopamine receptor agonist), as well as by α-adrenergic pathways. β-Adrenergic blockage induces basal GH and enhances GHRH- and insulin-evoked GH release.

ACTION The pattern of GH secretion may affect tissue responses. The higher GH pulsatility observed in males, as compared to the relatively continuous GH secretion in females, may be an important biologic determinant of linear growth patterns and liver enzyme induction.

The 70-kD peripheral GH receptor protein shares structural homology with the cytokine/hematopoietic superfamily. A fragment of the receptor extracellular domain generates a soluble GH binding protein (GHBP) that interacts with GH in the circulation. The liver contains the greatest number of GH receptors. GH binding induces receptor dimerization by making distinct contact through two separate binding domains of the hormone. The dimerized receptor interacts with members of the JAK/STAT family. The activated STAT proteins translocate to the nucleus, where they modulate expression of GH-regulated target genes. GH analogues that bind to the receptor, but are incapable of mediating receptor dimerization, are potent antagonists of GH action and are being investigated for potential use in the treatment of acromegaly and diabetic microangiopathy.

GH induces protein synthesis and nitrogen retention and impairs glucose tolerance by antagonizing insulin action. GH also stimulates lipolysis, leading to increased circulating fatty acid levels, reduced omental fat mass, and enhanced lean body mass. GH promotes sodium, potassium, and water retention and elevates serum levels of inorganic phosphate. Linear bone growth occurs as a result of complex hormonal and growth factor actions, including those of IGF-I. GH stimulates epiphyseal prechondrocyte differentiation. These precursor cells produce IGF-I locally and are also responsive to the growth factor.

INSULIN-LIKE GROWTH FACTORS Though GH exerts direct effects in target tissues, many of its physiologic effects are mediated indirectly through IGF-I, a potent growth and differentiation factor. The major source of circulating IGF-I is hepatic in origin. Peripheral tissue IGF-I exerts local paracrine actions that appear to be both dependent and independent of GH. Thus, GH administration induces circulating IGF-I level as well as stimulating IGF-I expression in multiple tissues.

Both IGF-I and -II are bound to one of six high-affinity circulating IGF-binding proteins (IGFBPs) that regulate IGF bioactivity. Levels of IGFBP3 are GH-dependent, and it serves as the major carrier protein for circulating IGF-I. GH deficiency and malnutrition are associated with low IGFBP3 levels. IGFBP1 and -2 regulate local tissue IGF action but do not bind appreciable amounts of circulating IGF-I.

Serum IGF-I concentrations are profoundly affected by various physiologic factors. Levels increase during puberty, peak at 16 years, and subsequently decline by >80% during the aging process. IGF-I concentrations are higher in females than in males. Because GH is the major determinant of hepatic IGF-I synthesis, abnormalities of GH synthesis or action (e.g., pituitary failure, GHRH receptor defect, or GH receptor defect) reduce IGF-I levels. Hypocaloric states are associated with GH resistance; IGF-I levels are therefore low with cachexia, malnutrition, and sepsis. In acromegaly, IGF-I levels are invariably high and reflect a log-linear relationship with GH concentrations.

IGF-I Physiology Though IGF-I is not an approved drug, investigational studies provide insight into its physiologic effects. High doses of injected IGF-I (100 μg/kg) induce hypoglycemia, primarily because of actions through the insulin receptor. Low IGF-I doses improve insulin sensitivity in patients with severe insulin resistance and diabetes. In cachectic subjects, IGF-I infusion (12 μg/kg per hour) enhances nitrogen retention and lowers cholesterol levels. Longer-term subcutaneous IGF-I injections exert a marked anabolic effect with enhanced protein synthesis. The impact of long-term IGF-I administration on bone mineral content is as yet unclear. Although bone formation markers are induced, bone turnover may also be stimulated by IGF-I.

Side effects of IGF-I are dose-dependent. An acute overdose may result in hypoglycemia and hypotension. Fluid retention, temporomandibular jaw pain, and increased intracranial pressure are reversible. Avascular necrosis of the femoral head has been reported. Chronic excess IGF-I would presumably result in features of acromegaly.

DISORDERS OF GROWTH AND DEVELOPMENT

Skeletal Maturation and Somatic Growth Linear growth is a function of endochrondral bone formation whereby cartilage is converted into bony skeleton in the long bones and vertebrae (Chap. 340). Ossification occurs within central diaphyseal and peripheral epiphyseal centers. A cartilaginous growth plate forms between the two centers, and chondrocytes proliferate within the growth plate. Linear bone growth ceases when this cartilage layer ossifies and fuses with epiphyseal and diaphyseal bone.

The growth plate is dependent on a variety of hormonal stimuli including GH, IGF-I, sex steroids, thyroid hormones, paracrine growth factors, and cytokines. GH directly stimulates prechondrocyte differentiation and clonal expansion, resulting in chondrocytes that express both IGF-I receptors and IGF-I protein. The growth-promoting process also requires caloric energy, amino acids, vitamins, and trace metals and consumes about 10% of normal energy production. Malnutrition impairs chondrocyte activity and reduces circulating IGF-I and IGFBP3 levels.

Bone age is delayed in patients with all forms of true GH deficiency or GH receptor defects that result in attenuated GH action. Rarely, GH excess accelerates growth, particularly in the setting of delayed bone age from concomitant hypogonadism. Thyroid hormone is permissive for GH synthesis and secretion as well as for maintaining normal circulating IGF-I and binding protein levels. Bone age is delayed by thyroid hormone deficiency. Consequently, congenital or acquired hypothyroidism is associated with stunted growth, which is partially reversed by thyroid hormone replacement (Chap. 330). Elevated pubertal sex steroid levels (especially estrogen) induce the GHRH-GH-IGF-I axis and also directly stimulate epiphyseal growth. High doses of estrogen lead to epiphyseal closure. A mutation of the estrogen receptor α prevented epiphyseal closure, confirming the important role of this pathway in bone maturation. Several pathologic conditions accompanied by increased levels of sex steroids, including precocious puberty, androgen exposure (exogenous or endogenous), congenital adrenal hyperplasia, and obesity, are associated with accelerated bone maturation. Thus, children with these conditions have accelerated early growth, but end up with reduced final height. In contrast to sex steroids, glucocorticoid excess inhibits linear growth. Glucocorticoids also stimulate SRIF and inhibit peripheral GH and IGF-I receptor signaling.

Linear bone growth rates are very high in infancy and are pituitary-dependent. Mean growth velocity is ~6 cm/year in later childhood and is usually maintained within a given range on a standardized percentile chart. Peak growth rates occur during midpuberty when bone age is 12 (girls) or 13 (boys) (Chap. 8). Secondary sexual development is associated with elevated sex steroids that cause progressive epiphyseal growth plate closure.

Short stature may occur as a result of constitutive intrinsic growth defects or because of acquired extrinsic factors that impair growth (Table 328-9). Genetic disorders, including pituitary transcription factor defects, mutations in growth-related genes, and pituitary hypoplasia syndromes, may all be associated with growth delay and short stature. In general, delayed bone age in a child with short stature is suggestive of a hormonal or systemic disorder, whereas normal bone age in a short child is more likely to be caused by a genetic growth plate disorder (Chap. 351). Other bone and cartilage dysplasia syndromes are associated with specific limb-body proportion phenotypes, and some involve associated calcium disorders (Chap. 343).

Intrauterine growth retardation results in short stature and may be caused by specific congenital anomalies (e.g., IGF-I deficiency, *Russell-Silver syndrome*, chromosomal disomy) or maternal factors such as diabetes mellitus, infections, hypoxia, drug addiction, or placental dysfunction. Long-term responses of these children to GH treatment are currently being evaluated.

Turner syndrome is caused by loss of all, or part, of an X chromosome in females (XO). It is characterized by short stature, in addition to gonadal dysgenesis and other characteristic features (Chap. 338). Short stature may be improved with a combination of GH and an anabolic steroid (oxandrolone); estrogen is required to induce and sustain sexual development. *Noonan syndrome* resembles Turner syndrome phenotypically, but patients have apparently normal sex chromosomes. These patients have delayed pubertal development but not primary gonadal failure.

GH Deficiency in Children • ***GH deficiency*** Isolated GH deficiency is characterized by short stature, micropenis, increased fat, high-pitched voice, and a propensity to hypoglycemia. The etiology of GH deficiency is not identifiable in most children with the disorder. Familial modes of inheritance are seen in one-third of these individuals and may be autosomal dominant, recessive, or X-linked, indicating that multiple genetic abnormalities can lead to GH deficiency. About 10% of children with growth hormone deficiency have mutations in the GH-N gene. These include gene deletions and a wide range of point mutations, including some that function in a dominant negative manner (heterozygous mutations) to impair the synthesis or function of GH expressed from the normal allele. Mutations in transcription factors Pit-1 and Prop-1, which control somatotrope development, cause GH deficiency in combination with other pituitary hormone deficiencies. The diagnosis of *idiopathic GH deficiency* (IGHD) should be made only after known molecular defects have been excluded.

GHRH receptor mutations Recessive mutations of the GHRH receptor gene have been described in several unrelated families with severe proportionate dwarfism. The low basal GH levels in these patients cannot be stimulated by exogenous GHRH, GHRP, or insulin-induced hypoglycemia, confirming the importance of the GHRH receptor for somatotrope cell proliferation and hormonal responsiveness.

Growth hormone insensitivity This is caused by defects of GH receptor structure or signaling. Homozygous or heterozygous exonic and intronic mutations of the GH receptor occur mainly in the extracellular ligand-binding domain and are associated with partial or complete GH insensitivity and growth failure (*Laron syndrome*). The diagnosis of this syndrome is based on normal or high GH levels, with decreased circulating GHBP, and low IGF-I levels. Very rarely, defective IGF-I, IGF-I receptor, or IGF-I signaling defects are also encountered.

Nutritional short stature Caloric deprivation and malnutrition, uncontrolled diabetes, and chronic renal failure represent secondary causes of abrogated GH receptor function. These conditions also stimulate the production of proinflammatory cytokines, including tumor necrosis factor (TNF) α and ILs, which can block GH-mediated signal transduction. Children with these conditions typically exhibit features of acquired short stature with elevated GH and low IGF-I levels. Circulating GH receptor antibodies may rarely cause peripheral GH insensitivity.

Psychosocial short stature Emotional and social deprivation lead to growth retardation accompanied by delayed speech, discordant hyperphagia, and attenuated response to administered GH. A nurturing environment restores growth rates.

Presentation and Diagnosis Short stature is commonly encountered in clinical practice, but the criteria for biochemical diagnosis of true GH deficiency have been difficult to define. The decision to evaluate these children requires clinical judgement in association with auxologic data and family history. Short stature should be comprehensively evaluated if a patient's height is >3 SD below the mean for age or if the growth rate has decelerated. Skeletal maturation is best evaluated by measuring a radiologic bone age, which is based mainly on the degree of growth plate fusion. Final height can be predicted using standardized scales (Bayley-Pinneau or Tanner-Whitehouse) or estimated by adding 6.5 cm (boys) or subtracting 6.5 cm (girls) from the midparental height.

Laboratory Investigation Because GH secretion is pulsatile, GH deficiency is best assessed by examining the response to provocative stimuli. Random GH measurements do not distinguish normal children from those with true GH deficiency. Adequate adrenal and thyroid hormone replacement should be assured before testing. Provocative stimuli such as exercise, insulin-induced hypoglycemia, and other pharmacologic tests normally increase GH to >7 μg/L in children. Insulin-induced hypoglycemia testing requires the blood sugar nadir to be <50% of baseline levels. This test should be performed under close supervision and is contraindicated in children with seizure disorders. IGF-I levels are not sufficiently sensitive or specific to make the diagnosis but can be useful to confirm GH deficiency; they must be controlled

Table 328-9 Etiology and Diagnosis of Short Stature

	Representative Conditions	Clinical and Laboratory Features
Genetic		
Normal variants	Familial intrinsic short stature	Family short stature, normal bone age; no clinical or laboratory abnormalities
	Constitutional delay in growth	Family history of delayed growth, delayed bone age; no clinical or laboratory abnormalities
Genetic disorders	Turner syndrome	Short, gonadal dysgenesis, variable phenotype, karyotype required
Chromosomal Aneuploidy		
SHOX mutations	Leri-Weill syndrome SHOX: short stature homeobox-containing gene Xp22, Yp11.3	Short stature with variable osteochondrosteosis, mesomelic dysplasia, and Madelung deformity; GH levels normal
Bone dysplasias	Achondroplasia	Abnormal body proportions, macrocephaly, short limbs, low nasal bridge, occasional hydrocephalus
Dysmorphic syndrome	Noonan's syndrome	Similar to Turner, normal karyotype, and present in both sexes
	Prader-Willi syndrome	Obesity, hypogonadism, hypotonia, intellectual and behavioral deficits, chromosome 15 abnormalities
	Pseudohypoparathyroidism (type 1A)	Hypocalcemia, moon facies, brachydactyly, mental retardation, abnormal Gsα
Intrauterine		
Growth retardation	Small for gestational age	Ongoing growth failure in a minority of nonsyndromic cases; diverse maternal, placental, and fetal disorders
	Russell-Silver syndrome	IUGR, relative macrocephaly, small triangular face, asymmetry
Nutritional		
Inadequate intake	Starvation Psychosocial feeding problems Anorexia due to chronic disease	Weight generally depressed more than height
Vitamin/mineral deficiency	Rickets	Nutritional deficiency in vitamin D is most common cause
Nutrient loss	Malabsorption	Gastrointestinal, liver, respiratory, or pancreatic disease
	Chronic vomiting	Gastrointestinal obstruction, achalasia of esophagus, electrolyte disturbances, increased intracranial pressure
Metabolic disorders	Uncontrolled diabetes mellitus	High glycohemoglobin, hepatomegaly
	Hyperthyroidism	Goiter, eye signs, elevated T_4 levels
Hormonal		
GH/IGF-I deficiency		
Congenital		May have neonatal hypoglycemia, midline defects; may have only short stature
Acquired		May have history of trauma, CNS insult, or abnormal CNS examination
Psychosocial deprivation		May show abnormal behavior, hyperphagia; may mimic panhypopituitarism; growth improves with better environment
Hypothyroidism		Growth failure may be only symptom; low T_4
Glucocorticoid excess		Supraphysiologic levels attenuate growth; often associated with obesity
Sex steroid deficiency		Deficiency after 10–11 years of age impairs growth
Chronic illness		May have features of chronic condition or short stature may be presenting feature; weight often impaired more than height

NOTE: GH, growth hormone; IGF, insulin-like growth factor; CNS, central nervous system; IUGR, intrauterine growth rate.
SOURCE: Adapted from RL Rosenfeld, L Cuttler, in LJ De Groot, JL Jameson (eds): *Somatic Growth and Maturation in Endocrinology*, 4th ed. Philadelphia, Saunders, 2000, with permission.

for age and gender. Pituitary MRI may reveal pituitary mass lesions or structural defects.

℞ **TREATMENT** Replacement therapy with recombinant GH (0.02 to 0.05 mg/kg per day subcutaneously) restores growth velocity in GH-deficient children to ~10 cm/year. If pituitary insufficiency is documented, other associated hormone deficits should be corrected—especially adrenal steroids. GH treatment is also moderately effective for accelerating growth rates in patients with Turner syndrome and chronic renal failure.

In patients with GH insensitivity and growth retardation due to mutations of the GH receptor, treatment with IGF-I bypasses the dysfunctional GH receptor. Growth rates have been maintained for several years, and this therapy now portends improved final adult stature in this group of patients.

ADULT GH DEFICIENCY (AGHD) This disorder is usually caused by hypothalamic or pituitary somatotrope damage. Acquired pituitary hormone deficiency follows a typical sequential pattern whereby loss of adequate GH reserve foreshadows subsequent hormone deficits. The sequential order of hormone loss is usually GH → FSH/LH → TSH → ACTH. The presence of documented central hypogonadism, hypothyroidism, and/or hypoadrenalism invariably assures the presence of GH deficiency. Conversely, ~40% of patients with incipient preclinical pituitary insufficiency already manifest GH deficiency, if rigorously tested.

Presentation and Diagnosis The clinical features of AGHD include changes in body composition, lipid metabolism, and quality of life and cardiovascular dysfunction (Table 328-10). Body composition changes are common and include reduced lean body mass, increased fat mass with selective deposition of intraabdominal visceral fat, and increased waist-to-hip ratio. Hyperlipidemia, left ventricular dysfunction, hypertension, and increase plasma fibrinogen levels may also be present. Bone mineral content is reduced, with resultant increased fracture rates. Patients may exhibit social isolation, depression, and difficulty in maintaining gainful employment. Adult hypopituitarism is associated with a three-fold increased cardiovascular mortality rate in comparison to age- and sex-matched controls, and this may be due to GH deficiency.

Laboratory Investigation AGHD is rare, and in light of the nonspecific nature of associated clinical symptoms, patients appropriate for testing should be carefully selected on the basis of well-defined criteria. With few exceptions, testing should be restricted to patients with the following predisposing factors: (1) pituitary surgery, (2) pituitary or hypothalamic tumor or granulomas, (3) cranial irradiation, (4) radiologic evidence of a pituitary lesion, (5) childhood requirement for GH replacement therapy, or, rarely, (6) unexplained low age- and sex-matched IGF-I level. The transition of the GH-deficient adolescent to adulthood requires retesting to document adult GH deficiency. Up to 20% of patients treated for childhood-onset GH deficiency are found to be GH-sufficient on repeat testing as adults.

A significant proportion (~25%) of truly GH-deficient adults have low-normal IGF-I levels. Thus, as in the evaluation of GH deficiency in children, valid age- and gender-matched IGF-I measurements provide a useful index of therapeutic responses but are not sufficiently sensitive for diagnostic purposes. AGHD is diagnosed by demonstrating a subnormal GH response (<3 μg/L) to a standard provocative test. None of the available stimulation tests provides standardized GH responses that clearly discriminate normal subjects from truly GH-deficient adults. The age-related decline of GH blurs this distinction further in elderly individuals. The most validated test to distinguish pituitary-sufficient patients from those with AGHD is insulin-induced (0.05 to 0.1 U/kg) hypoglycemia. After glucose reduction to ~40 mg/dL, most individuals experience neuroglycopenic symptoms (Chap. 334), and peak GH release occurs at 60 min and remains elevated for up to 2 h. About 90% of healthy adults exhibit GH responses >5 μg/L; AGHD is defined by a peak GH response to hypoglycemia of <3 μg/L. An attenuated GH response is observed in patients with pituitary damage, obesity, untreated hypothyroidism, depression, or chronic renal failure. Although an *insulin tolerance test* (ITT) is safe when performed under appropriate supervision, it is contraindicated in patients with diabetes, ischemic heart disease, cerebrovascular disease, or epilepsy and in elderly patients. Alternative stimulatory tests include L-dopa (500 mg orally) and intravenous arginine (30 g), GHRH (1 μg/kg), and GHRP-6 (90 μg). Combinations of these tests may evoke GH secretion in subjects not responsive to a single test.

Table 328-10 Features of Adult Growth Hormone Deficiency

Clinical	Imaging
Impaired quality of life	Pituitary: Mass or structural damage
Decreased energy and drive	Bone: Reduced bone mineral density
Poor concentration	Abdomen: Excess omental adiposity
Low self esteem	Laboratory
Social isolation	Evoked GH <3 ng/ml
Body composition changes	IGF-I and IGFBP3 low or normal
Increased body fat mass	Increased LDL-cholesterol
Central fat deposition	Concomitant gonadotropin, TSH, and/or ACTH reserve deficits may be present
Increased waist-hip ratio	
Decreased lean body mass	
Reduced exercise capacity	
Reduced maximum O_2 uptake	
Impaired cardiac function	
Reduced muscle mass	
Cardiovascular risk factors	
Impaired cardiac structure and function	
Abnormal lipid profile	
Decreased fibrinolytic activity	
Atherosclerosis	
Omental obesity	

NOTE: GH, growth hormone; IGF, insulin-like growth factor; IGFBP, IGF-binding proteins; LDL, low-density lipoprotein; TSH, thyroid-stimulating hormone; ACTH, adrenocorticotropin.

℞ **TREATMENT** Once the diagnosis of AGHD is unequivocally established, replacement of GH may be indicated. Contraindications to therapy include the presence of an active neoplasm, intracranial hypertension, or uncontrolled diabetes and retinopathy. The starting dose of 0.15 to 0.3 mg/d should be titrated (up to a maximum of 1.25 mg/d) to maintain IGF-I levels in the mid-normal range for age- and gender-matched controls (Fig. 328-8). Women require higher doses than men, and elderly patients require less GH. Long-term GH maintenance sustains normal IGF-I levels and is associated with persistent body composition changes (e.g., enhanced lean body mass and lower body fat). High-density lipoprotein cholesterol increases, but total cholesterol and insulin levels do not change significantly. Lumbar spine bone mineral density increases, but this response is gradual (>1 year). Many patients note significant improvement in quality of life when evaluated by standardized questionnaires. The effect of GH replacement on mortality rates in GH-deficient patients is currently the subject of long-term prospective investigation.

About 30% of patients exhibit reversible dose-related fluid retention, joint pain, and carpal tunnel syndrome, and up to 40% exhibit myalgias and paresthesias. Patients receiving insulin require careful monitoring for dosing adjustments, as GH is a potent counterregulatory hormone for insulin action. Patients with type 2 diabetes mellitus initially develop further insulin resistance. However, glycemic control improves with the sustained loss of abdominal fat associated with long-term GH replacement. Headache, increased intracranial pressure, hypertension, atrial fibrillation, and tinnitus occur rarely. Prevalence of pituitary tumor regrowth and potential progression of skin lesions are currently being assessed in long-term surveillance programs. To date, development of these potential side effects does not appear significant. For some patients, the expense of long-term GH replacement is prohibitive.

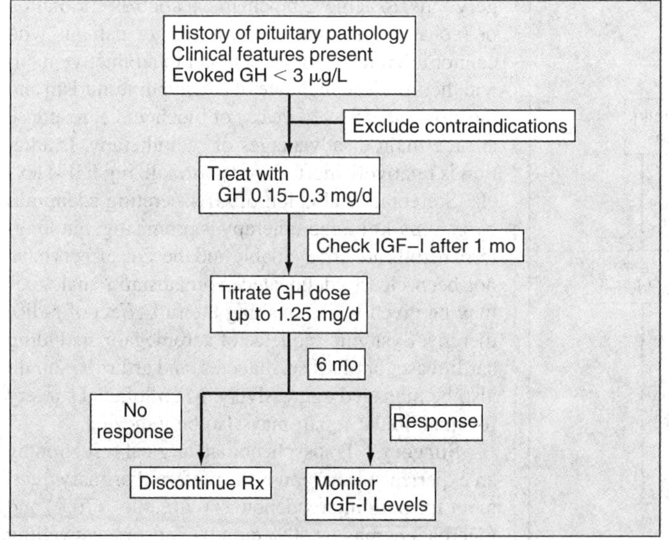

FIGURE 328-8 Management of adult growth hormone (GH) deficiency. (IGF, insulin-like growth factor.)

ACROMEGALY Etiology GH hypersecretion is usually the result of somatotrope adenomas but is also rarely caused by extrapituitary lesions (Table 328-11). In addition to typical GH-secreting somatotrope adenomas, mixed mammosomatotrope tumors and acidophilic stem-cell adenomas can secrete both GH and PRL. In patients with acidophilic stem-cell adenomas, features of hyperprolactinemia (hypogonadism and galactorrhea) predominate over the less clinically evident signs of acromegaly. Occasionally, mixed plurihormonal tumors are encountered that secrete ACTH, the glycoprotein hormone α subunit, or TSH, in addition to GH. Patients with partially empty sella may present with GH hypersecretion due to a small GH-secreting adenoma within the compressed rim of pituitary tissue; some of these may reflect the spontaneous necrosis of tumors that were previously larger. GH-secreting tumors rarely arise from ectopic pituitary tissue remnants in the nasopharynx or midline sinuses.

There are case reports of ectopic GH secretion by tumors of pancreatic, ovarian, or lung origin. Excess GHRH production may cause acromegaly because of chronic stimulation of somatotropes. These patients present with classic features of acromegaly, elevated GH levels, pituitary enlargement on MRI, and pathologic characteristics of pituitary hyperplasia. The most common cause of GHRH-mediated acromegaly is a chest or abdominal carcinoid tumor. Although these tumors usually express positive GHRH immunoreactivity, clinical features of acromegaly are evident in only a minority of patients with carcinoid disease. Excessive GHRH may also be elaborated by hypothalamic tumors, usually choristomas or neuromas.

Presentation and Diagnosis Protean manifestations of GH and IGF-I hypersecretion are indolent and often are not clinically diagnosed for 10 years or more. Acral bony overgrowth results in frontal bossing, increased hand and foot size, mandibular enlargement with prognathism, and widened space between the lower incisor teeth. In children and adolescents, initiation of GH hypersecretion prior to epiphyseal long bone closure is associated with the development of pituitary gigantism (Fig. 328-9). Soft tissue swelling results in increased heel pad thickness, increased shoe or glove size, ring tightening, characteristic coarse facial features, and a large fleshy nose. Other commonly encountered clinical features include hyperhidrosis, deep and hollow-sounding voice, oily skin, arthropathy, kyphosis, carpal tunnel syndrome, proximal muscle weakness and fatigue, acanthosis nigricans, and skin tags. Generalized visceromegaly occurs, including cardiomegaly, macroglossia, and thyroid gland enlargement.

Table 328-11 Causes of Acromegaly

	Prevalence, %
Excess growth hormone secretion	
Pituitary	98
Densely or sparsely granulated GH cell adenoma	60
Mixed GH cell and PRL cell adenoma	25
Mammosomatrope cell adenoma	10
Plurihormonal adenoma	
GH cell carcinoma or metastases	
Multiple endocrine neoplasia-1 (GH cell adenoma)	
McCune-Albright syndrome	
Ectopic sphenoid or parapharyngeal sinus pituitary adenoma	
Extrapituitary tumor	
Pancreatic islet cell tumor	<1
Excess growth hormone–releasing hormone secretion	
Central	<1
Hypothalamic hamartoma, choristoma, ganglioneuroma	<1
Peripheral	<1
Bronchial carcinoid, pancreatic islet cell tumor, small cell lung cancer, adrenal adenoma, medullary thyroid carcinoma, pheochromocytoma	

SOURCE: Adapted from S Melmed: N Engl J Med 322:966, 1990. Copyright © 1990, Massachusetts Medical Society. All rights reserved.

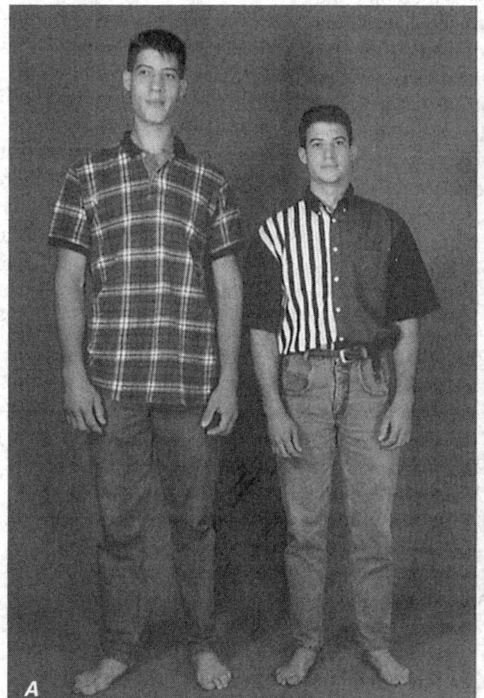

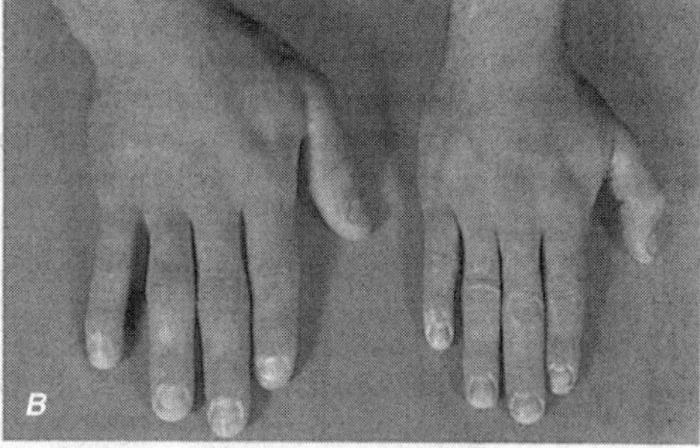

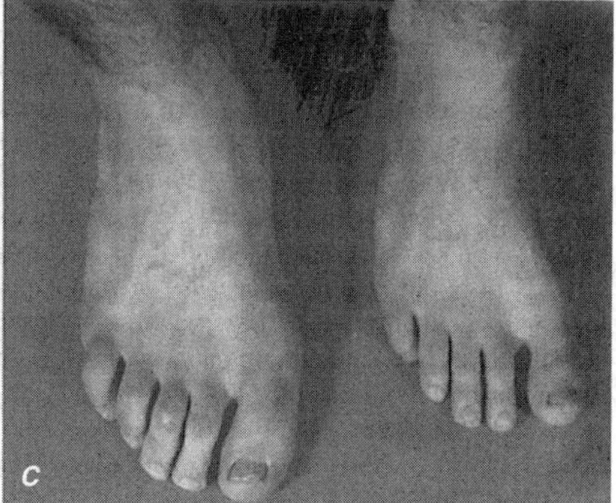

FIGURE 328-9 Features of acromegaly/gigantism. A 22-year-old man with gigantism due to excess growth hormone is shown to the left of his identical twin. The increased height and prognathism (*A*) and enlarged hand (*B*) and foot (*C*) of the affected twin are apparent. Their clinical features began to diverge at the age of approximately 13 years. *(Reproduced from R Gagel, IE McCutcheon: N Engl J Med 324:524, 1999, with permission.)*

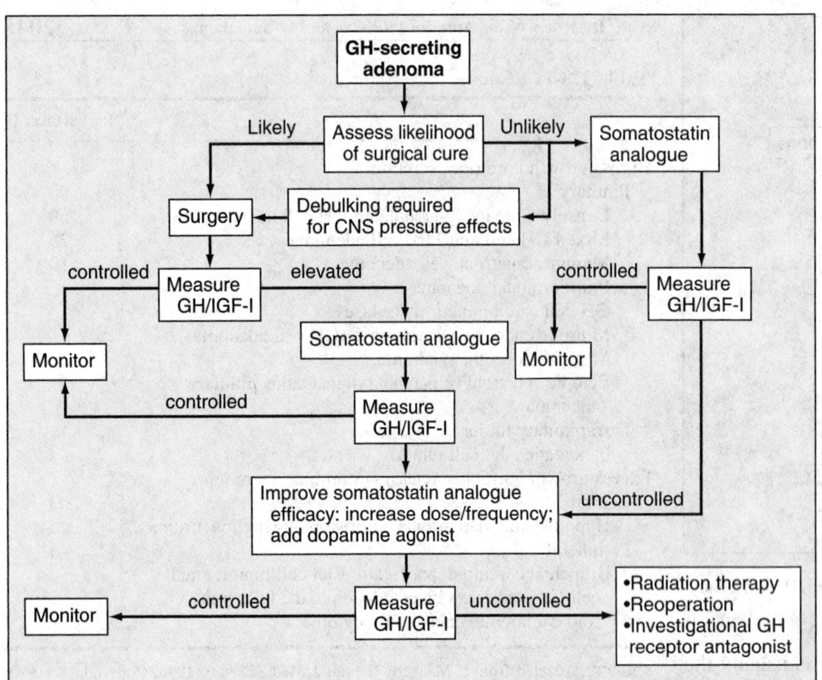

FIGURE 328-10 Management of acromegaly. (GH, growth hormone; CNS, central nervous system; IGF, insulin-like growth factor.) *(Adapted from S. Melmed et al: Current treatment guidelines for acromegaly. J Clin Endocrinol Metab 83:2646, 1998; © The Endocrine Society.)*

The most significant clinical impact of GH excess occurs with respect to the cardiovascular system. Coronary heart disease, cardiomyopathy with arrhythmias, left ventricular hypertrophy, decreased diastolic function, and hypertension occur in about 30% of patients. Upper airway obstruction with sleep apnea occurs in about 60% of patients and is associated with both soft tissue laryngeal airway obstruction and central sleep dysfunction. Diabetes mellitus develops in 25% of patients with acromegaly, and most patients are intolerant of a glucose load (as GH counteracts the action of insulin). Acromegaly is associated with an increased risk of colon polyps and colonic malignancy; polyps are diagnosed in up to one-third of acromegalic patients. Overall mortality is increased about three-fold and is due primarily to cardiovascular and cerebrovascular disorders, malignancy, and respiratory disease. Unless GH levels are controlled, survival is reduced by an average of 10 years compared with an age-matched control population.

Laboratory Investigation Age- and gender-matched serum IGF-I levels are invariably elevated in acromegaly. Consequently, an IGF-I level provides a useful laboratory screening measure when clinical features raise the possibility of acromegaly. Due to the pulsatility of GH secretion, measurement of a single random GH level is not useful for the diagnosis or exclusion of acromegaly and does not correlate with disease severity. The diagnosis of acromegaly is confirmed by demonstrating the failure of GH suppression to < 1 μg/L within 1 to 2 h of an oral glucose load (75 g). About 20% of patients exhibit a paradoxical GH rise after glucose. About 60% of patients with GH-secreting tumors may exhibit paradoxical GH responses to TRH administration. PRL should be measured as it is elevated in ~25% of patients with acromegaly. Thyroid function, gonadotropins, and sex steroids may be attenuated because of tumor mass effects. Because most patients will undergo surgery with glucocorticoid coverage, tests of ACTH reserve in asymptomatic patients are more efficiently deferred until after surgery.

℞ **TREATMENT** Surgical resection of GH-secreting adenomas is the initial treatment for most patients (Fig. 328-10). Somatostatin analogues are used as adjuvant treatment for preoperative shrinkage of large invasive macroadenomas, immediate relief of debilitating symptoms, and reduction of GH hypersecretion, in elderly patients experiencing morbidity, in patients who decline surgery, or, when surgery fails, to achieve biochemical control. Irradiation or repeat surgery may be required for patients who cannot tolerate or do not respond to adjunctive medical therapy. The high rate of late hypopituitarism and the slow rate (5 to 15 years) of biochemical response are the main disadvantages of radiotherapy. Irradiation is relatively ineffective in normalizing IGF-I levels. Stereotactic ablation of GH-secreting adenomas by gamma-knife radiotherapy is promising, but long-term results are not available and the side effects have not been clearly delineated. Somatostatin analogues may be given while awaiting the full effect of radiotherapy. Systemic sequelae of acromegaly, including cardiovascular disease, diabetes, and arthritis, should also be managed aggressively. Maxillofacial surgery for mandibular repair may also be indicated.

Surgery Transsphenoidal surgical resection by an experienced surgeon is the preferred primary treatment for both microadenomas (cure rate ~70%) and macroadenomas (<50% cured). Soft tissue swelling improves immediately after tumor resection. GH levels return to normal within an hour, and IGF-I levels are normalized within 3 to 4 days. In ~10% of patients, acromegaly may recur several years after apparently successful surgery; hypopituitarism develops in up to 15% of patients.

Somatostatin Analogues Somatostatin analogues exert their therapeutic effects through SSTR2 and -5 receptors, both of which are expressed by GH-secreting tumors. Octreotide acetate is an 8-amino-acid synthetic somatostatin analogue. In contrast to native somatostatin, the analogue is relatively resistant to plasma degradation. It has a 2-h serum half-life and possesses at least 40-fold greater potency than native somatostatin to suppress GH. These properties often allow effective pharmacologic control of GH hypersecretion without prior surgery or radiotherapy. Octreotide is administered by subcutaneous injection, beginning with 50 μg tid; the dose can be gradually increased up to 1500 μg/d. Fewer than 10% of patients do not respond to the analogue. Octreotide suppresses integrated GH levels to <5 μg/L in ~70% of patients and to <2 μg/L in up to 60% of patients. It normalizes IGF-I levels in ~75% of treated patients (Fig. 328-11). Prolonged use of the analogue is not associated with desensitization, even after ≥10 years of treatment. Rapid relief of headache and soft tissue swelling occurs in ~75% of patients within days to weeks of treatment initiation. Subjective clinical benefits of octreotide therapy occur more frequently than biochemical remission, and most patients report symptomatic improvement, including amelioration of headache, perspiration, obstructive apnea, and cardiac failure. Modest pituitary tumor size reduction occurs in about 40% of patients, but this effect is reversed when treatment is stopped.

Two long-acting somatostatin depot formulations, octreotide and lanreotide, are becoming the preferred medical treatment for acrome-

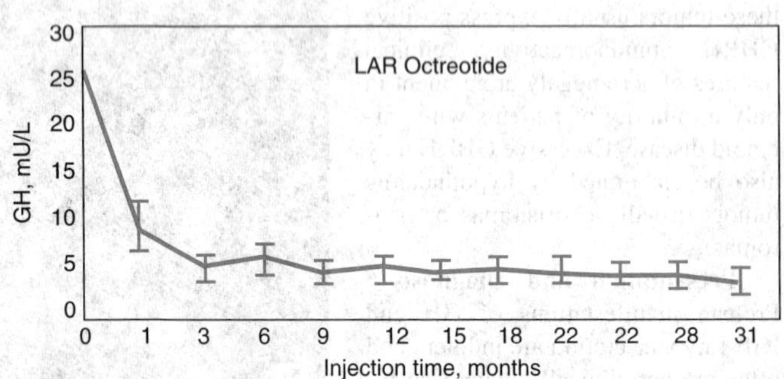

FIGURE 328-11 Medical therapy of acromegaly. Serum growth hormone (GH) levels in acromegaly following monthly LAR octreotide injections in 12 patients for 1 year, and 8 patients for 31 months. *(Reproduced from PH Davies, et al: Clin Endocrinol 48:311, 1998.)*

galic patients. *Sandostatin-LAR* is a sustained-release, long-acting formulation of octreotide incorporated into microspheres that sustain drug levels for several weeks after intramuscular injection. GH suppression occurs for as long as 6 weeks after a 30-mg injection; long-term monthly treatment sustains GH and IGF-I suppression and reduction of pituitary tumor size. *Lanreotide*, a slow-release depot somatostatin preparation, is a cyclic somatostatin octapeptide analogue that suppresses GH and IGF-I hypersecretion for 10 to 14 days after a 30-mg intramuscular injection. Long-term administration controls GH hypersecretion in two-thirds of treated patients and improves patient compliance because of the long interval required between drug injections.

Side effects Somatostatin analogues are well tolerated in most patients. Adverse effects are short-lived and mostly relate to drug-induced suppression of gastrointestinal motility and secretion. Nausea, abdominal discomfort, fat malabsorption, diarrhea, and flatulence occur in one-third of patients, though these symptoms usually remit within 2 weeks. Octreotide suppresses postprandial gallbladder contractility and delays gallbladder emptying; up to 30% of patients treated long-term develop echogenic sludge or asymptomatic cholesterol gallstones. Other side effects include mild glucose intolerance due to transient insulin suppression, asymptomatic bradycardia, hypothyroxinemia, and local pain at the injection site. The cost of chronic treatment may be prohibitive.

Dopamine Agonists Bromocriptine may suppress GH secretion in some acromegalic patients, particularly those with cosecretion of PRL. High doses (≥20 mg/d), administered as three to four daily doses, are usually required to lower GH, and therapeutic efficacy is modest. GH levels are suppressed to <5 μg/L in ~20% of patients, and IGF-I levels are normalized in only 10% of patients. Cabergoline also suppresses GH and decreases adenoma size when given at a relatively high dose of 0.5 mg/d. Combined treatment with octreotide and bromocriptine induces additive biochemical control compared to either drug alone.

GH Antagonists Investigational GH analogues antagonize endogenous GH action by blocking peripheral GH binding to its receptor. Consequently, serum IGF-I levels are suppressed, potentially reducing the deleterious effects of excess endogenous GH.

Radiation External radiation therapy or high-energy stereotactic techniques are used as adjuvant therapy for acromegaly. An advantage of radiation is that patient compliance with long-term treatment is not required. Tumor mass is reduced, and GH levels are attenuated over time. However, 50% of patients require at least 8 years for GH levels to be suppressed to <5 μg/L; this suboptimal level of GH reduction is achieved in about 90% of patients after 18 years. Patients may require interim medical therapy for several years prior to attaining maximal radiation benefits. Most patients also experience hypothalamic-pituitary damage, leading to gonadotropin, ACTH, and/or TSH deficiency within 10 years of therapy.

In summary, surgery is the preferred primary treatment for GH-secreting microadenomas (Fig. 328-10). The high frequency of GH hypersecretion after macroadenoma resection usually necessitates adjuvant or primary medical therapy for these larger tumors. Patients unable to receive or respond to medical treatment can be offered radiation.

ADRENOCORTICOTROPIN HORMONE

(See also Chap. 331)

SYNTHESIS ACTH-secreting corticotrope cells constitute about 20% of the pituitary cell population. ACTH (39 amino acids) is derived from the POMC precursor protein (266 amino acids) that also generates several other peptides, including β-lipotropin, β-endorphin, met-enkephalin, α melanocyte-stimulating hormone (MSH), and corticotropin-like intermediate lobe protein (CLIP). The POMC gene is located on chromosome 2 and possesses at least three different promoter regions that account for pituitary and peripheral tissue–specific POMC expression. A proximal promoter mediates POMC expression

in corticotropes. The gonads, placenta, gastrointestinal tissues, liver, kidney, adrenal medulla, lung, and lymphocytic tissue express shorter POMC transcripts derived from a downstream promoter region. Tumors arising from peripheral neuroendocrine tissues that secrete ectopic ACTH express the longer form of POMC. The POMC gene is powerfully suppressed by glucocorticoids and induced by CRH, arginine vasopressin (AVP), and gp 130 proinflammatory cytokines, including IL-6, and leukemia inhibitory factor.

CRH, a 41-amino-acid hypothalamic peptide synthesized in the paraventricular nucleus as well as in higher brain centers, is the predominant stimulator of ACTH synthesis and release. The CRH receptor is a GPCR that is expressed on the corticotrope. CRH signaling induces POMC transcription and is mediated by cyclic AMP, as well as mitogen activated protein (MAP) kinase–activator protein-1 (AP-1) cascades.

SECRETION ACTH secretion is pulsatile and exhibits a characteristic circadian rhythm, peaking at 6 A.M. and reaching a nadir about midnight. Adrenal glucocorticoid secretion, which is driven by ACTH, follows a parallel diurnal pattern. ACTH circadian rhymicity is determined by variations in secretory pulse amplitude rather than changes in pulse frequency. Superimposed on this endogenous rhythm, ACTH levels are increased by AVP, physical stress, exercise, acute illness, and insulin-induced hypoglycemia.

Loss of cortisol feedback inhibition, as occurs in primary adrenal failure, results in extremely high ACTH levels. Glucocorticoid-mediated negative regulation of the hypothalamo-pituitary-adrenal (HPA) axis occurs as a consequence of both hypothalamic CRH suppression and direct attenuation of pituitary POMC gene expression and ACTH release. Hypothalamic AVP stimulates the protein kinase C pathway and acts synergistically with CRH to enhance ACTH production.

Acute inflammatory or septic insults activate the HPA axis through the integrated actions of proinflammatory cytokines, bacterial toxins, and neural signals. The overlapping cascade of ACTH-inducing cytokines (TNF; IL-1, -2, and -6; and leukemia inhibitory factor) activates hypothalamic CRH and AVP secretion, pituitary POMC gene expression, and local paracrine pituitary cytokine networks. The resulting cortisol elevation restrains the inflammatory response and provides host protection. Concomitantly, cytokine-mediated central glucocorticoid receptor resistance impairs glucocorticoid suppression of the HPA. Thus, the neuroendocrine stress response reflects the net result of highly integrated hypothalamic, intrapituitary, and peripheral hormone and cytokine signals.

ACTION The major function of the HPA axis is to maintain metabolic homeostasis and to mediate the neuroendocrine stress response. Peripheral and central afferent signals, which are integrated by the pituitary corticotrope cell, ultimately affect the pattern and quantity of adrenal cortisol secretion. ACTH induces cortical steroidogenesis by maintaining adrenal cell proliferation and function. The receptor for ACTH, designated *melanocortin-2 receptor*, is a GPCR that activates cyclic AMP and MAP kinase pathways; it induces steroidogenesis by stimulating a cascade of steroidogenic enzymes (Chap. 331).

ACTH DEFICIENCY **Presentation and Diagnosis** Secondary adrenal insufficiency occurs as a result of pituitary ACTH deficiency. It is characterized by fatigue, weakness, anorexia, nausea, vomiting, and, occasionally, hypoglycemia (due to diminished insulin counterregulation). In contrast to primary adrenal failure, hypocortisolism associated with pituitary failure is not usually accompanied by pigmentation changes or mineralocorticoid deficiency. ACTH deficiency is commonly due to glucocorticoid withdrawal following treatment-associated suppression of the HPA axis. Isolated ACTH deficiency may occur after surgical resection of an ACTH-secreting pituitary adenoma that has suppressed the HPA axis; this phenomenon is suggestive of a surgical cure. The mass effects of other pituitary adenomas or sellar lesions may lead to ACTH deficiency, but usually in combination with other pituitary hormone deficiencies. Partial

ACTH deficiency may be unmasked in the presence of an acute medical or surgical illness, when clinically significant hypocortisolism reflects diminished ACTH reserve.

Laboratory Diagnosis Inappropriately low ACTH levels in the setting of low cortisol levels are characteristic of diminished ACTH reserve. Low basal serum cortisol levels are associated with blunted cortisol responses to ACTH provocative stimulation and impaired cortisol response to insulin-induced hypoglycemia, or testing with metyrapone or CRH. →*For description of provocative ACTH tests, see "Tests of Pituitary-Adrenal Responsiveness" in Chap. 331.*

℞ TREATMENT Glucocorticoid replacement therapy improves most features of ACTH deficiency. The total daily dose of hydrocortisone replacement should not exceed 30 mg daily, divided into two or three doses. Prednisone (5 mg each morning; 2.5 mg each evening) is longer acting and has fewer mineralocorticoid effects than hydrocortisone. Some authorities advocate lower maintenance doses in an effort to avoid cushingoid side effects. Doses should be increased several-fold during periods of acute illness or stress.

CUSHING'S DISEASE (ACTH-PRODUCING ADENOMA) (See also Chap. 331) **Etiology and Prevalence** Pituitary corticotrope adenomas account for 70% of patients with endogenous causes of Cushing's syndrome. However, it should be recalled that iatrogenic hypercortisolism is the most common cause of cushingoid features. Ectopic tumor ACTH production, cortisol-producing adrenal adenomas, carcinoma, and hyperplasia account for the other causes; rarely, ectopic tumor CRH production is encountered.

ACTH-producing adenomas account for about 10 to 15% of all pituitary tumors. Because the clinical features of Cushing's syndrome often lead to early diagnosis, most ACTH-producing pituitary tumors are relatively small microadenomas. However, macroadenomas are also seen, and some ACTH-secreting adenomas are clinically silent. Cushing's disease is 5 to 10 times more common in women than in men. These pituitary adenomas exhibit unrestrained ACTH secretion, with resultant hypercortisolemia. However, they retain partial suppressibility in the presence of high doses of administered glucocorticoids, providing the basis for dynamic testing to distinguish pituitary and nonpituitary causes of Cushing's syndrome.

Presentation and Diagnosis The diagnosis of Cushing's syndrome presents two great challenges: (1) to distinguish patients with pathologic cortisol excess from those with physiologic or other disturbances of cortisol production; and (2) to determine the etiology of cortisol excess, which can include iatrogenic administration of glucocorticoids, adrenal adenomas or carcinomas, pituitary adenomas, and ectopic sources of ACTH and CRH.

Typical features of chronic cortisol excess include thin, brittle skin, central obesity, hypertension, plethoric moon facies, purple striae and easy bruisability, glucose intolerance or diabetes mellitus, gonadal dysfunction, osteoporosis, proximal muscle weakness, signs of hyperandrogenism (acne, hirsutism), and psychologic disturbances (depression, mania, and psychoses) (Table 328-12). Hematopoietic features of hypercortisolism include leukocytosis, lymphopenia, and eosinopenia. Immune suppression includes delayed hypersensitivity. The protean manifestations of hypercortisolism make it challenging to decide which patients mandate formal laboratory evaluation. Certain features make pathologic causes of hypercortisolism more likely—these include characteristic central redistribution of fat, thin skin with striae and bruising, and proximal muscle weakness. In children and in young females, early osteoporosis may be particularly prominent. The primary cause of death is cardiovascular disease, but infections and risk of suicide are also increased.

Rapid development of features of hypercortisolism associated with skin hyperpigmentation and severe myopathy suggests the possibility of ectopic sources of ACTH. Hypertension, hypokalemic alkalosis, glucose intolerance, and edema are also more pronounced in these patients. Serum potassium levels <3.3 mmol/L are evident in ~70% of patients with ectopic ACTH secretion but are seen in <10% of patients with pituitary-dependent Cushing's disease.

Table 328-12 Clinical Features of Cushing's Syndrome (All Ages)

Symptoms/Signs	Frequency, %
Obesity or weight gain (>115% ideal body weight)	80
Thin skin	80
Moon facies	75
Hypertension	75
Purple skin striae	65
Hirsutism	65
Abnormal glucose tolerance	55
Impotence	55
Menstrual disorders (usually amenorrhea)	60
Plethora	60
Proximal muscle weakness	50
Truncal obesity	50
Acne	45
Bruising	45
Mental changes	45
Osteoporosis	40
Edema of lower extremities	30
Hyperpigmentation	20
Hypokalemic alkalosis	15
Diabetes mellitus	15

SOURCE: Adapted from MA Magiokou et al, in ME Wierman (ed), *Diseases of the Pituitary*. Totowa, NJ, Humana, 1997.

Laboratory Investigation The diagnosis of Cushing's syndrome is based on laboratory documentation of endogenous hypercortisolism. Measurements of 24-h urine free cortisol (UFC) is a precise and cost-effective screening test. Alternatively, the failure to suppress plasma cortisol after an overnight 1-mg dexamethasone suppression test can be used to identify patients with hypercortisolism. As nadir levels of cortisol occur at night, elevated midnight samples of cortisol are suggestive of Cushing's syndrome. Basal plasma ACTH levels often distinguish patients with ACTH-independent (adrenal or exogenous glucocorticoid) from those with ACTH-dependent (pituitary, ectopic ACTH) Cushing's disease. Mean basal ACTH levels are about eight-fold higher in patients with ectopic ACTH secretion compared to those with pituitary ACTH-secreting adenomas. However, extensive overlap of ACTH levels in these two disorders precludes using ACTH to make the distinction. Instead, dynamic testing, based on differential sensitivity to glucocorticoid feedback, or ACTH stimulation in response to CRH or cortisol reduction is used to discriminate ectopic versus pituitary sources of excess ACTH (Table 328-13). Very rarely, circulating CRH levels are elevated, reflecting ectopic tumor-derived secretion of CRH and often ACTH. →*For discussion of dynamic testing for Cushing's syndrome, see Chap. 331.*

Most ACTH-secreting pituitary tumors are <5 mm in diameter, and about half are undetectable by sensitive MRI. The high prevalence of incidental pituitary microadenomas diminishes the ability to distinguish ACTH-secreting pituitary tumors accurately by MRI.

Inferior petrosal venous sampling Because pituitary MRI with gadolinium enhancement is insufficiently sensitive to distinguish small (<2 mm) pituitary ACTH-secreting adenomas from ectopic ACTH-secreting tumors that may have similar clinical and biochemical characteristics, bilateral inferior petrosal sinus ACTH sampling before and after CRH administration may be required. Simultaneous assessment of ACTH concentrations in each inferior petrosal vein and in the peripheral circulation provides a strategy for confirming and localizing pituitary ACTH production. Sampling is performed at baseline and 2, 5, and 10 min after intravenous ovine CRH (1 μg/kg) injection. An increased ratio (>2) of inferior petrosal:peripheral vein ACTH confirms pituitary Cushing's disease. After CRH injection, peak petrosal: peripheral ACTH ratios of ≥3 confirm the presence of a pituitary ACTH-secreting tumor. The sensitivity of this test is 99%, with very rare false-positive results. False-negative results may be encountered in patients with aberrant venous anatomic drainage. Petrosal sinus

Table 328-13 Differential Diagnosis of ACTH-Dependent Cushing's Syndrome[a]

	ACTH-Secreting Pituitary Tumor	Ectopic ACTH Secretion
Etiology	Pituitary corticotrope adenoma Plurihormonal adenoma	Bronchial, abdominal carcinoid Small cell lung cancer Thymoma
Gender	F > M	M > F
Clinical features	Slow onset	Rapid onset Pigmentation Severe myopathy
Serum potassium <3.3 μg/L	<10%	75%
24-h urinary free cortisol (UFC)	High	High
Basal ACTH level	Inappropriately high	Very high
Dexamethasone suppression		
1 mg overnight		
Low dose (0.5 mg q6h)	Cortisol >5 μg/dL	Cortisol >5 μg/dL
High dose (2 mg q6h)	Cortisol >5 μg/dL	Cortisol >5 μg/dL
UFC > 80% suppressed	Microadenomas: 90% Macroadenomas: 50%	10%
Inferior petrosal sinus sampling (IPSS)		
Basal		
IPSS: peripheral	>2	<2
CRH-induced		
IPSS: peripheral	>3	<3

[a] ACTH-independent causes of Cushing's syndrome are diagnosed by suppressed ACTH levels and an adrenal mass in the setting of hypercortisolism. Iatrogenic Cushing's syndrome is excluded by history.

NOTE: ACTH, adrenocorticotropin hormone; F, female; M, male; CRH, corticotropin-releasing hormone.

catheterizations are technically difficult, and about 0.05% of patients develop neurovascular complications. The procedure should not be performed in patients with hypertension or in the presence of a well-visualized pituitary adenoma on MRI.

TREATMENT Selective transsphenoidal resection is the treatment of choice for Cushing's disease (Fig. 328-12). The remission rate for this procedure is ~80% for microadenomas but <50% for macroadenomas. After successful tumor resection, most patients experience a postoperative period of adrenal insufficiency that lasts for up to 12 months. This usually requires low-dose cortisol replacement, as patients experience steroid withdrawal symptoms as well as having a suppressed HPA axis. Biochemical recurrence occurs in approximately 5% of patients in whom surgery was initially successful.

When initial surgery is unsuccessful, repeat surgery is sometimes indicated, particularly when a pituitary source for ACTH is well documented. In older patients in whom growth and fertility are no longer important, hemi- or total hypophysectomy may be necessary if an adenoma is not recognized. Pituitary irradiation may be used after unsuccessful surgery, but it cures only about 15% of patients. Because radiation is slow and only partially effective in adults, steroidogenic inhibitors are used in combination with pituitary irradiation to block the adrenal effects of persistently high ACTH levels.

Mitotane (o,p'-DDD) suppresses cortisol hypersecretion by inhibiting 11β-hydroxylase and cholesterol side-chain cleavage enzymes and by destroying adrenocortical cells. Side effects of mitotane include gastrointestinal symptoms, dizziness, gynecomastia, hyperlipidemia, skin rash, and hepatic enzyme elevation. It may also lead to hypoaldosteronism. *Ketoconazole*, an imidazole derivative antimycotic agent, inhibits several P450 enzymes and effectively lowers cortisol in most patients with Cushing's disease when administered twice daily (600 to 1200 mg/d). Elevated hepatic transaminases, gynecomastia, impotence, gastrointestinal upset, and edema are common side effects.

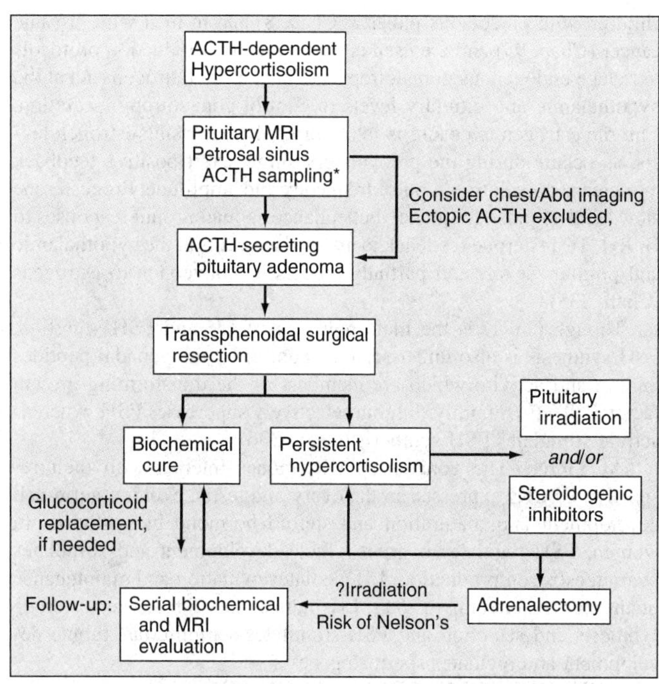

FIGURE 328-12 Management of Cushing's disease. (ACTH, adrenocorticotropin hormone; MRI, magnetic resonance imaging.) *, Not usually required.

Metyrapone (2 to 4 g/d) inhibits 11β-hydroxylase activity and normalizes plasma cortisol in up to 75% of patients. Side effects include nausea and vomiting, rash, and exacerbation of acne or hirsutism. Other agents include *aminoglutethimide* (250 mg tid), *trilostane* (200 to 1000 mg/d), *cyproheptadine* (24 mg/d), and IV *etomidate* (0.3 mg/kg per hour). Glucocorticoid insufficiency is a potential side effect of agents used to block steroidogenesis.

The use of steroidogenic inhibitors has decreased the need for bilateral adrenalectomy. Removal of both adrenal glands corrects hypercortisolism but may be associated with significant morbidity and necessitates permanent glucocorticoid and mineralocorticoid replacement. Adrenalectomy in the setting of residual corticotrope adenoma tissue predisposes to the development of *Nelson's syndrome*, a disorder characterized by rapid pituitary tumor enlargement and increased pigmentation secondary to high ACTH levels. Radiation therapy may be indicated to prevent the development of Nelson's syndrome after adrenalectomy.

GONADOTROPINS: FSH AND LH

SYNTHESIS AND SECRETION Gonadotrope cells comprise about 10% of anterior pituitary cells and produce two gonadotropins—LH and FSH. Like TSH and hCG, LH and FSH are glycoprotein hormones consisting of α and β subunits. The α subunit is common to these glycoprotein hormones; specificity is conferred by the β subunits, which are expressed by separate genes.

Gonadotropin synthesis and release are dynamically regulated. This is particularly true in females, in whom the rapidly fluctuating gonadal steroid levels vary throughout the menstrual cycle. Hypothalamic GnRH, a 10-amino-acid peptide synthesized in the preoptic region, regulates the synthesis and secretion of both LH and FSH. GnRH is secreted in discrete pulses every 60 to 120 min, which in turn elicit LH and FSH pulses (Fig. 328-3). GnRH acts through a GPCR to stimulate phospholipase C, protein kinase C, and calcium signaling pathways. The pulsatile mode of GnRH input is essential to its action; pulses prime gonadotrope responsiveness, whereas continuous GnRH exposure induces desensitization. Based on this phenomenon, long-acting GnRH agonists are used to suppress gonadotropin levels in children with precocious puberty (Chap. 8) and in men with prostate cancer (Chap. 95) and are used in some ovulation-induction protocols to reduce endogenous gonadotropins (Chap. 336). Estrogens act at the hypothalamic and pituitary levels to control gonadotropin secretion. Chronic estrogen exposure is inhibitory, whereas rising estrogen levels, as occurs during the preovulatory surge, exert positive feedback to increase gonadotropin pulse frequency and amplitude. Progesterone slows GnRH pulse frequency but enhances gonadotropin responses to GnRH. Testosterone feedback in males also occurs at the hypothalamic and pituitary levels and partially reflects its conversion to estrogens (Chap. 335).

Though GnRH is the main regulator of LH and FSH secretion, FSH synthesis is also under separate control by the gonadal peptides inhibin and activin, which are members of the transforming growth factor β (TGF-β) family. Inhibin selectively suppresses FSH, whereas activin stimulates FSH synthesis (Chap. 336).

ACTION The gonadotropin hormones interact with their respective GPCRs expressed in the ovary and testis, evoking germ-cell development and maturation and steroid hormone biosynthesis. In women, FSH regulates ovarian follicle development and stimulates ovarian estrogen production. LH mediates ovulation and maintenance of the corpus luteum. In men, LH induces Leydig cell testosterone synthesis and secretion and FSH stimulates seminiferous tubule development and regulates spermatogenesis.

GONADOTROPIN DEFICIENCY Hypogonadism is the most common presenting feature of adult hypopituitarism, even when other pituitary hormones are also deficient. It is often a harbinger of hypothalamic or pituitary diseases that impair GnRH production or delivery through the pituitary stalk. As noted above, hypogonadotropic hypogonadism is a common presenting feature of hyperprolactinemia.

A variety of inherited and acquired disorders are associated with *isolated hypogonadotropic hypogonadism* (IHH) (Chap. 335). Hypothalamic defects associated with GnRH deficiency include two X-linked disorders, Kallmann syndrome (see above) and mutations in the *DAX1* gene. GnRH receptor mutations and inactivating mutations of the LH β and FSH β subunit genes are rare causes of selective gonadotropin deficiency. Acquired forms of GnRH deficiency leading to hypogonadotropism are seen in association with anorexia nervosa (Chap. 78), stress, starvation, and extreme exercise, but may also be idiopathic. Hypogonadotropic hypogonadism in these disorders is reversed by removal of the stressful stimulus.

Presentation and Diagnosis In premenopausal women, hypogonadotropic hypogonadism presents as diminished ovarian function leading to oligomenorrhea or amenorrhea, infertility, decreased vaginal secretions, decreased libido, and breast atrophy. In hypogonadal adult males, secondary testicular failure is associated with decreased libido and potency, infertility, decreased muscle mass with weakness, reduced beard and body hair growth, soft testes, and characteristic fine facial wrinkles. Osteoporosis occurs in both untreated hyogonadal females and males.

Laboratory Investigation Central hypogonadism is associated with low or inappropriately low serum gonadotropin levels and low sex hormone concentrations (testosterone in males, estradiol in females). Three pooled serum samples drawn 20 min apart are used for accurate measurement of serum LH and FSH levels, thus allowing for the effects of hormone secretory pulses. Male patients have abnormal semen analysis.

Intravenous GnRH (100 μg) stimulates gonadotropes to secrete LH (which peaks within 30 min) and FSH (which plateaus during the ensuing 60 min). Normal responses vary according to menstrual cycle stage, age, and sex of the patient. Generally, LH levels increase about threefold, whereas FSH responses are less pronounced. In the setting of gonadotropin deficiency, a normal gonadotropin response to GnRH indicates intact gonadotrope function and suggests a hypothalamic abnormality. An absent response, however, cannot reliably distinguish pituitary from hypothalamic causes of hypogonadism. For this reason, GnRH testing usually adds little to the information gained from baseline evaluation of the hypothalamic-pituitary-gonadotrope axis, except in cases of isolated GnRH deficiency (e.g., Kallmann syndrome).

MRI examination of the sellar region and assessment of other pituitary functions are usually indicated in patients with documented central hypogonadism.

℞ **TREATMENT** In males, testosterone replacement is necessary to achieve and maintain normal growth and development of the external genitalia, secondary sex characteristics, male sexual behavior, and androgenic anabolic effects including maintenance of muscle function and bone mass. Testosterone may be administered by intramuscular injections every 1 to 4 weeks or using patches that are replaced daily (Chap. 335). Gonadotropin injections [hCG or human menopausal gonadotropin (hMG)] over 12 to 18 months are used to restore fertility. Pulsatile GnRH therapy (25 to 150 ng/kg every 2 h), administered by a subcutaneous infusion pump, is also effective for treatment of hypothalamic hypogonadism when fertility is desired.

In premenopausal women, cyclical replacement of estrogen and progesterone maintains secondary sexual characteristics and genitourinary tract integrity and prevents premature osteoporosis and possibly coronary artery disease (Chap. 336). Gonadotropin therapy is used for ovulation induction. Follicular growth and maturation are initiated using hMG or recombinant FSH; hCG is subsequently injected to induce ovulation. As in men, pulsatile GnRH therapy can be used to treat hypothalamic causes of gonadotropin deficiency.

NONFUNCTIONING AND GONADOTROPIN-PRODUCING PITUITARY ADENOMAS **Etiology and Prevalence** Nonfunctioning pituitary adenomas include those that secrete little or no pituitary hormones, as well as tumors that produce too little hormone to result in recognizable clinical features. They are the most common type of pituitary adenoma and are usually macroadenomas at the time of diagnosis because clinical features are inapparent until tumor mass effects occur. Based on immunohistochemistry, most clinically nonfunctioning adenomas can be shown to originate from gonadotrope cells. These tumors typically produce small amounts of intact gonadotropins (usually FSH) as well as uncombined α and LH β and FSH β subunits. Tumor secretion may lead to elevated α and FSH β subunits and, rarely, to increased LH β subunit levels. Some adenomas express α subunits without FSH or LH. TRH administration often induces an atypical increase of tumor-derived gonadotropins or subunits.

Presentation and Diagnosis Clinically nonfunctioning tumors may present with optic chiasm pressure and other symptoms of local expansion or be incidentally discovered on an MRI performed for another indication. Menstrual disturbances or ovarian hyperstimulation rarely occur in women with large tumors that produce FSH and LH. More commonly, adenoma compression of the pituitary stalk or surrounding pituitary tissue leads to attenuated LH and features of hypogonadism. Prolactin levels are usually slightly increased, also because of stalk compression. It is important to distinguish this circumstance from true prolactinomas, as most nonfunctioning tumors respond poorly to treatment with dopamine agonists.

Laboratory Investigation The goal of laboratory testing in clinically nonfunctioning tumors is to classify the type of the tumor, to identify hormonal markers of tumor activity, and to detect possible hypopituitarism. Free α subunit levels may be elevated in 10 to 15% of patients with nonfunctioning tumors. In female patients, peri- or postmenopausal basal FSH concentrations are difficult to distinguish from tumor-derived FSH elevation. Premenopausal women have cycling FSH levels, also preventing clear-cut diagnostic distinction from tumor-derived FSH. In men, gonadotropin-secreting tumors may be diagnosed because of slightly increased gonadotropins (FSH > LH) in the setting of a pituitary mass. Testosterone levels are usually low, despite the normal or increased LH level, perhaps reflecting reduced LH bioactivity or the loss of normal LH pulsatility. Because this pattern of hormone tests is also seen in primary gonadal failure and, to some extent, with aging (Chap. 335), the increased gonadotropins alone are insufficient for the diagnosis of a gonadotropin-secreting tumor. In the majority of patients with gonadotrope adenomas, TRH administration stimulates LH β subunit secretion; this response is not seen in normal individuals. GnRH testing is not helpful for making the diagnosis. For nonfunctioning and gonadotropin-secreting tumors, the diagnosis usually rests on immunohistochemical analyses of resected tumor tissue, as the mass effects of these tumors usually necessitate resection.

Although acromegaly or Cushing's syndrome usually presents with unique clinical features, clinically inapparent somatotrope or corticotrope adenomas can be excluded by a normal IGF-I value and normal 24-h urinary free cortisol levels. If PRL levels are <100 μg/L in a patient harboring a pituitary mass, a nonfunctioning adenoma causing pituitary stalk compression should be considered.

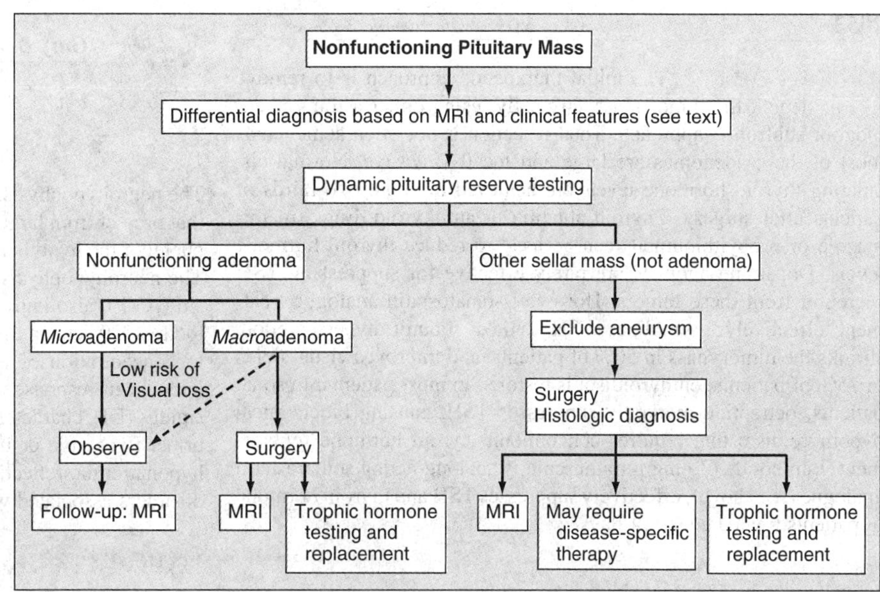

FIGURE 328-13 Management of a nonfunctioning pituitary mass.

TREATMENT Asymptomatic small nonfunctioning adenomas with no threat to vision may be followed with regular MRI and visual field testing without immediate intervention. However, for larger macroadenomas, transsphenoidal surgery is the only effective way to reduce tumor size and relieve mass effects (Fig. 328-13). Although it is not usually possible to remove all adenoma tissue surgically, vision improves in 70% of patients with preoperative visual field defects. Preexisting hypopituitarism that results from tumor mass effects commonly improves or may resolve completely. Early postoperative complications include diabetes insipidus and/or inappropriate antidiuretic hormone secretion. Beginning about 6 months postoperatively, MRI scans should be performed yearly to detect tumor regrowth. Within 5 to 6 years following successful surgical resection, ~15% of nonfunctioning tumors recur. When substantial tumor remains after transsphenoidal surgery, adjuvant radiotherapy may be indicated to prevent tumor growth. Radiotherapy may be deferred if no postoperative residual mass is evident.

Nonfunctioning pituitary tumors respond poorly to dopamine agonist treatment, with modest tumor shrinkage occurring in <10% of patients. Although SSTR subtypes 2 and 5 have been identified on nonfunctioning pituitary adenomas, octreotide does not shrink these tumors and only modestly suppresses gonadotropin and α subunit levels. Visual improvement sometimes occurs without evident reduction of tumor size by MRI, presumably reflecting relief of pressure on the optic tracts. The selective GnRH antagonist, Nal-Glu GnRH, suppresses FSH hypersecretion but has no effect on adenoma size.

THYROID-STIMULATING HORMONE

SYNTHESIS AND SECRETION TSH-secreting thyrotrope cells comprise 5% of the anterior pituitary cell population. TSH is structurally related to LH and FSH. It shares a common α subunit with these hormones but contains a specific TSH β subunit. TRH is a hypothalamic tripeptide (pyroglutamyl histidylprolinamide) that acts through a GPCR to stimulate phospholipase C, protein kinase C, and calcium pathways. TRH stimulates TSH synthesis and secretion; it also stimulates the lactotrope cell to secrete PRL. TSH secretion is stimulated by TRH, whereas thyroid hormones, dopamine, SRIF, and glucocorticoids suppress TSH by overriding TRH induction.

The thyrotrope is stimulated when TSH is released from the negative feedback inhibition of thyroid hormones. Thus, thyroid damage, including surgical thyroidectomy, radiation-induced hypothyroidism, chronic thyroiditis, or prolonged goitrogen exposure, are associated with increased TSH. Long-standing untreated hypothyroidism can lead to thyrotrope hyperplasia and pituitary enlargement, which may be evident on MRI.

ACTION TSH is secreted in pulses, though the excursions are modest in comparison to other pituitary hormones because of the relatively low amplitude of the pulses and the relatively long half-life of TSH. Consequently, single determinations of TSH suffice to assess its circulating levels. TSH binds to a GPCR on thyroid follicular cells to stimulate thyroid hormone synthesis and release (Chap. 330).

TSH DEFICIENCY Features of central hypothyroidism, due to TSH deficiency, mimic those seen whith primary hypothyroidism but are generally less severe. Pituitary hypothyroidism is characterized by low basal TSH levels in the setting of low free thyroid hormone. In contrast, patients with hypothyroidism of hypothalamic origin (presumably due to a lack of endogenous TRH) may exhibit normal or even slightly elevated TSH levels. There is evidence that the TSH produced in this circumstance has reduced biologic activity because of altered glycosylation.

TRH (200 μg) injected intravenously causes a two- to threefold increase in TSH (and PRL) levels within 30 min. Although TRH testing can be used to assess TSH reserve, abnormalities of the thyroid axis can usually be detected based on basal free T_4 and TSH levels, without the need for TRH testing.

Thyroid-replacement therapy should be initiated after establishing adequate adrenal function. Dose adjustment is based on thyroid hormone levels and clinical parameters rather than the TSH level.

TSH-SECRETING ADENOMAS TSH-producing macroadenomas are rare but are often large and locally invasive when they occur. Patients usually present with thyroid goiter and hyperthyroidism, reflecting overproduction of TSH. Diagnosis is based on demonstrating elevated serum free T_4 levels, inappropriately normal or high TSH secretion, and MRI evidence of a pituitary adenoma. An elevated free α subunit level occurs in about half of patients and supports the diagnosis of a TSH-secreting adenoma.

It is important to exclude other causes of inappropriate TSH secretion, such as resistance to thyroid hormone, an autosomal dominant disorder caused by mutations in the thyroid hormone β receptor (Chap. 330). The presence of a pituitary mass and elevated α subunit levels are suggestive of a TSH-secreting tumor. Dysalbuminemic hyperthyroxinemia syndromes, caused by various mutations in serum thyroid hormone binding proteins, are also characterized by elevated thyroid hormone levels, but with normal rather than suppressed TSH levels. However, free thyroid hormone levels are normal in these disorders, most of which are familial.

℞ TREATMENT The initial therapeutic approach is to remove or debulk the tumor mass surgically, using either a transsphenoidal or subfrontal approach. Total resection is not often achieved as most of these adenomas are large and locally invasive. Normal circulating thyroid hormone levels are achieved in about two-thirds of patients after surgery. Thyroid ablation or antithyroid drugs (methimazole or propylthiouracil) can be used to reduce thyroid hormone levels. Dopamine agonists are rarely effective for suppressing TSH secretion from these tumors. However, somatostatin analogue treatment effectively normalizes TSH and α subunit hypersecretion, shrinks the tumor mass in 50% of patients, and improves visual fields in 75% of patients; euthyroidism is restored in most patients. In some patients, octreotide markedly suppresses TSH, causing biochemical hypothyroidism that requires concomitant thyroid hormone replacement. Lanreotide (30 mg intramuscularly), a long-acting somatostatin analogue (see above), effectively suppresses TSH and thyroid hormone in patients treated every 14 days.

DIABETES INSIPIDUS

→*See Chap. 329 for diagnosis and treatment of diabetes insipidus.*

BIBLIOGRAPHY

BRUCKER-DAVIS F et al: Thyrotropin-secreting pituitary tumors: Diagnostic criteria, thyroid hormone sensitivity, and treatment outcome in 25 patients followed at the National Institutes of Health. J Clin Endocrinol Metab 84:476, 1999

Consensus guidelines for the diagnosis and treatment of adults with growth hormone deficiency: Summary statement of the Growth Hormone Research Society workshop on adult growth hormone deficiency. J Clin Endocrinol Metab 83:379, 1998

DELADOEY J et al: "Hot spot" in the PROP1 gene responsible for combined pituitary hormone deficiency. J Clin Endocrinol Metab 84:1645, 1999

GREENMAN Y, MELMED S: Diagnosis and management of nonfunctioning pituitary tumors. Ann Rev Med 47:95, 1996

HONEGGER J et al: Surgical treatment of craniopharyngiomas: Endocrinological results. J Neurosurg 90:251, 1999

KOJIMA M et al: Ghrelin is a growth-hormone-releasing acylated peptide from stomach. Nature 402:656, 1999

MELMED S et al: Current treatment guidelines for acromegaly. J Clin Endocrinol Metab 83:2646, 1998

MOLITCH ME: Diagnosis and treatment of prolactinomas. Adv Intern Med 44:117, 1999

NEWELL-PRICE J et al: The diagnosis and differential diagnosis of Cushing's syndrome and pseudo-Cushing's states. Endocr Rev 19:647, 1998

NEWMAN CB et al: Medical therapy of acromegaly. Endocrinol Metab Clin North Am 28:171, 1999

NIEMAN LK: Cushing's syndrome. Curr Ther Endocrinol Metab 6:161, 1997

SHALET SM et al: The diagnosis of growth hormone deficiency in children and adults. Endocr Rev 19:203, 1998

SHIMON I, MELMED S: Genetic basis of endocrine disease: Pituitary tumor pathogenesis. J Clin Endocrin Metab 82:1675, 1997

SHIN J et al: Cystic lesions of the pituitary: Clinicopathological features distinguishing craniopharyngioma, Rathke's cleft cyst, and arachnoid cyst. J Clin Endocrinol Metab 84:3972, 1999

SNYDER PJ: Gonadotrope adenomas. Curr Ther in Endocrinol Metab 6:56, 1997

SONINO N, BOSCARO M: Medical therapy for Cushing's disease. Endocrinol Metab Clin North Am 28:211, 1999

TREIER M et al: Multistep signaling requirements for pituitary organogenesis in vivo. Genes Dev 12:1691, 1998

TSIGOS C: Differential diagnosis and management of Cushing's syndrome. Ann Rev Med 47:443, 1996

WEBSTER J: A comparative review of the tolerability profiles of dopamine agonists in the treatment of hyperprolactemia and inhibition of lactation. Drug Safety 14:118, 1998

329 DISORDERS OF THE NEUROHYPOPHYSIS

Gary L. Robertson

The neurohypophysis, or posterior pituitary gland, is formed by axons that project from large cell bodies in the supraoptic and paraventricular nuclei of the hypothalamus to the posterior portion of the sella turcica. The neurohypophysis produces two hormones: (1) arginine vasopressin (AVP), also known as antidiuretic hormone (ADH); and (2) oxytocin. AVP acts on the renal tubules to induce water retention, leading to concentration of the urine. Oxytocin stimulates postpartum milk letdown in response to suckling. AVP deficiency causes diabetes insipidus (DI), characterized by the production of large amounts of dilute urine. Excessive or inappropriate production of AVP predisposes to hyponatremia, reflecting water retention. There are no known clinical disorders associated with oxytocin deficiency or excess.

VASOPRESSIN

ACTION AVP is a nonapeptide composed of a six-membered disulfide ring and a tripeptide tail on which the C-terminal carboxy group is amidated (Fig. 329-1). The most important, if not the only, physiologic action of AVP is to influence the rate of water excretion by promoting concentration of urine. This antidiuretic effect is achieved by increasing the hydroosmotic permeability of cells that line the distal tubule and medullary collecting ducts of the nephron. In the absence of AVP, these cells are impermeable to water and reabsorb little, if any, of the relatively large volume of dilute filtrate that enters from the cortical nephron. Low AVP concentration results in the production of large amounts of urine (as much as 0.2 mL/kg per minute) that is maximally dilute (specific gravity and osmolality ~1.000 and 50 mmol/L, respectively), a condition known as a *water diuresis.* In the presence of AVP, the luminal surface of the cells lining the terminal collecting duct becomes selectively permeable to water, allowing it to diffuse back down the osmotic gradient created by the hypertonic renal medulla. As a result, the dilute fluid passing through the tubules is concentrated and the rate of urine flow decreases. The magnitude of this antidiuretic effect varies in direct proportion to the plasma AVP concentration. It is mediated via binding of AVP to G protein–coupled V_2 receptors on the serosal surface of the cell, activation of adenyl cyclase, and insertion into the luminal surface of water channels composed of a protein known as *aquaporin 2* (Fig. 329-2). The genes encoding the V_2 receptors and aquaporin 2 have been cloned and appear to be expressed exclusively in the distal and collecting tubules of the kidney. Nonpeptide, as well as peptide, AVP analogues with potent agonist or antagonist actions at human V_2 receptors have been developed for treating disorders of water metabolism caused by deficient or excessive production of AVP (see below).

At high concentrations, AVP also has several other actions, including contraction of smooth muscle in blood vessels in the skin and gastrointestinal tract, glycogenolysis in the liver, and potentiation of adrenocorticotropic hormone (ACTH) release by corticotropin-releasing factor (CRF). These effects are mediated by V_{1a} or V_{1b} receptors that are coupled to phospholipase C. The genes that encode these receptors have also been cloned and sequenced and are expressed in

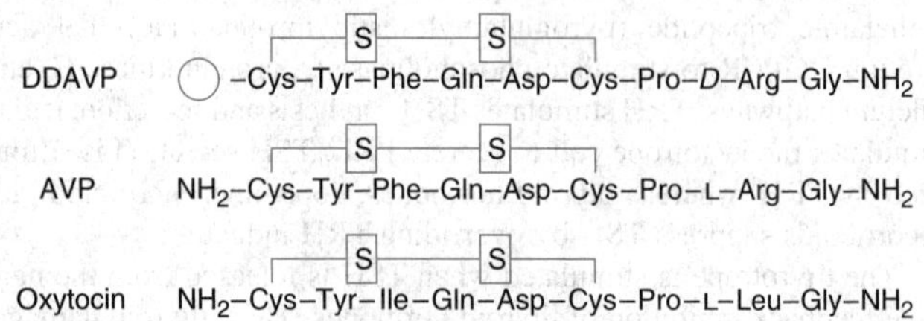

FIGURE 329-1 Primary structures of arginine vasopressin (AVP), oxytocin, and desamino-D-arginine-8 vasopressin (DDAVP).

many organs, including blood vessels, the anterior and posterior pituitary, and certain other areas of brain. Their role, if any, in human physiology/pathophysiology is still uncertain.

SYNTHESIS AVP is synthesized via a polypeptide precursor that includes a binding protein known as *neurophysin II* and a glycosylated peptide called *copeptin*. The gene encoding the AVP precursor is located on chromosome 20 and has three exons. It is expressed in distinct subpopulations of magno- and parvocellular neurons in the supraoptic and paraventricular nuclei. Like other peptide hormones destined for secretion, newly synthesized AVP–neurophysin II precursor is translocated from the cytosol to the endoplasmic reticulum, where the signal peptide is removed and the prohormone folds and oligomerizes before moving through the Golgi apparatus to the neurosecretory vesicles; there it is transported down the axons and further cleaved to AVP, neurophysin II, and copeptin. Stimulation of the neurons results in an influx of calcium, fusion of the neurosecretory vesicle with the cell membrane, and extrusion of its contents into the systemic circulation.

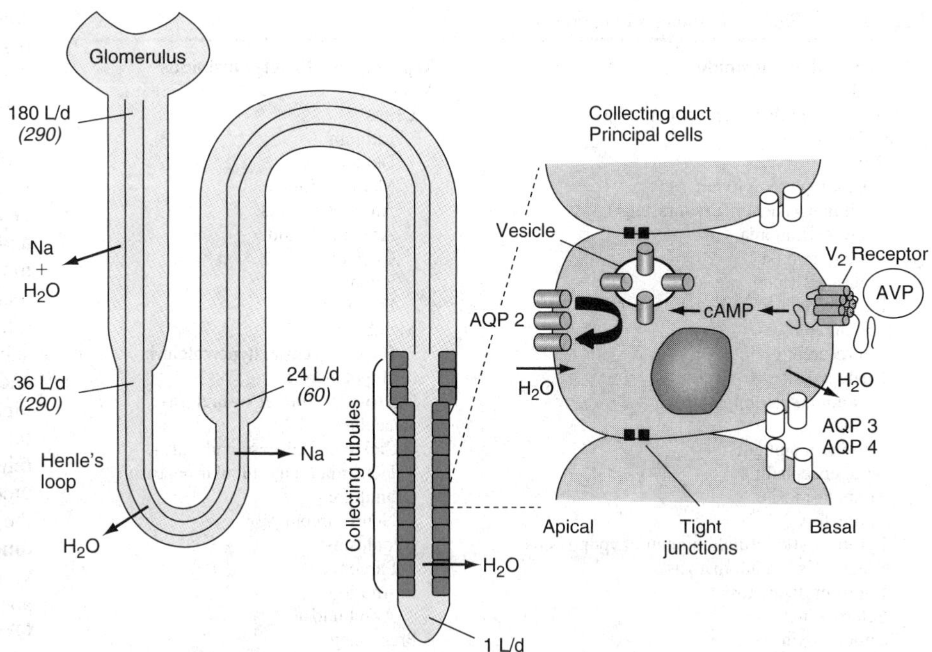

FIGURE 329-2 Antidiuretic effect of AVP in the regulation of urine volume. In a typical 70-kg adult, the kidney filters about 180 L /d of plasma. Of this, approximately 144 L (80%) is reabsorbed isosmotically in the proximal tubule and another 8 L (4 to 5%) is reabsorbed without solute in the descending limb of Henle's loop. The remainder is diluted to an osmolality of about 60 mmol/kg by selective reabsorption of sodium and chloride in the ascending limb. In the absence of AVP, the urine issuing from the loop passes largely unmodified through the distal tubules and collecting ducts, resulting in a maximum water diuresis. In the presence of AVP, solute-free water is reabsorbed osmotically through the principal cells of the collecting ducts, resulting in the excretion of a much smaller volume of concentrated urine. This antidiuretic effect is mediated via a G protein–coupled V_2 receptor that increases intracellular cyclic AMP, thereby inducing translocation of aquaporin 2 (AQP2) water channels into the apical membrane. The resultant increase in permeability permits an influx of water that diffuses out of the cell through AQP3 and AQP4 water channels on the basal-lateral surface. The net rate of flux across the cell is determined by the number of AQP2 water channels in the apical membrane and the strength of the osmotic gradient between tubular fluid and the renal medulla. Tight junctions on the lateral surface of the cells serve to prevent unregulated water flow.

SECRETION The secretion of AVP is regulated primarily by the "effective" osmotic pressure of body fluids. This control is mediated by specialized cells, known as *osmoreceptors*, which appear to be located in the anteromedial hypothalamus near the supraoptic nucleus. These osmoreceptors are extremely sensitive to small changes in the plasma concentration of sodium and certain other effective solutes such as mannitol but show little or no response to other solutes such as urea or glucose. They appear to have inhibitory as well as stimulatory components that function in concert to regulate AVP secretion around a specific set point. Thus, when plasma osmolality/sodium are depressed to a certain minimum or threshold level of ~280 mosmol/kg or 135 meq/L, respectively, plasma AVP is suppressed to low or undetectable levels and a water diuresis ensues. Conversely, when plasma osmolality/sodium rise above this "threshold," plasma AVP rises steeply in direct proportion, reaching a concentration sufficient to produce a maximum antidiuresis when plasma osmolality/sodium reach ~295 mosmol/kg and 143 meq/L. However, the exact "set" and "sensitivity" of this osmoregulatory system vary appreciably from person to person, apparently as a result of genetic influences, and change during pregnancy, the menstrual cycle, and normal aging; they can also be altered or disrupted by various pathologic conditions.

AVP secretion can also be influenced by acute changes in blood volume or pressure. This baroregulation is mediated largely by neuronal afferents that originate in transmural pressure receptors of the cardiac atria, aorta, and carotid arteries; project via the vagus and glossopharyngeal nerves to the nucleus tractus solitarius of the brain stem; and then ascend to the paraventricular and supraoptic nucleii of the hypothalmus. These pathways regulate AVP release by maintaining a tonic inhibitory tone that decreases when blood volume or pressure falls by >10 to 20%. This baroregulatory system is probably of minor importance in the physiology of AVP secretion because the hemodynamic changes required to affect it are larger than those usually occurring in the course of normal activities. Moreover, moderate hemodynamic stimuli do not disrupt or override the osmoregulatory system but do lower its threshold or set point by an amount proportional to the magnitude of the hypovolemia or hypotension. However, the baroregulatory system undoubtedly plays an important role in AVP secretion in patients with large, acute disturbances of hemodynamic function.

AVP secretion can also be stimulated by a variety of other nonosmotic variables including nausea, acute hypoglycemia, glucocorticoid deficiency, smoking, and, possibly, hyperangiotensinemia. The emetic stimuli are extremely potent since they typically elicit immediate, 50- to 100-fold increases in plasma AVP, even when the nausea is transient and unassociated with vomiting or other symptoms. They appear to act via the emetic center in the medulla and can be completely blocked by treatment with antiemetics such as fluphenazine. There is no evidence that pain or other noxious stresses have any affect on AVP unless they elicit a vasovagal reaction with its associated nausea and hypotension.

METABOLISM From the venous circulation, AVP distributes rapidly into a space roughly equal in size to the extracellular fluid volume. It is cleared irreversibly from this space with a $t_{1/2}$ of 10 to 30 min. Most AVP clearance is due to degradation in the liver and kidneys. Urinary clearance of the hormone is normally much less than creatinine clearance but can vary as much as tenfold, depending on individual differences and changes in total solute clearance. Therefore, measurement of urinary AVP excretion rates are not always a reliable indicator of changes in secretion or plasma levels of the hormone. During pregnancy, the metabolic clearance of AVP is increased three- to fourfold due to placental production of an N-terminal peptidase.

Table 329-1 Causes of Diabetes Insipidus

Pituitary diabetes insipidus

- Acquired
  - Head trauma (closed and penetrating)
  - Neoplasms
    - Primary
      - Craniopharyngioma
      - Pituitary adenoma (suprasellar)
      - Dysgerminoma
      - Meningioma
    - Metastatic (lung, breast)
    - Hematologic (lymphoma, leukemia)
  - Granulomas
    - Neurosarcoid
    - Histiocytosis
    - Xanthoma disseminatum
  - Infectious
    - Chronic meningitis
    - Viral encephalitis
    - Toxoplasmosis
  - Inflammatory
    - Lymphocytic infundibuloneurohypophysitis
    - Wegener's granulomatosis
    - Lupus erythematosus
    - Scleroderma
  - Chemical toxins
    - Tetrodotoxin
    - Snake venom
  - Vascular
    - Sheehan's syndrome
    - Aneurysm (internal carotid)
    - Aortocoronary bypass
    - Hypoxic encephalopathy
  - Pregnancy (vasopressinase)
  - Idiopathic
- Congenital malformations
  - Septooptic dysplasia
  - Midline craniofacial defects
  - Holoprosencephaly
  - Hypogensis, ectopia of pituitary
- Genetic
  - Autosomal dominant (AVP-neurophysin gene)
  - Autosomal recessive (AVP-neurophysin gene)
  - Autosomal recessive-Wolfram-(4p − WFS 1 gene)
  - X-linked recessive (Xq28)
  - Deletion chromosome 7q

Nephrogenic diabetes insipidus

- Acquired
  - Drugs
    - Lithium
    - Demeclocycline
    - Methoxyflurane
    - Amphotericin B
    - Aminoglycosides
    - Cisplatin
    - Rifampin
    - Foscarnet
  - Metabolic
    - Hypercalcemia, hypercalciuria
    - Hypokalemia
  - Obstruction (ureter or urethra)
  - Vascular
    - Sickle cell disease and trait
    - Ischemia (acute tubular necrosis)
  - Granulomas
    - Neurosarcoid
  - Neoplasms
    - Sarcoma
  - Infiltration
    - Amyloidosis
  - Pregnancy
  - Idiopathic
- Genetic
  - X-linked recessive (AVP receptor-2 gene)
  - Autosomal recessive (aquaporin-2 gene)
  - Autosomal dominant (aquaporin-2 gene)

Primary polydipsia

- Acquired
  - Psychogenic
    - Schizophrenia
    - Obsessive-compulsive disorder
  - Dipsogenic (abnormal thirst)
    - Granulomas
      - Neurosarcoid
    - Infectious
      - Tuberculous meningitis
    - Head trauma (closed and penetrating)
    - Demyelination
      - Multiple sclerosis
    - Drugs
      - Lithium
      - Carbamazepine
    - Idiopathic
  - Iatrogenic

THIRST Though AVP regulates the effective osmotic pressure of body fluids by varying the rate of urinary free-water excretion, it cannot reduce insensible or urinary water output below a certain minimum obligatory level. Thus, an additional mechanism—thirst—is essential to prevent hypertonic dehydration. Like AVP, thirst is regulated primarily by an osmostat that is located in the anteromedial hypothalamus and is able to detect very small changes in the plasma concentration of sodium and certain other effective solutes. It functions like the AVP osmostat except that it appears to be "set" slightly higher. This arrangement ensures that thirst, polydipsia, and dilution of body fluids do not occur until dehydration and the resultant rise in plasma osmolality start to exceed the defensive capacity of the antidiuretic mechanism.

OXYTOCIN

Oxytocin is also a nonapeptide and differs from AVP only at positions 3 and 8 (Fig. 329-1). However, it has relatively little antidiuretic effect and seems to act mainly on mammary ducts to facilitate milk letdown during nursing (Chap. 337). It may also help to initiate or facilitate labor by stimulating contraction of uterine smooth muscle, but it is not yet clear if this action is physiologic or necessary for normal delivery. Both the mammary and uterine effects are mediated by a G protein–coupled receptor that is linked to phospholipase C. Antagonists for this receptor have been developed and tested in humans for possible use in treating premature labor.

Oxytocin is also synthesized via a macromolecular precursor that is encoded by a gene located on chromosome 20, very near the AVP gene. However, it differs in orientation and size and encodes only a signal peptide, the hormone, and its associated neurophysin. Oxytocin is also expressed in different magnocellular neurons than AVP and, in humans, is not subject to any of the same regulatory influences. Indeed, with the possible exception of nipple stimulation in the postpartum period, no other stimuli are known to consistently induce release of the hormone in humans. Plasma oxytocin is not increased during pregnancy or at the initiation of labor, although the latter condition may be facilitated by upregulation of oxytocin receptors. The distribution and clearance of oxytocin are similar to those of AVP. Oxytocin is also degraded by the liver and kidneys and an N-terminal peptidase produced by the placenta.

DEFICIENCIES OF VASOPRESSIN SECRETION AND ACTION

DIABETES INSIPIDUS Clinical Characteristics Decreased secretion or action of AVP usually manifests as DI, a syndrome characterized by the production of abnormally large volumes of dilute urine. The 24-h urine volume is >50 mL/kg body weight and the osmolality is <300 mmol/kg. The polyuria produces symptoms of urinary frequency, enuresis, and/or nocturia, which may disturb sleep and cause mild daytime fatigue or somnolence. It is also associated with thirst and a commensurate increase in fluid intake (polydipsia). Clinical signs of dehydration are uncommon unless fluid intake is impaired.

Etiology Deficient secretion of AVP can be primary or secondary. The primary form usually results from agenesis or irreversible destruction of the neurohypophysis and is variously referred to as *neurohypophyseal DI, neurogenic DI, pituitary DI, cranial DI*, or *central DI*. It can be caused by a variety of congenital, acquired, or genetic disorders but almost half the time it is idiopathic (Table 329-1). The genetic form of neurohypophyseal DI is usually transmitted in an autosomal dominant mode and is caused by diverse mutations in the coding region of the AVP–neurophysin II gene. The mutant precursor cannot be processed properly or efficiently and eventually destroys the neuron, thereby accounting for the dominant mode of transmission and the delayed onset of the disorder. An X-linked recessive form also occurs. A primary deficiency of plasma AVP can also result from increased metabolism by an N-terminal aminopeptidase produced by the placenta. It is referred to as *gestational DI* since the signs and symptoms manifest during pregnancy and usually remit several weeks after delivery. However, a subclinical deficiency in AVP secretion can often be demonstrated in the nonpregnant state in these individuals, indicating that damage to the neurohypophysis may also contribute to the AVP deficiency. Finally, a primary deficiency of AVP can also result from malformation or destruction of the neurohypophysis by a variety of diseases or toxins (Table 329-1).

Secondary deficiencies of AVP result from inhibition of secretion by excessive intake of fluids. They are referred to as *primary polydip-*

sia and can be divided into three subcategories. One of them, called *dipsogenic DI*, seems to be caused by an inappropriate increase in thirst caused by a reduction in the "set" of the osmoregulatory mechanism. It sometimes occurs in association with multifocal diseases of the brain such as neurosarcoid, tuberculous meningitis, or multiple sclerosis but is often idiopathic. The second subtype, called *psychogenic polydipsia*, is not associated with thirst, and the polydipsia seems to be a feature of psychosis. The third subtype, which may be referred to as *iatrogenic polydipsia*, results from recommendations of health professionals or the popular media to increase fluid intake for its presumed preventive or therapeutic benefits for other disorders.

Primary deficiencies in the antidiuretic action of AVP result in *nephrogenic DI* (Table 329-1). It can be genetic, acquired, or caused by exposure to various drugs. The genetic form is usually transmitted in an X-linked mode and is caused by mutations in the coding region of the V_2 receptor gene. An autosomal recessive form is caused by mutations in the gene encoding the aquaporin protein that forms the water channels in the distal nephron.

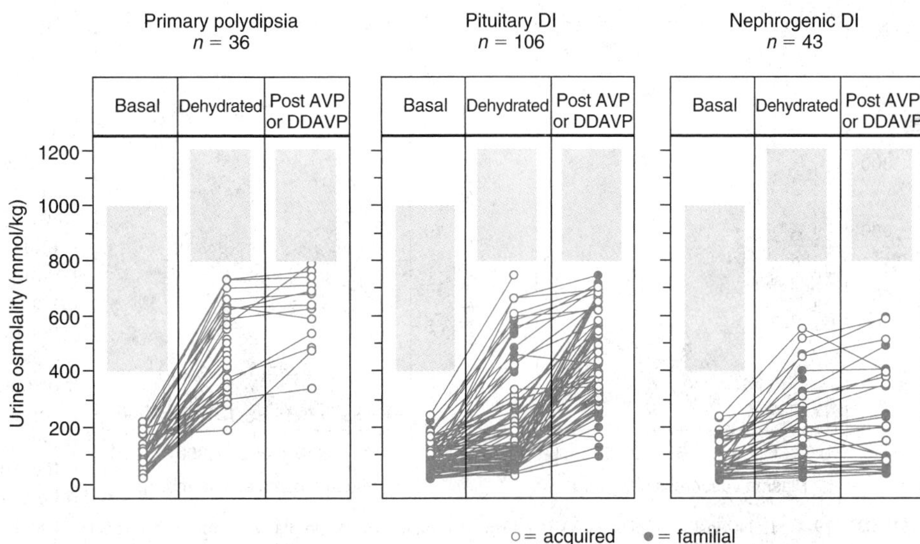

FIGURE 329-3 Urine osmolality under basal conditions of *ad libitum*/fluid intake, during fluid deprivation, and after the administration of AVP or DDAVP in patients with primary polydipsia (*left*), pituitary DI (*middle*), or nephrogenic DI (*right*). Normal ranges are depicted by shaded regions. DI, diabetes insipidus.

Secondary deficiencies in the antidiuretic response to AVP result from polyuria per se. They appear to be caused by washout of the medullary concentration gradient and/or suppression of aquaporin function. They usually resolve 24 to 48 h after the polyuria is corrected but often complicate interpretation of certain acute tests commonly used for differential diagnosis.

Pathophysiology When the net secretion or antidiuretic effect of AVP is decreased by >80 to 85%, the amount of hormone produced under basal conditions is insufficient to concentrate the urine and the rate of output increases exponentially to symptomatic levels. If the AVP defect is primary (e.g., the patient has pituitary, gestational, or nephrogenic DI), the polyuria results in a small (1 to 2%) decrease in body water and a commensurate increase in plasma osmolality and sodium concentration that stimulate thirst and a compensatory increase in water intake. As a result, *overt physical or laboratory signs of dehydration do not develop unless the patient also has a defect in thirst* (see below) *or fails to drink for some other reason.*

The severity of the defect in antidiuretic function varies markedly among patients with pituitary, gestational, or nephrogenic DI. In some, the deficiencies in AVP secretion or action are so severe that basal urine output approximates the maximum (10 to 15 mL/min); even an intense stimulus such as nausea or severe dehydration does not increase plasma AVP enough to concentrate the urine. In others, however, the deficiency in AVP secretion or action is less pronounced, and a modest stimulus such as a few hours of fluid deprivation, smoking, or a vasovagal reaction increases plasma AVP sufficiently to produce a profound antidiuresis. The maximum urine osmolality achieved in these patients is usually less than normal, largely because their maximal concentrating capacity is temporarily impaired by chronic polyuria per se. However, in a few patients with partial pituitary or nephrogenic DI, it can reach levels as high as 800 mosmol/kg (Fig. 329-3).

In primary polydipsia, the pathogenesis of the polydipsia and polyuria is the reverse of that in neurohypophyseal, nephrogenic, and gestational DI. Thus, the excessive intake of fluids slightly increases body water, thereby reducing plasma osmolality, AVP secretion, and urinary concentration. The latter results in a compensatory increase in urinary free-water excretion that varies in direct proportion to intake. Therefore, clinically appreciable overhydration is uncommon unless the compensatory water diuresis is impaired by a drug or disease that stimulates or mimics endogenous AVP.

In the dipsogenic form of primary polydipsia, fluid intake is excessive because the osmotic threshold for thirst appears to be reset to the left, often well below that for AVP release. As a result, thirst is abnormally increased and cannot be completely relieved because plasma AVP is suppressed and an offsetting water diuresis develops before plasma osmolality is reduced sufficiently to eliminate the dipsogenic stimulus. Typically, therefore, patients with dipsogenic DI present with complaints of chronic thirst, polydipsia, and polyuria indistinguishable from those in patients with pituitary, gestational, or nephrogenic DI. When deprived of fluids or subjected to some other acute osmotic or nonosmotic stimulus, they invariably increase plasma AVP normally, but the resultant increase in urine concentration is usually subnormal because their renal capacity to concentrate the urine is also blunted by chronic polyuria. Thus, their antidiuretic response to these stimuli may be indistinguishable from that in patients with partial pituitary, partial gestational, or partial nephrogenic DI (Fig. 329-3).

Differential Diagnosis When symptoms of urinary frequency, enuresis, nocturia, and/or persistent thirst are present, causes other than polyuria should be excluded. A 24-h urine output > 50 mL/kg per day (>3500 mL in a 70-kg man) is suspicious for DI. If the osmolality of the 24-h urine is >300 mosmol/kg, the patient has a solute diuresis and should be evaluated for uncontrolled diabetes mellitus or other less common causes of excessive solute excretion. However, if the 24-h urine osmolality is <300 mosmol/kg, the patient has a water diuresis and should be evaluated further to determine which type of DI is present.

In differentiating between the various types of DI, the history, physical examination, and routine laboratory tests may be helpful but are rarely sufficient because few, if any, of the findings are pathognomonic. Except in the rare patient who is clearly dehydrated under basal conditions of *ad libitum* fluid intake, this evaluation should begin with a *fluid deprivation test.* To minimize patient discomfort, avoid excessive dehydration, and maximize the information obtained, the test should be started in the morning and water balance should be monitored closely with hourly measurements of body weight, plasma osmolality and/or sodium concentration, and urine volume and osmolality.

If fluid deprivation does not result in urine concentration (osmolality >300 mosmol/kg, specific gravity >1.010) before body weight decreases by 5% or plasma osmolality/sodium exceed the upper limit of normal, primary polydipsia and a partial defect in AVP secretion or action are largely excluded (Fig. 329-3). In these patients, severe pituitary or nephrogenic DI can usually be distinguished by administering desmopressin (DDAVP, 0.03 μg/kg subcutaneously or intravenously) and repeating the measurement of urine osmolality 1 to 2 h

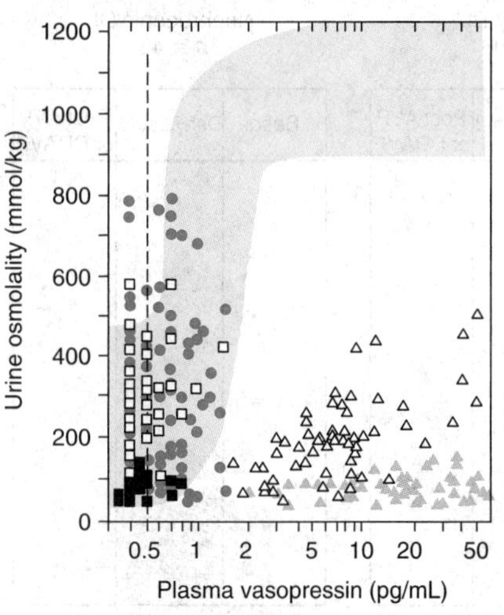

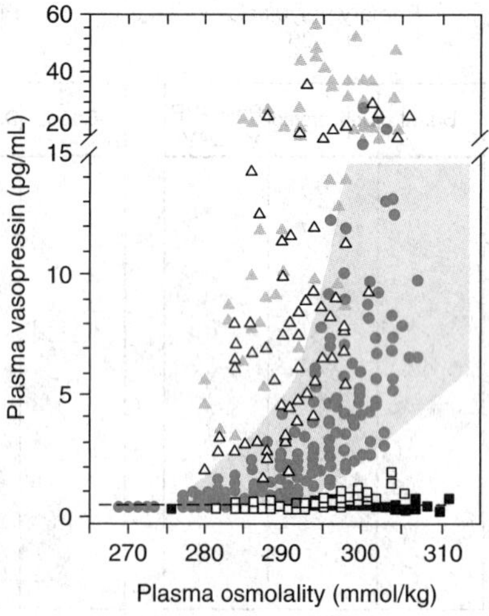

FIGURE 329-4 Relationship of plasma AVP to urine osmolality (*left*) and plasma osmolality (*right*) before and during fluid deprivation-hypertonic saline infusion test in patients with primary polydipsia (●), partial (□) or severe (■) pituitary diabetes insipidus (DI), or partial (△) or severe (▲) nephrogenic DI.

later. An increase of >50% indicates severe pituitary DI, whereas a smaller or absent response is strongly suggestive of nephrogenic DI.

However, these indirect criteria are not useful for diagnosis in patients who concentrate their urine during fluid deprivation, because the changes in urine osmolality are remarkably similar in primary polydipsia and partial pituitary and partial nephrogenic DI (Fig. 329-3). In this situation, the safest and most reliable way to differentiate these conditions is to measure plasma or urine AVP collected before and during the fluid deprivation test and analyze the result in relation to the concurrent plasma or urine osmolality (Fig. 329-4). This approach invariably differentiates partial nephrogenic DI from partial pituitary DI and primary polydipsia. It also differentiates pituitary DI from primary polydipsia if the hormone is measured when plasma osmolality or sodium is clearly above the normal range. However, the requisite level of hypertonic dehydration is difficult to produce by fluid deprivation alone when urine concentration occurs. Therefore, it is usually necessary to add an infusion of hypertonic (3%) saline and repeat the AVP measurements when plasma osmolality rises to >300 mmol/kg (Na^+ > 145 mmol/L). This endpoint is usually reached within 30 to 120 min if the hypertonic saline is infused at a rate of 0.1 mL/kg per minute and the fluid deprivation is maintained.

The differential diagnosis of DI may also be facilitated by magnetic resonance imaging (MRI) of the pituitary and hypothalamus. In most healthy adults and children, the posterior pituitary emits a hyperintense signal in T1 weighted mid-saggital images. This "bright spot" is almost invariably absent or abnormally small in patients with pituitary DI but is present in 80 to 90% of those with primary polydipsia. Thus, the presence of a normal bright spot virtually excludes pituitary DI, whereas its absence supports but does not prove this diagnosis. Therefore, the MRI findings must be interpreted with caution and only in conjunction with other diagnostic studies based on assays of AVP or the differential responses to treatment.

℞ **TREATMENT** The signs and symptoms of uncomplicated pituitary DI can be eliminated completely by treatment with DDAVP (Fig. 329-5). It is a synthetic analogue of AVP (Fig. 329-1) that acts selectively at V_2 receptors to increase urine concentration and decrease urine flow in a dose-dependent manner. However, it is more resistant to degradation than AVP and has a three- to fourfold longer duration of action. This property makes it particularly useful in the treatment of gestational DI or pituitary DI during pregnancy. DDAVP can be given by intravenous or subcutaneous injection, nasal inhalation, or oral tablet. The doses required to control pituitary DI completely vary widely, depending on the patient and the route of administration. However, they usually range from 1 to 2 μg qd or bid by injection, 10 to 20 μg bid or tid by nasal spray, and 100 to 400 μg bid or tid orally. The onset of action is rapid, ranging from as little as 15 min after injection to 60 min after oral administration. When given in doses sufficient to completely normalize urinary osmolality and flow, DDAVP produces a slight (1 to 3%) increase in total-body water and a commensurate decrease in plasma osmolality and sodium concentration that rapidly eliminates thirst and polydipsia. Consequently, water balance is maintained and hyponatremia does not develop unless the patient has an associated abnormality in the osmoregulation of thirst or ingests/receives excessive amounts of fluid for some other reason. Fortunately, abnormal thirst occurs in <10% of patients with pituitary DI, and the other causes of excessive intake can usually be eliminated by educating the patient about the risks of drinking for reasons other than thirst. Therefore, most patients with pituitary DI can take desmopressin in doses sufficient to maintain a normal urine output continuously and do not need to endure the inconvenience and discomfort of allowing intermittent escape to prevent water intoxication.

Pituitary DI can also be treated with chlorpropamide (Diabinese). The mechanism of its antidiuretic action is uncertain but may involve potentiation of the effect of small amounts of AVP or direct activation of the V_2 receptor. In patients with severe as well as partial pituitary DI, doses of chlorpropamide similar to those used in the treatment of diabetes mellitus (125 to 500 mg once daily) increase urine concentration and decrease urine flow, thirst, and polydipsia in a manner similar to DDAVP. The antidiuresis is usually less rapid and smaller than that produced by DDAVP but is almost always sufficient to re-

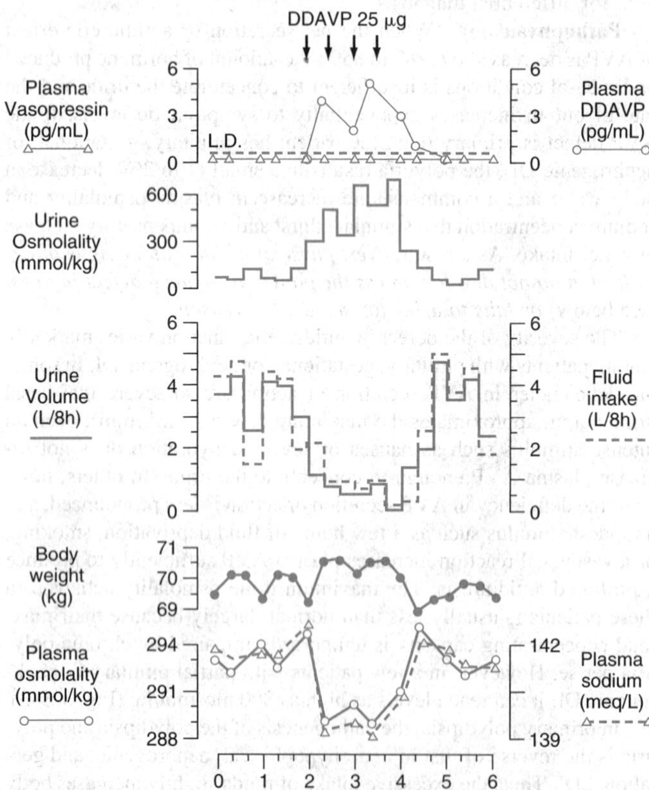

FIGURE 329-5 Effect of DDAVP therapy on water balance in patient with uncomplicated pituitary diabetes insipidus. Note that treatment rapidly reduces thirst and fluid intake as well as urine output to normal, with only a slight increase in body water (weight) and decrease in plasma osmolality/sodium. [*From Endocrinology and Metabolism, 4th e, P Felig, L Frohman (eds). New York, McGraw-Hill, 2001, with permission.*]

duce urine output by 30 to 70%. Moreover, its antidiuretic effect can be enhanced appreciably by cotreatment with a thiazide diuretic. The ability of water loading to reduce the antidiuretic effect of chlorpropamide makes it particularly useful in the treatment of patients who have pituitary DI and abnormal thirst since it is less likely than DDAVP to produce water intoxication. However, unlike DDAVP, chlorpropamide can have other side effects including hypoglycemia, which can be precipitated by severe reductions in caloric intake or heavy exercise, and it exhibits a disulfuram (Antabuse)-like reaction to ethanol. Chlorpropamide is contraindicated in the treatment of gestational DI because its teratogenicity is unknown.

Primary polydipsia cannot be treated with DDAVP in the usual way because a sustained inhibition of the compensatory water diuresis almost invariably results in the development of water intoxication within 24 to 48 h. This complication can also be caused by administration of a thiazide diuretic, smoking, or other nonosmotic stimuli to endogenous AVP secretion. Iatrogenic polydipsia can often be corrected by patient counseling; however, there is no effective treatment for either psychogenic or dipsogenic DI. In the latter, nocturia or nocturnal enuresis can often be controlled safely by administering a single small dose of DDAVP at bedtime. If the dose is adjusted carefully to provide no more than 8 to 10 h of antidiuresis, it will not result in water intoxication, because patients with dipsogenic, as well as other forms of DI, tend to drink less fluid at night than during the day. Family or other caregivers of patients with psychogenic or dipsogenic DI should also be warned about the hazards of water intoxication caused by a variety of diseases or drugs that can stimulate or mimic the antidiuretic effects of endogenous AVP (see below).

The symptoms and signs of nephrogenic DI are not affected by treatment with DDAVP or chlorpropamide but may be reduced by treatment with a thiazide diuretic and/or amiloride in conjunction with a low-sodium diet. Inhibitors of prostaglandin synthesis (e.g., indomethacin) are also effective in many patients.

ADIPSIC HYPERNATREMIA

Clinical Characteristics Adipsic hypernatremia is characterized by chronic or recurrent hypertonic dehydration and a deficient AVP response to osmotic stimulation. Despite their dehydration, the patients have little or no thirst and may even resist efforts to increase their oral intake of fluids. The hypernatremia varies in severity and is associated with commensurate signs of hypovolemia such as tachycardia, postural hypotension, azotemia, hyperuricemia, and hypokalemia. Muscle weakness, pain, rhabdomyolysis, hyperglycemia, hyperlipidemia, and acute renal failure may also occur. Most patients remain conscious unless they have severe hyperglycemia and/or hypertonicity or go on to develop hyponatremia as a result of excessive rehydration.

Etiology Adipsic hypernatremia is caused by agenesis or destruction of the hypothalamic osmoreceptors that normally regulate thirst and AVP secretion. The osmoreceptor deficiency can usually be traced to an identifiable congenital or acquired disease in the hypothalamus but is sometimes idiopathic (Table 329-2). The neurohypophysis and its other regulatory afferents are usually spared; an MRI typically shows a normal posterior pituitary bright spot, and the AVP response to nonosmotic stimuli is also normal. Occasionally, the neurohypophysis is also affected, resulting in a combined defect in water balance that is particularly severe and difficult to manage.

Pathophysiology Lack of thirst and failure to drink enough water to replenish renal and extrarenal losses decrease total-body water and increase plasma osmolality/sodium. Plasma renin activity and aldosterone secretion also increase, and plasma potassium falls due to increased urinary excretion. The severity, frequency, and speed with which hypertonic dehydration develops vary markedly from patient to patient, or from time to time in the same patient, owing largely to differences in the rate of insensible and/or renal loss.

The osmoregulation of AVP secretion is also impaired in nearly all patients with adipsic hypernatremia (Fig. 329-6). This deficiency is obvious when the hormone is measured in the presence of hypertonic dehydration but is rarely severe enough to produce DI. During rehy-

Table 329-2 Causes of Adipsic Hypernatremia

Acquired
Vascular: Occlusion anterior communicating artery
Tumors
Primary
Craniopharyngioma
Pinealoma, germinoma
Meningioma
Glioma
Metastatic (lung, breast)
Granulomas: Neurosarcoid
Histocytosis
Trauma: Closed
Penetrating (pituitary-hypothalamic surgery)
Psychogenic: Psychotic depression
Other: Hydrocephalus
Neurodegenerative
AIDS, cytomegalovirus encephalitis
Idiopathic
Congenital
Midline malformation (septum and corpus callosum)
Microcephaly
Genetic: Autosomal recessive (Schinzel-Giedion syndrome)

dration, however, some patients exhibit a further decrease in their plasma AVP and develop DI before their hypernatremia is fully corrected. In other patients, the osmoregulatory deficiency appears to be complete because basal plasma AVP remains relatively fixed, irrespective of whether plasma osmolality and sodium are above, within, or below the normal range. Thus, if overhydrated, these patients do not mount a compensatory water diuresis and quickly develop a hyponatremic syndrome that is clinically and biochemically indistinguishable from acute syndrome of inappropriate antidiuretic hormone, which is commonly referred to as SIADH (see below). In all but a few patients, the abnormality of AVP secretion is limited to the osmoregulatory system since the hormone responds normally to all nonosmotic stimuli, such as nausea.

Differential Diagnosis Adipsic hypernatremia should be distinguished from the hypernatremia that results from various other causes. These distinctions can usually be made from the history, physical examination, and routine laboratory tests. If a conscious patient denies thirst and/or does not drink vigorously in the presence of significant hypernatremia, the diagnosis of hypodipsia or adipsia can be made with confidence. This diagnosis is supported by laboratory evidence of hypovolemia (azotemia, hypokalemia, hyperuricemia, hyperreninemia) and a relative deficiency of plasma AVP. Close monitoring of these variables and urine osmolality during rehydration is useful for differentiating the patients who develop DI or SIADH in response to forced hydration. If the patient is obtunded or otherwise unable to answer questions or drink at the time of presentation, the possibility of adipsic hypernatremia can be evaluated after treatment by assessing the thirst and plasma AVP response to a controlled fluid deprivation–hypertonic saline infusion test similar to that described for evaluation of DI.

℞ **TREATMENT** Adipsic hypernatremia should be treated by administering water by mouth, if the patient is alert, or 0.45% saline by vein, if the patient is obtunded or uncooperative. The number of liters of free water that will be required to correct the deficit (ΔFW) can be estimated from body weight in kg (BW) and the serum sodium concentration in mmol/L (S_{Na}) by the formula $\Delta FW = 0.5BW \times [(S_{Na} - 140)/140]$. If serum glucose ($S_{Glu}$) is elevated, the measured S_{Na} should be corrected (S_{Na}*) by the formula $S_{Na}^* = S_{Na} + [(S_{Glu} - 90)/36]$. This amount plus an allowance for continuing insensible and urinary losses should be given over a 24- to 48-h period. If DI is present or develops during rehydration, DDAVP should also be given in standard doses to minimize urinary losses. If hyperglycemia and/or hypokalemia are present, insulin and/or potassium supplements should

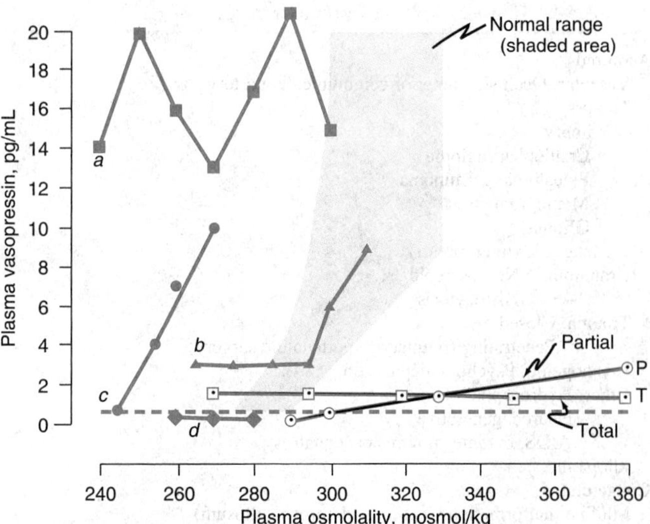

FIGURE 329-6 Heterogeneity of osmoregulatory dysfunction in adipsic hypernatremia (AH) and the syndrome of inappropriate antidiuretic hormone (SIADH). Each line depicts schematically the relationship of plasma AVP to plasma osmolality during water loading and/or infusion of 3% saline in a different patient with either AH (open symbols) or SIADH (closed symbols). The shaded area indicates the normal range of the relationship. The horizontal broken line indicates the plasma AVP level below which the hormone is undetectable and urinary concentration usually does not occur. Lines P and T represent patients with a selective deficiency in the osmoregulation of thirst and AVP that is either partial (○) or total (□). In the latter, plasma AVP does not change in response to increases or decreases in plasma osmolality but remains within a range sufficient to concentrate the urine even if overhydration produces hypotonic hyponatremia. In contrast, if the osmoregulatory deficiency is partial (○), rehydration of the patient suppresses plasma AVP to levels that result in urinary dilution and polyuria before plasma osmolality and sodium are reduced to normal. Lines *a–d* represent different defects in the osmoregulation of plasma AVP observed in patients with SIADH. In *a* (■), plasma AVP is markedly elevated and fluctuates widely without relation to changes in plasma osmolality, indicating complete loss of osmoregulation. In *b* (▲), plasma AVP remains fixed at a slightly elevated level until plasma osmolality reaches the normal range at which point it begins to rise appropriately, indicating a selective defect in the inhibitory component of the osmoregulatory mechanism. In *c* (●), plasma AVP rises in close correlation with plasma osmolality before the latter reaches the normal range, indicating downward resetting of the osmostat. In *d* (♦), plasma AVP appears to be osmoregulated normally, suggesting that the inappropriate antidiuresis is caused by some other abnormality.

be given. These variables plus urine output and plasma urea/creatinine should be monitored closely during treatment for signs of emerging DI, SIADH, or acute renal failure.

Once the acute fluid and electrolyte imbalances are corrected, an MRI of the brain and tests of anterior pituitary function should be performed. A long-term management plan to prevent or minimize recurrence of the fluid and electrolyte imbalance should also be developed, including a practical method that the patient can use to regulate fluid intake in accordance with day-to-day variations in water balance. The most effective way to accomplish these objectives is to prescribe DDAVP or chlorpropamide to completely control DI, if it is present, and teach the patient how to use day-to-day changes in body weight as a guide for adjusting fluid intake. Prescribing a constant fluid intake is less satisfactory because it does not take into account the large, uncontrolled variations in insensible loss that inevitably occur.

EXCESS VASOPRESSIN SECRETION AND ACTION

HYPONATREMIA (See also Chap. 49) **Clinical Characteristics** Excessive secretion or action of AVP results in the production of decreased volumes of more highly concentrated urine. If not accompanied by a commensurate reduction in fluid intake, the reduced suppressibility of AVP results in water retention and a decrease in plasma osmolality/sodium. If the hyponatremia develops gradually or has been present for more than a few days, it may be asymptomatic. However, if it develops acutely, it is almost always accompanied by symptoms and signs of water intoxication that may include mild headache, confusion, anorexia, nausea, vomiting, coma, and convulsions. Severe hyponatremia may be lethal. Depending on the cause of the increased antidiuresis, osmotically inappropriate thirst and/or fluid intake and other disturbances of fluid and electrolyte balance may also be present.

Etiology Osmotically inappropriate antidiuresis can be caused by a primary defect in AVP secretion or action or can be secondary to a recognized nonosmotic stimulus such as hypovolemia, hypotension, or glucocorticoid deficiency (Table 329-3). The primary forms are generally referred to as SIADH or euvolemic (type III) hyponatremia. They have many different causes, including ectopic production of AVP by lung cancer or other neoplasms, eutopic release by various diseases or drugs, and exogenous administration of AVP, DDAVP, or large doses of oxytocin. The ectopic forms result from abnormal and presumably unregulated expression of the AVP-NPII gene by primary or metastatic malignancies. They do not usually remit unless the ectopic source is eliminated. The eutopic forms manifest most often in patients with acute infections or strokes, but the mechanisms by which these diseases disrupt osmoregulation are not known. A form of acute or chronic hyponatremia very similar to SIADH can also result from stimulation of AVP secretion by protracted nausea or isolated glucocorticoid deficiency. In these patients the excess AVP secretion can be corrected quickly and completely by specific treatments (antiemetics or glucocorticoids) that are not useful in other forms of SIADH.

The secondary forms of osmotically inappropriate antidiuresis are usually divided into two groups: type I (hypervolemic) and type II (hypovolemic) hyponatremia. Type I occurs in sodium-retaining, edema-forming states such as congestive heart failure, cirrhosis, or nephrosis and is thought to be due to a reduction in "effective" blood volume. Type II occurs in sodium-depleted states such as severe gas-

Table 329-3 Causes of Syndrome of Inappropriate Antidiuretic Hormone (SIADH)

Neoplasms	Neurologic
Carcinomas	Guillain-Barré syndrome
Lung	Multiple sclerosis
Duodenum	Delerium tremens
Pancreas	Amytrophic lateral sclerosis
Ovary	Hydrocephalus
Bladder, ureter	Psychosis
Other neoplasms	Peripheral neuropathy
Thymoma	Congenital malformations
Mesothelioma	Agenesis corpus callosum
Bronchial adenoma	Cleft lip/palate
Carcinoid	Other midline defects
Gangliocytoma	Metabolic
Ewing's sarcoma	Acute intermittent porphyria
Head trauma (closed and penetrating)	Pulmonary
Infections	Asthma
Pneumonia, bacterial or viral	Pneumothorax
Abscess, lung or brain	Positive-pressure respiration
Cavitation (aspergillosis)	Drugs
Tuberculosis, lung or brain	Vasopressin or DDAVP
Meningitis, bacterial or viral	Chlorpropamide
Encephalitis	Oxytocin, high dose
AIDS	Vincristine
Vascular	Carbamazepine
Cerebrovascular occlusions, hemorrhage	Nicotine
Cavernous sinus thrombosis	Phenothiazines
	Cyclophosphamide
	Tricyclic antidepressants
	Monoamine oxidase inhibitors
	Serotonin reuptake inhibitors

troenteritis, diuretic abuse, or mineralocorticoid deficiency and is probably due to a reduction in blood volume and/or pressure.

Pathophysiology In SIADH, interference with the osmotic suppression of AVP results in significant expansion and dilution of body fluids only if water intake exceeds the rate of insensible and urinary output. These abnormalities in water intake often result from an associated defect in the osmoregulation of thirst but can also be due to psychogenic or iatrogenic factors, including the administration of intravenous fluids.

In SIADH, the defect in the osmoregulation of antidiuretic function can take any of four distinct forms (Fig. 329-6). In one of them, AVP secretion remains fully responsive to changes in plasma osmolality/sodium, but the threshold or set point of the osmoregulatory system is abnormally low. Patients with this kind of downward resetting of the osmostat differ from those with the other types of osmoregulatory defect in that they are able to maximally suppress plasma AVP and dilute their urine if their fluid intake is high enough to reduce their plasma osmolality/sodium to the new set point. Another, smaller subgroup (about 10% of the total) do not have a demonstrable defect in the osmoregulation of AVP (Fig. 329-6). Thus, their inappropriate antidiuresis may be due to other abnormalities such as enhanced renal sensitivity to the antidiuretic effect of normally low levels of AVP or activation of aquaporin 2 water channels by a mechanism that is independent of AVP and V_2 receptors.

The extracellular volume expansion that results from excessive retention of water in SIADH also produces an increase in atrial natriuretic hormone, suppression of plasma renin activity, and a compensatory increase in urinary sodium excretion that serves to reduce the hypervolemia but aggravates the hyponatremia. Thus, hyponatremia is due to a decrease in total-body sodium as well as an increase in total-body water. The acute retention of water and fall in plasma sodium also cause a rise in intracellular volume. The resultant brain swelling increases intracranial pressure and probably causes the acute symptoms of water intoxication. After several days, this intracellular volume expansion may be reduced by inactivation or elimination of intracellular solutes, resulting in the remission of symptoms that often occur with hyponatremia of this duration.

In type I (edematous) or type II (hypovolemic) hyponatremia, the osmotic inhibition of AVP and urine concentration is counteracted by a hemodynamic stimulus that results from a substantial reduction in effective or absolute blood volume. In both cases, the inadequate suppression of AVP appears to be due to downward resetting of the osmostat. The resultant antidiuresis is usually enhanced by decreased distal delivery of filtrate that results from increased reabsorption of sodium in proximal nephrons secondary to the hypovolemia. If it is not associated with a commensurate reduction in water intake, the marked reduction in urine output that ensues also leads to expansion and dilution of body fluids with symptoms of hyponatremia. This attenuates, but does not completely eliminate, the antidiuresis because the amount of water retained is usually insufficient to fully correct the effective or absolute hypovolemia. Unlike SIADH, therefore, plasma renin activity is elevated, causing secondary hyperaldosteronism and hypokalemia. The disturbance in salt and water balance that underlies the hyponatremia also differs from SIADH in that total-body sodium as well as water is increased in type I, whereas both are decreased in type II.

Differential Diagnosis When unexplained symptoms or signs consistent with water intoxication are present, serum sodium should be measured. If it is low and the reduction cannot be accounted for by an increase in plasma glucose or other solutes such as mannitol (e.g., plasma osmolality is also low), the type of hypotonic hyponatremia present can be determined by estimating extracellular fluid volume from the history, physical examination, and routine chemistries. If these findings are ambiguous or contradictory, measuring the rate of urinary sodium excretion or plasma renin activity may be helpful. These measurements can be misleading, however, if SIADH is stable or resolving or if the patient has type II hyponatremia due to a primary defect in renal conservation of sodium, surreptitious diuretic abuse, or hyporeninemic hypoaldosteronism. The latter may be suspected if serum potassium is elevated instead of low as is usually seen in types I and II hyponatremia. Measurements of plasma AVP are currently of no diagnostic value since they exhibit the same wide variation in abnormalities in all three types of hyponatremia. In patients who fulfill the clinical criteria for SIADH, plasma cortisol should also be measured to rule out unsuspected secondary adrenal insufficiency. If this is normal and there is no other obvious cause for SIADH, a careful search for occult lung cancer should also be undertaken.

℞ TREATMENT In acute SIADH, the keystone to treatment of hyponatremia is to restrict total fluid intake to less than the sum of insensible losses and urinary output. Total intake should include the water derived from food (300 to 500 mL/d). Because insensible losses in adults usually approximate 500 mL/d total discretionary intake (all water in liquid form) should be at least 500 mL less than urinary output. If achieved, this deficit usually reduces body water and increases serum sodium by about 1 to 2% per day. If more rapid correction of the hyponatremia is desired to eliminate severe symptoms or signs, the fluid restriction can be supplemented by intravenous infusion of hypertonic (3%) saline. This treatment has the advantage of correcting the sodium deficiency that is partly responsible for the hyponatremia as well as producing a solute diuresis that serves to remove some of the excess water. However, if the hyponatremia has been present for more than 24 to 48 h and is corrected too rapidly, the saline infusion also has the potential to produce central pontine myelinolysis, an acute, potentially fatal neurologic syndrome characterized by quadriparesis, ataxia, and abnormal extraocular movements (Chap. 376). The following guidelines appear to minimize, if not eliminate, the risk of this complication: the 3% saline should be infused a rate $\leq$0.05 mL/kg body weight per minute; the effect should be monitored continuously by STAT measurements of serum sodium at least once every hour; and the infusion should be stopped as soon as serum sodium increases by 12 mmol/L or to 130 mmol/L, whichever comes first. Urinary output should also be monitored continuously since spontaneous remission of the SIADH can result in an acute water diuresis that greatly accelerates the rate of rise in serum sodium produced by fluid restriction and 3% saline infusion.

In chronic SIADH, the hyponatremia can be minimized or eliminated by treatment with demeclocycline, 150 to 300 mg orally three or four times a day, or fludrocortisone, 0.05 to 0.2 mg orally twice a day. The effect of the demeclocycline manifests in 7 to 14 days and is due to production of a reversible form of nephrogenic DI. Potential side effects include phototoxicity and azotemia. The effect of fludrocortisone also manifests in 1 to 2 weeks and is partly due to increased retention of sodium and possibly inhibition of thirst. It also increases urinary potassium excretion, which may require replacement through dietary adjustments or supplements. Fludrocortisone may induce hypertension, occasionally necessitating discontinuation of the treatment.

One or more nonpeptide AVP antagonists that block the antidiuretic effect of AVP may soon be approved for use in the United States. Preliminary studies with these antagonists in acute or chronic SIADH indicate that they produce a dose-dependent increase in urinary free-water excretion, which, if combined with a modest restriction of fluid intake, gradually reduces body water and corrects the hyponatremia without any recognized adverse effect. Thus, they may become the treatment of choice for those forms of SIADH in which there is inappropriate secretion of AVP that cannot be corrected by other, more specific therapy such as antiemetics or glucocorticoids.

When an SIADH-like syndrome is due to protracted nausea and vomiting or isolated glucocorticoid deficiency, all abnormalities can be corrected quickly and completely by giving an antiemetic or hydrocortisone. As with other treatments, care must be taken to ensure that serum sodium does not rise too quickly or too far.

In type I hyponatremia, the only treatment currently available is severe fluid restriction, administration of urea or mannitol to produce a solute diuresis, and/or administration of cardiotonics or serum albumin to correct the effective hypovolemia. None of these treatments is particularly effective, and some (e.g., administration of mannitol or albumin) carry significant risks. Infusion of hypertonic saline is contraindicated because it worsens the sodium retention and edema and may precipitate cardiovascular decompensation. However, preliminary studies indicate that the AVP antagonists may be almost as effective and safe in type I hyponatremia as they are in SIADH. Thus, they may become the treatment of choice for this form of hyponatremia also.

In type II hyponatremia, the defect in AVP secretion and water balance can usually be corrected easily and quickly by stopping the loss of sodium and water and/or replacing the deficits by mouth or intravenous infusion of normal or hypertonic saline. As with the treatment of other forms of hyponatremia, care must be taken to ensure that plasma sodium does not increase too rapidly. Fluid restriction or administration of AVP antagonists is contraindicated as they would only aggravate the underlying volume depletion and could result in cardiovascular decompensation.

BIBLIOGRAPHY

BICHET DG: Vasopressin receptors in health and disease. Kidney Int 49:1706, 1996

———, FUJIWARA TM: Diversity of nephrogenic diabetes insipidus mutations and importance of early recognition and treatment. Clin Exp Nephrol 2:253, 1998

DRINCIC A, ROBERTSON GL: Treatment of diabetes insipidus, in *Hormone Replacement Therapy for Contemporary Endocrinology*, AW Miekle (ed). Totowa, NJ, Humana Press, 1999, pp 21–38

HANSEN LK et al: The genetic basis of familial neurohypophyseal diabetes insipidus. Trends Endocrinol Metab 8:363, 1997

KNEPPER MA: Molecular physiology of urinary concentrating mechanism: Regulation of aquaporin water channels by vasopressin. Am J Physiol 272:F3, 1997

KOVACS L, ROBERTSON GL: Syndrome of inappropriate antidiuresis. Endocrinol Metab Clin North Am 21:859, 1992

OHNISHI A et al: Potent aquaretic agent: A novel nonpeptide selective vasopressin 2 antagonist (OPC-31260) in men. J Clin Invest 92:2653, 1993

ROBERTSON GL: Disorders of thirst in man, in *Thirst: Physiological and Psychological Aspects*, D Ramsey (ed). London, Springer, 1991, pp 453–475

———: The use of vasopressin assays in vasopressin physiology and pathophysiology. Semin Nephrol 14:368, 1994

VERBALIS JG: Hyponatremia: Epidemiology, pathophysiology, and therapy. Curr Opin Nephrol Hypertens 2:636, 1993

330

J. Larry Jameson, Anthony P. Weetman

DISORDERS OF THE THYROID GLAND

AIT amiodarone-induced thyrotoxicosis	RTH resistance to thyroid hormone
ATC anaplastic thyroid cancer	RXRs retinoic acid X receptors
CT computed tomography	SES sick euthyroid syndrome
ESR erythrocyte sedimentation rate	SLE systemic lupus erythematosus
FNA fine-needle aspiration	TBG thyroxine-binding globulin
FTC follicular thyroid cancer	TBII TSH-binding inhibiting immunoglobulins
GPCR G protein–coupled receptor	Tg thyroglobulin
hCG human chorionic gonadotropin	TPO thyroid peroxidase
IFN interferon	TRH thyrotropin-releasing hormone
ILs interleukins	TRs thyroid hormone receptors
IRMAs immunoradiometric assays	TSH thyroid-stimulating hormone
MEN multiple endocrine neoplasia	TSH-R thyroid-stimulating hormone receptor
MNG multinodular goiter	TSI thyroid-stimulating immunoglobulins
MRI magnetic resonance imaging	TTF thyroid transcription factor
MTC medullary thyroid cancer	TTR transthyretin
NIS sodium iodide symporter	
PTC papillary thyroid cancer	

The thyroid gland produces two related hormones, thyroxine (T_4) and triiodothyronine (T_3) (Fig. 330-1). These hormones play a critical role in cell differentiation during development and help to maintain thermogenic and metabolic homeostasis in the adult. Thyroid hormones act through nuclear hormone receptors to modulate gene expression. Disorders of the thyroid gland result primarily from autoimmune processes that either stimulate the overproduction of thyroid hormones (*thyrotoxicosis*) or cause glandular destruction and underproduction of thyroid hormones (*hypothyroidism*). In addition, neoplastic processes in the thyroid gland can lead to benign nodules and various forms of thyroid cancer.

ANATOMY AND DEVELOPMENT

The thyroid gland is located in the neck, anterior to the trachea, between the cricoid cartilage and the suprasternal notch. The thyroid (Greek *thyreos*, shield, plus *eidos*, form) consists of two lobes that are connected by an isthmus. It is normally 12 to 20 g in size, highly vascular, and soft in consistency. Four parathyroid glands, which produce parathyroid hormone (Chap. 341), are located in the posterior region of each pole of the thyroid. The recurrent laryngeal nerves traverse the lateral borders of the thyroid gland and must be identified during thyroid surgery to avoid vocal cord paralysis.

The thyroid gland develops from the floor of the primitive pharynx during the third week of gestation. The gland migrates from the foramen cecum, at the base of the tongue, along the thyroglossal duct to reach its final location in the neck. This feature accounts for the rare ectopic location of thyroid tissue at the base of the tongue (lingual thyroid), as well as for the presence of thyroglossal duct cysts along this developmental tract. Thyroid hormone synthesis normally begins at about 11 weeks' gestation.

The parathyroid glands migrate from the third (inferior glands) and fourth (superior glands) pharyngeal pouches before becoming embedded in the thyroid gland. Neural crest derivatives from the ultimobranchial body give rise to thyroid medullary C cells that produce calcitonin, a calcium-lowering hormone. The C cells are interspersed throughout the thyroid gland, although their density is greatest in the juncture of the upper one-third and lower two-thirds of the gland.

Thyroid gland development is controlled by a series of developmental transcription factors. Thyroid transcription factor (TTF) 1 (also known as NKX2A), TTF-2 (also known as FKHL15), and paired homeobox-8 (PAX-8) are expressed selectively, but not exclusively, in the thyroid gland. In combination, they orchestrate thyroid cell development and the induction of thyroid-specific genes such as thyroglobulin (Tg), thyroid peroxidase (TPO), the sodium iodide symporter (NIS), and the thyroid-stimulating hormone receptor (TSH-R). Mutations in these developmental transcription factors or their downstream target genes are rare causes of thyroid agenesis or dyshormonogenesis and can cause congenital hypothyroidism (Table 330-1). Congenital hypothyroidism is common enough (approximately 1 in 3000 to 4000 newborns) that neonatal screening is now performed in most industrialized countries (see below). Though the underlying causes of most cases of congenital hypothyroidism are unknown, early treatment with thyroid hormone replacement precludes potentially severe developmental abnormalities.

The mature thyroid gland contains numerous follicles composed of thyroid follicular cells that surround secreted colloid, a proteinaceous fluid that contains large amounts of thyroglobulin, the protein precursor of thyroid hormones (Fig. 330-2). The thyroid follicular cells are polarized—the basolateral surface is apposed to the bloodstream and an apical surface faces the follicular lumen. Increased demand for thyroid hormone, usually signaled by thyroid-stimulating hormone (TSH) binding to its receptor on the basolateral surface of the follicular cells, leads to Tg reabsorption from the follicular lumen and proteolysis within the cell to yield thyroid hormones for secretion into the bloodstream.

REGULATION OF THE THYROID AXIS

TSH, secreted by the thyrotrope cells of the anterior pituitary, plays a pivotal role in control of the thyroid axis and serves as the most useful physiologic marker of thyroid hormone action. TSH is a 31-kDa hormone composed of α and β subunits; the α subunit is common to the other glycoprotein hormones [luteinizing hormone, follicle-stimulating hormone, human chorionic gonadotropin (hCG)], whereas the TSH β subunit is unique to TSH. The extent and nature of carbohydrate modification are modulated by thyrotropin-releasing hormone (TRH) stimulation and influence the biologic activity of the hormone. TSH has been produced recombinantly and is approved for use in the detection of residual thyroid cancer (see "Follow-up Whole-Body Scanning and Thyroglobulin Determinations," below).

Thyroxine (T4)
3,5,3′,5′-Tetraiodothyronine
Deiodinase 1 or 2 (5′-Deiodination)
Deiodinase 3>2 (5-Deiodination)
Tri-iodothyronine (T3)
3,5,3′-Triiodothyronine
Reverse T3 (rT3)
3,3′,5′-Triiodothyronine

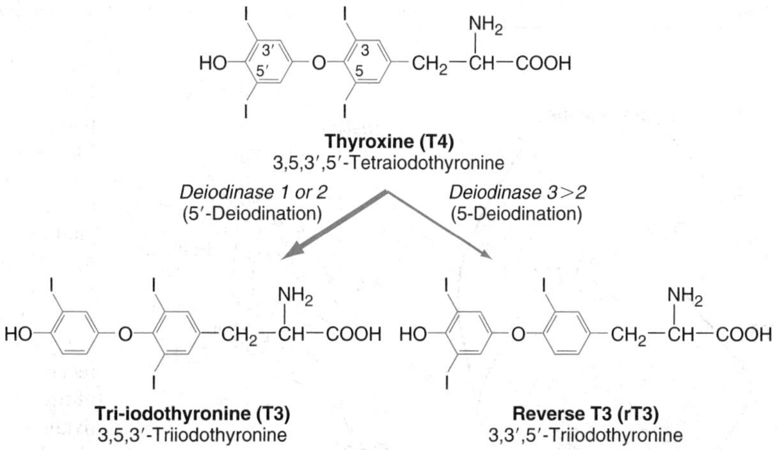

FIGURE 330-1 Structures of thyroid hormones. Thyroxine (T_4) contains four iodine atoms. Deiodination leads to production of the potent hormone, triiodothyronine (T_3), or the inactive hormone, reverse T_3.

The thyroid axis is a classic example of an endocrine feedback loop. Hypothalamic TRH stimulates pituitary production of TSH, which, in turn, stimulates thyroid hormone synthesis and secretion. Thyroid hormones feed back negatively to inhibit TRH and TSH production (Fig. 330-2). The "set-point" in this axis is established by TSH, the level of which is a sensitive and specific marker of thyroid function. TRH is the major positive regulator of TSH synthesis and secretion. TRH acts through a seven-transmembrane G protein–coupled receptor (GPCR) that activates phospholipase C to generate phosphatidylinositol turnover and the release of intracellular calcium. Peak TSH secretion occurs ~15 min after administration of exogenous TRH. Dopamine, glucocorticoids, and somatostatin suppress TSH but are not of major physiologic importance except when these agents are administered in pharmacologic doses. Reduced levels of thyroid hormone increase basal TSH production and enhance TRH-mediated stimulation of TSH. High thyroid hormone levels rapidly and directly suppress TSH and inhibit TRH-mediated stimulation of TSH, indicating that thyroid hormones are the dominant regulator of TSH production. Like other pituitary hormones, TSH is released in a pulsatile manner and exhibits a diurnal rhythm; its highest levels occur at night. However, these TSH excursions are modest in comparison to those of other pituitary hormones, in part because TSH has a relatively long plasma half-life (50 min). Consequently, single measurements of TSH are adequate for assessing its circulating level. TSH is measured using immunoradiometric assays that are highly sensitive and specific. These assays are capable of distinguishing between normal and suppressed TSH values, thus allowing TSH to be used for the diagnosis of hyperthyroidism (low TSH) as well as hypothyroidism (high TSH).

THYROID HORMONE SYNTHESIS, METABOLISM, AND ACTION

THYROID HORMONE SYNTHESIS Thyroid hormones are derived from Tg, a large iodinated glycoprotein. After secretion into the thyroid follicle, Tg is iodinated on selected tyrosine residues that are subsequently coupled via an ether linkage. Reuptake of Tg into the thyroid follicular cell allows proteolysis and the release of T_4 and T_3.

Iodine Metabolism and Transport Iodide uptake is a critical first step in thyroid hormone synthesis. Ingested iodine is bound to serum proteins, particularly albumin. Unbound iodine is excreted in the urine. The thyroid gland extracts iodine from the circulation in a highly efficient manner. For example, 10 to 25% of radioactive tracer (e.g., ^{123}I) is taken up by the normal thyroid gland over 24 h; this value can rise to 70 to 90% in Graves' disease.

Iodide uptake is mediated by the Na^+/I^- symporter (NIS), which is expressed at the basolateral membrane of thyroid follicular cells. NIS is most highly expressed in the thyroid gland but is also expressed at low levels in the salivary glands, lactating breast, and placenta. The iodide transport mechanism is highly regulated, allowing adaptation to variations in dietary supply. Low iodine levels increase the amount of NIS and stimulate uptake, whereas high iodine levels suppress NIS expression and uptake. The selective expression of the NIS in the thyroid allows isotopic scanning, treatment of hyperthyroidism, and ablation of thyroid cancer with radioisotopes of iodine, without significant effects on other organs. Mutation of the *NIS* gene is a rare cause of congenital hypothyroidism, underscoring its importance in thyroid hormone synthesis.

Iodine deficiency is prevalent in many mountainous regions and in central Africa, central South America, and northern Asia. In areas of relative iodine deficiency, there is an increased prevalence of goiter and, when deficiency is severe, hypothyroidism and cretinism. *Cretinism* is characterized by mental and growth retardation and occurs when children who live in iodine-deficient regions are not treated with iodine or thyroid hormone to restore normal thyroid hormone levels during early childhood. These children are often born to mothers with iodine deficiency, suggesting that maternal thyroid hormone deficiency worsens the condition. Concomitant selenium deficiency may also contribute to the neurologic manifestations of cretinism. Iodine supplemen-

Table 330-1 Genetic Causes of Congenital Hypothyroidism

Defective Gene Protein	Inheritance	Consequences
PROP-1	Autosomal recessive	Combined pituitary hormone deficiencies with preservation of ACTH
PIT-1	Autosomal recessive Autosomal dominant	Combined deficiencies of growth hormone, prolactin, thyroid-stimulating hormone (TSH)
TSHβ	Autosomal recessive	TSH deficiency
TTF-2	Autosomal recessive	Thyroid agenesis, choanal atresia, spiky hair
PAX-8	Autosomal dominant	Thyroid dysgenesis
TSH-receptor	Autosomal recessive	Resistance to TSH
$G_{s\alpha}$ (Albright hereditary osteodystrophy)	Autosomal dominant	Resistance to TSH
Na^+/I^- symporter	Autosomal recessive	Inability to transport iodide
Thyroid peroxidase	Autosomal recessive	Defective organification of iodide
Thyroglobulin	Autosomal recessive	Defective synthesis of thyroid hormone
Pendrin (anion transporter)	Autosomal recessive	Pendred's syndrome: sensorineural deafness and partial organification defect in thyroid
Dehalogenase	Autosomal recessive	Loss of iodide reutilization

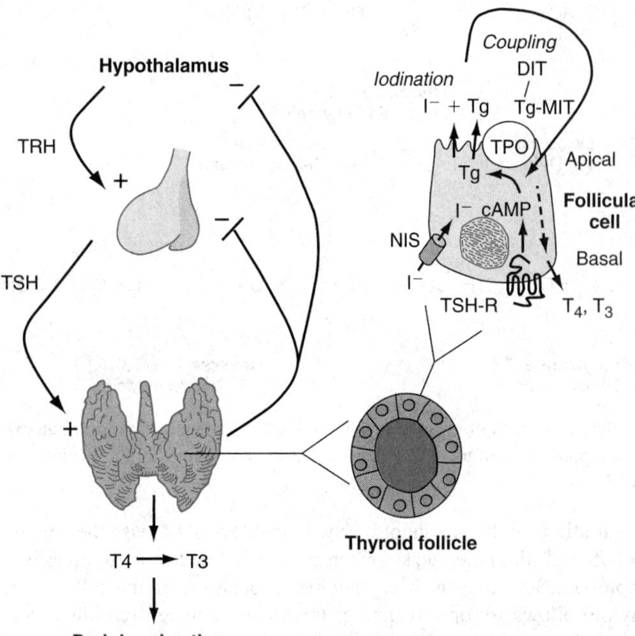

FIGURE 330-2 Regulation of thyroid hormone synthesis. *Left.* Thyroid hormones T_4 and T_3 feed back to inhibit hypothalamic production of thyrotropin-releasing hormone (TRH) and pituitary production of thyroid-stimulating hormone (TSH). TSH stimulates thyroid gland production of T_4 and T_3. *Right.* Thyroid follicles are formed by thyroid epithelial cells surrounding proteinaceous colloid, which contains thyroglobulin. Follicular cells, which are polarized, synthesize thyroglobulin and carry out thyroid hormone biosynthesis (see text for details). TSH-R, thyroid-stimulating hormone receptor; Tg, thyroglobulin; NIS, sodium-iodide symporter; TPO, thyroid peroxidase; DIT, di-iodotyrosine; MIT, monoiodotyrosine

tation of salt, bread, and other food substances has markedly reduced the prevalence of cretinism. Unfortunately, however, iodine deficiency remains the most common cause of preventable mental deficiency, often because of resistance to the use of food additives or the cost of supplementation. In addition to overt cretinism, mild iodine deficiency can lead to subtle reduction of IQ. Iodine intake is assessed by determination of excretion in a 24-h urine collection. Oversupply of iodine, through supplements or foods enriched in iodine (e.g., shellfish, kelp), is associated with an increased incidence of autoimmune thyroid disease. The recommended average daily intake of iodine is 150 μg/d for adults, 90 to 120 μg/d for children, and 200 μg/d for pregnant women.

Organification, Coupling, Storage, Release After iodide enters the thyroid, it is trapped and transported to the apical membrane of thyroid follicular cells where it is oxidized in an organification reaction that involves TPO and hydrogen peroxide. The reactive iodine atom is added to selected tyrosyl residues within Tg, a large (660 kDa) dimeric protein consisting of 2769 amino acids. The iodotyrosines in Tg are then coupled via an ether linkage in a reaction that is also catalyzed by TPO. Either T_4 or T_3 can be produced by this reaction, depending on the number of iodine atoms present in the iodotyrosines. After coupling, Tg is taken back into the thyroid cell where it is processed in lysosomes to release T_4 and T_3. Uncoupled mono- and diiodotyrosines (MIT, DIT) are deiodinated by the enzyme dehalogenase, thereby recycling any iodide that is not converted into thyroid hormones.

Disorders of thyroid hormone synthesis are rare causes of congenital hypothyroidism. The vast majority of these disorders are due to recessive mutations in TPO or Tg, but defects have also been identified in the TSH-R, NIS, the pendrin anion transporter, hydrogen peroxide generation, and in dehalogenase. Because of the biosynthetic defect, the gland is incapable of synthesizing adequate amounts of hormone, leading to increased TSH and a large goiter.

TSH Action TSH regulates thyroid gland function through the TSH-R, a seven-transmembrane GPCR. The TSH-R is coupled to the α subunit of stimulatory G protein ($G_{s\alpha}$) and activates adenylyl cyclase, leading to increased production of cyclic AMP. TSH also stimulates phosphatidylinositol turnover by activating phospholipase C. The functional role of the TSH-R has been underscored by naturally occurring mutations. Recessive loss-of-function mutations are a rare cause of thyroid hypoplasia and congenital hypothyroidism. Dominant gain-of-function mutations cause sporadic or familial nonautoimmune hyperthyroidism that is characterized by goiter, thyroid cell hyperplasia, and autonomous function. Most of these activating mutations involve in amino acid substitutions in the transmembrane domain of the receptor. They are thought to mimic conformational changes in the receptor similar to those induced by TSH binding or the interactions of thyroid-stimulating immunoglobulins (TSI) in Graves' disease. Activating TSH-R mutations also occur as somatic events and lead to clonal selection and expansion of the affected thyroid follicular cell (see below).

Factors that Influence Hormone Synthesis and Release TSH is the dominant hormonal regulator of thyroid gland growth and function. However, a variety of growth factors, most produced locally in the thyroid gland, also influence thyroid hormone synthesis. These include insulin-like growth factor I (IGF-I), epidermal growth factor, transforming growth factor β (TGF-β), endothelins, and various cytokines. The quantitative roles of these factors are not well understood, but they are important in selected disease states. In acromegaly, for example, increased levels of growth hormone and IGF-I are associated with goiter and predisposition to multinodular goiter. Certain cytokines and interleukins (ILs) produced in association with autoimmune thyroid disease induce thyroid growth, whereas others lead to apoptosis. As noted above, iodine is an important regulator of thyroid function. For example, iodine deficiency increases thyroid blood flow and stimulates uptake by the NIS. Excess iodide transiently inhibits thyroid iodide organification, a phenomenon known as the *Wolff-Chaikoff effect*. In individuals with a normal thyroid, the gland escapes from this inhibitory effect and iodide organification resumes; the suppressive action of high iodide may persist, however, in patients with underlying autoimmune thyroid disease.

THYROID HORMONE TRANSPORT AND METABOLISM **Serum Binding Proteins** T_4 is secreted from the thyroid gland in at least 20-fold excess over T_3 (Table 330-2). Both hormones circulate bound to plasma proteins, including thyroxine-binding globulin (TBG), transthyretin (TTR, formerly known as thyroxine-binding prealbumin, or TBPA), and albumin. The functions of serum-binding proteins are to increase the pool of circulating hormone, delay hormone clearance, and perhaps to modulate hormone delivery to selected tissue sites. The concentration of TBG is relatively low (1 to 2 mg/dL), but because of its high affinity for thyroid hormones ($T_4 > T_3$), it carries about 80% of the bound hormones. Albumin has relatively low affinity for thyroid hormones but has a high plasma concentration (~3.5 g/dL), and it binds up to 10% of T_4 and 30% of T_3. TTR also carries about 10% of T_4 but little T_3.

Table 330-2 Characteristics of Circulating T_4 and T_3

Hormone Property	T_4	T_3
Serum concentrations		
Total hormone	8 μg/dL	0.14 μg/dL
Fraction of total hormone in the free form	0.02%	0.3%
Free hormone	21×10^{-12} *M*	6×10^{-12} *M*
Serum half-life	7 d	0.75 d
Fraction directly from the thyroid	100%	20%
Production rate, including peripheral conversion	90 μg/d	32 μg/d
Intracellular hormone fraction	~20%	~70%
Relative metabolic potency	0.3	1
Receptor binding	10^{-10} *M*	10^{-11} *M*

When the effects of the various binding proteins are combined, approximately 99.98% of T_4 and 99.7% of T_3 are protein-bound. Because T_3 is less tightly bound than T_4, the amount of free T_3 is greater than free T_4, even though there is less total T_3 in the circulation. The unbound, or free, concentrations of the hormones are $\sim 2 \times 10^{-11}$ *M* for T_4 and $\sim 6 \times 10^{-12}$ *M* for T_3, which roughly correspond to the thyroid hormone receptor binding constants for these hormones (see below). Only the free hormone is biologically available to tissues. Therefore, homeostatic mechanisms that regulate the thyroid axis are directed towards maintenance of normal concentrations of free hormones.

Dysalbuminemic Hyperthyroxinemia A number of inherited and acquired abnormalities affect thyroid hormone binding proteins. X-linked TBG deficiency is associated with very low levels of total T_4 and T_3. However, because free hormone levels are normal, patients are euthyroid and TSH levels are normal. The importance of recognizing this disorder is to avoid efforts to normalize total T_4 levels, as this leads to thyrotoxicosis and is futile because of rapid hormone clearance in the absence of TBG. TBG levels are elevated by estrogen because of increased sialylation and delayed TBG clearance. Consequently, in women who are pregnant or taking estrogen-containing contraceptives, elevated TBG increases total T_4 and T_3 levels; however, free T_4 and T_3 levels are normal. Mutations in TBG, TTR, and albumin that increase binding affinity for T_4 and/or T_3 cause disorders known as *euthyroid hyperthyroxinemia* or *familial dysalbuminemic hyperthyroxinemia* (FDH) (Table 330-3). These disorders are usually dominantly transmitted and result in increased total T_4 and/or T_3, but free hormone levels are normal. The familial nature of the disorders, and the fact that TSH levels are normal rather than suppressed, should suggest the diagnosis. Free hormone levels (ideally measured by dialysis) are normal in FDH. The diagnosis can be confirmed, if necessary, by using tests that measure the affinities of radiolabeled hormone binding to specific transport proteins or by performing DNA sequence analyses of the abnormal transport protein genes.

Table 330-3 Conditions Associated with Euthyroid Hyperthyroxinemia

Disorder	Cause	Transmission	Characteristics
Familial dysalbuminemic hyperthyroxinemia (FDH)	Albumin mutations, usually R218H	AD	Increased T_4 Normal free T_4 Rarely increased T_3
TBG			
Familial excess	Increased TBG production	XL	Increased total T_4, T_3 Normal free T_4, T_3
Acquired excess	Medications (estrogen), pregnancy, cirrhosis, hepatitis	Acquired	Increased total T_4, T_3 Normal free T_4, T_3
Transthyretin[a]			
Excess	Islet tumors	Acquired	Usually normal T_4, T_3
Mutations	Increased affinity for T_4 or T_3	AD	Increased total T_4, T_3 Normal free T_4, T_3
Medications: propranolol, ipodate, iopanoic acid, amiodarone	Decreased $T_4 \rightarrow T_3$ conversion	Acquired	Increased T_4 Decreased T_3 Normal or increased TSH
Sick-euthyroid syndrome	Acute illness, especially psychiatric disorders	Acquired	Transiently increased free T_4 Decreased TSH T_4 and T_3 may also be decreased (see text)
Resistance to thyroid hormone (RTH)	Thyroid hormone receptor β mutations	AD	Increased free T_4, T_3 Normal or increased TSH Some patients clinically thyrotoxic

[a] Also known as thyroxine-binding prealbumin, TBPA.

NOTE: AD, autosomal dominant; TBG, thyroxine-binding globulin; TSH, thyroid-stimulating hormone; XL, X-linked.

Certain medications, such as salicylates and salsalate, can displace thyroid hormones from circulating binding proteins. Though these drugs transiently perturb the thyroid axis by increasing free thyroid hormone levels, TSH is suppressed until a new steady state is reached, thereby restoring euthyroidism. Circulating factors associated with acute illness may also displace thyroid hormone from binding proteins (see "Sick Euthyroid Syndrome," below).

Deiodinases In many respects, T_4 may be thought of as a precursor for the more potent T_3. T_4 is converted to T_3 by the deiodinase enzymes (Fig. 330-1). Type I deiodinase, which is located primarily in thyroid, liver, and kidney, has a relatively low affinity for T_4. Type II deiodinase has a higher affinity for T_4 and is found primarily in the pituitary gland, brain, brown fat, and thyroid gland. The presence of type II deiodinase allows it to regulate T_3 concentrations locally, a property that may be important in the context of levothyroxine (T_4) replacement. Type II deiodinase is also regulated by thyroid hormone—hypothyroidism induces the enzyme, resulting in enhanced $T_4 \rightarrow T_3$ conversion in tissues such as brain and pituitary. $T_4 \rightarrow T_3$ conversion may be impaired by fasting, systemic illness or acute trauma, oral contrast agents, and a variety of medications (e.g., propylthiouracil, propranolol, amiodarone, glucocorticoids). Type III deiodinase inactivates T_4 and T_3 and is the most important source of reverse T_3 (rT_3).

THYROID HORMONE ACTION Nuclear Thyroid Hormone Receptors Thyroid hormones act by binding to nuclear receptors, termed *thyroid hormone receptors* (TRs) α and β. Both TRα and TRβ are expressed in most tissues, but their relative levels of expression vary among organs; TRα is particularly abundant in brain, kidney, gonads, muscle, and heart, whereas TRβ expression is relatively high in the pituitary and liver. Both receptors are variably spliced to form unique isoforms. The TRβ2 isoform, which has a unique amino terminus, is selectively expressed in the hypothalamus and pituitary, where it appears to play a role in feedback control of the thyroid axis. The TRα2 isoform contains a unique carboxy terminus that prevents thyroid hormone binding; it may function to block the action of other TR isoforms.

The TRs contain a central DNA-binding domain and a C-terminal ligand-binding domain. They bind to specific DNA sequences, termed *thyroid response elements* (TREs), in the promoter regions of target genes (Fig. 330-3). The activated receptor can either stimulate gene transcription (e.g., myosin heavy chain α) or inhibit transcription (e.g., TSH β-subunit gene), depending on the nature of the regulatory elements in the target gene. The receptors bind as homodimers or as heterodimers with retinoic acid X receptors (RXRs) (Chap. 327).

Thyroid hormones bind with similar affinities to TRα and TRβ. However, T_3 is bound to its receptors with about 10 to 15 times greater affinity than T_4, which explains its increased hormonal potency. Though T_4 is produced in excess of T_3, receptors are occupied mainly by T_3, reflecting $T_4 \rightarrow T_3$ conversion by peripheral tissues, greater T_3 bioavailability in the plasma, and receptors' greater affinity for T_3. After binding to TRs, thyroid hormone induces conformational changes in the receptors that modify its interactions with accessory transcription factors. In the absence of thyroid hormone binding, the aporeceptors bind to corepressor proteins that inhibit gene transcription. Hormone binding dissociates the corepressors and allows the recruitment of coactivators that enhance transcription. The discovery of TR interactions with corepressors explains the fact that TR silences gene expression in the absence of hormone binding. Consequently,

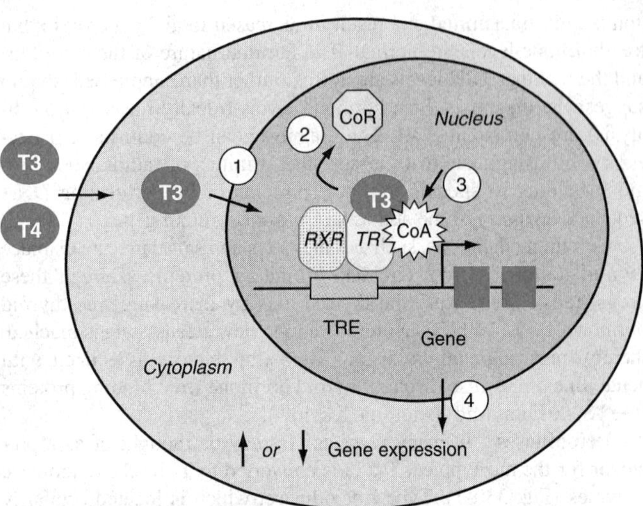

FIGURE 330-3 Mechanism of thyroid hormone receptor action. The thyroid hormone receptor (TR) and retinoid X receptor (RXR) form heterodimers that bind specifically to thyroid hormone response elements (TRE) in the promoter regions of target genes. In the absence of hormone, TR binds corepressor (CoR) proteins that silence gene expression. The numbers refer to a series of ordered reactions that occur in response to thyroid hormone: (1) T_4 or T_3 enters the nucleus; (2) T_3 binding dissociates CoR from TR; (3) Coactivators (CoA) are recruited to the T_3-bound receptor; (4) gene expression is altered.

hormone deficiency has a profound effect on gene expression because it causes active gene repression as well as loss of hormone-induced stimulation. This concept has been corroborated by the finding that targeted deletion of the TR genes in mice has a less pronounced phenotypic effect than hormone deficiency.

Thyroid Hormone Resistance Resistance to thyroid hormone (RTH) is an autosomal dominant disorder characterized by elevated free thyroid hormone levels and inappropriately normal or elevated TSH. Individuals with RTH do not, in general, exhibit signs and symptoms that are typical of hypothyroidism, apparently because hormone resistance is compensated by increased levels of thyroid hormone. The clinical features of RTH can include goiter, attention deficit disorder, mild reduction in IQ, delayed skeletal maturation, tachycardia, and impaired metabolic responses to thyroid hormone.

The disorder is caused by mutations in the TRβ receptor gene. These mutations, located in restricted regions of the ligand-binding domain, cause loss of receptor function. However, because the mutant receptors retain the capacity to dimerize with RXRs, bind to DNA, and recruit corepressor proteins, they function as antagonists of the remaining, normal TRβ and TRα receptors. This property, referred to as "dominant negative" activity, explains the autosomal dominant mode of transmission. The diagnosis is suspected when free thyroid hormone levels are increased without suppression of TSH. Similar hormonal abnormalities are common in other affected family members, though the TRβ mutation arises de novo in about 20% of patients. DNA sequence analysis of the TRβ gene provides a definitive diagnosis. RTH must be distinguished from other causes of euthyroid hyperthyroxinemia (e.g., familial dysalbuminemic hyperthyroxinemia) and inappropriate secretion of TSH by TSH-secreting pituitary adenomas (Chap. 328). In most patients, no treatment is indicated; the importance of making the diagnosis is to avoid inappropriate treatment of mistaken hyperthyroidism and to provide genetic counseling.

PHYSICAL EXAMINATION

In addition to the examination of the thyroid itself, the physical examination should include a search for signs of abnormal thyroid function and the extrathyroidal features of ophthalmopathy and dermopathy (see below). Examination of the neck begins by inspecting the seated patient from the front and side, and noting any surgical scars, obvious masses, or distended veins. The thyroid can be palpated with both hands from behind or the examiner can face the patient, using the thumbs to palpate each lobe. Most often it is best to use a combination of these methods, especially in cases of doubt or when there are small nodules. The patient's neck should be slightly flexed to relax the neck muscles. After locating the cricoid cartilage, the isthmus can be identified and followed laterally to locate either lobe (the right lobe is normally slightly larger than the left). By asking the patient to swallow sips of water, thyroid consistency can be better appreciated as the gland moves beneath the examiner's fingers.

Features to be noted include thyroid size, consistency, nodularity, and any tenderness or fixation. An estimate of thyroid size (normally 12 to 20 g) should be made, and a drawing is often the best way to record findings. However, ultrasound is the method of choice when it is important to determine thyroid size accurately. The size, location, and consistency of any nodules should also be depicted. A bruit over the gland indicates increased vascularity, as occurs in hyperthyroidism. If the lower borders of the thyroid lobes are not clearly felt, a goiter may be retrosternal. Large retrosternal goiters can cause venous distention over the neck and difficulty breathing, especially when the arms are raised (Pemberton's sign). With any central mass above the thyroid, the patient should be asked to stick out his or her tongue, as thyroglossal cysts then move upward. The thyroid examination is not complete without assessment for lymphadenopathy in the supraclavicular and cervical regions of the neck.

LABORATORY EVALUATION

MEASUREMENT OF THYROID HORMONES The enhanced sensitivity and specificity of *TSH assays* have greatly improved laboratory assessment of thyroid function. Because TSH levels change dynamically in response to alterations of free T_4 and T_3, a logical approach to thyroid testing is to determine first whether TSH is suppressed, normal, or elevated. With rare exceptions (see below), a normal TSH level excludes a primary abnormality of thyroid function. This strategy depends on the use of immunoradiometric assays (IRMAs) for TSH that are sensitive enough to discriminate between the lower limit of the reference range and the suppressed values that occur with thyrotoxicosis. Extremely sensitive (fourth generation) assays can detect TSH levels $\leq$0.004 mU/L, but for practical purposes assays sensitive to $\leq$0.1 mU/L are sufficient. The widespread availability of the TSH IRMA has rendered the TRH stimulation test virtually obsolete, as the failure of TSH to rise after an intravenous bolus of 200 to 400 μg TRH has the same implications as a suppressed basal TSH measured by IRMA.

The finding of an abnormal TSH level must be followed by measurements of circulating thyroid hormone levels to confirm the diagnosis of hyperthyroidism (suppressed TSH) or hypothyroidism (elevated TSH). Radioimmunoassays are widely available for serum *total* T_4 and *total* T_3. T_4 and T_3 are highly protein-bound, and numerous factors (illness, medications, genetic factors) can influence protein binding. It is useful, therefore, to measure the free or unbound hormone levels, which correspond to the biologically available hormone pool. Two direct methods are used to measure *free thyroid hormones*: (1) free thyroid hormone competition with radiolabeled T_4 (or an analogue) for binding to a solid-phase antibody, and (2) physical separation of the free hormone fraction by ultracentrifugation or equilibrium dialysis. Though early free hormone immunoassays suffered from artifacts, newer assays agree well with the results of the more technically demanding and expensive physical separation methods. An indirect method to estimate free thyroid hormone levels is to calculate the free T_3 or free T_4 index from the total T_4 or T_3 concentration and the *thyroid hormone binding ratio* (THBR). The latter is derived from the *T_3-resin uptake test*, which determines the distribution of radiolabeled T_3 between an absorbent resin and the unoccupied thyroid hormone binding proteins in the sample. The binding of the labeled T_3 to the resin is increased when there is reduced unoccupied protein binding sites (e.g., TBG deficiency) or increased total thyroid hormone in the sample; it is decreased under the opposite circumstances. The product of THBR and total T_3 or T_4 provides the *free T_3 or T_4 index.* In effect, the index corrects for anomalous total hormone values caused by abnormalities in hormone-protein binding.

Total thyroid hormone levels are elevated when TBG is increased due to estrogens (pregnancy, oral contraceptives, hormone replacement therapy, tamoxifen), and decreased when TBG binding is decreased (androgens, the nephrotic syndrome). Genetic disorders and acute illness can also cause abnormalities in thyroid hormone binding proteins, and various drugs (phenytoin, carbamazepine, salicylates, and nonsteroidal anti-inflammatory drugs) can interfere with thyroid hormone binding. Because free thyroid hormone levels are normal and the patient is euthyroid in all of these circumstances, assays that measure free hormone are preferable to those for total thyroid hormones.

For most purposes, the free T_4 level is sufficient to confirm thyrotoxicosis, but 2 to 5% of patients have only an elevated T_3 level (T_3 toxicosis). Thus, free T_3 levels should be measured in patients with a suppressed TSH but normal free T_4 levels. Free T_3 levels are normal in about 25% of patients with hypothyroidism and provide little useful information in this setting.

There are several clinical conditions in which the use of TSH as a screening test may be misleading, particularly without simultaneous free T_4 determinations. Any severe nonthyroidal illness can cause abnormal TSH levels (see below). Although hypothyroidism is the most common cause of an elevated TSH level, rare causes include a TSH-secreting pituitary tumor (Chap. 328), thyroid hormone resistance, and assay artifact. Conversely, a suppressed TSH level, particularly <0.1 mU/L, usually indicates thyrotoxicosis but may also be seen during the first trimester of pregnancy (due to hCG secretion), after treatment of hyperthyroidism (because TSH remains suppressed for several weeks), and in response to certain medications (e.g., high doses of glucocorticoids or dopamine). Importantly, secondary hypothyroidism, caused by hypothalamic-pituitary disease, is associated with a variable (low to high-normal) TSH level, which is inappropriate for the low free T_4 level. Thus, *TSH should not be used to assess thyroid function in patients with suspected or known pituitary disease.*

Tests for the end-organ effects of thyroid hormone excess or depletion, such as estimation of basal metabolic rate, tendon reflex speed, or serum cholesterol, are not useful as clinical determinants of thyroid function.

TESTS TO DETERMINE THE ETIOLOGY OF THYROID DYSFUNCTION Autoimmune thyroid disease is detected most easily by measuring circulating antibodies against TPO and Tg. As antibodies to Tg alone are rare, it is reasonable to measure only TPO antibodies. About 5 to 15% of euthyroid women and up to 2% of euthyroid men have thyroid antibodies; such individuals are at increased risk of developing thyroid dysfunction. Almost all patients with autoimmune hypothyroidism, and up to 80% of those with Graves' disease, have TPO antibodies, usually at high levels.

TSI are antibodies that stimulate the TSH-R in Graves' disease. They can be measured in bioassays or indirectly in assays that detect antibody binding to the receptor. The main use of these assays is to predict neonatal thyrotoxicosis caused by high maternal levels of TSI in the last trimester of pregnancy.

Serum Tg levels are increased in all types of thyrotoxicosis except thyrotoxicosis factitia. The main role for Tg measurement, however, is in the follow-up of thyroid cancer patients. After total thyroidectomy and radioablation, Tg levels should be undetectable; measurable levels (>1 to 2 ng/mL) suggest incomplete ablation or recurrent cancer.

RADIOIODINE UPTAKE AND THYROID SCANNING The thyroid gland selectively transports radioisotopes of iodine (^{123}I, ^{125}I, ^{131}I) and ^{99m}Tc pertechnetate, allowing thyroid imaging and quantitation of radioactive tracer fractional uptake.

Graves' disease is characterized by an enlarged gland and increased tracer uptake that is distributed homogeneously. Toxic adenomas appear as focal areas of increased uptake, with suppressed tracer uptake in the remainder of the gland. In toxic multinodular goiter, the

gland is enlarged—often with distorted architecture—and there are multiple areas of relatively increased or decreased tracer uptake. Subacute thyroiditis is associated with very low uptake because of follicular cell damage and TSH suppression. *Thyrotoxicosis factitia*, caused by self-administration of thyroid hormone, is also associated with low uptake.

Although the use of fine-needle aspiration (FNA) biopsy has diminished the use of thyroid scans in the evaluation of solitary thyroid nodules, the functional features of thyroid nodules have some prognostic significance. So-called cold nodules, which have diminished tracer uptake, are usually benign. However, these nodules are more likely to be malignant (~5 to 10%) than so-called hot nodules, which are almost never malignant.

Thyroid scanning is also used in the follow-up of thyroid cancer. After thyroidectomy and ablation using ^{131}I, there is diminished radioiodine uptake in the thyroid bed, allowing the detection of metastatic thyroid cancer deposits that retain the ability to transport iodine. Whole-body scans using 111 to 185 MBq (3 to 5 mCi) ^{131}I are typically performed after thyroid hormone withdrawal to raise the TSH level or after the administration of recombinant human TSH.

THYROID ULTRASOUND Ultrasonography is used increasingly to assist in the diagnosis of nodular thyroid disease, a reflection of the limitations of the physical examination and improvements in ultrasound technology. Using 10-MHz instruments, spatial resolution and image quality are excellent, allowing the detection of nodules and cysts >3 mm. In addition to detecting thyroid nodules, ultrasound is useful for monitoring nodule size, for guiding FNA biopsies, and for the aspiration of cystic lesions. Ultrasound is also used in the evaluation of recurrent thyroid cancer, including possible spread to cervical lymph nodes.

AUTOIMMUNE BASIS OF THYROID DISEASE

PREVALENCE Thyroid autoimmunity can cause several forms of thyroiditis and may lead to hypothyroidism as well as Graves' disease. Focal thyroiditis is present in 20 to 40% of autopsy cases and is associated with serologic evidence of autoimmunity, particularly the presence of TPO antibodies. These antibodies are 4 to 10 times more common in otherwise healthy women than men. About 5% of women experience self-limited *postpartum (silent) thyroiditis* in the months after pregnancy, often with transient clinical symptoms. This condition is associated with the presence of TPO antibodies ante-partum. Up to 20% of women with an episode of postpartum thyroiditis develop permanent hypothyroidism 5 to 10 years after delivery. Autoimmune-mediated hypothyroidism affects about 5 to 10% of middle-aged and elderly women, depending on diagnostic criteria and geographic location. Graves' disease is about one-tenth as common as hypothyroidism and tends to occur in younger individuals. Although seemingly diverse, these disorders have many pathophysiologic features in common, and patients may progress from one state to the other as the autoimmune process changes.

SUSCEPTIBILITY FACTORS As with most autoimmune disorders, susceptibility is determined by a combination of genetic and environmental factors. The concordance rate for Graves' disease in monozygotic twins is 20 to 30%. The risk of autoimmune thyroid disease is increased among siblings, who may exhibit features of either Graves' disease or autoimmune hypothyroidism. The autoimmune polyglandular syndrome type 2 (Chap. 339) involves the occurrence of autoimmune thyroid dysfunction with other autoimmune diseases (type 1 diabetes mellitus, Addison's disease, pernicious anemia, vitiligo). Shared genetic factors are likely in this group of autoimmune disorders.

HLA-DR3 is the best documented genetic risk factor for Graves' disease and autoimmune hypothyroidism in Caucasians, though different HLA associations exist for other racial groups, such as the Japanese and Chinese. A weak association with polymorphisms in the T cell regulatory gene CTLA-4 has been found in several racial groups. Other loci, including a region on chromosome 18q21, may be linked to Graves' disease as well as to several other autoimmune disorders such as type 1 diabetes mellitus, rheumatoid arthritis, and systemic lupus erythematosus (SLE). The female preponderance of thyroid autoimmunity is most likely due to the influence of sex steroids. Some studies suggest an association between antecedent major life events and Graves' disease, but a causal role for stress in the autoimmune process remains to be clearly established. Smoking is a minor risk factor for Graves' disease but a major risk factor for the development of ophthalmopathy. There is no convincing evidence for a role of infection in susceptibility, except for the congenital rubella syndrome, which is associated with a high frequency of autoimmune hypothyroidism. Viral thyroiditis does not induce subsequent autoimmune thyroid disease.

HUMORAL FACTORS The thyrotoxicosis of Graves' disease is caused by TSH-R-stimulating immunoglobulins that bind to the receptor and mimic the action of TSH. These TSI can cross the placenta and cause *transient neonatal thyrotoxicosis*, a phenomenon that complicates 1 to 2% of pregnancies in women with active or previous Graves' disease. However, the autoimmune response against the TSH-R can also result in antibodies that block TSH function, causing hypothyroidism. Stimulating and blocking antibodies bind to separate epitopes on the receptor. TSH-R blocking antibodies are found in about 20% of Asian patients with autoimmune hypothyroidism and are associated with thyroid atrophy; blocking antibodies are less common in Caucasians. Patients may have a mixture of TSH-R antibodies, and thyroid function can oscillate between hyperthyroidism and hypothyroidism as stimulating or blocking antibodies become dominant. Predicting the course of disease in such individuals is difficult, and close monitoring of thyroid function is required. Assays that measure the binding of antibodies to the receptor by competition with radiolabeled TSH [TSH-binding inhibiting immunoglobulins (TBII)] provide no information about functional effects and are used primarily to demonstrate the presence of TSH-R antibodies in atypical patients. Bioassays measure antibody-mediated stimulation of cyclic AMP production in cultured thyroid cells or cells transfected with the TSH-R. The use of these assays does not generally alter clinical management.

Antibodies to Tg and TPO, readily measured by immunofluorescence, hemagglutination, enzyme-linked immunosorbent assay, or radioimmunoassay, are clinically useful markers of thyroid autoimmunity, as discussed above. Any pathogenic effect is likely to be restricted to a secondary role in amplifying an ongoing autoimmune response. For instance, T cell– or cytokine-mediated injury to thyroid follicles could expose the enzyme on the apical border of follicles to TPO antibodies, which may then bind to the autoantigen and fix complement. There is evidence for intrathyroidal complement activation in both Graves' disease and autoimmune hypothyroidism. Tg antibodies do not fix complement, but could be involved in antibody-dependent, natural killer cell-mediated cytotoxicity. The NIS is also a target of autoantibody production in up to one-third of patients with autoimmune thyroid disease, but the functional consequences, if any, have not been established.

CELL-MEDIATED FACTORS Activated circulating T cells are increased in autoimmune thyroid disease, and the gland is infiltrated with CD4+ and CD8+ T cells. The latter are believed to mediate perforin-dependent cytotoxicity, leading ultimately to thyroid cell destruction. In addition, thyroid cells undergo apoptosis through cytokine-mediated upregulation of Fas and possibly Fas ligand. Cytokines produced by the infiltrating immune cells also induce expression of thyroid cell-surface molecules that lead to: (1) engagement by immune cells (e.g., adhesion molecules, HLA class I and II molecules); (2) induction of cytokine secretion by the thyroid cells themselves; (3) production of nitric oxide; and (4) reduction of thyroid hormone production through inhibition of TSH-R, TPO, and Tg synthesis. Administration of high concentrations of cytokines for therapeutic purposes [especially interferon (IFN)α] is associated with increased autoimmune thyroid disease, presumably via mechanisms similar to those that occur in sporadic autoimmune disease.

Cytokines appear to play a major role in thyroid-associated ophthalmopathy. There is infiltration of the extraocular muscles by activated T cells; the release of cytokines results in fibroblast activation and increased synthesis of glycosaminoglycans that trap water, thereby leading to characteristic muscle swelling. Late in the disease, there is fibrosis and only then do the muscle cells show evidence of injury. Orbital fibroblasts may be uniquely sensitive to cytokines, perhaps explaining the anatomic localization of the immune response. Though the pathogenesis of thyroid-associated ophthalmopathy remains unclear, there is mounting evidence that expression of the TSH-R may provide an important orbital autoantigen. In support of this idea, injection of TSH-R into certain strains of mice induces autoimmune hyperthyroidism, as well as features of ophthalmopathy. A variety of autoantibodies against orbital muscle and fibroblast antigens have been detected in patients with ophthalmopathy, but these antibodies most likely arise as a secondary phenomenon, dependent on T cell–mediated autoimmune responses.

HYPOTHYROIDISM

Iodine deficiency remains the most common cause of hypothyroidism worldwide. In areas of iodine sufficiency, autoimmune disease (Hashimoto's thyroiditis) and iatrogenic causes (treatment of hyperthyroidism) are most common (Table 330-4).

CONGENITAL HYPOTHYROIDISM **Prevalence** Hypothyroidism occurs in about 1 in 3000 to 4000 newborns. It may be transient, especially if the mother has TSH-R blocking antibodies or has received antithyroid drugs, but permanent hypothyroidism occurs in the majority. Neonatal hypothyroidism is due to thyroid gland dysgenesis in 85%, inborn errors of thyroid hormone synthesis in 10 to 15%, and is TSH-R antibody-mediated in 5% of affected newborns. The developmental abnormalities are twice as common in girls. Mutations that cause congenital hypothyroidism are being increasingly recognized, but the vast majority remain idiopathic (Table 330-1).

Clinical Manifestations The majority of infants appear normal at birth, and <10% are diagnosed based on clinical features, which include prolonged jaundice, feeding problems, hypotonia, enlarged tongue, delayed bone maturation, and umbilical hernia. Importantly, permanent neurologic damage results if treatment is delayed. Typical features of adult hypothyroidism may also be present (Table 330-5).

Table 330-4 Causes of Hypothyroidism

Primary
- Autoimmune hypothyroidism: Hashimoto's thyroiditis, atrophic thyroiditis
- Iatrogenic: ^{131}I treatment, subtotal or total thyroidectomy, external irradiation of neck for lymphoma or cancer
- Drugs: iodine excess (including iodine-containing contrast media and amiodarone), lithium, antithyroid drugs, *p*-aminosalicyclic acid, interferon-α and other cytokines, aminoglutethimide
- Congenital hypothyroidism: absent or ectopic thyroid gland, dyshormonogenesis, TSH-R mutation
- Iodine deficiency
- Infiltrative disorders: amyloidosis, sarcoidosis, hemochromatosis, scleroderma, cystinosis, Riedel's thyroiditis

Transient
- Silent thyroiditis, including postpartum thyroiditis
- Subacute thyroiditis
- Withdrawal of thyroxine treatment in individuals with an intact thyroid
- After ^{131}I treatment or subtotal thyroidectomy for Graves' disease

Secondary
- Hypopituitarism: tumors, pituitary surgery or irradiation, infiltrative disorders, Sheehan's syndrome, trauma, genetic forms of combined pituitary hormone deficiencies
- Isolated TSH deficiency or inactivity
- Bexarotene treatment
- Hypothalamic disease: tumors, trauma, infiltrative disorders, idiopathic

NOTE: TSH, thyroid-stimulating hormone; TSH-R, TSH receptor.

Table 330-5 Signs and Symptoms of Hypothyroidism (Descending Order of Frequency)

Symptoms	Signs
Tiredness, weakness	Dry coarse skin; cool peripheral extremities
Dry skin	Puffy face, hands and feet (myxedema)
Feeling cold	Diffuse alopecia
Hair loss	Bradycardia
Difficulty concentrating and poor memory	Peripheral edema
Constipation	Delayed tendon reflex relaxation
Weight gain with poor appetite	Carpal tunnel syndrome
Dyspnea	Serous cavity effusions
Hoarse voice	
Menorrhagia (later oligomenorrhea or amenorrhea)	
Paresthesias	
Impaired hearing	

Diagnosis and Treatment Because of the severe neurologic consequences of untreated congenital hypothyroidism, neonatal screening programs have been established in developed countries (Chap. 68). These are generally based on measurement of TSH or T_4 levels in heel-prick blood specimens. When the diagnosis is confirmed, T_4 is instituted at a dose of 10 to 15 μg/kg per day and the dosage is adjusted by close monitoring of TSH levels. T_4 requirements are relatively great during the first year of life, and a high circulating T_4 level is usually needed to normalize TSH. Early treatment with T_4 results in normal IQ levels, but subtle neurodevelopmental abnormalities may be detected in those with the most severe hypothyroidism at diagnosis or when treatment is suboptimal.

AUTOIMMUNE HYPOTHYROIDISM **Classification** Autoimmune hypothyroidism may be associated with a goiter (Hashimoto's, or *goitrous thyroiditis*) or, at the later stages of the disease, minimal residual thyroid tissue (*atrophic thyroiditis*). Because the autoimmune process gradually reduces thyroid function, there is a phase of compensation during which normal thyroid hormone levels are maintained by a rise in TSH. Though some patients may have minor symptoms, this state is called *subclinical hypothyroidism*. Later, free T_4 levels fall and TSH levels rise further; symptoms become more readily apparent at this stage (usually TSH $>$ 10 mU/L), which is referred to as *clinical hypothyroidism* (*overt hypothyroidism*).

Prevalence The mean annual incidence rate of autoimmune hypothyroidism is up to 4 per 1000 women and 1 per 1000 men. It is more common in certain populations, such as the Japanese, probably as a consequence of genetic factors and chronic exposure to a high-iodine diet. The mean age at diagnosis is about 60 years, and the prevalence of overt hypothyroidism increases with age. Subclinical hypothyroidism is found in 6 to 8% of women (10% over the age of 60) and 3% of men. The annual risk of developing clinical hypothyroidism is about 4% when subclinical hypothyroidism is associated with positive TPO antibodies.

Pathogenesis In Hashimoto's thyroiditis, there is a marked lymphocytic infiltration of the thyroid with germinal center formation, atrophy of the thyroid follicles accompanied by oxyphil metaplasia, absence of colloid, and mild to moderate fibrosis. In atrophic thyroiditis, the fibrosis is much more extensive, lymphocyte infiltration is less pronounced, and thyroid follicles are almost completely absent. Atrophic thyroiditis likely represents the end stage of Hashimoto's thyroiditis rather than a distinct disorder. Autoimmune features are similar in both types of hypothyroidism, though TSH-R blocking antibodies may be more frequent in Asian patients with atrophic thyroiditis. The mechanisms that result in thyroid follicular destruction are predominantly T cell mediated, but antibodies may also contribute to thyroid dysfunction by complement fixation or inhibition of thyroid cell function (see "Autoimmune Basis of Thyroid Disease," above).

Clinical Manifestations The main clinical features of hypothyroidism are summarized in Table 330-5. The onset is usually insidious, and the patient may become aware of symptoms only when euthyroidism is restored. Patients with Hashimoto's thyroiditis may present because of goiter rather than symptoms of hypothyroidism. The goiter may not be large but is usually irregular and firm in consistency. It is often possible to palpate a pyramidal lobe, normally a vestigial remnant of thyroglossal duct. Rarely, uncomplicated Hashimoto's thyroiditis is associated with pain.

Patients with atrophic thyroiditis, or the late stage of Hashimoto's thyroiditis, present with symptoms and signs of hypothyroidism. The skin is dry, and there is decreased sweating, thinning of the epidermis, and hyperkeratosis of the stratum corneum. Increased dermal glycosaminoglycan content traps water, giving rise to skin thickening without pitting (*myxedema*). Typical features include a puffy face with edematous eyelids and nonpitting pretibial edema (Fig. 330-4). There is pallor, often with a yellow tinge due to carotene accumulation. Nail growth is retarded, and hair is dry, brittle, difficult to manage, and falls out easily. In addition to diffuse alopecia, there is thinning of the outer third of the eyebrows.

Other common features include constipation and weight gain (despite a poor appetite). In contrast to popular perception, the weight gain is usually modest and due mainly to fluid retention in the myxedematous tissues. Libido is decreased in both sexes, and there may be oligomenorrhea or amenorrhea in long-standing disease, but menorrhagia is also common. Fertility is reduced and the incidence of miscarriage is increased. Prolactin levels are often modestly increased (Chap. 328) and may contribute to alterations in libido and fertility as well as causing galactorrhea.

Myocardial contractility and pulse rate are reduced, leading to a reduced stroke volume and bradycardia. Increased peripheral resistance may be accompanied by hypertension, particularly diastolic. Blood flow is diverted from the skin, producing the cool extremities. Pericardial effusions occur in up to 30% of patients but rarely compromise cardiac function. Though alterations in myosin heavy chain isoform expression have been documented, cardiomyopathy is unusual. Fluid may also accumulate in other serous cavities and in the middle ear, giving rise to conductive deafness. Pulmonary function is generally normal, but dyspnea may be due to pleural effusion, impaired respiratory muscle function, diminished ventilatory drive, or sleep apnea.

Carpal tunnel and other entrapment syndromes are common, as is impairment of muscle function with stiffness, cramps, and pain. On examination, there may be slow relaxation of tendon reflexes and pseudomyotonia. Memory and concentration are impaired. Rare neurologic problems include reversible cerebellar ataxia, dementia, psychosis, and myxedema coma. *Hashimoto's encephalopathy* is a rare and distinctive syndrome associated with myoclonus and slow-wave activity on electroencephalography, which can progress to confusion, coma, and

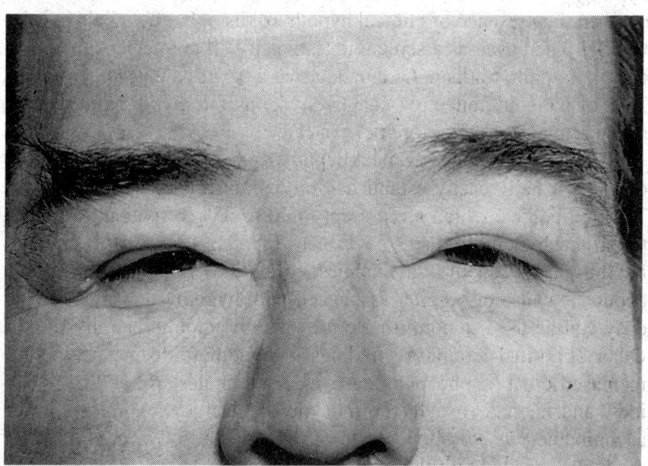

FIGURE 330-4 Facial appearance in hypothyroidism. Note puffy eyes and thickened, pale skin.

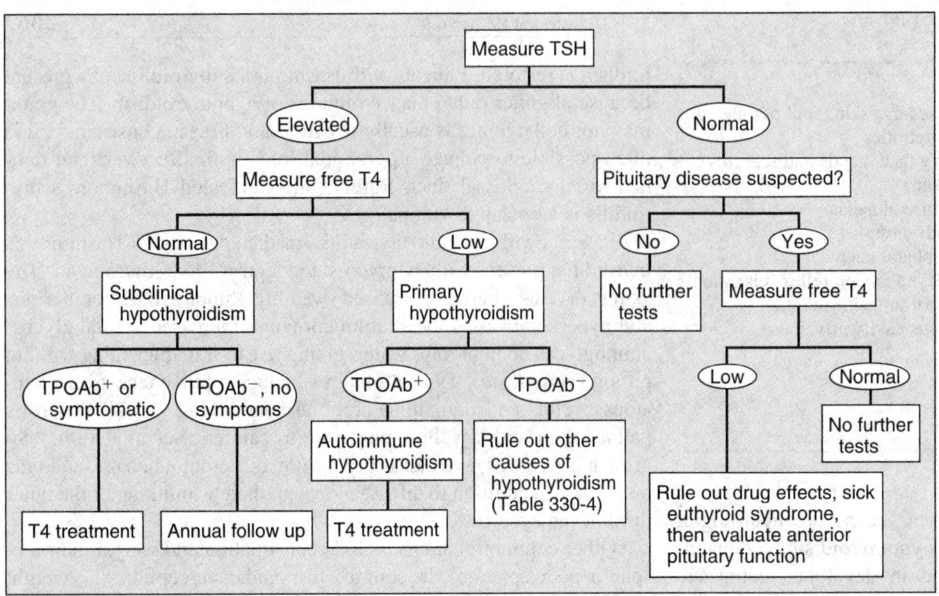

FIGURE 330-5 Evaluation of hypothyroidism. TPOAB$^+$, thyroid peroxidase antibodies present; TPOAB$^-$, thyroid peroxidase antibodies not present.

death. It is steroid-responsive and may occur in the presence of autoimmune thyroiditis, without hypothyroidism. The hoarse voice and occasionally clumsy speech of hypothyroidism are due to fluid accumulation in the vocal cords and tongue.

The features described above are due to a shortage of thyroid hormone. However, autoimmune hypothyroidism may be associated with signs or symptoms of other autoimmune diseases, particularly vitiligo, pernicious anemia, Addison's disease, alopecia areata, and type 1 diabetes mellitus. Less common associations include celiac disease, dermatitis herpetiformis, chronic active hepatitis, rheumatoid arthritis, SLE, and Sjögren's syndrome. Thyroid-associated ophthalmopathy, which usually occurs in Graves' disease (see below), occurs in about 5% of patients with autoimmune hypothyroidism.

Autoimmune hypothyroidism is uncommon in children and usually presents with slow growth and delayed facial maturation. The appearance of permanent teeth is also delayed. Myopathy, with muscle swelling, is more common than in adults. In most cases, puberty is delayed, but precocious puberty sometimes occurs. There may be intellectual impairment if the onset is before 3 years and the hormone deficiency is severe.

Laboratory Evaluation A summary of the investigations used to determine the existence and cause of hypothyroidism is provided in Fig. 330-5. A normal TSH level excludes primary (but not secondary) hypothyroidism. If the TSH is elevated, a free T_4 level is needed to confirm the presence of clinical hypothyroidism, but free T_4 is inferior to TSH when used as a screening test, as it will not detect subclinical or mild hypothyroidism. Circulating free T_3 levels are normal in about 25% of patients, reflecting adaptive responses to hypothyroidism. T_3 measurements are therefore not indicated.

Once clinical or subclinical hypothyroidism is confirmed, the etiology is usually easily established by demonstrating the presence of TPO antibodies, which are present in 90 to 95% of patients with autoimmune hypothyroidism. TBII can be found in 10 to 20% of patients, but these determinations are not needed routinely. If there is any doubt about the cause of a goiter associated with hypothyroidism, FNA biopsy can be used to confirm the presence of autoimmune thyroiditis. Other abnormal laboratory findings in hypothyroidism may include increased creatine phosphokinase, elevated cholesterol and triglycerides, and anemia (usually normocytic or macrocytic). Except when accompanied by iron deficiency, the anemia and other abnormalities gradually resolve with thyroxine replacement.

Differential Diagnosis An asymmetric goiter in Hashimoto's thyroiditis may be confused with a multinodular goiter or thyroid carcinoma, even when thyroid antibodies are present. Ultrasound can be used to show the presence of a solitary lesion or a multinodular goiter, rather than the heterogeneous thyroid enlargement typical of Hashimoto's thyroiditis. FNA biopsy is useful in the investigation of focal nodules. Other causes of hypothyroidism are discussed below but rarely cause diagnostic confusion (Table 330-4).

OTHER CAUSES OF HYPOTHYROIDISM *Iatrogenic hypothyroidism* is a common cause of hypothyroidism and can often be detected by screening before symptoms develop. In the first 3 to 4 months after radioiodine treatment, transient hypothyroidism may occur due to reversible radiation damage rather than to cellular destruction. Low-dose thyroxine treatment can be withdrawn if recovery occurs. Because TSH levels are suppressed by hyperthyroidism, free T_4 levels are a better measure of thyroid function than TSH in the months following radioiodine treatment. Mild hypothyroidism after subtotal thyroidectomy may also resolve after several months, as the gland remnant is stimulated by increased TSH levels.

Iodine deficiency is responsible for endemic goiter and cretinism but is an uncommon cause of adult hypothyroidism unless the iodine intake is very low or there are complicating factors, such as the consumption of thiocyanates in cassava or selenium deficiency. Though hypothyroidism due to iodine deficiency can be treated with thyroxine, public health measures to improve iodine intake should be advocated to eliminate this problem. Iodized salt or bread or the use of a single bolus of oral or intramuscular iodized oil have all been used successfully.

Paradoxically, chronic iodine excess can also induce goiter and hypothyroidism. The intracellular events that account for this effect are unclear, but individuals with autoimmune thyroiditis are especially susceptible. Iodine excess is responsible for the hypothyroidism that occurs in up to 13% of patients treated with amiodarone (see below). Other drugs, particularly lithium, may also cause hypothyroidism.

Secondary hypothyroidism is usually diagnosed in the context of other anterior pituitary hormone deficiencies; isolated TSH deficiency is very rare (Chap. 328). TSH levels may be low, normal, or even slightly increased in secondary hypothyroidism; the latter is due to secretion of immunoactive but bioinactive forms of TSH. The diagnosis is confirmed by detecting a low free T_4 level. The goal of treatment is to maintain free T_4 levels in the upper half of the reference range, as TSH levels cannot be used to monitor therapy.

Rx TREATMENT **Clinical Hypothyroidism** If there is no residual thyroid function, the daily replacement dose of levothyroxine is usually 1.5 μg/kg body weight (typically 100 to 150 μg). In many patients, however, lower doses suffice until residual thyroid tissue is destroyed. In patients who develop hypothyroidism after the treatment of Graves' disease, there is often underlying autonomous function, necessitating lower replacement doses (typically 75 to 125 μg/d).

Adult patients under 60 without evidence of heart disease may be started on 50 to 100μg levothyroxine (T_4) daily. The dose is adjusted on the basis of TSH levels, with the goal of treatment being a normal TSH, ideally in the lower half of the reference range. TSH responses are gradual and should be measured about 2 months after instituting treatment or after any subsequent change in levothyroxine dosage. The clinical effects of levothyroxine replacement are often slow to appear.

Patients may not experience full relief from symptoms until 3 to 6 months after normal TSH levels are restored. Adjustment of levothyroxine dosage is made in 12.5- or 25-μg increments if the TSH is high; decrements of the same magnitude should be made if the TSH is suppressed. Patients with a suppressed TSH of any cause, including T_4 overtreatment, have an increased risk of atrial fibrillation and reduced bone density.

Although dessicated animal thyroid preparations (thyroid extract USP) are available, they are not recommended as potency and composition vary between batches. Interest in using levothyroxine combined with liothyronine (triiodothyronine, T_3) has been revived, based on studies suggesting that patients feel better when taking the T_4/T_3 combination compared to T_4 alone. However, a long-term benefit from this combination is not established. There is no place for liothyronine alone as long-term replacement, because the short half-life necessitates three or four daily doses and is associated with fluctuating T_3 levels.

Once full replacement is achieved and TSH levels are stable, follow-up measurement of TSH is recommended at annual intervals and may be extended to every 2 to 3 years, if a normal TSH is maintained over several years. It is important to ensure ongoing compliance, however, as patients do not feel any difference after missing a few doses of levothyroxine, sometimes leading to self-discontinuation.

In patients of normal body weight who are taking ≥200 μg of levothyroxine per day, an elevated TSH level is often a sign of poor compliance. This is also the likely explanation for fluctuating TSH levels, despite a constant levothyroxine dosage. Such patients often have normal or high free T_4 levels, despite an elevated TSH, because they remember to take medication for a few days before testing; this is sufficient to normalize T_4 but not TSH levels. It is important to consider variable compliance, as this pattern of thyroid function tests is otherwise suggestive of disorders associated with inappropriate TSH secretion (Table 330-3). Because T_4 has a long half-life (7 days), patients who miss doses can be advised to take up to three doses of the skipped tablets at once. Other causes of increased levothyroxine requirements must be excluded, particularly malabsorption (e.g., celiac disease, small-bowel surgery) and drugs that interfere with T_4 absorption or clearance such as cholestyramine, ferrous sulfate, calcium supplements, lovastatin, aluminum hydroxide, rifampicin, amiodarone, carbamazepine, and phenytoin.

Subclinical Hypothyroidism By definition, subclinical hypothyroidism refers to biochemical evidence of thyroid hormone deficiency in patients who have few or no apparent clinical features of hypothyroidism. There are no generally accepted guidelines for the treatment of subclinical hypothyroidism. As long as excessive treatment is avoided, there is little risk in correcting a slightly increased TSH, and some patients likely derive modest clinical benefit from treatment. Moreover, there is some risk that patients will progress to overt hypothyroidism, particularly when TPO antibodies are present. Treatment is administered by starting with a low dose of levothyroxine (25 to 50 μg/d) with the goal of normalizing TSH.

Special Treatment Considerations Rarely, levothyroxine replacement is associated with pseudotumor cerebri in *children*. Presentation appears to be idiosyncratic and occurs months after treatment is begun. Women with a history or high risk of hypothyroidism should ensure that they are euthyroid prior to conception and during early pregnancy as maternal hypothyroidism may adversely affect fetal neural development. TSH and free T_4 levels should be measured once pregnancy is confirmed and at the beginning of the second and third trimesters. The dose of levothyroxine may need to be increased by ≥50% during pregnancy and returned to previous levels after delivery. In the *elderly*, especially patients with known coronary artery disease, the starting dose of levothyroxine is 12.5 to 25 μg/d with similar increments every 2 to 3 months until TSH is normalized. In some patients it may be impossible to achieve full replacement, despite optimal antianginal treatment. *Emergency surgery* is generally safe in patients with untreated hypothyroidism, although routine surgery in a hypothyroid patient should be deferred until euthyroidism is achieved.

Myxedema coma still has a high mortality rate, despite intensive treatment. Clinical manifestations include reduced level of consciousness, sometimes associated with seizures, as well as the other features of hypothyroidism (Table 330-5). Hypothermia can reach 23°C (74°F). There may be a history of treated hypothyroidism with poor compliance, or the patient may be previously undiagnosed. Myxedema coma almost always occurs in the elderly and is usually precipitated by factors that impair respiration, such as drugs (especially sedatives, anesthetics, antidepressants), pneumonia, congestive heart failure, myocardial infarction, gastrointestinal bleeding, or cerebrovascular accidents. Sepsis should also be suspected. Exposure to cold may also be a risk factor. Hypoventilation, leading to hypoxia and hypercapnia, plays a major role in pathogenesis; hypoglycemia and dilutional hyponatremia also contribute to the development of myxedema coma.

Levothyroxine can initially be administered as a single intravenous bolus of 500 μg, which serves as a loading dose. Although further levothyroxine is not strictly necessary for several days, it is usually continued at a dose of 50 to 100 μg/d. If a suitable intravenous preparation is not available, the same initial dose of levothyroxine can be given by nasogastric tube (though absorption may be impaired in myxedema). An alternative is to give liothyronine (T_3) intravenously or via nasogastric tube, in doses ranging from 10 to 25 μg every 8 to 12 h. This treatment has been advocated because $T_4 \rightarrow T_3$ conversion is impaired in myxedema coma. However, excess liothyroxine has the potential to provoke arrhythmias. Another commonly used option is to combine levothyroxine (200 μg) and liothyronine (25 μg) as a single, initial intravenous bolus followed by daily treatment with levothyroxine (50 to 100 μg/d) and liothyronine (10 μg every 8 h).

Supportive therapy should be provided to correct any associated metabolic disturbances. External warming is indicated only if the temperature is <30°C, as it can result in cardiovascular collapse (Chap. 17). Space blankets should be used to prevent further heat loss. Parenteral hydrocortisone (50 mg every 6 h) should be administered, as there is impaired adrenal reserve in profound hypothyroidism. Any precipitating factors should be treated, including the early use of broad-spectrum antibiotics, pending the exclusion of infection. Ventilatory support with regular blood gas analysis is usually needed during the first 48 h. Hypertonic saline or intravenous glucose may be needed if there is hyponatremia or hypoglycemia; hypotonic intravenous fluids should be avoided because they may exacerbate water retention secondary to reduced renal perfusion and inappropriate vasopressin secretion. The metabolism of most medications is impaired, and sedatives should be avoided if possible or used in reduced doses. Blood levels should be monitored, when available, to guide medication dosage.

THYROTOXICOSIS

Thyrotoxicosis is defined as the state of thyroid hormone excess and is not synonymous with *hyperthyroidism*, which is the result of excessive thyroid function. However, the major etiologies of thyrotoxicosis are hyperthyroidism caused by Graves' disease, toxic multinodular goiter, and toxic adenomas. Other causes are listed in Table 330-6.

GRAVES' DISEASE **Epidemiology** Graves' disease accounts for 60 to 80% of thyrotoxicosis, though the prevalence varies among populations, depending mainly on iodine intake (high iodine intake is associated with an increased prevalence of Graves' disease). Graves' disease occurs in up to 2% of women but is one-tenth as frequent in men. The disorder rarely begins before adolescence and typically occurs between 20 and 50 years of age, though it also occurs in the elderly.

Pathogenesis The hyperthyroidism of Graves' disease is caused by TSI that are directed to the TSH-R (see "Autoimmune Basis of Thyroid Disease," below). Other thyroid autoimmune responses coexist in these patients, and therefore there is no direct correlation between the levels of TSI and thyroid hormones. The extrathyroidal manifestations of Graves' disease—i.e., ophthalmopathy and dermo-

Table 330-6 Causes of Thyrotoxicosis

Primary hyperthyroidism
Graves' disease
Toxic multinodular goiter
Toxic adenoma
Functioning thyroid carcinoma metastases
Activating mutation of the TSH receptor (autosomal dominant)
Struma ovarii
Drugs: iodine excess (Jod-Basedow phenomenon)
Thyrotoxicosis without hyperthyroidism
Subacute thyroiditis
Silent thyroiditis
Other causes of thyroid destruction: amiodarone, radiation, infarction of adenoma
Ingestion of excess thyroid hormone (thyrotoxicosis factitia) or thyroid tissue
Secondary hyperthyroidism
TSH-secreting pituitary adenoma
Thyroid hormone resistance syndrome: occasional patients may have features of thyrotoxicosis
Chorionic gonadotropin-secreting tumors[a]
Gestational thyrotoxicosis[a]

[a] Circulating TSH levels are low in these forms of secondary hyperthyroidism.
NOTE: TSH, thyroid-stimulating hormone.

pathy—are due to immunologically mediated activation of fibroblasts in the extraocular muscles and skin, with accumulation of glycosaminoglycans, leading to the trapping of water and edema. Later, fibrosis becomes prominent. The fibroblast activation is caused by cytokines (IFN-γ, tumor necrosis factor, IL-1) derived from locally infiltrating T cells and macrophages.

Clinical Manifestations Signs and symptoms include features that are common to any cause of thyrotoxicosis (Table 330-7) as well as those specific for Graves' disease. The clinical presentation depends on the severity of thyrotoxicosis, the duration of the disease, individual susceptibility to excess thyroid hormone, and the age of the patient. In the elderly, features of thyrotoxicosis may be subtle or masked, and patients may present mainly with fatigue and weight loss, leading to *apathetic hyperthyroidism*.

Thyrotoxicosis may cause unexplained weight loss, despite an enhanced appetite, and is due to the increased metabolic rate. Weight gain occurs in 5 to 10% of patients, however, as a result of increased food intake. Other prominent features include hyperactivity, nervousness, and irritability, ultimately leading to a sense of easy fatiguability in some patients. Insomnia and impaired concentration are common; apathetic thyrotoxicosis may be mistaken for depression in the elderly. Fine tremor is a very frequent finding, best elicited by asking patients to stretch out the fingers and feeling the fingertips with the palm. Common neurologic manifestations include hyperreflexia, muscle wasting, and proximal myopathy without fasciculation. Chorea is a rare feature. Thyrotoxicosis is sometimes associated with a form of hypokalemic periodic paralysis; this disorder is particularly common in Asian males with thyrotoxicosis.

Table 330-7 Signs and Symptoms of Thyrotoxicosis (Descending Order of Frequency)

Symptoms	Signs[a]
Hyperactivity, irritability, dysphoria	Tachycardia; atrial fibrillation in the elderly
Heat intolerance and sweating	Tremor
Palpitations	Goiter
Fatigue and weakness	Warm, moist skin
Weight loss with increased appetite	Muscle weakness, proximal myopathy
Diarrhea	Lid retraction or lag
Polyuria	Gynecomastia
Oligomenorrhea, loss of libido	

[a] Excludes the signs of ophthalmopathy and dermopathy specific for Graves' disease.

The most common cardiovascular manifestation is sinus tachycardia, often associated with palpitations and sometimes due to supraventricular tachycardia. The high cardiac output produces a bounding pulse, widened pulse pressure, and an aortic systolic murmur, and can lead to worsening of angina or heart failure in the elderly or those with preexisting heart disease. Atrial fibrillation is more common in patients >50. Treatment of the thyrotoxic state alone reverts atrial fibrillation to normal sinus rhythm in fewer than half of patients, suggesting the existence of an underlying cardiac problem in the remainder.

The skin is usually warm and moist, and the patient complains of sweating and heat intolerance, particularly during warm weather. Palmar erythema; onycholysis; and, less commonly, pruritus, urticaria, and diffuse hyperpigmentation may be evident. Hair texture may become fine, and a diffuse alopecia occurs in up to 40% of patients, persisting for months after restoration of euthyroidism. Gastrointestinal transit time is decreased, leading to increased stool frequency, often with diarrhea and occasionally mild steatorrhea. Women frequently experience oligomenorrhea or amenorrhea; in men there may be impaired sexual function and, rarely, gynecomastia. The direct effect of thyroid hormones on bone resorption leads to osteopenia in long-standing thyrotoxicosis; mild hypercalcemia occurs in up to 20% of patients, but hypercalcuria is more common. There is a small increase in fracture rate in patients with a previous history of thyrotoxicosis.

In Graves' disease the thyroid is usually diffusely enlarged to two to three times its normal size. The consistency is firm, but less so than in multinodular goiter. There may be a thrill or bruit due to the increased vascularity of the gland and the hyperdynamic circulation.

Lid retraction, causing a staring appearance, can occur in any form of thyrotoxicosis and is the result of sympathetic overactivity. However, Graves' disease is associated with specific eye signs that comprise *Graves' ophthalmopathy* (Fig. 330-6A). This condition is also called *thyroid-associated ophthalmopathy*, as it occurs in the absence of Graves' disease in 10% of patients. Most of these individuals have autoimmune hypothyroidism or thyroid antibodies. The onset of Graves' ophthalmopathy occurs within the year before or after the diagnosis of thyrotoxicosis in 75% of patients but can sometimes precede or follow thyrotoxicosis by several years, accounting for some cases of euthyroid ophthalmopathy.

Many patients with Graves' disease have little clinical evidence of ophthalmopathy. However, the enlarged extraocular muscles typical of the disease, and other subtle features, can be detected in almost all patients when investigated by ultrasound or computed tomography (CT) imaging of the orbits. Unilateral signs are found in up to 10% of patients. The earliest manifestations of ophthalmopathy are usually a sensation of grittiness, eye discomfort, and excess tearing. About a third of patients have proptosis, best detected by visualization of the sclera between the lower border of the iris and the lower eyelid, with the eyes in the primary position. Proptosis can be measured using an exophthalmometer. In severe cases, proptosis may cause corneal exposure and damage, especially if the lids fail to close during sleep. Periorbital edema, scleral injection, and chemosis are also frequent. In 5 to 10% of patients, the muscle swelling is so severe that diplopia results, typically but not exclusively when the patient looks up and laterally. The most serious manifestation is compression of the optic nerve at the apex of the orbit, leading to papilledema, peripheral field defects, and, if left untreated, permanent loss of vision.

Many scoring systems have been used to gauge the extent and activity of the orbital changes in Graves' disease. The NO SPECS scheme is an acronym derived from the following classes of eye change:

0 = No signs or symptoms
1 = Only signs (lid retraction or lag), no symptoms
2 = Soft tissue involvement (periorbital edema)
3 = Proptosis (>22 mm)
4 = Extraocular muscle involvement (diplopia)
5 = Corneal involvement
6 = Sight loss

Although useful as a mnemonic, the NO SPECS scheme is inadequate to describe the eye disease fully, and patients do not necessarily progress from one class to another. When Graves' eye disease is active and severe, referral to an ophthalmologist is indicated and objective measurements are needed, such as lid fissure width; corneal staining with fluorescein; and evaluation of extraocular muscle function (e.g., Hess chart), intraocular pressure and visual fields, acuity, and color vision.

Thyroid dermopathy occurs in <5% of patients with Graves' disease (Fig. 330-6*B*), almost always in the presence of moderate or severe ophthalmopathy. Although most frequent over the anterior and lateral aspects of the lower leg (hence the term *pretibial myxedema*), skin changes can occur at other sites, particularly after trauma. The typical lesion is a noninflamed, indurated plaque with a deep pink or purple color and an "orange-skin" appearance. Nodular involvement can occur, and the condition can rarely extend over the whole lower leg and foot, mimicking elephantiasis. *Thyroid acropachy* refers to a form of clubbing found in <1% of patients with Graves' disease (Fig. 330-6*C*). It is so strongly associated with thyroid dermopathy that an alternative cause of clubbing should be sought in a Graves' patient without coincident skin and orbital involvement.

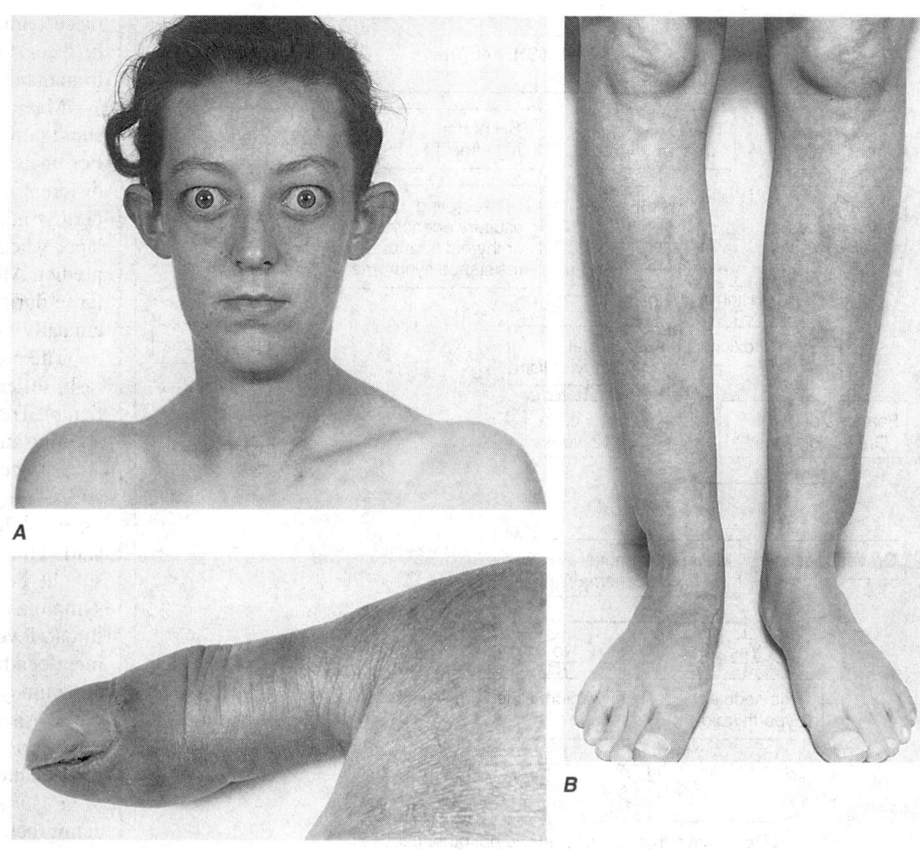

FIGURE 330-6 Features of Graves' disease. *A*. Facial appearance in Graves' disease; lid retraction, periorbital edema, and proptosis are marked. *B*. Thyroid dermopathy over the lateral aspects of the shins. *C*. Thyroid acropachy.

Laboratory Evaluation Investigations used to determine the existence and cause of thyrotoxicosis are summarized in Fig. 330-7. In Graves' disease, the TSH level is suppressed and free and total thyroid hormone levels are increased. In 2 to 5% of patients (and more in areas of borderline iodine intake), only T_3 is increased (T_3 toxicosis). The converse state of T_4 toxicosis, with elevated total and free T_4 and normal T_3 levels, is occasionally seen when hyperthyroidism is induced by excess iodine, providing surplus substrate for thyroid hormone synthesis. Measurement of TPO antibodies is useful in differential diagnosis, but assays for TSH-R antibodies are not usually needed. Associated abnormalities that may cause diagnostic confusion in thyrotoxicosis include elevation of bilirubin, liver enzymes, and ferritin. Microcytic anemia and thrombocytopenia occur less often.

Differential Diagnosis Diagnosis of Graves' disease is straightforward in a patient with biochemically confirmed thyrotoxicosis, diffuse goiter on palpation, ophthalmopathy, positive TPO antibodies, and often a personal or family history of autoimmune disorders. For patients with thyrotoxicosis who lack these features, the most reliable diagnostic method is a radionuclide (^{99m}Tc, ^{123}I, or ^{131}I) scan of the thyroid, which will distinguish the diffuse, high uptake of Graves' disease from nodular thyroid disease, destructive thyroiditis, ectopic thyroid tissue, and factitious thyrotoxicosis. In secondary hyperthyroidism due to a TSH-secreting pituitary tumor, there is also a diffuse goiter. The presence of a nonsuppressed TSH level, and the finding of a pituitary tumor on CT or magnetic resonance imaging (MRI) scan readily identify such patients.

Clinical features of thyrotoxicosis can mimic certain aspects of other disorders including panic attacks, mania, pheochromocytoma, and the weight loss associated with malignancy. The diagnosis of thyrotoxicosis can be easily excluded if the TSH level is normal. A normal TSH also excludes Graves' disease as a cause of diffuse goiter.

Clinical Course Clinical features generally worsen without treatment; mortality was 10 to 30% before the introduction of satisfactory therapy. Some patients with mild Graves' disease experience spontaneous relapses and remissions. Rarely, there may be fluctuation between hypo- and hyperthyroidism due to changes in the functional activity of TSH-R antibodies. About 15% of patients who enter remission after treatment with antithyroid drugs develop hypothyroidism 10 to 15 years later as a result of the destructive autoimmune process. The clinical course of ophthalmopathy does not follow that of the thyroid disease. Ophthalmopathy typically worsens over the initial 3 to 6 months, followed by a plateau phase over the next 12 to 18 months, with spontaneous improvement, particularly in the soft tissue changes. However, the course is more fulminant in up to 5% of patients, requiring intervention in the acute phase if there is optic nerve compression or corneal ulceration. Diplopia may appear late in the disease due to fibrosis of the extraocular muscles. Some studies suggest that radioiodine treatment for hyperthyroidism worsens the eye disease in a small proportion of patients (especially smokers). Antithyroid drugs or surgery have no adverse effects on the clinical course of ophthalmopathy. Thyroid dermopathy, when it occurs, usually appears 1 to 2 years after the development of Graves' hyperthyroidism; it may improve spontaneously.

℞ TREATMENT The *hyperthyroidism* of Graves' disease is treated by reducing thyroid hormone synthesis, using antithyroid drugs, or by reducing the amount of thyroid tissue with radioiodine (^{131}I) treatment or subtotal thyroidectomy. Antithyroid drugs are the predominant therapy in many centers in Europe and Japan, whereas radioiodine is more often the first line of treatment in North America. These differences reflect the fact that no single approach is optimal and that patients may require multiple treatments to achieve remission.

The main *antithyroid drugs* are the thionamides, such as propyl-

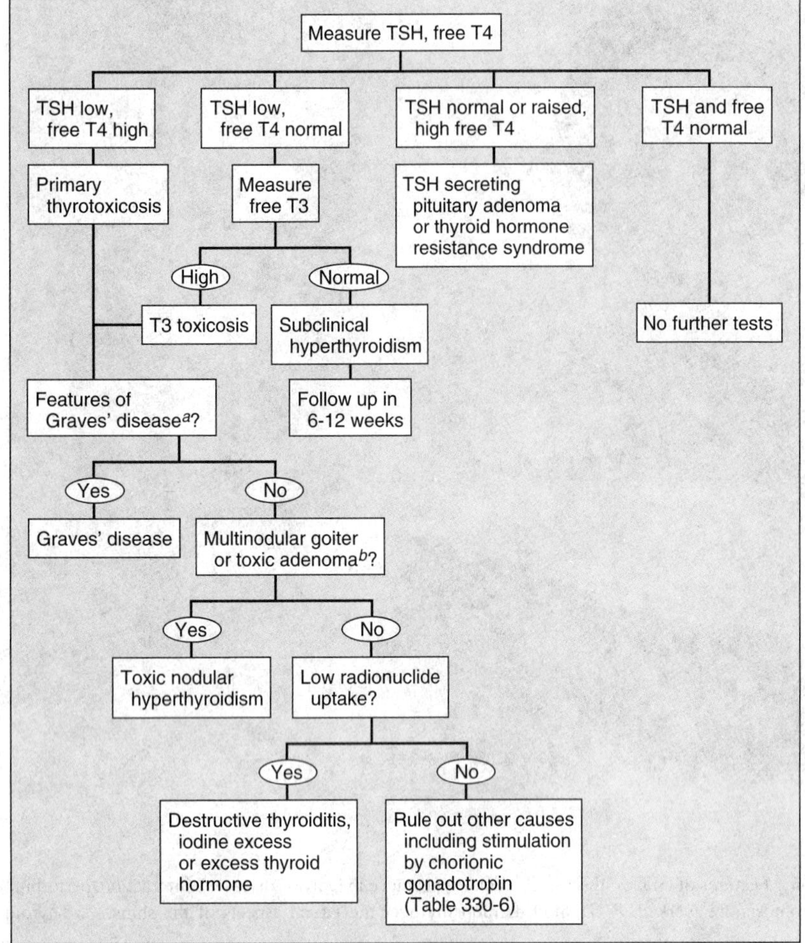

FIGURE 330-7 Evaluation of thyrotoxicosis. [a]Diffuse goiter, positive TPO antibodies, ophthalmopathy, dermopathy; [b] can be confirmed by radionuclide scan.

thiouracil, carbimazole, and the active metabolite of the latter, methimazole. All inhibit the function of TPO, reducing oxidation and organification of iodide. These drugs also reduce thyroid antibody levels by mechanisms that remain unclear, and they appear to enhance rates of remission. Propylthiouracil inhibits deiodination of $T_4 \rightarrow T_3$. However, this effect is of minor benefit, except in the most severe thyrotoxicosis, and is offset by the much shorter half-life of this drug (90 min) compared to methimazole (6 h).

There are many variations of antithyroid drug regimens. The initial dose of carbimazole or methimazole is usually 10 to 20 mg every 8 or 12 h, but once-daily dosing is possible after euthyroidism is restored. Propylthiouracil is given at a dose of 100 to 200 mg every 6 to 8 h, and divided doses are usually given throughout the course. Lower doses of each drug may suffice in areas of low iodine intake. The starting dose of antithyroid drugs can be gradually reduced (titration regimen) as thyrotoxicosis improves. Alternatively, high doses may be given combined with levothyroxine supplementation (block-replace regimen) to avoid drug-induced hypothyroidism. Initial reports suggesting superior remission rates with the block-replace regimen have not been reproduced in several other trials. The titration regimen is often preferred to minimize the dose of antithyroid drug and provide an index of treatment response.

Thyroid function tests and clinical manifestations are reviewed 3 to 4 weeks after starting treatment, and the dose is titrated based on free T_4 levels. Most patients do not achieve euthyroidism until 6 to 8 weeks after treatment is initiated. TSH levels often remain suppressed for several months and therefore do not provide a sensitive index of treatment response. The usual daily maintenance doses of antithyroid drugs in the titration regimen are 2.5 to 10 mg of carbimazole or methimazole and 50 to 100 mg of propylthiouracil. In the block-replace regimen, the initial dose of antithyroid drug is held constant and the dose of levothyroxine is adjusted to maintain normal free T_4 levels.

Maximum remission rates (up to 30 to 50% in some populations) are achieved by 18 to 24 months. For unclear reasons, remission rates appear to vary in different geographic regions. Patients with severe hyperthyroidism and large goiters are most likely to relapse when treatment stops, but outcome is difficult to predict. All patients should be followed closely for relapse during the first year after treatment and at least annually thereafter.

The common side effects of antithyroid drugs are rash, urticaria, fever, and arthralgia (1 to 5% of patients). These may resolve spontaneously or after substituting an alternative antithyroid drug. Rare but major side effects include hepatitis, an SLE-like syndrome, and, most importantly, agranulocytosis (<1%). It is essential that antithyroid drugs are stopped and not restarted if a patient develops major side effects. Patients should be given written instructions regarding the symptoms of possible agranulocytosis (e.g., sore throat, fever, mouth ulcers) and the need to stop treatment pending a complete blood count to confirm that agranulocytosis is not present. Management of agranulocytosis is described in Chap. 109. Most physicians do not prospectively monitor blood counts, as the onset of agranulocytosis is idiosyncratic and abrupt.

Propranolol (20 to 40 mg every 6 h) or longer acting beta blockers, such as atenolol, may be useful to control adrenergic symptoms, especially in the early stages before antithyroid drugs take effect. Anticoagulation with warfarin should be considered in all patients with atrial fibrillation. If digoxin is used, increased doses are often needed in the thyrotoxic state.

Radioiodine causes progressive destruction of thyroid cells and can be used as initial treatment or for relapses after a trial of antithyroid drugs. There is a small risk of thyrotoxic crisis (see below) after radioiodine, which can be avoided by pretreatment with antithyroid drugs for at least a month before treatment. Antecedent treatment with antithyroid drugs should be considered in all elderly patients, or in those with cardiac problems, to deplete thyroid hormone stores before administration of radioiodine. Antithyroid drugs must be stopped 3 to 5 days before radioiodine administration to achieve optimum iodine uptake.

Efforts to calculate an optimal dose of radioiodine that achieves euthyroidism, without a high incidence of relapse or progression to hypothyroidism, have not been successful. Some patients inevitably relapse after a single dose because the biologic effects of radiation vary between individuals, and hypothyroidism cannot be uniformly avoided even using accurate dosimetry. A practical strategy is to give a fixed dose based on clinical features, such as the severity of thyrotoxicosis, the size of the goiter (increases the dose needed), and the level of radioiodine uptake (decreases the dose needed). ^{131}I dosage generally ranges between 185 MBq (5 mCi) to 555 MBq (15 mCi). Incomplete treatment or early relapse is more common in males and in patients <40 years of age. Many authorities favor an approach aimed at thyroid ablation (as opposed to euthyroidism), given that levothyroxine replacement is straightforward and most patients ultimately progress to hypothyroidism over 5 to 10 years anyway, frequently with some delay in the diagnosis of hypothyroidism.

Certain radiation safety precautions are necessary in the first few days after radioiodine treatment, but the exact guidelines vary depending on local protocols. In general, patients need to avoid close, prolonged contact with children and pregnant women for several days because of possible transmission of residual isotope and excessive exposure to radiation emanating from the gland. Rarely there may be mild pain due to radiation thyroiditis 1 to 2 weeks after treatment.

Hyperthyroidism can persist for 2 to 3 months before radioiodine takes full effect. For this reason, β-adrenergic blockers or antithyroid drugs can be used to control symptoms during this interval. Persistent hyperthyroidism can be treated with a second dose of radioiodine, usually 6 months after the first dose. The risk of hypothyroidism after radioiodine depends on the dosage but is at least 10 to 20% in the first year and 5% per year thereafter. Patients should be informed of this possibility before treatment and require close follow-up during the first year and annual thyroid function testing thereafter.

Pregnancy and breast feeding are absolute contraindications to radioiodine treatment, but patients can conceive safely 6 to 12 months after treatment. The presence of severe ophthalmopathy requires caution, and some authorities advocate the use of prednisone, 40 mg/d, at the time of radioiodine treatment, tapered over 2 to 3 months to prevent exacerbation of ophthalmopathy. The overall risk of cancer after radioiodine treatment in adults is not increased, but many physicians avoid radioiodine in children and adolescents because of the theoretical risks of malignancy.

Subtotal thyroidectomy is an option for patients who relapse after antithyroid drugs and prefer this treatment to radioiodine. Some experts recommend surgery in young individuals, particularly when the goiter is very large. Careful control of thyrotoxicosis with antithyroid drugs, followed by potassium iodide (3 drops SSKI orally tid) is needed prior to surgery to avoid thyrotoxic crisis and to reduce the vascularity of the gland. The major complications of surgery—i.e., bleeding, laryngeal edema, hypoparathyroidism, and damage to the recurrent laryngeal nerves—are unusual when the procedure is performed by highly experienced surgeons. Recurrence rates in the best series are <2%, but the rate of hypothyroidism is only slightly less than that following radioiodine treatment.

The titration regimen of antithyroid drugs should be used to manage Graves' disease in *pregnancy*, as blocking doses of these drugs produce fetal hypothyroidism. Propylthiouracil is usually used because of relatively low transplacental transfer and its ability to block $T_4 \rightarrow T_3$ conversion. Also, carbimazole and methimazole have been associated with rare cases of fetal *aplasia cutis*. The lowest effective dose of propylthiouracil should be given, and it is often possible to stop treatment in the last trimester since TSH-R antibodies tend to decline in pregnancy. Nonetheless, the transplacental transfer of these antibodies rarely causes *fetal thyrotoxicosis* or *neonatal thyrotoxicosis*. Poor intrauterine growth, a fetal heart rate of >160 beats/min, and high levels of maternal TSH-R antibodies should suggest this complication. Antithyroid drugs given to the mother can be used to treat the fetus and may be needed for 1 to 3 months after delivery, until the maternal antibodies disappear from the baby's circulation. The postpartum period is a time of major risk for relapse of Graves' disease. Breast feeding is safe with low doses of antithyroid drugs. Graves' disease in *children* is best managed with antithyroid drugs, often given as a prolonged course of the titration regimen. Surgery may be indicated for severe disease. Radioiodine can also be used in children, though most experts defer this treatment until adolescence or later.

Thyrotoxic crisis, or *thyroid storm*, is rare and presents as a life-threatening exacerbation of hyperthyroidism, accompanied by fever, delirium, seizures, coma, vomiting, diarrhea, and jaundice. The mortality rate due to cardiac failure, arrhythmia, or hyperthermia is ~30%, even with treatment. Thyrotoxic crisis is usually precipitated by acute illness (e.g., stroke, infection, trauma, diabetic ketoacidosis), surgery (especially on the thyroid), or radioiodine treatment of a patient with partially treated or untreated hyperthyroidism. Management requires intensive monitoring and supportive care, identification and treatment of the precipitating cause, and measures that reduce thyroid hormone synthesis. Large doses of propylthiouracil (600-mg loading dose and 200 to 300 mg every 6 h) should be given orally or by nasogastric tube or per rectum; the drug's inhibitory action on $T_4 \rightarrow T_3$ conversion makes it the agent of choice. One hour after the first dose of propylthiouracil, stable iodide is given to block thyroid hormone synthesis via the Wolff-Chaikoff effect (the delay allows the antithyroid drug to prevent the excess iodine from being incorporated into new hormone).

A saturated solution of potassium iodide (5 drops SSKI every 6 h), or ipodate or iopanoic acid (0.5 mg every 12 h), may be given orally. (Sodium iodide, 0.25 g intravenously every 6 h is an alternative but is not generally available.) Propranolol should also be given to reduce tachycardia and other adrenergic manifestations (40 to 60 mg orally every 4 h; or 2 mg intravenously every 4 h). Although other β-adrenergic blockers can be used, high doses of propranolol have been documented to decrease $T_4 \rightarrow T_3$ conversion, and the doses can be easily adjusted. Caution is needed to avoid acute negative inotropic effects, but controlling the heart rate is important, as some patients develop a form of high-output heart failure. Additional therapeutic measures include glucocorticoids (e.g., dexamethasone, 2 mg every 6 h), antibiotics if infection is present, cooling, and intravenous fluids.

Ophthalmopathy requires no active treatment when it is mild or moderate, as there is usually spontaneous improvement. General measures include meticulous control of thyroid hormone levels, advice about cessation of smoking, and an explanation of the natural history of ophthalmopathy. Discomfort can be relieved with artificial tears (e.g., 1% methylcellulose) and the use of dark glasses with side frames. Periorbital edema responds to a more upright sleeping position. Corneal exposure during sleep can be avoided by taping the eyelids shut. Minor degrees of diplopia improve with prisms fitted to spectacles. Severe ophthalmopathy, with optic nerve involvement or chemosis resulting in corneal damage, is an emergency requiring joint management with an ophthalmologist. Short-term benefit can be gained in about two-thirds of patients by the use of high-dose glucocorticoids (e.g., prednisone, 40 to 80 mg daily), sometimes combined with cyclosporine. Glucocorticoid doses are tapered by 5 mg every 1 to 2 weeks, but the taper often results in reemergence of congestive symptoms. Pulse therapy with intravenous methylprednisolone (1 g of methylprednisolone in 250 mL of saline infused over 2 h daily for 1 week) followed by an oral regimen is also used. Once the eye disease has stabilized, surgery may be indicated for relief of diplopia and correction of the appearance of the eyes. Orbital decompression can be achieved by removing bone from any wall of the orbit, thereby allowing displacement of fat and swollen extraocular muscles. The transantral route is used most often, as it requires no external incision. Proptosis recedes an average of 5 mm, but there may be residual or even worsened diplopia. Alternatively, retroorbital tissue can be decompressed without removal of bony tissue. External beam radiotherapy of the orbits has been used for many years, but the objective evidence that this therapy is beneficial remains equivocal.

Thyroid dermopathy does not usually require treatment but can cause cosmetic problems or interfere with the fit of shoes. Surgical removal is not indicated. Treatment consists of topical, high-potency glucocorticoid ointment under an occlusive dressing. Octreotide may be beneficial.

OTHER CAUSES OF THYROTOXICOSIS Destructive thyroiditis (subacute or silent thyroiditis) typically presents with a short thyrotoxic phase due to the release of preformed thyroid hormones and catabolism of Tg (see "Subacute Thyroiditis," below). True hyperthyroidism is absent, as demonstrated by a low radionuclide uptake. Circulating Tg and IL-6 levels are usually increased. Other causes of thyrotoxicosis with low or absent thyroid radionuclide uptake include *thyrotoxicosis factitia*; iodine excess and, rarely, ectopic thyroid tissue, particularly teratomas of the ovary (*struma ovarii*); and functional metastatic follicular carcinoma. Whole-body radionuclide studies can demonstrate ectopic thyroid tissue, and thyrotoxicosis factitia can be distinguished from destructive thyroiditis by the clinical features and low levels of Tg. Amiodarone treatment is associated with thyrotoxicosis in up to 10% of patients, particularly in areas of low iodine intake.

TSH-secreting pituitary adenoma is a rare causes of thyrotoxicosis. It can be identified by the presence of an inappropriately normal or increased TSH level in a patient with hyperthyroidism, diffuse goiter, and elevated free T_4 and T_3 levels (Chap. 328). Elevated levels of the α subunit of TSH, released by the TSH-secreting adenoma, support this diagnosis, which can be confirmed by demonstrating the pituitary tumor on CT or MRI scan. A combination of transsphenoidal surgery, sella irradiation, and octreotide may be required to normalize TSH, as many of these tumors are large and locally invasive at the time of diagnosis. Radioiodine or antithyroid drugs can be used to control thyrotoxicosis.

Thyrotoxicosis caused by *toxic multinodular goiter* and *hyperfunctioning solitary nodules* is discussed below.

THYROIDITIS

A clinically useful classification of thyroiditis is based on the onset and duration of disease (Table 330-8).

ACUTE THYROIDITIS Acute thyroiditis is rare and is due to suppurative infection of the thyroid. In children and young adults, the most common cause is the presence of a piriform sinus, a remnant of the fourth branchial pouch that connects the oropharynx with the thyroid. Such sinuses are predominantly left sided. A long-standing goiter and degeneration in a thyroid malignancy are risk factors in the elderly. The patient presents with thyroid pain, often referred to the throat or ears, and a small, tender goiter that may be asymmetric. Fever, dysphagia, and erythema over the thyroid are common, as are systemic symptoms of a febrile illness and lymphadenopathy.

The differential diagnosis of *thyroid pain* includes subacute or, rarely, chronic thyroiditis, hemorrhage into a cyst, malignancy including lymphoma, and, rarely, amiodarone-induced thyroiditis or amyloidosis. However, the abrupt presentation and clinical features of acute thyroiditis rarely cause confusion. The erythrocyte sedimentation rate (ESR) and white cell count are usually increased, but thyroid function is normal. FNA biopsy shows infiltration by polymorphonuclear leukocytes; culture of the sample can identify the organism. Caution is needed in immunocompromised patients as fungal or *Pneumocystis* thyroiditis can occur in this setting. Antibiotic treatment is guided initially by Gram stain and subsequently by cultures of the FNA biopsy. Surgery may be needed to drain an abscess, which can be localized by CT scan or ultrasound. Tracheal obstruction, septicemia, retropharyngeal abscess, mediastinitis, and jugular venous thrombosis may complicate acute thyroiditis but are uncommon with prompt use of antibiotics.

SUBACUTE THYROIDITIS This is also termed *de Quervain's thyroiditis*, *granulomatous thyroiditis*, or *viral thyroiditis*. Many viruses have been implicated, including mumps, coxsackie, influenza, adenoviruses, and echoviruses, but attempts to identify the virus in an individual patient are often unsuccessful and do not influence management. The diagnosis of subacute thyroiditis is often overlooked because the symptoms can mimic pharyngitis. The peak incidence occurs at 30 to 50 years, and women are affected three times more frequently than men.

Table 330-8 Causes of Thyroiditis

Acute
Bacterial infection: especially *Staphylcoccus*, *Streptococcus*, and *Enterobacter*
Fungal infection: *Aspergillus*, *Candida*, *Coccidioides*, *Histoplasma*, and *Pneumocystis*
Radiation thyroiditis after ^{131}I treatment
Amiodarone (may also be subacute or chronic)
Subacute
Viral (or granulomatous) thyroiditis
Silent thyroiditis (including postpartum thyroiditis)
Mycobacterial infection
Chronic
Autoimmunity: focal thyroiditis, Hashimoto's thyroiditis, atrophic thyroiditis
Riedel's thyroiditis
Parasitic thyroiditis: echinococcosis, strongyloidiasis, cysticercosis
Traumatic: after palpation

Pathophysiology The thyroid shows a characteristic patchy inflammatory infiltrate with disruption of the thyroid follicles and multinucleated giant cells within some follicles. The follicular changes progress to granulomas accompanied by fibrosis. Finally, the thyroid returns to normal, usually several months after onset. During the initial phase of follicular destruction, there is release of Tg and thyroid hormones, leading to increased circulating free T_4 and T_3 and suppression of TSH (Fig. 330-8). During this destructive phase, radioactive iodine uptake is low or undetectable. After several weeks, the thyroid is depleted of stored thyroid hormone and a phase of hypothyroidism typically occurs, with low free T_4 (and sometimes T_3) and moderately increased TSH levels. Radioactive iodine uptake returns to normal or is even increased as a result of the rise in TSH. Finally, thyroid hormone and TSH levels return to normal as the disease subsides.

Clinical Manifestations The patient usually presents with a painful and enlarged thyroid, sometimes accompanied by fever. There may be features of thyrotoxicosis or hypothyroidism, depending on the phase of the illness. Malaise and symptoms of an upper respiratory tract infection may precede the thyroid-related features by several weeks. In other patients, the onset is acute, severe, and without obvious antecedent. Though the patient typically complains of a sore throat, examination reveals a small goiter that is exquisitely tender, and asymmetry is common. Pain is often referred to the jaw or ear. Complete resolution is the usual outcome, but permanent hypothyroidism can occur, particularly in those with coincidental thyroid autoimmunity. A prolonged course over many months, with one or more relapses, occurs in a small percentage of patients.

Laboratory Evaluation As depicted in Fig. 330-8, thyroid function tests characteristically evolve through three distinct phases over about 6 months: (1) thyrotoxic phase, (2) hypothyroid phase, and (3) recovery phase. In the thyrotoxic phase, T_4 and T_3 levels are increased, reflecting their discharge from the damaged thyroid cells, and TSH is suppressed. The T_4/T_3 ratio is greater than in Graves' disease or thyroid autonomy, in which T_3 is often disproportionately increased. The diagnosis is confirmed by a high ESR and low radioiodine uptake. Serum IL-6 levels increase during the thyrotoxic phase. The white blood cell count may be increased, and thyroid antibodies are negative. If the diagnosis is in doubt, FNA biopsy may be useful, particularly to distinguish unilateral involvement from bleeding into a cyst or neoplasm.

TREATMENT Relatively large doses of aspirin (e.g., 600 mg every 4 to 6 h) or nonsteroidal anti-inflammatory drugs are suf-

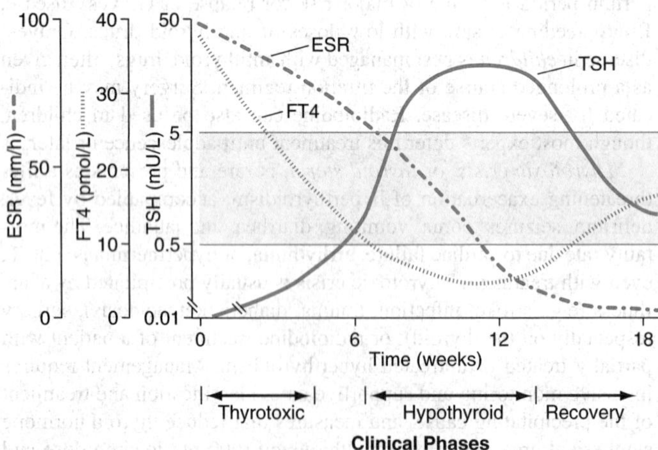

FIGURE 330-8 Clinical course of subacute thyroiditis. The release of thyroid hormones is initially associated with a thyrotoxic phase and suppressed TSH. A hypothyroid phase then ensues, with low T_4 and TSH levels that are initially low but gradually increase. During the recovery phase, increased TSH levels combined with resolution of thyroid follicular injury leads to normalization of thyroid function, often several months after the beginning of the illness.

ficient to control symptoms in most cases. If this treatment is inadequate, or if the patient has marked local or systemic symptoms, glucocorticoids should be given. The usual starting dose is 40 to 60 mg prednisone, depending on severity. The dose is gradually tapered over 6 to 8 weeks, in response to improvement in symptoms and the ESR. If a relapse occurs during glucocorticoid withdrawal, treatment should be started again and withdrawn more gradually. In these patients, it is useful to wait until the radioactive iodine uptake normalizes before stopping treatment. Thyroid function should be monitored every 2 to 4 weeks using TSH and free T_4 levels. Symptoms of thyrotoxicosis improve spontaneously but may be ameliorated by β-adrenergic blockers; antithyroid drugs play no role in treatment of the thyrotoxic phase. Levothyroxine replacement may be needed if the hypothyroid phase is prolonged, but doses should be low enough (50 to 100 μg daily) to allow TSH-mediated recovery.

SILENT THYROIDITIS *Painless thyroiditis*, or *"silent" thyroiditis*, occurs in patients with underlying autoimmune thyroid disease. It has a clinical course similar to that of subacute thyroiditis, except that there is little or no thyroid tenderness. The condition occurs most frequently 3 to 6 months after pregnancy and is then termed *postpartum thyroiditis*. Typically, patients have a brief phase of thyrotoxicosis, lasting 2 to 4 weeks, followed by hypothyroidism for 4 to 12 weeks, and then resolution; often, however, only one phase is apparent. As in subacute thyroiditis, the radioactive iodine uptake is initially suppressed. In addition to the painless goiter, silent thyroiditis can be distinguished from subacute thyroiditis by the normal ESR and the presence of TPO antibodies. Glucocorticoid treatment is not indicated for silent thyroiditis. Severe thyrotoxic symptoms can be managed with a brief course of propranolol, 20 to 40 mg three or four times daily. Thyroxine replacement may be needed for the hypothyroid phase but should be withdrawn after 6 to 9 months, as recovery is the rule. Annual follow-up thereafter is recommended, as a proportion of these individuals develop permanent hypothyroidism.

DRUG-INDUCED THYROIDITIS Patients receiving IFN-α, IL-2, or amiodarone may develop painless thyroiditis. INF-α, which is used to treat chronic hepatitis B or C, causes thyroid dysfunction in up to 5% of treated patients. It has been associated with painless thyroiditis, hypothyroidism, and Graves' disease. IL-2, which has been used to treat various malignancies, has also been associated with thyroiditis and hypothyroidism, though fewer patients have been studied. For discussion of amiodarone, see "Amiodarone Effects on Thyroid Function," below.

CHRONIC THYROIDITIS The most common cause of chronic thyroiditis is *Hashimoto's thyroiditis*, an autoimmune disorder that often presents as a firm or hard goiter of variable size (see above). *Riedel's thyroiditis* is a rare disorder that typically occurs in middle-aged women. It presents with an insidious, painless goiter with local symptoms due to compression of the esophagus, trachea, neck veins, or recurrent laryngeal nerves. Dense fibrosis disrupts normal gland architecture and can extend outside the thyroid capsule. Despite these extensive histologic changes, thyroid dysfunction is uncommon. The goiter is hard, nontender, often asymmetric and fixed, leading to suspicion of a malignancy. Diagnosis requires open biopsy as FNA biopsy is usually unhelpful. Treatment is surgical and directed to relief of compressive symptoms. There is an association between Riedel's thyroiditis and idiopathic fibrosis at other sites (retroperitoneum, mediastinum, biliary tree, lung, and orbit).

SICK EUTHYROID SYNDROME

Any acute, severe illness can cause abnormalities of circulating TSH or thyroid hormone levels in the absence of underlying thyroid disease, making these measurements potentially misleading. The major cause of these hormonal changes is the release of cytokines. Unless a thyroid disorder is strongly suspected, the routine testing of thyroid function should be avoided in acutely ill patients.

The most common hormone pattern in sick euthyroid syndrome

(SES) is a decrease in total and free T_3 levels (low T_3 syndrome) with normal levels of T_4 and TSH. The magnitude of the fall in T_3 correlates with the severity of the illness. T_4 conversion to T_3 via peripheral deiodination is impaired, leading to increased reverse T_3 (rT_3). Despite this effect, decreased clearance rather than increased production is the major basis for increased rT_3. Also, T_4 is alternately metabolized to the hormonally inactive T_3 sulfate. It is generally assumed that this low T_3 state is adaptive, as it can be induced in normal individuals by fasting. Teleologically, the fall in T_3 may provide a mechanism for limiting catabolism in starved or ill patients.

Very sick patients may have a fall in total T_4 and T_3 levels (low T_4 syndrome). This state has a poor prognosis. A key factor in the fall in T_4 levels is altered binding to TBG. Free T_4 assays usually demonstrate a normal free T_4 level in such patients, depending on the assay method used. Fluctuation in TSH levels also creates challenges in the interpretation of thyroid function in sick patients. TSH levels may range from <0.1 to >20 mU/L; these alterations reverse after recovery, confirming the absence of underlying thyroid disease. A rise in cortisol or administration of glucocorticoids may provide a partial explanation for decreased TSH levels. However, the exact mechanisms underlying the subnormal TSH seen in 10% of sick patients and the increased TSH seen in 5% remain unclear.

Any severe illness can induce changes in thyroid hormone levels, but certain disorders exhibit a distinctive pattern of abnormalities. Acute liver disease is associated with an initial rise in total (but not free) T_3 and T_4 levels, due to TBG release; these levels become subnormal with progression to liver failure. A transient increase in total and free T_4 levels, usually with a normal T_3 level, is seen in 5 to 30% of acutely ill psychiatric patients. TSH values may be transiently low, normal, or high in these patients. In the early stage of HIV infection, T_3 and T_4 levels rise, even if there is weight loss. T_3 levels fall with progression to AIDS, but TSH levels usually remain normal. Renal disease is often accompanied by low T_3 concentrations, but with normal rather than increased rT_3 levels, due to an unknown factor that increases uptake of rT_3 into the liver.

The diagnosis of the SES is challenging. Historic information may be limited, and patients often have multiple metabolic derangements. Useful features to consider include previous history of thyroid disease and thyroid function tests, evaluation of the severity and time course of the patient's acute illness, documentation of medications that may affect thyroid function or thyroid hormone levels, and measurements of rT_3 together with free thyroid hormones and TSH. The diagnosis of SES is frequently presumptive, given the clinical context and pattern of laboratory values; only resolution of the test results with clinical recovery can clearly establish this disorder. Treatment of SES with thyroid hormone (T_4 and/or T_3) is controversial, but most authorities recommend monitoring the patient's thyroid function tests during recovery, without administering thyroid hormone, unless there is historic or clinical evidence suggestive of hypothyroidism. Sufficiently large randomized controlled trials using thyroid hormone are unlikely to resolve this therapeutic controversy in the near future, because clinical presentations and outcomes are highly variable.

AMIODARONE EFFECTS ON THYROID FUNCTION

Amiodarone is a commonly used type III antiarrhythmic agent (Chap. 230). It is structurally related to thyroid hormone and contains 39% iodine by weight. Thus, typical doses of amiodarone (200 mg/d) are associated with very high iodine intake, leading to >40-fold increases in plasma and urinary iodine levels. Moreover, because amiodarone is stored in adipose tissue, high iodine levels persist for >6 months after discontinuation of the drug. Amiodarone inhibits deiodinase activity, and its metabolites function as weak antagonists of thyroid hormone action. Amiodarone has the following multiple effects on thyroid function: (1) acute, transient changes in thyroid function; (2) hypothyroidism in patients susceptible to the inhibitory effects of a high iodine load; and (3) thyrotoxicosis that may be caused by at least three mechanisms—a Jod-Basedow effect from the iodine load in the setting of multinodular goiter, a thyroiditis-like condition, and possibly induction of autoimmune Graves' disease.

The initiation of amiodarone treatment is associated with a transient decrease of T_4 levels, reflecting the inhibitory effect of iodine on T_4 release. Soon thereafter, most individuals escape from iodide-dependent suppression of the thyroid (Wolff-Chaikoff effect), and the inhibitory effects on deiodinase activity and thyroid hormone receptor action become predominant. These events lead to the following pattern of thyroid function tests: increased T_4, decreased T_3, increased rT_3, and a transient increase of TSH (up to 20 mU/L). TSH levels normalize or are slightly suppressed after about 1 to 3 months.

The incidence of hypothyroidism from amiodarone varies geographically, apparently correlating with iodine intake. Hypothyroidism occurs in up to 13% of amiodarone-treated patients in iodine-replete countries, such as the United States, but is less common (<6% incidence) in areas of lower iodine intake, such as Italy or Spain. The pathogenesis appears to involve an inability of the thyroid to escape from the high iodine load. Consequently, amiodarone-associated hypothyroidism is more common in women and individuals with positive TPO antibodies. It is usually unnecessary to discontinue amiodarone for this side effect, as levothyroxine can be used to normalize thyroid function. TSH levels should be monitored, because T_4 levels are often increased for the reasons described above.

The management of amiodarone-induced thyrotoxicosis (AIT) is complicated by the fact that there are several causes of thyrotoxicosis and because the increased thyroid hormone levels exacerbate underlying arrhythmias and coronary artery disease. Amiodarone treatment causes thyrotoxicosis in 10% of patients living in areas of low iodine intake and in 2% of patients in regions of high iodine intake. There are two major forms of AIT. Type 1 AIT is associated with an underlying thyroid abnormality (preclinical Graves' disease or nodular goiter). Thyroid hormone synthesis becomes excessive as a result of increased iodine exposure (Jod-Basedow phenomenon). Type 2 AIT occurs in individuals with no intrinsic thyroid abnormalities and is the result of drug-induced lysosomal activation leading to destructive thyroiditis with histiocyte accumulation in the thyroid. Mild forms of type 2 AIT can resolve spontaneously or can occasionally lead to hypothyroidism. Color-flow doppler thyroid scanning shows increased vascularity in type 1 but decreased vascularity in type 2 AIT; IL-6 levels are markedly raised in type 2 but only slightly increased in type 1 AIT. Thyroid scans are difficult to interpret in this setting, because the high endogenous iodine levels diminish tracer uptake. However, the presence of normal or increased uptake favors type 1 AIT.

In amiodarone-induced thyrotoxicosis the drug should be stopped, if possible, though this is often impractical because of the underlying cardiac disorder. Discontinuation of amiodarone will not have an acute effect because of its storage and prolonged half-life. High doses of antithyroid drugs can be used in type 1 AIT but are often ineffective. Potassium perchlorate, 200 mg every 6 h, has been used to reduce thyroidal iodide content. Perchlorate treatment has been associated with agranulocytosis, though the risk appears relatively low with short-term use. Glucocorticoids, administered as for subacute thyroiditis, are beneficial in type 2 AIT. Lithium blocks thyroid hormone release and can provide modest benefit. Near-total thyroidectomy rapidly decreases thyroid hormone levels and may be the most effective long-term solution, if the patient can undergo the procedure safely.

THYROID FUNCTION IN PREGNANCY

Three factors alter thyroid function in pregnancy: (1) the transient increase in hCG during the first trimester, which stimulates the TSH-R; (2) the estrogen-induced rise in TBG during the first trimester, which is sustained during pregnancy; and (3) increased urinary iodide excretion, which can cause impaired thyroid hormone production in areas of marginal iodine sufficiency. Women with a precarious iodine intake (<50 μg/d) are most at risk of developing a goiter during pregnancy, and iodine supplementation should be considered to prevent maternal and fetal hypothyroidism and the development of neonatal goiter.

The rise in circulating hCG levels during the first trimester is accompanied by a reciprocal fall in TSH that persists into the middle of pregnancy. This appears to reflect weak binding of hCG, which is present at very high levels, to the TSH-R. Rare individuals have been described with variant TSH-R sequences that enhance hCG binding and TSH-R activation. Occasionally these hCG-induced changes in thyroid function result in transient gestational hyperthyroidism and/or *hyperemesis gravidarum*, a condition characterized by severe nausea and vomiting and risk of volume depletion. Antithyroid drugs are rarely needed, and parenteral fluid replacement usually suffices until the condition resolves.

Maternal hypothyroidism occurs in 2 to 3% of women of child-bearing age and is associated with increased risk of developmental delay in the offspring. Thyroid hormone requirements are increased by 25 to 50 μg/d during pregnancy.

GOITER AND NODULAR THYROID DISEASE

Goiter refers to an enlarged thyroid gland. Biosynthetic defects, iodine deficiency, autoimmune disease, and nodular diseases can each lead to goiter, though by different mechanisms. Biosynthetic defects and iodine deficiency are associated with reduced efficiency of thyroid hormone synthesis, leading to increased TSH, which stimulates thyroid growth as a compensatory mechanism to overcome the block in hormone synthesis. Graves' disease and Hashimoto's thyroiditis are also associated with goiter. In Graves' disease, the goiter results mainly from the TSH-R-mediated effects of TSI. The goitrous form of Hashimoto's thyroiditis occurs because of acquired defects in hormone synthesis, leading to elevated levels of TSH and its consequent growth effects. Lymphocytic infiltration and immune system–induced growth factors also contribute to thyroid enlargement in Hashimoto's thyroiditis. Nodular disease is characterized by the disordered growth of thyroid follicles, often combined with the gradual development of fibrosis. The management of goiter differs in patients depending on the etiology, and the detection of thyroid enlargement on physical examination should prompt further evaluation to identify its cause.

Nodular thyroid disease is common, occurring in about 3 to 7% of adults when assessed by physical examination. Using more sensitive techniques, such as ultrasound, it is present in >25% of adults. Thyroid nodules may be solitary or multiple, and they may be functional or nonfunctional.

DIFFUSE NONTOXIC (SIMPLE) GOITER Etiology and Pathogenesis When diffuse enlargement of the thyroid occurs in the absence of nodules and hyperthyroidism, it is referred to as a *diffuse nontoxic goiter*. This is sometimes called *simple goiter*, because of the absence of nodules, or *colloid goiter*, because of the presence of uniform follicles that are filled with colloid. Worldwide, diffuse goiter is most commonly caused by iodine deficiency and is termed *endemic goiter* when it affects >5% of the population. In nonendemic regions, *sporadic goiter* occurs, and the cause is usually unknown. Thyroid enlargement in teenagers is sometimes referred to as *juvenile goiter*. In general, goiter is more common in women than men, probably because of the greater prevalence of underlying autoimmune disease and the increased iodine demands associated with pregnancy.

In *iodine-deficient areas*, thyroid enlargement reflects a compensatory effort to trap iodide and produce sufficient hormone under conditions in which hormone synthesis is relatively inefficient. Somewhat surprisingly, TSH levels are usually normal or only slightly increased, suggesting increased sensitivity to TSH or activation of other pathways that lead to thyroid growth. Iodide appears to have direct actions on thyroid vasculature and may indirectly affect growth through vasoactive substances such as endothelins and nitric oxide. Endemic goiter is also caused by exposure to environmental *goitrogens* such as cassava root, which contains a thiocyanate, vegetables of the Cruciferae family (e.g., brussels sprouts, cabbage, and cauliflower), and milk from regions where goitrogens are present in grass. Though relatively rare, inherited defects in thyroid hormone synthesis also lead to a diffuse nontoxic goiter. These involve abnormalities at each step in hormone synthesis including iodide transport (NIS), Tg synthesis, organification and coupling (TPO), and the regeneration of iodide (dehalogenase).

Clinical Manifestations and Diagnosis If thyroid function is preserved, most goiters are asymptomatic. Spontaneous hemorrhage into a cyst or nodule may cause the sudden onset of localized pain and swelling. Examination of a diffuse goiter reveals a symmetrically enlarged, nontender, generally soft gland without palpable nodules. Goiter is defined, somewhat arbitrarily, as a lateral lobe with a volume greater than the thumb of the individual being examined. If the thyroid is markedly enlarged, it can cause tracheal or esophageal compression. These features are unusual, however, in the absence of nodular disease and fibrosis. *Substernal goiter* may obstruct the thoracic inlet. *Pemberton's sign* refers to symptoms of faintness with evidence of facial congestion and external jugular venous obstruction when the arms are raised above the head, a maneuver that draws the thyroid into the thoracic inlet. Respiratory flow measurements and CT or MRI should be used to evaluate substernal goiter in patients with obstructive signs or symptoms.

Thyroid function tests should be performed in all patients with goiter to exclude thyrotoxicosis or hypothyroidism. It is not unusual, particularly in iodine deficiency, to find a low total T_4, with normal T_3 and TSH, reflecting enhanced $T_4 \rightarrow T_3$ conversion. A low TSH, particularly in older patients, suggests the possibility of thyroid autonomy or undiagnosed Graves' disease, causing subclinical thyrotoxicosis. TPO antibodies may be useful to identify patients at increased risk of autoimmune thyroid disease. Low urinary iodine levels (<100 μg/L) support a diagnosis of iodine deficiency. Thyroid scanning is not generally necessary but will reveal increased uptake in iodine deficiency and most cases of dyshormonogenesis. Ultrasound is not generally indicated in the evaluation of diffuse goiter, unless a nodule is palpable on physical examination.

℞ **TREATMENT** Iodine or thyroid hormone replacement induces variable regression of goiter in iodine deficiency, depending on how long it has been present and the degree of fibrosis that has developed. For other causes of nontoxic diffuse goiter, levothyroxine can be used in an attempt to reduce goiter size. Because of the possibility of underlying thyroid autonomy, caution should be exercised when instituting suppressive thyroxine therapy, particularly if the baseline TSH is in the low-normal range. In younger patients, the dose can be started at 100 μg/d and adjusted to suppress the TSH into the low-normal but detectable range. Treatment of elderly patients should be initiated at 50 μg/d. The efficacy of suppressive treatment is greater in younger patients and in those with soft goiters. Significant regression is usually seen within 3 to 6 months of treatment; after this time it is unlikely to occur. In older patients, and in those with some degree of nodular disease or fibrosis, fewer than one-third demonstrate significant shrinkage of the goiter. Surgery is rarely indicated for diffuse goiter. Exceptions include documented evidence of tracheal compression or obstruction of the thoracic inlet, which are more likely to be associated with substernal multinodular goiters (see below). Subtotal or near-total thyroidectomy for these or cosmetic reasons should be performed by an experienced surgeon to minimize complication rates, which occur in up to 10% of cases. Surgery should be followed by mild suppressive treatment with levothyroxine to prevent regrowth of the goiter. Radioiodine reduces goiter size by about 50% in the majority of patients. It is rarely associated with transient acute swelling of the thyroid, which is usually inconsequential unless there is severe tracheal narrowing. If not treated with levothyroxine, patients should be followed after radioiodine treatment for the possible development of hypothyroidism.

NONTOXIC MULTINODULAR GOITER **Etiology and Pathogenesis** Depending on the geographic region and the sensitivity of the methods used to detect the disorder, multinodular goiter (MNG) is common, occurring in between 1 and 12% of the population. MNG is more common in women than men and increases in prevalence with age. It is more common in iodine-deficient regions but also occurs in regions of iodine sufficiency, reflecting multiple genetic, autoimmune, and environmental influences on the pathogenesis.

Individual patients exhibit wide variation in nodule size. Histology reveals a spectrum of morphologies ranging from hypercellular regions to cystic areas filled with colloid. Fibrosis is often extensive, and areas of hemorrhage or lymphocytic infiltration may be seen. Using molecular techniques, most nodules within a MNG are polyclonal in origin, suggesting a hyperplastic response to locally produced growth factors and cytokines. TSH, which is usually not elevated, may play a permissive or contributory role. Monoclonal lesions also occur within a MNG, reflecting mutations in genes that confer a selective growth advantage to the progenitor cell.

Clinical Manifestations Most patients with nontoxic MNG are asymptomic and, by definition, euthyroid. MNG typically develops over many years and is detected on routine physical examination or because an individual notices an enlargement in the neck. If the goiter is large enough, it can ultimately lead to compressive symptoms including difficulty swallowing, respiratory distress (tracheal compression), or plethora (venous congestion), but these symptoms are uncommon. Symptomatic MNGs are usually extraordinarily large and/or develop fibrotic areas that cause compression. Sudden pain in a MNG is often caused by hemorrhage into a nodule but should raise the possibility of invasive malignancy. Hoarseness, reflecting laryngeal nerve involvement, also suggests malignancy.

Diagnosis On examination, thyroid architecture is distorted and multiple nodules of varying size can be appreciated. Substernal goiter is suggested by Pemberton's sign. Because many nodules are deeply embedded in thyroid tissue or reside in posterior or substernal locations, it is not possible to palpate all nodules. A TSH level should be measured to exclude subclinical hyper- or hypothyroidism, but thyroid function is usually normal. Tracheal deviation is common, but compression must usually exceed 70% of the tracheal diameter before there is significant airway compromise. Pulmonary function testing can be used to assess the functional effects of compression and to detect tracheomalacia, which characteristically causes inspiratory stridor. CT or MRI can be used to evaluate the anatomy of the goiter and the extent of substernal extension, which is often much greater than is apparent on physical examination. A barium swallow may reveal the extent of esophageal obstruction. MNG does not appear to predispose to thyroid carcinoma or to more aggressive carcinoma. For this reason, and because it is not possible to biopsy all nodular lesions, thyroid biopsies should only be performed if malignancy is suspected because of a dominant or enlarging nodule.

℞ **TREATMENT** Most nontoxic MNGs can be managed conservatively. T_4 suppression is rarely effective for reducing goiter size and introduces the risk of thyrotoxicosis, if there is underlying autonomy or if it develops during treatment. If levothyroxine is used, it should be started at low doses (50 μg) and advanced gradually while monitoring the TSH level to avoid excessive suppression. Contrast agents and other iodine-containing substances should be avoided because of the risk of inducing the *Jod-Basedow effect*, characterized by enhanced thyroid hormone production by autonomous nodules. Radioiodine is being used with increasing frequency because it often decreases goiter size and may selectively ablate regions of autonomy. Dosage of ^{131}I depends on the size of the goiter and radioiodine uptake but is usually about 3.7 MBq (0.1 mCi) per gram of tissue, corrected for uptake [typical dose, 370 to 1070 Mbq (10 to 29 mCi)]. Repeat treatment may be needed. It is possible to achieve a 40 to 50% reduction in goiter size in most patients. Earlier concerns about radiation-induced thyroid swelling and tracheal compression have diminished as recent studies have shown this complication to be rare. When acute compression occurs, glucocorticoid treatment or surgery may be needed. Radiation-induced hypothyroidism is less common than occurs after treatment for Graves' disease. However, posttreatment autoimmune thyrotoxicosis may occur in up to 5% of patients treated for nontoxic MNG. Surgery remains highly effective but is not without risk, particularly in older patients with underlying cardiopulmonary disease.

TOXIC MULTINODULAR GOITER The pathogenesis of toxic MNG appears to be similar to that of nontoxic MNG, the major difference being the presence of functional autonomy in toxic MNG. The molecular basis for autonomy in toxic MNG remains unknown. As in nontoxic goiters, many nodules are polyclonal, while others are monoclonal and vary in their clonal origins. Genetic abnormalities known to confer functional autonomy, such as activating TSH-R or $G_{s\alpha}$ mutations (see below), are not usually found in the autonomous regions of toxic MNG goiter.

In addition to features of goiter, the clinical presentation of toxic MNG includes subclinical hyperthyroidism or mild thyrotoxicosis. The patient is usually elderly and may present with atrial fibrillation or palpitations, tachycardia, nervousness, tremor, or weight loss. Recent exposure to iodine, from contrast dyes or other sources, may precipitate or exacerbate thyrotoxicosis. The TSH level is low. The T_4 level may be normal or minimally increased; T_3 is often elevated to a greater degree than T_4. Thyroid scan shows heterogeneous uptake with multiple regions of increased and decreased uptake; 24-h uptake of radioiodine may not be increased.

Rx **TREATMENT** The management of toxic MNG is challenging. Antithyroid drugs, often in combination with beta blockers, can normalize thyroid function and address clinical features of thyrotoxicosis. This treatment, however, often stimulates the growth of the goiter, and, unlike in Graves' disease, spontaneous remission does not occur. Radioiodine can be used to treat areas of autonomy, as well as to decrease the mass of the goiter. Usually, however, some degree of autonomy remains, presumably because multiple autonomous regions emerge as soon as others are treated. Nonetheless, a trial of radioiodine should be considered before subjecting patients, many of whom are elderly, to surgery. Surgery provides definitive treatment of underlying thyrotoxicosis as well as goiter. Patients should be rendered euthyroid using antithyroid drugs before operation.

HYPERFUNCTIONING SOLITARY NODULE A solitary, autonomously functioning thyroid nodule is referred to as *toxic adenoma.* The pathogenesis of this disorder has been unraveled by demonstrating the functional effects of mutations that stimulate the TSH-R signaling pathway. Most patients with solitary hyperfunctioning nodules have acquired somatic, activating mutations in the TSH-R (Fig. 330-9). These mutations, located primarily in the receptor transmembrane domain, induce constitutive receptor coupling to $G_{s\alpha}$, increasing cyclic AMP levels and leading to enhanced thyroid follicular cell proliferation and function. Less commonly, somatic mutations are identified in $G_{s\alpha}$. These mutations, which are similar to those seen in McCune-Albright syndrome (Chap. 336) or in a subset of somatotrope adenomas (Chap. 328), impair GTP hydrolysis, also causing constitutive activation of the cyclic AMP signaling pathway. In most series, activating mutations in either the TSH-R or the $G_{s\alpha}$ subunit genes are identified in >90% of patients with solitary hyperfunctioning nodules.

Thyrotoxicosis is usually mild. The disorder is suggested by the presence of the thyroid nodule, which is generally large enough to be palpable, and by the absence of clinical features suggestive of Graves' disease or other causes of thyrotoxicosis. A thyroid scan provides a definitive diagnostic test, demonstrating focal uptake in the hyper-

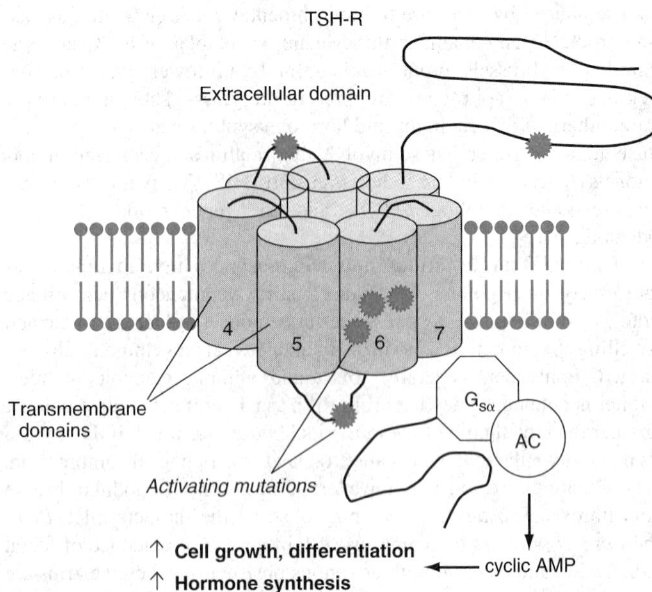

FIGURE 330-9 Activating mutations of the TSH-R. Mutations (*) that activate the thyroid-stimulating hormone receptor (TSH-R) reside mainly in transmembrane 5 and intracellular loop 3, though mutations have occurred in a variety of different locations. The effect of these mutations is to induce conformational changes that mimic TSH binding, thereby leading to coupling to stimulatory G protein ($G_{s\alpha}$) and activation of adenylate cyclase (AC), an enzyme that generates cyclic AMP (cAMP).

functioning nodule and diminished uptake in the remainder of the gland, as activity of the normal thyroid is suppressed.

Rx **TREATMENT** Radioiodine ablation is usually the treatment of choice. Because normal thyroid function is suppressed, ^{131}I is concentrated in the hyperfunctioning nodule with minimal uptake and damage to normal thyroid tissue. Relatively large radioiodine doses [e.g., 370 to 1110 MBq (10 to 29.9 mCi)^{131}I] have been shown to correct thyrotoxicosis in about 75% of patients within 3 months. Hypothyroidism occurs in <10% of patients over the next 5 years. Surgical resection is also effective and is usually limited to enucleation of the adenoma or lobectomy, thereby preserving thyroid function and minimizing risk of hypoparathyroidism or damage to the recurrent laryngeal nerves. Medical therapy using antithyroid drugs and beta blockers can normalize thyroid function but is not an optimal long-term treatment. Ethanol injection under ultrasound guidance has been used successfully in some centers to ablate hyperfunctioning nodules. Repeated injections (often more than 5 sessions) are required but reduce nodule size. Normal thyroid function can be achieved in most patients using this technique.

BENIGN NEOPLASMS

The various types of benign thyroid nodules are listed in Table 330-9. These lesions are common (5 to 10% adults) and often multiple, particularly when assessed by sensitive techniques such as ultrasound. The risk of malignancy is very low for *macrofollicular adenomas* and *normofollicular adenomas. Microfollicular, trabecular, and Hürthle cell variants* raise greater concern, partly because the histology is more difficult to interpret. About one-third of palpable nodules are *thyroid cysts.* These may be recognized by their ultrasound appearance or based on aspiration of large amounts of pink or straw-colored fluid (colloid). Many are mixed cystic/solid lesions, in which case it is desirable to aspirate cellular components under ultrasound or harvest cells after cytospin of cyst fluid. Cysts frequently recur, even after repeated aspiration, and may require surgical excision if they are large or if the cytology is suspicious. Sclerosis has been used with variable

Table 330-9 Classification of Thyroid Neoplasms

	Approximate Prevalence, %
Benign	
Follicular epithelial cell adenomas	
Macrofollicular (colloid)	
Normofollicular (simple)	
Microfollicular (fetal)	
Trabecular (embryonal)	
Hürtle cell variant (oncocytic)	
Malignant	
Follicular epithelial cell	
Well-differentiated carcinomas	
Papillary carcinomas	80–90
Pure papillary	
Follicular variant	
Diffuse sclerosing variant	
Tall cell, columnar cell variants	
Follicular carcinomas	5–10
Minimally invasive	
Widely invasive	
Hürthle cell carcinoma (oncocytic)	
Insular carcinoma	
Undifferentiated (anaplastic) carcinomas	
C cell (calcitonin-producing)	
Medullary thyroid cancer	10
Sporadic	
Familial	
MEN-2	
Other malignancies	
Lymphomas	1–2
Sarcomas	
Metastases	
Others	

NOTE: MEN, multiple endocrine neoplasia.

success but is often painful and may be complicated by infiltration of the sclerosing agent.

The treatment approach for benign nodules is similar to that for MNG. TSH suppression with levothyroxine decreases the size of about 30% of nodules and may prevent further growth. The TSH level should be suppressed into the low-normal range, assuming there are no contraindications; alternatively, nodule size can be monitored without suppression. If a nodule has not decreased in size after 6 to 12 months of suppressive therapy, treatment should be discontinued as little benefit is likely to accrue from long-term treatment.

THYROID CANCER

Thyroid carcinoma is the most common malignancy of the endocrine system. Malignant tumors derived from the follicular epithelium are classified according to histologic features. Differentiated tumors, such as papillary thyroid cancer (PTC) or follicular thyroid cancer (FTC), are often curable, and the prognosis is good for patients identified with early-stage disease. In contrast, anaplastic thyroid cancer (ATC) is aggressive, responds poorly to treatment, and is associated with a bleak prognosis.

The incidence of thyroid cancer (~9/100,000 per year) increases with age, plateauing after about age 50 (Fig. 330-10). Age is also an important prognostic factor—thyroid cancer at young age (<20) or in older persons (>65) is associated with a worse prognosis. Thyroid cancer is twice as common in women as men, but male sex is associated with a worse prognosis. Additional important risk factors include a history of childhood head or neck irradiation, large nodule size (≥4 cm), evidence for local tumor fixation or invasion into lymph nodes, and the presence of metastases (Table 330-10).

Several unique features of thyroid cancer facilitate its management: (1) thyroid nodules are readily palpable, allowing early detection and biopsy by FNA; (2) iodine radioisotopes can be used to diagnose

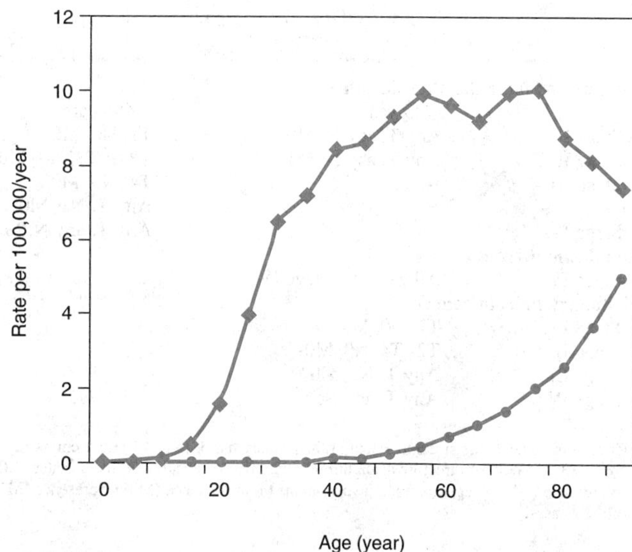

FIGURE 330-10 Age-associated incidence (—◆—) and mortality (—●—) rates for invasive thyroid cancer. *(Adapted from LAG Ries et al (eds): SEER Cancer Statistics Review, 1973–1996, Bethesda, National Cancer Institute, 1999.)*

(^{123}I) and treat (^{131}I) differentiated thyroid cancer, reflecting the unique uptake of this anion by the thyroid gland; and (3) serum markers allow the detection of residual or recurrent disease, including the use of Tg levels for PTC and FTC and calcitonin for medullary thyroid cancer (MTC).

CLASSIFICATION Thyroid neoplasms can arise in each of the cell types that populate the gland, including thyroid follicular cells, calcitonin-producing C cells, lymphocytes, and stromal and vascular elements, as well as metastases from other sites (Table 330-9). The American Joint Committee on Cancer (AJCC) has designated a staging system using the TNM classification (Table 330-11). Several other classification and staging systems are also widely used, some of which place greater emphasis on histologic features or risk factors such as age or gender.

PATHOGENESIS AND GENETIC BASIS **Radiation** Early studies of the pathogenesis of thyroid cancer focused on the role of external radiation, which predisposes to chromosomal breaks, presumably leading to genetic rearrangements and loss of tumor-suppressor genes. External radiation of the mediastinum, face, head, and neck region was administered in the past to treat an array of conditions including acne and enlargement of the thymus, tonsils, and adenoids. Radiation exposure increases the risk of benign and malignant thyroid nodules, is associated with multicentric cancers, and shifts the incidence of thyroid cancer to an earlier age group. Radiation from nuclear fallout also predisposes to thyroid cancer. Children seem more predisposed to the effects of radiation than adults. Of note, radiation derived from ^{131}I therapy appears to contribute little, if any, increased risk of thyroid cancer.

TSH and Growth Factors Thyroid growth is regulated primarily by TSH but also by a variety of growth factors and cytokines. Many

Table 330-10 Risk Factors for Thyroid Carcinoma in Patients with a Thyroid Nodule

History of head and neck irradiation	Family history of thyroid cancer or MEN-2
Age <20 or >70 years	Vocal cord paralysis, hoarse voice
Increased nodule size (>4 cm)	Nodule fixed to adjacent structures
New or enlarging neck mass	Suspected lymph node involvement
Male gender	Iodine deficiency (follicular cancer)

NOTE: MEN, multiple endocrine neoplasia.

Table 330-11 AJCC Staging System for Thyroid Cancers Using the TNM Classification[a]

Papillary or follicular thyroid cancers		
	<45 years	>45 years
Stage I	Any T, any N, M0	T1, N0, M0
Stage II	Any T, any N, M1	T2 or T3, N0, M0
Stage III	—	T4, N0, M0 Any T, N1, M0
Stage IV	—	Any T, any N, M1
Anaplastic thyroid cancer		
Stage IV	All cases are stage IV	
Medullary thyroid cancer		
Stage I	T1, N0, M0	
Stage II	T2–T4, N0, M0	
Stage III	Any T, N1, M0	
Stage IV	Any T, any N, M1	

[a] Criteria include: T, the size and extent of the primary tumor (T1 ≤ 1 cm; 1 cm < T2 ≤ 4 cm; T3 > 4 cm; T4 direct invasion through the thyroid capsule); N, the absence (N0) or presence (N1) of regional node involvement; M, the absence (M0) or presence (M1) of metastases.

differentiated thyroid cancers express TSH receptors and, therefore, remain responsive to TSH. This observation provides the rationale for T_4 suppression of TSH in patients with thyroid cancer. Residual expression of TSH receptors also allows TSH-stimulated uptake of ^{131}I therapy (see below).

Oncogenes and Tumor-Suppressor Genes Thyroid cancers are monoclonal in origin, consistent with the idea that they originate as a consequence of mutations that confer a growth advantage to a single cell. In addition to increased rates of proliferation, some thyroid cancers exhibit impaired apoptosis and features that enhance invasion, angiogenesis, and metastasis (Chap. 83). By analogy with the model of multistep carcinogenesis proposed for colon cancer (Chap. 81), thyroid neoplasms have been analyzed for a variety of genetic alterations, but without clear evidence of an ordered acquisition of somatic mutations as they progress from the benign to the malignant state. On the other hand, certain mutations are relatively specific for thyroid neoplasia, some of which correlate with histologic classification (Table 330-12). For example, activating mutations of the TSH-R and the $G_{s\alpha}$ subunit are associated with autonomously functioning nodules. Though these mutations induce thyroid cell growth, this type of nodule is almost always benign. A variety of rearrangements involving the *RET* gene on chromosome 10 bring this receptor tyrosine kinase under the control of other promoters, leading to receptor overexpression. *RET* rearrangements occur in 20 to 40% of PTCs in different series and were observed with increased frequency in tumors developing after the Chernobyl radiation disaster. Rearrangements in PTC have also been observed for another tyrosine kinase gene, *TRK1*, which is located on chromosome 1. To date, the identification of PTC with *RET* or *TRK1* rearrangements has not proven useful for predicting prognosis or treatment responses. *RAS* mutations are found in about 20 to 30% of thyroid neoplasms, including adenomas as well as PTC and FTC, suggesting that these mutations do not strongly affect tumor phenotype. Loss of heterozygosity (LOH), consistent with deletions of tumor-suppressor genes, is particularly common in FTC, often involving chromosomes 3p or 11q. Mutations of the tumor suppressor, p53, appear to play an important role in the development of ATC. Because p53 plays a role in cell cycle surveillance, DNA repair, and apoptosis,

Table 330-12 Genetic Alterations in Thyroid Neoplasia

Gene/Protein	Type of Gene	Chromosomal Location	Genetic Abnormality	Tumor
TSH receptor	GPCR receptor	14q31	Point mutations	Toxic adenoma, differentiated carcinomas
$G_{s\alpha}$	G protein	20q13.2	Point mutations	Toxic adenoma, differentiated carcinomas
RET/PTC	Receptor tyrosine kinase	10q11.2	Rearrangements PTC1: (inv(10)q11.2q21) PTC2: (t(10;17)(q11.2;q23)) PTC3: ELE1/TK	PTC
RET	Receptor tyrosine kinase	10q11.2	Point mutations	MEN-2, medullary thyroid cancer
TRK	Receptor tyrosine kinase	1q23-24	Rearrangements	Multinodular goiter, papillary thyroid cancer
RAS	Signal transducing p21	Hras 11p15.5 Kras 12p12.1; Nras 1p13.2	Point mutations	Differentiated thyroid carcinoma, adenomas
p53	Tumor suppressor, cell cycle control, apoptosis	17p13	Point mutations Deletion, insertion	Anaplastic cancer
APC	Tumor suppressor, adenomatous polyposis coli gene	5q21-q22	Point mutations	Anaplastic cancer, also associated with familial polyposis coli
p16 (MTS1, CDKN2A)	Tumor suppressor, cell cycle control	9p21	Deletions	Differentiated carcinomas
p21/WAF	Tumor suppressor, cell cycle control	6p21.2	Overexpression	Anaplastic cancer
MET	Receptor tyrosine kinase	7q31	Overexpression	Follicular thyroid cancer
c-MYC	Receptor tyrosine kinase	8q24.12.-13	Overexpression	Differentiated carcinoma
PTEN	Phosphatase	10q23	Point mutations	PTC in Cowden's syndrome (multiple hamartomas, breast tumors, gastrointestinal polyps, thyroid tumors)
Loss of heterozygosity (LOH)	?Tumor suppressors	3p; 11q13 Other loci	Deletions	Differentiated thyroid carcinomas, anaplastic cancer
PAX8-PPARγ1	Transcription factor Nuclear receptor fusion	t(2;3)(q13;p25)	Translocation	Follicular carcinoma

NOTE: TSH, thyroid-stimulating hormone; $G_{s\alpha}$, G-protein stimulating α-subunit; RET, rearranged during transfection proto-oncogene; PTC, papillary thyroid cancer; TRK, tyrosine kinase receptor; RAS, rat sarcoma proto-oncogene; p53, p53 tumor suppressor gene; MET, met proto-oncogene (hepatocyte growth factor receptor); c-MYC, cellular homologue of myelocytomatosis virus proto-oncogene; PTEN, phosphatase and tensin homologue; APC, adenomatous polyposis coli; MTS, multiple tumor suppressor; CDKN2A, cyclin-dependent kinase inhibitor 2A; P21, p21 tumor suppressor; WAF, wild-type p53 activated fragment; GPCR, G protein–coupled receptor; ELE1/TK, ret-activating gene ele1/tyrosine kinase; MEN-2, multiple endocrine neoplasia-2; PAX8, Paired domain transcription factor; PPARγ1, Peroxisome-proliferator activated receptor 81.

SOURCE: Adapted with permission from P Kopp, JL Jameson, in JL Jameson (ed): *Principles of Molecular Medicine*. Totowa, NJ, Humana Press, 1998.

its loss may contribute to the rapid acquisition of genetic instability as well as poor treatment responses (Chap. 82). The role of other tumor-suppressor genes in thyroid cancer is under investigation (Table 330-12).

MTC, when associated with multiple endocrine neoplasia (MEN) type 2, harbors an inherited mutation of the *RET* gene. Unlike the rearrangements of *RET* seen in PTC, the mutations in MEN-2 are point mutations that induce constitutive activity of the tyrosine kinase (Chap. 339). MTC is preceded by hyperplasia of the C cells, raising the likelihood that as-yet-unidentified "second hits" lead to cellular transformation. A subset of sporadic MTC contain somatic mutations that activate *RET*.

WELL-DIFFERENTIATED THYROID CANCER Papillary PTC is the most common type of thyroid cancer, accounting for 70 to 90% of well-differentiated thyroid malignancies. Microscopic PTC is present in as many 25% of thyroid glands at autopsy, but most of these lesions are very small (several millimeters) and are not clinically significant. Characteristic cytologic features of PTC help make the diagnosis by FNA or after surgical resection; these include psammoma bodies, cleaved nuclei with an "orphan-Annie" appearance caused by large nucleoli, and the formation of papillary structures.

PTC tends to be multifocal and to invade locally within the thyroid gland as well as through the thyroid capsule and into adjacent structures in the neck. It has a propensity to spread via the lymphatic system but can metastasize as well, particularly to bone and lung. Because of the relatively slow growth of the tumor, a significant burden of pulmonary metastases may accumulate, sometimes with remarkably few symptoms. The prognostic implication of lymph node spread is debated. Lymph node involvement by thyroid cancer can be remarkably well tolerated but probably increases the risk of recurrence and mortality, particularly in older patients. The staging of PTC by the TNM system is outlined in Table 330-11. Most papillary cancers are identified in the early stages (>80% stages I or II) and have an excellent prognosis, with survival curves similar to expected survival (Fig. 330-11*A*). Mortality is markedly increased in stage IV disease (distant metastases), but this group comprises only about 1% of patients. The treatment of PTC is described below.

Follicular The incidence of FTC varies widely in different parts of the world; it is more common in iodine-deficient regions. FTC is difficult to diagnose by FNA because the distinction between benign and malignant follicular neoplasms rests largely on evidence of invasion into vessels, nerves, or adjacent structures. FTC tends to spread by hematogenous routes leading bone, lung, and central nervous system metastases. Mortality rates associated with FTC are less favorable than for PTC, in part because a larger proportion of patients present with stage IV disease (Fig. 330-11*B*). Poor prognostic features include distant metastases, age >50 years, primary tumor size >4 cm, Hürthle cell histology, and the presence of marked vascular invasion.

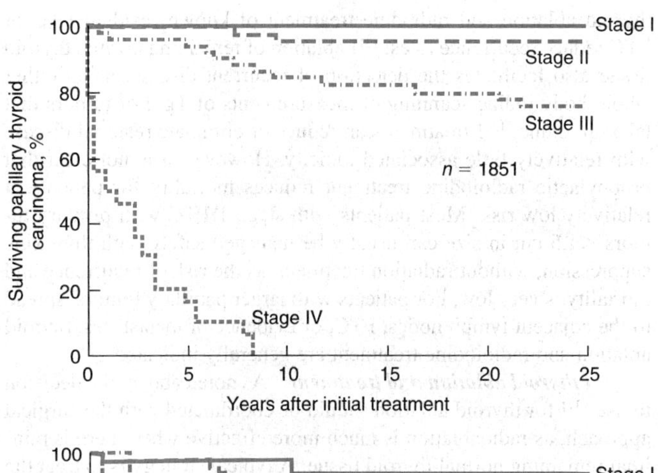

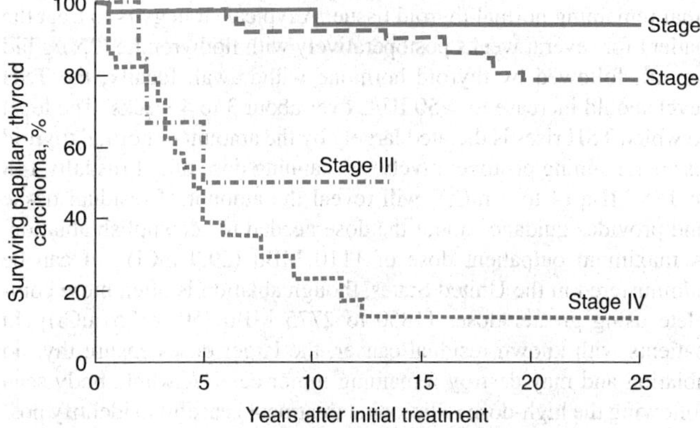

FIGURE 330-11 Survival rates in patients with differentiated thyroid cancer. *A.* Papillary cancer, cohort of 1851 patients. I, 1107 (60%), II, 408 (22%), III, 312 (17%), IV, 24 (1%); *n* = 1185. *B.* Follicular cancer, cohort of 153 patients. I, 42 (27%), II, 82 (54%), III, 6 (4%); IV, 23 (15%); *n* = 153. *(Adapted from Larsen et al.)*

℞ **TREATMENT Surgery** All well-differentiated thyroid cancers should be surgically excised. In addition to removing the primary lesion, surgery allows accurate histologic diagnosis and staging, and multicentric disease is commonly found in the contralateral lobe. Lymph node spread can also be assessed at the time of surgery, and involved nodes can be removed. Recommendations about the extent of surgery vary for stage I disease, as survival rates are similar for lobectomy and near-total thyroidectomy. Lobectomy is associated with a lower incidence of hypoparathyroidism and injury to the recurrent laryngeal nerves. However, it is not possible to monitor Tg levels or to perform whole-body ^{131}I scans in the presence of the residual lobe. Moreover, if final staging or subsequent follow-up indicates the need for radioiodine scanning or treatment, repeat surgery is necessary to remove the remaining thyroid tissue. The authors favor near-total thyroidectomy in almost all patients; complication rates are acceptably low if the surgeon is highly experienced in the procedure. This approach, in combination with postsurgical radioablation of the remnant thyroid tissue, facilitates the use of radioiodine scanning and Tg determinations to assess disease recurrence.

TSH Suppression Therapy As most tumors are still TSH-responsive, levothyroxine suppression of TSH is a mainstay of thyroid cancer treatment. Though TSH suppression clearly provides therapeutic benefit, there are no prospective studies that identify the optimal level of TSH suppression. A reasonable goal is to suppress TSH to as low as possible without subjecting the patient to unnecessary side effects from excess thyroid hormone, such as atrial fibrillation, osteopenia, anxiety, and other manifestations of thyrotoxicosis. For patients at low risk of recurrence, TSH should be suppressed into the low but detectable range (0.1 to 0.5 IU/L). For patients at high risk of recurrence, or with known metastatic disease, complete TSH suppression is indicated, if there are no strong contraindications to mild thyrotoxicosis. In this instance, free T_4 or free T_3 levels must also be monitored to avoid excessive treatment.

Radioiodine Treatment Well-differentiated thyroid cancer still incorporates radioiodine, though less efficiently than normal thyroid follicular cells. Radioiodine uptake is determined primarily by expression of the NIS and is stimulated by TSH, requiring expression of the TSH-R. The retention time for radioactivity is influenced by the extent to which the tumor retains differentiated functions such as iodide trapping and organification. After near-total thyroidectomy, substantial thyroid tissue remains, particularly in the thyroid bed and surrounding the parathyroid glands. Consequently, ^{131}I ablation is necessary to eliminate remaining normal thyroid tissue and may treat residual tumor cells.

Indications The use of therapeutic doses of radioiodine remains an area of controversy in thyroid cancer management. Postoperative thyroid ablation and radiodine treatment of known residual PTC or FTC reduce recurrence rates. ^{131}I ablation of remaining normal thyroid tissue also facilitates the detection of recurrent disease, using either whole-body iodine scanning or measurements of Tg. For tumors that take up iodine, ^{131}I treatment can reduce or eliminate residual disease with relatively little associated toxicity. However, it is not clear that prophylactic radioiodine treatment reduces mortality for patients at relatively low risk. Most patients with stage 1 PTC with primary tumors <1.5 cm in size can usually be managed safely with thyroxine suppression, without radiation treatment, as the risk of recurrence and mortality is very low. For patients with larger papillary tumors, spread to the adjacent lymph nodes, FTC, or evidence of metastases, thyroid ablation and radioiodine treatment are generally indicated.

^{131}I thyroid ablation and treatment As noted above, the decision to use ^{131}I for thyroid ablation should be coordinated with the surgical approach, as radioablation is much more effective when there is minimal remaining normal thyroid tissue. A typical strategy is to treat the patient for several weeks postoperatively with liothyronine (25 μg bid or tid), followed by thyroid hormone withdrawal. Ideally, the TSH level should increase to >50 IU/L over about 3 to 4 weeks. The level to which TSH rises is dictated largely by the amount of normal thyroid tissue remaining postoperatively. A scanning dose of ^{131}I [usually 148 to 185 MBq (4 to 5 mCi)] will reveal the amount of residual tissue and provides guidance about the dose needed to accomplish ablation. A maximum outpatient dose of 1110 MBq (29.9 mCi) ^{131}I can be administered in the United States, though ablation is often more complete using greater doses [1850 to 2775 MBq (50 to 75 mCi)]. In patients with known residual cancer, the larger doses ensure thyroid ablation and may destroy remaining tumor cells. A whole-body scan following the high-dose radioiodine treatment is useful to identify possible metastatic disease.

Follow-up whole-body thyroid scanning and thyroglobulin determinations An initial whole-body scan should be performed about 6 months after surgery and thyroid ablation. The strategy for follow-up management of thyroid cancer has been altered by the availability of recombinant human TSH (rhTSH) to stimulate ^{131}I uptake and by the improved sensitivity of Tg assays to detect residual or recurrent disease. A scheme for using either rhTSH or thyroid hormone withdrawal for thyroid scanning is summarized in Fig. 330-12. After thyroid ablation, rhTSH can be used to stimulate ^{131}I uptake without subjecting patients to thyroid hormone withdrawal and its associated symptoms of hypothyroidism and the risk of prolonged TSH-stimulated tumor growth. This approach is recommended for patients predicted to be at low risk of disease recurrence, since rhTSH is not currently approved for use in conjunction with therapeutic doses of ^{131}I. Alternatively, in patients who are likely to require ^{131}I treatment, the traditional approach of thyroid hormone withdrawal can be used to increase TSH. This involves switching patients from levothyroxine (T_4) to the more rapidly cleared hormone, liothyronine (T_3), thereby allowing TSH to increase more quickly. If residual disease is detected on the initial whole-body scan [148 to 185 MBq (4 to 5 mCi)], a larger treatment dose, usually between 2775 and 5550 MBq (75 and 150 mCi), can be administered depending on the degree of residual uptake and assessment of cancer risk. Because TSH stimulates Tg levels, Tg measurements should be obtained after administration of rhTSH or when TSH levels have risen after thyroid hormone withdrawal. If the initial whole-body scan is negative and Tg levels are low, a repeat scan should be performed 1 year later. If still negative, the patient can be managed with suppressive therapy and measurements of Tg every 6 to 12 months. If a second follow-up scan is negative, no further scanning may be necessary if the patient is at low risk and there is no clinical or laboratory evidence of recurrence. Many authorities advocate radioiodine treatment for scan-negative, Tg-positive (Tg >5 to 10 ng/mL) patients, as many derive therapeutic benefit from a large dose of ^{131}I.

In addition to radioiodine, external beam radiotherapy is also used

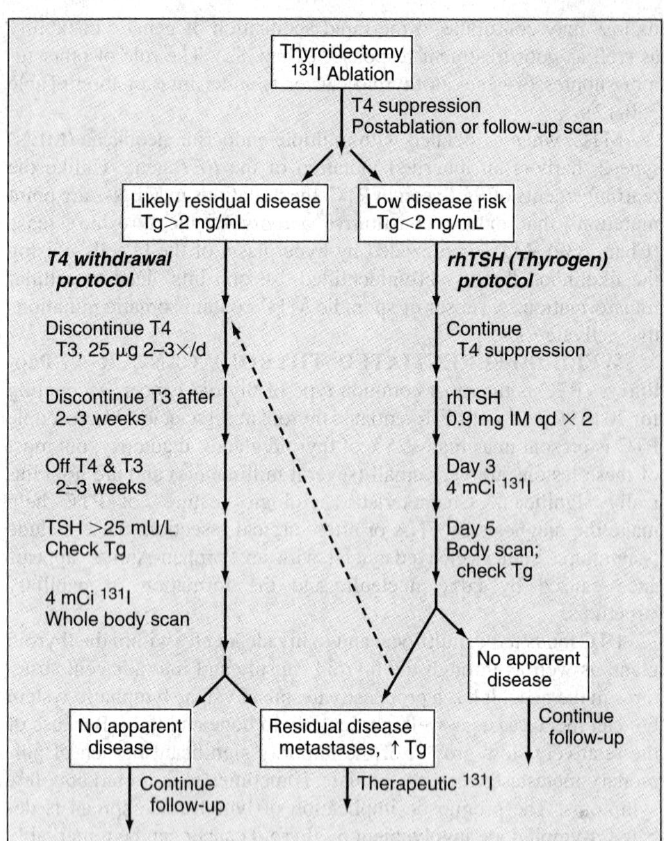

FIGURE 330-12 Use of recombinant thyroid-stimulating hormone (TSH) in the follow-up of patients with thyroid cancer.

to treat specific metastatic lesions, particularly when they cause bone pain or threaten neurologic injury (e.g., vertebral metastases).

ANAPLASTIC AND OTHER FORMS OF THYROID CANCER **Anaplastic Thyroid Cancer** As noted above, ATC is a poorly differentiated and aggressive cancer. The prognosis is poor, and most patients die within 6 months of diagnosis. Because of the undifferentiated state of these tumors, radioiodine uptake is usually negligible but can be used therapeutically if there is residual uptake. Chemotherapy has been attempted with multiple agents, including anthracyclines and paclitaxel, but is usually futile. External radiation therapy can be attempted and continued if tumors are responsive.

Thyroid Lymphoma Lymphoma in the thyroid gland often arises in the background of Hashimoto's thyroiditis. A rapidly expanding thyroid mass should suggest the possibility of this diagnosis. Diffuse large cell lymphoma is the most common type in the thyroid. Biopsies reveal sheets of lymphoid cells that can be difficult to distinguish from small cell lung cancer or ATC. These tumors are often highly sensitive to external radiation. Surgical resection should be avoided as initial therapy because it may spread disease that is otherwise localized to the thyroid. If staging indicates disease outside of the thyroid, treatment should follow guidelines used for other forms of lymphoma (Chap. 112).

MEDULLARY THYROID CARCINOMA MTC can be sporadic or familial and accounts for about 5 to 10% of thyroid cancers. There are three familial forms of MTC: MEN-2A, MEN-2B, and familial MTC without other features of MEN (Chap. 339). In general, MTC is more aggressive in MEN-2B than in MEN-2A, and familial MTC is more aggressive than sporadic MTC. Elevated serum calcitonin provides a marker of residual or recurrent disease. It is reasonable to test all patients with MTC for *RET* mutations, as genetic counseling and testing of family members can be offered to those individuals who test positive for mutations.

The management of MTC is primarily surgical. Unlike tumors derived from thyroid follicular cells, these tumors do not take up radioiodine. External radiation treatment and chemotherapy may provide palliation in patients with advanced disease (Chap. 339).

Approach to the Patient

Palpable thyroid nodules are found in about 5% of adults, though the prevalence varies considerably worldwide. Given this high prevalence rate, it is common for the practitioner to identify and evaluate thyroid nodules. The main goal of this evaluation is to identify, in a cost-effective manner, the small subgroup of individuals with malignant lesions.

As described above, nodules are more common in iodine-deficient areas, in women, and with aging. Most palpable nodules are >1 cm in diameter, but the ability to feel a nodule is influenced by its location within the gland (superficial versus deeply embedded), the anatomy of the patient's neck, and the experience of the examiner. More sensitive methods of detection, such as thyroid ultrasound and pathologic studies, reveal thyroid nodules in >20% of glands. These findings have led to much debate about how to detect nodules and which nodules to investigate further. Most authorities still rely on physical examination to detect thyroid nodules, reserving ultrasound for monitoring nodule size or as an aid in thyroid biopsy.

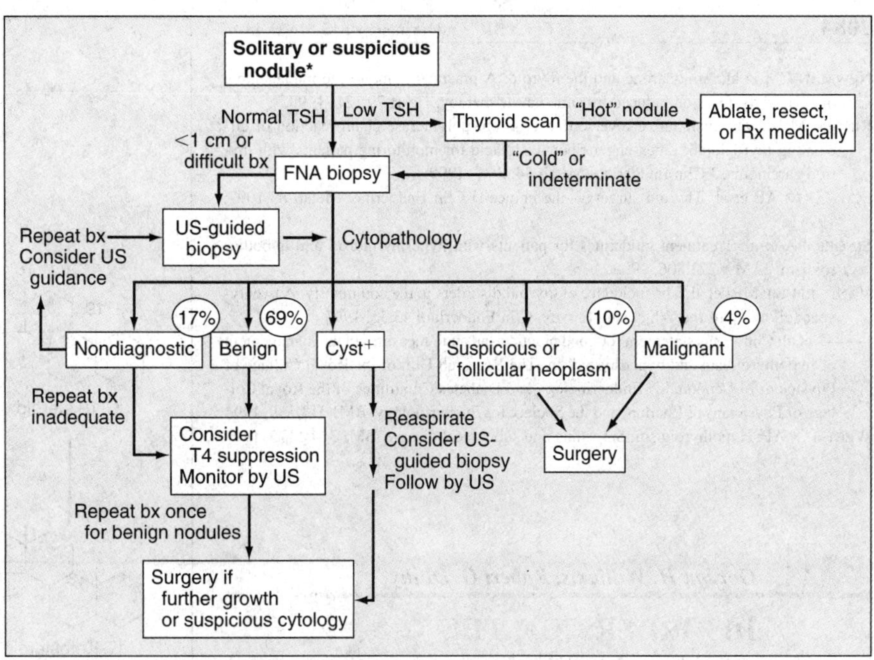

FIGURE 330-13 Approach to the patient with a thyroid nodule. *There are many exceptions to the suggested options. See text and references for details. †About one-third of nodules are cystic or mixed solid-cystic. US, ultrasound.

It is important to distinguish whether a patient presents with a solitary thyroid nodule or a prominent nodule in the context of a MNG, as the incidence of malignancy is greater in solitary nodules. An approach to the evaluation of a solitary nodule is outlined in Fig. 330-13. Most patients with thyroid nodules have normal thyroid function tests. Nonetheless, thyroid function should be assessed by measuring a TSH level, which may be suppressed by one or more autonomously functioning nodules. If the TSH is suppressed, a radionuclide scan is indicated to determine if the identified nodule is "hot," as lesions with increased uptake are almost never malignant and FNA is unnecessary. Otherwise, FNA biopsy should be the first step in the evaluation of a thyroid nodule. FNA has good sensitivity and specificity when performed by physicians familiar with the procedure and when the results are interpreted by experienced cytopathologists. The technique is particularly accurate for detecting PTC. The distinction of benign and malignant follicular lesions is often not possible using cytology alone.

In several large studies, FNA biopsies yield the following findings: 70% benign, 10% malignant or suspicious for malignancy, and 20% nondiagnostic or yielding insufficient material for diagnosis. Characteristic features of malignancy mandate surgery. A diagnosis of follicular neoplasm also warrants surgery, as benign and malignant lesions cannot be distinguished based on cytopathology or frozen section. The management of patients with benign lesions is more variable. Many authorities advocate TSH suppression, whereas others monitor nodule size without suppression. With either approach, thyroid nodule size should be monitored, either by palpation or ultrasound. Repeat FNA is indicated if a nodule enlarges, and most authorities recommend a second biopsy within 2 to 5 years to confirm the benign status of the nodule.

Nondiagnostic biopsies occur for many reasons, including a fibrotic reaction with relatively few cells available for aspiration, a cystic lesion in which cellular components reside along the cyst margin, or a nodule that may be too small for accurate aspiration. For these reasons, ultrasound-guided FNA is useful when the FNA is repeated. Ultrasound is also increasingly used for initial biopsies in an effort to enhance nodule localization and the accuracy of sampling.

The evaluation of a thyroid nodule is stressful for most patients. They are concerned about the possibility of thyroid cancer, whether verbalized or not. It is constructive, therefore, to review the diagnostic approach and to reassure patients when malignancy is not found. When a suspicious lesion or thyroid cancer is identified, an explanation of the generally favorable prognosis and available treatment options should be provided.

BIBLIOGRAPHY

ALLAHABADIA A et al: Age and gender predict the outcome of treatment for Graves' hyperthyroidism. J Clin Endocrinol Metab 85:1038, 2000

AMERICAN JOINT COMMITTEE ON CANCER: *Thyroid gland: AJCC Cancer Staging Manual*, 5th ed. Philadelphia, Lippincott-Raven, 1997, pp 59–64

BARTALENA L et al: Management of Graves' ophthalmopathy: Reality and perspectives. Endocr Rev 21:168, 2000

BRUCKER-DAVIES F et al: Thyrotropin-secreting pituitary tumors: Diagnostic criteria, thyroid hormone sensitivity, and treatment outcome in 25 patients followed at the National Institutes of Health. J Clin Endocrinol Metab 84:476, 1999

BUNEVICIUS R et al: Effects of thyroxine as compared with thyroxine plus triiodothyronine in patients with hypothyroidism. N Engl J Med 340:424, 1999

DELANGE F: Risks and benefits of iodine supplementation. Lancet 351:923, 1998

DEGROOT LJ et al: Thyroid gland (Part III), in *Endocrinology*, 4th ed, LJ DeGroot, JL Jameson (eds). Philadelphia, Saunders, 2000

FERRETTI E et al: Evaluation of the adequacy of levothyroxine replacement therapy in patients with central hypothyroidism. J Clin Endocrinol Metab 84:924, 1999

GHARIB H: Changing concepts in the diagnosis and management of thyroid nodules. Endocrinol Metab Clin North Am 26:777, 1997

HAUGEN BR et al: A comparison of recombinant human thyrotropin and thyroid hormone withdrawal for the detection of thyroid remnant or cancer. J Clin Endocrinol Metab 84:3877, 1999

KOPP P: Pendred's syndrome and genetic defects in thyroid hormone synthesis. Rev Endocrinol Metabol Dis 1:109, 2000

KOUTRAS DA: Subclinical hyperthyroidism. Thyroid 9:311, 1999

KROLL TG et al: PAX8-PPARγ1 fusion oncogene in human thyroid carcinoma. Science 289:1357, 2000

LARSEN PR et al: Thyroid, in *William's Textbook of Endocrinology*, 9th ed, JD Wilson et al (eds). Philadelphia, Saunders, 1998, pp 389–515

LAURBERG P et al: Guidelines for TSH-receptor antibody measurements in pregnancy: Results of an evidence-based symposium organized by the European Thyroid Association. Eur J Endocrinol 139:584, 1998

LEECH NJ, DAYAN CM: Controversies in the management of Graves' disease. Clin Endocrinol 49:273, 1998

LINDSAY RS, TOFT AD: Hypothyroidism. Lancet 349:413, 1997

MACCHIA PE: Recent advances in understanding the molecular basis of primary congenital hypothyroidism. Mol Med Today 6:36, 2000

MASIUKIEWICZ US, BURROW GN: Hyperthyroidism in pregnancy: Diagnosis and treatment. Thyroid 9:647, 1999

NEWMAN CM et al: Amiodarone and the thyroid: A practical guide to the management of thyroid dysfunction induced by amiodarone therapy. Heart 79:121, 1998

RINGEL MD et al: Quantitative reverse transcription–polymerase chain reaction of circulating thyroglobulin messenger ribonucleic acid for monitoring patients with thyroid carcinoma. J Clin Endocrinol Metab 84:4037, 1999

SCHWARTZ AE et al: Thyroid surgery—the choice. J Clin Endocrinol Metab 83:1097, 1998

SINGER PA et al: Treatment guidelines for patients with hyperthyroidism and hypothyroidism. JAMA 273:806, 1995

VANDERPUMP MPJ et al: The incidence of thyroid disorders in the community: A twenty-year follow-up of the Whickham Survey. Clin Endocrinol 43:55, 1995

——— et al: Consensus statement for good practice and audit measures in the management of hypothyroidism and hyperthyroidism. The Research Unit of the Royal College of Physicians of London, the Endocrinology and Diabetes Committee of the Royal College of Physicians of London, and the Society for Endocrinology. BMJ 313:539, 1996

WEETMAN AP: Hypothyroidism: Screening and subclinical disease. BMJ 314:1175, 1997

331

Gordon H. Williams, Robert G. Dluhy

DISORDERS OF THE ADRENAL CORTEX

ACE	angiotensin-converting enzyme	IL	interleukin
ACTH	adrenocorticotropic hormone	LDL	low-density lipoprotein
AVP	arginine vasopressin	β-LPT	β-lipotropin
CAH	congenital adrenal hyperplasia	MIF	migration-inhibiting factor
CBG	cortisol-binding globulin	MR	mineralocorticoid receptor
CMV	cytomegalovirus	MRI	magnetic resonance imaging
CRH	corticotropin-releasing hormone	PHA-I	pseudohypoaldosteronism type I
CT	computed tomography	POMC	pro-opiomelanocortin
DHEA	dehydroepiandrosterone	PRA	plasma renin activity
GABA	γ-aminobutyric acid	STAR	steroidogenic acute regulatory
GR	glucocorticoid receptor	TNF	tumor necrosis factor
GRA	glucocorticoid-remediable aldosteronism		
11β-HSD	hydroxysteroid dehydrogenase		

BIOCHEMISTRY AND PHYSIOLOGY

The adrenal cortex produces three major classes of steroids: (1) glucocorticoids, (2) mineralocorticoids, and (3) adrenal androgens. Consequently, normal adrenal function is important for modulating intermediary metabolism and immune responses through glucocorticoids; blood pressure, vascular volume, and electrolytes through mineralocorticoids; and secondary sexual characteristics (in females) through androgens. The adrenal axis plays an important role in the stress response by rapidly increasing cortisol levels. Adrenal disorders include hyperfunction (Cushing's syndrome) and hypofunction (adrenal insufficiency) as well as a variety of genetic abnormalities of steroidogenesis.

STEROID NOMENCLATURE Steroids contain as their basic structure a cyclopentenoperhydrophenanthrane nucleus consisting of three 6-carbon hexane rings and a single 5-carbon pentane ring (Fig. 331-1). The carbon atoms are numbered in a sequence beginning with ring A. Adrenal steroids contain either 19 or 21 carbon atoms. The C_{19} steroids have methyl groups at C-18 and C-19. C_{19} steroids with a ketone group at C-17 are termed *17-ketosteroids*; C_{19} steroids have predominantly androgenic activity. The C_{21} steroids have a 2-carbon side chain (C-20 and C-21) attached at position 17 and methyl groups at C-18 and C-19; C_{21} steroids with a hydroxyl group at position 17 are termed *17-hydroxycorticosteroids*. The C_{21} steroids have either glucocorticoid or mineralcorticoid properties.

BIOSYNTHESIS OF ADRENAL STEROIDS Cholesterol, derived from the diet and from endogenous synthesis, is the substrate for steroidogenesis. Uptake of cholesterol by the adrenal cortex is mediated by the low-density lipoprotein (LDL) receptor. With long-term stimulation of the adrenal cortex by adrenocorticotropic hormone (ACTH), the number of LDL receptors increases. The three major adrenal biosynthetic pathways lead to the production of glucocorticoids (cortisol), mineralocorticoids (aldosterone), and adrenal androgens (dehydroepiandrosterone). Separate zones of the adrenal cortex synthesize specific hormones (Fig. 331-2). This zonation is accompanied by the selective expression of the genes encoding the enzymes unique to the formation of each type of steroid: aldosterone synthase is normally expressed only in the outer (glomerulosa) cell layer, whereas 17-hydroxylase is expressed only in the (inner) faciculata-reticularis cell layers, which are the sites of cortisol and androgen biosynthesis, respectively.

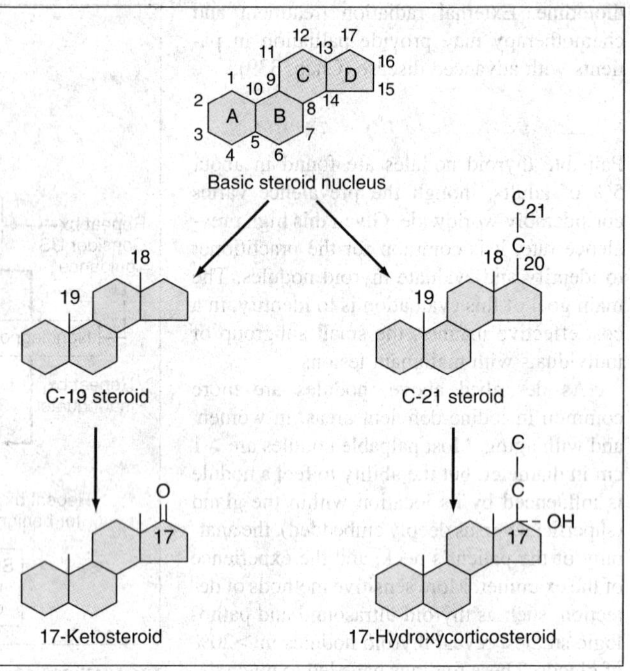

FIGURE 331-1 Basic steroid structure and nomenclature.

STEROID TRANSPORT Cortisol occurs in the plasma in three forms: free cortisol, protein-bound cortisol, and cortisol metabolites. *Free cortisol* is physiologically active hormone that is not protein-bound and, can act therefore, directly on tissue sites. Normally, <5% of circulating cortisol is free. Only the unbound cortisol and its metabolites are filterable at the glomerulus. Increased quantities of free steroid are excreted in the urine in states characterized by hypersecretion of cortisol, because the unbound fraction of plasma cortisol rises. Plasma has two cortisol-binding systems. One is a high-affinity, low-capacity α_2-globulin termed *transcortin* or *cortisol-binding globulin* (CBG), and the other is a low-affinity, high-capacity protein, *albumin*. The binding affinity of CBG for cortisol is reduced in areas of inflammation, thus increasing the local concentration of free cortisol. When the concentration of cortisol exceeds 700 nmol/(25 μg/dL), part of the excess binds to albumin, and a greater proportion than usual circulates unbound. The CBG level is increased in high-estrogen states (e.g., pregnancy, oral contraceptive administration). The rise in CBG is accompanied by a parallel rise in *protein-bound cortisol*, with the result that the plasma cortisol concentration is elevated. However, the free cortisol level probably remains normal, and manifestations of glucocorticoid excess are absent. Most synthetic glucocorticoid analogues bind less efficiently to CBG (~70% binding). This may explain the propensity of some synthetic analogues to produce cushingoid effects at low doses. *Cortisol metabolites* are biologically inactive and bind only weakly to circulating plasma proteins.

Aldosterone is bound to proteins to a smaller extent than cortisol, and an ultrafiltrate of plasma contains as much as 50% of the circulating concentration of aldosterone.

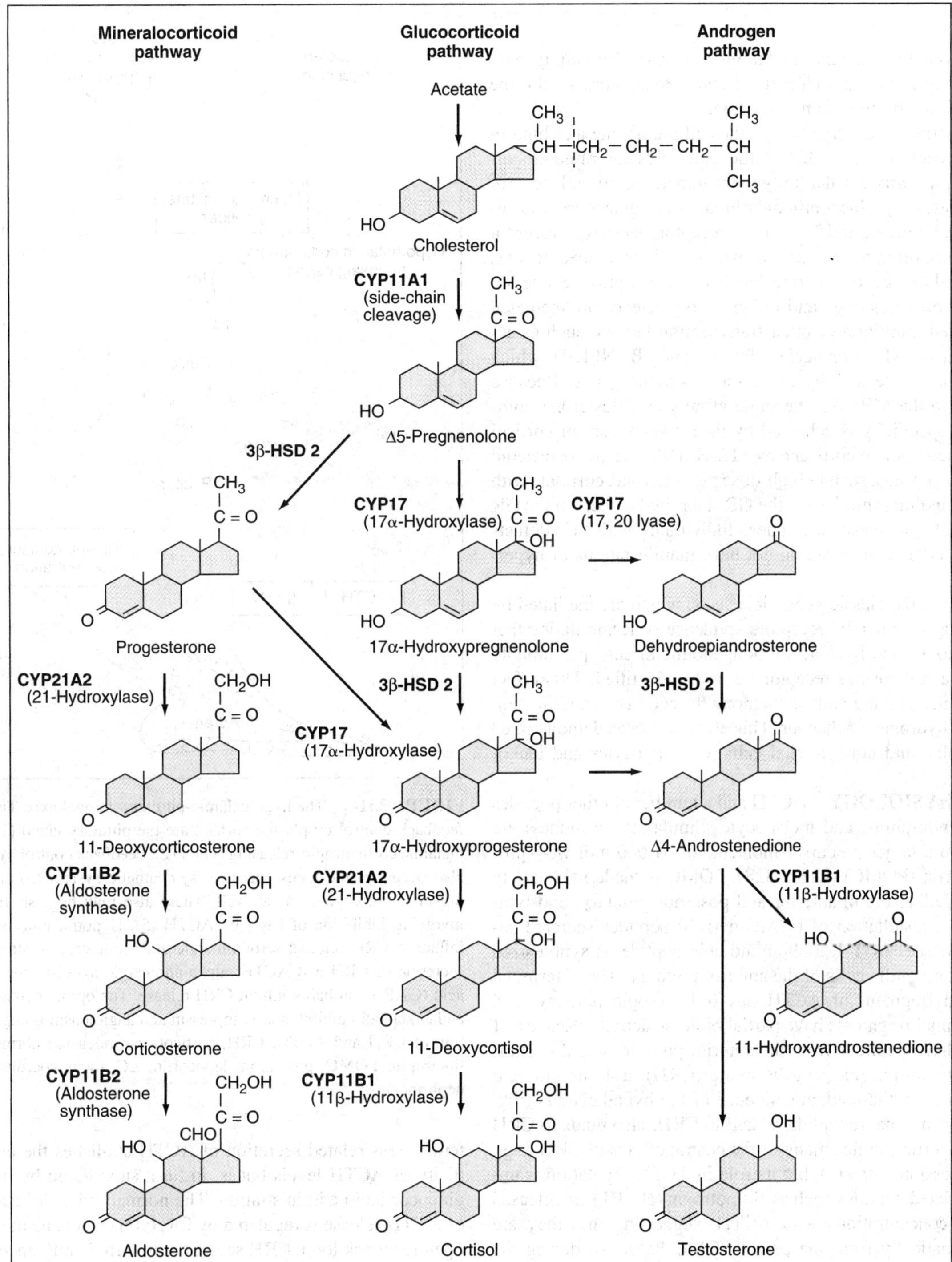

FIGURE 331-2 Biosynthetic pathways for adrenal steroid production; major pathways to mineralocorticoids, glucocorticoids, and androgens. 3β-HSD, 3β-hydroxysteroid dehydrogenase.

STEROID METABOLISM AND EXCRETION Glucocorticoids The daily secretion of cortisol ranges between 40 and 80 μmol (15 and 30 mg, 8–10 mg/m²), with a pronounced circadian cycle. The plasma concentration of cortisol is determined by the rate of secretion, the rate of inactivation, and the rate of excretion of free cortisol. The liver is the major organ responsible for steroid inactivation. A major enzyme regulating cortisol metabolism is 11β-hydroxysteroid dehydrogenase (11β-HSD). There are two isoforms: 11β-HSD I is primarily expressed in the liver and acts as a reductase, converting the inactive cortisone to the active glucocorticoid, cortisol; the 11β-HSD II isoform is expressed in a number of tissues and converts cortisol to the inactive metabolite cortisone. The oxidative reaction of 11β-HSD I is increased in hyperthyroidism.

Mineralocorticoids In normal individuals with a normal salt intake, the average daily secretion of aldosterone ranges between 0.1 and 0.7 μmol (50 and 250 μg). During a single passage through the liver, >75% of circulating aldosterone is normally inactivated by ring A reduction and conjugation with glucuronic acid because it is only weakly bound to proteins. However, under certain conditions, such as congestive failure, this rate of inactivation is reduced.

Adrenal Androgens The major androgen secreted by the adrenal is dehydroepiandrosterone (DHEA) and its sulfuric acid ester (DHEAS). From 15 to 30 mg of these compounds is secreted daily. Smaller amounts of androstenedione, 11β-hydroxyandrostenedione, and testosterone are secreted. DHEA is the major precursor of the urinary 17-ketosteroids. Two-thirds of the urine 17-ketosteroids in the male are derived from adrenal metabolites, and the remaining one-third comes from testicular androgens. In the female, almost all urine 17-ketosteroids are derived from the adrenal.

Steroids diffuse passively through the cell membrane and bind to intracellular receptors (Chap. 327). Glucocorticoids and mineralocorticoids bind with nearly equal affinity to the mineralocorticoid receptor (MR). However, only glucocorticoids bind to the glucocorticoid receptor (GR). After the steroid binds to the receptor, the steroid-receptor complex is transported to the nucleus, where it binds to specific sites on steroid-regulated genes, altering levels of transcription. Some actions of glucocorticoids (e.g., anti-inflammatory effects) are mediated by GR-mediated inhibition of other transcription factors, such as activating protein-1 (AP-1) or nuclear factor kappa-B (NFKB), which normally stimulate the activity of various cytokine genes. Because cortisol binds to the MR with the same affinity as aldosterone, mineralocorticoid specificity is achieved by local metabolism of cortisol to the inactive compound cortisone by 11β-HSDII. The glucocorticoid effects of other steroids, such as high-dose progesterone, correlate with their relative binding affinities for the GR. Inherited defects in the GR cause glucocorticoid resistance states. Individuals with GR defects have high levels of cortisol but do not have manifestations of hypercortisolism.

In addition to the classic genomic effects, which are mediated by steroids binding to cytosolic receptors, evidence is accumulating that mineralocorticoids also have acute, nongenomic effects, presumably by activating a cell-surface receptor yet to be identified. This effect uses a G-protein signaling pathway; among the actions is modification of the sodium-hydrogen exchanger. This effect has been demonstrated in both epithelial and nonepithelial cells, e.g., myocytes and leukocytes.

ACTH PHYSIOLOGY ACTH and a number of other peptides (lipotropins, endorphins, and melanocyte-stimulating hormones) are processed from a larger precursor molecule of 31,000 mol wt—pro-opiomelanocortin (POMC) (Chap. 328). POMC is made in a variety of tissues, including brain, anterior and posterior pituitary, and lymphocytes. The constellation of POMC-derived peptides secreted depends on the tissue. ACTH, a 39-amino acid peptide, is synthesized and stored in basophilic cells of the anterior pituitary. The *N*-terminal 18-amino acid fragment of ACTH has full biologic potency, and shorter *N*-terminal fragments have partial biologic activity. Release of ACTH and related peptides from the anterior pituitary gland is stimulated by corticotropin-releasing hormone (CRH), a 41-amino acid peptide produced in the median eminence of the hypothalamus (Fig. 331-3). Urocortin, a neuropeptide related to CRH, also binds to CRH receptors. Urocortin mimics many of the central effects of CRH (e.g., appetite suppression, anxiety), but its role in ACTH regulation is unclear. Some related peptides such as β-lipotropin (β-LPT) are released in equimolar concentrations with ACTH, suggesting that they are cleaved enzymatically from the parent POMC before or during the secretory process. However, β-endorphin levels may or may not correlate with circulating levels of ACTH, depending on the nature of the stimulus. The functions and regulation of secretion of the related peptides derived from POMC are poorly understood.

The major factors controlling ACTH release include CRH, the free cortisol concentration in plasma, stress, and the sleep-wake cycle (Fig. 331-3). The plasma level of ACTH varies during the day as a result of its pulsatile secretion, and it follows a circadian pattern with a peak just prior to waking and a nadir before sleeping. If a new sleep-wake cycle is adopted, the pattern changes over several days to conform to it. ACTH and cortisol levels also increase in response to eating. Stress (e.g., pyrogens, surgery, hypoglycemia, exercise, and severe emotional trauma) causes the release of CRH and arginine vasopressin (AVP) and activation of the sympathetic nervous system. These changes in turn enhance ACTH release, acting individually or in concert. For example, AVP release acts synergistically with CRH to amplify ACTH secretion; CRH also stimulates the locus coeruleus/sympathetic system. Stress-related secretion of ACTH abolishes the circadian periodicity of ACTH levels but is, in turn, suppressed by prior high-dose glucocorticoid administration. The normal pulsatile, circadian pattern of ACTH release is regulated by CRH; this mechanism is the so-called open feedback loop. CRH secretion, in turn, is influenced by hypothalamic neurotransmitters. For example, serotoninergic and cholinergic systems stimulate the secretion of CRH and ACTH; there is contradictory evidence regarding the inhibitory effects of α-adrenergic agonists and γ-aminobutyric acid (GABA) on CRH release. In addition, there may be direct pituitary effects of these neurotransmitters. There is also evidence for peptidergic regulation of ACTH release. For example, β-endorphin and enkephalin inhibit the secretion of ACTH, whereas vasopressin and angiotensin II augment it. The immune system also influences the hypothalamic-pituitary-adrenal axis (Fig. 331-4). For example, inflammatory cytokines [tumor necrosis factor (TNF)-α, interleukin (IL)-1α, IL-1β, and IL-6] produced by monocytes increase ACTH release by stimulating secretion of CRH and/or AVP. Finally, ACTH release is regulated by the level of free cortisol in plasma. Cortisol decreases the responsiveness of pituitary corticotropic cells to CRH; the response of the POMC mRNA to CRH is also inhibited by glucocorticoids. In addition, glucocorticoids inhibit the locus coeruleus/sympathetic system and CRH release. The latter ser-

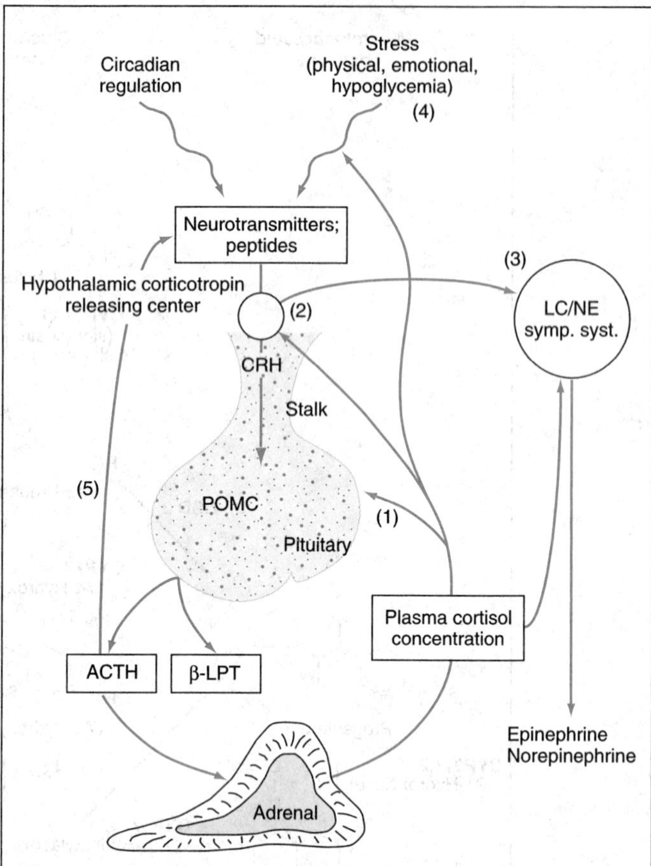

FIGURE 331-3 The hypothalamic-pituitary-adrenal axis. The main sites for feedback control by plasma cortisol are the pituitary gland (1) and the hypothalamic corticotropin-releasing center (2). Feedback control by plasma cortisol also occurs at the locus coeruleus/sympathetic system (3) and may involve higher nerve centers (4) as well. There also may be a short feedback loop involving inhibition of CRH by ACTH (5). Hypothalamic neurotransmitters influence CRH release; serotoninergic and cholinergic systems stimulate the secretion of CRH and ACTH; alpha-adrenergic agonists and γ-aminobutyric acid (GABA) probably inhibit CRH release. The opioid peptides β-endorphin and enkephalin inhibit, and vasopressin and angiotensin II augment, the secretion of CRH and ACTH. CRH, corticotropin-releasing hormone; β-LPT, β-lipotropin; POMC, pro-opiomelanocortin; LC, locus coeruleus; NE, norepinephrine.

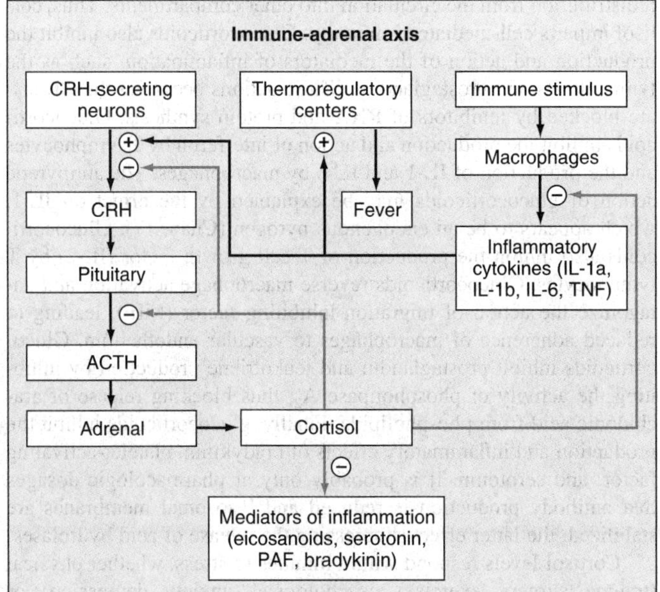

FIGURE 331-4 The immune-adrenal axis. Cortisol has anti-inflammatory properties that include effects on the microvasculature, cellular actions, and the suppression of inflammatory cytokines (the so-called immune-adrenal axis). A stress such as sepsis increases adrenal secretion, and cortisol in turn suppresses the immune response via this system. −, suppression; +, stimulation; CRH, corticotropin-releasing hormone; ACTH, adrenocorticotropin; IL, interleukin; TNF, tumor necrosis factor; PAF, platelet activating factor.

vomechanism establishes the primacy of cortisol in the control of ACTH secretion. The inhibition of ACTH occurs in two phases: (1) an early fast feedback, mediated via the MR, which lasts <10 min and depends on both the rate of increase of glucocorticoid levels and the specific glucocorticoid administered; and (2) a time-dependent, delayed feedback, likely mediated by the GR, which is probably due to inhibition of synthesis of the precursor protein. The suppression of ACTH secretion that results in adrenal atrophy following *prolonged* glucocorticoid therapy is caused primarily by suppression of hypothalamic CRH release, as exogenous CRH administration in this circumstance produces a rise in plasma ACTH. Cortisol also exerts feedback effects on higher brain centers (hippocampus, reticular system, and septum) and perhaps on the adrenal cortex (Fig. 331-4).

The biologic half-life of ACTH in the circulation is <10 min. The action of ACTH is also rapid; within minutes of its release, the concentration of steroids in the adrenal venous blood increases. ACTH stimulates steroidogenesis via activation of the membrane-bound adenyl cyclase. Adenosine-3′,5′-monophosphate (cyclic AMP), in turn, activates protein kinase enzymes, thereby resulting in the phosphorylation of proteins that activate steroid biosynthesis.

RENIN-ANGIOTENSIN PHYSIOLOGY (See also Chap. 246) Renin is a proteolytic enzyme that is produced and stored in the granules of the juxtaglomerular cells surrounding the afferent arterioles of glomeruli in the kidney. Renin exists in both active and inactive forms. Whether the inactive form is a precursor ("prorenin") or is a product formed after release is uncertain. Renin acts on the basic substrate angiotensinogen (a circulating α_2-globulin made in the liver) to form the decapeptide angiotensin I (Fig. 331-5). Angiotensin I is then enzymatically transformed by angiotensin-converting enzyme (ACE), which is present in many tissues (particularly the pulmonary vascular endothelium), to the octapeptide angiotensin II by the removal of the two C-terminal amino acids. Angiotensin II is a potent pressor agent and exerts its action by a direct effect on arteriolar smooth muscle. In addition, angiotensin II stimulates production of aldosterone by the zona glomerulosa of the adrenal cortex; the heptapeptide angiotensin III may also stimulate aldosterone production. The two major classes of angiotensin receptors are termed *AT1* and *AT2*; AT1 may exist as two subtypes α and β. Most of the effects of angiotensins II and III are mediated by the AT1 receptor. Angiotensinases rapidly destroy angiotensin II (half-life, approximately 1 min), while the half-life of renin is more prolonged (10 to 20 min). In addition to circulating renin-angiotensin, many tissues have a local renin-angiotensin system and the ability to produce angiotensin II. These tissues include the uterus, placenta, vascular tissue, heart, brain, and, particularly, the adrenal cortex and kidney. Although the role of locally generated angiotensin II is not established, it may be involved in the growth and modulation of function of the adrenal cortex and vascular smooth muscle.

The amount of renin released reflects the combined effects of four interdependent factors. The *juxtaglomerular cells*, which are specialized myoepithelial cells that cuff the afferent arterioles, act as miniature pressure transducers, sensing renal perfusion pressure and corresponding changes in afferent arteriolar perfusion pressures. For example, under conditions of a reduction in circulating blood volume, there is a corresponding reduction in renal perfusion pressure and, therefore, in afferent arteriolar pressure (Fig. 331-5). This change is perceived by the juxtaglomerular cells as a decreased stretch exerted on the afferent arteriolar walls. The juxtaglomerular cells then release more renin into the renal circulation. This results in the formation of angiotensin I, which is converted in the kidney and peripherally to angiotensin II by ACE. Angiotensin II influences sodium homeostasis via two major mechanisms: it changes renal blood flow so as to maintain a constant glomerular filtration rate, thereby changing the filtration fraction of sodium, and it stimulates the adrenal cortex to release aldosterone. Increasing plasma levels of aldosterone enhance renal sodium retention and thus result in expansion of the extracellular fluid volume, which, in turn, dampens the stimulus for renin release. In this context, the renin-angiotensin-aldosterone system regulates volume by modifying renal hemodynamics and tubular sodium transport.

A second control mechanism for renin release is centered in the *macula densa* cells, a group of distal convoluted tubular epithelial cells directly apposed to the juxtaglomerular cells. They may function as chemoreceptors, monitoring the sodium (or chloride) load presented to the distal tubule, and such information may be conveyed to the juxtaglomerular cells, where appropriate modifications in renin release take place. Under conditions of increased delivery of filtered sodium

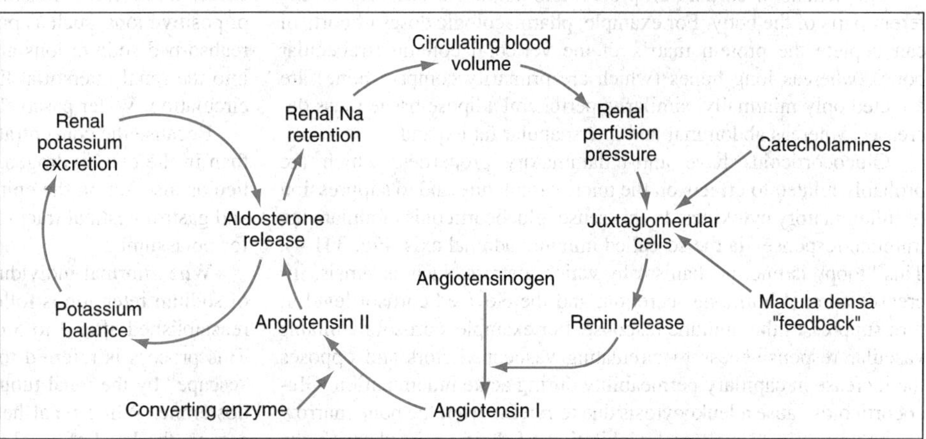

FIGURE 331-5 The interrelationship of the volume and potassium feedback loops on aldosterone secretion. Integration of signals from each loop determines the level of aldosterone secretion.

to the macula densa, increasing release of renin decreases the glomerular filtration rate, thereby reducing the filtered load of sodium.

The *sympathetic nervous system* regulates the release of renin in response to assumption of the upright posture. The mechanism is either a direct effect on the juxtaglomerular cell to increase adenyl cyclase activity or an indirect effect on either the juxtaglomerular or the macula densa cells via vasoconstriction of the afferent arteriole.

Finally, circulating factors influence renin release. Increased dietary intake of *potassium* decreases, and decreased potassium intake increases, renin release. The significance of these effects is unclear. *Angiotensin II* exerts negative feedback control on renin release that is independent of alterations in renal blood flow, blood pressure, or aldosterone secretion. *Atrial natriuretic peptides* also inhibit renin release. Thus, the control of renin release involves both *intrarenal* (pressor receptor and macula densa) and *extrarenal* (sympathetic nervous system, potassium, angiotensin, etc.) mechanisms. Steady-state renin levels reflect all these factors, with the intrarenal mechanism predominating.

GLUCOCORTICOID PHYSIOLOGY The division of adrenal steroids into glucocorticoids and mineralocorticoids is arbitrary in that most glucocorticoids have some mineralocorticoid-like properties. The descriptive term *glucocorticoid* is used for adrenal steroids whose predominant action is on intermediary metabolism. Their overall actions are directed at enhancing the production of the high-energy fuel, glucose, and reducing all other metabolic activity not directly involved in that process. Sustained activation, however, results in a pathophysiologic state, e.g., Cushing's syndrome. The principal glucocorticoid is cortisol (hydrocortisone). The effect of glucocorticoids on intermediary metabolism is mediated by the GR. Physiologic effects of glucocorticoids include the regulation of protein, carbohydrate, lipid, and nucleic acid metabolism. Glucocorticoids raise the blood glucose level by acting as an insulin antagonist and by suppressing the secretion of insulin, thereby inhibiting peripheral glucose uptake, which promotes hepatic glucose synthesis (gluconeogenesis) and increases hepatic glycogen content. The actions on protein metabolism are mainly catabolic in effect, resulting in an increase in protein breakdown and nitrogen excretion. In large part, these actions reflect a mobilization of glycogenic amino acid precursors from peripheral supporting structures, such as bone, skin, muscle, and connective tissue, due to protein breakdown and inhibition of protein synthesis and amino acid uptake. Hyperaminoacidemia also facilitates gluconeogenesis by stimulating glucagon secretion. Glucocorticoids act directly on the liver to stimulate the synthesis of certain enzymes, such as tyrosine aminotransferase and tryptophan pyrrolase. Glucocorticoids regulate fatty acid mobilization by enhancing the activation of cellular lipase by lipid-mobilizing hormones (e.g., catecholamines and pituitary peptides).

The actions of cortisol on protein and adipose tissue vary in different parts of the body. For example, pharmacologic doses of cortisol can deplete the protein matrix of the vertebral column (trabecular bone), whereas long bones (which are primarily compact bone) are affected only minimally; similarly, peripheral adipose tissue mass decreases, whereas abdominal and interscapular fat expand.

Glucocorticoids have anti-inflammatory properties, which are probably related to effects on the microvasculature and to suppression of inflammatory cytokines. In this sense, glucocorticoids modulate the immune response via the so-called immune-adrenal axis (Fig. 331-4). This "loop" is one mechanism by which a stress, such as sepsis, increases adrenal hormone secretion, and the elevated cortisol level in turn suppresses the immune response. For example, cortisol maintains vascular responsiveness to circulating vasoconstrictors and opposes the increase in capillary permeability during acute inflammation. Glucocorticoids cause a leukocytosis due to release from the bone marrow of mature cells as well as to inhibition of their egress through the capillary wall. Glucocorticoids produce a depletion of circulating eosinophils and of lymphoid tissue, specifically T cells, by causing a redistribution from the circulation into other compartments. Thus, cortisol impairs cell-mediated immunity. Glucocorticoids also inhibit the production and action of the mediators of inflammation, such as the lymphokines and prostaglandins. These actions occur via the GR and are blocked by inhibitors of RNA and protein synthesis. Glucocorticoids inhibit the production and action of interferon by T lymphocytes and the production of IL-1 and IL-6 by macrophages. The antipyretic action of glucocorticoids may be explained by the effect on IL-1, which appears to be an endogenous pyrogen (Chap. 17). Glucocorticoids also inhibit the production of T cell growth factor (IL-2) by T lymphocytes. Glucocorticoids reverse macrophage activation and antagonize the action of migration-inhibiting factor (MIF), leading to reduced adherence of macrophages to vascular endothelium. Glucocorticoids inhibit prostaglandin and leukotriene production by inhibiting the activity of phospholipase A_2, thus blocking release of arachidonic acid from phospholipids. Finally, glucocorticoids inhibit the production and inflammatory effects of bradykinin, platelet-activating factor, and serotonin. It is probably only at pharmacologic dosages that antibody production is reduced and lysosomal membranes are stabilized, the latter effect suppressing the release of acid hydrolases.

Cortisol levels respond within minutes to stress, whether physical (trauma, surgery, exercise), psychological (anxiety, depression), or physiologic (hypoglycemia, fever). The reasons why elevated glucocorticoid levels protect the organism under stress are not understood, but in conditions of glucocorticoid deficiency, such stresses may cause hypotension, shock, and death. Consequently, in individuals with adrenal insufficiency, glucocorticoid administration should be increased during stress.

Cortisol has major effects on body water. It helps regulate the extracellular fluid volume by retarding the migration of water into cells and by promoting renal water excretion, the latter effect mediated by suppression of vasopressin secretion, by an increase in the rate of glomerular filtration, and by a direct action on the renal tubule. The consequence is to prevent water intoxication by increasing solute-free water clearance. Glucocorticoids also have weak mineralocorticoid-like properties, and high doses promote renal tubular sodium reabsorption and increased urine potassium excretion. Glucocorticoids also can influence behavior; emotional disorders may occur with either an excess or a deficit of cortisol. Last, cortisol suppresses the secretion of pituitary POMC and its derivative peptides (ACTH, β-endorphin, and β-LPT) and the secretion of hypothalamic CRH and vasopressin.

MINERALOCORTICOID PHYSIOLOGY Mineralocorticoids are major regulators of extracellular fluid volume and the major determinant of potassium metabolism. These effects are mediated by the binding of aldosterone to the MR in target tissues, primarily the kidney. Volume is regulated through a direct effect on the collecting duct, where aldosterone causes an increase in sodium retention and an increase in potassium excretion. The reabsorption of sodium ions causes a fall in the transmembrane potential, thus enhancing the flow of positive ions, such as potassium, out of the cell into the lumen. The reabsorbed sodium ions are transported out of the tubular epithelium into the renal interstitial fluid and from there into the renal capillary circulation. Water passively follows the transported sodium.

Because the concentration of hydrogen ion is greater in the lumen than in the cell, hydrogen ion is also actively secreted. Mineralocorticoids also act on the epithelium of the salivary ducts, sweat glands, and gastrointestinal tract to cause reabsorption of sodium in exchange for potassium.

When normal individuals are given aldosterone, an initial period of sodium retention is followed by natriuresis, and sodium balance is reestablished after 3 to 5 days. As a result, edema does not develop. This process is referred to as the *escape phenomenon*, signifying an "escape" by the renal tubules from the sodium-retaining action of aldosterone. While renal hemodynamic factors may play a role in the escape, the level of atrial natriuretic peptide also increases. However, it is important to realize that there is no escape from the potassium-losing effects of mineralocorticoids.

There are additional nonclassic effects of mineralocorticoids, primarily on nonepithelial cells. These effects are likely genomic and therefore mediated through activation of the cytosolic MR, but they do not include a modification of sodium-potassium homeostasis. They are probably mediated by mineralocorticoids modifying the expression of several collagen genes and/or genes controlling tissue growth factors, e.g., transforming growth factor β (TGF-β) and plasminogen activator inhibitor (PAI-1). The resultant effects lead to microangiopathy, necrosis (acutely), and fibrosis in a variety of tissues, e.g., heart, kidney, and vasculature. Increased levels of aldosterone are not necessary to produce this damage; rather, an imbalance between the level of aldosterone and the volume and/or sodium balance state appears to be the critical factor.

Three primary mechanisms control aldosterone release—the renin-angiotensin system, potassium, and ACTH (Table 331-1). The renin-angiotensin system controls extracellular fluid volume via regulation of aldosterone secretion (Fig. 331-5). In effect, the renin-angiotensin system maintains the circulating blood volume constant by causing aldosterone-induced sodium retention during volume deficiency and by decreasing aldosterone-dependent sodium retention when volume is ample.

Potassium ion directly stimulates aldosterone secretion, independent of the circulating renin-angiotensin system, which it suppresses (Fig. 331-5). In addition to potassium's direct effect, it also modifies aldosterone secretion indirectly by activating the local renin-angiotensin system in the zona glomerulosa. This effect can be blocked by the administration of ACE inhibitors that reduce the local production of angiotensin II and thereby reduce the acute aldosterone response to potassium. An increase in serum potassium of as little as 0.1 mmol/L increases plasma aldosterone levels under certain circumstances. Oral potassium loading therefore increases aldosterone secretion, excretion, and plasma levels.

Physiologic amounts of ACTH stimulate aldosterone secretion acutely, but this action is not sustained unless ACTH is administered in a pulsatile fashion. Most studies relegate ACTH to a minor role in the control of aldosterone. For example, subjects receiving high-dose glucocorticoid therapy, and with presumed complete suppression of ACTH, have normal aldosterone secretion in response to sodium restriction.

Prior dietary intake of both potassium and sodium can alter the magnitude of the aldosterone response to acute stimulation. This effect results from a change in the expression and activity of aldosterone synthase. Increasing potassium intake or decreasing sodium intake sensitizes the response of the glomerulosa cells to acute stimulation by ACTH, angiotensin II, and/or potassium. Thus, regulation of aldosterone secretion occurs both early and late in its synthetic pathway.

Neurotransmitters (dopamine and serotonin) and some peptides, such as atrial natriuretic peptide, γ-melanocyte-stimulating hormone (γ-MSH), and β-endorphin, also participate in the regulation of aldosterone secretion (Table 331-1). Thus, the control of aldosterone secretion involves both stimulatory and inhibitory factors.

Table 331-1 Factors Regulating Aldosterone Biosynthesis

Factor	Effect
Renin-angiotensin system	Stimulation
Sodium ion	Inhibition (?physiologic)
Potassium ion	Stimulation
Neurotransmitters	
Dopamine	Inhibition
Serotonin	Stimulation
Pituitary hormones	
ACTH	Stimulation
Non-ACTH pituitary hormones (e.g., growth hormone)	Permissive (for optimal response to sodium restriction)
β-Endorphin	Stimulation
γ-Melanocyte-stimulating hormone	Permissive
Atrial natriuretic peptide	Inhibition
Ouabain-like factors	Inhibition
Endothelin	Stimulation

ANDROGEN PHYSIOLOGY Androgens regulate male secondary sexual characteristics and can cause virilizing symptoms in women (Chap. 53). Adrenal androgens have a minimal effect in males whose sexual characteristics are predominately determined by gonadal steroids (testosterone). In females, however, several androgen-like effects, e.g., sexual hair, are largely mediated by adrenal androgens. The principal adrenal androgens are DHEA, androstenedione, and 11-hydroxyandrostenedione. DHEA and androstenedione are weak androgens and exert their effects via conversion to the potent androgen testosterone in extraglandular tissues. DHEA also has poorly understood effects on the immune and cardiovascular systems. Adrenal androgen formation is regulated by ACTH, not by gonadotropins. It follows that adrenal androgens are suppressed by exogenous glucocorticoid administration.

LABORATORY EVALUATION OF ADRENOCORTICAL FUNCTION

A basic assumption is that measurements of the plasma or urinary level of a given steroid reflects the rate of adrenal *secretion* of that steroid. However, urine *excretion* values may not truly reflect the secretion rate because of improper collection or altered metabolism. Plasma levels reflect the level of secretion only at the time of measurement. The plasma level (*PL*) depends on two factors: the secretion rate (*SR*) of the hormone and the rate at which it is metabolized, i.e., its metabolic clearance rate (*MCR*). These three factors can be related as follows:

$$PL = \frac{SR}{MCR} \quad \text{or} \quad SR = MCR \times PL$$

BLOOD LEVELS Peptides The plasma levels of ACTH and angiotensin II can be measured by immunoassay techniques. Basal ACTH secretion shows a circadian rhythm, with lower levels in the early evening than in the morning. However, ACTH is secreted in a pulsatile manner, leading to rapid fluctuations superimposed on this circadian rhythm. Angiotensin II levels also vary diurnally and are influenced by dietary sodium and potassium intakes and posture. Both upright posture and sodium restriction elevate angiotensin II levels.

Most clinical determinations of the renin-angiotensin system, however, involve measurements of peripheral *plasma renin activity* (PRA) in which the renin activity is gauged by the generation of angiotensin I during a standardized incubation period. This method depends on the presence of sufficient angiotensinogen in the plasma as substrate. The generated angiotensin I is measured by radioimmunoassay. The PRA depends on the dietary sodium intake and on whether the patient is ambulatory. In normal humans, the PRA shows a diurnal rhythm characterized by peak values in the morning and decreases in activity in the afternoon. An alternative approach is to measure plasma active renin, which is easier and not dependent on endogenous substrate concentration. PRA and active renin correlate very well on low-sodium diets ($r = 0.85$ to 0.9) but less well on high-sodium diets.

Steroids Cortisol and aldosterone are both secreted episodically, and levels generally vary during the day, with peak values in the morning and low levels in the evening. In addition, the plasma level of aldosterone, but not of cortisol, is increased by dietary potassium loading, by sodium restriction, or by assumption of the upright posture. Measurement of the sulfate conjugate of DHEA may be a useful index of adrenal androgen secretion, as little DHEA sulfate is formed in the gonads and because the half-life of DHEA sulfate is 7 to 9 h. However, DHEA sulfate levels reflect both DHEA production and sulfatase activity.

URINE LEVELS For the assessment of glucocorticoid secretion, the urine *17-hydroxycorticosteroid* assay has been replaced by measurement of urinary free cortisol. Elevated levels of urinary free cortisol correlate with states of hypercortisolism, reflecting changes in the levels of unbound, physiologically active circulating cortisol. Normally, the rate of excretion is higher in the daytime (7 A.M. to 7 P.M.) than at night (7 P.M. to 7 A.M.).

Urinary *17-ketosteroids* originate in either the adrenal gland or the gonad. In normal women, 90% of urinary 17-ketosteroids is derived from the adrenal, and in men 60 to 70% is of adrenal origin. Urine 17-ketosteroid values are highest in young adults and decline with age.

A carefully timed urine collection is a prerequisite for all excretory determinations. Urinary creatinine should be measured simultaneously to determine the accuracy and adequacy of the collection procedure.

STIMULATION TESTS Stimulation tests are useful in the diagnosis of hormone deficiency states.

Tests of Glucocorticoid Reserve Within minutes after administration of ACTH, cortisol levels increase. This responsiveness can be used as an index of the functional reserve of the adrenal gland for production of cortisol. Under maximal ACTH stimulation, cortisol secretion increases tenfold, to 800 μmol/d (300 mg/d), but maximal stimulation can be achieved only with prolonged ACTH infusions.

A screening test (the so-called rapid ACTH stimulation test) involves the administration of 25 units (0.25 mg) of cosyntropin intravenously or intramuscularly and measurement of plasma cortisol levels before and 30 and 60 min after administration; the test can be performed at any time of the day. The most clear-cut criterion for a normal response is a stimulated cortisol level of >500 nmol/L (>18 μg/dL), and the minimal stimulated normal increment of cortisol is >200 nmol/L (>7 μg/dL) above baseline. Severely ill patients with elevated basal cortisol levels may show no further increases following acute ACTH administration.

Tests of Mineralocorticoid Reserve and Stimulation of the Renin-Angiotensin System Stimulation tests use protocols designed to create a programmed volume depletion, such as sodium restriction, diuretic administration, or upright posture. A simple, potent test consists of severe sodium restriction and upright posture. After 3 to 5 days of a 10-mmol/d sodium intake, rates of aldosterone secretion or excretion should increase two- to threefold over the control values. Supine morning plasma aldosterone levels are usually increased three- to sixfold, and they increase a further two- to fourfold in response to 2 to 3 h of upright posture.

When the dietary sodium intake is normal, stimulation testing requires the administration of a potent diuretic, such as 40 to 80 mg furosemide, followed by 2 to 3 h of upright posture. The normal response is a two- to fourfold rise in plasma aldosterone levels.

SUPPRESSION TESTS Suppression tests to document hypersecretion of adrenal hormones involve measurement of the target hormone response after standardized suppression of its tropic hormone.

Tests of Pituitary-Adrenal Suppressibility The ACTH release mechanism is sensitive to the circulating glucocorticoid level. When blood levels of glucocorticoid are increased in normal individuals, less ACTH is released from the anterior pituitary and less steroid is produced by the adrenal gland. The integrity of this feedback mechanism can be tested clinically by giving a glucocorticoid and judging the suppression of ACTH secretion by analysis of urine steroid levels and/or plasma cortisol and ACTH levels. A potent glucocorticoid such as dexamethasone is used, so that the agent can be given in an amount small enough not to contribute significantly to the pool of steroids to be analyzed.

The best *screening* procedure is the overnight dexamethasone suppression test. This involves the measurement of plasma cortisol levels at 8 A.M. following the oral administration of 1 mg dexamethasone the previous midnight. The 8 A.M. value for plasma cortisol in normal individuals should be <140 nmol/L (5 μg/dL).

The definitive test of adrenal suppressibility consists in administering 0.5 mg dexamethasone every 6 h for two successive days while collecting urine over a 24-h period for determination of creatinine and free cortisol and/or measuring plasma cortisol levels. In a patient with a normal hypothalamic-pituitary ACTH release mechanism, a fall in the urine free cortisol to <80 nmol/d (30 μg/d) or of plasma cortisol to <140 nmol/L (5 μg/dL) is seen on the second day of administration.

A normal response to either suppression test implies that the glucocorticoid regulation of ACTH and its control of the adrenal glands is physiologically normal. However, an isolated abnormal result, particularly to the overnight suppression test, does not in itself imply pituitary and/or adrenal disease.

Tests of Mineralocorticoid Suppressibility These tests rely on an expansion of extracellular fluid volume, which should decrease circulating plasma renin activity and decrease the secretion and/or excretion of aldosterone. Various tests differ in the rate at which extracellular fluid volume is expanded. One convenient suppression test involves the intravenous infusion of 500 mL/h of normal saline solution for 4 h, which normally suppresses plasma aldosterone levels to <220 pmol/L (<8 ng/dL) on a sodium-restricted diet or to <140 pmol/L (<5 ng/dL) on a normal sodium intake. Alternatively, a high-sodium diet can be administered for 3 days with 0.2 mg fludrocortisone twice daily. Aldosterone excretion is measured on the third day and should be <28 nmol/d (10 μg/d). These tests should not be performed in potassium-depleted individuals since they carry a risk of precipitating hypokalemia.

TESTS OF PITUITARY-ADRENAL RESPONSIVENESS Stimuli such as insulin-induced hypoglycemia, AVP, and pyrogens cause the release of ACTH from the pituitary by an action on higher neural centers or on the pituitary itself. Insulin-induced hypoglycemia is particularly useful, because it stimulates the release of both growth hormone and ACTH. In this test, regular insulin (0.05 to 0.1 U/kg body weight) is given intravenously as a bolus to reduce the fasting glucose level to at least 50% below basal. The normal cortisol response is a rise to more than 500 nmol/L (18 μg/dL).

One of the best ways to test the integrity of the pituitary-adrenal axis is the metyrapone test. Metyrapone inhibits 11β-hydroxylase in the adrenal. As a result, the conversion of 11-deoxycortisol (compound S) to cortisol is impaired, causing 11-deoxycortisol to accumulate in the blood and the blood level of cortisol to decrease (Fig. 331-2). The hypothalamic-pituitary axis responds to the declining cortisol blood levels by releasing more ACTH. Note that assessment of the response depends on both an intact hypothalamic-pituitary axis and an intact adrenal gland.

Although modifications of the original metyrapone test have been described, we believe the best involves administering 750 mg of the drug by mouth every 4 h over a 24-h period and comparing the control and postmetyrapone plasma levels of 11-deoxycortisol, cortisol, and ACTH. In normal individuals, plasma 11-deoxycortisol levels should exceed 210 nmol/L (7 μg/dL) and ACTH levels should exceed 17 pmol/L (75 pg/mL) following metyrapone administration. The metyrapone test does not accurately reflect ACTH reserve if subjects are ingesting exogenous glucocorticoids or drugs that accelerate the metabolism of metyrapone (e.g., phenytoin).

A direct and selective test of the pituitary corticotrophs can be achieved with CRH. The bolus injection of ovine CRH (corticorelin, ovine triflutate; 1 μg/kg body weight) stimulates secretion of ACTH and β-LPT in normal human subjects within 15 to 60 min. In normal individuals, the mean increment in ACTH is 9 pmol/L (40 pg/mL). However, the magnitude of the ACTH response is less than that produced by the insulin tolerance test, which implies that additional factors (such as vasopressin) augment stress-induced increases in ACTH secretion.

Although the rapid ACTH stimulation test is useful for the diagnosis of primary adrenal insufficiency, normal cortisol responsiveness may be seen in some patients with a partial ACTH deficit and absence of adrenal atrophy. These patients have an inadequate pituitary ACTH reserve and fail to increase ACTH secretion in response to a stress such as surgery or hypoglycemia. Because the use of a bolus of exogenous ACTH does not invariably exclude a diagnosis of secondary adrenocortical insufficiency, direct tests of pituitary ACTH reserve (metyrapone test, insulin tolerance testing) may be required in the appropriate clinical setting. Alternatively, ACTH at a physiologic dose (1 μg), the so-called low-dose ACTH test, may be used. Abnormal response is similar to the rapid ACTH test. However, levels need to be measured at 30 min, and the ACTH needs to be injected directly intravenously because it can be absorbed to plastic tubing. On the other hand, the rapid ACTH test can distinguish between primary and secondary adrenal insufficiency, because aldosterone secretion is preserved in secondary adrenal failure by the renin-angiotensin system and potassium. Cosyntropin (25 units) is given intravenously or intramuscularly, and plasma cortisol and aldosterone levels are measured before and 30 and 60 min after administration. The cortisol response is abnormal in both groups, but patients with secondary insufficiency show an increase in aldosterone levels by at least 140 pmol/L (5 ng/dL). No aldosterone response is seen in patients in whom the adrenal cortex is destroyed.

HYPERFUNCTION OF THE ADRENAL CORTEX

Excess cortisol is associated with Cushing's syndrome; excess aldosterone causes aldosteronism; and excess adrenal androgens cause adrenal virilism. These syndromes do not always occur in the "pure" form but may have overlapping features.

CUSHING'S SYNDROME **Etiology** Cushing described a syndrome characterized by truncal obesity, hypertension, fatigability and weakness, amenorrhea, hirsutism, purplish abdominal striae, edema, glucosuria, osteoporosis, and a basophilic tumor of the pituitary. As awareness of this syndrome has increased, the diagnosis of Cushing's syndrome has been broadened into the classification shown in Table 331-2. Regardless of etiology, all cases of endogenous Cushing's syndrome are due to increased production of cortisol by the adrenal. In most cases the cause is *bilateral adrenal hyperplasia* due to hypersecretion of pituitary ACTH or ectopic production of ACTH by a nonpituitary source. The incidence of pituitary-dependent adrenal hyperplasia is three times greater in women than in men, and the most frequent age of onset is the third or fourth decade. Most evidence indicates that the primary defect is the de novo development of a pituitary adenoma, as tumors are found in >90% of patients with pituitary-dependent adrenal hyperplasia. Alternatively, the defect may occasionally reside in the hypothalamus or in higher neural centers, leading to release of CRH inappropriate to the level of circulating cortisol. The consequence would be that a higher level of cortisol is required to reduce ACTH secretion to normal. This primary defect leads to hyperstimulation of the pituitary, resulting in hyperplasia or tumor formation. In surgical series, most individuals with hypersecretion of pituitary ACTH are found to have a microadenoma (<10 mm in diameter; 50% are ≤5 mm in diameter), but a pituitary macroadenoma (>10 mm) or diffuse hyperplasia of the corticotropic cells may be found. In some studies, the recurrence rate is >20%. Unfortunately, it may be difficult to distinguish between recurrence and inadequate primary therapy. Traditionally, only an individual who has an ACTH-producing pituitary tumor is defined as having *Cushing's disease*.

Table 331-2 Causes of Cushing's Syndrome

Adrenal hyperplasia
- Secondary to pituitary ACTH overproduction
  - Pituitary-hypothalamic dysfunction
  - Pituitary ACTH-producing micro- or macroadenomas
- Secondary to ACTH or CRH-producing nonendocrine tumors (bronchogenic carcinoma, carcinoid of the thymus, pancreatic carcinoma, bronchial adenoma)

Adrenal macronodular hyperplasia

Adrenal micronodular dysplasia
- Sporadic
- Familial (Carney's syndrome)

Adrenal neoplasia
- Adenoma
- Carcinoma

Exogenous, iatrogenic causes
- Prolonged use of glucocorticoids
- Prolonged use of ACTH

NOTE: CRH, corticotropin-releasing hormone.

Nonpituitary tumors may secrete polypeptides that are biologically, chemically, and immunologically indistinguishable from either ACTH or CRH and that cause bilateral adrenal hyperplasia (Chap. 100). The ectopic production of CRH results in clinical, biochemical, and radiologic features indistinguishable from those caused by hypersecretion of pituitary ACTH. The typical signs and symptoms of Cushing's syndrome may be absent or minimal with ectopic ACTH production, and hypokalemic alkalosis is a prominent manifestation. Most of these cases are associated with the primitive small cell (oat cell) type of bronchogenic carcinoma or with tumors of the thymus, pancreas, or ovary; medullary carcinoma of the thyroid; or bronchial adenomas. The onset of Cushing's syndrome may be sudden, particularly in patients with carcinoma of the lung, and this feature accounts in part for the failure of these patients to exhibit the classic manifestations. On the other hand, patients with carcinoid tumors or pheochromocytomas have longer clinical courses and usually exhibit the typical cushingoid features. The ectopic secretion of ACTH is also accompanied by the accumulation of ACTH fragments in plasma and by elevated plasma levels of ACTH precursor molecules. Because such tumors may produce large amounts of ACTH, baseline steroid values are usually markedly elevated, and increased skin pigmentation may be present. Indeed, hyperpigmentation in patients with Cushing's syndrome almost always points to an extraadrenal tumor, either in an extracranial location or within the cranium.

Approximately 20 to 25% of patients with Cushing's syndrome have an adrenal neoplasm. These tumors are usually unilateral, and about half are malignant. Occasionally, patients have biochemical features both of pituitary ACTH excess and of an adrenal adenoma. These individuals usually have *nodular hyperplasia* of both adrenal glands often the result of prolonged ACTH stimulation in the absence of a pituitary adenoma. Two additional entities cause nodular hyperplasia: a familial disorder in children or young adults (so-called pigmented micronodular dysplasia; see below) and an abnormal cortisol response to gastric inhibitory polypeptide or luteinizing hormone, probably secondary to expression of receptors for these hormones in the adrenal cortex.

The most common cause of Cushing's syndrome is *iatrogenic* administration of steroids for a variety of reasons. Although the clinical features bear some resemblance to those seen with adrenal tumors, these patients are usually distinguishable on the basis of history and laboratory studies.

Clinical Signs, Symptoms, and Laboratory Findings Many of the signs and symptoms of Cushing's syndrome follow logically from the known action of glucocorticoids (Table 331-3). Mobilization of

Table 331-3 Frequency of Signs and Symptoms in Cushing's Syndrome

Sign or Symptom	Percent of Patients
Typical habitus (centripetal obesity)[a]	97
Increased body weight	94
Fatigability and weakness	87
Hypertension (blood pressure >150/90)	82
Hirsutism[a]	80
Amenorrhea	77
Broad violaceous cutaneous striae[a]	67
Personality changes	66
Ecchymoses[a]	65
Proximal myopathy[a]	62
Edema	62
Polyuria, polydipsia	23
Hypertrophy of clitoris	19

[a] Features more specific for Cushing's syndrome.

peripheral supportive tissue causes muscle weakness and fatigability, osteoporosis, broad violaceous cutaneous striae, and easy bruisability. The latter signs are secondary to weakening and rupture of collagen fibers in the dermis. Osteoporosis may cause collapse of vertebral bodies and pathologic fractures of other bones. Decreased bone mineralization is particularly pronounced in children. Increased hepatic gluconeogenesis and insulin resistance can cause impaired glucose tolerance. Overt diabetes mellitus occurs in <20% of patients, who probably are individuals with a predisposition to this disorder. Hypercortisolism promotes the deposition of adipose tissue in characteristic sites, notably the upper face (producing the typical "moon" facies), the interscapular area (producing the "buffalo hump"), and the mesenteric bed (producing "truncal" obesity) (Fig. 331-6). Rarely, episternal fatty tumors and mediastinal widening secondary to fat accumulation occur. The reason for this peculiar distribution of adipose tissue is not known, but it is associated with insulin resistance and/or elevated insulin levels. The face appears plethoric, even in the absence of any increase in red blood cell concentration. Hypertension is common, and emotional changes may be profound, ranging from irritability and emotional lability to severe depression, confusion, or even frank psychosis. In women, increased levels of adrenal androgens can cause acne, hirsutism, and oligomenorrhea or amenorrhea. Some signs and symptoms in patients with hypercortisolism—i.e., obesity, hypertension, osteoporosis, and diabetes—are nonspecific and therefore are less helpful in diagnosing the condition. On the other hand, easy bruising, typical striae, myopathy, and virilizing signs (although less frequent) are, if present, more suggestive of Cushing's syndrome (Table 331-3).

Except in iatrogenic Cushing's syndrome, plasma and urine cortisol levels are variably elevated. Occasionally, hypokalemia, hypochloremia, and metabolic alkalosis are present, particularly with ectopic production of ACTH.

Diagnosis The diagnosis of Cushing's syndrome depends on the demonstration of increased cortisol production and failure to suppress cortisol secretion normally when dexamethasone is administered (Chap. 328). Once the diagnosis is established, further testing is designed to determine the etiology (Fig. 331-7 and Table 331-4).

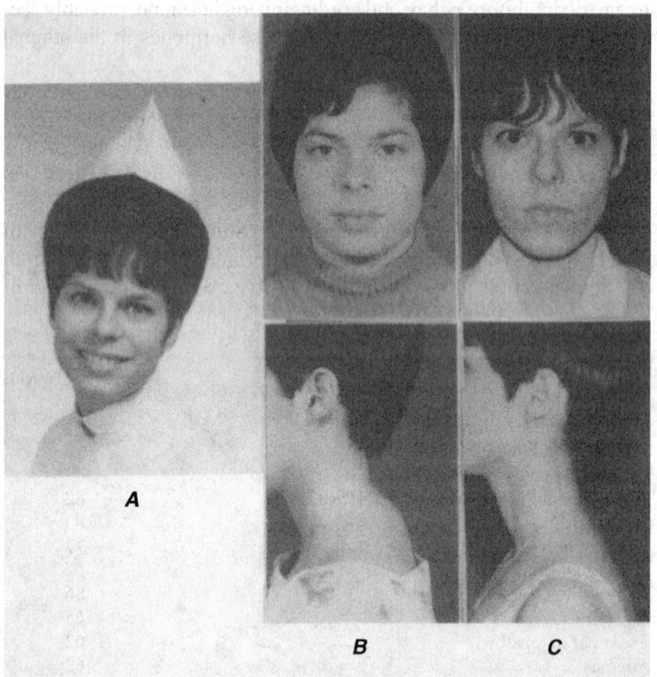

FIGURE 331-6 A woman with Cushing's syndrome due to a right adrenal cortical adenoma. *A*. Two years prior to surgery, age 18. *B*. One month prior to surgery, age 20. *C*. One year after surgery, age 21.

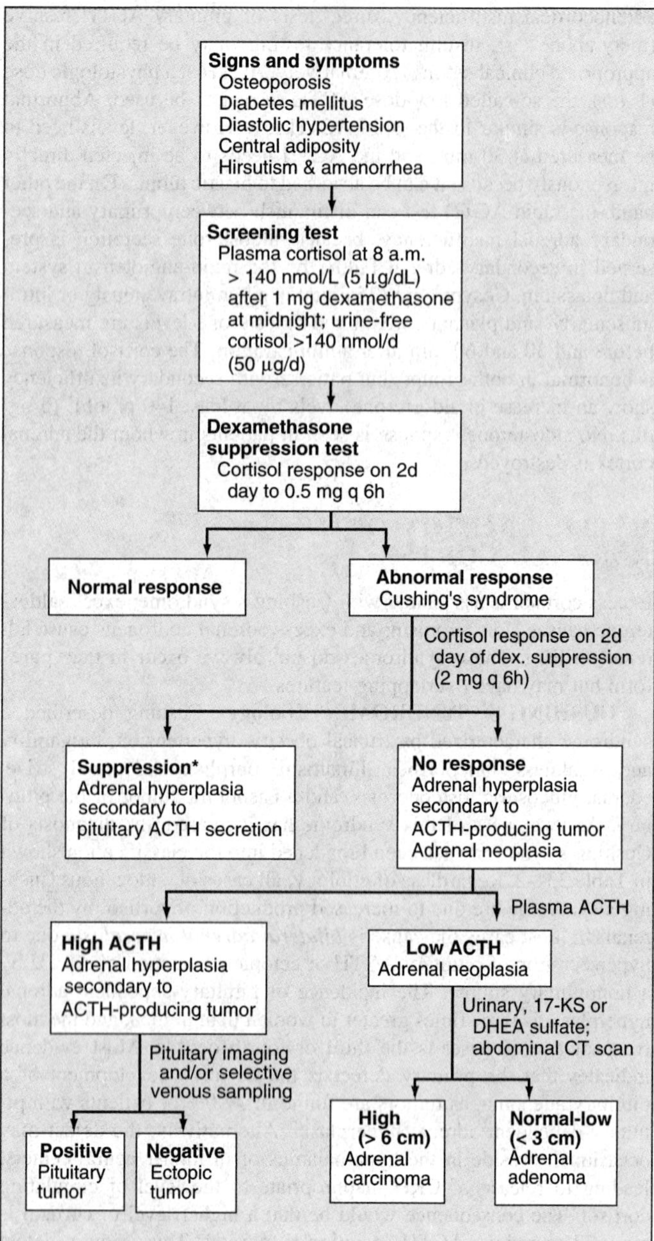

FIGURE 331-7 Diagnostic flowchart for evaluating patients suspected of having Cushing's syndrome. *This group probably includes some patients with pituitary-hypothalamic dysfunction and some with pituitary microadenomas. In some instances, a microadenoma may be visualized by pituitary MRI scanning. 17-KS, 17-ketosteroids; DHEA, dehydroepiandrosterone.

For initial screening, the overnight dexamethasone suppression test is recommended (see above). In difficult cases (e.g., in obese patients), measurement of a 24-h urine free cortisol also can be used as a screening test. A level >140 nmol/d (50 μg/d) is suggestive of Cushing's syndrome. The definitive diagnosis is then established by failure of urinary cortisol to fall to less than <25 nmol/d (10 μg/d) or of plasma cortisol to fall to <140 nmol/L (5 μg/dL) after a standard low-dose dexamethasone suppression test (0.5 mg every 6 h for 48 h). Owing to circadian variability, plasma cortisol and, to a certain extent, ACTH determinations are not meaningful when performed in isolation, but the absence of the normal fall of plasma cortisol at midnight is consistent with Cushing's syndrome.

The task of determining the etiology of Cushing's syndrome is complicated by the fact that all the available tests lack specificity and by the fact that the tumors producing this syndrome are prone to spontaneous and often dramatic changes in hormone secretion (periodic

Table 331-4 Diagnostic Tests to Determine the Type of Cushing's Syndrome

Test	Pituitary Macro-adenoma	Pituitary Micro-adenoma	Ectopic ACTH or CRH Production	Adrenal Tumor
Plasma ACTH level	↑ to ↑↑	N to ↑	↑ to ↑↑↑	↓
Percent who respond to high-dose dexamethasone	<10	95	<10	<10
Percent who respond to CRH	>90	>90	<10	<10

NOTE: CRH, corticotropin-releasing hormone; N, normal; ↑, elevated; ↓, decreased. See text for definition of a response.

hormonogenesis). No test has a specificity >95%, and it may be necessary to use a combination of tests to arrive at the correct diagnosis. A useful step to distinguish patients with an ACTH-secreting pituitary microadenoma or hypothalamic-pituitary dysfunction from those with other forms of Cushing's syndrome is to determine the response of cortisol output to administration of high-dose dexamethasone (2 mg every 6 h for 2 days). An alternative 8-mg, overnight high-dose dexamethasone test has been developed; however, this test has a lower sensitivity and specificity than the standard test. When the diagnosis of Cushing's syndrome is clear-cut on the basis of baseline urinary and plasma assays, the high-dose dexamethasone suppression test may be used without performing the preliminary low-dose suppression test. The high-dose suppression test provides close to 100% specificity if the criterion used is suppression of urinary free cortisol by >90%. Occasionally, in individuals with bilateral nodular hyperplasia and/or ectopic CRH production, steroid output is also suppressed. Failure of low- and high-dose dexamethasone administration to suppress cortisol production (Table 331-4) is usual in patients with adrenal hyperplasia secondary to an ACTH-secreting pituitary macroadenoma or an ACTH-producing tumor of nonendocrine origin and in those with adrenal neoplasms.

Plasma ACTH levels can be useful in distinguishing the various causes of Cushing's syndrome, particularly in separating ACTH-dependent from ACTH-independent causes. In general, measurement of plasma ACTH is useful in the diagnosis of ACTH-independent etiologies of the syndrome, since most adrenal tumors cause low or undetectable ACTH levels [<2 pmol/L (10 pg/mL)]. Furthermore, ACTH-secreting pituitary macroadenomas and ACTH-producing nonendocrine tumors usually result in elevated ACTH levels. In the ectopic ACTH syndrome, ACTH levels may be elevated to >110 pmol/L (500 pg/mL), and in most patients the level is >40 pmol/L (200 pg/mL). In Cushing's syndrome as the result of a microadenoma or pituitary-hypothalamic dysfunction, ACTH levels range from 6 to 30 pmol/L (30 to 150 pg/mL) [normal, <14 pmol/L (<60 pg/mL)], with half of values falling in the normal range. However, the main problem with the use of ACTH levels in the differential diagnosis of Cushing's syndrome is that ACTH levels may be similar in individuals with hypothalamic-pituitary dysfunction, pituitary microadenomas, ectopic CRH production, and ectopic ACTH production (especially carcinoid tumors) (Table 331-4).

Because of these difficulties, several additional tests have been advocated, such as the metyrapone and CRH infusion tests. The rationale underlying these tests is that steroid hypersecretion by an adrenal tumor or the ectopic production of ACTH will suppress the hypothalamic-pituitary axis so that inhibition of pituitary ACTH release can be demonstrated by either test. Thus, most patients with pituitary-hypothalamic dysfunction and/or a microadenoma have an increase in steroid or ACTH secretion in response to metyrapone or CRH administration, whereas most patients with ectopic ACTH-producing tumors do not. Most pituitary macroadenomas also respond to CRH, but their response to metyrapone is variable. However, false-positive and -negative CRH tests can occur in patients with ectopic ACTH and pituitary tumors.

The main diagnostic dilemma in Cushing's syndrome is to distinguish those instances due to microadenomas of the pituitary and/or pituitary-hypothalamic dysfunction from those due to tumors (e.g., carcinoids or pheochromocytoma) that produce CRH and/or ACTH ectopically. The clinical manifestations are similar unless the ectopic tumor produces other symptoms, such as diarrhea and flushing from a carcinoid tumor or episodic hypertension from a pheochromocytoma. Sometimes, one can distinguish between ectopic and pituitary ACTH production by using metyrapone or CRH tests, as noted above. In these situations, computed tomography (CT) of the pituitary gland is usually normal. Magnetic resonance imaging (MRI) with the enhancing agent gadolinium may be better than CT for this purpose but demonstrates pituitary microadenomas in only half of patients with Cushing's disease. In subjects with negative imaging studies, selective petrosal sinus venous sampling for ACTH is employed in some centers. Demonstration of an ACTH gradient between the petrosal sinus and peripheral blood localizes the source of ACTH overproduction to the pituitary gland but does not distinguish pituitary-dependent adrenal hyperplasia from pituitary hyperplasia secondary to a tumor producing CRH. CRH levels should be measured in the peripheral blood prior to petrosal sinus sampling. In centers where petrosal sinus sampling is performed frequently, it has proved useful for distinguishing pituitary and nonpituitary sources of ACTH excess. However, the catheterization procedure is technically difficult, and complications have occurred.

The diagnosis of a *cortisol-producing adrenal adenoma* is suggested by disproportionate elevations in baseline urine free-cortisol levels with only modest changes in urinary 17-ketosteroids or plasma DHEA sulfate. Adrenal androgen secretion is usually reduced in these patients owing to the cortisol-induced suppression of ACTH and subsequent involution of the androgen-producing zona reticularis.

The diagnosis of *adrenal carcinoma* is suggested by a palpable abdominal mass and by *markedly* elevated baseline values of *both* urine 17-ketosteroids and plasma DHEA sulfate. Plasma and urine cortisol levels are variably elevated. Adrenal carcinoma is usually resistant to both ACTH stimulation and dexamethasone suppression. Elevated adrenal androgen secretion often leads to virilization in the female. Estrogen-producing adrenocortical carcinoma usually presents with gynecomastia in men and dysfunctional uterine bleeding in women. These adrenal tumors secrete increased amounts of androstenedione, which is converted peripherally to the estrogens estrone and estradiol (Chap. 337). Adrenal carcinomas that produce Cushing's syndrome are often associated with elevated levels of the intermediates of steroid biosynthesis (especially 11-deoxycortisol), suggesting inefficient conversion of the intermediates to the final product. This feature also accounts for the characteristic increase in 17-ketosteroids. Approximately 20% of adrenal carcinomas are not associated with endocrine syndromes and are presumed to be nonfunctioning or to produce biologically inactive steroid precursors. In addition, the excessive production of steroids is not always clinically evident (e.g., androgens in adult men).

Differential Diagnosis • ***Pseudo-Cushing's Syndrome*** Problems in diagnosis include patients with obesity, chronic alcoholism, depression, and acute illness of any type. Extreme *obesity* is uncommon in Cushing's syndrome; furthermore, with exogenous obesity, the adiposity is generalized, not truncal. On adrenocortical testing, abnormalities in patients with exogenous obesity are usually modest. Basal urine steroid excretion levels in obese patients are also either normal or slightly elevated. Some patients have elevated conversion of secreted cortisol into excreted metabolites. Urinary and blood cortisol levels are usually normal, and the diurnal pattern in blood and urine levels is normal. Patients with *chronic alcoholism* and those with *depression* share similar abnormalities in steroid output: modestly elevated urine cortisol, blunted circadian rhythm of cortisol levels, and resistance to suppression using the overnight dexamethasone test. In contrast to alcoholic subjects, depressed patients do not have signs and

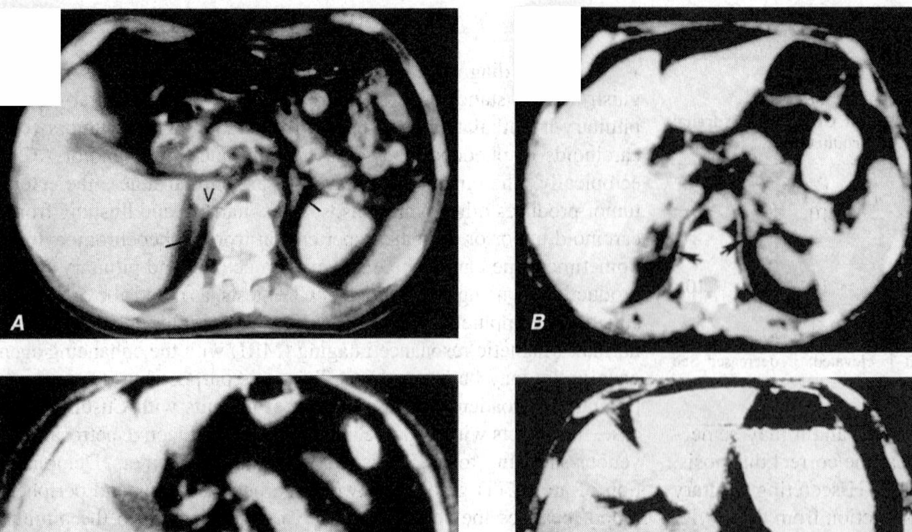

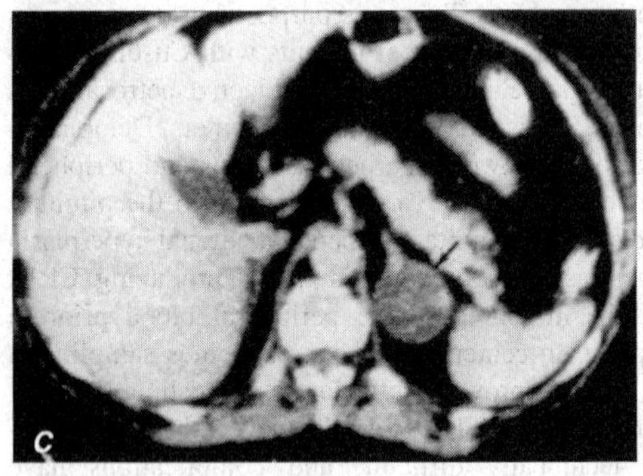

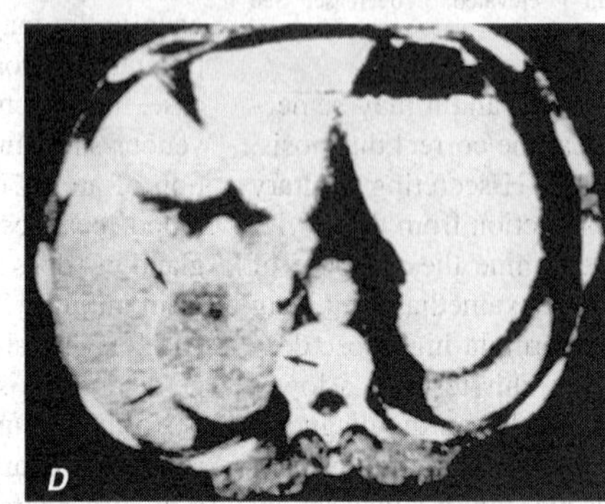

FIGURE 331-8 Computed tomography is the preferred method for visualizing the adrenal glands (*arrows*). *A*. The normal right adrenal gland is adjacent to the inferior vena cava (V) where it emerges from the liver. Approximately 90% of right adrenal glands appear as linear structures extending posteriorly from the inferior vena cava into the space between the right lobe of the liver and the crus of the diaphragm. The normal left adrenal gland is lateral to the left crus of the diaphragm and below the stomach. Most left adrenal glands are shaped like an inverted V or Y. *B*. Adrenal CT scan of a patient with ectopic ACTH production. Both adrenal glands (*arrows*) are enlarged (compare with *A*). In contrast, only 50% of patients with bilateral adrenal hyperplasia secondary to pituitary ACTH hypersecretion show enlargement of the adrenals when imaged by CT scan. *C*. CT scan of a patient with Cushing's syndrome with biochemical evidence only of cortisol overproduction. The left adrenal has been replaced by a racquet-shaped 2-cm tumor (*arrow*). Attenuation of the tumor is low because of its high lipid content. *D*. CT scan in a patient with Cushing's syndrome and biochemical evidence of an adrenal carcinoma. In contrast to the tumor in *C*, the right-sided mass in this patient is large and has a heterogeneous appearance—usual characteristics of an adrenal carcinoma.

symptoms of Cushing's syndrome. Following discontinuation of alcohol and/or improvement in the emotional status, results of steroid testing usually return to normal. One or more of three tests have been used to differentiate mild Cushing's syndrome and pseudo-Cushing's syndrome. The serum cortisol level following the standard 2-day low-dose dexamethasone test has very high sensitivity and specificity. While the CRH test alone is less useful, in combination with the low-dose dexamethasone test, there is nearly complete discrimination between these two conditions. Finally, a midnight cortisol level obtained in awake patients may have similar predictive value as the low-dose dexamethasone test if a cut-off of 210 nmol/L (7.5 μg/dL) is used. Patients with *acute illness* often have abnormal results on laboratory tests and fail to exhibit pituitary-adrenal suppression in response to dexamethasone, since major stress (such as pain or fever) interrupts the normal regulation of ACTH secretion. *Iatrogenic Cushing's syndrome*, induced by the administration of glucocorticoids or other steroids such as megestrol that bind to the glucocorticoid receptor, is indistinguishable by physical findings from endogenous adrenocortical hyperfunction. The distinction can be made, however, by measuring blood or urine cortisol levels in a basal state; in the iatrogenic syndrome these levels are low secondary to suppression of the pituitary-adrenal axis. The severity of iatrogenic Cushing's syndrome is related to the total steroid dose, the biologic half-life of the steroid, and the duration of therapy. Also, individuals taking afternoon and evening doses of glucocorticoids develop Cushing's syndrome more readily and with a smaller total daily dose than do patients taking morning doses only. The enzymatic disposition and binding of administered steroids differ among patients.

Radiologic Evaluation for Cushing's Syndrome The preferred radiologic study for visualizing the adrenals is a CT scan of the abdomen (Fig. 331-8). CT is of value both for localizing adrenal tumors and for diagnosing bilateral hyperplasia. All patients believed to have hypersecretion of pituitary ACTH should have a pituitary MRI scan with the contrast agent gadolinium. Even with this technique, small microadenomas may be undetectable; alternatively, false-positive masses due to cysts or nonsecretory lesions of the normal pituitary may be imaged. In patients with ectopic ACTH production, chest CT is a useful first step.

Evaluation of Asymptomatic Adrenal Masses With abdominal CT scanning, many incidental adrenal masses (so-called incidentalomas) are discovered. This is not surprising, since 10 to 20% of subjects at autopsy have adrenocortical adenomas. The first step in evaluating such patients is to determine whether the tumor is functioning by means of appropriate screening tests, e.g., measurement of 24-h urine catecholamines and metabolites and serum potassium and assessment of adrenal cortical function by dexamethasone-suppression testing. However, 90% of incidentalomas are nonfunctioning. If an extraadrenal malignancy is present, there is a 30 to 50% chance that the adrenal tumor is a metastasis. If the primary tumor is being treated and there are no other metastases, it is prudent to obtain a fine-needle aspirate of the adrenal mass to establish the diagnosis. In the absence of a known malignancy the next step is unclear. The probability of adrenal carcinoma is <0.01 percent, the vast majority of adrenal masses being benign adenomas. Features suggestive of malignancy include large size (a size >4 to 6 cm suggests carcinoma); irregular margins; and inhomogeneity, soft tissue calcifications visible on CT (Fig. 331-8), and findings characteristic of malignancy on a chemical-shift MRI image. If surgery is not performed, a repeat CT scan should be obtained in 3 to 6 months. Fine needle aspiration is not useful to distinguish between benign and malignant primary adrenal tumors.

℞ TREATMENT **Adrenal Neoplasm** When an adenoma or carcinoma is diagnosed, adrenal exploration is performed with excision of the tumor. Adenomas may be resected using laparoscopic techniques. Because of the possibility of atrophy of the contralateral adrenal, the patient is treated pre- and postoperatively as if for total adrenalectomy, even when a unilateral lesion is suspected, the routine being similar to that for an Addisonian patient undergoing elective surgery (see Table 331-8).

Despite operative intervention, most patients with adrenal carcinoma die within 3 years of diagnosis. Metastases occur most often to liver and lung. The principal drug for the treatment of adrenocortical carcinoma is mitotane (*o,p*′-DDD), an isomer of the insecticide DDT. This drug suppresses cortisol production and decreases plasma and urine steroid levels. Although its cytotoxic action is relatively selective for the glucocorticoid-secreting zone of the adrenal cortex, the zona glomerulosa may also be inhibited. Because mitotane also alters the extraadrenal metabolism of cortisol, plasma and urinary cortisol levels must be assessed to titrate the effect. The drug is usually given in divided doses three to four times a day, with the dose increased gradually to tolerability (usually <6 g daily). At higher doses, almost all patients experience side effects, which may be gastrointestinal (anorexia, diarrhea, vomiting) or neuromuscular (lethargy, somnolence, dizziness). All patients treated with mitotane should receive long-term glucocorticoid maintenance therapy, and, in some, mineralocorticoid replacement is appropriate. In approximately one-third of patients, both tumor and metastases regress, but long-term survival is not altered. In many patients, mitotane only inhibits steroidogenesis and does not cause regression of tumor metastases. Osseous metastases are usually refractory to the drug and should be treated with radiation therapy. Mitotane can also be given as adjunctive therapy after surgical resection of an adrenal carcinoma, although there is no evidence that this improves survival. Because of the absence of a long-term benefit with mitotane, alternative chemotherapeutic approaches based on platinum therapy have been used. However, there are no data presently available indicating a prolongation of life.

Bilateral hyperplasia Patients with hyperplasia have a relative or absolute increase in ACTH levels. Since therapy would logically be directed at reducing ACTH levels, the ideal primary treatment for ACTH- or CRH-producing tumors, whether pituitary or ectopic, is surgical removal. Occasionally (particularly with ectopic ACTH production) surgical excision is not possible because the disease is far advanced. In this situation, "medical" or surgical adrenalectomy may correct the hypercortisolism.

Controversy exists as to the proper treatment for bilateral adrenal hyperplasia when the source of the ACTH overproduction is not apparent. In some centers, these patients (especially those who suppress after the administration of a high-dose dexamethasone test) undergo surgical exploration of the pituitary via a transsphenoidal approach in the expectation that a microadenoma will be found. However, in most circumstances selective petrosal sinus venous sampling is recommended, and the patient is referred to an appropriate center if the procedure is not available locally. If a microadenoma is not found at the time of exploration, total hypophysectomy may be needed. Complications of transsphenoidal surgery include cerebrospinal fluid rhinorrhea, diabetes insipidus, panhypopituitarism, and optic or cranial nerve injuries.

In other centers, total adrenalectomy is the treatment of choice. The cure rate with this procedure is close to 100%. The adverse effects include the certain need for lifelong mineralocorticoid and glucocorticoid replacement and a 10 to 20% probability of a pituitary tumor developing over the next 10 years (Nelson's syndrome; Chap. 328). Many of these tumors require surgical therapy. It is uncertain whether they arise de novo in these patients or were present prior to adrenalectomy but were too small to be detected. Periodic radiologic evaluation of the pituitary gland by MRI as well as serial ACTH measurements should be performed in all individuals after bilateral adrenalectomy for Cushing's disease. Such pituitary tumors may become locally invasive and impinge on the optic chiasm or extend into the cavernous or sphenoid sinuses.

Except in children, pituitary irradiation is rarely used as primary treatment, being reserved rather for postoperative tumor recurrences. In some centers, high levels of gamma radiation can be focused on the desired site with less scattering to surrounding tissues by using stereotactic techniques. Side effects of radiation include ocular motor palsy and hypopituitarism. There is a long lag time between treatment and remission, and the remission rate is usually <50%.

Finally, in occasional patients in whom a surgical approach is not feasible, "medical" adrenalectomy may be indicated (Table 331-5). Inhibition of steroidogenesis may also be indicated in severely cushingoid subjects prior to surgical intervention. Chemical adrenalectomy may be accomplished by the administration of the inhibitor of steroidogenesis ketoconazole (600 to 1200 mg/d). In addition, mitotane (2 or 3 g/d) and/or the blockers of steroid synthesis aminoglutethimide (1 g/d) and metyrapone (2 or 3 g/d) may be effective either alone or in combination. Mitotane is slow to take effect (weeks). Mifepristone, a competitive inhibitor of the binding of glucocorticoid to its receptor, may be a treatment option. Adrenal insufficiency is a risk with all these agents, and replacement steroids may be required.

Table 331-5 Treatment Modalities for Patients with Adrenal Hyperplasia Secondary to Pituitary ACTH Hypersecretion

Treatments to reduce pituitary ACTH production
Transsphenoidal resection of microadenoma
Radiation therapy
Treatments to reduce or eliminate adrenocortical cortisol secretion
Bilateral adrenalectomy
Medical adrenalectomy (metyrapone, mitotane, aminoglutethimide, ketoconazole)[a]

[a] Not curative but effective as long as chronically administered in selected patients.

ALDOSTERONISM Aldosteronism is a syndrome associated with hypersecretion of the mineralocorticoid aldosterone. In *primary* aldosteronism the cause for the excessive aldosterone production resides within the adrenal gland; in *secondary* aldosteronism the stimulus is extraadrenal.

Primary Aldosteronism In the original case of excessive and inappropriate aldosterone production, the disease was the result of an *aldosterone-producing adrenal adenoma* (Conn's syndrome). Most cases involve a unilateral adenoma, which is usually small and may occur on either side. Rarely, primary aldosteronism is due to an adrenal carcinoma. Aldosteronism is twice as common in women as in men, usually occurs between the ages of 30 and 50, and is present in approximately 1% of unselected hypertensive patients. However, the prevalence may be as high as 10%, depending on the criteria and study population. Most of this difference is not secondary to the prevalence of patients with an aldosteronoma but rather because of the inclusion of those with bilateral hyperplasia. In many patients with clinical and biochemical features of primary aldosteronism, a solitary adenoma is not found at surgery. Instead, these patients have *bilateral cortical nodular hyperplasia*. In the literature, this disease is also termed *idiopathic hyperaldosteronism*, and/or *nodular hyperplasia*. The cause is unknown.

Signs and symptoms Hypersecretion of aldosterone increases the renal distal tubular exchange of intratubular sodium for secreted potassium and hydrogen ions, with progressive depletion of body potassium and development of hypokalemia. Most patients have diastolic hypertension, which may be very severe, and headaches. The hypertension is probably due to the increased sodium reabsorption and extracellular volume expansion. *Potassium depletion* is responsible for the muscle weakness and fatigue and is due to the effect of potassium depletion on the muscle cell membrane. The polyuria results from impairment of urinary concentrating ability and is often associated with polydipsia.

Electrocardiographic and roentgenographic signs of left ventricular enlargement are, in part, secondary to the hypertension. However, the left ventricular hypertrophy is disproportionate to the level of blood pressure when compared to individuals with essential hypertension, and regression of the hypertrophy occurs even if blood pressure is not reduced after removal of an aldosteronoma. Electrocardiographic signs of potassium depletion include prominent U waves, cardiac arrhythmias, and premature contractions. In the absence of associated congestive heart failure, renal disease, or preexisting abnormalities (such as thrombophlebitis), edema is characteristically absent. However, structural damage to the cerebral circulation, retinal vasculature, and kidney occurs more frequently than would be predicted based on the level and duration of the hypertension. Proteinuria may occur in as many as 50% of patients with primary aldosteronism, and renal failure occurs in up to 15%. Thus, it is probable that excess aldosterone production induces cardiovascular damage independent of its effect on blood pressure.

Laboratory findings Laboratory findings depend on both the duration and the severity of potassium depletion. An overnight concentration test often reveals impaired ability to concentrate the urine, probably secondary to the hypokalemia. Urine pH is neutral to alkaline because of excessive secretion of ammonium and bicarbonate ions to compensate for the metabolic alkalosis.

Hypokalemia may be severe (<3 mmol/L) and reflects body potassium depletion, usually >300 mmol. In mild forms of primary aldosteronism, potassium levels may be normal. *Hypernatremia* is due to sodium retention, a concomitant water loss from polyuria, and a resetting of the osmostat. Metabolic alkalosis and elevation of serum bicarbonate are a result of hydrogen ion loss into the urine and migration into potassium-depleted cells. The alkalosis is perpetuated by potassium deficiency, which increases the capacity of the proximal convoluted tubule to reabsorb filtered bicarbonate. If hypokalemia is severe, serum magnesium levels are also reduced.

Diagnosis The diagnosis is suggested by persistent hypokalemia in a nonedematous patient with a normal sodium intake who is not receiving potassium-wasting diuretics (furosemide, ethacrynic acid, thiazides). If hypokalemia occurs in a hypertensive patient taking a potassium-wasting diuretic, the diuretic should be discontinued and the patient should be given potassium supplements. After 1 to 2 weeks, the potassium level should be remeasured, and if hypokalemia persists, the patient should be evaluated for a mineralocorticoid excess syndrome (Fig. 331-9).

The criteria for the diagnosis of primary aldosteronism are (1) diastolic hypertension without edema, (2) hyposecretion of renin (as judged by low plasma renin activity levels) that fails to increase appropriately during volume depletion (upright posture, sodium depletion), and (3) hypersecretion of aldosterone that does not suppress appropriately in response to volume expansion.

Patients with primary aldosteronism characteristically *do not have edema*, since they exhibit an "escape" phenomenon from the sodium-retaining aspects of mineralocorticoids. Rarely, pretibial edema is present in patients with associated nephropathy and azotemia.

The estimation of plasma renin activity is of limited value in separating patients with primary aldosteronism from those with hypertension of other causes. Although failure of plasma renin activity to rise normally during volume-depletion maneuvers is a criterion for a diagnosis of primary aldosteronism, suppressed renin activity also occurs in about 25% of patients with essential hypertension.

Although a renin measurement alone lacks specificity, the ratio of serum aldosterone to plasma renin activity is a very useful screening test. A high ratio (>30), when aldosterone is expressed as ng/dL and plasma renin activity as ng/mL per hour, strongly suggests autonomy of aldosterone secretion. Aldosterone levels need to be >500 pmol/L (>15 ng/dL) and the salt intake not be restricted in making this assessment. Ultimately, it is necessary to demonstrate a lack of aldosterone suppression to diagnose primary aldosteronism (Fig. 331-9). The autonomy exhibited in these patients refers only to the resistance to suppression of secretion during volume expansion; aldosterone can and does respond in a normal or above-normal fashion to the stimulus of potassium loading or ACTH infusion.

Once hyposecretion of renin and failure of aldosterone secretion suppression are demonstrated, aldosterone-producing adenomas should be localized by abdominal CT scan, using a high-resolution scanner as many aldosteronomas are <1 cm in size. If the CT scan is negative, percutaneous transfemoral bilateral adrenal vein catheterization with adrenal vein sampling may demonstrate a two- to threefold increase in plasma aldosterone concentration on the involved side. In cases of hyperaldosteronism secondary to cortical nodular hyperplasia, no lateralization is found. It is important for samples to be obtained simultaneously if possible and for cortisol levels to be measured to ensure that false localization does not reflect dilution or an ACTH- or stress-induced rise in aldosterone levels. In a patient with an adenoma, the aldosterone/cortisol ratio lateralizes to the side of the lesion.

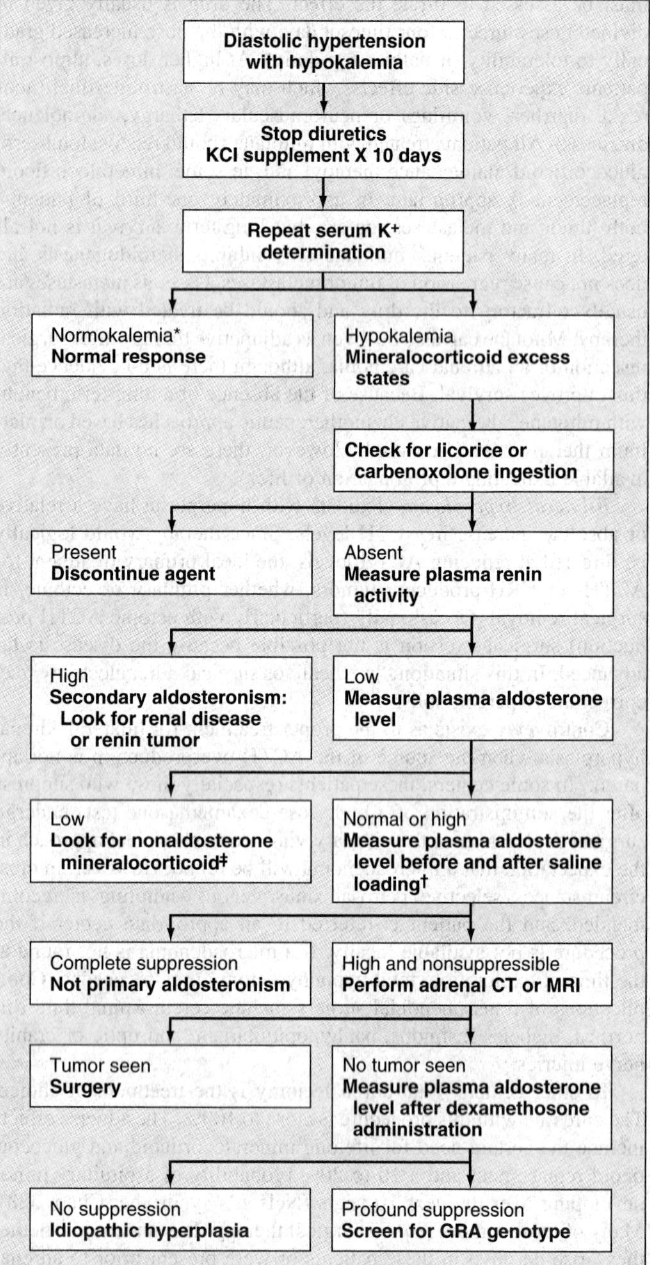

FIGURE 331-9 Diagnostic flowchart for evaluating patients with suspected primary aldosteronism. *Serum K^+ may be normal in some patients with hyperaldosteronism who are taking potassium-sparing diuretics (spironolactone, triamterene) or who have a low sodium intake and a high potassium intake. †This step should not be taken if hypertension is severe (diastolic pressure >115 mmHg) or if cardiac failure is present. Also, serum potassium levels should be corrected before the infusion of saline solution. Alternative methods that produce comparable suppression of aldosterone secretion include oral sodium loading (200 mmol/d) and the administration of fludrocortisone, 0.2 mg BID, for 3 days. (GRA, glucocorticoid-remediable aldosteronism.) ‡For example, Liddle's syndrome, apparent mineralocorticoid excess syndrome, or a deoxycorticosterone-secreting tumor.

Differential diagnosis Patients with hypertension and hypokalemia may have either primary or secondary hyperaldosteronism (Fig. 331-10). A useful maneuver to distinguish between these conditions is the measurement of plasma renin activity. Secondary hyperaldosteronism in patients with accelerated hypertension is due to elevated plasma renin levels; in contrast, patients with primary aldosteronism have suppressed plasma renin levels. Indeed, in patients with a serum potassium concentration of <2.5 mmol/L, a high ratio of plasma aldosterone to plasma renin activity in a random sample is usually suf-

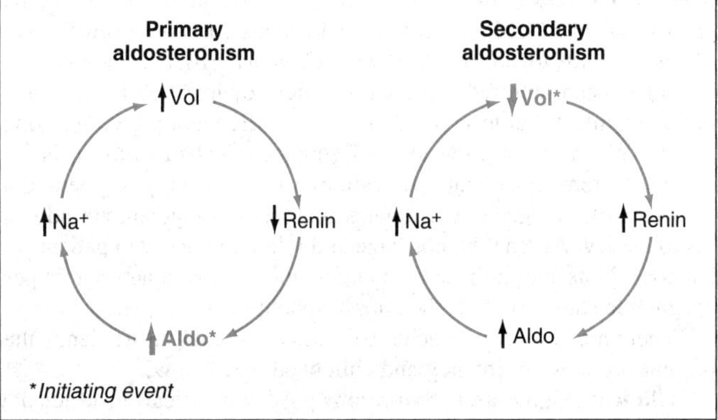

FIGURE 331-10 Responses of the renin-aldosterone volume control loop in primary versus secondary aldosteronism.

ficient to establish the diagnosis of primary aldosteronism without additional testing.

Primary aldosteronism must also be distinguished from other *hypermineralocorticoid states*. Nonaldosterone mineralocorticoid states will have suppressed plasma renin activity but low aldosterone levels. The most common problem is to distinguish between hyperaldosteronism due to an adenoma and that due to idiopathic bilateral nodular hyperplasia. This distinction is of importance because hypertension associated with idiopathic hyperplasia is usually not benefited by bilateral adrenalectomy, whereas hypertension associated with aldosterone-producing tumors is usually improved or cured by removal of the adenoma. Although patients with idiopathic bilateral nodular hyperplasia tend to have less severe hypokalemia, lower aldosterone secretion, and higher plasma renin activity than do patients with primary aldosteronism, differentiation is impossible solely on clinical and/or biochemical grounds. An anomalous postural decrease in plasma aldosterone and elevated plasma 18-hydroxycorticosterone levels are present in most patients with a unilateral lesion. However, these tests are also of limited diagnostic value in the individual patient, because some adenoma patients have an increase in plasma aldosterone with upright posture, so-called renin-responsive aldosteronoma. A definitive diagnosis is best made by radiographic studies, including bilateral adrenal vein catheterization, as noted above.

In a few instances, hypertensive patients with hypokalemic alkalosis have adenomas that secrete deoxycorticosterone (DOC). Such patients have reduced plasma renin activity levels, but aldosterone levels are either normal or reduced, suggesting the diagnosis of mineralocorticoid excess due to a hormone other than aldosterone. Several inherited disorders have clinical features similar to those of primary aldosteronism (see below).

℞ TREATMENT Primary aldosteronism due to an adenoma is usually treated by surgical excision of the adenoma. Where possible a laparoscopic approach is favored. However, dietary sodium restriction and the administration of an aldosterone antagonist, e.g., spironolactone, are effective in many cases. Hypertension and hypokalemia are usually controlled by doses of 25 to 100 mg spironolactone every 8 h. In some patients medical management has been successful for years, but chronic therapy in men is usually limited by side effects of spironolactone such as gynecomastia, decreased libido, and impotence.

When idiopathic bilateral hyperplasia is suspected, surgery is indicated only when significant, symptomatic hypokalemia cannot be controlled with medical therapy, e.g., by spironolactone, triamterene, or amiloride. Hypertension associated with idiopathic hyperplasia is usually not benefited by bilateral adrenalectomy.

Secondary Aldosteronism *Secondary aldosteronism* refers to an appropriately increased production of aldosterone in response to activation of the renin-angiotensin system (Fig. 331-10). The production rate of aldosterone is often higher in patients with secondary aldosteronism than in those with primary aldosteronism. Secondary aldosteronism usually occurs in association with the accelerated phase of hypertension or on the basis of an underlying edema disorder. Secondary aldosteronism in pregnancy is a normal physiologic response to estrogen-induced increases in circulating levels of renin substrate and plasma renin activity and to the antialdosterone actions of progestogens.

Secondary aldosteronism in hypertensive states is due either to a primary overproduction of renin (primary reninism) or to an overproduction of renin secondary to a decrease in renal blood flow and/or perfusion pressure (Fig. 331-10). Secondary hypersecretion of renin can be due to a narrowing of one or both of the major renal arteries by atherosclerosis or by fibromuscular hyperplasia. Overproduction of renin from both kidneys also occurs in severe arteriolar nephrosclerosis (malignant hypertension) or with profound renal vasoconstriction (the accelerated phase of hypertension). The secondary aldosteronism is characterized by hypokalemic alkalosis, moderate to severe increases in plasma renin activity, and moderate to marked increases in aldosterone levels (Chap. 246).

Secondary aldosteronism with hypertension can also be caused by rare renin-producing tumors (primary reninism). These patients have the biochemical characteristics of renal vascular hypertension, but the primary defect is renin secretion by a juxtaglomerular cell tumor. The diagnosis can be made by demonstration of normal renal vasculature and/or demonstration of a space-occupying lesion in the kidney by radiographic techniques and documentation of a unilateral increase in renal vein renin activity. Rarely, these tumors arise in tissues such as the ovary.

Secondary aldosteronism is present in many forms of *edema*. The rate of aldosterone secretion is usually increased in patients with edema caused by either cirrhosis or the nephrotic syndrome. In congestive heart failure, elevated aldosterone secretion varies depending on the severity of cardiac failure. The stimulus for aldosterone release in these conditions appears to be *arterial hypovolemia* and/or hypotension. Thiazides and furosemide often exaggerate secondary aldosteronism via volume depletion; hypokalemia and, on occasion, alkalosis can then become prominent features. On occasion secondary hyperaldosteronism occurs without edema or hypertension (Bartter's and Gitelman's syndromes, see below).

SYNDROMES OF ADRENAL ANDROGEN EXCESS Adrenal androgen excess results from excess production of DHEA and androstenedione, which are converted to testosterone in extraglandular tissues; elevated testosterone levels account for most of the virilization. Adrenal androgen excess may be associated with the secretion of greater or smaller amounts of other adrenal hormones and may, therefore, present as "pure" syndromes of virilization or as "mixed" syndromes associated with excessive glucocorticoids and Cushing's syndrome. *→For further discussion of hirsutism and virilization, see Chap. 53.*

HYPOFUNCTION OF THE ADRENAL CORTEX

Cases of adrenal insufficiency can be divided into two general categories: (1) those associated with primary inability of the adrenal to elaborate sufficient quantities of hormone, and (2) those associated with a secondary failure due to inadequate ACTH formation or release (Table 331-6).

PRIMARY ADRENOCORTICAL DEFICIENCY (ADDISON'S DISEASE) The original description of Addison's disease—"general languor and debility, feebleness of the heart's action, irritability of the stomach, and a peculiar change of the color of the skin"—summarizes the dominant clinical features. Advanced cases are usually easy to diagnose, but recognition of the early phases can be a real challenge.

Incidence Primary insufficiency is relatively rare, may occur at any age, and affects both sexes equally. Because of the common ther-

Table 331-6 Classification of Adrenal Insufficiency

PRIMARY ADRENAL INSUFFICIENCY

- Anatomic destruction of gland (chronic or acute)
  - "Idiopathic" atrophy (autoimmune, adrenoleukodystrophy)
  - Surgical removal
  - Infection (tuberculous, fungal, viral—especially in AIDS patients)
  - Hemorrhage
  - Invasion: metastatic
- Metabolic failure in hormone production
  - Congenital adrenal hyperplasia
  - Enzyme inhibitors (metyrapone, ketoconazole, aminoglutethimide)
  - Cytotoxic agents (mitotane)
- ACTH-blocking antibodies
- Mutation in ACTH receptor gene
- Adrenal hypoplasia congenita

SECONDARY ADRENAL INSUFFICIENCY

- Hypopituitarism due to hypothalamic-pituitary disease
- Suppression of hypothalamic-pituitary axis
  - By exogenous steroid
  - By endogenous steroid from tumor

apeutic use of steroids, secondary adrenal insufficiency is relatively common.

Etiology and Pathogenesis Addison's disease results from progressive destruction of the adrenals, which must involve >90% of the glands before adrenal insufficiency appears. The adrenal is a frequent site for chronic granulomatous diseases, predominantly tuberculosis but also histoplasmosis, coccidioidomycosis, and cryptococcosis. In early series, tuberculosis was responsible for 70 to 90% of cases, but the most frequent cause now is *idiopathic* atrophy, and an autoimmune mechanism is probably responsible. Rarely, other lesions are encountered, such as adrenoleukodystrophy, bilateral hemorrhage, tumor metastases, HIV, cytomegalovirus (CMV), amyloidosis, adrenomyeloneuropathy, familial adrenal insufficiency, or sarcoidosis.

Although half of patients with idiopathic atrophy have circulating adrenal antibodies, autoimmune destruction is probably secondary to cytotoxic T lymphocytes. Specific adrenal antigens to which autoantibodies may be directed include 21-hydroxylase (CYP21A2) and side chain cleavage enzyme but the significance of these antibodies in the pathogenesis of adrenal insufficiency is unknown. Some antibodies cause adrenal insufficiency by blocking the binding of ACTH to its receptors. Some patients also have antibodies to thyroid, parathyroid, and/or gonadal tissue (Chap. 339). There is also an increased incidence of chronic lymphocytic thyroiditis, premature ovarian failure, type 1 diabetes mellitus, and hypo- or hyperthyroidism. The presence of two or more of these autoimmune endocrine disorders in the same person defines the polyglandular autoimmune syndrome type II. Additional features include pernicious anemia, vitiligo, alopecia, nontropical sprue, and myasthenia gravis. Within families, multiple generations are affected by one or more of the above diseases. Type II polyglandular syndrome is the result of a mutant gene on chromosome 6 and is associated with the HLA alleles B8 and DR3.

The combination of parathyroid and adrenal insufficiency and chronic mucocutaneous moniliasis constitutes type I polyglandular autoimmune syndrome. Other autoimmune diseases in this disorder include pernicious anemia, chronic active hepatitis, alopecia, primary hypothyroidism, and premature gonadal failure. There is no HLA association; this syndrome is inherited as an autosomal recessive trait. It is caused by mutations in *a*utoimmune *p*oly*e*ndocrinopathy *c*andidiasis *e*ctodermal *d*ystrophy (APECED) located on chromosome 21q22.3. The gene encodes a transcription factor thought to be involved in lymphocyte function. The type I syndrome usually presents during childhood, whereas the type II syndrome is usually manifested in adulthood.

Clinical suspicion of adrenal insufficiency should be high in patients with AIDS (Chap. 309). CMV regularly involves the adrenal glands (so-called CMV necrotizing adrenalitis), and involvement with *Mycobacterium avium-intracellulare*, *Cryptococcus*, and Kaposi's sarcoma has been reported. Adrenal insufficiency in AIDS patients may not be manifest, but tests of adrenal reserve frequently give abnormal results. When interpreting tests of adrenocortical function, it is important to remember that medications such as rifampin, phenytoin, ketoconazole, megace, and opiates may cause or potentiate adrenal insufficiency. Adrenal hemorrhage and infarction occur in patients on anticoagulants and in those with circulating anticoagulants and hypercoagulable states, such as the antiphospholipid syndrome.

There are several rare genetic causes of adrenal insufficiency that present primarily in infancy and childhood (see below).

Clinical Signs and Symptoms Adrenocortical insufficiency caused by gradual adrenal destruction is characterized by an insidious onset of fatigability, weakness, anorexia, nausea and vomiting, weight loss, cutaneous and mucosal pigmentation, hypotension, and occasionally hypoglycemia (Table 331-7). Depending on the duration and degree of adrenal hypofunction, the manifestations vary from mild chronic fatigue to fulminating shock associated with acute destruction of the glands, as described by Waterhouse and Friderichsen.

Asthenia is the cardinal symptom. Early it may be sporadic, usually most evident at times of stress; as adrenal function becomes more impaired, the patient is continuously fatigued, and bed rest is necessary.

Hyperpigmentation may be striking or absent. It commonly appears as a diffuse brown, tan, or bronze darkening of parts such as the elbows or creases of the hand and of areas that normally are pigmented such as the areolae about the nipples. Bluish-black patches may appear on the mucous membranes. Some patients develop dark freckles, and irregular areas of vitiligo may paradoxically be present. As an early sign, tanning following sun exposure may be persistent.

Arterial hypotension with postural accentuation is frequent, and blood pressure may be in the range of 80/50 or less.

Abnormalities of gastrointestinal function are often the presenting complaint. Symptoms vary from mild anorexia with weight loss to fulminating nausea, vomiting, diarrhea, and ill-defined abdominal pain, which may be so severe as to be confused with an acute abdomen. Patients may have personality changes, usually consisting of excessive irritability and restlessness. Enhancement of the sensory modalities of taste, olfaction, and hearing is reversible with therapy. Axillary and pubic hair may be decreased in women due to loss of adrenal androgens.

Laboratory Findings In the early phase of gradual adrenal destruction, there may be no demonstrable abnormalities in the routine laboratory parameters, but adrenal reserve is decreased—that is, while basal steroid output may be normal, a subnormal increase occurs after stress. Adrenal stimulation with ACTH uncovers abnormalities in this stage of the disease, eliciting a subnormal increase of cortisol levels or no increase at all. In more advanced stages of adrenal destruction, serum sodium, chloride, and bicarbonate levels are reduced, and the

Table 331-7 Frequency of Symptoms and Signs in Adrenal Insufficiency

Sign or Symptom	Percent of Patients
Weakness	99
Pigmentation of skin	98
Weight loss	97
Anorexia, nausea, and vomiting	90
Hypotension (<110/70)	87
Pigmentation of mucous membranes	82
Abdominal pain	34
Salt craving	22
Diarrhea	20
Constipation	19
Syncope	16
Vitiligo	9

serum potassium level is elevated. The hyponatremia is due both to loss of sodium into the urine (due to aldosterone deficiency) and to movement into the intracellular compartment. This extravascular sodium loss depletes extracellular fluid volume and accentuates hypotension. Elevated plasma vasopressin and angiotensin II levels may contribute to the hyponatremia by impairing free water clearance. Hyperkalemia is due to a combination of aldosterone deficiency, impaired glomerular filtration, and acidosis. Basal levels of cortisol and aldosterone are subnormal and fail to increase following ACTH administration. Mild to moderate hypercalcemia occurs in 10 to 20% of patients for unclear reasons. The electrocardiogram may show nonspecific changes, and the electroencephalogram exhibits a generalized reduction and slowing. There may be a normocytic anemia, a relative lymphocytosis, and a moderate eosinophilia.

Diagnosis The diagnosis of adrenal insufficiency should be made only with ACTH stimulation testing to assess adrenal reserve capacity for steroid production (see above for ACTH test protocols). In brief, the best screening test is the cortisol response 60 min after 250 μg of cosyntropin given intramuscularly or intravenously. Cortisol levels should exceed 495 nmol/L (18 μg/dL). If the response is abnormal, then primary and secondary adrenal insufficiency can be distinguished by measuring aldosterone levels from the same blood samples. In secondary, but not primary, adrenal insufficiency the aldosterone increment will be normal [$\geq$150 pmol/l (5 ng/dL)]. Furthermore, in primary adrenal insufficiency, plasma ACTH and associated peptides (β-LPT) are elevated because of loss of the usual cortisol-hypothalamic-pituitary feedback relationship, whereas in secondary adrenal insufficiency, plasma ACTH values are low or "inappropriately" normal (Fig. 331-11).

Differential Diagnosis Since weakness and fatigue are common, diagnosis of early adrenocortical insufficiency may be difficult. However, the combination of mild gastrointestinal distress, weight loss, anorexia, and a suggestion of increased pigmentation makes it mandatory to perform ACTH stimulation testing to rule out adrenal insufficiency, particularly before steroid treatment is begun. Weight loss is useful in evaluating the significance of weakness and malaise. Racial pigmentation may be a problem, but a *recent* and progressive *increase* in pigmentation is usually reported by the patient with gradual adrenal destruction. Hyperpigmentation is usually absent when adrenal destruction is rapid, as in bilateral adrenal hemorrhage. The fact that hyperpigmentation occurs with other diseases may also present a problem, but the appearance and distribution of pigment in adrenal insufficiency are usually characteristic. When doubt exists, measurement of ACTH levels and testing of adrenal reserve with the infusion of ACTH provide clear-cut differentiation.

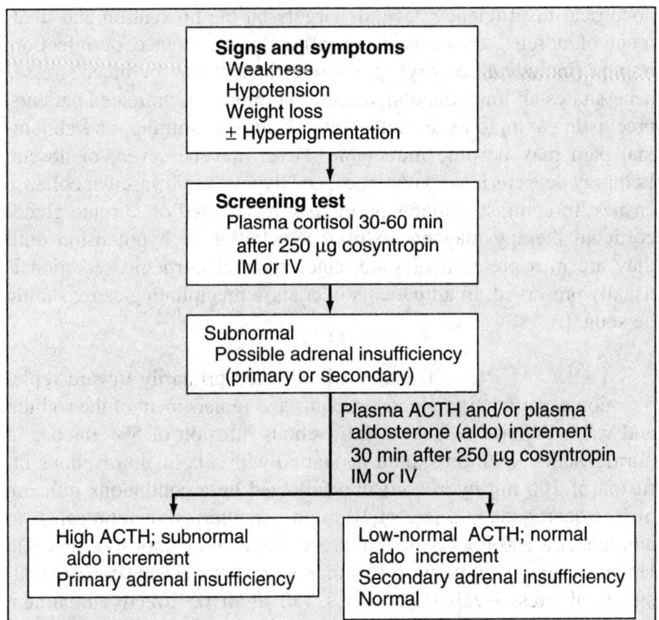

FIGURE 331-11 Diagnostic flowchart for evaluating patients with suspected adrenal insufficiency. Plasma ACTH levels are low in secondary adrenal insufficiency. In adrenal insufficiency secondary to pituitary tumors or idiopathic panhypopituitarism, other pituitary hormone deficiencies are present. On the other hand, ACTH deficiency may be isolated, as seen following prolonged use of exogenous glucocorticoids. Because the isolated blood levels obtained in these screening tests may not be definitive, the diagnosis may need to be confirmed by a continuous 24-h ACTH infusion. Normal subjects and patients with secondary adrenal insufficiency may be distinguished by insulin tolerance or metyrapone testing.

℞ TREATMENT All patients with adrenal insufficiency should receive specific hormone replacement. Like diabetics, these patients require careful education about the disease. Replacement therapy should correct both glucocorticoid and mineralocorticoid deficiencies. Hydrocortisone (cortisol) is the mainstay of treatment. The dose for most adults (depending on size) is 20 to 30 mg/d. Patients are advised to take glucocorticoids with meals or, if that is impractical, with milk or an antacid, because the drugs may increase gastric acidity and exert direct toxic effects on the gastric mucosa. To simulate the normal diurnal adrenal rhythm, two-thirds of the dose is taken in the morning, and the remaining one-third is taken in the late afternoon. Some patients exhibit insomnia, irritability, and mental excitement after initiation of therapy; in these, the dosage should be reduced. Other situations that may necessitate smaller doses are hypertension and diabetes mellitus. Obese individuals and those on anticonvulsive medications may require increased dosages. Measurements of plasma ACTH or cortisol or of urine cortisol levels do not appear to be useful in determining optimal glucocorticoid dosages.

Since the replacement dosage of hydrocortisone does not replace the mineralocorticoid component of the adrenal hormones, mineralocorticoid supplementation is usually needed. This is accomplished by the administration of 0.05 to 0.1 mg fludrocortisone per day by mouth. Patients should also be instructed to maintain an ample intake of sodium (3 to 4 g/d).

The adequacy of mineralocorticoid therapy can be assessed by measurement of blood pressure and serum electrolytes. Blood pressure should be normal and without postural changes; serum sodium, potassium, creatinine, and urea nitrogen levels should also be normal. Measurement of plasma renin levels may also be useful in titrating the dose.

In female patients with adrenal insufficiency, androgen levels are also low. Thus, some physicians believe that daily replacement with 25 to 50 mg of DHEA orally may improve quality of life and skeletal density.

Complications of glucocorticoid therapy, with the exception of gastritis, are *rare* at the dosages recommended for treatment of adrenal insufficiency. Complications of mineralocorticoid therapy include hypokalemia, hypertension, cardiac enlargement, and even congestive heart failure due to sodium retention. Periodic measurements of body weight, serum potassium level, and blood pressure are useful. All patients with adrenal insufficiency should carry medical identification, should be instructed in the parenteral self-administration of steroids, and should be registered with a medical alerting system.

Special Therapeutic Problems During periods of intercurrent illness, especially in the setting of fever, the dose of hydrocortisone should be doubled. With severe illness it should be increased to 75 to 150 mg/d. When oral administration is not possible, parenteral routes should be employed. Likewise, before surgery or dental extractions, supplemental glucocorticoids should be administered. Patients should also be advised to increase the dose of fludrocortisone and to add salt to their otherwise normal diet during periods of strenuous exercise with sweating, during extremely hot weather, and with gastrointestinal upsets such as diarrhea. A simple strategy is to supplement the diet

Table 331-8 Steroid Therapy Schedule for a Patient with Adrenal Insufficiency Undergoing Surgery[a]

	Hydrocortisone Infusion, Continuous, mg/h		Hydrocortisone (Orally) 8 A.M.	Hydrocortisone (Orally) 4 P.M.	Fludrocortisone (Orally), 8 A.M.
Routine daily medication			20	10	0.1
Day before operation			20	10	0.1
Day of operation	10				
Postoperative					
Day 1	5–7.5				
Day 2	2.5–5				
Day 3	2.5–5	*or*	40	20	0.1
Day 4	2.5–5	*or*	40	20	0.1
Day 5			40	20	0.1
Day 6			20	20	0.1
Day 7			20	10	0.1

[a] All steroid doses are given in milligrams. An alternative approach is to give 100 mg hydrocortisone as an intravenous bolus injection every 8 h on the day of the operation (see text).

one to three times daily with salty broth (1 cup of beef or chicken bouillon contains 35 mmol of sodium). For a representative program of steroid therapy for the patient with adrenal insufficiency who is undergoing major surgery, see Table 331-8. This schedule is designed so that on the day of surgery it will mimic the output of cortisol in normal individuals undergoing prolonged major stress (10 mg/h, 250 to 300 mg/d). Thereafter, if the patient is improving and is afebrile, the dose of hydrocortisone is tapered by 20 to 30% daily. Mineralocorticoid administration is unnecessary at hydrocortisone doses >100 mg/d because of the mineralocorticoid effects of hydrocortisone at such dosages.

SECONDARY ADRENOCORTICAL INSUFFICIENCY ACTH deficiency causes *secondary* adrenocortical insufficiency; it may be a selective deficiency, as is seen following prolonged administration of excess glucocorticoids, or it may occur in association with deficiencies of multiple pituitary hormones (panhypopituitarism) (Chap. 328). Patients with secondary adrenocortical hypofunction have many symptoms and signs in common with those having primary disease but are *characteristically not hyperpigmented*, since ACTH and related peptide levels are low. In fact, plasma ACTH levels distinguish between primary and secondary adrenal insufficiency, since they are elevated in the former and decreased to absent in the latter. Patients with total pituitary insufficiency have manifestations of multiple hormone deficiencies. An additional feature distinguishing primary adrenocortical insufficiency is the *near-normal level of aldosterone secretion* seen in pituitary and/or isolated ACTH deficiencies (Fig. 331-11). Patients with pituitary insufficiency may have hyponatremia, which can be dilutional or secondary to a subnormal increase in aldosterone secretion in response to severe sodium restriction. However, severe *dehydration*, *hyponatremia*, and *hyperkalemia* are characteristic of severe mineralocorticoid insufficiency and favor a diagnosis of primary adrenocortical insufficiency.

Patients receiving long-term steroid therapy, despite physical findings of Cushing's syndrome, develop adrenal insufficiency because of prolonged pituitary-hypothalamic suppression and adrenal atrophy secondary to the loss of endogenous ACTH. These patients have two deficits, a loss of adrenal responsiveness to ACTH and a failure of pituitary ACTH release. They are characterized by low blood cortisol and ACTH levels, a low baseline rate of steroid excretion, and abnormal ACTH and metyrapone responses. Most patients with steroid-induced adrenal insufficiency eventually recover normal hypothalamic-pituitary-adrenal responsiveness, but recovery time varies from days to months. The rapid ACTH test provides a convenient assessment of recovery of hypothalamic-pituitary-adrenal function. Because the plasma cortisol concentrations after injection of cosyntropin and during insulin-induced hypoglycemia are usually similar, the rapid ACTH test assesses the integrated hypothalamic-pituitary-adrenal function (see "Tests of Pituitary-Adrenal Responsiveness," above). Some investigators suggest using the low-dose (1 μg) ACTH test for suspected secondary ACTH deficiency. Additional tests to assess pituitary ACTH reserve include the standard metyrapone and insulin-induced hypoglycemia tests.

Glucocorticoid therapy in patients with secondary adrenocortical insufficiency does not differ from that for the primary disorder. Mineralocorticoid therapy is usually not necessary, as aldosterone secretion is preserved.

ACUTE ADRENOCORTICAL INSUFFICIENCY Acute adrenocortical insufficiency may result from several processes. On the one hand, *adrenal crisis* may be a rapid and overwhelming intensification of chronic adrenal insufficiency, usually precipitated by sepsis or surgical stress. Alternatively, acute hemorrhagic destruction of both adrenal glands can occur in previously well subjects. In children, this event is usually associated with septicemia with *Pseudomonas* or meningococcemia (Waterhouse-Friderichsen syndrome). In adults, anticoagulant therapy or a coagulation disorder may result in bilateral adrenal hemorrhage. Occasionally, bilateral adrenal hemorrhage in the newborn results from birth trauma. Hemorrhage has been observed during pregnancy, following idiopathic adrenal vein thrombosis, and as a complication of venography (e.g., infarction of an adenoma). The third and most frequent cause of acute insufficiency is the rapid withdrawal of steroids from patients with adrenal atrophy owing to chronic steroid administration. Acute adrenocortical insufficiency may also occur in patients with congenital adrenal hyperplasia or those with decreased adrenocortical reserve when they are given drugs capable of inhibiting steroid synthesis (mitotane, ketoconazole) or of increasing steroid metabolism (phenytoin, rifampin).

Adrenal Crisis The long-term survival of patients with adrenocortical insufficiency depends largely on the prevention and treatment of adrenal crisis. Consequently, the occurrence of infection, trauma (including surgery), gastrointestinal upsets, or other stresses necessitates an immediate increase in hormone. In untreated patients, preexisting symptoms are intensified. Nausea, vomiting, and abdominal pain may become intractable. Fever may be severe or absent. Lethargy deepens into somnolence, and hypovolemic vascular collapse ensues. In contrast, patients previously maintained on chronic glucocorticoid therapy may not exhibit dehydration or hypotension until they are in a preterminal state, since mineralocorticoid secretion is usually preserved. In all patients in crisis, a precipitating cause should be sought.

Rx TREATMENT Treatment is directed primarily toward repletion of circulating glucocorticoids and replacement of the sodium and water deficits. Hence an intravenous infusion of 5% glucose in normal saline solution should be started with a bolus intravenous infusion of 100 mg hydrocortisone followed by a continuous infusion of hydrocortisone at a rate of 10 mg/h. An alternative approach is to administer a 100-mg bolus of hydrocortisone intravenously every 6 h. However, only continuous infusion maintains the plasma cortisol constantly at stress levels [830 nmol/L (30 μg/dL)]. Effective treatment of hypotension requires glucocorticoid replacement and repletion of sodium and water deficits. If the crisis was preceded by prolonged nausea, vomiting, and dehydration, several liters of saline solution may be required in the first few hours. Vasoconstrictive agents (such as dopamine) may be indicated in extreme conditions as adjuncts to volume replacement. With large doses of steroid, e.g., 100 to 200 mg hydrocortisone, the patient receives a maximal mineralocorticoid effect, and supplementary mineralocorticoid is superfluous. Following improvement, the steroid dosage is tapered over the next few days to maintenance levels, and mineralocorticoid therapy is reinstituted if needed (Table 331-8).

HYPOALDOSTERONISM

Isolated aldosterone deficiency accompanied by normal cortisol production occurs in association with hyporeninism, as an inherited biosynthetic defect, postoperatively following removal of aldosterone-secreting adenomas, during protracted heparin or heparinoid administration, in pretectal disease of the nervous system, and in severe postural hypotension.

The feature common to all forms hypoaldosteronism is the inability to increase aldosterone secretion appropriately in response to salt restriction. Most patients have unexplained hyperkalemia, which often is exacerbated by restriction of dietary sodium intake. In severe cases, urine sodium wastage occurs at a normal salt intake, whereas in milder forms, excessive loss of urine sodium occurs only with salt restriction.

Most cases of isolated hypoaldosteronism occur in patients with a deficiency in renin production (so-called hyporeninemic hypoaldosteronism), most commonly in adults with diabetes mellitus and mild renal failure and in whom hyperkalemia and metabolic acidosis are out of proportion to the degree of renal impairment. Plasma renin levels fail to rise normally following sodium restriction and postural changes. The pathogenesis is uncertain. Possibilities include renal disease (the most likely), autonomic neuropathy, extracellular fluid volume expansion, and defective conversion of renin precursors to active renin. Aldosterone levels also fail to rise normally after salt restriction and volume contraction; this effect is probably related to the hyporeninism, since biosynthetic defects in aldosterone secretion usually cannot be demonstrated. In these patients, aldosterone secretion increases promptly after ACTH stimulation, but it is uncertain whether the magnitude of the response is normal. On the other hand, the level of aldosterone appears to be subnormal in relationship to the hyperkalemia.

Hypoaldosteronism can also be associated with high renin levels and low or elevated levels of aldosterone (see below). Severely ill patients may also have hyperreninemic hypoaldosteronism; such patients have a high mortality rate (80%). Hyperkalemia is not present. Possible explanations for the hypoaldosteronism include adrenal necrosis (uncommon) or a shift in steroidogenesis from mineralocorticoids to glucocorticoids, possibly related to prolonged ACTH stimulation.

Before the diagnosis of isolated hypoaldosteronism is considered for a patient with hyperkalemia, "pseudohyperkalemia" (e.g., hemolysis, thrombocytosis) should be excluded by measuring the *plasma* potassium level. The next step is to demonstrate a normal cortisol response to ACTH stimulation. Then, the response of renin and aldosterone levels to stimulation (upright posture, sodium restriction) should be measured. Low renin and aldosterone levels establish the diagnosis of hyporeninemic hypoaldosteronism. A combination of high renin levels and low aldosterone levels is consistent with an aldosterone biosynthetic defect or a selective unresponsiveness to angiotensin II. Finally, there is a condition that clinically and biochemically mimics hypoaldosteronism with elevated renin levels. However, the aldosterone levels are not low but high—so-called pseudohypoaldosteronism. This inherited condition is caused by a mutation in the epithelial sodium channel (see below).

℞ **TREATMENT** The treatment is to replace the mineralocorticoid deficiency. For practical purposes, the oral administration of 0.05 to 0.15 mg fludrocortisone daily should restore electrolyte balance if salt intake is adequate (e.g., 150 to 200 mmol/d). However, patients with hyporeninemic hypoaldosteronism may require higher doses of mineralocorticoid to correct hyperkalemia. This need poses a potential risk in patients with hypertension, mild renal insufficiency, or congestive heart failure. An alternative approach is to reduce salt intake and to administer furosemide, which can ameliorate acidosis and hyperkalemia. Occasionally, a combination of these two approaches is efficacious.

GENETIC CONSIDERATIONS **Glucocorticoid Diseases** • ***Congenital adrenal hyperplasia*** Congenital adrenal hyperplasia (CAH) is the consequence of recessive mutations that cause one of several distinct enzymatic defects (see below). Because cortisol is the principal adrenal steroid regulating ACTH elaboration and because ACTH stimulates adrenal growth and function, a block in cortisol synthesis may result in the enhanced secretion of adrenal androgens and/or mineralocorticids depending on the site of the enzyme block. In severe congenital virilizing hyperplasia, the adrenal output of cortisol may be so compromised as to cause adrenal deficiency despite adrenal hyperplasia.

CAH is the most common adrenal disorder of infancy and childhood (Chap. 338). Partial enzyme deficiencies can be expressed after adolescence, predominantly in women with hirsutism and oligomenorrhea but minimal virilization. Late-onset adrenal hyperplasia may account for 5 to 25% of cases of hirsutism and oligomenorrhea in women, depending on the population.

ETIOLOGY Enzymatic defects have been described in 21-hydroxylase (CYP21A2), 17α-hydroxylase/17,20-Lyase (CYP17), 11β-hydroxylase (CYP11B1), and in (3β-HSD2) (Fig. 331-2). Although the cDNAs for these enzymes have been cloned, the diagnosis of specific enzyme deficiencies with genetic techniques is not practical for routine use. CYP21A2 deficiency is closely linked to the HLA-B locus of chromosome 6 so that HLA typing and/or DNA polymorphism can be used to detect the heterozygous carriers and to diagnose affected individuals in some families (Chap. 306). The clinical expression in the different disorders is variable, ranging from virilization of the female (CYP2/A2) to feminization of the male (3β-HSD2) (Chap. 338).

Adrenal virilization in the female at birth is associated with ambiguous external genitalia (*female pseudohermaphroditism*). Virilization probably begins after the fifth month of intrauterine development. At birth there may be enlarged genitalia in the male infant and enlargement of the clitoris, partial or complete fusion of the labia, and sometimes a urogenital sinus in the female. If the labial fusion is nearly complete, the female infant has external genitalia resembling a penis with hypospadias. In the *postnatal* period, CAH is associated with virilization in the female and isosexual precocity in the male. The excessive androgen levels result in accelerated growth, so that bone age exceeds chronologic age. Because epiphyseal closure is hastened by excessive androgens, growth stops, but truncal development continues, the characteristic appearance being a short child with a well-developed trunk.

The most common form of CAH (95% of cases) is a result of impairment of CYP21A2. In addition to cortisol deficiency, aldosterone secretion is decreased in approximately one-third of the patients. Thus, with CYP21A2 deficiency, adrenal virilization occurs with or without a salt-losing tendency due to aldosterone deficiency (Fig. 331-2).

CYP11B1 deficiency causes a "hypertensive" variant of CAH. Hypertension and hypokalemia occur because of the impaired conversion of 11-deoxycorticosterone to corticosterone, resulting in the accumulation of 11-deoxycorticosterone, a potent mineralocorticoid. The degree of hypertension is variable. Increased shunting again occurs into the androgen pathway.

CYP17 deficiency is characterized by hypogonadism, hypokalemia, and hypertension. This rare disorder causes decreased production of cortisol and shunting of precursors into the mineralocorticoid pathway with hypokalemic alkalosis, hypertension, and suppressed plasma renin activity. Usually, 11-deoxycorticosterone production is elevated. Because CYP17 hydroxylation is required for biosynthesis of both adrenal androgens and gonadal testosterone and estrogen, this defect is associated with sexual immaturity, high urinary gonadotropin levels, and low urinary 17-ketosteroid excretion. Female patients have primary amenorrhea and lack of development of secondary sexual characteristics. Because of deficient androgen production, male patients have either ambiguous external genitalia or a female phenotype (*male pseudohermaphroditism*). Exogenous glucocorticoids can correct the hypertensive syndrome, and treatment with appropriate gonadal steroids results in sexual maturation.

With 3β-HSD2 deficiency, conversion of pregnenolone to progesterone is impaired, so that the synthesis of both cortisol and aldosterone is blocked, with shunting into the adrenal androgen pathway via 17α-hydroxypregnenolone and DHEA. Because DHEA is a weak androgen, and because this enzyme deficiency is also present in the gonad, the genitalia of the male fetus may be incompletely virilized or feminized. Conversely, in the female, overproduction of DHEA may produce partial virilization.

DIAGNOSIS The diagnosis of CAH should be considered in infants having episodes of acute adrenal insufficiency or salt-wasting or with hypertension. The diagnosis is further suggested by the finding of hypertrophy of the clitoris, fused labia, or a urogenital sinus in the female or of isosexual precocity in the male. In infants and children with a CYP21A2 defect, increased urine 17-ketosteroid excretion and increased plasma DHEA sulfate levels are typically associated with an increase in the blood levels of 17-hydroxyprogesterone and the excretion of its urinary metabolite pregnanetriol. Demonstration of elevated levels of 17-hydroxyprogesterone in amniotic fluid at 14 to 16 weeks of gestation allows prenatal detection of affected female infants.

The diagnosis of a *salt-losing form* of CAH due to defects in CYP21A2 is suggested by episodes of acute adrenal insufficiency with hyponatremia, hyperkalemia, dehydration, and vomiting. These infants and children often crave salt and have laboratory findings indicating deficits in both cortisol and aldosterone secretion.

With the *hypertensive form* of CAH due to CYP11B1 deficiency, 11-deoxycorticosterone and 11-deoxycortisol accumulate. The diagnosis is confirmed by demonstrating increased levels of 11-deoxycortisol in the blood or increased amounts of tetrahydro-11-deoxycortisol in the urine. Elevation of 17-hydroxyprogesterone levels does not imply a coexisting CYP21A2 deficiency.

Very high levels of urine DHEA with low levels of pregnanetriol and of cortisol metabolites in urine are characteristic of children with 3β-HSD2 deficiency. Marked salt-wasting may also occur.

Adults with *late-onset adrenal hyperplasia* (partial deficiency of CYP21A2, CYP11B1, or 3β-HSD2) are characterized by normal or moderately elevated levels of urinary 17-ketosteroids and plasma DHEA sulfate. A high basal level of a precursor of cortisol biosynthesis (such as 17-hydroxyprogesterone, 17-hydroxypregnenolone, or 11-deoxycortisol), or elevation of such a precursor after ACTH stimulation, confirms the diagnosis of a partial deficiency. Measurement of steroid precursors 60 min after bolus administration of ACTH is usually sufficient. Adrenal androgen output is easily suppressed by the standard low-dose (2 mg) dexamethasone test. ■

℞ TREATMENT Patients with CAH have a fundamental defect of cortisol deficiency with resultant excessive ACTH secretion, producing hyperplasia of the adrenal glands and causing additional shunting into the precursor steroid pathways. Therapy in these patients consists of daily administration of glucocorticoids to suppress pituitary ACTH secretion. Because of its cost and intermediate half-life, prednisone is the drug of choice except in infants, in whom hydrocortisone is usually used. In adults with late-onset adrenal hyperplasia, the smallest single bedtime dose of a long- or intermediate-acting glucocorticoid that suppresses pituitary ACTH secretion should be administered. The amount of steroid required by children with CAH is approximately 1 to 1.5 times the normal cortisol production rate of 27 to 35 μmol (10 to 13 mg) of cortisol per square meter of body surface per day and is given in divided doses two or three times per day. The dosage schedule is governed by repetitive analysis of the urinary 17-ketosteroids, plasma DHEA sulfate, and/or precursors of cortisol biosynthesis. Skeletal growth and maturation must also be monitored closely, as overtreatment with glucocorticoid replacement therapy retards linear growth.

Receptor Mutations Much less common than CAH are three syndromes secondary to mutation(s) in a key receptor involved in adrenal function. *Isolated glucocorticoid deficiency* is a rare autosomal recessive disease secondary to a mutation in the ACTH receptor. Usually mineralocorticoid function is normal. Adrenal insufficiency is manifest within the first 2 years of life usually as hyperpigmentation, convulsions, and/or frequent episodes of hypoglycemia. In some patients the adrenal insufficiency is associated with achalasia and alacrima—Allgrove's, or triple A, syndrome. However, in some triple A syndrome patients, no mutation in the ACTH receptor has been identified, suggesting that a distinct genetic abnormality causes this syndrome. *Adrenal hypoplasia congenita* is a rare X-linked disorder caused by a mutation in the *DAX1* gene located on the X chromosome. This gene encodes an orphan nuclear receptor that plays an important role in the development of the adrenal cortex and also the hypothalamic-pituitary-gonadal axis. Thus, patients present with signs and symptoms secondary to deficiencies of all three major adrenal steroids—cortisol, aldosterone, and adrenal androgens—as well as gonadotropin deficiency. Finally a rare cause of hypercortisolism without cushingoid stigmata is *primary cortisol resistance* due to mutations in the glucocorticoid receptor. The resistance is incomplete because patients do not exhibit signs of adrenal insufficiency. Thus, these three rare inherited disorders have in common an elevated ACTH. However, the clinical manifestations range from no evidence of adrenal insufficiency to only cortisol deficiency (similar to secondary adrenal insufficiency) to a clinical picture indistinguishable from classic Addison's disease.

Miscellaneous Conditions Adrenoleukodystrophy causes severe demyelination and early death in children, and adrenomyeloneuropathy is associated with a mixed motor and sensory neuropathy with spastic paraplegia in adults; both disorders are associated with elevated circulating levels of very long chain fatty acids and cause adrenal insufficiency. Autosomal recessive mutations in the *st*eroidogenic *a*cute *r*egulatory (STAR) protein gene cause congenital lipoid adrenal hyperplasia (Chap. 338), which is characterized by adrenal insufficiency and defective gonadal steroidogenesis. Because STAR mediates cholesterol transport into the mitochondrion, mutations in the protein cause massive lipid accumulation in steroidogenic cells, ultimately leading to cell toxicity. Thus, these three rare inherited disorders have in common an elevated ACTH. However, the clinical manifestations range from no evidence of adrenal insufficiency to only cortisol deficiency (similar to secondary adrenal insufficiency) to a clinical picture indistinguishable from classic Addison's disease.

MINERALOCORTICOID DISEASES Some forms of CAH have a mineralocorticoid component (see above). Others are caused by a mutation in other enzymes or ion channels important in mediating or mimicking aldosterone's action.

Hypermineralocorticoidism • ***Low plasma renin activity*** Rarely, hypermineralocorticoidism is due to a defect in cortisol biosynthesis, specifically 11- or 17-hydroxylation. ACTH levels are increased, with a resultant increase in the production of the mineralocorticoid 11-deoxycorticosterone. Hypertension and hypokalemia can be corrected by glucocorticoid administration. The definitive diagnosis is made by demonstrating an elevation of precursors of cortisol biosynthesis in the blood or urine or by direct demonstration of the genetic defect.

Glucocorticoid administration can also ameliorate hypertension or produce normotension even though a hydroxylase deficiency cannot be identified (Fig. 331-9). These patients have normal to slightly elevated aldosterone levels that do not suppress in response to saline but do suppress in response to 2 days of dexamethasone (2 mg/d). The condition is inherited as an autosomal dominant trait and is termed *glucocorticoid-remediable aldosteronism* (GRA). This entity is secondary to a chimeric gene duplication whereby the 11-β hydroxylase gene promoter (which is under the control of ACTH) is fused to the aldosterone synthase coding sequence. Thus, aldosterone synthase activity is ectopically expressed in the zona fasciculata and is regulated by ACTH, in a fashion similar to the regulation of cortisol secretion. Screening for this defect is best performed by assessing the presence or absence of the chimeric gene. Because the abnormal gene may be present in the absence of hypokalemia, its frequency as a cause of hypertension is unknown. Individuals with suppressed plasma renin levels and juvenile-onset hypertension or a history of early-onset hypertension in first-degree relatives should be screened for this disorder. Early hemorrhagic stroke also occurs in GRA-affected individuals.

Glucocorticoid-remediable hyperaldosteronism documented by genetic analysis may be treated with glucocorticoid administration or antimineralocorticoids, e.g., spironolactone, triamterene, or amiloride. Glucocorticoids should be used only in small doses to avoid inducing iatrogenic Cushing's syndrome. A combination approach is often necessary.

High plasma renin activity Bartter's syndrome is characterized by severe hyperaldosteronism (hypokalemic alkalosis) with moderate to marked increases in renin activity and hypercalciuria, but normal blood pressure and no edema; this disorder usually begins in childhood. Renal biopsy shows juxtaglomerular hyperplasia. The pathogenesis involves a defect in the renal conservation of sodium or chloride. The renal loss of sodium is thought to stimulate renin secretion and aldosterone production. Hyperaldosteronism produces potassium depletion, and hypokalemia further elevates prostaglandin production and plasma renin activity. In some cases, the hypokalemia may be potentiated by a defect in renal conservation of potassium. Increased production of prostaglandins is probably not a primary abnormality, since administration of inhibitors of prostaglandin synthesis reverses the features only temporarily (Chap. 276). Bartter's syndrome is caused by a mutation in the renal Na-K-2Cl co-transporter gene.

Gitelman's syndrome is an autosomal recessive trait characterized by renal salt wasting and as a result, as in Bartter's syndrome, activation of the renin-angiotensin-aldosterone system. As a consequence affected individuals have low blood pressure, low serum potassium, low serum magnesium, and high serum bicarbonate. In contrast to Bartter's syndrome, urinary calcium excretion is reduced. Gitelman's syndrome results from loss-of-function mutations of the renal thiazide-sensitive Na-Cl co-transporter.

Increased Mineralocorticoid Action Liddle's syndrome is a rare autosomal dominant disorder that mimicks hyperaldosteronism. The defect is in the genes encoding the β or γ subunits of the epithelial sodium channel. Both renin and aldosterone levels are low, owing to the constitutively activated sodium channel and the resulting excess sodium reabsorption in the renal tubule.

A rare autosomal recessive cause of hypokalemia and hypertension is 11β-HSD II deficiency, in which cortisol cannot be converted to cortisone and hence binds to the MR and acts as a mineralocorticoid. This condition, also termed *apparent mineralocorticoid excess syndrome*, is caused by a defect in the gene encoding the renal isoform of this enzyme, 11β-HSD II. Patients can be identified either by documenting an increased ratio of cortisol to cortisone in the urine or by genetic analysis. Patients with the 11β-HSD deficiency syndrome can be treated with small doses of dexamethasone. Although dexamethasone is a potent glucocorticoid that suppresses ACTH and endogenous cortisol production, it binds less well to the mineralocorticoid receptor than does cortisol.

The ingestion of candies or chewing tobacco containing certain forms of licorice produces a syndrome that mimics primary aldosteronism. The component of such agents that causes sodium retention is glycyrrhizinic acid, which inhibits the 11β-HSD II and hence allows cortisol to act as a mineralocorticoid and cause sodium retention, expansion of the extracellular fluid volume, hypertension, depressed plasma renin levels, and suppressed aldosterone levels. The diagnosis is established or excluded by a careful history.

Decreased Mineralocorticoid Production or Action In patients with these conditions, disorders of aldosterone biosynthesis or action are associated with high renin levels, salt wasting, and hyperkalemia. The aldosterone levels may be low or elevated. In patients with a deficiency in aldosterone biosynthesis, the transformation of corticosterone into aldosterone is impaired, owing to a mutation in the aldosterone synthase (CYP11B2) gene. These patients have low to absent aldosterone secretion, elevated plasma renin levels, and elevated levels of the intermediates of aldosterone biosynthesis (corticosterone and 18-hydroxycorticosterone).

Pseudohypoaldosteronism type I (PHA-I) is an autosomal recessive disorder that is seen in the neonatal period and is characterized by salt wasting, hypotension, hyperkalemia, and high renin and aldosterone levels. In contrast to the gain-of-function mutations in the epithelial sodium channel (ENaC) in Liddle's syndrome, mutations in PHA-I result in loss of ENaC function.

NONSPECIFIC CLINICAL USE OF ADRENAL STEROIDS

The widespread use of glucocorticoids emphasizes the need for a thorough understanding of the metabolic effects of these agents. Before adrenal hormone therapy is instituted, the expected gains should be weighed against undesirable effects.

HOW SERIOUS IS THE DISORDER? In a patient who has unexplained shock or in whom other measures have failed, the physician need not hesitate to employ high-dose steroid therapy. In contrast, one should exercise restraint in administering steroids to a patient with early rheumatoid arthritis for whom physiotherapy, anti-inflammatory agents, disease-modifying agents, and general medical care have not been tried (Chap. 312).

HOW LONG WILL GLUCOCORTICOID THERAPY BE REQUIRED? The use of intravenous steroids for 24 to 48 h for a life-threatening situation such as status asthmaticus or pseudotumor cerebri has few or no contraindications, in contrast to the initiation of chronic steroid therapy for asthma, arthritis, or psoriasis. In the latter instances, the almost certain development of some degree of Cushing's syndrome must be weighed against the potential benefit. These side effects should be minimized by a careful choice of steroid preparations, alternate-day or interrupted therapy; the use of topical steroids, e.g., inhaled, intranasal, or dermal, whenever possible; and the judicious use of supplementary adjuvants.

WHICH PREPARATION IS BEST? Several considerations should be taken into account in deciding which steroid preparation to use.

1. *The biologic half-life.* The rationale behind alternate-day therapy is to decrease the metabolic effects of the steroids for a significant part of each 48 h period while still producing a pharmacologic effect durable enough to be effective. Too long a half-life would defeat the first purpose, and too short a half-life would defeat the second. In general, the more potent the steroid, the longer its biologic half-life.
2. *The importance of the mineralocorticoid effects of the steroid.* Most synthetic steroids have less mineralocorticoid effect than hydrocortisone (Table 331-9).
3. *The biologically active form of the steroid.* Cortisone and prednisone have to be converted to biologically active metabolites before anti-inflammatory effects can occur. Because of this, in a condition for which steroids are known to be effective and when an adequate dose has been given without response, one should consider substituting hydrocortisone or prednisolone for cortisone or prednisone.
4. *The cost of the medication.* This is a serious consideration if chronic administration is planned. Prednisone is the least expensive of available steroid preparations.
5. *The type of formulation.* Topical steroids have the distinct advantage over oral steroids in reducing the likelihood of systemic side effects. In addition, some inhaled steroids have been designed to minimize side effects by increasing their hepatic inactivation if they are swallowed (Chap. 252). However, all topical steroids can be absorbed into the systemic circulation.

EVALUATION OF PATIENTS PRIOR TO INITIATING STEROID THERAPY (See Table 331-10) **Chronic Infection** Three issues demand attention: (1) Any active infection, particularly

Table 331-9 Glucocorticoid Preparations

	Estimated Potency[b]	
Commonly Used Name[a]	Glucocorticoid	Mineralocorticoid
SHORT-ACTING		
Hydrocortisone	1	1
Cortisone	0.8	0.8
INTERMEDIATE-ACTING		
Prednisone	4	0.25
Prednisolone	4	0.25
Methylprednisolone	5	<0.01
Triamcinolone	5	<0.01
LONG-ACTING		
Paramethasone	10	<0.01
Betamethasone	25	<0.01
Dexamethasone	30–40	<0.01

[a] The steroids are divided into three groups according to the duration of biologic activity. Short-acting preparations have a biologic half-life <12 h; long-acting, >48 h; and intermediate, between 12 and 36 h. Triamcinolone has the longest half-life of the intermediate-acting preparations.

[b] Relative milligram comparisons with hydrocortisone, setting the glucocorticoid and mineralocorticoid properties of hydrocortisone as 1. Sodium retention is insignificant for commonly employed doses of methylprednisolone, triamcinolone, paramethasone, betamethasone, and dexamethasone.

tuberculosis, should be identified. (2) If tuberculosis is present, steroid therapy should be employed only in conjunction with antituberculous chemotherapy. The chest film and tuberculin test provide baseline information for future comparison. Since high-dose steroids may impair the tuberculin reaction, serial chest roentgenograms may be necessary. (3) Infection due to opportunistic pathogens should be constantly considered in patients on steroid therapy, especially when combined with other immunosuppressive agents.

Diabetes Mellitus Prolonged glucocorticoid therapy may unmask or aggravate diabetes mellitus. The presence of diabetes mellitus or the demonstration of impaired glucose tolerance may affect the decision to institute glucocorticoid therapy.

Osteoporosis Patients receiving long-term steroid therapy are at risk for osteoporosis. Indeed, osteoporosis with vertebral fractures or compression is a dreaded complication for patients at high risk (postmenopausal women, elderly men, patients with restricted physical activity, and especially organ transplant patients who are maintained on high doses to prevent rejection). Alternate-day or interrupted steroid therapy does not prevent the risk of this complication (Table 331-11). Adjunctive therapies with antiresorptive agents, such as parenteral or oral bisphosphonates, have been shown to be effective in treating the osteoporosis (Chap. 342). Bone mineral density should be assessed periodically with dual-energy X-ray absorptiometry (DEXA) scans.

Peptic Ulcer, Gastric Hypersecretion, or Esophagitis In conventional doses (equivalent to ≤15 mg prednisone per day), glucocorticoids probably do not cause peptic ulceration; whether higher doses cause ulcer disease is not established and probably depends on duration, dose of treatment, and predisposing factors such as hypoalbuminemia or cirrhosis and also whether subjects are concomitantly ingesting nonsteroidal anti-inflammatory agents (NSAIDs). However,

Table 331-10 A Checklist for Use Prior to the Administration of Glucocorticoids in Pharmacologic Doses

- Presence of tuberculosis or other chronic infection (chest x-ray, tuberculin test)
- Evidence of glucose intolerance or history of gestational diabetes mellitus
- Evidence of preexisting osteoporosis (bone density assessment in organ transplant recipients or postmenopausal patients)
- History of peptic ulcer, gastritis, or esophagitis (stool guaiac test)
- Evidence of hypertension or cardiovascular disease
- History of psychological disorders

Table 331-11 Supplementary Measures to Minimize Undesirable Metabolic Effects of Glucocorticoids

- Monitor caloric intake to prevent weight gain.
- Restrict sodium intake to prevent edema and minimize hypertension and potassium loss.
- Provide supplementary potassium if necessary.
- Provide antacid, H_2 receptor antagonist, and/or H^+,K^+-ATPase inhibitor therapy.
- Institute alternate-day steroid schedule if possible. Patients receiving steroid therapy over a prolonged period should be protected by an appropriate increase in hormone level during periods of acute stress. A rule of thumb is to *double* the maintenance dose.
- Minimize osteopenia by
  - Administering gonadal hormone replacement therapy: 0.625–1.25 mg conjugated estrogens given cyclically with progesterone, unless the uterus is absent; testosterone replacement for hypogonadal men
- Ensuring high calcium intake (should be approximately 1200 mg/d)
- Administering supplemental vitamin D if blood levels of calciferol or $1,25(OH)_2$ vitamin D are reduced
- Administering bisphosphonate prophylactically, orally or parenterally, in high-risk patients

even at conventional doses, patients with a history of ulcer may experience aggravation of symptoms while receiving glucocorticoids. Consequently, all individuals with a positive history or with known risk factors should be managed with a vigorous antiulcer program (antacids, H_2 receptor antagonists, or ATPase inhibitors) along with glucocorticoids. *The development of anemia in a patient receiving glucocorticoids should suggest gastrointestinal bleeding as a cause.*

Hypertension or Cardiovascular Disease The capacity of many adrenal steroid preparations to promote sodium retention makes it necessary to exercise caution when using them in patients with preexisting hypertension or cardiovascular or renal disease. The use of preparations with minimal sodium-retaining activity, restriction of dietary sodium intake, and the use of diuretic agents and supplementary potassium salts minimize the mineralocorticoid effects of steroids. However, hypertension may be exacerbated by steroid-induced increases in renin substrate and angiotensin II levels and by reduction in vasodilator prostaglandin production. Steroids also accelerate atherogenesis by induction of hypertension, glucose intolerance, and unfavorable lipid profiles. Glucocorticoid-associated lipid abnormalities include hypertriglyceridemia, hypercholesterolemia, and increased LDL cholesterol levels.

Psychological Difficulties Steroid therapy may cause psychological disturbances. In general, these disturbances correlate better with the patient's personality than with the dose of hormone, although larger doses cause more serious reactions. There is no reliable method of predicting the psychological reaction to steroid therapy; moreover, previous tolerance of steroids does not necessarily ensure the safety of subsequent courses. Likewise, untoward psychological reactions on one occasion do not invariably mean that the patient will respond unfavorably to a second course. However, patients with depressive symptoms during a first course of steroids may benefit from prophylactic treatment prior to a second course.

Sleeplessness is common and can be minimized by using the shorter-acting steroids and by prescribing the total daily amount as a single early-morning dose.

ALTERNATE-DAY STEROID THERAPY The most effective way to minimize the cushingoid effects of glucocorticoids is to administer the total 48-h dose as a *single* dose of *intermediate-acting steroid* in the morning, *every other day*. If symptoms of the underlying disorder can be controlled by this technique, it offers distinct advantages. Three considerations deserve mention: (1) The alternate-day schedule may be approached through transition schedules that allow the patient to adjust gradually; (2) supplementary nonsteroid medications may be needed on the "off" day to minimize symptoms of the underlying disorder; and (3) many symptoms that occur during the off day (e.g., fatigue, joint pain, muscle stiffness or tenderness, and fever) may represent relative adrenal insufficiency rather than exacerbation of the underlying disease.

The alternate-day approach capitalizes on the fact that cortisol secretion and plasma levels normally are highest in the early morning and lowest in the evening. The normal pattern is mimicked by administering an intermediate-acting steroid in the morning (7 to 8 A.M.) (Table 331-9).

Initially, the steroid program often requires daily or more frequent doses of steroid to achieve the desired anti-inflammatory or immunity-suppressing action. *Only after this desired effect is achieved is an attempt made to switch to an alternate-day program.* A number of schedules can be used for transferring from a daily to an alternate-day program. The key points to be considered are flexibility in arranging a program and the use of supportive measures on the off day. One may attempt a gradual transition to the alternate-day schedule rather than an abrupt changeover. One approach is to keep the steroid dose constant on one day and gradually reduce it on the alternate day. Alternatively, the steroid dose can be increased on one day and reduced on the alternate day. In any case, it is important to anticipate that some increase in pain or discomfort may occur in the 36 to 48 h following the last dose.

WITHDRAWAL OF GLUCOCORTICOIDS FOLLOWING LONG-TERM USE It is possible to reduce gradually and eventually to discontinue a daily steroid dose, but under most circumstances withdrawal of steroids should be initiated by first implementing an alternate-day schedule. Patients who have been on an alternate-day program for a month or more experience less difficulty during termination regimens. The dosage is gradually reduced and finally discontinued after a replacement dosage has been reached (e.g., 5 to 7.5 mg prednisone). Complications rarely ensue unless undue stress is experienced, and patients should understand that for 1 year or longer after withdrawal from long-term high-dose steroid therapy, supplementary hormone should be given in the event of a serious infection, operation, or injury. A useful strategy in patients with symptoms of adrenal insufficiency on a tapering regimen is to measure plasma cortisol levels prior to the steroid dose. A level <140 nmol/L (5 μg/dL) indicates continuing suppression of the pituitary-adrenal axis and implies that a more cautious tapering of steroids is indicated.

In patients on high-dose daily steroid therapy, it is advised to reduce dosage to approximately 20 mg prednisone daily as a single morning dose before beginning the transition to alternate-day therapy. If a patient cannot tolerate an alternate-day program, consideration should be given to the possibility that the patient has developed primary adrenal insufficiency.

BIBLIOGRAPHY

AZZIZ R et al: Nonclassic adrenal hyperplasia: Current concepts. Clinical review 56. J Clin Endocrinol Metab 78:810, 1994

BARZON L et al: Risk factors and long-term follow-up of adrenal incidentalomas. J Clin Endocrinol Metab 84:520, 1999

BORNSTEIN SR et al: Adrenocortical tumors: Recent advances in basic concepts and clinical management. Ann Intern Med 130:579, 1999

BRAND E et al: Structural analysis and evaluation of the aldosterone synthase gene in hypertension. Hypertension 32:198, 1998

CONLIN PR et al: Disorders of the renin-angiotensin-aldosterone system, in *Renal and Electrolyte Disorders*, 5th ed, RW Schrier (ed). Boston, Little, Brown, 1997

DLUHY RG et al: Glucocorticoid-remediable aldosteronism. Endocrinol Metab Clin North Am 23:385, 1994

GANGULY A: Primary aldosteronism. N Engl J Med 339:1828, 1998

GHOSE R et al: Medical management of aldosterone-producing adenomas. Ann Intern Med 131:105, 1999

HABIBY RL et al: Adrenal hypoplasia congenita with hypogonadotropic hypogonadism: Evidence that DAX-1 mutations lead to combined hypothalamic and pituitary defects in gonadotropin production. J Clin Invest 98:1055, 1996

INVITTI C et al: Diagnosis and management of Cushing's syndrome: Results of an Italian multicentre study. J Clin Endocrinol Metab 84:440, 1999

JORGE P et al: X-linked adrenoleukodystrophy in patients with idiopathic Addison disease. Eur J Pediatr 153:594, 1994

KALTSAS GA et al: A critical analysis of the value of simultaneous inferior petrosal sinus sampling in Cushing's disease and the occult ectopic adrenocorticotropin syndrome. J Clin Endocrinol Metab 84:487, 1999

KEREM E et al: Pulmonary epithelial sodium-channel dysfunction and excess airway liquid in pseudohypoaldosteronism. N Engl J Med 341:156, 1999

KJELLMAN M et al: Molecular genetics of adrenal cortical tumors. Curr Opin Endocrinol Diabetes 6:70, 1999

KONG MF et al: Eighty-six cases of Addison disease. Clin Endocrinol 41:757, 1994

LIPWORTH B et al: Systemic adverse effects of inhaled corticosteroid therapy. Arch Intern Med 159:941, 1999

MORTENSEN RM, WILLIAMS GH: Aldosterone action (physiology), in *Endocrinology*, 4th ed, LJ DeGroot et al (eds). Philadelphia, Saunders, 2001

NEW M: Steroid 21-hydroxylase deficiency (congenital adrenal hyperplasia). Am J Med 98:2S, 1995

NEWELL-PRICE J et al: Diagnosis and management of Cushing's syndrome. Lancet 353: 2087, 1999

PAPANICOLAOU DA et al: A single midnight serum cortisol measurement distinguishes Cushing's syndrome from pseudo-Cushing's states. J Clin Endocrinol Metab 83:1163, 1998

ROGOFF D et al: The codon 213 of the 11beta-hydroxysteroid dehydrogenase type 2 gene is a hot spot for mutations in apparent mineralocorticoid excess. J Clin Endocrinol Metab 83:4391, 1998

SAMBROOK P et al: Prevention of corticosteroid osteoporosis. A comparison of calcium, calcitriol, and calcitonin. N Engl J Med 328:1747, 1993

SHIMKET RA et al: Liddle's syndrome: Heritable human hypertension caused by mutations in the beta subunit of the epithelial sodium channel. Cell 79:407, 1994

SWEARINGEN B et al: Long-term mortality after transsphenoidal surgery for Cushing's disease. Ann Intern Med 130:821, 1999

YOUNG MJ et al: Mineralocorticoids, salt hypertension: Effects on the heart. Steroids 61: 233, 1996

332 *Lewis Landsberg, James B. Young*

PHEOCHROMOCYTOMA

Pheochromocytomas produce, store, and secrete catecholamines. They are usually derived from the adrenal medulla but may develop from chromaffin cells in or about sympathetic ganglia (extraadrenal pheochromocytomas or paragangliomas). Related tumors that secrete catecholamines and produce similar clinical syndromes include chemodectomas derived from the carotid body and ganglioneuromas derived from the postganglionic sympathetic neurons.

The clinical features are due predominantly to the release of catecholamines and, to a lesser extent, to the secretion of other substances. Hypertension is the most common sign, and hypertensive paroxysms or crises, often spectacular and alarming, occur in over half the cases.

Pheochromocytoma occurs in approximately 0.1% of the hypertensive population but is, nevertheless, an important correctable cause of high blood pressure. Indeed, it is usually curable if properly diagnosed and treated, but it may be fatal if undiagnosed or mistreated. Postmortem series indicate that most pheochromocytomas are unsuspected clinically, even when the tumor is related to the fatal outcome.

PATHOLOGY **Location and Morphology** In adults, approximately 80% of pheochromocytomas are unilateral and solitary, 10% are bilateral, and 10% are extraadrenal. In children, a fourth of tumors are bilateral, and an additional fourth are extraadrenal. Solitary lesions inexplicably favor the right side. Although pheochromocytomas may grow to large size (over 3 kg), most weigh less than 100 g and are less than 10 cm in diameter. The tumors are highly vascular.

The tumors are made up of large, polyhedral, pleomorphic chromaffin cells. Less than 10% of these tumors are malignant. As with other endocrine tumors, malignancy cannot be determined from the histologic appearance; tumors that contain large numbers of aneuploid or tetraploid cells, as determined by flow cytometry, are more likely to recur. Local invasion of surrounding tissues or distant metastases indicate malignancy.

Extraadrenal pheochromocytomas Extraadrenal pheochromocytomas usually weigh 20 to 40 g and are <5 cm in diameter. Most are located within the abdomen in association with the celiac, superior mesenteric, and inferior mesenteric ganglia. Approximately 10% are in the thorax, 1% are within the urinary bladder, and <3% are in the neck, usually in association with the sympathetic ganglia or the extracranial branches of the ninth or tenth cranial nerves.

Catecholamine Synthesis, Storage, and Release Pheochromocytomas synthesize and store catecholamines by processes resembling those of the normal adrenal medulla (Chap. 72). Little is known about the mechanisms of catecholamine release from pheochromocytomas, but changes in blood flow and necrosis within the tumor may be the cause in some instances. These tumors are not innervated, and catecholamine release does not result from neural stimulation. Pheochromocytomas also store and secrete a variety of peptides, including endogenous opioids, adrenomedullin, endothelin, erythropoietin, parathyroid hormone–related protein, neuropeptide Y, and chromagranin A (Chap. 72). These peptides contribute to the clinical manifestations in selected cases, as noted below.

Epinephrine, norepinephrine, and dopamine Most pheochromocytomas contain and secrete both norepinephrine and epinephrine, and the percentage of norepinephrine is usually greater than in the normal adrenal. Most extraadrenal pheochromocytomas secrete norepinephrine exclusively. Rarely, pheochromocytomas produce epinephrine alone, particularly in association with multiple endocrine neoplasia (MEN). Although epinephrine-producing tumors may cause a preponderance of metabolic and beta-receptor effects, in general the major catecholamine secreted cannot be predicted from the clinical presentation. Increased production of dopamine and homovanillic acid (HVA) is uncommon with benign lesions but may occur with malignant pheochromocytoma.

FAMILIAL PHEOCHROMOCYTOMA In approximately 5% of cases, pheochromocytoma is inherited as an autosomal dominant trait either alone or in combination with other abnormalities such as MEN type 2a (Sipple's syndrome) or type 2b (mucosal neuroma syndrome) (Chap. 339), von Hippel–Lindau's retinal cerebellar hemangioblastomosis, or von Recklinghausen's neurofibromatosis. Bilateral adrenal pheochromocytomas are common in the familial syndromes; within MEN kindreds, over half of pheochromocytomas are bilateral. A familial syndrome should be suspected in any patient with bilateral pheochromocytomas.

GENETIC CONSIDERATIONS Several molecular genetic abnormalities have been identified in the familial pheochromocytoma syndromes. The MEN 2A and B syndromes are associated with abnormalities in the RET protooncogene located in pericentromeric region of chromosome 10 (Chap. 339). These mutations result in the constitutive activation of the receptor tyrosine kinase exposing adrenal medullary chromaffin cells and parafollicular C cells to hyperplasia and rendering them susceptible to malignant transformation. The RET mutations are located in the extracellular domain in MEN 2A and in the intracellular portion of the receptor in families with the MEN 2B syndrome. Interestingly, mutations at specific sites in the RET protooncogene are highly predictive of pheochromocytoma. The different phenotypic manifestations of the syndrome in different families, therefore, reflect differences in the specific mutations.

In the von Hippel–Landau (VHL) syndrome, mutation of one copy of the VHL tumor suppressor gene is associated with the development of tumors characteristic of the syndrome including pheochromocytomas. Loss of function of the VHL tumor suppressor gene promotes tumor formation by mechanisms that are incompletely understood but may involve mRNA transcript elongation. In the VHL syndrome, the frequency of pheochromocytoma varies considerably in different kindreds. As in the MEN 2 syndromes, certain VHL mutations are highly associated with the development of pheochromocytoma. Of further interest is the recent finding that the VHL mutation has been identified in some kindreds with familial pheochromocytoma as the sole manifestation without other clinical evidence of the VHL syndrome. Missense mutations, as opposed to deletions, insertions, or non-sense mutations, appear to be more commonly associated with pheochromocytoma. There is also a high incidence of germ-line VHL mutations in patients with thoracic extraadrenal pheochromocytomas.

Interestingly, neither the RET protooncogene nor the VHL mutation occurs commonly as a somatic mutation in sporadic pheochromocytomas. Screening apparently sporadic cases, however, may uncover a germ-line mutation and lead to the identification of an involved family that was unsuspected on clinical grounds. ■

CLINICAL FEATURES Pheochromocytoma occurs at all ages but is most common in young to midadult life. Some series show a slight female preponderance. Most patients come to medical attention as a result of hypertensive crisis, paroxysmal symptoms suggestive of seizure disorder or anxiety attacks, or hypertension that responds poorly to conventional treatment. Less commonly, unexplained hypotension or shock in association with surgery or trauma will suggest the diagnosis. Most patients have hypertension in association with headaches, excessive sweating, and/or palpitations.

Hypertension Hypertension is the most common manifestation. In approximately 60% of cases the hypertension is sustained, although significant blood pressure lability is usually present, and half of patients with sustained hypertension have distinct crises or paroxysms. The other 40% have blood pressure elevations only during an attack. The hypertension is often severe, occasionally malignant, and may be resistant to treatment with standard antihypertensive drugs.

Paroxysms or Crises The paroxysm or crisis occurs in over half of patients. In an individual patient, the symptoms are often similar with each attack. The paroxysms may be frequent or sporadic, occurring at intervals as long as weeks or months. With time, the paroxysms usually increase in frequency, duration, and severity.

The attack usually has a sudden onset. It may last from a few minutes to several hours or longer. Headache, profuse sweating, palpitations, and apprehension, often with a sense of impending doom, are common. Pain in the chest or abdomen may be associated with nausea and vomiting. Either pallor or flushing may occur during the attack. The blood pressure is elevated, often to alarming levels, and the elevation is usually accompanied by tachycardia.

The paroxysm may be precipitated by any activity that displaces the abdominal contents. In some cases a particular stimulus may induce an attack in a characteristic fashion, but in others no clearly defined precipitating event can be found. Although anxiety may accompany the attacks, mental or psychological stress does not usually provoke a crisis.

Other Distinctive Clinical Features Symptoms and signs of an increased metabolic rate, such as profuse sweating and mild to moderate weight loss, are common. Orthostatic hypotension is a consequence of diminished plasma volume and blunted sympathetic reflexes. Both these factors predispose the patient with unsuspected pheochromocytoma to hypotension or shock during surgery or trauma. Secretion of the hypotensive peptide adrenomedullin may contribute to the hypotension in some patients.

Cardiac manifestations Sinus tachycardia, sinus bradycardia, supraventricular arrhythmias, and ventricular premature contractions all have been noted. Angina and acute myocardial infarction may occur even in the absence of coronary artery disease. A catecholamine-induced increase in myocardial oxygen consumption and, perhaps, coronary spasm may play a role in these ischemic events. Electrocardiographic changes, including nonspecific ST-T wave changes, prominent U waves, left ventricular strain patterns, and right and left bundle branch blocks may be present in the absence of demonstrable ischemia or infarction. Cardiomyopathy, either congestive with myocarditis and myocardial fibrosis or hypertrophic with concentric or asymmetric hypertrophy, may be associated with heart failure and cardiac arrhythmias. Multiorgan system failure with noncardiogenic pulmonary edema may be the presenting manifestation. Elevated levels of amylase originating from damaged pulmonary endothelium and abdominal pain may suggest acute pancreatitis, although serum lipase levels are normal.

Carbohydrate intolerance Over half of patients have impaired carbohydrate tolerance due to suppression of insulin and stimulation of hepatic glucose output. The impaired glucose tolerance rarely requires treatment with insulin and disappears after removal of the tumor.

Hematocrit The elevated hematocrit is secondary to diminished plasma volume. Rarely, production of erythropoietin by the tumor may cause a true erythrocytosis.

Other manifestations Hypercalcemia has been attributed to the ectopic secretion of parathyroid hormone–related protein. Fever and an elevated erythrocyte sedimentation rate have been reported in association with the production of interleukin 6. Elevated temperature more commonly reflects catecholamine-mediated increases in metabolic rate and diminished heat dissipation secondary to vasoconstriction. Polyuria is an occasional finding, and rhabdomyolysis with myoglobinuric renal failure may result from extreme vasoconstriction with muscle ischemia.

Pheochromocytoma of the urinary bladder Pheochromocytoma in the wall of the urinary bladder may result in typical paroxysms in relation to micturition. The location in the bladder wall is responsible for the occurrence of symptoms while the tumors are quite small, and, consequently, catecholamine excretion may be normal or minimally elevated. Hematuria is present in over half of patients, and the tumor can often be visualized at cystoscopy.

Adverse Drug Interactions Severe and occasionally fatal paroxysms have been induced by opiates, histamine, adrenocorticotropin, saralasin, and glucagon. These agents appear to release catecholamines directly from the tumor. Indirect-acting sympathomimetic amines, including methyldopa (when administered intravenously), may cause an increase in blood pressure by releasing catecholamines from the augmented stores within nerve endings. Drugs that block neuronal uptake of catecholamines, such as tricyclic antidepressants or guanethidine, may enhance the physiologic effects of circulating catecholamines. Indeed, all medications should be considered carefully and administered cautiously in patients with known or suspected pheochromocytoma.

Associated Diseases Pheochromocytoma is associated with medullary carcinoma of the thyroid in the MEN syndrome types 2a and 2b and with hyperparathyroidism in MEN 2a (Chap. 339). Hypercalcemia, resolving after tumor resection, also has been described in the absence of parathyroid disease, as described above. Individuals at risk for MEN 2a and 2b should be screened periodically for pheochromocytoma by assay of a 24-h urine sample for catecholamines, including measurement of epinephrine. Pheochromocytoma should be excluded or removed before thyroid or parathyroid surgery.

The association of pheochromocytoma and neurofibromatosis is not common. Nevertheless, since incomplete forms of neurofibromatosis may be associated with pheochromocytoma, minor manifestations such as café au lait spots, vertebral abnormalities, or kyphoscoliosis should increase the suspicion of pheochromocytoma in a patient with hypertension. The incidence of pheochromocytoma in some kindreds with von Hippel–Lindau disease may be as high as 10 to 25%. Many of these are unsuspected clinically and diagnosed on a computed tomography (CT) scan or at postmortem.

The incidence of cholelithiasis is 15 to 20%. Cushing's syndrome is a rare association, usually a consequence of ectopic secretion of adrenocorticotropic hormone by the pheochromocytoma or, less commonly, by a coexistent medullary carcinoma of the thyroid.

Diagnosis The diagnosis is established by the demonstration of increased excretion of catecholamines or catecholamine metabolites. The diagnosis can usually be made by the analysis of a single 24-h urine sample, provided the patient is hypertensive or symptomatic at the time of collection.

Biochemical Tests The assays employed include those for vanillylmandelic acid (VMA), the metanephrines, and unconjugated or "free" catecholamines (Chap. 72). The VMA assay is both less sensitive and less specific than assays of metanephrines or catecholamines. Accuracy of diagnosis is improved when two of three determinations are employed. The following considerations apply to all the urinary tests: (1) Despite claims for the adequacy of determinations made on random urine samples, analysis of a full 24-h urine sample is preferable. Creatinine should also be determined to assess the adequacy of collection. (2) Where possible, the collection should be made when the patient is at rest, on no medication, and without recent exposure to radiographic contrast media. When it is not practical to discontinue all medications, drugs known specifically to interfere with these assays (as noted below) should be avoided. (3) The urine should be acidified and refrigerated during and after collection. (4) With high-quality assays, dietary restrictions are minimal and should be specified by the laboratory performing the analyses. (5) Although most patients with pheochromocytoma excrete increased amounts of catecholamines and catecholamine metabolites at all times, the yield is increased in patients with paroxysmal hypertension if a 24-h urine collection is initiated during a crisis.

Free catecholamines The upper limit of normal for total urinary catecholamines is between 590 and 885 nmol (100 and 150 μg) per 24 h. In most patients with pheochromocytoma, values in excess of 1480 nmol (250 μg) per day are obtained. Measurement of epinephrine is often of value, since increased epinephrine excretion [over 275 nmol (50 μg) per 24 h] is usually due to an adrenal lesion and may be the only abnormality in cases associated with MEN. False-positive increases in catecholamine excretion result from exogenous catecholamines and related drugs such as methyldopa, levodopa, labetalol, and sympathomimetic amines, which may elevate catecholamine excretion for up to 2 weeks. Endogenous catecholamines from stimulation of the sympathoadrenal system also may increase urinary catecholamine excretion. Relevant clinical situations that cause such increases include hypoglycemia, strenuous exertion, central nervous system disease with increased intracranial pressure, severe hypoxia, and clonidine withdrawal.

Metanephrines and VMA In most laboratories, the upper limit of normal is 7 μmol (1.3 mg) of total metanephrines and 35 μmol (7.0 mg) of VMA excretion per 24 h. In most patients with pheochromocytoma, the increase in these urinary metabolites is considerable, often to more than three times the normal range. Metanephrine excretion is increased by exogenous and endogenous catecholamines and by treatment with monoamine oxidase inhibitors; propranolol may cause a spurious increase in metanephrine excretion, since a propranolol metabolite interferes in the commonly used spectrophotometric assay. VMA is less affected by endogenous and exogenous catecholamines but is spuriously increased by a variety of drugs, including carbidopa. VMA excretion is decreased by monoamine oxidase inhibitors.

Plasma catecholamines Measurement of plasma catecholamines has a limited application. The care required in obtaining basal levels (Chap. 72) and the satisfactory results with urinary determinations make measurement of plasma catecholamines unnecessary in most cases. Plasma catecholamine levels are affected by the same drugs and physiologic perturbations that increase urinary catecholamine excretion. In addition, α- and β-adrenergic receptor blocking agents may elevate plasma catecholamines by impairing clearance.

When the clinical features suggest pheochromocytoma and the urinary assay results are borderline, measurement of plasma catecholamines may be worthwhile. Markedly elevated basal levels of total catecholamines support the diagnosis, although approximately one-third of patients with pheochromocytoma have normal or slightly elevated basal values. The usefulness of plasma catecholamine determinations may be increased by agents that suppress sympathetic nervous system activity. Clonidine and ganglionic blocking agents (Chap. 72) reduce plasma catecholamine levels in normal subjects and in patients with essential hypertension. These drugs have little effect on catecholamine levels in patients with pheochromocytoma. In patients with elevated or borderline basal catecholamine values, failure to suppress plasma or urinary levels with clonidine supports the diagnosis of pheochromocytoma.

Pharmacologic Tests Reliable methods for the measurement of catecholamines and catecholamine metabolites in urine have rendered obsolete both the provocative and adrenolytic tests, which are nonspecific and entail considerable risk. A modified version of the adrenolytic test may be of some use, however, as a therapeutic trial in a patient in hypertensive crisis with features suggestive of pheochromocytoma. A positive response to phentolamine (5-mg bolus following a test dose of 0.5 mg) is a reduction in blood pressure of at least 35/25 mmHg that peaks after 2 min and persists for 10 to 15 min. The pharmacologic response is never diagnostic, and biochemical confirmation is essential. Provocative tests in normotensive patients are potentially dangerous and rarely indicated. However, a glucagon provocative test may be of use in patients with paroxysmal hypertension and nondiagnostic basal catecholamine levels. Glucagon has a negligible effect on blood pressure or plasma catecholamine levels in normal or hypertensive subjects. In patients with pheochromocytoma, on the other hand, glucagon may increase both blood pressure and circulating catecholamine levels. The elevation in plasma catecholamine concentration, moreover, may occur without a blood pressure response. It must be emphasized, however, that life-threatening pressor crises have occurred after administration of glucagon to patients with pheochromocytoma, so the test should never be performed casually. Careful continuous monitoring of the blood pressure is required, intravenous access must be adequate, and phentolamine must be at hand to terminate the test if a significant pressor reaction ensues.

Differential Diagnosis Since the manifestations of pheochromocytoma can be protean, the diagnosis must be considered and excluded in many patients with suggestive clinical features. In patients with essential hypertension and "hyperadrenergic" features such as tachycardia, sweating, and increased cardiac output, and in patients with anxiety attacks associated with blood pressure elevations, analysis of a 24-h urine collection is usually decisive in excluding the diagnosis. Repeated determinations on urine collected during attacks may be necessary, however, before the diagnosis can be excluded with certainty. The clonidine suppression and glucagon stimulation tests may be helpful in excluding the diagnosis in difficult cases. Pressor crises associated with clonidine withdrawal and the use of cocaine or monoamine oxidase inhibitors (Chap. 72) may mimic the paroxysms of pheochromocytoma. Factitious crises may be produced by self-administration of sympathomimetic amines in psychiatrically disturbed patients.

Intracranial lesions, particularly posterior fossa tumors or subarachnoid hemorrhage, may cause hypertension and increased excretion of catecholamines or catecholamine metabolites. While this is most common in patients with an obvious neurologic catastrophe, the possibility of subarachnoid or intracranial hemorrhage secondary to pheochromocytoma should be considered. Diencephalic or autonomic epilepsy may be associated with paroxysmal spells, hypertension, and increased plasma catecholamine levels. This rare entity may be difficult to distinguish from pheochromocytoma, but an aura, an abnormal electroencephalogram, and a beneficial response to anticonvulsant medications will often suggest the proper diagnosis.

℞ TREATMENT **Preoperative Management** The induction of stable α-adrenergic blockade is the basis of preoperative management and provides the foundation for successful surgical treatment. Once the diagnosis is established, the patient should be placed on phenoxybenzamine to induce a long-lived, noncompetitive α-receptor blockade. The usual initial dose is 10 mg every 12 h with increments of 10 to 20 mg added every few days until the blood pressure is controlled and the paroxysms disappear. Because of the long duration of action, the therapeutic effects are cumulative, and the optimal dose must be achieved gradually with careful monitoring of supine and upright blood pressures. Most patients require between 40 and 80 mg phenoxybenzamine per day, although 200 mg or more may be necessary. Phenoxybenzamine should be administered for at least 10 to 14 days prior to surgery. Over this time, the combination of α-receptor blockade and a liberal salt intake will restore the contracted plasma volume to normal. Before adequate α-adrenergic blockade with phenoxybenzamine is achieved, paroxysms may be treated with oral prazosin or noncompetitive intravenous phentolamine. Selective α_1 antagonists have been employed for preoperative preparation, but their role in preparative management should be limited to the treatment of individual paroxysms. They may be useful as antihypertensive agents in patients with suspected pheochromocytoma while workup is in progress, since they are usually better tolerated than phenoxybenzamine and will prevent serious pressor crises if pheochromocytoma is present. Nitroprusside, calcium channel blocking agents, and possibly angiotensin-converting enzyme inhibitors reduce blood pressure in patients with pheochromocytoma. Nitroprusside may also be useful in the treatment of pressor crises.

β-Adrenergic receptor blocking agents should be given only after alpha blockade has been induced, since administration of such agents by themselves may cause a paradoxic increase in blood pressure by antagonizing beta-mediated vasodilation in skeletal muscle. Beta blockade is usually initiated when tachycardia develops during the induction of α-adrenergic blockade. Low doses often suffice, and a reasonable starting dose is 10 mg propranolol three to four times per day, increased as needed to control the pulse rate. Beta blockade is effective for catecholamine-induced arrhythmias, particularly those potentiated by anesthetic agents.

Preoperative Localization of the Tumor Surgical removal of pheochromocytoma is facilitated if the location of the tumor or tumors can be established preoperatively. Once pheochromocytoma is diagnosed, localization should be undertaken while the patient is being prepared for surgery. CT or magnetic resonance imaging (MRI) of the adrenals is usually successful in identifying intraadrenal lesions. Extraadrenal tumors within the chest can frequently be identified by conventional chest films or CT. MRI is useful in identifying extraadrenal tumors in the abdomen. If these studies are negative, abdominal aortography (once α-adrenergic blockade is complete) may identify extraadrenal pheochromocytomas in the abdomen, since these lesions are often supplied by a large aberrant artery. If aortography, CT, and MRI fail to localize the lesion, venous sampling at different levels of the inferior and superior vena cava may reveal catecholamine gradients in the region drained by the tumor; this area may then be restudied by selective angiography or scanning by CT or MRI. An additional localization technique involves a radionuclide scintiscan after administration of the radiopharmaceutical [^{131}I]metaiodobenzylguanidine (MIBG). This agent is concentrated by the amine uptake process and produces an external scintigraphic image at the site of the tumor. This type of scanning may be useful in characterizing lesions discovered by CT when biochemical confirmation is indeterminate, as well as in localizing extraadrenal pheochromocytomas. Percutaneous fine-needle aspiration of chromaffin tumors is contraindicated; indeed, pheochromocytoma should be considered before any adrenal lesions are aspirated.

Surgery Surgical treatment of pheochromocytoma is best performed in centers with experience in the preoperative, anesthetic, and intraoperative management of pheochromocytoma. In experienced hands, surgical mortality is $<$2 or 3%.

Monitoring during the surgical procedure should include continuous recording of arterial pressure and central venous pressure as well as electrocardiography; in the presence of cardiac disease or if congestive failure has been present, pulmonary capillary wedge pressure should be monitored. Adequate fluid replacement is crucial. Intraoperative hypotension responds better to volume replacement than to vasoconstrictors. Hypertension and cardiac arrhythmias are most likely during induction of anesthesia, intubation, and manipulation of the tumor. Intravenous phentolamine is usually sufficient to control the blood pressure, but nitroprusside may be required. Propranolol may be given in the treatment of tachycardia or ventricular ectopy.

Pheochromocytoma in pregnancy Spontaneous labor and vaginal delivery in unprepared patients are usually disastrous for mother and fetus. In early pregnancy, the patient should be prepared with phenoxybenzamine, and the tumor should be removed as soon as the diagnosis is confirmed. The pregnancy need not be terminated, but the operative procedure itself may result in spontaneous abortion. In the third trimester, treatment with adrenergic blocking agents should be undertaken; when the fetus is of sufficient size, cesarean section may be followed by extirpation of the tumor. Although the safety of adrenergic blocking drugs in pregnancy is not established, these agents have been administered in several cases without obvious adverse effect. Antepartum diagnosis and treatment lowers the maternal death rate to that approaching nonpregnant pheochromocytoma patients; fetal death rate, however, remains elevated.

Unresectable and malignant tumors In cases of metastatic or locally invasive tumor in patients with intercurrent illness that precludes surgery, long-term medical management is required. When the manifestations cannot be adequately controlled by adrenergic blocking agents, the concomitant administration of metyrosine may be required. This agent inhibits tyrosine hydroxylase, diminishes catecholamine production by the tumor, and often simplifies chronic management. Malignant pheochromocytoma frequently recurs in the retroperitoneum, and it metastasizes most commonly to bone and lung. Although these malignant tumors are resistant to radiotherapy, combination chemotherapy has had limited success in controlling them. Use of ^{131}I-MIBG has had limited success in the treatment of malignant pheochromocytoma, due to poor uptake of the radioligand.

PROGNOSIS AND FOLLOW-UP The 5-year survival rate after surgery is usually over 95%, the recurrence rate is <10%. After successful surgery, catecholamine excretion returns to normal in about 2 weeks and should be measured to ensure complete tumor removal. Catecholamine excretion should be assessed at the reappearance of suggestive symptoms or yearly if the patient remains asymptomatic. For malignant pheochromocytoma, the 5-year survival rate is <50%.

Complete removal cures the hypertension in approximately three-fourths of patients. In the remainder, hypertension recurs but is usually well controlled by standard antihypertensive agents. In this group, either underlying essential hypertension or irreversible vascular damage induced by catecholamines may cause the persistence of the hypertension.

BIBLIOGRAPHY

AVERBUCH SD et al: Malignant pheochromocytoma: Effective treatment with a combination of cyclophosphamide, vincristine, and dacarbazine. Ann Intern Med 109:267, 1988

BERNHARD BU et al: Functioning thoracic paraganglioma: Association with von Hippel–Landau syndrome. J Clin Endocrinol Metab 82:3356, 1997

DALY PA, LANDSBERG L: Phaeochromocytoma: Diagnosis and management. Baillieres Clin Endocrinol Metab 6:143, 1992

ENG C et al: Mutations in the RET proto-oncogene and the von Hippel–Landau disease tumor suppressor gene in sporadic and syndromic pheochromocytomas. J Med Genet 32:934, 1995

FRANK-RAUE K et al: Diagnosis and management of pheochromocytomas in patients with multiple endocrine neoplasis type 2: Relevance of specific mutations in the RET proto-oncogene. Eur J Endocrinol 135:222, 1996

GARCIA A et al: Molecular diagnosis of von Hippel–Lindau disease in a kindred with a predominance of familial phaeochromocytoma. Clin Endocrinol 46:359, 1997

GRAHAM PE et al: Laboratory diagnosis of pheochromocytoma: Which analyses should we measure? Ann Clin Biochem 30:129, 1993

KREMPF M et al: Use of m-(^{131}I) iodobenzylguanidine in the treatment of malignant pheochromocytoma. J Clin Endocrinol Metab 72:455, 1991

LANDSBERG L: Pheochromocytoma complicating pregnancy. Eur J Endocrinol 130:215, 1994

MACDOUGALL IC et al: Overnight clonidine suppression test in the diagnosis and exclusion of pheochromocytoma. Am J Med 84:993, 1988

MCCORKELL SJ, NILES NL: Fine-needle aspiration of catecholamine-producing adrenal masses: A possibly fatal mistake. Am J Roentgenol 145:113, 1985

MERIGIAN KS et al: Adrenergic crisis from crack cocaine ingestion: Report of five cases. J Emerg Med 12:485, 1994

NEUMANN HPH et al: Pheochromocytomas, multiple endocrine neoplasia type 2, and von Hippel-Lindau disease. N Engl J Med 329:1531, 1993

PANG L-C et al: Flow cytometric DNA analysis for the determination of malignant potential in adrenal and extra-adrenal pheochromocytomas or paragangliomas. Arch Pathol Lab Med 117:1142, 1993

REINIG JW, DOPPMAN JL: Magnetic resonance imaging of the adrenal. Radiologe 26: 186, 1986

SHEMIN D et al: Pheochromocytoma presenting as rhabdomyolysis and acute myoglobinuric renal failure. Arch Intern Med 150:2384, 1990

STEWART AF et al: Hypercalcemia in pheochromocytoma. Ann Intern Med 102:776, 1985

333 DIABETES MELLITUS

Alvin C. Powers

Diabetes mellitus (DM) comprises a group of common metabolic disorders that share the phenotype of hyperglycemia. Several distinct types of DM exist and are caused by a complex interaction of genetics, environmental factors, and life-style choices. Depending on the etiology of the DM, factors contributing to hyperglycemia may include reduced insulin secretion, decreased glucose usage, and increased glucose production. The metabolic dysregulation associated with DM causes secondary pathophysiologic changes in multiple organ systems that impose a tremendous burden on the individual with diabetes and on the health care system. In the United States, DM is the leading cause of end-stage renal disease, nontraumatic lower extremity amputations, and adult blindness. With an increasing incidence worldwide, DM will likely continue to be a leading cause of morbidity and mortality for the foreseeable future.

CLASSIFICATION

Recent advances in the understanding of the etiology and pathogenesis of diabetes have led to a revised classification (Table 333-1). Although all forms of DM are characterized by hyperglycemia, the pathogenic mechanisms by which hyperglycemia arises differ widely. Some forms of DM are characterized by an absolute insulin deficiency or a genetic defect leading to defective insulin secretion, whereas other forms share insulin resistance as their underlying etiology. Recent changes in classification reflect an effort to classify DM on the basis of the pathogenic process that leads to hyperglycemia, as opposed to criteria such as age of onset or type of therapy (Fig. 333-1).

The two broad categories of DM are designated type 1 and type 2. Type 1A DM results from autoimmune beta cell destruction, which usually leads to insulin deficiency. Type 1B DM is also characterized by insulin deficiency as well as a tendency to develop ketosis. However, individuals with type 1B DM lack immunologic markers indicative of an autoimmune destructive process of the beta cells. The mechanisms leading to beta cell destruction in these patients are unknown. Relatively few patients with type 1 DM fall into the type 1B idiopathic category; many of these individuals are either African-American or Asian in heritage.

Type 2 DM is a heterogeneous group of disorders usually characterized by variable degrees of insulin resistance, impaired insulin secretion, and increased glucose production. Distinct genetic and metabolic defects in insulin action and/or secretion give rise to the common phenotype of hyperglycemia in type 2 DM (see below). The identification of distinct pathogenic processes in type 2 DM has important potential therapeutic implications, as pharmacologic agents that target specific metabolic derangements become available.

Two features of the current classification of DM diverge from previous classifications. First, the terms *insulin-dependent diabetes mellitus* (IDDM) and *noninsulin-dependent diabetes mellitus* (NIDDM)

Table 333-1 Etiologic Classification of Diabetes Mellitus

I. Type 1 diabetes (β-cell destruction, usually leading to absolute insulin deficiency)
  A. Immune-mediated
  B. Idiopathic
II. Type 2 diabetes (may range from predominantly insulin resistance with relative insulin deficiency to a predominantly insulin secretory defect with insulin resistance)
III. Other specific types of diabetes
  A. Genetic defects of β-cell function characterized by mutations in:
    1. Hepatocyte nuclear transcription factor (HNF) 4α (MODY 1)
    2. Glucokinase (MODY 2)
    3. HNF-1α (MODY 3)
    4. Insulin promoter factor (IPF) 1 (MODY 4)
    5. HNF-1β (MODY 5)
    6. Mitochondrial DNA
    7. Proinsulin or insulin conversion
  B. Genetic defects in insulin action
    1. Type A insulin resistance
    2. Leprechaunism
    3. Rabson-Mendenhall syndrome
    4. Lipoatrophic diabetes
  C. Diseases of the exocrine pancreas—pancreatitis, pancreatectomy, neoplasia, cystic fibrosis, hemochromatosis, fibrocalculous pancreatopathy
  D. Endocrinopathies—acromegaly, Cushing's syndrome, glucagonoma, pheochromocytoma, hyperthyroidism, somatostatinoma, aldosteronoma
  E. Drug- or chemical-induced—Vacor, pentamidine, nicotinic acid, glucocorticoids, thyroid hormone, diazoxide, β-adrenergic agonists, thiazides, phenytoin, α-interferon, protease inhibitors, clozapine, beta blockers
  F. Infections—congenital rubella, cytomegalovirus, coxsackie
  G. Uncommon forms of immune-mediated diabetes—"stiff-man" syndrome, anti-insulin receptor antibodies
  H. Other genetic syndromes sometimes associated with diabetes—Down's syndrome, Klinefelter's syndrome, Turner's syndrome, Wolfram's syndrome, Friedreich's ataxia, Huntington's chorea, Laurence-Moon-Biedl syndrome, myotonic dystrophy, porphyria, Prader-Willi syndrome
IV. Gestational diabetes mellitus (GDM)

NOTE: MODY, maturity onset of diabetes of the young.
SOURCE: Adapted from American Diabetes Association, 2000

are obsolete. These previous designations reflected the observation that most individuals with type 1 DM (previously IDDM) have an absolute requirement for insulin treatment, whereas many individuals with type 2 DM (previously NIDDM) do not require insulin therapy to prevent ketoacidosis. However, because many individuals with type 2 DM eventually require insulin treatment for control of glycemia, the use of the latter term generated considerable confusion.

A second difference is that age is no longer used as a criterion in the new classification system. Although type 1 DM most commonly develops before the age of 30, an autoimmune beta cell destructive process can develop at any age. In fact, it is estimated that between 5 and 10% of individuals who develop DM after age 30 have type 1A DM. Likewise, although type 2 DM more typically develops with increasing age, it also occurs in children, particularly in obese adolescents.

OTHER TYPES OF DM Other etiologies for DM include specific genetic defects in insulin secretion or action, metabolic abnormalities that impair insulin secretion, and a host of conditions that impair glucose tolerance (Table 333-1). *Maturity onset diabetes of the young* (MODY) is a subtype of DM characterized by autosomal dominant inheritance, early onset of hyperglycemia, and impairment in insulin secretion (discussed below). Mutations in the insulin receptor cause a group of rare disorders characterized by severe insulin resistance.

DM can result from pancreatic exocrine disease when the majority of pancreatic islets (>80%) are destroyed. Several endocrinopathies can lead to DM as a result of excessive secretion of hormones that antagonize the action of insulin. Notable within this group are acromegaly and Cushing's disease, both of which may present with DM. Viral infections have been implicated in pancreatic islet destruction, but are an extremely rare cause of DM. Congenital rubella greatly increases the risk for DM; however, most of these individuals also have immunologic markers indicative of autoimmune beta cell destruction.

GESTATIONAL DIABETES MELLITUS (GDM) Glucose intolerance may develop and first become recognized during pregnancy. Insulin resistance related to the metabolic changes of late pregnancy increases insulin requirements and may lead to hyperglycemia or impaired glucose tolerance. GDM is seen in approximately 4% of pregnancies in the United States; most women revert to normal glucose tolerance post-partum but have a substantial risk (30 to 60%) of developing DM later in life.

EPIDEMIOLOGY

The worldwide prevalence of DM has risen dramatically over the past two decades. It is projected that the number of individuals with DM will continue to increase in the near future. Between 1976 and 1994, for example, the prevalence of DM among adults in the United States increased from 8.9% to 12.3%. These findings, based on national epidemiologic data, include individuals with a diagnosis of DM and those with undiagnosed DM (based on identical diagnostic criteria). Likewise, prevalence rates of impaired fasting glucose (IFG) increased from 6.5% to 9.7% over the same period. Although the prevalence of both type 1 and type 2 DM is increasing worldwide, the prevalence of type 2 DM is expected to rise more rapidly in the future because of increasing obesity and reduced activity levels.

There is considerable geographic variation in the incidence of both type 1 and type 2 DM. For example, Scandinavia has the highest rate of type 1 DM (in Finland, incidence is 35/100,000 per year). The

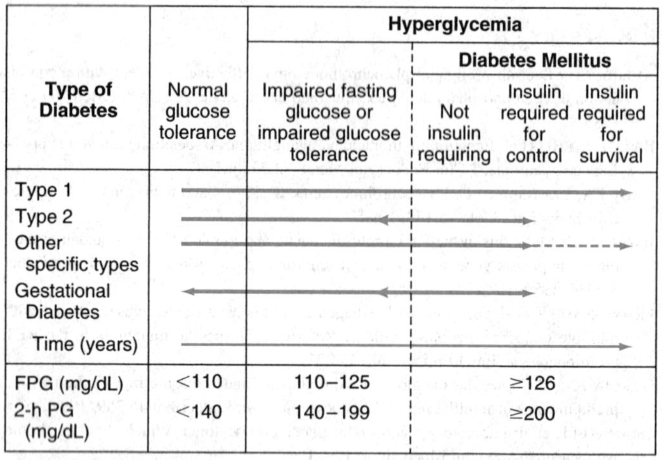

Type of Diabetes	Normal glucose tolerance	Hyperglycemia: Impaired fasting glucose or impaired glucose tolerance	Diabetes Mellitus: Not insulin requiring	Insulin required for control	Insulin required for survival
Type 1					
Type 2					
Other specific types					
Gestational Diabetes					
Time (years)					
FPG (mg/dL)	<110	110–125		≥126	
2-h PG (mg/dL)	<140	140–199		≥200	

FIGURE 333-1 Spectrum of glucose homeostasis and diabetes. The spectrum from normal glucose tolerance to diabetes in type 1 diabetes, type 2 diabetes, other specific types of diabetes, and gestational diabetes is shown from left to right. In most types of diabetes, the individual traverses from normal glucose tolerance to impaired glucose tolerance to frank diabetes. Arrows indicate that changes in glucose tolerance may be bi-directional in some types of diabetes. For example, individuals with type 2 diabetes may return to the impaired glucose tolerance category with weight loss; in gestational diabetes, diabetes may revert to impaired glucose tolerance or even normal glucose tolerance after delivery. The fasting plasma glucose (FPG) and 2-h plasma glucose (PG), after a glucose challenge for the different categories of glucose tolerance, are shown at the lower part of the figure (as defined by recent consensus panels—see text). These values do not apply to the diagnosis of gestational diabetes. Some types of diabetes may or may not require insulin for survival, hence the dotted line. (Conventional units are used in the figure.) *(Adapted from American Diabetes Association: Clinical Practice Guidelines, 2000)*

Pacific Rim has a much lower rate (in Japan and China, incidence is 1 to 3/100,000 per year) of type 1 DM; Northern Europe and the United States share an intermediate rate (8 to 17/100,000 per year). Much of the increased risk of type 1 DM is believed to reflect the frequency of high-risk HLA alleles among ethnic groups in different geographic locations.

The prevalence of type 2 DM and its harbinger, impaired glucose tolerance (IGT), is highest in certain Pacific islands, intermediate in countries such as India and the United States, and relatively low in Russia and China. This variability is likely due to both genetic and environmental factors. There is also considerable variation in DM prevalence among different ethnic populations within a given country.

In 1998, approximately 16 million individuals in the United States met the diagnostic criteria for DM. This represents ~6% of the population. About 800,000 individuals in the United States develop DM each year. The vast majority of these (>90%) have type 2 DM. The number of people with DM increases with the age of the population, ranging from an incidence of ~1.5% in individuals from 20 to 39 years to ~20% of individuals >75 years. The incidence of DM is similar in men and women throughout most age ranges but is slightly greater in men >60 years. The prevalence of DM is approximately twofold greater in African Americans, Hispanic Americans, and Native Americans than in non-Hispanic whites, and the onset of type 2 DM occurs, on average, at an earlier age in the former groups than in the non-Hispanic white population. The incidence of type 2 DM in these ethnic groups is rapidly increasing. The reasons for these differences are not yet clear.

DIAGNOSIS

Revised criteria for diagnosing DM have been issued by consensus panels of experts from the National Diabetes Data Group and the World Health Organization (Table 333-2). The revised criteria reflect new epidemiologic and metabolic evidence and are based on the following premises: (1) the spectrum of fasting plasma glucose (FPG) and the response to an oral glucose load varies in normal individuals, and (2) DM defined as the level of glycemia at which diabetes-specific complications are noted and not on the level of glucose tolerance from a population-based viewpoint. For example, the prevalence of retinopathy in Native Americans (Pima Indian population) begins to increase at a FPG > 6.4 mmol/L (116 mg/dL) (Fig. 333-2).

Glucose tolerance is classified into three categories based on the FPG: (1) FPG < 6.1 mmol/L (110 mg/dL) is considered normal; (2) FPG ≥ 6.1 mmol/L (110 mg/dL) but < 7.0 mmol/L (126 mg/dL) is defined as IFG; and (3) FPG ≥ 7.0 mmol/L (126 mg/dL) warrants the diagnosis of DM. IFG is a new diagnostic category defined by the Expert Committee on the Diagnosis and Classification of Diabetes Mellitus. It is analogous to IGT, which is defined as plasma glucose levels between 7.8 and 11.1 mmol/L (140 and 200 mg/dL) 2 h after a 75-g oral glucose load (Table 333-2). Individuals with IFG or IGT are at substantial risk for developing type 2 DM and cardiovascular disease in the future, though they may not meet the criteria for DM.

Table 333-2 Criteria for the Diagnosis of Diabetes Mellitus

- Symptoms of diabetes plus random blood glucose concentration ≥11.1 mmol/L (200 mg/dL)[a]

or

- Fasting plasma glucose ≥7.0 mmol/L (126 mg/dL)[b]

or

- Two-hour plasma glucose ≥11.1 mmol/L (200 mg/dL) during an oral glucose tolerance test[c]

In the absence of unequivocal hyperglycemia and acute metabolic decompensation, these criteria should be confirmed by repeat testing on a different day.

[a] Random is defined as without regard to time since the last meal.
[b] Fasting is defined as no caloric intake for at least 8 h.
[c] The test should be performed using a glucose load containing the equivalent of 75 g anhydrous glucose dissolved in water; not recommended for routine clinical use.
SOURCE: Adapted from American Diabetes Association, 2000.

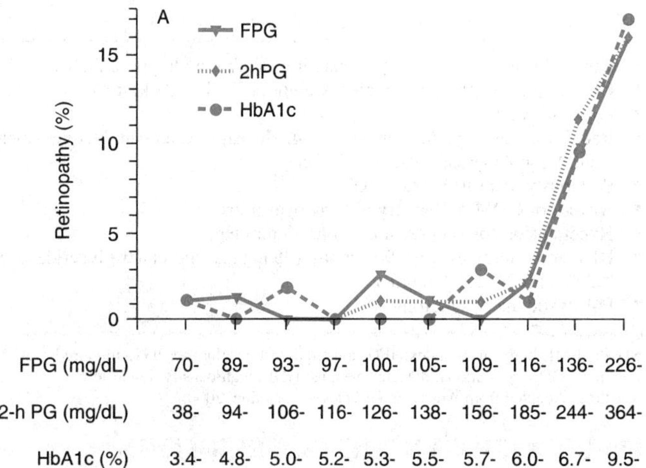

FIGURE 333-2 Relationship of diabetes-specific complication and glucose tolerance. This figure shows the incidence of retinopathy in Pima Indians as a function of the fasting plasma glucose (FPG), the 2-h plasma glucose after a 75-g oral glucose challenge (2hPG), or glycated hemoglobin (HbA1c). Note that the incidence of retinopathy greatly increases at a fasting plasma glucose >116 mg/dL, or a 2-h plasma glucose of 185 mg/dL, or a HbA1c >6.0%. (Conventional units are used in the figure.) *(From American Diabetes Association: Clinical Practice Guidelines, 2000, as adapted from McCance et al: BMJ 308:1323, 1994)*

The revised criteria for the diagnosis of DM emphasize the FPG as the most reliable and convenient test for diagnosing DM in asymptomatic individuals. A random plasma glucose concentration ≥11.1 mmol/L (200 mg/dL) accompanied by classic symptoms of DM (polyuria, polydipsia, weight loss) is sufficient for the diagnosis of DM (Table 333-2). Oral glucose tolerance testing, although still a valid mechanism for diagnosing DM, is not recommended as part of routine screening.

Some investigators have advocated the hemoglobin A1c (HbA1c) as a diagnostic test for DM. Though there is a strong correlation between elevations in the plasma glucose and the HbA1c (discussed below), the relationship between the FPG and the HbA1c in individuals with normal glucose tolerance or mild glucose intolerance is less clear, and the test is not universally standardized or available.

The diagnosis of DM has profound implications for an individual from both a medical and financial standpoint. Thus, the health care provider must be certain that these criteria are completely satisfied before assigning the diagnosis of DM to an individual. The revised criteria also allow for the diagnosis of DM to be withdrawn in situations where the FPG no longer exceeds these criteria. Abnormalities on screening tests for diabetes should be repeated before making a definitive diagnosis of DM, unless acute metabolic derangements or a markedly elevated plasma glucose are present (Table 333-2).

SCREENING Widespread use of the FPG as a screening test for type 2 DM is strongly encouraged because: (1) a large number of individuals who meet the current criteria for DM are unaware that they have the disorder, (2) epidemiologic studies suggest that type 2 DM may be present for up to a decade before diagnosis, and (3) as many as 50% of individuals with type 2 DM have one or more diabetes-specific complications at the time of their diagnosis. The Expert Committee suggests screening all individuals >45 years every 3 years and screening asymptomatic individuals with additional risk factors (Table 333-3) at an earlier age. In contrast to type 2 DM, it is rare for an individual to have a long asymptomatic period of hyperglycemia prior to the diagnosis of type 1 DM. A number of immunologic markers for type 1 DM are becoming available (discussed below), but their use is currently discouraged pending the identification of clinically beneficial interventions for individuals at high risk for developing type 1 DM.

Table 333-3 Risk Factors for Type 2 Diabetes Mellitus

- Family history of diabetes (i.e., parent or sibling with type 2 diabetes)
- Obesity (i.e., ≥20% desired body weight or BMI ≥ 27 kg/m²)
- Age ≥45 years
- Race/ethnicity (e.g., African American, Hispanic American, Native American, Asian American, Pacific Islander)
- Previously identified IFG or IGT
- History of GDM or delivery of baby over 9 lbs
- Hypertension (blood pressure ≥ 140/90 mm Hg)
- HDL cholesterol level ≤0.90 mmol/L (35 mg/dL) and/or a triglyceride level ≥2.82 mmol/L (250 mg/dL)
- Polycystic ovary syndrome

NOTE: BMI, body mass index; IFG, impaired fasting glucose; IGT, impaired glucose tolerance; GDM, gestational diabetes mellitus; HDL, high-density lipoprotein.
SOURCE: Adapted from American Diabetes Association, 2000.

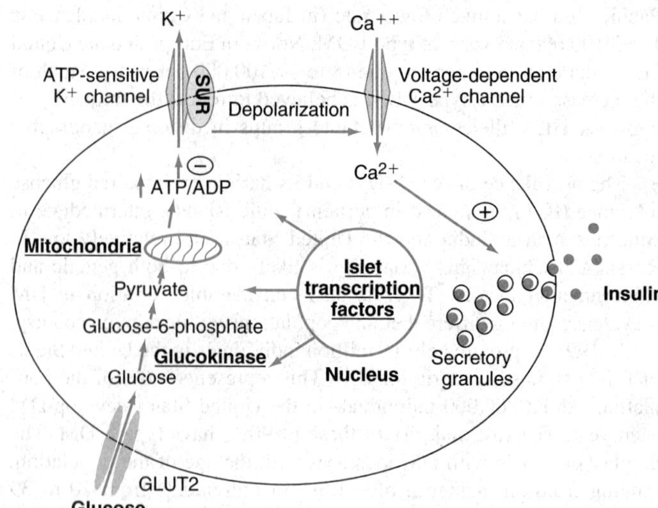

FIGURE 333-3 Diabetes and abnormalities in glucose-stimulated insulin secretion. Glucose and other nutrients regulate insulin secretion by the pancreatic beta cell. Glucose is transported by the GLUT2 glucose transporter; subsequent glucose metabolism by the beta cell alters ion channel activity, leading to insulin secretion. The SUR receptor is the binding site for oral hypoglycemic agents. Mutations in the events or proteins underlined are a cause of maturity onset diabetes of the young (MODY) or other forms of diabetes. SUR, sulfonylurea receptor; ATP, adenosine triphosphate; ADP, adenosine diphosphate. *(Adapted from Lowe, 1998.)*

INSULIN BIOSYNTHESIS, SECRETION, AND ACTION

BIOSYNTHESIS Insulin is produced in the beta cells of the pancreatic islets. It is initially synthesized as a single-chain 86-amino-acid precursor polypeptide, preproinsulin. Subsequent proteolytic processing removes the aminoterminal signal peptide, giving rise to proinsulin. Proinsulin is structurally related to insulin-like growth factors I and II, which bind weakly to the insulin receptor (Chap. 327). Cleavage of an internal 31-residue fragment from proinsulin generates the C peptide and the A (21 amino acids) and B (30 amino acids) chains of insulin, which are connected by disulfide bonds. The mature insulin molecule and C peptide are stored together and cosecreted from secretory granules in the beta cells. Because the C peptide is less susceptible than insulin to hepatic degradation, it is a useful a marker of insulin secretion and allows discrimination of endogenous and exogenous sources of insulin in the evaluation of hypoglycemia (Chap. 334). Human insulin is now produced by recombinant DNA technology; structural alterations at one or more residues are useful for modifying its physical and pharmacologic characteristics (see below).

SECRETION Glucose is the key regulator of insulin secretion by the pancreatic beta cell, although amino acids, ketones, various nutrients, gastrointestinal peptides, and neurotransmitters also influence insulin secretion. Glucose levels >3.9 mmol/L (70 mg/dL) stimulate insulin synthesis, primarily by enhancing protein translation and processing, as well as inducing insulin secretion. Glucose stimulates insulin secretion through a series of regulatory steps that begin with transport into the beta cell by the GLUT2 glucose transporter (Fig. 333-3). Glucose phosphorylation by glucokinase is the rate-limiting step that controls glucose-regulated insulin secretion.

Further metabolism of glucose-6-phosphate via glycolysis generates ATP, which inhibits the activity of an ATP-sensitive K^+ channel. This channel is a complex of two separate proteins, one of which is the receptor for certain oral hypoglycemics (e.g., sulfonylureas, meglitinides); the other subunit is an inwardly rectifying K^+ channel protein. Inhibition of this K^+ channel induces beta cell membrane depolarization, opening of voltage-dependent calcium channels (leading to an influx of calcium), and stimulation of insulin secretion. Careful studies of insulin secretory profiles reveal pulsatile pattern of hormone release, with small secretory bursts occurring about every 10 min, superimposed upon greater amplitude oscillations of about 80 to 150 min. Meals or other major stimuli of insulin secretion induce large (four- to fivefold increase versus baseline) bursts of insulin secretion that usually last for 2 to 3 h before returning to baseline. Derangements in these normal secretory patterns are one of the earliest signs of beta cell dysfunction in DM (see below).

ACTION Once insulin is secreted into the portal vein, ~50% is removed and degraded by the liver. Unextracted insulin enters the systemic circulation and binds to its receptor in target sites. The insulin receptor belongs to the tyrosine kinase class of membrane-bound receptors (Chap. 327). Insulin binding to the receptor stimulates intrinsic tyrosine kinase activity, leading to receptor autophosphorylation and the recruitment of intracellular signaling molecules, such as insulin receptor substrates (IRS) 1 and 2 (Fig. 333-4). These and other adaptor proteins initiate a complex cascade of phosphorylation and dephosphorylation reactions, ultimately resulting in the widespread metabolic and mitogenic effects of insulin. As an example, activation of the phosphatidylinositol-3′-kinase (PI-3 kinase) pathway stimulates translocation of glucose transporters (e.g., GLUT4) to the cell surface, an event that is crucial for glucose uptake by skeletal muscle and fat. Activation of other insulin receptor signaling pathways induces glycogen synthesis, protein synthesis, lipogenesis, and regulation of various genes in insulin-responsive cells.

Glucose homeostasis reflects a precise balance between hepatic glucose production and peripheral glucose uptake and utilization. Insulin is the most important regulator of this metabolic equilibrium, but the effects of other pathways including neural input, metabolic signals, and hormones (e.g., glucagon) result in integrated control of glucose supply and utilization (Chap. 334; Fig. 334-1). In the fasting state, low insulin levels promote hepatic gluconeogenesis and glycogenolysis to prevent hypoglycemia. Low insulin levels decrease glycogen synthesis, reduce glucose uptake in insulin-sensitive tissues, and promote mobilization of stored precursors. Reduced insulin levels are also permissive in allowing glucagon to stimulate glycogenolysis and gluconeogenesis by the liver and renal medulla. These processes are of critical importance to ensure an adequate glucose supply for the brain. Postprandially, a large glucose load elicits a rise in insulin and fall in glucagon, leading to a reversal of these processes. The major portion of postprandial glucose is utilized by skeletal muscle. Other tissues, most notably the brain, utilize glucose in an insulin-independent fashion.

PATHOGENESIS

TYPE 1 DM Type 1A DM develops as a result of the synergistic effects of genetic, environmental, and immunologic factors that ultimately destroy the pancreatic beta cells. The temporal development of type 1A DM is shown schematically as a function of beta cell mass in Fig. 333-5. Individuals with a genetic susceptibility have normal beta cell mass at birth but begin to lose beta cells secondary to autoimmune destruction that occurs over months to years. This autoimmune process is thought to be triggered by an infectious or environmental stimulus and to be sustained by a beta cell–specific molecule. In the majority of individuals, immunologic markers appear after the triggering event but before diabetes becomes clinically overt. Beta cell mass then begins to decline, and insulin secretion becomes progressively impaired, although normal glucose tolerance is maintained. The rate of decline in beta cell mass varies widely among individuals, with some patients progressing rapidly to clinical diabetes and others evolving more slowly. Features of diabetes do not become evident until a majority of beta cells are destroyed (~80%). At this point, residual functional beta cells still exist but are insufficient in number to maintain glucose tolerance. The events that trigger the transition from glucose intolerance to frank diabetes are often associated with increased insulin requirements, as might occur during infections or puberty. Following the initial clinical presentation of type 1A DM, a "honeymoon" phase may ensue during which time glycemic control is achieved with modest doses of insulin or, rarely, insulin is not needed. However, this fleeting phase of endogenous insulin production from residual beta cells disappears as the autoimmune process destroys the remaining beta cells, and the individual becomes completely insulin deficient.

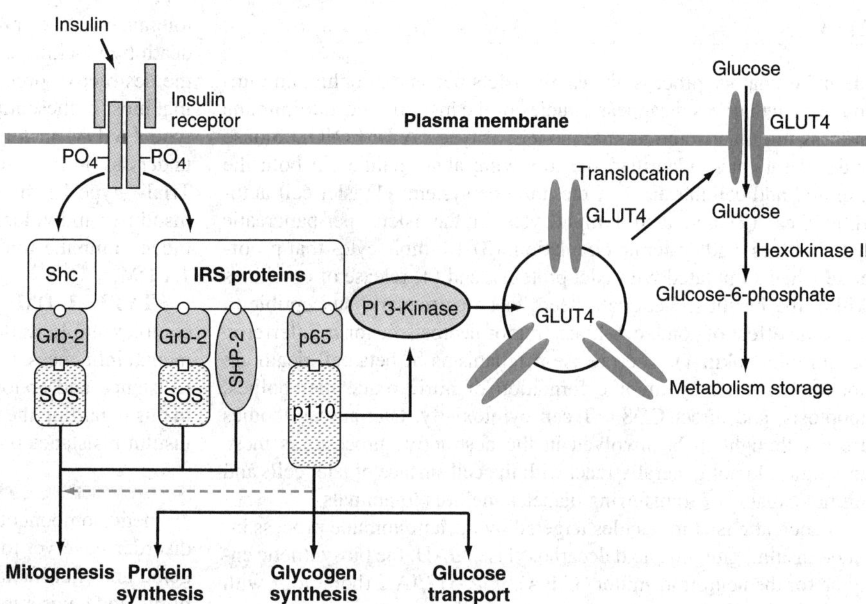

FIGURE 333-4 Insulin signal transduction pathway. The insulin receptor has intrinsic tyrosine kinase activity and interacts with insulin receptor substrates (IRS and Shc) proteins. A number of "docking" proteins bind to these cellular proteins and initiate the metabolic actions of insulin [GrB-2, SOS, SHP-2, p65, p110, and phosphoinositol phosphate 3-kinase (PI 3-kinase)]. Insulin increases glucose transport through PI 3-kinase, which promotes the translocation of intracellular vesicles containing GLUT4 glucose transporter to the plasma membrane. *(Adapted from Lowe, 1998; Virkamaki et al, 1999)*

Genetic Considerations The genetic contributions to type 1A DM involve multiple genes. The development of the disease appears to require inheritance of a sufficient complement of genes to confer susceptibility to the disorder. The concordance of type 1A DM in identical twins ranges between 30 and 70%, indicating that additional modifying factors must be involved in determining whether diabetes develops. The major susceptibility gene for type 1A DM is located in the HLA region on chromosome 6. Polymorphisms in the HLA complex appear to account for 40 to 50% of the genetic risk of developing type 1A DM. This region contains genes that encode the class II MHC molecules, which present antigen to helper T cells and thus are involved in initiating the immune response (Chaps. 305, 306, 307). The ability of class II MHC molecules to present antigen is dependent on the amino acid composition of their antigen-binding sites. Amino acid substitutions may influence the specificity of the immune response by altering the binding affinity of different antigens for the class II molecules.

Most individuals with type 1A DM have the HLA DR3 and/or DR4 haplotype. Refinements in genotyping of HLA loci have shown that the haplotypes DQA1*0301, DQB1*0302 and DQA1*501, DQB1*0201 have the strongest association with type 1A DM. These haplotypes are present in 40% of children with type 1A DM as compared to 2% of the normal U.S. population.

In addition to MHC class II associations, at least 17 different genetic loci may contribute susceptibility to type 1A DM. For example, polymorphisms in the promoter region of the insulin gene appear to account for ~10% of the predisposition to type 1A DM. Genes that confer protection against the development of the disease also exist. For example, the haplotype DQA1*0102, DQB1*0602 is present in 20% of the U.S. population but is extremely rare in individuals with type 1A DM (<1%).

Although type 1A DM is clearly associated with certain predisposing genotypes, most individuals with these haplotypes do not develop diabetes. In addition, most individuals with type 1A DM do not have a first-degree relative with this disorder. Nevertheless, the risk of developing type 1A DM for relatives of individuals with the disease is considerably higher compared to the risk for the general population. ■

Autoimmune Factors Although other islet cell types [alpha cells (glucagon-producing), delta cells (somatostatin-producing) or PP cells (pancreatic polypeptide-producing)] are functionally and embryologically similar to beta cells and express most of the same proteins as beta cells, they are inexplicably spared from the autoimmune process. Pathologically, the pancreatic islets are infiltrated with lymphocytes (in a process termed *insulitis*). After all beta cells are destroyed,

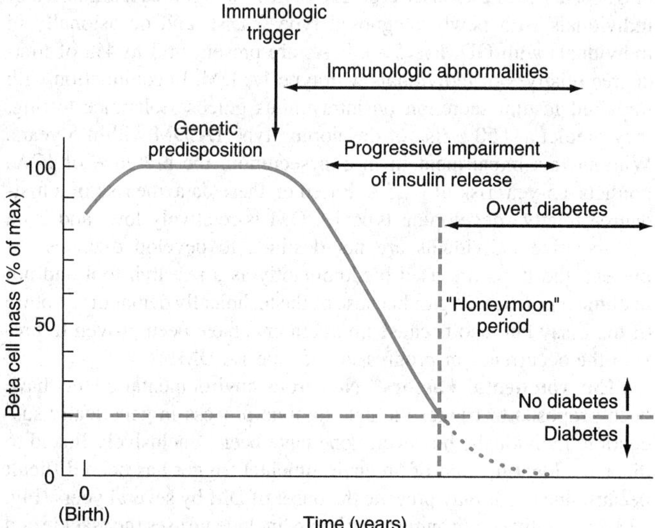

FIGURE 333-5 Temporal model for development of type 1 diabetes. Individuals with a genetic predisposition are exposed to an immunologic trigger that initiates an autoimmune process, resulting in a gradual decline in beta cell mass. The downward slope of the beta cell mass varies among individuals. This progressive impairment in insulin release results in diabetes when ~80% of the beta cell mass is destroyed. A "honeymoon" phase may be seen in the first 1 or 2 years after the onset of diabetes and is associated with reduced insulin requirements. *(Adapted from Medical Management of Type 1 Diabetes, 3d ed, JS Skyler (ed). Alexandria, VA, American Diabetes Association, 1998)*

the inflammatory process abates, the islets become atrophic, and immunologic markers disappear. Studies of the insulitis and autoimmune process in humans and animal models of type 1A DM (NOD mouse and BB rat) have identified the following abnormalities in both the humoral and cellular arms of the immune system: (1) islet cell autoantibodies; (2) activated lymphocytes in the islets, peripancreatic lymph nodes, and systemic circulation; (3) T lymphocytes that proliferate when stimulated with islet proteins; and (4) release of cytokines within the insulitis. Beta cells seem to be particularly susceptible to the toxic effect of some cytokines (tumor necrosis factor α, interferon γ, and interleukin 1). The precise mechanisms of beta cell death are not known but may involve formation of nitric oxide metabolites, apoptosis, and direct CD8+ T cell cytotoxicity. Islet autoantibodies are not thought to be involved in the destructive process, as these antibodies do not generally react with the cell surface of islet cells and are not capable of transferring diabetes mellitus to animals.

Pancreatic islet molecules targeted by the autoimmune process include insulin, glutamic acid decarboxylase (GAD; the biosynthetic enzyme for the neurotransmitter GABA), ICA-512/IA-2 (homology with tyrosine phosphatases), and phogrin (insulin secretory granule protein). Other less clearly defined autoantigens include an islet ganglioside and carboxypeptidase H. With the exception of insulin, none of the autoantigens are beta cell specific, which raises the question of how the beta cells are selectively destroyed. Current theories favor initiation of an autoimmune process directed at one beta cell molecule, which then spreads to other islet molecules as the immune process destroys beta cells and creates a series of secondary autoantigens. The beta cells of individuals who develop type 1A DM do not differ from beta cells of normal individuals, since transplanted islets are destroyed by a recurrence of the autoimmune process of type 1A DM.

Immunologic Markers Islet cell autoantibodies (ICAs) are a composite of several different antibodies directed at pancreatic islet molecules such as GAD, insulin, IA-2/ICA512, and an islet ganglioside and serve as a marker of the autoimmune process of type 1A DM. Testing for ICAs can be useful in classifying the type of DM as type IA and in identifying nondiabetic individuals at risk for developing type 1A DM. ICAs are present in the majority of individuals (>75%) diagnosed with new-onset type 1A DM, in a significant minority of individuals with newly diagnosed type 2 DM, and occasionally in individuals with GDM (<5%). ICAs are present in 3 to 4% of first-degree relatives of individuals with type 1A DM. In conjunction with impaired insulin secretion on intravenous glucose tolerance testing, they predict a >50% risk of developing type 1A DM within 5 years. Without this impairment in insulin secretion, the presence of ICAs predicts a 5-year risk of <25%. Based on these data, the risk of a first-degree relative developing type 1A DM is relatively low, and even ICA-positive individuals are not destined to develop diabetes. At present, the ICAs are used predominantly as a research tool and not in clinical practice, in part because of the technically demanding nature of the assay but also because no treatments have been proven to prevent the occurrence or progression of type 1A DM.

Environmental Factors Numerous environmental events have been proposed to trigger the autoimmune process in genetically susceptible individuals; however, none have been conclusively linked to diabetes. Identification of an environmental trigger has been difficult because the event may precede the onset of DM by several years (Fig. 333-5). Putative environmental triggers include viruses (coxsackie and rubella most prominently), early exposure to bovine milk proteins, and nitrosourea compounds. Epidemiologic studies have noted an association between bovine milk intake and type 1A DM; studies are ongoing to investigate a possible relationship between exposure to bovine milk and the autoimmune process of type 1A DM.

Prevention of Type 1A DM A number of interventions have successfully delayed or prevented diabetes in animal models. Some interventions have targeted the immune system directly (immunosuppression, selective T cell subset deletion, induction of immunologic tolerance to islet proteins), whereas others have prevented islet cell death by blocking cytotoxic cytokines or increasing islet resistance to the destructive process. Though results in animal models are promising, most of these interventions have not been successful in preventing type 1A DM in humans. Clinical trials of several interventions are underway in the United States and Europe. The Diabetes Prevention Trial—type 1 is being conducted to determine whether administering insulin to individuals at high risk for developing type 1A DM can induce immune tolerance and alter the autoimmune process of type 1A DM.

TYPE 2 DM Type 2 DM is a heterogeneous disorder with a complex etiology that develops in response to genetic and environmental influences. Central to the development of type 2 DM are insulin resistance and abnormal insulin secretion. Although controversy remains regarding the primary defect, most studies support the view that insulin resistance precedes insulin secretory defects.

GENETIC CONSIDERATIONS Type 2 DM has a strong genetic component. Although the major genes that predispose to this disorder have yet to be identified, it is clear that the disease is polygenic and multifactorial. Various genetic loci contribute to susceptibility, and environmental factors (such as nutrition and physical activity) further modulate phenotypic expression of the disease. The concordance of type 2 DM in identical twins is between 70 and 90%. Individuals with a parent with type 2 DM have an increased risk of diabetes; if both parents have type 2 DM, the risk in offspring may reach 40%. Insulin resistance, as demonstrated by reduced glucose utilization in skeletal muscle, is present in many nondiabetic, first-degree relatives of individuals with type 2 DM. However, definition of the genetic abnormalities of type 2 DM remains a challenge because the genetic defect in insulin secretion or action may not manifest itself unless an environmental event or another genetic defect, such as obesity, is superimposed.

The identification of individuals with mutations in various molecules involved in insulin action (e.g., the insulin receptor and enzymes involved in glucose homeostasis) has been useful for characterizing key steps in insulin action. However, mutations in these molecules account for a very small fraction of type 2 DM. Likewise, genetic defects in proteins involved in insulin secretion have not been found in most individuals with type 2 DM. Genome-wide scanning for mutations or polymorphisms associated with type 2 DM is being used in an effort to identify genes associated with type 2 DM. ■

Pathophysiology Type 2 DM is characterized by three pathophysiologic abnormalities: impaired insulin secretion, peripheral insulin resistance, and excessive hepatic glucose production. Obesity, particularly visceral or central, is very common in type 2 DM. Insulin resistance associated with obesity augments the genetically determined insulin resistance of type 2 DM. Adipocytes secrete a number of biologic products (leptin, tumor necrosis factor α, free fatty acids) that modulate processes such as insulin secretion, insulin action, and body weight and may contribute to the insulin resistance. In the early stages of the disorder, glucose tolerance remains normal, despite insulin resistance, because the pancreatic beta cells compensate by increasing insulin output. As insulin resistance and compensatory hyperinsulinemia progress, the pancreatic islets become unable to sustain the hyperinsulinemic state. IGT, marked by elevations in postprandial glucose, then develops. A further decline in insulin secretion and an increase in hepatic glucose production lead to overt diabetes with fasting hyperglycemia. Ultimately, beta cell failure may ensue.

Metabolic Abnormalities • ***Insulin resistance*** This is caused by the decreased ability of insulin to act effectively on peripheral target tissues (especially muscle and liver) and is a prominent feature of type 2 DM. This resistance is relative, since supernormal levels of circulating insulin will normalize the plasma glucose. Insulin dose-response curves exhibit a rightward shift, indicating reduced sensitivity, and a reduced maximal response, indicating an overall decrease in maximum glucose utilization (30 to 60% lower than normal individuals). Resistance to the action of insulin impairs glucose utilization by insulin-sensitive tissues and increases hepatic glucose output—both effects contributing to the hyperglycemia of diabetes. Increased hepatic glucose output predominantly accounts for increased FPG levels, whereas decreased peripheral glucose usage results in postprandial hyperglycemia. In skeletal muscle, there is a greater impairment in nonoxidative glucose usage (glycogen formation) than in oxidative glucose metabolism through glycolysis. Glucose usage in insulin-independent tissues is not decreased in type 2 DM.

The precise molecular mechanism of insulin resistance in type 2 DM has yet to be elucidated. Insulin receptor levels and tyrosine kinase activity in skeletal muscle are reduced, but these alterations are most likely secondary to hyperinsulinemia and are not a primary defect. Therefore, postreceptor defects are believed to play the predominant role in insulin resistance (Fig. 333-4). Polymorphisms in IRS-1 may be associated with glucose intolerance, raising the possibility that polymorphisms in various postreceptor molecules may combine to create an insulin-resistant state.

A current focus for the pathogenesis of insulin resistance focuses on a PI-3 kinase signaling defect, which causes reduced translocation of GLUT4 to the plasma membrane, among other abnormalities. Of note, not all insulin signal transduction pathways are resistant to the effects of insulin (e.g., those controlling cell growth and differentiation). Consequently, hyperinsulinemia may actually increase the insulin action through these pathways.

Another emerging theory proposes that elevated levels of free fatty acids, a common feature of obesity, may contribute to the pathogenesis of type 2 DM in several different ways. Free fatty acids can impair glucose utilization in skeletal muscle, promote glucose production by the liver, and impair beta cell function.

Impaired insulin secretion Insulin secretion and sensitivity are interrelated (Fig. 333-6). In type 2 DM, insulin secretion initially increases in response to insulin resistance in order to maintain normal glucose tolerance. Initially, the insulin secretory defect is mild and selectively involves glucose-stimulated insulin secretion. The response to other nonglucose secretagogues, such as arginine, is preserved. Eventually, the insulin secretory defect progresses to a state of grossly inadequate insulin secretion. Some endogenous insulin production continues, but the amount secreted is less than the amount secreted by normal individuals at the same plasma glucose concentration.

The reason(s) for the decline in insulin secretory capacity in type 2 DM is unclear. Despite the assumption that a second genetic defect—superimposed upon insulin resistance—leads to beta cell failure, intense genetic investigation has so far excluded mutations in islet candidate genes. Islet amyloid polypeptide or amylin is cosecreted by the beta cell and likely forms the amyloid fibrillar deposit found in the islets of individuals with longstanding type 2 DM. Whether such islet amyloid deposits are a primary or secondary event is not known. The metabolic environment may also impact islet function negatively. For example, chronic hyperglycemia paradoxically impairs islet function ("glucose toxicity") and leads to a worsening of hyperglycemia. Improvement in glycemic control is often associated with improved islet function. In addition, elevation of free fatty acid levels ("lipotoxicity") also worsens islet function.

Increased hepatic glucose production The liver maintains plasma glucose during periods of fasting through glycogenolysis and gluconeogenesis using substrates derived from skeletal muscle and fat (alanine, lactate, glycerol, and fatty acids). Insulin promotes the storage of glucose as hepatic glycogen and suppresses gluconeogenesis. In type 2 DM, insulin resistance in the liver arises from the failure of hyperinsulinemia to suppress gluconeogenesis, which results in fasting hyperglycemia and decreased glucose storage by the liver in the postprandial state. Increased hepatic glucose production occurs early in the course of diabetes, though likely after the onset of insulin secretory abnormalities and insulin resistance in skeletal muscle.

Insulin Resistance Syndromes It is likely that the insulin resistance condition comprises a spectrum of disorders, with hyperglycemia representing one of the most readily diagnosed features. *Syndrome X* is a term used to describe a constellation of metabolic derangements

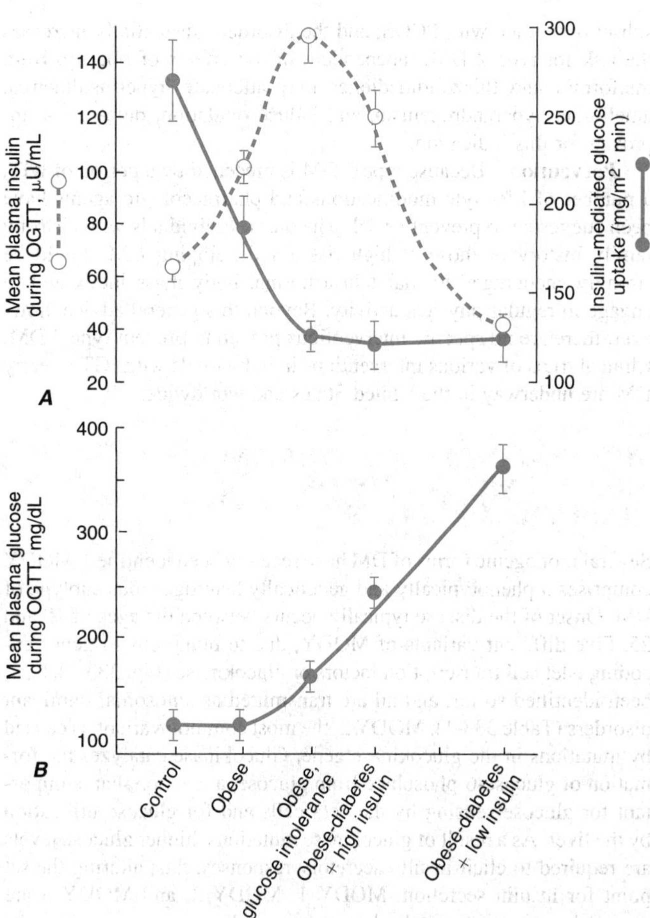

FIGURE 333-6 Metabolic changes during the development of type 2 diabetes. *A.* The mean plasma insulin and insulin-mediated glucose uptake during an oral glucose tolerance test (OGTT). *B.* The mean plasma glucose during an OGTT. On the x-axis are groups of: control individuals, obese individuals, obese and glucose intolerant individuals, obese individuals with diabetes and high insulin, and obese individuals with diabetes and low insulin. *(From RA DeFronzo: Lilly lecture. The triumvirate: Beta-cell, muscle, liver: A collusion responsible for NIDDM. Diabetes 37:667, 1998, with permission.)*

that includes insulin resistance, hypertension, dyslipidemia, central or visceral obesity, endothelial dysfunction, and accelerated cardiovascular disease. Epidemiologic evidence supports hyperinsulinemia as a marker for coronary artery disease risk, though an etiologic role has not been demonstrated.

A number of forms of severe insulin resistance may be associated with a phenotype similar to that in type 2 DM or IGT (Table 333-1). *Acanthosis nigricans* and signs of hyperandrogenism (hirsutism, acne, and oligomenorrhea) are common physical features. In addition to rare genetic syndromes seen in early childhood, two distinct syndromes of severe insulin resistance have been described in adults: (1) type A, which affects young women and is characterized by severe hyperinsulinemia, obesity, and features of hyperandrogenism; and (2) type B, which affects middle-aged women and is characterized by severe hyperinsulinemia, features of hyperandrogenism, and autoimmune disorders. Individuals with the type A insulin resistance syndrome have an undefined defect in the insulin signaling pathway; individuals with the type B insulin resistance syndrome have autoantibodies directed at the insulin receptor. These receptor autoantibodies may block insulin binding or may stimulate the insulin receptor, leading to intermittent hypoglycemia.

Polycystic ovary syndrome (PCOS) is a common disorder that affects premenopausal women and is characterized by chronic anovulation and hyperandrogenism. Insulin resistance is seen in a significant subset of women with PCOS, and the disorder substantially increases the risk for type 2 DM, independent of the effects of obesity. Both metformin and thiazolidinediones may attenuate hyperinsulinemia, ameliorate hyperandrogenism, and induce ovulation, but are not approved for this indication.

Prevention Because type 2 DM is preceded by a period of IGT, a number of life-style modifications and pharmacologic agents have been suggested to prevent or delay its onset. Individuals with a strong family history or those at high risk for developing DM should be strongly encouraged to maintain a normal body mass index and to engage in regular physical activity. Beyond this general advice, however, there are no specific interventions proven to prevent type 2 DM. Clinical trials of various interventions in individuals with IGT or early DM are underway in the United States and worldwide.

MODY: GENETICALLY DEFINED, MONOGENIC FORMS OF DIABETES MELLITUS

Several monogenic forms of DM have recently been identified. MODY comprises a phenotypically and genetically heterogeneous subtype of DM. Onset of the disease typically occurs between the ages of 10 and 25. Five different variants of MODY, due to mutations in genes encoding islet cell transcription factors or glucokinase (Fig. 333-3), have been identified so far, and all are transmitted as autosomal dominant disorders (Table 333-1). MODY 2, the most common variant, is caused by mutations in the glucokinase gene. Glucokinase catalyzes the formation of glucose-6-phosphate from glucose, a reaction that is important for glucose sensing by the beta cells and for glucose utilization by the liver. As a result of glucokinase mutations, higher glucose levels are required to elicit insulin secretory responses, thus altering the set point for insulin secretion. MODY 1, MODY 3, and MODY 5 are caused by mutations in the hepatocyte nuclear transcription factors HNF-4α, HNF-1α, and HNF-1β, respectively. As their names imply, these transcription factors are expressed in the liver but also in other tissues, including the pancreatic islets. The mechanisms by which such mutations lead to DM is not well understood, but it is likely that these factors affect islet development or the transcription of genes that are important in stimulating insulin secretion. MODY 4 is a rare variant caused by mutations in the insulin promoter factor (IPF-1), which is a transcription factor that regulates both pancreatic development and insulin gene transcription. Homozygous inactivating mutations lead to pancreatic agenesis, whereas heterozygous mutations result in early-onset DM. Studies of populations with type 2 DM suggest that mutations in the glucokinase gene and various islet cell transcription factors do not account for ordinary type 2 DM. Nevertheless, elucidation of the molecular genetics underlying these rare forms of DM has been important in identifying critical steps in the control of pancreatic beta cell function.

COMPLICATIONS OF DM

ACUTE COMPLICATIONS Diabetic ketoacidosis (DKA) and nonketotic hyperosmolar state (NKHS) are acute complications of diabetes. DKA is seen primarily in individuals with type 1 DM, and NKHS is seen in individuals with type 2 DM. Both disorders are associated with absolute or relative insulin deficiency, volume depletion, and altered mental status. DKA and NKHS exist along a continuum of hyperglycemia, with or without ketosis. The metabolic similarities and differences in DKA and NKHS are highlighted in Table 333-4. Both disorders are associated with potentially serious complications if not promptly diagnosed and treated.

DIABETIC KETOACIDOSIS **Clinical Features** The symptoms and physical signs of DKA are listed in Table 333-5. DKA may be the initial symptom complex that leads to a diagnosis of type 1 DM, but more frequently it occurs in individuals with established diabetes. Nausea and vomiting are often prominent, and their presence in an individual with diabetes warrants laboratory evaluation for DKA. Abdominal pain may be severe and sometimes suggests acute pancreatitis or ruptured viscous. Hyperglycemia leads to glucosuria, volume depletion, tachycardia, and possibly hypotension. Kussmaul respirations and an acetone odor on the patient's breath (both secondary to metabolic acidosis) are classic signs of the disorder. Lethargy and central nervous system depression may evolve into coma with severe DKA. Cerebral edema, an extremely serious complication of DKA, is seen most frequently in children. Signs of infection, which may precipitate DKA, should be sought on physical examination, even in the absence of fever.

Pathophysiology DKA results from insulin deficiency combined with counterregulatory hormone excess (glucagon, catecholamines, cortisol, and growth hormone). Both insulin deficiency and glucagon excess, in particular, are necessary for DKA to develop. The hyperglycemia of DKA results from increased hepatic glucose production (gluconeogenesis and glycogenolysis) and impaired peripheral glucose utilization. The decreased ratio of insulin to glucagon promotes gluconeogenesis, glycogenolysis, and ketone body formation in the liver, as well as increasing substrate delivery from fat and muscle (free fatty acids, amino acids) to the liver.

The combination of insulin deficiency and hyperglycemia reduces the hepatic level of fructose-2,6-phosphate, which alters the activity of phosphofructokinase and fructose-1,6-bisphosphatase. Glucagon excess decreases the activity of pyruvate kinase, whereas insulin deficiency increases the activity of phosphoenolpyruvate carboxykinase. These hepatic changes shift the handling of pyruvate toward glucose synthesis and away from glycolysis. Glycogenolysis is promoted by the increased levels of glucagon and catecholamines in the face of low insulin levels. Insulin deficiency also reduces levels of the GLUT4 glucose transporter, which impairs glucose uptake into skeletal muscle and fat and reduces intracellular glucose metabolism (Fig. 333-4).

Ketosis results from a marked increase in free fatty acid release from adipocytes, with a resulting shift toward ketone body synthesis in the liver. Reduced insulin levels, in combination with elevations in catecholamines and growth hormone, lead to an increase in lipolysis and release of free fatty acids. Normally, these free fatty acids are converted to triglycerides or very low density lipoproteins (VLDL) in the liver, but in DKA, hyperglucagonemia alters hepatic metabolism to favor ketone body formation, through activation of the enzyme carnitine palmitoyltransferase I. This enzyme is crucial for regulating fatty acid transport into

Table 333-4 Laboratory Values in Diabetic Ketoacidosis (DKA) and Nonketotic Hyperosmolar States (NKHS) (Representative Ranges at Presentation)

	DKA	NKHS
Glucose,[a] mmol/L (mg/dL)	16.7–33.3 (300–600)	33.3–66.6 (600–1200)
Sodium, meq/L	125–135	135–145
Potassium,[a] meq/L	Normal to ↑[b]	Normal
Magnesium [a]	Normal [b]	Normal
Chloride[a]	Normal	Normal
Phosphate[a]	↓	Normal
Creatinine, μmol/L (mg/dL)	Slightly ↑	Moderately ↑
Osmolality, mOsm/mL	300–320	330–380
Plasma ketones[a]	++++	+/−
Serum bicarbonate,[a] meq/L	<15 meq/L	Normal to slightly ↓
Arterial pH	6.8–7.3	>7.3
Arterial P_{CO_2}, mmHg	20–30	Normal
Anion gap[a] [Na − (Cl + HCO_3)], meq/L	↑	Normal to slightly ↑

[a] Large changes occur during treatment of DKA.
[b] Although plasma levels may be normal or high at presentation, total-body stores are usually depleted.

Table 333-5 Manifestations of Diabetic Ketoacidosis

Symptoms	Physical findings
Nausea/vomiting	Tachycardia
Thirst/polyuria	Dry mucous membranes/reduced skin turgor
Abdominal pain	Dehydration / hypotension
Altered mental function	Tachypnea / Kussmaul respirations/respiratory distress
Shortness of breath	Abdominal tenderness (may resemble acute pancreatitis or surgical abdomen)
Precipitating events	Fever
Inadequate insulin administration	Lethargy /obtundation / cerebral edema / possibly coma
Infection (pneumonia/UTI/gastroenteritis/sepsis)	
Infarction (cerebral, coronary, mesenteric, peripheral)	
Drugs (cocaine)	

NOTE: UTI, urinary tract infection.

the mitochondria, where beta oxidation and conversion to ketone bodies occurs. At physiologic pH, ketone bodies exist as ketoacids, which are neutralized by bicarbonate. As bicarbonate stores are depleted, metabolic acidosis ensues. Increased lactic acid production also contributes to the acidosis. The increased free fatty acids result in increased triglyceride production and increased hepatic production of VLDL. VLDL clearance is also reduced because the activity of insulin-sensitive lipoprotein lipase is decreased. Hypertriglyceridemia may be severe enough to cause pancreatitis.

DKA can be precipitated by inadequate levels of plasma insulin for a variety of reasons (Table 333-5). Most commonly, DKA is precipitated when relatively insufficient insulin is available when insulin requirements increase, as might occur during a concurrent illness. Failure to augment insulin therapy appropriately by the patient or health care team compounds the problem. Occasionally, complete omission of insulin by the patient or health care team (in a hospitalized patient with type 1 DM) precipitates DKA. Patients using insulin infusion devices with short-acting insulin have a greater potential for DKA, since even a brief interruption in insulin delivery (e.g., mechanical malfunction) quickly leads to insulin deficiency.

Laboratory Abnormalities and Diagnosis The timely diagnosis of DKA is crucial and allows for prompt initiation of therapy. DKA is characterized by hyperglycemia, ketosis, and metabolic acidosis (increased anion gap) along with a number of secondary metabolic derangements (Table 333-4)). Serum bicarbonate is frequently <10 mmol/L, and arterial pH ranges between 6.8 and 7.3, depending on the severity of the acidosis. Despite a total-body potassium deficit, the serum potassium at presentation is typically at the high end of the normal range or mildly elevated, secondary to the acidosis. Total-body stores of sodium, chloride, phosphorous, and magnesium are also reduced in DKA, but are not accurately reflected by their levels in the serum. Elevated blood urea nitrogen (BUN) and serum creatinine levels reflect intravascular volume depletion. Interference from acetoacetate may falsely elevate the serum creatinine measurement. Leukocytosis, hypertriglyceridemia, and hyperlipoproteinemia are commonly found as well. Hyperamylasemia may suggest a diagnosis of pancreatitis, especially when accompanied by abdominal pain. However, in DKA the amylase is usually of salivary origin and thus is not diagnostic of pancreatitis.

The measured serum sodium is reduced as a consequence of the hyperglycemia [1.6 meq (1.6 mmol/L) reduction in serum sodium for each 100 mg/dL (5.6 mmol/L) rise in the serum glucose]. A normal serum sodium in the setting of DKA indicates a more profound water deficit. In "conventional" units, the calculated serum osmolality [2 × (serum sodium + serum potassium) + plasma glucose (mg/dL)/18 + BUN/2.8] is mildly to moderately elevated, though to a lesser degree than that found in NKHS hyperosmolar state (see below).

In DKA, the ketone body, β-hydroxybutyrate, is synthesized at a threefold greater rate than acetoacetate; however, the latter ketone body is preferentially detected by a commonly used ketosis detection reagent (nitroprusside). Serum ketones are present at significant levels (usually positive at serum dilution of 1:8 or greater). The nitroprusside tablet, or stick, is often used to detect urine ketones; certain medications such as captopril or penicillamine may cause false-positive reactions. Serum or plasma assays for β-hydroxybutyrate more accurately reflect the true ketone body level.

The metabolic derangements of DKA exist along a spectrum, beginning with mild acidosis with moderate hyperglycemia evolving into more severe findings. The degree of acidosis and hyperglycemia do not necessarily correlate closely, as a variety of factors determine the level of hyperglycemia (oral intake, urinary glucose loss). Ketonemia is a consistent finding in DKA and distinguishes it from simple hyperglycemia.

℞ **TREATMENT** The management of DKA is outlined in Table 333-6. After initiating intravenous fluid replacement and insulin therapy, the agent or event that precipitated the episode of DKA should be sought and aggressively treated. If the patient is vomiting or has altered mental status, a nasogastric tube should be inserted to prevent aspiration of gastric contents. Central to successful treatment of DKA is careful patient monitoring and frequent reassessment to ensure that the patient and the metabolic derangements are improving. A comprehensive flow sheet should record chronologic changes in vital signs, fluid intake and output, and laboratory values as a function of insulin administered.

After the initial bolus of normal saline, replacement of the sodium and free water deficit is carried out over the next 24 h (fluid deficit is often 3 to 5 L). When hemodynamic stability and adequate urine output are achieved, intravenous fluids should be switched to 0.45% saline at a rate of 200 to 300 mL/h, depending on the calculated volume deficit. The change to 0.45% saline helps reduce the trend toward hyperchloremia later in the course of DKA. Alternatively, initial use of lactated Ringer's intravenous solution may reduce the hyperchloremia that commonly occurs with normal saline.

A bolus of intravenous or intramuscular insulin (10 to 20 units) should be administered immediately (Table 333-6)), and subsequent treatment should provide continuous and adequate levels of circulating insulin. Intravenous administration is preferred, because it assures

Table 333-6 Management of Diabetic Ketoacidosis

1. Confirm diagnosis (↑ plasma glucose, positive serum ketones, metabolic acidosis).
2. Admit to hospital; intensive-care setting may be necessary for frequent monitoring or if pH < 7.00 or unconscious.
3. Assess: Serum electrolytes (K^+, Na^+, Mg^{2+}, Cl^-, bicarbonate, phosphate)
   Acid-base status—pH, HCO_3^-, P_{CO_2}
   Renal function (creatinine, urine output)
4. Replace fluids: 2–3 L 0.9% saline over first 1–3 h (5–10 mL/kg per hour); subsequently, 0.45% saline at 150–300 mL/h; change to 5% glucose and 0.45% saline at 100–200 mL/h when plasma glucose reaches 14 mmol/L (250 mg/dL).
5. Administer regular insulin: 10–20 units IV or IM, then 5–10 units/h by continuous IV infusion; increase 2- to 10-fold if no response by 2–4 h.
6. Assess patient: What precipitated the episode (noncompliance, infection, trauma, infarction, cocaine)? Initiate appropriate workup for precipitating event [cultures, chest x-ray, electrocardiogram (ECG)]
7. Measure capillary glucose every 1–2 h; measure electrolytes (especially K^+, bicarbonate, phosphate) and anion gap every 4 h for first 24 h.
8. Monitor blood pressure, pulse, respirations, mental status, fluid intake and output every 1–4 h.
9. Replace K^+: 10 meq/h when plasma K^+ < 5.5 meq/L, ECG normal, urine flow, and normal creatinine documented; administer 40–80 meq/h when plasma K^+ < 3.5 meq/L or if bicarbonate is given.
10. Continue above until patient is stable; glucose goal is 8.3–13.9 mmol/L (150–250 mg/dL), until acidosis is resolved. Insulin infusion may be decreased to 1–4 units/h.
11. Administer intermediate or long-acting insulin as soon as patient is eating. Allow for overlap in insulin infusion and subcutaneous insulin injection.

SOURCE: Adapted from M Sperling, in *Therapy for Diabetes Mellitus and Related Disorders*, 1998.

rapid distribution and allows adjustment of the infusion rate as the patient responds to therapy. Intravenous insulin should be continued until the acidosis resolves and the patient is metabolically stable. As the acidosis and insulin resistance associated with DKA resolve, the insulin infusion rate can be decreased (to 1 to 4 units/h). Intermediate or long-acting insulin, in combination with subcutaneous regular insulin, should be administered as soon as the patient resumes eating, as this facilitates transition to an outpatient insulin regimen and reduces length of hospital stay. It is crucial to continue the insulin infusion until adequate insulin levels are achieved by the subcutaneous route. Even relatively brief periods of inadequate insulin administration in this transition phase may allow for DKA relapse.

Hyperglycemia usually improves at a rate of 4.2 to 5.6 mmol/L (75 to 100 mg/dL per hour) as a result of insulin-mediated glucose disposal, reduced hepatic glucose release, and rehydration. The latter reduces catecholamines, increases urinary glucose loss, and expands the intravascular volume. The decline in the plasma glucose within the first 1 to 2 h may be more rapid and is mostly related to volume expansion. When the plasma glucose reaches 13.9 mmol/L (250 mg/dL), glucose should be added to the 0.45% saline infusion to maintain the plasma glucose in the 11.1 to 13.9 mmol/L (200 to 250 mg/dL) range, and the insulin infusion should be continued. Ketoacidosis begins to resolve as insulin reduces lipolysis, increases peripheral ketone body use, suppresses hepatic ketone body formation, and promotes bicarbonate regeneration. However, the acidosis and ketosis resolve at a slower rate than does the hyperglycemia. As ketoacidosis improves, β-hydroxybutyrate is converted to acetoacetate. Ketone body levels may appear to increase if measured by laboratory assays that use the nitroprusside reaction, which only detects acetoacetate and acetone levels. The improvement in acidosis and anion gap, a result of bicarbonate regeneration and decline in ketone bodies, is reflected by a rise in the serum bicarbonate level and the arterial pH. Depending on the rise of serum chloride, the anion gap (but not bicarbonate) will normalize. A hyperchloremic acidosis [serum bicarbonate of 15 to 18 mmol/L (15 to 18 meq/L)] often follows successful treatment and is minimized by the use of hypotonic intravenous solutions. This gradually resolves as the kidney regenerates bicarbonate and excretes chloride.

Potassium stores are depleted in DKA [estimated deficit 3 to 5 mmol/kg (3 to 5 meq/kg)], but the serum potassium may be normal or even elevated at the time of presentation. During treatment with insulin and fluids, various factors contribute to the development of hypokalemia. These include insulin-mediated potassium transport into cells, resolution of the acidosis (which also promotes potassium entry into cells), and urinary loss of potassium salts of organic acids. Thus, potassium repletion should commence as soon as adequate urine output and a normal serum potassium are documented. If the initial serum potassium level is elevated, then potassium repletion should be delayed until the potassium falls into the normal range. Inclusion of 20 to 40 meq of potassium in each liter of intravenous fluid is reasonable, but additional potassium supplements may also be required. To reduce the amount of chloride administered, potassium phosphate or acetate can be substituted for the chloride salt. The goal is to maintain the serum potassium >3.5 mmol/L (3.5 meq/L).

Despite a bicarbonate deficit, bicarbonate replacement is not usually necessary or advisable. In fact, theoretical arguments suggest that bicarbonate administration and rapid reversal of acidosis may impair cardiac function, impair tissue oxygenation, and promote hypokalemia. The results of most clinical trials do not support the routine use of bicarbonate replacement. In the presence of severe acidosis (arterial pH < 7.0 or hypotension unresponsive to fluid resuscitation), some physicians administer bicarbonate [50 to 150 mmol/L (meq/L) of sodium bicarbonate in 250 mL of 0.45% saline over 1 to 2 h until the serum bicarbonate rises to approximately 10 mmol/L (meq/L)]. Hypophosphatemia may result from increased glucose usage, but randomized clinical trials have not demonstrated that phosphate replacement is beneficial in DKA. If the serum phosphate is < 0.32 mmol/L (1.0 mg/dl), then phosphate supplement should be considered and the serum calcium monitored. Hypomagnesemia may develop during DKA therapy and may also require supplementation.

With appropriate therapy, the mortality of DKA is low (<5%) and is related more to the underlying or precipitating event, such as infection or myocardial infarction. The major nonmetabolic complication of DKA therapy is cerebral edema, which most often develops in children as DKA is resolving. The etiology and optimal therapy for cerebral edema are not well established, but overreplacement of free water should be avoided. Venous thrombosis and adult respiratory distress syndrome occasionally complicate DKA.

Following successful treatment of DKA, the physician and patient should review the sequence of events that led to DKA to prevent future recurrences. Foremost is patient education about the symptoms of DKA, its precipitating factors, and the management of diabetes during a concurrent illness. During illness or when oral intake is compromised, patients should: (1) frequently measure the capillary blood glucose; (2) measure urinary ketones when the serum glucose >16.5 mmol/L (300 mg/dL); (3) drink fluids to maintain hydration; (4) continue or increase insulin; and (5) seek medical attention if dehydration, persistent vomiting, or uncontrolled hyperglycemia develop. In this way, early DKA can be detected and treated appropriately on an outpatient basis.

NONKETOTIC HYPEROSMOLAR STATE **Clinical Features** NKHS is most commonly seen in elderly individuals with type 2 DM. Its most prominent features include polyuria; orthostatic hypotension; and a variety of neurologic symptoms that include altered mental status, lethargy, obtundation, seizure, and possibly coma. The prototypical patient is a mildly diabetic, elderly individual with a several week history of polyuria, weight loss, and diminished oral intake that culminates in mental confusion, lethargy, or coma. The physical examination reflects profound dehydration and hyperosmolality and reveals hypotension, tachycardia, and altered mental status. Notably absent are symptoms of nausea, vomiting, and abdominal pain and the Kussmaul respirations characteristic of DKA. NKHS is often precipitated by a serious, concurrent illness such as myocardial infarction or stroke. Sepsis, pneumonia, and other serious infections are frequent precipitants and should be sought thoroughly. In addition, a debilitating condition (prior stroke or dementia) or social situation that compromises water intake may contribute to the development of the disorder. Finally, the development of NKHS can be associated with the use of certain medications (thiazide diuretics, glucocorticoids, phenytoin).

Pathophysiology Insulin deficiency and inadequate fluid intake are the underlying causes of NKHS. Insulin deficiency increases hepatic glucose production (through glycogenolysis and gluconeogenesis) and impairs glucose utilization in skeletal muscle (see above discussion under DKA). Hyperglycemia induces an osmotic diuresis that leads to profound intravascular volume depletion, which is exacerbated by inadequate fluid replacement. The absence of ketosis in NKHS is not completely understood. Presumably, the insulin deficiency is only relative and less severe than in DKA. Lower levels of counterregulatory hormones and free fatty acids have been found in NKHS than in DKA in some studies. It is also possible that the liver is less capable of ketone body synthesis or that the insulin/glucagon ratio does not favor ketogenesis.

Laboratory Abnormalities and Diagnosis The laboratory features in NKHS are summarized in Table 333-4. Most notable are the marked hyperglycemia [plasma glucose may be >55.5 mmol/L (1000 mg/dL)], hyperosmolality (>350 mosmol/L), and prerenal azotemia. The measured serum sodium may be normal or slightly low despite the marked hyperglycemia. The corrected serum sodium is usually increased [add 1.6 meq to measured sodium for each 5.6 mmol/L (100 mg/dL) rise in the serum glucose]. In contrast to DKA, acidosis and ketonemia are absent or mild. A small anion gap metabolic acidosis may be present secondary to increased lactic acid. Moderate ketonuria, if present, is secondary to starvation.

℞ **TREATMENT** Volume depletion and hyperglycemia are prominent features of both NKHS and DKA. Consequently, therapy of these disorders involves several shared elements (Table 333-6). In both disorders, careful monitoring of the patient's fluid status, laboratory values, and insulin infusion rate is crucial. Underlying or precipitating problems should be aggressively sought and treated. In NKHS, the volume depletion, free water deficit, and hyperosmolality are greater than in DKA. The patient with NKHS is usually older, more likely to have mental status changes, and thus more likely to have a life-threatening precipitating event with accompanying comorbidities. Even with proper treatment, NKHS has a substantially higher mortality than DKA (up to 50% in some clinical series).

Fluid replacement should initially stabilize the hemodynamic status of the patient (1 to 3 L of 0.9% normal saline over the first 2 to 3 h). Because the fluid deficit in NKHS is accumulated over a period of days to weeks, the rapidity of reversal of the hyperosmolar state must balance the need for free water repletion and the observation that too rapid a reversal may worsen neurologic function. If the serum sodium is >150mmol/L (150 meq/L), 0.45% saline should be used. After hemodynamic stability is achieved, the intravenous fluid administration is directed at reversing the free water deficit using hypotonic fluids (0.45% saline initially then 5% dextrose in water, D_5W). The calculated free water deficit (which averages 9 to 10 L) should be reversed over the next 1 to 2 days (infusion rates of 200 to 300 mL/h of hypotonic solution). Potassium repletion is usually necessary and should be dictated by repeated measurements of the serum potassium. In patients taking diuretics, the potassium deficit can be quite large and may be accompanied by magnesium deficiency. Hypophosphatemia may occur during therapy and can be improved by using KPO_4 and beginning nutrition.

As in DKA, rehydration and volume expansion lower the plasma glucose initially, but insulin is eventually required. In NKHS, patients tend to be more sensitive to insulin than in DKA and dose requirements are not usually as large. A reasonable regimen for NKHS begins with an intravenous insulin bolus of 5 to 10 units followed by intravenous insulin at a constant infusion rate (3 to 7 units/h). As in DKA, glucose should be added to intravenous fluid when the plasma glucose falls to 13.9 mmol/L (250 mg/dL), and the insulin infusion rate should be decreased to 1 to 2 units/h. The insulin infusion should be continued until the patient has resumed eating and can be transferred to a subcutaneous insulin regimen. The patient should be discharged from the hospital on insulin, though some patients can later undergo a trial of oral glucose-lowering agents.

CHRONIC COMPLICATIONS The chronic complications of DM affect many organ systems and are responsible for the majority of morbidity and mortality associated with the disease. Chronic complications can be divided into vascular and nonvascular complications (Table 333-7). The vascular complications of DM are further subdivided into microvascular (retinopathy, neuropathy, nephropathy) and macrovascular complications (coronary artery disease, peripheral vascular disease, cerebrovascular disease). Nonvascular complications include problems such as gastroparesis, sexual dysfunction, and skin changes. This division is rather arbitrary since it is likely that multiple pathogenic processes are involved in all forms of complications.

The risk of chronic complications increases as a function of the duration of hyperglycemia; they usually become apparent in the second decade of hyperglycemia. Since type 2 DM may have a long asymptomatic period of hyperglycemia, many individuals with type 2 DM have complications at the time of diagnosis.

The microvascular complications of both type 1 and type 2 DM result from chronic hyperglycemia. Randomized, prospective clinical trials involving large numbers of individuals with type 1 or type 2 DM have conclusively demonstrated that a reduction in chronic hyperglycemia prevents or reduces retinopathy, neuropathy, and nephropathy. Other incompletely defined factors also modulate the development of complications. For example, despite longstanding DM, some individuals never develop nephropathy or retinopathy. Many of these patients

Table 333-7 Chronic Complications of Diabetes Mellitus

Microvascular	Macrovascular
Eye disease	Coronary artery disease
Retinopathy (nonproliferative/ proliferative)	Peripheral vascular disease
Macular edema	Cerebrovascular disease
Cataracts	Other
Glaucoma	Gastrointestinal (gastroparesis, diarrhea)
Neuropathy	Genitourinary (uropathy/sexual dysfunction)
Sensory and motor (mono- and polyneuropathy)	Dermatologic
Autonomic	
Nephropathy	

have glycemic control that is indistinguishable from those who develop microvascular complications. Because of these observations, it is suspected that a genetic susceptibility for developing particular complications exists. However, the genetic loci responsible for these susceptibilities have not yet been identified.

Evidence implicating a causative role for chronic hyperglycemia in the development of macrovascular complications is less conclusive, but some results suggest a role for chronic hyperglycemia in the development of macrovascular disease. For example, coronary heart disease events and mortality are two to four times greater in patients with type 2 DM. These events correlate with fasting and postprandial plasma glucose levels as well as with the HbA1c. Other factors (dyslipidemia and hypertension) also play important roles in macrovascular complications.

MECHANISMS OF COMPLICATIONS Although chronic hyperglycemia is an important etiologic factor leading to complications of DM, the mechanism(s) by which it leads to such diverse cellular and organ dysfunction is unknown. Three major theories, which are not mutually exclusive, have been proposed to explain how hyperglycemia might lead to the chronic complications of DM (Fig. 333-7).

One hypothesis is that increased intracellular glucose leads to the formation of advanced glycosylation end products (AGEs) via the nonenzymatic glycosylaton of cellular proteins. Nonenzymatic glycosylation results from the interaction of glucose with amino groups on proteins. AGEs have been shown to cross-link proteins (e.g., collagen, extracellular matrix proteins), accelerate atherosclerosis, promote glomerular dysfunction, reduce nitric oxide synthesis, induce endothelial dysfunction, and alter extracellular matrix composition and structure. The serum level of AGEs correlates with the level of glycemia, and these products accumulate as glomerular filtration rate declines.

A second hypothesis proposed to explain how chronic hyperglycemia leads to complications of DM is based on the observation that hyperglycemia increases glucose metabolism via the sorbitol pathway. Intracellular glucose is predominantly metabolized by phosphorylation and subsequent glycolysis, but when intracellular glucose is increased, some glucose is converted to sorbitol by the enzyme aldose reductase. Increased sorbitol concentrations affect several aspects of cellular physiology (decreased myoinositol, altered redox potential) and may lead to cellular dysfunction. However, testing of this theory in humans, using aldose reductase inhibitors, has not demonstrated beneficial effects on clinical endpoints of retinopathy, neuropathy, or nephropathy.

A third hypothesis proposes that hyperglycemia increases the formation of diacylglycerol leading to activation of certain isoforms of protein kinase C (PKC), which, in turn, affect a variety of cellular events that lead to DM-related complications. For example, PKC activation by glucose alters the transcription of genes for fibronectin, type IV collagen, contractile proteins, and extracellular matrix proteins in endothelial cells and neurons in vitro. Growth factors appear to play an important role in DM-related complications. Vascular endothelial growth factor (VEGF) is increased locally in diabetic proliferative ret-

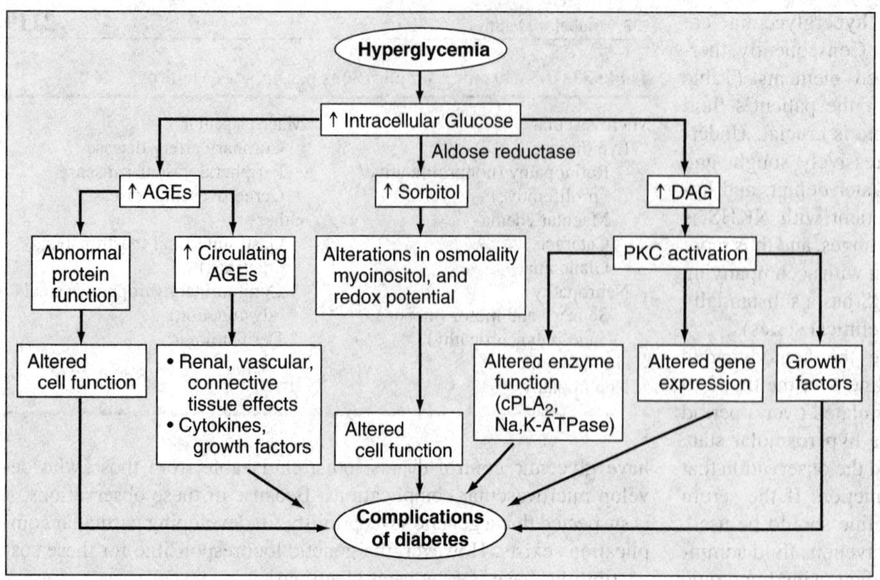

FIGURE 333-7 Possible molecular mechanisms of diabetes-related complications. AGEs, advanced glycation end products; PKC, protein kinase C; DAG, diacylglycerol; $cPLA_2$, phospholipase A_2; Na,K-ATPase, sodium-potassium ATPase.

inopathy and decreases after laser photocoagulation. Transforming growth factor β (TGF-β) is increased in diabetic nephropathy and appears to stimulate basement membrane production of collagen and fibronectin by mesangial cells. Other growth factors, such as platelet-derived growth factor, epidermal growth factor, insulin-like growth factor I, growth hormone, basic fibroblast growth factor, and even insulin, have been suggested to play a role in DM-related complications.

Although hyperglycemia serves as the initial trigger for complications of diabetes, it is still unknown whether the same pathophysiologic processes are operative in all complications or whether certain processes predominate in certain organs. Finally, oxidative stress and free radical generation, as a consequence of the hyperglycemia, may also promote the development of complications.

GLYCEMIC CONTROL AND COMPLICATIONS The Diabetes Control and Complications Trial (DCCT) provided definitive proof that reduction in chronic hyperglycemia can prevent many of the early complications of type 1 DM. This large multicenter clinical trial randomized over 1400 individuals with type 1 DM to either intensive or conventional diabetes management, and then evaluated the development of retinopathy, nephropathy, and neuropathy. Individuals in the intensive diabetes management group received multiple administrations of insulin each day along with intense educational, psychological, and medical support. Individuals in the conventional diabetes management group received twice daily insulin injections and quarterly nutritional, educational, and clinical evaluation. The goal in the former group was normoglycemia; the goal in the latter group was prevention of symptoms of diabetes. Individuals in the intensive diabetes management group achieved a substantially lower HbA1c (7.2%) than individuals in the conventional diabetes management group (HbA1c of 9.0%).

Results from the DCCT demonstrated that improvement of glycemic control reduced nonproliferative and proliferative retinopathy (47% reduction), microalbuminuria (39% reduction), clinical nephropathy (54% reduction), and neuropathy (60% reduction). Improved glycemic control also slowed the progression of early diabetic complications. There was a nonsignificant trend in reduction of macrovascular events. The results of the DCCT predicted that individuals in the intensive diabetes management group would gain 7.7 additional years of sight, 5.8 additional years free from end-stage renal disease (ESRD), and 5.6 years free from lower extremity amputations. If all complications of DM were combined, individuals in the intensive diabetes management group would experience 15.3 more years of life without significant microvascular or neurologic complications of DM as compared to individuals who received standard therapy. This translates into an additional 5.1 years of life expectancy for individuals in the intensive diabetes management group. The benefit of the improved glycemic control during the DCCT persisted even after the study concluded and glycemic control worsened.

The benefits of an improvement in glycemic control occurred over the entire range of HbA1c values (Fig. 333-8), suggesting that at any HbA1c level, an improvement in glycemic control is beneficial. Therefore, there is no threshold beneath which the HbA1c can be reduced and the complications of DM prevented. The clinical implication of this finding is that the goal of therapy is to achieve an HbA1c level as close to normal as possible, without subjecting the patient to excessive risk of hypoglycemia.

Considerable debate has emerged as to whether the DCCT findings are applicable to individuals with type 2 DM, in whom insulin resistance, hyperinsulinemia, and obesity predominate. Concerns have been raised that therapies associated with weight gain and additional insulin therapy may worsen underlying insulin resistance and hyperinsulinemia. Despite these concerns, most available data support extrapolation of the results of the DCCT to individuals with type 2 DM.

The United Kingdom Prospective Diabetes Study (UKPDS) studied the course of >5000 individuals with type 2 DM for >10 years. This complex and important study utilized multiple treatment regimens and monitored the effect of intensive glycemic control and risk factor treatment on the development of diabetic complications. Newly diagnosed individuals with type 2 DM were randomized to (1) intensive management using various combinations of insulin, a sulfonylurea, or metformin; or (2) conventional therapy using dietary modification and pharmacotherapy with the goal of symptom prevention. In addition, individuals were randomly assigned to different antihypertensive regimens. Individuals in the intensive treatment arm achieved an HbA1c of 7.0%, compared to a 7.9% HbA1c in the standard treatment group. The UKPDS demonstrated that each percentage point reduction in HbA1c was associated with a 35% reduction in microvascular complications, a 25% reduction in DM-related deaths, and a 7% reduction in all-cause mortality. As in the DCCT, there was a continuous relationship between glycemic control and development of complications. Although there was no statistically significant effect of

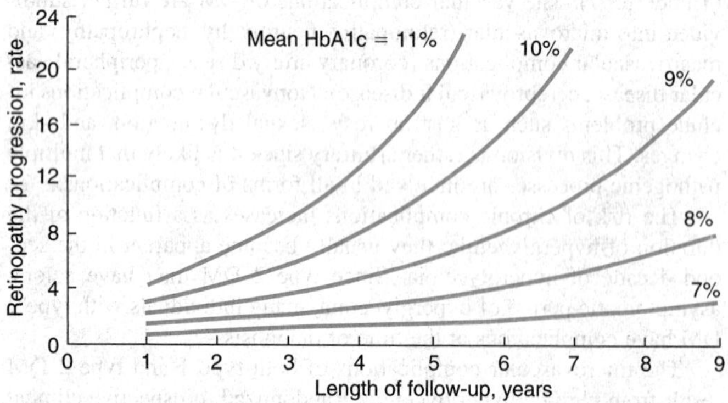

FIGURE 333-8 Relationship of glycemic control and diabetes duration to diabetic retinopathy. The progression of retinopathy in individuals in the Diabetes Control and Complications Trial is graphed as a function of the length of follow-up with different curves for different HbA1c values. *(Adapted from The Diabetes Control and Complications Trial Research Group, Diabetes 44: 968, 1995)*

glycemic control on cardiovascular complications, there was a 16% reduction in fatal and nonfatal myocardial infarctions.

One of the major findings of the UKPDS was the observation that strict blood pressure control significantly reduced both macro- and microvascular complications. In fact, the beneficial effects of blood pressure control were greater than the beneficial effects of glycemic control. Lowering blood pressure to moderate goals (144/82 mmHg) reduced the risk of DM-related death, stroke, microvascular end points, retinopathy, and heart failure (risk reductions between 32 and 56%). Improved glycemic control did not conclusively reduce (nor worsen) cardiovascular mortality but was associated with improvement with lipoprotein risk profiles, such as reduced triglycerides and increased high-density lipoprotein (HDL).

Similar reductions in the risks of retinopathy and nephropathy were also seen in a small trial of lean Japanese individuals with type 2 DM randomized to either intensive glycemic control or standard therapy with insulin (Kumamoto study). These results demonstrate the effectiveness of improved glycemic control in individuals of different ethnicity with a presumably different etiology of DM (i.e., phenotypically different from those in the DCCT and UKPDS).

The findings of the DCCT, UKPDS, and Kumamoto study support the idea that chronic hyperglycemia plays a causative role in the pathogenesis of diabetic microvascular complications. These landmark studies prove the value of metabolic control and emphasize the importance of (1) intensive glycemic control in all forms of DM, and (2) early diagnosis and strict blood pressure control in type 2 DM.

OPHTHALMOLOGIC COMPLICATIONS OF DIABETES MELLITUS DM is the leading cause of blindness between the ages of 20 and 74 in the United States. The gravity of this problem is highlighted by the finding that individuals with DM are 25 times more likely to become legally blind than individuals without DM. Blindness is primarily the result of progressive diabetic retinopathy and clinically significant macular edema. Diabetic retinopathy is classified into two stages: nonproliferative and proliferative. *Nonproliferative diabetic retinopathy* usually appears late in the first decade or early in the second decade of the disease and is marked by retinal vascular microaneurysms, blot hemorrhages, and cotton wool spots **(see Plate IV-15)**. Mild nonproliferative retinopathy progresses to more extensive disease, characterized by changes in venous vessel caliber, intraretinal microvascular abnormalities, and more numerous microaneurysms and hemorrhages. The pathophysiologic mechanisms invoked in nonproliferative retinopathy include loss of retinal pericytes, increased retinal vascular permeability, alterations in retinal blood flow, and abnormal retinal microvasculature, all of which lead to retinal ischemia.

The appearance of neovascularization in response to retinal hypoxia is the hallmark of *proliferative diabetic retinopathy*. These newly formed vessels may appear at the optic nerve and/or macula and rupture easily, leading to vitreous hemorrhage, fibrosis, and ultimately retinal detachment. Not all individuals with nonproliferative retinopathy develop proliferative retinopathy, but the more severe the nonproliferative disease, the greater the chance of evolution to proliferative retinopathy within 5 years. This creates a clear opportunity for early detection and treatment of diabetic retinopathy (discussed below). In contrast, *clinically significant macular edema* may appear when only nonproliferative retinopathy is present. Fluorescein angiography is often useful to detect macular edema, which is associated with a 25% chance of moderate visual loss over the next 3 years.

Duration of DM and degree of glycemic control are the best predictors of the development of retinopathy. Nonproliferative retinopathy is found in almost all individuals who have had DM for >20 years (25% incidence with 5 years, and 80% incidence with 15 years of type 1 DM). Although there is genetic susceptibility for retinopathy, it confers less influence on the development of retinopathy than either the duration of DM or the degree of glycemic control.

℞ TREATMENT The most effective therapy for diabetic retinopathy is prevention. Intensive glycemic control will greatly delay the development or slow the progression of retinopathy in individuals with either type 1 or type 2 DM. Paradoxically, during the first 6 to 12 months of improved glycemic control, established diabetic retinopathy may transiently worsen. Fortunately, this progression is temporary, and in the long term, improved glycemic control is associated with less diabetic retinopathy. Individuals with known retinopathy should be considered candidates for prophylactic photocoagulation when initiating intensive therapy. Once advanced retinopathy is present, improved glycemic control imparts less benefit, though adequate ophthalmologic care can prevent most blindness.

Equally as important as glycemic control are regular, comprehensive eye examinations for all individuals with DM. Most diabetic eye disease can be successfully treated if detected early. Routine, nondilated eye examinations by the primary care provider or diabetes specialist are *inadequate* to detect diabetic eye disease properly. The treatment of diabetic eye disease requires an ophthalmologist experienced in these disorders. Laser photocoagulation is very successful in preserving vision. Proliferative retinopathy is usually treated with panretinal laser photocoagulation, whereas macular edema is treated with focal laser photocoagulation. Although exercise has not been conclusively shown to worsen proliferative diabetic retinopathy, most ophthalmologists advise individuals with advanced diabetic eye disease to limit physical activities associated with repeated Valsalva maneuvers. Aspirin therapy (650 mg/d) does not appear to influence the natural history of diabetic retinopathy, but studies of other antiplatelet agents are under way.

RENAL COMPLICATIONS OF DIABETES MELLITUS Diabetic nephropathy is the leading cause of ESRD in the United States and a leading cause of DM-related morbidity and mortality. Proteinuria in individuals with DM is associated with markedly reduced survival and increased risk of cardiovascular disease. Individuals with diabetic nephropathy almost always have diabetic retinopathy also.

Like other microvascular complications, the pathogenesis of diabetic nephropathy is related to chronic hyperglycemia (Fig. 334-7). The mechanisms by which chronic hyperglycemia leads to ESRD, though incompletely defined, involve the following: interaction of soluble factors (growth factors, angiotensin II, endothelin, AGEs), hemodynamic alterations in the renal microcirculation (glomerular hyperfiltration, increased glomerular capillary pressure), and structural changes in the glomerulus (increased extracellular matrix, basement membrane thickening, mesangial expansion, fibrosis). Some of these effects may be mediated through angiotensin receptors. Smoking accelerates the decline in renal function.

The natural history of diabetic nephropathy is shown schematically in Fig. 333-9 and is characterized by a fairly predictable pattern of events. Although this sequence of events was defined for individuals with type 1 DM, a similar pattern is also likely in type 2 DM. Glomerular hyperfusion and renal hypertrophy occur in the first years after the onset of DM and are reflected by an increased glomerular filtration rate (GFR). During the first 5 years of DM, thickening of the glomerular basement membrane, glomerular hypertrophy, and mesangial volume expansion occur as the GFR returns to normal. After 5 to 10 years of type 1 DM, ~40% of individuals begin to excrete small amounts of albumin in the urine (microalbuminuria). *Microalbuminuria* is defined as 30 to 300 mg/d in a 24-h collection or 30 to 300 μg/mg creatinine in a spot collection. The appearance of microalbuminuria (incipient nephropathy) in type 1 DM is a very important predictor of progression to overt proteinuria (>300 mg/d). Blood pressure may rise slightly at this point but usually remains in the normal range. Once overt proteinuria is present, there is a steady decline in GFR, and ~50% of individuals reach ESRD in 7 to 10 years. The early pathologic changes and albumin excretion abnormalities are reversible with normalization of plasma glucose. However, once nephropathy becomes overt, the pathologic changes are likely irreversible.

The nephropathy that develops in type 2 DM differs from that of

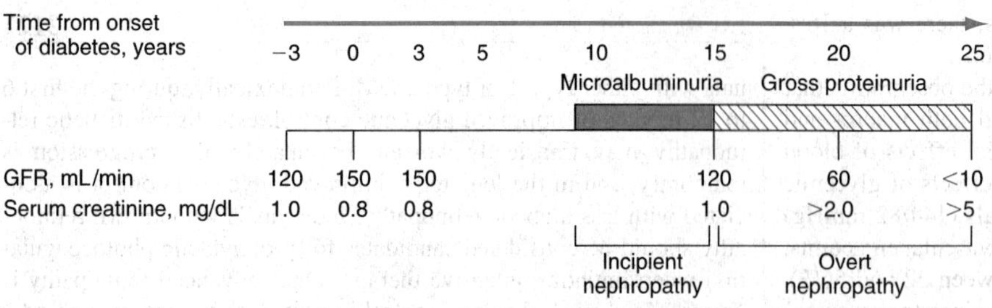

FIGURE 333-9 Time course of development of diabetic nephropathy. The relationship of time from onset of diabetes, the glomerular filtration rate (GFR), and the serum creatinine are shown. *(Adapted from DeFronzo RA, in Therapy for Diabetes Mellitus and Related Disorders, 1998)*

phase of declining renal function, insulin requirements may fall as the kidney is a site of insulin degradation. Furthermore, glucose-lowering medications (sulfonylureas and metformin) may accumulate and are contraindicated in renal insufficiency.

Many individuals with type 1 or type 2 DM develop hypertension. Numerous studies in both type 1 and type 2 DM demonstrate the effectiveness of strict blood pressure control in reducing albumin excretion and slowing the decline in renal function. Blood pressure should be maintained at <130/85 mmHg in diabetic individuals without proteinuria. A slightly lower blood pressure (120/80) should be targeted for individuals with microalbuminuria or overt nephropathy. Treatment of hypertension is discussed below.

type 1 DM in the following respects: (1) microalbuminuria or overt nephropathy may be present when type 2 DM is diagnosed, reflecting its long asymptomatic period; (2) hypertension more commonly accompanies microalbuminuria or overt nephropathy in type 2 DM; and (3) microalbuminuria may be less predictive of progression to overt nephropathy in type 2 DM. Finally, it should be noted that albuminuria in type 2 DM may be secondary to factors unrelated to DM, such as hypertension, congestive heart failure, prostate disease, or infection.

Other renal problems may also occur in individuals with DM. Type IV renal tubular acidosis (hyporeninemic hypoaldosteronism) occurs in many individuals with DM. These individuals develop a propensity to hyperkalemia, which may be exacerbated by medications [especially angiotensin-converting enzyme (ACE) inhibitors]. Patients with DM are predisposed to radiocontrast-induced nephrotoxicity. Individuals with DM undergoing radiographic procedures with contrast dye should be well hydrated before and after dye exposure, and the serum creatinine should be monitored for several days following the procedure.

℞ **TREATMENT** The optimal therapy for diabetic nephropathy is prevention. As part of comprehensive diabetes care, microalbuminuria should be detected at an early stage when effective therapies can be instituted. The recommended strategy for detecting microalbuminuria is outlined in Fig. 333-10. Interventions effective in slowing progression from microalbuminuria to overt nephropathy include: (1) near normalization of glycemia, (2) strict blood pressure control, and (3) administration of ACE inhibitors.

Improved glycemic control reduces the rate at which microalbuminuria appears and progresses in both type 1 and type 2 DM. However, once overt nephropathy exists, it is unclear whether improved glycemic control will slow progression of renal disease. During the

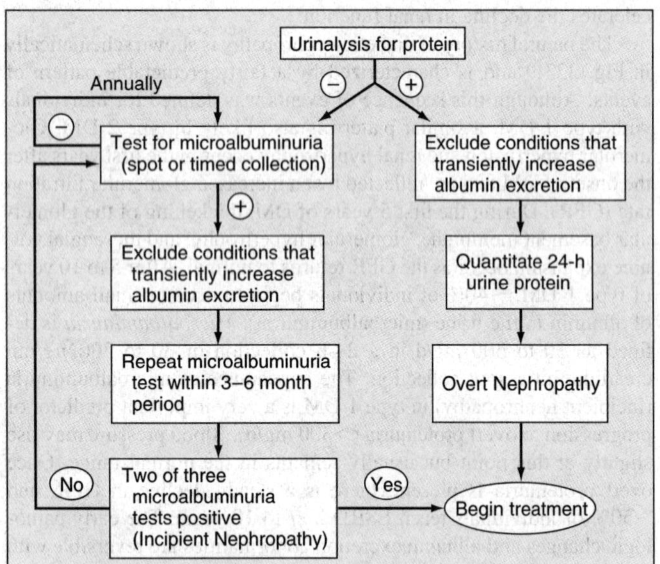

FIGURE 333-10 Screening for microalbuminuria. *(Adapted from DeFronzo RA, in Therapy for Diabetes Mellitus and Related Disorders, 1998)*

ACE inhibitors reduce the progression of overt nephropathy in individuals with type 1 or type 2 DM and should be prescribed in individuals with type 1 or type 2 DM and microalbuminuria. After 2 to 3 months of therapy, measurement of proteinuria should be repeated and the drug dose increased until either the albuminuria disappears or the maximum dose is reached. If an ACE inhibitor has an unacceptable side-effect profile (hyperkalemia, cough, and renal insufficiency), angiotensin II receptor blockers and calcium channel blockers (phenylalkylamine class) are alternatives. However, their efficacy in slowing the fall in glomerular filtration rate is not proven. Blood pressure control with any agent is extremely important, but a drug-specific benefit in diabetic nephropathy, independent of blood pressure control, has been shown only for ACE inhibitors.

A consensus panel of the American Diabetes Association (ADA) suggests modest restriction of protein intake in diabetic individuals with microalbuminuria (0.8 g/kg per day, which is the adult Recommended Daily Allowance, and about 10% of the daily caloric intake). Protein intake should be restricted further in individuals with overt diabetic nephropathy (0.6 g/kg per day), though conclusive proof of the efficacy of protein restriction is lacking.

Nephrology consultation should be considered after the diagnosis of early nephropathy. Once overt nephropathy ensues, the likelihood of ESRD is very high. As compared to nondiabetic individuals, hemodialysis in patients with DM is associated with more frequent complications, such as hypotension (autonomic neuropathy, loss of reflex tachycardia), more difficult vascular access, and accelerated progression of retinopathy. Survival after the onset of ESRD is shorter in the diabetic population compared to nondiabetics with similar clinical features. Atherosclerosis is the leading cause of death in diabetic individuals on dialysis, and hyperlipidemia should be aggressively treated. Renal transplantation from a living-related donor is the preferred therapy but requires chronic immunosuppression. Combined pancreas-kidney transplant offers the promise of normoglycemia but requires substantial expertise.

NEUROPATHY AND DIABETES MELLITUS Diabetic neuropathy occurs in approximately 50% of individuals with long-standing type 1 and type 2 DM. It may manifest as polyneuropathy, mononeuropathy, and/or autonomic neuropathy. As with other complications of DM, the development of neuropathy correlates with the duration of diabetes and glycemic control. Because the clinical features of diabetic neuropathy are similar to those of other neuropathies, the diagnosis of *diabetic* neuropathy should be made only after other possible etiologies are excluded (Chap. 378).

Polyneuropathy/Mononeuropathy The most common form of diabetic neuropathy is distal symmetric *polyneuropathy*. It most frequently presents with distal sensory loss. Hyperesthesia, parathesia, and pain also occur. Any combination of these symptoms may develop as neuropathy progresses. Physical examination reveals sensory loss, loss of ankle reflexes, and abnormal position sense. Parethesia is characteristically perceived as a sensation of numbness, tingling, sharpness, or burning that begins in the feet and spreads proximally. Neuropathic pain develops in some of these individuals, occasionally preceded by improvement in their glycemic control. Pain typically involves the lower extremities, is usually present at rest, and worsens at night. Both an acute (lasting <12 months) and a chronic form of painful diabetic neuropathy have been described. As diabetic neuropathy progresses, the pain subsides and eventually disappears, and a sensory deficit in the lower extremities persists.

Diabetic polyradiculopathy is a syndrome characterized by severe disabling pain in the distribution of one or more nerve roots. It may be accompanied by motor weakness. Intercostal or truncal radiculopathy causes pain over the thorax or abdomen. Involvement of the lumbar plexus or femoral nerve may cause pain in the thigh or hip and may be associated with muscle weakness in the hip flexors or extensors (diabetic amyotrophy). Fortunately, diabetic polyradiculopathies are usually self-limited and resolve over 6 to 12 months.

Mononeuropathy (dysfunction of isolated cranial or peripheral nerves) is less common than polyneuropathy in DM and presents with pain and motor weakness in the distribution of a single nerve. A vascular etiology is favored, but the pathogenesis is unknown. Involvement of the third cranial nerve is most common and is heralded by diplopia. Physical examination reveals ptosis and opthalmoplegia with normal papillary constriction to light. Sometimes cranial nerves IV, VI, or VII (Bell's palsy) are affected. Peripheral mononeuropathies or simultaneous involvement of more than one nerve (mononeuropathy multiplex) may also occur.

Autonomic Neuropathy Individuals with long-standing type 1 or 2 DM may develop signs of autonomic dysfunction involving the cholinergic, noradrenergic, and peptidergic (peptides such as pancreatic polypeptide, substance P, etc.) systems. DM-related autonomic neuropathy can involve multiple systems, including: the cardiovascular, gastrointestinal, genitourinary, sudomotor, and metabolic systems. Autonomic neuropathies affecting the cardiovascular system cause a resting tachycardia and orthostatic hypotension. Reports of sudden death have also been attributed to autonomic neuropathy. Gastroparesis and bladder-emptying abnormalities are also likely related to the autonomic neuropathy seen in DM (discussed below). Hyperhidrosis of the upper extremities and anhidrosis of the lower extremities result from sympathetic nervous system dysfunction. Anhidrosis of the feet can promote dry skin with cracking, which increases the risk of skin ulceration. Autonomic neuropathy may reduce counterregulatory hormone release, leading to an inability to sense hypoglycemia appropriately (*hypoglycemia unawareness*; Chap. 334), thereby subjecting the patient to the risk of severe hypoglycemia and complicating efforts to improve glycemic control.

℞ TREATMENT Treatment of diabetic neuropathy is less than satisfactory. Improved glycemic control should be pursued and will improve nerve conduction velocity, but the symptoms of diabetic neuropathy may not necessarily improve. Efforts to improve glycemic control may be confounded by autonomic neuropathy and hypoglycemia unawareness. Avoidance of neurotoxins (alcohol), supplementation with vitamins for possible deficiencies (B_{12}, B_6, folate; Chap. 75), and symptomatic treatment are the mainstays of therapy. Aldose reductase inhibitors do not currently offer significant symptomatic relief. Loss of sensation in the foot places the patient at risk for ulceration and its sequelae; consequently, prevention of such problems is of paramount importance. Since the pain of acute diabetic neuropathy may resolve over the first year, analgesics may be discontinued as progressive neuronal damage from DM occurs. Chronic, painful diabetic neuropathy is difficult to treat but may respond to tricyclic antidepressants (amitriptyline, desipramine, nortriptyline), gabapentin, nonsteroidal anti-inflammatory agents (avoid in renal dysfunction), and other agents (mexilitine, phenytoin, carbamazepine, capsaicin cream). Referral to a pain management center may be necessary.

Therapy of orthostatic hypotension secondary to autonomic neuropathy is difficult. A variety of agents have limited success (fludrocortisone, midodrine, clonidine, octreotide, and yohimbine) but have significant side effects. Nonpharmacologic maneuvers (adequate salt intake, avoidance of dehydration and diuretics, and lower extremity support hose) may offer some benefit.

GASTROINTESTINAL/GENITOURINARY DYSFUNCTION Long-standing type 1 and 2 DM may affect the motility and function of gastrointestinal (GI) and genitourinary systems. The most prominent GI symptoms are delayed gastric emptying (gastroparesis) and altered small- and large-bowel motility (constipation or diarrhea). *Gastroparesis* may present with symptoms of anorexia, nausea, vomiting, early satiety, and abdominal bloating. Nuclear medicine scintigraphy after ingestion of a radiolabeled meal is the best study to document delayed gastric emptying, but noninvasive "breath tests" following ingestion of a radiolabeled meal are under development. Though parasympathetic dysfunction secondary to chronic hyperglycemia is important in the development of gastroparesis, hyperglycemia itself also impairs gastric emptying. Nocturnal diarrhea, alternating with constipation, is a common feature of DM-related GI autonomic neuropathy. In type 1 DM, these symptoms should also prompt evaluation for celiac sprue because of its increased frequency. Esophageal dysfunction in long-standing DM is common but usually asymptomatic.

Diabetic autonomic neuropathy may lead to genitourinary dysfunction including cystopathy, erectile dysfunction, and female sexual dysfunction (reduced sexual desire, dyspareunia, reduced vaginal lubrication). Symptoms of diabetic cystopathy begin with an inability to sense a full bladder and a failure to void completely (Chap. 48). As bladder contractility worsens, bladder capacity and the postvoid residual increase, leading to symptoms of urinary hesitancy, decreased voiding frequency, incontinence, and recurrent urinary tract infections. Diagnostic evaluation includes cystometry and urodynamic studies.

Erectile dysfunction and retrograde ejaculation are very common in DM and may be one of the earliest signs of diabetic neuropathy. Erectile dysfunction, which increases in frequency with the age of the patient and the duration of diabetes, may occur in the absence of other signs of diabetic autonomic neuropathy.

℞ TREATMENT Current treatments for these complications of DM are inadequate. Improved glycemic control should be a primary goal, as some aspects (neuropathy, gastric function) may improve as near-normoglycemia is achieved. Smaller, more frequent meals that are easier to digest (liquid) and low in fat and fiber may minimize symptoms of gastroparesis. Cisapride (10 to 20 mg before each meal) is probably the most effective medication but has been removed from use in the U.S. market except under special circumstances. Other agents with some efficacy include dopamine agonists (metoclopramide, 5 to 10 mg, and domperidone, 10 to 20 mg, before each meal) and bethanechol (10 to 20 mg before each meal). Erythromycin interacts with the motilin receptor and may promote gastric emptying. Diabetic diarrhea in the absence of bacterial overgrowth is treated symptomatically with loperamide but may respond to clonidine at higher doses (0.6 mg tid) or octreotide (50 to 75 μg tid subcutaneously). Treatment of bacterial overgrowth with antibiotics is sometimes useful (Chap. 286).

Diabetic cystopathy should be treated with timed voiding or self-catherization. Medications (bethanechol) are inconsistently effective. The drug of choice for erectile dysfunction is sildenafil, but the efficacy in individuals with DM is slightly lower than in the nondiabetic population (Chap. 51). Sexual dysfunction in women may be improved with use of vaginal lubricants, treatment of vaginal infections, and systemic or local estrogen replacement.

CARDIOVASCULAR MORBIDITY AND MORTALITY Cardiovascular disease is increased in individuals with type 1 or type 2 DM. The Framingham Heart Study revealed a marked increase in several cardiovascular diseases in DM including peripheral vascular disease, congestive heart failure, coronary artery disease, myocardial infarction, and sudden death (risk increase from one- to fivefold). The American Heart Association recently designated DM as a major risk factor for cardiovascular disease (same category as smoking, hypertension, and hyperlipidemia). Because of the extremely high frequency of underlying cardiovascular disease in individuals with diabetes (especially in type 2 DM), evidence of atherosclerotic vascular disease should be sought in the individual with diabetes who has symptoms suggestive of cardiac ischemia, peripheral or carotid arterial disease, a resting electrocardiogram indicative of prior infarction, plans to initiate an exercise program, proteinuria, or two other cardiac risk factors (ADA recommendations). The absence of chest pain ("silent ischemia") is common in individuals with diabetes, and a thorough cardiac evaluation is indicated in individuals undergoing major surgical procedures.

The increase in morbidity and mortality appears to relate to the synergism of hyperglycemia with other cardiovascular risk factors. For example, after controlling for all known cardiovascular risk factors, type 2 DM increases the cardiovascular death rate by twofold in men and fourfold in women. Risk factors for macrovascular disease in diabetic individuals include dyslipidemia, hypertension, obesity, reduced physical activity, and cigarette smoking. Additional risk factors specific to the diabetic population include microalbuminuria, gross proteinuria, an elevation in serum creatinine, and altered platelet function. Insulin resistance, as reflected by elevated serum insulin levels, is associated with an increased risk of cardiovascular complications in individuals with and without DM. Individuals with insulin resistance and type 2 DM have elevated levels of plasminogen activator inhibitors (especially PAI-1) and fibrinogen, which enhances the coagulation process and impairs fibrinolysis, thus favoring the development of thrombosis.

Despite proof that improved glycemic control reduces microvascular complications in DM, it is possible that macrovascular complications may be unaffected or even worsened by such therapy. Concerns about the anabolic and atherogenic potential of insulin remain, since in nondiabetic individuals, higher serum insulin levels (indicative of insulin resistance) are associated with a greater risk of cardiovascular morbidity and mortality. In the DCCT, the number of cardiovascular events did not differ between the standard and intensively treated groups. However, the duration of DM in these individuals was relatively short, and the total number of events was very low. An improvement in the lipid profile of individuals in the intensive group [lower total and low-density lipoprotein (LDL) cholesterol, lower triglycerides] suggested that intensive therapy may reduce the risk of cardiovascular morbidity and mortality associated with DM. In the UKPDS, improved glycemic control did not conclusively reduce cardiovascular mortality. Importantly, treatment with insulin and the sulfonylureas did not appear to increase the risk of cardiovascular disease in individuals with type 2 DM, refuting prior claims about the atherogenic potential of these agents.

In addition to coronary artery disease, cerebrovascular disease is increased in individuals with DM (threefold increase in stroke). Individuals with DM have an increased incidence of congestive heart failure (diabetic cardiomyopathy). The etiology of this abnormality is probably multifactorial and includes factors such as myocardial ischemia from atherosclerosis, hypertension, and myocardial cell dysfunction secondary to chronic hyperglycemia.

℞ **TREATMENT** In general, the treatment of coronary disease is no different in the diabetic individual (Chap. 244), though overall prognosis after myocardial infarction is worse in the diabetic population. Revascularization procedures for coronary artery disease, including percutaneous transluminal coronary angioplasty (PTCA) and coronary artery bypass grafting (CABG), are less efficacious in the diabetic individual. Initial success rates of PTCA in diabetic individuals are similar to those in the nondiabetic population, but diabetic patients have higher rates of restenosis and lower long-term patency and survival rates. Perioperative mortality from CABG is not altered in DM, but both short- and long-term survival are reduced. Recent trials indicate that diabetic individuals with multivessel coronary artery disease or who recently suffered a Q-wave myocardial infarction have better long-term survival with CABG than PTCA.

Results of studies investigating the effect of intensive diabetes management on survival rates and cardiovascular events after myocardial infarction have been conflicting. In the face of conflicting data, the ADA has emphasized the importance of glycemic control and aggressive cardiovascular risk modification in all individuals with DM. Despite past trepidation about using beta blockers in individuals who have diabetes, these agents clearly benefit diabetic patients after myocardial infarction, analogous to the benefit in nondiabetic individuals. ACE inhibitors may also be particularly beneficial in reducing mortality after myocardial infarction in patients with DM.

Antiplatelet therapy reduces cardiovascular events in individuals with DM who have coronary artery disease. Current recommendations by the ADA suggest the use of aspirin as secondary prevention of additional coronary events. Although data demonstrating efficacy in primary prevention of coronary events are lacking, antiplatelet therapy should be considered, especially in diabetic individuals with other coronary risk factors such as hypertension, smoking, or hyperlipidemia. The aspirin dose (81 to 325 mg) is the same as that in nondiabetic individuals. Aspirin therapy does not have detrimental effects on renal function or hypertension, nor does it influence the course of diabetic retinopathy or maculopathy.

Cardiovascular Risk Factors • ***Dyslipidemia*** Individuals with DM may have several forms of dyslipidemia (Chap. 344). Because of the additive cardiovascular risk of hyperglycemia and hyperlipidemia, lipid abnormalities should be aggressively detected and treated as part of comprehensive diabetes care (Fig. 333-11). The most common pattern of dyslipidemia is hypertriglyceridemia and reduced HDL cholesterol levels. DM itself does not increase levels of LDL, but the small dense LDL particles found in type 2 DM are more atherogenic because they are more easily glycated and susceptible to oxidation.

According to guidelines of the ADA and the American Heart Association, the lipid profile in diabetic individuals without cardiovascular disease (primary prevention) should be: LDL < 3.4 mmol/L (130 mg/dL); HDL > 0.9 mmol/L (35 mg/dL) in men and >1.2 mmol/L

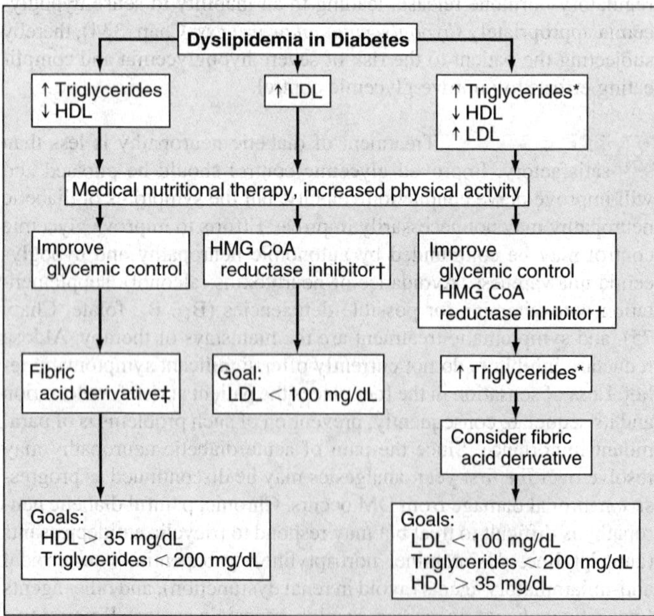

FIGURE 333-11 Dyslipidemia management in diabetes. *Triglycerides increased but <400 mg/dL. †Second line treatment: fibric acid derivative or bile acid–binding resin. ‡Alternative treatment: high dose HMG CoA reductase inhibitor. The level of HDL in women should be 10 mg/dl higher.

(45 mg/dL) in women; and triglycerides < 2.3 mmol/L (200 mg/dL). In diabetic individuals with cardiovascular disease, the LDL goal is < 2.6 mmol/L (100 mg/dL). Because of the risk of cardiovascular disease in diabetic individuals, many authorities recommend that optimal lipid levels for all individuals with DM (with or without cardiovascular disease) should be: LDL < 2.6 mmol/L (100 mg/dL), HDL > 1.15 mmol/L (45 mg/dL) in men and > 1.41 mmol/L (55 mg/dL) in women; and triglycerides < 2.3 mmol/L (200 mg/dL). The ADA recommends dietary modification in diabetic individuals without cardiovascular disease and a LDL cholesterol of 2.6 to 3.3 mmol/L (100 to 129 mg/dL). If multiple cardiovascular risk factors are present, the goal should be a LDL < 2.6 mmol/L (100 mg/dL) even without known cardiovascular disease.

Almost all studies of diabetic dyslipidemia have been performed in individuals with type 2 DM because of the greater frequency of dyslipidemia in this form of diabetes. Interventional studies have shown that the beneficial effects of LDL reduction are similar in the diabetic and nondiabetic populations. Large prospective trials of primary and secondary intervention for coronary heart disease have included a small number of individuals with type 2 DM, and subset analyses have consistently found that reductions in LDL reduce cardiovascular events and morbidity in individuals with DM. Most clinical trials used HMG CoA reductase inhibitors, although a fibric acid derivative was also beneficial in one trial. No prospective studies have addressed similar questions in individuals with type 1 DM.

Based on the guidelines provided by the ADA and the American Heart Association, the order of priorities in the treatment of hyperlipidemia is: (1) lower the LDL cholesterol, (2) raise the HDL cholesterol, and (3) decrease the triglycerides. A treatment strategy depends on the pattern of lipoprotein abnormalities (Fig. 333-11). Initial therapy for all forms of dyslipidemia should include dietary changes, as well as the same life-style modifications recommended in the nondiabetic population (smoking cessation, control of blood pressure, weight loss, increased physical activity). The dietary recommendations for individuals with DM are similar to those advocated by the National Cholesterol Education Program (Chap. 344) and include an increase in monounsaturated fat and carbohydrates and a reduction in saturated fats and cholesterol. Though viewed as important, the response to dietary alterations is often modest [<0.6-mmol/L (<25-mg/dL) reduction in the LDL]. Improvement in glycemic control will lower triglycerides and have a modest beneficial effect on raising HDL. Most medications that improve glycemic control are useful in lowering triglycerides and may raise the HDL slightly. Though fibric acid derivatives have some efficacy and are well tolerated, nicotinic acid may worsen glycemic control and increase insulin resistance; thus, niacin is relatively contraindicated in diabetic patients on oral glucose-lowering agents. As noted above, HMG CoA reductase inhibitors have proven benefit in patients with DM, even with modest elevations in LDL. Combination therapy with an HMG CoA reductase inhibitor and fibric acid derivative may be useful but increases the possibility of myositis. Bile acid–binding resins should not be used if hypertriglyceridemia is present.

Hypertension Hypertension can accelerate other complications of DM, particularly cardiovascular disease and nephropathy. Hypertension therapy should first emphasize life-style modifications such as weight loss, exercise, stress management, and sodium restriction (Chap. 35). Antihypertensive agents should be selected based on the advantages and disadvantages of the therapeutic agent in the context of an individual patient's risk factor profile. ACE inhibitors are glucose- and lipid-neutral and thus positively impact the cardiovascular risk profile. For example, captopril actually improves insulin resistance, reduces LDL slightly, and increases HDL slightly. In one study of nondiabetic individuals, the ACE inhibitor ramipril reduced the risk of developing type 2 DM. Other effective agents include α-adrenergic blockers (prazocin, terazosin, doxazosin), calcium channel blockers, beta blockers (both β_1 selective and nonselective), thiazide diuretics (hydrochlorothiazide and its derivatives), central adrenergic antagonists (clonidine, methyldopa), and vasodilators (minoxidil, hydralazine). DM-related considerations include the following:

1. α-Adrenergic blockers slightly improve insulin resistance and positively impact the lipid profile, whereas beta blockers and thiazide diuretics can increase insulin resistance, negatively impact the lipid profile, and slightly increase the risk of developing type 2 diabetes.
2. Beta blockers, often questioned because of the potential masking of hypoglycemic symptoms, are effective agents and hypoglycemic events are rare when cardioselective (β_1) agents are used.
3. Central adrenergic antagonists and vasodilators are lipid- and glucose-neutral.
4. Sympathetic inhibitors and α-adrenergic blockers may be associated with orthostatic hypotension in the diabetic individual with autonomic neuropathy.
5. Calcium channel blockers are glucose- and lipid-neutral, and some evidence suggests that they reduce cardiovascular morbidity and mortality in type 2 DM, particularly in elderly patients with systolic hypertension.

If microalbuminuria or overt albuminuria is present, the optimal antihypertensive agent is an ACE inhibitor. If albumin excretion is normal, then an ACE inhibitor or other antihypertensive agent may be used. Low-dose diuretics and beta blockers are sometimes preferred as initial agents because of their clear efficacy in the nondiabetic population. Since hypertension is often difficult to control with a single agent (especially in type 2 DM), multiple antihypertensive agents are usually required when blood pressure goals (<130/85 mmHg) are not achieved. In this setting, long-acting calcium channel antagonists should be considered as additional, or second-line, agents, as these drugs appear to provide protection against cardiovascular events. ACE inhibitors are contraindicated in pregnant diabetic patients and those anticipating pregnancy. Because of the high prevalence of atherosclerotic disease in individuals with DM, the possibility of renovascular hypertension should be considered when the blood pressure is not readily controlled.

LOWER EXTREMITY COMPLICATIONS DM is the leading cause of nontraumatic lower extremity amputation in the United States. Foot ulcers and infections are also a major source of morbidity in individuals with DM. The reasons for the increased incidence of these disorders in DM are complex and involve the interaction of several pathogenic factors: neuropathy, abnormal foot biomechanics, peripheral vascular disease, and poor wound healing. The peripheral sensory neuropathy interferes with normal protective mechanisms and allows the patient to sustain major or repeated minor trauma to the foot, often without knowledge of the injury. Disordered proprioception causes abnormal weight bearing while walking and subsequent formation of callus or ulceration. Motor and sensory neuropathy leads to abnormal foot muscle mechanics and to structural changes in the foot (hammer toe, claw toe deformity, prominent metatarsal heads). Autonomic neuropathy results in anhidrosis and altered superficial blood flow in the foot, which promote drying of the skin and fissure formation. Peripheral vascular disease and poor wound healing impede resolution of minor breaks in the skin, allowing them to enlarge and to become infected.

Approximately 15% of individuals with DM develop a foot ulcer, and a significant subset of those individuals will at some time undergo amputation (14 to 24% risk with that ulcer or subsequent ulceration). Risk factors for foot ulcers or amputation include: male sex, diabetes >10 years' duration, peripheral neuropathy, abnormal structure of foot (bony abnormalities, callus, thickened nails), peripheral vascular disease, smoking, and history of previous ulcer or amputation. Glycemic control is also a risk factor—each 2% increase in the HbA1c increases the risk of a lower extremity ulcer by 1.6 times and the risk of lower extremity amputation by 1.5 times.

℞ **TREATMENT** The optimal therapy for foot ulcers and amputations is prevention through identification of high-risk patients, education of the patient, and institution of measures to prevent ulceration. High-risk patients should be identified during the routine foot examination performed on all patients with DM (see "Ongoing Aspects of Comprehensive Diabetes Care," below). Patient education should emphasize: (1) careful selection of footwear, (2) daily inspection of the feet to detect early signs of poor-fitting footwear or minor trauma, (3) daily foot hygiene to keep the skin clean and moist, (4) avoidance of self-treatment of foot abnormalities and high-risk behavior (e.g., walking barefoot), and (5) prompt consultation with a health care provider if an abnormality arises. Patients at high risk for ulceration or amputation may benefit from evaluation by a foot care specialist. Interventions directed at risk factor modification include orthotic shoes and devices, callus management, nail care, and prophylactic measures to reduce increased skin pressure from abnormal bony architecture. Attention to other risk factors for vascular disease (smoking, dyslipidemia, hypertension) and improved glycemic control are also important.

Despite preventive measures, foot ulceration and infection are common and represent a potentially serious problem. Due to the multifactorial pathogenesis of lower extremity ulcers, management of these lesions must be multidisciplinary and often demands expertise in orthopedics, vascular surgery, endocrinology, podiatry, and infectious diseases. The plantar surface of the foot is the most common site of ulceration. Cellulitis without ulceration is also frequent and should be treated with antibiotics that provide broad-spectrum coverage, including anaerobes (see below).

An infected ulcer is a clinical diagnosis, since superficial culture of any ulceration will likely find multiple possible bacterial pathogens. The infection surrounding the foot ulcer is often the result of multiple organisms (gram-positive and -negative cocci and anaerobes), and gas gangrene may develop in the absence of clostridial infection. Cultures taken from the debrided ulcer base or from purulent drainage are most helpful. Wound depth should be determined by inspection and probing with a blunt-tipped sterile instrument. Plain radiographs of the foot should be performed to assess the possibility of osteomyelitis in chronic ulcers that have not responded to therapy. Nuclear medicine bone scans may be helpful, but overlying subcutaneous infection is often difficult to distinguish from osteomyelitis. Indium-labeled white cell studies are more useful in determining if the infection involves bony structures or only soft tissue, but they are technically demanding. Magnetic resonance imaging of the foot may be the most specific modality, although distinguishing bony destruction due to osteomyelitis from destruction secondary to Charcot arthropathy is difficult. If surgical debridement is necessary, bone biopsy and culture usually provide the answer.

Osteomyelitis is best treated by a combination of prolonged antibiotics and debridement of infected bone. The possible contribution of vascular insufficiency should be considered in all patients. Noninvasive blood-flow studies are often unreliable in DM, and angiography may be required, recognizing the risk of contrast-induced nephrotoxicity. Peripheral vascular bypass procedures are often effective in promoting wound resolution and in decreasing the need for amputation of the ischemic limb.

A growing number of possible treatments for diabetic foot ulcers exist, but they have yet to demonstrate clear efficacy in prospective, controlled trials. A recent consensus statement from the ADA identified six interventions with demonstrated efficacy in diabetic foot wounds: (1) off-loading, (2) debridement, (3) wound dressings, (4) appropriate use of antibiotics, (5) revascularization, and (6) limited amputation. Off-loading is the complete avoidance of weight bearing on the ulcer, which removes the mechanical trauma that retards wound healing. Bed rest and a variety of orthotic devices limit weight bearing on wounds or pressure points. Surgical debridement of neuropathic wounds is important and effective, but clear efficacy of other modalities for wound cleaning (enzymes, soaking, whirlpools) is lacking. Dressings promote wound healing by creating a moist environment and protecting the wound. Antiseptic agents and topical antibiotics should be avoided. Referral for physical therapy, orthotic evaluation, and rehabilitation may be useful once the infection is controlled.

Mild or non-limb-threatening infections can be treated with oral antibiotics (cephalosporin, clindamycin, amoxicillin/clavulanate, and fluoroquinolones), surgical debridement of necrotic tissue, local wound care (avoidance of weight bearing over the ulcer), and close surveillance for progression of infection. More severe ulcers may require intravenous antibiotics as well as bed rest and local wound care. Urgent surgical debridement may be required. Intravenous antibiotics should provide broad-spectrum coverage directed toward *Staphylococcus aureus*, streptococci, gram-negative aerobes, and anaerobic bacteria. Initial antimicrobial regimens include cefotetan, ampicillin/sulbactam, or the combination of clindamycin and a fluoroquinolone. Severe infections, or infections that do not improve after 48 h of antibiotic therapy, require expansion of antimicrobial therapy to treat methicillin-resistant *S. aureus* (e.g., vancomycin) and *Pseudomonas aeruginosa*. If the infection surrounding the ulcer is not improving with intravenous antibiotics, reassessment of antibiotic coverage and reconsideration of the need for surgical debridement or revascularization are indicated. With clinical improvement, oral antibiotics and local wound care can be continued on an outpatient basis with close follow-up. As infection improves, a comprehensive assessment of modifiable risk factors for foot ulceration should be performed and should involve health professionals with expertise in podiatry, orthotics, vascular surgery, and orthopedics.

New information about wound biology has led to a number of new technologies (e.g., living skin equivalents and growth factors such as basic fibroblast growth factor) that may prove useful. Recombinant platelet-derived growth factor has some benefit and complements the basic therapies of off-loading, debridement, and antibiotics. Hyperbaric oxygen has been used, but rigorous proof of efficacy is lacking.

INFECTIONS Individuals with DM exhibit a greater frequency and severity of infection. The reasons for this increase include incompletely defined abnormalities in cell-mediated immunity and phagocyte function associated with hyperglycemia, as well as diminished vascularization secondary to long-standing diabetes. Hyperglycemia likely aids the colonization and growth of a variety of organisms (*Candida* and other fungal species). Many common infections are more frequent and severe in the diabetic population, whereas several rare infections are seen almost exclusively in the diabetic population. Examples of this latter category includes rhinocerebral mucormycosis and malignant otitis externa, which is usually secondary to *P. aeruginosa* infection in the soft tissue surrounding the external auditory canal. Malignant otitis externa begins with pain and discharge and may progress rapidly to osteomyelitis and meningitis. These infections should be sought, in particular, in patients presenting with NKHS.

Pneumonia, urinary tract infections, and skin and soft tissue infections are all more common in the diabetic population. In general, the organisms that cause pulmonary infections are similar to those found in the nondiabetic population; however, gram-negative organisms, *S. aureus*, and *Mycobacterium tuberculosis* are more frequent pathogens. Urinary tract infections (either lower tract or pyelonephritis) are the result of common bacterial agents such as *Escherichia coli*, though several yeast species (*Candida* and *Torulopsis glabrata*) are commonly observed. Complications of urinary tract infections include emphysematous pyelonephritis and emphysematous cystitis. Bacteriuria occurs frequently in individuals with diabetic cystopathy. Susceptibility to furunculosis, superficial candidal infections, and vulvovaginitis is increased. Poor glycemic control is a common denominator in individuals with these infections. Diabetic individuals have an increased rate of colonization of *S. aureus* in the skin folds and nares. Diabetic patients also have a greater risk of postoperative wound infections.

DERMATOLOGIC MANIFESTATIONS The most common skin manifestations of DM are protracted wound healing and skin ulcerations. Diabetic dermopathy, sometimes termed *pigmented pretibial papules*, or "diabetic skin spots," begins as an erythematous area and evolves into an area of circular hyperpigmentation. These lesions result from minor mechanical trauma in the pretibial region and are more common in elderly men with DM. Bullous diseases (shallow ulcerations or erosions in the pretibial region) are also seen. *Necrobiosis lipoidica diabeticorum* is a rare disorder of DM that predominantly affects young women with type 1 DM, neuropathy, and retinopathy. It usually begins in the pretibial region as an erythematous plaque or papules that gradually enlarge, darken, and develop irregular margins, with atrophic centers and central ulceration. They may be painful. *Acanthosis nigricans* (hyperpigmented velvety plaques seen on the neck or extensor surfaces) is sometimes a feature of severe insulin resistance and accompanying diabetes. Generalized or localized *granuloma annulare* (erythematous plaques on the extremities or trunk) and *scleredema* (areas of skin thickening on the back or neck at the site of previous superficial infections) are more common in the diabetic population. *Lipoatrophy* and *lipohypertrophy* can occur at insulin injection sites but are unusual with the use of human insulin. Xerosis and pruritus are common and are relieved by skin moisturizers.

Approach to the Patient

DM and its complications produce a wide range of symptoms and signs; those secondary to acute hyperglycemia may occur at any stage of the disease, whereas those related to chronic complications begin to appear during the second decade of hyperglycemia. Individuals with previously undetected type 2 DM may present with chronic complications of DM at the time of diagnosis. The history and physical examination should assess for symptoms or signs of acute hyperglycemia and should screen for the chronic complications and conditions associated with DM.

History A complete medical history should be obtained with special emphasis on DM-relevant aspects such as weight, family history of DM and its complications, risk factors for cardiovascular disease, prior medical conditions, exercise, smoking, and ethanol use. Symptoms of hyperglycemia include polyuria, polydipsia, weight loss, fatigue, weakness, blurry vision, frequent superficial infections (vaginitis, fungal skin infections), and slow healing of skin lesions after minor trauma. Metabolic derangements relate mostly to hyperglycemia (osmotic diuresis, reduced glucose entry into muscle) and to the catabolic state of the patient (urinary loss of glucose and calories, muscle breakdown due to protein degradation and decreased protein synthesis). Blurred vision results from changes in the water content of the lens and resolves as the hyperglycemia is controlled.

In a patient with established DM, the initial assessment should also include special emphasis on prior diabetes care, including the type of therapy, prior HbA1c levels, self-monitoring blood glucose results, frequency of hypoglycemia, presence of DM-specific complications, and assessment of the patient's knowledge about diabetes. The chronic complications may afflict several organ systems, and an individual patient may exhibit some, all, or none of the symptoms related to the complications of DM (see above). In addition, the presence of DM-related comorbidities should be sought (cardiovascular disease, hypertension, dyslipidemia).

Physical Examination In addition to a complete physical examination, special attention should be given to DM-relevant aspects such as weight or body mass index, retinal examination, orthostatic blood pressure, foot examination, peripheral pulses, and insulin injection sites. Careful examination of the lower extremities should seek evidence of peripheral neuropathy, calluses, superficial fungal infections, nail disease, and foot deformities (such as hammer or claw toes and Charcot foot) in order to identify sites of potential skin ulceration. Vibratory sensation (128-MHz tuning fork at the base of the great toe) and the ability to sense touch with a monofilament (5.07, 10-g monofilament) are useful to detect moderately advanced diabetic neuropathy. Since dental disease is more frequent in DM, the teeth and gums should also be examined.

Classification of DM in an Individual Patient The etiology of diabetes in an individual with new-onset disease can usually be assigned on the basis of clinical criteria. Individuals with type 1 DM tend to have the following characteristics: (1) onset of disease prior to age 30; (2) lean body habitus; (3) requirement of insulin as the initial therapy; (4) propensity to develop ketoacidosis; and (5) an increased risk of other autoimmune disorders such as autoimmune thyroid disease, adrenal insufficiency, pernicious anemia, and vitiligo. In contrast, individuals with type 2 DM often exhibit the following features: (1) develop diabetes after the age of 30; (2) are usually obese (80% are obese, but elderly individuals may be lean); (3) may not require insulin therapy initially; and (4) may have associated conditions such as insulin resistance, hypertension, cardiovascular disease, dyslipidemia, or polycystic ovary syndrome. In type 2 DM, insulin resistance is often associated with abdominal obesity (as opposed to hip and thigh obesity) and hypertriglyceridemia. Although most individuals diagnosed with type 2 DM are older, the age of diagnosis appears to be declining in some ethnic groups, and there is a marked increase among overweight teenagers. On the other hand, some individuals (<10%) with the phenotypic appearance of type 2 DM do not have absolute insulin deficiency but have autoimmune markers suggestive of type 1 DM. Thus, despite the revised classification of DM, it is remains difficult to categorize some patients unequivocally. Individuals who deviate from the clinical profile of type 1 and type 2 DM, or who have other associated defects such as deafness, pancreatic exocrine disease, and other endocrine disorders, should be classified accordingly (Table 333-1).

Laboratory Assessment The laboratory assessment should first determine whether the patient meets the diagnostic criteria for DM (Table 333-2) and should then assess the degree of glycemic control (HbA1c, discussed below). In addition to the standard laboratory evaluation, the patient should be screened for DM-associated conditions (e.g., microalbuminuria, dyslipidemia, thyroid dysfunction). Individuals at high risk for cardiovascular disease should be screened for asymptomatic coronary artery disease by appropriate cardiac stress testing, when indicated.

The classification of the type of DM does not usually require laboratory assessments. Serum insulin or C-peptide measurements do not clearly distinguish type 1 from type 2 DM at the time of diabetes onset; a low C-peptide level merely confirms a patient's need for insulin. Conversely, many individuals with new-onset type 1 DM retain some C-peptide production. Measurement of islet cell antibodies at the time of diabetes onset may be useful if the type of DM is not clear based on the characteristics discussed above, but this knowledge does not usually alter therapy, which is based primarily on empirical metabolic features.

LONG-TERM TREATMENT

OVERALL PRINCIPLES The goals of therapy for type 1 or type 2 DM are to: (1) eliminate symptoms related to hyperglycemia, (2) reduce or eliminate the long-term microvascular and macrovascular complications of DM, and (3) allow the patient to achieve as normal a life-style as possible. To reach these goals, the physician should identify a target level of glycemic control for each patient, provide the patient with the educational and pharmacologic resources necessary to reach this level, and monitor/treat DM-related complications. Symptoms of diabetes usually resolve when the plasma glucose is <11.1 mmol/L (200 mg/dL), and thus most DM treatment focuses on achieving the second and third goals.

The care of an individual with either type 1 or type 2 DM requires a multidisciplinary team. Central to the success of this team are the patient's participation, input, and enthusiasm, all of which are essential for optimal diabetes management. Members of the health care team include the primary care provider and/or the endocrinologist or diabetologist, a certified diabetes educator, and a nutritionist. In addition, when the complications of DM arise, subspecialists (including neurologists, nephrologists, vascular surgeons, cardiologists, ophthalmologists, and podiatrists) with experience in DM-related complications are essential.

A number of names are sometimes applied to different approaches to diabetes care, such as intensive insulin therapy, intensive glycemic control, and "tight control." The current chapter, however, will use the term *comprehensive diabetes care* to emphasize the fact that optimal diabetes therapy involves more than plasma glucose management. Though glycemic control is central to optimal diabetes therapy, comprehensive diabetes care of both type 1 and type 2 DM should also detect and manage DM-specific complications and modify risk factors for DM-associated diseases.

In addition to assessing the physical aspects of the patient with DM, the physician and members of the diabetes management team should consider social, family, financial, cultural, and employment-related issues that may have an impact on diabetes care. With this information, the physician can work with the patient and his or her family to establish therapeutic goals and design a comprehensive and feasible plan for optimal diabetes care.

EDUCATION OF THE PATIENT ABOUT DM, NUTRITION, AND EXERCISE Patient participation is an essential component of comprehensive diabetes care. The patient with type 1 or type 2 DM should receive education about nutrition, exercise, care of diabetes during illness, and medications to lower the plasma glucose. Along with improved compliance, patient education allows individuals with DM to assume greater responsibility for their care. Patient education should be viewed as a continuing process with regular visits for reinforcement; it should *not* be a process that is completed after one or two visits to a nurse educator or nutritionist.

Diabetes Education The diabetes educator is a health care professional (nurse, dietician, or pharmacist) with specialized patient education skills who is certified in diabetes education (indicating demonstrated skills in diabetes knowledge and education and certification by the American Association of Diabetes Educators). The educator is a vital member of the comprehensive diabetes care program and educates the patient about a number of issues important for optimal diabetes care, including self-monitoring of blood glucose; urine ketone monitoring (type 1 DM); insulin administration; guidelines for diabetes management during illnesses; management of hypoglycemia; foot and skin care; diabetes management before, during, and after exercise; and risk factor–modifying activities.

Nutrition *Medical nutrition therapy* (MNT) is a term used by the ADA to describe the optimal coordination of caloric intake with other aspects of diabetes therapy (insulin, exercise, weight loss). Historically, nutrition has imposed restrictive, complicated regimens on the patient. Current practices have greatly changed, though many patients and health care providers still view the diabetic diet as monolithic and static. For example, modern MNT now includes foods with sucrose and seeks to modify other risk factors such as hyperlipidemia and hypertension rather than focusing exclusively on weight loss in individuals with type 2 DM. Like other aspects of DM therapy, MNT must be adjusted to meet the goals of the individual patient. Furthermore, MNT education is an important component of comprehensive diabetes care and should be reinforced by regular patient education. In general, the components of optimal MNT are similar for individuals with type 1 or type 2 DM (Table 333-8).

The goal of MNT in the individual with type 1 DM is to coordinate and match the caloric intake, both temporally and quantitatively, with the appropriate amount of insulin. MNT in type 1 DM and self-monitoring of blood glucose must be integrated to define the optimal insulin regimen. MNT must be flexible enough to allow for exercise, and the insulin regimen must allow for deviations in caloric intake. An important component of MNT in type 1 DM is to minimize the weight gain often associated with intensive diabetes management.

Table 333-8 Nutritional Recommendations for All Persons with Diabetes

- Protein to provide ~10–20% of kcal/d (~10% for those with nephropathy)
- Saturated fat to provide <10% of kcal/d (<7% for those with elevated LDL)
- Polyunsaturated fat to provide ≤10% of kcal
- Remaining calories to be divided between carbohydrate and monounsaturated fat, based on medical needs and personal tolerance
- Use of caloric sweeteners, including sucrose, is acceptable. Sugars must be accounted for so that the insulin demand they create is matched to available insulin
- Fiber (20–35 g/d) and sodium (≤3000 mg/d) levels as recommended for the general healthy population
- Cholesterol intake ≤300 mg/d
- The same precautions regarding alcohol use in the general population also apply to individuals with diabetes. In addition, alcohol may increase risk for hypoglycemia and therefore should be taken with food.

NOTE: LDL, low-density lipoprotein.
SOURCE: Adapted from Farkas-Hirsch, 1998.

The goals of MNT in type 2 DM are slightly different and address the greatly increased prevalence of cardiovascular risk factors (hypertension, dyslipidemia, obesity) and disease in this population. The majority of these individuals are obese, and weight loss is still strongly encouraged and should remain an important goal. Medical treatment of obesity is a rapidly evolving area and is discussed in Chap. 77. Hypocaloric diets and modest weight loss often result in rapid and dramatic glucose lowering in individuals with new-onset type 2 DM. Nevertheless, numerous studies document that long-term weight loss is uncommon. Therefore, current MNT for type 2 DM should emphasize modest caloric reduction, increased physical activity, and reduction of hyperlipidemia and hypertension. Increased consumption of soluble, dietary fiber may improve glycemic control in individuals with type 2 DM.

Exercise Exercise is an integral component of comprehensive diabetes care that can have multiple positive benefits (cardiovascular benefits, reduced blood pressure, maintenance of muscle mass, reduction in body fat, weight loss, etc.). For individuals with type 1 or type 2 DM, exercise is also useful for lowering plasma glucose (during and following exercise) and increasing insulin sensitivity.

Despite its benefits, exercise presents several challenges for individuals with DM because they lack the normal glucoregulatory mechanisms. Skeletal muscle is a major site for metabolic fuel consumption in the resting state, and the increased muscle activity during vigorous, aerobic exercise greatly increases fuel requirements. Individuals with type 1 DM are prone to either hyperglycemia or hypoglycemia during exercise, depending on the preexercise plasma glucose, the circulating insulin level, and the level of exercise-induced catecholamines. If the insulin level is too low, the rise in catecholamines may increase the plasma glucose excessively, promote ketone body formation, and possibly lead to ketoacidosis. Conversely, if the circulating insulin level is excessive, this relative hyperinsulinemia may reduce hepatic glucose production (decreased glycogenolysis, decreased gluconeogenesis) and increase glucose entry into muscle, leading to hypoglycemia.

To avoid exercise-related hyper- or hypoglycemia, individuals with type 1 DM should: (1) monitor blood glucose before, during, and after exercise; (2) delay exercise if blood glucose is >14 mmol/L (250 mg/dL), <5.5 mmol/L (100 mg/dL), or if ketones are present; (3) eat a meal 1 to 3 h before exercise and take supplemental carbohydrate feedings at least every 30 min during vigorous or prolonged exercise; (4) decrease insulin doses (based on previous experience) before exercise and inject insulin into a nonexercising area; and (5) learn individual glucose responses to different types of exercise and increase food intake for up to 24 h after exercise, depending on intensity and duration of exercise. In individuals with type 2 DM, exercise-related hypoglycemia is less common but can occur in individuals taking either insulin or sulfonylureas.

Because asymptomatic cardiovascular disease appears at a younger age in both type 1 and type 2 DM, formal exercise tolerance testing may be warranted in diabetic individuals with any of the following: age ≥35 years, long-standing type 1 DM (>20 to 25 years' duration), microvascular complications of DM (retinopathy, microalbuminuria, or nephropathy), peripheral vascular disease, other risk factors of coronary artery disease, or autonomic neuropathy. Untreated proliferative retinopathy is a relative contraindication to vigorous exercise, since this may lead to vitreous hemorrhage or retinal detachment.

MONITORING THE LEVEL OF GLYCEMIC CONTROL Optimal monitoring of glycemic control involves plasma glucose measurements by the patient and an assessment of long-term control by the physician (measurement of HbA1c and review of the patient's self-measurements of plasma glucose). These measurements are complementary: the patient's measurements provide a picture of short-term glycemic control, whereas the HbA1c reflects average glycemic control over the previous 2 to 3 months. Integration of both measurements provides an accurate assessment of the glycemic control achieved.

Self-Monitoring of Blood Glucose Self-monitoring of blood glucose (SMBG) is the standard of care in diabetes management and allows the patient to monitor his or her blood glucose at any time. In SMBG, a small drop of blood and an easily detectable enzymatic reaction allow measurement of the capillary plasma glucose. By combining glucose measurements with diet history, medication changes, and exercise history, the physician and patient can improve the treatment program.

The frequency of SMBG measurements must be individualized and adapted to address the goals of diabetes care as defined by the patient and the health care provider. Individuals with type 1 DM should routinely measure their plasma glucose four to eight times per day to estimate and select mealtime boluses of short-acting insulin and to modify long-acting insulin doses. Most individuals with type 2 DM require less frequent monitoring, though the optimal frequency of SMBG has not been clearly defined. Individuals with type 2 DM who are on oral medications should utilize SMBG as a means of assessing the efficacy of their medication and diet. Since plasma glucose levels fluctuate less in these individuals, one to two SMBG measurements per day (or fewer) may be sufficient. Individuals with type 2 DM who are on insulin should utilize SMBG more frequently than those on oral agents.

Two devices for continuous blood glucose monitoring have been recently approved by the U.S. Food and Drug Administration (FDA). The Glucowatch uses iontophoresis to assess glucose in interstitial fluid, whereas the Minimed device uses an indwelling subcutaneous catheter to monitor interstitial fluid glucose. Both devices utilize immobilized glucose oxidase to generate electrons in response to changing glucose levels. Though clinical experience with these devices is limited, they perform well in clinical trials and appear to provide useful short-term information about the patterns of glucose changes as well as an enhanced ability to detect hypoglycemic episodes.

Although urine glucose testing does not provide an accurate assessment of glycemic control, urine ketones are a sensitive indicator of early diabetic ketoacidosis and should be measured in individuals with type 1 DM when the plasma glucose is consistently 16.7 mmol/L (300 mg/dL); during a concurrent illness; or with symptoms such as nausea, vomiting, or abdominal pain.

Assessment of Long-Term Glycemic Control Measurement of glycated hemoglobin is the standard method for assessing long-term glycemic control. When plasma glucose is consistently elevated, there is an increase in nonenzymatic glycation of hemoglobin; this alteration reflects the glycemic history over the previous 2 to 3 months, since erythrocytes have an average life span of 120 days. There are numerous laboratory methods for measuring the various forms of glycated hemoglobin, and these have significant interassay variations. Because of its superior specificity and reliability, the HbA1c assay performed by the high-performance liquid chromatography (HPLC) method has become the standard reference method for most glycated hemoglobin measurements. Since glycated hemoglobin measurements are usually compared to prior measurements, it is essential for the assay results to be comparable. Depending on the assay methodology for HbA1c, hemoglobinopathies, hemolytic anemia, and uremia may interfere with the HbA1c result.

Glycated hemoglobin or HbA1c should be measured in all individuals with DM during their initial evaluation and as part of their comprehensive diabetes care. As the primary predictor of long-term complications of DM, the HbA1c should mirror, to a certain extent, the short-term measurements of SMBG. These two measurements are complementary in that recent intercurrent illnesses may impact the SMBG measurements but not the HbA1c. Likewise, postprandial and nocturnal hyperglycemia may not be detected by the SMBG of fasting and preprandial capillary plasma glucose but will be reflected in the HbA1c. When measured by HPLC, the HbA1c approximates the following mean plasma glucose values: an HbA1c of 6% is 6.6 mmol/L (120 mg/dL), 7% is 8.3 mmol/L (150 mg/dL), 8% is 10.0 mmol/L (180 mg/dL), etc. [A 1% rise in the HbA1c translates into a 1.7-mmol/L (30 mg/dL) increase in the mean glucose.] The degree of glycation of other proteins, such as albumin, has been used as an alternative indicator of glycemic control when the HbA1c is inaccurate (hemolytic anemia, hemoglobinopathies). The fructosamine assay (using albumin) is an example of an alternative measurement of glycemic control and reflects the glycemic status over the 2 to 4 prior weeks. Current consensus statements do not favor the use of alternative assays of glycemic control, as there are no studies to indicate whether such assays accurately predict the complications of DM.

℞ TREATMENT **Establishment of a Target Level of Glycemic Control** Because the complications of DM are related to glycemic control, normoglycemia or near normoglycemia is the desired, but often elusive, goal for most patients. However, normalization of the plasma glucose for long periods of time is extremely difficult, as demonstrated by the DCCT. Regardless of the level of hyperglycemia, improvement in glycemic control will lower the risk of diabetes complications (Fig. 333-8).

The target for glycemic control (as reflected by the HbA1c) must be individualized, and the health care provider should establish the goals of therapy in consultation with the patient after considering a number of medical, social, and life-style issues. Some important factors to consider include the patient's age, ability to understand and implement a complex treatment regimen, presence and severity of complications of diabetes, ability to recognize hypoglycemic symptoms, presence of other medical conditions or treatments that might alter the response to therapy, life-style and occupation (e.g., possible consequences of experiencing hypoglycemia on the job), and level of support available from family and friends.

The ADA has established suggested glycemic goals based on the premise that glycemic control predicts development of DM-related complications. In general, the target HbA1c should be <7.0% (Table 333-9). Other consensus groups (such as the Veterans Administration) have suggested HbA1c goals that take into account the patient's life expectancy at the time of diagnosis and the presence of microvascular complications. Such recommendations strive to balance the financial and personal costs of glycemic therapy with anticipated benefits (reduced health care costs, reduced morbidity). One limitation to this approach is that the onset of hyperglycemia in type 2 DM is difficult to ascertain and likely predates the diagnosis. Furthermore, though the life expectancy can be predicted for a patient population, the physician must treat an individual patient; consequently, the target HbA1c must be individualized to accommodate these other considerations.

Type 1 Diabetes Mellitus • *General aspects* Comprehensive diabetes care should be instituted in all individuals with type 1 DM and should involve attention to nutrition, exercise, and risk factor management in addition to insulin administration. The ADA recommendations for fasting and bedtime glycemic goals and HbA1c targets are summarized in Table 333-9. The goal is to design and implement insulin regimens that mimic physiologic insulin secretion. Because in-

Table 333-9 Ideal Goals for Glycemic Control[a]

Index	Normal Range	Goal	Additional Action Suggested
Average preprandial glucose, mmol/L (mg/dL)	<5.5 (100)	4.4–6.7 (80–120)	<4.4 (80) *or* >7.8 (140)
Average bedtime glucose, mmol/L (mg/dL)	<6.1 (110)	5.5–7.8 (100–140)	<5.5 (100) *or* >8.8 (160)
HbA1c, %	<6	<7	>8

[a] These values are for whole blood measurements, and home glucose-monitoring devices may report either whole blood or plasma glucose values. Plasma glucose values are 10–15% higher than whole blood values. The upper limit of the HbA1c reference range is 6.0% (mean 5.0%, with a standard deviation of 0.5%). These goals must be individualized for each patient and must consider the patient's age and other medical conditions.

SOURCE: Adapted from American Diabetes Association, 2000.

dividuals with type 1 DM lack endogenous insulin production, administration of basal, exogenous insulin is essential for regulating glycogen breakdown, gluconeogenesis, lipolysis, and ketogenesis. Likewise, postprandial insulin replacement should be appropriate for the carbohydrate intake and promote normal glucose utilization and storage.

Intensive management Intensive diabetes management is defined by the ADA as ". . . a mode of treatment for the person with DM that has the goal of achieving euglycemia or near-normal glycemia using all available resources to accomplish this goal." These resources include thorough and continuing patient education, comprehensive recording of plasma glucose measurements and nutrition intake by the patient, and a variable insulin regimen that matches glucose intake and insulin dose. Insulin regimens usually include multiple-component insulin regimens, multiple daily injections (MDI), or insulin infusion devices (all discussed below).

The benefits of intensive diabetes management and improved glycemic control include a reduction in the microvascular complications of DM and a possible delay or reduction in the macrovascular complications of DM. From a psychological standpoint, the patient experiences greater control over his or her diabetes and often notes an improved sense of well-being, greater flexibility in the timing and content of meals, and the capability to alter insulin dosing with exercise. In addition, intensive diabetes management in pregnancy reduces fetal malformation and morbidity. Intensive diabetes management is also strongly encouraged in newly diagnosed patients with type 1 DM because it may prolong the period of C-peptide production, which may result in better glycemic control and a reduced risk of serious hypoglycemia.

Although intensive management confers impressive benefits, it is also accompanied by significant personal and financial costs and is therefore not appropriate for all individuals. It requires a combination of dedication, persistence, and motivation on the part of the patient, as well as medical, educational, nursing, nutritional, and psychological expertise on the part of the diabetes management team. Circumstances in which intensive diabetes management should be strongly considered are listed in Table 333-10.

Insulin preparations Current insulin preparations are generated by recombinant DNA technology and consist of the amino acid sequence of human insulin. Animal insulin (beef or pork) is no longer used. Human insulin has been formulated with distinctive pharmacokinetics to mimic physiologic insulin secretion (Table 333-11). In the United States, all insulin is formulated as U-100 (100 units/mL), whereas in some other countries it is available in other units (e.g., U-40 = 40 units/mL). One short-acting insulin formulation, lispro, is an insulin analogue in which the 28th and 29th amino acids (lysine and proline) on the insulin B chain have been reversed by recombinant DNA technology. This insulin analogue has full biologic activity but less tendency toward subcutaneous aggregation, resulting in more rapid absorption and onset of action and a shorter duration of action. These characteristics are particularly advantageous for allowing entrainment of insulin injection and action to rising plasma glucose levels following meals, although improvement in HbA1c values have not been found consistently. The shorter duration of action also appears to be associated with a decreased number of hypoglycemic episodes, primarily because the decay of lispro action corresponds better to the decline in plasma glucose after a meal. Insulin glargine is a long-acting biosynthetic human insulin that differs from normal insulin in that asparagine is replaced by glycine at amino acid 21, and two arginine residues are added to the C-terminus of the B chain. Compared to NPH insulin, the onset of insulin glargine action is later, the duration of action is longer (~24 h), and there is no pronounced peak. A lower incidence of hypoglycemia, especially at night, was reported in one trial with insulin glargine when compared to NPH insulin. Since glargine has only recently approved, clinical experience is limited. Additional insulin analogues are currently under development.

Table 333-10 Indications for Intensive Diabetes Management

- Otherwise healthy adults with either type 1 or type 2 diabetes (selected adolescents and older children)
- Purposeful, therapeutic attempt to avoid or lessen microvascular complications
- All pregnant women with diabetes; all women with diabetes who are planning pregnancy
- Management of labile diabetes
- Availability of health care professionals with appropriate expertise
- Patients who have had kidney transplantation for diabetic nephropathy

SOURCE: Adapted from Farkas-Hirsch, 1998.

Basal insulin requirements are provided by intermediate (NPH or lente) or long-acting (ultralente or glargine) insulin formulations. These are usually combined with short-acting insulin in an attempt to mimic physiologic insulin release with meals. Although mixing of intermediate and short-acting insulin formulations is common practice, this mixing may alter the insulin absorption profile (especially those of short-acting insulins). For example, the absorption of regular insulin is delayed when mixed for even short periods of time (<5 min) with lente or ultralente insulin, but not when mixed with NPH insulin. Lispro absorption is delayed by mixing with NPH but not ultralente. Insulin glargine should not be mixed with other insulins. The miscibility of human regular and NPH insulin allows for the production of combination insulins that contain 75% NPH and 25% regular (75/25), 70% NPH and 30% regular (70/30), or equal mixtures of NPH and regular. These combinations of insulin are more convenient for the patient but prevent adjustment of only one component of the insulin formulation. The alteration in insulin absorption when the patient mixes different insulin formulation should not discourage the patient from mixing insulin. However, the following guidelines should be followed: (1) mix the different insulin formulations in the syringe immediately before injection (inject within 2 min after mixing); (2) if possible, do not store insulin as a mixture; and (3) follow the same routine in terms of insulin mixing and administration to standardize the physiologic response to injected insulin.

Insulin regimens Representations of the various insulin regimens that may be utilized in type 1 DM are illustrated in Fig. 333-12. Although the insulin profiles are depicted as "smooth," symmetric curves, there is considerable patient-to-patient variation in the peak and duration. In all regimens, long-acting insulins (NPH, lente, ultralente, or glargine insulin) supply basal insulin, whereas prandial insulin is provided by either regular or lispro insulin. Lispro should be injected just before a meal; regular insulin is given 30 to 45 min prior to a meal.

A shortcoming of current insulin regimens is that injected insulin immediately enters the systemic circulation, whereas endogenous insulin is secreted into the portal vein. Thus, exogenous insulin administration exposes the liver to subphysiologic insulin levels. No insulin regimen reproduces the precise insulin secretory pattern of the pancreatic islet. However, the most physiologic regimens entail more frequent insulin injections, greater reliance on short-acting insulin, and more frequent capillary plasma glucose measurements. In general, individuals with type 1 DM require 0.5 to 1.0 U/kg per day of insulin divided into multiple doses. Initial insulin-dosing regimens should be conservative; approximately 40 to 50% of the insulin should be given as basal insulin. A single daily injection of insulin is not appropriate therapy in type 1 DM.

Table 333-11 Pharmacokinetics of Insulin Preparations

Preparation	Time of Action: Onset, h	Peak, h	Effective Duration, h	Maximum Duration, h
Short-acting				
Lispro	<0.25	0.5–1.5	3–4	4–6
Regular	0.5–1.0	2–3	3–6	6–8
Intermediate-acting				
NPH	2–4	6–10	10–16	14–18
Lente	3–4	6–12	12–18	16–20
Long-acting				
Ultralente	6–10	10–16	18–20	20–24
Glargine	4	—[a]	24	>24
Combinations				
75/25–75% NPH, 25% regular	0.5–1	Dual	10–16	14–18
70/30–70% NPH, 30% regular	0.5–1	Dual	10–16	14–18
50/50–50% NPH, 50% regular	0.5–1	Dual	10–16	14–18

[a] Glargine has minimal peak activity.
SOURCE: Adapted from JS Skyler, in *Therapy for Diabetes Mellitus and Related Disorders*, 1998

One commonly used regimen consists of twice-daily injections of an intermediate insulin (NPH or lente) mixed with a short-acting insulin before the morning and evening meal (Fig. 333-12*A*). Such regimens usually prescribe two-thirds of the total daily insulin dose in the morning (with about two-thirds given as intermediate-acting insulin and one-third as short-acting) and one-third before the evening meal (with approximately one-half given as intermediate-acting insulin and one-half as short-acting). The drawback to such a regimen is that it enforces a rigid schedule on the patient, in terms of daily activity and the content and timing of meals. Although it is simple and effective at avoiding severe hyperglycemia, it does not generate near-normal glycemic control in most individuals with type 1 DM. Moreover, if the patient's meal pattern or content varies or if physical activity is increased, hyperglycemia or hypoglycemia may result. Moving the intermediate insulin from before the evening meal to bedtime may avoid nocturnal hypoglycemia and provide more insulin as glucose levels rise in the early morning (so-called dawn phenomenon). The insulin dose in such regimens should be adjusted based on SMBG results with the following general assumptions: (1) the fasting glucose is primarily determined by the prior evening intermediate-acting insulin; (2) the pre-lunch glucose is a function of the morning short-acting insulin; (3) the pre-supper glucose is a function of the morning intermediate-acting insulin; and (4) the bedtime glucose is a function of the pre-supper, short-acting insulin.

Multiple-component insulin regimens refer to the combination of basal insulin; preprandial short-acting insulin; and changes in short-acting insulin doses to accommodate the results of frequent SMBG, anticipated food intake, and physical activity. Sometimes also referred to as *multiple daily injections*, such regimens offer the patient maximal flexibility in terms of life-style and the best chance for achieving near normoglycemia. One such regimen, shown in Fig. 333-12*B*, consists of a basal insulin with ultralente twice a day and preprandial lispro. The lispro dose is based on individualized algorithms that integrate the preprandial glucose and the anticipated carbohydrate intake. An alternative multiple-component insulin regimen consists of bedtime intermediate insulin, a small dose of intermediate insulin at breakfast (20 to 30% of bedtime dose), and preprandial short-acting insulin. There are numerous variations of these regimens that can be optimized for individual patients. Frequent SMBG (four to 8 times per day) is absolutely essential for these types of insulin regimens.

Continuous subcutaneous insulin infusion (CSII) is another multiple-component insulin regimen (Fig. 333-12*C*). Sophisticated insulin infusion devices are now available that can accurately deliver small doses of insulin (microliters per hour). For example, multiple basal infusion rates can be programmed to: (1) accommodate nocturnal versus daytime basal insulin requirement, (2) alter infusion rate during periods of exercise, or (3) select different waveforms of insulin infusion. A preprandial insulin ("bolus") is delivered by the insulin infusion device based on instructions from the patient, which follow individualized algorithms that account for preprandial plasma glucose and anticipated carbohydrate intake. These devices require a health professional with considerable experience with insulin infusion devices and very frequent patient interactions with the diabetes management team. Insulin infusion devices present unique challenges, such as infection at the infusion site, unexplained hyperglycemia because the infusion set becomes obstructed, or diabetic ketoacidosis if the pump becomes disconnected. Since most physicians use lispro insulin in CSII, the extremely short half-life of this insulin quickly leads to

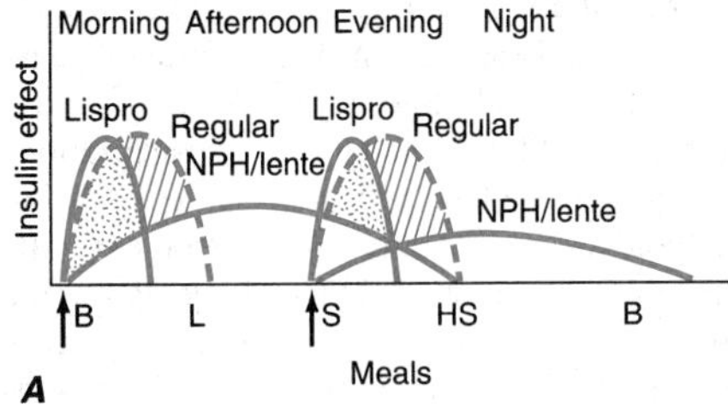

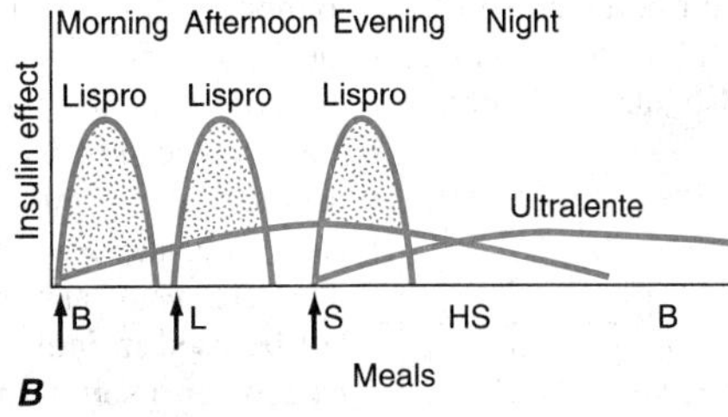

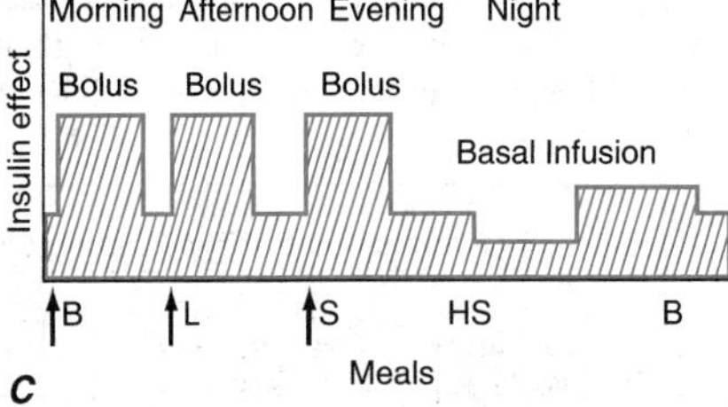

FIGURE 333-12 Representative insulin regimens for the treatment of diabetes. For each panel, the y-axis shows the amount of insulin effect and the x-axis shows the time of day. B, breakfast; L, lunch; S, supper; HS, bedtime; CSII, continuous subcutaneous insulin infusion. The time of insulin injection is shown with a vertical arrow. The type of insulin is noted above each insulin curve. *A*. The injection of two shots of intermediate-acting insulin (NPH or lente) and short-acting insulin (lispro or regular). Only one formulation of short-acting insulin is used. *B*: A multiple-component insulin regimen consisting of two shots of ultralente each day to provide basal insulin coverage and three shots of Lispro to provide glycemic coverage for each meal. The ultralente doses are usually 10 to 12 h apart. *C*: Insulin administration by insulin infusion device is shown with the basal insulin and a bolus injection at each meal. The basal insulin rate is decreased during the evening and increased slightly prior to the patient awakening in the morning. *(Adapted from Intensive Diabetes Management, 2d ed, R. Farkas-Hirsch (ed). Alexandria, VA, American Diabetes Association, 1998)*

insulin deficiency if the delivery system is interrupted. Essential to the safe use of infusion devices is thorough patient education about pump function and frequent SMBG.

Type 2 Diabetes Mellitus • ***General aspects*** The goals of therapy for type 2 DM are similar to those in type 1: improved glycemic control with near normalization of the HbA1c. While glycemic control tends to dominate the management of type 1 DM, the care of individuals with type 2 DM must also include attention to the treatment of conditions associated with type 2 DM (obesity, hypertension, dyslipidemia, cardiovascular disease) and detection/management of DM-related complications (Fig. 333-13). DM-specific complications may be present in up to 20 to 50% of individuals with newly diagnosed type 2 DM. Reduction in cardiovascular risk is of paramount importance as this is the leading cause of mortality in these individuals.

Diabetes management should begin with MNT (discussed above). An exercise regimen to increase insulin sensitivity and promote weight loss should also be instituted. After MNT and increased physical activity have been instituted, glycemic control should be reassessed; if the patient's glycemic target is not achieved after 3 to 4 weeks of MNT, pharmacologic therapy is indicated. Pharmacologic approaches to the management of type 2 DM include both oral glucose-lowering agents and insulin; most physicians and patients prefer oral glucose-lowering agents as the initial choice. Any therapy that improves glycemic control reduces "glucose toxicity" to the islet cells and improves endogenous insulin secretion.

Glucose-lowering agents Recent advances in the therapy of type 2 DM have generated considerable enthusiasm for oral glucose-lowering agents that target different pathophysiologic processes in type 2 DM. Based on their mechanisms of action, oral glucose-lowering agents are subdivided into agents that increase insulin secretion, reduce glucose production, or increase insulin sensitivity (Table 333-12). Oral glucose-lowering agents (with the exception of α-glucosidase inhibitors) are ineffective in type 1 DM and should not be used for glucose management of severely ill individuals with type 2 DM. Insulin is sometimes the initial glucose-lowering agent.

INSULIN SECRETAGOGUES Insulin secretagogues stimulate insulin secretion by interacting with the ATP-sensitive potassium channel on the beta cell (Fig. 333-1). These drugs are most effective in individuals with type 2 DM of relatively recent onset (<5 years), who have endogenous insulin production and tend to be obese. At maximum doses, first-generation sulfonylureas are similar in potency to second-generation agents but have a longer half-life, a greater incidence of hypoglycemia, and more frequent drug interactions (Table 333-13). Thus, second-generation sulfonylureas are generally preferred. An advantage to a more rapid onset of action is better coverage of the postprandial glucose rise, but the shorter half-life of such agents requires more than once-a-day dosing. Sulfonylureas reduce both fasting and postprandial glucose and should be initiated at low doses and increased at 1- to 2-week intervals based on SMBG. In general, sulfonylureas increase insulin acutely and thus should be taken shortly before a meal; with chronic therapy, though, the insulin release is more sustained. Replaglinide is not a sulfonylurea but also interacts with the ATP-sensitive potassium channel. Because of its short half-life, it is usually given with or immediately before each meal to reduce meal-related glucose excursions.

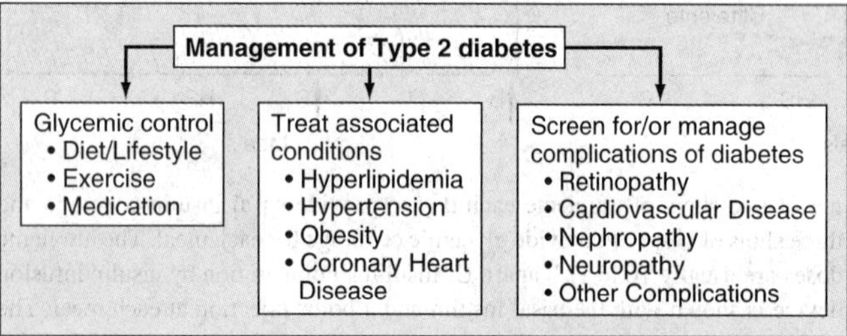

FIGURE 333-13 Essential elements in comprehensive diabetes care of type 2 diabetes.

Insulin secretagogues are well tolerated in general. All of these agents, however, have the potential to cause profound and persistent hypoglycemia, especially in elderly individuals. Hypoglycemia is usually related to delayed meals, increased physical activity, alcohol intake, or renal insufficiency. Individuals who ingest an overdose of these agents develop prolonged and serious hypoglycemia and should be monitored closely in the hospital (Chap. 334). Most sulfonylureas are metabolized in the liver to compounds that are cleared by the kidney. Thus, their use in individuals with significant hepatic or renal dysfunction is not advisable. Weight gain, a common side effect of sulfonylurea therapy, results from the increased insulin levels and improvement in glycemic control. Some sulfonylureas have significant drug interactions with other medications such as alcohol, warfarin, aspirin, ketoconazole, α-glucosidase inhibitors, and fluconazole. Despite prior concerns that use of sulfonylureas might increase cardiovascular risk, recent trials have refuted this claim.

BIGUANIDES Metformin is representative of this class of agents. It reduces hepatic glucose production through an undefined mechanism and may improve peripheral glucose utilization slightly (Table 333-12). Metformin reduces fasting plasma glucose and insulin levels, improves the lipid profile, and promotes modest weight loss. The initial starting dose of 500 mg once or twice a day can be increased to 850 mg tid or 1000 mg bid. Because of its relatively slow onset of action and gastrointestinal symptoms with higher doses, the dose should be escalated every 2 to 3 weeks based on SMBG measurements. The major toxicity of metformin, lactic acidosis, can be prevented by careful patient selection. Metformin should not be used in patients with renal insufficiency [serum creatinine >133 μmol/L (1.5 mg/dL) in men or >124 μmol/L (1.4 mg/dL) in women, with adjustments for age], any form of acidosis, congestive heart failure, liver disease, or severe hypoxia. Metformin should be discontinued in patients who are seriously ill, in patients who can take nothing orally, and in those receiving radiographic contrast material. Insulin should be used until metformin can be restarted. Though well tolerated in general, some individuals develop gastrointestinal side effects (diarrhea, anorexia, nausea, and metallic taste) that can be minimized by gradual dose escalation. Because the drug is metabolized in the liver, it should not be used in patients with liver disease or heavy ethanol intake.

α-GLUCOSIDASE INHIBITORS α-Glucosidase inhibitors (acarbose and miglitol) reduce postprandial hyperglycemia by delaying glucose absorption; they do not affect glucose utilization or insulin secretion (Table 333-12). Postprandial hyperglycemia, secondary to impaired hepatic and peripheral glucose disposal, contributes significantly to the hyperglycemic state in type 2 DM. These drugs, taken just before each meal, reduce glucose absorption by inhibiting the enzyme that cleaves oligosaccharides into simple sugars in the intestinal lumen. Therapy should be initiated at a low dose (25 mg of acarbose or miglitol) with the evening meal and may be increased to a maximal dose over weeks to months (50 to 100 mg for acarbose or 50 mg for miglitol with each meal). The major side effects (diarrhea, flatulence, abdominal distention) are related to increased delivery of oligosaccharides to the large bowel and can be reduced somewhat by gradual upward dose titration. α-Glucosidase inhibitors may increase levels of sulfonylureas and increase the incidence of hypoglycemia. Simultaneous treatment with bile acid resins and antacids should be avoided. These agents should not be used in individuals with inflammatory bowel disease, gastroparesis, or a serum creatinine >177 μmol/L (2.0 mg/dL). This class of agents is not as potent as other oral agents in lowering the HbA1c but is unique in that it reduces the postprandial glucose rise even in individuals with type 1 DM.

THIAZOLIDINEDIONES Thiazolidinediones represent a new class of agents that reduce insulin resistance. These drugs bind to a nuclear receptor (peroxisome proliferator-activated receptor, PPAR-γ) that regulates gene transcription. The PPAR-γ receptor is found at highest

Table 333-12 Oral Glucose-Lowering Therapies in Type 2 DM

	Mechanism of Action	Examples	Anticipated Reduction in HbA1c, %	Agent-Specific Advantages	Agent-Specific Disadvantages	Contraindications
Insulin secretagogues	↑ Insulin		1–2			
Sulfonylureas		See Table 333-13		Lower fasting blood glucose	Hypoglycemia weight gain, hyperinsulinemia	Renal/liver disease
Meglitinide		Repaglinide		Short onset of action, lower postprandial glucose	Hypoglycemia	Liver disease
Biguanides	↓ Hepatic glucose production, weight loss, ↑ glucose utilization	Metformin	1–2	Weight loss, improved lipid profile, no hypoglycemia	Lactic acidosis, diarrhea, nausea, possible increased cardiovascular mortality	Serum creatinine >1.5 mg/dL (men), >1.4 mg/dL (women), radiographic contrast studies, seriously ill patients, acidosis
α-Glucosidase inhibitors	↓ Glucose absorption	Acarbose, miglitol	0.5–1.0	No risk of hypoglycemia	GI flatulence, ↑ liver function tests	Liver/renal disease
Thiazolidinediones	↓ Insulin resistance, ↑ glucose utilization	Rosiglitazone, pioglitazone	1–2	↓ Insulin and sulfonylurea requirements, ↓ triglycerides	Frequent hepatic monitoring for idiosyncratic hepatocellular injury (see text)	Liver disease, congestive heart failure
Medical nutrition therapy and physical activity	↓ Insulin resistance	Low-calorie, low-fat diet, exercise	1–2	Other health benefits	Compliance difficult, long-term success low	

levels in adipocytes but is expressed at lower levels in many other insulin-sensitive tissues. Agonists of this receptor promote adipocyte differentiation and may reduce insulin resistance in skeletal muscle indirectly. Thiazolidinediones reduce the fasting plasma glucose by improving peripheral glucose utilization and insulin sensitivity (Table 333-12). Circulating insulin levels decrease with use of the thiazolidinediones, indicating a reduction in insulin resistance. Although direct comparisons are not available, the two currently available thiazolidinediones appear to have similar efficacy; the therapeutic range for pioglitazone is 15 to 45 mg/d in a single daily dose and for rosiglitazone the total daily dose is 2 to 8 mg/d administered either once daily or twice daily in divided doses. The ability of thiazolidinediones to influence other features of the insulin resistance syndrome is under investigation.

The prototype of this class of drugs, thiazolidinediones, was withdrawn from the U.S. market after reports of hepatotoxicity and an association with an idiosyncratic liver reaction that sometimes led to hepatic failure. The two other thiazolidinediones, rosiglitazone and pioglitazone, thus far do not appear to induce the liver abnormalities seen with troglitazone. However, long-term experience with the newer agents is limited. Consequently, the FDA recommends measurement of liver function tests prior to initiating therapy with a thiazolidinedione and at regular intervals (every two months for the first year and then periodically). The thiazolidinediones raise LDL and HDL slightly and lower triglycerides by 10 to 15%, but the clinical significance of these changes is not known. Thiazolidinediones are associated with minor weight gain (1 to 2 kg), a small reduction in the hematocrit, and a mild increase in plasma volume. Cardiac function is not affected, but the incidence of peripheral edema is increased. They are contraindicated in patients with liver disease or congestive heart failure (class III or IV). Thiazolidinediones have been shown to induce ovulation in premenopausal women with polycystic ovary syndrome (see "Insulin Resistance Syndromes," above). Women should be warned about the risk of pregnancy, since the safety of thiazolidinediones in pregnancy is not established.

Table 333-13 Characteristics of Agents that Increase Insulin Secretion

Generic Name	Approved Daily Dosage Range, mg	Duration of Action, h	Clearance
Sulfonylurea			
First generation			
Chlorpropamide	100–500	>48	Renal
Tolazamide	100–1000	12–24	Hepatic, renal
Tolbutamide	500–3000	6–12	Hepatic
Second generation			
Glimepiride	1–8	24	Hepatic, renal
Glipizide	2.5–40	12–18	Hepatic
Glipizide (extended release)	5–10	24	Hepatic
Glyburide	1.25–20	12–24	Hepatic, renal
Glyburide (micronized)	0.75–12	12–24	Hepatic, renal
Meglitinide			
Repaglinide	0.5–16	2–6	Hepatic

SOURCE: Adapted from Zimmerman, 1998.

INSULIN THERAPY IN TYPE 2 DM Modest doses of insulin are quite efficacious in controlling hyperglycemia in newly diagnosed type 2 DM. Insulin should be considered as the initial therapy in type 2 DM, particularly in lean individuals or those with severe weight loss, in individuals with underlying renal or hepatic disease that precludes oral glucose-lowering agents, or in individuals who are hospitalized or acutely ill. Insulin therapy is ultimately required by a substantial number of individuals with type 2 DM because of the progressive nature of the disorder and the relative insulin deficiency that develops in patients with long-standing diabetes.

Because endogenous insulin secretion continues and is capable of providing some coverage of mealtime caloric intake, insulin is usually initiated in a single dose of intermediate-acting insulin (0.3 to 0.4 U/

kg per day), given either before breakfast or just before bedtime (or ultralente at bedtime). Since fasting hyperglycemia and increased hepatic glucose production are prominent features of type 2 DM, bedtime insulin is more effective in clinical trials than a single dose of morning insulin. Some physicians prefer a relatively low, fixed starting dose of intermediate-acting insulin (~15 to 20 units in the morning and 5 to 10 units at bedtime) to avoid hypoglycemia. The insulin dose may then be adjusted in 10% increments as dictated by SMBG results. Both morning and bedtime intermediate insulin may be used in combination with oral glucose-lowering agents (biguanides, α-glucosidase inhibitors, or thiazolidinediones).

Choice of Initial Glucose-Lowering Agent Though insulin is an effective primary therapy for type 2 DM, most patients and physicians currently prefer oral glucose-lowering drugs as the initial pharmacologic approach. The level of hyperglycemia should influence the initial choice of therapy. Assuming maximal benefit of MNT and increased physical activity has been realized, patients with mild to moderate hyperglycemia [fasting plasma glucose <11.1 to 13.9 mmol/L (200 to 250 mg/dL)] often respond well to a single oral glucose-lowering agent. Patients with more severe hyperglycemia [fasting plasma glucose >13.9 mmol/L (250 mg/dL)] may respond partially but are unlikely to achieve normoglycemia with oral monotherapy. Nevertheless, many physicians prefer a stepwise approach that starts with a single agent and adds a second agent to achieve the glycemic target (see "Combination Therapy," below). Some physicians begin insulin in individuals with severe hyperglycemia [fasting plasma glucose >13.9 to 16.7 mmol/L (250 to 300 mg/dL)]. This approach is based on the rationale that more rapid glycemic control will reduce "glucose toxicity" to the islet cells, improve endogenous insulin secretion, and possibly allow oral glucose-lowering agents to be more effective. If this occurs, the insulin may be discontinued.

Insulin secretagogues, biguanides, α-glucosidase inhibitors, thiazolidinediones, and insulin are approved for monotherapy of type 2 DM. Although each class of oral glucose-lowering agents has unique advantages and disadvantages, certain generalizations apply: (1) insulin secretagogues, biguanides, and thiazolidinediones improve glycemic control to a similar degree (1 to 2% reduction in HbA1c) and are more effective than α-glucosidase inhibitors; (2) assuming a similar degree of glycemic improvement, no clinical advantage to one class of drugs has been demonstrated, and any therapy that improves glycemic control is beneficial; (3) insulin secretagogues and α-glucosidase inhibitors begin to lower the plasma glucose immediately, whereas the glucose-lowering effects of the biguanides and thiazolidinediones are delayed by several weeks to months; (4) not all agents are effective in all individuals with type 2 DM (primary failure); (5) biguanides, α-glucosidase inhibitors, and thiazolidinediones do not directly cause hypoglycemia; and (6) most individuals will eventually require treatment with more than one class of oral glucose-lowering agents, reflecting the progressive nature of type 2 DM.

Considerable clinical experience exists with sulfonylureas and metformin because they have been available for several decades. It is assumed that the α-glucosidase inhibitors and thiazolidinediones, which are newer classes of oral glucose-lowering drugs, will reduce DM-related complications by improving glycemic control, although long-term data are not yet available. The thiazolidinediones are theoretically attractive because they target a fundamental abnormality in type 2 DM, namely insulin resistance. However, these agents are currently more costly than others and require liver function monitoring.

A reasonable treatment algorithm for initial therapy proposes either a sulfonylurea or metformin as initial therapy because of their efficacy, known side-effect profile, and relatively low cost (Fig. 333-14). Metformin has the advantage that it promotes mild weight loss, lowers insulin levels, improves the lipid profile slightly, and may have a lower secondary failure rate. However, there is no difference in response rate or degree of glycemic control when metformin and

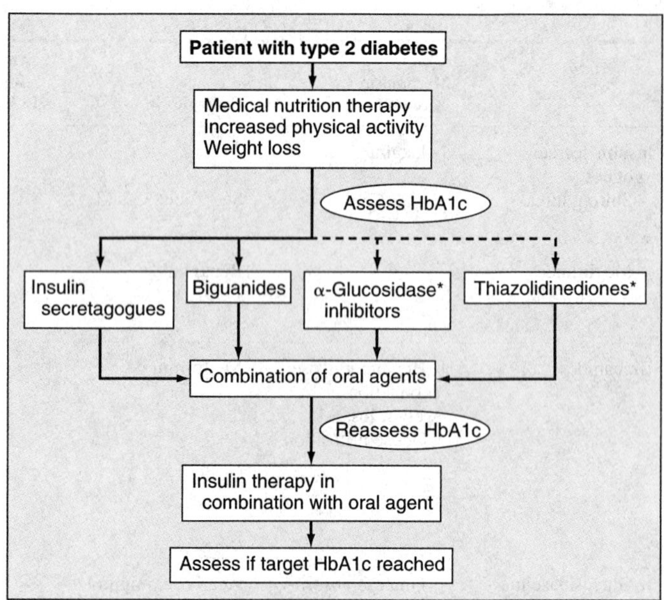

FIGURE 333-14 Glycemic management of type 2 diabetes. See text for discussion. *See text about use as monotherapy. The broken line indicates that biguanides or insulin secretagogues, but not α glucosidase inhibitors or thiazolidinediones, are preferred for initial therapy.

sulfonylureas are compared in randomized, prospective clinical trials. Based on SMBG results and the HbA1c, the dose of either the sulfonylurea or metformin should be increased until the glycemic target is achieved. α-Glucosidase inhibitors and thiazolidinediones are alternative, initial agents (Fig. 333-14).

When used as monotherapy, approximately one-third of individuals will reach their target glycemic goal with either a sulfonylurea or metformin. Approximately 25% of individuals will not respond to sulfonylureas or metformin; under these circumstances, the drug usually should be discontinued. Some individuals respond to one agent but not the other. The remaining individuals treated with either sulfonylureas or metformin alone will exhibit some improvement in glycemic control but will not achieve their glycemic target and should be considered for combination therapy.

Combination Therapy with Glucose-Lowering Agents A number of combinations of therapeutic agents are successful in type 2 DM, and the dosing of agents in combination is the same as when the agents are used alone. Because mechanisms of action of the first and second agents are different, the effect on glycemic control is usually additive. Commonly used regimens include: (1) insulin secretagogue with metformin or thiazolidinedione, (2) sulfonylurea with α-glucosidase inhibitor, and (3) insulin with metformin or thiazolidinedione. The combination of metformin and a thiazolidinedione is also effective and complementary. If adequate control is not achieved with two oral agents, bedtime insulin or a third oral agent may be added stepwise. However, long-term experience with any triple combination is lacking, and experience with two-drug combinations is relatively limited.

Insulin becomes required as type 2 DM enters the phase of relative insulin deficiency (as seen in long-standing DM) and is signaled by inadequate glycemic control on one or two oral glucose-lowering agents. Insulin can be used in combination with any of the oral agents in patients who fail to reach the glycemic target. For example, a single dose of intermediate-acting insulin at bedtime is effective in combination with metformin. As endogenous insulin production falls further, multiple injections of intermediate-acting and short-acting insulin regimens are necessary to control postprandial glucose excursions. These combination regimens are identical to the intermediate- and short-acting combination regimens discussed above for type 1 DM. Since the hyperglycemia of type 2 DM tends to be more "stable," these regimens can be increased in 10% increments every 2 to 3 days using SMBG results. The daily insulin dose required can become quite large (1 to 2 units/kg per day) as endogenous insulin production falls and insulin resistance persists. Individuals who require >1 unit/kg per day of intermediate-acting insulin should be considered for combination therapy with metformin or a thiazolidinedione. The addition of a thiazolidinedione can reduce insulin requirements in some individuals with type 2 DM, while maintaining or even improving glycemic control.

Intensive diabetes management (Table 333-10) is a treatment option in type 2 patients who cannot achieve optimal glycemic control and are capable of implementing such regimens. A recent study from the Veterans Administration found that intensive diabetes management is not associated with a greater degree of side effects (hypoglycemia, weight gain) than standard insulin therapy. The effect of higher insulin levels associated with intensive diabetes management on the prognosis of diseases commonly associated with type 2 DM (cardiovascular disease, hypertension) is still debated. In selected patients with type 2 DM, insulin pumps improve glycemic control and are well tolerated.

Emerging Therapies Whole pancreas transplantation (conventionally performed concomitantly with a renal transplant) may normalize glucose tolerance and is an important therapeutic option in type 1 diabetes, though it requires substantial expertise and is associated with the side effects of immunosuppression. Pancreatic islet transplantation has been plagued by limitations in pancreatic islet isolation and graft survival, but recent advances in specific immunomodulation have greatly improved the results. Islet transplantation is an area of active clinical investigation.

Advances in molecular biology and new insights into normal mechanisms of glucose homeostasis have led to a number of emerging therapies for diabetes and its complications. For example, glucagon-like peptide 1, a potent insulin secretagogue, may be efficacious in type 2 DM. Inhaled insulin and additional insulin analogues are in advanced stages of clinical trials. Aminoguanidine, an inhibitor of the formation of advanced glycosylation end products, and inhibitors of protein kinase C may reduce the complications of DM. Closed-loop pumps that infuse the appropriate amount of insulin in response to changing glucose levels are potentially feasible now that continuous glucose-monitoring technology has been developed.

COMPLICATIONS OF THERAPY FOR DIABETES MELLITUS

As with any therapy, the benefits of efforts directed towards glycemic control must be weighed against the risks of treatment. Side effects of intensive treatment include an increased frequency of serious hypoglycemia, weight gain, increased economic costs, and greater demands on the patient. In the DCCT, quality of life was very similar in the intensive therapy and standard therapy groups. The most serious complication of therapy for DM is hypoglycemia (Chap. 334). Weight gain occurs with most (insulin, insulin secretagogues, thiazolidinediones) but not all (metformin and α-glucosidase inhibitors) therapies that improve glycemic control due to the anabolic effects of insulin and the reduction in glucosuria. In the DCCT, individuals with the greatest weight gain exhibited increases in LDL cholesterol and triglycerides as well as increases in blood pressure (both systolic and diastolic) similar to those seen in individuals with type 2 DM and insulin resistance. These effects could increase the risk of cardiovascular disease in intensively managed patients. As discussed previously, improved glycemic control is sometimes accompanied by a transient worsening of diabetic retinopathy or neuropathy.

ONGOING ASPECTS OF COMPREHENSIVE DIABETES CARE

The morbidity and mortality of DM-related complications can be greatly reduced by timely and consistent surveillance procedures (Table 333-14). These screening procedures are indicated for all individuals with DM, but numerous studies have documented that most individuals with diabetes do not receive comprehensive diabetes care. Screening for dyslipidemia and hypertension should be performed annually. In addition to routine health maintenance, individuals with diabetes should also receive the pneumococcal and tetanus vaccines (at recommended intervals) and the influenza vaccine (annually).

Table 333-14 Guidelines for Ongoing Medical Care for Patients with Diabetes

- Self-monitoring of blood glucose (individualized frequency)
- HbA1c testing (2–4 times/year)
- Patient education in diabetes management (annual)
- Medical nutrition therapy and education (annual)
- Eye examination (annual)
- Foot examination (1–2 times/year by physician; daily by patient)
- Screening for diabetic nephropathy (annual; see Fig. 333-13)
- Blood pressure measurement (quarterly)
- Lipid profile (annual)

An annual comprehensive eye examination should be performed by a qualified optometrist or ophthalmologist. If abnormalities are detected, further evaluation and treatment require an ophthalmologist skilled in diabetes-related eye disease. Because many individuals with type 2 DM have had asymptomatic diabetes for several years before diagnosis, a consensus panel from the ADA recommends the following ophthalmologic examination schedule: (1) individuals with onset of DM at <29 years should have an initial eye examination within 3 to 5 years of diagnosis, (2) individuals with onset of DM at >30 years should have an initial eye examination at the time of diabetes diagnosis, and (3) women with DM who are contemplating pregnancy should have an eye examination prior to conception and during the first trimester.

An annual foot examination should: (1) assess blood flow, sensation, and nail care; (2) look for the presence of foot deformities such as hammer or claw toes and Charcot foot; and (3) identify sites of potential ulceration. Calluses and nail deformities should be treated by a podiatrist; the patient should be discouraged from self-care of even minor foot problems.

An annual microalbuminuria measurement is advised in individuals with type 1 or type 2 DM and no protein on a routine urinalysis (Fig. 333-10). If the urinalysis detects proteinuria, the amount of protein should be quantified by standard urine protein measurements. If the urinalysis was negative for protein in the past, microalbuminuria should be the annual screening examination. Routine urine protein measurements do not detect low levels of albumin excretion. Screening should commence 5 years after the onset of type 1 DM and at the time of onset of type 2 DM.

SPECIAL CONSIDERATIONS IN DIABETES MELLITUS

PSYCHOSOCIAL ASPECTS As with any chronic, debilitating disease, the individual with DM faces a series of challenges that affect all aspects of daily life. The individual with DM must accept that he or she may develop complications related to DM. Even with considerable effort, normoglycemia can be an elusive goal, and solutions to worsening glycemic control may not be easily identifiable. The patient should view him- or herself as an essential member of the diabetes care team and not as someone who is cared for by the diabetes team. Emotional stress may provoke a change in behavior so that individuals no longer adhere to a dietary, exercise, or therapeutic regimen. This can lead to the appearance of either hyper- or hypoglycemia. Depression and eating disorders (in women) are more common in individuals with type 1 or type 2 DM (Chap. 78).

MANAGEMENT IN THE HOSPITALIZED PATIENT Virtually all medical and surgical subspecialties may be involved in the care of hospitalized patients with diabetes. General anesthesia, surgery, and concurrent illness raise the levels of counterregulatory hormones (cortisol, growth hormone, catecholamines, and glucagon), and infection may lead to transient insulin resistance. These factors increase insulin requirements by increasing glucose production and impairing glucose utilization and thus may worsen glycemic control. On the other hand, the concurrent illness or surgical procedure may prevent the patient with DM from eating normally and may promote hypoglycemia. Glycemic control should be assessed (with HbA1c) and, if feasible, should be optimized prior to surgery. Electrolytes, renal function, and intravascular volume status should be assessed as well. The extremely high prevalence of asymptomatic cardiovascular disease in individuals with DM (especially in type 2 DM) may require preoperative cardiovascular evaluation.

The goals of diabetes management during hospitalization are avoidance of hypoglycemia, optimization of glycemic control, and transition back to the outpatient diabetes treatment regimen. Attention to each stage in this process requires integrating information regarding the plasma glucose, diabetes treatment regimen, and clinical status of the patient. For example, some surgical procedures utilizing local anesthesia or epidural anesthesia may have minimal effects on glycemic control. If the patient is eating soon after the procedure and there is no disruption of the patient's regular meal plans, then glycemic control is usually maintained.

The physician caring for an individual with diabetes in the perioperative period, during times of infection or serious physical illness, or simply when fasting for a diagnostic procedure must monitor the plasma glucose vigilantly, adjust the diabetes treatment regimen, and provide glucose infusion as needed. Several different treatment regimens (intravenous or subcutaneous insulin regimens) can be employed successfully. Individuals with type 1 DM require continued insulin administration to maintain the levels of circulating insulin necessary to prevent DKA. Prolongation of a surgical procedure or delay in the recovery room is not uncommon and may result in periods of insulin deficiency. Even relatively brief periods without insulin may lead to mild DKA. Individuals with type 1 DM who are undergoing general anesthesia and surgery, or who are seriously ill, should receive continuous insulin, either through an intravenous insulin infusion or by subcutaneous administration of a reduced dose of long-acting insulin. Short-acting insulin alone is insufficient.

Individuals with type 2 DM can be managed with either insulin infusion or a reduced dose of subcutaneous insulin. Oral glucose-lowering agents are discontinued at the time a combined insulin/glucose infusion is started. Oral agents such as sulfonylureas, metformin, acarbose, and thiazolidinediones are not useful in regulating the plasma glucose in clinical situations where the insulin requirements and glucose intake are changing rapidly. Moreover, these oral agents may be dangerous if the patient is fasting (e.g., hypoglycemia with sulfonylureas). Metformin should be withheld when radiographic contrast media will be given or if severe congestive heart failure, acidosis, or declining renal function is present.

Insulin infusions can effectively control plasma glucose in the perioperative period and when the patient is unable to take anything by mouth. The absorption of subcutaneous insulin may be variable in such situations because of changes in blood flow. The physician must consider carefully the clinical setting in which an insulin infusion will be utilized, including whether adequate ancillary personnel are available to monitor the plasma glucose frequently and whether they can adjust the insulin infusion rate, either based on an algorithm or in consultation with the physician. The initial rate for an insulin infusion may range from 0.5 to 5 units/h, depending on the degree of insulin resistance and the clinical situation. Based on hourly capillary glucose measurements, the insulin infusion rate is adjusted to maintain the plasma glucose within the desired range [5.6 to 11.1 mmol/L (100 to 200 mg/dL)]. Glucose infusion, initiated at the time the patient begins fasting, should be adjusted to deliver the equivalent of 50 to 150 mL of D_5W/h until the patient is reliably taking nutrition orally. The insulin infusion can be temporarily discontinued if hypoglycemia occurs and may be resumed at a lower infusion rate once the plasma glucose exceeds 5.6 mmol/L (100 mg/dL).

Insulin infusion is the preferred method for managing patients with type 1 DM in the perioperative period or when serious concurrent illness is present. Individuals with type 2 DM can be managed with an insulin infusion, but subcutaneous insulin in reduced doses can be used effectively as well. If the diagnostic or surgical procedure is brief and performed under local or regional anesthesia, a reduced dose of subcutaneous, long-acting insulin may suffice. This approach facilitates the transition back to the long-acting insulin after the procedure. The dose of long-acting insulin should be reduced by 30 to 40%, and short-acting insulin is either held or, likewise, reduced by 30 to 40%. Glucose should be infused to prevent hypoglycemia.

Total Parenteral Nutrition (See Chap. 76) Total parenteral nutrition (TPN) greatly increases insulin requirements. In addition, individuals not previously known to have DM may become hyperglycemic during TPN and require insulin treatment. Intravenous insulin infusion is the preferred treatment for hyperglycemia, and rapid titration to the required insulin dose is done most efficiently using a separate insulin infusion. After the total insulin dose has been determined, insulin may be added directly to the TPN solution. Often, individuals receiving either TPN or enteral nutrition receive their caloric loads continuously and not at "meal times"; consequently, subcutaneous insulin regimens must be adjusted.

GLUCOCORTICOIDS Glucocorticoids increase insulin resistance, decrease glucose utilization, increase hepatic glucose production, and impair insulin secretion. These changes lead to a worsening of glycemic control in individuals with DM and may precipitate diabetes in other individuals ("steroid-induced diabetes"). The effects of glucocorticoids on glucose homeostasis are dose-related, usually reversible, and most pronounced in the postprandial period. If the fasting plasma glucose is near the normal range, oral diabetes agents (sulfonylureas and acarbose) may be sufficient to reduce hyperglycemia. If the fasting plasma glucose >11.1 mmol/L (200 mg/dL), oral agents are usually not efficacious and insulin therapy is required. Short-acting insulin may be required to supplement long-acting insulin in order to control postprandial glucose excursions.

REPRODUCTIVE ISSUES Reproductive capacity in either men or women with DM appears to be normal. Menstrual cycles may be associated with alterations in glycemic control in women with DM. Pregnancy is associated with marked insulin resistance; the increased insulin requirements often precipitate DM and lead to the diagnosis of GDM. Glucose, which at high levels is a teratogen to the developing fetus, readily crosses the placenta, but insulin does not. Thus, hyperglycemia or hypoglycemia from the maternal circulation may stimulate insulin secretion in the fetus. The anabolic and growth effects of insulin may result in macrosomia. GDM complicates approximately 4% of pregnancies in the United States. The incidence of GDM is greatly increased in certain ethnic groups, including African Americans and Hispanic Americans, consistent with a similar increased risk of type 2 DM. Current recommendations advise screening for glucose intolerance between weeks 24 and 28 of pregnancy in women with high risk for GDM (≥25 years; obesity; family history of DM; member of an ethnic group such as Hispanic American, Native American, Asian American, African American, or Pacific Islander). Therapy for GDM is similar to that for individuals with pregnancy-associated diabetes and involves MNT and insulin, if hyperglycemia persists. Oral glucose-lowering agents have not been approved for use during pregnancy. With current practices, the morbidity and mortality of the mother with GDM and the fetus are no different from those in the nondiabetic population. Individuals who develop GDM are at marked increased risk for developing type 2 DM in the future and should be screened periodically for DM. After delivery, glucose homeostasis should be reassessed in the mother. Most individuals with GDM revert to normal glucose tolerance, but some will continue to have overt diabetes or impairment of glucose tolerance. In addition, children of women with GDM appear to be at risk for obesity and glucose intolerance and have an increased risk of diabetes beginning in the later stages of adolescence.

Pregnancy in individuals with known DM requires meticulous planning and adherence to strict treatment regimens. Intensive diabetes management and normalization of the HbA1c are the standard of care for individuals with existing DM who are planning pregnancy. The crucial period of glycemic control is extremely early following fertilization. The risk of fetal malformations is increased 4 to 10 times in individuals with uncontrolled DM at the time of conception. The goals are normal plasma glucose during the preconception period and throughout the periods of organ development in the fetus.

LIPODYSTROPHIC DM (See also Chap. 354) Lipodystrophy, or the loss of subcutaneous fat tissue, may be generalized in certain genetic conditions such as leprechaunism. Generalized lipodystrophy is associated with severe insulin resistance and is often accompanied by acanthosis nigricans and dyslipidemia. Localized lipodystrophy associated with insulin injections has been reduced considerably by the use of human insulin.

Protease Inhibitors and Lipodystrophy Protease inhibitors used in the treatment of HIV disease (Chap. 309) have been associated with a centripetal accumulation of fat (visceral and abdominal area), accumulation of fat in the dorsocervical region, loss of extremity fat, decreased insulin sensitivity (elevations of the fasting insulin level and reduced glucose tolerance on intravenous glucose tolerance testing), and dyslipidemia. Although many aspects of the physical appearance of these individuals resemble Cushing's syndrome, derangements in cortisol secretion have not been found consistently and do not appear to account for this appearance. Although some individuals have IGT, diabetes is not a common feature. The possibility remains that this is related to HIV infection by some undefined mechanism, since some features of the syndrome were observed before the introduction of protease inhibitors. Therapy for HIV-related lipodystrophy is not well established.

BIBLIOGRAPHY

General

ALBERTI KG, ZIMMET PZ: Definition, diagnosis and classification of diabetes mellitus and its complications. Part 1: Diagnosis and classification of diabetes, provisional report of a WHO Consultation. Diabet Med 15:539, 1997

AMERICAN DIABETES ASSOCIATION: Diabetes Care 23(Suppl 1), 2000

CARTER JS et al: Non-insulin-dependent diabetes mellitus in minorities in the United States. Ann Intern Med 125:221, 1996

HARRIS MI et al: Prevalence of diabetes, impaired fasting glucose, and impaired glucose tolerance in U.S. adults. The Third National Health and Nutrition Examination Survey, 1988–1994. Diabetes Care 21:518, 1998

REPORT OF THE EXPERT COMMITTEE ON THE DIAGNOSIS AND CLASSIFICATION OF DIABETES MELLITUS. Diabetes Care 20:1183, 1997

ROSENBLOOM AL et al: Emerging epidemic of type 2 diabetes in youth. Diabetes Care 22:345, 1999

Genetics/Pathogenesis

CLINE GW et al: Impaired glucose transport as a cause of decreased insulin-stimulated muscle glycogen synthesis in type 2 diabetes. N Engl J Med 341:240, 1999

DEFRONZO RA: Pathogenesis of type 2 diabetes. Diabetes Rev 5:177, 1997

FROGUEL P, VELHO G: Molecular genetics of maturity-onset diabetes of the young. Trends Endocrinol Metab 10:142, 1999

GERICH JE: The genetic basis of type 2 diabetes mellitus: Impaired insulin secretion versus impaired insulin sensitivity. Endocr Rev 19:491, 1998

LOWE WL: Genetics of diabetes, in *Principles of Molecular Medicine*, JL Jameson (ed). Totowa, NJ, Humana, 1998, pp 433–442

PUGLIESE A: Unraveling the genetics of insulin-dependent type 1A diabetes: The search must go on. Diabetes Rev 7:39, 1999

SCHRANZ DB, LERNMARK A: Immunology in diabetes: An update. Diabetes Metab Rev 14:3, 1998

SHEPHERD PR, KAHN BB: Glucose transporters and insulin action—implications for insulin resistance and diabetes mellitus. N Engl J Med 341:248, 1999

SHULMAN GI: Cellular mechanisms of insulin resistance in humans. Am J Cardiol 84:3J, 1999

TRITOS NA, MANTZOROS CS: Syndromes of severe insulin resistance. J Clin Endocrinol Metab 83:3025, 1998

VIRKAMAKI A et al: Protein-protein interaction in insulin signaling and the molecular mechanisms of insulin resistance. J Clin Invest 103:931, 1999

Complications of Diabetes

AIELLO LP et al: Diabetic retinopathy. Diabetes Care 21:143, 1998

CHEN YDI, REAVEN GM: Insulin resistance and atherosclerosis. Diabetes Rev 5:331, 1997

Consensus development conference on diabetic foot wound care. Diabetes Care 22:1354, 1999

DETRE KM et al: The effect of previous coronary-artery bypass surgery on the prognosis of patients with diabetes who have acute myocardial infarction. N Engl J Med 342: 989, 2000

DIABETES CONTROL AND COMPLICATIONS TRIAL RESEARCH GROUP: The relationship of glycemic exposure (HbAIC) to the risk of development and progression of retinopathy in the diabetes control and complications trial. Diabetes 44:968, 1995

GRUNDY SM et al: Diabetes and cardiovascular disease: A statement for healthcare professionals from the American Heart Association. Circulation 100:1134, 1999

MOGENSEN CE: Preventing end-stage renal disease. Diabet Med 15(Suppl 4):S51, 1998

RITZ E, ORTH SR: Nephropathy in patients with type 2 diabetes. N Engl J Med 341:1127, 1999

Therapy

ABRAIRA C et al: Cardiovascular events and correlates in the Veterans Affairs diabetes feasibility trial: Veterans Affairs diabetes cooperative study on glycemic control and complication in type II diabetes. Arch Intern Med 157:181, 1997

AMERICAN DIABETES ASSOCIATION: *Therapy for Diabetes Mellitus and Related Disorders*, 3d ed, HS Lebovitz (ed). Alexandria, VA, American Diabetes Association, 1998

———: Clinical Practice Guidelines 2000. Diabetes Care 23(Suppl):S1, 2000

BUSE JB: Overview of current therapeutic options in type 2 diabetes. Rationale for combining oral agents with insulin therapy. Diabetes Care 22(Suppl 3):C65, 1999

DAVIDSON MB, PETERS AL: An overview of metformin in the treatment of type 2 diabetes mellitus. Am J Med 102:99, 1997

DEFRONZO RA: Pharmacologic therapy for type 2 diabetes mellitus. Ann Intern Med 131: 281, 1999

DIABETES CONTROL AND COMPLICATIONS TRIAL RESEARCH GROUP: The effect of intensive treatment of diabetes on the development and progression of long-term complications in insulin-dependent diabetes mellitus. N Engl J Med 329:977, 1993

ESTACIO RO et al: The effect of nisoldipine as compared with enalapril on cardiovascular outcomes in patients with non-insulin-dependent diabetes and hypertension. N Engl J Med 338:645, 1998

FARKAS-HIRSCH R (ed): *Intensive Diabetes Management*, 2d ed. Alexandria VA, American Diabetes Association, 1998

JACOBER SJ, SOWERS JR: An update on perioperative management of diabetes. Arch Intern Med 159:2405, 1999

KREISBERG RA: Diabetic dyslipidemia. Am J Cardiol 82:67U, 1998

MARSHALL SM: Blood pressure control, microalbuminuria and cardiovascular risk in Type 2 diabetes mellitus. Diabet Med 16:358, 1999

OHKUBO Y et al: Intensive insulin therapy prevents the progression of diabetic microvascular complications in Japanese patients with non-insulin-dependent diabetes mellitus: A randomized prospective 6-year study. Diabetes Res Clin Pract 28:103, 1995

SKYLER JS (ed): *Medical Management of Type 1 Diabetes*, 3d ed. Alexandria VA, American Diabetes Association, 1998

TUOMILEHTO et al: Effects of calcium-channel blockade in older patients with diabetes and systolic hypertension. Systolic Hypertension in Europe Trial Investigators. N Engl J Med 340:677, 1999

UK PROSPECTIVE DIABETES STUDY GROUP: Intensive blood-glucose control with sulphonylureas or insulin compared with conventional treatment and risk of complications in patients with type 2 diabetes (UKPDS 33). Lancet 352:837, 1998

———: Effect of intensive blood-glucose control with metformin on complications in overweight patients with type 2 diabetes (UKPDS 34). Lancet 352:854, 1998

———: Tight blood pressure control and risk of macrovascular and microvascular complications in type 2 diabetes: UKPDS 38. BMJ 317:708, 1999

UMPIERREZ GE et al: Review: Diabetic ketoacidosis and hyperglycemic hyperosmolar nonketotic syndrome. Am J Med Sci 311:225, 1996

VETERANS HEALTH ADMINISTRATION: Clinical guidelines for management of patients with diabetes mellitus. www.VA.gov/health/diabetes, 1997

YKI-JARVINEN H et al: Comparison of bedtime insulin regimens in patients with type 2 diabetes mellitus: A randomized, controlled trial. Ann Intern Med 130:389, 1999

ZIMMERMAN BR (ed): *Medical Management of Type 2 Diabetes*, 4d ed. Alexandria VA, American Diabetes Association, 1998

334 HYPOGLYCEMIA

Philip E. Cryer

Hypoglycemia occurs most commonly as a result of treating patients with diabetes mellitus. However, a number of other disorders, including insulinoma, large mesenchymal tumors, end-stage organ failure, alcoholism, endocrine deficiencies, postprandial reactive hypoglycemic conditions, and inherited metabolic disorders, are also associated with hypoglycemia (Table 334-1). Hypoglycemia is sometimes defined as a plasma glucose level <2.5 to 2.8 mmol/L (<45 to 50 mg/dL). However, as discussed below, the glucose thresholds for hypoglycemia-induced symptoms and physiologic responses vary widely, depending on the clinical setting. Therefore, *Whipple's triad* provides an important framework for making the diagnosis of hypoglycemia: (1) symptoms consistent with hypoglycemia, (2) a low plasma glucose concentration, and (3) relief of symptoms after the plasma glucose level is raised. Hypoglycemia can cause significant morbidity and can be lethal, if severe or prolonged; it should be considered in any patient who presents with confusion, altered level of consciousness, or seizures.

SYSTEMIC GLUCOSE BALANCE AND COUNTERREGULATION

Glucose is an obligate metabolic fuel for the brain under physiologic conditions. By contrast, other organs can use fatty acids, in addition to glucose, to generate energy. The brain cannot synthesize glucose and stores only a few minutes' supply as glycogen. It therefore requires a continuous supply of glucose, which is delivered by facilitated diffusion from arterial blood. As the plasma glucose concentration falls below the physiologic range, blood-to-brain glucose transport becomes insufficient for adequate brain energy metabolism and functioning. It is therefore not surprising that redundant physiologic mechanisms prevent or rapidly correct hypoglycemia.

Table 334-1 Causes of Hypoglycemia

Drugs
Especially insulin, sulfonylureas, ethanol
Sometimes pentamidine, quinine
Rarely salicylates, sulfonamides, and others
Endogenous hyperinsulinism
Insulinoma
Other β cell disorders
Secretagogue (sulfonylurea)
Autoimmune (autoantibodies to insulin, insulin receptor, β cell?)
Ectopic insulin secretion
Critical illnesses
Hepatic, renal, or cardiac failure
Sepsis
Starvation and inanition
Endocrine deficiencies
Cortisol, growth hormone
Glucagon and epinephrine (type 1 diabetes)
Non-β-cell tumors
Fibrosarcoma, mesothelioma, rhabdomyosarcoma, liposarcoma, other sarcomas
Hepatoma, adrenocortical tumors, carcinoid
Leukemia, lymphoma, melanoma, teratoma
Disorders of infancy or childhood
Transient intolerance of fasting
Infants of diabetic mothers (hyperinsulinism)
Persistent hyperinsulinemic hypoglycemia of infancy
Inherited enzyme defects
Postprandial
Reactive (after gastric surgery)
Ethanol-induced
Autonomic symptoms without true hypoglycemia
Factitious
Insulin, sulfonylureas

Plasma glucose levels are maintained within a narrow range, usually between 3.3 and 8.3 mmol/L (60 and 150 mg/dL), despite wide variation in food intake and activity level. This delicate balance requires dynamic regulation of glucose influx into the circulation as glucose utilization in various tissues can change rapidly. The diet is normally a major source of glucose. However, between meals or during fasting, serum glucose levels are maintained primarily by the breakdown of glycogen in the liver and by gluconeogenesis (Fig. 334-1). In most people, hepatic glycogen stores are sufficient to maintain plasma glucose levels for 8 to 12 h, but this time period can be shorter if glucose demand is increased by exercise or if glycogen stores are depleted by illness or starvation.

As glycogen stores are depleted, glucose is generated by gluconeogenesis, which occurs primarily in the liver but also in the kidney. Gluconeogenesis requires a coordinated supply of precursors from liver, muscle, and adipose tissue. Muscle provides lactate, pyruvate, alanine, and other amino acids; triglycerides in adipose tissue are broken down into glycerol, which is a precursor for gluconeogenesis, and free fatty acids, which generate acetyl CoA for gluconeogenesis and provide an alternative fuel source to tissues other than brain.

The balance of glucose production and its uptake and utilization in peripheral tissues is exquisitely regulated by a network of hormones, neural pathways, and metabolic signals (Chap. 333). Among the factors that control glucose production and utilization, insulin plays a dominant and pivotal role. In the fasting state, insulin is suppressed, allowing increased gluconeogenesis in the liver and the kidney and enhancing glucose generation by the breakdown of liver glycogen. Low insulin levels also reduce glucose uptake and utilization in peripheral tissues and allow lipolysis and proteolysis to occur, leading to the release of precursors for gluconeogenesis and providing alternative energy sources. In the fed state, insulin release from the pancreatic β cells reverses these processes. Glycogenolysis and gluconeogenesis are inhibited, thereby reducing hepatic and renal glucose output; peripheral glucose uptake and utilization are enhanced; lipolysis and proteolysis are restrained; and energy storage is promoted by the conversion of substrates into glycogen, triglycerides, and proteins. Other hormones including glucagon, epinephrine, growth hormone, and cortisol play less important roles in the control of glucose flux during normal physiologic circumstances. However, as described below, these hormones are critically important in the response to hypoglycemia.

As glucose levels approach, and ultimately enter, the hypoglycemic range, a characteristic sequence of *counterregulatory hormone responses* occurs. Glucagon is the first and most important of these responses. It promotes glycogenolysis and gluconeogenesis. Epineph-

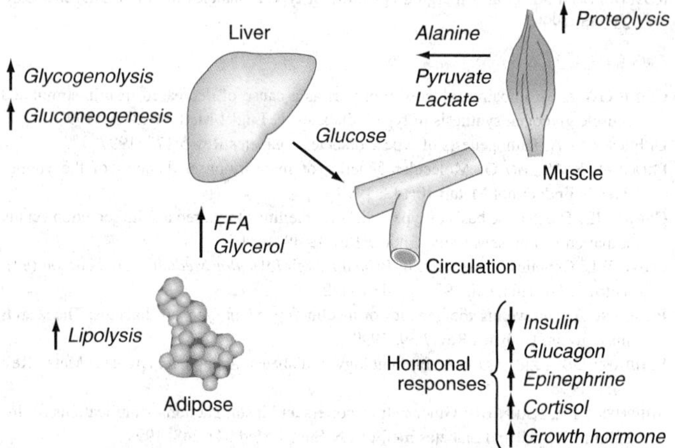

FIGURE 334-1 Overview of glucose metabolism and pathways of counterregulatory responses to fasting and hypoglycemia.

rine can also play an important role in the acute response to hypoglycemia, particularly when glucagon is insufficient. It, too, stimulates glycogenolysis and gluconeogenesis as well as limiting glucose utilization by insulin-sensitive tissues. When hypoglycemia is prolonged, growth hormone and cortisol also reduce glucose utilization and support its production.

The glucose thresholds at which various counterregulatory hormone responses occur are quite similar in healthy subjects (Table 334-2). Nonetheless, these thresholds are dynamic and can be influenced by recent metabolic events. A person with poorly controlled diabetes can have symptoms of hypoglycemia at higher-than-normal glucose levels. Recurrent hypoglycemia, as may occur in individuals with diabetes or in the setting of an insulinoma, shifts thresholds for symptoms and counterregulatory responses to lower glucose levels.

Table 334-2 Physiologic Responses to Decreasing Plasma Glucose Concentrations

Response	Glycemic Threshold, mmol/L (mg/dL)	Physiologic Effects	Role in the Prevention or Correction of Hypoglycemia (Glucose Counterregulation)
↓ Insulin	4.4–4.7 (80–85)	↑ R_a (↓ R_d)	Primary glucose regulatory factor/first defense against hypoglycemia
↑ Glucagon	3.6–3.9 (65–70)	↑ R_a	Primary glucose counterregulatory factor
↑ Epinephrine	3.6–3.9 (65–70)	↑ R_a, ↓ R_d	Involved, critical when glucagon is deficient
↑ Cortisol and growth hormone	3.6–3.9 (65–70)	↑ R_a, ↓ R_d	Involved, not critical
Symptoms	2.8–3.1 (50–55)	↑ Exogenous glucose	Prompt behavioral defense (food ingestion)
↓ Cognition	< 2.8 (< 50)	—	(Compromises behavioral defense)

NOTE: R_a, rate of glucose appearance, glucose production by the liver and kidneys; R_d, Rate of glucose disappearance, glucose utilization by insulin-sensitive tissues such as skeletal muscle, and by the central nervous system (where glucoregulatory hormones have no direct effect on glucose utilization).

CLINICAL MANIFESTATIONS

Symptoms of hypoglycemia can be divided into two categories, neuroglycopenic and neurogenic (or autonomic) responses. Neuroglycopenic symptoms are the direct result of central nervous system neuronal glucose deprivation. They include behavioral changes, confusion, fatigue, seizure, loss of consciousness, and, if hypoglycemia is severe and prolonged, death. Hypoglycemia-induced autonomic responses include adrenergic symptoms such as palpitations, tremor, and anxiety as well as cholinergic symptoms such as sweating, hunger, and paresthesia. Adrenergic symptoms are mediated by norepinephrine released from sympathetic postganglionic neurons and the release of epinephrine from the adrenal medullae. Increased sweating is mediated by cholinergic sympathetic nerve fibers. Patients with diabetes mellitus learn to recognize the characteristic symptoms of hypoglycemia, but these are less familiar to individuals with other causes of hypoglycemia. Symptoms may be less pronounced with repeated hypoglycemic episodes (see below).

Common signs of hypoglycemia include pallor and diaphoresis. Heart rate and the systolic blood pressure are typically raised, but these findings may not be prominent. The neuroglycopenic manifestations are valuable, albeit nonspecific, signs. Transient focal neurologic deficits occur occasionally.

CAUSES

Hypoglycemia is traditionally classified as *postprandial* or *fasting*. However, in the clinical setting, hypoglycemia most commonly results from the treatment of diabetes. This topic is therefore addressed before considering the other causes of hypoglycemia.

HYPOGLYCEMIA IN DIABETES **Frequency and Impact** Were it not for hypoglycemia, diabetes would be rather easy to treat by administering enough insulin (or any effective drug) to lower plasma glucose concentrations to, or below, the normal range. Because of imperfections in all current insulin-replacement regimens, individuals with type 1 diabetes are at ongoing risk for periods of relative hyperinsulinemia with resultant hypoglycemia. Those attempting to achieve near-normal glycemic control may experience several episodes of asymptomatic or symptomatic hypoglycemia each week. Plasma glucose levels may be <2.8 mmol/L (<50 mg/dL) as much as 10% of the time. At least 25% of such patients suffer an episode of severe, temporarily disabling hypoglycemia, often with seizure or coma, in a given year. Although seemingly complete recovery from the latter is the rule, the possibility of persistent cognitive deficits has been raised, but permanent neurologic defects are rare. About 2 to 4% of deaths associated with type 1 diabetes are estimated to result from hypoglycemia. Fear of hypoglycemia also can lead to disabling psychosocial morbidity.

Hypoglycemia is a less frequent problem in type 2 diabetes but occurs nevertheless in those treated with insulin or sulfonylureas. Transient, mild hypoglycemia may be seen with the shorter-acting sulfonylureas and repaglinide, which also acts by enhancing insulin secretion. Patients taking the long-acting sulfonylureas, chlorpropamide and glyburide, occasionally experience episodes of severe hypoglycemia that may last up to 24 to 36 h.

Conventional Risk Factors Insulin excess is the primary determinant of risk from iatrogenic hypoglycemia. Relative or absolute insulin excess occurs when: (1) insulin (or oral agent) doses are excessive, ill timed, or of the wrong type; (2) the influx of exogenous glucose is reduced, as during an overnight fast or following missed meals or snacks; (3) insulin-independent glucose utilization is increased, as during exercise; (4) insulin sensitivity is increased, as occurs with effective intensive therapy, in the middle of the night, late after exercise, or with increased fitness or weight loss; (5) endogenous glucose production is reduced, as following alcohol ingestion; and (6) insulin clearance is reduced, as in renal failure. However, analyses of the Diabetes Control and Complications Trial (DCCT) indicate that these conventional risk factors explain only a minority of episodes of severe iatrogenic hypoglycemia and that other causes are involved in the majority of episodes.

Hypoglycemia-Associated Autonomic Failure It is now clear that inadequate physiologic counterregulatory and behavioral responses greatly compound the problem of hypoglycemia caused by insulin excess. Hypoglycemia-associated autonomic failure has two main components: (1) reduced counterregulatory hormone responses, which result in impaired glucose generation; and (2) hypoglycemia unawareness, which precludes appropriate behavioral responses, such as eating.

Defective glucose counterregulation The counterregulatory hormone response is fundamentally altered in all people with established (e.g., absent C peptide) type 1 diabetes. As the patient becomes totally insulin-deficient over the first few months or years of the disease, circulating insulin levels are no longer tightly coordinated with glucose levels and are a passive function of administered insulin. Thus, insulin levels do not always decline as glucose levels fall; the first defense against hypoglycemia is lost. Over the same time frame, the glucagon response to falling glucose levels diminishes, and the second defense against hypoglycemia is lost. The cause of defective glucagon production by the pancreatic islet α cells is unknown, but it is tightly linked to the loss of insulin production by the β cells. It is a functional abnormality rather than an absolute deficiency of glucagon, as responses to stimuli other than hypoglycemia are intact. The third defense against hypoglycemia is compromised when the epinephrine response to hypoglycemia is reduced. In contrast to the absent glucagon response, epinephrine deficiency is a threshold abnormality; an epinephrine response can still be elicited, but a lower plasma glucose concentration is required. This threshold shift is largely the result of recent antecedent hypoglycemia, although an additional anatomic component may be present as well in patients affected by classic diabetic autonomic neuropathy. The development of a reduced epinephrine response is a critical pathophysiologic event. Prospective studies have shown that patients with combined deficiencies of glucagon and epinephrine suffer severe hypoglycemia at rates 25-fold or greater than individuals with absent glucagon but intact epinephrine responses.

Hypoglycemia unawareness Hypoglycemia unawareness refers to loss of the warning symptoms of hypoglycemia that normally alert individuals to the presence of hypoglycemia and prompt them to eat to abort the episode. Under these circumstances, the first manifestation of hypoglycemia is neuroglycopenia, and it is often too late for patients to treat themselves. Like defective counterregulation, the presence of hypoglycemia unawareness has been shown in prospective studies to be associated with a high frequency of severe hypoglycemia.

The interplay of factors involved in hypoglycemia-associated autonomic failure in type 1 diabetes, and consequent hypoglycemia unawareness, is summarized in Fig. 334-2. Periods of relative or absolute therapeutic insulin excess, in the setting of absent glucagon responses, lead to episodes of iatrogenic hypoglycemia. These episodes, in turn, cause reduced autonomic (including adrenomedullary) responses to falling glucose concentrations. These impaired autonomic responses result in reduced symptoms of impending hypoglycemia (e.g., hypoglycemia unawareness) and, because epinephrine responses are reduced in the setting of absent glucagon responses, impaired physiologic defense against developing hypoglycemia. Thus, a vicious cycle of recurrent hypoglycemia is created and perpetuated. The syndrome of hypoglycemia unawareness and the reduced epinephrine component of defective glucose counterregulation are reversible after as little as 2 weeks of scrupulous avoidance of hypoglycemia. This involves a shift of glycemic thresholds back to higher plasma glucose concentrations.

Hypoglycemia Risk Factor Reduction It is possible to minimize the risk of hypoglycemia by applying the principles of modern therapy—patient education and empowerment, frequent self-monitoring of blood glucose, flexible insulin (and other drug) regimens, rational glycemic goals, and ongoing professional guidance and support. With respect to the latter, the issue of hypoglycemia needs to be addressed in every patient contact. If hypoglycemia is a recognized problem, first consider each of the conventional risk factors summarized earlier and recommend the appropriate adjustments of medications, diet, and life-style. Nonselective beta blockers may attenuate the recognition of hypoglycemia and they impair glycogenolysis; a relatively selective β_1-antagonist (e.g., metoprolol or atenolol) is preferable when a beta blocker is indicated. One should consider the issue of compromised glucose counterregulation. Although it is possible to test for this abnormality using a low-dose insulin infusion test, this is not practical. A diagnosis of hypoglycemia unawareness can usually be made from the history. It should be remembered that hypoglycemia unawareness implies that previous episodes of hypoglycemia have occurred, whether these are documented or not. If low glucose levels are not apparent from the patient's self-monitoring log, one should suspect hypoglycemia during the night. The presence of clinical hypoglycemia unawareness makes defective glucose counterregulation quite likely. A 2 to 3 week period of conscientious avoidance of hypoglycemia is advisable.

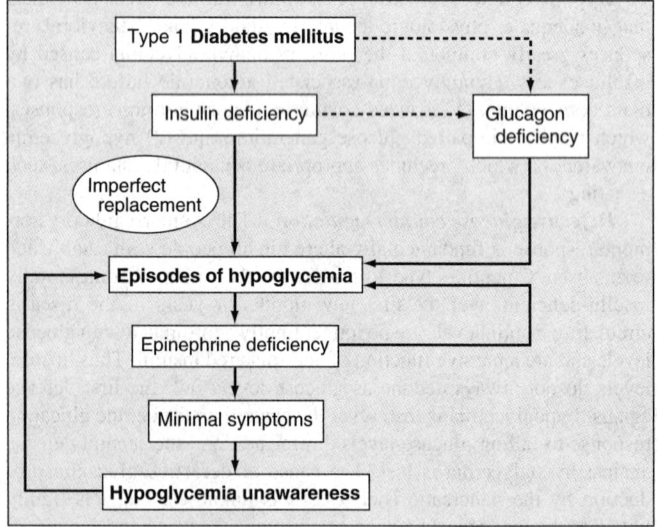

FIGURE 334-2 Hypoglycemia-associated autonomic failure and hypoglycemia unawareness in type 1 diabetes. *(Modified from PE Cryer: Diabetes 41: 255, 1992, with permission.)*

REACTIVE HYPOGLYCEMIA The postprandial (reactive) hypoglycemias occur only after meals, and hypoglycemia is self-limited. Postprandial hypoglycemia occurs in children with certain rare enzymatic defects in carbohydrate metabolism such as hereditary fructose intolerance and galactosemia (Chap. 350). Reactive hypoglycemia also occurs in some individuals who have undergone gastric surgery that results in the rapid passage of food from the stomach to the small intestine. This type of *alimentary hypoglycemia* causes a rapid postprandial rise in plasma glucose levels and the release of gut incretins, which induce an exuberant insulin response and subsequent hypoglycemia. Administration of an α-glucosidase inhibitor, which delays carbohydrate digestion and thus glucose absorption from the intestine, can be considered for treatment of reactive hypoglycemia, although its efficacy remains to be established in controlled trials.

If postprandial symptoms occur as an idiopathic disorder, caution should be exercised before labeling a person with the diagnosis of hypoglycemia. Indeed, a self-diagnosis of hypoglycemia has often been reinforced by the finding of a "low" venous glucose concentration late after glucose ingestion. An oral glucose tolerance test should not be used in this setting. Plasma glucose falls as low as 2.4 mmol/L (43 mg/dL) after a 100-g glucose load in 5% of normal asymptomatic individuals, making it difficult to identify hypoglycemia based on the results of this test. The diagnosis of postprandial hypoglycemia requires documentation of Whipple's triad after a typical mixed meal. The cause of repetitive postprandial symptoms in certain individuals is unknown, but they may be particularly sensitive to the normal autonomic responses that follow ingestion of a meal.

FASTING HYPOGLYCEMIA There are many causes of fasting hypoglycemia (Table 334-1). In addition to insulin and sulfonylureas used in the treatment of diabetes, ethanol use is a relatively common cause of hypoglycemia. Sepsis and renal failure are often complicated by hypoglycemia, but it is less common in other critical illnesses. Endocrine deficiencies, non-β-cell tumors, and endogenous hyperinsulinemia (including that caused by an insulinoma) are rare causes of hypoglycemia. Enzymatic metabolic errors that cause hypoglycemia are also rare but are being recognized more frequently in infants and children (Chaps. 350 and 352).

Drugs In contrast to the sulfonylureas and benzoic acid derivatives (e.g., repaglinide), other oral hypoglycemic agents—biguanides (e.g., metformin), α-glucosidase inhibitors (e.g., acarbose, miglitol), and thiazolidinediones (e.g., troglitazone, rosiglitazone, pioglitazone)—do not act by stimulating insulin secretion. Therefore, with these agents, insulin levels usually decrease appropriately as plasma glucose levels fall. Nonetheless, these drugs can contribute to hypoglycemia in other ways. Treatment with an α-glucosidase inhibitor alters the management of hypoglycemia; pure glucose should be used rather than ingestion of complex carbohydrates. Thiazolidinediones, as well as metformin, can predispose to hypoglycemia in patients receiving combined treatment with insulin or an insulin secretagogue.

Ethanol blocks gluconeogenesis but not glycogenolysis. Thus, alcohol-induced hypoglycemia typically occurs after a several-day ethanol binge during which the person eats little food, thereby causing glycogen depletion. Hypoglycemia in this setting can be profound, with mortality rates as high as 10%. Blood ethanol levels correlate poorly with plasma glucose concentrations at the time of diagnosis, as hypoglycemia occurs late in the sequence and often precludes further alcohol consumption.

Pentamidine, which is used to treat *Pneumocystis* pneumonia and other parasitic infections, is toxic to the pancreatic β cell. It causes insulin release initially, with hypoglycemia in about 10% of treated patients, and predisposes to the development of diabetes mellitus later. Quinine also stimulates insulin secretion. However, the relative contribution of hyperinsulinemia to the pathogenesis of hypoglycemia in quinine-treated patients who are critically ill with malaria is debated. Salicylates and sulfonamides can cause hypoglycemia but do so rarely. There are reports of hypoglycemia attributed to nonselective β-adrenergic antagonists (e.g., propranolol) and a variety of other drugs.

Critical Illness Rapid and extensive hepatic destruction (e.g., severe toxic hepatitis) causes fasting hypoglycemia because the liver is the major site of endogenous glucose production. The mechanism of hypoglycemia reported in patients with cardiac failure is unknown but likely involves hepatic congestion. Although the kidneys are a source of glucose production, it is perhaps too simplistic to attribute hypoglycemia in people with renal failure to this mechanism alone. The clearance of insulin is reduced substantially in renal failure, and reduced mobilization of gluconeogenic precursors has been reported.

Sepsis is sometimes complicated by hypoglycemia, which is multifactorial in origin. There is impaired endogenous glucose production, perhaps the result of hepatic hypoperfusion, and increased glucose utilization, which is induced by cytokines in macrophage-rich tissues such as the liver, spleen, and ileum and in muscle. Nutrition is also often inadequate in the setting of sepsis. Hypoglycemia can be seen with prolonged starvation, perhaps as a result of the loss of whole-body fat stores and the subsequent depletion of gluconeogenic precursors (e.g., amino acids), which necessitate increased glucose utilization.

Endocrine Deficiencies Neither cortisol nor growth hormone is critical to the prevention of acute hypoglycemia, at least in adults. Nonetheless, hypoglycemia can occur with prolonged fasting in patients with untreated primary adrenocortical failure (Addison's disease) or hypopituitarism. Anorexia and weight loss are typical features of chronic cortisol deficiency and likely result in glycogen depletion with increased reliance on gluconeogenesis. Cortisol deficiency is associated with low levels of gluconeogenic precursors, suggesting that substrate-limited gluconeogenesis, in the setting of glycogen depletion, is the cause of the impaired ability to tolerate fasting in cortisol-deficient individuals. Growth hormone deficiency can cause hypoglycemia in young children. In addition to extended fasting, high rates of glucose utilization (e.g., during exercise, pregnancy) or low rates of glucose production (e.g., following alcohol ingestion) can precipitate hypoglycemia in adults with hypopituitarism. Cortisol and growth hormone secretion should be evaluated in patients with fasting hypoglycemia when the history suggests pituitary or adrenal disease and when other causes of hypoglycemia are not apparent.

As discussed earlier, the combined loss of counterregulatory glucagon and epinephrine responses plays a central role in the pathogenesis of hypoglycemia in diabetes mellitus. However, hypoglycemia is not a feature of the epinephrine-deficient state that results from bilateral adrenalectomy when glucocorticoid replacement is adequate, nor does it occur during pharmacologic adrenergic blockage when other glucoregulatory systems are intact. There are case reports of fasting hypoglycemia attributed to isolated glucagon or epinephrine deficiency, although hyperinsulinemia was not excluded convincingly in the neonatal cases and other counterregulatory defects may have contributed in the adults. Thus, the regular assessment of glucagon and epinephrine secretion is not warranted.

Non-β-Cell Tumors Fasting hypoglycemia, often termed *non-islet cell tumor hypoglycemia*, occurs in some patients with large mesenchymal or other tumors (e.g., hepatoma, adrenocortical tumors, carcinoids). The glucose kinetic patterns resemble those of hyperinsulinism, but insulin secretion is suppressed appropriately during hypoglycemia. In most instances, hypoglycemia is due to overproduction of an incompletely processed form of insulin-like growth factor (IGF)II. Although total IGF-II levels are not consistently elevated, circulating free IGF-II levels are high. Hypoglycemia may result from IGF-II actions through the insulin or IGF-I receptors. Because of negative-feedback suppression of growth hormone secretion, IGF-I levels tend to be low, causing an increased IGF-II to IGF-I ratio.

Endogenous Hyperinsulinism Hypoglycemia due to excessive endogenous insulin secretion can be caused by: (1) a primary pancreatic islet β cell disorder, typically a β cell tumor (insulinoma), sometimes multiple insulinomas, or, especially in infants or young children, a functional β cell disorder without an anatomic correlate; (2) a β cell secretagogue, often a sulfonylurea, and, theoretically, a β cell–stimulating autoantibody; (3) an autoantibody to insulin; or (4) perhaps ectopic insulin secretion. None of these disorders is common. Endogenous hyperinsulinism is more likely in an overtly well individual without other apparent causes of hypoglycemia such as a relevant drug history, critical illness, endocrine deficiencies, or a non-β-cell tumor. Accidental, surreptitious, or even malicious administration of a sulfonylurea or insulin should also be considered in such individuals.

The fundamental pathophysiologic feature of endogenous hyperinsulinism is the failure of insulin secretion to fall to very low rates during hypoglycemia. This is assessed by measuring insulin, proinsulin, and C peptide, which is derived from the processing of proinsulin. The critical diagnostic findings are a plasma insulin concentration $\geq$36 pmol/L ($\geq$6 μU/mL) and a plasma C-peptide concentration $\geq$0.2 mmol/L ($\geq$0.6 ng/mL) when the plasma glucose concentration is $\leq$2.5 mmol/L ($\leq$45 mg/dL) in the fasting state with symptoms of hypoglycemia. Insulin and C-peptide levels do not need to be absolutely high (e.g., relative to euglycemic normal values) but only inappropriately high in the setting of fasting hypoglycemia. Plasma proinsulin concentrations are also inappropriately high, particularly in patients with an insulinoma. Sulfonylureas, because they stimulate insulin secretion, result in a pattern of glucose, insulin, and C-peptide levels that is indistinguishable from that produced by a primary β cell disorder. The measurement of sulfonylureas in plasma or urine distinguishes these conditions. Antibodies to insulin produce *autoimmune hypoglycemia* following the transition from the postprandial to the postabsorptive state, as insulin slowly dissociates from the antibodies. Total and free plasma insulin concentrations are inappropriately high. The distinguishing finding is the presence of circulating antibodies to insulin, but the need to measure these routinely is debated, since autoimmune hypoglycemia appears to be rare. Autoantibodies to the insulin receptor are another rare cause of hypoglycemia and usually occur in the context of other autoimmune diseases. A few cases of apparent ectopic secretion of insulin (from a non-β-cell tumor) have been reported.

Insulinoma and other primary β cell disorders Insulinomas are rare, but because approximately 90% are benign, they are a treatable cause of potentially fatal hypoglycemia. The yearly incidence is estimated to be 1 in 250,000. About 60% of cases occur in women. The median age at presentation is 50 years in sporadic cases, but it usually presents in the third decade when associated with multiple endocrine neoplasia type 1 (Chap. 339). Insulinomas arise within the substance of the pancreas in >99% of cases and are usually small (1 to 2 cm). About 5 to 10% of insulinomas are malignant, as evidenced by the presence of metastases.

Insulinomas almost always come to clinical attention because of hypoglycemia rather than mass effects. As noted earlier, unusually low plasma glucose concentrations may be required to produce symptoms and signs of hypoglycemia because recurrent hypoglycemia shifts the glycemic thresholds. Although symptomatic hypoglycemia can be seen after an overnight fast, it often follows exercise. Rarely, symp-

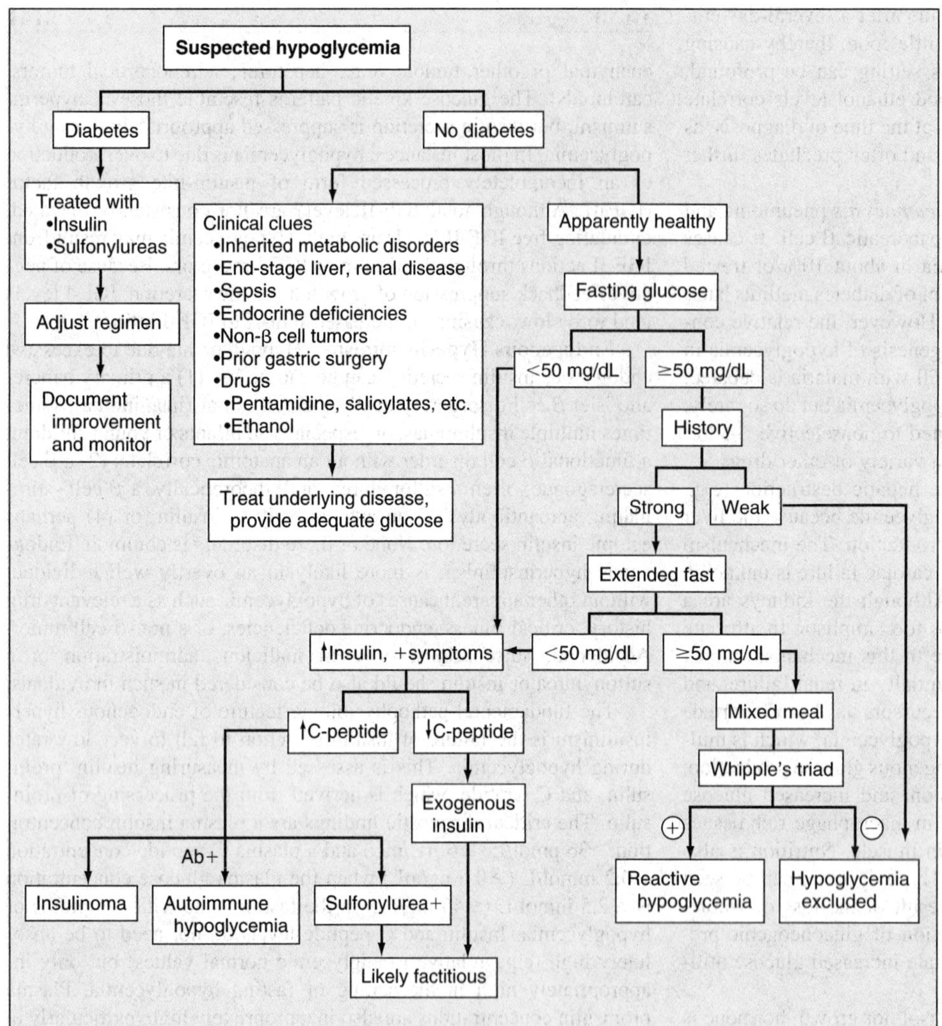

FIGURE 334-3 Diagnostic approach to a patient with suspected hypoglycemia based on a history of symptoms, a low plasma glucose concentration, or both.

tomatic hypoglycemia occurs following meals, but most such patients have evidence of fasting hypoglycemia as well.

Octreotide scans localize about half of insulinomas. Arteriography has been used extensively in the past, but false-negative and false-positive results occur, and it is generally preferable to use less invasive computed tomography (CT) or magnetic resonance imaging (MRI) scans, which detect 45 to 75% of tumors. Preoperative ultrasound is of value in some patients. Intraoperative ultrasonography has high sensitivity and may localize tumors not identified by palpation. Surgical resection of a solitary insulinoma is generally curative. Diazoxide, which inhibits insulin secretion, and the somatostatin analogue, octreotide, can be used to treat hypoglycemia in patients with unresectable insulinomas.

Factitious Hypoglycemia Factitious hypoglycemia, caused by malicious or self-administration of insulin or ingestion of a sulfonylurea, shares many clinical and laboratory features with insulinoma. It is most common among health care workers, patients with diabetes or their relatives, and people with a history of other factitious illnesses. When this diagnosis is suspected, it is useful to seek previous medical records, which may reveal admissions for similar episodes as well as relevant laboratory data. In individuals taking exogenous insulin, factitious hypoglycemia can be distinguished from insulinoma by the presence of high insulin levels without a concomitant increase in the C-peptide level, which is suppressed by the exogenous insulin. As noted above, sulfonylureas stimulate endogenous insulin and can therefore be detected only by measuring drug levels in plasma or urine. Factitious or surreptitious hypoglycemia should be considered in every patient requiring a fasting test for hypoglycemia. In addition to laboratory tests, observing the behavior of the patient may help make this diagnosis.

Approach to the Patient

In addition to recognition and documentation of hypoglycemia, and often urgent treatment, diagnosis of the hypoglycemic mechanism is critical for choosing a treatment that prevents, or at least minimizes, recurrent hypoglycemia. A diagnostic algorithm is shown in Fig. 334-3.

Recognition and Documentation

Urgent treatment is often necessary in patients with suspected hypoglycemia. Nevertheless, blood should be drawn, whenever possible, before the administration of glucose to allow documentation of the plasma glucose level. Convincing documentation of hypoglycemia requires the fulfillment of Whipple's triad. Thus, *the ideal time to test the plasma glucose is during an episode associated with hypoglycemic symptoms.* A normal plasma glucose concentration measured when the patient is free of symptoms does not exclude hypoglycemia at the time of earlier symptoms. When the cause of hypoglycemia is obscure, additional assays should include glucose, insulin, C peptide, sulfonylurea levels, cortisol, and ethanol.

Hypoglycemia is sometimes detected serendipitously. A distinctly low plasma glucose measurement in a person without a history of corresponding symptoms raises the possibility of a laboratory error caused by ongoing metabolism of glucose by the formed elements of the blood after the sample is drawn. This type of artifactually low glucose level is particularly likely when leukocyte, erythrocyte, or platelet counts are abnormally high, but it can also occur if separation of the plasma or serum from the formed elements is delayed.

Diagnosis of the Hypoglycemic Mechanism In an adult patient with documented hypoglycemia, a plausible hypoglycemic mechanism and further diagnostic evaluation can be guided by the history, physical examination, and available laboratory data (Fig. 334-3). Relevant historic elements include: drug history, particularly hypoglycemic agents or alcohol use; relevant critical illness (hepatic, renal, or cardiac failure, sepsis, or inanition); previous gastric surgery associated with postprandial hypoglycemia; features suggestive of cortisol or growth hormone deficiency; inherited enzyme deficiencies associated with hypoglycemia; or features of a non-β-cell tumor. Absent these, one must consider medication error, endogenous hyperinsulinism, or surreptitious sulfonylurea or insulin administration. In the absence of documented spontaneous hypoglycemia, overnight fasting, or food deprivation during observation in the outpatient setting, will sometimes elicit hypoglycemia and allow diagnostic evaluation. If these maneuvers do not reveal hypoglycemia, and there is a high degree of clinical suspicion, an extended fast lasting up to 72 h is often required to make these diagnoses. This procedure should be performed in the hospital with careful supervision and should be terminated if the plasma glucose drops to <2.5 mmol/L (<45 mg/dL) and the patient has symptoms. It is essential to draw blood samples for appropriate tests before administering glucose or allowing the patient to eat.

Urgent Treatment Oral treatment with glucose tablets or glucose-containing fluids, candy, or food is appropriate if the patient is able and willing to take these. A reasonable initial dose is 20 g of glucose. If neuroglycopenia precludes oral feedings, parenteral therapy is necessary. Intravenous glucose (25 g) should be given using a 50% solution followed by a constant infusion of 5 or 10% dextrose. If intravenous therapy is not practical, subcutaneous or intramuscular glucagon can be used, particularly in people with type 1 diabetes mellitus. Because it acts primarily by stimulating glycogenolysis, glucagon is ineffective in glycogen-depleted individuals (e.g., those with alcohol-induced hypoglycemia). These treatments raise plasma glucose concentrations only transiently, and patients should be encouraged to eat as soon as practical in order to replete glycogen stores.

Prevention of Recurrent Hypoglycemia Prevention of recurrent hypoglycemia requires an understanding of the hypoglycemic mechanism. Offending drugs can be discontinued or their doses reduced. It should be remembered that hypoglycemia caused by sulfonylureas may recur after a period of many hours or days. Underlying critical illnesses can often be treated. Cortisol and growth hormone can be replaced, if deficient. Surgical, radiotherapeutic, or chemotherapeutic reduction of a non-β-cell tumor can alleviate hypoglycemia, even if the tumor cannot be cured; glucocorticoid or growth hormone administration may also reduce hypoglycemic episodes in such patients. Surgical resection of an insulinoma is often curative; medical therapy with diazoxide or octreotide can be used if resection is not possible and in patients with a nontumor primary β cell disorder. The treatment of autoimmune hypoglycemia (e.g., with a glucocorticoid) is more problematic, but this disorder is often self-limited. Failing these treatments, frequent feedings and avoidance of fasting may be required. Uncooked cornstarch at bedtime or an overnight infusion of intragastric glucose may be necessary in some patients.

BIBLIOGRAPHY

CRYER PE: *Hypoglycemia: Pathophysiology, Diagnosis and Treatment.* New York, Oxford Univ Press, 1997

FRIER BM, FISHER BM. *Hypoglycaemia in Clinical Diabetes.* Chichester, Wiley, 1999

THE DIABETES CONTROL AND COMPLICATIONS TRIAL RESEARCH GROUP: Adverse events and their association with treatment regimens in the Diabetes Control and Complications Trial. Diabetes Care 18:1415, 1995

THE UNITED KINGDOM PROSPECTIVE DIABETES STUDY GROUP: UKPDS 24: A 6-year, randomized, controlled trial comparing sulfonylurea, insulin and metformin therapy in patients with newly diagnosed type 2 diabetes that could not be controlled with diet therapy. Ann Intern Med 128:165, 1998

SERVICE FJ: Hypoglycemic disorders. Endocrinol Metab Clin North Am 28:467, 1999

335

James E. Griffin, Jean D. Wilson

DISORDERS OF THE TESTES

The testes produce sperm and the steroid hormones that regulate male sexual function. Both processes are under complex feedback control by the hypothalamic-pituitary system so that the testes have biosynthetic and regulatory features similar to those of the ovary and the adrenal. Testicular hormones are also responsible for the formation of the basic male phenotype during embryogenesis (Chap. 338). Disorders that affect testicular function are common. Infertility occurs in about 5% of men; Klinefelter syndrome (XXY) occurs in 1 in 500 men and often escapes diagnosis; and various disorders cause hypogonadism, a condition that can be treated by hormone replacement. The testes are also a site of malignancies, most of which are highly responsive to radiation and/or chemotherapy (Chap. 96).

PHYSIOLOGY AND REGULATION OF TESTICULAR FUNCTION

The testis consists of two components—clusters of interstitial or Leydig cells, where androgenic steroids are synthesized, and a system of spermatogenic tubules for the production and transport of sperm. The components are regulated by the pituitary gonadotropins—luteinizing hormone (LH), which stimulates Leydig cell function, and follicle-stimulating hormone (FSH), which controls Sertoli cell function and spermatogenesis (Fig. 335-1).

GONADOTROPIN REGULATION AND TESTICULAR FUNCTION Gonadotropin-releasing hormone (GnRH), also called luteinizing hormone–releasing hormone (LHRH), regulates the production of the gonadotropins, LH and FSH (Chap. 328). Because hypothalamic GnRH is secreted in discrete pulses, the plasma concentrations of LH, FSH, and testosterone are not constant, but fluctuate in a pulsatile pattern that mirrors the secretion of GnRH (Fig. 335-2). Pulsatile secretion is most apparent for LH because it has a relatively short plasma half-life by comparison to FSH; pulsatile secretion of testosterone in response to LH is also apparent, although the pulses are dampened because of the need to stimulate steroid synthesis and secretion by the Leydig cell. In contrast to women, in whom the frequency and amplitude of LH pulses vary during the menstrual cycle, the frequency of LH pulses in adult men is relatively constant at about one pulse every 1 to 2 h.

Testosterone secretion is regulated primarily by pituitary LH. FSH may augment testosterone secretion by stimulating a Sertoli-cell derived factor that enhances testosterone production. Testosterone feeds back to regulate the hypothalamic-pituitary production of LH. It decreases hypothalamic GnRH pulse frequency and diminishes pituitary sensitivity to GnRH, leading to lower LH levels. Although the pituitary can convert testosterone to dihydrotestosterone and to estrogens, testosterone itself is the primary regulator of gonadotropin secretion by the pituitary. Under ordinary circumstances, LH secretion is exquisitely sensitive to the feedback effects of testosterone, with almost complete suppression after the administration of amounts of exogenous

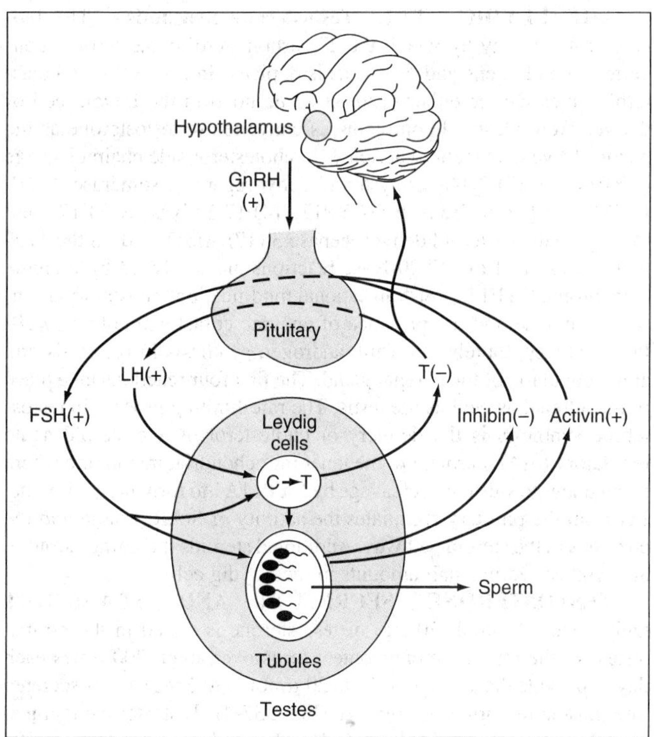

FIGURE 335-1 Regulation of testosterone and sperm production by LH and FSH. C, cholesterol; T, testosterone.

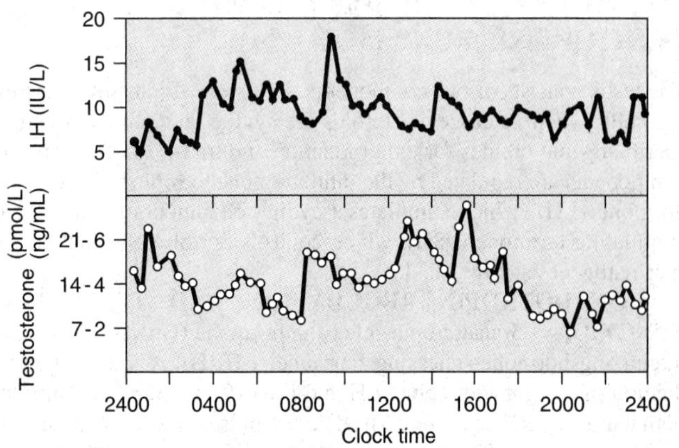

FIGURE 335-2 The 24-h pattern of plasma LH and testosterone in a normal man as samples every 20 min. *(From Griffin and Wilson.)*

androgen that approximate the normal daily secretory rate of testosterone (~20 μmol or 6 mg). However, prolonged elevation of plasma LH (as in testicular deficiency) renders the pituitary less sensitive to negative feedback control by androgen.

FSH is regulated by GnRH and also by the gonadal peptides—inhibins and activins. Inhibins A and B are heterodimeric proteins (composed of α-β_A or α-β_B subunits) that selectively suppress FSH without affecting LH; activins are homodimeric proteins (composed of β_A or β_B subunits) that selectively stimulate FSH production. Inhibin B, which is the major form of inhibin in the male, is produced by the Sertoli cell and provides feedback control of FSH production. Activins, which are produced in the pituitary as well as the gonad, stimulate FSH production through an autocrine-paracrine mechanism.

The interlocking system in which two pituitary hormones (LH and FSH) regulate testicular function provides a precise dual-control mechanism in which hormonal signals from Leydig cells and the spermatogenic tubules feed back on the hypothalamic-pituitary system to regulate their own function (Fig. 335-1).

THE LEYDIG CELL **Testosterone Synthesis** The biochemical pathway by which the 27-carbon sterol cholesterol is converted to androgens and estrogens is depicted in Fig. 335-3. Cholesterol, which can be either synthesized de novo in the Leydig cell or derived from plasma lipoproteins, is converted to testosterone as the result of five enzymatic reactions: (1) cholesterol side chain cleavage (CYP11A1); (2) 3β-hydroxysteroid dehydrogenase/isomerase 2 (3β-HSD2); (3) 17α-hydroxylase (CYP17); (4) 17,20-lyase (CYP17); and (5) 17β-hydroxysteroid dehydrogenase 3 (17β-HSD3). Both the 17α-hydroxylase and the 17,20-lyase reactions are catalyzed by a single cytochrome CYP17; post-translational modification (phosphorylation) of the enzyme and the presence of enzyme cofactors confers 17,20-lyase activity, thereby allowing androgen synthesis in the testis and zona reticularis of the adrenal gland. The first four reactions take place in the adrenal as well as the testis. The rate-limiting process in testosterone synthesis is the delivery of cholesterol by the steroid acute regulatory (StAR) protein to the inner mitochondrial membrane where it can undergo side chain cleavage by CYP11A1 to form pregnenolone. LH from the pituitary stimulates the activity of StAR protein and the enzymes in the steroid pathway. Additional steroids including estradiol are synthesized in small amounts in the Leydig cell.

TESTOSTERONE SECRETION AND TRANSPORT Only about 70 nmol (20 μg) of testosterone is stored in the normal testes, so the total hormone content turns over about 200 times each day to provide the average of 17 to 20 μmol (5 to 6 mg) that is secreted into plasma in normal young men (Fig. 335-4). Testosterone is transported in plasma bound to protein, largely to albumin and to a specific transport protein, sex hormone–binding globulin (SHBG), also called testosterone-binding globulin (TeBG). The bound and unbound

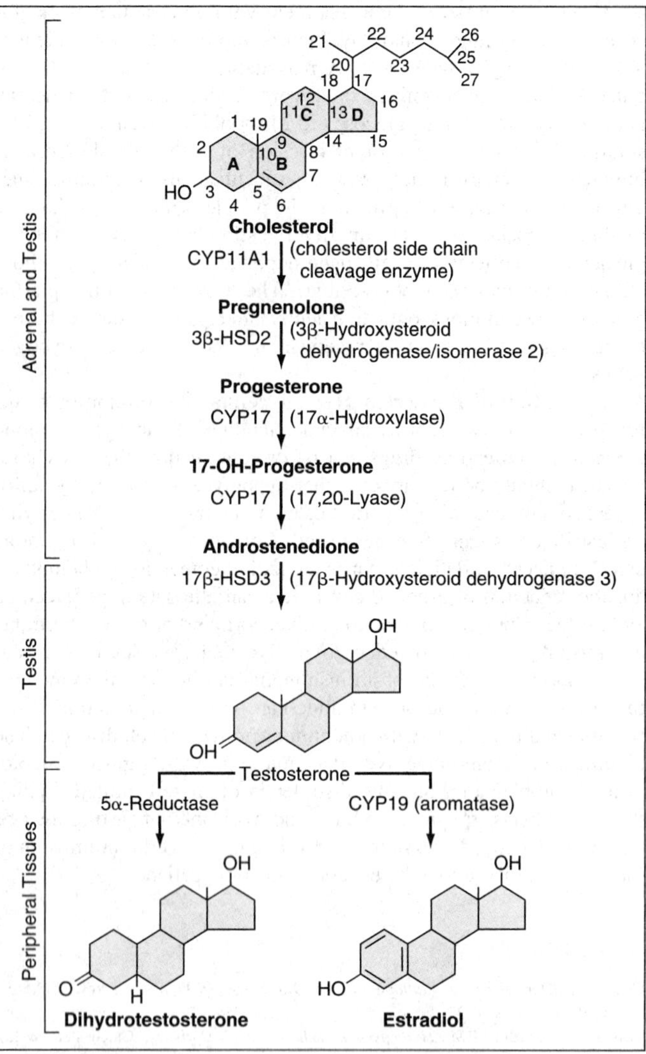

FIGURE 335-3 The biochemical pathway in the conversion of 27-carbon sterol cholesterol to androgens and estrogens.

fractions in plasma are in dynamic equilibrium, only ~1 to 3% being unbound. Because of rapid dissociation from albumin, the fraction of circulating testosterone available for entry into tissues (bioavailable testosterone) approximates the sum of the free and albumin-bound fractions or about half the total plasma level.

Peripheral Metabolism of Androgens Testosterone serves as a circulating precursor (or prohormone) for the formation of two other hormones that mediate many of the physiologic processes involved in androgen action (Fig. 335-3). Testosterone can be 5α-reduced to dihydrotestosterone, which is responsible for many of the differentiative, growth-promoting, and functional aspects of male sexual differentiation and virilization. Circulating testosterone (and androstenedione) also can be converted to estrogens by aromatase (CYP19) in extraglandular tissues (Fig. 335-4). All estrone production [averaging about 240 nmol (66 μg) per day] can be accounted for by formation from circulating precursors. The mean estradiol production is approximately 170 nmol (45 μg) per day; ~35% is derived from circulating testosterone, 50% is derived from the estrone, and 15% is secreted directly by the testes. When gonadotropin levels are elevated, estradiol secretion by the testes increases. Thus, the physiologic effects of testosterone are the result of the combined actions of testosterone itself plus those of the active androgen and estrogen metabolites of the parent molecule.

The 5α-reduced and estrogenic metabolites can exert local (paracrine) actions in the tissues in which they are formed or enter the circulation and act as hormones at other sites. Circulating dihydrotes-

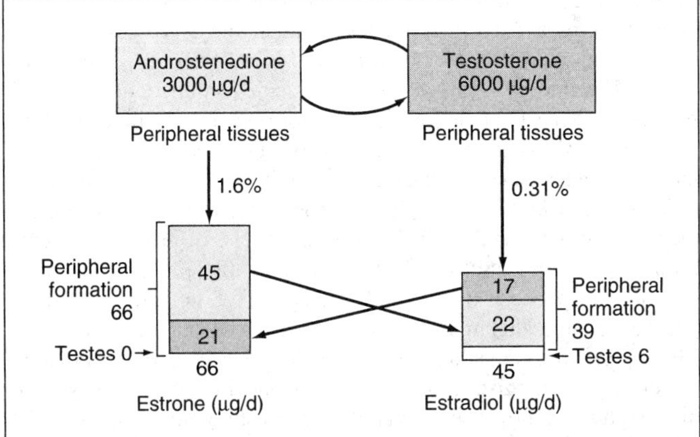

FIGURE 335-4 Androgen and estrogen production in normal young men. The average production of androsteredione and testosterone is shown in the top boxes, and the mean daily production of esterone and estradiol is shown in the lower boxes. Estrogen is formed by extraglandular aromatization (*braces*) or is secreted directly by the testes. *Vertical arrows* indicate the rates of extraglandular aromatization of androgens, and *horizontal arrows* indicate the interconversion of androgen and estrogens by 17β-hydroxysteroid dehydrogenase. Thus, estradiol arises from plasma testosterone, from estrone, and by direct secretion by the testes. *(Adapted from MacDonald et al.)*

tosterone is formed principally in the androgen target tissues; estrogen formation takes place in many tissues, the most significant being adipose tissue. The overall rate of extraglandular estrogen formation increases with age and with increased mass of adipose tissue.

Testosterone and its active metabolites are catabolized in the liver and excreted predominantly in the urine, approximately half in the form of urinary 17-ketosteroids (primarily androsterone and etiocholanolone) and half as polar metabolites (diols, triols, and conjugates).

Androgen Action The major functions of androgen are formation of the male phenotype during sexual differentiation, regulation of LH secretion, and induction of sexual maturation at puberty. The cellular process by which androgens perform these functions is schematized in Fig. 335-5. Testosterone enters the cell by passive diffusion and can be converted to dihydrotestosterone by either steroid 5α-reductase 1 or 2; 5α-reductase 2 is responsible for dihydrotestosterone formation in most androgen target tissues. Testosterone or dihydrotestosterone is then bound to the androgen-receptor protein in the nucleus. The hormone-receptor complex binds to specific DNA sequences to regulate the transcription of messenger RNA and, ultimately, the synthesis of cellular proteins. The androgen receptor, which is encoded by a gene on the long arm of the X chromosome, contains 917 amino acids and has a molecular mass of about 110 kDa. A polymorphic region in the amino terminus of the receptor, which contains a variable number of glutamine repeats, appears to modify the activity of the receptor. The androgen receptor is similar in structure to other steroid hormone receptors and has distinct hormone-binding, DNA-binding, and transcriptional regulatory domains (Chap. 327). Estradiol acts by a similar mechanism but has its own distinct estrogen receptors α and β (Chap. 336).

Although testosterone and dihydrotestosterone bind to the same receptor, their physiologic roles differ. The testosterone-receptor complex regulates gonadotropin secretion, spermatogenesis, and the virilization of the wolffian ducts during sexual differentiation (Chap. 338), whereas the dihydrotestosterone-receptor complex is responsible for external virilization during embryogenesis and for most androgen actions during sexual maturation and adult sexual life. The mechanism by which two hormones can interact with the same receptor but have different physiologic effects is not well understood. However, dihydrotestosterone binds to the receptor much more tightly than does testosterone, and hence its formation serves to amplify the hormonal signal.

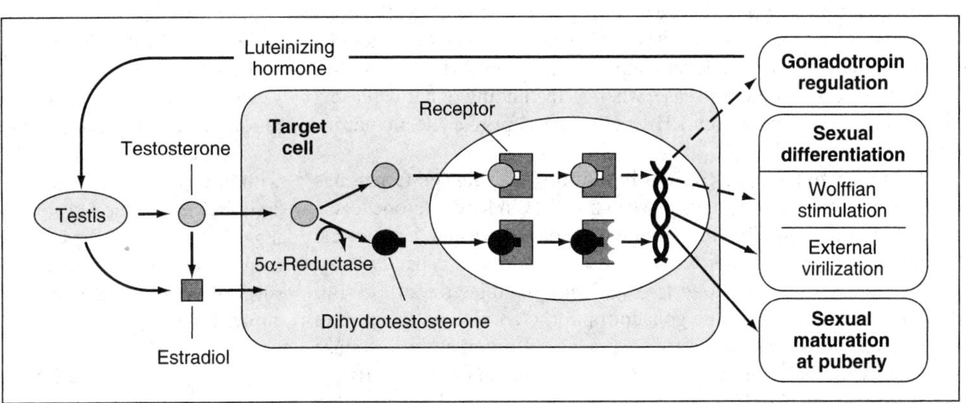

FIGURE 335-5 The mechanism of androgen action.

THE SEMINIFEROUS TUBULES AND SPERMATOGENESIS Spermatogenesis is dependent on both pituitary FSH and androgen production by the adjacent Leydig cells (Fig. 335-1). The function of FSH in gametogenesis has been clarified by rare, naturally occurring mutations in the *FSHβ* gene and in the FSH receptor. Females with these mutations are hypogonadal and infertile because ovarian follicles do not mature, whereas males with mutations in the FSH pathway exhibit variable degrees of impaired spermatogenesis. Thus, while FSH is not absolutely required for spermatogenesis, it increases the number and maturation of sperm. The major site of FSH action is the Sertoli cell, which regulates germ cell proliferation and maturation in the seminiferous tubules. Androgen, which reaches very high concentrations locally in the testis, appears to be essential for spermatogenesis, acting through receptors located in the seminiferous tubules. Several cytokines and growth factors are also involved in the regulation of spermatogenesis by paracrine and autocrine mechanisms. The normal adult testes produce >100 million sperm per day.

The Sertoli cell cannot synthesize steroid hormones de novo but can convert testosterone that diffuses from adjacent Leydig cells to estradiol and to dihydrotestosterone. The Sertoli cell also produces inhibin B. Damage to the seminiferous tubules (e.g., by radiation) reduces inhibin B production, causing a selective increase in FSH.

ASSESSMENT OF TESTICULAR FUNCTION

LEYDIG CELL FUNCTION History and Physical Examination The assessment of Leydig cell function and androgen status should include inquiry about the presence of developmental abnormalities of the urogenital tract; the timing and extent of sexual maturation at puberty; the rate of beard growth; and the current libido, sexual function, strength, and energy. Inadequate Leydig cell function or androgen action during embryogenesis may cause hypospadias, cryptorchidism, or microphallus. If Leydig cell failure occurs before puberty, sexual maturation will not occur, and the individual will develop the features termed *eunuchoidism*, including an infantile amount and distribution of body hair, poor development of skeletal muscles, and delayed closure of the epiphyses, so that the arm span is more than 5 cm greater than the height and the lower body segment (heel to pubic bone) is more than 5 cm longer than the upper body segment (pubic bone to crown). Detection of postpubertal Leydig cell failure requires a high index of suspicion and appropriate laboratory assessment because some functions that require androgens for initiation continue unabated when Leydig cell failure occurs, and functions that eventually regress may do so very slowly. For example, the frequency of shaving may not decrease for months or years because of slow decline in the rate of beard growth once established. Furthermore, decreased sexual function in adult men may be caused by nonendocrine as well as endocrine factors (Chap. 51).

Plasma Testosterone and Dihydrotestosterone Levels Plasma testosterone is measured by immunoassay. Testosterone is secreted into plasma in a pulsatile fashion every 60 to 90 min (Fig. 335-2). A single random testosterone sample provides a result within ±20% of the true mean value only two-thirds of the time; a pool of three samples spaced 15 to 20 min apart provides a more accurate assessment. The plasma testosterone level in normal adult men ranges from 10 to 35 nmol/L (3 to 10 ng/mL). However, in some normal men with long interpulse intervals of LH, testosterone levels can transiently fall below this normal range, emphasizing the importance of using pooled or repeated samples before making a diagnosis of testosterone deficiency. In adult men, plasma testosterone levels also vary somewhat throughout the day and at different times of the year. In young adult men the plasma testosterone level is ~30% higher in the morning than in the evening. Estimation of SHBG concentration by radioimmunoassay is sometimes useful in the interpretation of total plasma testosterone levels. Bioavailable testosterone in plasma can be estimated by measuring the non-SHBG-bound fraction of testosterone.

The plasma testosterone level is slightly higher in prepubertal boys than in girls, ranging in both from 0.2 to 0.7 nmol/L (0.05 to 0.2 ng/mL). The rise in plasma testosterone level at the start of male puberty begins as a result of sleep-related nocturnal gonadotropin surges, so that levels of plasma testosterone and LH are initially higher at night than during the day. Random daytime levels of plasma testosterone increase gradually as puberty progresses and reach adult levels at about age 17.

Dihydrotestosterone is also measured by immunoassay. In young men the plasma dihydrotestosterone level is about one-tenth the value for testosterone, averaging ~2 nmol/L (0.6 ng/mL). In older men with benign prostatic hyperplasia, plasma dihydrotestosterone levels average ~3 nmol/L (0.9 ng/mL).

Urinary 17-Ketosteroids The measurement of urinary 17-ketosteroids is not a valid way to assess testicular function because testosterone contributes only ~40% of urinary 17-ketosteroids in men, the bulk being derived from adrenal androgens.

Plasma LH Plasma LH is also measured by immunoassay. Dual-site immunometric assays have largely replaced radioimmunoassays. Because LH is secreted in a pulsatile fashion, assay of a pool of three samples drawn 15 to 20 min apart, as described above, provides a value approaching the true mean. In early puberty, plasma LH secretion increases only during sleep, but in the adult the pulsatile secretion is of similar magnitude during sleep and waking periods. The normal plasma LH values should be established for a given laboratory with an appropriate reference standard. A low plasma testosterone level can be interpreted correctly only if plasma LH is measured simultaneously, and, likewise, the "appropriateness" of a given plasma LH value must be interpreted in relation to the plasma testosterone level. For example, a low plasma testosterone level coupled with a low LH level implies hypothalamic or pituitary disease, whereas the finding of a low plasma testosterone level and a high LH level suggests primary testicular insufficiency.

Response to Gonadotropin Stimulation Leydig cell function is difficult to assess before puberty, when both LH and testosterone levels are low, but it is possible to measure response of plasma testosterone to gonadotropin stimulation as an index of Leydig cell capacity. Normal prepubertal boys respond to 3 to 5 days of injection of 1000 to 2000 IU of human chorionic gonadotropin (hCG) with an increase in the plasma testosterone level to ~7 nmol/L (2 ng/mL); the response increases with the initiation of puberty and peaks in early puberty.

Response to GnRH Before puberty, there is minimal response of plasma LH and FSH to the administration of GnRH because the pituitary has not been "primed" by previous exposure to GnRH or gonadal steroids. After pubertal development, the LH response to acute administration of GnRH increases, while the FSH response is less robust. The amount of LH released after acute administration of GnRH probably reflects the amount of stored hormone in the pituitary. When 100 μg GnRH is given subcutaneously or intravenously to normal men, LH levels usually increase four- to fivefold, with the peak level at 30 min. However, the range of response is broad, and some normal men exhibit less than a doubling of LH levels. In primary testicular failure, measurement of basal LH is usually sufficient, and assessment of GnRH response is of little aid in diagnosis. Since men with either pituitary or hypothalamic disease can have a normal or an abnormal LH response to acute administration of GnRH, a normal response does not clearly distinguish these causes of gonadal deficiency. A subnormal response is, however, of value in establishing that an abnormality exists, even though the site of the defect is not clearly determined. If pulsatile GnRH or daily infusions of GnRH for a week lead to the development of a normal acute LH response, a hypothalamic etiology is likely.

SEMINIFEROUS TUBULE FUNCTION **Examination of the Testes** Evaluation of the testes is an essential portion of the physical examination. The prepubertal testis measures about 2 cm in length and 2 mL in volume and grows during puberty to reach the adult proportions by age 16. When damage to the seminiferous tubules occurs before puberty, the testes are small and firm, whereas the testes are usually soft after postpubertal damage (the capsule, once enlarged, does not contract to its previous size). Testes in adult men average 4.6 cm in length (range, 3.5 to 5.5 cm), corresponding to a volume of 12 to 25 mL, and the seminiferous tubules account for ~60% of testicular mass. Advanced age does not influence testicular size, so the significance of small testes in the adult is the same at all ages. Asian men have smaller testes than western Europeans, independent of differences in body size. Because of its possible causal role in infertility, the presence of varicocele should be sought by palpation with the patient standing.

Semen Analysis Seminal fluid is analyzed on samples obtained by masturbation into a glass container after 24 to 36 h of abstinence. Analysis should be performed within an hour of collection. The normal ejaculate volume is 2 to 6 mL. Immediately after ejaculation, the seminal fluid coagulates, followed in 15 to 30 min by liquefaction. Motility should be assessed in undiluted seminal fluid; >60% of the sperm should be motile and of normal morphology. The normal range for sperm density is generally considered to be >20 million per milliliter, with a total count of >60 million per ejaculate, but the definition of a minimally adequate ejaculate is not clear. Some men with low sperm counts are nevertheless fertile. This uncertainty as to the lower level of sperm density, percent motility, and percent normal forms in fertile semen stems from two issues. First, the seminal fluid is routinely evaluated by tests that do not assess the functional capacity of sperm. Second, many factors produce temporary aberrations in sperm count; in men with semen of equivocal quality, it is necessary to examine three or more ejaculates to determine whether the abnormal findings are permanent.

Plasma FSH Plasma FSH, as measured by immunoassay, usually correlates inversely with spermatogenesis. When damage to the germinal epithelium is severe, plasma levels of inhibin B fall and plasma levels of FSH increase.

Testicular Biopsy Testicular biopsy is useful in some patients with oligospermia and azoospermia both as an aid in diagnosis and as an indication of the feasibility of treatment. For example, normal findings on testicular biopsy and a normal FSH level in an azoospermic man suggest obstruction of the vas deferens, which may be correctable surgically. In some men with severe oligospermia, testicular biopsy allows retrieval of sperm for intracytoplasmic sperm injections (ICSI) into oocytes (Chap. 54).

ESTROGENIC FUNCTION **Examination of the Breasts** Breast enlargement (gynecomastia) is the most consistent feature of feminizing states in men (Chap. 337). Gynecomastia is due to an increase in both glandular and adipose tissue. The presence of gynecomastia should be sought by examining the sitting patient, using the fingers to grasp glandular tissue. Early or minimal breast enlargement may be missed if the breast is palpated with the flat of the hand while the patient is supine. In obese men it is important to try to define the rim of the glandular tissue where it meets the adipose tissue of the chest wall.

Plasma Estrogen As discussed above, most of the estradiol and all of the estrone produced in normal men is formed by extraglandular aromatization of circulating androgens. The plasma level of estradiol usually is <180 pmol/L (50 pg/mL) in normal men; the plasma estrone level is somewhat higher but usually is <300 pmol/L (80 pg/mL). Elevations in estrogen production and estrogen plasma levels can be due to increases in plasma precursors (liver or adrenal disease), to increased extraglandular aromatization (obesity), or to increased production by the testes (testicular tumors, androgen resistance, gonadotropin stimulation).

PHASES OF NORMAL TESTICULAR FUNCTION

The phases of male sexual life can be defined in terms of the plasma testosterone value (Fig. 335-6). In the male embryo the production of testosterone by the testes commences at about 7 weeks of gestation and is stimulated in part by placental hCG. Shortly thereafter, plasma testosterone attains a high level that is maintained until late in gestation. The level then falls so that at the time of birth the plasma testosterone level is only slightly higher in males than in females. Shortly after birth, a transient increase of pituitary gonadotropins raises the plasma testosterone level in the male infant for ~3 months, before hormone levels again decrease to low levels by age 6 months to 1 year. The significance of the rise in plasma testosterone level during the first year of life is not certain. However, in other primates neonatal activation of the hypothalamic-pituitary-testicular axis is important for subsequent normal pubertal development. The testosterone concentration then remains low (but slightly higher in boys than in girls) until the onset of puberty, when it begins to rise in boys, reaching adult levels by about age 17. The level of bioavailable testosterone remains constant until the 40s when it begins to decline at a rate of ~1.2% per year; the level of SHBG increases by ~1.2% per year so that there is little decline in total testosterone until the later decades of life. During the third, or adult, phase of male sexual life, sperm production becomes sufficient to allow reproduction to take place. The physiologic events during these various phases differ, as do the pathologic consequences of derangements in testicular function. Male sexual differentiation during embryogenesis is considered in Chap. 338.

ABNORMALITIES OF TESTICULAR FUNCTION

PUBERTY The control of puberty is poorly understood and may reside in the hypothalamic-pituitary system, the testes, or the

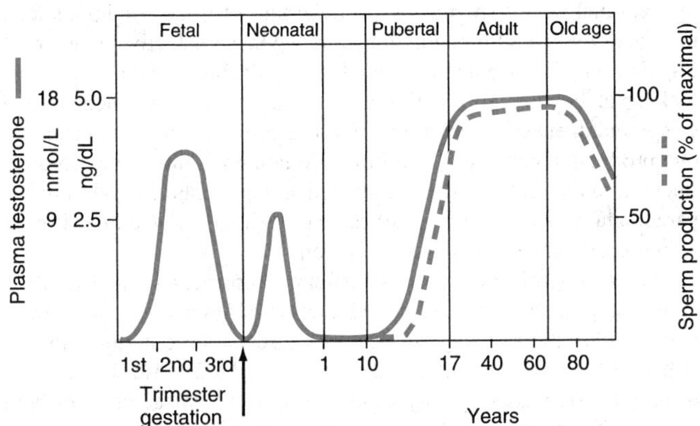

FIGURE 335-6 Phases of male sexual life. *(From Griffin and Wilson.)*

adrenals (Chap. 8). Before the onset of puberty, gonadotropin secretion by the pituitary is low, but prepubertal castration causes a rise in plasma gonadotropin levels. This finding suggests that before puberty the negative feedback control of gonadotropin secretion is exquisitely sensitive to the small amount of circulating testosterone. The onset of puberty is heralded by sleep-associated surges in gonadotropin secretion. Later in puberty the rises in LH and FSH levels persist throughout the day. Thus, with maturation, the hypothalamic-pituitary system becomes less sensitive to negative feedback control, and the consequences are higher mean plasma levels of testosterone and gonadotropins, maturation of the testes, and the onset of spermatogenesis. The rise in gonadotropin secretion is the consequence of an increase both in GnRH secretion and in the sensitivity of the pituitary to GnRH.

The somatic changes at the time of puberty are secondary to the rise in plasma testosterone, which induces the growth of the accessory organs of male reproduction (the penis, the prostate, the seminal vesicles, and the epididymides). Accelerated linear growth is accompanied by growth of muscle and connective tissue, which account for the major portion of nitrogen retention at puberty. The principal androgen-sensitive muscles are those of the pectoral region and the shoulder. The characteristic hair growth of male puberty involves development of mustache and beard; regression of the scalp line; appearance of body, extremity, and perianal hair; and extension of the pubic hair upward into a diamond-shaped pattern. Growth of axillary and pubic hair is initiated under the control of adrenal androgens and is promoted by testicular androgens. The larynx enlarges, and the vocal cords thicken, resulting in a lowering of the pitch of the voice. Hemoglobin levels increase by ~1 g/dL. These various androgen-mediated growth and maturation processes reach some limiting value, so that once puberty is completed, the administration of pharmacologic doses of androgen has no further effect. The entire process is heralded by testicular enlargement beginning at age 11 to 12 and is usually completed within 5 years, although some aspects of virilization, such as growth of the chest hair, may continue over a decade or more.

The events of normal male puberty are variable in onset, duration, and sequence. The central issue in dealing with disorders of puberty is separating true absence or precocity from the extremes of normal variation. The use of staging criteria that correlate developmental and anatomic landmarks with chronologic age is useful in making this distinction (Chap. 8).

Sexual Precocity Premature development of sexual characteristics that are phenotypically appropriate—i.e., virilization in boys—is termed *isosexual precocity*. *Heterosexual precocity* refers to feminizing syndromes in boys.

Isosexual precocity Sexual development before age 9 in boys is generally considered abnormal. *True precocious puberty* or *complete isosexual precocity* occurs when both virilization and spermatogenesis are premature. *Precocious pseudopuberty* or *incomplete isosexual precocity* refers to virilization unaccompanied by spermatogenesis. This distinction is blurred in practice, because pure virilizing syndromes may cause activation of gonadotropin secretion secondarily and thus be followed by development of spermatogenesis. Furthermore, local androgen production in the testis, as in Leydig cell tumors, can cause local areas of spermatogenesis and limited sperm production around the tumor. We therefore prefer a two-part classification: virilizing syndromes (in which hypothalamic-pituitary activity is appropriate for age) and premature activation of the hypothalamic-pituitary system.

Virilizing syndromes can result from Leydig cell tumors, hCG-secreting tumors, adrenal tumors, congenital adrenal hyperplasia (most commonly 21-hydroxylase deficiency), androgen administration, or Leydig cell hyperplasia. In these disorders plasma testosterone levels are inappropriately elevated for the age. Leydig cell tumors are rare in children but should be suspected when the testes are asymmetric in size (Chap. 96). Virilizing adrenal tumors mainly secrete androstenedione and dehydroepiandrosterone, some of which is converted to testosterone; consequently, they cause increased 17-ketosteroid excretion. Glucocorticoid administration does not reduce 17-ketosteroid excretion to normal in patients with testicular or adrenal tumors, in contrast to the prompt decrease that occurs after such treatment in patients with congenital adrenal hyperplasia. Congenital adrenal hyperplasia leads to elevated 17-hydroxyprogesterone levels and, as a consequence, elevated androgen levels (Chaps. 331 and 338). When this disorder is treated with glucocorticoids, true precocious puberty can then result if the increased androgen levels have caused sufficient hypothalamic maturation.

Gonadotropin-independent sexual precocity in boys may occur as a result of autonomous Leydig cell hyperplasia in the absence of a Leydig cell tumor. The disorder can occur sporadically or can be inherited as a male-limited autosomal disorder either from affected fathers or from mothers who are unaffected carriers. It is due to point mutations in the LH receptor that cause constitutive activation of the receptor in the absence of LH. Virilization usually begins by age 2. Testosterone levels are elevated, often to the adult male range; however, immunoreactive and bioactive LH levels and the LH response to GnRH are prepubertal. In the past many of these boys were mistakenly thought to have true precocious puberty because spermatogenesis may be present.

Premature activation of the hypothalamic-pituitary system Central precocious puberty may be "idiopathic" or due to central nervous system (CNS) tumors, infections, or injuries. Early hypothalamic-pituitary activation typically is associated with features of normal puberty, i.e., sleep-related gonadotropin secretion, elevated plasma bioactive LH, and enhanced gonadotropin response to GnRH. Since the diagnosis of idiopathic true precocious puberty is one of exclusion, patients may later prove to have been misclassified and to have a CNS abnormality. With improved means of diagnosis, such as magnetic resonance imaging, delays in diagnosis will probably be less frequent.

Management of sexual precocity due to steroid- or gonadotropin-producing tumors, congenital adrenal hyperplasia, or CNS abnormality is directed toward the primary disease. In boys with Leydig cell hyperplasia, attempts have been made to lower plasma testosterone with medroxyprogesterone acetate or ketoconazole, or to blunt hormone action with spironolactone, but treatment remains suboptimal. Idiopathic true precocious puberty and true precocious puberty due to inoperable CNS lesions are treated with long-acting GnRH analogue therapy, which inhibits gonadotropin production and testosterone synthesis, reversing pubertal maturation and decreasing the rate of skeletal development.

Heterosexual precocity Feminization in prepubertal boys can result from absolute or relative increases in estrogen due to a variety of causes (Chap. 337).

Delayed or Incomplete Puberty Separating failure of puberty from variants of normal development is one of the most difficult problems in endocrinology. Some boys fail to show the normal spurt of growth and sexual development at the usual time but eventually commence puberty by age 16 or older. Adolescence may then either progress rapidly, or slow pubertal development and growth may continue until age 20 to 22. Many men with delayed onset of puberty attain heights within the normal adult range. The history may reveal that a parent or sibling had a similar pattern of development. Panhypopituitarism and hypothyroidism can cause pubertal failure (Chaps. 328 and 330). Absent puberty also can result from primary testicular disease; this diagnosis is suspected on the basis of low plasma testosterone levels and elevated FSH and LH levels. Hereditary androgen resistance (in which plasma testosterone and LH levels are both high) usually causes male pseudohermaphroditism but in mild form may be manifested by absent or incomplete puberty (Chap. 338).

Most boys with absent puberty have low plasma levels of both testosterone and gonadotropins; in these boys it is necessary to distinguish delayed puberty from isolated gonadotropin deficiency or idiopathic *hypogonadotropic hypogonadism (Kallman syndrome)*. The manifestations of isolated gonadotropin deficiency vary from boys with eunuchoidal features and testes of prepubertal size to those with partial LH and/or FSH deficiency and some degree of testicular enlargement and pubertal development. Ansomia or hyposmia is caused by abnormal development of the olfactory tracts (which share progenitor cells with GnRH neurons) and is characteristically seen in Kallmann syndrome. X-linked *adrenal hypoplasia congenita (AHC)* is characterized by primary adrenal insufficiency, which usually presents in infancy, and hypogonadotropic hypogonadism, caused by deficient GnRH production and abnormal gonadotrope function. Congenital hypogonadotropic hypogonadism is frequently associated with cryptorchidism and a prepubertal manifestation can be microphallus, in which the size of the penis is below the fifth percentile for the age.

The pathogenesis of hypogonadotropic hypogonadism can involve several distinct abnormalities of GnRH formation or action. Some cases are inherited as an X-linked recessive trait associated with defects in a neural cell adhesion molecule (KAL) involved in the migration of GnRH neurons into the olfactory bulb. Other causes involve autosomal dominant disorders with variable expressivity; rare autosomal recessive cases are due to mutations that impair the GnRH receptor. Serum FSH and LH levels are usually below the normal male range, and plasma testosterone levels are low for age. The secretion of other pituitary hormones is normal. The administration of pulsatile GnRH corrects the endocrine abnormalities and initiates spermatogenesis in patients with GnRH deficiency; all patients respond to gonadotropin replacement. If untreated, these patients usually remain in the prepubertal state indefinitely.

It is particularly difficult to distinguish hypogonatropic hypogonadism from delayed puberty in boys of early or midpubertal age; the presence of microphallus, anosmia, or a family history may suggest the diagnosis. In the absence of such evidence, observation through the teenage years may be required before it becomes clear whether a patient has delayed puberty or a permanent form of hypogonadotropic hypogonadism. Since delayed puberty is associated with a decreased bone mass, therapy should not be delayed too long. In some cases the response of plasma LH to GnRH stimulation may be helpful in suggesting that puberty is imminent.

ADULTHOOD At the completion of puberty, plasma testosterone levels reach the adult level of 10 to 35 nmol/L (3 to 10 ng/mL) throughout the day, plasma gonadotropins are in the normal adult range, and sperm production is sufficient to allow reproduction. The adult pattern of hypothalamic-pituitary-gonadal regulation is sustained in the normal man for more than 40 years. However, the system is subject to a variety of influences, at the level of both the testes and the hypothalamic-pituitary system. Spermatogenesis is exquisitely sensitive to alterations in scrotal temperature, and brief increases in either systemic or local temperature (as in a hot bath) can be followed by temporary decreases in sperm production. The system also is influenced by diet, drugs, alcohol, environmental agents, and psychological stress, any of which may cause temporary decreases in sperm count.

Persistent abnormalities of testicular function in adult men can be due to hypothalamic-pituitary disorders (Chap. 328), testicular defects, or abnormalities of sperm transport. Certain of these conditions tend to affect Leydig cell function or spermatogenesis selectively, but most impair both androgenization and fertility (Table 335-1). The interlocking of Leydig cell function and fertility is due to the dependence of spermatogenesis on androgen. Even a partial decrease in testosterone production can cause infertility. Certain conditions (hyperprolactinemia, radiation therapy, cyclophosphamide therapy, autoimmunity, paraplegia, androgen resistance) can cause either isolated infertility or a combined defect in testicular function.

Hypothalamic-Pituitary Disorders Disorders of the hypothalamus and pituitary can impair the secretion of gonadotropins either as one manifestation of a generalized disease of the anterior pituitary (Chap. 328) or as an isolated defect. In the latter case the cause is usually hypogonadotropic hypogonadism, in which secretion of both LH and FSH are impaired. This disorder usually is congenital but may be acquired. Alternatively, gonadotropin secretion can be altered by

Table 335-1 Abnormalities of Adult Testicular Function

Infertility with Underandrogenization	Infertility with Normal Virilization
HYPOTHALAMIC-PITUITARY	
Panhypopituitarism	
Isolated gonadotropin deficiency	Isolated FSH deficiency
Adrenal hypoplasia congenita	Congenital adrenal hyperplasia
Cushing's syndrome	Hyperprolactinemia
Hyperprolactinemia	Androgen use
Hemochromatosis	
TESTICULAR	
Developmental and structural defects	
Klinefelter's syndrome[a]	AZF mutations of the Y chromosome
XX male	Germinal cell aplasia
	Cryptorchidism
	Varicocele
	Immotile cilia syndrome
Acquired defects	
Viral orchitis*	*Mycoplasma* infection
Trauma	
Radiation	Radiation
Drugs (spironolactone, alcohol, ketoconazole, cyclophosphamide)	Drugs (cyclophosphamide)
Environmental toxins	Environmental toxins
Autoimmunity	Autoimmunity
Granulomatous disease	
Associated with systemic diseases	
Liver disease	Febrile illness
Renal failure	Celiac disease
Sickle cell disease	
Immune disease (AIDS, rheumatoid arthritis)	
Neurologic disease (myotonic dystrophy, spinobulbar muscular atrophy, and paraplegia)	Neurologic disease (paraplegia)
Androgen resistance	Androgen resistance
SPERM TRANSPORT	
	Obstruction of the epididymis or vas deferens (cystic fibrosis, diethylstilbesterol exposure, congenital absence)

[a] The common testicular causes of underandrogenization and infertility in adults—Klinefelter's syndrome and viral orchitis—are associated with small testes.

factors other than hypothalamic-pituitary pathology. For example, elevation of plasma cortisol, as in the *Cushing syndrome*, can depress LH secretion independent of a space-occupying lesion of the pituitary. Critical illness also suppresses plasma gonadotropin levels. Some patients with uncontrolled *congenital adrenal hyperplasia* have elevated levels of adrenal androgens, suppressed gonadotropin secretion, and consequent infertility. Likewise, the use of *androgens* for purposes other than replacement therapy can inhibit gonadotropin secretion and impair sperm production (see below). *Hyperprolactinemia* (as the consequence either of pituitary adenomas or of drugs such as phenothiazines) can cause combined Leydig cell and seminiferous tubule dysfunction, presumably due to inhibition of LH and FSH secretion by prolactin. Occasionally, impaired fertility in hyperprolactinemia is associated with normal gonadotropin and androgen levels and is presumed to result from direct inhibition of spermatogenesis by prolactin. *Hemochromatosis* usually impairs testicular function as the result of effects on the pituitary; less often it affects the testis directly (Chap. 345). In some conditions, testosterone levels may be decreased in association with normal LH levels, and the mechanism is less clear. Men with massive obesity have decreased levels of SHBG and of total and bioavailable testosterone, which return toward normal with weight loss. Obesity may also contribute to the decreased testosterone levels in the subset of such men with Pickwickian syndrome (Chap. 263). Some men with temporal lobe seizures also have hypogonadotropic hypogonadism.

Testicular Defects Abnormalities of testicular function in the adult man can be grouped into several categories: developmental and structural defects of the testes, acquired testicular defects, and disorders secondary to systemic disease.

Developmental abnormalities The *Klinefelter syndrome* (*XXY*, both the classic and the mosaic forms) and the *XX male syndrome* are usually not recognized until after the time of expected puberty (Chap. 338). Some developmental defects cause infertility in the presence of normal androgen production. These include varicocele, germinal cell aplasia, deletions or mutations of the azoospermia factor (*AZF*) genes on the Y chromosome, and cryptorchidism. *Varicocele* may be of etiologic importance in as much as one-third of all cases of male infertility. It is caused by retrograde flow of blood into the internal spermatic vein that eventuates in progressive, often palpable dilation of the peritesticular pampiniform plexus of veins. Varicocele occurs in ~10 to 15% of men in the general population and in 20 to 40% of men with infertility. It is thought to result from incompetence of the valve between the internal spermatic vein and the renal vein and is more common on the left side (85%). Unilateral varicocele increases the blood flow and the temperature of both testes as a result of the extensive anastomoses of the venous systems. The increased scrotal (and testicular) temperature is believed to be the cause of the poor-quality semen and infertility (the testes no longer are 2°C cooler than the abdominal cavity). The findings on semen analysis are usually nonspecific, with all parameters showing some abnormality. Surgical repair of varicocele results in fertility in about half of men, with the best results (70% pregnancy rate) in those whose preoperative sperm counts are >10 million per milliliter.

Some patients with *germinal cell aplasia* (the Sertoli cell-only syndrome) have a positive family history and may constitute a specific group in whom the germinal epithelium is missing with resulting azoospermia; plasma testosterone and LH values are normal, and plasma FSH levels are elevated. Other patients with identical histologic and clinical findings have androgen resistance or a history of viral orchitis or cryptorchidism; microdeletions of one or more genes (e.g., *Deleted in Azoospermia, DAZ*) on the Y chromosome have been documented in 10 to 20% of men with azoospermia or oligospermia (many of whom have germinal cell aplasia), depending on the criteria used for selection.

Unilateral *cryptorchidism*, even when corrected before puberty, is associated with abnormal semen in many individuals, indicating that the testes can be bilaterally abnormal even in unilateral cryptorchidism.

The *immotile cilia syndrome* is an autosomal recessive defect characterized by immotility or poor motility of the cilia of the airways and of the sperm. Kartagener's syndrome is a subgroup of the immotile cilia syndrome associated with situs inversus, chronic sinusitis, and bronchiectasis (Chap. 256). The structural abnormality leading to impaired motility of cilia can usually be defined by the electron-microscopic appearance showing defects in the dynein arms, spokes, or microtubule doublets. Cilia from epithelia and sperm tails exhibit the same defects, but the pulmonary manifestations may be minor. Other less well understood structural defects can cause immotility of sperm without involvement of cilia in the lung.

Acquired testicular defects Acquired testicular failure in the adult man can be due to *viral orchitis*. The responsible viruses include mumps virus, echovirus, lymphocytic choriomeningitis virus, and group B arboviruses. The orchitis is due to actual infection of the tissue by virus rather than to indirect effects of infection. Orchitis occurs in as many as one-fourth of adult men with mumps; in about two-thirds the orchitis is unilateral, and in the remainder it is bilateral. Orchitis usually develops a few days after the onset of parotitis but may precede it. The testis may return to normal size and function or undergo atrophy. Atrophy is believed to be due both to direct effects of the virus on the seminiferous tubules and to ischemia secondary to pressure and edema within the taut tunica albuginea. Semen analysis returns to normal in three-fourths of men with unilateral involvement and in only one-third of men with bilateral orchitis. Atrophy is usually perceptible within 1 to 6 months after the acute illness, and the degree of atrophy is not necessarily proportional to the severity of the acute orchitis. Unilateral atrophy occurs in about one-third of patients, and bilateral atrophy occurs in about one-tenth.

Trauma, including torsion, can also cause secondary atrophy of the testes. The exposed position of the testes in the scrotum renders them susceptible to both thermal and physical trauma—particularly in men with hazardous occupations.

The testes are sensitive to *radiation damage*; decreased secretion of testosterone appears to be a consequence of diminished testicular blood flow. Doses >200 mGy (20 rad) cause increases in plasma FSH and LH levels and damage to the spermatogonia. After about 800 mGy (80 rad), oligospermia or azoospermia develops, and higher doses may obliterate the germinal epithelium, except for occasional stem and Sertoli cells. Fractionated radiation may have a more profound effect than single-dose radiation. Recovery of sperm density occurs in a dose-related fashion, and complete recovery of sperm density may require as long as 5 years. Permanent infertility can occur after radiation therapy for malignant lymphoma despite shielding of the testes. Permanent androgen deficiency in adult men is uncommon after therapeutic radiation; however, most boys given direct testicular radiation therapy for acute lymphoblastic leukemia have permanently low plasma testosterone levels. Sperm banking should be considered in patients before they undergo radiation treatment or chemotherapy.

In general, *drugs* interfere with testicular function in one of four ways—inhibition of testosterone synthesis, blockade of androgen action, enhancement of estrogen levels, or direct inhibition of spermatogenesis. Spironolactone and ketoconazole block the synthesis of androgen by interfering with the late steps in androgen biosynthesis. Spironolactone and cimetidine compete with androgen for binding to the androgen receptor and thus block androgen action in target cells. Testosterone levels may be low, and estradiol levels may be elevated in persons using marijuana, heroin, or methadone, although the exact reasons are unclear. Alcohol, when consumed in excess for prolonged periods, causes decreased plasma testosterone levels, independent of liver disease or malnutrition. Elevated plasma estradiol and decreased plasma testosterone levels may occur in men taking digitalis.

Antineoplastic and chemotherapeutic agents commonly interfere with spermatogenesis. Cyclophosphamide causes azoospermia or extreme oligospermia within a few weeks after the initiation of therapy. Cessation of therapy is followed by a return of spermatogenesis within 3 years in about half of patients. Combination chemotherapy for acute leukemia, Hodgkin's disease, and other malignancies also may impair Leydig cell function. In pubertal boys this impairment is manifested by decreased serum testosterone and elevated LH levels; in adult men testosterone levels do not decline, and the impaired Leydig cell function may be detected only as an enhanced LH response to GnRH. The alkylating agents in the chemotherapeutic regimens seem to be responsible for Leydig cell toxicity.

Because of the toxic effects of many physical and chemical agents on spermatogenesis, the occupational and recreational history should be carefully evaluated in all men with infertility. Known environmental hazards include microwaves, ultrasound, and chemicals such as the nematocide dibromochloropropane, cadmium, and lead. In some populations, sperm density is said to have declined by as much as 40% in the past 50 years, and it has been postulated that environmental estrogens or antiandrogens may be responsible.

Testicular failure also occurs as a part of *polyglandular autoimmune insufficiency* (Chap. 339). Sperm antibodies can cause isolated male infertility. In some instances these antibodies are secondary phenomena resulting from duct obstruction or vasectomy. *Granulomatous diseases* can destroy the testes, and testicular atrophy occurs in 10 to 20% of men with lepromatous leprosy owing to direct invasion of the tissue by the mycobacteria. The tubules are involved initially, followed by endarteritis and destruction of Leydig cells.

Testicular abnormalities associated with systemic disease In *cirrhosis of the liver*, a combined testicular and pituitary abnormality leads to decreased testosterone production independent of the direct toxic effects of ethanol. Although the plasma LH level is elevated, the level may be below the expected range given the degree of androgen deficiency. This situation most likely results from the inhibition of LH secretion by estrogen in patients with chronic liver disease. Increased estrogen production results from impaired hepatic extraction of adrenal androstenedione and subsequent increased extraglandular conversion to estrone and estradiol. In effect, estrogen precursors are shunted to sites of extraglandular aromatization. Testicular atrophy and gynecomastia are present in about half of men with cirrhosis, and many such men are impotent. Successful liver transplantation reverses the effects of cirrhosis on the pituitary-testicular axis.

In chronic *renal failure*, androgen synthesis and sperm production decrease despite elevated plasma gonadotropins. The elevated LH level is due to increased production and reduced clearance but does not restore normal testosterone production. In addition, about one-fourth of men with renal failure have hyperprolactinemia; the role of hyperprolactinemia in decreasing testosterone production is unclear. Low testosterone coupled with normal or increased plasma estrogen levels cause gynecomastia in about half of men on chronic hemodialysis, and about half of men on dialysis have decreased libido and/or impotence. Improvement in testosterone production with hemodialysis is incomplete, but successful transplantation may return testicular function to normal.

Men with *sickle cell anemia* usually have impaired secondary sexual development, and testicular atrophy is present in one-third of them. The defect may be at either the testicular or the hypothalamic-pituitary level. Abnormalities in Leydig cell function, frequently accompanied by decreased sperm density, have been noted in a variety of chronic systemic diseases, including protein-energy *malnutrition*, advanced *Hodgkin's disease* and *cancer* before chemotherapy, and *amyloidosis*. Most of these disorders cause a lowered plasma testosterone level coupled with a normal to increased plasma LH level, suggesting combined hypothalamic-pituitary and testicular defects. Similar hormone changes occur after *surgery*, *myocardial infarction*, and severe *burns* and thus may be a nonspecific effect of illness.

In HIV-infected men, elevation of gonadotropins (a compensated state of hypogonadism) may precede the development of overt hypogonadism, but 35 to 50% of men with AIDS eventually develop low testosterone levels. Elevation of SHBG levels may partially mask the fall in testosterone. Some of the hormonal changes in this disorder are likely nonspecific and related to severe illness. Whether testosterone deficiency contributes to the muscle wasting and weight loss characteristic of this disorder is unclear, but androgen replacement therapy may increase muscle and lean body mass.

Sperm density can decrease temporarily after *acute febrile illness* in the absence of a change in testosterone production. Infertility in men with *celiac disease* is associated with a hormonal pattern typical of androgen resistance, namely, elevated testosterone and LH levels. *Neurologic* diseases associated with altered testicular function include myotonic dystrophy, spinobulbar muscular atrophy, and paraplegia. In myotonic dystrophy, small testes may be associated with impairment of both spermatogenesis and Leydig cell function. Spinobulbar muscular atrophy is caused by an expansion of the glutamine repeat sequences in the amino-terminal region of the androgen receptor; this expansion impairs function of the androgen receptor, but it is unclear how the alteration is related to the neurologic manifestations. Men with spinobulbar muscular atrophy often have as a late manifestation underandrogenization and infertility and the hormonal features of androgen resistance (Chap. 338). *Spinal cord lesions* that cause paraplegia lead to a temporary decrease in testosterone levels and may cause persistent defects in spermatogenesis; some patients retain the capacity for penile erection and ejaculation.

Androgen resistance Defects of the androgen receptor cause resistance to the action of androgen, usually associated with defective male phenotypic development, infertility, and underandrogenization

(Chap. 338). Mutations of the androgen receptor that cause mild androgen resistance can cause infertility due to oligo- or azoospermia in otherwise phenotypically normal men.

Impairment of Sperm Transport Disorders of sperm transport may cause infertility in as many as 6% of infertile men with normal virilization. Obstruction of the ejaculatory system may be unilateral or bilateral, congenital or acquired. In men with unilateral obstruction, infertility may result from antisperm antibodies. Congenital defects of the vas deferens can occur as an isolated abnormality associated with absence of the seminal vesicles (and consequently absence of fructose in the ejaculate), in men whose mothers received *diethylstilbestrol* during pregnancy, and in men with *cystic fibrosis*. Furthermore, congenital bilateral absence of the vas deferens can be due to mutations in the cystic fibrosis conductance regulator (*CFTR*) gene; some of these mutations are distinct from those associated with the more typical pulmonary and gastrointestinal manifestations of cystic fibrosis. Acquired obstructive azoospermia can occur at the level of the epididymis in association with chronic infections of the paranasal sinuses and lungs and with tuberculosis, leprosy, and gonorrhea.

Empirical Therapy of Male Infertility Disorders for which there are logical or effective treatments (genital tract obstruction, sperm autoimmunity, gonadotropin deficiency) account for only 10% of infertile men, and pregnancies are infrequent when the male partner has genital tract obstruction or sperm autoimmunity. Severe oligospermia/azoospermia from other causes accounts for about one-fourth of cases of male infertility and has largely been considered untreatable. The other two-thirds of infertile men have a partial reduction in semen parameters and subfertility of a variable degree, and in this group spontaneous fertility may occur in untreated men (as high as 25% in one year). In the past various empirical therapies (e.g., testosterone rebound, gonadotropins, antiestrogens) have been tried without success. The only successful empirical therapy for men with mild to moderate defects in semen quality is in vitro fertilization. However, standard in vitro fertilization does not provide a good outcome in the presence of severe semen abnormalities, such as a sperm density of <5 million per milliliter, poor motility, and many abnormal forms. For such men the technique of intracytoplasmic sperm injection (ICSI) has been a major advance; indeed fertilization and pregnancy rates with this technique are similar to those for standard in vitro techniques in couples with fallopian tube pathology, e.g., a 50 to 70% fertilization rate and a 30% pregnancy rate per cycle. This technique is sometimes successful with spermatozoa recovered from testicular biopsies in men with azoospermia. →*The management of male infertility is discussed in Chap. 54.*

Fertility Control in Men (See also Chap. 54) A variety of approaches to fertility control in men have been tried, including use of the condom as an effective barrier that also prevents sexually transmitted diseases. Vasectomy, which involves transection or ligation of the vas deferens, has a high success rate and can be performed on an outpatient basis. The time required for azoospermia to occur after the operation depends on the number of sperm in the terminal vas deferens and ejaculatory ducts at the time of surgery, but it is usually less than 40 days. Azoospermia should be documented in each case to prove effectiveness. No deleterious effects on either testosterone production or the hypothalamic-pituitary axis have been documented. Despite reports of immune-complex–associated accelerated atherosclerosis in vasectomized nonhuman primates, there does not appear to be any association between vasectomy and atherosclerosis in men. Vasectomy should be recommended only for men requesting permanent sterilization. Only about 30 to 40% of men subjected to vasovasostomy for reanastomosis of the vas subsequently achieve fertility. Suppression of gonadotropins with long-acting GnRH analogues or GnRH antagonists causes marked reduction in sperm counts but requires concomitant androgen replacement. The efficacy and acceptance of this approach to male contraception remain to be established.

GONADAL FUNCTION DURING AGING Beginning at about age 40, mean plasma bioavailable testosterone concentrations decline gradually; about 40% of elderly men have low bioavailable testosterone levels. Although statistically lower than the levels in young men, the concentrations of total testosterone usually remain within the normal range, even in elderly men. The cause of the reduced testosterone level is likely a decreased number of Leydig cells. In older men seminiferous tubule function and sperm production also usually decline. Plasma LH and FSH levels are often slightly elevated, consistent with a decline in gonadal function. An increase in the conversion of androgen to estrogen in peripheral tissues results in a decrease in the effective ratio of androgen to estrogen. These latter hormonal changes may play a role in the development of prostatic hyperplasia and in the development of gynecomastia in aging men (Chaps. 95 and 337). Male sexual function gradually declines after early adulthood, but there is no convincing evidence that hormonal changes have any direct bearing on changes in sexual function with age in healthy men.

Prostatic Hyperplasia See Chap. 95.

Cancer of the Prostate See Chap. 95.

DISORDERS OF ALL AGES **Testicular Tumors** (See also Chap. 96) Low levels of hCG are present in normal testes may be elevated in persons with testicular tumors. Indeed, an elevated plasma level of the β subunit of hCG (hCG-β) is a sensitive and specific marker of tumor activity in some men with germ cell tumors. Plasma levels of hCG-β are elevated in all men with choriocarcinoma, in one-third of those with embryonal carcinomas and teratocarcinomas, and rarely in those with seminomas. Changes in hCG-β levels correlate with response to therapy.

Testicular tumors can cause elevated estradiol and testosterone levels by at least two mechanisms: (1) Trophoblastic, Leydig, and Sertoli cell tumors produce both hormones autonomously; pituitary gonadotropin secretion and hormone production by the uninvolved portions of the testes are depressed, and azoospermia is common; (2) hCG secretion by the tumors can increase estradiol and testosterone production in the unaffected areas of the testes; azoospermia is uncommon with such tumors. When estrogens and androgens are formed (directly or indirectly) by the tumors, feminization, virilization, or no obvious change may result, depending on the hormones produced and the age of the patient. α-Fetroprotein can provde another cellular marker of testicular tumor activity.

Gynecomastia See Chap. 337.

℞ TREATMENT **Androgens** • ***Pharmacologic preparations*** When testosterone is taken by mouth, it is absorbed into the portal blood and degraded promptly by the liver, so that only insignificant amounts reach the systemic circulation; when administered parenterally, testosterone is rapidly absorbed from the injection vehicle and rapidly degraded. As a consequence, effective androgen therapy requires the administration of either a slowly absorbed form of testosterone (dermal patches or micronized oral testosterone) or modified analogues. Chemical modifications either retard absorption or catabolism, or enhance the androgenic potency, so that full effects can be achieved at a lower blood level of drug. Three types of modification have had widespread clinical application (Fig. 335-7): (1) esterification of the 17β-hydroxyl group, (2) alkylation at the 17α position, and (3) alteration of the ring structure, particularly by substitutions at the 2, 9, and 11 positions. Most pharmacologic agents actually have combinations of ring structure alterations and either 17α-alkylation or esterification of the 17β-hydroxyl group. Esterification decreases the polarity of the molecule so that the steroid is more soluble in the fat vehicles used for injection, leading to slower release into the circulation. Most esters must be injected parenterally. The larger the acid esterified, the slower the release and the more prolonged the action. Esters such as testosterone cypionate and testosterone enanthate can be injected every 1 to 3 weeks, the usual regimen being 200 mg of either ester intramuscularly every 2 weeks. Because the esters are hydrolyzed before the hormones act, therapy can be monitored by assaying the plasma testosterone level at various times after administration.

The oral effectiveness of 17α-alkylated androgens (such as meth-

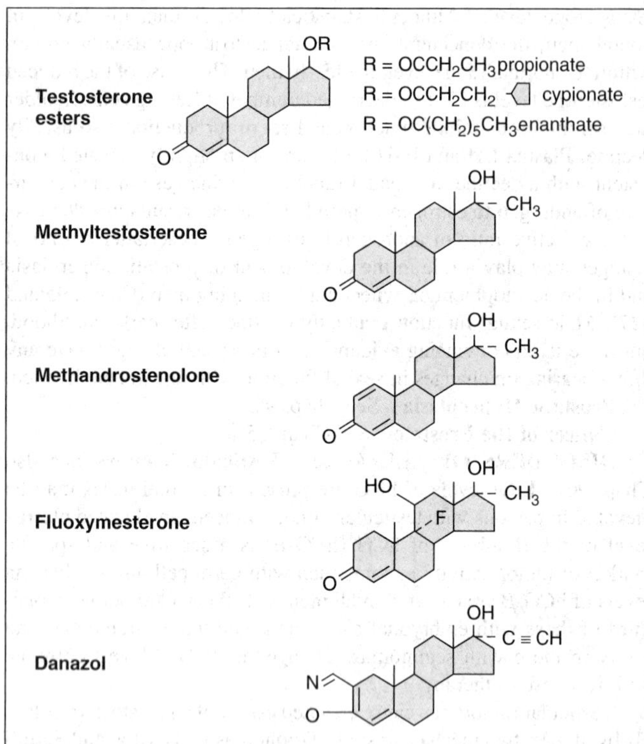

FIGURE 335-7 Some of the androgen preparations available for pharmacologic use.

yltestosterone and methandrostenolone) is due to slower hepatic catabolism, which allows the alkylated derivatives to reach the systemic circulation. For this reason, 17α-methyl or -ethyl substitution is a feature of most orally active androgens. Unfortunately, all 17α-alkylated steroids can cause abnormal liver function, and for this reason they have a limited role in therapy.

Other alterations of the ring structure have been adopted empirically; some slow the rate of inactivation, others enhance the potency of a given molecule, and some alter the conversion to other active metabolites. For example, the potency of fluoxymesterone may be due to the fact that, unlike most androgens, it is a poor precursor for conversion to estrogens in peripheral tissues.

Three transdermal preparations are available in which a testosterone-loaded patch is applied to the skin each day. One is a scrotal patch (Testoderm) that contains no permeation enhancers, which may irritate the skin, but it has a low rate of acceptance. The other two systems (Androderm, Testosterone TTS) are applied to the trunk, arms, or thighs. Each patch provides physiologic testosterone levels that mimic the normal diurnal variation with higher levels in the morning hours. High rates of dermatologic problems have been reported with the Androderm transdermal system.

Side effects of androgens All androgens carry the risk of inducing virilization in women. Early manifestations include acne, coarsening of the voice, hirsutism, and menstrual irregularities. If treatment is discontinued as soon as these effects develop, the manifestations may slowly subside. Long-term side effects such as male-pattern baldness, marked hirsutism, voice changes, and hypertrophy of the clitoris are largely irreversible. At physiologic replacement doses, testosterone esters have few toxic effects in mature men. At supraphysiologic doses, however, gonadotropin secretion is inhibited, the testes shrink, and the sperm count falls (indeed, androgen abuse can be associated with low sperm counts that may persist for 9 months or longer after cessation of the steroid). In some older men, testosterone therapy may cause polycythemia (hematocrit >52%); in men predisposed to obstructive sleep apnea, androgen therapy may initiate or worsen symptoms. In older men, the presence of benign prostatic hyperplasia is not a contraindication for androgen therapy, but such men should be screened for prostate cancer before initiating androgen replacement (Chap. 95).

The so-called toxic side effects vary among the different agents and with the clinical setting in which they are used. Retention of a limited amount of sodium is an inevitable consequence of androgen therapy and may lead to edema in patients with underlying heart disease or renal failure, or when androgens are administered in enormous amounts. Although androgens do not cause malignancy, they may promote the growth of and intensify pain from carcinomas of the prostate and breast in men.

The feminizing side effects of androgen therapy in men are poorly understood. Testosterone (but not 5α-reduced androgens) can be converted (aromatized) in extraglandular tissues to estradiol. The most common manifestation of feminization is the development of gynecomastia. Such breast enlargement is common in children given androgens, possibly because of a greater capacity to convert androgens to estrogens in childhood. The administration of testosterone esters to men results in an increase in plasma estrogen levels, but in men with normal liver function gynecomastia usually develops only after use of high doses.

All 17α-alkylated androgens can produce liver function abnormalities such as elevated plasma levels of alkaline phosphatase and conjugated bilirubin. The incidence of clinical liver disease probably depends on the previous integrity of the liver, but jaundice may occur in the absence of preexisting liver disease. 17α-Alkylated drugs also increase the levels of a variety of plasma proteins that are synthesized in the liver. The most serious complications of 17α-alkylated androgens are peliosis hepatis (blood-filled cysts in the liver) and hepatoma. These disorders were initially described in patients with aplastic anemia, many of whom had Fanconi anemia, itself a predisposing factor for the development of malignancy. However, both lesions can occur after administration of substituted androgens for other indications, including use by athletes. These tumors may either follow a benign course after discontinuation of the drugs or be rapidly fatal.

One indication for 17α-alkylated androgens is in the treatment of hereditary angioedema in which the desired therapeutic benefit (increased level of the inhibitor of the first component of complement) may actually be an effect of the 17-alkylated side chain rather than of the parent androgen. As a consequence, weak androgens such as danazol are effective in this disorder (Fig. 335-7). Danazol is also used in the management of endometriosis (Chap. 52).

Replacement therapy The aim of androgen therapy in hypogonadal men is to restore or bring to normal male secondary sexual characteristics (beard, body hair, external genitalia) and male sexual behavior and to mimic the hormonal effects on somatic development (hemoglobin, muscle mass, nitrogen balance, and epiphyseal closure). Since an assay for plasma testosterone is available for monitoring therapy, the treatment of androgen deficiency is almost universally successful. The parenteral administration of a long-acting testosterone ester such as 100 to 200 mg testosterone enanthate at 1- to 2-week intervals results in a sustained increase in plasma testosterone to the normal male range. Alternatively, testosterone may be administered transdermally. Testosterone patches, which are available in different doses, are replaced daily. If hypogonadism is primary and of long duration (as in the Klinefelter syndrome), suppression of plasma LH to the normal range may not occur for many weeks, if at all. There is considerable variability in the relation between plasma testosterone and male sexual behavior, but in cases of postpubertal testicular failure (even of many years duration), normal sexual activity usually is resumed after adequate replacement. Androgen administration does not restore spermatogenesis in hypogonadal states, but the volume of the ejaculate (derived largely from the prostate and seminal vesicles) and other male secondary sex characteristics return to normal. The effects of endogenous androgen on hemoglobin, nitrogen retention, and skeletal development are also reproduced.

In men of all ages in whom hypogonadism developed before expected puberty (such as men with isolated gonadotropin deficiency), it is appropriate to bring plasma testosterone into the adult range slowly. When therapy is commenced at the time of expected puberty in such men, the normal events of puberty proceed in the usual fashion. If therapy is delayed until after the time of usual puberty, the degree to which normal virilization will occur is variable, but many patients undergo a relatively complete anatomic and functional maturation. Intermittent low-dose androgen therapy is indicated in prepubertal hypogonadal boys with microphallus to bring the external genitalia into the normal range. If such patients are monitored closely and given androgens for only short periods, therapy usually has no adverse effects on somatic growth.

In boys of pubertal age with either isolated gonadotropin deficiency or primary testicular disease, the usual practice is to institute androgen therapy between the ages of 12 and 14 years, depending on the subjective need for sexual development. The initial administration of small doses of testosterone esters followed by a gradual increase to 100 to 150 mg/m^2 of body surface area every 1 to 3 weeks should result in a normal pubertal growth spurt. The time from the start of treatment to the appearance of secondary sex characteristics is variable. Penile development, deepening of the voice, and the appearance of other secondary sexual characteristics usually commence during the first year of treatment. In normal boys, puberty extends over several years, and treatment designed to replicate normal development does not shorten the process greatly.

Testosterone exerts its full action only in the presence of a balanced hormonal environment and, particularly, in the presence of adequate levels of growth hormone. Consequently, prepubertal boys with coexisting growth hormone and androgen deficiency respond poorly to androgens unless growth hormone is given simultaneously.

Pharmacologic uses Androgens have been used for a variety of disorders unassociated with hypogonadism in the hope that potential benefits from the nonvirilizing actions of the agents (such as increases in nitrogen retention, muscle mass, and hemoglobin) would outweigh any deleterious actions of the drugs. The most common nonreplacement uses of androgen have been attempts to improve nitrogen balance in catabolic states (e.g., AIDS), self-administration by athletes to increase muscle mass and/or athletic performance, attempts to enhance erythropoiesis in refractory anemias (including the anemia of renal failure), treatment of hereditary angioedema and endometriosis, and management of growth retardation of various etiologies. Most of the expected benefits in these disorders have not been realized for two reasons. First, modest pharmacologic doses of androgens have little physiologic effect in men when superimposed on normal testicular androgen, and in women the virilizing side effects of androgens are formidable. Second, no androgen has been devised that exhibits only the nonvirilizing effects of the hormone. This conclusion is not surprising in view of the fact that the physiologic actions of androgens are mediated by a single, high-affinity receptor (Fig. 335-5).

The most pervasive form of androgen abuse is by male athletes in the expectation that muscle development and athletic performance will be improved. In controlled studies using modest pharmacologic doses (two to four times the usual replacement doses), these agents do not improve performance consistently. However, at the doses frequently taken by athletes (which sometimes exceed 10 times the replacement dose), androgens do enhance nitrogen balance and muscle mass; since the drugs have multiple side effects at high doses, these benefits do not outweigh the risks associated with androgen abuse in man, and the use of androgens by female athletes is associated with disfiguring virilization. Thus this practice cannot be condemned too harshly. The only established indications for androgen therapy outside of male hypogonadism are in selected patients with anemia due to bone marrow failure or hereditary angioedema and as an adjunct to growth hormone therapy.

Gonadotropins Gonadotropin therapy is used to establish or restore fertility in patients with gonadotropin deficiency of any cause. Several gonadotropin preparations are available. Human menopausal gonadotropin (hMG) (purified from the urine of postmenopausal

women) contains 75 IU FSH and 75 IU LH per vial. hCG (purified from the urine of pregnant women) has little FSH activity and resembles LH in its ability to stimulate testosterone production by Leydig cells. Because of the expense of hMG, treatment is usually begun with hCG alone, and hMG is added later to promote the FSH-dependent stages of spermatid development. A high ratio of LH to FSH activity and treatment for 6 to 18 months may be necessary to bring about maturation of the prepubertal testes. Recombinant human FSH is also available and has been used mainly for ovulation induction in women. Trials are underway to examine its effects on spermatogenesis in men with hypogonadotropic hypogonadism. Once spermatogenesis is restored with combined FSH and LH therapy, hCG alone is often sufficient to maintain spermatogenesis.

The dose of hCG required to maintain a normal testosterone level varies from 1000 to 5000 IU weekly. A number of regimens have been used to induce maturation of spermatogenesis. Most involve starting with 2000 IU hCG three or more times a week until most of the clinical parameters, including plasma testosterone levels, are normal. hMG (usually one ampule) is then added three times a week to complete the development of spermatogenesis. The length of therapy required to restore spermatogenesis may be as long as 12 months.

GnRH and GnRH Analogues GnRH (gonadorelin) is available for endocrine testing and is used by some physicians for chronic therapy of the infertility of hypogonadotropic hypogonadism. In the latter instance, it is necessary to administer GnRH in frequent boluses (25 to 200 ng/kg of body weight every 2 h) with the use of portable infusion pumps, analogous to those used for insulin administration. In general, pulsatile GnRH does not appear to be more efficacious than gonadotropin in returning sperm counts to normal. GnRH analogues (leuprolide, nafarelin, histrelin) are available for the suppression of gonadotropin secretion, leading to hypogonadism. In prostatic cancer, testicular androgen production can be blocked by monthly injection of 7.5 mg leuprolide in depot form.

BIBLIOGRAPHY

BAKER HWG: Male infertility, in *Endocrinology*, 3d ed, LLJ deGroot (ed). Philadelphia, Saunders, 1995, pp 2404–2433

BHASIN S, SALEHIAN B: Gonadotropin therapy of men with hypogonadotropic hypogonadism, in *Current Therapy in Endocrinology and Metabolism*, 6th ed, CW Bardin (ed). St. Louis, Mosby, 1997, pp 349–352

CARR BR, GRIFFIN JE: Fertility control and its complications, in *Williams Textbook of Endocrinology*, 9th ed, JD Wilson, DW Foster (eds). Philadelphia, Saunders, 1998, pp 901–926

CHILLON M et al: Mutations in the cystic fibrosis gene in patients with congenital absence of the vas deferens. N Engl J Med 332:1475, 1995

DE KRETSER DM: Declining sperm counts. BMJ 312:457, 1996

DRINKA PJ et al: Polycythemia as a complication of testosterone therapy in nursing home men with low testosterone levels. J Am Geriat Soc 43:899, 1995

FORESTA C et al: Y-chromosome deletions in idiopathic severe testiculopathies. J Clin Endocrinol Metab 82:1075, 1997

GNESSI L et al: Gonadal peptides as mediators of development and functional control of the testis. Endocrine Rev 18:541, 1997

GOLDZIEHER JW et al: Improving the diagnostic reliability of rapidly fluctuating plasma hormone levels by optimized multiple-sampling techniques. J Clin Endocrinol Metab 43:824, 1976

GRAY A et al: Age, disease and changing sex hormone levels in middle-aged men: Results of the Massachusetts male aging study. J Clin Endocrinol Metab 73:1016, 1991

GRIFFIN JE, WILSON JD: Disorders of the testes and male reproductive tract, in *Williams Textbook of Endocrinology*, 9th ed, JD Wilson et al (eds). Philadelphia, Saunders, 1998, pp 819–876

GRINSPOON S et al: Sustained anabolic effects of long-term androgen administration in men with AIDS wasting. Clin Infect Dis 28:634, 1999

GRUMBACH MM, STYNE DM: Puberty: Ontogeny, neuroendocrinology, physiology, and disorders, in *Williams Textbook of Endocrinology*, 9th ed, JD Wilson et al (eds). Philadelphia, Saunders, 1998, pp 1509–1626

HANDELSMAN DJ: Testicular dysfunction in systemic disease. Endocrinol Metab Clin North Am 23:839, 1994

HAYES FJ et al: Differential control of gonadotropin secretion in the human: endocrine role of inhibin. J Clin Endocrinol Metab 83:1835, 1998

——— et al: Hypogonadotropic hypogonadism. Endocrinol Metab Clin North Am 27: 739, 1998

LESCHEK EW et al: Six year results of spironolactone and testolactone treatment of familial male-limited precocious puberty with addition of deslorelin after central puberty onset. J Clin Endocrinol Metab 84:175, 1999

MACDONALD PC et al: Origin of estrogen in normal men and in women with testicular feminization. J Clin Endocrinol Metab 49:905, 1979

MARSHALL WA, TANNER JM: Variation in the pattern of pubertal changes in boys. Arch Dis Child 45:13, 1970

NAJMABADI H et al: Substantial prevalence of microdeletions of the Y-chromosome in infertile men with idiopathic azoospermia and oligospermia detected using a sequence-tagged site-based mapping strategy. J Clin Endocrinol Metab 81:1347, 1996

PALERMO GD et al: Intracytoplasmic sperm injection: A novel treatment for all forms of male factor infertility. Fertil Steril 63:1231, 1995

PARKER S, ARMITAGE M: Experience with transdermal testosterone replacement therapy for hypogonadal men. Clin Endocrinol 50:57, 1999

RUGARLI EI, BALLABIO A: Kallmann syndrome. From genetics to neurobiology. JAMA 270:2713, 1993

SALEHIAN B et al: Testicular pathologic changes and the pituitary-testicular axis during human immunodeficiency virus infection. Endocr Pract 5:1, 1999

SCHNEIDER BK et al: Influence of testosterone on breathing during sleep. J Appl Physiol 61:618, 1986

SNYDER PF, LAWRENCE DA: Treatment of male hypogonadism with testosterone enanthate. J Clin Endocrinol Metab 51:1335, 1980

WHITCOMB RW, CROWLEY WF JR: Hypogonadotropic hypogonadism: Gonadotropin-releasing hormone therapy, in *Current Therapy in Endocrinology and Metabolism*, 6th ed, CW Bardin (ed). St Louis, Mosby, 1997, pp 353–355

336

Bruce R. Carr, Karen D. Bradshaw

DISORDERS OF THE OVARY AND FEMALE REPRODUCTIVE TRACT

ACTH	adrenocorticotropic hormone	HPV	human papilloma virus
CT	computed tomography	LH	luteinizing hormone
ER	estrogen receptor	MRI	magnetic resonance imaging
FSH	follicle-stimulating hormone	PCOS	polycystic ovarian syndrome
GnRH	gonadotropin-releasing hormone	TGF	transforming growth factor
hCG	Human chorionic gonadotropin	TSH	thyroid-stimulating hormone
hMG	human menopausal gonadotropin		

The ovary is the source of ova for reproduction and of the hormones that regulate female sexual life. The anatomic structure, response to hormonal stimuli, and secretory capacity of the ovary vary at different periods of life. This chapter will review normal ovarian physiology as a background for understanding ovarian abnormalities and will consider other disorders of the female reproductive tract.

DEVELOPMENT, STRUCTURE, AND FUNCTION OF THE OVARY

EMBRYOLOGY During the third week of gestation, the primordial germ cells differentiate from the endoderm lining the yolk sac at the caudal end of the embryo. The germ cells migrate to the genital ridge adjacent to the mesonephric kidney by the fifth week of gestation and undergo mitotic division. The gonads exist in an undifferentiated state until the seventh week of fetal life, at which time the primitive ovary can be distinguished from the testis (Chap. 338). Estrogen formation in the ovary commences between weeks 8 and 10, and by 10 to 11 weeks of gestation, oogonia in the ovarian cortex begin developing into primary oocytes. The ovary contains a finite number of germ cells, the number peaking at about 7 million oogonia by the fifth to sixth month of gestation. Subsequently, the germ cells decrease in number through a process of atresia so that only 1 million remain at birth, 400,000 are present at menarche, and only a few remain at menopause. Two normal X chromosomes are required for development of the ovary; in individuals with a 45,X karyotype, ovarian development occurs, but the rate of atresia is accelerated so that only a fibrous streak remains at birth (Chap. 338).

After the oogonia cease to proliferate, meiosis commences, continues until the diplotene stage of the first meiotic division is completed, and then is arrested until the onset of ovulation at puberty. From the fifth month of fetal life, the primordial follicle consists of the primary oocyte arrested in meiosis, a single surrounding layer of granulosa cells, and a basement membrane that separates the primordial follicle from surrounding stromal (interstitial) tissues.

PUBERTAL MATURATION The final maturation of ovarian follicles commences during puberty. The two major hormones that regulate follicular development are the pituitary gonadotropins—follicle-stimulating hormone (FSH) and luteinizing hormone (LH) (Fig. 336-1). During the second trimester of fetal development, the plasma gonadotropins rise to levels similar to those at menopause. This peak in gonadotropin levels may be responsible for the simultaneous peak in oocyte replication. After the second trimester, the hypothalamic-pituitary axis (the so-called gonadostat) becomes functional and is sensitive to negative feedback by steroid hormones, particularly estrogen and progesterone produced in the placenta. The levels of circulating gonadotropins consequently decrease, and gonadotropins are almost undetectable at the time of birth. In the neonate, concomitant with the decrease in estrogen and progesterone levels caused by separation from the placenta, there is a rebound increase in gonadotropin secretion for the first few months of life. With continued maturation of the hypothalamic-pituitary system, the gonadostat becomes exquisitely sensitive to negative feedback by low levels of circulating steroid hormones, and plasma gonadotropins again decrease.

As the time of puberty nears, a decrease in the sensitivity of the gonadostat allows for increased secretion of FSH and LH, possibly secondary to increased episodic or pulsatile secretion of gonadotropin-releasing hormone (GnRH) by the hypothalamus (Chap. 328). A sleep-induced, pulsatile pattern of LH secretion then ensues, the first step in the development of a cyclic pattern of gonadotropin secretion (Fig. 336-1). The increase in estrogen secretion exerts a positive feedback, which leads to an exaggeration of the pulsatile release of LH and eventually to menarche and ovulation, after which plasma gonadotropin concentrations reach adult values, which are similar during day and night. After the menopause, plasma gonadotropin levels rise, then plateau 5 to 10 years after menopause and remain fairly constant until the eighth to ninth decade of life, when the levels may fall. Although ovarian function is regulated primarily by LH and FSH, the ovary is a source of peptide and protein hormones and growth factors such as inhibin and activin that may play a role in ovarian function and regulation. The production of inhibin by the mature ovary accounts, in part, for the relative reduction in FSH that is seen during the reproductive years (Fig. 336-1).

With puberty the sensitivity of the hypothalamic-pituitary centers to circulating steroid hormones is decreased, GnRH release by the hypothalamus increases, gonadotropin secretion by the pituitary is enhanced, ovarian estrogen secretion increases, and the anatomic changes of puberty ensue. At age 10 to 11, the first secondary sexual characteristics begin to appear in girls, namely, development of the breast buds (thelarche), followed by the development of pubic hair (pubarche), and later by the development of axillary hair (adrenarche). The growth of pubic and axillary hair is believed to be initiated by adrenal androgens, the levels of which begin to rise at approximately 6 to 8 years of age. A growth spurt ensues, and peak growth rate is attained by age 12.

The culmination of puberty is the onset of predictable, cyclic menses. The average time between the beginning of breast development and the onset of menses (menarche) is 2 years. During the first few years after menarche, menstrual cycles are often irregular and unpredictable due to anovulation. The age of menarche is variable and is influenced by socioeconomic and genetic factors and by general health. In the United States, the mean age of menarche is believed to have

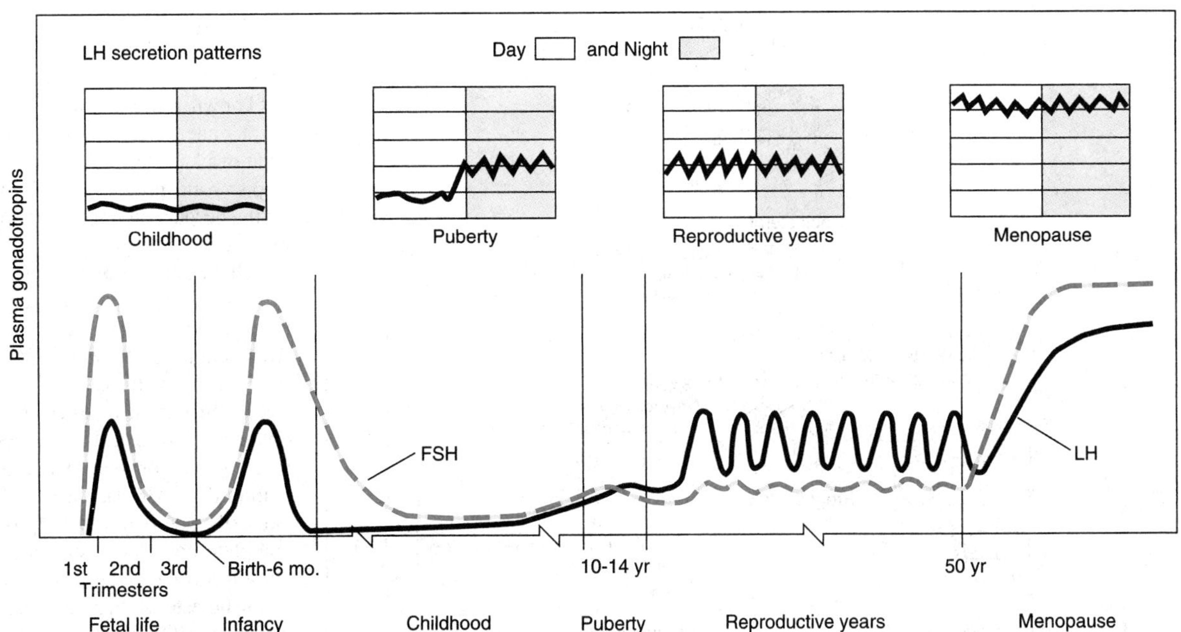

FIGURE 336-1 Pattern of gonadotropin secretion during different stages of life in women. FSH, follicle-stimulating hormone; LH, luteinizing hormone. The secretory patterns of LH during the waking hours (clear area) and night (stippled area) for each stage are indicated in the upper insets. *(After C Faiman et al: Clin Obstet Gynaecol 3:467, 1976.)*

decreased at a rate of 3 to 4 months per decade over the past 100 years and is now around 12 years, a change believed to be due to improved nutrition. A body weight of around 48 kg or some critical combination of weight, body water, and body fat is associated with development of hypothalamic insensitivity to feedback by steroids that leads to increased secretion of gonadotropins and finally to menarche. Obese girls have earlier menarche than girls with normal weights. In contrast, active participation in sports or ballet, malnutrition, and chronic debilitating disease can delay menarche.

MATURE OVARY **Morphology** The anatomic components and function of the adult ovary are illustrated schematically in Fig. 336-2. Under the influence of gonadotropins, a group of primary follicles are recruited, and by day 6 to 8 of the menstrual cycle, one follicle becomes mature or "dominant," a process characterized by accelerated growth of granulosa cells and enlargement of the fluid-filled antrum. The recruited follicles not destined to ovulate undergo degeneration, similar to the atresia that occurs in other follicles during embryogenesis. Just prior to ovulation, meiosis resumes in the ovum of the dominant follicle, and the first meiotic division results in formation of the first polar body. The antrum rapidly enlarges (up to 10 to 25 mm in size), follicular fluid increases in amount, and the follicular surface thins and forms a conical stigma. Ovulation from the dom-

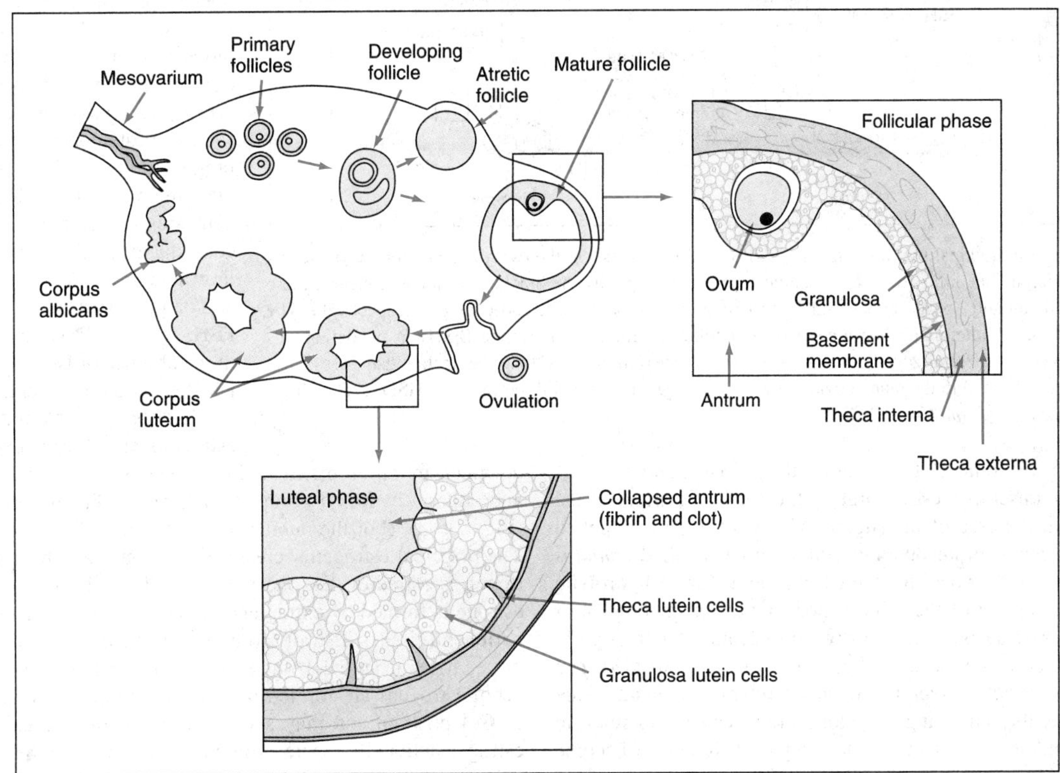

FIGURE 336-2 Developmental changes in the adult ovary during a complete 28-day cycle.

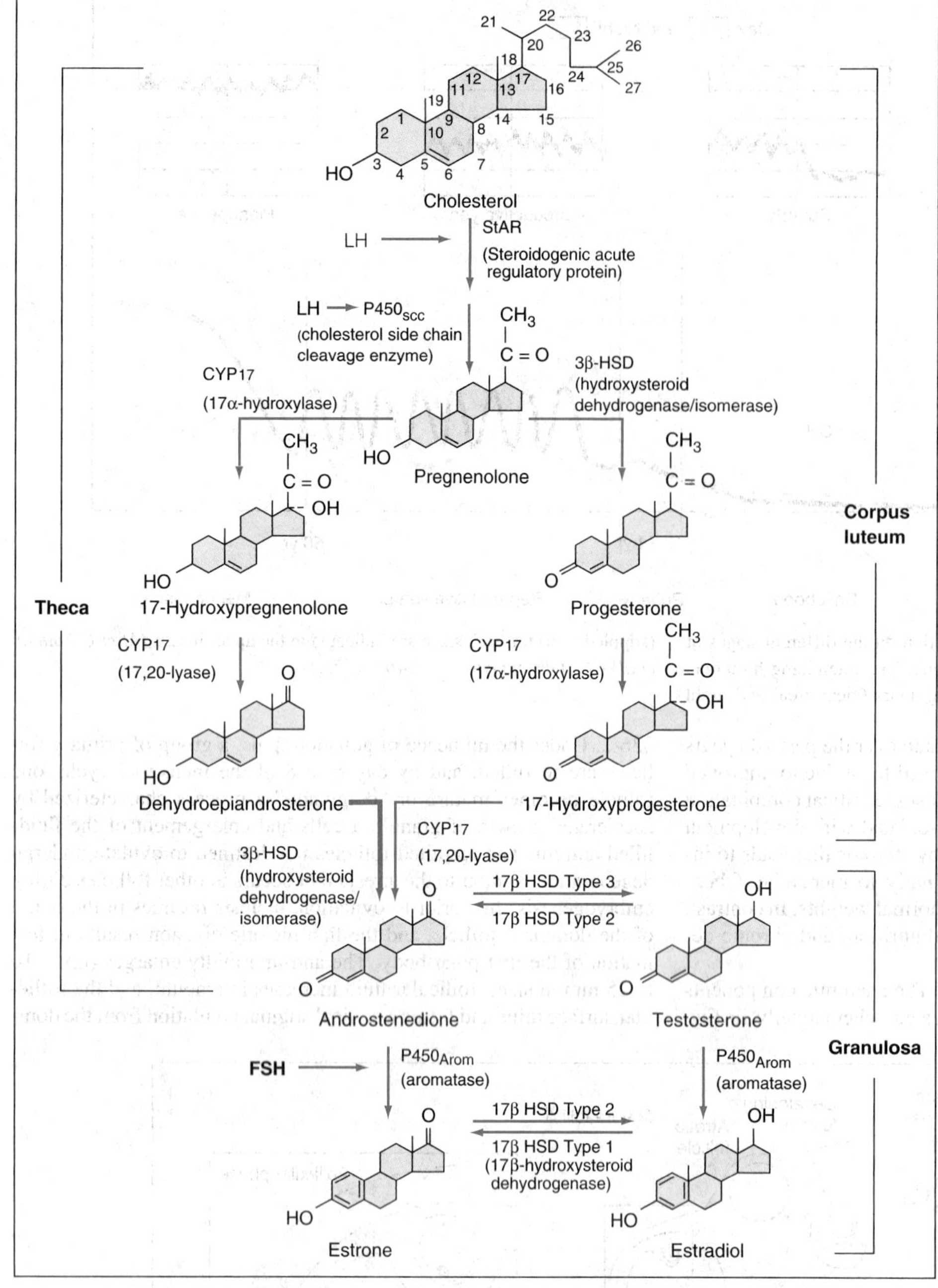

FIGURE 336-3 The principal pathway of steroid hormone biosynthesis in the ovary. The major enzyme complements for the corpus luteum, stroma, and granulosa cells are shown by the brackets; as a consequence, these cells produce predominantly progesterone and 17-OH progesterone, androgen, and estrogen, respectively. The major sites of action of luteinizing hormone (LH) and follicle-stimulating hormone (FSH) in mediating this pathway are shown in the horizontal arrows. The dotted line emphasizes that the metabolism of 17-hydroxyprogesterone is limited in the human ovary. StAR, steroidogenic regulatory protein. 17βHSD, 17β-hydroxysteroid dehydrogenase. *(From Carr, 1998.)*

inant follicle occurs some 16 to 23 h after the LH peak and some 24 to 38 h after the onset of the LH surge as the result of rupture of the follicular wall at the area of the stigma. The ovum is then expelled together with a mass of surrounding granulosa cells called *cumulus cells*. The rupture is believed to result from the action of hydrolytic enzymes on the surface of the follicle, possibly under the control of prostaglandins. The second meiotic division occurs after the egg is fertilized by a sperm, and the second polar body is then extruded. The formation of the *corpus luteum* begins in the retained remnant of the ovulated follicle; the remaining granulosa and theca cells increase in size and accumulate lipids and a yellow pigment, lutein, to become "luteinized." After a period of 14 ± 2 days (the functional life of the corpus luteum), the corpus luteum begins to atrophy, to be replaced in time by a fibrous scar, the *corpus albicans*. The factors that limit the life span of the human corpus luteum are not known, but if pregnancy occurs, the corpus luteum persists under the influence of placental or chorionic gonadotropins, and progesterone is produced by the corpus luteum for the support of pregnancy.

Hormone Formation • ***Steroid hormones*** Like other steroid hormones, ovarian steroids are derived from cholesterol (Fig. 336-3). The ovary can synthesize cholesterol de novo and can also utilize cholesterol obtained from circulating lipoproteins as substrate for steroid hormone formation (Fig. 336-4). Virtually all ovarian cells are believed to possess the complete complement of enzymes required for the synthesis of estradiol from cholesterol (Fig. 336-3); however, different cell types in the ovary contain different amounts of these enzymes so that the main steroids produced differ in different compartments. For example, the corpus luteum forms mainly progesterone and 17-hydroxyprogesterone, whereas theca and stromal cells convert cholesterol to androstenedione and testosterone. Granulosa cells are particularly rich in the aromatase enzyme responsible for estrogen synthesis and utilize as substrates for this process androgens synthesized in the granulosa cells and the adjacent theca cells.

The principal sites of action of LH and FSH are also illustrated in Figs. 336-3 and 336-4. LH acts primarily to regulate the early steps in steroid hormone biosynthesis, namely, the transport of cholesterol into the mitochondria by steroidogenic acute regulatory (StAR) protein and its conversion to pregnenolone. FSH acts mainly to regulate the final process by which androgens are aromatized to estrogens. As a consequence, LH enhances substrate flow and the formation of androgens and/or progesterone in the absence of FSH, whereas FSH action is impeded in the absence of LH because of diminished substrate for aromatization.

ESTROGENS Naturally occurring estrogens are 18-carbon steroids characterized by an aromatic A ring, a phenolic hydroxyl group at C-3, and either a hydroxyl group (estradiol) or a ketone (estrone) at C-17 (Fig. 336-3). (For the numbering of the steroid ring, see Fig. 335-1.) The principal estrogen secreted by the ovary and the most potent estrogen is estradiol. Estrone is also produced by the ovary, but most estrone is formed by extraglandular conversion of androstenedione in peripheral tissues. Estriol (16-hydroxyestradiol), the main estrogen in urine, arises from the 16-hydroxylation of estrone and estradiol. Catechol estrogens are formed by hydroxylation of estrogens at the C-2 or C-4 position and may act as the intracellular mediators of some estrogen action. Estrogens promote development of the secondary sexual characteristics in women and cause uterine growth, thickening of the vaginal mucosa, thinning of the cervical mucus, and development

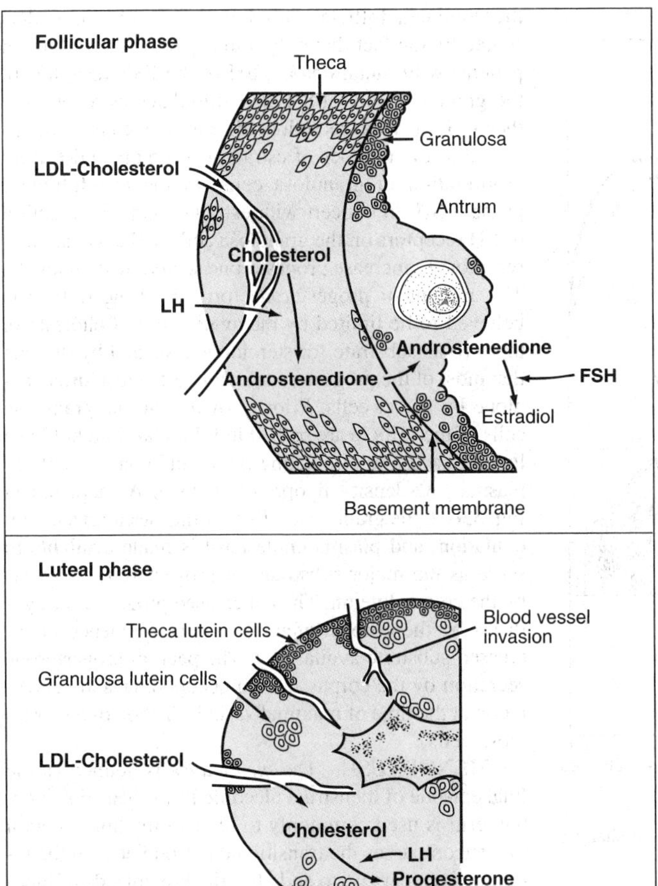

FIGURE 336-4 Cellular interactions in the ovary during the follicular phase (*top*) and luteal phase (*bottom*). LDL, low-density lipoprotein; FSH, follicle-stimulating hormone; LH, luteinizing hormone. *(From BR Carr et al: Fertil Steril 38:303, 1982.)*

of the ductule system of the breasts. Estrogens also alter lipid profiles and exert vascular effects that help prevent cardiovascular disease. The mechanism of estrogen action in target tissues is similar to that for other steroid hormones and involves binding to a nuclear steroid receptor—either estrogen receptor (ER)α or ERβ—and enhancement of the transcription of messenger RNA, which in turn causes increased protein synthesis in the cell cytoplasm (Chap. 327). These receptors have specific tissue site expression and bind various estrogens with different affinities, thereby conferring selective actions.

PROGESTERONE Progesterone, a 21-carbon steroid (Fig. 336-3), is the principal hormone secreted by the corpus luteum and is responsible for progestational effects, i.e., induction of secretory activity in the endometrium of the estrogen-primed uterus in preparation for implantation of the fertilized egg. Progesterone also induces a decidual reaction in endometrium. Other effects include inhibition of uterine contractions, an increase in the viscosity of cervical mucus, glandular development of the breasts, and an increase in basal body temperature (thermogenic effect).

ANDROGENS The ovary synthesizes a variety of 19-carbon steroids, including dehydroepiandrosterone, androstenedione, testosterone, and dihydrotestosterone, principally in stromal and thecal cells. The major ovarian 19-carbon steroid is androstenedione (Fig. 336-3), part of which is secreted into the plasma and part of which is converted to estrogen in granulosa cells or to testosterone in the interstitium. Androstenedione can also be converted to testosterone and estrogens in peripheral tissues. Only testosterone and dihydrotestosterone are true androgens that interact with the androgen receptor and induce virilizing signs in women (Chaps. 53 and 335).

Other hormones *Inhibin* is secreted in two forms (A and B) by the follicle and inhibits the release of FSH by the hypothalamic-pituitary unit. *Activin* is also secreted by the follicle and may enhance FSH secretion as well as having local effects on ovarian steroidogenesis. *Follistatin* is an activin-binding protein that attenuates the actions of activin and other members of the transforming growth factor (TGF)β family.

Some ovarian hormones play an uncertain role in human physiology. *Relaxin*, a polypeptide hormone produced by the human corpus luteum and by the decidua, causes softening of the cervix and loosening of the symphysis pubis in preparation for parturition in animals. *Oxytocin*, *vasopressin*, and other hypothalamic and pituitary hormones are also present in granulosa and/or luteal cells, but their function in these cells is unknown. *Follicle regulatory protein* (FRP), found in human follicular fluid, inhibits granulosa secretion and growth. *Gonadocrinins*, peptides purified from rat follicular fluid, stimulate the release of both FSH and LH from the pituitary in vitro and in vivo. Granulosa cells secrete *oocyte maturation inhibitor* (OMI), a factor that prevents premature ovulation. In addition, in the gonads of both sexes a *meiosis-inducing substance* (MIS) triggers the onset of meiosis, an event that occurs earlier in ovarian than in testicular development. Local growth factors [including insulin-like growth factors (IGFs) 1 and 2 and TGFα and -β] may also influence steroid secretion by the ovary.

The Normal Menstrual Cycle The menstrual cycle is divided into a follicular or proliferative phase and a luteal or secretory phase (Fig. 336-5). The secretion of FSH and LH is fundamentally under negative feedback control by ovarian steroids (particularly estradiol) and by inhibin (which selectively suppresses FSH), but the response of gonadotropins to different levels of estradiol varies. FSH secretion is inhibited progressively as estrogen levels increase—typical negative feedback. In contrast, LH secretion is suppressed maximally by sustained low levels of estrogen and is enhanced by a rising level of estradiol—positive feedback. Feedback of estrogen involves both the hypothalamus and pituitary. Negative feedback suppresses GnRH and inhibits gonadotropin production. Positive feedback is associated with an increased frequency of GnRH secretion and enhanced pituitary sensitivity to GnRH.

The length of the menstrual cycle is defined as the time from the onset of one menstrual bleeding episode to onset of the next. In women of reproductive age, the cycle averages 28 $\pm$ 3 days and the mean duration of flow is 4 $\pm$ 2 days. Longer menstrual cycles (usually characterized by anovulation) occur at menarche and near the onset of menopause. At the end of a cycle plasma levels of estrogen and progesterone fall, and circulating levels of FSH increase. Under the influence of FSH, follicular recruitment results in development of the follicle that will be dominant during the next cycle.

After the onset of menses, follicular development continues, but FSH levels decrease. Approximately 8 to 10 days prior to the midcycle LH surge, plasma estradiol levels begin to rise as the result of estradiol formation by the granulosa cells of the dominant follicle. During the second half of the follicular phase, LH levels also begin to rise (owing to positive feedback). Just before ovulation, estradiol secretion reaches a peak and then falls. Immediately thereafter, a further rise in the plasma level of LH mediates the final maturation of the follicle, followed by follicular rupture and ovulation 16 to 23 h after the LH peak. The rise in LH is accompanied by a smaller increase in the level of plasma FSH, the physiologic significance of which is unclear. The plasma progesterone level also begins to rise just prior to midcycle and facilitates the positive feedback action of estradiol on LH secretion.

At the onset of the luteal phase, plasma gonadotropins decrease and plasma progesterone increases. A secondary rise in estrogens causes further gonadotropin suppression. Near the end of the luteal phase, progesterone and estrogen levels fall, and FSH levels begin to rise to initiate the development of the next follicle (usually in the

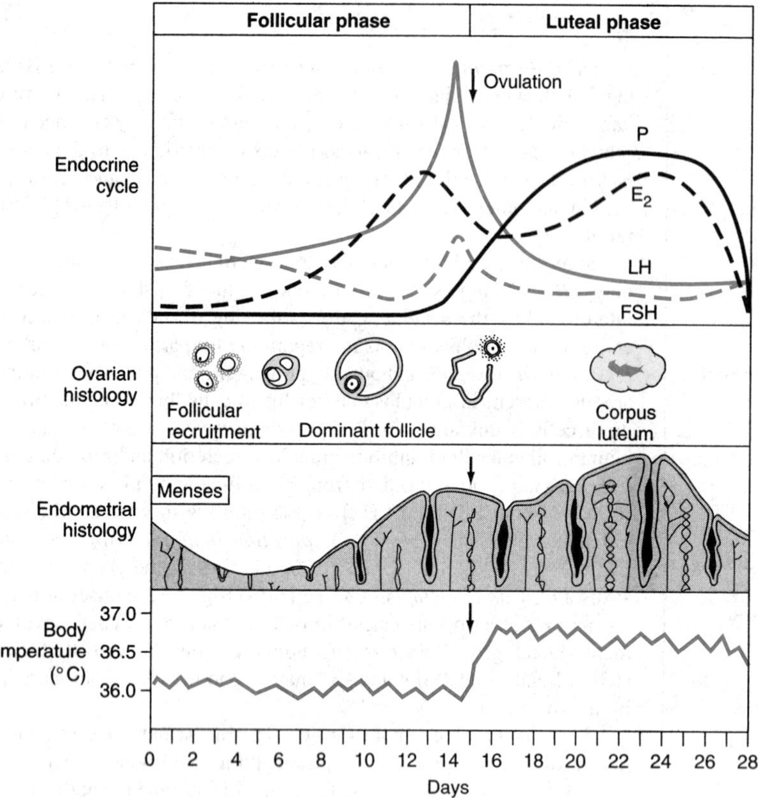

FIGURE 336-5 The hormonal, ovarian, endometrial, and basal body temperature changes and relationships throughout the normal menstrual cycle.

contralateral ovary) and the next menstrual cycle. Inhibin A levels are low in the follicular phase but reach a peak in the luteal phase. Inhibin B levels, in contrast, are increased in the follicular phase and low in the luteal phase.

The endometrium lining the uterine cavity undergoes marked alterations in response to the changing plasma levels of ovarian hormones (Fig. 336-5). Concurrent with the decrease in plasma estrogen and progesterone and the decline of corpus luteum function in the late luteal phase, intense vasospasm occurs in the spiral arterioles supplying blood to the endometrium, causing ischemic necrosis, endometrial desquamation, and bleeding. This vasospasm is caused by locally synthesized prostaglandins. The onset of bleeding marks the first day of the menstrual cycle. By the fourth to fifth day of the cycle, the endometrium is thin. During the proliferative phase, glandular growth of the endometrium is mediated by estrogen. After ovulation, increased progesterone levels lead to further thickening of the endometrium, but the rapid growth slows. The endometrium then enters the secretory phase, characterized by tortuosity of the glands, curling of the spiral arterioles, and glandular secretion. As corpus luteum function begins to wane in the absence of conception, the sequence of events leading to menstruation is again set into action.

Biphasic changes in basal body temperature are characteristic of the ovulatory cycle and are mediated by alterations in progesterone levels (Fig. 336-5). An increase in basal body temperature by 0.3 to 0.5°C begins after ovulation, persists during the luteal phase, and returns to the normal baseline (36.2 to 36.4°C) after the onset of the subsequent menses.

Cellular Interactions in the Ovary during the Normal Cycle LH stimulates thecal cells surrounding the follicle to form androgens, and androstenedione diffuses across the basement membrane of the follicle into granulosa cells, where it is aromatized to estrogen (Figs. 336-3 and 336-4).

The increase of FSH late in the preceding menstrual cycle stimulates growth and recruitment of the primary follicles by enhancing granulosa cell proliferation, resulting ultimately in the formation of the dominant follicle. This function of FSH is underscored by the fact that only primary follicles are seen in patients with mutations in FSH or the FSH receptor. In the granulosa cells, FSH also stimulates estrogen synthesis. Enhanced secretion of estradiol causes an increase in the number of estradiol receptors and further proliferation of granulosa cells. In the late follicular phase, FSH, in concert with estradiol, causes induction of LH receptors on the granulosa cells. LH acts via these receptors to increase progesterone secretion at midcycle. The amount of progesterone formed by the follicle is believed to be limited by the availability of cholesterol to serve as substrate for steroidogenesis and by the fact that most of the progesterone is converted to androstenedione by thecal cells. Prior to ovulation, the granulosa cells of the follicle are bathed in follicular fluid but have limited access to circulating blood and consequently to plasma low-density lipoprotein (LDL). As depicted in Fig. 336-4, the granulosa cells become vascularized after ovulation, and plasma cholesterol is made available to serve as the major substrate for progesterone synthesis by the corpus luteum. Thus, increased progesterone synthesis by the corpus luteum is the consequence of increased substrate availability. The peak in progesterone secretion by the corpus luteum occurs 8 days after ovulation at the time of maximal vascularization of the granulosa cells.

MENOPAUSE The *menopause* is defined as the final episode of menstrual bleeding in women. However, the term is used commonly to refer to the time interval that encompasses the transitional period between the reproductive years up to and after the last episode of menstrual bleeding. During this period, there is a progressive loss of ovarian function and a variety of endocrine, somatic, and psychological changes.

The median age of women at the time of cessation of menstrual bleeding is 50 to 51 years. Since the life expectancy of women is close to 80 years, approximately one-third of life occurs after cessation of reproductive function. Preceding the menopause, the pattern of menstrual cycles is variable, but the interval between menses usually becomes shorter, as follicular recruitment is hastened by increases in FSH. Day 3 FSH and E_2 levels are often elevated. Ovulatory cycles continue for some period of time, then anovulation becomes common.

The menopause is the consequence of the exhaustion of ovarian follicles. The decrease in the number of ova begins in intrauterine life; by the time of the menopause, few ova remain, and these appear to be nonfunctional. Only a small number of ova are lost as the result of ovulation during reproductive life; the majority are lost by atresia. The cessation of follicular development results in decreased production of estradiol, inhibin, and other hormones, which causes a loss of negative feedback on the hypothalamic-pituitary centers. In turn, the levels of plasma gonadotropins increase, with FSH levels rising earlier and higher than LH levels (Figs. 336-1 and 336-6). The higher concentration of FSH than LH in postmenopausal women may result from the decrease in inhibin secretion by the ovary, from the fact that FSH is cleared from plasma less rapidly than LH, and possibly from the loss of positive feedback on LH production by estradiol.

The ovaries of postmenopausal women are small and wrinkled, and the residual cells are predominantly stromal. Estrogen and androgen levels in plasma are reduced but not absent (Fig. 336-6). Before the menopause, plasma androstenedione is derived almost equally from the adrenals and the ovaries; after menopause the ovarian contribution ceases so that the plasma levels of androstenedione fall by 50% (Fig. 336-6). However, the menopausal ovary continues to secrete testosterone, presumably formed in stromal cells.

Circulating estrogens in the ovulating woman are derived from two sources. Some 60% of mean estrogen formation during the menstrual cycle is in the form of estradiol, formed primarily by ovaries, and the

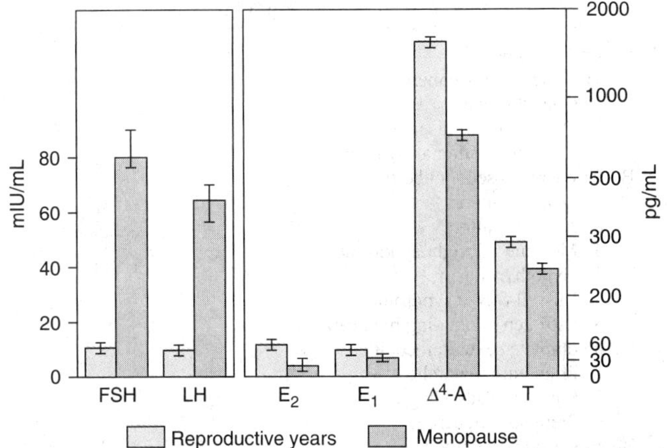

FIGURE 336-6 Differences in hormone concentration in women during the reproductive years and in women during the menopause. FSH, follicle-stimulating hormone; LH, luteinizing hormone; E_2, estradiol-17β; E_1, estrone; Δ^4-A, androstenedione; T, testosterone. *From SSC Yen et al (eds), Reproductive Endocrinology. Philadelphia, Saunders, 1999; and from DR Mishell Jr, V Dajavan (eds), Reproductive Endocrinology, Infertility, and Contraception, 2d ed, Philadelphia, Davis, 1986.*

remainder is estrone, formed mainly in extraglandular tissues from androstenedione. After menopause, extraglandular estrogen formation is the major pathway for estrogen synthesis. Because adipose tissue is a major site of extraglandular estrogen production, peripheral estrogen formation may actually be enhanced in obese postmenopausal women, so that total estrogen production rates may be as great or greater than in premenopausal women. The predominant estrogen formed is estrone rather than estradiol.

The most common menopausal symptoms are vasomotor instability (hot flashes), atrophy of the urogenital epithelium and skin, decreased size of the breasts, and osteoporosis. Approximately 40% of menopausal women develop symptoms serious enough to seek medical assistance.

The pathogenesis of the hot flash is uncertain. There is a close temporal relationship between the onset of the hot flash and pulses of LH secretion, which reflect hypothalamic secretion of GnRH. Alterations in catecholamine, prostaglandin, endorphin, or neurotensin metabolism may play a role in conjunction with low estrogen production. Symptoms associated with the hot flash, including nervousness, anxiety, irritability, and depression, may or may not be caused entirely by estrogen deficiency.

The decrease in size of the tissues of the female reproductive tract and breasts in the menopause is due to estrogen deficiency. The vaginal mucosa and the endometrium usually become thin and atrophic (although endometrial hyperplasia occurs in one-fifth of postmenopausal women).

Osteoporosis is one of the dread afflictions of aging, and there is a close relationship between estrogen deprivation and its development. Approximately one-fourth of aging women and one-tenth of elderly men sustain a vertebral or hip fracture between the ages of 60 and 90, and the incidence is highest in elderly white women. Such fractures are a major cause of loss of independence, death and morbidity, and the fracture-related mortality increases from <10% in the 60- to 64-year age group to >30% in patients over 80 (Chap. 342). Many factors affect the development of osteoporosis, including ethnic origin, diet, activity, smoking, and general health, and estrogen deprivation is of particular importance. White and Asian postmenopausal women are more predisposed to osteoporosis and its consequences because bone mass in this group is lower prior to menopause, so loss in bone density has more severe consequences. Further evidence that osteoporosis is a disease of estrogen deprivation is suggested by the early development of osteoporosis in women with premature menopause due to either natural causes or surgical castration. After the menopause women ex-

perience an increase in the incidence of cardiovascular disease as the result of a decrease in the level of high-density lipoprotein (HDL) cholesterol as well as the effects of hypoestrogenism on vascular endothelium and reactivity.

LABORATORY AND CLINICAL ASSESSMENT OF HORMONAL STATUS

The hormonal status of women can usually be assessed by history and physical examination. In general, the presence of secondary sexual characteristics such as normal female breast development indicates adequate estrogen secretion in the past, and the presence of regular, predictable, cyclic menses implies that ovulation and the production of gonadotropins, estrogen, progesterone, and androgens are adequate and that the outflow tract is intact. Such a history may be more valuable than laboratory tests in evaluating ovarian hormone status. However, laboratory tests provide valuable ancillary information in the evaluation of women with endocrine dysfunction or infertility (Chap. 54).

PITUITARY GONADOTROPINS Plasma gonadotropins are assessed by radioimmunoassay (RIA), fluoroimmunoassay (FIA), or immunoradiometric assay (IRMA). Because both FSH and LH are secreted in a pulsatile manner, the results obtained from a single serum sample may be difficult to interpret. Consequently, multiple samples taken at 20-min intervals over 2 h may be pooled to obtain a mean value. Serum gonadotropin measurements are of the most use in evaluating women with suspected ovarian failure and in supporting the diagnosis of polycystic ovarian syndrome (PCOS) and hypogonadotropic hypogonadism. The normal ranges for serum LH and FSH in ovulating women are 0.8 to 57 and 1.4 to 21 IU/L, respectively. FSH levels that are persistently >40 IU/L are diagnostic of ovarian failure, and an LH value <0.8 IU/L suggests hypogonadotropic hypogonadism. In practice, however, gonadotropin values may be equivocal and must be interpreted in light of the remainder of the findings.

OVARIAN HORMONES The mean plasma levels and production rates of the principal ovarian hormones are presented in Table 336-1.

Estrogen The presence of normal secondary sexual characteristics implies that estrogen production was adequate in the past. The current estrogen status can be estimated by pelvic examination. The presence of a moist, rugated vagina with copious, clear, thin cervical mucus that can be stretched and that exhibits arborization or ferning when spread on a slide is strong evidence of adequate estrogen production. Cytologic demonstration of mature vaginal epithelial cells and abundant cornified squamous epithelial cells with pyknotic nuclei confirms the presence of adequate estrogen levels.

The progesterone-withdrawal test provides a functional assessment

Table 336-1 Concentrations of the Major Ovarian Steroid Hormones in Blood of Ovulatory Women

Steroid	Binding[a]	Phase of Menstrual Cycle	Plasma Concentration, nmol/L (ng/mL)
Estradiol	SHBG and albumin	Follicular	0.07–2.6 (0.02–0.7)
		Luteal	0.7 (0.2)
Estrone	Albumin	Follicular	0.2–1.1 (0.05–0.3)
		Luteal	0.4 (0.1)
Progesterone	CBG and albumin	Follicular	3 (1)
		Luteal	16–80 (5–25)
Androstenedione	Albumin	—	5.6 (1.6)
Testosterone	SHBG and albumin	—	1.4 (0.4)

[a] SHBG, sex hormone binding globulin; CBG, cortisol-binding globulin.
SOURCE: Modified from MB Lipsett, in *Reproductive Endocrinology*, SSC Yen et al (eds). Philadelphia, Saunders, 1999.

of the endometrium, outflow tract, and estrogen status. If menses appear within a week to 10 days after the end of a trial of medroxyprogesterone acetate (10 mg by mouth once or twice a day for 5 days) or after a single intramuscular injection of progesterone (100 mg), then prior estrogen priming was adequate to allow withdrawal bleeding.

Owing to its variable level in plasma during the normal cycle and the difficulty of estimating the day of the cycle in women with abnormal cycles, the measurement of estrogen levels in plasma or urine is of little use in the routine assessment of estrogen status. Measurement of plasma estradiol is useful during attempts to induce ovulation with gonadotropins to prevent the development of the ovarian hyperstimulation syndrome and is used along with ultrasound assessment to monitor follicular growth in women who are to undergo in vitro fertilization.

Progesterone Cyclic, predictable menses also imply that adequate progesterone is secreted during the luteal phase of the menstrual cycle. Assessment of progesterone is useful to detect ovulation and to evaluate the adequacy of the luteal phase in infertile women. Several functional assays of progesterone can be used. The least expensive and most useful is the daily measurement of basal body temperature throughout a cycle. Owing to the thermogenic properties of progesterone, a normal biphasic monthly curve showing a temperature elevation lasting for approximately 2 weeks after ovulation is a valid indication of progesterone secretion during the luteal phase (Fig. 336-5). The presence of viscous cervical mucus that does not stretch or fern and of predominantly intermediate cells on vaginal cytology or demonstration of a secretory epithelium in an endometrial biopsy during the luteal phase on days 20 to 22 of the cycle provides additional assessment of progesterone secretion. In addition, serum progesterone can be measured to assess the function of the corpus luteum.

Androgen Under normal conditions, the ovary secretes androstenedione, testosterone, and dehydroepiandrosterone. In conditions of androgen excess, hirsutism and/or virilization are common. The evaluation of androgen excess is discussed in Chap. 53.

DIAGNOSIS OF PREGNANCY Pregnancy is usually recognized on the basis of the history and physical examination. That is, a woman with previously cyclic, predictable menses develops amenorrhea accompanied by breast tenderness, malaise, lassitude, and nausea, and on physical examination the uterus is soft and enlarged.

Assays of placental products facilitate the diagnosis of pregnancy. Human chorionic gonadotropin (hCG) is secreted by the trophoblastic cells of the placenta into the maternal plasma and excreted in the urine. Assays of the hCG content of serum or urine use antibodies against hCG and make it possible to detect pregnancies 8 to 10 days after ovulation, before the first missed menstrual period and long before pregnancy can be diagnosed by clinical assessments. Assay of the β subunit of hCG in serum or urine makes it possible to differentiate between excess LH and hCG, an important distinction in evaluating women with trophoblastic disease such as hydatidiform mole or choriocarcinoma. Sensitive and specific hCG-based pregnancy tests are now available for testing by patients at home.

DISORDERS OF OVARIAN FUNCTION

PREPUBERTAL YEARS Puberty is said to be *precocious* if breast budding begins before age 8 or if menarche occurs before age 9. Those disorders in which the developing sexual characteristics are appropriate for the genetic and gonadal sex—i.e., feminization in girls or virilization in boys—are termed *isosexual precocity*, whereas *heterosexual precocity* occurs when sexual characteristics are not in accord with the genetic sex, namely, virilization in girls or feminization in boys. Pubertal disorders of boys are described in Chap. 335.

Isosexual Precocious Puberty Isosexual precocious puberty in girls can be divided into three major categories (Table 336-2).

True precocious puberty True precocious puberty is characterized by an early but otherwise normal sequence of pubertal development, including increased secretion of gonadotropins and ovulatory menstrual cycles. Constitutional or idiopathic precocious puberty accounts for 90% of cases. In these individuals, no cause for the premature maturation of the central nervous system–hypothalamic-pituitary axis can be identified, and the diagnosis is confirmed by finding an adult pattern of LH and FSH release on a GnRH stimulation test. As many as half these individuals have abnormal findings on electroencephalograms. Premature appearance of secondary sexual characteristics and of ovulatory cycles with the accompanying risk of fertility may cause significant emotional disturbance. Therefore, prompt initiation of therapy is imperative. GnRH analogues suppress gonadotropins and inhibit estrogen synthesis, thereby blocking precocious puberty; they may also prevent premature closure of the epiphyses and the resulting short stature.

Table 336-2 Differential Diagnosis of Sexual Precocity

I. Isosexual precocity
   A. True precocious puberty
      1. Constitutional
      2. Organic brain disease
      3. Congenital adrenal hyperplasia
   B. Precocious pseudopuberty
      1. Ovarian tumors
      2. Adrenal tumors
      3. McCune-Albright syndrome
      4. Hypothyroidism
      5. Russell-Silver syndrome
      6. Estrogen-containing medications
   C. Incomplete sexual precocity
      1. Premature thelarche
      2. Premature adrenarche
      3. Premature pubarche
II. Heterosexual precocity
   A. Ovarian tumors
   B. Adrenal tumors
   C. Congenital adrenal hyperplasia

About 10% of cases are due to organic brain diseases, including brain tumors (hypothalamic gliomas, astrocytomas, ependymomas, germinomas, and hamartomas), encephalitis, meningitis, hydrocephalus, head injury, tuberous sclerosis, and neurofibromatosis. It is essential to distinguish this group of patients from those with the idiopathic disorder, and patients whose disorder is designated as idiopathic occasionally prove to have such tumors. Fortunately, most patients with organic lesions serious enough to cause precocious puberty have obvious neurologic signs and symptoms. Evaluation of all patients with precocious puberty should include, at a minimum, skull films and computed tomography (CT) or magnetic resonance imaging (MRI) of the brain. The success of treatment depends on the nature of the lesion, but surgical and radiation treatment of well-localized tumors is occasionally successful.

A rare cause of isosexual precocity is congenital adrenal hyperplasia due to 21-hydroxylase deficiency in girls in whom treatment is delayed until 4 to 8 years of age. After initiation of glucocorticoid replacement, such individuals may undergo isosexual precocious puberty (Chap. 331).

Precocious pseudopuberty Precocious pseudopuberty occurs when girls undergo feminization as a consequence of enhanced estrogen formation but do not ovulate or develop cyclic menses. Ovarian cysts or tumors that secrete estrogen (granulosa-theca cell tumors) are the most frequent cause of precocious pseudopuberty. Granulosa-theca cell tumors associated with intestinal polyps and pigmentation of the mucous membranes occur in the Peutz-Jeghers syndrome. Other ovarian tumors that secrete estrogens (or androgens that can be converted to estrogens at extraglandular sites) include dysgerminomas, teratomas, cystadenomas, and ovarian carcinomas (Chap. 97). Ovarian tumors can usually be detected by rectoabdominal examination or by sonography, CT, MRI, and/or laparoscopy. Ovarian teratomas and choriocarcinomas and other carcinomas that secrete hCG do not cause precocious puberty in girls unless they also secrete estrogen (hCG or

LH in the absence of FSH does not induce ovarian estrogen production). Rarely, feminizing tumors of the adrenal cause isosexual precocious puberty by direct formation of estrogens or by secretion of weak androgens, which are converted to estrogens in extraglandular tissues.

Other causes of precocious pseudopuberty include the following:

1. The McCune-Albright syndrome (polyostotic fibrous dysplasia) is due to an activating mutation in the G-protein, Gsα, that occurs during embryogenesis, leading to a mosaic pattern of expression in various tissues. It is characterized by café au lait spots, cystic fibrous dysplasia of bones, and sexual precocity. In the ovary, the Gsα mutation mimics the action of FSH, leading to autonomous follicle development and estrogen formation. Occasionally, this disorder leads to true precocious puberty (Chap. 343).
2. Primary hypothyroidism is occasionally associated with enhanced secretion of FSH, inducing ovarian estrogen secretion. High levels of thyroid-stimulating hormone (TSH) caused by hypothyroidism may also stimulate the FSH receptor.
3. The Russell-Silver syndrome, or congenital asymmetry, is associated with short stature and precocious feminization.
4. Estrogen-containing medications, including use of estrogen-containing creams for diaper rash or the ingestion of meat from estrogen-treated animals or poultry or of any estrogen by mouth, can cause this disorder.

Incomplete isosexual precocity This term is used to describe the premature development of a single pubertal event and encompasses several entities. Breast budding prior to age 7 (*premature thelarche*) without other evidence of estrogen secretion and without premature bone maturation is believed to be due to a transient increase in estrogen secretion or to a temporary increase in sensitivity to the small amounts of circulating estrogens formed prior to puberty. Usually, the disorder is self-limited and resolves spontaneously. Occasionally, axillary hair and/or pubic hair (*premature adrenarche* and *premature pubarche*) appear without any other secondary sexual development. The phenomenon is associated with adrenal androgen secretion in the range of normal puberty and can be distinguished from syndromes of virilization by the absence of clitoromegaly. It requires no treatment, and patients enter puberty at about the average time.

Heterosexual Precocity Virilization in a prepubertal female is usually due to congenital adrenal hyperplasia or to androgen secretion by an ovarian or adrenal tumor. The manifestations of virilization are described in Chaps. 53 and 331. Virilization in girls with congenital adrenal hyperplasia usually takes place in a background of variable sexual ambiguity (see Chap. 338).

Evaluation of Sexual Precocity The evaluation of sexual precocity involves a careful history and physical examination, including rectoabdominal examination, abdominal sonography, determination of bone age, and GnRH stimulation test, and measurement of thyroid hormones, TSH, and gonadotropins (and androgen or estrogen levels when appropriate). MRI and/or CT scans should be obtained if a neurologic disorder is suspected and no evidence of ovarian or adrenal tumor is found.

REPRODUCTIVE YEARS Disorders of the Menstrual Cycle • *Abnormal uterine bleeding* Between menarche and the menopause, almost every woman experiences one or more episodes of abnormal uterine bleeding, here defined as any bleeding pattern that differs in frequency, duration, or amount from the pattern observed during a normal menstrual cycle. A variety of descriptive terms (such as *menorrhagia*, *metrorrhagia*, and *menometrorrhagia*) have been used to characterize patterns of abnormal uterine bleeding. A more logical approach is to divide abnormal uterine bleeding into those patterns associated with ovulatory cycles and those associated with anovulatory cycles.

Ovulatory cycles Normal menstrual bleeding with ovulatory cycles is spontaneous, regular, cyclic, and predictable and is frequently associated with discomfort (*dysmenorrhea*). Deviations from this pattern associated with cycles that are still regular and predictable are most often due to organic disease of the outflow tract. For example, regular but prolonged and excessive bleeding episodes unassociated with bleeding dyscrasias (hypermenorrhea or menorrhagia) can result from abnormalities of the uterus such as submucous leiomyomas, adenomyosis, or endometrial polyps. Regular, cyclic, predictable menstruation characterized by spotting or light bleeding is termed *hypomenorrhea* and is due to obstruction of the outflow tract as from intrauterine synechiae or scarring of the cervix. Intermenstrual bleeding between episodes of regular, ovulatory menstruation is also often due to cervical or endometrial lesions. An exception to the association between organic disease and abnormal uterine bleeding is the occurrence of regular menstruation more frequently than 21 days apart (*polymenorrhea*). Such cycles may be a normal variant.

Anovulatory cycles Uterine bleeding that is unpredictable with respect to amount, onset, and duration and usually painless is described as *dysfunctional uterine bleeding*. This disorder is not due to abnormalities of the uterus but rather to chronic anovulation and occurs when there is interruption of the normal sequence of follicular and luteal phases under the influence of a dominant follicle and its resulting corpus luteum. As discussed above, uterine bleeding in ovulatory cycles is due to progesterone withdrawal and requires that the endometrium first be primed with estrogen. (When castrates or postmenopausal women are given progesterone, withdrawal bleeding usually does not occur.)

Dysfunctional uterine bleeding can occur in women who have a transient disruption of the synchronous hypothalamic-pituitary-ovarian patterns necessary for ovulatory cycles, most often at the extremes of the reproductive life—in the early menarche and in the perimenopausal period—but also after temporary stress or intercurrent illness.

Primary dysfunctional uterine bleeding can result from three disorders.

1. *Estrogen withdrawal bleeding* occurs when estrogen is given to a castrated or postmenopausal woman and then withdrawn. As in other types of dysfunctional uterine bleeding, this form of menstrual bleeding is usually painless.
2. *Estrogen breakthrough bleeding* occurs when there is continuous estrogen stimulation of the endometrium not interrupted by cyclic progesterone secretion and withdrawal. This is the most common type of dysfunctional uterine bleeding and is usually due to anovulation associated with chronic acyclic estrogen production, as in women with PCOS. Such women may have histories of irregular, unpredictable menses, oligomenorrhea, or amenorrhea (see below). Alternatively, estrogen breakthrough bleeding can occur in hypogonadal women given estrogens chronically rather than intermittently and in women with estrogen-secreting tumors of the ovary. Estrogen breakthrough bleeding may be profuse and is unpredictable with respect to duration, amount of flow, and time of occurrence. The endometrium is typically thin because its repair between episodes of bleeding is incomplete.
3. *Progesterone breakthrough bleeding* occurs in the presence of abnormally high ratios of progesterone to estrogen, e.g., in women using continuous low-dose oral contraceptives.

The approach to a patient with dysfunctional uterine bleeding begins with a careful history of menstrual patterns and prior hormonal therapy. Since not all urogenital tract bleeding is from the uterus, rectal, bladder, and vaginal or cervical sources must be excluded by physical examination. If the bleeding is from the uterus, a pregnancy-related disorder such as abortion or ectopic pregnancy must be ruled out.

℞ TREATMENT Once the diagnosis of dysfunctional uterine bleeding is established, a rational approach to management is as follows: During a first episode of dysfunctional bleeding the patient can simply be observed, provided the bleeding is not copious and no evidence of bleeding dyscrasia is present. If bleeding is moderately severe, control can be achieved with relatively high dose estrogen oral contraceptives for 3 weeks. Alternatively, a regimen of three or four low-dose oral contraceptive pills per day for 1 week followed by tapering to the usual dosage for up to 3 weeks is also effective. If uterine bleeding is more severe, hospitalization, bed rest, and intramuscular injections of estradiol valerate (10 mg) and hydroxyprogesterone caproate (500 mg) or intravenous or intramuscular conjugated estrogens (25 mg) usually control the bleeding. After initial treatment, iron replacement should be instituted, and recurrence can be prevented by cyclic oral contraceptives for 2 to 3 months (or more if pregnancy is not desired). Alternatively, menses can be induced every 2 to 3 months with medroxyprogesterone acetate, 10 mg by mouth once or twice a day for 10 days. If hormone therapy fails to control uterine bleeding, an endometrial biopsy, hysteroscopy, or dilatation and curettage may be required for diagnosis and therapy. Indeed, uterine sampling should be performed prior to hormone therapy in women at risk for endometrial cancer (i.e., in women who are approaching the age of menopause or are massively obese); endometrial cancer is rare in ovulatory women of reproductive age.

Amenorrhea An acceptable definition of amenorrhea is failure of menarche by age 15, irrespective of the presence or absence of secondary sexual characteristics, or the absence of menstruation for 6 months in a woman with previous periodic menses. However, women who do not fulfill these criteria should be evaluated if (1) the patient and/or her family are greatly concerned, (2) no breast development has occurred by age 13, or (3) any sexual ambiguity or virilization is present (Chap. 338). Amenorrhea is commonly categorized as either primary (the woman has never menstruated) or secondary (when menstruation has been present for a variable period of time in the past and has ceased). However, some disorders can cause either primary or secondary amenorrhea. For example, most women with gonadal dysgenesis have primary amenorrhea, but some have a few follicles and ovulate for short periods so that pregnancy occurs rarely. Furthermore, patients with chronic anovulation (PCOS) usually have secondary amenorrhea but on occasion have primary amenorrhea. For these reasons, categorization of amenorrhea into primary and secondary types is less helpful than a classification based on the underlying physiologic derangements: (1) anatomic defects, (2) ovarian failure, and (3) chronic anovulation with or without estrogen present.

ANATOMIC DEFECTS Anatomic or structural defects of the genital tract can preclude menstrual bleeding. Starting from the caudal end of the female genital tract, labial fusion is often associated with disorders of sexual development, particularly female pseudohermaphroditism (congenital adrenal hyperplasia or exposure to maternal androgens in utero; Chap. 338). Congenital defects of the vagina, imperforate hymen, and transverse vaginal septae can also cause amenorrhea. These women frequently have accumulation of menstrual blood behind the obstruction and may have cyclic, predictable episodes of abdominal pain.

More severe müllerian anomalies include müllerian agenesis (the Mayer-Rokitansky-Küster-Hauser syndrome; Chap. 338), second in frequency only to gonadal dysgenesis as a cause of primary amenorrhea. It can be caused by mutations in the genes encoding anti-müllerian hormone (AMH) or its receptor (AMHR). Women with this syndrome have a 46,XX karyotype, female secondary sex characteristics, and normal ovarian function, including cyclic ovulation, but have absence or hypoplasia of the vagina. The uterus usually consists of only rudimentary bicornuate cords, but if the uterus contains endometrium, cyclic abdominal pain and accumulation of blood may occur, as in other forms of outlet obstruction. One-third of women with this syndrome have abnormalities of the urogenital tract, and one-tenth have skeletal anomalies, usually involving the spine. The major diagnostic problem is distinguishing müllerian agenesis from complete testicular feminization, in which 46,XY genetic males with testes differentiate as phenotypic women but with a blind vaginal pouch and no uterus. Women with testicular feminization have feminized breasts but a paucity of pubic and axillary hair. The disorder is X-linked and is caused by mutations in the androgen receptor that result in profound resistance to the action of testosterone (Chap. 338). Testicular feminization can be diagnosed by demonstrating a male level of serum testosterone and a 46,XY karyotype, whereas demonstration of a 46,XX karyotype, the biphasic basal body temperature curve characteristic of ovulation, and elevated levels of progesterone during the luteal phase establish the diagnosis of müllerian agenesis.

A rare cause of absence of the uterus in 46,XY phenotypic women who are sexually infantile is the so-called testicular regression syndrome or testicular agenesis (Chap. 338).

Other abnormalities of the uterus that cause amenorrhea include obstruction due to scarring or stenosis of the cervix, often resulting from surgery, electrocautery, laser therapy, or cryosurgery. Such destruction of the endometrium (Asherman's syndrome) usually follows vigorous curettage for postpartum hemorrhage or after therapeutic abortion complicated by infection. This diagnosis is confirmed by hysterosalpingography or by direct visual examination of the endometrial scarring or synechiae using a hysteroscope.

Treatment of disorders of the outflow tract is surgical.

OVARIAN FAILURE Primary ovarian failure is associated with elevated plasma gonadotropin levels and can result from several causes. The most frequent cause is *gonadal dysgenesis*, in which the germ cells are absent and the ovary is replaced by a fibrous streak (Chaps. 65 and 338). Women with gonadal dysgenesis can be divided into two broad groups on the basis of chromosomal karyotype. The most common type is due to deletion of genetic material in the X chromosomes and accounts for about two-thirds of cases of gonadal dysgenesis. A 45,X karyotype is found in about half of women with this disorder, and most have somatic defects, including short stature, webbed neck, shield chest, and cardiovascular defects, collectively termed the *Turner phenotype*. The remainder of women with X chromosome abnormalities have chromosomal mosaicism with or without associated structural abnormalities of the X. The most common form of mosaicism is 45,X/46,XX. Gonadal tumors are rare in 45,X patients, but gonadal malignancies may occur in women with chromosomal mosaicism involving the Y chromosome. Therefore, chromosomal analysis should be performed in all cases of amenorrhea associated with ovarian failure, and the streak gonad should be removed if a Y chromosome is present. One means of identifying the presence of a Y chromosome is to amplify the sex-determining regions of the Y chromosome (SRY) by means of the polymerase chain reaction (Chap. 338). Approximately 90% of women with gonadal dysgenesis due to partial or complete deletion of the X never have menstrual bleeding, and the remaining 10% have sufficient follicles to experience menses and, rarely, fertility; the menstrual and reproductive lives of such individuals are invariably brief.

One-tenth of individuals identified as having bilateral streak gonads have a normal 46,XX or 46,XY karyotype and are said to have *pure gonadal dysgenesis*. These individuals have either normal or above-average stature, owing to failure of estrogen-mediated epiphyseal closure in the presence of a normal chromosomal constitution. Pure gonadal dysgenesis does not constitute a phenotypic or chromosomally homogeneous disorder (Chap. 338). Occasional women with a 46,XY karyotype develop signs of virilization, including clitoromegaly, and have an increased incidence of tumors in the gonadal streaks; as a consequence, gonadal streaks should be removed prophylactically, as discussed above, when a Y chromosome is present. Approximately two-thirds of women with 46,XX gonadal dysgenesis experience no menses, while the remainder have one or more menstrual episodes and are occasionally fertile.

Other causes of ovarian failure and amenorrhea include deficiency of the *CYP17* gene that encodes 17α-hydroxylase and 17,20-lyase activities, premature ovarian failure, the resistant-ovary syndrome, and ovarian failure secondary to chemotherapy or radiation therapy for malignancy. *17α-Hydroxylase deficiency* is characterized by primary amenorrhea, sexual infantilism, and hypertension, the latter due to increased production of desoxycorticosterone (DOC); whereas women with *17,20-lyase deficiency* have primary amenorrhea and sexual infantilism with normal blood pressure (Chaps. 331 and 338). The diagnosis of *premature ovarian failure* or *premature menopause* is applied to women who cease menstruating before age 40. The ovaries in such women are similar to the ovaries of postmenopausal women, containing few or no follicles as the result of accelerated follicular atresia. Premature ovarian failure due to ovarian antibodies may be one component of polyglandular failure, together with adrenal insufficiency, hypothyroidism, and other autoimmune disorders (Chap. 339). A rare form of ovarian failure is the *resistant-ovary syndrome*, in which the ovaries contain many follicles that are arrested in development prior to the antral stage, possibly because of resistance to the action of FSH in the ovary. A subset of these individuals have mutations in FSH or its receptor. To differentiate this disorder from the 46,XX variety of pure gonadal dysgenesis, which is also associated with sexual immaturity, it is necessary to perform ovarian biopsy. However, it is not clinically useful to make this distinction, since the conventional treatment of infertility in both conditions is usually unsuccessful. Women with ovarian failure who desire pregnancy have been treated with hormone replacement and transfer of donor embryos to the uterine cavity or fallopian tubes.

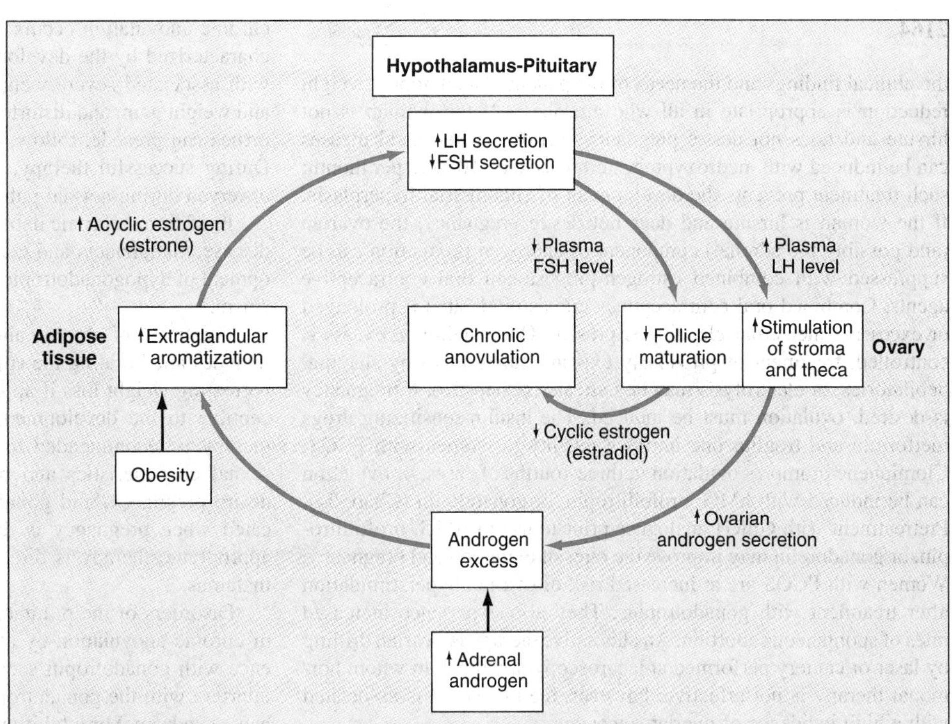

FIGURE 336-7 Proposed mechanism for the initiation and perpetuation of chronic anovulation in polycystic ovarian syndrome (PCOS). This cycle may be entered or initiated via adrenal androgen excess or obesity, both of which result in enhanced extraglandular formation of estrogens. The therapy of PCOS involves interruption of the cycle at any of several steps. *From SSC Yenet al (eds), Reproductive Endocrinology. Philadelphia, Saunders, 1999; and from U Goebelmann, in Reproductive Endocrinology, Infertility, and Contraception, 2d ed, DR Mishell Jr, V Davajan (eds), Philadelphia, Davis, 1986.*

Chronic anovulation At least 80% or more of gynecologic endocrine disorders result from chronic anovulation. Women with chronic anovulation fail to ovulate spontaneously but may ovulate with appropriate therapy. The ovaries of such women do not secrete estrogen in a normal cyclic pattern; it is clinically useful to differentiate those women who produce enough estrogen to have withdrawal bleeding after progestogen therapy from those who do not; the latter often have hypothalamic-pituitary dysfunction.

CHRONIC ANOVULATION WITH ESTROGEN PRESENT Women with chronic anovulation who experience withdrawal bleeding after progestogen administration are said to be in a state of "estrus" due to the acyclic production of estrogen, largely estrone, by extraglandular aromatization of circulating androstenedione. This disorder is commonly termed *polycystic ovarian syndrome* (PCOS) and is characterized by infertility, hirsutism, obesity, and amenorrhea or oligomenorrhea. When spontaneous uterine bleeding occurs in women with PCOS, it is unpredictable as to time of onset, duration, and amount; on occasion the bleeding can be severe. The dysfunctional uterine bleeding is usually due to estrogen breakthrough (see above).

The disorder, as originally described by Stein and Leventhal, was characterized by enlarged, polycystic ovaries, but it is now known to be associated with a variety of pathologic findings in the ovaries, only some of which result in enlargement and none of which are pathognomonic. The most common finding is a white, smooth, sclerotic ovary with a thickened capsule, multiple follicular cysts in various stages of atresia, a hyperplastic theca and stroma, and rare or absent corpora albicans. Other ovaries have hyperthecosis in which the ovarian stroma is hyperplastic and may contain lipid-laden luteal cells. Thus, the diagnosis of PCOS is a clinical one, based on the coexistence of chronic anovulation and varying degrees of androgen excess. The fundamental defect that causes PCOS is unknown, and it is likely to have several distinct causes.

In most women with PCOS, menarche occurs at the expected time, but uterine bleeding is unpredictable in onset, duration, and amount. Amenorrhea ensues after a variable period, although primary amenorrhea occurs in some women. Signs of androgen excess (hirsutism) usually become evident around the time of menarche. One scenario suggests that this disorder originates as an exaggerated adrenarche in obese girls (Fig. 336-7). The combination of elevated levels of adrenal androgens and obesity leads to increased formation of extraglandular estrogen. This estrogen exerts a positive feedback on LH secretion and negative feedback on FSH secretion, resulting in a ratio of LH to FSH levels in plasma that is characteristically greater than 2. The increased LH levels can then lead to hyperplasia of the ovarian stroma and theca cells and increased androgen production, which in turn provides more substrate for peripheral aromatization and perpetuates the chronic anovulation. In the advanced stage of the disorder, the ovary is the major site of androgen production, but the adrenal may continue to secrete excess androgen as well. The greater the obesity, the more strongly this sequence would be perpetuated because more androgen is converted to estrogen by adipose tissue stromal cells, which in turn exaggerates inappropriate LH release by positive feedback. Ovarian follicles from women with PCOS have low aromatase activity, but normal aromatase can be induced by treatment with FSH. An association exists between PCOS/hyperthecosis, virilization, acanthosis nigricans, and insulin resistance; in the ovary, insulin may interact via the insulin-like growth factor receptors to enhance androgen synthesis in insulin-resistant states.

℞ **TREATMENT** Treatment of PCOS is directed toward interrupting the self-perpetuating cycle and can be accomplished in several ways, such as by decreasing ovarian androgen secretion (by wedge resection or the use of oral contraceptive agents), decreasing peripheral estrogen formation (by weight reduction), or enhancing FSH secretion [by administration of clomiphene, human menopausal gonadotropin (hMG), GnRH (gonadorelin) by portable infusion pump, or purified FSH (urofollitropin)]. The choice of therapy depends on the clinical findings and the needs of the patient. An attempt at weight reduction is appropriate in all who are obese. If the woman is not hirsute and does not desire pregnancy, periodic withdrawal menses can be induced with medroxyprogesterone acetate 10 days per month; such treatment prevents the development of endometrial hyperplasia. If the woman is hirsute and does not desire pregnancy, the ovarian (and possibly the adrenal) component of androgen production can be suppressed with combined estrogen-progestogen oral contraceptive agents. Combined oral contraceptives are also indicated if prolonged or excessive menstrual bleeding is present. Once androgen excess is controlled, treatment of previously existing hair growth by shaving, depilatories, or electrolysis may be indicated (Chap. 53). If pregnancy is desired, ovulation must be induced. The insulin-sensitizing drugs metformin and troglitazone improve fertility in women with PCOS. Clomiphene promotes ovulation in three-fourths of cases, or ovulation can be induced with hMG, urofollitropin, or gonadorelin (Chap. 54). Pretreatment with GnRH analogues prior to use of hMG, urofollitropin, or gonadorelin may improve the rates of ovulation and pregnancy. Women with PCOS are at increased risk of ovarian hyperstimulation after treatment with gonadotropins. They also experience increased rates of spontaneous abortion. An alternative therapy is ovarian drilling by laser or cautery performed at laparoscopy in women in whom hormonal therapy is not effective; however, the procedure is associated with a high incidence of ovarian adhesions.

Chronic anovulation with estrogen present also may occur with tumors of the ovary. These include granulosa-theca cell tumors, Brenner tumors, cystic teratomas, mucous cystadenomas, and Krukenberg tumors (Chap. 97). Such tumors can either secrete excess estrogen themselves or produce androgens that are aromatized in extraglandular sites. Chronic anovulation and the clinical features of PCOS result. Occasionally, areas of the ovary not involved with tumors show the characteristic histologic changes of PCOS. Other causes of chronic anovulation with estrogen present include adrenal production of excess androgen (usually adult-onset adrenal hyperplasia due to partial 21-hydroxylase deficiency) and various thyroid disorders.

CHRONIC ANOVULATION WITH ESTROGEN ABSENT Women with chronic anovulation who have low or absent estrogen production and do not experience withdrawal bleeding after progestogen treatment usually have hypogonadotropic hypogonadism due to disease of either the pituitary or the central nervous system.

Isolated hypogonadotropic hypogonadism associated with defects of smell (olfactory bulb defects) is known as the *Kallmann syndrome* (Chaps. 328 and 335). Affected women are sexually infantile and have a defect in the synthesis and/or release of GnRH. Hypothalamic lesions that impair GnRH production and cause hypogonadotropic hypogonadism include craniopharyngioma, germinoma (pinealoma), glioma, Hand-Schüller-Christian disease, teratomas, endodermal-sinus tumors, tuberculosis, sarcoidosis, and metastatic tumors that cause suppression or destruction of the hypothalamus. Central nervous system trauma and irradiation can also cause hypothalamic amenorrhea and deficiencies in secretion of growth hormone, adrenocorticotropic hormone (ACTH), vasopressin, and thyroid hormone.

More commonly, gonadotropin deficiency leading to chronic anovulation is believed to arise from functional disorders of the hypothalamus or higher centers. A history of a stressful event in a young woman is frequent. For example, chronic anovulation can begin suddenly in a woman who leaves home for the first time or experiences the death of a loved one. Gonadotropin and estrogen levels are in the low to low-normal range as compared with normal women in the early follicular phase of the cycle. In addition, rigorous exercise, such as jogging or ballet, and diets that result in excessive weight loss may lead to chronic anovulation, particularly in girls with a history of prior menstrual irregularity. The amenorrhea in these women does not appear to be due to weight loss alone but to a combination of a decrease in body fat and chronic stress. An extreme form of weight loss with chronic anovulation occurs in anorexia nervosa. Anorexia nervosa is characterized by the development in a young woman of amenorrhea with associated severe weight loss, distorted attitudes toward eating and weight gain, and distorted body image. In anorexia nervosa amenorrhea can precede, follow, or coincide with weight loss (Chap. 78). During successful therapy, gonadotropin changes recapitulate those observed during normal puberty (Fig. 336-1).

In addition, chronic debilitating diseases such as end-stage kidney disease, malignancy, and malabsorption are believed to lead to development of hypogonadotropic hypogonadism via a hypothalamic mechanism.

Treatment of chronic anovulation due to hypothalamic disorders includes ameliorating the stressful situation, decreasing exercise, and correcting weight loss if appropriate. These women appear to be susceptible to the development of osteoporosis; estrogen replacement therapy is recommended to induce and maintain normal secondary sexual characteristics and prevent bone loss in those who do not desire pregnancy, and gonadotropin or gonadorelin therapy is indicated when pregnancy is desired (see "Treatment," below). When appropriate, therapy is directed at the primary disease of the hypothalamus.

Disorders of the pituitary can lead to the estrogen-deficient form of chronic anovulation by at least two mechanisms—direct interference with gonadotropin secretion by lesions that either obliterate or interfere with the gonadotropic cells (chromophobe adenomas, Sheehan's syndrome) or inhibition of gonadotropin secretion in association with excess prolactin (prolactinoma). *Pituitary tumors* make up approximately 10% of all intracranial tumors and may secrete no hormone, one hormone, or more than one hormone (Chap. 328). Prolactin levels are elevated in 50 to 70% of patients with pituitary tumors, either because of prolactin secretion by the tumor itself (in the case of prolactinomas) or because the tumor mass interferes with the normal hypothalamic inhibition of prolactin secretion.

Prolactinomas can be divided into microadenomas (<10 mm in diameter) and macroadenomas (>10 mm). Prolactin excess associated with low levels of LH and FSH constitutes a specific subtype of hypogonadotropic hypogonadism. One-tenth or more of amenorrheic women have increased levels of serum prolactin, and more than half of women with both galactorrhea and amenorrhea have elevated prolactin levels. The amenorrhea is most often associated with decreased or absent estrogen production, but prolactin-secreting tumors on occasion are associated with normal ovulatory menses or chronic anovulation with estrogen present. The increased frequency of diagnosis of prolactin-secreting adenomas is probably due to several factors, including increased awareness, improved radiographic detection methods, and availability of radioimmunoassays for prolactin. Since in older autopsy series a 9 to 23% prevalence of pituitary adenomas was observed in asymptomatic women, the clinical and prognostic significance of small microadenomas in asymptomatic individuals is unclear. However, when tumors of any size are associated with symptoms of amenorrhea or galactorrhea, particularly when visual field defects or severe headaches are present, bromocriptine therapy or neurosurgical evaluation is indicated. In the latter half of pregnancy, prolactin-secreting pituitary tumors may expand, leading to headaches, compression of the optic chiasm, bitemporal hemianopsia, and blindness. Therefore, before inducing ovulation for the purposes of achieving pregnancy, it is mandatory to exclude the presence of a pituitary tumor. →*The evaluation, differential diagnosis, and management of hyperprolactinemia are described in Chap. 328.*

Large pituitary tumors such as null cell adenomas—whether or not hyperprolactinemia is present—are likely to be associated with deficiency of hormones in addition to gonadotropins (Chap. 328).

Craniopharyngiomas, which are thought to arise from remnants of Rathke's pouch, account for 3% of intracranial neoplasms, occur most frequently in the second decade of life, and may extend into the suprasellar region. Many of these tumors calcify and can be diagnosed by conventional skull films. Patients often present with sexual infantilism, delayed puberty, and amenorrhea due to gonadotropin deficiency; secretion of TSH, ACTH, growth hormone, and vasopressin may also be impaired.

Panhypopituitarism can occur spontaneously, be caused by mutations in transcription factors (Pit1; Prop1) involved in pituitary gland development, result from surgical or radiation treatment of pituitary adenomas, or develop after postpartum hemorrhage (Sheehan's syndrome). Patients with the latter disorder characteristically have failure to lactate or ovulate, loss of genital and axillary hair, hypothyroidism, and adrenal insufficiency (Chap. 328).

Evaluation of amenorrhea A general scheme for the evaluation of women with amenorrhea is given in Fig. 336-8. On physical examination, attention should be given to three features: (1) the degree of maturation of the breasts, pubic and axillary hair, and external genitalia; (2) the current estrogen status; and (3) the presence or absence of a uterus. Pregnancy should be excluded in all women with amenorrhea; it is prudent to perform a suitable pregnancy screening test even when the history and physical examination are not suggestive. Once that is done, the cause of amenorrhea can frequently be diagnosed clinically. For example, Asherman's syndrome is suggested by a history of curettage in a woman who previously menstruated; in women with primary amenorrhea and sexual infantilism, the essential differential diagnosis is between gonadal dysgenesis and hypopituitarism, and the diagnosis of gonadal dysgenesis (Turner's syndrome) or of anatomic defects of the outflow tract (müllerian agenesis, testicular feminization, and cervical stenosis) is frequently suggested on the basis of physical findings. When a specific cause is suspected, it is appropriate to proceed directly to confirm the diagnosis (obtaining a chromosomal karyotype or measurement of plasma gonadotropins). It is also useful to measure serum prolactin and FSH levels during the initial evaluation.

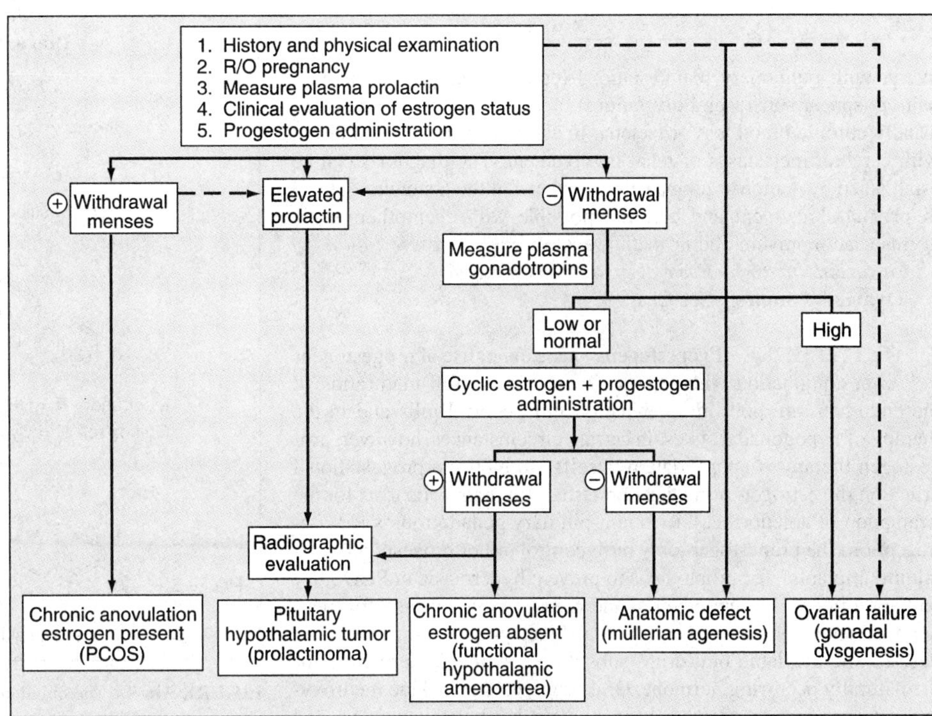

FIGURE 336-8 Flow diagram for the evaluation of women with amenorrhea. The most common diagnosis for each category is shown in parentheses. The dotted lines indicate that in some instances a correct diagnosis can be reached on the basis of history and physical examination alone.

Estrogen status is evaluated by determining if the vaginal mucosa is moist and rugated and if the cervical mucus can be stretched and shown to fern upon drying. If these criteria are indeterminate, a progestational challenge is indicated, most often the administration of 10 mg medroxyprogesterone acetate by mouth once or twice daily for 5 days or 100 mg progesterone in oil intramuscularly. (It should be emphasized that progestogen should never be administered until pregnancy is excluded.) If estrogen levels are adequate (and the outflow tract is intact), menstrual bleeding should occur within 1 week of ending the progestogen treatment. If withdrawal bleeding occurs, the diagnosis is chronic anovulation with estrogen present, usually caused by PCOS.

If no withdrawal bleeding or only minimal vaginal spotting occurs, the nature of the subsequent workup depends on the results of the initial prolactin assay. If plasma prolactin is elevated, or if galactorrhea is present, radiography of the pituitary should be undertaken. When the plasma prolactin level is normal in an anovulatory woman with estrogen absent and with elevated FSH levels, the diagnosis is ovarian failure. If the gonadotropins are in the low or normal range, the diagnosis is either hypothalamic-pituitary disorder or an anatomic defect of the outflow tract. As indicated previously, the diagnosis of outflow tract disorder is usually suspected or established on the basis of the history and physical findings. When the physical findings are not clear-cut, it is useful to administer cyclic estrogen plus progestogen (1.25 mg oral conjugated estrogens per day for 3 weeks, with 10 mg medroxyprogesterone acetate added for the last 7 to 10 days of estrogen treatment), followed by 10 days of observation. If no bleeding occurs, the diagnosis of Asherman's syndrome or another anatomic defect of the outflow tract is confirmed by hysterosalpingography or hysteroscopy. If withdrawal bleeding occurs following the estrogen-progestogen combination, the diagnosis of chronic anovulation with estrogen absent (functional hypothalamic amenorrhea) is suggested. Radiologic evaluations of the pituitary-hypothalamic areas may be indicated in the latter cases—irrespective of the prolactin level—because of the danger of overlooking a pituitary-hypothalamic tumor and because the diagnosis of functional hypothalamic amenorrhea is one of exclusion (Chap. 328).

Infertility Infertility, the failure to become pregnant after 1 year of unprotected intercourse, affects approximately 10 to 15% of couples and is a common reason for seeking gynecologic assistance (Chap. 54). Male factors account for 40% of infertility problems (Chap. 335). In women, failure of ovulation accounts for 30% of cases; pelvic factors, such as tubal disease or endometriosis, account for half; and a cervical factor is implicated in about one-tenth. In 10 to 20% of infertile women no etiology is found.

Medical Aspects of Pregnancy (See also Chap. 7) The possibility of pregnancy should be considered in all women of reproductive age who are evaluated for medical illness or considered for surgery. Procedures such as x-ray exposure, drugs, and anesthetics may be harmful to the developing fetus, and a variety of medical problems may worsen during pregnancy, including hypertension; diseases of the heart, lungs, kidney, and liver; and metabolic and endocrine disorders. Abnormal vaginal bleeding or amenorrhea during the reproductive years should prompt consideration of a complication of pregnancy, such as incomplete abortion, ectopic pregnancy, or trophoblastic disease (hydatidiform mole or choriocarcinoma). Women who present with these complications of pregnancy often have histories of abdominal pain and vaginal bleeding and may have evidence of intraabdominal hemorrhage.

Choriocarcinoma is a particular problem because of its protean manifestations. Half these malignancies follow pregnancies complicated by hydatidiform mole, and the remainder occur after spontaneous abortion, ectopic pregnancy, or normal deliveries. Patients may present with intraabdominal bleeding due to rupture of the uterus, liver, or ovary, with pulmonary manifestations (cough, hemoptysis, pleuritic pain, dyspnea, and respiratory failure) or gastrointestinal symptoms, usually chronic blood loss or melena. In addition, patients can present with cerebral metastases or renal involvement. The diagnosis can be established by demonstrating an elevated level of the β subunit of hCG in plasma. Treatment and cure are possible with chemotherapeutic agents (dactinomycin and/or methotrexate). →*The manifestations of choriocarcinoma in men are discussed in Chap. 96.*

Ovarian Tumors See Chap. 97

℞ TREATMENT **Progestogens** The major use of progestogens is in conjunction with estrogen to ensure the full maturation of the endometrium, both in combination birth control pills and in the therapy of hypogonadal states. In certain circumstances, however, progestogen therapy is appropriate by itself—to induce a progestational effect on the estrogen-primed endometrium (in diagnostic tests for the evaluation of amenorrhea), to inhibit pituitary gonadotropins for contraception (the progestogen-only birth control pill or progestogen-containing implants), for prophylaxis to prevent hyperplasia in PCOS, for palliation in cases of endometrial and breast carcinoma, and for treatment of endometriosis. Even when a direct progestational effect is desired, the available oral drugs substitute a synthetic derivative for the naturally occurring hormone. Oral progestogens include medroxyprogesterone acetate, megestrol acetate, norethindrone, norgestrel, and micronized progesterone. Parenteral agents include progesterone in oil, medroxyprogesterone acetate suspension, and 17-hydroxyprogesterone caproate. Vaginal progesterone suppositories are used for treatment of luteal-phase defects, and progestogen implants are available for long-term contraception.

The most common undesirable side effect is breakthrough bleeding, which occurs when progestogens are used continuously. Other complications include nausea, vomiting, and hirsutism. Abnormal liver function is a side effect of those derivatives with alkyl substitution in the 17α position. Synthetic progestogens are contraindicated if pregnancy is known or suspected, because of the risk of birth defects.

Estrogens Estrogens are used for the treatment of gonadal failure, the control of fertility, and the management of dysfunctional uterine bleeding. However, none of the available oral or parenteral hormones replaces the pattern of circulating estradiol levels characteristic of the normally cycling, premenopausal woman (Fig. 336-5). Estrogens that can be given by mouth are either nonsteroidal agents (such as diethylstilbestrol) that mimic the action of estradiol, estrogen conjugates that must be hydrolyzed before they become active (usually estrone sulfate from pregnant mare's urine), or estrogen analogues that cannot be metabolized to estradiol (mestranol, quinestrol; Fig. 336-9). Even when micronized estradiol is given orally, it is rapidly converted in the body to estrone. Because oral therapy neither replaces nor mimics the daily secretory pattern of the deficient hormone, such therapy must be viewed as a pharmacologic substitution rather than a physiologic replacement. Likewise, the use of parenteral estrogens rarely mimics the physiologic situation. Parenteral preparations of conjugated estrogens, like the oral derivatives, are poor precursors of estradiol, and estradiol esters (estradiol benzoate and valerate) rarely result in plasma estradiol levels that mimic the normal monthly secretory cycle of the hormone. Transdermal estradiol results in constant levels of blood estradiol and is effective in the treatment of menopausal symptoms. Estrogen vaginal rings and creams can be used for local treatment of vaginal atrophy, but systemic absorption is variable. The side effects of estrogen substitution differ at various times of life.

Hypoestrogenism In women with decreased estrogen production, whether due to disease of the ovaries (gonadal dysgenesis) or to hypogonadotropic hypogonadism, treatment with cyclic estrogens should be instituted at the time of expected puberty to induce the development and maintenance of female secondary sexual characteristics and to prevent osteoporosis. The most commonly used medications are conjugated estrogens (0.625 to 1.25 mg/d by mouth) together with medroxyprogesterone acetate (2.5 mg/d or 5 to 10 mg during the last several days of monthly estrogen treatment to prevent development of endometrial hyperplasia). Alternatively, oral contraceptives may be given (Chap. 54). Abnormal bleeding in women receiving estrogen replacement mandates histologic evaluation of the endometrium. Such substitution therapy or the use of oral contraceptives may also be used for the purpose of suppressing pituitary gonadotropins, as in women with PCOS, in whom the major therapeutic aim is suppression of ovarian androgen production.

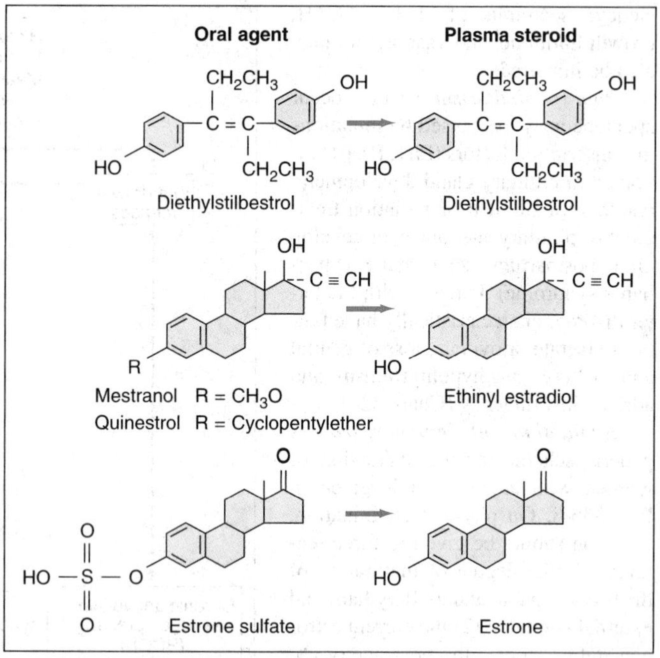

Oral agent | Plasma steroid

Diethylstilbestrol → Diethylstilbestrol

Mestranol R = CH_3O; Quinestrol R = Cyclopentylether → Ethinyl estradiol

Estrone sulfate → Estrone

FIGURE 336-9 The circulating forms of administered estrogenic drugs.

Temporary administration of estrogens in larger quantities (up to two times the usual adult maintenance dose) may be necessary to induce the full development of secondary sexual characteristics in girls and for the control of menopausal symptoms. Even larger doses of parenteral estrogens (10 mg estradiol valerate or 25 mg conjugated estrogen) in conjunction with progestogen may be required in some instances of dysfunctional uterine bleeding. In addition to the potential long-term side effects of all estrogens (see below), high doses may cause nausea, vomiting, and edema.

Contraceptives See Chap. 54

Estrogen Treatment of the Menopause The use of estrogens in postmenopausal women is based on evidence that they may relieve some of the complications of the postmenopausal state, including osteoporosis, and some manifestations of aging itself. In some parts of the United States, as many as half of women in the menopausal age group used one or more forms of estrogen replacement for a median period of 5 years.

The menopause is not, however, a state of simple estrogen deprivation, as some estrogens continue to be produced. It is instead a state of altered estrogen metabolism; the predominant estrogen becomes estrone, which is formed by extraglandular conversion of prehormone, rather than estradiol secreted by the ovary. As is true for all estrogen therapy, the estrogen treatment of the menopause is actually a pharmacologic substitution of one or another estrogen analogue for estradiol rather than a physiologic replacement of the missing steroid. The estrogens available for replacement therapy include conjugated estrogens, estrogen substitutes (diethylstilbestrol), synthetic estrogen (ethinyl estradiol or derivatives), micronized estradiol, estrogen-containing vaginal creams, and estrogen-containing dermal patches. Selective ER modulators (e.g., raloxifene) have estrogenic activity in the bone and the cardiovascular system but are antiestrogenic in breast and uterus. Raloxifene binds to the ER, with a conformational change in the domain of the receptor involved in transcription. Regimens associated with a low risk of complications include the following: (1) cyclic estrogen therapy in the lowest effective dose for 25 days per month or continuous estrogens given each day of the month, (2) estrogens plus the addition of progestogen during the last 10 to 14 days of estrogen therapy, (3) low-dose continuous progestogen plus estrogen given daily, and (4) daily selective ER modulators (SERM).

The most clear-cut early benefit of estrogen therapy in the menopause is the relief of vasomotor instability (hot flashes) and of atrophy of the urogenital epithelium and skin. Estrogen therapy ameliorates these symptoms in most cases. When estrogen therapy is intended to treat hot flashes alone, it should be continued for only a few years, since hot flashes tend to diminish after 3 to 4 years in untreated women. Selective ER modulators have no effect on hot flashes.

Several lines of evidence indicate that routine estrogen therapy is beneficial in preventing the complications of menopausal osteoporosis, especially in high-risk women (i.e., thin white women; Chap. 342). First, in women undergoing premature menopause, the incidence and complication rates of osteoporosis are increased, and long-term estrogen replacement appears to be beneficial. Second, estrogen therapy has short-term positive effects on calcium balance and long-term beneficial effects on bone density. Third, in women given estrogen therapy, the incidence of fractures is decreased.

Of the potential side effects, the possibility of an increased risk of endometrial carcinoma is perhaps most worrisome. The relative risk of developing endometrial adenocarcinoma in estrogen users is between six and eight times the risk in nonusers. This risk increases with increasing duration and dosage of estrogen but is largely negated in women given combination estrogen-progestogen therapy. Despite the large body of evidence linking endometrial carcinoma and estrogen use, the increased incidence primarily involves low-grade malignancies that may be difficult to distinguish histologically from hyperplasia. These forms of malignancy have little effect on life expectancy.

Apprehension concerning worsening of hypertension and thromboembolic disease appears to be due to reports of the effects of estrogen-progestogen oral contraceptives during the reproductive years and not to estrogen use in postmenopausal women. There is no conclusive evidence that low-dose estrogen therapy after menopause increases the incidence or the severity of breast cancer or hypertension, but the risk for venous thromboembolism is slightly increased. Low-dose estrogen treatment after menopause does not appear to influence the development of atherosclerosis, myocardial infarction, or stroke. Strong evidence suggests that, in fact, estrogens may decrease the incidence of death from myocardial infarction. There is a slightly increased risk for the development of gallbladder disease with postmenopausal estrogen use.

A reasonable approach to the postmenopausal use of estrogens is as follows: (1) For long-term use, estrogens should be given in the minimal effective doses (0.625 mg conjugated estrogen orally or 1.0 mg micronized estradiol or transdermal estradiol 0.05 to 1.0 mg in a formulation that is changed every 3.5 days or every week). For women with an intact uterus, it is the practice in some clinics to give estrogens alone for 15 days and estrogen plus a daily progestogen dose for the remainder of the month. The most common regimens involve continuous estrogen plus low-dose continuous progestogen. (2) Such replacement therapy is indicated routinely in women undergoing premature menopause (surgically induced or spontaneous). (3) Estrogen therapy is also indicated routinely in women of all ages who have severe hot flashes or symptomatic atrophy of the urogenital epithelium. Hot flashes rarely persist for longer than 7 years, so, if therapy is given for this purpose, its duration can be limited. (4) In women who have had a hysterectomy, the potential benefits of treatment appear to outweigh the dangers, and in such women cyclic or continuous estrogen without progestogen is recommended. Whether estrogens should be given routinely to all women with intact uteri is an unsettled question, but the authors prescribe it in the absence of contraindications in hopes of ameliorating osteoporosis and reducing the risk of cardiovascular disease. (5) Raloxifene is given as a 60-mg tablet daily when the goal is to provide protection against bone loss without incurring additional risk of estrogen-dependent breast cancer. Each woman receiving estrogens must be monitored indefinitely at yearly intervals.

Induction of Ovulation See Chap. 54

OTHER DISORDERS OF THE FEMALE REPRODUCTIVE TRACT

VULVA Most disorders of the vulva are due to venereal disease, most commonly syphilis (painless chancre), condylomata acuminata (venereal warts), and herpes vulvitis (painful ulcers; Chap. 132). All other lesions of the vulva, particularly in older women, must be biopsied. Early biopsy of cancer of the vulva is mandatory, because when it becomes symptomatic (pruritus and bleeding), it has often progressed to an advanced stage.

VAGINA Infections of the vagina usually present as vaginal discharge and pruritus. The most frequent organisms are *Trichomonas*, *Candida albicans*, and *bacterial vaginalis* (Chap. 132). The diagnosis is made by microscopic examination of the discharge, and appropriate therapy can be instituted using vaginal or oral antibiotics.

Abnormalities of the vagina and cervix in female offspring of women given diethylstilbestrol during pregnancy include adenosis of the vagina and structural abnormalities of the vagina, cervix, and uterus; the risk of developing a rare vaginal cancer (adenocarcinoma, clear cell type) is increased (2 per 10,000 exposed women). Periodic examination of women at risk should begin at age 12 to 14, and reexamination should be done after any episode of abnormal bleeding.

CERVIX Preinvasive lesions of the cervix (also known as *cervical intraepithelial neoplasia*) and invasive carcinoma of the cervix can be detected reliably by obtaining a Papanicolaou (Pap) smear.

Evaluation of the Pap Smear The incidence of invasive cervical cancer has declined as a result of Pap smear screening. In the United States, approximately 2 to 3 million abnormal Pap smears are found each year. Most represent low-grade lesions but require appropriate follow-up. The follow-up of abnormal Pap smears requires an understanding of the Bethesda system for evaluating such smears (see below) and of the limitations of cytologic screening systems. Further evaluation may require repeat cytologic examination, colposcopy, or both.

Current Screening Recommendations Risk factors for cervical neoplasia include a history of multiple sexual partners, coitus beginning at an early age, a history of infection with human papilloma virus (HPV), infection with HIV or another immunosuppressed state, and a history of cancer of the lower genital tract. Cervical cancer screening is recommended annually beginning at 18 years of age or when the woman becomes sexually active, if earlier than age 18. "Less frequent" screening is performed when three consecutive, negative, satisfactory annual Pap smears have been obtained or if the woman is in a low-risk category. There is no upper age limit for screening, because the prevalence of invasive cancer shows a linear increase with age, most of these cancers being diagnosed after age 50. Even after hysterectomy, annual screening should be performed if there is a history of abnormal Pap smears or other lower genital tract neoplasia.

The Bethesda System of Cytologic Examination Pap smears are evaluated in regard to the adequacy of the specimen (satisfactory for evaluation, satisfactory but limited, or unsatisfactory for evaluation because of a stated reason), the general diagnosis (normal or abnormal), and a descriptive diagnosis if the smear is abnormal. The descriptive diagnoses include benign cellular changes, reactive cellular changes, and epithelial cell abnormalities, the latter including (1) atypical squamous cells of undetermined significance (ASCUS); (2) low-grade squamous intraepithelial lesion (LSIL), which is further categorized to include HPV infection, cervical intraepithelial neoplasia (CIN 1), and high-grade squamous intraepithelial lesion (HSIL, which is itself subdivided into CIN 2 and CIN 3); and (3) squamous cell carcinoma.

Guidelines for the Management of Women with Abnormal Pap Smears For ASCUS smears that are unqualified or suggest a reactive process, a repeat smear should be obtained every 4 to 6 months for 2 years until three consecutive negative smears have been obtained. For ASCUS smears that are unqualified but have severe inflammation, any specific cause should be treated, and the smear should be repeated in 2 to 3 months; because invasive carcinoma can be obscured by severe inflammation, clinical evaluation is mandatory. For postmenopausal women not using hormone replacement, a course of topical estrogen should be given before the test is repeated. For LSIL smears, the Pap test is repeated every 4 to 6 months for 2 years until three consecutive negative smears have been obtained; treatment of HPV is of no established benefit, and there is a high rate of regression of LSIL, so that in compliant, low-risk individuals, the outcome is usually favorable. If LSIL is persistent, colposcopy with directed biopsy is performed, and endocervical curettage is undertaken if a specific diagnosis is made by biopsy. Cervical cone biopsy or loop electrosurgical excision procedures are performed for higher-grade lesions such as HSIL. If cervical cancer is diagnosed by biopsy, clinical staging is performed, and the patient is treated with radiation therapy or surgery.

UTERUS Only 40% of cases of endometrial adenocarcinoma are detected by Pap smear. In women at high risk for endometrial carcinoma (because of obesity, a history of chronic anovulatory cycles, diabetes mellitus, hypertension, or estrogen treatment), yearly endometrial sampling should be performed. Measurement of endometrial thickness by sonography can indicate which patients are at risk for endometrial pathology. Endometrial thickness <5 mm is rarely associated with either hyperplasia or cancer. Low-dose oral estrogen therapy rarely causes breakthrough or withdrawal bleeding in postmenopausal women. Therefore, irrespective of whether the patient is using estrogen therapy, the occurrence of postmenopausal bleeding makes it mandatory to obtain a tissue diagnosis by either endometrial sampling or curettage to exclude endometrial cancer.

One of the most common disorders of the uterus and the most frequent tumor of women (one of four women affected) is the uterine leiomyoma, or fibroid tumor. Three-fourths of women with leiomyoma are asymptomatic, and the diagnosis is made on routine pelvic examination. When the tumor is associated with excessive menstrual blood loss, is large or fast-growing, or causes significant pelvic pain (Chap. 52), the preferred treatment is hysterectomy if there is no desire for further childbearing. In young women, myomectomy is sometimes indicated when infertility or repeated fetal wastage is a manifestation or where future childbearing is desired.

FALLOPIAN TUBES AND OVARIES Infectious pelvic inflammatory disease is a common disorder of the fallopian tubes and usually becomes symptomatic after a menstrual period; the symptoms include fever, chills, abdominal pain, and vaginal discharge, and pelvic tenderness on physical examination is common. The initiating organism most often is *Chlamydia trachomatis* or *Neisseria gonorrhoeae*, but tuboovarian abscess and sterility are probably caused by mixed aerobic and anaerobic superinfections and require wide-spectrum antibiotic treatment (Chap. 133).

Endometriosis is a benign disorder characterized by the presence and proliferation of endometrial tissue (stroma and glands) outside the endometrial cavity. The clinical manifestations are variable. Endometriosis occurs most commonly between the ages of 30 and 40 and is found incidentally at the time of surgery in approximately one-fifth of all gynecologic operations. The fertility rate is reduced in affected women. The disorder usually involves the posterior cul-de-sac or the ovaries and can give rise to ovarian enlargement (endometriomas), although it may involve distant sites (lung, umbilicus). The major symptom is pelvic pain, characteristically dysmenorrhea (Chap. 52). However, the frequency and severity of symptoms correlate poorly with the extent of disease. Other manifestations include dyspareunia, pain with defecation, and infertility. The characteristic physical findings are multiple tender nodules palpable along the uterosacral ligament at the time of rectal-vaginal examination, a posteriorly fixed uterus, or enlarged, cystic ovaries. The diagnosis can only be confirmed by direct visualization, usually at diagnostic laparoscopy. Treatment depends on the degree of involvement and the desires of the patient and includes observation for mild disease with no associated infertility or pain, hormonal suppressive therapy, conservative surgery by laparoscopy or laparotomy if fertility is desired, or removal of the uterus, tubes, and ovaries in severe disease. Endometriosis is rare after the menopause.

Any adnexal mass that persists for more than 6 weeks or is larger than 6 cm must be evaluated. Although ovarian cysts and neoplasms are the most common pelvic adnexal masses (see above), tumors of the fallopian tubes, uterus, gastrointestinal tract, or urinary tract should also be considered. Sonography or radiographic evaluation is often helpful in identifying the nature of the adnexal mass prior to surgical exploration.

BIBLIOGRAPHY

ADASHI EV, LEUNG PCK: *The Ovary*. New York, Raven Press, 1993

BRZOSOWSKI AM et al: Molecular bases of agonist and antagonism in the oestrogen receptor. Nature 389:753, 1997

CARR BR: Disorders of the ovary and reproductive tract, in *Williams Textbook of Endocrinology*, 9th ed, JD Wilson et al (eds). Philadelphia, Saunders, 1998, pp 751–817

———, BLACKWELL RE (eds): *Textbook of Reproductive Medicine*. Stamford, CT, Appleton & Lange, 1998

CUNNINGHAM FG et al: *Williams' Obstetrics*, 20th ed. Stamford, CT, Appleton & Lange, 1993

DELMUS PD et al: Effects of raloxifene on bone mineral density, serum cholesterol concentrations, and uterine endometrium in postmenopausal women. N Engl J Med 337: 1641, 1997

FUTTERWEIT W: *Polycystic Ovarian Disease*. New York, Springer-Verlag, 1984

GRAVE GD, CUTLER GB: *Sexual Precocity*. New York, Raven Press, 1993

GRUMBACH MM, CONTE FA: Disorders of sex differentiation, in *Williams Textbook of Endocrinology*, 9th ed, JD Wilson et al (eds). Philadelphia, Saunders, 1998, pp 1303–1425

———, STYNE DM: Puberty: Ontogeny, neuroendocrinology, physiology and disorders, in *Williams Textbook of Endocrinology*, 9th ed, JD Wilson et al (eds). Philadelphia, Saunders, 1998, pp 1509–1625

HERBST AL et al: *Comprehensive Gynecology*, 2d ed. St. Louis, Mosby, 1992

KAPLAN SA (ed): *Clinical Pediatric Endocrinology*. Philadelphia, Saunders, 1990

KNOBIL E, NEILL JD (eds): *The Physiology of Reproduction*, 2d ed. New York, Raven Press, 1994

LOBO RA: *Treatment of the Menopausal Woman*. New York, Raven Press, 1994

MILLER WL, STYNE DM: Disorders of puberty in the male and female, in *Reproductive Endocrinology*, SSC Yen et al (eds). Philadelphia, Saunders, 4th ed. 1999, pp 388–412

NESTLER JE et al: Effects of metformin on spontaneous and clomiphene-induced ovulation in the polycystic ovarian syndrome. N Engl J Med 338:1876, 1998

ROCK JA et al: *Female Reproductive Surgery*. Baltimore, Williams & Wilkins, 1992

SEIBEL MM: A new era in reproductive technology. N Engl J Med 318:828, 1988

SODERSTROM RM: *Operative Laparoscopy*. New York, Raven Press, 1993

SPEROFF L et al: *Clinical Gynecologic Endocrinology and Infertility*, 5th ed. Baltimore, Williams & Wilkins, 1994

STUDD JWW, WHITEHEAD MI (eds): *The Menopause*. Oxford, Blackwell, 1988

THOMPSON JD, ROCK JA: *Te Lindes Operative Gynecology*. 8th ed. Philadelphia, Lippincott, 1992

YEN SSC et al (eds): *Reproductive Endocrinology*, 4th ed. Philadelphia, Saunders, 1999

337

Jean D. Wilson

ENDOCRINE DISORDERS OF THE BREAST

The breasts are the site of fatal and preventable cancer in women and provide clues to underlying systemic illness in both men and women. Consequently, examination of the breasts is an important part of the physical examination. It is the duty of every physician to distinguish the abnormal from the normal at the earliest possible stage and to seek referral if there is any doubt. →*For discussion of cancer of the breast, see Chap. 89.*

ENDOCRINE CONTROL OF THE BREAST There is no histologic or functional difference in the breasts of prepubertal boys and girls, but a profound sexual dimorphism in breast development ensues at the time of puberty. The endocrine control of female breast development is illustrated in Fig. 337-1. Growth of the female breast at puberty is mediated primarily by estradiol, which induces the enlargement, division, and elongation of the tubular duct system and maturation of the nipples. Administration of estrogen to men is equally effective in this regard. To produce true alveolar development at the ends of the ducts, however, the synergistic action of progesterone is required. Within the gland a variety of mediators influence epithelial cell division and differentiation, including stimulatory factors such as the insulin-like growth factors, transforming growth factor α, and epidermal growth factor and inhibitory factors such as transforming growth factor β. Once the anatomic development of the ducts and alveoli is complete, the continued action of estrogen and progesterone is not required for lactation itself.

The endocrine control of milk formation is complex, requiring, in addition to appropriate priming by estrogen and progesterone, lactogenic hormones and the permissive action of glucocorticoid, insulin, thyroxine, and, in some species, growth hormone. There are two lactogenic hormones: (1) human placental lactogen (hPL, or chorionic somatomammotropin) and (2) prolactin. hPL is secreted in large amounts by the placenta during the latter part of gestation and prepares the breast for milk production. It disappears from the maternal (and fetal) circulation shortly after termination of pregnancy. The secretion of pituitary prolactin (Chap. 328) rises during pregnancy and plays the critical role in the initiation and maintenance of lactation in the puerperium. During late pregnancy and lactation, 60 to 80% of the anterior pituitary may consist of prolactin-secreting lactotrope cells, reflecting the stimulatory effects of estrogen on these cells.

Unlike most pituitary hormones, prolactin secretion is controlled predominantly by tonic inhibition. Under basal conditions inhibitory hypothalamic hormones, the most important being dopamine, are delivered from the central nervous system to the pituitary via the hypothalamic portal system and inhibit the release of prolactin into the blood (Chap. 328). Most factors that influence prolactin secretion do so by affecting the synthesis or release of dopamine. Basal prolactin levels in the mother fall after delivery, but prolactin secretion is enhanced by stimulation of the breasts, such as the act of nursing (the so-called sucking reflex), a phenomenon that is probably mediated by the reflex release of oxytocin, which acts as a prolactin-releasing factor. Prolactin binds to specific receptors on the cell surface of the breast acinar cells and activates the JAK-STAT signal transduction cascade to stimulate the synthesis of β-casein, whey acidic protein, and other milk constituents. In the postgestational state, the normal lactating woman forms about a liter of milk per day containing 38 g fat, 70 g lactose, and 12 g protein. Lactation can be suppressed by the administration of estrogens or diethylstilbestrol, which inhibit milk production by direct effects on the breast, or dopamine agonists such as bromocriptine, which inhibit prolactin secretion by the pituitary. Alternatively, if a woman does not nurse or use breast pumps postpartum, lactation usually ceases in 1 to 2 weeks.

Stage	Duct system	Major hormones	Permissive hormones
Prepubertal		None	Unknown
Adult	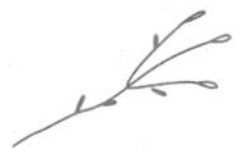	Estrogen (progesterone)	
Pregnancy	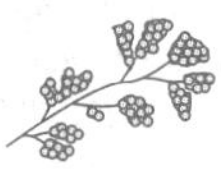	Estrogen Progesterone Prolactin Human placental lactogen	Insulin Thyroxine Glucocorticoids Growth hormone
Lactation	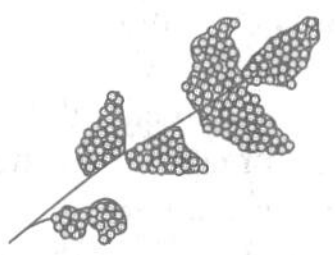	Prolactin Oxytocin	

FIGURE 337-1 Endocrine control of female breast development and function at various stages of life.

GALACTORRHEA *Galactorrhea* refers to the nonpuerperal discharge of milk-containing fluid from the breast. The definition of exactly what constitutes galactorrhea is not always clearly defined in the literature. According to the studies of Friedman and Goldfein, breast secretions are absent in normal, regularly menstruating nulligravid women. However, breast secretions can be demonstrated in a fourth of normal women who have been pregnant in the past; thus breast secretions in small amounts may be of no clinical significance in these instances. Spontaneous leakage of milk from the breasts is usually of more significance than milk that must be expressed. When the secretion is milky or white, it is safe to assume that it contains fat, casein, and lactose and is in fact milk; the concentration of milk constituents may increase after repeated sampling. When the secretion is brown or greenish, it rarely contains normal milk constituents and consequently may not result from an underlying endocrinopathy. Bloody discharges may be due to neoplasms of the breast. With these issues in mind, galactorrhea can be defined as inappropriate production of milk that is persistent or worrisome to the patient, recognizing that in some instances no underlying pathology may be demonstrated.

Since the action of a lactogenic hormone is necessary for the initiation of milk production, it is logical to consider galactorrhea as a consequence of deranged prolactin physiology. However, as indicated above, a complex hormonal milieu is necessary for lactation. Milk production does not take place in many instances in which prolactin is elevated, both in men and in women who have not been exposed to the necessary hormonal environment. As a consequence, hyperprolactinemia is more common than galactorrhea. Furthermore, while enhanced prolactin secretion is necessary for the initiation of lactation, continued production can be maintained in the presence of minimally or intermittently elevated prolactin levels so that basal plasma prolactin levels are not always elevated in patients with galactorrhea. In some such women prolactin levels may be elevated during sleep or with stimulation of the nipple; in others, hyperprolactinemia may have been present transiently. Perhaps the strongest evidence for a critical role for prolactin in galactorrhea is the fact that administration of dopaminergic agents that suppress plasma prolactin levels corrects galactorrhea even when the basal plasma prolactin levels are normal.

Differential Diagnosis Galactorrhea can be due to failure of the normal hypothalamic inhibition of prolactin release, to increased prolactin-releasing factor(s), or to autonomous prolactin secretion by tumors (Table 337-1). Pituitary stalk section, whether traumatic or secondary to the mass effects of sellar tumors, results in increases in prolactin secretion due to interruption in the delivery of dopamine to the pituitary. Likewise, many drugs that influence the central nervous system (CNS) (including virtually all psychotropic agents, methyldopa, reserpine, and antiemetics) enhance prolactin release, presumably by inhibiting synthesis, release, or action of dopamine. Estrogens increase prolactin secretion, but estrogen withdrawal (as in the discontinuation of oral contraceptives) may also trigger the onset of galactorrhea. CNS diseases outside the pituitary can cause galactorrhea presumably by interfering with the production or delivery of dopamine to the pituitary (CNS sarcoidosis, craniopharyngioma, pinealoma, encephalitis, meningitis, hydrocephalus, hypothalamic tumors).

In primary hypothyroidism, galactorrhea results from the enhanced production of thyrotropin-releasing hormone (TRH), which also stimulates prolactin release; thyroid hormone replacement corrects the galactorrhea. A similar mechanism, involving enhanced secretion of ox-

Table 337-1 Classification of Galactorrhea

I. Failure of normal hypothalamic inhibition of prolactin release
   A. Pituitary stalk section
   B. Drugs (phenothiazines, butyrophenones, methyldopa, tricyclic antidepressants, opiates, reserpine, verapamil, paroxetine, rispiradone, metoclopramide, sertraline)
   C. Central nervous system disease, including extrapituitary tumors and null cell adenomas of the pituitary
II. Enhanced prolactin release
   A. Hypothyroidism
   B. Sucking reflex and breast trauma
III. Autonomous prolactin release
   A. Pituitary tumors
      1. Prolactin-secreting tumors
      2. Mixed growth hormone and prolactin-secreting tumors
      3. Null cell adenomas
   B. Ectopic production of human placental lactogen and/or prolactin
      1. Hydatidiform moles and choriocarcinomas
      2. Bronchogenic carcinoma and hypernephroma
IV. Idiopathic

ytocin, may cause the galactorrhea that follows breast surgery or breast trauma.

Enhanced prolactin release can also occur from pituitary or nonpituitary tumors. Three types of pituitary tumors (Chap. 328) can cause galactorrhea: (1) pure prolactin-secreting micro- or macroadenomas, (2) mixed tumors that secrete both growth hormone and prolactin and cause acromegaly with galactorrhea, and (3) large null cell adenomas. The latter may interfere with the delivery of dopamine to the pituitary, either by mass effects on the hypothalamus or by compressing the pituitary stalk. Excess growth hormone secretion, in the absence of hyperprolactinemia, on occasion causes galactorrhea. Rarely, prolactin is secreted by bronchogenic carcinomas, and hydatidiform moles and choriocarcinomas may secrete placental lactogen.

In series involving several hundred patients with galactorrhea, a pituitary tumor was identified in about one-fourth, other known causes were identified in another fourth or fifth, and the remaining half fell into the idiopathic category. Many of the latter group ultimately developed prolactin-secreting pituitary tumors, some probably had subtle disorders of hypothalamic function, and in others a drug-related cause may have been missed. The fact remains that no satisfactory diagnosis is reached in many patients. When menses are normal, the likelihood of establishing a cause for galactorrhea is poor.

Galactorrhea is unusual in men, even in the presence of profound elevations of plasma prolactin; when it does occur, it is usually upon the background of a feminizing state (see below).

Diagnostic Evaluation If hyperprolactinemia is present, the evaluation is fundamentally that of a pituitary tumor once drug causes and hypothyroidism are excluded (Chap. 328). Even when a specific cause cannot be identified and the diagnosis of idiopathic galactorrhea is made by exclusion, it is necessary to remember that pituitary tumors may subsequently become manifest. The higher the prolactin values and the more persistent the galactorrhea, the greater is the likelihood of such a development.

℞ **TREATMENT** Breast binders can be effective in patients with mild galactorrhea of unknown etiology, presumably by preventing stimulation of the nipple and the consequent perpetuation of lactation. The aim of treatment in other instances is to correct the elevated prolactin level, and treatment of a pituitary tumor, cessation of causative drugs, or correction of hypothyroidism is often followed by the disappearance of galactorrhea. Dopamine agonists that suppress plasma prolactin have been used to treat idiopathic hyperprolactinemia, prolactin-secreting tumors of the pituitary (Chap. 328), and even normoprolactinemic galactorrhea. These drugs suppress lactation and may cause resumption of menstrual cycles (and even fertility) in women with amenorrhea and galactorrhea.

GYNECOMASTIA Enlargement of the male breast, or *gynecomastia*, can be a normal physiologic phenomenon at certain times of life or the result of several pathologic states (Table 337-2). A central issue in the evaluation of breast tissue in adult men is the separation of the normal from the abnormal, as gynecomastia can be an important indicator of underlying disease. It is sometimes difficult to distinguish true breast tissue enlargement from adipose tissue (*lipomastia*). True glandular tissue is often palpable, especially around the areolae, as it is firmer and contains cordlike features that are distinct from the texture of adipose tissue. In difficult cases, true gynecomastia can be identified by mammography or ultrasonography. In this discussion, we shall assume that any palpable breast tissue in men (except for the three physiologic states see below) can be due to an underlying endocrinopathy and deserves, at a minimum, a limited evaluation.

Early gynecomastia is characterized by proliferation in the breast of both the fibroblastic stroma and the duct system, which elongates, buds, and duplicates. As gynecomastia persists, progressive fibrosis and hyalinization are associated with regression of epithelial proliferation and, eventually, a decrease in the number of ducts. When the cause of the gynecomastia is corrected early in the course, resolution occurs by reduction in size and epithelial content with gradual disappearance of the ducts, leaving hyaline bands that eventually disappear.

Growth of the breast in men, as in women, is mediated by estrogen and results from an decrease in the ratio of active androgen to estrogen. As described in Chap. 335, estradiol formation in normal men occurs principally by the conversion of circulating androgen to estrogen in extraglandular tissues; the normal ratio of the two hormones in plasma is about 300:1. Growth of the breast ensues in men when the normal

Table 337-2 Differential Diagnosis of Gynecomastia

PHYSIOLOGIC GYNECOMASTIA

Newborn
Adolescence
Aging

PATHOLOGIC GYNECOMASTIA

I. Deficient production or action of testosterone
   A. Congenital anorchia
   B. Androgen resistance (testicular feminization and Reifenstein syndrome)
   C. Defects of testosterone synthesis
   D. Klinefelter syndrome
   E. Viral orchitis
   F. Trauma
   G. Castration
   H. Neurologic and granulomatous diseases
   I. Renal failure
II. Increased estrogen production
   A. Increased estrogen secretion
      1. Testicular tumors
      2. True hermaphroditism
      3. Carcinoma of the lung and other tumors producing hCG
   B. Increased substrate for extraglandular aromatase
      1. Adrenal disease
      2. Liver disease
      3. Malnutrition
      4. Hyperthyroidism
   C. Increase in extraglandular aromatase
III. Drugs
   A. Estrogens (diethylstilbestrol, birth control pills, digitalis, estrogen-containing cosmetics, estrogen-contaminated foods, phytoestrogens)
   B. Drugs that enhance endogenous estrogen secretion (gonadotropins, clomiphene)
   C. Inhibitors of testosterone synthesis and/or action (ketoconazole, metronidazole, alkylating agents, cisplatin, spironolactone, cimetidine, flutamide, etomidate)
   D. Unknown mechanisms (busulfan, isoniazid, methyldopa, tricyclic antidepressants, penicillamine, diazepam, omeprazole, calcium channel blockers, angiotensin-converting enzyme inhibitors, marijuana, heroin, finasteride, growth hormone, antiretroviral agents)
IV. Idiopathic

Note: hCG, human chorionic gonadotropin.

ratio decreases as the result of diminished testosterone production or action, enhanced estrogen formation, or both processes occurring simultaneously.

Physiologic Gynecomastia In the *newborn* transient enlargement of the breast is due to the action of maternal and/or placental estrogens. The enlargement usually disappears in a few weeks but may persist longer. *Adolescent* gynecomastia is common at some time during puberty. The median age of onset is 14; it is often asymmetric or transiently unilateral, frequently tender, and it regresses so that by age 20 only a small number of men have palpable vestiges of glandular tissue in one or both breasts. Although the origin of the excess estrogen has not been identified, the onset of gynecomastia correlates with the increase in adrenal androgens at adrenarche. In addition, the luteinizing hormone (LH) stimulation of androgen synthesis by the Leydig cell in early puberty may be associated with transient elevations of plasma estradiol so that the ratio of potent androgen to estrogen is low prior to the completion of puberty. *Gynecomastia of aging* also occurs in 40% or more of otherwise healthy elderly men. A likely explanation is the increase with age in the conversion of androgens to estrogens in extraglandular tissues. Abnormal liver function or drug therapy may be contributing causes in such men.

Pathologic Gynecomastia Pathologic gynecomastia can result from one of three basic mechanisms: deficiency in testosterone production or action (with or without a secondary increase in estrogen production), increase in estrogen production, or drugs (Table 337-2). Most of the disorders that cause primary and secondary testicular failure are discussed in Chap. 335. The fact that deficient testosterone production can cause gynecomastia is illustrated by the syndrome of congenital anorchia in which normal (or slightly low) estradiol levels, in the presence of profoundly decreased testosterone production, results in florid gynecomastia. Decreased testosterone production is also responsible for gynecomastia in some men with Klinefelter syndrome or testicular failure of other causes. In the disorders of androgen resistance, such as testicular feminization, deficient androgen action and increased testicular estrogen production are both present.

A primary increase in estrogen production can result from a variety of causes. Increased secretion of testicular estrogen may result from elevations in plasma gonadotropins, as in cases of aberrant production of chorionic gonadotropin by testicular tumors or by bronchogenic carcinomas, from the ovarian elements in the gonads of men with true hermaphroditism, or as the result of formation by testicular tumors (particularly Leydig and Sertoli cell tumors). Increased conversion of androgen to estrogens in extraglandular tissues can be due either to increased availability of substrate (androstenedione) for extraglandular estrogen formation (congenital adrenal hyperplasia, hyperthyroidism, and most feminizing adrenal tumors), or to diminished catabolism of androstenedione (liver disease) so that estrogen precursors are shunted to aromatase in peripheral sites. Extraglandular aromatase can be increased in tumors of the liver or adrenal gland and rarely as a result of an inherited disorder manifested by gynecomastia in affected males and macromastia in females.

Drugs can cause gynecomastia by several mechanisms. Many drugs either act directly as estrogens or cause an increase in plasma estrogen activity (e.g., in men receiving diethylstilbestrol for prostatic carcinoma and in transsexuals in preparation for sex-change operations). Boys and young men are particularly sensitive to estrogen and can develop gynecomastia after the use of dermal ointments containing estrogen or after the ingestion of milk or meat from estrogen-treated animals. The gynecomastia of digitalis ingestion is usually attributed to an estrogen-like side effect of the drug, but it occurs most commonly in men with abnormal liver function. A second mechanism of drug-induced gynecomastia is illustrated by clomiphene and human chorionic gonadotropin (hCG), which cause enhanced testicular secretion of estrogen. Other drugs cause gynecomastia by interfering with testosterone synthesis (ketoconazole and alkylating agents) and/or testosterone action, for instance, by blocking the binding of androgen to its receptor protein in target tissues (spironolactone and cimetidine). Finally, drugs that cause gynecomastia by mechanisms that have not been defined include busulfan, ethionamide, isoniazid, methyldopa, tricyclic antidepressants, penicillamine, omeprazole, calcium channel blocking agents, angiotensin-converting enzyme inhibitors, metoclopramide, antiretroviral agents, diazepam, marijuana, and heroin. In some instances, the feminization is due to effects of drugs on liver function. Treatment with growth hormone can cause gynecomastia even in prepubertal boys, suggesting that growth hormone itself or one of the insulin-like growth factors has a direct effect on the breast.

Diagnostic Evaluation The evaluation of patients with gynecomastia should include: (1) a careful drug history; (2) measurement and examination of the testes (if both are small, a chromosomal karyotype should be obtained; if the testes are asymmetric, a workup for testicular tumor should be instituted); (3) evaluation of liver function; and (4) endocrine workup to include measurement of serum androstenedione or 24-h urinary 17-ketosteroids (usually elevated in feminizing adrenal states), measurement of plasma estradiol and hCG (helpful if elevated but usually normal), and measurement of plasma LH and testosterone. If LH is high and testosterone is low, the diagnosis is usually testicular failure; if LH and testosterone are both low, the diagnosis is most likely increased primary estrogen production (e.g., a Sertoli cell tumor of the testis), provided hypogonadotropic hypogonadism has been excluded; and if both LH and testosterone are elevated, the diagnosis is either an androgen-resistance state or a gonadotropin-secreting tumor.

A satisfactory diagnosis can be made in only half or fewer of patients referred for gynecomastia. This implies either that the diagnostic techniques are not sufficiently refined to recognize mild disturbances, that many causes of gynecomastia are as yet undefined, that the causes may be transient and difficult to diagnose, or that gynecomastia may in some instances be normal rather than due to a pathologic state. Because of the problem of separating the normal from the abnormal, gynecomastia should probably be worked up routinely only if the drug history is negative, the breast is tender (indicating rapid growth), or the breast mass is >4 cm in diameter. However, the decision to perform an endocrine evaluation depends on the clinical context. For example, gynecomastia associated with signs of underandrogenization should always be evaluated. A firm or hard breast mass should raise suspicion of male breast cancer (Chap. 89).

℞ TREATMENT When the primary cause can be identified and corrected, the breast enlargement usually subsides promptly and eventually disappears. For example, androgen replacement therapy may produce dramatic improvement in men with testicular insufficiency. However, if the gynecomastia is of long duration (and fibrosis has replaced the original ductal hyperplasia), correction of the primary defect may not be followed by resolution. In such instances and when the primary cause cannot be corrected, surgery is the only effective therapy. Indications for surgery include several psychological and/or cosmetic problems, continued growth or tenderness, or suspected malignancy. Although the relative risk of carcinoma of the breast is increased in men with gynecomastia, it is rare nevertheless. Prophylactic radiation of the breasts prior to the institution of diethylstilbestrol or estrogen therapy is effective in preventing gynecomastia and has a low complication rate. In patients who have painful gynecomastia and who are not candidates for other therapy, treatment with antiestrogens such as tamoxifen may be indicated.

BIBLIOGRAPHY

GALACTORRHEA

ABDEL-GADIR A et al: The aetiology of galactorrhea in women with regular menstruation and normal prolactin levels. Human Reprod 7:912, 1992

BENJAMIN F: Normal lactation and galactorrhea. Clin Obstet Gynecol 37:887, 1994

EGBERTS AC et al: Non-puerperal lactation associated with antidepressant drug use. Br J Clin Pharmacol 44:277, 1997

FRANTZ AG, WILSON JD: Endocrine disorders of the breast, in *Williams Textbook of Endocrinology*, 9th ed, JD Wilson, DW Foster, HM Kronenberg, PR Larsen (eds). Philadelphia, Saunders, 1998, pp 877–900

FRIEDMAN S, GOLDFEIN A: Breast secretions in normal women. Am J Obstet Gynecol 104:846, 1969

HANEY AF: Galactorrhea, in *Current Therapy in Endocrinology and Metabolism*, 6th ed, CW Bardin (ed). St. Louis, Mosby, 1997, pp 393–396

JOHNSON DG et al: Prolactin secretion and biological activity in females with galactorrhoea and normal circulating prolactin concentrations at rest. Clin Endocrinol 22:661, 1985

KULSKI JK et al: Changes in the milk composition of nonpuerperal women. Am J Obstet Gynecol 139:597, 1981

LAURENCE DJ et al: The development of the normal human breast. Oxf Rev Reprod Biol 13:149, 1991

SAUER HJ: Physiology of lactation and factors affecting lactation. Obstet Gynecol Clin North Am 14:615, 1987

STRATAKIS CA et al: The aromatase excess syndrome is associated with feminization of both sexes and autosomal dominant transmission of aberrant P450 aromatase gene transcription. J Clin Endocrinol Metab 83:1348, 1998

TURKSOY RN et al: Diagnostic and therapeutic modalities in women with galactorrhea. Obstet Gynecol 56:323, 1980

YAZIGI RA et al: Prolactin disorders. Fertil Steril 67:215, 1997

GYNECOMASTIA

AGARWAL VR et al: Molecular basis of severe gynecomastia associated with aromatase expression in a fibrolamellar hepatocellular carcinoma. J Clin Endocrinol Metab. 83: 1797, 1998

APPELBAUM AH et al: Mammographic appearance of male breast disease. Radiographics 19:559, 1999

BLETHEN SL et al: Safety of recombinant deoxyribonucleic acid–derived growth hormone: The national cooperative growth study experience. J Clin Endocrinol Metab 81:1704, 1996

BRAUNSTEIN GD, GLASSMAN HA: Gynecomastia, in *Current Therapy in Endocrinology and Metabolism*, 6th ed, CW Bardin (ed). St Louis, Mosby, 1997, pp 401–404

CAVANAUGH J et al: Gynecomastia and cirrhosis of the liver. Arch Intern Med 150:563, 1990

DE GASPARO M et al: Antialdosterones: Incidence and prevention of sexual side effects. J Steroid Biochem 32:223, 1989

FELDMAN D: Ketoconazole and other imidazole derivatives as inhibitors of steroidogenesis. Endocr Rev 7:409, 1986

FRANTZ AG, WILSON JD: Endocrine disorders of the breast, in *Williams Textbook of Endocrinology*, 9th ed, JD Wilson, DW Foster, HM Kronenberg, PR Larsen (eds). Philadelphia, Saunders, 1998, pp 887–900

GEORGIADIS E et al: Incidence of gynaecomastia in 954 young males and its relationship to somatometric parameters. Ann Hum Biol 21:579, 1994

MABUCHI K et al: Risk factors for male breast cancer. J Natl Cancer Inst 74:371, 1985

MAHONEY CP: Adolescent gynecomastia: Differential diagnosis and management. Pediatr Clin North Am 37:1389, 1990

ROSE DP: Endocrine epidemiology of male breast cancer (review). Anticancer Res 8:845, 1988

SHER ES et al: Evaluation of boys with marked breast development at puberty. Clinic Pediatr (Phila) 37:367, 1998

STAIMAN VR, LOWE FC: Tamoxifen for flutamide/finasteride-induced gynecomastia. Urology 50:929, 1997

THOMPSON DF, CARTER R: Drug-induced gynecomastia. Pharmacotherapy 13:37, 1993

338

Jean D. Wilson, James E. Griffin

DISORDERS OF SEXUAL DIFFERENTIATION

Sexual differentiation is a sequential and ordered process. *Chromosomal sex*, established at the moment of fertilization, determines *gonadal sex*, and gonadal sex, in turn, causes the development of *phenotypic sex*, in which the male or female urogenital tract is formed (Fig. 338-1). A disturbance of any step in this process during embryogenesis may impair sexual differentiation (Table 338-1). Known causes of such disorders include environmental insults as in the ingestion of a virilizing drug during pregnancy, nonfamilial aberrations of the sex chromosomes as in 45,X gonadal dysgenesis, birth defects of multifactorial etiology as in most cases of hypospadias, and disorders due to single gene mutations as in the testicular feminization syndrome.

Limitations of knowledge make it necessary to make empirical assignments as to the type of derangement in some disorders, but specific diagnoses can usually be made as the result of genetic, endocrine, phenotypic, and chromosomal assessment. As a consequence, gender assignment in the newborn is usually appropriate, even in extreme instances of ambiguous genitalia.

NORMAL SEXUAL DIFFERENTIATION

The first event in sexual differentiation is the establishment of chromosomal sex, the heterogametic sex (XY) being male and the homogametic sex (XX) female. The embryos of both sexes then develop in an identical fashion until approximately 40 days of gestation.

The second phase of sexual differentiation is the conversion of the indifferent gonad into a testis or an ovary. No matter how many X chromosomes are present (as in 47,XXY, 48,XXXY, etc.), a testis will develop as long as a normal Y chromosome is present. Differentiation of the indifferent gonad into a testis is initiated by the actions of a single gene on the short arm of the Y chromosome (*SRY*); expression of an *SRY* transgene into female mice causes them to develop as males. The gene encodes a DNA-binding protein, but the mechanism by which *SRY* promotes testicular development remains poorly defined. At least four additional genes are also necessary for normal testicular development: (1) the Wilms' tumor–related gene (*WT1*), (2) steroidogenic factor 1 (*SF1*), (3) *SRY*-related HMG-box 9 (*SOX9*), and (4) *d*osage-sensitive sex reversal–*a*drenal hypoplasia congenita critical region on the *X* chromosome gene *1* (*DAX1*). These genes each encode putative transcription factors that regulate the expression of genes necessary for gonadal survival; mutations in *SRY* or any of the four downstream genes impair testicular development. It remains unclear if there are analogous "ovarian-determining genes," or if ovarian development is a default pathway in the absence of testicular determination genes. Mutations in some of the genes noted above (e.g., *SF1*) also prevent normal ovarian development.

The final process in sexual differentiation, the translation of gonadal sex into phenotypic sex (formation of the male or female urogenital tracts), is the consequence of the type of gonad formed and the endocrine secretions of the fetal gonads. The internal urogenital tract is derived from the wolffian and müllerian ducts that exist side by side in early embryos of both sexes (Fig. 338-1*A*). In the male the wolffian ducts give rise to the epididymides, vasa deferentia, and seminal vesicles, and the müllerian ducts disappear. In the female the müllerian ducts are converted into the fallopian tubes, uterus, and upper vagina, and the wolffian ducts regress. The external genitalia and urethra in the two sexes develop from common anlage—the urogenital sinus and the genital tubercle, folds, and swellings (Fig. 338-1*B*). The urogenital sinus gives rise to the prostate and prostatic urethra in the male and to the urethra and lower portion of the vagina in the female. The genital tubercle gives rise to the glans penis in the male and the clitoris in the female. The urogenital swellings become the scrotum or the labia majora, and the urethral folds form the labia minora or fuse to form the shaft of the penis and the male urethra.

In the absence of the testes, as in the normal female or in the male embryo castrated prior to the onset of gonadal differentiation, phenotypic sex develops along female lines. Thus, masculinization of the fetus is induced by hormones from the fetal testes, whereas female development does not require the presence of the ovary. Phenotypic sex normally conforms to chromosomal sex. That is, chromosomal sex determines gonadal sex, and gonadal sex, in turn, controls phenotypic sex.

Formation of the male phenotype is vested in the action of three hormones. Two—antimüllerian hormone (AMH) and testosterone—are secreted by the fetal testis. AMH [also termed *müllerian-inhibiting substance* (MIS)] is a protein that suppresses the müllerian ducts and prevents development of the uterus and fallopian tubes in the male. Testosterone acts directly to virilize the wolffian duct and is the precursor for the third embryonic male hormone, dihydrotestosterone (Chap. 335), which promotes development of the male urethra and prostate and formation of the penis and scrotum. Testosterone and dihydrotestosterone induce formation of the male urogenital tract during fetal life by acting through the same nuclear androgen receptor by which they act in postembryonic life (Chap. 335).

The secretion of testosterone by the fetal testes approaches a maximum by the tenth week of gestation, and formation of the sexual phenotypes is largely completed by the end of the first trimester. During the latter phases of gestation, the ovarian follicles develop and the vagina matures in the female, and testicular descent and phallic growth take place in the male.

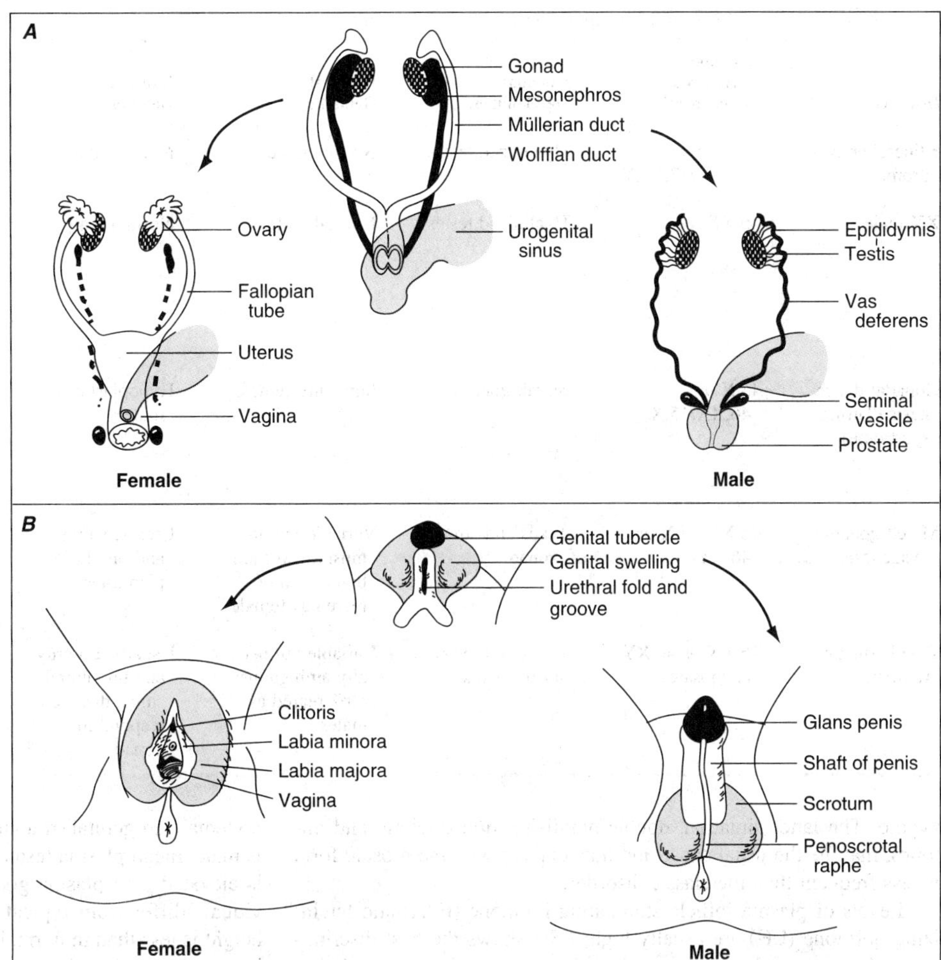

FIGURE 338-1 Normal sexual differentiation. *A.* Internal urogenital tract. *B.* External genitalia.

DISORDERS OF CHROMOSOMAL SEX

Disorders of chromosomal sex (Table 338-2) occur when the number or structure of the X or Y chromosomes is abnormal (Chap. 66).

KLINEFELTER SYNDROME

Clinical Features Klinefelter syndrome is characterized by small, firm testes, azoospermia, gynecomastia, and elevated levels of plasma gonadotropins in men with two or more X chromosomes. The common karyotype is either a 47,XXY chromosomal pattern (the classic form) or 46,XY/47,XXY mosaicism. It is the most frequent major abnormality of sexual differentiation, the incidence being around 1 in 500 men.

Prepubertally, the testes are small but otherwise appear normal. After puberty, the disorder is manifest as infertility, gynecomastia, or occasionally underandrogenization (Table 338-3). Hyalinization of the seminiferous tubules and azoospermia are consistent features of the 47,XXY variety. The small, firm testes are usually <2 cm and always <3.5 cm in length (corresponding to 2- and 12-mL volume, respectively). Longer legs cause increased mean height. Gynecomastia is common and ordinarily develops during adolescence, is generally bilateral and painless, and may become disfiguring (Chap. 337). Obesity and varicose veins occur in one-third to one-half, and leg ulcers are associated with deficiency of plasminogen activator inhibitor-1. The diagnosis is made most frequently in boys with developmental delay and/or learning disabilities and social maladjustment; abnormalities of thyroid function, diabetes mellitus, and pulmonary disease are also common. The risk of breast cancer is 20 times that of normal men (but only about a fifth that in women). Most have male psychosexual orientation and function sexually as normal men.

About 10% of the patients have the mosaic form, as estimated by chromosomal karyotypes on peripheral blood leukocytes. The frequency of this variant may be underestimated, since chromosomal mosaicism can be present in the testes when the peripheral leukocyte karyotype is normal. The mosaic form is usually not as severe as the 47,XXY variety, and the testes may be normal (Table 338-3). The endocrine abnormalities are less severe, and gynecomastia and azoospermia are less common, and occasional mosaic individuals are fertile. In some the diagnosis may not be suspected because the manifestations are so mild.

Approximately 30 additional variants of Klinefelter syndrome have been described, including those with uniform cell lines (such as 48,XXYY, 48,XXXY, and 49,XXXXY) and a variety of mosaicisms of the X chromosome with or without associated structural abnormalities of the X. In general, the greater the chromosomal abnormality the more severe the manifestations.

Pathophysiology The classic form is due to meiotic nondisjunction of the chromosomes during gametogenesis (Fig. 338-2). About 40% of the responsible meiotic nondisjunctions occur during spermatogenesis, and 60% occur during oogenesis. Advanced maternal age is a predisposing factor. The mosaic form is thought to result from chromosomal mitotic nondisjunction after fertilization of the zygote and can take place in either a 46,XY zygote (Fig. 338-2) or a 47,XXY

Table 338-1 Classification of Disorders of Sexual Development

Disorders of chromosomal sex
Klinefelter syndrome
XX male
Gonadal dysgenesis
Mixed gonadal dysgenesis
True hermaphroditism
Disorders of gonadal sex
Pure gonadal dysgenesis
Dysgenetic testes
Absent testis syndrome
Disorders of phenotypic sex
Female pseudohermaphroditism
Congenital adrenal hyperplasia
Nonadrenal female pseudohermaphroditism
Developmental disorders of müllerian ducts
Male pseudohermaphroditism
Abnormalities in androgen synthesis
Abnormalities in androgen action
Persistent müllerian duct syndrome
Development defects of male genitalia

Table 338-2 Clinical Features of the Disorders of Chromosomal Sex

Disorder	Common Chromosomal Complement	Gonadal Development	External Genitalia	Internal Genitalia	Breast Development	Comment
Klinefelter syndrome	47,XXY *or* 46,XY/47,XXY	Hyalinized testes	Normal male	Normal male	Gynecomastia	Most common disorder of sexual differentiation; tall stature.
XX male	46,XX	Hyalinized testes	Normal male	Normal male	Gynecomastia	Shorter than normal men; increased incidence of hypospadias. Similar to Klinefelter syndrome. May be familial.
Gonadal dysgenesis (Turner syndrome)	45,X *or* 46,XX/45,X	Streak gonads	Immature female	Hypoplastic female	Immature female	Short stature and multiple somatic abnormalities. May be 46,XX with structurally abnormal X chromosome.
Mixed gonadal dysgenesis	46,XY/45,X *or* 46,XY	Testis and streak gonad	Variable but almost always ambiguous; 60% reared as female	Uterus, vagina, and one fallopian tube	Usually male	Second most common cause of ambiguous genitalia in the newborn; tumors common.
True hermaphroditism	46,XX *or* 46,XY *or* mosaics	Testis and ovary or ovotestis	Variable but usually ambiguous; 60% reared as males	Usually a uterus and urogenital sinus; ducts correspond to gonad	Gynecomastia in 75%	May be familial.

zygote. The latter situation, double nondisjunction (meiotic and mitotic), may be the usual cause and thus explain why the mosaic form is less frequent than the classic disorder.

Levels of plasma follicle stimulating hormone (FSH) and luteinizing hormone (LH) are usually high; FSH shows the best discrimination because of the consistent damage to the seminiferous tubules. The plasma testosterone level averages half normal but may overlap the normal range. Mean plasma estradiol levels are elevated; early, estradiol secretion by the testes may increase in response to the elevated plasma LH level, but the testicular secretion of estradiol and testosterone eventually declines. Elevated plasma estradiol late in the course is probably due both to decreased metabolic clearance and increased conversion of testosterone to estradiol in extragonadal tissues. The net result both early and late is a variable degree of feminization and virilization. Feminization, including gynecomastia, depends on the ratio of circulating estrogen to androgen (relative or absolute), and individuals with low plasma testosterone and high plasma estradiol levels are more likely to develop gynecomastia (Chap. 337). Men with untreated Klinefelter syndrome may have enlarged pituitary glands, presumably due to hyperplasia of the gonadotrophs due to inadequate testosterone feedback.

℞ TREATMENT In men with some sperm production, or in whom spermatids can be recovered from testicular biopsy, fertility is possible with in vitro fertilization (Chap. 335). Gynecomastia should be treated surgically. Some underandrogenized men benefit from supplemental androgen, particularly in those with decreased bone density, but such treatment may worsen the gynecomastia, presumably by providing increased substrate for estrogen formation in peripheral tissues. Testosterone should be injected in the form of testosterone cypionate or testosterone enanthate or administered via the transdermal route (Chap. 335). Following the administration of testosterone, the plasma LH level returns to normal only after several months, if at all.

XX MALE SYNDROME A 46,XX karyotype is found in approximately 1 in 20,000 phenotypic males. The findings resemble those in Klinefelter syndrome: the testes are small and firm (generally <2 cm), gynecomastia is frequent, the penis is normal to small in size, azoospermia and hyalinization of the seminiferous tubules are usual, no female urogenital structures are present, psychosexual identification is male, mean plasma testosterone level is low, plasma estradiol level is elevated, and plasma gonadotropin levels are high. Affected individuals differ from typical Klinefelter patients only in that average height is less than in normal men, the incidence of cognitive problems is not increased, and the incidence of hypospadias is increased.

The majority of XX males have Y-related DNA (e.g., detected by polymerase chain reaction of the *SRY* gene); thus an X-Y or Y-autosome translocation appears to be the common cause. Some 46,XX males are negative for all Y-specific DNA, suggesting that their disorder is due to mutation in a downstream, autosomal or X-linked gene involved in development of the testes. The management is similar to that of Klinefelter syndrome.

GONADAL DYSGENESIS (TURNER SYNDROME) **Clinical Features** Gonadal dysgenesis is characterized by primary amenorrhea, sexual infantilism, short stature, multiple congenital anomalies, and bilateral streak gonads in phenotypic women with any of several defects of the X chromosome. This condition should be distinguished from (1) mixed gonadal dysgenesis in which a unilateral testis and a contralateral streak gonad may be present; (2) pure gonadal dysgenesis in which bilateral streak gonads are associated with a normal 46,XX or 46,XY karyotype, normal stature, and primary amenorrhea; and (3)

Table 338-3 Characteristics of Patients with Classic versus Mosaic Klinefelter Syndrome[a]

	47,XXY, %	46,XY/47,XXY, %
Abnormal testicular histology	100	94[b]
Decreased length of testis	99	73[b]
Azoospermia	93	50[b]
Decreased testosterone	79	33
Decreased facial hair	77	64
Increased gonadotropins	75	33[b]
Decreased sexual function	68	56
Gynecomastia	55	33[b]
Decreased axillary hair	49	46
Decreased length of penis	41	21

[a] Table based on 519 XXY patients and 51 XY/XXY patients.
[b] Significantly different at $p < .05$ or better.
SOURCE: After DL Gordon et al: Arch Intern Med 130:726, 1972.

the Noonan syndrome, an autosomal dominant disorder in both sexes characterized by webbed neck, short stature, congenital heart disease, cubitus valgus, and other congenital defects despite normal karyotypes and normal gonads.

The incidence is estimated at 1 in 3000 newborn females; the prenatal incidence may be as high as 2% of all human conceptuses, only a small fraction of whom survive to term. The diagnosis is made either at birth because of the associated anomalies or at puberty when amenorrhea and failure of sexual development are noted in conjunction with the associated anomalies. Gonadal dysgenesis is the most common cause of primary amenorrhea, accounting for a third of such patients. The external genitalia are unambiguously female but remain immature, and there is no breast development unless exogenous estrogen is given. The fallopian tubes and uterus are immature, and bilateral streak gonads are present in the broad ligaments. Primordial germ cells are present transiently during embryogenesis but disappear because of an accelerated rate of atresia (Chap. 336). After the age of expected puberty, these streaks lack identifiable follicles and ova and consist of fibrous tissue that is indistinguishable from normal ovarian stroma.

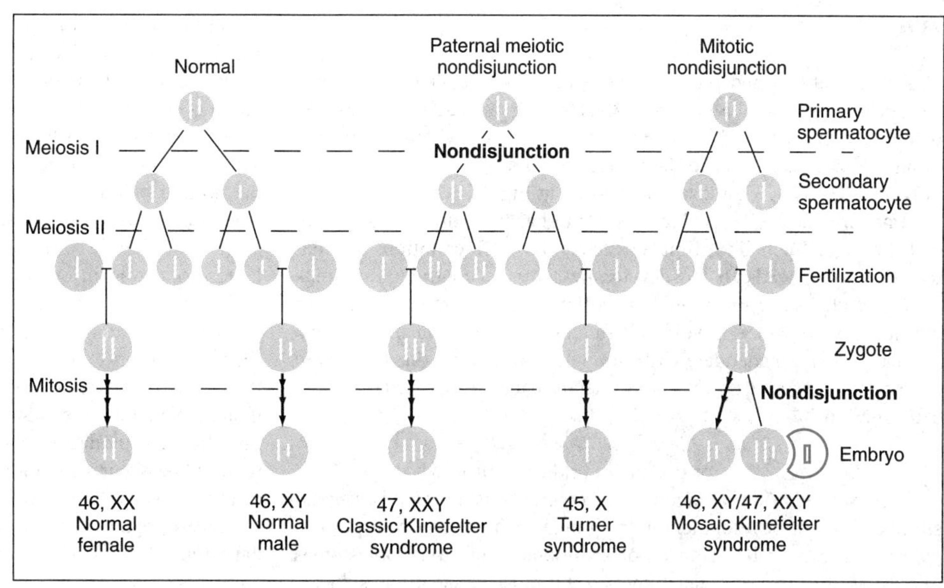

FIGURE 338-2 Schema for normal spermatogenesis and fertilization showing effects of meiotic and mitotic nondisjunction leading to classic Klinefelter syndrome, Turner syndrome, and mosaic Klinefelter. The schema would be similar if the abnormal events took place during oogenesis.

The somatic abnormalities primarily involve the skeleton and connective tissue. Lymphedema of the hands and feet, webbing of the neck, low hairline, redundant skin folds on the back of the neck, a shieldlike chest with widely spaced nipples, and growth retardation are features that suggest the diagnosis in infancy. Micrognathia, epicanthal folds, prominent low-set or deformed ears, a fishlike mouth, and ptosis may be present. Short fourth metacarpals are present in half, and 10 to 20% have coarctation of the aorta. In adults, the average height rarely exceeds 150 cm. Associated conditions include renal malformations, pigmented nevi, hypoplastic nails, tendency to keloid formation, perceptive hearing loss, unexplained hypertension, glucose intolerance, and autoimmune thyroid disease.

Pathophysiology About half have a 45,X karyotype, approximately one-fourth have mosaicism with no structural abnormality (46,XX/45,X), and the remainder have a structurally abnormal X chromosome with or without mosaicism (Chap. 66). The mechanism of chromosome loss is unknown and may occur during gametogenesis in either parent or as a mitotic error during one of the early cleavage divisions of the fertilized zygote (Fig. 338-2). Short stature and other somatic features result from haploinsufficiency of one or more genes encoded on the short arm of the X chromosome. Streak gonads result when genetic material is missing from either the long or short arm of the X. In individuals with mosaicism or structural abnormalities of the X, the phenotype on average is less severe than in the 45,X variety. In some patients with hypertrophy of the clitoris, an unidentified fragment of a chromosome is present and is assumed to be an abnormal Y; gonadoblastoma may develop in the streak gonads in this subset of patients. The Y-linked genes that predispose to gonadoblastoma are distinct from *SRY* because XY women with *SRY* deletions or mutations are also at risk for such tumors. Rarely, familial transmission of gonadal dysgenesis can be the result of a balanced X-autosome translocation (Chap. 66). Analysis of chromosomal karyotype is necessary to establish the diagnosis and to identify the group with Y chromosomal elements and hence a chance of developing malignancy in the streak gonads.

After the time of expected puberty, pubic and axillary hair remain sparse, the breasts are infantile, and no menses occur. Serum FSH is elevated in infancy, falls during midchildhood to the normal range, and increases to castrate levels at the age of 9 or 10. At this time, the serum LH level is also elevated, and plasma estradiol levels are low [<40 pmol/L (<10 pg/mL)]. Approximately 2% of 45,X and 12% of mosaic women have sufficient residual follicles to allow some menstruation, and occasionally minimally affected women become pregnant; the reproductive life in such individuals is brief.

℞ TREATMENT At the anticipated time of puberty, replacement therapy with estrogen should be instituted to induce maturation of the breasts, labia, vagina, uterus, and fallopian tubes (Chap. 336). Linear growth and bone maturation rates usually double during the first year of treatment with estradiol, but the eventual height rarely approaches the predicted height. Combination therapy with oxandrolone and/or growth hormone accelerates growth and increases final height. Streak gonads should be removed in all women who are virilized or have Y-chromosome sequences.

MIXED GONADAL DYSGENESIS **Clinical Features** Mosaicism for a Y-bearing cell line, usually the 45,X/46,XY karyotype, is responsible for most instances of mixed gonadal dysgenesis. Affected individuals usually have a testis on one side and a streak gonad on the other, but bilateral dysgenetic testes or bilateral streak gonads may be present. The incidence is unknown, but in most hospitals the disorder is the second most common cause of ambiguous genitalia in the neonate after congenital adrenal hyperplasia.

The phenotype varies depending on the proportion of XY cells and their distribution. About two-thirds of such children are reared as females. Many have ambiguous genitalia, including phallic enlargement, a urogenital sinus, and some labioscrotal fusion. In most the testis is intraabdominal; individuals with a testis in the inguinal or scrotal position are usually reared as males. A uterus, vagina, and at least one fallopian tube are almost invariably present.

The prepubertal testis appears relatively normal. The postpubertal testis contains abundant Leydig cells, but the seminiferous tubules lack germinal elements and contain only Sertoli cells. The streak gonad, a thin, pale, elongated structure located either in the broad ligament or along the pelvic wall, is composed of ovarian stroma. At puberty the testis secretes androgen, causing virilization and phallic enlargement. Feminization is rare; when it occurs, estrogen secretion from a gonadal tumor should be suspected.

Approximately a third of these individuals exhibit somatic features of 45,X gonadal dysgenesis. Approximately two-thirds have the 45,X/

46,XY karyotype, and the remainder have a 46,XY karyotype or a variant mosaicism. The origin of 45,X/46,XY mosaicism is best explained by the loss of a Y chromosome during an early mitotic division of an XY zygote similar to the postulated loss of the X chromosome in the 46,XY/47,XXY mosaicism shown in Fig. 338-2.

Pathophysiology It is assumed (but has been difficult to prove) that the 46,XY cell line stimulates testicular differentiation, whereas the 45,X stem leads to the development of the contralateral streak gonad. Both masculinization and müllerian duct regression in utero are incomplete. Since Leydig cell function may be that of a normal male at puberty, inadequate virilization in utero may be due to delayed development of a testis that is ultimately capable of normal Leydig cell function.

℞ TREATMENT For the older child or adult in whom gender is established prior to diagnosis, the central consideration is the possibility of tumor development in the gonads, which can occur prior to puberty. The overall incidence of seminomas and gonadoblastomas may be as high as 25%. Such tumors occur most frequently in subjects with a female phenotype who lack the somatic features of 45,X gonadal dysgenesis and are more common in testes than in the streak gonad. When the diagnosis is established in phenotypic females, prophylactic gonadectomy should be performed because gonadal tumors may occur in childhood and because the testes secrete androgen at puberty and thus cause virilization. Such women, like those with gonadal dysgenesis, are then given estrogen to induce and maintain feminization.

When the diagnosis is established in phenotypic males during late childhood or in adults, the management is more complicated. Men with mixed gonadal dysgenesis are infertile (no germinal elements are present in the testes) and have a high risk of developing gonadal tumors. In deciding which testes can be safely conserved the following observations apply: (1) tumors develop in scrotal streak gonads but not in scrotal testes, (2) tumors that develop in intraabdominal testes are always associated with ipsilateral müllerian duct structures, and (3) tumors in streak gonads are always associated with tumors in the contralateral abdominal testis. Based on these observations, it is recommended that (1) all streak gonads should be removed, (2) scrotal testes should be preserved, and (3) intraabdominal testes should be excised unless they can be relocated in the scrotum and are not associated with ipsilateral müllerian duct structures. Reconstructive surgery of the phallus should be performed when appropriate.

When the diagnosis is established in early infancy and the genitalia are ambiguous, gender assignment is usually female, and resection of the phallus and gonadectomy can be performed in infancy, sometimes in one procedure. If the decision is for male gender assignment, the same criteria apply as to which testes should be removed as in older males.

TRUE HERMAPHRODITISM **Clinical Features** True hermaphroditism is a condition in which both an ovary and a testis or one or more gonads with features of both (ovotestis) are present. To justify the diagnosis, both types of gonadal epithelium must be documented histologically, the presence of ovarian stroma without oocytes not being sufficient. The incidence is unknown, but more than 400 cases have been reported. Three categories are recognized: (1) one-fifth are bilateral—testicular and ovarian tissue (ovotestes) on each side; (2) two-fifths are unilateral—an ovotestis on one side and an ovary or a testis on the other; and (3) the remainder are lateral—a testis on one side and an ovary on the other.

The external genitalia exhibit all gradations of the male-to-female spectrum. Two-thirds of affected individuals are sufficiently masculinized to be reared as males, but fewer than one-tenth have normal male external genitalia; most have hypospadias and incomplete labioscrotal fusion. Two-thirds of phenotypic females have an enlarged clitoris, and most have a urogenital sinus. Differentiation of the internal ducts usually corresponds to the adjacent gonad. Although an epididymis usually develops adjacent to a testis, the vas deferens is usually incomplete. Of the patients with an ovotestis, three-fourths have an epididymis, two-thirds have a fallopian tube, one-tenth have a vas deferens, and one-tenth have both a vas deferens and a fallopian tube. The uterus may be hypoplastic or unicornuate. The ovary is usually in the normal position, but the testis or ovotestis may be found at any level along the route of testicular descent, frequently associated with an inguinal hernia. Testicular tissue is present in the scrotum or the labioscrotal fold in one-third, in the inguinal canal in one-third, and in the abdomen in one-third.

Variable feminization and virilization ensue at puberty; three-fourths develop gynecomastia, and about half menstruate. In phenotypic men, menstruation may cause cyclic hematuria. Ovulation occurs in approximately one-fourth and is more common than spermatogenesis. In men, ovulation may cause testicular pain. Fertility has been reported in women and more rarely in men. Congenital malformations of other systems are unusual.

Pathophysiology About two-thirds of individuals have a 46,XX karyotype, a tenth have a 46,XY karyotype, and the remainder are chimeras or mosaics in whom a Y cell line is present. The mechanism responsible for the abnormal gonadal development is unknown. Only 10% of 46,XX true hermaphrodites are *SRY* positive, presumably the consequence of mosaicism or translocation of a portion of the Y chromosome; the remainder are believed to result from gain-of-function mutations in downstream genes involved in *SRY* action. On occasion, multiple sibs with a 46,XX karyotype are affected, possibly the result of an autosomal or X-linked mutation.

Because corpora lutea are frequently present in the ovaries, it is presumed that the female neuroendocrine axis functions normally in such individuals. Feminization (gynecomastia and menstruation) is the result of secretion of estradiol by ovarian tissue. In masculinized patients, secretion of androgen predominates, and some produce sperm.

℞ TREATMENT When the diagnosis is made in early infancy, gender assignment depends on the anatomic features. In older children and adults, gonads and internal duct structures that are contradictory to the predominant phenotype (and the gender of rearing) should be removed, and the external genitalia should be modified when appropriate. Gonadal tumors are rare but have been reported in true hermaphrodites who carry Y chromosome sequences. Consequently, the possibility of future tumor development must be taken into account when the decision is made to preserve gonadal tissue.

DISORDERS OF GONADAL SEX

Disorders of gonadal sex result when chromosomal sex is normal but differentiation of the gonads is abnormal. Thus, gonadal sex does not correspond to chromosomal sex.

PURE GONADAL DYSGENESIS **Clinical Features** Pure gonadal dysgenesis is a disorder in which phenotypic females with gonads and genitalia characteristic of gonadal dysgenesis (bilateral streaks, infantile uterus and fallopian tubes, and sexual infantilism) have normal height, few if any somatic anomalies, and either a normal 46,XX or 46,XY karyotype. This disorder is about one-tenth as common as gonadal dysgenesis. It is genetically distinct but cannot be distinguished clinically from those instances of gonadal dysgenesis with minimal somatic abnormalities. The height is normal or greater than normal, some individuals being >170 cm. Estrogen levels vary from profound deficiency typical of 45,X gonadal dysgenesis to some breast development and menses that terminate in an early menopause. About 40% have some feminization. Axillary and pubic hair is scanty, and the internal genitalia consist of müllerian derivatives only. In both the 46,XX and the 46,XY forms the disorder prevents differentiation of ovary or testis, respectively; the development of the female phenotype and the elevation of gonadotropin secretion are due to failure of gonadal development.

Tumors may develop in the streak gonads, particularly dysgerminoma or gonadoblastoma in the 46,XY disorder. Such tumors may be heralded by the development of virilizing signs or a pelvic mass.

Pathophysiology Although chromosomal mosaicisms have been described under this nosology, the designation here is restricted to women with uniform 46,XX or 46,XY karyotypes. (Those with mosaicism are variants of gonadal dysgenesis or mixed gonadal dysgenesis, as described above.) The rationale for this restricted definition is based on the fact that both the XX and XY varieties can result from single gene mutations that are presumed to involve gene(s) essential for gonadal development. Several sibships have been reported in which more than one individual is affected with the 46,XX disorder, frequently the result of consanguineous matings, suggesting an autosomal recessive inheritance.

The 46,XY variety may occur in families; in some the disorder appears to be inherited as an X-linked trait, and in others the pattern suggests a male-limited autosomal recessive inheritance. About 15% of 46,XY women have either a deletion or a mutation in the *SRY* coding sequence. Other instances could be due to mutations in *SRY* outside the coding sequence, in other genes that influence *SRY* expression, or in the downstream genes that are controlled by *SRY*. Indeed, mutations in several genes that are downstream of *SRY* are now known to be a cause of the dysgenetic testes syndrome (also termed *dysgenetic male pseudohermaphroditism*; see below).

℞ TREATMENT The management of the estrogen deficiency is identical to that in gonadal dysgenesis; namely, appropriate estrogen replacement therapy is initiated at the time of expected puberty and maintained in adult life (Chap. 336). Because of the high frequency of gonadal tumors in the 46,XY variety, the streak gonads should be removed once the diagnosis is made; development of virilizing signs is indication for immediate surgery. The natural history of the gonadal tumors is uncertain, but the prognosis after surgical removal is usually good.

DYSGENETIC TESTES Individuals with these disorders are genetic males with disorders of testicular development that vary from streak gonads similar to those in gonadal dysgenesis to less severe defects. The disorders are frequently associated with systemic abnormalities, because many of the genes involved are also involved in the development of other tissues. The first of these genes to be identified was the Wilms' tumor gene *WT1*; mutations of this gene cause two disorders—the Denys-Drash and Frasier syndromes. *Denys-Drash syndrome* is an autosomal dominant disorder characterized by development of Wilms' tumors in males with a spectrum of gonadal defects ranging from streak gonads to less severely affected testes; urogenital defects include diffuse mesangial sclerosis of the kidneys. The underlying mutations in the zinc finger region of WT-1 are believed to inhibit the function of the wild-type protein and hence act as dominant negative mutations. Patients with *Frasier syndrome* have gonadal dysgenesis, impaired virilization, and focal sclerosis of the kidney but do not develop Wilms' tumors. Mutations in intron 9 of the *WT1* gene that cause Frasier syndrome interfere with the synthesis of specific splice variants of *WT1*.

A second downstream gene that is essential for differentiation of the testes is *SF1* (also known as *FTZF1*), a member of the nuclear hormone receptor superfamily. SF-1 regulates the expression of many genes involved in adrenal and gonadal development and steroidogenesis, as well as the *AMH* gene. Heterozygous mutation of this autosomal gene has been associated with 46,XY gonadal dysgenesis with adrenal insufficiency.

Another downstream gene is *SOX9*, a close relative of *SRY* that maps to chromosome 17q. This gene is expressed in high levels in the testes, where it is believed to be a key regulator of male differentiation. Heterozygous mutations of this gene cause 46,XY gonadal dysgenesis and skeletal abnormalities (*campomelic dysplasia*).

46,XY gonadal dysgenesis is also associated with duplication of the short arm of the X chromosome (Xp21), a phenomenon termed *dosage-sensitive sex reversal*. Loss-of-function mutations of the *DAX1* gene in this region of the X chromosome are associated with adrenal hypoplasia congenita and hypogonadotrophic hypogonadism. The DAX-1 protein inhibits the expression of SF-1-regulated genes, providing a potential mechanism by which an excess of DAX-1 could cause gonadal dysgenesis in genetic males with Xp21 duplications.

THE ABSENT TESTES SYNDROME (ANORCHIA, TESTICULAR REGRESSION, GONADAL AGENESIS, AGONADISM) Clinical Features A spectrum of phenotypes occurs in 46,XY males with absent or rudimentary testes but in whom unequivocal evidence exists that endocrine function of the testis (e.g., consistent müllerian duct regression and variable testosterone synthesis) was present at some time during embryonic life. In pure gonadal dysgenesis, in contrast, no evidence can be inferred for gonadal function during embryonic development. The manifestations vary from complete failure of virilization to incomplete virilization of the external genitalia to otherwise normal men with bilateral anorchia.

The purest form is represented by 46,XY females with absent testes, sexual infantilism, and absence of both müllerian duct derivatives and accessory organs of male reproduction. Such individuals differ from those with 46,XY pure gonadal dysgenesis in that no gonadal remnant can be identified, including no streak gonad and no müllerian derivatives. Testicular failure must have occurred, therefore, between the onset of AMH synthesis and the onset of testosterone secretion (e.g., after development of Sertoli cells but before the onset of Leydig cell function).

In others, testicular failure occurred later in gestation, and these individuals may constitute problems in gender assignment. In some, failure of müllerian regression is more pronounced than failure of testosterone secretion, but none exhibit normal müllerian development. In those with more extensive virilization, the external genitalia are phenotypically male, but rudimentary oviducts and vasa deferentia may coexist internally.

At the final extreme is the syndrome of bilateral anorchia in which phenotypic men have absence of müllerian structures and gonads but male wolffian duct derivatives and external genitalia. Microphallus implies that failure of testosterone secretion occurred late in embryogenesis after anatomic development of the male urethra was complete. Gynecomastia may or may not be present.

Pathophysiology The pathogenesis is not understood. Testicular regression could be the result of mutant genes, teratogen, or trauma, and the disorder may well be heterogeneous in origin. Several instances of agonadism have occurred in the same family, some unilateral and others bilateral. Some individuals in whom no testes can be identified at laparotomy have blood testosterone values above the castrate range, presumably derived from remnant testes.

℞ TREATMENT The management of the two extremes is clear-cut. Sexually infantile, phenotypic females should be given adequate estrogen to ensure appropriate feminization, and any coexisting vaginal agenesis should be treated by surgical or medical means. Likewise, phenotypic males with anorchia should be given androgen replacement to allow normal male secondary sexual development. Individuals with incomplete virilization or ambiguous external genitalia demonstrate a more complex problem and require careful assessment to determine appropriate gender assignment, hormonal therapy at the time of expected puberty, and surgical correction of the external genitalia when appropriate.

DISORDERS OF PHENOTYPIC SEX

Disorders of phenotypic sex occur in 46,XX or 46,XY individuals with appropriate gonadal sex but in whom development of the urogenital tract is inappropriate for the chromosomal/gonadal sex.

FEMALE PSEUDOHERMAPHRODITISM Female pseudohermaphroditism occurs in 46,XX women with bilateral ovaries but

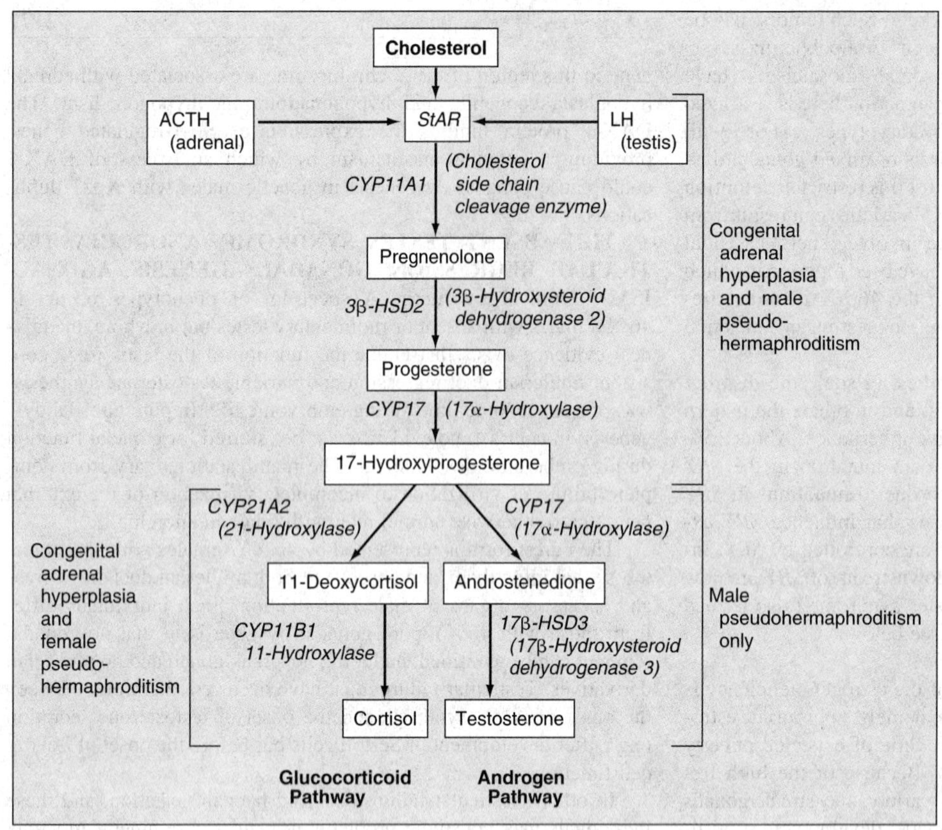

FIGURE 338-3 Pathways of glucocorticoid and androgen synthesis. Note abnormal conditions corresponding to impaired enzyme reactions.

with variable virilization of the urogenital tract because of androgen excess during fetal life.

Congenital Adrenal Hyperplasia • *Clinical features* The pathways by which glucocorticoids are synthesized in the adrenal gland and androgens are formed in the testis and adrenal are summarized in Fig. 338-3. Three reactions are common to both pathways (cholesterol side chain cleavage, 3β-hydroxysteroid dehydrogenase/isomerase, and 17α-hydroxylase); impairment of any of these reactions results in deficiency of glucocorticoid and androgen synthesis and consequently causes both congenital adrenal hyperplasia (due to enhanced ACTH levels) and defective virilization of the male embryo (male pseudohermaphroditism). Two reactions are involved exclusively in androgen synthesis (17,20-lyase and 17β-hydroxysteroid dehydrogenase); deficiency in either results in pure male pseudohermaphroditism with normal glucocorticoid synthesis. Deficiency of either of the terminal two enzymes of glucocorticoid synthesis (21-hydroxylase and 11β-hydroxylase) impairs formation of hydrocortisone; the compensatory increase in ACTH secretion causes adrenal hyperplasia and a secondary increase in androgen formation that virilizes the female and induces precocious masculinization in the male.

The major features of congenital adrenal hyperplasia are listed in Table 338-4. The *adrenal insufficiency* can be equally severe and life-threatening in both sexes and is described in Chap. 331. Some defects in steroidogenesis cause female pseudohermaphroditism, and some cause male pseudohermaphroditism. (3β-hydroxysteroid dehydrogenase/isomerase deficiency can cause either male or female pseudohermaphroditism, but since incomplete virilization of the male is more common, the disorder will be discussed under male pseudohermaphroditism.)

Congenital adrenal hyperplasia due to classic 21-hydroxylase deficiency is the most common cause of ambiguous genitalia in the newborn, with an incidence of between 1 in 5000 and 1 in 15,000 live births in Europe and the United States; it may or may not be associated with mineralocorticoid deficiency (salt loss) (Table 338-4). Virilization is usually apparent at birth in the female and within the first 2 to 3 years of life in the male. Manifestations in females include hypertrophy of the clitoris with ventral chordee, partial fusion of the labioscrotal folds, and variable virilization of the urethra. The uterus, fallopian tubes, and ovaries are normal, and the wolffian ducts do not virilize, probably because adrenal function begins relatively late in embryogenesis. The external appearance of an affected female newborn is similar to that of a male with bilateral cryptorchidism and hypospadias. The labioscrotal folds are bulbous and rugated and resemble a scrotum. Rarely, the virilization is so severe that development of a complete penile urethra and prostate results in errors in sex assignment at birth. Radiography following the injection of radiopaque dye into the external genital orifice is helpful in demonstrating the presence of vagina, uterus, and (sometimes) fallopian tubes. Occasionally, virilization of the female is slight or absent at birth and becomes evident in later infancy, adolescence, or adulthood (the so-called nonclassic or late-onset form of the disorder). In both sexes, rapid somatic maturation results in premature epiphyseal closure and a short adult height. The untreated female with the classic disorder grows rapidly during the first year of life and has progressive virilization. At the time of expected puberty

Table 338-4 Forms of Congenital Adrenal Hyperplasia

Deficiency	Cortisol	Aldosterone	Degree of Virilization of Females	Failure of Virilization in Males	Dominant Steroid Secreted	Comment
Classic 21-hydroxylase:						
Partial (simple virilizing or compensated)	Normal	↑	++++	none	17-Hydroxyprogesterone	Most common type (95% of total); from one- to two-thirds salt losers
Severe (salt-losing)	↓	↓	++++	none	17-Hydroxyprogesterone	
11β-Hydroxylase (hypertension)	↓	↓	++++	none	11-Deoxycortisol and 11-deoxycorticosterone	Hypertension
3β-Hydroxysteroid dehydrogenase/isomerase 2	↓	↓	+	++++	Δ^5-3β-OH compounds (dehydroepiandrosterone)	Probably second most common, usually salt loss
17α-Hydroxylase	↓	↓	none	++++	Corticosterone and 11-deoxycorticosterone	No feminization of female, hypertension
StAR protein	absent	absent	none	++++	Cholesterol(?)	Rare, usually salt loss

there is a failure of normal female sexual development and absence of menstruation.

Since male phenotypic differentiation is normal, the condition is usually not recognized at birth in boys in the absence of adrenal insufficiency. However, early maturation of the external genitalia, development of secondary sex characteristics, coarsening of the voice, frequent erections, and excessive muscular development are noticeable during the first few years of life. Virilization in the male can follow two patterns. Excessive adrenal androgens can inhibit gonadotropin production so that the testes remain infantile in size despite the acceleration of masculinization. Such untreated adult men are capable of erection and ejaculation but have no spermatogenesis. Alternatively, adrenal androgen secretion can induce premature maturation of the hypothalamic-pituitary axis and initiate a true precocious puberty including early maturation of spermatogenesis (Chap. 335). The untreated male is also subject to the development of ACTH-dependent "tumors" of the adrenal rest cells of the testes.

In classic 21-hydroxylase deficiency, which accounts for about 95% of congenital adrenal hyperplasia, decreased production of hydrocortisone leads to increased release of ACTH, enlargement of the adrenal glands, and partial or complete compensation of the defect in the secretion of hydrocortisone. In about half, the enzyme defect appears to be partial, and cortisol secretion is normal. This form is termed *simple virilizing*. When deficiency of the enzyme is more complete, the so-called salt-losing form of 21-hydroxylase deficiency, production of cortisol and aldosterone is inadequate, leading to severe salt wastage with anorexia, vomiting, volume depletion, and vascular collapse within the first few weeks of life. In untreated patients, there is overproduction of the cortisol precursors prior to the 21-hydroxylase step, causing an increase in plasma progesterone and 17-hydroxyprogesterone. These steroids are weak aldosterone antagonists at the receptor level; in the compensated state aldosterone production increases to attempt to maintain normal sodium balance. Increased substrate availability is also responsible for the enhanced androgen synthesis and hence for the virilization.

Female pseudohermaphroditism also occurs in 11β-hydroxylase deficiency. In this disorder, a block in hydroxylation at the 11-carbon results in the accumulation of 11-deoxycortisol and deoxycorticosterone (DOC), a potent salt-retaining hormone that causes hypertension rather than salt loss. The clinical features that stem from glucocorticoid deficiency and androgen excess are similar to those in 21-hydroxylase deficiency.

Pathophysiology Both disorders are due to autosomal recessive mutations. The carrier frequency for CYP21A2 deficiency is about 1 in 50. Because the gene is located on the sixth chromosome close to the HLA-B locus, heterozygous carriers and homozygotes within a given family can be identified on the basis of the HLA haplotype. At the molecular level the mutations that give rise to 21-hydroxylase deficiency are highly polymorphic; indeed, partial gene deletions (10 to 30%), conversion of the gene from a functional state to a form that is not transcribed normally (10%), and point mutations (60 to 75%) have been characterized in the disorder. The classic disorder is due to mutations that severely impair enzyme activity, and less severe mutations cause the nonclassic, or late-onset, variety. 11β-hydroxylase activity is encoded by two genes on chromosome 8; mutations of the *CYP11B1* gene are responsible for this disorder. The *CYP11B2* gene encodes aldosterone synthase. A late-onset variant of 11β-hydroxylase deficiency exists but has not been characterized at the molecular level.

Urinary excretion of 17-ketosteroids and of the metabolites that accumulate proximal to the enzymatic blocks is increased. Plasma ACTH is elevated. In CYP21A2 deficiency, 17-hydroxyprogesterone accumulates in blood and is excreted predominantly as pregnanetriol. In CYP11B1 deficiency, 11-deoxycortisol accumulates in blood and is excreted predominantly as tetrahydrocortexolone. →*For additional discussion of the endocrine pathology, see Chap. 331.*

℞ TREATMENT Gender assignment should correspond to the chromosomal and gonadal sex, and appropriate surgical correction of the external genitalia should be undertaken as early as possible. This is of importance because appropriately treated men and women are capable of fertility. However, if the correct diagnosis is made late (after 3 years of age), gender assignment should be changed only after careful consideration of the psychosexual background.

Treatment with appropriate glucocorticoids prevents the consequences of hydrocortisone deficiency, arrests the rapid virilization, and prevents premature somatic and epiphyseal maturation. The suppression of the abnormal steroid secretion corrects the hypertension in CYP11B1 deficiency and in both disorders allows normal onset of menses and development of female secondary sex characteristics. In males, glucocorticoid therapy suppresses adrenal androgens and results in normal gonadotropin secretion, testicular development, and spermatogenesis. The usual maintenance dose of hydrocortisone is 10 to 20 mg/m^2 per day, given in three divided doses. However, the dose must be adjusted on an individual basis to optimize ACTH suppression while avoiding glucocorticoid side effects, which include growth retardation as well as Cushingoid features. Measurements of plasma 17-hydroxyprogesterone, androstenedione, ACTH, and renin levels have all been used to assess adequacy of replacement therapy. In severe CYP21A2 deficiency associated with salt loss or elevated plasma renin activity, treatment with mineralocorticoids is also indicated, and plasma renin levels should be monitored to assess the adequacy of mineralocorticoid replacement. Trials are underway to assess the potential use of antiandrogens (e.g., spironolactone, cyproterone acetate, flutamide) or aromatase inhibitors (e.g., latrazole, testolactone) as adjunctive therapy that may allow reductions in glucocorticoid dose. Treatment of affected fetuses in utero (beginning at 4 to 6 weeks) has been accomplished by administering dexamethasone (which crosses the placenta) to the mother. Though this treatment can reduce the extent of virilization in some girls, it is associated with maternal side effects, and the long-term consequences have not been established.

Other Causes of Female Pseudohermaphroditism Placental aromatase deficiency due to mutations in the gene encoding aromatase (*CYP19*) causes virilization of female embryos because of defective conversion of androgens to estrogens in the placenta and the secondary increase in testosterone levels in the fetus; in postnatal life CYP19 deficiency in women causes hirsutism and development of polycystic ovaries. Female pseudohermaphroditism can also occur in babies born to mothers with virilizing tumors of the ovary (e.g., arrhenoblastomas or luteomas of pregnancy) and, rarely, to mothers with virilizing adrenal tumors. In the past, the administration to pregnant women of progestogens with androgenic side effects (such as 17α-ethinyl-19-nor-testosterone) to prevent abortion resulted in masculinization of female fetuses.

Developmental Disorders of Müllerian Ducts (Congenital Absence of the Vagina, Müllerian Agenesis) • ***Clinical features*** Congenital hypoplasia or absence of the vagina in combination with abnormal or absent uterus (the Mayer-Rokitansky-Kuster-Hauser syndrome) is second to gonadal dysgenesis as a cause of primary amenorrhea. Most patients are ascertained after the time of expected puberty because of failure to menstruate. The height is normal, and the breasts, axillary and pubic hair, and habitus are feminine in character. The uterus can vary from almost normal, lacking only a conduit to the introitus, to the characteristic rudimentary bicornuate cords with or without a lumen. In some patients cyclic abdominal pain indicates that sufficient functional endometrium is present to result in retrograde menstruation and/or hematometra.

About one-third have abnormal kidneys, most commonly agenesis, ectopy, fused kidneys of the horseshoe type, or solitary ectopic kidneys in the pelvis. Skeletal abnormalities are present in one-tenth; most involve the spine, and limb and rib defects account for the rest. Specific abnormalities include wedge vertebrae, fused rudimentary or asymmetric vertebral bodies, supernumerary vertebrae, and the Klippel-Feil syndrome (congenital fusion of the cervical spine, short neck, low posterior hairline, and painless limitation of cervical movement).

Pathophysiology The karyotype is 46,XX. Familial occurrence has been described, and the pattern of inheritance in most is consistent with a sex-limited autosomal dominant mutation. Sporadic cases may represent new mutations of the type responsible for the familial disorder or be multifactorial in etiology. In the familial cases, expressivity is variable; some have skeletal or renal abnormalities only, and some have other abnormalities of müllerian derivatives such as a double uterus. Bilateral renal aplasia in stillborn infants is commonly associated with absence of the uterus and vagina. Thus, the family history should be probed for isolated skeletal and renal abnormalities and for stillbirths that might result from congenital absence of both kidneys. Ovarian function is normal, and successful pregnancies have occurred after corrective vaginal surgery in patients with a normal uterus.

℞ TREATMENT Vaginal agenesis can be treated by surgical or nonsurgical means. Surgical repair generally utilizes a split-thickness skin graft around a solid rubber mold to create an artificial vagina. Medical therapy involves the repeated application of pressure against the vaginal dimple with a simple dilator to force development of adequate vaginal depth. In view of complication rates of 5 to 10% in surgical series, surgery should be reserved for patients in whom a well-formed uterus is present and the possibility of fertility exists. Frequent coitus or instrumental dilatation is essential for maintaining patency of neovaginas formed by either technique.

MALE PSEUDOHERMAPHRODITISM Defective virilization of the 46,XY embryo (male pseudohermaphroditism) can result from defects in androgen synthesis, defects in androgen action, defects in müllerian duct regression, and uncertain causes.

Abnormalities in Androgen Synthesis • ***Clinical features*** Enzymatic defects that result in defective testosterone synthesis (Fig. 338-3) account for only about a fifth of cases of male pseudohermaphroditism (Tables 338-4 and 338-5). Each of the defects blocks a step in the conversion of cholesterol to testosterone. Three enzymatic reactions are common to the synthesis of other adrenal hormones as well: cholesterol side chain cleavage, 3β-hydroxysteroid dehydrogenase/isomerase, and 17α-hydroxylase (CYP17). Consequently, their deficiency results in congenital adrenal hyperplasia (Table 338-4) as well as male pseudohermaphroditism. Two others (17,20-lyase and 17β-hydroxysteroid dehydrogenase 3) are unique to the pathway of androgen synthesis, and their deficiency results only in male pseudohermaphroditism. Since androgens are obligatory precursors of estrogens, synthesis of estrogen is also low in all but the terminal defect (17β-hydroxysteroid dehydrogenase 3 deficiency).

Adrenal dysfunction is described in Chap. 331, and the present discussion concerns the abnormal sexual development. In genetic males with defective testosterone synthesis, absence of the uterus and fallopian tubes indicates that müllerian duct inhibition was normal during embryogenesis. Masculinization of the urogenital tract and external genitalia and virilization at puberty vary from almost normal to absent, and, therefore, the manifestations vary from men with mild hypospadias to phenotypic women who prior to puberty resemble women with complete testicular feminization. This heterogeneity is the consequence of varying severity of the enzymatic defects, varying effects of the steroids that accumulate proximal to the various metabolic blocks, and the presence of alternative enzymatic pathways in some disorders. In patients with partial defects in whom the plasma testosterone level is normal, the diagnosis can only be made by measuring the steroids that accumulate proximal to the metabolic block.

Congenital lipoid adrenal hyperplasia is an autosomal recessive disorder in which virtually no urinary steroids (either 17-ketosteroids or 17-hydroxycorticoids) can be detected. Since the defect blocks the conversion of cholesterol to pregnenolone, a step catalyzed by the cholesterol side chain cleavage enzyme (CYP11A1), it was originally assumed that the defect must involve this enzyme. However, the disorder is instead caused by mutations in the *st*eroidogenic *a*cute *r*egulatory (*StAR*) gene, which encodes the protein that transports cholesterol from the cytosol to the inner mitochondrial membrane in the adrenal and gonads. Manifestations of the disorder include salt wasting and profound adrenal insufficiency, and most affected individuals die during infancy. At autopsy, the adrenals and testes are enlarged and infiltrated with lipid. Affected males are incompletely masculinized, whereas affected female infants have normal genital development because lipid accumulation in the ovary does not occur until there is follicular development and active steroidogenesis.

3β-Hydroxysteroid dehydrogenase/isomerase 2 deficiency causes varying failure of masculinization and the development of a vagina in male infants. Female infants may be modestly virilized at birth due to the weak androgenic potency of dehydroepiandrosterone, the major steroid secreted. If the enzyme is absent in both the adrenal and testis, no urinary steroids contain a Δ^4-3-keto configuration, whereas in patients in whom the defect is partial or affects only the testis, the urine may contain normal or elevated levels of Δ^4-3-ketosteroids. Most patients have marked salt wasting and profound adrenal insufficiency, and long-term survival in untreated cases occurs only in states of partial deficiency. Minimally affected males may experience an otherwise normal male puberty except for profound gynecomastia. In these boys, a low-normal blood testosterone level is accompanied by elevated Δ^5 precursor steroids. 3β-Hydroxysteroid dehydrogenase activity is catalyzed by more than one isoenzyme. The type 2 isoenzyme is expressed in adrenals and gonads; the disorder described above is due to any of several mutations in this enzyme. The coding sequence of this gene is said to be normal in several individuals with the late-onset variant of the disease, the pathophysiology of which is unclear.

17α-Hydroxylase-17,20-lyase (CYP17) *deficiency* impairs the introduction of the 17-hydroxyl and the scission of the C-17,20 carbon bond that convert pregnenolone and progesterone to dehydroepiandrosterone and androstenedione, respectively. These reactions are mediated by a single enzyme CYP17, which is encoded on chromosome 10; it remains unclear why both reactions occur in the ovary and testis, whereas in the adrenal 17-hydroxyprogesterone is largely converted to glucocorticoids and mineralocorticoids rather than the 19-carbon steroids. Of note, some patients appear to have selective impairment of either 17α-hydroxylase or 17,20-lyase activity. These mutations have identified enzyme domains proposed to undergo posttranslational modification and selective interactions with cofactors that switch enzymatic activity. Whatever the mechanism, the consequences of 17α-hydroxylase and 17,20-lyase deficiencies are different.

17α-Hydroxylase deficiency is characterized by hypogonadism, absence of secondary sex characteristics, hypokalemic alkalosis, hypertension, and virtually undetectable hydrocortisone secretion in phenotypic women. Formation of both corticosterone and DOC by the adrenal is elevated, and urinary 17-ketosteroids are low. Aldosterone secretion is low due to high plasma DOC and depressed angiotensin levels and returns to normal after suppressive doses of glucocorticoids. In 46,XX individuals, amenorrhea, absent sexual hair, and hypertension are common, but the phenotype is that of a normal prepubertal woman. In males, the deficiency results in defective virilization that varies from complete male pseudohermaphroditism to ambiguous genitalia with perineoscrotal hypospadias and, in some, gynecomastia. Adrenal insufficiency does not develop, since the secretion of both corticosterone (a weak glucocorticoid) and DOC (a mineralocorticoid) is elevated. Hypertension and hypokalemia are prominent (even in the neonatal period) and remit after suppression of the DOC secretion by glucocorticoid replacement. A variety of point mutations, deletions, and insertions in the *CYP17* gene have been characterized in affected individuals.

17,20-Lyase deficiency in males is associated with normal function of the adrenal cortex and a variable pattern of male pseudohermaphroditism. In the majority there is genital ambiguity at birth, with some virilization at the time of expected puberty. Rare 46,XY patients

Table 338-5 Anatomic, Genetic, and Endocrine Profile of Hereditary Male Pseudohermaphroditism

Disorder	Inheritance	Phenotype: Müllerian Ducts	Phenotype: Wolffian Ducts	Phenotype: Spermatogenesis	Phenotype: Urogenital Sinus	Phenotype: External Genitalia	Phenotype: Breast	Endocrine Profile Relative to Normal Male: Testosterone Production	Endocrine Profile Relative to Normal Male: Estrogen Production	Endocrine Profile Relative to Normal Male: LH
DEFECTS IN TESTOSTERONE SYNTHESIS										
Five enzymatic defects	Autosomal recessive	Absent	Variable development	Normal or decreased	Variable from male to female	Generally female	Usually male	Normal to decreased	Variable	High
DEFECTS IN ANDROGEN ACTION										
Steroid 5α-reductase 2 deficiency	Autosomal recessive	Absent	Male	Normal or decreased	Female	Clitoromegaly	Male	Normal	Normal	Normal or increased
Receptor disorders:										
Complete testicular feminization	X-linked recessive	Absent	Absent	Absent	Female	Female	Female	High	High	High
Incomplete testicular feminization	X-linked	Absent	Male	Absent	Female	Clitoromegaly and posterior fusion	Female	High	High	High
Reifenstein syndrome	X-linked recessive	Absent	Variable development	Absent	Variable from male to female	Incomplete male development	Female	High	High	High
Infertile or undervirilized fertile male	X-linked recessive	Absent	Male	Absent to normal	Male	Male	Usually male	Normal or high	Normal or high	Normal or high
DEFECTS IN MÜLLERIAN REGRESSION										
Persistent müllerian duct syndrome	Autosomal recessive	Rudimentary uterus and fallopian tubes	Male	Normal	Male	Male	Male	Normal	Normal	Normal

have had a female phenotype and no virilization at the time of expected puberty. The disorder has been recognized in one 46,XX woman with sexual infantilism. Mutations of *CYP17* that cause this disorder involve an area of the gene that is known to encode a binding site for the redox-partner of the enzyme.

17β-Hydroxysteroid dehydrogenase 3 (17β-HSD-3) *deficiency* involves the final step in testosterone biosynthesis, reduction of the 17-keto group of androstenedione. This is the most common enzymatic defect in testosterone synthesis. Affected 46,XY males usually have a female phenotype with a blind-ending vagina and absence of müllerian derivatives, but inguinal or abdominal testes and virilized wolffian duct structures are present. At the time of expected puberty, both virilization (with phallic enlargement and development of facial and body hair) and a variable degree of feminization take place. In some untreated patients, reversal of gender behavior from female to male occurs at puberty. Plasma testosterone level may be in the low-normal range, making it essential to document elevation in plasma androstenedione to make the diagnosis. Isoenzymes encoded by several different genes possess 17β-hydroxysteroid dehydrogenase activity, but the isoenzyme 3 is expressed in the testes. A variety of mutations have been characterized in the 17β-HSD-3 gene in affected individuals.

Pathophysiology These various disorders are inherited as autosomal recessive traits. The pattern of steroid secretion and excretion depends on the site of the various metabolic blocks (Fig. 338-3). In general, gonadotropin secretion is high, and many individuals with incomplete defects are able to compensate so that the steady-state levels of testosterone may be normal or almost normal.

In rare cases of male pseudohermaphroditism, testosterone formation is deficient for reasons other than a single enzyme defect in androgen synthesis. These include disorders in which Leydig cell agenesis is due to autosomal recessive loss-of-function mutations of the LH receptor or to the secretion of a biologically inactive LH molecule. In addition, as described above, several disorders, including familial 46,XY pure gonadal dysgenesis, sporadic dysgenetic testes, and the absent testis syndrome, are characterized by deficient testosterone production due to abnormal gonadal development.

Rx TREATMENT Therapy with glucocorticoids and in some instances mineralocorticoids is indicated in those disorders causing adrenal hyperplasia. The management of the genital abnormalities depends on the individual case. Fertility has not been reported, and its consideration does not enter into sex assignment. In genetic females there is no problem (except in diagnosis), in that affected individuals are raised appropriately as females and estrogen therapy is begun at the time of expected puberty to promote development of female secondary sex characteristics. Whether newborn males with ambiguous genitalia should be raised as males or females depends on the anatomic defect; in general, the more severely affected should be raised as females, and corrective surgery of the genitalia and removal of the testes should be undertaken as early as possible. In such women estrogen therapy is begun at the appropriate age to allow development of normal female secondary sex characteristics. In individuals raised as males, corrective surgery is indicated for any coexisting hypospadias, and plasma androgens should be monitored at the time of expected puberty to determine whether testosterone therapy is appropriate.

Abnormalities in Androgen Action Several disorders of male phenotypic development result from abnormalities of androgen action. The spectrum of phenotypes is described in Tables 338-4 and 338-5. In these disorders, testosterone formation and müllerian regression are normal, but male development is impaired because of resistance to androgen action in target tissues.

Steroid 5α-reductase 2 deficiency This autosomal recessive disorder is characterized by (1) severe perineoscrotal hypospadias; (2) a blind vaginal pouch of variable size opening either into the urogenital sinus or into the urethra; (3) testes with normal epididymides, vasa deferentia, and seminal vesicles, and termination of the ejaculatory ducts in the blind-ending vagina; (4) a female habitus with normal axillary and pubic hair but without female breast development; (5) the absence of uterus and fallopian tubes; (6) normal male plasma testosterone; and (7) masculinization to a variable degree at the time of puberty.

The realization that virilization during embryogenesis is defective only in the urogenital sinus and the external genitalia provided insight into the fundamental abnormality. Testosterone, the androgen secreted by the fetal testis, is responsible for conversion of the wolffian duct into the epididymis, vas deferens, and seminal vesicle, whereas dihydrotestosterone mediates virilization of the urogenital sinus and the external genitalia. Consequently, impairment of dihydrotestosterone formation in a male embryo would be expected to cause the phenotype in this disorder—normal male wolffian duct derivatives with defective masculinization of the external genitalia and urogenital sinus. Since testosterone itself regulates LH secretion (Chap. 335), plasma LH level is normal or minimally elevated. As a result, testosterone and estrogen production rates are those of normal men, and gynecomastia does not develop.

The fact that 5α-reductase 2 enzyme is deficient in this disorder was established by assay of biopsied tissues and cultured fibroblasts from affected individuals. Deletions or point mutations in the gene encoding steroid 5α-reductase 2 have been identified in most families studied. Approximately 40% are compound heterozygotes.

Receptor disorders The androgen receptor is a member of the steroid/thyroid family of receptors with steroid-binding, DNA-binding, and functional domains and is encoded by a gene on the long arm of the X chromosome. Mutations of this gene impair receptor function and hence impair male phenotypic differentiation and/or virilization.

CLINICAL FEATURES *Complete testicular feminization* (also called *complete androgen insensitivity*) is a common form of male pseudohermaphroditism; estimates of frequency vary from 1 in 20,000 to 1 in 64,000 male births. It is the third most common cause of primary amenorrhea after gonadal dysgenesis and congenital absence of the vagina. The features are characteristic. Namely, a woman is ascertained either because of inguinal hernia (prepubertal) or primary amenorrhea (postpubertal). The development of the breasts, the habitus, and the distribution of body fat are female in character so that most have a truly feminine appearance. Axillary and pubic hair is absent or scanty, but some vulval hair is usually present. Scalp hair is that of a normal woman, and facial hair is absent. The external genitalia are unambiguously female, and the clitoris is normal. The vagina is short and blind-ending and may be absent or rudimentary. All internal genitalia are absent except for testes that contain normal Leydig cells and seminiferous tubules without spermatogenesis. The testes may be located in the abdomen, along the course of the inguinal canal, or in the labia majora. Occasionally, remnants of müllerian or wolffian duct origin are present in the paratesticular fascia or in fibrous bands extending from the testis. Patients tend to be rather tall, and bone age is normal. Psychosexual development is unmistakably female with regard to behavior, outlook, and maternal instincts.

The major complication of undescended testes in this disorder, as in all forms of cryptorchidism, is the development of tumors (Chap. 96). Since affected individuals undergo normal pubertal growth and feminize at the time of expected puberty and since testicular tumors rarely develop until after puberty, it is usual to delay gonadectomy until after the time of expected puberty. Prepubertal gonadectomy is indicated if the testes are present in the inguinal region or labia majora and result in discomfort or hernia formation. (If hernia repair is indicated prepubertally, most physicians prefer to remove the testes at the same time to limit the number of operative procedures.) If the testes are removed prepubertally, estrogen therapy is required at the appropriate age to ensure normal growth and breast development. Postpubertal gonadectomy causes menopausal symptoms and other evidence of estrogen withdrawal, and suitable estrogen replacement is indicated (Chap. 336).

Incomplete testicular feminization is about one-tenth as frequent as the complete form. In this disorder there is minor virilization of the external genitalia (partial fusion of the labioscrotal folds and/or some degree of clitoromegaly), normal pubic hair, and mixed virilization and feminization at the time of expected puberty. The vagina is short and blind-ending, but in contrast to the complete form, the wolffian duct derivatives are often partially developed. Since women with the incomplete disorder virilize at the time of expected puberty, gonadectomy should be performed before the expected time of puberty in all prepubertal patients with clitoromegaly or posterior labial fusion.

Reifenstein syndrome (also called *partial androgen insensitivity*) is the term applied to forms of incomplete male pseudohermaphroditism initially described by a number of eponyms (Reifenstein syndrome, Gilbert-Dreyfus syndrome, Lubs syndrome). These syndromes are mutations that partially impair the function of the androgen receptor. The most common phenotype is a man with perineoscrotal hypospadias and gynecomastia, but the spectrum of defective virilization in affected families ranges from men with azoospermia to phenotypic women with pseudovaginas. Axillary and pubic hair is normal, but chest and facial hair is scanty. Cryptorchidism is common, the testes are small, and azoospermia is present. Some have defects in wolffian duct derivatives such as absence or hypoplasia of the vas deferens. Since the psychological development in most is unequivocally male, the hypospadias and cryptorchidism should be corrected surgically. The treatment of the gynecomastia is surgical removal.

A disorder of the androgen receptor that is not actually a form of male pseudohermaphroditism is manifested as *infertility and/or undervirilization in phenotypic men.* Some such individuals are minimally affected members of families with Reifenstein syndrome in whom azoospermia is the only manifestation of the receptor defect. The *undervirilized fertile male* is an even more subtle manifestation of androgen receptor defect. In these families, affected men have gynecomastia and undervirilization, and some are fertile. More commonly, however, individuals with negative family histories present with male infertility with or without undervirilization.

PATHOPHYSIOLOGY The karyotype is 46,XY, and the mutation is X-linked. The frequency of a positive family history varies from about two-thirds of patients with testicular feminization and Reifenstein syndrome to only occasional patients with the infertile male syndrome. The disorder in subjects with a negative family history is believed to be the result of new mutations.

Hormone dynamics are similar in all disorders of the androgen receptor. Plasma testosterone levels and rates of testosterone production by the testes are normal or high. Elevated testosterone production is caused by the high mean plasma level of LH, which, in turn, is due to defective feedback regulation caused by resistance to the action of androgen at the hypothalamic-pituitary level. Elevated LH concentration is responsible also for the increased estrogen production by the testes (Chap. 337). (In normal men, most estrogen is derived from peripheral formation from circulating androgens, but when the plasma LH level is elevated, the testes secrete increased amounts of estrogen into the circulation.) Thus resistance to the feedback regulation of LH secretion by circulating androgen results in elevated plasma LH levels, and this, in turn, results in the enhanced secretion of both testosterone and estradiol by the testes. Gonadotropin levels rise even higher (and menopausal symptoms may develop) when the testes are removed, indicating that gonadotropin secretion is under partial feedback control. Presumably, in the steady state and in the absence of an androgen effect, estrogen alone regulates LH secretion, a control purchased at the expense of an elevated plasma estrogen concentration for a male.

The hormonal changes in the infertile male syndrome are similar to those in the other receptor disorders but less marked. Some men with this syndrome do not have an elevation of plasma LH or plasma testosterone level.

Feminization in these disorders is the result of two interlocking phenomena. First, androgens and estrogens have antagonistic effects, and in the absence of androgen action, the cellular effect of estrogen is unopposed. Second, the testicular production of estradiol is greater than that of the normal male (although less than that of the normal female). Variable degrees of androgen resistance and enhanced estradiol production result in different degrees of defective virilization and enhanced feminization in the four clinical syndromes.

Each of these syndromes is the result of defects in the androgen receptor. In most families, the fundamental defect is due to point mutations in the coding sequence leading to premature termination codons or to amino acid substitutions in the hormone-binding domain. Such mutations impair receptor function to variable degrees. Some families with clinical syndromes typical of an androgen receptor disorder have normal androgen binding in fibroblasts; in most, point mutations in the DNA-binding domain of the androgen receptor are responsible for the androgen resistance.

℞ **TREATMENT** Individuals with 5α-reductase deficiency who are raised as females but elect at the time of expected puberty to change social sex to male or who are raised from the first as males should be monitored carefully and given supplemental androgens, preferably those such as nandrolone decanoate that do not require 5α-reduction for activation, when virilization is incomplete. Fertility has been reported in such an individual. Individuals with 5α-reductase deficiency who continue to function as females should be gonadectomized, given feminizing doses of estrogens indefinitely, and receive surgical correction of the introitus when appropriate. The management of subjects with androgen receptor defects depends on the phenotypic manifestations. Women with testicular feminization should be castrated (preferably after the completion of the pubertal growth spurt and the feminization of the breasts) to prevent tumor development in the testes and receive estrogen replacement to maintain feminization, prevent hot flashes, and protect the bones; shallow vaginal depth can usually be treated medically with the Frank technique. Men with the Reifenstein phenotype should have surgical correction of the hypospadias and may require surgery for gynecomastia; supplemental androgen therapy in these men rarely improves the incomplete virilization.

Persistent Müllerian Duct Syndrome Men with this uncommon disorder have testes and male phenotypic development and in addition have fallopian tubes and a uterus. In some, one or both testes are descended and the uterus and ipsilateral fallopian tube are in the inguinal canal or scrotum; both testes and fallopian tubes may be present in the hernia sac or can be drawn into it. In others, the testes are located high in the abdomen and hernias are not present. In both types, the vasa deferentia are embedded in the wall of the uterus, a feature that complicates surgical procedures designed to preserve potential fertility. Most individuals have uninformative family histories, but in some the condition is inherited as an autosomal recessive trait. Because the external genitalia are well developed and the subjects masculinize normally at puberty, it is assumed that during the critical stage of embryonic differentiation the fetal testes produce a normal amount of androgen. However, müllerian regression does not occur. Two types of mutations have been described in this disorder. In one the gene that encodes AMH is defective, and blood levels of AMH are usually low or undetectable; in the other the AMH receptor is defective, and blood levels of AMH are elevated. To minimize the chance of tumor development and to maintain virilization, orchiopexy should be performed. Malignancy in the uterus or vagina has not been described, and because the vasa deferentia are closely associated with the broad ligaments, the uterus and vagina should be left in place to avoid disruption of the vasa deferentia during removal and consequently to preserve possible fertility.

Developmental Defects of the Male Genitalia • ***Hypospadias*** Hypospadias is a congenital anomaly in which the urethra terminates in an abnormal position along the ventral midline of the penis at some site between the normal urethral meatus and the perineum. This malformation occurs in 0.5 to 0.8% of male births in the United States and is often associated with ventral contraction and bowing of the penis (chordee). It is common to categorize hypospadias as glandular (involving the glans penis), penile, or perineoscrotal. Since androgens control penile development, hypospadias is generally assumed to result from some unidentified defect in androgen formation or action during embryogenesis. Indeed, hypospadias occurs in most disorders of male sexual differentiation, and a rare cause of hypospadias is maternal ingestion of progestational agents early in pregnancy. However, the known causes (single-gene defects, chromosomal abnormalities, and maternal drug ingestion) account for only about one-fourth of cases, and the etiology of most is unknown. The management is surgical.

Cryptorchidism The control of testicular descent is poorly understood, both in regard to the nature of the forces that cause the movement and to the hormonal factors that regulate the process. In anatomic terms, testicular descent can be divided into three phases: (1) transabdominal movement of the testis from its site of origin above the kidney to the inguinal ring, (2) formation of the opening in the inguinal canal (processus vaginalis) through which the testis exits the abdominal cavity, and (3) actual movement of the testis through the inguinal canal to its permanent site in the scrotum. This process occurs over a 6- to 7-month period during gestation, beginning at about the sixth week, and is not completed in some until after birth. Impairment at any stage in this process can impair descent of one or both testes. About 3% of full-term and 30% of premature male infants have at least one cryptorchid testis at birth, but descent is usually completed within the first few weeks of life, so that the incidence of failure of descent by 6 to 9 months of age is only 0.6 to 0.7%. It is this latter category of maldescent that requires intervention.

Permanent cryptorchidism can be classified as intraabdominal (10%), canalicular (in the inguinal canal) (20%), high scrotal (40%), or obstructed (30%), in which maldescent is due to a physical barrier between the inguinal pouch and the inlet of the scrotum. These disorders must be distinguished from the temporarily retracted normal testis.

The cryptorchid testis functions poorly after puberty, but the extent to which maldescent is the result of an abnormality of the testis or the cause of abnormal function is unknown. Two general theories have been advanced as to the etiology—inadequate intraabdominal pressure and deficient endocrine function of the testis either because of deficient testosterone synthesis or inadequate formation of AMH. Indeed, defects that result in inadequate development of intraabdominal pressure or inadequate development of the testes can cause cryptorchidism. As in hypospadias, however, the known causes of cryptorchidism constitute only a small fraction of the cases, and the etiology in most remains to be identified. Two complications of cryptorchidism are important; spermatogenesis cannot occur at the temperature of the abdominal cavity, and it is necessary to correct the process as early as possible to allow possible fertility. The fact that infertility is common in men who have been treated for unilateral as well as bilateral cryptorchidism suggests that maldescent is usually the consequence rather than the cause of the testicular malfunction. There is also a greater frequency of malignancy in undescended testes, which should be surgically corrected for this reason (Chap. 96).

BIBLIOGRAPHY

ACHERMANN JC et al: A mutation in the gene encoding steroidogenic factor-1 causes XY sex reversal and adrenal failure in humans. Nat Genet 22:125, 1999

AFFARA NA et al: Analysis of the *SRY* gene in 22 sex-reversed XY females identifies four new point mutations in the conserved DNA binding domain. Hum Mol Genet 2:785, 1993

ANDERSSON S et al: Molecular genetics and pathophysiology of 17β-hydroxysteroid dehydrogenase 3 deficiency. J Clin Endocrinol Metab 81:130, 1996

BEHRINGER RR: The in vivo roles of mullerian-inhibiting substance. Curr Top Dev Biol 29:171, 1994

BOUCEKKINE C et al: Clinical and anatomical spectrum in XX sex reversed patients. Relationship to the presence of Y-specific DNA sequences. Clin Endocrinol 40:733, 1994

BULUN SE: Aromatase deficiency in women and men: Would you have predicted the phenotype? J Clin Endocrinol Metab 81:867, 1996

CHAN WY: Molecular genetic, biochemical, and clinical implications of gonadotropin receptor mutations. Mol Genet Metab 63:75, 1998

DONAHOE PA et al: Mixed gonadal dysgenesis, pathogenesis and management. J Pediatr Surg 14:287, 1979

——— et al: Congenital adrenal hyperplasia, in *The Metabolic and Molecular Bases of Inherited Disease*, 8th ed, CR Scriver et al (eds). New York, McGraw-Hill, 2001, pp 4077–4115

EDMAN CD et al: Embryonic testicular regression: A clinical spectrum of XY agonadal individuals. Obstet Gynecol 49:208, 1977

FOSTER JW et al: Campomelic dysplasia and autosomal sex reversal caused by mutations in an *SRY*-related gene. Nature 372:525, 1994

GEORGE FW, WILSON JD: Sex determination and differentiation, in *The Physiology of Reproduction*, 2d ed, E Knobil, JD Neill (eds). New York, Raven Press, 1994, vol 1, pp 3–28

GRIFFIN JE et al: Congenital absence of the vagina: The Mayer-Rokitansky-Kuster-Hauser syndrome. Ann Intern Med 85:224, 1976

——— et al: The androgen resistance syndromes: 5α-Reductase deficiency, and related disorders, in *The Metabolic and Molecular Bases of Inherited Disease,* 8th ed, CR Scriver et al (eds). New York, McGraw-Hill, 2001, pp 4117–4146

GRUMBACH MM, CONTE FA: Disorders of sexual differentiation, in *Williams Textbook of Endocrinology,* 9th ed, JD Wilson, et al (eds). Philadelphia, Saunders, 1998, pp 1303–1425

HAWKINS JR et al: Mutational analysis of *SRY*: Nonsense and missense mutations in XY sex reversal. Hum Genet 88:471, 1992

IMBEAUD S et al: A 27-base pair deletion of the anti-mullerian type II receptor gene is the most common cause of the persistent mullerian duct syndrome. Hum Mol Genet 5:1269, 1996

JOSSO N et al: Clinical aspects and molecular genetics of the persistent mullerian duct syndrome. Clin Endocrinol 47:137, 1997

KROB G et al: True hermaphroditism: Geographical distribution, clinical findings, chromosomes and gonadal histology. Eur J Pediatr 153:2, 1994

MILLER WL, STRAUSS JF III: Molecular pathology and mechanism of action of the steroidogenic acute regulatory protein, StAR. J Steroid Biochem Mol Biol 69:131, 1999

——— et al: The molecular basis of isolated 17,20 lyase deficiency. Endocrine Res 24: 817, 1998

MISHINA Y et al: Genetic analysis of the mullerian-inhibitory substance signal transduction pathway in mammalian sexual differentiation. Genes Dev 10:2577, 1996

PARKER KL et al: Gene interactions in gonadal development. Ann Rev Physiol 61:417, 1999

ROSENFELD R, GRUMBACH MM (eds): *Turner Syndrome.* New York, Marcel Dekker, 1990

ROVET J et al: The psychoeducational profile of boys with Klinefelter syndrome. J Learn Disabil 29:180, 1996

SIMARD J et al: Molecular biology and genetics of the 3β-hydroxysteroid dehydrogenase/Δ5-Δ4 isomerase gene family. J Endocrinol 150 (Suppl):S189, 1996

SMYTH CM, BREMNER WJ: Klinefelter syndrome. Arch Intern Med 158:1309, 1998

STRUBBE EH et al: The Mayer-Rokitansky-Kuster-Hauser (MRKH) syndrome without and with associated features: Two separate entities? Clin Dysmorphol 3:192, 1994

SWAIN A, LOVELL-BADGE R: Mammalian sex determination: A molecular drama. Genes Dev 13:755, 1999

YANASE T et al: 17α-Hydroxylase/17,20-lyase defects. J Steroid Biochem Mol Biol 53: 153, 1995

ZINN AR, ROSS JL: Turner syndrome and haploinsufficiency. Curr Opin Genet Dev 8: 322, 1998

339

Steven I. Sherman, Robert F. Gagel

DISORDERS AFFECTING MULTIPLE ENDOCRINE SYSTEMS

ACTH adrenocorticotropin	MEN multiple endocrine neoplasia
CT computed tomography	MRI magnetic resonance imaging
CRH corticotropin-releasing hormone	MTC medullary thyroid carcinoma
FHH familial hypocalciuric hypercalcemia	PGA polyglandular autoimmune
FMTC familial medullary thyroid carcinoma	POEMS polyneuropathy, organomegaly, endocrinopathy, M-proteins, and skin changes
GH growth hormone	TSH thyroid stimulating hormone
GHRH growth hormone–releasing hormone	VIP vasoactive intestinal peptide
	ZES Zollinger-Ellison syndrome

NEOPLASTIC DISORDERS AFFECTING MULTIPLE ENDOCRINE ORGANS

Several distinct genetic disorders predispose to endocrine gland neoplasia and cause hormone excess syndromes (Table 339-1). DNA-based genetic testing is now available for these disorders, but effective management requires an understanding of endocrine neoplasia and the range of clinical features that may be manifest in an individual patient.

MULTIPLE ENDOCRINE NEOPLASIA (MEN) TYPE 1

Clinical Manifestations MEN 1, or Wermer's syndrome, is characterized by neoplasia of parathyroid, pituitary, and pancreatic islet cells (Table 339-1). The syndrome is inherited as an autosomal dominant trait, so that each child of an affected parent has a 50% chance of inheriting the predisposing gene.

Several features of the pathogenesis of MEN 1 have important implications for its management. Though each tumor is derived from a single cell (clonal in origin), any endocrine cell within the affected organs can become transformed. Hyperplasia is the initiating lesion, followed later by adenomatous or carcinomatous changes. Consequently, the disease process within a single organ is multicentric. Neoplasia in one organ may affect the progression of disease in another organ. For example, the ectopic production of hypothalamic releasing hormones by a pancreatic tumor may stimulate the growth of a pituitary tumor. Because MEN 1 generally evolves over a 30- to 40-year period, the manifestations depend in part on when the disorder is identified.

Hyperparathyroidism is the most common manifestation of MEN 1. Hypercalcemia may be present during the teenage years, and most individuals are affected by age 40 (Fig. 339-1). Screening for hyperparathyroidism involves measurement of either an albumin-adjusted or ionized serum calcium level. The diagnosis is established by demonstrating elevated levels of serum calcium and intact parathyroid hormone. Manifestations of hyperparathyroidism in MEN 1 do not differ substantially from those in sporadic hyperparathyroidism and include calcium-containing kidney stones, bone abnormalities, and gastrointestinal and musculoskeletal complaints (Chap. 341).

Other familial disorders associated with hypercalcemia include familial parathyroid hyperplasia, familial adenomatous hyperparathyroidism, and familial hypocalciuric hypercalcemia (FHH). Calcium excretion is usually elevated in the patient with MEN 1 or other forms of primary hyperparathyroidism and low in FHH. Another distinguishing feature is that the serum calcium level is rarely elevated at birth in patients with MEN 1 but is frequently elevated in newborns with FHH. Differentiation of hyperparathyroidism of MEN 1 from other forms of familial primary hyperparathyroidism is usually based on family history, histologic features of resected parathyroid tissue, and, sometimes, long-term observation to determine whether other manifestations of MEN 1 develop. FHH is due to inactivating mutations of the calcium sensor, a transmembrane G protein–coupled receptor found in parathyroid tissue and kidney (Chap. 341).

Parathyroid hyperplasia is the common cause of hyperparathyroidism in MEN 1, although single and multiple adenomas have been described. Hyperplasia of one or more parathyroid glands is common in younger patients; adenomas are usually found in older patients or those with long-standing disease.

Neoplasia of the pancreatic islets is the second most common manifestation of MEN 1 and tends to occur in parallel with hyperparathyroidism (Fig. 339-1). Increased pancreatic islet cell hormones include pancreatic polypeptide (75 to 85%), gastrin [60%; Zollinger-Ellison syndrome (ZES)], insulin (25 to 35%), vasoactive intestinal peptide (VIP) (3 to 5%; Verner-Morrison or watery diarrhea syndrome), glucagon (5 to 10%), and somatostatin (1 to 5%). The tumors rarely produce adrenocorticotropin (ACTH), corticotropin-releasing hormone (CRH), growth hormone–releasing hormone (GHRH), calcitonin gene products, neurotensin, gastric inhibitory peptide, and others. Many of the tumors produce more than one peptide. The pancreatic neoplasms differ from the other components of MEN 1 in that approximately one-third of the tumors display malignant features, including hepatic metastases (Chap. 93).

Table 339-1 Disease Associations in the Multiple Endocrine Neoplasia (MEN) Syndromes

	MEN 2		
MEN 1	**MEN 2A**	**MEN 2B**	**Mixed Syndromes**
Parathyroid hyperplasia or adenoma Islet cell hyperplasia, adenoma, or carcinoma Pituitary hyperplasia or adenoma Other less common manifestations: foregut carcinoid, pheochromocytoma, subcutaneous or visceral lipomas, dermal angiofibromas or collagenomas	MTC Pheochromocytoma Parathyroid hyperplasia or adenoma Cutaneous lichen amyloidosis Hirschsprung disease FMTC	MTC Pheochromocytoma Mucosal and gastrointestinal neuromas Marfanoid features	Familial pheochromocytoma and islet cell tumor von Hippel–Lindau syndrome, pheochromocytoma, and islet cell tumor Neurofibromatosis with features of MEN 1 or 2 Myxomas, spotty pigmentation, and generalized endocrine overactivity in a single family

NOTE: MTC, medullary thyroid carcinoma; FMTC, familial MTC.

Pancreatic islet cell tumors are diagnosed by identification of a characteristic clinical syndrome, hormonal assays with or without provocative stimuli, or radiographic techniques. One approach involves annual screening of people at risk with measurement of basal and meal-stimulated levels of pancreatic polypeptide to identify the tumors as early as possible; the rationale of this screening strategy is the concept that surgical removal of islet cell tumors at an early stage will be curative. Other approaches to screening include measurement of serum gastrin and pancreatic polypeptide levels every 2 to 3 years, with the rationale that pancreatic neoplasms will be detected at a later stage but can be managed medically, if possible, or by surgery. High-resolution, early-phase computed tomography (CT) scanning provides the best noninvasive technique for identification of these tumors, but intraoperative ultrasonography is the most sensitive method for detection of small tumors.

ZES is caused by excessive gastrin production and occurs in more than half of MEN 1 patients with pancreatic islet cell tumors (Fig. 339-1) (Chap. 93). Clinical features include increased gastric acid production, recurrent peptic ulcers, diarrhea, and esophagitis. The ulcer diathesis is refractory to conservative therapy such as antacids. The diagnosis is made by finding increased gastric acid secretion, elevated basal gastrin levels in serum [generally >115 pmol/L (200 pg/mL)], and an exaggerated response of serum gastrin to either secretin or calcium. Other causes of elevated serum gastrin levels, such as achlorhydria, treatment with H_2 receptor antagonists or omeprazole, retained gastric antrum, small-bowel resection, gastric outlet obstruction, and hypercalcemia, should be excluded. Gastrin-producing carcinoid-like tumors are frequently present in the duodenal wall.

Insulinoma causes hypoglycemia in about one-third of MEN 1 patients with pancreatic islet cell tumors (Fig. 339-1). The tumors may be benign or malignant (25%). The diagnosis can be established by documenting hypoglycemia during a short fast with simultaneous inappropriate elevation of serum insulin and C-peptide levels. More commonly, it is necessary to subject the patient to a supervised 72-h fast to provoke hypoglycemia (Chap. 334). Large insulinomas may be identified by CT scanning; small tumors not detected by radiographic techniques may be localized by selective arteriographic injection of calcium into each of the arteries that supply the pancreas and sampling the hepatic vein for insulin to determine the anatomic region containing the tumor. Intraoperative ultrasonography can also be used to localize these tumors, but preoperative calcium injection data are helpful in guiding the subtotal pancreatectomy if multiple or no abnormalities are detected by intraoperative ultrasonography.

Glucagonoma in occasional MEN 1 patients causes a syndrome of hyperglycemia, skin rash (necrolytic migratory erythema), anorexia, glossitis, anemia, depression, diarrhea, and venous thrombosis. In about half of these patients the plasma glucagon level is high, leading to its designation as the *glucagonoma syndrome*, although elevation of plasma glucagon level in MEN 1 patients is not necessarily associated with these symptoms. The glucagonoma syndrome may represent a complex interaction between glucagon overproduction and the nutritional status of the patient.

The *Verner-Morrison* or *watery diarrhea syndrome* consists of watery diarrhea, hypokalemia, hypochlorhydria, and metabolic acidosis. The diarrhea can be voluminous and is almost always found in association with an islet cell tumor, prompting use of the term *pancreatic cholera*. However, the syndrome is not restricted to pancreatic islet tumors and has been observed with carcinoids or other tumors. This syndrome is believed to be due to overproduction of VIP, although plasma VIP levels may not be elevated. Hypercalcemia may

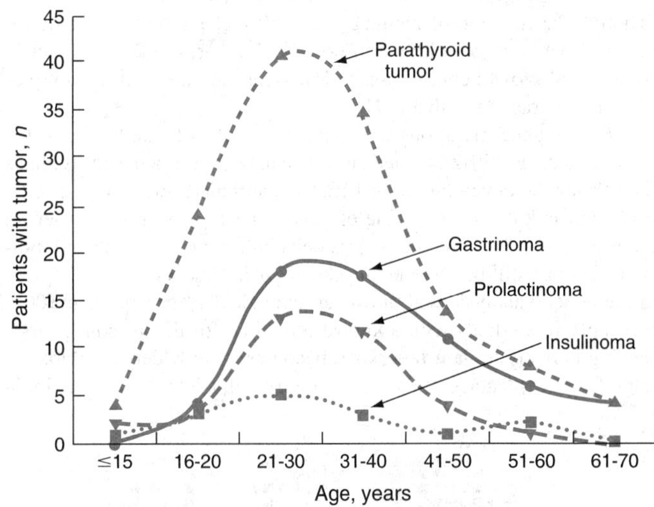

FIGURE 339-1 Age at onset of endocrine tumor expression in multiple endocrine neoplasia type 1 (MEN 1). Data derived from retrospective analysis for each endocrine organ hyperfunction in 130 cases of MEN 1. Age at onset is the age at first symptom or, with tumors not causing symptoms, age at the time of the first abnormal finding on a screening test. The rate of diagnosis of hyperparathyroidism increased sharply between ages 16 and 20 years. *(Reprinted with permission from Marx et al.)*

be induced by the effects of VIP on bone as well as by hyperparathyroidism.

Pituitary tumors occur in more than half of patients with MEN 1 and tend to be multicentric, making them difficult to resect (Chap. 328). Prolactinomas are most common (Fig. 339-1) and are diagnosed by finding serum prolactin levels >200 μg/L, with or without a pituitary mass evident by magnetic resonance imaging (MRI). Values <200 μg/L may be due to a prolactin-secreting neoplasm or to compression of the pituitary stalk by a different type of pituitary tumor. Acromegaly due to excessive growth hormone (GH) production is the second most common syndrome caused by pituitary tumors in MEN 1 (Chap. 328) but can rarely be due to production of GHRH by an islet cell tumor. Cushing's disease can be caused by ACTH-producing pituitary tumors or by ectopic production of ACTH or CRH by other tumors in the MEN 1 syndrome. Diagnosis of pituitary Cushing's disease is generally best accomplished by a high-dose dexamethasone suppression test or by petrosal venous sinus sampling for ACTH after intravenous injection of CRH (Chap. 328). Differentiation of a primary pituitary tumor from an ectopic CRH-producing tumor may be difficult because the pituitary is the source of ACTH in both disorders; documentation of CRH production by a pancreatic islet or carcinoid tumor may be the only method of proving ectopic CRH production. Adrenal cortical tumors are found in almost one-half of gene carriers but are rarely functional; malignancy in the cortical adenomas is uncommon.

Unusual manifestations of MEN 1 The rare carcinoid tumors in MEN 1 are of the foregut type and are derived from thymus, lung, stomach, or duodenum; they may metastasize or be locally invasive. These tumors usually produce serotonin, calcitonin, or CRH; the typical carcinoid syndrome with flushing, diarrhea, and bronchospasm is rare (Chap. 93). Subcutaneous or visceral lipomas and cutaneous leiomyomas may also be present but rarely undergo malignant transformation. Skin angiofibromas or collagenomas are seen in most patients with MEN 1 when carefully sought.

GENETIC CONSIDERATIONS MEN 1 is transmitted as an autosomal dominant trait, reflecting the fact that the *MEN1* gene, located on chromosome 11q13, encodes a tumor suppressor protein termed *menin* (Fig. 339-2). Affected individuals typically harbor a germline mutation in *MEN1* and acquire a "second hit" in the normal gene as a result of another mutation or, more commonly, loss of the portion of chromosome 11 that contains the *MEN1* locus (Chap. 81). Though the function of menin is not well understood, it is a nuclear protein that interacts with a transcriptional factor, Jun D, suggesting a role in cell growth control. Several missense mutations in menin prevent its interaction with Jun D.

MEN1 gene mutations are found in >90% of families with the syndrome (Fig. 339-2). Genetic testing can be performed in individuals at risk for the development of MEN 1, particularly when the specific mutation is known. The value of genetic testing for this disorder, in contrast to MEN 2 (see below), is debated because predisposed individuals must still be screened repeatedly using endocrine tests. A negative genetic analysis will, however, exclude disease with near 100% certainty in kindreds with a known mutation; for this reason, genetic testing is likely to gain favor as it becomes more widely available. A significant percentage of sporadic parathyroid, islet cell, and carcinoid tumors also have loss or mutation of *MEN1*. It is presumed that these mutations are somatic and occur in a single cell, leading to subsequent transformation. ■

Rx TREATMENT Almost everyone who inherits a mutant *MEN1* gene develops at least one clinical manifestation of the syndrome. Most develop hyperparathyroidism, 80% develop pancreatic islet cell tumors, and more than half develop pituitary tumors. For most of these tumors, initial surgery is not curative and patients frequently require multiple surgical procedures and surgery on two or more endocrine glands during a lifetime. For this reason, it is essential to establish clear goals for management of these patients rather than to recommend surgery casually each time a tumor is discovered. Ranges for acceptable management are discussed below.

Hyperparathyroidism Individuals with serum calcium levels >3.0 mmol/L (12 mg/dL), evidence of calcium nephrolithiasis or renal dysfunction, neuropathic or muscular symptoms, or bone involvement (including osteopenia) should undergo parathyroid exploration. In MEN 1 an additional criterion for parathyroid surgery is hypercalcemia associated with elevated gastrin levels, because elevated serum calcium may stimulate gastrin production and ZES, a condition that may be improved by return of calcium levels to normal. There is less agreement regarding the necessity for parathyroid exploration in individuals who do not meet these criteria, and observation may be appropriate in the MEN 1 patient with asymptomatic hyperparathyroidism.

When parathyroid surgery is indicated in MEN 1, all parathyroid tissue should be identified and removed at the time of primary operation, and parathyroid tissue should be implanted in the nondominant forearm. Thymectomy should also be performed because of the potential for later development of malignant carcinoid tumors. If reoperation is necessary, transplanted tissue can be resected under local anesthesia with titration of tissue removal to return the serum calcium level to normal. A less desirable approach is to remove 3 to 3½ parathyroid glands from the neck, carefully marking the location of residual tissue so that the remaining tissue can be located easily during subsequent surgery.

Pancreatic Islet Tumors (See Chap. 93 for discussion of pancreatic islet tumors not associated with MEN 1.) Two features of pancreatic islet cell tumors in MEN 1 complicate the management. First, the pancreatic islet cell tumors are multicentric, malignant about a third of the time, and cause death in 10 to 20% of patients. Second, removal of all pancreatic islets to prevent malignancy causes diabetes mellitus, a disease with severe long-term complications. These features make it difficult to formulate clear-cut guidelines, but some general concepts appear to be valid. First, islet cell tumors producing insulin, glucagon, VIP, GHRH, or CRH should be resected because medical therapy is generally ineffective. Second, gastrin-producing islet cell tumors that cause ZES are frequently multicentric. Recent experience suggests that a high percentage of ZES in MEN 1 is caused by duodenal wall tumors and that resection of these tumors improves the cure rate. Treatment with H_2 receptor antagonists (cimetidine or ranitidine) and the H^+,K^+-ATPase inhibitors (omeprazole or lansoprazole) provides an alternative to surgery for control of ulcer disease in patients with multicentric tumors or with hepatic metastases. Third, in families in which there is a high incidence of malignant islet cell tumors that cause death, total pancreatectomy at an early age may be justified to prevent malignancy.

Management of metastatic islet cell carcinoma is unsatisfactory.

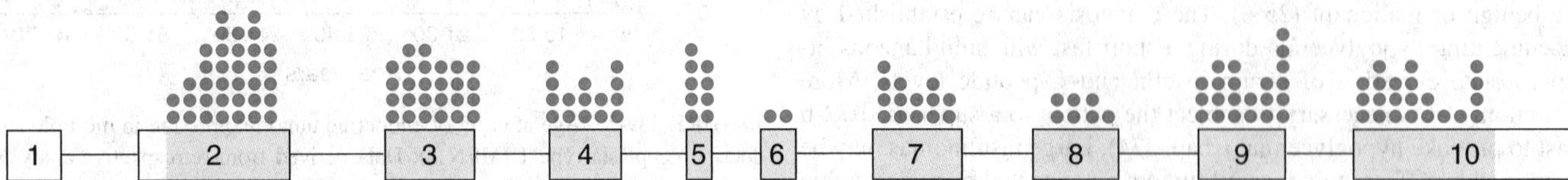

FIGURE 339-2 Schematic depiction of the *MEN1* gene and the distribution of mutations. The shaded areas show coding sequence. The closed circles show the relative distribution of mutations, mostly inactivating, in each exon. Mutation data are derived from the Human Gene Mutation Database from which more detailed information can be obtained (www.uwcm.ac.uk/uwcm/mg/hgmd0.html) *(From M Krawczak, DN Cooper: Trends Genet 13:1321, 1998.)*

Hormonal abnormalities can sometimes be controlled. For example, ZES can be treated with H_2 receptor antagonists or H^+,K^+-ATPase inhibitors; the somatostatin analogue, octreotide, is useful in the management of carcinoid and the watery diarrhea syndrome. Bilateral adrenalectomy may be required for ectopic ACTH syndrome if medical therapy is ineffective (Chap. 331). Islet cell carcinomas frequently metastasize to the liver but may grow slowly. Hepatic artery embolization or chemotherapy (5-fluorouracil, streptozocin, chlorozotocin, doxorubicin, or dacarbazine) may reduce tumor mass, control symptoms of hormone excess, and prolong life; however, these treatments are never curative.

Pituitary Tumors Treatment of prolactinomas with dopamine agonists (bromocriptine, cabergoline, or quinagolide) usually returns the serum prolactin level to normal and prevents further tumor growth (Chap. 328). Surgical resection of a prolactinoma is rarely curative but may relieve mass effects. Transsphenoidal resection is appropriate for neoplasms that secrete ACTH, GH, or the α-subunit of the pituitary glycoprotein hormones. Octreotide reduces tumor mass in one-third of GH-secreting tumors and reduces GH and insulin-like growth factor I levels in 75% of patients. Radiation therapy may be useful for large or recurrent tumors.

Improvements in the management of MEN 1, particularly islet cell and pituitary tumors, have improved outcome in these patients substantially. As a result, other neoplastic manifestations, such as carcinoid syndrome, are now seen with increased frequency.

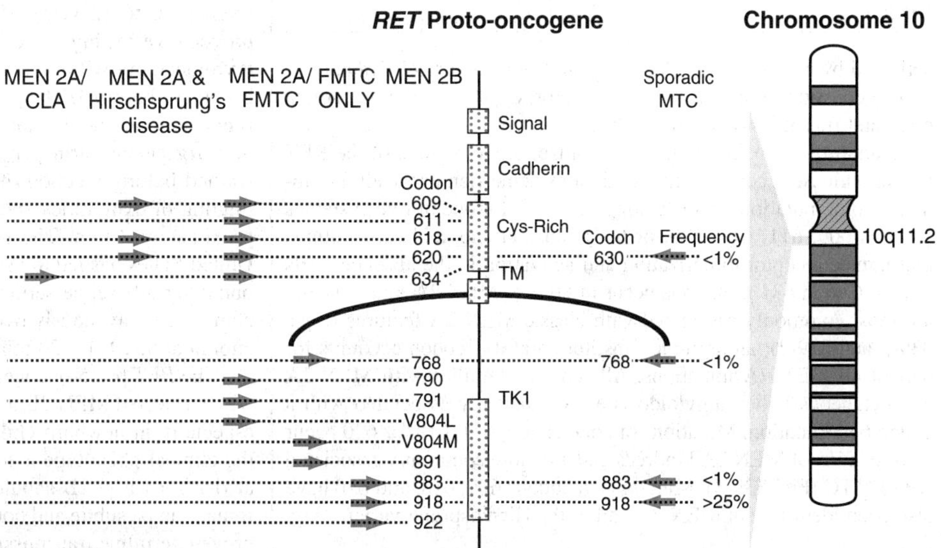

FIGURE 339-3 Schematic diagram of the *RET* proto-oncogene showing mutations found in MEN type 2 and sporadic medullary thyroid carcinoma (MTC). The *RET* proto-oncogene is located on the proximal arm of chromosome 10q (10q11.2). Activating mutations of two functional domains of RET tyrosine kinase receptor have been identified. The first affects a cysteine-rich (Cys-Rich) region in the extracellular portion of the receptor. Each germline mutation changes a cysteine at codons 609, 611, 618, 620, or 634 to another amino acid. The second region is the intracellular tyrosine kinase (TK) domain. Codon 634 mutations account for approximately 80% of all germline mutations. Mutations of codons 630, 768, 883, and 918 have been identified as somatic (nongermline) mutations that occur in a single parafollicular or C cell within the thyroid gland in sporadic MTC. A codon 918 mutation is the most common somatic mutation. Abbreviations: MEN 2, multiple endocrine neoplasia type 2; CLA cutaneous lichen amyloidosis; FMTC, familial medullary thyroid carcinoma; Signal, the signal peptide; Cadherin, a cadherin-like region in the extracellular domain; TM, transmembrane domain; TK, tyrosine kinase domain.

MULTIPLE ENDOCRINE NEOPLASIA TYPE 2 **Clinical Manifestations** Medullary thyroid carcinoma (MTC) and pheochromocytoma are associated in two major syndromes: MEN type 2A and MEN type 2B (Table 339-1). MEN 2A is the combination of MTC, hyperparathyroidism, and pheochromocytoma. Three subvariants of MEN 2A are familial medullary thyroid carcinoma (FMTC), MEN 2A with cutaneous lichen amyloidosis, and MEN 2A with Hirschsprung disease. MEN type 2B is the combination of MTC, pheochromocytoma, mucosal neuromas, intestinal ganglioneuromatosis, and marfanoid features.

Multiple endocrine neoplasia type 2A MTC is the most common manifestation. This tumor usually develops in childhood, beginning as hyperplasia of the calcitonin-producing cells (C cells) of the thyroid. MTC is typically located at the junction of the upper one-third and lower two-thirds of each lobe of the thyroid, reflecting the high density of C cells in this location; tumors >1 cm in size are frequently associated with local or distant metastases. Measurement of the serum calcitonin level after calcium or pentagastrin injection makes it possible to diagnose this disorder when the likelihood of metastasis is low (see below).

Pheochromocytoma occurs in approximately 50% of patients with MEN 2A and causes palpitations, nervousness, headaches, and sometimes sweating (Chap. 332). About half the tumors are bilateral, and >50% of patients who have had unilateral adrenalectomy develop a pheochromocytoma in the contralateral gland within a decade. A second feature of these tumors is a disproportionate increase in the secretion of epinephrine relative to norepinephrine. Capsular invasion is common, but malignant behavior is uncommon.

Hyperparathyroidism occurs in 15 to 20% of patients, with the peak incidence in the third or fourth decade. The manifestations of hyperparathyroidism do not differ from those in other forms of primary hyperparathyroidism (Chap. 341), with nephrolithiasis being common. Diagnosis is established by finding hypercalcemia, hypophosphatemia, hypercalciuria, and an inappropriately high serum level of intact parathyroid hormone. Multiglandular parathyroid hyperplasia is the most common histologic finding, although with long-standing disease adenomatous changes may be superimposed on hyperplasia.

Multiple endocrine neoplasia type 2B The association of MTC, pheochromocytoma, mucosal neuromas, and a marfanoid habitus is designated MEN 2B. MTC in MEN 2B develops earlier and is more aggressive than in MEN 2A. Metastatic disease has been described prior to 1 year of age, and death commonly occurs in the second or third decade of life. However, the prognosis is not invariably bad even in patients with metastatic disease, as evidenced by a number of multigenerational families with this disease.

Pheochromocytoma occurs in more than half of MEN 2B patients and does not differ from that in MEN 2A. Hypercalcemia is rare in MEN 2B, and there are no well-documented examples of hyperparathyroidism.

The mucosal neuromas and marfanoid body habitus are the most distinctive features and are recognizable in childhood. Neuromas are present on the tip of the tongue, under the eyelids, and throughout the gastrointestinal tract and are true neuromas, distinct from neurofibromas. Children may present with gastrointestinal symptoms, including increased gas, intermittent obstruction, and diarrhea caused by neuromas.

GENETIC CONSIDERATIONS Mutations of the *RET* proto-oncogene have been identified in 93 to 95% of patients with MEN 2 (Fig. 339-3). *RET* encodes a tyrosine kinase receptor that is normally activated by glial cell line–derived neurotropic factor. *RET* mutations induce constitutive activity of the receptor, explaining the autosomal dominant transmission of the disorder.

Naturally occurring mutations localize to two regions of the RET tyrosine kinase receptor. The first is a cysteine-rich extracellular domain; point mutations in the coding sequence for one of five cysteines (codons 609, 611, 618, 620, or 634) cause amino acid substitutions that induce receptor dimerization and activation in the absence of its ligand. Codon 634 mutations occur in 80% of MEN 2A kindreds and are most commonly associated with classic MEN 2A features (Figs. 339-3 and 339-2); an arginine substitution at this codon accounts for half of all MEN 2A mutations. All reported families with MEN 2A and cutaneous lichen amyloidosis are consistently associated with a codon 634 mutation. Mutations of codons 609, 611, 618, or 620 occur in 10 to 15% of MEN 2A kindreds and are more commonly associated with FMTC (Fig. 339-3). Mutations in codons 609, 618, and 620 have also been identified in MEN 2A and in the Hirschsprung variant (Fig. 339-3).

The second region of the RET tyrosine kinase that is mutated in MEN 2 is in the substrate recognition pocket at codon 918 (Fig. 339-3). This activating mutation is present in approximately 95% of patients with MEN 2B and accounts for 10 to 15% of all *RET* proto-oncogene mutations in MEN 2. Mutations of codon 883 and 22 have also been identified in a few patients with MEN 2B.

From 3 to 5% of kindreds with FMTC have no identifiable mutation of either of these regions. In a few such kindreds mutations of codons 768, 790, 791, 804, and 891 have been identified (Fig. 339-3).

Somatic mutations (found only in the tumor and not transmitted in the germline) of the *RET* proto-oncogene have been identified in sporadic MTC; 25 to 35% of sporadic tumors have codon 918 mutations, and somatic mutations in codons 630, 768, and 804 have also been identified (Fig. 339-3). Germline mutations of the *RET* proto-oncogene are present in about 6% of patients with apparent sporadic MTC, indicating that other family members may be at risk for the disease. ■

℞ TREATMENT **Screening for Multiple Endocrine Neoplasia Type 2** Death from MTC can be prevented by early thyroidectomy. The identification of *RET* proto-oncogene mutations and the application of DNA-based molecular diagnostic techniques to identify these mutations has simplified the screening process. During the initial evaluation of a kindred, a *RET* proto-oncogene analysis should be performed on an individual with proven MEN 2A. Establishment of the specific mutation in a kindred facilitates the subsequent analysis of other family members. Each family member at risk should be tested twice for the presence of the specific mutation; the second analysis should be performed on a new DNA sample and, ideally, in a second laboratory to exclude sample mix-up or technical error (see *endrcr06.mda.uth.tmc.edu* for a list of laboratory testing sites). Individuals in a kindred with a known mutation who have two normal analyses can be excluded from further screening.

There is general consensus that children with codon 883, 918, and 922 mutations, or those associated with MEN 2B, should have a total thyroidectomy and central lymph node dissection (level VI) performed during the first months of life or soon after identification of the syndrome. If local metastasis is discovered, a more extensive lymph node dissection (levels II to V) is generally indicated. In children with codon 611, 618, 620, 630, 634, and 891 mutations, thyroidectomy should be performed before the age of 6 years because of reports of local metastatic disease in children this age. Finally, there are kindreds with codon 609, 768, 790, 791, and 804 mutations where the phenotype of MTC appears to be less aggressive. In these kindreds, and in those with rare mutations, two management approaches have been suggested in association with genetic counseling: (1) perform a total thyroidectomy with or without central node dissection at some arbitrary age (perhaps 6 to 12 years of age), or (2) continue annual or biannual provocative testing for calcitonin release with performance of total thyroidectomy with or without central neck dissection when the test becomes abnormal. The pentagastrin test involves measurement of serum calcitonin basally and 2, 5, 10, and 15 min after a bolus injection of 5 μg pentagastrin per kilogram body weight. Patients should be warned before injection of epigastric tightness, nausea, warmth, and tingling of extremities and reassured that the symptoms will last approximately 2 min. The recent unavailability of pentagastrin in the United States has led to use of a short calcium infusion, performed by obtaining a baseline serum calcitonin and then infusing 150 mg calcium salt intravenously over 10 min with measurement of serum calcitonin at 5, 10, 15, 30 min after initiation of the infusion.

The *RET* proto-oncogene analysis should be performed in patients with suspected MEN 2B to detect codon 883, 918, and 922 mutations, especially in newborn children where the diagnosis is suspected but the clinical phenotype is not fully developed. Other family members at risk for MEN 2B should also be tested because the mucosal neuromas can be subtle and not always identified. In the rare families with proven germline transmission of MTC but no identifiable *RET* proto-oncogene mutation, annual pentagastrin or calcium-pentagastrin testing should be performed on members at risk.

Annual screening for pheochromocytoma in subjects with germline *RET* mutations should be performed by measuring basal plasma or 24-h urine catecholamines and metanephrines. The goal is to identify a pheochromocytoma before it causes significant symptoms or is likely to cause sudden death, an event most commonly associated with large tumors. Although there are kindreds with FMTC and specific *RET* mutations in which no pheochromocytomas have been identified (Fig. 339-3), it is not clear that a large enough experience has been gained to exclude pheochromocytoma screening in these individuals. Radiographic studies, such as MRI or CT scans, are generally reserved for individuals with abnormal screening tests or with symptoms suggestive of pheochromocytoma (Chap. 332). Women should be tested during pregnancy because undetected pheochromocytoma can cause maternal death during childbirth.

Measurement of serum calcium and parathyroid hormone levels every 2 to 3 years provides an adequate screen for hyperparathyroidism, except in those families in which hyperparathyroidism is a prominent component, where measurements should be made annually.

Treatment of Medullary Thyroid Carcinoma MTC is a multicentric disorder. Total thyroidectomy with a central lymph node dissection should be performed in children who carry the mutant genes. Incomplete thyroidectomy leaves the possibility of later transformation of residual long-term C cells. The goal of early therapy is cure, and a strategy that does not accomplish this goal is short-sighted. Long-term follow-up studies indicate an excellent outcome with approximately 90% of children free of disease 15 to 20 years after surgery. In contrast, 15 to 25% of patients in whom the diagnosis is made on the basis of a palpable thyroid nodule die from the disease within 15 to 20 years.

In adults with MTC >1 cm in size, metastases to regional lymph nodes are common. Total thyroidectomy with central lymph node dissection and selective dissection of other regional chains provide the best chance for cure. In patients with extensive local metastatic disease in the neck, external radiation may prevent local recurrence or reduce tumor mass but is not curative. Chemotherapy with combinations of adriamycin, vincristine, cyclophosphamide, and dacarbazine may provide palliation.

Treatment of Pheochromocytoma The long-term goal for management of pheochromocytoma is to prevent death and cardiovascular complications. Improvements in radiographic imaging of the adrenals make direct examination of the apparently normal contralateral gland during surgery less important, and the rapid evolution of laparoscopic surgery has simplified management of early pheochromocytoma. The major question is whether to remove both adrenal glands or to remove only the affected adrenal at the time of primary surgery. Issues to be considered in making this decision include the possibility of malignancy (<15 reported cases), the likelihood of developing pheochromocytoma in the apparently unaffected gland over an 8- to 10-year period, and the risks of adrenal insufficiency caused by removal of both glands (at least two deaths related to adrenal insufficiency in MEN 2 patients). Most clinicians recommend removing only the affected gland. If both adrenals are removed, glucocorticoid and mineralocorticoid replacement is mandatory. An alternative approach is to remove the pheochromocytoma and adrenal medulla, leaving the adrenal cortex behind. This approach is usually successful and eliminates the necessity for steroid hormone replacement, although the pheochromocytoma recurs in some.

Treatment of Hyperparathyroidism Hyperparathyroidism has been managed by one of two approaches. Removal of 3½ glands with maintenance of the remaining half gland in the neck is the usual procedure. In families in whom hyperparathyroidism is a prominent manifestation (almost always associated with a codon 634 *RET* mutation) and recurrence is common, total parathyroidectomy with transplantation of parathyroid tissue into the nondominant forearm is preferred. This approach is discussed above in the context of hyperparathyroidism associated with MEN 1.

OTHER GENETIC TUMOR SYNDROMES A number of mixed syndromes exist in which the neoplastic associations differ from those in MEN 1 or 2 (Table 339-1).

The cause of von Hippel–Lindau (VHL) syndrome, the association of central nervous system tumors, renal cell carcinoma, pheochromocytoma, and islet cell neoplasms, is mutations in the *VHL* tumor-suppressor gene. Germline-inactivating mutations of the *VHL* gene cause tumor formation when there is additional loss or somatic mutation of the normal *VHL* allele in brain, kidney, pancreatic islet, or adrenal medullary cells. A specific subset of mutations is more common in families with pheochromocytomas.

The molecular defect in type 1 neurofibromatosis inactivates neurofibromin, a cell membrane–associated protein that normally activates a GTPase. Inactivation of this protein impairs GTPase and causes continuous activation of p21 Ras and its downstream tyrosine kinase pathway. Endocrine tumors also form in less common neoplastic genetic syndromes. These include Cowden's disease, Carney complex, familial acromegaly, and familial carcinoid syndrome.

IMMUNOLOGIC SYNDROMES AFFECTING MULTIPLE ENDOCRINE ORGANS

When immune dysfunction affects two or more endocrine glands and other nonendocrine immune disorders are present, the *polyglandular autoimmune* (PGA) *syndromes* should be considered. The PGA syndromes are classified as two main types: the type I syndrome starts in childhood and is characterized by mucocutaneous candidiasis, hypoparathyroidism, and adrenal insufficiency; the type II, or *Schmidt syndrome*, is more likely to present in adults and most commonly comprises adrenal insufficiency, thyroiditis, and type 1 diabetes mellitus. However, the type II syndrome is heterogeneous and may consist of autoimmune thyroid disease along with a variety of other autoimmune endocrine disorders (Table 339-2).

POLYGLANDULAR AUTOIMMUNE SYNDROME TYPE I PGA type I is usually recognized in the first decade of life and requires two of three components for diagnosis: mucocutaneous candidiasis, hypoparathyroidism, and adrenal insufficiency. Mineralocorticoids and glucocorticoids may be lost simultaneously or sequentially. This disorder is also called *autoimmune polyendocrinopathy-candidiasis-ectodermal dystrophy* (APECED). Other endocrine defects can include gonadal failure, hypothyroidism, anterior hypophysitis, and, less commonly, destruction of the β cells of the pancreatic islets and development of insulin-dependent (type 1) diabetes mellitus. Additional features include hypoplasia of the dental enamel, ungual dystrophy, tympanic membrane sclerosis, vitiligo, keratopathy, and gastric parietal cell dysfunction resulting in pernicious anemia. Some patients develop autoimmune hepatitis, malabsorption (variably attributed to intestinal lymphangiectasia, IgA deficiency, bacterial overgrowth, or hypoparathyroidism), asplenism, achalasia, and cholelithiasis (Table 339-2). At the outset, only one organ may be involved, but the number increases with time so that patients eventually manifest two to five components of the syndrome.

Table 339-2 Features of Polyglandular Autoimmune (PGA) Syndromes

PGA I	PGA II
EPIDEMIOLOGY	
Autosomal recessive	Polygenic inheritance
Mutations in APECED gene	HLA-DR3 and HLA-DR4 associated
Childhood onset	Adult onset
Equal male:female ratio	Female predominance
DISEASE ASSOCIATIONS	
Mucocutaneous candidiasis	Adrenal insufficiency
Hypoparathyroidism	Hypothyroidism
Adrenal insufficiency	Graves' disease
Hypogonadism	Type 1 diabetes
Alopecia	Hypogonadism
Hypothyroidism	Hypophysitis
Dental enamel hypoplasia	Myasthenia gravis
Malabsorption	Vitiligo
Chronic active hepatitis	Alopecia
Vitiligo	Pernicious anemia
Pernicious anemia	Celiac disease

NOTE: APECED, autoimmune polyendocrinopathy-candidiasis-ectodermal dystrophy.

Most patients initially present with oral candidiasis in childhood; it is poorly responsive to treatment and relapses frequently. Chronic hypoparathyroidism usually occurs before adrenal insufficiency develops. More than 60% of postpubertal women develop premature hypogonadism. The endocrine components, including adrenal insufficiency and hypoparathyroidism, may not develop until the fourth decade, making continued surveillance necessary.

Type I PGA syndrome allows no HLA associations and is inherited as an autosomal recessive trait. The responsible gene, designated as either *APECED* or *AIRE*, encodes a transcription factor that is expressed in thymus and lymph nodes; a variety of different mutations have been reported.

POLYGLANDULAR AUTOIMMUNE SYNDROME TYPE II PGA type II is characterized by two or more of the endocrinopathies listed in Table 339-2. Most often these include primary adrenal insufficiency, Graves' disease or autoimmune hypothyroidism, type 1 diabetes mellitus, and primary hypogonadism. Because adrenal insufficiency is relatively rare, it is frequently used to define the presence of the syndrome. Among patients with adrenal insufficiency, type 1 diabetes mellitus coexists in 52% and autoimmune thyroid disease occurs in 69%. However, many patients with antimicrosomal and antithyroglobulin antibodies never develop abnormalities of thyroid function. Thus, increased antibody titers alone are poor predictors of future disease. Other associated conditions include hypophysitis, celiac disease, atrophic gastritis, and pernicious anemia. Vitiligo, caused by antibodies against the melanocyte (**see Plate IIA-11**), and alopecia are less common than in the type I syndrome. Mucocutaneous candidiasis does not occur. A few patients develop a late-onset, usually transient hypoparathyroidism caused by antibodies that compete with parathyroid hormone for binding to the parathyroid hormone receptor. Up to 25% of patients with myasthenia gravis, and an even higher percentage who have myasthenia and a thymoma, have PGA type II (Chap. 380).

The type II syndrome is familial in nature but does not exhibit a characteristic Mendelian pattern of transmission. Like many of the individual autoimmune endocrinopathies, certain HL-DR3 and HLA-

DR4 alleles increase disease susceptibility; several different genes probably contribute to the expression of this syndrome.

A variety of autoantibodies are seen in PGA type II, including antibodies directed against: (1) thyroid antigens such as thyroid peroxidase, thyroglobulin, or the thyroid stimulating hormone (TSH) receptor; (2) adrenal side chain cleavage enzyme, steroid 21-hydroxylase, or ACTH receptor; and (3) pancreatic islet glutamic acid decarboxylase or the insulin receptor, among others. The roles of cytokines such as interferon and cell-mediated immunity are unclear.

DIAGNOSIS The clinical manifestations of adrenal insufficiency often develop slowly, may be difficult to detect, and can be fatal if not diagnosed and treated appropriately. Thus, prospective screening should be performed routinely in all patients and family members at risk for PGA types I and II. The most effective screening test for adrenal disease is a cosyntropin stimulation test (Chap. 331). A fasting blood glucose level can be obtained to screen for hyperglycemia. Additional screening tests should include measurements of TSH, luteinizing hormone, follicle-stimulating hormone, and, in men, testosterone levels. In families with suspected type I PGA syndrome, calcium and phosphorus levels should be measured. These screening studies should be performed every 1 to 2 years up to about age 50 in families with PGA type II syndrome and until about age 40 in patients with type I syndrome. Screening measurements of autoantibodies against potentially affected endocrine organs are of uncertain prognostic value. The differential diagnosis of PGA syndrome should include the DiGeorge syndrome (hypoparathyroidism due to glandular agenesis and mucocutaneous candidiasis), Kearns-Sayre syndrome (hypoparathyroidism, primary hypogonadism, type 1 diabetes mellitus, and panhypopituitarism), Wolfram's syndrome (congenital diabetes insipidus and diabetes mellitus), and congenital rubella (type 1 diabetes mellitus and hypothyroidism).

℞ TREATMENT With the exception of Graves' disease, the management of each of the endocrine components of the disease involves hormone replacement and is covered in detail in the chapters on adrenal, thyroid, gonadal, and parathyroid disease (Chaps. 330, 331, 335, 336, and 341). One aspect of therapy deserves special emphasis. Namely, primary hypothyroidism can mask adrenal insufficiency by prolonging the half-life of cortisol; consequently, administration of thyroid hormone to a patient with unsuspected adrenal insufficiency can precipitate adrenal crisis. Thus, all patients with hypothyroidism in the context of PGA syndrome should be screened for adrenal disease and, if it is present, be treated with glucocorticoids prior to or concurrently with thyroid hormone therapy.

OTHER AUTOIMMUNE ENDOCRINE SYNDROMES

Insulin Receptor Antibodies Rare insulin-resistance syndromes occur in patients who develop antibodies that block the interaction of insulin with its receptor. Conversely, other classes of anti-insulin receptor antibodies can activate the receptor and can cause hypoglycemia; this disorder should be considered in the differential diagnosis of fasting hypoglycemia (Chap. 334).

Patients with insulin receptor antibodies and acanthosis nigricans are often middle-aged women who acquire insulin resistance in association with other autoimmune disorders such as systemic lupus erythematosus or Sjögren's syndrome. Vitiligo, alopecia, Raynaud's phenomenon, and arthritis may also be seen. Other autoimmune endocrine disorders, including thyrotoxicosis, hypothyroidism, and hypogonadism, occur rarely. Acanthosis nigricans, a velvety, hyperpigmented, thickened skin lesion, is prominent on the dorsum of the neck and other skin fold areas in the axillae or groin and often heralds the diagnosis in these patients. However, acanthosis nigricans also occurs in patients with obesity or polycystic ovarian syndrome, in which insulin resistance appears to be due to a postreceptor defect; thus acanthosis nigricans itself is not diagnostic of the immunologic form of insulin resistance.

Some patients with acanthosis nigricans have mild glucose intolerance, with a compensatory increase in insulin secretion that is only detected when insulin levels are measured. Others have severe diabetes mellitus requiring massive doses of insulin (several thousand units per day) to lower the blood glucose levels. The nature of the antibodies determines the manifestations; though insulin resistance is more common, fasting hypoglycemia can result from insulinomimetic antibodies.

Ataxia telangiectasia is an autosomal recessive disorder caused by mutations in *ATM*, a gene involved in cellular responses to ionizing radiation and oxidative damage (Chap. 364). This disorder is characterized by ataxia, telangiectasia, immune abnormalities, and an increased incidence of malignancies. Insulin-resistant diabetes mellitus occurs and is associated with anti-insulin antibodies.

Autoimmune Insulin Syndrome with Hypoglycemia This disorder typically occurs in patients with other autoimmune disorders and is caused by polyclonal insulin-binding autoantibodies that bind to endogenously synthesized insulin. If the insulin dissociates from the antibodies several hours or more after a meal, hypoglycemia can result. Most cases of the syndrome have been described from Japan, and there may be a genetic component. In plasma cell dyscrasias such as multiple myeloma, the plasma cells may produce monoclonal antibodies against insulin and cause hypoglycemia by a similar mechanism.

Antithyroxine Antibodies and Hypothyroidism Circulating autoantibodies against thyroid hormones in patients with both immune thyroid disease and plasma cell dyscrasias such as Waldenström's macroglobulinemia can bind thyroid hormones, decrease their biologic activity, and result in primary hypothyroidism. In other patients the antibodies simply interfere with thyroid hormone immunoassays and cause false elevations or decreases in measured hormone levels.

Crow-Fukase Syndrome The features of this syndrome are highlighted by an acronym that emphasizes its important features: *p*olyneuropathy, *o*rganomegaly, *e*ndocrinopathy, *M*-proteins, and *s*kin changes (POEMS). The most important feature is a severe, progressive sensorimotor polyneuropathy associated with a plasma cell dyscrasia. Localized collections of plasma cells (plasmacytomas) can cause sclerotic bone lesions and produce monoclonal IgG or IgA proteins. Endocrine manifestations include amenorrhea in women and impotence and gynecomastia in men, hypogonadism, hyperprolactinemia, type 2 diabetes mellitus, primary hypothyroidism, and adrenal insufficiency. Skin changes include hyperpigmentation, thickening of the dermis, hirsutism, and hyperhidrosis. Hepatomegaly and lymphadenopathy occur in about two-thirds of patients, and splenomegaly is seen in about one-third. Other manifestations include increased cerebrospinal fluid pressure with papilledema, peripheral edema, ascites, pleural effusions, glomerulonephritis, and fever. Five-year survival is about 60%.

The systemic nature of the disorder may cause confusion with other connective tissue diseases. The endocrine manifestations suggest an autoimmune basis of the disorder, but circulating antibodies against endocrine cells have not been demonstrated. Increased serum and tissue levels of interleukin 6, interleukin 1β, vascular endothelial growth factor, and tumor necrosis factor α are present, but the pathophysiologic basis for the POEMS syndrome is uncertain. Therapy directed against the plasma cell dyscrasia such as local radiation of bony lesions, chemotherapy, plasmapheresis, and treatment with all-*trans* retinoic acid may result in endocrine improvement.

MISCELLANEOUS DISORDERS WITH ENDOCRINE MANIFESTATIONS

A variety of other clinical and genetic disorders are associated with multiple endocrine manifestations are summarized in Table 339-3.

Table 339-3 Other Disorders with Common Polyglandular Manifestations

Condition	Clinical Features	Type of Endocrine Involvement: Hypothalamic-Pituitary	Thyroid	Parathyroid	Pancreas	Adrenal	Gonads	Inheritance/ Molecular Defect
Ataxia-telangiectasia	Early ataxia Oculocutaneous telangiectasia Immunologic deficiency	Occasional diminished pituitary reserve			Diabetes mellitus	Cortical hypoplasia	Dysgenetic gonads: gonadoblastomas later in females	Autosomal recessive Mutation of *ATM* gene
Pseudohypoparathyroidism	Short stature Short metacarpals and metatarsals Round facies Ectopic calcification	Variable deficiency of all pituitary hormones including prolactin	Hypo- or hyperthyroidism	Elevated parathyroid hormone levels with normo- or hypocalcemia	Diabetes mellitus		Ovarian failure	Mutation of the $G_{s\alpha}$
Myotonic dystrophy	Muscular dystrophy Premature baldness Mental retardation	Gonadotropin and growth hormone abnormalities, ? related to central integrative defect	Hypothyroidism		Diabetes mellitus		Primary gonadal failure	Insertion of unstable CTG repeat in myotonic dystrophy gene on chromosome 19
Noonan syndrome	Short stature Ptosis Webbed neck Pulmonary stenosis	Gonadotropin deficiency	Thyroiditis				Primary gonadal failure	Autosomal dominant
Fanconi syndrome	Short stature Bone marrow hypoplasia Abnormal skin pigmentation Radius malformations	Panhypopituitarism			Diabetes mellitus	Adrenal atrophy	Gonadal atrophy	Autosomal recessive Mutation of *FAA* gene
Werner syndrome	Premature aging Atropic skin Cataracts Early osteopenia		Papillary thyroid carcinoma		Diabetes mellitus		Gonadal atrophy	Autosomal recessive Mutation of *WRN* gene

NOTE: ATM, ataxia telangiectasia mutated; FAA, Fanconi anemia A; WRN, Werner.

BIBLIOGRAPHY

AGARWAL SK et al: Menin interacts with the AP1 transcription factor JunD and represses JunD-activated transcription. Cell 84:730, 1999

BETTERLE C et al: Clinical review 93: Autoimmune polyglandular syndrome type I. J Clin Endocrinol Metab 83:1049, 1998

BONI R et al: Somatic mutations of the MEN1 tumor suppressor gene detected in sporadic angiofibromas. J Invest Dermatol 111:539, 1998

CHANDRASEKHARAPPA SC et al: Positional cloning of the gene for multiple endocrine neoplasia-type 1. Science 276:404, 1997

DRALLE H et al: Prophylactic thyroidectomy in 75 children and adolescents with hereditary medullary thyroid carcinoma: German and Austrian experience. World J Surg 22:744, 1998

EISENHOFER G et al: Plasma normetanephrine and metanephrine for detecting pheochromocytoma in von Hippel–Lindau disease and multiple endocrine neoplasia type 2. N Engl J Med 340:1872, 9, 1999

GAGEL RF: Multiple endocrine neoplasia, in *Williams Textbook of Endocrinology*, 9th ed, JD Wilson, et al (eds). Philadelphia, Saunders, 1998

HEINO M et al: Mutation analyses of North American APS-1 patients. Hum Mutat 13:69, 1999

MARX S et al: Multiple endocrine neoplasia type 1: Clinical and genetic topics. Ann Intern Med 129:484, 1998

NORTON JA et al: Surgery to cure the Zollinger-Ellison syndrome. N Engl J Med 341: 635, 1999

SCOTT HS et al: Common mutations in autoimmune polyendocrinopathy-candidiasis-ectodermal dystrophy patients of different origins. Mol Endocrinol 12:1112, 1998

SOUBRIER MJ et al: POEMS syndrome: Study of 25 cases and a review of the literature. Am J Med 97:543, 1994

Section 2
DISORDERS OF BONE AND MINERAL METABOLISM

340 Michael F. Holick, Stephen M. Krane

INTRODUCTION TO BONE AND MINERAL METABOLISM

BONE STRUCTURE AND METABOLIM

(See also Chap. 343)

Bone is a dynamic tissue that is remodeled constantly throughout life. The arrangement of compact and cancellous bone provides a strength and density suitable for mobility. In addition, bone provides a reservoir for calcium, magnesium, phosphorus, sodium, and other ions necessary for homeostatic functions. The skeleton is highly vascular and receives about 10% of the cardiac output.

The extracellular components of bone consist of a solid mineral phase in close association with an organic matrix, of which 90 to 95% is type I collagen (Chap. 351). The noncollagenous portion of the organic matrix contains proteins derived from serum (albumin and α_2-HS glycoproteins), proteins containing α-carboxyglutamic acid (GLA) [*bone* GLA protein (BGP), *osteocalcin*, and a matrix GLA protein], the glycoprotein *osteonectin*, the phosphoprotein *osteopontin*, sialoproteins, *thrombospondin*, and other less well characterized proteins. Some of these proteins may function in initiating mineralization and in binding of the mineral phase to the matrix. The mineral phase is made up of calcium and phosphate and is best characterized as a poorly crystalline hydroxyapatite. The mineral phase of bone is deposited initially in intimate relation to the collagen fibrils and is found in specific locations in the "holes" between the collagen fibrils. This architectural arrangement of mineral and matrix results in a two-phase material well suited to withstand mechanical stresses.

Osteoblasts synthesize and secrete the organic matrix. Mineralization of the matrix, both in trabecular bone and in osteones of compact cortical bone (haversian systems), begins soon after the matrix is secreted (primary mineralization) but is not completed until after several weeks (secondary mineralization). Osteoblasts are derived from cells of mesenchymal origin (Fig. 340-1*A*). Although relatively little is known about the controls of osteoblast development, two genes have been shown to be important: core-binding factor A1 (*CBFA1*) and Indian hedgehog (*Ihh*). CBFA1 is a transcription factor and a homologue of the Drosophila factor, runt, and is expressed specifically in osteoblast progenitors and regulates the expression of several osteoblast-specific genes including osteopontin, bone sialoprotein, type I collagen, osteocalcin, and receptor-activator of NFκB (RANK) ligand. CBFA1 expression is regulated, in part, by bone morphogenic proteins (BMPs). *Cbfa1*-deficient mice are devoid of osteoblasts. Mice with a functional deletion of *Cbfa1* (*Cbfa1* $-/-$) have a cartilaginous skeleton but no osteoblasts and no bone, whereas mice with a deletion of only one allele (*Cbfa1* $+/-$) do have an osseous skeleton but have a delay in intramembranous bone formation of some cranial bones and the clavicles. The latter abnormalities are similar to those in the human disorder cleidocranial dysplasia, which maps to the locus that corresponds to *Cbfa1*.

The growth factor Ihh also plays a critical role in osteoblast development, as evidenced by the fact that Ihh-deficient mice lack osteoblasts in bone formed by endochondral ossification. Numerous other growth-regulatory factors affect osteoblast function, including transforming growth factor (TGF) β types I and II, acidic fibroblast growth factor (aFGF) and basic fibroblast growth factor (bFGF), platelet-derived growth factor (PDGF), and insulin-like growth factors (IGFs) I and II. Active osteoblasts are characterized by their location and morphology; the presence of a specific skeletal form of alkaline phosphatase; the presence of receptors for parathyroid hormone (PTH) and 1,25-dihydroxyvitamin D [$1,25(OH)_2D$]; and the ability to synthesize specific matrix proteins, such as type I collagen, osteocalcin, and osteopontin. As an osteoblast secretes matrix, which is then mineralized, the cell becomes an *osteocyte*, still connected with its blood supply through a series of canaliculi. Osteocytes are thought to be the mechanosensors in bone that communicate signals to surface osteoblasts and their progenitors through the canalicular network.

Resorption of bone is carried out mainly by *osteoclasts*, multinucleated cells that are formed by fusion of cells derived from hematopoietic stem cells related to the mononuclear phagocyte series. Multiple factors regulating osteoclast development have been identified (Fig. 340-1*B*). Macrophage colony stimulating factor (M-CSF) plays a critical role at several steps in the pathway that ultimately leads to fusion of osteoclast progenitor cells to form multinucleated, active osteoclasts. Discovery of the RANK signaling pathway provides new insight into the pathway that links osteoblast and osteoclast development (Fig. 343-2). RANK ligand is expressed on the surface of osteoblast progenitors and stromal fibroblasts. In a process involving cell-cell interactions, it binds to the RANK receptor on osteoclast progenitors, stimulating a signal transduction cascade that leads to osteoclast differentiation and activation. Al-

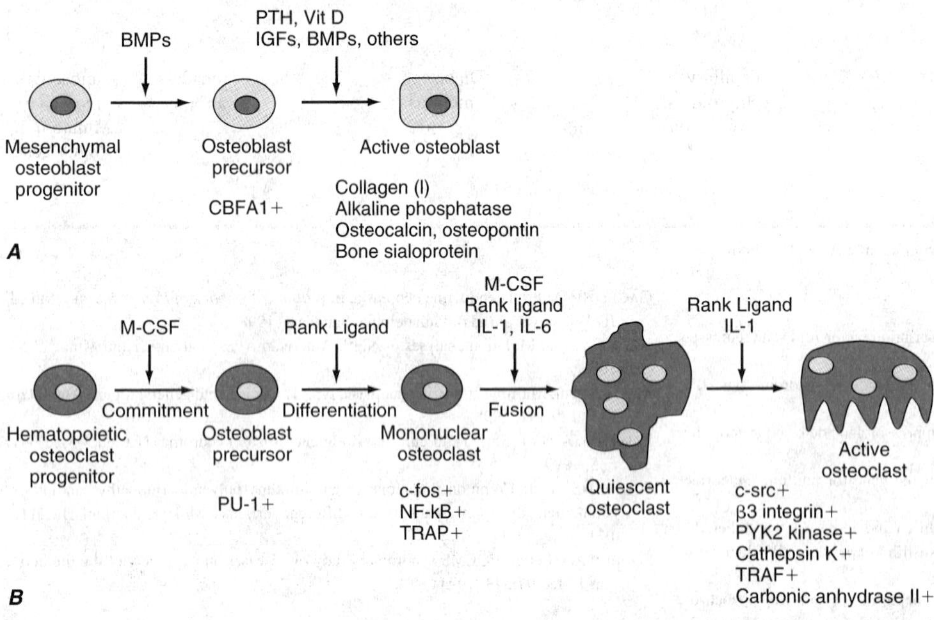

FIGURE 340-1 Pathways regulating development of (*A*) osteoblasts and (*B*) osteoclasts. Hormones, cytokines, and growth factors that control cell proliferation and differentiation are shown above the arrows. Transcription factors and other markers specific for various stages of development are depicted below the arrows. BMPs, bone morphogenic proteins; PTH, parathyroid hormone; Vit D, vitamin D; IGFs, insulin-like growth factors; CBFA1, core binding factor A1; M-CSF, macrophage colony stimulating factor; PU-1, a monocyte- and B lymphocyte–specific ets family transcription factor; NFκB, nuclear factor κB; TRAF, tumor necrosis factor receptor–associated factors; RANK ligand, receptor activator of NFκB ligand; IL-1, interleukin-1; IL-6, interleukin-6. *(Modified from Suda et al.)*

ternatively, a soluble decoy receptor, referred to as *osteoprotegerin* (OPG), can bind RANK ligand and inhibit osteoclast differentiation. Several growth factors and cytokines, including interleukins (IL) 1, 6, and 11, tumor necrosis factor (TNF), interferon γ, and M-CSF, modulate the osteoclast differentiation and function. Osteoclasts are also regulated indirectly by osteoblasts and adjacent stromal fibroblasts in the marrow. For example, PTH receptors are not found on mature osteoclasts, and PTH increases osteoclastic bone resorption by first acting on osteoblasts or stromal fibroblasts. $1,25(OH)_2D$ receptors are found in precursor cells that can differentiate into monocytes or osteoclasts, and $1,25(OH)_2D$ also promotes differentiation along the osteoclast pathway.

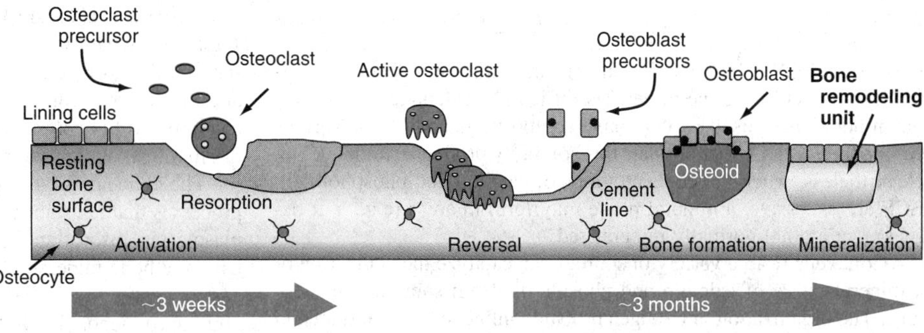

FIGURE 340-2 Schematic representation of bone remodeling. The cycle of bone remodeling is carried out by the basic multicellular unit (BMU), comprising a group of osteoclasts and osteoblasts. In cortical bone, the BMUs tunnel through the tissue, whereas in cancellous bone, they move across the trabecular surface. The process of bone remodeling is initiated by contraction of the lining cells and the recruitment of osteoclast precursors. These precursors fuse to form multinucleated, active osteoclasts that mediate bone resorption. Osteoclasts adhere to bone and subsequently remove it by acidification and proteolytic digestion. As the BMU advances, osteoclasts leave the resorption site and osteoblasts move in to cover the excavated area and begin the process of new bone formation by secreting osteoid, which is eventually mineralized into new bone. After osteoid mineralization, osteoblasts flatten and form a layer of lining cells over new bone.

In the embryo and in the growing child, bone develops by remodeling and replacing previously calcified cartilage (endochondral bone formation) or is formed without a cartilage matrix (intramembranous bone formation). The PTH/PTHrP receptor plays a central role in the control of chondrocyte differentiation at growth plates (Chap. 341). Ihh production by growth plate chondrocytes stimulates the production of PTH-related peptide (PTHrP), which slows the differentiation of chondrocytes. This pathway creates a local feedback system as Ihh is suppressed by the actions of PTHrP. Consistent with this mechanism, mice with null mutations of the PTH/PTHrP receptor or PTHrP exhibit growth plate chondrodysplasia that reflects accelerated differentiation of proliferating chondrocytes. In humans, homozygous inactivating mutations of the PTH/PTHrP receptor cause Blomstrand's chondrodysplasia.

New bone, whether formed in infants or in adults during repair, has a relatively high ratio of cells to matrix and is characterized by coarse fiber bundles of collagen that are interlaced and randomly dispersed (woven bone). In adults, the more mature bone is organized with fiber bundles regularly arranged in parallel or concentric sheets (lamellar bone). In long bones, deposition of lamellar bone in a concentric arrangement around blood vessels forms the haversian systems. Growth in length of bones is dependent on proliferation of cartilage cells and on the endochondral sequence at the growth plate. Growth in width and thickness is accomplished by formation of bone at the periosteal surface and by resorption at the endosteal surface, with the rate of formation exceeding that of resorption. In adults, after the epiphyses close, growth in length and endochondral bone formation cease, except for some activity in the cartilage cells beneath the articular surface. Even in adults, however, remodeling of bone (remodeling of haversian systems as well as trabecular bone) continues throughout life. In adults, ~4% of the surface of trabecular bone (such as iliac crest) is involved in active resorption, whereas 10 to 15% of trabecular surfaces is covered with osteoid. Radioisotope studies indicate that as much as 18% of the total skeletal calcium is deposited and removed each year. Thus, bone is an active metabolizing tissue that requires an intact blood supply.

The response of bone to fractures, infection, and interruption of blood supply and to expanding lesions is relatively limited. Dead bone must be resorbed, and new bone must be formed, a process carried out in association with growth of new blood vessels into the involved area. In injuries that disrupt the organization of the tissue, such as a fracture in which apposition of fragments is poor or when motion exists at the fracture site, the progenitor stromal cells differentiate into cells with functional capacities different from those of osteoblasts, and varying amounts of fibrous tissue and cartilage are formed. When there is good apposition with fixation and little motion at the fracture site, repair occurs predominantly by formation of new bone without other scar tissue.

Remodeling of bone occurs along lines of force modulated by the mechanical stresses to which it is subjected. The signals from these mechanical stresses are sensed by osteocytes, which then transmit other signals to osteoclasts (or their precursors) or osteoblasts (or their precursors). A bowing deformity increases new bone formation at the concave surface and resorption at the convex surface, seemingly designed to produce the strongest mechanical structure. Expanding lesions in bone, such as tumors, induce resorption at the surface in contact with the tumor. Even in a disorder as architecturally disruptive as Paget's disease, remodeling is dictated by mechanical forces. Thus, the plasticity of bone is due to the interaction of cells with each other and with the environment.

The cycle of bone resorption and formation is a highly orchestrated process carried out by the basic multicellular unit (BMU), composed of a group of osteoclasts and osteoblasts (Fig. 340-2). Osteoclast-mediated resorption of bone takes place in scalloped spaces (*Howship's lacunae*) where the osteoclasts are attached through a specific $\alpha v,\beta 3$ integrin to components of the bone matrix such as osteopontin. This clear zone contains contractile proteins. The resorbing end of the cell forms a specialized ruffled border, which is in contact with the bone. Proteins, including a specialized proton-pump ATPase, are found in the ruffled border membrane and contribute to the acid environment, which solubilizes the mineral phase. In addition to the proton pump, carbonic anhydrase (type II isoenzyme) is required to maintain the acid pH. Other features of active osteoclasts include expression of the proto-oncogene c-*src*, tartrate-resistant acid phosphatase, cell-surface receptors for calcitonin, sodium pumps of the kidney type, a bicarbonate/chloride exchanger of the band 3 family, and an ability to resorb mineralized bone. The bone matrix is resorbed in the acid environment adjacent to the ruffled border by proteinases that act at low pH, such as cathepsin K, following solubilization of the mineral phase.

Bone formation involves deposition of an organic matrix by osteoblasts followed by mineralization. The mineral phase is composed of calcium and phosphorus, and the concentration of these ions in the plasma and extracellular fluid (ECF) influences the rate at which mineral is formed. In vitro, mineralization can proceed and crystals of hydroxyapatite can grow at concentrations of calcium and phosphorus similar to those in an ultrafiltrate of plasma. The calcium phosphate solid phase at the inception of mineralization is brushite ($CaHPO_4 \cdot 2H_2O$). As mineralization progresses, the solid phase is a poorly crystalline hydroxyapatite with a relatively low (~1.2) calcium/phosphate molar ratio. With age and maturation, the perfection of the crystals and the calcium/phosphate ratio increase. Fluoride ions, when incorporated into the mineral phase, decrease the proportion of amorphous calcium phosphate and enhance the crystal structure.

There is a limit for the concentration of calcium and phosphorus ions in the ECF below which mineralization does not occur. A "solubility product" for bone mineral is difficult to calculate because (1) the mineral phase itself is of variable composition, and (2) the various components in ECF that regulate this solubility product are not known. Nevertheless, when the concentrations of calcium and phosphorus in ECF are excessive, a mineral phase may form in areas (e.g., soft tissues) that are not normally mineralized.

Collagens from a variety of sources can catalyze the nucleation of a mineral phase of calcium and phosphorus from solutions of these ions. The organization of collagen probably influences the amount and type of mineral phase formed in bone. The primary structures of type I collagen in skin and bone tissues are similar. There are differences, however, in posttranslational modifications of type I collagen, such as hydroxylations; glycosylations; and the type, number, and distribution of intermolecular cross-links (Chap. 351). In addition, the holes in the packing structure of the collagen are larger in mineralized collagen of bone and dentin than in unmineralized collagens such as tendon. Single amino-acid substitutions in the helical portion of either the $\alpha1$ or $\alpha2$ chain of type I collagen due to mutations in the *COL*1A1 or *COL*1A2 genes in osteogenesis imperfecta disrupt the organization of bone, and this indicates the importance of the fibrillar matrix in the structure of bone. At the time of their discovery, it was thought that some of the non-collagenous bone proteins—e.g., osteocalcin (bone-GLA protein), osteonectin, and osteopontin—played a role in mineralization, although such a role has not been established. Osteocalcin, a product exclusively of osteoblasts, is measurable by immunoassays in normal human serum, and its levels correlate with other measurements of bone formation. Matrix-GLA protein (MGP), a component of bone as well as non-osseous tissues, acts to inhibit mineralization in the non-osseous tissues. Thus, functional deletion of the MGP gene in mice results in massive soft tissue calcification, particularly in arterial walls.

Alkaline phosphatase is a marker for osteoblasts, and cellular levels of this enzyme correlate with rates of bone formation. Although mineralization defects occur in individuals with mutations that decrease alkaline phosphatase activity (hypophosphatasia), the function of alkaline phosphatase in mineralization is not completely understood. Other circulating markers of bone formation include osteocalcin and type I procollagen C-terminal peptides. Urinary markers for bone resorption are hydroxyproline, hydroxylysine and its glycosides, and the bone-specific hydroxypyridinium collagen cross-links (Chap. 342). Inorganic pyrophosphate is a potent inhibitor of mineralization at levels below those necessary to bind calcium ions.

CALCIUM METABOLISM

A total of 1 to 2 kg of calcium is present in the average adult, >98% of it in the skeleton. The calcium of the mineral phase at the surface of the crystals is in equilibrium with that in the ECF, but only a minor fraction of the total pool (~0.5%) is exchangeable. In normal adults plasma levels range from 2.2 to 2.6 mmol/L (8.8 to 10.4 mg/dL). The calcium in plasma is present as three forms: free ions, ions bound to plasma proteins, and, to a small extent, diffusible complexes. The concentration of free calcium ions, averaging 1.2 mmol/L (4.8 mg/dL), influences many cellular functions and is subjected to tight hormonal control, especially through PTH (Chap. 341). The concentration of serum proteins is an important determinant of calcium ion concentration; most calcium ion is bound to albumin. Ionized calcium can be measured directly with the use of calcium-specific electrodes. If ionized calcium cannot be measured, certain approximations can be used to estimate the protein-bound and ionized fractions. One formula that approximates the amount of calcium bound to protein is

$$\begin{aligned}\%\ \text{protein-bound Ca} &= 0.8 \times \text{albumin (g/L)}\\ &+ 0.2 \times \text{globulin (g/L)} + 3\end{aligned}$$

A simplified correction is sometimes used to assess whether the total serum calcium concentration is abnormal when serum proteins are low. The correction is to add 1 mg/dL to the serum calcium level for every 1 g/dL by which the serum albumin level is below 4.0 g/dL. If the serum calcium level, for example, is 7.8 mg/dL (a subnormal value) and the serum albumin level is only 3.0 g/dL, then the stated serum calcium level is corrected by adding 1 mg/dL; the corrected value of 8.8 mg/dL is within the normal range.

The concentration of calcium ions in the ECF is kept constant by processes that constantly add and remove calcium. Calcium enters the plasma via absorption from the intestinal tract and resorption of ions from the bone mineral. Calcium leaves the ECF via secretion into the gastrointestinal tract (~100 to 200 mg/d), urinary excretion (~50 to 300 mg/d), deposition in bone mineral, and losses in sweat (up to 100 mg/d). Bone resorption and formation are tightly coupled, with approximately 12 mmol (500 mg) calcium entering and leaving the skeleton daily (Fig. 340-3). Calcium ions inside the cell mediate a variety of cellular functions. The level of free calcium in the cell is very low, approximately 0.1 μmol/L; thus, the gradient between plasma and intracellular free calcium is about 10,000 to 1. This gradient is tightly regulated by various channels and ion pumps.

The average dietary calcium intake for most adults in the United States is approximately 15 to 20 mmol/d (0.6 to 0.8 g/d). However, with heightened awareness of the role of adequate calcium intake for the prevention of osteoporosis, many adults on supplements have an intake of 20 to 37 mmol/d (0.8 to 1.5 g/d). Less than half of dietary calcium is absorbed in adults. Calcium absorption increases during periods of rapid growth in children, in pregnancy, and in lactation and decreases with advancing age. Most of the calcium is absorbed in the proximal small intestine, and the efficiency of absorption decreases in the more distal intestinal segments. Both active transport and diffusion-limited absorption are involved; the former is more important in the upper intestine and the latter in the lower intestine. Both processes are influenced by vitamin D (see below). All forms of calcium in the diet are not equally absorbed; calcium as the chloride is probably absorbed more efficiently than that in other preparations. Secretion of calcium into the intestinal lumen is constant and independent of absorption. If calcium availability in the diet is low [<12 mmol/d (500 mg/d)], a positive calcium balance requires an efficiency of absorption >30 to 40%.

The urinary calcium excretion of normal adults having an average calcium intake ranges between 2.5 and 10 mmol/d (100 and 400 mg/d). When the dietary calcium level is <5 mmol/d (200 mg/d), urinary calcium excretion is usually <5 mmol/d (200 mg/d). However, in most normal individuals, wide variations in dietary intake have little effect on urinary calcium. Hence, when the diet is low in calcium, the

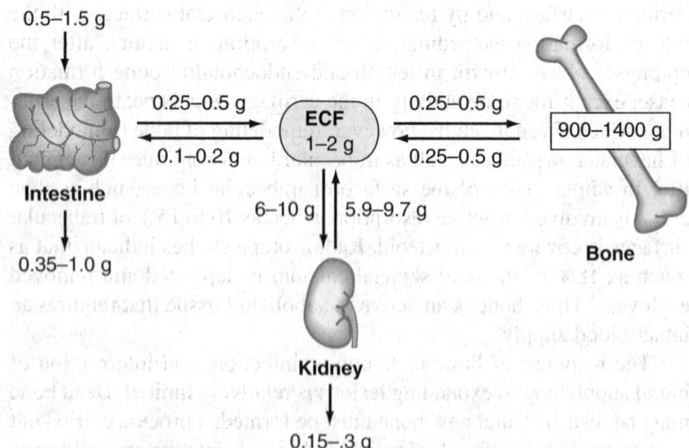

FIGURE 340-3 Calcium homeostasis. Schematic illustration of calcium content of extracellular fluid (ECF) and bone as well as of diet and feces; magnitude of calcium flux per day as calculated by various methods is shown at sites of transport in intestine, kidney, and bone. Ranges of values shown are approximate and chosen to illustrate certain points discussed in text. In conditions of calcium balance, rates of calcium release from and uptake into bone are equal.

relative inefficiency of renal calcium conservation leads to a negative calcium balance unless calcium absorption is maximal (Fig. 340-3).

The amount of calcium in the urine is small compared with that filtered by the glomerulus [~150 to 250 mmol/d (6 to 10 g/d)] because the rates of reabsorption of the filtered calcium are high. Reabsorption takes place predominantly in the proximal tubule (~60%) and in Henle's loop (~25%) and to a small extent in the distal tubule. The calcium-sensing receptor also plays a role in renal calcium excretion, though the mechanisms that regulate its function have not been fully defined (Chap. 341). The excretion of other electrolytes affects the urinary excretion of calcium. For example, urinary calcium is usually proportional to urinary sodium; sulfate also increases calcium excretion.

A deficiency of PTH or vitamin D, intestinal disease, or severe dietary calcium deprivation may provide challenges to calcium homeostasis that cannot be compensated adequately by renal calcium conservation, resulting in a negative calcium balance. Increased bone resorption may protect against ECF calcium depletion even in states of chronic negative calcium balance but only at the expense of progressive bone loss.

PATHOPHYSIOLOGY A decrease in the concentration of free calcium ions in plasma results in increased neuromuscular irritability and tetany. This syndrome is characterized by peripheral and perioral paresthesia, carpal spasm, pedal spasm, anxiety, seizures, bronchospasm, laryngospasm, Chvostek's sign, Trousseau's sign, and Erb's sign, and lengthening of the QT interval of the electrocardiogram. In infants tetany may be manifested only by irritability and lethargy. The level of calcium ions that determines which features of tetany will be manifested varies among individuals. Tetany is also influenced by other components of the ECF; e.g., hypomagnesemia and alkalosis lower whereas hypokalemia and acidosis raise the threshold for tetany.

Increases in total serum calcium concentration are usually accompanied by increases in free calcium levels and may be associated with anorexia, nausea, vomiting, constipation, hypotonia, depression, and occasionally lethargy and coma. Persistent hypercalcemia, especially when accompanied by normal or elevated levels of serum phosphate, may cause ectopic deposition of a solid phase of calcium and phosphate in walls of blood vessels, connective tissue about the joints, gastric mucosa, cornea, and renal parenchyma. Hypercalcemia per se alters renal function in addition to the pathologic effects of calcium phosphate deposition.

PHOSPHORUS METABOLISM

Phosphorus is a major component of bone and of all other tissues and in some form is involved in almost all metabolic processes, including energy storage, membrane transport, membrane composition, and signal transduction. About 600 g of phosphorus is present in the normal adult, of which 85% is present in the crystalline structure of the skeleton.

In plasma from fasting subjects, most of the phosphorus is present as inorganic orthophosphate in concentrations of approximately 0.75 to 1.45 mmol/L (2.5 to 4.5 mg/dL). In contrast to calcium, of which ~50% is bound, only ~12% of the phosphorus in plasma is bound to proteins. Free HPO_4^{2-} and $NaHPO_4^-$ normally account for ~75% of the total phosphorus, and free $H_2PO_4^-$ accounts for ~10%. Since so many species are present, depending on pH and other factors, concentrations are usually expressed in terms of elemental phosphorus, in units of mmol/L or mg/dL. The serum phosphorus, however, can vary based on age; young children have almost twice the serum phosphorus as adults due to the need for rapid skeletal mineralization. Postmenopausal women also have higher circulating phosphorus levels. After ingesting a meal containing carbohydrate, there is a decrease in serum phosphorus levels [by 0.3 to 0.5 mmol/dL (1.0 to 1.5 mg/dL)] in response to the increase in insulin secretion, which enhances cellular phosphorus uptake and utilization. An increase in serum pH will decrease serum phosphorus, whereas a decrease in pH increases phos-

phorus concentration. There is a circadian variation in phosphorus concentration even during a 24-h fast: the nadir occurs between 9:00 A.M. and noon followed by an increase to a plateau in the afternoon and another small peak after midnight.

Phosphorus is plentiful in the diet. Common sources include dairy products, meats, eggs, and carbonated beverages that contain phosphoric acid. Approximately 60 to 70% of phosphorus is passively absorbed in the small intestine (Fig. 340-4). $1,25(OH)_2D$ enhances phosphorus absorption along the entire small intestine, with the highest efficiency in the jejunum and ileum. Chronic low phosphorus intake (<2 mg/kg of body weight per day) decreases serum phosphorus levels. Low serum phosphorus stimulates the renal production of $1,25(OH)_2D$, which, in turn, increases the efficiency intestinal absorption up to 80 to 90%. $1,25(OH)_2D$ also decreases PTH secretion and, thereby reduces renal tubular loss of phosphorus.

The major control of phosphorus balance is exerted by the kidney. Approximately 90% of phosphorus in the circulation is filtered through the glomerulus and is largely absorbed by the proximal tubule such that only 10 to 15% of the filtered load is normally excreted. Urinary phosphorus excretion is reflective of dietary intake. Phosphorus absorption in the proximal tubule is coupled with sodium absorption. The primary regulation of phosphorus metabolism occurs in the distal convoluted tubule, and this mechanism is independent of sodium reabsorption. Volume expansion and decreased sodium reabsorption increase phosphorus clearance.

HYPOPHOSPHATEMIA Causes Although there are many potential causes for hypophosphatemia (Table 340-1), the most common etiologies include: (1) decreased intestinal phosphorus absorption, either due to vitamin D deficiency or the presence of a phosphorus-binding antacid; (2) urinary losses that are PTH- or alcohol-mediated; and (3) a shift of phosphorus from extracellular to intracellular compartments due to exogenous administration of insulin or consumption of nutrients that stimulate insulin release (e.g., carbohydrates). Increased renal clearance of phosphorus occurs in primary hyperparathyroidism, vitamin D deficiency, vitamin D–resistant and D–dependent rickets, hyperglycemic states, and oncogenic osteomalacia. In vitamin D deficiency, serum phosphorus is low because

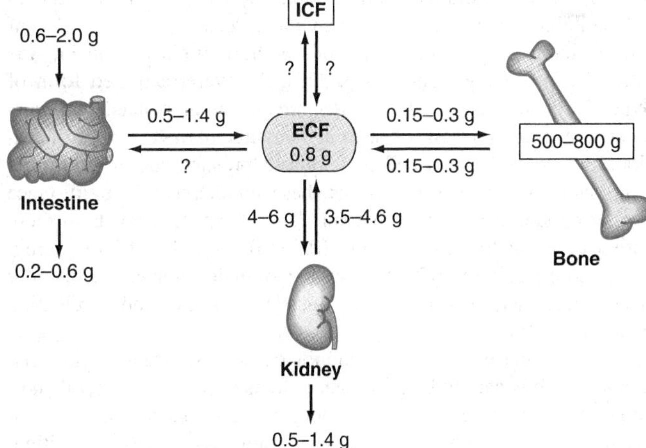

FIGURE 340-4 Phosphate homeostasis. Schematic illustration of inorganic phosphorus content (termed here *phosphate*) in extracellular fluid (ECF) and bone as well as diet and feces; magnitude of phosphorus flux per day as estimated by various methods is shown at transport sites in intestine, kidney, and bone. Range of values shown illustrates special features of phosphorus metabolism discussed in text. The compartment labeled ICF refers to intracellular phosphorus, both organic and inorganic; rapid shifts of phosphorus into cells (and corresponding, possibly slower, efflux of phosphorus from cells) contribute to changes in ECF phosphorus. These shifts between ECF and ICF and phosphorus release from and uptake by bone are equal in conditions of phosphorus balance.

Table 340-1 Causes of Hypophosphatemia

Decreased intestinal phosphate absorption
Vitamin D deficiency
Vitamin D–dependent rickets types I and II
Malabsorption
Phosphate-binding antacids
Extracellular shift of phosphorus to intracellular compartment
Increased renal phosphate excretion
Hyperparathyroidism
Vitamin D deficiency
Vitamin D–dependent rickets types I and II
X-linked hypophosphatemic rickets
Fanconi syndromes
Oncogenic osteomalacia
Hyperglycemic states
Alcoholism and alcohol withdrawal
Ketoacidosis
Other
Respiratory alkalosis
Blast crisis in leukemia
Starvation
Insulin therapy
Hungry bone syndrome after parathyroidectomy
Recovery from hypothermia
Sepsis

of decreased intestinal absorption as well as secondary hyperparathyroidism, which increases phosphorus losses in the urine. In X-linked hypophosphatemic rickets, there is a genetic defect in the *PHEX* gene, which encodes a neutral endopeptidase presumed to degrade the phosphaturia hormone known as *phosphatonin*. The disorder is associated with a severe renal leak of phosphorus into the urine. In addition, there is a defect in hypophosphatemia-mediated stimulation of 25(OH)D-1α-hydroxylase, resulting in decreased intestinal phosphorus absorption. Acidosis and hyperglycemic states associated with polyuria also cause excessive phosphorus loss in the urine. Ketoacidosis enhances intracellular and organic phosphorus degradation, thereby releasing large amounts of inorganic phosphorus into the circulation that is cleared into the urine. In ketosis, the serum phosphorus is often normal because of the continuous shift of phosphorus from intracellular to extracellular pools. However, when the ketosis is corrected, hypophosphatemia is apparent because of the return of phosphorus into the intracellular compartment (Chap. 333). A severe, acquired form of hypophosphatemia, *oncogenic osteomalacia*, is associated with vascular, mesenchymal tumors such as hemangiopericytomas but occasionally also with small cell lung cancer, prostate cancer, and other malignant tumors. It is likely that these tumors secrete a substance similar or identical to phosphatonin. The phosphorus levels in these patients are usually extremely low [0.4 to 0.5 mmol/L (1.2 to 1.5 mg/dL)], and the 1,25(OH)$_2$D levels are low or undetectable. The disorder is associated with severe fatigue, muscle weakness, and unrelenting bone discomfort.

Alcohol abuse is the most common cause of severe hypophosphatemia, which is caused by poor dietary intake of phosphorus, ethanol-enhanced urinary excretion of inorganic phosphorus, the use of calcium- or aluminum-containing antacids, and vomiting. Hypophosphatemia may transiently worsen with refeeding. Alcoholics may also have associated calcium and vitamin D deficiency and secondary hyperparathyroidism, which enhances phosphorus-wasting in the urine. Alcoholic ketoacidosis induces marked phosphaturia. Intense hyperventilation for prolonged periods may depress serum phosphorus levels due to associated alkalosis. Rapid correction of chronic respiratory acidosis has also been associated with hypophosphatemia and can lead to diaphragm weakness and an exacerbation of respiratory failure. Advanced leukemia with blast crisis (leukocyte counts usually >100,000) may cause severe hypophosphatemia; the likely cause is a rapid uptake of phosphorus into the rapidly dividing cells.

Laboratory and Clinical Findings Serum phosphorus levels should be determined in a fasting state. Mild hypophosphatemia is not usually associated with clinical symptoms. In severe hypophosphatemia [≤0.3 mmol/L (≤1.0 mg/dL)], multiple organ systems are affected. Patients become irritable, apprehensive, and hyperventilate, resulting in complaints of muscle weakness, numbness, and paresthesia. In the most severe form, they are confused or obtunded and suffer from seizures and coma, which can ultimately lead to death. This metabolic encephalopathy is often associated with slowing of the electroencephalogram.

Phosphorus is essential for muscle function because of the need for large amounts of ATP and creatine phosphate. Patients with severe hypophosphatemia often complain of fatigue, muscle weakness, myalgia, and myopathy. Hypophosphatemia can cause rhabdomyolysis, which is particularly common in chronic alcoholics or during alcohol withdrawal. Rhabdomyolysis can be precipitated during treatment for diabetic ketoacidosis or by hyperalimentation or refeeding in a malnourished patient. Cardiomyopathy can also occur, resulting in reduced cardiac output, impaired pressor responsiveness to catecholamines, hypotension, and ventricular arrhythmias. Restoration of phosphorus deficits can result in prompt reversal. Severe muscle weakness can lead to respiratory insufficiency.

Erythrocytes and leukocytes are highly dependent on phosphorus for their function. Chronic hypophosphatemia decreases 2,3-bisphosphoglycerate and ATP, enhancing oxygen dissociation from hemoglobin and leading to tissue hypoxia. Hypophosphatemia causes impaired phagocytosis and opsonization and, therefore, increases susceptibility to bacterial and fungal infections.

Chronic hypophosphatemia causes a mineralization defect of the skeleton. In children, this causes rickets. In adults, chronic hypophosphatemia (often due to vitamin D deficiency) causes osteomalacia (see below). Patients with severe renal phosphorus-wasting and severe chronic hypophosphatemia may have marked fatigue, muscle weakness, and severe bone pain, especially of their long bones and ribcage.

℞ TREATMENT Mild hypophosphatemia usually resolves spontaneously when the underlying cause is corrected. Oral phosphorus replacement is sufficient if serum phosphorus is >0.3 mmol/L (1 mg/dL) and the patient is asymptomatic. Milk is an excellent source of phosphorus as it contains 1 g of inorganic phosphorus per liter. Carbonated beverages that contain phosphoric acid provide another source of phosphorus, especially for patients with lactase deficiency. Pharmaceutical preparations of phosphorus, such as Neutraphos or KPhos, contain sodium and potassium salts of phosphate. Depending on the degree of hypophosphatemia, up to 3 g/d can be given in four to six divided doses per 24 h. These doses usually do not cause diarrhea; >5 g/d will induce diarrhea.

For severe hypophosphatemia, with serum phosphorus levels <0.2 to 0.3 mmol/L (<0.5 to 1.0 mg/dL), ≥3 g/d of phosphorus may be required over several days to replete body stores. In patients with severe symptomatic hypophosphatemia who are unable to eat, intravenous phosphorus can be given, up to 1 g in 1 L of fluid over 8 to 12 h. Some caution is necessary when giving phosphorus intravenously because of the potential for precipitating soft tissue calcification. A serum calcium × serum phosphorus product >70 markedly increases the risk of soft tissue calcification and nephrocalcinosis. Patients with chronic hypophosphatemia caused by inherited or acquired renal phosphorus leak require vigilance when receiving high doses of oral phosphorus. Transiently elevated serum phosphorus levels can decrease ionized calcium levels, resulting in chronic stimulation of the parathyroid gland and leading to autonomous, persistent hyperplasia of the parathyroid glands. Thus, it is best to give frequent divided doses of phosphorus (four to six times a day), equaling a total of 2 to 3 g/d.

Phosphorus should not be given intramuscularly or subcutaneously because it can cause soft tissue necrosis and severe discomfort. Intravenous sodium or potassium phosphate, 15 mmol (0.465 g) of elemental phosphorus given in 100 mL of 0.9% saline over 60 min, el-

Table 340-2 Causes of Hyperphosphatemia

Decreased renal phosphate excretion	Other
Acute renal failure	Vitamin D intoxication
Chronic renal failure	Acidosis, respiratory or metabolic
Hypoparathyroidism	Crush injuries
Pseudohypoparathyroidism	Rhabdomyolysis
Tumoral calcinosis	Cytotoxic therapy and tumor lysis
Bisphosphonates	Fulminant hepatitis
Acromegaly	Extracellular shift from intracellular compartment
	Artifactual due to hemolysis

evates serum phosphorus levels by an average of 0.6 to 1.2 mmol/L (1.75 to 3.8 mg/dL).

HYPERPHOSPHATEMIA In adults, hyperphosphatemia is defined as a serum phosphorus level >1.6 mmol/L (5 mg/dL). In children, this level is much higher. The most common causes of hyperphosphatemia are acute and chronic renal failure (Table 340-2). In renal failure, the loss of tubular function impairs phosphorus excretion. This results in a cascade of events that can also affect calcium and phosphorus metabolism. The increase in serum phosphorus levels reduces serum calcium levels and the production of $1,25(OH)_2D$, leading to decreased intestinal calcium absorption and secondary hyperparathyroidism. Patients with pseudohypoparathyroidism and tumoral calcinosis also have decreased renal phosphorus clearance that results in hyperphosphatemia. Hypothyroidism reduces renal phosphorus excretion and may increase circulating concentrations of phosphorus. Vitamin D intoxication, due to excessive ingestion of either vitamin D or one of its analogues, can cause hyperphosphatemia along with hypercalcemia. Severe hypothermia, crush injuries, nontrauma rhabdomyolysis, tumoral calcinosis, and cytotoxic therapy of hematologic malignancies such as acute lymphoblastic leukemia can be associated with hyperphosphatemia. The serum phosphorus level can be artifactually elevated due to hemolysis of the blood sample. Thrombocytosis and multiple myeloma can cause spuriously elevated serum phosphorus levels due to thrombocytolysis.

Laboratory and Clinical Findings A rapid elevation of serum phosphorus can cause hypocalcemia and symptoms of neuromuscular irritability and tetany. Chronic hyperphosphatemia in association with normocalcemia can result in nephrocalcinosis and soft tissue calcification.

℞ **TREATMENT** In addition to treating the underlying disorder, dietary phosphorus intake should be limited by restricting carbonated beverages containing phosphoric acid and decreasing milk and dairy product consumption. The dietary intake of phosphorus should be between 600 and 1000 mg a day with modest protein restriction. For control of chronic hyperphosphatemia, usually in patients with chronic renal failure, oral aluminum hydroxide or aluminum carbonate gels are indicated. Prolonged use of aluminum-containing compounds is not recommended because of aluminum toxicity causing adynamic bone disease, proximal myopathy, encephalopathy, and anemia. When hyperphosphatemia is due to vitamin D intoxication, calcium salts are contraindicated because the high efficiency of calcium absorption can lead to severe hypercalcemia, soft tissue calcification, and nephrocalcinosis.

MAGNESIUM METABOLISM

Magnesium is the most abundant intracellular divalent cation. It is an essential cofactor for a multitude of enzymatic reactions that are important for the generation of energy from ATP. Approximately 30% of magnesium in the serum is protein-bound, 55% is ionized, and the remaining 15% is complexed. Like calcium, magnesium is bound to albumin, and it is the ionized fraction that is important for physiologic processes including neuromuscular function and maintenance of cardiovascular tone.

The serum concentration of magnesium is tightly regulated within a narrow range of approximately 0.7 to 1.1 mmol/L (1.4 to 2.2 meq/L)(1.7 to 2.6 mg/dl) as a result of the efficient absorption of dietary magnesium by the small intestine and conservation of magnesium in the kidney. About 30% of dietary magnesium is absorbed in the small intestine, but this fraction increases markedly when intake is substantially reduced. Approximately 96% of filtered magnesium is reabsorbed along the nephron, and only 4% is excreted into the urine. Because there is no regulation of magnesium absorption in the distal tubule and because magnesium reabsorption is very efficient, an increase in distal delivery increases magnesium loss in the urine.

HYPOMAGNESEMIA Although magnesium deficiency is a common clinical problem, serum magnesium levels are often overlooked or not measured in patients at risk for the disorder. Approximately 10% of patients admitted to city hospitals are hypomagnesemic, and up to 65% of patients in intensive care units may be magnesium-deficient. Hypomagnesemia is caused primarily by renal or gastrointestinal losses or decreased efficiency of intestinal magnesium absorption (Table 340-3). Reduced renal reabsorption due to loop diuretics and alcohol use is a common cause of hypomagnesemia. Because magnesium excretion is tightly coupled to sodium and calcium excretion, intravenous fluid therapy and volume-expanded states, such as primary hyperaldosteronism, may result in hypomagnesemia. Hypercalcemia and hypercalciuria decrease tubular reabsorption of magnesium. Osmotic diuresis in diabetes mellitus is one of the more common causes of hypomagnesemia.

Vomiting and nasogastric suctioning can cause severe magnesium depletion because intestinal tract fluids contain ~0.5 mmol/L (1.2 mg/dL)(1 meq/L). Fluid loss from diarrhea can contain as much as 7.4 mmol/L (18 mg/dL)(15 meq/L). Consequently, ulcerative colitis, Crohn's disease, and intestinal or biliary fistulas can result in magnesium depletion. Hypomagnesemia is prevalent in alcoholics. Ethanol causes a transient loss of magnesium in the urine. In most alcoholics, however, the magnesium deficit is modest. A more profound fall in serum magnesium levels may occur during alcohol withdrawal, where the decrease is associated with falls in levels of serum phosphate and potassium, probably due to shifts of these ions into intracellular compartments. The use of loop diuretics, as well as aminoglycosides, cisplatin, cyclosporine, and amphotericin B can increase renal loss of magnesium.

The clinical manifestations of hypomagnesemia are similar to those of severe hypocalcemia. The signs and symptoms of hypomagnesemia include muscle weakness, prolonged PR and QT intervals, and cardiac arrhythmias. Positive Chvostek's and Trousseau's signs indicative of hypocalcemia are often positive in hypomagnesemic patients as well; carpopedal spasm can also occur with hypomagnesemia. Magnesium is important for effective PTH secretion as well as the

Table 340-3 Causes of Hypomagnesemia

Increased renal excretion	Metabolic and endocrine
Volume expansion	Diabetes mellitus
Hypercalcemia	Primary hyperparathyroidism
Osmotic diuresis	Primary aldosteronism
Renal disease with magnesium wasting	Hypoparathyroidism
Metabolic acidosis	Hyperthyroidism
Gitelman's syndrome	Phosphate depletion
Bartter's syndrome	Ketoacidosis with treatment
Increased intestinal losses	Acute and chronic diarrhea
Vomiting	Intestinal resection or bypass
Nasal-gastric suctioning	Drugs
Malabsorption syndromes	Diuretics
Ileitis	Aminoglycosides
Colitis	Cisplatin
Intestinal and biliary fistulas	Cyclosporine
Alcoholism	Amphotericin B
	Ethanol
	Pentamidine

Table 340-4 Causes of Hypermagnesemia

Renal failure receiving magnesium-containing antacid, laxative, or infusion
Acute renal failure with rhabdomyolysis
Ketoacidosis without treatment
Familial hypocalciuric hypercalcemia
Volume depletion
Lithium
Accidental Epsom salt (magnesium sulfate) ingestion

renal and skeletal responsiveness to PTH; thus, hypomagnesemia is often associated with hypocalcemia due to impaired PTH secretion and function (Chap. 341).

Low serum magnesium levels <0.7 mmol/L (1.8 mg/dL)(1.5 meq/L) are indicative of magnesium deficiency. For mild deficiency, oral magnesium replacement is effective. The major side effect is diarrhea. Symptoms often occur when the serum magnesium is <0.5 mmol/L (1.2 mg/dL)(1.0 meq/L). This level is indicative of significantly depleted total-body magnesium stores. Because most magnesium resides in the intracellular space, the total-body magnesium deficit is often ~200 mmol (4800 mg) by the time serum levels fall to <0.5 mmol/L (1.2 mg/dL)(1.0 meq/L). Parenteral magnesium administration is usually needed under these circumstances. Two grams of magnesium sulfate [8.0 mmol (192 mg)(16.2 meq) of magnesium] can be given intravenously, with a cumulative dose up to 24 mmol (576 mg) (48 meq) over 24 h. Alternatively, a 50% solution of 2 g of magnesium sulfate can be given every 8 h intramuscularly although these injections can be painful. Patients with severe hypomagnesemia and associated seizures or acute arrhythymias can be given 4 to 8 mmol (96 to 192 mg)(8 to 16 meq) of magnesium as an intravenous injection over 5 to 10 min, followed by 24 mmol/d (576 mg/d)(48 meq/d).

A normal serum magnesium concentration attained after acute magnesium repletion is not necessarily indicative of repletion of the total-body magnesium stores. Restoration of urinary magnesium excretion is a better indicator of magnesium repletion. Once urinary magnesium excretion increases, the body stores are usually replenished. Patients who have chronic magnesium loss from intestinal or renal sources may require continued oral magnesium supplementation on a daily basis of up to 12.5 mmol/d (300 mg/d) in divided doses. Patients with renal failure need to be monitored carefully to prevent hypermagnesemia.

HYPERMAGNESEMIA Hypermagnesemia is rare but can be seen in renal failure when patients are taking magnesium-containing antacids, laxatives, enemas, or infusions (Table 340-4). It can also be seen in acute rhabdomyolysis.

The most readily detected clinical sign of hypermagnesemia is the disappearance of deep tendon reflexes. Neuromuscular symptoms include depressed respiration and apnea due to paralysis of the voluntary muscles, prolonged PR intervals, and increased QRS duration and QT interval; complete heart block and cardiac arrest can occur. Hypocalcemia may occur because hypermagnesemia depresses PTH secretion and induces an end-organ resistance to PTH similar to the effect seen in hypomagnesemia.

Treatment includes stopping the antacid or other preparations that contain large amounts of magnesium. The excess magnesium is quickly excreted by the kidney. Renal failure patients may require dialysis against a low magnesium bath. For severe hypermagnesemia with associated life-threatening complications, intravenous calcium in doses of 100 to 200 mg (elemental) over 5 to 10 min will antagonize the toxic effects of magnesium.

VITAMIN D

Vitamin D is a hormone rather than a classic vitamin, since with adequate exposure to sunlight, no dietary supplements are needed. Vitamin D exerts its physiologic effects on bone, intestine, kidney, and the parathyroid glands to modulate calcium and phosphorus metabolism. The active principle of vitamin D is synthesized under metabolic control via successive hydroxylations in the liver and kidney and is transported through the blood to its main target tissues (the small intestine and bone), where it regulates calcium homeostasis.

PHOTOBIOGENESIS Vitamin D_3 is a derivative of 7-dehydrocholesterol (provitamin D_3), the immediate precursor of cholesterol. When skin is exposed to sunlight or certain artificial light sources, the ultraviolet radiation enters the epidermis and causes transformation of 7-dehydrocholesterol to vitamin D_3. Wavelengths between 290 and 315 nm are absorbed by the conjugated double bonds at C_5 and C_7 of 7-dehydrocholesterol to produce previtamin D_3 (Fig. 340-5). Vitamin D_3 is made in the skin from the previtamin for many hours after a single sun exposure (Fig. 340-5). Once vitamin D_3 is synthesized, it is translocated from the epidermis into the circulation by the vitamin D–binding protein. Melanin in the skin competes with 7-dehydrocholesterol for ultraviolet photons and thus can limit the synthesis of previtamin D_3. The photochemical isomerization of previtamin D_3 and vitamin D_3 to biologically inert products appears to be more important in preventing excessive production of previtamin D_3 and vitamin D_3 during prolonged exposure to the sun.

Aging decreases the capacity of the skin to produce vitamin D_3; this capacity is reduced more than fourfold after age 70. Topical sunscreens can reduce or prevent cutaneous production of vitamin D_3 by absorbing the solar radiation responsible for previtamin D_3 synthesis in the skin. Other factors that affect the cutaneous synthesis of vitamin D_3 include altitude, geographic location, time of day, and area exposed. Latitude has profound effects on the cutaneous synthesis of vitamin D_3. As the zenith angle of the sun increases with approaching winter, more of the high-energy ultraviolet photons responsible for formation of the previtamin are absorbed by the ozone layer. In an area such as Boston (42°N), the absorption of these photons is so complete that essentially no vitamin D_3 is made in the skin between the months of November through February.

When the entire body is exposed to sufficient sunlight to cause mild erythema, the increase in the blood vitamin D is approximately equivalent to consuming oral doses of 10,000 to 25,000 international units (1 IU = 0.025 μg) of vitamin D. Only when skin irradiation is insufficient to produce the required quantities of vitamin D_3 is dietary supplementation needed to prevent skeletal mineralization defects. The fortification of milk and some cereals with either crystalline vitamin D_2 (Fig. 340-5) or vitamin D_3 should prevent rickets and osteomalacia. A survey of the vitamin D content in milk from the United States and western Canada revealed, however, that 71% did not contain 80 to 120% of the amount of vitamin D on the label and that ~15% of skim milk did not contain detectable vitamin D.

In 1997, the Food and Nutrition Board for the Institute of the Medicine recommended 200 IU/d as the adequate intake of vitamin D for neonates, children, and adults up to 50 years. For adults 51 to 70 and >71 years, the committee recommended 400 and 600 IU/d, respectively. In the absence of adequate sunlight exposure, all children and adults require at least 400 to 600 IU/d.

METABOLISM In the liver, vitamin D is metabolized to 25-hydroxyvitamin D [25(OH)D] by hepatic mitochondrial and/or microsomal enzyme(s) (Fig. 340-5). 25(OH)D is one of the major circulating metabolites, and its half-life is about 21 days. The concentrations of 25(OH)D and some of its metabolites in the serum are measured using competitive binding assays. The normal serum 25(OH)D concentration varies among different laboratories from 20 to 200 nmol/L (8 to 80 ng/mL). Individuals exposed to excessive sunlight may have concentrations of 25(OH)D up to 250 nmol/L (100 ng/mL) without adverse effects on calcium metabolism. The serum 25(OH)D levels usually reflect both 25-hydroxyvitamin D_2 [25(OH)D_2] and 25-hydroxyvitamin D_3 [25(OH)D_3]. The ratio of these two 25-hydroxylated derivatives depends on the relative amounts of vitamins D_2 or D_3 present in the diet and the amount of previtamin D_3 produced by exposure to sunlight.

The hepatic 25-hydroxylation of vitamin D is regulated by a product feedback mechanism. This regulation, however, is not tight; an increase in dietary intake or endogenous production of vitamin D_3 increases 25(OH)D levels in the serum. The levels can rise to >1200 nmol/L (500 ng/mL) when the intake of vitamin D is excessive. Serum 25(OH)D levels are reduced in severe chronic liver disease (Table 340-5). 25(OH)D is probably not biologically active at physiologic levels in vivo but is active in vitro at high concentrations.

After formation in the liver, 25(OH)D is bound by the vitamin D–binding protein and transported to the kidney for an additional stereospecific hydroxylation on either C_1 or C_{24} (Fig. 340-5). The kidney plays a pivotal role in the metabolism of 25(OH)D to the biologically active metabolite. The renal mitochondrial 25(OH)D-1-hydroxylase activity is enhanced by hypocalcemia to increase the rate of conversion of 25(OH)D to $1,25(OH)_2D$. Hypocalcemia may not control this hydroxylation directly, however. Any decrease in the serum concentration of calcium below normal is a stimulus for increased secretion of PTH, which increases the synthesis of $1,25(OH)_2D$ in the renal proximal convoluted tubule. The renal production of $1,25(OH)_2D$ enhances the effects of PTH in lowering circulating concentrations (and presumably renal intracellular concentrations) of phosphate (Fig. 340-6). $1,25(OH)_2D$ also influences the renal metabolism of 25(OH)D by diminishing 25(OH)D-1α-hydroxylase activity and enhancing the metabolism of 25(OH)D to 24*R*,25-dihydroxyvitamin D [$24,25(OH)_2D$].

$24,25(OH)_2D$ is normally present in serum at a concentration of 1 to 10 nmol/L (0.5 to 5.0 ng/mL). $24,25(OH)_2D$ is also a substrate for renal 25(OH)D-1α-hydroxylase and is converted to 1α,24*R*,25-trihydroxyvitamin D [$1,24,25(OH)_3D$], which, in turn, is metabolized to the biologically inactive substance calcitroic acid (Fig. 340-5). Cultured cells that possess nuclear receptors for $1,25(OH)_2D$, such as chondrocytes, skin keratinocytes and fibroblasts, and intestinal and melanoma cells, also metabolize 25(OH)D to $24,25(OH)_2D$. Studies of the vitamin D-24-hydroxylase null mice indicate that the major role of 24-hydroxylation is in the regulation of levels of $1,25(OH)_2D$.

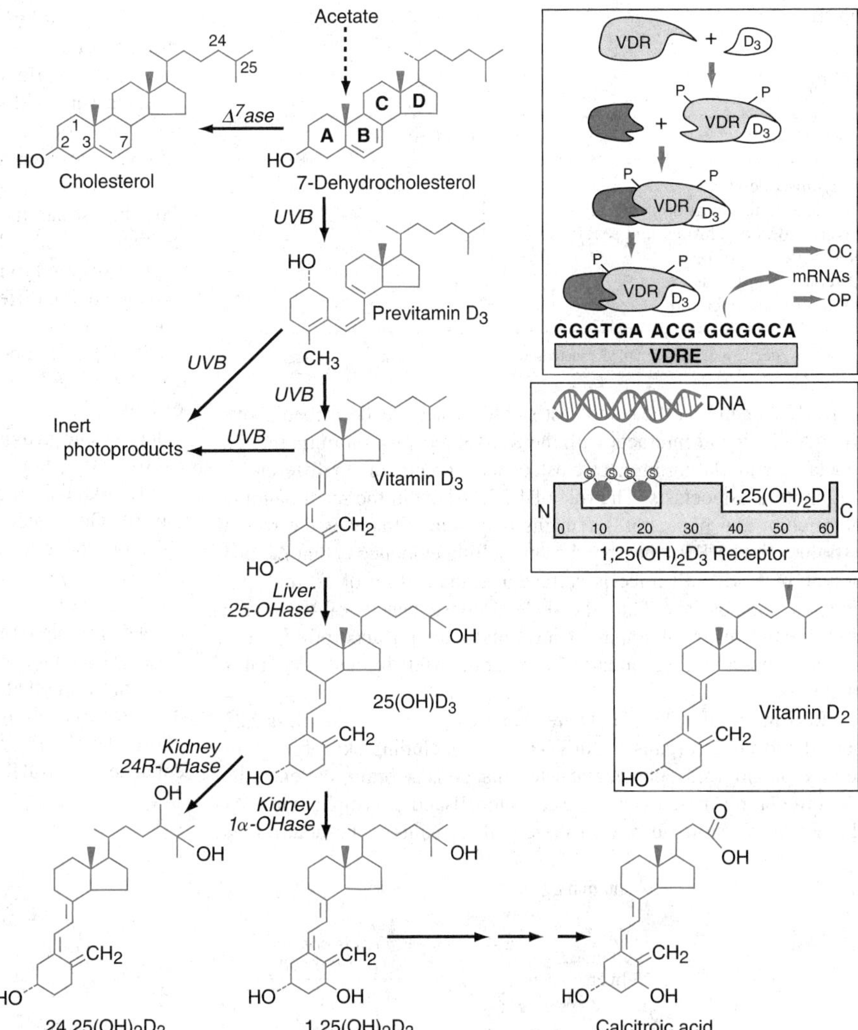

FIGURE 340-5 The photobiogenesis and metabolism of vitamin D. 7-Dehydrocholesterol can be either reduced by 7-dehydrocholesterol reductase (Δ^7ase) to cholesterol or photolyzed in the skin by solar ultraviolet B radiation (UVB) to previtamin D_3. Once formed, previtamin D_3 thermally isomerizes to vitamin D_3. Exposure of previtamin D_3 and vitamin D_3 to UVB radiation results in the generation of a variety of biologically inert photoproducts. Vitamin D_3 enters the circulation and is hydroxylated by the hepatic vitamin D-25-hydroxylase (step 25) to 25-hydroxyvitamin D_3, shown as $25(OH)D_3$. 25-Hydroxyvitamin D_3 can be metabolized by a 25(OH)D-24-hydroxylase (step 24R) to 24,25-dihydroxyvitamin D_3, i.e., $24,25(OH)_2D_3$. 25-Hydroxyvitamin D_3 is converted in the kidney by the 25-OH-D-1α-hydroxylase (step 1α) to its biologically active form, 1,25-dihydroxyvitamin D_3, i.e., $1,25(OH)_2D_3$. As shown in the top two inserts, the vitamin D receptor (VDR), a member of the steroid superfamily of receptors, interacts with $1,25(OH)_2D_3$ (identified as D_3), resulting in the phosphorylation of the $1,25(OH)_2D_3$–VDR complex. This complex interacts with the retinoic acid X receptor (RXR) to form a heterodimer, which, in turn, interacts with the vitamin D–responsive element (VDRE) in the promoters of target genes. In the bone, this interaction increases the expression of mRNAs for osteocalcin (OC) and osteopontin (OP). 1,25-Dihydroxyvitamin D_3 can undergo multiple hydroxylations in its side chain that may ultimately result in the formation of the water-soluble biologically inactive calcitroic acid.The lower insert is the structure for vitamin D_2. It is structurally different from vitamin D_3 in having a double bond between C_{22} and C_{23} and a methyl group on C_{24}.

PHYSIOLOGY $1,25(OH)_2D$, produced by the kidney and the placenta, is the only known important metabolite of vitamin D; the potential roles of other metabolites have not been clarified. $1,25(OH)_2D$ bound to a vitamin D–binding protein is delivered to various target organs, where the free form is taken up by cells and transported to a specific nuclear receptor protein. The vitamin D receptor (VDR) belongs to the nuclear receptor superfamily of steroid-retinoid-thyroid hormone-vitamin D transcription regulatory factors (Chap. 327). The VDR interacts with the retinoic acid X receptor (RXR) to form a heterodimeric (RXR-VDR) complex that binds to specific DNA sequences, termed the *vitamin D response elements* (VDREs). After $1,25(OH)_2D$ binds to the receptor, it induces conformational changes that result in the recruitment of a multitude of transcriptional coactivators that stimulate the transcription of target genes. In the intestine, the activated VDR stimulates calcium-binding protein synthesis; in bone, it stimulates production of osteocalcin, osteopontin, and alkaline phosphatase. $1,25(OH)_2D$ also may have nonnuclear effects on its target tissues; $1,25(OH)_2D$ increases the transport of calcium from the extracellular to intracellular space, and it can mobilize calcium from intracellular calcium pools and enhance phosphatidylinositol metabolism. In the intestine, the net effect of $1,25(OH)_2D$ is to stimulate calcium and phosphate transport from the lumen of the small intestine into the circulation (Fig. 340-6). The effect of $1,25(OH)_2D$ on the enhancement of bone resorption is synergistic with that of PTH. Mature osteoclasts do not possess receptors for either PTH or $1,25(OH)_2D$. Both PTH and $1,25(OH)_2D$ interact with their specific receptors on osteoblasts or stromal fibroblasts to induce the production

Table 340-5 Serum Concentrations of 25(OH)D in Disorders of Calcium, Phosphorus, and Bone Metabolism

Disease States	Serum 25(OH)D
Vitamin D deficiency	↓
Intestinal malabsorption syndromes	↓
Liver disorders (chronic and severe)	↓
Nephrotic syndrome	↓
Osteopenia in the aged	N or ↓
Vitamin D intoxication	↑

NOTE: ↓, decreased; N, normal; ↑, increased.

of RANK ligand on the osteoblast's cell surface. As described above, the RANK ligand interacts with the RANK receptor on immature osteoclasts, stimulating immature osteoclastic precursors to differentiate into mature osteoclasts. The role of $1,25(OH)_2D$ in the renal handling of calcium and phosphorus remains uncertain. Whatever the role of extraintestinal VDRs may be, the compelling evidence is that the phenotype of VDR null mice is corrected in the setting of normal mineral ion homeostasis. Thus the skeletal consequences of VDR ablation are the result of impaired intestinal calcium absorption and/or the accompanying secondary hyperparathyroidism and hypophosphatemia.

Receptors for $1,25(OH)_2D$ are also present in cells not classically considered target organs for this hormone, including skin, breast, pituitary, parathyroids, pancreatic beta cells, gonads, brain, skeletal muscle, circulating monocytes, and activated B and T lymphocytes. Although its physiologic role in these cells remains to be determined,

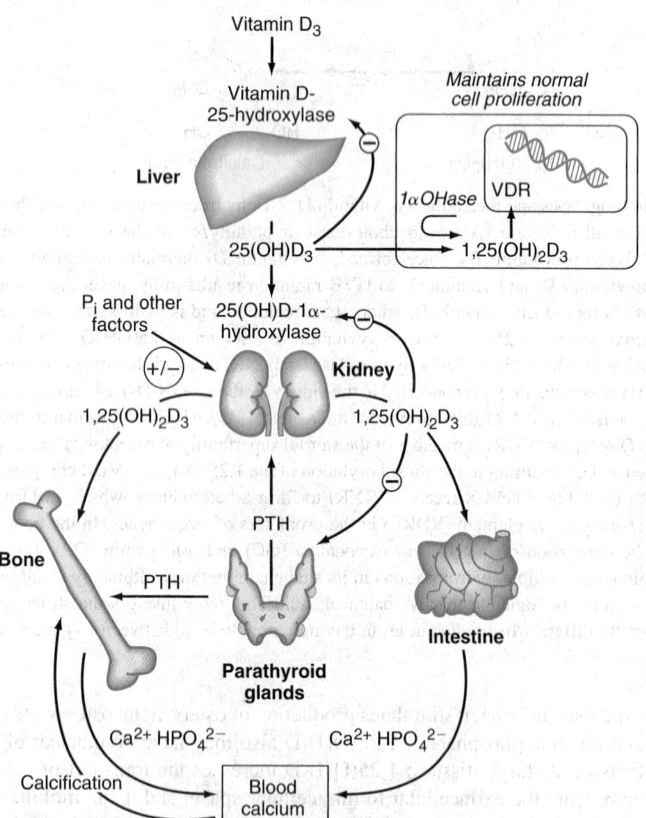

FIGURE 340-6 Schematic representation of the hormonal control loop for vitamin D metabolism and function. A reduction in the serum calcium level below ~2.2 mmol/L (8.8 mg/dL) prompts a proportional increase in the secretion of parathyroid hormone (PTH) and so mobilizes additional calcium from the bone. PTH promotes the synthesis of $1,25(OH)_2D$ in the kidney, which, in turn, stimulates the mobilization of calcium from bone and intestine and regulates the synthesis of PTH by negative feedback.

$1,25(OH)_2D$ inhibits proliferation of keratinocytes and fibroblasts, stimulates terminal differentiation of keratinocytes, induces monocytes to produce interleukin (IL)1 and to differentiate into macrophages and osteoclast-like cells, inhibits the production of PTH, and inhibits the production of IL-2 and immunoglobulin by activated T and B lymphocytes, respectively.

In addition, a variety of tumor cell lines, including lines derived from breast carcinomas, melanomas, and promyeloblasts, possess receptors for $1,25(OH)_2D$. Tumor cell lines that have $1,25(OH)_2D$ receptors respond to the hormone by decreasing the rate of proliferation and enhancing differentiation. For example, when malignant receptor-positive human promyelocytic cells (HL-60) are exposed to $1,25(OH)_2D$, the cells mature into functioning macrophages within 1 week. Although calcitriol [$1,25(OH)_2D$] is not useful for the treatment of leukemia, the antiproliferative effects of calcitriol and its analogue calcipotriene provide the rationale for their use in the treatment of psoriasis.

$1,25(OH)_2D$ regulates PTH synthesis by negative feedback (Fig. 340-6). This effect is the rationale for giving $1,25(OH)_2D_3$, and its less calcemic-inducing analogue 19-nor-1,25-dihydroxyvitamin D_3 (Fig. 340-7), to lower circulating levels of PTH in patients with chronic renal failure (Chap. 341).

The principal physiologic mechanism regulating the production of $1,25(OH)_2D$ appears to involve changes in serum extracellular calcium concentrations that result in reciprocal changes in secretion of PTH, the latter controlling, possibly through actions on serum or tissue phosphorus levels, the rate of $1,25(OH)_2D$ production. Other factors that enhance $1,25(OH)_2D$ production include estrogen, prolactin, and

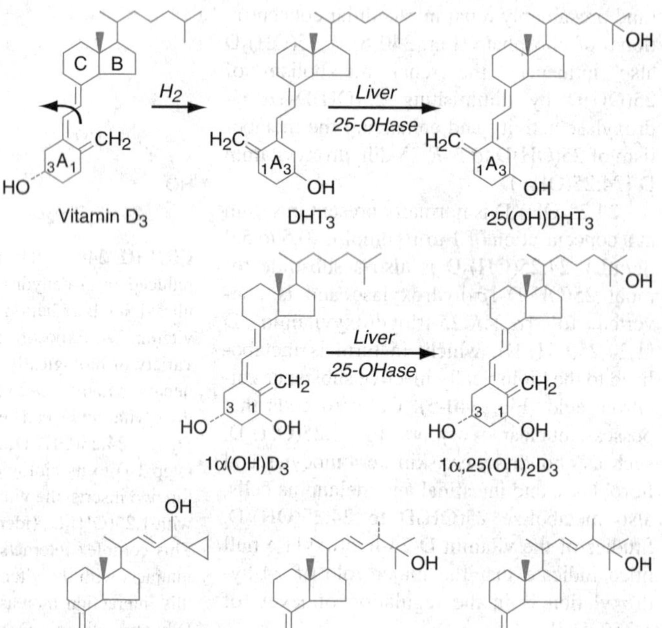

FIGURE 340-7 Structure of 1,25-dihydroxyvitamin D_3, i.e., $1\alpha,25(OH)_2D_3$, and some of its clinically important analogues. When vitamin D_3 is hydrogenated, its A ring is rotated 180°, placing the 3β-OH in a pseudo 1α spatial orientation. This analogue, dihydrotachysterol (DHT_3) is metabolized by a liver 25-hydroxylase (step 25) to 25-hydroxydihydrotachysterol, i.e., $25(OH)DHT_3$. It is believed that $25(OH)DHT_3$ is the biologically active form that mimics $1,25(OH)_2D_3$ in its activity. Two clinically important analogues of $1\alpha,25(OH)_2D_3$ include its 25-deoxy derivative 1α-hydroxyvitamin D_3, i.e., $1\alpha(OH)D_3$, and calcipotriene. $1\alpha(OH)D_3$ is metabolized in the liver by 25-hydroxylase to $1\alpha,25(OH)D_3$. Calcipotriene is an analogue that is currently being used in Europe for the topical treatment of psoriasis.

growth hormone. Humans adapt to increased calcium requirements during growth, pregnancy, and lactation by increasing the efficiency of intestinal calcium absorption, possibly by enhancing 25(OH)D-1α-hydroxylase activity. During the first two trimesters of pregnancy, the levels of 1,25$(OH)_2$D increase in proportion to the concentration of the vitamin D–binding protein; levels of free 1,25$(OH)_2$D do not change. During the last trimester, the need for calcium for mineralization of the fetal skeleton is met by an increase in the concentrations of free 1,25$(OH)_2$D and enhanced maternal intestinal calcium absorption.

Most measurements of circulating 1,25$(OH)_2$D in various physiologic or pathologic states utilize a receptor/competitive binding assay. Serum levels of vitamin D and 25(OH)D vary with the season and with vitamin D intake, whereas levels of 1,25$(OH)_2$D appear to be unaltered by seasonal variation, by increases in dietary vitamin D, or by exposure to sunlight (Table 340-6); as long as vitamin D supplies and circulating concentrations of 25(OH)D are sufficient, metabolic influences control the renal 25(OH)D-1α-hydroxylase to ensure a closely regulated circulating concentration of 1,25$(OH)_2$D. The serum concentration of 1,25$(OH)_2$D ranges from 40 to 160 pmol/L (16 to 65 pg/mL), and its serum half-life is from 3 to 6 h.

PHARMACOLOGY Casual exposure to sunlight provides most people with adequate vitamin D. In elderly individuals, exposure of hands, face, and arms to a suberythemal dose of sunlight two to three times a week is usually adequate. A variety of over-the-counter vitamin preparations contain 400 IU of either vitamin D_2 (ergocalciferol) or vitamin D_3 (cholecalciferol). More potent preparations of vitamin D (calciferol) are available in capsule and tablet form (50,000 IU), as oil (500,000 IU/mL), and in oral solution (8000 IU/mL). A single oral dose of 50,000 IU of vitamin D_2 increases the circulating concentration of vitamin D from <25 nmol/L (10 ng/mL) to 130 to 260 nmol/L (50 to 100 ng/mL) within 12 to 24 h; the plasma half-life is about 2 days. Serum concentrations of 25(OH)D and 1,25$(OH)_2$D are not changed by these doses of vitamin D. For treatment of vitamin D deficiency, 50,000 IU of vitamin D once a week for 8 weeks raises the circulating concentration of 25(OH)D into the normal range; in the presence of secondary hyperparathyroidism, the circulating concentrations of 1,25$(OH)_2$D can increase to supranormal levels [up to 600 pmol/L (250 pg/mL)]. 25(OH)D_3 (calcifediol) available in capsules containing either 20 or 50 μg may be useful in treating vitamin D deficiency [low 25(OH)D concentrations] in patients with severe liver dysfunction. Pharmacologic doses are used to treat disorders of 25(OH)D metabolism; in pharmacologic doses, 25(OH)D_3 is believed to act via interaction with the VDR. Calcitriol is available in capsules containing 0.25 or 0.5 μg and as a solution for intravenous use (1.0 and 2.0 μg/mL). Calcitriol is efficacious in a variety of disorders (Chap. 341), but even low doses can cause hypercalcemia, leading to attempts to develop analogues with less calcemic activity. Two such calcitriol analogues have been approved in the United States for the treatment of renal osteodystrophy; 19-nor-1,25-dihydroxyvitamin D_2, and 24-epi-1,25-dihydroxyvitamin D_2 (Fig. 340-7). 1α-Hydroxyvitamin D_3 [1(OH)D_3] is a potent 1,25$(OH)_2D_3$ agonist that is used in Europe and Japan. The structure of this analogue is identical to that of the natural renal hormone with the exception that it lacks a C_{25} OH. In humans, this analogue is rapidly metabolized by the liver to 1,25$(OH)_2D_3$. Topical preparations of calcitriol (3 μg/g) in Europe and calcipotriene (50 μg/g) in Europe and the United States are used for the treatment of psoriasis. When applied over a large surface area, both can potentially cause hypercalcemia and hypercalciuria. Oral calcitriol is also effective for psoriasis and psoriatic arthritis.

When vitamin D is chemically manipulated to rotate the A ring through 180°, the C_3 β-OH assumes a geometric position that mimics the C_1 α-OH (Fig. 340-7). These compounds, called *pseudo-1α-hydroxyvitamin D analogues*, include the clinically useful dihydrotachysterol (DHT). This analogue is less effective in stimulating intestinal calcium transport on a weight basis than either vitamin D or 1,25$(OH)_2$D. Because it does not require 1α-hydroxylation to be active on intestinal calcium transport, it is 3 to 10 times more potent than vitamin D in disease states that impair renal 25(OH)D-1α-hydroxylase, such as hypoparathyroidism and chronic renal failure. Dihydrotachysterol is efficiently metabolized in the liver to 25-hydroxy-DHT, which is the biologically active form.

Table 340-6 Serum Concentrations of 1,25$(OH)_2$D in Disorders of Calcium, Phosphorus, and Bone Metabolism

Disease States	Serum 1,25$(OH)_2$D
Vitamin D deficiency	↓ [a]
Renal failure:	
GFR > 30 (mL/min)/1.7 m^2	↓ or N
GFR < 30 (mL/min)/1.7 m^2	↓
Hypoparathyroidism	↓ or N
Pseudohypoparathyroidism	↓ or N
Vitamin D–dependent rickets:	
Type I	↓
Type II	↑
X-linked vitamin D–resistant rickets	↓ or N
Tumor-induced osteomalacia	↓
Oncogenic hypercalcemia	↓
Some lymphomas	↑
Hyperparathyroidism	↑
Sarcoidosis, tuberculosis, silicosis	↑
Idiopathic hypercalciuria	N or ↑
Williams' syndrome	↑
Vitamin D intoxication	N or ↑

[a] Serum 1,25$(OH)_2$D concentrations are normal or elevated in occasional patients with biopsy-proven osteomalacia and undetectable or low circulating concentrations of 25(OH)D. These patients also have secondary hyperparathyroidism and may represent a partially treated state; if a small amount of vitamin D is obtained from the diet or generated in the skin in these patients, the vitamin is efficiently converted to 1,25$(OH)_2$D. The net effect is low or undetectable circulating concentrations of 25(OH)D along with normal or elevated concentrations of 1,25$(OH)_2$D. However, in extreme vitamin D deficiency, circulating concentrations of 1,25$(OH)_2$D are low or undetectable.

NOTE: ↓ decreased; N, normal; ↑, increased; GFR, glomerular filtration rate.

RICKETS AND OSTEOMALACIA

Rickets and osteomalacia are disorders in which mineralization of the organic matrix of the skeleton is defective. These disorders are caused by a number of different conditions associated with vitamin D deficiency or resistance (Table 340-7). In *rickets*, the growing skeleton is involved; defective mineralization occurs both in the bone and cartilaginous matrix of the growth plate. The term *osteomalacia* is usually used for this mineralization disorder in the adults in whom the epiphyseal growth plates are closed.

For normal skeletal mineralization, sufficient calcium and phosphate must be present at the mineralization sites. In addition, intact metabolic and transport functions of osteoblasts and chondrocytes and adequate production of cross-linked collagen matrix are required. In cartilage, the initial mineral phase is enclosed in membrane-bound extracellular vesicles. If the osteoblast continues to produce matrix components that cannot be mineralized adequately, rickets or osteomalacia results. A characteristic feature of these disorders is therefore an increase in osteoid volume and thickness (the latter being normally <12 to 14 μm) and a decrease in calcification of the mineralization front. This can be detected in unmineralized sections by the fluorescence of previously ingested tetracyclines or by special stains. The inadequate mineralization of the matrix of cartilage in growing children leads to a widening of the epiphyseal plates of the long bones due to a disorganization of the otherwise highly ordered columns of hypertrophied cartilage cells. In addition, the poorly mineralized long bones are incapable of withstanding usual mechanical stresses and tend to undergo bowing deformities. Growth of the epiphyseal plates is diminished, stunting the growth of the long bones. Osteomalacia also compromises the architectural structure and strength of the skeleton in adults, causing an increase in fractures.

Table 340-7 Classification of Rickets and Osteomalacia

- Vitamin D deficiency
  - Dietary deficiency
  - Deficient endogenous synthesis
- Gastrointestinal disorders
  - Small-intestinal diseases with malabsorption
  - Partial or total gastrectomy
  - Hepatobiliary disease
  - Chronic pancreatic insufficiency
- Disorders of vitamin D metabolism
  - Hereditary: pseudovitamin D deficiency or vitamin D dependency types I and II
  - Acquired: Anticonvulsants
    - Chronic renal failure
    - Tumor-associated (oncogenic) rickets and osteomalacia
- Acidosis
  - Distal renal tubular acidosis (classic or type I)
  - Secondary forms of renal acidosis
  - Ureterosigmoidostomy
  - Drug-induced disease: Chronic acetazolamide ingestion
    - Chronic ammonium chloride ingestion
- Chronic renal failure
- Phosphate depletion
  - Dietary: low phosphate intake plus ingestion of nonabsorbable antacids
  - Impaired renal tubular phosphate reabsorption
    - Hereditary
      - X-linked hypophosphatemic rickets (vitamin D–resistant rickets)
      - Adult-onset vitamin D–resistant hypophosphatemic osteomalacia
    - Acquired
      - Sporadic hypophosphatemic osteomalacia (phosphate diabetes)
      - Tumor-associated (oncogenic) rickets and osteomalacia
      - Neurofibromatosis
      - Fibrous dysplasia
- Generalized renal tubular disorders (Fanconi's syndrome)
  - Primary renal
  - Associated with systemic metabolic abnormality
    - Cystinosis
    - Glycogenosis
    - Lowe's syndrome
  - Systemic disorder with associated renal disease
    - Hereditary
    - Inborn errors: Wilson's disease
      - Tyrosinemia
    - Neurofibromatosis
  - Acquired: Multiple myeloma
    - Nephrotic syndrome
    - Transplanted kidney
  - Intoxications: Cadmium
    - Lead
    - Outdated tetracycline
- Primary mineralization defects
  - Hereditary: hypophosphatasia
  - Acquired: Disodium etidronate treatment (Note: Of the bisphosphonates, only etidronate has this effect)
    - Fluoride treatment
- States of rapid bone formation with or without a relative defect in bone resorption
  - Postoperative hyperparathyroidism with osteitis fibrosa cystica
  - Osteopetrosis
- Defective matrix synthesis: fibrogenesis imperfecta ossium
- Miscellaneous: Magnesium-dependent conditions
  - Axial osteomalacia
  - Parenteral alimentation
  - Aluminum intoxication

PATHOPHYSIOLOGY A large number of disorders are associated with rickets or osteomalacia, primarily through alterations of vitamin D nutrition or metabolism or because of phosphate wasting (Table 340-7). *Hypovitaminosis D* results from inadequate endogenous production of vitamin D_3 in the skin, from insufficient dietary supplementation, and/or from an inability of the small intestine to absorb adequate amounts of the vitamin from the diet. Resistance to the effects of vitamin D can result from (1) use of drugs that antagonize vitamin D action, (2) alterations in the metabolism of vitamin D, or (3) deficient or defective receptors for $1,25(OH)_2D$. The consequences of hypovitaminosis D include (1) disturbances of mineral ion metabolism and secretion of PTH, and (2) mineralization defects in the skeleton (e.g., rickets in children, osteomalacia in adults). With an adequate glomerular filtration rate (GFR), the main changes are hypophosphatemia, normal or near-normal serum calcium levels, increased levels of PTH, and low levels of 25(OH)D (Table 340-5).

With regard to calcium metabolism, lack of vitamin D action leads to insufficient intestinal calcium absorption and hypocalcemia. The latter stimulates the secretion of PTH (secondary hyperparathyroidism), which enhances calcium release from bone, decreases calcium clearance by the kidney, and tends to blunt the hypocalcemia; as a consequence, most patients have a normal or low-normal serum calcium level. (Late in the course of untreated hypovitaminosis D, severe hypocalcemia develops.) Hypophosphatemia is more marked than hypocalcemia, especially in early stages of the deficiency. The efficiency of intestinal phosphate absorption is also decreased. The increased secretion of PTH, although partially effective in minimizing hypocalcemia, leads to urinary phosphate wasting because of decreased renal tubular reabsorption. This latter effect is the most significant factor in causing hypophosphatemia. Aging decreases the responsiveness of the renal 25(OH)D-1-hydroxylase to PTH, decreasing circulating levels of $1,25(OH)_2D$ and contributing to decreased calcium absorption in the elderly.

Although the conversion of vitamin D to 25(OH)D is impaired in severe chronic liver disease, there is not a strong correlation between low serum 25(OH)D levels and osteopenia. Patients with nephrotic syndrome with >4 g/d of proteinuria may have low 25(OH)D levels owing to loss in the urine of the vitamin D–binding protein with its associated tightly bound 25(OH)D. Circulating levels of 25(OH)D may also be decreased when the metabolism of 25(OH)D to $1,25(OH)_2D$ is increased, as in sarcoidosis and hyperparathyroidism. Chronic anticonvulsant therapy can also cause the development of osteomalacia or rickets; mineralization defects are worse in patients receiving multiple drug therapy and when vitamin D intake or exposure to sunlight is inadequate. Anticonvulsant drugs have multiple effects on calcium metabolism. Phenobarbital induces hepatic microsomal enzymes, alters the kinetics of the vitamin D-25-hydroxylase, and stimulates bile secretion, resulting in decreased serum concentrations of vitamin D and 25(OH)D. Phenytoin and phenobarbital inhibit intestinal calcium transport and bone mineral mobilization, independent of effects on vitamin D metabolism.

Glucocorticoids in high doses cause osteoporosis but do not induce osteomalacia and rickets (Chap. 342). Glucocorticoids directly inhibit vitamin D–mediated intestinal calcium absorption and bone mineral mobilization. Patients receiving glucocorticoids chronically may have depressed circulating levels of $1,25(OH)_2D$; the mechanism(s) is unknown. Glucocorticoids also exert direct effects to induce apoptosis of osteoblasts and osteocytes.

A genetic defect in the hepatic 25-hydroxylation of vitamin D has not been described, but in one inherited disorder of calcium and bone metabolism, renal production of $1,25(OH)_2D$ is defective because of recessive mutations 25(OH)D-1α-hydroxylase activity. In this syndrome of pseudovitamin D–deficient rickets (also known as vitamin D–dependent rickets type I), renal production of $1,25(OH)_2D$ is impaired, circulating levels of $1,25(OH)_2D$ are low, but the therapeutic response to physiologic doses of calcitriol (0.25 to 1.0 μg/d) is normal. In patients with a similar phenotype, pseudovitamin D–resistant rickets (vitamin D–dependent rickets type II), mutations in the vitamin D receptor impair its function by altering the binding of the hormone to the receptor or by altering the binding of the receptor heterodimer complex to DNA. Individuals with this disorder have high circulating levels of $1,25(OH)_2D$, but the hormone is ineffective because of the receptor defect. Alopecia is another feature of this disorder, suggesting a role for the VDR in hair follicle development.

Inherited forms of phosphate wasting disorders include X-linked hypophosphatemic rickets and autosomal dominant hypophosphatemic rickets. The gene responsible for the autosomal form is unknown but has been mapped to chromosome 12p13. The X-linked disorder is caused by mutations in the *PHEX* (phosphate-regulating gene with homology to endopeptidases on the X-chromosome) gene. The *PHEX* gene is postulated to encode an osteoblast protein that inactivates phosphatonin, a phosphaturic factor. Consequently, inactivating mutations result in phosphate wasting. The gene is expressed in heterozygotes, suggesting that the disorder is caused by haploinsufficiency. In patients with X-linked hypophosphatemic rickets, serum concentrations of $1,25(OH)_2D$ are normal or low. Since hypophosphatemia is a potent stimulator of the renal 25(OH)D-1α-hydroxylase, levels of $1,25(OH)_2D$ should be high, which suggests the existence of a functional defect in the 25(OH)D-1α-hydroxylase in this disorder. Therefore, the combination of calcitriol and phosphate supplements is more effective than therapy with phosphate supplements alone.

Patients with hypocalcemia due to hypoparathyroidism or pseudohypoparathyroidism have lower-than-normal mean serum concentrations of $1,25(OH)_2D$, although individual values may be in the normal range. In these patients, small replacement doses of calcitriol (0.25 to 1.0 μg/d) are effective even when the serum 25(OH)D concentrations are elevated. These observations indicate that absent or ineffective action of PTH decreases the activity of renal 25(OH)D-1α-hydroxylase. It is not known whether serum $1,25(OH)_2D$ levels would be restored if the hyperphosphatemia were controlled.

Patients with tumor-induced (oncogenic) osteomalacia have low levels of serum phosphorus and $1,25(OH)_2D$. Some of these tumors, especially malignant carcinomas, produce PTHrP (Chap. 341), leading to hypercalcemia as well as hypophosphatemia. Other tumors, particularly more benign neoplasms of vascular or mesenchymal origin, may be responsible for severe hypophosphatemia in the presence of normocalcemia. The mechanism for inhibition of $1,25(OH)_2D$ synthesis remains unknown; after removal of the tumor, however, the serum phosphorus and $1,25(OH)_2D$ levels return to normal.

It has been suggested that alteration of vitamin D receptor levels in target tissues (such as intestine) could affect calcium and bone metabolism, and bone mineral density appears to be associated with specific polymorphisms of the VDR gene. These polymorphisms affect the noncoding intervening DNA sequences (introns) or the coding sequence in a way that does not alter the amino acid sequence of the VDR. Some reports suggest that polymorphisms involving the endonucleases Bsm-I and Taq-I (bb, TT) are associated with higher bone mineral density; other studies have not confirmed these findings. The genetic contribution of VDR polymorphic variants to bone mineral density, as well as a number of other diseases with which they have been associated, require additional, larger-scale studies.

CLINICAL FEATURES The clinical manifestations of rickets are the result of skeletal deformities, susceptibility to fractures, weakness and hypotonia, and disturbances in growth. As the disorder progresses, particularly that associated with vitamin D deficiency, children are unable to walk without support due to the skeletal deformities in the lower limbs and severe muscle weakness (Fig. 340-8). Abnormal parietal flattening and frontal bossing develops in the skull. The calvariae are softened (*craniotabes*) and sutures may be widened. Prominence of the costochondral junctions is called the *rachitic rosary* and the indentation of the lower ribs at the site of attachment of the diaphragm is known as *Harrison's groove*. If untreated, deformities of the pelvis and extremities progress, with bowing being particularly common in the tibia, femur, radius, and ulna. For women, the flattening of the pelvis increases the risk of maternal and infant morbidity and mortality during childbirth. Fractures are frequent, dental eruption is often delayed, and enamel defects are common.

The presentation of osteomalacia in adults is usually more insidious. Bone pain and muscle weakness are common complaints and may be overlooked as indicators of vitamin D deficiency. It is estimated in the United States and Europe that >40% of the adult population over the age of 50 are vitamin D deficient. Although the standard lower limit of the normal range for 25(OH)D is 10 ng/mL, several studies suggest that the cutoff for vitamin D deficiency should be increased to 20 ng/mL. This suggestion is based on PTH responses to various serum levels of 25(OH)D. For example, elevated levels of PTH are frequently seen in individuals with 25(OH)D levels between 10 and 20 ng/mL, and administration of vitamin D (50,000 units of vitamin D once a week for 8 weeks) lowers PTH levels. Defects in skeletal mineralization may accompany these disturbances in vitamin D and mineral metabolism.

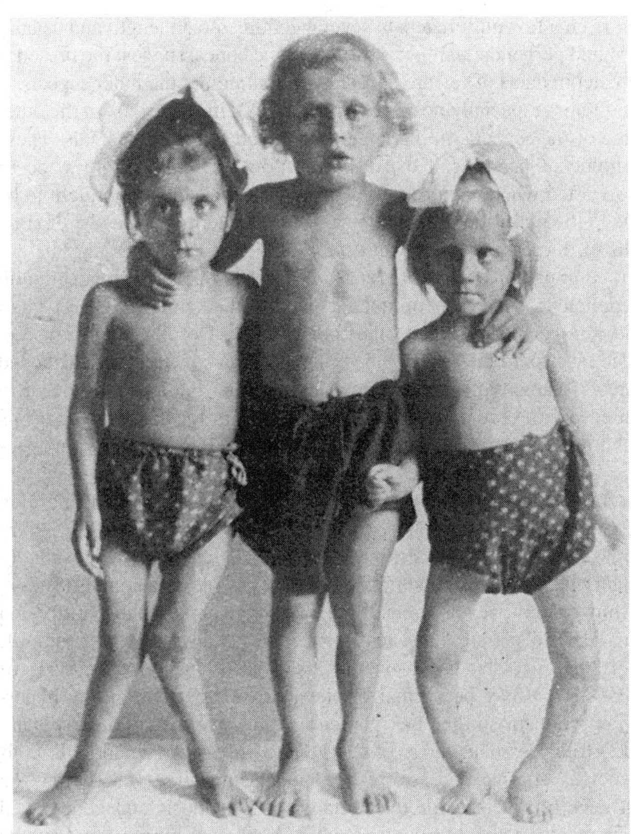

FIGURE 340-8 Typical clinical features of rickets. The child in the middle is normal; the children on either side have severe muscle weakness and bony deformities including bowed legs (right) or knock knees (left). *[Reproduced with permission from F Bicknell, F Prescott: in W Heineman (ed) The Vitamins in Medicine, 2nd ed. London, Random House UK, 1948.]*

Pain in the hips may result in an antalgic gait. Muscle weakness is often associated with osteomalacia but is difficult to distinguish from hesitancy to move because of skeletal pain. Proximal weakness may mimic that of primary muscle disorders and contribute to the waddling gait. Many factors, including secondary hyperparathyroidism, hypophosphatemia, and vitamin D deficiency, contribute to the myopathy. Fractures of the involved bones may occur with minimal trauma. When the ribs are involved, severe deformities may develop in the thorax, and the collapse of the vertebral bodies may produce loss of height.

RADIOLOGIC FEATURES In rickets, the most prominent radiologic alteration is evident at the growth plate (physis) which is increased in thickness, cupped, and hazy at the metaphyseal border owing to decreased calcification of the hypertrophic zone and inadequate mineralization of the primary spongiosa. The trabecular pattern of the metaphysis is abnormal, the cortices of the diaphysis may be thinned, and the shafts may be bowed.

In osteomalacia, a decrease in bone density is usually associated with loss of trabeculae and thinning of the cortices. Radiologic and bone densitometric changes are indistinguishable from those in osteoporosis (Chap. 342). Trabecular patterns may be blurred, producing a homogeneous "ground glass" appearance. Radiolucent bands, ranging from a few millimeters to several centimeters in length and usually oriented perpendicular to the surface of the bones, suggest the presence of osteomalacia. They are particularly common at the inner aspects of the femur (especially near the femoral neck), in the pelvis, in the outer edge of the scapula, in the upper fibula, and in the metatarsals. These radiolucent bands, called *pseudofractures* or *Looser's zones*, occur most often where major arteries cross the bones and are thought to be due to the pulsation of these vessels in the undermineralized area (Fig. 340-9). Increased rather than decreased density of bones may be observed in patients who have renal tubular disorders rather than vitamin D deficiency and may produce a striking thickening of the cortices and a trabecular pattern of the spongy bone. Despite the increase in bone mass per unit volume, the trabeculae are covered with thickened osteoid seams typical of osteomalacia. Similar findings may occur in patients with chronic renal failure. The reason for the hyperostosis is unknown; the bone is architecturally abnormal and is subject to fracture with minimal trauma.

LABORATORY FINDINGS Changes in serum concentration of calcium, inorganic phosphorus, 25(OH)D, and $1,25(OH)_2D$ vary with the different disorders. In vitamin D deficiency, whether due to dietary lack, inadequate sunlight exposure, or intestinal malabsorption, serum calcium levels are normal or low, whereas phosphorus and 25(OH)D levels are consistently low, the latter usually <15 nmol/L (<10 ng/mL) depending on the assay used. In contrast, levels of $1,25(OH)_2D$ may be normal or elevated owing to secondary hyperparathyroidism and the fact that circulating levels of $1,25(OH)_2D$ are 1000-fold less than those of 25(OH)D. Only when vitamin D deficiency is chronic and severe is hypocalcemia observed. It may be sufficiently severe to produce tetany. Mild acidosis and generalized aminoaciduria result from secondary hyperparathyroidism. Patients with renal tubular disorders have normal serum calcium levels and hypophosphatemia. Other laboratory findings such as glucosuria, aminoaciduria, acidosis, and hypouricemia reflect variable degrees of disturbance of proximal tubular function or are features of underlying disease (e.g., low plasma ceruloplasmin in Wilson's disease or abnormalities of immunoglobulins in multiple myeloma). In chronic renal failure, hyperphosphatemia and hypocalcemia are usually accompanied by normal 25(OH)D and low $1,25(OH)_2D$ levels. In nephrotic syndrome, serum 25(OH)D levels can be low owing primarily to urinary losses of vitamin D binding protein–bound 25(OH)D. Serum phosphorus levels are also normal or elevated in hypophosphatasia. Markers of bone resorption increase when secondary hyperparathyroidism and excessive bone resorption are associated with the defect in mineralization. Alkaline phosphatase levels in serum are usually elevated in rickets and osteomalacia.

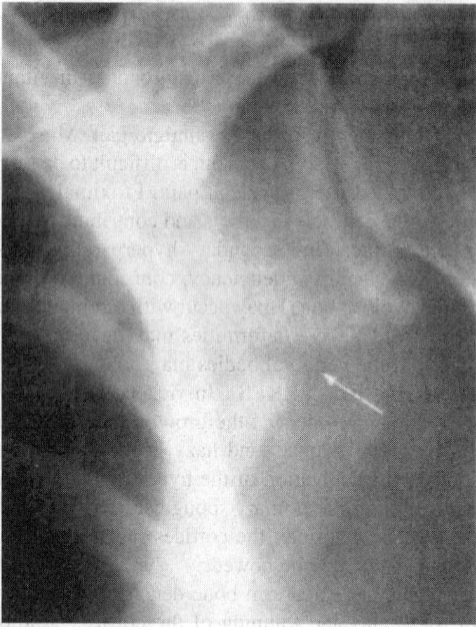

FIGURE 340-9 Radiograph of the scapula of a 58-year-old woman with phosphate diabetes as a cause of osteomalacia. The presence of a pseudofracture or Looser's zone is indicated by an arrow.

℞ **TREATMENT** In rickets and osteomalacia due to dietary absence of vitamin D or inadequate exposure to sunlight, vitamin D_2 (ergocalciferol) or vitamin D_3 (cholecalciferol) is given orally in doses of 800 to 4000 IU (0.02 to 0.1 mg) daily for 6 to 12 weeks, followed by daily supplements of 200 to 600 IU, which are adequate to prevent the development of the disorder in otherwise normal persons. In elderly persons with vitamin D deficiency, the administration of 50,000 IU vitamin D by mouth once each week for 8 weeks raises the serum levels of 25(OH)D into the mid-normal range. In infants and children, such treatment causes improvement in muscle tone and strength, an increase in serum calcium and phosphorus levels, and a decrease in alkaline phosphatase levels after several weeks. Radiologic evidence of healing appears within weeks, and healing may be complete by a few months. Calcium supplements and larger initial doses of vitamin D may be necessary in infants and children with tetany. In adults with nutritional osteomalacia, healing of pseudofractures may be evident within 3 to 4 weeks after therapy with as little as 2000 IU (0.5 mg) vitamin D daily. Healing is usually complete by 6 months.

Patients with osteomalacia due to intestinal malabsorption do not respond to small doses of vitamin D. In the presence of active steatorrhea, daily oral doses of vitamin D of 50,000 to 100,000 IU (1.25 to 2.5 mg) and large doses of calcium (e.g., 15 g calcium lactate or 4 g calcium carbonate orally per day) may be required. In some instances, oral vitamin D is ineffective, and the parenteral route is required (e.g., 10,000 IU/d intramuscularly). Another approach is the use of artificial ultraviolet B radiation or exposure to sunlight in addition to supplemental calcium. Small doses of calcitriol (0.5 to 1.0 μg daily) are also usually effective in this form of osteomalacia. Inorganic phosphate therapy is not indicated either in deficiency or in intestinal malabsorption of the vitamin, since hypocalcemia will develop and intestinal calcium absorption will remain inadequate. In all patients in whom large doses of vitamin D are used, serum calcium and 25(OH)D levels should be monitored periodically. Semiquantitative urinary calcium measurements are inadequate.

In patients treated with multiple anticonvulsant agents, it is usually necessary to continue the drugs while adding 1000 IU/d of vitamin D and to monitor levels of serum calcium and serum 25(OH)D until a therapeutic response (evidence of radiologic healing, improvement in symptoms) is obtained.

Treatment of rickets and osteomalacia in the presence of renal tubular disorders is more difficult. Oral supplements of inorganic phosphate in divided doses of phosphorus (as elemental P), 1.0 to 3.6 g/d (50 mg/kg body weight per day for children), and calcitriol, 0.5 to 2.0 μg/d (30 ng/kg body weight per day for children), constitute the best regimen to restore skeletal growth and heal the bone disease. Patients with nephrotic syndrome and low serum 25(OH)D levels benefit from modest vitamin D supplementation (800 to 1000 IU/d). Small doses of calcitriol are equally effective in treating hypocalcemia and osteodystrophy resulting from chronic renal failure. The recommended initial dose of calcitriol is 0.25 μg/d. If after 2 to 4 weeks on this dose the biochemical parameters are unaltered, the dose is increased by 0.25 μg/d every 2 to 4 weeks until a satisfactory clinical biochemical response (including elevation of serum calcium levels and decrease in PTH levels) is obtained. The usual dose is 0.5 to 1.0 μg/d. Calcitriol may also be administered intravenously (1.0 to 2.5 μg three times weekly) to patients on dialysis, particularly to treat refractory osteitis fibrosa. Serum calcium levels should be monitored frequently during the first 1 to 2 months of therapy and less frequently once a stable dose has been established.

In patients who have had rickets in childhood, the abnormal mechanical stress of severe deformities may contribute to the development of degenerative joint disease, particularly in the hips and knees. Osteotomies at the proper time after healing may prevent this complication and the requirement for more extensive arthroplasties later in life.

BIBLIOGRAPHY

Bone Structure and Metabolism

Avioli LV, Krane SM (eds): *Metabolic Bone Disease*, 3d ed. San Diego, Academic Press, 1998

Burger EH, Klein-Nulend J: Mechanotransduction in bone—role of the lacunocanalicular network. FASEB J 13:S101, 1999

Ducy P et al: Osf2/Cbfa1: A transcriptional activator of osteoblast differentiation. Cell 89:677, 1997

——— et al: Leptin inhibits bone formation through a hypothalamic relay: A central control of bone mass. Cell 100:197, 2000

Karsenty G: The genetic transformation of bone biology. Genes Dev 13:3037, 1999

Kronenberg HM et al: Functional analysis of the PTH/PTHrP network of ligands and receptors. Recent Prog Horm Res 53:283, 1998

Li J et al: RANK is the intrinsic hematopoietic cell surface receptor that controls osteoclastogenesis and regulation of bone mass and calcium metabolism. Proc Natl Acad Sci USA 97:1566, 2000

Manolagas SC: Birth and death of bone cells: Basic regulatory mechanisms and implications for the pathogenesis and treatment of osteoporosis. Endocrine Rev 21:115, 2000

Mundlos S et al: Mutations involving the transcription factor CBFA1 cause cleidocranial dysplasia. Cell 89:773, 1997

Russell RG et al: The pharmacology of bisphosphonates and the new insights into their mechanisms of action. J Bone Miner Res 14(Suppl 2):53, 1999

Soriano P et al: Targeted disruption of the c-*src* proto-oncogene leads to osteopetrosis in mice. Cell 64:693, 1991

Suda T et al: Modulation of osteoclast differentiation and function by the new members of the tumor necrosis factor receptor and ligand families. Endocrine Rev 20:345, 1999

Zhang P et al: A homozygous inactivating mutation in the parathyroid hormone/parathyroid hormone-related peptide receptor causing Blomstrand chondrodysplasia. J Clin Endocrinol Metab 83:3365, 1998

Calcium, Phosphorus, and Magnesium

Bringhurst FR: Regulation of calcium and phosphate homeostasis, in *Endocrinology*, 4th ed, LJ DeGroot, JL Jameson (eds). Philadelphia, Saunders, 2000

Bryant RJ et al: The new dietary reference intakes for calcium: Implications for osteoporosis. J Am Coll Nutr 18(5Suppl):406S, 1999

Dresner MK; *PHEX* gene and hypophosphatemia. Kidney Int 57:9, 2000

Econs MJ: New insights into the pathogenesis of inherited phosphate wasting disorders. Bone 25:131, 1999

Holick MF: Evaluation and treatment of disorders in calcium, phosphorus, and magnesium metabolism, in *Primary Care and General Medicine*, 2d ed, J Noble (ed). St. Louis, Mosby, 1996, pp 545–557

Hruska KA, Lederer ED: Hyperphosphatemia and hypophosphatemia, in *Primer on Metabolic Bone Diseases and Disorders of Mineral Metabolism*, 4th ed, MJ Favus (ed). Philadelphia, Lippincott-Raven, 1999, pp 245–253

Matkovic V: Calcium intake and peak bone mass. N Engl J Med 327:119, 1992

Rude RK: Magnesium depletion and hypermagnesemia, in *Primer on Metabolic Bone Diseases and Disorders of Mineral Metabolism*, 4th ed, MJ Favus (ed). Philadelphia, Lippincott-Raven, 1999, pp 241–245

Scheinman SJ et al: Isolated hypercalciuria with mutation in CLCN5: Relevance to idiopathic hypercalciuria. Kidney Int 57:232, 2000

Yamaguchi T et al: G protein–coupled extracellular Ca^{2+} (Ca^{2+})-sensing receptor (CaR) in cell signaling and control of diverse cellular functions. Adv Pharmacol 47:209, 2000

Vitamin D

Bouillon R: The many faces of rickets. N Engl J Med 338:681, 1998

———: Vitamin D: From photosynthesis, metabolism, and action, to clinical applications, in *Endocrinology*, 4th ed, LJ DeGroot, JL Jameson (eds). Philadelphia, Saunders, 2000

Darwin H, DeLuca H: Vitamin D-regulated gene expression. Crit Rev Eukaryotic Gene Expr 3:89, 1993

Holick MF (ed): *Vitamin D—Physiology, Molecular Biology and Clinical Applications*. Totowa, NJ, Humana Press, 1998

———, Adams JS: Vitamin D metabolism and biological function, in *Metabolic Bone Disease*, 3rd ed, LV Avioli, SM Krane (eds). San Diego, Academic Press, 1998, pp 123–163

Kitanaka S et al: Inactivating mutations in the 25-hydroxyvitamin D_3 1α-hydroxylase gene in patients with pseudovitamin D-deficiency rickets. N Engl J Med 338:653, 1998

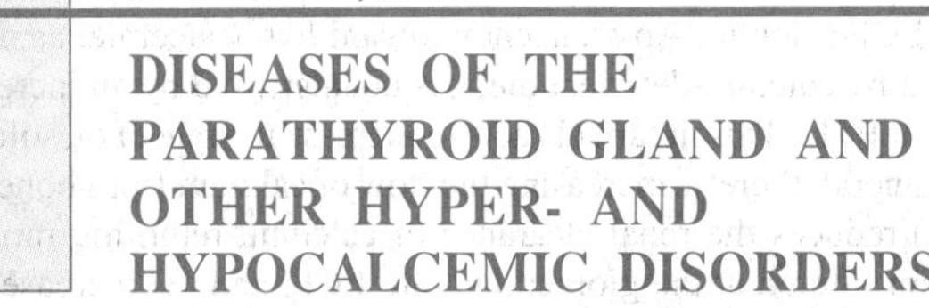

341 DISEASES OF THE PARATHYROID GLAND AND OTHER HYPER- AND HYPOCALCEMIC DISORDERS

John T. Potts, Jr

AHO Albright's hereditary osteodystrophy	IP_3 inositol triphosphate
CGRP calcitonin gene–related peptide	MEN multiple endocrine neoplasia
CT computed tomography	PTH parathyroid hormone
DAG diacylglycerol	PTHrP parathyroid hormone–related peptide
ECF extracellular fluid	PHP pseudohypoparathyroidism
FHH familial hypocalciuric hypercalcemia	PPHP pseudopseudohypoparathyroidism
GPCR G protein–coupled receptor	SERMs selective estrogen receptor modulators

The four parathyroid glands are located posterior to the thyroid gland. They produce parathyroid hormone (PTH), which is the primary regulator of calcium physiology. PTH acts directly on bone, where it induces calcium resorption, and on the kidney, where it stimulates calcium reabsorption and synthesis of 1,25-dihydroxyvitamin D [$1,25(OH)_2D$], a hormone that stimulates gastrointestinal calcium absorption. Serum PTH levels are tightly regulated by a negative feedback loop. Calcium, acting through the calcium-sensing receptor, and vitamin D, acting through its nuclear receptor, inhibit PTH synthesis and release. Understanding the hormone pathways that regulate calcium levels and bone metabolism is essential for effective diagnosis and management of a wide array of hyper- and hypocalcemic disorders.

Hyperparathyroidism, characterized by excess production of PTH, is a common cause of hypercalcemia and is usually the result of autonomously functioning adenomas or hyperplasia. Surgery for this disorder is highly effective and has been shown recently to reverse some of the deleterious effects of long-standing PTH excess on bone density. Hypercalcemia of malignancy is also common and is usually due to the overproduction of parathyroid hormone–related peptide (PTHrP) by cancer cells. The similarities in the biochemical characteristics of hyperparathyroidism and hypercalcemia of malignancy, first noted by Albright in 1941, are now known to reflect the actions of PTH and PTHrP through the same G protein–coupled (GPC) PTH/PTHrP receptor.

Clarification over the past decade of genetic influences on parathyroid gland and bone cell function helps in constructing a logical approach to hyper- and hypocalcemic disorders. Advances that have occurred include elucidation of the genetic basis of multiple endocrine neoplasia (MEN) types 1 and 2, familial hypocalciuric hypercalcemia (FHH), the different forms of pseudohypoparathyroidism (PHP), Jansen's syndrome, disorders of vitamin D synthesis and action, and the molecular events associated with parathyroid gland neoplasia. The advent of new drugs, including bisphosphonates and selective estrogen receptor modulators (SERMs), offers new avenues for the treatment and prevention of metabolic bone disease. PTH analogues are promising therapeutic agents for the treatment of postmenopausal or senile osteoporosis, and calcimimetic agents, which act through the calcium-sensing receptor, may provide new approaches for PTH suppression.

PARATHYROID HORMONE

PHYSIOLOGY The primary function of PTH is to maintain the extracellular fluid (ECF) calcium concentration within a narrow normal range. The hormone acts directly on bone and kidney and indirectly on intestine through its effects on synthesis of $1,25(OH)_2D$ to increase serum calcium concentrations; in turn, PTH production is closely regulated by the concentration of serum ionized calcium. This feedback system is the critical homeostatic mechanism for maintenance of ECF calcium. Any tendency toward hypocalcemia, as might be induced by calcium-deficient diets, is counteracted by an increased secretion of PTH. This in turn (1) acts to increase the rate of dissolution of bone mineral, thereby increasing the flow of calcium from bone into blood; (2) reduces the renal clearance of calcium, returning more of the calcium filtered at the glomerulus into ECF; and (3) increases the efficiency of calcium absorption in the intestine. Immediate control of blood calcium is probably due to effects of the hormone on bone and, to a lesser extent, on renal calcium clearance. Maintenance of steady-state calcium balance, on the other hand, probably results from the effects of $1,25(OH)_2D$ on calcium absorption (Chap. 340). The renal actions of the hormone are exerted at multiple sites and include inhibition of phosphate transport (proximal tubule), increased reabsorption of calcium (distal tubule), and stimulation of the renal 25(OH)D-1α-hydroxylase. As much as 12 mmol (500 mg) calcium is transferred between the ECF and bone each day (a large amount in relation to the total ECF calcium pool), and PTH has a major effect on this transfer. The homeostatic role of the hormone can preserve calcium concentration in blood acutely at the cost of bone destruction.

PTH has multiple actions on bone, some direct and some indirect. It increases the rate of calcium release from bone into blood acutely; PTH-mediated changes in bone calcium release can be seen within minutes. The chronic effects of PTH are to increase the number of bone cells, both osteoblasts and osteoclasts, and to increase the remodeling of bone; these effects are apparent within hours after the hormone is given and persist for hours after PTH is withdrawn. Continuous exposure to elevated levels of PTH for days (as in hyperparathyroidism or long-term infusions in animals) leads to increased osteoclast-mediated bone resorption. However, the administration of PTH intermittently over days in animals or osteoporotic patients leads to a net stimulation of bone formation rather than bone breakdown. Striking increases, especially in trabecular bone in the spine and hip, have been reported with the use of PTH in combination with estrogen. PTH as monotherapy caused a highly significant reduction in fracture incidence in a worldwide placebo-controlled trial.

Osteoblasts (or stromal cell precursors), which have PTH receptors, are crucial to this bone-forming effect of PTH; osteoclasts, which appear to lack PTH receptors, mediate bone breakdown. PTH-mediated stimulation of osteoclasts is believed to be indirect, acting in part through cytokines released from osteoblasts to activate osteoclasts; in experimental studies of bone resorption in vitro, osteoblasts must be present for PTH to activate osteoclasts to resorb bone. The nature of the cytokines that stimulate osteoclasts is a subject of major interest. Insulin-like growth factor 1, interleukin 6, granulocyte-macrophage colony stimulating factor, and possibly other agents are candidates, but the definitive messenger(s) has not been determined. Direct cell-to-cell contact between osteoblasts (stromal cells) and osteoclast precursors is also key to osteoclast function. Cell-associated ligands and receptors, as well as soluble decoy receptors, are involved in these interactions (Chap. 340).

STRUCTURE PTH is an 84-amino-acid single-chain peptide. The amino acid sequence of PTH has been characterized in multiple mammalian species, revealing marked conservation in the amino-terminal portion, which is critical for many biologic actions of the molecule. Synthetic fragments of the amino-terminal sequence as small as 1–14 residues are sufficient to activate the major receptor (see below). Biologic roles for the carboxyl-terminal region of PTH are under investigation; a separate receptor may exist for this region of the molecule. Fragments shortened or modified at the amino terminus still bind to the PTH receptor but lose the capacity to stimulate biologic responses. For example, the peptide composed of sequences 7–34 is a competitive inhibitor of active hormone binding to receptors in vitro but is a weak inhibitor in vivo.

BIOSYNTHESIS, SECRETION, AND METABOLISM

Synthesis Parathyroid cells have multiple methods of adapting to increased needs for PTH production. Most rapid (within minutes) is secretion of preformed hormone in response to hypocalcemia. Second, within hours, changes in gene activity and increased PTH mRNA are induced by sustained hypocalcemia. Finally, protracted challenge leads within days to cellular replication to increase gland mass.

PTH is initially synthesized as a larger molecule (preproparathyroid hormone, consisting of 115 amino acids), which is then reduced in size by a second cleavage (proparathyroid hormone, 90 amino acids) before secretion as the 84-amino-acid peptide. The hydrophobic regions of the preproparathyroid hormone serve a role in guiding transport of the polypeptide from sites of synthesis on polyribosomes through the endoplasmic reticulum to secretory granules. In one kindred with hypoparathyroidism, a mutation in the preprotein region of the gene disrupts this critical hydrophobic sequence and interferes with hormone secretion.

Studies with cloned and expressed PTH genes in vitro have demonstrated DNA regions involved in transcriptional control, including sites for interaction and regulation by the vitamin D receptor, as well as sites through which ambient calcium regulates transcription. Suppression of PTH gene activity at the transcriptional level by calcium is nearly maximal at physiologic concentrations; hypercalcemia results in no significant change. Hypocalcemia, however, increases transcriptional activity within hours. $1,25(OH)_2D_3$ strongly suppresses PTH gene transcription, though not when chronic hypocalcemia is induced experimentally in animals. In patients with renal failure, however, intravenous administration of supraphysiologic levels of $1,25(OH)_2D_3$ or analogues of the active metabolite can dramatically suppress PTH overproduction, which is sometimes difficult to control due to severe secondary hyperparathyroidism. Control over hormone stores is exerted by variation in the rates of proteolytic destruction of preformed hormone under the control of ECF calcium; high calcium increases and low calcium inhibits the proteolytic destruction of hormone stores. Regulation of hormone precursor processing and proteolytic destruction of preformed hormone (posttranslational regulation of hormone production) is an important mechanism for mediating rapid (minutes) changes in hormone availability.

Regulation of PTH Secretion PTH secretion increases steeply to a maximum value of five times the basal rate of secretion as calcium concentration falls from normal to the range of 1.9 to 2.0 mmol/L (7.5 to 8.0 mg/dL) (measured as total calcium). The ionized fraction of blood calcium is the important determinant of hormone secretion. Magnesium may influence hormone secretion in the same direction as calcium. It is unlikely, however, that physiologic variations in magnesium concentration affect PTH secretion. Severe intracellular magnesium deficiency impairs PTH secretion (see below).

The level of ECF calcium controls PTH secretion by interaction with a calcium sensor, a GPCR for which Ca^{2+} ions act as the ligand (see below). This receptor is a member of a distinctive subfamily of the GPCR superfamily that is characterized by a large extracellular domain suitable for "clamping" the small-molecule ligand. Stimulation of the receptor by high calcium levels leads to suppression of PTH secretion. The intracellular signals generated by the active receptor appear to be inositol triphosphate (IP_3) and diacylglycerol (DAG) formed by activation of phospholipase. The receptor is present in parathyroid glands and the calcitonin-secreting cells (C cells) of the thyroid, brain, and kidney. Genetic evidence has revealed a key biologic role for the calcium-sensing receptor in parathyroid gland responsiveness to calcium and, unexpectedly, in renal calcium clearance. Point mutations associated with loss of function cause a syndrome resembling hyperparathyroidism (FHH) but with hypocalciuria. On the other hand, gain-of-function mutations cause a form of hypocalcemia resembling hypoparathyroidism (see below).

Metabolism The secreted form of PTH is indistinguishable by immunologic criteria and by molecular size from the 84-amino-acid peptide (PTH 1–84) extracted from glands. However, much of the immunoreactive material found in the circulation is smaller than the extracted or secreted hormone. The principal circulating fragments of immunoreactive hormone lack a portion of the critical amino-terminal sequence required for biologic activity and, hence, are biologically inactive fragments (so-called middle- and carboxyl-terminal fragments). Much of the proteolysis of hormone occurs in the liver and kidney. However, fragments corresponding to the middle- and carboxyl-terminal portions have also been detected in effluent blood from the parathyroids and in the peripheral circulation; there is no convincing evidence, however, for circulating amino-terminal fragments. Peripheral metabolism of PTH does not appear to be regulated by physiologic states (high versus low calcium, etc.); hence peripheral metabolism of hormone, although responsible for rapid clearance of secreted hormone, appears to be a high-capacity, metabolically invariant catabolic process.

The rate of clearance of the secreted 84-amino-acid peptide from blood is more rapid than the rate of clearance of the biologically inactive fragment(s) corresponding to the middle- and carboxyl-terminal regions of PTH. Consequently, the interpretation of PTH immunoassays is influenced by the nature of the peptide fragments detected by the antibodies. Before the introduction of double-antibody assays designed to detect intact, biologically active hormone, most immunoassays also measured biologically inert long-lived fragments. Changes in the rate of production or clearance of fragments therefore alter the concentration of immunoreactive hormone.

Although the problems inherent in PTH measurements have been largely circumvented by use of double-antibody assays that detect only the intact molecule, new evidence has revealed the existence of a hitherto unappreciated larger PTH fragment that may affect the interpretation of most currently available double-antibody assays as well. A large amino-terminally truncated form of PTH, possibly PTH(7–84), is present in normal and uremic individuals in addition to PTH(1–84). The concentration of the putative 7–84 fragment relative to that of intact PTH(1–84) is higher with induced hypercalcemia (e.g., in uremic patients) than in eucalcemic or hypocalcemic conditions. The large fragment almost certainly cannot have (on the basis of structure-activity studies with PTH discussed above) much, if any, of the biologic potency of PTH. The suggestion that the PTH(7–84)-like fragment might act as an inhibitor of PTH action remains to be clarified. The identification of this fragment has clinical significance, particularly in renal failure, as efforts to prevent secondary hyperparathyroidism by a variety of measures (vitamin D analogues, higher calcium intake, and phosphate-lowering strategies) may have led to oversuppression of biologically active intact PTH when the presence of the amino-terminally truncated PTH was not appreciated. The role, if any, of excessive PTH suppression due to inaccurate measurement of PTH in adynamic bone disease in renal failure (see below) is unknown. Newer assays with extreme amino-terminal epitopes are being studied intensively.

PARATHYROID HORMONE–RELATED PROTEIN

The paracrine factor termed *PTHrP* is responsible for most instances of hypercalcemia of malignancy, a syndrome that resembles hyperparathyroidism. Many different cell types produce PTHrP, including brain, pancreas, heart, lung, mammary tissue, placenta, endothelial cells, and smooth muscle. In fetal animals, PTHrP directs transplacental calcium transfer, and high concentrations of PTHrP are produced in mammary tissue and secreted into milk. Human and bovine milk, for example, contain very high concentrations of the hormone; the biologic significance of the latter is unknown. PTHrP may also play a role in uterine contraction and other biologic functions, still being clarified in other tissue sites.

PTH and PTHrP, although distinctive products of different genes, exhibit considerable functional and structural homology (Fig. 341-1) and may have evolved from a shared ancestral gene. The structure of the gene for human PTHrP, however, is more complex than that of PTH, containing multiple exons and multiple sites for alternate splicing patterns during formation of the mRNA. Protein products of 141, 139, and 173 amino acids are produced, and other molecular forms may result from tissue-specific degradation at accessible internal cleavage sites. The biologic roles of these various molecular species and the nature of the circulating forms of PTHrP are unclear. It is uncertain whether PTHrP circulates at any significant level in normal human adults; as a paracrine factor, PTHrP may be produced, act, and be destroyed locally within tissues. In adults PTHrP appears to have little influence on calcium homeostasis, except in disease states, when large tumors, especially of the squamous cell type, lead to massive overproduction of the hormone (Fig. 341-1).

PTH AND PTHrP HORMONE ACTION Because PTHrP shares a significant homology with PTH in the critical amino terminus, it binds to and activates the PTH/PTHrP receptor, indistinguishably from effects seen with PTH. The 500-amino-acid PTH/PTHrP receptor (also known as the PTH1 receptor) belongs to a subfamily of GPCR that includes those for glucagon, secretin, and vasoactive intestinal peptide. The extracellular regions are involved in hormone binding, and the intracellular domains, after hormone activation, bind G protein subunits to transduce hormone signaling into cellular responses through stimulation of second messengers (Fig. 341-2). A second PTH receptor (PTH2 receptor) is expressed in brain, pancreas, and several other tissues. Its amino acid sequence and the pattern of its binding and stimulatory response to PTH and PTHrP differ from those of the PTH1 receptor. The PTH/PTHrP receptor responds equivalently to PTH and PTHrP, whereas the PTH2 receptor responds only to PTH. The endogenous ligand and the physiologic significance of this receptor are not completely defined.

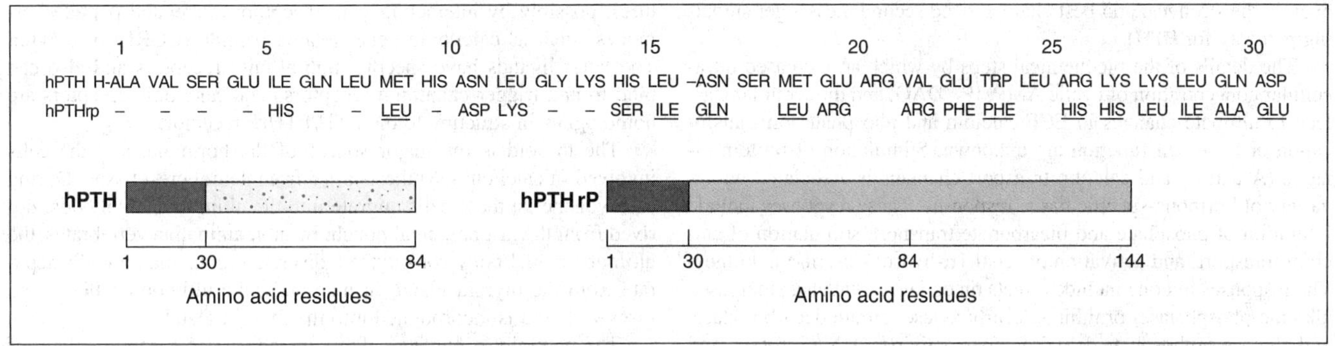

FIGURE 341-1 Schematic diagram to illustrate similarities and differences in structure of human parathyroid hormone (PTH) and human PTH-related peptide (PTHrP). Close structural (and functional) homology exists between the first 30 amino acids of hPTH and hPTHrP. The PTHrP sequence may be 144 amino acid residues in length or longer. PTH is only 84 residues long; after residue 30, there is little structural homology between the two. Dashed lines in the PTHrP sequence indicate homology; underlined residues, although different from those of PTH, still represent conservative changes (charge or polarity preserved). Eleven amino acids are identical, and a total of 21 of 30 are homologues.

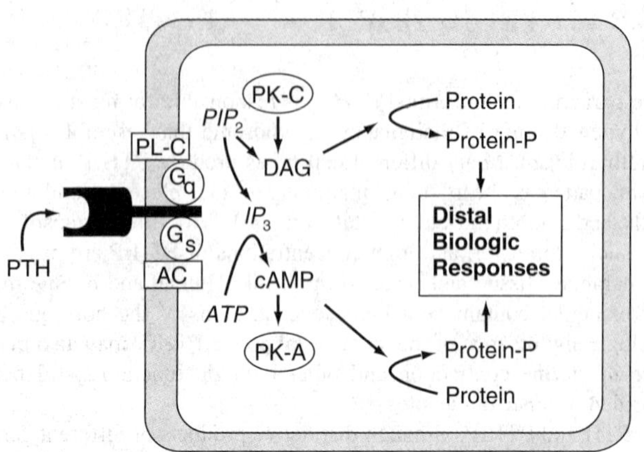

FIGURE 341-2 Schematic model of parathyroid hormone (PTH) action. Only one PTH receptor has been identified in bone and kidney. Different G proteins—G_s, G_q, etc.—activate a cellular second messenger pathway involving either an effect on adenyl cyclase (AC) to enhance cyclic AMP (cAMP) or phospholipase C (PL-C) activation of diacylglycerol (DAG) and inositol triphosphate (IP_3). These second messengers then activate protein kinase A (PK-A) or protein kinase C (PK-C). Phosphorylation of specific proteins, mostly still unidentified, leads to distal biologic responses. Cellular specificity or other factors (e.g., hormone levels, receptor expression levels) must determine which pathway is activated predominantly in a given cell type. Although only one form of receptor appears to be present in kidney and bone, another receptor (PTH2 receptor) has been described in brain, and others may exist.

The PTH1 and PTH2 receptors can be traced backward in evolutionary time to fish. The zebrafish PTH1 and PTH2 receptors exhibit the same selective responses to PTH and PTHrP as do the human PTH1 and PTH2 receptors. The evolutionary conservation of structure and function suggests unique biologic roles for these receptors. Recently, a 39-amino-acid hypothalamic peptide, tubular infundibular peptide (TIP-39), has been characterized and is a likely natural ligand of the PTH2 receptor.

G proteins of the G_s class link the PTH/PTHrP receptor to adenylate cyclase, an enzyme that generates cyclic AMP, leading to activation of protein kinase A. Coupling to G proteins of the G_q class links hormone action to phospholipase C, an enzyme that generates inositol phosphates (e.g., IP_3) and DAG, leading to activation of protein kinase C and intracellular calcium release (Fig. 341-2). Studies using the cloned PTH/PTHrP receptor confirm that it can be coupled to more than one G protein and second-messenger kinase pathway, apparently explaining the multiplicity of pathways stimulated by PTH. Incompletely characterized second-messenger responses may be independent of phospholipase C or adenylate cyclase stimulation (the latter, however, is the strongest and best characterized second messenger signaling pathway for PTH).

The details of the biochemical steps by which an increased intracellular concentration of cyclic AMP, IP_3, DAG, and intracellular Ca^{2+} lead to ultimate changes in ECF calcium and phosphate ion translocation or bone cell function are unknown. Stimulation of protein kinases (A and C) and calcium transport channels is associated with a variety of hormone-specific tissue responses. These responses include inhibition of phosphate and bicarbonate transport, stimulation of calcium transport, and activation of renal 1α-hydroxylase in the kidney. The responses in bone include effects on collagen synthesis; increased alkaline phosphatase, ornithine decarboxylase, citrate decarboxylase, and glucose-6-phosphate dehydrogenase activities; DNA, protein, and phospholipid synthesis; and calcium and phosphate transport. Ultimately, these biochemical events lead to an integrated hormonal response in bone turnover and calcium homeostasis.

PTH also activates Na^+/Ca^{2+} exchanges in renal distal tubular sites and stimulates translocation of preformed calcium transport channels, moving them from the interior to the apical surface to mediate in-

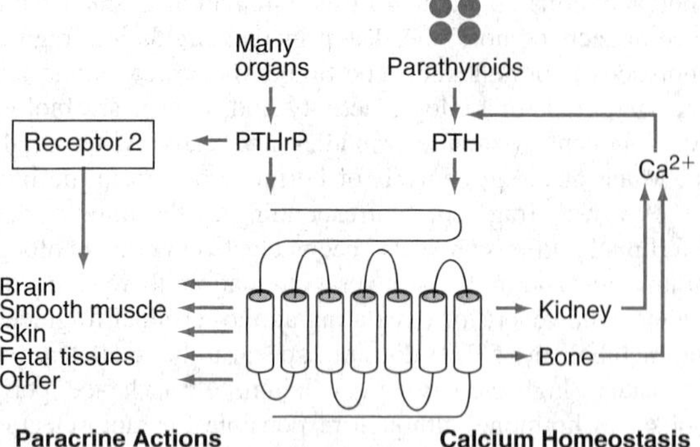

FIGURE 341-3 Dual role for the actions of the PTH/PTHrP receptor. Parathyroid hormone (PTH; endocrine-calcium homeostasis) and PTH-related peptide (PTHrP; paracrine–multiple tissue actions including growth plate cartilage in developing bone) use the single receptor for their disparate functions.

creased tubular uptake of calcium. PTH-dependent stimulation of phosphate excretion (blocking reabsorption—the opposite effect from actions on calcium in the kidney) involves the sodium-dependent phosphate cotransporter, NPT-2, lowering its apical membrane content (and therefore function). Similar shifts may be involved in other renal tubular transport effects of PTH.

PTHrP exerts important developmental influences on fetal bone development and in adult physiology. A homozygous knockout of the PTHrP gene (or the gene for the PTH receptor) in mice causes a lethal deformity in which animals are born with severe skeletal deformities resembling chondrodysplasia (Fig. 341-3).

CALCITONIN (See also Chap. 339)

Calcitonin is a hypocalcemic peptide hormone that in several mammalian species acts as the physiologic antagonist to PTH. Calcitonin seems to be of limited physiologic significance in humans, at least in calcium homeostasis, as contrasted with a clearly definable role in calcium metabolism in many other mammalian species. Calcitonin is of medical significance, however, because of its role as a tumor marker in sporadic and hereditary cases of medullary carcinoma and its medical use as an adjunctive treatment in severe hypercalcemia and in Paget's disease of bone.

The hypocalcemic activity of calcitonin is accounted for primarily by inhibition of osteoclast-mediated bone resorption and secondarily by stimulation of renal calcium clearance. These effects are mediated by receptors on osteoclasts and renal tubular cells. Calcitonin exerts additional effects through receptors present in brain, gastrointestinal tract, and the immune system. The hormone, for example, exerts analgesic effects directly on cells in the hypothalamus and related structures, possibly by interacting with receptors for related peptide hormones, such as calcitonin gene–related peptide (CGRP) or amylin. The latter ligands have specific high-affinity receptors and also can bind to and trigger calcitonin receptors. The calcitonin receptors are homologous in structure to the PTH/PTHrP receptor.

The thyroid is the major source of the hormone, and the cells involved in calcitonin synthesis arise from neural crest tissue. During embryogenesis, these cells migrate into the ultimobranchial body, derived from the last branchial pouch. In submammalian vertebrates, the ultimobranchial body constitutes a discrete organ, anatomically separate from the thyroid gland; in mammals, the ultimobranchial gland fuses with and is incorporated into the thyroid gland.

The naturally occurring calcitonins consist of a peptide chain of 32 amino acids. There is considerable sequence variability among species. Calcitonin from salmon is 10 to 100 times more potent than mammalian forms in lowering serum calcium in animals. Calcitonin is synthesized as a precursor molecule that is four times larger than calcitonin itself. Analysis of the sequence of the coding portions of the gene for rat calcitonin indicates that at least two peptides flank calcitonin. It is likely (by analogy with the common precursor for adrenocorticotropic hormone and endorphin) that these peptides, of still uncharacterized biologic function, are released along with calcitonin.

There are two calcitonin genes, α and β, located on chromosome 11 in the general region of the β-globulin and PTH genes; the transcriptional control of these genes is complex. Two different mRNA molecules are transcribed from the α gene; one is translated into the precursor for calcitonin, and the other message is translated into an alternative product, CGRP. CGRP is synthesized wherever the calcitonin mRNA is expressed, e.g., in medullary carcinoma of the thyroid. The β, or CGRP-2, gene is transcribed into the mRNA for CGRP in the central nervous system (CNS); this gene does not produce calcitonin, however. CGRP has cardiovascular actions and may serve as a neurotransmitter or play a developmental role in the CNS.

The secretion of calcitonin is under the direct control of blood calcium. The circulating level of calcitonin in humans is lower than that in many other species. In humans, changes in calcium and phosphate metabolism are not seen despite extreme variations in calcitonin production; no definite effects are attributable to calcitonin deficiency (totally thyroidectomized patients receiving only replacement thyroxine) or excess (patients with medullary carcinoma of the thyroid, a calcitonin-secreting tumor) (Chap. 339). Although there are no obvious abnormalities in calcium metabolism in patients with elevated calcitonin levels, bone remodeling is chronically suppressed. Calcitonin has been a useful pharmacologic agent to suppress bone resorption in Paget's disease (Chap. 343), has had limited use in the treatment of osteoporosis (Chap. 342), and is useful in early phases of treatment of severe hypercalcemia (see below).

HYPERCALCEMIA

Hypercalcemia can be a manifestation of a serious illness such as malignancy or can be detected coincidentally by laboratory testing in a patient with no obvious illness. The number of patients recognized with asymptomatic hypercalcemia, usually hyperparathyroidism, increased in the late twentieth century but is now declining somewhat, perhaps due to decreased use of routine blood calcium measurements or for other unknown reasons.

Whenever hypercalcemia is confirmed, a definitive diagnosis must be established. Although hyperparathyroidism, a frequent cause of asymptomatic hypercalcemia, is a chronic disorder in which manifestations, if any, may be expressed only after months or years, hypercalcemia can also be the earliest manifestation of malignancy, the second most common cause of hypercalcemia in the adult. The causes of hypercalcemia are numerous (Table 341-1), but hyperparathyroidism and cancer account for 90% of cases.

Before undertaking a workup, it is essential to be sure that true hypercalcemia, not a false-positive laboratory test, is present. A false-positive diagnosis of hypercalcemia is usually the result of inadvertent hemoconcentration during blood collection or elevation in serum proteins such as albumin. Hypercalcemia is a chronic problem, and it is cost-effective to obtain several serum calcium measurements; these tests need not be in the fasting state.

Clinical features are helpful in differential diagnosis. Hypercalcemia in an adult who is asymptomatic is usually due to primary hyperparathyroidism. In malignancy-associated hypercalcemia the disease is usually not occult; rather, symptoms of malignancy bring the patient to the physician, and hypercalcemia is discovered during the workup. In such patients the interval between detection of hypercalcemia and death is often <6 months. Accordingly, if an asymptomatic individual has had hypercalcemia or some manifestation of hypercalcemia, such as kidney stones, for >1 or 2 years, it is unlikely that malignancy is the cause. Nevertheless, differentiating primary hyperparathyroidism from *occult* malignancy can occasionally be difficult, and careful evaluation is required, particularly when the duration of the hypercalcemia is unknown. Hypercalcemia not due to hyperparathyroidism or malignancy can result from excessive vitamin D action,

high bone turnover from any of several causes, or from renal failure (Table 341-1). Dietary history and a history of ingestion of vitamins or drugs are often helpful in diagnosing some of the less frequent causes. PTH immunoassays based on double-antibody methods serve as the principal laboratory test in differential diagnosis.

Hypercalcemia from any cause can result in fatigue, depression, mental confusion, anorexia, nausea, vomiting, constipation, reversible renal tubular defects, increased urination, a short QT interval in the electrocardiogram, and, in some patients, cardiac arrhythmias. There is a variable relation from one patient to the next between the severity of hypercalcemia and the symptoms. Generally, symptoms are more common at calcium levels >2.9 to 3 mmol/L (11.5 to 12.0 mg/dL), but some patients, even at this level, are asymptomatic. When the calcium level is >3.2 mmol/L (13 mg/dL), calcification in kidneys, skin, vessels, lungs, heart, and stomach occurs and renal insufficiency may develop, particularly if blood phosphate levels are normal or elevated due to impaired renal function. Severe hypercalcemia, usually defined as ≥3.7 to 4.5 mmol/L (15 to 18 mg/dL) can be a medical emergency; coma and cardiac arrest can occur.

Except in malignancy-associated hypercalcemia, acute management of the hypercalcemia is usually successful prior to definitive therapy. The type of treatment is based on the severity of the hypercalcemia and the nature of associated symptoms.

PRIMARY HYPERPARATHYROIDISM Natural History and Incidence Primary hyperparathyroidism is a generalized disorder of calcium, phosphate, and bone metabolism due to an increased secretion of PTH. The elevation of circulating hormone usually leads to hypercalcemia and hypophosphatemia. There is great variation in the manifestations. Patients may present with multiple signs and symptoms, including recurrent nephrolithiasis, peptic ulcers, mental changes, and, less frequently, extensive bone resorption. However, with greater awareness of the disease and wider use of multiphasic screening tests, including blood calcium assays, the diagnosis is frequently made in patients who have no symptoms and minimal, if any, signs of the disease other than hypercalcemia and elevated levels of PTH. The manifestations may be subtle, and the disease may have a benign course for many years or a lifetime. Rarely, hyperparathyroidism develops or worsens abruptly and causes severe complications, such as marked dehydration and coma, so-called hypercalcemic parathyroid crisis.

The annual incidence of the disease is estimated to be as high as 0.2% in patients >60, with an estimated prevalence, including undis-

Table 341-1 Classification of Causes of Hypercalcemia

I. Parathyroid-related
   A. Primary hyperparathyroidism
      1. Solitary adenomas
      2. Multiple endocrine neoplasia
   B. Lithium therapy
   C. Familial hypocalciuric hypercalcemia
II. Malignancy-related
   A. Solid tumor with metastases (breast)
   B. Solid tumor with humoral mediation of hypercalcemia (lung, kidney)
   C. Hematologic malignancies (multiple myeloma, lymphoma, leukemia)
III. Vitamin D–related
   A. Vitamin D intoxication
   B. ↑ $1,25(OH)_2D$; sarcoidosis and other granulomatous diseases
   C. Idiopathic hypercalcemia of infancy
IV. Associated with high bone turnover
   A. Hyperthyroidism
   B. Immobilization
   C. Thiazides
   D. Vitamin A intoxication
V. Associated with renal failure
   A. Severe secondary hyperparathyroidism
   B. Aluminum intoxication
   C. Milk-alkali syndrome

covered asymptomatic patients, of ≥1%. The disease has a peak incidence between the third and fifth decades but occurs in young children and in the elderly.

Etiology • ***Solitary adenomas*** The cause of hyperparathyroidism is one or more hyperfunctioning glands. The traditional view has been that a single abnormal gland is the cause in approximately 80% of patients; the abnormality in the gland is usually a benign neoplasm or adenoma and rarely a parathyroid carcinoma. Some surgeons and pathologists report that the enlargement of multiple glands is common; double adenomas are reported. In approximately 15% of patients, all glands are hyperfunctioning; *chief cell parathyroid hyperplasia* is usually hereditary and frequently associated with other endocrine abnormalities.

Multiple endocrine neoplasia Hereditary hyperparathyroidism can occur without other endocrine abnormalities but is usually part of a *multiple endocrine neoplasia* syndrome (Chap. 339). MEN 1 (Wermer's syndrome) consists of hyperparathyroidism and tumors of the pituitary and pancreas, often associated with gastric hypersecretion and peptic ulcer disease (Zollinger-Ellison syndrome). MEN 2A is characterized by pheochromocytoma and medullary carcinoma of the thyroid, as well as hyperparathyroidism; MEN 2B has additional associated features such as multiple neuromas but usually lacks hyperparathyroidism. Each of these MEN syndromes is transmitted in an autosomal dominant manner.

Pathology Adenomas are most often located in the inferior parathyroid glands, but in 6 to 10% of patients, parathyroid adenomas may be located in the thymus, the thyroid, the pericardium, or behind the esophagus. Adenomas are usually 0.5 to 5 g in size but may be as large as 10 to 20 g (normal glands weigh 25 mg on average). Chief cells are predominant in both hyperplasia and adenoma. The adenoma is sometimes encapsulated by a rim of normal tissue. With chief cell hyperplasia, the enlargement may be so asymmetric that some involved glands appear grossly normal. If generalized hyperplasia is present, however, histologic examination reveals a uniform pattern of chief cells and disappearance of fat even in the absence of an increase in gland weight. Thus, microscopic examination of biopsy specimens of several glands is essential to interpret findings at surgery. When an adenoma is present, the other glands are usually normal and contain a normal distribution of all cell types (rather than only chief cells) and normal amounts of fat.

Parathyroid carcinoma is usually not aggressive in character. Long-term survival without recurrence is common if at initial surgery the entire gland is removed without rupture of the capsule. Recurrent parathyroid carcinoma is usually slow-growing with local spread in the neck, and surgical correction of recurrent disease may be feasible. Occasionally, however, parathyroid carcinoma is more aggressive, with distant metastases (lung, liver, and bone) found at the time of initial operation. It may be difficult to appreciate initially that a primary tumor is carcinoma; increased numbers of mitotic figures and increased fibrosis of the gland stroma may precede invasion. The diagnosis of carcinoma is often made in retrospect. Hyperparathyroidism from a parathyroid carcinoma may be indistinguishable from other forms of primary hyperparathyroidism; a potential clue to the diagnosis, however, is provided by the degree of calcium elevation. Calcium values of 3.5 to 3.7 mmol/L (14 to 15 mg/dL) are frequent with carcinoma and may alert the surgeon to remove the abnormal gland with care to avoid capsular rupture.

GENETIC CONSIDERATIONS **Defects Associated with Hyperparathyroidism** As in many other types of neoplasia, two fundamental types of genetic defects have been identified in parathyroid gland tumors: (1) overactivity of protooncogenes, and (2) loss of function of tumor suppressor genes. The former, by definition, can lead to uncontrolled cellular growth and function by activation (gain-of-function mutation) of a single allele of the responsible gene, whereas the latter requires loss of function of both allelic copies.

Mutations in the *MENIN* gene locus on chromosome 11q13 are responsible for causing MEN 1; the normal allele of this gene fits the definition of a tumor suppressor gene. A mutation of one allele is inherited; loss of the other allele via somatic cell mutation leads to monoclonal expansion and tumor development in tissues such as the parathyroids. In approximately 20% of sporadic parathyroid adenomas, the *MENIN* locus on chromosome 11 appears to be deleted, implying that the same defect responsible for MEN 1 can also cause the sporadic disease (Fig. 341-4*A*). Consistent with the Knudson hypothesis for two-step neoplasia in certain inherited cancer syndromes (Chap. 81), the earlier onset of hyperparathyroidism in the hereditary syndromes reflects the statistical probability of only one mutational event triggering the monoclonal outgrowth. In sporadic adenomas, typically occurring later in life, two different somatic events must occur before the *MENIN* gene is silenced.

The *MENIN* gene codes for a novel protein consisting of 610 amino acids. The protein has a nuclear localization signal and appears to interact with the transcription factor Jun D. Most of the mutations are clearly of the inactivating type (nonsense, deletions); there is not, however, a good correlation between clinical features in different kindreds and the specific mutation detected (e.g., penetrance or age of onset of pituitary or pancreatic tumors). This is in contrast to the correlation between genotype and phenotype in MEN 2 (see below).

Other presumptive antioncogenes involved in hyperparathyroidism include a gene mapped to chromosome 1p seen in 40% of sporadic parathyroid adenomas and a gene mapped to chromosome Xp11 in patients with secondary hyperparathyroidism and renal failure, who progressed to "tertiary" hyperparathyroidism, now known to reflect monoclonal outgrowths within previously hyperplastic glands.

The *Rb* gene, a tumor suppressor gene located on chromosome 13q14, was initially associated with retinoblastomas but has since been implicated in many other forms of neoplasia including parathyroid carcinoma. Allelic deletion (with a presumed point mutation in the second allele) has been identified in all parathyroid carcinomas examined; there is also an abnormal staining pattern of the protein product of the gene. Allelic deletion is also seen in 10% of parathyroid adenomas, although the abnormal staining pattern of the Rb protein is not seen. Other gene loci on chromosome 13 may be involved in addition to the *Rb* locus.

There are two rare syndromes associated with hyperparathyroidism that involve one or more genes located on chromosome 1q. The hereditary hyperparathyroidism jaw tumor (HPT-JT) syndrome shows an autosomal dominant inheritance pattern; the jaw tumors are benign, but the parathyroid pathology may involve carcinoma as well as adenoma. Parathyroid carcinoma may also appear in the other syndrome, familial isolated primary hyperparathyroidism (FIPH). Both syndromes have been mapped through linkage studies to the chromosome 1q21-q31 region. Certain findings have led to speculation that this chromosome region might contain a protooncogene rather than an antioncogene.

In some parathyroid adenomas, activation of a protooncogene has been identified (Fig. 341-4*B*). A reciprocal translocation involving chromosome 11 has been identified that juxtaposes the PTH gene promoter upstream of a gene product termed *PRAD-1*, a cyclin D protein that plays a key role in normal cell division. This translocation is found in as many as 15% of parathyroid adenomas, usually in larger tumors. Targeted overexpression of cyclin D_1 in the parathyroid glands of transgenic mice causes the development of hyperparathyroidism, consistent with the role of this cell cycle control protein in parathyroid neoplasia.

A mutated protooncogene, *RET*, is involved in each of the clinical variants of MEN2 (Chap. 339). *RET* encodes a tyrosine kinase–type receptor; specific mutations lead to constitutive activity of the receptor, thereby explaining the autosomal dominant mode of transmission and the relatively early onset of neoplasia. ■

Signs and Symptoms Half or more of patients with hyperparathyroidism are asymptomatic. In series in which patients are followed without operation, as many as 80% are classified as without symptoms.

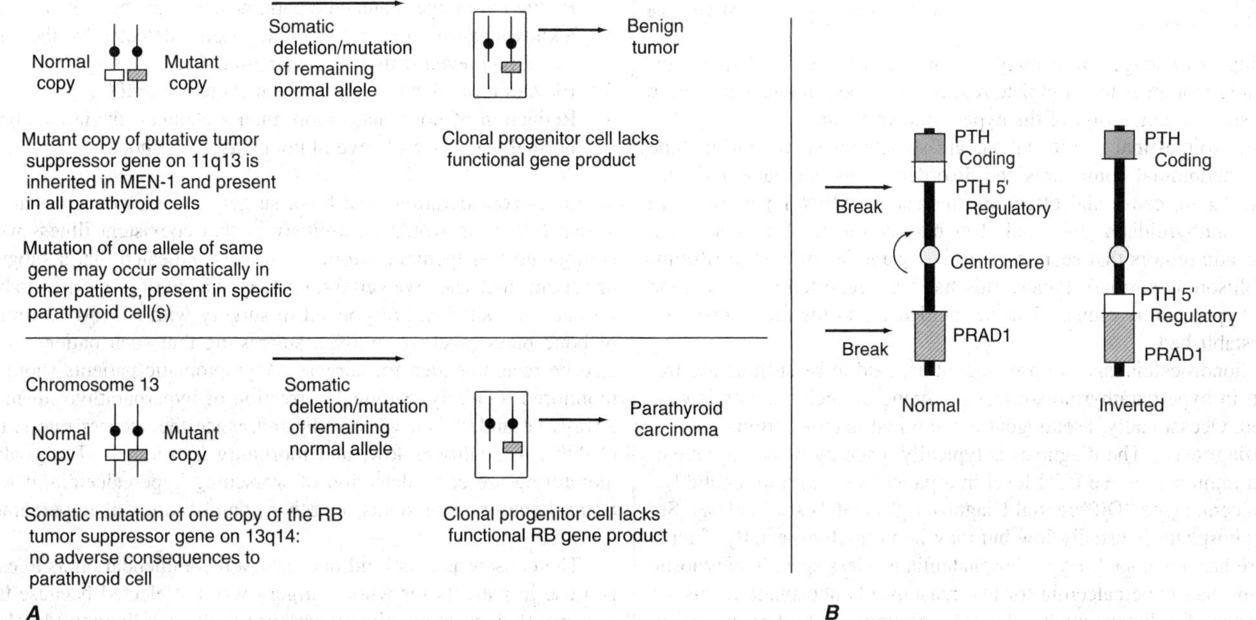

FIGURE 341-4 *A.* Schematic diagram indicating concept of autosomal recessive rather than autosomal dominant inheritance of tumor susceptibility. The patient with the hereditary abnormality (multiple endocrine neoplasia, or MEN) is envisioned as having one defective gene (mutant receptor) inherited from the affected parent on chromosome 11, but one copy of the normal gene is present from the other parent. In the monoclonal tumor (benign tumor), a somatic event, here partial chromosomal deletion, removes the remaining normal gene from a cell. In nonhereditary tumors, two successive somatic mutations must occur, a process that takes a longer time. By either pathway, the cell, deprived of growth-regulating influence from this gene, has unregulated growth and becomes a tumor. A different genetic locus also involving loss of a tumor suppressor gene on chromosome 13 is involved in the pathogenesis of parathyroid carcinoma. *B.* Schematic illustration of the mechanism and consequences of gene rearrangement and overexpression of the PRAD 1 proto-oncogene (pericentromeric inversion of chromosome 11) in parathryoid adenomas. The excessive expression of PRAD 1 (a cell cycle control protein, cyclin D_1) by the highly active PTH gene promoter in the parathyroid cell contributes to excess cellular proliferation. *(From Habener et al, with permission.)*

Manifestations of hyperparathyroidism involve primarily the kidneys and the skeletal system. Kidney involvement, due either to deposition of calcium in the renal parenchyma or to recurrent nephrolithiasis, was present in 60 to 70% of patients prior to 1970. With earlier detection, renal complications occur in <20% of patients in many large series. Renal stones are usually composed of either calcium oxalate or calcium phosphate. In occasional patients, repeated episodes of nephrolithiasis or the formation of large calculi may lead to urinary tract obstruction, infection, and loss of renal function. Nephrocalcinosis may also cause decreased renal function and phosphate retention.

The distinctive bone manifestation of hyperparathyroidism is *osteitis fibrosa cystica*, which in series reported 50 years ago occurred in 10 to 25% of patients. In recent years, osteitis fibrosa cystica is very rare in primary hyperparathyroidism, probably due to the increased incidence of mild disease. Histologically, the pathognomonic features are an increase in the giant multinucleated osteoclasts in scalloped areas on the surface of the bone (Howship's lacunae) and a replacement of the normal cellular and marrow elements by fibrous tissue. X-ray changes include resorption of the phalangeal tufts and replacement of the usually sharp cortical outline of the bone in the digits by an irregular outline (subperiosteal resorption).

With the use of multiple markers of bone turnover, such as formation indices (bone-specific alkaline phosphatase, osteocalcin, and type I procollagen peptides) and bone resorption indices (including hydroxypyridinium collagen cross-links and telopeptides of type I collagen), increased skeletal turnover is detected in essentially all patients with established hyperparathyroidism.

Computed tomography (CT) scan and dual-energy x-ray absorptiometry (DEXA) of the spine provide reproducible quantitative estimates (within a few percent) of spinal bone density (Chap. 342). Similarly, cortical bone density in the extremities can be quantified by single-photon densitometry, usually of the distal radius at a site chosen to be primarily cortical. Studies reveal that cortical bone density is reduced while cancellous bone density, especially in the spine, is relatively preserved. Serial studies in patients who choose to be followed without surgery have indicated that in the majority there is little further change over a number of years, consistent with laboratory data indicating relatively unchanged blood calcium and PTH levels. After an initial loss of bone mass in patients with mild asymptomatic hyperparathyroidism, a new equilibrium may be reached, with bone density and biochemical manifestations of the disease remaining relatively unchanged. This clinical course has led to the recommendations (discussed below) that asymptomatic patients may be safely followed with medical supervision. Certain recent findings have raised questions about the impact of asymptomatic hyperparathyroidism on the skeleton, however. In one careful, long-term study, parathyroidectomy led to improvements in bone density in the spine and hip in 10 to 15% of patients; the improved bone density has been maintained for a number of years of follow-up. Another group compared fracture incidence in a large cohort of hyperparathyroid patients followed for years without surgery versus those seen in an age- and sex-matched control population. The incidence of fractures of the spine, wrist, and ribs was significantly increased in the hyperparathyroid group (although there were no data available on bone density).

In symptomatic patients, dysfunctions of the central nervous system, peripheral nerve and muscle, gastrointestinal tract, and joints also occur. An awareness of the signs and symptoms of hyperparathyroidism may give the initial clue to the diagnosis. It has been reported that severe neuropsychiatric manifestations may be reversed by parathyroidectomy; it remains unclear, in the absence of controlled studies, whether this improvement has a defined cause-and-effect relationship. Generally, the fact that hyperparathyroidism is common in elderly patients, in whom there are often other problems, suggests the possibility that such coexisting problems as hypertension, renal deterioration, and depression may not be parathyroid-related and suggests caution in recommending parathyroid surgery as a cure for these conditions.

Neuromuscular manifestations may include proximal muscle weakness, easy fatigability, and atrophy of muscles and may be so striking as to suggest a primary neuromuscular disorder. The distinguishing feature is the complete regression of neuromuscular disease after surgical correction of the hyperparathyroidism.

Gastrointestinal manifestations are sometimes subtle and include vague abdominal complaints and disorders of the stomach and pancreas. Again, cause and effect are unclear. In MEN 1 patients with hyperparathyroidism, duodenal ulcer may be the result of associated pancreatic tumors that secrete excessive quantities of gastrin (Zollinger-Ellison syndrome). Pancreatitis has been reported in association with hyperparathyroidism, but the incidence and the mechanism are not established.

Chondrocalcinosis and pseudogout are said to be sufficiently frequent in hyperparathyroidism that screening of such patients is warranted. Occasionally, pseudogout is the initial manifestation.

Diagnosis The diagnosis is typically made by detecting an elevated immunoreactive PTH level in a patient with asymptomatic hypercalcemia (see "Differential Diagnosis: Special Tests," below). Serum phosphate is usually low but may be normal, especially if renal failure has developed. Hypophosphatemia is a less specific diagnostic finding than hypercalcemia for two reasons: (1) phosphate levels are influenced by dietary intake, diurnal variations, and other factors; to be useful, samples must be obtained in the morning under fasting conditions; and (2) patients with severe hypercalcemia of any cause may have a low serum phosphate.

Many tests based on renal responses to excess PTH (renal calcium and phosphate clearance; blood phosphate, chloride, magnesium; urinary or nephrogenous cyclic AMP) were used in earlier decades. These tests have low specificity for hyperparathyroidism and are therefore not cost-effective; they have been replaced by PTH immunoassays.

℞ TREATMENT **Medical Treatment** Management of hyperparathyroidism involves two separate issues. The critical question is whether the disease should be treated surgically. If severe hypercalcemia [3.7 to 4.5 mmol/L (15 to 18 mg/dL)] is present, surgery is mandatory as soon as the diagnosis can be confirmed by a PTH immunoassay. However, in most patients with hyperparathyroidism, hypercalcemia is mild and does not require urgent surgical or medical treatment.

Several hundred patients have been closely followed without surgery in attempts to define the natural history of the disease and the benefits of surgery versus the risks of medical observation. Large-scale randomized, prospective clinical trials have not been undertaken, however. Rather, the long-term effects of hyperparathyroidism have been assessed in patients who do not have kidney stones, osteitis fibrosa cystica, or other clear-cut symptoms. Progressive loss of bone mass is a worrisome problem in women who face the problem of age-dependent and estrogen-deficient bone loss in the absence of hyperparathyroidism. The principal concern is that such patients, even though asymptomatic, will suffer sufficient bone loss due to PTH excess to make them more vulnerable to developing symptomatic osteoporosis.

The National Institutes of Health held a Consensus Conference on Management of Asymptomatic Hyperparathyroidism in 1991. *Asymptomatic hyperparathyroidism* was defined as documented (presumptive) hyperparathyroidism without signs or symptoms attributable to the disease. The consensus was that patients <50 should undergo surgery, given the long surveillance that would be required. Patients >50 are appropriate for medical monitoring if certain criteria are met and the patients wish to avoid surgery. Guidelines for recommending surgery in patients with asymptomatic hyperparathyroidism include the following:

1. Elevation of serum calcium, >0.25 to 0.40 mmol/L (1 to 1.6 mg/dL) above the upper limit of normal for the test laboratory.
2. History of life-threatening hypercalcemia, such as an episode induced by dehydration and recurring illness.
3. Reduction of age-matched creatinine clearance by >30% without a known cause. Presence of kidney stones detected by abdominal radiograph even if they are asymptomatic.
4. Elevation of 24-h urinary calcium excretion >400 mg.
5. Reduction of bone mass more than 2 standard deviations below normal using one of several noninvasive methods.

Other considerations that favor surgery include concern that consistent follow-up would be unlikely or that coexistent illness would complicate management. More recent data indicated that a subgroup of patients had selective vertebral osteopenia out of proportion to bone loss at other sites and responded to surgery with striking restoration of bone mass (average >20%), suggesting that such patients might also be recommended for surgery. Asymptomatic patients should be monitored regularly. Surgical correction of hyperparathyroidism can always be undertaken when indicated, since the success rate is high (>90%), mortality is low, and morbidity is minimal. The goals of monitoring are early detection of worsening hypercalcemia, deteriorating bone or renal status, or other complications of hyperparathyroidism.

The consensus panel did not make a recommendation as to estrogen use in patients for whom surgery was not elected because there was insufficient cumulative experience with such therapy to balance theoretical risks (breast and endometrial cancer) versus benefits. New medical therapies may change the approach to the disease in the future. Raloxifene (Evista), the first of the SERMS, has been shown to have many of the bone protective effects of estrogen in osteoporotic subjects yet at the same time lowers the incidence of breast cancer; use of this agent has not yet been reported in a series of hyperparathyroid patients, however. Early experience with calcimimetics, drugs that selectively stimulate the calcium sensor and suppress PTH secretion, indicates that these agents decrease PTH levels for several hours after a single dose.

European investigators have reported serious cardiovascular complications in patients with hyperparathyroidism that reverse, at least in part, after surgery. They also found an increased incidence of malignancy and an absolute increase in age-adjusted mortality due to hyperparathyroidism. These reports clearly describe experiences in a group of patients with more advanced disease, at least based on laboratory tests such as blood PTH levels, than the patients followed in the United States. In fact, a recent long-term epidemiologic study of a large cohort of patients in the United States, with a milder form of the disease (fitting the criteria for medical surveillance listed above), had an age-adjusted mortality no different than that of euparathyroid patients and no increased incidence of malignancy.

Surgical Treatment Parathyroid exploration is challenging and is best undertaken by an experienced surgeon with the help of an experienced pathologist. Certain features help in predicting the pathology (e.g., multiple abnormal glands in familial cases). However, some critical decisions regarding management can be made only during the operation. The examination by frozen section of tissue removed at surgery helps direct the subsequent course of the operation.

As discussed above, there are many unresolved issues to consider in surgery for this disease. At the extreme of conservatism, the surgical approach is based on the view that typically only one gland (the adenoma) is abnormal. If an enlarged gland is found, a normal gland should be sought. In this view, if a biopsy of a normal-sized second gland confirms its histologic (and presumed functional) normality, no further exploration, biopsy, or excision is needed. At the other extreme is the minority viewpoint that all four glands be sought and that most of the total parathyroid tissue mass should be removed. The concern with the former approach is that the recurrence rate of hyperparathyroidism may be high if a second abnormal gland is missed; the latter approach could involve unnecessary surgery and an unacceptable rate of hypoparathyroidism. The majority viewpoint, judged by surgical reviews, is in favor of conservative surgery, i.e., removal of what is usually only one enlarged gland but only after four-gland exploration to eliminate the possibility that more than one gland is abnormal.

When normal glands are found in association with one enlarged gland, excision of the single adenoma usually leads to cure or symptom-free disease, although long-term follow-up studies are limited.

Surgical management has been enhanced recently by the use of preoperative ^{99m}Tc sestamibi scans to predict the location of an abnormal gland and intraoperative sampling of PTH before and at 5- to 15-min intervals after removal of a suspected adenoma to confirm a rapid fall (>50%) in PTH levels. In several centers, a combination of preoperative sestamibi imaging, cervical block anesthesia, minimal surgical incision, and intraoperative PTH measurements has allowed successful outpatient surgical management with a clear-cut cost benefit compared to general anesthesia and more extensive neck surgery. The use of these minimally invasive approaches requires clinical judgment to select patients unlikely to have multiple gland disease (e.g., MEN or secondary hyperparathyroidism).

Multiple gland hyperplasia, as predicted in familial cases, poses more difficult questions of surgical management. Once a diagnosis of hyperplasia is established, all the glands must be identified. Two schemes have been proposed for surgical management. One is that three glands be totally removed and the fourth gland be partially excised; care is taken to leave a good blood supply for the remaining gland. Other surgeons advocate total parathyroidectomy with immediate transplantation of a portion of a removed, minced parathyroid gland into the muscles of the forearm, with the view that surgical excision is easier from the ectopic site in the arm if there is recurrent hyperfunction. When parathyroid carcinoma is encountered, the tissue should be widely excised; care must be taken to avoid rupture of the capsule to prevent local seeding of tumor cells.

In a minority of cases, if no abnormal parathyroid glands are found in the neck, the issue of further exploration must be decided. There are documented cases of five or six parathyroid glands and of unusual locations for adenomas, such as in the mediastinum. A variety of techniques have been developed to aid in the preoperative localization of the abnormal parathyroid tissue. Usually these techniques are reserved for patients with initial unsuccessful neck explorations, since the combined success of the localization techniques is not better than that of an experienced parathyroid surgeon in finding the abnormal tissue at the first operation. Noninvasive or minimally invasive techniques include ultrasound, CT scan of the neck and mediastinum, and differential scanning after technetium-sestamibi administration.

When a second parathyroid exploration is indicated, the minimally invasive techniques such as ultrasound, CT scan, and isotope scanning should probably be combined with venous sampling and/or selective digital arteriography in one of the centers specializing in these techniques. Intraoperative monitoring of PTH levels by rapid PTH immunoassays may be useful in guiding the surgery, especially in patients who are reexplored after an initial unsuccessful operation. At one center, long-term cures have been achieved with selective embolization or injection of large amounts of contrast material into the end-arterial circulation feeding the parathyroid tumor.

A decline in serum calcium occurs within 24 h after successful surgery; usually blood calcium falls to low-normal values for 3 to 5 days until the remaining parathyroid tissue resumes hormone secretion. Severe postoperative hypocalcemia is likely only if osteitis fibrosa cystica is present or if injury to all the normal parathyroid glands occurs during surgery.

In general, patients who do not have symptomatic bone disease or a large deficit in bone mineral and who have good renal and gastrointestinal function have few problems with postoperative hypocalcemia. The extent of postoperative hypocalcemia varies with the surgical approach. If all glands are biopsied, hypocalcemia may be transiently symptomatic and more prolonged. Hypocalcemia is more likely to be symptomatic after second parathyroid explorations, particularly when normal parathyroid tissue was removed at the initial operation and when the manipulation and/or biopsy of the remaining normal glands is more extensive in the search for the missing adenoma.

Patients with hyperparathyroidism have efficient intestinal calcium absorption due to the increased levels of $1,25(OH)_2D$ stimulated by PTH excess. Once hypocalcemia signifies successful surgery, patients can be put on a high-calcium intake or be given oral calcium supplements. Despite mild hypocalcemia, most patients do not require parenteral therapy. If the serum calcium falls to <2 mmol/L (8 mg/dL), *and if the phosphate level rises simultaneously*, the possibility that surgery has caused hypoparathyroidism must be considered. Coexistent hypomagnesemia should be checked for, as it interferes with PTH secretion and causes functional hypoparathyroidism (see below). Parenteral calcium replacement at a low level should be instituted when hypocalcemia is symptomatic. Such indications include a general sense of anxiety and positive Chvostek and Trousseau signs coupled with serum calcium consistently <2 mmol/L (8 mg/dL). For parenteral therapy, calcium (gluconate or chloride) solutions are prepared at a concentration of 1 mg/mL in 5% dextrose in water. The rate and duration of intravenous therapy are determined by the severity of the symptoms and the response of the serum calcium. An infusion of 0.5 to 2 (mg/kg)/h or 30 to 100 mL/h of a 1-mg/mL solution usually suffices to relieve symptoms. Usually, parenteral therapy is required for only a few days. If symptoms worsen or if parenteral calcium is needed for >2 to 3 days, therapy with a vitamin D analogue and/or oral calcium (2 to 4 g/d) should be started (see below). It is cost-effective to use calcitriol (doses of 0.5 to 1.0 μg/d) because of the rapidity of onset and rapidity of cessation of action, in comparison to other forms of vitamin D (see below). A rise in blood calcium after several months of vitamin D replacement may indicate restoration of parathyroid function to normal. It is also appropriate to monitor serum PTH serially to estimate gland function in such patients.

Magnesium deficiency may also complicate the postoperative course. Magnesium deficiency impairs the secretion of PTH, and so hypomagnesemia should be corrected whenever detected. Magnesium chloride is effective by mouth, but this compound is not widely available. Repletion is usually parenteral. Because the depressant effect of magnesium on central and peripheral nerve functions does not occur at levels <2 mmol/L (normal range 0.8 to 1.2 mmol/L), parenteral replacement can be given rapidly. A cumulative dose as great as 0.5 to 1 mmol/kg of body weight can be administered if severe hypomagnesemia is present; often, however, total doses of 20 to 40 mmol are sufficient. The magnesium is given either as an intravenous infusion over 8 to 12 h or in divided doses intramuscularly (magnesium sulfate, USP).

OTHER PARATHYROID-RELATED CAUSES OF HYPERCALCEMIA **Lithium Therapy** Lithium, used in the management of bipolar depression and other psychiatric disorders, causes hypercalcemia in approximately 10% of treated patients. The hypercalcemia is dependent on continued lithium treatment, remitting and recurring when lithium is stopped and restarted. The parathyroid adenomas reported in some hypercalcemic patients with lithium therapy may reflect the presence of an independently occurring parathyroid tumor; a permanent effect of lithium on parathyroid gland growth need not be implicated as most patients have complete reversal of hypercalcemia when lithium is stopped. However, long-standing stimulation of parathyroid cell replication by lithium may predispose to development of adenomas (as is documented in secondary hyperparathyroidism and renal failure).

The presence of hypercalcemia does not correlate with plasma lithium level, but the frequency with which hypercalcemia occurs is sufficiently high to support a causal relationship between lithium and the hypercalcemia, particularly the dependence of the hypercalcemia on the continuation of the lithium. At the levels achieved in blood in treated patients, lithium can be shown in vitro to shift the PTH secretion curve in response to calcium to the right; i.e., higher calcium levels are required to lower PTH secretion, probably acting at the calcium sensor (see below). It is logical to assume that this effect can cause elevated PTH levels and consequent hypercalcemia in otherwise normal individuals. If persistent hypercalcemia is detected during lithium therapy, it may be necessary to try alternative medication for the underlying psychiatric illness. Parathyroid surgery should not be recommended unless hypercalcemia and elevated PTH levels persist after lithium is discontinued.

GENETIC DISORDERS CAUSING HYPERPARATHYROID-LIKE SYNDROMES **Familial Hypocalciuric Hypercalcemia** FHH (also called *familial benign hypercalcemia*) is inherited as an autosomal dominant trait. Affected individuals are discovered because of asymptomatic hypercalcemia. This disorder and Jansen's disease (discussed below) are variants of hyperparathyroidism. FHH involves excessive secretion of PTH, whereas Jansen's disease is caused by excessive biologic activity of the PTH receptor in target tissues. Neither disorder, however, involves a primary growth disorder of the parathyroids.

The pathophysiology of FHH is now understood. The primary defect is abnormal sensing of the blood calcium by the parathyroid gland and renal tubule, causing inappropriate secretion of PTH and excessive renal reabsorption of calcium (Fig. 341-5). The calcium sensor is a member of the third family of GPCR (type C or III) and is located on chromosome 3. The receptor responds to the ECF calcium concentration, suppressing PTH secretion through second messenger signaling, thereby providing negative-feedback regulation of PTH secretion. More than 20 different mutations in the calcium-sensing receptor have been identified in patients with FHH (Fig. 341-6). These mutations lower the capacity of the sensor to bind calcium, and the mutant receptors function as though blood calcium levels are low; excessive secretion of PTH occurs from an otherwise normal gland. Approximately two-thirds of patients with FHH have mutations within the protein-coding region of the gene. The remaining one-third of kindreds may have mutations in the gene promoter or in other regions of the genome identified through mapping studies (e.g., chromosome 19).

Even before elucidation of the pathophysiology of FHH, abundant clinical evidence served to separate the disorder from primary hyperparathyroidism. Patients with primary hyperparathyroidism have <99% renal calcium reabsorption, whereas most patients with FHH have >99% reabsorption. The hypercalcemia in FHH is often detectable in affected members of the kindreds in the first decade of life, whereas hypercalcemia rarely occurs in patients with primary hyperparathyroidism or the MEN syndromes who are <10. PTH may be elevated in FHH, but the values are usually normal or lower for the same degree of calcium elevation than in patients with primary hyperparathyroidism. Parathyroid surgery in a few patients with FHH led

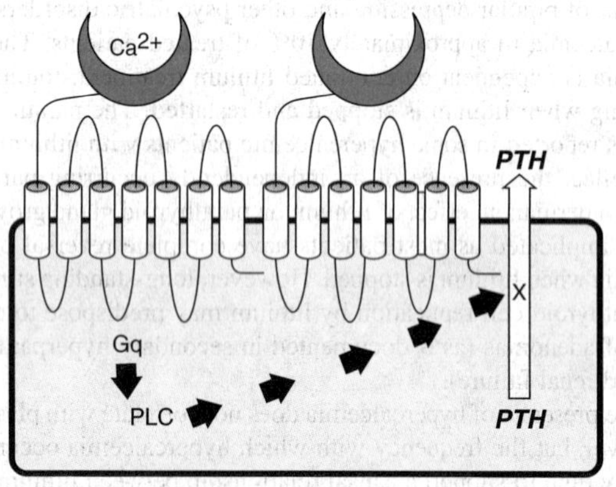

FIGURE 341-5 The calcium sensor's role in parathyroid hormone (PTH) secretion and calcium homeostasis. The extracellular domain closes upon binding to calcium. PLC, phospholipase C; the G protein is shown as G_q (the subclass of G protein thought to activate PLC). When calcium in the blood is low, the sensor is less active and suppression of PTH secretion is lowered (i.e., more PTH is secreted). *(From BR Conklin, HR Bourne: Nature 367:22, 1994, with permission.)*

to permanent hypoparathyroidism, but hypocalciuria persisted nevertheless, establishing that hypocalciuria, therefore, is not PTH-dependent (now known to be due to the abnormal calcium sensor in the kidney).

Few clinical signs or symptoms are present in patients with FHH, and other endocrine abnormalities are not present. Most patients are detected as a result of family screening after hypercalcemia is detected in a proband. In those patients inadvertently operated upon, the parathyroids appeared normal or moderately hyperplastic. Parathyroid surgery is not appropriate, nor, in view of the lack of symptoms, does medical treatment seem needed to lower the calcium. Calcimimetic agents that bind to the calcium sensor and elevate the set point are under investigation.

One striking exception to the rule against parathyroid surgery in this syndrome is the occurrence, usually in consanguinous marriages (due to the rarity of gene), of a homozygous or compound heterozygote state, resulting in complete loss of the calcium sensor function. In this condition, neonatal severe hypercalcemia, total parathyroidectomy is mandatory.

Jansen's Disease Mutations in the PTH/PTHrP receptor have been identified as responsible for this rare autosomal dominant syndrome. Because the mutations lead to constitutive receptor function, one abnormal copy of the mutant receptor is sufficient to cause the disease, thereby accounting for its dominant mode of transmission. The disorder leads to short-limbed dwarfism due to abnormal regulation of the bone growth plate. In adult life, there are numerous abnormalities in bone, including multiple cystic resorptive areas resembling those seen in severe hyperparathyroidism. Hypercalcemia and hypophosphatemia with undetectable or low PTH levels are typically seen. The pathogenesis of the disease has been confirmed by transgenic experiments in which targeted expression of the mutant receptor to the growth plate emulated several features of the disorder.

MALIGNANCY-RELATED HYPERCALCEMIA **Clinical Syndromes and Mechanisms of Hypercalcemia** Hypercalcemia due to malignancy is common (occurring with 10 to 15% of certain types of tumor, such as lung carcinoma), often severe and difficult to manage, confusing as to etiology, and sometimes difficult to distinguish from primary hyperparathyroidism. Although malignancy is often clinically obvious, hypercalcemia can occasionally be due to an occult tumor. Previously, hypercalcemia associated with malignancy was thought to be due to local invasion and destruction of bone by tumor cells; many cases are now known to result from the elaboration by the malignant cells of humoral mediators of hypercalcemia. PTHrP is the responsible humoral agent in most cases.

The histologic character of the tumor is more important than the extent of skeletal metastases in predicting hypercalcemia. Small cell carcinoma (oat cell) and adenocarcinoma of the lung, although the most common lung tumors associated with skeletal metastases, rarely cause hypercalcemia. By contrast, as many as 10% of patients with squamous cell carcinoma of the lung develop hypercalcemia. Histologic studies of bone in patients with squamous cell or epidermoid carcinoma of the lung, in sites invaded by tumor as well as areas remote from tumor invasion, reveal bone remodeling, including osteoclastic and osteoblastic activity. In contrast, minimal skeletal metabolic activation occurs even if there are extensive skeletal metastases of small cell (oat cell) carcinoma.

Two main mechanisms of hypercalcemia are operative in cancer hypercalcemia. Many solid tumors associated with hypercalcemia, particularly squamous cell and renal tumors, produce and secrete humoral factors that cause increased bone resorption and mediate the hypercalcemia through systemic actions on the skeleton. Alternatively, direct bone marrow invasion occurs with hematologic malignancies such as leukemia, lymphoma, and multiple myeloma. Lymphokines and cytokines produced by cells involved in the marrow response to the tumors promote resorption of bone through local destruction. Several hormones, hormone analogues, cytokines, and growth factors have been implicated as the result of clinical assays, in vitro tests, or chemical isolation. In some lymphomas, typically B cell lymphomas, there is an increased blood level of $1,25(OH)_2D$, which is probably produced by lymphocytes. The etiologic factor produced by activated normal lymphocytes and by myeloma and lymphoma cells, termed *osteoclast activation factor*, now appears to represent the biologic action of several different cytokines, probably interleukin 1 and lymphotoxin or tumor necrosis factor.

The more common mechanism, humoral hypercalcemia of malignancy, occurs with cancers of the lung and kidney, in particular, in which bone metastases are absent, minimal, or not detectable clinically. The clinical picture resembles primary hyperparathyroidism (hypophosphatemia accompanies hypercalcemia), and elimination or regression of the primary tumor leads to disappearance of the hypercalcemia. The disorder is due to secretion by the tumors of the PTH-like factor, PTHrP, that activates the PTH/PTHrP receptor (see above).

As in hyperparathyroidism, patients with the humoral hypercalcemia of malignancy have elevated urinary nephrogenous cyclic AMP excretion, hypophosphatemia, and increased urinary phosphate clearance. However, in humoral hypercalcemia of malignancy, immunoreactive PTH is undetectable or suppressed, making the differential diagnosis easier. Other features of the disorder differ from those of true hyperparathyroidism. Patients may have high, rather than low, renal calcium clearance (relative to serum calcium when compared to true hyperparathyroidism, unlike the expected elevation) and low to normal levels of $1,25(OH)_2D$. The reason that the humoral syndrome differs from hyperparathyroidism in these parameters is unclear since the biologic actions of PTH and PTHrP are presumably exerted through the same receptor. Other cytokines elaborated by the malignancy may be responsible for these variations from hyperparathyroidism. In some patients with the humoral hypercalcemia of malignancy, osteoclastic resorption is unaccompanied by an osteoblastic or bone-forming response, implying inhibition of the normal coupling of bone formation and resorption. Thus the interaction of more than one substance may determine whether hypercalcemia develops in a particular patient.

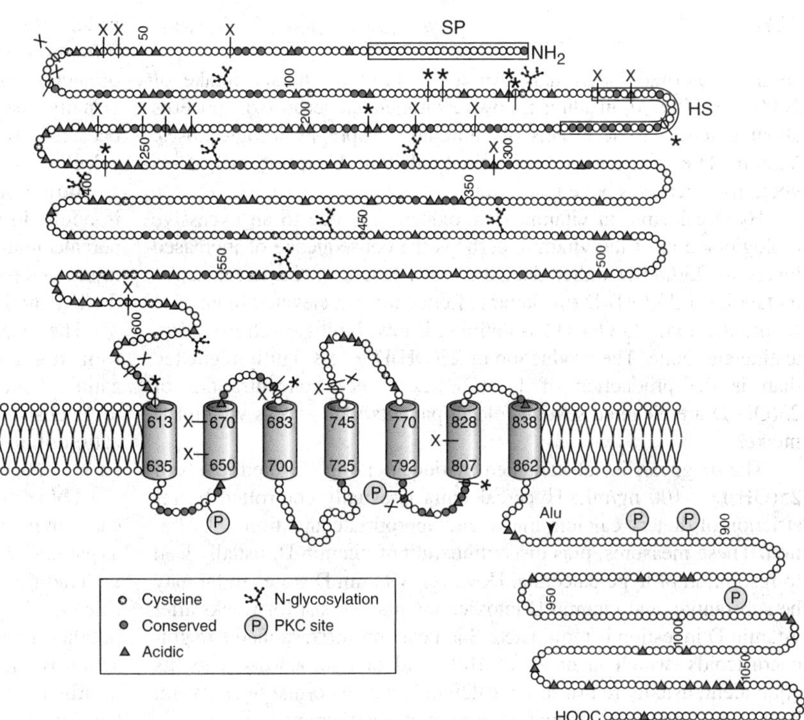

FIGURE 341-6 Mutations in the calcium sensor receptor. The identified sequence alterations (X) cause loss of function and lead to inadequate suppression of parathyroid hormone release and, therefore, mild hypercalcemia (FHH); ♦, a gain-of-function mutation that causes hypocalcemia; S, a stop codon that is a loss of function mutation; •, conserved residues; ▲, acidic residues. *(From EM Brown et al: J Nutr 125:1965S, 1995, with permission.)*

Several different assays (single- or double-antibody, different epitopes) have been developed to detect PTHrP. Most data indicate that circulating PTHrP levels are undetectable (or low) in normal individuals, elevated in most cancer patients with the humoral syndrome, and high in human milk. Despite the discovery of PTHrP, identifying the etiologic mechanisms in cancer hypercalcemia is often complex. For example, in breast carcinoma (metastatic to bone) and in a distinctive type of T cell lymphoma/leukemia initiated by human T cell lymphotropic virus I, hypercalcemia is caused by direct local lysis of bone as well as by a humoral mechanism involving excess production of PTHrP.

Diagnostic Issues Levels of PTH measured by the double-antibody technique are undetectable or extremely low in tumor hypercalcemia, as would be expected with the mediation of the hypercalcemia by a factor other than PTH (the hypercalcemia suppresses the normal parathyroid glands). In a patient with minimal symptoms referred for hypercalcemia, low or undetectable PTH and elevated PTHrP levels would focus attention on occult malignancy.

Ordinarily, the diagnosis of cancer hypercalcemia is not difficult because tumor symptoms are prominent when hypercalcemia is detected. Indeed, hypercalcemia may be noted incidentally during the workup of a patient with known or suspected malignancy. Clinical suspicion that malignancy is the cause of the hypercalcemia is heightened when there are other paraneoplastic signs or symptoms, such as weight loss, fatigue, muscle weakness, or unexplained skin rash, or when symptoms specific for a particular tumor are present. Squamous cell tumors are most frequently associated with hypercalcemia, particularly tumors of the lung, kidney, head and neck, and urogenital tract. Radiologic examinations can focus on these areas when clinical evidence is unclear. Bone scans with technetium-labeled bisphosphonate are useful for detection of osteolytic metastases; the sensitivity is high, but specificity is low; results must be confirmed by conventional x-rays to be certain that areas of increased uptake are due to osteolytic metastases per se. Bone marrow biopsies are helpful in patients with anemia or abnormal peripheral blood smears.

℞ TREATMENT Treatment of the hypercalcemia of malignancy is first directed to control of the tumor; reduction of tumor mass usually corrects hypercalcemia. If a patient has severe hypercalcemia yet has a good chance for effective tumor therapy, treatment of the hypercalcemia should be vigorous while awaiting the results of definitive therapy. If hypercalcemia occurs in the late stages of a tumor that is resistant to therapy, the treatment of the hypercalcemia should be judicious as high calcium levels can have a mild sedating effect. Standard therapies for hypercalcemia (discussed below) are applicable to patients with malignancy.

VITAMIN D–RELATED HYPERCALCEMIA Hypercalcemia caused by vitamin D can be due to excessive ingestion or abnormal metabolism of the vitamin. Abnormal metabolism of the vitamin is usually acquired in association with a widespread granulomatous disorder. Vitamin D metabolism is carefully regulated, particularly the activity of renal 1α-hydroxylase, the enzyme responsible for the production of $1,25(OH)_2D$ (Chap. 340). The regulation of 1α-hydroxylase and the normal feedback suppression by $1,25(OH)_2D$ seem to work less well in infants than in adults and to operate poorly, if at all, in sites other than the renal tubule; these phenomena explain the occurrence of hypercalcemia secondary to excessive $1,25(OH)_2D_3$ production in infants with Williams' syndrome (see below) and in adults with sarcoidosis or lymphoma.

Vitamin D Intoxication Chronic ingestion of 50 to 100 times the normal physiologic requirement of vitamin D (amounts >50,000 to 100,000 U/d) is usually required to produce significant hypercalcemia in normal individuals. An upper limit of dietary intake of 2000 U/d (50 μg/d) in adults is now recommended because of concerns about potential toxic effects of cumulative supraphysiologic doses. Vitamin D excess increases intestinal calcium absorption and, if severe, also increases bone resorption.

Hypercalcemia in vitamin D intoxication is due to an excessive biologic action of the vitamin, perhaps the consequence of increased levels of 25(OH)D rather than increased levels of the usual active metabolite 1,25$(OH)_2$D (the latter is frequently not elevated in vitamin D intoxication). 25(OH)D has definite, if low, biologic activity in intestine and bone. The production of 25(OH)D is less tightly regulated than is the production of 1,25$(OH)_2$D. Hence concentrations of 25(OH)D are elevated several-fold in patients with excess vitamin D intake.

The diagnosis is substantiated by documenting elevated levels of 25(OH)D >100 ng/mL. Hypercalcemia is usually controlled by restriction of dietary calcium intake and appropriate attention to hydration. These measures, plus discontinuation of vitamin D, usually lead to resolution of hypercalcemia. However, vitamin D stores in fat may be substantial, and vitamin D intoxication may persist for weeks after vitamin D ingestion is terminated. Such patients are responsive to glucocorticoids, which in doses of 100 mg/d of hydrocortisone or its equivalent, usually return serum calcium levels to normal over several days; severe intoxication may require intensive therapy.

Sarcoidosis and Other Granulomatous Diseases In patients with sarcoidosis and other granulomatous diseases, such as tuberculosis and fungal infections, excess 1,25$(OH)_2$D is synthesized in macrophages or other cells in the granulomas. Indeed, increased 1,25$(OH)_2$D levels have been reported in anephric patients with sarcoidosis and hypercalcemia. Macrophages obtained from granulomatous tissue convert 25(OH)D to 1,25$(OH)_2$D at an increased rate. There is a positive correlation in patients with sarcoidosis between 25(OH)D levels (reflecting vitamin D intake) and the circulating concentrations of 1,25$(OH)_2$D, whereas normally there is no increase in 1,25$(OH)_2$D with increasing 25(OH)D levels due to multiple feedback controls on renal 1α-hydroxylase (Chap. 340). The usual regulation of active metabolite production by calcium or PTH does not operate in these patients; hypercalcemia does not lead to a reduction in the blood levels of 1,25$(OH)_2$D in patients with sarcoidosis. Clearance of 1,25$(OH)_2$D from blood may be decreased in sarcoidosis as well. PTH levels are usually low and 1,25$(OH)_2$D levels are elevated, but primary hyperparathyroidism and sarcoidosis may coexist in some patients.

Management of the hypercalcemia can often be accomplished by avoiding excessive sunlight exposure and limiting vitamin D and calcium intake. Presumably, however, the abnormal sensitivity to vitamin D and abnormal regulation of 1,25$(OH)_2$D synthesis will persist as long as the disease is active. Alternatively, glucocorticoids in the equivalent of ≤100 mg/d of hydrocortisone control hypercalcemia. Glucocorticoids appear to act by blocking excessive production of 1,25$(OH)_2$D as well as the response to it in target organs.

Idiopathic Hypercalcemia of Infancy This rare disorder, usually referred to as *Williams' syndrome*, is an autosomal dominant disorder characterized by multiple congenital development defects, including supravalvular aortic stenosis, mental retardation, and an elfin facies, in association with hypercalcemia due to abnormal sensitivity to vitamin D. The syndrome was first recognized in England after the fortification of milk with vitamin D. Levels of 1,25$(OH)_2$D are elevated, ranging from 46 to 120 nmol/L (150 to 500 pg/mL). The mechanism of the abnormal sensitivity to vitamin D and of the increased circulating levels of 1,25$(OH)_2$D is still unclear. Studies suggest that mutations involving the elastin locus and perhaps other genes on chromosome 7 may play a role in the pathogenesis.

HYPERCALCEMIA ASSOCIATED WITH HIGH BONE TURNOVER **Hyperthyroidism** As many as 20% of hyperthyroid patients have high-normal or mildly elevated serum calcium concentrations; hypercalciuria is even more common. The hypercalcemia is due to increased bone turnover, with bone resorption exceeding bone formation. Severe calcium elevations are not typical, and the presence of such suggests a concomitant disease such as hyperparathyroidism. Usually, the diagnosis is obvious, but signs of hyperthyroidism may occasionally be occult, particularly in the elderly (Chap. 330). Hypercalcemia is managed by treatment of the hyperthyroidism.

Immobilization Immobilization is a rare cause of hypercalcemia in adults in the absence of an associated disease but may cause hypercalcemia in children and adolescents, particularly after spinal cord injury and paraplegia or quadriplegia. With resumption of ambulation, the hypercalcemia in children usually returns to normal.

The mechanism appears to involve a disproportion between bone formation and bone resorption. Hypercalciuria and increased mobilization of skeletal calcium can develop in normal volunteers subjected to extensive bed rest, although hypercalcemia is unusual. Immobilization of an adult with a disease associated with high bone turnover, such as Paget's disease, may cause hypercalcemia.

Thiazides Administration of benzothiadiazines (thiazides) can cause hypercalcemia in patients with high rates of bone turnover, such as patients with hypoparathyroidism treated with high doses of vitamin D. Traditionally, thiazides are associated with aggravation of hypercalcemia in primary hyperparathyroidism, but this effect can be seen in other high-bone-turnover states as well. The mechanism of thiazide action is complex. Chronic thiazide administration leads to reduction in urinary calcium; the hypocalciuric effect appears to reflect the enhancement of proximal tubular resorption of sodium and calcium in response to sodium depletion. Some of this renal effect is due to augmentation of PTH action and is more pronounced in individuals with intact PTH secretion. However, thiazides cause hypocalciuria in hypoparathyroid patients on high-dose vitamin D and oral calcium replacement if sodium intake is restricted. This finding is the rationale for the use of thiazides as an adjunct to therapy in hypoparathyroid patients, as discussed below. Thiazide administration to normal individuals causes a transient increase in blood calcium (usually within the high-normal range) that reverts to preexisting levels after a week or more of continued administration. If hormonal function and calcium and bone metabolism are normal, homeostatic controls are reset to counteract the calcium-elevating effect of the thiazides. In the presence of hyperparathyroidism or increased bone turnover from another cause, homeostatic mechanisms are ineffective. The abnormal effects of the thiazide on calcium metabolism disappear within days of cessation of the drug.

Vitamin A Intoxication Vitamin A intoxication is a rare cause of hypercalcemia and is most commonly a side effect of dietary faddism (Chap. 75). Calcium levels can be elevated into the 3 to 3.5 mmol/L (12 to 14 mg/dL) range after the ingestion of 50,000 to 100,000 units of vitamin A daily (10 to 20 times the minimum daily requirement). Typical features of severe hypercalcemia include fatigue, anorexia, and, in some, severe muscle and bone pain. Excess Vitamin A intake is presumed to increase bone resorption.

The diagnosis can be established by history and by measurement of vitamin A levels in serum, which may be severalfold above normal. Occasionally, skeletal x-rays reveal periosteal calcifications, particularly in the hands. Withdrawal of the vitamin is usually associated with prompt disappearance of the hypercalcemia and reversal of the skeletal changes. As in vitamin D intoxication, administration of 100 mg/d hydrocortisone or its equivalent leads to a rapid return of the serum calcium to normal.

HYPERCALCEMIA ASSOCIATED WITH RENAL FAILURE **Severe Secondary Hyperparathyroidism** Secondary hyperparathyroidism occurs when partial resistance to the metabolic actions of PTH leads to excessive production of the hormone. Parathyroid gland hyperplasia occurs because resistance to the normal level of PTH leads to hypocalcemia, which, in turn, is a stimulus to parathyroid gland enlargement. This concept is supported by studies of the treatment of patients treated with bisphosphonates, which block the skeletal resorptive response. Because a portion of PTH secretion by each parathyroid cell is not suppressible by any degree of elevation of blood calcium, larger glands (more cells) have a higher hormone output at the hypercalcemic end of the dose-response curve.

Secondary hyperparathyroidism occurs not only in patients with renal failure but also in those with osteomalacia due to multiple causes (Chap. 340), including deficiency of vitamin D action, and PHP (deficient response to PTH at the level of the receptor). Hypocalcemia seems to be the common denominator in initiating secondary hyperparathyroidism. Only in patients with renal failure, however, is hypercalcemia sometimes encountered despite appropriate medical management regimens (see below). Primary and secondary hyperparathyroidism can be distinguished conceptually by the autonomous growth of the parathyroid glands in primary hyperparathyroidism (presumably irreversible) and the adaptive response of the parathyroids in secondary hyperparathyroidism (typically reversible). In fact, reversal over weeks from an abnormal pattern of secretion, presumably accompanied by involution of parathyroid gland mass to normal, occurs in patients who have been treated effectively to reverse the resistance to PTH (such as with calcium and vitamin D in osteomalacia).

Patients with secondary hyperparathyroidism may develop bone pain, ectopic calcification, and pruritus. The bone disease seen in patients with secondary hyperparathyroidism and renal failure is termed *renal osteodystrophy*. Osteomalacia (predominantly due to vitamin D and calcium deficiency) and/or osteitis fibrosa cystica (excessive PTH action on bone) may occur.

Two other skeletal disorders are associated with long-term dialysis in patients with renal failure. Aluminum deposition (see below) is associated with an osteomalacia-like picture. The other entity is a low-bone-turnover state termed "aplastic" or "adynamic" bone disease; PTH levels are lower than in typical secondary hyperparathyroidism. It is believed that the condition is caused, at least in part, by excessive PTH suppression, which may be even greater than previously appreciated in light of evidence that some of the immunoreactive PTH detected by most commercially available PTH assays is not the full-length biologically active molecule (as discussed above).

℞ **TREATMENT** Medical therapy to reverse secondary hyperparathyroidism includes reduction of excessive blood phosphate by restriction of dietary phosphate, the use of nonabsorbable antacids, and careful, selective addition of calcitriol (0.25 to 2.0 μg/d); calcium carbonate is preferred over aluminum-containing antacids to prevent aluminum toxicity. Intravenous calcitriol, administered as several pulses each week, helps control secondary hyperparathyroidism. Aggressive but carefully administered medical therapy can often, but not always, reverse hyperparathyroidism and its symptoms and manifestations.

Occasional patients develop severe manifestations of secondary hyperparathyroidism, including hypercalcemia, pruritus, extraskeletal calcifications, and painful bones, despite aggressive medical efforts to suppress the hyperparathyroidism. PTH hypersecretion no longer responsive to medical therapy, a state of severe hyperparathyroidism in patients with renal failure that requires surgery, has been referred to as *tertiary hyperparathyroidism*. Parathyroid surgery is necessary to control this condition. Based on genetic evidence from examination of tumor samples in these patients, the emergence of autonomous parathyroid function is due to a monoclonal outgrowth of one or more previously hyperplastic parathyroid glands.

Aluminum Intoxication Aluminum intoxication (and often hypercalcemia as a complication of medical treatment) may occur in patients on chronic dialysis; manifestations include acute dementia and unresponsive and severe osteomalacia. Bone pain, multiple nonhealing fractures, particularly of the ribs and pelvis, and a proximal myopathy may occur. Hypercalcemia develops when these patients are treated with vitamin D or calcitriol because of impaired skeletal responsiveness. Aluminum is present at the site of osteoid mineralization, osteoblastic activity is minimal, and calcium incorporation into the skeleton is impaired. Prevention is accomplished by avoidance of aluminum excess in the dialysis regimen; treatment of established disease involves mobilizing aluminum through the use of the chelating agent deferoxamine (Chap. 348).

Milk-Alkali Syndrome The milk-alkali syndrome is due to excessive ingestion of calcium and absorbable antacids such as milk or calcium carbonate. It is much less frequent since nonabsorbable antacids and other treatments became available for peptic ulcer disease. However, the increased use of calcium carbonate in the management of osteoporosis has led to reappearance of the syndrome. Several clinical presentations—acute, subacute, and chronic—have been described, all of which feature hypercalcemia, alkalosis, and renal failure. The chronic form of the disease, termed *Burnett's syndrome*, is associated with irreversible renal damage. The acute syndromes reverse if the excess calcium and absorbable alkali are stopped.

Individual susceptibility is important in the pathogenesis, as many patients are treated with calcium carbonate alkali regimens without developing the syndrome. One variable is the fractional calcium absorption as a function of calcium intake. Some individuals absorb a high fraction of calcium, even with intakes as high as 2 g or more of elemental calcium per day, instead of reducing calcium absorption with high intake, as occurs in most normal individuals. Resultant mild hypercalcemia after meals in such patients is postulated to contribute to the generation of alkalosis. Development of hypercalcemia causes increased sodium excretion and some depletion of total-body water. These phenomena and perhaps some suppression of endogenous PTH secretion due to mild hypercalcemia lead to increased bicarbonate resorption and to alkalosis in the face of continued calcium carbonate ingestion. Alkalosis per se selectively enhances calcium resorption in the distal nephron, thus aggravating the hypercalcemia. The cycle of mild hypercalcemia → bicarbonate retention → alkalosis → renal calcium retention → severe hypercalcemia perpetuates and aggravates hypercalcemia and alkalosis as long as calcium and absorbable alkali are ingested.

DIFFERENTIAL DIAGNOSIS: SPECIAL TESTS Differential diagnosis of hypercalcemia is best achieved by using clinical criteria, but the immunoassay for PTH is especially useful in distinguishing among major causes (Fig. 341-7). The clinical features that deserve emphasis are the presence or absence of symptoms or signs of disease and evidence of chronicity. If one discounts fatigue or depression, >90% of patients with primary hyperparathyroidism have *asymptomatic hypercalcemia*; symptoms of malignancy are usually present in cancer-associated hypercalcemia. Disorders other than hyperparathyroidism and malignancy cause <10% of cases of hypercalcemia, and some of the nonparathyroid causes are associated with clear-cut manifestations such as renal failure.

Hyperparathyroidism is the likely diagnosis in patients with *chronic hypercalcemia*. If hypercalcemia has been manifest for >1 year, malignancy can usually be excluded as the cause. A striking feature of malignancy-associated hypercalcemia is the rapidity of the course, whereby signs and symptoms of the underlying malignancy are evident within months of the detection of hypercalcemia. A careful history of dietary supplements and drug use may suggest intoxication with vitamins D or vitamin A or the use of thiazides.

Although clinical considerations are helpful in arriving at the correct diagnosis of the cause of hypercalcemia, appropriate laboratory testing is essential for definitive diagnosis. The immunoassay for PTH should separate hyperparathyroidism from all other causes of hypercalcemia. Patients with hyperparathyroidism have elevated PTH levels despite hypercalcemia, whereas patients with malignancy and the other causes of hypercalcemia (except for disorders mediated by PTH such as lithium-induced hypercalcemia) have levels of hormone below normal or undetectable. Assays based on the double-antibody method for PTH exhibit very high sensitivity (especially if serum calcium is simultaneously evaluated) and specificity for the diagnosis of primary hyperparathyroidism (Fig. 341-8).

In summary, PTH values are elevated in >90% of parathyroid-

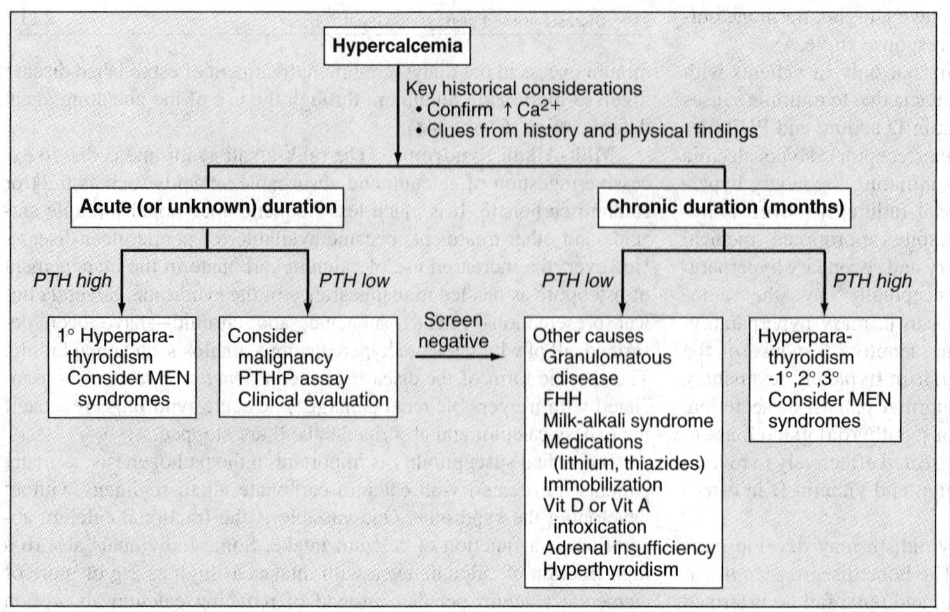

FIGURE 341-7 Algorithm for the evaluation of patients with hypercalcemia. See text for details. FHH, familial hypocalciuric hypercalcemia; MEN, multiple endocrine neoplasia; PTH, parathyroid hormone; PTHrP, parathyroid hormone–related peptide.

related causes of hypercalcemia, undetectable or low in malignancy-related hypercalcemia, and undetectable or normal in vitamin D–related and high-bone-turnover causes of hypercalcemia. In view of the specificity of the PTH immunoassay and the high frequency of hyperparathyroidism in hypercalcemic patients, it is cost-effective to measure the PTH level in all hypercalcemic patients unless malignancy or a specific nonparathyroid disease is obvious. False-positive PTH assay results are rare. There are very rare reports of ectopic production of excess PTH by nonparathyroid tumors. Immunoassays for PTHrP are helpful in diagnosing certain types of malignancy-associated hypercalcemia. Although FHH is parathyroid-related, the disease should be managed distinctively from hyperparathyroidism. Clinical features and the low urinary calcium excretion can help make the distinction. Because the incidence of malignancy and hyperparathyroidism both increase with age, they can coexist as two independent causes of hypercalcemia.

$1,25(OH)_2D$ levels are elevated in many (but not all) patients with primary hyperparathyroidism. In other disorders associated with hypercalcemia, concentrations of $1,25(OH)_2D$ are low or, at the most, normal. However, this test is of low specificity and is not cost-effective, as not all patients with hyperparathyroidism have elevated $1,25(OH)_2D$ levels, and not all nonparathyroid hypercalcemic patients have suppressed $1,25(OH)_2D$. Measurement of $1,25(OH)_2D$ is, however, critically valuable in establishing the cause of hypercalcemia in sarcoidosis and certain B cell lymphomas.

A useful general approach is outlined in Fig. 341-7. If the patient is *asymptomatic* and there is evidence of *chronicity* to the hypercalcemia, hyperparathyroidism is almost certainly the cause. If PTH levels (usually measured at least twice) are elevated, the clinical impression is confirmed and little additional evaluation is necessary. If there is only a short history or no data as to the duration of the hypercalcemia, *occult malignancy* must be considered; if the PTH levels are not elevated, then a thorough workup must be undertaken for malignancy, including chest x-ray, CT of chest and abdomen, and bone scan. Immunoassays for PTHrP may be especially useful in such situations. Attention should also be paid to clues for underlying hematologic disorders such as anemia, increased plasma globulin, and abnormal serum immunoelectrophoresis; bone scans can be negative in some patients with metastases, such as in multiple myeloma. Finally, if a patient with chronic hypercalcemia is asymptomatic and malignancy therefore seems unlikely on clinical grounds, but PTH values are not elevated, it is useful to search for other chronic causes of hypercalcemia, such as occult sarcoidosis.

℞ TREATMENT Hypercalcemic States

The approach to medical treatment of hypercalcemia varies with its severity. Mild hypercalcemia, <3.0 mmol/L (12 mg/dL), can be managed by hydration. More severe hypercalcemia [levels of 3.2 to 3.7 mmol/L (13 to 15 mg/dL)] must be managed aggressively; above that level, hypercalcemia can be life-threatening and requires emergency measures. By using a combination of approaches, the serum calcium concentration can be decreased by 0.7 to 2.2 mmol/L (3 to 9 mg/dL) within 24 to 48 h in most patients, enough to relieve acute symptoms, prevent death from hypercalcemic crisis, and permit diagnostic evaluation. Therapy can then be directed at the underlying disorder—the second priority.

Hypercalcemia develops because of excessive skeletal calcium release, increased intestinal calcium absorption, or inadequate renal calcium excretion. Understanding the particular pathogenesis helps guide therapy. For example, hypercalcemia in patients with malignancy is primarily due to excessive skeletal calcium release and is, therefore, minimally improved by restriction of dietary calcium. On the other hand, patients with vitamin D hypersensitivity

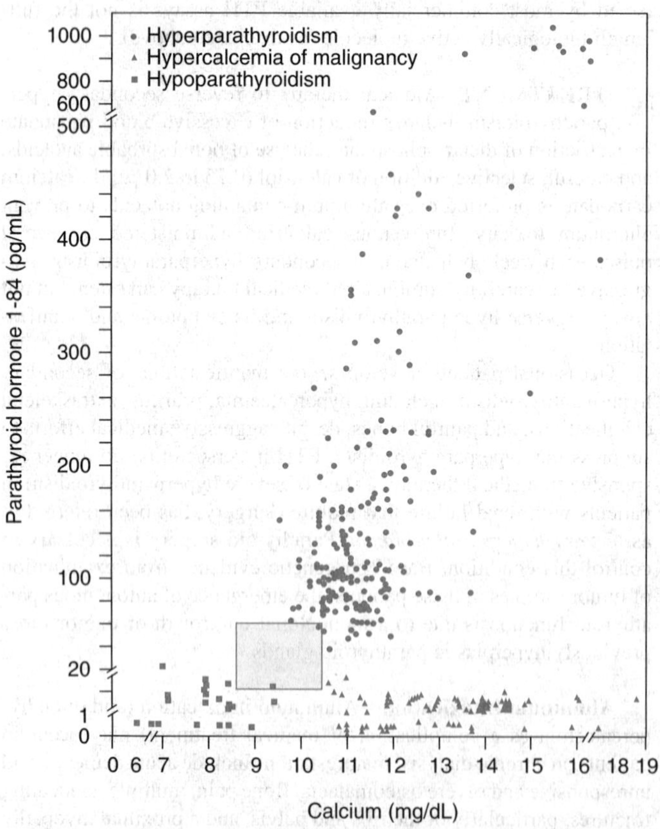

FIGURE 341-8 Levels of immunoreactive parathyroid hormone (PTH) detected in patients with primary hyperparathyroidism, hypercalcemia of malignancy, and hypoparathyroidism. Boxed area represents the upper and normal limits of blood calcium and/or immunoreactive PTH. *(From Nussbaum and Potts, with permission.)*

or vitamin D intoxication have excessive intestinal calcium absorption, and restriction of dietary calcium is beneficial. Decreased renal function or ECF depletion decreases urinary calcium excretion. In such situations, rehydration may rapidly reduce or reverse the hypercalcemia, even though increased bone resorption persists. As outlined below, the more severe the hypercalcemia, the greater the number of combined therapies that should be used. Rapid acting (hours) approaches—rehydration, forced diuresis, and calcitonin—can be used with the most effective antiresorptive agents, such as bisphosphonates (since severe hypercalcemia usually involves excessive bone resorption).

Hydration, increased salt intake, mild and forced diuresis The first principle of treatment is to restore normal hydration. Many hypercalcemic patients are dehydrated because of vomiting, inanition, and/or hypercalcemia-induced defects in urinary concentrating ability. The resultant drop in glomerular filtration rate is accompanied by an additional decrease in renal tubular sodium and calcium clearance. Restoring a normal ECF volume corrects these abnormalities and increases urine calcium excretion by 2.5 to 7.5 mmol/d (100 to 300 mg/d). Increasing urinary sodium excretion to 400 to 500 mmol/d increases urinary calcium excretion even further than simple rehydration. After rehydration has been achieved, saline can be administered or furosemide or ethacrynic acid can be given twice daily to depress the tubular reabsorptive mechanism for calcium (care must be taken to prevent dehydration). The combined use of these therapies can increase urinary calcium excretion to ≥12.5 mmol/d (500 mg/d) in most hypercalcemic patients. Since this is a substantial percentage of the exchangeable calcium pool, the serum calcium concentration usually falls 0.25 to 0.75 mmol/L (1 to 3 mg/dL) within 24 h. Precautions should be taken to prevent potassium and magnesium depletion; calcium-containing renal calculi are a potential complication.

Under life-threatening circumstances, the preceding approach can be pursued more aggressively, giving as much as 6 L isotonic saline (900 mmol sodium) daily plus furosemide or equivalent in doses up to 100 mg every 1 to 2 h or ethacrynic acid in doses to 40 mg every 1 to 2 h. Urinary calcium excretion may exceed 25 mmol/d (1000 mg/d), and the serum calcium may decrease by ≥1 mmol/L (4 mg/dL) within 24 h. Depletion of potassium and magnesium is inevitable unless replacements are given; pulmonary edema can be precipitated. The potential complications can be reduced by careful monitoring of central venous pressure and plasma or urine electrolytes; catheterization of the bladder may be necessary. This treatment approach should be supplemented with agents to block bone resorption. Though these agents do not become effective for several days, forced diuresis is difficult to sustain even in patients with good cardiopulmonary and renal function.

Bisphosphonates The bisphosphonates are analogues of pyrophosphate, with high affinity for bone, especially in areas of increased bone turnover, where they are powerful inhibitors of bone resorption. These bone-seeking compounds are stable in vivo because phosphatase enzymes cannot hydrolyze the central carbon-phosphorus-carbon bond. The bisphosphonates are concentrated in areas of high bone turnover and are taken up by and inhibit osteoclast action; the mechanism of action is complex. Bisphosphonates alter osteoclast proton pump function or impair the release of acid hydrolases into the extracellular lysosomes contiguous with mineralized bone. They may also inhibit the differentiation of monocyte-macrophage precursors into osteoclasts and possibly have effects on osteoblasts as well. The bisphosphonate molecules that contain amino groups in the side chain structure (see below) interfere with prenylation of proteins and can lead to cellular apoptosis. The highly active non-amino group–containing bisphosphonates are also metabolized to cytotoxic products.

The initial bisphosphonate widely used in clinical practice, etidronate, was effective but had several disadvantages, including the capacity to inhibit bone formation as well as blocking resorption. Subsequently, a number of second-generation compounds have become the mainstays of antiresorptive therapy for treatment of hypercalcemia. The most widely used, pamidronate, is a potent inhibitor of osteoclast-mediated skeletal resorption yet does not cause mineralization defects at ordinary doses. Several additional bisphosphonates (alendronate, tiludronate, and risedronate) are potent and also have a highly favorable ratio of blocking resorption versus inhibiting bone formation. Though the bisphosphonates have similar structures, the routes of administration, efficacy, toxicity, and side effects vary. The potency of the compounds for inhibition of bone resorption varies a thousandfold in the order of etidronate, tiludronate, pamidronate, alendronate, and risedronate. Oral alendronate is approved for the therapy of osteoporosis in the United States, and in Europe oral preparations of these bisphosphonates are used in the chronic treatment of hypercalcemia. Only the intravenous use of pamidronate is approved for this purpose in the United States; between 30 and 90 mg pamidronate, given as a single intravenous dose over a few hours, returns serum calcium to normal within 24 to 48 h with an effect that lasts for weeks in 80 to 100% of patients.

Pamidronate causes low-grade fever in as many as 20% of patients, likely related to release of cytokines from osteoclasts, monocytes, and macrophages (Table 341-2). This effect is usually seen only with the initial doses. Etidronate causes hyperphosphatemia through a direct renal mechanism, whereas hypophosphatemia is seen after therapy with other bisphosphonates. Overall, second-generation bisphosphonates are now the agents of choice in severe hypercalcemia, particularly that associated with malignancy. Zoledronate, a third-generation bisphosphonate, is claimed to be 100 to 800 times more potent than pamidronate and to normalize calcium more quickly and for longer periods.

Calcitonin Calcitonin acts within a few hours of its administration, through receptors on osteoclasts, to block bone resorption and, in addition, to increase urinary calcium excretion by inhibition of renal tubular calcium reabsorption. However, calcitonin leads to variable and usually minimal lowering of calcium. Tachyphylaxis, a known phenomenon with this drug, may explain the variable results. However, in life-threatening hypercalcemia, calcitonin can be used effectively within the first 24 h in combination with rehydration and saline diuresis while waiting for more sustained effects from a simultaneously administered bisphosphonate such as pamidronate. Usual doses of calcitonin are 2 to 8 U/kg of body weight intravenously, subcutaneously, or intramuscularly every 6 to 12 h.

Other therapies *Plicamycin* (mithramycin), which inhibits bone resorption, has been a useful therapeutic agent but is now little used because of the effectiveness of bisphosphonates. Plicamycin must be given intravenously, either as a bolus injection or by slow infusion. The usual dose is 25 μg/kg body weight. Major side effects include thrombocytopenia, hepatocellular necrosis with increased lactic acid dehydrogenase (LDH) and aspartate aminotransferase (AST) levels, and decreased levels of clotting factors with resultant epistaxis, bruising, hemorrhage, and bleeding gums.

Gallium nitrate exerts a hypocalcemic action by inhibiting bone resorption and altering the structure of bone crystals. Major disadvantages include the 5-day duration of infusion and the potential for nephrotoxicity and relatively shorter duration of action than bisphosphonates. Accordingly it is not often used because of superior alternatives.

Glucocorticoids increase urinary calcium excretion and decrease intestinal calcium absorption when given in pharmacologic doses, but they also cause negative skeletal calcium balance. In normal individuals and in patients with primary hyperparathyroidism, glucocorticoids neither increase nor decrease the serum calcium concentration. In patients with hypercalcemia due to certain osteolytic malignancies, however, glucocorticoids may be effective as a result of antitumor effects. The malignancies in which hypercalcemia responds to glucocorticoids include multiple myeloma, leukemia, Hodgkin's disease, other lymphomas, and carcinoma of the breast, at least early in the course of the disease. Glucocorticoids are also effective in treating hypercalcemia due to vitamin D intoxication and sarcoidosis. In all the preceding situations, the hypocalcemic effect develops over several days,

Table 341-2 Therapies for Severe Hypercalcemia

Treatment	Onset of Action	Duration of Action	Advantages	Disadvantages
MOST USEFUL THERAPIES				
Hydration with saline	Hours	During infusion	Rehydration invariably needed	Volume overload, cardiac decompensation, intensive monitoring, electrolyte disturbance, inconvenience
Forced diuresis; saline plus loop diuretic	Hours	During treatment	Rapid action	
Bisphosphonates 1st generation: etidronate	1–2 days	5–7 days in doses used	First available bisphosphonate; intermediate onset of action	Less effective than other bisphosphonates
2d generation: pamidronate	1–2 days	10–14 days to weeks	High potency; intermediate onset of action	Fever in 20% hypophosphatemia, hypocalcemia, hypomagnesemia
Calcitonin	Hours	1–2 days	Rapid onset of action; useful as adjunct in severe hypercalcemia	Rapid tachyphylaxis
SPECIAL USE THERAPIES				
Phosphate Oral	24 h	During use	Chronic management (with hypophosphatemia); low toxicity if P < 4 mg/dL	Limited use except as adjuvant or chronic therapy
Intravenous	Hours	During use and 24–48 h afterward	Rapid action, highly potent but *rarely used* except with severe hypercalcemia and cardiac and renal decompensation present	Ectopic calcification; renal damage, fatal hypocalcemia
Glucocorticoids	Days	Days, weeks	Oral therapy, antitumor agent	Active only in certain malignancies; glucocorticoid side effects
Dialysis	Hours	During use and 24–48 h afterward	Useful in renal failure; onset of effect in hours; can immediately reverse life-threatening hypercalcemia	Complex procedure, reserved for extreme or special circumstances

and the usual glucocorticoid dosage is 40 to 100 mg prednisone (or its equivalent) daily in four divided doses. The side effects of chronic glucocorticoid therapy may be acceptable in some circumstances.

Dialysis is often the treatment of choice for hypercalcemia complicated by renal failure, which is difficult to manage. Peritoneal dialysis with calcium-free dialysis fluid can remove 5 to 12.5 mmol (200 to 500 mg) of calcium in 24 to 48 h and lower the serum calcium concentration by 0.7 to 3 mmol/L (3 to 12 mg/dL). Large quantities of phosphate are lost during dialysis, and serum inorganic phosphate concentrations usually fall, thus aggravating hypercalcemia. Therefore, the serum inorganic phosphate concentration should be measured after dialysis, and phosphate supplements should be added to the diet or to dialysis fluids if necessary.

Phosphate therapy, oral or intravenous, has a limited role in certain circumstances. Patients with primary hyperparathyroidism are frequently hypophosphatemic, and hypercalcemia of other causes also may be complicated by hypophosphatemia. Hypophosphatemia decreases the rate of calcium uptake into bone, increases intestinal calcium absorption, and directly and indirectly stimulates bone breakdown. These effects aggravate hypercalcemia, and correcting hypophosphatemia lowers the serum calcium concentration. The usual treatment is 1 to 1.5 g phosphorus per day for several days, given in four divided doses to minimize the chances of developing hyperphosphatemia. Such therapy has been administered for prolonged periods in selected patients. It is generally believed, but not established, that toxicity does not occur if therapy is limited to restoring serum inorganic phosphate concentrations to normal.

Raising the serum inorganic phosphate concentration above normal decreases serum calcium levels, sometimes strikingly. Intravenous phosphate is one of the most dramatically effective treatments available for severe hypercalcemia but is toxic and even dangerous (fatal hypocalcemia). For these reasons, it is used rarely and only in severely hypercalcemic patients with cardiac or renal failure. A phosphate phosphorus dose of ≥1500 mg intravenously over 6 to 8 h leads to a prompt decrease in serum calcium of as much as 1.2 to 2.5 mmol/L (5 to 10 mg/dL) in patients with initially normal serum inorganic phosphate concentrations. This therapy should be employed only in extreme emergencies. Inorganic phosphate is commercially available for oral use in liquid, powder, and capsule form and as a liquid for intravenous use. It is important to calculate doses in terms of phosphate phosphorus.

Summary The various therapies for hypercalcemia are listed in Table 341-2. The choice depends on the underlying disease, the severity of the hypercalcemia, the serum inorganic phosphate level, and the renal, hepatic, and bone marrow function. Mild hypercalcemia [≤3 mmol/L (12 mg/dL)] can usually be managed by hydration. Severe hypercalcemia [3.7 mmol/L (15 mg/dL)] requires rapid correction. Calcitonin should be given for its rapid, albeit short-lived, blockade of bone resorption, and intravenous pamidronate should be administered, although its onset of action is delayed for 1 to 2 days. In addition, for the first 24 to 48 h, aggressive sodium-calcium diuresis with intravenous saline and large doses of furosemide and ethacrynic acid following initial hydration should be initiated, but only if appropriate monitoring is available and cardiac and renal function are adequate. Otherwise, dialysis may be necessary. Intermediate degrees of hypercalcemia between 3.0 and 3.7 mmol/L (12 and 15 mg/dL) should be approached with vigorous hydration and then the most appropriate selection for the patient of the combinations used with severe hypercalcemia.

HYPOCALCEMIA

PATHOPHYSIOLOGY OF HYPOCALCEMIA: CLASSIFICATION BASED ON MECHANISM *Chronic hypocalcemia* is less common than hypercalcemia; causes include chronic renal failure, hereditary and acquired hypoparathyroidism, vitamin D deficiency, PHP, and hypomagnesemia.

Critically ill patients may have transient hypocalcemia with severe sepsis, burns, acute renal failure, and extensive transfusions with citrated blood. Acute hypocalcemia with certain medications is usually transient and may produce no symptoms. Although as many as half of patients in an intensive care setting are reported to have calcium concentrations <2.1 mmol/L (8.5 mg/dL), <10% have a reduction in ionized calcium. Patients with severe sepsis may have a decrease in ionized calcium (true hypocalcemia), but in other severely ill individuals, hypoalbuminemia is the primary cause of the reduced total calcium concentration. Alkalosis increases calcium binding to proteins, and in this setting direct measurements of ionized calcium should be made.

Medications such as protamine, heparin, and glucagon may cause transient hypocalcemia. These forms of hypocalcemia are usually not associated with tetany and resolve with improvement in the overall medical condition. The hypocalcemia after repeated transfusions of citrated blood usually resolves quickly.

Patients with *acute pancreatitis* have hypocalcemia that persists during the acute inflammation and varies in degree with the severity of the pancreatitis. The cause of hypocalcemia remains unclear. PTH values are reported to be low, normal, or elevated, and both resistance to PTH and impaired PTH secretion have been postulated. Occasionally, a chronic low total calcium and low ionized calcium concentration are detected in an elderly patient without obvious cause and with a paucity of symptoms; the pathogenesis is unclear.

Chronic hypocalcemia, however, is usually symptomatic and requires treatment. Neuromuscular and neurologic manifestations of chronic hypocalcemia include muscle spasms, carpopedal spasm, facial grimacing, and, in extreme cases, laryngeal spasm and convulsions. Respiratory arrest may occur. Increased intracranial pressure occurs in some patients with long-standing hypocalcemia, often in association with papilledema. Mental changes include irritability, depression, and psychosis. The QT interval on the electrocardiogram is prolonged, in contrast to its shortening with hypercalcemia. Arrhythmias occur, and digitalis effectiveness may be reduced. Intestinal cramps and chronic malabsorption may occur. Chvostek's or Trousseau's sign can be used to confirm latent tetany.

The classification of hypocalcemia shown in Table 341-3 is based on the premise that PTH is responsible for minute-to-minute regulation of plasma calcium concentration and, therefore, that the occurrence of hypocalcemia must mean a failure of the homeostatic action of PTH. Failure of the PTH response can occur due to hereditary or acquired parathyroid gland failure, if PTH is ineffective in target organs, or if the action of the hormone is overwhelmed by the loss of calcium from the ECF at a rate faster than it can be replaced.

PTH ABSENT Whether hereditary or acquired, hypoparathyroidism has a number of common components. Acute and chronic symptoms of untreated hypocalcemia are shared by both types of hypoparathyroidism, although the onset of hereditary hypoparathyroidism is more gradual and is often associated with other developmental defects. Basal ganglia calcification and extrapyramidal syndromes are more common and earlier in onset in hereditary hypoparathyroidism. In earlier decades, acquired hypoparathyroidism secondary to surgery in the neck was more common than hereditary hypoparathyroidism, but the frequency of surgically induced parathyroid failure has diminished as a result of improved surgical techniques that spare the parathyroid glands and increased use of nonsurgical therapy for hyperthyroidism. PHP, an example of ineffective PTH action rather than a failure of parathyroid gland production, may share several features with hypoparathyroidism, including extraosseous calcification and extrapyramidal manifestations such as choreoathetotic movements and dystonia.

Papilledema and raised intracranial pressure may occur in both hereditary or acquired hypoparathyroidism, as do chronic changes in fingernails and hair and lenticular cataracts, the latter usually reversible with treatment of hypocalcemia. Certain skin manifestations, including alopecia and candidiasis, are characteristic of hereditary hypoparathyroidism associated with autoimmune polyglandular failure (Chap. 339).

Hypocalcemia associated with hypomagnesemia is associated with both deficient PTH release and impaired responsiveness to the hormone. Patients with hypocalcemia secondary to hypomagnesemia have absent or low levels of circulating PTH, indicative of diminished hormone release despite maximum physiologic stimulus by hypocalcemia. Plasma PTH levels return to normal with correction of the hypomagnesemia. Thus hypoparathyroidism with low levels of PTH in blood can be due to hereditary gland failure, acquired gland failure, or acute but reversible gland dysfunction (hypomagnesemia).

Genetic Abnormalities and Hereditary Hypoparathyroidism Hereditary hypoparathyroidism can occur as an isolated entity without other endocrine or dermatologic manifestations (idiopathic hypoparathyroidism); more typically, it occurs in association with other abnormalities such as defective development of the thymus or failure of function of other endocrine organs such as the adrenal, thyroid, or ovary (Chap. 339). Idiopathic and hereditary hypoparathyroidism are often manifest within the first decade but may appear later.

A rare form of hypoparathyroidism associated with defective development of both the thymus and the parathyroid glands is termed the *DiGeorge syndrome* (DGS), or the *velocardiofacial syndrome* (VCFS). Congenital cardiovascular, facial, and other developmental defects are present, and most patients die in early childhood with severe infections, hypocalcemia and seizures, or cardiovascular complications. Some survive into adulthood, and milder, incomplete forms occur. Most cases are sporadic, but an autosomal dominant form involving microdeletions of chromosome 22q11.2 has been described. Smaller deletions in this region are seen in incomplete forms of the DGS syndrome, appearing in childhood or adolescence, that are manifest primarily by parathyroid gland failure.

Hypoparathyroidism can occur in association with a complex hereditary autoimmune syndrome involving failure of the adrenals, the ovaries, the immune system, and the parathyroids in association with recurrent mucocutaneous candidiasis, alopecia, vitiligo, and pernicious anemia (Chap. 339). The responsible gene on chromosome 21q22.3 has been identified. The protein product, which resembles a transcription factor, has been termed the *AIRE* (autoimmune regulator). A stop codon mutation occurs in many Finnish families with the disorder, commonly referred to as *polyglandular autoimmune type 1 deficiency*.

Gain-of-function mutations in the calcium-sensing receptor cause *autosomal dominant hypocalcemia* (ADH). These mutations induce constitutive receptor functions that lead to features that are the inverse of FHH. The activated receptor suppresses PTH, leading to hypocalcemia; receptor activation in the kidney results in excessive renal calcium excretion. Recognition of the syndrome is important because efforts to treat the hypocalcemia of these patients with vitamin D analogues and increased oral calcium exacerbate the already excessive urinary calcium secretion (several grams or more per 24 h), leading to irreversible renal damage from stones and ectopic calcification.

Table 341-3 Functional Classification of Hypocalcemia (Excluding Neonatal Conditions)

PTH ABSENT	
Hereditary hypoparathyroidism Acquired hypoparathyroidism	Hypomagnesemia
PTH INEFFECTIVE	
Chronic renal failure Active vitamin D lacking ↓ Dietary intake or sunlight Defective metabolism: Anticonvulsant therapy Vitamin D–dependent rickets type I	Active vitamin D ineffective Intestinal malabsorption Vitamin D–dependent rickets type II Pseudohypoparathyroidism
PTH OVERWHELMED	
Severe, acute hyperphosphatemia Tumor lysis Acute renal failure Rhabdomyolysis	Osteitis fibrosa after parathyroidectomy

NOTE: PTH, parathyroid hormone.

Hypoparathyroidism is seen in two disorders associated with mitochondrial dysfunction and myopathy, one termed the *Kearns-Sayre syndrome* (KSS), with ophthalmaplegia and pigmentary retinopathy, and the other termed the *MELAS syndrome*, *m*itochondrial *e*ncephalopathy, *l*actic *a*cidosis, and *s*troke-like episodes. Mutations or deletions in mitochondrial genes have been identified (Chap. 67).

The two other rare forms of hypoparathyroidism with other multisystem developmental abnormalities follow either an autosomal dominant pattern, with deafness and/or renal dysplasia, or an autosomal recessive pattern, with growth retardation and dysmorphic features.

Hereditary hypoparathyroidism occurs also as an isolated entity without any other defects. The pattern of inheritance varies and includes autosomal dominant, autosomal recessive, and X-linked inheritance patterns. In one family in which the disorder is transmitted as an autosomal dominant trait, a structural abnormality in the PTH gene has been identified. A defect in the signal sequence needed for processing of the hormone impairs PTH secretion. In another kindred with autosomal recessive inheritance, the mutant allele in the first intron of the PTH gene causes a splicing defect in mRNA production. An X-linked recessive form of hypoparathyroidism has been described in males from two kindreds that are probably related. The locus of the defect has been located to chromosome Xq26-q27.

Acquired Hypoparathyroidism *Acquired chronic hypoparathyroidism* is usually the result of inadvertent surgical removal of all the parathyroid glands; in some instances, not all the tissue is removed, but the remainder undergoes vascular supply compromise secondary to fibrotic changes in the neck after surgery. In the past, the most frequent cause of acquired hypoparathyroidism was surgery for hyperthyroidism. Hypoparathyroidism now usually occurs after surgery for hyperparathyroidism when the surgeon, facing the dilemma of removing too little tissue and thus not curing the hyperparathyroidism, removes too much. Parathyroid function may not be totally absent in all patients with postoperative hypoparathyroidism.

Even rarer causes of acquired chronic hypoparathyroidism include radiation-induced damage subsequent to radioiodine therapy of hyperthyroidism and glandular damage in patients with hemochromatosis or hemosiderosis after repeated blood transfusions. Infection may involve one or more of the parathyroids but usually does not cause hypoparathyroidism because all four glands are rarely involved.

Transient hypoparathyroidism is frequent following surgery for hyperparathyroidism. After a variable period of hypoparathyroidism, normal parathyroid function may return due to hyperplasia or recovery of remaining tissue. Occasionally, recovery occurs months after surgery.

℞ **TREATMENT** Treatment of acquired and hereditary hypoparathyroidism involves replacement with vitamin D or $1,25(OH)_2D_3$ (calcitriol) combined with a high oral calcium intake. In most patients, blood calcium and phosphate levels are satisfactorily regulated, but some patients show resistance and a brittleness with a tendency to alternate between hypocalcemia and an overshoot hypercalcemia. For many patients, vitamin D in doses of 1 to 3 mg/d (40,000 to 120,000 U/d) combined with ≥1 g elemental calcium is satisfactory. The wide dosage range reflects the variation encountered from patient to patient; precise regulation of each patient is required. Compared to typical daily requirements in euparathyroid patients of 200 U/d, the high dose of vitamin D reflects the reduced conversion of vitamin D to $1,25(OH)_2D$. Many physicians now use 0.5 to 1.0 μg of calcitriol in management of such patients, especially if they are difficult to control. When vitamin D (because of storage in fat) is withdrawn, weeks are required for the disappearance of the biologic effects, compared with a few days for calcitriol, which has a rapid turnover.

Oral calcium and vitamin D restore the overall calcium-phosphate balance but do not reverse the lowered urinary calcium reabsorption typical of hypoparathyroidism. Therefore, care must be taken to avoid excessive urinary calcium excretion after vitamin D and calcium replacement therapy; otherwise, kidney stones can develop. Thiazide diuretics lower urine calcium by as much as 100 mg/d in hypoparathyroid patients on vitamin D, provided they are maintained on a low-sodium diet. Use of thiazides seems to be of benefit in mitigating hypercalciuria and easing the daily management of these patients.

Hypomagnesemia Severe hypomagnesemia is associated with hypocalcemia (Chap. 340). Restoration of the total-body magnesium deficit leads to rapid reversal of hypocalcemia. There are at least two causes of the hypocalcemia—impaired PTH secretion and reduced responsiveness to PTH.

Hypomagnesemia is generally classified as primary or secondary; primary hypomagnesemia is due to hereditary defects in intestinal absorption or renal reabsorption of magnesium. Secondary hypomagnesemia, a more common condition, occurs on a nutritional basis or as a result of acquired intestinal or renal disorders. The most common causes of the secondary disorder are chronic alcoholism with poor nutritional intake, intestinal malabsorption syndromes, and parenteral nutrition when magnesium replacement is omitted.

The effects of magnesium on PTH secretion are similar to those of calcium; hypermagnesemia suppresses and hypomagnesemia stimulates PTH secretion. The effects of magnesium on PTH secretion are normally of little significance, however, because the calcium effects dominate. Greater change in magnesium than in calcium is needed to influence hormone secretion. Nonetheless, hypomagnesemia might be expected to increase hormone secretion. It is therefore surprising to find that severe hypomagnesemia is associated with blunted secretion of PTH. The explanation for the paradox is that severe, chronic hypomagnesemia leads to intracellular magnesium deficiency, which interferes with secretion and peripheral responses to PTH. The mechanism of the cellular abnormalities caused by hypomagnesemia is unknown, although effects on adenylate cyclase (for which magnesium is a cofactor) have been proposed.

Serum magnesium must usually fall below 0.4 mmol/L (1.0 mg/dL) to cause hypocalcemia. PTH levels are undetectable or inappropriately low despite the stimulus of severe hypocalcemia, and acute repletion of magnesium leads to a rapid increase in PTH level. Serum phosphate levels are often not elevated, in contrast to the situation with acquired or idiopathic hypoparathyroidism, probably because phosphate deficiency is a frequent accompaniment of hypomagnesemia.

Diminished peripheral responsiveness to PTH also occurs in some patients, as documented by subnormal response in urinary phosphorus and urinary cyclic AMP excretion after administration of exogenous PTH to patients who are hypocalcemic and hypomagnesemic. Both blunted PTH secretion and lack of renal response to administered PTH can occur in the same patient. When acute magnesium repletion is undertaken, the restoration of PTH levels to normal or supranormal may precede restoration of normal serum calcium by several days.

℞ **TREATMENT** Repletion of magnesium cures the condition, and attention must be given to restoring the intracellular deficiency, which may be considerable. Repletion should be parenteral. After intravenous magnesium administration, serum magnesium may return transiently to the normal range, but unless replacement therapy is adequate serum magnesium will again fall. If renal function is normal, urinary magnesium excretion is a useful indicator of magnesium repletion, as magnesium is retained by the kidney until the deficiency is corrected. Intracellular deficits can be ≥50 mmol. Parenteral administration of 10 to 14 mmol magnesium usually reverses the signs of magnesium deficiency, but greater amounts may occasionally be required if the deficit is large. If the cause of the hypomagnesemia is renal magnesium wasting, magnesium may have to be given chronically to prevent recurrence (Chap. 340).

PTH INEFFECTIVE PTH is ineffective when the hormone receptor–guanyl nucleotide–binding protein complex is defective (PHP, discussed below), when PTH action to promote calcium absorption from the diet is impaired because of vitamin D deficiency or because vitamin D is ineffective (receptor or synthesis defects), or in chronic renal failure in which the calcium-elevating action of PTH is impaired.

Typically, hypophosphatemia is more severe than hypocalcemia in vitamin D deficiency states because of the increased secretion of PTH, which, although only partly effective in elevating blood calcium, is capable of promoting phosphaturia.

PHP, on the other hand, has a pathophysiology different from the other disorders of ineffective PTH action. PHP resembles hypoparathyroidism (in which PTH synthesis is deficient) and is manifested by hypocalcemia and hyperphosphatemia. The cause of the disorder is defective hormone activation of guanyl nucleotide–binding proteins, resulting in failure of PTH to increase intracellular cyclic AMP (see below).

Chronic Renal Failure Improved medical management of chronic renal failure and/or a more indolent course of the renal disease now allow many patients to survive long enough to develop features of renal osteodystrophy. Phosphate retention and impaired production of $1,25(OH)_2D$ are the principal factors that cause calcium deficiency, secondary hyperparathyroidism, and bone disease. The uremic state also causes impairment of intestinal absorption by mechanisms other than defects in vitamin D metabolism. Nonetheless, treatment with supraphysiologic amounts of vitamin D or calcitriol corrects the impaired calcium absorption.

Hyperphosphatemia in renal failure lowers blood calcium levels by several mechanisms, including extraosseous deposition of calcium and phosphate, impairment of the bone-resorbing action of PTH, and reduction in $1,25(OH)_2D$ production by remaining renal tissue. Low levels of $1,25(OH)_2D$ due to hyperphosphatemia and destruction of renal tissue and are critical in the development of hypocalcemia.

℞ TREATMENT Therapy of chronic renal failure (Chap. 270) involves appropriate management of patients prior to dialysis and adjustment of regimens once dialysis is initiated. Attention should be paid to restriction of phosphate in the diet; use of calcium-containing salts as phosphate-binding antacids is preferable, rather than aluminum, to avoid the problem of aluminum intoxication; provision of an adequate calcium intake by mouth, usually 1 to 2 g/d; and supplementation with 0.25 to 1.0 μg/d calcitriol. Each patient must be monitored closely. The aim of therapy is to restore normal calcium balance to prevent osteomalacia and secondary hyperparathyroidism. Reduction of hyperphosphatemia and restoration of normal intestinal calcium absorption by calcitriol can improve blood calcium levels and reduce the manifestations of secondary hyperparathyroidism. Since adynamic bone disease can occur in association with low PTH levels, it is important to avoid excessive suppression of the parathyroid glands while recognizing the beneficial effects of controlling the secondary hyperparathyroidism. These patients should probably be closely monitored with PTH assays that detect only the full-length PTH 1–84 to avoid interference by biologically inactive amino-terminally truncated PTH.

Vitamin D Deficiency due to Inadequate Diet and/or Sunlight Vitamin D deficiency due to inadequate intake of dairy products enriched with vitamin D, lack of vitamin supplementation, and reduced sunlight exposure in the elderly, particularly during winter in northern latitudes, is more common in the United States than previously recognized. Biopsies of bone in elderly patients with hip fracture (documenting osteomalacia) and abnormal levels of vitamin D metabolites, PTH, calcium, and phosphate indicate that vitamin D deficiency may occur in as many as 25% of elderly patients, particularly in areas where there is little ambient sunlight. Concentrations of 25(OH)D are low or low-normal in these patients. Quantitative histomorphometry of bone biopsy specimens reveals widened osteoid seams consistent with osteomalacia. PTH hypersecretion compensates for the tendency for the blood calcium to fall but also induces renal phosphate wasting and results in osteomalacia.

Treatment involves adequate replacement with vitamin D and cal-

cium until the deficiencies are corrected. Severe hypocalcemia rarely occurs in moderately severe vitamin D deficiency of the elderly, but vitamin D deficiency must be considered in the differential diagnosis of mild hypocalcemia.

Defective Vitamin D Metabolism • ***Anticonvulsant therapy*** Anticonvulsant therapy with any of several agents induces acquired vitamin D deficiency by increasing the conversion of vitamin D to inactive compounds. The more marginal the vitamin D intake in the diet, the more likely that anticonvulsant therapy will lead to abnormal mineral and bone metabolism (Chap. 340).

Although $1,25(OH)_2D$ levels are lower in patients treated with chronic anticonvulsants than in the normal population, there is a great deal of variation. The greater prevalence of the disorder in some European populations and in the mentally retarded may reflect the lower vitamin D intake of those groups. Restoration of bone mineral mass and reversal of hypocalcemia can be accomplished with vitamin D replacement plus oral calcium. Administration of 50,000 units of vitamin D monthly may be preventive if anticonvulsant therapy needs to be given chronically.

Vitamin D–dependent rickets type I Rickets can be due to *resistance to the action* of vitamin D as well as to vitamin D deficiency. Vitamin D–dependent rickets type I, previously termed *pseudo-vitamin D–resistant rickets*, differs from true vitamin D–resistant rickets (vitamin D-dependent rickets type II, see below) in that it is less severe and the biochemical and radiographic abnormalities can be reversed with appropriate doses of the vitamin or the active metabolite, $1,25(OH)_2D_3$.

Clinical features include hypocalcemia, often with tetany or convulsions, hypophosphatemia, secondary hyperparathyroidism, and osteomalacia, often associated with skeletal deformities and increased alkaline phosphatase. Physiologic amounts of calcitriol cure the disease (Chap. 340). This finding fits with the pathophysiology as the disorder, which is autosomal recessive, is now known to be caused by a series of mutations in the gene for the 25(OH)D-1α-hydroxylase. Over 20 different mutations have been identified. All patients have both alleles inactivated, but often the genetic pattern is that of a compound heterozygote. Response to high doses of vitamin D or calcifediol, as noted in prior years, is probably due to direct effects of 25(OH)D at high levels. Treatment begins with 1 to 2 μg/d calcitriol, but maintenance is satisfactory with physiologic doses of calcitriol (0.5 to 1.0 μg/d). Careful adjustment of calcitriol dose is required, particularly during growth periods.

Vitamin D Ineffective • ***Intestinal malabsorption*** Mild hypocalcemia, secondary hyperparathyroidism, severe hypophosphatemia, and a variety of nutritional deficiencies occur with gastrointestinal diseases. Hepatocellular dysfunction can lead to reduction in 25(OH)D levels, as in portal or biliary cirrhosis of the liver, and malabsorption of vitamin D and its metabolites, including $1,25(OH)_2D$, may occur in a variety of bowel diseases, hereditary or acquired. Hypocalcemia itself can lead to steatorrhea, due to deficient production of pancreatic enzymes and bile salts. Depending on the disorder, vitamin D or its metabolites can be given parenterally, guaranteeing adequate blood levels of active metabolites.

Vitamin D–dependent rickets type II Vitamin D–dependent rickets type II results from end-organ resistance to the active metabolite $1,25(OH)_2D_3$. The clinical features resemble those of the type I disorder and include hypocalcemia, hypophosphatemia, secondary hyperparathyroidism, and rickets. A clear distinction is partial or total alopecia in type II. Plasma levels of $1,25(OH)_2D$ are at least three times normal, in keeping with the refractoriness of the end organs. Some patients respond to very high doses of vitamin D or vitamin D metabolites (e.g., 17 to 20 μg/d calcitriol). Earlier suggestions that there were both receptor and postreceptor defects are incorrect. All of the genetically characterized phenotypes have mutations in the gene for the vitamin D receptor. Nineteen mutations have been identified that affect different regions of the receptor primarily in the DNA binding

Table 341-4 Classification of Pseudohypoparathyroidism (PHP) and Pseudopseudohypoparathyroidism (PPHP)

Type	Hypocalcemia, Hyperphosphatemia	Response of Urinary cAMP to PTH	Serum PTH	$G_{s\alpha}$ Subunit Deficiency	AHO	Resistance to Hormones in Addition to PTH
PHP-Ia	Yes	↓	↑	Yes	Yes	Yes
PHP-Ib	Yes	↓	↑	No	No	No
PHP-II	Yes	Normal	↑	No	No	No
PPHP	No	Normal	Normal	Yes	Yes	±

NOTE: ↓, decreased; ↑, increased; AHO, Albright's hereditary osteodystrophy; PTH, parathyroid hormone.

domain (with normal ligand binding: these were the so-called postreceptor defects detected by earlier indirect methods) or in the ligand-binding domain (classified previously as receptor negative).

Pseudohypoparathyroidism PHP is a hereditary disorder characterized by symptoms and signs of hypoparathyroidism, typically in association with distinctive skeletal and developmental defects. The hypoparathyroidism is due to a deficient end-organ response to PTH. Hyperplasia of the parathyroids, a response to hormone resistance, causes elevation of PTH levels. Studies, both clinical and basic, have clarified some aspects of this syndrome, including the variable clinical spectrum, the pathophysiology, the genetic defects, and the inheritance.

A working classification of the various forms of PHP is given in Table 341-4. The classification scheme is based on the signs of ineffective PTH action (low calcium and high phosphate), urinary cyclic AMP response to exogenous PTH, the presence or absence of *Albright's hereditary osteodystrophy* (AHO), and assays of the concentration of the $G_s\alpha$ subunit of the adenylate cyclase enzyme. Using these criteria, there are four types: PHP type I, subdivided into a and b categories; PHP-II; and pseudopseudohypoparathyroidism (PPHP).

PHP-Ia and PHP-Ib Individuals with PHP-I, the most common of the disorders, show a deficient urinary cyclic AMP response to administration of exogenous PTH. Patients with PHP-I are divided into type a, who have reduced amounts of $G_s\alpha$ in vitro assays with erythrocytes, and type b, with normal amounts of $G_s\alpha$ in erythrocytes. There is a third type (PHP-Ic, reported in a few patients) that differs from PHP-Ia only in having normal erythroycte levels of $G_s\alpha$ despite having AHO, hypocalcemia, and decreased urinary cyclic AMP responses to PTH (presumably with a post-$G_s\alpha$ defect in adenyl cyclase stimulation).

Most patients show characteristic features of AHO, consisting of short stature, round face, skeletal anomalies (brachydactyly), and heterotopic calcification. Patients have low calcium and high phosphate levels, as with true hypoparathyroidism. PTH levels, however, are elevated, reflecting resistance to hormone action.

Amorphous deposits of calcium and phosphate are found in the basal ganglia in about half of patients. The defects in metacarpal and metatarsal bones are sometimes accompanied by short phalanges as well, possibly reflecting premature closing of the epiphyses. The typical findings are short fourth and fifth metacarpals and metatarsals. The defects are usually bilateral. Exostoses and radius curvus are frequent. Impairments in olfaction and taste and unusual dermatoglyphic abnormalities have been reported.

PPHP The initial view that the defect responsible for PHP-Ia was simply the deficiency of $G_s\alpha$ subunits was temporarily confounded by the subsequent discovery that the same 50% reduction in $G_s\alpha$ subunits was seen in patients with PPHP, who have typical features of the hereditary osteodystrophy syndrome despite normal serum calcium levels and normal response of urinary cyclic AMP to exogenous PTH.

Multiple defects have now been identified in the *GNAS-1* gene in PHP-Ia and PPHP patients. This gene, which is located on chromosome 20q13, encodes the stimulatory G protein subunit $G_s\alpha$, among other products (see below). Mutations include abnormalities in splice junctions associated with deficient mRNA production and point mutations that result in a protein with defective function as well as the 50% reduction in $G_s\alpha$ levels in erythrocytes.

Detailed analyses of disease transmission in affected kindreds have clarified many features of PHP-Ia, PPHP, and PHP-Ib (Fig. 341-9). The former two entities, traced through multiple kindreds, have an inheritance pattern consistent with gene imprinting—only females, not males, can transmit the full disease with hypocalcemia—and PHP and PPHP do not coexist in the same generation. The phenomenon of gene imprinting involves selective inactivation of either the maternal or the paternal allele (Chap. 65). In the case of the $G_s\alpha$ gene, it is paternally imprinted (silenced) so that the disease PHP-Ia is never inherited from the father carrying the defective allele but only from the mother. On the other hand, the defective allele is not imprinted or silenced in all tissues. It seems possible, therefore, that the AHO phenotype recognized in PPHP as well as PHP-Ia reflects haplotype insufficiency. In the renal cortex, however, it is postulated that only the maternal allele is normally active, such that lack of activity from a defective paternal allele is not of consequence. This explains the occurrence in PHP-Ia of hypocalcemia, hyperphosphatemia, and other stigmata such as variable resistance to other hormones (if similar tissue-specific imprinting occurs in other organs). Strong evidence favoring this overall hypothesis comes from gene knockout studies in the mouse (ablating exon 2 of the gene). Mice inheriting the mutant allele from the female had undetectable $G_s\alpha$ protein in renal cortex and were hypocalcemic and resistant to renal actions of PTH. Offspring inheriting the mutant allele from the male showed no evidence of PTH resistance or hypercalcemia.

The complex mechanisms that control the GNAS-1 gene also con-

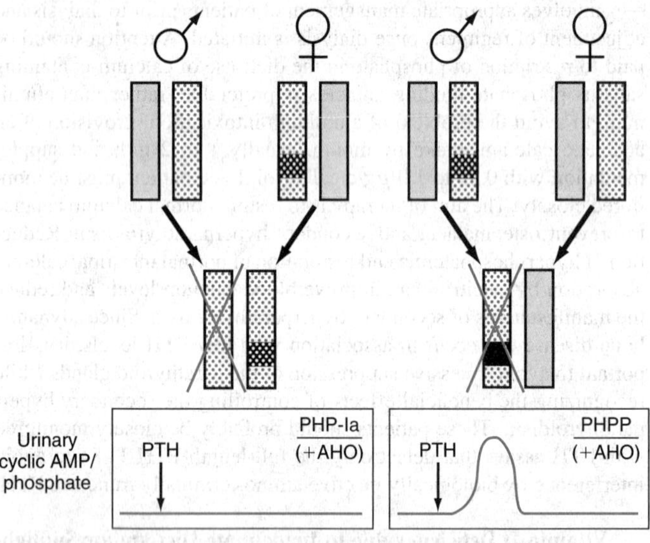

FIGURE 341-9 Paternal imprinting of renal parathyroid hormone (PTH) resistance (*GNAS-1* gene for $G_s\alpha$ subunit) in pseudohypoparathyroidism (PHP). An impaired excretion of urinary cyclic AMP and phosphate is observed in patients with PHP. In the renal cortex, there is selective silencing of the paternal $G_s\alpha$ gene mRNA. The disease becomes manifest only in patients who inherit the defective gene from an obligate female carrier (*left*). If the genetic defect is inherited from an obligate male gene carrier, there is no biochemical abnormality; administration of PTH causes an appropriate increase in the urinary cyclic AMP and phosphate concentration [pseudo-PHP (PPHP); *right*]. Both patterns of inheritance lead to Albright's hereditary osteodystrophy (AHO), perhaps because of haplotype insufficiency—i.e., both copies of $G_s\alpha$ must be active in the fetus for normal bone development. If an abnormal allele is inherited from a father with AHO (PPHP), PTH resistance is not transmitted to offspring, but they have AHO (haplotype insufficiency); if the abnormal allele comes from the mother (with the normal paternal allele silenced in the kidney cortex), the full disease spectrum results.

tribute to challenges involved in unraveling the pathogenesis of these disorders. Alternative splicing patterns produce three different transcripts that encode distinct proteins. In addition to $G_s\alpha$, this gene encodes a second protein product with a unique NH_2-terminus (the XL exon); $XL_\alpha s$ includes exons 2–13. It is unknown whether this protein can function as a stimulatory G protein, but the mRNA encoding it is expressed in numerous endocrine tissues and is transcribed from only the paternal allele. A third transcript is transcribed from only the maternal allele and encodes the protein product, NESP55, which contains no homology with $XL_\alpha s$ or $G_s\alpha$.

PHP-Ib, lacking the AHO phenotype, shares with PHP-Ia the resistance to PTH action and a blunted urinary cyclic AMP response to administered PTH, a standard test for hormone resistance (Table 341-4). PHP-Ib patients, however, show normal levels of $G_s\alpha$ in erythrocytes. Bone responsiveness may be excessive rather than blunted in PHP-Ib compared to PHP-Ia patients, based on case reports that have emphasized an osteitis fibrosa–like pattern in some PHP patients who lack the AHO phenotype. The inheritance patterns in PHP-Ib kindreds are clearly consistent with paternal imprinting and lack male transmission of symptomatic disease; gene cloning studies have narrowed the responsible region to chromosome 20, close to—if not within—the *GNAS-1* gene locus. Elucidation of the responsible genetic and pathogenetic mechanisms in this disorder may further illuminate the function of the complex *GNAS-1* gene and the role of its products in hormonal signaling.

PHP-II refers to patients with hypocalcemia and hyperphosphatemia who have a normal urinary cyclic AMP response to PTH. These patients are assumed to have a defect in the response to PTH at a locus distal to cyclic AMP production, although at least some patients may instead have occult vitamin D deficiency.

The diagnosis of these hormone-resistant states can usually be made without difficulty when there is a positive family history for developmental defects and/or the presence of developmental anomalies, including brachydactyly, in association with the signs and symptoms of hypoparathyroidism. In all categories—PHP-Ia, -Ib, and -II—serum PTH levels are elevated, particularly when patients are hypocalcemic. However, patients with PHP-Ib or PHP-II do not have phenotypic abnormalities, only hypocalcemia with high PTH levels, confirming hormone resistance. In PHP-Ib, the response of urinary cyclic AMP to the administration of exogenous PTH is blunted. Levels of $G_s\alpha$ subunits in erythrocyte membranes are, however, normal in those with PHP-Ib. The diagnosis of PHP-II is more complex, in that cyclic AMP responses in urine are, by definition, normal. Since vitamin D deficiency itself can dissociate phosphaturic and urinary cyclic AMP responses to exogenous PTH, vitamin D deficiency must be excluded before the diagnosis of PHP-II can be entertained.

℞ TREATMENT Treatment of PHP is similar to that of hypoparathyroidism, except that the doses of vitamin D and calcium are usually lower than those required in true hypoparathyroidism, presumably because the defect in PHP is only partial because of imprinting in specific tissues (renal cortex vs. renal medulla). Variability in response makes it necessary to establish the optimal regimen for each patient, based on maintaining the appropriate blood calcium level and urinary calcium excretion.

PTH Overwhelmed Occasionally, loss of calcium from the ECF is so severe that PTH cannot compensate. Such situations include acute pancreatitis and severe, acute hyperphosphatemia, often in association with renal failure, conditions in which there is rapid efflux of calcium from extracellular fluid. Severe hypocalcemia can occur quickly; PTH rises in response to hypocalcemia but does not return blood calcium to normal.

Severe, Acute Hyperphosphatemia Severe hyperphosphatemia is associated with extensive tissue damage or cell destruction (Chap. 340). The combination of increased release of phosphate from muscle and impaired ability to excrete phosphorus because of renal failure causes moderate to severe hyperphosphatemia, the latter causing calcium loss from the blood and mild to moderate hypocalcemia. Hypocalcemia is usually reversed with tissue repair and restoration of renal function as phosphorus and creatinine values return to normal. There may even be a mild hypercalcemic period in the oliguric phase of renal function recovery. This sequence, severe hypocalcemia followed by mild hypercalcemia, reflects widespread deposition of calcium in muscle and subsequent redistribution of some of the calcium to the ECF after return of phosphate levels to normal.

Other causes of hyperphosphatemia include hypothermia, massive hepatic failure, and hematologic malignancies, either because of high cell turnover of malignancy or because of cell destruction by chemotherapy.

℞ TREATMENT Treatment is directed toward lowering of blood phosphate by the administration of phosphate-binding antacids or dialysis, often needed for the management of renal failure. Although calcium replacement may be necessary if hypocalcemia is severe and symptomatic, calcium administration during the hyperphosphatemic period tends to increase extraosseous calcium deposition and aggravate tissue damage. The levels of $1,25(OH)_2D$ may be low during the hyperphosphatemic phase and return to normal during the oliguric phase of recovery.

Osteitis Fibrosis after Parathyroidectomy Severe hypocalcemia after parathyroid surgery is less common now that osteitis fibrosa cystica is an infrequent manifestation of hyperparathyroidism. When osteitis fibrosa cystica is severe, however, bone mineral deficits can be large. After parathyroidectomy, hypocalcemia can persist for days if calcium replacement is inadequate. Treatment may require parenteral administration of calcium; addition of calcitriol and oral calcium supplementation is sometimes needed for weeks to a month or two until bone defects are filled (which, of course, is of therapeutic benefit in the skeleton), making it possible to discontinue parenteral calcium and/or reduce the amount.

DIFFERENTIAL DIAGNOSIS OF HYPOCALCEMIA Care must be taken to ensure that true hypocalcemia is present; in addition, acute transient hypocalcemia can be a manifestation of a variety of severe, acute illnesses, as discussed above. *Chronic hypocalcemia*, however, can usually be ascribed to a few disorders associated with absent or ineffective PTH. Important clinical criteria include the duration of the illness, signs or symptoms of associated disorders, and the presence of features that suggest a hereditary abnormality. A nutritional history can be helpful in recognizing a low intake of vitamin D and calcium in the elderly, and a history of excessive alcohol intake may suggest magnesium deficiency.

Hypoparathyroidism and PHP are typically lifelong illnesses, usually (but not always) appearing by adolescence; hence a recent onset of hypocalcemia in an adult is more likely due to nutritional deficiencies, renal failure, or intestinal disorders that result in deficient or ineffective vitamin D. Neck surgery, even long past, however, can be associated with a delayed onset of postoperative hypoparathyroidism. A history of seizure disorder raises the issue of anticonvulsive medication. Developmental defects, particularly in childhood and adolescence, may point to the diagnosis of PHP. Rickets and a variety of neuromuscular syndromes and deformities may indicate ineffective vitamin D action, either due to defects in vitamin D metabolism or to vitamin D deficiency.

A pattern of *low calcium with high phosphorus* in the absence of renal failure or massive tissue destruction almost invariably means hypoparathyroidism or PHP. A *low calcium and low phosphorus* points to absent or ineffective vitamin D, thereby impairing the action of PTH on calcium metabolism (but not phosphate clearance). The relative ineffectiveness of PTH in vitamin D deficiency, anticonvulsant therapy, gastrointestinal disorders, and hereditary defects in vitamin D metabolism leads to secondary hyperparathyroidism as a compensation. The relatively unopposed action of the excess PTH on renal tubule phosphate transport, which is less dependent on vitamin D than calcium transport, accounts for renal phosphate wasting and hypophosphatemia.

Exceptions to these patterns may occur. Most forms of hypomagnesemia are due to long-standing nutritional deficiency as seen in chronic alcoholics. Despite the fact that the hypocalcemia is principally due to an acute absence of PTH, phosphate levels are usually low, rather than elevated as in hypoparathyroidism. Chronic renal failure is often associated with hypocalcemia and hyperphosphatemia, despite secondary hyperparathyroidism.

Diagnosis is usually established by application of the PTH immunoassay, tests for vitamin D metabolites, and measurements of the urinary cyclic AMP response to exogenous PTH. In hereditary and acquired hypoparathyroidism and in severe hypomagnesemia, PTH is either undetectable or in the normal range. This finding in a hypocalcemic patient is supportive of hypoparathyroidism, as distinct from ineffective PTH action, in which even mild hypocalcemia is associated with elevated PTH levels. Hence a failure to detect elevated PTH levels establishes the diagnosis of hypoparathyroidism; elevated levels suggest the presence of secondary hyperparathyroidism, as found in many of the situations in which the hormone is ineffective due to associated abnormalities in vitamin D action. Assays for 25(OH)D and $1,25(OH)_2D$ can be helpful. Low or low normal 25(OH)D indicates vitamin D deficiency due to lack of sunlight, inadequate vitamin D intake, or intestinal malabsorption. A low level of $1,25(OH)_2D$ in the presence of elevated concentrations of PTH suggests ineffective PTH action in disorders such as chronic renal failure, severe vitamin D deficiency, vitamin D–dependent rickets type I, and PHP. Recognition that mild hypocalcemia, rickets, and hypophosphatemia are due to anticonvulsant therapy is made by history.

℞ TREATMENT **Hypocalcemic States** The management of hypoparathyroidism, PHP, chronic renal failure, and hereditary defects in vitamin D metabolism involves the use of vitamin D or vitamin D metabolites and calcium supplementation. Vitamin D itself is the least expensive form of vitamin D replacement and is frequently used in the management of uncomplicated hypoparathyroidism and some disorders associated with ineffective vitamin D action. When vitamin D is used prophylactically, as in the elderly or in those with chronic anticonvulsant therapy, there is a wider margin of safety than with the more potent metabolites. However, most of the conditions in which vitamin D is administered chronically for hypocalcemia require amounts 50 to 100 times the daily replacement dose because the formation of $1,25(OH)_2D$ is deficient. In such situations, vitamin D is no safer than the active metabolite because intoxication can occur with high-dose therapy (because of storage in fat). Calcitriol is more rapid in onset of action and also has a short biologic half-life.

Vitamin D (5 μg/d) or calcifediol and lower doses of calcitriol (0.25 to 1.0 μg/d) are required to prevent rickets in normal individuals. In contrast, 1 to 3 mg (1000 to 3000 μg of vitamin D_2 or D_3 is typically required in hypoparathyroidism; doses of calcifediol are also high (several hundred micrograms per day). The dose of calcitriol is unchanged in hypoparathyroidism, since the defect is in hydroxylation by the 25(OH)D-1α-hydroxylase.

Patients with hypoparathyroidism should be given 2 to 3 g elemental calcium by mouth each day. The two agents, vitamin D or calcitriol and oral calcium, can be varied independently. If hypocalcemia alternates with episodes of hypercalcemia in more brittle patients with hypoparathyroidism, administration of calcitriol and use of thiazides, as discussed above, may make management easier.

BIBLIOGRAPHY

ARNOLD A et al: Monoclonality of parathyroid tumors in chronic renal failure and in primary parathyroid hyperplasia. J Clin Invest 95:2047, 1995

BASTEPE M, JÜPPNER H: Pseudohypoparathyroidism: New insights into an old disease. Endocrinol Metab Clin North Am, in press, 2000

BODY JJ et al: A dose-finding study of zoledronate in hypercalcemic cancer patients. J Bone Miner Res 14:1557, 1999

CHEN H et al: Outpatient minimally invasive parathyroidectomy: A combination of sestamibi-SPECT localization, cervical block anesthesia, and intraoperative parathyroid hormone assay. Surgery 126:1021, 1999

CHOU Y-H W et al: Mutations in the human Ca^{2+}-sensing-receptor gene that cause hypocalciuric hypercalcemia. Am J Hum Genet 56:1075, 1995

CRYNS VL et al: Frequent loss of chromosome arm 1p DNA in parathyroid adenomas. Genes Chromosomes Cancer 13:9, 1995

HABENER J et al: Hyperparathyroidism, in *Endocrinology*, 4th ed, L DeGroot et al (eds). Philadelphia, Saunders, 2000

HERBERT SC et al: Role of the Ca^{2+}-sensing receptor in divalent mineral ion homeostasis. J Exp Biol 200:295, 1997

JÜPPNER H et al: The gene responsible for pseudohypoparathyroidism type Ib is paternally imprinted and maps in four unrelated kindreds to chromosome 20q13.3 Proc Natl Acad Sci USA 95:11798, 1998

MALLETTE LE, EICHORN E: Effects of lithium carbonate on human calcium metabolism. Arch Intern Med 146:770, 1986

NEMETH EF et al: Calcimimetics with potent and selective activity on the parathyroid calcium receptor. Proc Natl Acad Sci USA 95:4040, 1998

NUSSBAUM SR, POTTS JT JR: Medical management of hyperparathyroidism and hypercalcemia, in *Endocrinology*, 4th ed, L DeGroot et al (eds). Philadelphia, Saunders, 2000

PIERCE SH et al: A familial syndrome of hypocalcemia with hypercalciuria due to mutations in the calcium-sensing receptor (see comments). N Engl J Med 335:1115, 1996

POLLAK MR et al: Familial hypocalciuric hypercalcemia and neonatal severe hyperparathyroidism. Effects of mutant gene dosage on phenotype. J Clin Invest 93:1108, 1994

POTTS JT JR et al (eds): Proceedings of the NIH Consensus Development Conference on Diagnosis and Management of Asymptomatic Primary Hyperparathyroidism. J Bone Miner Res 6 (Suppl 2):S1, 1991

——— et al: Parathyroid hormone and parathyroid hormone–related peptide in calcium homeostasis, bone metabolism, and bone development: The proteins, their genes, and receptors, in *Metabolic Bone Disease*, LV Avioli, SM Krane (eds.). New York, Academic, 1997, p 51

SALUSKY IB et al: The renal osteodystrophies, in *Endocrinology*, 4th ed, L DeGroot et al (eds). Philadelphia, Saunders, 2000

SCHWINDINGER WF et al: Targeted disruption of *Gnas* in embryonic stem cells. Endocrinology 138:4058, 1997

SEGRE GV, POTTS JT JR: Differential diagnosis of hypercalcemia, in *Endocrinology*, 4th ed., L DeGroot et al (eds). Philadelphia, Saunders, 2000

SILVERBERG SJ et al: Longitudinal measurements of bone density and biochemical indices in untreated primary hyperparathyroidism. J Clin Endocrinol Metab 80:723, 1995

——— et al: Primary hyperparathyroidism: 10-year course with or without parathyroid surgery. N Engl J Med 341:1249, 1999

STEWART AF et al: Malignancy-associated hypercalcemia, in *Endocrinology*, 4th ed, L DeGroot et al (eds). Philadelphia, Saunders, 2000

THAKKER RV: Molecular genetics of parathyroid disease. Curr Opin Endocrinol Diab 3: 521, 1996

WERMERS RA et al: Survival after the diagnosis of hyperparathyroidism. Am J Med 104: 115, 1998

YU S et al: Variable and tissue-specific hormone resistance in heterotrimeric Gs protein α-subunit ($G_s\alpha$) knockout mice is due to tissue-specific imprinting of the $G_s\alpha$ gene. Proc Natl Acad Sci USA 95:8715, 1998

ZHANG P et al: A homozygous inactivating mutation in the parathyroid hormone/parathyroid hormone–related peptide receptor causing Blomstrand chondrodysplasia. J Clin Endocrinol Metab 83:3365, 1998

342

Robert Lindsay, Felicia Cosman

OSTEOPOROSIS

Osteoporosis, characterized by decreased bone strength, is prevalent among postmenopausal women but also occurs in men and women with underlying conditions or major risk factors associated with bone demineralization. Its chief clinical manifestations are vertebral and hip fractures. Osteoporosis affects >10 million individuals in the United States, but only 10 to 20% are diagnosed and treated.

DEFINITION *Osteoporosis* is defined as a reduction of bone mass (or density) or the presence of a fragility fracture. This reduction in bone tissue is accompanied by deterioration in the architecture of the skeleton, leading to a markedly increased risk of fracture. Osteoporosis is defined operationally as a bone density that falls 2.5 standard deviations (SD) below the mean—also referred to as a *T-score* of −2.5. Those who fall at the lower end of the young normal range (a T-score of >1 SD below the mean) have low bone density and are considered to be at increased risk of osteoporosis.

EPIDEMIOLOGY In the United States, as many as 8 million women and 2 million men have osteoporosis (T-score < −2.5), and an additional 18 million individuals have bone mass levels that put them at increased risk of developing osteoporosis (e.g., bone mass T-score <−1.0). Osteoporosis occurs more frequently with increasing age as bone tissue is progressively lost. In women, the loss of ovarian function at menopause (typically after age 50) precipitates rapid bone loss such that most women meet the criteria for osteoporosis by age 70.

The epidemiology of fractures follows similar trends as the loss of bone density. Fractures of the distal radius increase in frequency before age 50 and plateau by age 60, with only a modest age-related increase thereafter. In contrast, incidence rates for hip fractures double every 5 years after age 70 (Fig. 342-1). This distinct epidemiology may be related to the way people fall as they age, with fewer falls on an outstretched hand. At least 1.5 million fractures occur each year in the United States as a consequence of osteoporosis. As the population continues to age, the total number of fractures will continue to escalate.

About 300,000 hip fractures occur each year in the United States, most of which require hospital admission and surgical intervention. The probability that a 50-year-old white individual will have a hip fracture during his or her lifetime is 14% for women and 5% for men; the risk for African Americans is much lower (about half these rates). Hip fractures are associated with a high incidence of deep vein thrombosis and pulmonary embolism (20 to 50%) and a mortality rate between 5 and 20% during the few months after surgery.

There are about 500,000 vertebral crush fractures per year in the United States. Only a fraction of these are recognized clinically, since many are relatively asymptomatic and are identified incidentally during radiography for other purposes (Fig. 342-2). Vertebral fractures rarely require hospitalization but are associated with long-term morbidity and a slight increase in mortality. Multiple fractures lead to height loss (often of several inches), kyphosis, and secondary pain and discomfort related to altered biomechanics of the back. Thoracic fractures can be associated with restrictive lung disease, whereas lumbar fractures are associated with abdominal symptoms including distention, early satiety, and constipation.

Approximately 200,000 wrist fractures occur in the United States each year. Fractures of other bones also occur with osteoporosis, which is not surprising given that bone loss is a systemic phenomenon. Fractures of the pelvis and proximal humerus are clearly associated with osteoporosis. Although some fractures are clearly the result of major trauma, the threshold for fracture is reduced for an osteoporotic bone (Fig. 342-3). A list of common risk factors for osteoporotic fractures is summarized in Table 342-1. Prior fractures, a family history of osteoporotic fractures, and low body weight are each independent predictors of fracture. Chronic diseases that increase the risk of falling or frailty, including dementias, Parkinson's disease, and multiple sclerosis, also increase fracture risk.

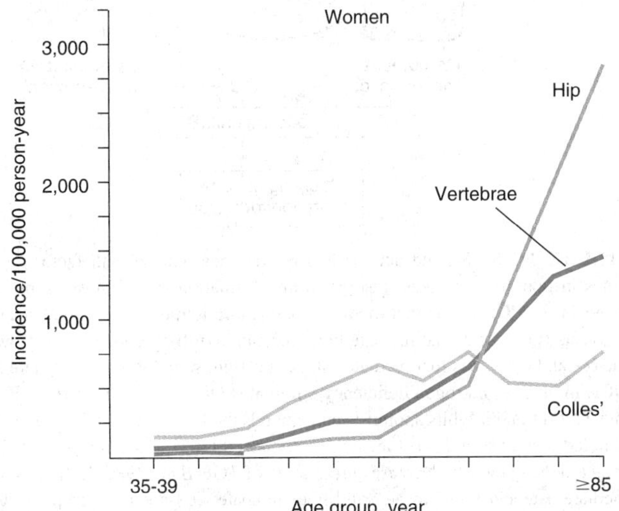

FIGURE 342-1 Epidemiology of vertebral, hip, and Colles' fractures with age. *(Adapted from LJ Melton III, in BL Riggs, LJ Melton II (eds): Osteoporosis: Etiology, Diagnosis and Management, 2d ed. Rochester, MN, Mayo Foundation, 1995.)*

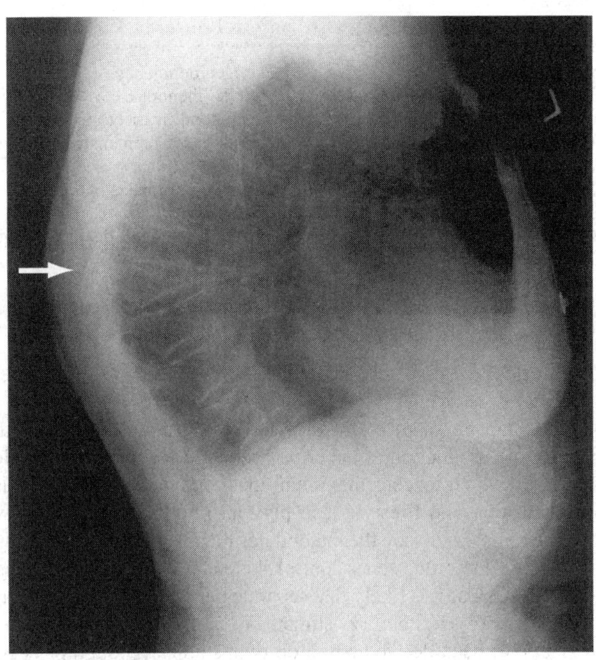

FIGURE 342-2 Lateral spine x-ray showing severe osteopenia and a severe wedge-type deformity (severe anterior compression).

In the United States and Europe, osteoporosis-related fractures are more common among women than men, presumably due to a lower peak bone mass as well as postmenopausal bone loss in women. However, this gender difference in bone density and age-related increase in hip fractures is not as apparent in some other cultures, possibly due to genetics, physical activity level, or diet.

PATHOPHYSIOLOGY **Bone Remodeling** Osteoporosis results from bone loss due to normal age-related changes in bone remodeling as well as extrinsic and intrinsic factors that exaggerate this process. These changes may be superimposed on a low peak bone mass. Consequently, the bone remodeling process is fundamental for understanding the pathophysiology of osteoporosis (Chap. 340). The skeleton increases in size by linear growth and by apposition of new bone tissue on the outer surfaces of the cortex (Fig. 342-4). This latter process is the phenomenon of modeling, which also allows the long

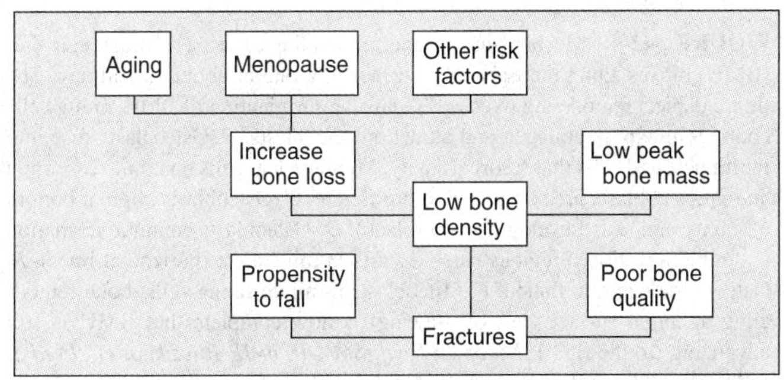

FIGURE 342-3 Factors leading to osteoporotic fractures.

Table 342-1 Risk Factors for Osteoporosis Fracture

Nonmodifiable	Estrogen deficiency
Personal history of fracture as an adult	Early menopause (<45 years) or bilateral ovariectomy
History of fracture in first-degree relative	Prolonged premenstrual amenorrhea (>1 year)
Female sex	Low calcium intake
Advanced age	Alcoholism
Caucasian race	Impaired eyesight despite adequate correction
Dementia	Recurrent falls
Potentially modifiable	Inadequate physical activity
Current cigarette smoking	Poor health/frailty
Low body weight [<58 kg (127 lb)]	

bones to adapt in shape to the stresses placed upon them. Increased sex hormone production at puberty is required for maximum skeletal maturation, which reaches maximum mass and density in early adulthood. Nutrition and lifestyle also play an important role in growth, though genetic factors are the major determinants of peak skeletal mass and density. Numerous genes control skeletal growth, peak bone mass, and body size, but it is likely that separate genes control skeletal structure and density. Heritability estimates of 50 to 80% for bone density and size have been derived based on twin studies. Though peak bone mass is often lower among individuals with a family history of osteoporosis, association studies of candidate genes [vitamin D receptor; Type I collagen, the estrogen receptor (ER), interleukin (IL) 6; and insulin-like growth factor (IGF) I] have not been consistently replicated. Linkage studies suggest that a genetic locus on chromosome 11 is associated with high bone mass.

Once peak skeletal mass has been attained, the process of remodeling becomes the principal metabolic activity of the skeleton. This process has three primary functions: (1) to repair microdamage within the skeleton, (2) to maintain skeletal strength, and (3) to supply calcium from the skeleton to maintain serum calcium. Acute demands for calcium involve osteoclast-mediated resorption as well as calcium transport by osteocytes. The activation of remodeling may be induced by microdamage to bone due to excessive or accumulated stress.

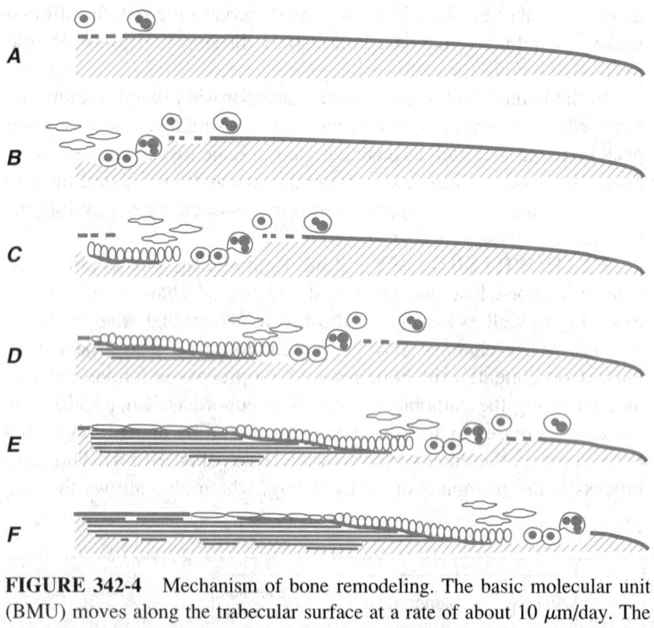

Bone remodeling is also regulated by several circulating hormones, including estrogens, androgens, vitamin D, and parathyroid hormone (PTH), as well as locally produced growth factors such as IGF-I and -II, transforming growth factor (TGF) β, parathyroid hormone-related peptide (PTHrP), ILs, prostaglandins, tumor necrosis factor (TNF), and osteoprotegrin ligand (Fig. 342-5). Additional influences include include nutrition (particularly calcium intake) and physical activity level. The end result of this remodeling process is that the resorbed bone is replaced by an equal amount of new bone tissue. Thus, the mass of the skeleton remains constant after peak bone mass is achieved in adulthood. After age 30 to 45, however, the resorption and formation processes become imbalanced, and resorption exceeds formation. This imbalance may begin at different ages and varies at different skeletal sites; it becomes exaggerated in women after menopause. Excessive bone loss can be due to an increase in osteoclastic activity and/or a decrease in osteoblastic activity. In addition, an increase in remodeling activation frequency can magnify the small imbalance seen at each remodeling unit.

In trabecular bone, if the osteoclasts are sufficiently aggressive to penetrate trabeculae, they leave no template for new bone formation to occur and, consequently, may cause rapid bone loss. In cortical bone, increased activation of remodeling creates more porous bone. The effect of this increased porosity on cortical bone strength may be modest if the overall diameter of the bone is not changed. However, decreased apposition of new bone on the periosteal surface coupled

FIGURE 342-4 Mechanism of bone remodeling. The basic molecular unit (BMU) moves along the trabecular surface at a rate of about 10 μm/day. The figure depicts remodeling over ~120 days. *A.* Origination of BMU-lining cells contract to expose collagen and attract preosteoclasts. *B.* Osteoclasts fuse into multinucleated cells that resorb a cavity. Mononuclear cells continue resorption and preosteoblasts are stimulated to proliferate. *C.* Osteoblasts align at bottom of cavity and start forming osteoid (black). *D.* Osteoblasts continue formation and mineralization. Previous osteoid starts to mineralize (horizontal lines). *E.* Osteoblasts begin to flatten. *F.* Osteoblasts turn into lining cells; bone remodeling at initial surface (left of drawing) is now complete, but BMU is still advancing (to the right). *[Adapted from: SM Ott, in JP Bilezikian et al (eds): Principles of Bone Biology, vol. 18. San Diego, Academic Press, 1996, pp 231–241.]*

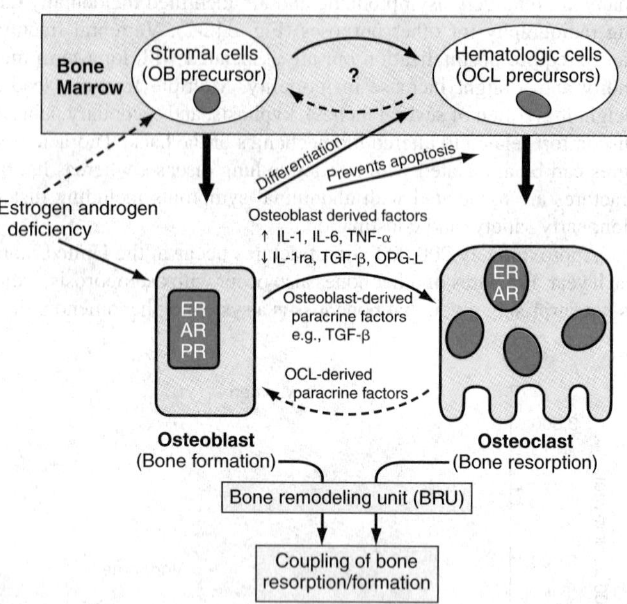

FIGURE 342-5 Steroid actions and interactions with growth factors/cytokines in bone cells at bone resorption and formation sites. Estrogen inhibits osteoclasts (OCL), cells that mediate bone resorption; estrogen stimulates osteoblasts (OB), cells that mediate bone formation. OBs produce many growth factors and cytokines that mediate estrogen action, some of which regulate the OCL indirectly. Estrogen deficiency stimulates OB production of IL-1, IL-6, and TNFα (and inhibits apoptosis and extends the life span of OCLs. Estrogen deficiency decreases IL-1ra leading to enhanced OCL sensitivity to IL-1. Estrogen deficiency also decreases production of TGF-β and OPG-L, factors that mediate osteoclast apoptosis. Solid lines indicate well-documented pathways. Dashed lines indicate less well defined pathways. ER, estrogen receptor; AR, androgen receptor; OPG, osteoprotegerin; OPG-L, osteoprotegerin-ligand; IL, interleukin; IL-1ra, interleukin 1 receptor antagonist; TGF-β, transforming growth factor β; TNFα, tumor necrosis factor α. *(Adapted from TC Spelsberg et al: Mol Endocrinol 13:819, 1999.)*

with increased endocortical resorption of bone decreases the biomechanical strength of long bones. Even a slight exaggeration in normal bone loss patterns increases the risk of osteoporotic fracture.

Calcium Nutrition Peak bone mass may be impaired by inadequate calcium intake during growth, thereby leading to increased risk of osteoporosis in later life. During the adult phase of life, calcium deprivation induces secondary hyperparathyroidism and an increase in the rate of remodeling. PTH stimulates the hydroxylation of vitamin D in the kidney, leading to increased levels of 1,25-dihydroxyvitamin D [1,25$(OH)_2$D] and enhanced gastrointestinal calcium absorption. PTH also reduces renal calcium loss. Though these are appropriate short-term homeostatic responses for improving calcium economy, the long-term effects are detrimental to the skeleton because of the ongoing imbalance at remodeling sites.

Total daily calcium intakes of <400 mg are likely to be detrimental to the skeleton, but there is more doubt about intakes in the 600- to 800-mg range, which is the average intake among adults in the United States. The recommended daily required intake of 1000 to 1200 mg for adults accomodates population heterogeneity in controlling calcium balance (Chap. 73).

Vitamin D (See also Chap. 340) Severe vitamin D deficiency causes rickets in children or osteomalacia in adults. There is accumulating evidence that vitamin D deficiency may be more prevalent than previously thought, particularly among individuals at increased risk, such as the elderly; those living in northern latitudes; and in individuals with poor nutrition, malabsorption, or chronic liver or renal disease. Modest vitamin D deficiency leads to compensatory secondary hyperparathyroidism and is an important risk factor for osteoporosis and fractures. Some studies have shown that >50% of inpatients on a general medical service exhibit biochemical features of vitamin D deficiency, including increased levels of PTH and alkaline phosphatase and lower levels of ionized calcium. In women living in northern latitudes, it has been shown that vitamin D levels decline during the winter months. This is associated with a striking seasonal bone loss, reflecting increased bone turnover. Treatment with vitamin D and calcium supplementation prevents this seasonal effect on bone metabolism. Reduced fracture rates have also been documented among individuals in northern latitudes who have greater vitamin D intake and have higher 25-hydroxyvitamin D [25(OH)D] levels (see below).

Estrogen Status Estrogen deficiency probably causes bone loss by two distinct but interrelated mechanisms: (1) activation of new bone remodeling sites, and (2) exaggeration of the imbalance between bone formation and resorption. The change in activation frequency causes a transient bone loss until a new steady state between resorption and formation is achieved. The remodeling imbalance, however, results in a permanent decrement in mass that can only be corrected by a remodeling event during which bone formation exceeds resorption. In addition, the very presence of more remodeling sites in the skeleton increases the probability that trabeculae will be penetrated, thereby eliminating the template upon which new bone can be formed and accelerating the loss of bony tissue.

The most frequent estrogen-deficient state is the cessation of ovarian function at the time of menopause, which occurs on average at the age of 51. Thus, with current life expectancy, an average woman will spend about 30 years without ovarian supply of estrogen. The mechanism by which estrogen deficiency causes bone loss is summarized in Fig. 342-5. Marrow cells (macrophages, monocytes, osteoclast precursors, mast cells) as well as bone cells (osteoblasts, osteocytes, osteoclasts) express ERs α and β. The net effect of estrogen deficiency is increased osteoclast recruitment and perhaps activity. Estrogen may also play an important role in determining the life span of bone cells by controlling the rate of apoptosis. Thus, in situations of estrogen deprivation, the life span of osteoblasts may be decreased whereas the longevity of osteoclasts is increased.

Since remodeling is initiated at the surface of bone, it follows that trabecular bone—which has a considerably larger surface area (80% of the total) than cortical bone—will be preferentially affected by estrogen deficiency. Fractures occur earliest at sites where trabecular bone contributes most to bone strength; consequently, vertebral fractures are the most common early consequence of estrogen deficiency.

Physical Activity Inactivity, such as prolonged bed rest or paralysis, results in significant bone loss. Concordantly, athletes have higher bone mass than the general population. These changes in skeletal mass are most marked when the stimulus begins during growth and before the age of puberty. Adults are less capable than children of increasing bone mass following restoration of physical activity. Epidemiologic data support the beneficial effects on the skeleton of chronic high levels of physical activity. Fracture risk is lower in rural communities and in countries where physical activity is maintained into old age. However, when exercise is initiated during adult life, the effects of moderate exercise are modest, with a bone mass increase of 1 to 2%. It is argued that more active individuals are less likely to fall and are more capable of protecting themselves upon falling, thereby reducing fracture risk.

Chronic Disease Various genetic and acquired diseases are associated with an increase in the risk of osteoporosis (Table 342-2). Mechanisms that contribute to bone loss are unique for each disease and typically result from multiple factors including nutrition, reduced physical activity levels, and factors that affect bone-remodeling rates.

Medications A large number of medications used in clinical practice have potentially detrimental effects on the skeleton (Table 342-3). *Glucocorticoids* are a common cause of medication-induced osteoporosis. It is often not possible to determine the extent to which osteoporosis is related to the glucocorticoid or to other factors, as treatment is superimposed on the effects of the primary disease, which may itself be associated with bone loss (e.g., rheumatoid arthritis). Excessive doses of thyroid hormone can accelerate bone remodeling and result in bone loss.

Other medications have less detrimental effects upon the skeleton than pharmacologic doses of glucocorticoids. *Anticonvulsants* are thought to increase the risk of osteoporosis, although many affected individuals have concomitant vitamin D insufficiency, as anticonvulsants that induce the cytochrome P450 system alter vitamin D metabolism. Patients undergoing transplantation are at high risk for rapid bone loss and fracture not only from glucocorticoids but also from

Table 342-2 Diseases Associated with an Increased Risk of Generalized Osteoporosis in Adults

Hypogonadal states	Hematologic disorders/malignancy
Turner syndrome	Multiple myeloma
Klinefelter syndrome	Lymphoma and leukemia
Anorexia nervosa	Malignancy-associated parathyroid hormone–related (PTHrP) production
Hypothalamic amenorrhea	Mastocytosis
Hyperprolactinemia	Hemophilia
Other primary or secondary hypogonadal states	Thalassemia
Endocrine disorders	Selected inherited disorders
Cushing's syndrome	Osteogenesis imperfecta
Hyperparathyroidism	Marfan syndrome
Thyrotoxicosis	Hemochromatosis
Insulin-dependent diabetes mellitus	Hypophosphatasia
Acromegaly	Glycogen storage diseases
Adrenal insufficiency	Homocystinuria
Nutritional and gastrointestinal disorders	Ehlers-Danlos syndrome
Malnutrition	Porphyria
Parenteral nutrition	Menkes' syndrome
Malabsorption syndromes	Epidermolysis bullosa
Gastrectomy	Other disorders
Severe liver disease, especially biliary cirrhosis	Immobilization
Pernicious anemia	Chronic obstructive pulmonary disease
Rheumatologic disorders	Pregnancy and lactation
Rheumatoid arthritis	Scoliosis
Ankylosing spondylitis	Multiple sclerosis
	Sarcoidosis
	Amyloidosis

Table 342-3 Drugs Associated with an Increased Risk of Generalized Osteoporosis in Adults

Glucocorticoids	Excessive thyroxine
Cyclosporine	Aluminum
Cytotoxic drugs	Gonadotropin-releasing hormone agonists
Anticonvulsants	Heparin
Excessive alcohol	Lithium

treatment with other *immunosuppressants*, such as cyclosporine and tacrolimus (FK506). In addition, these patients often have underlying metabolic abnormalities, such as hepatic or renal failure, that predispose to osteopenia.

Cigarette Consumption The use of cigarettes over a long period has detrimental effects on bone mass. These effects may be mediated directly, by toxic effects on osteoblasts, or indirectly by modifying estrogen metabolism. On average, cigarette smokers reach menopause 1 to 2 years earlier than the general population. Cigarette smoking also has secondary effects on bone growth, such as illness, frailty, decreased exercise, and the need for additional medications (e.g., glucocorticoids for lung disease).

MEASUREMENT OF BONE MASS Several noninvasive techniques are now available for estimating skeletal mass or density. These include dual-energy x-ray absorptiometry (DXA), single-energy xray absorptiometry (SXA), quantitative computed tomography (CT), and ultrasound.

DXA is a highly accurate x-ray technique that has become the standard for measuring bone density in most centers. Though it can be used for measurements of any skeletal site, clinical determinations are usually made of the lumbar spine and hip. Portable DXA machines have been developed that measure the heel (calcaneus), forearm (radius and ulna), or finger (phalanges), and DXA can also be used to measure body composition. In the DXA technique, two x-ray energies are used to estimate the area of mineralized tissue, and the mineral content is divided by the area, which partially corrects for body size. However, this correction is only partial since DXA is a two-dimensional scanning technique and cannot estimate the depths or posteroanterior length of the bone. Thus, small people tend to have lower-than-average bone mineral density (BMD). Bone spurs, which are frequent in osteoarthritis, tend to falsely increase bone density of the spine. Because DXA instrumentation is provided by several different manufacturers, the output varies in absolute terms. Consequently, it has become standard practice to relate the results to "normal" values using T-scores, which compare individual results to those in a young population that is matched for race and gender. Alternatively, Z-scores compare individual results to those of an age-matched population that is also matched for race and gender. Thus, a 60-year-old woman with a Z-score of −1 (1 SD below mean for age) could have a T-score of −2.5 (2.5 SD below mean for a young control group) (Fig. 342-6).

CT is used primarily to measure the spine, and peripheral CT is used to measure bone in the forearm or tibia. Research into the use of CT for measurement of the hip is ongoing. The results obtained from CT are different from all others currently available since this technique specifically analyzes trabecular bone and can provide a true density (mass of bone per unit volume) measurement. However, CT remains expensive, involves greater radiation exposure, and is less reproducible.

Ultrasound is used to measure bone mass by calculating the attenuation of the signal as it passes through bone or the speed with which it traverses the bone. It is unclear whether ultrasound assesses bone quality, but this may be an advantage of the technique. Because of its relatively low cost and mobility, ultrasound is amenable for use as a screening procedure.

All of these techniques for measuring BMD have been approved by the U.S. Food and Drug Administration (FDA) based upon their capacity to predict fracture risk. The hip is the preferred site of measurement in most individuals, since it directly assesses bone mass at an important fracture site. When hip measurements are performed by DXA, the spine can be measured at the same time. In younger individuals, such as perimenopausal women, spine measurements may be the most sensitive indicator of bone loss.

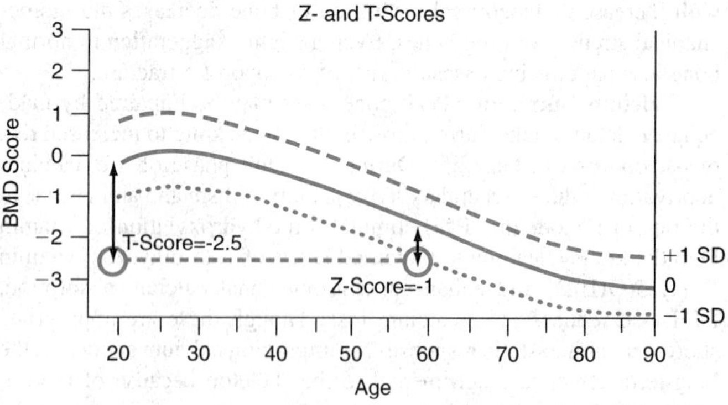

FIGURE 342-6 Relationship between Z-scores and T-scores in a 60-year-old woman. (BMD, bone mineral density; SD, standard deviation.)

When to Measure Bone Mass Clinical guidelines developed by the National Osteoporosis Foundation recommend bone mass measurements in postmenopausal women, assuming they have risk factors for osteoporosis in addition to age, gender, and estrogen deficiency. The guidelines further recommend that bone mass measurement be considered in *all* women by age 60 to 65. Criteria approved for Medicare reimbursement of BMD are summarized in Table 342-4.

When to Treat Based Upon Bone Mass Results The guidelines developed by the National Osteoporosis Foundation suggest that patients be considered for treatment when BMD > 2.5 SD below the mean value for young adults (T-score ≤ −2.5). Treatment should also be considered in women with risk factors in addition to menopause, if measurement of BMD of the hip gives a T score < −2.0. Because the fracture risk increases continuously as T-scores decline, there is no critical threshold and treatment decisions must be individualized. Cost-benefit analyses in this area are changing rapidly because of the availability of new drugs [e.g., bisphosphonates, selective estrogen receptor modulators (SERMs)] and the results of trials [e.g., the Heart and Estrogen-Progestin Replacement Study (HERS)] examining the long-term cardiovascular effects of hormone replacement therapy (HRT).

Approach to the Patient

The perimenopausal transition is a good opportunity to initiate discussion about risk factors for osteoporosis and to consider indications for a BMD test. A careful history and physical examination should be performed to identify risk factors for osteoporosis. As noted above, a low Z-score increases the suspicion of a secondary disease. Height loss >2.5 to 3.8 cm (1 to 1.5 in.) is an indication for radiography to rule out asymptomatic vertebral fractures, as is the presence of significant kyphosis or back pain, particularly if it began after menopause. For patients who present with fractures, it is important to ensure that the fractures are truly due to trauma or osteoporosis and not to secondary underlying malignancy. Usually this is clear on routine radi-

Table 342-4 FDA-Approved Indications for BMD Tests[a]

Estrogen deficient women at clinical risk of osteoporosis
Vertebral abnormalities on x-ray suggestive of osteoporosis (osteopenia, vertebral fracture)
Glucocorticoid treatment equivalent to ≥7.5 mg of prednisone, or duration of therapy >3 months
Primary hyperparathyroidism
Monitoring response to an FDA-approved medication for osteoporosis
Repeat BMD evaluations at >23-month intervals, or more frequently, if medically justified

[a] Criteria adapted from the 1998 Bone Mass Measurement Act.
NOTE: FDA, U.S. Food and Drug Administration; BMD, bone mineral density.

ography, but on occasion, CT, magnetic resonance imaging, or radionuclide scans may be helpful. Severe unremitting back pain also raises the suspicion of other causes such as malignancy (especially myeloma).

Routine Laboratory Evaluation There is no established algorithm for the evaluation of women presenting with osteoporosis. A general evaluation that includes complete blood count, serum calcium, and perhaps urine calcium is helpful for identifying selected secondary causes of low bone mass, particularly for women with fractures or very low Z-scores. An elevated serum calcium level suggests hyperparathyroidism or malignancy, whereas a reduced serum calcium level may reflect malnutrition and osteomalacia. In the presence of hypercalcemia, a serum PTH level differentiates between hyperparathyroidism (PTH ↑) and malignancy (PTH ↓), and a high PTHrP level can help document the presence of humoral hypercalcemia of malignancy (Chap. 341). A low urine calcium (<50 mg/24 h) suggests osteomalacia, malnutrition, or malabsorption; a high urine calcium (>300 mg/24 h) is indicative of hypercalciuria and must be investigated further. Hypercalciuria occurs primarily in three situations: (1) a renal calcium leak, which is more frequent in males with osteoporosis; (2) absorptive hypercalciuria, which can be idiopathic or associated with increased $1,25(OH)_2D$ in granulomatous disease; or (3) hematologic malignancies or conditions associated with excessive bone turnover such as Paget's disease, hyperparathyroidism, and hyperthyroidism.

When there is clinical suspicion of hyperthyroidism or Cushing's syndrome, thyroid stimulating hormone (TSH) or urinary free cortisol levels should be measured. When bowel disease, malabsorption, or malnutrition is suspected, serum albumin, cholesterol, and a complete blood count should be checked. Asymptomatic malabsorption might be suspected if there is anemia (macrocytic—vitamin B_{12} or folate deficiency; or microcytic—iron deficiency), or low serum cholesterol or urinary calcium levels. If these or other features suggest malabsorption, further evaluation is required. Asymptomatic celiac sprue with selective malabsorption is not uncommon; the diagnosis requires antigliadin and antiendomysial antibody tests and often a small-bowel biopsy. A trial of a gluten-free diet may be confirmatory (Chap. 286).

Myeloma can masquerade as generalized osteoporosis, although it more commonly presents with bone pain and characteristic "punched-out" lesions on radiography. Serum and urine electrophoresis and evaluation for light chains in urine are required to exclude this diagnosis. A bone marrow biopsy may be required to rule out myeloma (in patients with equivocal electrophoretic results) and can also be used to exclude mastocytosis, leukemia, and other marrow infiltrative disorders, such as Gaucher's disease.

Bone Biopsy Although the use of bone biopsy is rarely required today, it remains an important tool in clinical research. Tetracycline labeling of the skeleton allows determination of the rate of remodeling as well as evaluation for other metabolic bone diseases. The current use of BMD tests, in combination with hormonal evaluation and biochemical markers of bone remodeling, has largely replaced bone biopsy.

Biochemical Markers Several biochemical tests are now available that provide an index of the overall rate of bone remodeling (Table 342-5). Biochemical markers are usually characterized as those related primarily to *bone formation* or *bone resorption*. These tests measure the overall state of bone remodeling at a single point in time. Clinical use of these tests has been hampered by biologic variability (in part related to circadian rhythm) as well as to analytical variability.

For the most part, remodeling markers do not predict rates of bone loss well enough to use this information clinically. However, markers of bone resorption may help in the prediction of fracture risk, particularly in older individuals. In women ≥65 years, when bone density results are greater than the usual treatment thresholds noted above, a high level of bone resorption should prompt consideration of treatment. The primary use of biochemical markers is for monitoring the response to treatment. With the introduction of antiresorptive therapeutic agents, bone remodeling declines rapidly, with the fall in resorption occurring earlier than the fall in formation. Inhibition of bone

Table 342-5 Biochemical Markers of Bone Metabolism in Clinical Use

Bone formation
Serum bone-specific alkaline phosphatase
Serum osteocalcin
Serum propeptide of type I procollagen
Bone resorption
Urine and serum cross-linked N-telopeptide
Urine and serum cross-linked C-telopeptide
Urine total free deoxypyridinoline
Urine hydroxyproline
Serum tartrate-resistant acid phosphatase
Serum bone sialoprotein
Urine hydroxylysine glycosides

resorption is maximal within 3 to 6 months. Thus, measurement of bone resorption prior to initiating therapy and 4 to 6 months after starting therapy provides an earlier estimate of patient response than does bone densitometry. A decline in resorptive markers can be ascertained after treatment with bisphosphonates and HRT; this effect is less marked after treatment with either raloxifene or intranasal calcitonin. A biochemical marker response to therapy is particularly useful for asymptomatic patients and helps to ensure long-term compliance. When agents that stimulate bone formation become available, bone remodeling markers may be useful to help select therapy. However, since all current therapeutic approaches reduce bone turnover, this strategy currently has little value.

Rx TREATMENT Management of Osteoporotic Fractures

Treatment of the patient with osteoporosis frequently involves management of acute fractures as well as treatment of the underlying disease. Hip fractures almost always require surgical repair if the patient is to become ambulatory again. Depending on the location and severity of the fracture, condition of the neighboring joint, and general status of the patient, procedures may include open reduction and internal fixation with pins and plates, hemiarthroplasties, and total arthroplasties. These surgical procedures are followed by intense rehabilitation in an attempt to return patients to their prefracture functional level. Long bone fractures often require either external or internal fixation. Other fractures (e.g., vertebral, rib, and pelvic fractures) are usually managed with only supportive care, requiring no specific orthopedic treatment.

Only ~25 to 30% of vertebral compression fractures present with sudden-onset back pain. For acutely symptomatic fractures, treatment with analgesics is required, including nonsteroidal anti-inflammatory agents and/or acetaminophen, sometimes with the addition of a narcotic agent (codeine or oxycodone). A few small, randomized clinical trials have demonstrated that calcitonin may reduce pain related to acute vertebral compression fracture. A recently developed, but still experimental, technique involves percutaneous injection of artificial cement (polymethylmethacrylate) into the vertebral body (vertebroplasty or kyphoplasty); this has been reported to offer significant immediate pain relief in the majority of patients. Short periods of bed rest may be helpful for pain management, but, in general, early mobilization is recommended as it helps prevent further bone loss associated with immobilization. Occasionally, use of a soft elastic-style brace may facilitate earlier mobilization. Muscle spasms often occur with acute compression fractures and can be treated with muscle relaxants and heat treatments.

Severe pain usually resolves within 6 to 10 weeks. Chronic pain is probably not bony in origin; instead, it is related to abnormal strain on muscles, ligaments, and tendons and to secondary facet-joint arthritis associated with alterations in thoracic and/or abdominal shape. Chronic pain is difficult to treat effectively and may require analgesics, sometimes including narcotic analgesics. Frequent intermittent rest in a supine or semireclining position is often required to allow the soft tissues, which are under tension, to relax. Back-strengthening exercises (paraspinal) may be beneficial. Heat treatments help relax muscles and reduce the muscular component of discomfort. Various physical modalities, such as ultrasound and transcutaneous nerve stimulation, may be beneficial in some patients. Pain also occurs in the neck region, not as a result of compression fractures (which almost never occur in the cervical spine as a result of osteoporosis) but because of chronic strain associated from trying to elevate the head in a person with a severe thoracic kyphosis.

Multiple vertebral fractures are often associated with psychological symptoms, not always commonly appreciated. The changes in body configuration and back pain can lead to marked loss of self-image and a secondary depression. Altered balance, precipitated by the kyphosis and the anterior movement of the body's center of gravity, leads to a fear of falling, a consequent tendency to remain indoors, and the onset of social isolation. These symptoms can sometimes be alleviated by family support and/or psychotherapy. Medication may be necessary when depressive features are present.

Management of the Underlying Disease • ***Risk factor reduction*** Patients should be thoroughly educated to reduce the likelihood of any risk factors associated with bone loss and falling. Medications should be reviewed to ensure that any glucocorticoid medication is truly indicated and is being given in doses as low as possible. For those on thyroid hormone replacement, TSH testing should be performed to ensure that an adequate, but not excessive, dose is being used, as excess can be associated with increased bone loss. In patients who smoke, efforts should be made to facilitate smoking cessation. Reducing risk factors for falling also includes alcohol abuse treatment and a review of the medical regimen for any drugs that might be associated with orthostatic hypotension and/or sedation, including hypnotics and anxiolytics. If nocturia occurs, the frequency should be reduced, if possible (e.g., by decreasing or modifying diuretic use), as arising in the middle of sleep is a common precipitant of a fall. Patients should be instructed about environmental safety with regard to eliminating exposed wires, curtain strings, slippery rugs, and mobile tables. Avoiding stocking feet on wood floors, checking carpet condition (particularly on stairs), and providing good light in paths to bathrooms and outside the home are good preventive measures. Treatment for impaired vision is recommended, particularly a problem with depth perception, which is specifically associated with increased falling risk. Elderly patients with neurologic impairment (e.g., stroke, Parkinson's disease, Alzheimer's disease) are particularly at risk of falling and require specialized supervision and care.

Nutritional recommendations • *CALCIUM* A large body of data indicates that optimal calcium intake reduces bone loss and suppresses bone turnover. Recommended intakes from a recent report from the Institute of Medicine are shown in Table 342-6. The National Health and Nutritional Evaluation Studies (NHANES) have consistently documented that average calcium intakes fall considerably short of these recommendations. The preferred source of calcium is from dairy products and other foods, but many patients require additional calcium supplementation. Food sources of calcium are dairy products (milk, yogurt, and cheese) and fortified foods such as certain cereals, waffles, snacks, juices, and crackers. Some of these fortified foods contain as much calcium per serving as milk.

If a calcium supplement is required, it should be taken in doses ≤600 mg at a time, as the calcium absorption fraction decreases at higher doses. Calcium supplements should be calculated based on the elemental calcium content of the supplement, not the weight of the calcium salt (Table 342-7). Calcium supplements containing carbonate are best taken with food since they require acid for solubility. Calcium citrate supplements can be taken at any time.

Several controlled clinical trials of calcium plus vitamin D have confirmed reductions in clinical fractures, including fractures of the hip (~20 to 30% risk reduction). All recent studies of pharmacologic agents have been conducted in the context of calcium replacement (± vitamin D). Thus, it is standard practice to ensure an adequate calcium and vitamin D intake in patients with osteoporosis, whether they are receiving additional pharmacologic therapy or not.

Although side effects from supplemental calcium are minimal, individuals with a history of kidney stones should have a 24-h urine calcium determination before starting increased calcium to avoid hypercalciuria. Furthermore, a thiazide-containing diuretic might be indicated in some patients to increase renal tubular calcium reabsorption and to reduce urine calcium levels.

VITAMIN D Vitamin D is synthesized in skin under the influence of heat and ultraviolet light (Chap. 340). However, large segments of the population do not obtain sufficient vitamin D to maintain what is now considered an adequate supply [serum 25(OH)D consistently >15 to 20 ng/mL]. Since vitamin D supplementation at doses that would achieve these serum levels is safe and inexpensive, it is now routine to recommend supplemental vitamin D. The Institute of Medicine recommends daily intakes of 200 IU for adults <50 years of age, 400 IU for those from 50 to 70 years, and 600 IU for those >70 years. Multivitamin tablets usually contain 400 IU, and many calcium supplements also contain vitamin D.

OTHER NUTRIENTS Other nutrients such as salt and caffeine may have modest effects on calcium excretion or absorption. Adequate vitamin K states is required for optimal carboxylation of osteocalcin. States in which vitamin K nutrition or metabolism is impaired, such as with long-term coumadin therapy, have been associated with reduced bone mass.

Magnesium is abundant in foods, and magnesium deficiency is quite rare in the absence of a serious chronic disease. Magnesium supplementation may be warranted in patients with inflammatory bowel disease, celiac sprue, chemotherapy, severe diarrhea, malnutrition, or alcoholism. Phytoestrogens may impact skeletal health, although the degree of this effect is unclear. Dietary phytoestrogens, which are derived primarily from soy products and legumes (e.g., garbanzo beans, chickpeas, and lentils), are insufficiently potent to justify their use in place of a pharmacologic agent in the treatment of osteoporosis.

Patients with hip fracture are often frail and relatively malnourished. Some data suggest an improved outcome in such patients when they are provided calorie and protein supplementation.

Exercise Exercise in young individuals increases the likelihood that they will attain the maximal genetically determined peak bone

Table 342-6 Adequate Calcium Intake

Life Stage Group	Estimated Adequate Daily Calcium Intake, mg/d
Young Children (1–3 years)	500
Older children (4–8 years)	800
Adolescents and young adults (9–18 years)	1300
Men and women (19–50 years)	1000
Men and women (51 and older)	1200

NOTE: Pregnancy and lactation needs are the same as for nonpregnant women (e.g., 1300 mg/d for adolescents/young adult and 1000 mg/d for ≥19 years.)

SOURCE: Adapted from the Standing Committee on the Scientific Evaluation of Dietary Reference Intakes. Food and Nutrition Board. Institute of Medicine. Washington, DC, 1997. National Academy Press.

Table 342-7 Elemental Calcium Content of Various Oral Calcium Preparations

Calcium Preparation	Elemental Calcium Content
Calcium citrate	60 mg/300 mg
Calcium lactate	80 mg/600 mg
Calcium gluconate	40 mg/500 mg
Calcium carbonate	400 mg/g
Calcium carbonate + 5 μg vitamin D_2 (OsCal 250)	250 mg/tablet
Calcium carbonate (Tums 500)	500 mg/tablet

SOURCE: SM Krane and MF Holick, Chap. 355 in HPIM, 14 ed, 1998.

mass. Meta-analyses of studies performed in postmenopausal women indicate that weight-bearing exercise prevents bone loss but does not appear to result in substantial bone gain. When the exercise is discontinued, any effects on bone mass wane. It is important to note, however, that exercise also has beneficial effects on neuromuscular function. Exercise can improve coordination, balance, and strength and thereby reduce the risk of falling, as well as the severity of injury upon a fall. Therefore, the beneficial effects of exercise on muscle mass and reduced risk of falling justify its recommendation for all age groups. A walking program is a practical way to start. Other activities such as dancing, racquet sports, cross-country skiing, and use of gym equipment are also recommended, depending on the patient's personal preference. Even women who cannot walk benefit from swimming or water exercises, not so much for the effects on bone, which are quite minimal, but because of effects on muscle. Exercise habits should be consistent, optimally at least three times a week.

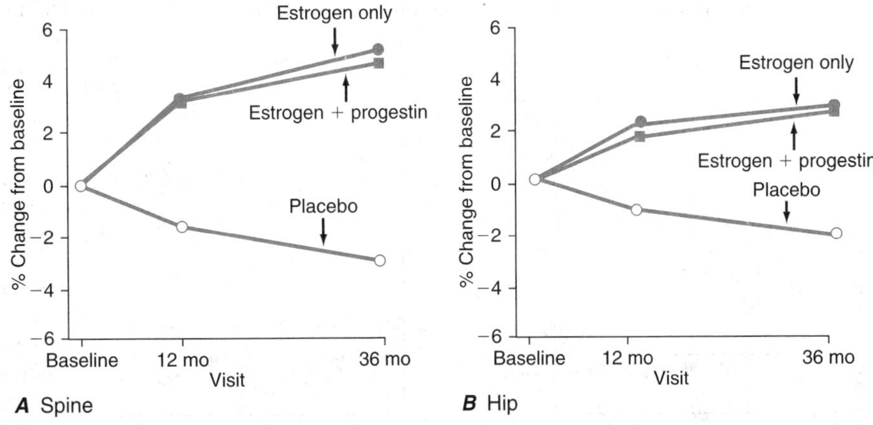

FIGURE 342-7 Results of hormone-replacement therapy (HRT) regimens on bone mineral density (BMD) of the spine (*A*) and hip (*B*). Unadjusted mean percent change in BMD in the hip by treatment assignment and visit: adherent PEPI participants only. Results From the Postmenopausal Estrogen/Progestin Interventions (PEPI) Trial. Estrogen, conjugated equine estrogen 0.625 mg/d; Progestin, medroxyprogesterone acetate 10 mg/d. *(Adapted from TL Bush et al: JAMA 276:1389, 1996.)*

Pharmacologic Therapies Until fairly recently, estrogen treatment, either by itself or in concert with a progestin, was the primary therapeutic agent for prevention or treatment of osteoporosis. Over the past 5 years, a number of new drugs have appeared, and more are expected in the near future. Some are agents that specifically treat osteoporosis (bisphosphonates, calcitonin); others, such as tissue-selective estrogens (or SERMs), have broader effects. The availability of these drugs allows therapy to be tailored to the needs of an individual patient. The evidence supporting the effectiveness of each remedy is variable, in part because these treatments are new.

Estrogens A large body of clinical trial data indicates that various types of estrogens (conjugated equine estrogens, estradiol, estrone, esterified estrogens, ethinyl estradiol, and mestranol) reduce bone turnover, prevent bone loss, and induce small increases in bone mass of the spine, hip, and total body. The effects of estrogen are seen in women with natural or surgical menopause and in late postmenopausal women with or without established osteoporosis. Estrogens are efficacious when administered orally, buccally, vaginally, percutaneously, subcutaneously, and transdermally. For both oral and transdermal routes of administration, combined estrogen/progestin preparations are now available in many countries, obviating the problem of taking two tablets or using a patch and oral progestin. One large study, referred to as PEPI (Postmenopausal Estrogen/ Progestin Intervention Trial), indicated that C-21 progestins alone do not augment the effect of estrogen on bone mass (Fig. 342-7).

DOSE OF ESTROGEN For oral estrogens, the recommended dose is 0.3 mg/d for esterified estrogens, 0.625 mg/d for conjugated equine estrogens, and 5 μg/d for ethinyl estradiol. For transdermal estrogen, the commonly used dose supplies 50 μg estradiol per day, but a lower dose may be appropriate for some individuals. Dose-response data are not available for other routes of administration.

FRACTURE DATA In contrast to the body of clinical trial data evaluating the effects of estrogen on bone mass, its effects on fracture occurrence have been less well studied. Epidemiologic databases indicate that women who take estrogen replacement have a 50% reduction, on average, of osteoporotic fractures, including hip fractures. The beneficial effect of estrogen is greatest among those who start replacement early and continue the treatment; the benefit wanes after discontinuation such that there is no residual protective effect against fracture by 10 years after discontinuation. There are no clinical trial data confirming that estrogen administration reduces the risk of hip fracture. In fact, the HERS trial of women with established coronary artery disease showed no reduction in the risk of hip or clinical fractures in the estrogen-progestin arm relative to the placebo group. These data may not be definitive, however, since the women were not chosen for osteoporosis risk and were at unknown risk of osteoporotic fracture. Furthermore, radiographic vertebral fractures were not assessed in this study. One clinical study which looked at all nonvertebral fractures suggested a reduction in HRT-treated women.

A few clinical trials have evaluated spine fracture occurrence as an outcome with estrogen therapy. One that used high doses of estrogen (2.5 mg conjugated equine estrogen per day) indicated marked vertebral fracture reduction in estrogen-treated women. Several other small studies, using lower estrogen doses, have consistently shown that estrogen treatment reduces the incidence of vertebral compression fracture. The ongoing Women's Health Initiative will provide additional data about the effects of estrogen on the risk of other osteoporosis-related fractures.

Long-term estrogen use may be associated with an increase in the risk of venous thromboembolism and gallbladder, uterine, and breast cancer; in observational studies, estrogens have been associated with a significant reduction in myocardial infarction, although this was not so in HERS. The WHI will provide further information.

MODE OF ACTION Two subtypes of ERs, α and β, have been identified in bone and other tissues. Cells of monocyte lineage express both ERα and -β, as do osteoblasts. Estrogen-mediated effects vary depending on the receptor type. Using ER knockout mouse models, elimination of ERα produces a modest reduction in bone mass, whereas ERβ null animals had very little abnormality, except greater cortical bone mass. A male patient with a homozygous mutation of ERα had markedly decreased bone density as well as abnormalities in epiphyseal closure, confirming the important role of ERα in bone biology. The mechanism of estrogen action in bone is an area of active investigation (Fig. 342-5). Though data are conflicting, estrogens appear to inhibit osteoclasts directly. However, the majority of estrogen (and androgen) effects on bone resorption are mediated indirectly through paracrine factors produced by osteoblasts. These actions include: (1) increasing IGF-1 and TGF-β, and (2) suppressing IL-1 (α and β), IL-6, TNF-α, and osteocalcin synthesis. The consequence of these effects is primarily to decrease bone resorption.

Progestins In women with a uterus, daily progestin or cyclical progestins at least 12 days per month are prescribed in combination with estrogens to reduce the risk of uterine cancer. Medroxyprogesterone acetate and norethindrone acetate blunt the high-density lipoprotein response to estrogen, but micronized progesterone does not. Neither medroxyprogesterone acetate nor micronized progesterone appears to have an independent effect on bone; at lower doses, norethindrone acetate might have an additive benefit. On breast tissue, progestins may increase the risk of breast cancer, though this is by no means definite.

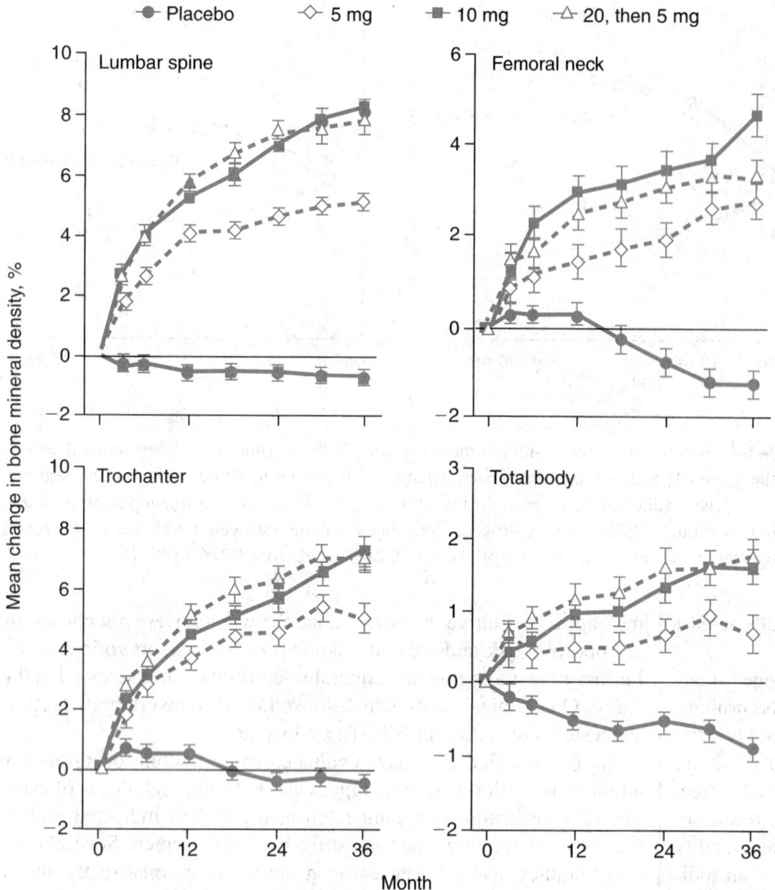

FIGURE 342-8 Alendronate treatment. Percentage change in bone mineral density in women receiving alendronate or placebo over 3 years. *(From UA Liberman et al: N Engl J Med 333:1437, 1995.)*

Tissue-selective estrogens, or SERMs Two SERMs are currently being used in postmenopausal women: raloxifene, which is approved for prevention and treatment of osteoporosis, and tamoxifen, which is approved for the prevention and treatment of breast cancer.

Tamoxifen reduces bone turnover and bone loss in postmenopausal women compared to placebo groups. These findings support the concept that tamoxifen acts as an estrogenic agent in bone. There are limited data on the effect of tamoxifen on fracture risk, but the Breast Cancer Prevention study indicated a possible reduction in clinical vertebral, hip, and Colles' fractures. The major benefit of tamoxifen is on breast cancer occurrence. The breast cancer prevention trial indicated that tamoxifen administration over 4 to 5 years reduced the incidence of new invasive and noninvasive breast cancer by approximately 45% in women at increased risk of breast cancer. The incidence of ER-positive breast cancers was reduced by 65%.

Raloxifene (60 mg/d) has effects on bone turnover and bone mass that are very similar to those of tamoxifen, indicating that this agent is also estrogenic on the skeleton. The effect of raloxifene on bone density (+1.4 to 2.8% versus placebo in the spine, hip, and total body) is somewhat less than that seen with standard doses of estrogens. Raloxifene reduces the occurrence of vertebral fracture by 30 to 50%, depending on the subpopulation.

Raloxifene, like tamoxifen and estrogen, has effects throughout other organ systems. The most positive effect appears to be a reduction in invasive breast cancer (mainly decreased ER-positive) occurrence of about 70% in women who take raloxifene compared to placebo. In contrast to tamoxifen, raloxifene is not associated with an increase in the risk of uterine cancer or benign uterine disease. Raloxifene increases the occurrence of hot flashes. Although raloxifene reduces serum total and low-density lipoprotein cholesterol, lipoprotein(a), and fibrinogen, no studies including cardiovascular disease or cerebrovascular disease endpoints are available.

MODE OF ACTION OF SERMS All SERMs bind to the ER, but each agent produces a unique receptor conformation. As a result, specific coactivator or corepressor proteins are bound to the receptor (Chap. 327), resulting in differential effects on gene transcription that vary according to other transcription factors present in the cell. Another aspect of selectivity is the affinity of each SERM for the different ERα and β subtypes, which are expressed differentially in various tissues. These tissue-selective effects of SERMs offer the possibility of tailoring estrogen therapy to best meet the needs and risk factor profile of an individual patient.

Bisphosphonates Both alendronate and risedronate are approved for the prevention and treatment of postmenopausal osteoporosis and treatment of steroid-induced osteoporosis. Risedronate is also approved for the prevention of steroid-induced osteoporosis.

Alendronate has been shown to have dramatic effects in patients with osteoporosis, decreasing bone turnover and increasing bone mass in the spine by up to 8% versus placebo and by 6% versus placebo in the hip (Fig. 342-8). Multiple trials have evaluated the effect of alendronate on fracture occurrence. The Fracture Intervention Trial provided evidence in over 2000 women with prevalent vertebral fractures that daily alendronate treatment (5 mg/d for 2 years and 10 mg/d for 9 months afterwards) reduces vertebral fracture risk by about 50%, multiple vertebral fractures by up to 90%, and hip fractures by up to 50% (Fig. 342-9). Several subsequent trials have confirmed these findings. For example, in a study of >1900 women with low bone mass treated with alendronate (10 mg/d) versus placebo, the incidence of all nonvertebral fractures was reduced by ~47% after just 1 year.

Alendronate (5 to 10 mg/d) should be given with a full glass of water before breakfast, as bisphosphonates are poorly absorbed. Because of the potential for esophageal irritation, alendronate is contraindicated in patients who have stricture or inadequate emptying of the esophagus. It is recommended that patients remain upright for at least 30 min after taking the medication to avoid esophageal irritation. Cases of esophagitis, esophageal ulcer, and esophageal stricture have been described, but the incidence appears to be low. In clinical trials, overall gastrointestinal symptomatology was no different with alendronate compared to placebo.

Risedronate produces a dramatic reduction in bone turnover and an increase in bone mass. Controlled clinical trials have demonstrated >40% reduction in vertebral fracture risk over 3 years, accompanied by a 33% reduction in clinical nonspine fractures. Reports from several studies show a 40% reduction in hip fracture in patients with osteoporosis, with a somewhat greater effect in patients with prevalent vertebral fractures. Patients should take risedronate (5.0 mg orally) with a full glass of plain water [0.18 to 0.25 L (6 to 8 oz)], to facilitate delivery to the stomach, and should not lie down for 30 min after taking the drug. The incidence of gastrointestinal side effects in these trials with risedronate was similar to that of placebo.

Etidronate was the first bisphosphonate to be approved, initially for use in Paget's disease and hypercalcemia. This agent has also been used in osteoporosis trials of smaller magnitude than those performed for alendronate and risedronate. Etidronate probably has some efficacy against vertebral fracture when given as an intermittent cyclical regimen (2 weeks on, 2 1/2 months off).

MODE OF ACTION Bisphosphonates are structurally related to pyrophosphates, compounds that are incorporated into bone matrix. Through mechanisms that remain to be fully elucidated, bisphosphonates specifically impair osteoclast function and reduce osteoclast number, in part by the induction of apoptosis. Recent evidence suggests that the nitrogen-containing bisphosphonates also inhibit protein pren-

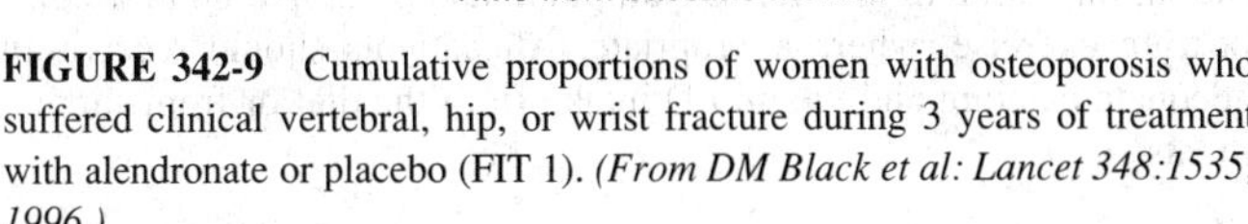

FIGURE 342-9 Cumulative proportions of women with osteoporosis who suffered clinical vertebral, hip, or wrist fracture during 3 years of treatment with alendronate or placebo (FIT 1). *(From DM Black et al: Lancet 348:1535, 1996.)*

ylation, one of the end products in the mevalonic acid pathway. This effect disrupts intracellular protein trafficking and may ultimately lead to apoptosis. Bisphosphonates have very long retention in the skeleton and may exert long-term effects.

Calcitonin Calcitonin is a polypeptide hormone produced by the thyroid gland (Chap. 341). Its physiologic role is unclear as no skeletal disease has been described in association with calcitonin deficiency or calcitonin excess. Calcitonins are approved by the FDA approved for Paget's disease, hypercalcemia, and osteoporosis in women >5 years past menopause.

Injectable calcitonin produces small increments in bone mass of the lumbar spine. However, difficulty of administration and frequent reactions, including nausea and facial flushing, make general use limited. In 1995, a nasal spray containing calcitonin (200 IU/d) was approved for treatment of osteoporosis in postmenopausal women. Several studies indicate that nasal calcitonin produces small increments in bone mass and a small reduction in new vertebral fractures in calcitonin-treated patients versus those on calcium alone.

Calcitonin is not indicated for prevention of osteoporosis and is not sufficiently potent to prevent bone loss in early postmenopausal women. As mentioned above, calcitonin might have an analgesic effect on bone pain, both in the subcutaneous and possibly the nasal form.

Mode of Action Calcitonin suppresses osteoclast activity by direct action on the osteoclast calcitonin receptor. Osteoclasts exposed to calcitonin cannot maintain their active ruffled border, which normally maintains close contact with underlying bone. Calcitonin also affects osteoclast mobility and the movement of enzyme-containing cytoplasmic granules.

Experimental agents • *Parathyroid Hormone* Endogenous PTH is an 84-amino-acid peptide that is largely responsible for calcium homeostasis (Chap. 341). Although chronic elevation of PTH, as occurs in hyperparathyroidism, is associated with bone loss (particularly cortical bone), PTH can also exert anabolic effects on bone. Consistent with this, some observational studies have indicated that mild elevations in PTH are associated with maintenance of trabecular bone mass. On the basis of these findings, preclinical and early clinical studies have been performed using an exogenous PTH analogue (1-34 PTH). The first randomized controlled trial in postmenopausal women showed that PTH, when superimposed on ongoing estrogen therapy, produced substantial increments in bone mass (13% over a 3-year period compared to estrogen alone). This increment in bone mass was also associated with a reduction in risk of vertebral compression deformity (Fig. 342-10). More recent studies have confirmed the ability of combined treatment with estrogen and PTH to induce striking increases in bone mass.

PTH use may be limited by its mode of administration, which currently requires subcutaneous injection. Alternative modes of delivery are being investigated, including transdermal and inhalation routes. The optimal frequency of administration also remains to be established, and it is possible that PTH might also be effective when used in high doses, 1 month out of every 3.

Mode of Action Exogenously administered PTH appears to have direct actions on osteoblast activity, with biochemical and histomorphometric evidence of de novo bone formation early in response to PTH, prior to activation of bone resorption. Subsequently, PTH activates bone remodeling but still appears to favor bone formation over bone resorption. PTH stimulates IGF-I and collagen production and appears to increase osteoblast number by inhibiting apoptosis and stimulating replication.

Fluoride Fluoride has been available for many years and is a potent stimulator of osteoprogenitor cells when studied in vitro. It has been used in multiple osteoporosis studies with conflicting results, in part related to use of varying doses and preparations. Fluoride produces marked effects on bone mass, especially in the spine, where gains of around 10% per year have been observed. However, despite increments in bone mass, there is no consistent effect of fluoride on vertebral or nonvertebral fracture, which might actually increase when high doses of fluoride are used. Furthermore, animal data suggest that there is reduced biomechanical strength when fluoride is incorporated into bone as fluoroapatite, with excess osteoid accumulation and evidence of woven rather than lamellar bone formation, especially at high doses. For these reasons, fluoride remains an experimental agent, despite its long history and multiple studies.

Other Potential Anabolic Agents Several small studies of growth hormone (GH), alone or in combination with other agents, have not shown consistent or substantial positive effects on skeletal mass. Many of these studies are relatively short-term, and the effects of GH

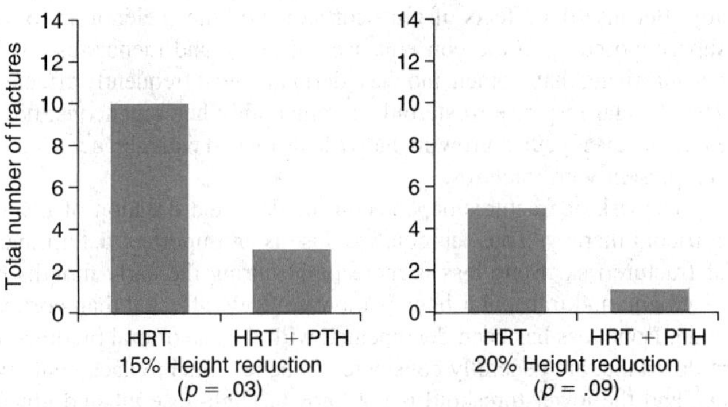

FIGURE 342-10 Number of incident vertebral deformities (15% and 20% reductions) in women with osteoporosis on HRT, compared to HRT + PTH over 3 years. (HRT, hormone-replacement therapy; PTH, parathyroid hormone.) *(From Lindsay et al.)*

and the IGFs are still under investigation. Anabolic steroids, mostly derivatives of testosterone, act primarily as antiresorptive agents to reduce bone turnover but may also stimulate osteoblastic activity. Effects on bone mass remain unclear but appear weak, in general, and use is limited by masculinizing side effects. Several recent observational studies suggest that the statin drugs, currently used to treat hypercholesterolemia, may be associated with increased bone mass and reduced fractures, but there are not clinical trial data.

Nonpharmacologic Approaches Protective pads worn around the outer thigh, which cover the trochanteric region of the hip can prevent hip fractures in elderly residents in nursing homes. The use of hip protectors is limited largely by compliance and comfort, but new devices are being developed that may circumvent these problems and provide adjunctive treatments.

Treatment Monitoring There are currently no well-accepted guidelines for monitoring treatment of osteoporosis. Because most osteoporosis treatments produce small or moderate bone mass increments on average, it is reasonable to consider BMD as a monitoring tool. As with any biologic or assay determination, there is precision error with repeated measurements. Changes must exceed ~4% in the spine and 6% in the hip to be considered significant in any individual. The hip is the preferred site due to larger surface area and greater reproducibility. Medication-induced increments may require several years to produce changes of this magnitude (if they do at all). Consequently, it can be argued that BMD should not be repeated at intervals <2 years. Only significant BMD reductions should prompt a change in medical regimen, as it is expected that many individuals will not show responses greater than the detection limits of the current measurement techniques.

Biochemical markers of bone turnover may prove useful for treatment monitoring, but there is currently little hard evidence to support this concept; it remains unclear which endpoint is most useful. If bone turnover markers are used, a determination should be made before starting therapy and repeated ≥4 months after therapy is initiated. In general, a change in bone turnover markers must be 30 to 40% lower than the baseline to be significant because of the biologic and technical variability in these tests. A positive change in biochemical markers and/or bone density can be useful to help patients adhere to treatment regimens.

GLUCOCORTICOID-INDUCED OSTEOPOROSIS Osteoporotic fractures are a well-characterized consequence of the hypercortisolism associated with Cushing's syndrome. However, the therapeutic use of glucocorticoids is by far the most common form of glucocorticoid-induced osteoporosis. Glucocorticoids are widely used in the treatment of a variety of disorders, including chronic lung disorders, rheumatoid arthritis and other connective tissue diseases, inflammatory bowel disease, and posttransplantation. Osteoporosis and related fractures are serious side effects of chronic glucocorticoid therapy. Because the effects of glucocorticoids on the skeleton are often superimposed upon the consequences of aging and menopause, it is not surprising that women and the elderly are most frequently affected. The skeletal response to steroids is remarkably heterogeneous, however, and even young, growing individuals treated with glucocorticoids can present with fractures.

The risk of fractures depends on the dose and duration of glucocorticoid therapy. Thus, cumulative dose is an important determinant of fracture risk. Bone loss is more rapid during the early months of treatment, and trabecular bone is more severely affected than cortical bone. Bone loss has been documented with the use of oral prednisone at doses that are generally considered to be less than replacement levels, and the lower threshold is not known. High-dose inhaled glucocorticoids can produce systemic effects on the skeleton, as can intra-articular injections. Alternate-day delivery does not appear to ameliorate the skeletal effects of glucocorticoids. The prevalence of vertebral fractures in asthmatic patients treated for 1 year with glucocorticoids is 11%, and increased risk of fractures has been demonstrated in most other disease states treated with glucocorticoids.

Pathophysiology Glucocorticoids increase bone loss by multiple mechanisms including: (1) inhibition of osteoblast function and potential increase in osteoblast apoptosis, resulting in impaired synthesis of new bone; (2) stimulation of bone resorption, probably as a secondary effect; (3) impairment of the absorption of calcium across the intestine, probably by a vitamin D–independent effect; (4) increase of urinary calcium loss and induction of some degree of secondary hyperparathyroidism; (5) reduction of adrenal androgens and suppression of ovarian and testicular secretion of estrogens and androgens; and (6) potential induction of glucocorticoid myopathy, which may exacerbate effects on skeletal and calcium homeostasis, as well as increase the risk of falls.

Evaluation of the Patient Because of the prevalence of glucocorticoid-induced osteopenia, it is important to evaluate the status of the skeleton in all patients being initiated on or already receiving long-term glucocorticoid therapy. Modifiable risk factors should be identified, including those for falls. Examination should include height and muscle strength testing. Laboratory evaluation should include an assessment of 24-h urinary calcium. A task force of the American College of Rheumatology recommends that all patients who are being initiated on glucocorticoids and patients already on long-term (>6 months) glucocorticoids have measurement of bone mass at both the spine and hip using DXA. If only one skeletal site can be measured, it is best to assess the spine in individuals <60 years and the hip for those >60 years.

Prevention Bone loss caused by glucocorticoids can be prevented, and the risk of fractures significantly reduced. Strategies must include using the lowest dose of glucocorticoid for disease management. Topical and inhaled routes of administration are preferred, where appropriate. Risk factor reduction is important, including smoking cessation, limitation of alcohol consumption, and participation in weight-bearing exercise, where appropriate. All patients should receive an adequate calcium and vitamin D intake from the diet or from supplements.

℞ **TREATMENT** Only bisphosphonates have been demonstrated in large clinical trials to reduce the risk of fractures in patients being treated with glucocorticoids. Risedronate has been shown to prevent bone loss and to reduce vertebral fracture risk by about 70%. Similar beneficial effects are observed in studies of alendronate and etidronate. Controlled trials of HRT have shown bone-sparing effects, and calcitonin also has some protective effect. Thiazides reduce urine calcium loss, but their role in prevention of fractures is unclear.

BIBLIOGRAPHY

Berard A et al: Meta-analysis of the effectiveness of physical activity for the prevention of bone loss in postmenopausal women. Osteoporos Int 7:331, 1997

Cauley JA et al: Estrogen replacement therapy and fractures in older women. Study of Osteoporotic Fractures Research Group. Ann Intern Med 122:9, 1995

Chapuy MC et al: Effect of calcium and cholecalciferol treatment for three years on hip fractures in elderly women. BMJ 308:1081, 1994

Collaborative Group on Hormonal Factors in Breast Cancer: Breast cancer and hormone replacement therapy: Collaborative reanalysis of data from 51 epidemiological studies of 52705 women with breast cancer and 108411 women without breast cancer. Lancet 350:1047, 1997

Cosman F, Lindsay R Selective estrogen receptors modulators: Clinical spectrum. Endocr Rev 20: 418, 1999

Cummings SR et al: The effect of raloxifene on risk of breast cancer in postmenopausal women: Results from the MORE randomized trial. Multiple Outcomes of Raloxifene Evaluation. JAMA 281:2189, 1999

Early Breast Cancer Trialists Collaborative Group: Tamoxifen for early breast cancer: An overview of the randomised trials. Lancet 351:1451, 1998

Eastell RD: Treatment of postmenopausal osteoporosis. N Engl J Med 338:736, 1998

Ettinger B et al: Reduction of vertebral fracture risk in postmenopausal women with osteoporosis treated with raloxifene: Results from a 3-year randomized clinical trial. Multiple Outcomes of Raloxifene Evaluation (MORE) Investigators. JAMA 282:637, 1999

Gregg EW et al: Physical activity and osteoporotic fracture risk in older women. Ann Intern Med 129:81, 1998

HARRIS ST et al: Effects of risedronate treatment on vertebral and nonvertebral fractures in women with postmenopausal osteoporosis: A randomized controlled trial. Vertebral Efficacy with Risedronate Therapy (VERT) Study Group. JAMA 282:1344, 1999
HOSKING D et al: Prevention of bone loss with alendronate in postmenopausal woman under 60 years of age. N Engl J Med 338: 485, 1998
HULLEY S et al: Randomized trial of estrogen plus progestin for secondary prevention of coronary heart disease in postmenopausal women. Heart and Estrogen/progestin Replacement Study (HERS) Research Group. JAMA 280:605, 1998
LINDSAY R: Clinical utility of biochemical markers. Osteoporos Int 9 (Suppl): S29, 1999
——— et al: Randomized controlled study of effect of parathyroid hormone on vertebral-bone mass and fracture incidence among postmenopausal women on estrogen with osteoporosis. Lancet 350:550, 1997
MARCUS R et al: *Osteoporosis*. San Diego, Academic, 1996, pp. 1–1373
OVERGAARD K et al: Effect of calcitonin given intranasally on bone mass and fracture rates in a dose response study. BJM 305:556, 1992
PAK CY et al: Treatment of postmenopausal osteoporosis with slow release sodium fluoride. Final report of a randomized controlled trial. Ann Intern Med 123:401, 1995
POLS HAP et al: Multinational, placebo-controlled, randomized trial of the effects of alendronate on bone density and fracture risk in postmenopausal women with low bone mass: Results of the FOSIT study. Fosamax International Trial Study Group. Osteoporosis Int 9: 461, 1999
SAAG KG et al: Alendronate for the prevention and treatment of glucocorticoid-induced osteoporosis. Glucocorticoid-Induced Osteoporosis Intervention Study Group. N Engl J Med 339:292, 1998
WASNICH RD et al: Antifracture efficacy of antiresorptive agents are related to changes in bone density. J Clin Endocrinol Metab 85: 231, 2000

343

Stephen M. Krane, Alan L. Schiller

PAGET'S DISEASE AND OTHER DYSPLASIAS OF BONE

PAGET'S DISEASE OF BONE

Paget's disease of bone (osteitis deformans) is characterized by excessive resorption of bone by osteoclasts, followed by the replacement of normal marrow by vascular, fibrous connective tissue. At some stage and to a variable degree, the resorbed bone is replaced by coarse-fibered, dense trabecular bone organized in haphazard fashion. The irregular and often rapid deposition of this new bone, to a great extent still lamellar, results in an increase in the number of prominent, irregular cement lines that give the bone its characteristic "mosaic" pattern. Most lesions show both excessive resorption and chaotic new bone formation. The disorder is usually focal but may be widespread.

INCIDENCE The prevalence is difficult to determine because the disease is often asymptomatic. It is frequently detected when roentgenograms are obtained for other reasons or because of a high level of alkaline phosphatase on routine blood screening. On the basis of autopsy examination, the incidence is estimated to be about 3% in individuals over age 40; the likelihood of occurrence increases with age. The incidence varies in different parts of the world. Radiologic surveys indicate that the frequency in adults is <1% in the United States, Great Britain, and Australia. In India, Japan, the Middle East, and Scandinavia, the disease is rare.

ETIOLOGY The cause is unknown. Some of the manifestations can be suppressed with glucocorticoids, salicylates, and cytotoxic drugs, but there is no convincing evidence that the fundamental lesion is inflammatory. Intranuclear inclusions have been found by electron microscopy in osteoclasts in pagetic bone. Some of the inclusions resemble nucleocapsids of viruses belonging to the measles group. Indirect immunofluorescence studies using antibodies to measles virus suggest that the inclusions are indeed measles virus nucleocapsids. The presence of mutations in specific regions of the viral genome is consistent with persistent infection. In some individuals with Paget's disease, osteoclasts and bone marrow mononuclear cells contain nucleocapsids of respiratory syncytial virus alone or in addition to nucleocapsids of measles virus; in some areas of Britain, canine distemper virus sequences have been identified in pagetic bone cells. Thus, different paramyxoviruses may have roles in the initiation or propagation of Paget's disease. Further evidence supporting the potential role of measles virus in the pathogenesis of the excessive bone resorption in Paget's disease has been obtained from studies of osteoclast precursors in vitro. Normal bone marrow–derived CD34+ cells transduced with a measles virus nucleocapsid gene differentiate into abnormal multinucleated osteoclasts that can resorb bone.

There is renewed interest in genetic factors that might be important in the predisposition to and pathogenesis of Paget's disease. Several large kindreds have been identified in which Paget's disease affects two or more generations with a pattern of inheritance consistent with autosomal dominant transmission. A rare Paget's disease–like disorder, familial expansile osteolysis, has been mapped to chromosome 18q21-22; Paget's disease was mapped to the same locus in several families. However, in other families with Paget's disease, there is no linkage to 18q21-22, indicating genetic heterogeneity. In some sporadic osteosarcomas, there is constitutional loss of heterozygosity mapped to the same region of chromosome 18, and the rare sarcomas associated with Paget's disease (see below) also exhibit loss of heterozygosity in this region. It is of great interest that the gene within the 18q21-22 locus (*TNFRS-F11A* gene) responsible for familial expansile osteolysis encodes the receptor activator of NfκB (RANK), a member of the tumor necrosis factor (TNF) superfamily crucial for osteoclast differentiation (see below). The mutation results in constitutive activation of RANK. It is unknown whether similar mutations occur in some individuals with Paget's disease.

PATHOPHYSIOLOGY The characteristic feature is increased resorption of bone accompanied by an increase in bone formation. In the early phase, bone resorption predominates (e.g., in the variant *osteoporosis circumscripta*) and the bones are very vascular. This has been termed the *osteoporotic*, *osteolytic*, or *destructive phase* of disease. Body calcium balance may be negative. Commonly, the excessive resorption is followed closely by formation of new pagetic bone. In this so-called mixed phase of the disease, the rate of bone formation is so geared to that of bone resorption that the magnitude of the increase in bone turnover is not reflected in the overall calcium balance. As the activity decreases, the resorptive rate may decline progressively relative to formation, eventually leading to development of hard, dense, less vascular bone (the so-called *osteoplastic* or *sclerotic phase*) and a positive calcium balance. The rates of bone turnover may be increased enormously in the early phases of the disease, occasionally more than 20 times normal.

Increased generation and overactivity of osteoclasts are considered the major abnormality. The osteoclasts are larger than normal and contain multiple pleomorphic nuclei. Increased numbers of osteoclast-like multinucleated cells are generated from hematopoietic precursors in long-term marrow cultures from individuals with Paget's disease. Production of interleukin (IL) 6 by the pagetic bone (marrow) cells is increased, and the cells are more sensitive than normal to the pro-resorptive effects of $1{,}25(OH)_2D_3$.

The calcification rate is characteristically increased in pagetic bone. Bone turnover correlates with the increased plasma level of bone alkaline phosphatase, which is higher in Paget's disease than in any other condition except for hereditary hyperphosphatasia. Although increased bone resorption enhances release of calcium and phosphate ions from bone, the plasma concentrations of these ions are usually normal, presumably because of mineral deposition in new bone and because of feedback control of parathyroid hormone secretion. The concentration of phosphate in the plasma is normal or slightly elevated. When the imbalance between bone formation and resorption favors resorption, as after prolonged immobilization or fractures, urinary calcium excretion may be increased and on occasion hypercalcemia may occur. If, on the other hand, bone formation exceeds resorption (relatively uncommon), circulating levels of parathyroid hormone may be increased. Significant increases in trabecular bone resorption and osteoid surfaces in normal bone from patients with Paget's disease may be due to compensatory, secondary hyperparathyroidism. Resorption involves both the organic and mineral phases of bone. While the inorganic ions of the mineral phase are reutilized for bone formation, amino acids such as hydroxyproline and hydroxylysine and the hydroxypyridinium cross-link compounds are released during resorption of the collagen matrix of bone and are not reutilized for collagen biosynthesis. The increased urinary excretion of small peptides containing hydroxyproline reflects increased bone resorption. The pyridinium cross-link compounds pyridinoline (Pyr) and deoxypyridinoline (D-Pyr) are released from bone collagen during osteoclastic bone resorption and can be measured in urine by several commercial assays. The C- and N-telopeptide measurements are also useful for monitoring therapy, but measurements of serum alkaline phosphatase activity alone are usually sufficient.

RADIOLOGIC CHANGES The pelvic bones are most commonly involved, followed by the femur, skull, tibia, lumbosacral spine, dorsal spine, clavicles, and ribs; small bones are not as frequently diseased. The lytic phase of the disease may be overlooked except when it occurs in the skull as osteoporosis circumscripta, with areas of sharply demarcated radiolucency in the frontal, parietal, and occipital bones. In the long bones, the lytic areas are usually first seen at one end and progress toward the other end with a V-shaped advancing edge. The lesion may cause expansion of the cortex and exhibit features suggesting malignancy. Usually lysis is followed by a zone of increased density, representing the new bone formation of the mixed phase of the disease. In general, the bone enlarges with an irregularly widened cortex in a coarse, striated pattern and with increased density, occasionally focal in distribution. Perpendicular lines of radiolucency (cortical infractions) are frequent and occur on the convex side of bowed long bones, particularly the femur and tibia. The remodeling of the pagetic bone usually follows the lines of stress produced by muscle pull or gravity, accounting for the characteristic lateral bowing of the femur or anterior bowing of the tibia and the tendency for most of the dense bone to be deposited on the concave side of the bowed bone. In the mixed stage, there is enlargement and thickening of the skull, especially of the outer table, with irregular, spotty areas of increased density (Fig. 343-1). The changes in the pelvis reflect the varying degrees of bone resorption and new bone formation and are frequently accompanied by a characteristic thickening of the pelvic brim. In the sclerotic phase of the disease, the bone may show uniform increase in density, often in the absence of striations. This feature is common in the facial bones but occasionally occurs in the vertebrae, where a homogeneous, dense pattern gives an "ivory" appearance similar to that typical of Hodgkin's disease, although the involved vertebrae in Hodgkin's disease are not enlarged. Computed tomography (CT) and magnetic resonance imaging (MRI) are useful in defining atypical lesions, particularly when neoplastic involvement is suspected. Technetium 99m diphosphonate bone scans are useful in documenting the extent of disease when therapy is contemplated or to confirm the diagnosis when radiologic findings are inconclusive.

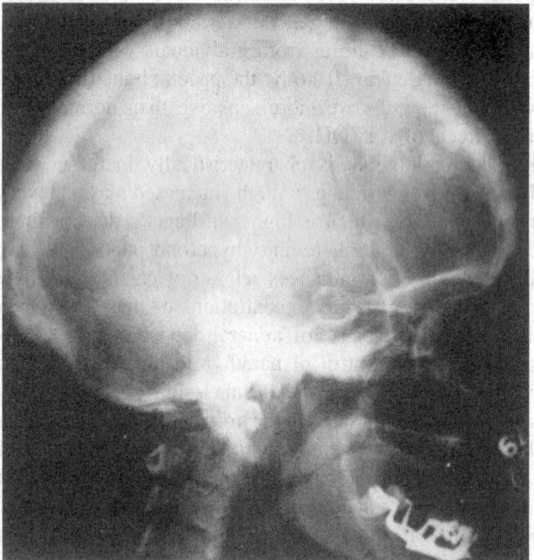

FIGURE 343-1 Lateral roentgenogram of the skull from a 58-year-old woman with Paget's disease of bone.

CLINICAL MANIFESTATIONS The clinical presentation is a function of the extent of the disease, the particular bones involved, and the presence of complications. Many patients are asymptomatic. In these individuals the disorder is discovered during radiologic examination of the pelvis or spine for another problem or because of the finding of an elevated level of plasma alkaline phosphatase. Other individuals may gradually become aware of a swelling or deformity of a long bone or develop a disturbance in gait due to unequal length of the lower extremities. Enlargement of the skull is often not noticed by the patients, except by awareness of increasing hat size. Facial pain and headache are initial complaints in some; backache and leg pain are common. The pain is usually dull but may be shooting or knifelike. Back pain is most common in the lumbar region and may radiate into the buttocks or lower extremities. This pain can be due to the pagetic process itself, to distortion of articular facets, or to secondary osteoarthritis. Pain in the lower extremities may be associated with the transverse cortical infractions along the convex lateral surface of the femur or the anterior surface of the tibia. New lytic lesions detected on bone scan may be the most painful. Pain may also be due to involvement of the hip joint resembling degenerative joint disease, which is characterized by narrowing of the joint space, bony lipping at the margin of the acetabulum, and deepening of the acetabulum. Angioid streaks may be present in the retina. Hearing loss can be due to direct involvement of the ossicles of the inner ear, involvement of bone in the region of the cochlea, or impingement on the eighth cranial nerve in the auditory foramen. More serious neurologic complications can result from overgrowth of bone at the base of the skull (platybasia) and compression of the brainstem. Compression of the spinal cord can cause paraplegia, particularly with involvement of the mid-dorsal spine. Pathologic fractures of vertebrae may also produce spinal cord lesions.

COMPLICATIONS Blood flow may be markedly increased in extremities involved with Paget's disease. There is proliferation of blood vessels in pagetic bone, but anatomic and functional studies have not confirmed the presence of arteriovenous fistulas. Although blood flow is increased in bone, cutaneous vasodilatation in the pagetic extremities accounts for the increased warmth noted clinically. When the disease is widespread, involving one-third or more of the skeleton, the increased blood flow raises *cardiac output* and rarely leads to high-output heart failure. However, heart disease in individuals with Paget's disease is usually due to the same conditions that occur in other patients of similar age. *Pathologic fracture* may occur at any stage but is more common in the destructive phase of the disease. In the weight-bearing bones fractures are often incomplete, multiple, and on the convex side of the bone. They may occur spontaneously or after slight trauma. Though many lesions heal with no major disability, more serious fractures also occur. Complete fractures are often transverse as if the bone was snapped like a piece of chalk.

There is no characteristic level of urinary calcium excretion, but it tends to be higher when the resorptive phase predominates, possibly accounting for the somewhat higher incidence of *urinary stones* in these patients. *Hyperuricemia* and gout are common in men with Paget's disease, and calcific periarthritis may occur.

Sarcoma is the dread complication. The incidence is probably ≤1%, although higher incidence has been noted in series that include many patients with polyostotic involvement. The sarcomas most frequently arise in the femur, humerus, skull, facial bones, and pelvis and rarely in the vertebrae. Pagetic osteosarcomas are lytic in appearance on radiographs, in contrast to the sclerotic appearance of radiation-induced osteosarcomas. The tumors are multicentric in about 20% of patients. Fibrosarcomas and chondrosarcomas have also been found.

Pain and swelling are the common complaints that lead to recognition of the sarcomas. The extent and character of the neoplastic involvement are established by CT and/or MRI. In occasional patients, an "explosive rise" of the phosphatase level may accompany the growth of the sarcoma, whereas in patients with limited Paget's disease, phosphatase levels may be only slightly elevated and give no clue to the development of the malignant lesion. The prognosis is poor following the development of sarcomas, and ablative surgery is rarely successful. In contrast to the successful treatment of some osteosarcomas in children, chemotherapy has little effect on survival of patients with pagetic osteosarcomas. Reparative granulomas resembling giant cell tumors may cause local destruction, but they do not metastasize.

℞ **TREATMENT** Most patients require no treatment, since the disease is localized and does not cause symptoms. Indications for therapy include persistent pain in involved bones, neural compression, rapidly progressive deformity resulting in disabling disturbance of posture and/or gait, high-output congestive heart failure, hypercalcemia, severe hypercalciuria with or without formation of renal stones, repeated fractures or nonunion, and preparation for major orthopedic surgery. Nonsteroidal anti-inflamatory drugs, such as one of the COX2 inhibitors or acetaminophen, may be useful to relieve pain, especially that involving the hip joints. Patients with severe hip or knee pain, unrelieved by analgesics and not responsive to therapy with agents that inhibit bone resorption, are candidates for total joint replacement. Results of joint replacement are often excellent, although patients with Paget's disease have an increased risk of ectopic bone formation around the operative site. Osteotomies are also useful in patients with bowing deformities of the tibia. In patients who have undergone surgical procedures, early ambulation and adequate fluid intake are important to prevent the development of hypercalciuria and hypercalcemia.

Potent bisphosphonates can inhibit bone resorption and are usually well tolerated. They appear to act by adsorbing to the surface of the calcium/phosphate mineral phase of bone and inhibiting osteoclast function. Bisphosphates are chemically stable analogues of inorganic pyrophosphate and are available in two classes: nitrogen-containing and non-nitrogen-containing. The non-nitrogen-containing bisphosphates (e.g., clodronate and etidronate) are metabolically incorporated into nonhydrolyzable analogues of ATP that may inhibit ATP-mediated reactions. The nitrogen-containing bisphosphates (e.g., pamidronate, alendronate, and risedronate) do not form ATP compounds, but they do inhibit enzymes in the mevalonate pathway, particularly enzymes involved in the synthesis of farnesyl pyrophosphate and geranylgeranyl pyrophosphate. The latter compounds are involved in protein prenylation reactions.

The first bisphosphate available for treatment of Paget's disease in the United States, editronate, was moderately effective in alleviating symptoms but did not decrease biochemical indices to the normal range. Editronate also inhibits mineralization of bone and produces osteomalacia. The newer bisphosphonates such as alendronate, pamidronate, risedronate, and tiludronate are more potent than etidronate and do not produce mineralization defects. Consequently, editronate is no longer indicated for treatment of Paget's disease. In the United States, pamidronate is approved for intravenous use, and alendronate and risedronate are approved for oral administration.

The bisphosphonates as a class are poorly absorbed from the gastrointestinal tract. Alendronate should be given orally with water after an overnight fast 30 to 60 min before breakfast; the dose is 40 mg/d for 6 months. Risedronate is administered at 30 mg/d for 2 to 3 months. Gastric irritability and rarely esophageal ulcerations may occur. Several regimens are advocated for the intravenous administration of pamidronate. For example, pamidronate is used intravenously as an infusion of 30 mg/d over 3 to 4 h in 5% glucose in water or normal saline on three or four successive days. Responses are usually rapid, with decreases in urinary excretion of hydroxyproline and pyridinium cross-link compounds within days to weeks, followed by a fall in levels of serum alkaline phosphatase. Flulike symptoms accompanied by fever may occur but usually subside rapidly.

Patients given bisphosphonates should also be given daily calcium supplements of 1 to 1.5 g and approximately 400 IU of vitamin D. Clinical and biochemical improvement often lasts for more than a year after bisphosphonate therapy. Clinical evaluation and assessment of alkaline phosphatase levels at 3-month intervals are useful for assessing the need for retreatment. Radiographs at 6-month intervals may be indicated for evaluation of lytic lesions, which usually heal with these agents.

Calcitonin therapy has largely been replaced by bisphosphonates for primary treatment of severe disease, but calcitonin may still be useful in patients who cannot tolerate alendronate or residronate because of gastrointestinal side effects or who prefer to avoid intravenous therapy with pamidronate. The administration of porcine, salmon, and human *calcitonins* for prolonged periods decreases plasma alkaline phosphatase and urinary hydroxyproline excretion. Treatment with calcitonin variably decreases bone pain due to suppression of the pagetic lesion as well as to an independent, centrally mediated analgesic effect. The calcitonins are probably most useful in patients with pain in areas of pagetic involvement not due to associated joint disease. The dose of salmon calcitonin is 50 to 100 MRC units daily given subcutaneously. In most cases, it is possible to reduce the dose to three times weekly. Some patients develop a sensation of warmth and/or nausea 30 min to several hours after injection. Nasal spray formulations of calcitonin can be administered at doses of 200 IU/d. Cytotoxic drugs such as plicamycin and dactinomycin no longer have a place in therapy.

Although the bisphosphonates and calcitonins act primarily to decrease bone resorption, the rate of new bone formation subsequently falls. As a result, the state of high bone turnover is shifted to a state of lower turnover, where rates of formation and resorption are still apparently geared to each other. In this lower turnover state, collagen fibers of the bone matrix are deposited in a more orderly fashion similar to normal bone.

HYPEROSTOSIS

A number of disease states have in common an increase in the mass of bone per unit volume (*hyperostosis*) (Table 343-1). This increase in bone mass is often associated with disturbance in the architecture of the tissue. The additional bone may be located at the periosteum, within the compact bone of the cortex, or in the trabeculae of the cancellous regions. In some diseases, the increase in bone mass may be spotty, as in osteopoikilosis, whereas in others, most of the skeleton may be involved, as in the malignant form of osteopetrosis in children. The increase in mass is usually not due to an excessive amount of mineral relative to matrix, except in disorders where islands of calcified cartilage may persist such as osteopetrosis. In some diseases, such as the osteosclerosis of untreated renal insufficiency, bone mass and radiodensity may be increased, even though the new bone formed is poorly mineralized and contains widened osteoid seams.

Although hyperostosis is usually due to decreased numbers of osteoclasts or altered osteoclast function, dysfunction of osteoblasts can also occur. For example, an engineered null mutation of the osteocalcin gene in mice results in a higher bone mass due to increased bone formation without change in bone resorption. Infection of newborn mice also produces an osteopetrosis-like phenotype in which osteoblast progenitors appear to induce increased bone formation. In human osteopetrosis of the relatively benign and sporadic type, viral nucleocapsid particles have been found in osteoclasts, and it is possible that viral infection accounts for the excessive bone mass.

OSTEOPETROSIS Also known as Albers-Schönberg or marble bone disease, osteopetrosis is clinically, biochemically, and genetically heterogeneous. Although osteopetrosis has many causes, a defect in bone resorption is always the underlying mechanism.

Table 343-1 Causes of Hyperostosis

Endocrine disorders
- Primary hyperparathyroidism
- Hypothyroidism
- Acromegaly

Radiation osteitis
Chemical poisoning
- Fluoride
- Elemental phosphorus
- Beryllium
- Arsenic
- Vitamin A intoxication
- Lead
- Bismuth

Osteomalacia
- Renal tubular osteomalacia (vitamin D resistance or phosphate diabetes)
- Chronic renal glomerular failure

Osteosclerosis (localized) associated with chronic infection
Osteosclerotic phase of Paget's disease
Osteosclerosis associated with carcinomatous metastases, malignant lymphoma, and hematologic disorders (myeloproliferative disorders, sickle cell disease, leukemia, multiple myeloma, systemic mastocytosis)
Osteosclerosis of erythroblastosis fetalis
Osteopetrosis
- Infantile (malignant, autosomal recessive form)
- Adult (benign, dominant form)
- Intermediate form with carbonic anhydrase II deficiency and renal tubular acidosis

Unclassified disorders
- Pyknodysostosis
- Osteomyelosclerosis
- Hyperostosis corticalis generalisata
- Hyperostosis generalisata with pachydermia
- Hereditary hyperphosphatasia
- Progressive diaphyseal dysplasia (osteopathia hyperostotica multiplex infantilis; Camurati-Engelmann disease)
- Melorheostosis
- Osteopoikilosis
- Hyperostosis frontalis interna

Several inherited forms of osteopetrosis occur in rodents, some of which can be cured by bone marrow transplantation from a normal littermate and are probably due to stem cell defects. The osteopetrosis in *op/op* mice and in *tl/tl* toothless rats is not cured by bone marrow transplantation, however. These animals have few osteoclasts, and those that are present appear to be defective. The *op/op* mice have a defect in the coding region of the gene for macrophage colony stimulating factor (M-CSF). The skeletal defects in these animals and in *tl/tl* rats can be reversed by treatment with M-CSF. Another form of osteopetrosis has been produced in mice by targeted disruption of the c-*src* gene, which is normally expressed at high levels in osteoclasts. These *src*−/− mice still have osteoclasts on bone surfaces, but they fail to form a ruffled border at the bone-resorbing surface. Disruption of the c-*fos* gene results in osteopetrosis in which osteoclasts are absent.

Important advances have also been made in understanding the interactions between osteoblasts/stromal cells and hemopoietic osteoclast precursor cells that lead to osteoclastogenesis (Fig. 343-2). A novel member of the TNF receptor superfamily, referred to as *osteoprotegerin* (OPG; also known as *osteoclastogenesis inhibitory factor*, OCIF) functions as a soluble decoy receptor that binds, and presumably neutralizes, RANK ligand, a transmembrane ligand expressed on osteoblasts/stromal cells. RANK ligand binds to RANK, a transmembrane receptor on hemopoietic osteoclast precursor cells, to activate osteoclast differentiation and function (Chap. 340). The RANK receptor binds to intracellular signaling molecules called *TNF receptor–associated factors* (TRAFs) that activate NFκB, a transcription factor known to be required for normal osteoclast function. Genetic models in mice are beginning to unravel this complex signaling pathway. Expression of a soluble version of RANK ligand stimulates osteoclast differentiation. Overexpression of OPG in transgenic mice leads to osteopetrosis, apparently by blocking RANK ligand. Mice deficient in RANK lack osteoclasts and develop severe osteopetrosis (as well as T cell immunologic defects). TRAF6-deficient mice also develop osteopetrotic features because of defective osteoclast function. It is clear, based on these and other lines of evidence, that the RANK ligand/OPG/RANK/TRAF/NFκB pathway plays a pivotal role in the control of osteoclast development and function.

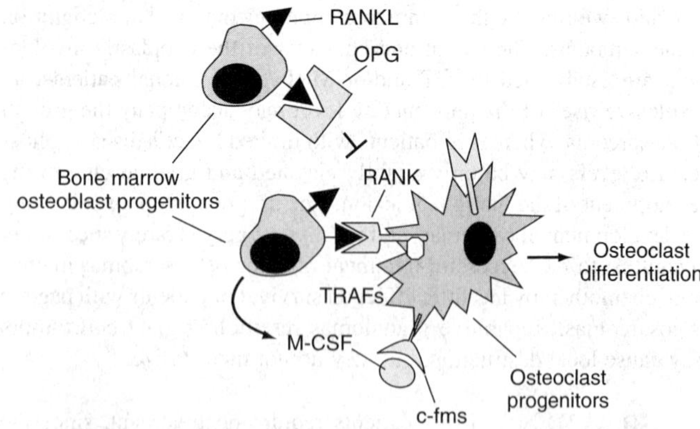

FIGURE 343-2 Role of the RANK pathway in osteoclast differentiation and function. Stromal bone marrow cells produce multiple growth factors and cytokines, including macrophage colony stimulating factor (M-CSF), to modulate osteoclastogenesis. RANKL (receptor activator of NFκB ligand) is produced by osteoblast progenitors. It can bind to a soluble decoy receptor known as OPG (osteoprotegerin) to inhibit action of the RANKL. Alternatively, a cell-cell interaction between osteoblast and osteoclast progenitors allows RANKL to bind to its membrane-bound receptor, RANK, thereby stimulating osteoclast differentiation and function. RANK binds intracellular proteins called TRAFs (tumor necrosis factor receptor–associated factors) that mediate receptor signaling through transcription factors such as NFκB. M-CSF binds to its receptor, c-fms, the cellular homologue of the *fms* oncogene. See text for the potential role of these pathways in disorders of osteoclast function such as osteopetrosis.

In humans the infantile autosomal recessive form of osteopetrosis, until recently, has been of unknown cause. It is a severe bone disease that is usually fatal within the first decade of life. Osteoclasts are usually present in normal or increased numbers. In addition, since bone resorption is markedly suppressed, it has been assumed that the defect is not in genes responsible for osteoclast differentiation but in those responsible for osteoclast function. This form of osteopetrosis is manifested in utero and progresses after birth with anemia, hepatosplenomegaly, hydrocephalus, cranial nerve involvement, and death, often due to infections. Transplantation of bone marrow from allogeneic donors to provide normal osteoclast precursor cells has been successful in several patients, in whom osteopetrotic bone was repopulated with donor osteoclasts that produced radiologic and/or bone-biopsy evidence of bone resorption. Nearly 100 bone marrow transplantations have been reported over the past 15 years. If the transplants are successful, markers of donor cells can be found in bone resorbing areas and skeletal improvement persists for years. Although restoration of visual acuity usually does not occur with successful transplantation, this is the only means of approaching cure even in mild cases. The genetic defect in about half of the subjects studied has now been identified. The gene in the human disease was mapped to chromosome 11q13, a region that contains several potential candidate genes. In mice, introduction of a null mutation in one of the genes in this region, *Tcirg1*, that encodes the osteoclast-specific (*OC116*) subunit of the vacuolar proton pump ([V]-type H^+-ATPase) responsible for acidification of the extracellular compartment adjacent to the brush border, results in osteopetrosis with abundant osteoclasts. Furthermore a deletion of the 5′ portion of the gene is the cause for the defect in *oc/oc* mice with spontaneous osteopetrosis. In approximately half of the human subjects with the autosomal recessive form of osteopetrosis so far examined, missense, frameshift, or potential splicing mutations have just been identified in the homologous gene, *TC1RG1*. Thus, mutations in *TG1RG1* are a frequent, although not the sole, cause of this form of osteopetrosis.

Less fulminant forms of osteopetrosis occur in older children and adults. In some the disorder appears to be sporadic, and in others the osteopetrosis is inherited as an autosomal dominant trait and progresses with age; anemia is not as severe, neurologic abnormalities are not as frequent, and recurrent pathologic fractures are the main feature. Although the disorder is most common in infants and children, the diagnosis may be made in adults when roentgenograms are obtained because of fractures or unrelated diseases.

An "intermediate" form of autosomal recessive osteopetrosis has been described in kindreds in which the skeletal abnormality is associated with renal tubular acidosis and cerebral calcification. This form is compatible with long survival and is associated with profound impairment of the activity of one of the isoenzymes of carbonic anhydrase (carbonic anhydrase II). Carbonic anhydrase II is a major component of the system that generates the acid environment adjacent to the ruffled border of the osteoclast. Deficiency of the enzyme impairs bone resorption. The defect in remodeling results in disorganization of bone structure, with thickened cortices and lack of funnelization of metaphyses. Despite increased density, the bone may be abnormal mechanically and can fracture readily. Osteomalacia or rickets is sometimes a component of osteopetrosis in children.

Roentgenograms reveal uniformly dense, sclerotic bone, often with no distinction between the cortical and cancellous regions (Fig. 343-3). In the severe infantile form, there is persistence of the primary spongiosa with central calcified cartilage cores surrounded by woven bone. Osteoclasts may be increased in number but do not function normally due to the acidification defect that results from the mutated vacuolar proton pump. In other forms of osteopetrosis, there may be different morphologic abnormalities such as loss of ruffled borders. The variability may reflect heterogeneity in this syndrome, as in the osteopetrosis in rodents. The long bones are usually involved, with increased density along the entire shaft. The metaphyses have a characteristic clubbed or splayed appearance. Alternating horizontal bands of increased and decreased density in the long bones and vertebrae suggest that the defect is intermittent during periods of growth. The skull, pelvis, ribs, and other bones may be involved. The phalanges and the distal humerus are usually spared.

Encroachment of bone on the marrow cavity, particularly in the severe infantile disorder, is associated with anemia of the myelophthisic type with extramedullary hematopoiesis in liver, spleen, and lymph nodes and enlargement of these organs. Neurologic abnormalities caused by encroachment on cranial nerves include optic atrophy, nystagmus, papilledema, exophthalmos, and impairment of extraocular muscles. Facial paralysis and deafness are frequent; trigeminal lesions and anosmia are less common. In infants, macrocephaly, hydrocephalus, and convulsions may occur, and infections such as osteomyelitis are frequent. Renal tubular acidosis is a feature of the osteopetrosis associated with carbonic anhydrase II deficiency.

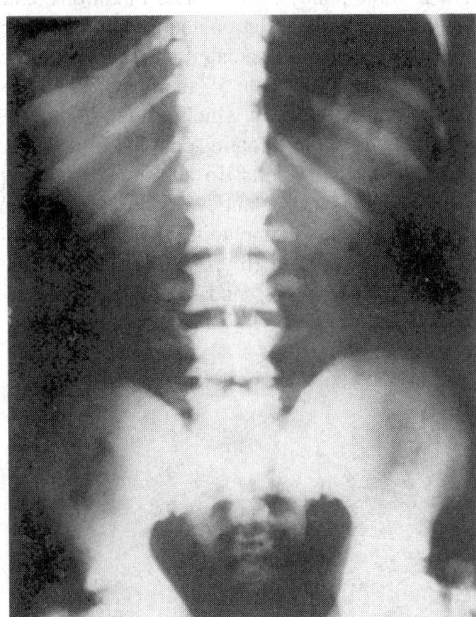

FIGURE 343-3 Roentgenogram of the spine and pelvis of a 55-year-old man with the more benign, dominant form of osteopetrosis.

In the less severe forms, about half of patients have no symptoms, and the disorder is discovered incidentally on roentgenograms. Others present with fractures, bone pain, osteomyelitis, and cranial nerve palsies.

Fractures may occur with trivial trauma. Healing of such fractures is usually slow but satisfactory. When the disease is manifested first in adult life, fractures may be the only clinical problem. Levels of calcium and alkaline phosphatase in the plasma are usually normal in adults, but hypophosphatemia and moderate hypocalcemia may occur in children. Serum acid phosphatase levels are usually increased.

As mentioned, in children with severe osteopetrosis, bone marrow transplantation from allogeneic donors or HLA-identical siblings has resulted in histologic and radiologic increases in bone resorption and variable improvement in anemia, vision, hearing, and growth and development. Unfortunately, it is not always possible to find appropriate donors, or patients may not be good candidates for bone marrow transplantation. In some patients with the lethal forms of the disorder, calcitriol therapy is associated with the appearance of osteoclasts with normal ruffled borders and other evidence of increased bone resorption.

PYKNODYSOSTOSIS Pyknodysostosis is an autosomal recessive form of osteosclerosis that superficially resembles osteopetrosis. It is a form of short-limbed dwarfism associated with bone fragility and a tendency to fracture with minimal trauma. Nevertheless, life span is usually normal. In addition to a generalized increase in bone density, features include short stature; separated cranial sutures; hypoplasia of the mandible; kyphoscoliosis and deformities of the trunk; persistence of deciduous teeth; progressive acroosteolysis of the terminal phalanges; high, arched palate; proptosis; blue sclerae; and a pointed, beaked nose. Patients usually present because of frequent fractures. The disorder is caused by mutations in a gene on chromosome 1q21 that encodes cathepsin K, a cysteine protease that is expressed in normal osteoclasts. Null mutations in the cathepsin K gene in mice result in a phenotype with many features of pyknodysostosis. Osteoclasts are present but do not function normally since there is no proteinase secreted into the area adjacent to the ruffled border where bone collagen resorption normally takes place.

OSTEOMYELOSCLEROSIS In osteomyelosclerosis, the marrow cells are replaced by diffuse fibroplasia, occasionally accompanied by osseous metaplasia and increased skeletal density on roentgenograms. In early stages woven bone may be found in intratrabecular locations, whereas in more advanced stages, woven bone is observed in the medulla. The disorder is probably a phase in the course of the myeloproliferative disorders and is characteristically accompanied by extramedullary hematopoiesis.

Hyperostosis corticalis generalisata (van Buchem's disease) is characterized by osteosclerosis of the skull (base and calvaria), lower jaw, clavicles, and ribs and thickening of the diaphyseal cortices of the long and short bones. Alkaline phosphatase levels in the serum are elevated, and the disorder may be due to increased formation of bone of normal structure. The major manifestations are due to neural compression and consist of optic atrophy, facial paralysis, and perception deafness. In *hyperostosis generalisata with pachydermia* (Uehlinger), the sclerosis is due to increased formation of subperiosteal spongy bone and involves the epiphyses, metaphyses, and diaphyses. Pain, swelling of joints, and thickening of the skin of the lower arms are common.

HEREDITARY HYPERPHOSPHATASIA This disorder is characterized by structural deformities of the skeleton, with increased thickness of the calvaria, increased density at the base of the skull, and widening and loss of normal architecture of the shafts and the epiphyses of the long and short bones. The failure to deposit normal bone and the haphazard orientation of lamellae suggest active remodeling that resembles that of Paget's disease. Osteoclasts with multiple nuclei characteristic of Paget's disease and the typical "mosaic" pattern of faceted units of lamellar bone are not found, however. Levels of plasma alkaline phosphatase and urinary excretion of hydroxyproline peptides and other collagen-degradation products are increased. The disorder is apparently inherited as an autosomal recessive trait. Treatment with bisphosphonates or calcitonin therapy may be of value.

PROGRESSIVE DIAPHYSEAL DYSPLASIA (CAMURATI-ENGELMANN DISEASE) This is an autosomal dominant disorder in which a symmetric thickening and increased diameter of the diaphyses of long bones occurs, particularly in the femur, tibia, fibula, radius, and ulna. Pain over affected areas, fatigue, abnormal gait, and muscle wasting are the major manifestations. Serum alkaline phosphatase levels may be elevated, and, on occasion, hypocalcemia and hyperphosphatemia may be found. Other abnormalities include anemia, leukopenia, and an elevated erythrocyte sedimentation rate. Linkage studies have localized a candidate gene (*DPD1*) to chromosome 19q13.2. Clinical and biochemical improvement may result from the use of glucocorticoids.

MELORHEOSTOSIS This rare, sporadic condition usually begins in childhood and is characterized by a slowly progressive linear hyperostosis in one or more bones of one limb, usually in a lower extremity. All segments of the bone may be involved, with sclerotic areas that have a "flowing" distribution. The involved limb is often extremely painful. Soft tissue masses, not connected to bone, are often mineralized and are composed of osseous or cartilaginous tissue. Other types of soft tissue masses are associated with joint contractures or consist of fibrofatty, lymphatic, or vascular tissue.

OSTEOPOIKILOSIS This is a benign autosomal dominant trait usually discovered by chance. In some families, the occurrence of melorheostosis suggests that these disorders may involve the same genetic locus. Osteopoikilosis is characterized by dense spots of trabecular bone <1 cm in diameter, usually of uniform density, located in the epiphyses and adjacent parts of the metaphyses. All bones may be involved except the skull, ribs, and vertebrae.

HYPEROSTOSIS FRONTALIS INTERNA This is an abnormality of the inner table of the frontal bones of the skull consisting of smooth, rounded enostoses covered by dura and projecting into the cranial cavity. These enostoses are usually <1 cm at their greatest diameter and do not extend posteriorly beyond the coronal suture. The abnormality is found almost exclusively in women who are frequently obese, hirsute, and may have a variety of neuropsychiatric complaints (Morgagni-Stewart-Morel syndrome). The disorder also occurs in women with no obvious illness or particular associated disease. The finding in the skull may be a manifestation of a generalized metabolic disorder.

FIBROUS DYSPLASIA (MCCUNE-ALBRIGHT SYNDROME)

The bony lesions of fibrous dysplasia are characterized by proliferation of fibroblast-like cells that in some areas have features of osteoblasts, with production of an extracellular matrix that may be calcified and have the appearance of woven bone. In other areas the cells have features of chondrocytes and produce a cartilage-like extracellular matrix. The lesions of fibrous dysplasia are usually focal and have a radiolucent appearance; they may be monostotic or polyostotic. The disorder occurs with equal frequency in both sexes. Some individuals have distinctive areas of skin pigmentation and precocious puberty (McCune-Albright syndrome) (Chap. 336). These diverse manifestations are the consequence of postzygotic mutations in the gene encoding the regulatory $G_{s\alpha}$ proteins.

INCIDENCE The monostotic form is the most common type of fibrous dysplasia. The lesions can be asymptomatic, can be associated with local pain, or predispose to pathologic fracture. Most of the lesions are in the ribs or in the craniofacial bones, especially the maxillae. Other bones that may be affected include metaphyseal or diaphyseal portions of the proximal femurs or tibias. Monostotic fibrous dysplasia is most often diagnosed in patients between 20 and 30 years of age. There are usually no associated skin lesions. Approximately one-quarter of the individuals with the polyostotic form have more than half the skeleton involved by disease. One side of the body may be affected, and the lesions may be distributed segmentally in a limb, particularly in the lower extremities. Craniofacial lesions are present in approximately half of patients with the polyostotic form. Whereas the monostotic form is usually detected in young adults, fractures and skeletal deformities occur in childhood in the polyostotic form; early-onset disease is generally more severe. Lesions, especially monostotic lesions, can become quiescent at puberty and worsen during pregnancy. McCune-Albright syndrome (polyostotic fibrous dysplasia, multiple café au lait spots, and sexual precocity) is more common (10:1) in females. Short stature is due to premature closure of the epiphyses.

PATHOPHYSIOLOGY Histologically, the lesions contain benign-appearing fibroblastic tissue arranged in a loose whorled pattern (Fig. 343-4). Malignant transformation of either monostotic or polyostotic fibrous dysplasia occurs with a frequency of $<1\%$. The malignant change is usually detected in the third or fourth decade in individuals who have had lesions first identified in childhood. In about one-third of the cases the neoplasms arise in previously irradiated lesions. Ossifying fibroma of long bones is a peculiar fibroosseous cortical lesion that may be a variant of fibrous dysplasia. It is most common in the tibial shaft in teenagers. Although benign, the lesion has a tendency to recur if not adequately excised.

Fibrous dysplasia and McCune-Albright syndrome represent a phenotypic spectrum of disorders caused by activating mutations in the *GNAS1* gene, which encodes the $G_{s\alpha}$ protein. Because these postzygotic mutations occur at different stages in early development, the extent and type of tissues affected by the mutations are variable, explaining the mosaic pattern of skin and bone changes. The mutations occur in regions (e.g., Arg 201) of $G_{s\alpha}$ that selectively inhibit its GTPase activity. Because the GTP-bound form of the regulatory protein confers its active state (Chap. 341), the mutations confer constitutive stimulation of the cyclic AMP–protein kinase A signal transduction pathway. The mutations in *GNAS1* are also found in patients with fibrous dysplasia without manifestations of the McCune-Albright syndrome. Thus, in the boney lesions these mutations result in abnormalities in osteoblastic differentiation and the production of abnormal bone. In addition, there is an associated increase in osteoclastic bone resorption that provides a rationale for therapy with the bisphosphonate, pamidronate. Other tissues in which growth control and function are strongly regulated by $G_{s\alpha}$ protein–coupled receptors are particularly susceptible to the mutations. In addition to bone (parathyroid hormone receptor) and skin (melanocyte-stimulating hormone receptor), various endocrine glands, including the ovary (follicle-stimulating hormone receptor), thyroid (thyroid-stimulating hormone receptor), adrenal (ACTH-receptor), and pituitary (growth hormone–

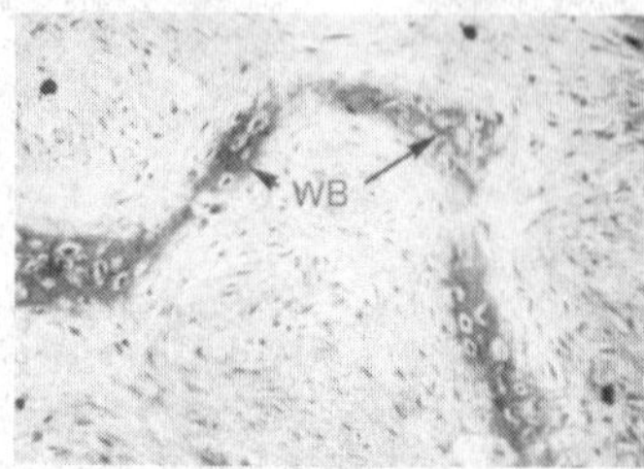

FIGURE 343-4 Photomicrograph of the lesion of fibrous dysplasia. Note spicules of dark-staining woven bone (WB) surrounded by loose fibroblastic tissue.

releasing hormone receptor), are commonly affected by the $G_{s\alpha}$ mutations. It is of interest that the genetic abnormality in Albright's hereditary osteodystrophy (pseudohypoparathyroidism) is the opposite of that found in the McCune-Albright syndrome. In the former, alterations in $G_{s\alpha}$ function or expression result in *deficient* activity and decreased responsiveness to hormones that function through cyclic AMP–mediated signal transduction pathways (Chap. 341).

RADIOLOGIC CHANGES The roentgenographic appearance of the lesions is that of a radiolucent area with a well-delineated, smooth or scalloped border, typically associated with focal thinning of the cortex of the bone (Fig. 343-5). Fibrous dysplasia can cause bones to become larger than normal, a feature characteristic of Paget's disease as well. The "ground-glass" appearance is due to the thin spicules of calcified woven bone. Deformities can include coxa vara, shepherd's-crook deformity of the femur, bowing of the tibia, Harrison's grooves, and protrusio acetabuli. Involvement of facial bones, usually with lesions of increased radiodensity, may create a leonine appearance (*leontiasis ossea*). Fibrous dysplasia of the temporal bones can cause progressive loss of hearing and obliteration of the external ear canal. Advanced skeletal age in girls is correlated with sexual precocity but can occur in boys without sexual precocity. Occasionally, a focus of fibrous dysplasia may undergo cystic degeneration, with an enormous distortion of the shape of the bone, and mimic the so-called aneurysmal bone cyst.

CLINICAL MANIFESTATIONS The clinical course is variable. Skeletal lesions are usually detected because of localized pain, deformities, or fractures. Other symptoms ascribable to bone involvement are headache, seizures, cranial nerve abnormalities, hearing loss, narrowing of the external ear canal, or even spontaneous scalp hemorrhages if there is craniofacial bone disease. On rare occasions the onset of sexual precocity is the first clinical manifestation of the McCune-Albright syndrome. Serum calcium and phosphorus values are usually normal. In approximately one-third of patients with the polyostotic form, bone turnover is increased, as reflected by high levels of serum alkaline phosphatase and increased urinary excretion of collagen breakdown products. In some patients high cardiac output resembles that in extensive Paget's disease. Widespread disease does not usually develop when the disease is mild at the outset.

The cutaneous pigmentation in most patients with McCune-Albright syndrome consists of isolated dark-brown to light-brown mac-

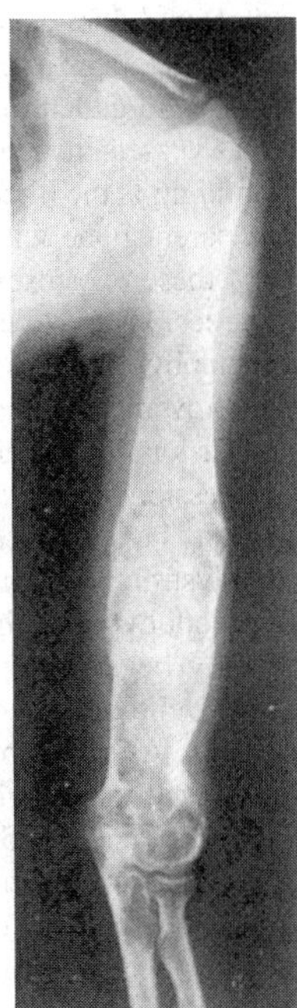

FIGURE 343-5 Roentgenogram of the upper extremity from a 33-year-old woman with fibrous dysplasia of bone. Typical lesions involve the entire humerus as well as the scapula and proximal ulna.

ules that tend to be located on one side of the midline (Fig. 343-6). The border is usually, although not always, irregular or jagged ("coast of Maine"), in contrast to the smooth borders of the pigmented macules of neurofibromatosis ("coast of California"). As a rule, there are fewer than six of the lesions, which range in size from 1 cm to very large lesions, covering areas such as the back, buttocks, or sacral regions. When the lesions are in the scalp, the overlying hair may be more deeply pigmented. Localized alopecia is associated with osteomas of the skin, and such lesions tend to overly skeletal lesions. The pigmentation also tends to be on the same side as the skeletal lesions and actually to overlie them. Occasionally, neurofibromatosis and fibrous dysplasia coexist.

Sexual precocity occurs more commonly in girls than in boys. Premature vaginal bleeding, breast development, and growth of axillary and pubic hair are the usual features. Sexual precocity is due to autonomous end-organ activity, not to pituitary or hypothalamic dysfunction. Thus, girls have high estrogen levels and low or undetectable gonadotropins. The characteristic pigmented macules are usual but not invariable. Hyperthyroidism occurs with increased frequency, and rare associations include Cushing's syndrome, acromegaly, pulmonary lesions, and soft tissue myxomas. Hypophosphatemic osteomalacia may also accompany fibrous dysplasia and resembles the disorder associated with other skeletal and nonskeletal tumors.

Although the lytic lesions of fibrous dysplasia resemble the brown tumors of hyperparathyroidism, the age of the patient, normal calcium levels, increased density of bone in the skull, and areas of cutaneous pigmentation identify the former condition. Fibrous dysplasia and hyperparathyroidism may coexist, however. Neurofibromas may involve bone and produce cutaneous pigmentation as well as nodules in the skin. The pigmented macules of neurofibromatosis are more numerous and more widely distributed than in fibrous dysplasia, usually have smooth borders, and tend to involve areas such as the axillary folds. Other lesions that have roentgenographic features similar to those of isolated fibrous dysplasia are unicameral bone cysts, aneurysmal bone cysts, and nonossifying fibromas. Leontiasis ossea is most often due to fibrous dysplasia, although other disorders may also produce this appearance, such as craniometaphyseal dysplasia, hyperphosphatasia, and, in adults, Paget's disease.

℞ **TREATMENT** Fibrous dysplasia is not curable. The skeletal lesions, however, can be improved by orthopedic procedures such as casting, osteotomy with internal fixation, curettage, and bone grafting, depending on the lesion and the age of the patient. Indications for such procedures include progressive deformity, nonunion of fractures,

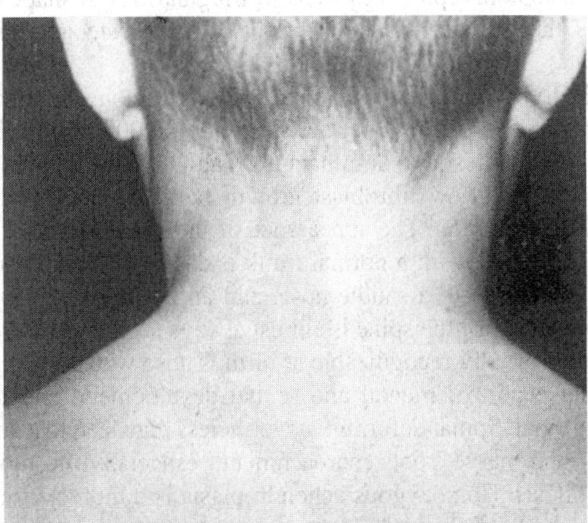

FIGURE 343-6 Typical pigmented café au lait lesion of the skin in an 11-year-old boy with polyostotic fibrous dysplasia. The border has the jagged "coast of Maine" appearance that is characteristic of McCune-Albright's syndrome. Note that the lesion is limited to one side (left) of the body.

and pain unresponsive to conservative treatment. Calcitonin may be effective in treatment of widespread disease associated with bone pain and high serum alkaline phosphatase levels. Pamidronate (0.5 to 1 mg/kg per day intravenously for 2 to 3 days) at 6-month or yearly intervals has been shown to reduce bone pain with refilling of osteolytic lesions in about half of patients and to decrease elevated levels of serum alkaline phosphatase and urinary hydroxyproline excretion. Precocious puberty does not respond to long-acting gonadotropin-releasing hormone (GnRH) analogues, consistent with the autonomous function of the gonads. Aromatase inhibitors, such as testolactone (22 mg/kg per day), have been used to block estrogen production, but with limited efficacy. Promising initial results have been seen with estrogen antagonists, such as tamoxifen. In addition to preventing pubertal progression, blockade of estrogen action is helpful to prevent early epiphyseal closure and short stature.

OTHER DYSPLASIAS OF BONE AND CARTILAGE

A variety of diseases of bone and cartilage have been called *dystrophies* or *dysplasias*. The *osteochondrodysplasias* are heritable disorders of connective tissue characterized by primary abnormalities of cartilage that lead to disturbances in cartilage and bone growth and development. They comprise several hundred distinct entities, which can be distinguished on the basis of clinical, genetic, and radiologic features. The molecular defects in a number of these disorders have been identified utilizing positional cloning and screening of candidate genes. Several of the disorders are due to mutations in collagen genes. →*For discussion of chondrodysplasias, see Chap. 351.*

SPONDYLOEPIPHYSEAL DYSPLASIA The *spondyloepiphyseal dysplasias* are disorders in which abnormalities of growth occur in various bones, including the vertebrae, pelvis, carpal and tarsal bones, and the epiphyses of tabular bones. On the basis of roentgenographic findings, this group can be divided into (1) those with generalized platyspondyly, (2) those with multiple epiphyseal dysplasias, and (3) those with epiphysometaphyseal dysplasias. *Morquio's syndrome*, in which there is a defect in degradation of glycosaminoglycans (therefore, a "mucopolysaccharidosis"), is inherited as an autosomal recessive trait and is associated with corneal opacities, dental defects, variable disturbances in intellect, and increased urinary excretion of keratosulfate; it belongs in the first group (Chap. 349). Other forms of spondyloepiphyseal dysplasia, some of which are accounted for by defects in type II collagen, may not be recognized until late in childhood or young adult life. Flat vertebral bodies are associated with other abnormalities in shape and alignment. The disordered development of the capital femoral epiphyses leads to irregularities in shape and flattening of the femoral heads and early onset of osteoarthritis of the hips.

ACHONDROPLASIA This disorder is among the more common types of dwarfism (1 in 15,000 to 1 in 40,000 live births). It is inherited as an autosomal dominant trait, although most cases are sporadic and due to new fibroblast growth factor receptor 3 (FGFR3) mutations (see below). The appearance of short limbs, particularly the proximal portions, with a normal trunk is characteristically accompanied by a large head, a saddle nose, and an exaggerated lumbar lordosis. The length of the spine is almost always normal. Features of the disorder are usually recognizable at birth. Those who survive infancy usually have normal mental and sexual development, and life span may be normal. Spinal deformity nevertheless may lead to a cord compression and nerve root encroachment, especially in those with kyphoscoliosis. Homozygous achondroplasia is a more serious disorder and a cause of neonatal death.

The most common mutation responsible for achondroplasia substitutes an arginine for glycine in the transmembrane domain of FGFR3 and causes a gain-of-function, implying that fibroblast growth factor normally acts via the FGFR3 to inhibit chondrocyte proliferation in the growth plate. The abnormal proliferation at the growth plate, leaving other areas relatively unaffected in the tubular bones, causes production of short bones that are proportionately thick. Formation and maturation of the secondary ossification centers and articular cartilage are not disturbed. Appositional growth at the metaphysis continues, with resulting flare in this region of the bone; intramembranous bone formation at the periosteum is normal. Consistent with the inhibitory role of the FGFR3, a null mutation of the *Fgfr3* gene in mice causes increased growth in the physis. Mutations in other domains of the *FGFR3* gene have been described in thanatophoric dysplasia, the most severe and lethal dysplasia. In several types of the so-called craniosynostosis syndromes (Pfeiffer, Crouzon, Jackson-Weiss, and Apert syndromes), mutations have been identified in the *FGFR1* or *FGFR2* genes.

Pseudoachondroplasia clinically resembles achondroplasia with respect to the limb deformities but there are no skull abnormalities. Affected individuals have mutations in the gene encoding a non-collagenous component of cartilage called cartilate oligomeric matrix protein (COMP). Mutations in the *COMP* gene have also been described in one of the less severe forms of multiple epiphyseal dysplasia (EDM1).

ENCHONDROMATOSIS (DYSCHONDROPLASIA, OLLIER'S DISEASE) This is also a disorder of the growth plate in which the hypertrophic cartilage is not resorbed and ossified normally. It results in masses of cartilage with disorderly arrangement of the chondrocytes showing variable proliferative and hypertrophic changes. These masses are located in the metaphyses in close association with the growth plate in children but may be diaphyseal in teenagers and young adults. The disorder is usually recognized in childhood by the appearance of deformities or retardation in growth. The most common sites of involvement are the ends of long bones, usually in the region where rate of growth is most marked. The pelvis is often involved, but ribs, sternum, and skull are seldom affected. There is a tendency toward unilateral involvement. Chondrosarcoma develops occasionally in the enchondromata. The association of enchondromatosis and cavernous hemangiomata in the soft tissues including the skin is known as *Maffucci's syndrome*. Both Ollier's disease and Maffuci's syndrome have been associated with other primary malignancies as diverse as granulosa cell tumor of the ovary and cerebral gliomas.

MULTIPLE EXOSTOSES (DIAPHYSEAL ACLASIS OR OSTEOCHONDROMATOSIS) This is a disorder of the metaphysis, transmitted in an autosomal dominant manner, in which areas of the growth plate become displaced, presumably by growing through a defect in the perichondrium, or so-called ring of Ranvier. The spongiosa forms within the mass as vessels invade the cartilage. Therefore, the diagnostic radiographic finding is the direct continuity of the mass to the marrow cavity of the parent bone with absence of underlying cortex. Usually the growth of these exostoses ceases when growth of the adjacent plate ceases. The lesions may be solitary or multiple and are usually located in the metaphyseal areas of long bones, with the apex of the exostosis directed toward the diaphysis. Often the lesions produce no symptoms, but occasionally, interference with the function of a joint or tendon or compression of nerves may result. Dwarfism may occur. The metacarpals may be shortened, resembling those seen in Albright's hereditary osteodystrophy. Multiple exostoses are sometimes seen in patients with pseudohypoparathyroidism.

An exostosis may suddenly begin to enlarge long after growth should have ceased, and rarely, chondrosarcomas may develop from the cartilage cap of an exostosis. Although pregnancy may stimulate growth of an exostosis that clinically may mimic malignancy, the lesion merely undergoes exuberant endochondral ossification and cartilage hyperplasia without malignant changes.

Multiple inactivating mutations or deletions have been identified in the *EXT1* or *EXT2* genes in patients with hereditary multiple exostoses. The *EXT* genes probably function normally as a tumor suppressor, and mutations in *EXT* could contribute both to the development of the exostoses and to the malignant transformation to chondrosarcoma that sometimes occurs. Mutations in *EXT* genes apparently cause abnormal processing the cytoskeletal proteins in chondrocytes.

BIBLIOGRAPHY

BERNARD MA et al: Cytoskeletal abnormalities in chondrocytes with EXT1 and EXT2 mutations. J Bone Miner Res 15:442, 2000

BIANCO P et al: Mutations of the *GNAS1* gene, stromal cell dysfunction, and osteomalacic changes in non-McCune-Albright fibrous dysplasia of bone. J Bone Miner Res 15: 120, 2000

CHAPURLAT RD, MEUNIER PJ: Fibrous dysplasia of bone. Baillieres Best Pract Res Clin Rheumatol 14:385, 2000

COOPER HA et al: SPONASTRIME dysplasia: Report of an 11-year-old boy and review of the literature. Am J Med Genet 92:33, 2000

DEERE M et al: Identification of nine novel mutations in cartilage oligomeric matrix protein in patients with pseudoachondroplasia and multiple epiphyseal dysplasia. Am J Hum Genet 85:486, 1999

DINI G et al: Long-term follow-up of two children with a variant of mild autosomal recessive osteopetrosis undergoing bone marrow transplantation. Bone Marrow Transplant 26:219, 2000

DREZNER MK: Proceeding of the third international symposium on Paget's disease. Napa, California, USA, November 29–30, 1998. J Bone Miner Res. 14(Suppl 2):1, 1999

EUGSTER EA et al: Tamoxifen treatment of progressive precocious puberty in a patient with McCune-Albright syndrome. J Pediatr Endocrinol Metab 12:681, 1999

FISHER JE et al: Alendronate mechanism of action: Geranylgeraniol, an intermediate in the mevalonate pathway, prevents inhibition of osteoclast formation, bone resorption, and kinase activation in vitro. Proc Natl Acad Sci USA 96:133, 1999

FRATTINI A et al: Defects in TCIRG1 subunit of the vacuolar proton pump are responsible for a subset of human autosomal recessive osteopetrosis. Nature Genet 25:343, 2000

GELB BD et al: Pycnodysostosis, a lysosomal disease caused by cathepsin K deficiency. Science 273:1236, 1996

GLASER RL et al: Paternal origin of *FGFR2* mutations in sporadic cases of Crouzon syndrome and Pfeiffer syndrome. Am J Hum Genet 66:768, 2000

HOCKING L et al: Familial Paget's disease of bone: Patterns of inheritance and frequency of linkage to chromosome 18q. Bone 26:577, 2000

HUGHES AE et al: Mutations in *TNFRS11A*, affecting the signal peptide of RANK, cause familial expansile osteolysis. Nat Genet 24:45, 2000

JANSSENS K et al: Localisation of the gene causing diaphyseal dysplasia Camurati-Engelmann to chromosome 19q13. J Med Genet 37:245, 2000

KARSENTY G: The genetic transformation of bone biology. Genes Dev 13:3037, 1999

KORNAK U et al: Mutations in the $\alpha 3$ subunit of the vacuolar H^+-ATPase cause infantile malignant osteopetrosis. Hum Mol Genet 9:2059, 2000

KURIHARA N et al: Osteoclasts expressing the measles virus nucleocapsid gene display a pagetic phenotype. J Clin Invest 105:607, 2000

LALA R et al: Pamidronate treatment of bone fibrous dysplasia in nine children with McCune-Albright syndrome. Acta Paediatr 89:188, 2000

LI J et al: RANK is the intrinsic hematopoietic cell surface receptor that controls osteoclastogenesis and regulation of bone mass and calcium metabolism. Proc Natl Acad Sci USA 97:1566, 2000

NELLISSERY MJ et al: Evidence for a novel osteosarcoma tumor-suppressor gene in the chromosome 18 region genetically linked with Paget disease of bone. Am J Hum Genet 63:817, 1998

NEVIN NC et al: Melorheostosis in a family with autosomal dominant osteopoikilosis. Am J Med Genet 82:409, 1999

RINGEL MD et al: Clinical implications of genetic defects in G proteins. The molecular basis of McCune-Albright syndrome and Albright hereditary osteodystrophy. Medicine 75:171, 1996

SAFTIG P et al: Functions of cathepsin K in bone resorption. Lessons from cathepsin K deficient mice. Adv Exp Biol 477:293, 2000

SILVE C: Hereditary hypophosphatasia and hyperphosphatasia. Curr Opin Rheumatol 6: 336, 1994

SINGER FR, KRANE SM: Paget's disease of bone, in *Metabolic Bone Disease and Clinically Related Disorders*, LV Avioli, SM Krane (eds). San Diego, Academic Press, 1998, pp 545–603

VAJO Z et al: The molecular and genetic basis of fibroblast growth factor receptor 3 disorders: The achondrodysplasia family of skeletal dysplasias, Muenke craniosynostosis, and Crouzon syndrome with acanthosis nigricans. Endocrine Rev 21:23, 2000

WHYTE MP, MURPHY WA: Osteopetrosis and other sclerosing bone disorders, in *Metabolic Bone Disease and Clinically Related Disorders*, LV Avioli, SM Krane (eds). San Diego, Academic Press, 1998

WUYTS W, VAN HUL W: Molecular basis of muliple exostoses: Mutations in the *EXT1* and *EXT2* genes. Hum Mutat 15:220, 2000

Section 3
DISORDERS OF INTERMEDIARY METABOLISM

344

Henry N. Ginsberg,, Ira J. Goldberg

DISORDERS OF LIPOPROTEIN METABOLISM

CETP cholesteryl ester transfer protein	LCAT lecithin:cholesterol acyltransferase
CHD coronary heart disease	LDL low-density lipoprotein
CPK creatine phosphokinase	LPL lipoprotein lipase
DM diabetes mellitus	LRP LDL receptor–related protein
FCHL familial combined hyperlipidemia	NCEP National Cholesterol Education Program
FH familial hypercholesterolemia	PLTP phospholipid transfer protein
HDL high-density lipoproteins	TSH thyroid-stimulating hormone
HTGL hepatic triglyceride lipase	VLDL very low density lipoproteins
IDL intermediate-density lipoproteins	

Lipoproteins are macromolecular complexes that carry hydrophobic plasma lipids, particularly cholesterol and triglyceride, in the plasma. More than half of the coronary heart disease (CHD) in the United States is attributable to abnormalities in the levels and metabolism of plasma lipids and lipoproteins. Some premature CHD is due to mutations in major genes involved in lipoprotein metabolism. However, elevated lipoprotein levels in most patients with CHD reflect the adverse impact of a sedentary lifestyle, excess body weight, and diets high in total and saturated fat superimposed on a genetic background that confers susceptibility to increased circulating lipids. A large body of evidence indicates that lifestyle changes and drug treatment strategies that correct hyperlipidemias reduce CHD risk (Chap 242). More than 70 clinical trials examining the effects of cholesterol reduction have been reported, including several large-scale studies using the potent cholesterol-lowering HMG-CoA reductase inhibitors (also known as statins). These studies unequivocally demonstrate that lowering low-density lipoprotein (LDL) cholesterol reduces fatal and nonfatal heart attacks (Table 344-1).

This chapter focuses on the major lipid disorders, including both the dyslipoproteinemias caused by single-gene defects and the disorders that are likely to be multifactorial in origin. A practical approach is provided to assist in the identification, evaluation, and treatment of patients with increased risk of CHD.

LIPID AND LIPOPROTEIN TRANSPORT

LIPOPROTEIN STRUCTURE Lipoproteins are spherical particles made up of hundreds of lipid and protein molecules. They are smaller than red blood cells and visible only by electron microscopy. However, when the larger, triglyceride-rich lipoproteins are present in high concentration, plasma can appear turbid or milky to the naked eye. The major lipids of the lipoproteins are cholesterol, triglycerides, and phospholipids. Triglycerides and the esterified form of cholesterol (cholesteryl esters) are nonpolar lipids that are insoluble in aqueous environments (hydrophobic) and comprise the core of the lipoproteins. Phospholipids and a small quantity of free (unesterified)

Table 344-1 Summary of Selected Major Lipid-Lowering Trials Investigating Effects on CHD

Trial [a]	Year Published	Treatment	Lipid Characteristics	1° or 2° [b]	Results
Los Angeles VA	1968	Unsaturated fat diet	—	1	↓ MI
Oslo	1981	Diet and smoking	—	1	↓ Reduced sudden death and MI
LRC Trial	1984	Cholestyramine	—	2	↓ Cardiac events[c]
Coronary Drug Project	1985	Niacin	—	2	↓ Cardiac death over 15 years
Helsinki	1987	Gemfibrozil	—	1	↓ Cardiac events
POSCH	1990	Ileal bypass	—	1	↓ Cardiac events
FATS	1990	Combination	—	2	↓ Cardiac events
4S	1994	Simvastatin	High cholesterol	2	↓ Death, cardiac events, and stroke
WOSCOPS	1995	Pravastatin	High cholesterol	1	↓ Cardiac events
CARE	1996	Pravastatin	Average LDL	2	↓ Cardiac events and stroke
LIPID	1998	Pravastatin	Variable LDL	2	↓ Cardiac events
AFCAPS/TexCAPS	1998	Mevacor	Average LDL Low HDL	1	↓ Cardiac events
VA HIT	1999	Gemfibrozil	Low-normal LDL Low HDL	2	↓ Cardiac events
AVERT	1999	Atorvastatin	—	2	↓ Time to new events compared to angioplasty

[a] LRC, Lipid Research Clinics; 4S, Scandanavian Simvastatin Survival Study; WOSCOPS, West of Scotland Coronary Prevention Study; CARE, Cholesterol and Recurrent Events Trial; AFCAPS/TexCAPS, Air Force/Texas Coronary Atherosclerosis Prevention Study; POSCH, Program on the Surgical Control of the Hyperlipidemias; FATS, Familial Atherosclerosis Treatment Study; LIPID, Long-Term Intervention with Pravastatin in Ischemic Disease; VA HIT, Veterans Administration-HDL Intervention Trial; AVERT, Atorvastatin versus Revascularization Treatments.

[b] 1°, Primary prevention trial in population without known CHD; 2°, secondary prevention trial in population with established (CHD) assessed for recurrent clinical episodes.

[c] Cardicac events, fatal and nonfatal CHD.

NOTE: CHD, coronary heart disease; MI, myocardial infarction; LDL, low-density lipoprotein; HDL, high-density lipoprotein.

cholesterol, which are soluble in both lipid and aqueous environments (amphipathic), cover the surface of the particles, where they act as the interface between the plasma and core components. A family of proteins, the apolipoproteins, also occupies the surface of the lipoproteins; the apolipoproteins play crucial roles in the regulation of lipid transport and lipoprotein metabolism.

Lipoproteins have been classified on the basis of their densities into five major classes:(1) chylomicrons, (2) very low density lipoproteins (VLDL), (3) intermediate-density lipoproteins (IDL), (4) LDL, and (5) high-density lipoproteins (HDL). The physical-chemical characteristics of the major lipoprotein classes are presented in Table 344-2.

APOLIPOPROTEINS The apolipoproteins (apos) provide structural stability to the lipoproteins and determine the metabolic fate of the particles upon which they reside. They were named in an arbitrary alphabetical order and, for the purposes of this discussion, will be described in relation to their association with lipoprotein classes (Table 344-3).

There are two forms of apo B—apo B100 and apo B48. Apo B100 is the major apolipoprotein of VLDL, IDL, and LDL, comprising approximately 30, 60, and 95% of the protein in these lipoproteins, respectively. Apo B100 has a molecular mass of about 545 kDa and is synthesized in the liver. It is essential for the assembly and secretion of VLDL from the liver and is the ligand for the removal of LDL by the LDL receptor. The LDL receptor is a cell-surface protein that binds and internalizes lipoproteins that contain apo B100 or apo E. The LDL receptor binding domain of apo B100 is the sequence between amino acids 3200 and 3600, a region that is absent in apo B48.

Apo B48 is essential for the assembly and secretion of chylomicrons. Apo B48 is encoded by the same gene and messenger ribonucleic acid (mRNA) as Apo B100. However, the mRNA is edited in an unusual way: A cytidine deaminase in the intestine changes a cytidine to a uridine in base 6666 of the apo B100 mRNA to produce a stop codon so that apo B48 contains only the N-terminal 48% of the full-length apo B100. In contrast, the apo B100 mRNA in human liver is not edited. The role of apo B48 in the metabolism of chylomicrons in plasma is unclear. Individuals with mutations that interfere with the normal synthesis of apo B have absent or very low levels of chylomicrons, VLDL, IDL and LDL.

The apolipoproteins of the C series are synthesized in the liver and are present in all plasma lipoproteins (trace amounts in LDL). Individual apo Cs have different metabolic roles, but all inhibit the removal of plasma chylomicrons and VLDL remnants by the liver. Overexpression of apo CI in transgenic mice inhibits the uptake of chylomicron and VLDL remnants by the liver. Apo CI under- or overexpression has not been described in humans. Apo CII is an essential activator of the enzyme lipoprotein lipase (LPL), which hydrolyzes triglycerides in chylomicrons and VLDL; individuals lacking apo CII have severe hypertriglyceridemia. Apo CIII inhibits LPL, and apo CIII overexpression in transgenic mice causes severe hypertriglyceridemia. Humans who lack apo CIII have accelerated rates of VLDL triglyceride lipolysis.

Apo E is synthesized mainly in hepatocytes but is also made in other cells, including macrophages, neurons, and glial cells. It is found in chylomicrons, IDL, VLDL, and HDL and mediates the uptake of these lipoproteins in the liver by both the LDL receptor and the LDL receptor–related protein (LRP). Apo E also binds to heparin-like proteoglycan molecules on the surface of all cells. There are three major apo E alleles: E2, E3, and E4; these isoforms differ in sequence at two positions and have frequencies of about 0.12, 0.75, and 0.13, respectively, in the general population. Apo E2 binds to the LDL receptor with lower affinity than apo E3 or E4. Individuals who are homozygous for apo E2 may develop severe hyperlipidemia (type III dysbetalipoproteinemia); complete absence of apo E increases plasma levels of chylomicron and VLDL remnants and causes early atherosclerosis.

Apo AI, apo AII, and apo AIV are found primarily on HDL. Apo AI and apo AII are synthesized in the small intestine and the liver; apo AIV is made only in the intestine. Apo AI comprises about 70 to 80% of the protein of HDL and plays a critical structural role in HDL particles. Individuals with a profound deficiency of apo AI also lack HDL. Apo AI activates the enzyme lecithin:cholesterol acyl-

Table 344-2 Physical-Chemical Characteristics of the Major Lipoprotein Classes

Lipoprotein	Density, g/dL	Molecular Mass, kDa	Diameter, nm	Lipid, %[a]		
				TG	Chol	PL
Chylomicrons	0.95	400×10^3	75–1200	80–95	2–7	3–9
VLDL	0.95–1.006	$10–80 \times 10^3$	30–80	55–80	5–15	10–20
IDL	1.006–1.019	$5–10 \times 10^3$	25–35	20–50	20–40	15–25
LDL	1.019–1.063	2.3×10^3	18–25	5–15	40–50	20–25
HDL	1.063–1.210	$1.7–3.6 \times 10^2$	5–12	5–10	15–25	20–30

[a] The remaining percent composition is made up of the apoproteins.

NOTE: TG, triglyceride; Chol, the sum of free and esterified cholesterol; PL, phospholipid; VLDL, very low density lipoprotein; IDL, intermediate density lipoprotein; LDL, low-density lipoprotein; HDL, high-density lipoprotein.

transferase (LCAT), which esterifies free cholesterol in plasma. Plasma levels of HDL cholesterol and apo AI are inversely related to risk for CHD, and some patients with apo AI deficiency develop early, severe atherosclerosis. Transgenic mice that overexpress human apo AI are resistant to atherosclerosis. Apo AII is the second most abundant apoprotein in HDL, but its function has not been determined; transgenic mice that overexpress apo AII have high plasma levels of both HDL cholesterol and triglycerides but may be susceptible to atherosclerosis. Apo AII knockout mice have low levels of HDL, indicating that apo AII is also necessary for the integrity of HDL particles. Apo AIV, a minor component of HDL and chylomicrons may play a role in the activation of LCAT.

Apoprotein(a), a large glycoprotein that shares a high degree of sequence homology with plasminogen, is made by hepatocytes and is secreted into plasma where it forms a covalent linkage with the apo B100 of LDL to form lipoprotein(a). The physiologic role of lipoprotein(a) is not known, but elevated levels are associated with an increased risk for atherosclerosis.

Table 344-3 Characteristics of the Major Apolipoproteins

Apolipoprotein	Molecular Mass, Da	Lipoproteins	Metabolic Functions
Apo AI	28,016	HDL, chylomicrons	Structural component of HDL; LCAT activator
Apo AII	17,414	HDL, chylomicrons	Unknown
Apo AIV	46,465	HDL, chylomicrons	Unknown: possibly facilitates transfer of other apos between HDL and chylomicrons
Apo B48	264,000	Chylomicrons	Necessary for assembly and secretion of chylomicrons from the small intestine
Apo B100	540,000	VLDL, IDL, LDL	Necessary for assembly and secretion of VLDL from the liver; structural protein of VLDL, IDL, LDL; ligand for LDL receptor
Apo CI	6630	Chylomicrons, VLDL, IDL, HDL	May inhibit hepatic uptake of chylomicron and VLDL remnants
Apo CII	8900	Chylomicrons, VLDL, IDL, HDL	Activator of lipoprotein lipase
Apo CIII	8800	Chylomicrons, VLDL, IDL, HDL	Inhibitor of lipoprotein lipase; may inhibit hepatic uptake of chylomicron and VLDL remnants
Apo E	34,145	Chylomicrons, VLDL, IDL, HDL	Ligand for binding of several lipoproteins to the LDL receptor, to LRP, and possibly to a separate hepatic apo E receptor

NOTE: HDL, high-density lipoprotein; LCAT, lecithin:cholesterol acyltransferase; VLDL, very low density lipoprotein; IDL, intermediate-density lipoprotein; LDL, low-density lipoprotein; LRP, LDL receptor–related protein.

ENZYMES INVOLVED IN LIPOPROTEIN METABOLISM LPL is synthesized in fat and muscle, secreted into the interstitial space, transported across endothelial cells, and bound to proteoglycans on the luminal surfaces in the adjacent capillary beds. LPL mediates the hydrolysis of the triglycerides of chylomicrons and VLDL to generate free fatty acids and glycerol. The free fatty acids diffuse into adjacent tissues to be burned for energy or stored as fat. Most circulating LPL is associated with LDL. Insulin stimulates the synthesis and secretion of LPL; reduced LPL activity in diabetes mellitus can lead to impaired triglyceride clearance. Homozygotes for mutations that impair LPL have severe hypertriglyceridemia that usually manifests in childhood (type I hyperlipidemia). Heterozygotes for LPL defects have mild to moderate fasting hypertriglyceridemia but may have marked hypertriglyceridemia after consuming a high-fat meal. LPL is also expressed in macrophages, including cholesteryl ester–laden macrophages (foam cells) in atherosclerotic lesions. In this setting, secreted LPL may associate with LDL, causing retention of the lipoprotein in the subendothelial space.

Hepatic triglyceride lipase (HTGL), a member of a family of enzymes that includes LPL and pancreatic lipase, is synthesized in the liver and interacts with lipoproteins in hepatic sinusoids. HTGL removes triglycerides from VLDL remnants (IDL), thus promoting the conversion of VLDL to LDL. It may also play a role in the clearance of chylomicron remnants and in the conversion of HDL_2 to HDL_3 in the liver by hydrolyzing the triglyceride and phospholipid in HDL (see below). Severe hypertriglyceridemia in individuals with genetic deficiency of HTGL is due to the accumulation of chylomicron and VLDL remnants in plasma. In contrast to most patients with hypertriglyceridemia, however, individuals with HTGL deficiency have normal levels of HDL.

LCAT is synthesized in the liver and secreted into plasma where it is bound predominantly to HDL. LCAT mediates the transfer of linoleate from lecithin to free cholesterol on the surface of HDL to form cholesteryl esters that are then transferred to VLDL and eventually LDL. Apo AI is a cofactor for esterification of free cholesterol by LCAT. Deficiency of LCAT can be caused by mutations in the enzyme or in Apo A1. LCAT deficiency causes low levels of cholesteryl esters and HDL, and it can lead to corneal clouding and renal insufficiency.

Cholesteryl ester transfer protein (CETP) is synthesized primarily in the liver and circulates in plasma in association with HDL. CETP mediates the exchange of cholesteryl esters from HDL with triglyceride from chylomicrons or VLDL. This exchange can explain much of the inverse relationship between plasma levels of triglycerides and HDL cholesterol. LDL cholesteryl ester can also be exchanged with triglyceride from chylomicrons and VLDL, leading to the generation of small, dense LDL. Individuals who are homozygotes for mutations in the CETP gene have marked elevations of HDL cholesterol and apo AI. Heterozygotes for these mutations have slight elevations of HDL, indicating that CETP plays an important role in the removal of cholesteryl esters from HDL.

Phospholipid transfer protein (PLTP) is synthesized in the liver and lung. The production of mature HDL particles depends on PLTP, which provides phospholipid to the enlarging particles.

TRANSPORT OF EXOGENOUS (DIETARY) LIPIDS Exogenous lipid transport in chylomicrons and chylomicron remnants is depicted in Fig. 344-1*A*. In western societies, where individuals ordinarily consume 50 to 100 g of fat and 0.5 g of cholesterol during three or four meals, transport of dietary fats is essentially continual. Normolipidemic individuals dispose of most dietary fat in the bloodstream within 8 h of the last meal, but some individuals with dyslipidemia, particularly those with elevated fasting levels of VLDL triglyceride, have measurable levels of intestinally derived lipoproteins in the circulation as long as 24 h after the last meal.

In the intestinal mucosa dietary triglyceride and cholesterol are incorporated into the core of nascent chylomicrons. The surface coat of the chylomicron is composed of phospholipid, free cholesterol, apo B48, apo AI, apo AII, and apo AIV. The chylomicron, essentially a fat droplet containing 80 to 95% triglycerides, is secreted into lacteals and transported to the circulation via the thoracic duct. In the plasma, apo C proteins are transferred to the chylomicron from HDL. Apo CII mediates hydrolysis of triglycerides by activating LPL on capillary endothelial cells in fat and muscle. After the triglyceride core has been hydrolyzed, apo CII and apo CIII recirculate back to HDL. The addition of apo E allows the chylomicron remnant to bind first to heparan sulfate proteoglycans within the space of Disse and then to hepatic LDL receptors and/or LDL receptor-related protein. As a consequence, dietary triglyceride is delivered to adipocytes and muscle cells as fatty acids, and dietary cholesterol is taken up by the liver where it can be used for bile acid formation, incorporated into membranes, resecreted as lipoprotein cholesterol back into the circulation, or excreted as cho-

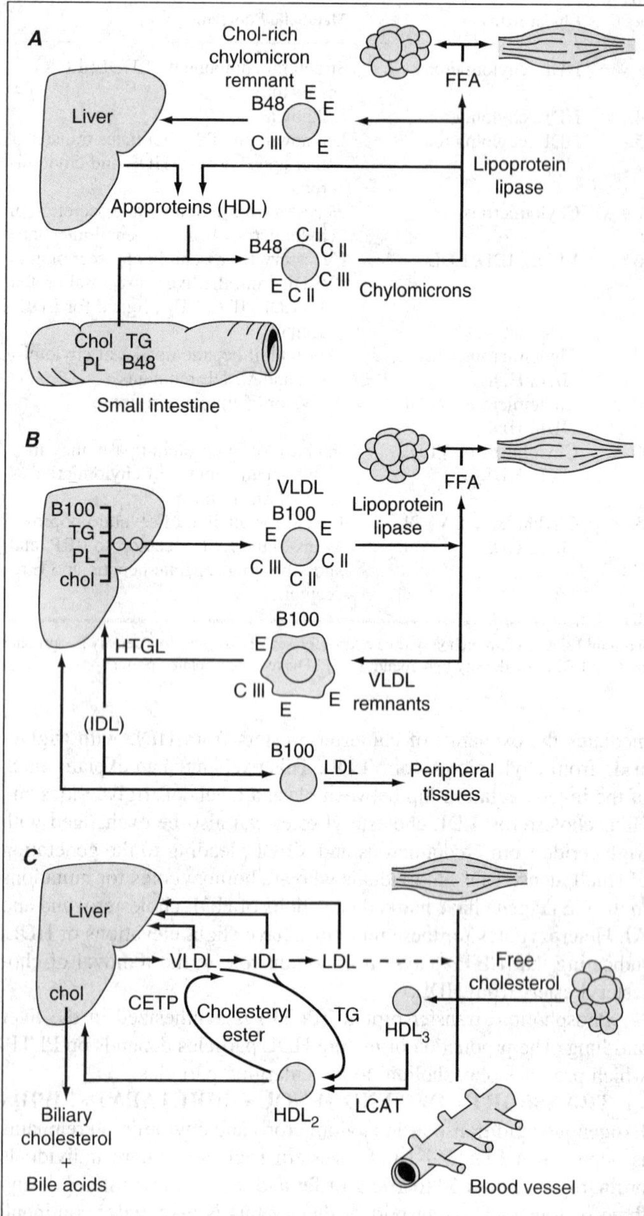

FIGURE 344-1 *A.* Transport of endogenous hepatic lipids via VLDL, IDL, and LDL. Note the relative and absolute changes in apoproteins, other than apo B100, as VLDL is converted to IDL and LDL. The sites of action of the two lipases, LPL and HTGL, are denoted as well, though the role of HTGL has not been completely defined. *B.* A schematic depiction of the transport of exogenously derived lipids from the intestine to peripheral tissues and liver via the chylomicron system. The cyclic movement of several apoproteins between HDL and chylomicrons is also represented. *C.* Simplified representation of HDL metabolism and the role of HDL in reverse cholesterol transport. Free cholesterol is accepted from peripheral tissues by HDL_3 and, after esterification, may be transferred to apo B100 lipoproteins. Cholesteryl ester may also be delivered to the liver by HDL itself. The significance of each of the three possible transport systems for cholesterol in overall reverse cholesterol transport is unknown. CETP, cholesteryl ester transfer protein; FFA, free fatty acids; HDL, high-density lipoprotein; HTGL, hepatic triglyceride lipase; IDL, intermediate-density lipoprotein; LDL, low-density lipoprotein; LPL, lipoprotein lipase; PL, phospholipase; TG, triglyceride; VLDL, very low density lipoprotein. *[From HN Ginsberg, Endocrinol Metab Clin North Am 19(2): 211, 1990.]*

lesterol into bile. Dietary cholesterol also regulates endogenous hepatic cholesterol synthesis.

Abnormal transport and metabolism of chylomicrons may predispose to atherosclerosis, and postprandial hyperlipidemia may be a risk factor for CHD. Chylomicrons and their remnants can be taken up by cells of the vessel wall, including monocyte-derived macrophages that migrate into the vessel wall from plasma. Cholesteryl ester accumulation by these macrophages transforms them into foam cells, the earliest cellular lesion of the atherosclerotic plaque (Chap. 241). If the postprandial levels of chylomicrons or their remnants are elevated, or if their removal from plasma is prolonged, cholesterol delivery to the artery wall may be increased.

TRANSPORT OF ENDOGENOUS LIPIDS The endogenous lipid transport system, which conveys lipids from the liver to peripheral tissues and from peripheral tissues back to the liver, can be separated into two subsystems: the apo B100 lipoprotein system (VLDL, IDL, and LDL) and the apo AI lipoprotein system (HDL).

The Apo B100 Lipoprotein System (See Fig. 344-1*B*) In the liver, triglycerides are made from fatty acids that are either taken up from plasma or synthesized de novo within the liver. Cholesterol can also be synthesized by the liver or delivered to the liver via lipoproteins, particularly chylomicron remnants. These core lipids are packaged together with apo B100 and phospholipids into VLDL and secreted into plasma where apos CI, CII, CIII, and E are added to the nascent VLDL particles. Triglycerides make up the bulk of the VLDL (55 to 80% by weight), and the size of the VLDL is determined by the amount of triglyceride available. Hence, very large triglyceride-rich VLDL are secreted in situations where excess triglycerides are synthesized, such as in states of caloric excess, in diabetes mellitus, and after alcohol consumption. Small VLDL are secreted when fewer triglycerides are available. Although VLDL are the principal hepatic lipoprotein secreted by most individuals, VLDL and cholesteryl ester–enriched IDL and/or LDL-like particles may be secreted by the liver in individuals with combined hyperlipidemia (see below).

In the plasma, triglycerides are hydrolyzed by LPL and VLDL particles are converted to VLDL remnants (IDL). In contrast to chylomicron remnants, VLDL remnants can either enter the liver or give rise to LDL. Larger VLDL particles carry more triglycerides and are likely to be removed directly from plasma without being converted to LDL; apo E in the VLDL remnants binds to the LDL receptor to mediate removal from the plasma. Smaller, more dense VLDL particles are more efficiently converted to LDL; apo E and HTGL play important roles in this process. Individuals with deficiency of either apo E2 or HTGL accumulate IDL in plasma. Apo B100 is the only protein that remains on the surface of the LDL particle.

The half-life of LDL in plasma is determined principally by the availability (or "activity") of LDL receptors. Most plasma LDL is taken up by the liver, and the remainder is delivered to peripheral tissues, including the adrenals and gonads, which utilize cholesterol as a precursor for steroid hormone synthesis. The adrenals have the highest concentration of LDL receptors per cell in the body. Overall, about 70 to 80% of LDL catabolism occurs via LDL receptors, and the remainder is removed by fluid endocytosis and possibly by other receptors.

The LDL receptor, a glycoprotein with a molecular mass of approximately 160 kDa, is present on the surfaces of nearly all cells in the body. Goldstein and Brown characterized the molecular genetics and cell biology of the LDL receptor and defined its role in cholesterol metabolism. They showed that cholesterol delivered to the cytoplasm by LDL regulates both the rate of cholesterol synthesis in the liver and the number of LDL receptors on the surface of hepatocytes. LDL receptor synthesis is mediated by sterol response element regulatory proteins (SREBPs). These transcription factors are activated in the absence of cholesterol, proteolytically cleaved, and transferred from the endoplasmic reticulum into the nucleus where they stimulate LDL receptor gene expression. Though the LDL receptor is a major factor in determining plasma LDL cholesterol levels, the rates of entry of VLDL into plasma and the efficiency with which VLDL is converted to LDL also influence steady-state LDL concentrations in plasma.

Increased levels of plasma LDL cholesterol and apo B100 are risk factors for atherosclerosis. Normal LDL does not cause foam cell formation when incubated with cultured macrophages or smooth-muscle cells. But, when LDL undergoes lipid peroxidation, it becomes a ligand for alternative, scavenger receptors that are present on endothelial cells and macrophages. Uptake of modified (oxidized) lipoproteins by these receptors in macrophages results in formation of cholesterol-laden foam cells. In addition to inducing foam cell formation, oxidized LDL acts in the vessel wall to stimulate the secretion of cytokines and growth factors by endothelial cells, smooth-muscle cells, and monocyte-derived macrophages (Chap. 242). The consequence is recruitment of more monocytes to the lesion and proliferation of smooth-muscle cells, which synthesize and secrete increased amounts of extracellular matrix, such as collagen. The critical role of LDL in atherosclerosis has been confirmed in genetically altered mice. Although mice are normally resistant to atherosclerosis, increased plasma levels of remnant lipoproteins or LDL lead to atherosclerosis in this species.

The role of VLDL in atherogenesis is less certain. The major reason for this uncertainty derives from the inverse relationship between elevated levels of triglyceride-rich lipoproteins and reduced levels of the antiatherogenic HDL cholesterol. It is possible, for example, that hypertriglyceridemia may not be directly atherogenic but rather the surrogate of other lipoprotein abnormalities. If postprandial hyperlipidemia is a risk factor for CHD, individuals who have normal fasting plasma triglyceride levels but develop postprandial hypertriglyceridemia after consumption of a fat load would be misclassified as "normal" in studies in which only fasting blood samples are analyzed. It is clear that cholesteryl ester–enriched VLDL, isolated from cholesterol-fed animals, can be taken up by receptors on macrophages and smooth-muscle cells and cause foam cell formation. These cholesteryl ester–laden VLDLs are enriched in apo E and are probably representative of VLDL remnants. Thus, the risk of atherosclerosis from hypertriglyceridemia and elevated VLDL levels may be determined by the level of cholesteryl ester–enriched VLDL remnants. The atherogenic potential of IDL is probably similar to that of VLDL remnants.

Apo AI–Containing Lipoproteins (See Fig. 344-1*C*) In contrast to atherogenic apo B lipoproteins, the apo AI–containing HDL appear to be antiatherogenic. In fact, in some studies, HDL cholesterol levels are as strong an indicator of protection from CHD as LDL cholesterol levels are an indicator of risk. Although a great deal is known about the HDL transport system, the mechanism by which these lipoproteins protect against atherosclerosis is poorly defined.

HDL particles are formed in plasma from the coalescence of individual phospholipid-apolipoprotein complexes. Apo AI appears to be the crucial, structural apoprotein for HDL, and apo AI/phospholipid complexes probably fuse with other phospholipid vesicles that contain apo AII and apo AIV to form the various types of HDL. The C apoproteins can be added to HDL after their secretion as phospholipid complexes or by their transfer from triglyceride-rich lipoproteins. This may involve the action of PLTP. These small, cholesterol-poor HDL particles are heterogeneous in size and content and are referred to as HDL_3. Free cholesterol is transferred from cell membranes to HDL_3; a cholesterol transporter called ABC1 mediates this important first step in reverse cholesterol transport. Free cholesterol in HDL_3 is converted to cholesteryl ester by LCAT, and the cholesteryl ester moves into the core of the HDL. Formation of cholesteryl ester increases the capacity of the HDL_3 to accept more free cholesterol and enlarge to form the more buoyant class of HDL particles termed *HDL_2*. HDL_2 can be metabolized by two pathways: (1) cholesteryl esters can be transferred from HDL_2 to apo B lipoproteins or cells, or (2) the entire HDL_2 particle can be removed from plasma. The transfer of cholesteryl ester from HDL to triglyceride-rich apo B lipoproteins (chylomicrons and VLDL in the fed and fasted states, respectively) is mediated by CETP. Triglyceride is transferred to HDL in this process and is a substrate for lipolysis by LPL and/or HTGL. As a result, HDL_2 is converted back into HDL_3. When the apo B lipoproteins are removed by the liver, reverse cholesterol transfer is complete. HDL cholesteryl ester may also be transferred selectively to cells via interaction of HDL with the scavenger receptor B-1, a receptor expressed by hepatocytes and steroid-producing cells. HDL-mediated reverse cholesterol transport (from peripheral tissues to the liver) is thought to be the primary mechanism by which HDL protects against atherosclerosis.

Rarely, low plasma HDL is due to a genetic deficiency of one of the structural components of HDL (such as apo AI). However, low HDL cholesterol levels are usually the secondary consequence of increased plasma levels of VLDL and IDL (or chylomicrons and their remnants). Mutations in the *ABC1* gene (see above) are associated with Tangier's disease, a rare form of low HDL. Low levels of HDL cholesterol and apo AI may increase atherosclerosis risk by any of several mechanisms. HDL could remove cholesterol from foam cells in atherosclerotic lesions or protect LDL from oxidative modification. Alternatively, the atherosclerotic risk of low HDL may be due to the commonly associated elevations of apo B–containing lipoproteins, which accept HDL cholesteryl esters and deliver cholesteryl esters to the vessel wall.

THE HYPERLIPOPROTEINEMIAS (See Table 344-4)

HYPERCHOLESTEROLEMIA Elevated levels of fasting plasma total cholesterol in the presence of normal levels of triglycerides are almost always associated with increased concentrations of plasma LDL cholesterol (type IIa), as LDL carries about 65 to 75% of total plasma cholesterol. A rare individual with markedly elevated HDL cholesterol may also have increased plasma total cholesterol levels. Elevations of LDL cholesterol can result from single-gene defects, polygenic disorders, or from the secondary effects of other disease states.

Familial Hypercholesterolemia (FH) FH is a codominant genetic disorder that occurs in the heterozygous form in approximately 1 in 500 individuals. FH is due to mutations in the gene for the LDL receptor and is genetically heterogeneous, >200 different mutations in the gene having been described. Plasma levels of LDL cholesterol are elevated at birth and remain so throughout life. In untreated adults, total cholesterol levels range from 7 to 13 mmol/L (275 to 500 mg/dL). Plasma triglyceride levels are typically normal, and HDL cholesterol levels are normal or reduced. As would be expected of a disorder with decreased numbers of LDL receptors, the fractional clearance of LDL apo B is reduced. LDL production is increased because the liver secretes more VLDL and IDL and more IDL particles are converted to LDL rather than taken up by the hepatic LDL receptors. FH heterozygotes usually develop severe atherosclerosis in early or middle age. *Tendon xanthomas*, which are due to both intracellular and extracellular deposits of cholesterol, most commonly involve the Achilles tendons and the extensor tendons of the knuckles; they are found in about 75% of adults with FH. *Tuberous xanthomas*, which are softer, painless nodules on the elbows and buttocks, and *xanthelasmas*, which are barely elevated deposits of cholesterol on the eyelids, are common in heterozygous FH. CHD develops in men by the fourth decade of life or earlier.

The homozygous form of FH occurs in 1 out of 1 million individuals and is associated with a marked increase of plasma cholesterol levels (>13 mmol/L; >500 mg/dL), large xanthelesmas, and prominent tendon and planar xanthomas. These individuals have severe, premature CHD that can be manifested in childhood.

Familial Defective Apo B100 This autosomal dominant disorder is a phenocopy of FH and is due to a missense mutation at amino acid 3500 that reduces the affinity of LDL for the LDL receptor and, thus, impairs LDL catabolism. The prevalence and manifestations of both the heterozygous and homozygous forms are similar to those produced by mutations of the LDL receptor.

Polygenic Hypercholesterolemia Most moderate hypercholesterolemia [plasma cholesterol levels between 6.5 and 9 mmol/L (240

Table 344-4 Characteristics of Common Hyperlipidemias

Lipid Phenotype	Plasma Lipid Levels, mmol/L (mg/dL)	Lipopoteins Elevated	Phenotype	Clinical Signs
ISOLATED HYPERCHOLESTEROLEMIA				
Familial hypercholesterolemia	Heterozygotes: total chol = 7–13 (275–500)	LDL	IIa	Usually develop xanthomas in adulthood and vascular disease at 30–50 years
	Homozygotes: total chol > 13 (>500)	LDL	IIa	Usually develop xanthomas and vascular disease in childhood
Familial defective apo B100	Heterozygotes: total chol = 7–13 (275–500)	LDL	IIa	
Polygenic hypercholesterolemia	Total chol = 6.5–9.0 (250–350)	LDL	IIa	Usually asymptomatic until vascular disease develops; no xanthomas
ISOLATED HYPERTRIGLYCERIDEMIA				
Familial hypertriglyceridemia	TG = 2.8–8.5 (250–750) (plasma may be cloudy)	VLDL	IV	Asymptomatic; may be associated with increased risk of vascular disease
Familial lipoprotein lipase deficiency	TG > 8.5 (>750) (plasma may be milky)	Chylomicrons	I, V	May be asymptomatic; may be associated with pancreatitis, abdominal pain, hepatosplenomegaly
Familial apo CII deficiency	TG > 8.5 (>750) (plasma may be milky)	Chylomicrons	I, V	As above
HYPERTRIGLYCERIDEMIA AND HYPERCHOLESTEROLEMIA				
Combined hyperlipidemia	TG = 2.8–8.5 (250–750) Total chol 6.5–13.0 (250–500)	VLDL, LDL	IIb	Usually asymptomatic until vascular disease develops; familial form may also present as isolated high TG or an isolated high LDL cholesterol
Dysbetalipoproteinemia	TG = 2.8–5.6 (250–500) Total chol 6.5–13.0 (250–500)	VLDL, IDL; LDL normal	III	Usually asymptomatic until vascular disease develops; may have palmar or tuboeruptive xanthomas

NOTE: total chol, the sum of free and esterified cholesterol; LDL, low-density lipoprotein; TG, triglycerides; VLDL, very low density lipoproteins; IDL, intermediate-density lipoprotein.

and 350 mg/dL)] is polygenic in origin. Multiple genes interact with environmental factors to contribute to the hypercholesterolemia, and both overproduction and reduced catabolism of LDL are thought to play roles in the pathophysiology. The severity is probably affected by the consumption of saturated fat and cholesterol, age, and the level of physical activity. Plasma triglyceride and HDL cholesterol levels are usually normal. These individuals are at increased risk of atherosclerosis. Tendon xanthomas are not present. Genes involved in cholesterol and bile acid metabolism may be involved in the pathogenesis.

HYPERTRIGLYCERIDEMIA The diagnosis of hypertriglyceridemia is made by determining plasma lipids after an overnight fast. Because of the less certain association of triglycerides with CHD (compared to LDL cholesterol), plasma concentrations greater than the 90th or 95th percentile for age and sex have been used to define hypertriglyceridemia. Some studies show, however, that plasma triglyceride levels >130 to 150 mg/dL are associated with low HDL cholesterol levels and small, dense LDL particles. Furthermore, a meta-analysis of several prospective population studies confirms that triglyceride concentrations are independent predictors of CHD risk. Isolated elevations of plasma triglycerides can be due to increased levels of VLDL (type IV) or combinations of VLDL and chylomicrons (type V). Rarely, only chylomicron levels are elevated (type I). Plasma is usually clear when triglyceride levels are <4.5 mmol/L (<400 mg/dL) and cloudy when levels are higher and VLDL (and/or chylomicron) particles become large enough to scatter light. When chylomicrons are present, a creamy layer floats to the top of plasma after refrigeration for several hours. Tendon xanthomas and xanthelasmas do not occur with isolated hypertriglyceridemia, but eruptive xanthomas (small orange-red papules) can appear on the trunk and extremities when triglyceride levels are >11.5 mmol/L (>1000 mg/dL) (i.e., when chylomicronemia is present). At these high levels of triglycerides, the retinal vessels can appear to be orange-yellow in color (lipemia retinalis). Pancreatitis is the major risk associated with plasma triglyceride concentrations >11 mmol/L (>1000 mg/dL).

Elevations in plasma triglycerides are usually associated with increased synthesis and secretion of VLDL triglycerides by the liver. Hepatic triglyceride synthesis is regulated by substrate flow (the availability of free fatty acids), energy balance (the level of glycogen stores in the liver), and hormonal status (the balance between insulin and glucagon). Obesity, excessive consumption of simple sugars and saturated fats, inactivity, alcohol consumption, and insulin resistance are commonly associated with hypertriglyceridemia. In most of these situations, increased free fatty acid flux from adipose tissue to the liver stimulates the assembly and secretion of VLDL. When VLDL triglyceride levels are markedly elevated [>11.5 mmol/L (>1000 mg/dL)], LPL may be saturated so that an acquired LPL deficiency develops during the postprandial period even if there is no underlying genetic disorder. The addition of chylomicrons to the circulation may cause dramatic increases in plasma triglycerides.

Familial Hypertriglyceridemia Familial hypertriglyceridemia appears to be transmitted as an autosomal dominant disorder, though the underlying mutation(s) have not been identified. The pathophysiology is complex: both reduced catabolism of triglyceride-rich lipoproteins and overproduction of VLDL have been reported. Elevated levels of fasting plasma triglycerides in the range of 2.3 to 8.5 mmol/L (200 to 750 mg/dL) are usually associated with increased levels of VLDL triglycerides only. When VLDL triglyceride levels are markedly elevated (regardless of etiology), chylomicron triglycerides can also be present, even after a 14-h fast. A 20-year follow-up of individuals with familial hypertriglyceridemia demonstrated a moderate increase in CHD risk.

Familial Lipoprotein Lipase Deficiency This autosomal recessive disorder is due to the severe impairment or absence of LPL, leading to massive accumulation of chylomicrons in plasma. Manifestations begin in infancy and include pancreatitis, eruptive xanthomas, hepatomegaly, splenomegaly, foam cell infiltration of the bone marrow, and, when the level of triglycerides is >11 mmol/L (1000 mg/dL), lipemia retinalis. Atherosclerosis is not accelerated. The diagnosis is suspected by finding a creamy layer (chylomicrons) at the top of plasma that has incubated overnight at 4°C; it is confirmed by demonstrating that LPL levels in plasma do not increase after the administration of heparin (which normally releases LPL from endothelial surfaces). Manifestations recede dramatically when patients are placed on fat-free diets.

LPL levels are within the normal range in most patients with moderate hypertriglyceridemia [2.8 to 5.6 mmol/L (250 to 500 mg/dL)]. Heterozygous mutations in the LPL gene are present in 5 to 10% of hypertriglyceridemic individuals; LPL activity may be reduced by 20 to 50% in these individuals. Heterozygotes for LPL deficiency may also present with severe hypertriglyceridemia if they have poorly controlled diabetes, are pregnant, consume excessive quantities of alcohol, take exogenous estrogen, or are obese.

Familial Apoprotein CII Deficiency This rare autosomal recessive disorder causes a functional deficiency of LPL and clinical manifestations similar to those of familial LPL deficiency. Deficiency of apoprotein CII impairs hydrolysis of chylomicrons and VLDL so that either, or both, lipoproteins accumulate in blood. The diagnosis is suspected in children or adults with recurrent attacks of pancreatitis and confirmed by demonstrating the absence of apo CII on gel electrophoresis and that plasma transfusion (which contains abundant apo CII) causes a dramatic fall in plasma triglycerides. Heterozygotes have half-normal levels of apo CII, may have mild elevations of triglycerides, and are asymptomatic. Dietary fat restriction should be lifelong.

Hepatic Lipase Deficiency Total deficiency of HTGL is a rare autosomal recessive disorder that impairs the final catabolism and/or remodeling of small VLDL and IDL. Subjects with HTGL deficiency often have elevated levels of VLDL remnants; HDL_2 levels may be elevated because HTGL participates in the conversion of HDL_2 to HDL_3. HTGL activity is frequently increased in hypertriglyceridemic individuals, but the meaning of this association is unclear.

HYPERCHOLESTEROLEMIA WITH HYPERTRIGLYCERIDEMIA Concomitant hypercholesterolemia and hypertriglyceridemia occurs in two disorders—familial combined hyperlipidemia (FCHL) and dysbetalipoproteinemia.

Familial Combined Hyperlipidemia FCHL is transmitted as an autosomal dominant disorder. Probands (the initial case discovered within a family) typically have combined hyperlipidemia, isolated hypertriglyceridemia, or isolated elevated levels of LDL cholesterol. The diagnosis requires documentation at some time of combined hyperlipidemia in the proband or, if the proband has isolated hypercholesterolemia or hypertriglyceridemia, the various lipid phenotypes in first-degree relatives at risk. The lipoprotein phenotype in affected individuals may change over time. The underlying defect in this disorder is not known, though mutations or polymorphisms in the LPL gene and in the gene cluster for apo AI, apo CIII, and apo AIV may contribute to the disorder in some families. Insulin resistance is present in many individuals with FCHL; the link may result from increased free fatty acid flux driving assembly and secretion of apo B100 lipoproteins.

FCHL is associated with increased secretion of VLDL particles, as determined by the flux of VLDL apo B. The lipoprotein patterns associated with the disorder are most likely determined by genetic polymorphisms in genes that regulate the metabolism of VLDL. For example, if the affected individual also has a defect in LPL, hypertriglyceridemia will be present. Since the hydrolysis of VLDL triglycerides also regulates the generation of LDL in plasma, individuals with FCHL who have inefficient catabolism of VLDL may also have reduced levels of LDL cholesterol and high VLDL cholesterol. Finally, individuals with FCHL who synthesize normal quantities of triglycerides and secrete VLDL that carries normal amounts of triglyceride generate increased numbers of LDL particles and present with isolated elevations of plasma LDL cholesterol. These variations in VLDL catabolism, together with additional genetic heterogeneity and environmental variability, form the basis for the variable phenotype in this disorder. FCHL may occur in as many as 0.5 to 1.0% of Americans and is the most common familial lipid disorder in survivors of myocardial infarction. The increased risk for atherosclerosis is due to the presence of increased numbers of small, atherogenic VLDLs and the conversion of VLDL to the more atherogenic IDL and LDL. Persons with FCHL usually have clear plasma and do not have xanthomas or xanthelasma.

Dysbetalipoproteinemia This rare disorder affects 1 in 10,000 persons and is due to homozygosity for apo E2, the binding-defective form of apo E. Because apo E plays a crucial role in the catabolism of chylomicron and VLDL remnants, affected individuals have elevations in both VLDL triglyceride and VLDL cholesterol, and chylomicron remnants are present in fasting plasma. The ratio of total cholesterol to triglyceride approximates 1.0, and the ratio of VLDL cholesterol to triglyceride is greater than 0.25. LDL and HDL cholesterol levels are usually low. Although 1% of the population is homozygous for apo E2, most have normal plasma triglyceride and cholesterol levels. Thus, a second defect in lipid metabolism must be present in the 0.01% of individuals with dysbetalipoproteinemia. These individuals may have tuberous xanthomas and deposits of cholesterol in the palmar creases (striae palmaris); the latter, appearing as yellow-orange lines, are specific for dysbetalipoproteinemia. The risk for atherosclerosis and its complications is increased, with onset in the fourth and fifth decades. The incidence of peripheral vascular disease is higher than in FH.

REDUCED HDL CHOLESTEROL Low levels of HDL cholesterol can be defined as <0.9 mmol/L (<35 mg/dL) in men and <1 to 1.2 mmol/L (<40 to 45 mg/dL) in women. Low concentrations of HDL cholesterol are usually associated with coexistent hypertriglyceridemia, though "primary hypoalphalipoproteinemia" has been identified in both individuals and families. The relationship between hypertriglyceridemia and low HDL levels probably derives from: (1) CETP-mediated transfer of cholesteryl ester from the core of HDL to VLDL; (2) shift of surface components, particularly phospholipids apo CII, and apo CIII, from HDL to VLDL; and (3) increased fractional catabolism of the cholesteryl ester–poor apoAI that results from the first two processes. The complexity of the relationship between HDL and triglyceride levels is highlighted by the fact that HDL levels do not return to normal when fasting plasma triglycerides are reduced in most persons with hypertriglyceridemia and low HDL cholesterol levels. Low HDL is clinically silent, and the plasma is usually clear (it can be cloudy or creamy if there is concomitant hypertriglyceridemia).

Primary hypoalphalipoproteinemia refers to the state where HDL cholesterol concentrations are markedly reduced but plasma triglyceride concentrations are normal. Many individuals with this phenotype have had hypertriglyceridemia in the past or have an older (or more obese) first-degree relative who has both low HDL and increased triglyceride levels. Hence, both family studies and long-term follow-up may be required to identify individuals with primary reductions in HDL cholesterol. Rare mutations have been described in the apo AI gene that lead to reductions in apo AI synthesis or increases in catabolism. One mutation that is common in Italy, apo AI-Milano, is associated with a high fractional clearance rate of apo AI but is not associated with increased risk for atherosclerosis.

Some rare genetic disorders of lipid metabolism are summarized in Table 344-5.

SECONDARY CAUSES OF HYPERLIPOPROTEINEMIA (See Table 344-6) **Diabetes Mellitus** Diabetes can affect lipid and lipoprotein metabolism through several mechanisms (Chap. 333). In type 1 diabetes mellitus (DM) (formerly called insulin-dependent di-

Table 344-5 Rare Genetic Disorders of Lipid Metabolism

Disorder	Typical Age of Onset	Plasma Lipid Abnormality	Major Clinical Manifestations	Pathogenesis	Treatment
Hypobetalipoproteinemia, abetalipoproteinemia	Early childhood	Very low cholesterol and triglyceride levels	Malabsorption of fat, ataxia, neuropathy, retinitis pigmentosa, acanthocytosis	Defective synthesis or secretion of apo B leads to low or absent chylomicrons, VLDL, and LDL in plasma	Vitamin E
Tangier disease	Childhood	Low cholesterol; triglycerides, normal to slightly elevated	Large orange tonsils, corneal opacities, relapsing polyneuropathy No premature atherosclerosis	Defect in ABC transporter 1; abnormal cholesterol uptake into and/or efflux from macrophages; increased apo AI clearance	None
Lecithin: cholesterol acyltransferase (LCAT) deficiency (fish-eye disease)	Young adult	Total plasma cholesterol level variable with marked decrease in esterified cholesterol and increase in unesterified cholesterol; elevated VLDL level; structure of all lipoproteins is abnormal	Corneal opacities, hemolytic anemia, renal insufficiency, premature atherosclerosis	Decreased LCAT activity in plasma leads to accumulation of excess unesterified cholesterol in plasma and body tissues	Fat-restricted diet, kidney transplantation
Cerebrotendinous xanthomatosis	Young adult	None	Progressive cerebellar ataxia, dementia and spinal cord paresis; subnormal intelligence, tendon xanthomas, cataracts	Defect in sterol 27 hydroxylase; defective synthesis of primary bile acids in liver leads to increased hepatic synthesis of cholesterol and cholestanol, which accumulate in brain, tendons, and other tissues	Chenodeoxycholic acid
Sitosterolemia	Childhood	Elevated levels of plant sterols in plasma, elevated or normal levels of cholesterol, normal triglyceride levels	Tendon xanthomas	Increased intestinal absorption of dietary cholesterol, sitosterol, and other plant sterols with accumulation in plasma and tendons	Diet low in plant sterols and cholesterol

NOTE: VLDL, very low density lipoprotein; LDL, low-density lipoprotein.
SOURCE: Modified from MS Brown and JL Goldstein in *Harrison's Principles of Internal Medicine*, 13th ed, KJ Isselbacher et al (eds), New York, McGraw-Hill, 1994.

Table 344-6 Secondary Causes of Lipoprotein Abnormalities

HYPERCHOLESTEROLEMIA	
Hypothyroidism	Acute intermittent porphyria
Obstructive liver disease	Drugs: progestogens, cyclosporine, thiazides
Nephrotic syndrome	
Anorexia nervosa	
HYPERTRIGLYCERIDEMIA	
Obesity	Pregnancy
Diabetes mellitus	Drugs: estrogen, isotretinoin, beta blockers, glucocorticoids, bile acid–binding resins, thiazides
Chronic renal failure	
Lipodystrophy	
Glycogen storage disease	Acute hepatitis
Alcohol	Systemic lupus erythematosus
Ileal bypass surgery	Monoclonal gammopathy: multiple myeloma, lymphomas
Stress	
Sepsis	AIDS: protease inhibitors
HYPOCHOLESTEROLEMIA	
Malnutrition	Monoclonal gammopathy
Malabsorption	Chronic liver disease
Hyperthyroidism	
Myeloproliferative diseases	
Chronic infectious diseases: AIDS, tuberculosis	
LOW HDL	
Malnutrition	Beta blockers
Obesity	Anabolic steroids
Cigarette smoking	

NOTE: HDL, high-density lipoprotein.

abetes mellitus), plasma lipids are usually normal when control of diabetes with insulin is adequate. In diabetic ketoacidosis, hypertriglyceridemia can be severe due to increases in both VLDL and chylomicrons. These abnormalities are associated with overproduction of VLDL and LPL deficiency secondary to insulinopenia. They usually improve with tight control of the diabetes. In type 2 DM (formerly called non-insulin-dependent diabetes mellitus), insulin resistance and obesity combine to cause mild to moderate hypertriglyceridemia and low HDL cholesterol levels. In general, this pattern of dyslipidemia is due to overproduction of VLDL. LDL cholesterol is usually normal in type 2 DM, though the LDLs are small, dense, and perhaps more atherogenic. Treatment of type 2 DM and weight reduction improve, but usually do not completely correct, the dyslipidemia (particularly the low HDL cholesterol levels). Therapy of hyperlipidemia should not be delayed in patients with type 2 DM, as they are at increased risk for CHD. It is recommended that patients with diabetes should be treated as if they already have CHD, i.e., the treatment goal is to reduce their LDL to <2.6 mmol/L (<100 mg/dL) (Fig. 344-2).

Hypothyroidism Hypothyroidism accounts for about 2% of all cases of hyperlipidemia and is second only to DM as a cause of secondary hyperlipidemia. Levels of LDL cholesterol can be elevated, even in patients with subclinical disease in whom thyroid-stimulating hormone (TSH) levels are elevated but other thyroid function tests are normal. Hypertriglyceridemia can occur if obesity is present. Hypothyroidism is also associated with increased levels of HDL cholesterol, probably because of reduced HTGL activity. Correction of hypothyroidism reverses the lipid abnormalities.

Renal Disease Renal disease causes a wide range of lipid abnormalities. The nephrotic syndrome can be accompanied by elevations in LDL, VLDL, or both. The severity of the hyperlipidemia cor-

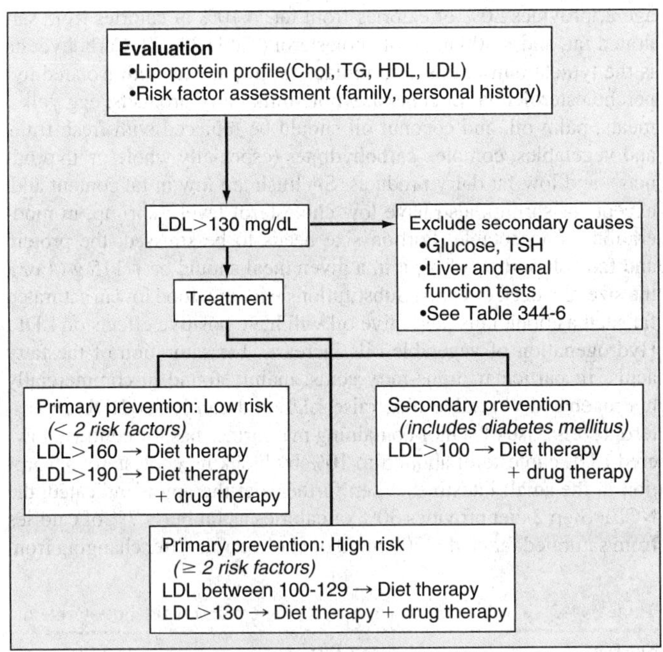

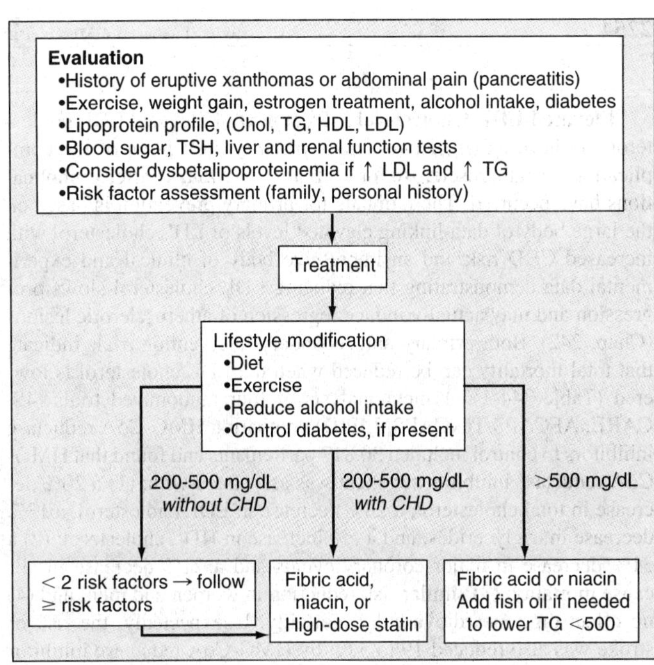

FIGURE 344-2 Algorithms for the evaluation and treatment of hypercholesterolemia (*A*) and hypertriglyceridemia (*B*). Statin, HMG-CoA reductase inhibitor; Chol, cholesterol; HDL, high-density lipoprotein; LDL, low-density lipoprotein; TG, triglyceride; TSH, thyroid-stimulating hormone; CHD, coronary heart disease.

relates with the degree of hypoproteinemia. Renal failure is associated with hypertriglyceridemia and low HDL cholesterol concentrations.

Ethanol The metabolism of ethanol enhances the level of NADH in the liver which, in turn, stimulates the synthesis of fatty acids and their incorporation into triglycerides. Moderate ethanol consumption raises plasma VLDL levels, with the degree of elevation dependent on the baseline level. Severe hypertriglyceridemia and pancreatitis usually develop on the background of a genetic hyperlipidemia and heavy alcohol intake. Because ethanol also stimulates the synthesis of apo AI and inhibits CETP, ethanol-associated hypertriglyceridemia is usually accompanied by normal or elevated levels of HDL cholesterol.

Liver Disease Primary biliary cirrhosis and extrahepatic biliary obstruction can cause hypercholesterolemia and elevated levels of plasma phospholipids associated with increased levels of an abnormal lipoprotein (lipoprotein X; Chap. 299) and LDL. Severe liver injury often leads to a decrease in levels of both cholesterol and triglyceride. Acute hepatitis can cause elevated levels of VLDL and impairment of LCAT formation.

AIDS Use of protease inhibitor therapies has been associated with a generalized metabolic syndrome that includes hypertriglyceridemia, alterations in fat distribution, and occasionally type 2 DM (Chap. 309).

DIAGNOSIS Although the initial indication of an abnormality in lipoprotein metabolism is via blood measurements of triglyceride and cholesterol, the disorders are due to abnormalities of specific lipoproteins. Thus, lipoprotein analysis should assess VLDL, LDL, and HDL levels. Direct measurements of plasma LDL require laborious centrifugation techniques. However, LDL cholesterol concentrations can be estimated indirectly in individuals with triglyceride levels <4.5 mmol/L (<400 mg/dL) by subtracting the HDL and VLDL cholesterol from the total plasma cholesterol. HDL cholesterol is determined after chemical precipitation of VLDL and LDL. VLDL cholesterol is estimated to be the plasma triglyceride level divided by five. Therefore

$$\text{LDL cholesterol} = \text{total cholesterol} - (\text{HDL} + \text{triglycerides}/5)$$

where all values are measured in milligrams per deciliter.

In persons with triglyceride levels >4.5 mmol/L (>400 mg/dL), the ratio of triglyceride to cholesterol in VLDL is >5, and this equation cannot be used to calculate the plasma LDL cholesterol level. The other disorder that is not detected with this method is dysbetalipoproteinemia because the ratio of triglyceride to cholesterol in the VLDL is ≪5. In these two situations, direct measurement of LDL cholesterol must be performed in ultracentrifuged plasma. Commercial methods for the measurement of "direct LDL" are available. Although these methods appear to be precise and accurate, the measured values for LDL cholesterol are 0.06 to 0.17 mmol/L (5 to 15 mg/dL) less than estimated LDL because the estimated value is actually the combination of IDL and LDL. If a "direct LDL" measurement is used, the National Cholesterol Education Program (NCEP) guidelines (based on estimated LDL) must be adjusted before therapeutic decisions are made.

Because plasma triglyceride levels rise and both HDL and LDL cholesterol levels fall modestly after a fat-containing meal (due to the action of CETP), it is preferable to measure plasma lipids after a 12-h fast. Measuring cholesterol levels alone will not detect individuals with isolated low HDL; screening for CHD should therefore include measurement of HDL. Because serum lipid levels vary from day to day, at least two to three measurements should be made days or weeks apart before initiating therapy. Some experts advocate the use of total cholesterol/HDL ratios as a better assessment of individual risk. This is a reasonable approach provided both the patient and physician are aware that the treatment goal is to reduce LDL. In addition, rare patients with very high or very low levels of both LDL and HDL have ratios that are not interpretable on the basis of population studies. Although some laboratories offer measurements of individual apoproteins (e.g., apo B100 and apo AI), or size estimates of LDL, this information is not generally helpful in decision-making. Measurement of lipoprotein (a) levels can provide an indication of risk that cannot be gleaned from lipid measurements. Lipoprotein electrophoresis is not useful except for the diagnosis of dysbetalipoproteinemia, a diagnosis that otherwise requires ultracentrifugation methods. Apo E genotyping is also helpful in the diagnosis of dysbetalipoproteinemia (although rarely the disorder can be due to other defects in the apo E gene).

Both LDL and HDL cholesterol levels are temporarily decreased for several weeks after myocardial infarction or acute inflammatory states but can be accurately measured if blood is obtained within 8 h of the event.

Approach to the Patient

Elevated LDL Cholesterol Treatment of elevated LDL cholesterol can have either of two aims—*primary prevention* of the complications of atherosclerosis or *secondary treatment* after complications have occurred. The rationale for primary prevention is based on the large body of data linking elevated levels of LDL cholesterol with increased CHD risk and an impressive body of clinical and experimental data demonstrating that reducing LDL cholesterol slows progression and may actually induce regression of atherosclerotic lesions (Chap. 242). Both primary and secondary intervention trials indicate that total mortality can be reduced when the LDL cholesterol is lowered (Table 344-1). A meta-analysis of four randomized trials (4S, CARE, AFCAPS/TexCAPS, LIPID) comparing HMG-CoA reductase inhibitors to control included 30,817 participants and found that HMG-CoA reductase inhibitor treatment was associated with: (1) a 20% decrease in total cholesterol, a 28% decrease in LDL cholesterol, a 13% decrease in triglycerides, and a 5% increase in HDL cholesterol; (2) a 31% decrease in major coronary events and a 21% decrease in all-cause mortality; (3) similar risk reduction in women and men; and (4) no effect on noncardiovascular mortality. Unexpectedly, the risk of stroke was also reduced 19 to 32% by HMG-CoA reductase inhibitor treatment, even though previous observational studies show a relatively weak association between cholesterol level and stroke risk.

Dietary Alterations A fundamental starting point for both primary prevention and secondary treatment involves counseling to modify diet, exercise, smoking, and other life-style factors that increase the risk of CHD. The typical American diet derives about 35% of its calories from fat (14 to 15% from saturated fat) and contains 400 to 500 mg/d of cholesterol. Individuals with hyperlipidemia should be encouraged to eat a diet lower in cholesterol and saturated fat. The NCEP Step 1 diet, which is recommended for all Americans above age 2, provides 30% of calories from fat, <10% of calories from saturated fat, and <300 mg/d of cholesterol (Table 344-7). Carbohydrate is the typical nutrient used to replace fat in patients with isolated hypercholesterolemia. In general, whole-milk dairy products, egg yolks, meats, palm oil, and coconut oil should be replaced with fresh fruits and vegetables, complex carbohydrates (especially whole-grain products), and low-fat dairy products. Shellfish are low in fat content and, except for shrimp, also have low cholesterol levels; shrimp, in moderation, is acceptable. Portion size needs to be stressed; the protein and fat-rich portion of meat in a given meal should be <115 g (4 oz), the size of a deck of cards. Substitutions with any food low in saturated fat such as bran, nuts, and olive oil will have positive effects on LDL. Hydrogenation of vegetable oils increases the saturation of the fatty acids. In particular, trans-fatty acids, mainly found in commercially hydrogenated vegetable oils, raise LDL and can lower HDL cholesterol levels. Use of stanol-containing margarines has, by contrast, lowered LDL cholesterol about 5 to 10% by blocking cholesterol absorption in the small intestine. When further diet therapy is indicated, the NCEP Step 2 diet provides 30% of calories as fat but <7% of calories from saturated fat, and <200 mg/d of cholesterol. After changing from

Table 344-7 The Two-Step Approach to Treating Hypercholesterolemia

Nutrient	Step 1 Diet	Step 2 Diet
Total fat	<30% calories	<30% calories
Fatty acids		
Saturated	<10% calories	<7% calories
Polyunsaturated	≤10% calories	≤10% calories
Monounsaturated	10–15% calories	10–15% calories
Carbohydrates	50–60% calories	50–60% calories
Protein	10–20% calories	10–20% calories
Cholesterol	<300 mg/d	<200 mg/d

[a] Total calories: to achieve and maintain desirable body weight.

Table 344-8 Hypolipidemic Drugs

Drugs	Mode of Action	Lipoprotein Class Affected
HMG-CoA reductase inhibitors Lovastatin (Mevacor) 10–80 mg/d Pravastatin (Pravachol) 10–40 mg/d Simvastatin (Zocor) 5–40 mg/d Fluvastatin (Lescol) 20–40 mg/d Atorvastatin (Lipitor) 10–80 mg/d Cerivastatin (Baycol) 0.3–0.4 mg/d	↓ Cholesterol synthesis ↑ LDL receptors	↓ LDL 25–55% ↓ VLDL, ↓ TG 10–20% ↑ HDL 5–10%
Nicotinic acid Niacin 50–100 mg tid initially, then increase to 1.0–2.5 g tid Niaspan 1–2 g/d	↓ Synthesis of VLDL and LDL; mechanism not defined	↓ TG 25–35% ↓ VLDL 25–35% ↓ LDL 15–25% ↑ HDL 15–30%
Bile acid–binding resins Cholestyramine (Questran) 8–12 g bid or tid Cholestipol (Cholestid) 10–15 g bid or tid	Interruption of the enterohepatic recycling of bile acids; ↑ Synthesis of new bile acids from cholesterol ↑ LDL receptors	↓ LDL 20–30% ↑ HDL 5% ↑ TG 10%
Fibric acid derivatives Clofibrate (Atromid) 1000 mg bid Gemfibrozil (Lopid) 600 mg bid Fenofibrate (Tricor) 200 mg qd	↑ LPL and ↑ triglyceride hydrolysis; ↓ VLDL synthesis ↑ LDL catabolism	↓ TG 25–40% ↑ or ↓ LDL ↑ HDL 5–15%
Probucol Probucol (Lorelco) 500 mg bid	↑ LDL clearance from plasma ↓ Apo A I synthesis Antioxidant	↓ LDL 10–15% ↓ HDL 20–25%

NOTE: LDL, low-density lipoprotein; VLDL, very low density lipoprotein; TG, triglycerides; HDL, high-density lipoprotein; LPL, lipoprotein lipase; CPK, creative phosphokinase.

the average American diet to the Step 1 diet, the LDL cholesterol usually drops 8 to 10%; an additional reduction of 5 to 7% can be achieved by advancing to the Step 2 diet. There is, however, great individual variability in diet responsiveness, and several values should be obtained before judging the efficacy of any diet treatment.

Primary Prevention The NCEP Adult Treatment Panel recommends measuring plasma cholesterol in all adults older than age 20 at least every 5 years. Ideally, this testing involves a lipoprotein profile to allow better risk stratification. Primary prevention goals include LDL cholesterol <3.36 mmol/L (<130 mg/dL), triglycerides <1.7 mmol/L (<150 mg/dL), and HDL cholesterol >1.03 mmol/L (>40 mg/dL) for men and >1.29 mmol/L (>50 mg/dL) for women. In individuals without DM or known CHD, treatment recommendations for primary prevention are outlined in Fig. 344-2. Assessment of risk factors in addition to LDL cholesterol is an essential part of this decision-making process. Risk factors include: (1) family history of premature CHD (<55 years in a male parent or sibling or <65 in female relatives), (2) hypertension (even if it is controlled with medications), (3) cigarette smoking (>10 cigarettes per day), (4) DM, and (5) low HDL [<0.9 mmol/L (<35 mg/dL)]. In addition, because CHD is more prevalent in older individuals, age (men >45 years, women >55 years, or younger women with premature menopause without estrogen replacement) is also an important risk factor. HDL cholesterol >1.6 mmol/L (>60 mg/dL) is a negative risk factor, i.e., one other risk factor can be negated by a high HDL cholesterol level.

In individuals with fewer than two risk factors, life-style modifications alone and follow-up testing may be used if LDL is <4.14 mmol/L (<160 mg/dL). For those with LDL >4.91 mmol/L (>190 mg/dL), drug treatment is indicated. If two or more risk factors are present, drug treatment in addition to life-style modifications should be instituted if LDL cholesterol is >3.36 mmol/L (>130 mg/dL). HMG-CoA reductase inhibitors are first-line medications for most patients; niacin and resins are second-line treatments (see below).

Secondary Prevention The NCEP guidelines are stringent for the secondary treatment of patients with CHD. Patients with CHD should be screened for lipid abnormalities during and after their initial diagnoses. A goal of lowering plasma LDL concentrations to <2.6 mmol/L (<100 mg/dL) is advocated for such individuals as well as for patients with DM (Fig. 344-2). As described below, this requires modifications of diet in addition to the use of one or more medications.

If a patient with CHD has only a modestly elevated LDL cholesterol level [e.g., <3.36 mol/L (<130 mg/dL)], a 4- to 6-week period of Step 1 diet therapy can precede the addition of drugs. In such a patient, moving to the Step 2 diet, which provides the same total fat but <7% of calories from saturated fat, can be useful. If, however, the LDL cholesterol is >3.36 mmol/L (>130 mg/dL), drug therapy should be instituted along with diet therapy (Fig. 344-2).

High Triglycerides and Low HDL The evidence that treatment to reduce plasma triglyceride levels or increase levels of HDL cholesterol leads to long-term health benefits is less compelling than that for treatment of high LDL levels. Two recent clinical trials have shown, however, that lowering triglycerides (using fibric acids) or lowering LDL (HMG-CoA reductase inhibitors) decreases CHD events in these patients. There have been no intervention trials in which only increases in HDL cholesterol concentrations have been achieved. Beneficial effects of niacin have been attributed, in part, to its HDL-raising effect and its action to reduce triglycerides and LDL. Even with drugs that primarily affect LDL cholesterol levels, such as bile acid–binding resins and HMG-CoA reductase inhibitors, some of the benefits achieved may be related to increases in HDL cholesterol levels.

In patients with isolated elevations of triglyceride levels or with hypertriglyceridemia and high LDL cholesterol, life-style modifications should be introduced as described above, and weight reduction

Common Side Effects	Contraindications	Drug Interactions	Combined Use
Hepatic dysfunction <2%, severe myositis <1%, ↑ CPK, len opacities may occur	Risk of myositis increased by impaired renal function and in combination with gemfibrozil or nicotinic acid	Fibric acid derivatives, niacin, ketoconazole, cyclosporine, erythromycin, coumadin	Bile acid resins; increased myositis risk when combined with gemfibrozil, niacin
Flushing (may be relieved by aspirin), hepatic dysfunction, tachycardia, atrial arrythmias, pruritus, dry skin, nausea, diarrhea, glucose intolerance, hyperuricemia	Peptic ulcer disease, cardiac arrhythmias, hepatic disease, gout, diabetes mellitus	Synergistic with ganglionic blocking agents used to treat hypertension	Bile acid resins, HMG-CoA reductase inhibitors, fibric acid derivatives
Constipation, gastric discomfort, nausea, hemorrhoidal bleeding, theoretical ↑ lithogenicity of bile	Biliary tract obstruction, gastric outlet obstruction	↓ Absorption of phenylbutazone, phenobarbital, thyroid hormone, digoxin, coumadin, thiazide diuretics, and some antibiotics; binds fat-soluble vitamins (A,D,E,K);	Nicotinic acid, HMG-CoA reductase inhibitors, fibric acid derivatives
↑ Lithogenicity of bile, gallstones, nausea, hepatic dysfunction, myositis <1%, cardiac arrythmias	Hepatic or biliary disease, renal insufficiency associated with ↑ risk of myositis	↑ Anticoagulant activity of coumadin	Bile acid resins
Diarrhea, nausea, abdominal pain, cardiac arrhythmias	Prolonged QT interval, primary biliary cirrhosis		Bile acid resins

should be strongly encouraged if obesity is present. Fat intake should be decreased, but the concomitant increase in carbohydrate intake may raise triglyceride and lower HDL cholesterol levels. If this occurs, replacing some of the saturated fat with monounsaturated fat, which will not raise LDL cholesterol, may be valuable. Severe hypertriglyceridemia and hyperchylomicronemia require very low fat diets, avoidance of free sugars, and decreased alcohol intake. Patients with genetic LPL deficiency are instructed to prepare their food using medium-chain triglycerides, which are not incorporated into chylomicrons. Fish oils decrease triglyceride synthesis, and high doses may be used for severe hypertriglyceridemia.

The management of hypertriglyceridemia focuses on the associated LDL and HDL concentrations as guidelines for therapy. Thus, the overall risk profile can be used to set goals for LDL cholesterol, using a low HDL level (commonly associated with hypertriglyceridemia) as a concomitant major risk factor for atherosclerosis. However, when triglyceride levels are >5.6 mmol/L (>500 mg/dL), the risk of developing pancreatitis increases, and a direct focus on lowering triglycerides is recommended. Thus, triglyceride levels >5.6 mmol/L (>500 mg/dL) are generally treated with drugs, whereas lower levels [2.2 to 5.6 mmol/L (200 to 500 mg/dL)] are not treated unless other CHD risk factors are present (Fig. 344-2).

℞ TREATMENT Three classes of lipid-lowering agents are recommended as first-line therapy against hypercholesterolemia: (1) the HMG-CoA reductase inhibitors; (2) niacin; and (3) the bile acid–binding resins (Table 344-8). Fibric acid derivatives are second-line agents for hypercholesterolemia and are most effective for lowering triglycerides.

HMG-CoA Reductase Inhibitors This class of drugs, which include lovastatin, simvastatin, pravastatin, fluvastatin, atorvastatin, and cerivastatin, inhibits the rate-limiting step in hepatic cholesterol biosynthesis (the conversion of HMG-CoA to mevalonate), causing an increase in LDL receptor levels in hepatocytes and enhanced receptor-mediated clearance of LDL cholesterol from the circulation. At usual doses, the HMG-CoA reductase inhibitors decrease total cholesterol by 20 to 30% and LDL cholesterol by 25 to 40%. Larger reductions may be achieved with higher doses. Treatment with reductase inhibitors often reduces triglycerides by 10 to 20%, possibly due to reduced secretion of VLDL by the liver. Higher doses of more potent reductase inhibitors, which can lower LDL cholesterol by 45 to 60%, can lower triglycerides by 30 to 45%. HDL cholesterol levels rise about 5 to 10%. In comparison with other lipid-lowering agents, HMG-CoA reductase inhibitors are relatively free of side effects. Mild, transient elevations in liver enzymes occur with all of the agents at the highest doses, but elevations in serum aminotransferases to more than three times the upper limits of normal occur in <2% of patients. Therapy should be discontinued when elevations of this magnitude occur. A rare but potentially serious adverse effect of HMG-CoA reductase inhibitors is myopathy, manifest by muscle pain with elevation of serum creatine phosphokinase (CPK). This occurs in <1% of patients treated with reductase inhibitors alone but is more common (about 2 to 3%) when used in combination with gemfibrozil, niacin, or cyclosporine.

Niacin The mechanism of action of niacin is not fully understood, but it appears to inhibit the secretion of lipoproteins containing apo B100 from the liver. Niacin decreases both total and LDL cholesterol approximately 15 to 25%, reduces VLDL levels by 25 to 35%, and raises HDL cholesterol levels by as much as 15 to 25%. Thus, niacin exerts favorable changes on the three major lipoproteins (VLDL, LDL, and HDL). Efficacy of monotherapy was confirmed in a long-term secondary prevention trial in which niacin significantly reduced the incidence of myocardial infarction. An even longer-term follow-up of that study (15 years total) showed an 11% decrease in all-cause mortality among patients randomized to niacin. Because of its ability to reduce VLDL synthesis, niacin is also a first-line drug for treatment of hypertriglyceridemia.

Niacin is safe, having been in use for almost 30 years, but unpleasant side effects, including cutaneous flushing with or without pruritus, may limit patient acceptability. The cutaneous symptoms tend to subside after several weeks and may be minimized by initiating therapy at low doses or by administering aspirin 30 min before the niacin dose. Less common adverse effects include elevations of liver enzymes, gastrointestinal distress, impaired glucose tolerance, and elevated serum uric acid levels with or without gouty arthritis. Liver enzymes may be elevated in 3 to 5% of patients on full doses of niacin (>2 g/d). Because of its propensity to worsen the control of blood sugar, niacin should be used with caution in patients with DM. Niaspan, an intermediate-release form of niacin, appears to exhibit lipid-altering activity similar to regular niacin.

Bile Acid–Binding Resins Cholestyramine and colestipol have been in use as lipid-lowering agents for almost three decades. These drugs interfere with reabsorption of bile acids in the intestine, resulting in a compensatory increase in bile acid synthesis and upregulation of LDL receptors in hepatocytes. The bile acid sequestrants are useful in the treatment of patients with elevated levels of LDL cholesterol and normal triglycerides. Sequestrants produce dose-dependent decreases on the order of 15 to 25% in total cholesterol and of 20 to 35% in LDL cholesterol. The agents cause modest increases in HDL cholesterol. A limitation of the sequestrants is their tendency to raise triglyceride levels through compensatory increases in hepatic synthesis of VLDL; they should not be given to hypertriglyceridemic individuals. Bile acid–binding resins are efficacious and safe and are recommended for young adult men and premenopausal women with moderate cholesterol elevations. Patient compliance is low, in part because of the need to dissolve these powdered agents in fluid; the availability of colestipol as a tablet may alleviate this problem. Gastrointestinal side effects include constipation, bloating, and gas.

Combination Therapy Combinations of bile acid–binding resins and reductase inhibitors are effective for the treatment of severe, isolated elevations of LDL cholesterol. Combinations of reductase inhibitors and niacin, or resins and niacin, are useful for the treatment of high LDL and low HDL cholesterol levels, though the former combination carries an increased risk of myositis (2 to 3%). If triglyceride and LDL levels are both elevated (HDL is usually reduced as well), resins and niacin are an excellent combination, with resins and gemfibrozil (see below) as an alternative. The combination of a reductase inhibitor and gemfibrozil can be useful when LDL cholesterol is very high in the face of concomitant hypertriglyceridemia, but the risk of myositis (about 2 to 3%) must be considered. Combinations of reductase inhibitors with either niacin or gemfibrozil might best be reserved for patients with CHD and combined hyperlipidemia.

LDL Apheresis In patients with homozygous FH and in ordinary FH patients who respond poorly to diet and drug therapy or who cannot tolerate drugs, apheresis at 7- to 14-day intervals can cause profound lowering of LDL cholesterol levels. Diet and drug regimens are continued during treatment. This approach should be considered for patients with few therapeutic options.

Fibric Acids Gemfibrozil and fenofibrate stimulate the activity of a liver transcription factor termed *PPARα* that increases LPL activity and production of apo AI. Moreover, these drugs reduce VLDL triglyceride entry into plasma and reduce synthesis of apo CIII, which might improve LPL-induced lipolysis or reduce VLDL secretion. Stimulation of peroxisomal fatty acid oxidation by fibrates may also contribute to the triglyceride-lowering actions. Gemfibrozil and fenofibrate treatment is associated with 25 to 40% reductions in plasma triglyceride levels. Postprandial triglyceride levels, which are linked to fasting concentrations, are also reduced. HDL cholesterol levels increase 5 to 15% with fibrate treatment. Fibric acids and a low-fat diet are particularly useful in the treatment of dysbetalipoproteinemia and are first-line therapy for this disorder except in postmenopausal women, who should initially be given estrogen replacement (if not contraindicated).

Significant increases in LDL cholesterol can accompany otherwise potentially beneficial falls in triglycerides and increases in HDL cholesterol during fibrate therapy. Such rises may require a change to another drug or addition of a second agent.

In the short term, these drugs are well tolerated; mild gastrointestinal distress in the form of epigastric pain is the major side effect. Elevations of liver enzymes occur in 2 to 3% of patients but do not usually require cessation of treatment. Rarely, hepatitis can occur. Fibrates appear to make the bile more lithogenic, and long-term use is probably associated with a twofold increase in gallstone formation. Myopathy with myositis is a rare occurrence with the fibrates, either alone or in combination with HMG CoA reductase inhibitors.

Fish Oils Large doses of omega-3 fatty acids reduce triglyceride levels by diminishing their production. In the United States, omega-3 fatty acid capsules contain 40 to 60% omega-3 fatty acids; the rest of the fatty acids are omega-6. Therefore, to consume 2 to 4 g of omega-3 fatty acids, an individual must take 5 to 10 capsules per day.

HYPOCHOLESTEROLEMIA

A low total cholesterol concentration [<2.6 mmol/L (<100 mg/dL)] in an adult can be due to rare hereditary traits or secondary to a number of diseases. As described earlier, mutations in the gene for apo B100 that disrupt synthesis or produce truncated forms of apo B100 are associated with hypobetalipoproteinemia. These mutations are inherited as codominant traits; heterozygotes have plasma cholesterol levels in the range of 1.3 to 2.6 mmol/L (50 to 100 mg/dL), with reduced LDL cholesterol levels but normal plasma HDL cholesterol levels. Heterozygotes are asymptomatic, whereas hypolipoproteinemia homozygotes (or compound heterozygotes) have even lower total and LDL cholesterol concentrations and may have malabsorption of fats and fat-soluble vitamins similar to that in abetalipoproteinemia.

Abetalipoproteinemia (Table 344-5) is a rare, autosomal recessive disorder in which there are mutations in the microsomal triglyceride transfer protein (MTP) gene. Individuals who are homozygous for this disorder have total cholesterol levels <1.3 mmol/L (<50 mg/dL) and essentially no VLDL, IDL, LDL, or chylomicrons. Because dietary fat and vitamins A and E are transported from the intestine in chylomicrons, these patients may have malabsorption of fat and fat-soluble vitamins. Vitamin E deficiency in infancy and early childhood can result in neurologic problems (Chap. 75). If vitamin replacement is adequate, individuals with abetalipoproteinemia can live normal, healthy lives.

Moderately low levels of total cholesterol may also be associated with extreme reductions in HDL cholesterol. As noted above, these are almost always secondary to mutations in the gene for apo AI and a lack of apo AI in plasma.

A number of systemic diseases can cause low cholesterol concentrations. Malnutrition, often associated with alcoholism or gastrointestinal disease, can cause low levels of total and LDL cholesterol. Hyperthyroidism, particularly when severe, can reduce cholesterol levels. Patients with uncontrolled AIDS may have total cholesterol levels <2.1 mmol/L (<80 mg/dL), usually associated with severe wasting, diarrhea, and a poor prognosis. Several neoplasms, particularly those involving the hematopoietic system, are associated with hypocholesterolemia. Patients with acute and chronic myelogenous leukemia and myeloid metaplasia with splenomegaly can have severe reductions in both LDL and HDL levels. Other diseases with concomitant splenomegaly, including lipid storage diseases such as Gaucher's disease and Niemann-Pick disease, can cause very low LDL and HDL cholesterol concentrations due to increased lipoprotein catabolism.

BIBLIOGRAPHY

GOLDSTEIN JL et al: Familial hypercholesterolemia, in *The Metabolic and Molecular Bases of Inherited Disease*, 8th ed, CR Scriver et al (eds). New York, McGraw-Hill, 2001, pp 2863–2913

GOTTO AM Jr.: Triglyceride as a risk factor for coronary artery disease. Am J Cardiol 82: 22Q, 1998

GRUNDY SM: Primary prevention of coronary heart disease: Integrating risk assessment with intervention. Circulation 100:988, 1999

KNOPP RH: Drug treatment of lipid disorders. N Engl J Med 341:498, 1999

KRAUSS RM et al: Dietary guidelines for healthy American adults. A statement for health professionals from the Nutrition Committee, American Heart Association. Circulation 94:1795, 1996

LAROSA JC et al: Effect of statins on risk of coronary disease: A meta-analysis of randomized controlled trials. JAMA 282:2340, 1999

RIFKIND BM: Clinical trials of reducing low-density lipoprotein concentrations. Endocrinol Metab Clin North Am 27:585, 1998

STEINBERG D, GOTTO AM: Preventing coronary artery disease by lowering cholesterol levels: Fifty years from bench to bedside. JAMA 282:2043, 1999

Summary of the Second Report of the National Cholesterol Education Program expert panel on detection, evaluation, and treatment of high blood cholesterol in adults. JAMA 269:3015, 1993

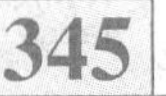

345

Lawrie W. Powell, Kurt J. Isselbacher

HEMOCHROMATOSIS

DEFINITION Hemochromatosis is a common disorder of iron storage in which an appropriate increase in intestinal iron absorption results in deposition of excessive amounts of iron in parenchymal cells with eventual tissue damage and impaired function of organs, especially the liver, pancreas, heart, joints, and pituitary. The disease was termed *hemochromatosis* and the iron-storage pigment was called *hemosiderin* because it was believed that the pigment was derived from the blood. The terms *hemosiderosis* and *siderosis* are often used to describe the presence of stainable iron in tissues, but tissue iron must be quantified to assess body iron status (see below and Chap. 105). *Hemochromatosis* implies potentially severe progressive iron overload leading to fibrosis and organ failure. Cirrhosis of the liver, diabetes mellitus, arthritis, cardiomyopathy, and hypogonadotrophic hypogonadism are common manifestations.

Although there is debate about definitions, it seems logical to use the following terminology:

1. *Hereditary* or *genetic hemochromatosis*: This disorder is most often caused by inheritance of a mutant *HFE* gene, which is tightly linked to the HLA-A locus on chromosome 6p (see below). The genetic disease can be recognized during its early stages when iron overload and organ damage are minimal. At this stage the disease is best referred to as *early* or *precirrhotic hemochromatosis* (Fig. 345-1).

2. *Secondary iron overload*: Tissue injury usually occurs secondary to an iron-loading anemia such as thalassemia or sideroblastic anemia, in which increased erythropoiesis is ineffective. In the acquired iron-loading disorders, massive iron deposits in parenchymal tissues can lead to the same clinical and pathologic features as in hemochromatosis.

PREVALENCE Hemochromatosis is one of the most common genetic diseases, although its prevalence varies in different ethnic groups. It is most common in populations of northern European extraction in whom approximately 1 in 10 persons are heterozygous carriers and 0.3 to 0.5% are homozygotes. However, expression of the disease is modified by several factors, especially dietary iron intake, blood loss associated with menstruation and pregnancy, and blood donation. The clinical expression of the disease is 5 to 10 times more frequent in men than in women. Nearly 70% of affected patients develop the first symptoms between ages 40 and 60. The disease is rarely evident before age 20, although with family screening (see below) and periodic health examinations, asymptomatic subjects with iron overload can be identified, including young menstruating women. A recent study in a European non-blood bank population revealed that 30% of homozygous individuals did not have evidence of iron overload. Thus, the penetrance of the mutation is variable.

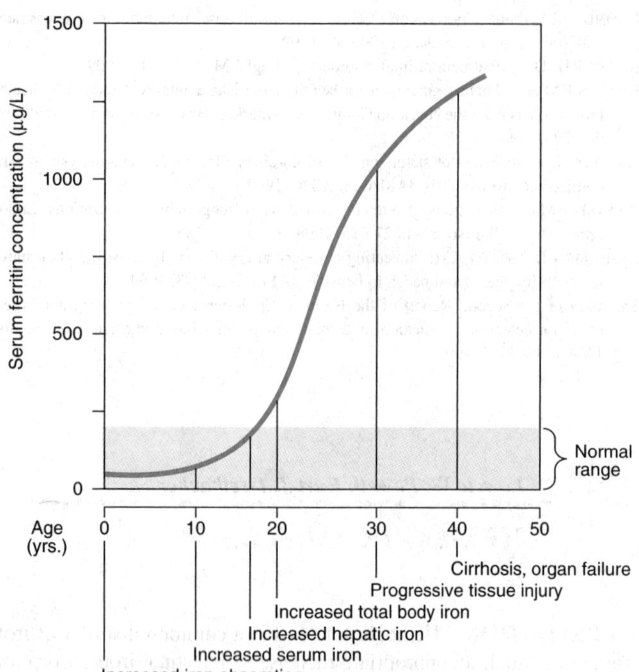

FIGURE 345-1 Sequence of events in genetic hemochromatosis and their correlation with the serum ferritin concentration. Increased iron absorption is present throughout life. Overt, symptomatic disease usually develops between ages 40 and 60, but latent disease can be detected long before this.

GENETIC BASIS AND MODE OF INHERITANCE The gene involved in the most common form of hemochromatosis was cloned in 1996 and is termed *HFE*. A homozygous G→A mutation resulting in a cysteine to tyrosine substitution at position 282 (C282Y) is the most common mutation. It was identified in 85 to 100% of patients with hereditary hemochromatosis in populations of northern European descent but was found in only 60% of cases from Mediterranean populations (e.g., southern Italy). A second, relatively common *HFE* mutation has also been identified. This results in an amino acid substitution of histidine to aspartic acid at position 63 (H63D). Some compound heterozygotes (e.g., one copy each of C282Y and H63D) have increased body iron stores. Thus, *HFE*-associated hemochromatosis is inherited as an autosomal recessive trait; heterozygotes have no, or minimal, increase in iron stores. However, in some cases this slight increase in hepatic iron acts as a cofactor that aggravates other diseases such as porphyria cutanea tarda (PCT) and nonalcoholic steatohepatitis.

Mutations in other genes, currently unidentified, are responsible for non-*HFE* associated hemochromatosis, including juvenile hemochromatosis, which affects subjects in the second and third decade of life (Table 345-1).

PATHOGENESIS Normally, the body iron content of 3 to 4 g is maintained such that intestinal mucosal absorption of iron is equal to iron loss. This amount is approximately 1 mg/d in men and 1.5 mg/d in menstruating women. In hemochromatosis, mucosal absorption is inappropriate to body needs and amounts to 4 mg/d or more. The progressive accumulation of iron causes an early elevation in plasma iron, an increased saturation of transferrin, and progressive elevation of plasma ferritin level (Fig. 345-1).

The *HFE* gene encodes a 343 amino acid protein that is structurally related to MHC class I proteins. The basic defect in hemochromatosis is a lack of cell surface expression of HFE (due to the C282Y mutation). The normal (wild type) HFE protein forms a complex with β_2-microglobulin and transferrin, and the C282Y mutation completely abrogates this interaction. As a result, the mutant HFE protein remains trapped intracellularly, reducing transferrin receptor-mediated iron uptake by the intestinal crypt-cell. This is postulated to upregulate the divalent metal transporter (DMT-1) on the brush border of the villous cells, leading to inappropriately increased intestinal iron absorption. In advanced disease, the body may contain 20 g or more of iron that is deposited mainly in parenchymal cells of the liver, pancreas, and heart. Iron may be increased 50- to 100-fold in the liver and pancreas and 5- to 25-fold in the heart. Iron deposition in the pituitary causes hypogonadotropic hypogonadism in both men and women. Tissue injury may result from disruption of iron-laden lysosomes, from lipid peroxidation of subcellular organelles by excess iron, or from stimulation of collagen synthesis by activated stellate cells.

Table 345-1 Classification of Iron Overload States

Hereditary hemochromatosis
Hemochromatosis, *HFE*-related
C282Y homozygosity
C282Y/H63D compound heterozygosity
Hemochromatosis non-*HFE*-related
Juvenile hemochromatosis
Autosomal dominant hemochromatosis (Solomon Islands)
Acquired iron overload
Iron-loading anemias
Thalassemia major
Sideroblastic anemia
Chronic hemolytic anemias
Transfusional and parenteral iron overload
Dietary iron overload
Chronic liver disease
Hepatitis C
Alcoholic cirrhosis, especially when advanced
Nonalcoholic steatohepatitis
Porphyria cutanea tarda
Dysmetabolic iron overload syndrome
Post portacaval shunting
Miscellaneous
Iron overload in sub-Sahara Africa
Neonatal iron overload
Aceruloplasminemia
Congenital atransferrinemia

Secondary iron overload with deposition in parenchymal cells occurs in chronic disorders of erythropoiesis, particularly in those due to defects in hemoglobin synthesis or ineffective erythropoiesis such as sideroblastic anemia and thalassemia (Chap. 106). In these disorders, the absorption of iron is increased. Moreover, these patients require blood transfusions and are also frequently treated inappropriately with iron. PCT, a disorder characterized by a defect in porphyrin biosynthesis (Chap. 346), is also sometimes associated with excessive parenchymal iron deposits. The magnitude of the iron load in PCT is usually insufficient to produce tissue damage. However, recent reports have found that many patients with PCT also have mutations in the *HFE* gene, and some have associated hepatitis C infection. Although the relationship among these disorders remains to be clarified, iron overload accentuates the inherited enzyme deficiency in PCT and should be avoided along with other agents (alcohol, estrogens, haloaromatic compounds) that may exacerbate PCT. Another cause of hepatic parenchymal iron overload is hereditary aceruloplasminemia. In this disorder, impairment of iron mobilization due to deficiency of ceruloplasmin (a ferroxidase) causes iron overload in hepatocytes.

Alcoholic subjects with end-stage chronic liver disease may have increased tissue iron stores of the degree seen in hemochromatosis. The increased iron may be caused by cell death and uptake of the released iron, as well as by hemolysis associated with spur-cell anemia (Chap. 108). Hemochromatosis in a heavy drinker can be distinguished from alcoholic liver disease by the presence of the C282Y mutation.

Excessive iron ingestion over many years rarely results in hemochromatosis. An important exception has been reported in South Africa among groups who brew fermented beverages in vessels made of iron. Hemochromatosis has on occasion been described in apparently normal subjects who have taken medicinal iron over many years, but such individuals probably have a genetic disorder.

The common denominator in all patients with hemochromatosis is *excessive amounts of iron in parenchymal tissues.* Parenteral administration of iron in the form of blood transfusions or iron preparations results predominantly in reticuloendothelial cell iron overload. This appears to lead to less tissue damage than iron loading of parenchymal cells.

PATHOLOGY At autopsy, the enlarged nodular liver and pancreas are rusty in color. Histologically, iron is increased in amount in many organs, particularly in the liver, heart, and pancreas, and to a lesser extent in the endocrine glands. The epidermis of the skin is thin, and melanin is increased in the cells of the basal layer. Deposits of iron are present around the synovial lining cells of the joints.

In the liver of patients with hemochromatosis, parenchymal iron is in the form of ferritin and hemosiderin. In the early stages these deposits are seen in the periportal parenchymal cells, especially within lysosomes in the pericanalicular cytoplasm of the hepatocytes. This stage progresses to perilobular fibrosis and eventually to deposition of iron in bile duct epithelium, Kupffer cells, and fibrous septa. In the advanced stage, a macronodular or mixed macro- and micronodular cirrhosis develops.

CLINICAL MANIFESTATIONS Initial symptoms include weakness, lassitude, weight loss, change in skin color, abdominal pain, loss of libido, and symptoms of diabetes mellitus. Hepatomegaly, increased pigmentation, spider angiomas, splenomegaly, arthropathy, ascites, cardiac arrhythmias, congestive heart failure, loss of body hair, testicular atrophy, and jaundice are prominent in advanced disease.

The *liver* is usually the first organ to be affected, and hepatomegaly is present in more than 95% of symptomatic patients. Hepatic enlargement may exist in the absence of symptoms or of abnormal liver function tests. Indeed, over half of patients with symptomatic hemochromatosis have little laboratory evidence of functional impairment of the liver, in spite of hepatomegaly and fibrosis. Loss of body hair, palmar erythema, testicular atrophy, and gynecomastia are common. Manifestations of portal hypertension and esophageal varices occur less commonly than in cirrhosis from other causes. Hepatocellular carcinoma develops in about 30% of patients with cirrhosis, and it is the most common cause of death in treated patients; hence the importance of early diagnosis and therapy. Its incidence increases with age, is more common in men, and occurs almost exclusively in cirrhotic patients. Splenomegaly occurs in approximately half of symptomatic cases.

Excessive skin pigmentation is present in over 90% of symptomatic patients at the time of diagnosis. The characteristic metallic or slate gray hue is sometimes referred to as bronzing and results from increased melanin and iron in the dermis. Pigmentation usually is diffuse and generalized, but it may be more pronounced on the face, neck, extensor aspects of the lower forearms, dorsa of the hands, lower legs, genital regions, and in scars.

Diabetes mellitus occurs in about 65% of patients and is more likely to develop in those with a family history of diabetes, suggesting that direct damage to the pancreatic islets by iron deposition occurs in combination with a genetic predisposition. The management is similar to that of other forms of diabetes, although pronounced insulin resistance is more common in association with hemochromatosis. Late complications are the same as seen in other causes of diabetes mellitus.

Arthropathy develops in 25 to 50% of patients. It usually occurs after age 50, but may occur as a first manifestation, or long after therapy. The joints of the hands, especially the second and third metacarpophalangeal joints, are usually the first joints involved, a feature that helps to distinguish the chondrocalcinosis associated with hemochromatosis from the idiopathic form (Chap. 322). A progressive polyarthritis involving wrists, hips, ankles, and knees also may ensue. Acute brief attacks of synovitis may be associated with deposition of calcium pyrophosphate (chondrocalcinosis or pseudogout), mainly in the knees. Radiologic manifestations include cystic changes of the subchondral bones, loss of articular cartilage with narrowing of the joint space, diffuse demineralization, hypertrophic bone proliferation, and calcification of the synovium. The arthropathy tends to progress despite removal of iron by phlebotomy. Although the relation of these abnormalities to iron metabolism is not known, the fact that similar changes occur in other forms of iron overload suggests that iron is directly involved.

Cardiac involvement is the presenting manifestation in about 15% of patients. The most common manifestation is congestive heart failure, which occurs in about 10% of young adults with the disease, especially those with juvenile hemochromatosis. Symptoms of congestive failure may develop suddenly, with rapid progression to death if untreated. The heart is diffusely enlarged and may be misdiagnosed as idiopathic cardiomyopathy if other overt manifestations are absent. Cardiac arrhythmias include premature supraventricular beats, paroxysmal tachyarrhythmias, atrial flutter, atrial fibrillation, and varying degrees of atrioventricular block.

Hypogonadism occurs in both sexes and may antedate other clinical features. Manifestations include loss of libido, impotence, amenorrhea, testicular atrophy, gynecomastia, and sparse body hair. These changes are primarily the result of decreased production of gonadotropins due to impairment of hypothalamic-pituitary function by iron deposition; however, primary testicular dysfunction may be seen in some cases. Adrenal insufficiency, hypothyroidism, and hypoparathyroidism may also occur.

DIAGNOSIS The association of (1) hepatomegaly, (2) skin pigmentation, (3) diabetes mellitus, (4) heart disease, (5) arthritis, and (6) hypogonadism should suggest the diagnosis. However, a parenchymal iron overload of comparatively short duration or modest degree may exist with none or only some of these manifestations [e.g., in young subjects (Fig. 345-1)]. Therefore, a high index of suspicion is needed to make the diagnosis early. This is particularly important because treatment before there is permanent organ damage can reverse the iron toxicity and restore life expectancy to normal (see below).

The history should be particularly detailed in regard to disease in other family members, alcohol ingestion, iron intake, and ingestion of large doses of ascorbic acid, which promotes iron absorption (Chap. 75). Appropriate tests should be performed to exclude iron deposition due to hematologic disease. The presence of liver, pancreatic, cardiac, and joint disease should be confirmed by physical examination, roentgenography, and standard function tests of these organs. The degree of increase in total-body iron stores should be assessed with particular attention to an increase in parenchymal iron concentration, with or without tissue damage.

The methods available for assessing parenchymal iron stores include (1) measurement of serum iron and the percent saturation of transferrin (or the unsaturated iron-binding capacity); (2) measurement of serum ferritin concentration; (3) liver biopsy with measurement of the iron concentration and calculation of the hepatic iron index (Table 345-2), (4) estimation of chelatable iron stores following the administration of deferoxamine; and (5) computed tomography (CT) and/or magnetic resonance imaging (MRI) of the liver. Each has its advantages and limitations. The serum iron level and percent saturation of transferrin are elevated early in the course, but their specificity is reduced by significant false-positive and false-negative rates. For example, serum iron concentration may be increased in patients with alcoholic liver disease without iron overload; in this situation, however, the hepatic iron index is usually not increased as in hemochromatosis (Table 345-1). In otherwise healthy persons, a fasting serum transferrin saturation greater than 50% is abnormal and suggests homozygosity for hemochromatosis.

The serum ferritin concentration is usually a good index of body iron stores, whether decreased or increased. In fact, an increase of 1 μg/L in serum ferritin level reflects an increase of about 65 mg in body stores. In most untreated patients with hemochromatosis, the serum ferritin level is greatly increased (Fig. 345-1 and Table 345-1). However, in patients with inflammation and hepatocellular necrosis, serum ferritin levels may be elevated out of proportion to body iron stores due to increased release from tissues. A repeat determination of serum

Table 345-2 Representative Iron Values in Normal Subjects, Patients with Hemochromatosis, and Patients with Alcoholic Liver Disease

Determination	Normal	Symptomatic Hemochromatosis	Homozygotes with Early, Asymptomatic Hemochromatosis	Heterozygotes	Alcoholic Liver Disease
Plasma iron, μmol/L (μg/dL)	9–27 (50–150)	32–54 (180–300)	Usually elevated	Elevated or normal	Often elevated
Total iron-binding capacity, μmol/L (μg/dL)	45–66 (250–370)	36–54 (200–300)	36–54 (200–300)	Elevated or normal	45–66 (250–370)
Transferrin saturation, percent	22–46	50–100	50–100	Normal or elevated	27–60
Serum ferritin, μg/L	10–200	900–6000	200–500	Usually <500	10–500
Urinary iron,[a] mg/24 h	0–2	9–23	2–5	2–5	Usually <5
Liver iron, μg/g dry wt	300–1400	6000–18,000	2000–4000	300–3000	300–2000
Hepatic iron index (μg/g dry wt) / 56 × age	<1.0	>2	Usually >2	<2	<2

[a] After intramuscular administration of 0.5 g deferoxamine.

ferritin should therefore be carried out after acute hepatocellular damage has subsided, e.g., in alcoholic liver disease. Ordinarily, the combined measurements of the percent transferrin saturation and serum ferritin level provide a simple and reliable screening test for hemochromatosis, including the precirrhotic phase of the disease. If either of these tests is abnormal, genetic testing for hemochromatosis should be performed (Fig. 345-2).

The role of liver biopsy in the diagnosis and management of hemochromatosis is being reassessed as a result of the widespread availability of genetic testing for the C282Y mutation. The absence of severe fibrosis can be accurately predicted in most patients using clinical and biochemical variables. Thus, there is virtually no risk of severe fibrosis in a C282Y homozygous subject with: (1) serum ferritin level less than 1000 μg/L; (2) normal serum alanine amino transaminase values; (3) no hepatomegaly; and (4) no excess alcohol intake. However, it should be emphasized that liver biopsy is the only reliable method for establishing or excluding the presence of hepatic cirrhosis, which is the critical factor determining prognosis and the risk of developing hepatocellular carcinoma. Biopsy also permits histochemical estimation of tissue iron and measurement of hepatic iron concentration. Increased density of the liver due to iron deposition can be demonstrated by CT or MRI. A retrospective assessment of body iron storage is also provided by performing weekly phlebotomy and calculating the amount of iron removed before iron stores are exhausted (1 mL blood = approximately 0.5 mg iron).

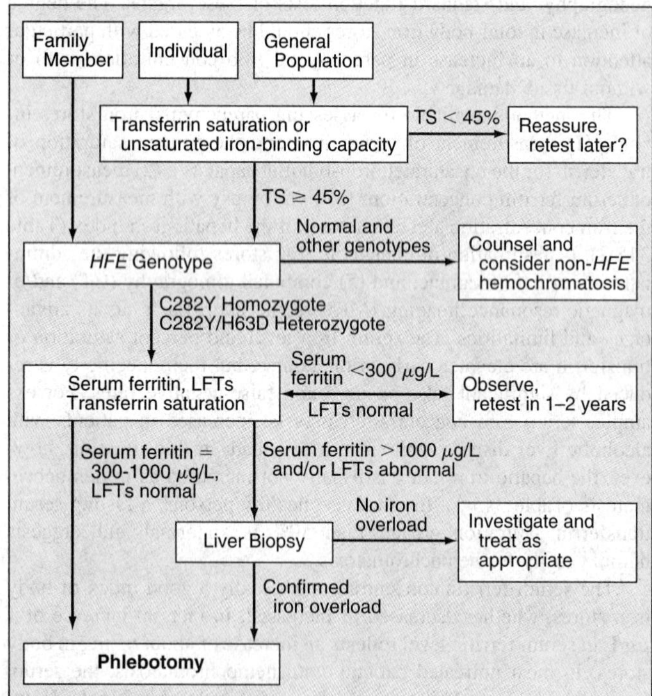

FIGURE 345-2 Algorithm for screening for *HFE*-associated hemochromatosis. LFT, liver function tests; TS, transferrin saturation. (*With permission from The Canadian Journal of Gastroenterology.*)

SCREENING FOR HEMOCHROMATOSIS When the diagnosis of hemochromatosis is established, it is important to counsel and screen other family members (Chap. 68). Asymptomatic as well as symptomatic family members with the disease usually have an increased saturation of transferrin and an increased serum ferritin concentration. These changes occur even before the iron stores are greatly increased (Fig. 345-1). All first-degree relatives of patients with hemochromatosis should be tested for the C282Y and H63D mutations and advised appropriately. In affected individuals, it is important to confirm or exclude the presence of cirrhosis, and begin therapy as early as possible. When children of a proband are affected, a homozygote-heterozygote mating is most likely.

The role of population screening for hemochromatosis is controversial. Hemochromatosis fulfills the criteria established by the World Health Organization for population screening, and DNA testing could, in principle, be performed along with other neonatal tests. However, because iron overload does not develop until the second, third, or fourth decades, and the degree of penetrance is still uncertain, screening by phenotypic expression is more practical at present (Fig. 345-2).

℞ **TREATMENT** The therapy of hemochromatosis involves removal of the excess body iron and supportive treatment of damaged organs. Iron removal is best begun by weekly or twice-weekly phlebotomy of 500 mL. Although there is an initial modest decline in the volume of packed red blood cells to about 35 mL/dL, the level stabilizes after several weeks. The plasma transferrin saturation remains increased until the available iron stores are depleted. In contrast, the plasma ferritin concentration falls progressively, reflecting the gradual decrease in body iron stores. Since one 500-mL unit of blood contains 200 to 250 mg iron and about 25 g iron should be removed, weekly phlebotomy may be required for 1 or 2 years. When the transferrin saturation and ferritin level become normal, phlebotomies are performed at appropriate intervals to maintain levels within the normal range. The measurements promptly become abnormal with iron reaccumulation. Usually one phlebotomy every 3 months will suffice.

Chelating agents such as deferoxamine, when given parenterally, remove 10 to 20 mg iron per day, which is much less than that mobilized by once-weekly phlebotomy. Phlebotomy is also less expensive, more convenient, and safer for most patients. However, chelating agents are indicated when anemia or hypoproteinemia is severe enough to preclude phlebotomy. Subcutaneous infusion of deferoxamine using a portable pump is the most effective means of administration.

The management of hepatic failure, cardiac failure, and diabetes mellitus is similar to conventional therapy for these conditions. Loss of libido and change in secondary sex characteristics are partially relieved by parenteral testosterone or gonadotropin therapy (Chap. 335).

PROGNOSIS The principal causes of death in untreated patients are cardiac failure (30%), hepatocellular failure or portal hypertension (25%), and hepatocellular carcinoma (30%).

Life expectancy is improved by removal of the excessive stores of iron and maintenance of these stores at near-normal levels. The 5-year survival rate with therapy increases from 33 to 89%. With repeated phlebotomy, the liver and spleen decrease in size, liver function improves, pigmentation of skin decreases, and cardiac failure may be reversed. Diabetes improves in about 40%, but removal of excess iron has little effect on hypogonadism or arthropathy. Hepatic fibrosis may decrease, but cirrhosis is irreversible. End-stage liver disease can be treated with orthotopic liver transplantation, but the results are suboptimal unless excess iron stores are first corrected. Hepatocellular carcinoma usually occurs as a late sequela in patients who are cirrhotic at presentation. The apparent increase in its incidence in treated patients is probably related to their increased life span. Hepatocellular carcinoma does not appear to develop if the disease is treated in the precirrhotic stage. Indeed, the life expectancy of homozygotes treated before the development of cirrhosis is normal.

The importance of family screening and early therapy cannot be emphasized too strongly. Asymptomatic subjects detected by family studies should have phlebotomy therapy if iron stores are moderately to severely increased. Assessment of iron stores at appropriate intervals is also important. With this management approach, most manifestations of the disease can be prevented.

BIBLIOGRAPHY

ADAMS PC: Population screening for hemochromatosis. Hepatology 29:1324, 1999

BACON BR et al: Molecular medicine and hemochromatosis: At the crossroads. Gastroenterology 116:193, 1999

BONKOVSKY HL et al: Porphyria cutanea tarda, hepatitis C and HFE gene mutations in North America. Hepatology 27:1661, 1998

BROCK J et al: *Iron Metabolism in Health and Disease*. London, Saunders, 1994

CAMASCHELLA C et al: Juvenile and adult hemochromatosis are distinct genetic disorders. Eur J Hum Genet 5:371, 1997

EDWARDS CQ et al: Prevalence of hemochromatosis among 11,065 presumably healthy blood donors. N Engl J Med 318:1355, 1988

FEDER JN et al: A novel MHC class I-like gene is mutated in patients with hereditary hemochromatosis. Nat Genet 13:399, 1996

FEDER JN et al: The hemochromatosis founder mutation in HLA-H disrupts β_2 microglobulin interaction and cell surface expression. J Biol Chem 272:14025, 1997

GUYADER D et al: Noninvasive prediction of fibrosis in C282Y homozygous hemochromatosis. Gastroenterology 115:929, 1998

LUDWIG K et al: Hemosiderosis in cirrhosis: A study of 447 native livers. Gastroenterology 112:882, 1997

NEIDERAU C et al: Long-term survival in patients with hereditary hemochromatosis. Gastroenterology, 110:1107, 1996

OLYNYK JK et al: A population based study of the clinical expression of the hemochromatosis gene. N Engl J Med 341:718, 1999

346

Robert J. Desnick

THE PORPHYRIAS

AIP	acute intermittent porphyria	HMB	hydroxymethylbilane
ALA	δ-aminolevulinic acid	PBG	porphobilinogen
CEP	congenital erythropoietic porphyria	PCT	porphyria cutanea tarda
COPRO	coproporphyrinogen	PROTO	protoporphyrinogen
EPP	erythropoietic protoporphyria	URO	uroporphyrinogen
HCP	hereditary coproporphyria	VP	variegate porphyria
HEP	hepatoerythropoietic porphyria	XLSA	X-linked sideroblastic anemia

The porphyrias are inherited or acquired disorders of specific enzymes in the heme biosynthetic pathway (Fig. 346-1). These disorders are classified as either *hepatic* or *erythropoietic* depending on the primary site of overproduction and accumulation of the porphyrin precursor or porphyrin (Tables 346-1 and 346-2), although some have overlapping features. The major manifestations of the hepatic porphyrias are neurologic, including neuropathic abdominal pain, neuropathy, and mental disturbances, whereas the erythropoietic porphyrias characteristically cause cutaneous photosensitivity. The reason for neurologic involvement in the hepatic porphyrias is poorly understood. Cutaneous sensitivity to sunlight is due to the fact that excitation of excess porphyrins in the skin by long-wave ultraviolet light leads to cell damage, scarring, and deformation. Steroid hormones, drugs, and nutrition influence the production of porphyrin precursors and porphyrins, thereby precipitating or increasing the severity of some porphyrias. Thus, the porphyrias are multifactorial genetic disorders, in which environmental, physiologic, and genetic factors interact to cause disease (Chap. 68).

Because many symptoms of the porphyrias are nonspecific, diagnosis is often delayed. Laboratory testing is required to confirm or exclude the various types of porphyria (Table 346-2). Urinary δ-aminolevulinic acid (ALA) and porphobilinogen (PBG) are easily quantitated by chemical methods; the urinary porphyrin isomers can be separated and quantitated by high-performance liquid chromatography. The diagnostic profile of accumulated precursors and/or porphyrins in each disorder can also be defined by extraction and thin-layer chromatography of fecal porphyrins. However, a definite diagnosis requires demonstration of the specific enzyme deficiency or gene defect. The isolation and characterization of the cDNAs encoding the heme biosynthetic enzymes have permitted identification of the genetic basis of each porphyria. Molecular genetic analyses now make it possible to provide precise heterozygote identification and prenatal diagnoses in families with known mutations or with informative polymorphisms.

HEME BIOSYNTHESIS The first and last three enzymes in the heme biosynthetic pathway are located in the mitochondrion, whereas the other four are in the cytosol (Fig. 346-1). The first enzyme, δ-aminolevulinate synthase (ALA synthase), catalyzes the condensation of glycine, activated by pyridoxal phosphate and succinyl coenzyme A, to form ALA. In the liver, this rate-limiting enzyme can be induced by a variety of drugs, steroids, and other chemicals. Distinct erythroid-specific and nonerythroid (e.g., housekeeping) forms of ALA synthase are encoded by separate genes; defects in the erythroid form cause X-linked sideroblastic anemia (XLSA).

The second enzyme, δ-aminolevulinate dehydratase (ALA dehydratase), catalyzes the condensation of two molecules of ALA to form PBG. Four molecules of PBG condense to form the tetrapyrrole uroporphyrinogen (URO) III by a two-step process catalyzed by hydroxymethylbilane (HMB) synthase (also known as PBG deaminase or URO I synthase) and URO III synthase. HMB synthase catalyzes the head-to-tail condensation of four PBG molecules by a series of deaminations to form the linear tetrapyrrole HMB. URO synthase catalyzes the rearrangement and rapid cyclization of HMB to form the asymmetric, physiologic, octacarboxylate porphyrinogen URO III isomer.

The fifth enzyme in the pathway, URO decarboxylase, catalyzes the sequential removal of the four carboxyl groups from the acetic acid side chains of URO III to form coproporphyrinogen (COPRO) III, a tetracarboxylate porphyrinogen. This compound then enters the mitochondrion, where COPRO oxidase, the sixth enzyme, catalyzes the decarboxylation of two of the four propionic acid groups to form the two vinyl groups of protoporphyrinogen (PROTO) IX, a dicarboxylate porphyrinogen. Next, PROTO oxidase oxidizes PROTO IX to protoporphyrin IX by the removal of six hydrogen atoms. The product of the reaction is a porphyrin (oxidized form), in contrast to the preceding tetrapyrrole intermediates, which are porphyrinogens (reduced forms). Finally, ferrous iron is inserted into protoporphyrin IX to form heme, a reaction catalyzed by the eighth enzyme in the pathway, ferrochelatase (also known as heme synthetase or protoheme ferrolyase).

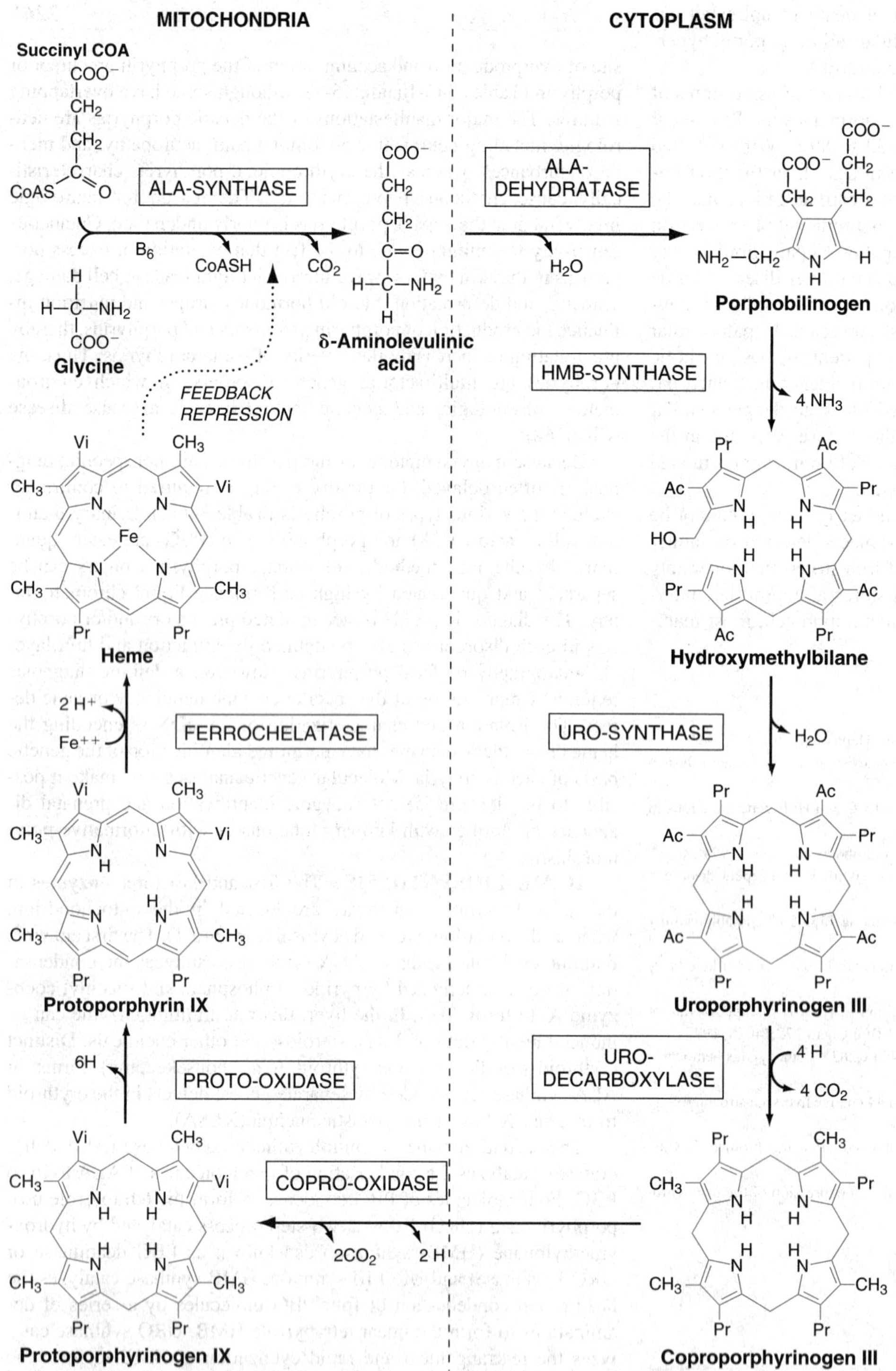

FIGURE 346-1 The human heme biosynthetic pathway.

Each of the heme biosynthetic enzymes is encoded by a separate gene. Full-length human cDNAs for each of the enzymes, including those for both forms of ALA synthase, have been isolated and sequenced, and the chromosomal locations of the genes have been identified (Table 346-3).

REGULATION OF HEME BIOSYNTHESIS About 85% of the heme produced in the body is synthesized in erythroid cells to provide heme for hemoglobin; most of the remainder is produced in the liver, where the biosynthetic pathway is under negative feedback control (Chap. 104). "Free" heme in the liver regulates the synthesis and mitochondrial translocation of the housekeeping form of ALA synthase. Heme represses the synthesis of the ALA synthase mRNA and interferes with the transport of the enzyme from the cysotol into mitochondria. ALA synthase is increased by many of the same chemicals that induce the cytochrome P450 enzymes in the endoplasmic reticulum of the liver. Because most of the heme in the liver is used for the synthesis of cytochrome P450 enzymes, hepatic ALA synthase and the cytochrome P450s are regulated in a coordinated fashion.

Different regulatory mechanisms control production of heme for hemoglobin. The erythroid-specific ALA synthase encoded on the X chromosome is expressed at higher levels than the hepatic enzyme, and an erythroid-specific control mechanism regulates iron transport into erythroid cells. During erythroid differentiation, the activities of the heme biosynthetic enzymes are increased.

THE HEPATIC PORPHYRIAS

The acute hepatic porphyrias are characterized by the rapid onset of neurologic manifestations. During the acute attack, individuals have markedly elevated plasma and urinary concentrations of the porphyrin precursors ALA and PBG, which originate from the liver.

ALA DEHYDRATASE–DEFICIENT PORPHYRIA This is a rare autosomal recessive disorder that has been described in only a few patients. Onset and severity of the disease are variable, presumably depending on the amount of residual ALA dehydratase activity. Treatment and prevention of the neurologic complications are the same as for other acute porphyrias (see below).

Clinical Features The clinical presentation is variable. The first reported cases were in two unrelated German men who had clinical onset during adolescence of abdominal pain and neuropathy, resembling acute intermittent porphyria (AIP; see below). A Swedish infant presented with failure to thrive and required transfusions and parenteral nutrition. Presumably, the earlier age of onset and more severe manifestations reflect a more complete enzyme deficiency. A Belgian man developed an acute motor polyneuropathy and polycythemia at age 63. Recently a Japanese woman was described who had her first acute attack and the syndrome of inappropriate secretion of antidiuretic hormone at age 69.

Diagnosis Patients have increased urinary levels of ALA and coproporphyrin. ALA dehydratase activity in erythrocytes is <5% of normal. Because either succinylacetone (which accumulates in hereditary tyrosinemia and is structurally similar to ALA) or lead can inhibit ALA dehydratase, increase urinary excretion of ALA, and cause manifestations that resemble those of the acute porphyrias, lead intoxication and hereditary tyrosinemia (fumarylacetoacetase deficiency) should be considered in the differential diagnosis of ALA dehydratase–deficient porphyria. Immunologic studies in the reported cases demonstrated the presence of nonfunctional enzyme proteins that cross-reacted with anti-ALA dehydratase antibodies. DNA analysis revealed different missense mutations that resulted in the amino acid substitutions G133R and V275M in the infantile-onset patient, and R240W and A274T in a juvenile-onset patient.

Heterozygotes are clinically asymptomatic and do not excrete increased levels of ALA, but they can be detected by demonstration of intermediate levels of erythrocyte ALA dehydratase activity or by demonstrating a specific mutation in the *ALA dehydratase* gene. Prenatal diagnosis of this disorder has not been achieved but should be possible by determination of the ALA dehydratase activity in cultured chorionic villi or amniocytes.

℞ **TREATMENT** Treatment is similar to that of AIP (see below). The severely affected infant was supported by hyperalimentation and periodic blood transfusions. Continued failure to thrive led to liver transplantation, which did not improve the hematologic manifestations.

Table 346-1 Classification of the Human Porphyrias

Type/Porphyria	Deficient Enzyme	Inheritance[a]	Photosensitivity	Neurovisceral Symptoms
HEPATIC PORPHYRIAS				
ALA dehydratase deficiency (ADP)	ALA dehydratase	AR	–	+
Acute intermittent porphyria (AIP)	HMB synthase	AD	–	+
Porphyria cutanea tarda (PCT)	URO decarboxylase	AD	+++	–
Hereditary coproporphyria (HCP)	COPRO oxidase	AD	+	+
Variegate porphyria (VP)	PROTO oxidase	AD	+	+
ERYTHROPOIETIC PORPHYRIAS				
X-linked sideroblastic anemia (XLSA)	ALA synthase	XLR	–	–
Congenital erythropoietic porphyria (CEP)	URO synthase	AR	+++	–
Erythropoietic protoporphyria (EPP)	Ferrochelatase	AD	+	–

[a] AR, autosomal recessive; AD, autosomal dominant; XLR, X-linked recessive.

NOTE: ALA, δ-aminolevulinic acid; HMB, hydroxymethylbilane; URO, uroporphyrinogen; COPRO, copoporphyrinogen; PROTO, protoporphyrinogen.

ACUTE INTERMITTENT PORPHYRIA This hepatic porphyria is an autosomal dominant condition resulting from the half-normal level of HMB synthase (also termed PBG deaminase) activity. The disease is widespread but is especially common in Scandinavia and perhaps Great Britain. The enzyme deficiency can be demonstrated in most heterozygous individuals, but clinical expression is highly variable. Activation of the disease is related to environmental or hormonal factors, such as drugs, diet, and steroid hormones, which can precipitate the manifestations. Attacks can be prevented by avoiding known precipitating factors.

Clinical Features Most heterozygotes remain clinically asymptomatic (latent) unless exposed to factors that increase the production of porphyrins. Endogenous and exogenous gonadal steroids, porphyrinogenic drugs, alcohol ingestion, and low-calorie diets, usually instituted for weight loss, are common precipitating factors. Table 346-4 lists the major drugs that are harmful in AIP [and also in hereditary coproporphyria (HCP) and variegate porphyria (VP)] and some drugs and anesthetic agents known to be safe. More extensive lists of drugs considered harmful or safe are available (see the bibliography), but information is incomplete for many of them. Attacks also can be provoked by infections and by surgery.

Because the neurovisceral symptoms rarely occur before puberty and are often nonspecific, a high index of suspicion is required to make the diagnosis. The disease can be disabling but is rarely fatal. Abdominal pain, the most common symptom, is usually steady and poorly localized but may be cramping. Ileus, abdominal distention, and decreased bowel sounds are common. However, increased bowel sounds and diarrhea may occur. Abdominal tenderness, fever, and leukocytosis are usually absent or mild because the symptoms are neurologic rather than inflammatory. Nausea, vomiting, constipation, tachycardia, hypertension, mental symptoms, pain in the limbs, head, neck, or chest, muscle weakness, sensory loss, dysuria, and urinary retention are characteristic. Tachycardia, hypertension, restlessness, tremors, and excess sweating are due to sympathetic overactivity.

The peripheral neuropathy is due to axonal degeneration (rather than demyelinization) and primarily affects motor neurons. Significant neuropathy does not occur with all acute attacks; abdominal symptoms are usually more prominent. Motor neuropathy affects the proximal muscles initially, more often in the shoulders and arms. The course and degree of involvement are variable. Deep tendon reflexes may be normal or hyperactive but are usually decreased or absent with advanced neuropathy. Motor weakness can be asymmetric and focal and may involve cranial nerves. Sensory changes such as paresthesia and loss of sensation are less prominent. Progressive muscle weakness can lead to respiratory and bulbar paralysis and death when diagnosis and

Table 346-2 The Major Metabolites Accumulated in the Human Porphyrias

Type/Porphyria	Increased Erythrocyte Porphyrins	Porphyrin Excretion	
		Urine	Stool
HEPATIC PORPHYRIAS			
ALA dehydratase deficiency (ADP)	PROTO	ALA, COPRO III	—
Acute intermittent porphyria (AIP)	—	ALA, PBG	—
Porphyria cutanea tarda (PCT)	—	URO I, 7-carboxylate porphyrin	ISOCOPRO
Hereditary coproporphyria (HCP)	—	ALA, PBG, COPRO III	COPRO III
Variegate porphyria (VP)	—	ALA, PBG COPRO III	PROTO IX, 5-carboxylate porphyrin
ERYTHROPOIETIC PORPHYRIAS			
X-linked sideroblastic anemia (XLSA)	—	—	—
Congenital erythropoietic porphyria (CEP)	URO I	URO I	COPRO I, URO I
Erythropoietic protoporphyria (EPP)	PROTO IX	—	PROTO IX

NOTE: ALA, δ-aminolevulinic acid; PBG, porphobilinogen; COPRO I, coproporphyrinogen; ISOCOPRO, isocoproporphyrin; URO, uroporphyrinogen; PROTO, protoporphyrinogen.

Table 346-3 The Human Heme Biosynthesis Genes and Their Chromosomal Location[a]

Gene	Chromosome Location	cDNA/ Protein	Genomic Organization Length/# Exons
δ-Aminolevulinate synthase			
Housekeeping	3p21.1	2,199 bp/640 aa	17 kb/11 exons
Erythroid-specific	Xp11.21	1,937 bp/587 aa	22 kb/11 exons
δ-Aminolevulinate dehydratase	9q34		
Housekeeping		1,149 bp/330 aa	15.9 kb/exons 1A, 2–12
Erythroid-specific		1,154 bp/330 aa	15.9 kb/exons 1B, 2–12
Hydroxymethylbilane synthase	11q23.3		
Housekeeping		1,086 bp/361 aa	11 kb/exons 1, 3–15
Erythroid-specific		1,035 bp/344 aa	11 kb/exons 2–15
Uroporphyrinogen III synthase	10q25.2→q26.3		
Housekeeping		1,296 bp/265 aa	34 kb/exons 1, 2B–10
Erythroid-specific		1,216 bp/265 aa	34 kb/exons 2A, 2B–10
Uroporphyrinogen decarboxylase	1p34	1,104 bp/367 aa	3 kb/10 exons
Coproporphyrinogen oxidase	3q12	1,062 bp/354 aa	14 kb/7 exons
Protoporphyrinogen oxidase	1q23	1,431 bp/477 aa	5.5 kb/13 exons
Ferrochelatase	18q21.3	1,269 bp/423 aa	45 kb/11 exons

[a] cDNA basepairs (bp), number of encoded amino acids (aa), genomic length in kilobases (kb), and number of exons are indicated.

treatment are delayed. Sudden death may result from sympathetic overactivity and cardiac arrhythmia.

Mental symptoms such as anxiety, insomnia, depression, disorientation, hallucinations, and paranoia can occur in acute attacks. Seizures can be due to neurologic effects or to hyponatremia. Treatment of seizures is difficult because virtually all antiseizure drugs (except bromides) may exacerbate AIP (clonazepam may be safer than phenytoin or barbiturates). Hyponatremia results from hypothalamic involvement and inappropriate vasopressin secretion or from electrolyte depletion due to vomiting, diarrhea, poor intake, or excess renal sodium loss. Persistent hypertension and impaired renal function may occur. When an attack resolves, abdominal pain may disappear within hours, and paresis begins to improve within days and may continue to improve over several years.

Diagnosis ALA and PBG levels are increased in plasma and urine during acute attacks. Urinary PBG excretion is usually 220 to 880 μmol/d (50 to 200 mg/d) [normal, 0 to 18 μmol/d (0 to 4 mg/d)], and urinary ALA excretion is 150 to 760 μmol/d (20 to 100 mg/d) [normal, 8 to 53 μmol/d (1 to 7 mg/d)]. The excretion of these compounds generally decreases with clinical improvement, particularly after hematin infusions (see below). A normal urinary PBG level effectively excludes AIP as a cause for current symptoms. Fecal porphyrins are usually normal or minimally increased in AIP, in contrast to HCP and VP. Most asymptomatic ("latent") heterozygotes with HMB synthase deficiency have normal urinary excretion of ALA and PBG. Therefore, measurement of HMB synthase in erythrocytes is useful to confirm the diagnosis and to screen asymptomatic family members.

The enzyme deficiency is detectable in erythrocytes from most AIP heterozygotes (*classic AIP*). Note that the activity is higher in young erythrocytes and may increase into the normal range in AIP when erythropoiesis is increased due to a concurrent condition. However, patients with the rare erythroid form of AIP (*erythroid, or variant, AIP*) have normal enzyme levels in erythrocytes and deficient activity in nonerythroid tissues (see below). The erythroid and housekeeping forms of HMB synthase are encoded by a single gene, which has two promoters: one promoter generates the ubiquitously expressed housekeeping mRNA; the other promoter transcribes the erythroid-specific mRNA. Several deletions and over 150 different point mutations have been found in the coding region of the gene in unrelated AIP families (Fig. 346-2). These mutations alter the kinetic properties and/or stability of the mutant enzymes or create premature termination codons. Mutations that cause erythroid AIP variants with half-normal enzyme in nonerythroid tissues, but normal activity in erythrocytes, include point mutations in the initiation methionine codon (which prevent translation) or in the 5′ donor splice site of intron 1 (which cause abnormal splicing of the HMB synthase transcript).

Heterozygotes can be identified using various polymorphic sites in the *HMB synthase* gene. Efforts are now under way to identify the specific mutations in the *HMB synthase* gene in all AIP families; this information will make it possible to identify all heterozygotes in affected families and to advise them to avoid the factors that cause acute attacks. The prenatal diagnosis of a fetus at risk can be made with cultured amniotic cells or chorionic villi.

Table 346-4 Categories of Unsafe and Safe Drugs in AIP, HCP, and VP

Unsafe	Safe
Barbiturates	Narcotic analgesics
Sulfonamide antibiotics	Aspirin
Meprobamate	Acetaminophen
Glutethimide	Phenothiazines
Methyprylon	Penicillin and derivatives
Ethchlorvynol	Streptomycin
Mephenytoin	Glucocorticoids
Succinimides	Bromides
Carbamazepine	Insulin
Valproic acid	Atropine
Pyrazolones	
Griseofulvin	
Ergots	
Synthetic estrogens and progestogens	
Danazol	
Alcohol	

NOTE: AIP, acute intermittent porphyria; HCP, hereditary coproporphyria; VP, variegate porphyria.

℞ **TREATMENT** During acute attacks, narcotic analgesics may be required for abdominal pain, and phenothiazines are useful for nausea, vomiting, anxiety, and restlessness. Chloral hydrate can be given for insomnia, and benzodiazepines are probably safe in low doses, if a minor tranquilizer is required. Although intravenous glucose (at least 300 g/d) can be effective in acute attacks of porphyria, a more complete parenteral nutritional regimen may be beneficial if oral feeding is not possible for a prolonged period. However, intravenous heme is more effective than glucose in reducing porphyrin precursor excretion and probably leads to more rapid recovery. The response to heme therapy is reduced if therapy is delayed. Therefore, 3 to 4 mg of heme, in the form of hematin (Abbott Laboratories), heme albumin, or heme arginate (Leiras Oy, Turku, Finland), may be infused daily for 4 days beginning as soon as possible after onset of an attack. Heme arginate and heme albumin are chemically stable and are less likely than hematin to produce phlebitis or an anticoagulant effect. The rate of recovery from an acute attack depends on the degree of neuronal damage and may be rapid (1 to 2 days) with prompt therapy. Recovery from severe motor neuropathy may require months or years. Identification and avoidance of inciting factors can hasten recovery from an attack and prevent future attacks. Multiple inciting factors may contribute to a symptomatic episode. Frequent clear-cut cyclical attacks occur in some women and can be prevented with a long-acting gonadotropin-releasing hormone analogue (this indication is not approved by the U.S. Food and Drug Administration) (Chap. 336).

PORPHYRIA CUTANEA TARDA Porphyria cutanea tarda (PCT), the most common of the porphyrias, can be sporadic (type I) or familial (types II and III) and can also develop after exposure to halogenated aromatic hydrocarbons. Hepatic URO decarboxylase is deficient in all types of PCT. In type I PCT, URO decarboxylase activity is normal in erythrocytes. In type II PCT, an autosomal dominant disorder, the enzyme is deficient in erythrocytes and other tissues. In type III PCT, deficiency of the enzyme is limited to the liver. Deficient hepatic URO decarboxylase and a porphyrin pattern resembling PCT can be produced by exposure of normal individuals to a number of halogenated aromatic hydrocarbons. Hepatoerythropoietic porphyria (HEP) is an autosomal recessive form of porphyria that results from marked systemic deficiency of URO decarboxylase activity.

Clinical Features Cutaneous photosensitivity is the major clinical feature. Neurologic manifestations are not observed. Fluid-filled vesicles and bullae develop on sun-exposed areas such as the face, the dorsa of the hands and feet, the forearms, and the legs. The skin in these areas is friable, and minor trauma may lead to the formation of bullae. The appearance of small white plaques, termed *milia,* may precede or follow vesicle formation. Bullae and denuded skin heal slowly and are subject to infection. Other features include hypertrichosis and hyperpigmentation, especially of the face, and thickening, scarring, and calcification resembling the cutaneous changes of systemic sclerosis.

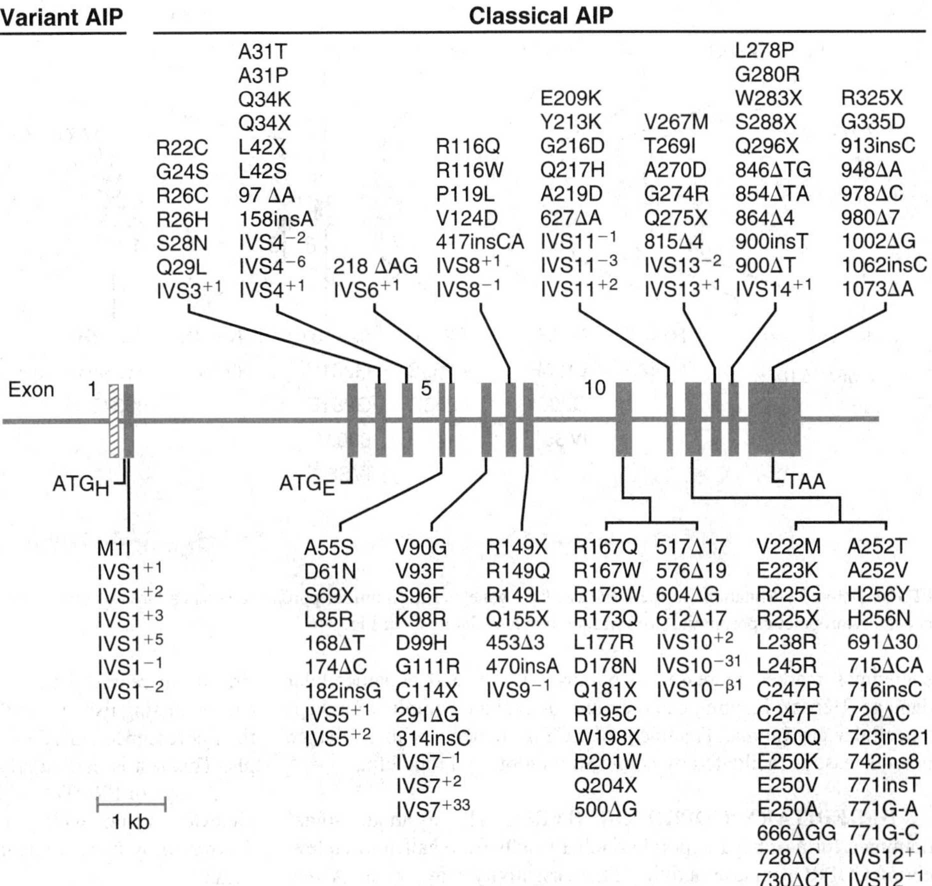

FIGURE 346-2 Mutations in the *HMB synthase* gene causing acute intermittent porphyria. Mutation nomenclature: letters, one-letter code for amino acids; numbers, codon positions.

A number of factors contribute to the development of hepatic URO decarboxylase deficiency, including excess alcohol, iron, and estrogens. The importance of excess hepatic iron as a precipitating factor is underscored by the finding that the incidence of the common hemochromatosis-causing mutations, *HFE* C282Y and H63D, are increased in patients with types I and II PCT (Chap. 345). Various chemicals can also induce PCT; an epidemic of PCT occurred in eastern Turkey in the 1950s as a consequence of wheat contaminated with the fungicide hexachlorobenzene. PCT also occurs after exposure to other chemicals, including di- and trichlorophenols and 2,3,7,8-tetrachlorodibenzo-(*p*)-dioxin (TCDD, dioxin). Patients with PCT characteristically have liver damage and are at risk for hepatocellular carcinoma. These carcinomas do not produce porphyrins.

HEP resembles congenital erythropoietic porphyria (CEP) and usually presents with blistering skin lesions, hypertrichosis, scarring, and red urine in infancy or childhood.

Diagnosis Porphyrins are increased in the liver, plasma, urine, and stool. The urinary ALA level may be slightly increased, but the PBG level is normal. Urinary porphyrins consist mostly of uroporphyrin and 7-carboxylate porphyrin, with lesser amounts of coproporphyrin and 5- and 6-carboxylate porphyrins. Plasma porphyrins are also increased in a pattern that resembles that in urine. Isocoproporphyrins are increased in feces and sometimes in plasma and urine. The finding of increased isocoproporphyrins is diagnostic for a deficiency of hepatic URO decarboxylase.

Type II PCT and HEP can be distinguished by finding decreased URO decarboxylase in erythrocytes. URO decarboxylase activity in liver, erythrocytes, and cultured skin fibroblasts in type II PCT is approximately 50% of normal in affected individuals and in family members with latent disease. In HEP, the URO decarboxylase activity is markedly deficient, with typical levels of 3 to 10% of normal. Several point mutations have been identified in the coding region of the *URO decarboxylase* gene from unrelated type II PCT and HEP patients (Fig. 346-3). Excess hepatic iron contributes to development of sporadic and familial forms of PCT. As noted above, coinheritance of *HFE* mutations that cause hemochromatosis increases susceptibility to PCT-precipitating factor. In the familial forms (types II and III), iron inhibits the residual normal enzyme, so that enzymatic activity in liver is <50% of normal. In type I PCT the decreased hepatic URO decarboxylase activity is not accompanied by a decrease in the amount of enzyme protein, suggesting that the enzyme is present in an inactive form; hepatic URO decarboxylase activity gradually increases after a remission is induced by phlebotomy.

℞ TREATMENT Alcohol, estrogens, iron supplements, and, if possible, any drugs that may exacerbate the disease should be discontinued, but this step does not always lead to improvement. A complete response can almost always be achieved by repeated phlebotomy to reduce hepatic iron. A unit (450 mL) of blood can be removed every 1 to 2 weeks. Because iron overload is not marked in most cases, remission may occur after only five or six phlebotomies. Hemoglobin levels or hematocrits and serum ferritin should be followed closely to prevent development of iron deficiency and anemia. After remission, continued phlebotomy may not be needed even if ferritin levels return to normal. Relapses are treated by additional phlebotomy.

PCT can also be treated with chloroquine or hydroxychloroquine, both of which complex with the excess porphyrins and promote their excretion. Small doses (e.g., 125 mg chloroquine phosphate twice weekly) should be given, because standard doses can induce transient,

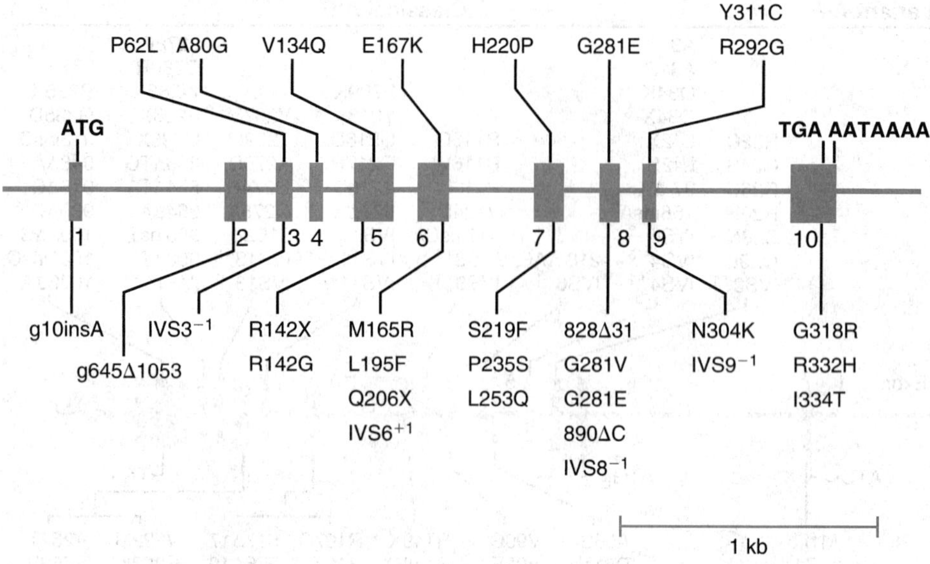

FIGURE 346-3 Mutations in the *URO synthase* gene causing familial porphyria cutanea tarda (*bottom*) and hepatoerythropoietic porphyria. (*top*) Mutation nomenclature as in Fig. 346-2.

sometimes marked increases in photosensitivity and hepatocellular damage. Hepatic imaging can diagnose or exclude complicating hepatocellular carcinoma. Treatment of PCT in patients with end-stage renal disease is facilitated by administration of erythropoietin.

HEREDITARY COPROPORPHYRIA HCP is an autosomal dominant form of hepatic porphyria that results from half-normal levels of COPRO oxidase activity. Photosensitivity may occur. A few cases of homozygous HCP have been reported.

Clinical Features HCP is influenced by the same factors that cause attacks in AIP. The disease is latent before puberty, and symptoms are more common in women. Neurovisceral symptoms and other manifestations are virtually identical to those of AIP. Photosensitivity may resemble that in PCT and VP. Cutaneous lesions may begin in childhood in rare homozygous cases.

Diagnosis Coproporphyrin is markedly increased in the urine and feces in symptomatic disease and sometimes when there are no symptoms. Urinary ALA and PBG levels are increased during acute attacks but may return to normal when symptoms resolve. Although the diagnosis can be confirmed by measuring COPRO oxidase activity, these assays are not widely available and require cells other than erythrocytes.

℞ TREATMENT Neurologic symptoms are treated as in AIP (see above). Phlebotomy and chloroquine are ineffective when cutaneous lesions are present.

VARIEGATE PORPHYRIA VP, a hepatic porphyria that results from the deficient activity of PROTO oxidase, is transmitted in an autosomal dominant manner and can present with neurologic symptoms, photosensitivity, or both.

Clinical Features Neurovisceral signs and symptoms develop after puberty and are similar to those of AIP or HCP (see above). Attacks are provoked by the same drugs, steroids, and nutritional factors that are detrimental in AIP. Skin manifestations are more common than in HCP but usually occur apart from the neurovisceral symptoms. Because the skin lesions in VP, HCP, and PCT are not distinguishable by clinical examination or biopsy, these conditions must be diagnosed by assay of porphyrins and porphyrin precursors in blood, urine, and feces.

VP is particularly common in South Africa, where 3 of every 1000 whites have the disorder. Most are descendants of a couple who emigrated from Holland to South Africa in 1688. Homozygous VP is associated with photosensitivity, neurologic symptoms, and developmental disturbances, including growth retardation, in infancy or childhood; all cases had increased erythrocyte levels of zinc protoporphyrin, a characteristic finding in all homozygous porphyrias so far described.

Dual porphyria, the simultaneous occurrence of VP and familial PCT, has been documented in several kindreds. *Chester porphyria* was described in a large British family in which individuals had acute porphyric attacks and deficiency of both PROTO oxidase and HMB synthase. Photosensitivity was not observed. It is unclear whether Chester porphyria is a variant of VP or AIP.

Diagnosis When VP is symptomatic, levels of fecal protoporphyrin and coproporphyrin and of urinary coproporphyrin are increased. Urinary ALA and PBG levels are increased during acute attacks. Plasma levels of porphyrins are increased, particularly when there are cutaneous lesions. VP can be distinguished rapidly from all other porphyrias by examining the fluorescence emission spectrum of porphyrins in plasma at neutral pH. This test is particularly useful for differentiating VP from PCT.

Assays of PROTO oxidase activity in cultured fibroblasts or lymphocytes are not widely available. Some latent cases of VP can be diagnosed by measurement of fecal porphyrins in relatives of VP patients.

℞ TREATMENT Acute attacks are treated with hematin as in AIP. Other than avoiding sun exposure, there are few effective measures for treating the skin lesions. β-Carotene, phlebotomy, and chloroquine are not helpful.

THE ERYTHROPOIETIC PORPHYRIAS

In the erythropoietic porphyrias, porphyrins from bone marrow erythrocytes and plasma are deposited in the skin and lead to cutaneous photosensitivity.

X-LINKED SIDEROBLASTIC ANEMIA XLSA results from the deficient activity of the erythroid form of ALA synthase and is associated with ineffective erythropoiesis, weakness, and pallor.

Clinical Features Typically, males with XLSA develop refractory hemolytic anemia, pallor, and weakness during infancy. They have secondary hypersplenism, become iron overloaded, and can develop hemosiderosis. The severity depends on the level of residual erythroid ALA synthase activity and on the responsiveness of the specific mutation to pyridoxal 5′-phosphate supplementation (see below). Peripheral blood smears reveal a hypochromic, microcytic anemia with striking anisocytosis, poikilocytosis, and polychromasia; the leukocytes and platelets appear normal. Hemoglobin content is reduced, and the mean corpuscular volume and mean corpuscular hemoglobin concentration are decreased. Patients with milder, late-onset disease have been reported recently.

Diagnosis Bone marrow examination reveals hypercellularity with a left shift and megaloblastic erythropoiesis with an abnormal maturation. A variety of Prussian blue–staining sideroblasts are observed. Levels of urinary porphyrin precursors and of both urinary and fecal porphyrins are normal. The level of erythroid ALA synthase is decreased in bone marrow, but this enzyme is difficult to measure in the presence of the normal ALA synthase housekeeping enzyme. Definitive diagnosis requires the demonstration of mutations in the *erythroid ALA synthase* gene.

℞ **TREATMENT** The severe anemia may respond to pyridoxine supplementation. This cofactor is essential for ALA synthase activity, and mutations in the pyridoxine binding site of the enzyme have been found in several responsive patients. Cofactor supplementation may make it possible to eliminate or reduce the frequency of transfusion. Unresponsive patients may be transfusion-dependent and require chelation therapy.

CONGENITAL ERYTHROPOIETIC PORPHYRIA CEP is an autosomal recessive disorder, also known as *Gunther's disease*, that is due to the markedly deficient activity of URO synthase; it is associated with hemolytic anemia and cutaneous lesions. CEP is characterized by accumulation of uroporphyrin I and coproporphyrin I isomers.

Clinical Features Severe cutaneous photosensitivity begins in early infancy. The skin over sun-exposed areas is friable, and bullae and vesicles are prone to rupture and infection. Skin thickening, focal hypo- and hyperpigmentation, and hypertrichosis of the face and extremities are characteristic. Secondary infection of the cutaneous lesions can lead to disfigurement of the face and hands. Porphyrins are deposited in teeth and in bones. As a result, the teeth are reddish brown and fluoresce on exposure to long-wave ultraviolet light. Hemolysis is probably due to the marked increase in erythrocyte porphyrins and leads to splenomegaly. Adults with a milder form of the disease have been described.

Diagnosis Uroporphyrin and coproporphyrin (mostly type I isomers) accumulate in the bone marrow, erythrocytes, plasma, urine, and feces. The diagnosis should be confirmed by demonstration of markedly deficient URO synthase activity. The disease can be detected in utero by measuring porphyrins in amniotic fluid and URO synthase activity in cultured amniotic cells or chorionic villi. Molecular analyses of the mutant alleles from over 20 unrelated patients have revealed the presence of gene rearrangements, an mRNA processing defect, and several point mutations that cause amino acid substitutions.

℞ **TREATMENT** The transfusion of sufficient blood to suppress erythropoiesis is effective but results in iron overload. Splenectomy may reduce hemolysis and decrease transfusion requirements. Protection from sunlight and from minor skin trauma is important. β-Carotene may be of some value. Complicating bacterial infections should be treated promptly. Recently, bone marrow transplantation has proven effective in several transfusion-dependent children, providing the rationale for stem-cell gene therapy.

ERYTHROPOIETIC PROTOPORPHYRIA Erythropoietic protoporphyria (EPP) is an autosomal dominant disorder due to the partial deficiency of ferrochelatase activity. Protoporphyrin accumulates in erythroid cells and plasma and is excreted in bile and feces. EPP is the most common erythropoietic porphyria and, after PCT, the second most common porphyria.

Clinical Features Skin photosensitivity usually begins in childhood. The skin manifestations differ from those of other porphyrias. Vesicular lesions are uncommon. Redness, swelling, burning, and itching can develop within minutes of sun exposure and resemble angioedema. Symptoms may seem out of proportion to the visible skin lesions. Sparse vesicles and bullae occur in 10% of cases. Chronic skin changes may include lichenification, leathery pseudovesicles, labial grooving, and nail changes. Severe scarring is rare, as are pigment changes, friability, and hirsutism.

The primary source of excess protoporphyrin is the bone marrow reticulocyte. Erythrocyte protoporphyrin is free (not complexed with zinc) and is mostly bound to hemoglobin. In plasma, protoporphyrin is bound to albumin. Hemolysis and anemia are usually absent or mild.

Liver function is usually normal, but in some patients accumulation of protoporphyrin causes chronic liver disease that can progress to liver failure and death. The hepatic complications are often preceded by increasing levels of erythrocyte and plasma protoporphyrin and probably result, in part, from protoporphyrin accumulation in the liver. Protoporphyrin is insoluble, forms crystalline structures in liver cells, and can decrease hepatic bile flow. Gallstones composed at least in part of protoporphyrin occur in some patients.

Some obligate heterozygotes are asymptomatic and have little or no increase in erythrocyte protoporphyrin. Thus there is phenotypic variation in this disease.

Diagnosis Protoporphyrin levels are increased in bone marrow, circulating erythrocytes, plasma, bile, and feces. Urinary levels of porphyrin and porphyrin precursors are normal. Ferrochelatase activity in cultured lymphocytes or fibroblasts is decreased.

℞ **TREATMENT** Oral β-carotene (120 to 180 mg/d) improves tolerance to sunlight in many patients. The dosage may need to be adjusted to maintain serum carotene levels in the recommended range of 10 to 15 μmol/L (600 to 800 μg/dL). Mild skin discoloration due to carotenemia is the only significant side effect. The beneficial effects of β-carotene may involve quenching of singlet oxygen or free radicals. Unfortunately, this drug is less effective in other forms of porphyria associated with photosensitivity.

Treatment of hepatic complications is difficult. However, cholestyramine and other porphyrin absorbents such as activated charcoal may interrupt the enterohepatic circulation of protoporphyrin and promote its fecal excretion, leading to some improvement. Splenectomy may be helpful when the disease is accompanied by hemolysis and significant splenomegaly. Caloric restriction and drugs or hormones that may induce the heme pathway or impair hepatic excretory function should be avoided. Iron deficiency should be prevented or treated. Transfusions or intravenous heme therapy may suppress erythroid and hepatic protoporphyrin production and are sometimes beneficial. Liver transplantation has been carried out in some patients with severe liver complications.

BIBLIOGRAPHY

ANDERSON KE et al: Disorders of heme biosynthesis: X-linked sideroblastic anemia and the porphyrias, in *The Metabolic and Molecular Bases of Inherited Disease*, 8th ed, CR Scriver et al (eds). New York, McGraw-Hill, 2001, pp 2991–3062

BONKOVSKY HL et al: Porphyria cutanea tarda, hepatitis C and HFE gene mutations in North America. Hepatology 27:1661, 1998

DE SIERVI A et al: Identification and characterization of hydroxymethylbilane synthase mutations causing acute intermittent porphyria: Evidence for an ancestral founder of the common G111R mutation. Am J Med Genet 86:366, 1999

DESNICK RJ, ANDERSON KE: Heme biosynthesis and its disorders: Porphyrias and sideroblastic anemias, in *Hematology: Basic Principles and Practices*, 2d ed, R Hoffman et al (eds). New York, Churchill Livingstone, 1995, pp 523–545

——— et al: Molecular genetics of congenital erythropoietic porphyria. Semin Liver Dis 18:77, 1998

LINDBERG RL et al: Motor neuropathy in porphobilinogen deaminase–deficient mice imitates the peripheral neuropathy of human acute porphyria. J Clin Invest 103:1127, 1999

MAY A, BISHOP DF: The molecular biology and pyridoxine responsiveness of X-linked sideroblastic anaemia. Haematologica 83:56, 1998

MENDEZ M et al: Familial prophyria cutanea tarda: Characterization of seven novel uroporphyrinogen decarboxylase mutations and frequency of common hemochromatosis alleles. Am J Hum Genet 63:1363, 1998

MOORE MR et al: *Disorders of Porphyrin Metabolism*. New York, Plenum, 1987

TEZCAN I et al: Congenital erythropoietic porphyria successfully treated by allogeneic bone marrow transplantation. Blood 92:4053, 1998

XU W et al: Congenital erythropoietic porphyria: Identification and expression of 10 mutations in the uroporphyrinogen III synthase gene. J Clin Invest 95:905, 1995

347

Robert L. Wortmann

DISORDERS OF PURINE AND PYRIMIDINE METABOLISM

amidoPRT	amidophosphoribosyltransferase	5-FU	5-fluorouracil
AMP	adenosine monophosphate	GMP	guanosine monophosphate
APRT	adenine phosphoribosyltransferase	HPRT	hypoxanthine phosphoribosyltransferase
DPD	dihydropyrimidine dehydrogenase	IMP	inosine monophosphate
		PRPP	phosphoribosylpyrophosphate
		UMP	uridine-5′-monophosphate

Purines and pyrimidines are the bases that, when linked to sugars (ribose or deoxyribose) and phosphate groups, create the nucleic acids that comprise the building blocks of RNA and DNA. The main purine bases are adenine and guanine; the pyrimidine bases include cytosine, thymine, and uracil. In addition, purines participate in diverse cellular functions, including intracellular energy metabolism (e.g., ATP), cell signaling pathways (e.g., GTP), and intercellular communication (e.g., adenosine). The nucleotides therefore serve fundamental roles in the replication of genetic material, gene transcription, protein synthesis, and cellular metabolism. Disorders that involve abnormalities of nucleotide metabolism range from relatively common diseases such as hyperuricemia and gout, in which there is increased production or impaired excretion of a metabolic end product of purine metabolism (uric acid), to rare enzyme deficiencies that affect purine and pyrimidine synthesis or degradation. Understanding these biochemical pathways has led, in some instances, to the development of specific forms of treatment, such as the use of allopurinol to reduce uric acid production.

URIC ACID METABOLISM

Uric acid is the final breakdown product of purine degradation in humans. It is a weak acid with pK_as of 5.75 and 10.3. Urates, the ionized forms of uric acid, predominate in plasma extracellular fluid and synovial fluid, with approximately 98% existing as monosodium urate at pH 7.4. Monosodium urate is easily dialyzed from plasma. Binding of urate to plasma proteins has little physiologic significance.

Plasma is saturated with monosodium urate at a concentration of 415 μmol/L (6.8 mg/dL) at 37°C. At higher concentrations, plasma is therefore supersaturated, creating the potential for urate crystal precipitation. However, precipitation sometimes does not occur even at plasma urate concentrations as high as 4800 μmol/L (80 mg/dL), perhaps because of the presence of solubilizing substances in plasma.

Uric acid is more soluble in urine than in water, possibly because of the presence of urea, proteins, and mucopolysaccharides. The pH of urine greatly influences its solubility. At pH 5.0, urine is saturated with uric acid at concentrations ranging from 360 to 900 μmol/L (6 to 15 mg/dL). At pH 7.0, saturation is reached at concentrations between 9480 and 12,000 μmol/L (158 and 200 mg/dL). Ionized forms of uric acid in urine include mono- and disodium, potassium, ammonium, and calcium urates.

Although purine nucleotides are synthesized and degraded in all tissues, urate is produced only in tissues that contain xanthine oxidase, primarily the liver and small intestine. The amount of urate in the body is the net result of the amount produced and the amount excreted (Fig. 347-1). Urate production varies with the purine content of the diet and the rates of purine biosynthesis, degradation, and salvage. Normally, two-thirds to three-fourths of urate is excreted by the kidneys, and most of the remainder is eliminated through the intestines. A four-component model describes the renal handling of uric acid in humans and includes: (1) glomerular filtration, (2) tubular reabsorption, (3) secretion, and (4) postsecretory reabsorption (Fig. 347-2). Approximately 8 to 12% of urate filtered by the glomeruli is excreted in the urine as uric acid. After filtration, 98 to 100% of the urate is reabsorbed; about half the reabsorbed urate is secreted back into the proximal tubule, and about 40% of that is again reabsorbed.

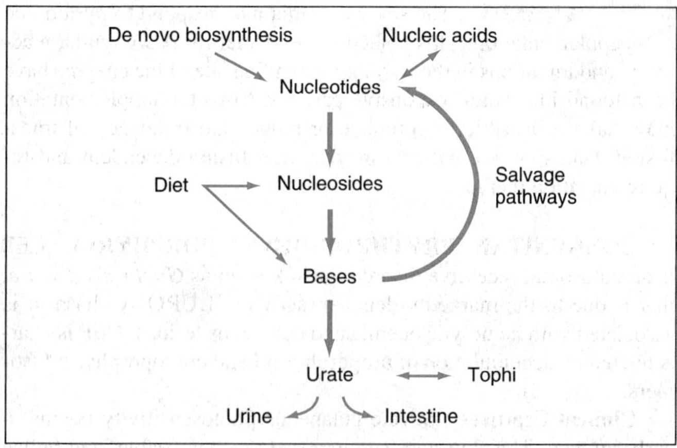

FIGURE 347-1 The total-body urate pool is the net result between urate production and excretion. Urate production is influenced by dietary intake of purines and the rates of de novo biosynthesis of purines from nonpurine precursors, nucleic acid turnover, and salvage by phosphoribosyltransferase activities. The formed urate is normally excreted by urinary and intestinal routes. Hyperuricemia can result from increased production, decreased excretion, or a combination of both mechanisms. When hyperuricemia exists, urate can precipitate and deposit in tissues as tophi.

Serum urate levels vary with age and sex. Most children have serum urate concentrations of 180 to 240 μmol/L (3.0 to 4.0 mg/dL). Levels begin to rise during puberty in males but remain low in females until menopause. Although the cause of this gender variation is not completely understood, it is due in part to a higher excretion of urate in females. Mean serum urate values of adult men and premenopausal women are 415 and 360 μmol/L (6.8 and 6.0 mg/dL), respectively. After menopause, values for women increase to approximate those of men. In adulthood, concentrations rise steadily over time and vary with height, body weight, blood pressure, renal function, and alcohol intake.

HYPERURICEMIA

Hyperuricemia can result from increased production or decreased excretion of uric acid or from a combination of the two processes. When sustained hyperuricemia exists, plasma and extracellular fluids are supersaturated with respect to urate, and total body urate is increased. Sustained hyperuricemia predisposes some individuals to develop clinical manifestations including gouty arthritis (Chap. 322) and renal dysfunction (see below).

Hyperuricemia may be defined as a plasma (or serum) urate concentration >420 μmol/L (7.0 mg/dL). This definition is based on physicochemical, epidemiologic, and disease-related criteria. Physicochemically, hyperuricemia is the concentration of urate in the blood that exceeds the solubility limits of monosodium urate in plasma, 415 μmol/L (6.8 mg/dL). In epidemiologic studies, hyperuricemia is defined as the mean plus 2 standard deviations of values determined from

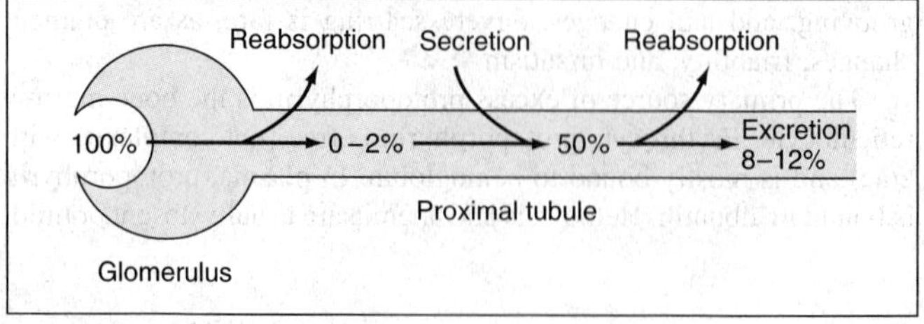

FIGURE 347-2 Schematic for handling of uric acid by the kidney. Components are illustrated with the percentage of filtered urate.

a randomly selected healthy population. When measured in unselected individuals, 95% have serum urate concentrations <420 μmol/L (7.0 mg/dL). Finally, hyperuricemia can be defined in relation to the risk of disease. The risk of developing gouty arthritis or urolithiasis increases with urate levels >420 μmol/L (7.0 mg/dL) and escalates in proportion to the degree of elevation. Hyperuricemia is present in between 2.0 and 13.2% of ambulatory adults and somewhat more frequently in hospitalized individuals.

CAUSES OF HYPERURICEMIA Hyperuricemia may be classified as primary or secondary depending on whether the cause is innate or is the result of an acquired disorder (Table 347-1). However, it is more useful to classify hyperuricemia in relation to the underlying pathophysiology, i.e., whether it results from increased production, decreased excretion, or a combination of the two (Fig. 347-1, Table 347-2).

Increased Urate Production Diet provides an exogenous source of purines and, accordingly, contributes to the serum urate in proportion to its purine content. Strict restriction of purine intake reduces the mean serum urate level by about 60 μmol/L (1.0 mg/dL) and urinary uric acid excretion by approximately 1.2 mmol/d (200 mg/d). Because about 50% of ingested RNA purine and 25% of ingested DNA purine appear in the urine as uric acid, foods high in nucleic acid content have a significant effect on the serum urate level. Such foods include liver, "sweetbreads" (i.e., thymus and pancreas), kidney, and anchovy.

Endogenous sources of purine production also influence the serum urate level (Fig. 347-3). De novo purine biosynthesis, the formation of a purine ring from nonring structures, is an 11-step process that results in formation of inosine monophosphate (IMP). The first step combines phosphoribosylpyrophosphate (PRPP) and glutamine and is catalyzed by amidophosphoribosyltransferase (amidoPRT). The rates of purine biosynthesis and urate production are determined, for the most part, by this enzyme. AmidoPRT is regulated by the substrate PRPP, which drives the reaction forward, and by the end products of biosynthesis (IMP and other ribonucleotides), which provide feedback inhibition. A secondary regulatory pathway is the salvage of purine bases by hypoxanthine phosphoribosyltransferase (HPRT). HPRT catalyzes the combination of the purine bases hypoxanthine and guanine with PRPP to form the respective ribonucleotides IMP and guanosine monophosphate (GMP). Increased salvage activity thus retards de novo synthesis by reducing PRPP levels and increasing concentrations of inhibitory ribonucleotides.

Serum urate levels are closely coupled to the rates of de novo purine biosynthesis, which is driven in part by the level of PRPP, as evidenced by two inborn errors of purine metabolism. Both increased PRPP synthetase activity and HPRT deficiency are associated with overproduction of purines, hyperuricemia, and hyperuricaciduria (see below for clinical descriptions). An X-linked disorder that causes an increase in activity of the enzyme PRPP synthetase leads to increased

Table 347-1 Classification of Hyperuricemia by Cause

- Primary
  - No recognized cause
  - Hypoxanthine phosphoribosyltransferase deficiency
  - Increased phosphoribosyl pyrophosphatase activity
- Secondary
  - Hereditary fructose intolerance
  - Glycogen storage disease
  - Myeloproliferative disease
  - Lymphoproliferative disease
  - Hemolytic anemia
  - Psoriasis
  - Obesity
  - Renal insufficiency
  - Lead intoxication
  - Chronic beryllium disease
  - Sarcoidosis
  - Drugs
    - Low-dose salicylates
    - Diuretics
    - Pyrazinamide
    - Ethambutol
    - Nicotinamide
    - Ethanol

Table 347-2 Classification of Hyperuricemia by Pathophysiology

URATE OVERPRODUCTION		
Primary idiopathic HPRT deficiency PRPP synthetase overactivity Hemolytic processes Lymphoproliferative diseases	Myeloproliferative diseases Polycythemia vera Psoriasis Paget's disease Glycogenosis III, V, and VII	Rhabdomyolysis Exercise Alcohol Obesity Purine-rich diet
DECREASED URIC ACID EXCRETION		
Primary idiopathic Renal insufficiency Polycystic kidney disease Diabetes insipidus Hypertension Acidosis Lactic acidosis Diabetic ketoacidosis	Starvation ketosis Berylliosis Sarcoidosis Lead intoxication Hyperparathyroidism Hypothyroidism Toxemia of pregnancy Bartter's syndrome Down syndrome	Drug ingestion Salicylates (>2 g/d) Diuretics Alcohol Levodopa Ethambutol Pyrazinamide Nicotinic acid Cyclosporine
COMBINED MECHANISM		
Glucose-6-phosphatase deficiency	Fructose-1-phosphate aldolase deficiency	Alcohol Shock

NOTE: HPRT, hypoxanthine phosphoribosyltransferase; PRPP, phosphoribosylpyrophosphate.

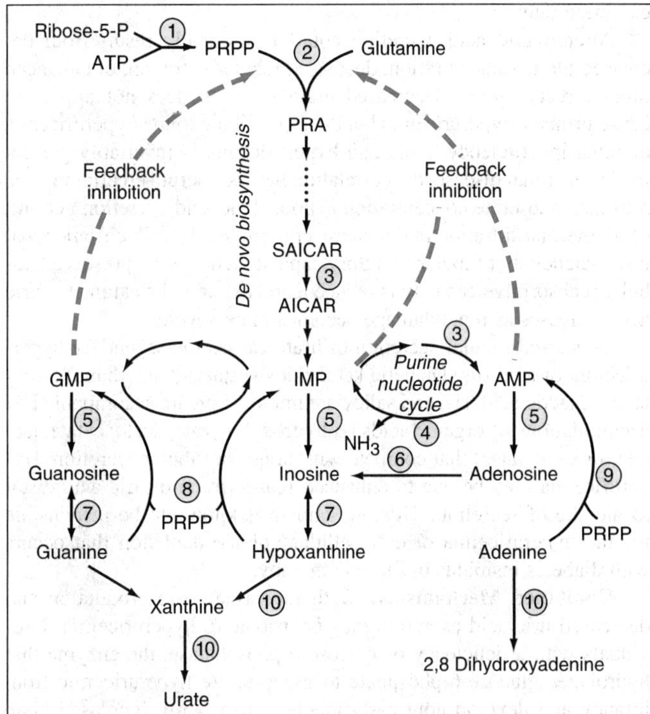

FIGURE 347-3 Abbreviated scheme of purine metabolism. (1) Phosphoribosylpyrophosphate (PRPP) synthetase, (2) amidophosphoribosyltransferase (amidoPRT), (3) adenylosuccinate lyase, (4) adenylate (AMP) deaminase, (5) 5′-nucleotidase, (6) adenosine deaminase, (7) purine nucleoside phosphorylase, (8) hypoxanthine phosphoribosyltransferase (HPRT), (9) adenine phosphoribosyltransferase (APRT), and (10) xanthine oxidase. PRA, phosphoribosylamine; SAICAR, succinylaminoimidazole carboxamide ribotide; AICAR, aminoimidazole carboxamide ribotide; GMP, guanylate; IMP, inosinate.

PRPP production and accelerated de novo biosynthesis. PRPP is a substrate and allosteric activator of amidoPRT, the first enzyme in the de novo pathway. HPRT deficiency is also X-linked and enhances urate biosynthesis in two ways. PRPP is accumulated as a result of decreased utilization in the salvage pathway and, in turn, provides increased substrate for amidoPRT and de novo biosynthesis. In addition, decreased formation of the nucleoside monophosphates, IMP and GMP, via the salvage pathway impairs feedback inhibition on amidoPRT, further enhancing de novo biosynthesis.

Accelerated purine nucleotide degradation can also cause hyperuricemia, i.e., with conditions of rapid cell turnover, proliferation, or cell death, as in leukemic blast crises, cytotoxic therapy for malignancy, hemolysis, or rhabdomyolysis. Nucleic acids released from cells are hydrolyzed by the sequential activities of nucleases and phosphodiesterases, forming nucleoside monophosphates, which in turn are degraded to nucleosides, bases, and urate. Hyperuricemia can result from excessive degradation of skeletal muscle ATP after strenuous physical exercise or status epilepticus and in glycogen storage diseases types III, V, and VII (Chap. 350). The hyperuricemia of myocardial infarction, smoke inhalation, and acute respiratory failure may also be related to accelerated breakdown of ATP.

Decreased Uric Acid Excretion Over 90% of individuals with sustained hyperuricemia have a defect in the renal handling of uric acid. In hyperuricemia with gout the renal defect is evidenced by a lower than normal ratio of urate clearance to glomerular filtration rate (or urate to insulin clearance rate) over a wide range of filtered loads. As a result, gouty individuals excrete approximately 40% less uric acid than nongouty individuals for any given plasma urate concentration. Uric acid excretion increases in gouty and nongouty individuals when plasma urate levels are raised by purine ingestion or infusion, but in those with gout, plasma urate concentrations must be 60 to 120 μmol/L (1 to 2 mg/dL) higher than normal to achieve equivalent uric acid excretion rates.

Altered uric acid excretion could theoretically result from decreased glomerular filtration, decreased tubular secretion, or enhanced tubular reabsorption. Decreased urate filtration does not appear to cause primary hyperuricemia but does contribute to the hyperuricemia of renal insufficiency. Although hyperuricemia is invariably present in chronic renal disease, the correlation between serum creatinine, urea nitrogen, and urate concentration is poor. Uric acid excretion per unit of glomerular filtration rate increases progressively with chronic renal insufficiency, but tubular secretory capacity tends to be preserved, tubular reabsorptive capacity is reduced, and extrarenal clearance of uric acid increases as renal damage becomes more severe.

Decreased tubular secretion of urate causes the secondary hyperuricemia of acidosis. Diabetic ketoacidosis, starvation, ethanol intoxication, lactic acidosis, and salicylate intoxication are accompanied by accumulations of organic acids (β-hydroxybutyrate, acetoacetate, lactate, or salicylates) that compete with urate for tubular secretion. Hyperuricemia may be due to enhanced reabsorption of uric acid distal to the site of secretion. This mechanism is known to be responsible for the hyperuricemia of extracellular volume depletion that occurs with diabetes insipidus or diuretic therapy.

Combined Mechanisms Both increased urate production and decreased uric acid excretion may contribute to hyperuricemia. Individuals with a deficiency of glucose-6-phosphatase, the enzyme that hydrolyzes glucose-6-phosphate to glucose, are hyperuricemic from infancy and develop gout early in life (Chap. 350). Increased urate production results from accelerated ATP degradation during fasting or hypoglycemia. In addition, the lower levels of nucleoside monophosphates decrease feedback inhibition of amidoPRT, thereby accelerating de novo biosynthesis. Glucose-6-phosphatase–deficient individuals may also develop hyperlacticacidemia, which blocks uric acid excretion by decreasing tubular secretion.

Patients with hereditary fructose intolerance caused by fructose-1-phosphate aldolase deficiency also develop hyperuricemia by both mechanisms. In homozygotes, vomiting and hypoglycemia after fructose ingestion can lead to hepatic failure and proximal renal tubular dysfunction. Ingestion of fructose, the substrate for the enzyme, causes accumulation of fructose-1-phosphate. This action results in ATP depletion, accelerated purine nucleotide catabolism, and hyperuricemia. Both lactic acidosis and renal tubular acidosis contribute to urate retention. Heterozygous carriers develop hyperuricemia, and perhaps one-third develop gout. The heterozygous state has a prevalence of 0.5 to 1.5%, suggesting that fructose-1-phosphate aldolase deficiency may be a relatively common cause of familial gout.

Alcohol also promotes hyperuricemia by both mechanisms. Excessive alcohol consumption accelerates hepatic breakdown of ATP and increases urate production. Alcohol consumption can also induce hyperlacticacidemia, which blocks uric acid secretion. The higher purine content in some alcoholic beverages such as beer may also be a factor.

EVALUATION OF HYPERURICEMIA Hyperuricemia does not necessarily represent a disease, nor is it a specific indication for therapy. Rather, the finding of hyperuricemia is an indication to determine its cause. The decision to treat depends on the cause and the potential consequences of the hyperuricemia in each individual.

Quantification of uric acid excretion can be used to determine whether hyperuricemia is caused by overproduction or decreased excretion. On a purine-free diet, men with normal renal function excrete <3.6 mmol/d (600 mg/d). Thus, the hyperuricemia of individuals who excrete uric acid above this level while on a purine-free diet is due to purine overproduction, whereas it is due to decreased excretion in those who excrete lower amounts on the purine-free diet. If the assessment is performed while the patient is on a regular diet, the level of 4.2 mmol/d (800 mg/d) can be used as the discriminating value. With renal insufficiency, less urate is filtered in the glomeruli and less uric acid appears in the urine. Consequently, a lower 24-h urinary uric acid value in the presence of renal insufficiency does not necessarily rule out urate overproduction, but an elevated value provides strong evidence of urate overproduction. Spuriously high values can occur if a uricosuric agent is being taken at the time of urine collection. Glucocorticoids, ascorbic acid, salicylates in doses >2 g/d, and other agents that promote urate excretion interfere with the interpretation of results.

Assessment of the ratio of uric acid to creatinine (or the ratio of uric acid clearance to creatinine clearance) in spot or random urine samples is not a reliable method to screen for urate overproduction. However, this is a useful tool for evaluating individuals with acute renal failure suspected of having acute uric acid nephropathy (see below).

Pyrazinamide, which has a suppressive action on tubular secretion, can be used to investigate presecretory reabsorption of uric acid. Probenecid, an agent that inhibits postsecretory reabsorption, can be used to evaluate tubular secretion and postsecretory reabsorption.

COMPLICATIONS OF HYPERURICEMIA The most recognized complication of hyperuricemia is *gouty arthritis*. In the general population the prevalence of hyperuricemia ranges between 2.0 and 13.2%, and the prevalence of gout is between 1.3 and 3.7%. The higher the serum urate level, the more likely an individual is to develop gout. In one study, the incidence of gout was 4.9% for individuals with serum urate concentrations >540 μmol/L (9.0 mg/dL) compared with 0.5% for those with values between 415 and 535 μmol/L (7.0 and 8.9 mg/dL). The complications of gout correlate with both the duration and severity of hyperuricemia. →***For further discussion of gout, see Chap. 322.***

Hyperuricemia also causes several renal problems: (1) nephrolithiasis; (2) urate nephropathy, a rare cause of renal insufficiency attributed to monosodium urate crystal deposition in the renal interstitium; and (3) uric acid nephropathy, a reversible cause of acute renal failure resulting from deposition of large amounts of uric acid crystals in the renal collecting ducts, pelvis, and ureters.

Nephrolithiasis Uric acid nephrolithiasis occurs most commonly, but not exclusively, in individuals with gout. In gout, the prevalence of nephrolithiasis correlates with the serum and urinary uric acid levels, reaching approximately 50% with serum urate levels of 770 μmol/L (13 mg/dL) or urinary uric acid excretion >6.5 mmol/d (1100 mg/d).

Uric acid stones can develop in individuals with no evidence of arthritis, only 20% of whom are hyperuricemic. Uric acid can also play a role in other types of kidney stones. Some nongouty individuals with calcium oxalate or calcium phosphate stones have hyperuricemia or hyperuricaciduria. Uric acid may act as a nidus on which calcium oxalate can precipitate or lower the formation product for calcium oxalate crystallization.

Urate Nephropathy Urate nephropathy, sometimes referred to as *urate nephrosis*, is a late manifestation of severe gout and is characterized histologically by deposits of monosodium urate crystals surrounded by a giant cell inflammatory reaction in the medullary interstitium and pyramids. The disorder is now rare and cannot be diagnosed in the absence of gouty arthritis. The lesions may be clinically silent or cause proteinuria, hypertension, and renal insufficiency.

Uric Acid Nephropathy This reversible cause of acute renal failure is due to precipitation of uric acid in renal tubules and collecting ducts that causes obstruction to urine flow. Uric acid nephropathy develops following sudden urate overproduction and marked hyperuricaciduria. Factors that favor uric acid crystal formation include dehydration and acidosis. This form of acute renal failure occurs most often during an aggressive "blastic" phase of leukemia or lymphoma prior to or coincident with cytolytic therapy but has also been observed in individuals with other neoplasms, following epileptic seizures, and after vigorous exercise with heat stress. Autopsy studies have demonstrated intraluminal precipitates of uric acid, dilated proximal tubules, and normal glomeruli. The initial pathogenic events are believed to include obstruction of collecting ducts with uric acid and obstruction of distal renal vasculature.

If recognized, uric acid nephropathy is potentially reversible. Appropriate therapy has reduced the mortality from about 50% to practically nil. Serum levels cannot be relied on for diagnosis because this condition has developed in the presence of urate concentrations varying from 720 to 4800 μmol/L (12 to 80 mg/dL). The distinctive feature is the urinary uric acid concentration. In most forms of acute renal failure with decreased urine output, urinary uric acid content is either normal or reduced, and the ratio of uric acid to creatinine is <1. In acute uric acid nephropathy the ratio of uric acid to creatinine in a random urine sample or 24-h specimen is >1, and a value that high is essentially diagnostic.

℞ TREATMENT **Asymptomatic Hyperuricemia** Hyperuricemia is present in approximately 5% of the population and in up to 25% of hospitalized individuals. The vast majority are asymptomatic with regard to their hyperuricemia and are at no clinical risk because of it. Elevated serum urate concentrations have been associated with insulin resistance, obesity, hypertension, dyslipidemia (sometimes referred to as syndrome X), and atherosclerotic disease. However, urate does not appear to have a causal role in the development of coronary heart disease or death from cardiovascular disease. In the past, the association of hyperuricemia with cardiovascular disease and renal failure led to the use of urate-lowering agents for people with asymptomatic hyperuricemia. This practice is no longer recommended with the exception of individuals receiving cytolytic therapy for neoplastic disease, in which treatment is given in an effort to prevent uric acid nephropathy.

Hyperuricemic individuals are at risk to develop gouty arthritis, especially those with higher serum urate levels. However, treatment of asymptomatic hyperuricemia to prevent the first attack of gouty arthritis is not indicated because most hyperuricemic people never develop gout. Furthermore, neither structural kidney damage nor tophi are identifiable before the first attack. Reduced renal function cannot be attributed to asymptomatic hyperuricemia, and treatment of asymptomatic hyperuricemia does not alter the progression of renal dysfunction in patients with renal disease. Although nephrolithiasis is common in gouty patients, and a number of individuals with nephrolithiasis are hyperuricemic, increased risk of stone formation in people with asymptomatic hyperuricemia is not established.

Thus, because treatment with antihyperuricemic agents entails inconvenience, cost, and potential toxicity, routine treatment of asymptomatic hyperuricemia cannot be justified other than for prevention of acute uric acid nephropathy. In addition, routine screening for asymptomatic hyperuricemia is not recommended. If hyperuricemia is diagnosed, however, the cause should be determined. Causal factors should be corrected if the condition is secondary, and associated problems such as hypertension, hypercholesterolemia, diabetes mellitus, and obesity should be treated.

Symptomatic Hyperuricemia (See Chap. 322 for treatment of gout) • ***Nephrolithiasis*** Antihyperuricemic therapy is recommended for the individual who has both gouty arthritis and either uric acid– or calcium-containing stones, both of which may occur in association with hyperuricaciduria. Regardless of the nature of the calculi, fluid ingestion should be sufficient to produce a daily urine volume >2 L. Alkalinization of the urine with sodium bicarbonate or acetazolamide may be justified to increase the solubility of uric acid. Specific treatment of uric acid calculi requires reducing the urine uric acid concentration with allopurinol. Allopurinol administration decreases the serum urate concentration and the urinary excretion of uric acid in the first 24 h, with a maximum reduction occurring within 2 weeks. The average effective dose of allopurinol is 300 mg/d. Allopurinol can be given once a day because of the long half-life (18 h) of its active metabolite oxypurinol. The drug is effective in patients with renal insufficiency, but the dose should be reduced. Allopurinol is also useful in reducing the recurrence of calcium oxalate stones in gouty patients and in nongouty individuals with hyperuricemia or hyperuricaciduria. Potassium citrate (30 to 80 mmol/d orally in divided doses) is an alternative therapy for patients with uric acid stones alone or mixed calcium/uric acid stones. Allopurinol is also indicated for the treatment of 2,8-dihydroxyadenine kidney stones.

Uric acid nephropathy Uric acid nephropathy is often preventable, and immediate, appropriate therapy has greatly reduced the mortality rate. Vigorous intravenous hydration and diuresis with furosemide dilute the uric acid in the tubules and promote urine flow to ≥100 mL/h. The administration of acetazolamide, 240 to 500 mg every 6 to 8 h, and sodium bicarbonate, 89 mmol/L, intravenously enhances urine alkalinity and thereby solubilizes more uric acid. It is important to ensure that the urine pH remains >7.0 and to watch for circulatory overload. In addition, antihyperuricemic therapy in the form of allopurinol in a single dose of 8 mg/kg is administered to reduce the amount of urate that reaches the kidney. If renal insufficiency persists, subsequent daily doses should be reduced to 100 to 200 mg because oxypurinol, the active metabolite of allopurinol, accumulates in renal failure. Despite these measures, hemodialysis may be required.

HYPOURICEMIA

Hypouricemia, defined as a serum urate concentration <120 μmol/L (2.0 mg/dL) can result from decreased production of urate, increased excretion of uric acid, or a combination of both mechanisms. It occurs in <0.2% of the general population and <0.8% of hospitalized individuals. Hypouricemia causes no symptoms or pathology and therefore requires no therapy. It is, however, a sign of potential pathology, and its cause should be determined.

Most hypouricemia results from increased renal uric acid excretion. The finding of normal amounts of uric acid in a 24-h urine collection in an individual with hypouricemia is evidence for a renal cause. Medications with uricosuric properties (Table 347-3) include aspirin (at doses >2.0 g/d), x-ray contrast materials, and glycerylguaiacholate. Total parenteral hyperalimentation can also cause hypouricemia, possibly a result of the high glycine content of the infusion formula. Other causes of increased urate clearance include conditions

Table 347-3 Medications with Uricosuric Activity

Acetohexamide	Glyceryl guaiacolate
ACTH	Glycopyrrolate
Ascorbic acid	Halofenate
Azauridine	Meclofenamate
Benzbromarone	Phenolsulfonphthalein
Calcitonin	Phenylbutazone
Chlorprothixene	Probenecid
Citrate	Radiographic contrast agents
Dicumarol	Salicylates (>2 g/2d)
Diflunisal	Sulfinpyrazone
Estrogens	Tetracycline that is outdated
Glucocorticoids	Zoxazolamine

such as neoplastic disease, hepatic cirrhosis, diabetes mellitus, and inappropriate secretion of vasopressin; defects in renal tubular transport such as primary Fanconi syndrome and Fanconi syndromes caused by Wilson's disease, cystinosis, multiple myeloma, and heavy metal toxicity; and isolated congenital defects in the bidirectional transport of uric acid.

Hypouricemia from decreased production of urate is accompanied by very low urinary uric acid levels. Accumulation of other purine nucleosides and bases may occur depending on the specific defect. Individuals treated with allopurinol and some patients with neoplastic disease or severe hepatic dysfunction are hypouricemic and excrete increased quantities of hypoxanthine and xanthine in the urine. Xanthine oxidase deficiency can be inherited or acquired. Inherited forms include isolated xanthine oxidase deficiency and combined xanthine oxidase and sulfite oxidase deficiencies. Both cause hypouricemia and xanthinuria. Affected individuals excrete essentially no uric acid and may develop xanthine nephrolithiasis. Individuals with purine nucleoside phosphorylase deficiency, an inborn error of metabolism causing T cell–deficient immune dysfunction, are hypouricemic and excrete increased quantities of guanosine, deoxyguanosine, inosine, and deoxyinosine in the urine.

INBORN ERRORS OF PURINE METABOLISM

(See also Table 347-4, Fig. 347-3)

HPRT DEFICIENCY A complete deficiency of HPRT, the Lesch-Nyhan syndrome, is characterized by hyperuricemia, self-mutilative behavior, choreoathetosis, spasticity, and mental retardation. A partial deficiency of HPRT, the Kelley-Seegmiller syndrome, is associated with hyperuricemia but no central nervous system manifestations. In both disorders, the hyperuricemia results from urate overproduction and can cause uric acid crystalluria, nephrolithiasis, obstructive uropathy, and gouty arthritis. Early diagnosis and appropriate therapy with allopurinol can prevent or eliminate all the problems attributable to hyperuricemia but have no effect on the behavioral or neurologic abnormalities.

HPRT catalyzes the reaction that combines PRPP and the purine bases hypoxanthine and guanine to form the respective nucleoside monophosphate IMP or GMP and pyrophosphate. The enzyme is encoded by a single gene located on the X chromosome in region q26-q27. Consequently, affected males are hemizygous for the trait and inherit the mutant allele from their asymptomatic mother, who is a carrier, or are the result of spontaneous gene mutations. The deficiency state is generally the result of point mutations, small deletions or insertions, or endoduplication of exons rather than major gene alterations.

INCREASED PRPP SYNTHETASE ACTIVITY Cells from individuals with increased PRPP synthetase activity contain elevated levels of PRPP. The high substrate content drives de novo purine synthesis, causing overproduction of uric acid. Like the HPRT deficiency states, PRPP synthetase overactivity is X-linked and results in gouty arthritis and uric acid nephrolithiasis. Nerve deafness occurs in some families.

ADENINE PHOSPHORIBOSYLTRANSFERASE (APRT) DEFICIENCY Individuals with a deficiency of APRT develop kidney stones composed of 2,8-dihydroxyadenine. APRT catalyzes the conversion of adenine to adenosine monophosphate (AMP). In the absence of APRT, adenine is converted by xanthine oxidase to 2,8-dihydroxyadenine, which is insolable in urine. Reports of 2,8-dihydroxyadenine stones are rare, most likely because of its chemical similarity to uric acid. Analysis by x-ray powder diffraction is necessary for correct identification. Because this technique is rarely employed, many 2,8-dihydroxyadenine stones are incorrectly called uric acid. The consequence of this misidentification is not deleterious, as allopurinol therapy is the correct treatment for each type of stone.

APRT deficiency is inherited as an autosomal recessive trait. Caucasians with the disorder have a complete deficiency (type I), whereas Japanese subjects have some measurable enzyme activity (type II). Expression of the defect is similar in the two populations, as is the frequency of the heterozygous state (0.4 to 1.1 per 100).

HEREDITARY XANTHINURIA A deficiency of xanthine oxidase causes all purine in the urine to occur in the form of hypoxanthine and xanthine. About two-thirds of deficient individuals are asymptomatic. The remainder develop kidney stones composed of xanthine. A very small number of symptomatic individuals also have myopathy or recurrent polyarteritis. Xanthinuria appears to be inherited in an autosomal recessive pattern.

In a second form of inherited xanthinuria, the deficiency of xanthine oxidase is associated with a deficiency of sulfite oxidase. Neurologic symptoms attributable to the sulfite oxidase deficiency predominate over those of xanthinuria in individuals with the combined deficiency.

MYOADENYLATE DEAMINASE DEFICIENCY Adenylate deaminase (AMP deaminase) catalyzes the conversion of AMP to IMP with the release of ammonia and is an integral component of the purine nucleotide cycle, which plays an important role in skeletal muscle energy metabolism. Both primary (inherited) and secondary (acquired) forms of myoadenylate deaminase deficiency have been described. Myoadenylate deaminase is the only activity affected in the inherited form, whereas other muscle enzymes (creatine kinase and

Table 347-4 Inborn Errors of Purine Metabolism

Enzyme	Activity	Inheritance	Clinical Features
Hypoxanthine phosphoribosyltransferase	Complete deficiency	X-linked	Self-mutilation, choreoathetosis, hyperuricemia, gout, and uric acid lithiasis
	Partial deficiency	X-linked	Hyperuricemia, gout, and uric acid lithiasis
Phosphoribosylpyrophosphate synthetase	Overactivity	X-linked	Hyperuricemia, gout, uric acid lithiasis, and deafness
Adenine phosphoribosyltransferase	Deficiency	Autosomal recessive	2,8-Dihydroxyadenine lithiasis
Xanthine oxidase	Deficiency	Autosomal recessive	Xanthinuria and xanthine lithiasis
Adenylosuccinate lyase	Deficiency	Autosomal recessive	Autism and psychomotor retardation
Myoadenylate deaminase	Deficiency	Autosomal recessive	Myopathy with exercise intolerance or asymptomatic
Adenosine deaminase	Deficiency	Autosomal recessive	Severe combined immunodeficiency disease and chrondro-osseous dysplasia
Purine nucleoside phosphorylase	Deficiency	Autosomal recessive	T cell–mediated immunodeficiency

myokinase) are also decreased in the acquired deficiencies. In contrast, mRNA abundance is low in muscle from patients with acquired deficiencies, suggesting a different molecular basis for this form.

The primary form is inherited as an autosomal recessive trait. Clinically, this form does not appear to cause disease, and most individuals with this defect may be asymptomatic. Another explanation for the myopathy should be sought in symptomatic patients with this deficiency. The acquired deficiency occurs in association with a wide variety of neuromuscular disease, including muscular dystrophies, neuropathies, inflammatory myopathies, and collagen vascular diseases.

ADENYLOSUCCINATE LYASE DEFICIENCY Adenylosuccinate lyase participates in the synthesis of purine nucleotides in two ways. It catalyzes the conversion of succinylaminoimidazole carboxamide ribotide (SAICAR) to aminoimidazole carboxamide ribotide (AICAR) in the de novo pathway and in the conversion of AMP succinate to AMP in the purine nucleotide cycle. Deficiency of this enzyme is due to an autosomal recessive trait and causes profound psychomotor retardation, seizures, and other movement disorders. All individuals with this deficiency are mentally retarded, and most are autistic.

ADENOSINE DEAMINASE DEFICIENCY AND PURINE NUCLEOSIDE PHOSPHORYLASE DEFICIENCY See Chap. 308.

PYRIMIDINE DISORDERS

The pyrimidine, cytidine, is found in both DNA and RNA; it is a complementary base pair for guanine. Thymidine is found only in DNA where it is paired with adenine. Uridine is found only in RNA and can pair with either adenine or guanine in RNA secondary structures. Pyrimidines can be synthesized by a de novo pathway (Fig. 347-4) or reused in a salvage pathway. More than 25 different enzymes are involved in pyrimidine synthesis, salvage, and degradation pathways. Nonetheless, disorders of pyrimidine metabolism are rare. They are more difficult to recognize than purine disorders because of het-

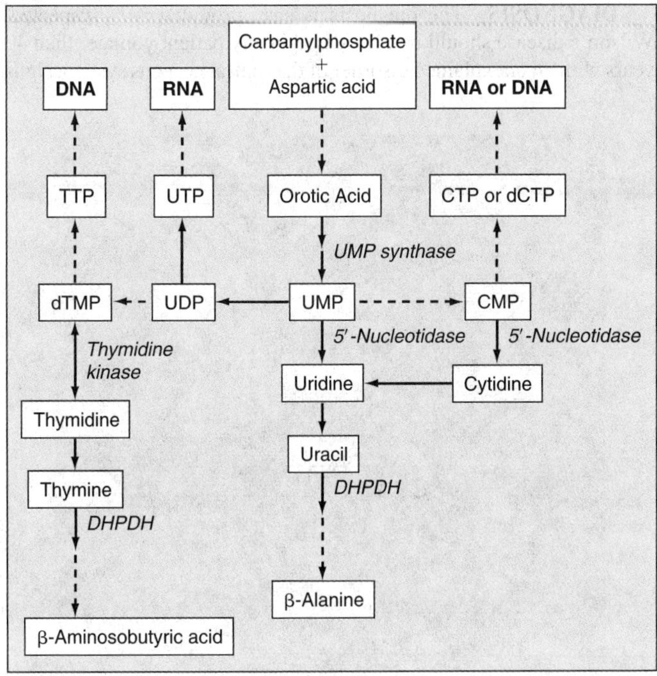

FIGURE 347-4 Abbreviated scheme of pyrimidine metabolism. Deficiency of uridine-5′-monophosphate (UMP) synthase causes orotic aciduria. Deficiency of pyrimidine-5′-nucleotidase causes a form of hemolytic anemia. Dihydropyrimidine dehydrogenase (DHPDH) deficiency impairs degradation of thymine and uracil, leading to seizure disorders and cerebral dysfunction. This enzyme is also required for metabolism of 5-fluorouracil. DTMP, deoxythymidine-5′-monophosphate; CMP, cytidine-5′-monophosphate.

erogeneous phenotypes and the absence of readily detected biochemical markers. Three disorders of pyrimidine metabolism are discussed below.

OROTIC ACIDURIA Hereditary orotic aciduria is an autosomal recessive disorder caused by mutations in a bifunctional enzyme, uridine-5′-monophosphate (UMP) synthase, which converts orotic acid to UMP in the de novo synthesis pathway (Fig. 347-4). The same protein encodes two distinct enzymatic activities. The disorder is characterized by hypochromic megaloblastic anemia that is unresponsive to vitamin B_{12} and folic acid, growth retardation, and neurologic abnormalities. Increased excretion of orotic acid causes crystalluria and obstructive uropathy. Replacement of uridine (100 to 200 mg/kg per day) corrects the anemia, reduces orotic acid excretion, and improves the other sequelae of the disorder.

PYRIMIDINE 5′-NUCLEOTIDASE DEFICIENCY Pyrimidine 5′-nucleotidase catalyzes the removal of the phosphate group from pyrimidine ribonucleoside monophosphates (cytidine-5′-monophosphate or UMP) (Fig. 347-4). Deficiency of this enzyme is transmitted as a recessive trait and causes hemolytic anemia with prominent basophilic stippling of erythrocytes. The accumulation of pyrimidines or cytidine diphosphate choline (CDPC) is thought to induce hemolysis. The enzyme deficiency alters nucleoside composition and thereby generates a characteristic ultraviolet spectrum in deproteinized erythrocytes. There is no specific treatment.

DIHYDROPYRIMIDINE DEHYDROGENASE DEFICIENCY Dihydropyrimidine dehydrogenase (DPD) is the rate-limiting enzyme in the pathway of uracil and thymine degradation (Fig. 347-4). Deficiency of this enzyme causes excessive urinary excretion of uracil and thymine. DPD deficiency is transmitted in a recessive manner and causes nonspecific cerebral dysfunction with convulsive disorders, motor retardation, and mental retardation. A splice donor site mutation, which causes deletion of exon 14, accounts for 52% of mutant alleles. No specific treatment is available. DPD is also involved in the degradation of 5-fluorouracil (5-FU), a chemotherapeutic agent that inhibits thymidylate synthase. Consequently, deficiency of this enzyme is associated with 5-FU neurotoxicity.

MEDICATION EFFECTS ON PYRIMIDINE METABOLISM In addition to the role of DPD in 5-FU degradation (see above), other medications can influence pyrimidine metabolism. Leflunomide, which is used to treat rheumatoid arthritis, inhibits de novo pyrimidine synthesis by inhibiting dihydroorotate dehydrogenase, resulting in an antiproliferative effect on T cells. Allopurinol, an inhibitor of xanthine oxidase and purine synthesis, also inhibits orotidine-5′-phosphate decarboxylase, a step in UMP synthesis. Consequently, allopurinol use is associated with increased excretion of orotidine and orotic acid; there are no known clinical effects of this inhibition.

BIBLIOGRAPHY

Becker MA et al: Purines and pyrimidines, in *The Metabolic and Molecular Bases of Inherited Disease*, 7th ed, CR Scriver et al (eds). New York, McGraw-Hill, 1995, pp 1655–1841

Culleton BF et al: Serum uric acid risk for cardiovascular disease and death: The Framingham heart study. Ann Intern Med 131:7, 1999

Seegmiller JE et al: Metabolism of purines and genetic defects leading to hyperuricemia and gout, in *Gout, Hyperuricemia, and Other Crystal-Associated Arthropathies*, CJ Smyth, VM Holers (eds). New York, Marcel Dekker, 1999, p 127

Suchi M et al: Molecular cloning of the human UMP synthase gene and characterization of point mutations in two hereditary orotic aciduria families. Am J Hum Genet 60: 525, 1997

Van Kuilenburg ABP et al: Genotype and phenotype in patients with dihydropyrimidine dehydrogenase deficiency. Hum Genet 104:1, 1999

Webster DR et al: Hereditary orotic aciduria and other disorders of pyrimidine metabolism, in *The Metabolic and Molecular Bases of Inherited Disease*, 8th ed, CR Scriver et al (eds). New York, McGraw-Hill, 2001, pp 2663–2702

Wortmann RL: Gout and hyperuricemia, in *Kelly's Textbook of Rheumatology*, 6th ed, ED Harris, Jr, S Ruddy, CB Sledge (eds). Philadelphia, Saunders, 2000, in press

———, Bentzel CJ: Renal handling of uric acid, in *Textbook of Nephrology*, 4th ed, SG Massary, RJ Glassrock (eds). Philadelphia, Lippincott Williams & Wilkins, in press

348 WILSON'S DISEASE

I. Herbert Scheinberg

Wilson's disease is an inherited disorder of copper metabolism in individuals with two mutant *ATP7B* genes. Impairment of the normal excretion of hepatic copper results in toxic accumulation of the metal in liver, brain, and other organs. The disease occurs in every ethnic and geographic population, with a worldwide prevalence of ~1 in 30,000, and a heterozygous carrier frequency of ~1 in 90.

NATURAL HISTORY The average concentrations of ceruloplasmin and hepatic copper are indistinguishable in normal neonates and in patients with Wilson's disease. In normal infants, however, the ceruloplasmin concentration increases and the hepatic copper concentration falls to adult levels during the first 3 months of life. In infants with Wilson's disease, the neonatal deficiency of ceruloplasmin and excess of hepatic copper persist indefinitely. Clinical manifestations are rare before age 6, occur most frequently in mid-adolescence, and eventually develop in all untreated patients.

In about half of patients any of four types of hepatic disturbances may herald the clinical onset. *Acute hepatitis* is usually self-limited, is often mistaken for viral hepatitis or infectious mononucleosis, and may be forgotten later in life. *Parenchymal liver disease* may persist after acute hepatitis or may develop insidiously without prior acute disease into a histologic and clinical picture indistinguishable from chronic active hepatitis and cirrhosis. In other patients *cirrhosis* may develop insidiously after a lapse of decades with no prior sign or symptom of liver disease. *Fulminant hepatitis*, generally fatal, is characterized by progressive jaundice, ascites, encephalopathy, hypoalbuminemia, hypoprothrombinemia, moderately elevated plasma levels of liver enzymes, and Coombs-negative hemolytic anemia.

In most other patients neurologic or psychiatric disturbances are the first clinical signs and are always accompanied by Kayser-Fleischer rings **(Plate III-16)**. These golden deposits of copper in Descemet's membrane of the cornea do not interfere with vision but indicate that copper has been released from the liver and has probably caused brain damage. If a patient with frank neurologic or psychiatric disease does not have Kayser-Fleischer rings when examined by a trained observer using a slit lamp, the diagnosis of Wilson's disease can be excluded. Rarely, Kayser-Fleischer rings may be accompanied by sunflower cataracts.

The neurologic manifestations include resting and intention tremors, spasticity, rigidity, chorea, drooling, dysphagia, and dysarthria. Babinski responses may be present, and abdominal reflexes are often absent. Inexplicably—in view of the ubiquity of copper excess in the brain—sensory changes never occur, except for headache.

Psychiatric disturbances are present in most patients with neurologic symptoms. Schizophrenia, manic-depressive psychoses, and classic neuroses may occur, but the commonest disturbances are bizarre behavioral patterns that defy classification. Improvement in the psychiatric state can occur with pharmacologic reduction of the copper excess, but psychotherapy and additional pharmacotherapy may be required.

In about 5% of patients the clinical onset reflects neither a hepatic nor a central nervous system disturbance. The first manifestation may be primary or secondary amenorrhea or repeated and unexplained spontaneous abortions, perhaps due to excess free copper in intrauterine secretions. Kayser-Fleischer rings may occasionally first be discovered during routine ophthalmologic examination.

PATHOGENESIS The metabolic defect in Wilson's disease is an inability to maintain a near-zero balance of copper. Dietary copper is generally in excess of the small amount that is essential to life. Normally, any excess absorbed copper is excreted by the liver; in patients with Wilson's disease, copper accumulates in the liver, reaching a mean level of about 1000 μg/g dry weight—40 times normal.

Fatty infiltration of the hepatic parenchyma and nuclear glycogen deposits are the earliest findings by light microscopy (Fig. 348-1). With electron microscopy, characteristic mitochondrial abnormalities appear to be specific for Wilson's disease. Later, necrosis, inflammation, fibrosis, bile duct proliferation, and cirrhosis ensue. Abnormalities in liver chemistries, particularly elevations in aminotransferases, may be seen at any stage. The capacity of hepatocytes to store copper is eventually exceeded, and copper is released into blood and taken up into extrahepatic tissues with disastrous effects in the brain (Table 348-1).

With magnetic resonance imaging, the effects of copper toxicity in the brain are seen most frequently in the lenticular nuclei and less commonly in the pons, medulla, thalamus, cerebellum, and cerebral cortex. Opalski and Alzheimer type II cells are present early in the course, although neither is specific for Wilson's disease, and neuronal necrosis and cavitation develop later.

An increased copper concentration in the kidney produces little, if any, structural change and usually does not alter renal function. Microscopic hematuria and/or minimal proteinuria occur occasionally; and nephrocalcinosis, renal calculi, and renal tubular acidosis are rare. Pathologic effects in other organs and tissues are minor.

GENETIC CONSIDERATIONS The autosomal recessive Wilson disease gene, *ATP7B*, and the X-linked Menkes disease gene, *ATP7A*, are membrane-bound, P-type, copper-transporting ATPases containing 6 copper-binding sites (Chap. 353). The amino acid sequences of these genes are 54% identical. In liver the Wilson protein incorporates copper ions into apoceruloplasmin to form ceruloplasmin whose catabolism is accompanied by biliary excretion of its copper ions. In fetal liver the Menkes protein incorporates copper ions into apoceruloplasmin to form fetal ceruloplasmin whose catabolism is accompanied by hepatic retention of its copper ions. In Wilson's disease, ceruloplasmin that is synthesized in the presence of the *ATP7B* mutant is catabolized like fetal ceruloplasmin, leading to hepatic retention of its copper ions. ■

DIAGNOSIS The diagnosis is easy provided it is suspected. Wilson's disease should be considered in any patient younger than 40 years with an unexplained disorder of the central nervous system, signs

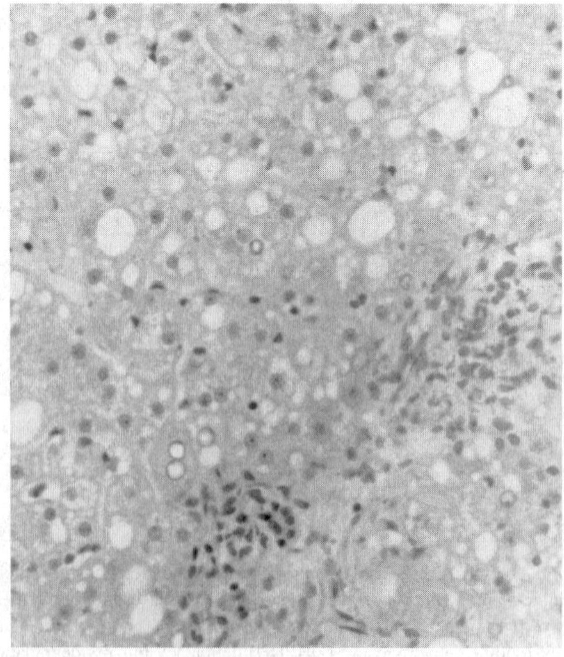

FIGURE 348-1 Macro- and microvesicular fatty changes, glycogen deposits in nuclei, and cellular infiltrates in a hematoxylin- and eosin-stained section of liver from an asymptomatic boy with Wilson's disease.

Table 348-1 Summary of Analytic Data for Patients with Wilson's Disease, Heterozygous Carriers, and Control Subjects

	Serum Ceruloplasmin		Hepatic Copper Concentration	
Group	No. of Patients	Mean ± SD, mg/dL	No. of Patients	Mean ± SD, μg/g Dry Weight
Wilson's disease				
Asymptomatic	31	3.6 ± 5.3	36	983.5 ± 368
Symptomatic	84	5.9 ± 7.1	33	588.3 ± 304
Heterozygous carriers	95[a]	28.4 ± 8.5	14	117.0 ± 51
Control subjects	180	30.7 ± 3.5	16	31.5 ± 6.8

[a] 71 parents of patients with Wilson's disease and 24 children, each of whom had one parent with Wilson's disease.

SOURCE: Sternlieb and Scheinberg, 1968.

or symptoms of hepatitis, chronic active hepatitis, unexplained persistent elevations of serum aminotransferase, hemolytic anemia in the presence of hepatitis, or unexplained cirrhosis and in any patient who has a relative with Wilson's disease.

The diagnosis is confirmed by the demonstration of either (1) a serum ceruloplasmin level <20 mg/dL *and* Kayser-Fleischer rings or (2) a serum ceruloplasmin level <20 mg/dL *and* a concentration of copper in a liver biopsy sample >250 μg/g dry weight. Most symptomatic patients excrete >100 μg copper per day in urine and have histologic abnormalities on liver biopsy.

℞ **TREATMENT** Treatment consists of removing and detoxifying the deposits of copper as rapidly as possible and must be instituted once the diagnosis is secure whether the patient is ill or asymptomatic. Penicillamine is administered orally in an initial dose of 1 g daily in a single or divided doses at least 30 min before and 2 h after eating. Because penicillamine has an antipyridoxine effect, 25 mg/d of pyridoxine is also given. In ~10% of patients sensitivity to penicillamine develops early, making it necessary to monitor the body temperature and skin daily. White blood cell and platelet counts should be assessed and urinalysis performed several times during the first month of treatment. Penicillamine should be discontinued and replaced by trientine, if rash, fever, leukopenia, thrombocytopenia, lymphadenopathy, or proteinuria develops, or if neurologic worsening accompanies the institution of penicillamine and persists for a week or more.

After therapy with penicillamine has been successfully instituted, the patient should be seen at 1- to 3-month intervals to assess the effectiveness of therapy and monitor for late drug toxicity. The history and the physical examination should focus on hepatic, neurologic, and psychiatric signs and symptoms. Slit-lamp examination of the corneas should be performed by an ophthalmologist if neurologic or psychiatric disturbances appear or worsen. White blood cell and platelet counts, transaminase levels, albumin, bilirubin, and free serum copper (total serum copper minus ceruloplasmin-bound copper) should be measured, the aim being a concentration of free copper less than ~0.2 μmol/dL (10 μg/dL). A persistent concentration >0.4 μmol/dL (20 μg/dL) indicates that the dose of penicillamine is too low or that the patient is noncompliant. For patients who are asymptomatic or who have improved maximally after several years on 1 g/d of penicillamine, the usual effective maintenance dose is 0.75 g/d taken 45 min before breakfast.

At any time, even after years of uneventful penicillamine administration, granulocytopenia, thrombocytopenia, the nephrotic syndrome, Goodpasture's syndrome, systemic lupus erythematosus, severe arthralgias, myasthenia, mammary gigantism, or elastosis perforans serpiginosa may supervene. Except for transient thrombocytopenia or granulocytopenia, these reactions mandate the replacement of penicillamine with trientine.

The dose of trientine is 1g/d on an empty stomach. Most patients find it convenient to take four 250-mg capsules, delaying breakfast for about an hour. Pyridoxine need not be given. Although the only reported toxic reaction to trientine is sideroblastic anemia, the same clinical procedures and laboratory determinations should be performed during its administration as are used during penicillamine therapy. Except for systemic lupus erythematosus and, occasionally, elastosis perforans serpiginosa, the other late penicillamine-induced toxic reactions disappear or improve with trientine therapy. Moreover, trientine is as effective therapeutically as penicillamine.

Zinc acetate or gluconate are effective as maintenance therapy, at doses of 150 mg/d of elemental zinc, for patients who are asymptomatic or have improved maximally on penicillamine or trientine. Zinc must *not*, however, be given together with penicillamine or trientine, both of which can chelate zinc and form complexes that are therapeutically ineffective.

Treatment must be continued for life. Inadequate treatment or interruption of therapy can be fatal or cause irreversible relapse. Indeed, of 11 patients who voluntarily discontinued penicillamine after years of successful treatment, 8 died after an average of 2.6 years of noncompliance. In contrast, of 13 patients in whom trientine was substituted because of an adverse reaction to penicillamine, 1 died accidentally, 5 were lost to follow-up, and 7 are alive and well 11 to 23 years later.

Prophylactic treatment of more than 100 asymptomatic patients with a documented diagnosis of Wilson's disease has shown that continual therapy with penicillamine or trientine can maintain the asymptomatic state indefinitely. Several such patients have been treated with penicillamine for >30 years.

Patients with severe neurologic disease who do not improve with penicillamine or trientine therapy that has reduced serum free copper to <0.3 μmol/dL (15 μg/dL) may benefit significantly from treatment with dimercaprol. Intramuscular injections of 3 mL (containing 300 mg of dimercaprol) are given on five successive weekdays for 4 weeks. Treatment is interrupted for 1 week, and a second 4-week course is given. If there is neurologic improvement, additional courses are given as long as improvement continues. If no improvement is seen after two courses, it is unlikely that additional courses will be effective.

The simultaneous occurrence of fulminant hepatitis and Coombs-negative hemolytic anemia may be the initial clinical manifestation of Wilson's disease or may occur in a noncompliant patient. The syndrome is almost always fatal, usually within a week or two, unless liver transplantation is performed. Transplantation is also indicated if progressive hepatic insufficiency occurs despite adequate treatment with penicillamine or trientine.

More than 150 women with Wilson's disease treated with penicillamine and more than 20 women treated with trientine have had successful and uneventful pregnancies.

BIBLIOGRAPHY

BREWER GJ et al: Treatment of Wilson's disease with zinc: XI. Interaction with other anticopper agents. J Am Coll Nutr 12:26, 1993

KRESSNER MS et al: Origins of biliary copper. Hepatology 4:867, 1984

PETRUKHIN K et al: Mapping, cloning and genetic characterization of the region containing the Wilson disease gene. Nat Genet 5:338, 1993

SCHEINBERG IH, STERNLIEB I: Wilson's and Menkes' Diseases. Cambridge, Harvard University Press (in preparation)

———, ———: Treatment of the neurological manifestations of Wilson's disease. Arch Neurol 52:339, 1995

———, ———: The use of trientine in preventing the effects of interrupting penicillamine therapy in Wilson's disease. N Engl J Med 317:209, 1987

SCHILSKY ML et al: Liver transplantation for Wilson's disease: Indications and outcome. Hepatology 19:583, 1994

STERNLIEB I, SCHEINBERG IH: Prevention of Wilson's disease in asymptomatic patients. N Engl J Med 278:352, 1968

VULPE C et al: Isolation of a candidate gene for Menkes disease and evidence that it encodes a copper-transporting ATPase. Nat Genet 3:7, 1993

349

Gregory A. Grabowski

LYSOSOMAL STORAGE DISEASES

GENERAL FEATURES

Lysosomes are heterogeneous subcellular organelles containing specific hydrolyases that allow targeted processing or degradation of proteins, nucleic acids, carbohydrates, and lipids. There are >30 different lysosomal storage diseases, and they vary greatly in the types of metabolic abnormalities that occur as well as in their clinical manifestations. Nonetheless, these disorders are considered together because they share a related pathophysiology that involves the accumulation of specific macromolecules within cells that normally process large amounts of these substrates. The disorders are classified based on the nature of the stored material and include mucopolysaccharidoses (MPS), gangliosidoses, glycosphingolipidoses, glycoproteinoses, mucolipidoses, leukodystrophies, and lipid storage disorders (Table 349-1). The most prevalent lysosomal storage diseases in adults are Fabry disease, Gaucher disease, and Niemann Pick disease (NPD).

Lysosomal storage diseases should be considered in the differential diagnosis of patients with neurologic or muscular degeneration, unexplained hepatomegaly or splenomegaly, or skeletal dysplasias and deformations. Physical findings are disease-specific, and definitive diagnosis is made by enzyme assays.

PHYSIOLOGY OF LYSOSOMES Lysosomal biogenesis is a continuous process that involves ongoing synthesis of lysosomal hydrolases, membrane constitutive proteins, and new membranes. Lysosomes originate from the fusion of *trans*-golgi network (TGN) vesicles with late endosomes. Progressive vesicular acidification accompanies the maturation of TGN vesicles, which contain various hydrolases, into lysosomes. Early endosomes have an internal pH of ~6.0 to 6.2; late endosomes and lysosomes have a pH of ~5.5 to 6.0 and ≤5, respectively. This gradient facilitates the pH-dependent dissociation of receptors and ligands [e.g., the mannose-6-phosphate (M6P) receptor and M6P-containing oligosaccharides] as well as activating lysosomal hydrolase function. This dynamic system, which has supplanted the static view of the lysosome, is consistent with the presence of heterogeneous populations of similar organelles whose contents differ significantly in time and location within the cell.

The accurate sorting, targeting, and activation of lysosomal enzymes is essential for maintaining normal cellular function. Abnormalities at several steps along the biosynthetic pathway can impair enzyme activation and lead to a lysosomal storage disorder. After cleavage of the hydrophobic signal peptide in the endoplasmic reticulum (ER) membrane, *N*-glycosylation occurs cotranslationally in the lumen of the ER. Complex oligosaccharide modifications occur during transit through the Golgi. The M6P modification of high-mannose oligosaccharide chains of many soluble lysosomal hydrolases occurs early in this process. Defects of this modification result in inappropriate extracellular secretion of most soluble lysosomal hydrolases, leading to severe phenotypes (I-cell disease). Lysosomal integral or associated membrane proteins (LIMPS or LAMPS) are sorted to the membrane or interior of the lysosome by several different signals. Phosphorylation, sulfation, additional proteolytic processing, and macromolecular assembly of heteromers occur concurrently and are critical to enzyme function. Defects in the latter can result in multiple enzyme/protein deficiencies.

PATHOGENESIS OF LYSOSOMAL STORAGE DISEASES The final common pathway for lysosomal storage diseases is the accumulation of specific macromolecules within tissues and cells that normally have a high flux of these substrates. The majority of lysosomal enzyme deficiencies result from point mutations or genetic rearrangements at a locus that encodes a single lysosomal hydrolase. However, some mutations cause deficiencies of several different lysosomal hydrolases by altering the enzymes/proteins involved in targeting, active site modifications, or macromolecular association or trafficking. All are inherited as autosomal recessive disorders, except Hunter (MPS II) and Fabry diseases, which are X-linked. Lysosomal distortion, which is caused by substrate accumulation, probably has significant pathologic consequences. However, abnormal amounts of metabolites may also have pharmacologic effects important to disease pathophysiology.

For many lysosomal diseases, the accumulated substrates are endogenously synthesized within particular tissue sites of pathology. Other diseases have greater exogenous substrate supplies; that is, they are delivered by low-density lipoprotein receptor–mediated uptake in Fabry and cholesteryl ester storage diseases or by phagocytosis in Gaucher disease type 1.

The concept of the *threshold hypothesis* has important implications for disease classification, pathophysiology, and treatment. It implies a threshold of enzyme activity below which disease develops. Consequently, small changes in enzyme activity near the threshold can lead to or prevent disease. A critical element of this model is that enzymatic activity can be challenged by changes in substrate flux based on genetic background, cell turnover, recycling, or metabolic demands. Thus, a set level of residual enzyme may be adequate for substrate in some tissues or cells, but not in others. For some lysosomal storage diseases [e.g., metachromatic leukodystrophy (MLD), Tay-Sachs disease, Gaucher disease], genotype-phenotype correlations may help to predict the severity of clinical consequences associated with certain levels of enzyme activity. Defining enzyme activity thresholds may also be useful for predicting dose-response relationships for treatment and for the evaluation of exogenous enzyme replacement therapy.

SPECIFIC DISORDERS

MUCOPOLYSACCHARIDOSES (MPS) The various forms of MPS result from deficiencies of lysosomal enzymes needed for glycosaminoglycan (GAG) catabolism. GAGs are long-chain, complex carbohydrates that are linked to proteins in connective tissue. They are components of proteoglycans and include: chondroitin-4-sulfate, chondroitin-6-sulfate, heparan sulfate, dermatan sulfate, keratan sulfate, and hyaluronic acid. The particular accumulated GAG is determined by the specific enzyme deficiency. GAG accumulation in various tissues produces a spectrum of clinical features that can include skeletal abnormalities, corneal clouding, organomegaly, joint stiffness, hernias, short stature, and, in some disorders, mental retardation. Vacuolated lymphocytes in the peripheral smear and excessive urinary GAGs are typical findings. Clinical and laboratory features overlap among the MPS diseases and are not diagnostic. The MPS diseases occur with individual frequencies of about 1/50,000 to 1/100,000 in most populations.

The diagnosis is established by specific enzyme assays or, when known, DNA mutation analysis. Prenatal diagnosis is conducted most frequently with cultured amniotic cells. Mutation studies for carriers can be performed, if the mutation is known.

Treatment of the MPS diseases requires comprehensive, multisystem evaluations. Symptomatic therapies currently include corneal transplantation, correction of nerve entrapment, and heart valve replacement. Physical therapy for joint contractures is needed in all but MPS IV. In MPS III variants, psychotropic drugs are used to control behavior. For patients with MPS IH and IV, cervical myelopathy can be prevented by prospective cervical spinal fusion. The efficacy of bone marrow transplantation and enzyme replacement is under investigation.

MPS IH (Hurler Disease) This a severe autosomal recessive disorder that results from numerous different mutations of α-L-iduronidase. Progressive mental retardation, hepatosplenomegaly, skeletal malformations, and cardiopulmonary compromise typically lead to death during the first decade. Affected individuals appear normal at birth but exhibit accelerated growth and mild coarsening of facial features in the first year. Subsequently, there is slowing of growth, leading to short stature. In the first 2 years, clinical diagnosis is suggested by hepatosplenomegaly, corneal clouding, coarse features, large tongue, joint stiffness, and characteristic dysostosis multiplex on skeletal x-rays. Instability of the cervical vertebral bodies can lead to paralysis, particularly with subluxation on hyperextension. Developmental delay is apparent by 12 to 28 months, with subsequent slow mental regression. Additional features of this multisystem disease include hearing loss, chronic respiratory infections, valvular heart disease, and brain ventricular enlargement. The latter occurs from involvement of the arachnoid granulations.

MPS (Scheie Disease) and MPS I H/S (Hurler-Scheie Disease) These MPS variants are less severe than MPS IH (Hurler disease). They result from allelic mutations in the α-L-iduronidase gene, presumably with a less severe effect on enzyme function. Patients with MPS IS can survive into late adulthood with normal intelligence, though with severe progressive skeletal disease that resembles osteoarthritis. Bone marrow transplantation in MPS IH, if instituted before substantial central nervous system CNS involvement, has shown therapeutic promise. Preliminary intravenous enzyme administration has led to improvement in hepatosplenomegaly and connective tissue involvement.

MPS II (Hunter Syndrome) This is an X-linked recessive disorder that results from deletions and point mutations in the gene encoding iduronate sulfatase. Clinically, MPS IH and II are similar, though corneal clouding is absent in MPS II. Clinical manifestations range from severe CNS and visceral involvement with death in late childhood to milder forms with normal CNS function and survival into adulthood. Bone marrow transplantation has not been successful for treating the severe variants, and experience in the less severe variants is too limited to permit conclusions. Enzyme therapy trials are imminent.

MPS IIIA, IIIB, IIIC, and IIID (the Sanfilippo Syndromes) These autosomal recessive disorders are caused by various enzymatic deficiencies as summarized in Table 349-1. Skeletal defects and hepatosplenomegaly are less pronounced in this group of MPS variants, though progressive behavioral problems, mental retardation, and seizures are present. Affected patients can survive into the third or fourth decade with progressive CNS disease.

MPS IV (Morquio Syndrome) These MPS variants are autosomal recessive disorders characterized by severe skeletal diseases that resemble the spondyloepiphyseal dysplasias. There is extreme shortening of the trunk due to multiple vertebral collapses. The long bones are relatively spared. Joint laxity can lead to osteoarthritis-like destruction of the joints. Upper cervical spinal cord compression due to atlantoaxial instability predisposes to subluxation and paralysis. Many patients have mitral valve insufficiency that can be functionally significant. The A and B variants are distinguished clinically by more severe skeletal disease, *N*-acetylgalactosamine-6-sulfate sulfatase deficiency in A, than in β-galactosidase defects in B. Enzyme therapy trials will begin in the near future.

MPS VI (Maroteaux-Lamy Disease) Mutations in the arylsulfatase B gene cause this autosomal recessive disorder. Although clinically variable, the general phenotype resembles Hurler disease. Intelligence is normal, and the life span can extend beyond three decades. Cardiac valvular disease and progressive pulmonary hypertension are frequent causes of death. Bone marrow transplantation may be useful in diminishing these manifestations.

GM_2 GANGLIOSIDOSES The Tay-Sachs and Sandhoff disease variants are caused by defects in β-hexosaminidase (Hex) A and/or B. Hex A is a heteromeric protein with α and β chains, whereas Hex B contains only β chains. The α and β chains are encoded by different genes. Infantile, juvenile, and adult-onset variants are distinguished by age at onset and rate of progression.

In addition to other clinical manifestations described below, specific neurologic features, such as the retinal cherry red spot, suggest the diagnosis of Tay-Sachs and Sandhoff diseases. Diagnosis is confirmed by Hex A and/or B levels in blood plasma or nucleated cells. Screening for Tay-Sachs disease carriers in the Ashkenazi Jewish population is recommended.

Tay-Sachs Disease About 1 in 30 Ashkenazi Jews is a carrier for Tay-Sachs disease, which is caused by total Hex A deficiency. The infantile form is a fatal neurodegenerative disease that is characterized by macrocephaly, loss of motor skills, increased startle reaction, and macular pallor with cherry red spot on retinal examination. The juvenile-onset form presents with ataxia and dementia, with death by age 10 to 15 years. The adult-onset disorder is characterized by clumsiness in childhood; progressive motor weakness in adolescence; and additional spinocerebellar, lower motor neuron symptoms, and dysarthria in adulthood. Intelligence declines slowly, and psychosis is also common.

Sandhoff Disease Sandhoff disease is nearly identical to Tay-Sachs disease, though hepatosplenomegaly and bony dysplasias are present in the former. The later onset variants are characterized by progressive visceral and CNS disease. Treatment is supportive.

NEUTRAL GLYCOSPHINGOLIPID LIPID STORAGE DISORDERS **Fabry Disease** This is an X-linked disorder that results from a variety of mutations in the α-galactosidase gene. This enzyme cleaves the terminal α-galactosyl moiety from globotriaosylceramide (trihexosylceramide, THC), a key step in glycosphingolipid metabolism. Clinically, the disease manifests with angiokeratomas (telangiectatic skin lesions); hypohidrosis; corneal and lenticular opacities; acroparesthesia; and small-vessel disease of the kidney, heart, and brain. The estimated prevalence of hemizygous males with Fabry disease is 1/40,000.

The angiokeratomas and acroparesthesia may appear in childhood and lead to early diagnosis, if suspected. Angiokeratomas are punctate, dark red to blue-black, flat or slightly raised, usually symmetric, and do not blanch with pressure. They range from barely visible to several millimeters in diameter and have a tendency to increase in size and number with age. Characteristically, they are most dense between the umbilicus and knees—"the bathing suit area"—but may occur anywhere, including the mucosal surfaces. Corneal and lenticular lesions, detectable on slit-lamp examination, are present in affected men and ~70% of heterozygous women. Tortuosity of the conjunctival and retinal vessels is common. The acroparesthesia can be debilitating in childhood and adolescence, with a tendency to decrease after the third decade. Episodic agonizing, burning pain of the hands, feet, and proximal extremities can last from minutes to days and can be precipitated by exercise, fatigue, or fever. Abdominal pain can resemble that from appendicitis or renal colic.

Casts and microscopic hematuria can occur early, whereas proteinuria, isosthenuria, and progressive renal dysfunction occur in the second to fourth decades. Progressive renal failure occurs and requires transplantation. Hypertension, left ventricular hypertrophy, anginal chest pain with or without myocardial ischemia or infarction, and congestive heart failure can occur in the third to fourth decades. Leg lymphedema without hypoproteinemia and episodic diarrhea also occur. Death is due to renal failure or cardiovascular or cerebrovascular disease in untreated patients. Variants with residual α-galactosidase activity may have late-onset manifestations limited to the cardiovascular system that resemble hypertrophic myocardiopathies. Heterozygous females may exhibit some of these clinical manifestations but usually not the severe organ involvement.

Acroparesthesia, hypohidrosis or anhidrosis, angiokeratomas, and the typical corneal and lenticular lesions provide a presumptive diagnosis in males. Angiokeratomas are not diagnostic, however, and also occur in Fordyce scrotal angiokeratoma and several other lysosomal storage diseases.

Phenytoin and carbamazepine diminish the chronic and episodic acroparesthesia. Chronic hemodialysis or kidney transplantation can be lifesaving in patients with renal failure. Initial enzyme therapy results are promising.

Table 349-1 Selected Lysosomal Storage Diseases

Disorder[a]	Enzyme Deficiency	Stored Material	Clinical Types (Onset)	Inheritance	Neurologic
MUCOPOLYSACCHARIDOSES (MPS)					
MPS I H, Hurler (136)	α-L-Iduronidase	Dermatan sulfate Heparan sulfate	Infantile	AR	Mental retardation
MPS I H/S, Hurler/Scheie			Intermediate		Mental retardation
MPS I S, Scheie			Adult		None
MPS II, Hunter (136)	Iduronate sulfatase	Dermatan sulfate Heparan sulfate	Severe infantile Mild juvenile	X-linked	Mental retardation, less in mild form
MPS III A, Sanfilippo A (136)	Heparan-*N*-sulfatase	Heparan sulfate	Late infantile	AR	Severe mental retardation
MPS III B, Sanfilippo B	*N*-Acetyl-α-glucosaminidase	Heparan sulfate	Late infantile	AR	Severe mental retardation
MPS III C, Sanfilippo C	Acetyl-CoA: α-glucosaminide *N*-acetyltransferase	Heparan sulfate	Late infantile	AR	Severe mental retardation
MPS III D, Sanfilippo D	*N*-Acetylglucosamine-6-sulfate sulfatase	Heparan sulfate	Late infantile	AR	Severe mental retardation
MPS IV A, Morquio (136)	*N*-Acetylgalactosamine-6-sulfate sulfatase	Keratan sulfate Chondroitin-6 sulfate	Childhood	AR	None
MPS VI B, Morquio (136)	β-Galactosidase		Childhood	AR	None
MPS VI, Maroteaux-Lamy (136)	Arylsulfatase B	Dermatan sulfate	Late infantile	AR	None
MPS VII (136)	β-Glucuronidase	Dermatan sulfate Heparan sulfate	Neonatal Infantile Adult	AR	Mental retardation, absent in some adults
GM_2 GANGLIOSIDOSES					
Tay-Sachs' disease (153)	β-Hexosaminidase A	GM_2 gangliosides	Infantile Juvenile	AR	Mental retardation, seizures, later juvenile form
Sandhoff's disease (153)	β-Hexosaminidases A and B	GM_2 gangliosides	Infantile	AR	Mental retardation, seizures
NEUTRAL GLYCOSPHINGOLIPIDOSES					
Fabry disease (150)	α-Galactosidase A	Globotriaosylceramide	Childhood	X-linked	Painful acroparesthesias
Gaucher disease (146)	Acid β-Glucosidase	Glucosylceramide	Type 1 Type 2 Type 3	AR	None ++++ ++
Niemann-Pick disease (144) A and B	Sphingomyelinase	Sphingomyelin	Neuronopathic, type A Nonneuronopathic, type B	AR	Mental retardation and seizures
GLYCOPROTEINOSES					
Fucosidosis (140)	α-Fucosidase	Glycopeptides, oligosaccharides	Infantile Juvenile	AR	Mental retardation
α-Mannosidosis (140)	α-Mannosidase	Oligosaccharides	Infantile Milder variant	AR	Mental retardation
β-Mannosidosis (140)	β-Mannosidase	Oligosaccharides		AR	Seizures, mental retardation
Aspartylglucosaminuria (140)	Aspartylglucosaminidase	Aspartylglucosamine, glycopeptides	Young adult onset	AR	Mental retardation
Sialidosis (140)	Neuraminidase	Sialyloligosaccharides	Type I, congenital Type II, infantile and juvenile forms	AR	Myoclonus, mental retardation
MUCOLIPIDOSES (ML)					
ML-II, I-cell disease (138)	UDP-*N*-Acetylglucosamine-1-phosphotransferase	Glycoprotein, glycolipids	Infantile	AR	Mental retardation
ML-III, pseudo-Hurler polydystrophy (138)	UDP-*N*-Acetylglucosamine-1-phosphotransferase	Glycoprotein, glycolipids	Late infantile	AR	Mild mental retardation
LEUKODYSTROPHIES					
Krabbe's disease (147)	Galactosylceramidase	Galactosylceramide, Galactosyl sphingosine	Infantile	AR	Mental retardation
Metachromatic leukodystrophy (148)	Arylsulfatase A	Cerebroside sulfate	Infantile Juvenile Adult	AR	Mental retardation, dementia, and psychosis in adult
Multiple sulfatase deficiency (149)	Active site cysteine to C_α-formylglycine-converting enzyme	Sulfatides, mucopolysaccharides	Late infantile	AR	Mental retardation
DISORDERS OF NEUTRAL LIPIDS					
Wolman disease (142)	Acid lysosomal lipase	Cholesterol esters, triglycerides	Infantile	AR	Mild mental retardation
Cholesteryl ester storage disease (142)	Acid lysosomal lipase	Cholesteryl esters	Childhood	AR	None
Farber disease (142)	Acid ceramidase	Ceramide	Infantile Juvenile	AR	Occasional mental retardation

[a] Numbers in parentheses refer to the chapters in Scriver et al, 8th edition, for detailed reviews.
NOTE: AR, autosomal recessive.

Clinical Features				
Liver and/or Spleen Enlargement	**Skeletal Disease**	**Ophthalmologic**	**Hematologic**	**Unique Features**
+++	++++	Corneal clouding	Vacuolated lymphocytes	Coarse facies, cardiovascular involvement, joint stiffness
+++	++++	Retinal degeneration, no corneal clouding	Granulated lymphocytes	Coarse facies, cardiovascular, joint stiffness, distinctive pebbly skin lesions
+	+	None	Granulated lymphocytes	Mild coarse facies
+	+	None	Granulated lymphocytes	Mild coarse facies
+	+	None	Granulated lymphocytes	Mild coarse facies
+	+	None	Granulated lymphocytes	Mild coarse facies
+	++++	Corneal clouding	Granulated neutrophils	Distinctive skeletal deformity, odontoid hypoplasia, aortic valve disease
±	++++			
++	++++	Corneal clouding	Granulated neutrophils and lymphocytes	Coarse facies, valvular heart disease
+++	+++	Corneal clouding	Granulated neutrophils	Coarse facies, vascular involvement, hydrops fetalis in neonatal form
None	None	Cherry red spot in infantile form	None	Macrocephaly, hyperacusis in infantile form
++	±	Cherry red spot	None	Macrocephaly, hyperacusis
None	None	Corneal dystrophy, vascular lesions	None	Cutaneous angiokeratomas, hypohydrosis
++++	++++	None	Gaucher cells in bone marrow, cytopenias	Adult form highly variable
+++	+	Eye movements		
++++	++++	Eye movements		
++++	None	Macular degeneration	Foam cells in bone marrow	Pulmonary infiltrates
	Osteo-Porosis			Lung failure
++	++	None	Vacuolated lymphocytes, foam cells	Coarse facies, angiokeratomas in juvenile form
+++	++	Cataracts, corneal clouding	Vacuolated lymphocytes, granulated neutrophils	Coarse facies, enlarged tongue
	++	None	Vacuolated lymphocytes, foam cells	Angiokeratomas
±	++	None	Vacuolated lymphocytes, foam cells	Coarse facies
++, less in type I	++ less in type I	Cherry red spot	Vacuolated lymphocytes	MPS phenotype in type II
±	++++	Corneal clouding	Vacuolated and granulated neutrophils	Coarse facies, absence of mucopolysacchariduria, gingival hypoplasia
None	+++	Corneal clouding, mild retinopathy, hyperopic astigmatism		Coarse facies, stiffness of hands and shoulders
None	None	None	None	White matter globoid cells
None	None	Optic atrophy	None	Gait abnormalities in late infantile form
+	++	Retinal degeneration	Vacuolated and granulated cells	Absent activity of all known cellular sulfatases
+++	None	None	None	Adrenal calcification
Hepatomegaly	None	None	None	Cirrhosis
+/−	None	Macular degeneration	None	Arthropathy, subcutaneous nodules

Gaucher Disease This is an autosomal recessive disorder that results from defective activity of acid β-glucosidase; >175 mutations have been described. This enzyme cleaves glucosylceramide, the parent compound of many glycosphingolipids and related glucolipids. Disease variants are classified based on the absence or presence and severity of neuronopathic involvement.

Type 2 Gaucher disease is a rare, severe CNS disease that leads to death by 2 years of age; it will not be addressed here.

Type 3 Gaucher disease has highly variable manifestations in the CNS and viscera. It can present in early childhood with rapidly progressive, massive visceral disease and slowly progressive to static CNS involvement; in adolescence with dementia; or in early adulthood with rapidly progressive, uncontrollable myoclonic seizures and mild visceral disease. Variants that span this spectrum also occur. Visceral disease in type 3 is nearly identical to that in type 1 but is generally more severe (see below). Early CNS findings may be limited to defects in lateral gaze tracking, which may remain static for decades. Mental retardation can be slowly progressive or static. This variant is most frequent among individuals of Swedish descent.

Type 1 Gaucher disease is a highly variable nonneuronopathic disease that can present in childhood to adulthood with slowly to rapidly progressive visceral disease. There is marked variability in age at onset and degree and progression of visceral involvement. In general, earlier diagnoses are associated with worse prognosis. The average age at diagnosis is ~20 years in Caucasian populations and somewhat younger in other groups. This pattern of presentation is distinctly bimodal, however, with peaks at <10 to 15 years and at ~25 years. Younger patients tend to have a greater degree of hepatosplenomegaly and accompanying blood cytopenias. In contrast, the older group has a greater tendency for chronic bone disease. Hepatosplenomegaly occurs in virtually all symptomatic patients and can be minor or massive. Accompanying anemia and thrombocytopenia are variable and are not linearly related to liver or spleen volume. Severe liver dysfunction is unusual, though minor liver function abnormalities are common. Splenic infarctions can resemble an acute abdomen. Pulmonary hypertension and alveolar Gaucher cell accumulation are uncommon, but life-threatening, and can occur at any age.

Though it is more common in adult patients, clinically evident skeletal disease in children can be devastating, resulting in massive destruction of the axial and peripheral skeleton. All patients with Gaucher disease have nonuniform infiltration of bone marrow by lipid-laden macrophages, termed *Gaucher cells*. This can lead to marrow packing with subsequent infarction, ischemia, necrosis, and cortical bone destruction. Bone marrow involvement spreads from proximal to distal in the limbs and can involve the axial skeleton extensively, causing vertebral collapse. In addition to bone marrow involvement, bone remodeling is defective, with loss of total bone calcium leading to osteopenia, osteonecrosis, avascular infarction, and vertebral compression fractures and spinal cord involvement. Aseptic necrosis of the femoral head is common, as is fracture of the femoral neck. The mechanism by which diseased bone marrow macrophages interact with osteoclasts and/or osteoblasts to lead to this complex bone disease is not well understood.

Affected patients experience chronic, ill-defined bone pain that can be debilitating and poorly correlated with radiographic findings. These are treated symptomatically. Some patients have one or more "bone crises" in their lifetimes that are associated with localized, excruciating pain, and, on occasion, local erythema, fever, and leukocytosis. Some patients have frequent crises, whereas other patients experience only one. Any bone can be involved, though the femurs and vertebral bodies are affected most often. These crises represent acute infarctions of bone, as evidenced in nuclear scans by localized absent uptake of pyrophosphate agents. X-rays are usually negative initially but may show lytic lesions 4 to 6 months after the acute phase. Osteomyelitis should be excluded by appropriate cultures. Bone cultures should be obtained only under sterile operating room conditions to minimize the chance of seeding an infection.

The diagnosis of Gaucher disease is established by demonstrating decreased acid β-glucosidase activity (0 to 20% of normal) in nucleated cells. The enzyme is not present in bodily fluids. The sensitivity of enzyme testing is poor for detecting heterozygous carriers; molecular testing is preferred when the mutations are known. The disease frequency varies from about 1 in 1000 in Ashkenazi Jews to <1 in 100,000 in some other populations. About 1 in 12 to 15 Ashkenazi Jews carries a Gaucher disease allele. Four common mutations account for ~90 to 95% of the mutations in affected patients: N370S (1226G), 84GG (a G insertion at cDNA position 84), L444P (1448C), and IVS-2 (an intron 2 splice junction mutation).

Genotype/phenotype studies indicate a significant correlation, though not absolute, between disease type and severity and the acid β-glucosidase genotype. For example, the most common mutation in the Ashkenazi Jewish population (N370S) shares a 100% association (to date) with nonneuronopathic, type 1 Gaucher disease, possibly because the N370S enzyme retains significant activity. The N370S/N370S and N370S/other mutant allele genotypes are associated with later onset/less severe and earlier onset/severe disease, respectively. The other alleles are L444P (very low activity), 84GG (null), or IVS-2 (null), and rare/private or uncharacterized alleles. As many as 50 to 60% of N370S/N370S patients are discovered as asymptomatic family members. The N370S/other mutant allele genotypes have disease onset about 2 decades earlier than those with N370S/N370S. The L444P/L444P patients almost always have life-threatening to very severe/early-onset disease, and many, though not all, develop CNS involvement in the first 2 decades of life. Some patients with this genotype have lethal neuronopathic disease at <1 year (type 2). Thus, this genotype is prognostic of very severe disease, with or without obvious CNS involvement.

Symptomatic management of the blood cytopenias and joint replacement surgeries continue to have important roles in the treatment of affected patients. However, enzyme therapy is currently the treatment of choice in significantly affected patients. Cerezyme, a recombinantly produced mannose-terminated (macrophage-targeted) acid β-glucosidase, has proved highly efficacious and safe in diminishing the hepatosplenomegaly and improving bone marrow involvement and hematologic findings.

Niemann-Pick Disease NPD is an autosomal recessive trait that occurs as several variants. Types A and B result from defects in acid sphingomyelinase; various mutations have been detected at this locus. Other variants, including NPD C, result from defective transport of cholesterol across the lysosomal membrane. Only NPD variants A and B will be considered here.

NPD A and B are distinguished primarily by an early age of onset and progressive CNS disease in A. NPD A typically has onset in the first 6 months, with rapidly progressive CNS deterioration, spasticity, failure to thrive, and massive hepatosplenomegaly. In contrast, NPD B has a later, more variable onset and progression of hepatosplenomegaly, with eventual development of cirrhosis and hepatic replacement by foam cells. Affected patients develop progressive pulmonary disease with dyspnea, hypoxemia, and a reticular infiltrative pattern on chest x-ray. Foam cells are present in alveoli, lymphatic vessels, and pulmonary arteries. Progressive hepatic or lung disease with associated bronchopneumonia, pulmonary hypertension, cor pulmonale, and decreased diffusion capacities lead to demise in adolescence to early adulthood.

The diagnosis is established by markedly decreased (1 to 10% of normal) sphingomyelinase activity in nucleated cells. Enzyme assays to detect NPD A or B carriers are unreliable. In families with known mutations, the molecular defect in heterozygotes can be identified by DNA analysis.

There is no specific treatment for NPD. The efficacy of hepatic or bone marrow transplantation has not been proven. Clinical trials using enzyme therapy are anticipated to begin soon.

THE LEUKODYSTROPHIES Globoid cell leukodystrophy and metachromatic leukodystrophy variants are autosomal recessive disorders that primarily involve CNS white matter and myelinated peripheral nervous system tracts.

Globoid Cell Leukodystrophy (GCL) The GCL variants are due to mutations in the galactosylceramidase gene. The term *globoid cell* is derived from the presence of characteristic multinucleated cells filled with galactosylceramide in the brains of affected patients. Infantile GCL (Krabbe disease) is a rapidly progressive, fatal disorder; patients succumb in the first 2 years. Juvenile and adult variants present with more slowly progressive dementia. For all variants, manifestations are confined to the CNS and peripheral nervous system. Diagnosis is confirmed by demonstrating defective galactosylceramidase activity in nucleated cells. Treatment is supportive, but bone marrow transplantation has shown some promise in the later onset variants.

Metachromatic Leukodystrophy MLD is due to defects in arylsulfatase A and accumulation of its substrate, galactosylceramide sulfate or sulfatide. The late-infantile form presents in the second year with progressive regression of developmental milestones and intellectual development. The disease is fatal in the first decade. The juvenile and adult forms have variable manifestations and present with gait disturbances, ataxia, mental regression, peripheral neuropathy, and/or seizures. In adults, behavioral disturbances, psychosis, and dementia tend to predominate. These later onset diseases may respond to bone marrow transplantation.

The diagnosis is established by demonstrating a deficiency of arylsulfatase A in nucleated cells. Homozygosity for a null allele (splicing defect in intron 2) produces severe infantile disease, whereas P426L homozygotes develop adult-onset disease. Compound heterozygotes, such as null and P426L alleles, have juvenile-onset variants. The diagnosis of MLD is complicated by the presence of a very frequent (10 to 15%) "pseudodeficiency allele" for arylsulfatase A. Although in vitro activity with synthetic substrates is deficient, cleavage of sulfatide is low-normal in vivo. Compound heterozygotes for the pseudodeficiency allele and true MLD alleles therefore appear to have deficient arylsulfatase A activity, diagnostic of MLD, but these individuals are not affected by the disease. MLD-causing mutations also occur on the background of the pseudodeficient allele, emphasizing the importance of careful genetic testing.

GLYCOGEN STORAGE DISEASE TYPE II (See also Chap. 350) Glycogen storage disease type II is an autosomal recessive disorder due to defects in acid α-glucosidase that lead to lysosomal glycogen accumulation. Numerous mutations have been found at this locus in affected patients. Skeletal and cardiac muscles are primarily involved. The infantile form (Pompe disease) is a fatal disorder characterized by hypertrophic cardiomegaly, macroglossia, and hypotonia due to glycogen accumulation in muscle. The juvenile form has progressive proximal muscle weakness, including impairment of respiratory function. Adult patients have phenotypes resembling slowly progressive muscular dystrophies. Prenatal diagnosis can be performed. Treatment is supportive, and enzyme trials are underway.

MUCOLIPIDOSES Mucolipidoses II (I-cell) and III (pseudo-Hurler polydystrophy) are rare autosomal recessive diseases. Both are caused by defective targeting of lysosomal hydrolases that require the M6P signal for sorting to the lysosome. As a result, >20 enzymes are secreted out of the cell and their substrates accumulated in specific cell types. *N*-acetylglucosamine-1-phosphotransferase activity, which is necessary for developing the M6P signal, is defective in these diseases. I-cell disease has a phenotype similar to MPS IH, whereas mucolipidosis-III is more similar to MPS IH/S; mental retardation is a feature of both. Diagnosis is suspected based on the characteristic phenotype and is established by demonstrating greatly elevated serum levels of lysosomal enzymes, as well as their deficiency in cells. Specific enzyme assays can also be performed. Carrier detection is possible but is not straightforward. Prenatal diagnosis can be performed using amniotic fluid and cells in at-risk families. Treatment is supportive.

BIBLIOGRAPHY

BEIGHTON P (ed): *McKusick's Heritable Disorders of Connective Tissue*, 5th ed. St. Louis, Mosby, 1993

SCRIVER CR et al (eds): *The Metabolic and Molecular Bases of Inherited Diseases*, 8th ed. New York, McGraw-Hill, 2000

WATTS RWE, GIBBS DA (eds): *Lysosomal Storage Diseases: Biochemical and Clinical Aspects*. Philadelphia, Taylor and Francis, 1986

350

Yuan-Tsong Chen

GLYCOGEN STORAGE DISEASES AND OTHER INHERITED DISORDERS OF CARBOHYDRATE METABOLISM

Carbohydrate synthesis and degradation play a vital role in cellular function by providing the energy required for most metabolic processes. The carbohydrates to be discussed include three monosaccharides: glucose, galactose, and fructose, and a polysaccharide, glycogen; the relevant biochemical pathways involved in the metabolism of these carbohydrates are shown in Fig. 350-1. Glucose is the principle substrate of energy metabolism in humans. Metabolism of glucose generates ATP via glycolysis and mitochondrial oxidative phosphorylation. A continuous source of glucose from dietary intake, gluconeogenesis, and degradation of glycogen maintain normal blood glucose levels. Sources of glucose in our diet are obtained by ingesting polysaccharides, primarily starch, and disaccharides including lactose, maltose, and sucrose. Galactose and fructose are two other monosaccharides that provide fuel for cellular metabolism; however, their role as fuel sources is much less significant than that of glucose. Galactose is derived from lactose (galactose + glucose), which is found in milk and milk products. If necessary, galactose can be incorporated into glycogen and thus becomes a source of glucose. Galactose is also an important component for certain glycolipids, glycoproteins, and glycosaminoglycans. The two dietary sources of fructose are sucrose (fructose + glucose), a commonly used sweetener, and fructose itself, which is found in fruits, vegetables, and honey.

This chapter is devoted to the inherited disorders of carbohydrate metabolism caused by defects in enzymes or transport proteins involved in glycogen metabolism, gluconeogenesis, and glycolysis (Table 350-1). Defects in glycogen metabolism typically cause an accumulation of glycogen in the tissues; hence, the name *glycogen storage diseases*. The defects in gluconeogenesis or glycolytic pathways including galactose and fructose metabolism do not usually result in glycogen accumulation.

Clinical manifestations of the various disorders of carbohydrate metabolism differ markedly. The symptoms range from harmless to lethal. Unlike disorders of lipid metabolism, mucopolysaccharidoses, or other storage diseases, dietary therapy has been effective in many of the carbohydrate disorders. Almost all the genes responsible for the inherited defects of carbohydrate metabolism have been cloned, and mutations have been identified. Advances in our understanding of the molecular basis of these diseases are being used to improve diagnosis and management, and some of these disorders are candidates for early trials of gene therapy.

Glycogen, the storage form of glucose in animal cells, is composed of glucose residues joined in straight chains by α1-4 linkages and branched at intervals of 4 to 10 residues with α1-6 linkages. The tree-like molecule can have a molecular weight of many millions and may aggregate to form structures recognizable by electron microscopy. In muscle, glycogen forms β particles, which are spherical and contain

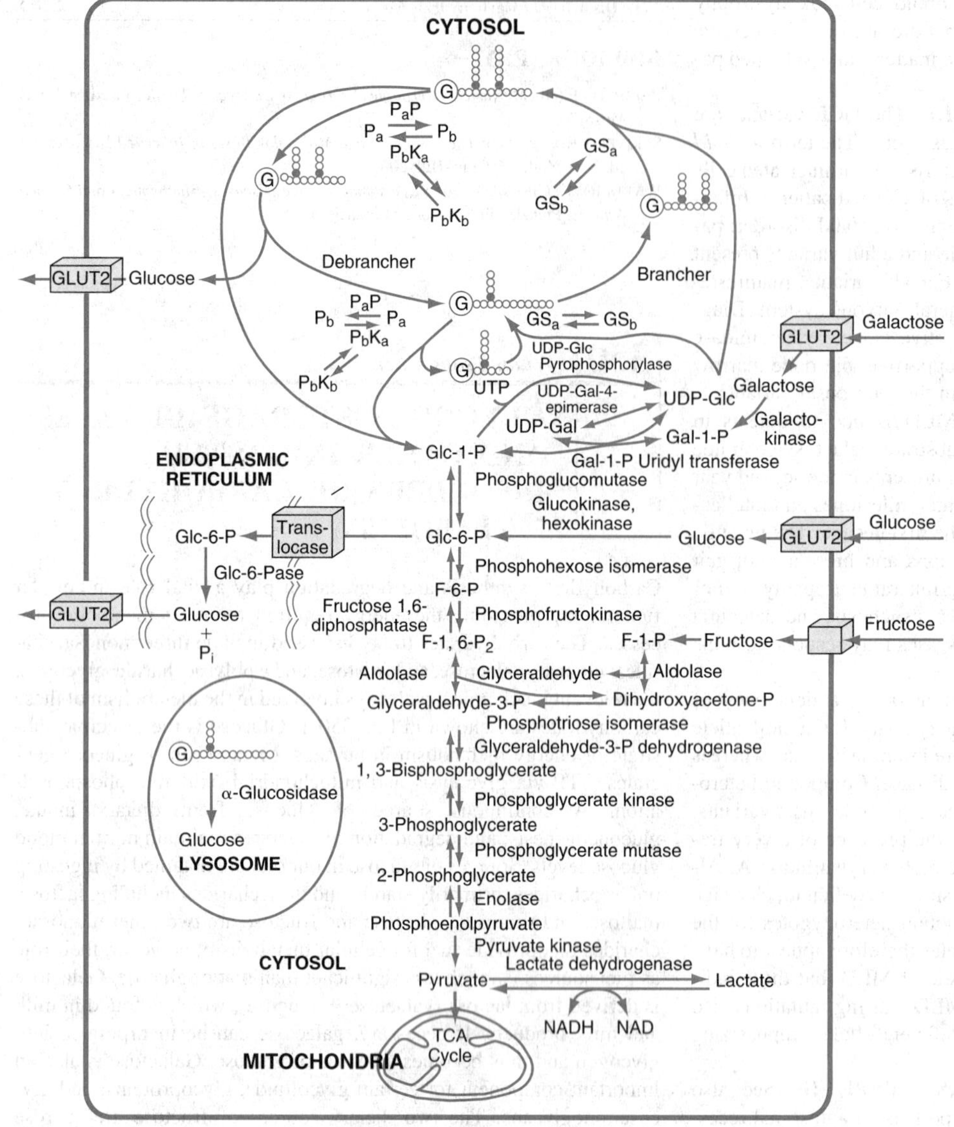

FIGURE 350-1 Metabolic pathways related to glycogen storage diseases and galactose and fructose disorders. Nonstandard abbreviations are as follows: GS_a, active glycogen synthase; GS_b, inactive glycogen synthase; P_a, active phosphorylase; P_b, inactive phosphorylase; P_aP, phosphorylase *a* phosphatase; P_bK_a, active phosphorylase *b* kinase; P_bK_b, inactive phosphorylase *b* kinase; G, glycogenin, the primer protein for glycogen synthesis. *[Modified from AR Beaudet: Glycogen storage disease, in KJ Isselbacher et al. (ed): Harrison's Principles of Internal Medicine, 13th ed., New York, McGraw-Hill, 1994, p 1855.]*

up to 60,000 glucose residues. Each β particle contains a covalently linked protein called *glycogenin*. Liver contains β particles and rosettes of glycogen called α particles, which appear to be aggregated β particles.

The primary function of glycogen varies in different tissues. In skeletal muscle, stored glycogen is a source of fuel that is used for short-term, high-energy consumption during muscle activity; in the brain, the small amount of stored glycogen is used during brief periods of hypoglycemia or hypoxia as an emergency supply of energy. In contrast, the liver takes up glucose from the bloodstream after a meal and stores it as glycogen. When blood glucose levels start to fall, the liver converts glycogen back into glucose and releases it into the blood for use by tissues such as brain and erythrocytes that cannot store significant amounts of glycogen.

Glycogen storage diseases are inherited disorders that affect glycogen metabolism. Disorders in virtually every enzyme involved in the synthesis or degradation of glycogen and its regulation cause some type of glycogen storage disease (Fig. 350-1) in which glycogen is abnormal in quantity, quality, or both. Excluded from this chapter are those conditions in which tissue glycogen accumulation is secondary, such as overtreatment of diabetes mellitus with insulin or administration of pharmacologic amounts of glucocorticoids.

Historically, the glycogen storage diseases were categorized numerically in the order in which the enzymatic defects were identified. They can also be classified by the organs involved and clinical manifestations, the system followed in this chapter (Table 350-1).

Because liver and muscle have abundant glycogen, they are the most commonly and seriously affected tissues. The hepatic glycogen storage diseases can be divided into two groups, with some overlap. The first is characterized by hepatomegaly and hypoglycemia. Because carbohydrate metabolism in the liver controls plasma glucose levels, the disorders of hepatic glycogen degradation and glucose release cause fasting hypoglycemia. Diseases in this group include glucose-6-phosphatase deficiency (type I), debranching enzyme deficiency (type III), liver phosphorylase deficiency (type VI), phosphorylase kinase deficiency (type IX), glycogen synthase deficiency (type 0), and glucose transporter-2 defects (type XI). The second group, characterized by cirrhosis of the liver and hepatomegaly, is associated with accumulation of abnormal forms of glycogen, which may be the cause of the hepatocellular injury. This group is represented by branching enzyme deficiency (type IV).

The role of glycogen in muscle is to provide substrates for the generation of sufficient ATP for muscle contraction. The muscle glycogen storage diseases can also be divided into two groups. The first is a muscle-energy disorder characterized by muscle pain, exercise intolerance, myoglobinuria, and susceptibility to fatigue. This group includes type V (McArdle disease), a muscle phosphorylase deficiency, and deficiencies of phosphofructokinase (type VII), phosphoglycerate kinase, phosphoglycerate mutase, lactase dehydrogenase, fructose 1,6-biphosphate aldolase A, and pyruvate kinase. Some of these latter enzyme deficiencies are associated with a compensated hemolysis, suggesting a more generalized defect in glucose metabolism. The second group of muscle disorders is characterized by progressive skeletal muscle weakness and atrophy and/or cardiomyopathy; it includes a lysosomal enzyme deficiency (acid α-glucosidase, type II) and deficiency of cardiac-specific phosphorylase kinase. Some glycogen storage diseases such as debranching enzyme deficiency (type IIIa) and branching enzyme deficiency (type IV) involve both muscle and liver.

The overall frequency of all forms of glycogen storage disease is approximately 1 in 20,000 live births; most are inherited as autosomal recessive traits, but phosphoglycerate kinase deficiency and one form of phosphorylase kinase deficiency are X-linked disorders. The most common childhood disorders are glucose-6-phosphatase deficiency (type I), lysosomal acid α-glucosidase deficiency (type II), debrancher deficiency (type III), and liver phosphorylase kinase deficiency (type IX). The most common adult disorder is myophosphorylase deficiency

Table 350-1 Features of Glycogen Storage Diseases and Galactose and Fructose Disorders

Type/Common Name	Basic Defect	Clinical Features	Comments
LIVER GLYCOGENOSES			
Disorders with hepatomegaly and hypoglycemia			
Ia/von Gierke	Glucose-6-phosphatase	Growth retardation, enlarged liver and kidney, hypoglycemia, elevated blood lactate, cholesterol, triglycerides, and uric acid	Common, severe hypoglycemia
Ib	Glucose-6-phosphate translocase	As for Ia, with additional findings of neutropenia and neutrophil dysfunction	~10% of type I
IIIa/Cori or Forbes	Liver and muscle debranching enzyme	Childhood: Hepatomegaly, growth retardation, muscle weakness, hypoglycemia, hyperlipidemia, elevated liver transaminases; liver symptoms improve with age Adulthood: muscle atrophy and weakness; onset: third to fourth decades; variable cardiomyopathy	Common, intermediate severity of hypoglycemia Liver cirrhosis can occur in adulthood
IIIb	Liver debranching enzyme (normal muscle debrancher activity)	Liver symptoms same as in type IIIa; no muscle symptoms	~15% of type III
VI/Hers	Liver phosphorylase	Hepatomegaly, mild hypoglycemia, hyperlipidemia and ketosis; symptoms improve with age	Rare, ''benign'' glycogenosis
IX/phosphorylase kinase deficiency	Liver phosphorylase kinase α subunit	As for VI	Common, ''benign glycogenosis,'' X-linked
0/glycogen synthase deficiency	Glycogen synthase	Fasting hypoglycemia and ketosis, elevated lactic acid and hyperglycemia after glucose load	Decreased glycogen stores
XI/Fanconi-Bickel	Glucose transporter-2	Failure to thrive, rickets, hepatomegaly, proximal renal tubular dysfunction, impaired glucose and galactose utilization	Rare, consanguinity in 70%
Disorders associated with liver cirrhosis			
IV/Andersen	Branching enzyme	Failure to thrive, hypotonia, hepatomegaly, splenomegaly, progressive liver cirrhosis and failure (death usually before fifth year); some without progression	One of the rarer glycogenoses; other neuromuscular variants exist
MUSCLE GLYCOGENOSES			
Disorders with muscle-energy impairment			
V/McArdle	Muscle phosphorylase	Exercise intolerance, muscle cramps, myoglobinuria on strenuous exercise, increased CK	Common, male predominance
VII/Tarui	Phosphofructokinase—M subunit	As for type V, with additional findings of a compensated hemolysis	Prevalent in Ashkenazi Jews and Japanese
Phosphoglycerate kinase deficiency	Phosphoglycerate kinase	As for type V, with additional findings of a hemolytic anemia and CNS dysfunction	Rare, X-linked
Phosphoglycerate mutase deficiency	Phosphoglycerate mutase—M subunit	As for type V	Rare; most patients are African American
Lactate dehydrogenase deficiency	Lactic acid dehydrogenase—M subunit	As for type V, with additional findings of erythematous skin eruption and uterine stiffness resulting in childbirth difficulty in female	Rare
Fructose 1,6-bisphosphate aldolase A deficiency	Fructose 1,6-bisphosphate aldolase A	As for type V, with additional finding of hemolytic anemia	Rare
Pyruvate kinase deficiency	Pyruvate kinase—muscle isozyme	Muscle cramps and/or fixed muscle weakness	Rare
Muscle phosphorylase kinase deficiency	Muscle-specific phosphorylase kinase	As for type V, some patients may have muscle weakness and atrophy	Rare, autosomal recessive
Disorders with progressive skeletal myopathy and/or cardiomyopathy			
II/Pompe	Lysosomal acid α-glucosidase	Infantile: hypotonia, muscle weakness, cardiac enlargement and failure, fatal early Juvenile and adult: progressive skeletal muscle weakness and atrophy, proximal muscle and respiratory muscle are seriously affected	Common, undetectable, or very low level of enzyme activity in infantile form; residual enzyme activity in late-onset
Cardiac phosphorylase kinase deficiency	Cardiac-specific phosphorylase kinase	Severe cardiomyopathy and early heart failure	Very rare
GALACTOSE DISORDERS			
Galactosemia with uridyl transferase deficiency	Galactose 1-phosphate uridyl transferase	Vomiting, hepatomegaly, jaundice, cataracts, amino aciduria, failure to thrive	Long-term complications exist despite early diagnosis and treatment
Galactokinase deficiency	Galactokinase	Cataracts	Benign
Uridine diphosphate galactose 4-epimerase deficiency	Uridine diphosphate galactose 4-epimerase	Similar to transferase deficiency with additional findings of hypotonia and nerve deafness	Benign variant exists

(continued)

Table 350-1 Features of Glycogen Storage Diseases and Galactose and Fructose Disorders—*(continued)*

Type/Common Name	Basic Defect	Clinical Features	Comments
FRUCTOSE DISORDERS			
Essential fructosuria	Fructokinase	Asymptomatic, positive urine reducing substance	Benign
Hereditary fructose intolerance	Fructose 1-phosphate aldolase B	Vomiting, lethargy, failure to thrive, hepatic failure	Prognosis good with early diagnosis and fructose restriction
Fructose 1,6-diphosphatase deficiency	Fructose 1,6-diphosphatase	Episodic hypoglycemia and lactic acidosis	Avoid fasting, good prognosis

NOTE: CK, creatine kinase; M, muscle; CNS, central nervous system.

(type V, or McArdle disease). In the past, the prognosis for many glycogen storage diseases was guarded. However, early diagnosis and better management have improved the survival rates, and many affected children are now adults.

GLYCOGEN STORAGE DISEASES: LIVER GLYCOGENOSES

DISORDERS WITH HEPATOMEGALY AND HYPOGLYCEMIA Type I Glycogen Storage Disease (Glucose-6-Phosphatase or Translocase Deficiency, von Gierke Disease) Type I glycogen storage disease is due to a defect in glucose-6-phosphatase in liver, kidney, and intestinal mucosa. It can be divided into two subtypes: type Ia, in which the glucose-6-phosphatase enzyme is defective, and type Ib, which is due to a defect in the translocase that transports glucose-6-phosphate across the microsomal membrane. The defects in both subtypes lead to inadequate conversion in the liver of glucose-6-phosphate to glucose and thus make affected individuals susceptible to fasting hypoglycemia.

GENETIC CONSIDERATIONS Type I glycogen storage disease is an autosomal recessive disorder. Both types Ia and Ib disease have been reported in many ethnic groups, but type Ia is rarely seen in blacks. The structural gene for glucose-6-phosphatase is located on chromosome 17q21; three common mutations (R83C, 130X, Q347X) are responsible for 70% of the known disease alleles. The structural gene for glucose 6-phosphate translocase is located on chromosome 11q23; two mutations, G339C and 1211delCT, appear to be prevalent in Caucasian patients, while W118R appears to be most common in Japanese patients. Carrier detection and prenatal diagnosis are possible with the use of molecular techniques. ■

Clinical and laboratory findings Persons with type I disease may develop hypoglycemia and lactic acidosis during the neonatal period, but, more commonly, they present at 3 to 4 months of age with hepatomegaly and/or hypoglycemia. These children often have doll-like faces with fat cheeks, relatively thin extremities, short stature, and a protuberant abdomen that is due to massive hepatomegaly; the kidneys are enlarged, but the spleen and heart are of normal size.

The hallmarks of the disease are hypoglycemia, lactic acidosis, hyperuricemia, and hyperlipidemia. Hypoglycemia and lactic acidosis can develop after a short fast. Hyperuricemia is present in young children, but gout rarely develops before puberty. Despite hepatomegaly, liver enzymes are usually normal or near normal. Intermittent diarrhea may occur (the mechanism is not known). Easy bruising and epistaxis are associated with a prolonged bleeding time as a result of impaired platelet aggregation/adhesion.

Hypertriglyceridemia may cause the plasma to appear "milky," and cholesterol and phospholipids are also elevated. The lipid abnormality resembles type IV hyperlipidemia and is characterized by increased levels of very low-density lipoprotein (VLDL); low-density lipoprotein (LDL); increased levels of apoliproteins B, C, and E; and normal or reduced levels of apoliproteins A and D. The hepatocytes are distended by glycogen and fat with large and prominent lipid vacuoles. There is little associated fibrosis.

All these findings apply to both types Ia and Ib disease, but type Ib has the additional feature of recurrent bacterial infections due to neutropenia and impaired neutrophil function. Oral and intestinal mucosa ulcerations are common, and inflammatory bowel disease may occur.

Long-term complications Although type I glycogen storage disease mainly affects the liver, multiple organ systems are also involved. Gout usually becomes symptomatic around puberty as a result of the long-term hyperuricemia. Puberty is often delayed, but fertility appears to be normal. Hypertriglyceridemia causes an increased risk of pancreatitis, but premature atherosclerosis has not been documented. Impaired platelet aggregation may reduce the risk of atherosclerosis.

By the second or third decade of life, most patients with type I glycogen storage disease develop hepatic adenomas that can hemorrhage and, in rare cases, may become malignant. Other complications include pulmonary hypertension and osteoporosis.

Renal disease is a late complication, and almost all patients older than 20 years have proteinuria. Many have hypertension, kidney stones, nephrocalcinosis, and altered creatinine clearance. Glomerular hyperfiltration, increased renal plasma flow, and microalbuminuria can occur before the onset of gross proteinuria. In young patients, hyperfiltration and hyperperfusion may be the only signs of renal abnormalities. With advanced renal disease, focal segmental glomerulosclerosis and interstitial fibrosis are evident on biopsy. In some patients, renal function deteriorates and progresses to failure, requiring dialysis or transplantation. Other abnormalities in renal function include amyloidosis, Fanconi-like syndrome, and distal renal tubular acidification defect. The increases in renal perfusion and maternal blood volume that normally occur in pregnancy can exacerbate renal problems. In addition, hypoglycemia may also become more difficult to control.

Diagnosis The diagnosis of type I disease can be suspected on the basis of clinical presentation and abnormal plasma lactate and lipid values. In addition, administration of glucagon or epinephrine causes little or no rise in blood glucose but increases lactate levels significantly. Before the glucose 6-phosphatase and glucose 6-phosphate translocase genes were cloned, a definitive diagnosis required a liver biopsy to demonstrate a deficiency. Gene-based mutation analysis now provides a noninvasive way of diagnosis for most patients with types Ia and Ib disease.

Rx TREATMENT Treatment is designed to maintain normal blood glucose levels and is achieved by continuous nasogastric infusion of glucose or oral administration of uncooked cornstarch. Nasogastric drip feeding in early infancy may consist of an elemental enteral formula or may contain only glucose to maintain normoglycemia during the night; frequent feedings with a high-carbohydrate content are given during the day.

Uncooked cornstarch acts as a slow-release form of glucose and can be given at a dose of 1.6 g/kg every 4 h for infants younger than 2 years. As the child grows older, the cornstarch regimen can be changed to every 6 h, and it can be given by mouth as a liquid (1:2, weight:volume) at a dose of 1.75 to 2.5 g/kg of body weight. Because fructose and galactose cannot be converted to free glucose, their dietary intake should be restricted, and dietary supplements of multivitamins and calcium are required. Allopurinol is given to lower the levels of uric acid. In patients with type Ib disease, granulocyte and granulocyte-macrophage colony stimulating factors have been used successfully to correct the neutropenia, decrease the severity of bacterial infection, and improve the chronic inflammatory bowel disease.

Before surgery, the bleeding status of the patient should be evaluated, and good metabolic control should be established. Prolonged bleeding time can be corrected by the administration of a constant intravenous glucose infusion for 24 to 48 h before surgery. Vasopressin can be given during surgery to reduce bleeding complications, and normal glucose levels should be maintained throughout surgery.

Prognosis In the past, many patients with type I glycogen storage disease died, and the prognosis was guarded for those who survived. The long-term complications discussed above occur mostly in adults whose disease was not adequately treated during childhood. Early diagnosis and initiation of effective treatment have improved the outcome, but it is not known if all long-term complications can be avoided through good metabolic control.

Type III Glycogen Storage Disease (Debrancher Deficiency, Limit Dextrinosis) Type III glycogen storage disease is caused by a deficiency of glycogen debranching enzyme. Debranching enzyme and phosphorylase are responsible for complete degradation of glycogen; when debranching enzyme is defective, glycogen breakdown is incomplete, and an abnormal glycogen accumulates that has short outer chains and resembles limit dextrin.

GENETIC CONSIDERATIONS The type III glycogenoses are inherited as autosomal recessive traits. The disease has been reported in many different ethnic groups, and the frequency is relatively high in non-Ashkenazi Jews of North African descent. The gene for debranching enzyme is located on chromosome 1p21. At least 20 different mutations that cause type III disease have been identified. Two mutations (17delAG and Q6X), both located in exon 3 at amino acid codon 6, are exclusively found in the subtype IIIb. Carrier detection and prenatal diagnosis are possible with DNA-based linkage or mutation analysis. ■

Clinical and laboratory findings Deficiency of glycogen debranching enzyme causes hepatomegaly, hypoglycemia, short stature, variable skeletal myopathy, and cardiomyopathy. The disorder usually involves both liver and muscle and is termed *type IIIa glycogen storage disease*. However, in about 15% of patients, the disease appears to involve only the liver and is classified as *type IIIb*.

During infancy and childhood, the disease may be almost indistinguishable from type I disease because hepatomegaly, hypoglycemia, hyperlipidemia, and growth retardation are common features of both. Splenomegaly may be present, but the kidneys are not enlarged in type III disease. Remarkably, hepatomegaly and hepatic symptoms in most patients with type III disease improve with age and usually disappear after puberty. However, progressive liver cirrhosis with failure may occur and seems especially common in Japanese patients.

In patients with muscle involvement (type IIIa), muscle weakness is usually minimal during childhood but can become severe during the third or fourth decade of life, as evidenced by slowly progressive weakness and muscle wasting. Electromyographic (EMG) changes are consistent with a widespread myopathy, and nerve conduction may be abnormal. Ventricular hypertrophy is frequent, but overt cardiac dysfunction is rare. Hepatic symptoms may be so mild that the diagnosis is not made until adulthood, when neuromuscular disease becomes manifest. Polycystic ovaries appear to be a common finding in female patients; fertility, however, does not seem to be affected.

Hypoglycemia, hyperlipidemia, and elevated liver transaminases occur in children. In contrast to type I disease, fasting ketosis is prominent, and blood lactate and uric acid concentrations are usually normal. The administration of glucagon 2 h after a carbohydrate meal causes a normal rise of blood glucose, but after an overnight fast glucagon may provoke no change in blood glucose. Serum creatine kinase levels can sometimes be used to identify patients with muscle involvement, but normal levels do not rule out muscle enzyme deficiency.

The histology of the liver is characterized by a universal distention of hepatocytes by glycogen and by the presence of fibrous septa. The fibrosis and the paucity of fat distinguish type III from type I glycogenosis. The fibrosis can range from minimal periportal fibrosis to micronodular cirrhosis.

Diagnosis In type IIIa glycogen storage disease, deficient debranching enzyme activity can be demonstrated in liver, skeletal muscle, and heart. In contrast, patients with type IIIb have debranching enzyme deficiency in the liver but not in muscle. In the past, definitive assignment of subtype required enzyme assays in both liver and muscle. DNA-based analyses now provide a noninvasive way of subtyping these disorders in most patients.

℞ TREATMENT Dietary management of type III disease is less demanding than that of type I. If hypoglycemia is present, frequent high-carbohydrate meals with cornstarch supplements or nocturnal gastric drip feedings are usually effective. A high-protein diet during the day plus overnight protein enteral infusion may be tried in patients with myopathy, but it is not established whether such a regimen is effective. Patients do not need to restrict dietary intake of fructose and galactose, as do those with type I disease.

Prognosis Liver symptoms improve with age and usually disappear after puberty. Cirrhosis of the liver may occur later in life. In type IIIa disease, muscle weakness and atrophy worsen during adulthood.

Type VI Glycogen Storage Disease [Liver Phosphorylase Deficiency (Hers Disease)] The number of patients with enzymatically documented liver phosphorylase deficiency is small. It appears that patients with liver phosphorylase deficiency have a benign course. These patients present with hepatomegaly and growth retardation early in childhood. Hypoglycemia, hyperlipidemia, and hyperketosis are usually mild if present. Plasma lactic acid and uric acid levels are normal. The heart and skeletal muscles are not involved. The hepatomegaly and growth retardation improve with age and usually disappear at puberty. Treatment is symptomatic. A high-carbohydrate diet and frequent feeding are effective in preventing hypoglycemia, but most patients require no specific treatment. The liver phosphorylase gene is located on chromosome 14q21. A splicing site mutation in intron 13 has been identified in a large Mennonite kindred, and four other mutations have been found in patients with different ethnic backgrounds.

Type IX Glycogen Storage Disease (Liver Phosphorylase Kinase Deficiency) Defects of phosphorylase kinase cause a heterogeneous group of glycogenoses. The heterogeneity is due to the complexity of the phosphorylase kinase enzyme complex. It consists of four subunits (α, β, γ, and δ), each encoded by different genes (X chromosome as well as autosomes) that are differentially expressed in various tissues. Phosphorylase kinase deficiency can be divided into several subtypes on the basis of the gene/subunit involved, the tissues that are primarily affected, and the mode of inheritance.

Subtypes of phosphorylase kinase deficiency • *X-LINKED LIVER PHOSPHORYLASE KINASE DEFICIENCY* X-linked liver phosphorylase kinase deficiency is one of the most common liver glycogenoses. Phosphorylase kinase activity may also be deficient in erythrocytes and leukocytes but is normal in muscle. Typically, a child between the ages of 1 and 5 years presents with growth retardation and hepatomegaly. Levels of cholesterol, triglycerides, and liver enzymes are mildly elevated. Ketosis may occur after fasting. Lactic and uric acid levels are normal. Hypoglycemia is mild, if present. The rise in the blood glucose level after the administration of glucagon is normal. Hepatomegaly and abnormal blood chemistries gradually return to normal with age. Most adults achieve a normal final height and are practically asymptomatic, despite a persistent phosphorylase kinase deficiency.

Liver histology shows glycogen-distended hepatocytes. The accumulated glycogen (α particles, rosette form) has a frayed or burst appearance and is less compact than in type I or type III disease. Fibrous septa and low-grade inflammatory changes may be present.

The structural gene for the liver isoform of the phosphorylase kinase α-subunit is located on chromosome Xp22, and mutations of this gene have been found in the disorder. Subtle mutations tend to retain the phosphorylase kinase activity in blood cells, whereas nonsense mutations cause enzyme deficiency in both liver and blood cells.

AUTOSOMAL LIVER AND MUSCLE PHOSPHORYLASE KINASE DEFICIENCY An autosomal recessive form of liver and muscle phosphorylase kinase deficiency has been reported in several patients. As in the X-linked form of the disorder, hepatomegaly and growth retardation are the predominant symptoms in early childhood. Some patients also exhibit muscle hypotonia and have reduced activity of phosphorylase kinase in muscle. This form of the phosphorylase kinase deficiency is caused by mutations in the β-subunit of the gene located on chromosome 16q12-13.

AUTOSOMAL LIVER PHOSPHORYLASE KINASE DEFICIENCY In contrast to the benign course of X-linked phosphorylase kinase deficiency, patients with the autosomal recessive form of liver phosphorylase kinase deficiency have more severe phenotypes and often develop liver cirrhosis. This form of phosphorylase kinase deficiency is due to mutations in the testis/liver isoform of the γ-subunit gene located on chromosome 16p.

MUSCLE-SPECIFIC PHOSPHORYLASE KINASE DEFICIENCY Muscle-specific phosphorylase kinase deficiency causes cramps and myoglobinuria on exercise or progressive muscle weakness and atrophy. The activity of the enzyme is decreased in muscle but normal (when determined) in liver and blood cells. There is no hepatomegaly or cardiomegaly. The disorder may be due to mutation in the muscle isoform of the α-subunit located on the X chromosome.

CARDIAC-SPECIFIC PHOSPHORYLASE KINASE DEFICIENCY Several sporadic cases of cardiac-specific phosphorylase kinase deficiency have been reported. All patients died during infancy from cardiac failure due to massive glycogen deposition in the myocardium. The molecular basis has not been defined.

Diagnosis Definitive diagnosis of phosphorylase kinase deficiency requires demonstration of the enzymatic defect in affected tissues. Although phosphorylase kinase can be measured in leukocytes and erythrocytes, the enzyme has many tissue-specific isozymes, and the diagnosis can be missed without studies of the liver, muscle, or heart.

Rx TREATMENT The treatment for liver phosphorylase or phosphorylase kinase deficiency is based on symptoms. A high-carbohydrate diet and frequent feedings are effective in preventing hypoglycemia, but most patients require no specific treatment. Prognosis is usually good; adult patients have normal stature and minimal hepatomegaly. There is no treatment for the fatal form of isolated cardiac phosphorylase kinase deficiency.

Type 0 Glycogen Storage Disease (Glycogen Synthase Deficiency) Strictly speaking, type 0 is not a glycogen storage disease, as the deficiency of the enzyme leads to decreased glycogen stores. The patients present in early infancy with morning drowsiness and fatigue and sometimes convulsions associated with hypoglycemia and hyperketonemia. There is no hepatomegaly or hyperlipidemia. Prolonged hyperglycemia and elevated lactate levels with normal insulin levels after administration of glucose suggest a possible diagnosis of glycogen synthase deficiency. Definitive diagnosis requires a liver biopsy to measure the enzyme activity. Treatment is symptomatic and involves frequent feedings rich in protein and nighttime supplements of uncooked cornstarch to alleviate hypoglycemia. Prognosis is good as patients survive to adulthood with a resolution of hypoglycemia except during pregnancy. Mutations in the liver glycogen synthase gene (located on chromosome 12p12.2) that cause glycogen synthase deficiency have been identified.

Type XI Glycogen Storage Disease (Hepatic Glycogenosis with Renal Fanconi Syndrome, Fanconi-Bickel Syndrome) This rare autosomal recessive disease is caused by defects in the facilitative glucose transporter 2 (GLUT-2) which transports glucose in and out of hepatocytes, pancreatic cells, and the baso-lateral membranes of intestinal and renal epithelial cells. The disease is characterized by proximal renal tubular dysfunction, impaired glucose and galactose utilization, and accumulation of glycogen in liver and kidney.

GENETIC CONSIDERATIONS The low prevalence of Fanconi-Beckel syndrome (fewer than 100 cases reported worldwide) is underscored by the fact that consanguinity is found in 70% of the patients with a detectable GLUT-2 mutation. The gene for GLUT-2 is located on chromosome 3q26 and most mutations detected so far cause premature termination of translation. ■

Clinical and laboratory findings The affected child presents in the first year of life with failure to thrive, rickets, and a protuberant abdomen due to liver and kidney enlargement. Laboratory findings include glucosuria, phosphaturia, generalized aminoaciduria, bicarbonate wasting, hypophosphatemia, increased serum alkaline phosphatase levels, and radiologic findings of rickets. Mild fasting hypoglycemia and hyperlipidemia may be present. Liver transaminases, plasma lactate, and uric acid levels are usually normal. Oral galactose or glucose tolerance tests show intolerance to these sugars, which may be caused by the functional loss of GLUT-2, which prevents liver uptake of these sugars. Tissue biopsies show marked accumulation of glycogen in hepatocytes and proximal renal tubular cells, presumably due to the altered transport of glucose out of these organs.

Rx TREATMENT There is no specific therapy. Growth retardation persists through adulthood. Symptomatic replacement of water, electrolytes, and vitamin D, restriction of galactose intake, and a diabetes mellitus-like diet, presented in frequent and small meals with a cornstarch supplement, may improve growth.

DISORDERS ASSOCIATED WITH LIVER CIRRHOSIS

Type IV Glycogen Storage Disease (Branching Enzyme Deficiency, Amylopectinosis, or Andersen Disease) Deficiency of branching enzyme activity results in accumulation of an abnormal glycogen with poor solubility. The disease is referred to as *type IV glycogen storage disease or amylopectinosis*, because the abnormal glycogen has fewer branch points, more 1-4 linked glucose units, and longer outer chains, resulting in a structure resembling amylopectin.

GENETIC CONSIDERATIONS Type IV glycogen storage disease is a rare autosomal recessive disease. Prenatal diagnosis is available with use of cultured amniocytes or chorionic villi to measure the level of enzymatic activity. The glycogen branching enzyme gene is located on chromosome 3p12. Both hepatic and neuromuscular forms of the disease are caused by mutations in the same branching enzyme gene; its characterization in individual patients may be useful in predicting the clinical course. ■

Clinical and laboratory findings This disorder is clinically variable. The most common form is characterized by progressive cirrhosis of the liver and is manifest in the first 18 months of life as hepatosplenomegaly and failure to thrive. The cirrhosis progresses to cause portal hypertension, ascites, esophageal varices, and liver failure that leads to death by age 5. Less frequently, patients survive without progression of liver disease.

Tissue deposition of amylopectin-like materials can be demonstrated in liver, heart, muscle, skin, intestine, brain, spinal cord, and peripheral nerve. The histologic findings in the liver are characterized by both micronodular cirrhosis and faintly stained basophilic inclusions in the hepatocytes. The inclusions consist of coarsely clumped, stored material that is periodic acid Schiff-positive and partially resistant to diastase digestion. Electron microscopy shows, in addition to the conventional χ and β glycogen particles, an accumulation of fibrillar aggregations typical of amylopectin. Definitive diagnosis requires demonstration that branching enzyme activity is deficient in liver, muscle, cultured skin fibroblasts, or leukocytes.

A neuromuscular form of type IV glycogen storage disease has also been reported. Patients with this disease may present (1) at birth with severe hypotonia, muscle atrophy, and neuronal involvement and die during the neonatal period; (2) in late childhood with myopathy or cardiomyopathy; or (3) as adults with diffuse central and peripheral nervous system dysfunction accompanied by accumulation of polyglucosan bodies in the nervous system (so-called adult polyglucosan body disease). Definitive diagnosis of the adult disease requires assay of the branching enzyme in leukocytes or nerve biopsy, as the deficiency is limited to those tissues.

℞ TREATMENT There is no specific treatment for type IV glycogen storage disease. For progressive hepatic failure, liver transplantation has been performed. However, caution should be taken in selecting patients for liver transplantation because a nonprogressive hepatic form of the disease exists, and extra hepatic manifestations of the disease may occur after transplantation.

GLYCOGEN STORAGE DISEASES: MUSCLE GLYCOGENOSES

DISORDERS WITH MUSCLE-ENERGY IMPAIRMENT

Type V Glycogen Storage Disease (Muscle Phosphorylase Deficiency, McArdle Disease) Deficiency of muscle phosphorylase is the prototype muscle-energy disorder. Deficiency of this enzyme in muscle limits ATP generation by glycogenolysis and results in glycogen accumulation.

GENETIC CONSIDERATIONS Type V glycogen storage disease is an autosomal recessive disorder that does not appear to have ethnic predilection. The gene for muscle phosphorylase is located on chromosome 11q13. The most common mutation in patients in the United States is a nonsense mutation that changes an arginine to a stop codon (R49X), and the most common mutation in the Japanese is deletion of a single codon (F708). These features allow DNA-based diagnosis and carrier detection in these two populations. ■

Clinical and laboratory findings Symptoms usually develop first in adulthood and are characterized by exercise intolerance with muscle cramps. Two types of activity tend to cause symptoms: (1) brief exercise of great intensity, such as sprinting or carrying heavy loads; and (2) less intense but sustained activity, such as climbing stairs or walking uphill. Moderate exercise, such as walking on level ground, can be performed by most patients for long periods. Many patients experience a characteristic "second wind" phenomenon; if they rest briefly at the first appearance of muscle pain, they can resume exercise with more ease. About half of patients report burgundy-colored urine after exercise, the consequence of myoglobinuria secondary to rhabdomyolysis. Intense myoglobinuria after vigorous exercise may cause renal failure. Although most patients are diagnosed in the second or third decade, many report weakness and lack of endurance since childhood. In rare cases, EMG findings may suggest an inflammatory myopathy, and the diagnosis can be confused with polymyositis.

The level of serum creatine kinase is usually elevated at rest and increases more after exercise. Exercise also increases the levels of blood ammonia, inosine, hypoxanthine, and uric acid. The latter abnormalities are attributed to accelerated recycling of muscle purine nucleotides in the face of insufficient ATP production.

Diagnosis Lack of an increase in blood lactate and exaggerated blood ammonia elevations after an ischemic exercise test are indicative of muscle glycogenosis and suggest a defect in the conversion of glycogen or glucose to lactate. The abnormal exercise response, however, is not limited to type V disease and can occur with other defects in glycogenolysis or glycolysis, such as deficiencies of muscle phosphofructokinase or debranching enzyme (when the test is done after fasting). Definitive diagnosis is made by enzymatic assay in muscle tissue or by mutation analysis of the myophosphorylase gene.

℞ TREATMENT In general, avoidance of strenuous exercise can prevent major episodes of rhabdomyolysis. Exercise tolerance can be augmented by aerobic training or by ingestion of glucose or fructose. A high-protein diet may increase exercise endurance in some patients. Longevity does not appear to be affected.

Type VII Glycogen Storage Disease (Muscle Phosphofructokinase Deficiency, Tarui Disease) Type VII disease is caused by a deficiency of muscle phosphofructokinase, which catalyzes the conversion of fructose-6-phosphate to fructose-1,6-diphosphate and is a key regulatory enzyme of glycolysis.

Phosphofructokinase is composed of three isozyme subunits (M, muscle; L, liver; and P, platelet), which are encoded by different genes and are differentially expressed in tissues. Skeletal muscle contains only M isozyme, and red blood cells contain a hybrid of L and M forms. Type VII disease is due to defective M isoenzyme, which causes complete enzyme deficiency in muscle and partial deficiency in red blood cells.

GENETIC CONSIDERATIONS Type VII glycogen storage disease is inherited as an autosomal recessive trait. The disease appears to be rare, and most reported patients are either Ashkenazi Jews or Japanese. The gene for the M isoenzyme is located on chromosome 12q13.3. In Ashkenazi Jews, 95% of mutant alleles are either a splicing defect or a nucleotide deletion. ■

Clinical and laboratory findings The features are similar to those in type V disease, namely, early onset of fatigue and pain with exercise. Vigorous exercise causes severe muscle cramps and myoglobinuria. However, several features of type VII disease are distinctive. (1) Exercise intolerance is usually evident in childhood, is more severe than in type V disease, and may be associated with nausea and vomiting. (2) A compensated hemolysis occurs as evidenced by an increased level of serum bilirubin and reticulocyte count. (3) Hyperuricemia is common and becomes more marked after exercise. (4) An abnormal glycogen resembling amylopectin is present in muscle fibers; it is periodic acid Schiff-positive and resistant to diastase digestion. (5) Exercise intolerance is particularly acute after meals rich in carbohydrate because glucose cannot be utilized in muscle and because the ingested glucose inhibits lipolysis and thus deprives muscle of fatty acid and ketone substrates. In contrast, patients with type V disease can metabolize glucose derived from either liver glycogenolysis or exogenous glucose. Indeed, glucose infusion improves exercise tolerance in patients with type V disease.

Two rare type VII variants have been reported. One begins in infancy with hypotonia and limb weakness, and a rapidly progressive myopathy leads to death by age 4. The other occurs in adults and is characterized by a slowly progressive, fixed muscle weakness rather than by cramps and myoglobinuria.

Diagnosis The M isoenzyme defect must be demonstrated in muscle, red blood cells, or cultured skin fibroblasts by biochemical or histochemical techniques.

℞ TREATMENT There is no specific treatment. Avoidance of strenuous exercise prevents acute attacks of muscle cramps and myoglobinuria.

Other Muscle Glycogenoses with Muscle-Energy Impairment Five additional enzyme defects produce muscle glycogenoses, namely, deficiencies in phosphoglycerate kinase, phosphoglycerate mutase, lactate dehydrogenase, fructose 1,6-bisphosphate aldolase A, and pyruvate kinase. All five enzymes affect terminal glycolysis, and deficiency causes muscle-energy impairment similar to that in type V and type VII disease. The failure of blood lactate to increase in response to exercise can be used to separate muscle glycogenoses from disorders of lipid metabolism, such as carnitine palmitoyl transferase II deficiency and very long chain acyl-coenzyme A dehydrogenase deficiency, which also cause muscle cramps and myoglobinuria. Muscle glycogen levels may be normal in the disorders affecting terminal glycolysis, and definitive diagnosis is made by assaying the enzymatic activity in muscle.

DISORDERS WITH PROGRESSIVE SKELETAL MUSCLE MYOPATHY AND/OR CARDIOMYOPATHY Type II Glycogen Storage Disease (Acid α-1,4 Glucosidase Deficiency, Pompe Disease) (See also Chap. 349) Type II disease is caused by a deficiency of lysosomal acid α-1,4 glucosidase (acid maltase), an enzyme responsible for the degradation of glycogen in lysosomal vacuoles. It is characterized by the accumulation of glycogen in lysosomes as opposed to its accumulation in cytoplasm in the other glycogenoses.

GENETIC CONSIDERATIONS Pompe disease is an autosomal recessive disorder and does not appear to have an ethnic predilection. The gene for acid α-glucosidase is on chromosome 17q25. A splice site mutation (IVS1-13TG) is common in patients with adult-onset disease. Prenatal diagnosis with amniocytes or chorionic villi is available. ■

Clinical and laboratory findings The disorder encompasses a range of phenotypes, each including myopathy but differing in age of onset, organ involvement, and clinical severity. The most severe is the infantile-onset disease with cardiomegaly, hypotonia, and death before 1 year of age. Infants appear normal at birth but soon develop generalized muscle weakness with feeding difficulties, macroglossia, hepatomegaly, and congestive heart failure due to a hypertrophic cardiomyopathy. Electrocardiographic findings include a high-voltage QRS complex and a shortened PR interval. Death usually occurs from cardiorespiratory failure.

The juvenile or late-childhood form is characterized by skeletal muscle manifestations, usually without cardiac involvement, and a slowly progressive course. The juvenile form typically presents as delayed motor milestones (if age of onset is early enough) and difficulty in walking; these manifestations are followed by swallowing difficulties, proximal muscle weakness, and respiratory muscle involvement. This form can cause death before the end of the second decade.

An adult form of type II disease presents as a slowly progressive myopathy without cardiac involvement and has its onset between the second and seventh decades. The clinical picture is dominated by slowly progressive proximal muscle weakness with truncal involvement. The pelvic girdle, paraspinal muscles, and the diaphragm are most seriously affected. The initial symptoms may be respiratory insufficiency manifested by somnolence, morning headache, orthopnea, and exertional dyspnea.

Laboratory findings include elevated levels of serum creatine kinase, aspartate transaminase, and lactate dehydrogenase, particularly in infants. Muscle biopsy shows the presence of vacuoles that stain positively for glycogen, and muscle acid phosphatase is increased, presumably from a compensatory increase of lysosomal enzymes. Electron microscopy reveals the glycogen accumulation. EMG reveals myopathic features with irritability of muscle fibers and pseudomyotonic discharges. Serum creatine kinase is not always elevated in adults and, depending on the muscle biopsied or tested, muscle histology or EMG may not be abnormal. It is prudent to examine affected muscle.

Diagnosis Diagnosis can be established by demonstration of the absence or reduced levels of acid α-glucosidase activity in muscle or cultured skin fibroblasts. Deficiency is usually more severe in the infantile form than in the juvenile and adult disorders.

Rx TREATMENT No effective treatment for the infantile form is currently available. Enzyme replacement is a promising therapy for this fatal lysosomal storage disease, and clinical trials are ongoing to test its safety and efficacy. A high-protein diet may be useful for the juvenile and adult forms. Nocturnal ventilatory support can improve the quality of life.

DISORDERS OF GALACTOSE METABOLISM

GALACTOSE 1-PHOSPHATE URIDYL TRANSFERASE DEFICIENCY GALACTOSEMIA "Classic" galactosemia is a serious disease with an early onset of symptoms; the incidence is 1 in 60,000. The newborn infant normally receives up to 20% of caloric intake as lactose, which consists of glucose and galactose. Without the transferase, the infant is unable to metabolize galactose 1-phosphate (Fig. 350-1), the accumulation of which results in injury to parenchymal cells of the kidney, liver, and brain.

GENETIC CONSIDERATIONS Galactosemia caused by transferase deficiency is inherited as an autosomal recessive trait; there are several enzymatic variants. The Duarte variant exhibits diminished red cell enzyme activity that is usually of no clinical significance. Some African-American patients have milder symptoms despite the absence of measurable transferase activity in erythrocytes; these patients retain 10% of the enzyme activity in liver and intestinal mucosa. Most Caucasian patients have no detectable enzyme activity in any of these tissues. The gene for galactose-1 phosphate uridyl transferase is located on chromosome 9p13. In African Americans, 48% of the mutant alleles are represented by the S135L substitution, perhaps accounting for the milder phenotype. In the Caucasian population, 70% of mutant alleles are represented by the Q188R substitution. Carrier testing and prenatal diagnosis can be carried out by direct enzyme analysis of amniocytes or chorionic villi. DNA-based testing can also be performed. ■

Clinical and laboratory findings The clinical manifestations of uridyl transferase deficiency are myriad, necessitating a high index of suspicion if the diagnosis is to be made. Clinical features may include: jaundice, hepatomegaly, vomiting, hypoglycemia, convulsions, lethargy, irritability, feeding difficulties, poor weight gain, aminoaciduria, cataracts, vitreous hemorrhage, hepatic cirrhosis, ascites, splenomegaly, or mental retardation. Patients with galactosemia are at increased risk for *Escherichia coli* neonatal sepsis; the onset of sepsis often precedes the diagnosis of galactosemia. When the diagnosis is not made at birth, damage to the liver (cirrhosis) and brain (mental retardation) becomes increasingly severe and irreversible. For this reason, routine neonatal screening tests for galactosemia have been instituted in many parts of the world.

Diagnosis The preliminary diagnosis of galactosemia is made by demonstrating a reducing substance (by Clinitest) in urine specimens collected while the patient is receiving human or cow's milk or another formula containing lactose. The reducing substance found in urine, which is negative in a glucose oxidase test, can be identified as galactose with chromatography or an enzymatic test specific for galactose. Definitive diagnosis requires the demonstration of deficient activity of galactose-1-phosphate uridyl transferase in erythrocytes or other tissues, which also exhibit increased concentrations of galactose-1-phosphate.

Rx TREATMENT Because of widespread newborn screening for galactosemia, patients are now being identified and treated early. Elimination of galactose from the diet reverses growth failure, renal, and hepatic dysfunction. Cataracts regress and most patients have no impairment of eyesight. Early diagnosis and treatment have improved the prognosis of galactosemia; on long-term follow-up, however, patients still have ovarian failure manifest as primary or secondary amenorrhea, as well as developmental delay and learning disabilities, which increase in severity with age. In addition, most patients have speech disorders and a smaller number demonstrate poor growth and impaired motor function and balance (with or without overt ataxia). The relative control of galactose-1-phosphate levels does not always correlate with long-term outcome, suggesting that other factors, such as uridine diphosphate (UDP)-galactose deficiency (a donor for galacto-lipids and proteins), may be responsible for some of the metabolic consequences of the disease.

GALACTOKINASE DEFICIENCY In contrast to the multiple systems that are affected in uridyl transferase deficiency, cataracts are usually the sole manifestation of galactokinase deficiency. The affected infant is otherwise asymptomatic. This disorder is characterized by elevated blood galactose levels with normal uridyl transferase activity and an absence of galactokinase activity in erythrocytes. Treatment is dietary restriction of galactose intake. Mutations leading to galactokinase deficiency have been identified in the gene coding for galactokinase (located on chromosome 17q24).

URIDINE DIPHOSPHATE GALACTOSE 4-EPIMERASE (UDP GAL 4-EPIMERASE) DEFICIENCY The abnormally accumulated metabolites in this disorder are very much like those seen in uridyl transferase deficiency; however, there is also an increase in cellular UDP galactose. There are two distinct forms of epimerase deficiency. A benign form was discovered incidentally as a result of the neonatal screening program. Affected persons in this case are healthy; the enzyme deficiency is limited to leukocytes and erythrocytes, without deranged metabolism in other tissues, and no treatment is required. The second form of epimerase deficiency is severe with clinical manifestations resembling uridyl transferase deficiency. Additional features include hypotonia and nerve deafness. The enzyme deficiency is generalized, and clinical symptoms respond to restriction of dietary galactose. Although this form of galactosemia is very rare, it must be considered in a symptomatic patient who has normal transferase activity. The gene for epimerase is located on chromosome 1p35-36; mutations responsible for both forms of the epimerase deficiency have been identified.

DISORDERS OF FRUCTOSE METABOLISM

DEFICIENCY OF FRUCTOKINASE (BENIGN FRUCTOSURIA) This condition is not associated with any clinical manifestations. It is an incidental finding, usually made through the detection of fructose as a reducing substance in the urine. No treatment is necessary.

DEFICIENCY OF FRUCTOSE 1,6-BISPHOSPHATE ALDOLASE (ALDOLASE B) (HEREDITARY FRUCTOSE INTOLERANCE) This is a severe disease of infants that appears with the ingestion of fructose-containing food. It is caused by deficiency of fructose 1,6-bisphosphate aldolase B activity in the liver, kidney, and intestine. The enzyme catalyzes the hydrolysis of fructose 1-phosphate and fructose 1,6-bisphosphate into the 3-carbon sugars, dihydroxyacetone phosphate, glyceraldehyde-3-phosphate, and glyceraldehyde (Fig. 350-1). Deficiency of this enzyme activity causes rapid accumulation of fructose 1-phosphate and initiates severe toxic symptoms when exposed to fructose.

GENETIC CONSIDERATIONS The true incidence of hereditary fructose intolerance is not known but may be as high as 1 in 23,000. The gene for aldolase B is on chromosome 9q22.3. Several mutations causing heredity fructose intolerance have been identified. A single missense mutation, which results in substitution of proline for alanine at position 149, is the most common mutation identified in northern Europeans. This mutation plus two other point mutations account for approximately 80 to 85% of hereditary fructose intolerance in Europe and the United States. The diagnosis of hereditary fructose intolerance can thus be made in most cases by direct DNA analysis. Prenatal diagnosis should be possible from either amniocentesis or chorionic villi with the use of DNA for mutational or linkage analysis. ■

Clinical and laboratory findings Patients with fructose intolerance are healthy and asymptomatic until fructose or sucrose (table sugar) is ingested (usually from fruit, fruit juice, or sweetened cereal). Clinical manifestations may resemble those of galactosemia and include jaundice, hepatomegaly, vomiting, lethargy, irritability, and convulsions. Laboratory findings include prolonged clotting time, hypoalbuminemia, elevation of bilirubin and transaminases, and proximal renal tubular dysfunction. If the disease is not diagnosed and intake of the noxious sugar persists, hypoglycemic episodes recur, and liver and kidney failure progress, eventually leading to death.

Diagnosis Suspicion of the enzyme deficiency is suggested by the presence of a reducing substance in the urine during an attack. The diagnosis is supported by an intravenous fructose tolerance test, which will cause a rapid decline of serum phosphate, followed by blood glucose, and a subsequent rise of uric acid and magnesium. An oral tolerance test should not be performed as patients may become acutely ill. Definitive diagnosis is made by assay of fructaldoase B activity in the liver.

℞ TREATMENT Treatment consists of the complete elimination of all sources of sucrose, fructose and sorbitol from the diet. With this treatment, liver and kidney dysfunction improve, and catch-up growth is common. Intellectual development is usually unimpaired. As the patient matures, symptoms become milder, even after fructose ingestion, and the long-term prognosis is good. Owing to dietary avoidance of sucrose, affected patients have few dental caries.

FRUCTOSE 1,6-DIPHOSPHATASE DEFICIENCY Fructose 1,6-diphosphatase deficiency is a defect in gluconeogenesis. The disease is characterized by life-threatening episodes of acidosis, hypoglycemia, hyperventilation, convulsions, and coma. These episodes are triggered by febrile infections and gastroenteritis when oral food intake decreases. Laboratory findings include low blood glucose, high lactate and uric acid levels, and a blood gas picture of metabolic acidosis. In contrast to hereditary fructose intolerance, there is usually no aversion to sweets, and renal tubular and liver functions are normal. Treatment of acute attacks consists of correction of hypoglycemia and acidosis by intravenous infusion; the response is usually rapid. Later, avoidance of fasting and elimination of fructose and sucrose from the diet prevent further episodes. For long-term prevention of hypoglycemia, a slowly released carbohydrate such as cornstarch is useful. Patients who survive childhood seem to develop normally.

Diagnosis The diagnosis is established by demonstrating enzyme deficiency in either the liver or an intestinal biopsy specimen. The enzyme defect may also be demonstrated in leukocytes in some cases. The gene coding for fructose 1,6-diphosphatase is located on chromosome 9q22. In patients with known mutations, carrier detection and prenatal diagnosis are possible by DNA-based testing.

BIBLIOGRAPHY

ALI M et al: Hereditary fructose intolerance. J Med Genet 35:353, 1998

CHEN Y-T: Glycogen storage diseases, in *The Metabolic and Molecular Bases of Inherited Disease*, 8th ed, CR Scriver et al (eds). New York, McGraw-Hill, 2001, pp 1521–1551

DIMAURO S, BRUNO C: Glycogen storage disease of muscle. Curr Opin Neurol 11:477, 1998

ELPELEG ON: The molecular background of glycogen metabolism disorders. J Ped Endocrinol Metab 12:363, 1999

FERNANDEZ J, CHEN Y-T: The glycogen storage diseases, in *Inborn Metabolic Disease: Diagnosis and Treatment*, J Fernandez et al (eds). Berlin, New York, Springer-Verlag, 1995, p 71–87

HIRSCHHORN R, REUSER AJ: Glycogen storage disease type II: Acid α-glucosidase (acid maltase) deficiency, in *The Metabolic and Molecular Bases of Inherited Disease*, 8th ed, CR Scriver et al (eds). New York, McGraw-Hill, 2001, pp 1389–1420

KIKUCHI T et al: Clinical and metabolic correction of Pompe disease by enzyme therapy in acid maltase deficient quail. J Clin Invest 101:827, 1998

SEGAL S, BERRY GT: Disorders of galactose metabolism, *The Metabolic and Molecular Bases of Inherited Disease*, 7th ed, CR Scriver et al (eds). New York, McGraw-Hill, 1995, pp 967–1000

SANTER R et al: Mutations in *GLUT2*, the gene for the liver-type glucose transporter, in patients with Fanconi-Bickel syndrome. Nat Genet 17:324, 1997

SHEN J-J et al: Mutations in exon 3 of the glycogen debranching enzyme gene are associated with glycogen storage disease type III that is differentially expressed in liver and muscle. J Clin Invest 98:352, 1996

VEIGA DA CUNHA M et al: A gene on chromosome 11q23 coding for a putative glucose 6-phosphate translocase is mutated in glycogen storage disease type Ib and type Ic. Am J Hum Genet 63:976, 1998

WALTER JH et al: Recommendations for the management of galactosemia. UK Galactosemia Steering Group. Arch Dis Child 80:93, 1999

351 Darwin J. Prockop, Helena Kuivaniemi, Gerard Tromp, Leena Ala-Kokko

INHERITED DISORDERS OF CONNECTIVE TISSUE

Heritable disorders that involve the major connective tissues of the body such as bone, skin, cartilage, blood vessels, and basement membranes are among the most common genetic diseases in human beings. Here we will focus primarily on those disorders that can have severe manifestations, are relatively common, and are sufficiently understood at the molecular level to provide useful paradigms: osteogenesis imperfecta (OI), the Ehlers-Danlos syndrome (EDS), chondrodysplasias (CDs), the Marfan syndrome (MFS), epidermolysis bullosa (EB), and the Alport syndrome (AS).

THE CHALLENGE OF CLASSIFYING THE DISEASES The original classification of connective tissue diseases was based on the pattern of inheritance, the cluster of signs and symptoms, the histologic changes in tissues, and limited information about the molecular defects involved. This classification included about a dozen types and subtypes for OI, about the same number for the EDS, and over 150 for the CDs. Several limitations in these original classifications are now apparent. One is that the same mutation does not always produce the same disease phenotype in terms of severity of the condition or its clinical course. Such phenotypic variation occurs in many genetic diseases, including the connective tissue disorders, in which some members of a family are severely affected, whereas others with the same mutation have a mild disorder.

Most patients with classic features of a severe connective tissue disease have a mutation in a gene or genes coding for a single protein. For example, the majority of patients with OI have a mutation in one of the two genes coding for type I procollagen. Similarly, most patients with MFS have mutations in a gene for fibrillin. For other disease categories, the situation is more complex. In EDS, for example, the type IV variant is usually caused by mutations in the gene for type III procollagen, the type VI variant by defects in the gene for lysyl hydroxylase, and the type VII variant by defects that impair the processing of type I procollagen to type I collagen.

Classifications of these disorders also tend to overemphasize the etiologic differences between severe genetic diseases that are apparent in infants and the more common diseases that appear much later in life. Single-gene defects can cause subsets of late-onset diseases such as osteoporosis, aneurysms, and osteoarthritis. For example, a small subset of patients with postmenopausal osteoporosis have mutations in the genes for procollagen I similar to the mutations in the same genes that produce lethal variants of OI. Likewise, a subset of patients with familial aortic aneurysms have mutations in the gene for procollagen III similar to the mutations in the same gene that cause lethal variants of type IV EDS, and occasional patients with osteoarthritis have mutations in the gene for procollagen II similar to the mutations in the same gene that cause lethal CDs. There is disagreement as to the best diagnosis for such patients in that some investigators feel that after a mutation similar to those seen in the early-onset diseases is identified, the patients should be reclassified as having mild forms of OI, EDS, or CD, even though they do not have definitive evidence of the early-onset diseases or seek medical attention until adulthood. Therefore, the category of diseases referred to as *inherited disorders of connective tissue* may have to be expanded as we obtain additional information about more common diseases.

DEFINITION AND COMPOSITION OF CONNECTIVE TISSUES Connective tissues are composed of specific macromolecules, many of which are also constituents of the lung, the kidney, the walls of blood vessels, the vitreous gel of the eye, and the synovial fluid. Indeed, most organs and tissues contain small amounts of the same macromolecules assembled into membranes and septa. Therefore, virtually all structures contain some connective tissue.

The distinguishing feature of connective tissues is that the component macromolecules are assembled into an insoluble extracellular matrix (Table 351-1). The macromolecules include at least 19 different types of collagens, the related fibrous proteins known as *elastin* and *fibrillin*, a series of proteoglycans, and components whose structure and function are only partially defined.

Differences in the connective tissues of bone, skin, and cartilage are in part explained by differences in the content of specific components (Table 351-1). For example, tendons and ligaments consist primarily of type I collagen fibrils and small amounts of other components that help organize the type I fibrils into fibers and fiber bundles. Cartilage consists primarily of fibrils of type II collagen in the form of arcades that are distended by highly charged proteoglycans. The extracellular matrix of the aorta contains collagens that provide tensile strength and elastin that provides elasticity. Differences among the connective tissues also depend on the three-dimensional organization of the molecular components. The type I collagen fibrils in tendon are packed into thick, parallel bundles of fibers, whereas type I collagen fibrils in skin are randomly oriented. In cortical bone, helical arrays of type I collagen fibrils are deposited around haversian canals.

Table 351-1 Constituents of Connective Tissues in Various Tissues

Connective Tissue	Major Constituents	Approximate Amounts, % dry wt	Characteristics or Functions
Dermis, ligaments, tendons	Type I collagen	80	Bundles of fibrils
	Type III collagen	5–15	Thin fibrils
	Type IV collagen, laminin, nidogen	<5	In basal laminae under epithelium and endothelium
	Types V, VI, and VII collagens	<5	VII forms anchoring fibrils; others unknown
	Elastin, fibrillin	<5	Provides elasticity
	Fibronectin	<5	Associated with collagen fibers and cell surfaces
	Proteoglycans,[a] hyaluronate	0.5	Provide resiliency
Bone (demineralized)	Type I collagen	90	Complex fibril network
	Type VI collagen	1–2	Function unclear
	Proteoglycans[a]	1	Function unclear
	Osteonectin, osteopontin, osteocalcin, α2-glycoprotein, sialoproteins	1–5	May regulate mineralization
Aorta	Type I collagen	20–40	Fibril network
	Type III collagen	20–40	Thin fibrils
	Elastin, fibrillin	20–40	Provide elasticity
	Type IV collagen, laminin, nidogen	<5	Form basal lamina
	Types V and VI collagens	<2	Functions unclear
	Proteoglycans[a]	<3	Provide resiliency
Cartilage	Type II collagen	40–50	Arcades of thin fibrils
	Type IX collagen	5–10	Links type II fibrils
	Type X collagen	5–10	Surrounds hypertrophic cells
	Type XI collagen	<10	Function unclear
	Proteoglycans,[a] hyaluronate	15–50	Provides resiliency

[a] As discussed in text, >30 proteoglycans have now been identified. They differ in the structures of their core proteins and their contents of glycosaminoglycans side chains of chondroitin-4-sulfate, chondroitin-6-sulfate, dermatan sulfate, and keratin sulfate. Basal lamina contain a proteoglycan with a side chain of heparan sulfate that resembles heparin.

BIOSYNTHESIS OF CONNECTIVE TISSUE Connective tissues form primarily by a process of self-assembly, in which a molecule of the correct size, shape, and surface properties binds to other molecules with the same or similar structure in a spontaneous but ordered manner. The molecular mechanisms and driving forces are similar to those involved in crystal formation.

Collagen Synthesis The self-assembly of connective tissue is illustrated by the assembly of collagen into fibrils. The collagen molecule that forms fibrils is a long, thin rod consisting of three polypeptide α chains wrapped into a rigid, ropelike triple helix (Fig. 351-1). The molecule has a triple-helical conformation, because each of the three α chains has a simple, repetitive amino acid sequence of about 1000 amino acids in which glycine (Gly) appears as every third amino acid. Therefore, the sequence of each α chain can be designated as $(\text{-Gly-X-Y-})_{333}$, where X and Y represent amino acids other than glycine. To fold into a triple helix, every third amino acid in an α chain must be glycine, the smallest amino acid, since this residue must fit in a sterically restricted space where the three chains of the triple helix come together. Many of the X- and Y-position amino acids are proline and hydroxyproline, which provide rigidity to the triple helix. The remaining amino acids form clusters of hydrophobic and charged regions on the surface of the molecule that direct how one molecule spontaneously binds to other collagen molecules and thereby self-assembles into the large collagen fibrils in tissues (see Fig. 351-1).

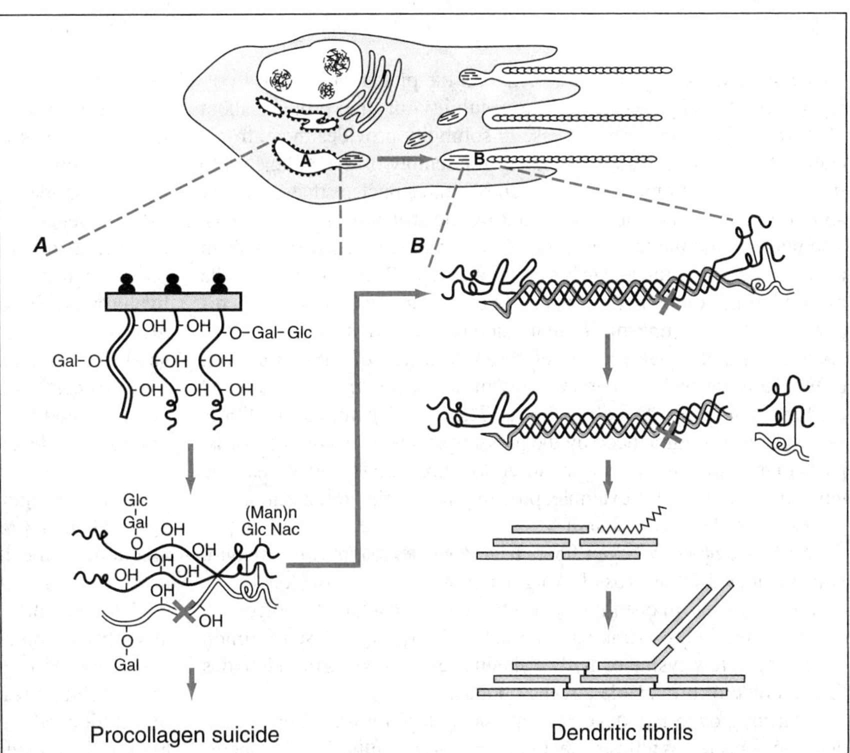

FIGURE 351-1 Schematic representation of synthesis of a type I collagen fibril by a fibroblast. *A*. Intracellular steps in the assembly of the procollagen molecule. Hydroxylations and glycosylations of the proα chains begin soon after the amino termini pass into the cisternae of the rough endoplasmic reticulum and continue after the three chains associate through their carboxy-terminal propeptides and become disulfide linked. *B*. Cleavage of procollagen to collagen, self-assembly of the collagen molecule into quarter-staggered fibrils, and cross-linking of the molecules in the fibrils. Cleavage of the propeptides may occur within crypts of the fibroblast, as shown here, or some distance from the cell. Mutations (depicted by X) cause the synthesis of structurally abnormal proα1(I) or proα2(I) chains of type I procollagen by interfering either with protein assembly (procollagen suicide) (*A*) or with processing to normal collagen fibrils (*B*). *(From DJ Prockop et al, Am J Med Genet 34:60, 1989, with permission.)*

More than 19 different collagens have been identified. Most are minor constituents that probably have highly specialized functions. The fibrillar collagens are found in tissues as long, highly ordered fibrils with a characteristic banding pattern by electron microscopy. Type I collagen, the most abundant, is found as cross-striated fibrils in a large number of tissues (Table 351-1). It is composed of two identical α chains called α1(I) and a third called α2(I). Type II collagen, another fibrillar collagen of cartilage, is composed of three identical α chains called α1(II). Type III collagen is found in small amounts in many tissues that contain type I collagen and in large amounts in large blood vessels; it is composed of three identical chains called α1(III). The nonfibrillar collagens are similar to the fibrillar collagens in that they contain -Gly-X-Y- sequences of amino acids that form triple-helical domains, but they also contain large globular domains. Self-assembly of most of the nonfibrillar collagens usually involves binding between the globular domains to form networks. For example, the type IV collagen in basement membranes self-assembles into a complex three-dimensional network that provides a diffusion barrier in the renal glomerulus and pulmonary alveolus. The network also provides support for epithelial and endothelial cells in these tissues and in skin, the gastrointestinal tract, and blood vessels. Some nonfibrillar collagens bind to the surface of fibrils formed by the more abundant collagens and alter the lateral growth of the fibrillar collagens or prevent the fibrils from coalescing into fiber bundles.

Because the molecules or monomers fibrillar collagens spontaneously self-assemble into fibrils, they are first synthesized as larger and more soluble precursors called *procollagens* and composed of proα chains. As the proα chains of procollagen are synthesized on ribosomes, the free ends move into the cisternae of the rough endoplasmic reticulum (Fig. 351-1). Hydrophobic signal peptides at the N termini are cleaved, and additional posttranslational reactions begin. Proline residues in the Y position of the repeating -Gly-X-Y- sequences are converted to hydroxyproline by prolyl hydroxylase in a reaction requiring ascorbic acid. Lysine residues in the Y position are similarly hydroxylated to hydroxylysine by lysyl hydroxylase. Many of the hydroxylysine residues are glycosylated with galactose or with galactose and glucose. A large mannose-rich oligosaccharide is assembled on the C-terminal propeptide of each chain. The association of the proα chains is directed by the structure and the surface properties of the globular C-propeptides. After the C-propeptides assemble correctly, the structure is locked in place by the formation of interchain disulfide bonds. Posttranslational modifications of the proα chains continue until each chain acquires about 100 hydroxyproline residues. Then a few of the hydroxyproline-rich -Gly-X-Y- sequences at the C terminus of the protein fold into a triple helix. The short region of triple helix becomes a nucleus for self-assembly of the triple helix of the whole protein, much like a nucleus for crystallization, in that the triple-helical conformation in one -Gly-X-Y- sequence induces the next -Gly-X-Y- sequence to fold into the same conformation. As a result, the conformation is propagated in a zipper-like fashion from the C terminus to the N terminus of the molecule, and the entire α-chain domain becomes a continuous triple helix. The protein then passes from the rough endoplasmic reticulum to other compartments and is secreted. The requirement for ascorbic acid in the hydroxylation of prolyl residues explains why wounds fail to heal in scurvy (Chap. 75). If sufficient proline residues are not converted to hydroxyproline, collagen cannot fold into a triple helix that is stable at body temperature. The abnormal protein accumulates in the cisternae of the rough endoplasmic reticulum and is slowly degraded.

After secretion, procollagen is processed to collagen by cleavage of the N-propeptides by procollagen N-proteinase and of the C-propeptides by procollagen C-proteinase. The processing of type I procollagen by the two proteinases converts the precursor to type I collagen and thereby decreases the solubility of the protein about 1000-fold. The 1000-fold decrease in solubility provides the entropic energy that drives the spontaneous self-assembly of the collagen into fibrils. Collagen monomers first assemble into a nucleus that grows by addition of monomers as determined by the structure of the nucleus. The nucleus and the final fibril can be assembled spontaneously from a single kind of collagen such as type I or type II. Fibrils can also be assembled as copolymers in which two or more collagens are incorporated into the same fibril simultaneously. Alternatively, a second collagen or a proteoglycan can bind to the surface of a growing fibril or to a fully formed fibril and thereby influence the final structure and the functional properties of the fibrils. The final structure of the fibrils in tissues is also influenced by the pressure and tensions on the fibrils, particularly after their tips are inserted into muscle and bone. The tension on tendons, for example, probably makes the initial thin fibrils coalesce into large fiber bundles.

Self-assembled collagen fibers have considerable tensile strength, which is increased by cross-linking reactions that form covalent bonds between α chains in one molecule and α chains in adjacent molecules. The first step in cross-linking is oxidation by lysyl oxidase of amino groups on a few lysine or hydroxylysine residues to form aldehydes that interact to form stable covalent bonds.

During growth and development, the collagen fibrils in all tissues undergo repeated synthesis, degradation, and resynthesis. The degradation of collagen fibers in tissues is initiated by specific collagenases found in leukocytes, fibroblasts, synovial cells, or related cell types. The collagenases cleave the collagen molecule at a point about three-quarters of the distance from its N terminus. The cleavage apparently triggers unfolding of the molecules on the surface of a fibril and further degradation by other proteinases.

Collagen fibers in most tissues of normal adults undergo very little metabolic turnover. One exception to this is the collagen fibrils that are degraded and resynthesized as part of the continual remodeling of bone. Although the collagen in many adult tissues is metabolically stable, the rate of turnover changes under some circumstances. In starvation, a large fraction of the collagen in skin and other connective tissues is degraded, thus providing amino acids for gluconeogenesis. Large losses of collagen also occur in most connective tissues during immobilization or prolonged periods of low-gravitational stress. In rheumatoid arthritis, pannus invasion causes a rapid degradation of collagen in the articular cartilage. Glucocorticoids decrease the collagen content of most connective tissues, including bone, by decreasing the rate of collagen synthesis. Decreases in collagen weaken tissues. In many pathologic states, however, collagen is deposited in excess. With injury to tissue, inflammation is usually followed by increased deposition primarily of type I collagen fibrils in the form of fibrotic tissue and scars. The deposition of collagen fibrils during the repair process is largely irreversible and is a major feature of the pathologic changes in hepatic cirrhosis, pulmonary fibrosis, atherosclerosis, and nephrosclerosis and in the scarring in skin and ligaments after surgery or trauma.

Elastin Synthesis Elastin assembly appears to be closely related to that of collagen, since a few of the prolines in the protein are hydroxylated to hydroxyproline by prolyl hydroxylase. The elastin monomer, however, is a single polypeptide that does not fold into a defined three-dimensional structure and is not synthesized as a larger precursor molecule. Instead, it is slowly secreted from cells into extracellular compartments, where it forms amorphous deposits around previously deposited microfibrils. The elastin deposits then become covalently cross-linked through oxidation of lysine residues to aldehydes by the same lysyl oxidase that initiates the cross-linking of collagen. The microfibrils in elastin deposits are largely composed of fibrillin, a large protein that forms beadlike strands.

Proteoglycan Synthesis The synthesis of proteoglycans begins in the cisternae of the rough endoplasmic reticulum with assembly of a core protein that then undergoes modification by sugar and sulfate transferases that generate large side chains of glycosaminoglycans. At least 30 proteoglycans have been identified by differences in the structures of their core proteins. The major proteoglycan of cartilage, called *aggrecan*, has a core protein of about 2000 amino acids to which are bound multiple side chains of chondroitin sulfate and keratin sulfate, polysaccharides consisting of highly charged and repetitive disaccharide sequences. After secretion from cells, the aggrecan monomer binds to a smaller protein called a *link protein*. The complex of core protein and link protein then spontaneously binds to a long chain of hyaluronic acid to form a huge copolymer called a *proteoglycan aggregate*. The highly charged proteoglycan aggregate binds water and small ions and thereby provides a large swelling pressure and resiliency to cartilage. Smaller proteoglycans such as decorin, biglycan, and fibromodulin have smaller core proteins with fewer and different polysaccharide side chains. They do not form large aggregates with hyaluronate but bind to fibrils of collagen or fibronectin and may thereby help regulate the assembly or spatial orientation of fibrils. One group of small proteoglycans known as *syndecans* binds to the plasma membranes of cells and may have a role in cell migration along fibrils or in signal transduction.

The assembly of bone follows much the same principles as the assembly of other connective tissues (Chap. 340). The first step is deposition of osteoid tissue that consists largely of type I collagen fibrils. Mineralization of osteoid occurs by steps that are still incompletely defined; proteins such as osteopontin and osteocalcin probably bind to the collagen fibrils and chelate calcium to initiate mineralization. Small proteoglycans such as decorin or fibromodulin may also play a role.

MUTATIONS THAT PRODUCE DISEASES OF CONNECTIVE TISSUES Because of the large number of tissue-specific macromolecules present in connective tissues, a large number of gene-protein systems are candidates for mutations that might cause disease of the tissues.

The most complete data on mutations causing heritable disorders of connective tissue are available on OI. Most patients with severe OI (types II and III) have mutations in either the gene for the proα1(I) chain or the gene for the proα2(I) chain of type I procollagen (the COL1A1 and COL1A2 genes). In patients with mild disease, many of the mutations decrease expression of protein from one allele of the genes. Most of the mutations in patients with severe OI cause synthesis of a structurally abnormal but partially functional proα chain. Mutations that cause synthesis of structurally abnormal proα chains include partial gene deletions, partial gene duplications, and RNA splicing mutations. The most common mutations, however, cause the substitution of single amino acids with bulky side chains for the glycine residues that appear as every third amino acid in the triple helix of a proα chain (Fig. 351-2). The structurally abnormal proα chains exert their effects primarily through one of three mechanisms (Fig. 351-1). First, the presence of an abnormal proα chain in a procollagen molecule containing two normal proα chains can prevent folding of the protein into a triple-helical conformation and lead to degradation of the whole molecule in a process called *procollagen suicide*. Similar dominant negative mutations are seen with other multisubunit proteins. The net result of procollagen suicide is accumulation of the unfolded protein in the rough endoplasmic reticulum of cells and a reduction in the amount of collagen available for fibril assembly. Second, the presence of one abnormal proα chain in a procollagen molecule can interfere with cleavage of the N-propeptide from the protein. The persistence of the N-propeptide on a fraction of the molecules interferes with the self-assembly of normal collagen so that thin and irregular collagen fibrils are formed. Third, the substitution of a bulkier amino acid for glycine can produce a change in the conformation of the molecule and result in the assembly of collagen fibrils that are abnormally branched or abnormally thick and short. Also, copolymerization of the mutated collagen with normal collagen can slow fibril assembly and decrease the total amount of collagen incorporated into fibrils.

Over 300 mutations in the two genes for type I procollagen have been found in patients with OI (Fig. 351-2). Initially, there was concern that many of the mutations might be neutral variations in the structure of the genes and not the cause of the disease phenotypes. However, the causal relationship between most of the mutations and the disease has been established by several kinds of evidence: (1) DNA linkage studies in families with mild variants of OI showed that specific mutated alleles were coinherited with the disease phenotypes. (2) Probands with lethal variants of OI were shown to have new mutations not found in the normal parents or in only a few cells from a mosaic parent (see below). (3) Studies with cultured skin fibroblasts from patients demonstrated that the mutations either produced specific disruptions in the biosynthesis of type I procollagen or caused synthesis of a type I procollagen that formed abnormal collagen fibrils (Fig. 351-1). (4) The mutations in probands with OI were not found in normal alleles for the genes. (5) Expression of several of the mutated genes for type I procollagen in transgenic mice generated disease phenotypes similar to those seen in patients who inherited the mutated genes (Fig. 351-3).

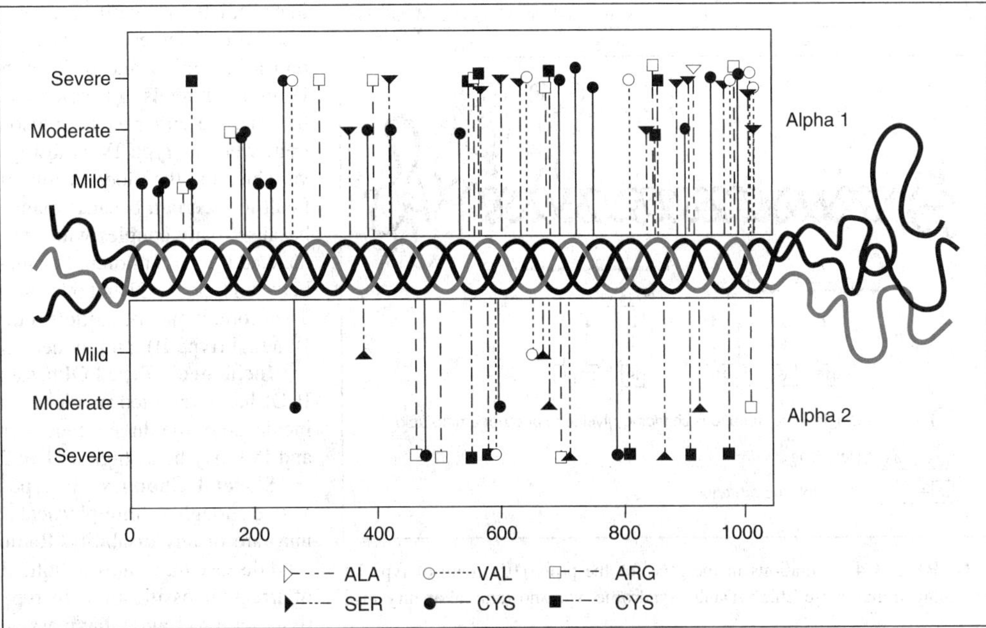

FIGURE 351-2 Examples of single-base mutations found in type I procollagen in patients with osteogenesis imperfecta (OI) and osteoporosis. Mild refers to type I OI, severe to type II OI, and moderate to type III or type IV OI.

The data on mutations in type I procollagen that cause OI have been used as a paradigm for defining other mutations in other collagen and procollagen genes that cause other disorders of connective tissue. For example, similar mutations in the gene for type III procollagen occur in patients with the type IV variant of EDS, which causes early death because of rupture of the aorta or other hollow organs (Fig. 351-4). Also, similar mutations in the gene for type II procollagen (COL2A1) are found in a number of patients with CDs (Fig. 351-5). In addition, transgenic mice expressing mutated genes for type II procollagen develop phenotypes resembling the CDs. Similar mutations in the gene for type VII collagen (COL7A1) are found in patients with the dystrophic form of EB, and mutations in the genes for type IV collagen are found in many patients with AS. As discussed below, the paradigm for defining the consequences of mutations in procollagen genes also helps explain findings on mutations in a fibrillin gene that cause MFS and mutations in keratin genes that cause the simplex variant of EB.

Several generalizations can be made about mutations in collagen genes. One is that unrelated patients rarely have the same mutation in the same gene. Another is that mutations that cause the most severe disease are usually new mutations in one allele that occur either during the generation of the germline in one of the parents or during meiosis in the fertilized egg (Chap. 65). Still another generalization is that most mild variants are caused by mutations that are specific or "private" to a given family. Indeed, the number of recurrent mutations in structural genes are so infrequent that there are, in effect, no common mutations responsible for the disorders in unrelated patients and no "hot spots" that contain most of the mutations.

Another general trend is that similar mutations in the same gene can produce different disease syndromes in terms of both severity and the major tissues involved. One reason for heterogeneity in pathologic manifestations is that different regions of a large molecule may be more important for its function in some connective tissues than in others. For example, some regions of the type I collagen molecule may be essential for the binding of mineralizing proteins in bone so that mutations in these regions cause fragile bones but do not impair function in skin and other nonmineralizing tissues. It is more difficult, however, to explain how the same mutation can produce a severe phenotype in some and a mild phenotype in other members of the same family. Such phenotypic variation appears to be characteristic of OI, where some subjects are short and have multiple fractures from minor trauma, whereas others in the same family can be of normal stature and free of fractures. In the past, such phenotypic variation was explained by undefined variations in the genetic background of different family members. Studies in transgenic mice, however, demonstrated similar phenotypic variation with expression of a mutated collagen gene in an inbred strain of mice in whom the genetic background is uniform. Therefore, the phenotypic variation is probably caused by undefined stochastic or chance events during embryonic and fetal development. Although dramatic phenotypic variations are relatively rare in OI and related disorders, it is important to consider in counseling families about the consequences of inherited mutations.

OSTEOGENESIS IMPERFECTA OI is an inherited disorder that causes a generalized decrease in bone mass (osteopenia) and makes the bones brittle. The disorder is frequently associated with blue sclerae, dental abnormalities (dentinogenesis imperfecta), progressive hearing loss, and a positive family history. The most severe forms cause death in utero, at birth, or shortly thereafter. The course of mild and moderate forms is more variable. Some patients appear normal at

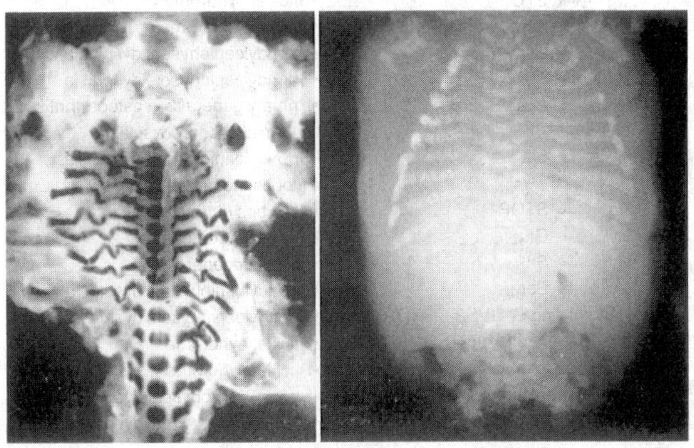

FIGURE 351-3 Similarities of the phenotypes in transgenic mice with mutated type I procollagen and in a child with osteogenesis imperfecta. Note in both pictures the waviness of the ribs due to fractures in utero.

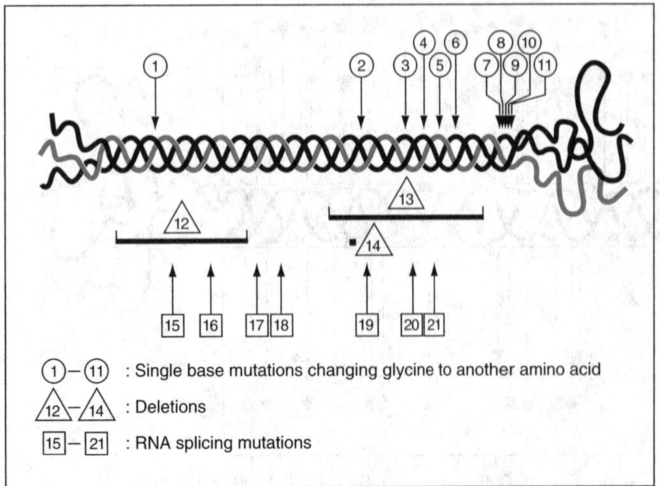

FIGURE 351-4 Mutations in the gene for the proα1(III) chain of type III procollagen that cause Ehlers-Danlos syndrome type and familial aneurysms.

birth and become progressively worse. Some have multiple fractures in infancy and childhood, improve after puberty, and fracture more frequently later in life. Women are particularly prone to fracture during pregnancy and after menopause. A few women from families with mild variants of OI do not develop fractures until after menopause, and their disease may be difficult to distinguish from postmenopausal osteoporosis.

Classification The most common classification for OI was developed by Sillence (Table 351-2). Type I, the mildest form, is inherited as an autosomal dominant trait. Most patients have distinctly blue sclerae. Type I is subdivided into types IA and IB depending on whether or not dentinogenesis imperfecta is present. Type II is lethal in utero or shortly after birth. Radiographic criteria can be used to subdivide type II into five groups, with subgroup 1 showing the most severe changes and subgroup 5 the least. Types III and IV OI are intermediate in severity between types I and II. They differ from type I because of lesser severity and because the sclerae are only slightly bluish in infancy and white in adulthood. Type III differs from type IV in that it tends to become more severe with age. Also, type III can be inherited either as an autosomal recessive or autosomal dominant trait, whereas type IV is always dominant. The clinical courses are variable, and the mode of inheritance in types III and IV may be difficult to ascertain because many patients have sporadic mutations and because many couples with one child severely affected by OI do not have additional children. For these and related reasons, the distinction between type IV OI and other severe variants of OI may not be helpful. Therefore, it may be sufficient to classify patients simply as mild (type I), lethal (type II), and moderately severe (type III).

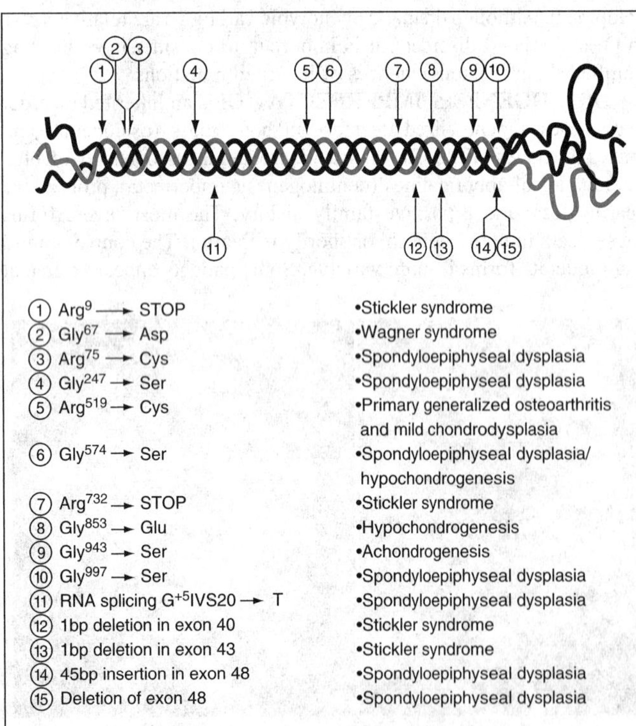

FIGURE 351-5 Mutations in the gene for the proα1(II) chain of type II procollagen that cause chondrodysplasia and related disorders.

Incidence Type I OI has a frequency of about 1 in 30,000. Type II OI has a reported incidence at birth of about 1 in 60,000, but the incidence of the three severe forms recognizable at birth (types II, III, and IV) may be as high as 1 in 20,000.

Skeletal Changes In type I OI, the fragility of bones may be severe enough to limit physical activity or so mild that individuals are unaware of any disability. Radiographs of the skull of patients with mild disease may show a mottled appearance because of small islands of irregular ossification. In type II OI, bones and other connective tissues are so fragile that massive injuries can occur in utero or during delivery (Fig. 351-3). Ossification of many bones is frequently incomplete. Continuously beaded or broken ribs and crumpled long bones (accordina femora) may be present. For unclear reasons, the long bones may be either thick or thin. In types III and IV, multiple fractures from minor physical stress can produce severe deformities. Kyphoscoliosis can impair respiration, cause cor pulmonale, and predispose to pulmonary infections. The appearance on radiographs of "popcorn-like" deposits of mineral on the ends of long bones is an ominous sign. Progressive neurologic symptoms may result from basilar compression and communicating hydrocephalus.

In all forms of OI, bone mineral density in unfractured bone is decreased. However, the degree of osteopenia may be difficult to evaluate because recurrent fractures limit exercise and thereby worsen the decrease in bone mass. Surprisingly, fractures appear to heal normally.

Ocular Changes The sclerae can be normal, slightly bluish, or bright blue. The color is probably caused by a thinness of the collagen layers of the sclerae that allows the choroid layers to be seen. Blue sclerae, however, are an inherited trait in some families who do not have increased bone fragility.

Dentinogenesis Imperfecta The teeth may be normal, moderately discolored, or grossly abnormal. The enamel generally appears normal, but the teeth may have a characteristic amber, yellowish brown, or translucent bluish gray color because of improper deposition or deficiency of dentin. The deciduous teeth are usually smaller than normal, whereas permanent teeth are frequently bell-shaped and restricted at the base. In some patients, the teeth readily fracture and need to be extracted. The defect in dentin is directly attributable to the fact that normal dentin is rich in type I collagen. Similar tooth defects, however, can be inherited without any evidence of OI.

Hearing Loss Hearing loss usually begins during the second decade of life and occurs in over 50% of subjects over age 30. The loss can be conductive, sensorineural, or mixed and varies in severity. The middle ear usually exhibits maldevelopment, deficient ossification, persistence of cartilage in areas that are normally ossified, and abnormal calcium deposits.

Associated Features Other connective tissue involvement can include thin skin that scars extensively, joint laxity with permanent dislocations indistinguishable from those of EDS, and, occasionally, cardiovascular manifestations such as aortic regurgitation, floppy mitral valves, mitral incompetence, and fragility of large blood vessels. For unknown reasons, some patients develop a hypermetabolic state with elevated serum thyroxine levels, hyperthermia, and excessive sweating.

Molecular Defects Most patients with OI have mutations in one of the two genes that encode type I procollagen. Over 90% of patients with type I OI and blue sclerae have mutations in the proα1(I) gene that decrease the steady-state levels of the mRNA for proα1(I) chains and decrease the rates of synthesis of proα1(I) chains relative to those for proα2(I) chains. In more severe forms (types II, III, and IV), the effects of mutations that cause synthesis of abnormal proα chains are amplified by the three mechanisms discussed above (Fig. 351-1). Mutations that change the structure of the protein near the N-proteinase cleavage site cause accumulation of a partially processed procollagen and produce lax joints similar to those in type VII EDS that is caused by mutations in the gene for the N-proteinase. Mutations that change the structure in the middle or near the C terminus of the molecule tend to cause severe or lethal variants of OI. It is difficult, however, to correlate the site or nature of the mutation and the clinical phenotype (Fig. 351-2). Most patients are heterozygotes with mutations in a single allele, but rare patients are homozygotes with two mutated alleles for proα1(I) or proα2(I) chains.

Table 351-2 Classification of Osteogenesis Imperfecta (OI)

Type	Bone Fragility	Blue Sclerae	Abnormal Dentition	Hearing Loss	Inheritance[a]
I	Mild	Present	Absent in IA, present in IB	Present in most	AD
II	Extreme	Present	Present in some	Unknown	S, rarely AR
III	Severe	Bluish at birth	Present in some	High incidence	AR or AD
IV	Variable	Absent	Absent in IVA, present in IVB	High incidence	AD

[a] AD, autosomal dominant; AR, autosomal recessive; S, sporadic.

Mosaicism in Germ-Line Cells and in Somatic Cells Most lethal OI is the result of new autosomal dominant mutations. The frequency of a second child with lethal OI in the same family, however, is about 7% because of germ-line mosaicism in one of the parents. The presence of germ-line mosaicism has been demonstrated in several fathers of patients with type II OI by demonstrating the mutated gene in a fraction of their sperm. Apparently normal parents of children with severe OI may also have somatic cell mosaicism in which the mutated allele is present in a fraction of somatic cells such as fibroblasts, leukocytes, and hair root cells. Because of the possibility of germ-line mosaicism, asymptomatic parents of a child with severe OI should be counseled that recurrence can occur.

Diagnosis The diagnosis is usually made on the basis of clinical criteria. The presence of fractures together with blue sclerae, dentinogenesis imperfecta, or family history of the disease is usually sufficient to make the diagnosis. Other causes of pathologic fractures must be excluded, including the battered child syndrome, nutritional deficiencies, malignancies, and other inherited disorders such as CDs and hypophosphatasia (Table 351-3). X-rays usually reveal a decrease in bone density that can be verified by photon or x-ray absorptiometry. There is no consensus, however, as to whether the diagnosis can be made by microscopy of bone. A molecular defect in type I procollagen can be demonstrated in half or more of patients by incubating skin fibroblasts with radioactive amino acids and then analyzing the proα chains by polyacrylamide gel electrophoresis. The analysis detects decreases in the rate of synthesis of proα1(I) chains relative to proα2(I) chains, abnormally long proα chains, abnormally short proα chains, and proα chains with abnormal posttranslational modification because of an amino acid substitution that impairs folding of the triple helix. The mutations themselves can be defined in most patients by sequencing of genomic DNA. Because each proband and family usually has a "private" mutation, extensive analysis of about 10,000 bases in each of the two genes is required to identify the exact mutation. After a mutation in a type I procollagen gene is identified, a test based on the polymerase chain reaction can be used to screen family members at risk and for prenatal diagnosis.

℞ **TREATMENT** Many patients with OI have successful careers despite severe deformities. Those with mild disorder may need little treatment when fractures decrease after puberty, but women require special attention during pregnancy and after menopause, when fractures again increase. More severely affected children require a comprehensive program of physical therapy, surgical management of fractures and skeletal deformities, and vocational education.

Many of the fractures are only slightly displaced and have little soft tissue swelling. Therefore, they can be treated with minimal support or traction for a week or two followed by a light cast. If fractures are relatively painless, physical therapy can be initiated early. A judicious amount of exercise prevents loss of bone mass secondary to physical inactivity. Some physicians advocate insertion of steel rods into long bones to correct limb deformities; the risk/benefits and cost/benefits of such procedures are difficult to evaluate. Aggressive conventional intervention is usually warranted for pneumonia and cor pulmonale. For severe hearing loss, stapedectomy or replacement of the stapes with a prosthesis may be successful. Moderately to severely affected patients should be evaluated periodically to anticipate possible neurologic problems. About half of children have a substantial increase in growth when given growth hormone. Treatment with bisphosphonates to decrease bone loss has been introduced on an experimental basis. Initial results are promising, but the long-term effects of decreasing bone resorption are unknown. Also, a clinical trial has been initiated to use stromal cells from bone marrow that can differentiate into osteoblasts after systemic infusion. In the first phase of the trial, three children with severe OI (type III) showed clinical improvement after marrow ablation and transplantation of whole bone marrow from an HLA-compatible sibling.

A program for careful orthotic management developed by Bleck and a program for compressive management developed by Marini are useful. Counseling and emotional support are important for patients and parents, and lay organizations in some countries provide help in these areas. Prenatal ultrasonography will detect severely affected fetuses at about 16 weeks of pregnancy. Diagnosis by demonstrating synthesis of abnormal proα chains or by DNA sequencing can be carried out in chorionic villa biopsies at 8 to 12 weeks of pregnancy.

EHLERS-DANLOS SYNDROME EDS is characterized by hyperelasticity of the skin and hypermobile joints.

Classification Five types of EDS were initially defined based primarily on the extent to which the skin, joints, and other tissues are

Table 351-3 Differential Diagnosis of Osteogenesis Imperfecta

Age	Diagnosis	Distinguishing Features
At birth	Hypophosphatasia	Unmineralized skull
	Achondrogenesis	Unmineralized vertebrae
	Thanatophoric dwarfism	H-shaped vertebrae
	Asphyxiating thoracic dystrophy	Cylindrical thorax
	Achondroplasia	Large head, short, tubular bones
Infancy	Battered child syndrome	Skull and rib fractures more common; soft tissue bruises
	Immobilization osteogenesis	
	Scurvy	
	Congenital syphilis	
	Infantile cortical hyperostosis (Coffey's disease)	
	Pyknodystosis	
	Osteopetrosis	
Childhood	Homocystinuria	Marfanoid appearance and mental deficiency
	Celiac disease	Steatorrhea, anemia
	Adrenal cortical tumor	
	Glucocorticoid therapy	
	Juvenile osteoporosis	
	Fibrous dysplasia	
	Sarcoma	

SOURCE: After R Smith et al: *The Brittle Bone Syndrome: Osteogenesis Imperfecta*. London, Butterworth, 1983.

Table 351-4 Clinical Features, Mode of Inheritance, and Biochemical Defects in Ehlers-Danlos Syndrome

Type	Clinical Features	Inheritance[a]	Biochemical Defects
I, gravis	Soft, velvety, hyperextensible skin; easy bruising; "cigarette paper" scars; hypermobile joints; varicose veins; prematurity	AD	Some in $\alpha 1(V)$ and $\alpha 2(V)$ chains of type V collagen
II, mitis	Similar to type I but less severe	AD	Some in $\alpha 1(V)$ chain of type V collagen
III, familial hypermobility	Soft skin, no scarring, marked hypermobility	AD	Not known
IV, acrogeric, ecchymotic, vascular	Thin, translucent skin with visible veins; increased bruisability, skin and joints have normal extensibility; arterial, bowel, and uterine rupture	AD	Mutations in type III procollagen (see Fig. 351-4)
V, X-linked	Similar to type II	XLR	Not known
VI, ocular-scoliotic	Soft, velvety, hyperextensible skin; hypermobile joints; scoliosis; ocular fragility and keratoconus	AR	Lysyl hydroxylase deficiency
VII, arthrochalasis multiplex congenita	Marked joint hypermobility, soft skin with normal scarring	AD	A. Structural defect in the pro$\alpha 1$(I) chain
		AD	B. Structural defect in the pro$\alpha 2$(I) chain
		AR	C. Procollagen N-proteinase deficiency
VIII, periodontal	Generalized periodontitis, skin similar to type II but fragile and scars	AD	Not known
IX, cutis laxa occipital horn syndrome	Vacant, now recategorized as a disorder of copper transport		
X	Similar to type II	AR	Possible defect in fibronectin
XI, familial joint instability	Vacant, now recategorized with familial articular hypermobility syndromes		Not known

[a] AD, autosomal dominant; AR, autosomal recessive; XLR, X-linked recessive.

SOURCE: Adapted from Steinmann et al; A De Paepe et al: Am J Hum Genet 60, 547, 1997; and K. Michalickova et al: Hum Mol Genet 7:249, 1998.

involved, but the classification has now been extended (Table 351-4). Type I is the classic, severe form of the disease, with both severe joint hypermobility and skin that is velvety in texture, hyperextensible, and easily scarred. Type II is similar to type I but milder. In type III joint hypermobility is more prominent than skin changes. In type IV the skin changes are more prominent than joint changes. However, type IV patients are predisposed to sudden death from rupture of large blood vessels or other hollow organs. Type V is similar to type II but is inherited as an X-linked trait. Type VI is characterized by scoliosis, ocular fragility, and a cone-shaped deformity of the cornea (keratoconus). Type VII is characterized by marked joint hypermobility that is difficult to distinguish from type III except by the specific molecular defects in the processing of type I procollagen to collagen. Type VIII is distinguished by periodontal changes. Types IX, X, and XI were defined on the basis of preliminary biochemical and clinical data, but these classifications have not proven useful. Because of overlapping signs and symptoms, many patients and families with some of the features of EDS cannot be assigned to any of the defined types.

Incidence The incidence of EDS is difficult to establish, largely because patients with mild skin or joint symptoms rarely seek medical attention. It is also difficult to define the normal range of variation for joint mobility or skin elasticity. The incidence may be about 1 in 5000 births, although a higher value has been reported for blacks. Types I, II, and III account for most diagnoses.

Skin The changes vary from thin and velvety skin to skin that is either dramatically hyperextensible ("rubber man" syndrome) or easily torn or scarred. Type I patients develop characteristic "cigarette-paper" scars. In type IV extensive scars and hyperpigmentation develop over bony prominences, and the skin may be so thin that subcutaneous blood vessels are visible. In type VIII the skin is more fragile than hyperextensible, and it heals with atrophic, pigmented scars. Easy bruisability occurs in several types of EDS.

Ligament and Joint Changes Laxity and hypermobility of joints vary from mild to unreducible dislocations of hips and other large joints. In mild forms patients learn to reduce dislocations themselves and to avoid them by limiting physical activity. In more severe forms, surgical repair may be required. Some patients have progressive difficulty with age, but severe joint laxity is compatible with a normal life span.

Associated Changes Mitral valve prolapse and hernias occur, particularly in type I. Pes planus and mild to moderate scoliosis are common. Extreme joint laxity and repeated dislocations may lead to degenerative arthritis. In type VI the eye may rupture with minimal trauma, and kyphoscoliosis can cause respiratory impairment. Sclerae may be blue in type VI.

Molecular Defects Mutations in two of the three genes for type V collagen have been found in patients with types I and II EDS. The mutations include glycine substitutions in the triple-helical domain, RNA splicing mutations, exon skipping mutations, a small deletion of 7 bp, and a substitution of serine for cysteine in the C-propeptide. Mutations in both the $\alpha 1(V)$ and $\alpha 2(V)$ chain are found in patients with type I EDS, but to date only mutations in the $\alpha 1(V)$ chain have been found in patients with type II EDS. Electron microscopy of skin from some patients with types I, II, or III EDS are consistent with mutations in a low-abundance collagen such as types III or V that either copolymerize with or bind to the surface of type I fibrils. However, irregular fibrils are not seen in all patients, and similar irregular fibrils can be seen in normal skin.

Most patients with type IV EDS have a defect either in the synthesis or structure of type III procollagen, a finding consistent with the fact that these patients are prone to spontaneous rupture of the aorta and intestines, tissues rich in type III collagen. The thinness and scarring of skin are more difficult to explain, since type III constitutes a small fraction of the collagen in skin (Table 351-1). The >50 mutations identified in the type III procollagen gene include partial gene deletions, RNA splicing mutations, and single-base mutations that cause substitution of glycine by amino acids with bulkier side chains (Fig. 351-4). In effect, most of the mutations lead to synthesis of abnormal but partially functional pro$\alpha 1$(III) chains that produce procollagen suicide or alter fibril formation by the same mechanisms that amplify the effects of mutations in the genes for type I procollagen. Similar mutations in type III procollagen can cause aortic aneurysms in some individuals without other evidence of EDS type IV, MFS, or other inherited disorders of connective tissue.

Type VI EDS is caused by mutations in the gene that encodes lysyl hydrolase. In one series, all the patients were homozygous or compound heterozygotes for the mutated genes, and all the mutations caused profound deficiency of lysyl hydroxylase, a decrease in the hydroxylysine content of collagen, and a decrease in the cross-links in collagen fibers. The decrease in cross-links is explained by the observation that some cross-links are less stable if formed from lysine instead of hydroxylysine.

Type VII EDS is due to a defect in the conversion of procollagen to collagen caused either by mutations that make type I procollagen resistant to cleavage by procollagen N-proteinase or by mutations that decrease the activity of the enzyme. The type VIIA mutations alter the cleavage site in the proα1(I) chain, and the type VIIB mutations alter the cleavage site in the proα2(I) chain. Both types are dominantly inherited. Type VIIC is caused by mutations that decrease the activity of procollagen N-proteinase and is inherited as an autosomal recessive trait. In all three forms of type VII EDS, the persistence of the N-propeptide causes the formation of collagen fibrils that are thin and irregular. Since most patients do not have clinical osteopenia, the thin and irregular fibrils apparently suffice for the mineralization of bone but do not provide the necessary tensile strength for ligaments and joint capsules. However, some patients fracture easily and are difficult to distinguish from variants of OI.

The cause of type VIII EDS is unknown. Type IX is a disorder of copper transport. The syndrome, also referred to as *Menkes' syndrome*, is due to an X-linked defect and is associated with cutis laxa, hypopigmentation, unusual hair ("kinky"), vascular aneurysms, neurologic degeneration, and mental retardation. Mutations in a gene coding for a copper-transporting ATPase cause the disease (Chaps. 348 and 353). Type X EDS may be caused by defects in fibronectin, but no specific mutations have been defined.

Diagnosis The diagnosis is based on clinical criteria. Biochemical assays and gene analyses for known molecular defects in EDS are difficult and time-consuming, but specific diagnostic tests should be available in the future for families in which the genes at fault have been defined.

℞ **TREATMENT** There is no specific therapy. Surgical repair and tightening of joint ligaments require careful evaluation of individual patients, as the ligaments frequently do not hold sutures. Patients with easy bruisability should be evaluated for other bleeding disorders. Patients with type IV EDS and members of their families should probably be evaluated at regular intervals by sonography and related techniques for early detection of aneurysms. Surgical repair of aneurysms may be difficult because of increased friability of tissues, and there is limited experience with elective surgery in such patients. Also, women with type IV EDS should be counseled about the increased risk of uterine rupture, bleeding, and other complications of pregnancy.

Table 351-5 Some Gene Mutations in Chondrodysplasias (CD)

Disease	Major Findings	Gene	Protein
SED congenita	Short-trunk dwarfism, hearing loss, cleft palate	COL2A1	Type II collagen
Achondrogenesis II/hypochondrogenesis	Short-limb dwarfism, large head, lethal	COL2A1	Type II collagen
Stickler syndrome			
Classic	Myopia, vitreoretinal degeneration, hearing loss, cleft palate, arthropathy	COL2A1/COL11A1	Type II or type XI collagen
Nonocular	Same as above, but no eye findings	COL11A2	Type XI collagen
Marshall syndrome	Similar to classic Stickler but less severe eye changes and more severe hearing loss	COL11A1	Type XI collagen
Kniest dysplasia	Short limbs and trunks, enlarged joints, myopia, hearing loss, cleft palate	COL2A1	Type II collagen
Metaphyseal CD, Schmidt type	Short limb dwarfism, flaring of metaphyses	COL10A1	Type X collagen
Pseudochondrodysplasia	Short stature, early OA	COMP	Cartilage oligomeric matrix protein
Multiple epiphyseal dysplasia	Short stature (variable), early OA	COMP COL9A2 COL9A3	Cartilage oligomeric matrix protein/type IX collagen
OA with mild CD	Early onset OA with mild epiphyseal changes	COL2A1	Type II collagen

NOTE: OA, osteoarthritis; SED, spondyloepiphyseal dysplasia: spondylo-, spinal changes including irregular endplates, flattened or wedge-shaped vertebrae; -epiphyseal, widening or irregularities of epiphyses; -metaphyseal, flared, cupped, irregularly mineralized or fragmented metaphyses.

CHONDRODYSPLASIAS (See also Chap. 343) The CDs are inherited skeletal disorders that cause dwarfism and abnormal body proportions. The category also includes some individuals with normal stature and body proportions who have features such as ocular changes or cleft palate that are common in more severe CDs. Many patients develop degenerative joint changes, and mild CD in adults may be difficult to differentiate from primary generalized osteoarthritis. Some authors refer to the disorders as "skeletal dysplasias," but CD is a more widely used term.

Classification Over 150 distinct types and subtypes have been defined (Table 351-5) based on criteria such as "bringing death" (thanatophoric), causing "twisted" bones (diastrophic), affecting metaphyses (metaphyseal), affecting epiphyses (epiphyseal), and producing histologic changes such as an apparent increase in the fibrous material in the epiphyses (fibrochondrogenesis). Also, a number of eponyms are based on the first or most comprehensive case reports. Severe forms of the diseases produce gross distortions of most cartilaginous structures and of the eye. Mild forms are more difficult to classify. Among the features are cataracts, degeneration of the vitreous and retinal detachment, high forehead, hypoplastic facies, cleft palate, short extremities, and gross distortions of the epiphyses, metaphyses, and joint surfaces.

Incidence Data on the frequency of most CDs are not available, but the incidence of the Stickler syndrome may be as high as 1 in 10,000. Therefore, the diseases are probably among the more common heritable disorders of connective tissue.

Molecular Defects The first mutations shown to cause CDs were in the COL2A1 gene for type II collagen, the most abundant protein in cartilage. A number of mutations in this gene have now been reported in variants of CD ranging from mild to lethal (Fig. 351-5). A large fraction of patients with lethal CDs, a smaller number of patients with moderately severe CDs, and about 2% of families with early-onset generalized osteoarthritis have mutations in the same gene. However, similar phenotypes can also be caused by mutations in other genes, including genes for three other collagens, additional components of the cartilage matrix, growth factors, growth factor receptors, and transcription factors (see Table 351-6 for selected examples). The number of mutated genes reported does not necessarily reflect the incidence of such mutations in the diseases themselves but rather the complexity of the genes and the technical difficulties in searching the complete gene for mutations. Also, it reflects the availability of large families for DNA linkage analysis and the vigor with which investigators have pursued their interest in a given gene. It is likely that mutations in additional genes will be found.

Mutations in the COL2A1 gene were first found in patients with severe CDs characterized by gross deformities of bones and cartilage such as spondyloepiphyseal dysplasia congenita, hypochondrogenesis/achondrogenesis II, and the Kniest syndrome. However, mutations in the COL2A1 gene have been found in a few families in which few if any symptoms are present in childhood but in which joint stiffness, joint pain, and degenerative changes of osteoarthritis develop in midlife. The mutations in the COL2A1 gene are similar to the mutations in the genes for types I and III procollagens (Fig. 351-5), and the

Table 351-6 Examples of Genetic Mutations in Signaling Pathways and Developmental Genes

Category	Mutated Gene	Consequences	Clinical Phenotype
Transcription factor/extracellular signaling	Deficiency of GLI-3 transcription factor	Upregulation of sonic hedgehog pathway	Polysyndactyly and bifid phalanges with craniofacial defects (Greig syndrome)
	Truncation of GLI-3 transcription factor	Downregulation of sonic hedgehog pathway	Polydactyly, short limbs, imperforate anus, laryngeal cleft, and hypothalamic hamartoblastoma (Pallister-Hall syndrome)
Receptors	Missense in FGF-3 receptor	Increased FGF signaling	Short-trunk dwarfism (achondrodysplasia; hypochondrodysplasia; thanatrophoric dysplasia)
Developmental genes	HOXD-13	Inactivation of homeobox gene	Polysyndactyly
	PAX-3	Inactivation of paired-box gene	Hearing loss, abnormal pigmentation, craniofacial changes (Waardenburg syndrome)
Transcription factor	SOX-9	Slowed chondrocyte differentiation, decreased expression of type II collagen	Sex reversal, abnormal skeletal development (campomelic dysplasia)

correlations between genotype and the severity of the phenotype are equally difficult. In addition, mutations that change a codon for a Y-position amino acid in the -Gly-X-Y- repeat sequence from an arginine to cystine were found in families with early-onset osteoarthritis and minimal evidence of CDs. Stickler syndrome and related syndromes are caused by mutations in three different genes: the COL2AI gene for type II collagen and the COL11A1 and COL11A2 genes for type XI collagen. A series of mutations that introduce premature terminal signals in the COL2A1 gene lead to classic Stickler syndrome. However, some patients with classic Stickler syndrome have glycine substitutions in COL11A1. RNA splicing mutations in the COL11A1 gene are found in patients with the Marshall syndrome, which is similar to classic Stickler syndrome but with milder eye changes and more severe hearing loss. Patients classified as having nonocular Stickler syndrome have RNA splicing mutations in the COL11A2 gene.

Many individuals with the Schmid metaphyseal CD, characterized by short stature, *coxa vara*, flaring metaphyses, and waddling gait, have mutations in the gene for the type X collagen, a short, network-forming collagen found primarily in the hypertrophic zone of endochondral cartilage.

Mutations in the receptor for fibroblast growth factor 3 (FGFR-3) are present in most patients with achondroplasia, the most common cause of short-limbed dwarfism accompanied by macrocephaly and dysplasias of the metaphyses of long bones (Table 351-6). The same single-base mutation in the gene that converts glycine to arginine at position 380 is present in >90% of patients. Most patients represent sporadic new mutations, and this nucleotide change must be one of the most common recurring mutations in the human genome. The mutation causes unregulated signal transduction through the receptor and inappropriate development of cartilage. Mutations that alter other domains of FGFR-3 have been found in patients with the more severe disorders hypochondroplasia and thanatophoric dysplasia and in a few families with a variant of craniosynostosis. However, most patients with craniosynostosis appear to have mutations in the related gene FGFR-2 gene.

Mutations in the gene for the cartilage oligomeric matrix protein (COMP) have been found in patients with multiple epiphyseal dysplasia or pseudoachondroplasia, and in related syndromes characterized by short limbs and degenerative arthritis. However, some families with multiple epiphyseal dysplasia had a mutation in the gene for the $\alpha2$(IX) or $\alpha3$(IX) chain of type IX collagen (COL9A2 and COL9A3). All the known mutations in these two type IX collagen genes in patients with multiple epiphyseal dysplasia cause splicing out of the codons of exon 3. A mutation in the COL9A2 gene was also found in patients with the common condition of sciatica and herniations of vertebral discs. About 4% of Finnish probands with the phenotype had a single base substitution that converted a codon for glutamate to tryptophan in the $\alpha2$(IX) chain of type IX collagen.

Diagnosis The diagnosis of severe forms of CD is made on the basis of the physical appearance, x-ray findings, histologic changes, and clinical course (Table 351-5).

℞ **TREATMENT** No definitive therapy is available. Symptomatic treatment is directed to secondary features such as degenerative arthritis. Many patients require joint replacement surgery and corrective surgery for cleft palate. The eyes should be monitored carefully for the development of cataracts and for the need for laser therapy to prevent retinal detachment. Patients should probably be advised to avoid obesity and contact sports. Counseling for the psychological problems of short stature is critical, and support groups have formed in many countries. Ultrasonography is sometimes successful for prenatal diagnosis but less frequently than with OI. Specific DNA tests are available for the CDs caused by mutations in the genes for types II, X, and XI collagens.

MARFAN SYNDROME Severe MFS is characterized by a triad of features: (1) long, thin extremities frequently associated with other skeletal changes, such as loose joints and arachnodactyly; (2) reduced vision as the result of dislocations of the lenses (ectopia lentis); and (3) aortic aneurysms that typically begin at the base of the aorta.

Classification The clinical diagnosis is frequently problematic because some affected members of families with MFS present with only one or two features of the typical clinical trial. Also, many patients present with one or two of the features of MFS without a family history, apparently because they represent sporadic mutations. Therefore, it is frequently difficult to determine on the basis of clinical data alone whether a patient with ectopia lentis or the characteristic body habitus of MFS is at risk for developing a life-threatening aortic aneurysm. The new DNA diagnostic tests for mutations in the fibrillin-1 and fibrillin-2 genes can probably resolve most, but not all, of these problems. Most patients who are prone to develop an aortic aneurysm as a component of MFS can be identified by detection of mutations in the fibrillin-1 gene. Some of these patients develop aortic aneurysms because of a mutation in the fibrillin-1 gene without the skeletal or ocular changes characteristic of MFS. Patients with the rarer form of MFS that is characterized by contractural arachnodactyly instead of loose joints can usually be identified by detection of a mutation in the fibrillin-2 gene that is similar in structure to the gene for fibrillin-1. Preliminary data suggest that patients with mutations in the fibrillin-2 gene are not prone to develop aneurysms. However, affected members of some rare families with a mutation in the fibrillin-1 gene also do not develop aortic aneurysms, even though they may show the skeletal or ocular changes. Therefore, the DNA tests are most helpful if: (1) a mutation is detected in either of the two genes, and (2) informative data are available on the clinical symptoms that the same mutation produces in the patient's family or in other families with similar clinical features.

Incidence and Inheritance MFS has an incidence of about 1 in 10,000 in most racial and ethnic groups. The disorder is inherited as an autosomal dominant trait; at least one-fourth of patients do not have an affected parent, and their cases are probably due to new mutations.

Skeletal Changes Patients are usually tall compared with other members of the same family and have long limbs. The ratio of the upper segment (top of the head to top of the pubic ramus) to the lower segment (top of the pubic ramus to the floor) is usually 2 SDs below mean for age, race, and sex. The fingers and hands are long and slender and have a spider-like appearance (arachnodactyly). Many patients have severe chest deformities, including depression (pectus excavatum), protrusion (pectus carinatum), or asymmetry. Scoliosis is frequent and usually accompanied by kyphosis. High-arched palate and high pedal arches or pes planus are common. A few patients have severe joint hypermobility similar to EDS.

Cardiovascular Changes Cardiovascular abnormalities are the major source of morbidity and mortality (Chap. 247). Mitral valve prolapse develops early in life and in about one-quarter progresses to mitral valve regurgitation of increasing severity because of redundancy of the leaflets, stretching of the chordae tendineae, and dilatation of the valvulae annulus. Dilatation of the root of the aorta and the sinuses of Valsalva are characteristic and ominous features of the disease that can develop at any age and in rare instances may be detected by echocardiography in utero. The rate of dilatation is unpredictable, but it can lead to aortic regurgitation, dissection of the aorta, and rupture. Dilatation is probably accelerated by physical and emotional stress, as well as by pregnancy.

Ocular Changes Dislocations of the lens may be readily apparent, but diagnosis usually requires pupillary dilatation and slit-lamp examination. The displacement is usually not progressive but may contribute to the formation of cataracts. The ocular globe is frequently elongated, most patients are myopic, and some develop retinal detachment. A few patients have lattice degeneration and retinal tears; most have adequate vision.

Associated Changes Striae may occur over the shoulders and buttocks. Otherwise the skin is normal. A number of patients develop spontaneous pneumothorax. Inguinal and incisional hernias are common. Marked dilatation of the dural sac is seen frequently in computed tomography scans, but the condition is usually asymptomatic. Patients are typically thin with little subcutaneous fat, but adults may develop centripetal obesity.

Molecular Defects Most patients with the classic features of MFS are heterozygotes for mutations in a gene on chromosome 15 that encodes fibrillin-1, a glycoprotein of 350 kDa that is a major component of elastin-associated microfibrils. These microfibrils are abundant in large blood vessels and the suspensory ligaments of the lens. Mutations in the fibrillin-1 gene include missense, nonsense, in-frame deletions, and RNA splicing mutations. Many of the mutations are single amino acid substitutions in the epidemal growth factor-like domains of the molecule that may be involved with calcium binding. Mutations in the fibrillin-2 gene that cause the MFS variant characterized by contractures appear to follow a similar pattern. As with most genetic diseases, the nature and location of mutations in the genes are only an approximate guide to the severity of the phenotype unless the same mutation has been seen in other members of the same family or in similar unrelated patients. However, there is a clustering of mutations in the middle portion of the molecule of fibrillin-1 encoded by exons 23 to 32 that causes the most severe phenotype, referred to as *neonatal lethal MFS*. The function of fibrillin has not been defined, but the data suggest that fibrillin self-assembles into a fibrillar structure and that the conformation and surface properties of the entire molecule are critical for normal assembly. Therefore, the functional consequences of mutations that change the amino acid sequence of fibrillin may be similar to the effects of mutations that change the conformation of a fibrillar collagen.

Diagnosis The diagnosis is easily established if the patient and other members of the family have dislocated lenses, aortic dilatation, and long and thin extremities together with kyphoscoliosis or other chest deformities. The diagnosis is frequently made if ectopia lentis and an aneurysm of the ascending aorta occur in the absence of a Marfan habitus or a positive family history. All patients in whom the diagnosis is suspected should have a slit-lamp examination and an echocardiogram. Also, homocystinuria (Table 351-3) should be ruled out by a negative cyanide-nitroprusside test for disulfides in the urine (Chap. 352). A few patients with types I, II, and III EDS have ectopia lentis but lack the Marfan habitus and instead have characteristic skin changes not present in MFS. Patients with familial aortic aneurysms tend to develop aneurysms at the base of the abdominal aorta. The location of the aneurysms, however, is somewhat variable, and the high incidence of aortic aneurysms in the general population (1 in 100) makes the differential diagnosis difficult unless other features of MFS are clearly present. A few families with familial aortic aneurysms have mutations in the gene for type III procollagen (Fig. 351-4).

℞ TREATMENT There is no established treatment, but several investigators have recommended use of propranolol or other β-adrenergic blocking agents to lower blood pressure and thereby delay or prevent aortic dilatation. Surgical replacement of the aorta, aortic valve, and mitral valve has been successful in some patients, and all patients should be followed carefully with echocardiography and other techniques for evaluation of cardiovascular changes (Chap. 247). Patients should probably be advised of the risks of severe physical and emotional stress and of pregnancy.

The scoliosis tends to be progressive and should be treated by mechanical bracing and physical therapy if >20° or by surgery if it progresses to >45°. Estrogen has been tried in girls with scoliosis, but the results are inconclusive. Dislocated lenses rarely require surgical removal, but patients should be followed closely for retinal detachment.

Diagnostic tests based on detection of fibrillin defects in cultured skin fibroblasts or DNA analysis of the gene are now available from several laboratories.

DISEASES RELATED TO ELASTIN As may be expected from the role of elastin in maintaining the elasticity of skin, mutations in the elastin gene cause *cutis laxa*, a rare and heterogeneous group of disorders characterized by skin that is both lax and inelastic. Three different frame-shift mutations were found in three unrelated families with dominant forms of the disease. Surprisingly, other mutations in the elastin gene produce phenotypes that primarily involve the aorta, whose elasticity also depends on the presence of elastin. A large deletion that includes the elastin gene and probably several adjacent genes causes the *Williams syndrome*, characterized by supravalvular aortic stenosis, growth retardation, characteristic facies, and an unusual mental phenotype of low intelligence quotient together with a high degree of sociability.

EPIDERMOLYSIS BULLOSA EB consists of a group of similar disorders in which the skin and related epithelial tissues break and blister as the result of minor trauma. As with most heritable disorders of connective tissues, the clinical manifestations range from lethal to mild.

Classification Four types of EB are defined on the basis of the level at which blistering occurs: EB simplex for blistering in the epidermis, EB hemidesmosomal for fissures between kerotinocytes and between kerotinocytes and the basal lamina, EB junctional for blistering in the dermal-epidermal junction, and EB dystrophica for blistering in the dermis (Table 351-7).

Incidence The incidence of EB in the United States is estimated to be 1 in 50,000.

Molecular Defects The molecular basis of several specific variants of EB has been defined. A series of patients with EB simplex were found to have mutations in either keratin 14 or keratin 5, two of the major keratins in basal epithelial cells. Patients with the related

Table 351-7 Clinical Variants of Epidermolysis-Bullosa (EB)

EB Variant	Level of Tissue Separation	Mutated Gene
Simplex	Intraepidermal	KRT5
		KRT14
Hemidesmosomal[a]	Basal keratinocyte/ lamina lucida interface	
GABEB		COL17A1
EB-PA		ITGA6
		ITGB4
EB-MD		PLEC1
Junctional	Lamina lucida	LAMA3
		LAMB3
		LAMC2
Dystrophic	Sub-lamina densa	COL7A1

[a] GABEB, generalized atrophic benign EB; EB-PA, EB with pyloric artresia; EB-MD, EB with late-onset muscular dystrophy.
SOURCE: Modified from Pulkkinen and Uitto.

syndrome, epidermolytic icthyosis, have mutations in keratin 1 and keratin 10. The new disease phenotype of hemidesmosomal EB has three clinical variants that are caused by mutations in one of four genes (Table 351-7): (1) A generalized atrophic and benign form of EB is caused by mutations in the COL17A1 gene for type XVII collagen; (2) a variant with EB associated with pyloric atresia and other intestinal abnormalities is caused by mutations in either the gene for the $\alpha 6$ integrin (ITG A6) or the gene for the $\beta 4$ integrin (ITG B4); and (3) another variant characterized by relatively mild blistering at birth but associated with late-onset muscular dystrophy is caused by mutations in the gene for plectin (PLEC-1). Junctional EB is caused by mutations in any one of three genes for laminin (LAMA-3, LAMB-3, LAMC-2). The most severe dystrophic form of EB is caused by mutations in the gene for type VII collagen (COL7A1).

Diagnosis The diagnosis is based on skin that readily breaks and forms blisters. EB simplex and EB hemidesmosomal are generally milder than EB junctional or EB dystrophica. EB dystrophica variants usually cause large and prominent scars. Precise classification within subtypes usually requires electron microscopy. The treatment is symptomatic.

ALPORT SYNDROME (See also Chap. 275) AS is an inherited disorder characterized by hematuria. Four forms of the disease are now recognized: (1) classic AS, which is inherited as an X-linked disorder with hematuria, sensorineural deafness, and conical deformation of the anterior surface of the lens (lenticonus); (2) a subtype of the X-linked form associated with diffuse leiomyomatosis; (3) an autosomal recessive form; and (4) an autosomal dominant form. The two autosomal forms can cause renal disease without deafness or lenticonus.

Incidence The incidence of AS is about 1 in 10,000 in the general population and as high as 1 in 5000 in some ethnic groups. About 80% of AS patients have the X-linked variant.

Molecular Defects Electron microscopy of kidneys from patients with classic AS demonstrates that the glomerular basement membrane is up to five times thicker than normal and that the lamina densa is distorted and split. The X-linked and autosomal recessive forms are caused primarily by mutations in genes for the $\alpha 3$(IV), $\alpha 4$(IV), $\alpha 5$(IV), or $\alpha 6$(IV) chains of type IV collagen, a major component of basement membranes. The type IV collagen in most membranes consists primarily of $\alpha 1$(IV) and $\alpha 2$(IV) chains folded into a large, rodlike molecule with globular ends and a long triple-helical domain that is interrupted by short sequences that do not form triple helices. The molecules self-assemble through both the globular ends and the long triple-helical domain to form a complex three-dimensional network. The four additional α chains of type IV collagen are minor components of basement membranes, similar in structure, and are probably incorporated into the same or similar molecules. The six genes for the proteins are arranged in tandem pairs on different chromosomes in a head-to-head orientation and with overlapping promoters, i.e., the $\alpha 1$(IV) and $\alpha 2$(IV) genes are head-to-head on chromosome 13q34, the $\alpha 3$(IV) and $\alpha 4$(IV) genes are on chromosome 2q35-37, and the $\alpha 5$(IV) and $\alpha 6$(IV) genes are on chromosome Xq22. An X-linked variant is caused by mutations in the COL4A5 gene, and the X-linked variant associated with leiomyomatosis is caused by deletions that involve both the COL4A5 gene and the nearby COL4A6 gene. The autosomal recessive variants are caused by mutations in either the COL4A3 or COL4A4 genes. The mutations responsible for the autosomal dominant variants are still unknown, but they have been mapped to the same locus as the COL4A3 and COL4A4 genes.

Diagnosis The diagnosis of classic AS is based on X-linked inheritance of hematuria, sensorineural deafness, and lenticonus. Because of the X-linked transmission, women are usually less severely affected than men and are generally underdiagnosed. The hematuria progresses to nephritis and may cause renal failure in late adolescence in affected males and at older ages in some women. The sensorineural deafness is primarily in the high-tone range. It can frequently be detected only by an audiogram and is usually not progressive. The lenticonus can occur without nephritis but is generally considered to be pathognomonic of classic AS.

℞ **TREATMENT** There is no known treatment, but renal transplantation is usually successful.

BIBLIOGRAPHY

BYERS PH: Osteogenesis imperfecta, in *Connective Tissue and Its Heritable Disorders*, PM Royce, B Steinmann (eds). New York, Wiley-Liss, 1993, p 317

DE PAEPE A et al: Revised diagnostic criteria for the Marfan syndrome. Am J Med Genet 62:417, 1996

GLORIEUX FH et al: Cyclic administration of pamidronate in children with severe osteogenesis imperfecta. N Engl J Med 339:947, 1998

HORTON WA, HECHT JT: The chondrodysplasias, in *Connective Tissue and Its Heritable Disorders*, PM Royce, B Steinmann (eds). New York, Wiley-Liss, 1993, p 641

INTERNATIONAL WORKING GROUP ON CONSTITUTIONAL DISEASES OF BONE: International nomenclature and classification of the osteochondrodysplasias (1997). Am J Med Genet 79:376, 1998

KASHTAN CE: Alport syndrome: An inherited disorder of renal, ocular, and cochlear basement membranes. Medicine 78:838, 1999

KUIVANIEMI H et al: Mutations in the fibrillar collagens (types I, II, III, IX and XI), and fibril-associated collagen, and the network-forming collagen (type X) cause a spectrum of diseases of bone, cartilage and blood vessels. Hum Mutat, 9:300, 1997

MANOUVRIER-HANU S et al: Genetics of limb anomalies in humans. Trends Genet 15: 409, 1999

MARINI JC: Osteogenesis imperfecta. Comprehensive management. Adv Pediatr 35:391, 1988

MUNDLOS S, OLSEN BR: Heritable diseases of the skeleton. Part II: Molecular insights into skeletal development-matrix components and their homeostasis. FASEB J 11: 227, 1997

PEPIN M et al: Clinical and genetic features of Ehlers-Danlos syndrome type IV, the vascular type. N Engl J Med 342:673, 2000

PROCKOP DJ: Mutations in collagen genes as a cause of connective-tissue diseases. N Engl J Med 326:540, 1992

———, KIVIRIKKO KI: Collagen: Molecular biology, diseases and potentials for therapy. Annu Rev Biochem 64:403, 1996

PULKKINEN L, UITTO J: Mutations analysis and molecular genetics of epidermolysis bullosa. Matrix Biol 18:29, 1999

RAMIREZ F et al: Marfan syndrome: New clues to genotype-phenotype correlations. Ann Med 31:202, 1999

STEINMANN B et al: The Ehlers-Danlos syndrome, in *Connective Tissue and Its Heritable Disorders*, PM Royce, B Steinmann (eds). New York, Wiley-Liss, 1993, p 351

TASSABEHJI M et al: An elastin gene mutation producing abnormal tropoelastin and abnormal elastic fibres in a patient with autosomal dominant cutis laxa. Hum Mol Genet 7:1021, 1998

352

Nicola Longo

INHERITED DISORDERS OF AMINO ACID METABOLISM AND STORAGE

All polypeptides and proteins are polymers of amino acids. Eight amino acids, referred to as *essential*, cannot be synthesized by humans and must be obtained from dietary sources. The others are formed endogenously. Although most of the body's amino acids are "tied up" in proteins, small intracellular pools of *free* amino acids are in equilibrium with extracellular reservoirs in plasma, cerebrospinal fluid, and the lumina of the gut and kidney. Physiologically, amino acids are more than mere "building blocks" of proteins. Some (glycine, glutamate, γ-aminobutyric acid) are neurotransmitters. Others (phenylalanine, tyrosine, tryptophan, glycine) are precursors of hormones, coenzymes, pigments, purines, or pyrimidines. Each has a unique degradative pathway by which its nitrogen and carbon components are used for the synthesis of other amino acids, carbohydrates, and lipids.

More than 70 disorders of amino acid metabolism are now known. The catabolic and storage defects (approximately 60) discussed in this chapter far outnumber the transport abnormalities (approximately 10) considered in Chap. 353. Each of these disorders is rare—the incidences range from 1 in 10,000 for cystinuria or phenylketonuria to 1 in 200,000 for homocystinuria or alkaptonuria. Collectively, however, they occur in perhaps 1 in 500 to 1 in 1000 live births. Almost all are transmitted as autosomal recessive traits.

The features of inherited disorders of amino acid catabolism are summarized in Table 352-1. In general, these disorders are named for the compound that accumulates to highest concentration in blood (*-emias*) or urine (*-urias*). For many conditions (often called *aminoacidopathies*), the parent amino acid is found in excess; for others, generally referred to as *organic acidemias*, products in the catabolic pathway accumulate. Which compound(s) accumulates depends, of course, on the site of the enzymatic block, the reversibility of the reactions proximal to the lesion, and the availability of alternative pathways of metabolic "runoff." For some amino acids, such as the sulfur-containing or branched-chain molecules, defects have been described at nearly each step in the catabolic pathway. For others, only small numbers of defective reactions have been described. Biochemical and genetic heterogeneity is common. Four distinct forms of hyperphenylalaninemia, seven forms of homocystinuria, and seven types of methylmalonic acidemia are recognized. Such heterogeneity reflects the presence of an even larger array of molecular defects.

The manifestations of these conditions differ widely (Table 352-1). Some, such as sarcosinemia or hyperprolinemia, produce no clinical consequences. At the other extreme, complete deficiency of ornithine transcarbamylase or of branched-chain keto acid dehydrogenase is lethal in the untreated neonate. Central nervous system (CNS) dysfunction, in the form of developmental retardation, seizures, alterations in sensorium, or behavioral disturbances, is present in more than half the disorders. Protein-induced vomiting, neurologic dysfunction, and hyperammonemia occur in many disorders of urea cycle intermediates. Metabolic ketoacidosis, often accompanied by hyperammonemia, is a frequent presenting finding in the disorders of branched-chain amino acid metabolism. Occasional disorders produce focal tissue or organ involvement such as liver disease, renal failure, cutaneous abnormalities, or ocular lesions.

The clinical manifestations in many of these conditions can be prevented or mitigated if diagnosis is achieved early and appropriate treatment (i.e., dietary protein or amino acid restriction or vitamin supplementation) is instituted promptly. For this reason, several aminoacidopathies and organic acidemias are routinely screened in newborns using an array of chemical and microbiologic techniques. Once a presumptive diagnosis is made, confirmation can be provided by direct enzyme assay on extracts of leukocytes, erythrocytes, or cultured fibroblasts. DNA-based testing is possible for several disorders including phenylketonuria, ornithine transcarbamylase deficiency, citrullinemia, gyrate atrophy of the retina, propionic acidemia, and methylmalonic acidemia. As additional mutations are defined, DNA-based analysis may allow better predictions of outcome and improved therapeutic plans.

Several of these disorders (including branched-chain ketoaciduria, isovaleric acidemia, propionic acidemia, methylmalonic acidemia, homocystinuria, cystinosis, phenylketonuria, ornithine transcarbamylase deficiency, citrullinemia, argininosuccinic aciduria) can be diagnosed prenatally by chemical analysis of amniotic fluid or by chemical, enzymatic, or DNA-based studies of fresh or cultured amniotic fluid cells. In addition to predicting genotype and alleviating parental anxiety, prenatal diagnosis has led to improved treatment of affected newborns.

The focus of this chapter is on selected disorders that illustrate the principles, properties, and problems presented by the disorders of amino acid metabolism.

THE HYPERPHENYLALANINEMIAS

DEFINITION The hyperphenylalaninemias (Table 352-1) result from impaired conversion of phenylalanine to tyrosine. The most common and clinically important is *phenylketonuria*, which is characterized by an increased concentration of phenylalanine in blood, increased concentrations of phenylalanine and its by-products (notably phenylpyruvate, phenylacetate, phenyllactate, and phenylacetylglutamine) in urine, and severe mental retardation if untreated in infancy.

GENETIC CONSIDERATIONS Each of the hyperphenylalaninemias results from reduced activity of phenylalanine hydroxylase. In humans, this complete enzyme system is expressed only in liver. Phenylalanine and molecular oxygen are substrates, and a reduced pteridine, tetrahydrobiopterin, is a cofactor (Fig. 352-1). Tyrosine and dihydrobiopterin are the products of this catalytic system, the latter being reconverted to tetrahydrobiopterin by two enzymes, pterin-4α-carbinolamine dehydratase and dihydropteridine reductase.

Abnormalities in phenylalanine metabolism are autosomal recessive traits that occur in about 1 in 10,000 births. Phenylketonuria type I is widely distributed among whites and Orientals. It is rare in blacks. Phenylalanine hydroxylase activity in obligate heterozygotes is low but higher than in affected homozygotes. Adult heterozygous carriers are clinically well but can be identified by an increased ratio of phenylalanine/tyrosine in plasma in the semifasting state. They may have transient cognitive impairment after phenylalanine loads. Hyperphenylalaninemias are caused by mutations in the gene encoding phenylalanine hydroxylase (*PAH*) or in genes encoding enzymes involved in tetrahydrobiopterin synthesis or recycling. In the vast majority of patients, mutations occur in the *PAH* gene (causing phenylketonuria type I), and >300 mutations have been identified. Mutations causing a complete impairment of enzyme activity, such as the R408W, are associated with a more severe outcome requiring stringent dietary restriction of phenylalanine. Mutations causing a less complete deficiency of the enzyme, such as the I65T, are associated with milder forms of phenylketonuria.

In fewer than 2% of patients with phenylketonuria, mutations occur in other genes, including dihydrobiopterin reductase (*DHPR*) (30%), 6-pyruvoyl-tetrahydropterin synthase (*6-PTS*) (60%), GTP cyclohydrolase I (*GTP-CH*) (5%), and pterin-4α-carbinolamine dehydratase (*PCD*) (5%). In these cases, the impairment in phenylalanine hydroxylation results from tetrahydrobiopterin deficiency due to blocks in the pathway by which tetrahydrobiopterin is synthesized from GTP (phenylketonuria type III and malignant hyperphenylalaninemia) or deficiency of dihydropterine reductase (phenylketonuria type II), the enzyme that regenerates tetrahydrobiopterin from dihydrobiopterin (Fig. 352-1). Tyrosine hydroxylase and tryptophan hy-

Table 352-1 Inherited Disorders of Amino Acid Catabolism

Amino Acid(s) Affected	Disorder or Condition	Enzyme Defect	Clinical Manifestations[a]: Mental Retardation	Neuro-psychiatric Dysfunction	Protein Intolerance	Metabolic Ketoacidosis	Ammonia Intoxication	Other	Inheritance Pattern[b]
AROMATIC—HETEROCYCLIC									
Phenylalanine	Phenylketonuria type I (severe to mild)	Phenylalanine hydroxylase	+	+	−	−	−	Hypopigmented skin and hair, eczema	AR
	Phenylketonuria type II	Dihydropteridine reductase	+	+	−	−	−		AR
	Phenylketonuria type III	6-Pyruvoyl-tetrahydropterin synthase	+	+	−	−	−		AR
	Malignant hyperphenylalaninemia	GTP cyclohydrolase	+	+	−	−	−		AR
	Hyperphenylalaninemia with primapterinuria	Pterin-4α-carbinolamine dehydratase	−	±	−	−	−	Transient hyperphenylalaninemia	AR
Tyrosine	Tyrosinemia type I (hepatorenal)	Fumarylacetoacetate hydrolase	−	−	±	−	−	Cirrhosis, hepatic failure, renal tubular defects, rickets	AR
	Tyrosinemia type II (oculocutaneous)	Tyrosine transaminase	±	−	−	−	−	Palmoplantar keratosis, painful corneal erosions with photophobia	AR
	Tyrosinemia type III	4-Hydroxyphenylpyruvate dioxygenase	−	−	−	−	−		AR
	Hawkinsinuria	4-Hydroxyphenylpyruvate dioxygenase	−	−	−	−	−	Failure to thrive, metabolic acidosis in infancy, fine hairs	AD
	Alkaptonuria	Homogentisic acid oxidase	−	−	−	−	−	Ochronosis, arthritis	AR
	Albinism (oculocutaneous)	Tyrosinase	−	−	−	−	−	Hypopigmentation of hair, skin, and optic fundus	AR
	Albinism (ocular)	Unknown	−	−	−	−	−	Hypopigmentation of optic fundus	XL, AR
Tryptophan	Tryptophanuria	Unknown	+	+	−	−	−	Photosensitive skin rash	AR
	Xanthurenic aciduria	Kynureninase	?	−	−	−	−		?
Histidine	Histidinemia	Histidine-ammonia lyase	±	±	−	−	−	Hearing and speech deficit	AR
	Urocanic aciduria	Urocanase	+	+	−	−	−		?
	Formiminoglutamic aciduria	Formiminotransferase	?	+	−	−	−		(AR)
GLYCINE-IMINO ACIDS									
Glycine	Hyperglycinemia	Glycine cleavage	+	+	−	−	−		AR
	Sarcosinemia	Sarcosine dehydrogenase	−	−	−	−	−		AR
	Hyperoxaluria (type I)	Alanine: glyoxylate amino-transferase	−	−	−	−	−	Calcium oxalate nephrolithiasis, renal failure	AR
	Hyperoxaluria (type II)	D-Glyceric acid dehydrogenase/glyoxylate reductase	−	−	−	−	−	Calcium oxalate nephrolithiasis, renal failure	AR

(continued)

Amino Acid(s) Affected	Disorder or Condition	Enzyme Defect	Clinical Manifestations[a]						Inheritance Pattern[b]
			Mental Retardation	Neuro-psychiatric Dysfunction	Protein Intolerance	Metabolic Ketoacidosis	Ammonia Intoxication	Other	
Imino acids	Hyperprolinemia (type I)	Proline oxidase	–	–	–	–	–		AR
	Hyperprolinemia (type II)	Δ′-Pyrroline dehydrogenase	–	–	–	–	–		AR
	Hyperhydroxyprolinemia	Hydroxyproline reductase	–	–	–	–	–		AR
	Iminopeptiduria	Prolidase	+	–	–	–	–	Crusting erythematous, ecchymotic dermatitis, recurrent infections	AR
SULFUR-CONTAINING									
Methionine	Hypermethioninemia	Methionine adenosyltransferase	–	–	–	–	–		?
Homocystine	Homocystinuria	Cystathionine β-synthase	±	±	–	–	–	Dislocated lenses, osteoporosis, thrombotic vascular disease	AR
	Homocystinuria	5,10-Methylenetetrahydrofolate reductase	+	+	–	–	–		AR
	Homocystinuria and methylmalonic acidemia (cblC, -D)[c]	Cobalamin (vitamin B_{12}) reductase (cytosol)	+	+	–	–	–	Megaloblastic anemia	AR
	Homocystinuria and methylmalonic acidemia (cblF)	Lysosomal efflux	+	+	–	–	–		(?)
	Homocystinuria (cblE, -G)	Methionine synthase (MS) and MS reductase	+	+	–	–	–	Megaloblastic anemia	AR
Cystathionine	Cystathioninuria	Cystathionase		–	–	–	–		AR
Cystine	Cystinosis	Lysosomal efflux	–	–	–	–	–	Fanconi syndrome, renal failure, photophobia	AR
S-Sulfo-L-cysteine	*S*-Sulfo-L-cysteine, sulfite, thiosulfaturia	Sulfite oxidase	+	+	–	–	–	Dislocated lenses	AR
CATIONIC									
Lysine	Hyperlysinemia	α-Aminoadipic semialdehyde synthase			–	–	–		AR
	Saccharopinuria	δ-Aminoadipic semialdehyde synthase	–	–	–	–	–		?
	α-Ketoadipic aciduria	α-Ketoadipic acid dehydrogenase			–	–	–		?
	Glutaric aciduria (type I)	Glutaryl CoA dehydrogenase	–	+	–	–	–	Progressive dystonia and athetosis	AR
	Glutaric aciduria (type II)	Electron transfer flavoprotein; or ETF-ubiquinone oxidoreductase	–	+	–	+	–	Hypoglycemia, acidosis, ''sweaty feet'' odor, hypotonia, fatty degeneration of liver and kidney	AR

(continued)

Table 352-1 Inherited Disorders of Amino Acid Catabolism—*(continued)*

Amino Acid(s) Affected	Disorder or Condition	Enzyme Defect	Clinical Manifestations[a]: Mental Retardation	Neuro-psychiatric Dysfunction	Protein Intolerance	Metabolic Ketoacidosis	Ammonia Intoxication	Other	Inheritance Pattern[b]
Ornithine	Hyperornithinemia, hyperammonemia, homocitrullinuria	Mitochondrial ornithine transporter-1	+	+	+	−	+		AR
	Hyperornithinemia	Ornithine-D-aminotransferase	−	−	−	−	−	Gyrate atrophy of choroid and retina	AR
UREA CYCLE									
Carbamyl-phosphate	Hyperammonemia (type I)	Carbamylphosphate synthetase I	+	+	+	−	+		AR
N-acetyl-glutamate	Hyperammonemia (type IA)	*N*-acetylglutamate synthetase	±	+	+	−	+		AR
Ornithine	Hyperammonemia (type II)	Ornithine transcarbamylase	+	+	+	−	+		XL
Citrulline	Citrullinemia-1	Argininosuccinate synthetase	+	+	+	−	+		AR
	Citrullinemia-2	Activating protein (?)	±	+	−	−	+		AR
Argininosuccinic acid	Argininosuccinic aciduria	Argininosuccinase	+	+	+	−	+		AR
Arginine	Argininemia	Arginase	+	+	+	−	+		AR
BRANCHED-CHAIN									
Valine	Hypervalinemia	Valine aminotransferase	+	+	+	−	−		AR
Leucine, isoleucine	Hyperleucine-isoleucinemia	Leucine-isoleucine aminotransferase	+	+	+	−	−		?
Valine, leucine, isoleucine	Classic branched-chain ketoaciduria	Branched-chain ketoacid dehydrogenase	+	+	+	±	−	"Maple syrup" odor	AR
	Intermittent branched-chain ketoaciduria	Branched-chain ketoacid dehydrogenase	±	−	+	+	−		AR
Leucine	Isovaleric acidemia	Isovaleryl CoA dehydrogenase	±	±	+	+	±	"Sweaty feet" odor	AR
	β-Methylcrotonyl glycinuria	β-Methylcrotonyl CoA carboxylase	+	+	−	+	−	"Cat's urine" odor	AR
	β-Hydroxy-β-methylglutaric aciduria	β-Hydroxy-β-methylglutaryl CoA lyase	−	+	+	+	−		AR
Isoleucine, valine	α-Methylacetoacetic aciduria	β-Ketothiolase	±	±	+	+	+		AR
	Propionic acidemia (pcc A, B, C)[c]	Propionyl CoA carboxylase	±	±	+	+	+		AR
	Propionic acidemia (bio)[c]	Holocarboxylase synthetase; biotinidase	+	±	+	+	−		AR
	Methylmalonic acidemia (mut)[c]	Methylmalonyl CoA mutase	±	±	+	+	+		AR
	Methylmalonic acidemia (cbl A)[c]	Cobalamin (vitamin B_{12}) reductase (mitochondrial) (?)	±	±	+	+	+		AR
	Methylmalonic acidemia (cbl B)[c]	Cobalamin (vitamin B_{12}): ATP adenosyltransferase	±	±	+	+	+		AR

[a] +, Regularly present; ±, sometimes present; −, absent; ?, uncertain; all designations refer to manifestations in untreated disorder.

[b] AR, autosomal recessive; XL, X-linked; (AR), probably autosomal recessive.

[c] Designations in parentheses refer to complementation groups assigned by genetic analysis with cultured cells.

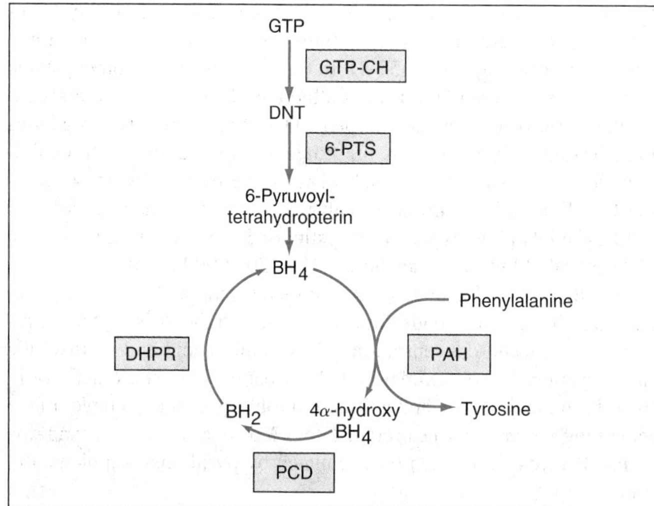

FIGURE 352-1 Pathways, enzymes, and coenzymes involved in the hyperphenylalaninemias. Blocked-in symbols highlight points of etiologic or therapeutic significance to the various genetic defects underlying these disorders. Abbreviations: GTP, guanosine triphosphate; GTP-CH, guanosine triphosphate cyclohydrolase; DNT, dihydroneopterin triphosphate; 6-PTS, 6-pyruvoyl-tetrahydropterin synthase; BH4, tetrahydrobiopterin; BH2, dihydrobiopterin; DHPR, dihydropteridine reductase; PAH, phenylalanine hydroxylase; PCD, pterin-4α–carbinolamine dehydratase.

droxylase also require tetrahydrobiopterin. Their products (L-dopa and 5-hydroxytryptophan) are essential for the synthesis of neurotransmitters. Heterozygotes for these conditions do not have hyperphenylalaninemia, but carriers of mutations in GTP cyclohydrolase have a peculiar form of dystonia, transmitted as a dominant trait with variable expressivity and higher penetrance in females; it is exquisitely responsive to levodopa. Neurotransmitter levels are not altered in transient hyperphenylalaninemia (sometimes called *transient phenylketonuria*), which has been described in some patients with pterin-4α-carbinolamine dehydratase deficiency. ■

Etiology and Pathogenesis Phenylalanine accumulation in blood and urine and reduced tyrosine formation are direct consequences of the impaired hydroxylation. In untreated phenylketonuria and in its tetrahydrobiopterin-deficient variants, plasma concentrations of phenylalanine become sufficiently high [1 mmol/L (16 mg/dL)] to activate alternative pathways of metabolism and lead to formation of phenylpyruvate, phenylacetate, phenyllactate, and other derivatives that are rapidly cleared by the kidney and excreted in urine. The severe brain damage is due to several consequences of phenylalanine accumulation: competitive inhibition of transport of other amino acids required for protein synthesis, impaired polyribosome formation or stabilization, reduced synthesis and increased degradation of myelin, and inadequate formation of norepinephrine and serotonin. Phenylalanine is a competitive inhibitor of tyrosinase, a key enzyme in the pathway of melanin synthesis. This block, plus reduced availability of the melanin precursor tyrosine, accounts for the hypopigmentation of hair and skin.

Clinical Manifestations No abnormalities are apparent at birth, but untreated children with classic phenylketonuria fail to attain early developmental milestones, develop microcephaly, and demonstrate progressive impairment of cerebral function. Hyperactivity, seizures, and severe mental retardation are major clinical problems later in life. Electroencephalographic abnormalities; "mousy" odor of skin, hair, and urine (due to phenylacetate accumulation); and a tendency to hypopigmentation and eczema complete the devastating clinical picture. In contrast, affected children who are detected at birth and treated promptly show none of these abnormalities. Children with tetrahydrobiopterin deficiency, however, suffer a worse clinical course. Seizures appear early, followed by progressive cerebral and basal ganglia dysfunction (rigidity, chorea, spasms, hypotonia). Most succumb to secondary infection within a few years despite early diagnosis and vigorous treatment.

A number of women with phenylketonuria who have been treated since infancy have reached adulthood and become pregnant. If maternal phenylalanine levels are not strictly controlled before and during pregnancy, their offspring are at risk, even if they are heterozygous, for *maternal phenylketonuria*. Affected children have microcephaly and an increased risk of congenital defects. After birth, these children have severe neurodevelopmental delay and growth retardation.

Diagnosis Plasma phenylalanine concentrations are usually normal at birth in the hyperphenylalaninemias but rise rapidly after institution of protein feedings. To prevent mental retardation, diagnosis and initiation of dietary treatment of classic phenylketonuria must occur before the child is 3 weeks of age. For this reason, most newborns in North America and Europe are screened by determinations of blood phenylalanine concentration using the Guthrie bacterial inhibition assay. Abnormal values are confirmed using quantitative analysis of plasma amino acids. Prenatal diagnosis of type I phenylketonuria is now feasible using DNA-based tests that detect specific mutations or polymorphic markers that are linked to the *PAH* gene.

In newborns with type I phenylketonuria, plasma levels depend on the amount of phenylalanine in the diet and the degree of impairment of phenylalanine hydroxylase. Dietary phenylalanine restriction is usually instituted if blood phenylalanine levels are >250 μmol/L (4 mg/dL). Careful monitoring of these infants reveals the degree of phenylalanine hydroxylase impairment and dictates the degree of dietary phenylalanine restriction.

Deficiency of tetrahydrobiopterin, which occurs in 1 to 2% of newborns with increased blood phenylalanine, is excluded by screening the urinary pteridine profile and by assay of dihydropteridine reductase activity on dried blood specimens. Dihydropteridine reductase deficiency and the blocks in tetrahydrobiopterin synthesis can be detected in utero using assays on cultured amniocytes. Tetrahydrobiopterin deficiency manifests with hyperphenylalaninemia and progressive neurologic impairment despite prompt dietary restriction of phenylalanine.

℞ **TREATMENT** Phenylketonuria is the first inherited metabolic disease in which a strategy of reducing the accumulation of the offending metabolite prevented the dire clinical consequences. This was accomplished by a special diet low in phenylalanine and supplemented with tyrosine. Tyrosine becomes an essential amino acid in phenylalanine hydroxylase deficiency. Sufficient phenylalanine is provided for new protein synthesis and normal growth. This amount varies with age and requires frequent adjustments, especially early in life. Ordinarily, plasma phenylalanine concentrations are maintained between 120 and 360 μmol/L (2 and 6 mg/dL). Such diet therapy must be instituted during the first 3 weeks of life. Even then, modest CNS dysfunction may occur with more deleterious mutations or after excess protein intake. Because uncontrolled hyperphenylalaninemia results in brain damage, dietary restriction should be continued and monitored indefinitely, recognizing that transient phenylketonuria may not require lifelong therapy. An enteric-coated formulation of phenylalanine ammonia lyase, which degrades phenylalanine in the gut, is under investigation for its potential to reduce the strain imposed by the special diet.

Children with tetrahydrobiopterin deficiency deteriorate despite dietary phenylalanine restriction. Such patients may be helped, however, by a regimen in which dietary phenylalanine restriction is combined with tetrahydrobiopterin supplements, levodopa, 5-hydroxytryptophan, and carbidopa. Finally, the deleterious consequences of maternal phenylketonuria can be minimized by continuing lifelong phenylalanine-restricted diets in females with phenylketonuria and assuring strict phenylalanine restriction prior to conception and throughout gestation.

THE HOMOCYSTINURIAS (HYPERHOMOCYSTEINEMIAS)

The homocystinurias are seven biochemically and clinically distinct disorders (Table 352-1), each characterized by increased concentration of the sulfur-containing amino acid homocystine in blood and urine. The most common form results from reduced activity of cystathionine β-synthase (CBS), an enzyme in the transsulfuration pathway that converts methionine to cysteine (Fig. 352-2). The other forms are the result of impaired conversion of homocysteine to methionine, a reaction catalyzed by homocysteine:methyltetrahydrofolate methyltransferase (also known as *methionine synthase*) and two essential cofactors, methyltetrahydrofolate and methylcobalamin (methyl-vitamin B_{12}). Depending on the underlying disorder, some patients show chemical and, in some instances, clinical improvement following administration of specific vitamin supplements (pyridoxine, folate, or cobalamin) (Chap. 75). In classic homocystinuria, the levels of free homocystine in plasma increase and result in homocystinuria. *Hyperhomocysteinemia* refers to increased total plasma concentration of homocysteine in the sulfhydryl and disulfide form, free and protein-bound. Hyperhomocysteinemia, in the absence of significant homocystinuria, is found in individuals who are heterozygous or homozygous for certain genetic defects that impair folate or vitamin B_{12} metabolism or cause cystathionine synthase deficiency. Changes of homocysteine levels are also observed with increasing age; in postmenopausal women; in patients with renal failure, hypothyroidism, leukemias, or psoriasis; and during therapy with drugs such as methotrexate, nitrous oxide, isoniazid, and some antiepileptic agents.

Homocysteine acts as an atherogenic and thrombophilic agent. An increase in total plasma homocysteine represents an independent risk factor for coronary, cerebrovascular, and peripheral arterial disease as well as for deep-vein thrombosis (Chap. 241). Homocysteine is synergistic with hypertension and smoking, and it is additive with other risk factors that predispose to peripheral arterial disease. In addition, hyperhomocysteinemia and folate and vitamin B_{12} deficiency have been associated with an increased risk of neural tube defects in pregnant women.

CYSTATHIONINE β-SYNTHASE DEFICIENCY Definition Deficiency of this enzyme leads to increased concentrations of methionine and homocystine in body fluids and to decreased concentrations of cysteine and cystine. Clinical hallmarks include dislocation of optic lenses (usually downward and medially), mental retardation, marfanoid habitus, osteoporosis, and thrombotic vascular disease.

GENETIC CONSIDERATIONS The sulfur atom of the essential amino acid methionine is transferred to cysteine by the transsulfuration pathway (Fig. 352-2). In one of these steps, homocysteine condenses with serine to form cystathionine. This reaction is catalyzed by the pyridoxal phosphate–dependent enzyme CBS. Heterogenous mutations in the *CBS* gene are present in different families. The G307S mutation is associated with lack of response to pyridoxine, whereas the I278T mutation correlates with pyridoxine-responsiveness and a milder clinical phenotype. Homocystinuria is common in Ireland (1 in 60,000 births) but rare elsewhere (<1 in 200,000 births). ■

Etiology and Pathogenesis Homocysteine and methionine accumulate in cells and body fluids; cysteine synthesis is impaired, resulting in reduced concentrations of this amino acid and its disulfide form, cystine. In approximately half of patients, synthase activity in liver, brain, leukocytes, and cultured fibroblasts is undetectable. In the remaining patients, tissues retain 1 to 5% of normal activity, and this residual activity can often be stimulated by pyridoxine supplementation.

Homocysteine interferes with the normal cross-linking of collagen, an effect that likely plays an important role in the ocular, skeletal, and vascular complications. Altered collagen in the suspensory ligament of the optic lens and in bone matrix may account for the dislocated lenses and osteoporosis. Similarly, interference with normal ground substance metabolism in vascular walls may predispose to the arterial and venous thrombotic diathesis. Increased platelet adhesiveness may result from homocysteine accumulation, thereby contributing to the thrombotic occlusive disease so often observed. Recurrent cerebrovascular accidents secondary to thrombotic disease may account for the mental retardation, but direct chemical effects on cerebral cell metabolism have not been excluded.

Clinical Manifestations More than 80% of homozygotes for complete CBS deficiency develop dislocated optic lenses. This abnormality usually appears by 3 to 4 years of age and often results in glaucoma and impaired visual acuity. Mental retardation occurs in about half of such patients, often accompanied by ill-defined behavioral disturbances. Osteoporosis is a common radiologic finding (seen in two-thirds of patients by age 15) but rarely causes clinical disease. Life-threatening vascular complications, probably initiated by damage to vascular endothelium, are the major cause of morbidity and mortality. Occlusion of coronary, renal, and cerebral arteries with attendant tissue infarction can occur during the first decade of life. Nearly a fourth of patients die of vascular disease before age 30. These vascular complications seem to be exacerbated by angiographic procedures. Importantly, pyridoxine-responsive patients have milder clinical manifestations in all regards and may escape newborn screening and present with ectopia lentis or premature vascular occlusion. Hetero-

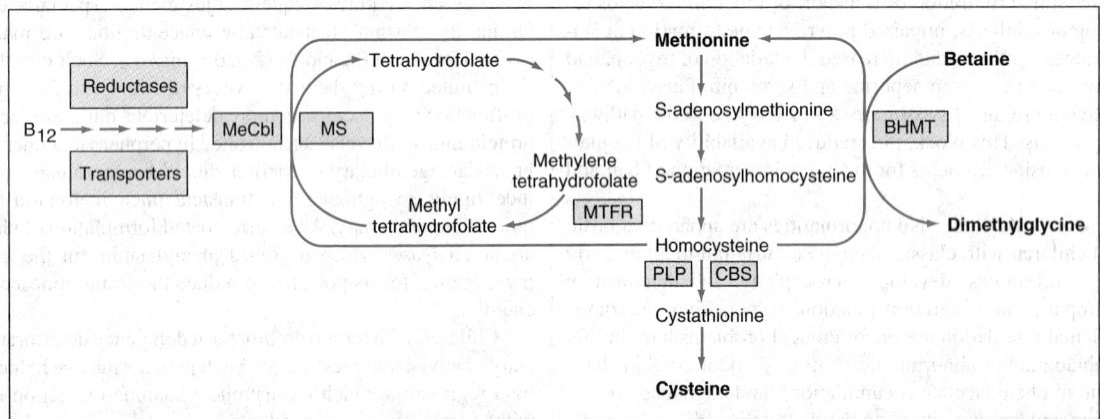

FIGURE 352-2 Pathways, enzymes, and coenzymes involved in the homocystinurias. Blocked-in symbols highlight specific moieties of particular etiologic or therapeutic significance to the various genetic defects underlying these disorders. Abbreviations: B_{12}, hydroxocobalamin; MeCbl, methylcobalamin; MTFR, methylenetetrahydrofolate reductase; PLP, pyridoxal phosphate; CBS, cystathionine β-synthase; BHMT, betaine:homocysteine methyl transferase; MS, methionine synthase (5-methyltetrahydrofolate:homocysteine transferase).

zygous carriers for *CBS* deficiency (about 1 in 70 in the population) may have hyperhomocysteinemia, with an increased risk for premature coronary, peripheral, and cerebral occlusive vascular disease.

Diagnosis The cyanide-nitroprusside test is a simple way of demonstrating increased excretion of sulfhydryl-containing compounds in urine. This is confirmed by measurement of free plasma methionine and homocystine. Plasma methionine tends to be increased in synthase-deficient patients and normal or low in those with other causes of homocystinuria and impaired methionine formation (see below). Diagnostic confirmation depends on measurements of CBS activity in tissue extracts or cells cultured from patients. Heterozygotes can be identified by measurement of peak serum homocystine after an oral methionine load (100 mg/kg) and by measurement of tissue synthase activity.

℞ TREATMENT As with classic phenylketonuria, effective treatment depends on early diagnosis. A number of infants diagnosed in the newborn period have been treated successfully with methionine-restricted, cystine-supplemented diets. In approximately half of patients, oral pyridoxine (25 to 500 mg/d) produces a fall in plasma and urinary methionine and homocystine and an increase in cystine concentration in body fluids. This effect probably reflects a modest increase in CBS activity in cells of patients in whom the defect is characterized either by reduced affinity for cofactor or by accelerated degradation of mutant enzyme. Vitamin supplementation at these doses is apparently harmless and should be tried in all patients. Folate deficiency should be prevented by adequate supplementation. Betaine has also been effective in reducing homocystine levels in pyridoxine-unresponsive patients.

5,10-METHYLENETETRAHYDROFOLATE REDUCTASE (MTFR) DEFICIENCY Definition Hyperhomocysteinemia with normal or decreased methionine levels is caused by deficiency of MTFR, the enzyme involved in the synthesis of 5-methyltetrahydrofolate, a cofactor in the enzymatic formation of methionine from homocysteine (Fig. 352-2). CNS dysfunction and premature vascular occlusion may occur.

Genetic Basis and Pathogenesis 5-Methyltetrahydrofolate:homocysteine methyltransferase (methionine synthase) catalyzes the conversion of homocysteine to methionine. A primary defect in MTFR activity results, secondarily, in deficient methyltransferase activity and impaired conversion of homocysteine to methionine. This series of reactions is critical to normal DNA and RNA synthesis. Methionine deficiency and impaired nucleic acid synthesis may contribute to CNS dysfunction, while homocystine accumulation may predispose to thrombosis.

Hyperhomocysteinemia is inherited as an autosomal recessive trait and is caused by mutations in the MTFR (*MTHFR*) gene, which is located on chromosome 1p36.3. A thermolabile variant form of this enzyme, which has reduced activity, may be a common cause of hyperhomocysteinemia associated with increased risk of vascular disease in young adults.

Clinical Manifestations More than 30 patients with homocystinuria due to MTFR deficiency have been reported. The most severely affected have developmental retardation and cerebral atrophy early in life. Others have behavioral disturbances (catatonia) during the second decade or mild retardation. The severity of the clinical manifestations reflects the severity of the reductase deficiency.

Diagnosis Increased concentrations of free homocystine in body fluids with normal or decreased concentrations of methionine suggest severe MTFR deficiency. Total plasma homocysteine levels slightly above the normal range suggest milder dysfunction of this enzyme. Serum folate concentration is low in some patients. Confirmation requires direct MTFR assays in cultured fibroblasts.

℞ TREATMENT Therapeutic experience is limited. Folate, vitamin B_{12}, methionine, or betaine supplementation decrease homocystine urinary excretion and improve the clinical manifestations in some patients.

DEFICIENCY OF COBALAMIN (VITAMIN B_{12}) COENZYME SYNTHESIS Definition Five other forms of homocystinuria also reflect impaired conversion of homocysteine to methionine. The primary defects in these entities, however, are in the synthesis of methylcobalamin, a cobalamin (vitamin B_{12}) coenzyme required by methionine synthase (MS) (Fig. 352-2). In some, methylmalonic acid accumulates in body fluids because of impaired synthesis of a second coenzyme, adenosylcobalamin, required for isomerization of methylmalonyl coenzyme A (CoA) to succinyl CoA. These disorders are designated cblC, -D, -E, -F, and -G.

Etiology and Pathogenesis As with MTFR deficiency, each disorder impairs remethylation of homocysteine. Since methylcobalamin is required for methyl-group transfer from methyltetrahydrofolate to homocysteine, impaired cobalamin metabolism leads to deficient methyltransferase activity. The defects responsible for impaired synthesis of methylcobalamin involve one of several steps in lysosomal or cytosolic activation of the vitamin precursor (Fig. 352-2). Somatic cell genetic studies indicate that each of the five abnormalities (cblC to -G) is distinct and imply that all are inherited as autosomal recessive traits.

Clinical Manifestations More than 45 patients—mostly children—with these defects in cobalamin metabolism have been described. Although clinical manifestations vary, abnormalities include developmental delay, dementia, spasticity, megaloblastic anemia, and pancytopenia. It is not possible to define a specific clinical syndrome for each of the defects in cobalamin metabolism.

Diagnosis Homocystinuria, homocysteinemia, and hypomethioninemia are the chemical hallmarks. Methylmalonic acidemia, too, has been noted in those defects resulting from defective synthesis of both cobalamin coenzymes. These findings may also be present in juvenile- or adult-onset pernicious anemia in which intestinal cobalamin absorption is impaired. Measurement of serum cobalamin concentrations, low in pernicious anemia and normal in patients with defective conversion of cobalamin vitamin to coenzymes, helps in the differential diagnosis. Definitive diagnosis depends on demonstrating impaired coenzyme synthesis in cultured cells.

℞ TREATMENT Treatment of affected children with hydroxycobalamin injections (1 to 2 mg/QD) and betaine supplements decreases homocystine and methylmalonate excretion; the hematologic and neurologic deficits have also been diminished to variable degrees in some patients. Intervention early in life seems to offer the best long-term prognosis.

ALKAPTONURIA

Definition Alkaptonuria is a rare disorder of tyrosine catabolism in which deficiency of homogentisate 1,2-dioxygenase (also known as *homogentisic acid oxidase*) leads to excretion of large amounts of homogentisic acid in urine and accumulation of oxidized homogentisic acid pigment in connective tissues (*ochronosis*). After many years, ochronosis produces a distinctive form of degenerative arthritis.

Genetic Basis and Pathogenesis Alkaptonuria was the first human disease shown to be inherited as an autosomal recessive trait. Affected homozygotes occur with a frequency of about 1 in 200,000. Heterozygous carriers are clinically well and excrete no homogentisic acid in urine, even after loading doses of tyrosine. The gene for homogentisate 1,2-dioxygenase (*HGD*) maps to chromosome 3q21-q23 and encodes a 445 amino acid protein expressed not only in liver and kidney but also in small intestine, colon, and prostate. Expression in this latter organ is consistent with accumulation of black calculi of homogentisic acid in the prostate of patients with alkaptonuria, sometimes requiring prostatectomy.

Patients have minimally increased concentrations of homogentisic acid in blood because it is rapidly cleared by the kidney. However, homogentisic acid accumulates in cells and body fluids. Its oxidized polymers bind to collagen, leading to the progressive deposition of a gray to bluish-black pigment. The mechanism(s) by which this deposition causes degenerative changes in cartilage, intervertebral disk, and other connective tissues is unknown but may involve direct chemical irritation, impaired collagen cross-linking, disturbed articular chondrocyte metabolism, or some combination of factors.

Clinical Manifestations Alkaptonuria may go unrecognized until middle life when degenerative joint disease develops. Prior to this time, the tendency of the patient's urine to darken on standing may go unnoticed, as may slight pigmentation of the sclerae and ears. The latter manifestations are generally the earliest external evidence of the disorder and develop after age 20 to 30. Foci of gray-brown scleral pigment and generalized darkening of the concha, anthelix, and finally, helix of the ear are typical. Ear cartilages may be irregular and thickened. *Ochronotic arthritis* is heralded by pain, stiffness, and some limitation of motion of the hips, knees, and shoulders. Acute arthritis may resemble rheumatoid arthritis, but small joints are usually spared. Limitation of motion and ankylosis of the lumbosacral spine are common late manifestations. Pigmentation of heart valves, larynx, tympanic membranes, and skin occurs, and occasional patients develop pigmented renal or prostatic calculi. Degenerative cardiovascular disease may be increased in older patients.

Diagnosis A patient whose urine darkens to blackness on standing must be suspected of having alkaptonuria, but this may not be observed with the use of modern plumbing conditions. The diagnosis is usually made from the triad of degenerative arthritis, ochronotic pigmentation, and urine that turns black upon alkalinization. Homogentisic acid in urine may be identified presumptively by other tests: after addition of ferric chloride, a purple-black color is observed; treatment with Benedict's reagent yields a brown color; addition of a saturated silver nitrate solution produces an intermediate black color. These screening tests can be confirmed by chromatographic, enzymatic, or spectrophotometric determinations of homogentisic acid. X-rays of the lumbar spine show degeneration and dense calcification of the intervertebral disks and narrowing of the intervertebral spaces (bamboo-like appearance).

℞ TREATMENT There is no specific treatment for ochronotic arthritis. Joint manifestations might be mitigated if homogentisic acid accumulation and deposition could be curbed by dietary restriction of phenylalanine and tyrosine, but the long-term nature of the disease discourages such therapeutic attempts. Ascorbic acid impedes oxidation and polymerization of homogentisic acid in vitro, but the efficacy of this form of treatment has not been established. Symptomatic treatment is similar to that for osteoarthritis (Chap. 321).

CYSTINOSIS

Definition Cystinosis is a rare disorder characterized by the intralysosomal accumulation of free cystine in body tissues. This results in the appearance of cystine crystals in the cornea, conjunctiva, bone marrow, lymph nodes, leukocytes, and internal organs. Three variants have been identified: an infantile (nephropathic) form leading to the Fanconi syndrome and renal insufficiency in the first decade, a juvenile (intermediate) form in which renal disease is manifest during the second decade, and an adult (benign) form characterized by deposition of cystine in the cornea but not in the kidney.

GENETIC CONSIDERATIONS All types are inherited as autosomal recessive traits. The gene for the infantile form of nephropathic cystinosis encodes an integral membrane protein, which is a putative lysosomal cystine transporter. The gene is located on chromosome 17p13 and is designated *CTNS*. It is highly expressed in the pancreas, kidney, skeletal muscle, placenta, and heart. A common 65-kb deletion accounts for the majority of patients of European ancestry with infantile cystinosis. The juvenile- and adult-onset forms of nephropathic cystinosis are allelic with the infantile form. Obligate heterozygotes have intracellular cystine concentrations intermediate between those of normal persons and affected patients, but they are free of clinical abnormalities.

The basic defect involves impaired efflux of cystine from lysosomes rather than an abnormality in cystine catabolism. Lysosomal cystine efflux is an active, ATP-dependent process. The cystine content of tissues may be more than 100 times normal in the infantile form and more than 30 times normal in the adult form. Intracellular cystine in lysosomes does not exchange with other intra- or extracellular pools of this amino acid. Neither plasma nor urinary concentrations of cystine are particularly elevated. Cystine accumulation in the kidney causes renal insufficiency in the infantile and juvenile forms. Patchy depigmentation and degeneration of the peripheral retina occur in the infantile and juvenile forms. Cystine crystals may also be deposited in the cornea, ocular conjunctiva, or uvea. ■

Clinical Manifestations In the infantile form, abnormalities are usually apparent by 6 to 10 months of age. Growth retardation, vomiting, fever, vitamin D–resistant rickets, polyuria, dehydration, and metabolic acidosis are prominent. Generalized proximal tubular dysfunction (the Fanconi syndrome) leads to hyperphosphaturia and hypophosphatemia, renal glycosuria, generalized amino aciduria, low plasma carnitine, hypouricemia, and often hypokalemia. Death due to uremia or intercurrent infection usually occurs before age 10. Ocular manifestations are prominent. Photophobia is usually demonstrable within the first years of life due to cystine deposits in the cornea, and retinal degeneration may appear even earlier. Hypothyroidism, insulin-dependent diabetes mellitus, and delayed puberty are often observed in older patients.

In contrast, patients with the adult form have only ocular abnormalities. Photophobia, headache, and burning or itching of the eyes are major complaints. Glomerular and tubular function and the integrity of the retina are preserved. The findings in the juvenile variant fall between these extremes. Ocular and renal manifestations do not become significant until the second decade. The renal lesion, albeit milder than that in the infantile form, eventually leads to renal insufficiency.

Diagnosis Cystinosis must be considered in any child with vitamin D–resistant rickets, the Fanconi syndrome, or glomerular insufficiency. Hexagonal or rectangular cystine crystals can be detected in the cornea (by slit-lamp examination), in leukocytes from peripheral blood or bone marrow, or in biopsies of rectal mucosa. Diagnosis is confirmed by measurement of cystine in leukocytes. The infantile form has been diagnosed prenatally by the demonstration of increased cystine content in cultured amniotic fluid cells.

℞ TREATMENT The adult form is benign and requires no treatment. Symptomatic treatment of renal disease in the infantile or juvenile form includes maintenance of adequate fluid intake to prevent dehydration; correction of the metabolic acidosis; administration of supplementary calcium, phosphate, and vitamin D to heal the rickets; and carnitine supplements (100 mg/kg per day) to correct the increased urinary losses. Specific therapy with the free thiol cysteamine slows the progression of renal dysfunction and improves growth. This compound acts in lysosomes by forming a mixed disulfide with cysteine, allowing it to be transported out of the organelle by an unrelated transporter not affected by the disease. Treatment is more effective if initiated before the patient is 2 years of age. Eye drops containing cysteamine can remove corneal crystals but requires frequent applications (10 to 14 times a day).

Children with nephropathic cystinosis and end-stage renal disease benefit from kidney transplantation. Patients who tolerate the procedure and do not develop immunologic problems have return of kidney function toward normal. The transplanted kidneys have not developed the functional abnormalities typical of cystinosis (i.e., the Fanconi syndrome or glomerular insufficiency). Patients may, however, continue to accumulate cystine in the cornea and other organs (thyroid, brain, and muscle).

PRIMARY HYPEROXALURIA

Definition Primary hyperoxaluria is the designation for two rare autosomal recessive disorders characterized by chronic excessive urinary excretion of oxalic acid and by calcium oxalate nephrolithiasis and nephrocalcinosis. Typically, patients with both forms develop renal insufficiency early in life and die of uremia. Calcium oxalate deposits are widespread in renal and extrarenal tissues, causing a condition referred to as *oxalosis*.

GENETIC CONSIDERATIONS The metabolic basis for the primary hyperoxalurias involves pathways of glyoxylate metabolism. In type I hyperoxaluria, urinary excretion of oxalate and of the oxidized and reduced forms of glyoxylate is increased. The excessive synthesis of these substances results from a block in glyoxylate metabolism. The primary defect in most patients is deficiency of the hepatic peroxisomal enzyme alanine:glyoxylate amino transferase. The gene (*AGXT*) for this enzyme maps to 2q36-37, and several distinct mutations have been defined in patients with type I hyperoxaluria. Some of these mutations misdirect the enzyme to mitochondria and render it nonfunctional.

In type II hyperoxaluria, L-glyceric acid is excreted in excess along with oxalate. In this condition, activity of D-glyceric acid dehydrogenase, which catalyzes the reduction of hydroxypyruvate to D-glyceric acid in the catabolic pathway of serine metabolism, is absent in leukocytes (and presumably other tissues). The accumulated hydroxypyruvate is instead reduced by lactic dehydrogenase to the L-isomer of glycerate, which is excreted in the urine. The same enzyme possesses glyoxylate reductase activity, and its deficiency promotes the oxidation of glyoxylate to oxalate, thus causing the formation of increased oxalate.

Stone formation, nephrocalcinosis, and oxalosis are due to insolubility of calcium oxalate. Extrarenal deposits of oxalate are prominent in the heart, walls of arteries and veins, male urogenital tract, and bone, particularly in type I hyperoxaluria. ■

Clinical Manifestations Nephrolithiasis and oxalosis may be manifest during the first year of life. Most patients experience renal colic or hematuria between ages 2 and 10 and succumb to uremia before age 20. With the onset of uremia, patients may develop severe peripheral arterial spasm and necrosis with resulting vascular insufficiency. Oxalate excretion falls as renal failure worsens. In patients with delayed onset of symptoms, survival to age 50 or 60 has been reported, despite recurrent nephrolithiasis. Type II hyperoxaluria is a milder disease with less involvement of extrarenal organs and delayed impairment of kidney function.

Diagnosis Oxalate excretion in normal children or adults is <0.5 mmol (60 mg) per 1.73 m^2 surface area per day. Patients with type I or type II hyperoxaluria excrete two to four times this amount. Distinction between the two types depends on the identification of the other organic acids that identify them: glycolic acid in type I and L-glyceric acid in type II. Since patients with pyridoxine deficiency or chronic ileal disease may excrete excessive amounts of oxalate, these conditions must be excluded.

TREATMENT There is no satisfactory treatment. Increasing the volume of urine can transiently reduce urinary oxalate concentration. Large doses of pyridoxine (100 mg/d) may reduce urinary oxalate in some patients, but long-term effects are not dramatic. A diet high in phosphate content seems to reduce the frequency of attacks of renal colic, but oxalate excretion is unaffected. Combined liver-kidney transplantation can correct the enzyme deficiency and replace the damaged organs. Liver transplantation seems promising in patients diagnosed before the onset of kidney failure.

ACKNOWLEDGMENT
This chapter includes the contributions of Dr. Leon E. Rosenberg and Dr. Louis J. Elsas from previous editions.

BIBLIOGRAPHY

DANPURE CJ: Primary hyperoxaluria, in *The Molecular and Metabolic Bases of Inherited Disease*, 8th ed, CR Scriver et al (eds). New York, McGraw-Hill, 2001, pp 3323–3367

ELSAS LJ, ACOSTA PB: Nutritional support of inherited metabolic diseases, in *Modern Nutrition in Health and Disease*, 9th ed, ME Shils et al (eds). Baltimore, Williams & Wilkins, 1998, Chap 61

GAHL WA: Cystinosis: A disorder of lysosomal membrane transport, in *The Molecular and Metabolic Bases of Inherited Disease*, 8th ed, CR Scriver et al (eds). New York, McGraw-Hill, 2001, pp 5085–5108

LA DU BN: Alkaptonuria, in *The Molecular and Metabolic Bases of Inherited Disease*, 8th ed, CR Scriver et al (eds). New York, McGraw-Hill, 2001, pp 2109–2123

MUDD SH et al: Disorders of transsulfuration, in *The Molecular and Metabolic Bases of Inherited Disease*, 8th ed, CR Scriver et al (eds). New York, McGraw-Hill, 2001, pp 2007–2056

NYHAN WL, OZAND PT: *Atlas of Metabolic Diseases*. London, Chapman & Hall Medical, 1998

ROSENBERG LE, SCRIVER CR: Disorders of amino acid metabolism, in *Metabolic Control and Disease*, 8th ed, PK Bondy, LE Rosenberg (eds). Philadelphia, Saunders, 1980, pp 583–776

ROSENBLATT DS, FENTON WA: Inherited disorders of folate and cobalamin transport and metabolism, in *The Molecular and Metabolic Bases of Inherited Disease*, 8th ed, CR Scriver et al (eds). New York, McGraw-Hill, 2001, pp 3897–3933

SCRIVER CR, KAUFMAN S: Hyperphenylalaninemia: Phenylalanine hydroxylase deficiency, in *The Molecular and Metabolic Bases of Inherited Disease*, 8th ed, CR Scriver et al (eds). New York, McGraw-Hill, 2001, pp 1667–1724

353

Nicola Longo

INHERITED DEFECTS OF MEMBRANE TRANSPORT

Specific membrane transporters mediate the passage of a wide variety of substances across plasma cell membranes. Classes of substrates represented include amino acids, sugars, cations, anions, vitamins, and water. The disorders considered in this chapter have three features in common: each is characterized by a specific defect in the transport of one or more compounds; each is inherited as a dominant or recessive trait, implying that variation in a single genetic locus is involved; and each is presumed to reflect a primary alteration in a specific membrane protein. Many of these defects have been well characterized physiologically and genetically. Inherited defects impairing the transport of amino acids, hexoses, and chloride are discussed here as examples of the abnormalities encountered; others are considered elsewhere in this text.

The number of inherited disorders of membrane transport continues to increase with the identification of new transporters and the clarification of the molecular basis of diseases with previously unknown pathophysiology. The first transport disorders identified affected the gut or the kidney, but transport processes are now proving essential for the normal function of every organ. Mutations in transporter molecules have been demonstrated in disorders of the heart, muscle, brain, and endocrine and sensory organs (see examples in Table 353-1). In some cases, the same phenotype can be caused by mutations in different genes (*nonallelic heterogeneity*), often because they encode interacting proteins. In other cases, distinct mutations in the same gene (*allelic heterogeneity*) can cause different diseases depending on the degree of functional inactivation caused by the mutation, the presence of dominant-negative effects, or paradoxical activation of function.

Table 353-1 Genetic Disorders of Membrane Transport

Class of Substance and Disorder	Individual Substrates	Tissues Manifesting Transport Defect	Proposed Molecular Basis of Defect	Major Clinical Manifestations	Mode of Inheritance	Location of Discussion
AMINO ACIDS						
Classic cystinuria	Cystine, lysine, arginine, ornithine	Proximal renal tubule, jejunal mucosa	Shared dibasic-cystine transport protein	Cystine nephrolithiasis	Autosomal recessive	Chap. 353
Dibasic aminoaciduria	Lysine, arginine, ornithine	Proximal renal tubule, jejunal mucosa	Dibasic transport protein	Type I: Benign Type II: Protein intolerance, hyperammonemia, retardation	Autosomal recessive	Chap. 353
Hypercystinuria	Cystine	Proximal renal tubule	Cystine transport protein	Some risk of cystine nephrolithiasis	Autosomal recessive	Chap. 353
Lysinuria	Lysine	Proximal renal tubule, jejunal mucosa	Lysine transport protein	Seizures, physical and mental retardation	Possible autosomal recessive	Chap. 353
Hartnup disease	Neutral amino acids	Proximal renal tubule, jejunal mucosa	Shared neutral amino acid transport protein	Constant neutral aminoaciduria, intermittent symptoms of pellagra	Autosomal recessive	Chap. 353
Tryptophan malabsorption	Tryptophan	Jejunal mucosa	Tryptophan transport protein	Indoluria, ?hypercalcemia, ?nephrocalcinosis	Probable autosomal recessive	Chap. 353
Methionine malabsorption	Methionine	Jejunal mucosa	Methionine transport protein	α-Hydroxybutyricaciduria, white hair, mental retardation, convulsions, hyperpneic attacks, edema	Probable autosomal recessive	Chap. 353
Histidinuria	Histidine	Proximal renal tubule, jejunal mucosa	Histidine transport protein	Mental retardation	Autosomal recessive	Chap. 353
Iminoglycinuria	Glycine, proline, hydroxyproline	Proximal renal tubule, jejunal mucosa	Shared glycine–imino acid transport protein	None	Autosomal recessive	Chap. 353
Dicarboxylicaminoaciduria	Glutamic acid, aspartic acid	Proximal renal tubule, jejunal mucosa	Shared dicarboxylic amino acid transport protein	None	Probable autosomal recessive	Chap. 353
Cystinosis	Cystine	Lysosomal membranes	Cystine transport protein	Renal failure, hypothyroidism, blindness	Autosomal recessive	Chap. 352
HEXOSES						
Renal glycosuria	D-Glucose	Proximal renal tubule	D-glucose transport protein (Na^+-dependent)	Glycosuria with normal blood glucose	Autosomal recessive	Chap. 353
Glucose-galactose malabsorption	D-Glucose D-Galactose	Jejunal mucosa, proximal renal tubule	Shared Na^+-dependent glucose-galactose transport protein	Watery diarrhea on feeding glucose, lactose, sucrose, or galactose	Autosomal recessive	Chaps. 286, 352
Glucose-transporter protein syndrome	D-Glucose	Ubiquitous	Facilitative glucose transporter GLUT1	Seizures, mental retardation	Autosomal recessive	Chap. 353
Fanconi-Bickel syndrome	D-Glucose	Liver, kidney, pancreas, intestine	Facilitative glucose transporter GLUT2	Growth retardation rickets, hepatorenal glycogenosis, hypo- and hyperglycemia	Autosomal recessive	Chap. 353
Glycogen storage disease type ID (?)	D-Glucose	Liver microsomes	Facilitative glucose transporter GLUT7	Hypoglycemia, neutropenia, glycogen storage disease	Autosomal recessive	Chap. 350
LIPIDS						
Familial hypercholesterolemia	Cholesterol	Fibroblasts, lymphoid lines, leukocytes	Membrane LDL–cholesterol receptor protein	Hypercholesterolemia, tendon xanthomas, arcus corneae, coronary artery atherosclerosis	Autosomal dominant	Chap. 344

(continued)

Table 353-1—*(continued)*

Class of Substance and Disorder	Individual Substrates	Tissues Manifesting Transport Defect	Proposed Molecular Basis of Defect	Major Clinical Manifestations	Mode of Inheritance	Location of Discussion
Defect in transport of long-chain fatty acids	Long-chain fatty acids	Liver	Fatty acid transporter	Nonketotic hypoglycemia, acute liver failure	Autosomal recessive	
URATE						
Hypouricemia	Uric acid	Proximal renal tubule	Urate transport protein	Hypouricemia, hyperuricosuria, ?hypercalciuria	Autosomal recessive	Chap. 278
ANIONS						
Familial hypophosphatemic rickets	Inorganic phosphate	Proximal renal tubule, jejunal mucosa	Phosphate-regulator homologue to endopeptidases PHEX	Hypophosphatemia, phosphaturia, phosphatopenic rickets/ osteomalacia	X-linked dominant	Chap. 342
Congenital chloridorrhea	Chloride, sulfate	Ileal and colonic mucosa	Cl^-/HCO_3^- exchange pump carrier protein (DRA)	Hydramnios, watery diarrhea, elevated fecal chloride, achloriduria, metabolic alkalosis with volume depletion, hyperaldosteronism	Autosomal recessive	Chaps. 286, 353
Dent's syndrome, X-linked recessive hypophosphatemic rickets and nephrocalcinosis	Chloride, phosphate	Proximal renal tubule	Voltage-gated Cl^- channel CLCN5	Proteinuria, hypercalciuria, nephrocalcinosis, nephrolithiasis, rickets	X-linked recessive	Chap. 342
Hypophosphatemic rickets with hypercalciuria	Phosphate	Renal tubule	Phosphate transporter	Hypophosphatemic rickets, hypercalciuria	Autosomal recessive	Chap. 342
Bartter's syndrome	Sodium, chloride	Renal tubule	Na,K,2·Cl cotransporter, apical ATP-regulated K^+ channel, basolateral Cl^- channel	Hypochloremic metabolic alkalosis, hypercalciuria, hyperaldosteronism	Autosomal recessive	Chaps. 49, 276
Gitelman's syndrome	Sodium, chloride	Distal convoluted tubule	Na^+/Cl^- cotransporter SLC12A3	Hypokalemic metabolic alkalosis, hypomagnesemia, hypocalciuria	Autosomal recessive	Chaps. 49, 276
Congenital myotonia	Chloride	Muscle	Cl^- channel CLCN1	Myotonia, muscle cramps	Autosomal dominant and recessive	Chap. 383
Pendred syndrome	Iodide, chloride	Thyroid, cochlea	Na^+-independent I^- and Cl^- transporter	Deafness, ± goiter	Autosomal recessive	Chap. 330
Cystic fibrosis	Chloride	Lung, pancreas, sweat gland	Ion channel protein	Pulmonary, pancreatic destruction	Autosomal recessive	Chap. 257
Distal renal tubular acidosis (type I—gradient)	Chloride, bicarbonate	Distal renal tubule, erythrocytes	Anion exchanger SLC4A1	Hyperchloremic acidosis, hypokalemia, acquired nephrocalcinosis, hypercalciuria, elliptocytosis	Autosomal dominant	Chap. 276
Familial goiter	Inorganic iodide	Thyroid gland, salivary gland, gastric mucosa	Iodide transport protein	Congenital hypothyroidism (cretinism), goiter	Probable autosomal recessive	Chap. 330
Achondrogenesis type 1B, astelosteogenesis type 2, diatrophic dysplasia	Sulfate	Osteoblasts, chondrocytes	Sulfate transporter	Skeletal dysplasia, dwarfism, deformities	Autosomal recessive	Chap. 343
Dubin-Johnson syndrome	Bile acids	Liver	Biliary organic anion transporter ABCC2	Jaundice, hepatomegaly, conjugated hyperbilirubinemia	Autosomal recessive	Chap. 294

(continued)

Table 353-1 Genetic Disorders of Membrane Transport—*(continued)*

Class of Substance and Disorder	Individual Substrates	Tissues Manifesting Transport Defect	Proposed Molecular Basis of Defect	Major Clinical Manifestations	Mode of Inheritance	Location of Discussion
CATIONS						
Proximal renal tubular acidosis (type II—HCO^{3-} wasting)	Hydrogen ion	Proximal renal tubule	Proximal tubule H^+ pump carrier protein	Hyperchloremic acidosis, bicarbonate wasting	Probable autosomal recessive	Chap. 276
Menkes' disease	Copper	Most tissues except liver	Copper-transporting ATPase (ATP7A)	Severe mental retardation, pili torti (kinky hair), typical facies, arterial tortuosity, excess Wormian bones, thermal instability	X-Linked recessive	Chap. 355
Distal renal tubular acidosis	Hydrogen ion	Distal nephron, cochlea	H^+ ATPase ATP6B1	Hyperchloremic acidosis, growth retardation, sensineural deafness	Autosomal recessive	Chaps. 49, 276
Liddle's syndrome	Sodium	Collecting tubule	Epithelial Na^+ channel SCNN1 (activation)	Hypertension, hypokalemia, metabolic alkalosis	Autosomal dominant	Chaps. 49, 276
Type I pseudohypoaldosteronism	Sodium	Collecting tubule	Epithelial Na^+ channel SCNN1 (inactivation)	Hyponatremia, growth retardation, hyperkalemia	Autosomal recessive	Chaps. 49, 331
Hyperkalemic periodic paralysis, paramyotonia congenita	Sodium	Muscle	Muscle Na^+ channel α subunit SCN4A	Periodic paralysis, muscle wasting, variable myotonia	Autosomal dominant	Chap. 383
Nesidioblastosis of pancreas	Potassium	Pancreatic β cell	Sulfonylurea receptor SUR1, K^+ channel KCNJ11	Neonatal hypoglycemia, hyperinsulinemia	Autosomal recessive	Chap. 334
Wilson's disease	Copper	Liver and kidney	Copper-transporting ATPase (ATP7B)	Motor and psychiatric disturbances, hepatolenticular degeneration	Autosomal recessive	Chap. 348
Darier disease	Calcium	Keratinocytes, muscle, brain	Sarcoplasmic Ca^{2+}-ATPase ATP2A2	Keratotic skin papules, bullous lesions, psychosis	Autosomal dominant	Chap. 57
Long QT syndrome	Potassium, sodium	Heart	Voltage-gated K^+ channels KCNQ1, KCNH2, KCNE2, Na^+ channel SCN5A	Syncope, arrhythmia, sudden death	Autosomal dominant	Chap. 230
Jervell and Lange-Nielsen syndrome	Potassium	Heart, inner ear	Voltage-gated K^+ channels KCNQ1, KCNE1	Syncope, arrhythmia, sudden death, deafness	Autosomal recessive	Chap. 234
Benign familial neonatal epilepsy	Potassium	Brain	Voltage-gated K^+ channels KCNQ2, KCNQ3	Neonatal convulsions normal development	Autosomal dominant	Chap. 360
WATER						
Nephrogenic diabetes insipidus (AVP-resistant)	Water	Distal renal tubule	AVP receptor	Polyuria, polydipsia, hyposthenuria	X-linked recessive	Chap. 276, 329
Nephrogenic diabetes insipidus	Water	Collecting tubule	Aquaporin 2 (water channel)	Polyuria, dehydration, hyposthenuria	Autosomal recessive and dominant	Chap. 329
VITAMINS						
Juvenile pernicious anemia	Cobalamin (vitamin B_{12})	Ileal mucosa	Receptor for intrinsic factor–cobalamin complex	Megaloblastic anemia	Autosomal recessive	Chap. 107
Folate malabsorption	Folic acid	Small bowel	Folate transport protein	Megaloblastic anemia	Autosomal recessive	Chap. 107

(continued)

Table 353-1—*(continued)*

Class of Substance and Disorder	Individual Substrates	Tissues Manifesting Transport Defect	Proposed Molecular Basis of Defect	Major Clinical Manifestations	Mode of Inheritance	Location of Discussion
Rogers' syndrome	Thiamine	Ubiquitous	Thiamine transporter SLC19A2	Megaloblastic anemia, diabetes, deafness	Autosomal recessive	Chap. 75
OTHER						
Sialic acid storage	Sialic acid (monosaccharide)	Lysosomes	Sialic acid transport protein AST	Retardation	Autosomal recessive	Chap. 349
Carnitine transport	Carnitine	Muscle, kidney, fibroblasts	High-affinity carnitine transporter OCTN2	Hypoketotic hypoglycemia, cardiomyopathy, hypotonia	Autosomal recessive	Chap. 334
Benign recurrent and progressive familial intrahepatic cholestasis	Bile salts	Liver	Phosphatidylcholine transporter MDR3, phospholipid transporter FIC1, bile salt export pump	Cholestasis, hepatomegaly, cirrhosis, liver failure	Autosomal recessive	Chap. 294
Primary bile acid malabsorption	Bile salts	Gut	Na^+-dependent bile acid transporter	Congenital diarrhea, steatorrhea	Autosomal recessive	Chap. 294
Glycogen storage disease type Ib	D-Glucose	Liver microsomes	Glucose-6-phosphate transporter	Hypoglycemia, neutropenia, glycogen storage disease	Autosomal recessive	Chap. 350

DISORDERS OF AMINO ACID TRANSPORT

As listed in Table 353-1, 10 disorders of amino acid transport have been described. Five (cystinuria, dibasic aminoaciduria, Hartnup disease, iminoglycinuria, and dicarboxylic aminoaciduria) show transport abnormalities for structurally related amino acids, thereby implying the existence of group-specific membrane receptors or carriers. With the exception of iminoglycinuria and dicarboxylic aminoaciduria, the defects have important clinical consequences. The remaining five disorders affect the transport of only one amino acid, implying the existence of substrate-specific transport systems. Each of these conditions affects transport in the kidney, gut, or both; none has been shown to alter transport in other tissues.

CYSTINURIA **Definition** Cystinuria, the most common inborn error of amino acid transport, is characterized by impaired renal tubular reabsorption and excessive urinary excretion of the dibasic amino acids lysine, arginine, ornithine, and cystine. A similar transport defect exists in the intestinal mucosa. Because cystine is the least soluble of the naturally occurring amino acids, its overexcretion predisposes to the formation of renal, ureteral, and bladder stones. Such stones are responsible for the signs and symptoms of the disorder.

GENETIC CONSIDERATIONS Cystinuria is among the most common inborn errors, with a frequency of 1 in 10,000 to 1 in 15,000 in many ethnic groups. The disorder is transmitted as an autosomal recessive trait and results from impaired function of membrane carrier proteins in the apical brush border of proximal renal tubule and small intestinal cells.

There are three genetic variants of cystinuria. The urinary excretion patterns and renal clearance abnormalities in each type are similar in homozygotes, but the three variants are distinguished by studies of intestinal transport in homozygotes and urinary excretion patterns in heterozygotes. Type I homozygotes lack mediated intestinal transport of cystine, lysine, arginine, and ornithine; heterozygotes have normal urinary amino acid excretion patterns. Type II homozygotes lack mediated lysine transport in the gut but retain some capacity for cystine transport; heterozygotes have moderately increased urinary excretion of each of the four amino acids. Type III homozygotes retain some capacity for mediated intestinal transport of the four involved substrates; heterozygotes have modestly increased urinary lysine and cystine. The gene for type I cystinuria (*SLC3A1*) encodes solute carrier family 3 and maps to chromosome 2p16.3. The other two types of cystinuria (types II and III) are caused by mutations in *SLC7A9*, which maps to chromosome 19q13 and encodes the light subunit needed for the correct processing of SLC3A1. ■

Clinical Manifestations Massive excretion of cystine and the other disbasic amino acids occurs in homozygotes with classic cystinuria. Cystine stones account for 1 to 2% of all urinary tract calculi but are the most common cause of stones in children. The maximum solubility of cystine in the physiologic urinary pH range of 4.5 to 7.0 is about 1200 μmol/L (300 mg/L). Since affected homozygotes regularly excrete 2400 to 7200 μmol (600 to 1800 mg) daily, crystalluria and stone formation are a constant threat. Stone formation usually becomes manifest in the second or third decade but may occur in the first year of life or as bladder calculi at birth. Symptoms and signs are those typical of urolithiasis: hematuria, flank pain, renal colic, obstructive uropathy, and infection (Chap. 279). Recurrent urolithiasis may lead to progressive renal insufficiency.

Diagnosis The presence of cystine in a urinary tract stone is pathognomonic of cystinuria. However, because half the stones in cystinuric individuals are of mixed composition, and because the cystine core in as many as 10% may not be detected, a urinary nitroprusside test should be performed on all patients with urolithiasis to exclude this diagnosis. The nitroprusside test is also positive (appearance of a cherry red color) in some heterozygotes for cystinuria and in patients with hypercystinuria, homocystinuria, and mercaptolactate-cysteine disulfiduria. When cystine content exceeds 1000 μmol/L (250 mg/L), cystine crystals may be seen in the sediment of acidified, concentrated, chilled urine. These hexagonal crystals are pathognomonic of cystine overexcretion in patients not taking sulfonamides.

Diagnostic confirmation of cystinuria depends on demonstration of the characteristic amino acid excretion pattern in the urine. Selective overexcretion of cystine, lysine, arginine, and ornithine can be demonstrated by qualitative and quantitative chromatography. Quantitation is important for differentiating heterozygotes from homozygotes and for following free cystine excretion during therapy.

TREATMENT Management is aimed at preventing cystine crystal formation by reducing the concentration of cystine in urine. This aim is accomplished by increasing urinary volume and by maintaining an alkaline urine pH. Fluid ingestion in excess of 4 L/d is essential, and 5 to 7 L/d is optimal. Urinary cystine concentration should be <1000 to 1200 μmol/L (250 to 300 mg/L). The daily fluid ingestion necessary to maintain this dilution of excreted cystine should be spaced over 24 h, with one-third of the total volume ingested between bedtime and 2 to 3 A.M. Stones can be prevented and even dissolved by such hydration. It must be made clear to individuals with cystinuria that water is a necessary drug for them. Solubility of cystine in urine rises sharply above pH 7.5, and urinary alkalinization can be therapeutic in some situations. Vigorous administration of sodium bicarbonate, acetazolamide, and polycitrates is required to maintain a persistently alkaline pH, but this measure introduces the danger of inducing formation of calcium oxalate, calcium phosphate, and magnesium ammonium phosphate stones and of producing nephrocalcinosis.

Another treatment involves administration of penicillamine, which undergoes sulfhydryl-disulfide exchange with cystine to form the mixed disulfide of penicillamine and cysteine. Since this disulfide is more than 50 times as soluble as cystine, penicillamine (1 to 3 g/d) reduces free cystine excretion markedly, thereby preventing new stone formation and promoting dissolution of existing calculi. Unfortunately, side effects include acute serum sickness, agranulocytosis, pancytopenia, immune glomerulitis, and the Goodpasture syndrome. Thus its use should be reserved for patients who fail to respond to hydration alone or who are in a high-risk category (one remaining kidney, renal insufficiency). Tiopronin (α-mercaptopropionylglycine, 800 to 1200 mg/d in four divided doses) has a mechanism of action similar to that of penicillamine, has lower toxicity, and is a suitable alternative. Captopril, a sulfhydryl-containing antihypertensive agent, has limited efficacy to reduce cystine excretion. When medical management fails, urologic surgery is required, but it should be a last resort as cystine stones reform more easily in scarred epithelium. Small (<1.5 cm) cystine stones can be treated with extracorporeal shock wave lithotripsy. Ureteroscopic removal is effective for ureteral stones, while larger or branched cystine stones require percutaneous nephrostolithotomy, sometimes associated with other procedures. All these procedures may produce smaller fragments, which can cause severe renal colic. Occasional patients progress to renal failure and require kidney transplantation.

DIBASIC AMINOACIDURIA This disorder is characterized by a defect in renal tubular reabsorption of the three dibasic amino acids lysine, arginine, and ornithine but *not* cystine. There are two variants, transmitted as autosomal recessive traits. In the common form of dibasic aminoaciduria (type II), also known as *lysinuric protein intolerance*, homozygotes show defective intestinal transport of dibasic amino acids as well as exaggerated renal losses. It is most common in Finland (1 in 60,000) and is rare elsewhere. The transport defect affects basolateral rather than luminal membrane transport and is associated with impairment of the urea cycle. The defective gene (*SLC7A7*) in this condition maps to chromosome 14q11.2 and encodes a unique membrane transporter, y^+LAT, that associates with the cell-surface glycoprotein 4F2 heavy chain to form the complete sodium-independent transporter y^+L. The requirement for multiple gene products in the formation of this dimeric transporter probably explains part of the intrafamilial variability observed in lysinuric protein intolerance.

Manifestations are related to the losses of ornithine, arginine, and lysine. Affected patients present in childhood with hepatosplenomegaly, protein intolerance, and episodic ammonia intoxication. Older patients may present with severe osteoporosis, impairment of kidney function, or interstitial changes in the lungs. Plasma concentrations of lysine, arginine, and ornithine are reduced, whereas urinary excretion of lysine and orotic acid are increased. Hyperammonemia may develop after the ingestion of protein loads or with infections, probably due to insufficient amounts of arginine and ornithine to maintain proper function of the urea cycle. The clinical features have been attributed to the hyperammonemia and to insufficient amounts of lysine to support protein synthesis during growth.

Type I dibasic aminoaciduria has been described in a large French-Canadian kindred. Type I patients have profound mental retardation without hyperammonemia and protein intolerance. The condition also differs from type II by the presence of a modest excess of dibasic amino acids in the urine of asymptomatic heterozygotes. Type I disease may involve the same transport system as that impaired in the more common type II dibasic aminoaciduria.

℞ TREATMENT Dietary protein should be restricted in conjunction with supplementation of citrulline (2 to 8 g/d), a neutral amino acid that fuels the urea cycle when metabolized to arginine and ornithine. Carnitine supplements may improve growth by sparing lysine and by enhancing fatty acid oxidation. Pulmonary disease responds to glycocorticoids in some patients.

HARTNUP DISEASE Pellagra-like skin lesions, variable neurologic manifestations, and neutral or aromatic aminoaciduria characterize this disease. Alanine, serine, threonine, valine, leucine, isoleucine, phenylalanine, tyrosine, tryptophan, glutamine, asparagine, and histidine are excreted in urine in quantities 5 to 10 times normal, and intestinal transport of these same amino acids is defective. The clinical manifestations result from nutritional deficiency of the essential amino acid tryptophan, caused by its intestinal and renal malabsorption. Manifestations are episodic, related in part to metabolic demands for tryptophan. Only a small fraction of patients with the chemical findings of this disorder develop a pellagra-like syndrome, implying that manifestations depend on other factors in addition to the transport defect.

Hartnup disease is inherited as an autosomal recessive trait, and the gene has been mapped to chromosome 11q13. Homozygotes occur with a frequency of about 1 in 24,000 births. Heterozygotes exhibit no clinical or chemical abnormalities. In patients with Hartnup disease, the renal and intestinal transport defect for tryptophan leads to niacin deficiency. Tryptophan metabolism leads to the synthesis of niacin and nicotinamide-adenine dinucleotide and supplies about half the daily niacin needs. The transport defect likely reflects abnormalities of a group-specific system for neutral amino acids. Some residual reabsorptive capacity persists for each involved amino acid. This suggests that they are transported by other carrier systems as well, a conclusion supported by the identification of patients with substrate-specific transport defects for tryptophan, methionine, and histidine.

The diagnosis of Hartnup disease should be suspected in any patient with clinical features of pellagra without a history of dietary niacin deficiency (Chap. 75). The neurologic and psychiatric manifestations range from attacks of cerebellar ataxia to mild emotional lability to frank delirium and are usually accompanied by exacerbations of the erythematous, eczematoid skin rash. Fever, sunlight, stress, and sulfonamide therapy provoke clinical relapses. Diagnosis is made by detection of the neutral aminoaciduria, which does not occur in dietary niacin deficiency. Treatment is directed at niacin repletion and includes a high-protein diet and daily nicotinamide supplementation (50 to 250 mg). Tryptophan ethyl esters can also bypass the absorption defect.

IMINOGLYCINURIA This benign autosomal recessive trait is characterized by excessive urinary excretion of glycine and the imino acids proline and hydroxyproline. Homozygotes occur with a frequency of about 1 in 16,000. The enhanced excretion of glycine, proline, and hydroxyproline reflects a defect in the tubular transport system shared by these three compounds. An intestinal transport defect may also be present. This suggests that more than one mutation may lead to iminoglycinuria, a thesis corroborated by the demonstration that obligate heterozygotes from some, but not all, families have glycinuria. No consistent clinical abnormalities have been reported in homozygotes that are usually detected by urinary amino acid screening programs.

DICARBOXYLIC AMINOACIDURIA Selective urinary loss and exaggerated endogenous renal clearance of glutamic and aspartic acids have been described in two unrelated children. Intestinal absorption of these dicarboxylic amino acids was impaired in one. This patient suffered from recurrent hypoglycemia; the other was asymptomatic.

SUBSTRATE-SPECIFIC DEFECTS IN AMINO ACID TRANSPORT Rare pedigrees exist in which individuals have defective renal tubular reabsorption and/or impaired intestinal absorption of a single free amino acid (Table 353-1). These disorders, each apparently inherited as an autosomal recessive trait, suggest that transport of amino acids is catalyzed by substrate-specific as well as group-specific transport mechanisms. Examples include hypercystinuria, lysinuria, histidinuria, and selective malabsorption of methionine or tryptophan.

DISORDERS OF HEXOSE TRANSPORT

D-Glucose is the major carbohydrate used by the cell for energy production and many other anabolic purposes. A number of transporter proteins work together to maintain glucose homeostasis in the intact organism by coordinating absorption and utilization of D-glucose by all cells in the body. Two main classes of glucose transporters have been identified in humans: active Na^+-glucose cotransporters (SGLT) and the facilitative glucose transporters (GLUT). Na^+-glucose cotransporters actively concentrate glucose inside intestinal and renal cells using the electrochemical potential of Na^+ as their energy source. Defects in this class of transporters cause renal glycosuria (SGLT2) and intestinal glucose-galactose malabsorption (SGLT1). Facilitative glucose transporters allow glucose to enter cells using its own concentration gradient. This process is essential for the delivery of glucose to the cell for energy production. Defects in facilitative transporters cause the glucose-transporter protein syndrome (GLUT1) and the Fanconi-Bickel syndrome (GLUT2) and may be involved in one subtype of glycogen storage disorder (GLUT7).

DISORDERS OF CONCENTRATIVE GLUCOSE TRANSPORTERS *Renal glycosuria* is characterized by the urinary excretion of glucose at normal concentrations of blood glucose. The renal tubular malabsorption is specific for glucose. Unlike generalized tubular dysfunction, other compounds such as phosphate and amino acids are transported normally. The genetic basis for this condition is not known at present. The condition is benign, but occasionally glycosuria may be severe enough to cause polyuria and polydipsia. Even more rarely, dehydration or ketosis may develop under conditions of stress such as pregnancy or starvation.

In normal persons, glucose is present in the glomerular filtrate at a concentration equal to that in plasma water and is reabsorbed throughout the proximal renal tubule by a sodium-dependent, phlorizin-inhibitable transport process. Reabsorptive capacity exceeds normal plasma glucose concentration. The plasma concentration at which filtered glucose begins to escape proximal tubular reabsorption is usually around 10 mmol/L (200 mg/dL). Maximal renal absorptive capacity is exceeded at a filtered load of around 2 mmol (325 mg)/min per 1.73 m^2 body surface area, and this value is defined as the tubular maximum for glucose (TmG).

Two patterns of glycosuria are recognized: type A, characterized by a reduced tubular maximum reabsorptive capacity, and type B, showing a reduced threshold for glycosuria, an increased "splay" in the titration curve, and a normal TmG. Renal glycosuria occurs in homozygotes with either of these recessively inherited mutations and in compound heterozygotes with these presumably allelic mutations. Modest reduction in renal threshold or TmG is present in heterozygotes in some families; modest glycosuria occurs in such family members when plasma glucose is elevated. In the few patients studied, renal glycosuria was not associated with impaired intestinal transport.

Glucose-galactose malabsorption is characterized by profuse, watery diarrhea in infants fed milk or foods containing lactose, sucrose, glucose, or galactose. The primary defect involves the sodium-hexose cotransporter in the intestinal and renal brush border. A specific defect in intestinal absorption of glucose and galactose can be demonstrated by oral tolerance tests that produce little or no increase in plasma glucose or galactose. Active D-glucose and D-galactose transport is absent in affected children, and intermediate transport capacity is present in their parents. Fructose-containing or carbohydrate-free formulas are well tolerated. Treatment with a glucose- and galactose-free diet leads to resolution of symptoms in childhood. Although the basic transport defect is present throughout life, most patients show an improved tolerance for glucose and galactose with age.

A number of these patients have renal glycosuria at normal plasma glucose concentrations. Renal titration studies generally demonstrate a reduced threshold for glucose reabsorption (type B renal glycosuria) and a normal TmG. Urinary glucose loss is not as severe as in isolated renal glycosuria. This finding suggests the presence of multiple glucose transport proteins in the kidney. One, whose gene remains to be identified, is responsible for the bulk of glucose reabsorption in the proximal convoluted tubule and is believed to be abnormal in renal glycosuria. Another transporter, SGLT1, is shared by glucose and galactose and is responsible for the reabsorption of the least traces of glucose in the late proximal straight tubule. Its function is abnormal in glucose-galactose malabsorption, and heterogeneous mutations have been found in the *SGLT1* gene on chromosome 22q. In glucose-galactose malabsorption, as in renal glycosuria, transport of sugars in other tissues is normal, reflecting the multiplicity and tissue specificity of hexose transporters.

DISORDERS OF FACILITATIVE GLUCOSE TRANSPORTERS At least five different facilitative glucose transporters (GLUT1, -2, -3, -4, and -7) mediate the influx and efflux of glucose in mammalian cells. Disease-causing mutations have been identified in two of these transporters (GLUT1 and GLUT2). The tissue specificity and redundancy of facilitative glucose transporters in different tissues helps to explain the clinical manifestations that result from their defective function. De novo mutations in the gene encoding the ubiquitous GLUT1 transporter cause the glucose-transporter protein syndrome. Patients present with seizures, developmental delay, and acquired microcephaly. These patients have normal blood glucose concentration but markedly decreased concentration of glucose in their cerebrospinal fluid. GLUT1 is the predominant glucose transporter in the blood-brain barrier. Haploinsufficiency reduces the transfer of glucose through the blood-brain barrier, restricting the energy supply to the brain. This defect is expressed in other cells, such as erythrocytes and fibroblasts, that have less stringent energy requirements or express additional glucose transporters, preventing cellular damage and clinical sequelae. Therapy in the glucose-transporter protein syndrome consists of using a ketogenic diet to deliver alternative fuels to the brain.

The GLUT2 transporter is expressed mainly in liver, pancreatic β cells, and in the basolateral membrane of gut and renal tubular cells. Truncating mutations in the *GLUT2* transporter gene have been identified in the autosomal recessive disorder Fanconi-Bickel syndrome. Patients present early in life with failure to thrive and polydipsia, with prominent glycosuria and aminoaciduria, rickets, fasting hypoglycemia with ketonuria, and prolonged postprandial hyperglycemia. Glycogen is accumulated in the liver and kidney, reflecting the inability to release glucose through the GLUT2 transporter. This results in fasting hypoglycemia and ketonuria and in generalized renal tubular dysfunction. The prolonged postprandial hyperglycemia is due to decreased sugar uptake by the liver and by the pancreatic β cell, the latter resulting in defective insulin synthesis and release. Affected patients do not develop diabetes because human pancreatic β cells have alternative glucose transporters (GLUT1 and GLUT3) that can partially compensate for the absence of GLUT2 transporters. Therapy consists of symptomatic replacement of the renal losses of water and electrolytes, vitamin D replacement, and a diet plan consisting of frequent meals rich in complex carbohydrates to prevent hypoglycemia, analogous to the treatment of patients with glycogen storage diseases (Chap. 350).

DEFECTIVE ANION TRANSPORT: CHLORIDORRHEA

This rare, autosomal recessive disease results from impairment of active transport of chloride in the ileum and colon. Absence of chloride-bicarbonate ion exchange causes profound symptoms even before birth (polyhydramnios and absence of meconium). Massive watery diarrhea is apparent from the first days of life. This fluid loss, with its attendant impairment of electrolyte homeostasis, is life-threatening. A hypokalemic, hypochloremic, hyponatremic metabolic alkalosis develops with dehydration and secondary hyperaldosteronism. Fecal fluid contains an excess of chloride ion over the sum of the accompanying cations sodium and potassium. Fecal chloride concentration always exceeds 90 mmol/L when volume and serum electrolyte disturbances are corrected, and this chloridorrhea is diagnostic. Renal chloride transport is normal. Decreased urine chloride results from the kidney's attempts to conserve salt and water. The defective gene in this condition, called *DRA* (for downregulated in adenoma), maps to chromosome 7q and encodes an anion transporter, which is expressed only in the gastrointestinal tract. A deletion of the Val 317 codon in the *DRA* gene is responsible for the Finnish form of congenital chloride diarrhea.

Treatment requires adequate, lifelong repletion of electrolyte and fluid losses. Exact replacement of water, sodium chloride, and potassium chloride can prevent the growth and psychomotor retardation and the development of progressive renal damage. The renal lesion, with hyalinized glomeruli, juxtaglomerular hyperplasia, calcifications, and arteriolar changes, is probably a result of chronic volume depletion. Treatment of hyperreninemia and hypokalemia with prostaglandin inhibitors may reduce renal damage but does not alter intestinal symptoms or the need for chronic sodium chloride repletion. Omeprazole, while not decreasing the need for adequate oral replacement of electrolytes, may decrease stool output and improve the social life of patients.

ACKNOWLEDGMENT

This chapter includes the contributions of Dr. Leon E. Rosenberg and Dr. Louis J. Elsas from previous editions.

BIBLIOGRAPHY

BORSANI G et al: SLC7A7, encoding a putative permease-related protein, is mutated in patients with lysinuric protein intolerance. Nat Genet 21:297, 1999

DESJEUX J-F et al: Congenital selective Na^+ D-glucose cotransport defects leading to renal glycosuria and congenital selective intestinal malabsorption of glucose and galactose, in *The Molecular and Metabolic Bases of Inherited Disease*, 7th ed, CR Scriver et al (eds). New York, McGraw-Hill, 1995, pp 3563–3580

ELSAS LJ, ROSENBERG LE: Renal glycosuria, in *Strauss and Welt's Diseases of the Kidney*, 3d ed, LE Earley, CW Gottschalk (eds). Boston, Little, Brown, 1979, pp 1021–1028

LEVY HL: Hartnup disorder, in *The Molecular and Metabolic Bases of Inherited Disease*, 8th ed, CR Scriver et al (eds). New York, McGraw-Hill, 2001, pp 4957–4969

LONGO N, ELSAS LJ: Human glucose transporters. Adv Pediatr 45:293, 1998

PALACIN M et al: Cystinuria, in *The Molecular and Metabolic Bases of Inherited Disease*, 8th ed, CR Scriver et al (eds). New York, McGraw-Hill, 2001, pp 4909–4932

SHORT EM, ROSENBERG LE: Renal aminoaciduria, in *Strauss and Welt's Diseases of the Kidney*, 3d ed, LE Earley, CW Gottschalk (eds). Boston, Little, Brown, 1979, pp 975–1020

TORRENTS D et al: Identification of SLC7A7, encoding y+LAT-1, as the lysinuric protein intolerance gene. Nat Genet 21:293, 1999

Abhimanyu Garg

THE LIPODYSTROPHIES AND OTHER PRIMARY DISORDERS OF ADIPOSE TISSUE

The distribution and quantity of adipose tissue are controlled by multiple factors, including genetic background, diet, hormones, and exercise. The lipodystrophies are a heterogeneous group of adipose tissue disorders characterized by a selective loss of body fat (Tables 354-1 and 354-2). Patients with lipodystrophies have a propensity to develop insulin resistance, hypertriglyceridemia, diabetes mellitus, and fatty liver.

FAMILIAL OR GENETIC LIPODYSTROPHIES

CONGENITAL GENERALIZED LIPODYSTROPHY (BERARDINELLI-SEIP SYNDROME) ***Clinical features*** The primary diagnostic features of congenital generalized lipodystrophy (CGL) include a near-total lack of body fat and a marked muscular appearance from birth (Fig. 354-1*A*). On careful physical examination, however, fat can be detected in the palms and soles; with magnetic resonance imaging (MRI), normal amounts of fat can also be visualized in the orbits, scalp, perineum, and juxtaarticular and epidural regions (where the cushioning or protective functions of adipose tissue are critical). MRI studies also reveal a near-complete absence of metabolically active adipose tissue from most subcutaneous areas, intra-abdominal and intrathoracic regions, and bone marrow.

Children exhibit accelerated linear growth and advanced bone age, but plasma levels of growth hormone or insulin-like growth factor I (IGF-I) are normal. Their basal metabolic rate is relatively high. It is unclear, however, whether hypermetabolism results from a primary increase in sympathetic nervous system activity or whether it is a compensatory response to protect against excessive heat loss due to extreme lack of body fat. Other features include acanthosis nigricans, prominent umbilicus or hernia, and an acromegalic appearance with coarse facial features and large hands and feet. Occasionally, excess body hair and hyperhidrosis have been noted. Fatty liver has been noted during infancy and can lead to cirrhosis and its complications. Liver, spleen, and kidney enlargement can cause abdominal protuberance. A few patients develop hypertrophic cardiomyopathy, but it rarely leads to heart failure.

Postpubertal women may have clitoromegaly, mild hirsutism, polycystic ovaries, and oligomenorrhea. Successful pregnancy in affected women is rare, whereas affected males have normal reproductive potential. Penile enlargement may be noted in childhood. After puberty, the skeleton appears sclerotic and focal lytic lesions develop in the appendicular bones. Some patients develop goiter.

Metabolic abnormalities Patients with CGL have markedly elevated fasting serum insulin and C-peptide concentrations, as well as extreme insulin resistance. Diabetes mellitus appears during the pubertal years, and pancreatic pathology reveals severe amyloidosis of

Table 354-1 Classification of Lipodystrophies

FAMILIAL OR GENETIC FORMS
Congenital generalized lipodystrophy (CGL; Berardinelli-Seip Syndrome)
Familial partial lipodystrophy
Dunnigan variety (FPLD)
Köbberling variety
Mandibuloacral dysplasia variety
Other types
ACQUIRED FORMS
Acquired generalized lipodystrophy (Lawrence syndrome)
Acquired partial lipodystrophy (Barraquer-Simons syndrome)
HIV-1 protease inhibitor–induced lipodystrophy
Localized lipodystrophies

Table 354-2 Distinguishing Features of Various Lipodystrophies

Feature	Congenital Generalized	Familial Partial (Dunnigan)	Acquired Generalized	Acquired Partial	HIV-1 Protease Inhibitor–induced
Pathogenesis	Genetic, autosomal recessive	Genetic, autosomal dominant	Autoimmune or post-viral infection	Autoimmune or post-viral infection	Drug-induced
Age of onset	Birth	Puberty	Childhood	Childhood	All ages
Sex incidence	Equal	Equal	Female preponderance	Female preponderance	Male preponderance
Areas with fat loss	Face, neck, trunk, limbs, intraabdominal, intrathoracic, bone marrow	Trunk, limbs	Face, neck, trunk, limbs, palms, soles	Face, neck, upper trunk, and upper limbs	Face, trunk, limbs
Areas with excess fat	None	Face, neck, intraabdominal	None	Lower abdomen, hips, lower limbs	Neck, upper back, intraabdominal
Insulin resistance	Severe	Mild to moderate	Severe	Usually absent	Mild to moderate
Diabetes mellitus	During teenage	After 2nd decade	During teenage	Rare	Occasional
Hypertriglyceridemia	Moderate to severe	Moderate to severe	Moderate to severe	Rare	Moderate to severe
Fatty liver, hepatomegaly	Severe	Mild to moderate	Severe	Usually absent	Mild
Acanthosis nigricans	Severe	Absent or mild	Absent or mild	Absent	Absent
Polycystic ovaries, menstrual abnormalities	Frequent	In one-fifth	None	None	None
Umbilical hernia	Present	Absent	Absent	Absent	Absent
Kidney pathology	Nephromegaly; diabetic nephropathy later	Diabetic nephropathy later	Diabetic nephropathy later	Membranocapillary glomerulonephritis	None
Autoimmune diseases	None	None	Relatively common	Relatively common	None

the pancreatic islets with loss of β cells. Plasma leptin concentrations are low, as expected in view of the reduced adipose tissue. Fasting plasma free fatty acid concentrations are normal. Hypertriglyceridemia may be observed during childhood, and patients can develop chylomicronemia, eruptive xanthomas, and acute pancreatitis. Low concentrations of high-density lipoprotein (HDL) cholesterol are also common.

Course Patients with CGL are at risk of early mortality from cirrhosis and its complications, acute pancreatitis, or diabetic nephropathy. They also may develop diabetic retinopathy. Despite long-standing hypertriglyceridemia and hyperglycemia, atherosclerotic vascular complications are rare.

GENETIC CONSIDERATIONS Approximately 120 patients of various ethnic backgrounds have been reported with this autosomal recessive form of lipodystrophy. The absence of fat could result from agenesis, failure of differentiation of preadipocytes, or an inability of mature adipocytes to synthesize and/or store triglycerides. Numerous candidate genes have been excluded, including the insulin receptor, β_3-adrenergic receptor, fatty acid binding protein 2, IGF-I receptor, insulin receptor substrate-1, hormone-sensitive lipase, leptin, and peroxisome proliferator–activated receptor γ. Genome-wide linkage analysis of 17 families revealed genetic heterogeneity, but a candidate *CGL1* gene was localized to chromosome 9q34; the defective *CGL* gene(s) have yet to be identified. ■

FAMILIAL PARTIAL LIPODYSTROPHY Dunnigan Variety • ***Clinical features*** Patients with familial partial lipodystrophy, Dunnigan variety (FPLD) appear normal during childhood. During puberty, however, these patients begin to lose subcutaneous fat from the limbs and trunk, while exhibiting "increased muscularity" (Fig. 354-1*B*). Many patients accumulate excess fat in the face and neck, often resulting in a double chin, supraclavicular humps, and round face. Occasionally, fat accumulates in the axillae. Labia majora appear prominent in women. MRI demonstrates excess fat inside the abdomen and in the intermuscular fasciae. Bone marrow and fat in certain mechanical locations, such as the orbits and joints, are normal. Acanthosis nigricans, hirsutism, menstrual abnormalities, and polycystic ovaries are infrequent. Hepatomegaly due to fatty liver is common, but progression to cirrhosis has not been reported.

Metabolic abnormalities Patients with FPLD have mild to moderate insulin resistance, and diabetes mellitus develops, usually after the second decade. Patients have low serum HDL cholesterol and can develop severe hypertriglyceridemia. Fasting plasma free fatty acid concentrations may be elevated.

Course Major causes of morbidity and mortality in patients with FPLD include coronary heart disease, other atherosclerotic vascular complications, and acute pancreatitis.

GENETIC CONSIDERATIONS This rare autosomal dominant disorder has been reported in 35 Caucasian families and one Indian family comprising approximately 200 affected individuals. The *FPLD* locus has been mapped to chromosome 1q21-22. Recently, several missense mutations in the gene encoding the nuclear envelope protein lamin A/C (*LMNA*) have been found to be responsible for FPLD. Alternative splicing of *LMNA* produces Lamins A and C, members of the intermediate filament multigene family. All mutations causing typical FPLD cluster in exon 8 of *LMNA*, affecting the globular C-terminal tail of the Lamin A/C protein except one in exon 11 that only affects Lamin A and causes an atypical mild FPLD. The loss of subcutaneous adipose tissue in the limbs and trunk in FPLD may be due to adipocyte apoptosis and degeneration. Fat accumulation in the face and neck may be a secondary phenomenon, since it is not always present. ■

Köbberling Variety Characteristic features include loss of fat from the limbs with preservation of facial fat; truncal subcutaneous fat may be excessive. Most patients have hypertriglyceridemia and diabetes mellitus. Still unknown are the pattern of inheritance, age of onset, and whether this disorder is a distinct entity or a variant of the Dunnigan variety. Only a few women from two small pedigrees and four sporadic cases have been reported; it is not yet clear whether men can also be affected.

Mandibuloacral Dysplasia Variety This autosomal recessive disorder is characterized by short stature, high-pitched voice, mandibular and clavicular hypoplasia, dental abnormalities, acroosteolysis, stiff joints, and ectodermal defects. A few patients have also exhibited loss of limb fat. Insulin resistance and diabetes mellitus are rare.

OTHER TYPES An autosomal dominant type of generalized lipodystrophy with acromegaloid features has been reported in a pedigree from Brazil. The onset of lipodystrophy occurred after 18 years of age. In another form of lipodystrophy, marked loss of subcutaneous fat from the limbs, face, palms, and soles, but excess subcutaneous fat in the neck and trunk has been noted.

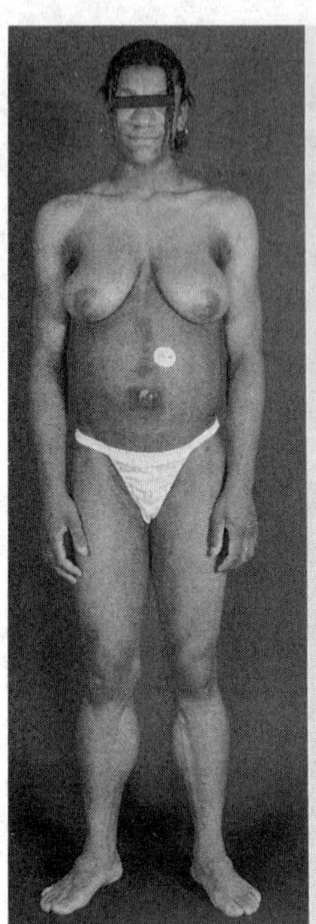
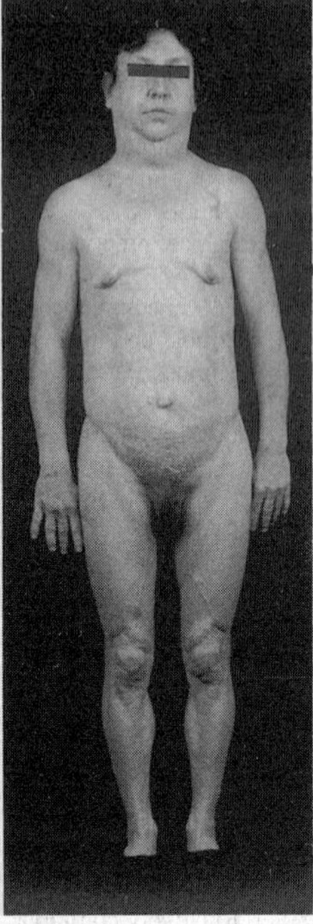
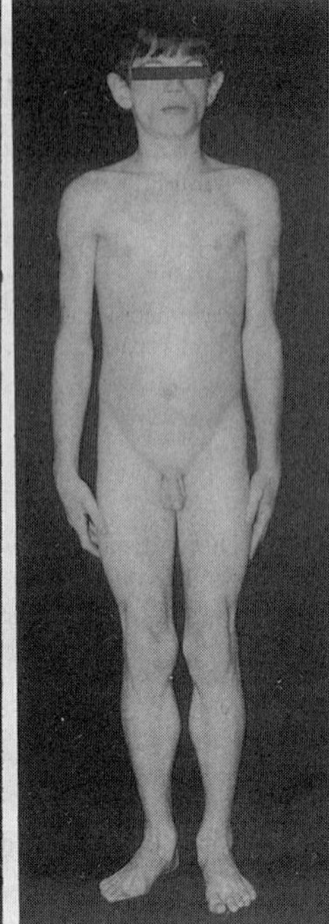
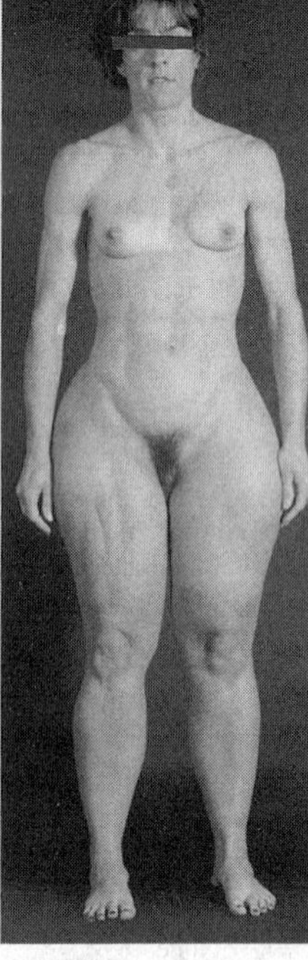

FIGURE 354-1 Anterior view of patients with different forms of lipodystrophy. *A.* Congenital generalized lipodystrophy: a 16-year-old girl with generalized loss of fat, acromegaloid features, severe acanthosis nigricans affecting axillae and abdomen, umbilical hernia. *B.* Familial partial lipodystrophy, Dunnigan variety: a 43-year-old woman with marked loss of subcutaneous fat from both the limbs and trunk and excess fat deposition in the face, chin, supraclavicular area, and labia majora. *C.* Acquired generalized lipodystrophy: a 10-year-old boy who developed generalized loss of fat that also affected the palms and soles after panniculitis at the age of 3 months. *D.* Acquired partial lipodystrophy: a 30-year-old woman with onset of lipodystrophy at age 14 years shows loss of fat from the face, neck, upper limbs, trunk, and anterior thighs. There is accumulation of excess fat in the hips and other regions of lower limbs. *(Parts A and B are reproduced with permission from the Endocrine Society and Nature Genetics.)*

ACQUIRED LIPODYSTROPHIES

ACQUIRED GENERALIZED LIPODYSTROPHY (LAWRENCE SYNDROME) This form of lipodystrophy has been reported in approximately 50 patients and is characterized by a generalized disappearance of fat, mostly during childhood or adolescence. It is three times more common in females than males.

Clinical features Fat loss affects the face, neck, trunk, and extremities and usually occurs over several months or years; superficial veins and muscles become prominent (Fig. 354-1*C*). Fat loss can include the palms and soles. In some, the onset of the disorder was reported after infections such as varicella, measles, pertussis, diphtheria, pneumonia, osteomyelitis, parotitis, infectious mononucleosis, or hepatitis. In others, lipodystrophy starts with painful, purple-brown subcutaneous nodules that leave depressed areas with loss of subcutaneous fat. Adipose tissue may show infiltration with lymphocytes, mononuclear macrophages, fat-cell necrosis, and fat-filled macrophages; this infiltration is consistent with a type of acute panniculitis. Almost one-third of these patients develop acanthosis nigricans, and some have mild hirsutism. Hepatomegaly due to fatty infiltration is a consistent finding and can lead to cirrhosis. Splenomegaly has also been reported.

Metabolic abnormalities Ketosis-resistant diabetes mellitus usually occurs after the onset of lipodystrophy, and metabolic abnormalities are similar to those in CGL. Severely hyperglycemic patients may have elevated plasma free fatty acids.

Pathogenesis It is not yet known whether preceding infections play a causal role in this disorder. Some patients reportedly develop autoimmune diseases, including childhood dermatomyositis, juvenile rheumatoid arthritis, Hashimoto's thyroiditis, vitiligo, hemolytic anemia, or chronic active hepatitis. Autoantibodies against adipocyte membranes have been reported; it seems likely that antibody- and/or cell-mediated adipocyte lysis causes fat loss in these patients.

ACQUIRED PARTIAL LIPODYSTROPHY (BARRAQUER-SIMONS SYNDROME) This form of lipodystrophy affects females three times more often than males and has been reported in about 200 patients. The onset usually occurs during childhood or adolescence. Fat loss typically affects the face, neck, upper limbs, thorax, and upper abdomen, and there is increased fat deposition in the hips and lower extremities (Fig. 354-1*D*).

Clinical features Fat loss occurs gradually over 1 to 2 years and initially affects the face; other areas are affected later. In most cases, the lower abdomen, hips, and lower extremities are spared. In general, patients do not develop insulin resistance and other metabolic abnormalities, acanthosis nigricans, hirsutism, or menstrual problems. Approximately one-third of patients develop mesangiocapillary glomerulonephritis, usually 10 years after disease onset. Systemic lupus erythematosus and other autoimmune diseases have also been reported, including childhood dermatomyositis, thyroiditis, pernicious anemia, celiac disease, dermatitis herpetiformis, rheumatoid arthritis, Sjögren's syndrome, temporal arteritis, and leukocytoclastic vasculitis. In addition, many patients have serum antinuclear and anti-double-stranded DNA antibodies.

Pathogenesis C3 nephritic factor (C3NeF), a polyclonal IgG immunoglobulin, can be detected in the serum of up to 90% of these patients. Serum C3 is universally low, but C1q, C4, C5, C6, factor B, and properdin concentrations are usually normal (which suggests activation of the alternative complement pathway). Loss of fat may be due to C3NeF-induced lysis of adipocytes that express factor D. C3NeF also binds and inactivates factor H, which can induce glomerulonephritis by mechanisms similar to those seen in genetic factor H deficiency.

HIV-1 PROTEASE INHIBITOR–INDUCED LIPODYSTROPHY Highly active antiretroviral therapy (HAART) therapy for HIV, a combination which includes HIV-1 protease inhibitors, is associated with the development of lipodystrophy in the majority of patients after 18 months to 2 years of treatment (Chap. 309). It is characterized by marked reduction in subcutaneous fat from the face, trunk, and limbs, resulting in an appearance of "increased muscularity." Excess fat may also accumulate around the neck (double chin and buffalo hump) and inside the abdomen. Patients are prone to develop insulin resistance, diabetes mellitus, and hypertriglyceridemia. It is unclear whether this disorder is caused by a side effect of one or more of the drugs (most likely a protease inhibitor) or by a metabolic response to dramatic reduction of viral load. Hormonal causes, such as hypercortisolism, have been excluded.

LOCALIZED LIPODYSTROPHIES These disorders are characterized by a loss of subcutaneous adipose tissue from small areas or parts of a limb. Fat loss may occur secondary to injections of insulin, glucocorticoids, antibiotics, iron dextrans, or diphtheria/pertussis/tetanus vaccine. Repeated pressure against any body part, such as the thigh or chin, can cause lipodystrophy. In some patients, acute panniculitis causes localized lipodystrophy without progressing further. *Centrifugal lipodystrophy* begins in the abdomen, groin, and axillae of children under the age of 3, and eventually spreads to involve the entire abdomen. The surrounding areas show slightly erythematous and scaly changes with an accumulation of lymphocytes and histiocytes on histology. Complete or partial improvement occurs spontaneously after 8 to 10 years.

TREATMENT Patients with lipodystrophies have cosmetic problems that warrant judicious treatment. Facial reconstruction can be accomplished with free flaps, transposition of facial muscle, and silicone or other implants. In acquired partial lipodystrophy, adipose tissue transplantation from the thigh to face lasts for only 2 to 5 years. In FPLD, excess fat in the face and neck may require liposuction or lipectomy. Etretinate and fish oil have improved acanthosis nigricans in some patients with generalized lipodystrophy.

Dietary fat should be restricted for patients with severe hypertriglyceridemia. Reduced energy intake and increased physical activity can mitigate insulin resistance. In children, however, enough energy should be provided to allow for normal growth and development. Medium chain triglycerides have been reported to benefit some patients with acquired generalized lipodystrophy.

In patients with CGL, diabetes control may require extremely high doses of insulin. Oral hypoglycemic agents may also be used (Chap. 333). Glycemic control can mitigate dyslipidemia and prevent diabetic complications. Severe hypertriglyceridemia should be treated with fibrates and/or omega-3 polyunsaturated fatty acids. Niacin worsens glycemic control and should not be used. Estrogens should be avoided because they may accentuate hypertriglyceridemia and can cause acute pancreatitis.

LIPOMATOSIS

MULTIPLE SYMMETRIC LIPOMATOSIS (MADELUNG DISEASE) This type of lipomatosis affects men 4 to 15 times more frequently than women. It is characterized by a symmetric, progressive growth of nonencapsulated subcutaneous adipose tissue, primarily in the neck (bull neck with buffalo hump and double chin) and supraclavicular and shoulder regions. Fat may also accumulate in the trunk and proximal limbs, though the distal arms and legs are spared. Rarely, laryngeal, tracheal, or vena caval compression may occur from deep lipomatous infiltration in the neck and mediastinum. Many patients also have peripheral neuropathy; hypertriglyceridemia and hyperuricemia are uncommon. Serum HDL cholesterol levels are usually elevated, and diabetes mellitus has not been reported.

Most of these patients have a preceding history of heavy ethanol intake. The underlying mechanisms and predisposing factors for the disorder, however, remain unknown. The lipomatous tissue contains small adipocytes (but not brown fat) with increased lipoprotein lipase activity and reduced catecholamine-stimulated lipolysis. In several families and in some sporadic cases, mitochondrial DNA mutations A-to-G and G-to-A transitions at nucleotides 8344 and 8363, respectively, or deletions in the $tRNA^{Lys}$ gene have been reported. Most of these patients had multiple, discrete, and encapsulated lipomas in the neck and trunk, which is distinct from the features of typical patients with multiple symmetric lipomatosis. These patients also have associated peripheral neuropathy, myopathy, cerebellar ataxia, myoclonus, or hearing loss. Mitochondrial DNA mutations have not been found in many patients with typical multiple symmetric lipomatosis.

Surgical resection may be required to relieve compression or for cosmetic reasons. Cessation of alcohol intake does not result in regression but may slow growth rate.

OTHER FORMS OF LIPOMATOSIS *Mediastinal lipomatosis* is characterized by local overgrowth of adipose tissue in the mediastinum. It occurs in patients with Cushing's syndrome and can occasionally cause tracheal compression.

Pelvic lipomatosis is characterized by overgrowth of pelvic fat, causing bladder dysfunction (frequency, dysuria, and nocturia), constipation, and lower abdominal pain. Bilateral ureteral obstruction may also occur. The male:female ratio is 18:1. The etiology is not known, but the condition may result from a localized manifestation of obesity. Surgery may be needed to relieve urinary tract obstruction.

Epidural lipomatosis occurs in obese patients or in those receiving exogenous steroid therapy. Fat deposition most often occurs in the thoracic or lumbar spine, causing back pain, radicular pain, or spinal cord compression. Laminectomy may be indicated for cord compression. Weight loss or discontinuation of steroid therapy may also be helpful.

ADIPOSIS DOLOROSA (DERCUM DISEASE)

This is a rare disease of unknown etiology that mainly affects obese postmenopausal women (female:male ratio, 30:1). It is characterized by the presence of multiple circumscribed or diffuse painful subcutaneous fat deposits on the trunk and limbs, particularly near the knees. Patients also report weakness, fatigue, and emotional lability. Relief of pain is difficult; intravenous lidocaine, glucocorticoids, surgical excision, and liposuction are sometimes helpful.

ACUTE PANNICULITIS

A variety of systemic diseases including collagen vascular diseases such as systemic lupus erythematosus and scleroderma are associated with *acute panniculitis*, or *nodular fat necrosis* (Chap. 311). Panniculitis may also occur as a manifestation of lymphoproliferative disorders (Chap. 112).

Disseminated fat necrosis is usually associated with acute pancreatitis or pancreatic carcinoma. It may be caused by the release of pancreatic enzymes into the circulation (Chap. 304).

HORMONAL EFFECTS ON ADIPOSE DISTRIBUTION

A variety of hormones influence the distribution of adipose tissue. Growth hormone, for example, reduces truncal fat but can increase fat in the palms and soles. Insulin enhances lipogenesis and fat storage. Thyroid hormones increase metabolic rate, including energy expenditure by fat tissue. Estrogens induce fat accumulation in the hips, legs, breasts and other subcutaneous regions. Glucocorticoids redistribute adipose tissue from peripheral to central locations. In Cushing's syndrome, characteristic features include buffalo hump, increased supraclavicular and truncal fat.

BIBLIOGRAPHY

BRODOVSKY J et al: Adiposis dolorsa (Dercum's disease): 10 year follow-up. Ann Plast Surg 33:664, 1994

CARR A et al: A syndrome of peripheral lipodystrophy, hyperlipidaemia and insulin resistance in patients receiving HIV protease inhibitors. AIDS 2:F51, 1998

GAMEZ J et al: Familial multiple symmetric lipomatosis associated with the A8344G mutation of mitochondrial DNA. Neurology 51:258, 1998

GARG A: Lipodystrophies. Am J Med 108:143, 2000

GARG A et al: Adipose tissue distribution pattern in patients with familial partial lipodystrophy (Dunnigan variety). J Clin Endocrinol Metab 84:170, 1999

——— et al: A gene for congenital generalized lipodystrophy maps to human chromosome 9q34. J Clin Endocrinol Metab 84:3390, 1999

KOBBERLING J et al: Lipodystrophy of the extremities. A dominantly inherited syndrome associated with lipoatrophic diabetes. Humangenetik 29:111, 1975

PETERS JM et al: Localization of the gene for familial partial lipodystrophy (Dunnigan variety) to chromosome 1q21-22. Nat Genet 18:292, 1998

SEIP M, TRYGSTAD O: Generalized lipodystrophy, congenital and acquired (lipoatrophy). Acta Paediatr Suppl 413:2, 1996

SPECKMAN RA et al: Mutational and haplotype analyses of families with familial partial lipodystrophy (Dunnigan variety) reveal recurrent missense mutations in the globular C-terminal domain of lamin A/C. Am J Hum Genet 66:1192, 2000

NOBEL PRIZE IN PHYSIOLOGY OR MEDICINE, 1923

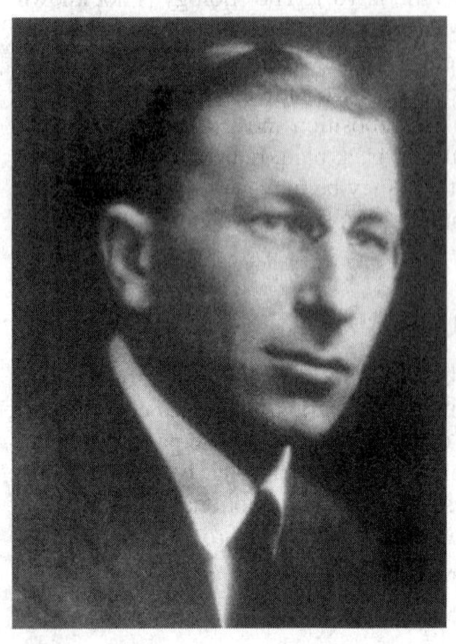

Frederick G. Banting was born on November 14, 1891, in Alliston, Ontario, Canada. He was the youngest of five children born to Margaret and William Banting, hard-working farmers. After high school Banting was accepted to theUniversity of Toronto to study for the Methodist ministry; however, at the end of the first year he switched to medicine. In 1917, after completion of medical school, he saw service in World War I in France, where he was wounded and received the Military Cross. After the war he sought a permanent position in surgery at the University of Toronto based on his wartime experiences but was unsuccessful; he therefore entered private practice. He obtained, however, an appointment as a demonstrator at the University of Western Ontario, where he became interested in medical research. Banting's private practice did not flourish, and he became quite frustrated. On the background of a faltering practice, Banting had two other possibilities—accompany an oil exploration to Northwest Canada as a doctor or find a laboratory in which to pursue his ideas about diabetes.

It is said that his interest in diabetes occurred at an early age when he lost a childhood friend to the disease. Banting had read an article about the pancreas and diabetes in which two areas of the pancreas were discussed: one produced exocrine substances for food digestion in the intestine, and the other, the islets of Langerhans, appeared to be degenerated in diabetic patients. However, multiple researchers had failed to treat diabetic patients successfully with various pancreatic extracts. Banting reasoned that if the pancreatic ducts were ligated, the exocrine portion of the pancreas would atrophy, thereby facilitating the isolation of the endocrine extract that was lacking in the diabetic patient. Banting contacted John J.R. Macleod, Professor of Physiology at the University of Toronto, with his idea. The senior Macleod was quite skeptical, in part because of Banting's lack of research experience. Nevertheless, Macleod thought it was worth a try and appointed Charles Best, who was in his final undergraduate year in physiology and biochemistry, as Banting's assistant.

After many dogs had died, Banting and Best finally had an animal whose pancreatic ducts had been tied and the exocrine portion of the pancreas had degenerated. The extract of the remaining portion of the pancreas rapidly lowered the blood and urine sugar in a pancreatectomized diabetic dog. A second diabetic dog was near coma and actually awakened and walked on administration of the pancreatic extract (figure). Both dogs, however, died one day later. James Collip, a biochemist with expertise in processing tissue extracts, was then enlisted to provide a purer pancreatic extract for administration to humans with diabetes. In January, 1922, a 14-year-old diabetic boy received the first purified extract; he improved immediately. Similar results were obtained with six other diabetic patients. In 1923 Banting shared the Nobel Prize in Physiology or Medicine with John Macleod for his discovery of insulin. He shared the monetary award of the prize with Charles Best.

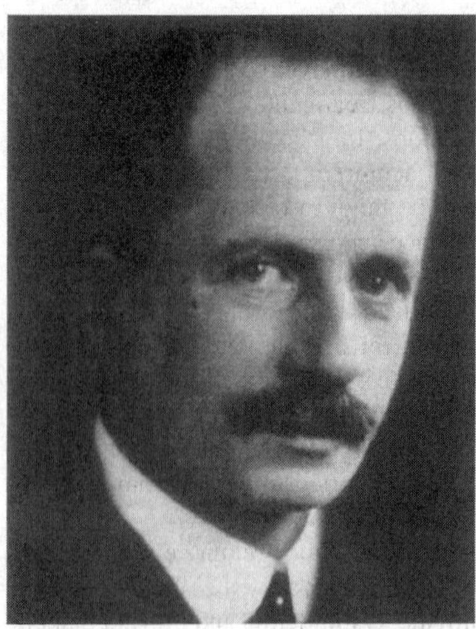

John J. R. Macleod was born on September 6, 1876, in Cluny, Perthshire, Scotland to Jane and Robert Macleod, a minister. Macleod received his early schooling at Aberdeen Gramar School and then matriculated into the University of Aberdeen to study medicine. He graduated with honors, then studied biochemistry at the University of Leipzig in Germany. Macleod then was a demonstrator in physiology and later a lecturer in biochemistry. In 1903 he was appointed Professor of Physiology at Western Reserve University in the United States where he commenced his studies in diabetes mellitus. In 1918 he was appointed Professor and Head of the Physiology Department at the University of Toronto in Canada where Frederick G. Banting contacted him about conducting research in diabetes. Prior to this time, Macleod had focused his research predominantly on non-pancreatic aspects of glucose regulation, particularly the role of the liver and the central nervous system. With the discovery of insulin and the award of the Nobel Prize to Banting and Macleod, there was substantial debate about what role Macleod had played in the discovery. He certainly had lent the facilities of his department for Best's and Banting's research. As Banting shared his prize money with Best, Macleod shared his prize money with James Collip who had purified the pancreatic extract.

REFERENCES

1. Aaseng N: *The Disease Fighters*. Minneapolis, Lerner Publications, 1987
2. Magill FN (ed): *Nobel Prize Winners: Physiology and Medicine*, vol 1. Pasadena, Salem Press, 1993
3. Schrier RW: *A Salute to Nobel Laureates in Physiology and Medicine*
4. Sourkes TL: *Nobel Prize Winners in Medicine and Physiology 1901–1965*. London, Abelard-Schuman, 1967

Robert W. Schrier, MD

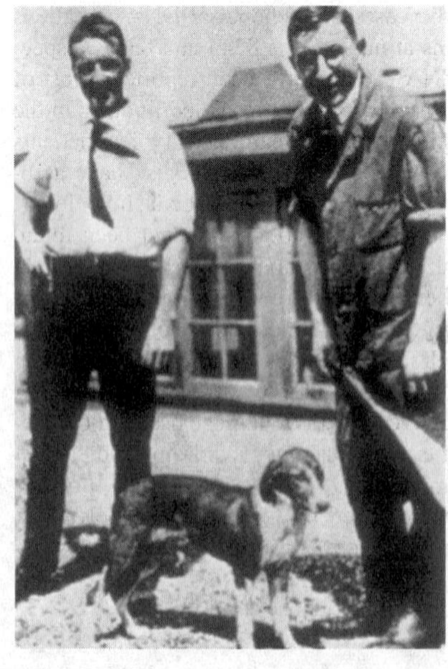

Best and Banting with pancreatectomized dog, Marjorie, whose diabetic coma was treated with insulin. (Reprinted with permission from Ref. 1.)

PART FOURTEEN

NEUROLOGIC DISORDERS

Section 1
DIAGNOSIS OF NEUROLOGIC DISORDERS

355 *Stephen L. Hauser, M. Flint Beal*

NEUROBIOLOGY OF DISEASE

The human nervous system is the organ of consciousness, cognition, ethics, and behavior; as such, it is the most intricate structure known to exist. One-third of the ~35,000 genes encoded in the human genome is expressed in the nervous system. Each mature brain is composed of 100 billion neurons, several million miles of axons and dendrites, and more than 10^{15} synapses. Neurons exist within a dense parenchyma of multifunctional glial cells that synthesize myelin, preserve homeostasis, and regulate immune responses. Measured against this background of complexity, the achievements of molecular neuroscience have been extraordinary. Advances in cell biology and genetics have provided new tools to explore the pathophysiology of nervous system diseases, clarifying their underlying causes, revealing new unanticipated groupings, and raising realistic hope that novel therapies and prevention strategies will be possible. This chapter reviews selected themes in neurobiology that provide a context for understanding fundamental mechanisms underlying neurologic disorders. →*The reader is also referred to related discussions of neurogenetic disorders (Chap. 359) and the neurobiology of addiction (Chap. 386), and to the individual chapters on specific disorders.*

ION CHANNELS AND CHANNELOPATHIES The resting potential of neurons and the action potentials responsible for impulse conduction are generated by ion currents and ion channels. Most ion channels are gated, meaning that they can transition between conformations that are open or closed to ion conductance. Individual ion channels are distinguished by the specific ions they conduct; by their kinetics; and by whether they directly sense voltage, are linked to receptors for neurotransmitters or other ligands such as neurotrophins, or are activated by second messengers. The diverse characteristics of different ion channels provide a means by which neuronal excitability can be exquisitely modulated at both the cellular and the subcellular levels. Mutations in ion channels—channelopathies—are responsible for a growing list of human neurologic disorders (Table 355-1). One example is epilepsy, a syndrome of diverse causes characterized by repetitive, synchronous firing of neuronal action potentials. Action potentials are normally generated by the opening of sodium channels and the inward movement of sodium ions down the intracellular concentration gradient. Depolarization of the neuronal membrane opens potassium channels, resulting in outward movement of potassium ions, repolarization, closure of the sodium channel, and hyperpolarization. Sodium or potassium channel subunit genes have long been considered candidate disease genes in inherited epilepsy syndromes, and recently such mutations have been identified (Chap. 360). These mutations appear to alter the normal gating function of these channels, increasing the inherent excitability of neuronal membranes in regions where the abnormal channels are expressed.

Whereas the specific clinical manifestations of channelopathies are quite variable, one common feature is that manifestations tend to be intermittent or paroxysmal, such as occurs in epilepsy, migraine, ataxia, myotonia, or periodic paralysis. Exceptions are clinically progressive channel disorders such as spinocerebellar ataxia type 6 (SCA6) and autosomal dominant hearing impairment. The neurologic channelopathies identified to date are all uncommon disorders caused by obvious mutations in channel genes. As the full repertoire of human ion channels and related proteins are identified, it is likely that additional channelopathies will be discovered. In addition to rare disorders that result from obvious mutations, it is possible that subtle allelic variations in channel genes or in their pattern of expression might underlie susceptibility to some common forms of epilepsy, migraine, or other disorders.

NEUROTRANSMITTERS AND NEUROTRANSMITTER RECEPTORS Synaptic neurotransmission is the predominant means by which neurons communicate with each other. Classic neurotransmitters are synthesized in the presynaptic region of the nerve terminal; stored in vesicles; and released into the synaptic cleft, where they bind to receptors on the postsynaptic cell. Secreted neurotransmitters are eliminated by reuptake into the presynaptic neuron (or glia), by diffusion away from the synaptic cleft, and/or by specific inactivation. In addition to the classic neurotransmitters, many neuropeptides have been identified as definite or probable neurotransmitters; these include substance P, neurotensin, enkephalins, β-endorphin, histamine, vasoactive intestinal polypeptide, cholecystokinin, neuropeptide Y, and somatostatin. Peptide neurotransmitters are synthesized in the cell body rather than the nerve terminal and may colocalize with classic neurotransmitters in single neurons. Nitric oxide and carbon monoxide are gases that appear also to function as neurotransmitters, in part by signaling in a retrograde fashion from the postsynaptic to the presynaptic cell.

Neurotransmitters modulate the function of postsynaptic cells by binding to specific neurotransmitter receptors, of which there are two major types. *Ionotropic receptors* are direct ion channels that open after engagement by the neurotransmitter. *Metabotropic receptors* interact with G proteins, stimulating production of second messengers and activating protein kinases, which modulate a variety of cellular events. Ionotropic receptors are multiple subunit structures, whereas

Table 355-1 Examples of Neurologic Channelopathies

Category	Disorder	Channel Type	Gene	Chap. Ref.
Ataxias	Episodic ataxia-1	K	*KCNAI*	364
	Episodic ataxia-2	Ca	*CACNLIAd*	
	Spinocerebellar ataxia-6	Ca	*CACNLIAd*	
Migraine	Familial hemiplegic migraine	Ca	*CACNLIAd*	15
Epilepsy	Benign neonatal familial convulsions	K	*KCNQ2, KCNQ3*	360
	Generalized epilepsy with febrile convulsions plus	Na	*SCNIβ*	
Periodic paralysis	Hyperkalemic periodic paralysis	Na	*SCN4A*	383
	Hypokalemic periodic paralysis	Ca	*CACNLIA3*	
Myotonia	Myotonia congenita	Cl	*CLCN1*	383
	Paramyotonia congenita	Na	*SCN4A*	
Deafness	Jorvell and Lange-Nielsen syndrome (deafness, prolonged QT interval, and arrythmia)	K	*KCNQ1, KCNE1*	29
	Autosomal dominant progressive deafness	K	*KCNQ4*	

metabotropic receptors are composed of single subunits only. One important difference between ionotropic and metabotropic receptors is that the kinetics of ionotropic receptor effects are fast (generally less than a millisecond) because neurotransmitter binding directly alters the electrical properties of the postsynaptic cell, whereas metabotropic receptors function over longer time periods. These different properties contribute to the potential for selective and finely modulated signaling by neurotransmitters.

Individual neurotransmitter systems are perturbed in a large number of clinical disorders, examples of which are highlighted in Table 355-2. One example is the involvement of dopaminergic neurons originating in the substantia nigra of the midbrain and projecting to the striatum (nigrostriatal pathway) in Parkinson's disease and in heroin addicts after the ingestion of the toxin MPTP (1-methyl-4-phenyl-1,2,5,6-tetrahydropyridine) (Chap. 363). A second important dopaminergic system arising in the subtantia nigra is the mesolimbic pathway, which influences behavior and appears to be important in the pathogenesis of addiction. Addictive drugs share the property of increasing dopamine release, and blockade of dopamine in the nucleus accumbens (a part of the mesolimbic pathway) terminates the rewarding effects of addictive drugs (Chap. 386).

CELL TO CELL COMMUNICATION THROUGH GAP JUNCTIONS Not all cell-to-cell communication in the nervous system occurs via neurotransmission. Gap junctions provide for direct neuron-neuron electrical conduction and also create openings for the diffusion of ions and metabolites between cells. In addition to neurons, gap junctions are also widespread in glia, creating a syncytium that protects neurons by removing glutamate and potassium from the extracellular environment. Gap junctions consist of membrane-spanning proteins termed connexins that pair across adjacent cells. Mechanisms

Table 355-2 Principal Classic Neurotransmitters

Neurotransmitter	Anatomy	Clinical Aspects
Acetylcholine (Ach) $CH_3-C(=O)-O-CH_2-CH_2-N-(CH_3)_3$	Motor neurons in spinal cord → neuromuscular junction	Acetylcholinesterases (nerve gases) Myasthenia gravis (antibodies to Ach receptor) Congenital myasthenic syndromes (mutations in Ach receptor subunits) Lambert-Eaton syndrome (Antibodies to Ca channels impair Ach release) Botulism (toxin disrupts Ach release by exocytosis)
	Basal forebrain → widespread cortex	Alzheimer's disease (selective cell death) Autosomal dominant frontal lobe epilepsy (mutations in CNS Ach receptor)
	Interneurons in striatum	Parkinson's disease (tremor)
	Autonomic nervous system (preganglionic and postganglionic sympathetic)	
Dopamine HO, HO–(benzene ring)–$CH_2-CH_2-NH_2$	Substantia nigra → striatum (nigrostriatal pathway)	Parkinson's disease (selective cell death) MPTP parkinsonism (toxin transported into neurons)
	Substantia nigra → limbic system and widespread cortex	Addiction, behavioral disorders
	Arcuate nucleus of hypthalamus → anterior pituitary (via portal veins)	Inhibits prolactin secretion
Norepinephrine (NE) HO, HO–(benzene ring)–$CH(OH)-CH_2-NH_2$	Locus ceruleus (pons) → limbic system, hypothalamus, cortex Medulla → locus ceruleus, spinal cord Postganglionic neurons of sympathetic nervous system	Mood disorders (MAO-A inhibitors and tricyclics increase NE and improve depression) Anxiety Orthostatic tachycardia syndrome (mutations in NE transporter)
Serotonin HO–(indole, N–H)–$CH_2-CH_2-NH_2$	Pontine raphe nuclei → widespread projections	Mood disorders (SSRIs improve depression) Migraine pain pathway
	Medulla/pons → dorsal horn of spinal cord	Pain pathway
γ-aminobutyric acid (GABA) $H_2N-CH_2-CH_2-CH_2-COOH$	Major inhibitory neurotransmitter in brain; widespread cortical interneurons and long projection pathways	Stiff person syndrome (antibodies to glutamic acid decarboxylase, the biosynthetic enzyme for GABA) Epilepsy (Gabapentin and valproic acid increase GABA)
Glycine H_2N-CH_2-COOH	Major inhibitory neurotransmitter in spinal cord	Spasticity Hyperekplexia (myoclonic startle syndrome) due to mutations in glycine receptor
Glutamate $H_2N-CH(COOH)-CH_2-CH_2-COOH$	Major excitatory neurotransmitter; located throughout CNS, including cortical pyramidal cells	Seizures due to ingestion of domoic acid (a glutamate analogue) Rasmussen's encephalitis (antibody against glutamate receptor 3) Excitotoxic cell death

that involve gap junctions have been related to a variety of neurologic disorders. Mutations in connexin 32, a gap junction protein expressed by Schwann cells, are responsible for the X-linked form of Charcot-Marie-Tooth disease (Chap. 379). Mutations in either of two gap junction proteins expressed in the inner ear—connexin 26 and connexin 31—result in autosomal dominant progressive hearing loss (Chap. 29). Glial calcium waves mediated through gap junctions also appear to explain the phenomenon of spreading depression associated with migraine auras and the march of epileptic discharges. Spreading depression is a neural response that follows a variety of different stimuli and is characterized by a circumferentially expanding negative potential that propagates at a characteristic speed of 20 μm/s and is associated with an increase in extracellular potassium.

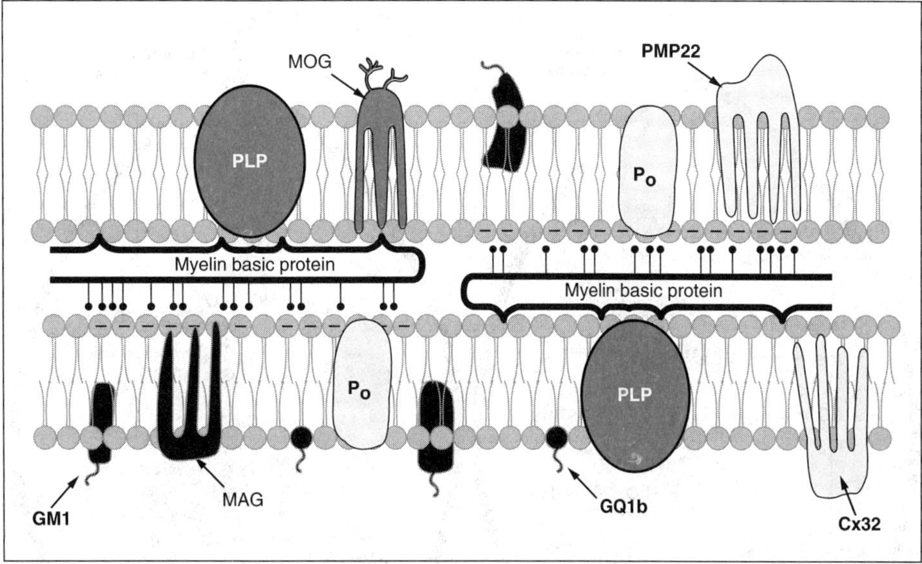

FIGURE 355-1 The molecular architecture of the myelin sheath illustrating the most important disease-related proteins. The illustration represents a composite of CNS and PNS myelin. Proteins restricted to CNS myelin are shown in dark blue, proteins of PNS myelin are light blue, and proteins present in both CNS and PNS are black.

In the CNS, the X-linked allelic disorders, Pelizaeus Merzbacher disease and one variant of familial spastic paraplegia, are caused by mutations in the gene for proteolipid protein (PLP) that normally promotes extracellular compaction between adjacent myelin lamellae. The homologue of PLP in the PNS is the P_0 protein, mutations in which cause the neuropathy Charcot-Marie-Tooth disease (CMT) type 1B. The most common form of CMT is the 1A subtype caused by a duplication of the *PMP22* gene; deletions in *PMP22* are responsible for another inherited neuropathy termed hereditary liability to pressure palsies (Chap. 379).

In multiple sclerosis (MS), myelin basic protein (MBP) and the quantitatively minor CNS protein, myelin oligodendrocyte glycoprotein (MOG), are likely T cell and B cell antigens, respectively (Chap. 371). The location of MOG at the outermost lamella of the CNS myelin membrane may facilitate its targeting by autoantibodies. In the PNS, autoantibodies against myelin gangliosides are implicated in a variety of disorders, including GQ1b in the Fisher variant of Guillain-Barré syndrome, GM1 in multifocal motor neuropathy, and sulfatide constituents of myelin-associated glycoprotein (MAG) in peripheral neuropathies associated with monoclonal gammopathies (Chap. 378).

SIGNALING PATHWAYS AND GENE TRANSCRIPTION The fundamental issue of how memory, learning, and thinking are encoded in the nervous system is likely to be clarified by identifying the signaling pathways involved in neuronal differentiation, axon guidance, and synapse formation, and by understanding how these pathways are modulated by experience. Many families of transcription factors, each comprising multiple individual components, are expressed in the nervous system. Elucidation of these signaling pathways has already begun to provide insights into the cause of a variety of neurologic disorders, including inherited disorders of cognition such as X-linked mental retardation. This syndrome affects approximately 1 in 500 males, and linkage studies in different families suggest that as many as 60 different X-chromosome encoded genes may be responsible. A number of disease genes have now been identified. Three encode proteins that regulate members of the ras family of GTP-binding proteins thought to have roles in regulation of the actin cytoskeleton and in neurite outgrowth (*OPHN1*, *PAK3*) or synaptic vesicle transport and neurotransmitter release (*GDI1*); one (*IL1RAPL*) has homology to an interleukin (IL)1 receptor accessory protein involved in IL-1 signaling; and one (*FMR2*) functions as a nuclear transcriptional regulatory protein. Rett syndrome, a common cause of (dominant) X-linked progressive mental retardation in females, is also due to a mutation in a gene (*MECP2*) encoding a DNA-binding protein involved in transcriptional repression. As the X chromosome comprises only approximately 3% of germline DNA, then by extrapolation the number of genes that potentially contribute to clinical disorders affecting intelligence in humans must be potentially very large.

MYELIN Myelin is the multilayered insulating substance that surrounds axons and speeds impulse conduction by permitting action potentials to jump between naked regions of axons (nodes of Ranvier) and across myelinated segments. A single oligodendrocyte usually ensheaths multiple axons in the central nervous system (CNS), whereas in the peripheral nervous system (PNS) each Schwann cell typically myelinates a single axon. Myelin is a lipid-rich material formed by a spiraling process of the membrane of the myelinating cell around the axon, creating multiple membrane bilayers that are tightly apposed (compact myelin) by charged protein interactions. A number of clinically important neurologic disorders are caused by inherited mutations in myelin proteins of the CNS or PNS. Constituents of myelin also have a propensity to be targeted as autoantigens in autoimmune demyelinating disorders (Fig. 355-1).

NEUROTROPHIC FACTORS Neurotrophic factors (Table 355-3) are secreted proteins that modulate neuronal growth, differentiation, repair, and survival; some have additional functions, including roles in neurotransmission and in the synaptic reorganization involved in learning and memory. Because of their survival promoting and anti-apoptotic effects, neurotrophic factors are in theory outstanding candidates for therapy of disorders characterized by premature death of neurons such as occurs in amyotrophic lateral sclerosis (ALS) and other degenerative motor neuron disorders. Knockout mice lacking receptors for ciliary neurotrophic factor (CNTF) receptor or brain-derived neurotrophic factor (BDNF) show loss of motor neurons, and experimental motor neuron death can be rescued by treatment with various neurotrophic factors including CNTF and BDNF. However, in phase 3 clinical trials both CNTF and BDNF were ineffective in human ALS, and two other trials of insulin-like growth factor 1 yielded con-

Table 355-3 Neurotrophic Factors

Neurotrophin family	Transforming growth factor β family
Nerve growth factor	Glial-derived neurotrophic family
Brain-derived neurotrophic factor	Neurturin
Neurotrophin-3	Persephin
Neurotrophin-4	Fibroblast growth factor family
Neurotrophin-6	Hepatocyte growth factor
Cytokine family	Insulin-like growth factor (IGF) family
Ciliary neurotrophic factor	IGF-1
Leukemia inhibitory factor	IGF-2
Interleukin-6	
Cardiotrophin-1	

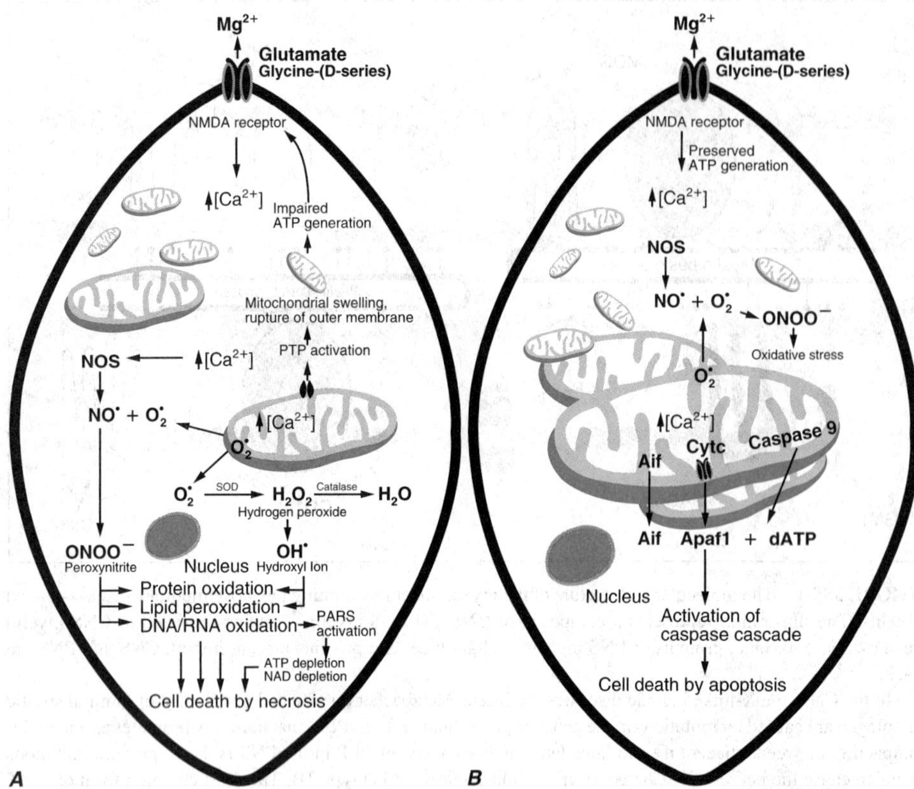

FIGURE 355-2 Involvement of mitochondria in cell death. A severe excitotoxic insult (*A*) results in cell death by necrosis, whereas a mild excitotoxic insult (*B*) results in apoptosis. After a severe insult (such as ischemia), there is a large increase in glutamate activation of NMDA receptors, an increase in intracellular Ca^{2+} concentrations, activation of nitric oxide synthase (NOS), and increased mitochondrial Ca^{2+} and superoxide generation followed by the formation of $ONOO^-$. This sequence results in damage to cellular macromolecules including DNA, leading to activation of poly-ADP-ribose polymerase (PARS). Both mitochondrial accumulation of Ca^{2+} and oxidative damage lead to activation of the permeability transition pore (PTP) that is linked to excitotoxic cell death.

A mild excitotoxic insult can occur due either to an abnormality in an excitotoxicity amino acid receptor, allowing more Ca^{2+} flux, or to impaired functioning of other ionic channels or of energy production, which may allow the voltage-dependent NMDA receptor to be activated by ambient concentrations of glutamate. This event can then lead to increased mitochondrial Ca^{2+} and free radical production, yet relatively preserved ATP generation. The mitochondria may then release cytochrome c (Cyt c), caspase 9, apoptosis-inducing factor (Aif), and perhaps other mediators that lead to apoptosis. The precise role of the PTP in this mode of cell death is still being clarified, but there does appear to be involvement of the adenine nucleotide transporter that is a key component of the PTP.

flicting results with little evidence of clinically significant efficacy. Current understanding of the redundancy and diversity of neurotrophic factor activities at different stages in the life and health of individual neurons is extremely limited, and data obtained in rodent systems are not always applicable to humans. For example, CNTF knockout mice show a partial loss of motoneurons, yet humans who have homozygous mutations that inactivate the gene for CNTF gene are asymptomatic.

STEM CELLS AND TRANSPLANTATION The nervous system is traditionally considered to be a nonmitotic organ, in particular with respect to neurons. These concepts have been challenged by the finding that neural progenitor or stem cells exist in the adult CNS that are capable of differentiation, migration over long distances, and extensive axonal arborization and synapse formation with appropriate targets. These capabilities also indicate that the repertoire of factors required for growth, survival, differentiation, and migration of these cells exist in the mature nervous system. The poor outcome associated with many neurologic disorders, however, clearly indicates that any potential for functional neuronal reconstitution after injury must be extremely limited in most clinical contexts. In rodents, neural stem cells, defined as progenitor cells capable of differentiating into mature cells of neural or glial lineage, have been experimentally propagated from fetal CNS and neuroectodermal tissues, and also from adult germinal matrix and ependyma regions. Human fetal CNS tissue is also capable of differentiation into cells with neuronal, astrocyte, and oligodendrocyte morphology when cultured in the presence of particular growth factors. Impressively, such cells could be stably engrafted into mouse CNS tissue, creating neural chimeras. Once the repertoire of signals required for cell type specification are better understood, differentiation into specific neural or glial subpopulations can be directed in vitro; such cells could also be engineered to express therapeutic molecules.

Experimental transplantation of human fetal dopaminergic neurons in patients with Parkinson's disease has shown that these transplanted cells can survive within the host striatum. Studies of transplantation for patients with Huntington's disease have also reported encouraging, although very preliminary, results. Oligodendrocyte precurser cells transplanted into mice with a dysmyelinating disorder effectively migrated in the new environment, interacted with axons, and mediated myelination; such experiments raise hope that similar transplantation strategies may be feasible in human disorders of myelin such as multiple sclerosis. Enthusiasm for transplantation therapy must be tempered by unresolved concerns over safety (including the theoretical risk of malignant transformation of transplanted cells), ethics (particularly with respect to use of fetal tissue), and efficacy.

CELL DEATH—EXCITOTOXICITY AND APOPTOSIS Excitotoxicity refers to neuronal cell death caused by activation of excitatory amino acid receptors (Fig. 355-2). Compelling evidence for a role of excitotoxicity, especially in ischemic neuronal injury, is derived from experiments in animal models. Experimental models of stroke are associated with increased extracellular concentrations of the excitatory amino acid neurotransmitter glutamate, and neuronal damage is attenuated by denervation of glutamine-containing neurons or the administration of glutamate receptor antagonists. The distribution of cells sensitive to ischemia corresponds closely with that of *N*-methyl-D-aspartate (NMDA) receptors (except for cerebellar Purkinje cells, which are vulnerable to hypoxia-ischemia but lack NMDA receptors); and competitive and noncompetitive NMDA antagonists are effective in preventing focal ischemia. In global cerebral ischemia, non-NMDA receptors (kainic acid and AMPA) are activated, and antagonists to these receptors are protective. Experimental brain damage induced by hypoglycemia is also attenuated by NMDA antagonists.

Excitotoxicity is not a single event but rather a cascade of cell injury. Excitotoxicity causes influx of calcium into cells and much of the calcium is sequestered in mitochondria rather than in the cytoplasm. Increased mitochondrial calcium causes metabolic dysfunction and free radical generation; activates protein kinases, phospholipases, nitric oxide synthase, proteases, and endonucleases; and inhibits protein synthesis. Activation of nitric oxide synthase generates nitric oxide ($NO^•$), which can react with superoxide ($O_2^•$) to generate peroxynitrite ($ONOO^-$), which may play a direct role in neuronal injury. Another critical pathway is activation of poly-ADP-ribose polymerase, which occurs in response to free radical-mediated DNA damage. Experimentally, mice with knockout mutations of neuronal nitric oxide synthase or poly-ADP-ribose polymerase, or those that overexpress superoxide dismutase, are resistant to focal ischemia.

Apoptosis, or programmed cell death, plays an important role in both physiologic and pathologic conditions. During embryogenesis, apoptotic pathways operate to destroy neurons that fail to differentiate appropriately or reach their intended targets. There is mounting evidence for an increased rate of apoptotic cell death in a variety of acute and chronic neurologic diseases. Apoptosis is characterized by neuronal shrinkage, chromatin condensation, and DNA fragmentation, whereas necrotic cell death is associated with cytoplasmic and mitochondrial swelling followed by dissolution of the cell membrane. Apoptotic and necrotic cell death can coexist or be sequential events depending on the severity of the initiating insult. Cellular energy reserves appear to have an important role in these two forms of cell death, with apoptosis favored under conditions in which ATP levels are preserved. Evidence of DNA fragmentation has been found in a number of degenerative neurologic disorders, including Alzheimer's disease, Huntington's disease, and ALS. The best characterized genetic neurologic disorder related to apoptosis is infantile spinal muscular atrophy (Werdnig-Hoffmann disease), in which two genes thought to be involved in the apoptosis pathways are causative.

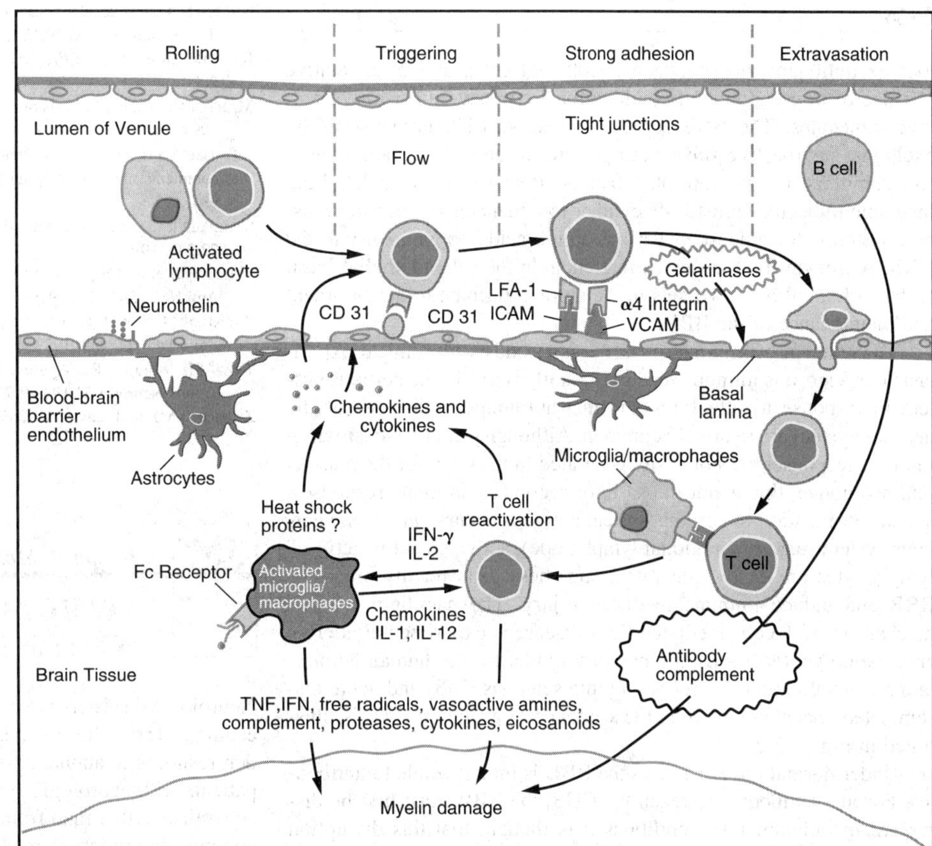

FIGURE 355-3 A model for experimental allergic encephalomyelitis (EAE). Crucial steps for disease initiation and progression include peripheral activation of preexisting autoreactive T cells; homing to the CNS and extravasation across the blood-brain barrier; reactivation of T cells by exposed autoantigens; secretion of cytokines; activation of microglia and astrocytes and recruitment of a secondary inflammatory wave; and immune-mediated myelin destruction. ICAM, intercellular adhesion molecule; LFA-1, leukocyte function-associated antigen-1; VCAM, vascular cell adhesion molecule; IFN, interferon; IL, interleukin; TNF, tumor necrosis factor.

Mitochondria are essential in controlling specific apoptosis pathways. The redistribution of cytochrome c from mitochondria during apoptosis leads to the activation of a cascade of intracellular proteases known as caspases. Redistribution of cytochrome c is prevented by overproduction of the apoptotic protein BCL2 and is promoted by the proapoptotic protein BAX. These pathways may be triggered by activation of a large pore in the mitochondrial inner membrane known as the permeability transition pore. Recent studies suggest that blocking this pore reduces both hypoglycemic and ischemic cell death.

PROTEIN AGGREGATION AND NEURODEGENERATION The possibility that protein aggregation plays a role in the pathogenesis of neurodegenerative diseases is a major focus of current research. Protein aggregation is a major histopathologic hallmark of neurodegenerative diseases. Deposition of β-amyloid is strongly implicated in the pathogenesis of Alzheimer's disease. Genetic mutations in familial Alzheimer's disease produce increased amounts of β-amyloid with 42 amino acids, which has an increased propensity to aggregate, as compared to β-amyloid with 40 amino acids. Mutations in genes encoding the microtubule associated protein tau lead to altered splicing of tau and the production of neurofibrillary tangles in frontotemporal dementia and progressive supranuclear palsy. Familial Parkinson's disease is associated with mutations in α-synuclein and the ubiquitin carboxy-terminal hydrolase. The characteristic histopathologic feature of Parkinson's disease is the Lewy body, an eosinophilic cytoplasmic inclusion that contains both neurofilaments and α-synuclein. Huntington's disease and cerebellar degenerations are associated with expansions of polyglutamine repeats in proteins, which aggregate to produce neuronal intranuclear inclusions. Familial ALS is associated with superoxide dismutase mutations and cytoplasmic inclusions containing superoxide dismutase. In autosomal dominant neurohypophyseal diabetes insipidus, mutations in vasopressin result in abnormal protein processing, accumulation in the endoplasmic reticulum, and cell death (Chap. 329).

The major scientific question presently is whether protein aggregates contribute to neuronal death or whether they are merely a secondary bystander. Protein aggregates are usually ubiquinated, which targets them for degradation by the 26S component of the proteosome. An inability to degrade protein aggregates could lead to cellular dysfunction, impaired axonal transport, and cell death by apoptotic mechanisms.

In experimental models of Huntington's disease and cerebellar degeneration, protein aggregates are not well correlated with neuronal death. A number of compounds have been developed to block β-amyloid production and/or aggregation, and these agents are being studied in early clinical trials in humans.

NEUROIMMUNOLOGY The nervous system is traditionally considered to be an immunologically privileged organ, a concept originally derived from observations that tissue grafts implanted in the brain were not rejected efficiently. In this context, immune privilege of the CNS may be maintained by a variety of mechanisms including: the lack of an efficient surveillance function by T cells; the absence of a traditional lymphoid system; limited expression of major histocompatibility complex (MHC) molecules required for T cell recognition of antigen; effects of regulatory cytokines secreted spontaneously or in response to mediators such as nerve growth factor (NGF), creating an immunosuppressive milieu; and also from expression of fas ligand that can induce apoptosis of fas-expressing immune cells that enter the brain. The blood-brain barrier (BBB) partially isolates the brain from the peripheral environment and contributes to immune privilege. Anatomically, the barrier is created by the presence of impermeable tight junctions between endothelial cells, and by a relative absence of transendothelial conduits for the passive diffusion of soluble molecules. The BBB serves to preserve CNS homeostasis by excluding neuroactive substances present in the serum, such as neurotransmitters and neurotrophic factors. Because of the BBB, lipid insoluble molecules must utilize either ion channels or specific transport systems (for glucose or various amino acids) to gain entry to the CNS. Astrocyte foot processes that encircle the subendothelial basal surface of small blood vessels in the brain contribute to development and maintenance of the BBB.

The concept of immune privilege is at odds with clinical experience that vigorous immune reactions readily occur in the nervous system in response to infections and that autoimmune diseases of the nervous system are relatively common. Although primary (sensitizing) immune responses are not easily generated in the CNS for the reasons outlined above, this is not the case for secondary immune responses. When sensitization to nervous system antigens occurs *outside* the nervous system (e.g., in a regional lymph node), activated autoreactive T lymphocytes are easily generated, and these cells readily cross the BBB and induce immune mediated injury. The paradigm for this mechanism of T cell–mediated CNS disease is experimental allergic encephalomyelitis (EAE), a laboratory model for the human autoimmune demyelinating disorders multiple sclerosis (MS) and acute disseminated encephalomyelitis; the sequence of events in EAE is illustrated in Fig. 355-3.

Under normal circumstances the BBB is impermeable to antibodies. For autoantibodies to reach the CNS, the BBB must first be disrupted. In inflammatory conditions it is thought that this disruption most often occurs via actions of proinflammatory cytokines elaborated within the brain consequent to interactions between pathogenic T cells and antigen-presenting cells (APCs). In contrast to the BBB, in the PNS the blood-nerve barrier is incomplete. Endothelial tight junctions are lacking, and the capacity of charged molecules, including antibodies, to cross the barrier appears to be greatest in two regions of the PNS: proximally in the spinal roots and distally at neuromuscular junctions. This anatomic feature is likely to contribute to the propensity of antibody-mediated autoimmune disorders of the PNS to target proximal nerves (Guillain-Barré syndrome) or the neuromuscular junction (myasthenia gravis, Eaton-Lambert syndrome).

The major APCs in the CNS are microglial cells and macrophages; both cell types express MHC class 2 molecules as well as costimulatory molecules required for antigen presentation. Neurons do not express MHC class 2 molecules; however, some neurons express MHC class 1 proteins, which may be further increased in response to neuronal activity. Neuronal MHC class 1 molecules may function as retrograde postsynaptic signaling molecules that interact with presynaptic CD3ζ molecules to stabilize active synapses and transynaptically modulate neuronal function. Studies in mice also indicate that MHC class 1 molecules influence the mating behavior of females; a hierarchichal pattern of preference is determined by the specific class 1 alleles expressed by potential male suitors. This behavior appears to be mediated by distinctive odors imparted either by the class 1 molecules themselves or by other families of molecules controlled by class 1 alleles. Thus, it appears likely that MHC molecules subserve a variety of signaling and adhesion functions that influence nervous system function far beyond their well-established roles as mediators of APC-T lymphocyte interactions.

BIBLIOGRAPHY

ALBRIGHT TD et al: Neural science: A century of progress and the mysteries that remain. Cell 25:S1, 2000

BERKE JD, HYMAN SE: Addiction, dopamine, and the molecular mechanisms of memory. Neuron 25:515, 2000

COOPER EC, JAN LY: Ion channel genes and human neurological disease: Recent progress, prospects, and challenges. Proc Natl Acad Sci USA 96:4759, 1999

DARNELL RB: Immunologic complexity in neurons. Neuron 21:947, 1998

GREEN T et al: Molecular neurobiology and genetics: Investigation of neural function and dysfunction. Neuron 20:427, 1998.

KANDEL ER et al (eds): *Principles of Neural Science*, 4th ed. New York, McGraw-Hill, 2000

MARTIN JB: Molecular basis of the neurodegenerative disorders. N Engl J Med 340:1970, 1999

MITSUMOTO H, TSUZAKA K: Neurotrophic factors and neuromuscular disease: 1. General comments, the neurotrophin family, and neuropoietic cytokines. Muscle/Nerve 22: 983, 1999

SCHEFFLER B et al: Marrow-mindedness: A perspective on neuropoiesis. Trends Neurosci 22:348, 1999

SCHULZ JB et al: Caspases as treatment targets in stroke and neurodegenerative diseases. Ann Neurol 45:421, 1999

SVENDSEN CN et al: Human neural stem cells: Isolation, expansion and transplantation. Brain Pathol 9:499, 1999

TRAN PB, MILLER RJ: Aggregates in neurodegenerative disease: Crowds and power? Trends Neurosci 22:194, 1999

ZIGMOND MJ et al (eds): *Molecular neuroscience*. London, Academic Press, 1999

356

Joseph B. Martin, Stephen L. Hauser

APPROACH TO THE PATIENT WITH NEUROLOGIC DISEASE

Neurologic disorders are common and costly. According to one recent estimate, 180 million Americans suffer from a nervous system disorder, resulting in annual cost of 634 billion dollars (Table 356-1). Most patients with neurologic symptoms seek care from internists and other generalists rather than from neurologists, and this situation is likely to continue as primary care–based health care systems become increasingly prevalent and access to specialists is reduced. Because useful therapies now exist for many neurologic disorders, a skillfull approach to their diagnosis is important. Many errors result from an over-reliance on neuroimaging and other laboratory tests at the expense of a primary focus on the history and examination. These errors can be avoided by adherence to an approach in which the patient's illness is defined first in *anatomic* and then in *pathophysiologic* terms; only then should a specific diagnosis be entertained. Arrival at a diagnosis permits the physician to institute therapy and to inform and counsel patients and their families about the expected disease course.

THE NEUROLOGIC METHOD OF CLINICAL EVALUATION

LOCATE THE LESION(S) The first priority is to define the anatomic substrate responsible for the patient's illness by seeking to determine what part of the neural axis is likely to be involved in causing the neurologic symptoms. Can the disorder be mapped to one specific site in the nervous system, is it multifocal, or is there evidence of a more diffuse neurologic disease? Is the disorder restricted to the nervous system, or does it arise in the context of a systemic illness? Is it in the central nervous system (CNS), the peripheral nervous system (PNS), or both? If in the CNS, is the process restricted to the cerebral cortex, or is there evidence of basal ganglia, brainstem, cerebellum, and/or spinal cord involvement? Are the pain-sensitive meninges involved? If in the PNS, could the disorder be located in peripheral nerves and, if so, are motor or sensory nerves primarily affected, or is a lesion in the neuromuscular junction or muscle more likely?

The first clues to defining the anatomic area of involvement appear in the history, and the examination is then directed to confirm or rule out these impressions and to clarify uncertainties suggested by the history. A more detailed examination of a particular region of the CNS or PNS is often indicated. For example, the examination of a patient who presents with a history of ascending paresthesias and weakness should be directed toward deciding, among other things, if the location of the lesion is in the spinal cord or peripheral nerves. Focal back pain,

Table 356-1 Impact of Neurologic and Psychiatric Diseases in the United States

Disorder	Patients in Millions	Cost in $ Billions
Addiction	17.5	160
Alzheimer's disease	4	100
Blindness/vision loss	13	38.4
Deafness/hearing loss	28	56
Depression/manic depressive illness	17.5	47.3
Developmental disorders	8.6	30
Epilepsy	2.5	3.5
Head injury	2	25
Huntington's disease	0.03	—
Multiple sclerosis	0.3	2.5
Pain	80	100
Parkinson's disease	1	6
Schizophrenia	2	30
Spinal cord injury	0.25	5
Stroke	3	30
Total	180	634

SOURCE: Modified from Dana Alliance for Brain Initiatives.

a spinal cord sensory level, and incontinence suggest a spinal cord origin, whereas a stocking-glove pattern of sensory loss suggests peripheral nerve disease; areflexia usually indicates peripheral neuropathy but may also be present with spinal shock in acute spinal cord disorders.

Deciding "where the lesion is" accomplishes the task of limiting the possible etiologies to a manageable, finite number. In addition, this strategy safeguards against making tragic errors. Symptoms of recurrent vertigo, diplopia, and nystagmus should not trigger "multiple sclerosis" as an answer (etiology) but "brainstem" or "pons" (location); then a diagnosis of brainstem arteriovenous malformation will not be missed for lack of consideration. Similarly, the combination of optic neuritis and spastic ataxic paraparesis should initially suggest optic nerve and spinal cord disease; multiple sclerosis, CNS syphilis, and vitamin B_{12} deficiency are treatable disorders that can produce this syndrome. Once the question, "Where is the lesion?" is answered, then the question, "What is the lesion?" can be addressed.

DEFINE THE PATHOPHYSIOLOGY Clues to the pathophysiology of the disease process may also be present in the history. Primary neuronal (gray matter) disorders may present as early cognitive disturbances, movement disorders, or seizures, whereas white matter involvement produces predominantly "long tract" disorders of motor, sensory, visual and cerebellar pathways. Progressive and symmetric symptoms often have a metabolic or degenerative origin; in such cases lesions are usually not sharply circumscribed. Thus, a patient with paraparesis and a clear spinal cord sensory level is unlikely to have vitamin B_{12} deficiency as the explanation. A Lhermitte symptom (electric shock–like sensations evoked by neck flexion) is due to ectopic impulse generation in white matter pathways and occurs with demyelination in the cervical spinal cord. Symptoms that worsen after exposure to heat or exercise may indicate conduction block in demyelinated axons and suggest a diagnosis of multiple sclerosis. Slowly advancing visual scotoma with luminous edges, termed fortification spectra, are diagnostic of spreading cortical depression, such as occurs in migraine.

ESTABLISH AN ETIOLOGIC DIAGNOSIS The clinical data obtained from the history and the examination are assembled into one of the known syndromes and are interpreted and translated in terms of neuroanatomy and neurophysiology. From the syndrome the physician should be able to determine the anatomic localization(s) that best explains the clinical findings. The proper selection of laboratory tests is important to arrive at an anatomic, but more particularly an etiologic, diagnosis. The laboratory assessment of a patient with positive neurologic findings may include (1) serum electrolytes, complete blood count, and renal, liver, and endocrine studies; (2) cerebrospinal fluid (CSF) examination (see below); (3) neuroimaging studies (Chap. 358); or (4) electrophysiologic studies (Chap. 357). The anatomic localization, mode of onset and course of illness, other medical data, and laboratory findings are then integrated to establish an etiologic diagnosis.

THE NEUROLOGIC HISTORY

Attention to the description of the symptoms as experienced by the patient and substantiated by family members or friends often permits an accurate localization and determination of the probable cause of the complaints even before the neurologic examination is undertaken. Two principles should be followed. First, each complaint should be pursued as far as possible in an effort to delineate where the lesion might be or, more importantly, to formulate a set of questions to be answered by the examination. A patient complains of weakness of the right arm. What are the associated features? Is this weakness for brushing the hair (proximal) or opening a twist-top bottle (distal)? Second, negative associations may also be crucial. A patient with a right hemiparesis without a language deficit likely has a lesion (and likely an etiology) different from that of a patient with a right hemiparesis and aphasia. Additional features of the history include the following:

1. *Temporal course of the illness.* It is important to ascertain the precise time of appearance and rate of progression of the symptoms experienced by the patient. The rapid onset of a neurologic complaint, occurring within seconds or minutes, usually indicates a cerebrovascular event, a seizure, or rarely migraine. The onset of sensory symptoms located in one extremity that spread over a few seconds to adjacent portions of that extremity and then to the other limb or to the face suggests a seizure. A more gradual onset and less well localized sensory symptoms point to the possibility of a transient ischemic attack (TIA). A similar but slower temporal march of a sensory change occurring with headache, nausea, or visual disturbance suggests migraine. In general, the march of migraine is slower than that of seizure, and a TIA tends to be more generalized in location on the side of the body or extremities. The presence of "positive" sensory symptoms (e.g., tingling) or involuntary motor movements suggests a seizure; in contrast, transient loss of function (negative symptoms) suggests a TIA. A stuttering onset where symptoms appear, stabilize, and then progress over hours or days also suggests cerebrovascular disease; an additional history of transient remission or regression indicates that the process is due to ischemia and not hemorrhage. On occasion, a demyelinating process may also produce new symptoms that evolve rapidly over the course of a few hours. Progressing symptoms associated with the systemic manifestations of fever, stiff neck, and altered level of consciousness raise the possibility of an infectious process. Relapsing and remitting symptoms involving different levels of the neuraxis suggest multiple sclerosis. Slowly progressive symptoms without remissions are characteristic of neurodegenerative disorders.

2. *Subjective descriptions of the complaint.* The same words often mean different things to different patients. "Dizziness" may imply impending syncope, a sense of giddiness, or true spinning vertigo. "Numbness" may mean a complete loss of feeling, a positive sensation of tingling, or paralysis. "Blurred vision" may be used to describe unilateral visual loss, as in transient monocular blindness, or diplopia. It is important to define the contextual meaning of the patient's complaint to understand its true significance.

3. *Corroboration of the history by others.* It is often useful to obtain additional information from family, friends, or observers to corroborate or expand the patient's description. Memory loss, aphasia, loss of insight, drug or alcohol abuse, and other factors may impair the patient's capacity to communicate normally with the examiner or prevent openness about factors that have contributed to the illness. Episodes of loss of consciousness that may be due to syncope or seizures necessitate that details be sought from observers to ascertain the exact circumstances.

4. *Family history*. Many neurologic disorders have an underlying genetic component. The presence of a Mendelian disorder, such as Huntington's disease or Charcot-Marie-Tooth neuropathy, is often obvious if appropriate family data are available. In polygenic disorders such as multiple sclerosis or migraine, a positive family history, when present, may be helpful. It is important to elicit family history about all illnesses, in addition to neurologic and psychiatric disorders. A familial propensity to hypertension or heart disease may be relevant to a patient who presents with a stroke. Many inherited neurologic illnesses are associated with multisystem manifestations that may provide clues to the correct diagnosis (e.g., the phakomatoses, hepatocerebral disorders, neuro-ophthalmic syndromes).

5. *Medical illnesses*. Many neurologic illnesses occur in the context of systemic disorders. Disorders such as diabetes mellitus, hypertension, and abnormalities of blood lipids predispose to cerebrovascular disease. Marfan's syndrome and related collagen disorders predispose to dissection of the cranial arteries and also to aneurysmal subarachnoid hemorrhage; the latter may also occur with polycystic kidney disease. A recent onset of asthma suggests the possibility of polyarteritis nodosa. Various neurologic disorders occur with dysthyroid states. A solitary mass lesion may be a brain abscess in a patient with valvular heart disease, a primary hemorrhage in a patient with a coagulopathy, a metastasis in a patient with underlying cancer, or a lymphoma or toxoplasmosis in a patient with AIDS. The presence of systemic diseases that are associated with peripheral neuropathy should be explored. Most patients with coma in a hospital setting can be shown to have a metabolic, toxic, or infectious process.

6. *The patient's perception of the disease*. It is frequently helpful to ask patients what they perceive to be wrong. Patients who complain of failing memory are often concerned that they have early symptoms of Alzheimer's disease; more often they are found to suffer from depression. Patients with headaches may fear that a tumor or an impending stroke is a possibility. Patients with sensory symptoms frequently are concerned about the possibility of multiple sclerosis. The patient may seek medical attention because a relative or friend has been diagnosed with a serious neurologic illness.

7. *Drug use and abuse and toxin exposure*. It is essential to inquire about the history of drug use, both prescribed and illicit. Digitalis use may provoke complaints of yellow vision. Excessive vitamin ingestion may lead to disease; for example, vitamin A and pseudotumor cerebri, or pyridoxine and peripheral neuropathy. Aminoglycoside antibiotics may exacerbate symptoms of weakness in patients with disorders of neuromuscular transmission, such as myasthenia gravis. Dizziness may be secondary to ototoxicity caused by aminoglycosides. Many patients are unaware that over-the-counter sleeping pills, cold preparations, and diet pills are actually drugs. Alcohol, the most prevalent neurotoxin, is often not recognized as such by patients. A history of environmental or industrial exposure to neurotoxins may provide an essential clue; consultation with the patient's family or employer may be required.

8. *History of malignancy*. Patients with malignancy may present with nervous system metastases, a paraneoplastic syndrome (Chap. 101), or complications from chemotherapy or radiotherapy.

9. *Formulating an impression of the patient*. Use the opportunity while taking the history to form an impression of the patient. Is there evidence of anxiety, depression, hypochondriasis? Are there any clues to defects of language, memory, inappropriate behavior, or secondary gain? The neurologic assessment begins as soon as the patient walks into the room and the first introduction is made.

THE NEUROLOGIC EXAMINATION

A systematic neurologic examination should encompass a survey of all functions from the cerebrum to the peripheral nerve and muscle, i.e., from the mental status examination to the simplest reflexes. Physicians should acquire skills that come only from the repeated use of the same techniques and instruments on a large number of individuals with and without neurologic disease. Errors and serious omissions are avoided if the examination procedure is orderly and systematic, beginning with mental (cerebral) functions and continuing with cranial nerves; then with motor, reflex, and sensory functions of the arms, trunk, and legs; and finishing with an analysis of posture and gait (Table 356-2).

This detailed examination is undertaken only if there are symptoms of disturbed nervous system functioning. If none are present, it suffices to do an abbreviated examination that includes evaluation only of pupils, ocular movements, optic fundi, facial movements, speech, strength of arm and leg muscles, tendon and plantar reflexes, pain and vibratory sensation in hands and feet, and gait. All this can be completed in 3 to 5 min.

Several additional points about the examination are worth noting. First, in recording observations, it is important to describe what is found rather than to apply a poorly defined medical term (i.e., "patient groans to sternal rub" rather than "obtunded"). Second, if the patient's complaint is brought out by some activity, reproduce the activity in the office. If the complaint is of dizziness when raising the right arm and turning the head to the left, have the patient do it. If pain occurs after walking two blocks, have the patient demonstrate it, and repeat the examination. Finally, the use of tests that are individually tailored to the patient's problem can be of value in assessing changes over time. Tests of walking a 25-ft distance (normal, 5 to 6 s; note assistance, if any), repetitive finger or toe tapping (normal, 20 to 25 taps in 5 s), or handwriting are examples.

The neurologic examination may be normal even in patients with a serious neurologic disease, such as one that causes seizures or syncope. A comatose patient may arrive with no available history; the examination proceeds along the lines described in Chap. 24. An inadequate history may be compensated for to some extent by a succession of examinations from which the course of the illness may be plotted.

LUMBAR PUNCTURE

The clinical indications for lumbar puncture (LP) are listed in Table 356-3. In experienced hands, LP is a safe procedure. The patient is asked to lie on his or her side facing away from the examiner. The back is positioned at the edge of the bed or table near the examiner. The patient is asked to "roll up into a ball"—the neck is gently flexed and the knees drawn up to the abdomen. Proper positioning is essential for success; the examiner should ensure that the shoulders and pelvis are vertically aligned without forward or backward tilt. A pillow is placed under the neck for comfort and a blanket offered for warmth. Because the spinal cord terminates at approximately the L1 vertebral level, the LP is performed below this level; i.e., at or below the L2–L3 interspace. A useful anatomic guidepost is the iliac crest which corresponds to the L3–L4 interspace. The interspace is chosen after gentle palpation to identify the spinous processes at each lumbar level. The skin is cleansed with an antibacterial liquid and alcohol, and the area is draped with sterile cloths. Local anesthetic, typically 1% lidocaine, is injected into the subcutaneous tissue; a topical anesthetic cream (lidocaine 2.5%/prilocaine 2.5%) applied 90 min before the procedure can eliminate pain associated with injection. Approximately 5 min after the lidocaine injection, the LP needle (typically 22 gauge) is inserted in the midline between two spinous processes and slowly advanced at a slightly cephalic angle aiming at the umbilicus. The bevel of the needle should be maintained in a horizontal position, parallel to the direction of the dural fibers; this minimizes injury to the fibers as the dura is penetrated. In most adults, the needle is advanced 4 to 5 cm (1½ to 2 in.) before the subarachnoid space is reached, and the examiner usually recognizes entry as a sudden release of resistance. Some examiners prefer to remove the stylet periodically as the needle is advanced to look for CSF flow. If the needle cannot be advanced because bone is hit, if the patient experiences sharp radiating pain

Mental Status Examination (See also Chaps. 24 to 26)

These tests are designed to evaluate attention, orientation, memory, insight, judgment, and grasp of general information. A series of numbers can be recited and the patient asked to respond every time a specific item recurs (attention). The patient can be asked his or her name, the place, the day, and the date. Retentive memory and immediate recall can be tested by determining the number of digits that can be repeated in sequence. Recent memory is evaluated by testing recall of a series of objects after defined times (e.g., 5 and 15 min). More remote memory is evaluated by assessment of the patient's ability to provide a coherent chronologic history of his or her illness or personal life events. Recall of major historical or current events can be used to assess the fund of general knowledge. If answers suggest that there may be a problem with insight, the patient should be asked whether anything is wrong with his or her health. Interpretation of proverbs (e.g., "People who live in glass houses. . ."; A bird in the hand. . . .") can provide information relative to judgment and capacity to reason in an abstract manner. Specific higher cortical functions can be tested when clinical circumstances suggest that deficits may be present. Evaluation of language function should include assessment of spontaneous speech, naming, repetition, reading, writing, and comprehension. Calculations, identification of right from left, identification of fingers, praxis (whistling, brushing teeth, combing hair, saluting), and ability to draw and copy figures may also be assessed.

Cranial Nerve (CN) Examination (See also Chaps. 28, 29, and 367)

CNI Occlude each nostril sequentially. Use a mild test stimulus such as soap, toothpaste, coffee, or lemon oil. With the eyes closed, the patient sniffs and tries to identify the stimulus.

CNII Check visual acuity (with eyeglasses or pinhole correction) using a Snellen chart (distance) or Jaeger's test type (near). Map visual fields by confrontation testing in each quadrant of the visual field for each eye individually. The best method is to sit facing the patient [0.6 to 1.0 m (2 to 3 ft) apart] and ask him or her to gently cover one eye and fix the uncovered eye on the examiner's nose. A small object (e.g., a white hatpin or cotton-tipped applicator) is then moved from the periphery of the field toward the center until appreciated by the patient. The patient's visual field should be mapped against the examiner's for comparison. The size of the blind spot can also be estimated in this manner; for central vision, use of a red pin will improve sensitivity of the study. Formal perimetry and tangent screen examinations may be required to identify and delineate small defects. Optic fundi should be examined with an ophthalmoscope, and the color, size, and degree of swelling or elevation of the optic disc recorded. The retinal vessels should be checked for size, regularity, arterial-venous nicking at crossing points, hemorrhage, exudates, aneurysms, etc. Normally, 8 to 12 vessels course over the disc margin, and the darker arterioles are approximately two-thirds the size of the lighter colored venules.

CN III, IV, VI Describe the size and shape of pupils and direct and consensual pupillary reactions to light. Check for pupillary accommodation with convergence (ask the patient to follow a small object as it moves towards the bridge of the nose). Check for lid droop, lag, or retraction. Ask the patient to follow a small object (e.g., a hatpin) at a distance of 0.6 m (2 ft). Move the target slowly in both horizontal and vertical planes; observe any paresis, nystagmus, or abnormality of smooth pursuit (saccades, oculomotor ataxia, etc.). Horizontal nystagmus is best assessed at 45° and not at extreme lateral gaze. Incomplete eye movements may result from a nuclear or supranuclear cause; a supranuclear cause is present if full eye movements are present with doll's-head maneuver (gentle, rapid side-to-side or up-and-down movements of the neck).

CN V Feel the masseter and temporalis muscles as the patient bites down. Test jaw opening, protrusion, and lateral motion against resistance. Examine sensation over the entire face and corneals using a light wisp of cotton.

CN VII Look for facial asymmetry at rest and with spontaneous movements. Test eyebrow elevation, forehead wrinkling, eye closure, smiling, frowning, cheek puff, whistle, lip pursing, and chin muscle contraction. Look in particular for differences in strength of the lower versus upper facial muscles. Taste on the anterior two-thirds of the tongue may be impaired by lesions of the nerve proximal to the chordi tympani. Test taste for sweet (sugar), salt, sour (lemon), and bitter (quinine) using cotton-tipped applicators moistened in the appropriate solution and placed on the lateral margin of the protruded tongue halfway back from the tip.

CN VIII Check the ability to hear a tuning fork, finger rub, watch tick, and whispered voice with each ear. Check for air versus mastoid bone conduction (Rinne) and lateralization of a tuning fork placed on the center of the forehead (Weber). Examine the tympanic membranes. Quantitative testing of hearing requires formal audiometry.

CN IX, X Check for symmetric elevation of the palate-uvula with phonation ("aah") as well as the position of the uvula and palatal arch at rest. Sensation in the region of the tonsils, posterior pharynx, and tongue may also require testing in some patients. Pharyngeal ("gag") reflex is evaluated by stimulating the posterior pharyngeal wall on each side with a blunt object (e.g., tongue blade). Direct examination of vocal cords by laryngoscopy may be necessary.

CN XI Check shoulder shrug (trapezius muscle) and head rotation to each side (sternocleidomastoid muscle) against resistance.

CN XII Examine the bulk and power of the tongue. Look for atrophy, deviation from midline with protrusion, tremor, and small flickering or twitching movements (fibrillations, fasciculations).

Motor Examination (See also Chap. 22)

Inspection Muscles are examined for atrophy or hypertrophy. Fasciculations may be observed as fine twitching that occurs spontaneously or is induced by light percussion. Involuntary movements may be present at rest (e.g., tics, myoclonus, choreoathetosis, ballismus), during maintained posture (pill-rolling tremor of Parkinson's disease), or with voluntary action (intention tremor of cerebellar disease or familial tremor).

Tone Muscle tone is tested by resistance to passive motion of a relaxed limb. During testing, it is useful to distract the patient from the examination to minimize active movements. In the upper limbs, tone is assessed by repetitive pronation and supination of the forearm and by rolling the hand at the wrist. In the lower limbs, the examiner's hands are placed behind the thighs and rapidly raised; with normal tone the ankles drag along the table surface for a variable distance before rising, whereas increased tone results in an immediate lift of the heel off the surface. Decreased tone is most commonly due to lower motor neuron, peripheral nerve, or cerebellar pathway disorders. Increased tone may be evident as spasticity (resistance determined by the angle and direction of motion; corticospinal tract disease), rigidity (similar resistance at all angles of motion; extrapyramidal disease), or paratonia/Gegenhalten (fluctuating changes in resistance to repetitive passive movements; frontal lobe pathways). One frequently observed type of rigidity is the cogwheel rigidity of Parkinson's disease, in which passive motion elicits jerky interruptions in resistance.

Strength Muscle strength is tested by evaluating flexion, extension, adduction, and abduction at each joint, and recorded using the following scale:

0 = no movement
1 = flicker or trace of contraction but no associated movement at a joint
2 = movement with gravity eliminated
3 = movement against gravity but not against resistance
4− = movement against a mild degree of resistance
4 = movement against moderate resistance
4+ = movement against strong resistance
5 = full power

Reflexes

Muscle Stretch Reflexes Commonly tested are the biceps (**C5**, C6), brachioradialis (C5, **C6**), triceps (**C7**, C8), and finger flexor (**C8**) reflexes in the upper limbs and the patellar or quadriceps (**L3**, L4) and Achilles (**S1**, S2) reflexes in the lower limbs. Stretch reflexes are best elicited in a relaxed limb. It is sometimes useful to use conversation to distract the patient during reflex testing. Reflexes may be enhanced by asking the patient to voluntarily contract other, distant muscle groups (Jendrassik maneuver). For example, upper limb reflexes may be reinforced by voluntary teeth-clenching, and the Achilles reflex by hooking the flexed fingers of the two hands together and by attempting to pull them apart. For each reflex tested, left and right limbs should be similarly positioned and the two sides tested sequentially. It is more useful to determine the smallest stimulus required to elicit a reflex rather than the maximum response that can be obtained.

(continued)

Table 356-2 The Neurologic Examination—*(continued)*

Reflexes are graded according to the following scale:

0 = absent
1 = present but diminished
2 = normoactive
3 = exaggerated
4 = clonus

Clonus refers to repetitive rhythmic contractions evoked by a stretch stimulus; it is most commonly noted at the Achilles tendon. Occasional normal individuals will have two or three beats of physiologic ankle clonus, but sustained ankle clonus is an abnormal finding that signifies hyperactivity of the motor unit resulting from an upper motor neuron lesion.

Cutaneous Reflexes The plantar reflex is elicited by stroking, with a noxious stimulus (i.e., a key or tongue blade), the lateral surface of the sole beginning near the heel and moving across the ball of the foot to the great toe. The normal reflex consists of plantar flexion of the toes. With upper motor neuron lesions above the S1 level of the spinal cord, a paradoxical extension of the great toe is noted, associated with fanning and extension of the other toes (extensor plantar response or Babinski sign); a prominent extensor plantar response may be accompanied by triple flexion at the ankle, knee, and hip. In some patients with corticospinal tract lesions, the great toe on the involved side may assume an extensor posture at rest or after movement of the foot. Some patients may voluntarily withdraw from the plantar stroke, simulating an extensor response. In these situations, the true direction of the plantar response may be determined by pressure applied to the anterior tibia, stroking towards the ankle (Oppenheim sign), pressure applied to the calf (Gordon sign) or ankle (Schaefer sign), or pricking of the dorsum of the great toe (Bing sign).

Superficial abdominal reflexes are elicited by lightly stroking the abdominal wall with a sharp object (e.g., a pin) and observing movement of the umbilicus. The upper abdominal reflex (spinal cord level T9) is elicited by stroking the upper lateral corner of the abdomen towards the umbilicus, whereas the lower abdominal reflex (T12) is elicited by a stimulus beginning at the lower lateral abdomen. The normal response consists of diagonal movement of the umbilicus toward the origin of the stimulus. With upper motor neuron lesions, these reflexes are absent. They are most helpful when there is preservation of upper but not lower abdominal reflexes, indicating a spinal lesion between T9 and T12, or when the response is asymmetric. Obese individuals or multiparous women may lack visible superficial abdominal reflexes. Other useful cutaneous reflexes include the cremasteric (ipsilateral elevation of the testicle following stroking of the medial thigh), anal (contraction of the anal sphincter following pinprick stimulation of the perianal region), and bulbocavernosus (contraction of urethra and anal sphincter after a stimulus to the glans penis) reflexes.

Primitive Reflexes In disease of the frontal lobe pathways, several primitive reflexes not normally present in the adult may appear. The suck response is elicited by lightly touching the center of the lips, and the root response the corner of the lips, with a tongue blade; the patient will move the lips to suck or root in the direction of the stimulus. The grasp reflex is elicited by touching the palm, and in particular the area between the thumb and index finger, with the examiner's fingers; a positive (abnormal) response consists of a forced grasp of the stimulated hand. The palmomental response consists of contraction of the mentalis muscle ipsilateral to a scratch stimulus diagonally applied to the palm.

Sensory Examination (See also Chap. 23)

Five primary sensory modalities—vibration, joint position, light touch, pinprick, and temperature—are routinely tested in each limb. Vibration testing generally utilizes a 128-Hz weighted tuning fork applied to the terminal phalynx of the great toe or middle finger just below the nail bed. The examiner compares the patient's threshold of vibration perception with his or her own or compares distal and proximal thresholds in the patient. For joint position testing, the examiner grasps the limb laterally and distal to the joint to be assessed; small 1–2 mm excursions are normally appreciated. Light touch is best assessed with a wisp of cotton, pinprick with a new pin (compare sharp versus blunt end), and temperature initially with a tuning fork immersed in cold and warm water. Patients with lesions above the level of the thalamus may have disorders of "discriminative sensation," resulting in an inability to perceive double simultaneous stimuli, to localize stimuli accurately, to identify closely approximated stimuli as separate (two-point discrimination), to identify objects by touch alone (stereognosis), or identify letters or numbers written on the skin surface (graphesthesia).

Coordination (See also Chap. 22)

The patient is asked to touch his or her index finger repetitively to the nose and then to the examiner's outstretched finger; the examiner's finger can be moved with each repetition. Another useful test is to ask the patient to alternate tapping the palm then the back of one hand on the thigh. To test coordination in the legs, in the supine position the patient is asked to slide the heel (not the arch!) of each foot from the knee down the shin of the other leg, and to raise the leg and touch with the great toe the examiner's index finger. For all these movements, the accuracy, speed, and rhythm are noted.

Gait (See also Chap. 22)

Gait testing is essential; unexpected abnormalities may be detected that prompt the examiner to return, in more detail, to other aspects of the examination. Normal gait requires that multiple systems—including power, sensation, coordination, and praxis—function in a coordinated fashion. The ability to rise from the sitting or lying position, to walk, turn, and heel-toe walk along a straight line should be noted. A positive Romberg test consists of an ability to stand with feet together and eyes open but not with eyes closed, and usually signifies a proprioceptive sensory deficit. The examination may reveal decreased arm swing on one side (corticospinal tract disease), a stooped posture and short-stepped gait (parkinsonism), a broad-based unstable gait (ataxia), scissoring (spasticity), or a high-stepped, slapping gait (posterior column or peripheral nerve disease), or the patient may appear to be stuck in place (apraxia).

down one leg, or if the tap is "dry," the needle is removed completely and repositioned.

Once the subarachnoid space is reached, a manometer is attached to the needle and the CSF pressure is measured. The examiner should look for normal oscillations in CSF pressure associated with pulse and respirations. Depending on the clinical indication, fluid is then obtained for studies that include the following: (1) cell count, differential, and presence of microorganisms—it is often useful to repeat the cell count in the first and last tube; (2) protein, glucose, and other chemical measurements; (3) cytology; (4) bacteriologic cultures and virus isolation; (5) VDRL, cryptococcal antigen, and serologic and genetic tests for other microorganisms as appropriate; (6) immunoelectrophoresis for determination of gamma globulin level (paired serum sample essential), oligoclonal banding, and other special biochemical tests (NH_3, pH, CO_2, enzymes). Normal values of CSF constituents are shown in Appendix A. Under most conditions, the physician should not be concerned about removing too large a quantity of CSF. A sufficient volume to obtain all the data required is essential. In particular, adequate volumes for cytology, when indicated, should be removed.

Failure to enter the lumbar subarachnoid space after two or three trials can usually be corrected by repositioning the patient in the sitting position and then assisting them to lie on their side. The "dry tap" is more often due to an improperly placed needle than to a pathologic obliteration of subarachnoid space by a compressive lesion of the spinal cord or by chronic adhesive arachnoiditis. A bloody tap due to penetration of a meningeal vessel may be confused with subarachnoid hemorrhage. In these situations a specimen of CSF should be centrifuged immediately after it is obtained; clear supernatant CSF after centrifugation supports the diagnosis of a bloody tap, whereas xanthochromic supernatant suggests subarachnoid hemorrhage. In

Table 356-3 Indications for Diagnostic Lumbar Puncture

Absolute Indications
- Meningitis
- Encephalitis
- Meningeal cancer
- Guillain-Barré syndrome
- Acute demyelinating disorders
  - Acute disseminated encephalomyelitis
  - Transverse myelitis
  - Brainstem encephalomyelitis
- Benign intracranial hypertension (pseudotumor cerebri)
- Unexplained neurologic disorders
  - Seizure
  - Stroke
  - Polyneuropathy
  - Dementia
  - Altered level of consciousness

Possible indications (Depending on the clinical situation)
- Multiple sclerosis
- Subarachnoid hemorrhage (if CT negative)

general, bloody CSF due to a meningeal vessel puncture clears gradually in successive tubes, whereas blood due to a subarachnoid hemorrhage does not. In addition to subarachnoid hemorrage, xanthochromic CSF may also be present in patients with liver disease or when the level of CSF protein is elevated [>1.5 to 2.0 g/L (150 to 200 mg/dL)].

There are several absolute or relative contraindications to LP. The procedure should be undertaken with particular care in patients with thrombocytopenia or disorders of blood coagulation because serious hemorrhage into the extradural or intradural space may occur. In these situations, it is prudent whenever possible to transfuse platelets, administer fresh frozen plasma, or reverse therapeutic anticoagulation before the procedure. Patients receiving low-molecular-weight heparin may be at risk of hemorrhage unless doses are held for 24 h. An LP through areas of cutaneous or soft tissue infection may spread infection to the meninges; thus LP at these sites should be avoided.

In patients with elevated CSF pressure, potentially fatal cerebellar or tentorial herniation may follow LP. This possibility should be considered in all patients with focal neurologic findings, altered mental status, or papilledema. If CSF examination is required in such cases, it is wise to first obtain a neuroimaging scan to exclude a mass lesion. An exception to this rule is suspected meningitis, where immediate CSF examination is indicated. In this situation, the LP may be performed with a fine-bore (24-gauge) needle. If the pressure is >400 mmHg, the minimum required sample of fluid should be obtained, the needle removed, and, according to the suspected clinical disease and the patient's condition, intravenous mannitol administered in a dose of 0.75 to 1.0 mg/kg; unless contraindicated, dexamethasone may also be started in a dose of 4 to 6 mg every 6 h.

After LP, the patient is normally positioned in a comfortable, recumbant position for 1 h before rising. The principal complication of LP is headache, occurring in 10 to 30% of patients, caused by a drop in CSF pressure related to persistent leakage of CSF. Such headaches typically begin 12 to 48 h after the procedure and may last from several days to 2 weeks, rarely longer. These headaches are strikingly positional in character; they are worsened by an upright posture and are relieved by lying flat. →***Therapy is discussed in Chap. 15.***

BIBLIOGRAPHY

ADAMS RD et al: *Principles of Neurology*, 6th ed. New York, McGraw-Hill, 1997

AMERICAN ACADEMY OF NEUROLOGY: Practice parameter: Lumbar puncture (summary statement). Report of the Quality Standards Subcommittee. Neurology 43:625, 1993

DANA ALLIANCE FOR BRAIN INITIATIVES: *Delivery Results: A Progress Report on Brain Research*. New York, Dana Press, 1996

FISHMAN RA: *Cerebrospinal Fluid in Diseases of the Nervous System*, 2d ed. Philadelphia, Saunders, 1992

FULLER G: Neurological examination made easy. New York. Churchill Livingstone, 1999

GOPAL AK et al: Cranial computed tomography before lumbar puncture: a prospective clinical evaluation. Arch Int Med 159:2681, 1999

HAERER AF: *DeJong's The Neurologic Examination*. Philadelphia, Lippincott, 1992

QUINT DJ: Indications for emergent MRI of the central nervous system. JAMA 283:853, 2000

357

Michael J. Aminoff

ELECTROPHYSIOLOGIC STUDIES OF THE CENTRAL AND PERIPHERAL NERVOUS SYSTEMS

ELECTROENCEPHALOGRAPHY

The electrical activity of the brain [the *electroencephalogram* (EEG)] is easily recorded from electrodes placed on the scalp. The potential difference between pairs of electrodes on the scalp (bipolar derivation) or between individual scalp electrodes and a relatively inactive common reference point (referential derivation) is amplified and displayed on paper or the screen of an oscilloscope. The findings depend on the patient's age and level of arousal. The rhythmic activity normally recorded represents the postsynaptic potentials of vertically oriented pyramidal cells of the cerebral cortex and is characterized by its frequency. In normal awake adults lying quietly with the eyes closed, an 8- to 13-Hz alpha rhythm is seen posteriorly in the EEG, intermixed with a variable amount of generalized faster (beta) activity, and it is attenuated when the eyes are opened (Fig. 357-1). During drowsiness, the alpha rhythm is also attenuated; with light sleep, slower activity in the theta (4 to 7 Hz) and delta (<4 Hz) ranges becomes more conspicuous.

The EEG is best recorded from several different electrode arrangements (montages) in turn, and activating procedures are generally undertaken in an attempt to provoke abnormalities. Such procedures commonly include hyperventilation (for 3 or 4 min), photic stimulation, sleep, and the deprivation of sleep on the night prior to the recording.

Electroencephalography is relatively inexpensive and may aid clinical management in several different contexts.

THE EEG AND EPILEPSY The EEG is most useful in evaluating patients with suspected epilepsy. The presence of *electrographic seizure activity*, i.e., of abnormal, repetitive, rhythmic activity having an abrupt onset and termination, clearly establishes the diagnosis. The absence of such electrocerebral accompaniment does not exclude a seizure disorder, however, because there may be no change in the scalp-recorded EEG during simple or complex partial seizures. With generalized tonic-clonic seizures, however, the EEG is always abnormal during the episode. It is often not possible to obtain an EEG during clinical events that may represent seizures, especially when such events occur unpredictably or infrequently. The development of portable equipment to record the EEG continuously on cassettes for 24 h or longer in ambulatory patients has made it easier to capture the electrocerebral accompaniments of such clinical episodes, and monitoring by this means is sometimes helpful in confirming that seizures are occurring, characterizing the nature of clinically equivocal episodes, and determining the frequency of epileptic events.

The EEG findings may also be helpful in the interictal period by showing certain abnormalities that are strongly supportive of a diagnosis of epilepsy. Such *epileptiform activity* consists of bursts of abnormal discharges containing spikes or sharp waves. The presence of epileptiform activity is not specific for epilepsy, but it has a much greater prevalence in epileptic patients than in normal individuals. When epileptiform activity is found in the EEG of a patient with ep-

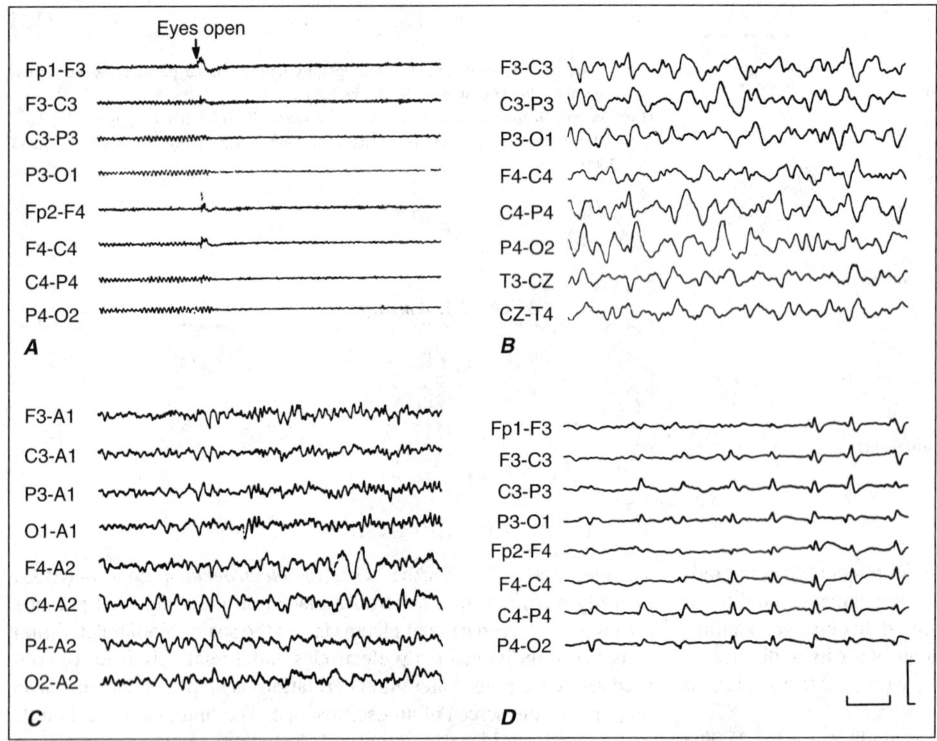

FIGURE 357-1 *A.* Normal EEG showing a posteriorly situated 9-Hz alpha rhythm that attenuates with eye opening. *B.* Abnormal EEG showing irregular diffuse slow activity in an obtunded patient with encephalitis. *C.* Irregular slow activity in the right central region, on a diffusely slowed background, in a patient with a right parietal glioma. *D.* Periodic complexes occurring once every second in a patient with Creutzfeldt-Jakob disease. Horizontal calibration: 1 s; vertical calibration: 200 μV in A, 300 μV in other panels. *(From Aminoff, 1999.)* In this and the following figure, electrode placements are indicated at the left of each panel and accord with the international 10:20 system. A, earlobe; C, central; F, frontal; Fp, frontal polar; P, parietal; T, temporal; O, occipital. Right-sided placements are indicated by even numbers, left-sided placements by odd numbers, and midline placements by Z.

isodic behavioral disturbances that clinically might be epileptic in nature, the likelihood that epilepsy is the correct diagnosis is markedly increased.

The EEG findings have also been used in classifying seizure disorders and selecting appropriate anticonvulsant medication for individual patients (Fig. 357-2). The episodic generalized spike-wave activity that occurs during and between seizures in patients with typical absences (petit mal epilepsy) contrasts with the normal findings, focal interictal epileptiform discharges, or ictal patterns found in patients with complex partial seizures. These latter seizures may have no correlates in the scalp-recorded EEG or may be associated with abnormal rhythmic activity of variable frequency, a localized or generalized distribution, and a stereotyped pattern that varies with the patient. Focal or lateralized epileptogenic lesions are important to recognize, especially if surgical treatment is contemplated. Intensive long-term monitoring of clinical behavior and the EEG is required for operative candidates, however, and this generally also involves recording from intracranially placed electrodes (which may be subdural, extradural, or intracerebral in location).

The findings in the routine scalp-recorded EEG may indicate the prognosis of seizure disorders: in general, a normal EEG implies a better prognosis than otherwise, whereas an abnormal background or profuse epileptiform activity suggests a poor outlook. The EEG findings are not helpful in determining which patients with head injuries, stroke, or brain tumors will go on to develop seizures, because in such circumstances epileptiform activity is commonly encountered regardless of whether seizures occur. The EEG findings are sometimes used to determine whether anticonvulsant medication can be discontinued in epileptic patients who have been seizure-free for several years, but the findings provide only a general guide to prognosis: further seizures may occur after withdrawal of anticonvulsant medication despite a normal EEG or, conversely, may not occur despite a continuing EEG abnormality. The decision to discontinue anticonvulsant medication is made on clinical grounds, and the EEG does not have a useful role in this context except for providing guidance when there is clinical ambiguity or the patient requires reassurance about a particular course of action.

The EEG has no role in the management of tonic-clonic status epilepticus except when there is clinical uncertainty whether seizures are continuing in a comatose patient. In patients treated by pentobarbital-induced coma for refractory status epilepticus, the EEG findings are useful in indicating the level of anesthesia and whether seizures are occurring. During status epilepticus, the EEG shows repeated electrographic seizures or continuous spike-wave discharges. In nonconvulsive status epilepticus, a disorder that may not be recognized unless an EEG is performed, the EEG may also show continuous spike-wave activity ("spike-wave stupor") or, less commonly, repetitive electrographic seizures (complex partial status epilepticus).

THE EEG AND COMA In patients with an altered mental state or some degree of obtundation, the EEG tends to become slower as consciousness is depressed, regardless of the underlying cause (Fig. 357-1). Other findings may also be present and may suggest diagnostic possibilities, as when electrographic seizures are found or there is a focal abnormality indicating a structural lesion. The EEG generally slows in metabolic encephalopathies, and triphasic waves may be present. The findings do not permit differentiation of the underlying metabolic disturbance but help to exclude other encephalopathic processes by indicating the diffuse extent of cerebral dysfunction. The response of the EEG to external stimulation is helpful prognostically because electrocerebral responsiveness implies a lighter level of coma than a nonreactive EEG. Serial records provide a better guide to prognosis than a single record and supplement the clinical examination in following the course of events. As the depth of coma increases, the EEG becomes nonreactive and may show a burst-suppression pattern, with bursts of mixed-frequency activity separated by intervals of relative cerebral inactivity. In other instances there is a reduction in amplitude of the EEG until eventually electrocerebral activity cannot be detected. Such electrocerebral silence does not necessarily reflect irreversible brain damage, because it may occur in hypothermic patients or with drug overdose. The prognosis of electrocerebral silence, when recorded using an adequate technique, depends upon the clinical context in which it is found. In patients with severe cerebral anoxia, for example, electrocerebral silence in a technically satisfactory record implies that useful cognitive recovery will not occur.

In patients with clinically suspected brain death, an EEG, when recorded using appropriate technical standards, may be confirmatory by showing electrocerebral silence. However, complicating disorders that may produce a similar but reversible EEG appearance (e.g., hypothermia or drug intoxication) must be excluded. The presence of residual EEG activity in suspected brain death fails to confirm the diagnosis but does not exclude it. The EEG is usually normal in patients with locked-in syndrome and helps in distinguishing this dis-

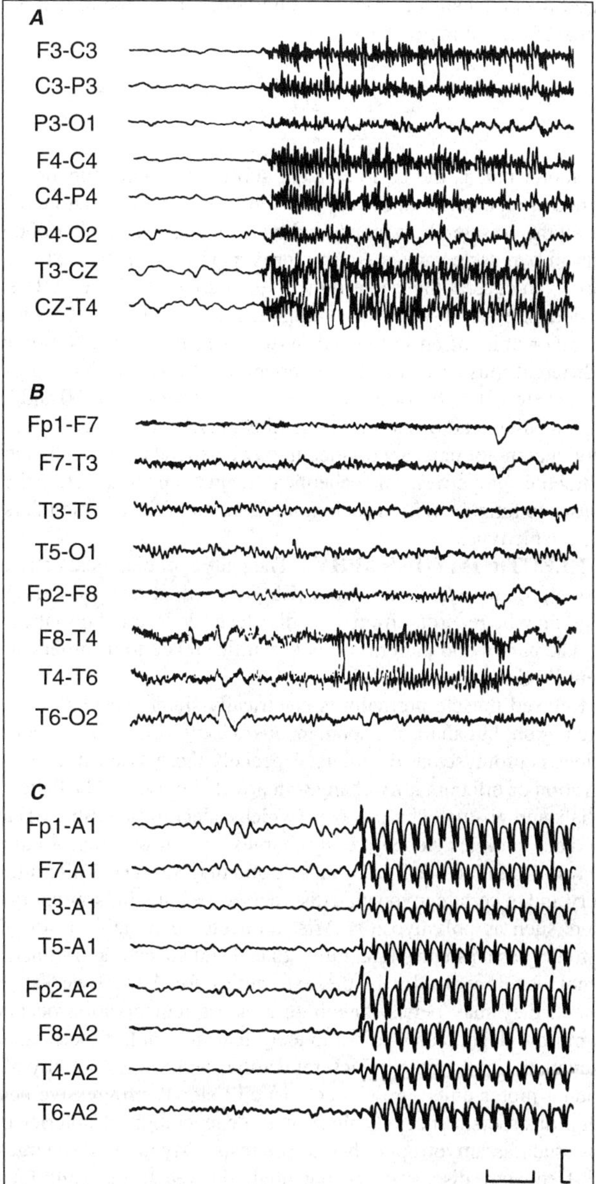

FIGURE 357-2 Electrographic seizures. *A*. Onset of a tonic seizure showing generalized repetitive sharp activity with synchronous onset over both hemispheres. *B*. Burst of repetitive spikes occurring with sudden onset in the right temporal region during a clinical spell characterized by transient impairment of external awareness. *C*. Generalized 3-Hz spike-wave activity occurring synchronously over both hemispheres during an absence (petit mal) attack. Horizontal calibration: 1 s; vertical calibration: 400 μV in A, 200 μV in B, and 750 μV in C. *(From Aminoff, 1999.)*

order from the comatose state with which it is sometimes confused clinically.

THE EEG IN OTHER NEUROLOGIC DISORDERS In the developed countries, computed tomography (CT) scanning and magnetic resonance imaging (MRI) have taken the place of EEG as a noninvasive means of screening for focal structural abnormalities of the brain, such as tumors, infarcts, or hematomas (Fig. 357-1). Nonetheless, the EEG is still used for this purpose in many parts of the world, although infratentorial or slowly expanding lesions may fail to cause any abnormalities. Focal slow-wave disturbances, a localized loss of electrocerebral activity, or more generalized electrocerebral disturbances are common findings but provide no reliable indication about the nature of the underlying pathology.

In patients with an acute encephalopathy, focal or lateralized periodic slow-wave complexes, sometimes with a sharpened outline, suggest a diagnosis of herpes simplex encephalitis, and periodic lateralized epileptiform discharges (PLEDs) are commonly found with acute hemispheric pathology such as a hematoma, abscess, or rapidly expanding tumor. The EEG findings in dementia are usually nonspecific and do not distinguish between the different causes of cognitive decline except in rare instances when the presence of complexes occurring with a regular repetition rate (so-called periodic complexes) in dementing disorders, for example, supports a diagnosis of Creutzfeldt-Jakob disease (Fig. 357-1) or subacute sclerosing panencephalitis. In most patients with dementias, the EEG is normal or diffusely slowed, and the EEG findings alone cannot indicate whether a patient is demented or distinguish between dementia and pseudodementia.

EVOKED POTENTIALS

SENSORY EVOKED POTENTIALS The noninvasive recording of spinal or cerebral potentials elicited by stimulation of specific afferent pathways is an important means of monitoring the functional integrity of these pathways but does not indicate the pathologic basis of lesions involving them. Such evoked potentials (EPs) are so small compared to the background EEG activity that the responses to a number of stimuli have to be recorded and averaged with a computer in order to permit their recognition and definition. The background EEG activity, which has no fixed temporal relationship to the stimulus, is averaged out by this procedure.

Visual evoked potentials (VEPs) are elicited by monocular stimulation with a reversing checkerboard pattern and are recorded from the occipital region in the midline and on either side of the scalp. The component of major clinical importance is the so-called P100 response, a positive peak having a latency of approximately 100 ms. Its presence, latency, and symmetry over the two sides of the scalp are noted. Amplitude may also be measured, but changes in size are much less helpful for the recognition of pathology. VEPs are most useful in detecting dysfunction of the visual pathways anterior to the optic chiasm. In patients with acute severe optic neuritis, the P100 is frequently lost or grossly attenuated; as clinical recovery occurs and visual acuity improves, the P100 is restored but with an increased latency that generally remains abnormally prolonged indefinitely. The VEP findings are therefore helpful in indicating previous or subclinical optic neuritis. They may also be abnormal with ocular abnormalities and with other causes of optic nerve disease, such as ischemia or compression by a tumor. Normal VEPs may be elicited by flash stimuli in patients with cortical blindness.

Brainstem auditory evoked potentials (BAEPs) are elicited by monaural stimulation with repetitive clicks and are recorded between the vertex of the scalp and the mastoid process or earlobe. A series of potentials, designated by roman numerals, occurs in the first 10 ms after the stimulus and represents in part the sequential activation of different structures in the pathway between the auditory nerve (wave I) and the inferior colliculus (wave V) in the midbrain. The presence, latency, and interpeak latency of the first five positive potentials recorded at the vertex are evaluated. The findings are helpful in screening for acoustic neuromas, detecting brainstem pathology, and evaluating comatose patients. The BAEPs are normal in coma due to metabolic/toxic disorders or bihemispheric disease but abnormal in the presence of brainstem pathology.

Somatosensory evoked potentials (SEPs) are recorded over the scalp and spine in response to electrical stimulation of a peripheral (mixed or cutaneous) nerve. The configuration, polarity, and latency of the responses depend on the nerve that is stimulated and on the recording arrangements. SEPs are used to evaluate proximal (otherwise inaccessible) portions of the peripheral nervous system and the integrity of the central somatosensory pathways.

Clinical Utility of Sensory Evoked Potentials EP studies may detect and localize lesions in afferent pathways in the central nervous system (CNS). They have been used particularly to investigate patients with suspected multiple sclerosis (MS), the diagnosis of which requires the recognition of lesions involving several different regions of the central white matter. In patients with clinical evidence of only one lesion, the electrophysiologic recognition of abnormalities in other sites helps to suggest or support the diagnosis but does not establish it unequivocally. Multimodality EP abnormalities are not specific for MS; they may occur in AIDS, Lyme disease, systemic lupus erythematosus, neurosyphilis, spinocerebellar degenerations, familial spastic paraplegia, and deficiency of vitamin E or B_{12}, among other disorders. The diagnostic utility of the electrophysiologic findings therefore depends upon the circumstances in which they are found. Abnormalities may aid in the localization of lesions to broad areas of the CNS, but attempts at precise localization on electrophysiologic grounds are misleading because the generators of many components of the EP are unknown.

The EP findings are sometimes of prognostic relevance. Bilateral loss of SEP components that are generated in the cerebral cortex implies that cognition may not be regained in posttraumatic or postanoxic coma, and EP studies may also be useful in evaluating patients with suspected brain death. In patients who are comatose for uncertain reasons, preserved BAEPs suggest either a metabolic-toxic etiology or bihemispheric disease. In patients with spinal cord injuries, SEPs have been used to indicate the completeness of the lesion—the presence or early return of a cortically generated response to stimulation of a nerve below the injured segment of the cord indicates an incomplete lesion and thus a better prognosis for functional recovery than otherwise. In surgery, intraoperative EP monitoring of neural structures placed at risk by the procedure may permit the early recognition of dysfunction and thereby permit a neurologic complication to be averted or minimized.

Visual and auditory acuity may be determined using EP techniques in patients whose age or mental state precludes traditional ophthalmologic or audiologic examinations.

COGNITIVE EVOKED POTENTIALS Certain EP components depend upon the mental attention of the subject and the setting in which the stimulus occurs, rather than simply on the physical characteristics of the stimulus. Such "event-related" potentials (ERPs) or "endogenous" potentials are related in some manner to the cognitive aspects of distinguishing an infrequently occurring target stimulus from other stimuli occurring more frequently. For clinical purposes, attention has been directed particularly at the so-called P3 component of the ERP, which is also designated the P300 component because of its positive polarity and latency of approximately 300 to 400 ms after onset of an auditory target stimulus. The P3 component is prolonged in latency in many patients with dementia, whereas it is generally normal in patients with depression or other psychiatric disorders that might be mistaken for dementia. ERPs are therefore sometimes helpful in making this distinction when there is clinical uncertainty, although a response of normal latency does not exclude a dementing disorder.

MOTOR EVOKED POTENTIALS The electrical potentials recorded from muscle or the spinal cord following stimulation of the motor cortex or central motor pathways are referred to as *motor evoked potentials.* For clinical purposes such responses are recorded most often as the compound muscle action potentials elicited by transcutaneous magnetic stimulation of the motor cortex. A strong but brief magnetic field is produced by passing a current through a coil, and this induces stimulating currents in the subjacent neural tissue. The procedure is painless and apparently safe. Abnormalities have been described in several neurologic disorders with clinical or subclinical involvement of central motor pathways, including MS and motor neuron disease. In addition to a possible role in the diagnosis of neurologic disorders or in evaluating the extent of pathologic involvement, the technique provides information of prognostic relevance (e.g., in suggesting the likelihood of recovery of motor function after stroke) and is useful as a means of monitoring intraoperatively the functional integrity of central motor tracts.

ELECTROPHYSIOLOGIC STUDIES OF MUSCLE AND NERVE

The motor unit is the basic element subserving motor function. It is defined as an anterior horn cell, its axon and neuromuscular junctions, and all the muscle fibers innervated by the axon. The number of motor units in a muscle ranges from approximately 10 in the extraocular muscles to several thousand in the large muscles of the legs. There is considerable variation in the average number of muscle fibers within the motor units of an individual muscle, i.e., in the innervation ratio of different muscles. Thus the innervation ratio is less than 25 in the human external rectus or platysma muscle and between 1600 and 1700 in the medial head of the gastrocnemius muscle. The muscle fibers of individual motor units are divided into two general types by distinctive contractile properties, histochemical stains, and characteristic responses to fatigue. Within each motor unit, all of the muscle fibers are of the same type.

ELECTROMYOGRAPHY The pattern of electrical activity in muscle [i.e., the *electromyogram* (EMG)], both at rest and during activity, may be recorded from a needle electrode inserted into the muscle. The nature and pattern of abnormalities relate to disorders at different levels of the motor unit.

Relaxed muscle normally is electrically silent except in the end-plate region, but abnormal spontaneous activity (Fig. 357-3) occurs in various neuromuscular disorders, especially those associated with denervation or inflammatory changes in affected muscle. Fibrillation potentials and positive sharp waves (which reflect muscle fiber irritability) and complex repetitive discharges are most often—but not always—found in denervated muscle and may also occur after muscle injury and in certain myopathic disorders, especially inflammatory disorders such as polymyositis. After an acute neuropathic lesion they are found earlier in proximal rather than distal muscles and sometimes do not develop distally in the extremities for 4 to 6 weeks; once present, they may persist indefinitely unless reinnervation occurs or the muscle degenerates so completely that no viable tissue remains. Fasciculation potentials (which reflect the spontaneous activity of individual motor units) are characteristic of slowly progressive neuropathic disorders, especially those with degeneration of anterior horn cells (such as amyotrophic lateral sclerosis). Myotonic discharges—high-frequency discharges of potentials derived from single muscle

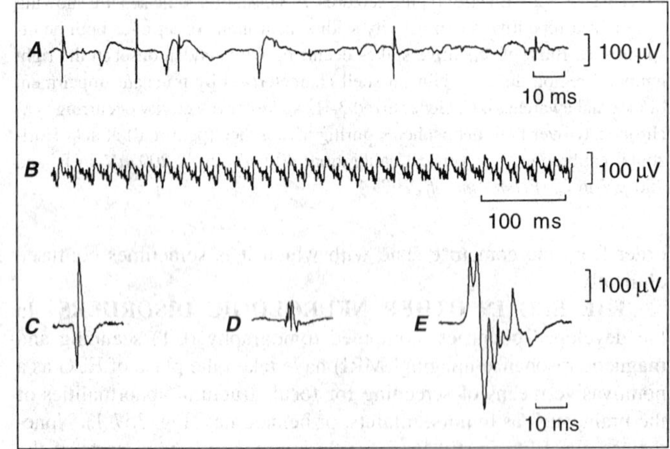

FIGURE 357-3 Activity recorded during EMG. *A.* Spontaneous fibrillation potentials and positive sharp waves. *B.* Complex repetitive discharges recorded in partially denervated muscle at rest. *C.* Normal triphasic motor unit action potential. *D.* Small, short-duration, polyphasic motor unit action potential such as is commonly encountered in myopathic disorders. *E.* Long-duration polyphasic motor unit action potential such as may be seen in neuropathic disorders.

fibers that wax and wane in amplitude and frequency—are the signature of myotonic disorders such as myotonic dystrophy or myotonia congenita but occur occasionally in polymyositis or other, rarer, disorders.

Slight voluntary contraction of a muscle leads to activation of a small number of motor units. The potentials generated by any muscle fibers of these units that are within the pick-up range of the needle electrode will be recorded (Fig. 357-3). The parameters of normal motor unit action potentials depend on the muscle under study and age of the patient, but their duration is normally between 5 and 15 ms, amplitude is between 200 μV and 2 mV, and most are bi- or triphasic. The number of units activated depends on the degree of voluntary activity. An increase in muscle contraction is associated with an increase in the number of motor units that are activated (recruited) and in the frequency with which they discharge. With a full contraction, so many motor units are normally activated that individual motor unit action potentials can no longer be distinguished, and a complete interference pattern is said to have been produced.

The incidence of small, short-duration, polyphasic motor unit action potentials (i.e., having more than four phases) is usually increased in myopathic muscle, and an excessive number of units is activated for a specified degree of voluntary activity. By contrast, the loss of motor units that occurs in neuropathic disorders leads to a reduction in number of units activated during a maximal contraction and an increase in their firing rate, i.e., there is an incomplete or reduced interference pattern; the configuration and dimensions of the potentials may also be abnormal, depending on the duration of the neuropathic process and on whether reinnervation has occurred. The surviving motor units are initially normal in configuration but, as reinnervation occurs, they increase in amplitude and duration and become polyphasic (Fig. 357-3).

Action potentials from the same motor unit sometimes fire with a consistent temporal relationship to each other, so that double, triple, or multiple discharges are recorded, especially in tetany, hemifacial spasm, or myokymia.

Electrical silence characterizes the involuntary, sustained muscle contraction that occurs in phosphorylase deficiency, which is designated a *contracture*.

EMG enables disorders of the motor units to be detected and characterized as either neurogenic or myopathic. In neurogenic disorders, the pattern of affected muscles may localize the lesion to the anterior horn cells or to a specific site as the axons traverse a nerve root, limb plexus, and peripheral nerve to their terminal arborizations. The findings do not enable a specific etiologic diagnosis to be made, however, except in conjunction with the clinical findings and results of other laboratory studies.

The findings may provide a guide to the severity of an acute disorder of a peripheral or cranial nerve (by indicating whether denervation has occurred and the completeness of the lesion), and whether the pathologic process is active or progressive in chronic or degenerative disorders such as amyotrophic lateral sclerosis. Such information is important for prognostic purposes.

Various quantitative EMG approaches have been developed. The most common is to determine the mean duration and amplitude of 20 motor unit action potentials using a standardized technique. The technique of macro-EMG provides information about the number and size of muscle fibers in a larger volume of the motor unit territory and has also been used to estimate the number of motor units in a muscle. Scanning EMG is a computer-based technique that has been used to study the topography of motor unit action potentials and, in particular, the spatial and temporal distribution of activity in individual units. The technique of single-fiber EMG is discussed separately below.

NERVE CONDUCTION STUDIES Recording of the electrical response of a muscle to stimulation of its motor nerve at two or more points along its course (Fig. 357-4) permits conduction velocity to be determined in the fastest-conducting motor fibers between the points of stimulation. The latency and amplitude of the electrical re-

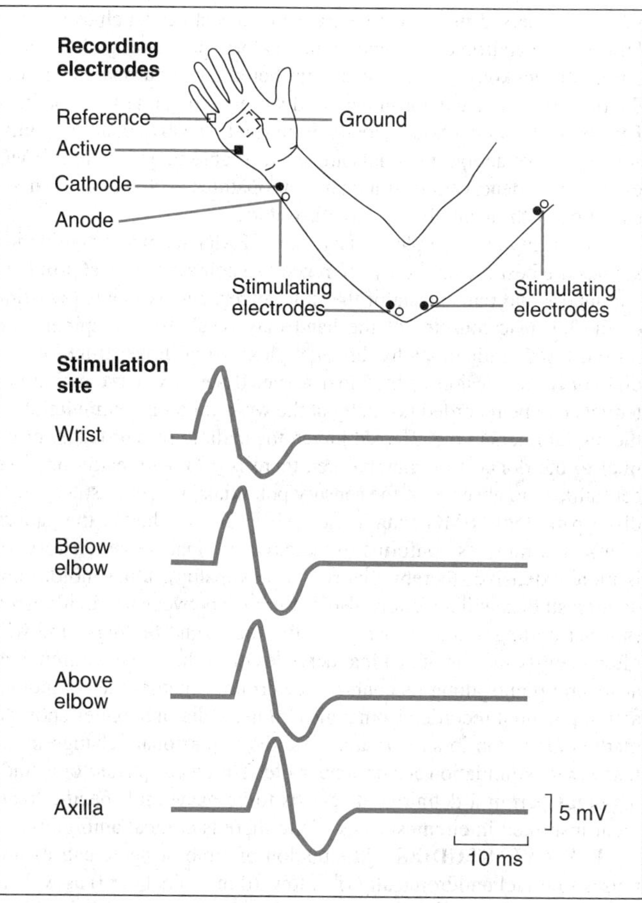

FIGURE 357-4 Arrangement for motor conduction studies of the ulnar nerve. Responses are recorded with a surface electrode from the abductor digiti minimi muscle to supramaximal stimulation of the nerve at different sites, and are shown in the lower panel. *(From Aminoff, 1998.)*

sponse of muscle (i.e., of the compound muscle action potential) to stimulation of its motor nerve at a distal site are also compared with values defined in normal subjects. Sensory nerve conduction studies are performed by determining the conduction velocity and amplitude of action potentials in sensory fibers when these fibers are stimulated at one point and the responses are recorded at another point along the course of the nerve. In adults, conduction velocity in the arms is normally between 50 and 70 m/s, and in the legs is between 40 and 60 m/s.

Nerve conduction studies complement the EMG examination, enabling the presence and extent of peripheral nerve pathology to be determined. They are particularly helpful in determining whether sensory symptoms are arising from pathology proximal or distal to the dorsal root ganglia (in the former instance, peripheral sensory conduction studies will be normal) and whether neuromuscular dysfunction relates to peripheral nerve disease. In patients with a mononeuropathy, they are invaluable as a means of localizing a focal lesion, determining the extent and severity of the underlying pathology, providing a guide to prognosis, and detecting subclinical involvement of other peripheral nerves. They enable a polyneuropathy to be distinguished from a mononeuropathy multiplex when this is not possible clinically, an important distinction because of the etiologic implications. Nerve conduction studies provide a means of following the progression and therapeutic response of peripheral nerve disorders and are being used increasingly for this purpose in clinical trials. They may suggest the underlying pathologic basis in individual cases. Conduction velocity is often markedly slowed, terminal motor latencies are prolonged, and compound motor and sensory nerve action potentials may be dispersed in the demyelinative neuropathies (such as in Guillain-Barré syndrome, chronic inflammatory polyneuropathy, metachromatic leukodystrophy, or certain hereditary neuropathies); conduction block is frequent in acquired varieties of these neuropathies. By contrast, conduction velocity is normal or slowed only mildly, sensory nerve action potentials are small or absent, and there is EMG evidence of denervation in axonal neuropathies such as occur in association with metabolic or toxic disorders.

The utility and complementary role of EMG and nerve conduction studies are best illustrated by reference to a common clinical problem. Numbness and paresthesia of the little finger, and associated wasting of the intrinsic muscles of the hand may result from a spinal cord lesion, C8/T1 radiculopathy, brachial plexopathy (lower trunk or medial cord), or a lesion of the ulnar nerve. If sensory nerve action potentials can be recorded normally at the wrist following stimulation of the digital fibers in the affected finger, the pathology is probably proximal to the dorsal root ganglia, i.e., there is a radiculopathy or more central lesion; absence of the sensory potentials, by contrast, suggests distal pathology. EMG examination will indicate whether the pattern of affected muscles conforms to radicular or ulnar nerve territory, or is more extensive (thereby favoring a plexopathy); ulnar motor conduction studies will generally also distinguish between a radiculopathy (normal findings) and ulnar neuropathy (abnormal findings) and will often identify the site of an ulnar nerve lesion—the nerve is stimulated at several points along its course to determine whether the compound action potential recorded from a distal muscle that it supplies shows a marked alteration in size or area, or a disproportionate change in latency, with stimulation at a particular site. The electrophysiologic findings thus permit a definitive diagnosis to be made and specific treatment instituted in circumstances where there is clinical ambiguity.

F WAVE STUDIES Stimulation of a motor nerve causes impulses to travel antidromically (i.e., toward the spinal cord) as well as orthodromically (to the nerve terminals). Such antidromic impulses cause a few of the anterior horn cells to discharge, producing a small motor response that occurs considerably later than the direct response elicited by nerve stimulation. The F wave so elicited is sometimes abnormal (absent or delayed) with proximal pathology of the peripheral nervous system, such as a radiculopathy, and may therefore be helpful in detecting abnormalities when conventional nerve conduction studies are normal. In general, however, the clinical utility of F wave studies has been disappointing, except perhaps in Guillain-Barré syndrome, where they are often absent or delayed.

H REFLEX STUDIES The H reflex is easily recorded only from the soleus muscle (S1) in normal adults. It is elicited by low-intensity stimulation of the tibial nerve and represents a monosynaptic reflex in which spindle (Ia) afferent fibers constitute the afferent arc and alpha motor axons the efferent pathway. The H reflexes are often absent bilaterally in elderly patients or with polyneuropathies and may be lost unilaterally in S1 radiculopathies.

MUSCLE RESPONSE TO REPETITIVE NERVE STIMULATION The size of the electrical response of a muscle to supramaximal electrical stimulation of its motor nerve relates to the number of muscle fibers that are activated. Neuromuscular transmission can be tested by several different protocols, but the most helpful is to record with surface electrodes the electrical response of a muscle to supramaximal stimulation of its motor nerve by repetitive (2 to 3 Hz) shocks delivered before and at selected intervals after a maximal voluntary contraction.

There is normally little or no change in size of the compound muscle action potential following repetitive stimulation of a motor nerve at 2 to 3 Hz with stimuli delivered at intervals after voluntary contraction of the muscle for about 20 to 30 s, even though preceding activity in the junctional region influences the release of acetylcholine and thus the size of the endplate potentials elicited by a test stimulus. This is because more acetylcholine is normally released than is required to bring the motor endplate potentials to the threshold for generating muscle fiber action potentials. In disorders of neuromuscular transmission this safety factor is reduced. Thus, in myasthenia gravis repetitive stimulation, particularly at a rate of between 2 and 5 Hz, may lead to a depression of neuromuscular transmission, with a decrement in size of the response recorded from affected muscles. Similarly, immediately after a period of maximal voluntary activity, single or repetitive stimuli of the motor nerve may elicit larger muscle responses than before, indicating that more muscle fibers are responding. This postactivation facilitation of neuromuscular transmission is followed by a longer-lasting period of depression, maximal between 2 and 4 min after the conditioning period and lasting for as long as 10 min or so, during which responses are reduced in size.

Decrementing responses to repetitive stimulation at 2 to 5 Hz are common in myasthenia gravis but may also occur in the congenital myasthenic syndromes. In Lambert-Eaton myasthenic syndrome, in which there is defective release of acetylcholine at the neuromuscular junction, the compound muscle action potential elicited by a single stimulus is generally very small. With repetitive stimulation at rates of up to 10 Hz, the first few responses may decline in size, but subsequent responses increase. If faster rates of stimulation are used (20 to 50 Hz), the increment may be dramatic so that the amplitude of compound muscle action potentials eventually reaches a size that is several times larger than the initial response. In patients with botulism, the response to repetitive stimulation is similar to that in Lambert-Eaton syndrome, although the findings are somewhat more variable and not all muscles are affected.

SINGLE-FIBER ELECTROMYOGRAPHY The technique is particularly helpful in detecting disorders of neuromuscular transmission. A special needle electrode is placed within a muscle and positioned to record action potentials from two muscle fibers belonging to the same motor unit. The time interval between the two potentials will vary in consecutive discharges, and this is called the *neuromuscular jitter*. The jitter can be quantified as the mean difference between consecutive interpotential intervals and is normally between 10 and 50 μs. This value is increased when neuromuscular transmission is disturbed for any reason, and in some instances impulses in individual muscle fibers may fail to occur because of impulse blocking at the neuromuscular junction. Single-fiber EMG is more sensitive than repetitive nerve stimulation or determination of acetylcholine receptor antibody levels in diagnosing myasthenia gravis.

Single-fiber EMG can also be used to determine the mean fiber density of motor units (i.e., mean number of muscle fibers per motor unit within the recording area) and to estimate the number of motor units in a muscle, but this is of less immediate clinical relevance.

BLINK REFLEXES Electrical or mechanical stimulation of the supraorbital nerve on one side leads to two separate reflex responses of the orbicularis oculi—an ipsilateral R1 response having a latency of approximately 10 ms and a bilateral R2 response with a latency in the order of 30 ms. The trigeminal and facial nerves constitute the afferent and efferent arcs of the reflex, respectively. Abnormalities of either nerve or intrinsic lesions of the medulla or pons may lead to uni- or bilateral loss of the response, and the findings may therefore be helpful in identifying or localizing such pathology.

BIBLIOGRAPHY

AMINOFF MJ: *Electromyography in Clinical Practice: Electrodiagnostic Aspects of Neuromuscular Disease*, 3d ed. New York, Churchill Livingstone, 1998

——— (ed): *Electrodiagnosis in Clinical Neurology*, 4th ed. New York, Churchill Livingstone, 1999

BRIL V et al: Electrophysiological monitoring in clinical trials. Muscle Nerve 11:1368, 1998

DALY DD, PEDLEY TA (eds): *Current Practice of Clinical Electroencephalography*, 2d ed. New York, Raven Press, 1990

DUMITRU D: *Electrodiagnostic Medicine*. Philadelphia, Hanley and Belfus, 1995

EBERSOLE JS (ed): *Ambulatory EEG Monitoring*. New York, Raven Press, 1988

KIMURA J: *Electrodiagnosis in Diseases of Nerve and Muscle*, 2d ed. Philadelphia, Davis, 1989

NIEDERMEYER E, LOPES DA SILVA F (eds): *Electroencephalography*, 3d ed. Baltimore, Urban & Schwarzenberg, 1993

358

William P. Dillon

NEUROIMAGING IN NEUROLOGIC DISORDERS

A dramatic increase in the role of imaging in diagnosis of neurologic diseases occurred with the development of computed tomography (CT) in the early 1970s and of magnetic resonance imaging (MRI) in the 1980s. MRI has gradually replaced CT for many indications and has also reduced the indications for invasive neuroimaging techniques, such as myelography and angiography. In general, MRI is more sensitive than CT for the evaluation of most lesions affecting the central nervous system, particularly those in the spinal cord, cranial nerves, and posterior fossa. CT is more sensitive than MRI for visualizing fine osseous detail, such as temporal bone anatomy and fractures. Recent developments, such as helical CT, CT angiography (CTA), MR angiography (MRA), positron emission tomography (PET), Doppler ultrasound, and interventional angiography have continued to advance diagnosis and guide therapy. Conventional angiography is reserved for cases in which small-vessel detail is essential for diagnosis (Table 358-1).

COMPUTED TOMOGRAPHY Technique The CT image is a computer-generated cross-sectional representation of anatomy created by an analysis of the attenuation of x-ray beams passed through various points around a section of the body. As the x-ray source, collimated to the desired slice thickness, rotates around the patient, sensitive x-ray detectors aligned 180° from the source detect x-rays attenuated by the patient's anatomy. A computer calculates a "back projection" image from the 360° x-ray attenuation profile. Greater x-ray attenuation, as caused by bone, results in areas of high "density," while soft tissue structures, which attenuate x-rays less, are lower in density. The resolution of an image depends on the radiation dose, the collimation (slice thickness), the field of view, and the matrix size of the display. A typical modern CT scanner is capable of obtaining sections 1 to 2, 5, and 10 mm thick at a speed of 1 to 3 s per section; complete studies of the brain can be completed in <2 to 3 min.

Intravenous contrast is often administered prior to or during a CT study to identify vascular structures and to detect defects in the blood-brain barrier (BBB) associated with disorders such as tumors, infarcts, and infections. An intact BBB prevents contrast molecules, which are large, from exiting the intravascular compartment. In the normal central nervous system, only vessels and those structures not having a BBB (e.g., the pituitary gland, choroid plexus, and dura) enhance. The use of contrast agents carries a risk of allergic reaction, increases the dose of radiation when both noncontrast and contrast CT scans are to be obtained, adds expense, and may mask hemorrhage; thus, before contrast is administered, the indication for its use should always be considered carefully.

Helical CT is a new technique in which continuous three-dimensional CT information is obtained. In the helical scan mode, the table moves continuously through the rotating x-ray beam, generating a "helix" of information that can be reformatted into various slice thicknesses. Advantages include shorter scan times, reduced patient and organ motion, and the ability to acquire images during the infusion of intravenous contrast. The contrast images can be used to construct CT angiograms of vascular structures. CTA images require a workstation to threshold and segment CT images for display (Fig. 358-1). CTA has proven useful in assessing the carotid bifurcation and intracranial arterial anatomy in selected instances in which a contraindication to MRA exists. Newer "multidetector" scanners allow multiple sections to be obtained with each revolution of the gantry. These scanners have further decreased the time per examination and permit rapid assessment of vascular anatomy (Fig. 358-2).

Indications The indications for CT have decreased since the development of MRI. While MRI gives greater soft tissue contrast and is more sensitive than CT in detecting early brain damage, CT is useful in imaging osseous structures of the spine, skull base, and temporal bones. CT is also more sensitive and specific than MRI for acute subarachnoid hemorrhage. In the spine, CT is useful in evaluating patients

Table 358-1 Guidelines for the Use of CT, Ultrasound, and MRI

Condition	Recommended Technique
Hemorrhage	
Acute parenchymal	CT > MRI
Subacute/chronic	MRI
Subarachnoid hemorrhage	CT, lumbar puncture → angiography
Aneurysm	Angiography > ?MRA
Ischemic infarction	
Hemorrhagic infarction	CT or MRI
Bland infarction	MRI > CT
Carotid or vertebral dissection	MRI/MRA
Vertebral basilar insufficiency	MRI/MRA
Carotid stenosis	Doppler ultrasound, MRA, CTA
Suspected mass lesions	
Neoplasm, primary or metastatic	MRI + contrast
Infection/abscess	MRI + contrast
Immunosuppression with focal findings	MRI + contrast
Vascular malformations	MRI ± angiography
White matter disorders	MRI
Demyelinating disease	MRI ± contrast
Dementia	MRI or CT
Trauma	
Acute trauma	CT (noncontrast)
Shear injury/chronic hemorrhage	MRI
Headache/migraine	CT (noncontrast) or MRI
Seizure	
First time, no focal neurologic deficits	MRI > CT as screen
Partial complex/refractory	MRI + coronal T2W imaging
Cranial neuropathy	MRI + contrast
Meningeal disease	MRI + contrast
SPINE	
Low back pain	
No neurologic deficits	Conservative therapy, consider MRI or CT after 4 weeks
With focal deficits	MRI > CT
Spinal stenosis	MRI or CT
Cervical spondylosis	MRI or CT myelography
Infection	MRI + contrast > CT
Myelopathy	MRI + contrast, consider myelography if MRI negative
Arteriovenous malformations	MRI, myelography/angiography

NOTE: CT, computed tomography; MRI, magnetic resonance imaging; MRA, MR angiography; CTA, CT angiography; T2W, T2-weighted.

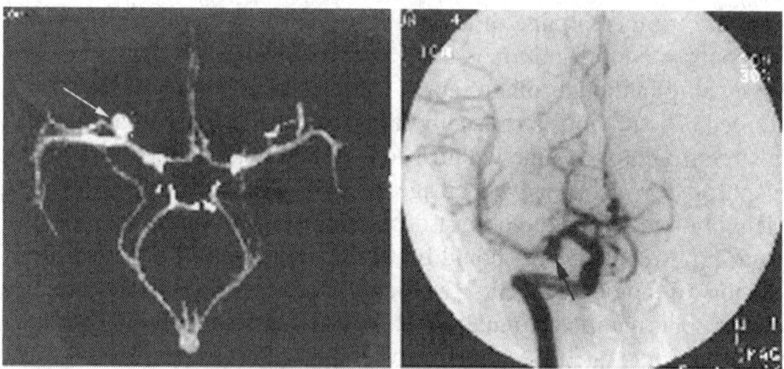

FIGURE 358-1 CT angiography (CTA) of middle cerebral aneurysm. A right middle cerebral aneurysm (*arrow*) is shown on CTA (*left image*) and confirmed by conventional internal carotid angiography (*right image*). CTA image is produced by helical scans or 1-mm CT scans performed during a rapid bolus infusion of intravenous contrast medium. Subtraction of background nonenhancing brain results in the CTA image. *(From RA Alberico et al: Am J Neuroradiol 16:1571, 1995.)*

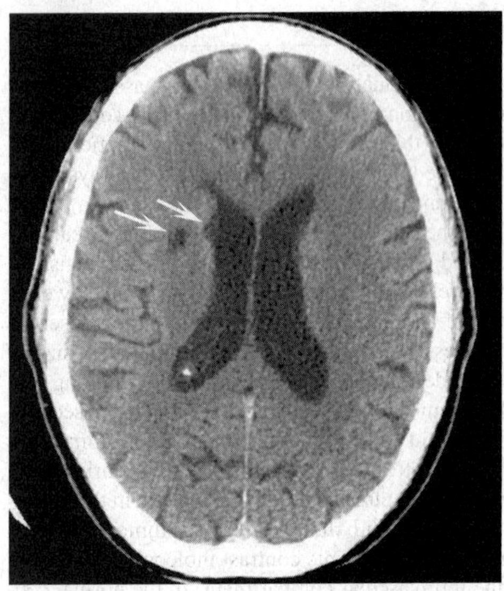

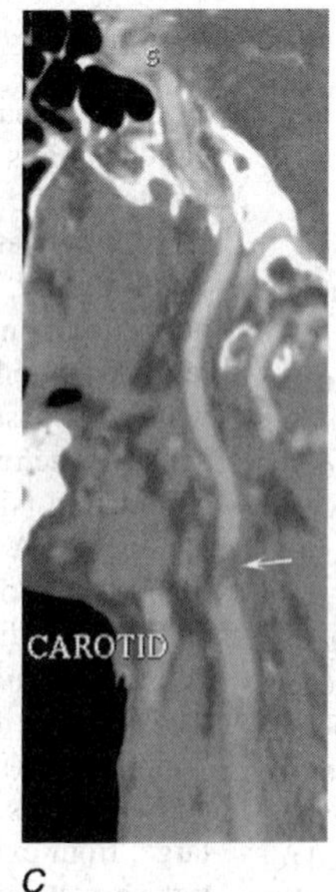

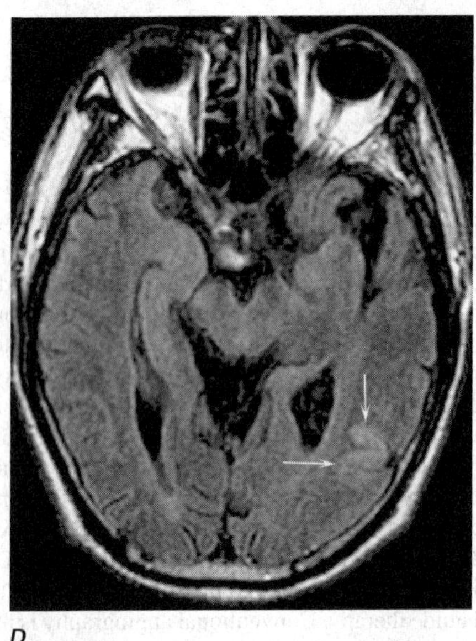

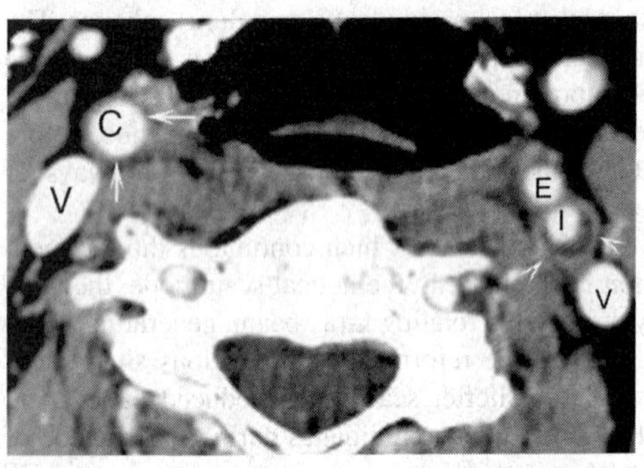

FIGURE 358-2 A 65-year-old man with aphasia of 5 h duration. Prior right lacunar infarctions were noted by history. *A.* Noncontrast CT scan through the lateral ventricles demonstrates two low-density foci representing old cerebral infarctions on the right. No pathology is seen in the left hemisphere, the site of his acute symptoms. B. Single axial CT image from a CT angiography (CTA) examination obtained in 45 s through the entire supraortic vasculature, cervical carotids, and circle of Willis. Normal right common carotid artery is homogeneously opacified (*arrows*). Left internal carotid artery lumen is narrowed by eccentric low-density atherosclerotic plaque (*arrowheads*), which narrows the lumen to approximately 40%. (C, common carotid artery; V, internal jugular vein; I, internal carotid artery; E, external carotid artery.) *C.* Sagittal reformation through the cervical carotid vasculature from the CTA data set demonstrates the plaque at the origin of the internal carotid artery (*arrow*). *D.* Axial T2-weighted FLAIR (fluid-attenuated inversion recovery) MR image 7 h following onset of aphasia demonstrates a focal cortical high signal intensity (*arrows*) consistent with a small infarction in the posterior temporal lobe. Following anticoagulation, patient improved to his baseline status.

with osseous spinal stenosis and spondylosis, but MRI is often preferred in those with neurologic deficits. CT can also be obtained following intrathecal contrast injection to evaluate the intracranial cisterns for cerebrospinal fluid (CSF) fistula, as well as the spinal subarachnoid space.

Complications CT is safe and reliable. Radiation exposure is between 3 and 5 cGy per examination. The most frequent complications are associated with use of intravenous contrast agents. Two broad categories of contrast media, ionic and nonionic, are in use. Ionic agents are relatively safe and inexpensive but cause a higher incidence of toxicity reactions than nonionic agents.

Nephrotoxicity caused by contrast administration (*contrast nephropathy*) may result from hemodynamic changes, tubular obstruction and cell damage, or immunologic reactions to contrast agents. A rise in serum creatinine of at least 85 μmol/L (1 mg/dL) within 48 h of contrast administration is often used as a definition of contrast nephropathy, although other causes of acute renal failure must be excluded. The prognosis is usually favorable, with serum creatinine levels returning to baseline within 1 to 2 weeks. Risk factors for contrast nephropathy include advanced age, preexisting renal disease, diabetes, dehydration, and high contrast dose. Patients with diabetes and those with mild renal failure should be well hydrated prior to the administration of nonionic agents. Nonionic, low-osmolar media produce fewer abnormalities in renal blood flow and less endothelial cell damage than ionic agents (see guidelines on p. 2339).

A sensation of heat, pain, nausea, and *vomiting* are well-known side effects following intravenous administration of ionic contrast media, and they become more important as studies require longer imaging times and repeated contrast injections. Pain and the sensation of heat are probably due to the osmolality of the agent and vasodilation. These side effects are less intense or nonexistent with nonionic contrast media.

Anaphylactoid reactions to intravenous contrast media range from mild hives to bronchospasm to acute anaphylaxis and death. The pathogenesis of these allergic reactions is not fully understood, but it is thought to include the release of mediators such as histamine, antibody-antigen reactions, and complement activation. Severe allergic reactions occur in approximately 0.04% of patients receiving nonionic media, sixfold fewer than with ionic media. Risk factors include a history of prior contrast reaction, allergy (asthma and hay fever), and cardiac disease. In these patients, a noncontrast CT or MRI procedure should be considered as an alternative to contrast administration. If contrast is absolutely required, a nonionic agent should be used in conjunction with pretreatment with glucocorticoids and antihistamines (Table 358-2 and guidelines on p. 2339). Patients with allergic reactions to iodinated contrast material do not usually react against gadolinium-based magnetic resonance (MR) contrast material, although it would be wise to pretreat in a similar fashion prior to MR contrast administration.

MAGNETIC RESONANCE IMAGING Technique The phenomenon of magnetic resonance is a complex interaction between protons in biologic tissues, a static and alternating magnetic field (the magnet), and energy in the form of radiofrequency waves of a specific frequency (Rf), introduced by coils placed next to the body part of interest. The energy state of the hydrogen protons is transiently excited. The subsequent return to equilibrium (*relaxation*) of the protons results in a release of Rf energy (the *echo*), which can be measured by the same surface coils that delivered the Rf pulses. The complex Rf signal, or echo, is transformed by Fourier analysis into the information used to form an MR image.

T1 and T2 relaxation times The rate of return to equilibrium of perturbed protons is called the *relaxation rate*. The relaxation rate is different for different normal and pathologic tissues. The relaxation rate of a hydrogen proton in a tissue is influenced by surrounding

Guidelines for Use of Intravenous Contrast in Patients with Impaired Renal Function

Serum Creatinine Level, μmol/L (mg/dL)[a]	Recommendations
<133 (<1.5)	Use either ionic or nonionic contrast at 2 mL/kg to 150 mL total
133–177 (1.5–2.0)	Use nonionic contrast; hydrate diabetics
>177 (>2.0)	Consider noncontrast CT or MRI; use nonionic contrast if required
177–221 (2.0–2.5)	Use nonionic contrast only if required (as above); contraindicated in diabetics
>265 (>3.0)	Nonionic contrast given only to patients undergoing dialysis within 24 h

[a] Risk is greatest in patients with rising creatinine levels.
NOTE: CT, computed tomography; MRI, magnetic resonance imaging.

molecular environment and atomic neighbors. Two relaxation rates, the T1 and T2 relaxation times, are measurable. The T1 relaxation rate is the time for 63% of the protons to return to their normal equilibrium state, while the T2 relaxation rate is the time for 63% of the protons to become dephased owing to interactions among adjacent protons. The intensity of the signal, and thus the image contrast, can be modulated by altering certain parameters, such as the interval between Rf pulses (TR) and the time between the Rf pulse and the signal reception (TE). So-called T1-weighted (T1W) images are produced by keeping the TR and TE relatively short. Under these conditions, contrast between structures is based primarily on their T1 relaxation differences. T2-weighted (T2W) images are produced by using longer TR and TE times. Fat and subacute hemorrhage have short T1 relaxation rates and a high signal intensity on T1W images. Watery media, such as CSF and edematous tissue, have long T1 and T2 relaxation rates, a low signal intensity on T1W images, and a high signal intensity on T2W images. As white matter contains more lipid (due to myelin), it contains 10 to 15% less water than gray matter. These two chemical differences account for much of the contrast difference between gray and white matter on MRI (Fig. 358-3). T2W images are more sensitive than T1W images to edema or myelin destruction (Fig. 371-2).

MR images can be generated in sagittal, coronal, axial, and oblique planes without changing the patient's position. Each plane obtained requires a separate sequence lasting 5 to 10 min. Unlike CT, movement of the patient during a sequence will distort *all* the images; therefore, patient cooperation is important. Approximately 5% of the population experience claustrophobia in the MR environment. This can be reduced by mild sedation. Three-dimensional volumetric imaging is also possible with MR, resulting in data that can be reformatted in any plane and manipulated in a real-time fashion to highlight certain disease processes. Fluid-attenuated inversion recovery, or FLAIR, is a pulse sequence that produces T2W images in which the CSF signal is suppressed. FLAIR images are more sensitive than standard spine echo images for cortical lesions and meningeal processes (Fig. 358-2*D*).

Table 358-2 Indications for the Use of Nonionic Contrast Media

- Prior adverse reaction to contrast media, with the exception of heat, flushing, or an episode of nausea or vomiting
- Asthma or other serious lung disease
- History of atopic allergies (pretreatment with glucocorticoids and antihistamines recommended)
- Age under 2 years old
- Renal failure or a creatinine level >177 μmol/L (>2.0 mg/dL)
- Cardiac dysfunction, including cardiac failure, severe arrhythmias, unstable angina pectoris, recent myocardial infarction, or pulmonary hypertension
- Diabetes
- Severe debilitation

Guidelines for the Premedication of Patients with Prior Allergic Reaction to Contrast Agents

12 h before examination:
Prednisone, 40 mg PO *or* methylprednisolone, 32 mg PO
2 h before examination:
Prednisone, 40 mg PO *or* methylprednisolone, 32 mg PO
and
Cimetidine, 300 mg PO *or* ranitidine, 150 mg PO
Immediately before examination:
Benadryl, 50 mg IV (alternatively, can be given PO 2 h before exam)

Contrast material The heavy-metal element *gadolinium* forms the basis of all current intravenous MR contrast agents. Gadolinium is a paramagnetic substance, which means that it reduces the T1 and T2 relaxation times of nearby water protons, resulting in a high signal on T1W images. The metal is chelated to an agent such as DTPA, which allows renal excretion without toxicity. Approximately 0.2 mL/kg body weight is administered intravenously (10 to 15 mL for the average-sized adult); the cost is approximately $60 per 20 mL. Gadolinium contrast does not cross a normal BBB, and thus it causes enhancement of brain tissue only at sites of abnormalities in the BBB (Fig. 371-2*D*) and in areas of the brain that normally have no BBB, such as the pituitary gland. Allergic reactions are extremely rare; renal failure does not occur. These agents can be administered safely to children as well as adults.

MAGNETIC RESONANCE ANGIOGRAPHY Flowing blood exhibits complex MR signals that range from bright to dark relative to background stationary tissue (Fig. 358-3). Fast-flowing blood, such as arterial blood, shows no signal on routine MR images. Slower flow, as in veins or distal to arterial stenoses, may appear high in signal. It is possible, by varying the MR image parameters, to assess blood flow either qualitatively or quantitatively. This is the basis of MRA, which capitalizes on the differences in signal between moving blood and stationary tissue on gradient echo images (Fig. 358-4). *Gradient echo images* differ from standard spin echo images in being more sensitive to blood products, calcification, and other susceptibility artifacts. The suppression of background signal achieved in short-flip-angle gradient echo images provides the contrast needed for flowing blood to appear bright in signal on MRA images.

It is important to understand that MRA provides a *vascular flow map* rather than the anatomic map given by conventional angiography. Two MRA techniques, time-of-flight (TOF) and phase-contrast, are used. TOF, currently the technique used most frequently, relies on the suppression of nonmoving tissue to provide a background for the high signal intensity of flowing blood. A typical TOF angiography sequence results in a series of contiguous thin MR sections (0.9 mm thick), which can be viewed as a stack to create an angiographic image data set that can be reformatted or viewed in various planes and angles to reveal the vascular relationships (Fig. 358-4). Either arterial (MRA) or venous (MRV) structures may be highlighted.

Phase-contrast MRA has a longer acquisition time than TOF MRA but reveals the velocity and direction of blood flow in addition to providing anatomic information similar to that of TOF imaging. Through the selection of different imaging parameters, differing blood velocities can be highlighted; selective venous and arterial MRA images thus can be obtained. One advantage of phase-contrast MRA is the excellent suppression of background signal.

MRA has lower resolution than conventional angiography and therefore cannot detect small-vessel detail, such as is needed in the workup of vasculitis. It is also less sensitive to slow flow and thus may not differentiate occlusive disease from near-occlusive disease. Motion, either by the patient or by anatomic structures, may distort the images, creating artifacts that may be misinterpreted as stenoses

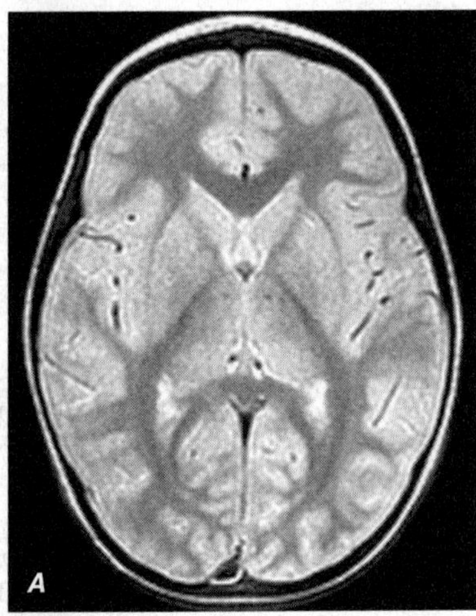

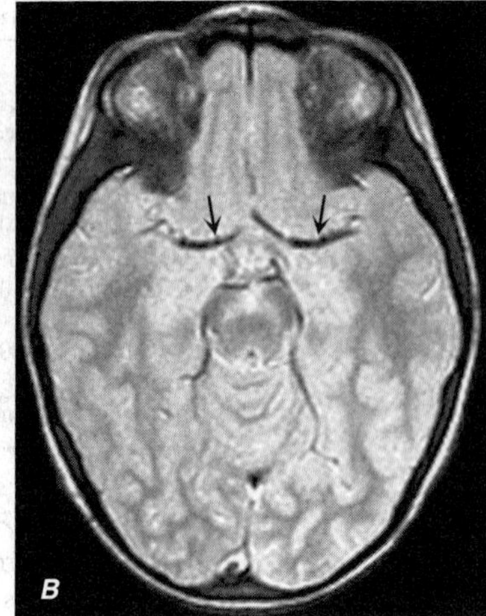

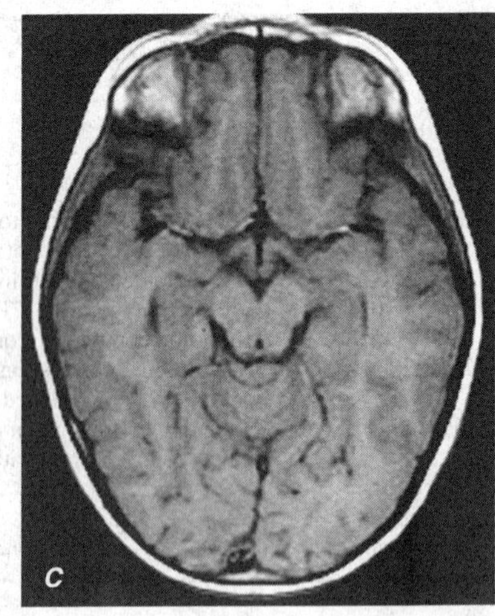

FIGURE 358-3 MRI scans of the normal brain. *A, B.* Axial T2-weighted images through (*A*) the lateral ventricles and (*B*) the circle of Willis. Note that gray matter is slightly higher in signal intensity than white matter. Cerebrospinal fluid (CSF) has a bright signal intensity owing to its free mobile water content. Moving protons in arterial structures demonstrate a signal void (*arrows*). *C.* T1-weighted image. Less contrast is visible between gray and white matter structures; however, white matter appears slightly higher in signal intensity than gray matter owing to a shorter T1 relaxation time. Signal flow voids are seen in arterial structures and CSF spaces.

or occlusions. These limitations notwithstanding, MRA has proved useful in evaluation of the cervical carotid artery and larger-caliber intracranial arterial and venous structures. It has also proved useful in the noninvasive detection of intracranial aneurysms (Fig. 361-13) and vascular malformations.

ECHO-PLANAR MR IMAGING Recent improvements in gradients, software, and high-speed computer processors now permit MR imaging of the brain on the order of milliseconds. With echo-planar MRI (EPI), fast gradients are switched on and off at high speeds to create the information used to form an image. In routine spin echo imaging, images of the brain can be obtained in 5 to 10 min. With EPI, all of the information required for processing an image is accumulated in 50 to 150 ms, and the information for the entire brain is obtained in 5 to 10 s. EPI allows motion-free imaging, as well as perfusion imaging, diffusion imaging (Fig. 358-4*A*), functional MRI, and kinematic motion studies.

EPI techniques are making their way into clinical practice. The hope for these techniques is that they will provide useful functional data in addition to exquisite anatomic images. EPI *perfusion imaging* and *diffusion imaging* are useful in early detection of ischemic injury of the brain, and may be useful in demonstrating "tissue at risk" of further infarction (Fig. 358-4*A*). Diffusion imaging may also be useful in the characterization of white matter tracts. *Functional MRI* of the brain is a technique that localizes regions of activity in the brain following task activation. Tasks alter the balance of oxyhemoglobin and deoxyhemoglobin within specific regions of the activated cortex. Repetitive actions such as finger tapping elicit an increase in the amount of blood flow delivered to a specific region of the brain, resulting in a slight increase in oxyhemoglobin and a 2 to 3% change in signal intensity. Further work will determine whether these techniques are cost-effective or clinically useful, but currently somatosensory and auditory cortex localization are possible.

Complications of MRI and Patient Safety MRI is considered safe for patients, even at very high field strengths. Serious injuries have been caused, however, by the high magnetic fields used. Ferromagnetic (metal) objects are attracted to the magnet and may act as missiles if brought too close to the magnet. Likewise, ferromagnetic aneurysm clips may torque within the magnet, causing hemorrhage and even death. Metallic foreign bodies in the eye have moved and caused hemorrhage, so screening for ocular metallic fragments is indicated in those with a history of ocular metallic foreign bodies. Implanted cardiac pacemakers are a contraindication to MRI owing to the risk of induced arrhythmias. All personnel and patients must be screened and educated thoroughly to prevent such disasters. Table 358-3 lists several of the more common contraindications for MRI.

POSITRON EMISSION TOMOGRAPHY PET relies on the detection of positrons emitted during the decay of a radionuclide that has been injected into a patient. The most frequently used moiety is 2-[^{18}F]fluoro-2-deoxy-D-glucose (FDG), which is an analogue of glucose and is taken up by cells competitively with 2-deoxyglucose. Multiple images of glucose uptake activity are formed after 45 to 60 min. Images reveal differences in regional glucose activity among normal and pathologic brain structures. FDG PET scanning has been used to assist in differentiating radiation necrosis from active neoplasm following therapy, in localizing temporal lobe epileptic foci, and in detecting metastatic disease and determining cardiac viability. A lower activity of FDG in the parietal lobes has been associated with Alzheimer's disease (Fig. 362-1).

MYELOGRAPHY Technique Myelography involves the intrathecal instillation of 8 to 15 mL of water-soluble iodinated contrast medium (180 to 300 mg/mL) into the lumbar or cervical subarachnoid space via a percutaneously placed spinal needle (22 gauge or smaller). Contrast is maneuvered into the area of interest by fluoroscopic guidance and patient rotation. *Conventional myelography* involves a relatively high concentration and volume of contrast material and visualization by x-ray "spot films" and formal "overhead" plain films. The radiation exposure during conventional myelography is 4 to 8 cGy, making it one of the more radiation-intense procedures. The gonads should be shielded if possible, although doing so is sometimes difficult. CT scanning is often performed after myelography (*CT myelography*), to better demonstrate the spinal cord and roots as filling defects in the opacified subarachnoid space. CT myelography alone, in which CT is performed after the subarachnoid injection of a small amount of relatively dilute contrast material, has replaced conventional myelography for many indications, thereby reducing exposure to radiation and contrast media. CT slices 3 mm thick are routinely obtained through the area of interest.

Indications For diagnosis of diseases of the spinal canal and cord, myelography has been largely replaced by CT, CT myelography, and MRI (Table 358-1). The remaining indications for conventional plain film myelography include the evaluation of suspected meningeal or arachnoid cysts and the localization of spinal dural arteriovenous fistulas and CSF fistulas. Conventional myelography and CT myelog-

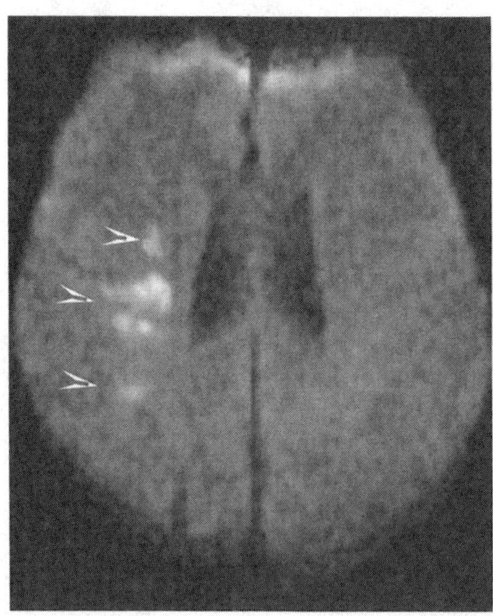
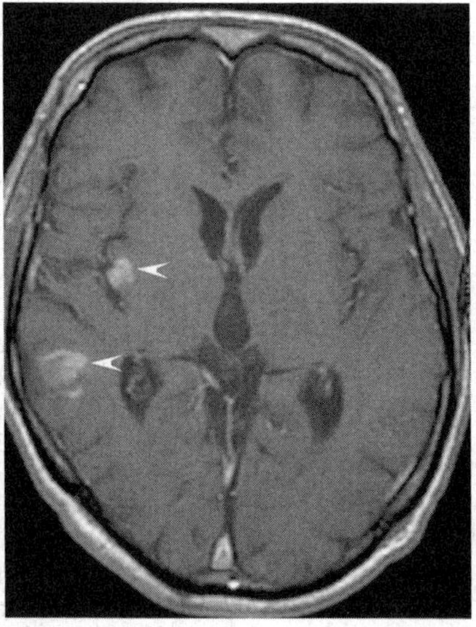
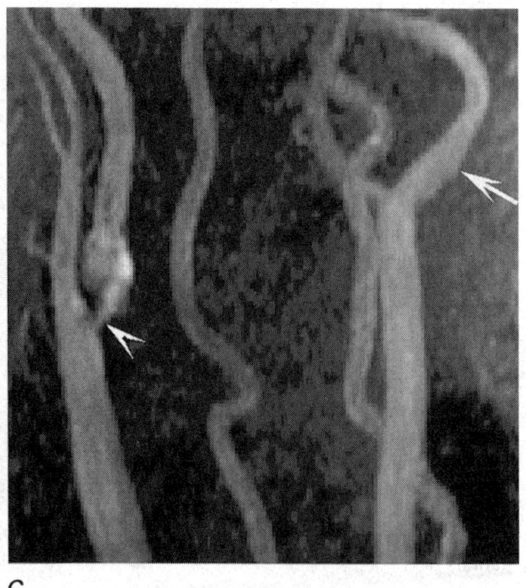

A B C

FIGURE 358-4 *A.* Axial echo-planar diffusion-weighted MR image demonstrates three foci of reduced diffusion consistent with acute cerebral ischemia (*arrowheads*) located in the subcortical white matter of the frontal lobe. Reduced diffusion is consistent with cytotoxic edema and is most commonly associated with acute cerebral infarction. *B.* Axial postcontrast T2-weighted image demonstrates two foci of subcortical enhancement consistent with subacute cerebral ischemia. *C.* A 15° projection from a three-dimensional time-of-flight magnetic resonance angiogram through the cervical carotid arteries. Note the normal internal carotid artery on the left (*arrow*). The right internal carotid artery demonstrates a high-grade stenosis at the carotid bifurcation and origin of the internal carotid artery (*arrowhead*).

raphy provide the most precise information in patients with prior spinal fusion and spinal fixation hardware.

Contraindications Myelography is relatively safe. However, it should be performed with caution in any patient with suspected herniation, elevated intracranial pressure, or a history of allergic reaction to intrathecal contrast media. In patients with a suspected spinal block, only a small amount of contrast medium should be instilled below the level of the block to minimize the risk of deterioration. Lumbar puncture is to be avoided in patients with bleeding disorders, including patients receiving anticoagulant therapy (Chap. 356).

Complications Complications resulting from myelography are related to the needle puncture and to reactions to intrathecal contrast material.

Vasovagal syncope may occur during lumbar puncture; it is accentuated by the upright position used during lumbar myelography. Adequate hydration before and after myelography will reduce the incidence of this complication.

Headache, *nausea*, and *vomiting* are the most frequent complications of dural puncture and myelography, occurring in up to 38% of patients. These symptoms are thought to result from neurotoxic effects of the contrast agent, persistent leakage of CSF at the puncture site, or psychological reactions to the procedure. The incidence of headache has been reduced with the use of smaller-gauge spinal needles and nonionic, water-soluble contrast agents.

Postural headache (post–lumbar puncture headache) is generally due to prolonged leakage of CSF from the puncture site, resulting in CSF hypotension. Intravenous hydration may be helpful, and an autologous epidural blood patch is indicated in patients with persistent headache 48 h after myelography (Chap. 15).

Hearing loss is a rare complication. It may result from a direct toxic effect of the contrast medium or from an alteration of the pressure equilibrium between CSF and perilymph in the inner ear.

Puncture of the spinal cord is a rare but serious complication of cervical (C1-2) and high lumbar puncture. The cervical approach requires proper alignment of the patient and is best performed in the prone position using fluoroscopic guidance. Direct puncture of the spinal cord, laceration of epidural and vertebral venous and arterial structures, and hyperextension of the neck are reported complications. Injection of contrast material into the spinal cord can precipitate acute neurologic decline or subacute hemorrhagic necrosis of the gray matter. The risk of cord puncture is greatest in patients with spinal stenosis or conditions that reduce CSF volume. In these settings, a low-dose lumbar injection followed by thin-section CT is a safer alternative to cervical puncture.

Intrathecal contrast reactions are rare, but aseptic meningitis and encephalopathy may occur. The latter is usually dose-related and associated with contrast entering the intracranial subarachnoid space. *Seizures* occur following myelography in 0.1 to 0.3% of patients. Risk factors include a preexisting seizure disorder and the use of a total iodine dose of >4500 mg. Other reported symptoms include headache, hyperthermia, hallucinations, depression, and anxiety states. These neurotoxic side effects have been reduced by the development of nonionic, water-soluble contrast agents, as well as by head elevation and generous hydration following myelography.

Arachnoiditis, or inflammation of the leptomeninges, has also been ascribed to the use of contrast agents for myelography. Pantopaque, an oil-soluble contrast agent no longer used, was first noted to cause arachnoiditis, especially in cases where myelography resulted in subarachnoid bleeding (i.e., traumatic tap). The incidence of arachnoiditis with new water-soluble, nonionic contrast agents is much lower than with Pantopaque and with ionic, water-soluble agents (metrizamide). Other variables that increase the likelihood of arachnoiditis include trauma, infection, and subarachnoid hemorrhage.

ANGIOGRAPHY **Technique** Angiography is essential in the diagnostic evaluation of many patients with vascular pathology. However, it carries the greatest risk of morbidity of all diagnostic imaging procedures, owing to the necessity of inserting a catheter into a blood vessel, directing the catheter to the required location, injecting contrast material to visualize the vessel, and removing the catheter while maintaining hemostasis. Therapeutic transcatheter procedures (see below) have become important options for the treatment of some cerebrovascular diseases. The decision to undertake a diagnostic or therapeutic angiographic procedure requires careful assessment of the goals of the investigation and its attendant risks.

Patients undergoing angiography should be well hydrated before and after the procedure to better tolerate the contrast agents. Since the

Table 358-3 Common Contraindications for MRI[a]

Cardiac pacemaker or permanent pacemaker leads
Internal defibrillatory devices
Cochlear prostheses
Bone growth stimulators
Implanted spinal cord stimulators
Electronic infusion devices
Intracranial aneurysm clips (some but not all)
Ocular implants (some) or ocular metallic foreign body
McGee stapedectomy piston prosthesis
Omniphase penile implant
Swan-Ganz catheter
Magnetic stoma plugs
Magnetic dental implants
Magnetic sphincters
Ferromagnetic IVC filters, coils, stents—considered safe at 6 weeks after implantation
Tattooed eyeliner (contains ferromagnetic material and may result in eye irritation)

[a] For a complete list, see Shellock and Kanal.

femoral route is used most commonly, the femoral artery must be compressed after the procedure to prevent a hematoma from developing. The puncture site and distal pulses should be evaluated carefully after the procedure; complications can include thigh hematoma or distal emboli.

Indications Table 358-1 lists some of the indications for conventional angiography. Over the past 20 years, angiography has been replaced for many indications by CT or MRI. However, it is still used today for evaluating intracranial small-vessel pathology (such as vasculitis), for assessing vascular malformations and aneurysms, and in intravascular therapeutic procedures.

Complications The vast majority of aortic arch, carotid, and vertebral arteriograms are carried out via transfemoral arterial access. A common femoral arterial puncture provides retrograde access via the aorta to the aortic arch and great vessels. The most feared complication of cerebral angiography is stroke. Thrombus can form on or inside the tip of the catheter, and atherosclerotic thrombus or plaque can be dislodged by the catheter or guidewire or by the force of injection and can embolize distally in the cerebral circulation. The duration and extent of the resulting ischemic neurologic deficit depends on the size and length of the embolus, its composition (fresh thrombus is thought to fragment more readily), its location, and the available collateral circulation. Risk factors for ischemic complications include limited experience on the part of the angiographer, atherosclerosis, vasospasm, low cardiac output, decreased oxygen-carrying capacity, advanced age, and possibly migraine. The risk of a neurologic complication varies but is approximately 4% for transient ischemic attack and stroke, 1% for permanent deficit, and <0.1% for death.

Ionic contrast material injected into the cerebral vasculature can be neurotoxic if the BBB is breached, either by an underlying disease or by the injection of hyperosmolar contrast agent. Ionic contrast media are less well tolerated than nonionic media, probably because they can induce changes in cell membrane electrical potentials. Patients with dolichoectasia of the basilar artery can suffer reversible brainstem dysfunction and acute short-term memory loss during angiography owing to the slow percolation of the contrast material and the consequent prolonged exposure of the brain. Rarely, an intracranial aneurysm ruptures during an angiographic contrast injection, causing subarachnoid hemorrhage, perhaps as a result of injection under high pressure.

Spinal Angiography Spinal angiography may be indicated to evaluate vascular malformations and tumors and to identify the artery of Adamkiewicz prior to aortic aneurysm repair. The procedure is lengthy and requires the use of relatively large volumes of contrast; the incidence of serious complications, including paraparesis, subjective visual blurring, and altered speech, is approximately 2%.

Interventional Neuroradiology This rapidly developing field is providing new therapeutic options for patients with difficult neurovascular problems. Available procedures include detachable coil therapy for aneurysms, particulate or liquid adhesive embolization of arteriovenous malformations, balloon angioplasty and stenting of stenosis or vasospasm, transarterial or transvenous embolization of dural arteriovenous fistulas, balloon occlusion of carotid-cavernous and vertebral fistulas, endovascular treatment of vein-of-Galen malformations, preoperative embolization of tumors, and thrombolysis of acute arterial or venous thrombosis. Many of these disorders place the patient at high risk of cerebral hemorrhage, stroke, or death. The therapeutic risks are comparable to those of neurosurgery rather than routine diagnostic radiographic procedures.

The highest complication rates are found with the therapies designed to treat the highest-risk diseases. In a large series of surgically difficult intracranial aneurysms treated with detachable balloons, Higashida and colleagues reported a 7.4% incidence of stroke and a 9.8% death rate. These figures must be considered in light of the high morbidity and mortality associated with untreated and surgically unapproachable aneurysms (Chap. 361). The advent of the electrolytically detachable coil has reduced these rates and ushered in a new era in the treatment of cerebral aneurysms. It remains to be determined what the role of coils will be relative to surgical options, but in many centers, coiling of aneurysms has become standard therapy for many aneurysms.

BIBLIOGRAPHY

GONZÁLEZ RG et al: Diffusion-weighted MR imaging: Diagnostic accuracy in patients imaged within 6 hours of stroke symptom onset. Radiology 210:155, 1999

HIGASHIDA RT et al: Intracranial aneurysms: Interventional neurovascular treatment with detachable balloons—results in 215 cases. Radiology 178:663, 1991

MULLER M et al: Ischemia after carotid endarterectomy: Comparison between transcranial Doppler sonography and diffusion-weighted MR imaging (see comments). AJNR Am J Neuroradiol 21:47, 2000

PROVENZALE JM, SORENSON AG: Diffusion-weighted MR imaging in acute stroke: Theoretic considerations and clinical applications. AJR Am J Roentgenol 173:1459, 1999

SORENSEN AG et al: Hyperacute stroke: Evaluation with combined multisection diffusion-weighted and hemodynamically weighted echo-planar MR imaging. Radiology 199(2):391, 1996

YOSHIURA T et al: Advanced MR techniques: Diffusion MR imaging, perfusion MR imaging, and spectroscopy. Neuroimaging Clin North Am 9:439, 1999

359

Joseph B. Martin, Frank M. Longo

MOLECULAR DIAGNOSIS OF NEUROLOGIC DISORDERS

AD Alzheimer's disease	HD Huntington's disease
ALS amyotrophic lateral sclerosis	HYPP hyperkalemic periodic paralysis
BMD Becker muscular dystrophy	OMIM Online Mendelian Inheritance in Man
CMT1A Charcot-Marie-Tooth	PCR polymerase chain reaction
DM dystrophia myotonica	SCA spinocerebellar ataxia
DMD Duchenne muscular dystrophy	UTR untranslated region
FA Friedreich's ataxia	

Completion of the Human Genome Project, along with evolving strategies for linking disease phenotypes with gene loci, will increase the rate at which genes responsible for neurologic disorders are discovered. The widespread availability of DNA testing has already changed traditional diagnostic approaches and raised novel ethical issues. For example, the discovery of "susceptibility" genes that do not directly cause disease but modify the age of disease onset or rate of disease progression creates complexity in the application of molecular diagnosis, particularly in guiding the use of preventative therapies. In this chapter we review molecular diagnostic approaches relevant to neurologic disease and illustrate how they contribute to patient care.

DNA-BASED DIAGNOSIS OF NEUROLOGIC DISORDERS Appropriate use of DNA testing in the clinical setting requires that the clinician have a general understanding of the available molecular diagnostic approaches and the limitations in their application and interpretation. For many of the disorders listed in Table 359-1, the identification of specific disease-causing mutations has made direct DNA diagnosis possible. Most disease-causing mutations consist of single base substitutions leading to amino acid substitutions (missense mutations), premature translation stop signals (nonsense mutations), or abnormal RNA transcript splicing. Other mutations result from DNA deletions, DNA duplications, or instability of trinucleotide repeats. The ability to detect a mutation eliminates the need for additional diagnostic studies. For disorders that have been linked to specific gene loci but for which specific mutations have not been identified, DNA diagnosis may be possible by family linkage analysis. Linkage analysis requires that family relationships (such as paternity) are correctly established, that informative markers are available, and that an adequate number of family members are genotyped and clinically evaluated. For many patients, lack of this information makes DNA diagnosis impossible.

Approaches for Detection of DNA Mutations • ***Direct sequencing of patient DNA*** These methods generally require amplification of DNA by the polymerase chain reaction (PCR). With most current sequencing methods, only 300 to 400 DNA bases are determined in each sequencing reaction; therefore, sequencing-based strategies are best applied when a limited region contains the majority of potential mutation sites. Direct DNA sequencing allows novel mutations to be detected and decreases the chances of a false-negative result. In some cases, the significance of previously uncharacterized missense mutations will be difficult to interpret. While they may code for harmless amino acid polymorphisms, in other cases they may be the cause of the disease. The segregation of the same mutation with the disease phenotype within a family or the substitution of nonconserved amino acids, especially in critical protein regions, suggests the latter.

Allele-specific oligonucleotide hybridization This technique, in which sequence-specific oligonucleotides differentially recognize DNA segments with normal or mutated sequence, is best suited for detecting known mutations and can be applied to a large number of samples.

Differential restriction endonuclease patterns of PCR-amplified DNA DNA is digested with restriction enzymes that recognize either normal or mutated DNA sequence; the size pattern of resulting DNA fragments indicates whether the DNA sample contains normal or variant sequence (Chap. 65). This method is directed toward detecting known mutations.

Analysis of unstable repeats The number of trinucleotide (or other sized) repeats at a specific DNA locus can be counted by amplifying the DNA segment using PCR and then applying electrophoresis to determine the repeat number present in the amplified DNA. Large repeat expansions such as occur in myotonic dystrophy often prevent reliable application of PCR and require Southern blot analysis for detection.

Analysis of single-stranded conformation polymorphisms Gene segments of several hundred bases are PCR-amplified and electrophoresed under denaturing conditions. Mutation-induced alterations of DNA structure lead to altered electrophoretic patterns. This approach can detect novel mutations directly. Large numbers of samples, either covering many exons of a large gene or from many patients, can be analyzed using this method.

Detection of DNA deletions by fluorescence in situ hybridization DNA deletions are detected by hybridizing chromosomes with a fluorescent probe corresponding to the gene of interest. Fluorescence in situ hybridization (FISH) can detect deletions smaller than the 2000- to 3000-kb minimum detected by banding techniques.

Detection of DNA deletions or duplications by pulsed-field electrophoresis with Southern blot analysis DNA deletions and duplications can also be detected using an electrophoresis technique (pulsed-field) optimized for separation of large DNA segments. This method is used for the detection of chromosome 17p11.2-12 duplications or deletions in the diagnosis of Charcot-Marie-Tooth disease type 1A (CMT1A) and hereditary neuropathy with liability to pressure palsies (HNPP), respectively.

Cytogenetic testing Chromosomes isolated from peripheral blood lymphocytes or tissue are stained, allowing identification of insertions, deletions, other chromosome imbalances, and assessment of chromosomal number (Chap. 66).

Some disorders such as Duchenne muscular dystrophy (DMD), Becker muscular dystrophy (BMD), neurofibromatosis (type 1 and 2), and familial amyotrophic lateral sclerosis (ALS) can be caused by dozens of different mutations within one gene. Heterogeneity over a wide region of a given gene is common for many genes involved in metabolic diseases. Many methods of DNA analysis focus on recurring point mutations or relatively short segments of DNA. Using such focused DNA analysis, mutations are found in only about two-thirds of DMD, BMD, and neurofibromatosis type 2 patients and in fewer than half of those with neurofibromatosis type 1. Advances in multiplex PCR and single-strand chain polymorphism analysis have increased this yield, but the clinician should be aware of the sensitivity of each DNA analysis.

Detection of Protein Abnormalities For some applications, diagnostic methods based on protein properties or function are more effective and efficient than DNA-based tests. Traditional enzyme activity–based assays continue to be useful for diagnosis of many metabolic diseases, and additional protein functions can be used to detect other disorders. For example, immunostaining or western blot analysis using dystrophin antibodies may reveal decreased protein levels or aberrant distribution of dystrophin in a muscle biopsy of a patient in whom no DNA mutations are detected.

COMPLICATIONS AND LIMITATIONS OF GENETIC TESTING The limitations of DNA testing must be considered. If the presumed diagnosis is in error or if the phenotype overlaps with other disorders, the failure to detect a given mutation does not rule out other phenotype-causing mutations in the same gene or other genes. Different mutations in the same gene can result in different phenotypes (*allelic heterogeneity*), and mutations in different genes can result in the same phenotype (*nonallelic genetic heterogeneity*). Other phenomena such as phenocopies, incomplete penetrance, age-dependent onset of phenotype, polygenic inheritance, imprinting, mitochondrial inheritance, and dynamic mutations (trinucleotide repeats) may also make interpretation of genetic testing difficult.

Nonallelic Genetic Heterogeneity Nonallelic genetic heterogeneity (also known simply as genetic heterogeneity) exists when individuals or families have similar pathologic and/or clinical syndromes caused by mutations in different genes, as in the multiple demyelinating forms of CMT disease (Table 359-1). For CMT type 1A the locus is 17p11.2, and mutations are present in the *PMP-22* gene encoding the peripheral myelin protein. CMT type 1B, which is clinically similar to CMT 1A but less common, is caused by a mutation on chromosome 1q22 in the *PMZ* gene encoding the P_0 protein, a component of compact myelin. Familial Alzheimer's disease (AD) is caused by mutations in genes located on chromosome 14 (*presenilin 1*, causing 70 to 80% of early-onset AD), 1 (*presenilin 2*), and 21 (*amyloid precursor protein*). Type I autosomal dominant spinocerebellar ataxias (SCAs) are caused by mutations in at least 10 different genes. The phenotypically similar limb-girdle muscular dystrophies (LGMD) are also caused by mutations in a large number of distinct genes, several of which encode products in distinct protein families. As disease-causing mutations continue to be identified, genetic heterogeneity is emerging as a common theme.

An intriguing basis of genetic heterogeneity consists of mutations in distinct genes encoding proteins that function via direct interaction in common mechanistic pathways. The phenotypically similar X-

Table 359-1 Selected Neurogenetic Diseases

Disorder	Chromosomal Localization	Principal Clinical Findings—Phenotype	Mode of Inheritance	Gene Product/Function	Chapter or Reference (OMIN)
DEMENTIAS					
Alzheimer's disease, early onset, familial (AD1)	21q21.3-22.05	Rare cause of early-onset AD	AD	Point mutations in gene encoding the APP protein alter APP metabolism	362, Selkoe (104760)
Alzheimer's disease, late onset, familial and sporadic (AD2)	19q13.2	Memory loss, dementia	Co-Dom	ε4 allele of the ApoE gene associated with increased risk and earlier onset	362 (107741)
Alzheimer's disease, early onset, familial (AD3)	14q24.3	Dementia, memory loss, typical AD	AD	Mutations in gene encoding presenilin-1 lead to elevated Aβ42 production	362 (104311)
Alzheimer's disease, early onset, familial (AD4)	1q31-42	Dementia, memory loss, typical AD	AD	Mutations in gene encoding presenilin-2 lead to elevated Aβ42 production	362 (600759)
Familial Creutzfeldt-Jakob disease	20pter-p12	Spongiform encephalopathy with dementia, myoclonus	AD	Mutations in gene encoding the prion protein	375 (123400)
Fatal familial insomnia	20pter-p12	Adult-onset insomnia	AD	Mutations in gene encoding the prion protein	27, 375 (600072)
Gerstmann-Straüssler-Scheinker	20pter-p12	Spongiform encephalopathy with dementia, myoclonus	AD	Mutations in gene encoding the prion protein	375 (137440)
Hereditary frontotemporal dementia (FTD)	17q21.2	Insidious mood and behavioral changes beginning prior to dementia; some cases with ALS/parkinsonism	AD	Mutations in the gene encoding the tau protein; changes in protein structure alter tau-microtubule interactions	362, Wilhelmsen et al. Lee and Trojanowski (601630)
MOVEMENT DISORDERS					
Dystonia DYT1	9q34	Early onset, generalized dystonia, starts in a limb	AD	A 3-bp (GAG) deletion in the gene encoding torsin A; homology to heat-shock/chaperone proteins	363, Ozelius et al. Klein et al. (128100)
Dystonia DYT2	Unknown	Early onset, generalized or segmental	AR	Unknown	(224500)
Dystonia DYT3	Xq13.1	~50% of cases with parkinsonism	XL-R	Unknown	(314250)
Dystonia DYT4	Unknown	Whispering dysphonia	AD	Unknown	(128101)
Dystonia DYT5a	14q22.1-22.2	Onset in first decade; starts in distal lower extremity and spreads; diurnal fluctuation; responds to levodopa	AD	Mutations in gene encoding GTP cyclohydrolase I	(128230)
Dystonia DYT5b	11p15.5	Dopa-responsive dystonia	AR	Mutations in gene encoding tyrosine hydroxylase	(191290)
Dystonia DYT6	8p21-22	Onset in adolescence, segmental	AD	Unknown	(602629)
Dystonia DYT7	18p	Adult onset, focal (writer's cramp, toricollis, dysphonia, blepharospasm)	AD	Unknown	(602124)
Dystonia DYT8	2q33-25	Paroxysmal dystonia-choreoathetosis precipitated by stress, fatigue, alcohol	AD	Unknown	(118800)
Dystonia DYT9	1p21-13.8	Paroxysmal dystonia; paresthesias, diplopia; spastic paraplegia between attacks	AD	Unknown	(118800)
Dystonia DYT10	Unknown	Paroxysmal dystonia-choreoathetosis precipitated by sudden movements	AD	Unknown	(128200)
Dystonia DYT11	11q23	Myoclonus combined with dystonia	AD	Unknown	(159900)
Dystonia DYT12	19q	Rapid-onset dystonia and parkinsonism		Mutations in gene encoding D_2 dopamine receptor	(128235)
Familial Parkinson's disease (PD), Park 1	4q21-23	Family of Italian descent; very rare familial cause of PD	AD	Point mutation in gene encoding α-synuclein	363, Spacy and Wood (601508)
Familial Parkinson's disease, Park 2	6q25.2-27	Juvenile-onset parkinsonism and a marked response to levodopa	AR	Point mutations or deletions in *parkin* gene	363 (602544)
Huntington's disease	4p16.3	Chorea, depression, dementia; rigidity and epilepsy in juvenile patients	AD	Expansion of CAG repeat in ORF of gene encoding huntingtin	362 (143100)
Wilson's disease	13q14.3	Extrapyramidal signs, psychiatric disorder	AR	Mutations in gene encoding a P-type ATPase regulating copper transport	348 (277900)

(continued)

Table 359-1—*(continued)*

Disorder	Chromosomal Localization	Principal Clinical Findings—Phenotype	Mode of Inheritance	Gene Product/Function	Chapter or Reference (OMIN)
ATAXIAS					
Ataxia telangiectasia	11q22.3	Cerebellar degeneration, choreoathetosis, ocular apraxia, oculocutaneous tenalgiectasia, immunodeficiency, endocrinopathy	AR	Mutations in *ATM* gene which encodes P1-3 kinase signaling protein; regulates cell cycle and differentiation	364 (208900)
Ataxia with vitamin E deficiency (AVED)	8q13	Same as Friedreich's ataxia but with severe vitamin E deficiency	AR	Mutations in gene encoding α-tocopherol transfer protein	364 (600415)
Dentatorubral-pallidoluysian atrophy (DRPLA)	12p12.3-13.1	Ataxia, choreoathetosis, myoclonus, dementia, seizures	AD	Expansion of CAG repeat in ORF of gene encoding DRPLA (atrophin) protein	364 (125370)
Episodic ataxia type 1 (EA-1)	12p13	Ataxic episodes, seconds to minutes, myokymia, paroxysmal kinesogenic choreoathetosis, acetazolamide and phenytoin responsive	AD	Mutations in gene encoding the KCNA1 potassium channel	364 (160120)
Episodic ataxia type 2 (EA-2)	19p13	Ataxic episodes lasting hours to days, downgaze nystagmus, headache, progressive cerebellar signs and atrophy, acetazolamide responsive	AD	Mutations in gene encoding α1A voltage-gated calcium channel; allelic with familial hemiplegic migraine and spinocerebellar ataxia type 6	364 (108500)
Friedreich's ataxia	9q13-21.1	Onset during puberty, ataxia, dysarthria, absent reflexes, decreased vibration, joint position sense, cardiomyopathy, diabetes mellitus	AR	Expansion of trinucleotide repeat (GAA) in intron of *frataxin* gene	364 (229300)
Spinocerebellar ataxia-1 (SCA1)	6p22-23	Ataxia, ophthalmoparesis, spasticity, onset 3rd or 4th decade	AD	Expansion of CAG repeat in ORF of gene encoding ataxin-1	364 (164400)
Spinocerebellar ataxia-2 (SCA2)	12q23-24.1	Features similar to SCA1, can include hypotonia and ophthalmoplegia	AD	Expansion of CAG repeat in ORF of gene encoding ataxin-2	364 (183090)
Spinocerebellar ataxia-3 (SCA3), Machado-Joseph disease (MJD)	14q32-24.3	Ataxia, ophthalmoparesis, bulging eyes, corticospinal signs, dystonia-rigidity, amyotrophy	AD	Expansion of CAG repeat in ORF of *MJD1* gene	364 (109150)
Spinocerebellar ataxia-4 (SCA4)	16q22.1	Ataxia, sensory axonal neuropathy, normal eye movements, corticospinal signs	AD	Unknown	364 (600223)
Spinocerebellar ataxia-5 (SCA5)	11p11-q11 (centromeric)	Ataxia, dysarthria; mild	AD	Unknown	364 (600224)
Spinocerebellar ataxia-6 (SCA6)	19p13	Slowly progressive ataxia; predominant cerebellar signs, gaze-evoked and vertical nystagmus	AD	Expansion of CAG repeat in ORF of gene encoding α1A calcium channel; allelic with familial hemiplegic migraine and episodic ataxia type 2	364 (184086)
Spinocerebellar ataxia-7 (SCA7)	3p13-12	Ataxia, retinal degeneration	AD	Expansion of CAG repeat in ORF of gene encoding ataxin-7	364 (164500)
Spinocerebellar ataxia-8 (SCA8)	13q21	Ataxia, bulbar findings, sensory neuropathy	AD	Expansion of CTG repeat in 3′ UTR of antisense *SCA8* transcripts; CTG repeat not found in sense *SCA8* transcripts; whether expansions are causative or polymorphic remains to be established.	364, Koob et al. (603680)
Spinocerebellar ataxia-10 (SCA10)	22q13	Ataxia, epilepsy	AD	Unknown	364, Zu et al. (603516)
Spinocerebellar ataxia-11 (SCA11)	15q15-21.3	Slowly progressive ataxia; predominant cerebellar signs; similar to SCA6	AD	Unknown	364 (604432)

(continued)

Table 359-1 Selected Neurogenetic Diseases—*(continued)*

Disorder	Chromosomal Localization	Principal Clinical Findings—Phenotype	Mode of Inheritance	Gene Product/Function	Chapter or Reference (OMIN)
Spinocerebellar ataxia-12 (SCA12)	5q31-33	Ataxia, corticospinal signs, abnormal eye movements	AD	Expansion of CAG repeat in 5′UTR region of *PPP2R2B* gene encoding a brain-specific regulator subunit of the protein phosphatase PP2A	364, Holmes et al. (604326)
SPASTIC PARAPLEGIAS					
Autosomal dominant hereditary spastic paraplegias (AD-HSP)	SPG3:14q11-22 SPG4:2p21-22 SPG6:15q11.1 SPG8: 8q23-24	"Uncomplicated" spastic paraplegia primarily involving corticospinal tracts; SPG4 locus accounts for 40–50% of AD-HSP families	AD	In 2p21-22-linked forms, mutations present in gene coding spastin, a ubiquitously expressed ATPase	365, Fink and Hedera Hazan et al. (182600; 182601; 600363; 603563)
Autosomal recessive hereditary spastic paraplegias (AR-HSP)	SPG5:8q11-13 SPG7: 16q24.3 SPG9:15q13-15	Either pure spastic paraplegia or including involvement of other CNS systems	AR	In 16q-linked forms, mutations present in the gene encoding paraplegin, a mitochondrial metalloprotease	365, Pearce (270800; 602783; 601162)
X-linked hereditary spastic paraplegias	SPG1: Xq28 SPG2: Xq21-22	Initial pure spastic paraplegia; involvement of entire CNS over years;	X-LR	SPG1: mutations in L1CAM gene; allelic with X-linked hydrocephalus and MASA syndrome; SPG2: mutations in proteolipid protein (PLP) gene; allelic with Pelizaeus-Merzbacher disease	365, Fransen et al. (312900; 312920)
VASCULAR DISEASES					
Cerebral autosomal dominant arteriopathy with subcortical infarcts and leukoencephalopathy (CADASIL)	19p13.1	Multiple subcortical infarcts, leukoencephalopathy, vascular dementia	AD	Mutations in gene encoding the Notch3 protein, a transmembrane signal transduction protein	361, Dichgans et al. Joutel et al. (125310)
Cerebral cavernous malformation (CCM1)	7q11.2-21	Headache, intracerebral hemorrhage, seizures, neurologic deficits	AD	Unknown	Craig et al. (116860)
Cerebral cavernous malformation (CCM2)	7p13-15	Headache, intracerebral hemorrhage, seizures, neurologic deficits	AD	Unknown	(603284)
Cerebral cavernous malformation (CCM3)	3q25.2-27	Headache, intracerebral hemorrhage, seizures, neurologic deficits	AD	Unknown	(603285)
Familial cerebral amyloid angiopathy (Dutch type)	21q21.3-22.05	Cerebral hemorrhage	AD	Mutation in gene encoding APP	Watson et al. (104760)
Familial hemiplegic migraine	19p13	Onset 5–30 years, aura with unilateral paresis and other focal symptoms lasting 30–60 min; headache, ± cerebellar signs	AD	Mutations in gene encoding α1A voltage-gated calcium channel; allelic with EA-2 and SCA6	15, Lehmann-Horn and Jurkat-Rott Davies and Hanna (141500)
EPILEPSY SYNDROMES					
Autosomal dominant nocturnal frontal lobe epilepsy (ADNFLE)	20q13.2	Seizures begin in childhood, occur at night; predominantly motor and occasionally violent	AD	Mutations in gene encoding the α_4 subunit of the neuronal nicotinic acetylcholine receptor (CHRNA4)	360, McNamara (600513)
Benign neonatal epilepsy-1 (EBN1)	20q13.3	Generalized seizures, neonatal onset, benign course, usually resolving at 6–12 months, 10–15% have seizures later in life	AD	Mutations in gene encoding the KCNQ2 potassium channel	360, McNamara (121200)
Benign neonatal epilepsy-2 (EBN2)	8q24	Clinically indistinguishable from EBN1	AD	Mutations in gene encoding the KCNQ3 potassium channel	360, McNamara (121201)
Epilepsy, progressive myoclonic (Unverricht-Lundborg type) (EPM1)	21q22.3	Generalized seizures, stimulus-reactive myoclonus, onset age 6–15, progressive	AD	Most common mutation is expansion of a dodecamer repeat in the 5′ UTR of the gene encoding cystatin B, an inhibitor of cystein protease	360, Serratosa et al. (254800)
Epilepsy, progressive myoclonic (Lafora disease) (EPM2A)	6q24	Onset of seizures and myoclonus at age 15 followed by myoclonus; intracellular Lafora bodies	AR	Mutations in *EPM2A* gene which encodes a protein tyrosine phosphatase	(254780)

(continued)

Disorder	Chromosomal Localization	Principal Clinical Findings—Phenotype	Mode of Inheritance	Gene Product/Function	Chapter or Reference (OMIN)
Generalized epilepsy with febrile seizures plus (GEFS+)	19q13.1	Febrile seizures before 3 months of age or after 3 years of age	AD	Mutations in gene encoding the β_1 subunit of the voltage-gated sodium channel (SCN1B)	360, McNamara (604236)
Progressive epilepsy with mental retardation (EPMR)	8pter-p22	Normal at birth, generalized seizures onset age 5–10 years, severe mental retardation after seizure onset	AR	Mutations in *CLN8* gene, encoding a putative transmembrane protein	360, Ranta et al. (600143)
MOTOR NEURON DISEASES					
Familial amyotrophic lateral sclerosis, adult, dominant (ALS1)	21q22.1	Weakness, muscle atrophy, spasticity, increased TRDs; about 10% of cases are familial, indistinguishable clinically from sporadic form	AD	Point mutations in gene encoding Cu, Zn-superoxide dismutase (SOD1) in some families (20%); altered SOD1 protein structure may lead to aberrant and toxic copper-mediated catalysis	365, Cleveland (105400)
Familial amyotrophic lateral sclerosis, juvenile, recessive (ALS2)	2q33-34	Earlier onset and slower progression than ALS1	AR	Unknown; mapped to a 8-Mb region	365 (205100)
Familial amyotrophic lateral sclerosis, adult, dominant (ALS3)	22q12.2	Similar to ALS1	AD	Mutations in neurofilament protein heavy chain gene in ~1% of "sporadic" cases; disruption of neurofilament cross-linking; mutations might be either causative or constitute risk factors	365 (162230)
Spinobulbar muscular atrophy (SBMA; Kennedy syndrome)	Xq12	Muscular weakness and atrophy	X-LR	Expansion of CAG repeat in ORF of gene encoding androgen receptor	365 (313200)
Spinal muscular atrophy I–III (SMA)	5q13	SMA I: infantile, Werdnig-Hoffman disease—present by 3 mos., hypotonia, proximal weakness, areflexia SMA II: childhood onset, limb-girdle weakness, areflexia, 70% never ambulate independently SMA III: juvenile, Kugelberg-Welander disease—onset after age 2, slowly progressive symmetric proximal muscle weakness sparing bulbar muscles	AR	All three types of SMA are caused by mutations in the survival motor neuron (SMN1) gene; most cases show homozygous absence of specific SMN1 exons; severity of phenotype may be related to SMH1 protein levels	365, Wirth (253300; 253550; 253400)
NEUROPATHIES					
Charcot-Marie-Tooth disease, type 1A (CMT1A)	17p11.2	HMSN I: Variable onset, motor > sensory neuropathy, distal muscle atrophy, absent reflexes, high arches in feet, decreased nerve conduction velocities, +/− nerve enlargement; (~50% of hereditary neuropathy)	AD	Majority with 1.5 Mb duplication in gene encoding peripheral myelin protein (PMP-22), a component of compact myelin; point mutations also found.	379, Chance Warner et al (118220)
Charcot-Marie-Tooth disease, type 1B (CMT1B)	1q22-23	Similar to HMSN I (~40 families identified)	AD	Mutations in *MPZ* gene encoding P_o protein, a component of compact myelin	379 (118200)
Charcot-Marie-Tooth disease, types 1,2,3 X-linked (CMTX1,2,3)	CMTX1: Xq13.1 CMTX2: Xp22.2 CMTX3:Xq26	HMSN I (~10–15% of hereditary neuropathy)	X-linked dominant	CMTX1: mutations in gene encoding connexin32, a gap junction protein localized to uncompacted peripheral myelin at the nodes of Ranvier and Schmidt-Lanterman clefts; CMTX2,3: genes unknown	379 (302800) (302801) (302802)
Charcot-Marie-Tooth disease, type 2A (CMT2A)	1p35-36	HMSNII: Later onset, sensorimotor axonal neuropathy, near-normal nerve conduction velocities (20–50% of hereditary neuropathy)	AD	Unknown	379 (118210)

(continued)

Disorder	Chromosomal Localization	Principal Clinical Findings—Phenotype	Mode of Inheritance	Gene Product/Function	Chapter or Reference (OMIN)
Charcot-Marie-Tooth disease, type 2B (CMT2B)	3q13-22	HSMNII (several families)	AD	Unknown	379 (600882)
Charcot-Marie-Tooth disease, type 4A (CMT4A)	8q13-21.1	HMSN I (few families; Tunisia)	AR	Unknown	379 (214400)
Congenital hypomyelinating neuropathy (CH)	10q21.1-22.1 1q22-23	Neonatal hypomyelinating neuropathy with extremely slow nerve conduction velocities	AD and AR	Cases mapped to 10q21.1-22.1 demonstrate mutations in the *EGR2* gene encoding a zinc finger DNA binding protein; cases mapped to 1q22-23 show mutations in the *MPZ* gene coding P_o protein, a component of compact myelin	379 (129010; 159440)
Déjerine-Sottas disease (DSDA)	17p11.2-12 1q22-23	HSMNIII: Onset birth/infancy, slowly progressive sensorimotor deficits, high arches, scoliosis, ataxia, enlarged nerves, markedly decreased conduction velocities	AD	17p-linked: mutations in gene encoding PMP22 (see above) 1q-linked: mutations in *MPZ* gene encoding P_o (see above)	379 (145900)
Familial amyloidotic polyneuropathy (FAP)	18q11.2-12.1 and other loci	Sensory/autonomic peripheral neuropathy, cardiomyopathy	AD	Mutations in gene encoding transthyretin; amyloid formation	379 (176300)
Hereditary neuropathy with pressure palsies (HNPP)	17p11.2	Recurrent entrapment/pressure neuropathies, segmental demyelination (relatively frequent, 1:10,000; underrecognized)	AD	Deletions or point mutations in gene encoding PMP-22; HNPP and CMT1A may result from reciprocal products of unequal crossover	379 Stogbauer et al. (162500)
NEUROMUSCULAR JUNCTION DISORDERS					
Congenital myasthenic syndrome type Ia (familial infantile myasthenia)	17p12-11	Onset at birth to early childhood, myasthenic weakness and possible respiratory distress	AR	Loss-of-function mutations in gene encoding the ε subunit of the acetylcholine receptor (AChR) cause decreased response to ACh or decreased levels of the AChR	380, Engel et al. (254210)
Congenital myasthenic syndrome type II ("slow-channel" syndrome)	2q24-32 17p12-11	Onset at birth to early childhood, myasthenic weakness and possible respiratory distress	AD	Gain-of-function mutations in genes encoding the α, β, or ε subunits of the AChR cause increased response to ACh	380, Engel et al. (601462)
MYOPATHIES					
Central core disease (CCD)	19q13.1	Nonprogressive primarily proximal myopathy, onset in infancy	AD	Mutation in ryanodine receptor gene (RYR1); allelic with malignant hyperthermia syndrome (MHS1)	383 (117000)
Congenital muscular dystrophy (merosin deficient) (CMD)	6q22-23	Weakness and hypotonia at birth, limb contractures at birth or later	AR	Mutations in *LAMA2* gene encoding merosin	383 (156225)
Duchenne/Becker muscular dystrophy (DMD/BMD)	Xp21.2	DMD: onset of muscular weakness early in life, progressive; BMD: later onset, less severe	X-LR	Mutations in dystrophin gene resulting in complete absence or major deletions of dystrophin (DMD), or less severe derangement of dystrophin structure (BMD)	383, Hoffman (310200)
Emery-Dreifuss muscular dystrophy	Xq28 1q21.2	Childhood onset, benign course with early contractures; progressive muscle wasting with humeral/peroneal predominance, cardiac conduction defects; X-linked and AD forms have similar phenotype	X-LR AD	Xq28: mutations in gene encoding emerin, an inner nuclear membrane protein; 1q11-q23: mutations in gene encoding the lamin A/C protein; main A/C interaction with emerin may be involved in targeting emerin to the nuclear envelope	383, Bonne et al. (310300; 181350)

(continued)

Table 359-1—*(continued)*

Disorder	Chromosomal Localization	Principal Clinical Findings—Phenotype	Mode of Inheritance	Gene Product/Function	Chapter or Reference (OMIN)
Facioscapulohumeral dystrophy	4q35	Weakness, atrophy; face and shoulder muscles	AD	Associated with deletion of variable number of 3.3 kb repeat units; more severe phenotype with larger deletions; nature of gene products affected by deletion are unknown	383, Fitzsimons (158900)
Fukuyama-type congenital muscular dystrophy (FCMD)	9q31	Weakness and hypotonia at birth, cerebral and cerebellar polymicrogyria and cerebellar cysts, ocular anomalies; overlaps with Walker-Warberg syndrome	AR	3 kb retrotransposal insertion in the 3′UTR of the gene encoding fukutin, a putative secreted protein of unknown function; severe phenotypes including Walker-Warburg syndrome associated with compound heterozygotes	383, Kondo-Iida et al. Toda (253800)
Hyperkalemic periodic paralysis (HYPP)	17q23.1-25.3	Myotonia, periodic areflexic paralysis	AD	Mutations in gene encoding α subunit, sodium channel (SCN4A); allelic with paramyotonia congenita (PC)	383 (170500)
Hypokalemic periodic paralysis (HOKPP)	1q32	Similar to HYPP, but attacks accompanied by hypokalemia, triggered by insulin or glucose	AD	Loss-of-function mutations in α_1 subunit of the dihydropyridine (DHP)–sensitive calcium channel	383 (170400)
Limb-girdle muscular dystrophy, autosomal dominant forms	LGMD1A: 5q31 LGMD1B: 1q11-21 LGMD1C: 3p25	Late (third decade) onset muscular dystrophy, sparing the face; slow progression	AD	LGMD1C: mutations in gene encoding caveolin-3; genes unknown for LGMD1A and LGMD1B	383 (601253)
Limb-girdle muscular dystrophy, autosomal recessive forms (clinical and genetic overlap with severe childhood autosomal recessive muscular dystrophy, SCARMD)	LGMD2A: 15q LGMD2B: 2p16-13 LGMD2C: 13q LGMD2D: 17q LGMD2E: 4q LGMD2F: 5q LGMD2G: 17q LGMD2H: 9q	Heterogeneous group of myopathies with progressive weakness of shoulder and pelvic muscles; severe forms with onset in first decade and milder forms with later onset; disorders caused by mutations in genes encoding sarcoglycan are also known as "sarcoglycanopathies"	AR	Mutations in genes encoding: calpain 3 (LGMD2A); dysferlin (LGMD2B); telethonin (LGMD2G). Sarcoglycanopathies: γ-sarcoglycan (LGMD2C); α-sarcoglycan (adhalin) (LGMD2D); β-sarcoglycan (LGMD2E); δ-sarcoglycan (LGMD2F)	383, Bushby Moreira et al. Vainzof et al. (253600)
Malignant hyperthermia (MHS1) and central core disease (CCD)	19q13.1 Other candidate loci: 1q, 3q, 5p, 7q, 17q	Sensitivity to volatile anesthetics, muscle contraction	AD	In 19q-linked forms (~50% of cases) mutations in gene encoding ryanodine receptor (RYR1) cause disturbances in calcium flux	383, Jurkat-Rott et al. (145600)
Desmin-related myopathy (myofibrillar myopathy; hereditary distal myopathy)	2q35 11q22.3-23.1 and other loci	Proximal and distal weakness, cardiomyopathy, neuropathy	AR and AD	2q35-linked forms: mutations in gene encoding desmin 11q21-linked forms: mutations in gene encoding αB-crystallin, a chaperone for desmin	383, Engel (601419)
Myotonia congenita (dominant myotonia congenita, Thomsen's disease)	7q35	Onset in first decade, muscle stiffness/myotonia, muscle hypertophy without weakness	AD	Mutations in gene encoding the ClC-1 chloride channel lead to a dominant loss of function within the homomultimeric channel	383 (160800)
Myotonia congenita (recessive myotonia congenita, Becker)	7q35	Similar to dominant myotonia congenita	AR	Loss-of-function mutations in gene encoding the ClC-1 chloride channel	383 (160800)
Myotonic dystrophy	19q13.3	Multisystem disorder; cataracts, myotonia, weakness, frontal baldness, mental retardation	AD	CTG repeats 3′ UTR of gene encoding myotonin protein kinase, localized to membranes of neuromuscular and myotendinous junctions; expression of adjacent genes may also be affected	383 (160900)

(continued)

Disorder	Chromosomal Localization	Principal Clinical Findings—Phenotype	Mode of Inheritance	Gene Product/Function	Chapter or Reference (OMIN)
Nemaline myopathy	1q22-23 2q21.2-22 1q42.1	Most commonly congenital nonprogressive or slowly progressive myopathy; forms range from severe congenital to mild adult	AD and AR	Dominant 1p22-linked form: mutations in α-tropomyosin gene (*TPM3*) leading to increased tropomyosin-actin affinity; 2q21-linked form: mutations in gene encoding nebulin; 1q42 linked form: mutations in gene coding α-actin (*ACTA1*)	383, Nowak et al. Wallgren-Pettersson et al. (161800)
Oculopharyngeal muscular dystrophy (OPMD)	14q11.2-13	Onset usually after age 50, ptosis, dysphagia, and proximal limb weakness	AD	Mutation in gene encoding the poly(A) binding protein 2 (PABP2); a GCG repeat encoding a polyalanine tract expands from 6 to 8–13 repeats	383, Brais et al. (164300)
Paramyotonia congenita (PC)	17q23.1-25.3	Cold-induced muscle stiffness (myotonia) and weakness, occasional periodic paralysis	AD	Mutations in gene encoding α subunit, sodium channel (SCN4A); allelic with HYPP	383 (168300)
Startle disease (hyperexplexia)	5q21-31	Exaggerated startle, neonatal hypertonia, nocturnal myoclonus	AD, AR	Mutations in gene coding the α_1 subunit of the inhibitory glycine receptor	22 (149400)
Walker-Warburg syndrome (WWS)	9q33-31	Congenital muscular dystrophy, lissencephaly, ocular anomalies, hydrocephalus, callosal hypoplasia, septal agenesis	AR	Mutation in gene encoding fukutin; often compound heterozygote mutations; allelic with Fukuyama-type congenital muscular dystrophy (FCMD)	(236670)
NEUROCUTANEOUS SYNDROMES					
Neurofibromatosis, type 1 (NF1) (Von Recklinghausen's disease)	17q11.2	Café au lait spots, neurofibromas, axillary or inguinal freckling, Lisch nodules in iris; affects 1 in 4000 individuals	AD	Mutations in the gene encoding neurofibromin, a member of the Ras-GTPase activating protein (GAP) family	370 (162200)
Neurofibromatosis, type 2 (NF2)	22q12.2	Acoustic neuromas, bilateral meningiomas; affects 1 in 50,000 individuals	AD	Deletions in the gene that encodes merlin, a membrane-cytoskeletal linkage protein	370 (101000)
Tuberous sclerosis, type 1 (TSC1)	9q34	Epilepsy, facial angiofibromas, mental retardation; ~50% of TSC families linked to TSCI and ~50% to TSC2; two-thirds of TCS cases arise from spontaneous mutations, with the majority TSC2-linked	AD	Mutations in gene encoding hamartin, a putative membrane-associated protein that forms cytosolic complexes with tuberin	370, Crino and Henske Nellist et al. (191100)
Tuberous sclerosis, type 2 (TSC2)	16p13.3	Epilepsy, facial angiofibromas, mental retardation	AD	Mutations in gene encoding tuberin, which has homology to GTPase activating proteins; tuberin binds to hamartin, possibly acting as a chaperon	370 (191092)

NOTE: OMIN web site www3.ncbi.nlm.nih.gov/omin/ AD, autosomal dominant; ALS, amyotrophic lateral sclerosis; APP, amyloid precursor protein; AR, autosomal recessive; CNS, central nervous system; Co-Dom, codominant; TRDs, trinucleotide repeat disorders; HMSN, hereditary motor and sensory neuropathy; MASA, mental retardation, aphasia, shuffling gait, adducted thumbs; ORF, open reading frame; X-LR, X-linked recessive; UTR, untranslated region.

linked and autosomal dominant Emery-Dreifuss muscular dystrophies are caused by mutations in genes encoding emerin and lamin A/C, respectively. Emerin and lamin A/C interaction is likely to be important for targeting emerin to the nuclear envelope. Tuberous sclerosis types 1 and 2 are caused by mutations in the genes encoding tuberin and hamartin, respectively. Evidence suggests that tuberin binds to hamartin, possibly acting as a chaperon.

Allelic Heterogeneity Different mutations in the same gene (allelic mutations) can cause markedly distinct clinical phenotypes. Mutations in the α1A voltage-gated calcium channel subunit can cause either familial hemiplegic migraine, SCA type 6, or episodic ataxia type 2 (EA-2). Familial Creutzfeldt-Jakob disease, fatal familial insomnia, and Gerstmann-Sträussler-Scheinker disease are all caused by allelic mutations in the prion protein gene (20pter-p12), each of which results in distinct aberrant protein isoforms or alterations in expression. Mutations in the gene encoding the L1 cell adhesion molecule (L1CAM) can cause either isolated hydrocephalus or MASA syndrome (mental retardation, aphasia, shuffling gait, and adducted thumbs). Mutations in the sodium channel α subunit (SCN4A) can cause either hyperkalemic periodic paralysis (HYPP) or paramyotonia congenita (PC). In cases of allelic heterogeneity, different mutations cause distinct alterations in protein structure and function, resulting in separate phenotypes.

Phenocopies Patients may have a clinical presentation that resembles the phenotype of a genetic disorder but that has a nongenetic cause. Examples include vascular dementia appearing as familial AD, toxin- or drug-induced chorea mimicking Huntington's disease (HD), and vitamin E deficiency resembling Friedreich's ataxia (FA).

Variable Expressivity Variable expressivity occurs when the severity of a trait resulting from a mutant allele varies from mild to severe. Expression of the disease phenotype can be modified by other factors such as predisposing alleles of other genes, environmental agents, sex, and age. Variation in expression can also occur following somatic variations in trinucleotide repeats, as occurs in myotonic dystrophy (dystrophia myotonica, or DM).

Incomplete Penetrance Penetrance refers to the all-or-none expression of a mutant genotype. If a disease is expressed in <100% of individuals carrying the abnormal allele, it is said to have incomplete penetrance.

Polygenic Inheritance and Complex Traits The majority of diseases listed in Table 359-1 are caused by mutations in single genes. In disorders such as "sporadic" AD, Parkinson's disease, and multiple sclerosis, it is likely that disease onset is determined by concomitant mutations or polymorphisms in large numbers of genes. Genetic testing for susceptibility or diagnosis will require assessment of multigene "panels."

INFLUENCE OF GENETIC BACKGROUND Machado-Joseph disease (MJD) and SCA type 3 are autosomal dominant ataxias originally described in different ethnic backgrounds with distinct features. MJD occurs in families, often of Portuguese-Azorean origin, and is manifest as hereditary ataxia with dystonia, rigidity, faciolingual fasciculation, and bulging eyes. In French families with a syndrome of progressive ataxia and dysarthria recognizably distinct from that found in Portuguese-Azorean families, the SCA3 gene was mapped to a site on chromosome 14q near the MJD locus. It is now clear that MJD and SCA3 are both caused by expansion of the same tract of CAG repeats in the same gene (*MJD1*) at 14q32.1. Although expansions in *MJD1* are the most common mutations in German SCA patients, the diagnosis of MJD had not previously been considered in this population. The extent to which different genetic background causes phenotypic heterogeneity will require further studies.

SUSCEPTIBILITY GENES Allelic variations or mutations can cause increased susceptibility to specific diseases. Detection of such DNA polymorphisms can influence differential diagnosis, as in the genotyping of *APOE* alleles in the diagnosis of AD. Apolipoprotein E (apoE) is a 299-amino-acid protein involved in mobilization and reutilization of lipoprotein cholesterol. ApoE secreted by astrocytes appears to be internalized by neurons via low-density lipoprotein-related receptors where it contributes to neuronal function. The three isoforms of apoE (apoE2, apoE3, and apoE4) are derived from three corresponding alleles of the *APOE* gene located at 19q13.2; the apoE4 allele is overrepresented in sporadic and familial AD and is a significant risk factor for the disease. In contrast, the apoE2 allele is underrepresented and thus may have a "protective" effect (Chap. 362).

The increased incidence of the *APOE4/4* genotype in AD patients has raised the possibility that ascertainment of *APOE* genotype might be useful in the diagnostic assessment of patients with dementia. For example, since AD accounts for some two-thirds of late-onset dementia, the prior probability of an elderly patient with dementia having AD is approximately 0.66. In many populations the probability of a demented patient with the *APOE4/4* genotype having AD increases to >0.90. However, since the relationship between *APOE4* genotype and probability of AD changes with age, gender, and ethnic background, application of population-based probabilities to specific individuals is limited. If a 25-year-old presents with dementia and has the *APOE4/4* genotype, it is very unlikely that this patient has AD. Since individuals with all *APOE* genotypes can have AD, genotypes cannot absolutely rule in or rule out this diagnosis. Even if genotyping increases the odds that a given patient has AD, it does not rule out the possibility that a treatable cause of dementia is present. Current diagnostic studies for demented patients are focused on detecting reversible causes of dementia (Chap. 26) *APOE* genotype results would not change the diagnostic evaluation and should not be ordered on a routine basis. Nevertheless, *APOE* genotyping might eventually be combined with

yet-to-be developed diagnostic tests to form a "panel" of data with acceptable sensitivity and specificity for diagnosis (Chap. 362).

The availability of *APOE* genotyping raises questions about the use of predictive testing in asymptomatic individuals. Until preventive therapy is available, many clinicians would consider such predictive testing unethical. Moreover, useful predictions of age of onset based solely on *APOE* genotyping are not possible. For the 2% of the population with the high-risk *E4/E4* genotype, the period of risk extends from the fifties to beyond the nineties.

APPROACHES TO GENETIC TESTING One indication for DNA analysis is to confirm the diagnosis of a specific disease already suggested by clinical assessment. DNA testing can also be used to narrow the differential diagnosis in cases with multiple diagnostic possibilities. DNA testing for HD allows patients to avoid neuroimaging and other diagnostic studies. When a patient presents with a well-established and relatively specific clinical phenotype, such as that of HD, initial genetic testing can focus on a single gene. In other disorders, such as the SCAs, the high degree of phenotypic overlap calls for concomitant testing of a panel of genes (*SCA1*, *SCA2*, *SCA3*, *SCA6*, and *SCA7*). Another application of genetic analysis is presymptomatic testing in members of families known or suspected to have a specific disorder. In these cases the most common reasons for testing are life management issues, reproductive planning decisions, and eliminating the stress of unknown carrier status. Development of new therapies that delay onset or progression of neurodegenerative diseases will provide additional indications for presymptomatic testing.

Genetic testing should be conducted only in the context of comprehensive genetic counseling, in which the implications of potential test results are fully explained and adequate support services are available. Clinicians ordering genetic studies should be familiar with issues regarding informed consent, suicide risk, ongoing patient support, insurance, employment discrimination, testing of minors, and testing of fetal tissue.

A directory of diseases for which DNA diagnostic testing is available, along with a listing of testing sites, on the www.genetests.org, web site. This site was developed at the University of Washington, Seattle, and is supported by the U.S. National Library of Medicine and Maternal and Child Health Bureau.

CLINICAL AND GENETIC CLASSIFICATION OF GENE DISORDERS Neurogenetic disorders have traditionally been classified and subtyped on the basis of clinical and pathophysiologic concepts. Their complexity, phenotypic variability, and overlapping features limit the resolution of phenotype-based classification and confound nosology. Identification of tightly linked disease markers and discovery of disease-causing mutations have provided a basis for refining such classifications. For example, the clinical distinction between neurofibromatosis type 1 and type 2 has been upheld by the discovery that they are caused by mutations in different genes, encoding the GTPase-activating protein and the merlin (schwannomin) cytoskeletal protein, respectively. In contrast, the finding that DMD and BMD are caused by mutations in the same gene points to shared pathophysiologic mechanisms and blurs the distinctions between these disorders. Mutations in different genes can lead to overlapping clinical syndromes as in the inherited ataxias. In other instances, phenotypically dissimilar disorders are caused by mutations in the same gene, as described above for the α1A voltage-gated calcium channel subunit gene.

Neurogenetic disorders with known chromosomal gene localization are organized primarily by clinical phenotype in Table 359-1. As in any clinical classification, there is frequent overlap in specific phenotypic features. Reference numbers from the Online Mendelian Inheritance in Man (OMIM) database (described below) are included to facilitate access to continuously updated disease information.

Different modes of inheritance occur in each of these categories. Neurologic genetic disorders inherited in Mendelian autosomal dominant mutations include HD, familial AD, ALS, DM, CMT, familial HYPP, SCA, and tuberous sclerosis. Autosomal recessive disorders include FA, Wilson's disease, and ataxia telangiectasia. X-linked recessive traits include DMD, spinobulbar muscular atrophy (Kennedy syndrome), and fragile X syndrome. Non-Mendelian patterns of transmission such as maternal inheritance can result from mitochondrial mutations (Chap. 383) and unstable trinucleotide repeats (see below).

The types of mutations causing neurologic genetic disorders include gene deletions (the most common finding in DMD), insertions (e.g., Fukuyama-type congenital muscular dystrophy), duplications (e.g., CMT1A), translocations that interrupt the gene (neurofibromatosis type 1), and point mutations (e.g., in the superoxide dismutase gene in ALS). Point mutations, either missense or nonsense, are considered "static" mutations because they generally remain stable during meiosis and provide the basis for classic Mendelian inheritance. Unstable trinucleotide repeats cause "dynamic" mutations and account for the clinical phenomenon of anticipation.

GENETICALLY INDUCED MECHANISMS OF CELL DEATH Three general mechanisms of cell death in genetic disorders have been proposed: loss of function, dominant-negative effects, and gain of function.

In *loss-of-function disorders*, the mutation causes a deficiency in an enzyme or protein resulting in cellular dysfunction. The best defined examples are the lysosomal storage disorders in which enzymatic deficiencies in complex lipid metabolism lead to accumulation of normal or abnormal cellular constituents. The mode of inheritance in these disorders is most often autosomal recessive, but it can also be X-linked or the combined result of an inherited germline mutation and an acquired somatic mutation ("second hit") that knocks out both alleles (such as the loss of a growth-suppressor gene in tumors such as retinoblastoma). It is less common for loss-of-function disorders to result from autosomal dominant mutations.

In the case of a *dominant-negative effect*, the abnormal mutation competes with or abolishes the normal allelic function at either the DNA, RNA, or protein level. A dominant-negative mechanism in DM has been suggested by observations that RNA transcripts with expanded CTG repeats precipitate normal RNA transcripts. In myotonia congenita, abnormal protein isoforms combined with normal isoforms of the CLC-1 chloride channel disrupt overall homomultimeric channel function.

In *gain-of-function effects*, the abnormal cellular function exerted by the mutation at one allele in some way renders the cell susceptible to toxic effects, whether or not the normal allele is expressed.

True dominant disorders such as HD and SCA1, in which the heterozygote genotype elicits the full disease phenotype, could be the result of (1) dominant-negative effects, in which proteins with expanded polyglutamine tracts would form oligomers with normal protein isoforms and thereby interfere with their function; or (2) toxic gain-of-function effects.

DISORDERS ASSOCIATED WITH TRINUCLEOTIDE REPEATS An important group of neurologic disorders is caused by abnormal expansions of trinucleotide repeats (Table 359-2). A useful way of organizing repeat diseases and understanding their mechanisms is based on the location of the repeat expansions within the gene. Expansions can occur in the 5′ untranslated region (UTR), within the open reading frame (translated portion of the gene), within the 3′ UTR, or within introns.

The first category of trinucleotide repeat disorders in which repeats are located in the 5′ UTR includes fragile X syndrome and SCA12. Expansions in this region lead to impaired transcription with subsequent loss of protein expression.

The second category of trinucleotide diseases consists of neurodegenerative disorders in which expansion of a CAG repeat in the open reading frame encodes an aberrant protein with an expanded polyglutamine tract. The stretches of CAG repeats, which vary between 5 and 37 in the normal alleles of each gene, are increased two- to fourfold in the mutation. There is a striking correlation between larger numbers of repeats and both increased severity of the neurologic disorder and earlier age of onset. HD patients homozygous for the disease allele have phenotypes similar to heterozygous patients.

These observations suggest a model in which a gain of function is toxic to neurons. One possibility is that expanded polyglutamine tracts provide a substrate for aberrant protein–protein interactions. Such interactions might lead to a loss of function of a critical protein or toxic accumulations of protein aggregates. Several lines of evidence support such a protein-based hypothesis. Open reading frame CAG repeats are indeed translated into protein. Transgenic mice expressing a human *SCA1* gene with an expanded CAG repeat develop the characteristic phenotype only when the transgene is expressed. One study has suggested that polyglutamine tracts of the proteins that cause HD and dentatorubral-pallidoluysian atrophy (DRPLA) interact with glyceraldehyde-3-phosphate dehydrogenase and thereby might have a deleterious effect on neuronal energy metabolism.

Table 359-2 Neurologic Diseases Caused by Expansion of Trinucleotide Repeats

Disorder	Site of Repeat/*Gene*	Effect on Gene Expression or Protein Structure
Fragile X	CGG repeat in 5′ UTR/*FMR1*	Decreased transcript expression and loss of FMRP protein
Spinocerebellar ataxia SCA-12	CAG repeat in 5′UTR/*PPP2R2B*	Likely decreased transcript expression and loss of regulator subunit of the protein phosphatase PP2A
Huntington's disease	CAG repeat in ORF/*IT15 (HD)*	Expanded polyglutamine tract in huntingtin protein
Dentatorubropallidoluysian atrophy (DRPLA)	CAG repeat in ORF/*atrophin-1*	Expanded polyglutamine tract in atrophin-1 protein
Spinal and bulbar muscular atrophy (SBMA)	CAG repeat in ORF/*AR*	Expanded polyglutamine tract in androgen receptor
Spinocerebellar ataxia (SCA)		
SCA-1	CAG repeat in ORF/*SCA-1*	Expanded polyglutamine tract in ataxin-1 protein
SCA-2	CAG repeat in ORF/*SCA-2*	Expanded polyglutamine tract in ataxin-2 protein
SCA-3 (MJD)	CAG repeat in ORF/*MJD*	Expanded polyglutamine tract in MJD protein
SCA-6	CAG repeat in ORF/*CACNL1A4*	Expanded polyglutamine tract in α1A calcium channel
SCA-7	CAG repeat in ORF/*SCA-7*	Expanded polyglutamine tract in ataxin-7 protein
Oculopharyngeal muscular dystrophy (OPMD)	GCG repeat in ORF/*PABP2*	Expanded polyalanine tract in poly(A) binding protein 2
SCA-8	CTG repeat in 3′UTR/*SCA-8*	CTG repeat found in antisense but not sense transcripts; may lead to decreased levels of sense transcripts
Myotonic dystrophy	CTG repeat in 3′UTR/*DMPK*	Possible alterations in DMPK transcript processing, functions of 3′UTR-binding proteins, and expression of adjacent *DMR-N9* and *DMAHP* genes
Friedreich's ataxia	GAA repeat in intron/*X25*	Altered gene structure interferes with transcription leading to loss of frataxin protein

NOTE: MJD, Machado-Joseph disease; ORF, open reading frame; UTR, untranslated region.

Gain-of-function models of polyglutamine tract diseases must also reconcile the observations that each neurodegenerative disease affects only regionally specific populations of neurons, yet proteins associated with these disorders are widely expressed. One possibility is that each of these polyglutamine tract proteins interacts with yet-to-be discovered proteins that are indeed cell-type specific. The huntingtin-associated protein (HAP1) is one such candidate. HAP1 is selectively expressed in brain tissue and demonstrates enhanced association with forms of huntingtin protein with increased lengths of glutamine repeats. Another potential mechanism of cell-type specificity is that somatic instability of CAG repeats leads to greater expansions in specific cell populations. However, the relatively small variations of three to five in the number of triplet repeats in the HD gene in different regions of the brain makes this explanation less likely.

In the third category of trinucleotide repeat disorders, repeat expansion occurs in the 3′ UTR. In DM, a GTC (CAG in the antisense) repeat in the 3′ UTR of the DM kinase gene expands manyfold, from 5 to 40 repeats in normal alleles to up to 2700 in severe cases. The repeat expansion is variable in different tissues, indicating that errors in DNA replication can occur during meiosis and during somatic cell mitosis. Since DNA sequence motifs in the 3′ UTR of RNA transcripts regulate transcript stability and processing, expansions in this region might affect transcript levels and alter DM kinase protein levels. Quantitative analysis of messenger RNA in muscle biopsies has demonstrated marked disease-specific decreases in DM kinase mRNA in adult-onset DM patients. Levels of normal as well as mutant DM transcripts were decreased, suggesting a novel mechanism of a dominant-negative mutation occurring at the RNA level.

A second potential mechanism in DM is that expansion of the GTC repeat could inhibit expression of the adjacent *DMR-N9* (telomeric) and *DMAHP* (centromeric) genes. Disruption of adjacent chromatin structure by repeat expansion is one mechanism by which expression of adjacent genes could be inhibited. Alternatively, repeat expansions at one locus might affect expression of more than one gene by a *cis*-acting effect, and expansion-containing transcripts may alter levels of transcripts derived from a separate allele by a *trans*-acting effect.

A fourth category of trinucleotide repeat disease occurs with repeat expansion in an intron. FA is caused by the expansion of a GAA triplet in intron 1 of the *X25* gene. Repeat expansions with associated alterations in DNA structure are likely to impair *X25* transcription. Consistent with an autosomal recessive pattern of inheritance and a loss-of-function disease mechanism, the majority of FA patients tested to date demonstrate homozygosity for expanded alleles, while a smaller number are heterozygous with a combination of one expanded allele and point mutations in the other allele. FA is not associated with anticipation (see below) and manifests more often during adolescence rather than middle age, distinguishing it from other trinucleotide repeat diseases.

The discovery of triplet repeats has given molecular precision to old concepts such as *anticipation* (earlier onset of the disease in successive generations, which is associated with further expansion of the abnormal repeats in more severely affected individuals) and has helped to account for variations in gene expression. Variations in trinucleotide repeats in HD, and particularly in DM have given a molecular explanation for *variable expression*, where variations in repeats occurring among individual members of the family can lead to earlier onset or more severe symptoms and signs, as occurs in juvenile HD. Studies suggesting that other neurologic and psychiatric disorders involve anticipation raise the possibility that additional trinucleotide repeat diseases will be discovered.

ONLINE MENDELIAN INHERITANCE IN MAN The OMIM catalogue contains a frequently updated listing of all known genetic traits. For each disease it includes information on clinical manifestations, mapping studies and identity (if available) of the relevant gene, and status of genetic testing. OMIM is administered by the National Center for Biotechnologic Information and is on the Internet at www3.ncbi.nlm.nih.gov/omim/.

BIBLIOGRAPHY

Bird TD: Apolipoprotein E genotyping in the diagnosis of Alzheimer's disease: A cautionary view. Ann Neurol 38:2, 1995

———: Risks and benefits of DNA testing for neurogenetic disorders. Semin Neurol 19: 253, 1999

Bonne G et al: Mutations in the gene encoding lamin A/C cause autosomal dominant Emery-Dreifuss muscular dystrophy. Nat Genet 21:285, 1999

Brais B et al: Short GCG expansions in the PABP2 gene cause oculopharyngeal muscular dystrophy. Nat Genet 18:164, 1998

Bushby KMD: Making sense of the limb-girdle muscular dystrophies. Brain 122:1403, 1999

Chance PF: Molecular genetics of hereditary neuropathies. J Child Neurol 14:43, 1999

Cleveland DW: From Charcot to SOD1: Mechanisms of selective motor neuron death in ALS. Neuron 24:515, 1999

Craig HD et al: Multilocus linkage identifies two new loci for a Mendelian form of stroke, cerebral cavernous malformation, at 7p15-13 and 3q25.2-27. Hum Mol Genet 7:1851, 1998

Crino PB, Henske EP: New developments in the neurobiology of the tuberous sclerosis complex. Neurology 53:1384, 1999

Davies NP, Hanna MG: Neurological channelopathies: Diagnosis and therapy in the new millennium. Ann Med 31:406, 1999

Dichgans M et al: The phenotypic spectrum of CADASIL: Clinical findings in 102 cases. Ann Neurol 44:731, 1998

Engel AG: Myofibrillar myopathy. Ann Neurol 46:681, 1999

——— et al: Congenital myasthenic syndromes. Arch Neurol 56:163, 1999

Figlewicz DA, Bird TD: "Pure" hereditary spastic paraplegias. The story becomes complicated. Neurology 53:5, 1999

Fink JK: Approach to patients with inherited neurological disorders. Semin Neurol 18: 211, 1998

———, Hedera P: Hereditary spastic paraplegia: Genetic heterogeneity and genotype-phenotype correlation. Semin Neurol 19:301, 1999

Fitzsimons RB: Facioscapulohumeral muscular dystrophy. Curr Opin Neurol 12:501, 1999

Fransen E et al: Genotype-phenotype correlation in L1 associated diseases. J Med Genet 35:399, 1998

Hazan J et al: Spastin, a new AAA protein, is altered in the most frequent form of autosomal dominant spastic paraplegia. Nat Genet 23:296, 1999

Hoffman EP: Muscular dystrophy: Identification and use of genes for diagnostics and therapeutics. Arch Pathol Lab Med 123:1050, 1999

Hoh HH, Ott J: Complex inheritance and localizing disease genes. Hum Hered 50:85, 2000

Holmes SE et al: Expansion of a novel CAG trinucleotide repeat in the 5′ region of *PPP2R2B* is associated with SCA12. Nat Genet 23:391, 1999

Joutel A et al: *Notch3* mutations in CADASIL, a hereditary adult-onset condition causing stroke and dementia. Nature 383:707, 1996

Jurkat-Rott K et al: Genetics and pathogenesis of malignant hyperthermia. Muscle Nerve 23:4, 2000

Klein C et al: Genetics of primary dystonia. Semin Neurol 19:271, 1999

Kondo-Iida E et al: Novel mutations and genotype-phenotype relationships in 107 families with Fukuyama-type congenital muscular dystrophy (FCMD). Hum Mol Genet 8:2303, 1999

Koob MD et al: An untranslated CTG expansion causes a novel form of spinocerebellar ataxia (SCA8). Nat Genet 21:379, 1999

Lee VM-Y, Trojanowski JQ: Neurodegenerative tauopathies: Human disease and transgenic mouse models. Neuron 24:507, 1999

Lehmann-Horn F, Jurkat-Rott K: Voltage-gated ion channels and hereditary disease. Physiol Rev 79:1317, 1999

Lin X et al: Expanding our understanding of polyglutamine diseases through mouse models. Neuron 24:499, 1999

Martin JB: Molecular basis of the neurodegenerative disorders. N Engl J Med 340:1970, 1999

McNamara JO: Emerging insights into the genesis of epilepsy. Nature 399:A15, 1999

Moreira ES et al: Limb-girdle muscular dystrophy type 2G is caused by mutations in the gene encoding the sarcomeric protein telethonin. Nat Genet 24:163, 2000

Nellist M et al: Characterization of the cytosolic tuberin-hamartin complex. J Biol Chem 274:35647, 1999

Nowak KJ et al: Mutations in the skeletal muscle a-actin gene in patients with actin myopathy and nemaline myopathy. Nat Genet 23:208, 1999

Ozelius LJ et al: The TOR1A (DYT1) gene family and its role in early onset torsion dystonia. Genomics 62:377, 1999

Pandolfo M: Friedreich's ataxia: Clinical aspects and pathogenesis. Semin Neurol 19: 311, 1999

PEARCE DA: Hereditary spastic paraplegia: Mitochondrial metalloproteases of yeast. Hum Genet 104:443, 1999

RANTA S et al: The neuronal ceroid lipfuscinoses in human EPMR and mnd mutant mice are associated with mutations in CLN8. Nat Genet 23:233, 1999

REDDY PH et al: Recent advances in understanding the pathogenesis of Huntington's disease. Trends Neurosci 22:248, 1999

SELKOE DJ: Translating cell biology into therapeutic advances in Alzheimer's disease. Nature 399:A23, 1999

SERRATOSA JM et al: The molecular genetic bases of the progressive myoclonus epilepsies. Adv Neurol 79:383, 1999

SPACY SD, WOOD NW: The genetics of Parkinson's disease. Curr Opin Neurol 12:427, 1999

STEVANIN G et al: Are (CTG)n expansions at the SCA8 locus rare polymorphisms? Nat Genet 24:213, 2000

STOGBAUER F et al: Hereditary recurrent focal neuropathies. Neurology 54:546, 2000

THOMSON G, ESPOSITO MS: The genetics of complex diseases. Trends Cell Biol 9:M17, 1999

TIMCHENKO LT, CASKEY CT: Triplet repeat disorders: Discussion of molecular mechanisms. Cell Mol Life Sci 55:1432, 1999

TODA T et al: Fukuyama-type congenital muscular dystrophy: The first human disease to be caused by an ancient retrotransposal integration. J Mol Med 77:816, 1999

TOURNIER-LASSERVE E: *CACNA1A* mutations. Hemiplegic migraine, episodic ataxia type 2 and the others. Neurology 53:3, 1999

VAINZOF M et al: Sarcoglycanopathies are responsible for 68% of severe autosomal recessive limb-girdle muscular dystrophy in the Brazilian population. J Neurol Sci 164: 44, 1999

VNENCAK-JONES CL: Molecular testing for inherited diseases. Am J Clin Pathol 112:S19, 1999

WALLGREN-PETTERSSON C et al: Clinical and genetic heterogeneity in autosomal recessive nemaline myopathy. Neuromuscul Disord 9:564, 1999

WARNER LE et al: Hereditary peripheral neuropathies: Clinical forms, genetics, and molecular mechanisms. Annu Rev Med 50:263, 1999

WATSON DJ et al: Effects of the amyloid precursor protein Glu693Gln 'Dutch' mutation on the production and stability of amyloid beta-protein. Biochem J 340:703, 1999

WILHELMSEN KC et al: Tau mutations in frontotemporal dementia. Dement Geriatr Cogn Disord 10:S88, 1999

WIRTH B: An update of the mutation spectrum of the survival motor neuron gene (SMN1) in autosomal recessive spinal muscular atrophy (SMA). Hum Mutat 15:228, 2000

WORTH PF et al: Large, expanded repeats in SCA8 are not confined to patients with cerebellar ataxia. Nat Genet 34:214, 2000

ZU L et al: Mapping of a new autosomal dominant spinocerebellar ataxia to chromosome 22. Am J Hum Genet 64:594, 1999

Section 2
DISEASES OF THE CENTRAL NERVOUS SYSTEM

360

Daniel H. Lowenstein

SEIZURES AND EPILEPSY

CT	computed tomography	MRI	magnetic resonance imaging
CNS	central nervous system	MTLE	mesial temporal lobe epilepsy
EEG	electroencephalogram	PET	positron emission tomography
GABA	γ-aminobutyric acid	SPECT	single photon emission computed tomography
ILAE	International League Against Epilepsy	VNS	vagus nerve stimulation
JME	juvenile myoclonic epilepsy		

A *seizure* (from the Latin *sacire*, "to take possession of") is a paroxysmal event due to abnormal, excessive, hypersynchronous discharges from an aggregate of central nervous system (CNS) neurons. Depending on the distribution of discharges, this abnormal CNS activity can have various manifestations, ranging from dramatic convulsive activity to experiential phenomena not readily discernible by an observer. Although a variety of factors influence the incidence and prevalence of seizures, approximately 5 to 10% of the population will have at least one seizure during their lifetime, with the highest incidence occurring in early childhood and late adulthood. Because seizures are common, this clinical problem is encountered frequently during medical practice in a variety of settings.

The meaning of the term seizure needs to be carefully distinguished from that of epilepsy. *Epilepsy* describes a condition in which a person has *recurrent* seizures due to a chronic, underlying process. This definition implies that a person with a single seizure, or recurrent seizures due to correctable or avoidable circumstances, does not necessarily have epilepsy. Epilepsy refers to a clinical phenomenon rather than a single disease entity, since there are many forms and causes of epilepsy. However, among the many causes of epilepsy there are various *epilepsy syndromes* in which the clinical and pathologic characteristics are distinctive and suggest a specific underlying etiology.

Using the definition of epilepsy as two or more unprovoked seizures, the incidence of epilepsy is approximately 0.3 to 0.5% in different populations throughout the world, and the prevalence of epilepsy has been estimated at 5 to 10 persons per 1000.

CLASSIFICATION OF SEIZURES

An essential step in the evaluation and management of a patient with a seizure is to determine the type of seizure that has occurred. The importance of this cannot be overemphasized—classifying the seizure is essential for focusing the diagnostic approach on particular etiologies, selecting the appropriate therapy, and providing potentially vital information regarding prognosis. In 1981, the International League Against Epilepsy (ILAE) published a modified version of the International Classification of Epileptic Seizures that has continued to be a useful classification system (Table 360-1). This system is based on the clinical features of seizures and associated electroencephalographic findings. Other potentially distinctive features such as etiology or cellular substrate are not considered in this classification system, although this will undoubtedly change in the future as more is learned about the pathophysiologic mechanisms that underlie specific seizure types.

The main characteristic that distinguishes the different categories of seizures is whether the seizure activity is partial (synonymous with focal) or generalized. *Partial seizures* are those in which the seizure activity is restricted to discrete areas of the cerebral cortex. *General-*

Table 360-1 Classification of Seizures

1. Partial seizures
   a. Simple partial seizures (with motor, sensory, autonomic, or psychic signs)
   b. Complex partial seizures
   c. Partial seizures with secondary generalization
2. Primarily generalized seizures
   a. Absence (petit mal)
   b. Tonic-clonic (grand mal)
   c. Tonic
   d. Atonic
   e. Myoclonic
3. Unclassified seizures
   a. Neonatal seizures
   b. Infantile spasms

ized seizures involve diffuse regions of the brain simultaneously in a bilaterally symmetric fashion. Partial seizures are often associated with structural abnormalities of the brain. In contrast, generalized seizures may result from cellular, biochemical, or structural abnormalities that have a more widespread distribution.

PARTIAL SEIZURES Partial seizures occur within discrete regions of the brain. If consciousness is fully preserved during the seizure, the clinical manifestations are considered relatively simple and the seizure is termed a *simple partial seizure*. If consciousness is impaired, the symptomatology is more complex and the seizure is termed a *complex partial seizure*. An important additional subgroup comprises those seizures that begin as partial seizures and then spread diffusely throughout the cortex, i.e., *partial seizures with secondary generalization*.

Simple Partial Seizures Simple partial seizures cause motor, sensory, autonomic, or psychic symptoms without an obvious alteration in consciousness. For example, a patient having a partial motor seizure arising from the right primary motor cortex in the vicinity controlling hand movement will note the onset of involuntary movements of the contralateral, left hand. These movements are typically clonic (i.e., repetitive, flexion/extension movements) at a frequency of approximately 2 to 3 Hz; pure tonic posturing may be seen as well. Since the cortical region controlling hand movement is immediately adjacent to the region for facial expression, the seizure may also cause abnormal movements of the face synchronous with the movements of the hand. The electroencephalogram (EEG) recorded with scalp electrodes during the seizure (i.e., an ictal EEG) may show abnormal discharges in a very limited region over the appropriate area of cerebral cortex if the seizure focus involves the cerebral convexity (Chap. 357). Seizure activity occurring within deeper brain structures is often not recorded by the standard EEG, however, and may require intracranial electrodes for its detection.

Three additional features of partial motor seizures are worth noting. First, in some patients the abnormal motor movements may begin in a very restricted region such as the fingers and gradually progress (over seconds to minutes) to include a larger portion of the extremity. This phenomenon was originally described by Hughlings Jackson and is known as a "Jacksonian march," representing the spread of seizure activity over a progressively larger region of motor cortex. Second, patients may experience a localized paresis (Todd's paralysis) for minutes to many hours in the involved region following the seizure. Third, in rare instances the seizure may continue for hours or days. This condition, termed *epilepsia partialis continua*, is often quite refractory to medical therapy.

Other forms of simple partial seizures include those that cause changes in somatic sensation (e.g., paresthesias), vision (flashing lights or formed hallucinations), equilibrium (sensation of falling or vertigo), or autonomic function (flushing, sweating, piloerection). Simple partial seizures arising from the temporal or frontal cortex may also cause alterations in hearing, olfaction, or higher cortical function (psychic symptoms). This includes the sensation of unusual, intense odors (e.g., burning rubber or kerosene) or sounds (crude or highly complex sounds), or an epigastric sensation that rises from the stomach or chest to the head. Some patients describe odd, internal feelings such as fear, a sense of impending change, detachment, depersonalization, déjà vu, or illusions that objects are growing smaller (micropsia) or larger (macropsia). When such symptoms precede a complex partial or secondarily generalized seizure, these simple partial seizures serve as a warning, or *aura*.

Complex Partial Seizures Complex partial seizures are characterized by focal seizure activity accompanied by a transient impairment of the patient's ability to maintain normal contact with the environment. Operationally this means that the patient is unable to respond appropriately to visual or verbal commands during the seizure and has impaired recollection or awareness of the ictal phase. The seizures frequently begin with an aura (i.e., a simple partial seizure) that is stereotypic for the patient. The start of the ictal phase is often a sudden behavioral arrest or motionless stare, and this marks the onset of the event for which the patient will be amnestic. The behavioral arrest is usually accompanied by automatisms, which are involuntary, automatic behaviors that have a wide range of manifestations. Automatisms may consist of very basic behaviors such as chewing, lip smacking, swallowing, or "picking" movements of the hands, or more elaborate behaviors such as a display of emotion or running. The patient is typically confused following the seizure, and the transition to full recovery of consciousness may range from seconds up to an hour. Careful examination of the patient immediately following the seizure may show an anterograde amnesia or, in cases involving the dominant hemisphere, a postictal aphasia.

The routine, interictal (i.e., between seizures) EEG in patients with complex partial seizures is often normal, or may show brief discharges termed *epileptiform spikes*, or *sharp waves*. Since complex partial seizures can arise from the medial temporal lobe or inferior frontal lobe, i.e., regions distant from the scalp, the EEG recorded during the seizure may be nonlocalizing. However, the seizure focus is often detected using special electrodes such as sphenoidal or surgically placed intracranial electrodes.

The range of potential clinical behaviors linked to complex partial seizures is so broad that extreme caution is advised before concluding that stereotypic episodes of bizarre or atypical behavior are not due to seizure activity. In such cases it is imperative to consider more detailed EEG studies to determine whether the behaviors are caused by a seizure disorder.

Partial Seizures with Secondary Generalization Partial seizures can spread to involve both cerebral hemispheres and produce a generalized seizure, usually of the tonic-clonic variety (discussed below). Secondary generalization is observed frequently following simple partial seizures, especially those with a focus in the frontal lobe, but may also be associated with partial seizures occurring elsewhere in the brain. A partial seizure with secondary generalization is often difficult to distinguish from a primarily generalized tonic-clonic seizure, since bystanders tend to emphasize the more dramatic, generalized convulsive phase of the seizure and overlook the more subtle, focal symptoms present at onset. In some cases, the focal onset of the seizure becomes apparent only when a careful history identifies a preceding aura (i.e., simple partial seizure). Often, however, the focal onset is not clinically evident and may be established only through careful EEG analysis. Nonetheless, distinguishing between these two entities is extremely important, as there may be substantial differences in the evaluation and treatment of partial versus generalized seizure disorders.

GENERALIZED SEIZURES By definition, generalized seizures arise from both cerebral hemispheres simultaneously. However, it is currently impossible to exclude entirely the existence of a focal region of abnormal activity that initiates the seizure prior to rapid secondary generalization. For this reason, generalized seizures may be practically defined as bilateral clinical and electrographic events without any detectable focal onset. Fortunately, a number of the subtypes of generalized seizures have distinctive features that facilitate clinical diagnosis.

Absence Seizures (Petit Mal) Absence seizures are characterized by sudden, brief lapses of consciousness without loss of postural control. The seizure typically lasts for only seconds, consciousness returns as suddenly as it was lost, and there is no postictal confusion. Although the brief loss of consciousness may be clinically inapparent or the sole manifestation of the seizure discharge, absence seizures are usually accompanied by subtle, bilateral motor signs such as rapid blinking of the eyelids, chewing movements, or small-amplitude, clonic movements of the hands.

Absence seizures usually begin in childhood (ages 4 to 8) or early adolescence and are the main seizure type in 15 to 20% of children with epilepsy. The seizures can occur hundreds of times per day, but the child may be unaware of or unable to convey their existence. This can lead to a situation in which the patient is constantly struggling to piece together experiences that have been interrupted by the seizures. Since the clinical signs of the seizures are subtle, especially to new parents, it is not surprising that the first clue to absence epilepsy is often unexplained "daydreaming" and a decline in school performance recognized by a teacher.

The electrophysiologic hallmark of typical absence seizures is a generalized, symmetric, 3-Hz spike-and-wave discharge that begins and ends suddenly on a normal EEG background (Chap. 357). Periods of spike-and-wave discharges lasting more than a few seconds usually correlate with the clinical signs, but the EEG often shows many more periods of abnormal cortical activity than were suspected clinically. Hyperventilation tends to provoke these electrographic discharges and even the seizures themselves and is routinely used when recording the EEG.

Typical absence seizures are often associated with generalized, tonic-clonic seizures, but patients usually have no other neurologic problems and respond well to treatment with specific anticonvulsants. Although estimates vary, approximately 60 to 70% of such patients will have a spontaneous remission during adolescence.

Atypical Absence Seizures Atypical absence seizures have features that deviate from both the clinical and EEG features of typical absence seizures. For example, the lapse of consciousness is usually of longer duration and less abrupt in onset and cessation, and the seizure is accompanied by more obvious motor signs that may include focal or lateralizing features. The EEG shows a generalized, slow spike-and-wave pattern with a frequency of ≤2.5/s, as well as other abnormal activity. Atypical absence seizures are usually associated with diffuse or multifocal structural abnormalities of the brain and therefore may accompany other signs of neurologic dysfunction such as mental retardation. Furthermore, the seizures are less responsive to anticonvulsants compared to typical absence seizures.

Generalized, Tonic-Clonic Seizures (Grand Mal) Primarily generalized, tonic-clonic seizures are the main seizure type in approximately 10% of all persons with epilepsy. They are also the most common seizure type resulting from metabolic derangements and are therefore frequently encountered in many different clinical settings. The seizure usually begins abruptly without warning, although some patients describe vague premonitory symptoms in the hours leading up to the seizure. This prodrome should be distinguished from the stereotypic auras associated with focal seizures that secondarily generalize. The initial phase of the seizure is usually tonic contraction of muscles throughout the body, accounting for a number of the classic features of the event. Tonic contraction of the muscles of expiration and the larynx at the onset will produce a loud moan or cry. Respirations are impaired, secretions pool in the oropharynx, and the patient becomes cyanotic. Contraction of the jaw muscles may cause biting of the tongue. A marked enhancement of sympathetic tone leads to increases in heart rate, blood pressure, and pupillary size. After 10 to 20 s, the tonic phase of the seizure typically evolves into the clonic phase, produced by the superimposition of periods of muscle relaxation on the tonic muscle contraction. The periods of relaxation progressively increase until the end of the ictal phase, which usually lasts no more than 1 min. The postictal phase is characterized by unresponsiveness, muscular flaccidity, and excessive salivation that can cause stridorous breathing and partial airway obstruction. Bladder or bowel incontinence may occur at this point as well. Patients gradually regain consciousness over minutes to hours, and during this transition there is typically a period of postictal confusion. Patients will subsequently complain of headache, fatigue, and muscle ache that can last for many hours. The duration of impaired consciousness in the postictal phase can be extremely long, i.e., many hours, in patients with prolonged seizures or underlying CNS diseases such as alcoholic cerebral atrophy.

The EEG during the tonic phase of the seizure shows a progressive increase in generalized low-voltage fast activity, followed by generalized high-amplitude, polyspike discharges. In the clonic phase, the high-amplitude activity is typically interrupted by slow waves to create a spike-and-wave pattern. The postictal EEG shows diffuse slowing that gradually recovers as the patient awakens.

There are many variants of the generalized tonic-clonic seizure, including pure tonic and pure clonic seizures. Brief tonic seizures lasting only a few seconds are especially noteworthy since they are usually associated with known epileptic syndromes having mixed seizure phenotypes, such as the Lennox-Gastaut syndrome (discussed below).

Atonic Seizures Atonic seizures are characterized by sudden loss of postural muscle tone lasting 1 to 2 s. Consciousness is briefly impaired, but there is usually no postictal confusion. A very brief seizure may cause only a quick head drop or nodding movement, while a longer seizure will cause the patient to collapse. This can be quite dramatic and extremely dangerous, since there is a substantial risk of direct head injury with the fall. The EEG shows brief, generalized spike-and-wave discharges followed immediately by diffuse slow waves that correlate with the loss of muscle tone. Similar to pure tonic seizures, atonic seizures are usually seen in association with known epileptic syndromes.

Myoclonic Seizures Myoclonus is a sudden and brief muscle contraction that may involve one part of the body or the entire body. A normal, common physiologic form of myoclonus is the sudden jerking movement observed while falling asleep. Pathologic myoclonus is most commonly seen in association with metabolic disorders, degenerative CNS diseases, or anoxic brain injury (Chap. 22). Although the distinction from other forms of myoclonus is imprecise, myoclonic seizures are considered to be true epileptic events since they are caused by cortical (versus subcortical or spinal) dysfunction. The EEG shows bilaterally synchronous spike-and-wave discharges. Myoclonic seizures usually coexist with other forms of generalized seizure disorders but are the predominant feature of juvenile myoclonic epilepsy (discussed below).

UNCLASSIFIED SEIZURES Not all seizure types can be classified as partial or generalized. This appears to be especially true of seizures that occur in neonates and infants. The distinctive phenotypes of seizures at these early ages likely result, in part, from differences in neuronal function and connectivity in the immature versus mature CNS.

EPILEPSY SYNDROMES

In addition to recognizing the patterns of different types of seizures, it is also useful to be familiar with some of the more common epilepsy syndromes, since this often helps in the determination of therapy and prognosis. Epilepsy syndromes are disorders in which epilepsy is a predominant feature, and there is sufficient evidence (e.g., through clinical, EEG, radiologic, or genetic observations) to suggest a common underlying mechanism. Three important epilepsy syndromes are listed below; additional examples with a known genetic basis are shown in Table 360-2.

JUVENILE MYOCLONIC EPILEPSY Juvenile myoclonic epilepsy (JME) is a generalized seizure disorder of unknown cause that appears in early adolescence and is usually characterized by bilateral myoclonic jerks that may be single or repetitive. The myoclonic seizures are most frequent in the morning after awakening and can be provoked by sleep deprivation. Consciousness is preserved unless the myoclonus is especially severe. Many patients also experience generalized tonic-clonic seizures, and up to one-third have absence seizures. The condition is otherwise benign, and although complete remission is uncommon, the seizures respond well to appropriate anticonvulsant medication. There is often a family history of epilepsy, and genetic linkage studies suggest a polygenic cause.

LENNOX-GASTAUT SYNDROME Lennox-Gastaut syndrome occurs in children and is defined by the following triad: (1) multiple seizure types (usually including generalized tonic-clonic, atonic, and atypical absence seizures); (2) an EEG showing slow (<3 Hz) spike-and-wave discharges and a variety of other abnormalities; and (3) impaired cognitive function in most but not all cases. Lennox-Gastaut syndrome is associated with CNS disease or dysfunc-

Table 360-2 Examples of Genes Associated with Epilepsy Syndromes[a]

Gene (Locus)	Function of Gene	Clinical Syndrome	Comments
CHRNA4 (20q13.2)	Nicotinic acetylcholine receptor subunit; mutations cause a decrease in Ca^{2+} flux through the receptor; this may reduce amount of GABA release in presynaptic terminals	Autosomal dominant nocturnal frontal lobe epilepsy (ADNFLE); childhood onset; brief, nighttime seizures with prominent motor movements; often misdiagnosed as primary sleep disorder	Rare; first identified in a large Australian family; additional CHRNA4 mutation found in a Norweigan family with similar phenotype; second ADNFLE locus found on 15q24
KCNQ2 (20q13.3) KCNQ3 (8q24)	Voltage-gated potassium channel subunits; mutation in pore regions may cause a 20–40% reduction of potassium currents, which will lead to impaired repolarization	Benign familial neonatal convulsions (BFNC); autosomal dominant inheritance; onset in 1st week of life in infants who are otherwise normal; remission usually within weeks to months; long-term epilepsy in 10–15%	Rare; sequence and functional homology to KCNQ1, mutations of which cause long QT syndrome and a cardiac-auditory syndrome
SCN1B (19q12.1)	β-subunit of a voltage-gated sodium channel; mutation disrupts disulfide bridge that is crucial for structure of extracellular domain; mutated β-subunit leads to slower sodium channel inactivation	Generalized epilepsy with febrile seizures plus (GEFS+); autosomal dominant inheritance; presents with febrile seizures at either <3 months or >3 years, then variable seizure types not associated with fever	Incidence uncertain; GEFS+ identified in other families without SCN1B mutations; significant phenotypic heterogeneity within same family, including members with febrile seizures only
CSTB (21q22.3)	Cystatin B, a noncaspase cysteine protease inhibitor; normal protein may block neuronal apoptosis by inhibiting caspases directly or indirectly (via cathepsins), or controlling proteolysis	Progressive myoclonus epilepsy (PME) (Unverricht-Lundborg disease); autosomal recessive inheritance; age of onset between 6–15 years, myoclonic seizures, ataxia, and progressive cognitive decline; brain shows neuronal degeneration	Overall rare, but relatively common in Finland and Western Mediterranean (>1 in 20,000); precise role of cystatin B in human disease unknown, although mice with null mutations of cystatin B have similar syndrome
EPM2A (6q24)	Laforin, a protein tyrosine phosphatase (PTP); may influence glycogen metabolism, which is known to be regulated by phosphatases	Progressive myoclonus epilepsy (Lafora's disease); autosomal recessive inheritance; onset age 6–19 years, death within 10 years; brain degeneration associated with polyglucosan intracellular inclusion bodies in numerous organs	Most common PME in Southern Europe, Middle East, Northern Africa, and Indian subcontinent; genetic heterogeneity; unknown whether seizure phenotype due to degeneration or direct effects of abnormal laforin expression.
Doublecortin (Xq21-24)	Doublecortin, expressed primarily in frontal lobes; function unknown; potentially an intracellular signalling molecule	Classic lissencephaly associated with severe mental retardation and seizures in males; subcortical band heterotopia with more subtle findings in females (presumably due to random X-inactivation); X-linked dominant	Relatively rare but of uncertain incidence, recent increased ascertainment due to improved imaging techniques; relationship between migration defect and seizure phenotype unknown

[a] The first three syndromes listed in the table (ADNFLE, BFNC, and GEFS+) are all the currently known idiopathic generalized epilepsies associated with identified gene mutations. The last three syndromes are examples of the numerous Mendelian disorders in which seizures are one part of the phenotype.
NOTE: GABA, γ-aminobutyric acid.

tion from a variety of causes, including developmental abnormalities, perinatal hypoxia/ischemia, trauma, infection, and other acquired lesions. The multifactorial nature of this syndrome suggests that it is a nonspecific response of the brain to diffuse neural injury. Unfortunately, many patients have a poor prognosis due to the underlying CNS disease and the physical and psychosocial consequences of severe, poorly controlled epilepsy.

MESIAL TEMPORAL LOBE EPILEPSY SYNDROME Mesial temporal lobe epilepsy (MTLE) is the most common syndrome associated with complex partial seizures and is an example of a symptomatic, partial epilepsy. Distinctive clinical, electroencephalographic, and pathologic features define this syndrome (Table 360-3). High-resolution magnetic resonance imaging (MRI) can detect the characteristic hippocampal sclerosis that appears to be an essential element in the pathophysiology of MTLE for many patients (Fig. 360-1). Recognition of this syndrome is especially important because it tends to be refractory to treatment with anticonvulsants but responds extremely well to surgical intervention. Major advances in the understanding of basic mechanisms of epilepsy have come through studies of experimental models of MTLE, discussed below.

Table 360-3 Characteristics of the Mesial Temporal Lobe Epilepsy (MTLE) Syndrome

History	
History of febrile seizures	Seizures may remit and reappear
Positive family history of epilepsy	Seizures often intractable
Early onset	
Rare secondarily generalized seizures	
Clinical Observations	
Aura common	Postictal disorientation, memory loss, dysphasia (with focus in dominant hemisphere)
Behavioral arrest/stare	
Complex automatisms	
Unilateral posturing	
Laboratory Studies	
Unilateral or bilateral anterior temporal spikes on EEG	
Hypometabolism on interictal PET	
Hypoperfusion on interictal SPECT	
Material-specific memory deficits on intracranial amobarbital (Wada) test	
MRI findings	
Small hippocampus with increased signal on T2-weighted sequences	
Small temporal lobe	
Enlarged temporal horn	
Pathologic findings	
Highly selective loss of specific cell populations within hippocampus in most cases	

NOTE: EEG, electroencephalogram; PET, positron emission tomography; SPECT, single photon emission computed tomography.

THE CAUSES OF SEIZURES AND EPILEPSY

Seizures are a result of a shift in the normal balance of excitation and inhibition within the CNS. Given the numerous properties that control

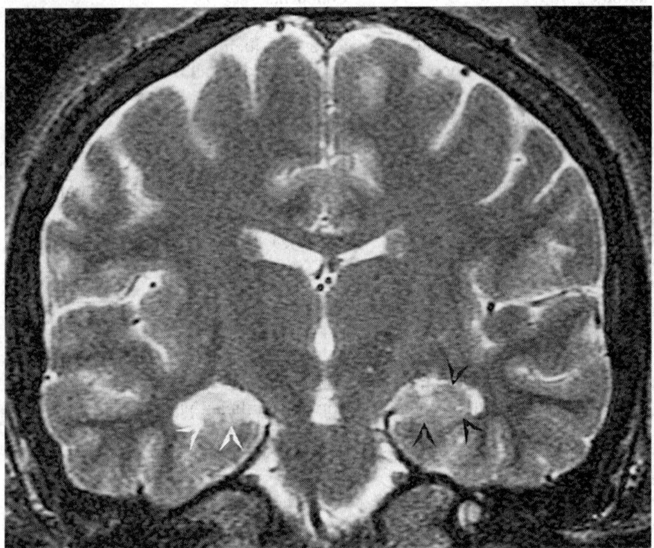

FIGURE 360-1 Mesial temporal lobe epilepsy. The EEG suggested a right temporal lobe focus. Coronal high-resolution T2-weighted fast spin echo magnetic resonance image obtained through the body of the hippocampus demonstrates abnormal high signal intensity in the right hippocampus (white arrows; compare with the normal hippocampus on the left, black arrows) consistent with mesial temporal sclerosis.

neuronal excitability, it is not surprising that there are many different ways to perturb this normal balance, and therefore many different causes of both seizures and epilepsy. Our understanding of the basic mechanisms involved remains very limited, and consequently there is not a rigorous, mechanistic-based framework for organizing all the etiologies. Conceptually, however, three important clinical observations emphasize how a variety of factors determine why certain conditions may cause seizures or epilepsy in a given patient.

1. *The normal brain is capable of having a seizure under the appropriate circumstances, and there are differences between individuals in the susceptibility or threshold for seizures.* For example, seizures may be induced by high fevers in children who are otherwise normal and who never develop other neurologic problems, including epilepsy. However, febrile seizures occur only in a relatively small proportion of children. This implies there are various underlying, *endogenous factors* that influence the threshold for having a seizure. Some of these factors are clearly genetic, as it has been shown that a family history of epilepsy will influence the likelihood of seizures occurring in otherwise normal individuals. Normal development also plays an important role, since the brain appears to have different seizure thresholds at different maturational stages.

2. *There are a variety of conditions that have an extremely high likelihood of resulting in a chronic seizure disorder.* One of the best examples of this is severe, penetrating head trauma, which is associated with up to a 50% risk of subsequent epilepsy. The high propensity for severe traumatic brain injury to lead to epilepsy suggests that the injury results in a long-lasting, pathologic change in the CNS that transforms a presumably normal neural network into one that is abnormally hyperexcitable. This process is known as *epileptogenesis,* and the specific changes that result in a lowered seizure threshold can be considered *epileptogenic factors.* Other processes associated with epileptogenesis include stroke, infections, and abnormalities of CNS development. Likewise, the genetic abnormalities associated with epilepsy likely involve processes that trigger the appearance of specific sets of epileptogenic factors.

3. *Seizures are episodic.* Patients with epilepsy have seizures intermittently and, depending on the underlying cause, many patients are completely normal for months or even years between seizures. This implies there are important provocative or *precipitating factors* that induce seizures in patients with epilepsy. Similarly, precipitating factors are responsible for causing the single seizure in someone without epilepsy. Precipitants include those due to intrinsic physiologic processes, such as psychological or physical stress, sleep deprivation, or hormonal changes associated with the menstrual cycle. They also include exogenous factors such as exposure to toxic substances and certain medications.

These observations emphasize the concept that the many causes of seizures and epilepsy result from a dynamic interplay between endogenous factors, epileptogenic factors, and precipitating factors. The potential role of each needs to be carefully considered when determining the appropriate management of a patient with seizures. For example, the identification of predisposing factors (e.g., family history of epilepsy) in a patient with febrile seizures may increase the necessity for closer follow-up and a more aggressive diagnostic evaluation. Finding an epileptogenic lesion may help in the estimation of seizure recurrence and duration of therapy. Finally, removal or modification of a precipitating factor may be an effective and safer method for preventing further seizures than the prophylactic use of anticonvulsant drugs.

CAUSES ACCORDING TO AGE In practice, it is useful to consider the etiologies of seizures based on the age of the patient, as age is one of the most important factors determining both the incidence and likely causes of seizures or epilepsy (Table 360-4). During the *neonatal period and early infancy*, potential causes include hypoxic-ischemic encephalopathy, trauma, CNS infection, congenital CNS abnormalities, and metabolic disorders. Babies born to mothers using neurotoxic drugs such as cocaine, heroin, or ethanol are susceptible to drug-withdrawal seizures in the first few days after delivery. Hypoglycemia and hypocalcemia, which can occur as secondary complications of perinatal injury, are also causes of seizures early after delivery. Seizures due to inborn errors of metabolism usually present once regular feeding begins, typically 2 to 3 days after birth. Pyridox-

Table 360-4 The Causes of Seizures

Neonates (<1 month)	Perinatal hypoxia and ischemia Intracranial hemorrhage and trauma Acute CNS infection Metabolic disturbances (hypoglycemia, hypocalcemia, hypomagnesemia, pyridoxine deficiency) Drug withdrawal Developmental disorders Genetic disorders
Infants and children (>1 mo and <12 years)	Febrile seizures Genetic disorders (metabolic, degenerative, primary epilepsy syndromes) CNS infection Developmental disorders Trauma Idiopathic
Adolescents (12–18 years)	Trauma Genetic disorders Infection Brain tumor Illicit drug use Idiopathic
Young adults (18–35 years)	Trauma Alcohol withdrawal Illicit drug use Brain tumor Idiopathic
Older adults (>35 years)	Cerebrovascular disease Brain tumor Alcohol withdrawal Metabolic disorders (uremia, hepatic failure, electrolyte abnormalities, hypoglycemia) Alzheimer's disease and other degenerative CNS diseases Idiopathic

NOTE: CNS, central nervous system.

ine (vitamin B_6) deficiency, an important cause of neonatal seizures, can be effectively treated with pyridoxine replacement. The idiopathic or inherited forms of benign neonatal convulsions are also seen during this time period.

The most common seizures arising in *late infancy and early childhood* are febrile seizures, which are seizures associated with fevers but without evidence of CNS infection or other defined causes. The overall prevalence is 3 to 5% and even higher in some parts of the world, such as Asia. Patients often have a family history of febrile seizures or epilepsy. Febrile seizures usually occur between 3 months and 5 years of age and have a peak incidence between 18 and 24 months. The typical scenario is a child who has a generalized, tonic-clonic seizure during a febrile illness in the setting of a common childhood infection such as otitis media, respiratory infection, or gastroenteritis. The seizure is likely to occur during the rising phase of the temperature curve (i.e., during the first day) rather than well into the course of the illness. A *simple* febrile seizure is a single, isolated event, brief, and symmetric in appearance. *Complex* febrile seizures have repeated seizure activity, last >15 min, or have focal features. Approximately one-third of patients with febrile seizures will have a recurrence, but <10% have three or more episodes. Recurrences are much more likely when the febrile seizure occurs in the first year of life. Simple febrile seizures are not associated with an increase in the risk of developing epilepsy, while complex febrile seizures have a risk of 2 to 5%; other risk factors include the presence of preexisting neurologic deficits and a family history of nonfebrile seizures.

Childhood marks the age at which many of the well-defined epilepsy syndromes present. Some children who are otherwise normal develop idiopathic, generalized tonic-clonic seizures without other features that fit into specific syndromes. Temporal lobe epilepsy usually presents in childhood and may be related to mesial temporal lobe sclerosis (as part of the MTLE syndrome) or other focal abnormalities such as cortical dysgenesis. Other types of partial seizures, including those with secondary generalization, may be the relatively late manifestation of a developmental disorder, an acquired lesion such as head trauma, CNS infection (especially viral encephalitis), or very rarely a CNS tumor.

The period of *adolescence and early adulthood* is one of transition during which the idiopathic or genetically based epilepsy syndromes, including JME and juvenile absence epilepsy, become less common, while epilepsies secondary to acquired CNS lesions begin to predominate. Seizures that begin in patients in this age range may be associated with head trauma, CNS infections (including parasitic infections such as cysticercosis), brain tumors, congenital CNS abnormalities, illicit drug use, or alcohol withdrawal.

Head trauma is a common cause of epilepsy in adolescents and adults. The head injury can be caused by a variety of mechanisms, and the likelihood of developing epilepsy is strongly correlated with the severity of the injury. A patient with a penetrating head wound, depressed skull fracture, intracranial hemorrhage, or prolonged posttraumatic coma or amnesia has a 40 to 50% risk of developing epilepsy, while a patient with a closed head injury and cerebral contusion has a 5 to 25% risk. Recurrent seizures usually develop within 1 year after head trauma, although intervals of 10 years or longer are well known. In controlled studies, mild head injury, defined as a concussion with amnesia or loss of consciousness of <30 min, was not found to be associated with an increased likelihood of epilepsy. Nonetheless, most epileptologists know of patients who have partial seizures within hours or days of a mild head injury and subsequently develop chronic seizures of the same type; such cases may represent rare examples of chronic epilepsy resulting from mild head injury.

The causes of seizures in *older adults* include cerebrovascular disease, trauma (including subdural hematoma), CNS tumors, and degenerative diseases. Cerebrovascular disease may account for approximately 50% of new cases of epilepsy in patients older than 65. Acute seizures (i.e., occurring at the time of the stroke) are seen more often with embolic rather than hemorrhagic or thrombotic stroke. Chronic seizures typically appear months to years after the initial event and are associated with all forms of stroke.

Table 360-5 Drugs and Other Substances that Can Cause Seizures

Antimicrobials/antivirals	Psychotropics
β-lactam and related compounds	Antidepressants
Quinolones	Antipsychotics
Acyclovir	Lithium
Isoniazid	Radiographic contrast agents
Ganciclovir	Theophylline
Anesthetics and Analgesics	Sedative-hypnotic drug withdrawal
Meperidine	Alcohol
Tramadol	Barbiturates
Local anesthetics	Benzodiazepines
Class 1B agents	Drugs of abuse
Immunomodulatory drugs	Amphetamine
Cyclosporine	Cocaine
OKT3 (monoclonal antibodies to T cells)	Phencyclidine
Tacrolimus (FK-506)	Methylphenidate
Interferons	Flumazenil[a]

[a] In benzodiazepine-dependent patients.

Metabolic disturbances such as electrolyte imbalance, hypo- or hyperglycemia, renal failure, and hepatic failure may cause seizures at any age. Similarly, endocrine disorders, hematologic disorders, vasculitides, and many other systemic diseases may cause seizures over a broad age range. A wide variety of medications and abused substances are known to precipitate seizures as well (Table 360-5).

BASIC MECHANISMS

MECHANISMS OF SEIZURE INITIATION AND PROPAGATION Partial seizure activity can begin in a very discrete region of cortex and then spread to neighboring regions, i.e., there is a *seizure initiation* phase and a *seizure propagation* phase. Studies of experimental models of these phases suggest that the initiation phase is characterized by two concurrent events in an aggregate of neurons: (1) high-frequency bursts of action potentials, and (2) hypersynchronization. The bursting activity is caused by a relatively long-lasting depolarization of the neuronal membrane due to influx of extracellular calcium (Ca^{2+}), which leads to the opening of voltage-dependent sodium (Na^+) channels, influx of Na^+, and generation of repetitive action potentials. This is followed by a hyperpolarizing afterpotential mediated by γ-aminobutyric acid (GABA) receptors or potassium (K^+) channels, depending on the cell type. The synchronized bursts from a sufficient number of neurons result in a so-called spike discharge on the EEG.

Normally, the spread of bursting activity is prevented by intact hyperpolarization and a region of surrounding inhibition created by inhibitory neurons. With sufficient activation there is a recruitment of surrounding neurons via a number of mechanisms. Repetitive discharges lead to the following: (1) an increase in extracellular K^+, which blunts the extent of hyperpolarization and depolarizes neighboring neurons; (2) accumulation of Ca^{2+} in presynaptic terminals, leading to enhanced neurotransmitter release; and (3) depolarization-induced activation of the *N*-methyl-D-aspartate (NMDA) subtype of the excitatory amino acid receptor, which causes more Ca^{2+} influx and neuronal activation. The recruitment of a sufficient number of neurons leads to a loss of the surrounding inhibition and propagation of seizure activity into contiguous areas via local cortical connections, and to more distant areas via long commissural pathways such as the corpus callosum.

Many factors control neuronal excitability, and thus there are many potential mechanisms for altering a neuron's propensity to have bursting activity. Examples of mechanisms *intrinsic* to the neuron include changes in the conductance of ion channels, response characteristics of membrane receptors, cytoplasmic buffering, second-messenger systems, and protein expression as determined by gene transcription, translation, and posttranslational modification. Mechanisms *extrinsic* to the neuron include changes in the amount or type of neurotransmitters present at the synapse, modulation of receptors by extracellular ions and other molecules, and temporal and spatial properties of both synaptic and nonsynaptic input. Nonneural cells, such as astrocytes and oligodendrocytes, have an important role in many of these mechanisms as well.

Certain known causes of seizures are explained by these mechanisms. For example, accidental ingestion of domoic acid, which is an analogue of glutamate (the principal excitatory neurotransmitter in the brain), causes profound seizures via direct activation of excitatory amino acid receptors throughout the CNS. Penicillin, which can lower the seizure threshold in humans and is a potent convulsant in experimental models, reduces inhibition by antagonizing the effects of GABA at its receptor. The basic mechanisms of other precipitating factors of seizures, such as sleep deprivation, fever, alcohol withdrawal, hypoxia, and infection, are not as well understood but presumably involve analogous perturbations in neuronal excitability. Similarly, the endogenous factors that determine an individual's seizure threshold may relate to these properties as well.

Knowledge of the mechanisms responsible for the initiation and propagation of most generalized seizures (including tonic-clonic, myoclonic, and atonic types) remains rudimentary and reflects the limited understanding of the connectivity of the brain at a systems level. Much more is understood about the origin of generalized spike-and-wave discharges in absence seizures. These appear to be related to oscillatory rhythms that are normally generated during sleep by circuits connecting the thalamus and cortex. This oscillatory behavior involves an interaction between $GABA_B$receptors, T-type Ca^{2+} channels, and K^+ channels located within the thalamus. Pharmacologic studies indicate that modulation of these receptors and channels can induce absence seizures, and there is speculation that the genetic forms of absence epilepsy may be associated with mutations of components of this system.

MECHANISMS OF EPILEPTOGENESIS Epileptogenesis refers to the transformation of a normal neuronal network into one that is chronically hyperexcitable. For example, there is often a delay of months to years between an initial CNS injury such as trauma, stroke, or infection and the first seizure. The injury appears to initiate a process that gradually lowers the seizure threshold in the affected region until a spontaneous seizure occurs. In many genetic and idiopathic forms of epilepsy, epileptogenesis is presumably determined by developmentally regulated events.

Pathologic studies of the hippocampus from patients with temporal lobe epilepsy have led to the suggestion that some forms of epileptogenesis are related to *structural changes in neuronal networks.* For example, many patients with MTLE syndrome have a highly selective loss of neurons that has been proposed to contribute to inhibition of the main excitatory neurons within the dentate gyrus. There is also evidence that, in response to the loss of neurons, there is reorganization or "sprouting" of surviving neurons in a way that affects the excitability of the network. Some of these changes can be seen in experimental models of prolonged electrical seizures or traumatic brain injury. Thus, an initial injury such as head injury may lead to a very focal, confined region of structural change that causes local hyperexcitability. The local hyperexcitability leads to further structural changes that evolve over time until the focal lesion produces clinically evident seizures. Similar models have also provided strong evidence for long-term alterations in *intrinsic, biochemical properties of cells* within the network, such as chronic changes in glutamate receptor function.

GENETIC CAUSES OF EPILEPSY The most important recent progress in epilepsy research has been the identification of genetic mutations associated with a variety of epilepsy syndromes. Table 360-2 describes some of these in further detail. Although all of the mutations identified to date cause rare forms of epilepsy, they have led to extremely important conceptual advances. For example, it appears that many of the inherited, idiopathic epilepsies (i.e., the relatively "pure" forms of epilepsy in which seizures are the phenotypic abnormality and brain structure and function are otherwise normal) are due to mutations affecting ion channel function. These syndromes are therefore part of the larger group of "channelopathies" causing paroxysmal disorders such as cardiac arrhythmias, episodic ataxia, periodic weakness, and familial hemiplegic migraine (Chap. 15). In contrast, gene mutations observed in symptomatic epilepsies (i.e., disorders in which other neurologic abnormalities, such as cognitive impairment, coexist with seizures) are proving to be associated with pathways influencing CNS development or neuronal homeostasis. A current challenge is to identify the multiple susceptibility genes that underlie the more common forms of idiopathic epilepsies.

MECHANISMS OF ACTION OF ANTIEPILEPTIC DRUGS Currently available antiepileptic drugs appear to act primarily by blocking the initiation or spread of seizures. This occurs through a variety of mechanisms, and in most cases the drugs have pleiotropic effects. The mechanisms include inhibition of Na^+-dependent action potentials in a frequency-dependent manner (e.g., phenytoin, carbamazepine, topiramate, zonisamide), inhibition of voltage-gated Ca^{2+}channels (phenytoin), decrease of glutamate release (lamotrigine), potentiation of GABA receptor function (benzodiazepines and barbiturates), and increase in the availability of GABA (valproic acid, gabapentin, tiagabine). The two most effective drugs for absence seizures, ethosuximide and valproic acid, probably act by inhibiting T-type Ca^{2+} channels in thalamic neurons.

In contrast to the relatively large number of antiepileptic drugs that can attenuate seizure activity, there are currently no drugs known to prevent the formation of a seizure focus following CNS injury in humans. The eventual development of such "antiepileptogenic" drugs will provide an important means of preventing the emergence of epilepsy following injuries such as head trauma, stroke, and CNS infection.

EVALUATION OF THE PATIENT WITH A SEIZURE

When a patient presents shortly after a seizure, the first priorities are attention to vital signs, respiratory and cardiovascular support, and treatment of seizures if they resume (see "Treatment"). Life-threatening conditions such as CNS infection, metabolic derangement or drug toxicity must be recognized and managed appropriately.

When the patient is not acutely ill, the evaluation will initially focus on whether or not there is a history of earlier seizures (Fig. 360-2). If this is the patient's first seizure, then the emphasis will be to (1) establish whether the reported episode was a seizure rather than another paroxysmal event, (2) determine the cause of the seizure by identifying risk factors and precipitating events, and (3) decide whether anticonvulsant therapy is required in addition to treatment for any underlying illness.

In the patient with prior seizures or a known history of epilepsy, the evaluation is directed toward (1) identification of the underlying cause and precipitating factors, and (2) determination of the adequacy of the patient's current therapy.

HISTORY AND EXAMINATION The history should first determine whether the event was truly a seizure. It is essential to take the time to gather an in-depth history, for *in many cases the diagnosis of a seizure is based solely on clinical grounds—the examination and laboratory studies are often normal.* Keeping in mind the characteristics of different seizure types, questions need to focus precisely on the symptoms before, during, and after the episode in order to discriminate a seizure from other paroxysmal events (see "Differential Diagnosis of Seizures"). Seizures frequently occur out-of-hospital, and the patient may be unaware of the ictal and immediate postictal phases; thus witnesses to the event should be interviewed carefully.

The history should also focus on risk factors and predisposing events. Clues for a predisposition to seizures include a history of febrile seizures, earlier auras or brief seizures not recognized as such, and a family history of seizures. Epileptogenic factors such as prior head trauma, stroke, tumor, or vascular malformation should be identified. In children, a careful assessment of developmental milestones may provide evidence for underlying CNS disease. Precipitating factors such as sleep deprivation, systemic diseases, electrolyte or metabolic derangements, acute infection, drugs that lower the seizure threshold (Table 360-5), or alcohol or illicit drug use should also be identified.

The general physical examination includes a search for signs of infection or systemic illness. Careful examination of the skin may reveal signs of neurocutaneous disorders, such as tuberous sclerosis or neurofibromatosis, or chronic liver or renal disease. A finding of organomegaly may indicate a metabolic storage disease, and limb asymmetry may provide a clue for brain injury early in development. Signs of head trauma and use of alcohol or illicit drugs should be sought. Auscultation of the heart and carotid arteries may identify an abnormality that predisposes to cerebrovascular disease.

All patients require a complete neurologic examination, with particular emphasis on eliciting signs of cerebral hemispheric disease (Chap. 356). Careful assessment of mental status (including memory, language function, and abstract thinking) may suggest lesions in the anterior frontal, parietal, or temporal lobes. Testing of visual fields will help screen for lesions in the optic pathways and occipital lobes. Screening tests of motor function such as pronator drift, deep tendon reflexes, gait, and coordination may suggest lesions in motor (frontal) cortex, and cortical sensory testing (e.g., double simultaneous stimulation) may detect lesions in the parietal cortex.

LABORATORY STUDIES

Routine blood studies are indicated to identify the more common metabolic causes of seizures, such as abnormalities in electrolytes, glucose, calcium, or magnesium, and hepatic or renal disease. A screen for toxins in blood and urine should also be obtained from all patients in the appropriate risk groups, especially when no clear precipitating factor has been identified. A lumbar puncture is indicated if there is any suspicion of meningitis or encephalitis and is mandatory in all patients infected with HIV, even in the absence of symptoms or signs suggesting infection.

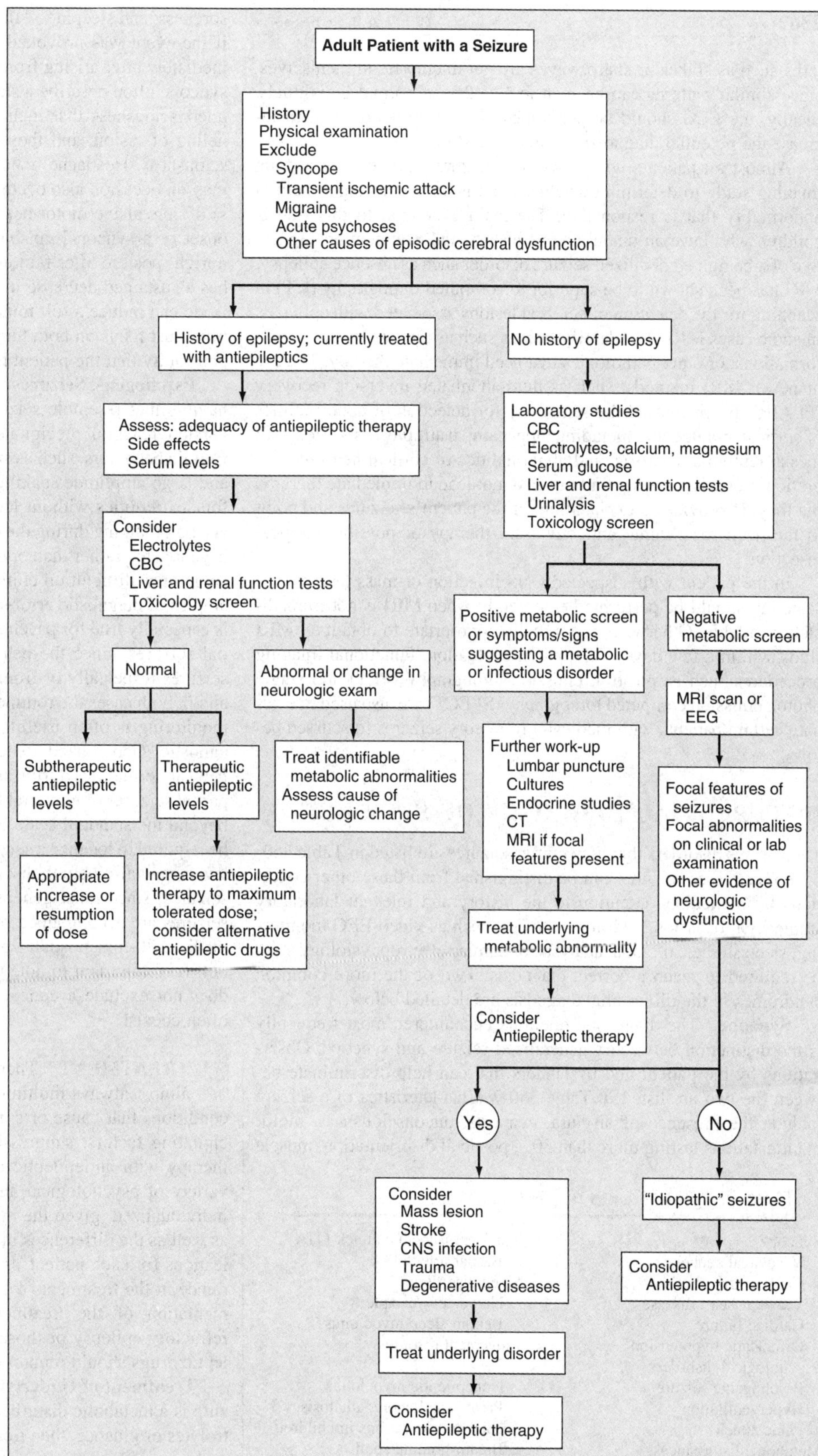

FIGURE 360-2 Evaluation of the adult patient with a seizure. CBC, complete blood count; CT, computed tomography; MRI, magnetic resonance imaging; EEG, electroencephalogram; CNS, central nervous system.

All patients who have a possible seizure disorder should be evaluated with an EEG (Chap. 357) as soon as possible. The EEG may help to establish the diagnosis of epilepsy, classify the seizure type, and provide evidence for the existence of a particular epilepsy syndrome. If the patient is having frequent seizures, such as a child with absence epilepsy, the EEG may confirm the presence of seizures and help to identify the seizure type. In patients with infrequent seizures, the EEG may reveal potentially abnormal interictal activity that, when combined with clinical or radiologic data, aids in establishing the diagnosis. However, the existence of epileptiform patterns such as spikes or sharp waves are not diagnostic in themselves, since similar patterns can be seen in 1 to 2% of normal individuals. Ideally, the EEG should be performed after sleep deprivation to increase the potential diagnostic yield of the study.

Almost all patients with new-onset seizures should have a brain imaging study to determine whether there is an underlying structural abnormality that is responsible. The main exception to this rule is children who have an unambiguous history and examination suggestive of a benign, generalized seizure disorder such as absence epilepsy. MRI has been shown to be superior to computed tomography (CT) in scanning for the detection of cerebral lesions associated with epilepsy. In some cases MRI will identify lesions such as tumors, vascular malformations, or other pathologies that need immediate therapy. The use of newer MRI methods, such as fluid-attenuated inversion recovery (FLAIR), has increased the sensitivity for detection of abnormalities of cortical architecture, including hippocampal atrophy associated with mesial temporal sclerosis, and abnormalities of cortical neuronal migration. In such cases the findings may not lead to immediate therapy, but they do provide an explanation for the patient's seizures and point to the need for chronic anticonvulsant therapy or possible surgical resection.

In the patient with suspected CNS infection or mass lesions, CT scanning should be performed emergently when MRI is not immediately available. Otherwise, it is usually appropriate to obtain an MRI study within a few days of the initial evaluation. Functional imaging procedures such as positron emission tomography (PET) and single photon emission computed tomography (SPECT) are also used to evaluate certain patients with medically refractory seizures (discussed below).

DIFFERENTIAL DIAGNOSIS OF SEIZURES

The various disorders that may mimic seizures are listed in Table 360-6. In most cases seizures can be distinguished from these other conditions by meticulous attention to the history and relevant laboratory studies. On occasion, additional studies, such as video-EEG monitoring, sleep studies, tilt table analysis, or cardiac electrophysiology, may be required to reach a correct diagnosis. Two of the more common syndromes in the differential diagnosis are detailed below.

Syncope The diagnostic dilemma encountered most frequently is the distinction between a generalized seizure and syncope. Observations by the patient and bystanders that can help discriminate between the two are listed in Table 360-7. Characteristics of a seizure include the presence of an aura, cyanosis, unconsciousness, motor manifestations lasting more than 30 s, postictal disorientation, muscle soreness, and sleepiness. In contrast, a syncopal episode is more likely if the event was provoked by acute pain or anxiety or occurred immediately after arising from the lying or sitting position. Patients with syncope often describe a stereotyped transition from consciousness to unconsciousness that includes tiredness, sweating, nausea, and tunneling of vision, and they experience a relatively brief loss of consciousness. Headache or incontinence usually suggests a seizure but may on occasion also occur with syncope. A brief period (i.e., 1 to 10 s) of convulsive motor activity is frequently seen immediately at the onset of a syncopal episode, especially if the patient remains in an upright posture after fainting (e.g., in a dentist's chair) and therefore has a sustained decrease in cerebral perfusion. Rarely, a syncopal episode can induce a full tonic-clonic seizure. In such cases the evaluation must focus on both the cause of the syncopal event as well as the possibility that the patient has a propensity for recurrent seizures.

Table 360-6 The Differential Diagnosis of Seizures

Syncope	Transient ischemic attack (TIA)
Vasovagal syncope	Basilar artery TIA
Cardiac arrhythmia	Sleep disorders
Valvular heart disease	Narcolepsy/cataplexy
Cardiac failure	Benign sleep myoclonus
Orthostatic hypotension	Movement disorders
Psychological disorders	Tics
Psychogenic seizure	Nonepileptic myoclonus
Hyperventilation	Paroxysmal choreoathetosis
Panic attack	Special considerations in children
Metabolic disturbances	Breath-holding spells
Alcoholic blackouts	Migraine with recurrent abdominal pain and cyclic vomiting
Delirium tremens	Benign paroxysmal vertigo
Hypoglycemia	Apnea
Hypoxia	Night terrors
Psychoactive drugs (e.g., hallucinogens)	Sleepwalking
Migraine	
Confusional migraine	
Basilar migraine	

Psychogenic Seizures Psychogenic seizures are nonepileptic behaviors that resemble seizures. The behavior is often part of a conversion reaction precipitated by underlying psychological distress. Certain behaviors, such as side-to-side turning of the head, asymmetric and large-amplitude shaking movements of the limbs, twitching of all four extremities without loss of consciousness, pelvic thrusting, and crying or talking during the event, are more commonly associated with psychogenic rather than epileptic seizures. However, the distinction is sometimes difficult on clinical grounds alone, and there are many examples of diagnostic errors made by experienced epileptologists. This is especially true for psychogenic seizures that resemble complex partial seizures, since the behavioral manifestations of complex partial seizures (especially of frontal lobe origin) can be extremely unusual, and in both cases the routine surface EEG may be normal. Video-EEG monitoring is often useful when the clinical observations are nondiagnostic. Generalized tonic-clonic seizures always produce marked EEG abnormalities during and after the seizure. For suspected complex partial seizures of temporal lobe origin, the use of additional electrodes beyond the standard scalp locations (e.g., sphenoidal electrodes) may be required to localize a seizure focus. Measurement of serum prolactin levels may also help to discriminate between organic and psychogenic seizures, since most generalized seizures and many complex partial seizures are accompanied by rises in serum prolactin (during the immediate 30-min postictal period), whereas psychogenic seizures are not. It is important to note that the diagnosis of psychogenic seizures does not exclude a concurrent diagnosis of epilepsy, since the two often coexist.

℞ **TREATMENT** Therapy for a patient with a seizure disorder is almost always multimodal and includes treatment of underlying conditions that cause or contribute to the seizures, avoidance of precipitating factors, suppression of recurrent seizures by prophylactic therapy with antiepileptic medications or surgery, and addressing a variety of psychological and social issues. Treatment plans must be individualized, given the many different types and causes of seizures as well as the differences in efficacy and toxicity of antiepileptic medications for each patient. In almost all cases a neurologist with experience in the treatment of epilepsy should design and oversee implementation of the treatment strategy. Furthermore, patients with refractory epilepsy or those who require polypharmacy with antiepileptic drugs should remain under the regular care of a neurologist.

Treatment of Underlying Conditions If the sole cause of a seizure is a metabolic disturbance such as an abnormality of serum electrolytes or glucose, then treatment is aimed at reversing the metabolic problem and preventing its recurrence. Therapy with antiepileptic drugs is usually unnecessary unless the metabolic disorder cannot be corrected promptly and the patient is at risk of having further seizures. If the apparent cause of a seizure was a medication (e.g., theophylline) or illicit drug use (e.g., cocaine), then appropriate therapy is avoidance of the drug and there is usually no need for antiepileptic medications unless subsequent seizures occur in the absence of these precipitants.

Seizures caused by a structural CNS lesion such as a brain tumor, vascular malformation, or brain abscess may not recur after appropriate treatment of the underlying lesion. However, despite removal of the structural lesion, there is a risk that the seizure focus will remain in the surrounding tissue or develop de novo as a result of gliosis and other processes induced by surgery, radiation, or other therapies. Most patients are therefore maintained on an antiepileptic medication for at least 1 year, and an attempt is made to withdraw medications only if the patient has been completely seizure-free. If the seizures are refractory to medication, the patient may benefit from surgical removal of the epileptic brain region (see "Surgical Treatment of Refractory Epilepsy").

Avoidance of Precipitating Factors Unfortunately, little is known about the specific factors that determine precisely when a seizure will occur in a patient with epilepsy. Some patients can identify particular situations that appear to lower their seizure threshold; these situations should be avoided. For example, a patient who has seizures in the setting of sleep deprivation should obviously be advised to maintain a normal sleep schedule. Many patients note an association between alcohol intake and seizures, and they should be encouraged to modify their drinking habits accordingly. There are also relatively rare cases of patients with seizures that are induced by highly specific stimuli such as a video game monitor, music, or an individual's voice ("reflex epilepsy"). If there is an association between stress and seizures, stress reduction techniques such as physical exercise, meditation, or counseling may be helpful.

Table 360-7 Clinical Features of a Generalized Tonic-Clonic Seizure Versus Syncope

Features	Seizure	Syncope
Immediate precipitating factors	Usually none	Emotional stress, valsalva, orthostatic hypotension, cardiac etiologies
Premonitory symptoms	None or aura (e.g., odd odor)	Tiredness, nausea, diaphoresis, tunneling of vision
Posture at onset	Variable	Usually erect
Transition to unconsciousness	Often immediate	Gradual over seconds[a]
Duration of unconsciousness	Minutes	Seconds
Duration of tonic or clonic movements	30–60 s	Never more than 15 s
Facial appearance during event	Cyanosis, frothing at mouth	Pallor
Disorientation and sleepiness after event	Many minutes to hours	<5 min
Aching of muscles after event	Often	Sometimes
Biting of tongue	Sometimes	Rarely
Incontinence	Sometimes	Unusual
Headache	Sometimes	Rarely

[a] May be sudden with certain cardiac arrhythmias.

Antiepileptic Drug Therapy Antiepileptic drug therapy is the mainstay of treatment for most patients with epilepsy. The overall goal is to completely prevent seizures without causing any untoward side effects, preferably with a single medication and a dosing schedule that is easy for the patient to follow. Seizure classification is an important element in designing the treatment plan, since some antiepileptic drugs have different activities against various seizure types. However, there is considerable overlap between many antiepileptic drugs, such that the choice of therapy is often determined more by specific needs of the patient, especially the patient's assessment of side effects.

When to initiate antiepileptic drug therapy Antiepileptic drug therapy should be started in any patient with recurrent seizures of unknown etiology or a known cause that cannot be reversed. Whether to initiate therapy in a patient with a single seizure is controversial. Patients with a single seizure due to an identified lesion such as a CNS tumor, infection, or trauma, in which there is strong evidence that the lesion is epileptogenic, should be treated. The risk of seizure recurrence in a patient with an apparently unprovoked or idiopathic seizure is uncertain, with estimates ranging from 31 to 71% in the first 12 months after the initial seizure. This uncertainty arises from differences in the underlying seizure types and etiologies in various published epidemiologic studies. Generally accepted risk factors associated with recurrent seizures include the following: (1) an abnormal neurologic examination, (2) seizures presenting as status epilepticus, (3) postictal Todd's paralysis, (4) a strong family history of seizures, or (5) an abnormal EEG. Most patients with one or more of these risk factors should be treated. Issues such as employment or driving may influence the decision whether or not to start medications as well. For example, a patient with a single, idiopathic seizure and whose job depends on driving may prefer taking antiepileptic drugs rather than risking a seizure recurrence and the potential loss of driving privileges.

Selection of antiepileptic drugs The choices of antiepileptic drugs in the United States for different seizure types are shown in Table 360-8, and the main pharmacologic characteristics of commonly used drugs are listed in Table 360-9. Older medications such as phenytoin, valproic acid, carbamazepine, and ethosuximide are generally used as first-line therapy for most seizure disorders since, overall, they are as effective as recently marketed drugs and significantly less expensive. Of the new drugs that have become available in the United States in the past decade, most are currently being used as add-on or alternative therapy.

In addition to efficacy, other factors influencing the specific choice of an initial medication for a patient include the relative convenience of dosing schedule (e.g., once daily versus three or four times daily) and potential side effects. Almost all of the commonly used antiepileptic drugs can cause similar, dose-related side effects such as sedation, ataxia, and diplopia. Close follow-up is required to ensure these are promptly recognized and reversed. Most of the drugs may also cause idiosyncratic toxicity such as rash, bone marrow suppression, or hepatotoxicity. Although rare, these side effects need to be carefully considered during drug selection, and patients require laboratory tests (e.g., complete blood count and liver function tests) prior to the institution of a drug (to establish baseline values) and during initial dosing and titration of the agent.

ANTIEPILEPTIC DRUG SELECTION FOR PARTIAL SEIZURES Carbamazepine or phenytoin is currently the initial drug of choice for the treatment of partial seizures, including those that secondarily generalize. Overall they have very similar efficacy, but differences in phar-

Table 360-8 Antiepileptic Drugs of Choice

	Primary Generalized Tonic-Clonic	Partial[a]	Absence	Atypical Absence, Myoclonic, Atonic
First-Line	Valproic acid Lamotrigine	Carbamazepine Phenytoin Valproic acid Lamotrigine	Ethosuximide Valproic acid	Valproic acid
Alternatives	Phenytoin Carbamazepine Topiramate Primidone Phenobarbital Felbamate	Gabapentin[b] Topiramate[b] Tiagabine[b] Primidone Phenobarbital	Lamotrigine Clonazepam	Lamotrigine Topiramate[b] Clonazepam Felbamate

[a] Includes simple partial, complex partial, and secondarily generalized seizures.
[b] As adjunctive therapy.

Table 360-9 Commonly Used Antiepileptic Drugs

Generic Name	Trade Name	Principal Uses	Typical Dosage and Dosing Intervals	Half-Life	Therapeutic Range	Adverse Effects: Neurologic	Adverse Effects: Systemic	Drug Interactions
Phenytoin (diphenylhydantoin)	Dilantin	Tonic-clonic (grand mal) Focal-onset	300–400 mg/d (3–6 mg/kg, adult; 4–8 mg/kg, child) qd-bid	24 h (wide variation, dose-dependent)	10–20 μg/mL	Dizziness Diplopia Ataxia Incoordination Confusion	Gum hyperplasia Lymphadenopathy Hirsutism Osteomalacia Facial coarsening Skin rash	Level increased by isoniazid, sulfonamides Level decreased by enzyme-inducing drugs[a] Altered folate metabolism
Carbamazepine	Tegretol Carbatrol	Tonic-clonic Focal-onset	600–1800 mg/d (15–35 mg/kg, child) bid-qid	10–17 h	6–12 μg/mL	Ataxia Dizziness Diplopia Vertigo	Aplastic anemia Leukopenia Gastrointestinal irritation Hepatotoxicity Hyponatremia	Level decreased by enzyme-inducing drugs[a] Level increased by erythromycin, propoxyphene, isoniazid, cimetidine
Valproic acid	Depakene Depakote	Tonic-clonic Absence Atypical absence Myoclonic Focal-onset	750–2000 mg/d (20–60 mg/kg) bid-qid	15 h	50–150 μg/mL	Ataxia Sedation Tremor	Hepatotoxicity Thrombocytopenia Gastrointestinal irritation Weight gain Transient alopecia Hyperammonemia	Level decreased by enzyme-inducing drugs[a]
Lamotrigine	Lamictal	Focal-onset Tonic-clonic Atypical absence Myoclonic Lennox-Gastaut syndrome	150–500 mg/d bid	25 h 14 h (with enzyme-inducers) 59 h (with valproic acid)	Not established	Dizziness Diplopia Sedation Ataxia Headache	Skin rash Stevens-Johnson syndrome	Level decreased by enzyme-inducing drugs[a] Level increased by valproic acid
Ethosuximide	Zarontin	Absence (petit mal)	750–1250 mg/d (20–40 mg/kg) qd-bid	60 h, adult 30 h, child	40–100 μg/mL	Ataxia Lethargy Headache	Gastrointestinal irritation Skin rash Bone marrow suppression	
Gabapentin	Neurontin	Focal-onset	900–2400 mg/d tid-qid	5–9 h	Not established	Sedation Dizziness Ataxia Fatigue	Gastrointestinal irritation	No known significant interactions
Topiramate	Topamax	Focal-onset Tonic-clonic	400 mg/d bid	20–30 h	Not established	Psychomotor slowing Sedation Speech or language problems Fatigue Paresthesias	Renal stones (avoid use with other carbonic anhydrase inhibitors)	Level decreased by enzyme-inducing drugs[a]

(continued)

Table 360-9—*(continued)*

Generic Name	Trade Name	Principal Uses	Typical Dosage and Dosing Intervals	Half-Life	Therapeutic Range	Adverse Effects: Neurologic	Adverse Effects: Systemic	Drug Interactions
Tiagabine	Gabatril	Focal-onset Tonic-clonic Lennox-Gastaut syndrome	32–56 mg/d bid-qid	7–9 h	Not established	Confusion Sedation Depression Dizziness Speech or language problems Paresthesias Psychosis	Gastrointestinal irritation	Level decreased by enzyme-inducing drugs[a]
Phenobarbital	Luminol	Tonic-clonic Focal-onset	60–180 mg/d (1–4 mg/kg, adult); (3–6 mg/kg, child) qd	90 h (70 h in children)	10–40 μg/mL	Sedation Ataxia Confusion Dizziness Decreased libido Depression	Skin rash	Level increased by valproic acid, phenytoin Enhances metabolism of other drugs via liver enzyme induction
Primidone	Mysoline	Tonic-clonic Focal-onset	750–1000 mg/d (10–25 mg/kg) bid-tid	Primidone, 8–15 h Phenobarbital, 90 h	Primidone, 4–12 μg/mL Phenobarbital, 10–40 μg/mL	Same as phenobarbital		
Clonazepam	Klonopin	Absence Atypical absence Myoclonic	1–12 mg/d (0.1–0.2 mg/kg) qd-tid	24–48 h	10–70 ng/mL	Ataxia Sedation Lethargy	Anorexia	Level decreased by enzyme-inducing drugs[a]
Felbamate	Felbatol	Focal-onset Lennox-Gastaut syndrome	2400–3600 mg/d, (45 mg/kg, child) tid-qid	16–22 h	Not established	Insomnia Dizziness Sedation Headache	Aplastic anemia Hepatic failure Weight loss Gastrointestinal irritation	Increases phenytoin, valproic acid, active carbamazepine metabolite
Levetiracetam	Keppra	Focal-onset	1000–3000 mg/d bid	6–8 h	Not established	Sedation Fatigue Incoordination Psychosis	Anemia Leukocytopenia	None known
Zonisamide	Zonegran	Focal-onset	200–800 mg/d	50–68 h	Not established	Sedation Dizziness Confusion Headache	Anorexia Renal stones	Level decreased by enzyme-inducing drugs[a]
Oxcarbazepine	Trileptal	Focal-onset	900–2400 mg/d bid	10–17 h (for active metabolite)	6–12 μg/mL	Fatigue Ataxia Dizziness Diplopia Vertigo Headache	See carbamazepine	Level decreased by enzyme-inducing drugs[a] May increase phenytoin

[a] Phenytoin, carbamazepine, phenobarbital

macokinetics and toxicity are the main determinants for use in a given patient. Phenytoin has a relatively long half-life and offers the advantage of once or twice daily dosing compared to two or three times daily dosing for carbamazepine (although a more expensive, extended-release form of carbamazepine is now available). An advantage of carbamazepine is that its metabolism follows first-order pharmacokinetics, and the relationship between drug dose, serum levels, and toxicity is linear. By contrast, phenytoin shows properties of saturation kinetics, such that small increases in phenytoin doses above a standard maintenance dose can precipitate marked side effects. This is one of the main causes of acute phenytoin toxicity. Long-term use of phenytoin is associated with untoward cosmetic effects (e.g., hirsutism, coarsening of facial features, and gingival hypertrophy), so it is often avoided in young patients who are likely to require the drug for many years. Carbamazepine can cause leukopenia, aplastic anemia, or hepatotoxicity and would therefore be contraindicated in patients with predispositions to these problems.

Valproic acid is an effective alternative for some patients with partial seizures, especially when the seizures secondarily generalize. Gastrointestinal side effects are fewer when using the valproate semisodium formulation (Depakote). Valproic acid also rarely causes reversible bone marrow suppression and hepatotoxicity, and laboratory testing is required to monitor toxicity. This drug should generally be avoided in patients with preexisting bone marrow or liver disease. Irreversible, fatal hepatic failure appearing as an idiosyncratic rather than dose-related side effect is a relatively rare complication; its risk is highest in children <2 years old, especially those taking other antiepileptic drugs or with inborn errors of metabolism. Valproic acid therapy should therefore only be used in infants and young children when the benefits clearly exceed this risk.

Lamotrigine, gabapentin, topiramate, tiagabine, and phenobarbital are additional drugs currently used for the treatment of partial seizures with or without secondary generalization. Lamotrigine appears to have an overall efficacy profile similar to the more standard drugs and is now being used as monotherapy. All patients, particularly children, need to be monitored closely for a lamotrigine-induced rash during the initiation of therapy. Also, lamotrigine must be started very slowly when used as add-on therapy with valproic acid, since valproic acid can inhibit its metabolism, thereby substantially prolonging its half-life. Gabapentin is unique in not having any significant drug interactions. This makes it potentially useful as add-on therapy, especially in patients who are particularly susceptible to side effects of other medications. Until recently, phenobarbital and other barbiturate compounds were commonly used as first-line therapy for many forms of epilepsy. However, the barbiturates frequently cause sedation in adults, hyperactivity in children, and other more subtle cognitive changes; thus, their use should be limited to situations in which no other suitable treatment alternatives exist.

Antiepileptic Drug Selection For Generalized Seizures Valproic acid is currently considered the best initial choice for the treatment of primarily generalized, tonic-clonic seizures and lamotrigine, followed by carbamazepine and phenytoin, are suitable alternatives. Valproic acid is also particularly effective in absence, myoclonic, and atonic seizures and is therefore the drug of choice in patients with generalized epilepsy syndromes having mixed seizure types. Ethosuximide remains the preferred drug for the treatment of uncomplicated absence seizures, but it is not effective against tonic-clonic or partial seizures. Ethosuximide rarely causes bone marrow suppression, so that periodic monitoring of blood cell counts is required. Although approved for use in partial seizure disorders, lamotrigine appears to be effective in epilepsy syndromes with mixed, generalized seizure types such as JME and Lennox-Gastaut syndrome.

Initiation and monitoring of therapy Because the response to any antiepileptic drug is unpredictable, patients should be carefully educated about the approach to therapy. Patients need to understand that the goal is to prevent seizures and minimize the side effects of therapy; determination of the optimal dose is often a matter of trial and error. This process may take months or longer if the baseline seizure frequency is low. Most anticonvulsant drugs need to be introduced relatively slowly to minimize side effects, and patients should expect that minor side effects such as mild sedation, slight changes in cognition, or imbalance will typically resolve within a few days. Starting doses are usually the lowest value listed under the dosage column in Table 360-9. Subsequent increases should be made only after achieving a steady state with the previous dose (i.e., after an interval of five or more half-lives).

Monitoring of serum antiepileptic drug levels can be very useful for establishing the initial dosing schedule. However, the published therapeutic ranges of serum drug concentrations are only an approximate guide for determining the proper dose for a given patient. The key determinants are the clinical measures of seizure frequency and presence of side effects, not the laboratory values. Conventional assays of serum drug levels measure the total drug (i.e., both free and protein-bound), yet it is the concentration of free drug that reflects extracellular levels in the brain and correlates best with efficacy. Thus, patients with decreased levels of serum proteins (e.g., decreased serum albumin due to impaired liver or renal function) may have an increased ratio of free to bound drug, yet the concentration of free drug may be adequate for seizure control. These patients may have a "subtherapeutic" drug level, but the dose should be changed only if seizures remain uncontrolled, not just to achieve a "therapeutic" level. It is also useful to monitor free drug levels in such patients. In practice, other than during the initiation or modification of therapy, monitoring of antiepileptic drug levels is most useful for documenting compliance.

If seizures continue despite gradual increases to the maximum tolerated dose and documented compliance, then it becomes necessary to switch to another antiepileptic drug. This is usually done by maintaining the patient on the first drug while a second drug is added. The dose of the second drug should be adjusted to decrease seizure frequency without causing toxicity. Once this is achieved, the first drug can be gradually withdrawn (usually over weeks unless there is significant toxicity). The dose of the second drug is then further optimized based on seizure response and side effects.

When to discontinue therapy Overall, about 70% of children and 60% of adults who have their seizures completely controlled with antiepileptic drugs can eventually discontinue therapy. Clinical studies suggest that the following patient profile yields the greatest chance of remaining seizure-free after drug withdrawal: (1) complete medical control of seizures for 1 to 5 years; (2) single seizure type, either partial or generalized; (3) normal neurologic examination, including intelligence; and (4) normal EEG. The appropriate seizure-free interval is unknown and undoubtedly varies for different forms of epilepsy. However, it seems reasonable to attempt withdrawal of therapy after 2 years in a patient who meets all of the above criteria, is motivated to discontinue the medication, and clearly understands the potential risks and benefits. In most cases it is preferable to reduce the dose of the drug gradually over 2 to 3 months. Most recurrences occur in the first 3 months after discontinuing therapy, and patients should be advised to avoid potentially dangerous situations such as driving or swimming during this period.

Treatment of refractory epilepsy Approximately one-third of patients with epilepsy do not respond to treatment with a single antiepileptic drug, and it becomes necessary to try a combination of drugs to control seizures. Patients who have focal epilepsy related to an underlying structural lesion or those with multiple seizure types and developmental delay are particularly likely to require multiple drugs. There are currently no clear guidelines for rational polypharmacy, but in most cases the initial combination therapy combines first-line drugs, i.e., carbamazepine, phenytoin, valproic acid, and lamotrigine. If these drugs are unsuccessful, then the addition of a newer drug such as topiramate or gabapentin is indicated. Patients with myoclonic seizures resistant to valproic acid may benefit from the addition of clonazepam, and those with absence seizures may respond to a combination of valproic acid and ethosuximide. The same principles concerning the monitoring of therapeutic response, toxicity, and serum levels for monotherapy apply to polypharmacy, and potential drug interactions need to be recognized. If there is no improvement, a third drug can be added while the first two are maintained. If there is a response, the least effective of the first two drugs should be gradually withdrawn.

Surgical Treatment of Refractory Epilepsy Approximately 20% of patients with epilepsy are resistant to medical therapy despite efforts to find an effective combination of antiepileptic drugs. For some, surgery can be extremely effective in substantially reducing seizure frequency and even providing complete seizure control. Understanding the potential value of surgery is especially important when, at the time of diagnosis, a patient has an epilepsy syndrome that is considered likely to be drug-resistant. Rather than submitting the patient to years of unsuccessful medical therapy and the associated psychosocial trauma of ongoing seizures, the patient should have an efficient but relatively brief attempt at medical therapy and then be referred for surgical evaluation.

The most common surgical procedure for patients with temporal lobe epilepsy involves resection of the anteromedial temporal lobe (temporal lobectomy) or a more limited removal of the underlying hippocampus and amygdala. Focal seizures arising from extratemporal regions may be suppressed by a focal neocortical resection or precise removal of an identified lesion (lesionectomy). When the cortical region cannot be removed, multiple subpial transection, which disrupts intracortical connections, is sometimes used to prevent seizure spread. Hemispherectomy or multilobar resection is useful for some patients with severe seizures due to hemispheric abnormalities such as hemimegaloencephaly or other dysplastic abnormalities, and corpus callosotomy has been shown to be effective for disabling tonic or atonic seizures, usually when they are part of a mixed-seizure syndrome (e.g., Lennox-Gastaut syndrome).

Presurgical evaluation is designed to identify the functional and structural basis of the patient's seizure disorder. Inpatient video-EEG monitoring is used to define the anatomic location of the seizure focus and to correlate the abnormal electrophysiologic activity with behavioral manifestations of the seizure. Routine scalp or scalp-sphenoidal recordings are usually sufficient for localization, and advances in neuroimaging have made the use of invasive electrophysiologic monitoring such as implanted depth electrodes or subdural electrodes much less common. A high-resolution MRI scan is routinely used to identify structural lesions. Functional imaging studies such as SPECT and PET are adjunctive tests that may help verify the localization of an apparent epileptogenic region with an anatomic abnormality. Once the presumed location of the seizure onset is identified, additional studies, including neuropsychological testing and the intracarotid amobarbital test (Wada test) may be used to assess language and memory localization and to determine the possible functional consequences of surgical removal of the epileptogenic region. In some cases, the exact extent of the resection to be undertaken is determined by performing cortical mapping at the time of the surgical procedure. This involves electrophysiologic recordings and cortical stimulation in the awake patient to identify the extent of epileptiform disturbances and the function of cortical regions in question.

Advances in presurgical evaluation and microsurgical techniques have led to a steady increase in the success of epilepsy surgery. Clinically significant complications of surgery are $<5\%$, and the use of functional mapping procedures has markedly reduced the neurologic sequelae due to removal or sectioning of brain tissue. For example, about 70% of patients treated with temporal lobectomy will become seizure-free, and another 15 to 25% will have at least a 90% reduction in seizure frequency. Marked improvement is also usually seen in patients treated with hemispherectomy for catastrophic seizure disorders due to large hemispheric abnormalities. Postoperatively, patients generally need to remain on antiepileptic drug therapy, but the marked reduction of seizures following surgery can have a very beneficial effect on their quality of life.

Vagus Nerve Stimulation (VNS) VNS is a new treatment option for patients with medically refractory epilepsy who are not candidates for resective brain surgery. The procedure involves placement of a bipolar electrode on the midcervical portion of the left vagus nerve. The electrode is connected to a small, subcutaneous generator located in the infraclavicular region, and the generator is programmed to deliver intermittent electrical pulses to the vagus nerve. The precise mechanism of action of VNS is unknown, although experimental studies have shown that stimulation of vagal nuclei leads to widespread

activation of cortical and subcortical pathways and an associated increased seizure threshold. In practice, the efficacy of VNS appears to be no greater than recently introduced anticonvulsant medications. Adverse effects of the surgery are rare, and stimulation-induced side effects, including transient hoarseness, cough, and dyspnea, are usually mild and well tolerated.

STATUS EPILEPTICUS Status epilepticus refers to continuous seizures or repetitive, discrete seizures with impaired consciousness in the interictal period. The duration of seizure activity sufficient to meet the definition of status epilepticus has traditionally been specified as 15 to 30 min. However, a more practical definition is to consider status epilepticus as a situation in which the duration of seizures prompts the acute use of anticonvulsant therapy, typically when seizures last beyond 5 min.

Status epilepticus is an emergency and must be treated immediately, since cardiorespiratory dysfunction, hyperthermia, and metabolic derangements can develop as a consequence of prolonged seizures, and these can lead to irreversible neuronal injury. Furthermore, CNS injury can occur even when the patient is paralyzed with neuromuscular blockade but continues to have electrographic seizures. The most common causes of status epilepticus are anticonvulsant withdrawal or noncompliance, metabolic disturbances, drug toxicity, CNS infection, CNS tumors, refractory epilepsy, and head trauma.

Generalized status epilepticus is obvious when the patient is having overt convulsions. However, after 30 to 45 min of uninterrupted seizures, the signs may become increasingly subtle. Patients may have mild clonic movements of only the fingers, or fine, rapid movements of the eyes. There may be paroxysmal episodes of tachycardia, hypertension, and pupillary dilation. In such cases, the EEG may be the only method of establishing the diagnosis. Thus, if the patient stops having overt seizures, yet remains comatose, an EEG should be performed to rule out ongoing status epilepticus.

The first step in the management of a patient in status epilepticus is to attend to any acute cardiorespiratory problems or hyperthermia, perform a brief medical and neurologic examination, establish venous access, and send samples for laboratory studies to identify metabolic abnormalities. Anticonvulsant therapy should then begin without delay; a treatment approach is shown in Fig. 360-3.

BEYOND SEIZURES: OTHER MANAGEMENT ISSUES

Interictal Behavior The adverse effects of epilepsy often go beyond the occurrence of clinical seizures, and the extent of these effects depends largely upon the etiology of the seizure disorder, the degree to which the seizures are controlled, and the presence of side effects from antiepileptic therapy. Many patients with epilepsy are completely normal between seizures and able to live highly successful and productive lives. In contrast, patients with seizures secondary to developmental abnormalities or acquired brain injury may have impaired cognitive function and other neurologic deficits. Frequent interictal EEG abnormalities have been shown to be associated with subtle dysfunction of memory and attention. Patients with many seizures, especially those emanating from the temporal lobe, often note an impairment of short-term memory that may progress over time.

Patients with epilepsy are at risk of developing a variety of psychiatric problems including depression, anxiety, and psychosis. This risk varies considerably depending on many factors, including the etiology, frequency, and severity of seizures and the patient's age and previous history. Depression occurs in approximately 20% of patients, and the incidence of suicide is higher in epileptic patients than in the general population. Depression should be treated through counseling or medication. The selective serotonin reuptake inhibitors typically

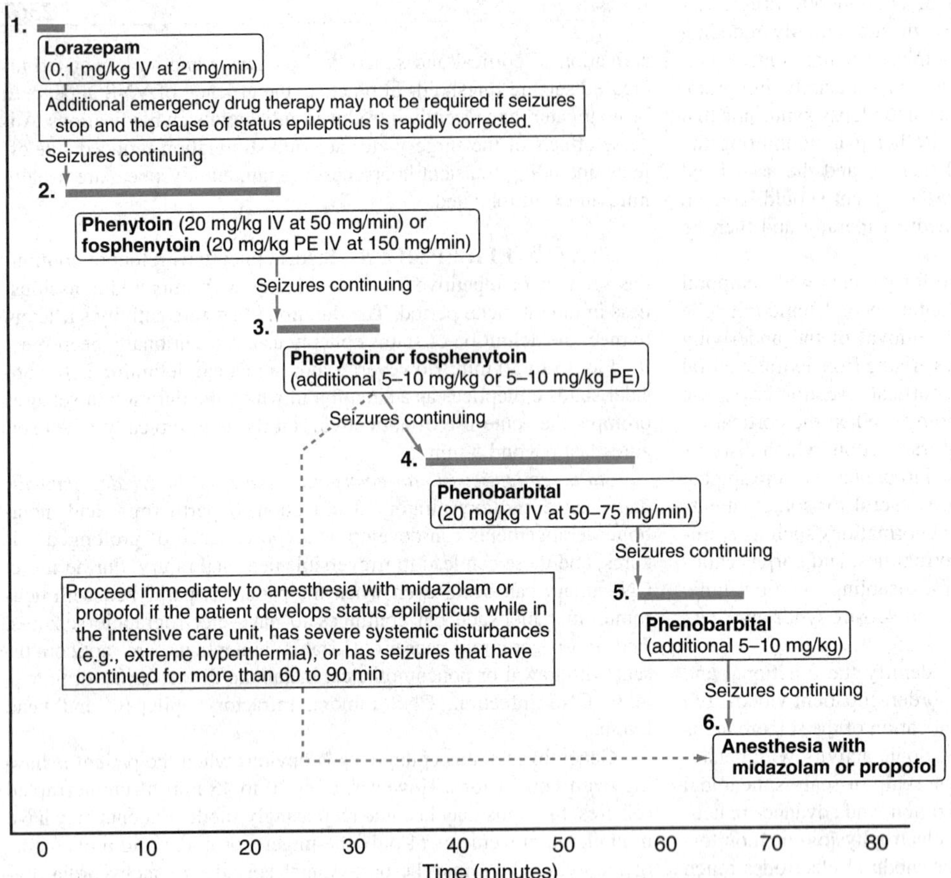
1.
Lorazepam
(0.1 mg/kg IV at 2 mg/min)
Additional emergency drug therapy may not be required if seizures stop and the cause of status epilepticus is rapidly corrected.
Seizures continuing
2.
Phenytoin (20 mg/kg IV at 50 mg/min) or
fosphenytoin (20 mg/kg PE IV at 150 mg/min)
Seizures continuing
3.
Phenytoin or fosphenytoin
(additional 5–10 mg/kg or 5–10 mg/kg PE)
Seizures continuing
4.
Phenobarbital
(20 mg/kg IV at 50–75 mg/min)
Seizures continuing
5.
Proceed immediately to anesthesia with midazolam or propofol if the patient develops status epilepticus while in the intensive care unit, has severe systemic disturbances (e.g., extreme hyperthermia), or has seizures that have continued for more than 60 to 90 min
Phenobarbital
(additional 5–10 mg/kg)
Seizures continuing
6.
Anesthesia with midazolam or propofol
0
10
20
30
40
50
60
70
80
Time (minutes)

FIGURE 360-3 Pharmacologic treatment of generalized tonic-clonic status epilepticus in adults. IV, intravenous; PE, phenytoin equivalents. The horizontal bars indicate the approximate duration of drug infusions.

have no effect on seizures, while the tricyclic antidepressants may lower the seizure threshold. Anxiety can appear as a manifestation of a seizure, and anxious or psychotic behavior can sometimes be observed as part of a postictal delirium. Interictal psychosis is a rare phenomenon that typically occurs after a period of increased seizure frequency. There is usually a brief lucid interval lasting up to a week, followed by days to weeks of agitated, psychotic behavior. The psychosis will usually resolve spontaneously but may require treatment with antipsychotic or anxiolytic medications.

There is ongoing controversy as to whether some patients with epilepsy (especially temporal lobe epilepsy) have a stereotypical "interictal personality." The predominant view is that the unusual or abnormal personality traits observed in such patients are, in most cases, not due to epilepsy but result from an underlying structural brain lesion, the effects of antiepileptic drugs, or psychosocial factors.

Mortality of Epilepsy Patients with epilepsy have an increased risk of death that is roughly two to three times greater than what would be expected in a matched population without epilepsy. Most of the increased mortality is due to the underlying etiology of epilepsy, i.e., more widespread neurologic or systemic diseases in children and tumors or strokes in older adults. However, a small number of patients die from a syndrome known as *sudden unexpected death in epileptic patients* (SUDEP), which usually affects young people with convulsive seizures and tends to occur at night. The cause(s) remain unknown, although the leading theories propose brainstem-mediated effects of seizures on cardiac rhythms or pulmonary function.

Psychosocial Issues There continues to be a cultural stigma about epilepsy, although it is slowly declining in societies with effective health education programs. Because of this stigma, many patients with epilepsy harbor fears, such as the fear of becoming mentally retarded or dying during a seizure. These issues need to be carefully addressed by educating the patient about epilepsy and by ensuring that family members, teachers, fellow employees, and other associates are equally well informed. The Epilepsy Foundation of America (1-800-EFA-1000) is a patient advocacy organization and a useful source of educational material.

Employment and Driving Many patients with epilepsy face difficulty in obtaining or maintaining employment, even when their seizures are well controlled. Federal and state legislation is designed to prevent employers from discriminating against patients with epilepsy, and patients should be encouraged to understand and claim their legal rights. Patients in these circumstances also benefit greatly from the assistance of health providers who act as strong patient advocates.

Loss of driving privileges is one of the most disruptive social consequences of epilepsy. Physicians should be very clear about local regulations concerning driving and epilepsy, since the laws vary considerably among states and countries. In all cases, it is the physician's responsibility to warn patients of the danger imposed on themselves and others while driving if their seizures are uncontrolled (unless the seizures are not associated with impairment of consciousness or motor control). In general, most states allow patients to drive after a seizure-free interval (on or off medications) between 3 months and 2 years.

SPECIAL ISSUES RELATED TO WOMEN AND EPILEPSY

Catamenial Epilepsy Some women experience a marked increase in seizure frequency around the time of menses. This is thought to reflect either the effects of estrogen and progesterone on neuronal excitability or changes in antiepileptic drug levels due to altered protein binding. Acetazolamide (250 to 500 mg/d) may be effective as adjunctive therapy in some cases when started 7 to 10 days prior to the onset of menses and continued until bleeding stops. Some patients may benefit from increases in antiepileptic drug dosages during this time or from control of the menstrual cycle through the use of oral contraceptives.

Pregnancy Most women with epilepsy who become pregnant will have an uncomplicated gestation and deliver a normal baby. However, epilepsy poses some important risks to a pregnancy. Seizure frequency during pregnancy will remain unchanged in approximately 50% of women, increase in 30%, and decrease in 20%. Changes in seizure frequency are attributed to endocrine effects on the CNS, variations in antiepileptic drug pharmacokinetics (such as acceleration of hepatic drug metabolism or effects on plasma protein binding), and changes in medication compliance. It is therefore useful to see patients at more frequent intervals during pregnancy and monitor serum antiepileptic drug levels. Measurement of the unbound drug concentrations may be useful if there is an increase in seizure frequency or worsening of side effects of antiepileptic drugs.

The overall incidence of fetal abnormalities in children born to mothers with epilepsy is 5 to 6%, compared to 2 to 3% in healthy women. Part of the higher incidence is due to teratogenic effects of antiepileptic drugs, and the risk increases with the number of medications used (e.g., 10% risk of malformations with three drugs). A syndrome comprising facial dysmorphism, cleft lip, cleft palate, cardiac defects, digital hypoplasia, and nail dysplasia was originally ascribed to phenytoin therapy, but it is now known to occur with other first-line antiepileptic drugs (i.e., valproic acid and carbamazepine) as well. Also, valproic acid and carbamazepine are associated with a 1 to 2% incidence of neural tube defects compared with a baseline of 0.5 to 1%. Little is currently known about the safety of newer drugs.

Since the potential harm of uncontrolled seizures on the mother and fetus is considered greater than the teratogenic effects of antiepileptic drugs, it is currently recommended that pregnant women be maintained on effective drug therapy. When possible, it seems prudent to have the patient on monotherapy at the lowest effective dose, especially during the first trimester. Patients should also take folate (1 to 4 mg/d), since the antifolate effects of anticonvulsants are thought to play a role in the development of neural tube defects, although the benefits of this treatment remain unproved in this setting.

Enzyme-inducing drugs such as phenytoin, phenobarbital, and primidone cause a transient and reversible deficiency of vitamin K–dependent clotting factors in approximately 50% of newborn infants. Although neonatal hemorrhage is uncommon, the mother should be treated with oral vitamin K (20 mg daily) in the last 2 weeks of pregnancy, and the infant should receive an intramuscular injection of vitamin K (1 mg) at birth.

Contraception Special care should be taken when prescribing antiepileptic medications for women who are taking oral contraceptive agents. Drugs such as carbamazepine, phenytoin, phenobarbital, and topiramate can significantly antagonize the effects of oral contraceptives via enzyme induction and other mechanisms. Patients should be advised to consider alternative forms of contraception, or their contraceptive medications should be modified to offset the effects of the antiepileptic medications.

Breast Feeding Antiepileptic medications are excreted into breast milk to a variable degree. The ratio of drug concentration in breast milk relative to serum is approximately 80% for ethosuximide, 40 to 60% for phenobarbital, 40% for carbamazepine, 15% for phenytoin, and 5% for valproic acid. Given the overall benefits of breast feeding and the lack of evidence for long-term harm to the infant by being exposed to antiepileptic drugs, mothers with epilepsy should be encouraged to breast feed. This should be reconsidered, however, if there is any evidence of drug effects on the infant, such as lethargy or poor feeding.

BIBLIOGRAPHY

BATE L, GARDINER M: Genetics of inherited epilepsies. Epileptic Disorders 1:7, 1999

BRODIE MJ, DICHTER MA: Antiepileptic drugs. N Engl J Med 334:168, 1996

CHADWICK D: Seizures and epilepsy after traumatic brain injury. Lancet 355:334, 2000

DEVINSKY O: Patients with refractory seizures. N Engl J Med 340:1565, 1999

ENGEL J JR: Surgery for seizures. N Engl J Med 334:647, 1996

KOTAGAL P, LUDERS HO (eds): *The Epilepsies: Etiologies and Prevention*. San Diego, Academic Press, 1999

LOWENSTEIN DH, ALLDREDGE BK: Status epilepticus. N Engl J Med 338:970, 1998

MCNAMARA JO: Emerging insights into the genesis of epilepsy. Nature 339(6738 Suppl): A15, 1999

SACKELLARES JC, BERENT S (eds): *Psychological Disturbances in Epilepsy*. Boston, Butterworth-Heinemann, 1997

SCHILLER Y et al: Discontinuation of antiepileptic drugs after successful epilepsy surgery. Neurology 54:346, 2000

WYLLIE E (ed): *The Treatment of Epilepsy: Principles and Practice*, 2d ed. Baltimore, Williams & Wilkins, 1997

361

Wade S. Smith, Stephen L. Hauser, J. Donald Easton

CEREBROVASCULAR DISEASES

Cerebrovascular diseases occur predominately in the middle and late years of life. They cause approximately 200,000 deaths in the United States each year, as well as considerable neurologic disability. The incidence of stroke increases with age; thus the disability affects many people in their "golden years," a segment of the population that is growing rapidly in Western countries. Categories of cerebrovascular diseases include ischemia-infarction and intracranial hemorrhage (Table 361-1). Many of the arterial and cardiac disorders underlying these diseases are preventable; the morbidity and mortality from cerebrovascular diseases has been diminishing in recent years, apparently because of better recognition and treatment of hypertension.

Most cerebrovascular diseases are manifest by the abrupt onset of a focal neurologic deficit. The deficit may remain fixed or may rapidly improve or progressively worsen. It is this abrupt onset of a nonconvulsive and focal neurologic deficit that defines a *stroke*, or cerebrovascular accident (CVA).

Cerebral ischemia is caused by a reduction in blood flow that lasts for several seconds to a few minutes. Neurologic symptoms are manifest within 10 s because neurons lack glycogen and suffer rapid energy failure. When blood flow is rapidly restored brain tissue can recover fully, and the patient's symptoms are only transient: a transient ischemic attack (TIA) is said to have occurred. Typically the neurologic signs and symptoms of TIA last for 5 to 15 min but, by definition, must last <24 h. If the cessation of flow lasts for more than a few minutes, *infarction* or death of brain tissue results. Stroke has occurred if the neurologic signs and symptoms last for >24 h. A *generalized* reduction in cerebral blood flow due to systemic hypotension (e.g., cardiac arrhythmia, myocardial infarction, or hemorrhagic shock) usually produces syncope (Chap. 21). If low cerebral blood flow is maintained for a longer duration, then infarction in the border zones between the major cerebral artery distributions or widespread brain necrosis develops. This process is termed *global hypoxia-ischemia* and a patient with cognitive sequelae is said to have *hypoxic-ischemic encephalopathy* (Chap. 376). *Focal* ischemia or infarction, on the other hand, is usually caused by thrombosis of the cerebral vessels themselves or by emboli from a proximal arterial source or the heart. A comprehensive list of causes of ischemia-infarction is shown in Table 361-2.

Cerebral hemorrhage produces neurologic symptoms by producing a mass effect on neural structures or from the toxic effects of blood itself; debate exists as to how much injury occurs from tamponade of surrounding blood vessels. As with ischemia-infarction, the causes are numerous (Tables 361-1 and 361-7).

When faced with an acute stroke, the clinician must rapidly differentiate between ischemia-infarction and hemorrhage, because the method of emergency treatment depends on cause. The clinician should focus on two goals: (1) to prevent or reverse acute brain injury, and (2) to prevent future neurologic injury. The first goal involves identifying those patients who may benefit from thrombolysis and attending to acute medical issues of airway, blood pressure, and concomitant organ failure; the second goal is achieved once the mechanism of stroke is elucidated and the proper secondary prevention strategy prescribed.

ISCHEMIC STROKE

MECHANISMS AND DEFINITIONS Several pathophysiologic processes may produce cerebral ischemia and infarction. A common form is atherosclerotic damage to the aortic arch, carotid bifurcation, or intracranial vessels that produces local thrombosis and distal

Table 361-1 Pathophysiologic Classification of Cerebrovascular Diseases

Stroke Subtype	Frequency, %	CT Findings	Causes
Ischemic	85		
Thrombotic	25		
Lacunar stroke	20–25	Hypodensity usually <1 cm^3	Lipohyalinosis of small vessels
Large vessel	1–5	Varies	Atherosclerosis of intracranial arteries
Embolic	75		
Cardioembolic	20	Wedge-shaped cortical/subcortical hypodensity	See Table 361-2
Artery-artery	15	Wedge-shaped cortical/subcortical hypodensity	Aortic, carotid or intracranial atherosclerosis
Cryptogenic	30	Wedge-shaped cortical/subcortical hypodensity	Extensive workup reveals no cause
Other	10	Varies	
Hemorrhagic	15		
Intraparenchymal	10	Hyperdensity within brain substance	Hypertension, AVM, amyloid angiopathy
Subdural	<1	Hyperdensity within subdural space	Trauma
Epidural	<1	Hyperdensity within epidural space	Trauma
Subarachnoid	1–2	Hyperdensity within subarachnoid space	Ruptured aneurysm, trauma

NOTE: AVM, arteriovenous malformation; CT, computed tomography.

embolism of the clot. The released clot travels until it occludes a distal vessel and prevents distal cerebral blood flow. Such strokes are called *atherothromboembloic strokes*, or simply *embolic strokes*, and are a subset of *artery-artery embolic strokes*. Stroke produced by thrombosis of large (~0.5 to 3 mm) intracranial vessels in situ from atherosclerosis is termed *atherothrombotic stroke*. Unlike coronary arteries in which vascular occlusion may be sudden and complete, sudden thrombosis of intracranial vessels occurs less frequently. It may be more likely that atherosclerosis of an intracranial vessel will produce stroke by distal embolism rather than by occlusion. Stenosis of an extra- or intracranial vessel may produce a *low-flow stroke* or TIA if cardiac output or systemic blood pressure is reduced below some threshold. This mechanism was thought to be the cause of stroke from carotid atherosclerosis, but it is now clear that carotid disease produces stroke primarily by an embolic mechanism. True flow-related TIAs and stroke are rare, but it is important to identify them since they will respond to revascularization procedures rather than standard antithrombotic treatment. Thrombotic occlusion of smaller intracranial vessels (~30 to 100 μm), in contrast to larger vessel thrombosis, is a frequent cause of stroke. These end-arteries typically supply a small volume of brain tissue, and their occlusion may result in a *lacunar syndrome*, of which there are >30 types. A patient who has a stroke from this event is said to have *lacunar stroke*. The underlying pathology of this form of stroke is usually lipohyalinosis or microatheromata with thrombosis of the vascular lumen.

Clinically, thrombotic strokes are more gradual in onset or may stutter. It is common for a person to experience several TIAs of the lacunar type prior to eventual stroke. *Crescendo TIAs*—the occurrence of increasing number and frequency of TIAs—have a particularly high likelihood of evolving to stroke. *Stroke in progression* is said to be present if a patient suffers progressive neurologic deficits over a few hours or days that are not accounted for by cerebral edema. This may happen as a small vessel slowly thromboses or, more ominously, as a larger intracranial vessel such as the basilar artery progressively thromboses, producing an ever enlarging region of cerebral ischemia. Heparin and thrombolytic treatment may arrest progression, but it has been difficult to demonstrate in clinical trials whether or not such treatments improve outcome.

Embolism from a cardiac source is most commonly from red atrial thrombi but can arise from numerous sources. In most cases the clinician does not observe clot within the heart and makes the diagnosis by associating a known cardiac cause (e.g., atrial fibrillation, recent myocardial infarction) with a sudden large-vessel occlusion in the brain. Such strokes are called *cardioembolic strokes*. Some patients, however, may develop sudden occlusion of a large intracranial vessel, and despite extensive evaluation, no cause is apparent. These strokes are called *cryptogenic strokes*.

Clinically, embolic events usually produce a sudden onset of neurologic dysfunction that is maximum at onset. The extent of neuronal ischemia is determined by the location of the occlusion and the degree to which collateral flow is offered to the ischemic tissue bed, the blood pressure and body temperature, and other factors. Embolic strokes have a higher risk of transforming into hemorrhagic stroke in which petechial bleeding or frank hemorrhage occurs into the infarcted tissue hours or days following the initial embolic occlusion. This natural history risk of spontaneous hemorrhage must be taken into account in acute stroke trials testing the safety of thrombolytic treatment.

RISK FACTORS FOR ISCHEMIC STROKE Older age, family history of thrombotic stroke, diabetes mellitus, hypertension, tobacco smoking, elevated blood cholesterol levels, and other factors are risk factors for atherosclerosis and

Table 361-2 Causes of Stroke

Common Causes	Uncommon Causes
Thrombosis	Hypercoagulable disorders
Lacunar stroke (small vessel)	Protein C deficiency
Large vessel thrombosis	Protein S deficiency
Dehydration	Antithrombin III deficiency
Embolic occlusion	Antiphospholipid syndrome
Artery-to-artery	Factor V Leiden mutation[a]
Carotid bifurcation	Prothrombin G20210 mutation[a]
Aortic arch	Systemic malignancy
Arterial dissection	Sickle cell anemia
Cardioembolic	β-Thalassemia
Atrial fibrillation	Polycythemia vera
Mural thrombus	Systemic lupus erythematosus
Myocardial infarction	Homocysteinemia
Dilated cardiomyopathy	Thrombotic thrombocytopenic purpura
Valvular lesions	Disseminated intravascular coagulation
Mitral stenosis	Dysproteinemias
Mechanical valve	Nephrotic syndrome
Bacterial endocarditis	Inflammatory bowel disease
Paradoxical embolus	Oral contraceptives
Atrial septal defect	Venous sinous thrombosis[b]
Patent foramen ovale	Fibromuscular dysplasia
Atrial septal aneurysm	Vasculitis
Spontaneous echo contrast	Systemic vasculitis (PAN, Wegner's, Takayasu's, giant cell arteritis)
	Primary CNS vasculitis
	Meningitis (syphilis, tuberculosis, fungal, bacterial, zoster)
	Cardiogenic
	Mitral valve calcification
	Atrial myxoma
	Intracardiac tumor
	Marantic endocarditis
	Libman-Sacks endocarditis
	Subarachnoid hemorrhage vasospasm
	Drugs: cocaine, amphetamine
	Moyamoya disease
	Eclampsia

[a] Chiefly cause venous sinus thrombosis.
[b] May be associated with any hypercoagulable disorder.
NOTE: CNS, central nervous system; PAN, polyarteritis nodosa.

hence either proven or probable risk factors for ischemic stroke. Risk of second stroke is strongly influenced by prior stroke or TIA (Table 361-3). Many cardiac conditions predispose to stroke, including atrial fibrillation and recent myocardial infarction. Oral contraceptives may increase stroke risk slightly, and certain inherited and acquired hypercoagulable states predispose to stroke. Identification of modifiable risk factors and prophylactic interventions to lower risk is probably the best treatment for stroke overall, as the total number of strokes could be reduced substantially by these means. (See below for recommendations for risk factor modification.)

ACUTE STROKE **Clinical Encounter** Patients with acute stroke often do not seek medical assistance on their own, perhaps because it is rarely painful but also because they may lose the appreciation that something is wrong with them (*anosognosia*). It is often a family member or a bystander who calls for help, and many gain entry into the medical system through emergency medical services, such as the 911 system in the United States. Use of such a system allows rapid evaluation of patients for consideration for time-sensitive treatments such as thrombolysis. Patients at risk for stroke should be counseled to call emergency medical services if they experience the sudden onset of any of the following: loss of sensory and/or motor function on one half of the body; change in vision, gait, or ability to speak or understand; or a sudden, severe headache.

The differential diagnosis of neurologic symptoms of sudden onset includes stroke (ischemic or hemorrhagic), TIA, seizure with postictal Todd's paralysis, intracranial tumor, migraine, and metabolic encephalopathy (Table 361-4). An adequate history from an observer that no convulsive activity occurred at the onset reasonably excludes seizure. Tumors may present with acute neurologic symptoms due to hemorrhage, seizure, or hydrocephalus. Surprisingly, migraine can mimic cerebral ischemia, even in patients without a significant migraine history. When it develops without head pain (*acephalgic migraine*), the diagnosis may remain elusive. Elderly patients without any prior history of complicated migraine may develop acephalgic migraine after age 65. The sensory disturbance is often prominent, and the sensory deficit, as well as any motor deficits, tends to migrate slowly across a limb over minutes. The diagnosis of migraine becomes more likely as the cortical disturbance begins to cross vascular boundaries. At times it may be difficult to make the diagnosis until multiple episodes have occurred leaving behind no residual stroke or brain imaging abnormality. Classically, metabolic encephalopathies produce a fluctuating mental status without focal neurologic findings. However, in the setting of prior stroke or brain injury, a patient with fever or sepsis will manifest hemiparesis, which clears rapidly when the infection is remedied. The metabolic process serves to "unmask" a prior deficit.

STROKE SYNDROMES A careful history and neurologic examination can often localize the region of brain dysfunction; if this region corresponds to a particular arterial distribution, the possible causes responsible for the syndrome can be narrowed. This is of particular importance when the patient presents with a TIA and a normal examination. For example, if a patient develops language loss and a right homonymous hemianopia, a search for causes of left middle cerebral emboli should be performed. A finding of an isolated stenosis of the right internal carotid artery in that patient suggests an asymptomatic carotid stenosis, which carries a significantly lower risk than symptomatic stenosis (i.e., stenosis of the left internal carotid artery). The following sections describe the clinical findings of arterial ischemia associated with cerebral vascular territories depicted in Figs. 361-1 through 361-9. Stroke syndromes are divided into: (1) large vessel stroke within the anterior circulation, (2) large vessel stroke within the posterior circulation, and (3) small vessel disease of either vascular bed.

Table 361-3 Annual Vascular Event Rates for Patients with Atherosclerotic Cerebral Vascular Disease

	Annual Probability, %, of		
Cerebrovascular Features	**Stroke**	**Vascular Death**	**All Death**
General elderly male population	0.6		
Asymptomatic carotid disease	1.3	3.4	6.0
Transient monocular blindness	2.2	3.5	4.3
Transient ischemic attack	3.7	2.3	4.0
Minor stroke	6.1	3.2	4.9
Major stroke	9.0	3.5	7.6
Symptomatic carotid stenosis, >70%	15.0	2.0	

SOURCE: Modified with permission from JL Wilterdink, JD Easton: Outcome rates for vascular events in patients with atherosclerotic cerebral vascular disease. Arch Neurol 49: 857, 1992.

Table 361-4 Clinical Management of Acute Stroke

New onset of neurologic deficit: Stroke or TIA?	Differential diagnosis of new focal deficit Stroke or TIA Seizure with postictal Todd's paresis Tumor Migraine Metabolic encephalopathy Fever/infection and old stroke Hyperglycemia Hypercalcemia Hepatic encephalopathy
Initial assessment and management	ABCs, serum glucose Noncontrast head CT Hemorrhage Medical and surgical management Tumor or other CNS process Treat accordingly Normal or hypodense area consistent with acute ischemic stroke Consider thrombolysis, heparin, aspirin Maintain blood pressure and hydrate Admit patient to appropriate level of care depending on concomitant medical problems and airway
Subsequent hospital management	Establish cause of stroke and risk factors Plan for secondary prophylaxis (drugs, risk factor modifications) Obtain physical, occupational, and speech therapy consultation and social work as appropriate Establish nutrition Discharge planning should include prescriptions for risk factor reduction, including when to institute antihypertensive treatment, and antithrombotic medication prophylaxis

NOTE: ABCs, airway management, breathing, cardiac status; CNS, central nervous system; CT, computed tomography; TIA, transient ischemic attack.

Large Vessel Stroke within the Anterior Circulation • ***Pathophysiology*** The internal carotid artery and its branches comprise the anterior circulation of the brain. These vessels can be occluded by intrinsic disease of the vessel (e.g., atherosclerosis or dissection) or by embolic occlusion from a proximal source. The causes of occlusion are enumerated here, and the clinical manifestations are listed in the next section.

EXTRACRANIAL INTERNAL CAROTID ARTERY The origin of the internal carotid artery is probably the most common site of atherosclerosis that leads to TIA or stroke. Atherosclerosis is usually most severe in the first 2 cm and arises from the posterior wall, often extending downward into the common carotid artery. Atherosclerosis at this site is often manifested by a TIA or minor stroke, presumably caused by embolism or, less frequently, low flow.

Dissection of the carotid artery produces cerebral ischemia by distal embolization and/or low flow to the anterior circulation. When low flow is the mechanism, there is presumably inadequate collateral flow through the circle of Willis. Fibromuscular dysplasia of the carotids may produce distal emboli or dissection.

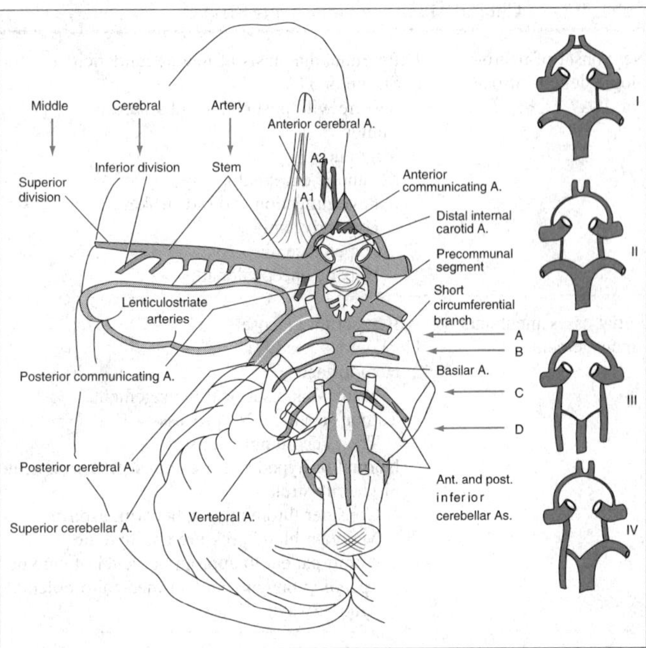

FIGURE 361-1 Diagram of the brainstem, cerebellum, inferior right frontal lobe, and transected temporal lobe. Principal branches of the vertebral basilar arterial system are pictured. The stem of the middle cerebral artery with its small, deep penetrating lenticulostriate arteries and the circle of Willis with its small, deep penetrating branches are shown. Roman numerals I, II, III, and IV represent some of the possible variations of the circle of Willis due to atresia of one or more of its arterial components. *A, B, C,* and *D* arrows indicate the four levels of the brainstem diagrammed below (*D*, Fig. 361-6; *A*, Fig. 361-7; *B*, Fig. 361-8; *C*, Fig. 361-9). Although typical vascular syndromes of the pons and medulla have been designated by the shaded areas in Figs. 361-6 to 361-9, the shading is approximate only. Great variability in infarct size and location occurs when the basilar or vertebral arteries or one of their penetrating branches becomes occluded. This variability is because of variation in arterial anatomic location and available collateral circulation. Thus the stroke syndromes produced are often atypical, incomplete, or merge with one another. *(Courtesy of CM Fisher, MD.)*

Rarely a large embolus will lodge in the common or internal carotid artery. Emboli of a size sufficient to block the internal carotid most often originate from pulmonary veins or extensive atrial or myocardial thrombi. *Takayasu's arteritis* (Chap. 317) is the most common form of vasculitis that affects the carotid artery.

INTRACRANIAL INTERNAL CAROTID ARTERY Atheromatous disease at the petrous inlet, the siphon (S-shaped portion of the internal carotid artery in the cavernous sinus), or the proximal segment of the middle or anterior cerebral arteries may produce distal embolization. These intracranial sites predominate in African Americans, Hispanics, and Asians. *Moyamoya syndrome* results from progressive stenosis and occlusion of the distal internal carotid artery and/or proximal middle and anterior cerebral arteries. It is idiopathic in children and acquired secondary to atherosclerosis in adults. Ischemia is produced by breakdown in lenticulostriate collaterals that form to reconstitute flow in the middle cerebral artery (MCA) or by progressive sclerosis of cortical vessels. Capsular hemorrhage may occur from rupture of the enlarged lenticulostriate vessels.

MIDDLE CEREBRAL ARTERY In contrast to the internal carotid artery, occlusion of the proximal MCA or one of its major branches is most often due to an embolus (artery-to-artery, cardiac, or of unknown source) rather than intracranial atherothrombosis. Atherosclerosis of the proximal MCA may cause distal emboli to the middle cerebral territory or, less commonly, may produce low-flow TIAs. Collateral formation via leptomeningeal vessels often prevents MCA stenosis from becoming symptomatic.

ANTERIOR CEREBRAL ARTERY Atheromatous deposits in the proximal segment of the anterior cerebral artery rarely cause symptoms because the effects of occlusion are usually circumvented by collateral circulation through the anterior communicating artery. If the anterior communicating artery is congenitally atretic or the atheromatous lesion occurs distally in the anterior cerebral artery, TIAs and stroke may occur. The anterior cerebral artery is rarely the recipient of emboli.

Clinical manifestations • *MIDDLE CEREBRAL ARTERY* The cortical branches of the MCA supply the lateral surface of the hemisphere except for (1) the frontal pole and a strip along the superomedial border of the frontal and parietal lobes supplied by the anterior cerebral artery and (2) the lower temporal and occipital pole convolutions supplied by the posterior cerebral artery (Figs. 361-2, 361-4, and 361-5).

The proximal MCA (M1 segment) gives rise to penetrating branches (termed *lenticulostriate arteries*) that supply the putamen, outer globus pallidus, posterior limb of the internal capsule above the plane of the upper border of the globus pallidus, the adjacent corona radiata, and the body and upper and lateral head of the caudate nucleus. In the sylvian fissure, the middle cerebral artery in most patients divides into *superior* and *inferior* divisions (M2 branches). Branches of the inferior division supply the inferior parietal and temporal cortex, and those from the superior division supply the frontal and superior parietal cortex (Fig. 361-3). There is considerable variability in the parietal lobe supply between the two divisions, with about two-thirds of individuals having an inferior division that supplies regions above the angular gyrus.

If the entire MCA is occluded at its origin (blocking both its penetrating and cortical branches) and the distal collaterals are limited, the clinical findings are contralateral hemiplegia, hemianesthesia, homonymous hemianopia, and a day or two of gaze preference to the ipsilateral side. When the dominant hemisphere is involved, global aphasia is present also, and when the nondominant hemisphere is affected, anosognosia, constructional apraxia, and neglect are found (Fig. 361-3). Dysarthria may also occur.

Complete MCA syndromes occur most often when an embolus occludes the stem of the artery. Cortical collateral blood flow and differing arterial configurations are probably responsible for the development of many partial syndromes. Partial syndromes also may be due to emboli that enter the proximal MCA without complete occlusion, occlude distal MCA branches, or fragment and move distally.

Partial syndromes due to embolic occlusion of a single branch include hand, or arm and hand, weakness alone (brachial syndrome) or facial weakness with nonfluent (expressive, Broca) aphasia (Chap 25), with or without arm weakness (frontal opercular syndrome). A

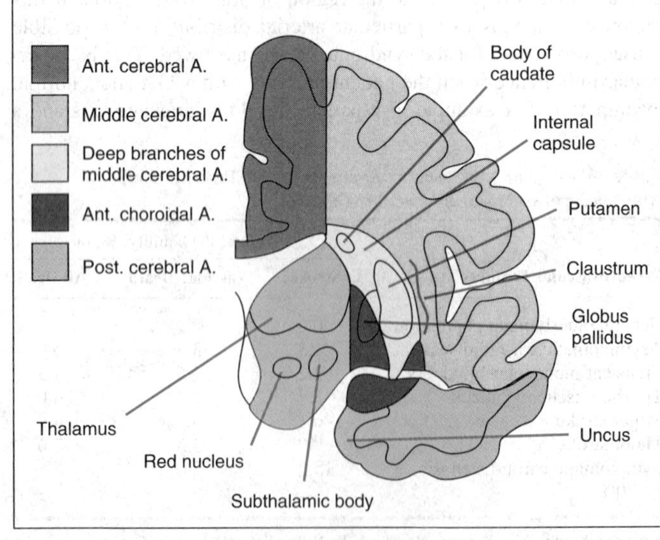

FIGURE 361-2 Diagram of a cerebral hemisphere in coronal section showing the territories of the major cerebral vessels. *(Courtesy of C M Fisher, MD.)*

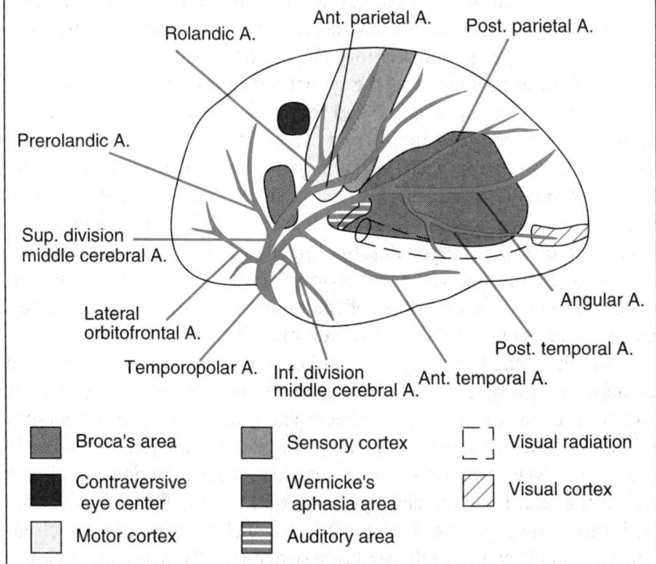

FIGURE 361-3 Diagram of a cerebral hemisphere, lateral aspect, showing the branches and distribution of the middle cerebral artery and the principal regions of cerebral localization. Note the bifurcation of the middle cerebral artery into a superior and inferior division. *(Courtesy of CM Fisher, MD.)*

Signs and symptoms: *Structures involved*

Paralysis of the contralateral face, arm, and leg; sensory impairment over the same area (pinprick, cotton touch, vibration, position, two-point discrimination, stereognosis, tactile localization, barognosis, cutaneographia): *Somatic motor area for face and arm and the fibers descending from the leg area to enter the corona radiata and corresponding somatic sensory system*

Motor aphasia: *Motor speech area of the dominant hemisphere*

Central aphasia, word deafness, anomia, jargon speech, sensory agraphia, acalculia, alexia, finger agnosia, right-left confusion (the last four comprise the Gerstmann syndrome): *Central, suprasylvian speech area and parietooccipital cortex of the dominant hemisphere*

Conduction aphasia: *Central speech area (parietal operculum)*

Apractognosia of the minor hemisphere (amorphosynthesis), anosognosia, hemiasomatognosia, unilateral neglect, agnosia for the left half of external space, dressing "apraxia," constructional "apraxia," distortion of visual coordinates, inaccurate localization in the half field, impaired ability to judge distance, upside-down reading, visual illusions (e.g., it may appear that another person walks through a table): *Nondominant parietal lobe (area corresponding to speech area in dominant hemisphere); loss of topographic memory is usually due to a nondominant lesion, occasionally to a dominant one*

Homonymous hemianopia (often homonymous inferior quadrantanopia): *Optic radiation deep to second temporal convolution*

Paralysis of conjugate gaze to the opposite side: *Frontal contraversive field or projecting fibers*

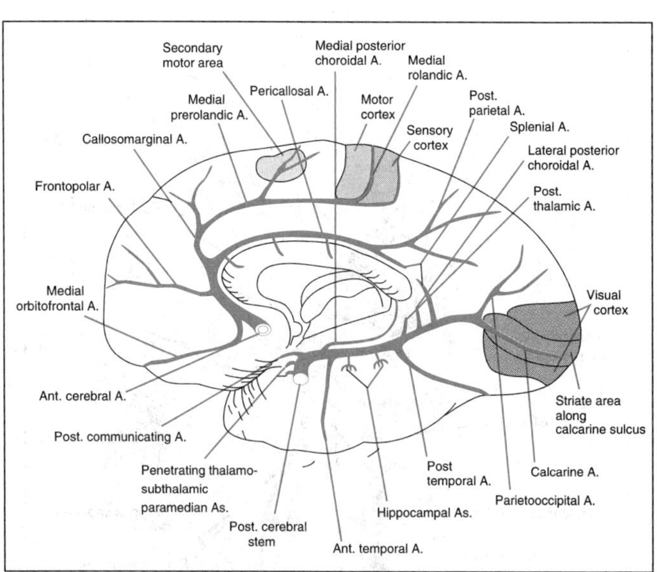

FIGURE 361-4 Diagram of a cerebral hemisphere, medial aspect, showing the branches and distribution of the anterior cerebral artery and the principal regions of cerebral localization. *(Courtesy of CM Fisher, MD.)*

Signs and symptoms: *Structures involved*

Paralysis of opposite foot and leg: *Motor leg area*

A lesser degree of paresis of opposite arm: *Arm area of cortex or fibers descending to corona radiata*

Cortical sensory loss over toes, foot, and leg: *Sensory area for foot and leg*

Urinary incontinence: *Sensorimotor area in paracentral lobule*

Contralateral grasp reflex, sucking reflex, gegenhalten (paratonic rigidity): *Medial surface of the posterior frontal lobe (?) supplemental motor area*

Abulia (akinetic mutism), slowness, delay, intermittent interruption, lack of spontaneity, whispering, reflex distraction to sights and sounds: *Uncertain localization—probably cingulate gyrus and medial inferior portion of frontal, parietal, and temporal lobes*

Impairment of gait and stance (gait apraxia): *Frontal cortex near leg motor area*

Dyspraxia of left limbs, tactile aphasia in left limbs: *Corpus callosum*

combination of sensory disturbance, motor weakness, and nonfluent aphasia suggests that an embolus has occluded the proximal superior division and infarcted large portions of the frontal and parietal cortices (Fig. 361-3). If a fluent (Wernicke's) aphasia occurs without weakness, the inferior division of the MCA supplying the posterior part (temporal cortex) of the dominant hemisphere is probably involved (Fig. 361-3). Jargon speech and an inability to comprehend written and spoken language are prominent features, often accompanied by a contralateral, homonymous superior quadrantanopia. Hemineglect or spatial agnosia without weakness indicates that the inferior division of the MCA in the nondominant hemisphere is involved.

ANTERIOR CEREBRAL ARTERY The anterior cerebral artery is divided into two segments: the precommunal (A1) circle of Willis, or stem, which connects the internal carotid artery to the anterior communicating artery, and the postcommunal (A2) segment distal to the anterior communicating artery (Figs. 361-1 and 361-4). The A1 segment gives rise to several deep penetrating branches that supply the anterior limb of the internal capsule, the anterior perforate substance, amygdala, anterior hypothalamus, and the inferior part of the head of the caudate nucleus (Fig. 361-2).

Occlusion of the proximal anterior cerebral artery is usually well tolerated because of collateral flow. Occlusion of a single A2 segment results in the contralateral symptoms noted in the legend of Fig. 361-4. If both A2 segments arise from a single anterior cerebral stem (contralateral A1 segment atresia), the occlusion affects both hemispheres. Profound abulia (a delay in verbal and motor response) and bilateral pyramidal signs with paraparesis and urinary incontinence result.

ANTERIOR CHOROIDAL ARTERY This artery arises from the internal carotid artery and supplies the posterior limb of the internal capsule and the white matter posterolateral to it, through which pass some of the geniculocalcarine fibers (Figs. 361-2 and 361-5). The complete syndrome of anterior choroidal artery occlusion consists of contralateral hemiplegia, hemianesthesia (hypesthesia), and homonymous hemianopia. However, because this territory is also supplied by penetrating vessels of the proximal MCA and the posterior communicating and posterior choroidal arteries, minimal deficits may occur, and patients frequently recover substantially.

INTERNAL CAROTID ARTERY The clinical picture of internal carotid occlusion varies depending on whether the cause of ischemia is propagated thrombus, embolism, or low flow. The cortex supplied by the middle cerebral territory is affected most often. With a competent circle of Willis, occlusion may go unnoticed. If the thrombus propagates up the internal carotid artery into the MCA, or embolizes it, symptoms are identical to proximal MCA occlusion (see above).

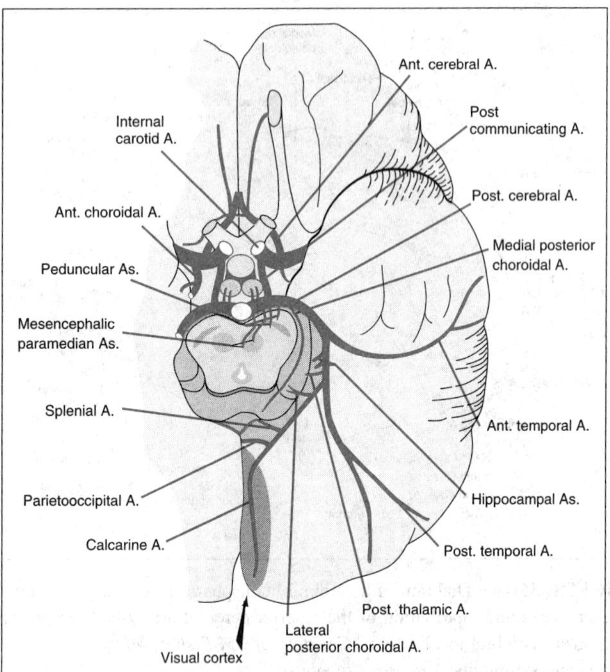

FIGURE 361-5 Inferior aspect of the brain with the branches and distribution of the posterior cerebral artery and the principal anatomic structures shown. *(Courtesy of CM Fisher, MD.)*

Signs and Symptoms: *Structures involved*

1. Peripheral territory (see also Fig. 361-4). Homonymous hemianopia (often upper quadrantic): *Calcarine cortex or optic radiation nearby.* Bilateral homonymous hemianopia, cortical blindness, awareness or denial of blindness; tactile naming, achromatopia (color blindness), failure to see to-and-fro movements, inability to perceive objects not centrally located, apraxia of ocular movements, inability to count or enumerate objects, tendency to run into things that the patient sees and tries to avoid: *Bilateral occipital lobe with possibly the parietal lobe involved.* Verbal dyslexia without agraphia, color anomia: *Dominant calcarine lesion and posterior part of corpus callosum.* Memory defect: *Hippocampal lesion bilaterally or on the dominant side only.* Topographic disorientation and prosopagnosia: *Usually with lesions of nondominant, calcarine, and lingual gyrus.* Simultagnosia, hemivisual neglect: *Dominant visual cortex, contralateral hemisphere.* Unformed visual hallucinations, peduncular hallucinosis, metamorphopsia, teleopsia, illusory visual spread, palinopsia, distortion of outlines, central photophobia: *Calcarine cortex.* Complex hallucinations: *Usually nondominant hemisphere.*
2. Central territory. Thalamic syndrome: sensory loss (all modalities), spontaneous pain and dysesthesias, choreoathetosis, intention tremor, spasms of hand, mild hemiparesis: *Posteroventral nucleus of thalamus; involvement of the adjacent subthalamus body or its afferent tracts.* Thalamoperforate syndrome: crossed cerebellar ataxia with ipsilateral third nerve palsy (Claude's syndrome): *Dentatothalamic tract and issuing third nerve.* Weber's syndrome: third nerve palsy and contralateral hemiplegia: *Third nerve and cerebral peduncle.* Contralateral hemiplegia: *Cerebral peduncle.* Paralysis or paresis of vertical eye movement, skew deviation, sluggish pupillary responses to light, slight miosis and ptosis (retraction nystagmus and "tucking" of the eyelids may be associated): *Supranuclear fibers to third nerve, interstitial nucleus of Cajal, nucleus of Darkschewitsch, and posterior commissure.* Contralateral rhythmic, ataxic action tremor; rhythmic postural or "holding" tremor (rubral tremor): *Dentatothalamic tract (?).*

Sometimes there is massive infarction of the entire deep white matter and cortical surface. When the origins of both the anterior and middle cerebral arteries are occluded at the top of the carotid artery, abulia or stupor occurs with hemiplegia, hemianesthesia, and aphasia or anosognosia. When the posterior cerebral artery arises from the internal carotid artery (an unusual configuration called a *fetal posterior cerebral artery*), it also may become occluded and give rise to symptoms referable to its peripheral territory (Figs. 361-4 and 361-5).

In addition to supplying the ipsilateral brain, the internal carotid artery perfuses the optic nerve and retina via the ophthalmic artery. In about 25% of symptomatic internal carotid disease, recurrent transient monocular blindness (TMB or amaurosis fugax) warns of the lesion. Patients typically describe a horizontal shade that sweeps down or up across the field of vision. They may also complain that their vision was blurred in that eye or that the upper or lower half of vision disappeared. In most cases, these symptoms last only a few minutes. Rarely, ischemia or infarction of the ophthalmic artery or central retinal arteries occurs at the time of cerebral TIA or infarction.

A high-pitched prolonged carotid bruit fading into diastole is often associated with tightly stenotic lesions. As the stenosis grows tighter and flow distal to the stenosis becomes reduced, the bruit becomes fainter and may disappear when occlusion is imminent. A stenosis is said to be *asymptomatic* if the patient has never experienced TIA or stroke that can be explained by the carotid lesion. The risk of stroke with this finding is low. *Symptomatic carotid stenosis*, in distinction, carries a significantly higher risk for stroke (see "Treatment," below).

COMMON CAROTID ARTERY All symptoms and signs of internal carotid occlusion may also be present with occlusion of the common carotid artery. Bilateral common carotid artery occlusions at their origin may occur in Takayasu's arteritis (Chap. 317).

Large Vessel Stroke within the Posterior Circulation The posterior circulation is composed of the paired vertebral arteries, the basilar artery, and the paired posterior cerebral arteries. The vertebral arteries join to form the basilar artery at the pontomedullary junction. The basilar artery divides into two posterior cerebral arteries in the interpeduncular fossa (Fig. 361-1). These major arteries gives rise to long and short circumferential branches and to smaller deep penetrating branches that supply the cerebellum, medulla, pons, midbrain, subthalamus, thalamus, hippocampus, and medial temporal and occipital lobes. Occlusion of each vessel produces its own distinctive syndrome.

Pathophysiology • *POSTERIOR CEREBRAL ARTERY* In 75% of cases, both posterior cerebral arteries arise from the bifurcation of the basilar artery; in 20%, one has its origin from the ipsilateral internal carotid artery via the posterior communicating artery; in 5%, both originate from the respective ipsilateral internal carotid arteries (Fig. 361-1). The precommunal, or P1, segment of the true posterior cerebral artery is atretic in such cases.

Atheroma formation or emboli that lodge at the top of the basilar artery or along the P1 segment may cause symptoms by occluding one or more of the small brainstem-penetrating branches (Figs. 361-1 and 361-5) that supply the middle cerebral peduncles, the substantia nigra, red nucleus, oculomotor nuclei, midbrain reticular formation, subthalamic nucleus, decussation of the superior cerebellar peduncles, the medial longitudinal fasciculus, and the medial lemniscus. The *artery of Percheron* arises from either the right or the left precommunal segment of the posterior cerebral artery; it divides in the subthalamus to supply the inferomedial and anterior portions of the thalamus and subthalamus bilaterally. The *thalamogeniculate branches*, which also originate from the precommunal portion of the posterior cerebral artery, supply the dorsal, dorsomedial, anterior and inferior thalamus, and the medial geniculate body. The *medial posterior choroidal artery* supplies the superior dorsomedial and dorsoanterior thalamus and the medial geniculate body in addition to the tela choroidea of the third ventricle. The *lateral posterior choroidal artery* supplies the choroid plexus of the lateral ventricle.

Occlusions in the posterior cerebral artery distal to the junction with the posterior communicating artery (P2 segment) (Fig. 361-5) may disrupt small circumferential branches that course around the midbrain to supply the lateral part of the cerebral peduncles, medial lemniscus, tegmentum of the midbrain, superior colliculi, lateral geniculate body, and posterolateral nucleus of the thalamus, choroid plexus, and hippocampus. On the rare occasions when atheroma occur more distally in the posterior cerebral artery (Fig. 361-5), occlusion may produce ischemia in the inferomedial temporal lobe, parahippocampal and hippocampal gyri, and occipital lobe—including the primary visual cortex and the visual association areas.

In addition to atherothrombosis and embolism, posterior circulation disease may also be caused by dissection of either vertebral artery and fibromuscular dysplasia.

Vertebral And Posterior Inferior Cerebellar Arteries The vertebral artery, which arises from the innominate artery on the right and the subclavian artery on the left, divides into four anatomic segments. The first (V1) extends from its origin to its entrance into the sixth or fifth transverse vertebral foramen. The second segment (V2) transverses the vertebral foramina from C6 to C2. The third (V3) passes through the transverse foramen and circles around the arch of the atlas to pierce the dura at the foramen magnum. The fourth (V4) segment courses upward to join the other vertebral artery to form the basilar artery; only the fourth segment gives rises to branches that supply the brainstem and cerebellum. The *posterior inferior cerebellar artery* (PICA) in its proximal segment supplies the lateral medulla and, in its distal branches, the inferior surface of the cerebellum. Anastomotic channels exist among the ascending cervical arteries, the thyrocervical arteries, the occipital artery (branch of the external carotid artery), and the second segment of the vertebral artery.

Atherothrombotic lesions have a predilection for V1 and V4 segments of the vertebral artery. The first segment may become diseased at the origin of the vessel and may produce posterior circulation emboli; collateral flow from the contralateral vertebral artery or the ascending cervical, thyrocervical, or occipital arteries is usually sufficient to prevent low-flow TIAs or stroke. When one vertebral artery is atretic and an atherothrombotic lesion threatens the origin of the other, the collateral circulation, which may also include retrograde flow down the basilar artery, is often insufficient (Figs. 361-1 and 361-5). In this setting, low-flow TIAs may occur, consisting of syncope, vertigo, and alternating hemiplegia; this state also sets the stage for thrombosis. Disease of the distal fourth segment of the vertebral artery can promote thrombus formation manifest as embolism or with propagation as basilar artery thrombosis. Stenosis proximal to the origin of the posterior inferior cerebellar artery can threaten the lateral medulla and posterior inferior surface of the cerebellum.

If the subclavian artery is occluded proximal to the origin of the vertebral artery, there is a reversal in the direction of blood flow in the ipsilateral vertebral artery. Exercise of the ipsilateral arm may increase demand on vertebral flow, producing posterior circulation TIAs, or "subclavian steal."

Although atheromatous disease rarely narrows the second and third segments of the vertebral artery, this region is subject to dissection, fibromuscular dysplasia, and, rarely, encroachment by osteophytic spurs within the vertebral foramina.

Basilar Artery Branches of the basilar artery supply the base of the pons and superior cerebellum and fall into three groups: (1) paramedian, 7 to 10 in number, which supply a wedge of pons on either side of the midline; (2) short circumferential, 5 to 7 in number, which supply the lateral two-thirds of the pons and middle and superior cerebellar peduncles; and (3) bilateral long circumferential (superior cerebellar and anterior inferior cerebellar arteries), which course around the pons to supply the cerebellar hemispheres.

Atheromatous lesions can occur anywhere along the basilar trunk but are most frequent in the proximal basilar and distal vertebral segments. Typically, lesions occlude either the proximal basilar and one or both vertebral arteries. The clinical picture varies depending on the availability of retrograde collateral flow from the posterior communicating arteries. Rarely, dissection of a vertebral artery may involve the basilar artery and, depending on the location of true and false lumen, may produce multiple penetrating artery strokes.

Although atherothrombosis occasionally occludes the distal portion of the basilar artery, emboli from the heart or proximal vertebral or basilar segments are more commonly responsible for "top of the basilar" syndromes.

Clinical manifestations • *Posterior Cerebral Artery* Embolic occlusion is the usual cause of stroke in this vascular territory. Two syndromes are commonly observed: (1) midbrain, subthalamic, and thalamic signs, which are due to disease of the P1 segment or of its penetrating branches; and (2) cortical temporal and occipital lobe signs, due to occlusion of the P2 segment.

1. *P1 syndromes*. If the P1 segment is occluded, infarction usually occurs in the ipsilateral subthalamus and medial thalamus and in the ipsilateral cerebral peduncle and midbrain (Fig. 361-5). A third nerve palsy with contralateral ataxia (Claude's syndrome) or with contralateral hemiplegia (Weber's syndrome) may result. The ataxia indicates involvement of the red nucleus or dentatorubrothalamic tract; the hemiplegia is localized to the cerebral peduncle. If the subthalamic nucleus is involved, contralateral hemiballismus may occur. Occlusion of the artery of Percheron produces paresis of upward gaze and drowsiness, and often abulia. Extensive infarction in the midbrain and subthalamus occurring with bilateral proximal posterior cerebral artery occlusion presents as coma, unreactive pupils, bilateral pyramidal signs, and decerebrate rigidity.

Atheromatous occlusion of the penetrating branches of thalamic and thalamogeniculate arteries produces less extensive thalamic and thalamocapsular lacunar syndromes. The *thalamic Déjerine-Roussy syndrome* is the best known. Its main feature is contralateral hemisensory loss followed later by an agonizing, searing or burning pain in the affected areas. It is persistent and responds poorly to analgesics. Anticonvulsants (carbamazepine or gabapentin) or tricyclic antidepressants may be beneficial. Associated motor signs include hemiparesis, hemiballismus, choreoathetosis, intention tremor, incoordination, and posturing of the hand and arm, particularly while walking.

2. *P2 syndromes* (see also Fig. 361-5). Occlusion of the distal posterior cerebral artery causes infarction of the medial temporal and occipital lobes. Contralateral homonymous hemianopia with macula sparing is the usual manifestation. Occasionally, only the upper quadrant of visual field is involved. If the visual association areas are spared and only the calcarine cortex is involved, the patient may be aware of visual defects. Medial temporal lobe and hippocampal involvement may cause an acute disturbance in memory, particularly if it occurs in the dominant hemisphere. The defect usually clears because memory has bilateral representation. If the dominant hemisphere is affected and the infarct extends to involve the splenium of the corpus callosum, the patient may demonstrate alexia without agraphia. Visual agnosia for faces, objects, mathematical symbols, and colors and anomia with paraphasic errors (amnestic aphasia) may also occur in this setting, even without callosal involvement. Occlusion of the posterior cerebral artery can produce *peduncular hallucinosis* (visual hallucinations of brightly colored scenes and objects).

Bilateral infarction in the distal posterior cerebral arteries produces cortical blindness (blindness with preserved pupillary light reaction). The patient is often unaware of the blindness or may even deny it (*Anton's syndrome*). Tiny islands of vision may persist, and the patient may report that vision fluctuates as images are captured in the preserved portions. Rarely, only peripheral vision is lost and central vision is spared, resulting in "gun-barrel" vision. A constellation of symptoms termed *Balint's syndrome* can occur, usually with bilateral visual association area lesions. It includes optic ataxia (inability to visually guide limb movements), ocular ataxia (inability to direct eyes to a precise point in the visual field), inability to enumerate objects in a picture (simultagnosia) or extract meaning from a picture, and inability to avoid objects in one's path. Balint's syndrome occurs most often with infarctions secondary to low flow in the "watershed" between the distal posterior and middle cerebral artery territories, as occurs after cardiac arrest. Patients may even experience persistence of a visual image for several minutes despite gazing at another scene (*palinopia*). Embolic occlusion of the top of the basilar artery can produce any or all of the central or peripheral territory symptoms. The hallmark is the sudden onset of bilateral signs, including ptosis, pupillary asymmetry or lack of reaction to light, and somnolence.

VERTEBRAL AND POSTERIOR INFERIOR CEREBELLAR ARTERIES Embolic occlusion or thrombosis of a V4 segment causes ischemia of the lateral medulla. The constellation of vertigo, numbness of the ipsilateral face and contralateral limbs, diplopia, hoarseness, dysarthria, dysphagia, and ipsilateral Horner's syndrome is called the lateral medullary (or Wallenberg's) syndrome (Fig. 361-6). Most cases result from ipsilateral vertebral artery occlusion; in the remainder, PICA occlusion is responsible. Occlusion of the medullary penetrating branches of the vertebral artery or PICA results in partial syndromes. *Hemiparesis is not a feature of vertebral artery occlusion.*

Rarely, a *medial medullary syndrome* occurs with infarction of the pyramid and contralateral hemiparesis of the arm and leg, sparing the face. If the medial lemniscus and emerging hypoglossal nerve fibers are involved, contralateral loss of joint position sense and ipsilateral tongue weakness occur.

Cerebellar infarction with edema can lead to *sudden respiratory arrest* due to raised intracranial pressure (ICP) in the posterior fossa. Drowsiness, Babinski signs, dysarthria, and bifacial weakness may be absent, or present only briefly, before respiratory arrest ensues. Gait unsteadiness, dizziness, nausea, and vomiting may be the only early symptoms and signs and should arouse suspicion of this impending complication, which may require neurosurgical decompression, often with an excellent outcome.

BASILAR ARTERY Because the brainstem contains many structures in close apposition, a diversity of clinical syndromes may emerge with ischemia, reflecting involvement of the corticospinal and corticobulbar tracts, ascending sensory tracts, and cranial nerve nuclei (Figs. 361-7, 361-8, and 361-9).

The symptoms of transient ischemia or infarction in the territory of the basilar artery often do not indicate whether the basilar artery itself or one of its branches is diseased, yet this distinction has important implications for therapy. *The picture of complete basilar occlusion, however, is easy to recognize as a constellation of bilateral long tract signs (sensory and motor) with signs of cranial nerve and cerebellar dysfunction.* A "locked-in" state of preserved consciousness with quadriplegia and cranial nerve signs suggest complete pontine and lower midbrain infarction. The therapeutic goal is to identify *impending* basilar occlusion before devastating infarction occurs. A series of TIAs and a slowly progressive, fluctuating stroke are extremely significant as they often herald an atherothrombotic occlusion of the distal vertebral or proximal basilar artery.

TIAs in the proximal basilar distribution may produce dizziness (often described by patients as "swimming," "swaying," "moving," "unsteadiness" or "light-headedness"). Other symptoms that warn of basilar thrombosis include diplopia, dysarthria, facial or circumoral numbness, and hemisensory symptoms. In general, symptoms of basilar branch TIAs affect one side of the brainstem, whereas symptoms of basilar artery TIAs usually affect both sides, though a "herald" hemiparesis has been emphasized as an initial symptom of basilar occlusion. Most often TIAs, whether due to impending occlusion of the basilar artery or a basilar branch, are short-lived (5 to 30 min) and repetitive, occurring several times a day. The pattern suggests intermittent reduction of flow. Many neurologists treat with heparin to prevent clot propagation.

Atherothrombotic occlusion of the basilar artery with infarction usually causes *bilateral* brainstem signs. A gaze paresis or internuclear ophthalmoplegia associated with ipsilateral hemiparesis may be the only manifestations of bilateral brainstem ischemia. More often, unequivocal signs of bilateral pontine disease are present. Complete basilar thrombosis carries a high mortality.

Occlusion of a branch of the basilar artery usually causes *unilateral* symptoms and signs involving motor, sensory, and cranial nerves. As long as symptoms remain unilateral, concern over pending basilar occlusion should be reduced.

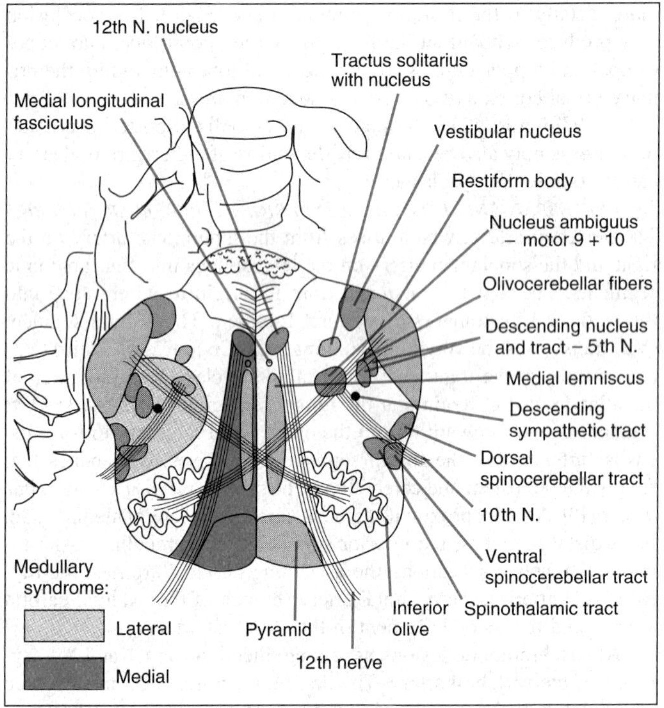

FIGURE 361-6 *(Courtesy of CM Fisher, MD.)*

Signs and Symptoms: *Structures involved*

1. Medial medullary syndrome (occlusion of vertebral artery or of branch of vertebral or lower basilar artery)
   On side of lesion
      Paralysis with atrophy of half the tongue: *Ipsilateral twelfth nerve*
   On side opposite lesion
      Paralysis of arm and leg sparing face; impaired tactile and proprioceptive sense over half the body: *Contralateral pyramidal tract and medial lemniscus*
2. Lateral medullary syndrome (occlusion of any of five vessels may be responsible—vertebral, posterior inferior cerebellar, superior, middle, or inferior lateral medullary arteries)
   On side of lesion
      Pain, numbness, impaired sensation over half the face: *Descending tract and nucleus fifth nerve*
      Ataxia of limbs, falling to side of lesion: *Uncertain—restiform body, cerebellar hemisphere, cerebellar fibers, spinocerebellar tract (?)*
      Nystagmus, diplopia, oscillopsia, vertigo, nausea, vomiting: *Vestibular nucleus*
      Horner's syndrome (miosis, ptosis, decreased sweating): *Descending sympathetic tract*
      Dysphagia, hoarseness, paralysis of palate, paralysis of vocal cord, diminished gag reflex: *Issuing fibers ninth and tenth nerves*
      Loss of taste: *Nucleus and tractus solitarius*
      Numbness of ipsilateral arm, trunk, or leg: *Cuneate and gracile nuclei*
   On side opposite lesion
      Impaired pain and thermal sense over half the body, sometimes face: *Spinothalamic tract*
3. Total unilateral medullary syndrome (occlusion of vertebral artery): Combination of medial and lateral syndromes
4. Lateral pontomedullary syndrome (occlusion of vertebral artery): Combination of lateral medullary and lateral inferior pontine syndromes
5. Basilar artery syndrome (the syndrome of the lone vertebral artery is equivalent): A combination of the various brainstem syndromes plus those arising in the posterior cerebral artery distribution
   Bilateral long tract signs (sensory and motor; cerebellar and peripheral cranial nerve abnormalities): *Bilateral long tract; cerebellar and peripheral cranial nerves*
   Paralysis or weakness of all extremities, plus all bulbar musculature: *Corticobulbar and corticospinal tracts bilaterally;*

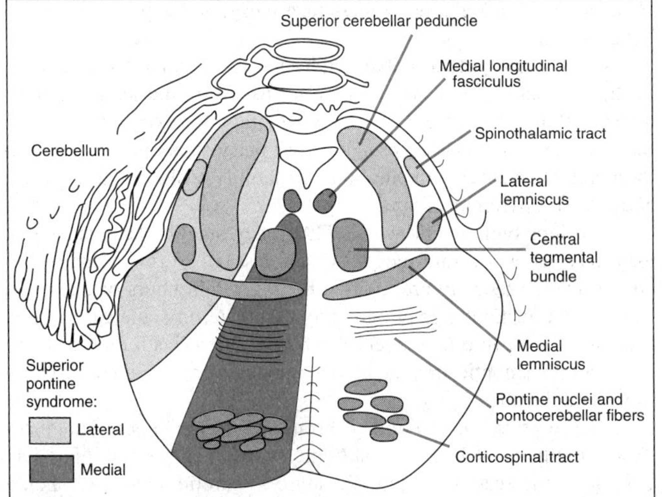

FIGURE 361-7 *(Courtesy of CM Fisher, MD.)*

Signs and Symptoms: *Structures involved*

1. Medial superior pontine syndrome (paramedian branches of upper basilar artery)
   - On side of lesion
     - Cerebellar ataxia (probably): *Superior and/or middle cerebellar peduncle*
     - Internuclear ophthalmoplegia: *Medial longitudinal fasciculus*
     - Myoclonic syndrome, palate, pharynx, vocal cords, respiratory apparatus, face, oculomotor apparatus, etc.: *Localization uncertain—central tegmental bundle (?), dentate projection (?), inferior olivary nucleus (?)*
   - On side opposite lesion
     - Paralysis of face, arm, and leg: *Corticobulbar and corticospinal tract*
     - Rarely touch, vibration, and position are affected: *Medial lemniscus*
2. Lateral superior pontine syndrome (syndrome of superior cerebellar artery)
   - On side of lesion
     - Ataxia of limbs and gait, falling to side of lesion: *Middle and superior cerebellar peduncles, superior surface of cerebellum, dentate nucleus*
     - Dizziness, nausea, vomiting; horizontal nystagmus: *Vestibular nucleus;*
     - Paresis of conjugate gaze (ipsilateral): *Pontine contralateral gaze*
     - Skew deviation: *Uncertain*
     - Miosis, ptosis, decreased sweating over face (Horner's syndrome): *Descending sympathetic fibers*
     - Tremor: *Dentate nucleus (?), superior cerebellar peduncle (?)*
   - On side opposite lesion
     - Impaired pain and thermal sense on face, limbs, and trunk: *Spinothalamic tract*
     - Impaired touch, vibration, and position sense, more in leg than arm (there is a tendency to incongruity of pain and touch deficits): *Medial lemniscus (lateral portion)*

Superior Cerebellar Artery Occlusion results in severe ipsilateral cerebellar ataxia, nausea and vomiting, dysarthria, and contralateral loss of pain and temperature sensation over the extremities, body, and face (spino- and trigeminothalamic tract). Partial deafness, ataxic tremor of the ipsilateral upper extremity, Horner's syndrome, and palatal myoclonus may occur rarely. Partial syndromes occur frequently (Fig. 361-7). With large strokes, swelling and mass effects may compress the midbrain or produce hydrocephalus; these symptoms may evolve rapidly. Neurosurgical intervention may be lifesaving in such cases.

Anterior Inferior Cerebellar Artery Occlusion produces variable degrees of infarction because the size of this artery and the territory it supplies vary inversely with those of the PICA. The principal symptoms include: (1) ipsilateral deafness, facial weakness, vertigo, nausea and vomiting, nystagmus, tinnitus, cerebellar ataxia, Horner's syndrome, and paresis of conjugate lateral gaze; and (2) contralateral loss of pain and temperature sensation. An occlusion close to the origin of the artery may cause corticospinal tract signs (Fig. 361-9).

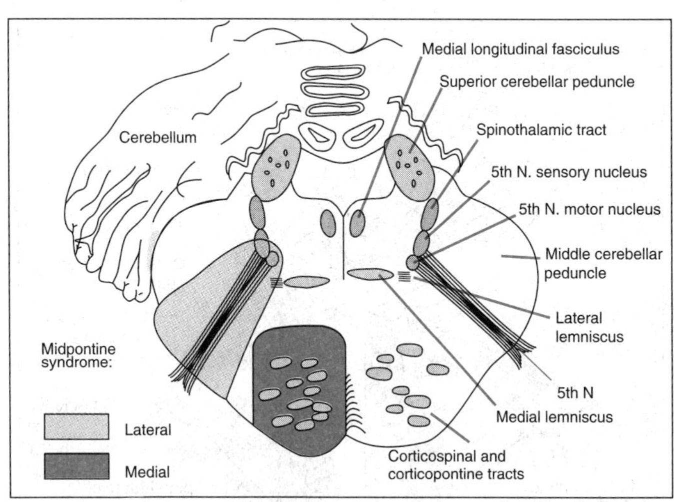

FIGURE 361-8 *(Courtesy of CM Fisher, MD.)*

Signs and Symptoms: *Structures involved*

1. Medial midpontine syndrome (paramedian branch of midbasilar artery)
   - On side of lesion
     - Ataxia of limbs and gait (more prominent in bilateral involvement): *Pontine nuclei*
   - On side opposite lesion
     - Paralysis of face, arm, and leg: *Corticobulbar and corticospinal tract*
     - Variable impaired touch and proprioception when lesion extends posteriorly: *Medial lemniscus*
2. Lateral midpontine syndrome (short circumferential artery)
   - On side of lesion
     - Ataxia of limbs: *Middle cerebellar peduncle*
     - Paralysis of muscles of mastication: *Motor fibers or nucleus of fifth nerve*
     - Impaired sensation over side of face: *Sensory fibers or nucleus of fifth nerve*
   - On side opposite lesion
     - Impaired pain and thermal sense on limbs and trunk: *Spinothalamic tract*

Occlusion of one of the short circumferential branches of the basilar artery affects the lateral two-thirds of the pons and middle or superior cerebellar peduncle, whereas occlusion of one of the paramedian branches affects a wedge-shaped area on either side of the medial pons (Figs. 361-7 to 361-9).

Small Vessel "Lacunar" Stroke The term *lacunar infarction* refers to infarction following atherothrombotic or lipohyalinotic occlusion of one of the small, penetrating branches of the circle of Willis, middle cerebral artery stem, or vertebral and basilar arteries. The term *small vessel stroke* denotes occlusion of a small penetrating artery, regardless of mechanism.

Pathophysiology The middle cerebral artery stem, the arteries comprising the circle of Willis (A1 segment, anterior and posterior communicating arteries, and P1 segment), and the basilar and vertebral arteries all give rise to 100- to 300-μm branches that penetrate the deep gray and white matter of the cerebrum or brainstem (Fig. 361-1). Each of these small branches can occlude either by atherothrombotic disease at its origin or by the development of lipohyalinotic thickening. Thrombosis of these vessels causes small infarcts that are referred to as *lacunes* (Latin for "lake" of fluid noted at autopsy). They range in size from 3 or 4 mm to 1 or 2 cm. Hypertension and age are the principal risk factors. Lacunar infarcts cause approximately 20% of all strokes.

Clinical manifestations The most common *lacunar syndromes* are the following: (1) Pure motor hemiparesis from an infarct in the posterior limb of the internal capsule or basis pontis; the face, arm and leg are almost always involved. (2) Pure sensory stroke from an infarct in the ventrolateral thalamus. (3) Ataxic hemiparesis from an infarct

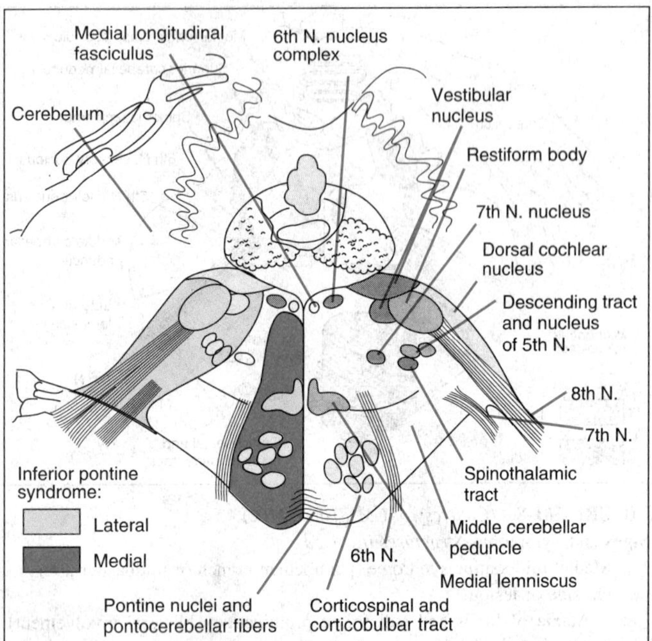

FIGURE 361-9 *(Courtesy of CM Fisher, MD.)*

Signs and symptoms: *Structures involved*

1. Medial inferior pontine syndrome (occlusion of paramedian branch of basilar artery)
   - On side of lesion
     - Paralysis of conjugate gaze to side of lesion (preservation of convergence): *"Center" for conjugate lateral gaze*
     - Nystagmus: *Vestibular nucleus*
     - Ataxia of limbs and gait: *Middle cerebellar peduncle (?)*
     - Diplopia on lateral gaze: *Abducens nerve*;
   - On side opposite lesion
     - Paralysis of face, arm, and leg: *Corticobulbar and corticospinal tract in lower pons*
     - Impaired tactile and proprioceptive sense over half of the body: *Medial lemniscus*
2. Lateral inferior pontine syndrome (occlusion of anterior inferior cerebellar artery)
   - On side of lesion
     - Horizontal and vertical nystagmus, vertigo, nausea, vomiting, oscillopia: *Vestibular nerve or nucleus*
     - Facial paralysis: *Seventh nerve*
     - Paralysis of conjugate gaze to side of lesion: *"Center" for conjugate lateral gaze*
     - Deafness, tinnitus: *Auditory nerve or cochlear nucleus*
     - Ataxia: *Middle cerebellar peduncle and cerebellar hemisphere*
     - Impaired sensation over face: *Descending tract and nucleus fifth nerve*
   - On side opposite lesion
     - Impaired pain and thermal sense over half the body (may include face): *Spinothalamic tract*

in the base of the pons. (4) Dysarthria and a clumsy hand or arm due to infarction in the base of the pons or in the genu of the internal capsule. (5) Pure motor hemiparesis with "motor (Broca's) aphasia" due to thrombotic occlusion of a lenticulostriate branch supplying the genu and anterior limb of the internal capsule and adjacent white matter of the corona radiata.

Syndromes 1 and 2 often overlap. Syndromes resulting from occlusion of the penetrating arteries of the proximal posterior cerebral artery were discussed above. Syndromes resulting from occlusion of the penetrating arteries of the basilar artery (Figs. 361-7 to 361-9) include ipsilateral ataxia and contralateral crural (leg) paresis, hemiparesis with horizontal gaze palsy, and hemiparesis with a crossed sixth nerve palsy. Lower basilar branch syndromes include internuclear ophthalmoplegia, horizontal gaze palsy, and appendicular cerebellar ataxia.

An anarthric pseudobulbar syndrome due to bilateral infarctions in the internal capsule can occur from disease in the lenticulostriate arteries. Before the advent of effective therapy for hypertension, multiple lacunes often caused pseudobulbar palsy (predominantly dysarthria and dysphagia) with emotional instability, a slowed abulic state, and bilateral pyramidal signs.

Transient symptoms (lacunar TIAs) may herald a lacunar infarct; they may occur several times a day and last only a few minutes. Recovery from a lacunar stroke often begins within hours or days, and over weeks or months may be nearly complete; in some cases, however, there is severe permanent disability. Often, institution of combined antithrombotic treatments does not prevent eventual stroke in "stuttering lacunes."

A large vessel source (either thrombosis or embolism) may manifest initially as a lacunar syndrome with small vessel infarction. Therefore, the search for embolic sources (carotid and heart) should not be abandoned in the evaluation of these patients.

FINDING THE CAUSE OF STROKE The clinical presentation, temporal profile, and signs found on examination often establish the cause or narrow the possibilities to a few. Judicious use of laboratory testing and imaging studies complete the initial evaluation. For stroke without an identified cause (cryptogenic stroke), the exact diagnosis may be made months or years later as new symptoms develop. Unfortunately, nearly 30% of strokes remains unexplained despite extensive evaluation; nevertheless, they occur in patients with the same clinical profiles as those whose strokes are due to atherothrombosis.

Clinical examination should be focused on the peripheral vascular system (carotid auscultation for bruits, blood pressure, and pressure comparison between arms), the heart (dysrhythmia, murmurs), extremities (peripheral emboli), and retina [effects of hypertension and cholesterol emboli (Hollenhorst plaques)]; with a complete neurologic examination to localize the site of stroke. A chest x-ray, electrocardiogram (ECG), urinalysis, complete blood count, erythrocyte sedimentation rate, serum electrolytes, blood urea nitrogen, creatinine, blood sugar, serologic test for syphilis, serum lipid profile, prothrombin time, and partial thromboplastin time should be evaluated in all patients. An ECG may demonstrate conduction abnormalities and arrhythmias or reveal evidence of recent myocardial infarction. A lumbar puncture (LP) will generally confirm or exclude subarachnoid hemorrhage (SAH) and can reveal meningitis as a cause for stroke. However, an LP should not be performed on patients with a possible intracranial mass lesion and therefore should generally be avoided in patients with a suspected stroke who are comatose or who have lateralizing neurologic signs with indications of increased ICP. Finally, an imaging study of the brain is nearly always performed and is required for patients being considered for thrombolysis.

BRAIN IMAGING (See also Chap. 358) **Computed Tomographic Scans** Computed tomography (CT) images identify or exclude hemorrhage as the cause of stroke, and they identify extraparenchymal hemorrhages, neoplasms, abscesses, and other conditions masquerading as stroke. Scans obtained in the first several hours after an infarction generally show no abnormality, and the infarct may not be seen reliably for 24 to 48 h. Even later, CT may fail to show small ischemic strokes in the posterior fossa because of bone artifact and may also miss small infarcts on the cortical surface. The CT scan documents most supratentorial lacunar infarcts. Lacunar infarction is diagnosed when the infarct size is <2 cm and its location is consistent with occlusion of a small penetrating branch of a major artery at the base of the brain. Larger deep white matter infarcts in the territory of the MCA may present as a lacunar syndrome but are caused by occlusions of large vessels and compensatory collateral perfusion.

Contrast-enhanced CT scans add specificity by showing contrast enhancement of subacute infarcts and allow visualization of venous structures. Coupled with newer generation scanners, administration of intravenous contrast allows visualization of large cerebral arteries.

Such "CT angiograms" may be useful in acute stroke management to reveal the presence or absence of large vessel pathology.

Magnetic Resonance Imaging (MRI) MRI reliably documents the extent and location of infarction in all areas of the brain, including the posterior fossa and cortical surface, if appropriate imaging sequences are obtained. It also identifies intracranial hemorrhage and other abnormalities. The higher the field strength, the more reliable and precise the image. Diffusion-weighted imaging is more sensitive for early brain infarction than standard magnetic resonance (MR) sequences (Fig. 361-10) as is FLAIR (fluid-attenuated inversion recovery) imaging (Chap. 358). MR angiography is highly sensitive for extracranial internal carotid plaque as well as intracranial stenosis of large vessels. With higher degrees of stenosis, MR angiography tends to overestimate the degree of stenosis when compared to conventional x-ray angiography. MRI with fat saturation is an imaging sequence used to visualize extra- or intracranial arterial dissection. This sensitive technique images clotted blood within the dissected vessel wall and has revealed carotid or vertebral dissection as the cause of stroke in a sizable fraction of young patients (age <45). Stroke with neck, jaw, or retroauricular pain, with or without Horner's syndrome, should prompt this imaging modality or conventional x-ray angiography.

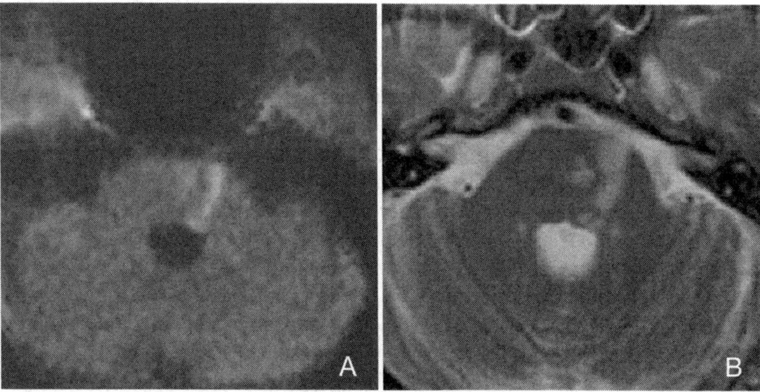

FIGURE 361-10 Magnetic resonance imaging of acute stroke. *A.* Diffusion-weighted image of the posterior fossa in a woman with sudden-onset left palate and tongue weakness, showing restricted diffusion in the left basis pontis. T2-weighted MRI at the same time as image *A* showed no evidence of infarction (not shown). *B.* T2-weighted image 2 days later clearly defines the area of infarct.

MRI is less sensitive for acute blood products than CT and is more expensive and less readily available. Claustrophobia also limits its application. Most acute stroke protocols use CT because of these limitations. However, outside this setting, MRI provides superior information compared with CT in nearly every case of stroke.

Cerebral Angiography Conventional x-ray cerebral angiography is the "gold standard" for identifying and quantifying atherosclerotic stenoses of the cerebral arteries and other pathologies, including aneurysm, vasospasm, intraluminal thrombi, fibromuscular dysplasia, arteriovenous fistula, vasculitis, and collateral channels of blood flow. Endovascular techniques, which are evolving rapidly, can be used to deploy stents within delicate intracranial vessels and perform balloon angioplasty of stenotic lesions. Recent studies have documented that intraarterial delivery of thrombolytic agents to patients with acute MCA stroke can effectively recanalize vessels and improve clinical outcomes. Although investigational in many centers, use of cerebral angiography coupled with endovascular techniques for cerebral revascularization may become routine in the near future.

Ultrasound Techniques Stenosis at the origin of the internal carotid artery can be identified and quantified reliably by ultrasonography that combines a B-mode ultrasound image with a Doppler ultrasound assessment of flow velocity ("Duplex" ultrasound). Transcranial Doppler (TCD) assessment of middle, anterior, and posterior cerebral artery flow and of vertebrobasilar flow is also useful. This latter technique can detect stenotic lesions in the middle cerebral stem, the distal vertebral arteries, and the basilar artery because such lesions increase systolic flow velocity. When there is an occlusion or hemodynamically significant stenosis at the origin of the internal carotid artery or in the carotid siphon, TCD assesses collateral flow across the anterior or posterior circle of Willis. In many cases, MR angiography combined with carotid and transcranial ultrasound studies eliminates the need for conventional x-ray angiography in evaluating carotid artery lesions for surgery. The combination of the two studies is less expensive than x-ray angiography and reduces the risk of stroke secondary to the procedure.

Ultrasound cannot distinguish reliably between complete and near-complete carotid occlusion; this distinction can be made reliably only by x-ray angiography.

Other Techniques Both xenon techniques (principally xenon-CT) and positron emission tomography (PET) can quantify cerebral blood flow. These tools are generally used for research (Chap. 358) but can be useful for determining the significance of arterial stenosis and planning for revascularization surgery. Single photon emission tomography (SPECT), CT-perfusion, and MR-perfusion techniques report relative cerebral blood flow and currently are research tools.

FINDING EMBOLIC SOURCES If the clinical syndrome of stroke suggests large vessel ischemia or is sudden in onset or if imaging studies reveal infarction consistent with embolism, a search for the cause of embolism is warranted. Documentation of the exact embolic source can direct therapy that can lessen mortality and morbidity. Embolic stroke is classified by the artery involved (e.g., embolic MCA stroke, as discussed above) or by the source of embolism, either from another artery (artery-to-artery embolic stroke) or cardioembolic. Both causes of embolic stroke are discussed below.

Cardioembolic Stroke • *Pathophysiology* Cardioembolism causes approximately 20% of all ischemic strokes. Stroke caused by heart disease is primarily due to embolism of thrombotic material forming on the atrial or ventricular wall or the left heart valves. These thrombi then detach and embolize the arterial circulation. The thrombus may fragment or lyse quickly, producing only TIA. Alternatively, the arterial occlusion may last longer, producing stroke. Subsequent thrombosis distal to the obstruction may occur, producing stroke in progression.

Emboli from the heart most often lodge in the MCA or one of its branches; infrequently, the anterior cerebral artery territory is involved. Emboli large enough to occlude the stem of the MCA (3 to 4 mm) lead to large infarcts that involve both deep gray and white matter and some portions of the cortical surface and its underlying white matter. A smaller embolus may occlude a small cortical or penetrating arterial branch. The location and size of an infarct within a vascular territory often depend on the extent of the collateral circulation.

Vascular congestion of varying degree is common to all ischemic strokes, but extravasation of blood is often associated with embolic infarcts. Because emboli migrate and lyse, recirculation into the infarcted brain may cause petechial hemorrhages. Sometimes there is enough seepage of blood into the infarct to cause visible hemorrhagic infarction on a CT scan. This *hemorrhagic transformation* of a pale infarct typically occurs from 12 to 36 h after embolization and is often asymptomatic. Frank hemorrhage into the infarct sometimes occurs and almost always causes clinical worsening. This is more likely to occur when the stem of the MCA is occluded and a large infarct develops in the territory of the lenticulostriate arteries before recirculation occurs. Edema invariably accompanies the tissue necrosis. In large infarcts, massive edema may compress adjacent tissue, adding to the ischemic process; it also increases ICP and may cause herniation of the brain from one intracranial compartment to another.

The most frequent causes of cardioembolic stroke in most of the world are nonrheumatic (often called nonvalvular) atrial fibrillation, myocardial infarction, prosthetic valves, rheumatic heart disease, and ischemic cardiomyopathy (Table 361-2). Cardiac disorders causing brain embolism are discussed in the respective chapters on heart diseases. A few pertinent aspects are highlighted here.

Nonrheumatic atrial fibrillation is the most common cause of cerebral embolism. Patients with atrial fibrillation have an average annual risk of stroke of ~5%. The risk varies according to the presence of certain risk factors, including older age, hypertension, poor left ventricular function, prior cardioembolism, diabetes, and thyrotoxicosis. Patients younger than 60 with none of these risk factors have an annual risk for stroke of about 0.5%, while those with most of the factors have a rate of about 15%. Guidelines for the use of warfarin are based on risk factors (Table 361-5). The presumed stroke mechanism is thrombus formation in the fibrillating atrium or atrial appendage with subsequent embolization. Left atrial enlargement and congestive heart failure are additional risk factors for formation of atrial thrombi. Rheumatic heart disease usually causes ischemic stroke when there is prominent mitral stenosis or atrial fibrillation.

The cardioembolic causes of stroke are enumerated in Table 361-2. A recent myocardial infarction may be a source of emboli, especially when transmural and involving the anteroapical ventricular wall. Mitral valve prolapse is not usually a source of emboli unless the prolapse is severe.

Paradoxical embolization occurs when venous thrombi migrate to the arterial circulation, usually via a patent foramen ovale or atrial septal defect, which may be occult. Bubble-contrast echocardiography (intravenous injection of agitated saline coupled with either transthoracic or transesophageal echocardiography) can demonstrate a right-to-left shunt, revealing the conduit for paradoxical embolization. Alternatively, a right-to-left shunt is implied if immediately following intravenous injection of agitated saline, high-intensity transients (HITs) can be observed during TCD insonation of the MCA. Both techniques are highly sensitive for detection of right-to-left shunts. Fat and tumor emboli, bacterial endocarditis, and air and amniotic fluid emboli associated with delivery may occasionally be responsible.

Bacterial endocarditis causes valvular vegetations that can give rise to multiple septic emboli (Chap. 126). The appearance of multifocal or diffuse symptoms and signs in a patient with stroke makes bacterial endocarditis a more likely consideration. Infarcts of microscopic size occur, and large septic infarcts may evolve into brain abscesses. Large septic emboli may cause hemorrhage into the infarct, which usually precludes use of anticoagulation or thrombolytics. Mycotic aneurysms caused by septic emboli give rise to SAH or intracerebral hemorrhage.

Clinical manifestations The stroke is nearly always sudden and maximal at onset. Certain neurologic syndromes suggest embolism, often cardioembolism, as their cause. In the MCA territory these include (1) the frontal opercular syndrome, with facial weakness and severe aphasia or dysarthria; (2) the brachial or hand plegia syndrome, in which the arm or hand is paralyzed with or without cortical sensory abnormalities; (3) Broca's or Wernicke's aphasia alone; or (4) left visual neglect, when the nondominant parietal lobe is involved. Sudden hemianopia suggests a posterior cerebral artery embolus, and sudden foot and shoulder weakness suggests an anterior cerebral embolus.

Table 361-5 Consensus Recommendation for Antithrombotic Prophylaxis in Atrial Fibrillation

Age	Risk Factors[a]	Recommendation
Age ≤65	≥1	Warfarin INR 2–3
	0	Aspirin or no treatment
Age 65–75	≥1	Warfarin INR 2–3
	0	Warfarin INR 2–3 or aspirin
Age >75		Warfarin INR 2–3

[a] Risk factors include previous transient ischemic attack or stroke, hypertension, heart failure, diabetes, clinical coronary artery disease, mitral stenosis, prosthetic heart valves, or thyrotoxicosis.

SOURCE: Modified from Laupacis et al.

Sudden sleepiness and inability to look up associated with bilateral ptosis suggest an embolus to the top of the basilar artery, specifically to the artery of Percheron (see above).

Seizures at the time of stroke occur in 3 to 5% of infarctions, are more often associated with embolic stroke rather than thrombosis, and are usually associated with supratentorial cortical surface infarctions. Another 3 to 5% of patients develop epilepsy 6 to 18 months after stroke. Many cases of idiopathic epilepsy in the elderly are probably the result of silent cortical infarction.

Artery-to-Artery Stroke Thrombus formation on atherosclerotic plaques may embolize to distant arteries. The most common source is the carotid bifurcation, but any diseased vessel may be a source, including the aortic arch and common carotid, internal carotid, and vertebral-basilar arteries.

Dissection of the internal carotid or vertebral arteries or even vessels beyond the circle of Willis is a common source of embolic stroke in young patients. The dissection is usually painful and precedes stroke by several hours or days. Extracranial dissections rarely cause hemorrhage because of the tough adventitia of these vessels. Intracranial dissections, on the other hand, may produce SAH because the adventitia of intracranial vessels is thin, and pseudoaneurysms may form, requiring treatment to prevent rerupture. The cause of dissection is usually unknown and recurrence is rare. Ehlers-Danlos type IV, Marfan's disease, cystic medial necrosis, and fibromuscular dysplasia are associated with dissections. Trauma (usually a motor vehicle accident or a sports injury) can cause carotid and vertebral artery dissections. Chiropractic neck manipulation is also associated with dissection and stroke.

Laboratory and Imaging Evaluation for Embolic Stroke A thorough cardiac evaluation should be undertaken in patients in whom the suspicion of cardioembolism is high. This includes the young, those with a history of heart disease, those with multifocal or hemorrhagic infarcts, and those with seizures at onset. Continuous ECG monitoring may reveal intermittent atrial fibrillation. An echocardiogram may disclose mitral valve disease, an intracardiac thrombus or tumor, or a dyskinetic area of myocardium. Spontaneous echo contrast within the atrial appendage is associated with stroke and may represent a tendency for spontaneous clotting of blood within the atrium. Transesophageal echocardiography is superior to the transthoracic technique for visualization of valves, left atrium, and aortic arch. Intravenous bubble contrast should be administered to all patients undergoing echocardiography in search of an embolic source. The presence of atrial fibrillation alone is sufficient to establish cause, even in the absence of a left atrial clot.

Embolic infarction may appear as a single low-density area compatible with pale infarction on CT imaging. Petechial hemorrhages within the area may be seen as well and are more likely a day or two after the infarction. MRI scanning better documents infarction both supra- and infratentorially; when coupled with MR angiography, it can help identify arterial sources of emboli from either the extra- or intracranial vessels. MRI with fat saturation should be performed on patients with neck pain preceding stroke, as this technique is highly sensitive for detecting arterial dissection. Carotid ultrasonography and TCD techniques may reveal carotid atherosclerosis or intracranial stenosis, respectively. Conventional x-ray angiography is rarely indicated.

Arterial imaging (CT or MR angiography or TCD) performed in the early hours of stroke often shows occlusion of one or more vessels. Complete lysis of emboli often occurs, and angiography performed after several days may be normal.

LESS COMMON CAUSES OF STROKE (Table 361-2) *Hypercoagulable disorders* (Chap. 62) primarily cause increased venous thrombotic risk and therefore may cause venous sinus thrombosis. Protein S deficiency and homocysteinemia may cause arterial thromboses as well. Systemic lupus erythematosus with Libman-Sacks endocarditis can be a cause of embolic stroke. These conditions overlap with the antiphospholipid syndrome, which probably requires long-term anticoagulation to prevent further stroke.

Venous sinus thrombosis of the lateral or sagittal sinus or of small cortical veins (cortical vein thrombosis) occurs as a complication of pregnancy and the postpartum period, sepsis, and intracranial infections (meningitis). It is seen with increased incidence in patients with laboratory-confirmed thrombophilia (Table 361-2) including polycythemia, sickle cell anemia, proteins C and S deficiency, factor V Leiden mutation (resistance to activated protein C), antithrombin III deficiency, homocysteinemia, and the prothrombin G20210 mutation. Women who take oral contraceptives and have the prothrombin G20210 mutation may be at high risk for sinus thrombosis. Patients present with headache, focal neurologic signs (especially paraparesis), and seizures. Often, CT imaging is normal unless an intracranial venous hemorrhage has occurred, but the venous sinus occlusion is readily visualized using MR venography or conventional x-ray angiography. With greater degrees of sinus thrombosis, the patient may develop signs of increased ICP and coma. Intravenous heparin, regardless of the presence of intracranial hemorrhage, has been shown to reduce morbidity and mortality, and the long-term outcome is generally good. Heparin prevents further thrombosis and reduces venous hypertension and ischemia. If an underlying hypercoagulable state is not found, many physicians treat with warfarin for 3 to 6 months then convert to aspirin, depending on the degree of resolution of the venous sinus clot, and continue indefinite anticoagulation if thrombophilia is diagnosed.

Fibromuscular dysplasia affects the cervical arteries and occurs mainly in women. The carotid or vertebral arteries show multiple rings of segmental narrowing alternating with dilatation. Occlusion is usually incomplete. The process is often asymptomatic but occasionally is associated with an audible bruit, TIAs, or stroke. The cause and natural history of fibromuscular dysplasia is unknown (Chap. 248). TIA or stroke generally occurs only when the artery is severely narrowed or dissects. Anticoagulation or antiplatelet therapy may be helpful.

Temporal (giant cell) arteritis (Chap. 317) is a relatively common affliction of elderly persons in which the external carotid system, particularly the temporal arteries, becomes the site of a subacute granulomatous inflammation with giant cells. Occlusion of posterior ciliary arteries derived from the ophthalmic artery results in blindness in one or both eyes and can be prevented with glucocorticoids. It rarely causes stroke as the internal carotid artery is usually not inflamed. Idiopathic giant cell arteritis involving the great vessels arising from the aortic arch (Takayasu's arteritis) may cause carotid or vertebral thrombosis; it is rare in the western hemisphere.

Necrotizing (or granulomatous) arteritis, occurring alone or in association with generalized polyarteritis nodosa or Wegener's granulomatosis, involves the distal small branches (<2 mm diameter) of the main intracranial arteries and produces small ischemic infarcts in the brain, optic nerve, and spinal cord. The cerebrospinal fluid often shows pleocytosis, and the protein level is elevated. *Primary central nervous system vasculitis* is rare; small or medium-sized vessels are usually affected. Brain biopsy or high-resolution conventional x-ray angiography is usually required to make the diagnosis. Patients with any form of vasculitis may present with insidious progression of combined white and gray matter infarctions, prominent headache, and cognitive decline. Aggressive immunosuppression with glucocorticoids, and often cyclophosphamide, is usually necessary to reverse the ischemia. Depending upon the duration of the disease, many patients can make an excellent recovery.

Drugs, in particular amphetamines and perhaps cocaine, may cause stroke on the basis of acute hypertension and drug-induced vasculitis. Abstinence appears to be the best treatment, as no data exist on use of any treatment.

Arteritis can also occur as a consequence of bacterial, tuberculous, and syphilitic meningitis.

Moyamoya disease is a poorly understood occlusive disease involving large intracranial arteries, especially the distal internal carotid artery and the stem of the middle and anterior cerebral arteries. Vascular inflammation is absent. The lenticulostriate arteries develop a rich collateral circulation around the occlusive lesion, which gives the impression of a "puff of smoke" ("moyamoya" in Japanese) on conventional x-ray angiography. Other collaterals include transdural anastomoses between the cortical surface branches of the meningeal and the scalp arteries. The disease occurs mainly in Asian children or young adults but can occur in adults who have atherosclerosis. The etiology of the childhood form is unknown. Because of the occurrence of SAH from rupture of the transdural anastomotic channels, anticoagulation is risky. Breakdown of dilated lenticulostriate arteries may produce parenchymal hemorrhage, and progressive occlusion of large surface arteries can occur, producing large artery distribution strokes. Bypass of extracranial carotid arteries to the dura or MCAs may prevent stroke and hemorrhage.

Reversible widespread cerebral segmental vasoconstriction is hypothesized to occur in certain patients with headache and fluctuating neurologic symptoms and signs. Sometimes cerebral infarction ensues. The cause is unknown. Head injury, migraine, sympathomimetic drug use, eclampsia, and the postpartum period have all been associated with this entity. Conventional x-ray angiography is the only means of establishing the diagnosis, but because angiography itself can cause spasm of vessels, even the existence of this vascular entity is debated.

Binswanger's disease (chronic progressive subcortical encephalopathy) is a rare condition in which infarction of the subcortical white matter occurs subacutely. CT or MRI scans detect periventricular white matter infarcts and gliosis. There is lipohyalinosis in the small arteries of the deep white matter, as in hypertension. There are usually associated lacunar infarcts. Binswanger's disease may represent a type of border zone ischemic infarction in the deep white matter between the penetrating arteries of the circle of Willis and of the cortex. The pathophysiologic basis of the disease is unclear, but it typically occurs in older patients with severe long-standing hypertension.

CADASIL (cerebral autosomal dominant arteriopathy with subcortical infarcts and leukoencephalopathy) is an inherited disorder that presents as small vessel strokes, progressive dementia, and extensive symmetric white matter changes visualized by MRI. Approximately 40% of patients have migraine with aura, often manifest as transient motor or sensory deficits. Onset is usually in the fourth or fifth decade of life. This autosomal dominant condition is caused by a missense mutation in Notch-3, a member of a highly conserved gene family characterized by epidermal growth factor repeats in its extracellular domain. Definitive diagnosis is made by brain biopsy revealing typical osmophilic inclusions within smooth-muscle cells of blood vessels; these inclusions may also be present in skin biopsy sections. CADASIL is the only monogenic ischemic stroke syndrome so far described. Genetic testing is not currently available except on a research basis.

℞ TREATMENT **Acute Stroke Management** After the clinical diagnosis of stroke is made, an orderly process of evaluation and treatment should follow (Table 361-4). The first goal is to prevent or reverse brain injury. After initial stabilization, an emergency noncontrast head CT scan should be performed to differentiate ischemic from hemorrhagic stroke; there are no reliable clinical findings that conclusively separate ischemia from hemorrhage, although a more depressed level of consciousness and higher initial blood pressure favor hemorrhage, and a deficit that remits suggests ischemia. The second goal is to obtain an accurate understanding of the stroke mechanism so one can halt progression of brain injury or begin to prevent a second stroke. Often this is done during an acute hospitalization, but depending on stroke severity, it may be performed in the outpatient setting. There exists no consensus on the rate with which this evaluation should proceed, primarily because there are few data on the daily risks of recurrence following an initial stroke.

General principles During focal brain ischemia, a gradation in brain perfusion exists such that a core of tissue is infarcted within minutes but a shell of surrounding tissue is only marginally ischemic.

This *ischemic penumbra* may progress to infarction within minutes to hours depending on a number of factors (Chap. 376). Salvage of this "at risk" tissue is the goal of emergency stroke therapy. The penumbral tissue will infarct with only minor drops in systemic blood pressure because cerebral autoregulation within this zone is impaired. *Therefore, a patient's blood pressure at presentation should not be lowered* unless it is >185/110 and thrombolytic therapy will be given (see below). Revascularization of the parent vessel occlusion can restore blood flow to the penumbra and prevent infarction. This concept fuels research into intravenous and intraarterial thrombolysis as well as mechanical means of arterial thrombectomy.

Treatments designed to reverse or lessen the amount of tissue infarction fall within five categories: (1) medical support, (2) thrombolysis, (3) anticoagulation, (4) antiplatelet agents, and (5) neuroprotection.

Medical support When cerebral infarction occurs, the immediate goal is to optimize cerebral perfusion in the surrounding ischemic area. Attention is also directed toward preventing the common complications of bedridden patients—infections (pneumonia, urinary tract, and skin) and deep venous thrombosis with pulmonary embolism.

Elevated blood pressure should not be lowered unless there is malignant hypertension (Chap. 246) or concomitant myocardial ischemia. When faced with the competing demands of myocardium and brain, heart rate lowering with the β_1-adrenergic blocker esmolol can be a first step to decrease cardiac work and maintain blood pressure. If the blood pressure is low, raising it is advisable, using intravenous fluids or vasopressor drugs to enhance perfusion within the ischemic penumbra. Fever is detrimental and should be treated with antipyretics.

Between 5 and 10% of patients develop enough cerebral edema to cause obtundation or brain herniation. Edema peaks on the second or third day but causes mass effect for 10 days. The larger the infarct, the greater the likelihood that clinically significant edema will develop. Even small amounts of cerebellar edema can acutely increase ICP in the posterior fossa. The resulting brainstem compression may result in coma and respiratory arrest and require emergency surgical decompression. Water restriction and intravenous mannitol may be used to raise the serum osmolarity, but hypovolemia should be avoided as this may contribute to hypotension and worsening infarction. Trials are under way to test the clinical benefits of craniotomy and elevation of the skull (hemicraniectomy) for large hemispheric infarcts with marked cerebral edema.

Thrombolysis The use of thrombolytic agents in acute cerebral infarction has been studied extensively. Angiography performed within a few hours of infarction frequently demonstrates arterial occlusions corresponding to patients' presenting signs and symptoms. It is this association of arterial occlusion with acute neurologic symptoms that prompted the study of thrombolytic agents in stroke patients.

Three early intravenous streptokinase trials were stopped because of a higher death rate in the streptokinase-treated patients, mainly due to symptomatic intracranial bleedings. These trials enrolled patients several hours into the stroke process, which may account for the high hemorrhage rates.

The European Cooperative Acute Stroke Study (ECASS) tested intravenous recombinant tissue plasminogen activator (rtPA; 1.1 mg/kg to a 100 mg max.; 10% as a bolus, then the remainder over 60 min) vs. placebo in patients with ischemic stroke within 6 h of onset of symptoms. The median time to treatment was 4 h. Overall, thrombolysis was not beneficial because of an excess of cerebral hemorrhage. However, in those patients who had no signs of major infarction on the initial CT scan, the functional outcome was improved.

The National Institute of Neurological Disorders and Stroke (NINDS) rtPA Stroke Study showed a clear benefit for rtPA in selected patients with acute stroke. The NINDS study used intravenous rtPA (0.9 mg/kg to a 90 mg max.; 10% as a bolus, then the remainder over 60 min) vs. placebo in patients with ischemic stroke within 3 h of onset. Half of the patients were treated within 90 min. Symptomatic intracerebral hemorrhage occurred in 6.4% of patients on rtPA and 0.6% on placebo. There was a nonsignificant 4% reduction in mortality on rtPA, (21% on placebo and 17% on rtPA) and a significant 12% absolute increase in the number of patients with only minimal disability (32% on placebo and 44% on rtPA.) Thus, despite an increased incidence of symptomatic intracerebral hemorrhage, treatment with intravenous rtPA within 3 h of the onset of ischemic stroke improved clinical outcome. A lower dose of rtPA was used than in the ECASS, and half of the patients were treated within 90 min of stroke onset. These two features may account for much of the increase in benefit and decrease in bleeding hazard compared to the results seen in ECASS.

Finally, ECASS-II tested the NINDS dose of rtPA (0.9 mg/kg, maximum dose 90 mg) but allowed patients to receive drug up to the sixth hour, as in ECASS-I. No significant benefit was found, but improvement was found in post hoc analyses.

Because of the marked differences in trial design, including drug and dose used, time to thrombolysis, and severity of stroke, the precise efficacy of intravenous thrombolytics for acute ischemic stroke remains unclear. The risk of intracranial hemorrhage appears to rise with larger strokes, longer times from onset of symptoms, and higher doses of rtPA administered. The established dose of 0.9 mg/kg administered intravenously within 3 h of stroke onset appears safe. Many hospitals have developed expert stroke teams to facilitate this treatment. The drug is now approved in the United States and Canada for acute stroke when given within 3 h from the time the stroke symptoms began, and efforts should be made to give it as early in this 3-h window as possible. The time of stroke onset is defined as the time the patient's symptoms began or the time the patient was last seen as normal. A patient who awakens with stroke has the onset defined as when they went to bed. Table 361-6 summarizes eligibility criteria and instructions for administration of rtPA.

A recent trial of the fibrinolytic agent ancrod provides further evidence that this approach is effective in acute ischemic stroke.

There is growing interest in using thrombolytics via an intraarterial

Table 361-6 Administration of Intravenous Recombinant Tissue Plasminogen Activator (rtPA) for Acute Ischemic Stroke[a]

Indication	Contraindication
Clinical diagnosis of stroke	Sustained BP > 185/110
Onset of symptoms to time of drug administration ≤3 h	Platelets < 100,000; HCT < 25%; glucose < 50 or > 400
CT scan showing no hemorrhage or significant edema	Use of heparin within 48 h and prolonged PTT, or elevated INR
Age ≥18 years	Rapidly improving symptoms
Consent by patient or surrogate	Prior stroke or head injury within 3 months; prior intracranial hemorrhage
	Major surgery in preceding 14 days
	Minor stroke symptoms
	Gastrointestinal bleeding in preceding 21 days
	Recent myocardial infarction
	Coma or stupor

Administration of rtPA
- Intravenous access with two peripheral IV lines (avoid arterial or central line placement)
- Review eligibility for rtPA
- Administer 0.9 mg/kg intravenously (maximum 90 mg) IV as 10% of total dose by bolus, followed by remainder of total dose over 1 h
- Continous cuff blood pressure monitoring
- No other antithrombotic treatment for 24 h
- For decline in neurologic status or uncontrolled blood pressure, stop infusion, give cryoprecipitate, and reimage brain emergently
- Avoid urethral catheterization for ≥2 h

[a] See Activase (tissue plasminogen activator) package insert for complete list of contraindications and dosing.

NOTE: BP, blood pressure; CT, computed tomography; HCT, hematocrit; INR, international normalized ratio; PTT, partial thromboplastin time.

route to increase the concentration of drug at the clot and minimize systemic bleeding complications. Two recent trials [PROACT and PROACT II (prolyse in acute cerebral thromboembolism)] using intraarterial thrombolysis for acute MCA occlusions up to the sixth hour following onset of stroke showed benefit. Nevertheless, intraarterial use in ischemic stroke is not approved by the FDA. Intraarterial treatment of basilar artery occlusions may also be beneficial for selected patients, but all intraarterial therapy remains experimental.

Anticoagulation The role of anticoagulation in atherothrombotic cerebral ischemia is uncertain. Several recent trials have investigated antiplatelet versus anticoagulant medications given within 12 to 24 h of the initial event. The U.S. Trial of Organon 10172 in Acute Stroke Treatment (TOAST), an investigational low-molecular-weight heparin, failed to show any benefit over aspirin. Use of subcutaneous unfractionated heparin versus aspirin was tested in two trials, the International Stroke Trial (IST) and the Chinese Acute Stroke Trial (CAST). Taken together, the trials, which studied an aggregate of 40,541 patients, showed a reduction in stroke and death by 1% within 2 to 4 weeks in patients treated with aspirin rather than placebo. Heparin given subcutaneously [without monitoring the partial thromboplastin time (PTT)] afforded no additional benefit over aspirin and increased bleeding rates. Therefore, trials do not support the use of heparin for patients with atherothrombotic stroke of ≥12 h duration.

The use of antiplatelet or anticoagulant medication in acute stroke (i.e., <6 h) is less well studied. Heparin is widely used for crescendo TIAs, despite the absence of data from controlled studies regarding this indication. In approximately 20% of patients with acute stroke, deficits will progress over several hours to 1–2 days. Many physicians heparinize all patients with recent mild ischemic stroke in order to prevent some of this worsening. Theoretically, heparin may prevent propagation of clot within a thrombosed vessel or may prevent more emboli from occurring. Some neurologists use heparin until carotid and intracranial vessel patency can be assessed then convert to aspirin if the large vessels are patent. The bleeding complication rate for 7 days of heparin is about 10% with a serious bleed rate of ~2%. Clearly the value of this approach must be clarified.

Heparinization is generally accomplished by beginning an infusion without bolus and is monitored to maintain the activated PTT at approximately twice normal. This regimen is maintained for 2 to 5 days. During this time the patient is monitored for hemorrhagic complications, the evaluation is completed, and a decision is made regarding the need for carotid endarterectomy, long-term anticoagulation, or an antiplatelet therapy. If long-term anticoagulation is chosen, warfarin is administered and heparin discontinued when the international normalized ratio (INR) is in the range of 2 to 3.

Antiplatelet agents Aspirin is the only antiplatelet agent that has been prospectively studied for the treatment of acute ischemic stroke. The recent large trials, IST and CAST, found that the use of aspirin within 48 h of stroke onset reduced both stroke recurrence risk and mortality minimally. Among 19,435 patients in IST, those allocated to aspirin had slightly fewer deaths within 14 days (9.0 vs. 9.4%), significantly fewer recurrent ischemic strokes (2.8 vs. 3.9%), no excess of hemorrhagic strokes (0.9 vs. 0.8%), and a trend towards a reduction in death or dependence at 6 months (61.2 vs. 63.5%). In CAST, 21,106 patients with ischemic stroke received 160 mg/d of aspirin or a placebo for up to 4 weeks. There were very small reductions in the aspirin group in early mortality (3.3 vs. 3.9%), recurrent ischemic strokes (1.6 vs. 2.1%), and dependency at discharge or death (30.5 vs. 31.6%). These trials demonstrate that the use of aspirin in the treatment of acute ischemic stroke is safe and produces a small but definite net benefit. For every 1000 acute strokes treated with aspirin, about 9 deaths or nonfatal stroke recurrences will be prevented in the first few weeks and approximately 13 fewer patients will be dead or dependent at 6 months.

Agents that act at the glycoprotein IIb/IIIa receptor are undergoing clinical trials in acute stroke treatment.

Neuroprotection Neuroprotection is the concept of providing a treatment that prolongs the brain's tolerance to ischemia long enough to allow other measures to be employed to mitigate ischemia. Hypothermia is probably the most powerful neuroprotectant but is only now the subject of clinical trials. Drugs that block the excitatory amino acid pathways have been shown to protect neurons and glia in animals, but despite multiple clinical trials they have not yet been proven to be beneficial in humans.

Primary and Secondary Prevention • ***General principles*** A number of medical and surgical interventions, as well as life-style modifications, are available for preventing stroke. Some of these can be widely applied because of their low cost and minimal risk; others are expensive and carry substantial risk, but may be valuable for selected high-risk patients.

Evaluation of a patient's *clinical risk profile* can help determine which preventive treatments to offer. In addition to known risk factors for ischemic stroke (above), certain clinical characteristics also contribute to an increased risk of stroke (Table 361-3). The North American Symptomatic Carotid Endarterectomy Trial (NASCET; see below) found that even in patients with the same degree of carotid artery stenosis, specifically 70 to 99%, nine prospectively selected risk factors predicted the risk of vascular outcomes in the medically treated patients. The overall risk of stroke was much greater in a high-risk group (those with more than six risk factors) than in a low-risk group (those with fewer than six risk factors). Fully 39% of patients in the high-risk group treated medically experienced an ipsilateral stroke within 2 years. The rate for the low-risk group was less than half that but was still 17%.

Atherosclerosis risk factors The relationship of various factors to the risk of atherosclerosis is described in Chap. 241. Older age, family history of thrombotic stroke, diabetes mellitus, hypertension, tobacco smoking, elevated blood cholesterol, and other factors are either proven or probable risk factors for ischemic stroke, largely by their link to atherosclerosis. Hypertension is the most significant of the risk factors; in general, all hypertension should be treated. The presence of known cerebrovascular disease is not a contraindication to treatment aimed at achieving normotension. Also, the value of treating systolic hypertension in older patients has been clearly established. Care must be taken to avoid overtreatment of hypertension, however; the treatment goal is to achieve normotension gradually.

Treatment of hypercholesterolemia has been well established for coronary artery disease but has been studied little in the prevention of stroke. In several recent studies, statin drugs were found to lower stroke risk. Since coronary artery disease is the most common cause of death in patients with cerebrovascular disease, treatment of hypercholesterolemia seems prudent for both the heart and brain. Tobacco smoking should be discouraged in all patients (Chap. 390). Whether or not tight control of blood sugar in patients with diabetes lowers stroke risk is uncertain.

Antiplatelet agents • ATHEROTHROMBOTIC STROKE *Platelet antiaggregation agents* can prevent atherothrombotic events, including TIA and stroke, by inhibiting the formation of intraarterial platelet aggregates. These can form on diseased arteries, induce thrombus formation, and occlude the artery or embolize into the distal circulation. Aspirin, clopidogrel, and the combination of aspirin plus extended-release dipyridamole are the antiplatelet agents used most for this purpose. Ticlopidine has been largely abandoned because of its adverse effects.

Aspirin is the most widely studied antiplatelet agent. Its antiplatelet effect is accomplished by acetylating the cyclooxygenase enzyme in platelets. This irreversibly inhibits the formation in platelets of thromboxane A_2, a platelet aggregating and vasoconstricting prostaglandin. This effect is permanent and lasts for the usual 8-day life of the platelet. Paradoxically, aspirin also inhibits the formation in endothelial cells of prostacyclin, an antiaggregating and vasodilating prostaglandin. This effect is transient. As soon as the aspirin is cleared from the blood, the nucleated endothelial cells again produce prostacyclin. Aspirin in low doses given once daily inhibits the production of thromboxane A_2 in platelets without substantially inhibiting prostacyclin formation. The FDA recommends 50 to 325 mg of aspirin daily for stroke prevention.

Ticlopidine blocks the ADP receptor on platelets and thus prevents the cascade resulting in activation of the glycoprotein IIb/IIIa receptor that leads to fibrinogen binding to the platelet and consequent platelet aggregation. Ticlopidine is more effective than aspirin; however, it has the disadvantage of causing diarrhea, skin rash, a low incidence of neutropenia, and thrombotic thrombocytopenic purpura. Clopidogrel works by the same mechanism as ticlopidine and is not associated with these important side effects. Although many physicians have accepted clopidogrel as equivalent to ticlopidine in stroke prevention, the CAPRIE (Clopidogrel versus Aspirin in Patients at Risk of Ischemic Events) trial, which led to FDA approval, showed less robust efficacy. Studies of clopidogrel in combination with aspirin are in progress in both cerebrovascular and cardiovascular patients.

Dipyridamole is an antiplatelet agent that inhibits the uptake of adenosine by a variety of cells, including those of the vascular endothelium. The accumulated adenosine is an inhibitor of aggregation. At least in part through its effects on platelet and vessel wall phosphodiesterases, dipyridamole also potentiates the antiaggregatory effects of prostacyclin and nitric oxide produced by the endothelium and acts by inhibiting platelet phosphodiesterase, which is responsible for the breakdown of cyclic AMP. The resulting elevation in cyclic AMP inhibits aggregation of platelets. Dipyridamole has a controversial history in stroke prevention. The European Stroke Prevention Study-2 showed efficacy of both 50 mg daily of aspirin and extended-release dipyridamole in preventing stroke, and a significantly better risk reduction when the two agents were combined. A combination capsule of extended-release dipyridamole and aspirin is approved for prevention of stroke.

Many large clinical trials have demonstrated clearly that most antiplatelet agents reduce the risk of all important vascular atherothrombotic events (i.e., ischemic stroke, myocardial infarction, and death due to all vascular causes) in patients at risk for these events. The overall *relative* reduction in risk of nonfatal stroke is about 25 to 30% and of all vascular events is about 25%. The *absolute* reduction varies considerably depending on the particular patient's risk. Individuals at very low risk for stroke seem to experience the same relative reduction, but their risk may be so low that the "benefit" is meaningless. On the other hand, individuals with a 10 to 15% risk of vascular events per year experience a reduction to about 7.5 to 11%.

Aspirin is inexpensive, can be given in low doses, and could be recommended for all adults to prevent both stroke and myocardial infarction. However, it causes epigastric discomfort, gastric ulceration, and gastrointestinal hemorrhage, which may be asymptomatic or life-threatening. Consequently, not every 40- or 50-year old should be advised to take aspirin regularly because the risk of atherothrombotic stroke is extremely low and is outweighed by the risk of adverse side effects. Conversely, every patient who has experienced an atherothrombotic stroke and has no contraindication should be taking an antiplatelet agent regularly because the average annual risk of another stroke is 8 to 10%; another few percent will experience a myocardial infarction or vascular death. Clearly, the likelihood of benefit far outweighs the risks of treatment.

The choice of antiplatelet agent, and dose, similarly must balance the risk of stroke against the risks and cost of the treatments against the expected benefits. But these data are less definitive, and opinions therefore vary. Many authorities believe low-dose (30 to 75 mg daily) and high-dose (650 to 1300 mg daily) aspirin are about equally effective. Some advocate very low doses to avoid adverse effects, and still others advocate very high doses to be sure the benefit is maximal. Most physicians in North America recommend 325 mg daily, while most Europeans recommend 50 to 100 mg. Similarly, the choice of aspirin, clopidogrel, or dipyridamole plus aspirin must balance the fact that the latter are more effective than aspirin but the cost is higher.

EMBOLIC STROKE Although warfarin is more effective than aspirin in preventing ischemic stroke associated with atrial fibrillation, some patients with atrial fibrillation have a low rate of ischemic stroke, and others have a high risk of hemorrhage and lose all of the expected benefit of anticoagulation by this complication. Still others are at such high risk for ischemic stroke that the benefits of warfarin override even the high hemorrhage rate. Preventive treatment depends on knowing the relative risks and benefits for the particular patient.

The Stroke Prevention in Atrial Fibrillation II trial showed that in "low-risk" patients (those without hypertension, recent heart failure, or prior thromboembolism) younger than 75 years given aspirin, the thromboembolism rate was only 0.5% per year. Consequently, one could reasonably recommend that patients <75 years with no risk factors be treated with aspirin only (Table 361-5).

Anticoagulation therapy • *ATHEROTHROMBOTIC STROKE* There are few data to support the use of long-term warfarin for preventing atherothrombotic stroke, either intracranially or extracranially. Several large trials are in progress.

EMBOLIC STROKE Several recent trials demonstrated that anticoagulation (INR range 2 to 3) in patients with chronic nonvalvular (nonrheumatic) atrial fibrillation prevents cerebral embolism and is safe. For primary prevention and for patients who have experienced stroke or TIA, anticoagulation with warfarin reduces the risk by about 65% and clearly outweighs the 1% per year rate of major bleeding complication.

The decision to use anticoagulation for primary prevention is based primarily on risk factors (Table 361-5). The presence of any risk factor tips the balance in favor of anticoagulation.

Because of the high annual stroke risk in untreated rheumatic heart disease, primary prophylaxis against stroke has not been studied in a double-blind fashion. These patients generally receive long-term anticoagulation.

Anticoagulation also reduces the risk of embolism in acute myocardial infarction. Most clinicians recommend a 3-month course of anticoagulation when there is anterior Q-wave infarction, substantial left ventricular dysfunction, congestive heart failure, mural thrombosis, or atrial fibrillation. Warfarin is recommended long-term if atrial fibrillation persists.

Thromboembolism is one of the most serious complications of prosthetic heart valve implantation. Anticoagulation has been proven effective for preventing strokes in this situation, while antiplatelet therapy alone has not. However, coupled with warfarin anticoagulation, aspirin adds substantial benefit. A greater degree of anticoagulation (INR of 3 to 4, depending on valve type) is recommended for prosthetic heart valve patients.

If the embolic source cannot be eliminated, anticoagulation should in most cases be continued indefinitely. Many neurologists recommend combining antiplatelet agents with anticoagulants for patients who "fail" one form of therapy (i.e., have another stroke of TIA). This empirical approach subjects the patient to an increased bleeding risk.

Secondary prophylaxis for ischemic stroke of unknown origin is controversial. Some physicians prescribe anticoagulation for 3 to 6 months followed by antiplatelet treatment. The results of ongoing stroke trials may help to clarify the best treatment.

SURGICAL THERAPY Surgery for atherosclerotic occlusive disease is largely limited to *carotid endarterectomy* for plaques located at the origin of the internal carotid artery in the neck (see below).

Balloon angioplasty coupled with stenting is being used with increasing frequency to open stenotic carotid arteries and maintain their patency. This method has not been compared prospectively with endarterectomy. Concern exists about distal embolization of plaque during vessel dilation. Some neurointerventional centers are treating *intracranial* atherosclerotic disease with angioplasty and stenting. Surgery in the proximal common carotid, the subclavian, and the vertebral arteries is uncommon and is being replaced by endovascular stenting and angioplasty. Extracranial to intracranial bypass surgery has been proven ineffective for atherosclerotic stenoses that are inaccessible to conventional carotid endarterectomy. Although experimental, bypass surgery may have a role in patients with moyamoya disease or the unusual patient with intracranial stenosis and flow-related TIA.

Carotid disease Carotid endarterectomy is a proven effective prophylaxis against stroke and TIA. Approximately 100,000 of these procedures are performed annually in the United States to remove obstructing atherosclerotic plaques. The most important clinical distinction is between symptomatic and asymptomatic carotid stenosis. Symptomatic stenosis is defined as carotid stenosis ipsilateral to the vascular distribution of a stroke or TIA; e.g., a left carotid stenosis in a patient with transient expressive aphasia. Asymptomatic carotid stenosis is defined by the absence of clinical signs or symptoms of stroke or TIA relevant to the carotid lesion. The distinction is important because the natural history of these conditions is markedly different.

Symptomatic carotid stenosis was studied in the NASCET and the European Carotid Surgery Trial (ECST). Both showed a substantial benefit for surgery in patients with a stenosis of >70%. In NASCET, the average cumulative ipsilateral stroke rate at 2 years was 26% for patients treated medically and 9% for those receiving the same medical treatment plus a carotid endarterectomy. This 17% *absolute* reduction in the surgical group is a 65% *relative* risk reduction favoring surgery. NASCET also showed a significant benefit for patients with 50 to 70% stenosis, although less robust. ECST found harm for patients with stenosis in the 0 to 30% range treated surgically.

A patient's risk of stroke and possible benefit from surgery is related to the presence of retinal versus hemispheric symptoms, degree of arterial stenosis, extent of associated medical conditions, institutional surgical morbidity and mortality, and other factors. A patient with multiple atherosclerosis risk factors, symptomatic hemispheric ischemia, very high grade stenosis in the appropriate internal carotid artery, and an institutional perioperative morbidity and mortality rate of ≤6% generally should undergo carotid endarterectomy. If the perioperative stroke rate is >6% for any particular surgeon, however, the benefits of carotid endarterectomy are lost.

The indications for surgical treatment of *asymptomatic carotid disease* have been clarified by the results of the Asymptomatic Carotid Atherosclerosis Study (ACAS), which randomized patients with ≥60% stenosis to medical treatment with aspirin or the same medical treatment plus carotid endarterectomy. The surgical group had a risk over 5 years for ipsilateral stroke (and any perioperative stroke or death) of 5.1%, compared to a risk in the medical group of 11%. While this demonstrates a 53% *relative* risk reduction, the *absolute* risk reduction is only 5.9% over 5 years, or 1.2% annually. The perioperative complication rate was higher in women, so they received only a 17% relative risk reduction over 5 years. Nearly half of the strokes in the surgery group were caused by preoperative angiograms.

The natural history of asymptomatic stenosis is an approximate 2% per year stroke rate, while symptomatic patients experience a 13% per year risk of stroke. Whether to recommend carotid revascularization for an asymptomatic patient remains controversial and depends on many factors including patient preference, age, and comorbidities. Medical therapy for reduction of atherosclerosis risk factors and aspirin, 325 mg/d, are generally recommended for patients with asymptomatic carotid stenosis. As with atrial fibrillation, it is imperative to counsel the patient about TIAs so their therapy can be revised if they become symptomatic.

Stroke Centers and Rehabilitation Comprehensive stroke units that care for the acute patient followed by rehabilitation services have been shown to improve neurologic outcomes and reduce mortality. Use of clinical pathways and dedicating staff to the stroke patient can improve the efficacy of care. Stroke teams that provide emergency 24-h evaluation of acute stroke patients for consideration of thrombolysis and acute medical management are essential components of the care process.

Proper rehabilitation of the stroke patient includes early physical, occupational, and speech therapy. It is directed toward educating the patient and family about the patient's neurologic deficit, preventing the complications of immobility (e.g., pneumonia, deep vein thrombosis and pulmonary embolism, pressure sores of the skin, muscle contractures), and providing encouragement and instruction in overcoming the deficit. The goal of rehabilitation is to return the patient to home and to maximize recovery by providing a safe, progressive regimen suited to the individual patient.

Table 361-7 Causes of Intracranial Hemorrhage

Cause	Location	Comments
Head trauma	Intraparenchymal: frontal lobes, anterior temporal lobes; subarachnoid	Coup and contracoup injury during brain deceleration
Hypertensive hemorrhage	Putamen, globus pallidus, thalamus, cerebellar hemisphere, pons	Chronic hypertension produces hemorrhage from small (~100 μm) vessels in these regions
Transformation of prior ischemic infarction	Basal ganglion, subcortical regions, lobar	Occurs in 1–6% of ischemic strokes with predilection for large hemispheric infarctions
Metastatic brain tumor	Lobar	Lung, choriocarcinoma, melanoma, renal cell carcinoma, thyroid, atrial myxoma
Coagulopathy	Any	Uncommon cause; often associated with prior stroke or underlying vascular anomaly
Drug	Lobar, subarachnoid	Cocaine, amphetamine
Arteriovenous malformation	Lobar, intraventricular, subarachnoid	Risk is approximately 2–4% per year for bleeding
Aneurysm	Subarachnoid, intraparenchymal, rarely subdural	Mycotic and nonmycotic forms of aneurysms
Amyloid angiopathy	Lobar	Degenerative disease of intracranial vessels; linkage to Alzheimer's disease, rare in patients <60
Cavernous angioma	Intraparenchymal	Multiple cavernous angiomas linked to chromosome 7q
Dural arteriovenous fistula	Lobar, rarely subarachnoid	Produces bleeding by venous hypertension
Capillary telangiectasias	Usually brainstem	Rare cause of hemorrhage

INTRACRANIAL HEMORRHAGE

Blood can extravasate anywhere within the cranial vault or spinal column. Hemorrhages are classified by their location and the underlying vascular pathology. Bleeding into subdural and epidural spaces is principally produced by trauma (Chap. 369). Intraparenchymal, intraventricular, and subarachnoid hemorrhage will be considered here.

DIAGNOSIS Intracranial hemorrhage is often discovered on noncontrast CT imaging of the brain during the acute evaluation of stroke. CT is more sensitive than routine MRI for acute blood. The location of hemorrhage narrows the differential diagnosis to a few entities. Table 361-7 lists the causes and anatomic spaces involved in hemorrhages.

EMERGENCY MANAGEMENT Close attention should be paid to airway management since a reduction in the level of consciousness is common. The initial blood pressure should be maintained until the results of the CT scan are reviewed. Patients with acute SAH should have blood pressure lowered to a normal range with nonvasodilating agents such as labetalol or esmolol. Patients with cerebellar hemorrhages or with depressed mental status and radiographic evidence of hydrocephalus should undergo urgent neurosurgical evaluation. Based on the clinical examination and CT findings, further imaging studies may be necessary, including MRI or conventional x-ray angiography. Stuporous or comatose patients generally are treated presumptively for elevated ICP, with tracheal intubation and hyperventilation, mannitol administration, and elevation of the head of the bed while surgical consultation is obtained (Chap. 376).

INTRAPARENCHYMAL HEMORRHAGE Intraparenchymal hemorrhage is the most common type of intracranial hemorrhage. It is an important cause of stroke, especially in Asians and blacks. Hypertension, trauma, and cerebral amyloid angiopathy cause the majority of these hemorrhages. Advanced age and heavy alcohol consumption increase the risk, and cocaine use is one of the most important causes in the young.

Hypertensive Intraparenchymal Hemorrhage • ***Pathophysiology*** Hypertensive parenchymal hemorrhage (hypertensive hemorrhage or hypertensive intracerebral hemorrhage) usually results from spontaneous rupture of a small penetrating artery deep in the brain. The most common sites are the basal ganglia (putamen, thalamus, and adjacent deep white matter), deep cerebellum, and pons. When hemorrhages occur in other brain areas or in nonhypertensive patients, greater consideration should be given to hemorrhagic disorders, neoplasms, vascular malformations, and other causes. The small arteries in these areas seem most prone to hypertension-induced vascular injury. The hemorrhage may be small or a large clot may form and compress adjacent tissue, causing herniation and death. Blood may dissect into the ventricular space, which substantially increases morbidity and may cause hydrocephalus. If the patient survives, the clot liquefies, is absorbed, and leaves only a small residual cleft.

Most hypertensive intraparenchymal hemorrhages develop over 30 to 90 min, whereas those associated with anticoagulant therapy may evolve for as long as 24 to 48 h. Within 48 h macrophages begin to phagocytize the hemorrhage at its outer surface. After 1 to 6 months, the hemorrhage is generally resolved to a slitlike orange cavity lined with glial scar and hemosiderin-laden macrophages.

Clinical manifestations Although not particularly associated with exertion, intracerebral hemorrhages almost always occur while the patient is awake and sometimes when stressed. The hemorrhage generally presents as the abrupt onset of focal neurologic deficit. Seizures are uncommon. The focal deficit typically worsens steadily over 30 to 90 min and is associated with a diminishing level of consciousness and signs of increased ICP, such as headache and vomiting.

The putamen is the most common site for hypertensive hemorrhage, and the adjacent internal capsule is invariably damaged (Fig. 361-11). Contralateral hemiparesis is therefore the sentinel sign. When mild, the face sags on one side over 5 to 30 min, speech becomes slurred, the arm and leg gradually weaken, and the eyes deviate away from the side of the hemiparesis. The paralysis may worsen until the affected limbs become flaccid or extend rigidly with a Babinski sign on the same side. When hemorrhages are large, drowsiness gives way to stupor as signs of upper brainstem compression appear. Coma ensues, accompanied by deep, irregular, or intermittent respiration; a dilated and fixed ipsilateral pupil; bilateral Babinski signs; and decerebrate rigidity. In milder cases, edema in adjacent brain tissue may cause progressive deterioration over 12 to 72 h.

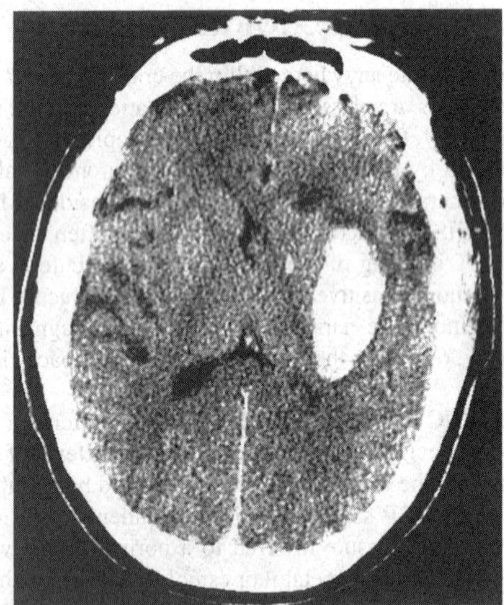

FIGURE 361-11 Acute onset of right hemiparesis. Transaxial noncontrast CT scan through the region of the basal ganglia reveals a hematoma involving the left putamen. This is a typical hypertensive hemorrhage.

Thalamic hemorrhages also produce a contralateral hemiplegia or hemiparesis from pressure on, or dissection into, the adjacent internal capsule. A prominent sensory deficit involving all modalities is usually present. Aphasia, often with preserved verbal repetition, may occur after hemorrhage into the dominant thalamus, and apractognosia or mutism occurs in some cases of nondominant hemorrhage. There may also be a homonymous visual field defect. Thalamic hemorrhages cause several typical ocular disturbances by virtue of extension medially into the upper midbrain. These include deviation of the eyes downward and inward so that they appear to be looking at the nose, unequal pupils with absence of light reaction, skew deviation with the eye opposite the hemorrhage displaced downward and medially, ipsilateral Horner's syndrome, absence of convergence, paralysis of vertical gaze, and retraction nystagmus. Patients may later develop a chronic, contralateral pain syndrome (see Déjerine-Roussy syndrome, above).

In pontine hemorrhages, deep coma with quadriplegia usually occurs over a few minutes. There is often prominent decerebrate rigidity and "pin-point" (1 mm) pupils that react to light. There is impairment of reflex horizontal eye movements evoked by head turning (doll's-head or oculocephalic maneuver) or by irrigation of the ears with ice water (Chap. 24). Hyperpnea, severe hypertension, and hyperhidrosis are common. Death usually occurs within a few hours, but there are occasional survivors.

Cerebellar hemorrhages usually develop over several hours and are characterized by occipital headache, repeated vomiting, and ataxia of gait. In mild cases there may be no other neurologic signs other than gait ataxia. Dizziness or vertigo may be prominent. There is often paresis of conjugate lateral gaze toward the side of the hemorrhage, forced deviation of the eyes to the opposite side, or an ipsilateral sixth nerve palsy. Less frequent ocular signs include blepharospasm, involuntary closure of one eye, ocular bobbing, and skew deviation. Dysarthria and dysphagia may occur. There are no Babinski signs until late in the evolution of the hemorrhage as it compresses or dissects into the ventral brainstem. As the hours pass, the patient often becomes stuporous and then comatose from brainstem compression or obstructive hydrocephalus; immediate surgical evacuation may be lifesaving.

Laboratory and Imaging Evaluation The CT scan reliably detects acute focal hemorrhages in the supratentorial space. Small pontine hemorrhages may not be identified because of motion and bone-induced artifact that obscure structures in the posterior fossa. After the first 2 weeks, x-ray attenuation values of clotted blood diminish until they become isodense with surrounding brain. Mass effect and edema may remain. In some cases, a surrounding rim of contrast enhancement appears after 2 to 4 weeks and may persist for months. MRI, though more sensitive for delineating posterior fossa lesions, is generally not necessary in most instances. Images of flowing blood on MRI scan may identify arteriovenous malformations (AVMs) as the cause of the hemorrhage. MRI and conventional x-ray angiography are used when the cause of intracranial hemorrhage is uncertain, particularly if the patient is young or not hypertensive and the hematoma is not in one of the four usual sites for hypertensive hemorrhage. For example, hemorrhage into the temporal lobe suggests rupture of a MCA saccular aneurysm.

Since these patients typically have focal neurologic signs and obtundation, and often show signs of increased ICP, an LP should be avoided as it may induce cerebral herniation.

℞ TREATMENT **Acute Management** Nearly 50% of patients with a hypertensive intracerebral hemorrhage die. The volume and location of the hematoma determine the prognosis. In general, supratentorial hematomas with volumes <30 mL have a good prognosis, 30 to 60 mL an intermediate prognosis, and >60 mL a poor prognosis during initial hospitalization. Infratentorial pontine hematomas >3 cm are usually fatal. Extension into the ventricular system, especially the fourth ventricle, worsens the prognosis. Except in patients who are on therapeutic anticoagulation or who have a bleeding disorder, little can be done about the hemorrhage itself. Hematomas may expand for several hours following the initial hemorrhage, so treating severe hypertension seems reasonable to prevent hematoma progression. As with ischemic stroke, lowering blood pressure too much or too quickly might cause cerebral ischemia around the hemorrhage cavity.

Evacuation of the hematoma is usually not helpful, except in cerebellar hemorrhages. For cerebellar hemorrhages, a neurosurgeon should be consulted immediately to assist with the evaluation; most cerebellar hematomas >3 cm in diameter will require surgical evacuation. If the patient is alert without focal brainstem signs and if the hematoma is <1 cm in diameter, surgical removal is usually unnecessary. Patients with hematomas between 1 and 3 cm require careful observation for signs of impaired consciousness, which usually means surgery is required.

Tissue surrounding hematomas is displaced and compressed but not necessarily infarcted. Hence, in survivors, major improvement commonly results as the hematoma is reabsorbed and the adjacent tissue regains its function. Careful management of the patient during the acute phase of the hemorrhage can lead to considerable recovery.

Surprisingly, despite large intraparenchymal hemorrhages, ICP is often not elevated. However, if the hematoma causes marked midline shift of structures with consequent obtundation or coma or hydrocephalus, osmotic agents coupled with induced hyperventilation can be instituted to lower ICP (Chap. 376). These maneuvers will provide enough time to place a ventriculostomy or ICP monitor. Once ICP is recorded, further hyperventilation and osmotic therapy can be tailored to the individual patient. For example, if ICP is found to be high, cerebrospinal fluid (CSF) can be drained from the ventricular space and osmotic therapy continued; persistent or progressive elevation in ICP may prompt surgical evacuation of the clot or withdrawal of support. Alternately, if ICP is normal or only mildly elevated, induced hyperventilation can be reversed and osmotic therapy tapered. Since hyperventilation may actually produce ischemia by cerebral vasoconstriction, as a general management principal induced hyperventilation should be limited to acute resuscitation of the patient with presumptive high ICP and eliminated once other treatments (osmotic therapy or surgical treatments) have been instituted. Glucocorticoids are not helpful for the edema from intracerebral hematoma.

Prevention Hypertension is the leading cause of primary intracerebral hemorrhage. Prevention is aimed at reducing hypertension, excessive alcohol use, and use of illicit drugs such as cocaine and amphetamines.

OTHER CAUSES OF INTRACEREBRAL HEMORRHAGE *Cerebral amyloid angiopathy* is a disease of the elderly in which arteriolar degeneration occurs and amyloid is deposited in the walls of the cerebral arteries but not elsewhere. Amyloid angiopathy causes both single and recurrent lobar hemorrhages and is probably the most common cause of lobar hemorrhage in the elderly. It accounts for some intracranial hemorrhages associated with intravenous thrombolysis given for myocardial infarction. This disorder can be suspected in patients who present with multiple hemorrhages (and infarcts) over several months or years, but it is definitively diagnosed by demonstration of Congo red staining of amyloid in cerebral vessels.

Cocaine-induced stroke is an important cause of stroke, particularly in patients <40. Intracerebral hemorrhage, ischemic stroke, and SAH are all associated with cocaine use. Angiographic findings vary from completely normal arteries to large vessel occlusion or stenosis, vasospasm, or changes consistent with vasculitis. The mechanism of cocaine-related stroke is not known, but cocaine enhances sympathetic activity causing acute, sometimes severe, hypertension, and this may lead to hemorrhage. Slightly more than half of cocaine-related intracranial hemorrhages are intracerebral, and the rest are subarachnoid. In cases of SAH, a saccular aneurysm is usually identified. Presumably, acute hypertension causes aneurysmal rupture.

Head injury often causes intracranial bleeding. The common sites are intracerebral (especially temporal and inferior frontal lobes) and into the subarachnoid, subdural, and epidural spaces. Trauma must be considered in any patient with an unexplained acute neurologic deficit (hemiparesis, stupor, or confusion), particularly if the deficit occurred in the context of a fall (Chap. 369).

Intracranial hemorrhages associated with *anticoagulant therapy* can occur at any location; they are often lobar or subdural. Anticoagulant-related intracerebral hemorrhages may evolve slowly, over 24 to 48 h. Coagulopathy should be reversed with fresh-frozen plasma and vitamin K to limit the volume of hemorrhage. When intracerebral hemorrhage is associated with thrombocytopenia (platelet count <50,000/μl), transfusion of fresh platelets is indicated. Intracerebral hemorrhage associated with *hematologic disorders* (leukemia, aplastic anemia, thrombocytopenic purpura) can occur at any site and may present as multiple intracerebral hemorrhages. Skin and mucous membrane bleeding is usually evident and offers a diagnostic clue.

Hemorrhage into a *brain tumor* may be the first manifestation of neoplasm. Choriocarcinoma, malignant melanoma, renal cell carcinoma, and bronchogenic carcinoma are among the most common metastatic tumors associated with intracerebral hemorrhage. Glioblastoma multiforme in adults and medulloblastoma in children may also have areas of intracerebral hemorrhage.

Hypertensive encephalopathy is a complication of malignant hypertension. In this acute syndrome, severe hypertension is associated with headache, nausea, vomiting, convulsions, confusion, stupor, and coma. Focal or lateralizing neurologic signs, either transitory or permanent, may occur but are infrequent and therefore suggest some other vascular disease (hemorrhage, embolism, or atherosclerotic thrombosis). There are retinal hemorrhages, exudates, papilledema (hypertensive retinopathy grade IV), and evidence of renal and cardiac disease. In most cases ICP and CSF protein levels are elevated. The hypertension may be essential or due to chronic renal disease, acute glomerulonephritis, acute toxemia of pregnancy, pheochromocytoma, or other causes. Lowering the blood pressure reverses the process, but stroke can occur. Neuropathologic examination reveals multifocal to diffuse cerebral edema and hemorrhages of various sizes from petechial to massive. Microscopically, there are necrosis of arterioles, minute cerebral infarcts, and hemorrhages. The term *hypertensive encephalopathy* should be reserved for this syndrome and not for chronic recurrent headaches, dizziness, recurrent TIAs, or small strokes that often occur in association with high blood pressure.

Primary intraventricular hemorrhage is rare. It usually begins within the substance of the brain and dissects into the ventricular system without leaving signs of intraparenchymal hemorrhage. Vasculitis, usually polyarteritis nodosa or lupus erythematosus, can produce hemorrhage into any region of the central nervous system; most hemorrhages are associated with hypertension, but the arteritis itself may cause bleeding by disrupting the vessel wall. *Sepsis* can cause small petechial hemorrhages throughout the cerebral white matter. *Moyamoya disease*, mainly an occlusive arterial disease that causes ischemic symptoms, may on occasion produce multiple small aneurysms that rupture. Hemorrhages into the spinal cord are usually the result of an AVM or metastatic tumor. *Epidural spinal hemorrhage* produces a rapidly evolving syndrome of spinal cord or nerve root compression (Chap. 368).

Clinical Manifestations Symptoms and signs appear over several minutes. Most lobar hemorrhages are small and cause a restricted clinical syndrome that simulates an embolus to an artery supplying one lobe. For example, the major neurologic deficit with an occipital hemorrhage is hemianopia; with a left temporal hemorrhage, aphasia and delirium; with a parietal hemorrhage, hemisensory loss; and with frontal hemorrhage, arm weakness. Large hemorrhages may be associated with stupor or coma if they compress the thalamus or midbrain. Most patients with lobar hemorrhages have focal headaches, and more than half vomit or are drowsy. Stiff neck and seizures are uncommon. Spinal hemorrhages usually present with sudden back pain and some manifestation of myelopathy.

Laboratory and Imaging Evaluation CT scanning reliably detects even very small supratentorial hemorrhages. MRI is more sensitive for delineating associated abnormalities, such as aneurysm, vascular malformation, and neoplasm, and is superior for imaging the posterior fossa and spinal column. MRI with gadolinium contrast enhancement is useful for revealing tumors and AVMs. Using special sequences sensitive for hemosiderin, MRI may show evidence of multiple prior hemorrhages, suggesting amyloid angiopathy and vascular anomalies. Repeating an MRI scan at 4 to 8 weeks may be necessary to reveal the underlying cause of hemorrhage, as the acute hematoma may obscure an underlying vascular anomaly or tumor. Conventional x-ray angiography is used when the cause of hemorrhage is uncertain, especially in the young and the middle-aged, or when better delineation of vascular anomalies is necessary.

Treatment The recommendations for management of hypertensive intracerebral hemorrhage generally apply. If a causative lesion is found, it is treated appropriately.

SUBARACHNOID HEMORRHAGE Excluding head trauma, the most common cause of SAH is rupture of a saccular aneurysm. Other causes include bleeding from a vascular anomaly and extension into the subarachnoid space from a primary intracerebral hemorrhage. Many idiopathic SAHs are localized to the perimesencephalic cisterns and are benign; they probably have a venous or capillary source, and angiography is unrevealing.

Saccular Aneurysm Autopsy studies have found that 3 to 4% of the population harbor aneurysms, for a prevalence of 8 to 10 million people in the United States. The incidence of bleeding is only 25,000 to 30,000 cases per year. The mortality rate for patients who arrive alive at hospital is about 50% during the first month. Of those who survive, more than half are left with major neurologic deficits as a result of the initial hemorrhage, cerebral vasospasm with infarction, or hydrocephalus. If the patient survives but the aneurysm is not obliterated, the annual rebleed rate is about 3%. Given these alarming figures, the major therapeutic emphasis is on preventing the predictable early complications of the rupture.

Unruptured, asymptomatic aneurysms are much less dangerous than a recently ruptured aneurysm. The annual risk of rupture for aneurysms <10 mm in size is approximately 0.1%, and for aneurysms ≥10 mm in size is approximately 0.5%; the surgical morbidity far exceeds these percentages. As more data become available, a true risk-benefit analysis for treating these aneurysms will result.

Giant aneurysms, those >2.5 cm in diameter, occur at the same sites (see below) as small aneurysms and account for 5% of cases. The three most common locations are the terminal internal carotid artery, MCA bifurcation, and top of the basilar artery. Their risk of rupture is about 6% in the first year after identification and may remain high indefinitely. They often cause symptoms by compressing the adjacent brain or cranial nerves.

Mycotic aneurysms are usually located distal to the first bifurcation of major arteries of the circle of Willis. Most result from infected emboli due to bacterial endocarditis causing septic degeneration of arteries and subsequent dilatation and rupture. Whether these lesions should be sought and repaired prior to rupture, or left to heal spontaneously, is controversial.

Pathophysiology Saccular aneurysms occur at the bifurcations of the large arteries at the base of the brain; rupture is into the subarachnoid space in the basal cisterns and often into the parenchyma of the adjacent brain. Approximately 85% of aneurysms occur in the anterior circulation, mostly on the circle of Willis. Common sites include the junction of the anterior communicating artery with the anterior cerebral artery, the junction of the posterior communicating artery with the internal carotid artery, the bifurcation of the MCA, the top of the basilar artery, the junction of the basilar artery and the superior cerebellar artery or the anterior inferior cerebellar artery, and the junction of the vertebral artery and the posterior inferior cerebellar artery. About 20% of patients have multiple aneurysms, many at mirror sites bilaterally. As an aneurysm develops, it typically forms a neck with a dome. The length of the neck and the size of the dome vary greatly and are factors that are important in planning both neurosurgical obliteration or endovascular embolization. The arterial internal elastic lamina disappears at the base of the neck. The media thins, and connective tissue replaces smooth-muscle cells. At the site of rupture (most often the dome) the wall thins, and the tear that allows bleeding is often no more than 0.5 mm long. It is not currently possible to predict which aneurysms are likely to rupture, but limited data suggest that most ruptured aneurysms are >7 mm in diameter.

Clinical manifestations Most aneurysms present as a sudden SAH. At the moment of aneurysmal rupture with major SAH, the ICP suddenly rises. Abrupt, severe, and generalized vasospasm may occur transiently. These events may account for the sudden transient loss of consciousness that occurs in nearly half of patients. Sudden loss of consciousness may be preceded by a brief moment of excruciating headache, but most patients first complain of headache upon regaining consciousness. In 10% of cases, aneurysmal bleeding is severe enough to cause loss on consciousness for several days. In about 45% of cases, severe headache associated with exertion is the presenting complaint. The patient often calls the headache "the worst headache of my life." However, the clinician should be sensitive to the less dramatic features of sudden onset of headache or to a new or different headache than what the patient has ever experienced. The headache is usually generalized, and vomiting is common.

Although sudden headache in the absence of focal neurologic symptoms is the hallmark of aneurysmal rupture, focal neurologic deficits may occur. Anterior communicating artery or middle cerebral bifurcation aneurysms may rupture into the adjacent brain or subdural space and form a hematoma large enough to produce mass effect. The common deficits that result include hemiparesis, aphasia, and abulia.

Occasionally, prodromal symptoms suggest the location of a progressively enlarging unruptured aneurysm. A third cranial nerve palsy, particularly when associated with pupillary dilatation, loss of light reflex, and focal pain above or behind the eye, may occur with an expanding aneurysm at the junction of the posterior communicating artery and the internal carotid artery. A sixth nerve palsy may indicate an aneurysm in the cavernous sinus, and visual field defects can occur with an expanding supraclinoid carotid or anterior cerebral artery aneurysm. Occipital and posterior cervical pain may signal a posterior inferior cerebellar artery or anterior inferior cerebellar artery aneurysm. Pain in or behind the eye and in the low temple can occur with an expanding MCA aneurysm. Growing aneurysms rarely cause head pain in the absence of neurologic symptoms and signs.

Aneurysms can undergo small ruptures and leaks of blood into the subarachnoid space, so-called sentinel bleeds. Sudden unexplained headache at any location should raise suspicion of SAH and be investigated because a major hemorrhage may be imminent.

DELAYED NEUROLOGIC DEFICITS There are four major causes of delayed neurologic deficits; rerupture, hydrocephalus, vasospasm, and hyponatremia.

1. *Rerupture* The incidence of rerupture of an untreated aneurysm in the first month following SAH is about 30% with the peak at 7 days. It is associated with a 60% mortality and poor outcome. Early treatment eliminates this risk.

2. *Hydrocephalus* Acute hydrocephalus can cause stupor and coma. More often, subacute hydrocephalus develops over a few days or weeks and causes progressive drowsiness or slowed mentation (abulia) with incontinence. Differentiating hydrocephalus from cerebral vasospasm is accomplished with a CT scan, TCD ultrasound, or con-

ventional x-ray angiography. Hydrocephalus may clear spontaneously or require temporary ventricular drainage. Chronic hydrocephalus may develop weeks to months after SAH and manifest as gait difficulty, incontinence, or impaired mentation. Subtle signs may be a lack of initiative in conversation or a failure to recover independence.

3. *Vasospasm* Narrowing of the arteries at the base of the brain following SAH occurs regularly. This vasospasm causes symptomatic ischemia and infarction in approximately 30% of patients and is the major cause of delayed morbidity or death. Signs of ischemia appear 4 to 14 days after the hemorrhage, most frequently at about 7 days. The severity and distribution of vasospasm determine whether infarction will occur.

The mechanism of delayed vasospasm is likely to be related to direct effects of clotted blood and its breakdown products on the artery. In general, the more blood that surrounds the arteries, the greater the chance of symptomatic vasospasm. Spasm of the MCA typically causes contralateral hemiparesis and dysphasia (dominant hemisphere). Proximal anterior cerebral artery vasospasm causes abulia and incontinence, while severe vasospasm of the posterior cerebral artery causes hemianopia. Severe spasm of the basilar or vertebral arteries occasionally produces focal brainstem ischemia. All of these focal symptoms may present abruptly, fluctuate, or develop over a few days.

Vasospasm can be detected reliably with conventional x-ray angiography, but this invasive procedure is expensive and carries risk of stroke and other complications. TCD ultrasound is based on the principle that the velocity of blood flow within an artery will rise as the lumen diameter is narrowed. By directing the probe along the MCA and proximal anterior cerebral, carotid terminus, vertebral, and basilar arteries on a daily or every-other-day basis, vasospasm can be reliably detected noninvasively and treatments initiated to prevent cerebral ischemia (see below).

Severe cerebral edema in patients with infarction from vasospasm may increase the ICP enough to reduce cerebral perfusion pressure. Treatment is with mannitol and hyperventilation (Chap. 376).

4. *Hyponatremia* Hyponatremia may be profound and develop quickly in the first 2 weeks following SAH. It usually results from inappropriate secretion of vasopressin (Chap. 329) and secretion of atrial and brain natriuretic factors, which produce a natriuresis. This "cerebral salt-wasting syndrome" clears over the course of 1 to 2 weeks and, in the setting of SAH, arguably should not be treated with free-water restriction (see below).

Laboratory evaluation and imaging (Fig. 361-12) The hallmark of aneurysmal rupture is blood in the CSF. More than 95% of cases have enough blood to be visualized on a high-quality noncontrast CT scan obtained within 72 h. If the scan fails to establish the diagnosis of SAH and no mass lesion or obstructive hydrocephalus is found, an LP should be performed to establish the presence of subarachnoid blood. Lysis of the red blood cells and subsequent conversion of hemoglobin to bilirubin stains the spinal fluid yellow within 6 to 12 h of SAH. This xanthochromic spinal fluid peaks in intensity at 48 h and lasts for 1 to 4 weeks, depending on the amount of subarachnoid blood.

The extent and location of subarachnoid blood on noncontrast CT scan help locate the underlying aneurysm, identify the cause of any neurologic deficit, and predict delayed vasospasm. A high incidence of symptomatic vasospasm in the middle and anterior cerebral arteries has been found when early CT scans show subarachnoid clots $>5 \times 3$ mm in the basal cisterns or layers of blood >1 mm thick in the cerebral fissures. CT scans less reliably predict vasospasm in the vertebral, basilar, or posterior cerebral arteries.

LP prior to scanning is indicated only if a CT scan is not available at the time of the suspected SAH. Once the diagnosis of hemorrhage from a ruptured saccular aneurysm is suspected, four-vessel conventional x-ray angiography (both carotids and both vertebrals) is generally performed to localize and define the anatomic details of the aneurysm and to determine if other unruptured aneurysms exist. At certain centers, the ruptured aneurysm can be treated using endovascular techniques at the time of the initial angiogram (see following treatment).

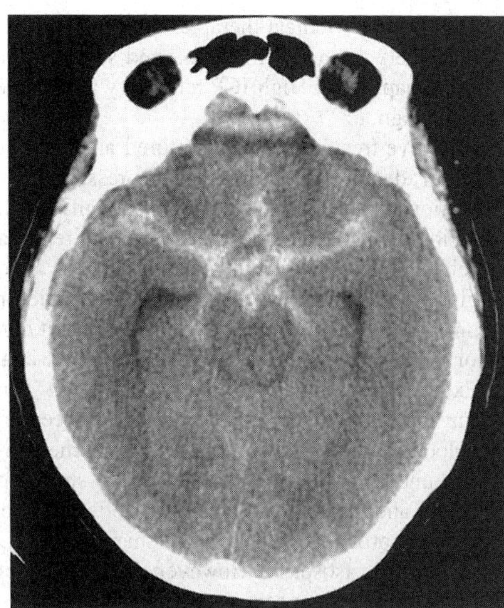

FIGURE 361-12 Subarachnoid hemorrhage. Sudden onset of headache and altered mental status. Noncontrast CT scan at the level of the suprasellar cistern revealed subarachnoid hemorrhage. Communicating hydrocephalus is present, indicated by dilation of the temporal horns of the lateral ventricle. Angiography demonstrated an aneurysm of the anterior communicating artery, which had ruptured.

The ECG frequently shows ST-segment and T-wave changes similar to those associated with cardiac ischemia. Prolonged QRS complex, increased QT interval, and prominent "peaked" or deeply inverted symmetric T waves are usually secondary to the intracranial hemorrhage. The cause of these changes is debated, but there is evidence that structural myocardial lesions produced by circulating catecholamines may occur after SAH.

Serum electrolytes are obtained because hyponatremia may develop. Close monitoring (daily or twice daily) of serum sodium is important since hyponatremia can occur precipitously during the first 2 weeks following SAH (see above).

TCD ultrasound assessment of proximal middle, anterior, and posterior cerebral and basilar artery flow is helpful in detecting the onset of vasospasm and in following its course and response to therapy.

℞ TREATMENT Aneurysm rerupture is common in the early days after SAH and is associated with a 60% incidence of death or poor outcome. Early aneurysm repair prevents future hemorrhage and allows the safe application of techniques to improve blood flow (e.g., induced hypertension and hypervolemia) should symptomatic vasospasm develop. An aneurysm can be "clipped" by a neurosurgeon or "coiled" by a neurointerventional radiologist. Surgical repair involves placing a metal clip across the aneurysm neck, with the advantage that rebleeding risk is eliminated immediately. This approach requires craniotomy and brain retraction, which is associated with neurologic deficits. The newer endovascular technique involves placing platinum coils within the aneurysm via a catheter from the femoral artery. The aneurysm is packed tightly to enhance thrombosis and over time is walled-off from the circulation. The safety and efficacy of these two techniques are being compared in an ongoing European trial.

The medical management of SAH centers on airway protection, blood pressure management before and after aneurysm treatment, preventing rebleeding prior to treatment, managing vasospasm, treating hydrocephalus, and treating hyponatremia.

Intracranial hypertension following aneurysmal rupture occurs secondary to subarachnoid blood, parenchymal hematoma, acute hydrocephalus, or loss of vascular autoregulation. Patients who are stuporous should undergo emergent ventriculostomy to prevent cerebral ischemia from high ICP. Medical therapies designed to combat raised ICP (e.g., mild hyperventilation, mannitol, and sedation) can also be used as needed (Chap. 376). High ICP refractory to treatment carries a poor prognostic sign.

Prior to definitive treatment of the ruptured aneurysm, care is required to maintain adequate cerebral perfusion pressure while avoiding excessive elevation of arterial pressure. Occasionally an intracranial hematoma causing neurologic deterioration requires removal.

Because rebleeding is common, all patients who are not candidates for early surgical treatment are put on bed rest in a quiet, preferably darkened, room and are given stool softeners to prevent constipation. If headache or neck pain is severe, mild sedation and analgesia are prescribed. Extreme sedation is avoided because it can obscure changes in neurologic status. Adequate hydration is necessary to avoid a decrease in blood volume predisposing to brain ischemia.

Seizures are uncommon at the onset of aneurysmal rupture. The quivering, jerking, and extensor posturing that often accompany loss of consciousness are probably related to the sharp rise in ICP or, perhaps, acute generalized vasospasm. However, phenytoin is often given as prophylactic therapy since a seizure may promote rebleeding.

Glucocorticoids may help reduce the head and neck ache caused by the irritative effect of the subarachnoid blood. There is no good evidence they reduce cerebral edema, are neuroprotective, or reduce vascular injury, and their routine use therefore is controversial.

Antifibrinolytic agents are not routinely prescribed but may be considered in patients in whom aneurysm treatment cannot proceed immediately. They are associated with a reduced incidence of aneurysmal rerupture but are also associated with an increased incidence of delayed cerebral infarction and deep venous thrombosis.

Vasospasm remains the leading cause of morbidity and mortality following aneurysmal SAH and treatment of the aneurysm. Treatment with the calcium channel antagonist nimodipine (60 mg orally q6h) has been reported to be beneficial, but the effects seem to be modest. Nimodipine can cause significant hypotension in some patients, which may worsen cerebral ischemia in patients with vasospasm. The most widely accepted therapy for symptomatic cerebral vasospasm is to increase the cerebral perfusion pressure by raising mean arterial pressure through plasma volume expansion and the judicious use of vasopressor agents, usually phenylephrine or dopamine. Raised perfusion pressure has been associated with clinical improvement in many patients, but high arterial pressure may promote rebleeding in unprotected aneurysms. Treatment with induced hypertension and hypervolemia generally requires monitoring of arterial and central venous pressures and in severe cases, the pulmonary artery wedge pressure. Volume expansion helps prevent hypotension, augments cardiac output, and reduces blood viscosity by reducing hematocrit. This method is called "triple-H" (hypertension, hemodilution, and hypervolemic) therapy.

If symptomatic vasospasm persists despite optimal medical therapy, intraarterial papaverine and percutaneous transluminal angioplasty are considered. Vasodilatation following angioplasty appears to be permanent, allowing triple-H therapy to be tapered sooner. The vasodilating effects of papaverine do not last more than 12 to 24 h.

Acute hydrocephalus can cause stupor or coma. It may clear spontaneously or require temporary ventricular drainage. When chronic hydrocephalus develops, ventricular shunting is the treatment of choice.

Free-water restriction is contraindicated in patients with SAH at risk for vasospasm because hypovolemia and hypotension may occur and precipitate cerebral ischemia. Many patients continue to experience a decline in serum sodium despite normal saline parenteral fluids. Frequently, supplemental oral salt coupled with normal saline will mitigate hyponatremia, but often patients will need hypertonic saline in addition. Care must be taken to not correct serum sodium too quickly in patients with marked hyponatremia of several days' duration, as central pontine myelinolysis (Chap. 376) may occur. All patients should have pneumatic compression stockings applied to prevent pulmonary embolism. Systemic heparin is contraindicated in patients with ruptured and untreated aneurysms; it is a relative contraindication following craniotomy, and it may delay thrombosis of a coiled aneurysm.

Vascular Anomalies Vascular anomalies can be divided into congenital vascular malformations and acquired vascular lesions.

Congenital vascular malformations True AVMs, venous anomalies, and capillary telangiectasias are congenital lesions that usually remain clinically silent through life.

True *arteriovenous malformations* are congenital shunts between the arterial and venous systems that may present as headache, focal seizures, and intracranial hemorrhage. AVMs consist of a tangle of abnormal vessels across the cortical surface or deep within the brain substance. AVMs vary in size from a small blemish a few millimeters in diameter to a huge mass of tortuous channels composing an arteriovenous shunt of sufficient magnitude to raise cardiac output. The blood vessels forming the tangle interposed between arteries and veins are usually abnormally thin and do not have a normal structure. AVMs occur in all parts of the cerebral hemispheres, brainstem, and spinal cord, but the largest ones are most frequently in the posterior half of the hemispheres, commonly forming a wedge-shaped lesion extending from the cortex to the ventricle.

Although the lesion is present from birth, bleeding or other symptoms are most common between the ages of 10 and 30, occasionally as late as the fifties. AVMs are more frequent in men, and rare familial cases have been described.

Headache (without bleeding) may be hemicranial and throbbing, like migraine, or diffuse. Focal seizures, with or without generalization, occur in about 30% of cases. Half of AVMs become evident as intracerebral hemorrhages. In most, the hemorrhage is mainly intraparenchymal with a small amount of spillage into the subarachnoid space. Blood is usually not deposited in the basal cisterns, and symptomatic cerebral vasospasm is rare. The threat of rerupture in the early weeks is low. Hemorrhages may be massive, leading to death, or may be as small as 1 cm in diameter, leading to minor focal symptoms or no deficit. The AVM may be large enough to steal blood away from adjacent normal brain tissue or to increase venous pressure significantly to produce venous ischemia locally and in remote areas of the brain. This is seen most often with large AVMs in the territory of the MCA.

Large AVMs of the anterior circulation may be associated with a systolic and diastolic bruit (sometimes self-audible) over the eye, forehead, or neck and a bounding carotid pulse. Headache at the onset of AVM rupture is not generally as explosive as with aneurysmal rupture. MRI is better than CT for diagnosis, although contrast CT scanning sometimes detects calcification of the AVM.

Surgical treatment of symptomatic AVMs, often with preoperative embolization to reduce operative bleeding, is generally indicated for accessible lesions. Sterotaxic radiation, an alternative to surgery, can produce a slow sclerosis of arterial channels over 1 to 2 years.

Most data suggest that patients with asymptomatic AVMs have a low risk for hemorrhage; the risk increases after a first hemorrhage to about 2 to 3% annually. Several angiographic features of the AVM can be used to help predict future bleeding risk. Paradoxically, smaller lesions seem to have a higher hemorrhage rate. The mortality rate with each bleed is about 15%.

Venous anomalies are the result of development of anomalous cerebral, cerebellar, or brainstem drainage. These structures, unlike AVMs, are functional venous channels. They are of little clinical significance and should be ignored if found incidentally on brain imaging studies. Surgical resection of these anomalies may result in venous infarction and hemorrhage. Venous anomalies may be associated with cavernous malformations (see below), which do carry some bleeding risk. If resection of a cavernous malformation is attempted, the venous anomaly should not be disturbed.

Capillary telangiectasias are true capillary malformations that often form extensive vascular networks through an otherwise normal brain structure. The pons and deep cerebral white matter are typical locations, and these capillary malformations can be seen in patients with hereditary hemorrhagic telangiectasia (Osler-Rendu-Weber) syndrome. If bleeding does occur, it rarely produces mass effect or significant symptoms. No treatment options exist.

Acquired vascular lesions *Cavernous angiomas* are tufts of capillary sinusoids that form within the deep hemispheric white matter and brainstem with no normal intervening neural structures. The pathogenesis is unclear. Familial cavernous angiomas have been mapped to several different chromosomal loci; the gene responsible for 7q-linked form encodes a protein that interacts with a member of the RAS family of GTPases. Cavernous angiomas are typically <1 cm in diameter and are often associated with a venous anomaly. Bleeding is usually of small volume, causing slight mass effect only. The bleeding risk for single cavernous malformations is 0.7 to 1.5% per year and may be higher for patients with prior clinical hemorrhage or multiple malformations. Seizures may occur if the malformation is located near the cerebral cortex. Surgical resection eliminates bleeding risk and may reduce seizure risk, but it is reserved for those malformations that form near the brain surface. Radiation treatment has not been shown to be of benefit.

Dural arteriovenous fistulas are acquired connections usually from a dural artery to a dural sinus. Patients may complain of a pulse-synchronous cephalic bruit ("pulsatile tinnitus") and headache. Depending on the magnitude of the shunt, venous pressures may rise high enough to cause cortical ischemia or venous hypertension and hemorrhage. Surgical and endovascular techniques are usually curative. These fistulas may form because of trauma, but most are idiopathic. There is an association between fistulas and dural sinus thrombosis. Fistulas have been observed to appear months to years following venous sinus thrombosis, suggesting that angiogenesis factors elaborated from the thrombotic process may cause these anomalous connections to form. Alternatively, dural arteriovenous fistulas can produce venous sinus occlusion over time, perhaps from the high pressure and high flow through a venous structure.

BIBLIOGRAPHY

ALBERS GW et al: Antithrombotic and thrombolytic therapy for ischemic stroke. Fifth ACCP Consensus Conference on Antithrombotic Therapy. Chest 114:683S, 1998

BARNETT HJ et al: Benefit of carotid endarterectomy in patients with symptomatic moderate or severe stenosis. North American Symptomatic Carotid Endarterectomy Trial Collaborators. N Engl J Med 339:1415, 1998

BILLER J et al: *Guidelines for Carotid Endarterectomy*. A statement for healthcare professionals from a Special Writing Group of the Stroke Council, American Heart Association. Circulation 97:501, 1998

CAPRIE STEERING COMMITTEE: A randomised, blinded, trial of clopidogrel versus aspirin in patients at risk of ischaemic events (CAPRIE). Lancet 348:1329, 1996

CAST: Randomised placebo-controlled trial of early aspirin use in 20,000 patients with acute ischaemic stroke. CAST (Chinese Acute Stroke Trial) Collaborative Group. Lancet 349:1641, 1997

EUROPEAN CAROTID SURGERY TRIALISTS' COLLABORATIVE GROUP: MRC European Carotid Surgery Trial: Interim results for symptomatic patients with severe (70–99%) or with mild (0–29%) carotid stenosis. Lancet 337:1235, 1991

EXECUTIVE COMMITTEE FOR THE ASYMPTOMATIC CAROTID ATHEROSCLEROSIS STUDY: Endarterectomy for asymptomatic carotid artery stenosis. JAMA 273:1421, 1995

GORTER JW: Major bleeding during anticoagulation after cerebral ischemia: Patterns and risk factors. Stroke Prevention In Reversible Ischemia Trial (SPIRIT). European Atrial Fibrillation Trial (EAFT) study groups. Neurology 53:1319, 1999

HACKE W et al: Randomised double-blind placebo-controlled trial of thrombolytic therapy with intravenous alteplase in acute ischaemic stroke (ECASS II). Second European-Australasian Acute Stroke Study Investigators. Lancet 352:1245, 1998

INTERNATIONAL STUDY OF UNRUPTURED INTRACRANIAL ANEURYSMS INVESTIGATORS: Unruptured intracranial aneurysms—risk of rupture and risks of surgical intervention. N Engl J Med 339:1725, 1998

INZITARI D et al: The causes and risk of stroke in patients with asymptomatic internal-carotid-artery stenosis. N Engl J Med 342:169, 2000

LABERGE-LE COUTEULX CS et al: Truncating mutations in CCM1, encoding KRIT1, cause hereditary cavernous angiomas. Nat Genet 23:189, 1999

LAUPACIS A et al: Antithrombotic therapy for atrial fibrillation. Chest 114:579S, 1998

PLEHN JF et al: Reduction of stroke incidence after myocardial infarction with pravastatin: The Cholesterol and Recurrent Events (CARE) study. The Care Investigators. Circulation 99:216, 1999

SHERMAN DG et al: Intravenous ancrod for treatment of acute ischemic stroke. The STAT study: A randomized controlled trial. JAMA 283:2395, 2000

THE INTERNATIONAL STROKE TRIAL (IST): A randomised trial of aspirin, subcutaneous heparin, both, or neither among 19,435 patients with acute ischaemic stroke. International Stroke Trial Collaborative Group. Lancet 349:1569, 1997

THE NATIONAL INSTITUTE OF NEUROLOGICAL DISORDERS AND STROKE RT-PA STROKE STUDY GROUP: Tissue plasminogen activator for acute ischemic stroke. N Engl J Med 333:1581, 1995

THE PUBLICATIONS COMMITTEE FOR THE TRIAL OF ORG 10172 IN ACUTE STROKE TREATMENT (TOAST) INVESTIGATORS: Low molecular weight heparinoid, ORG 10172 (danaparoid), and outcome after acute ischemic stroke: A randomized controlled trial. JAMA 279:1265, 1998

THE STROKE PREVENTION IN REVERSIBLE ISCHEMIA TRIAL (SPIRIT) STUDY GROUP: A randomized trial of anticoagulants versus aspirin after cerebral ischemia of presumed arterial origin. Ann Neurol 42:857, 1997

TURPIE AGG et al: A comparison of aspirin with placebo in patients treated with warfarin after heart-valve replacement. N Engl J Med 329:534, 1993

WILTERDINK JL, EASTON JD: Dipyridamole plus aspirin in cerebrovascular disease. Arch Neurol 56:1087, 1999

362

Thomas D. Bird

ALZHEIMER'S DISEASE AND OTHER PRIMARY DEMENTIAS

AD Alzheimer's disease
ALS amyotrophic lateral sclerosis
APP amyloid precursor protein
CAT choline acetyltransferase
CJD Creutzfeldt-Jakob disease
CSF cerebrospinal fluid
CT computed tomography
EEG electroencephalogram
FAD familial AD
FTD frontotemporal dementia
HD Huntington's disease
MRI magnetic resonance imaging
NFTs neurofibrillary tangles
NPH normal-pressure hydrocephalus
PET positron emission tomography
SSRIs selective serotonin reuptake inhibitors

ALZHEIMER'S DISEASE Alzheimer's disease (AD) is the most common cause of dementia in western countries. Approximately 10% of all persons over the age of 70 have significant memory loss; in more than half the cause is AD. This translates into approximately 3 to 4 million persons with AD in the United States, with a total health care cost of more than $80 billion per year. It is estimated that the annual total cost of caring for a single AD patient in an advanced stage of the disease is $47,000. The disease also exacts a heavy emotional toll on family members and caregivers. AD was first described in 1907 in a 55-year-old woman by Professor Alois Alzheimer in Germany. The condition was initially thought to represent a relatively uncommon form of presenile dementia. However, it has become clear that AD can occur in any decade of adulthood and is the most common cause of dementia in the elderly. The disease is defined as a clinical-pathologic entity. Clinically, AD most often presents with subtle onset of memory loss followed by a slowly progressive dementia that has a course of several years. Pathologically there is gross, diffuse atrophy of the cerebral cortex with secondary enlargement of the ventricular system. Microscopically there are extracellular neuritic plaques containing Aβ amyloid, silver-staining neurofibrillary tangles in neuronal cytoplasm, and accumulation of Aβ amyloid in arterial walls of cerebral blood vessels (see "Pathogenesis," below). The recent identification of four different susceptibility genes for AD has provided a foundation for rapid progress in understanding the biologic basis of the disease.

Clinical Manifestations In the early stages of the disease, the memory loss may go unrecognized or may be ascribed to benign forgetfulness. Slowly the cognitive problems begin to interfere with daily activities, such as keeping track of finances, following instructions on the job, driving, shopping, and housekeeping. Some patients are un-

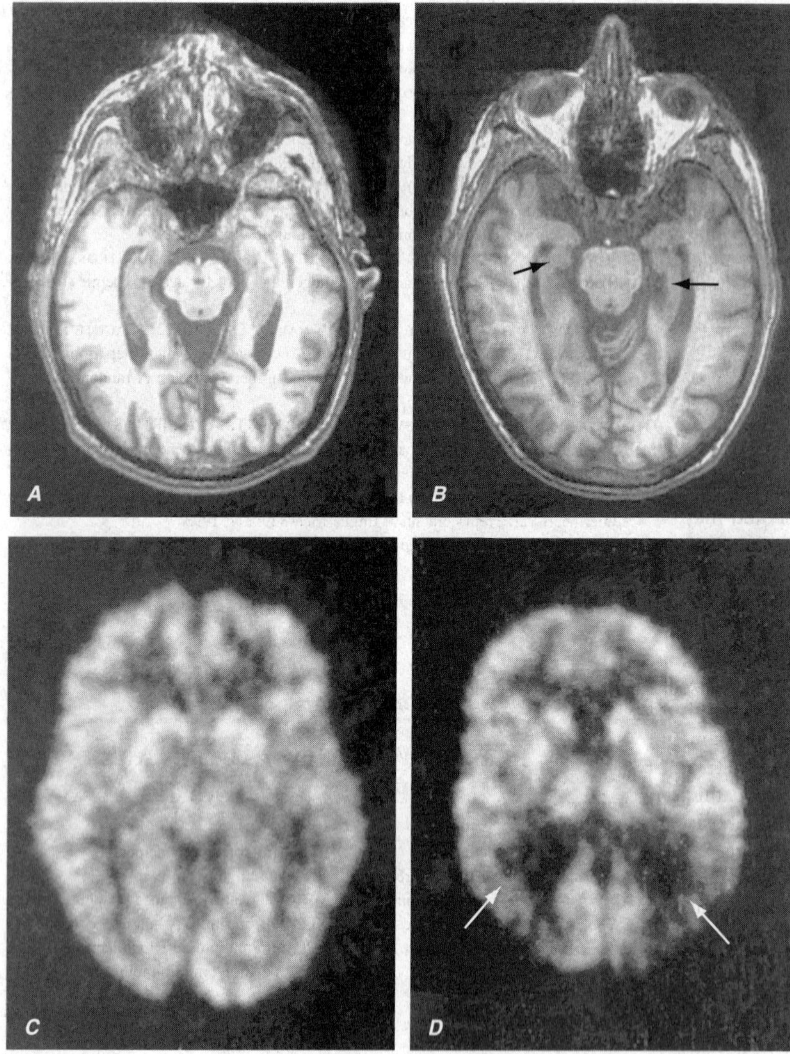

FIGURE 362-1 Alzheimer's disease. Axial T1-weighted MR images through the midbrain of a normal 86-year-old athletic individual (*A*) and a 77-year-old male (*B*) with Alzheimer's disease. Note that both individuals have prominent sulci and slight dilatation of the lateral ventricles. However, there is a reduction in the volume of the hippocampus of the patient with Alzheimer's disease (*arrows*) compared with the normal-for-age hippocampus of the older individual. Below, fluorodeoxyglucose positron emission tomographic scans of a normal control (*C*) and a patient with Alzheimer's disease (*D*). Note that the patient has decreased activity in the parietal lobes bilaterally (*arrows*), a typical finding in this condition. *(Images courtesy of TF Budinger, University of California.)*

aware of these difficulties (agnosognosia), and others have considerable insight, resulting in frustration and anxiety. These major differences in insight have no clear explanation. Change of environment may be bewildering, and the patient may become lost on walks or while driving an automobile. In the middle stages of the disease, the patient is unable to work, is easily lost and confused, and requires daily supervision. Social graces, routine behavior, and superficial conversation may be surprisingly retained. Language may be impaired, especially comprehension and naming of objects. In some patients, aphasia is an early and prominent feature. Word-finding difficulties and circumlocution may be a problem even when formal testing demonstrates intact naming and fluency. Although confrontation naming is frequently deficient, there are often other language deficits as well, including impairments in fluency, comprehension, and repetition. Various apraxias are also common, i.e., deficits in performing sequential motor tasks such as dressing, eating, solving simple puzzles, and copying geometric figures. Patients may be unable to do simple calculations or tell time. Rarely, AD patients may have a form of cortical blindness in which they deny their inability to see. This correlates at autopsy with severe neuropathologic changes in the visual cortex. In the late stages of the disease, some persons remain ambulatory but wander aimlessly and may have complete loss of judgment, reason, and cognitive abilities. Hallucinations and delusions are common; they are usually concrete and not too complex or bizarre. For example, patients may falsely accuse a spouse of infidelity, not recognize an old friend, think a visitor is a burglar, or become frightened of their own image in a mirror. Loss of inhibitions and belligerence may occur and may even alternate with passivity and social withdrawal. Sleep-wake patterns may be disturbed, and nighttime wandering may be very disruptive to the household. Some patients develop a shuffling gait with generalized muscle rigidity associated with slowness and awkwardness of movement. The patients often look parkinsonian but rarely have a rapid, rhythmic, resting tremor. In end-stage AD, patients frequently, but not always, become rigid, mute, incontinent, and bedridden. Help may be needed with the simplest tasks, such as eating, dressing, and toilet function. They may show hyperactive tendon reflexes and primitive sucking and snouting reflexes. Myoclonic jerks (sudden brief contractions of various muscles or the whole body) may occur spontaneously or in response to physical or auditory stimulation. This phenomenon raises the possibility of Creutzfeldt-Jakob disease (CJD) (Chap. 375), but the course of AD is much more prolonged. Generalized seizures may also occur. Death usually results from malnutrition, secondary infections, or heart disease. The typical duration of AD is 8 to 10 years, but the course can range from 1 to 25 years. For unknown reasons, some AD patients show a steady downhill decline in function, while others have prolonged plateaus without major deterioration.

Differential Diagnosis Early in the disease course, other etiologies of dementia should be excluded. These include treatable entities such as thyroid disease, vitamin deficiencies, brain tumor, drug and medication intoxication, chronic infection, and severe depression (pseudodementia) (see Chap. 26). Neuroimaging studies [computed tomography (CT) and magnetic resonance imaging (MRI)] are not specific for AD and may be normal early in the course of the disease. However, neuroimaging helps to exclude other disorders, such as primary and secondary neoplasms, multi-infarct dementia, diffuse white matter disease, and normal-pressure hydrocephalus. As AD progresses, diffuse cortical atrophy becomes apparent, and detailed MRI scans show atrophy of the hippocampus (Fig. 362-1*A*). The electroencephalogram (EEG) in AD may be normal or show nonspecific slowing. Routine spinal fluid examination gives normal results. Research studies have indicated a general decrease in cerebrospinal fluid (CSF) Aβ amyloid levels with an increase in tau protein. There is considerable overlap of these levels with those of the normal aged population, and the usefulness of these measurements in diagnosis remains unclear. Combining the results of both measurements may prove to be most helpful. The use of blood apolipoprotein (Apo) E genotyping is discussed under "Pathogenesis," below. Slowly progressive decline in memory and orientation, normal results on laboratory tests, and an MRI or CT scan showing only diffuse cortical atrophy including the hippocampus is highly suggestive of AD. A clinical diagnosis of AD reached after careful evaluation is confirmed at autopsy 80 to 90% of the time. The misdiagnosed cases usually represent one of the other dementing disorders described later in this chapter. Relatively simple clinical clues are useful in the differential diagnosis. Early prominent gait disturbance with only mild memory loss suggests normal-pressure hydrocephalus (see below). Resting tremor with stooped posture, bradykinesia, and masked face suggests

Parkinson's disease (Chap. 363). Chronic alcoholism suggests vitamin deficiency. Loss of sensibility to position and vibration stimuli accompanied by Babinski responses suggests vitamin B_{12} deficiency (Chap. 368). Early onset of a seizure suggests a metastatic or primary brain neoplasm (Chap. 370). A past history of long-term depression suggests pseudodementia (see below). A history of treatment for insomnia, anxiety, psychiatric disturbance, or epilepsy suggests chronic drug intoxication. Rapid progression over a few weeks or months associated with ataxia, rigidity, and myoclonus suggests CJD (Chap. 375). Prominent behavioral changes with intact memory and lobar atrophy on brain imaging suggests frontotemporal dementia (FTD). A positive family history of dementia suggests either one of the familial forms of AD or one of the other genetic disorders associated with dementia, such as Huntington's disease (see below), familial FTD (see below), familial forms of prion diseases, or rare forms of hereditary ataxias (Chap. 364).

Pathogenesis The most important risk factors for AD are old age and a positive family history. The frequency of AD increases with each decade of adult life to reach 20 to 40% of the population over the age of 85. A positive family history of dementia suggests a genetic cause of AD, as discussed below. Female gender may also be a risk factor independent of the greater longevity of women. Unconfirmed studies have suggested that postmenopausal estrogen use is associated with a decreased frequency of AD. Some AD patients have a past history of head trauma with concussion, but this appears to be a relatively minor risk factor. There is some suggestion that AD is more common in groups with lower educational attainment, but education influences test-taking ability, and it is clear that AD can affect persons of all intellectual levels. One unconfirmed study found that the capacity to express complex written language in early adulthood correlated with a decreased risk for AD. Numerous environmental factors, including aluminum, mercury, viruses, and prions, have been proposed as causes of AD, but none has been proved to play a role. Preliminary studies have suggested that inflammation may play some role in the pathogenesis of AD, as the use of nonsteroidal anti-inflammatory agents is associated with decreased risk. Vascular disease does not seem to be a direct cause of AD, even though there is an associated amyloid angiopathy.

Positron emission tomography (PET) has indicated that the earliest metabolic changes in AD occur in parietal cortex (Fig. 362-1*C, D*). At autopsy, the most severe pathology is usually seen in the hippocampus, temporal cortex, and nucleus basalis. The most important microscopic findings are neuritic "senile" plaques and cytoplasmic neurofibrillary tangles (NFTs). These two lesions accumulate in small numbers during normal aging of the brain but occur in quantitative excess in the dementia of AD. The neuritic plaques contain a central core that includes Aβ amyloid, proteoglycans, Apo E, α_1 antichymotrypsin, and other proteins. Aβ amyloid is a 4.2-kDa protein of 39 to 42 amino acids that is derived proteolytically from a larger transmembrane protein (amyloid precursor protein, APP) through cleavage by two enzymes termed β and γ secretase. The normal function of Aβ amyloid is unknown. APP has been shown to have neurotrophic and neuroprotective activities. The plaque core is surrounded by the debris of degenerating neurons, microglia, and macrophages. The accumulation of Aβ amyloid in cerebral arterioles is termed *amyloid angiopathy*. The NFTs were first noted by Alzheimer. They are silver-staining, twisted neurofilaments in neuronal cytoplasm that represent abnormally phosphorylated tau (τ) protein and appear as paired helical filaments by electron microscopy. Tau is a microtubule-associated protein that may function to assemble and stabilize the microtubules that convey cell organelles, glycoproteins, and other important materials through the neuron. The ability of tau protein to bind to microtubule segments is determined partly by the number of phosphate groups attached to it. Increased phosphorylation of tau protein may disturb this normal process. Biochemically, AD is associated with a decrease in the cerebral cortical levels of several proteins and neurotransmitters, especially acetylcholine, its synthetic enzyme choline acetyltransferase (CAT), and nicotinic cholinergic receptors. Reduction of acetylcholine may be related in part to degeneration of cholinergic neurons in the nucleus basalis of Meynert that project to many areas of cortex. There is also reduction in norepinephrine levels in brainstem nuclei such as the locus coeruleus.

Several genetic factors are known to play important roles in the pathogenesis of at least some cases of AD. One is the *APP* gene on chromosome 21. Adults with trisomy 21 (Down's syndrome) consistently develop the typical neuropathologic hallmarks of AD if they survive beyond age 40. Many also develop a progressive dementia superimposed on their baseline mental retardation. APP is a membrane-spanning protein that is subsequently processed into smaller units, including the Aβ amyloid that is deposited in the neuritic plaques of AD. Presumably the extra dose of the *APP* gene on chromosome 21 is the initiating cause of AD in adult Down's syndrome and eventually results in an excess of cerebral Aβ amyloid. Furthermore, a few families with early-onset familial AD (FAD) have been discovered to have point mutations in the *APP* gene. Although very rare, these families were the first indication of a single-gene autosomal dominant transmission of AD. The most frequent of these *APP* mutations is substitution of valine for isoleucine at position 717. Elevated plasma Aβ peptide may be a risk factor for developing AD in the general population.

Investigation of large families with multigenerational FAD led subsequently to the discovery of two additional AD genes, termed the *presenilins*. Presenilin-1 (*PS-1*) is on chromosome 14 and encodes a protein called S182. Mutations in this gene cause an early-onset AD (onset before age 60 and often before age 50) that is transmitted in an autosomal dominant, highly penetrant fashion. More than 40 different mutations have been found in the *PS-1* gene in families from a wide range of ethnic backgrounds. Presenilin-2 (*PS-2*) is on chromosome 1 and encodes a protein called STM2. A mutation in the *PS-2* gene was first found in a group of American families with Volga German ethnic background. The two genes (*PS-1* and *PS-2*) are highly homologous and encode similar proteins that at first appeared to have seven transmembrane domains (hence the designation *STM*), but subsequent studies have suggested eight such domains with a ninth submembrane region. The normal function of these proteins and the means by which mutations affecting them result in AD is unknown. Both S182 and STM2 are cytoplasmic neuronal proteins that are widely expressed throughout the nervous system. They are homologous to a cell-trafficking protein, sel 12, that is found in the nematode *Coenorhabditis elegans*. Knockout of the *PS-1* gene in mice causes embryonic death, but PS-2 knockout mice have only mild pulmonary pathology, suggesting very different primary functions of the two proteins. The AD pathology in transgenic mice carrying both APP and PS-1 mutations is worse than that in mice with only a single mutation. Also, the mutant human *PS-1* gene protects PS-1 knockout mice from embryonic lethality, and this observation fits with the idea that *PS-1* mutations cause disease by a toxic gain of function. Patients with mutations in these genes have elevated plasma levels of Aβ amyloid, suggesting a possible link between the presenilins and APP. There is evidence that presenilin-1 may normally cleave APP at the γ secretase site, and mutations in either gene (*PS-1* or *APP*) may disturb this function. Mutations in *PS-1* have thus far proved to be the most common cause of early-onset FAD, representing 40 to 70% of this relatively rare syndrome. Mutations in *PS-1* tend to produce AD with an earlier age of onset (mean, 45 years) and a shorter, more rapidly progressive course (mean duration, 6 to 7 years) than the disease caused by mutations in *PS-2* (onset, 53 years; duration, 11 years). Some carriers of uncommon *PS-2* mutations have had onset of dementia after the age of 70. Mutations in the presenilins are rarely involved in the more common sporadic cases of late-onset AD occurring in the general population. Molecular DNA blood testing for these uncommon mutations is now possible on a research basis, and mutation analysis of *PS-1* is commercially available. Such testing is likely to be positive only in early-onset cases of FAD. Any testing of asymptomatic persons at risk must be done in the context of formal, thoughtful genetic counseling (Chap. 359).

A discovery of great importance has implicated the *Apo E* gene on chromosome 19 in the pathogenesis of late-onset familial and sporadic forms of AD. Apo E is involved in cholesterol transport (Chap. 344) and has three alleles: ε2, ε3, and ε4. The ε4 allele of *Apo E* shows a strong association with AD in the general population, including sporadic and late-onset familial cases. Approximately 24 to 30% of the normal white population has at least one ε4 allele (12 to 15% allele frequency), and about 2% are ε4/4 homozygotes. In a group of AD patients, approximately 40 to 65% have at least one ε4 allele, a highly significant difference compared with controls. On the other hand, many AD patients have no ε4 allele, and individuals with ε4 may never develop AD. Therefore, ε4 is neither necessary nor sufficient as a cause of AD. Nevertheless, it is clear that the Apo E ε4 allele, especially in the homozygous 4/4 state, is an important risk factor for AD. It appears to act as a dose-dependent modifier of age of onset, with the earliest onset associated with the ε4/4 homozygous state. One study found a 45% risk for developing AD by age 73 in females who were 4/4 homozygotes. It is unknown how Apo E functions as a risk factor modifying age of onset. Apo E is present in the neuritic amyloid plaques of AD, and may also be involved in NFT formation, because it binds to tau protein. Apo E4 decreases neurite outgrowth in cultures of dorsal root ganglion neurons. There is suggestive evidence that the ε2 allele may be "protective." Interesting but unconfirmed reports suggest that AD patients with an ε4 allele may be less responsive cholinesterase inhibitor drugs. The use of Apo E testing in the diagnosis of AD is controversial. It is not indicated as a predictive test in normal persons, because its precise predictive value is unclear, and many individuals with the ε4 allele never develop dementia. However, some cognitively normal ε4/4 homozygotes have been found by PET to have decreased cerebral cortical metabolic rates, suggesting possible presymptomatic abnormalities compatible with the earliest stage of AD. Studies show that in demented persons who meet clinical criteria for AD, the finding of an ε4 allele increases the reliability of diagnosis. However, the absence of an ε4 allele does not eliminate the diagnosis of AD. Furthermore, all patients with dementia, including those with an ε4 allele, require a search for reversible causes of their cognitive impairment. Nevertheless, Apo E remains the single most important biologic marker associated with risk for AD, and studies of its functional role and diagnostic usefulness are progressing rapidly. Its association (or lack thereof) with other dementing illnesses needs to be fully evaluated. The ε4 allele is not associated with the dementia of Parkinson's disease, FTD, or CJD.

Additional genes are also likely to be involved in AD, including a potential candidate on chromosome 12 (α_2-macroglobulin).

℞ TREATMENT The management of Alzheimer's disease is difficult and frustrating, because there is no specific treatment and the primary focus is on long-term amelioration of associated behavioral and neurologic problems. Building rapport with the patient, family members, and other caregivers is essential to successful management.

Tacrine (tetrahydroaminoacridine) and donepezil (Aricept) are the only drugs presently approved by the U.S. Food and Drug Administration (FDA) for treatment of AD. Their pharmacologic action is presumed to be inhibition of cholinesterase, with a resulting increase in cerebral levels of acetylcholine. Double-blind, placebo-controlled, crossover studies with cholinesterase inhibitors have shown them to be associated with improved caregiver ratings of patients' functioning and with an apparent decreased rate of decline in cognitive test scores over periods of up to 2 years. Such studies are difficult to perform because of the subjective nature of many of the observations and the lack of a uniform rate of decline among patients. Nevertheless, a small but important minority of AD patients (approximately 10 to 20%) appear to show a modest response to these agents and tolerate their side effects (which include dose-related nausea, vomiting, diarrhea, bradycardia, and dizziness). Even without actual improvement these agents may provide stabilization of the patient's condition for a period of months. There is no evidence that these drugs are beneficial in the late stages of AD. Tacrine may be hepatotoxic, necessitating frequent testing of liver function and adjustment of the dose. Donepezil is not hepatotoxic and can be administered once daily (5 to 10 mg). Contraindications for cholinesterase inhibitor treatment include liver disease, alcoholism, peptic ulcer disease, chronic obstructive pulmonary disease; and bradycardia. Clinical trials of other anticholinesterase drugs are in progress.

In a recent prospective observational study, the use of estrogen replacement therapy appeared to protect—by about 50%—against development of AD in women. This study appeared to confirm the results of two earlier case-controlled studies. On the other hand, a prospective treatment study of women with AD found no difference between estrogen and placebo. The mechanism of possible estrogen effects on Alzheimer's disease is unknown but may result from direct effects on cholinergic neurons, antioxidant properties, or a lowering of levels of Apo E. A prospective randomized clinical trial of estrogen replacement therapy in women is underway.

In patients with moderately advanced AD, a prospective trial of the antioxidants selegiline, α tocopherol (vitamin E), or both demonstrated no significant benefit on primary outcomes of progression. However, a modest beneficial effect of each treatment compared to placebo was present in secondary analyses that controlled for intergroup difference in baseline dementia scores. These possible beneficial effects are small in magnitude and require confirmation.

A randomized, double-blind, placebo-controlled trial of an extract of *Ginkgo biloba* found modest improvement in cognitive function in subjects with AD and vascular dementia. This study requires confirmation before *G. biloba* is considered an effective treatment for dementia, because there was a high subject dropout rate and no improvement on a clinician's judgment scale.

As noted above, several retrospective studies have also suggested a protective effect on dementia of nonsteroidal anti-inflammatory agents. Controlled prospective studies are in progress.

In an APP mutation mouse model of AD, weekly immunization with Aβ peptide both prevented the occurrence and reversed the accumulation of amyloid plaques in the brain. The possible benefit of this treatment strategy in humans is unknown and is under evaluation. In addition, the identification of a protease that acts as the APP β secretase has raised the possibility that inhibiting this enzyme might decrease amyloid accumulation in brain, another potential therapeutic strategy for AD.

Mild to moderate depression is common in the early stages of AD and may respond to antidepressant medication. Selective serotonin reuptake inhibitors (SSRIs) are commonly used, as are tricyclic antidepressants with low anticholinergic side effects (desipramine and nortriptyline). Generalized seizures should be treated with an appropriate anticonvulsant, such as phenytoin or carbamazepine. Agitation, insomnia, hallucinations, and belligerence are especially troublesome characteristics of some AD patients and often are responsible for nursing home placement. Mild sedation with benadryl may help insomnia, and agitation has been variously treated with phenothiazines (such as thioridazine), haloperidol, risperidone, and benzodiazepines (such as lorazepam). These medications frequently have untoward side effects, including sedation, confusion, increased muscle tone, and adventitious movements. Low-dose haloperidol (0.5 to 2 mg), trazodone, buspirone, propranolol, and olanzapine may be the most helpful and have the fewest side effects. The few controlled studies comparing drugs with behavioral intervention in the treatment of agitation suggest that both approaches are equally effective. However, careful, daily, nondrug behavior management is often not available, rendering medication necessary. In the early stages of AD, memory aids such as notebooks and posted daily reminders are helpful. Common sense and clinical studies have shown that family members should emphasize activities that are pleasant and deemphasize those that are unpleasant. Kitchens, bathrooms, and bedrooms need to be made safe, and patients eventually must stop driving. Loss of independence and change of environment may worsen confusion, agitation, and anger. Communication and repeated calm reassurance are necessary. Caregiver "burnout" is common, often resulting in nursing home placement of the patient and respite breaks for the caregiver help to maintain successful long-term management of the patient. Use of adult daycare centers can be most helpful. Local and national support groups, such as the Alzheimer's Disease and Related Disorders Association, are valuable resources.

VASCULAR DEMENTIA Dementia associated with cerebral vascular disease can be divided into two general categories: multi-infarct dementia and diffuse white matter dementia (also called subcortical arteriosclerotic encephalopathy or Binswanger's disease). Cerebral vascular disease appears to be a more common cause of dementia in Asia than in Europe and North America. Individuals who have had several strokes may develop chronic cognitive deficits, commonly called *multi-infarct dementia*. The strokes may be large or small (sometimes lacunar) and usually involve several different brain regions. In fact, one study has shown that lacumar stroke is the most common stroke subtype associated with dementia. The occurrence of dementia seems to depend partly on the total volume of damaged cortex, but it is also more common in individuals with left-hemisphere lesions, independent of any language disturbance, and when the stroke involves the hippocampus. Subcortical infarction has been associated with both frontal and global cerebral hypometabolism, which may in turn lead to dementia. The patients give a history of episodes of sudden neurologic deterioration. Multi-infarct dementia patients usually also have a history of hypertension, diabetes, coronary artery disease, or other manifestations of diffuse atherosclerosis. Physical examination usually reveals focal neurologic deficits such as hemiparesis, unilateral Babinski reflex, a visual field defect, or pseudobulbar palsy. The recurrent strokes result in a stepwise progression of disease. Neuroimaging studies clearly show the multiple areas of infarction. Thus, the history and neuroimaging findings differentiate this condition from AD. However, AD and multiple infarctions are both common and sometimes occur together. With normal aging, there is also an accumulation of amyloid in cerebral blood vessels, leading to a condition called *cerebral amyloid angiopathy of aging* (not associated with dementia), which predisposes older persons to hemorrhagic lobar stroke. AD patients with amyloid angiopathy and hypertension also appear to be at increased risk of cerebral infarction. Apo E ε4 has been reported to be a risk factor for amyloid angiopathy independent of AD.

Some persons with dementia are discovered on MRI studies to have bilateral abnormalities of subcortical white matter, termed *diffuse white matter disease* (or leukoaraiosis) (Fig. 362-2). The dementia may be of subtle onset and slow progression, features that distinguish it from multi-infarct dementia. (A few such patients have been described with apparently sudden onset of cognitive impairment.) Early symptoms are mild confusion, apathy, change in personality, and memory deficit. Marked difficulties in judgment and orientation and dependence on others for daily activities develop later. Euphoria, elation, or aggressive behavior are common. A mixed picture of pyramidal and cerebellar signs may be present in the same patient. Lateralizing motor signs are uncommon. A gait disorder appears in at least half the patients. In advanced cases, urinary incontinence and dysarthria with or without pseudobulbar features are frequent. Seizures and myoclonic jerks appear in a minority of patients. This disorder appears to be the result of chronic ischemia due to occlusive disease of small penetrating cerebral arteries and arterioles (microangiopathy). The patients usually, but not always, have a history of hypertension, but any disease causing stenosis of small cerebral vessels may be the critical underlying factor. An association with abnormalities of the coagulation-fibrinolysis pathway has been reported. Binswanger described several patients with this condition, but the term *Binswanger's disease* should be used with caution, because it does not really identify a single entity. Other rare causes of white matter disease may also present with dementia, such as adult metachromatic leukodystrophy and progressive multifocal leukoencephalopathy (papovavirus infection). The term *CADASIL* refers to an inherited form of diffuse white matter disease described as *c*erebral *a*utosomal *d*ominant *a*rteriopathy with *s*ubcortical *i*nfarcts and *l*eukoencephalopathy. Clinically there is a progressive dementia developing in the fifth to seventh decades in multiple family members who may also have a history of migraine and recurrent stroke without hypertension. Skin biopsy may show characteristic dense bodies in the media of arterioles. The disease is caused by mutations in the notch 3 gene, but there is no commercially available genetic test. The frequency of this disorder is unknown.

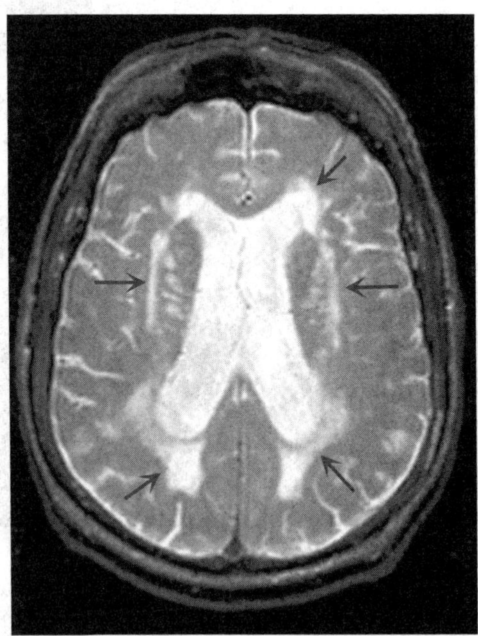

FIGURE 362-2 Diffuse white matter disease (Binswanger's disease). Axial T2-weighted MR image through the lateral ventricles reveals multiple areas of abnormal high signal intensity involving the periventricular white matter as well as the corona radiata and lentiform nuclei (*arrows*). While seen in some individuals with normal cognition, this appearance is more pronounced in patients with dementia of a vascular etiology.

Treatment of vascular dementia must be focused on the underlying causes, such as hypertension, atherosclerosis, and diabetes. Recovery of lost cognitive function is not likely to occur.

FRONTOTEMPORAL DEMENTIA AND PICK'S DISEASE FTD may be the cause of as many as 10% of all cases of dementia and an even greater proportion of presenile onset (<65 years) cases. The patients are often irritable; have loss of inhibitions; and do better on construction, copying, and calculation tasks than patients with AD. Memory is often intact early in the disease. Patients may be socially inappropriate or remote and withdrawn. Hoarding, overeating, and weight gain are common. Rigidity and mutism often occur late in the disease. Imaging studies reveal atrophy confined to the frontal or frontal and temporal lobes. The condition is heterogeneous, and the broad designation FTD usually includes Pick's disease (discussed below) as a subcategory. An autosomal dominant genetic form of FTD has been linked to DNA markers on chromosome 17. Some of these families have disinhibition dementia associated with motor neuron disease, whereas others display parkinsonian features. Cytoplasmic aggregations of tau protein are found in many neurons of cortex, striatum, and substantia nigra. These aggregates sometimes resemble those found in progressive supranuclear palsy (Chap. 363) or AD. This con-

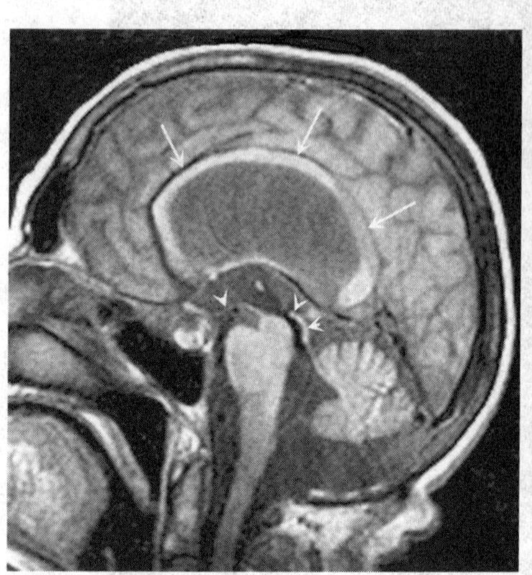

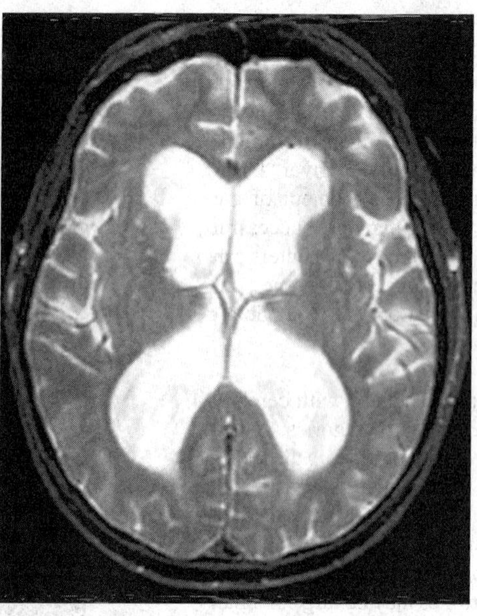

A B

FIGURE 362-3 Normal pressure hydrocephalus. *A.* Sagittal T1-weighted MR image demonstrates dilatation of the lateral ventricle and stretching of the corpus callosum (*arrows*), depression of the floor of the third ventricle (*single arrowhead*), and enlargement of the aqueduct (*double arrowheads*). Note the diffuse dilatation of the lateral, third, and fourth ventricles with a patent aqueduct, typical of communicating hydrocephalus. *B.* Axial T2-weighted MR images demonstrate dilatation of the lateral ventricles without cortical atrophy. This patient underwent successful ventriculoperitoneal shunting.

dition is referred to as *frontotemporal dementia with parkinsonism linked to chromosome 17* (FTDP-17). Many FTDP-17 families have been found to inherit missense mutations in the tau gene that disturb the microtubule-binding function of tau or alter the carefully regulated alternative splicing of the gene. Recent studies show that only a small portion of sporadic FTD patients have tau mutations, which are more commonly found in familial FTD cases with known tau neuropathology at autopsy.

Pick's disease is a commonly discussed disorder that is difficult to differentiate clinically from AD and is less well defined as a distinct entity. The major distinguishing hallmark is marked symmetric lobar atrophy of temporal and/or frontal lobes, which can be visualized by neuroimaging studies (CT, MRI, or single photon emission CT) and is readily apparent at autopsy. The atrophy is sometimes asymmetric and may involve the basal ganglia. Microscopic findings include gliosis, neuronal loss, and swollen or ballooned neurons, which frequently contain silver-staining cytoplasmic inclusions referred to as *Pick bodies*. Pick bodies consist of straight and constricted fibrils that share antigenic determinants with the NFTs of AD, including the microtubule-associated protein tau, suggesting that Pick bodies derive from altered components of the neuronal cytoskeleton. Onset is usually in the fifth through seventh decades. Clinically, there is a slowly progressive dementia often associated with hyper-oral behavior, bulimia, language disturbance, emotional disinhibition, irritability, and persistent aimless wandering. In the early stages the behavioral changes are more prominent than memory loss. The language disturbance may be aphasia or forced repetitive speech patterns, sometimes progressing to echolalia, language impoverishment, and mutism. These clinical characteristics may sometimes occur in AD, so that the clinical diagnosis of Pick's disease often requires confirmation at autopsy. Some brains containing Pick bodies may also have varying quantities of amyloid plaques and NFTs, blurring the distinction from AD. Examples of familial Pick's disease that display an autosomal dominant-like pattern of inheritance have been reported. There is no specific treatment.

DIFFUSE LEWY BODY DISEASE Lewy bodies are intraneuronal cytoplasmic inclusions that stain with periodic acid–Schiff and ubiquitin. They are composed of straight neurofilaments 7 to 20 nm long with surrounding amorphous material. They contain epitopes recognized by antibodies against phosphorylated and nonphosphorylated neurofilament proteins, ubiquitin, and a presynaptic protein called α-synuclein. Lewy bodies are traditionally found in the substantia nigra of patients with idiopathic Parkinson's disease (Chap. 363). Large numbers of such inclusions have also been discovered in cortical neurons in patients with dementia. In patients without other pathologic features, the condition is referred to as *diffuse Lewy body disease.* In patients whose brains also contain amyloid plaques and NFTs, the condition is called the *diffuse Lewy body variant of Alzheimer's disease.* The quantity of Lewy bodies required to establish the diagnosis is uncertain. The diagnosis is primarily a neuropathologic entity; however, there is some evidence that there is a characteristic clinical syndrome. In addition to chronic progressive dementia, these patients often also have parkinsonian features, in particular rigidity, which may be combined with an intention tremor. Frequent fluctuations of behavior, cognitive ability, and level of alertness may occur. These fluctuations can be marked, with the occurrence of episodic confusion and lucid intervals suggesting delirium. However, despite the fluctuating pattern, the clinical features persist over a long period, unlike a typical transient delirium. Delusions and visual hallucinations are common, and auditory hallucinations may also occur. Repeated unexplained falls are often noted. Frequently there is an unusual sensitivity to neuroleptic medications and benzodiazepines, with exaggerated adverse responses to standard doses. In most patients, this condition is difficult to distinguish from AD or Parkinson's disease with dementia. The population prevalence of diffuse Lewy body disease is not known, but it is now more commonly diagnosed than in the past because of the use of ubiquitin staining during neuropathologic studies. At autopsy, 10 to 30% of demented patients may show cortical Lewy bodies. It is not yet clear what role Apo E may play in Lewy body disease without AD changes. There is no specific treatment.

NORMAL-PRESSURE HYDROCEPHALUS Normal-pressure hydrocephalus (NPH) is a syndrome with distinct clinical, physiologic, and neuroimaging characteristics. The clinical triad includes an abnormal gait (ataxic or apractic), dementia (usually mild to moderate), and urinary incontinence. Neuroimaging studies of the brain reveal enlarged lateral ventricles (hydrocephalus) with little or no cortical atrophy. This is a communicating hydrocephalus with a patent aqueduct of Sylvius and upward stretching of the corpus callosum (Fig. 362-3). Lumbar puncture opening pressure is in the high normal range, and the CSF protein and sugar concentrations and cell count are normal. NPH is presumed to be caused by obstruction to normal flow of CSF over the cerebral convexity and delayed absorption into the venous system. The indolent nature of the process results in enlarged lateral ventricles but relatively little increase in CSF pressure. There is presumably stretching and distortion of white matter tracts in the corona radiata, but the exact physiologic cause of the clinical syndrome is unclear. Some patients with NPH have a history of conditions producing scarring of the basilar meninges (blocking upward flow of CSF) such as previous meningitis, subarachnoid hemorrhage, or head trauma. Most patients seem to have no pertinent past history. In contrast to patients with AD, the patient with NPH has an early and prominent gait disturbance and no evidence of cortical atrophy on CT or MRI. A number of attempts have been made to use various special studies to improve the diagnosis of NPH and predict the success of ventricular shunting. These include radionuclide cisternography (showing a delay in CSF absorption over the convexity) and various attempts to monitor and alter CSF flow dynamics, including a constant-pressure infusion test. None of these studies has proven to be specific or consistently useful. There is sometimes a transient improvement in gait or cognition following lumbar puncture (or serial punctures) with removal of 30 to 50 mL of CSF, but this finding also has not proved to be consistently predictive of post-shunt improvement. One study determined that no more than 1 to 2% of a large group of demented patients had NPH. AD often masquerades as NPH, because the gait may be abnormal in AD and cortical atrophy is sometimes difficult to determine by CT or MRI early in the disease. Hippocampal atrophy on MRI may be a clue suggesting AD (Fig. 362-1). Approximately 30 to 50% of patients identified by careful diagnosis as having NPH will show improvement with a ventricular shunting procedure. Gait may improve more than memory. Transient, short-lasting improvement is common. Patients should be carefully selected for this operation, because subdural hematoma and infection are known complications. A recent study limited to four patients showed benefit from aggressive siphoning of CSF to reduce ventricular size, but there were frequent perioperative complications.

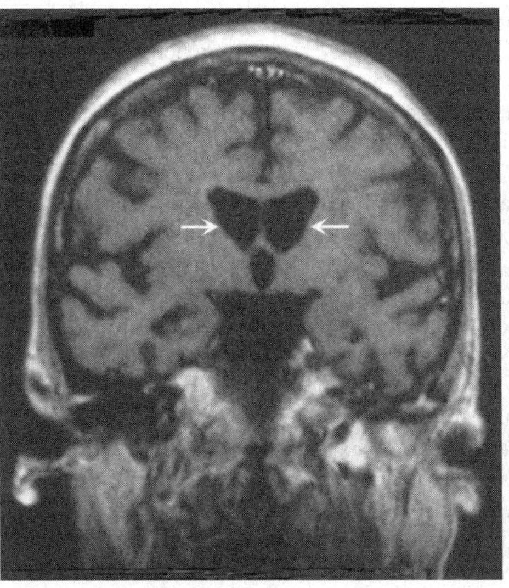

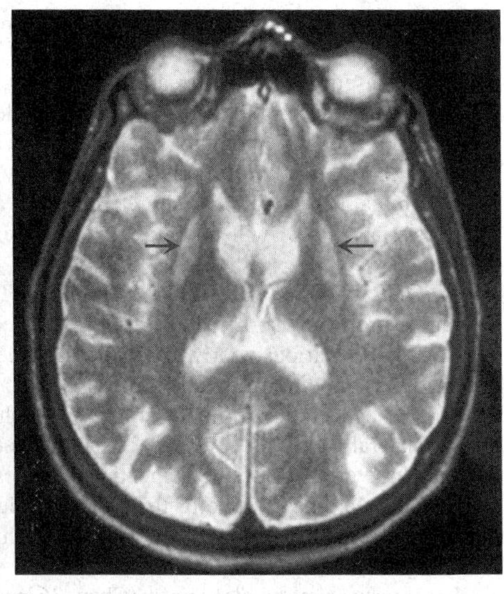

FIGURE 362-4 Huntington's disease *A*. Sagittal T1-weighted MRI shows enlargement of the lateral ventricles reflecting typical caudate atrophy (*arrows*). *B*. Axial T2-weighted image demonstrates abnormal high signal intensity in the putamen (*arrows*).

HUNTINGTON'S DISEASE Huntington's disease (HD) is a genetic, autosomal dominant, degenerative brain disorder. It has a population frequency of about 10/100,000. The two clinical hallmarks of the disease are chorea and behavioral disturbance. The illness may begin with either or both of these symptoms predominating. Onset is usually in the fourth or fifth decade, but there is a wide range in age of onset, from childhood to >75 years. The chorea begins as subtle fidgeting that may be unrecognized by the patient and family. However, the movement disorder is usually slowly progressive and eventually may become disabling. There are frequent, irregular, sudden jerks and movements of any of the limbs or trunk. Grimacing, grunting, and poor articulation of speech may be prominent. The gait is disjointed and poorly coordinated and has a so-called dancing (choreic) quality. Memory is frequently not impaired until late in the disease, but attention, judgment, awareness, and executive functions may be seriously deficient at an early stage. Depression, apathy, social withdrawal, irritability, and intermittent disinhibition are common. Delusions and obsessive-compulsive behavior may occur. Schizophrenia is occasionally the initial diagnosis. The disease duration is typically about 15 years but also shows a wide range. Early onset before the age of 20 (juvenile HD) is associated with rigidity, ataxia, cognitive decline, and more rapid progression, with a typical duration of about 8 years. Seizures are rare with adult-onset HD but more common with juvenile-onset disease. There is no specific treatment, but the adventitious movements and behavioral changes may partially respond to phenothiazines, haloperidol, benzodiazepines, or olanzepine. SSRIs may help with the frequently associated depression.

Neuropathologically, the disease predominantly strikes the striatum. Atrophy of the caudate nuclei, which form the lateral margins of the lateral ventricles, can be visualized on neuroimaging studies in the middle and late stages of the disease (Fig. 362-4). More diffuse cortical atrophy can be seen late in the disease. Microscopically there are no dramatic pathologic characteristics, such as the plaques and tangles seen with AD. However, there is gliosis and neuronal loss, especially of medium-sized spiny neurons in the caudate and putamen. Some neurons contain intranuclear inclusions that stain with antibodies to polyglutamine. There is relative sparing of large cholinergic aspiny neurons. (Treatment with 3-nitroproprionic acid, a succinate dehydrogenase inhibitor, has produced HD-like pathologic changes in experimental animals). Neurochemically there is a marked decrease of γ-aminobutyric acid (GABA) and its synthetic enzyme glutamic acid decarboxylase throughout the basal ganglia. The levels of other neurotransmitters, including substance P and enkephalins, are also reduced. Magnetic resonance spectroscopy (MRS) in living subjects with HD has shown elevated levels of lactate in the basal ganglia.

The HD gene, called *IT15*, is located on chromosome 4p, contains a CAG trinucleotide repeat expansion, and codes for a protein called *huntingtin*. The protein is found in neurons throughout the brain; its normal function is unknown. Inactivation of the homologous gene in mice causes embryonic death in homozygotes, but heterozygotes are phenotypically normal. Transgenic mice with an expanded CAG repeat in the HD gene develop a progressive movement disorder. The CAG repeat codes for a long polyglutamine domain in the expressed protein. The disease process may result from a toxic gain of function (Chap. 359). One hypothesis is that these polyglutamine tracts cause abnormal protein-binding reactions, which then interfere with other cell processes such as mitochondrial activity. The HD mutation may lead to abnormal cleavage of the huntingtin protein, passage of protein fragments from cytoplasm to nucleus, and interference of nuclear mechanisms leading to apoptosis and neuronal death.

The DNA repeat expansion forms the basis of a diagnostic blood test for the disease gene. Persons having 38 or more CAG repeats in the HD gene have inherited the disease mutation and will eventually develop symptoms if they live to an advanced age. Each of their children has a 50% risk of also inheriting the abnormal gene. There is a rough correlation between a larger number of repeats and an earlier age of onset, but most patients fall into a range of intermediate repeat numbers (40 to 49 repeats) in which this correlation is not clinically useful. For unclear reasons, juvenile onset with a large repeat expansion most often occurs when the father is the affected parent (a form of genetic anticipation). There is a CAG repeat range (about 26 to 37) in the HD gene that is rarely associated with clinical symptoms, but it is unstable and may expand to a symptomatic range when passed to a child. Asymptomatic adult children at risk for HD should receive careful genetic counseling prior to DNA testing, because a positive result may have serious emotional and social consequences. Detailed testing and counseling protocols have been published. In addition to use in genetic counseling of persons at risk for HD, the DNA test can also be used in differential diagnosis. For example, some persons with late-onset, apparently sporadic "senile" chorea have been found to carry the HD mutation. Also, disorders that may mimic HD, such as schizophrenia, benign familial chorea, inherited ataxias, neural acanthocytosis, and FAD, will not show the CAG expansion in the HD gene.

OTHER DEGENERATIVE DEMENTIAS Several other primary neurologic disorders have been associated with dementia and are the result of various poorly understood degenerative neuronal processes. These conditions include progressive supranuclear palsy, cortical basal degeneration, primary progressive aphasia, and the amyotrophic lateral sclerosis (ALS)/parkinsonian/dementia complex of Guam. These are progressive dementing illnesses of unknown cause whose names are descriptive of the typical clinical signs or the anatomic brain areas that are involved with nonspecific atrophy and neuronal degeneration.

Progressive supranuclear palsy (Chap. 363) is a degenerative disease that involves both the brainstem and neocortex with diffuse NFTs. Clinically, this disorder begins with vertical supranuclear gaze paresis and progresses slowly to include symmetric rigidity and dementia. Stiff, unstable posture with hyperextension of the neck and slow gait with frequent falls are common. Early in the disease, the patients have difficulty with downgaze and lose vertical opticokinetic nystagmus on downward movement of the target. Although the patients have very limited voluntary eye movements, their eyes still retain oculocephalic reflexes (doll's head maneuver). The dementia is considered to be of the subcortical type, with slowed thought processes, impaired verbal fluency, and difficulty with sequential actions and with shifting from one task to another. Seizures and sleep apnea may occur. There is only a limited response to L-dopa, and there is no other effective treatment. Death occurs within 5 to 10 years. At autopsy, the NFTs are found in multiple subcortical structures (including the subthalamus, globus pallidus, substantia nigra, locus coeruleus, periaqueductal gray matter, superior colliculi, and oculomotor nuclei) as well as in the neocortex. The NFTs have similar staining characteristics to those of AD, but on electron microscopy they generally are seen to consist of straight tubules rather than the paired helical filaments found in AD.

Progressive supranuclear palsy is often confused with idiopathic *Parkinson's disease* (Chap. 363). Although elderly Parkinson's patients may have some difficulty with upgaze, they do not develop significant downgaze paresis or progressive supranuclear palsy, and neurologic findings in Parkinson's disease are more likely to be asymmetric. However, dementia does occur in approximately 20% of Parkinson's disease patients. The occurrence of dementia in Parkinson's disease is more likely with increasing age, increasing severity of extrapyramidal signs, and the presence of depression. These patients may also show cortical atrophy on brain imaging. Neuropathologically, there may be Alzheimer changes in the cortex (amyloid plaques and NFTs), neuronal Lewy body inclusions in both the substantia nigra and the cortex, or no specific microscopic changes other than gliosis and neuronal loss.

Cortical basal ganglionic degeneration is a slowly progressive dementing illness associated with severe gliosis and neuronal loss in both the neocortex and basal ganglia (substantia nigra and striatum). There is often a unilateral onset with rigidity, dystonia, and apraxia of one arm and hand ("alien hand" syndrome). Eventually the condition becomes bilateral and includes dysarthria, slow gait, action tremor, and dementia. The microscopic features include enlarged, achromatic neurons in the cortex, and there may also be NFTs and amyloid plaques. The condition is rarely familial; the cause is unknown; and there is no specific treatment.

Another entity is *primary progressive aphasia* (Chap. 25). Patients with this disorder have aphasia associated with asymmetric atrophy of the left hemisphere and occasionally go on to develop dementia. Neuroimaging studies show the left hemisphere atrophy. Some patients are nonfluent, with hesitant, telegraphic speech associated with impaired comprehension and naming. Neuropathologic studies have shown a heterogeneous group of abnormalities, including Pick's disease, AD, CJD, and nonspecific gliosis.

The *ALS/parkinsonian/dementia complex of Guam* is a rare degenerative disease that occurs in the Chamorro natives on the island of Guam. Individual patients may have any combination of parkinsonian features, dementia, and motor neuron disease. The most characteristic pathologic features are the presence of NFTs in degenerating neurons of the cortex and substantia nigra and loss of motor neurons in the spinal cord. Epidemiologic evidence supports a probable environmental cause, such as exposure to a neurotoxin with a long latency period. One interesting but unproven candidate neurotoxin occurs in the seed of the false palm tree (cycad), which Guamanians traditionally used to make flour. The possibility of a contributing genetic factor has not been excluded. The ALS syndrome is decreasing in frequency on Guam, but a dementing illness with rigidity continues to be seen.

Finally, rare forms of degenerative dementia continue to be reported, such as dementia lacking specific histologic features and an early-onset hereditary dementia caused by mutations in neuroserpin, a type of serine protease inhibitor.

BIBLIOGRAPHY

BIRD TD, BENNETT RL: Why do DNA testing? Practical and ethical implications of new neurogenetic tests. Ann Neurol 38:141, 1995

BOWEN J et al: Progression to dementia in patients with isolated memory loss. Lancet 349:763, 1998

BREITNER JCS et al: Apo E-ε4 count predicts age when prevalence of AD increases, then declines. Neurology 53:321, 1999

CAPLAN LR: Binswanger's disease—revisited. Neurology 45:626, 1995

DANIEL SE et al: The clinical and pathological spectrum of Steele-Richardson-Olszewski syndrome (progressive supranuclear palsy): A reappraisal. Brain 118:759, 1995

DUBINSKY RM et al: Practice parameter: Risk of driving and Alzheimer's disease (an evidence-based review). Report of the Quality Standards Subcommittee of the American Academy of Neurology. Neurology 54:2205, 2000

LENDON C et al: Exploring the etiology of Alzheimer disease using molecular genetics. JAMA 277:825, 1997

LIM A et al: Clinico-neuropathological correlation of Alzheimer's disease in a community-based case series. J Am Geriatr Soc 47:564, 1999

MALM J et al: The predictive value of cerebrospinal fluid dynamic tests in patients with the idiopathic adult hydrocephalus syndrome. Arch Neurol 52:783, 1995

MARTIN JB: Molecular basis of the neurodegenerative disorders. N Engl J Med 340:1970, 1999

MAYEUX R et al: Utility of the apolipoprotein E genotype in the diagnosis of Alzheimer's disease. N Engl J Med 338:506, 1998

MAYEUX R, SANO M: Treatment of Alzheimer's Disease. N Engl J Med 341:1670, 1999

MCKEITH IG et al: An evaluation of the predictive validity and inter-rater reliability of clinical diagnostic criteria for senile dementia of Lewy body type. Neurology 44:872, 1994

MENDEZ MF et al: Pick's disease versus Alzheimer's disease: A comparison of clinical characteristics. Neurology 43:289, 1993

RABER J et al: Apolipoprotein E and cognitive performance. Nature 404:352, 2000

RAFTOPOULOS C et al: Cognitive recovery in idiopathic normal pressure hydrocephalus: A prospective study. Neurosurgery 35:397, 1994

REIMAN EM et al: Preclinical evidence of Alzheimer's disease in persons homozygous for the ε4 allele for apolipoprotein E. N Engl J Med 334:752, 1996

SCHENK D et al: Immunization with amyloid-β attenuates Alzheimer disease-like pathology in the PDAPP mouse. Nature 400:173, 1999

SHERRINGTON R et al: Cloning of a gene bearing missense mutations in early-onset familial Alzheimer's disease. Nature 375:754, 1995

TATEMICHI TK et al: Dementia after stroke: Baseline frequency, risks, and clinical features in a hospitalized cohort. Neurology 42:1185, 1992

TERRY RD et al: *Alzheimer Disease*, 2d ed. New York, Lippincott Williams & Wilkins, 1999

TISON F et al: Dementia in Parkinson's disease: A population-based study in ambulatory and institutionalized individuals. Neurology 45:705, 1995

VANNESTE JAL: Three decades of normal pressure hydrocephalus: Are we wiser now? J Neurol Neurosurg Psychiatry 57:1021, 1994

VASSAR R et al: β-Secretase cleavage of Alzheimer's amyloid precursor protein by the transmembrane aspartic protease BACE. Science 286:735, 1999

WILHELMSEN KC: Frontotemporal dementia genetics. J Geriatr Psychiatry Neurol 11:55, 1998

363 PARKINSON'S DISEASE AND OTHER EXTRAPYRAMIDAL DISORDERS

Michael J. Aminoff

PARKINSON'S DISEASE Parkinsonism is a syndrome consisting of a variable combination of tremor, rigidity, bradykinesia, and a characteristic disturbance of gait and posture. Parkinson's disease is a chronic, progressive disorder in which idiopathic parkinsonism occurs without evidence of more widespread neurologic involvement.

Parkinson's disease generally commences in middle or late life and leads to progressive disability with time. The disease occurs in all ethnic groups, has an equal sex distribution, and is common, with a prevalence of 1 to 2 per 1000 of the general population and 2 per 100 among people older than 65 years. Signs of parkinsonism are extremely common in the elderly; one survey indicated that 15% of individuals between 65 and 74 years of age, and more than half of all individuals after age 85, have abnormalities on examination consistent with the presence of an extrapyramidal disorder.

Neuroanatomy Symptoms of Parkinson's disease are caused by loss of nerve cells in the pigmented substantia nigra pars compacta and the locus coeruleus in the midbrain. Cell loss also occurs in the globus pallidus and putamen. Eosinophilic intraneural inclusion granules (Lewy bodies) are present in the basal ganglia, brainstem, spinal cord, and sympathetic ganglia.

Pars compacta neurons of the substantia nigra provide dopaminergic input to the striatum, which is part of the basal ganglia (Fig. 22-4*A*). In Parkinson's disease, loss of pars compacta neurons leads to striatal dopamine depletion and ultimately to reduced thalamic excitation of the motor cortex (Fig. 22-4*B*). Other neurotransmitters, such as norepinephrine, are also depleted, with clinical consequences that are uncertain but perhaps contribute to depression, dysautonomia, and "freezing" episodes of marked akinesia. →*The neural pathways that modulate motor activity are considered in detail in Chap. 22.*

Pathogenesis Parkinsonism can be induced in primates by exposure to 1-methyl-4-phenyl-1,2,3,6-tetrahydropyridine (MPTP), which is converted by monoamine oxidase B to *N*-methyl-4-phenylpyridinium (MPP^+), an active toxin. MPP^+ is taken up by dopaminergic nigral neurons through an active transport system that is normally involved in dopamine reuptake, and then inhibits oxidative phosphorylation, possibly at the level of complex I in the respiratory chain. This results in the death of nigrostriatal neurons, dopamine depletion in the basal ganglia, and parkinsonism. In addition to energy failure, MPP^+ may also generate free radicals and oxidative stress.

The cause of Parkinson's disease is unknown. One suggested cause is exposure to an unrecognized environmental toxin, perhaps structurally similar to MPTP. Such exposure may have occurred years before the onset of any clinical disturbance, because symptoms will not develop until the cumulative cell loss from toxin exposure and natural aging approximates 80% of the original cell population. Alternatively or additionally, endogenous toxins may be responsible. In particular, the normal neurotransmitter dopamine readily oxidizes to produce free radicals, which can cause cell death. Although the precise role of dopamine itself remains unclear, the evidence relating Parkinson's disease to damage by free radicals is compelling.

Oxidative stress is likely when dopamine turnover is increased, glutathione is reduced (leaving neurons more vulnerable to oxidant stress), and reactive iron is increased (promoting the generation of potentially toxic hydroxyl radicals). A mitochondrial complex 1 defect occurs in Parkinson's disease and may contribute to neuronal vulnerability and loss through free radical generation.

Accumulating evidence suggests a genetic susceptibility to the disease. An increased incidence of parkinsonism has been noted in the monozygotic twins of patients developing Parkinson's disease prior to the age of 50. First-degree relatives of patients are twice as likely to develop the disease as controls. Approximately 5% of parkinsonian patients have a familial form of the disorder. Three genes for the parkinsonian phenotype have recently been identified. Two different mutations of the α synuclein gene (in the q21-23 region of chromosome 4) have been identified in dominantly inherited parkinsonism; the α synuclein protein is of uncertain function but is abundant in neurons, especially at synaptic terminals, and in Lewy bodies. Homozygous deletions of the parkin gene (6q25.2-q27) have been associated with autosomal recessive parkinsonism; parkin is a protein expressed in the substantia nigra. Finally, a heterozygous missense mutation of the gene for ubiquitin carboxy-terminal hydrolase L1 has been identified in a parkinsonian family. The mechanism by which these mutations leads to parkinsonism remains to be determined, but the phenotype clearly has genetic heterogeneity.

Clinical Manifestations The 4- to 6-Hz *tremor* is typically most conspicuous at rest and worsens with emotional stress. It often begins with rhythmic flexion-extension of the fingers, hand, or foot, or with rhythmic pronation-supination of the forearm, and may be confined initially to one limb or to the two limbs on one side before becoming more generalized. It may also involve the mouth and chin. In 10 to 15% of patients, however, the tremor is faster (7 to 8 Hz) and postural, resembling essential tremor (see below) both clinically and in its response to pharmacotherapy.

Rigidity, defined as an increase in resistance to passive movement (Chap. 22), is a common clinical feature that accounts for the flexed posture of many patients. The most disabling feature, however, is *bradykinesia* (or, in its most severe form, akinesia), a slowness of voluntary movement and an associated reduction in automatic movements, such as swinging of the arms when walking. There is a fixity of facial expression, with widened palpebral fissures and infrequent blinking. There may be blepharoclonus (fluttering of the closed eyelids), blepharospasm (involuntary closure of the eyelids), and drooling of saliva from the mouth. The voice is hypophonic and poorly modulated. Power is preserved, but fine or rapidly alternating movements are impaired. The combination of tremor, rigidity, and bradykinesia results in small, tremulous, and often illegible handwriting. Patients have difficulty in rising from bed or an easy chair and tend to assume a flexed posture when erect. Walking is often difficult to initiate, and patients may have to lean forward increasingly until they can advance. They walk with small, shuffling steps, have no arm swing, are unsteady (especially on turning), and may have difficulty in stopping. Some patients walk with a *festinating gait*, i.e., at an increasing speed to prevent themselves from falling because of their abnormal center of gravity.

The tendon reflexes are unaltered, and the plantar responses are flexor. Repetitive tapping (at about 2 Hz) over the glabella produces a sustained blink response (Myerson's sign), in contrast to the response of normal subjects. A depressed mood is common, and an impairment of cognitive function—sometimes amounting to a frank dementia—is frequently evident in advanced cases.

Differential Diagnosis Parkinsonism is simulated by certain disorders. *Depression* is associated with changes in the voice and facial appearance and a poverty of spontaneous activity, such as occur in Parkinson's disease. A trial of treatment with antidepressant drugs helps to clarify the diagnosis if uncertainty persists and other signs of parkinsonism are absent. *Essential (benign, familial) tremor* may be mistaken for parkinsonian tremor, but a family history of tremor is common; alcohol in small quantities may ameliorate the tremor, and other neurologic signs are lacking. Moreover, essential tremor commonly involves the head (with a nodding or no-no tremor), whereas parkinsonism spares the head but affects the face and lips. *Normal-pressure hydrocephalus* (Chap. 362) causes an apraxic gait disturbance (sometimes resembling the gait of parkinsonism), urinary incontinence, and dementia. Imaging studies reveal dilation of the ventricular system without cortical atrophy, and surgical shunting procedures to

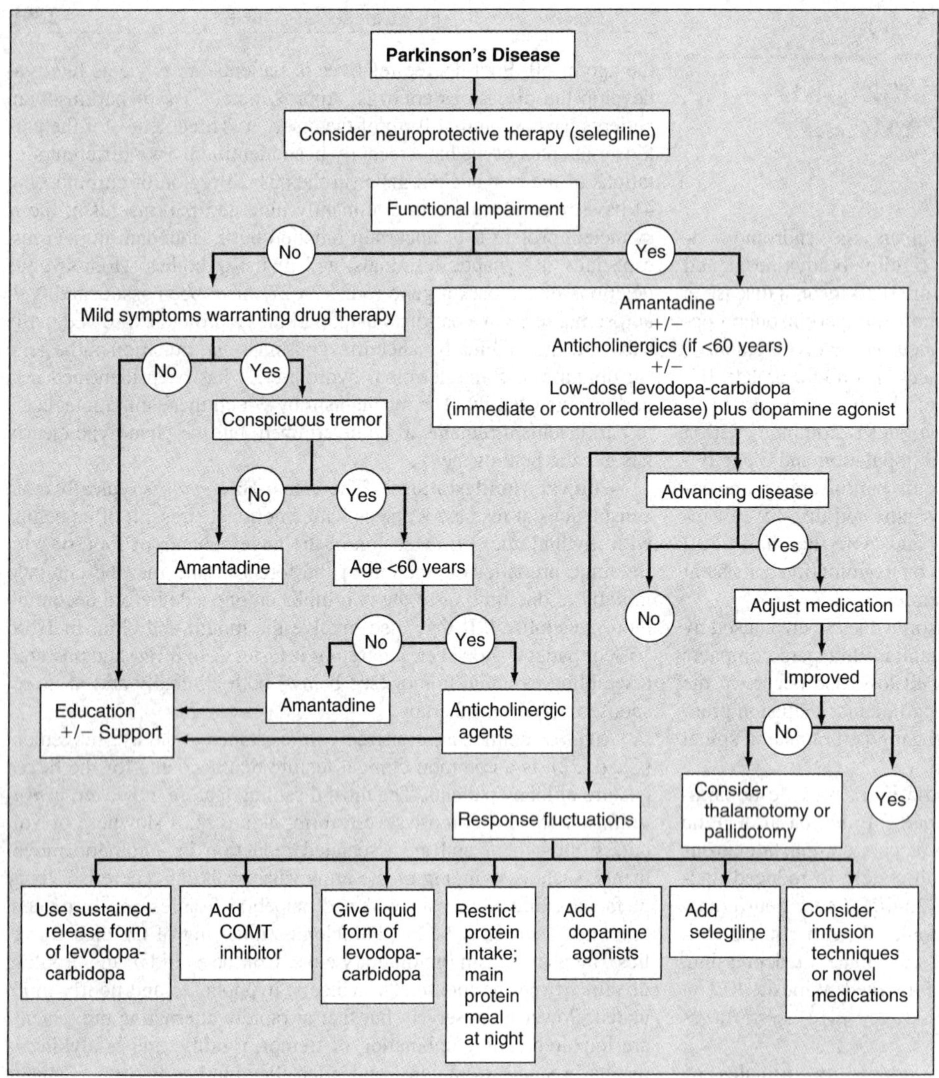

FIGURE 363-1 Algorithm for the management of patients with Parkinson's disease.

bypass any obstruction to the flow of cerebrospinal fluid (CSF) may be helpful.

Parkinsonism may occur as part of various neurologic diseases that are important to distinguish from Parkinson's disease for prognostic and therapeutic purposes. In *Wilson's disease* (Chap. 348), other abnormal movements are also usually present. The family history, early age of onset, associated Kayser-Fleischer rings, and low serum copper and ceruloplasmin levels distinguish it from Parkinson's disease. *Huntington's disease* (Chap. 362) sometimes presents with rigidity and akinesia, but the family history and any accompanying dementia point to the correct diagnosis, which can be confirmed by genetic studies. The *Shy-Drager syndrome* (Chap. 366) is a degenerative disorder characterized by parkinsonism, impaired autonomic function (resulting in postural hypotension, abnormal thermoregulatory sweating, disturbances of bladder and bowel control, impotence, and gastroparesis) and by signs of more widespread neurologic involvement (pyramidal, cerebellar, or lower motor neuron signs). There is generally no treatment except for the postural hypotension, which may respond to the measures discussed in Chap. 366. The response to antiparkinsonian agents is usually disappointing. *Striatonigral degeneration* (see below) leads to bradykinesia and rigidity, but tremor is usually inconspicuous. Cerebellar deficits sometimes occur (multisystem atrophy), and there may be autonomic insufficiency (Shy-Drager syndrome). Antiparkinsonian drugs are generally ineffective. *Progressive supranuclear palsy* (discussed separately, below) causes bradykinesia and rigidity, but conspicuous abnormalities of voluntary eye movements (especially vertical gaze), dementia, pseudobulbar palsy, and axial dystonia distinguish it from Parkinson's disease. There is little or no response to antiparkinsonian drugs. *Cortical-basal ganglionic degeneration* may be mistaken for Parkinson's disease, but intellectual decline, aphasia, apraxia, sensory neglect, and other evidence of cortical dysfunction should suggest the correct diagnosis. In *diffuse Lewy body disease*, parkinsonism is joined with a conspicuous dementia and with evidence of more widespread neurologic involvement. In *Creutzfeldt-Jakob disease*, any parkinsonian features are overshadowed by the rapidly progressive dementia; myoclonus is common, ataxia or pyramidal signs may occur, visual disturbances are sometimes conspicuous, and the electroencephalographic findings are often characteristic. Similarly, in *Alzheimer's disease* there may be minor extrapyramidal deficits, but these are generally inconsequential compared with the marked cognitive impairment that characterizes the disorder. →***Alzheimer's disease and diffuse Lewy body disease are considered in Chap. 362, and Creutzfeldt-Jakob disease is discussed in Chap. 375.***

Parkinsonism sometimes occurs as a consequence of a systemic disorder. Drug-induced *secondary parkinsonism* is especially common (discussed below). MPTP-induced parkinsonism has occurred in several humans who inadvertently took this meperidine analogue for recreational purposes. The mechanisms involved are discussed above, and the history of exposure, unusually early age of onset, and rapid progression should suggest the correct diagnosis. Exposure to various toxins, such as manganese dust or carbon disulfide, also causes parkinsonism, and the diagnosis is suggested by an accurate occupational history. Parkinsonism sometimes occurs as a result of severe carbon monoxide poisoning or develops after an encephalitic illness. Postencephalitic parkinsonism was especially common after the outbreak of encephalitis lethargica that occurred in an early part of the twentieth century.

℞ TREATMENT Approaches to treatment are summarized in Fig. 363-1.

Symptomatic Pharmacologic Treatment Nonselective muscarinic antagonists (*anticholinergic drugs*) are sometimes helpful, especially in relieving tremor. Various preparations are available, including trihexyphenidyl, benztropine, procyclidine, and orphenadrine. The usual maintenance doses are shown in Table 363-1. Common side effects include dryness of the mouth, constipation, urinary retention, and blurred vision. Narrow-angle glaucoma may be aggravated. Con-

Table 363-1 Commonly Used Muscarinic Antagonists (Anticholinergic Drugs) for the Treatment of Parkinson's Disease

Generic Name	Proprietary Name	Tablet Strength	Usual Dose, mg
Benztropine	Cogentin	0.5, 1, 2	0.5–2 tid
Biperiden	Akineton	2	1–3 qid
Orphenadrine	Disipal	100	100 tid
Procyclidine	Kemadrin	5	2.5–10 tid
Trihexyphenidyl	Artane	2, 5	2–5 tid

fusion and hallucinations are especially troublesome in the elderly. Treatment is started with the preparation of choice in a small initial dose that is gradually increased, depending on response and tolerance. If the drug is unhelpful, another anticholinergic preparation is substituted.

Amantadine, either alone or combined with an anticholinergic agent, is sometimes helpful for mild parkinsonism; it acts by potentiating the release of endogenous dopamine. It may improve all major clinical features of the disorder, has relatively uncommon side effects (restlessness, confusion, skin rashes, edema, disturbances of cardiac rhythm), and is given in a standard dose (100 mg twice daily). However, many patients derive only transient, if any, benefit from it.

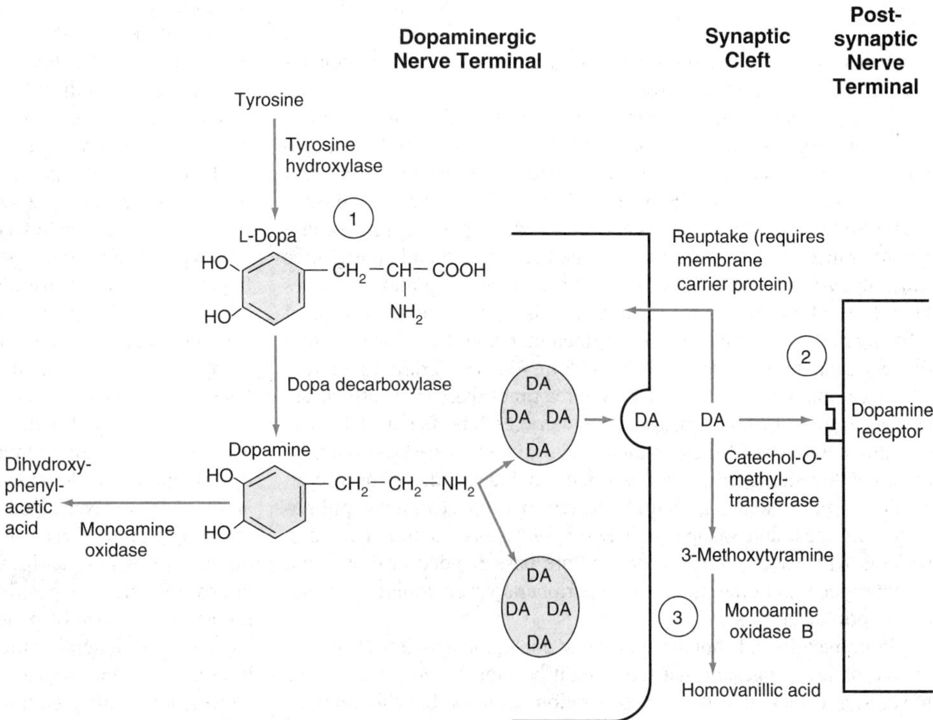

FIGURE 363-2 Diagrammatic representation of a dopaminergic nerve terminal and the associated postsynaptic dopamine receptors. The metabolic pathways for the synthesis and breakdown of dopamine are shown. The circled numbers indicate the site of action of several drugs used in the treatment of Parkinson's disease: ①, the site of action of levodopa (L-dopa); ②, that of dopamine agonist drugs; and ③, that of selegiline. DA, dopamine.

Levodopa, the metabolic precursor of dopamine (Fig. 363-2), provides symptomatic benefit in most patients with parkinsonism and is often particularly helpful in relieving bradykinesia. The presence in the intestinal mucosa of dopa decarboxylase, which converts levodopa to dopamine, means that most of an ingested dose of levodopa is lost before it even enters the general circulation. Administration of levodopa in combination with an extracerebral dopa-decarboxylase inhibitor reduces the extracerebral metabolism of levodopa and also reduces the incidence of peripheral side effects. Levodopa is therefore administered routinely in combination with a peripheral dopa-decarboxylase inhibitor (carbidopa in the United States; benserazide in Europe). In the United States, the combination of carbidopa and levodopa (in 1:10 and 1:4 ratios) is available commercially as Sinemet. Standard formulations are Sinemet 25/100, 10/100, and 25/250 mg. A common starting dose is 25/100 mg three times daily, which is increased gradually to 25/250 mg three or four times daily, taken 1 h before or 2 h after meals to maximize absorption and transport across the blood-brain barrier.

There was initially concern that the early introduction of levodopa might accelerate the death of nigrostriatal neurons because of a hypothetical increase in dopamine-mediated neurotoxity. It is now clear that levodopa should be introduced as soon as is warranted by the patient's clinical state, rather than postponed out of concern for this theoretical possibility. However, initial treatment with a dopamine agonist may provide similar benefit to levodopa and thus allow introduction of the latter to be postponed; in consequence, emergence of late side effects may be delayed. The most common initial side effects of levodopa are nausea, vomiting, postural hypotension, and, occasionally, cardiac arrhythmias. Abnormal movements (dyskinesias), restlessness (akathisia), and confusion tend to occur somewhat later and are dose-related. Dyskinesias may be present during most of the day, occur only when plasma levodopa levels peak, or develop when the plasma levodopa concentration reaches a certain submaximal level. Management depends on distinguishing these possibilities by the temporal profile of the dyskinesia. When dyskinesias occur only at a certain submaximal blood level of levodopa, adjustment of the daily dose to produce higher or lower blood levels may alleviate them; dyskinesias related to peak blood levels of levodopa are helped by a reduction in dose.

Important late complications of levodopa therapy are the wearing-off effect (transient deterioration shortly before the next dose is due) and the "on-off" phenomenon—abrupt but transient fluctuations in clinical state that occur frequently during the day, without warning or an obvious relationship to dosing schedule, resulting in alternating periods of marked akinesia or greater mobility accompanied by iatrogenic dyskinesias. Response fluctuations can be controlled in part by reducing dosing intervals, administering levodopa 1 h before meals and restricting dietary protein intake (to reduce any competition by various amino acids with levodopa for the active carrier system that transports it into the blood and from the blood into the brain), or treatment with dopamine agonists. The addition of selegiline (5 mg at breakfast and lunch), a monoamine oxidase B inhibitor, reduces the metabolic breakdown of dopamine and may also be helpful (see "Neuroprotective Treatment," below).

Response fluctuations to oral levodopa may also be reduced or eliminated by catechol-*O*-methyltransferase (COMT) inhibitor agents or by frequent or continuous administration of levodopa intravenously, intraduodenally, or by intragastric infusion. A commercially available controlled-release formulation of Sinemet (Sinemet CR 25/100 or 50/200 mg) sometimes helps in reducing the dosing frequency and maintaining steady blood levels of levodopa, but it is of only limited benefit in reducing response fluctuations. Surgical treatment is also effective (see later). The pathogenesis of the on-off phenomenon is obscure, but proposed mechanisms relate to the pharmacokinetics of levodopa, degeneration of presynaptic dopaminergic nerve terminals, altered sensitivity of dopamine receptors, and abnormalities of nondopaminergic neurotransmitter systems.

Dopamine agonist drugs may produce symptomatic benefit by direct stimulation of dopamine receptors (Fig. 363-2). There are five major dopamine-receptor subtypes classified into two groups. The D_1 group is made of the D_1 and D_5 subtypes, and the D_2 group consists of D_2, D_3, and D_4 subtypes. Drug efficacy and toxicity may relate to receptor specificity of dopamine agonists. The absorption and cerebral distribution of dopamine agonist drugs are less erratic than with levodopa, and they do not require enzymatic conversion to an active metabolite. Their early introduction either prior to Sinemet or in conjunction with low-dose Sinemet therapy (25/100 mg three times daily) yields sustained benefit and a lower incidence of late complications (such as response fluctuations and dyskinesias) than when levodopa is used alone and in a higher dose.

The agonists initially available were bromocriptine and pergolide, which are ergot derivatives. Bromocriptine, which stimulates dopamine D_2 receptors (Fig. 22-4), is introduced in a dose of 1.25 mg/d for 1 week and 2.5 mg/d for the next week, after which the daily dose is increased by 2.5-mg increments every 2 weeks, depending on response and tolerance. Maintenance doses range between 2.5 and 10 mg three times daily when the drug is taken with Sinemet. Pergolide activates both D_1 and D_2 dopamine receptors. It is introduced in a dose of 0.05 mg daily for 2 days; the dose is then increased by 0.1 to 0.15 mg/d every 3 days for 12 days and by 0.25 mg/d every 3 days thereafter. The usual maintenance dose is 1 mg three times daily. Side effects are similar to those of levodopa, but psychiatric effects such as delusions or hallucinations are more common, and dyskinesias are less common, than with levodopa. Other adverse effects include headache, nasal congestion, erythromelalgia, pleural and retroperitoneal fibrosis, pulmonary infiltrates, and vasospasm. These agonists are contraindicated in patients with psychotic disorders and are best avoided in those with recent myocardial infarction, severe peripheral vascular disease, or active peptic ulceration.

Pramipexole and ropinirole are new dopamine agonists. Their selective nature suggested that they might be more effective and have fewer side effects that the first-generation agonists, but this remains uncertain from the few studies comparing them to bromocriptine or pergolide. Because of their non-ergoline structure, adverse effects such as erythromelalgia, vasospasm, and pleural or retroperitoneal fibrosis are unlikely. Both agents, however, may cause postural hypotension, lassitude, sleep disturbances, peripheral edema, constipation, nausea, dyskinesias, and confusion. Excessive or uncontrollable somnolence may require withdrawal of the medication.

Pramipexole, an aminobenzthiazol-derived selective D_3 agonist, provides worthwhile benefit when used alone for mild parkinsonism or when taken together with Sinemet for advanced disease. It permits a reduction in Sinemet dosage and smooths response fluctuations. It may also benefit associated affective symptoms. Pramipexole is absorbed rapidly from the gastrointestinal tract, reaches peak plasma concentrations in about 2 h, and is excreted by the kidneys; renal failure may therefore necessitate reduction in daily dose. The starting dose is 0.125 mg three times daily, with doubling of the dose after 1 week, and again after another week. The daily dose is then increased by 0.75 mg at weekly intervals depending on need and tolerance. The usual maintenance dose is 0.5 to 1.5 mg three times daily. Ropinirole, a selective D_2 agonist, is also effective for mild or advanced disease. It is started at 0.25 mg three times daily; total daily dose is increased by 0.75 mg at weekly intervals until the fourth week and then by 1.5 mg as needed. The usual maintenance dose is between 2 and 8 mg three times daily. It is metabolized by CYP1A2, and its clearance may be reduced by drugs undergoing hepatic metabolism.

Various new dopamine agonists are being evaluated, and new means of administering them (e.g., by subcutaneous infusion pump or transdermally) may lead to a steadier clinical response.

Selective COMT inhibitors such as tolcapone and entacapone enhance the benefits of levodopa therapy by reducing the conversion of levodopa to 3-*O*-methyldopa (which competes with levodopa for an active carrier mechanism) and by increasing the availability in the brain of levodopa. They are helpful in patients with response fluctuations to Sinemet, leading to a smoother response, greater "on" time, and reduction in daily levodopa requirement. Both agents are absorbed rapidly, bound to plasma proteins, and metabolized before being excreted. Both have peripheral effects, but tolcapone is also active centrally. Tolcapone is slightly more potent, has a longer duration of action, and is usually taken in a dose of 100 mg (rarely, 200 mg) three times daily, whereas entacapone (200 mg) is taken with each dose of Sinemet and may thus be taken four to six times daily. When COMT inhibitors are introduced, the daily dose of Sinemet may have to be reduced by up to 30% in the first 48 h to prevent or minimize such complications as dyskinesias, nausea, and confusion. Other adverse effects include diarrhea, abdominal pain, postural hypotension, sleep disturbances, and discolored urine. Acute hepatic failure has occurred in rare patients receiving tolcapone, and a transient increase in liver enzymes is not uncommon. Accordingly, when tolcapone is prescribed, a consent form should be signed by the patient and liver function monitored every 2 weeks for the first year and less frequently thereafter, as recommended by the manufacturer.

Experimental studies suggest that glutamate antagonists may benefit patients with Parkinson's disease, and clinical studies of such agents are planned. G_{M1} ganglioside and various neurotrophic factors influence dopaminergic nigrostriatal cells, and work is continuing to develop delivery systems that will permit their use in the treatment of Parkinson's disease.

Surgical Treatment Destructive neurosurgical procedures were used for some years to treat parkinsonism, but their use declined with the advent of levodopa. Unilateral posteroventral pallidotomy or thalamotomy was resurrected in the 1990s as a therapeutic approach for relieving rigidity, bradykinesia, and tremor in patients with advanced disease in whom antiparkinsonian medication was ineffective or poorly tolerated. A positive (but incomplete) response to surgery is reported in >90% of patients; the beneficial effect predominates on the side contralateral to the procedure. Complications include cerebral infarction or hemorrhage, dysarthria or hypophonia, cognitive disturbances, and—after pallidotomy—visual field defects. Bilateral procedures have a higher morbidity and are generally discouraged. Such surgery is being replaced in some centers by high-frequency stimulation of selected locations in the brain, using an implanted electrode and stimulator, to induce a functional but reversible lesion. Thalamic stimulation is very effective in relieving tremor, and preliminary studies suggest that stimulation of the globus pallidus internus or subthalamic nucleus increases "on" time and improves clinical status in those with advanced parkinsonism and response fluctuations. Brain stimulation surgery has a lower morbidity than ablative surgery, but neither approach is warranted in patients with secondary or atypical parkinsonism or dementia.

There is ongoing interest in transplantation of fetal midbrain dopaminergic (nigral) cells into the putamen of patients with Parkinson's disease. Survival of engrafted cells has been documented by enhancement of fluorodopa uptake as visualized by positron emission tomography (PET), and in one autopsy study there was extensive striatal reinnervation by the transplanted cells. Fetal nigral transplantation remains an experimental procedure, and the nature of any long-term benefit is uncertain. Transplantation of autologous adrenal medullary tissue has also been attempted for Parkinson's disease, with mixed results; benefit seems most likely to occur in individuals younger than 50 years of age.

Neuroprotective Treatment Selective inhibitors of monoamine oxidase B such as selegiline (Eldepryl; Deprenyl) may reduce oxidative damage and thus slow disease progression, but the evidence for this effect is incomplete. In a large multicenter study, treatment with selegiline delayed the need for symptomatic therapy in patients with untreated parkinsonism, suggesting that progression of the disease had been retarded, but it was subsequently found that selegiline itself has a mild effect on symptoms. Thus, the basis of the observed effect is uncertain. The use of selegiline for protective purposes should probably be discussed with all patients unless they have end-stage disease or are very elderly, but the uncertainty of any benefit should be indicated. Selegiline in a standard dose (5 mg with breakfast and 5 mg with lunch) is not associated with the hypertensive ("cheese") effect of nonselective monoamine oxidase inhibitors. Acute toxic interactions may, however, occur with meperidine, tricyclic drugs, or serotonin reuptake inhibitors, and selegiline should not be prescribed to patients receiving those medications. Selegiline is metabolized to amphetamine and methamphetamine, so some patients may experience anxiety or insomnia. Moreover, an increased mortality rate has recently been found among patients receiving selegiline, raising concerns about its long-term safety. Patients must understand that selegiline is not intended to relieve symptoms and that there is no means of determining whether it is affecting disease progression in individual cases. Other inhibitors of monamine oxidase B are currently being evaluated for their effect on the natural history of Parkinson's disease and may clarify the issue.

Tocopherol (vitamin E) is an important scavenger of free radicals, but in a large study it failed to provide any protective benefit when taken in a dose of 2000 units daily. The extent to which it penetrates the brain, however, is not clear.

General Measures Physical therapy and speech therapy may help patients with moderately severe parkinsonism. In advanced cases, the quality of life can be improved by certain aids to daily living, such as extra rails or banisters placed in the home, table cutlery with large handles, nonslip table mats, voice amplifiers, and chairs that can gently eject the occupant.

FAMILIAL OR BENIGN ESSENTIAL TREMOR A postural tremor (Chap. 22) may develop in otherwise normal individuals, sometimes on a familial basis with autosomal dominant inheritance. The pathophysiologic basis of the disorder is unknown.

Symptoms can develop at any age but often do not appear until middle or later life. Typically one or both hands, the head, and the voice are affected in any combination; the legs are generally spared. Apart from the tremor, no other abnormalities are present on neurologic examination. The tremor may worsen with time and ultimately become an embarrassment, but it generally causes no disability except when it disturbs handwriting or performance of fine tasks with the hands. A small quantity of alcohol sometimes relieves the tremor for a short period.

℞ TREATMENT Treatment is often unnecessary and is best delayed for as long as possible because, once initiated, it generally needs to be continued indefinitely. Propranolol, 40 to 120 mg orally twice daily, may reduce the amplitude of the tremor. A single oral dose (40 to 120 mg) may be taken in anticipation of known precipitating circumstances. Primidone is also effective but has to be introduced gradually. Other agents that may be helpful include alprazolam and mirtazapine. Thalamic stimulation (discussed earlier) may be helpful for severe tremor unresponsive to medical treatment.

PROGRESSIVE SUPRANUCLEAR PALSY Progressive supranuclear palsy (also referred to as *Steele-Richardson-Olszewski syndrome*) is a sporadic degenerative disorder characterized pathologically by neuronal loss, gliosis, and neurofibrillary tangles in the midbrain, pons, basal ganglia, and dentate nuclei of the cerebellum. The neurofibrillary tangles of this disorder are distinct from those of Alzheimer's disease in that they are composed of straight filaments rather than paired helical filaments. The microtubule-associated protein tau is a constituent of the tangles, and a genetic association between an intrinsic polymorphism of tau and progressive supranuclear palsy has recently been reported. Thus, progressive supranuclear palsy may represent a tau pathologic process. There are also decreased concentrations of dopamine and homovanillic acid in the caudate nucleus and putamen.

Clinical Manifestations This uncommon disorder generally begins between the ages of 45 and 75 years; it affects men twice as frequently as women. Supranuclear ophthalmoplegia is characteristic. There is conspicuous failure of voluntary saccadic gaze (and of the fast phase of optokinetic nystagmus) in a vertical plane, especially downward, with later involvement of horizontal gaze. Eventually, smooth pursuit movements are also affected. Oculocephalic (e.g., doll's-head) and oculovestibular (caloric) reflexes are intact. Axial dystonia in extension, especially of the neck, is common and is frequently accompanied by limb rigidity and bradykinesia that may mimic Parkinson's disease. Tremor, however, is unusual. The combination of supranuclear ophthalmoplegia and axial rigidity accounts for the common presenting complaint of frequent falls. There may be facial weakness, dysarthria, dysphagia, and exaggerated jaw jerk and gag reflexes (pseudobulbar palsy) as well as exaggerated and inappropriate emotional responses (pseudobulbar affect). Brisk tendon reflexes, extensor plantar responses, and cerebellar signs are sometimes encountered. A global impairment of intellectual function is frequent, but focal cortical dysfunction is rare.

Progressive supranuclear palsy should be considered whenever a middle-aged or elderly person with repeated falls has an extrapyramidal syndrome accompanied by nuchal dystonia and paralysis of voluntary downgaze. The marked impairment of voluntary downward and horizontal gaze distinguishes this disorder from Parkinson's disease, as does the extended rather than flexed dystonic posturing of the axial musculature, the absence of tremor, and the poor response to antiparkinsonian medications.

℞ TREATMENT The course is generally progressive, with aspiration or inanition leading to a fatal outcome within 10 years. Dopaminergic preparations sometimes reduce rigidity and bradykinesia, and anticholinergic (trihexyphenidyl, 6 to 15 mg/d) or tricyclic drugs (amitriptyline, 50 to 75 mg at bedtime) may benefit speech, gait, and pseudobulbar affect, but any benefit is limited and not sustained.

CORTICAL-BASAL GANGLIONIC DEGENERATION This rare sporadic disorder typically begins in middle or later life with functional impairment of one or more limbs. Examination reveals signs of parkinsonism, but the extrapyramidal abnormalities are generally insufficient to account for the clinical deficit, which results from apraxia. As the disorder progresses, other evidence of cortical dysfunction also appears, such as aphasia, agnosia, sensory inattention, and mild dementia. Pathologically there is cell loss and gliosis in the cerebral cortex as well as the substantia nigra. The response to antiparkinsonian medication is disappointing, and the course is generally progressive, with increasing disability and dependence leading ultimately to death.

STRIATONIGRAL DEGENERATION In a few patients with seemingly classic Parkinson's disease, there is little or no response to dopaminergic medication, and pathologic study at autopsy reveals neuronal loss and gliosis in the putamen, globus pallidus, caudate and subthalamic nuclei, and substantia nigra. This disorder has therefore been called *striatonigral degeneration*. It has an age and gender distribution similar to those of Parkinson's disease. Clinical examination reveals the findings of parkinsonism, but tremor is usually relatively inconspicuous. Cognitive function is preserved.

There may be an accompanying impairment of autonomic function (Shy-Drager syndrome; Chap. 366), and examination in such cases often reveals that a combination of pyramidal and cerebellar signs is also present. Indeed, in some cases the cerebellar findings are so conspicuous that the disorder is more properly called *spinocerebellar ataxia type 1* (olivopontocerebellar atrophy; Chap. 364).

The management of patients with striatonigral degeneration is difficult. Antiparkinsonian medications generally are prescribed but are usually ineffective.

MACHADO-JOSEPH DISEASE (SPINOCEREBELLAR ATAXIA TYPE 3) Machado-Joseph disease is an autosomal dominant form of striatonigral degeneration that generally begins in the third or fourth decade. Most affected individuals are of Portuguese ancestry. There may be only mild parkinsonian signs, whereas spasticity, hyperreflexia, extensor plantar responses, cerebellar findings, external ophthalmoplegia and, sometimes, peripheral neuropathy are conspicuous. Cognitive function is preserved. Pathologically the findings are similar to those of striatonigral degeneration, but the dentate nucleus of the cerebellum is also involved. There is no specific treatment. →***The different clinical subtypes of the disease, their genetic basis, and related autosomal dominant ataxias with some extrapyramidal features are discussed in Chap. 364.***

IDIOPATHIC TORSION DYSTONIA The occurrence of dystonic movements and postures without other neurologic signs in patients with a normal birth and developmental history is designated *idiopathic torsion dystonia*. The pathophysiologic and biochemical basis of this entity is unknown. Pathologic examination reveals no specific abnormalities, but the disorder is attributed to basal ganglia dysfunction partly because of observations made in cases of secondary dystonia. Other possible causes of dystonia (Chap. 22) should be excluded before this diagnosis is made. The disorder may occur on a sporadic or hereditary basis. In cases with onset in childhood or adolescence, inheritance is commonly autosomal dominant, with the gene, designated DYT1, localized to 9q32-34 and involving a GAG deletion. The gene codes for the protein Torsin A, the function of which is unclear. Onset is typically in a limb (commonly the leg), with subsequent spread to the other limbs and trunk, but sparing of the cranial muscles. Other autosomal dominant forms present in children or adults and begin in limb, axial, or cranial muscles; cranial involvement (facial, laryngeal, cervical) is common. This gene (DYT6) has been mapped to chromosome 8 in certain families. In a few families with autosomal dominant, adult-onset cranial, cervical, or upper limb dystonia, the responsible gene (DYT7) has been mapped to chromosome 18p. In other families, other unmapped genetic loci appear to be involved. Autosomal recessive and X-linked recessive (Xq21.3) forms are also described. Onset in childhood is associated with a positive family history, symptoms that begin in the legs, and greater disability than with later onset. About one-third of patients eventually become chair- or bedbound.→*A summary of the genetic loci responsible for the various dystonic disorders is provided in Table 359-1.*

Examination reveals the abnormal movements and sustained postures that characterize the disorder. There may be involvement of the neck, trunk, limbs, and face (blepharospasm or oromandibular dystonia). A description of these various motor abnormalities is provided in Chap. 22. Initially they may be brought out by voluntary activity, but eventually they are present constantly, leading to deformity and disability.

Occasional patients have *dopa-responsive dystonia*, which is inherited in an autosomal dominant manner with incomplete penetrance. The responsible gene (DYT5) maps to chromosome 14q. Onset is usually in childhood, and examination typically reveals associated bradykinesia and rigidity. The response to low-dose levodopa therapy is dramatic.

℞ TREATMENT Treatment is symptomatic and is often unsatisfactory. Anticholinergic drugs in high doses (e.g., trihexyphenidyl, 30 to 50 mg/d) are probably the most effective means of providing some relief of the abnormal movements and postures. They are introduced in a low dose and built up gradually, depending on response and tolerance. Phenothiazines or haloperidol are sometimes helpful but usually cause mild parkinsonism. Diazepam, baclofen, and carbamazepine are helpful occasionally. Stereotactic thalamotomy may be beneficial when dystonia is predominantly unilateral and involves the limbs.

FOCAL TORSION DYSTONIA Dystonia may occur as an isolated phenomenon affecting a discrete part of the body, rather than having the more generalized distribution described above. Such focal or segmental dystonias probably represent variants of idiopathic torsion dystonia; its genetic basis was discussed earlier. Both *blepharospasm* (spontaneous, involuntary forced closure of the eyelids) and *oromandibular dystonia* can occur as isolated focal dystonias. Oromandibular dystonia consists of involuntary contractions of the masticatory, lingual, and perioral muscles, leading to opening or closure of the mouth; pouting, pursing, or retraction of the lips; and roving or protruding movements of the tongue. The combination of blepharospasm and oromandibular dystonia is called *Meige syndrome*.

Spasmodic torticollis is characterized by a tendency for the head to turn to one side. The designation *anterocollis* indicates that the head is flexed forward, and *retrocollis* that it is pulled backward. These cervical dystonias are often intermittent initially, but eventually the head is held continuously in the abnormal position. Spontaneous remission occurs occasionally, especially in the first few months after onset, but thereafter the disorder is likely to be permanent and may worsen with time.

℞ TREATMENT Pharmacotherapy is usually unrewarding, but the drugs used in treating idiopathic torsion dystonia are helpful in some patients. Local injection of botulinum toxin into the overactive muscles often produces a benefit lasting several weeks or months by producing a temporary presynaptic block of neuromuscular transmission, and injections can be repeated as needed. This is the most effective treatment available for most focal dystonias. Selective section of the spinal accessory nerve (cranial nerve XI) and the upper cervical nerve roots is sometimes helpful for patients with cervical dystonia unresponsive to other measures.

TASK-SPECIFIC FOCAL DYSTONIA Writer's cramp is a task-specific dystonia in which abnormal posturing of the hand and forearm occurs when the hand is used for writing. As the disorder worsens, abnormal posturing may also occur with other tasks, such as applying cosmetics, shaving, or using table cutlery. Drug treatment is usually unrewarding, and it is often necessary for patients to learn to use the other hand for these tasks. Injections of botulinum toxin into the involved muscles are sometimes helpful, but function usually remains impaired. Other task-specific dystonias include violinist's cramp, barber's cramp, and telegrapher's cramp, in each of which dystonic posturing occurs when the hand is used for a skilled, occupationally related function. The pathophysiologic basis of these disorders is uncertain, but recent work relates it to abnormal processing of sensory input from the affected extremity during the activity.

DRUG-INDUCED MOVEMENT DISORDERS **Parkinsonism** Parkinsonism is a frequent complication of treatment with dopamine-depleting agents such as reserpine or antipsychotic dopamine antagonists such as the phenothiazines or butyrophenones. The antipsychotic drugs most likely to cause parkinsonism are those that are potent D_2 receptor antagonists having little anticholinergic effect, such as piperazine phenothiazines, haloperidol, and thiothixene. Women and the elderly have an increased risk of this complication. In comparison with Parkinson's disease, tremor is less common and bradykinesia is typically symmetric, but the two disorders are sometimes impossible to distinguish except by the history of drug ingestion. Signs usually develop within 3 months of starting the causal agent and may persist for several months (or longer) after its withdrawal. Drug-induced parkinsonism is best managed by discontinuing the antipsychotic drug when possible, substituting an antipsychotic with greater anticholinergic potency, or adding an anticholinergic drug such as trihexyphenidyl. Levodopa should not be prescribed—it is of no help if the offending neuroleptic agent is continued, and it may worsen the underlying psychotic disorder.

Acute Dystonia or Dyskinesia Acute dystonia (such as blepharospasm or torticollis) or dyskinesia (such as chorea or facial grimacing) may complicate treatment with a dopamine receptor antagonist. It typically commences within 1 week of the introduction of such medication, usually in the first 48 h, and is more common in young patients. Its pathophysiologic basis is uncertain. Treatment with an anticholinergic drug (e.g., benztropine, 2 mg, or diphenhydramine, 50 mg intravenously) is usually helpful.

Tardive Akathisia *Akathisia* denotes a motor restlessness. Patients are unable to sit still and feel obliged to move about. It is commonly induced by chronic antipsychotic drug treatment, especially in women, and is treated like drug-induced parkinsonism.

Tardive Dyskinesia or Dystonia Tardive dyskinesia or dystonia is a common complication of long-term antipsychotic drug treatment (with dopamine receptor antagonists). The risk of its development increases with advancing age, but its pathogenesis is unclear. One suggestion is that it is related to drug-induced supersensitivity of striatal dopamine receptors. However, although supersensitivity is an inevitable accompaniment of chronic antipsychotic drug treatment, tardive dyskinesia does not always occur. Moreover, the time courses of the two phenomena are different. Supersensitivity occurs relatively early during treatment and reverses when medication is withdrawn, whereas tardive dyskinesia usually requires exposure for at least 6 months before it develops and may persist indefinitely. Another suggestion is that it involves an abnormality of γ-aminobutyric acid (GABA)-ergic neurons. This is supported by observations that GABA and glutamic acid decarboxylase (its synthesizing enzyme) are depleted in the basal ganglia by long-term administration of antipsychotic drugs to animals and that CSF levels of GABA are reduced in patients with tardive dyskinesia.

The clinical features of tardive dyskinesia include abnormal choreoathetoid movements, especially involving the face and mouth in adults and the limbs in children. Tardive dystonia may be focal, producing, for example, blepharospasm, torticollis, or oromandibular dystonia, or it may affect contiguous body parts (e.g., the face and neck or arm and trunk). Generalized dystonia is uncommon, especially in older patients. It may be impossible to distinguish these disturbances from those of Huntington's disease (Chap. 362), Sydenham's chorea (Chap. 235), or idiopathic torsion dystonia except by the history of drug exposure. The iatrogenic disorder often resolves spontaneously in children or young adults but frequently persists in middle-aged or older individuals.

℞ **TREATMENT** Treatment of the established disorder is often unsatisfactory. It is therefore important that antipsychotic drugs be prescribed only when necessary and that their long-term use be accompanied by periodic drug holidays to determine whether treatment is still required. Drug holidays may actually unmask incipient dyskinesias, which often worsen on withdrawal of the causal agent. In such circumstances, permanent withdrawal of the antipsychotic medication, if this is possible, may lead to remission of the dyskinesia. Treatment with antidopaminergic agents such as haloperidol or phenothiazines (which cause the disorder) often suppresses the dyskinesias at least for a period, but these agents are best avoided, because they may exacerbate the underlying problem. Treatment with dopamine-depleting agents, such as reserpine, 0.25 mg gradually increased to 2 to 4 mg/d, or tetrabenazine (in countries where it is available), 12.5 mg gradually increased to as much as 200 mg/d, is sometimes worthwhile in reducing the severity of the dyskinesia. Other pharmacologic approaches are unrewarding in most instances. Tardive dystonia may respond to tetrabenazine (if available) or to anticholinergic drugs used as for idiopathic torsion dystonia.

Tardive tic resembles Gilles de la Tourette's syndrome (see below) and is best treated with clonidine or clonazepam.

Neuroleptic Malignant Syndrome Rigidity, hyperthermia, altered mental status resembling catatonia, labile blood pressure, and autonomic dysfunction characterize this serious complication of treatment with antipsychotic (neuroleptic) agents, especially haloperidol. Associated clinical features include tachycardia, tachypnea, metabolic acidosis, and myoglobinuria that may be fatal. The cause is unknown, but antagonism of dopamine is a likely contributor. The prevalence of this syndrome among patients receiving neuroleptics is $<2\%$, with the disorder occurring most commonly in young adults. Symptoms evolve over 1 to 2 days. The syndrome can develop at any time during exposure to the medication, but it usually occurs within the first 30 days of use.

The differential diagnosis includes infection, malignant hyperthermia, and alcohol- or drug-withdrawal states. Drug-induced parkinsonism may be similar but is not associated with fever or the autonomic features described above.

℞ **TREATMENT** Treatment includes immediate withdrawal of antipsychotic drugs and also of lithium and anticholinergic agents, which may increase the risk of developing the disorder. Symptomatic treatment is also necessary and includes antipyretics and artificial cooling, rehydration, and measures to maintain the blood pressure. Serum potassium should be monitored. Dantrolene, bromocriptine or another dopamine agonist, levodopa, amantadine, or benzodiazepines are sometimes helpful, but the mortality rate is on the order of 5 to 20%. Subcutaneous heparin administration reduces the risk of venous thrombosis. Most survivors recover completely, but potential complications include renal failure, pulmonary embolism, and a chronic cerebellar syndrome (related to the hyperthermia). Recovery generally occurs over 2 to 3 weeks.

Other Drug-Induced Movement Disorders Dyskinesia or dystonia may complicate therapy with levodopa or dopamine agonists as a dose-related phenomenon that is reversed by withdrawal of the medication or reduction of the dose. Reversible chorea may also complicate treatment with anticholinergic drugs, phenytoin, carbamazepine, amphetamines, lithium, and oral contraceptives; dystonia may follow treatment with lithium, carbamazepine, and metoclopramide; and postural tremor from theophylline, caffeine, lithium, thyroid hormone, tricyclic antidepressants, valproic acid, and isoproterenol.

GILLES DE LA TOURETTE'S SYNDROME Gilles de la Tourette's syndrome, which has a prevalence in the United States of approximately 0.05%, consists of chronic multiple motor and phonic tics that have no known cause. The disorder is not related to social or ethnic background or to perinatal abnormalities. Symptoms typically begin between 5 and 15 years of age and follow a relapsing and remitting course. A family history is sometimes obtained, and partial expression of the trait may occur in siblings or offspring of patients. In most families with chronic tic disorders, there is an autosomal dominant mode of inheritance with variable penetrance that is gender related. Boys are affected much more commonly than girls.

The pathophysiology is obscure, and no structural pathology has been recognized. A dopaminergic excess has been suggested by the clinical observation that the tics may respond to treatment with dopamine-blocking drugs.

Clinical Manifestations The first signs consist of single or multiple motor tics in 80% of cases and of phonic tics in 20%. Motor tics commonly affect the face and may consist of repetitive sniffing, winking, blinking, elevation of the eyelids, eye closure, pursing of the lips, or facial twitching. Patients eventually develop several different motor and phonic tics, the latter frequently taking the form of grunts, barks, hisses, sighs, throat-clearing, coughing, and verbal utterances that may involve coprolalia (involuntary and inappropriate swearing or obscene speech), echolalia (involuntary repetition of the phrases of others), and palilalia (repetition of words or phrases). The tics may change in location, severity, complexity, and character with time; are worsened by emotional stress; and can be suppressed voluntarily for short periods. In some cases, tics are complex (such as jumping up in the air) or involve repetitive self-mutilating activities (such as nail-biting, hair-pulling, or lip-biting). Tics that involve repetitive sensory phenomena, such as pressure, tickle, or thermal sensations, also occur. Many patients have associated behavioral abnormalities, especially obsessive-compulsive disorder and attention deficit hyperactivity disorder.

Apart from the presence of tics, physical examination typically reveals no other abnormalities, but the incidence of left-handedness or ambidexterity is greater than among normal persons, and many patients have nonspecific electroencephalographic abnormalities of no diagnostic significance.

The diagnosis is often delayed for years, the symptoms sometimes being attributed to psychiatric illness. Patients may be subjected to unnecessary and expensive treatment before the correct diagnosis is made. Depression, sometimes leading to suicide, may result from social embarrassment caused by the tics.

Differential Diagnosis Many children develop transient or chronic simple tics, and these have a benign prognosis and require no treatment. In some instances, simple or multiple tics persist for several years but resolve in late adolescence. Wilson's disease, a treatable cause of dyskinesias and tics, is generally associated with hepatic and renal involvement, Kayser-Fleischer corneal rings, low serum copper and ceruloplasmin levels, and increased 24-h urinary copper excretion (Chap. 348). The associated dementia, the character of the abnormal movements, and genetic studies distinguish Huntington's disease (Chap. 362). Sydenham's chorea (Chap. 235) may be confused with Gilles de la Tourette's syndrome when a history of rheumatic fever or polyarthritis is lacking and there is no cardiac involvement, but it usually resolves over 3 to 6 months. Tics may also occur in postencephalitic syndromes and as a side effect of stimulant or neuroleptic medication.

℞ **TREATMENT** Treatment is symptomatic and may need to be continued indefinitely.

Clonidine alleviates motor and phonic tics in some children, possibly by reducing activity in noradrenergic neurons of the locus coeruleus. The initial dose is 2 to 3 μg/kg per day, increased after 2 weeks to 4 μg/kg per day and then, if required, to 5 μg/kg per day. There may be a transient fall in blood pressure when this agent is introduced. Other side effects are sedation, reduced or excessive salivation, and diarrhea.

Haloperidol has been used widely for many years. It is introduced in a low daily dose (0.25 mg), which is gradually increased by 0.25 mg every 5 days, depending on response and tolerance. The optimal dose is usually 2 to 8 mg/d. Side effects include extrapyramidal movement disorders, sedation, xerostomia, blurred vision, and gastrointestinal disturbances. Pimozide, another dopaminergic-receptor antagonist, may be of benefit when haloperidol is unhelpful or poorly tolerated. It may produce widening of the QT interval and sudden death at high doses, so the electrocardiogram should be monitored routinely. Its long-term safety is unknown. It is introduced in a dose of 1 mg/d, and the dose is then increased by 2 mg every 10 days; most patients require 7 to 16 mg/d. The total dose should not exceed 0.3 mg/kg per day. Phenothiazines such as fluphenazine sometimes help, but patients unresponsive to haloperidol do not usually benefit from these drugs. Clonazepam or carbamazepine can also be tried. Family counseling and psychotherapy are sometimes helpful.

RESTLESS LEGS SYNDROME The restless legs syndrome is a common, chronic disorder that often has a familial basis, with evidence of autosomal dominant inheritance. It is characterized by a need to move because of unpleasant creeping sensations that arise deep within the legs and occasionally also in the arms, especially when patients are relaxed. For this reason, there is often difficulty in settling down to sleep at night. Periodic leg movements may also occur during sleep and can be documented by polysomnography. The cause is unknown, although the disorder is common during pregnancy and is sometimes associated with uremic or diabetic neuropathy, primary amyloidosis, or malignancy. Clinical examination may reveal evidence of underlying systemic disease or mild peripheral neuropathy but is more often normal. Symptoms may respond to correction of coexisting iron-deficiency anemia or to treatment with dopaminergic medication (such as levodopa, bromocriptine, or pergolide), benzodiazepines (diazepam or clonazepam), or opiates (codeine, propoxyphene, or oxycodone).

BIBLIOGRAPHY

BENNETT DA et al: Prevalence of parkinsonian signs and associated mortality in a community population of older people. N Engl J Med 334:771, 1996

DUNNETT SB, BJORKLUND A: Prospects for new restorative and neuroprotective treatments in Parkinson's disease. Nature 399:A32, 1999

FINE J et al: Long-term follow-up of unilateral pallidotomy in advanced Parkinson's disease. N Engl J Med 342:1708, 2000

GRATZ SS, SIMPSON GM: Neuroleptic malignant syndrome. Diagnosis, epidemiology and treatment. CNS Drugs 2:429, 1994

HYDE TM, WEINBERGER DR: Tourette's syndrome: A model neuropsychiatric disorder. JAMA 273:498, 1995

IANNACCONE S et al: Evidence of peripheral axonal neuropathy in primary restless legs syndrome. Mov Disord 10:2, 1995

JANKOVIC J: New and emerging therapies for Parkinson disease. Arch Neurol 56:785, 1999

KOLLER W et al: High-frequency unilateral thalamic stimulation in the treatment of essential and parkinsonian tremor. Ann Neurol 42:292, 1997

KORDOWER JH et al: Neuropathological evidence of graft survival and striatal reinnervation after the transplantation of fetal mesencephalic tissue in a patient with Parkinson's disease. N Engl J Med 332:1118, 1995

KURTH MC et al: Tolcapone improves motor function and reduces levodopa requirement in patients with Parkinson's disease experiencing motor fluctuations: A multicenter, double-blind, randomized, placebo-controlled trial. Neurology 48:81, 1997

LANG AE, LOZANO AM: Parkinson's disease. N Engl J Med 339:1044, 1130, 1998

——— et al: Posteroventral medial pallidotomy in advanced Parkinson's disease. N Engl J Med 337:1036, 1997

LIMOUSIN P et al: Electrical stimulation of the subthalamic nucleus in advanced Parkinson's disease. N Engl J Med 339:1105, 1998

MARTIN JB: Molecular basis of the neurodegenerative disorders. N Engl J Med 340:1970, 1999

NYGAARD TG et al: Linkage mapping of dopa-responsive dystonia (DRD) to chromosome 14q. Nat Genet 5:386, 1993

OLANOW CW, TATTON WG: Etiology and pathogenesis of Parkinson's disease. Annu Rev Neurosci 22:123, 1999

OZELIUS LJ et al: The early-onset torsion dystonia gene (DYT1) encodes an ATP-binding protein. Nat Genet 17:40, 1997

PARKINSON STUDY GROUP: Effects of tocopherol and deprenyl on the progression of disability in early Parkinson's disease. N Engl J Med 328:176, 1993

———: Impact of deprenyl and tocopherol treatment on Parkinson's disease in DATATOP subjects not requiring levodopa. Ann Neurol 39:29, 1996

POLYMEROPOULOS MH et al: Mapping of a gene for Parkinson's disease to chromosome 4q21-q23. Science 274:1197, 1996

QUINN N: Drug treatment of Parkinson's disease. BMJ 310:575, 1995

SCHUURMAN PR et al: A comparison of continuous thalamic stimulation and thalamotomy for suppression of severe tremor. N Engl J Med 342:461, 2000

STARR PA et al: Ablative surgery and deep brain stimulation for Parkinson's disease. Neurosurgery 43:989, 1998

TANNER CM et al: Parkinson disease in twins: An etiologic study. JAMA 281:341, 1999

UITTI RJ et al: Unilateral pallidotomy for Parkinson's disease: Comparison of outcome in younger versus older patients. Neurology 49:1072, 1997

364

Roger N. Rosenberg

ATAXIC DISORDERS

AT ataxia telangiectasia
AVED Ataxia of the Friedreich's phenotype with vitamin E deficiency
CNS central nervous system
CT computed tomography
DRPLA dentratorubropallidoluysian atrophy
EA episodic ataxia
MJD Machado-Joseph disease
MRI magnetic resonance imaging
mtDNA mitochondrial DNA
MTP microsomal triglyceride transfer protein
SCAs spinocerebellar ataxias
VLDL very-low-density lipoprotein

Approach to the Patient

Ataxia is a common and important neurologic finding. Symptoms and signs of ataxia consist of gait impairment, unclear ("scanning") speech, visual blurring due to nystagmus, hand incoordination, and tremor with movement (Chap. 22). These result from the involvement of the cerebellum and its afferent and efferent pathways including the spinocerebellar pathways, and the frontopontocerebellar pathway originating in the rostral frontal lobe (Brodmann's area 10). True cerebellar ataxia must be distinguished from ataxia associated with vestibular nerve or labyrinthine disease, as the latter results in a disorder of gait associated with a significant degree of dizziness, light-headedness, or the perception of movement (Chap. 21). True cerebellar ataxia is devoid of these vertiginous complaints and is clearly an unsteady gait due to imbalance. Weakness of proximal leg muscles and a variant of acute idiopathic polyneuritis (Miller-Fisher syndrome) can on occasion simulate the imbalance of cerebellar disease. In the patient who presents with ataxia, the rate and pattern of the development of cerebellar symptoms are important in determining the diagnostic possibilities (Table 364-1). A gradual and progressive increase in symptoms with bilateral and symmetric involvement suggests a biochemical, metabolic, immune, or toxic etiology. Conversely, focal, unilateral symptoms with headache and impaired level of consciousness accompanied by ipsilateral cranial nerve palsies and contralateral weakness imply a space-occupying cerebellar lesion.

Symmetric Ataxia Progressive and symmetric ataxia can be classified with respect to onset as acute (over hours or days), subacute (weeks or months), or chronic (months to years). Acute and reversible ataxias include those caused by intoxication with alcohol, phenytoin, lithium, barbiturates, and other drugs. Intoxication caused by toluene exposure, gasoline sniffing, glue sniffing, spray painting, or exposure to methyl mercury or bismuth are additional causes of acute or subacute ataxia, as is treatment with cytotoxic chemotherapeutic drugs such as flourouracil and paclitaxel. Children with a postinfectious syndrome (especially after varicella) may develop gait ataxia and mild dysathria, which are both reversible (Chap. 371). Rare infectious causes of acquired ataxia include poliovirus, coxsackievirus, echovirus, Epstein-Barr virus, toxoplasmosis, *Legionella*, and the prion protein responsible for Creutzfeldt-Jakob disease. The subacute development of ataxia of gait over weeks to months (acute cerebellar degeneration of the vermis) may be due to the combined effects of alcoholism and malnutrition, particularly with deficiencies of vitamins B_1 and B_{12}. Hyponatremia has also been associated with ataxia. A paraneoplastic syndrome, which may be associated with myoclonus and opsoclonus, may present as incapacitating gait ataxia. Specific autoantibodies (Yo, Ri, and PCD) have been identified that are responsible for cerebellar degeneration involving principally the midline or vermis (Chap. 101). Female patients may present with cerebellar ataxia before the identification of a breast or ovarian carcinoma. Removal of the tumor may prevent further progression of symptoms and in some patients result in gait improvement. Chronic symmetric gait ataxia of months' to years' duration suggests an inherited ataxia (discussed below), a metabolic disorder, or a chronic infection. Hypothyroidism must always be considered as a readily treatable and reversible form of gait ataxia. Infectious diseases that can present with ataxia are meningovascular syphilis and tabes dorsalis due to degeneration of the posterior columns and spinocerebellar pathways in the spinal cord. Lyme disease may cause ataxic symptoms.

Focal Ataxia Acute focal ataxia commonly results from cerebrovascular disease, usually ischemic infarction, hemorrhagic infarction, or cerebellar hemorrhage. These lesions typically produce cerebellar symptoms ipsilateral to the injured cerebellum and may be associated with an impaired level of consciousness due to brainstem compression and increased intracranial pressure; ipsilateral pontine signs, including sixth and seventh nerve palsies, may be present. Focal and worsening signs of acute ataxia should also prompt consideration of a posterior fossa subdural hematoma, bacterial abscess, primary or metastatic cerebellar tumor, or acute demyelinating lesion of multiple sclerosis. Computed tomography (CT) or magnetic resonance imaging (MRI) studies will reveal clinically significant processes of this type, which may require surgical decompression. Many of these lesions represent true neurologic emergencies, as sudden herniation, either rostrally through the tentorium or caudal herniation of cerebellar tonsils through the foramen magnum can occur and is usually devastating (Chap. 376). Lymphoma or progressive multifocal leukoencephalopathy (PML) in a patient with AIDS may present with an acute or subacute focal cerebellar syndrome. Chronic etiologies of ataxia include multiple sclerosis and congenital lesions such as the Chiari type I malformation, and congenital cysts of the posterior fossa (Dandy-Walker syndrome).

Table 364-1 Etiology of Cerebellar Ataxia

Symmetrical and Progressive Signs			Focal and Ipsilateral Cerebellar Signs		
Acute (Hours to Days)	Subacute (Days to Weeks)	Chronic (Months to Years)	Acute (Hours to Days)	Subacute (Days to Weeks)	Chronic (Months to Years)
Intoxication: alcohol, lithium, diphenylhydantoin, barbiturates (positive history and toxicology screen) Acute viral cerebellitis (CSF supportive of acute viral infection) Postinfection syndrome	Intoxication: mercury, solvents, gasoline, glue; cytotoxic chemotherapeutic drugs Alcoholic-nutritional (vitamin B_1 and B_{12} deficiency) Lyme disease	Paraneoplastic syndrome Hypothyroidism Inherited diseases Tabes dorsalis (tertiary syphilis)	Vascular: Cerebellar infarction, hemorrhage, or subdural hematoma Infectious: cerebellar abscess (positive mass lesion on MRI/CT, positive history in support of lesion)	Neoplastic: cerebellar glioma or metastatic tumor (positive for neoplasm on MRI/CT) Demyelinating: Multiple sclerosis (history, CSF and MRI are consistent) AIDS-related multifocal leukoencephalopathy (positive HIV test and CD4+ cell count for AIDS)	Stable gliosis secondary to vascular lesion or demyelinating plaque (stable lesion on MRI/CT older than several months) Congenital lesion: Chiari or Dandy-Walker malformations (malformation noted on MRI/CT)

ABBREVIATIONS: CSF, cerebrospinal fluid; CT, computed tomography; MRI, magnetic resonance imaging.

THE INHERITED ATAXIAS

Of the syndromes that constitute the inherited ataxias, some show autosomal dominant or autosomal recessive modes of inheritance, and some are caused by mitochondrial mutations and thus show a maternal mode of inheritance. Substantial progress has been made in recent years in identifying the molecular basis of these syndromes (Table 364-2), so that a genomic classification is superseding previous ones based on clinical expression alone.

Although the clinical manifestations and neuropathologic findings of cerebellar disease dominate the clinical picture, there may also be characteristic changes in the basal ganglia, brainstem, spinal cord, optic nerves, retina, and peripheral nerves. In large families with dominantly inherited disease, there are many gradations from purely cerebellar manifestations to mixed cerebellar and brainstem disorders, cerebellar and basal ganglia syndromes, and spinal cord or peripheral nerve disease. Rarely, dementia is present as well. The clinical picture may be consistent within a family with dominantly inherited ataxia, but sometimes most affected family members show one characteristic syndrome, while one or several members have an entirely different phenotype.

The autosomal spinocerebellar ataxias (SCAs) are caused by CAG triplet repeat expansions in different genes including SCA1, SCA2, MJD, SCA6, SCA7, and SCA13. SCA8 is due to a CTG repeat expansion (Table 364-2). The clinical phenotypes of these SCAs overlap. A single phenotype can result from several different genotypes, and conversely a single genotype can be associated with more than one different phenotype. The genotype has become the gold standard for diagnosis and classification. CAG encodes glutamine, and these expanded CAG triplet repeat expansions result in expanded polyglutamine proteins, termed *ataxins*, that produce a toxic gain of function with

Table 364-2 Genotype Classification of the Spinocerebellar Ataxias

Name	Locus	Phenotype
SCA1 (autosomal dominant type 1)	6p22-p23 with CAG repeats (exonic) Ataxin-1	Ataxia with ophthalmoparesis, pyramidal and extrapyramidal findings
SCA2 (autosomal dominant type 2)	12q23-q24.1 with CAG repeats (exonic) Ataxin-2	Ataxia with slow saccades and minimal pyramidal and extrapyramidal findings
Machado-Joseph disease/SCA3 (autosomal dominant type 3)	14q24.3-q32 with CAG repeats (exonic) MJD–ataxin-3	Ataxia with ophthalmoparesis and variable pyramidal, extrapyramidal, and amyotrophic signs
SCA4 (autosomal dominant type 4)	16q24-ter	Ataxia with normal eye movements, sensory axonal neuropathy, and pyramidal signs
SCA5 (autosomal dominant type 5)	Centromeric region of chromosome 11	Ataxia and dysarthria; family descended from paternal grandparents of President Lincoln
SCA6 (autosomal dominant type 6)	19p13 with CAG repeats in α_{1A}-voltage–dependent calcium channel gene (exonic)	Ataxia and dysarthria, nystagmus, mild proprioceptive sensory loss
SCA7 (autosomal dominant type 7)	3p14.1-p21.1 with CAG repeats (exonic) Ataxin-7	Ophthalmoparesis, visual loss, ataxia, dysarthria, extensor plantar response, pigmentary retinal degeneration; severity varies from asymptomatic to late onset/mild to early onset/aggressive
SCA8 (autosomal dominant type 8)	13q21 with CTG repeats (untranslated)	Gait ataxia, dysarthria, nystagmus; leg spasticity and reduced vibratory sensation
SCA10 (autosomal dominant type 10)	22q	Gait ataxia, dysarthria, nystagmus; partial complex and generalized motor seizures
SCA11 (autosomal dominant type 11)	15q14-q21.3 by linkage	Slowly progressive gait and extremity ataxia, dysarthria, vertical nystagmus, hyperreflexia
SCA12 (autosomal dominant type 12)	5q31-q33 by linkage	Tremor, decreased movement, increased reflexes, dystonia, ataxia, dysautonomia, dementia
SCA13 (single case)	6q27 with CAG repeats in the TATA binding-protein gene	Gait and extremity ataxia, hyperreflexia, extensor plantar responses, dysarthria, dysphagia, severe mental retardation
Dentatorubropallidoluysian atrophy (autosomal dominant)	12p12-ter with CAG repeats (exonic) Atrophin	Ataxia, choreoathetosis, dystonia, seizures, myoclonus, dementia
Friedreich's ataxia (autosomal recessive)	9q13-q21.1 with intronic GAA repeats Frataxin	Ataxia, areflexia, extensor plantar responses, position sense deficits, cardiomyopathy, diabetes mellitus, scoliosis, foot deformities; defective iron transport from mitochondria
Friedreich's ataxia (autosomal recessive)	8q13.1-q13.3; α-TTP deficiency	Same as phenotype that maps to 9q but associated with vitamin E deficiency
Kearns-Sayre syndrome (sporadic)	mtDNA deletion and duplication mutations	Ptosis, ophthalmoplegia, pigmentary retinal degeneration, cardiomyopathy, diabetes mellitus, deafness, heart block, increased CSF protein, ataxia
Myoclonus epilepsy and ragged red fiber syndrome (MERRF) (maternal inheritance)	Mutation in mtDNA of the $tRNA^{lys}$ at 8344; also mutation at 8356	Myoclonic epilepsy, ragged red fiber myopathy, ataxia
Mitochondrial encephalopathy, lactic acidosis, and stroke syndrome (MELAS) (maternal inheritance)	$tRNA^{leu}$ mutation at 3243; also at 3271 and 3252	Headache, stroke, lactic acidosis, ataxia
Leigh's disease; subacute necrotizing encephalopathy (maternal inheritance or autosomal recessive)	mtDNA complex V defect (ATPase gene at 8993) or mitochondrial protein synthesis defect (both maternally inherited); or complex IV defect (autosomal recessive)	Obtundation, hypotonia, cranial nerve defects, respiratory failure, hyperintense signals on T2-weighted magnetic resonance images in basal ganglia, cerebellum, or brainstem; ataxia
Episodic ataxia, type 1 (EA-1) (autosomal dominant)	12p; potassium channel gene, KCNA1	Episodic ataxia for minutes; provoked by startle or exercise; with facial and hand myokymia; cerebellar signs are not progressive; responds to phenytoin
Episodic ataxia, type 2 (EA-2) (autosomal dominant)	19p13(CACNA1A) (allelic with SCA6) (α_{1a}-voltage–dependent calcium channel subunit)	Episodic ataxia for days; provoked by stress, fatigue; with down-gaze nystagmus; cerebellar atrophy results; progressive cerebellar signs; responds to acetazolamide
Ataxia telangiectasia (autosomal recessive)	11q22-q23; ATM gene for regulation of cell cycle; mitogenic signal transduction and meiotic recombination	Telangiectasia, ataxia, dysarthria, pulmonary infections, neoplasms of lymphatic system; IgA and IgG deficiencies; diabetes mellitus, breast cancer
Infantile-onset spinocerebellar ataxia of Nikali et al. (autosomal recessive)	10q23.3-q24.1	Infantile ataxia, sensory neuropathy; athetosis, hearing deficit, ophthalmoplegia, optic atrophy; primary hypogonadism in females

autosomal dominant inheritance. Although the phenotype is variable for any given disease gene, a pattern of neuronal loss with gliosis is produced that is relatively unique for each ataxia. Immunohistochemical and biochemical studies have shown cytoplasmic (SCA2), neuronal (SCA1, MJD, SCA7), and nucleolar (SCA7) accumulation of the specific mutant polyglutamine containing ataxin proteins. Expanded polyglutamine ataxins with more than approximately 40 glutamines are potentially toxic to neurons for a variety of reasons including the following: high levels of gene expression for the mutant polyglutamine ataxin in affected neurons; conformational change of the aggregated protein to a β-pleated structure; abnormal transport of the ataxin into the nucleus (SCA1, MJD, SCA7); binding to other polyglutamine proteins, including the TATA-binding transcription protein and the CREB-binding protein, impairing their functions; altering the efficiency of the ubiquitin-proteosome system of protein turnover; and inducing neuronal apoptosis. An earlier age of onset (anticipation) and more aggressive disease in subsequent generations are due to further expansion of the CAG triplet repeat and increased polyglutamine number in the mutant ataxin. A new classification based on the genotype and its specific mutant ataxin is presented in Table 364-2, and the salient features of the most common disorders are discussed below.

AUTOSOMAL DOMINANT ATAXIAS The new genomic classification of the dominantly inherited ataxias includes SCA type 1 through SCA13, dentatorubropallidoluysian atrophy (DRPLA), and episodic ataxia (EA) types 1 and 2 (Table 364-2).

SCA1 SCA1 was previously referred to as *olivopontocerebellar atrophy*, but genomic data have shown that that entity represents several different genotypes with overlapping clinical features.

Symptoms and signs SCA1 is characterized by the development in early or middle adult life of progressive cerebellar ataxia of the trunk and limbs, impairment of equilibrium and gait, slowness of voluntary movements, scanning speech, nystagmoid eye movements, and oscillatory tremor of the head and trunk. Dysarthria, dysphagia, and oculomotor and facial palsies may also occur. Extrapyramidal symptoms include rigidity, an immobile face, and parkinsonian tremor. The reflexes are usually normal, but knee and ankle jerks may be lost, and extensor plantar responses may occur. Dementia may be noted but is usually mild. Impairment of sphincter function is common, with urinary and sometimes fecal incontinence. Cerebellar and brainstem atrophy are evident on MRI (Fig. 364-1).

Marked shrinkage of the ventral half of the pons, disappearance of the olivary eminence on the ventral surface of the medulla, and atrophy of the cerebellum are evident on gross postmortem inspection of the brain. Variable loss of Purkinje cells, reduced numbers of cells in the molecular and granular layer, demyelination of the middle cerebellar peduncle and the cerebellar hemispheres, and severe loss of cells in the pontine nuclei and olives are found on histologic examination. Degenerative changes in the striatum, especially the putamen, and loss of the pigmented cells of the substantia nigra may be found in cases with extrapyramidal features. More widespread degeneration in the central nervous system (CNS), including involvement of the posterior columns and the spinocerebellar fibers, is often present, especially in the cases with autosomal dominant inheritance.

GENETIC CONSIDERATIONS SCA1 was mapped positionally to chromosome 6 (6p22-p23), and the causal gene was found to contain CAG expanded DNA repeats (Chap. 359). The mutant allele has >40 CAG repeats, whereas alleles from unaffected individuals have ≤36 repeats. A few patients with 38 to 40 CAG repeats have been described. There is a direct correlation between a larger number of repeats and a younger age of onset for SCA1. Juvenile patients have higher numbers of repeats, and anticipation is present in subsequent generations. The SCA1 gene is 450 kilobases (kb) long and has nine exons, with the first seven exons located in a 5′ untranslated region and the last two exons containing the coding region. The SCA1 transcript contains 10,660 bases and is transcribed from both the wild-type allele and SCA1 alleles. The CAG repeat, which codes for a polyglutamine tract, lies within the coding region. The SCA1 gene product, called ataxin-1, is a novel protein of unknown function. Recently, polyglutamine aggregates bound to ubiquitin have been described in neuronal nuclei that are undergoing degeneration. Similar neuronal nuclear inclusions have been seen in cerebellar Purkinje cells of transgenic mice overexpressing an expanded variant of the ataxin-1 gene that causes human SCA1. Other transgenic mice carrying the SCA1 gene but with the self-association region deleted, so that polyglutamine aggregation did not occur, still developed ataxia and Purkinje cell pathology. Thus, although nuclear localization of ataxin-1 is necessary, nuclear aggregation of ataxin-1 is not required to initiate pathogenesis in transgenic mice. ■

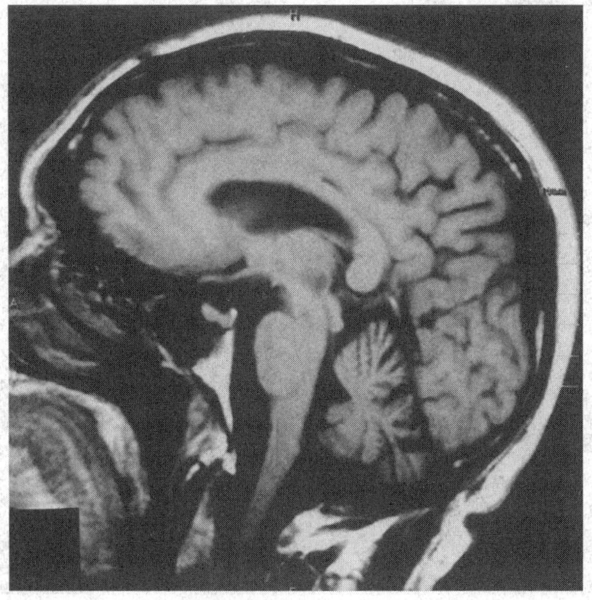

FIGURE 364-1 Sagittal MRI of the brain of a 60-year-old man with gait ataxia and dysarthria due to SCA1, illustrating cerebellar atrophy.

SCA2 • *Symptoms and signs* Another clinical phenotype, SCA2, has been described in Cubans. These patients probably are descendants of a common ancestor, and the population may be the largest homogeneous group of patients with ataxia yet described. The age of onset ranges from 2 to 65 years, and there is considerable clinical variability within families. Although neuropathologic and clinical findings are compatible with a diagnosis of SCA1, including parkinsonian rigidity, optic disk pallor, mild spasticity, and retinal degeneration, it appears that SCA2 is a unique form of cerebellar degenerative disease.

GENETIC CONSIDERATIONS The gene in SCA2 families has been mapped to 12q23-q24.1. Thus, the similar clinical phenotypes of SCA1 and SCA2, mapped respectively to 6p and 12q, represent different genotypes. The gene has recently been identified, and it also contains CAG repeat expansions coding for a polyglutamine-containing protein, ataxin-2. Normal alleles contain 15 to 24 repeats; mutant alleles have 35 to 59 repeats. ■

Machado-Joseph Disease/SCA3 Machado-Joseph disease (MJD) is an autosomal dominant spinocerebellar degenerative disease first described among the Portuguese and their descendants in New England and California. Subsequently, MJD has been found in families from Portugal, Australia, Brazil, Canada, China, England, France, India, Israel, Italy, Japan, Spain, Taiwan, and the United States. In most populations, it is the most common inherited autosomal dominant ataxia.

Symptoms and signs MJD has been classified into three clinical types. In type I MJD (amyotrophic lateral sclerosis–parkinsonism–dystonia type), neurologic deficits appear in the first two decades and involve weakness and spasticity of extremities, especially the legs, often with dystonia of the face, neck, trunk, and extremities. Patellar and ankle clonus are common, as are extensor plantar responses. The gait is slow and stiff, with a slightly broadened base and lurching from side to side; this gait results from spasticity, not true ataxia. There is no truncal titubation. Pharyngeal weakness and spasticity cause difficulty with speech and swallowing. Of note is the prominence of horizontal and vertical nystagmus, loss of fast saccadic eye movements, hypermetric and hypometric saccades, and impairment of upward vertical gaze. Facial fasciculations, facial myokymia, lingual fasciculations without atrophy, ophthalmoparesis, and ocular prominence are common and early manifestations.

In type II MJD (ataxic type), true cerebellar deficits appear, including dysarthria and gait and extremity ataxia, beginning in the second to fourth decades, along with corticospinal and extrapyramidal deficits of spasticity, rigidity, and dystonia. Type II is the most common form of MJD. Ophthalmoparesis, upward vertical gaze deficits, and facial and lingual fasciculations are also present. Type II MJD must be distinguished from the clinically similar disorders SCA1 and SCA2.

Type III MJD (ataxic-amyotrophic type) presents in the fifth to the seventh decades with a pancerebellar disorder that includes dysarthria and gait and extremity ataxia. Distal sensory loss involving pain, touch, vibration, and position senses and distal atrophy are prominent, indicating the presence of peripheral neuropathy. The deep tendon reflexes are depressed to absent, and there are no corticospinal or extrapyramidal findings.

The mean age of onset of symptoms in MJD is 25 years. Neurologic deficits invariably progress and lead to death from debilitation within 15 years of onset, especially in patients with types I and II disease. Usually, patients retain full intellectual function.

The major pathologic findings are variable loss of neurons and glial replacement in the corpus striatum and severe loss of neurons in the pars compacta of the substantia nigra. A moderate loss of neurons occurs in the dentate nucleus of the cerebellum and in the red nucleus. Purkinje cell loss and granule cell loss occur in the cerebellar cortex. Cell loss also occurs in the dentate nucleus and in the cranial nerve motor nuclei. Sparing of the inferior olives distinguishes MJD from other dominantly inherited ataxias.

GENETIC CONSIDERATIONS The gene locus for MJD has been mapped to 14q24.3-q32. The genes from families with MJD in Japan and North and South America all map to the same locus. Unstable CAG repeat expansions are present in the MJD gene coding for a polyglutamine-containing protein named ataxin-3 or MJD-ataxin. An earlier age of onset is associated with longer repeats. Alleles from normal individuals have between 12 and 37 CAG repeats, and MJD alleles have 60 to 84 CAG repeats. A patient with autonomic dysfunction and ataxia has been described with 56 CAG repeats. Polyglutamine-containing aggregates of ataxin-3 (MJD-ataxin) have been described in neuronal nuclei undergoing degeneration. ■

SCA6 Genomic screening for CAG repeats in other families with autosomal dominant ataxia and vibratory and proprioceptive sensory loss have yielded another locus. Of interest is that different mutations in the same gene for the α_{1A} voltage-dependent calcium channel subunit (CACNLIA4) (also referred to as the CACNA1A gene) at 19p13 result in different clinical disorders. CAG repeat expansions (21 to 27 in patients; 4 to 16 triplets in normal individuals) result in late onset progressive ataxia with cerebellar degeneration. Missense mutations in this gene result in familial hemiplegic migraine. Non-sense mutations resulting in termination of protein synthesis of the gene product yield hereditary paroxysmal cerebellar ataxia or episodic ataxia. Some patients with familial hemiplegic migraine develop progressive ataxia and also have cerebellar atrophy.

Dentatorubropallidoluysian Atrophy DRPLA is a disorder of variable clinical presentation that is characterized by progressive ataxia, choreoathetosis, dystonia, seizures, myoclonus, and dementia. DRPLA is due to unstable CAG triplet repeats in the open reading frame of a gene named atrophin located on chromosome 12p12-ter. Larger expansions are found in patients with earlier onset. The number of repeats is ≥49 in patients with DRPLA; it is ≤26 in normal individuals. Anticipation occurs; successive generations in individual families show progressively earlier onset of disease in association with an increasing CAG repeat number. Larger expansions occur in children who inherit the disease from their father.

Episodic Ataxia Types 1 and 2 are two rare dominantly inherited disorders that have been mapped to chromosomes 12p (a potassium channel gene) for type 1 and 19p for type 2. Patients with EA-1 have brief episodes of ataxia with myokymia and nystagmus that last only minutes. Startle, sudden change in posture, and exercise can induce episodes. Acetazolamide or anticonvulsants may be therapeutic. Patients with EA-2 have episodes of ataxia with nystagmus that can last for hours or days. Stress, exercise, or excessive fatigue may be precipitants. Acetazolamide may be therapeutic and can reverse the relative intracellular alkalosis detected by MR spectroscopy. Stop codon, non-sense mutations causing EA-2 have been found in the CACNA1A gene, encoding the α_{1A} voltage-dependent calcium channel subunit (see SCA6 above). See Table 364-2 for details.

AUTOSOMAL RECESSIVE ATAXIAS Friedreich's Ataxia This is the most common form of inherited ataxia, comprising one-half of all hereditary ataxias. It can occur in a classic form or in association with a genetically determined vitamin E deficiency syndrome; the two forms are clinically indistinguishable.

Symptoms and signs Friedreich's ataxia presents before 25 years of age with progressive staggering gait, frequent falling, and titubation. The lower extremities are more severely involved than the upper ones. Dysarthria occasionally is the presenting symptom; and rarely progressive scoliosis, foot deformity, nystagmus, or cardiopathy are initial signs.

The neurologic examination reveals nystagmus, loss of fast saccadic eye movements, truncal titubation, dysarthria, dysmetria, and ataxia of extremity and truncal movements. Extensor plantar responses (with normal tone in trunk and extremities), absence of deep tendon reflexes, and weakness (greater distally than proximally) are usually found. Loss of vibratory and proprioceptive sensation occurs. The median age of death is 35 years. Women have a significantly better prognosis than men; the 20-year survival rate is 100% in women and 63% in men.

Cardiac involvement occurs in 90% of patients. Cardiomegaly, symmetric hypertrophy, murmurs, and conduction defects are reported. Idebenone, a free-radical scavenger, has been shown in preliminary studies to protect heart muscle from iron-induced injury and to decrease myocardial hypertrophy. Iron chelators and antioxidant drugs are potentially harmful. Moderate mental retardation or psychiatric syndromes are present in a small percentage of patients. A high incidence of diabetes mellitus (20%) is found and is associated with insulin resistance and pancreatic β-cell dysfunction. However, no linkage is reported between the Friedreich's ataxia gene and loci predisposing to diabetes mellitus. Musculoskeletal deformities are common and include pes cavus, pes equinovarus, and scoliosis. MRI of the spinal cord shows significant cord atrophy in affected patients (Fig. 364-2).

The primary sites of pathology are the spinal cord, dorsal root ganglion cells, and the peripheral nerves. Slight atrophy of the cerebellum and cerebral gyri may occur. Sclerosis and degeneration occur

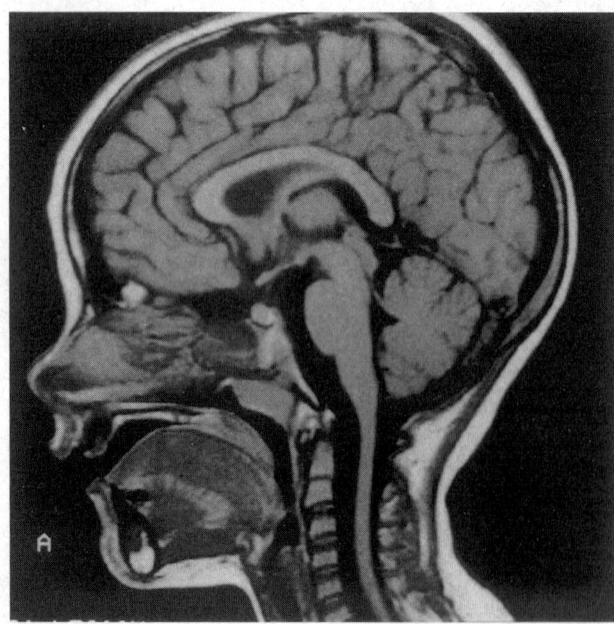

FIGURE 364-2 Sagittal MRI of the brain and spinal cord of a patient with Friedreich's ataxia, demonstrating spinal cord atrophy

predominantly in the spinocerebellar tracts, lateral corticospinal tracts, and posterior columns. Degeneration of the glossopharyngeal, vagus, hypoglossal, and deep cerebellar nuclei is described. The cerebral cortex is histologically normal except for loss of Betz cells in the precentral gyri. The peripheral nerves are extensively involved, with a loss of large myelinated fibers. The density of small myelinated fibers is normal, but axonal size and myelin thickness are diminished. Cardiac pathology consists of myocytic hypertrophy and fibrosis, focal vascular fibromuscular dysplasia with subintimal or medial deposition of periodic acid–Schiff (PAS)-positive material, myocytopathy with unusual pleomorphic nuclei, and focal degeneration of myelinated and unmyelinated nerves and cardiac ganglia.

GENETIC CONSIDERATIONS The classic form of Friedreich's ataxia has been mapped to 9q13-q21.1, and the mutant gene, frataxin, contains expanded GAA triplet repeats in the first intron. There is homozygosity for expanded GAA repeats in most patients. Normal persons have 7 to 22 GAA repeats, and patients have 200 to 900 GAA repeats. Patients with Friedreich's ataxia have undetectable or extremely low levels of frataxin mRNA, as compared with carriers and unrelated individuals; thus, disease appears to be caused by a loss of expression of the frataxin protein. Frataxin is a mitochondrial protein involved in iron homeostasis. Mitochondrial iron accumulation due to loss of the iron transporter coded by the mutant frataxin gene results in oxidized intramitochondrial iron. Excess oxidized iron results in turn in the oxidation of cellular components and irreversible cell injury.

Two forms of hereditary ataxia associated with abnormalities in the interactions of vitamin E (α-tocopherol) with very-low-density lipoprotein (VLDL) have been delineated. Ataxia of the Friedreich's phenotype with vitamin E deficiency (AVED) and abetalipoproteinemia (Bassen-Kornzweig syndrome) have both been clarified at the molecular genetic level. Abetalipoproteinemia is caused by mutations in the gene coding for the larger subunit of the microsomal triglyceride transfer protein (MTP). Defects in MTP result in impairment of formation and secretion of VLDL in liver. This defect results in a deficiency of delivery of vitamin E to tissues, including the central and peripheral nervous system, as VLDL is the transport molecule for vitamin E and other fat-soluble substitutes. AVED is due to mutations in the gene for α-tocopherol transfer protein (α-TTP) on chromosome 8 (8q13). These patients have an impaired ability to bind vitamin E into the VLDL produced and secreted by the liver, resulting in a deficiency of vitamin E in peripheral tissues. Hence, either absence of VLDL (abetalipoproteinemia) or impaired binding of vitamin E to VLDL (AVED) causes an ataxic syndrome. Once again, a genotype classification has proved to be essential in sorting out the various clinical forms of the Friedreich's disease syndrome. ■

Ataxia Telangiectasia • ***Symptoms and signs*** Patients present in the first decade of life with progressive telangiectatic lesions associated with deficits in cerebellar function and nystagmus. The neurologic manifestations correspond to those in Friedreich's disease, which should be included in the differential diagnosis. Truncal ataxia, extremity ataxia, dysarthria, extensor plantar responses, myoclonic jerks, areflexia, and distal sensory deficits may develop. There is a high incidence of recurrent pulmonary infections and neoplasms of the lymphatic and reticuloendothelial system in patients with ataxia telangiectasia (AT) as well as an increased incidence of cancer. Thymic hypoplasia with cellular and humoral (IgA and IgG2) immunodeficiencies, premature aging, and endocrine disorders such as insulin-dependent diabetes mellitus are described. There is an increased incidence of lymphomas, Hodgkin's disease, and acute leukemias of the T cell type. There is also an increased incidence of breast cancer in women who are heterozygous for AT. The immunologic defects and increased susceptibility to cancer have been causally linked to cellular disorders in AT. Exposure of cultured cells to ionizing radiation slows the rate of DNA replication and increases the frequency of chromosomal aberrations.

The most striking neuropathologic changes include loss of Purkinje, granule, and basket cells in the cerebellar cortex as well as of neurons in the deep cerebellar nuclei. The inferior olives of the medulla also may have neuronal loss. There is a loss of anterior horn neurons in the spinal cord and of dorsal root ganglion cells associated with posterior column spinal cord demyelination. A poorly developed or absent thymus gland is the most consistent defect of the lymphoid system.

GENETIC CONSIDERATIONS The gene for AT (the *ATM* gene) has been positionally mapped to chromosome 11q22-q23. *ATM*, which has a 12-kb transcript, was mutated in AT patients from all complementation groups described previously. A partial *ATM* cDNA clone of 5.9 kb encodes a protein that is similar to several yeast and mammalian phosphatidylinositol-3′-kinases involved in mitogenic signal transduction, meiotic recombination, and cell cycle control. Defective DNA repair in AT fibroblasts exposed to ultraviolet light has been demonstrated. The discovery of *ATM* will make possible the identification of heterozygotes who are at risk for cancer (e.g., breast cancer) and permit early diagnosis. ■

Mitochondrial Ataxias Spinocerebellar syndromes have been identified with mutations in mitochondrial DNA (mtDNA). Thirty pathogenic mtDNA point mutations and >60 different types of mtDNA deletions are known, several of which cause or are associated with ataxia (Chap. 383).

Xeroderma Pigmentosum Xeroderma pigmentosum is a rare autosomal recessive neurocutaneous disorder caused by the inability to repair damage to DNA, such as that produced by ultraviolet radiation. In addition to skin lesions, patients may show progressive mental deterioration, microcephaly, ataxia, spasticity, choreoathetosis, and hypogonadism. Nerve deafness, peripheral neuropathy (predominantly axonal), electroencephalographic abnormalities, and seizures are reported. Neuronal death occurs in pyramidal cells, cerebellar Purkinje cells, the deep nuclei of the cerebellum, the brainstem, the spinal cord, and peripheral nerves.

Cockayne Syndrome This is a rare autosomal recessive disorder first described by Cockayne in 1936. Clinical features are mental retardation, optic atrophy, dwarfism, neural deafness, hypersensitivity of skin to sunlight, cataracts, and retinal pigmentary degeneration. Cerebellar, pyramidal, and extrapyramidal deficits and peripheral neuropathy may occur, with a "bird-headed" facial appearance and normal-pressure hydrocephalus. Skin fibroblasts exposed to ultraviolet light demonstrate defective DNA repair.

Marinesco-Sjögren Syndrome This rare syndrome, in which progressive cerebellar deficits begin early in childhood, is another example in which a Friedreich's syndrome is associated with additional specific features. In this case, cataracts, mental retardation, multiple skeletal abnormalities, hypogonadotropic hypogonadism, and severe cerebellar atrophy are associated. The syndrome is likely a lysosomal storage disorder caused by an enzymatic defect, but the pathophysiology is unknown.

Rx TREATMENT The physician's most important task in the management of patients with ataxia is to identify treatable disease entities. Malignancies may present with chronic progressive ataxia either directly with a mass effect in the posterior fossa or indirectly by paraneoplastic degeneration. Other mass lesions can be treated appropriately. Malabsorption syndromes leading to vitamin E deficiency may lead to ataxia. The vitamin E deficiency form of Friedreich's ataxia must be considered, and serum vitamin E levels measured. Vitamin E therapy is indicated for these rare patients. There is preliminary evidence that idebenone, a free-radical scavenger, is therapeutic for patients with classic Friedreich ataxia by reducing myocardial hypertrophy. There is no current evidence that it improves neurologic function. Iron chelators and antioxidant drugs are potentially harmful as they may increase heart muscle injury. Vitamin B_1 and B_{12} levels in serum must be measured, and the vitamins should be administered to patients having deficient levels. The deleterious effects of diphenylhydantoin and alcohol on the cerebellum are well known. Hypothyroidism is easily treated. Aminoacidopathies, leukodystrophies, urea-cycle abnormalities, and mitochondrial encephalomyopathies may produce ataxia, and some dietary or metabolic therapies are available. The cerebrospinal fluid should be tested for a syphilitic infection in patients with progressive ataxia and other features of tabes dorsalis. Similarly, antibody titers for Lyme disease and *Legionella* should be measured, and appropriate antibiotic therapy should be instituted in antibody-positive patients. There is no proven therapy for the dominant ataxias (SCA1 to 13). The identification of gene defects will, it is hoped, lead to specific pharmacologic therapy. At present, identification of an at-risk person's genotype, together with appropriate family and genetic counseling, can reduce the incidence of these cerebellar syndromes (Chaps. 68, 359).

BIBLIOGRAPHY

BRADLEY JL et al: Clinical, biochemical and molecular genetic correlations in Friedreich's ataxia. Hum Mol Genetics 9(2):275, 2000

CONNER KE, ROSENBERG RN: The hereditary ataxias, in *The Molecular and Genetic Basis of Neurological Disease*, 2d ed, RN Rosenberg et al (eds). Boston, Butterworth-Heinemann, 1997, pp 503–544

HOLMES SE et al: A novel CAG trinucleotide repeat expansion adjacent to a gene encoding a subunit of protein phosphatase 2A is associated with a progressive neurological disorder. Soc Neurosci 25:1096, 1999

MATSUURA T et al: Mapping of the gene for a novel spinocerebellar ataxia with pure cerebellar signs and epilepsy. Ann Neurol 45:407, 1999

PANDOLFO M, MONTERMINI L: Molecular genetics of the hereditary ataxias. Adv Genet 38:31, 1998

PAULSON HL: Human Genetics '99: Trinucleotide repeats: Protein fate in neurodegenerative proteinopathies: Polyglutamine diseases join the (Mis)fold. Am J Hum Genet 64:339, 1999

ROSENBERG RN: Autosomal dominant cerebellar phenotypes: The genotype has settled the issue. Neurology 45:1, 1995

TERRY JB, ROSENBERG RN: Frontal lobe ataxia. Surg Neurol 44:583, 1995

365

Robert H. Brown, Jr.

AMYOTROPHIC LATERAL SCLEROSIS AND OTHER MOTOR NEURON DISEASES

AMYOTROPHIC LATERAL SCLEROSIS Amyotrophic lateral sclerosis (ALS) is the most common form of progressive motor neuron disease. It is a prime example of a neuronal system disease and is arguably the most devastating of the neurodegenerative disorders.

Pathology The pathology of motor neuron degenerative disorders involves lower motor neurons (consisting of anterior horn cells in spinal cord and their brainstem homologues innervating bulbar muscles) and upper, or corticospinal, motor neurons (emanating from layer five of motor cortex to descend via the pyramidal tract to synapse with lower motor neurons, either directly or indirectly via interneurons; (Chap. 22). Although at its onset ALS may involve selective loss of function of only upper or lower motor neurons, it ultimately causes progressive loss of both categories of motor neurons. Indeed, in the absence of clear involvement of both motor neuron types, the diagnosis of ALS is questionable.

Other motor neuron diseases involve only particular subsets of motor neurons (Tables 365-1 and 365-2). Thus, in bulbar palsy and spinal muscular atrophy (SMA, also called progressive muscular atrophy), the lower motor neurons of brainstem and spinal cord, respectively, are most severely involved. By contrast, pseudobulbar palsy, primary lateral sclerosis (PLS), and familial spastic paraplegia (FSP) affect only upper motor neurons innervating the brainstem and spinal cord.

Table 365-1 Sporadic Motor Neuron Diseases

CHRONIC
Upper and lower motor neurons
Amyotrophic lateral sclerosis
Predominantly upper motor neurons
Primary lateral sclerosis
Predominantly lower motor neurons
Multifocal motor neuropathy with conduction block
Motor neuropathy with paraproteinemia or cancer
Motor-predominant peripheral neuropathies
Other
Associated with other degenerative disorders
Secondary motor neuron disorders (see Table 365-3)
ACUTE
Poliomyelitis
Herpes zoster
Coxsackie virus

In each of these diseases, the affected motor neurons undergo shrinkage, often with accumulation of the pigmented lipid (lipofuscin) that normally develops in these cells with advancing age. In ALS, the motor neuron cytoskeleton is typically affected early in the illness. Focal enlargements are frequent in proximal motor axons; ultrastructurally, these "spheroids" are composed of accumulations of neurofil-

Table 365-2 Genetic Motor Neuron Diseases

Disease	Locus	Gene
I. Upper and lower motor neurons (familial ALS)		
A. Autosomal dominant	21q	Superoxide dismutase
	22q	Neurofilament heavy subunit
	X_{cent}	Unknown
B. Autosomal recessive (juvenile)	2q	Unknown
	15q	Unknown
C. Mitochondrial	mtDNA	Cytochrome c oxidase
II. Upper motor neurons		
A. Familial spastic paraplegia (FSP)		
1. Autosomal dominant	2p	Spastin
	14q	Unknown
2. Autosomal recessive	8p	Unknown
	16q	Paraplegin
3. X-linked	Xq21	Proteolipid protein
	Xq28	L1 CAM
B. Adrenomyeloneuropathy	Xq21	Adrenoleukodystrophy protein
III. Lower motor neurons		
A. Spinal muscular atrophies	5q	Survival motor neuron protein
1. Infantile: Werdnig-Hoffmann disease		Survival motor neuron protein
2. Childhood		Survival motor neuron protein
3. Adolescent: Kugelberg-Welander disease		Survival motor neuron protein
B. X-linked spinobulbar muscular atrophy	Xq	Androgen receptor
C. G_{M2} gangliosidosis		
1. Adult Tay-Sach's disease	15q	Hexosaminidase A
2. Sandhoff disease	5q	Hexosaminidase B
3. AB variant	5q	GM2 activator protein
IV. ALS-plus syndromes		
A. ALS with frontotemporal dementia	9q	Unknown
B. Amyotrophy with behavioral disorder and parkinsonian features	17q	Tau protein

aments. Beyond some astroglial proliferation, which is the inevitable accompaniment of all degenerative processes in the central nervous system (CNS), the interstitial and supportive tissues and the macrophage system remain largely inactive, and there is no inflammation.

The death of the peripheral motor neurons in the brainstem and spinal cord leads to denervation and consequent atrophy of the corresponding muscle fibers. Histochemical and electrophysiologic evidence indicates that in the early phases of the illness denervated muscle can be reinnervated by sprouting of nearby distal motor nerve terminals, although reinnervation in this disease is considerably less extensive than in most other disorders affecting motor neurons (e.g., poliomyelitis, peripheral neuropathy). As denervation progresses, muscle atrophy is readily recognized in muscle biopsies and on clinical examination. This is the basis for the term *amyotrophy* in the name for the disease. The loss of cortical motor neurons results in thinning of the corticospinal tracts that travel via the internal capsule and brainstem to the lateral and anterior white matter columns of the spinal cord. The loss of fibers in the lateral columns and resulting fibrillary gliosis impart a particular firmness (*lateral sclerosis*) (Fig. 365-1). A remarkable feature of the disease is the selectivity of neuronal cell death. By light microscopy, the entire sensory apparatus, the regulatory mechanisms for the control and coordination of movement, and the components of the brain that are needed for cognitive processes remain intact. However, immunostaining indicates that neurons bearing ubiquitin, a marker for degeneration, are also detected in nonmotor systems. Moreover, studies of glucose metabolism in the illness also indicate that there is neuronal dysfunction outside of the motor system. Within the motor system, there is some selectivity of involvement. Thus, motor neurons required for ocular motility remain unaffected, as do the parasympathetic neurons in the sacral spinal cord (the nucleus of Onufrowicz, or Onuf) that innervate the sphincters of the bowel and bladder.

Clinical Manifestations The manifestations of ALS are somewhat variable depending on whether corticospinal or lower motor neurons in the brainstem and spinal cord are more prominently involved. Typically, with lower motor neuron dysfunction and early denervation, the initial sign of the disease is insidiously developing asymmetric weakness, usually first evident distally in one of the limbs. A detailed history often discloses recent development of cramping with volitional movements, typically in the early hours of the morning (e.g., while stretching in bed). Weakness caused by denervation is associated with progressive wasting and atrophy of muscles and, particularly early in the illness, spontaneous twitching of motor units, or fasciculations. In the hands, a preponderance of extensor over flexor weakness is common. When the initial denervation involves bulbar rather than limb muscles, the problem at onset is difficulty with chewing, swallowing, and movements of the face and tongue. Early involvement of the muscles of respiration may lead to death before the disease is far advanced elsewhere.

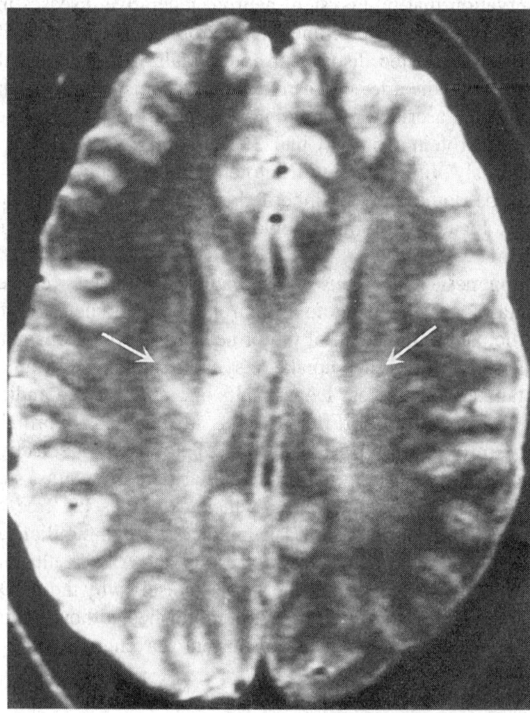

FIGURE 365-1 Amyotrophic lateral sclerosis. Axial T2-weighted MRI scan through the lateral ventricles of the brain reveals abnormal high signal intensity within the corticospinal tracts (*arrows*). This MRI feature represents an increase in water content in myelin tracts undergoing Wallerian degeneration secondary to cortical motor neuronal loss. This finding is commonly present in ALS, but can also be seen in AIDS-related encephalopathy, infarction, or other disease processes that produce corticospinal neuronal loss in a symmetric fashion.

With prominent corticospinal involvement, there is hyperactivity of the muscle-stretch reflexes (tendon jerks) and, often, spastic resistance to passive movements of the affected limbs. Patients with significant reflex hyperactivity complain of muscle stiffness often out of proportion to weakness. Degeneration of the corticobulbar projections innervating the brainstem results in dysarthria and exaggeration of the motor expressions of emotion. The latter leads to involuntary excess in weeping or laughing (so-called pseudobulbar affect).

Virtually any muscle group may be the first to show signs of the disease, but, as time passes, more and more muscles become involved until ultimately the disorder takes on a symmetric distribution in all regions. It is characteristic of ALS that, regardless of whether the initial disease involves upper or lower motor neurons, both will eventually be implicated. Even in the late stages of the illness, sensory, bowel and bladder, and cognitive functions are preserved. Even when there is severe brainstem disease, ocular motility is spared until the very late stages of the illness. Dementia is not a component of sporadic ALS. In some families, ALS is co-inherited with frontotemporal dementia, characterized by early behavioral abnormalities with prominent behavioral features indicative of frontal lobe dysfunction.

A committee of the World Federation of Neurology has established diagnostic guidelines for ALS. Essential for the diagnosis is the presence of simultaneous upper and lower motor neuron involvement with progressive weakness, and the exclusion of all alternative diagnoses. The disorder is classified as "definite" ALS when three or four of the following sites are involved: bulbar, cervical, thoracic, and lumbosacral motor neurons. When two sites are involved, the diagnosis is "probable"; when only one site is implicated, the diagnosis is "possible." An exception is made for those who have progressive upper and lower motor neuron signs at only one site and a mutation in the gene encoding superoxide dismutase (below).

Epidemiology The illness is relentlessly progressive, leading to death from respiratory paralysis; the median survival is from 3 to 5 years. There are very rare reports of stabilization or even regression of ALS. In most societies there is an incidence of 1 to 3 per 100,000 and a prevalence of 3 to 5 per 100,000. Several endemic foci of higher prevalence exist in the western Pacific (e.g., in specific regions of Guam or Papua New Guinea). In the United States and Europe, males are somewhat more frequently affected than females. While ALS is overwhelmingly a sporadic disorder, some 5 to 10% of cases are inherited as an autosomal dominant trait.

Familial ALS Several forms of selective motor neuron disease are heritable (Table 365-2). Two involve both corticospinal and lower motor neurons. The most common is familial ALS (FALS). Apart from its inheritance as an autosomal dominant trait, it is clinically indistinguishable from sporadic ALS. Genetic studies have identified mutations in the gene encoding the cytosolic enzyme superoxide dismutase (SOD1) as the cause of one form of FALS. However, this accounts for only 20% of inherited cases of ALS; there clearly are other ALS genes to be identified. There is a juvenile-onset, dominantly inherited form of ALS that is genetically mapped to the long-arm of chromosome 9. Two recessively inherited forms of juvenile-onset ALS with long survival map to chromsomes 2 and 15. Another familial, adult-onset disorder that may mimic aspects of ALS is Kennedy's syndrome, described below.

Differential Diagnosis Because ALS is currently untreatable, it is imperative that potentially remediable causes of motor neuron dysfunction be excluded (Table 365-3). This is particularly true in cases that are atypical by virtue of (1) restriction to either upper or lower motor neurons, (2) involvement of neurons other than motor neurons, and (3) evidence of motor neuronal conduction block on electrophysiologic testing. Compression of the cervical spinal cord or cervicomedullary junction from tumors in the cervical regions or at the foramen magnum or from cervical spondylosis with osteophytes projecting into the vertebral canal can produce weakness, wasting, and fasciculations in the upper limbs and spasticity in the legs, closely resembling ALS. The absence of cranial nerve involvement may be helpful in differentiation, although some foramen magnum lesions may compress the twelfth cranial (hypoglossal) nerve, with resulting paralysis of the tongue. Absence of pain or of sensory changes, normal bowel and bladder function, normal roentgenographic studies of the spine, and normal cerebrospinal fluid (CSF) all favor ALS. Where doubt exists, magnetic resonance imaging (MRI) scans should be performed to visualize the cervical spinal cord.

Table 365-3 Etiology and Investigation of Motor Neuron Disorders

Diagnostic Categories	Investigations
Structural lesions	MRI scan of head (including foramen magnum), cervical spine[a]
Parasagittal or foramen magnum tumors	
Cervical spondylosis	
Chiari malformation or syrinx	
Spinal cord arteriovenous malformation	
Infections	CSF exam, culture[a]
Bacterial—tetanus, Lyme	Lyme antibody titer[a]
Viral—poliomyelitis, herpes zoster	Antiviral antibody titers (e.g., enteroviruses)
Retroviral myelopathy	HTLV-1, HTLV-2 titers
Intoxications, physical agents	
Toxins—lead, aluminum, other metals	24-h urine for heavy metals[a] Serum and urine for lead, aluminum
Drugs—strychnine, phenytoin	
Electric shock, x-irradiation	
Immunologic mechanisms	Complete blood count[a]
Plasma cell dyscrasias	Sedimentation rate[a]
Autoimmune polyradiculoneuropathy	Immunoprotein electrophoresis[a] Anti-G_{M1} antibodies[a]
Motor neuropathy with conduction block	
Paraneoplastic	Anti-Hu antibody
Paracarcinomatous/lymphoma	MRI scan, bone marrow biopsy
Metabolic	
Hypoglycemia	Fasting blood sugar (FBS), routine chemistries including calcium[a]
Hyperparathyroidism	PTH, calcium, phosphate
Hyperthyroidism	Thyroid functions[a]
Deficiency of folate, vitamins B_{12}, E, and folate	Vitamin B_{12}, vitamin E, folate levels[a]
Malabsorption	24-h stool fat, carotene, prothrombin time
Mitochondrial dysfunction	Fasting lactate, pyruvate, ammonia Consider mtDNA analysis
Hereditary biochemical disorders	
Superoxide dismutase 1 mutation	White blood cell DNA analysis
Androgen receptor defect (Kennedy's disease)	Abnormal CAG insert in androgen receptor gene
Hexosaminidase deficiency	Lysosomal enzyme screen
Infantile (α-glucosidase deficiency (Pompe's disease)	
Hyperlipidemia	Lipid electrophoresis
Hyperglycinuria	Urine and serum amino acids
Methylcrotonylglycinuria	CSF amino acids

[a] Denotes studies that should be obtained in all cases.

NOTE: CSF, cerebrospinal fluid; HTLV, human T cell leukemia virus; MRI, magnetic resonance imaging.

Another important entity in the differential diagnosis of ALS is multifocal motor neuropathy (MMN) with conduction block, discussed below and in Chap. 378. A diffuse, lower motor axonal neuropathy mimicking ALS sometimes evolves in association with hematopoietic disorders such as lymphoma (Chap. 101). The underlying marrow pathology is often signaled by the presence of an M-component in serum which, in this clinical setting, should prompt consideration of a bone marrow biopsy. Lyme infection may also cause an axonal, lower motor neuropathy.

Other treatable disorders that occasionally mimic ALS are chronic lead poisoning and thyrotoxicosis. These disorders may be suggested by the patient's social or occupational history or by unusual clinical features. When the family history is positive, disorders involving the genes encoding SOD1, hexosaminidase A, or α-glucosidase deficiency must be excluded (Chap. 349). These are readily identified by appropriate laboratory tests. Benign fasciculations are occasionally a source of concern because on inspection they resemble the fascicular twitchings that accompany motor neuron degeneration. The absence of weakness, atrophy, or denervation phenomena on electrophysiologic examination usually excludes ALS or other serious neurologic disease. Patients who have recovered from poliomyelitis may experience a delayed deterioration of motor neurons that presents clinically with progressive weakness, atrophy, and fasciculations. Its cause is unknown but is thought to reflect sublethal prior injury to motor neurons by poliovirus (Chap. 193).

Rarely, ALS develops concurrently with features indicative of more widespread neurodegeneration. Thus, one infrequently encounters otherwise typical ALS patients with a Parkinsonian movement disorder or dementia. It remains unclear whether this reflects the unlikely simultaneous occurrence of two disorders or a primary defect triggering two forms of neurodegeneration. The latter is suggested by the observation that multisystem neurodegenerative diseases may be inherited. For example, prominent amyotrophy has been described as a dominantly inherited disorder in individuals with bizarre behavior and a movement disorder suggestive of parkinsonism; many such cases have now been ascribed to mutations that alter the expression of isoforms of tau protein in brain (Chap. 362). In other cases, ALS develops simultaneously with a striking frontotemporal dementia. These disorders may be dominantly co-inherited; in some families, this trait is linked to a locus on chromosome 9q, although the underlying genetic defect is not established.

Pathogenesis The cause of sporadic ALS is not well defined. Some data suggest that excitotoxic neurotransmitters such as glutamate may participate in the death of motor neurons in ALS. This may be a consequence of diminished uptake of synaptic glutamate by an astroglial glutamate transporter, EAAT2. In one study of sporadic ALS brains, this loss of transport function was attributed to abnormal splicing of the mRNA transcript for the EAAT2 transporter selectively in motor cortex. It is striking that one cellular defense against such excitotoxicity is the enzyme SOD1, which detoxifies the free radical superoxide anion. Because SOD1 is mutated in some familial cases of ALS, it may be that glutamate excitotoxicity and ALS result from free radical accumulations in motor neurons. Precisely why the SOD1 mutations are toxic to motor nerves is not established, although it is clear that the effect is not simply loss of normal scavenging of the superoxide anion.

℞ **TREATMENT** There is no treatment capable of arresting the underlying pathologic process in ALS. The drug riluzole was approved for use in ALS because it produces a modest lengthening of survival. In one trial, the survival rate at 18 months with riluzole (100 mg/d) was similar to placebo at 15 months. The mechanism of this effect is not known with certainty; it may reduce excitotoxicity by diminishing glutamate release. Side effects of riluzole may include nausea, dizziness, weight loss, and elevated liver enzymes. In a single study, insulin-like growth factor (IGF-1) was found to slow the progression of ALS modestly; because this effect was not confirmed in a second trial, IGF-1 is not routinely available as an ALS treatment at this time. Clinical trials of several other agents are in progress, including brain-derived neurotrophic factor, glial-derived neurotrophic factor, the anti-glutamate compound topiramate, and creatine. Creatine has proven to be beneficial in SOD-1 transgenic ALS mice, perhaps by augmenting intracellular ATP stores. In a single study in France, vitamin E was beneficial in sporadic ALS. It is also modestly beneficial in the ALS mice and thus is now used empirically by many individuals with ALS. On the basis of successful animal experiments, trials of neural stem therapy of the spinal cord are also being developed in ALS.

In the absence of a primary therapy for ALS, a variety of rehabilitative aids may substantially assist ALS patients. Foot-drop splints facilitate ambulation by avoiding tripping on a floppy foot and obviating excessive hip flexion. Finger-extension splints can potentiate grip. Respiratory support may be life-sustaining. For patients electing against long-term ventilation by tracheostomy, positive-pressure ventilation by mouth or nose provides transient (several weeks) relief from hypercarbia and hypoxia. Also extremely beneficial for some patients is a respiratory device (In-exsufflator, Emerson) that produces an artificial cough. This is highly effective in clearing airways and preventing aspiration pneumonia. When bulbar disease prevents normal chewing and swallowing, gastrostomy is uniformly helpful, restoring normal nutrition and hydration. Fortunately, an increasing variety of speech synthesizers are now available to augment speech when there is advanced bulbar palsy. Because they facilitate oral communication and may be effective for telephone use, such devices are helpful in preserving patient autonomy.

In contrast to ALS, several of the disorders (Table 365-2) that bear some clinical resemblance to ALS are treatable; for this reason, a careful search for such forms of secondary motor neuron disease is warranted.

SELECTED DISORDERS OF THE LOWER MOTOR NEURON In the varieties of motor neuron disease grouped under this heading, the peripheral motor neurons are affected without evidence of involvement of the corticospinal motor system (Table 365-1).

X-Linked Spinobulbar Muscular Atrophy (Kennedy's Disease) This is an X-linked lower motor neuron disorder in which progressive weakness and wasting of limb and bulbar muscles begins in males in midadult life and is conjoined with androgen insensitivity manifested by gynecomastia and reduced fertility (Chap. 335). In addition to gynecomastia, which may be subtle, two findings distinguishing this disorder from ALS are the absence of signs of pyramidal tract disease (spasticity) and the presence of a subtle sensory neuropathy in some patients. The underlying molecular defect is an expanded trinucleotide repeat (-CAG-) in the first exon of the androgen receptor gene on the X chromosome; this may be readily screened from DNA from blood. An inverse correlation appears to exist between the number of -CAG- repeats and the age of onset of the disease (Chap. 359).

Adult Tay-Sach's Disease Several reports have described adult-onset, predominantly lower motor neuropathies arising from deficiency of the enzyme β-hexosaminidase (hex A). These tend to be distinguishable from ALS because they are very slowly progressive; dysarthria and radiographically evident cerebellar atrophy may be prominent. In rare cases, spasticity may also be present, although it is generally absent (Chap. 349).

Spinal Muscular Atrophy The SMAs are a family of selective lower motor neuron diseases of early onset. Despite some phenotypic variability (largely in age of onset), the defect in the majority of families with SMA is genetically linked to a locus on the proximal long arm of chromosome 5. The affected gene at this locus is a putative motor neuron survival protein (SMN, for survival motor neuron) that is important in the formation and trafficking of RNA complexes across the nuclear membrane. All types of SMA are transmitted as traits. Neuropathologically these disorders are characterized by extensive loss of large motor neurons; muscle biopsy reveals evidence of denervation atrophy. Several clinical forms are described.

Infantile SMA (SMA I, Werdnig-Hoffmann Disease) has the earliest onset and most rapidly fatal course. In some instances it is apparent even before birth, as indicated by decreased fetal movements late in the third trimester. Though alert, afflicted infants are weak and floppy (hypotonic) and lack muscle stretch reflexes. Death generally ensues within the first year of life. When the family history is unclear, it is difficult in the early weeks and months to distinguish SMA I from benign congenital hypotonia. An electromyogram is often particularly helpful as SMA I usually demonstrates fulminant denervation; in congenital hypotonia the electromyogram is often myopathic or normal.

Chronic childhood SMA (SMA II) begins later in childhood and evolves with a more slowly progressive course. *Juvenile SMA* (SMA III, Kugelberg-Welander disease) manifests during late childhood and runs a slow, indolent course. Unlike most denervating diseases, in this chronic disorder weakness is greatest in the proximal muscles; indeed, the pattern of clinical weakness can suggest a primary myopathy such as limb-girdle dystrophy. Electrophysiologic and muscle biopsy evidence of denervation distinguish SMA III from the myopathic syndromes.

Multifocal Motor Neuropathy with Conduction Block In this disorder lower motor neuron function is regionally and chronically disrupted by remarkably focal blocks in conduction. Many patients have elevated serum titers of mono- and polyclonal antibodies to ganglioside G_{M1}; it is hypothesized that the antibodies produce selective, focal, paranodal demyelination of motor neurons. MMN is not typically associated with corticospinal signs. In contrast to ALS, MMN may respond dramatically to therapy such as intravenous immunoglobulin or chemotherapy; it is thus imperative that MMN be excluded when considering a diagnosis of ALS. →*A detailed discussion of this condition can be found in Chap. 378.*

Other Forms of Lower Motor Neuron Disease In individual families, other syndromes characterized by selective lower motor neuron dysfunction in an SMA-like pattern have been described. There are rare X-linked and autosomal dominant forms of apparent SMA. There is an ALS variant of juvenile onset, the Fazio-Londe syndrome, which involves mainly the musculature innervated by the brainstem. A component of lower motor neuron dysfunction is also found in degenerative disorders such as Machado-Joseph disease and the related olivopontocerebellar degenerations (Chap. 364).

SELECTED DISORDERS OF THE UPPER MOTOR NEURON **Primary Lateral Sclerosis** This exceedingly rare disorder arises sporadically in adults in mid- to late life. Clinically PLS is characterized by progressive spastic weakness of the limbs, preceded or followed by spastic dysarthria and dysphagia, indicating combined involvement of the corticospinal and corticobulbar tracts. Fasciculations, amyotrophy, and sensory changes are absent; neither electromyography nor muscle biopsy shows denervation. On neuropathologic examination there is selective loss of the large pyramidal cells in the precentral gyrus and degeneration of the corticospinal and corticobulbar projections. The peripheral motor neurons and other neuronal systems are spared. The course of PLS is variable; while long-term survival is documented, the course may be as aggressive as in ALS, with approximately 3-year survival from onset to death. Early in its course, PLS raises the question of multiple sclerosis or other demyelinating diseases such as adrenoleukodystrophy as diagnostic considerations. A myelopathy suggestive of PLS is infrequently seen with infection with the human T cell leukemia virus (HTLV-I) (Chap. 368). The clinical course and laboratory testing will distinguish these possibilities.

Familial Spastic Paraplegia In its pure form, FSP is usually transmitted in families as an autosomal dominant trait; most adult-onset cases are dominantly inherited. It arises in the third or fourth decade and is characterized by progressive spastic weakness beginning in the distal lower extremities. Patients with FSP typically have long survival, presumably because respiratory function is spared. Late in the illness there may be urinary urgency and incontinence and sometimes fecal incontinence; sexual function tends to be preserved. In pure forms of FSP, ataxia, posterior column sensory loss, and amyotrophy are absent or minimal; however, in some patients, minor sensory changes (impaired vibration and position sense) may be observed in late stages. Some family members may show isolated spasticity without other clinical symptoms. Neuropathologically, in FSP there is degeneration of the corticospinal tracts, which appear nearly normal in the brainstem but show increasing atrophy at more caudal levels in the spinal cord. It is now apparent that defects at several different loci underlie both dominantly and recessively inherited forms of FSP (Table 365-2). An infantile-onset form of X-linked, recessive FSP arises from mutations in the gene for proteolipid protein. This is an example of rather striking allelic variation, as most other mutations in the same gene cause not FSP but Pelizaeus-Merzbacher disease, a disorder of CNS myelin. Defects in two other genes encoding the proteins "spastin" and "paraplegin" have recently been associated, respectively, with dominantly and recessively inherited FSP. The latter gene is of particular interest as it has homology to metalloproteases that are important in mitochondrial function in yeast.

Rarely, FSP may arise concomitantly with significant involvement of other regions of the nervous system. Thus, it has been described concurrently with amyotrophy, mental retardation, mental retardation with skin thickening, optic atrophy, and sensory neuropathy. In some cases there is loss of fibers in the ascending posterior columns and the spinocerebellar tracts, features reminiscent of Friedreich's ataxia. These complicated forms of FSP emphasize the challenge inherent in classifying the neurodegenerative disorders; there may be considerable overlap of the clinical phenotypes in diseases otherwise classified as distinct. Fortunately, it is likely that increasingly available genetic testing will clarify these nosologic difficulties.

WEB SITES Several web sites provide valuable information on ALS including those offered by the Muscular Dystrophy Association (www.mdausa.org), the Amyotrophic Lateral Sclerosis Association (www.alsa.org), and the World Federation of Neurology (www.wfnals.org).

BIBLIOGRAPHY

BROWN RH et al: *Amyotrophic Lateral Sclerosis*. London, Martin Dunitz, 1999

CASARI G: Spastic paraplegia and OXPHOS impairment caused by mutations in paraplegin, a nuclear-encoded mitochondrial metalloprotease. Cell 93:973, 1998

CLEVELAND DW: From Charcot to SOD1: Mechanisms of selective motor neuron death in ALS. Neuron 24:515, 1999

COMI GP et al: Cytochrome c oxidase subunit I microdeletion in a patient with motor neuron disease. Ann Neurol 43:110, 1998

LACOMBLEZ L et al: Dose-ranging study of riluzole in amyotrophic lateral sclerosis. Lancet 347:1425, 1997

LAI EC et al: Effect of recombinant human insulin-like growth factor-1 on progression of ALS. A placebo-controlled study. Neurol 49:1621, 1997

MARTIN JB: Molecular basis of the neurodegenerative disorders. N Engl J Med 340:1970, 1999

MILLER RG et al: The ALS patient care database: Goals, design and early results. Neurology 54:53, 2000

PELLIZZONI L et al: A novel function of SMN, the spinal muscular atrophy disease gene product, in pre-mRNA splicing. Cell 95:615, 1998

ROSEN DR et al: Mutations in Cu/Zn superoxide dismutase gene are associated with familial amyotrophic lateral sclerosis. Nature 362:59, 1993

TRAYNOR BJ et al: Amyotrophic lateral sclerosis mimic syndromes: A population based study. Arch Neurol 54:109, 2000

366

John W. Engstrom, Joseph B. Martin

DISORDERS OF THE AUTONOMIC NERVOUS SYSTEM

Rapid adjustments in vital physiologic mechanisms critical to survival are accomplished by the autonomic nervous system (ANS). The importance of this regulation is emphasized by the extent and severity of disability resulting from compromised ANS function. This chapter describes the clinical manifestations, diagnosis, and treatment of ANS disorders. →*The functional anatomy and relevant pharmacology of the sympathetic and parasympathetic components of the ANS are discussed in Chap. 72. Hypothalamic disorders that cause disturbances in homeostasis are discussed in Chaps. 17 and 328.*

CLINICAL MANIFESTATIONS Classification Disorders of the ANS may result from central nervous system (CNS) or peripheral nervous system (PNS) causes (Table 366-1). In many instances, the clinical signs and symptoms are due to interruption of a reflex arc controlling autonomic responses. The interruption can occur in the afferent limb, CNS processing centers, or efferent limb of the reflex arc. For example, a lesion of the medulla produced by a posterior fossa tumor can impair blood pressure (BP) responses to postural changes and result in orthostatic hypotension. Hypotension can also be caused by lesions of the spinal cord or peripheral vasomotor nerve fibers (diabetes mellitus). Diagnosis of the site of reflex interruption is dependent on the clinical context, ANS tests, and neuroimaging. Important elements of the clinical context include the presence or absence of CNS signs (pathophysiology and prognosis differ), association with sensory or motor polyneuropathy, family history, and pathologic findings. Some syndromes do not fit easily into any classification scheme because little is known about etiology, pathology, or treatment.

Table 366-1 Classification of ANS Disorders

I. With CNS signs
   - Multiple system atrophy
   - Spinal cord disorders (multiple sclerosis, tabes dorsalis, trauma, syrinx, hereditary degenerations)
   - Parkinson's disease
   - Huntington's disease
   - Tumors, multiple cerebral infarcts
   - Hypothalamic disorders
   - Wernicke's encephalopathy

II. Without CNS signs
   - Diabetes mellitus
   - Other peripheral neuropathies (alcoholism, amyloidosis, porphyria, uremia, collagen vascular disease, leprosy, Chagas disease, vitamin B_{12} deficiency, HIV)
   - Pure autonomic failure
   - Acute pandysautonomia
   - Chronic idiopathic anhidrosis
   - Familial dysautonomia—Riley-Day syndrome
   - Guillain-Barré syndrome
   - Toxic neuropathies (vincristine, heavy metals, propafenone, uremia)
   - Paraneoplastic (sensory neuropathy, enteric neuropathy)
   - Tangier's and Fabry's diseases
   - Neuromuscular junction (botulism, Lambert-Eaton syndrome)

III. Miscellaneous
   - Postural orthostatic tachycardia syndrome (POTS)
   - Prolonged bed rest or space flight
   - Raynaud's syndrome
   - Advanced age
   - Dopamine β-hydroxylase deficiency
   - Monamine oxidase deficiency

IV. Focal ANS disorders
   - Complex regional pain syndrome type I (reflex sympathetic dystrophy, shoulder–hand syndrome)
   - Complex regional pain syndrome type II (causalgia)
   - Radiculopathy
   - Horner's syndrome
   - Adie's syndrome
   - Reinnervation anomalies ("crocodile" tears)

COLOR ATLASES

I. Atlas of Cardiology

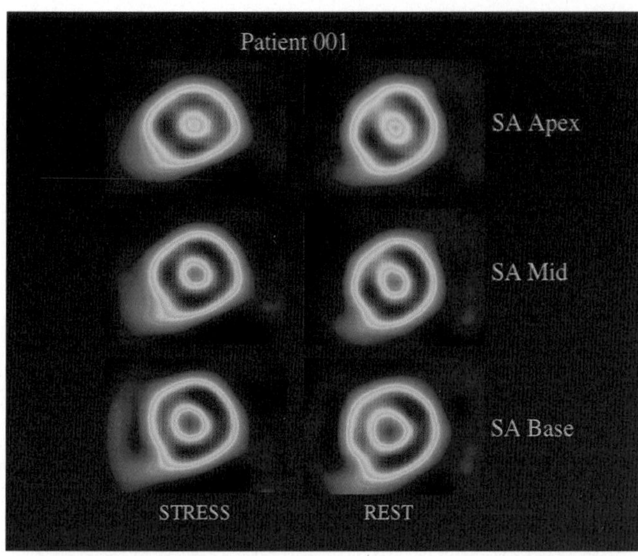

I-1A **Exercise sestamibi study** on a 71-year-old, white female with atypical angina. *Left:* stress images; *right:* rest images. The images are normal. There is even sestamibi update throughout the myocardium at rest and during stress. SA, short axis. Mid, middle of the left ventricle. VLA, vertical long axis. HLA, horizontal long axis.

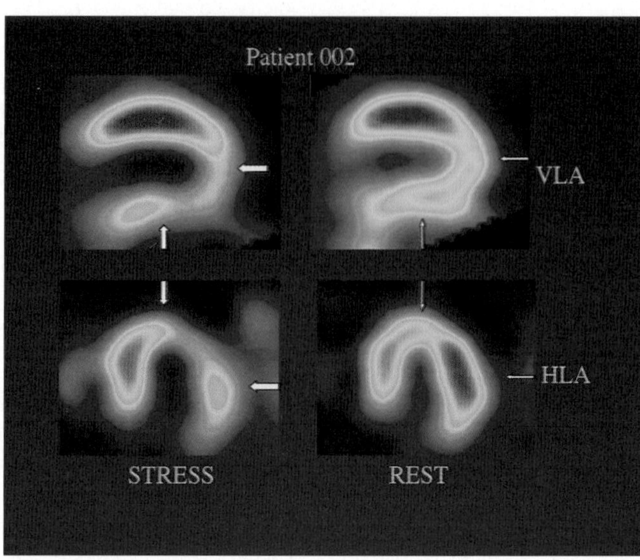

I-1B **Exercise sestamibi study** on a 75-year-old male with a history of typical angina. *Left:* stress images; *right:* rest images. The stress images show a large defect involving the apex, lateral, and inferior walls (*thick arrows*), which improves at rest (*thin arrows*). Subsequent coronary angiography demonstrates severe three-vessel coronary artery disease.

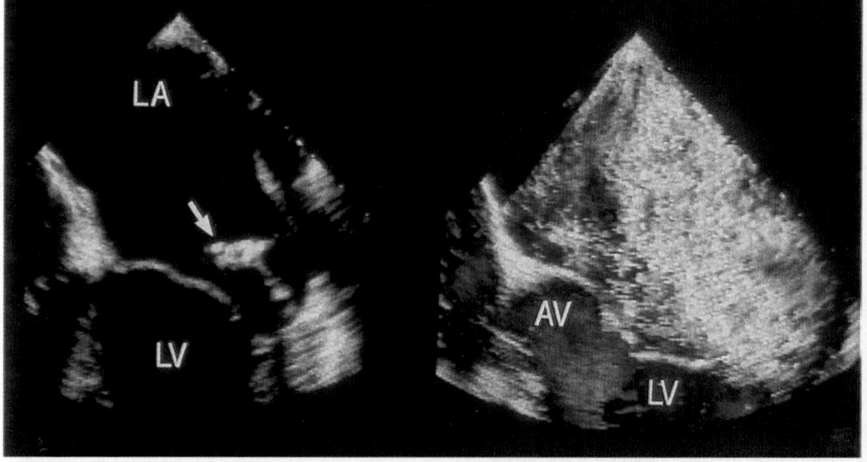

I-2 **Transesophageal echocardiographic view** of a patient with severe mitral regurgitation due to a flail posterior leaflet. The *arrow* points to the portion of the posterior leaflet that is unsupported and moves into the left atrium during systole. *Right:* color flow imaging demonstrating a large mosaic jet of mitral regurgitation during systole. LA, left atrium; LV, left ventricle; AV, aortic valve.

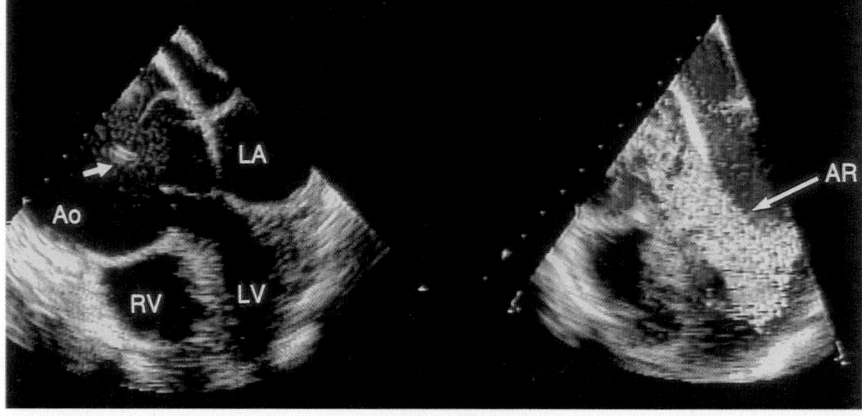

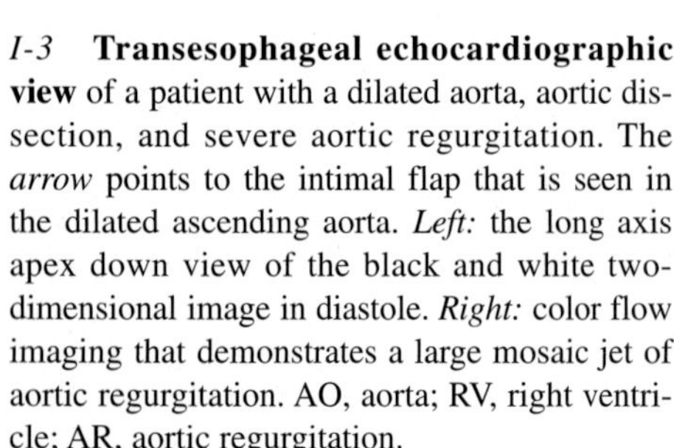

I-3 **Transesophageal echocardiographic view** of a patient with a dilated aorta, aortic dissection, and severe aortic regurgitation. The *arrow* points to the intimal flap that is seen in the dilated ascending aorta. *Left:* the long axis apex down view of the black and white two-dimensional image in diastole. *Right:* color flow imaging that demonstrates a large mosaic jet of aortic regurgitation. AO, aorta; RV, right ventricle; AR, aortic regurgitation.

II. Atlas of Dermatology

Stephen F. Templeton / Thomas J. Lawley

A. Common Skin Diseases and Lesions

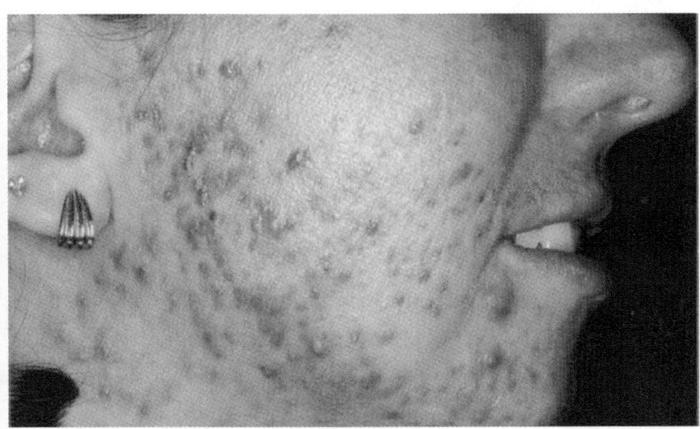

IIA-1 **Acne vulgaris** with inflammatory papules, pustules, and comedones

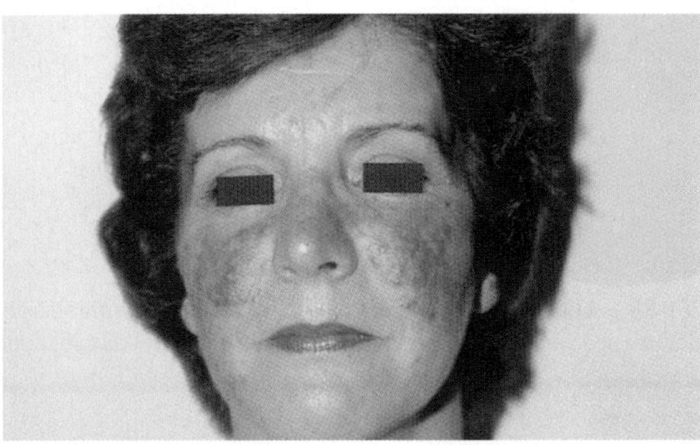

IIA-2 **Acne rosacea** with prominent facial erythema, telangiectasias, scattered papules, and small pustules.

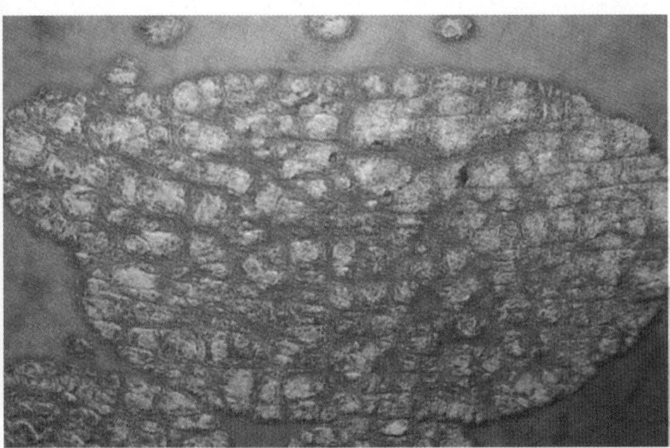

IIA-3 **Psoriasis** is characterized by small and large erythematous plaques with adherent silvery scale.

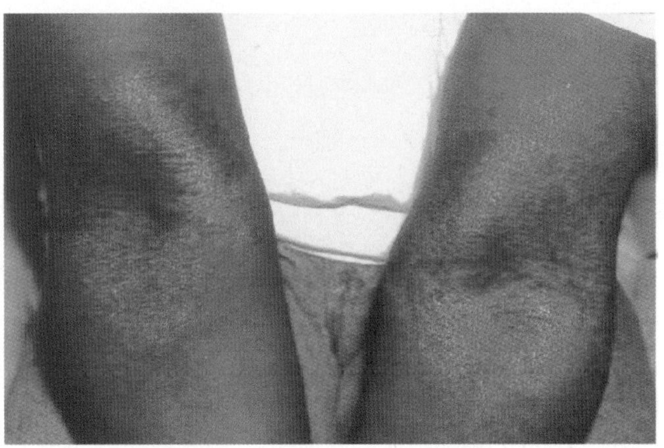

IIA-4 **Atopic dermatitis** with hyperpigmentation, lichenification, and scaling in the antecubital fossae.

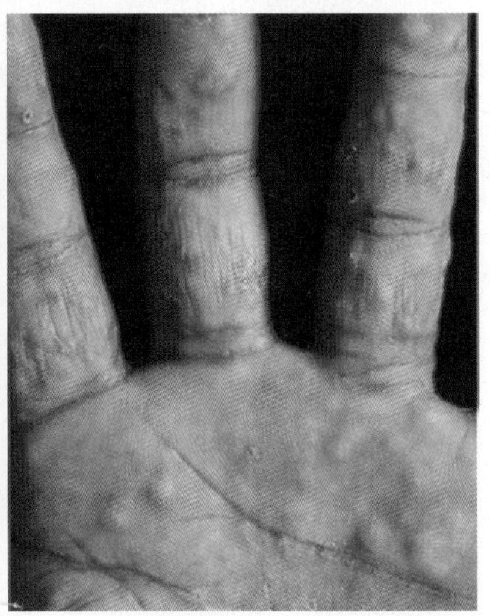

IIA-5 **Dyshidrotic eczema,** characterized by deep-seated vesicles and scaling on palms and lateral fingers, is often associated with an atopic diathesis.

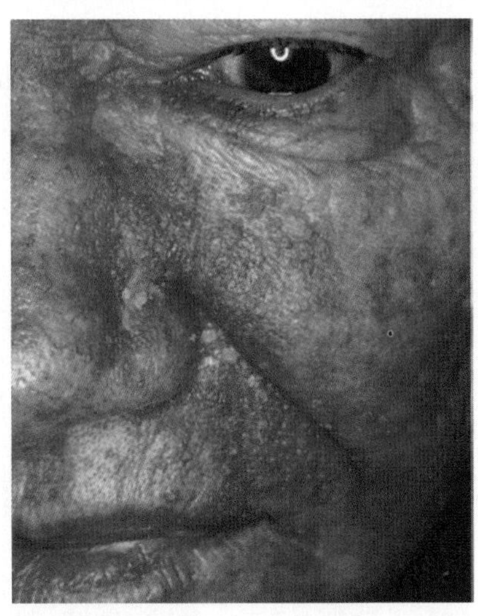

IIA-6 **Seborrheic dermatitis** showing central facial erythema with overlying greasy, yellowish scale.

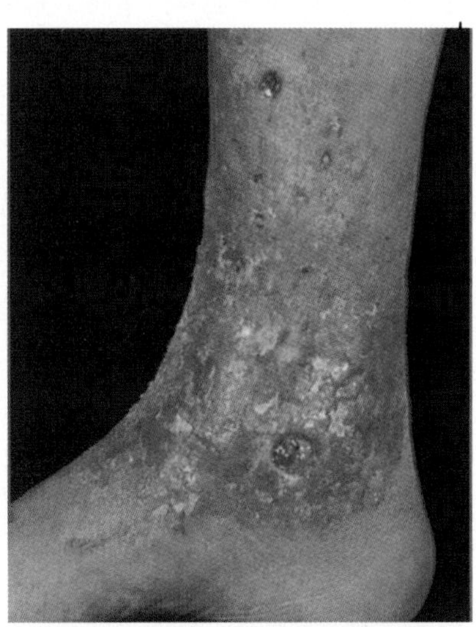

IIA-7 **Stasis dermatitis** showing erythematous, scaly, and oozing patches over the lower leg. Several stasis ulcers are also seen in this patient.

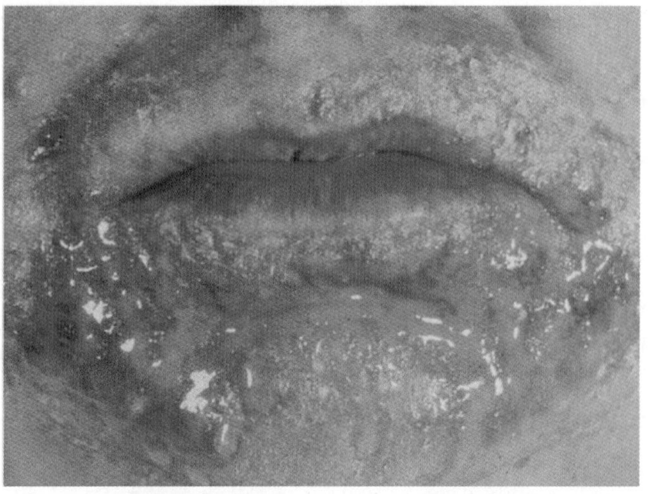

IIA-8A **Allergic contact dermatitis,** acute phase, with sharply demarcated, weeping, eczematous plaques in a perioral distribution.

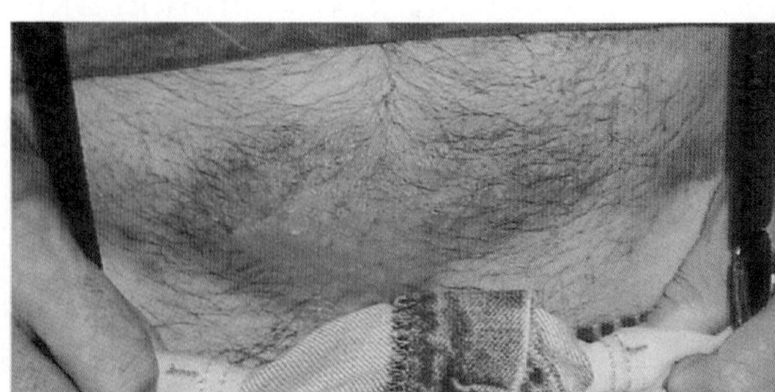

IIA-8B **Allergic contact dermatitis** to nickel, chronic phase demonstrating an erythematous, lichenified, weeping plaque on skin chronically exposed to a metal snap.

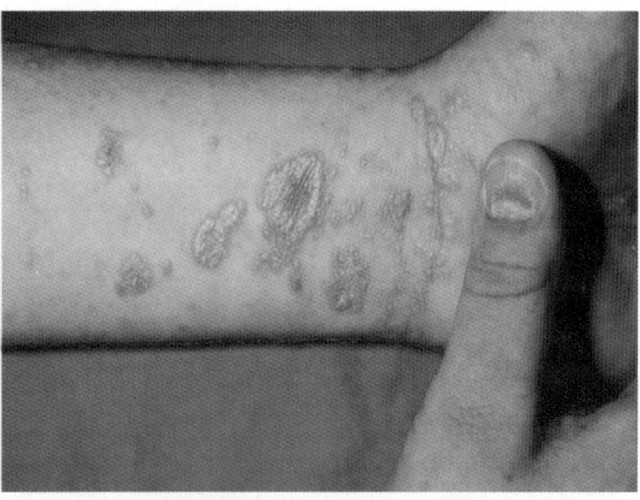

IIA-9 **Lichen planus** showing multiple flat-topped, violaceous papules and plaques. Nail dystrophy as seen in this patient's thumbnail may also be a feature.

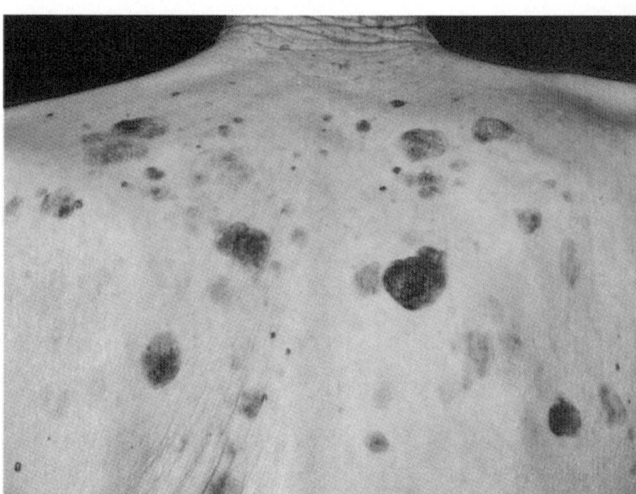

IIA-10 **Seborrheic keratoses** are seen as "stuck on," waxy, verrucous papules and plaques with a variety of colors ranging from light tan to black.

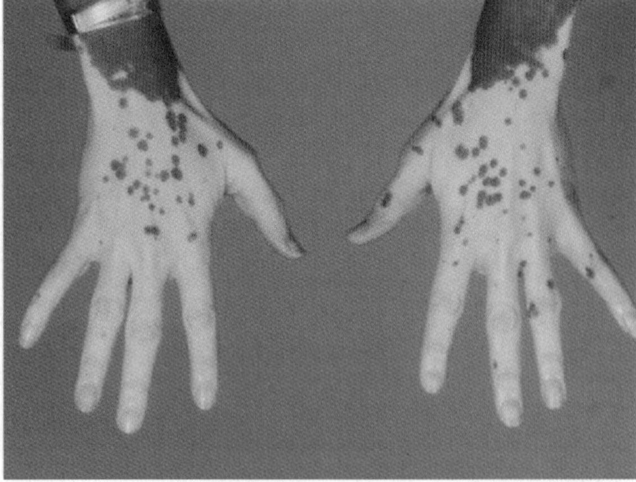

IIA-11 **Vitiligo** in a typical acral distribution demonstrating striking cutaneous depigmentation, as a result of loss of melanocytes.

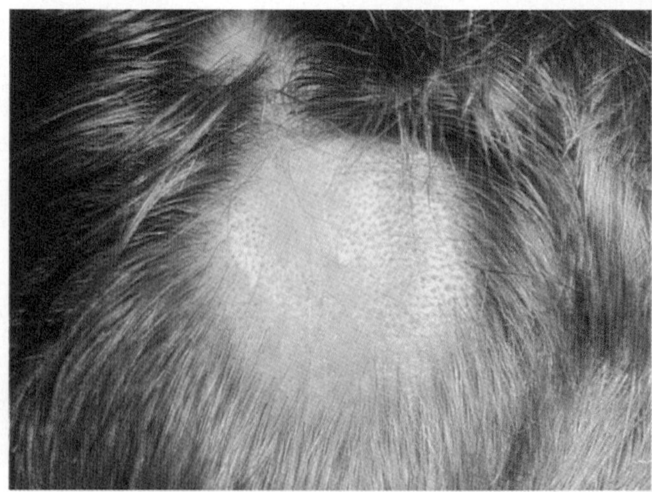

IIA-12 **Alopecia areata** characterized by a sharply demarcated circular patch of scalp completely devoid of hairs. Follicular orifices are preserved, indicating a nonscarring alopecia.

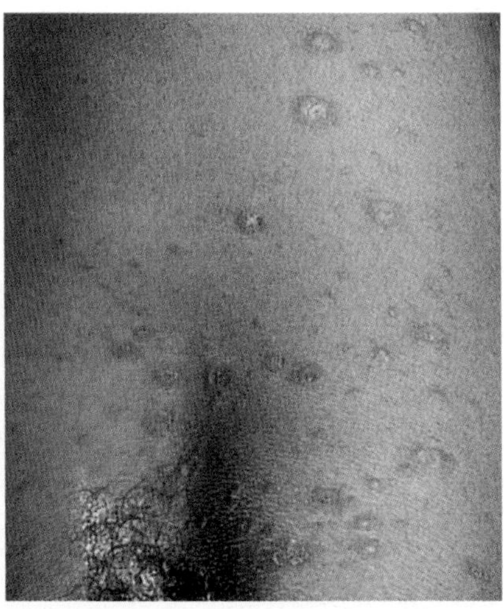

IIA-13 **Pityriasis rosea** Multiple round to oval erythematous patches with fine central scale are distributed along the skin tension lines on the trunk.

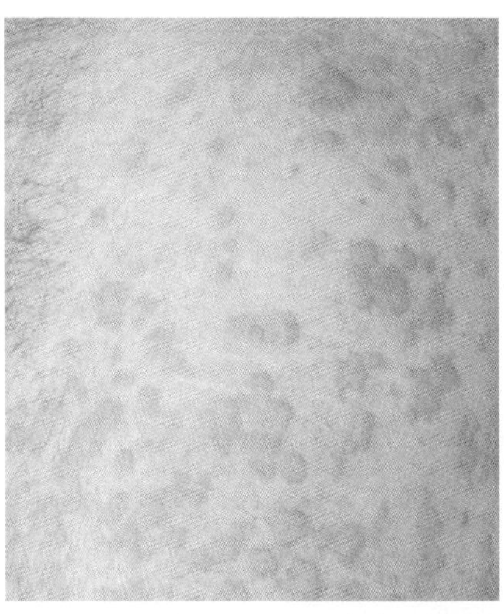

IIA-14A **Urticaria** showing characteristic discrete and confluent, edematous, erythematous papules and plaques.

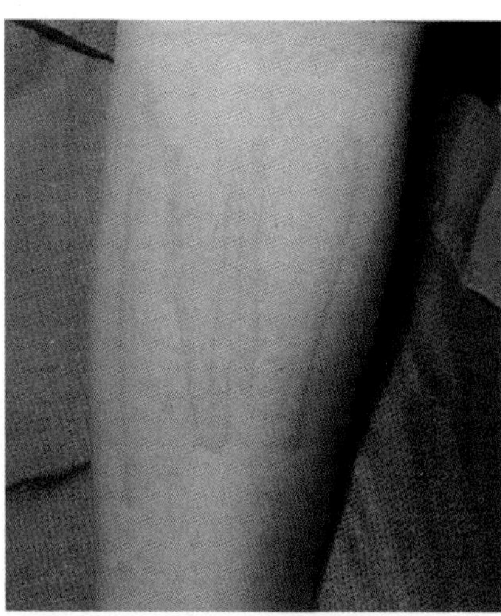

IIA-14B **Dermatographism** Erythema and whealing that developed after firm stroking of the skin.

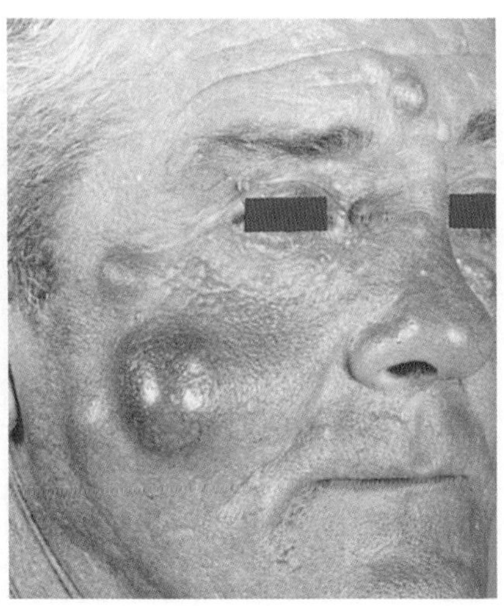

IIA-15 **Epidermoid cysts** Several inflamed and noninflamed firm, cystic nodules are seen in this patient. Often a patulous follicular punctum is observed on the overlying epidermal surface.

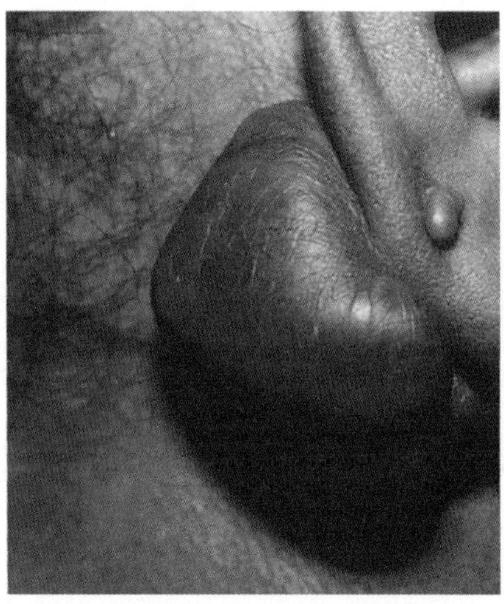

IIA-16 **Keloids** resulting from ear piercing, with firm exophytic flesh-colored to erythematous nodules of scar tissue.

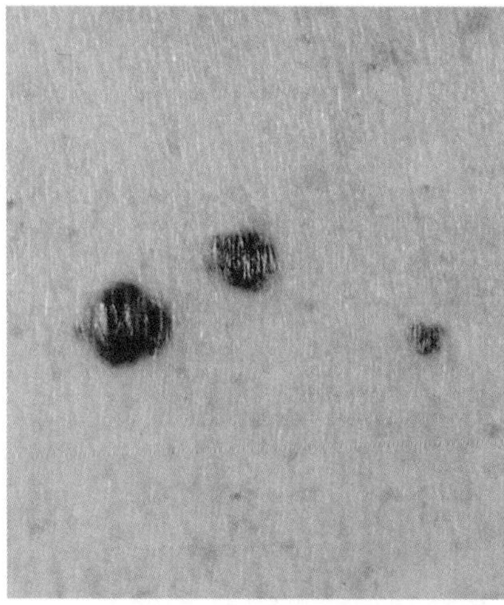

IIA-17 **Cherry hemangiomas** are very common and arise in middle-aged to older adults. They are characterized by multiple erythematous to dark purple papules usually located on the trunk.

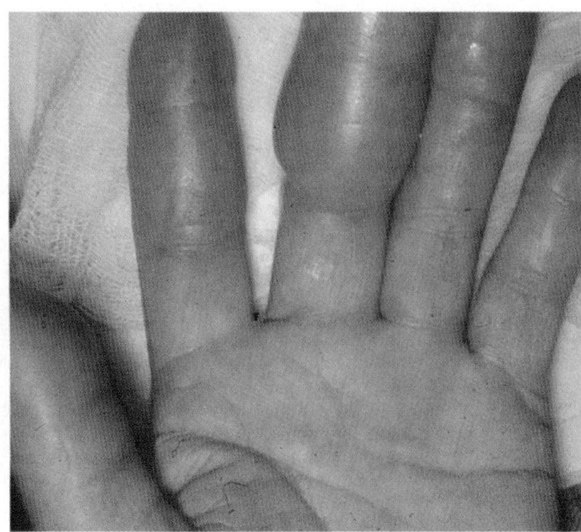

IIA-18 **Frostbite** with vesiculation, surrounded by edema and erythema.

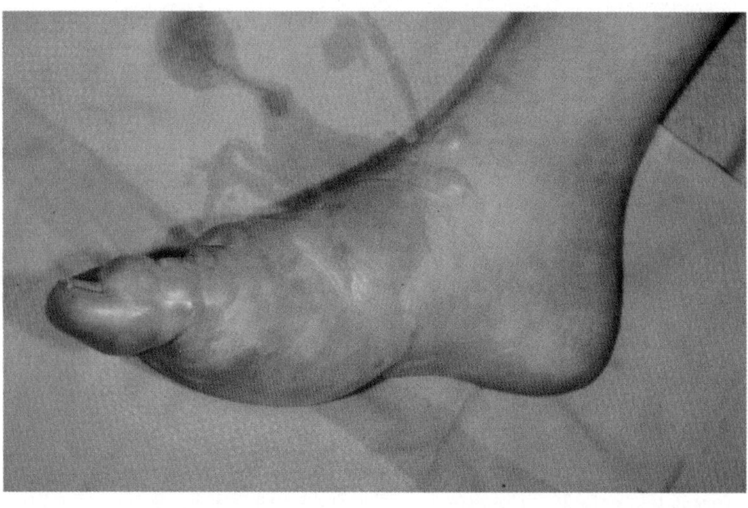

IIA-19 **Frostbite** with vesiculation, surrounded by edema and erythema.

B. Cutaneous Neoplasms

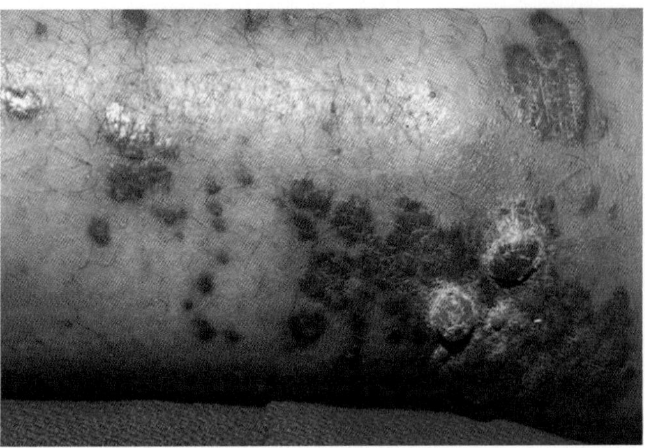

IIB-20 **Kaposi's sarcoma** in a patient with AIDS demonstrating patch, plaque, and tumor stages.

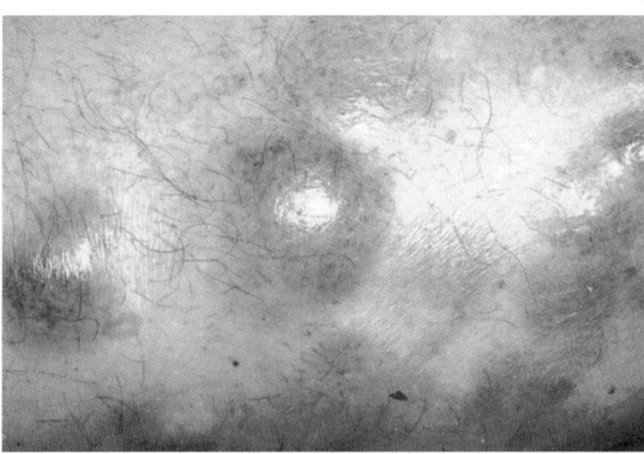

IIB-21 **Non-Hodgkin's lymphoma** involving the skin with typical violaceous, "plum-colored" nodules.

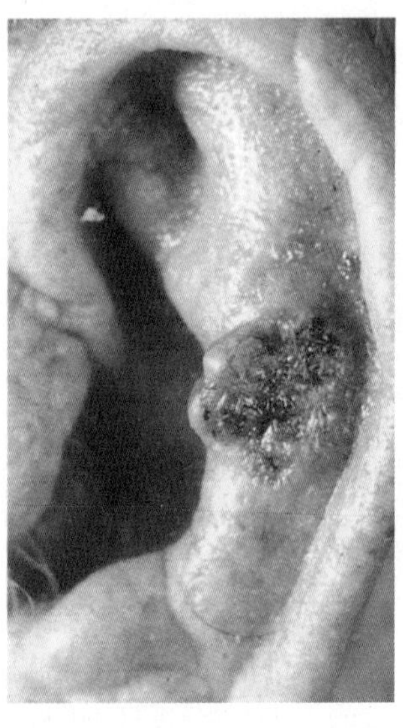

IIB-22 **Basal cell carcinoma** showing central ulceration and a pearly, rolled, telangiectatic tumor border.

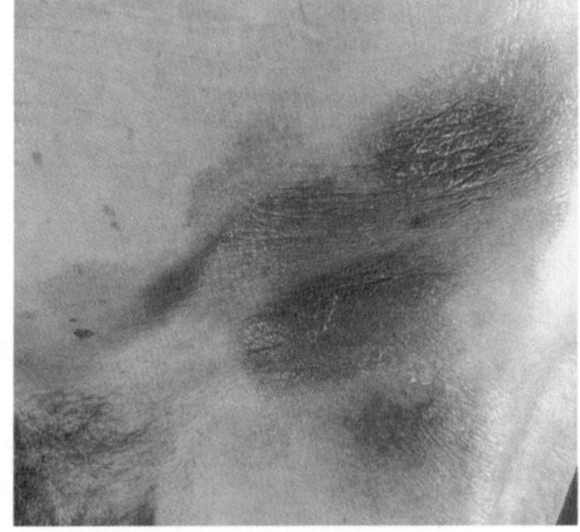

IIB-23 **Mycosis fungoides** is a cutaneous T cell lymphoma, and plaque stage lesions are seen in this patient.

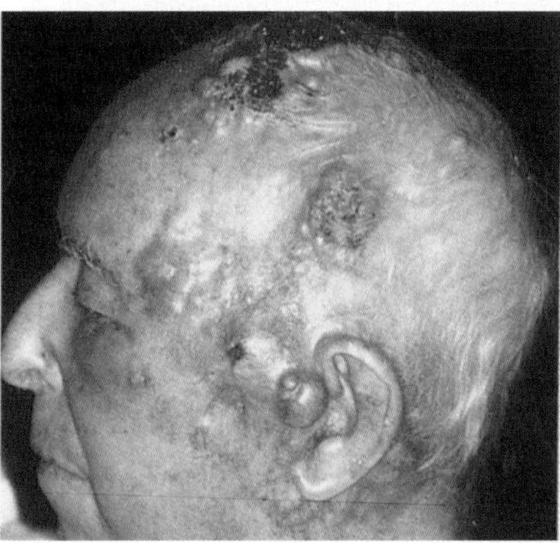

IIB-24 **Metastatic carcinoma** to the skin is characterized by inflammatory, often ulcerated dermal nodules.

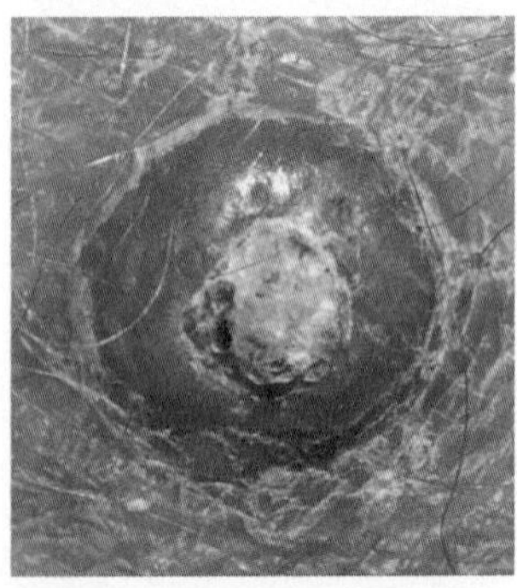

IIB-25 **Keratoacanthoma** is a low-grade squamous cell carcinoma that presents as an exophytic nodule with central keratinous debris.

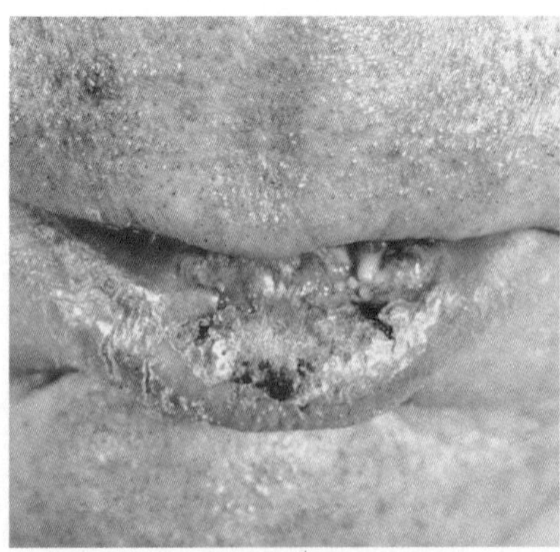

IIB-26 **Squamous cell carcinoma** seen here as a hyperkeratotic crusted and somewhat eroded plaque on the lower lip. Sun-exposed skin such as the head, neck, hands, and arms are other typical sites of involvement.

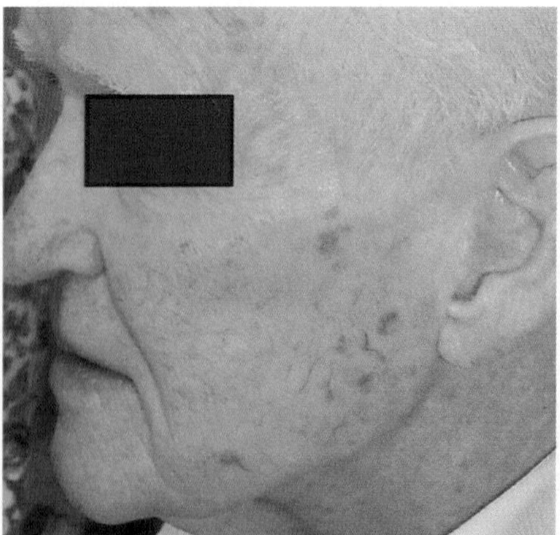

IIB-27 **Actinic keratoses** consists of hyperkeratotic erythematous papules and patches on sun-exposed skin. They arise in middle-aged to older adults and have some potential for malignant transformation.

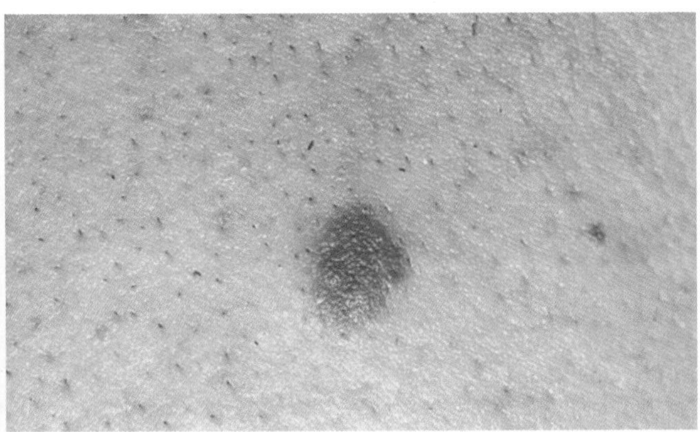

IIC-28 **Nevus** Nevi are benign proliferations of nevomelanocytes characterized by regularly shaped hyperpigmented macules or papules of a uniform color.

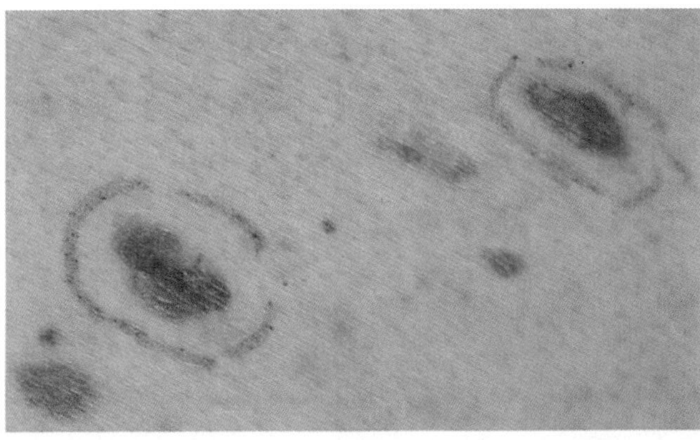

IIC-29 **Dysplastic nevi** are irregularly pigmented and shaped nevomelanocytic lesions which may be associated with familial melanoma.

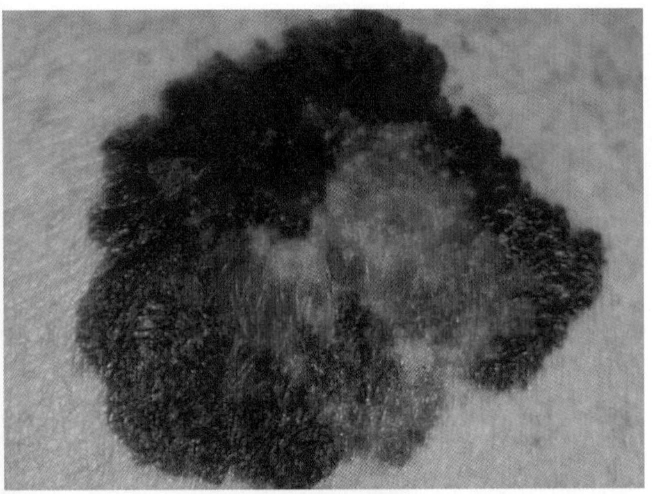

IIC-30 **Superficial spreading melanoma** is the most common type of malignant melanoma and demonstrates color variegation (black, blue, brown, pink, and white) and irregular borders.

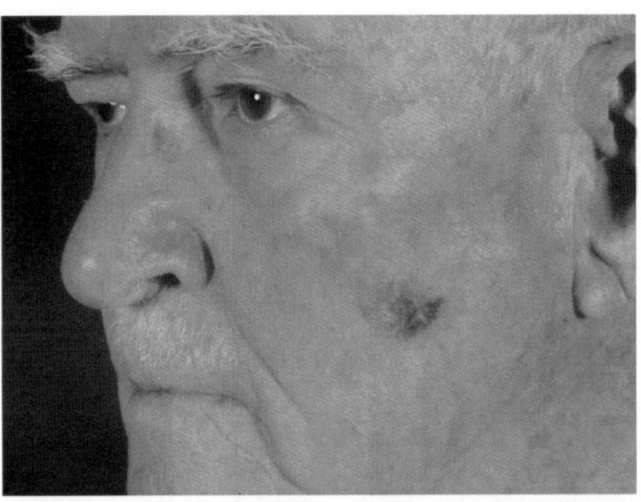

IIC-31 **Lentigo maligna melanoma** occurs on sun-exposed skin as a large, hyperpigmented macule or plaque with irregular borders and variable pigmentation.

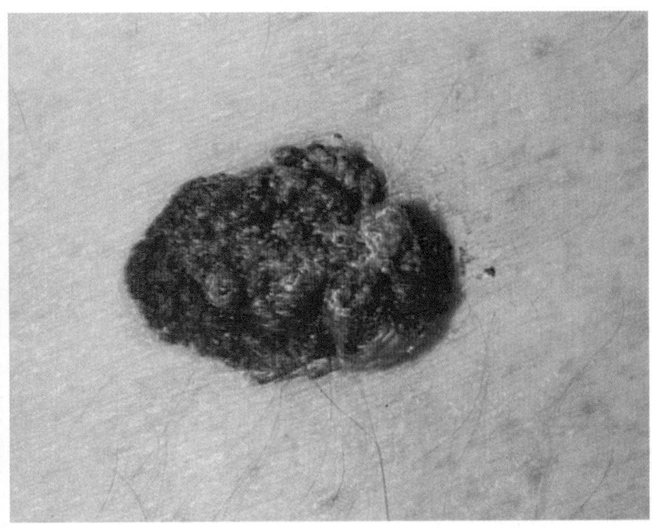

IIC-32 **Nodular melanoma** most commonly manifests itself as a rapidly growing, often ulcerated or crusted black nodule.

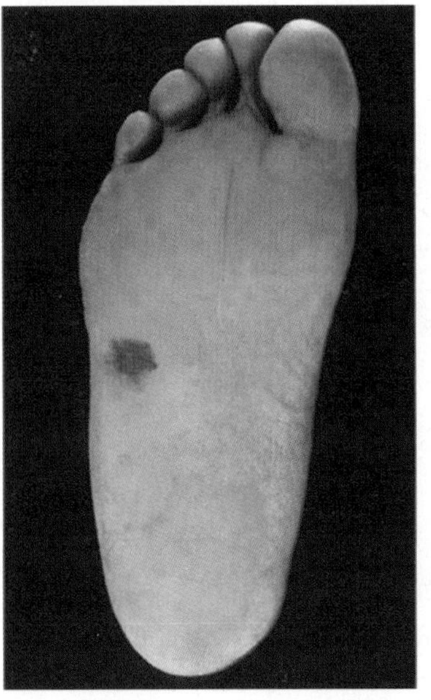

IIC-33 **Acral lentiginous melanoma** is more common in blacks, Asians, and Hispanics and occurs as an enlarging hyperpigmented macule or plaque on the palms and soles. Lateral pigment diffusion is present.

D. Infectious Disease and the Skin

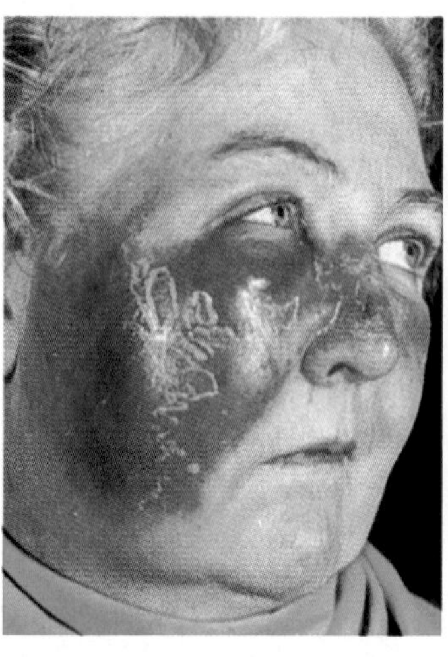

IID-34 **Erysipelas** is a streptococcal infection of the superficial dermis and consists of well-demarcated, erythematous, edematous, warm plaques.

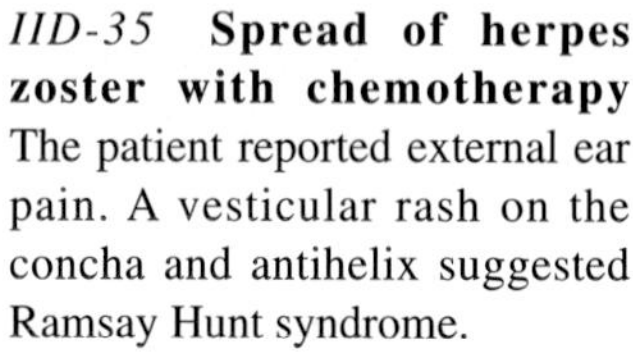

IID-35 **Spread of herpes zoster with chemotherapy** The patient reported external ear pain. A vesticular rash on the concha and antihelix suggested Ramsay Hunt syndrome.

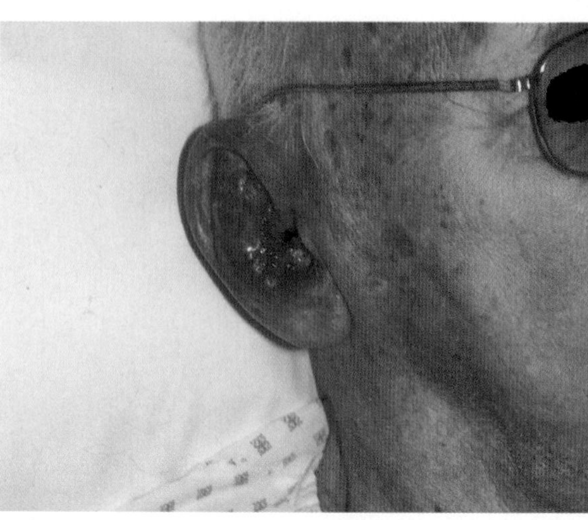

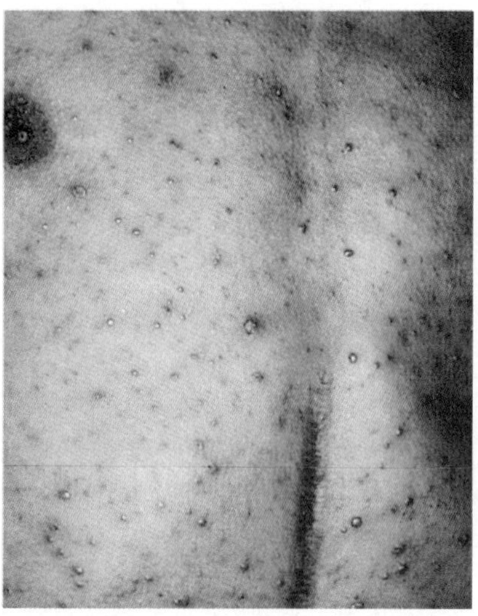

IID-36 **Varicella** showing numerous lesions in various stages of evolution: vesicles on an erythematous base, umbilicated vesicles, and crusts.

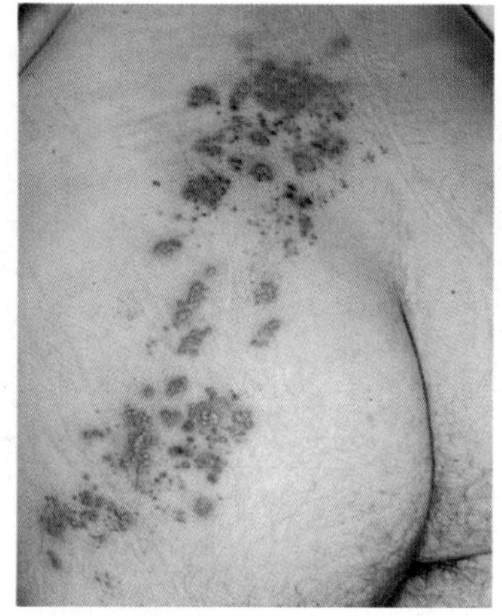

IID-37 **Herpes zoster** is seen in this HIV-infected patient as hemorrhagic vesicles and pustules on an erythematous base grouped in a dermatomal distribution.

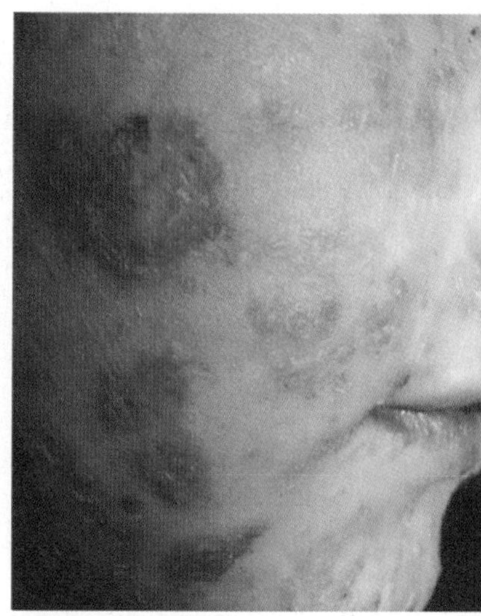

IID-38 **Impetigo contagiosa** is a superficial streptococcal or *Staphylococcus aureus* infection consisting of honey-colored crusts and erythematous weeping erosions. Occasionally, bullous lesions may be seen.

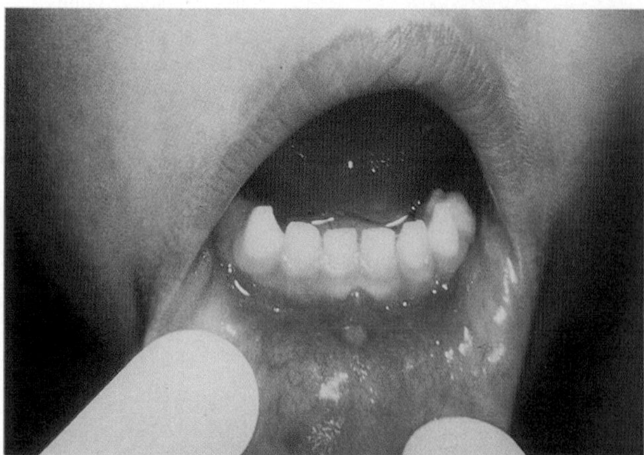

IID-39 **Tender vesicles and erosions** in the mouth of a patient with hand-foot-and-mouth disease.

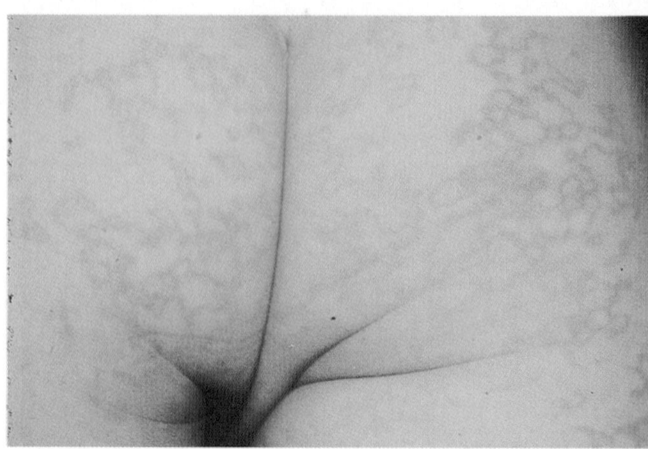

IID-40 **Lacy reticular rash of erythema infectiosum** (fifth disease).

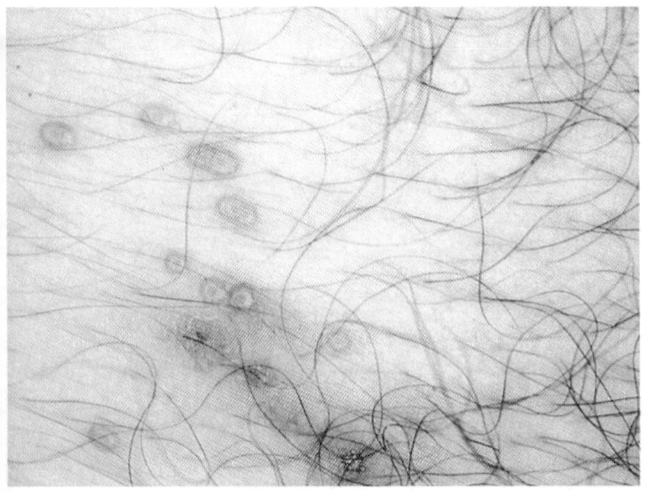

IID-41 **Molluscum contagiosum** is a cutaneous poxvirus infection characterized by multiple umbilicated flesh-colored or hypopigmented papules.

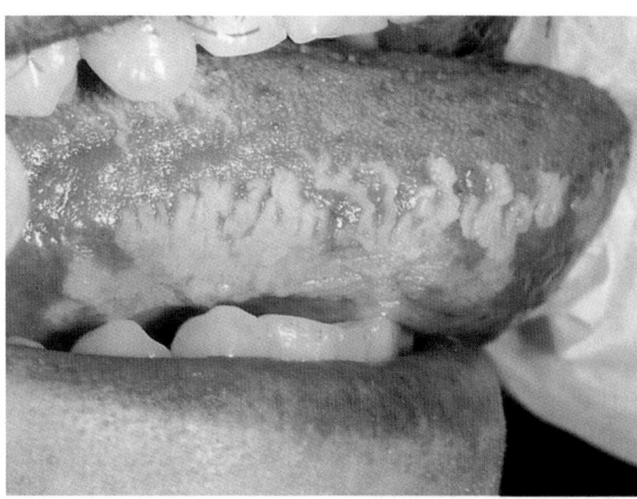

IID-42 **Oral hairy leukoplakia** often presents as white plaques on the lateral tongue and is associated with Epstein-Barr virus infection.

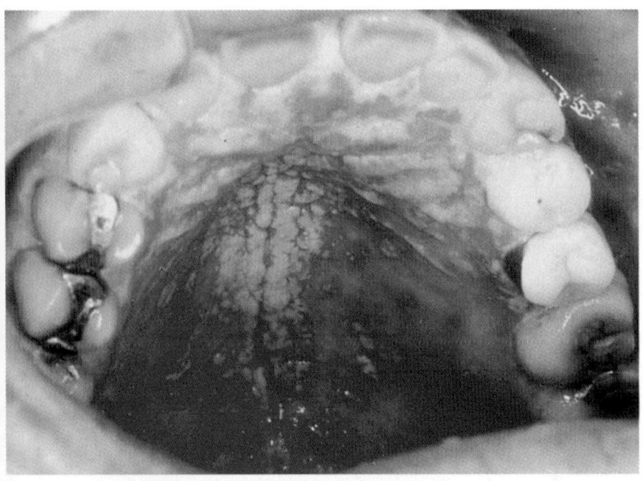

IID-43 **Pseudomembranous oral candidiasis** Adherent white, mucoid plaques with an erythematous halo seen here on the palate often indicate an immunocompromised state.

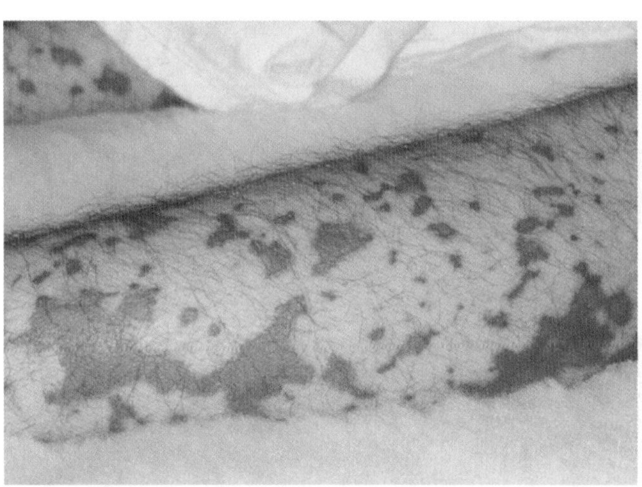

IID-44 **Fulminant meningococcemia** with extensive angular purpuric patches.

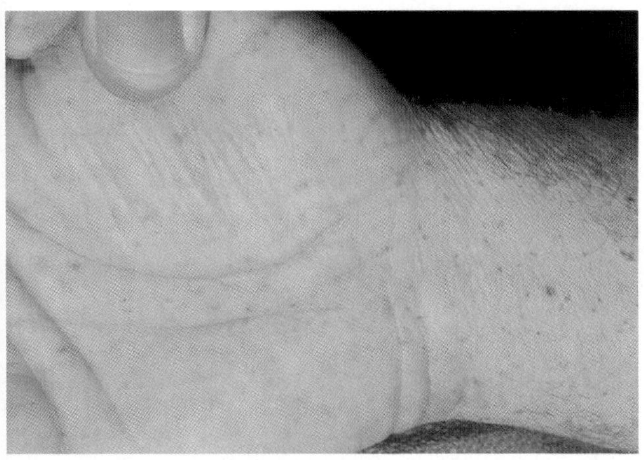

IID-45 **Rocky Mountain spotted fever** demonstrating pinpoint petechial lesions on the palm and volar aspect of the wrist.

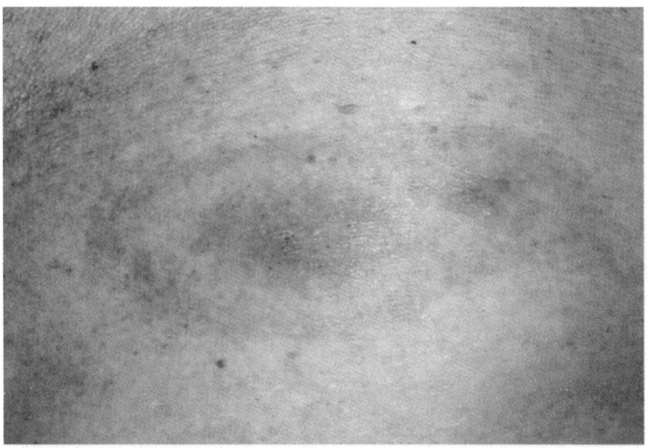

IID-46 **Erythema chronicum migrans** is the early cutaneous manifestation of Lyme disease and is characterized by erythematous annular patches, often with a central erythematous papule at the tick bite site.

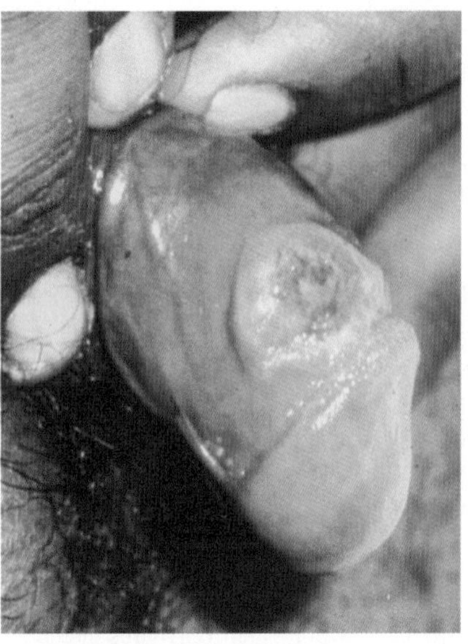

IID-47 **Primary syphilis** with a firm, nontender chancre.

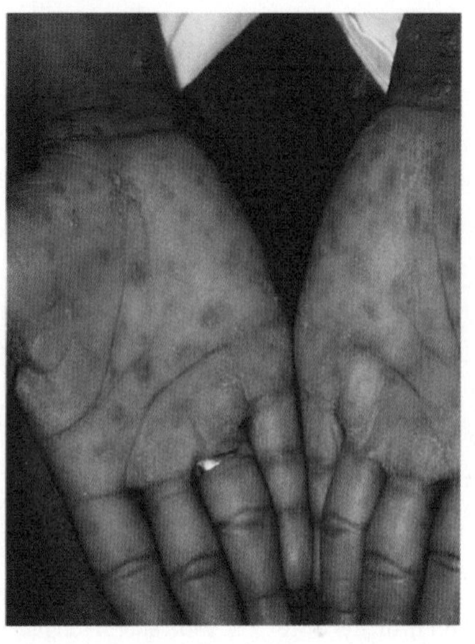

IID-48 **Secondary syphilis** commonly affects the palms and soles with scaling, firm, red-brown papules.

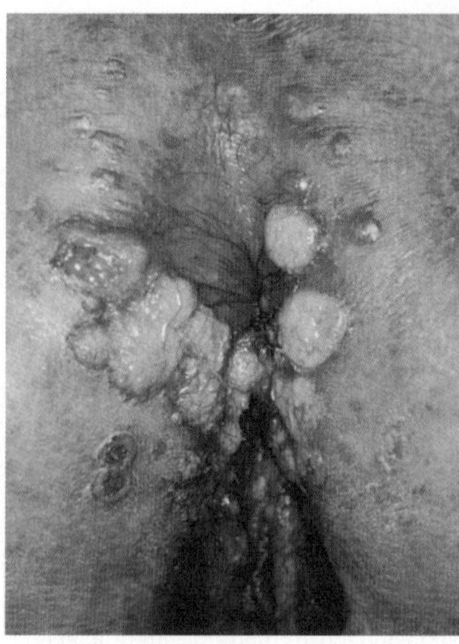

IID-49 **Condylomata lata** are moist, somewhat verrucous intertriginous plaques seen in secondary syphilis.

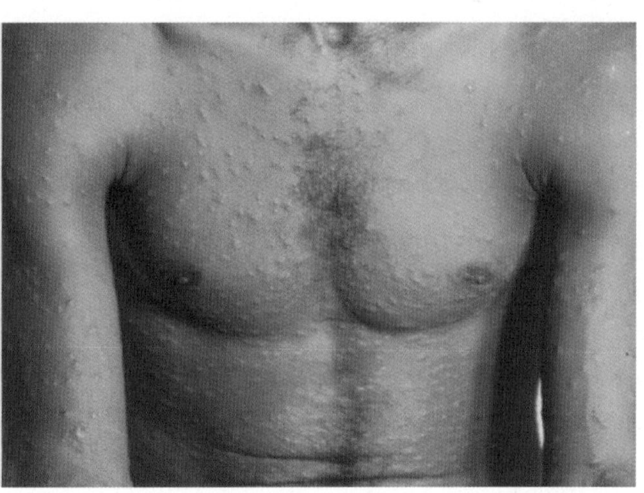

IID-50 **Secondary syphilis** demonstrating the papulosquamous truncal eruption.

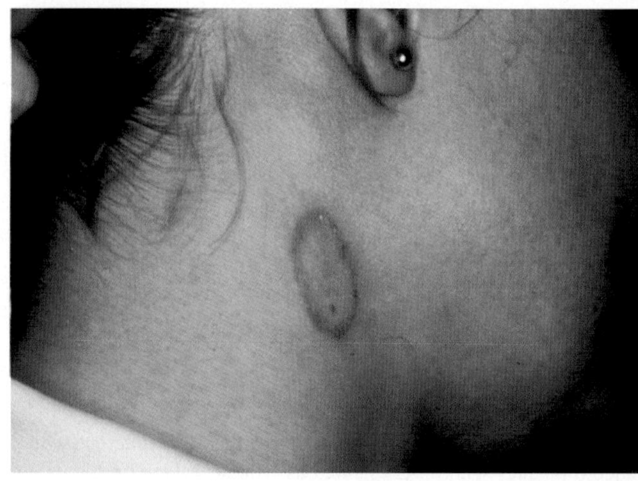

IID-51 **Tinea corporis** is a superficial fungal infection, seen here as an erythematous annular scaly plaque with central clearing.

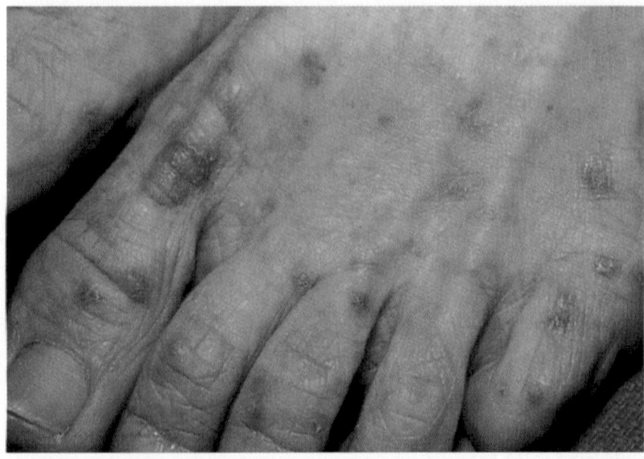

IID-52 **Scabies** showing typical scaling erythematous papules and few linear burrows.

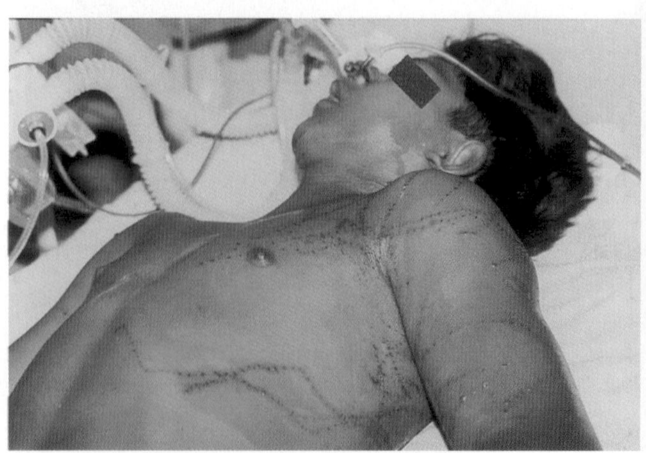

IID-53 **Skin lesions** caused by *Chironex fleckeri* sting.

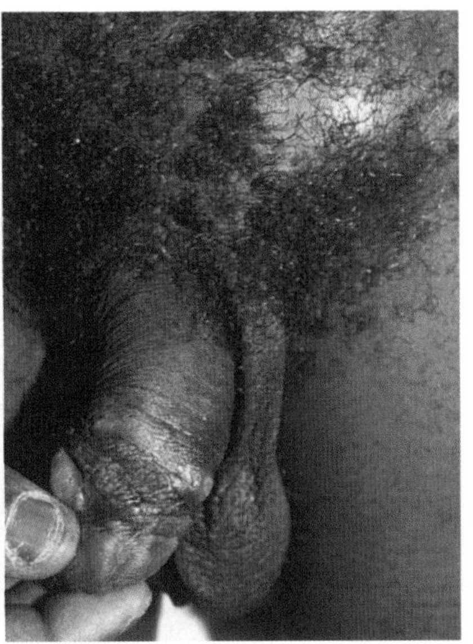

IID-54 **Chancroid** with characteristic penile ulcers and associated left inguinal adenitis (bubo).

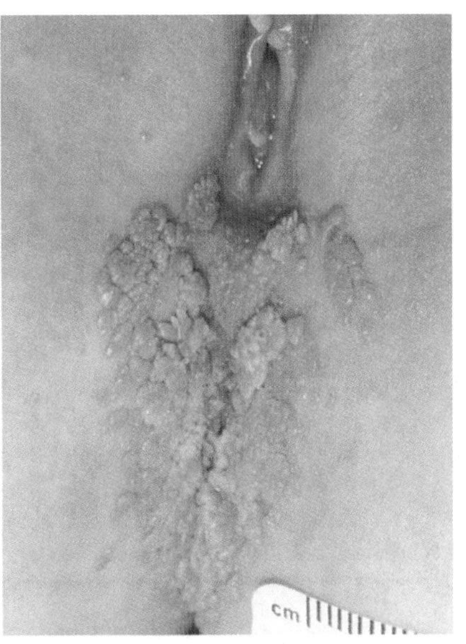

IID-55 **Condylomata acuminata** are lesions induced by human papillomavirus and in this patient are seen as multiple verrucous papules coalescing into plaques.

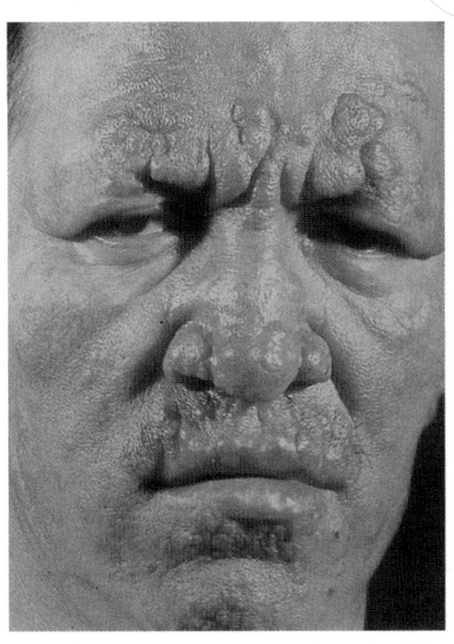

IID-56 **A patient with features of polar lepromatous leprosy;** multiple nodular skin lesions, particularly of the forehead, and loss of eyebrows.

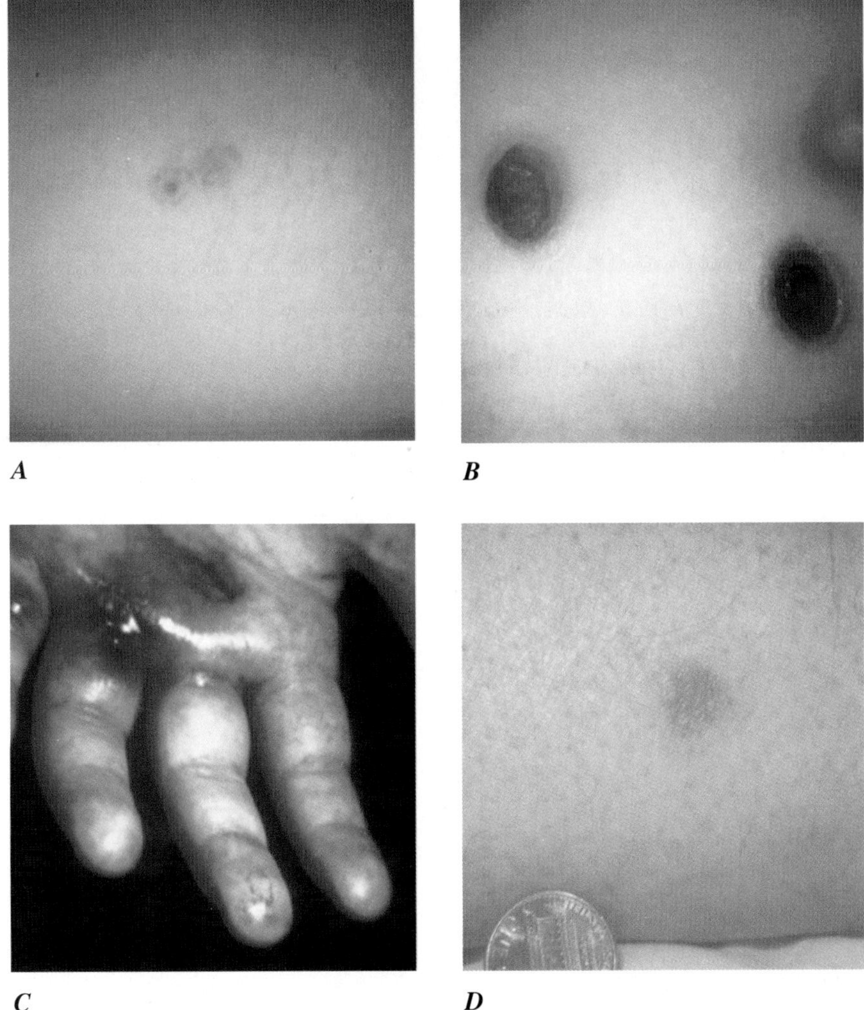

IID-57 **Skin lesions of neutropenic patients** *A.* Papules related to *Escherichia coli* bacteremia in a neutropenic patient with acute lymphocytic leukemia. *B.* The same lesion the following day. *C.* Ecthyma gangrenosum in a neutropenic patient with *Pseudomonas aeruginosa* bacteremia. *D.* Papule in a neutropenic patient with *Candida tropicalis* fungemia.

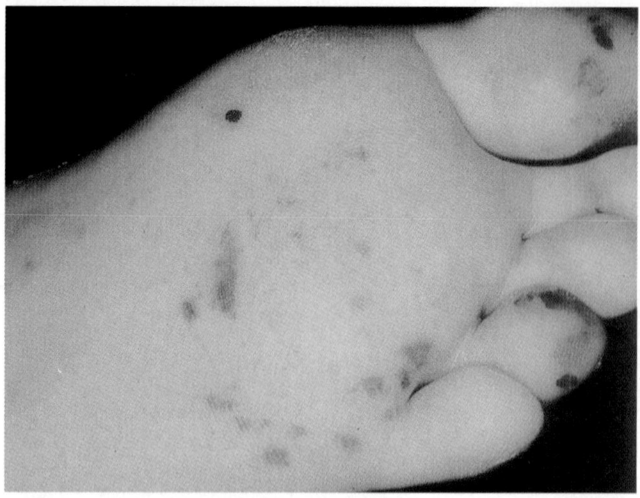

IID-58 **Septic emboli** with hemorrhage and infarction due to acute *Staphylococcus aureus* endocarditis.

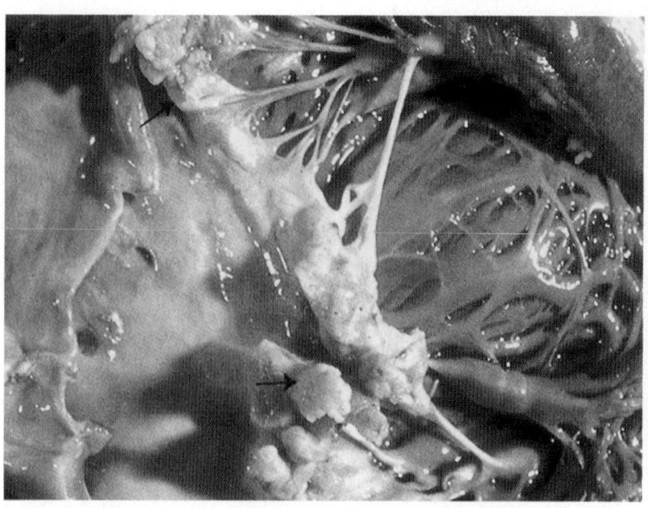

IID-59 Vegetations (*arrows*) due to viridans streptococcal endocarditis involving the mitral valve.

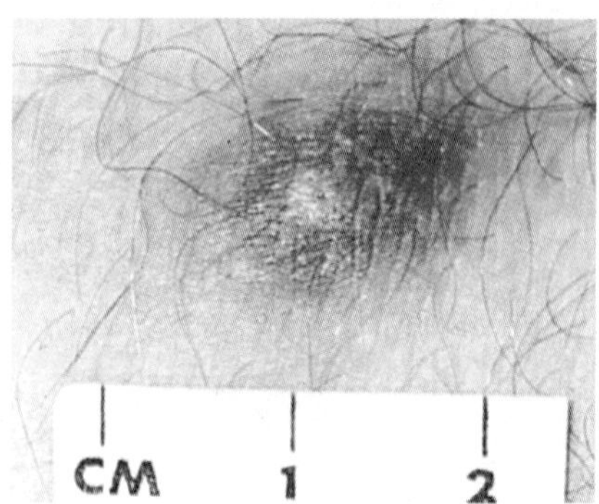

IID-60 **Disseminated gonococcemia** in the skin is seen as hemorrhagic papules and pustules with purpuric centers in an acral distribution.

IIE-61A **Systemic lupus erythematosus** showing prominent, scaly, malar erythema. Involvement of other sun-exposed sites is also common.

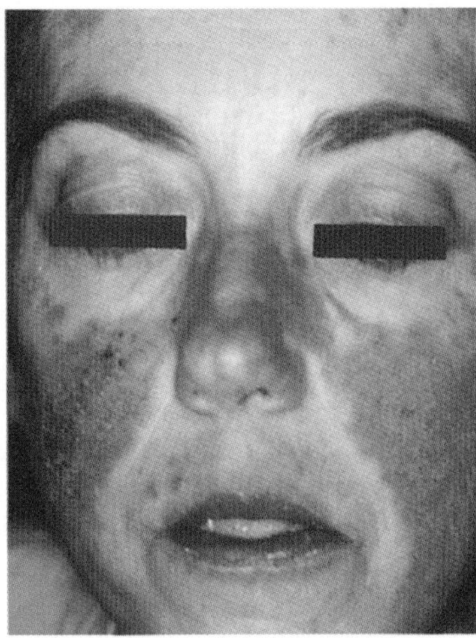

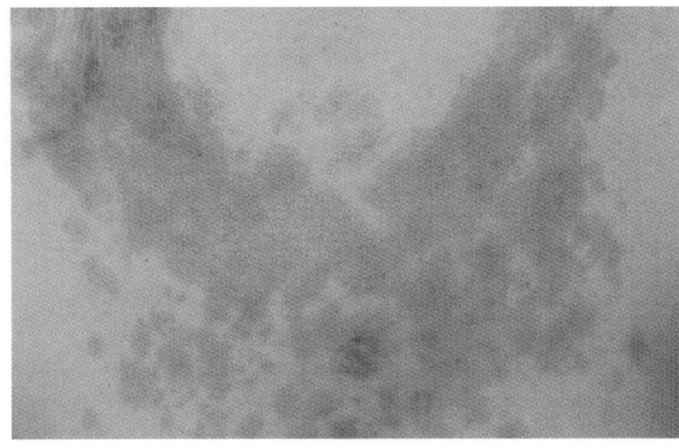

IIE-61B **Acute LE** on the upper chest demonstrating brightly erythematous and slightly edematous coalescence papules and plaques.

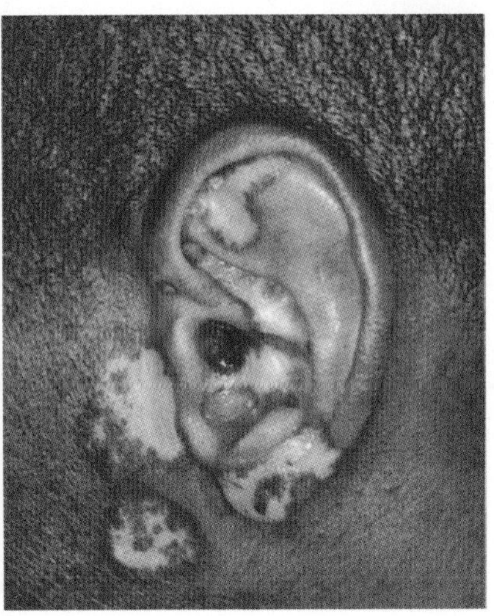

IIE-62 **Discoid lupus erythematosus** Violaceous, hyperpigmented, atrophic plaques, often with evidence of follicular plugging, which may result in scarring, are characteristic of this cutaneous form of lupus.

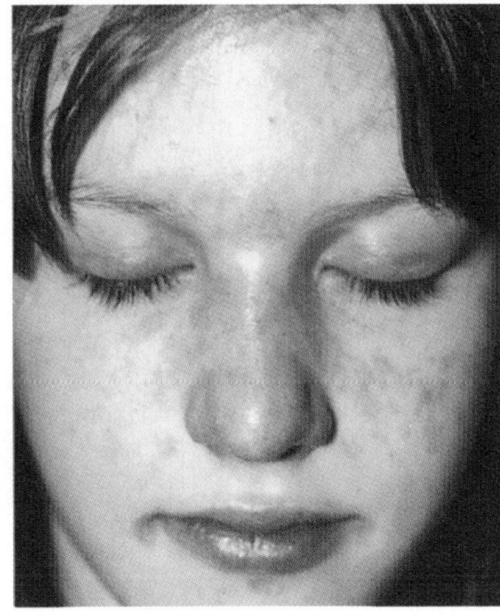

IIE-63 **Dermatomyositis** Periorbital violaceous erythema characterizes the classic heliotrope rash.

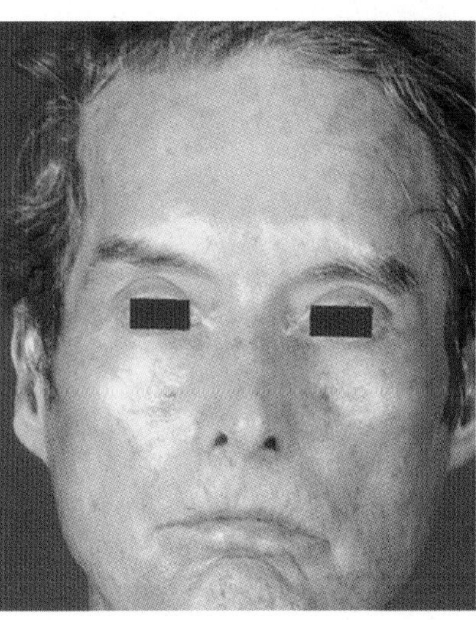

IIE-64 **Scleroderma** characterized by typical expressionless, mask-like facies.

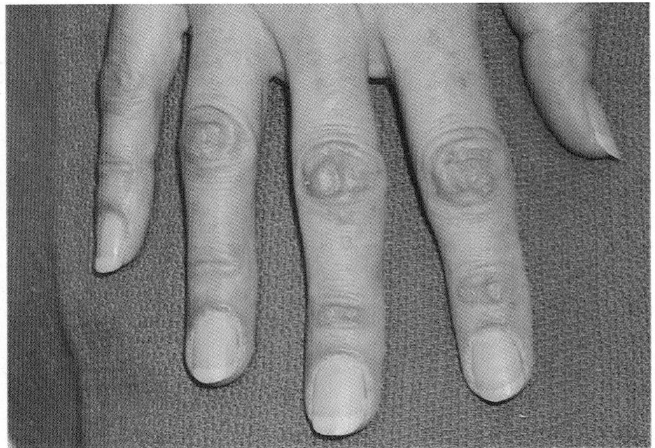

IIE-65 **Dermatomyositis** often involves the hands as erythematous flat-topped papules over the knuckles (Gottron's sign) and periungal telangiectasias.

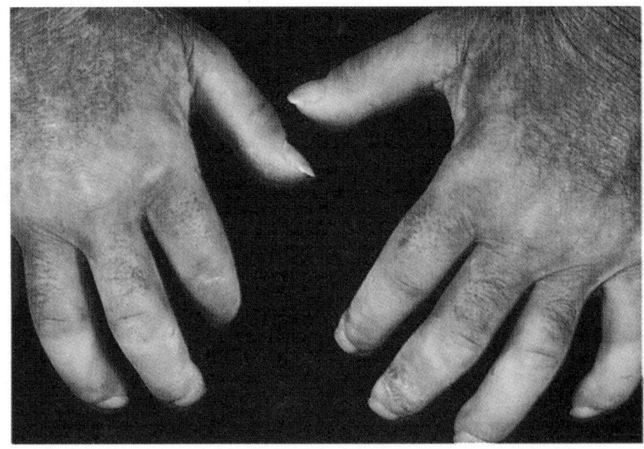

IIE-66 **Scleroderma** showing acral sclerosis and focal digital ulcers.

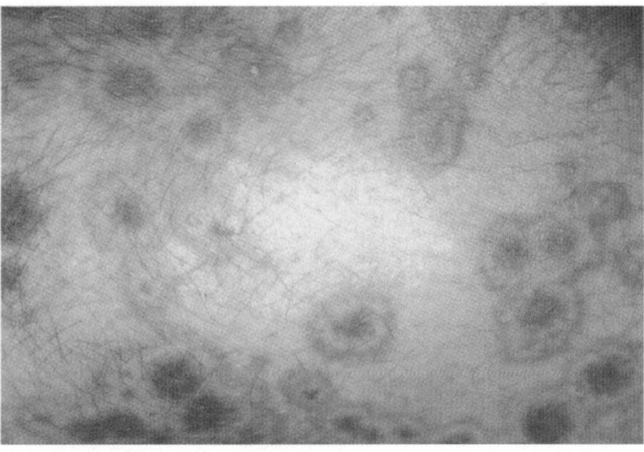

IIE-67 **Erythema multiforme** is characterized by multiple erythematous plaques with a target or iris morphology and usually represents a hypersensitivity reaction to drugs or infections (especially herpes simplex virus).

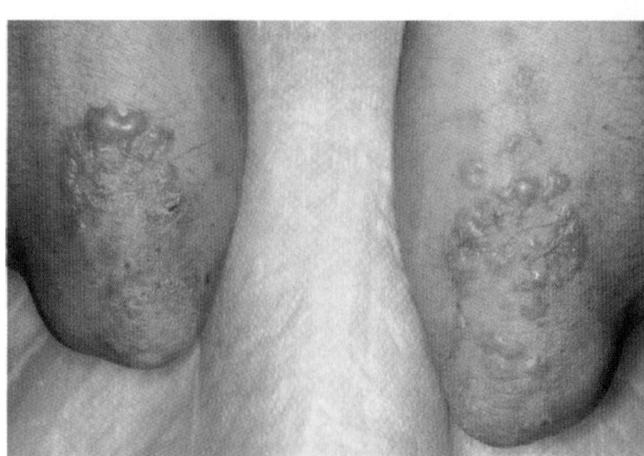

IIE-68 **Dermatitis herpetiformis** manifested by pruritic, grouped vesicles in a typical location. The vesicles are often excoriated and may occur on knees, buttocks, and posterior scalp.

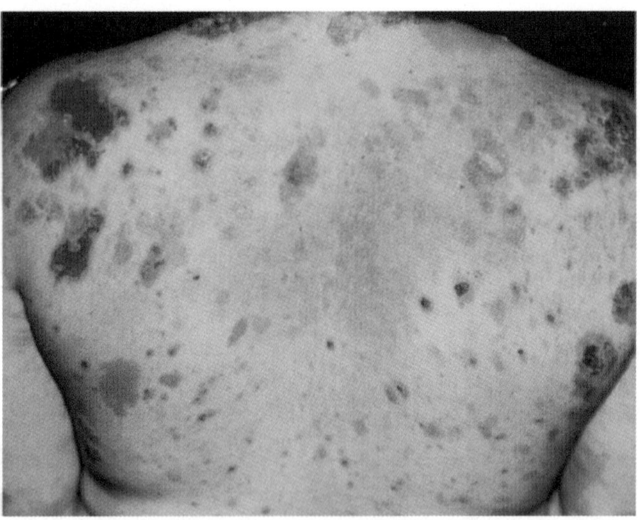

IIE-69A **Pemphigus vulgaris** demonstrating flaccid bullae that are easily ruptured, resulting in multiple erosions and crusted plaques.

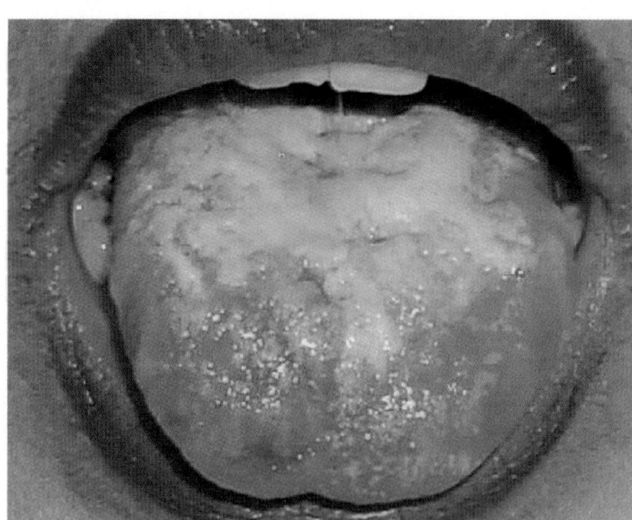

IIE-69B **Pemphigus vulgaris** almost invariably involves the oral mucosa and may present with erosions involving the gingiva, buccal mucosa, palate, posterior pharynx, or the tongue.

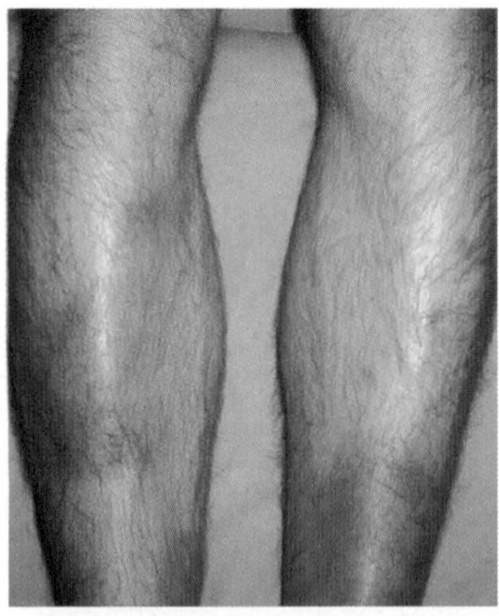

IIE-70 **Erythema nodosum** is a panniculitis characterized by tender deep-seated nodules and plaques usually located on the lower extremities.

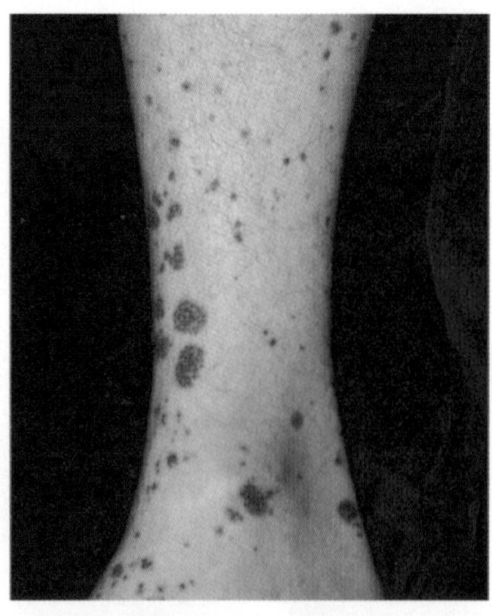

IIE-71 **Vasculitis** Palpable purpuric papules on the lower legs are seen in this patient with cutaneous small vessel vasculitis.

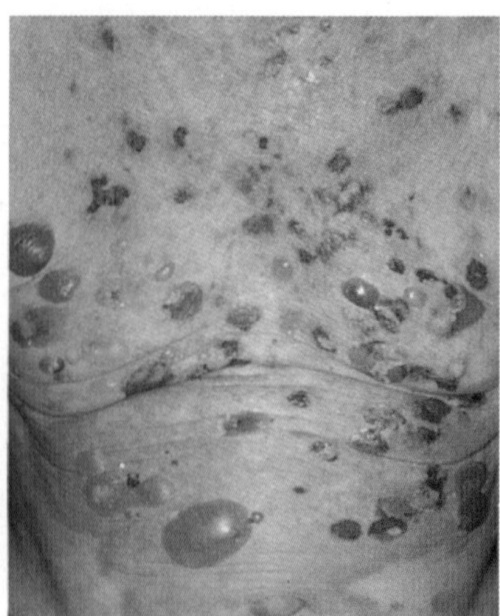

IIE-72 **Bullous pemphigoid** with tense vesicles and bullae on an erythematous, urticarial base.

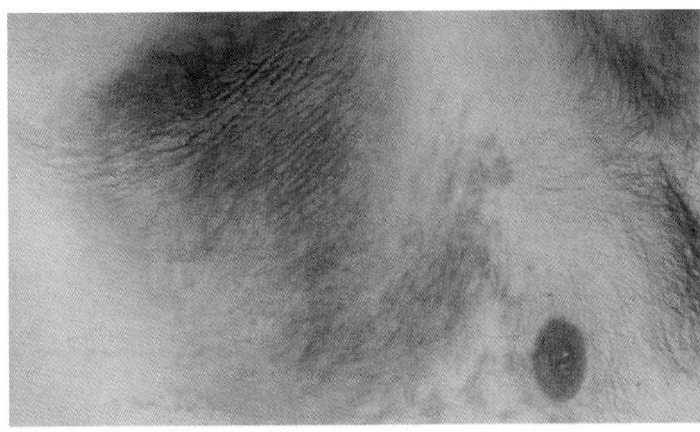

IIF-73 **Acanthosis nigricans** demonstrating typical hyperpigmented axillary plaques with a velvet-like, verrucous surface.

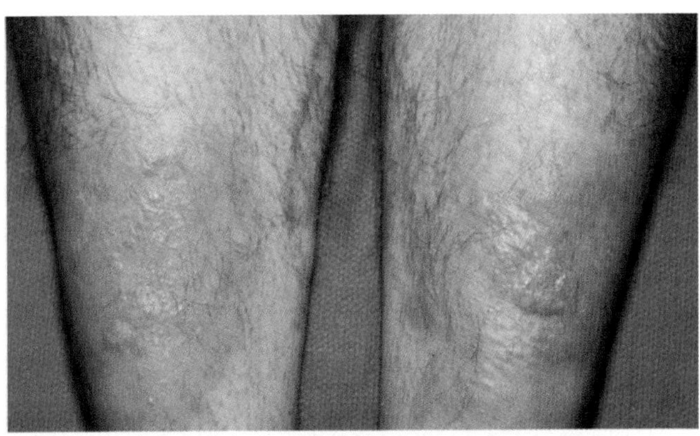

IIF-74 **Pretibial myxedema** manifesting as waxy, infiltrated plaques in a patient with Graves' disease.

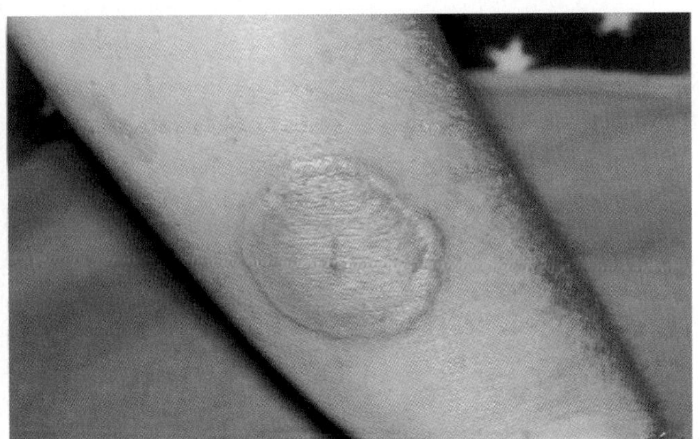

IIF-75 **Plaque of Sweet's syndrome** demonstrating an erythematous indurated plaque with a pseudo-vesicular border.

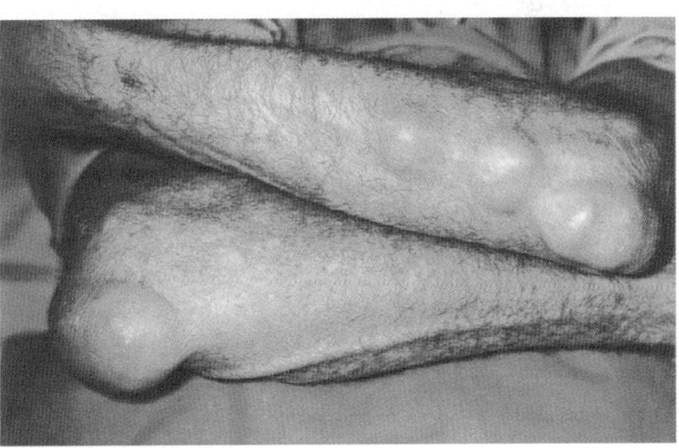

IIF-76 **Bilateral rheumatoid nodules** of the upper extremities.

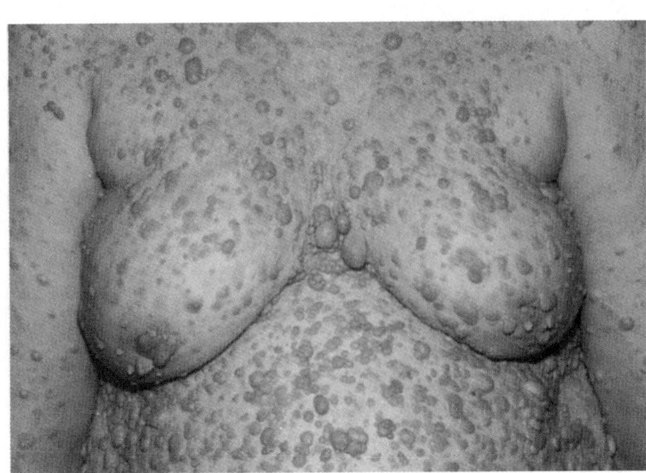

IIF-77 **Neurofibromatosis** demonstrating numerous flesh-colored cutaneous neurofibromas.

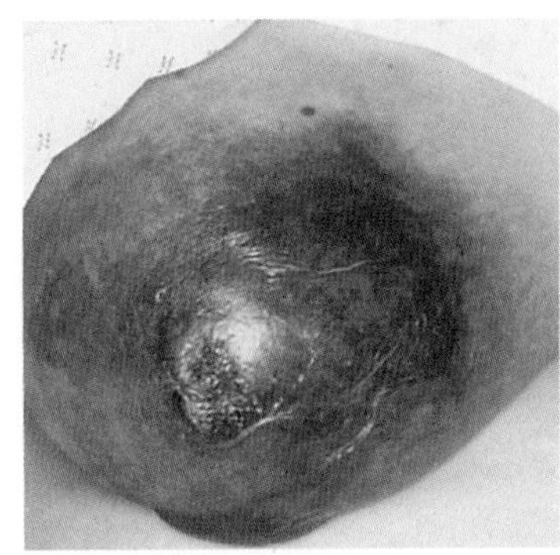

IIF-78 **Coumarin** necrosis showing cutaneous and subcutaneous necrosis of a breast. Other fatty areas such as buttocks and thighs are also common sites of involvement.

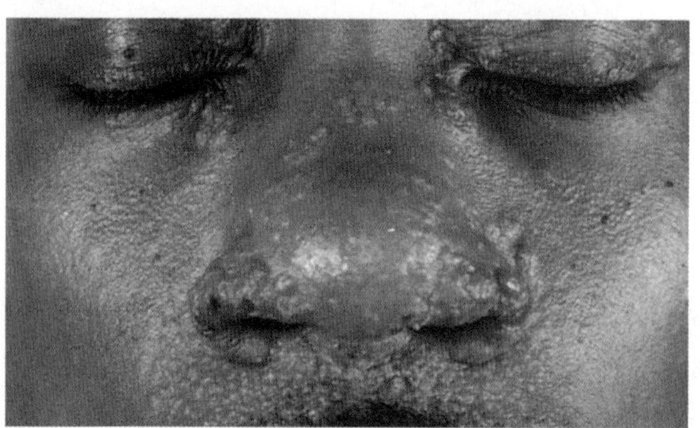

IIF-79A **Sarcoid** Infiltrated papules and plaques of variable color are seen in a typical paranasal and periorbital location.

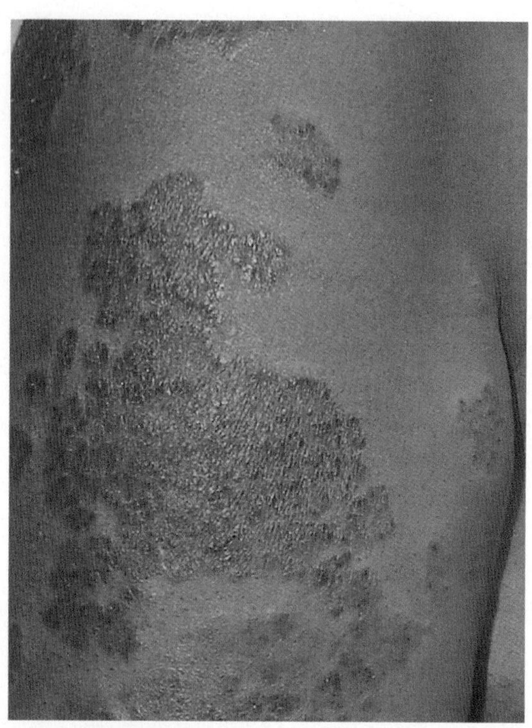

IIF-79B **Sarcoid** Infiltrated, hyperpigmented, and slightly erythematous coalescent papules and plaques on the upper arm.

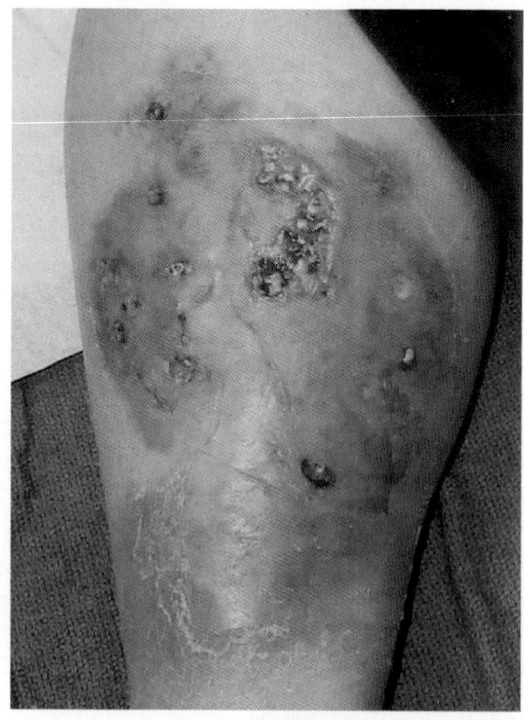

IIF-80 **Pyoderma gangrenosum** on the posterior-lateral aspect of the lower leg demonstrating multiple purulent draining ulcers on an infiltrated erythematous plaque.

III. Atlas of Endoscopic Findings

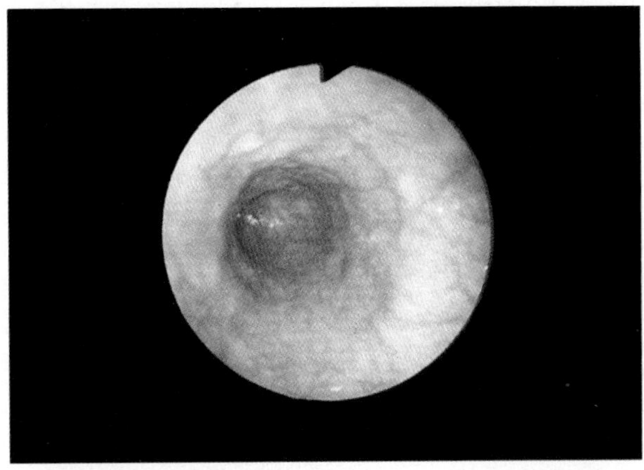

III-1 **Normal esophagus** Fine vasculature can be seen.

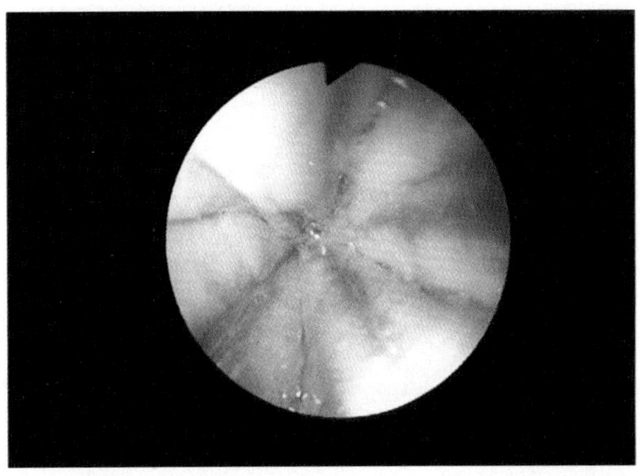

III-2 **Peptic regurgitant esophagitis** Linear red streaks with a central white streak extend up the esophagus.

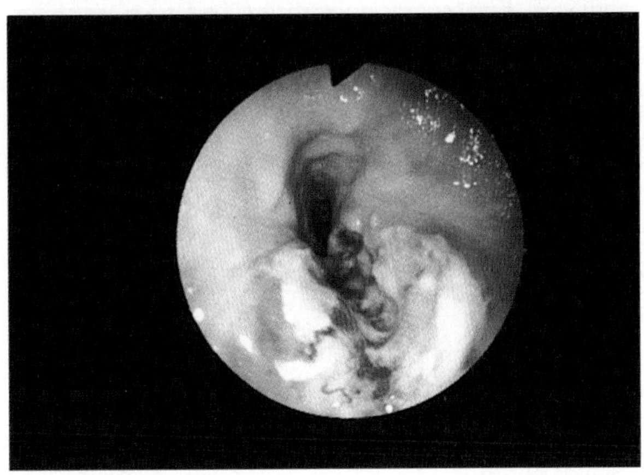

III-3 **Ulcerated squamous cell carcinoma,** with a depressed center, involving one wall of the esophagus.

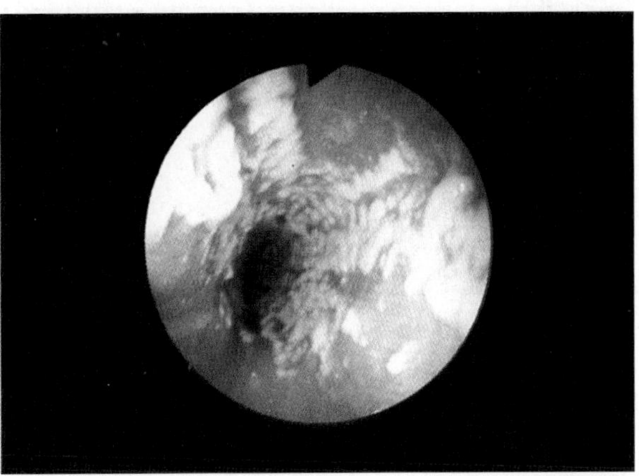

III-4 **Moniliasis of the esophagus** A white exudate is seen with underlying erythematous mucosa.

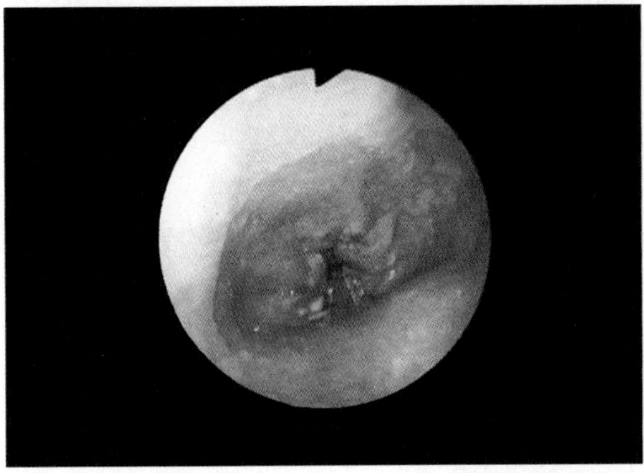

III-5 **Barrett's metaplasia of the esophagus with an adenocarcinoma** The squamocolumnar junction is noted in the proximal esophagus. A mucosal irregularity in the center of the photograph was an adenocarcinoma.

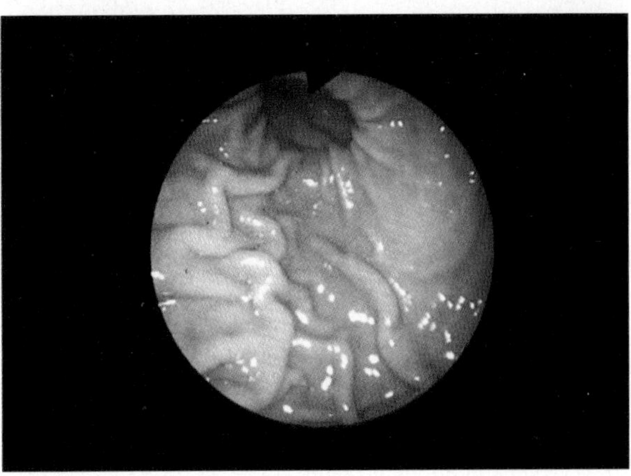

III-6 **Normal body of the stomach with rugal folds**

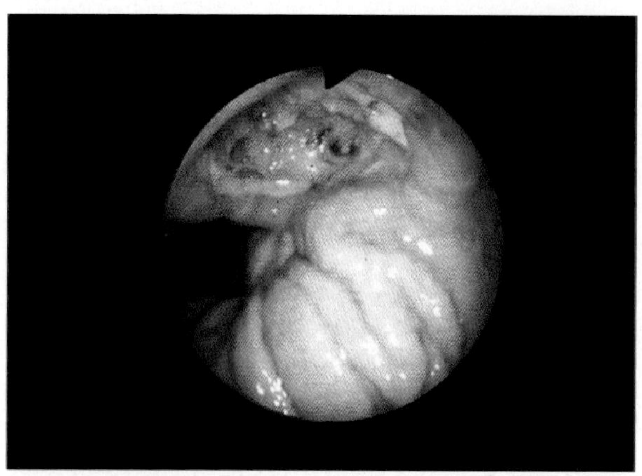

III-7 **Large, benign, lesser curve gastric ulcer** The folds end at the ulcer margin.

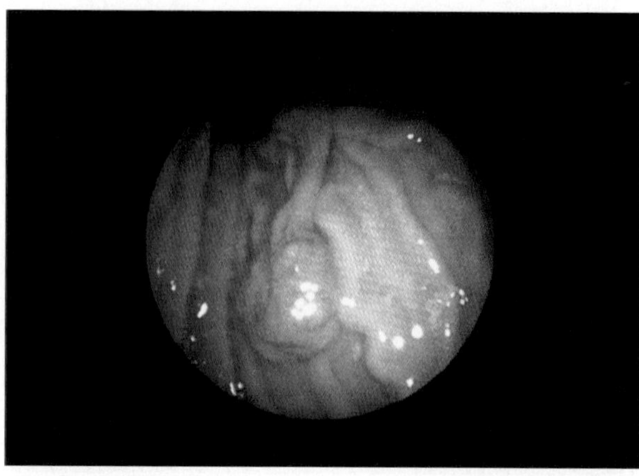

III-8 **Gastric polyp** The histologic type must be determined by excision and pathologic examination.

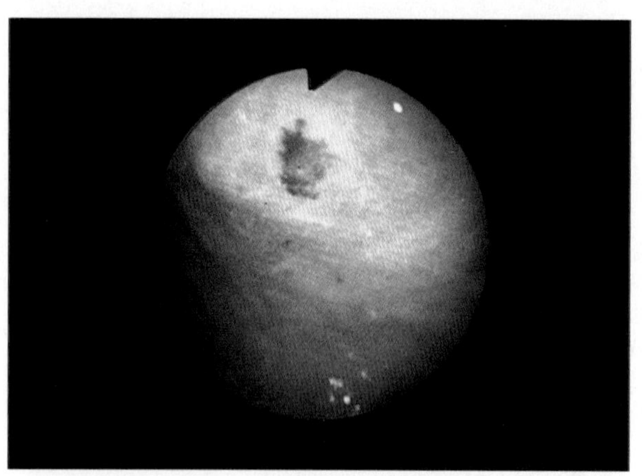

III-9 **Arteriovenus malformation of the gastric mucosa**

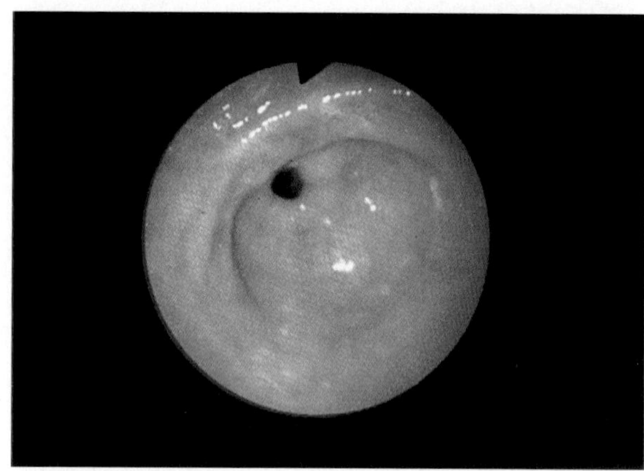

III-10 **Normal pylorus** Note the absence of gastric rugal folds in the antrum proximal to the pylorus.

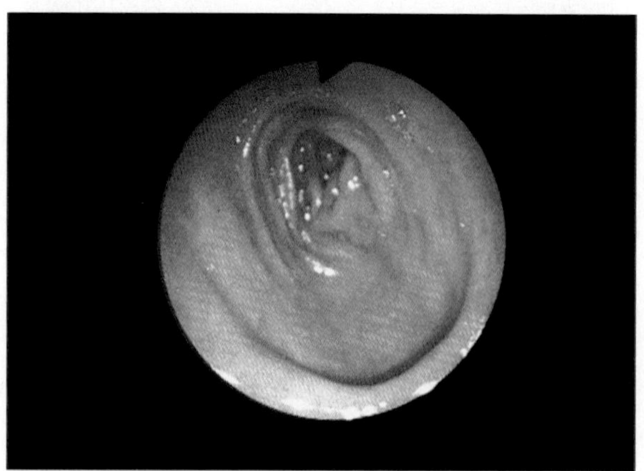

III-11 **Normal duodenal bulb**

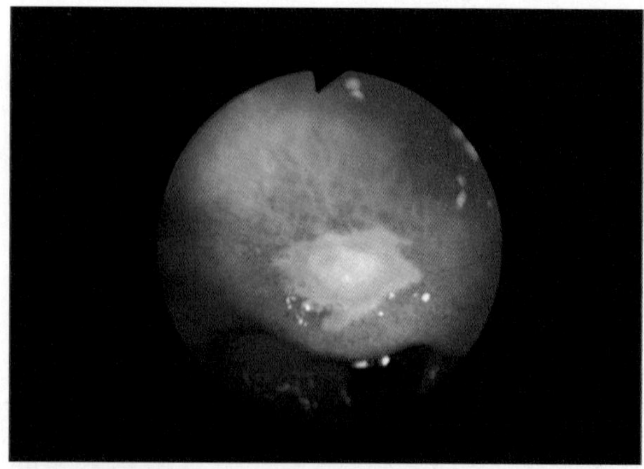

III-12 **Duodenal ulcer** A typical ulcer with a clean base is seen on the anterior surface of the duodenal bulb.

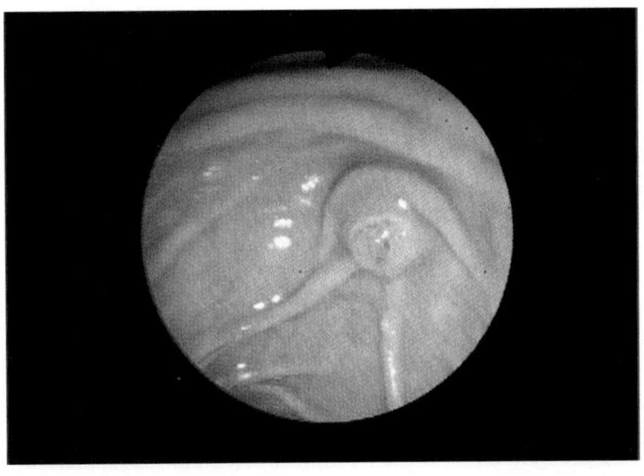

III-13 **Normal papilla of Vater** The fold pattern surrounding the papilla is normal; bile is seen adjacent to the papilla.

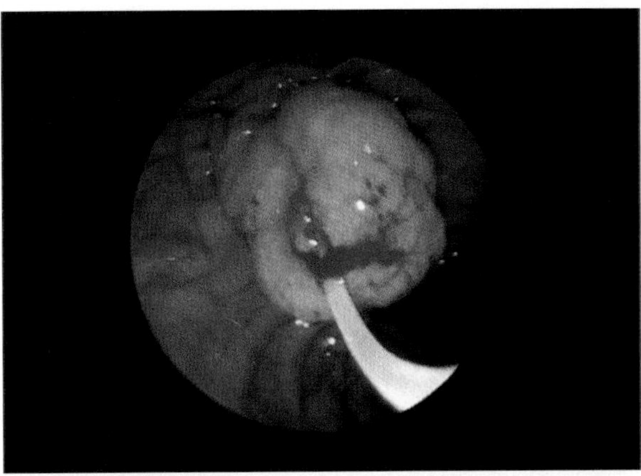

III-14 **Periampullary carcinoma** The mass at the papilla of Vater has been catheterized during ERCP.

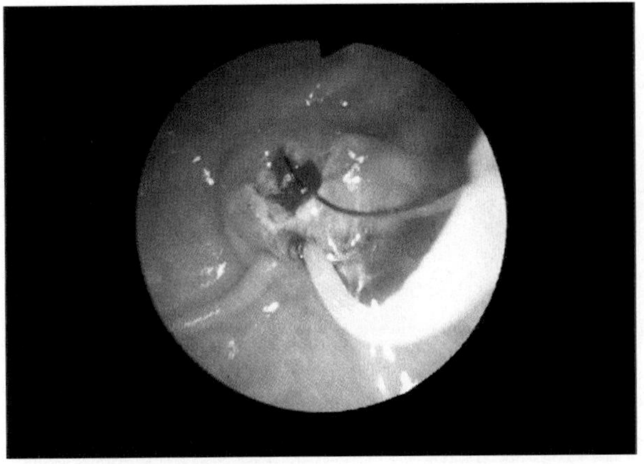

III-15 **Endoscopic papillotomy** A papillotome has been passed into the papilla, the wire bowed, and an incision made, with electrosurgical current, in the superior aspect of the papilla.

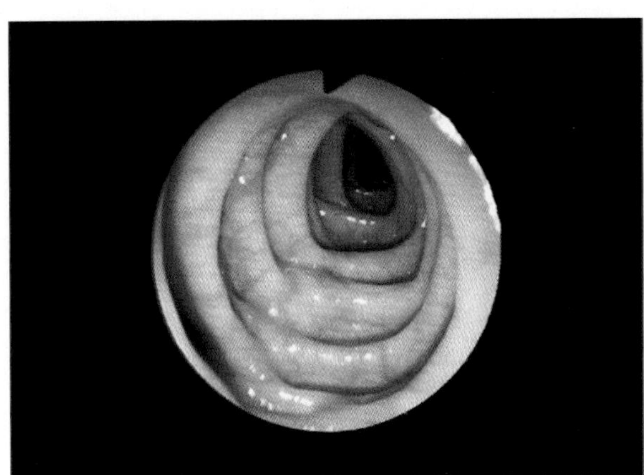

III-16 **Normal colon** Typical folds and vascular pattern can be seen.

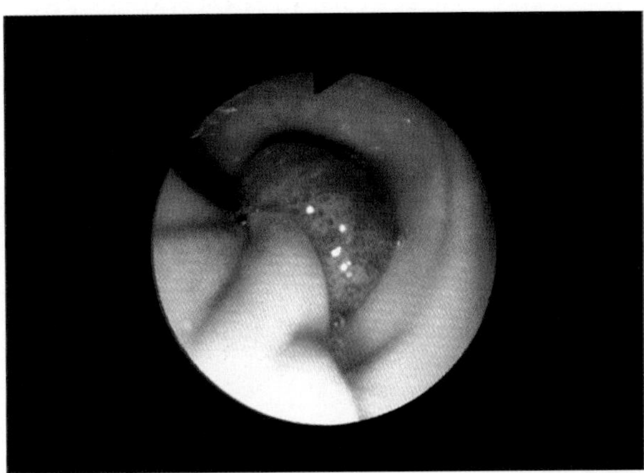

III-17 **Colonic adenomatous polyp** The polyp is erythematous; a stalk is seen covered with normal mucosa.

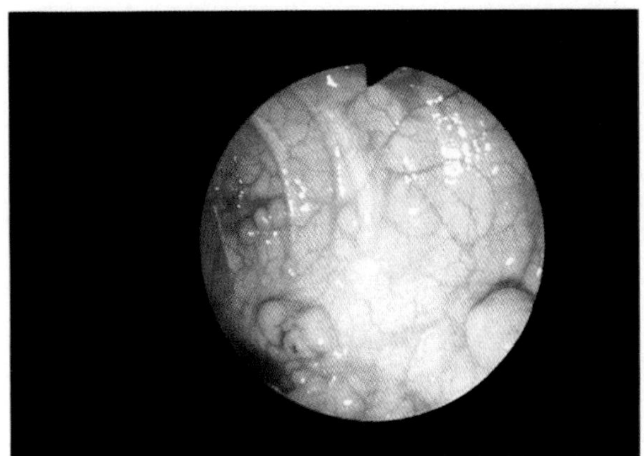

III-18 **Multiple, small, colonic adenomatous polyps in a case of familial polyposis coli** This colon must be removed to prevent the development of cancer.

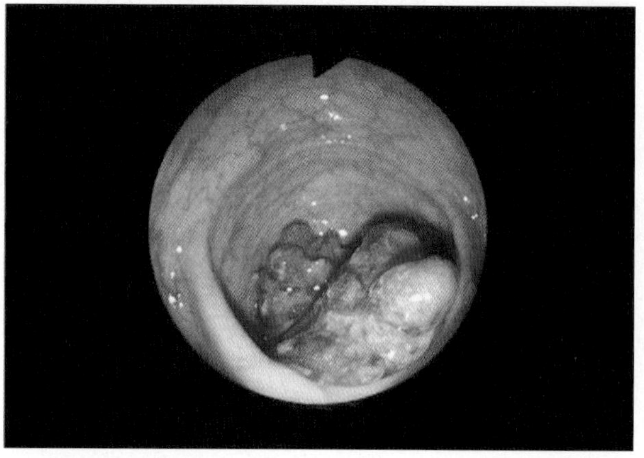

III-19 **Colon adenocarcinoma** The cancer is multilobed and growing into the lumen.

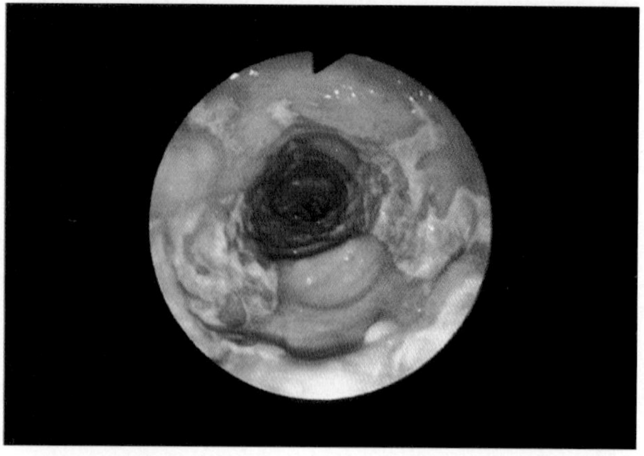

III-20 **Crohn's colitis** with linear, serpiginous, white-based ulcers surrounded by colonic mucosa which is relatively normal.

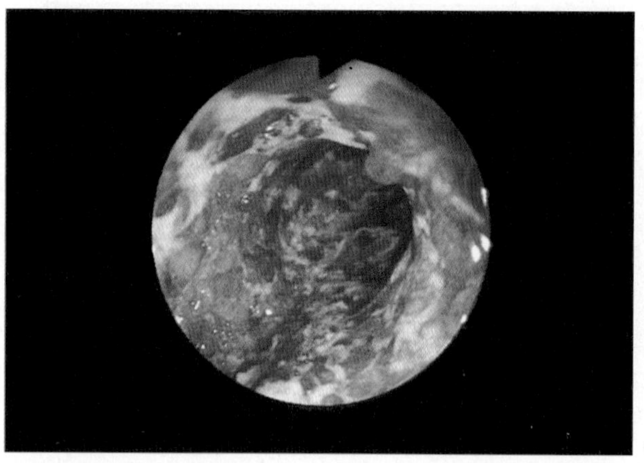

III-21 **Severe ulcerative colitis** with diffuse ulceration, bleeding, and exudation.

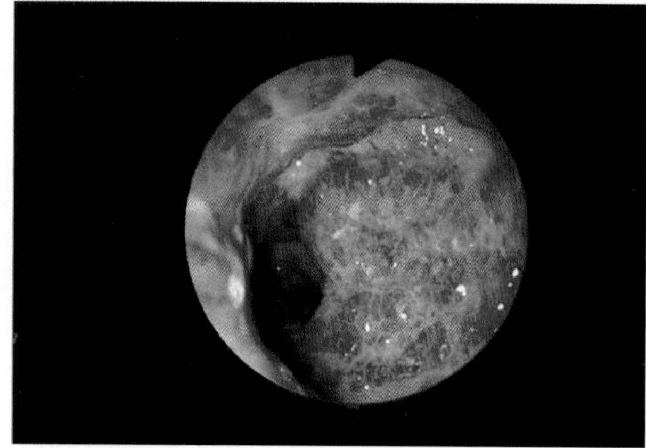

III-22 **Kaposi's sarcoma involving the colon in a patient with AIDS** The erythematous lesions involve most of the colonic mucosa in the photograph.

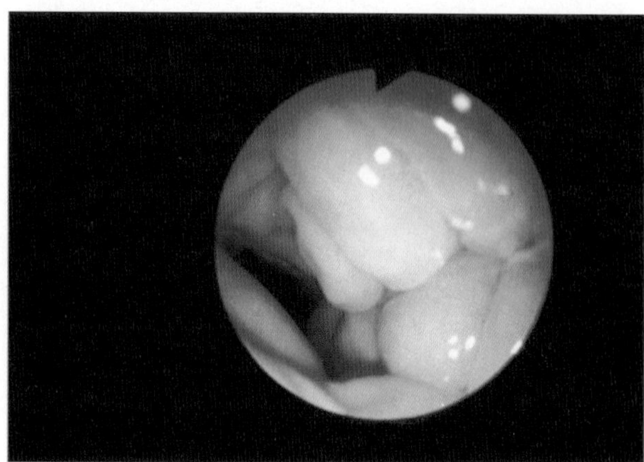

III-23 **Colonic varices** Multiple, serpiginous, subephithelial structures impinge on the colonic lumen.

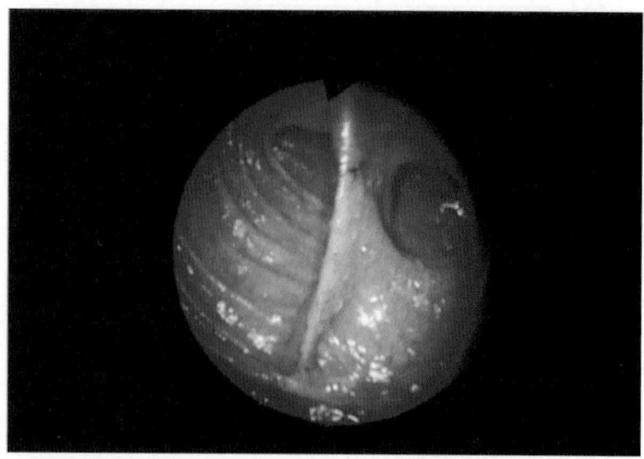

III-24 **Ileal pouch** The mucosa appears normal in this pouch reconstructed from ileum to provide a reservoir after total proctocolectomy and ileoanal anastomosis.

IV. Atlas of Funduscopic Findings

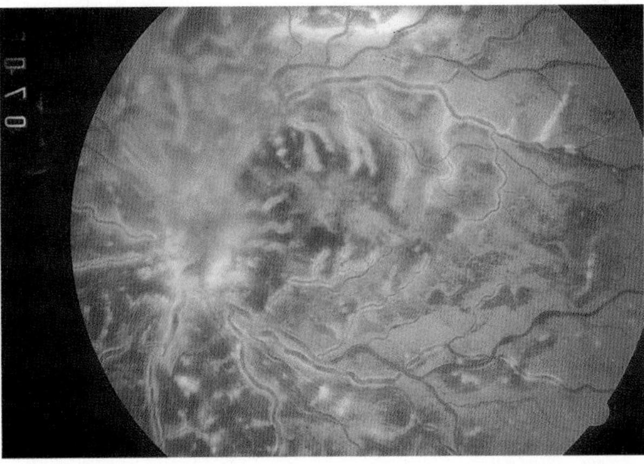

IV-1 **Retinal vasculitis, uveitis, and hemorrhage** in a 32-year-old woman with Crohn's disease. Note that the veins are frosted with a white exudate. Visual acuity improved from 20/400 to 20/20 following treatment with intravenous methylprednisolone.

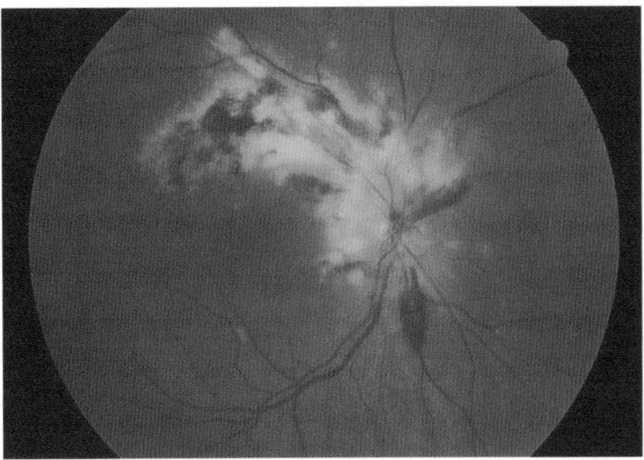

IV-2 **Cytomegalovirus** in a patient with AIDS appears as an arcuate zone of retinitis with hemorrhages and optic disc swelling. Often CMV is confined to the retinal periphery, beyond view of the direct ophthalmoscope.

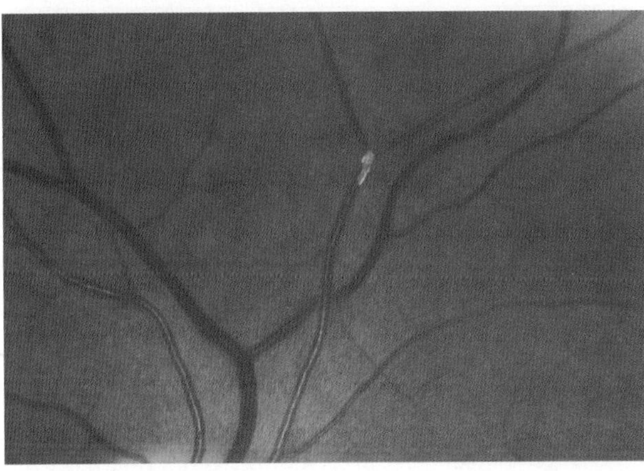

IV-3 **Hollenhorst plaque** lodged at the bifurcation of a retinal arteriole proves that a patient is shedding emboli from either the carotid artery, great vessels, or heart.

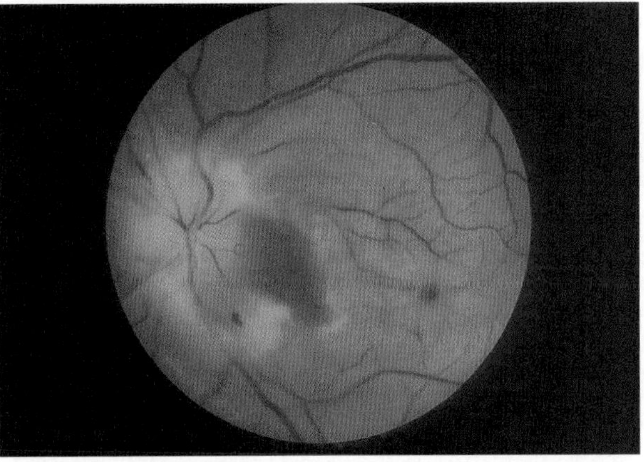

IV-4 **Central retinal artery occlusion** combined with ischemic optic neuropathy in a 19-year-old woman with an elevated titer of anticardiolipin antibodies. Note the orange dot (rather than cherry red) corresponding to the fovea and the spared patch of retina just temporal to the optic disc.

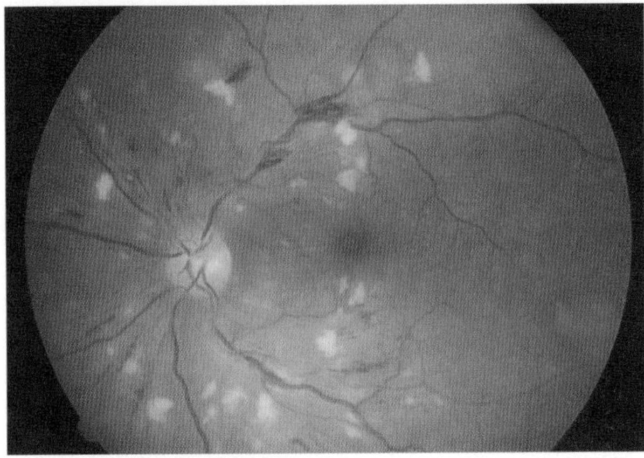

IV-5 **Hypertensive retinopathy** with scattered flame (splinter) hemorrhages and cotton wool spots (nerve fiber layer infarcts) in a patient with headache and a blood pressure of 234/120.

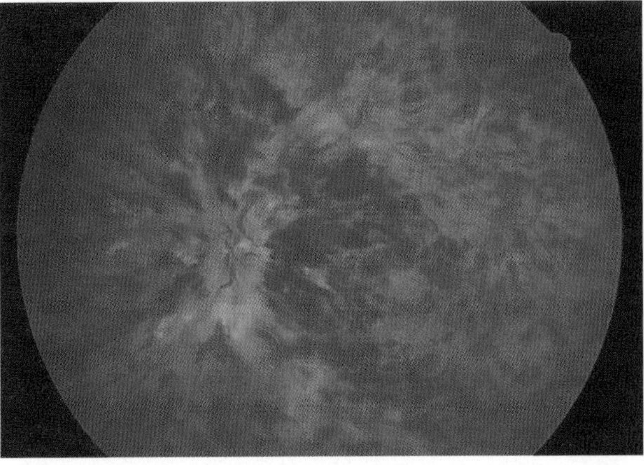

IV-6 **Central retinal vein occlusion** can produce massive retinal hemorrhage ("blood and thunder"), ischemia, and vision loss.

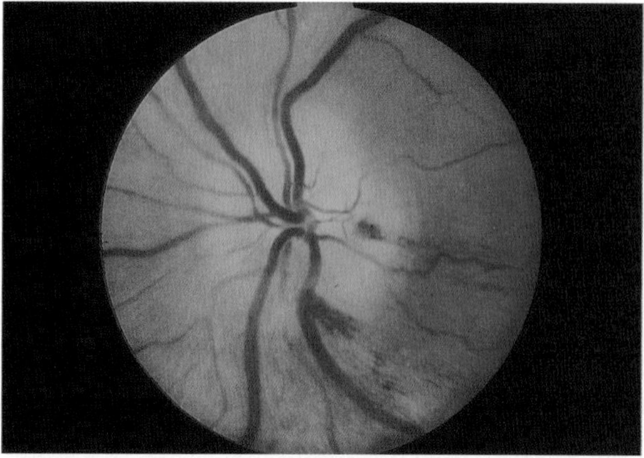

IV-7 **Anterior ischemic optic neuropathy** from temporal arteritis in a 78-year old woman with pallid disc swelling, hemorrhage, visual loss, myalgia, and an erythrocyte sedimentation rate of 86 mm/h..

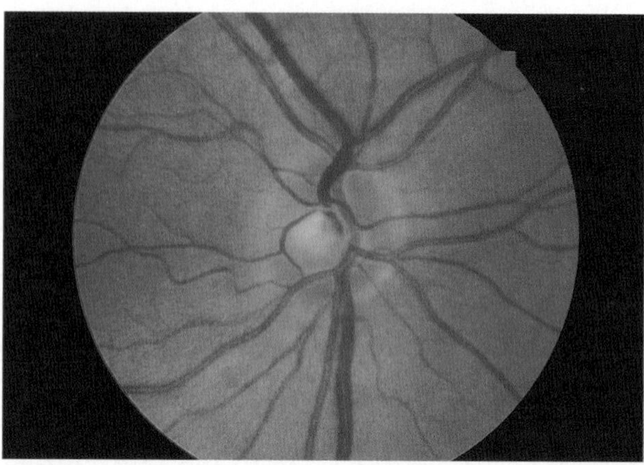

IV-8 **Retrobulbar optic neuritis** is characterized by a normal fundus examination initially, hence the rubric, "the doctor sees nothing, and the patient sees nothing." Optic atrophy develops after severe or repeated attacks.

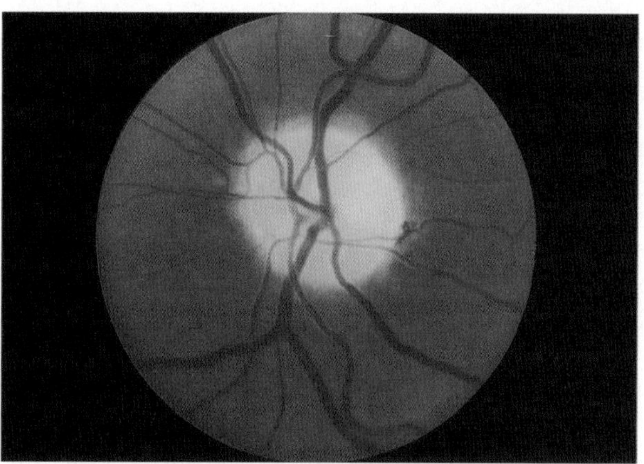

IV-9 **Optic atrophy** is not a specific diagnosis, but refers to the combination of optic disc pallor, arteriolar narrowing, and nerve fiber layer destruction produced by a host of eye diseases, especially optic neuropathies.

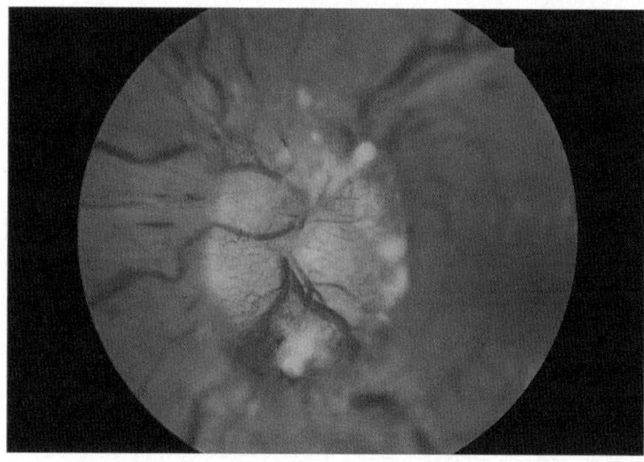

IV-10 **Papilledema** means optic disc edema from raised intracranial pressure. This obese young woman with pseudotumor cerebri was misdiagnosed as a migraineur until fundus examination was performed, showing optic disc elevation, hemorrhages, and cotton wool spots.

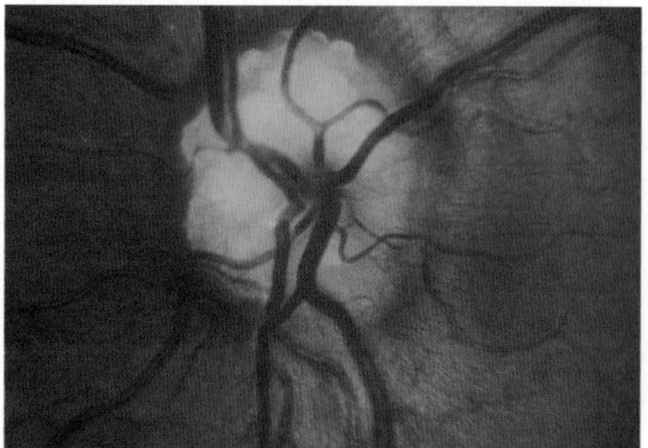

IV-11 **Optic disc drusen** are calcified deposits of unknown etiology within the optic disc. They are sometimes confused with papilledema.

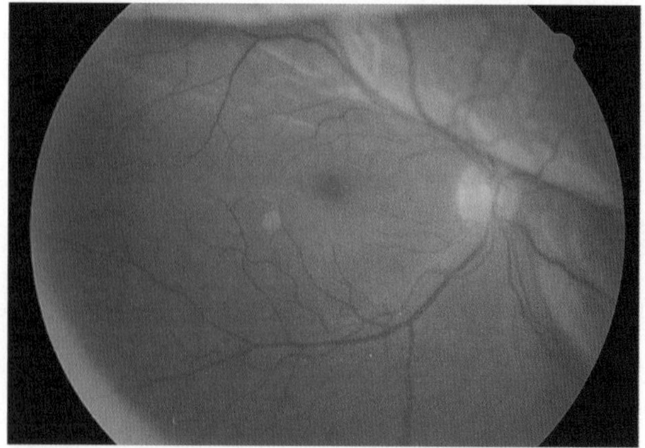

IV-12 **Retinal detachment** appears as an elevated sheet of retinal tissue with folds. In this patient the fovea was spared, so acuity was normal, but a superior detachment produced an inferior scotoma.

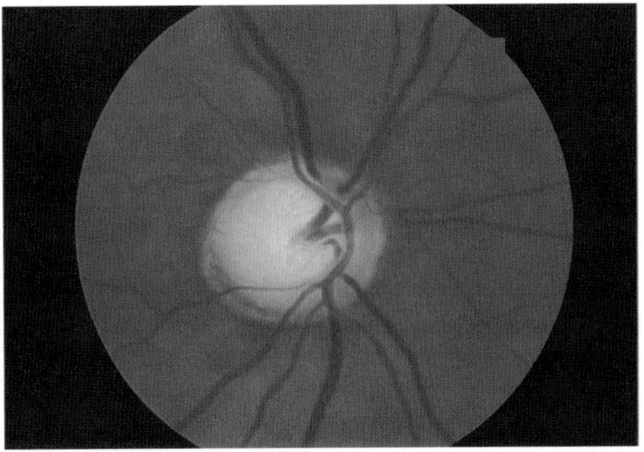

IV-13 **Glaucoma** results in "cupping" as the neural rim is destroyed and the central cup becomes enlarged and excavated. The cup-to-disc ratio is about 0.7/1.0 in this patient.

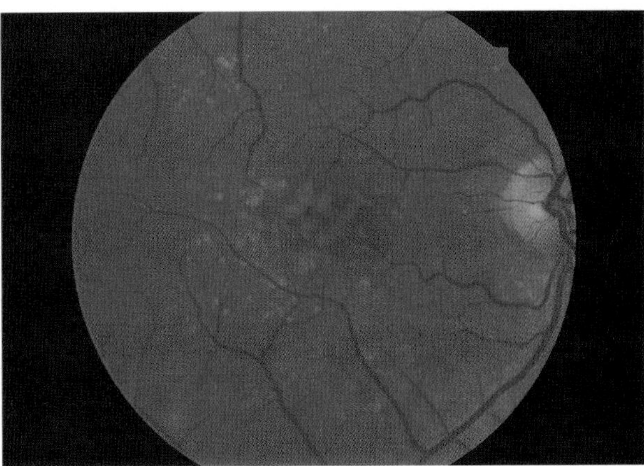

IV-14 **Age-related macular degeneration** begins with the accumulation of drusen within the macula. They appear as scattered yellow subretinal deposits.

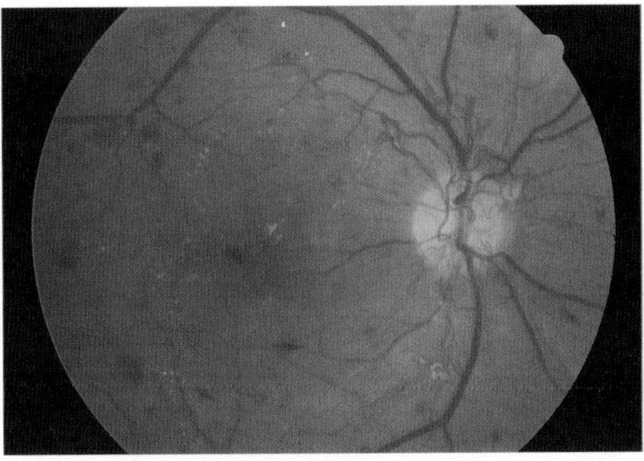

IV-15 **Diabetic retinopathy** results in scattered hemorrhages and yellow exudates. This patient has neovascular vessels proliferating from the optic disc, requiring urgent pan retinal laser photocoagulation.

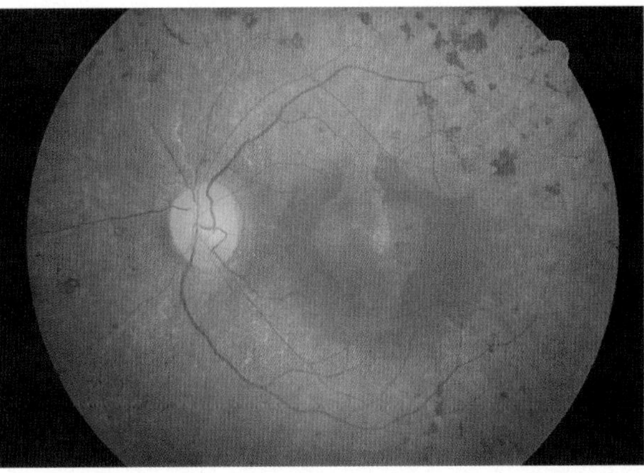

IV-16 **Retinitis pigmentosa** with black clumps of pigment in the retinal periphery known as "bone spicules." There is also atrophy of the retinal pigment epithelium, making the vasculature of the choroid easily visible.

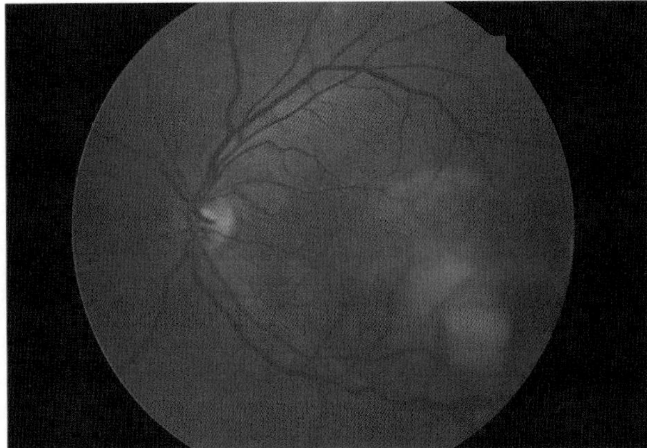

IV-17 **Melanoma of the choroid,** appearing as an elevated dark mass in the inferior temporal fundus, just encroaching upon the fovea.

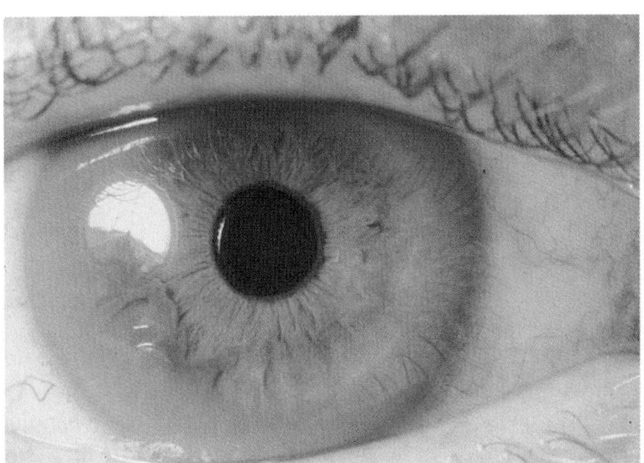

IV-18 **Kayser-Fleischer ring** develops in Wilson's disease from copper deposition in Descemet's membrane, producing brownish discoloration of the peripheral cornea. It should not be confused with the yellow-white lipid ring of arcus senilis, which is common in the elderly and occasionally signifies hyperlipidemia, especially when it appears at a young age.

V. Atlas of Hematology

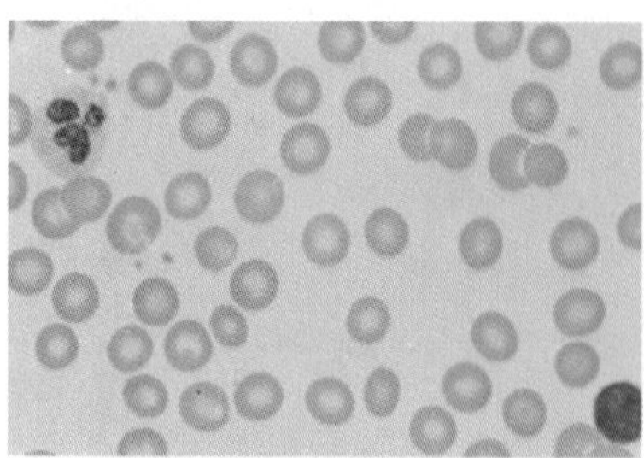

V-1 **Normal blood smear** Normal red blood cells are round, possess an area of central pallor, appear slightly smaller than the nucleus of a mature lymphocyte, and vary little in size (anisocytosis) or in shape (poikilocytosis).

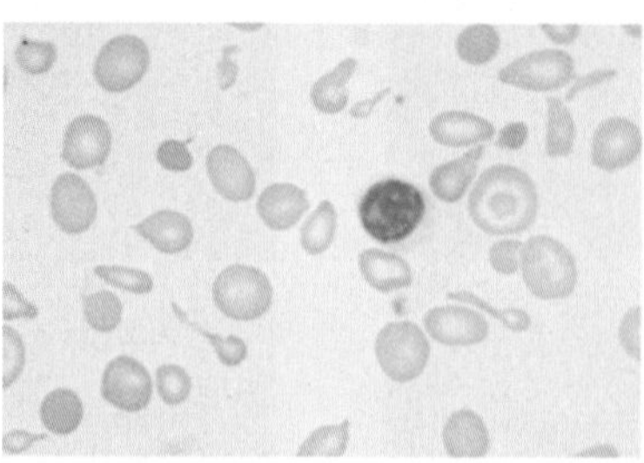

V-2 **β-Thalassemia intermedia** Microcytic and hypochromic red blood cells are seen that resemble the red blood cells of severe iron deficiency anemia shown in Fig. IV-4. Many elliptical and teardrop-shaped red blood cells are noted.

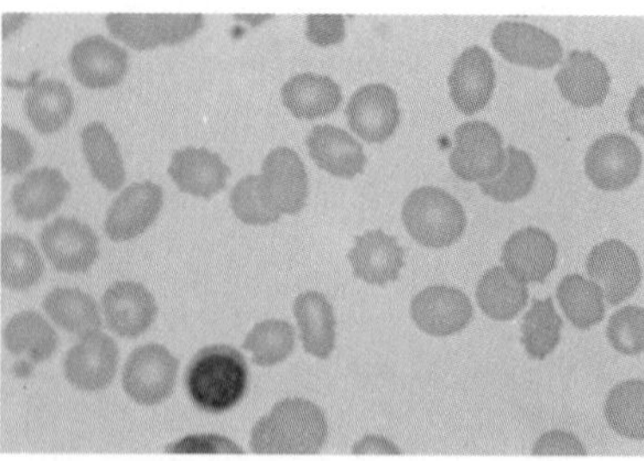

V-3 **Uremia** The red blood cells in uremia may acquire numerous, regularly spaced, small spiny projections. Such cells, called burr cells or echinocytes, are readily distinguishable from irregularly spiculated acanthocytes shown in Fig. V-27.

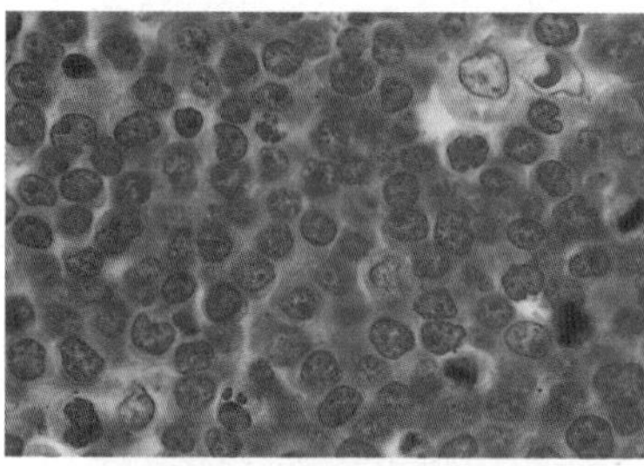

V-4 **Burkitt's lymphoma** The neoplastic cells are homogenous, medium-sized B cells with frequent mitotic figures, a morphologic correlate of high growth fraction. Reactive macrophages are scattered through the tumor and their pale cytoplasm in a background of blue-staining tumor cells gives the tumor a so-called "starry sky" appearance.

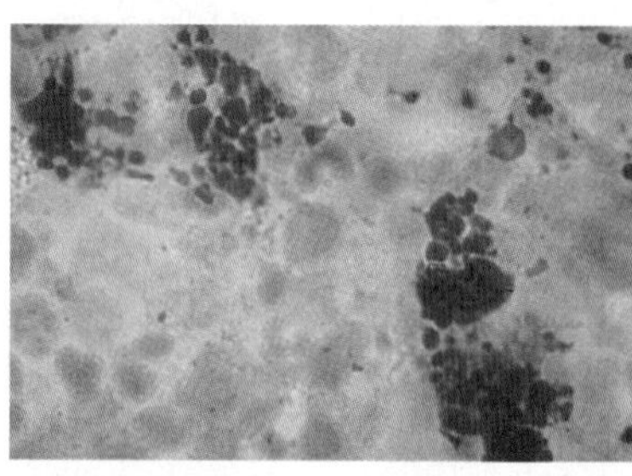

V-5 **Marrow iron stores** This marrow section is stained with Prussian blue. Iron takes up the stain and is concentrated in reticuloendothelial cells. This picture shows normal iron stores. In iron deficiency states, no stainable iron is detectable. In the anemia of chronic disease, iron is present but cytokines prevent its mobilization and utilization in heme synthesis.

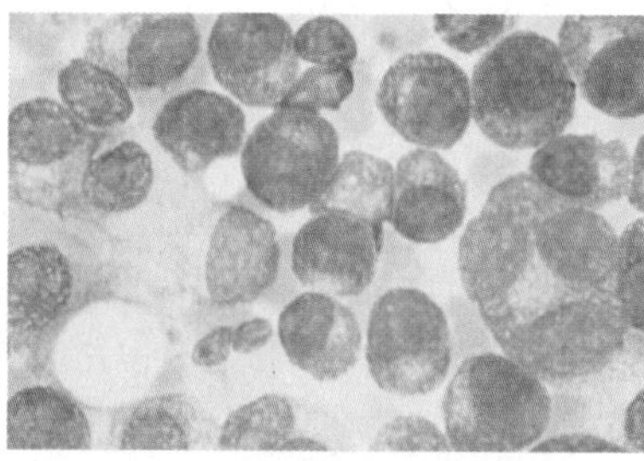

V-6 **Multiple myeloma (marrow)** The cells bear characteristic morphologic features of plasma cells, round or oval cells with an eccentric nucleus composed of coarsely clumped chromatin, a densely basophilic cytoplasm, and a perinuclear clear zone (hof) containing the Golgi apparatus. Binucleate and multinucleate malignant plasma cells also can be seen.

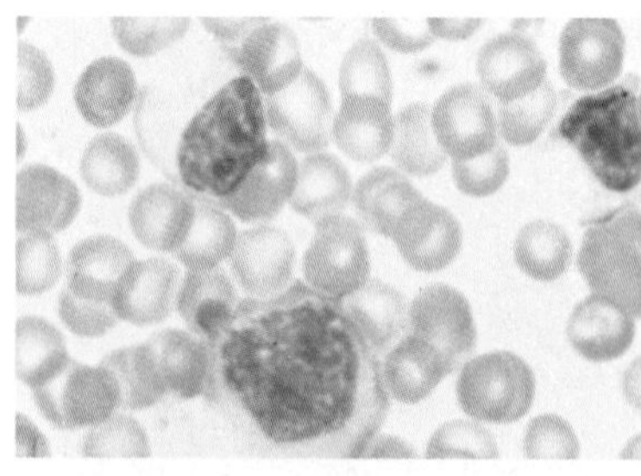

V-7 **Reactive lymphocytes (infectious mononucleosis)** Reactive lymphocytes are usually large and contain abundant cytoplasm. The nucleus may be eccentrically placed and may have irregular borders and indentations (not seen on this plate). The cytoplasm contains areas that stain a darker blue due to their increased content of RNA. The cytoplasm may be indented where it abuts against a red blood cell.

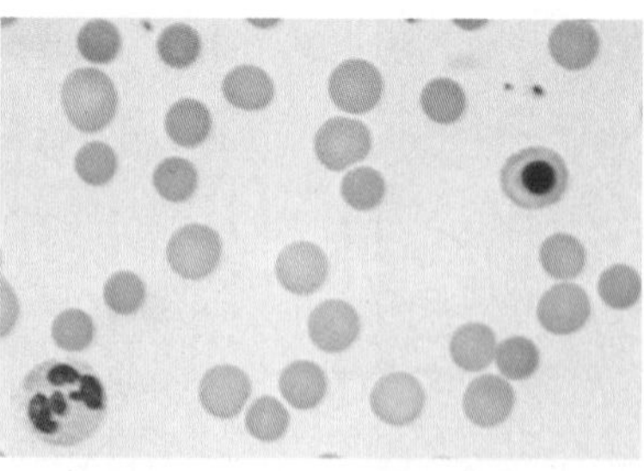

V-8 **Immunohemolytic anemia** Microspherocytes are seen on this blood smear along with several macrocytes with a slight purple tinge (polychromasia). The latter represent new red blood cells released early from the bone marrow. The microspherocytes seen in immunohemolytic anemia may be indistinguishable from the microspherocytes seen in hereditary spherocytosis (Fig. V-26).

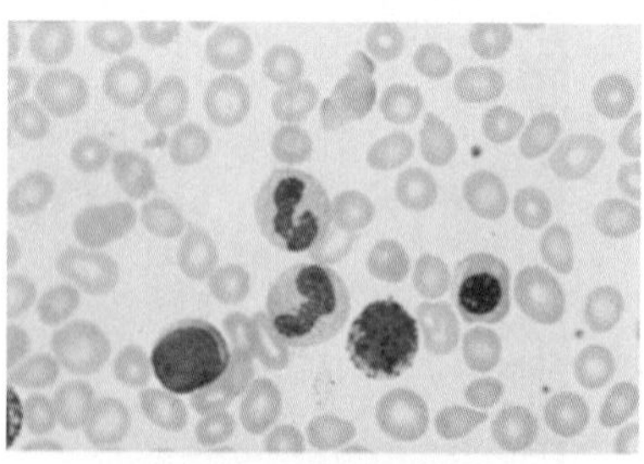

V-9 **Leukoerythroblastic smear** Teardrop-shaped red blood cells indicative of membrane damage from collagen fibers, a nucleated red blood cell indicative of premature release of erythroid precursors, and immature myeloid cells indicative of extramedullary hematopoiesis are noted. This peripheral blood smear is related to marrow fibrosis, either primary myelofibrosis or secondary myelophthisis.

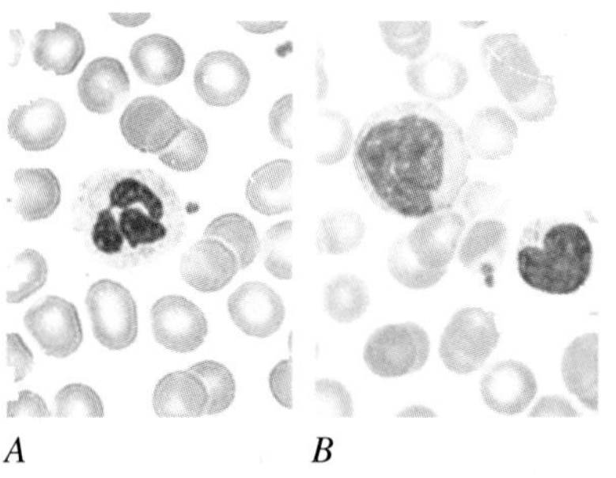

V-10 A. **Normal granulocyte** The normal granulocyte has a segmented nucleus with heavy, clumped chromatin; fine neutrophilic granules are dispersed throughout its cytoplasm. *B.* **Normal monocyte and lymphocyte** The normal monocyte is a large cell with an indented or folded nucleus containing loose, strand-like chromatin; the cytoplasm is a blue-gray color and usually contains fine azurophilic granules. The normal lymphocyte is a smaller cell. Its nucleus is usually round but may be indented, as in the cell shown in this plate. The nuclear chromatin has a smudgy appearance; the cytoplasm is blue.

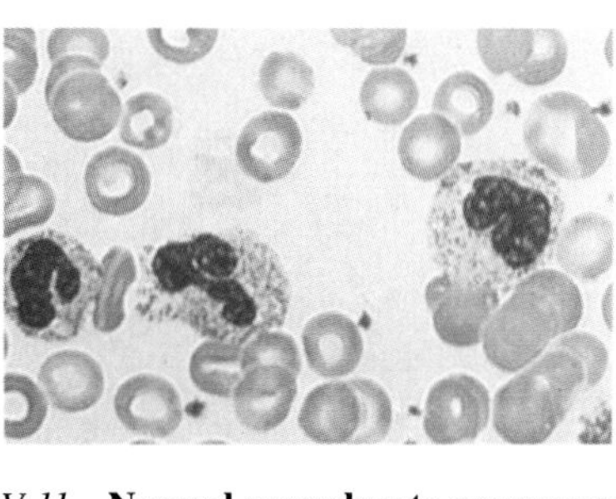

V-11 **Normal granulocyte precursors in marrow** The earliest granulocytic precursor (myeloblast) possesses a round nucleus with fine, punctate chromatin and one or more nucleoli; the cytoplasm is blue. As nuclear differentiation proceeds, the nucleoli disappear, the chromatin coarsens, and the nucleus becomes increasingly indented and finally segmented. As cytoplasmic differentiation proceeds, azurophilic granules appear and cytoplasm changes color from blue to the yellow-pink-gray hue of the mature granulocyte, and as this occurs the azurophilic granules become obscured by fine neutrophilic granules.

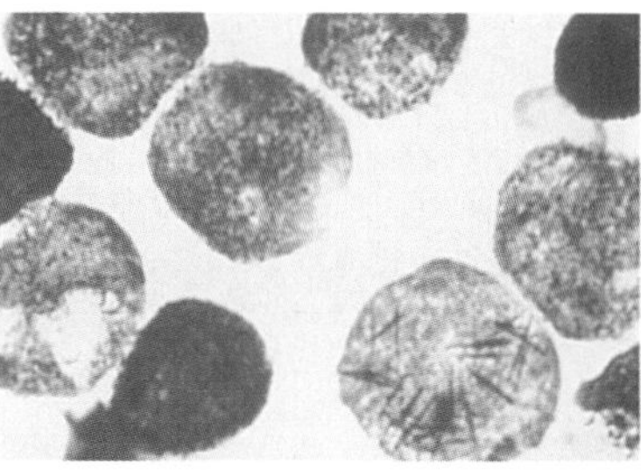

V-12 **Leukemic cell in acute promyelocytic leukemia** Note multiple Auer rods.

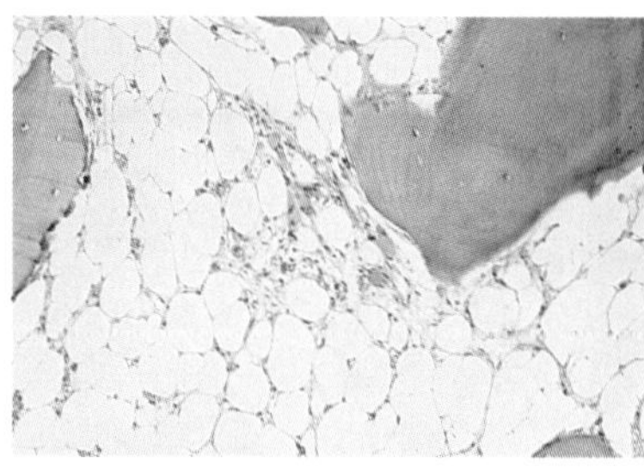

V-13 **Aplastic anemia** This marrow section shows only fat with nearly complete absence of hematopoietic tissue.

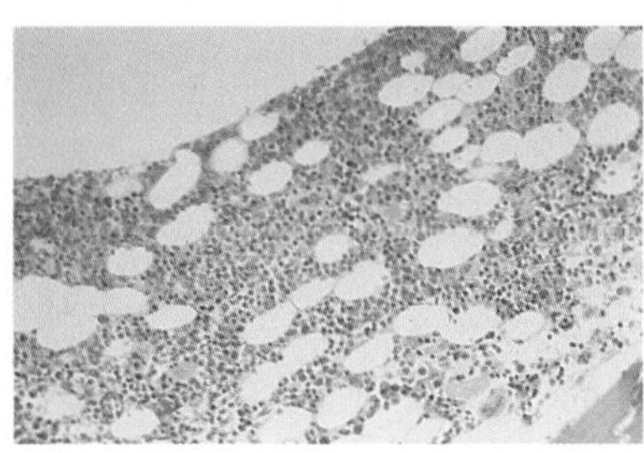

V-14 **Normal bone marrow biopsy** This a low power view of an H&E-stained section of normal marrow. Note that the nucleated cellular elements account for about 40 to 50 percent and the fat *(clear areas)* accounts for about 50 to 60 percent of the area.

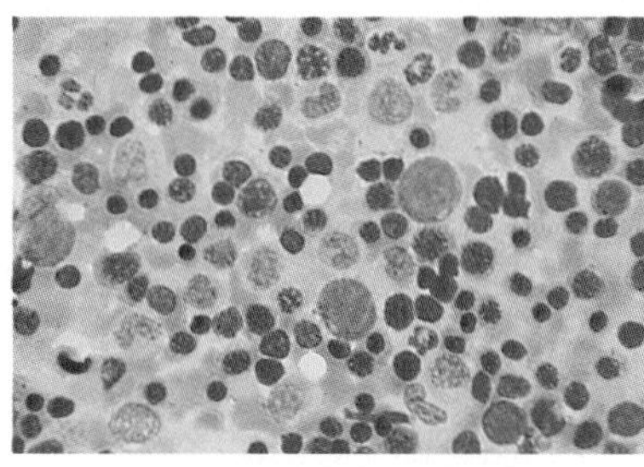

V-15 **Erythroid hyperplasia** This marrow section shows an increase in the fraction of cells in the erythroid lineage as might be seen in a healthy marrow compensating for acute blood loss or hemolysis. The E/G ratio is greater than 1/1.

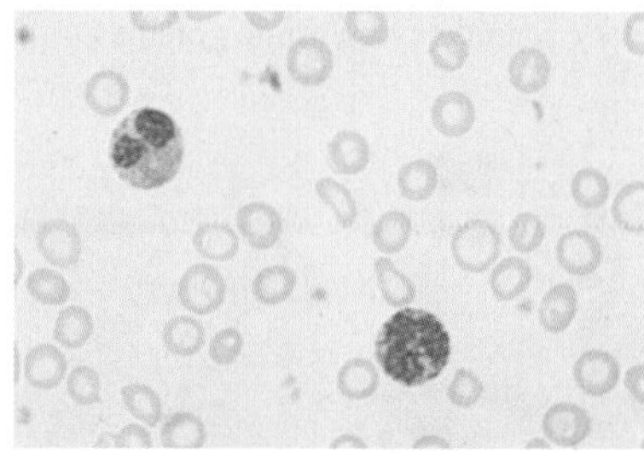

V-16 **Iron-deficiency anemia** In severe iron deficiency, the red blood cells are smaller than normal (microcytosis), and their central area of pallor is expanded (hypochromia) so that the cells appear to have only a thin rim of hemoglobin.

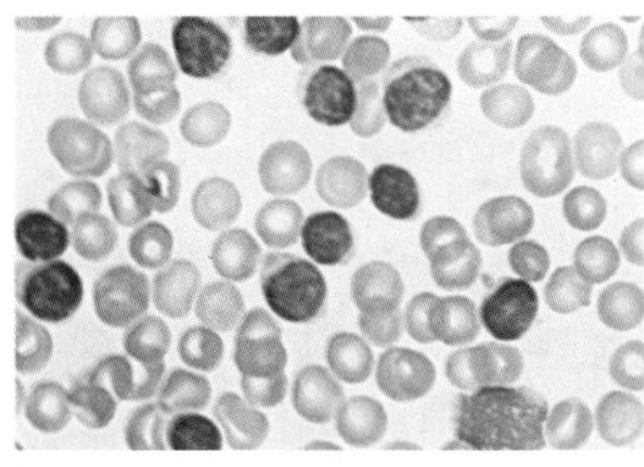

V-17 **Chronic lymphocytic leukemia** The peripheral WBC count is high due to increased numbers of small, well-differentiated lymphocytes. However, the leukemic lymphocytes are fragile, and substantial numbers of broken, smudged cells are usually also present on the blood smear.

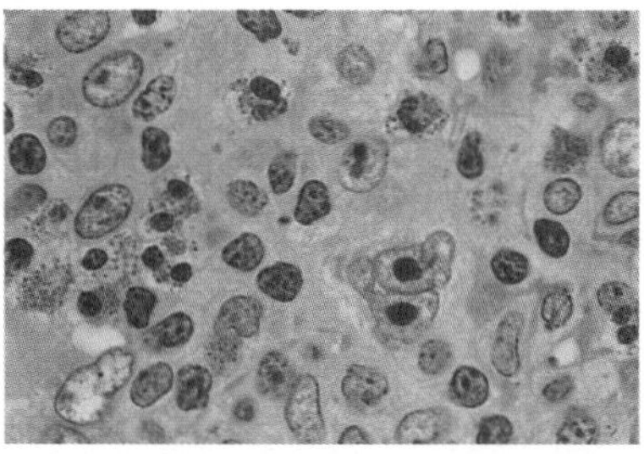

V-18 **Hodgkin's disease, mixed cellularity** A Reed-Sternberg cell is present near the center of the field; a large cell with a bilobed nucleus and prominent nucleoli. The majority of the cells are normal lymphocytes, neutrophils, and eosinophils that form a pleiomorphic cellular infiltrate.

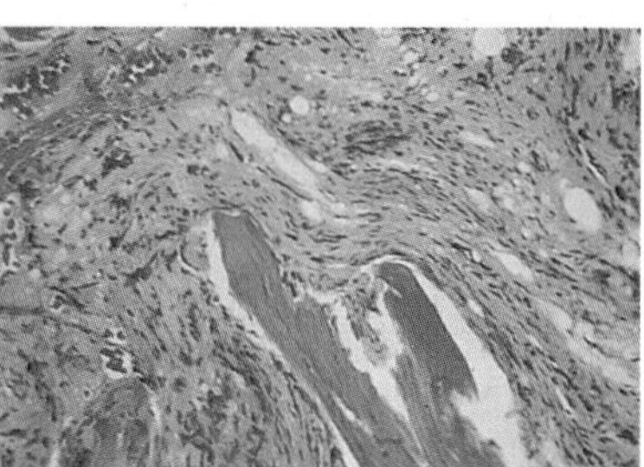

V-19 **Marrow fibrosis** This marrow section shows the marrow cavity replaced by fibrous tissue composed of reticulin fibers and collagen. When this fibrosis is due to a primary hematologic process, it is called *myelofibrosis*. When the fibrosis is secondary to a tumor or a granulomatous process, it is called *myelophthisis*.

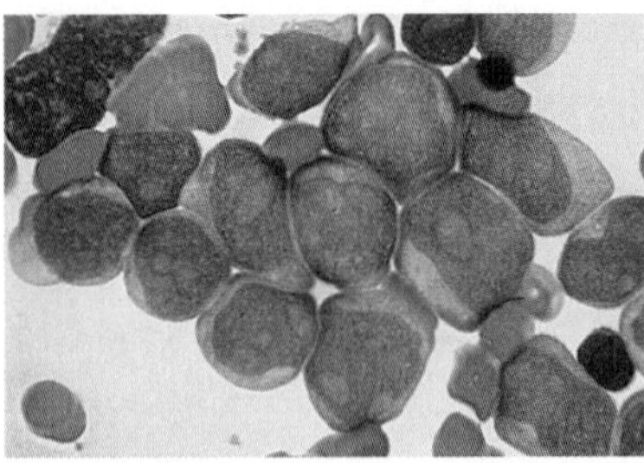

V-20 **Acute myelocytic leukemia** This marrow section shows sheets of primitive myeloblasts with numerous large nucleoli.

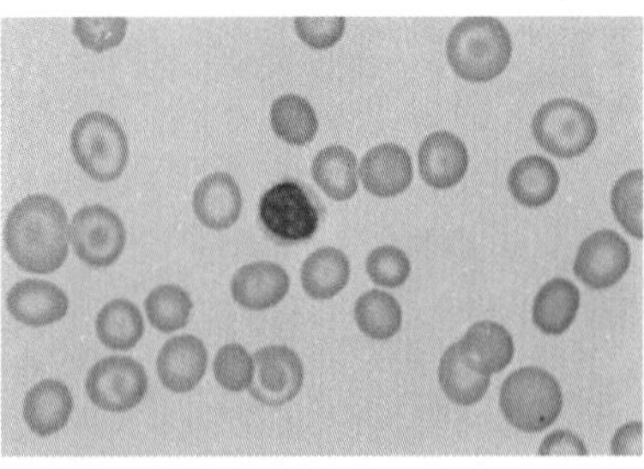

V-21 **Liver disease** Round macrocytes of rather uniform size are seen. Many of the macrocytes are also target cells.

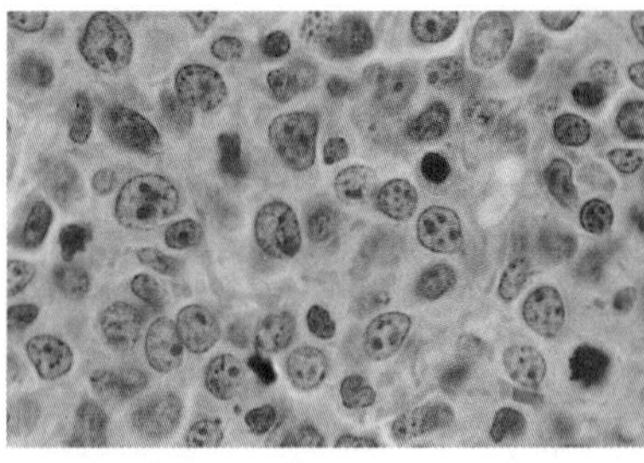

V-22 **Diffuse large B cell lymphoma** The neoplastic cells are large with vesicular nuclear chromatin and prominent nucleoli.

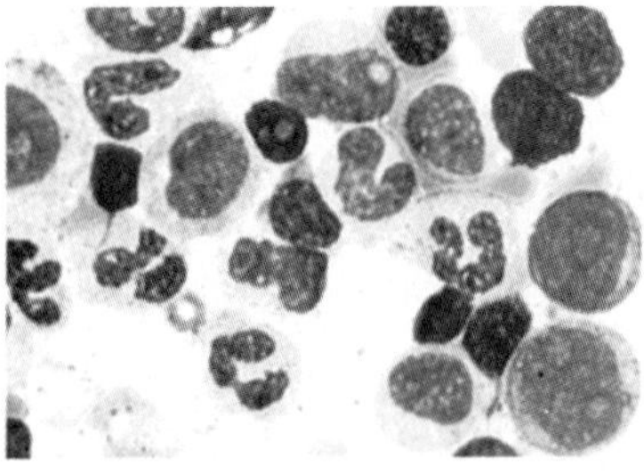

V-23 **Neutrophils with toxic granulation** In infection and other toxic states, azurophilic granules may become visible in mature granulocytes as coarse, dark-staining cytoplasmic granules.

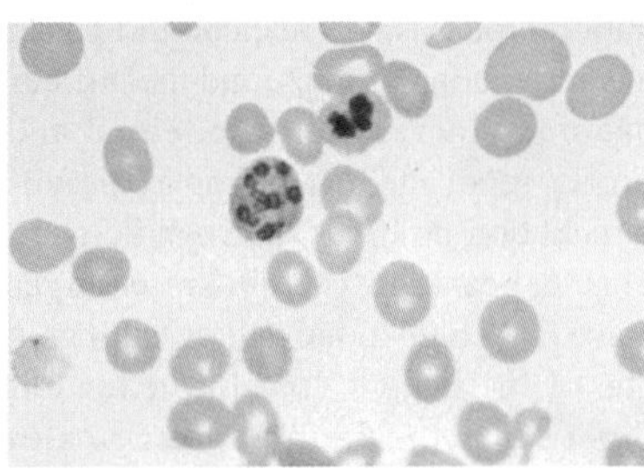

V-24 **Megaloblastic anemia** Oval macrocytes, well filled with hemoglobin, are admixed with lesser numbers of small teardrop-shaped red blood cells. Note also hypersegmented granulocyte.

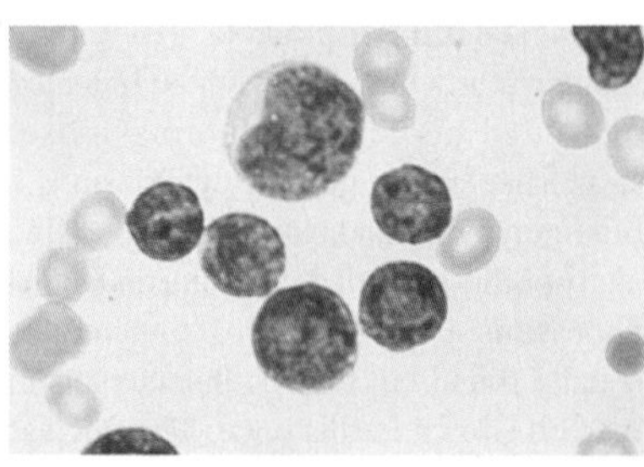

V-25 **Leukemic cells in acute lymphoblastic leukemia** characterized by round or convoluted nuclei, high nuclear/cytoplasmic ratio and absence of cytoplasmic granules.

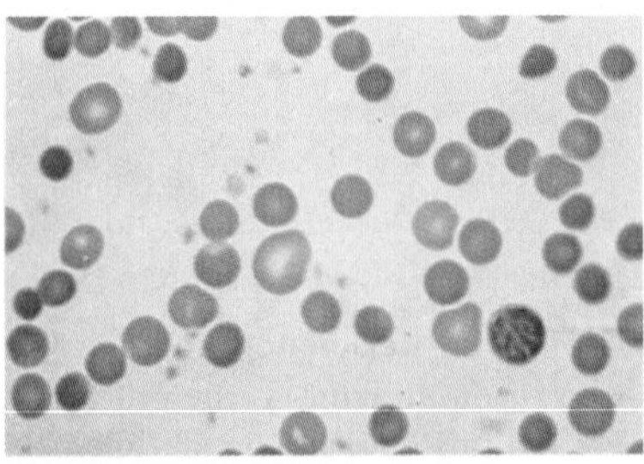

V-26 **Hereditary spherocytosis** Small, densely staining red blood cells are seen that have lost their central area of pallor (microsherocytes). Microspherocytes may also be found in other hemolytic disorders (Fig. V-8).

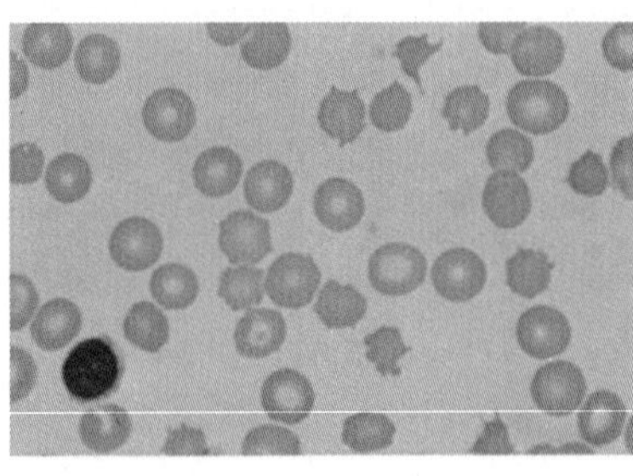

V-27 **Spur cell anemia** Spur cells are recognized as distorted red blood cells containing several irregularly distributed thornlike projections. Cells with this morphologic abnormality are also called acanthocytes.

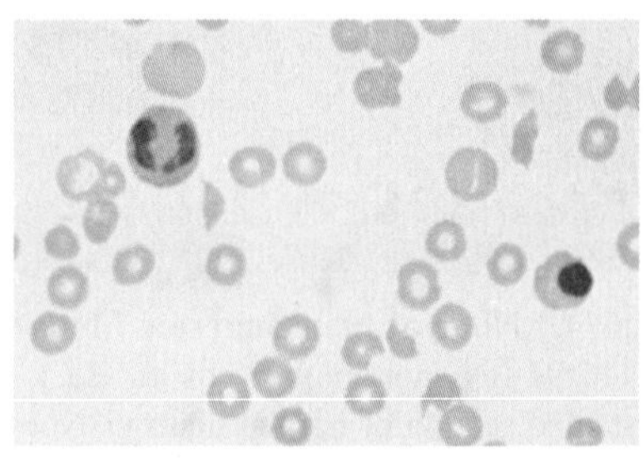

V-28 **Traumatic hemolysis** The helmet-shaped red blood cell and the small triangular-shaped red blood cells seen on this smear represent morphologic evidence of mechanical damage to red blood cells within the blood vessels.

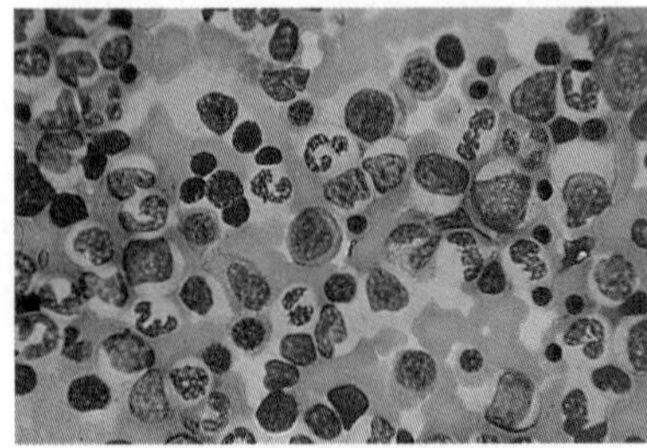

V-29 **Granulocytic hyperplasia** This marrow section shows an increase in the fraction of cells in the myeloid or granulocytic lineage as might be seen in a healthy marrow responding to infection. The E/G ratio is less than 1/3.

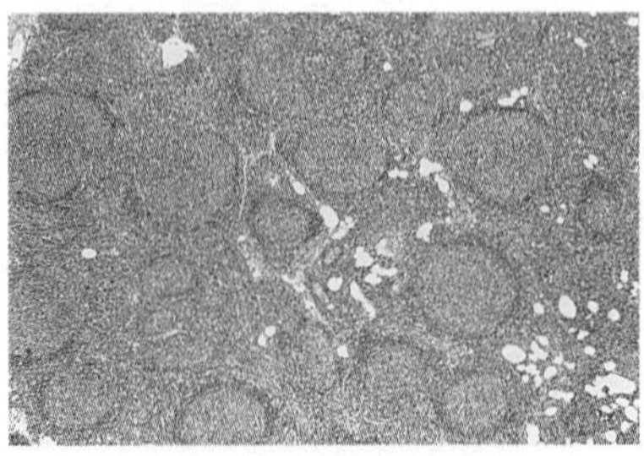

V-30 **Follicular lymphoma** The normal nodal architecture is effaced by nodular expansions of tumor cells. Nodules vary in size and mimic normal lymphoid follicles.

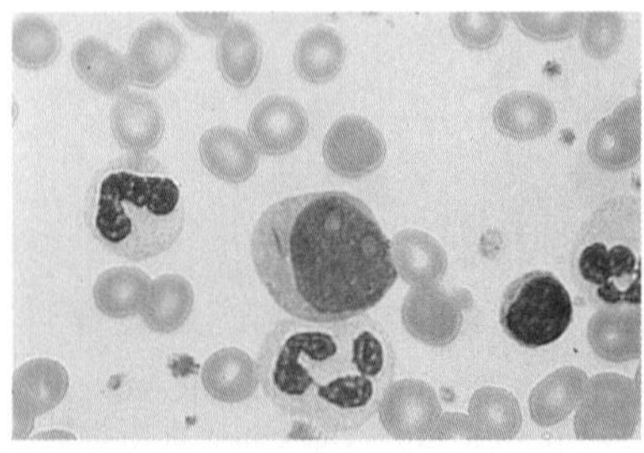

V-31 **Auer rod** This peripheral blood smear shows a myeloblast with a single Auer rod in the cytoplasm. Auer rods, when present, are usually seen in acute myelocytic leukemia.

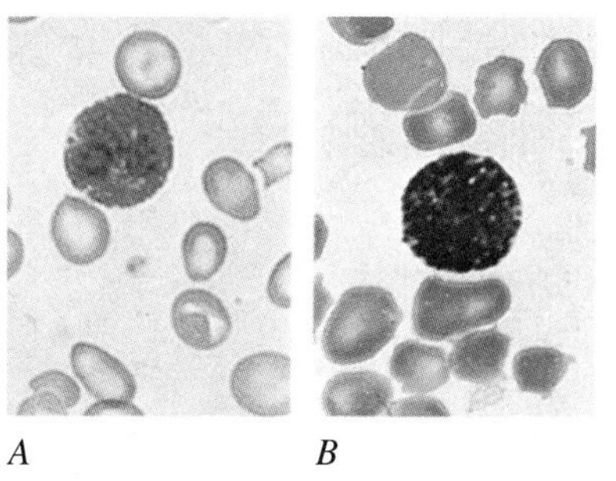

A *B*

V-32 A. **Normal eosinophil** The eosinophil contains large, bright-orange granules; the nucleus is bilobed. *B.* **Basophil** The basophil contains large, purple-black granules that fill the cell and obscure the nucleus.

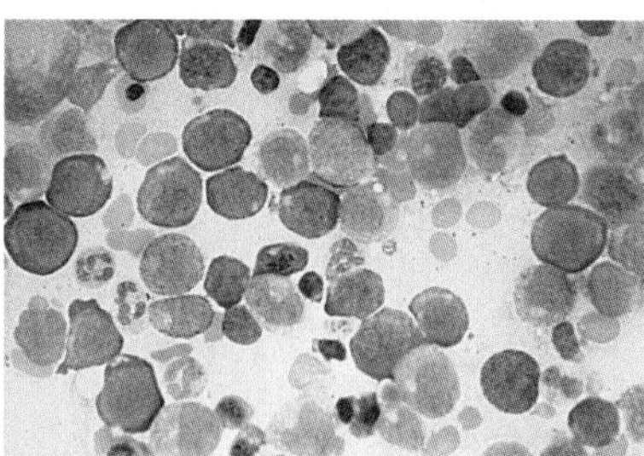

V-33 **Megaloblastic erythropoiesis** This marrow section demonstrates so-called nuclear-cytoplasmic dissociation; the cytoplasm of erythroblasts is filled with hemoglobin demonstrating nearly complete maturation while the nuclei have loose chromatin characteristic of more immature erythroid cells. The slow nuclear maturation is related to a decrease in DNA synthesis related to an insufficient supply of reduced folate to synthesize thymidylate. DNA synthesis inhibitors can produce this picture, as can folate and B_{12} deficiency.

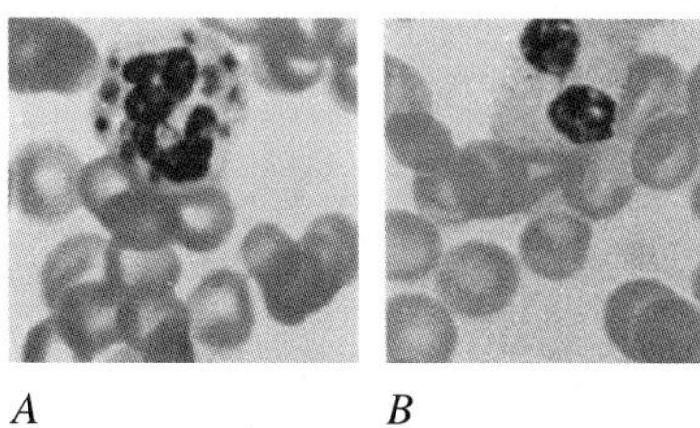

A *B*

V-34 A. **Chédiak-Higashi anomaly** In this ultimately fatal disorder, the granulocytes contain huge cytoplasmic granules, formed from aggregation and fusion of azurophilic and specific granules. Large abnormal granules are found in other granule-containing cells throughout the body. *B.* **Pelger-Hüet anomaly** In this benign disorder, the majority of granulocytes are bilobed. The nucleus frequently has a spectacle-like or "pince-nez" configuration.

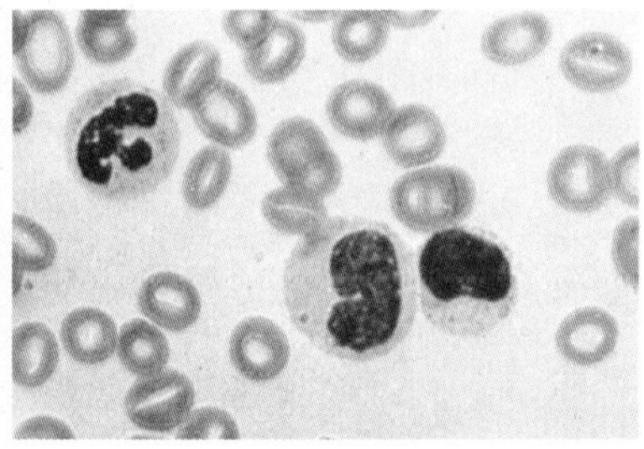

V-35 **Band with Döhle body** (center) Döhle bodies are discrete, blue-staining non-granular areas found in the periphery of the cytoplasm of the neutrophil in infections and other toxic states. They represent aggregates of rough endoplasmic reticulum.

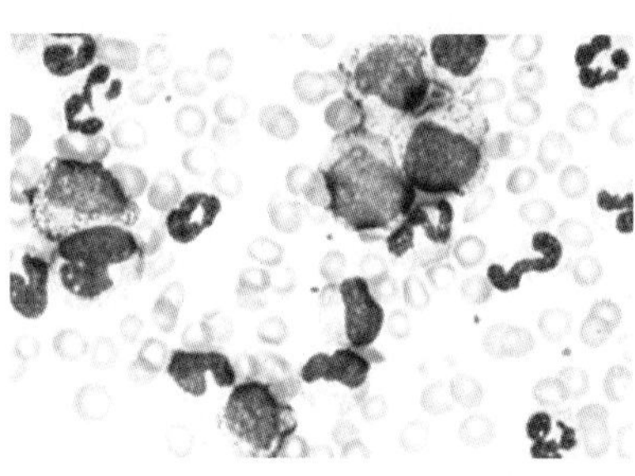

V-36 **Chronic granulocytic leukemia** The peripheral WBC count is high due to increased numbers of granulocytes and their precursors. The majority of the WBCs are segmented granulocytes or band forms, but myelocytes (as seen on this plate) and promyeloblasts (not seen on this plate) may also be found on review of the blood smear.

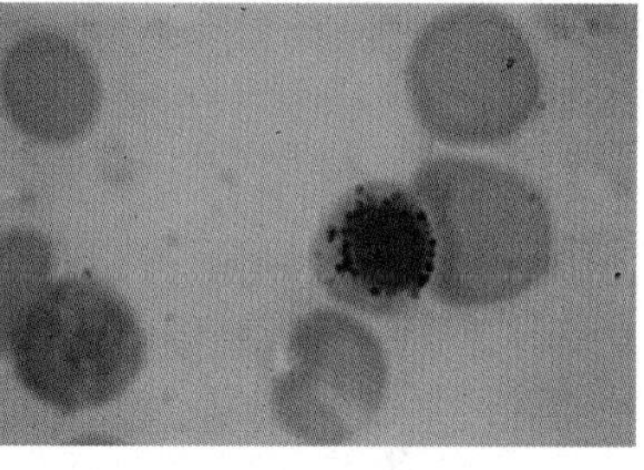

V-37 **Ringed sideroblast** Refractory anemia with ringed sideroblasts (RARS) is in the spectrum of myelodysplastic syndromes. This marrow Prussian blue stain shows an orthochromatic normoblast with a collar of blue granules surrounding the nucleus. The blue granules represent iron-laden mitochondria.

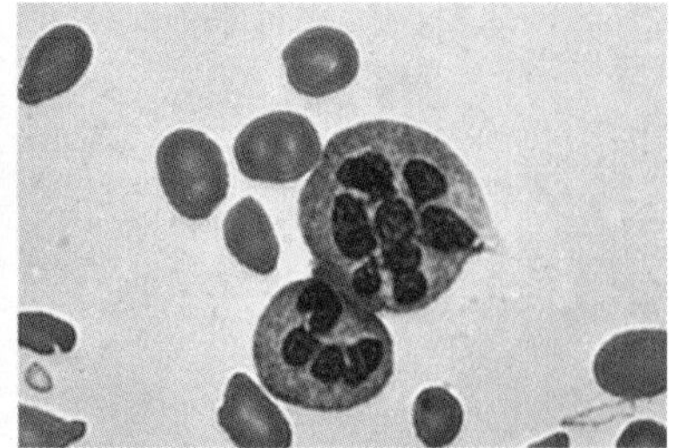

V-38 **Hypersegmentation** Frequent five-lobed granulocytes on a blood smear or granulocytes with more than five lobes are evidence of hypersegmentation, an important clue to the diagnosis of megaloblastic anemia.

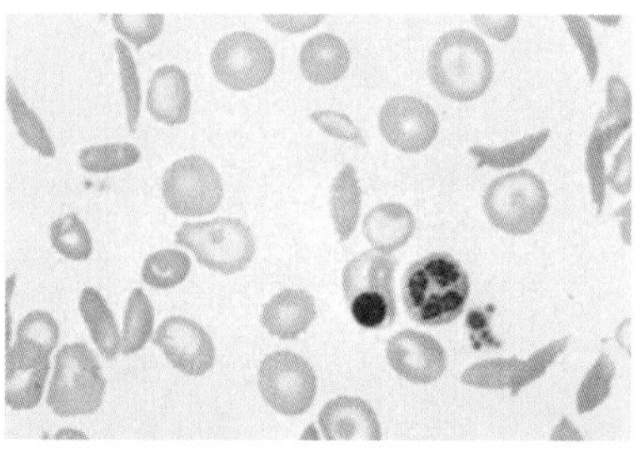

V-39 **Sickle cell anemia** The elongated and crescent-shaped red blood cells seen on this smear represent circulating irreversibly sickled cells. Target cells and a nucleated red blood cell are also seen.

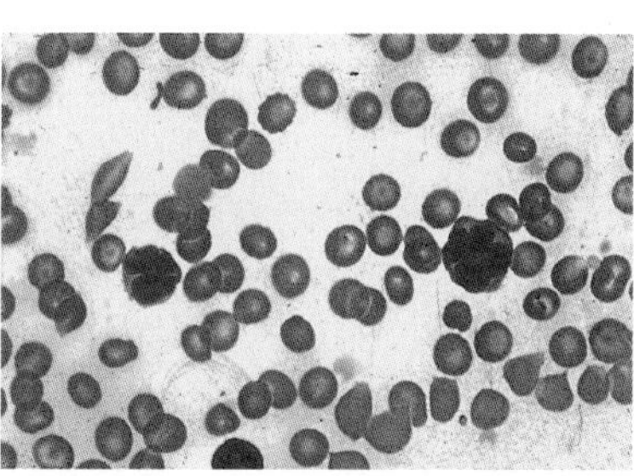

V-40 **Adult T cell leukemia/lymphoma** This peripheral blood smear reveals leukemia cells with the typical "flower-shaped" nucleus.

VI. Atlas of Diagnostic Microbiology

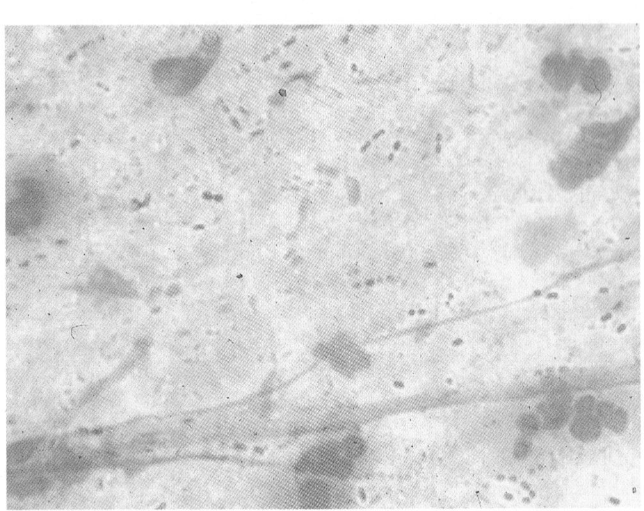

VI-1 **Gram-stained sputum** from a patient with acute purulent tracheobronchitis. Many polymorphonuclear neutrophils and a few macrophages are seen along with many gram-negative cocci, (*Moraxella catarrhalis*), a few of which appear as pairs. Nearly all organisms are cell associated and probably have been taken up by phagocytes, consistent with the notion that *Moraxella* is a lower-grade pathogen than organisms such as *Streptococcus pneumoniae*.

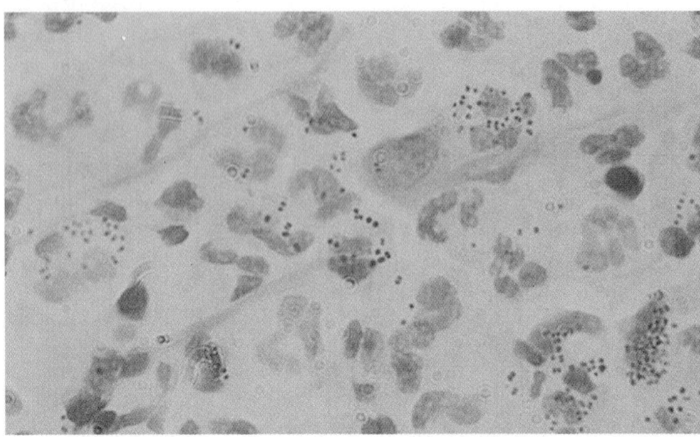

VI-2 The microbiologist can easily identify *Streptococcus pneumoniae* as the etiologic agent of pneumonia when microscopic examination of Gram-stained sputum specimen reveals this kind of picture.

Plates VI-3 through VI-33 are photomicrographs reproduced from "Benchaids for the Diagnosis of Malaria Infections," 2d ed, with the permission of the World Health Organization.

P. falciparum—thin film

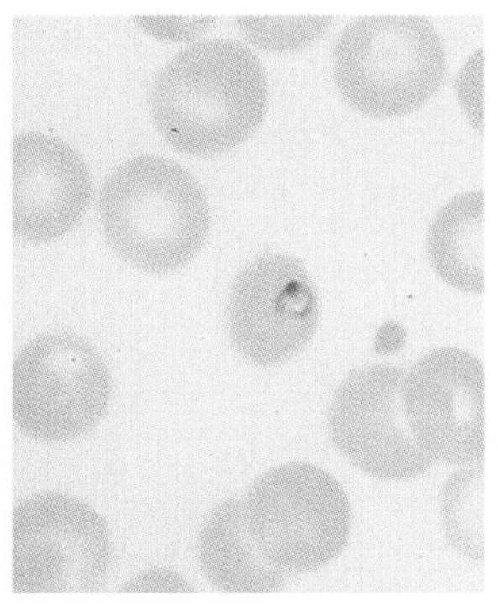

VI-3 Trophozoites–young

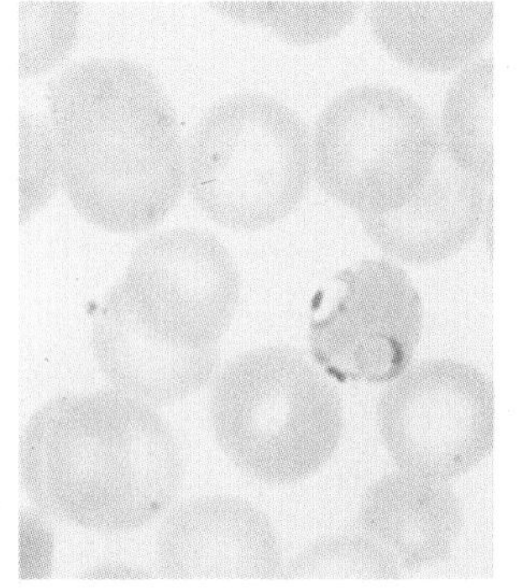

VI-4 Trophozoites–old

VI-5 Pigment in polymorphonuclear cell and trophozoites

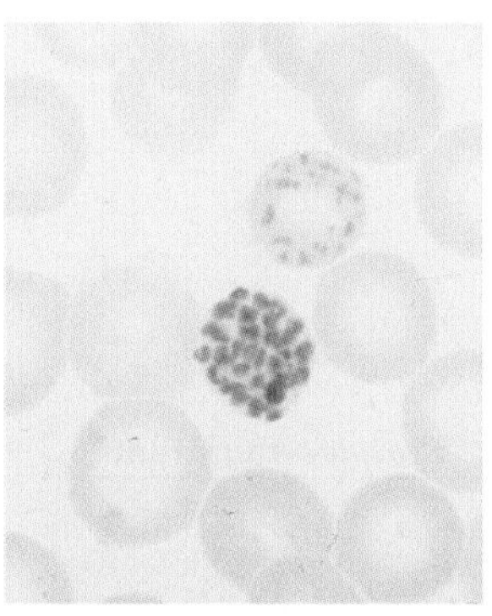

VI-6 Schizonts–mature

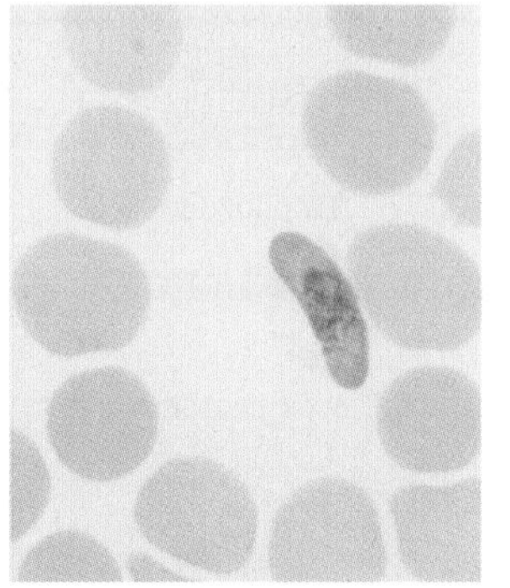

VI-7 Gametocytes–female

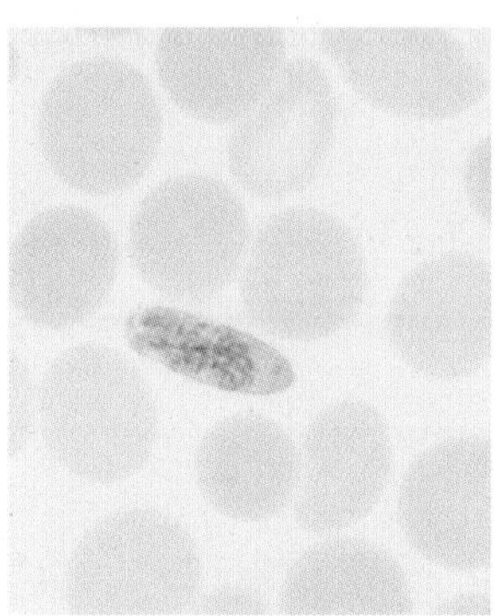

VI-8 Gametocytes–male

P. vivax—thin film

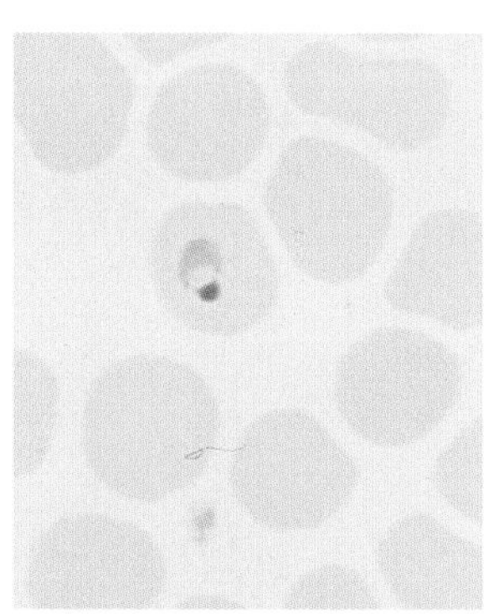

VI-9 Trophozoites–young

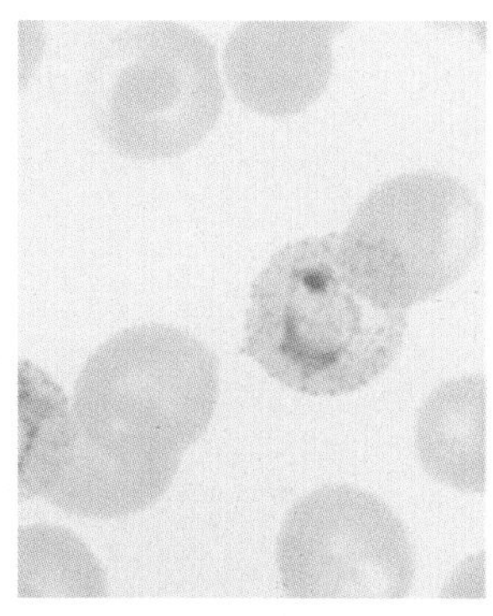

VI-10 Trophozoites–old

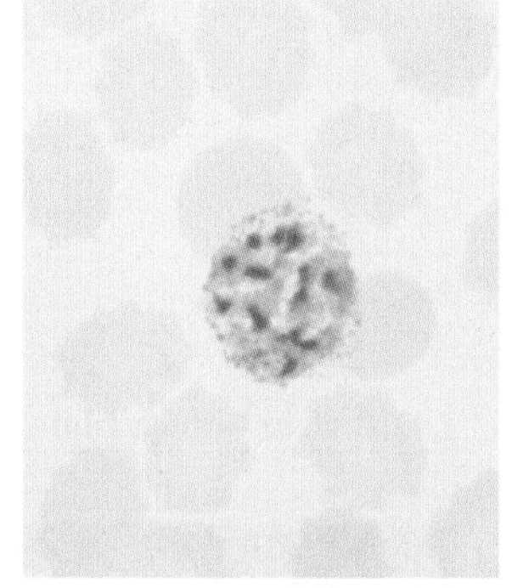

VI-11 Schizonts–mature

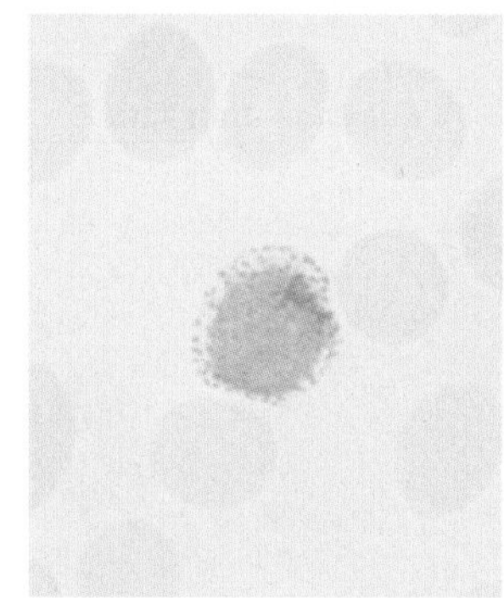

VI-12 Gametocytes–female

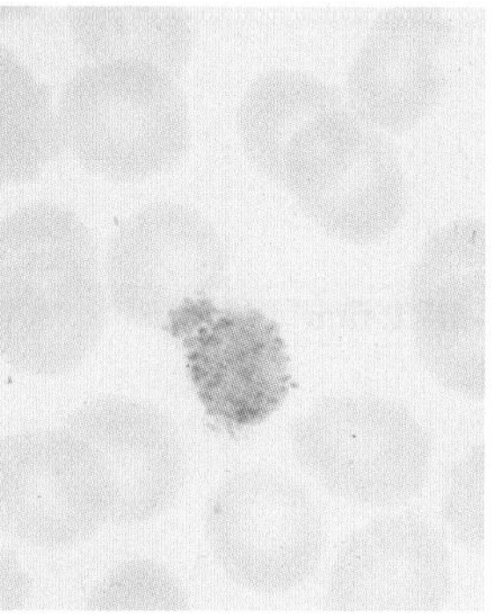

VI-13 Gametocytes–male

P. ovale—thin film

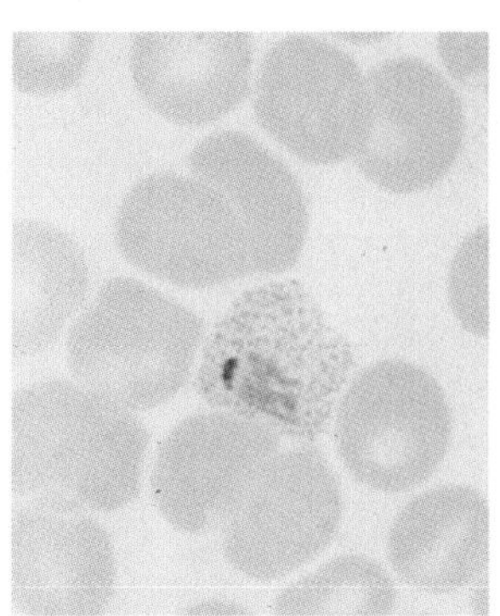

VI-14 Trophozoites–old

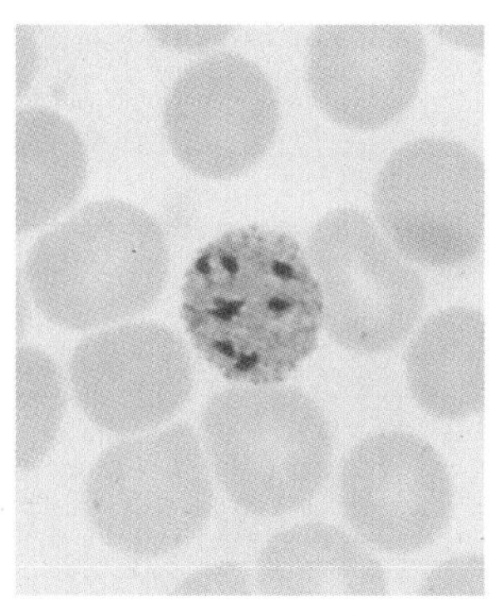

VI-15 Schizonts–mature

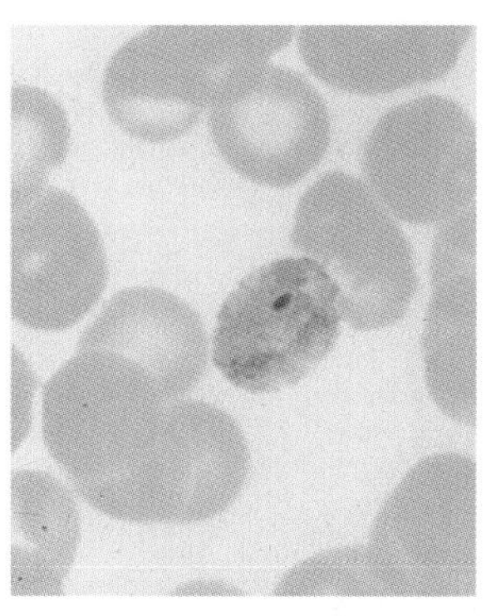

VI-16 Gametocytes–male

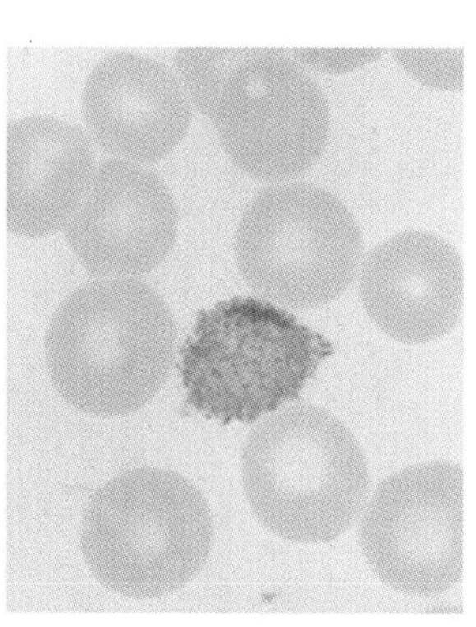

VI-17 Gametocytes–female

P. malariae—thin film

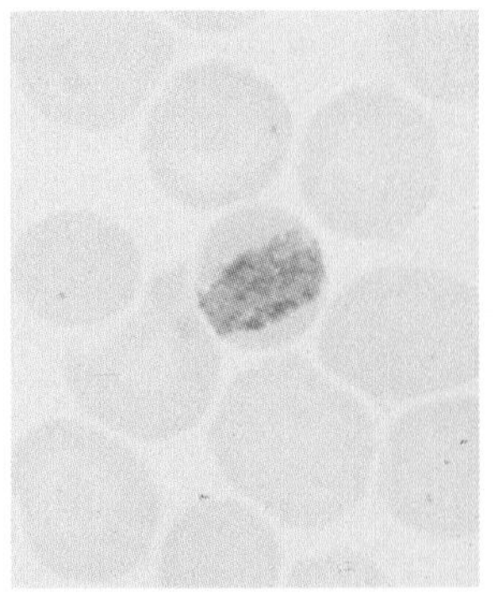
VI-18 Trophozoites–old

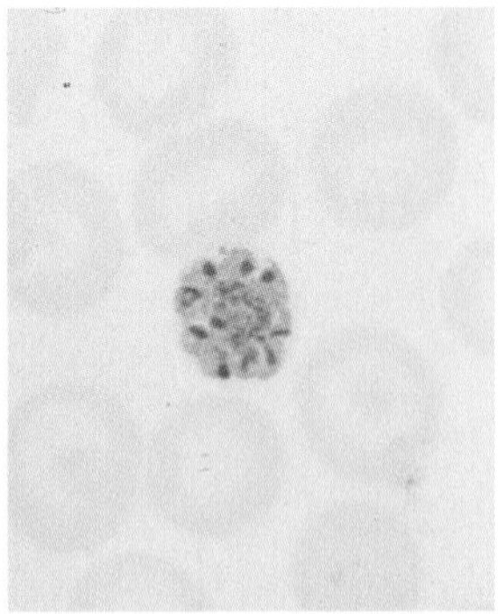
VI-19 Schizonts–mature

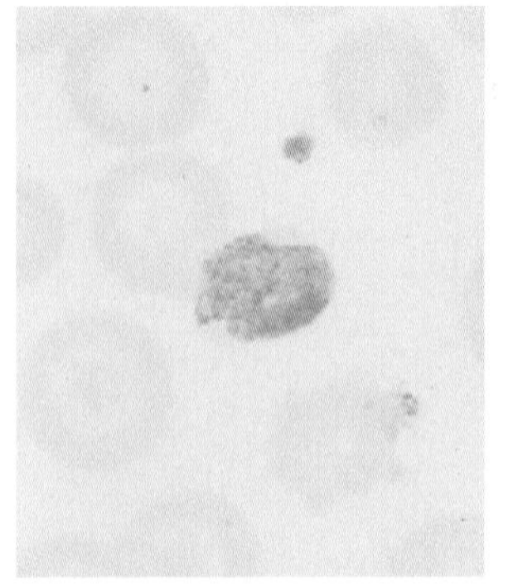
VI-20 Gametocytes–male

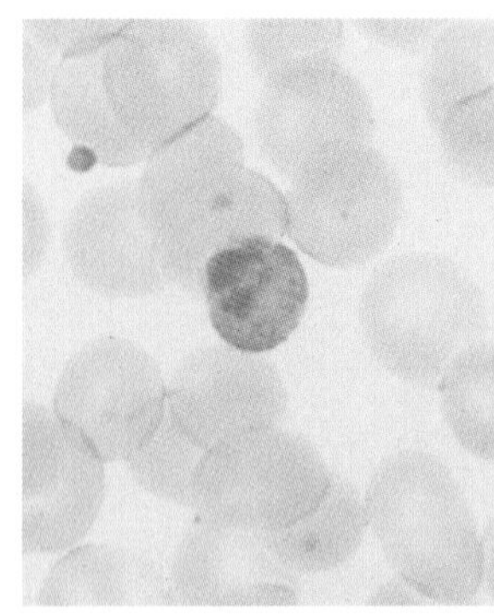
VI-21 Gametocytes–female

Babesia—thin film

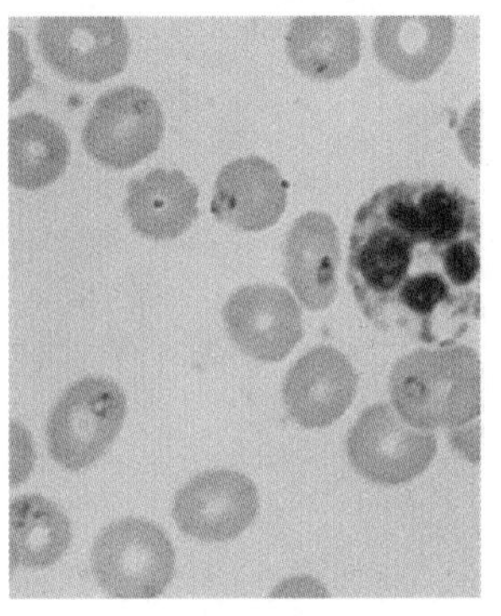
VI-22 Trophozoites

P. falciparum—thick film

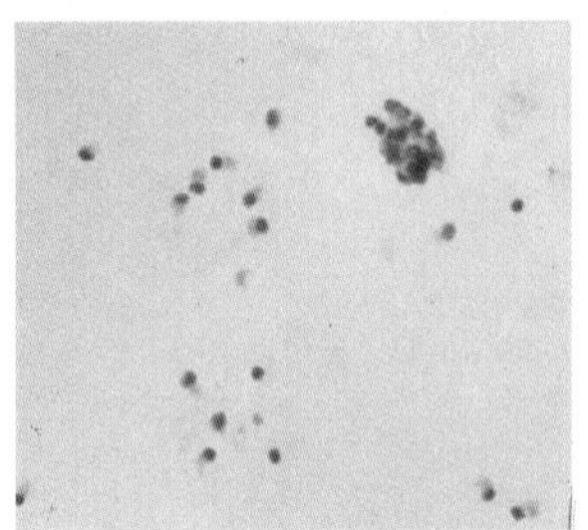
VI-23 Trophozoites

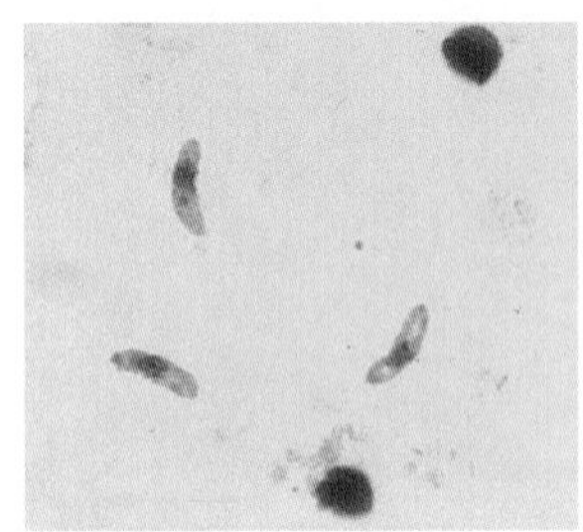
VI-24 Gametocytes

P. vivax—thick film

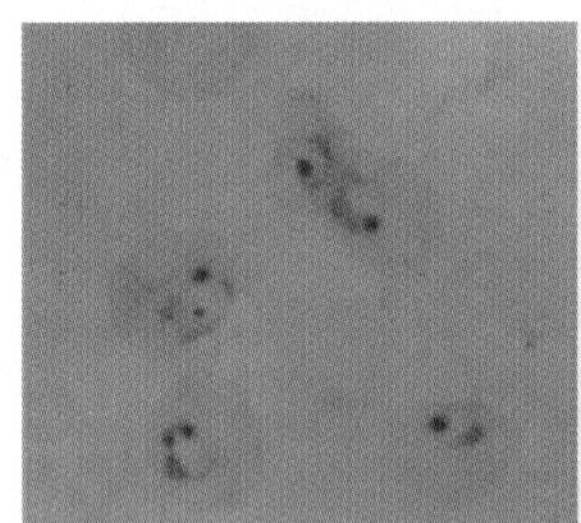
VI-25 Trophozoites

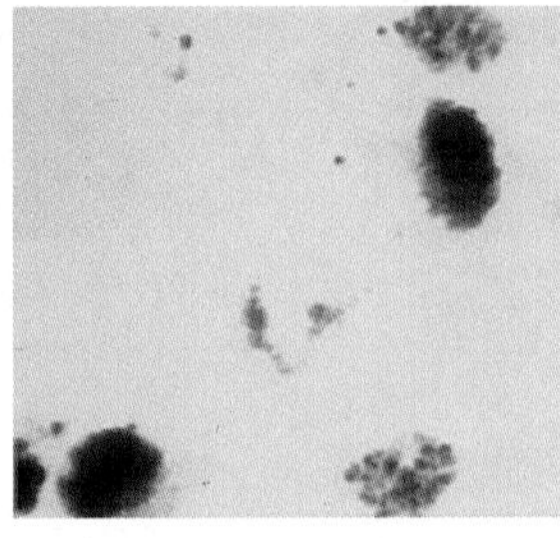
VI-26 Schizonts

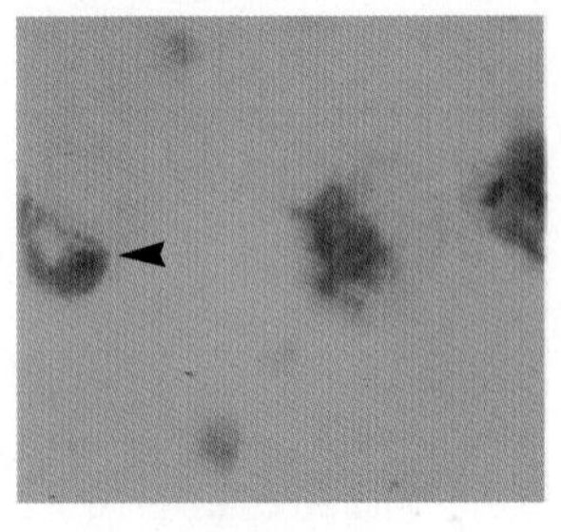
VI-27 Gametocytes

P. ovale—thick film

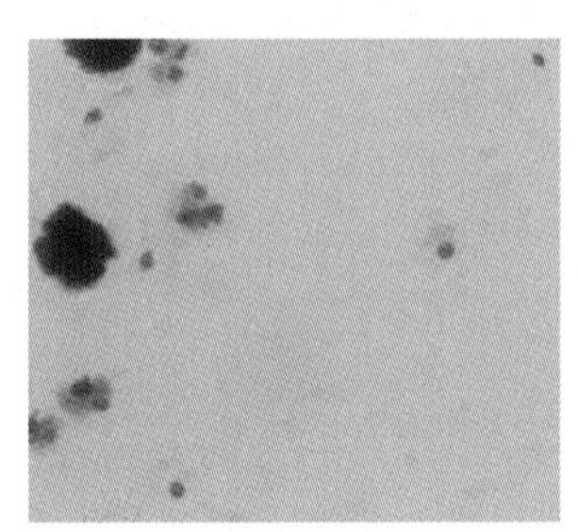
VI-28 Trophozoites

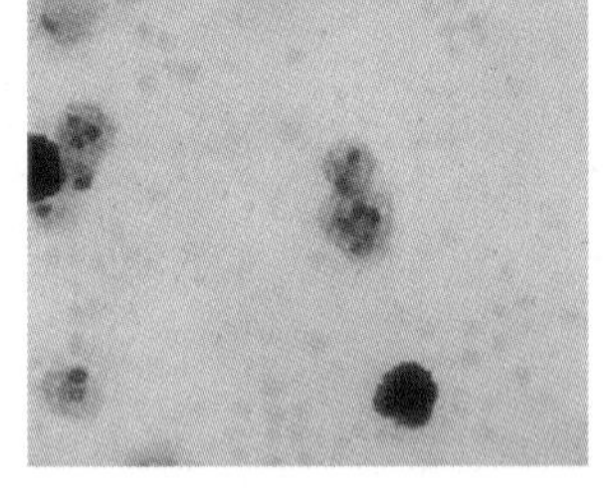
VI-29 Schizonts

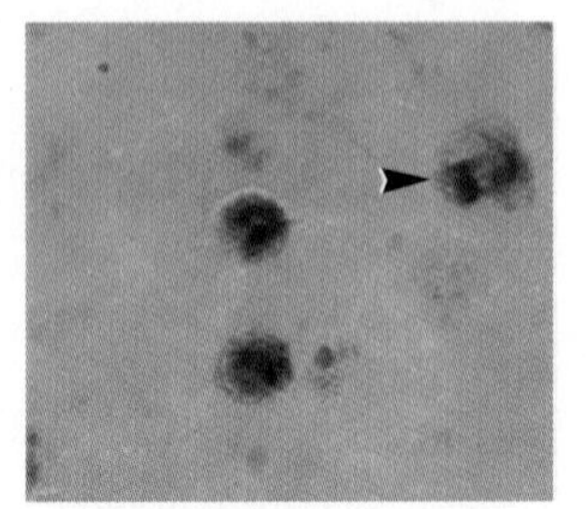
VI-30 Gametocytes

P. malariae—thick film

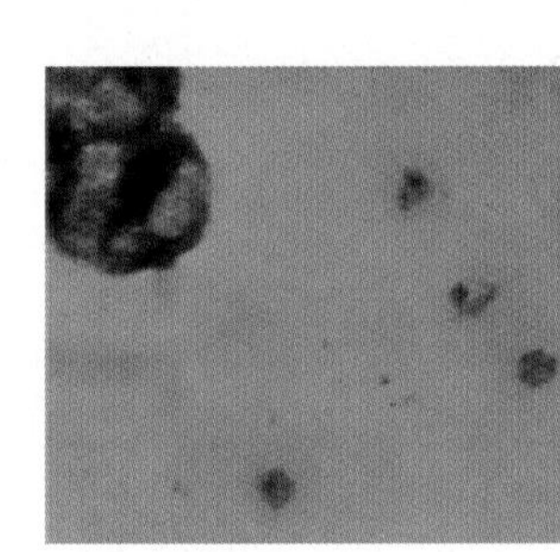
VI-31 Trophozoites

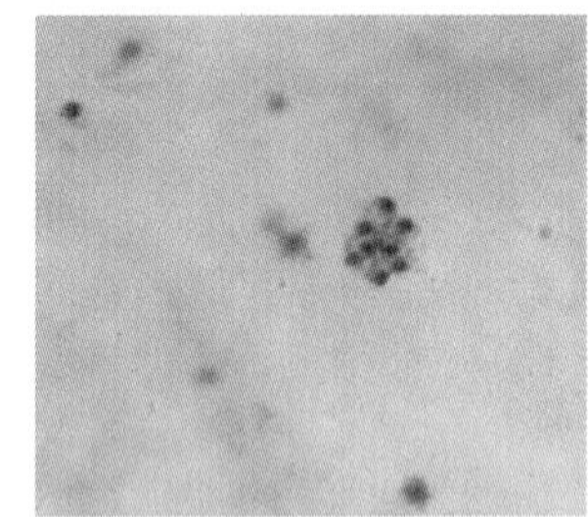
VI-32 Schizonts

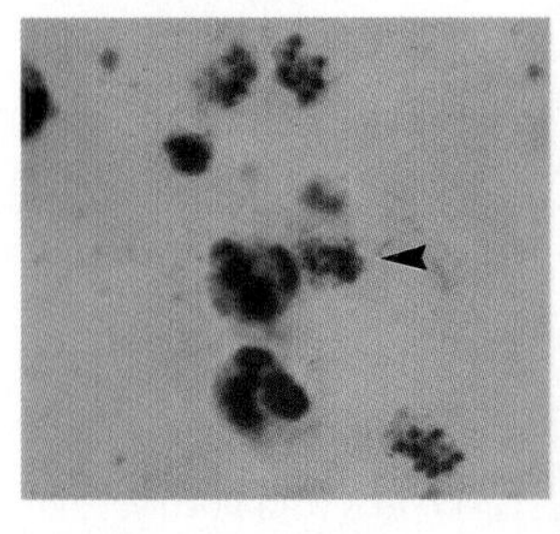
VI-33 Gametocytes

SOURCES OF PHOTOGRAPHS

I. CARDIOLOGY

R. Gibbons, MD I-1A, I-1B Exercise sestamibi study

II. DERMATOLOGY

L. Baden, MD IID-58 Septic emboli
Jean Bolognia, MD IIA-6 Seborrheic dermatitis; IIB-21 Non-Hodgkin's lymphoma
S. Wright Caughman, MD IIC-32 Nodular melanoma; IID-55 Condylomata acuminatum
Gregory Cox, MD IID-47 Primary syphilis
Daniel F. Danzl, MD IIA-18, IIA-19 Frostbite
Robert Gelber, MD IID-56 Polar lepromatous leprosy
Stephen E. Gellis, MD IID-39 Hand foot-and-mouth disease; IID-44 Fulminant meningococcemia
John Greenspan, PhD IID-42 Oral hairy leukoplakia; IID-43 Pseudomembranous oral candidiasis
Robert Hartman, MD IID-36 Varicella
A.W. Kerchner, MD IID-59 Veridans streptococcal endocarditis
James Krell, MD IIE-63 Dermatomyositis
Marilynne McKay, MD IIE-62 Discoid lupus erythematosus
V. Pranava Murthy, MD IID-53 Skin lesions
Daniel M. Musher, MD IID-60 Disseminated gonococcemia
Alvin Solomon, MD IIC-31 Lentigo maligna melanoma; IID-48 Secondary syphilis of the palms
Mary Spraker, MD IID-38 Impetigo contagiosa
Robert Swerlick, MD IIA-2 Acne rosacea; IIA-4 Atopic dermatitis; IIA-8*B* Allergic contact dermatitis; IIA-9 Lichen planus; IIA-12 Alopecia areata; IIA-14*B* Dermatographism; IIB-27 Actinic keratoses; IID-37 Disseminated herpes zoster; IID-45 Rocky Mountain spotted fever; IIE-61*B* Acute lupus erythematosus; IIE-63 Dermatomyositis; IIE-69*B* Pemphigus vulgaris; IIE-70 Erythema nodosum; IIE-71 Vasculitis; IIF-75 Sweet's syndrome; IIF-76 Rheumatoid nodules; IIF-79B Sarcoid; IIF-80 Pyoderma gangrenosum
Kalman Watsky, MD IIA-1 Acne vulgaris
Yale Resident's Slide Collection IID-41 Molluscum contagiosum; IID-46 Erythema chronicum migrans; IID-49 Condylomata lata; IIE-67 Erythema multiforme; IIE-72 Bullous pemphigoid
Kim Yancey, MD IIF-78 Coumarin necrosis

III. ENDOSCOPIC FINDINGS

FE Silverstein and **GN Tytgat** *Atlas of Gastrointestinal Endoscopy,* New York, Gower Medical Publishing, 1987. All photographs except III-12, III-23, III-24
GN Tytgat III-12; III-23; III-24

IV FUNDUSCOPIC FINDINGS

Jonathan C. Horton, MD, PhD IV-1 to IV-18

V. HEMATOLOGY

Robert S. Hillman, MD, and **Kenneth A. Ault, MD** *Hematology in General Practice,* New York, McGraw-Hill, 1995. Courtesy of the American Society of Hematology Slide Bank. V-30 to V-39
Elaine Jaffe, MD V-25 to V-29

VI. DIAGNOSTIC MICROBIOLOGY

Elil Renganathan, MD, WHO, Geneva VI-3 to VI-33

Symptoms of Autonomic Dysfunction The clinical manifestations of autonomic lesions are influenced by the organ involved, the normal balance of sympathetic–parasympathetic innervation, the nature of the underlying illness, and the severity and stage of progression. *Impotence* often heralds autonomic failure in men and may precede other symptoms by more than a decade (Chap. 51). A decrease in the frequency of spontaneous early morning erections may occur months before loss of nocturnal penile tumescence and development of total impotence. *Bladder dysfunction* may appear early in men and women, particularly in those with CNS involvement. Brain and spinal cord disease above the level of the lumbar spine results first in urinary frequency and small bladder volumes, and eventually in incontinence (*upper motor neuron* or *spastic bladder*). Disease of PNS autonomic nerve fibers to and from the bladder results in large bladder volumes, urinary frequency, and overflow incontinence (*lower motor neuron bladder* or *flaccid bladder*). Measurement of bladder volume (postvoid residual) is a useful bedside test for distinguishing between upper and lower motor neuron bladder dysfunction. *Gastrointestinal autonomic dysfunction* typically presents as severe constipation. Diarrhea occurs occasionally (as in diabetes mellitus) due to rapid transit of contents or uncoordinated small bowel motor activity, or on an osmotic basis from bacterial overgrowth associated with small bowel stasis. Impaired glandular secretory function may cause difficulty with food intake due to decreased salivation or eye irritation due to decreased lacrimation. Occasionally, temperature elevation and vasodilation can result from *anhidrosis* because sweating is normally important for heat dissipation (Chap. 17).

Orthostatic hypotension (OH) (also called "postural hypotension") is the most disabling feature of autonomic dysfunction. OH can cause a variety of symptoms, including dimming or loss of vision, lightheadedness, diaphoresis, diminished hearing, pallor, and weakness. Syncope results when the drop in BP impairs cerebral perfusion. Other manifestations of impaired cardiovascular control from baroreflex dysfunction include supine hypertension, a heart rate that is fixed regardless of posture, and postprandial hypotension. The most common causes of OH are not neurologic in origin (Table 366-2) and must be distinguished from neurogenic etiologies (Table 366-1). →*Neurocardiogenic and cardiac syncope are considered in Chap. 20.*

Approach to the Patient

The most common, clinically significant autonomic disorders present with symptoms of OH. The first step in the evaluation of symptomatic orthostasis is the exclusion of treatable causes. The history should include a review of current medications which may cause OH (e.g., diuretics, antihypertensives, antidepressants, phenothiazines, ethanol, narcotics, insulin, barbiturates, and β-adrenergic and calcium channel blockers). Exaggerated responses to medications may be the first sign of an underlying autonomic disorder. The history may reveal a potential underlying cause for symptoms (e.g., diabetes, Parkinson's disease) or may reveal specific underlying mechanisms (e.g., cardiac pump failure, reduced intravascular volume). Inappropriate or extreme venous pooling may contribute to symptomatic OH. The relationship of symptoms to meals (splanchnic shunting of blood), or standing on awakening in the morning (due to relative intravascular volume depletion) should be sought.

Physical examination includes measurement of supine and standing pulse and BP, with a period of at least 2 min between positions. Sustained drops in systolic (>20 mmHg) or diastolic (>10 mmHg) BP after standing for at least 2 min that are not associated with an increase in pulse rate of >15 beats per minute suggest an autonomic deficit. In nonneurogenic causes of OH, the BP drop is accompanied by a compensatory increase in heart rate of >15 beats per minute. The requirement that the hypotension is sustained differentiates autonomic failure from sluggish baroreceptor responses that are common in the elderly. Other common signs of ANS dysfunction include supine hypertension or postprandial hypotension. Neurologic evaluation should include a mental status examination (to exclude neurodegenerative disorders), cranial nerve examination (to detect the impaired downgaze found with progressive supranuclear palsy), motor examination (for Parkinson's disease and parkinsonian syndromes), and sensory examination (for polyneuropathies). In patients without a clear initial diagnosis, follow-up neurologic evaluations performed over years may reveal an evolution of neurologic findings that makes it possible to reach a specific diagnosis.

Table 366-2 Nonneurogenic Causes of Orthostatic Hypotension

Cardiac pump failure	Venous pooling
Myocardial infarction	Alcohol
Myocarditis	Postprandial dilation of splanchnic vessel beds
Constructive pericarditis	Vigorous exercise with dilation of skeletal vessel beds
Aortic stenosis	Heat: hot environment, hot showers and baths, fever
Tachyarrhythmias	Prolonged recumbancy or standing
Bradyarrhythmias	Sepsis
Salt-losing nephropathy	Medications
Adrenal insufficiency	Antihypertensives
Diabetes insipidus	Diuretics
Venous obstruction	Vasodilators: nitrates, hydralazine
Reduced intravascular volume	Alpha- and beta-blocking agents
Straining of heavy lifting, urination, defecation	CNS sedatives: barbiturates, opiates
Dehydration	Tricylic antidepressants
Diarrhea, emesis	Phenothiazines
Hemorrhage	
Burns	
Metabolic	
Adrenocortical insufficiency	
Hypoaldosteronism	
Pheochromocytoma	
Severe potassium depletion	

Disorders of autonomic function should be considered in the differential diagnosis of patients with symptoms of altered sweating (hyperhidrosis or hypohidrosis), constipation, impotence, or bladder dysfunction (urinary frequency, hesitancy, or incontinence). An initial practical approach to the patient with OH or autonomic symptoms is summarized in Table 366-3.

Autonomic Testing (See also Chap. 357) Autonomic function tests are helpful when the history and physical examination findings are inconclusive, when detection of subclinical involvement is important to evaluate the extent and severity of abnormalities, or to monitor the effects of therapy. Both physiologic and pharmacologic tests are available to assess the functional characteristics of the ANS. Commonly used physiologic tests assess autonomic aspects of cardiovascular function. These tests are noninvasive and provide quantitative and regional data about autonomic function. Pharmacologic tests can elucidate pathophysiologic abnormalities and guide the development of rational therapy.

Heart rate variation with deep breathing This is a test of parasympathetic influence on cardiovascular function. Results are influenced by the subject's posture, rate and depth of respiration [5 to 6 breaths per minute and a forced vital capacity (FVC) >1.5 L are optimal], age, medications, and hypocapnea. Interpretation of results requires comparison of test data with results from normal individuals collected under the same test conditions. For example, the lower limit of normal heart rate variation with deep breathing in persons younger than 20 years is >15 to 20 beats/min, but for persons over age 60 it is 5 to 8 beats/min. Heart rate variation with deep

Table 366-3 Initial Evaluation of OH or ANS Symptoms

Review medication use
Review coexisting medical disorders
Determine the relationship of OH to meals, exercise, straining, and standing up from bed in the morning
Record supine and standing BP and pulse
Complete neurologic examination

Table 366-4 Normal Blood Pressure and Heart Rate Changes during the Valsalva Maneuver

Phase	Maneuver	Blood Pressure	Heart Rate	Comments
I	Onset of expiration against a partially closed glottis	Rises due to aortic compression	Decreases	
II *early*	Continued expiration	Falls due to decreased venous return	Increases	
II *late*	Continued expiration	Total peripheral vascular resistance increases (increased sympathetic discharge and plasma epinephrine)	Increases at slower rate	Requires efferent sympathetic response
III	End of expiration	Falls due to increased capacitance of pulmonary bed	Increases further	
IV	Recovery	Increases ("overshoot") due to vasoconstriction and increased cardiac output	Compensatory bradycardia	Requires efferent sympathetic response

breathing (respiratory sinus arrhythmia) is abolished by the administration of atropine.

Valsalva response This response assesses integrity of the afferent limb, central processing, and efferent limb of the baroreceptor reflex (Table 366-4). The response is obtained with the subject sitting or supine. A constant expiratory pressure of 40 mmHg is maintained for 15 s while changes in heart rate and beat-to-beat BP are measured. There are four phases of BP and heart rate response to the Valsalva maneuver. Phases I and III are mechanical and related to changes in intrathoracic and intraabdominal pressure. In early phase II, reduced stroke volume and venous return results in a fall in BP, reflex tachycardia, and increased total peripheral resistance. Increased total peripheral resistance arrests the BP drop approximately 5 to 8 s after the onset of the maneuver. Late phase II begins with a progressive rise in BP toward baseline. Venous return and cardiac output return to normal in phase IV. Persistent peripheral arteriolar vasoconstriction results in a temporary BP overshoot and phase IV bradycardia (mediated by the baroreceptor reflex).

Autonomic function during the Valsalva maneuver can be measured in several ways. The *Valsalva ratio* is calculated from heart rate changes during the maneuver and is defined as the maximum phase II tachycardia divided by the minimum phase IV bradycardia. The ratio reflects the integrity of the entire baroreceptor reflex arc and of sympathetic efferents to blood vessels; sympathetic efferent function is assessed in the phase II BP response and the BP overshoot. Test results depend on the age and posture of the subject, the expiratory pressure, the duration of expiration, the FVC, and medications. Noninvasive recording of beat-to-beat BP changes provides a direct measure of sympathetic efferent input to blood vessels during phases II and IV that does not depend on the presence of a normal baroreceptor reflex arc.

Sudomotor function The capacity to produce sweat can be assessed quantitatively or qualitatively. Sweating is induced by release of acetylcholine from sympathetic postganglionic fibers. The *quantitative sudomotor axon reflex test* (QSART) is a measure of regional autonomic function mediated by acetylcholine-induced sweating. A reduced or absent response indicates a lesion of the postganglionic sudomotor axon. For example, sweating may be reduced in the legs as a result of peripheral neuropathy (e.g., in diabetes) before other signs of autonomic dysfunction emerge. The *thermoregulatory sweat test* (TST) is a *qualitative* measure of regional sweat production in response to an elevation of body temperature. An indicator powder placed on the anterior body surface changes color with sweat production during temperature elevation. The pattern of color changes is a measure of regional sweat secretion. The pattern of sweat abnormality may suggest a peripheral or central cause for the deficit. For example, a unilateral decrease over half the body suggests a central lesion. Measurement of galvanic skin responses in the limbs after an induced electrical potential is another qualitative test for detecting the presence or absence of sweating. The response is simple to measure, but habituation occurs.

Orthostatic blood pressure recordings Beat-to-beat BP measurements determined in supine, 80° tilt, and tilt-back positions are useful to quantitate orthostatic failure of BP control. It is important to allow a 20-min period of supine rest before assessing changes in BP during tilting. The test can be useful for the evaluation of patients with unexplained syncope and to detect vagally mediated syncope.

Cold pressor test The cold pressor test assesses sympathetic function. The individual immerses one hand in ice water (1° to 4°C) and BP is measured at 30 s and 1 min. The systolic and diastolic pressures normally rise by 10 to 20 mmHg. The afferent pathway is spinothalamic and thus is distinct from the afferent limb of the baroreceptor reflex arc. When spinothalamic pathways are intact, an abnormal response indicates an abnormality of autonomic central processing or sympathetic efferent function. When the response to the cold pressor test is normal and the Valsalva response is abnormal, the lesion is located in the afferent limb of the baroreceptor reflex arc.

Pharmacologic tests Pharmacologic assessments can help localize an autonomic defect to the CNS or the PNS. The test is controlled for time of day, position of the patient, level of patient activity, and food intake. Measures should be taken to minimize patient stress. Measurement of plasma levels of neurotransmitter metabolites and BP responses to infused drugs helps to distinguish between central and peripheral causes of autonomic dysfunction (Table 366-5); however, these studies are not routine clinical tools.

SPECIFIC SYNDROMES OF ANS DYSFUNCTION **Multiple System Atrophy** Multiple system atrophy (MSA) is an uncommon entity that comprises several overlapping clinical syndromes, including striatonigral degeneration (Shy-Drager syndrome), progressive supranuclear palsy (Chap. 363), and olivopontocerebellar atrophy (Chap. 364). The clinical syndrome can include various combinations of symptoms of autonomic dysfunction (OH, impotence, bladder and bowel dysfunction, and defective sweating), as well as additional symptoms of CNS disease such as rigidity, tremor, loss of associative movements, or abnormal eye movements. Most patients present with autonomic dysfunction alone, and other neurologic manifestations usually develop within 5 years. Patients with the striatonigral variant exhibit a form of parkinsonism in which bradykinesia and rigidity are more prominent than tremor. Patients with either a pure cerebellar

Table 366-5 Pharmacology Testing of Central and Peripheral Causes of Autonomic Failure

	Central	Peripheral	Intact
Supine plasma NE level	Normal	Low	Normal
Standing plasma NE level	No change	Low	Doubles
Blood pressure response to infused NE	Normal/increased	Exaggerated response	Normal/increased

syndrome or striatonigral degeneration may also develop pyramidal tract involvement. Some patients have features of both subtypes.

These disorders progress relentlessly to death 7 to 10 years after onset. Pharmacologic differences distinguish MSA from peripheral causes of autonomic failure (Table 366-4). Neuropathologic changes include primary neuronal degeneration with loss of neurons and gliosis in many CNS regions, including the brainstem, the cerebellum, the striatum, and the intermediolateral cell column of the thoracolumbar spinal cord. ANS abnormalities are also associated with Parkinson's disease and Huntington's disease.

Spinal Cord Lesions Spinal cord lesions from any cause may result in focal autonomic deficits or autonomic hyperreflexia. Descending pathways from the brain normally modulate organized patterns of sympathetic activity and modulate segmental autonomic reflexes. Spinal cord transection or hemisection may be attended by autonomic hyperreflexia affecting bowel, bladder, sexual, temperature-regulation, or cardiovascular functions. Dangerous increases or decreases in body temperature may result from inability to experience the sensory accompaniments of heat or cold exposure below the level of the injury. Quadriparetic patients exhibit both supine hypertension and OH after upward tilting. Markedly increased autonomic discharge can be elicited by bladder pressure or stimulation of the skin or muscles; suprapubic palpation of the bladder, catheter insertion, catheter obstruction, or urinary infection are common and correctable precipitants. This phenomenon, termed autonomic dysreflexia, affects 85% of patients with a traumatic spinal cord lesion above the C6 level. In patients with supine hypertension, BP can be lowered by tilting the head upward. Vasodilator drugs may be used to treat acute elevations in BP. Clonidine is used prophylactically to reduce the hypertension resulting from bladder stimulation. Sudden, dramatic increases in BP can lead to intracranial hemorrhage and death.

Peripheral Nerve and Neuromuscular Junction Disorders Peripheral neuropathies (Chap. 377) are the most common cause of chronic autonomic insufficiency. Neuropathies that affect small myelinated and unmyelinated fibers of the sympathetic and parasympathetic nerves occur in diabetes mellitus, amyloidosis, chronic alcoholism, porphyria, and Guillain-Barré syndrome. Neuromuscular junction disorders include botulism and Lambert-Eaton syndrome.

Diabetes mellitus Autonomic involvement in diabetes may begin at any stage in the disease (Chap. 333) and often presents with asymptomatic abnormalities in vagal function that can be detected as reduced heart rate variation with deep breathing. Loss of small myelinated and unmyelinated nerve fibers in the splanchnic distribution, carotid sinus, and vagus nerves is characteristic. Widespread enteric neuropathy can cause profound disturbances in gut motility (gastroparesis), nausea and vomiting, malnutrition, achlorhydria, and bowel incontinence. Other symptoms may include impotence, urinary incontinence, pupillary abnormalities, and OH. Typical symptoms and signs of hypoglycemia may fail to appear because damage to the sympathetic innervation of the adrenal gland can result in a lack of epinephrine release. Insulin excess may also cause profound hypotension. Autonomic dysfunction may lengthen the QT interval and enhance the risk of sudden death. Hyperglycemia appears to be one risk factor for autonomic involvement. Biochemical and pharmacologic studies in diabetic neuropathy are compatible with autonomic failure localized to the PNS [low supine plasma norepinephrine (NE) levels and exaggerated pressor responsiveness].

Amyloidosis Autonomic neuropathy occurs in both sporadic and familial forms of amyloidosis (Chap. 319). Although patients usually present with a distal painful neuropathy accompanied by sensory loss, autonomic insufficiency can precede the development of the polyneuropathy. Death is usually due to cardiac or renal impairment. Postmortem studies reveal amyloid deposition in many organs, including two sites that contribute to autonomic failure: intraneural blood vessels and autonomic ganglia. Pathologic examination reveals a loss of unmyelinated and myelinated nerve fibers.

Alcoholic neuropathy Abnormal parasympathetic vagal and efferent sympathetic function occurs in individuals with chronic alcoholism. Pathologic changes can be demonstrated in the parasympathetic (vagus) and sympathetic fibers and in ganglia. Impotence is a major problem, but concurrent gonadal hormone abnormalities may obscure the parasympathetic component to this symptom. Clinical symptoms of autonomic failure generally appear when the polyneuropathy is severe. OH may also be prominent in Wernicke's encephalopathy (Chap. 376). Autonomic involvement may contribute to the high mortality rates associated with alcoholism (Chap. 387).

Porphyria Although each of the porphyrias can cause autonomic dysfunction, the condition is most extensively documented in the acute intermittent type (Chap. 346). Autonomic symptoms include tachycardia, sweating, urinary retention, and hypertension or, less commonly, hypotension. Other prominent symptoms include anxiety, abdominal pain, nausea, and vomiting. Abnormal autonomic function can occur both during acute attacks and during remissions. Elevated catecholamine levels during acute attacks correlate with the degree of tachycardia and hypertension.

Guillain-Barré syndrome BP fluctuations and arrhythmias can be severe (Chap. 378). It is estimated that 2 to 10% of seriously ill patients with Guillain-Barré syndrome suffer fatal cardiovascular collapse. Abnormal sweating, sphincter disturbance, and pupillary dysfunction also occur. Demyelination has been described in the vagus and glossopharyngeal nerves, the sympathetic chain, and the white rami communicantes. The presence of autonomic involvement is not clearly related to the severity of motor or sensory involvement.

Botulism The toxin binds presynaptically to cholinergic nerve terminals and, after uptake into the cytosol, blocks acetycholine release by digesting key proteins involved in neurotransmitter release. Manifestations of this blockade consist of motor paralysis and autonomic disturbances, including blurred vision, dry mouth, nausea, unreactive or sluggishly reactive pupils, constipation, and urinary retention (Chap. 144).

Pure Autonomic Failure (PAF) This sporadic syndrome consists of postural hypotension, impotence, bladder dysfunction, and defective sweating. The disorder begins in the middle decades and occurs in women more than in men. The symptoms can be disabling, but the disease does not shorten life span. The clinical and pharmacologic characteristics suggest a primary involvement of postganglionic sympathetic neurons. There is a severe reduction in the density of neurons within sympathetic ganglia, resulting in low supine plasma NE levels and noradrenergic supersensitivity (Table 366-5). The clinical diagnosis may be difficult in early stages because patients may present with isolated OH, raising a question of PAF, but they later develop signs of multiple system atrophy (discussed above).

Postural Orthostatic Tachycardia Syndrome (POTS) This syndrome is characterized by symptomatic orthostatic intolerance (*not* OH) and an increase in heart rate to >120 beats per minute or by 30 beats per minute with standing. The condition affects young adult women most commonly, but it can occur over a wide age range. Associated symptoms include light-headedness, shortness of breath, and exercise intolerance. The pathogenesis is unclear in most cases; hypovolemia, venous pooling, impaired brainstem regulation, or β-receptor supersensitivity may play a role. In one affected individual, a mutation in the NE transporter resulting in impaired NE clearance from synapses was responsible. Only one-fourth of patients eventually resume their usual daily activities. Expansion of fluid volume and postural training are initial approaches to treatment. If the response to treatment is inadequate, then fludrocortisone, phenobarbital, beta blockers, and clonidine have been used with some success.

Postprandial Hypotension The importance of postprandial hypotension (PPH) among healthy elderly persons, hypertensive patients, and elderly patients in nursing homes has probably been underestimated. Abnormally reduced peripheral vasoconstriction in response to shunting of blood to the splanchnic circulation after a meal contributes to PPH. The wisdom of administering cardiovascular medications that have hypotensive effects at mealtimes to healthy and hypertensive elderly patients is questionable. PPH is also associated with diabetes, Parkinson's disease, renal failure treated with hemodialysis, cardiovascular disease, paraplegia, and autonomic failure.

Inherited Disorders Riley-Day syndrome (familial dysautonomia) is an autosomal recessive disorder of infants and children that occurs among Ashkenazi Jews. The defective gene, located on the long arm of chromosome 9, has not been identified. Decreased tearing, hyperhidrosis, reduced sensitivity to pain, areflexia, absent fungiform papillae on the tongue, and labile BP may be present. Episodic abdominal crises and fever are common. Increased sensitivity to intraocular methacholine and absent axon flare response to intradermal histamine injection are useful diagnostic markers. Normal resting plasma NE levels that do not increase on standing are consistent with an afferent lesion. Pathologic examination of nerves reveals a loss of small myelinated and unmyelinated nerve fibers.

Primary Hyperhidrosis This syndrome presents with excess sweating of the palms of the hands and soles of the feet. The disorder affects 0.6 to 1.0% of the population; the etiology is unclear (there may be a genetic component). While not dangerous, the condition can be socially embarrassing (e.g., shaking hands) or disabling (e.g., inability to write without soiling the paper). Onset of symptoms is usually in adolescence; the condition tends to improve with age. Topical antiperspirants (e.g., Drysol) are occasionally helpful. T2 ganglionectomy or sympathectomy is successful in >90% of patients with palmar hyperhidrosis. The advent of endoscopic transaxillary T2 sympathectomy has lowered the complication rate of the procedure. The most common complication is compensatory hyperhidrosis, which improves spontaneously over months; other potential complications include recurrent hyperhidrosis (16%), Horner's syndrome (<2%), gustatory sweating, wound infection, hemothorax, and intercostal neuralgia. Local injection of botulinum toxin has been used to block cholinergic, post-ganglionic sympathetic fibers to sweat glands in patients with palmar hyperhidrosis; however, the technique is limited by the need for repetitive injections (the effect usually lasts 4 months before waning), pain with injection, the high cost of botulinum toxin, and the possibility of temporary intrinsic hand muscle weakness. Tap water iontophoresis has been successful for some patients.

Miscellaneous The importance of autoimmunity in the pathogenesis of autonomic failure has been underestimated; autoantibodies against acetylcholine receptors in autonomic ganglia have been found in some patients with acute pandysautonomia and paraneoplastic autonomic neuropathy. Other conditions associated with autonomic failure include infections, poisoning (organophosphates), malignancy, and aging. Disorders of the hypothalamus can affect autonomic function and produce abnormalities in temperature control, satiety, sexual function, and circadian rhythms (Chap. 328).

Reflex Sympathetic Dystrophy and Causalgia The failure to identify a primary role of the ANS in the pathogenesis of these disorders has resulted in a change of nomenclature. *Complex regional pain syndrome* (CRPS) *types I* and *II* are now used in place of reflex sympathetic dystrophy (RSD) and causalgia, respectively.

CRPS type I is a regional pain syndrome that usually develops after tissue trauma. Examples of associated trauma include myocardial infarction, minor shoulder or limb injury, and stroke. *Allodynia* (the perception of a nonpainful stimulus as painful), *hyperpathia* (an exaggerated pain response to a mildly painful stimulus), and spontaneous pain occur; these symptoms are unrelated to the severity of the initial trauma and are not confined to the distribution of a single peripheral nerve. CRPS type II is a regional pain syndrome that develops after injury to a peripheral nerve. Spontaneous pain initially develops within the territory of the affected nerve but eventually may spread outside the nerve distribution.

Pain is the primary clinical feature of CRPS. Vasomotor abnormalities, sudomotor abnormalities, or focal edema may occur alone or in combination, but must be present for diagnosis. Limb pain syndromes that do not meet these criteria are best classified as "limb pain—not otherwise specified (NOS)". In CRPS, localized sweating (increased resting sweat output) and changes in blood flow may produce temperature differences between affected and unaffected limbs.

CRPS type I (RSD) has classically been divided into three clinical phases but is now considered to be more variable than previously thought. Phase I consists of pain and swelling in the distal extremity occurring within weeks to 3 months after the precipitating event. The pain is diffuse, spontaneous, and either burning, throbbing, or aching in quality. The involved extremity is warm and edematous, and the joints are tender. Increased sweating and hair growth are present. In phase II (3 to 6 months after onset), thin, shiny, cool skin appears. After an additional 3 to 6 months (phase III), atrophy of the skin and subcutaneous tissue plus flexion contractures complete the clinical picture.

Therapy for both types of CRPS is unsatisfactory. The desire to provide relief for these severely disabling pain syndromes has produced a variety of surgical and medical treatments with conflicting reports of efficacy. Clinical trials suggest that early mobilization with physical therapy or a brief course of steroids may be helpful for CRPS type I. The long-term results of this treatment are unclear. Other medical treatments have included the use of adrenergic blockers, nonsteroidal anti-inflammatory drugs (NSAIDs), calcium channel blockers, phenytoin, opioids, and calcitonin. Stellate ganglion blockade is a commonly used invasive therapeutic technique. Although stellate ganglion blocks often provide temporary pain relief, the efficacy of repetitive blocks is uncertain.

℞ **TREATMENT** Management of autonomic failure is usually limited to alleviating the disability caused by symptoms. Treatment of the primary disorder does not generally improve autonomic function. The history and examination are key to the identification of easily reversible conditions (Table 366-3).

OH is often severely disabling but may be mild. Neurogenic OH should be treated only if symptoms are present that limit activities of daily living. Nonpharmacologic interventions can be helpful. Patients should avoid sodium depletion or dehydration by maximizing salt intake (eating salty foods) and deliberately drinking at least 2 to 2.5 L/d of water. Sleeping in a head-up tilt position reduces nocturnal diuresis, morning postural hypotension and hypovolemia, and minimizes supine hypertension. Patients are often advised to sit with legs dangling over the edge of the bed for several minutes before attempting to stand in the morning. Isotonic exercise is desirable, but vigorous exercise or prolonged recumbency should be avoided. Circumstances that accentuate vasodilation (alcohol intake, high ambient temperature) may precipitate severe hypotension. Nonprescription medicines containing sympathomimetics must be used carefully because they may cause severe hypertension in the setting of autonomic failure accompanied by denervation supersensitivity. Compressive garments are of questionable value.

Most patients require pharmacologic therapy for the management of OH. Fludrocortisone is the initial drug of choice; at doses between 0.1 mg/d and 0.3 mg bid orally, it enhances renal sodium conservation and increases the sensitivity of arterioles to norepinephrine. Susceptible patients may develop fluid overload, congestive heart failure, supine hypertension, or hypokalemia; with chronic administration, potassium supplements are often necessary. Sustained elevations of supine BP above 200/110 should be avoided.

OH of moderate severity can be treated with a combination of fludrocortisone and the α_1-receptor agonist midodrine. Midodrine is well absorbed when given orally and causes arteriolar and venous constriction without CNS or cardiac stimulation. It is administered orally 30 to 45 min before meals at an initial dose of 5 mg tid, increasing to a maximum of 10 mg q4h. Side effects include pruritus, uncomfortable piloerection, and supine hypertension.

OH with a postprandial component may respond to several measures. Frequent, small, low-carbohydrate meals may diminish splanchnic shunting of blood after meals and reduce PPH. Prostaglandin inhibitors (ibuprofen or indomethacin) taken with meals can prevent

PPH. Caffeine (250 mg or two cups of coffee) can be given once per day, usually in the morning. The somatostatin analogue octreotide can be useful in the treatment of postprandial syncope by inhibiting the release of gastrointestinal peptides that have vasodilator and hypotensive effects. The dose ranges from 25 μg subcutaneously bid to 100 to 200 μg subcutaneously tid. Despite the lack of a pressor effect, octreatide may also be useful for preventing the PPH that occurs in normal elderly patients.

OH accompanied by diarrhea may respond to the α_2 agonist clonidine; coincident causes of nonneurogenic OH must be excluded before this treatment is begun because the risk of associated hypotension is significant. Initial doses are 0.1 to 0.2 mg orally every morning; the dose is gradually increased if drowsiness, dry mouth, constipation, supine hypertension, or hypotension are not dose-limiting. Octreotide may also be useful for some patients with this condition.

OH associated with anemia may respond to erythropoietin. One study found that systolic BP increased by 20 mmHg and orthostatic symptoms improved with normalization of the hematocrit. Erythropoietin is administered subcutaneously at doses of 25 to 75 U/kg three times per week. The hematocrit increases after 2 to 6 weeks. A weekly maintenance dose is usually necessary. The increased intravascular volume that accompanies the rise in hematocrit can exacerbate supine hypertension.

Many patients with ANS failure exhibit exaggerated sensitivity to various drugs. Compounds with hypotensive actions should generally be avoided. For example, anticholinergic agents are a better initial choice than dopaminergic compounds for parkinsonism. Anesthetic management poses unique problems since these patients may have abnormal baroreceptor reflexes, impaired sympathetic innervation of peripheral arterioles, exaggerated pharmacologic responses, abnormal fluid balance, or adrenal medullary insufficiency. More important than the choice of anesthetic is awareness by the physician of the implications that autonomic failure may have for peri- and postoperative monitoring and management.

BIBLIOGRAPHY

BRAUS DF et al: The shoulder-hand syndrome after stroke: A prospective clinical trial. Ann Neurol 36:728, 1994

JANSEN RW, LIPSITZ LA: Postprandial hypotension: Epidemiology, pathophysiology, and clinical management. Ann Intern Med 122:286, 1995

LOW PA (ed): *Clinical Autonomic Disorders*, 2d ed. New York, Lippincott-Raven, 1997

——— et al: Efficacy of midodrine vs. placebo in neurogenic orthostatic hypotension. JAMA 277:1046, 1997

MATHIAS CJ: Orthostatic hypotension: Causes, mechanisms, and influencing factors. Neurology 45(Suppl 5):S6, 1995

MCLEOD JG: Autonomic dysfunction in peripheral nerve disease. Invited review. Muscle Nerve 15:3, 1992

POLINSKY RJ: Clinical autonomic neuropharmacology. Neurol Clin 8:77, 1990

ROBERTSON D, DAVIS TL: Recent advances in the treatment of orthostatic hypotension. Neurology 45(Suppl 5):S26, 1995

SHANNON JR et al: Orthostatic intolerance and tachycardia associated with norepinephrine-transporter deficiency. N Engl J Med 342:541, 2000

STOLMAN LP: Treatment of hyperhidrosis. Dermatol Clin 16:863–67, 1998

VELDMAN PHJM et al: Signs and symptoms of reflex sympathetic dystrophy: Prospective study of 829 patients. Lancet 342:1012, 1993

VERNINO S et al: Autoantibodies to ganglionic acetylcholine receptors in autoimmune autonomic neuropathies. N Engl J Med 343:847, 2000

367

M. Flint Beal, Stephen L. Hauser

COMMON DISORDERS OF THE CRANIAL NERVES

Symptoms and signs of cranial nerve pathology are common in internal medicine. They often develop in the context of a widespread neurologic disturbance, and in such situations cranial nerve involvement may represent the initial manifestation of the illness. In other disorders, involvement is largely restricted to one or several cranial nerves; these distinctive disorders are reviewed in this chapter. Disorders of ocular movement are discussed in Chap 28; disorders of smell, taste, and hearing in Chap 29; and vertigo and disorders of vestibular function in Chap 21.

DISORDERS OF FACIAL SENSATION

The trigeminal (fifth cranial) nerve supplies sensation to the skin of the face and anterior half of the head (Fig. 367-1). Its motor part innervates the masseter and pterygoid masticatory muscles.

TRIGEMINAL NEURALGIA (TIC DOULOUREUX) The most striking disorder of trigeminal nerve function is tic douloureux, a condition characterized by excruciating paroxysms of pain in the lips, gums, cheek, or chin and, very rarely, in the distribution of the ophthalmic division of the fifth nerve. The disorder occurs almost exclusively in middle-aged and elderly persons. The pain seldom lasts more than a few seconds or a minute or two but may be so intense that the patient winces, hence the term *tic*. The paroxysms recur frequently, both day and night, for several weeks at a time. Another characteristic feature is the initiation of pain by stimuli applied to certain areas on the face, lips, or tongue ("trigger zones") or by movement of these parts. *Objective signs of sensory loss cannot be demonstrated*. The adequate stimulus to a trigger zone for precipitating an attack is a tactile one and possibly tickle, rather than a noxious or thermal stimulus. Usually a spatial and temporal summation of impulses is necessary to trigger an attack, which is followed by a refractory period of up to 2 or 3 min.

The *diagnosis* of this disorder rests on these strict clinical criteria, and the condition must be distinguished from other forms of facial and cephalic neuralgia and pain arising from diseases of the jaw, teeth, or sinuses (Chap. 15). Tic douloureux is usually without assignable cause; in typical cases, neuroimaging studies are not necessary. On occasion, when trigeminal neuralgia develops in a younger adult, it may be due to a plaque of multiple sclerosis at the root entry zone of the fifth nerve in the pons. Very rarely it occurs with herpes zoster or a tumor. To a degree that remains uncertain, pain of tic douloureux may be caused by a redundant or tortuous blood vessel in the posterior fossa, causing an irritative lesion of the nerve or its root. Usually, however, lesions such as aneurysms, neurofibromas, or meningiomas affecting the nerve produce a loss of sensation (trigeminal neuropathy, see below).

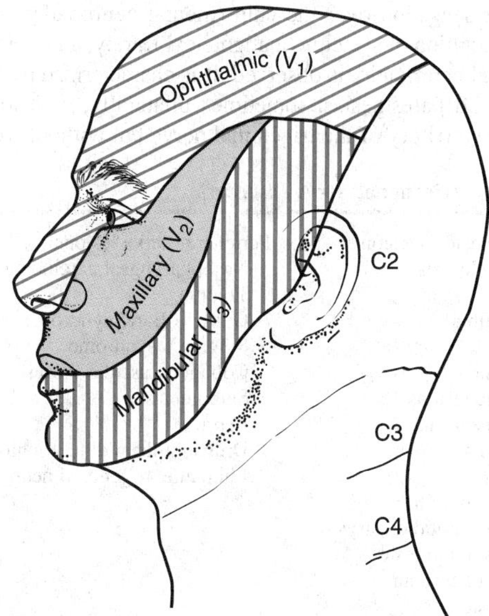

FIGURE 367-1 The three major sensory divisions of the trigeminal nerve consist of the ophthalmic, maxillary, and mandibular nerves.

℞ TREATMENT Drug therapy with carbamazepine is the initial treatment of choice and is effective in approximately 50 to 75% of patients. Carbamazepine should be started as a single daily dose of 100 mg taken with food, and increased gradually (by 100 mg daily every 1 to 2 days) until substantial (>50%) pain relief is achieved. Most patients require a maintenance dose of 200 mg qid. Doses >1200 mg daily provide no additional benefit. Dizziness, imbalance, sedation, and rare cases of agranulocytosis are the most important side effects of carbamazepine. If treatment is effective, it is usually continued for approximately 1 month and then tapered as tolerated. If carbamazepine is not well tolerated or is ineffective, phenytoin, 300 to 400 mg daily, can be tried. Baclofen may also be administered, either alone or in combination with carbamazepine or phenytoin. The initial dose is 5 to 10 mg tid, gradually increasing as needed to 20 mg qid.

If drug treatment fails, surgical therapy should be offered. The most widely applied procedure creates a heat lesion of the trigeminal (gasserian) ganglion or nerve, a method termed *radiofrequency thermal rhizotomy*. Injection of glycerol in Meckel's cave is a method preferred by some surgeons. Either procedure produces short-term relief in >95% of patients; however, long-term studies indicate that pain recurs in a substantial percentage of treated patients in some series. Complications and morbidity are infrequent in experienced hands. These procedures result in partial numbness of the face and carry a risk of corneal denervation with secondary keratitis when used for the rare instances of first-division trigeminal neuralgia.

A third treatment, microvascular decompression, requires a suboccipital craniectomy, a major procedure requiring several days of hospitalization. It has an 80% efficacy rate, but the pain may recur, and, in a small number of cases, there is damage to the eighth or seventh nerve.

TRIGEMINAL NEUROPATHY A variety of diseases in addition to tic douloureux may affect the trigeminal nerve (Table 367-1). Most present with sensory loss on the face or with weakness of the jaw muscles. Deviation of the jaw on opening indicates weakness of the pterygoids on the side to which the jaw deviates. Tumors of the middle cranial fossa (meningiomas), of the trigeminal nerve (schwannomas), or of the base of the skull (metastatic tumors) may cause a combination of motor and sensory signs. Lesions in the cavernous sinus can affect the first and second divisions of the trigeminal nerve, and lesions of the superior orbital fissure can affect the first (ophthalmic) division. The accompanying corneal anesthesia increases the risk of ulceration (neurokeratitis).

Loss of sensation over the chin (mental neuropathy) can be the only manifestation of systemic malignancy. Rarely, an idiopathic form of trigeminal neuropathy is observed. It is characterized by feelings of numbness and paresthesias, sometimes bilaterally, with loss of sensation in the territory of the trigeminal nerve but without weakness of the jaw. Recovery is the rule, but the symptoms may be troublesome for many months, or even years. Leprosy may involve the trigeminal nerves.

Tonic spasm of the masticatory muscles, known as *trismus*, is symptomatic of tetanus (Chap. 143). It may also occur as an idiosyncratic reaction in patients treated with phenothiazine drugs; lesser degrees may be associated with disease of the pharynx, temporomandibular joint, teeth, and gums.

Table 367-1 Trigeminal Nerve Disorders

Nuclear (brainstem) lesions, preganglionic and gasserian ganglion lesions	Peripheral nerve lesions
Nuclear (brainstem) lesions	Peripheral nerve lesions
Multiple sclerosis	Nasopharyngeal carcinoma
Stroke	Trauma
Syringobulbia	Guillain-Barré syndrome
Glioma	Sjögren's syndrome
Lymphoma	Collagen-vascular diseases
Preganglionic lesions	Sarcoidosis
Acoustic neuroma	Leprosy
Meningioma	Drugs (stilbamidine, trichloroethylene)
Metastasis	Idiopathic trigeminal neuropathy
Chronic meningitis	
Cavernous carotid aneurysm	
Gasserian ganglion lesions	
Trigeminal neuroma	
Herpes zoster	
Infection (spread from otitis media or mastoiditis)	

DISORDERS OF THE FACIAL NERVE

The seventh cranial nerve supplies all the muscles concerned with facial expression. The sensory component is small (the nervus intermedius); it conveys taste sensation from the anterior two-thirds of the tongue and probably cutaneous impulses from the anterior wall of the external auditory canal. The motor nucleus of the seventh nerve lies anterior and lateral to the abducens nucleus. After leaving the pons, the seventh nerve enters the internal auditory meatus with the acoustic nerve. The nerve continues its course in its own bony channel, the facial canal, and exits from the skull via the stylomastoid foramen. It then passes through the parotid gland and subdivides to supply the facial muscles.

A complete interruption of the facial nerve at the stylomastoid foramen paralyzes all muscles of facial expression. The corner of the mouth droops, the creases and skin folds are effaced, the forehead is unfurrowed, and the eyelids will not close. Upon attempted closure of the lids, the eye on the paralyzed side rolls upward (Bell's phenomenon). The lower lid sags also, and the punctum falls away from the conjunctiva, permitting tears to spill over the cheek. Food collects between the teeth and lips, and saliva may dribble from the corner of the mouth. The patient complains of a heaviness or numbness in the face, but sensory loss is rarely demonstrable and taste is intact.

If the lesion is in the middle ear portion, taste is lost over the anterior two-thirds of the tongue on the same side. If the nerve to the stapedius is interrupted, there is hyperacusis (painful sensitivity to loud sounds). Lesions in the internal auditory meatus may also affect the adjacent auditory and vestibular nerves, causing deafness, tinnitus, or dizziness. Intrapontine lesions that paralyze the face usually affect the abducens nucleus as well, and often the corticospinal and sensory tracts.

If the peripheral facial paralysis has existed for some time and recovery of motor function is incomplete, a continuous diffuse contraction of facial muscles may appear. The palpebral fissure becomes narrowed, and the nasolabial fold deepens. Attempts to move one group of facial muscles may result in contraction of all of them (associated movements, or *synkinesis*). Facial spasms may develop and persist indefinitely, being initiated by every facial movement (*hemifacial spasm*). This condition may represent a transient or permanent sequela to a Bell's palsy but may also be due to an irritative lesion of the facial nerve (e.g., an acoustic neuroma, an aberrant artery that compresses the nerve and is relieved by surgery, or a basilar artery aneurysm). However, in the most common form of hemifacial spasm, the cause and pathology are unknown. Anomalous regeneration of the seventh nerve fibers may result in other troublesome phenomena. If fibers originally connected with the orbicularis oculi come to innervate the orbicularis oris, closure of the lids may cause a retraction of the mouth, or if fibers originally connected with muscles of the face later innervate the lacrimal gland, anomalous tearing ("crocodile tears") may occur with any activity of the facial muscles, such as eating. Yet another unusual facial synkinesia is one in which jaw opening causes a closure of the eyelids on the side of the facial palsy (jaw-winking).

BELL'S PALSY The most common form of facial paralysis is idiopathic, i.e., *Bell's palsy*. The incidence rate of this disorder is about 23 per 100,000 annually, or about 1 in 60 or 70 persons in a lifetime. The pathogenesis of the paralysis is unproven, but an association with herpes simplex virus type 1 DNA in endoneurial fluid and posterior auricular muscle has been documented.

Clinical Manifestations The onset of Bell's palsy is fairly abrupt, maximal weakness being attained by 48 h as a general rule. Pain behind the ear may precede the paralysis for a day or two. Taste sensation may be lost unilaterally, and hyperacusis may be present. In some cases there is mild cerebrospinal fluid (CSF) lymphocytosis. Magnetic resonance imaging (MRI) may reveal swelling and uniform enhancement of the geniculate ganglion and facial nerve, and, in some cases, entrapment of the swollen nerve in the temporal bone is noted. Fully 80% of patients recover within a few weeks or months. Electromyography may be of some prognostic value; evidence of denervation after 10 days indicates that there has been axonal degeneration and that there will be a long delay (3 months, as a rule) before regeneration occurs and that it may be incomplete. The presence of incomplete paralysis in the first week is the most favorable prognostic sign.

Differential Diagnosis There are many other causes of facial palsy that must be considered in the differential diagnosis of idiopathic Bell's palsy. Tumors that invade the temporal bone (carotid body, cholesteatoma, dermoid) may produce a facial palsy, but the onset is insidious and the course progressive. The *Ramsay Hunt syndrome*, presumably due to herpes zoster of the geniculate ganglion, consists of a severe facial palsy associated with a vesicular eruption in the pharynx, external auditory canal, and other parts of the cranial integument; often the eighth cranial nerve is affected as well. *Acoustic neuromas* frequently involve the facial nerve by local compression. Infarcts, demyelinating lesions of multiple sclerosis, and tumors are the common pontine lesions that interrupt the facial nerve fibers; other signs of brainstem involvement are usually present. Bilateral facial paralysis (facial diplegia) occurs in *Guillain-Barré syndrome* (Chap. 378) and also in a form of sarcoidosis known as *uveoparotid fever* (*Heerfordt syndrome*). Lyme disease is a frequent cause of facial palsies in endemic areas. The *Melkersson-Rosenthal syndrome* consists of a rarely encountered triad of recurrent facial paralysis, recurrent—and eventually permanent—facial (particularly labial) edema, and less constantly, plication of the tongue; its cause is unknown. Leprosy frequently involves the facial nerve, and facial neuropathy may also occur in diabetes mellitus.

All these forms of nuclear or peripheral facial palsy must be distinguished from the supranuclear type. In the latter, the frontalis and orbicularis oculi muscles are involved less than those of the lower part of the face, since the upper facial muscles are innervated by corticobulbar pathways from both motor cortices, whereas the lower facial muscles are innervated only by the opposite hemisphere. In supranuclear lesions there may be a dissociation of emotional and voluntary facial movements, and often some degree of paralysis of the arm and leg or an aphasia (in dominant hemisphere lesions) is conjoined.

Laboratory Evaluation The diagnosis of Bell's palsy can usually be made clinically in patients with (1) a typical presentation, (2) no risk factors or preexisting symptoms for other causes of facial paralysis, (3) absence of cutaneous lesions of herpes zoster in the external ear canal, and (4) a normal neurologic examination with the exception of the facial nerve. Particular attention to the eighth cranial nerve, which courses near to the facial nerve in the pontomedullary junction and in the temporal bone, and to other cranial nerves is essential. In atypical or uncertain cases, an erythrocyte sedimentation rate, testing for diabetes mellitus, a Lyme titer, chest x-ray for possible sarcoidosis, or MRI scanning may be indicated.

℞ TREATMENT Symptomatic measures include (1) the use of paper tape to depress the upper eyelid during sleep and prevent corneal drying, and (2) massage of the weakened muscles. A course of glucocorticoids, given as prednisone 60 to 80 mg daily during the first 5 days and then tapered over the next 5 days, appears to shorten the recovery period and modestly improve the functional outcome. In one double-blind study, patients treated within 3 days of onset with both prednisone and acyclovir (400 mg five times daily for 10 days) had a better outcome than patients treated with prednisone alone.

OTHER FACIAL DISORDERS *Facial hemiatrophy* occurs mainly in females and is characterized by a disappearance of fat in the dermal and subcutaneous tissues on one side of the face. It usually begins in adolescence or early adult years and is slowly progressive. In its advanced form, the affected side of the face is gaunt, and the skin is thin, wrinkled, and rather brown. The facial hair may turn white and fall out, and the sebaceous glands become atrophic. The muscles and bones are not involved as a rule. Sometimes the atrophy becomes bilateral. The condition is a form of lipodystrophy. Treatment is cosmetic, consisting of transplantation of skin and subcutaneous fat.

Facial myokymia refers to a fine rippling activity of the facial muscles; it may be caused by a plaque of multiple sclerosis. *Blepharospasm* is an involuntary recurrent spasm of both eyelids that occurs in elderly persons as an isolated phenomenon or with varying degrees of spasm of other facial muscles. Severe, persistent cases of blepharospasm or hemifacial spasm can be treated by local injection of botulinus toxin into the orbicularis oculi; the spasms are relieved for 3 to 4 months, and the injections can be repeated.

GLOSSOPHARYNGEAL NERVE DISORDERS

GLOSSOPHARYNGEAL NEURALGIA This form of neuralgia resembles trigeminal neuralgia in many respects but is much less common. The pain is intense and paroxysmal; it originates in the throat, approximately in the tonsillar fossa. In some cases the pain is localized in the ear or may radiate from the throat to the ear because of involvement of the tympanic branch of the glossopharyngeal nerve. Spasms of pain may be initiated by swallowing. There is no demonstrable sensory or motor deficit. Cardiac symptoms—bradycardia, hypotension, and fainting—have been reported. A trial of carbamazepine or phenytoin is the recommended therapy, but if that is unsuccessful, division of the glossopharyngeal nerve near the medulla is the definitive treatment. Percutaneous rhizotomy of glossopharyngeal and vagal fibers in the jugular foramen alleviates pain in some patients.

Very rarely, herpes zoster involves the glossopharyngeal nerve. Glossopharyngeal neuropathy in conjunction with vagus and accessory nerve palsies may also occur with a tumor or aneurysm in the posterior fossa or in the jugular foramen. Hoarseness due to vocal cord paralysis, some difficulty in swallowing, deviation of the soft palate to the intact side, anesthesia of the posterior wall of the pharynx, and weakness of the upper part of the trapezius and sternocleidomastoid muscles make up the syndrome (Table 367-2, jugular foramen syndrome).

DISORDERS OF THE VAGUS NERVE

DYSPHAGIA AND DYSPHONIA Complete interruption of the intracranial portion of one vagus nerve results in a characteristic paralysis. The soft palate droops ipsilaterally and does not rise in phonation. There is loss of the gag reflex on the affected side, as well as of the "curtain movement" of the lateral wall of the pharynx, whereby the faucial pillars move medially as the palate rises in saying "ah." The voice is hoarse and slightly nasal, and the vocal cord lies immobile midway between abduction and adduction. There may also be a loss of sensibility at the external auditory meatus and the posterior pinna.

The pharyngeal branches of both vagi may be affected in diphtheria; the voice has a nasal quality, and regurgitation of liquids through the nose occurs during the act of swallowing.

The vagus nerve may be involved at the meningeal level by neoplastic and infectious processes and within the medulla by tumors, vascular lesions (e.g., the lateral medullary syndrome of Wallenberg), and motor neuron disease. This nerve may be involved by the inflammatory lesion of herpes zoster. Polymyositis and dermatomyositis, which cause hoarseness and dysphagia by direct involvement of laryngeal and pharyngeal muscles, may be confused with diseases of the vagus nerves. Also, dysphagia is a symptom in some patients with

Table 367-2 Cranial Nerve Syndromes

Site	Cranial Nerves Involved	Usual Cause
Sphenoid fissure (superior orbital)	III, IV, first division V, VI	Invasive tumors of sphenoid bone; aneurysms
Lateral wall of cavernous sinus	III, IV, first division V, VI, often with proptosis	Infection, thrombosis, aneurysm, or fistula of cavernous sinus; invasive tumors from sinuses and sella turcica; benign granuloma responsive to glucocorticoids
Retrosphenoid space	II, III, IV, V, VI	Large tumors of middle cranial fossa
Apex of petrous bone	V, VI	Petrositis; tumors of petrous bone
Internal auditory meatus	VII, VIII	Tumors of petrous bone (dermoids, etc.); infectious processes; acoustic neuroma
Pontocerebellar angle	V, VII, VIII, and sometimes IX	Acoustic neuroma; meningioma
Jugular foramen	IX, X, XI	Tumors and aneurysms
Posterior laterocondylar space	IX, X, XI, XII	Tumors of parotid gland and carotid body and metastatic tumors
Posterior retroparotid space	IX, X, XI, XII and Horner syndrome	Tumors of parotid gland, carotid body, lymph nodes; metastatic tumor; tuberculous adenitis

myotonic dystrophy. →*See Chap. 40 for discussion of nonneurologic forms of dysphagia.*

The recurrent laryngeal nerves, especially the left, are most often damaged as a result of intrathoracic disease. Aneurysm of the aortic arch, an enlarged left atrium, and tumors of the mediastinum and bronchi are much more frequent causes of an isolated vocal cord palsy than are intracranial disorders.

When confronted with a case of laryngeal palsy, the physician must attempt to determine the site of the lesion. If it is intramedullary, there are usually other signs, such as ipsilateral cerebellar dysfunction, loss of pain and temperature sensation over the ipsilateral face and contralateral arm and leg, and an ipsilateral Horner syndrome. If the lesion is extramedullary, the glossopharyngeal and spinal accessory nerves are frequently involved (see jugular foramen syndrome, Table 367-2). If it is extracranial in the posterior laterocondylar or retroparotid space, there may be a combination of ninth, tenth, eleventh, and twelfth cranial nerve palsies and a Horner syndrome (Table 367-2). If there is no sensory loss over the palate and pharynx and no palatal weakness or dysphagia, the lesion is below the origin of the pharyngeal branches, which leave the vagus nerve high in the cervical region; the usual site of disease is then the mediastinum.

DISORDERS OF THE ACCESSORY NERVE

Isolated involvement of the accessory, or eleventh cranial, nerve can occur anywhere along its route, resulting in partial or complete paralysis of the sternocleidomastoid and trapezius muscles. More commonly, involvement occurs in combination with deficits of the ninth and tenth cranial nerves in the jugular foramen or after exit from the skull (Table 367-2). An idiopathic form of accessory neuropathy, akin to Bell's palsy, has been described, and it may be recurrent in some cases. Most but not all patients recover.

DISORDERS OF THE HYPOGLOSSAL NERVE

The twelfth cranial nerve supplies the ipsilateral muscles of the tongue. The nucleus of the nerve or its fibers of exit may be involved by intramedullary lesions such as tumor, poliomyelitis, or most often motor neuron disease. Lesions of the basal meninges and the occipital bones (platybasia, invagination of occipital condyles, Paget's disease) may compress the nerve in its extramedullary course or in the hypoglossal canal. Isolated lesions of unknown cause can occur. Atrophy and fasciculation of the tongue develop weeks to months after interruption of the nerve.

MULTIPLE CRANIAL NERVE PALSIES

Several cranial nerves may be affected by the same disease process. In this situation, the main clinical problem is to determine whether the lesion lies within the brainstem or outside it. Lesions that lie on the surface of the brainstem are characterized by involvement of adjacent cranial nerves (often occurring in succession) and late and rather slight involvement of the long sensory and motor pathways and segmental structures lying within the brainstem. The opposite is true of intramedullary, intrapontine, and intramesencephalic lesions. The extramedullary lesion is more likely to cause bone erosion or enlargement of the foramens of exit of cranial nerves. The intramedullary lesion involving cranial nerves often produces a crossed sensory or motor paralysis (cranial nerve signs on one side of the body and tract signs on the opposite side).

Involvement of multiple cranial nerves outside the brainstem is frequently the result of diabetes or trauma (sudden onset), localized infections such as herpes zoster (acute onset), infectious and noninfectious causes of meningitis (Chap. 374) or granulomatous diseases such as Wegener's granulomatosis (subacute onset), Behçet's disease, or tumors and enlarging saccular aneurysms (chronic development). Of the tumors, lymphomas, neurofibromas, meningiomas, chordomas, cholesteatomas, carcinomas, and sarcomas have all been observed to involve a succession of lower cranial nerves. Owing to their anatomic relationships, the multiple cranial nerve palsies form a number of distinctive syndromes, listed in Table 367-2. Sarcoidosis is the cause of some cases of multiple cranial neuropathy, and chronic glandular tuberculosis (scrofula) the cause of a few others. Midline granuloma of the nasopharynx may also affect multiple cranial nerves, as do nasopharyngeal tumors, platybasia, basilar invagination of the skull, and the adult Chiari malformation. A purely motor disorder without atrophy always raises the question of myasthenia gravis (Chap. 380). Guillain-Barré syndrome commonly affects the facial nerves bilaterally (facial diplegia). In the Fisher variant of the Guillain-Barré syndrome, oculomotor paresis occurs with ataxia and areflexia in the limbs (Chap. 378). Wernicke encephalopathy can cause a severe ophthalmoplegia combined with other brainstem signs.

The *cavernous sinus syndrome* is a distinctive and frequently life-threatening disorder. It often presents as orbital or facial pain; orbital swelling and chemosis due to occlusion of the ophthalmic veins; fever; oculomotor neuropathy affecting the third, fourth, and sixth cranial nerves; and trigeminal neuropathy affecting the ophthalmic (V_1) and occasionally the maxillary (V_2) divisions of the trigeminal nerve. Cavernous sinus thrombosis, often secondary to infection from orbital cellulitis (frequently *Staphylococcus aureus*), a cutaneous source on the face, or sinusitis (especially with mucormycosis in diabetic patients), is the most frequent cause; other etiologies include aneurysm of the carotid artery, a carotid-cavernous fistula (orbital bruit may be present), meningioma, nasopharyngeal carcinoma or other tumor, or an idiopathic granulomatous disorder (Tolosa-Hunt syndrome). Due to the anatomy of the cavernous sinus (Fig. 367-2) the syndrome may extend to become bilateral. Early diagnosis is essential, especially in cases due to infection, and treatment depends upon the underlying etiology. In infectious cases, prompt administration of broad-spectrum antibiotics, drainage of any abcess cavities, and identification of the offending organism is essential. Anticoagulant therapy may benefit cases of primary thrombosis. Repair or occlusion of the carotid artery may be required for treatment of fistulas or aneurysms. The Tolosa-Hunt syndrome generally responds to glucocorticoids.

An idiopathic form of multiple cranial nerve involvement on one or both sides of the face is occasionally seen (see Juncos and Beal). The syndrome consists of a subacute onset of boring facial pain, followed by paralysis of motor cranial nerves. The clinical features over-

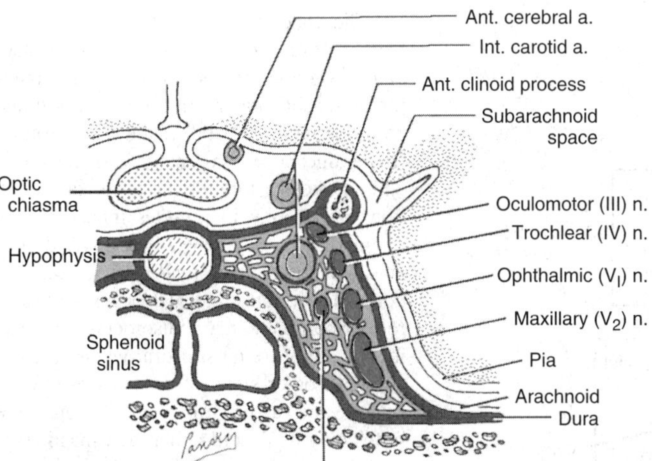

FIGURE 367-2 Anatomy of the cavernous sinus in coronal section, illustrating the location of the cranial nerves in relation to the vascular sinus, internal carotid artery (which loops anteriorly to the section), and surrounding structures.

lap those of the Tolosa-Hunt syndrome and appear to be due to idiopathic inflammation of the dura mater, which may be visualized by MRI. The syndrome is frequently responsive to glucocorticoids.

ACKNOWLEDGMENT

The authors acknowledge the contributions of Dr. Joseph B. Martin and Dr. Maurice Victor to this chapter in previous editions.

BIBLIOGRAPHY

ADAMS RD, VICTOR M: *Principles of Neurology*, 6th ed. New York, McGraw-Hill, 1997, chap 47, pp 1370–1385

ADOUR KK et al: Bell's palsy treatment with acyclovir and prednisone compared with prednisone alone: A double-blind, randomized, controlled trial. Ann Otol Rhinol Laryngol 105:371, 1996

BARKER FG et al: The long-term outcome of microvascular decompression for trigeminal neuralgia. N Engl J Med 334:1077, 1996

CHALK C, ISAACS H: Recurrent spontaneous accessory neuropathy. J Neurol Neurosurg Psychiatry 53:621, 1990

DELZELL JE, GRELLE AR: Trigeminal neuralgia: New treatment options for a well-known cause of facial pain. Arch Fam Med 8:264, 1999

FURUTA Y et al: Reactivation of herpes simplex virus type 1 in patients with Bell's palsy. J Med Virol 54:162, 1998

JACKSON CG, VON DOERSTEN PG: The facial nerve. Current trends in diagnosis, treatment, and rehabilitation. Med Clin North Am 83:179, 1999

JANKOVIC J, BRIN MF: Therapeutic uses of botulinum toxin. N Engl J Med 324:1186, 1991

JUNCOS JL, BEAL MF: Idiopathic cranial polyneuropathy. Brain 110:197, 1987

KEANE JR: Bilateral seventh nerve palsy: Analysis of 43 cases and review of the literature. Neurology 44:1198, 1994

KEANE JR: Fourth nerve palsy: Historical review and study of 215 inpatients. Neurology 43:2439, 1993

———: Twelfth-nerve palsy. Arch Neurol 53:561, 1996

LECKY BRF et al: Trigeminal sensory neuropathy. Brain 110:1463, 1987

LOSSOS A, SIEGAL T: Numb chin syndrome in cancer patients: Etiology, response to treatment, and prognostic significance. Neurology 42:1181, 1992

MIWA H et al: Recurrent cranial neuropathy as a clinical presentation of idiopathic inflammation of the dura mater: A possible relationship to Tolosa-Hunt syndrome and cranial pachymeningitis. J Neurol Sci 154:101, 1998

PHATOUROS CC et al: Carotid artery cavernous fistulas. Neurosurg Clin N Am 11:67, 2000

STEINER I, MATTAN Y: Bell's palsy and herpes viruses: to (acyclo)vir or not to (acyclo)vir? J Neurol Sci 170:19, 1999

WANG A, JANKOVIC J: Hemifacial spasm: Clinical findings and treatment. Muscle Nerve 21:1740, 1998

YOON KB et al: Long-term outcome of thermocoagulation for trigeminal neuralgia. Anaesthesia 54:803, 1999

368

Stephen L. Hauser

DISEASES OF THE SPINAL CORD

Diseases of the spinal cord are frequently devastating. They can produce quadriplegia, paraplegia, and sensory deficits far beyond the damage they would inflict elsewhere in the nervous system because the spinal cord contains, in a small cross-sectional area, almost the entire motor output and sensory input systems of the trunk and limbs. Many spinal cord diseases are reversible if recognized and treated at an early stage (Table 368-1); thus, they are among the most critical of neurologic emergencies. The efficient use of diagnostic procedures, guided by a working knowledge of the relevant anatomy and clinical features of common spinal cord diseases, is often the key to a successful outcome.

Approach to the Patient

Spinal Cord Anatomy Relevant to Clinical Signs The spinal cord is a thin, tubular extension of the central nervous system contained within the bony spinal canal. It originates at the medulla and continues caudally to terminate at the filum terminale, a fibrous extension of the conus medullaris that terminates at the coccyx. The adult spinal cord is approximately 18 inches long, oval or round in shape, and enlarged in the cervical and lumbar regions, where neurons that innervate the upper and lower extremities, respectively, are located. The white matter tracts containing ascending sensory and descending motor pathways are located peripherally, whereas nerve cell bodies are clustered in an inner region shaped like a four-leaf clover that surrounds the central canal (anatomically an extension of the fourth ventricle). The membranes that cover the spinal cord—the pia, arachnoid, and dura—are continuous with those of the brainstem and cerebral hemispheres.

The spinal cord is somatotopically organized, consisting of 31 segments, each containing an exiting ventral motor root and entering dorsal sensory root (Fig. 368-1). During embryologic development, growth of the cord lags behind that of the vertebral column, and in the adult the spinal cord ends at approximately the first lumbar vertebral body. The lower spinal nerves take an increasingly downward course to exit via the appropriate intervertebral foramina. The first seven pairs of cervical spinal nerves exit above the same-numbered vertebral bodies, whereas all the subsequent nerves exit below the same-numbered vertebral bodies; this situation is due to the presence of eight cervical spinal cord segments but only seven cervical vertebrae. The approxi-

Table 368-1 Some Treatable Spinal Cord Disorders

Compressive
Epidural, intradural, or intramedullary neoplasm
Epidural abscess
Epidural hemorrhage
Cervical spondylosis
Herniated disc
Posttraumatic compression by fractured or displaced vertebra or hemorrhage
Vascular
Arteriovenous malformation
Inflammatory
Transverse myelitis
Multiple sclerosis
Infectious
Viral: Herpes simplex type 2
Bacterial: Syphilis, tuberculosis, listeria, other
Parasitic: Schistosomiasis, toxoplasmosis
Developmental
Syringomyelia
Metabolic
Subacute combined degeneration

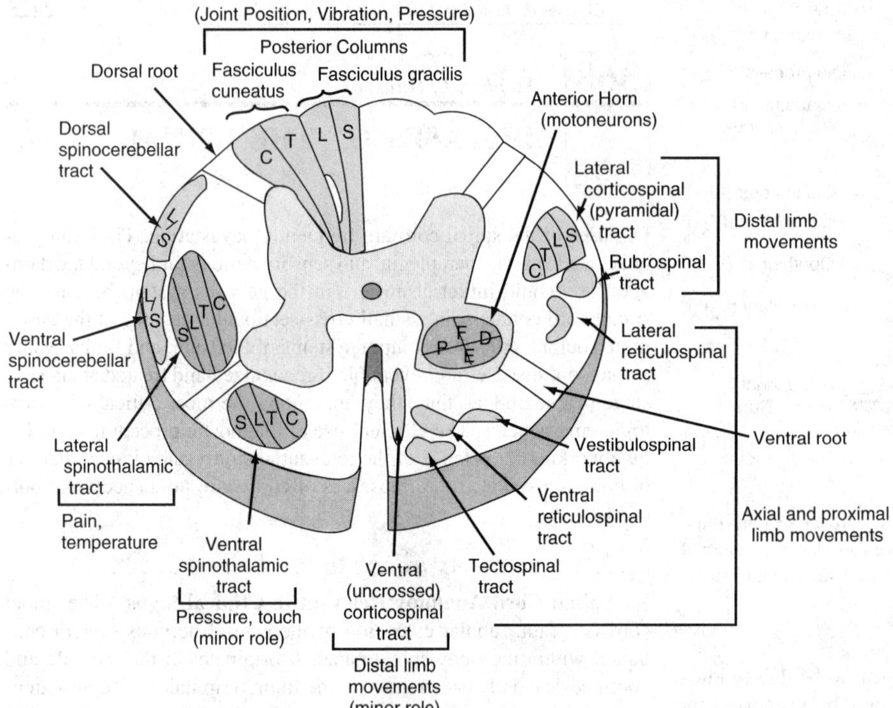

FIGURE 368-1 Transverse section through the spinal cord, composite representation, illustrating the principal ascending (*left*) and descending (*right*) pathways. The lateral and ventral spinothalamic tracts (*dark-blue*) ascend contralateral to the side of the body that is innervated. C, cervical; T, thoracic; L, lumbar; S, sacral; P, proximal; D, distal; F, flexors; E, extensors.

mate relationship between spinal cord segments and the corresponding vertebral bodies is shown in Table 368-2. These relationships assume importance for localization of lesions that cause spinal cord compression; a T10 spinal cord level, for example, indicates involvement of the cord adjacent to the seventh or eighth thoracic vertebral body.

Level of the lesion The presence of a *level* below which sensory, motor, and/or autonomic function is disturbed is a hallmark of spinal cord disease. A sensory level is sought by asking the patient to identify as sharp a pinprick stimulus or as cool a cold stimulus (a dry tuning fork after immersion in cold water) applied to the low back and sequentially moved up toward the neck on each side. In general, a sensory level to pinprick or temperature, indicating damage to the spinothalamic tract, is located one to two segments below the actual level of a unilateral spinal cord lesion, but it may be at the level of the lesion when bilateral. That is because sensory fibers enter the cord at the dorsal root, synapse in the dorsal horn, and then ascend ipsilaterally for several segments before crossing just anterior to the central canal to join the opposite spinothalamic tract. Lesions that disrupt descending corticospinal and bulbospinal tracts cause paraplegia or quadriplegia, with increased muscle tone, exaggerated deep tendon reflexes, and extensor plantar signs. Such lesions also typically produce autonomic disturbances, with disturbed sweating and bladder, bowel, and sexual dysfunction. A sweat level may be determined by drawing a spoon up the torso. There will be little resistance to movement of the spoon along the dry, nonsweating skin; at the level at which sweating begins, resistance will suddenly increase.

Table 368-2 Spinal Cord Levels Relative to the Vertebral Bodies

Spinal Cord Level	Corresponding Vertebral Body
Upper cervical	Same as cord level
Lower cervical	1 level higher
Upper thoracic	2 levels higher
Lower thoracic	2 to 3 levels higher
Lumbar	T10–T12
Sacral	T12–L1
Coccygeal	L1

The uppermost level of a spinal cord lesion is often localized by attention to *segmental signs* corresponding to disturbed motor or sensory innervation by an individual cord segment. A band of altered sensation (hyperalgesia or hyperpathia) at the upper end of the sensory disturbance, fasciculations or atrophy in muscles innervated by one or several segments, or a single diminished or absent deep tendon reflex may be noted. These signs may also occur with focal root or peripheral nerve disorders; thus, segmental signs are most useful when they occur with other signs of cord disease. With severe and acute transverse lesions, the limbs may be flaccid rather than spastic (so-called spinal shock). This state may last for several days, rarely for weeks, and may be initially mistaken for extensive damage to many segments of the cord (as in ascending necrotic myelopathy associated with cancer) or as polyneuropathy. Brief clonic or myoclonic movements of the limbs often precede paralysis in acute transverse lesions, particularly those due to cord infarction.

Patterns of spinal cord disease The location of the major ascending and descending pathways of the spinal cord are shown in Fig. 368-1. Most fiber tracts—including the posterior columns and the spinocerebellar and pyramidal tracts—travel ipsilateral to the side of the body they innervate. As noted above, afferent fibers mediating pain and temperature sensation are unusual in that they ascend contralaterally as the spinothalamic tract. The anatomic relationships of these various fiber tracts and nuclei produce distinctive clinical syndromes that are pathognomonic of spinal cord disease and that often provide clues to the underlying disease process.

BROWN-SEQUARD HEMICORD SYNDROME This syndrome consists of ipsilateral weakness (pyramidal tract) and loss of joint position and vibratory sense (posterior column), with contralateral loss of pain and temperature sense (spinothalamic tract) below the lesion. The sensory level for pain and temperature is one or two levels below the lesion. Segmental signs, such as radicular pain, muscle atrophy, or loss of a deep tendon reflex, when they occur, are unilateral. Pure examples of hemicord syndromes are rare; partial or bilateral forms are more common. Partial syndromes may involve the dorsal (posterior) quadrant, producing ipsilateral loss of vibration and position sense, or ventral (anterior) quadrant with ipsilateral paralysis and contralateral loss of pain and temperature sense.

CENTRAL CORD SYNDROME The central cord syndrome results from disorders of gray matter nerve cells and crossing spinothalamic tracts near the central canal. In the cervical cord, the central cord syndrome produces arm weakness out of proportion to leg weakness and a "dissociated" sensory loss consisting of loss of pain and temperature sense in a cape distribution over the shoulders, lower neck, and upper trunk with intact light touch, joint position, and vibration sense. Trauma, syringomyelia, tumors, and anterior spinal artery ischemia are common causes of the central cord syndrome.

ANTERIOR TWO-THIRDS SYNDROME This syndrome results from extensive bilateral disease of the spinal cord that spares the posterior columns. All spinal cord functions—motor, sensory and autonomic—are lost below the level of the lesion, with the striking exception of intact vibration and position sensation. The etiology is vascular, either thromboembolism of the anterior spinal artery or compression of this vessel by mass lesions within the spinal canal.

INTRAMEDULLARY AND EXTRAMEDULLARY SYNDROMES The diagnosis of spinal cord disorders frequently requires that intramedullary processes, which arise within the substance of the cord, be distinguished from extramedullary processes that compress the spinal cord or its vascular supply. Distinguishing features are relative and serve only as rough guides to clinical decision making. With extramedullary lesions, radicular pain is often prominent, and there is early sacral sensory loss (lateral spinothalamic tract) and spastic weakness in the legs (corticospinal tract) due to the superficial location of these fibers in the lateral spinal cord, which renders them susceptible to external compression. Intramedullary lesions tend to produce poorly localized burning pain rather than radicular pain and spare sensation in the perineal and sacral areas; corticospinal tract signs may appear late. With extramedullary lesions, the distinction between extradural and intradural masses is important, as the former are generally malignant and the latter benign; a long duration of symptoms favors an intradural origin.

Specific localizing signs • *CERVICAL CORD* High cervical cord lesions are frequently life-threatening, producing quadriplegia and weakness of respiratory muscles innervated by the phrenic nerve (C3-C5). There is diaphragmatic paralysis, and breathing is possible only by use of accessory muscles of respiration. Extensive lesions near the junction of the cervical cord and medulla are usually fatal owing to involvement of adjacent medullary centers, which results in vasomotor and respiratory collapse. Partial lesions in this area, generally due to trauma, may interrupt decussating pyramidal tract fibers destined for the legs, which cross below those of the arms, resulting in a "crural paresis" of the lower limbs. Compressive lesions near the foramen magnum may produce weakness of the ipsilateral shoulder and arm followed by weakness of the ipsilateral leg, then the contralateral leg, and finally the contralateral arm; the patient may complain of suboccipital pain spreading to the neck and shoulders. Lesions at C4-C5 produce quadriplegia with preserved respiratory function. At the mid-cervical (C5-C6) level, there is relative sparing of shoulder muscles and loss of biceps and brachioradialis reflexes. Lesions at C7 spare the biceps but produce weakness of finger and wrist extensors and loss of the triceps reflex. Lesions at C8 paralyze finger and wrist flexion, and the finger flexor reflex is lost. In general, cervical cord disorders are best localized by the pattern of weakness that ensues, whereas sensory deficits have less localizing value. A Horner's syndrome (miosis, ptosis, and facial hypohidrosis) may also occur ipsilateral to cervical cord lesions at any level.

THORACIC CORD Lesions of the thoracic cord are best localized by identification of a sensory level on the trunk. Sensory dermatomes of the body are shown in Fig. 23-2; useful markers are at the nipples (T4) and umbilicus (T10). Weakness of the legs and disturbances of bladder, bowel, or sexual function may also accompany damage to the thoracic cord. The abdominal wall musculature, supplied by the lower thoracic cord, is observed during movements of respiration or coughing or by asking the patient to interlock the fingers behind the head in the supine position and attempt to sit up. Lesions at T9-T10 paralyze the lower, but spare the upper, abdominal muscles, resulting in upward movement of the umbilicus when the abdominal wall contracts (Beevor's sign) and in loss of lower, but not upper, superficial abdominal reflexes (Chap. 356). With unilateral lesions, attempts to contract the abdominal wall produce movement of the umbilicus to the normal side; superficial abdominal reflexes are absent on the involved side. Midline back pain is a useful localizing sign in the thoracic region.

LUMBAR CORD The lumbar and sacral cord segments progressively decrease in size, and focal lesions of these segments are less easily localized than in cervical and thoracic regions. Lesions at L2-L4 paralyze flexion and adduction of the thigh, weaken leg extension at the knee, and abolish the patellar reflex. Lesions at L5-S1 paralyze movements of the foot and ankle, flexion at the knee, and extension of the thigh, and abolish the ankle jerk (S1). A cutaneous reflex useful in localization of lumbar cord disease is the cremasteric reflex (Chap. 356), which is segmentally innervated at L1-L2.

SACRAL CORD/CONUS MEDULLARIS The conus medullaris is the tapered caudal termination of the spinal cord, comprising the lower sacral and single coccygeal segments. Isolated lesions of the conus medullaris spare motor and reflex functions in the legs. The conus syndrome is distinctive, consisting of bilateral saddle anesthesia (S3-S5), prominent bladder and bowel dysfunction (urinary retention and incontinence with lax anal tone), and impotence. The bulbocavernosus (S2-S4) and anal (S4-S5) reflexes are absent (Chap. 356). Muscle strength is largely preserved. Lesions of the conus medullaris must be distinguished from those of the cauda equina, the cluster of nerve roots derived from the lower cord as they descend to their exits in the intervertebral foramina. Cauda equina lesions are characterized by severe low back or radicular pain, asymmetric leg weakness or sensory loss, variable areflexia in the lower extremities, and relative sparing of bowel and bladder function. Mass lesions in the lower spinal canal may produce a mixed clinical picture in which elements of both cauda equina and conus medullaris syndromes coexist. →*Cauda equina syndromes are discussed in Chap. 16.*

ACUTE AND SUBACUTE SPINAL CORD DISEASES

Acute and subacute spinal cord disorders are commonly due to extramedullary compression (tumor, infection, spondylosis, or trauma), infarction or hemorrhage, or inflammation. In this category are some of the most dangerous—and treatable—disorders in clinical practice. Early recognition is the key to successful management. Epidural compression due to malignancy often presents with warning signs, generally neck or back pain, bladder disturbances, or sensory symptoms, that precede the development of paralysis. Infarction, hemorrhage, or spinal subluxation is more likely to produce sudden "strokelike" myelopathy without antecedent symptoms.

NEOPLASTIC SPINAL CORD COMPRESSION Neoplasms of the spinal canal may be extramedullary (epidural or intradural) or intramedullary. In adults, most neoplasms are epidural in origin, resulting from metastases to the adjacent vertebral body, spinous or transverse process, or pedicle. Vertebral metastases are essentially bone-marrow metastases, and the propensity of solid tumors to metastasize to the vertebral column probably reflects the high percentage of bone marrow located in the axial skeleton of older individuals. Retroperitoneal neoplasms (especially lymphomas or sarcomas) may enter the spinal canal through the intervertebral foramina; typically they produce radicular pain and other signs of root involvement prior to cord compression. Almost any malignant tumor can metastasize to the spinal canal, although breast, lung, prostate, kidney, lymphoma, and plasma cell dyscrasia are particularly frequent. The thoracic cord is most commonly involved; exceptions are metastases from prostate and ovarian cancer, which occur disproportionately in the sacral and lumbar vertebrae, perhaps resulting from spread through Batson's plexus, a network of veins along the anterior surface of the spinal cord in the epidural space.

Pain is the initial symptom; it may be either aching and localized or sharp and radiating in quality. Pain indicates displacement of pain-sensitive structures, especially periosteum and meninges. The pain worsens with movement, coughing, or sneezing and may awaken patients at night. The recent onset of back pain, particularly if in the thoracic spine (which is uncommonly involved by spondylosis), should prompt consideration of vertebral metastasis. Rarely, pain is mild or absent. Pain typically precedes signs of cord compression by weeks or even months, but once cord compression occurs, it is always progressive and may advance rapidly. Therapy is effective only if administered early, when signs of cord dysfunction are mild or absent; therapy will not reverse a complete paralysis that has been present for >48 h. These realities highlight the importance of prompt recognition and efficient management of these lesions.

Plain radiographs of the spine and radionuclide bone scans have only a limited role in diagnosis because they fail to identify 15 to 20% of metastatic vertebral lesions and may miss paravertebral masses that reach the epidural space by growth through the intervertebral foramina.

Magnetic resonance imaging (MRI) provides excellent anatomic resolution of the site and extent of the tumor (Fig. 368-2); at most centers, MRI has largely replaced computed tomography (CT) and myelography in the diagnosis of epidural masses. MRI can often distinguish between malignant lesions and other masses—epidural abscess, tuberculoma, or epidural hemorrhage, among others—that present in a similar fashion. Vertebral metastases are usually hypointense relative to a normal bone marrow signal on T1-weighted MRI scans; after the administration of gadolinium, contrast enhancement may "normalize" the appearance of the tumor by increasing its intensity to that of normal bone marrow. In contrast to infection, vertebral metastases typically do not cross the disk space. Nonetheless, it can be difficult to distinguish between infection and malignancy by MRI.

Because imaging resources are scarce, and both cancer and back pain are common, it is important to convey to the radiologist an estimate of the urgency of the imaging procedure requested. If signs of spinal cord involvement are present, imaging should be obtained on an emergency basis. If there are radicular symptoms but no evidence of myelopathy, it is usually safe to defer imaging for 24 to 48 h. With back or neck pain only, imaging studies should be obtained within a few days. Finally, up to 40% of patients who present with symptomatic disease at one level are found to have asymptomatic epidural disease elsewhere; thus, the entire spine should be imaged in all patients with epidural malignancy.

℞ **TREATMENT** Management includes glucocorticoids to reduce interstitial edema, local radiotherapy (initiated as early as possible) to the symptomatic lesion, and specific therapy for the underlying tumor type. Glucocorticoids (dexamethasone, 40 mg daily) can be administered before the imaging study if the clinical suspicion is strong and continued at a lower dose (20 mg daily in divided doses) until radiotherapy (a total of 3000 cGy administered in 15 daily fractions) is completed. Radiotherapy appears to be as effective as surgery, even for classically radioresistant metastases. Biopsy of the epidural mass is usually unnecessary in patients with known preexisting cancer, but biopsy is indicated if a history of underlying cancer is lacking. Surgery, either decompression or vertebral body resection, should be considered when signs of cord compression worsen despite radiotherapy, when the maximum tolerated dose of radiotherapy has been delivered previously to the site, or when a vertebral compression fracture contributes to cord compression. A good response to radiotherapy can be expected in individuals who are ambulatory at presentation; new weakness is prevented, and some recovery of motor function occurs in approximately half of treated patients. Fixed motor deficits—paraplegia or quadriplegia—do not usually respond to either radiotherapy or surgery.

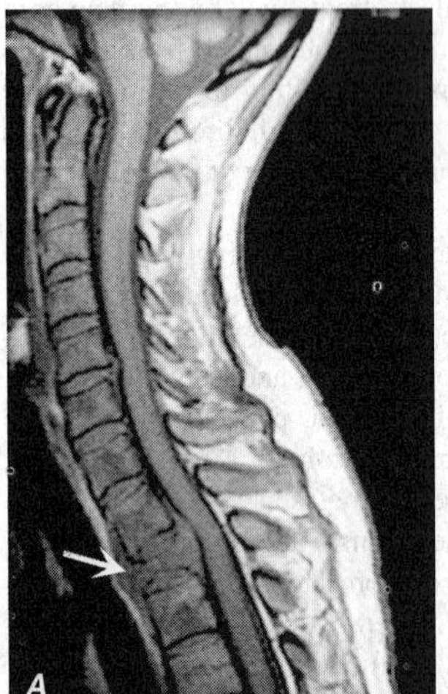

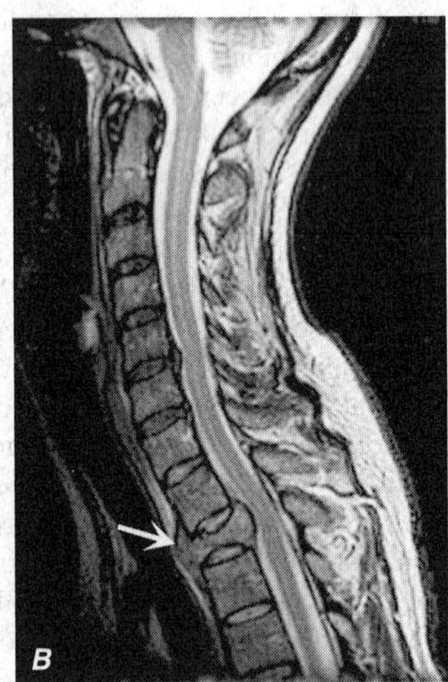

FIGURE 368-2 Epidural spinal cord compression due to breast carcinoma. Sagittal T1-weighted (*A*) and T2-weighted (*B*) MRI scans through the cervicothoracic junction reveal a compression fracture of the second thoracic vertebral body with posterior displacement and compression of the upper thoracic spinal cord. The low-intensity bone marrow signal in *A* signifies replacement by tumor.

In contrast to tumors of the epidural space, most intradural mass lesions are slow-growing and benign. Meningiomas and neurofibromas account for most of these lesions, with occasional cases representing chordoma, lipoma, dermoid, or sarcoma. Meningiomas (Fig. 368-3) are often located posterior to the thoracic cord or near the foramen magnum, although they can arise from the meninges anywhere along the spinal canal. Neurofibromas are benign tumors of the nerve sheath that typically arise near the posterior root; when multiple, neurofibromatosis (Chap. 370) is the likely etiology. Symptoms usually begin with radicular sensory symptoms followed by an asymmetric, progressive spinal cord syndrome. Therapy is surgical resection.

Primary intramedullary tumors of the spinal cord are uncommon. They typically present as central cord or hemicord syndromes, often in the cervical region; there may be poorly localized burning pain in the extremities and sparing of sacral sensation. In adults, most of these lesions are either ependymomas, hemangioblastomas, or low-grade astrocytomas (Fig. 368-4). Complete resection of an intramedullary ependymoma is often possible with microsurgical techniques. Debulking of an intramedullary astrocytoma can also be helpful, as these are often slowly growing lesions; the value of adjunctive radiotherapy is uncertain. Secondary (metastatic) intramedullary tumors are rare.

SPINAL CORD INFARCTION The spinal cord is supplied by three arteries that course vertically over its surface, a single anterior spinal artery, and paired posterior spinal arteries. At each segment, paired penetrators branching from the anterior spinal artery supply the anterior two-thirds of the spinal cord; the posterior spinal arteries, which often become less distinct below the midthoracic level, supply the posterior columns. Rostrally, the spinal arteries arise from the vertebral arteries. During embryogenesis, arterial feeders arise at each segmental level, but most involute before birth; generally, between

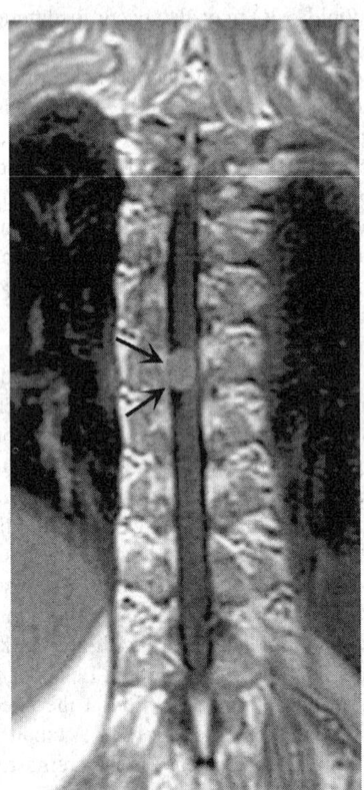

FIGURE 368-3 MRI of a thoracic meningioma. Coronal T1-weighted postcontrast image through the thoracic spinal cord demonstrates intense enhancement of a well-circumscribed extramedullary mass (*arrows*) which displaces the spinal cord to the left, widening the cistern adjacent to the mass.

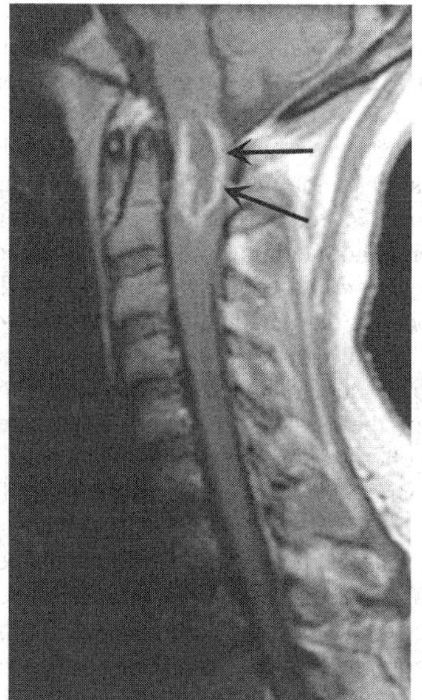

FIGURE 368-4 MRI of an intramedullary astrocytoma. Sagittal T1-weighted postcontrast image through the cervical spine demonstrates expansion of the upper cervical spine by a mass lesion emanating from within the spinal cord at the cervicomedullary junction. Irregular peripheral enhancement occurs within the mass (*arrows*).

three and eight major feeders remain, arising from the vertebral, subclavian, intercostal (off the aorta), iliac, and sacral arteries. In addition to the vertebral arteries, in adults, anterior spinal artery feeders often occur at C6, at an upper thoracic level, and at T11-L2 (artery of Adamkiewicz). Feeders from the aorta are more likely to arise from the left side.

Spinal cord ischemia can occur at any level. The signs are determined by the level of the lesion and by the individual vascular anatomy, including areas of watershed flow and potential for anastomosis. The anterior spinal artery is discontinuous in some individuals, increasing the importance of feeders to the lower cord. With systemic hypotension, cord infarction occurs at the level of greatest ischemic risk, often T3-T4, and also at boundary zones between the anterior and posterior spinal artery territories. The latter may result in an acute—or more commonly progressive—syndrome of weakness and spasticity with little sensory change resembling amyotrophic lateral sclerosis (ALS).

Acute infarction in the territory of the anterior spinal artery produces paraplegia or quadriplegia, dissociated sensory loss affecting pain and temperature sense but sparing vibration and position sense, and loss of sphincter control. Onset may be sudden and dramatic or progressive over minutes or hours. Sharp midline or radiating back pain localized to the area of ischemia is frequently noted. Partial infarction of one anterior hemicord (hemiplegia or monoplegia and crossed pain and temperature loss) may also occur. Areflexia due to spinal shock is often present initially; with time, hyperreflexia and spasticity appear.

The acute onset of pain, sparing of posterior column function, and sharply demarcated spinal cord level distinguish anterior spinal artery infarction from epidural spinal cord compression, in which pain is often chronic, posterior column sense is impaired, and a cord level is indistinct. An exception to this rule is when epidural tumors compress or invade vascular structures, resulting in an anterior spinal artery syndrome. Infarction in the territory of the posterior spinal arteries, resulting in loss of posterior column function, also occurs and may be underrecognized as a cause of loss of position and vibration sense.

Spinal cord infarction is associated with aortic atherosclerosis, dissecting aortic aneurysm (chest or back pain with diminished pulses in legs), or hypotension from any cause. Cardiogenic emboli, vasculitis related to collagen vascular disease, and surgical clipping of aortic aneurysms are other predisposing conditions. Occasional cases de-

velop either during pregnancy or after acute back trauma or exercise that by an unknown mechanism leads to embolism of nucleus pulposus material into spinal vessels. In a substantial number of cases, no cause can be found, and thromboembolism in arterial feeders is suspected.

MRI is often normal but is useful to exclude other causes of acute myelopathy, in particular epidural compression, spinal cord hemorrhage (hematomyelia), infectious myelitis, or transverse myelitis. Lumbar puncture is indicated whenever the underlying cause has not been clarified by MRI. Other useful laboratory studies include a sedimentation rate to search for an underlying vasculitis, Venereal Disease Research Laboratories test, and evaluation for aortic or cardiac disease or for a hypercoagulable state.

Therapy is directed at treatment of any predisposing condition. In cord infarction due to presumed thromboembolism, anticoagulation is probably not indicated, with the exception of the unusual transient ischemic attack or incomplete infarction with a stuttering or progressive course.

EPIDURAL HEMATOMA Hemorrhage into the epidural (or subdural) space can compress the spinal cord or roots. Presenting symptoms are the acute onset of focal or radicular pain followed by variable signs of a spinal cord or conus medullaris disorder. Trauma, tumor, or blood dyscrasias are predisposing conditions. Rare cases complicate lumbar puncture or epidural anesthesia, sometimes in association with use of low-molecular-weight heparin. Epidural hematoma can also occur on an idiopathic basis. MRI confirms the clinical suspicion and can delineate the extent of the bleed. Extrinsic spinal cord compression from any cause is a medical emergency, and appropriate treatment consists of prompt recognition, reversal of any underlying clotting disorder, and emergency surgical decompression. Surgery may be followed by substantial recovery, especially in patients with some preservation of motor function preoperatively. Because of the risk of hemorrhage, lumbar puncture should be avoided whenever possible in patients with thrombocytopenia or other coagulopathics (including those due to therapeutic anticoagulation) until the underlying bleeding disorder is reversed.

HEMATOMYELIA Hemorrhage into the substance of the spinal cord is rare. It may result from trauma, an intraparenchymal vascular malformation (see below), vasculitis due to polyarteritis nodosa or lupus erythematosus, bleeding disorders, or spinal cord infection or neoplasm. Hematomyelia presents as an acute painful transverse myelopathy. With large lesions, extension into the subarachnoid space may occur, resulting in subarachnoid hemorrhage (Chap. 361). Diagnosis is best made by MRI. Therapy is supportive, and surgical intervention is generally not useful. An exception is hematomyelia due to an underlying vascular malformation; in such cases, selective spinal angiography may be indicated, followed by acute surgical intervention to evacuate the clot and remove the underlying vascular lesion.

EPIDURAL ABSCESS Spinal epidural abscess presents as a clinical triad of pain, fever, and rapidly progressive weakness. Prompt recognition of this distinctive and treatable medical emergency will in most cases prevent severe and permanent sequelae. Epidural abscesses can form anywhere along the spinal canal. Pain is almost always present, either midline along the spine or radicular in type. The duration of pain prior to presentation is generally two weeks or less, but in some chronic cases it may be several months or longer. Fever is common, often accompanied by an elevated white blood cell count or sedimentation rate. As the abscess expands, spinal cord injury results from venous congestion and thrombosis, thrombophlebitis of the epidural space, spinal artery disease, or cord compression. Once weakness and other signs of myelopathy appear, progression is often rapid, although it may be gradual.

Risk factors include impaired immune status (diabetes mellitus, renal failure, alcoholism, malignancy), intravenous drug abuse, and infections of the skin or other tissues. Two-thirds of epidural infections result from hematogenous spread from the skin (furunculosis), soft tissue (pharyngeal or dental abscesses), or deep viscera (bacterial endocarditis). One-third result from direct extension of a local infection to the subdural space; examples of local predisposing conditions are vertebral osteomyelitis, decubitus ulcers, or iatrogenic complications of lumbar puncture, epidural anesthesia, or spinal surgery.

Most cases are due to *Staphylococcus aureus*; gram-negative bacilli, *Streptococcus*, anaerobes, and fungi can also cause epidural abscesses. Tuberculosis from an adjacent vertebral source remains an important cause in the underdeveloped world. As the population ages and the number of immunosuppressed individuals increases, an increase in the incidence of spinal epidural abscess (currently 2 per 1000 hospital admissions) has been noted.

MRI scans (Fig. 368-5) localize the abscess and exclude a primary intraparenchymal lesion, for example, transverse myelitis or hematomyelia. Lumbar puncture is often not required but may be indicated if encephalopathy or other clinical signs raise the question of associated meningitis, which is present in fewer than 25% of cases. In such situations, the level of the tap should be planned carefully to minimize the risk of inducing either meningitis by passage of the needle through infected tissue or herniation from decompression below an area of obstruction to the flow of cerebrospinal fluid (CSF). A high cervical tap is often the safest approach. CSF abnormalities in subdural abscess consist of pleocytosis with a preponderance of polymorphonuclear cells, an elevated protein level, and a reduced glucose level. Blood cultures are positive in <25% of cases.

℞ TREATMENT Treatment is emergency decompressive laminectomy with debridement combined with long-term antibiotic treatment. Surgical evacuation prevents development of paralysis and may improve or reverse paralysis in evolution, but it is unlikely to improve deficits of more than several days duration. Antibiotics should be started empirically before surgery, modified on the basis of culture results, and usually continued for at least 4 weeks. If surgery is contraindicated or if there is a fixed paraplegia or quadriplegia that is unlikely to improve following surgery, long-term administration of systemic and oral antibiotics can be used; in such cases, coverage may be guided by results of positive blood cultures. However, paralysis may develop or progress during antibiotic therapy; thus, initial surgical management remains the treatment of choice.

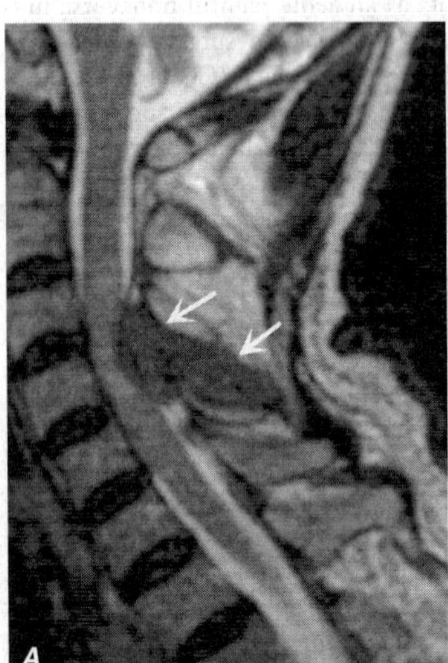

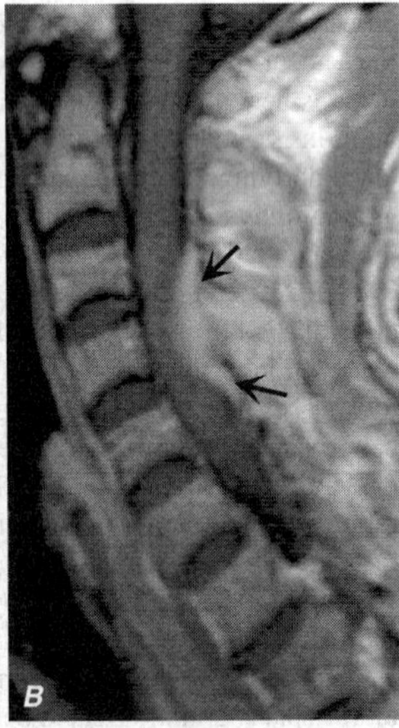

FIGURE 368-5 MRI of a spinal epidural abscess due to tuberculosis. *A.* Sagittal T2-weighted free spin-echo MR sequence. A hypointense mass replaces the posterior elements of C3 and extends epidurally to compress the spinal cord (*arrows*). *B.* Sagittal T1-weighted image after contrast administration reveals a diffuse enhancement of the epidural process (*arrows*) with extension into the epidural space.

TRANSVERSE MYELITIS Transverse myelitis is an acute or subacute, generally monophasic, inflammatory disorder of the spinal cord. The initial symptom is focal neck or back pain, followed by various combinations of paresthesias, sensory loss, motor weakness, and sphincter disturbance evolving within hours to several days. There may be mild sensory symptoms only, or a devastating functional transection of the cord. Partial forms may selectively involve posterior columns, anterior spinothalamic tracts, or one hemicord. Dysesthesias may begin in the feet and ascend either symmetrically or asymmetrically, earlier in one leg than in the other; these symptoms may initially raise a question of Guillain-Barré syndrome, but involvement of the trunk with a sharply demarcated spinal cord level indicates the myelopathic nature of the process. In severe cases, areflexia indicating spinal shock may be present, but hyperreflexia soon supervenes; persistent areflexic paralysis indicates necrosis over multiple segments of the spinal cord.

Up to 40% of cases are associated with an antecedent infection or recent vaccination. Many infectious agents have been implicated, including influenza, measles, varicella, rubeola, mumps, and Epstein-Barr virus and cytomegalovirus, as well as *Mycoplasma*. As in the related disorder acute disseminated encephalomyelitis (Chap. 371), transverse myelitis often begins as the patient appears to be recovering from the infection, and infectious agents have not been isolated from the nervous system of affected individuals. These features suggest that transverse myelitis results from an autoimmune response triggered by infection and not from direct infection of the spinal cord.

Multiple sclerosis (MS) (see below) may present initially as transverse myelitis. MS-associated transverse myelitis usually is not associated with an antecedent infection or vaccination. Devic's disease (Chap. 371) is a demyelinating disorder that presents as transverse myelitis associated with optic neuritis that is typically bilateral. Transverse myelitis, at times recurrent, has also been associated with systemic lupus erythematosus and other collagen-vascular diseases, Sjögren's syndrome, and Behçet's disease; sarcoidosis may produce a subacute transverse myelopathy with severe cord swelling.

MRI findings consist of variable swelling of the cord and diffuse or multifocal areas of abnormal bright signal on T2-weighted sequences, often extending over several cord segments. Contrast enhancement, indicating disruption in the blood-brain barrier associated with perivenous inflammation, is present in acute cases. MRI is also useful to exclude cord compression. A brain MRI should be obtained in all cases to assess the likelihood that the transverse myelitis represents an initial attack of MS. A normal scan indicates that the risk of evolution to MS is low—approximately 5% over 3 to 5 years; by contrast, the finding of multiple periventricular T2-bright lesions indicates a risk of 50% or greater over the same time period. CSF may be normal, but more often there is pleocytosis, with up to several hundred mononuclear cells per microliter; in severe or rapidly evolving cases, polymorphonuclear cells may be present. CSF protein levels are normal or at most mildly elevated; oligoclonal banding is a variable finding but, when present, is associated with future evolution to MS.

There are no prospective trials of therapy. Intravenous methylprednisolone (500 mg qd for 3 days) followed by oral prednisone (1 mg/kg per day for several weeks, then gradual taper) is used for treatment of moderate to severe symptoms.

ACUTE INFECTIOUS MYELOPATHIES These inflammatory disorders result from direct invasion of the spinal cord by infectious agents. Bacterial etiologies are rare; almost any pathogenic species may be responsible and in one recent review *Listeria monocytogenes* was most frequently identified. Poliomyelitis is the prototypic virus that produces acute infection of the spinal cord. Herpes zoster is currently the most common viral cause of acute myelitis; cytomegalovirus, herpes simplex virus type 1, Epstein-Barr virus, and rabies virus have been identified in occasional cases. Herpes simplex virus type 2 may produce a recurrent sacral myelitis, which could be mistaken for MS, in association with outbreaks of genital herpes. →*Viral infections of the spinal cord are discussed in Chap. 373.*

Schistosomiasis (Chap. 222) is an important cause of parasitic myelitis worldwide. The myelitis is intensely inflammatory and granulomatous in nature, caused by a local response to tissue-digesting enzymes produced by ova from the parasite. Toxoplasmosis (Chap. 217) can cause a focal myelopathy, and this diagnosis should be considered in patients with AIDS owing to the high frequency of nervous system toxoplasmosis in this population.

CHRONIC MYELOPATHIES

SPONDYLITIC MYELOPATHY Neck and shoulder pain with stiffness are early symptoms; pressure on nerve roots results in radicular arm pain, most often in a C5 or C6 distribution. Compression of the cervical cord produces a slowly progressive spastic paraparesis, at times asymmetric, and often accompanied by paresthesias in the feet and hands. Vibratory sense is frequently diminished in the legs, and occasionally there is a sensory level for vibration on the upper thorax. Coughing or straining often produces leg weakness or radiating arm or shoulder pain. Dermatomal sensory loss in the arms, atrophy of intrinsic hand muscles, increased deep tendon reflexes in the legs, and extensor plantar responses are common. Urinary urgency or incontinence occurs in advanced cases. Reflexes in the arms are often diminished at some level, often the biceps (C5-C6). In individual cases, radicular, myelopathic, or combined signs may predominate. The diagnosis should be considered in cases of progressive cervical myelopathy, paresthesias of the feet and hands, or wasting of the hands. Spondylitic myelopathy is also one of the most common causes of gait difficulty in the elderly.

Diagnosis is best made by MRI. Extrinsic compression is appreciated on axial views, and T2-weighted sequences may reveal abnormal areas of high signal intensity within the cord adjacent to the site of compression. Definitive therapy consists of surgical relief of the compression, generally by posterior laminectomy. When that is not feasible, an anterior approach with resection of the protruded disc material may be required.→*Cervical spondylosis and related degenerative diseases of the spine are discussed in Chap. 16.*

VASCULAR MALFORMATIONS Although uncommon, vascular malformations are important lesions because they represent a treatable cause of progressive myelopathy. Arteriovenous malformations (AVMs) are most often located posteriorly, within the dura or along the surface of the cord, at or below the midthoracic level. The typical presentation is a middle-aged man with a progressive myelopathy. The myelopathy may worsen slowly or rapidly or may have periods of apparent remission with superimposed worsenings resembling MS. Acute deterioration due to hemorrhage into the spinal cord or subarachnoid space may also occur. At presentation, most patients have sensory, motor, and bladder disturbances. The motor disorder may predominate and produce a mixture of upper and lower motoneuron signs, simulating ALS. Pain, either dysesthesias or radicular pain, is also common. Other symptoms suggestive of AVM include intermittent claudication (symptoms that appear with exercise and are relieved by rest), or an effect of posture, menses, or fever on symptoms. A rare AVM syndrome presents as a progressive thoracic myelopathy with paraparesis developing over weeks or several months, associated with abnormally thick, hyalinized vessels (Foix-Alajouanine syndrome).

AVMs located at cervical or upper thoracic levels are distinctive; they occur equally in males and females, tend to be located anterior rather than posterior to the cord, often have an intramedullary component to the malformation, and may bleed (see "Hematomyelia," above).

Examination of the skin overlying the spine may reveal a vascular lesion, lipoma, or area of altered pigmentation, all clues to a spinal cord AVM. Bruits are rare but should be sought at rest or after exercise. High-resolution MRI with contrast administration detects most AVMs (Fig. 368-6). A small number of AVMs not detected by MRI may be visualized by CT myelography as enlarged vessels along the surface of the cord. Definitive diagnosis requires selective spinal angiography, which will also define the vascular feeders and extent of the malfor-

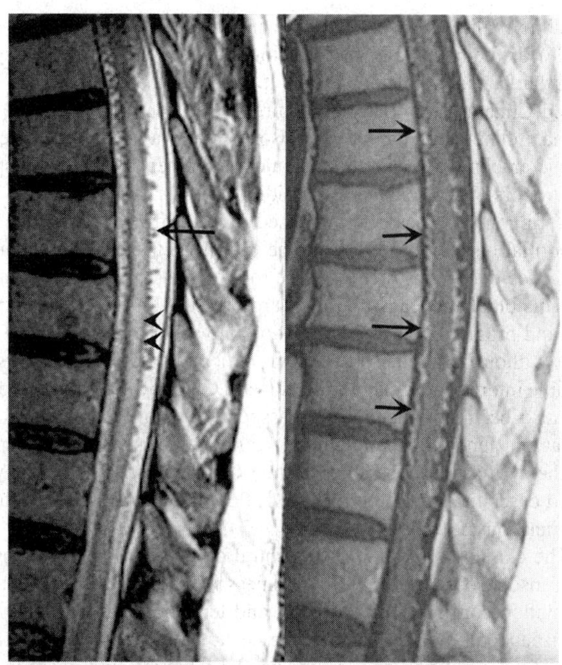

FIGURE 368-6 Arteriovenous malformation. Sagittal MR scans of the thoracic spinal cord: T2 fast spin-echo technique (*left*) and T1 post-contrast image (*right*). On the T2-weighted image (*left*), abnormally high signal intensity is noted in the central aspect of the spinal cord (*arrowheads*). Numerous punctate flow voids indent the dorsal and ventral spinal cord (*arrow*). These represent the abnormally dilated venous plexus supplied by a dural arteriovenous fistula. After contrast administration (*right*), multiple, serpentine, enhancing veins (*arrows*) on the ventral and dorsal aspect of the thoracic spinal cord are visualized, diagnostic of arteriovenous fistula. This patient was a 54-year-old man with a 4-year history of progressive paraparesis.

mation. Embolization with occlusion of the major feeding vessels may stabilize a progressive neurologic deficit or produce a gradual recovery.

RETROVIRUS-ASSOCIATED MYELOPATHIES The myelopathy associated with the human T cell lymphotropic virus type I (HTLV-I) presents as a slowly progressive spastic paraparesis with variable sensory and bladder disturbance. The myelopathy is typically thoracic. Approximately half of patients have back or leg pain. Signs may be asymmetric, may lack a well-defined sensory level, and may spare upper extremity function, although hyperreflexia in the arms is common. Onset is generally insidious, and the tempo of progression is variable, but most patients are nonambulatory within 10 years of onset. This presentation may resemble primary progressive MS or a thoracic AVM. Diagnosis is made by demonstration of HTLV-I–specific antibody in serum by enzyme-linked immunosorbent assay (ELISA), confirmed by radioimmunoprecipitation or Western blot analysis of specific antibody directed against protein products of the viral *gag* and *env* genes. There is no effective treatment; symptomatic therapy for spasticity and bladder symptoms may be helpful. →*HTLV-I infections of the nervous system are discussed in Chap. 373.*

A progressive myelopathy may also occur in AIDS, characterized by vacuolar degeneration of the posterior and lateral tracts resembling subacute combined degeneration (see below).

SYRINGOMYELIA Syringomyelia is a cavitary expansion of the spinal cord that may produce a progressive myelopathy. Syrinxes commonly occur in the lower cervical/high thoracic region or in the high cervical region, where they may extend rostrally to the medulla or pons (syringobulbia); any region of the spinal cord may be involved. More than half of all cases are associated with Chiari malformations. In the Chiari type 1 malformation, the cerebellar tonsils protrude through the foramen magnum and into the cervical spinal canal; when this abnormality is associated with protrusion of meninges (meningocele) or meninges and cord (meningomyelocele) through a spinal canal that has incompletely closed, it is designated a Chiari type 2 (or Arnold-Chiari) malformation. Acquired cases are often associated with trauma, inflammatory spinal cord disorders such as transverse myelitis, chronic arachnoiditis due to tuberculosis or other etiologies, or spinal cord tumors. Occasional cases are idiopathic.

Syringomyelia has been proposed to result from interference with the normal outflow of CSF from the fourth ventricle to the subarachnoid space due to obstruction of the foramina of Luschka and Magendie. This blockage leads to downward pressure on the cervical spinal cord and progressive syrinx formation. However, syringomyelia may occur without foraminal obstruction, indicating that other factors, for example interference with normal upward CSF flow in the spinal canal, may also be important. Syrinxes associated with Chiari type 1 malformations generally communicate freely with the subarachnoid space, and the syrinx fluid resembles normal CSF; by contrast, in many acquired cases the syrinx cavities do not communicate, and the fluid is proteinaceous.

The classic presentation is a central cord syndrome with dissociated sensory loss and areflexic weakness in the upper limbs. The sensory deficit consists of loss of pain and temperature sensation which is "suspended" over the nape of the neck, shoulders, and upper arms in a cape distribution or is in the hands; vibration and position sensation is largely preserved. Most cases begin asymmetrically with unilateral sensory loss. Muscle wasting in the lower neck, shoulders, arms, and hands with asymmetric or absent reflexes reflects extension of the cavity to the anterior horns. As the lesion enlarges, spasticity and weakness of the legs, bladder and bowel dysfunction, and, in some cases, a Horner's syndrome appear. Thoracic kyphoscoliosis is a frequent additional finding. Some patients develop numbness and sensory loss on the face from damage to the descending tract of the trigeminal nerve (C2 level or above). With Chiari malformations, cough headache, and neck, arm, or facial pain are common. Syringobulbia may present as palatal or vocal cord paralysis, dysarthria, horizontal or vertical nystagmus, episodic dizziness, and/or tongue weakness.

Symptoms typically begin insidiously in adolescence or early adulthood, progress irregularly, and may undergo spontaneous arrest for several years. Onset or sudden deterioration may follow trauma, neck manipulation or extension, or severe cough. Symptoms of syringobulbia may progress rapidly.

MRI scans accurately identify syrinx cavities and associated spinal cord enlargement (Fig. 368-7). In all cases, MRI scans of the brain and the entire spinal cord should be obtained to delineate the full extent of the syrinx, assess posterior fossa structures, and determine whether hydrocephalus is present. If a Chiari malformation is not found, a contrast-enhanced MRI scan should be obtained to search for abnormal enhancement from an associated spinal cord tumor.

℞ **TREATMENT** Treatment is surgical. Syringomyelia associated with tonsillar herniation is treated with posterior fossa decompression, generally consisting of suboccipital craniectomy, upper cervical laminectomy, and placement of a dural graft. If obstruction of fourth ventricular outflow is present, flow is reestablished by enlargement of the opening. If the syrinx cavity is large, some surgeons recommend direct decompression of the fluid cavity, but the added benefit of this procedure is uncertain, and morbidity may occur. With Chiari malformations, shunting of hydrocephalus should generally precede any attempt to correct the syrinx. Surgical results are often excellent, with stabilization of the neurologic deficit in most cases; some patients have improvement postoperatively. Syringomyelia secondary to trauma or infection is treated with a decompression and drainage procedure in which a small shunt is inserted between the syrinx cavity and the subarachnoid space. Finally, syringomyelia due to an intramedullary spinal cord tumor is managed by resection of the tumor if feasible; decompression of the cyst cavity may produce temporary relief, but recurrence is common.

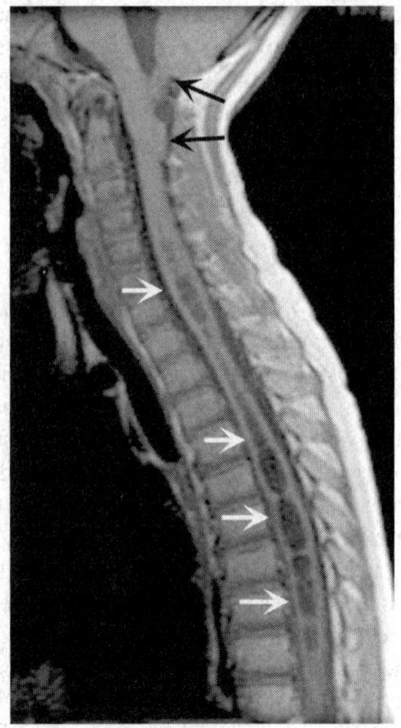

FIGURE 368-7 MRI of a syringomyelia associated with a Chiari malformation. Sagittal T1-weighted image through the cervical and upper thoracic spine demonstrates descent of the cerebellar tonsils and vermis below the level of the foramen magnum (*black arrows*). Within the substance of the cervical and thoracic spinal cord, a CSF collection dilates the central canal (*white arrows*).

MULTIPLE SCLEROSIS Spinal cord involvement is common in MS. It may develop acutely as an exacerbation in a patient with known MS or appear as the presenting manifestation of the disease (see "Transverse Myelitis," above). Chronic progressive myelopathy is the most frequent cause of disability in both primary progressive and secondary progressive forms of MS. Involvement is typically asymmetric, producing motor, sensory, and bladder/bowel disturbances. Diagnosis is facilitated by identification of earlier attacks that may not be initially recalled by the patient; by MRI, CSF and evoked response testing; and by exclusion of other conditions. The diagnosis may be particularly difficult to establish in patients with primary progressive MS. Therapy with interferon β or glatiramer acetate is indicated for many patients with MS-related myelopathy that is not due to primary progressive MS. →*MS is discussed in Chap. 371.*

SUBACUTE COMBINED DEGENERATION (VITAMIN B_{12} DEFICIENCY) This treatable myelopathy presents with paresthesias in the hands and feet, early loss of vibration and position sensation, and a progressive spastic and ataxic weakness. Loss of reflexes due to a superimposed peripheral neuropathy, present in many patients, is an important diagnostic clue. Optic atrophy and irritability and other mental changes may be prominent in advanced cases and on occasion are the presenting symptoms (megaloblastic madness). The myelopathy of subacute combined degeneration tends to be diffuse rather than focal; signs are generally symmetric and reflect predominant involvement of the posterior and lateral tracts. The diagnosis is confirmed by the finding of a low serum B_{12} concentration, elevated levels of homocysteine and methylmalonic acid in uncertain cases, and a positive Schilling test (Chap. 75).

TABES DORSALIS Tabes dorsalis and meningovascular syphilis of the spinal cord are presently rare but must be considered in the differential diagnosis of spinal cord syndromes, in particular those that arise in individuals infected with HIV. The most common symptoms of tabes are characteristic fleeting and repetitive, lancinating pains, which occur mostly in the legs and less commonly in the back, thorax, abdomen, arms, and face. Ataxia of the legs and gait due to loss of position sense occurs in half of patients. Paresthesias, bladder disturbances, and acute abdominal pain with vomiting (visceral crisis) occur in 15 to 30% of patients. The cardinal signs of tabes are loss of reflexes in the legs, impaired position and vibratory sense, Romberg's sign, and bilateral Argyll Robertson pupils, which fail to constrict to light but react with accommodation.

FAMILIAL SPASTIC PARAPLEGIA Occasional cases of progressive myelopathy occur on a familial basis. Most present with progressive spasticity and weakness in the legs. Sphincter disturbances and mild degrees of sensory loss may also be present. On examination, a sharply defined spinal cord level is not detected, in contrast to many focal spinal cord disorders. In some families, whose condition is referred to as "complicated" familial spastic paraplegia, additional neurologic signs, for example, nystagmus, ataxia, or optic atrophy, occur. Onset may be as early as the first year of life or as late as middle adulthood. The genetic basis of several forms of familial spastic paraplegia is now known (Table 368-3). No disease-modifying therapy exists.

Table 368-3 Inherited (Monogenic) Myelopathies[a]

Designation	Clinical Presentation	Genetics
Autosomal recessive	Early onset (age 1–20), progressive spasticity of legs, mild loss of vibration and position sense, bladder symptoms	Linkage to chromosome 16q; encodes paraplegin, a mitochondrial ATPase involved in diverse cellular functions. Additional loci exist at 8q and 15q.
Autosomal dominant	Most common form; families have either early or late onset (before or after age 35)	Linkage to chromosome 2p for both early and late onset; encodes spastin, an ATPase that may be involved in function of nuclear protein complexes. Other loci exist at 14q, 15q, and 8q.
X-linked	Early childhood onset as pure spastic paraplegia or ''complicated'' with nystagmus, ataxia, or other neurologic signs	''Complicated'' form due to mutation of proteolipid protein gene; differs from the dysmyelinating disorder Pelizaeus-Merzbacher disease in that the allelic protein DM20, essential for oligodendrocyte development, is normal
X-linked	Pure or ''complicated''	Mutations in neural cell adhesion molecule L1CAM. Allelic disorders X-linked hydrocephalus and MASA syndrome (mental retardation, aphasia, shuffling gait, adducted thumbs).

[a] See also Chap. 359.

ADRENOMYELONEUROPATHY This X-linked disorder, a variant of adrenoleukodystrophy, most commonly presents as a progressive spastic paraparesis beginning in early adulthood; some patients also have a mild peripheral neuropathy. Affected males usually have a history of adrenal insufficiency beginning in childhood. Rare heterozygous females may also present with adult-onset myelopathy. Diagnosis is usually made by demonstration of elevated levels of very long chain fatty acids in plasma and in cultured fibroblasts. The responsible gene, located at Xq17-28, encodes a protein involved in peroxysomal transport. Steroid replacement is indicated if hypoadrenalism is present, and bone marrow transplantation has been attempted for this condition without clear evidence of efficacy.

OTHER CHRONIC MYELOPATHIES Primary lateral sclerosis (Chap. 365) is characterized by progressive spasticity with weakness, often accompanied by dysarthria and dysphonia. Sensory function is spared. The disorder resembles ALS, but there is no evidence of a lower motor neuron disturbance. Toxic causes include (1) lathyrism due to ingestion of chick peas containing the excitotoxin β-*N*-oxalylaminoalanine (BOAA) and seen primarily in the undeveloped world, and (2) nitrous oxide inhalation producing a myelopathy identical to subacute combined degeneration. Systemic lupus erythematosus (Chap. 311) and Sjögren's syndrome (Chap. 314) have both been associated with progressive myelopathy. Cancer-related causes include chronic paraneoplastic myelopathy (Chap. 101) or radiation injury (Chap. 370). Finally, in some patients the etiology of a chronic myelopathy may not be determined initially. A cause can ultimately be identified in most idiopathic cases and thus periodic reassessment is essential.

→*Traumatic spinal cord lesions are discussed in Chap. 369.*

MEDICAL REHABILITATION OF SPINAL CORD DISORDERS

The prospects for significant recovery from an acute spinal cord lesion fade after approximately 4 months. There are currently no effective means to promote repair of injured spinal cord tissue; promising experimental approaches include the use of factors that influence reinnervation by axons of the corticospinal tract or nerve graft bridges that promote reinnervation across spinal cord lesions. The disability associated with irreversible spinal cord damage is determined primarily by the level of the lesion and by whether the disturbance in function is complete or incomplete (Table 368-4). Even a complete high cervical cord lesion may be compatible with a productive life. Development of a rehabilitation plan framed by realistic expectations, and attention to the neurologic, medical, and psychological complications that commonly arise, are primary goals of treatment.

The usual symptoms associated with medical illnesses may be lacking, because of the destruction of afferent pain pathways in the cord. Unexplained fever, worsening of spasticity, or deterioration in neurologic function should prompt search for an underlying cause such as infection, thrombophlebitis, or an intraabdominal pathology; these etiologies are far more likely to be responsible than primary neurologic events such as meningitis, secondary syringomyelia, or chronic arachnoiditis. The loss of normal thermoregulation and inability to maintain normal body temperature can produce recurrent fever (*quadriplegic fever*), although most episodes of fever are due to infection of the urinary tract, lung, skin, or bone.

Bladder dysfunction generally results from loss of supraspinal innervation of the detrusor muscle of the bladder wall and the sphincter musculature. Detrusor spasticity is treated with anticholinergic drugs (oxybutinin, 2.5 to 5 mg qid) or tricyclic antidepressants with anticholinergic properties (imipramine, 25 to 200 mg/d). Failure of the sphincter muscle to relax during bladder emptying (urinary dyssynergia) may be managed with the α-adrenergic blocking agent terazosin

Table 368-4 Expected Neurologic Function Following Complete Cord Lesions

Level	Self-Care	Transfers	Maximum Mobility
High quadriplegia (C1-C4)	Dependent on others; requires respiratory support	Dependent on others	Motorized wheelchair
Low quadriplegia (C5-C8)	Partially independent with adaptive equipment	May be dependent or independent	May use manual wheelchair, drive an automobile with adaptive equipment
Paraplegia (below T1)	Independent	Independent	Ambulates short distances with aids

SOURCE: Adapted from Ditunno and Formal.

hydrochloride (1 to 2 mg tid or qid), with intermittent catheterization, or, if that is not feasible, by use of a condom catheter in men or a permanent indwelling catheter. Surgical options include the creation of an artificial bladder by isolating a segment of intestine that can be catheterized intermittently (enterocystoplasty) or can drain continuously to an external appliance (urinary conduit). Bladder areflexia due to acute spinal shock or conus lesions is best treated by catheterization.

Bladder dysfunction predisposes the patient to urinary tract infection. Bacteriuria due to asymptomatic colonization is extremely common and is generally not treated. Prophylaxis with antiseptics or antibiotics is of little value. Urinary tract infections may present only as foul-smelling urine or a change in voiding pattern; the development of high fever or other systemic signs often indicates pyelonephritis. Bowel regimens and disimpaction are necessary in most patients to ensure at least biweekly evacuation and avoid colonic distention or obstruction.

High cervical cord lesions cause various degrees of mechanical respiratory failure requiring artificial ventilation. In cases of incomplete respiratory failure, chest physical therapy is useful, and a negative-pressure cuirass may alleviate atelectasis, particularly if the major lesion is below C4. With severe respiratory failure, tracheal intubation, followed by tracheotomy, provides tracheal access for ventilation and suctioning. Phrenic nerve pacing may be useful in some patients with lesions at C5 or above.

Patients with acute cord injury are at high risk for venous thrombosis and pulmonary embolism. During the first two weeks, use of calf-compression devices and anticoagulation with heparin (5000 U subcutaneously every 12 h) or warfarin (INR, 2 to 3) are recommended. In cases of persistent paralysis, anticoagulation should probably be continued for 3 months.

Prophylaxis against decubitus ulcers should involve frequent changes in position in a chair or bed, the use of special mattresses, and cushioning of areas where pressure sores often develop, such as the sacral prominence and heels. Early treatment of ulcers with careful cleansing, surgical or enzyme debridement of necrotic tissue, and appropriate dressing and drainage may prevent infection of adjacent soft tissue or bone.

Spasticity (Chap. 22) is often a late manifestation of spinal cord disease, occurring weeks or even months after the initial insult. Stretching exercises are useful to maintain mobility of joints. Drug treatment is effective but may result in reduced function, as some patients use their spasticity as an aid to stand, transfer, or walk. Baclofen (15 to 240 mg/d in divided doses) is the most effective drug available; it acts by facilitating GABA-mediated inhibition of motor reflex arcs. Diazepam acts by a similar mechanism and is useful for leg spasms that interrupt sleep (2 to 4 mg at bedtime). For nonambulatory patients, the direct muscle inhibitor dantrolene (25 to 100 mg qid) may be used, but it is potentially hepatotoxic. In severe cases, intrathecal baclofen administered via an implanted pump, botulinum toxin injections, or dorsal rhizotomy may be required to control spasticity.

Paroxysmal autonomic hyperreflexia may occur following lesions above the major splanchnic sympathetic outflow at T6. Headache, flushing, and diaphoresis above the level of the lesion, and hypertension with bradycardia or tachycardia, are the major symptoms. The trigger is typically a noxious stimulus—for example, bladder or bowel distention, a urinary tract infection, or a decubitus ulcer—below the level of the cord lesion. Ascending sensory fibers are thought to activate, via interneurons, sympathetic neurons of the intermediolateral nuclei in the thoracic spinal cord, producing vasoconstriction, tachycardia, and systemic hypertension. Reflex pathways, activated by carotid and aortic baroreceptors and projecting to the central nervous system via the vagus and glossopharyngeal nerves, then inhibit sympathetic activity above the cord lesion, producing vasodilation, but below the lesion descending pathways are blocked and sympathetic hyperactivity continues. Treatment consists of removal of offending stimuli; ganglionic blocking agents (mecamylamine, 2.5 to 5 mg) or other short-acting antihypertensive drugs are useful in some patients (see review by Colachis).

BIBLIOGRAPHY

BLAIVAS JG: Bladder function in the SCI patient. J Neurol Rehab 8:47, 1994

CHAN CT, GOLD WL: Intramedullary abcess of the spinal cord in the antibiotic era: Clinical features, microbial etiologies, trends in pathogenesis, and outcomes. Clin Infect Dis 27:619, 1998

COLACHIS SC: Autonomic hyperreflexia with spinal cord injury. J Am Paraplegia Soc 15(3):172, 1992

CRISTANTE L, HERRMANN H-D: Surgical management of intramedullary spinal cord tumors: Functional outcome and sources of morbidity. Neurosurgery 35:69, 1994

DAROUICHE RO et al: Bacterial spinal epidural abscess: Review of 43 cases and literature survey. Medicine 71:369, 1992

DITUNNO JF, FORMAL CS: Chronic spinal cord injury. N Engl J Med 330:550, 1994

HAZAN J et al: Spastin, a new AAA protein, is altered in the most frequent form of autosomal dominant spastic paraplegia. Nat Genet 23:296, 1999

KATZ JD, ROPPER AH: Progressive necrotic myelopathy: Clinical course in 9 patients. Arch Neurol 57:355, 2000

MILHORAT TH et al: Chiari1 malformation redefined: Clinical and radiologic findings for 364 symptomatic patients. Neurosurgery 44:1005, 1999

SCOTT TF et al: Transverse myelitis: Comparison with spinal cord presentations of multiple sclerosis. Neurology 50:429, 1998

SMALL JA, SHERIDAN PH: Research priorities for syringomyelia: A National Institute of Neurologic Disorders and Stroke workshop summary. Neurology 46:577, 1996

SMYTH MD, PEACOCK WH: The surgical treatment of spasticity. Muscle Nerve 23:153, 2000

369

Allan H. Ropper

TRAUMATIC INJURIES OF THE HEAD AND SPINE

Head injuries are frequent in industrialized countries and affect many individuals in the prime of life. Almost 10 million head injuries occur annually in the United States alone, about 20% of which are serious enough to cause brain damage. Among men under 35 years, accidents, usually motor vehicle collisions, are the chief cause of death, and >70% of these involve head injury. Minor head injuries are so common that almost all physicians encounter patients requiring immediate care or suffering from various sequelae. Traumatic spinal cord injuries often occur in conjunction with head injury. The two are best considered together in the context of trauma to the nervous system.

A recent decline in mortality from head and spinal cord injuries can be attributed mainly to the use of seat belts and motorcycle helmets and the development of ambulance systems with trained personnel. In addition, a systematic approach to the evaluation of patients with head and spine trauma, beginning at the scene of the accident, has contributed to the improvement in outcome. Also, the wide availability of computed tomography (CT) and magnetic resonance imaging (MRI) has contributed to advances in diagnosis and intensive care treatment and an understanding of the pathologic lesions that are produced by trauma.

TYPES OF HEAD INJURIES

SKULL FRACTURES A blow to the skull causes a fracture if the elastic tolerance of the bone is exceeded. Intracranial lesions accompany two-thirds of skull fractures, and the presence of a skull fracture increases manyfold the chances of an underlying subdural or epidural hematoma. Consequently, fractures are important primarily as markers of the site and severity of injury. They are also the cause of cranial nerve injuries and the source of entry pathways to the cerebrospinal fluid (CSF) for bacteria (meningitis), air (pneumocephalus), and leakage of CSF.

Fractures are classified as *linear*, *basilar*, *compound*, or *depressed*.

Linear fractures, which are most often associated with subdural or epidural hematomas, account for 80% of all skull fractures. They are usually oriented from the point of impact toward the base of the skull. Basilar skull fractures are often extensions of adjacent fractures over the convexity of the skull but may occur independently owing to stresses on the floor of the middle cranial fossa or occiput. They are usually located parallel to the petrous bone or along the sphenoid bone toward the sella turcica and ethmoidal groove. Although most are uncomplicated, basilar skull fractures can cause CSF leakage, pneumocephalus, and cavernous-carotid fistulas. Hemotympanum (blood behind the tympanic membrane), delayed ecchymosis over the mastoid process (Battle's sign), or periorbital ecchymosis ("racoon sign") all signify fracture of the basilar skull. Because routine x-ray examination may fail to disclose basilar fractures, they should be suspected if these clinical signs are present. CSF may leak through the cribriform plate or the adjacent sinus and manifest as a watery discharge from the nose (CSF rhinorrhea). Persistent rhinorrhea and recurrent meningitis are indications for surgical repair of torn dura underlying the fracture. The precise site of the leak is often difficult to determine, but useful diagnostic tests include the instillation of water-soluble contrast into the CSF followed by CT with the patient in various positions, and injection of radionuclide compounds or fluorescein into the CSF with an assessment of uptake of these compounds by absorptive nasal pledgets. The site of an intermittent leak is rarely delineated, and most resolve spontaneously. Sellar fractures, even ones associated with serious neuroendocrine dysfunction, are sometimes radiologically occult. Fractures of the dorsum sella may cause sixth or seventh nerve palsies or optic nerve damage. An air-fluid level in the sphenoid sinus suggests a fracture of the sellar floor.

Petrous bone fractures, especially those oriented along the long axis of the bone, may be associated with facial palsy, disruption of ear ossicles, and CSF otorrhea. Transverse petrous fractures are less common; they almost always damage the cochlea or labyrinths and often the facial nerve. External bleeding from the ear is usually from local abrasion of the external canal but can also result from petrous fracture.

Fractures of the frontal bone are often depressed, involving the frontal and paranasal sinuses and the orbits; permanent anosmia results if the olfactory filaments in the cribriform plate are disrupted. Depressed skull fractures are typically compound, but they are often neurologically asymptomatic because the impact energy is dissipated in breaking the bone; however, some are associated with brain contusions and focal neurologic signs caused by damage to the underlying cortical area. Prompt debridement and exploration of compound fractures are required in order to avoid infection.

CRANIAL NERVE INJURIES The cranial nerves likely to be injured with head trauma include the olfactory, optic, oculomotor, and trochlear nerves; the first and second branches of the trigeminal nerve; and the facial and auditory nerves. Anosmia and an apparent loss of taste (actually a loss of perception of aromatic flavors, with elementary tastes retained) occur in ~10% of persons with serious head injuries, particularly with falls on the back of the head. This sequela results from displacement of the brain and shearing of the olfactory nerve filaments and may occur in the absence of a fracture. Recovery is the rule, leaving residual hyposmia, but if bilateral anosmia persists for several months, the prognosis is poor. Fractures of the sphenoid bone may rarely bruise or transect the optic nerve, resulting in unilateral partial or complete blindness and an unreactive pupil, usually equal in size to that of the other side and with a preserved consensual light response. Partial optic nerve injuries from closed trauma result in blurring of vision, central or paracentral scotomas, or sector defects. Direct orbital injury may cause short-lived blurred vision for close objects and pupillary paralysis because of reversible iridoplegia. Diplopia limited to downward gaze, which suggests trochlear nerve damage, occurs as an isolated problem after minor injury and can develop after a delay of several days; it may also result from fracture of the lesser wing of the sphenoid bone. The diplopia is corrected if the head is tilted away from the affected eye. Direct facial nerve injury by a basal fracture is present immediately in 3% of severe injuries; it may also be delayed 5 to 7 days. Fractures through the petrous bone, particularly the less common transverse type, are liable to produce this injury. Delayed facial palsy, the mechanism of which is unknown, has a good prognosis. Injury to the eighth cranial nerve from a fracture of the petrous bone causes loss of hearing, vertigo, and nystagmus immediately after injury. Deafness from nerve injury must be distinguished from that due to rupture of the eardrum, blood in the middle ear, or disruption of the ossicles from fracture through the middle ear. A high-tone hearing loss occurs with direct cochlear concussion.

SEIZURES *Convulsions* are surprisingly uncommon immediately after a head injury, but a brief period of tonic extensor posturing or a few clonic movements of the limbs just after the moment of impact may occur. However, the superficial cortical scars that evolve from contusions are highly epileptogenic and may later manifest as seizures, even after many years (Chap. 360). The severity of injury determines the risk of future seizures. It has been estimated that 17% of individuals with brain contusion, subdural hematoma, or prolonged loss of consciousness will develop a seizure disorder and that this risk extends for an indefinite period of time, whereas the risk is only 2% after mild injury; the majority of convulsions in the latter group occur within 5 years of injury.

CONCUSSION *Concussion* refers to an immediate but transient loss of consciousness that is associated with a short period of amnesia and described as the experience or appearance of being dazed or "star struck." It typically occurs after a blunt impact that creates a sudden deceleration of the cranium and a movement of the brain within the skull. Severe concussion may precipitate a brief convulsion or autonomic signs such as facial pallor, bradycardia, faintness with mild hypotension, or sluggish pupillary reaction, but most patients are neurologically normal. Higher primates are particularly susceptible to concussion; in contrast, billy goats, rams, and woodpeckers can tolerate impact velocity and deceleration 100-fold greater than that experienced by humans. The mechanism of loss of consciousness in concussion is believed to be a transient electrophysiologic dysfunction of the reticular activating system in the upper midbrain caused by rotation of the cerebral hemispheres on the relatively fixed brainstem (Chap. 24).

Gross and light-microscopic changes in the brain are usually absent following concussion, but biochemical and ultrastructural changes, such as mitochondrial ATP depletion and local disruption of the blood-brain barrier, suggest that complex abnormalities occur. CT and MRI scans are usually normal; however, approximately 3% of patients will be found to have an intracranial hemorrhage of some type.

The amnesia of concussion typically follows at least a few moments of unresponsiveness, but rarely there is no loss of consciousness. The memory loss spans the time of, and moments before, mild impact injuries but may encompass previous weeks (rarely months) in cases of more severe trauma. The extent of retrograde amnesia has been suggested as a rough measure of the severity of injury. Any anterograde amnesia is usually brief and disappears rapidly in alert patients. Memory is regained in an orderly way from the most distant to recent memories, with islands of amnesia occasionally remaining in severe cases. The mechanism of peritraumatic amnesia is not known. Hysterical posttraumatic amnesia is not uncommon and should be suspected when inexplicable abnormalities of behavior occur, such as recounting events that cannot be recalled on later testing, a bizarre affect that emulates the lay notion of amnesia or psychosis (Ganser syndrome), forgetting one's own name, or a persistent anterograde deficit that is excessive in comparison with the degree of injury.

A single, uncomplicated head injury only infrequently produces permanent neurobehavioral changes in patients who are free of preexisting psychiatric problems and substance abuse. However, there has been increasing attention to minor problems in memory and concentration that may have an anatomic correlate in small shearing or other microscopic lesions (see below).

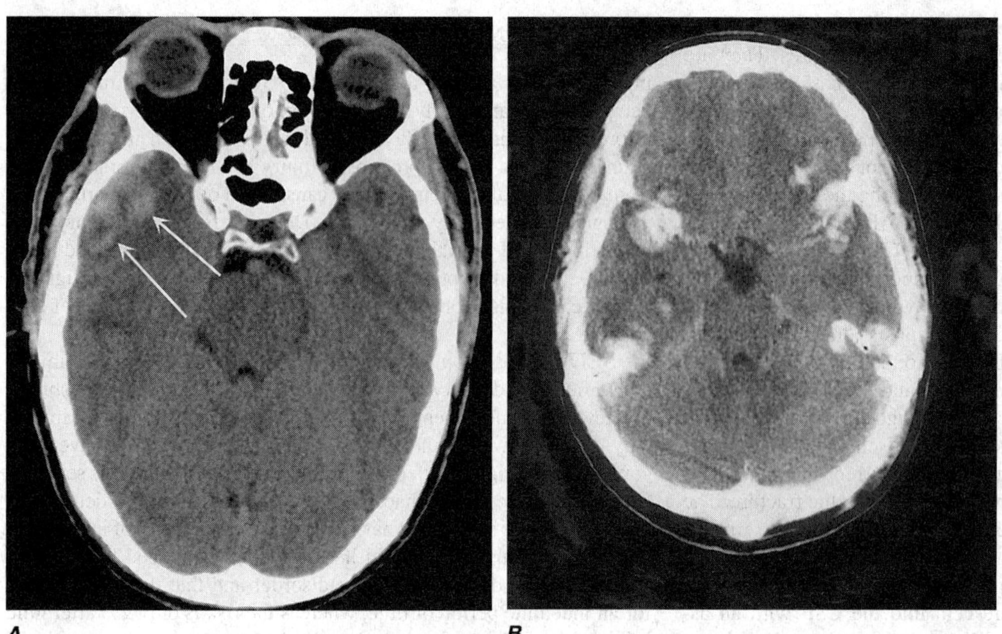

FIGURE 369-1 *A.* Traumatic cerebral contusion. Noncontrast CT scan demonstrating a hyperdense hemorrhagic region in the anterior temporal lobe. *B.* Cerebral contusions adjacent to the bony prominences of the skull. Hemorrhagic areas are seen in the basal frontal and temporal regions where the brain is impelled against the sphenoid and petrous bones.

CONTUSION, BRAIN HEMORRHAGE, AND SHEARING LESIONS A surface bruise of the brain, or *contusion*, consists of varying degrees of petechial hemorrhage, edema, and tissue destruction. Contusions and deeper hemorrhages result from mechanical forces that displace the hemispheres forcefully relative to the skull by deceleration of the brain against the inner skull, either under a point of impact (coup lesion) or, as the brain swings back, in the antipolar area (contrecoup lesion). Trauma sufficient to cause prolonged unconsciousness usually produces some degree of contusion. Because the motion of the hemispheres brings them into contact with the prominences of the sphenoid and other frontal basal bones, blunt impact, as from an automobile dashboard or from falling forward while drunk, typically causes contusions on the orbital surfaces of the frontal lobes and the anterior and basal portions of the temporal lobes. With lateral forces, as from the doorframe of a car, the contusions are situated on the lateral convexity of the hemispheres. In both instances there may be obverse contrecoup contusions.

Contusions are visible on CT and MRI scans, appearing early as inhomogeneous hyperdensities on CT and as hyperintensities on MRI; the signal changes reflect small scattered areas of cortical and subcortical blood and localized brain edema (Fig. 369-1); there is also some degree of subarachnoid bleeding, which may be detected by scans or lumbar puncture. Confluent, roughly spherical contusions can be distinguished from cerebral hemorrhages by their involvement of the cortical surface. Contusions may acquire a surrounding ringlike contrast enhancement after a week that may be mistaken for tumor or abscess. Glial and macrophage reactions begin within 2 days and result years later in scarred, hemosiderin-stained depressions on the surface (*plaques jaunes*) that are one source of posttraumatic epilepsy.

The clinical signs produced by contusions vary with their location and size; a hemiparesis or gaze preference, similar to the signs of a middle cerebral artery stroke, is fairly typical. Large bilateral contusions produce coma with extensor posturing. Contusions limited to the frontal lobes produce an abulic-taciturn state and those in the temporal lobe may cause an aggressive, combative, or delirous syndrome, described below. The secondary effects of progressive edema are the most threatening aspect of contusion injury and lead to coma and signs of secondary brainstem compression (pupillary enlargement).

Deep hemorrhages in the central white matter may result from confluent contusions in the depths of a sulcus. However, ganglionic, diencephalic, and other deep hematomas due to torsion or shearing forces in the brain occur independently of surface damage. Large single hemorrhages after minor trauma may bring to attention a bleeding diathesis or cerebrovascular amyloidosis in the elderly. For unexplained reasons, deep cerebral hemorrhages may not develop until several days after severe injury. Sudden neurologic deterioration in a comatose patient or an unexplained rise in intracranial pressure (ICP) should therefore prompt investigation with a CT scan.

Another type of deep white matter lesion consists of widespread acute disruption, or "shearing," of axons at the time of impact. Characteristically there are small areas of tissue disruption in the corpus callosum and dorsolateral pons, but these areas may not be appreciated in scans. The presence of widespread axonal damage of both hemispheres, a state called *diffuse axonal injury*, has been proposed as the explanation of persistent coma or vegetative state, but small ischemic-hemorrhagic lesions in the midbrain and low diencephalon are as often the cause. Only severe shearing lesions that contain blood are visualized by CT, usually in the corpus callosum and centrum semiovale (Fig. 369-2); however, within days of the injury, MRI scan demonstrates such lesions throughout the white matter, especially with the use of gradient echo MRI sequences.

On occasion, especially in children, cranial trauma causes diffuse brain swelling within a few hours after injury, even though CT may not reveal focal contusions or hemorrhages. The swelling creates a mass effect with disastrous consequences. Swelling is likely due to microvascular disruption and greatly increased cerebral blood flow. Episodes of moderate hypotension after the injury may play a role in this complication.

Residual symptoms and signs of primary or secondary compressive brainstem hemorrhages or ischemic lesions include cerebellar tremor, pupillary enlargement, eye movement abnormalities, and the "locked-in" syndrome (Chap. 24).

SUBDURAL AND EPIDURAL HEMATOMAS Hemorrhages beneath the dura (subdural) or between the dura and skull (epidural) may be associated with contusions and other injuries, making it difficult to determine their relative contribution to the clinical state. However, subdural and epidural hematomas more often occur as the sole manifestation of injury, and each has characteristic clinical and radiologic features. Because the mass effect and the rise in ICP caused by these hemorrhages may be life threatening, it is imperative that they be identified immediately by CT or MRI scan and evacuated when appropriate.

Acute Subdural Hematoma These lesions become symptomatic minutes or hours after injury. Up to one-third of patients have a lucid interval before coma supervenes, but most are drowsy or comatose from the moment of injury. Direct cranial trauma is not required for acute subdural hemorrhage to occur; acceleration forces alone, as from whiplash, are adequate, especially in the elderly and those taking anticoagulant medications. A unilateral headache and slightly enlarged pupil on the same side are frequently but not invar-

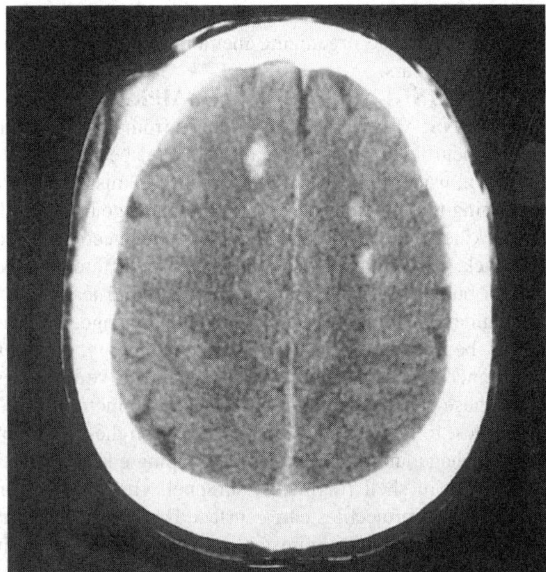

FIGURE 369-2 Multiple small areas of hemorrhage and tissue disruption in the white matter of the frontal lobes on noncontrast CT scan. These appear to reflect an extreme type of the "diffuse axonal shearing" lesions that occur with closed head injury.

iably found. Stupor or coma, a hemiparesis, and unilateral pupillary enlargement are the typical signs of larger hematomas; pupillary dilation is contralateral to the hematoma in 5 to 10%. In an acutely deteriorating patient with diminished alertness and with pupillary enlargement, burr (drainage) holes or an emergency craniotomy are appropriate, at times even without prior radiographic confirmation of subdural hematoma. Small subdural hematomas may be asymptomatic and usually do not require therapy. A more subacute syndrome from subdural hematoma occurs days to weeks after injury with drowsiness, headache, confusion, or mild hemiparesis; it is seen in alcoholics and in the elderly. Chronic subdural hematoma is described below.

Most subdural hematomas appear as crescentic collections over the convexity of the hemisphere and are located over the frontotemporal region, less often in the inferior middle fossa or over the occipital poles (Fig. 369-3). The degree of midline shift is disproportionately greater than the apparent size of the clot in any one axial CT scan, but the guidelines relating shift to the level of consciousness outlined in Chap. 24 remain useful. Less common instances of interhemispheric, posterior fossa, or bilateral convexity clots are difficult to diagnose clinically, although drowsiness and the signs expected for each region can be detected (Chap 25). Larger clots are thought to be primarily venous in origin, though additional arterial bleeding sites are often found; some large clots, when explored surgically, appear to be exclusively arterial.

Acute Epidural Hematoma Epidural hematomas evolve more rapidly than subdural hematomas and are therefore more treacherous. They occur in up to 10% of severe trauma cases and are less often associated with underlying cortical damage than are subdural hematomas. Most patients are unconscious when first seen. A "lucid interval" of several minutes to hours before coma supervenes is said to be most characteristic of epidural hemorrhage, although it is not common, and epidural hemorrhage by no means is the only cause of this temporal profile.

An epidural hematoma located over the convexity of either lateral temporal lobe is explained by its origin from a torn dural vessel, most commonly the middle meningeal artery, which is transected by a fracture of the squamous portion of the temporal bone. Frontal, inferior temporal, or occipitoparietal epidural hematomas are less frequent, occurring when fractures disrupt branches of the middle meningeal

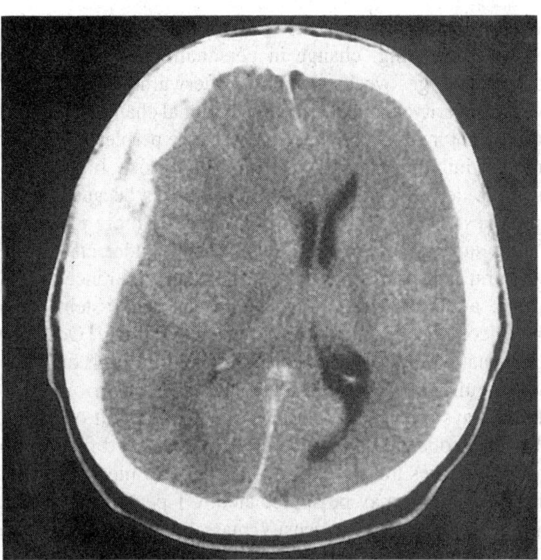

FIGURE 369-3 Acute subdural hematoma in a noncontrast CT scan. The hyperdense clot has an irregular border with the brain and typically causes more horizontal displacement (mass effect) than might be expected from its thickness. The disproportionate mass effect is the result of the large rostral-caudal extent of these hematomas. Compare to Fig. 369-4.

artery. The hematoma strips the tightly attached dura from the inner table of the skull, producing a characteristic lenticular shaped clot on CT (Fig. 369-4). Epidural hematomas may be less frequent in the elderly because of the tighter attachment of dura to skull that occurs with aging. Posterior fossa epidural hematomas are rare and difficult to detect clinically; most result from surgery in that region, such as resection of an acoustic schwannoma.

Chronic Subdural Hematoma A history of trauma may or may not be elicited; 20 to 30% of patients recall no head injury, particularly the elderly and those with a bleeding diathesis. The causative injury may be trivial (striking the head against the branch of a tree, a sudden stop in a car, or minor head contact during a fall or faint) and is often

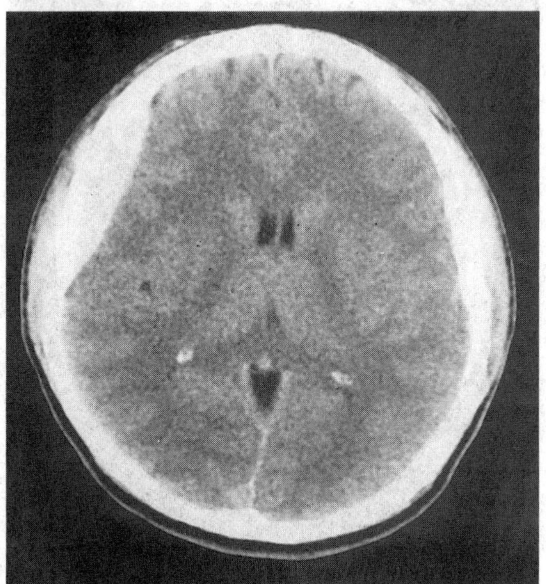

FIGURE 369-4 Acute epidural hematoma. The typical lenticular shape is due to the dura, which is tightly adherent to the skull. Epidural hematomas are usually caused by disruption of the middle meningeal artery following fracture of the temporal bone.

forgotten because it was remote. Headaches (common but not invariable), slowed thinking, change in personality, a seizure, or a mild hemiparesis emerges weeks or months afterwards. The headache may fluctuate in severity, sometimes with positional changes. Many chronic subdural hematomas are bilateral and produce perplexing clinical syndromes. The initial clinical impression is of a stroke, brain tumor, drug intoxication, depression, or a dementing illness because drowsiness, inattentiveness, and incoherence of thought are more prominent than focal signs such as hemiparesis. Patients with undetected small bilateral subdural hematomas seem to have a low tolerance for surgery, anesthesia, and drugs that depress the nervous system, remaining drowsy or confused for long periods postoperatively. Occasionally a chronic hematoma causes brief episodes of hemiparesis or aphasia that are indistinguishable from transient ischemic attacks.

Skull x-rays are usually normal except for a shift of the calcified pineal body to one side or an occasional unexpected fracture. In very long-standing cases the irregular calcification of membranes that surround the collection may be appreciated. CT performed without contrast infusion shows a low-density mass over the convexity of the hemisphere (Fig. 369-5), but between 2 to 6 weeks after the initial bleeding the clot appears isodense compared to adjacent brain. Bilateral chronic hematomas may fail to be detected because of the absence of lateral tissue shifts; this circumstance is suggested by a "hypernormal" CT scan with fullness of the cortical sulci and small ventricles in an older patient. CT with contrast demonstrates the vascular fibrous capsule surrounding the clot; MRI can reliably identify either a subacute or chronic clot. Lumbar puncture is not recommended for diagnosis because of the risk of worsening tissue shifts but, if performed, shows xanthochromia of the spinal fluid and a variable number of red blood cells. Chronic subdural hematomas can expand gradually and clinically resemble tumors of the brain.

Clinical observation and serial imaging are reasonable in patients with few symptoms and small subdural collections. Treatment with glucocorticoids alone is sufficient in some cases, but surgical evacuation is more often successful. The fibrous membranes that grow from the dura and encapsulate the region require surgical resection to prevent recurrent fluid accumulation. Small hematomas are largely resorbed, leaving only the organizing membranes, which become calcified after many years.

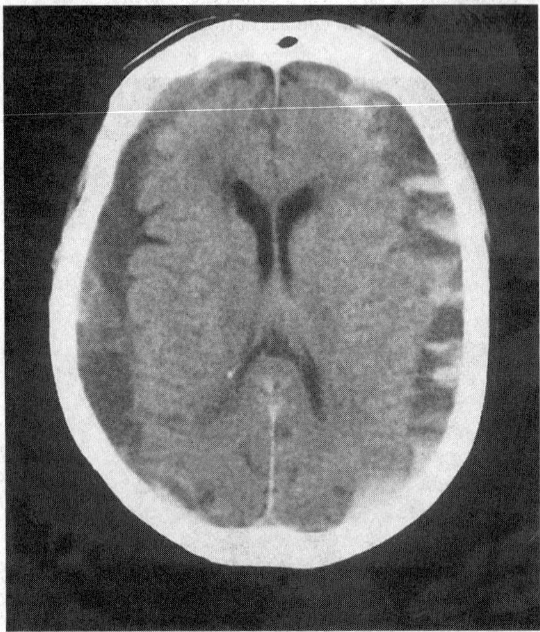

FIGURE 369-5 CT scan of chronic bilateral subdural hematomas of different ages. The collections began as acute hematomas and have become hypodense (called *hygromas*) in comparison to the adjacent brain after a period during which they were isodense and difficult to appreciate. Some areas of resolving blood are contained on the more recently formed collection on the left.

PENETRATING INJURIES, COMPRESSIONS, AND LACERATIONS Tangential scalp wounds from bullets are capable of producing neurologic signs or delayed seizures because small hemorrhages or contusions arise even in the absence of missile penetration. Bullets entering the brain cause considerable damage because of their tremendous kinetic energy. A cylindrical area of necrosis surrounds the bullet track, but the nature of injury differs for different projectiles. Soft civilian bullets typically shatter on impact and leave a track of metallic fragments with moderate parenchymal damage, whereas military bullets, because of their high velocity and energy, disrupt tissue at great distances from the track and produce massive brain destruction. All of these penetrating injuries cause a rapid increase in ICP for several minutes, followed by a drop depending on the volume of secondary hemorrhage and the degree of developing edema. Infection is a risk mainly from shell fragments, shrapnel, grenades, and mines, because such small projectiles carry surface bacteria and dirt into the brain. Most neurosurgeons administer systemic antibiotics prophylactically and perform local debridement for all types of penetrating injuries. Aneurysms may form as a result of disruption of vessel walls from the shock wave of the passing projectile; facial-orbital entrance wounds have the highest incidence of this complication. The aneurysms have an unpredictable course, but most that rupture do so in the first month. The prognosis for survival after missile injuries is good if consciousness is preserved and poor if coma is present from the outset.

In civilian practice, intracranial foreign bodies such as knives, picks, studgun staples, or high-speed tool bits may be missed unless skull x-rays are taken after what are seemingly minor penetrating injuries. Surgical removal of the object, debridement, and extensive exploration for hemorrhage and necrotic tissue are required.

TRAUMATIC VASCULAR DISSECTION AND OCCLUSION The kinetic energy of minor or more severe head or neck trauma can produce dissection of the internal carotid or vertebral arteries by stripping the intima or the media. Chiropractic neck manipulation accounts for some cases. Severe blunt impacts to the neck can initiate a dissection several centimeters above the origins of the internal carotid or vertebral arteries. There is usually local neck pain over the affected carotid artery, a Horner's syndrome, and headache over the ipsilateral anterior cranium. Some patients with carotid dissection subsequently have large middle cerebral artery strokes with hemiplegia after a period of fluctuating hemiparesis. In drowsy or comatose patients, evidence of dissection or subsequent stroke is difficult to determine, but its presence is suggested by unexplained hemiplegia, unilateral miosis, or appearance of cerebral infarction on CT scan.

Traumatic vertebral artery dissection causes vertigo, vomiting, suboccipital or supraorbital headache, and other signs of lateral medullary or cerebellar ischemia. These symptoms may be attributed erroneously to vestibular concussion. In comatose patients, the only indication may be inferior cerebellar infarction on imaging studies. Vasospasm from traumatic subarachnoid blood may also be involved in the development of infarction after head injury.

Cavernous sinus arteriovenous fistulas are rare but serious complications in patients who survive severe head injury. The problem is first evident as a self-audible bruit (many are also audible to the examiner), proptosis, conjunctival injection, or visual impairment. Angiography shows early filling of the cavernous sinus and its draining tributaries. The fistula enlarges, causing increasingly severe local changes around the eye and orbit and decreased chances of visual recovery. About 10%, mostly small fistulas, resolve spontaneously. Many surgical approaches have been tried, including ligation of the carotid artery and direct obliteration of the fistula or cavernous sinus, but a detachable balloon that is delivered by an intravascular catheter has proved most successful.

INTRACRANIAL PRESSURE AND CEREBRAL BLOOD FLOW

Raised ICP arising from contusion, hematoma, and subsequent progressive edema accounts for at least 50% of deaths after head injury; outcome is inversely related to the level of ICP. Aggressive treatment of raised ICP in modern intensive care units is believed to contribute to improved survival after severe head injury, but many other factors pertain, and the role of direct monitoring of ICP to guide therapy, while favored in many centers, is still uncertain.

For several minutes to an hour after acute head injury, cerebral blood flow increases in most patients, although metabolic demands and oxygen consumption of the cerebrum are diminished. Autoregulation—the ability of the cerebral vasculature to maintain a constant blood flow in response to decreased or increased perfusion pressure—is impaired globally and even more so in damaged regions. The rise in cerebral blood volume caused by the failure of autoregulation is thought to account for approximately two-thirds of the rise in ICP after severe head injury. The blood-brain barrier also becomes more permeable in contused regions, promoting edema formation. Resting ICP is spontaneously interrupted by rises in ICP, termed *plateau waves*, which arise as a result of a loss of cerebrovascular tone and a resultant increase in cerebral blood volume. Plateau waves may be precipitated by iatrogenic maneuvers such as suctioning, physical therapy, excess fluid administration, or pain but also by mild, often unnoticed hypotension that causes cerebrovascular dilation. Signs of clinical deterioration, such as pupillary enlargement, may occur after plateau waves; occasionally, brain death ensues. Other secondary systemic phenomena after severe head injury, particularly hypotension and hypoxia, cause brain damage and greatly alter outcome. →*The regulation of ICP and its relationship to cerebral blood flow (CBF) are discussed in Chap. 376.*

CLINICAL SYNDROMES AND TREATMENT OF HEAD INJURY

MINOR INJURY The patient who is fully alert and attentive after head injury but who has one or more symptoms of headache, faintness, nausea, a single episode of emesis, difficulty with concentration, or slight blurring of vision has a good prognosis with little risk of subsequent deterioration. Such patients have usually sustained a concussion and are expected to have a brief amnestic epoch. Children and young adults are particularly prone to drowsiness, vomiting, and irritability, which is sometimes delayed for several hours after apparently minor injuries. Occasionally, vasovagal syncope occurs several minutes to an hour after the injury and may cause undue concern. Constant generalized or frontal headache is common in the days following trauma; it may be migrainous (throbbing and hemicranial) in nature. After several hours of observation, patients with this category of injury may be accompanied home and observed by a family member or friend. Most patients with a minor syndrome do not have a skull fracture on skull x-ray or hemorrhage on CT. The decision to perform these tests depends largely on clinical signs suggesting that the impact was severe (e.g., prolonged concussion, periorbital or mastoid hematoma, repeated vomiting), on the seriousness of other bodily injuries, and on the degree of surveillance that can be expected at home. Persistent severe headache and repeated vomiting in the context of normal alertness and no focal neurologic signs are usually benign, but radiologic studies should be obtained and observation in the hospital is justified.

INJURY OF INTERMEDIATE SEVERITY Patients who are not comatose but who have persistent confusion, behavioral changes, subnormal alertness, extreme dizziness, or focal neurologic signs such as hemiparesis should be admitted to the hospital and soon thereafter have a CT scan. Usually a contusion or hematoma is found. The clinical syndromes most common in this group, in addition to postconcussive headache, dizziness, and vomiting, include (1) delirium with a disinclination to be examined or moved, expletive speech, and resistance if disturbed (anterior temporal lobe contusions); (2) a quiet, disinterested, slowed mental state (abulia) with dull facial appearance and irascibility (inferior frontal and frontopolar contusions); (3) a focal deficit such as aphasia or mild hemiparesis (due to subdural hematoma or convexity contusion, or, less often, carotid artery dissection); (4) confusion with inattention, poor performance on simple mental tasks, and fluctuating or slightly erroneous orientation (associated with several types of injuries, including the first two described above as well as medial frontal contusions and interhemispheric subdural hematoma); (5) repetitive vomiting, nystagmus, drowsiness, and unsteadiness (usually labyrinthine concussion, but occasionally due to a posterior fossa subdural hematoma or vertebral artery dissection); and (6) diabetes insipidus (damage to the median eminence or pituitary stalk). It needs to be emphasized that intermediate-grade injuries are often complicated by drug or alcohol intoxication.

Clinical observation is necessary to detect increasing drowsiness, change in respiratory pattern, or pupillary enlargement and to ensure restriction of free water (unless there is diabetes insipidus). Asymmetry in limb posture, limb movement, or gaze preference suggests a subdural or epidural hematoma or large contusion. Most patients in this category improve over several days. During the first week, the state of alertness, memory, and other cognitive performance often fluctuate, and irascibility or agitation is common. Behavioral changes are worst at night, as with most other encephalopathies, and may be treated with small doses of antipsychotic medications. Subtle abnormalities of attention, intellect, spontaneity, and memory tend to return to normal weeks or months after the injury, sometimes surprisingly abruptly; persistent losses in cognition are discussed below.

SEVERE INJURY Patients who are comatose from the onset require immediate neurologic attention and often resuscitation. After intubation, with care taken to avoid deforming the cervical spine, the depth of coma, pupillary size and reactivity, limb movements, and Babinski responses are assessed. As soon as vital functions permit and cervical spine x-rays and a CT scan have been obtained, the patient should be transported to a critical care unit. The finding of an epidural or subdural hematoma or large intracerebral hemorrhage is an indication for prompt surgery and intracranial decompression in otherwise salvageable patients. Subsequent treatment is probably best guided by direct measurement of ICP but may proceed on a presumptive basis using clinical status and CT scan as guides. All potential exacerbating factors must be eliminated. Hypoxia, hyperthermia, hypercarbia, awkward head positions, and high mean airway pressures from mechanical ventilation all increase cerebral blood volume and ICP. Many, but not all, patients will have lower ICP when the head and trunk are elevated. Active management of raised ICP includes hyperosmolar dehydration with 20% mannitol (0.25 to 1 g/kg every 3 to 6 h), preferably using directly measured ICP as a guide. Otherwise, a serum osmolality of ~300 mosmol/L is desirable. It is customary to restrict free water administration in order to maintain high serum osmolarity, but there is no rationale for a reduction in the total volume of fluids administered if they are iso- or hyperosmolar, e.g., normal saline. Induced hypocarbia to an initial level of 28 to 33 mmHg P_{CO_2} is rapidly effective in reducing ICP, but its duration of effect is limited and its use has fallen out of favor, perhaps excessively so.

Persistently raised ICP after inception of this conservative therapy generally indicates a poor outcome. Although the addition of high-dose barbiturates may further lower ICP, there is no beneficial effect on overall outcome. In many instances, barbiturates cause a parallel reduction in ICP and BP without a net improvement in cerebral perfusion. Systolic BP should be maintained >100 mmHg by vasopressor agents, if necessary. Mean BP levels >110 to 120 mmHg may exaggerate brain edema, but some neurosurgeons allow the BP to rise above normal on the basis that this may abort plateau waves. A conventional approach to extreme hypertension utilizes diuretics and β-adrenergic blocking agents, angiotensin-converting enzyme inhibitors, or intermittent doses of barbiturates. A number of other antihypertensive drugs, including some calcium channel blockers and nitrates, are said to be relatively contraindicated because they may raise ICP. Antacids administered by nasogastric tube or direct-acting drugs are utilized to keep gastric pH >3.5 and prevent gastrointestinal bleeding as described below. The use of large doses of glucocorticoids in severe head injury does not improve outcome. Several studies suggest that early nutritional support results in faster neurologic recovery from head injury. If the patient remains comatose, it is worthwhile to repeat the CT or MRI scan to exclude a delayed surface or intracerebral hemorrhage. Intensive care salvages some critically ill head-injured patients by concentrating efforts on simple treatments that avoid medical complications, particularly pneumonia and sepsis and preventable increases in ICP.

SYSTEMIC DERANGEMENTS RESULTING FROM SEVERE HEAD TRAUMA Injuries outside the cranium should be searched for at the outset, because they are likely to be forgotten if not initially noted. In particular, associated spinal, long bone, and abdominal injuries may cause delayed difficulties in management. Over half of patients who persist in coma for 24 h after head injury develop *abnormalities of electrolytes or fluid balance*. Diabetes insipidus should be suspected if urine output increases and urine specific gravity is low (Chap. 329). Replacement of water losses suffices for mild cases, but vasopressin may be required. Secretion of aldosterone and antidiuretic hormone (vasopressin, AVP) in response to stress favor the retention of sodium and free water, respectively. The latter usually predominates, leading to mild hypervolemic hyponatremia, but this is obscured if osmotic dehydrating agents have been used.

Some patients with head injuries suffer *hypoxia* acutely after injury without obvious pulmonary infiltrates. Aspiration pneumonia presents a great risk; lung injury from aspirated gastric contents, infection, and atelectasis may combine to produce the adult respiratory distress syndrome (ARDS) and severe arteriovenous shunting (Chap. 265). ARDS also occurs owing to disseminated intravascular coagulopathy, fat embolism, or, rarely, "neurogenic" pulmonary edema (see below). The effect of positive end-expiratory pressure (PEEP) on ICP is complex, but PEEP should not be withheld if necessary for oxygenation. *Atelectasis* is common in all poorly responsive patients and is treated with chest physical therapy and adequate ventilator tidal volumes. *Pulmonary embolism* is also a major threat to bedridden patients, and intermittent pneumatic calf compression or modest doses of subcutaneous heparin may be useful prophylaxis. The latter has not predisposed to intracerebral or gastrointestinal bleeding. Early recognition of deep leg vein thrombosis and aggressive treatment by occlusion of the inferior vena cava may prevent later emboli.

Patients with severe long bone injuries are subject to widespread *cerebral fat embolism*. For uncertain reasons, this complication is seen less often than previously, perhaps because of better fluid replacement. In the typical case, head injury is a minor part of the overall trauma; nonetheless, severe cranial injury masks the syndrome. Several days after the bone fractures occur, restlessness, delirium or drowsiness progressing to coma in severe cases, seizures, generalized brain edema, and hypoxia develop. About half the patients have retinal and punctate conjunctival hemorrhages or fat that is visible in retinal vessels. A petechial rash (prominent in the anterior axillary folds and supraclavicular fossae), diffuse interstitial infiltrates on the chest x-ray, fat in the urine, and/or renal failure occur in some patients. Severe reduction in arterial oxygen content is common from widespread lung injury (ARDS). Cerebral fat embolism causes a cerebral purpura, mainly in the white matter, due to capillary occlusion by fat globules. There is evidence that patients in whom this complication is recognized and treated early have a better prognosis. Massive doses of glucocorticoids and administration of positive-pressure ventilation with high end-expiratory pressures have been claimed to be useful.

Most patients with severe head injuries develop gastric erosions, but only a few have clinically significant hemorrhages. *Gastrointestinal bleeding* usually occurs in the first days to 1 week after injury. Unlike the majority of patients in shock or with stress ulceration, head-trauma patients often have elevated gastric acidity. Prophylactic treatment with gastric coating agents as discussed above, with H_2 receptor blockers, or with frequent antacid administration probably reduces gastric hemorrhage in other stress states and is commonly used in head trauma.

Acute head trauma may cause transient apnea and cardiac arrest. In the absence of overwhelming brain damage, recovery from the arrest is the rule. Subsequently, a sympathoadrenal discharge or raised ICP causes *systemic hypertension*, either with the classically associated bradycardia of the Cushing response or, almost as frequently, with tachycardia. Cardiac arrhythmias are common, most notably sinus bradycardia, supraventricular tachycardias, nodal rhythm, and heart block. T-wave inversion and alterations in the ST segment may simulate subendocardial ischemia. In some instances these changes are due to cardiac muscle contusion.

Neurogenic pulmonary edema is a form of respiratory failure in which the alveoli fill with fluid, as in congestive heart failure, but left ventricular end-diastolic pressure is normal after the infiltrates are established. The nature of this pulmonary vascular leak is not settled, but it may be the result of a sudden shift of intravascular volume from the systemic to the pulmonary circulation or there may be a direct cerebral neurogenic influence on the pulmonary microvasculature. The alveolar capillary leak may continue despite a return of pulmonary vascular pressure to normal.

Many patients demonstrate a mild *coagulopathy*, and 5 to 10% have various degrees of disseminated intravascular coagulation, a harbinger of poor outcome. There is a correlation between the severity of injury and the level of increased fibrin degradation products in blood, and one cause of the coagulopathy may be the release of highly thromboplastic material from damaged brain tissue.

PROGNOSIS Extensive work by Jennet's group in Glasgow and by the Traumatic Coma Data Bank has provided data on the outcome in severe head injury. Verbal output, eye opening, and the best motor response of the limbs have been found to be predictive of outcome and are summarized using the "Glasgow Coma Scale" (Table 369-1). Over 85% of patients with aggregate scores of 3 or 4 die within 24 h. However, a number of patients with slightly higher scores but a poor initial prognosis, including absent pupillary light responses, survive, suggesting that an initially aggressive approach is justified in most patients. Patients <20 years, particularly children, may make remarkable recoveries after having grave early neurologic signs. In

Table 369-1 Glasgow Coma Scale for Head Injury

Eye opening (E)	
Spontaneous	4
To loud voice	3
To pain	2
Nil	1
Best motor response (M)	
Obeys	6
Localizes	5
Withdraws (flexion)	4
Abnormal flexion posturing	3
Extension posturing	2
Nil	1
Verbal response (V)	
Oriented	5
Confused, disoriented	4
Inappropriate words	3
Incomprehensible sounds	2
Nil	1

NOTE: Coma score = E + M + V. Patients scoring 3 or 4 have an 85 percent chance of dying or remaining vegetative, while scores above 11 indicate only a 5 to 10 percent likelihood of death or vegetative state and 85 percent chance of moderate disability or good recovery. Intermediate scores correlate with proportional chances of recovery.

one large study of severe head injury, 55% of children had a good outcome at 1 year, compared with 21% of adults. Older age, increased ICP, hypoxia and hypotension, and CT scan evidence of compression of the cisterns surrounding the brainstem and shift of midline structures are all poor prognostic signs. Delayed evacuation of large intracerebral clots is also associated with a poor prognosis.

Evoked potentials have prognostic value in head injury, similar to their use in ischemic-hypoxic brain injury, and their accuracy in predicting a poor outcome probably exceeds that of purely clinical methods. The results obtained from somatosensory evoked potentials are clearest, with the bilateral absence of cortical potentials (more caudal potentials present) predicting death or a vegetative state in over 90% of patients. A normal or mildly abnormal test, however, does not reliably predict a good functional outcome.

NEUROPSYCHOLOGICAL OUTCOME AFTER HEAD INJURY

A structural basis has been sought for the posttraumatic nervous instability termed the *postconcussion syndrome*, which consists of fatigue, dizziness, headache, and difficulty in concentration after mild or moderate injury. Most instances are difficult to distinguish from asthenia and depression. However, with intermediate-grade injury there is probably a substantial incidence of difficulty with attention and memory as well as other subtle cognitive deficits. Based on experimental models, some investigators believe that subtle axonal shearing lesions or biochemical alterations account for these symptoms despite normal findings on brain imaging, evoked potentials, and electroencephalogram. In moderate and severe trauma, neuropsychological changes are found routinely, but some of these deficits identified in formal testing are not important in daily functioning. Test scores tend to improve rapidly during the first 6 months after injury, then more slowly for years.

SPINAL CORD TRAUMA

Approximately 10,000 patients a year in the United States, mostly young and otherwise healthy, become paraplegic or quadriplegic because of spinal cord injuries; there are an estimated 200,000 quadriplegics in the nation. Most spinal cord injuries in civilian life result from fracture or dislocation of the surrounding vertebral column. Vertical compression with flexion is the main mechanism of injury in the thoracic cord, and hyperextension or flexion is the main cause of injury in the cervical cord. Preexisting spondylosis, a congenitally narrowed spinal canal, hypertrophied ligamentum flavum (Chap. 16), and instability of the apophyseal joints from diseases such as rheumatoid arthritis predispose to severe spinal cord damage even after minor degrees of injury.

PATHOPHYSIOLOGY AND PATHOLOGY OF SPINAL CORD INJURY Considerable spinal cord damage results from secondary phenomena that arise in the minutes and hours following injury. Even when a complete transverse myelopathy is evident immediately after impact, some secondary changes and the resultant damage may be reversible. The immediate compression of the cord causes pericapillary hemorrhages that coalesce and enlarge, particularly in the gray matter. Infarction of gray matter and early white matter edema are evident within 4 hours of experimental blunt injury. Eight hours after injury, there is global infarction at the traumatized level, and only at this point does necrosis of white matter and paralysis below the level of the lesion become irreversible. The necrosis and central hemorrhages enlarge to occupy one or two levels above and below the point of primary impact. Gliosis progresses over several months, and the affected regions may cavitate, causing a syringomyelic syndrome.

A large number of interventions for acute spinal compression injury have been of uncertain benefit, but high doses of methylprednisolone (typically 30 mg/kg followed by 5.4 mg/kg hourly for 23 h) administered within 8 hours of injury is associated with a slightly improved outcome. The critical factor for recoverable function is the time from injury to the institution of any therapy.

MANAGEMENT OF SPINAL CORD INJURY SYNDROMES Any patient with an injury that involves the spine or head potentially has an associated instability of the spinal column. The care of such patients begins at the scene of the accident: the neck should be immobilized, and care should be taken during transport and during the physical and radiologic examinations to prevent extension or rotation of the neck and torsion-rotation of the thoracic spine. Intubation, if necessary, can be accomplished by a blind nasotracheal technique or over an endoscope in order to avoid neck extension. High thoracic or cervical cord transection causes hypotension and bradycardia because of a functional sympathectomy (sometimes corroborated by bilateral ptosis and miosis—Horner's syndrome), which responds to infusion of crystalloid or colloid.

The neurologic assessment in the awake patient with possible spinal injury focuses on neck or back pain, diminished limb power, a sensory level on the trunk, and on deep tendon reflexes, which are usually absent below the level of acute cord injury. The level of injury can be approximated from the upper dermatome of sensory loss. Injuries above C5 cause quadriplegia and respiratory failure. At C5 and C6 the biceps are weak, whereas the deltoid and the supra- and infraspinatus are spared. C7 injuries cause weakness of the triceps, wrist extensors, and forearm pronators. Injuries at T1 and below cause paraplegia. Compression in the lower thoracic and lumbar spine causes a conus medullaris or cauda equina syndrome. Cauda equina injuries are usually incomplete, involving peripheral nerves rather than spinal cord, and therefore are surgically remediable for longer periods after injury than spinal cord compression. In a comatose patient, absent reflexes, especially with small pupils or paradoxical breathing and hypotension, signify a high cervical cord injury. →***The principles of spinal cord localization are considered in detail in Chap. 368.***

Reversible and preventable causes of spinal cord compression must be detected and surgically remedied. These include dislocation of a vertebral body, or an unstable vertebral fracture that can lead to misalignment and cord compression in the future. Treatment of fractures through the pedicles, facets, or vertebral bodies varies; some fractures heal with immobilization and time, usually 2 to 3 months, while others require surgical fusion to ensure stability. Many traumatic myelopathies have no clearly associated fracture or dislocation, but there is generally rupture of the supporting ligaments that has produced transient cord compression during the impact. If x-rays suggest any aberration in the position of vertebrae, then realignment should generally be undertaken quickly. CT or MRI exam is the most useful for demonstrating spinal misalignment and fractures. The role of myelography is not as compelling as it was in the past, but many neurosurgeons choose to instill a few drops of water-soluble contrast medium into the spinal subarachnoid space to demonstrate a block to the flow of CSF by CT or conventional myelography. Decompression within 2 hours of severe injury may lead to some recovery of spinal cord function. With incomplete myelopathies, especially if the limbs are becoming progressively weaker, early realignment is performed even many hours after injury. The surgical approaches to decompressing the spinal column depend on the specific nature of the injury. In complete transverse myelopathies beyond 6 to 12 hours after injury, decompressive laminectomies are usually unsuccessful in restoring function.

Atlantoaxial dislocation can cause immediate death from respiratory failure, an event that may occur unexpectedly even without other neurologic signs. Rheumatoid arthritis predisposes to this injury. Atlantooccipital dislocations occur predominantly in children and are almost always fatal. "Jefferson's fractures" are burst fractures of the ring of the atlas resulting from a force descending on the vertex of the skull, as in diving accidents; they are usually asymptomatic. "Hangman's fractures" are produced by hyperextension and longitudinal distraction of the upper cervical spine, as occurs with penal hanging or striking the chin on a steering wheel in a head-on collision. These are usually fractures through the pedicles of C2 with subluxation anteriorly of C2 on C3. Traction reduction and prolonged immobilization usually allow proper healing.

Hyperflexion dislocation of the cervical vertebrae commonly causes quadriplegia. Occasionally, a markedly displaced injury is unassociated with neurologic dysfunction, presenting only with neck pain. Any degree of subluxation must be considered as potentially unstable.

Compression fracture of the cervical spine can cause neurologic damage if a bone fragment is driven backward (burst fracture) into the spinal cord. "Teardrop fractures" with crushing of a vertebral body, leaving a fragment of bone anteriorly, are usually associated with ligamentous disruption and spinal instability. Single compression fractures of the thoracic spine are usually stable because the thoracic cage provides support, but they may be associated with anterior spinal cord compression and require decompression and stabilization with the insertion of metal rods.

Mild *cervical hyperextension* injuries may cause only disruption of supporting ligamentous structures and can be well tolerated. More severe injuries cause vertebral displacement and cord compression. The "central cord syndrome" is produced by brief compression of the cervical cord and disruption of the central gray matter. It usually occurs in patients with an already narrow spinal canal, either congenitally or from cervical spondylosis. There is weakness of the arms with pinprick loss over the arms and shoulders, and relative sparing of leg power and sensation on the trunk and legs. Abnormality of bladder function is variable. The prognosis for recovery is good.

Thoracolumbar fracture is produced by impact in the high or middle back, usually while the patient is bent over. Impingement on the spinal canal results in a complex combination of cauda equina and conus medullaris dysfunction. Purely lumbar fractures with displacement of a vertebral body produce cauda equina compression. Surgical decompression is usually recommended, even with severe neurologic deficits, because there is considerable potential for recovery of the nerve roots of the cauda.

The subsequent care of patients with spinal cord injury is best undertaken in specialized centers. →***General principles of medical and urologic management are discussed in Chap. 368.***

BIBLIOGRAPHY

ANNEGERS JF et al: A population-based study of seizures after traumatic brain injury. N Engl J Med 338:20, 1998

COLLINS MW et al: Current issues in managing sports-related concussion. JAMA 282: 2283, 1999

DACEY RG et al: Neurosurgical complications after apparently minor head injury. J Neurosurg 65:203, 1986

EISENBERG HM et al: Report of the Traumatic Coma Data Bank. J Neurosurg 75(Suppl): S1, 1991

GOLDSTEIN M: Traumatic brain injury: A silent epidemic. Ann Neurol 27:327, 1990

LANGFITT TW, GENARELLI TA: Can the outcome from head injury be improved? J Neurosurg 56:19, 1982

LEVIN HS et al: Neurobehavioral outcome following minor head injury: A three center study. J Neurosurg 66:234, 1987

MCCRORY PR, BERKOVIC SF: Video analysis of acute motor and convulsive manifestations in sport-related concussion. Neurology 54:1488, 2000

ROPPER AH (ed): *Neurological and Neurosurgical Intensive Care*, 3d ed. New York, Raven, 1993

ROSNER MJ et al: Cerebral perfusion pressure: Management protocol and clinical results. J Neurosurg 83:949, 1995

RUFF RM et al: Predictors of outcome following severe head trauma: Follow-up data from the Traumatic Coma Data Bank. Brain Inj 7:101, 1993

STEIN SC et al: Delayed and progressive brain injury in closed-head trauma: Radiological demonstration. Neurosurgery 32:25, 1993

370

Stephen M. Sagar, Mark A. Israel

PRIMARY AND METASTATIC TUMORS OF THE NERVOUS SYSTEM

CEA carcinonembryonic antigen	PET positron emission tomography
CNS central nervous system	PNET primitive neuroectodermal tumors
CSF cerebrospinal fluid	SPECT single-photon emission computed tomography
CT computed tomography	VHL von Hippel–Lindau
EEG electroencephalography	
MRI magnetic resonance imaging	

Malignant primary tumors of the central nervous system (CNS) occur in approximately 18,000 individuals and account for an estimated 13,300 deaths in the United States annually, a mortality rate of 5 per 100,000. An almost equal number of benign tumors of the CNS were diagnosed, with a much lower mortality rate. Glial tumors account for 50 to 60% of primary brain tumors, meningiomas account for about 25%, schwannomas for about 10%, and all other CNS tumors for the remainder. An increase in the frequency of diagnosis of malignant gliomas in the elderly has been reported in recent years. It is unclear if this change represents a true increased incidence or is the result of more frequent use of modern neuroimaging techniques.

Brain and vertebral metastases from systemic tumors are more prevalent than primary CNS tumors. About 15% of patients who die of cancer (80,000 individuals each year in the United States) have symptomatic brain metastases; an additional 5% suffer spinal cord involvement. These tumors, therefore, pose a major problem in the management of systemic cancer.

BRAIN TUMORS

Approach to the Patient

Clinical Features Brain tumors usually present with one of three syndromes: (1) subacute progression of a focal neurologic deficit; (2) seizure; or (3) nonfocal neurologic disorder such as headache, dementia, personality change, or gait disorder. The presence of systemic symptoms such as malaise, weight loss, anorexia, or fever suggests a metastatic rather than a primary brain tumor.

Progressive focal neurologic deficits result from compression of neurons and white matter tracts by expanding tumor and surrounding edema. Less commonly, a brain tumor may present with a stroke-like onset of focal neurologic deficit. Although this presentation may be caused by hemorrhage into the tumor, often no hemorrhage can be demonstrated and the mechanism is obscure. Tumors frequently associated with hemorrhage include high-grade astrocytomas and metastatic melanoma and choriocarcinoma.

Seizures may result from disruption of cortical circuits. Tumors that invade or compress the cerebral cortex, even small meningiomas, are more likely to be associated with seizures than subcortical neoplasms. Nonfocal neurologic dysfunction usually reflects increased intracranial pressure, hydrocephalus, or diffuse tumor spread. Tumors in some areas of the brain may produce subtle deficits; for example, frontal lobe tumors may present with personality change, dementia, or depression.

Headache may result from focal irritation or displacement of pain-sensitive structures (Chap. 15) or from a generalized increase in intracranial pressure. A headache that worsens rather than abates with recumbency is suggestive of a mass lesion. The headache of increased intracranial pressure has a characteristic pattern. Early on, these headaches are usually holocephalic and episodic, occurring more than once a day. They typically develop rapidly over several minutes, persist for 20 to 40 min, and subside quickly. They may awaken the patient from a sound sleep, generally 60 to 90 min after retiring, or may be precipitated by coughing, sneezing, or straining. Vomiting may occur with severe headaches. As elevated intracranial pressure becomes sustained, the headache becomes continuous but varying in intensity. Elevated intracranial pressure may cause papilledema (Chap. 28), although it is often not present in patients over 55 years old.

Infrequent but characteristic brain tumor presentations include anosmia from a meningioma arising along the cribiform plates and olfactory tracts and unilateral hearing loss from schwannomas of the eighth cranial nerve. Asymptomatic brain tumors, most often meningiomas, are commonly discovered incidentally on imaging studies obtained for unrelated purposes.

The Karnofsky performance scale is useful in assessing and following patients with brain tumors (Chap. 79). A score ≥70 indicates that the patient is ambulatory and independent in self-care activities; it has often been taken as a level of function justifying aggressive therapy.

Table 370-1 Hereditary Syndromes Associated with Brain Tumors

Syndrome	Gene (Locus)	Gene Product (Function)	Nervous System Neoplasms
Neurofibromatosis type 1 (von Recklinghausen's Disease)[a]	*NF1* (17q)	Neurofibromin (GTPase activating protein)	Neuroma, schwannoma, meningioma, optic glioma
Neurofibromatosis type 2[a]	*NF2* (22q)	Merlin (cytoskeletal protein)	Schwannoma, glioma, ependymoma, meningioma
Tuberous sclerosis	*TSC1* (9q) *TSC2* (16p)	Hamartin (unknown function) Tuberin (GTPase activating protein)	Astrocytoma
von Hippel-Lindau[a]	*VHL* (3p)	pVHL (modulator of mRNA elongation)	Hemangioblastoma of retina, cerebellum and spinal cord; pheochromocytoma
Li-Fraumeni[a]	*p53* (17p)	TP53 (cell cycle and transcriptional regulator)	Malignant glioma
Retinoblastoma[a]	*RB1* (13q)	RB (cell cycle regulator)	Retinoblastoma, pineoblastoma, malignant glioma
Turcot	*APC* (5q) (adenomatous polyposis coli)	APC (cell adhesion)	Medulloblastoma, malignant glioma
Gorlin (basal cell nevus syndrome)	*PTCH* (9q) (patched)	PTH (developmental regulator)	Medulloblastoma
Multiple endocrine neoplasia 1 (Werner syndrome)[a]	*MEN1* (11q13)	Menin (cofactor for transcription)	Pituitary adenoma, malignant schwannoma

[a] Genetic testing possible.

Laboratory Examination Primary brain tumors typically do not produce serologic abnormalities such as an elevated sedimentation rate or tumor-specific antigens associated with systemic cancers. In contrast, metastases to the nervous system, depending on the type and extent of the primary tumor, may be associated with systemic signs of malignancy (Chap. 83). Lumbar puncture may precipitate brain herniation in patients with mass lesions, and should be performed only in patients with suspected CNS infection or meningeal metastasis. Findings in the cerebrospinal fluid (CSF) of patients with primary and metastatic nervous system tumors may include raised opening pressure, elevated protein level, and a mild lymphocytic pleocytosis. Astrocytomas that extend to the ventricular surface, or the rupture of an epidermoid cyst, can occasionally produce an intense CSF inflammatory reaction simulating infectious meningitis. The CSF rarely contains malignant cells, with the important exceptions of leptomeningeal metastases, primary CNS lymphoma and primitive neuroectodermal tumors, including medulloblastoma.

Neuroimaging Computed tomography (CT) and magnetic resonance imaging (MRI) reveal mass effect and contrast enhancement. Mass effect reflects the volume of neoplastic tissue as well as surrounding edema. Brain tumors typically produce a vasogenic pattern of edema, with accumulation of excess water in white matter. The normal blood-brain barrier results from tight junctions between endothelial cells that prevent entry of most charged molecules into the nervous system. Contrast enhancement reflects a breakdown of the blood-brain barrier within the tumor, permitting leakage of contrast agent. Low-grade gliomas typically do not exhibit contrast enhancement.

Positron emission tomography (PET) and single-photon emission tomography (SPECT) have ancillary roles in the imaging of brain tumors, primarily in distinguishing tumor recurrence from tissue necrosis that can occur after irradiation (see below). Electroencephalography (EEG) has a role in the evaluation of patients with possible seizures. Functional imaging with PET, MRI, or magnetoencephalography may be of use in surgical or radiosurgical planning to define the anatomic relationship of the tumor to critical brain regions such as the primary motor cortex.

℞ TREATMENT **Symptomatic** Glucocorticoids decrease the volume of edema surrounding brain tumors and improve neurologic function; dexamethasone (12 to 20 mg/d in divided doses orally or intravenously) is used because it has relatively little mineralocorticoid activity.

Tumors that involve the cerebral cortex or hippocampus may produce epilepsy. Anticonvulsants are therefore used therapeutically and prophylactically; phenytoin, carbamazepine, and valproic acid are equally effective (Chap. 360). If the tumor is subcortical in location, prophylactic anticonvulsants are unnecessary.

Gliomas are associated with an increased risk for deep vein thrombosis and pulmonary embolism, probably because these tumors secrete procoagulant factors into the systemic circulation. Whether this risk extends to other brain tumors is unknown. Even though hemorrhage within gliomas is a frequent histopathologic finding, patients with gliomas appear to be at no increased risk for symptomatic intracranial bleeding following treatment with an anticoagulant. Prophylaxis with low-dose subcutaneous heparin should be considered for patients with gliomas who have lower limb immobility, which places them at risk for deep venous thrombosis.

PRIMARY BRAIN TUMORS

ETIOLOGY Exposure to ionizing radiation is the only well-documented environmental risk factor for the development of brain tumors. A number of hereditary syndromes are associated with an increased risk of brain tumors (Table 370-1). Genes that contribute to the development of brain tumors, as well as other malignancies, fall into two general classes, *tumor-suppressor genes* and *proto-oncogenes* (Chap. 81). Whereas germ line mutations of tumor suppressor genes are rare, somatic mutations are almost invariably found in malignant tumors, including brain tumors. Likewise, the over-expression of proto-oncogenes is frequent in brain tumors as well as systemic malignancies. Moreover, cytogenetic analysis often reveals characteristic changes. In astrocytic tumors, DNA is commonly lost on chromosomes 10p, 17p, 13q, and 9. Oligodendrogliomas frequently have deletions of 1p and 19q. In meningiomas portions of 22q, which contains the gene for neurofibromatosis type 2, are often lost. Less frequently there is evidence of amplification of specific genes, for example *EGFR* in some astrocytomas.

The particular constellation of genetic alterations varies among individual gliomas, even those that are histologically indistinguishable. Moreover, gliomas are genetically unstable, genetic abnormalities tend to accumulate with time, and these changes correspond with increasingly aggressive malignant behavior. There appear to be at least two genetic routes for the development of malignant glioma (Fig. 370-1). One route involves the progression, generally over years, from a low grade astrocytoma with early deletions of chromosome 17 and inactivation of the p53 gene to a malignant glioma with additional chromosomal deletions. The second route is characterized by the de novo appearance of a malignant glioma with amplification of the *EGFR* gene and an intact p53 gene. In both pathways, inactivation of the *PTEN* gene as a result of the loss of chromosome 10 occurs frequently.

ASTROCYTOMAS Tumors derived from astrocytes are the most common primary intracranial neoplasms (Fig. 370-2). Their neuropathologic appearance is highly variable. The most widely used histologic grading system is the World Health Organization (WHO) four-tiered grading system. Grade I is reserved for special histologic variants of astrocytoma that have an excellent prognosis after surgical excision. These include *juvenile pilocytic astrocytoma*, *subependymal giant cell astrocytoma* (which occurs in patients with tuberous sclerosis), and *pleiomorphic xanthoastrocytoma*. At the other extreme is grade IV, *glioblastoma multiforme*, a clinically aggressive tumor. *Astrocytoma* (grade II) and *anaplastic astrocytoma* (grade III) are intermediate. The histologic features associated with higher grade are hypercellularity, nuclear and cytoplasmic atypia, endothelial proliferation, mitotic activity, and necrosis. Endothelial proliferation and necrosis are especially robust predictors of aggressive behavior.

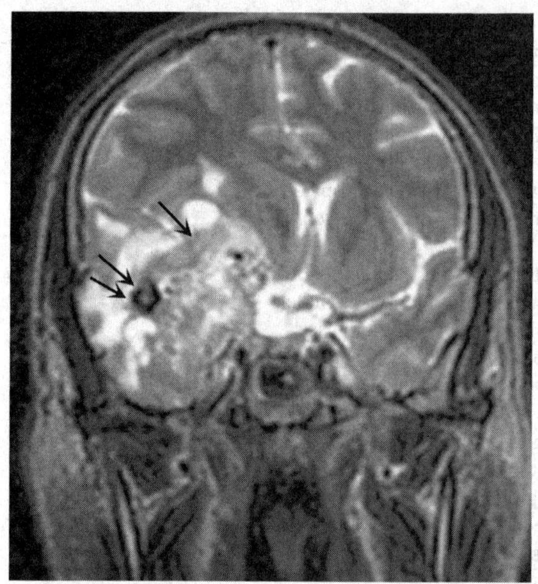

FIGURE 370-2 Malignant astrocytoma (glioblastoma). Coronal proton density-weighted MR scan through the temporal lobes demonstrates a heterogeneous right temporal lobe mass (*arrows*) compressing the third and lateral ventricles. The area of hypointense signal (*double arrows*) indicates either hemorrhage or calcification. Heterogeneous MR signal intensity is typical of glioblastoma.

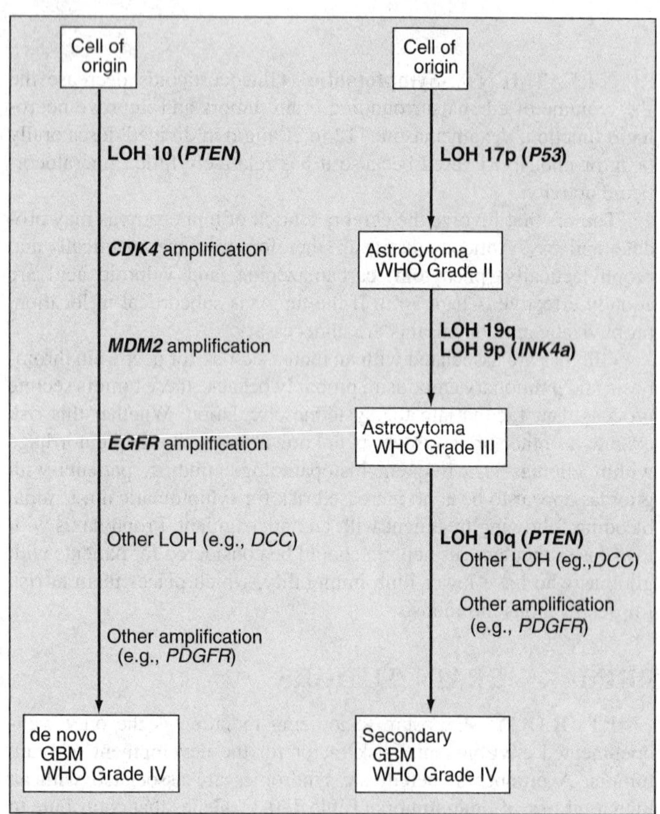

FIGURE 370-1 Proposed model for the pathogenesis of human astrocytoma. The highest grade of astrocytoma, glioblastoma multiforme (GBM), typically presents without evidence of a precursor lesion, although it is associated with multiple genetic alterations. The most diagnostic of these is amplification of the epidermal growth factor receptor (*EGFR*). Tumors with such a presentation are referred to as de novo GBM. Less commonly, GBM arises in association with progressive genetic alterations after the diagnosis of a lower grade astrocytoma. These tumors are referred to as secondary GBM. The most widely described alterations are mutations of *P53* and *INK4a*. Other genes implicated in the development of these primary brain tumors include *CDK4*, *MDM2*, *DDC*, and *PDGFR*. LOH, loss of heterozygosity.

A limitation of all grading schemes, especially when applied to a single biopsy, is that astrocytic tumors are histologically variable from region to region, and their histopathology may change with time. It is common for low-grade astrocytomas to progress over time to a higher histopathologic grade and a more aggressive clinical course.

Quantitative measures of mitotic activity also correlate with prognosis. The proliferation index can be determined by immunohistochemical staining with antibodies to the proliferating cell nuclear antigen (PCNA) or with a monoclonal antibody termed *Ki-67*, which recognizes a histone protein expressed in proliferating but not quiescent cells. These measures provide estimates of DNA synthesis and correlate with malignant clinical behavior of the tumor.

The overall prognosis is poor. In a representative Finnish population, the median survival was 93.5 months for patients with grade I or II astrocytomas, 12.4 months for patients with grade III (anaplastic astrocytoma), and 5.1 months for patients with grade IV (glioblastoma) tumors. In the United States, the median survival of patients with high-grade brain tumors is approximately 12 months. In addition to histopathology, features that correlate with poor prognosis include age over 65 and a poor functional status, as defined by the Karnofsky performance scale (see Table 79-2).

Low-Grade Astrocytoma Low-grade astrocytomas are more common in children than adults. Pilocytic astrocytoma, named for its characteristic spindle-shaped cells, is the most common childhood brain tumor. It frequently occurs in the cerebellum. Typically, this tumor is cystic and well demarcated from adjacent brain. Complete surgical excision usually produces long-term, disease-free survival.

The optimal management of other low-grade astrocytomas, termed fibrillary astrocytomas, is controversial. For patients who are symptomatic from mass effect or poorly controlled epilepsy, surgical excision can relieve symptoms. For patients who are asymptomatic or minimally symptomatic at presentation, a diagnostic biopsy should be performed and, when surgically feasible, the tumor may be resected. The indications for postoperative radiation therapy are uncertain. In many centers, when only a biopsy or partial resection is possible, postoperative external beam radiation therapy is administered, whereas it is not used if a gross total tumor resection can be achieved. Other centers reserve radiation therapy for tumor recurrence or progression, at which time the tumor may display a more malignant phenotype. No role for chemotherapy in the management of low-grade astrocytoma has been defined.

High-Grade Astrocytoma The large majority of astrocytomas arising in adults are high grade, supratentorial, and do not have a clearly defined margin. Neoplastic cells migrate away from the main tumor mass and infiltrate adjacent brain, often tracking along white matter pathways. Imaging studies do not indicate the full extent of the tumor. These tumors are eventually fatal, although prolonged survival occurs in a few patients. Longer survival correlates with younger age, better performance status, and greater extent of surgical resection. Late in their course, gliomas, especially those located in the posterior fossa, can metastasize along CSF pathways to the spine. Metastases outside the CNS are rare.

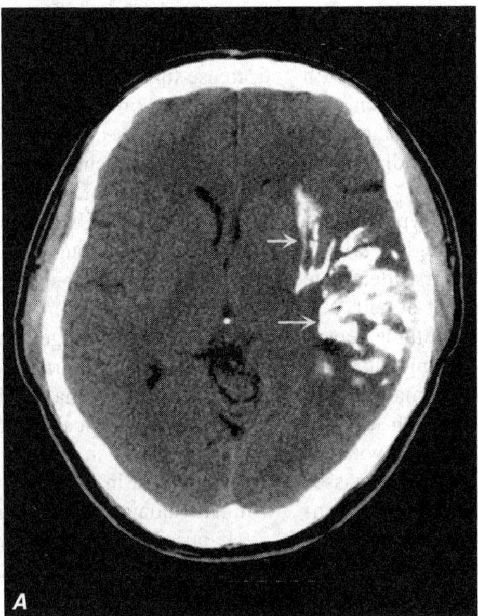

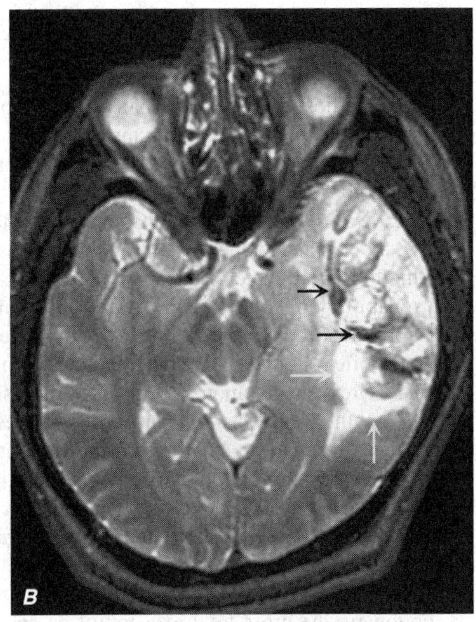

FIGURE 370-3 Oligodendroglioma. *A.* Noncontrast CT scan reveals a calcified mass involving the left temporal lobe (*arrows*) associated with mild mass effect but little edema. *B.* An MR T2-weighted image demonstrates a heterogeneous mass with hypointense signal (*black arrows*) surrounded by a zone of higher signal intensity (*white arrows*), consistent with a calcified temporal lobe mass. The tumor extends into the left medial temporal lobe and compresses the midbrain.

High-grade astrocytomas are managed with glucocorticoids, surgery, radiation therapy, and chemotherapy. Dexamethasone is generally administered at the time of diagnosis and continued for the duration of radiation therapy. After completion of radiotherapy, the dose of dexamethasone is tapered to the lowest tolerated dose.

Because astrocytomas infiltrate adjacent normal brain, total surgical excision is not possible. Surgery is indicated to obtain tissue for pathologic diagnosis and to control mass effect. Moreover, retrospective studies indicate that the extent of tumor resection correlates with survival, at least in younger patients. Therefore, accessible astrocytomas are resected aggressively in patients younger than 65 years old who are in good general medical condition.

Postoperative radiation therapy prolongs survival and improves quality of life, although the duration of benefit is only a few months. Treated with dexamethasone alone following surgery, the mean survival of patients under 65 years of age with glioblastoma is 7 to 9 months. Survival is prolonged to 11 to 13 months with radiation therapy. Focal brain irradiation is less toxic and is as effective as whole-brain radiation for the treatment of primary glial tumors. Radiation is generally administered to the tumor mass, as defined by contrast enhancement on a CT or MRI scan, plus a 3- to 4-cm margin. A total dose of 5000 to 7000 cGy is administered in 25 to 35 equal fractions, 5 days per week.

The roles of stereotaxic radiosurgery and interstitial brachytherapy in glioma treatment are uncertain. *Stereotaxic radiosurgery* is the administration of a focused high dose of radiation to a precisely defined volume of tissue in a single treatment, usually using the gamma knife. Stereotaxic radiosurgery can potentially achieve tumor ablation without surgery. A major limitation of stereotaxic radiosurgery is that it can be used for only relatively small tumors, generally less than 3 cm in maximum diameter. *Interstitial brachytherapy*, the implantation of radioactive beads into the tumor mass, is generally reserved for tumor recurrence because of its associated toxicity—in particular, necrosis of adjacent brain tissue.

Chemotherapy is marginally effective and is often used as an adjuvant following surgery and radiation therapy. Nitrosoureas, including carmustine (BCNU) and lomustine (CCNU), are the most effective available agents. Since a typical glioma infiltrates normal brain where the blood-brain barrier is relatively intact, lipid-soluble agents such as the nitrosoureas, which cross the blood-brain barrier, may reach more malignant cells than water-soluble agents. Experimental approaches include intraarterial infusion of chemotherapy, the implantation of chemotherapy-releasing wafers or injection of chemotherapeutic agents into the tumor resection cavity, administration of chemotherapy after disruption of the blood-brain barrier, and intensive chemotherapy regimens supported by autologous bone marrow transplantation.

Gliomatosis cerebri is a rare form of astrocytoma in which there is diffuse infiltration of the brain by malignant astrocytes without a focal enhancing mass. It generally presents as a multifocal CNS syndrome or a more generalized disorder including dementia, personality change, or seizures. Neuroimaging studies are often nonspecific, and biopsy is required to establish the diagnosis. Gliomatosis is treated with whole-brain radiation therapy and, in selected patients, with systemic chemotherapy.

OLIGODENDROGLIOMAS Oligodendrogliomas have a more benign course and are more responsive to cytotoxic treatment than astrocytomas. Five-year survival is greater than 50%, and 10-year survival is 25 to 34%.

Oligodendrogliomas occur chiefly in supratentorial locations; in adults about 30% contain areas of calcification (Fig. 370-3). Many gliomas contain mixtures of cells with astrocytic and oligodendroglial features. If this mixed histology is prominent, the tumor is termed a *mixed glioma* or an *oligoastrocytoma*. The greater the oligodendroglial component, the more benign the clinical course. As a rule, oligodendrogliomas are less infiltrative than astrocytomas, permitting more complete surgical excision. The histologic features of mitoses, necrosis, and nuclear atypia are associated with a more aggressive clinical course. If these features are prominent, the tumor is termed an *anaplastic oligodendroglioma*.

The optimal management of oligodendrogliomas has not been defined. Surgery, at minimum a stereotaxic biopsy, is necessary to establish a diagnosis. Many oligodendrogliomas are amenable to gross total surgical resection. In addition, oligodendrogliomas may respond dramatically to systemic combination chemotherapy with procarbazine, lomustine and vincristine (PCV). Oligodendrogliomas with deletions of chromosomes 1p and 19q typically respond to PCV, but only about 25% of oligodendrogliomas lacking these genetic markers respond to chemotherapy. Chemotherapy may be used as the initial treatment, and residual tumor can be surgically excised or treated with stereotaxic radiosurgery. An alternative approach is to first excise the accessible tumor mass, then administer systemic chemotherapy and finally, employ stereotaxic radiosurgery or external beam radiation for residual tumor.

EPENDYMOMAS In adults ependymomas are typically located in the spinal canal, especially in the lumbosacral region, arising from the filum terminale of the spinal cord. These tumors often have a myxopapillary histology, with a papillary arrangement of cells and mucin production. In children, ependymomas occur within the ventricles, most often the fourth ventricle, and may exhibit diagnostic ependymal rosettes. Ependymomas with histologic signs of malignancy, including cellular atypia, frequent mitotic figures, or a high labeling index, virtually always recur after surgical resection. Imaging with CT or MRI scans reveals ependymomas as uniformly enhancing masses that are relatively well demarcated from adjacent neural tissue. Ependymomas may metastasize via CSF pathways: brain tumor metastases that spread to the spinal cord by this means are termed *drop metastases*.

Following the gross total excision of an ependymoma, the prognosis is excellent. The 5-year disease-free survival is >80%. However, many ependymomas cannot be totally excised, and postoperative focal external beam radiation or stereotaxic radiosurgery is used. Whether focal radiation is adequate or whether the entire neuraxis needs to be irradiated is not resolved.

GERMINOMAS These tumors most commonly present during the second decade of life, generally at sites within or adjacent to the third ventricle including the pineal region. Germinomas are the most frequent variety of *germ cell tumor*, a tumor type arising in midline structures and including *teratoma*, yolk sac tumor (*endodermal sinus tumor*), *embryonal carcinoma*, and *choriocarcinoma*. Germinomas of the CNS may be benign but are more often aggressive and invasive. Due to their location, patients frequently present with hypothalamic-pituitary dysfunction including diabetes insipidus, visual field deficits, disturbances of memory or mood, or hydrocephalus (Chap. 328). Neuroimaging demonstrates germinomas to be uniformly enhancing masses with or without well-defined borders. The treatment of choice is complete surgical resection. For unresectable tumors, a stereotaxic biopsy is performed for diagnosis, and focal radiation is the primary therapy. When the extent of disease or very young age precludes radiotherapy as primary treatment, platinum-based chemotherapy may decrease tumor size and facilitate subsequent radiation therapy of residual disease or recurrent tumor. Prognosis depends on the histology and surgical resectability of the tumor. Germinomas are generally radiosensitive and chemosensitive, and 5-year survival is >85%.

MEDULLOBLASTOMAS AND PRIMITIVE NEUROECTODERMAL TUMORS (PNET) These highly cellular malignant tumors are thought to arise from neural precursor cells. Medulloblastomas of the posterior fossa are the most frequent malignant brain tumor of children. If the tumor is not disseminated at presentation, the prognosis is generally favorable; subsets of pediatric patients have >70% survival rates at 5 years, although <50% of all children with medulloblastoma survive to adulthood. PNET is a term applied to tumors histologically indistinguishable from medulloblastoma but occurring either in adults or supratentorially in children. In adults, >50% present in the posterior fossa, but these tumors frequently disseminate along CSF pathways.

If possible, these tumors should be surgically excised, although outcome is not related to the extent of surgery. In adults, surgical excision of a PNET should be followed by chemotherapy and irradiation of the entire neuraxis, with a boost in radiation dose to the primary tumor. Aggressive treatment can result in prolonged survival, although half of adult patients relapse within 5 years of treatment.

CNS LYMPHOMA **Primary CNS Lymphoma** These are B cell malignancies of intermediate to high grade that present within the neuraxis without evidence of systemic lymphoma. They occur most frequently in immunocompromised individuals, specifically organ transplant recipients or patients with AIDS (Chap. 309), but the incidence of primary CNS lymphoma is increasing in both immunocompetent and immunocompromised patients. In immunocompromised patients, CNS lymphomas are invariably associated with Epstein-Barr virus (EBV) infection of the tumor cells. Chromosomal translocations involving the c-*myc* gene occur in EBV-associated lymphomas outside the CNS (Chap. 112) but not in primary CNS lymphoma.

In immunocompetent patients, neuroimaging studies most often reveal a uniformly enhancing mass lesion. In immunocompromised patients, primary CNS lymphoma is likely to be multicentric and exhibit ring enhancement or to arise in the meninges (Fig. 370-4). Stereotaxic needle biopsy can be used to establish the diagnosis. Leptomeningeal involvement is present in approximately 15% of patients

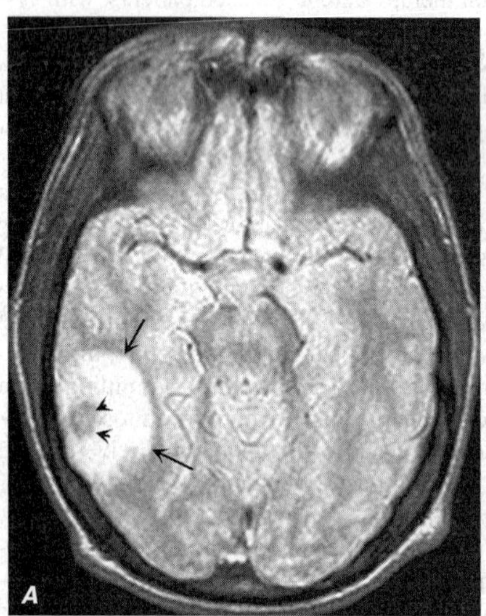

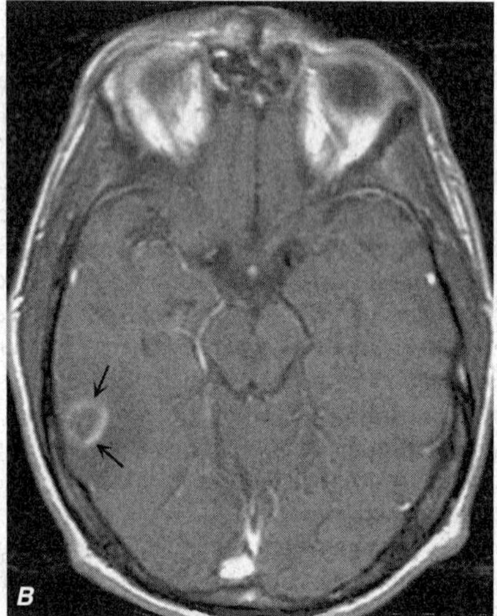

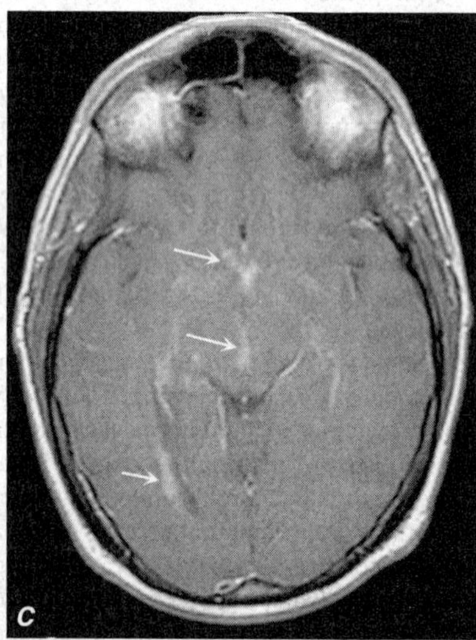

FIGURE 370-4 CNS lymphoma. *A.* Proton density–weighted MR image through the temporal lobe demonstrates a low signal intensity nodule (*small arrows*) surrounded by a ring of high signal intensity edema (*larger arrows*). *B.* T1-weighted contrast-enhanced axial MRI demonstrates ring enhancement surrounded by a nonenhanced rim of edema. In this patient with AIDS, a solitary lesion of this type is consistent with either lymphoma or toxoplasmosis; the presence of multiple lesions favors toxoplasmosis. *C.* In a different patient with lymphomatous meningitis, an axial postcontrast T1-weighted MRI through the midbrain demonstrates multiple areas of abnormal enhancement in periventricular and subependymal regions (*arrows*). Lymphoma tends to spread subependymally at interfaces of CSF and brain parenchyma.

at presentation and in 50% at some time during the course of the illness. Moreover, the disease extends to the eyes in up to 15% of patients. Therefore, a slit-lamp examination and, if indicated, anterior chamber paracentesis or vitreous biopsy is necessary before radiation therapy to define radiation ports.

The prognosis of primary CNS lymphoma is poor compared to histologically similar lymphoma occurring outside the CNS. Many patients experience a favorable clinical and radiographic response to glucocorticoids that may be dramatic; however, it is invariably transient and relapse occurs within weeks. Radiotherapy has been the mainstay of treatment, but systemic combination chemotherapy including high-dose methotrexate is also effective. Intrathecal chemotherapy with methotrexate should also be used if leptomeningeal disease is present. Despite aggressive therapy, >90% of patients develop recurrent CNS disease. Historically, the survival of immunocompetent patients with CNS lymphoma has been approximately 18 months, and may now be longer with the use of systemic chemotherapy. In organ transplant recipients, reversal of the immunosuppressed state can improve outcome. Survival with AIDS-related primary CNS lymphoma is very poor, generally ≤3 months; pretreatment performance status, the degree of immunosuppression, and the extent of CNS dissemination at diagnosis all appear to influence outcome.

Secondary CNS Lymphoma Secondary CNS lymphoma almost always occurs in association with progressive systemic disease in adults with B cell lymphoma or B cell leukemia who have tumor involvement of bone, bone marrow, testes, or the cranial sinuses. Leptomeningeal lymphoma is usually detectable with contrast-enhanced CT or gadolinium-enhanced MRI of the brain and spine or by CSF examination. Treatment consists of systemic chemotherapy, intrathecal chemotherapy, and CNS irradiation. It is usually possible to effectively suppress the leptomeningeal disease, although the overall prognosis is determined by the course of the systemic lymphoma.

PITUITARY ADENOMAS See Chap. 328.

MENINGIOMAS Meningiomas are derived from mesoderm, probably from cells giving rise to the arachnoid granulations. These tumors are usually benign and attached to the dura. They may invade the skull but only infrequently invade the brain. Meningiomas most often occur along the sagittal sinus, over the cerebral convexities, in the cerebellar-pontine angle, and along the dorsum of the spinal cord. They are more frequent in women than men, with a peak incidence in middle age.

Meningiomas may be found incidentally on a CT or MRI scan or may present with a focal seizure, a slowly progressive focal deficit, or symptoms of raised intracranial pressure. The radiologic image of a dural-based, extra-axial mass with dense, uniform contrast enhancement is essentially diagnostic, although a dural metastasis must also be considered (Fig. 370-5). A meningioma may have a "dural tail," a streak of dural enhancement flanking the main tumor mass; however, this finding may be present with other dural tumors.

Total surgical resection of benign meningiomas is curative. If a total resection cannot be achieved, local external beam radiotherapy reduces the recurrence rate to <10%. For meningiomas that are not surgically accessible, targeted radiosurgery with the gamma knife or heavy particle radiation should be considered. Small asymptomatic meningiomas incidentally discovered in older patients can safely be followed radiologically; these tumors grow at an average rate of approximately 0.24 cm in diameter per year and only rarely become symptomatic.

Rare meningiomas invade the brain or have histologic evidence of malignancy such as nuclear pleomorphism and cellular atypia. A high mitotic index is also predictive of aggressive behavior. *Hemangiopericytoma*, although not strictly a meningioma, is a meningeal tumor with an especially aggressive behavior. Meningiomas with features of aggressiveness and hemangiopericytomas, even if totally excised by gross inspection, frequently recur and should receive postoperative radiotherapy. Chemotherapy has no proven benefit.

SCHWANNOMAS These tumors are also called *neuromas*, *neurinomas*, or *neurolemmomas*. They arise from Schwann cells of

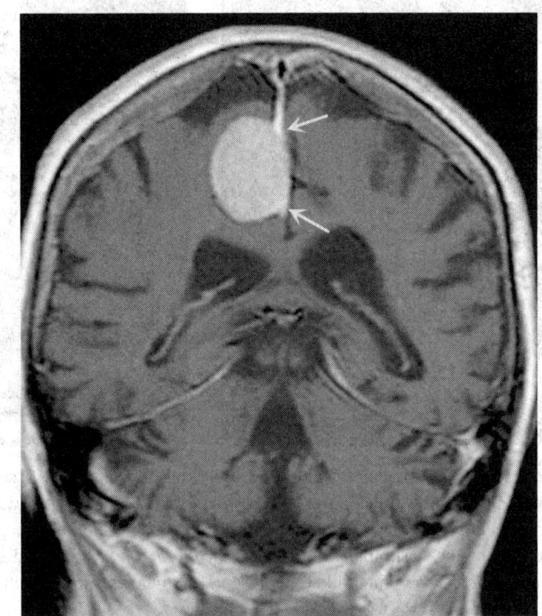

FIGURE 370-5 Meningioma. Coronal postcontrast T1-weighted MR image demonstrates an enhancing extraaxial mass arising from the falx cerebri (*arrows*).

nerve roots, most frequently in the eighth cranial nerve (vestibular schwannoma, formerly termed acoustic schwannoma). The fifth cranial nerve is the second most frequent site; however, schwannomas may arise from any cranial or spinal root except the optic and olfactory nerves, which are myelinated by oligodendroglia rather than Schwann cells. Neurofibromatosis (NF) type 2 (see below) strongly predisposes to vestibular schwannoma. Schwannomas of spinal nerve roots are also seen in these patients as well as patients with NF type 1.

Eighth nerve schwannomas typically arise from the vestibular division of the nerve. Because the vestibular system adapts to slow destruction of the eighth nerve, vestibular schwannomas characteristically present as progressive unilateral hearing loss rather than with dizziness or other vestibular symptoms. Unexplained unilateral hearing loss always merits evaluation, including audiometry and either brainstem auditory evoked potentials or an MRI scan (Chap. 29). As a vestibular schwannoma grows, it can compress the cerebellum, pons, or facial nerve, producing associated symptoms. With rare exceptions schwannomas are histologically and clinically benign. They appear as dense and uniformly enhancing neoplasms on MRI (Fig. 370-6). Vestibular schwannomas enlarge the internal auditory canal, an imaging feature that helps distinguish them from other cerebellopontine angle masses.

Whenever possible, schwannomas should be surgically excised. When the tumors are small, it is usually possible to preserve hearing in the involved ear. In the case of large tumors, the patient is usually deaf at presentation; nonetheless, surgery is indicated to prevent further compression of posterior fossa structures. Gamma knife treatment is also effective for schwannoma but is equivalent in cost and complication rate to surgery. Moreover, the long-term consequences of stereotaxic radiosurgery, including the possibility of secondary radiation-induced neoplasms, are unknown.

OTHER BENIGN BRAIN TUMORS *Epidermoid tumors* are cystic tumors with proliferative epidermal cells at the periphery and more mature epidermal cells towards the center of the cyst. The mature cells desquamate into the liquid center of the cyst. Epidermoid tumors are thought to arise from embryonic epidermal rests within the cranium. They occur extraaxially near the midline, in the middle cranial fossa, the suprasellar region, or the cerebellopontine angle. Epidermoid cysts are well-demarcated lesions that are amenable

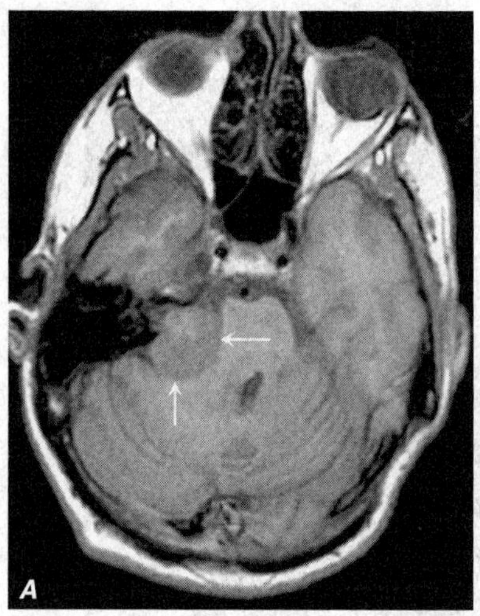

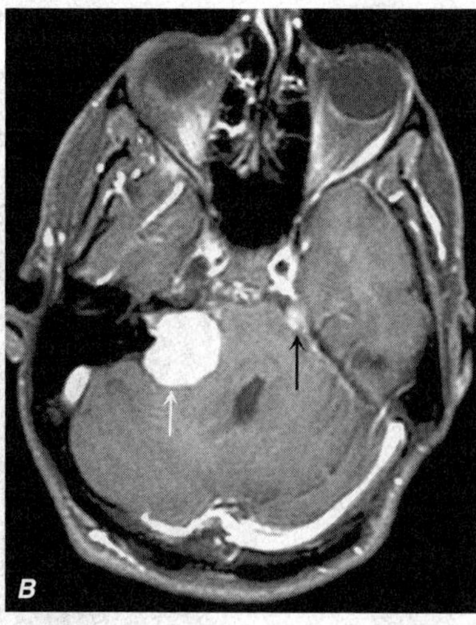

FIGURE 370-6 Vestibular schwannoma. *A.* Axial noncontrast MR scan through the cerebellopontine angle demonstrates an extraaxial mass that extends into a widened internal auditory canal, displacing the pons (*arrows*). *B.* Postcontrast T1-weighted image demonstrates intense enhancement of the vestibular schwannoma (*white arrow*). Abnormal enhancement of the left fifth nerve (*black arrow*) most likely represents another schwannoma in this patient with neurofibromatosis type 2.

to complete surgical excision. Postoperative radiation therapy is unnecessary.

Dermoid cysts are thought to arise from embryonic rests of skin tissue trapped within the CNS during closure of the neural tube. The most frequent locations are in the midline supratentorially or at the cerebellopontine angle. Histologically, they are composed of all elements of the dermis, including epidermis, hair follicles, and sweat glands; they frequently calcify. Treatment is surgical excision.

Craniopharyngiomas are thought to arise from remnants of Rathke's pouch, the mesodermal structure from which the anterior pituitary gland is derived (Chap. 328). Craniopharyngiomas typically present as suprasellar masses. Histologically, craniopharyngiomas resemble epidermoid tumors; they are usually cystic, and in adults 80% are calcified. Because of their location, they may present as growth failure in children, endocrine dysfunction in adults, or visual loss in either age group. Treatment is surgical excision; postoperative external beam radiation or stereotaxic radiosurgery is added if total surgical removal cannot be achieved.

Colloid cysts are benign tumors of unknown cellular origin that occur within the third ventricle and can obstruct CSF flow. *Rare benign primary brain tumors* include neurocytomas, subependymomas, and pleomorphic xanthoastrocytomas. Surgical excision of these neoplasms is the primary treatment and can be curative.

NEUROCUTANEOUS SYNDROMES

This group of genetic disorders, also known as the *phakomatoses*, produces a variety of developmental abnormalities of skin along with an increased risk of nervous system tumors (Table 370-1). These disorders are inherited as autosomal dominant conditions with variable penetrance.

NEUROFIBROMATOSIS TYPE 1 (VON RECKLINGHAUSEN'S DISEASE) NF1 is characterized by cutaneous *neurofibromas*, pigmented lesions of the skin called *café au lait spots*, freckling in non-sun exposed areas such as the axilla, hamartomas of the iris termed Lisch nodules, and pseudoarthrosis of the tibia. Neurofibromas are benign peripheral nerve tumors composed of proliferating Schwann cells and fibroblasts. They present as multiple, palpable, rubbery, cutaneous tumors. They are generally asymptomatic; however, if they grow in an enclosed space, e.g., the intervertebral foramen, they may produce a compressive radiculopathy or neuropathy. Aqueductal stenosis with hydrocephalus, scoliosis, short stature, hypertension, epilepsy, and mental retardation may also occur.

Mutation of the *NF1* gene on chromosome 17 causes von Recklinghausen's disease. The *NF1* gene is a tumor suppressor gene; it encodes a protein, *neurofibromin*, which modulates signal transduction through the *ras* GTPase pathway. Patients with NF1 are at increased risk of developing nervous system neoplasms, including plexiform neurofibromas, optic gliomas, ependymomas, meningiomas, astrocytomas, and pheochromocytomas. Neurofibromas may undergo secondary malignant degeneration and become sarcomas.

NEUROFIBROMATOSIS TYPE 2 NF2 is characterized by the development of bilateral vestibular schwannomas in >90% of individuals who inherit the gene. Patients with NF2 also have a predisposition for the development of meningiomas, gliomas, and schwannomas of cranial and spinal nerves. In addition, a characteristic type of cataract, juvenile posterior subcapsular lenticular opacity, occurs in NF2. Multiple café au lait spots and peripheral neurofibromas occur rarely.

In patients with NF2, vestibular schwannomas usually present with progressive unilateral deafness early in the third decade of life. Bilateral vestibular schwannomas are generally detectable by MRI at that time (Fig. 370-6). Surgical management, designed to treat the underlying tumor and preserve hearing as long as possible, is difficult.

The *NF2* gene on chromosome 22q codes for a protein called *neurofibromin 2*, *schwannomin*, or *merlin*, with homology to a family of cytoskeletal proteins that includes moesin, ezrin, and radixin.

TUBEROUS SCLEROSIS (BOURNEVILLE'S DISEASE) Tuberous sclerosis is characterized by cutaneous lesions, seizures, and mental retardation. The cutaneous lesions include adenoma sebaceum (facial angiofibromas), ash leaf–shaped hypopigmented macules (best seen under ultraviolet illumination with a Wood's lamp), shagreen patches (yellowish thickenings of the skin over the lumbosacral region of the back), and depigmented nevi. On neuroimaging studies, the presence of subependymal nodules, which may be calcified, is characteristic. Patients inheriting the tuberous sclerosis gene are at increased risk of developing ependymomas and childhood astrocytomas, of which >90% are *subependymal giant cell astrocytomas*. These are benign neoplasms that may develop in the retina or along the border of the lateral ventricles. They may obstruct the foramen of Monro and produce hydrocephalus. Rhabdomyomas of the myocardium and angiomyomas of the kidney, liver, adrenals, and pancreas may also occur.

Treatment is symptomatic. Anticonvulsants for seizures, shunting for hydrocephalus, and behavioral and educational strategies for mental retardation are the mainstays of management. Severely affected individuals generally die before age 30.

Mutations at both 9q(TSC-1) and 16p(TSC-2) are associated with tuberous sclerosis. The mutated genes code for *tuberins*, proteins that modulate the GTPase activity of other cellular proteins.

VON HIPPEL–LINDAU SYNDROME This syndrome consists of retinal, cerebellar, and spinal hemangioblastomas, which are slowly growing cystic tumors. Hypernephroma, renal cell carcinoma, pheochromocytoma, and cysts of the kidneys, pancreas, epididymis, or liver may also occur. Erythropoietin production by hemangioblastomas may result in polycythemia. The von Hippel–Lindau (VHL) tumor suppressor gene on chromosome 3p encodes a protein that appears to suppress transcription elongation by RNA polymerase II.

TUMORS METASTATIC TO BRAIN

MECHANISMS OF BRAIN METASTASES The large majority of brain metastases disseminate by hematogenous spread. The anatomic distribution of brain metastases generally parallels regional cerebral blood flow, with a predilection for the gray matter–white matter junction and for the border zone between middle cerebral and posterior cerebral artery distributions. The lung is the most common origin of brain metastases; both primary lung cancer and cancers metastatic to the lung can metastasize to the brain. Breast cancer has a propensity to metastasize to the cerebellum and the posterior pituitary gland. This propensity could be explained by patterns of retrograde venous flow from the thorax into the skull or by an especially hospitable environment for breast cancer cells provided by the cerebellum and pituitary (the "seed and soil" hypothesis).

Lung cancer (adenocarcinoma and small cell lung cancer), breast cancer (especially ductal carcinoma), gastrointestinal malignancies, and melanoma are common tumors that metastasize to brain (Table 370-2). Certain less common tumors have a special propensity to metastasize to brain, including germ cell tumors and thyroid cancer. By contrast, prostate cancer, ovarian cancer, and Hodgkin's disease rarely metastasize to the brain. Moreover, breast cancer that metastasizes to bone tends not to metastasize to the brain. Therefore, the cellular environment of the brain is hospitable to only a subset of systemic cancers. Parenchymal spinal cord metastases are rare.

EVALUATION OF METASTASES FROM KNOWN CANCER On MRI scans brain metastases typically appear as well-demarcated, approximately spherical lesions that are hypointense or isointense relative to brain on T1-weighted images and bright on T2-weighted images. They invariably enhance with gadolinium, reflecting extravasation of gadolinium through tumor vessels that lack a blood-tumor barrier (Fig. 370-7). Small metastases often enhance uniformly. Larger metastases typically produce ring enhancement surrounding a central mass of nonenhancing necrotic tissue that develops as the metastasis outgrows its blood supply. Metastases are surrounded by variable amounts of edema. Blood products may also be seen, reflecting hemorrhage of abnormal tumor vessels.

The radiologic appearance of a brain metastasis is not specific. The differential diagnosis of ring-enhancement lesions includes brain abscess, radiation necrosis, toxoplasmosis, granulomas (tuberculosis, sarcoidosis), demyelinating lesions, primary brain tumors, primary CNS lymphoma, stroke, hemorrhage, and trauma. Contrast-enhanced CT scanning is less sensitive than MRI for the detection of brain metastases. Cytologic examination of the CSF is not indicated, since intraparenchymal brain metastases almost never shed cells into CSF. Measuring CSF levels of tumor markers such as carcinoembryonic antigen (CEA) is rarely helpful in management.

BRAIN METASTASES WITHOUT A KNOWN PRIMARY TUMOR In general hospital populations, up to one-third of patients presenting with brain metastases do not have a known underlying cancer. These patients generally present with either a seizure or a progressive neurologic deficit. Neuroimaging studies demonstrate one or multiple ring-enhancement lesions. In individuals who are not immunocompromised and not at risk for brain abscesses, this radiologic pattern is most likely due to brain metastasis.

Diagnostic evaluation begins with a search for the primary tumor. Blood tests should include CEA and liver function tests. A careful examination of the skin for melanoma and the thyroid gland for masses should be carried out. A CT scan of the chest, abdomen, and pelvis should be obtained. If these are all negative, further imaging studies, including bone scan, other radionuclide scans, and upper and lower gastrointestinal barium studies, are unlikely to be productive. The search for a primary cancer most often discloses lung cancer, particularly small cell lung cancer, or melanoma. In 30% of patients no primary tumor can be identified even after extensive evaluation.

A tissue diagnosis is essential. If a primary tumor is found, it will usually be more accessible to biopsy than a brain lesion. If a single brain lesion is found in a surgically accessible location, if a primary tumor is not found, or if the primary tumor is in a location difficult to biopsy, the brain metastasis should be biopsied or resected.

Table 370-2 Frequency of Primary Tumors that Metastasize to the Nervous System

Site of Primary Tumor	Brain Metastases, %	Leptomeningeal Metastases, %	Spinal Cord Compression, %
Lung	40	24	18
Breast	19	41	24
Melanoma	10	12	4
Gastrointestinal tract	7	13	6
Genitourinary tract	7		18
Other	17	10	30

℞ **TREATMENT** Once a systemic cancer metastasizes to the brain it is, with rare exception, incurable. Therapy is therefore palliative, designed to prevent disability and suffering and, if possible, to prolong life. Published outcome studies have focused on survival as the primary end point, leaving questions regarding quality of life unanswered. There is, however, widespread agreement that glucocorticoids, anticonvulsants, and radiation therapy improve the quality of life for many patients. The roles of surgery and chemotherapy are less well established.

General Measures High-dose glucocorticoids frequently ameliorate symptoms of brain metastases. Improvement is often dramatic, occurs within 6 to 24 h, and is sustained with continued administration, although the toxicity of glucocorticoids is cumulative. Therefore, if possible, a more definitive therapy for metastases should be instituted to permit withdrawal of glucocorticoid therapy. One-third of patients with brain metastases have one or more seizures. Anticonvulsants are empirically used for seizure prophylaxis when supratentorial metastases are present.

Specific Measures • ***Radiation therapy*** Radiation is the primary treatment for brain metastases. Since multiple microscopic deposits of tumor cells throughout the brain are likely to be present in addition to metastases visualized by neuroimaging studies, whole-brain irradiation is usually used. Its benefit has been established in controlled studies, but no clear dose response has been shown. Usually, 30–37.5 Gy is administered in 10 to 15 fractions; an additional dose

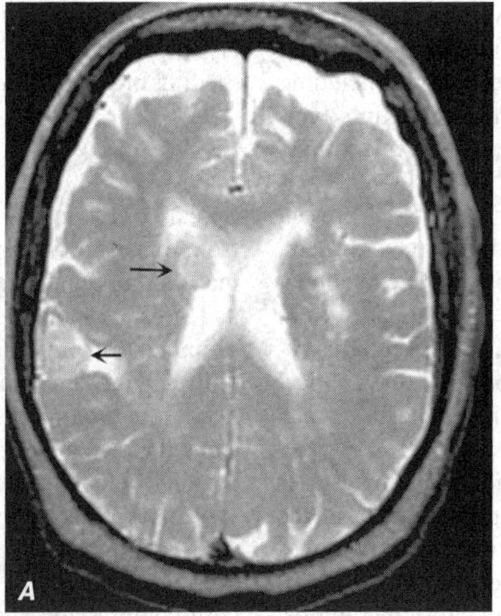

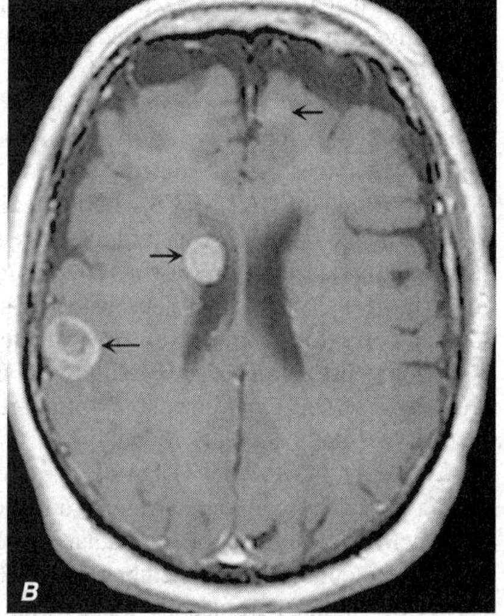

FIGURE 370-7 Brain metastasis. *A.* Axial T2-weighted MRI through the lateral ventricles reveals two isodense masses, one in the subependymal region and one near the cortex (*arrows*). *B.* T1-weighted postcontrast image at the same level as *A* reveals enhancement of the two masses seen on the T2-weighted image as well as a third mass in the left frontal lobe (*arrows*).

("boost") of focal irradiation to a single or large metastasis may also be administered.

Surgery Up to 40% of patients with brain metastases have only a single tumor mass identified by CT. Accessible single metastases are usually surgically excised as a palliative measure. If the systemic disease is under control, total resection of a single brain lesion has been demonstrated to improve survival and minimize disability. Survival appears to be improved if surgery is followed by whole-brain irradiation.

Chemotherapy Brain metastases of certain tumors, including breast cancer, small cell lung cancer, and germ cell tumors, are often responsive to systemic chemotherapy. Although metastases frequently do not respond as well as the primary tumor, dramatic responses to systemic chemotherapy or hormonal therapy may occur in some cases. In patients who are neurologically stable, two to four cycles of systemic chemotherapy may be administered initially to reduce tumor mass and render the residual tumor more amenable to radiation therapy. Even if a complete radiologic remission is achieved from chemotherapy, whole-brain irradiation should then be administered.

Experimental therapies These include stereotaxic radiosurgery, gene therapy, immunotherapy, intraarterial chemotherapy, and chemotherapy administered following osmotic disruption of the blood-brain barrier.

LEPTOMENINGEAL METASTASES

Leptomeningeal metastases are also called *carcinomatous meningitis, meningeal carcinomatosis*, and, in the cases of specific tumors, *leukemic meningitis* or *lymphomatous meningitis*. Clinical evidence of leptomeningeal metastases is present in 8% of patients with metastatic solid tumors; at necropsy, the prevalence is as high as 19%. Among solid tumors, adenocarcinomas of the breast and lung and melanoma are most often responsible (Table 370-2). In one-quarter of patients the systemic cancer is under control; thus effective control of leptomeningeal disease can improve the quality and duration of life.

Pathologically, three patterns of tumor involvement may be seen: (1) a diffuse coating of the leptomeninges by a thin layer of tumor cells, (2) nodular growth of macroscopic tumor metastases in meninges and on nerve roots, or (3) plaque-like metastases in the leptomeninges with many cells shed into the subarachnoid space and extension of tumor into Virchow-Robin spaces. Leptomeningeal metastases may coexist with parenchymal CNS metastases.

Cancer usually metastasizes to the meninges via the bloodstream. Alternatively, a superficially located parenchymal metastasis may shed cells directly into the subarachnoid space. Some tumors, including squamous cell carcinoma of the skin and some non-Hodgkin's lymphomas, have a propensity to grow along peripheral nerves and may seed the meninges by that route.

CLINICAL FEATURES Leptomeningeal metastases present with signs and symptoms at multiple levels of the nervous system, most often in a setting of known systemic malignancy. Encephalopathy is frequent, and cranial neuropathy or spinal radiculopathy from nodular nerve root compression is characteristic. Hydrocephalus results from obstruction of CSF outflow in the posterior fossa. Focal neurologic deficits from coexisting intraparenchymal metastases may occur.

LABORATORY EVALUATION Leptomeningeal metastases are diagnosed by cytologic demonstration of malignant cells in the CSF, by MRI demonstration of nodular tumor deposits in the meninges or diffuse meningeal enhancement (Fig. 370-8), or by meningeal biopsy. CSF findings are usually those of an inflammatory meningitis, consisting of lymphocytic pleocytosis, elevated protein levels, and normal or low CSF glucose. A complete MRI examination of the neuraxis may demonstrate hydrocephalus due to obstruction of CSF pathways and identify nodular meningeal metastases.

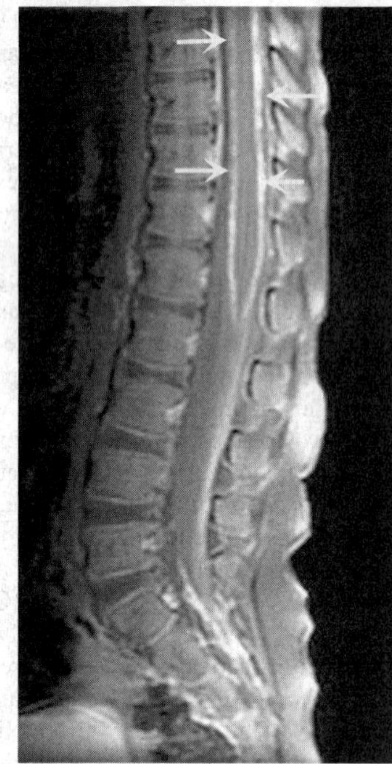

FIGURE 370-8 Carcinomatous meningitis. Sagittal postcontrast MRI through the lower thoracic region demonstrates diffuse pial enhancement along the surface of the spinal cord (*arrows*), typical of CSF spread of neoplasm.

℞ **TREATMENT** In selected patients, intrathecal chemotherapy and focal external beam radiotherapy to sites of leptomeningeal disease are the mainstays of management. Although the prognosis of leptomeningeal metastases is poor, approximately 20% of patients aggressively treated for leptomeningeal metastases can expect a sustained response of approximately 6 months. Intrathecal therapy exposes meningeal tumor to high concentrations of chemotherapy with minimal systemic toxicity. Methotrexate can be safely administered intrathecally and is effective against leptomeningeal metastases from a variety of solid tumors and lymphoma; ara-C and thio-TEPA are alternative agents. Intrathecal chemotherapy may be administered either by repeated lumbar puncture or through an indwelling Ommaya reservoir, which consists of a catheter in one lateral ventricle attached to a reservoir implanted under the scalp. If there is a question of patency of CSF pathways, a radionuclide flow study may be performed.

Large deposits of tumor on the meninges or along nerve roots are unlikely to respond to intrathecal chemotherapy, as the barrier to diffusion is too great. Therefore, external beam radiation is employed. Hydrocephalus is treated with a ventriculoperitoneal shunt, although seeding of the peritoneum by tumor is a risk.

MALIGNANT SPINAL CORD COMPRESSION

Spinal cord compression from solid tumor metastases usually results from expansion of a vertebral metastasis into the epidural space. Primary tumors that frequently metastasize to bone include lung, breast, and prostate cancer. Back pain is usually the first symptom and is prominent at presentation in 90% of patients. The pain is typically dull, aching, and may be associated with localized tenderness. If a nerve root is compressed, radicular pain is also present. The neurologic signs that accompany spinal cord compression are determined by the spinal level of the lesion; the thoracic cord is most often affected. Weakness, sensory loss, and autonomic dysfunction (urinary urgency and incontinence, fecal incontinence, and sexual impotence in men) are the hallmarks of spinal cord compression. Once signs of spinal cord compression appear, they tend to progress rapidly. It is thus essential to recognize and treat this devastating complication of malignancy at the earliest possible time in order to prevent irreversible neurologic deficits. →***Diagnosis and management are discussed in Chap. 368.***

METASTASES TO THE PERIPHERAL NERVOUS SYSTEM

Systemic cancer may compress or invade peripheral nerves. Compression of the brachial plexus may occur by direct extension of Pancoast's tumors (cancer of the apex of the lung) or by extension of local lymph node metastases of breast or lung cancer or lymphoma. The lumbosacral plexus may be compressed by the retroperitoneal spread of prostate or ovarian cancer or lymphoma. Skull metastases may compress cranial nerve branches as they pass through the skull, and pituitary metastases may extend into the cavernous sinus. The epineurium generally provides an effective barrier to invasion of the peripheral nerves by solid tumors, but certain tumors characteristically invade and spread along peripheral nerves. Squamous cell carcinoma of the skin may spread along branches of the trigeminal nerve and extend intracranially. Non-Hodgkin's lymphoma may be neurotrophic and cause a syndrome resembling mononeuropathy multiplex. Focal external beam radiation may reduce pain, prevent irreversible loss of peripheral nerve function, and possibly restore function.

In patients with cancer who have brachial or lumbosacral plexopathy, it may be difficult to distinguish tumor invasion from radiation injury. High radiation dose or the presence of myokymia (rippling contractions of muscle) suggests radiation injury, whereas pain suggests tumor. Radiographic imaging studies may be equivocal, and surgical exploration is sometimes required.

COMPLICATIONS OF THERAPY

RADIATION TOXICITY The nervous system is vulnerable to delayed injury by therapeutic radiation. The mechanism of injury is unknown, but radiation-induced free radical production is probably contributory. Histologically, there is demyelination, hyaline degeneration of small arterioles, and eventually brain infarction and necrosis. However, radiation injury can occur without vasculopathy, suggesting that ischemia is a late manifestation and does not account entirely for the tissue damage.

Radiation injury to the brain is classified by the time of its occurrence. *Acute radiation injury* occurs during or immediately after therapy. It is rarely seen with current protocols of external beam radiation but may occur after stereotaxic radiosurgery. Manifestations include headache, sleepiness, and worsening of preexisting neurologic deficits. *Early delayed radiation injury* occurs within 4 months of therapy. It is associated with an increased white matter T2 signal on MRI scans. In children, the *somnolence syndrome* is a common form of early delayed radiation injury in which somnolence and ataxia develop after whole-brain irradiation. Irradiation of the cervical spine may cause Lhermitte's phenomenon, an electricity-like sensation evoked by neck flexion (Chap. 368). Acute and early delayed radiation injury are steroid-responsive and self-limited disorders and do not appear to increase the risk of late radiation injury.

Late delayed radiation injury produces permanent damage to the nervous system. It occurs more than 4 months (generally 8 to 24 months) after completion of therapy; onset 15 years after therapy has been described. After whole-brain irradiation, progressive dementia can occur, sometimes accompanied by gait apraxia. White matter signal abnormalities are present on MRI studies (Fig. 370-9). Following focal brain irradiation, radiation necrosis occurs within the radiation field, producing a contrast-enhanced mass, frequently with ring enhancement. MRI or CT scans are often unable to distinguish radiation necrosis from recurrent tumor, but PET or SPECT scans may demonstrate that glucose metabolism is increased in tumor tissue but decreased in radiation necrosis. Biopsy is frequently required to establish the correct diagnosis. Peripheral nerves, including the brachial and lumbosacral plexuses, may also develop late delayed radiation injury over a time span similar to that observed in the CNS.

If untreated, radiation necrosis of the CNS may act as an expanding mass lesion, although it may resolve spontaneously or after steroid treatment. Progressive radiation necrosis is best treated with surgical resection if the patient has a life expectancy of at least 6 months and a good Karnofsky performance score. There are anecdotal reports that anticoagulation with heparin or coumadin may be beneficial. Radiation injury also accelerates the development of atherosclerosis in large arteries, but an increase in the risk of stroke becomes significant only years after radiation treatment.

Endocrine dysfunction frequently follows exposure of the hypothalamus or pituitary gland to therapeutic radiation. Growth hormone is the pituitary hormone most sensitive to radiation therapy, and thyroid-stimulating hormone is the least sensitive; ACTH, prolactin, and the gonadotropins have an intermediate sensitivity.

Development of a second neoplasm is another risk of therapeutic radiation that generally occurs many years after radiation exposure. Depending on the irradiated field, the risk of gliomas, meningiomas, sarcomas, and thyroid cancer is increased.

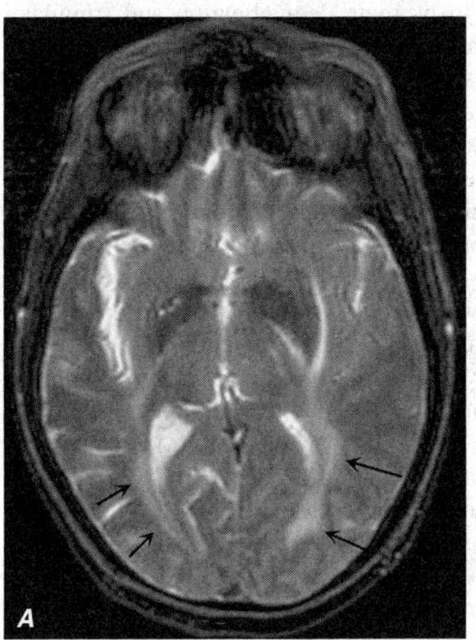

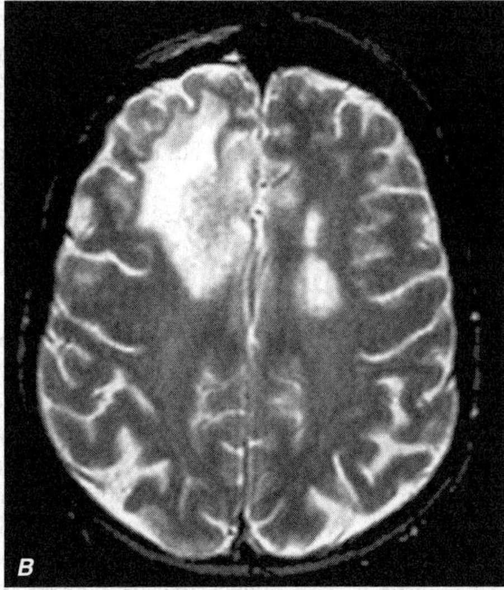

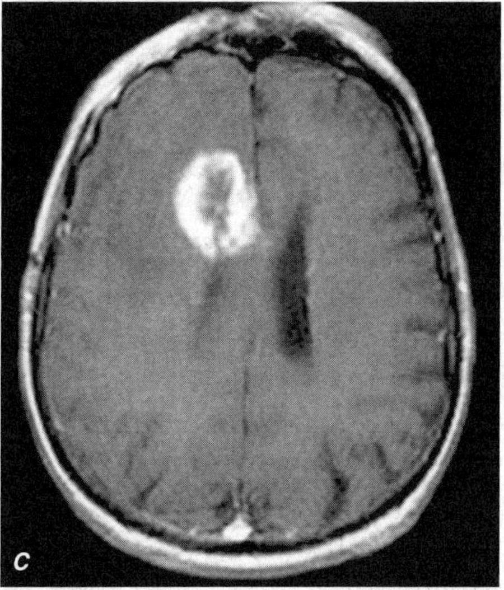

FIGURE 370-9 Radiation injury. *A.* Late-delayed radiation injury 1 year after whole-brain radiation (5500 cGy). T2-weighted MR image at the level of the temporal lobes reveals high signal intensity abnormality in periventricular white matter (*arrows*). *B* and *C.* Focal radiation necrosis 3 years after radiotherapy (7000 cGy) for carcinoma of the nasopharynx. Axial T2-weighted MRI (*B*) demonstrates a mass in the right frontal lobe with surrounding vasogenic edema. Abnormal signal changes are also present on the left. T1-weighted postcontrast MRI (*C*) reveals a heterogeneously enhancing mass in the right cingulate gyrus.

COMPLICATIONS OF CHEMOTHERAPY Chemotherapy regimens used to treat primary brain tumors have generally included a nitrosourea and are well tolerated. Infrequently, nitrosoureas and other drugs used to treat CNS neoplasms cause altered mental states (e.g., confusion, depression), ataxia, and seizures. Chemotherapy for systemic malignancy is a more frequent cause of nervous system toxicity. Cisplatin commonly produces tinnitus and high-frequency bilateral hearing loss, especially in younger patients. At cumulative doses >450 mg/m^2, cisplatin can produce a symmetric, large fiber axonal predominantly sensory neuropathy; paclitaxel (Taxol) produces a similar picture. Fluorouracil and high-dose cytosine arabinoside can cause cerebellar dysfunction that resolves after discontinuation of therapy. Vincristine, which is commonly used to treat lymphoma, may cause an acute ileus and is frequently associated with development of a progressive distal, symmetric sensory-motor neuropathy with foot drop and paresthesias.

BIBLIOGRAPHY

BIGNER DD, MCLENDON RE, BRUNER JM (eds): *Russell and Rubinstein's Pathology of Tumors of the Nervous System*. New York, Oxford Univ Press, 1998

BIGNER SH: Cerebrospinal fluid cytology: Current status and diagnostic applications. J Neuropath Exp Neurol 51:235, 1992

BYRNE TN: Spinal cord compression from epidural metastases. N Engl J Med 327:614, 1992

CAIRNCROSS JG et al: Specific genetic predictors of chemotherapeutic response and survival in patients with anaplastic oligodendrogliomas. J Natl Cancer Inst 90:1473, 1998

GUTMANN DH et al: The diagnostic evaluation and multidisciplinary management of neurofibromatosis 1 and neurofibromatosis 2. JAMA 278:51, 1997

KORI SH et al: Brachial plexus lesions in patients with cancer: 100 cases. Neurology 31:45, 1981

MAHER ER, KAELIN WG: von Hippel-Lindau disease. Medicine 76:381, 1997

MCKUSICK VA (ed): *Online Mendelian Inheritance in Man*. URL: www.ncbi.nlm.nih.gov/Omim/. Washington, DC, National Library of Medicine, 1999

MECKLING S et al: Malignant supratentorial glioma in the elderly: Is radiotherapy useful? Neurology 47:901, 1996

NG H-K, LAM PYP: The molecular genetics of central nervous system tumors. Pathology 30:196, 1998

OLSON JD et al: Long-term outcome of low-grade oligodendroglioma and mixed glioma. Neurology 54:1442, 2000

PATCHELL RA et al: A randomized trial of surgery in the treatment of single metastases to the brain. N Engl J Med 322:494, 1990

POSNER JB: *Neurologic Complications of Cancer*. Philadelphia, FA Davis, 1995

SKLAR CA, CONSTINE LS: Chronic neuroendocrinological sequelae of radiation therapy. Int J Radiation Oncol Biol Phys 31:1113, 1995

VON DEIMLING A et al: Molecular pathways in the formation of gliomas. Glia 15:328, 1995

WILSON CB: Meningiomas: Genetics, malignancy, and the role of radiation in induction and treatment. J Neurosurg 81:666, 1994

371

Stephen L. Hauser, Donald E. Goodkin

MULTIPLE SCLEROSIS AND OTHER DEMYELINATING DISEASES

ADEM acute disseminated encephalomyelitis	MOG myelin oligodendrocyte glycoprotein
CNS central nervous system	MRI magnetic resonance imaging
CSF cerebrospinal fluid	MS multiple sclerosis
EAE experimental allergic encephalomyelitis	PNS peripheral nervous system
IFN interferon	PPMS primary progressive MS
IL interleukin	RRMS relapsing-remitting MS
MBP myelin basic protein	SPMS secondary progressive MS
MHC major histocompatibility complex	TNF tumor necrosis factor

The demyelinating diseases occupy a unique place in neurology owing to their frequency; tendency to strike young adults; diversity of manifestations; and range of fundamental questions in neurobiology, immunology, virology, and genetics that arise regarding their pathogenesis. These disorders share features of inflammation and selective destruction of central nervous system (CNS) myelin; the peripheral nervous system (PNS) is spared. No specific tests for the demyelinating diseases exist, and diagnosis is based on recognition of the distinctive clinical patterns of CNS injury they produce.

MULTIPLE SCLEROSIS

Multiple sclerosis (MS) is characterized by (1) a relapsing-remitting or progressive course and (2) a pathologic triad of CNS inflammation, demyelination, and gliosis (scarring). Lesions of MS are classically said to be *disseminated* in time and space. MS affects approximately 350,000 Americans and 1.1 million individuals worldwide. In Western societies, MS is second only to trauma as a cause of neurologic disability arising in early to middle adulthood. Current evidence indicates that MS is an autoimmune disease that develops in genetically susceptible individuals who have resided in certain permissive environments. Manifestations of MS vary from a benign illness to a rapidly evolving and incapacitating disease requiring profound adjustments in life-style and goals for patients and their families. Complications from MS affect multiple body systems; hence, a multidisciplinary approach is recommended to optimize clinical care.

PATHOGENESIS Anatomy MS derives its name from the multiple scarred areas visible on macroscopic examination of the brain. These lesions, termed *plaques*, are sharply demarcated gray or pink areas easily distinguished from surrounding white matter. Plaques vary in size from 1 or 2 mm to several centimeters. The acute MS lesion, rarely found at autopsy, consists of perivenular cuffing by inflammatory mononuclear cells, predominantly T lymphocytes and macrophages, which also infiltrate white matter tissue and appear to orchestrate demyelination. At sites of inflammation, the blood-brain barrier is disrupted but the vessel wall itself is preserved, distinguishing the MS lesion from vasculitis. In some inflammatory lesions, a distinctive pattern of myelin damage, termed *vesicular demyelination*, can be appreciated. This change consists of dissolution of the multilamellated compact myelin sheaths that surround axon cylinders and their reconstitution as a lattice-like network of myelin membrane fragments. Myelin-specific autoantibodies (see "Immunology," below) are bound to the vesiculated myelin membranes, at least in some patients; these autoantibodies are thought to promote demyelination and stimulate macrophages and microglial cells (specialized CNS phagocytes of bone marrow origin) that scavenge the myelin debris. As lesions evolve, astrocytes proliferate extensively (gliosis). Oligodendrocytes, the myelin-producing cells, also proliferate initially in most MS lesions, but these cells are often destroyed as the infiltration and gliosis progress. Surviving oligodendrocytes or those that newly differentiate from a precurser pool may partially remyelinate naked axons, resulting in *shadow plaques*. MS lesions may enlarge by gradual concentric outward growth; some chronic plaques display histologic gradations of increasing acuity from the center to the lesion edge.

The correspondence between number and size of plaques ("plaque burden") and the severity of clinical symptoms is imprecise. Hence, an extensive plaque burden may be associated with mild symptoms; or, conversely, seemingly minor pathologic changes may be present in some severely disabled individuals. Occasional cases either are clinically silent or produce "nonspecific" isolated symptoms such as facial pain, and evidence of MS is found unexpectedly at autopsy.

Recent ultrastructural studies of MS lesions suggest that different underlying pathologies may be present in different patients. Heterogeneity has been identified both in terms of the fate (i.e., death or survival) of oligodendrocytes in plaques and by the presence or absence of antibody and complement deposition. In primary progressive MS (PPMS; see below), a distinctive oligodendroglial cytopathy has been reported based on examination of a limited number of cases; if confirmed, this finding would suggest that PPMS is a unique disorder. Finally, although selective demyelination with sparing of axon cylinders is the hallmark of MS, partial or total axonal destruction, and in extreme cases cavitation, may also occur. The extent of axonal loss appears to correlate with irreversible neurologic disability. Axonal loss and cavitation are particularly prominent in the subtype of MS known as neuromyelitis optica or Devic's syndrome (see below).

Physiology Demyelination may have either negative or positive effects on axonal conduction. *Negative conduction abnormalities* consist of slowed axonal conduction, variable conduction block that occurs in the presence of high- but not low-frequency volleys of impulses, or complete conduction block. Conduction block in demyelinated fibers may also occur in response to raised temperature or metabolic derangements. The mechanism of conduction block appears to involve a hyperpolarization of the resting axon potential due to the exposure of voltage-dependent potassium channels that are normally buried underneath the myelin sheath. *Positive conduction abnormalities* include generation of ectopic impulses, spontaneously or after mechanical deformation, and abnormal "crosstalk" between demyelinated axons. Variable conduction block may explain the fluctuations in function that vary from hour to hour and from day to day in many patients and the characteristic worsening that is associated with fever or exercise. Ectopic impulse generation or "crosstalk" might give rise to Lhermitte's symptom, paroxysmal symptoms, or paresthesias (see below). Experimental therapies designed to alleviate conduction abnormalities in MS have included the use of calcium channel blockers to reduce the threshold for impulse generation and pharmacologic blockade (with 4-aminopyridine) of potassium channels.

Epidemiology MS is approximately twice as common in females as in males. In both sexes, the incidence rises steadily from adolescence to age 35 and declines gradually thereafter. The mean age of onset is slightly later in men than in women, due in part to a relative overrepresentation of males in PPMS, which has a later mean age of onset. MS beginning as early as age two years or as late as the eighth decade of life is rare but well documented. Various epidemiologic observations, summarized below, support of the role of an environmental exposure of some type in MS.

Location and risk MS is primarily a disease of individuals living in temperate climates. The prevalence increases with increasing distance from the equator; this finding appears to be true in both the northern and southern hemispheres. Prevalence rates and north-south gradients are generally similar in North America and Europe. The highest known prevalence (250 per 100,000) occurs in the Orkney islands, located north of the mainland of Scotland, and MS is also common throughout Scandinavia and northern Europe. Numerous studies also suggest that location influences MS risk. For example, the prevalence of MS is low in Japan (2 per 100,000) but moderate (15 per 100,000) in Japanese Americans.

Changes in prevalence Studies from the United States, Europe, and Australia suggest that the prevalence of MS may have increased during the twentieth century, however these findings could represent an artifact due to improved detection of cases in the modern era.

Reported clusters Several possible point epidemics of MS have been described, the most convincing of which occurred in the Faeroe Islands off the coast of Denmark after the British occupation during World War II.

GENETIC CONSIDERATIONS An inherent genetic susceptibility to MS exists, as summarized by the following observations:

Risk in Different Ethnic Groups The prevalence of MS differs among ethnic groups that reside in the same environment. In the United States, the prevalence of MS is higher in Caucasians than in other racial groups, consistent with observations in other parts of the world.

Familial Aggregation First-, second-, and third-degree relatives of patients with MS are at increased risk for the disease. Siblings of affected individuals have a lifetime risk of ~5%, whereas the risk to parents or children of affected individuals is somewhat lower. Studies of adoptees, half-siblings, and spouses of patients with MS strongly indicate that familial aggregation is primarily determined by shared genetic, and not environmental, factors.

Twin Studies The most compelling evidence for a genetic effect on MS is derived from twin studies, which demonstrate concordance rates of ~30% in monozygotic twins and 5% in dizygotic twins (similar to the risk in nontwin siblings).

The inheritance of MS cannot be explained with a simple genetic model. A single-gene hypothesis is at odds with concordance estimates in twin and family studies and with the observed nonlinear decrease in disease risk as the genetic distance from the MS proband is increased. It is likely that susceptibility is determined by multiple independent genetic loci (polygenic inheritance), each with a relatively small contribution to the overall risk. It is also possible that different genetic causes of susceptibility to MS (genetic heterogeneity) may exist. Linkage and association studies have identified the major histocompatibility complex (MHC) on chromosome 6 as one genetic determinant for MS. This complex encodes the histocompatibility antigens (the HLA system) that present peptide antigens to T cells. The class II (HLA-D) region of the MHC is most strongly associated with MS, and susceptibility appears to result from the presence of the DR2 allele and its corresponding haplotype, defined by molecular criteria as DRB1*1501, DQA1*0102, DQB1*0602. Other genetic regions implicated in MS susceptibility include loci on chromosomes 3, 5, 16, and 19. ■

Immunology MS appears to be an autoimmune disease mediated, at least in part, by T lymphocytes. Evidence in support of this concept is derived from analogy to the laboratory model experimental allergic encephalomyelitis (EAE) and from direct studies of the immune system of MS patients.

Autoreactive T lymphocytes Myelin basic protein (MBP) is an important T cell antigen in EAE and probably also in human MS. In patients with MS but not in unaffected individuals activated MBP-reactive T cells can be identified in the peripheral blood. In cerebrospinal fluid (CSF), the frequency of T cells reactive against MBP (and other myelin proteins) is also higher in patients with MS than in unaffected individuals. Direct evidence that MBP-reactive T cells are present in MS lesions has also been suggested by sequence analysis of the antigen-binding domain of T cell receptor molecules cloned from plaque tissue. The susceptibility gene DR2 may influence the immune response to MBP because it binds with high affinity to a fragment of MBP spanning amino acids 89 to 101; this region of MBP appears to be immunodominant for T cell responses in DR2-positive individuals.

Autoantibodies Increasing evidence suggests that autoantibodies play some role in MS, probably acting in concert with a pathogenic T cell response. In EAE, autoantibodies directed against myelin oligodendrocyte glycoprotein (MOG), a quantitatively minor myelin protein, were found to mediate MS-like demyelinating lesions; and recently anti-MOG antibodies were also detected in actively demyelinating MS lesions. MOG is thus a good candidate as a humoral autoantigen in MS. Evidence of an abnormal humoral immune response is present in the CSF of patients with MS. Membrane attack complexes can be detected in the CSF, suggesting a role for complement-mediated antibody damage. Elevated levels of immunoglobulin are easily measured and are characteristic of CSF in MS. Oligoclonal antibody—derived from expansion of a small number of different molecules—is also present in most cases. Oligoclonal immunoglobulin is also detected in other chronic inflammatory responses, including infections, and thus is not specific to MS. It is synthesized locally, and the specific pattern is unique to each patient. Attempts to identify an antigen against which most oligoclonal immunoglobulin is directed have been unsuccessful.

Cytokines Numerous cytokines and chemokines have been detected in brain, CSF, and peripheral blood of patients with MS, and it is probable that these molecules regulate many of the cellular interactions that operate in this disease (Chap. 305). By analogy to EAE T_H1 cytokines that regulate cellular immunity, including interleukin (IL) 2, tumor necrosis factor (TNF) α, and interferon (IFN) γ have traditionally been thought to be central to MS pathogenesis. TNF-α or IFN-γ may contribute directly to tissue damage by injuring oligodendrocytes or the myelin membrane. Unfortunately, treatment strategies designed to blunt the T_H1 response have thus far not been successful in treating MS. Furthermore, a recent clinical trial with a humanized antibody to TNF-α appeared to worsen MS. The identification of autoantibodies in MS suggests that T_H2 cytokines (including IL-4, IL-5, and IL-10) may play a pathogenic role in MS, and may explain why the results of T_H1-based approaches have been disappointing.

Triggers Magnetic resonance imaging (MRI) scans indicate that many patients with relapsing forms of MS have bursts of multifocal inflammation that occur approximately monthly, or 7 to 10 times more frequently than clinical attacks. This finding suggests the presence of a large reservoir of subclinical disease in MS. Bursts appear to be associated with the migration of activated T cells from the peripheral blood across the blood-brain barrier and into brain; the triggers responsible for these bursts are not known. Patients may experience relapses after nonspecific upper respiratory infections, suggesting that molecular mimicry between viruses and myelin antigens may trigger attacks, or that some viruses may function as superantigens capable of activating disease-inducing T cells in MS (Chap. 305).

Microbiology As noted above, epidemiologic evidence supports the role of an environmental exposure in MS. MS risk also correlates with high socioeconomic status, which may reflect improved sanitation and delayed initial exposures to infectious agents. Some viruses, e.g., poliomyelitis and measles viruses, produce neurologic sequelae more frequently when the age of initial infection is delayed. The most widely studied experimental model of virus-induced demyelinating disease is infection with Theiler virus, a murine coronavirus similar to measles virus and canine distemper virus. Infection with some Theiler strains produces a chronic infection of oligodendrocytes with multifocal perivascular lymphocytic infiltration and demyelination, closely resembling lesions of MS.

In patients with MS, high antibody titers have been reported in serum and CSF against many viruses, including measles, herpes simplex, varicella, rubella, Epstein-Barr, and influenza C and some parainfluenza strains. Furthermore, numerous viruses and bacteria (or their genomic sequences) have been recovered from MS tissues and fluids. The most recent claims have involved human herpes virus type 6 (HHV-6) and chlamydia pneumoniae. A causal role for any infectious agent in MS remains unproven.

CLINICAL MANIFESTATIONS The onset of MS may be abrupt or insidious. Symptoms may be severe or seem so trivial that a patient may not seek medical attention for months or years. Initial symptoms are commonly one or more of the following: weakness or diminished dexterity in one or more limbs, a disturbance of gait, optic neuritis, sensory disturbance, diplopia, and ataxia (Table 371-1).

Weakness of the limbs may manifest as fatigue, disturbance of gait, or loss of dexterity. Initially, weakness may be detected only after physical exertion. Weakness is frequently accompanied by pyramidal signs including increased motor tone (spasticity), hyperreflexia, an extensor plantar response, and an absent superficial abdominal reflex. Occasionally, a tendon reflex may be lost (simulating a peripheral nerve lesion) if afferent fibers of the motor reflex arc are disrupted by a lesion in the dorsal root entry zone.

Table 371-1 Initial Symptoms of MS

Symptom	Percent of Cases	Symptom	Percent of Cases
Weakness	35	Lhermitte	3
Sensory loss	37	Pain	3
Paresthesias	24	Dementia	2
Optic neuritis	36	Visual loss	2
Diplopia	15	Facial palsy	1
Ataxia	11	Impotence	1
Vertigo	6	Myokymia	1
Paroxysmal attacks	4	Epilepsy	1
Bladder	4	Falling	1

SOURCE: After WB Matthews et al, *McAlpine's Multiple Sclerosis*, New York, Churchill Livingstone, 1991.

Optic neuritis generally presents as diminished acuity, dimness, or color desaturation in the central field of vision. These symptoms may be mild or progress over hours or days to severe visual loss, or rarely to complete loss of light perception. Visual symptoms are generally monocular but may occur bilaterally. Periorbital pain frequently precedes or accompanies diminished visual acuity and may be aggravated by eye movement. An afferent pupillary defect (Fig. 28-2) may be detected by a swinging flashlight test. Funduscopic examination may be normal or reveal swelling of the optic disc (papillitis). Venous sheathing of retinal vessels, due to the transendothelial migration of lymphocytes, is occasionally present. Pallor of the optic disc (optic atrophy) commonly follows an episode of optic neuritis. Uveitis occurs rarely.

Visual blurring in MS may result from optic neuritis or diplopia. These two causes are distinguished by asking the patient to cover each eye sequentially and observing whether the visual difficulty clears. *Diplopia* may result from an internuclear ophthalmoplegia (INO) or extraocular muscle weakness of the sixth (or rarely the third or fourth) cranial nerves. An INO consists of impaired or slowed adduction of one eye from a lesion in the ipsilateral medial longitudinal fasciculus. This tract connects the sixth cranial nerve nucleus with the contralateral third nerve nucleus. Prominent nystagmus is often observed in the abducting eye, along with a small skew deviation. An INO can resemble an isolated medial rectus palsy. Convergence is often preserved in INO, helping to differentiate between these two entities. The finding of bilateral INO is highly suggestive of MS. Other common gaze disturbances in MS include a horizontal gaze palsy due to an ipsilateral lesion in the abducens nucleus or the paramediam pontine reticular formation, a "one and a half" syndrome from a horizontal gaze palsy plus an INO, and acquired pendular nystagmus.

Sensory symptoms commonly include paresthesias (tingling, "pins and needles," or painful burning) or hypesthesia (numbness or a "dead" feeling). Complaints of unpleasant feelings of "swollen," "wet,", "raw", or "tightly wrapped" body parts are common. Sensory symptoms often begin in a focal area of a limb, the torso, or the head and spread over hours or days to adjacent ipsilateral or contralateral areas of the body. Involvement of the trunk with a "cord level" is diagnostically helpful because it identifies the spinal cord and not the PNS as the origin of the sensory symptoms.

Ataxia of gait and limbs reflects demyelination in the cerebellum or cerebellar pathways. In advanced MS cerebellar dysarthria (scanning speech) is common. The true extent of cerebellar involvement may be uncertain when motor and sensory deficits coexist.

Bladder dysfunction manifests as urgency or hesitancy in voiding, incomplete emptying, or incontinence. Constipation is also common. One or more of these symptoms occurs at some time in most patients with MS and may be present at onset. Fecal urgency or bowel incontinence occur less commonly.

Cognitive dysfunction may be recognized early or late in the course of MS. Cognitive deficits most commonly include memory loss, impaired attention, problem-solving difficulties, slowed information processing, and difficulties in shifting between cognitive tasks. Impaired judgment and emotional liability may be evident. These symptoms impair activities of daily living in as many as 20% of patients.

Depression is experienced by ~60% of patients during the course of the illness. Suicide is 7.5-fold more common than in age-matched controls.

Fatigue occurs in most patients with MS. It may be maximum during mid-afternoon or continuous throughout the day. Symptoms of fatigue include generalized motor weakness, limited ability to concentrate or read, lassitude, and sleepiness.

Heat sensitivity is experienced as the appearance of new symptoms or the worsening of preexisting symptoms on exposure to heat. For example, transient visual blurring may become apparent during a hot shower or with physical exercise. It is a common phenomenon for symptoms of MS to worsen transiently, sometimes in a dramatic fashion, during the course of a febrile illness (see pseudoexacerbation, below).

Ancillary Symptoms *Lhermitte's symptom* is the sensation of a momentary electric current or shock evoked by neck flexion, other neck movements, or cough. The symptom typically radiates down the spine into the legs, but it may radiate into the arms or be provoked by movements of the lumbar spine. Lhermitte's symptom is not specific to MS; it also occurs with other spinal cord disorders, including cervical spondylosis.

Paroxysmal symptoms are brief and stereotypic. Tonic spasms consist of an unpleasant tingling or other sensation association with tonic contraction of a limb, face, or trunk. Other paroxysmal symptoms include dysarthria and ataxia, diplopia, transient unilateral paralysis, hemifacial spasm, paresthesias, and pain. Attacks may be momentary or persist for ≥30 s. They generally begin in clusters, occurring many times throughout the day, and the patient may identify precipitating factors such as hyperventilation or particular movements.

Trigeminal neuralgia, a lancinating facial pain, may also occur; features that suggest MS rather than an idiopathic etiology (Chap. 367) include onset before 50 years of age, bilateral occurrence, objective facial sensory loss, and constant rather than paroxysmal pain.

Facial weakness may resemble idiopathic Bell's palsy; however, facial weakness due to MS is generally not associated with ipsilateral loss of taste sensation or retroauricular pain (Chap. 367).

Facial myokymia, or chronic flickering contractions of the facial musculature, are also common. The movements commonly involve the orbicularis oculus muscle and appear under the eye. Facial myokymia may arise from lesions of the corticobulbar tracts or brainstem course of the facial nerve.

Vertigo may appear suddenly and in dramatic fashion with gait unsteadiness and vomiting, resembling acute labyrinthitis. A brainstem rather than end-organ origin of vertigo is suggested by the presence of coexisting trigeminal or facial nerve involvement, vertical nystagmus, or nystagmus that is unaccompanied by latency of onset, direction reversal, or fatigue (Chap. 21). Hearing loss may also occur but is uncommon.

DISEASE COURSE Approximately 85% of patients with MS experience an abrupt onset of symptoms and signs at disease onset. Thereafter, the clinical course may be characterized by acute episodes of worsening (exacerbations or relapses), gradual progression of disability, or combinations of both. Four clinical patterns are recognized by international consensus. Patients with *relapsing-remitting MS* (RRMS) experience relapses with or without complete recovery and are clinically stable between these episodes (Fig. 371-1, A and B). Approximately 50% of patients with RRMS convert to *secondary progressive MS* (SPMS) within 10 years of disease onset. The secondary progressive phase is characterized by gradual progression of disability with or without superimposed relapses (Fig. 371-1, C and D). In contrast, patients with *primary progressive MS* (PPMS) experience gradual progression of disability from onset without superimposed relapses (Fig. 371-1, E and F). Approximately 10% of patients with MS experience this clinical pattern. Patients with *progressive relapsing MS* experience gradual progression of disability from disease onset later accompanied by one or more relapses; this clinical pattern affects ~5% of patients (Fig. 376-1G).

DIAGNOSIS There is no definitive diagnostic test. Diagnostic criteria for clinically definite MS require documentation of two or more episodes of symptoms and two or more signs that reflect pathology in anatomically noncontiguous white matter tracts of the CNS (Table 371-2). Symptoms must last more than one day and occur as distinct episodes that are separated by 28 or more days. At least one of the two required signs must be present on neurological examination. The second may be documented as an abnormal paraclinical test, either

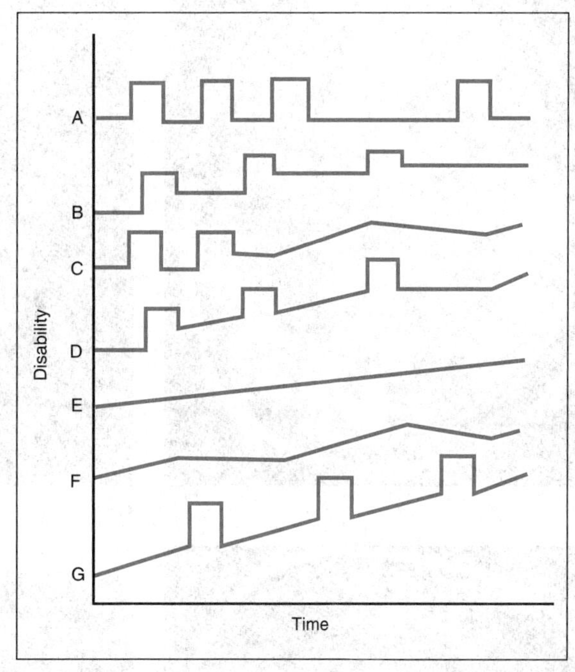

FIGURE 371-1 Clinical patterns of MS. A, B, relapsing-remitting; C, D, secondary progressive; E, F, primary progressive; G, progressive relapsing.

Table 371-2 Diagnostic Criteria for MS

1. Examination must reveal *objective* abnormalities of the CNS.
2. Involvement must reflect predominantly disease of white matter long tracts, usually including (a) pyramidal pathways, (b) cerebellar pathways, (c) medial longitudinal fasciculus, (d) optic nerve, and (e) posterior columns.
3. Examination or history must implicate involvement of two or more areas of the CNS.
   a. MRI may be used to document a *second* lesion when only one site of abnormality has been demonstrable on examination. A confirmatory MRI must have either four lesions involving the white matter or three lesions if one is periventricular in location. Acceptable lesions must be >3 mm in diameter. For patients older than 50 years, two of the following criteria must also be met: (a) lesion size >5 mm, (b) lesions adjacent to the bodies of the lateral ventricles, and (c) lesion(s) present in the posterior fossa.
   b. Evoked response testing may be used to document a *second* lesion not evident on clinical examination.
4. The clinical pattern must consist of (a) two or more separate *episodes* of worsening involving different sites of the CNS, each lasting at least 24 h and occurring at least 1 month apart, or (b) gradual or stepwise *progression* over at least 6 months if accompanied by increased CSF IgG synthesis or two or more oligoclonal bands.
5. Age of onset between 15 and 60 years.
6. The patient's neurologic condition could not better be attributed to another disease. Laboratory testing that may be advisable in certain cases includes (a) CSF analysis, (b) MRI of the head or spine, (c) serum vitamin B_{12} level, (d) human T cell lymphotropic virus type I (HTLV-I) titer, (e) erythrocyte sedimentation rate, (f) rheumatoid factor, antinuclear, anti-DNA antibodies (SLE), (g) serum VDRL, (h) angiotensin-converting enzyme (sarcoidosis), (i) *Borrelia* serology (Lyme disease), (j) very-long-chain fatty acids (adrenoleukodystrophy), and (k) serum or CSF lactate, muscle biopsy, or mitochondrial DNA analysis (mitochondrial disorders).

DIAGNOSTIC CATEGORIES

1. *Definite MS:* All six criteria fulfilled.
2. *Probable MS:* All six criteria fulfilled except (a) only one objective abnormality despite two symptomatic episodes or (b) only one symptomatic episode despite two or more objective abnormalities.
3. *At risk for MS:* All six criteria fulfilled except only one symptomatic episode and one objective abnormality.

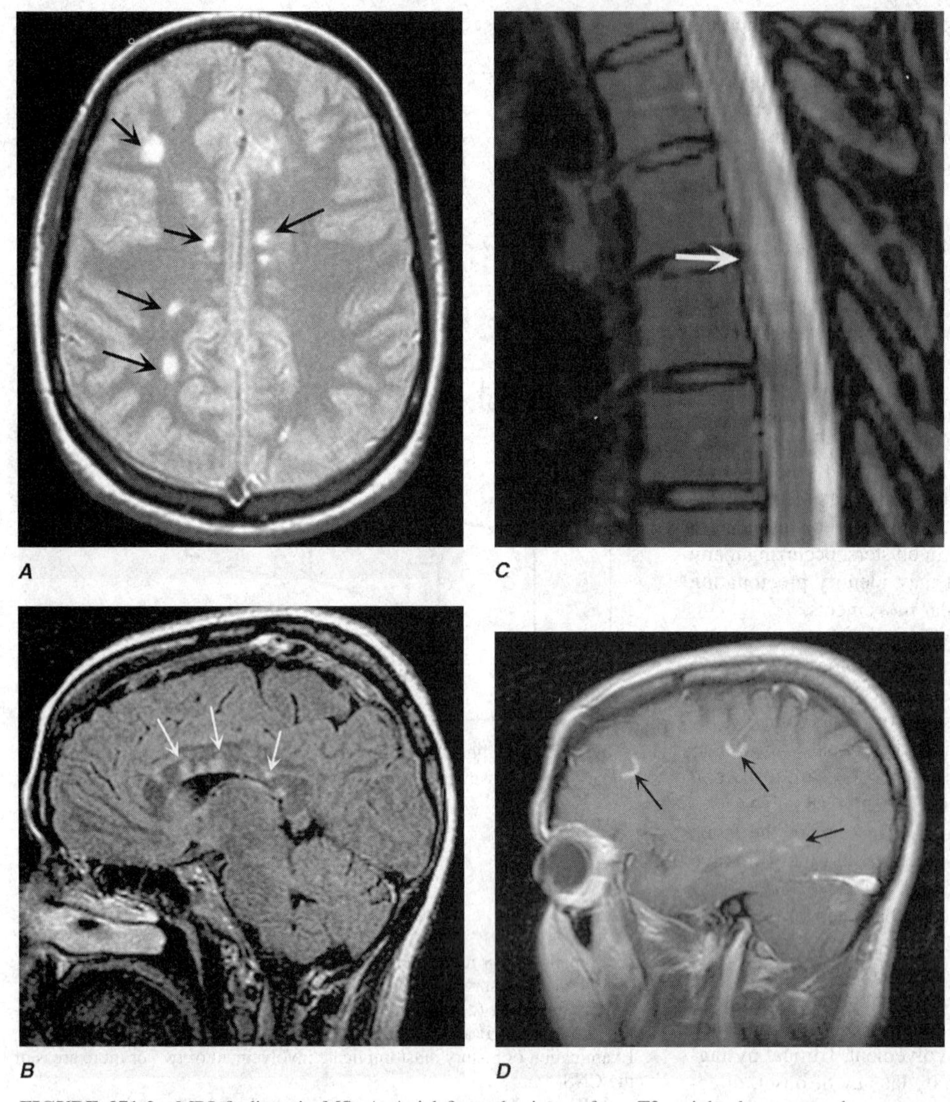

FIGURE 371-2 MRI findings in MS. *A.* Axial first-echo image from T2-weighted sequence demonstrates multiple bright signal abnormalities in white matter, typical for MS. *B.* Sagittal T2-weighted FLAIR (fluid attenuated inversion recovery) image in which the high signal of CSF has been suppressed. CSF appears dark, while areas of brain edema or demyelination appear high in signal as shown here in the corpus callosum (*arrows*). Lesions in the anterior corpus callosum are frequent in MS and rare in vascular disease. *C.* Sagittal T2-weighted fast spin echo image of the thoracic spine demonstrates a fusiform high signal intensity lesion in the mid thoracic spinal cord. *D.* Sagittal T1-weighted image obtained afer the intravenous administration of gadolinium DTPA reveals focal areas of blood-brain barrier disruption, identified as high-signal-intensity regions (*arrows*).

brain or spinal cord MRI, or visual, auditory, or somatosensory evoked electrical response. In patients who experience gradual progression of disability for 6 or more months without superimposed relapses, documentation of intrathecal IgG may be used to support the diagnosis.

DIAGNOSTIC TESTS **Magnetic Resonance Imaging** Widespread availability of brain and spinal cord MRI has revolutionized the diagnosis and management of MS. Disease-related changes are detected by MRI (Fig. 371-2) in >95% of patients who otherwise meet diagnostic criteria for definite MS (Table 371-2). An increase in vascular permeability, detected by leakage of the intravenous contrast agent gadolinium DPTA into the brain, appears to be a very early event in the formation of new MS lesions and perhaps is a marker of inflammation. Gadolinium enhancement persists for 2 to 8 weeks; and the residual mixture of edema, inflammation, demyelination, axonal loss, and gliosis in the MS plaque remains visible as a focal area of hyperintensity on spin-echo (T2-weighted) and proton-density images. Lesions often appear to extend outward from the ventricular surface, corresponding to a pattern of perivenous demyelination that is observed pathologically in MS (Dawson's fingers). Lesions are also commonly found within the brainstem, corpus callosum, cerebellum, and spinal cord. Lesions of the anterior corpus callosum are particularly useful diagnostically because this site is usually spared in cerebrovascular disease. Specific criteria for the use of MRI in support of a diagnosis of MS have been proposed (Table 371-2).

The correlation between the total volume of T2-weighted signal abnormality—the "lesion burden"—and clinical measures of disability is poor. Approximately one-third of hyperintense T2-weighted lesions appear hypointense on T1-weighted imaging sequences. These "black holes" provide more specific imaging markers of irreversible demyelination and axonal loss that correlate more robustly with clinical measures of disability. The correlation between MRI measures and clinical status is even stronger with emerging imaging techniques, including magnetization transfer imaging and proton-magnetic resonance spectroscopic imaging, which can distinguish irreversible demyelination and axonal loss from reversible edema and inflammation.

Evoked Responses Evoked response testing may detect slowed or absent conduction in visual, auditory, somatosensory, or motor pathways (Chap. 357). These tests use computer averaging techniques to record the electrical response evoked in the nervous system after repetitive sensory stimuli. One or several evoked responses are abnormal in 80 to 90% of patients with MS. Abnormalities in evoked responses occur with a variety of neurologic disorders that disrupt pathways being measured; thus, they are not specific to MS. Testing is of diagnostic value when it provides evidence of a subclinical second lesion in a patient who manifests only one abnormality on neurologic examination (Table 371-2).

Cerebrospinal Fluid (CSF) CSF abnormalities consist of abnormally increased levels of intrathecally synthesized IgG, oligoclonal banding, and mononuclear cell pleocytosis. Various formulas are used to distinguish intrathecally synthesized IgG from serum IgG that may have entered the CNS passively across a disrupted blood-brain barrier. One formula expresses the ratio of IgG to albumin in the CSF divided by the ratio in the serum ("the CSF IgG index"). Oligoclonal banding of CSF IgG is detected by agarose gel electrophoresis techniques. Two or more oligoclonal bands are found in 75 to 90% of patients with MS. Oligoclonal banding may be absent at the onset of MS, and in individual patients the number of bands present may increase with time. It is important that paired serum samples be studied to exclude a systemic origin of the oligoclonal bands.

Other CSF abnormalities also occur but are less specific for MS. In one large series, CSF mononuclear pleocytosis (>5 cells/μL) was present in 25% of patients with MS. CSF cell counts are generally <20/μL in patients with MS, and counts >50/μL are unusual but may occur with acute myelopathy. Pleocytosis of >75 cells/μL or a finding of polymorphonuclear leukocytes in CSF makes the diagnosis of MS unlikely. Pleocytosis is more common in young patients with relapsing-remitting MS than in older patients with progressive forms of MS. The total CSF protein content is usually normal or only slightly increased. A protein elevation >100 mg/dL is rare and should prompt consideration of alternative diagnosis such as an infection or tumor.

DIFFERENTIAL DIAGNOSIS Numerous diagnostic formulas have been proposed for MS (Table 371-2); although useful, they cannot replace sound clinical judgment. No single clinical sign or test is diagnostic of MS. The diagnosis is usually easily made in a young adult with relapsing and remitting symptoms referable to different areas of CNS white matter. The possibility of an alternate diagnosis should be considered when (1) symptoms are localized exclusively to the posterior fossa, craniocervical junction, or spinal cord; (2) the patient is younger than 15 or older than 60 years; (3) the clinical course is progressive from onset; and (4) the patient has never experienced visual, sensory or bladder symptoms. Diagnosis may also be difficult in patients with a rapid or even explosive onset suggesting a cerebrovascular accident, or mild symptoms only and a normal neurologic examination. In such situations, the patient should be questioned carefully for a history of prior attacks that may not be recalled initially. Rarely, a mass lesion resulting from intense inflammation and swelling may occur in MS and may mimic a primary or metastatic tumor.

Examination reveals evidence of neurologic disease in most patients. Abnormal signs are often more widespread than expected from the interview. For example, a patient with MS may present with symptoms in one leg and signs in both. This type of finding is helpful when it permits exclusion of a single focal lesion as the source of a patient's symptoms. Conversely, the presence of features that are uncommon or rare in MS should call the diagnosis into question. These include aphasia, extrapyramidal syndromes suggesting parkinsonism, chorea, isolated dementia, amyotrophy with fasciculations, peripheral neuropathy, fever, headache, seizures, or coma.

Systemic lupus erythematosus (SLE) rarely produces a relapsing or progressive disorder that mimics MS; other manifestations of SLE are usually present (Chap. 311). Behçet's syndrome may produce a chronic illness with optic neuropathy and myelopathy but more often presents as an acute or subacute multifocal CNS disorder; characteristic oral and genital lesions, uveitis, and an elevated ESR are distinguishing features (Chap. 316). Relapsing-remitting CNS syndromes have also been described in Sjögren's syndrome. Sarcoidosis may produce cranial nerve palsies (especially of the seventh cranial nerve), progressive optic atrophy, or myelopathy (Chap. 318). Systemic involvement helps to distinguish these conditions from MS. Lyme borreliosis may involve the optic nerve, brainstem, or spinal cord in the absence of characteristic rash, fever, or meningoradiculitis (Chap. 176). Other chronic infections, including meningovascular syphilis and infection with HIV, may need to be considered. HTLV type I–associated myelopathy (HAM; tropical spastic paraparesis) is characterized by back pain, progressive spasticity affecting predominantly the lower limbs, and bladder symptoms (Chap. 373). Diagnosis is based on identification of specific antibody to HTLV-I in serum and CSF and by direct virus isolation. Infection with the HTLV-II retrovirus may cause a progressive myelopathy similar to that caused by HTLV-I.

As noted above, the acute onset of a focal CNS disturbance in a previously healthy individual may suggest a stroke or migraine. Progressive focal deficits should always prompt consideration of a compressive lesion. Primary CNS lymphoma may produce single or multiple lesions that contrast-enhance on MRI and may resemble acute lesions of MS. A progressive or relapsing brainstem disturbance may be due to a vascular malformation in the posterior fossa. Pontine glioma is distinguished from MS by its tendency to produce progressive deficits that involve contiguous structures. Chiari malformations presenting in adulthood may cause cerebellar ataxia, nystagmus, and spastic weakness of the limbs; headache, lower cranial nerve palsies, and a syringomyelic syndrome are useful distinguishing features. Progressive myelopathies may result from cervical spondylosis, spinal cord tumor, or arteriovenous malformation (Chap. 368).

A positive family history, neurologic signs suggesting diffuse symmetric demyelination, and lack of characteristic CSF changes raise the possibility of a metabolic or genetic condition that may mimic MS. Subacute combined degeneration due to vitamin B_{12} deficiency may produce an MS-like syndrome in the absence of megaloblastic anemia (Chap. 368). Uncommon genetic disorders that may mimic MS include Krabbe's disease, metachromatic leukodystrophy, methylenetetrahydrofolate reductase deficiency, biotinidase deficiency, adrenomyeloneuropathy, familial spastic paraparesis, spinocerebellar ataxia, mitochondrial encephalopathy with lactic acidosis and stroke (MELAS), Leber's disease, and subacute necrotizing encephalomyelopathy (Leigh's disease).

PROGNOSIS Most patients with MS experience progressive disability. Fifteen years after diagnosis, fewer than 20% of patients with MS have no functional limitation, 50 to 60% require assistance when ambulating, 70% are limited or unable to perform major activities of daily living, and 75% are not employed. In 1998, it was estimated that the total annual economic burden of MS in the United States exceeded 6.8 billion. The following clinical and brain MRI features may confer a more favorable prognosis: presentation with isolated optic neuritis or sensory symptoms, complete recovery from a first attack, age of onset younger than 40 years, female sex, relapsing-remitting clinical course, and fewer than two relapses in the first year of illness. In general, patients who experience minimal neurologic impairment 5 years after the first symptoms are least likely to be severely disabled 10 to 15 years later. By comparison, patients with persistent truncal ataxia, severe action tremor, or a disease course that is progressive from the onset are more likely to experience progression of disability.

In patients who experience an initial attack of monosymptomatic optic neuritis, brainstem signs, or myelopathy, brain MRI provides useful prognostic information. If the brain MRI reveals multiple T2-weighted lesions, the risk of developing definite MS within a 10-year period of follow-up is 70 to 80%. Conversely, if the brain MRI is normal, <10% of patients will experience a second episode of symptoms consistent with MS within 10 years.

℞ **TREATMENT** The treatment of MS may be divided into two categories: (1) treatments designed to modify the disease process and (2) symptomatic management. Longitudinal scoring of the functional consequences of MS is essential for treatment decisions. The Kurtzke Expanded Disability Status Score (EDSS) is the most widely used measure of neurologic impairment in MS (Table 371-3).

Disease Modifying Therapies for RRMS (Fig. 371-3) Three treatment options for patients with RRMS are approved for use in the United States: (1) IFN-β1b (Betaseron), (2) IFN-β1a (Avonex), and (3) glatiramer acetate (Copaxone). Each of these treatments is also prescribed for patients with SPMS who experience frequent exacerbations because this clinical pattern cannot be distinguished reliably from RRMS with incomplete recovery from exacerbations. In Phase III clinical trials, recipients of IFN-β1b, IFN-β1a, and glatiramer acetate experienced ~30% fewer clinical exacerbations and significantly fewer new MRI lesions compared to placebo recipients. IFN-β1b and IFN-β1a also convincingly delayed time to onset of sustained progression of disability. Furthermore, IFN-β1a was found to delay the development of clinically definite MS in patients who experience a single episode of demyelination and have MRI findings indicating prior subclinical disease.

Treatment effects with IFN-β1b and IFN-β1a may be mediated by down regulating (1) expression of MHC molecules on the surface of antigen-presenting cells, (2) actions of proinflammatory cytokines, and

Table 371-3 Scoring Systems for MS

KURTZKE EXPANDED DISABILITY STATUS SCORE (EDSS)

0.0 = Normal neurologic exam [all grade 0 in functional status (FS)]
1.0 = No disability, minimal signs in one FS (i.e., grade 1)
1.5 = No disability, minimal signs in more than one FS (more than one grade 1)
2.0 = Minimal disability in one FS (one FS grade 2, others 0 or 1)
2.5 = Minimal disability in two FS (two FS grade 2, others 0 or 1)
3.0 = Moderate disability in one FS (one FS grade 3, others 0 or 1) or mild disability in three or four FS (three/four FS grade 2, others 0 or 1) though fully ambulatory
3.5 = Fully ambulatory but with moderate disability in one FS (one grade 3) and one or two FS grade 2; or two FS grade 3; or five FS grade 2 (others 0 or 1)
4.0 = Ambulatory without aid or rest for ≥ 500 m
4.5 = Ambulatory without aid or rest for ≥ 300 m
5.0 = Ambulatory without aid or rest for ≥ 200 m
5.5 = Ambulatory without aid or rest for ≥ 100 m
6.0 = Unilateral assistance required to walk about 100 m with or without resting
6.5 = Constant bilateral assistance required to walk about 20 m without resting
7.0 = Unable to walk beyond about 5 m even with aid; essentially restricted to wheelchair; wheels self and transfers alone
7.5 = Unable to take more than a few steps; restricted to wheelchair; may need aid to transfer
8.0 = Essentially restricted to bed or chair or perambulated in wheelchair, but out of bed most of day; retains many self-care functions; generally has effective use of arms
8.5 = Essentially restricted to bed much of the day; has some effective use of arm(s); retains some self-care functions
9.0 = Helpless bed patient; can communicate and eat
9.5 = Totally helpless bed patient; unable to communicate or eat
10.0 = Death due to MS

FUNCTIONAL STATUS (FS) SCORE

A. Pyramidal functions
0 = Normal
1 = Abnormal signs without disability
2 = Minimal disability
3 = Mild or moderate paraparesis or hemiparesis, or severe monoparesis
4 = Marked paraparesis or hemiparesis, moderate quadriparesis, or monoplegia
5 = Paraplegia, hemiplegia, or marked quadriparesis
6 = Quadriplegia

B. Cerebellar functions
0 = Normal
1 = Abnormal signs without disability
2 = Mild ataxia
3 = Moderate truncal or limb ataxia
4 = Severe ataxia all limbs
5 = Unable to perform coordinated movements due to ataxia

C. Brainstem functions
0 = Normal
1 = Signs only
2 = Moderate nystagmus or other mild disability
3 = Severe nystagmus, marked extraocular weakness, or moderate disability of other cranial nerves
4 = Marked dysarthria or other marked disability
5 = Inability to swallow or speak

D. Sensory functions
0 = Normal
1 = Vibration or figure-writing decrease only, in 1 or 2 limbs
2 = Mild decrease in touch or pain or position sense, and/or moderate decrease in vibration in 1 or 2 limbs, or vibratory decrease alone in 3 or 4 limbs
3 = Moderate decrease in touch or pain or position sense, and/or essentially lost vibration in 1 or 2 limbs, or mild decrease in touch or pain, and/or moderate decrease in all proprioceptive tests in 3 or 4 limbs
4 = Marked decrease in touch or pain or loss of proprioception, alone or combined, in 1 or 2 limbs or moderate decrease in touch or pain and/or severe proprioceptive decrease in more than 2 limbs
5 = Loss (essentially) of sensation in 1 or 2 limbs or moderate decrease in touch or pain and/or loss of proprioception for most of the body below the head
6 = Sensation essentially lost below the head

E. Bowel and bladder functions
0 = Normal
1 = Mild urinary hesitancy, urgency, or retention
2 = Moderate hesitancy, urgency, retention of bowel or bladder, or rare urinary incontinence
3 = Frequent urinary incontinence
4 = In need of almost constant catheterization
5 = Loss of bladder function
6 = Loss of bowel and bladder function

F. Visual (or optic) functions
0 = Normal
1 = Scotoma with visual acuity (corrected) better than 20/30
2 = Worse eye with scotoma with maximal visual acuity (corrected) of 20/30 to 20/59
3 = Worse eye with large scotoma, or moderate decrease in fields, but with maximal visual acuity (corrected) of 20/60 to 20/99
4 = Worse eye with marked decrease of fields and maximal acuity (corrected) of 20/100 to 20/200; grade 3 plus maximal acuity of better eye of 20/60 or less
5 = Worse eye with maximal visual acuity (corrected) less than 20/200; grade 4 plus maximal acuity of better eye of 20/60 or less
6 = Grade 5 plus maximal visual acuity of better eye of 20/60 or less

G. Cerebral (or mental) functions
0 = Normal
1 = Mood alteration only (does not affect EDSS score)
2 = Mild decrease in mentation
3 = Moderate decrease in mentation
4 = Marked decrease in mentation
5 = Chronic brain syndrome—severe or incompetent

SOURCE: After JF Kurtzke, Neurology 33:1444, 1983.

(3) expression of vascular endothelial adhesion molecules and matrix metalloproteinases that mediate trafficking of activated lymphocytes and macrophages into the CNS. Glatiramer acetate, a synthetic polypeptide designed to resemble MBP, may act by (1) inducing antigen-specific suppressor T cells as a result of shared determinants between copolymer 1 and MBP and (2) binding to MHC molecules on the surface of antigen-presenting cells.

IFN-β1b, 8.0 million international units (MIU), is administered by subcutaneous injection every other day. IFN-β1a, 6.0 MIU, is administered by intramuscular injection once every week. Glatiramer acetate, 20 mg, is administered by subcutaneous injection every day. IFN-β1b, IFN-β1a and glatiramer acetate are generally well tolerated. Erythematous reactions at the injection site are common with IFN-β1b and glatiramer acetate. Transient flu-like symptoms frequently occur at the beginning of IFN-β treatment; these symptoms, which usually resolve within several months, can be managed with ibuprofen, acetaminophen or other analgesic medications. Approximately 15% of glatiramer acetate recipients experience one or more episodes of flushing, chest tightness, dyspnea, palpitations, and anxiety after injection. This systemic reaction is unpredictable, self-limited, and generally lasts <1 h. Approximately 40% of IFN-β1b recipients and 5 to 25% of IFN-β1a recipients develop neutralizing antibodies within 12 months of initiating therapy. Data suggest that neutralizing antibodies may degrade clinical efficacy, but this relationship is not apparent in all patients. The clinical usefulness of commercially available tests for neutralizing antibodies is unclear.

In the United States, ~90% of treated patients with RRMS receive one of the interferons as first-line therapy, and the remaining 10%

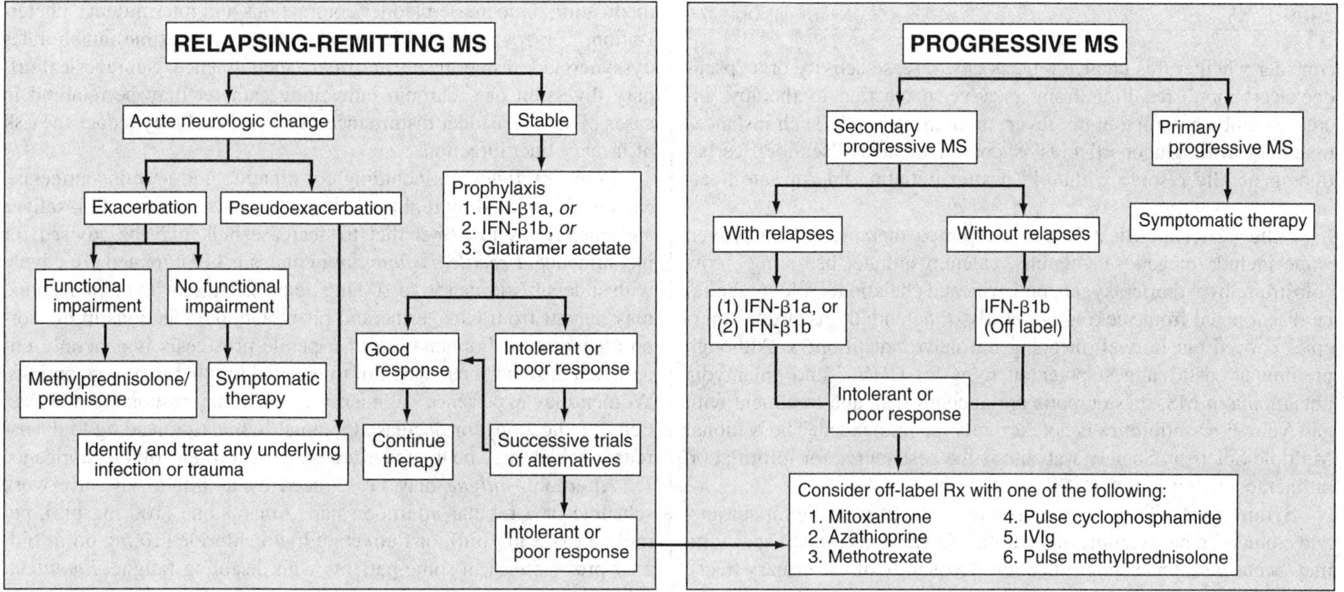

FIGURE 371-3 Therapeutic decision making for MS.

receive glatiramer acetate. Irrespective of the agent chosen, treatment should probably be discontinued in patients who continue to experience frequent clinical exacerbations or gradual progression of disability for ≥6 months. It is unknown whether patients who fail to respond adequately to treatment with any one of these interventions will respond more favorably to another; thus, it is reasonable to try a second agent (Fig. 371-3). The value of combination therapy is also unknown at this time.

Disease Modifying Therapies for SPMS IFN-β1b (Betaferon) and mitoxantrone (novantrone) were each shown to reduce annual exacerbation rates and MRI activity and delay time to onset of sustained progression of disability in patients with SPMS. Applications for approval of use of these drugs are filed in the United States. IFN-β1b is currently approved for treatment of SPMS in Canada and Europe. IFN-β1b, 8.0 MIU, is administered subcutaneously every other day. Mitoxantrone, 12 mg/m^2, is administered by intravenous infusion every third month. It may act as a T and B cell immunosuppressant and an enhancer of suppressor cell function. Mitoxantrone may cause mild nausea, slight hair thinning, leukopenia, thrombocytopenia and irreversible amennorhea. Dose-related cardiac toxicity is of concern, and treatment with mitoxantrone should be considered only in patients with normal ventricular ejection fractions; periodic echocardiograms are advised if cumulative doses of mitoxantrone exceed 100 mg/m^2.

Other Off-Label Treatment Options for RRMS and SPMS *Azathioprine*, 2 to 3 mg/kg body weight, is administered orally each day. This drug modestly reduces annual exacerbation rates in patients with RRMS and SPMS. Its effect on sustained progression of disability is less convincing

Methotrexate, 7.5 mg, is administered orally once each week. This drug, when administered for up to 2 years, modestly reduces disease activity in patients with SPMS as assessed by MRI and standardized tests of manual dexterity. An important practical advantage of methotrexate is the simplicity of a weekly oral dosing schedule.

Cyclophosphamide (CTX) reduces progression of disability in patients with SPMS when compared to ACTH. However, this observation has not been convincingly demonstrated in a placebo-controlled trial. Some investigators advocate pulse CTX therapy for young adults with aggressive forms of MS who fail to respond to approved treatment options.

Intravenous immunoglobulin (IVIg), 0.15 to 0.20 g/kg body weight, administered monthly for up to 2 years convincingly reduced annual exacerbation rates, but its effects on disability and MRI activity were not investigated. At higher doses, 1g/kg body weight daily for 2 days every 6 months, IVIg significantly reduced new MRI activity. Use of this treatment will probably be limited because of its high cost, questions about optimal dose, and uncertainty about the effect of long-term treatment on disability.

Methylprednisolone administered in bimonthly cycles at high doses modestly delays time to onset of sustained progression of disability.

2-Chlorodeoxyadenosine (2-CDA, cladribine) significantly reduces MRI activity in patients with SPMS. However, significant clinical benefits were not observed during 12 months of therapy in a Phase III clinical trial. In the absence of convincing clinical benefit, it is unlikely that 2-CDA will be commonly prescribed.

Disease-Modifying Therapies for PPMS No approved therapies for PPMS exist at this time. The results of ongoing trials of IFN-β1a, glatiramer acetate, and mitoxantrone in PPMS are awaited.

Therapy for Exacerbations The severity and duration of acute exacerbations of MS are reduced by treatment with glucocorticoids. Although methylprednisolone (MePDN) is most commonly prescribed, there is no consensus for the optimal dose and route of administration. Clinical exacerbations that impair activities of daily living can be treated with MePDN, 1000 mg, administered intravenously each day for 3 days followed by oral prednisone, 60 mg daily for 5 days, then tapering by 10 mg each day thereafter. A similar approach is employed for treatment of initial attacks of demyelinating disease. With the exception of severe attacks that jeopardize patient safety, treatment can generally be administered in an outpatient setting. Physical and occupational therapy should be prescribed when impaired mobility or decreased manual dexterity impair activities of daily living.

Common side effects of short-term glucocorticoid therapy include fluid retention, potassium loss, weight gain, gastric disturbances, acne, and emotional lability. Salt and fluid retention are managed with a low-salt, potassium-rich diet and avoidance of potassium-wasting diuretics. In patients who have heart disease or require concurrent diuretic therapy, oral potassium supplementation is advised. Lithium carbonate (300 mg orally bid) may provide effective prophylaxis for patients who experience emotional lability and insomnia associated with glucocorticoid therapy. For patients with a history of peptic ulcer disease, cimetidine (400 mg bid) or ranitidine (150 mg bid) is advised.

In one small controlled trial, plasma exchange (7 treatments given over 2 weeks) was effective in some patients with unusually fulminant attacks of demyelination unresponsive to glucocorticoids.

When patients experience an acute deterioration, it is important to consider whether this change reflects new disease activity or a "pseudoexacerbation" resulting from an adverse reaction to therapy, increased ambient temperature, fever, or an infection. In such instances treatment with glucocorticoids is contraindicated. Pseudoexacerbations generally resolve within 48 h after initiating appropriate treatment.

Other Therapeutic Claims Purported therapies of no proven value include megadose vitamins, calcium orotate, bee stings, cow colostrum, hyperbaric oxygen, procarin, and chelation. Patients should be discouraged from seeking out costly or potentially hazardous therapies carried out by well-meaning but naive practitioners. Although preliminary data suggest potential roles for HHV-6 and chlamydia pneumonia in MS, these reports are unconfirmed, and treatment with gancyclovir or antibiotics is not currently recommended. The National Multiple Sclerosis Society web site is the best source for information on therapeutic options for MS.

Symptomatic Therapy *Spasticity* with stiffness, flexor spasms, and clonus can be disabling and painful. Acute worsening of spasticity may occur with underlying infection (frequently of the urinary tract), obstipation, bedsores, other painful lesions, or injuries. Although the mechanisms are poorly understood, spasticity may also worsen following IFN-β therapy. These potential precipitants should be considered and treated specifically. All medications for spasticity have limited efficacy and may produce symptomatic worsening in patients who rely upon spasticity to provide leg strength necessary for effective ambulation. Baclofen (15 to 80 mg/d in divided doses) is the most useful drug available. In refractory cases, baclofen administered orally in higher doses (up to 240 mg/d) or intrathecally via an indwelling catheter may be effective. Tizanidine (2 to 8 mg tid) and diazepam (1 to 2 mg bid or tid) are particularly effective for painful nocturnal spasms, but daytime use is often limited by excessive somnolence. Cyclobenzaprine hydrochloride (5 to 10 mg bid or tid), clonazepam (0.5 to 1.0 mg tid, including a bedtime dose), and clonidine hydrochloride (0.1 to 0.2 mg tid, including a bedtime dose) may be useful for patients who otherwise fail to respond. Dantrolene may produce unacceptable weakness, and its use is usually reserved for nonambulatory patients. A course of glucocorticoids may be given in exceptional cases where other agents have failed, but benefits seldom last more than 2 to 3 weeks.

Pain, including trigeminal neuralgia and painful dysesthesias, may respond to carbamazepine (100 to 1200 mg/d in divided, escalating doses), gabapentin (300–3600 mg/d), dilantin (300–400 mg/d), amitriptyline (25–150 mg/d), or baclofen (10–80 mg/d). In patients with unilateral leg pain, it may be difficult to distinguish dysesthesias due to MS from radiculopathy due to lumbar disk disease; nonsurgical therapy is justified in the absence of convincing signs of nerve root compression.

Paroxysmal symptoms respond to carbamazepine (up to 1200 mg in divided doses), gabapentin (100 to 600 mg tid), or acetazolamide (125 to 250 mg tid). Although no treatment for tremor is satisfactory, slight improvement is occasionally seen with clonazepam (0.5 to 1.0 mg bid or tid), primidone (125 to 250 mg bid or tid), ondansetron (4 to 8 mg bid or tid), and isoniazid (up to 1200 mg in divided doses). Stereotaxic thalamotomy may be considered in cases of disabling tremor in which a unilateral reduction in symptoms is required, but the general experience with this procedure has been disappointing.

Because specific symptoms of *bladder dysfunction* correlate poorly with physiologic findings, urodynamic evaluation is often required. The pathophysiology of abnormal micturition also may change over time in MS. Bladder hyperreflexia is treated with anticholinergics: oxybutynin (5 mg bid or tid), tolterodine (1 to 2 mg bid), or propantheline (7.5 to 15 mg qid). Urinary retention due to bladder hyporeflexia may respond to the cholinergic drug bethanecol (10 to 50 mg tid or qid). Dyssynergia between detrusor and external sphincter muscles may be treated effectively with a combination of anticholinergic medication to decrease bladder contractions and intermittent catheterization. Terazosin hydrochloride (1 to 5 mg at bedtime) ameliorates dyssynergia but may result in urinary incontinence. Supravesical urinary diversion or a chronic indwelling catheter may be required in cases of severe bladder disturbance. Ascorbic acid may reduce the risk of urinary tract infections.

Bowel dysfunction, including constipation and urge incontinence, can be ameliorated by regimentation of bowel function with laxatives and enemas. A low-fiber diet to decrease bulk may be advised for incontinence. *Erectile dysfunction* in males is often treated effectively with sildenafil citrate (50 to 100 mg po prn). Those who fail to respond may benefit from papaverine and phentolamine injections in the corpora cavernosa. Implantation of a penile prosthesis is generally undertaken only for those who fail to respond to other treatment options. Women may experience vaginismus, which may respond to antispasticity medications, or decreased vaginal lubrication leading to dyspareunia, which may be treated effectively with water soluble lubricants.

Afternoon *fatigue* may be reduced by a shift to an early work schedule or a regular afternoon nap. Amantadine (100 mg bid), pemoline (37.5 mg bid), or fluoxetine hydrochloride (20 mg qd or bid) may prove useful in some patients with disabling fatigue. *Emotional lability* often responds to amitriptyline (25 to 75 mg/d) or fluoxetine (20 mg/d). It is essential to be vigilant for clinical evidence of *depression*, since the risk of suicide is increased in patients with MS. Occupational counseling and other support services may assist patients and their families in coping with the effects of the disease. Health maintenance should be emphasized, including stress reduction, a balanced diet, avoidance of rapid change in weight, and adequate rest. Although there is little evidence linking vaccination with relapses of MS, it is prudent to avoid unnecessary immunizations. Swimming is an ideal form of exercise for many patients because of the buoyant support and hypothermia that is achieved.

Pregnancy may affect the course of MS. Compared with nonpregnant MS patients, pregnant patients experience fewer attacks during gestation but more attacks in the first 3 months after parturition. The two effects appear to be roughly similar in magnitude; thus, no effect of pregnancy on disability or on the overall disease course has been identified. Although it has been hypothesized that high levels of prolactin induced in the postpartum period and maintained by breast feeding result in immune stimulation that predisposes to relapses of MS, studies indicate no effect of breast feeding on attack frequency in the postpartum period. The advisability of childbearing should be determined primarily by the patient's physical state and available social support.

CLINICAL VARIANTS OF MS *Neuromyelitis optica (Devic's syndrome)* is characterized by separate attacks of acute optic neuritis and myelitis. Optic neuritis may be unilateral or bilateral and precede or follow an attack of myelitis by days, months, or years. Respiratory failure may result from cervical cord lesions. CSF neutrophil counts $>50/\mu L$ are reported to occur in as many as 20% of patients. In contrast to patients with MS, patients with Devic's syndrome do not experience brainstem, cerebellar, and cognitive involvement, and the brain MRI is normal. Characteristically, MRI demonstrates a transiently enhancing focal region of swelling and cavitation that extends over three or more spinal cord segments. In contrast to MS, histopathology of these lesions may reveal areas of necrosis and thickening of blood vessel walls. Thus, it remains uncertain whether Devic's syndrome is a variant of MS or a separate entity. The role of disease-modifying therapies for MS has not been rigorously studied in patients with Devic's syndrome. This syndrome is unusual in Caucasians but appears to be more common in Asians. The 5-year survival rate in the Mayo Clinic series was ~70%.

Acute MS (Marburg's variant) is a rare acute fulminant process that generally ends in death from brainstem involvement within one year. There are no remissions. Diagnosis can be established only at postmortem examination; widespread demyelination, axonal loss, edema, and macrophage infiltration are characteristic, and discrete plaques may also be seen. In contrast to postinfectious encephalomyelitis (see below), this disorder does not follow exanthematous infection or vaccination. It has been suggested that acute MS may be associated with an immature form of myelin that is more susceptible to breakdown. As with Devic's syndrome, it is unclear whether this syndrome represents an extreme form of MS or another disease altogether.

ACUTE DISSEMINATED ENCEPHALOMYELITIS

In contrast to MS, acute disseminated encephalomyelitis (ADEM) is distinguished by a monophasic course and a frequent association with antecedent immunization (postvaccinal encephalomyelitis) or infection (postinfectious encephalomyelitis). The pathologic hallmark of ADEM is the presence of widely scattered small foci of perivenular inflammation and demyelination. In its most explosive form, acute hemorrhagic leukoencephalitis, lesions are vasculitic and hemorrhagic, and the clinical course is devastating.

Postvaccinal encephalomyelitis may follow the administration of smallpox and certain rabies vaccines. Postinfectious encephalomyelitis is most frequently associated with the viral exanthems of childhood. Natural infection with measles virus is the most common antecedent (1 in 1000 cases). Worldwide, measles encephalomyelitis remains a common illness, but in developed countries use of the live measles vaccine has dramatically reduced its incidence. An ADEM-like illness rarely follows vaccination with live measles vaccine (1 to 2 in 10^6 immunizations). ADEM is now most frequently associated with varicella (chickenpox) infections (1 in 4000 to 10,000 cases). It also may follow infection with rubella, mumps, influenza, parainfluenza, and infectious mononucleosis viruses and with *Mycoplasma*. Some patients may have a nonspecific upper respiratory infection or no known antecedent illness.

An autoimmune response to MBP can be detected in the CSF from many patients with ADEM. This response has been most clearly established after rabies vaccination and infection with measles virus. With measles infection, the induction of immune responses to a variety of CNS antigens may occur, but only the response to MBP correlates with the development of ADEM. Many cases of postvaccinal encephalomyelitis may result from sensitization with brain material that contaminates the viral vaccines. Attempts to demonstrate direct viral invasion of the CNS have been unsuccessful. The molecular mechanism responsible for virus-induced triggering of an autoimmune response to MBP is not known but may include molecular mimicry due to antigens shared between the virus and host determinants or to virus-mediated CNS injury with secondary sensitization to MBP.

CLINICAL MANIFESTATIONS The severity of ADEM varies. In severe cases, the onset is abrupt, and progression is rapid (hours to days). In postinfectious ADEM, the neurologic syndrome generally begins late in the course of the viral illness as the exanthem is fading. Fever reappears, and headache, meningismus, and lethargy progressing to coma may develop. Seizures are common. Signs of disseminated neurologic disease are consistently present. Motor findings may include hemiparesis or quadriparesis and extensor plantar responses. Tendon reflexes may be lost initially, later to become hyperactive. Variable degrees of sensory loss and of brainstem involvement may occur. In ADEM due to complications from chickenpox, cerebellar involvement is often prominent. CSF protein is modestly elevated (50 to 150 mg/dL). Lymphocytic pleocytosis, generally $\leq$200 cells per microliter, occurs in 80% of patients. Occasional patients have higher counts or a mixed polymorphonuclear-lymphocytic pattern during the initial days of the illness. Transient CSF oligoclonal banding has been reported. MRI may reveal extensive gadolinium enhancement of white matter in brain and spinal cord.

DIAGNOSIS The diagnosis is easily established when there is a history of recent vaccination or exanthematous illness. In severe cases with predominantly cerebral involvement, acute encephalitis due to infection with herpes simplex or other viruses may be difficult to exclude. In the absence of a specific viral prodrome or of immunization, it may not be possible to distinguish ADEM from acute MS. The simultaneous onset of disseminated symptoms and signs indicating optic nerve, brain, and spinal cord involvement is common in ADEM and rare in MS. Similarly, meningismus, drowsiness or coma, or seizures suggest ADEM. Optic nerve involvement is generally bilateral in ADEM and unilateral in MS, and transverse myelopathy is usually complete in the former and partial in the latter. The CSF protein level is normal in most patients with MS; lymphocyte counts are rarely >50 cells/μL, and polymorphonuclear leukocytes are not present. MRI findings that may support a diagnosis of ADEM include extensive and relatively symmetric white matter abnormalities and diffuse gadolinium enhancement of all abnormal areas, indicating active disease and a monophasic course.

Rx **TREATMENT** Therapy consists of intravenous methylprednisolone as employed for exacerbations of MS. Uncontrolled studies have found ACTH and plasmapheresis also to be of benefit. Occasional patients show evidence of relapse shortly after termination of therapy, and for them, reinstitution of therapy may be useful. The prognosis reflects the severity of the underlying acute illness. Measles encephalomyelitis is associated with a mortality rate of 5 to 20%, and most survivors have permanent neurologic sequelae. Children who recover may have persistent seizures and behavioral and learning disorders.

BIBLIOGRAPHY

ARCHELOS JJ et al: The role of B cells and autoantibodies in multiple-sclerosis. Ann Neurol 47:694, 2000

CONFAVREUX C et al: Rate of pregnancy-related relapse in multiple sclerosis. N Engl J Med 339:285, 1998

EUROPEAN STUDY GROUP ON INTERFERON β-1B IN SECONDARY PROGRESSIVE MS. Placebo-controlled multicentre randomised trial of interferon β-1b in treatment of secondary progressive multiple sclerosis. Lancet 352:1491, 1998

FAZEKAS F et al: Randomized placebo-controlled trial of monthly intravenous immunoglobin therapy in relapsing-remitting multiple sclerosis. Lancet 349:589, 1997

GENAIN C et al: Identification of autoantibodies associated with myelin damage in multiple sclerosis. Nat Med 5:2, 1999

JACOBS LD et al: Intramuscular interferon beta 1a initiated during a first demyelinating event in multiple sclerosis. N Engl J Med 343:898, 2000

JOHNSON KP et al: Extended use of glatiramer acetate (copaxone) is well tolerated and maintains its clinical effect on multiple sclerosis relapse rate and degree of disability. Neurology 50:701, 1998

LUCCHINETTI C et al: Heterogeneity of multiple sclerosis lesions: Implications for the pathogenesis of demyelination. Ann Neurol 47:707, 2000

THE MULTIPLE SCLEROSIS GENETICS GROUP: Linkage of the MHC to familial multiple sclerosis suggests genetic heterogeneity. Hum Mol Gen 7:8, 1998

NOSEWORTHY JH et al: Medical progress: multiple sclerosis. N Engl J Med 343:938, 2000

THE OWIMS STUDY GROUP: Evidence of interferon β-1a dose response in relapsing-remitting MS. Neurology 53:679, 1999

OKSENBERG JR, HAUSER SL: The molecular pathogenesis of multiple sclerosis, in *Molecular Neurology*, JB Martin (ed). New York, Scientific American Medicine, 1998

PRISMS STUDY GROUP: Randomised double-blind placebo-controlled study of interferon β-1a in relapsing-remitting multiple sclerosis. Lancet 352:1498, 1998

RUDICK RA, GOODKIN DE (eds): *Multiple Sclerosis Therapeutics*. London, Martin Dunitz, 1999

STUVE O, ZAMVIL S: Pathogenesis, diagnosis, and treatment of acute disseminated encephalomyelitis (ADEM). Curr Opin Neurol 12:395, 1999

WEINSHENKER BG et al: A randomized trial of plasma exchange in acute central nervous system inflammatory disease. Ann Neurol 46:878, 1999

ZHAO GJ et al: Effect of interferon beta-1b in MS: Assessment of annual accumulation of PD/T2 activity on MRI. UBC MS/MRI Analysis Group and the MS Study Group. Neurology 54:200, 2000

372

Karen L. Roos, Kenneth L. Tyler

BACTERIAL MENINGITIS AND OTHER SUPPURATIVE INFECTIONS

CNS	central nervous system	LPS	lipopolysaccharide
CPP	cerebral perfusion pressure	MAP	mean arterial pressure
CSF	cerebrospinal fluid	MIC	minimal inhibitory concentration
CT	computed tomography	MRI	magnetic resonance imaging
EEG	electroencephalogram	PCR	polymerase chain reaction
Hib	*H. influenzae* type b	PMNs	polymorphonuclear neutrophils
HSV	herpes simplex virus	SAH	subarachnoid hemorrhage
ICP	intracranial pressure	SDE	subdural empyema
IL	interleukin	TNF	tumor necrosis factor
LA	latex particle agglutination		

ACUTE BACTERIAL MENINGITIS

DEFINITION Bacterial meningitis is an acute purulent infection within the subarachnoid space. It is associated with a central nervous system (CNS) inflammatory reaction that may result in decreased consciousness, seizures, raised intracranial pressure, and stroke. The meninges, the subarachnoid space, and the brain parenchyma are all involved in the inflammatory reaction; as such, *meningoencephalitis* is the more accurate descriptive term.

EPIDEMIOLOGY Bacterial meningitis is the most common form of suppurative intracranial infection, with an annual incidence >2.5 cases/100,000 population. The epidemiology of bacterial meningitis has changed in recent years. Currently, the organisms most commonly responsible for community-acquired bacterial meningitis are *Streptococcus pneumoniae* (~50%), *Neisseria meningitidis* (~25%), group B streptococci (~10%), and *Listeria monocytogenes* (~10%). *Haemophilus influenzae* was once the most common cause of bacterial meningitis in the United States. The incidence of *H. influenzae* meningitis declined precipitously following the introduction of the *H. influenzae* type b (Hib) vaccine in 1987, and *H. influenzae* now accounts for <10% of bacterial meningitis cases. There have also been major changes in the epidemiology of pneumococcal disease, with the global emergence and increasing prevalence of penicillin- and cephalosporin-resistant strains of *S. pneumoniae*. As of 1998, ~44% of clinical isolates of *S. pneumoniae* in the United States had intermediate or high levels of resistance to penicillin. In the past several years, there has been an increase in the incidence of meningococcal infections on college campuses and an increase in the incidence of meningococcal disease in North America and Europe due to the emergence of a virulent strain of serogroup C, serotype 2a *N. meningitidis*. An increasing incidence of *N. meningitidis* strains with moderate or relative resistance to penicillin and a decreased susceptibility to ampicillin has been reported worldwide, but the clinical significance of these strains is still unknown. Annual meningitis epidemics, caused primarily by the serogroup A meningococcus, continue to occur in the meningitis belt of sub-Saharan Africa. Epidemics due to the serogroup B meningococcus continue to occur in Europe, Latin America, and New Zealand. Group B streptococcus or *S. agalactiae* was previously responsible for meningitis predominantly in neonates, but it has been reported with increasing frequency in individuals >50 years, particularly those with underlying diseases. *L. monocytogenes* has emerged as an important cause of bacterial meningitis in the elderly and in individuals with impaired cell-mediated immunity.

ETIOLOGY *S. pneumoniae* (Chap. 140) is the most common cause of meningitis in adults >20 years. There are a number of predisposing conditions that increase the risk of pneumococcal meningitis, the most important of which is pneumococcal pneumonia. Additional risk factors include coexisting acute or chronic otitis media, alcoholism, diabetes, splenectomy, hypogammaglobulinemia, complement deficiency, and head trauma with basilar skull fracture and cerebrospinal fluid (CSF) rhinorrhea.

N. meningitidis (Chap. 146) accounts for nearly 60% of bacterial meningitis cases in children and young adults between the ages of 2 and 20. The nasopharynx is initially colonized by this organism, resulting in either an asymptomatic carrier state or invasive meningococcal disease. The risk of invasive disease following nasopharyngeal colonization depends on both bacterial virulence factors and host immune defense mechanisms, including the host's capacity to produce antimeningococcal antibodies and to lyse meningococci by both the classic and alternative complement pathways. Individuals with deficiencies of any of the complement components, including properdin, are highly susceptible to meningococcal infections.

Enteric gram-negative bacilli are the causative organisms of meningitis that is associated with chronic and debilitating diseases such as diabetes, cirrhosis or alcoholism, and chronic urinary tract infections and following neurosurgical procedures, particularly craniotomy or craniectomy.

Resistance to infection with *L. monocytogenes* requires effective cell-mediated immunity. As a result, elderly individuals and those with impaired cell-mediated immunity due to organ transplantation, pregnancy, malignancy, chronic illness, or immunosuppressive therapy are all at increased risk for listerial meningitis. Infection is acquired by ingesting foods contaminated by this organism. Foodborne human listerial infection has been reported from contaminated coleslaw, milk, deli meat, and soft cheeses.

The frequency of *H. influenzae* type b meningitis in children has declined dramatically since the introduction of the Hib conjugate vaccine, although rare cases of Hib meningitis in vaccinated children have been reported. More frequently, *H. influenzae* causes meningitis in unvaccinated children and adults.

Staphylococcus aureus and coagulase-negative staphylococci are predominant organisms causing meningitis that follows invasive neurosurgical procedures, particularly shunting procedures for hydrocephalus, or occurs as a complication of the use of subcutaneous Ommaya reservoirs for the administration of intrathecal chemotherapy.

PATHOPHYSIOLOGY The most common bacteria that cause meningitis, *S. pneumoniae* and *N. meningitidis*, initially colonize the nasopharynx by attaching to nasopharyngeal epithelial cells. Bacteria are transported across epithelial cells in membrane-bound vacuoles to the intravascular space or invade the intravascular space by creating separations in the apical tight junctions of columnar epithelial cells. Once the bacteria gain access to the bloodstream, they are able to avoid phagocytosis by neutrophils and classic complement–mediated bactericidal activity because of the presence of a polysaccharide capsule. Once in the bloodstream, bacteria can reach the intraventricular choroid plexus. Infection of choroid plexus epithelial cells allows bacteria direct access to the CSF. Some bacteria, such as *S. pneumoniae*, can adhere directly to cerebral capillary endothelial cells and subsequently migrate through or between these cells to reach the CSF. Bacteria are able to multiply rapidly within CSF because of the absence of effective host immune defenses. Normal CSF contains few white blood cells (WBCs) and relatively small amounts of complement proteins and immunoglobulins. The paucity of the latter two prevents effective opsonization of bacteria, an essential prerequisite for bacterial phagocytosis by neutrophils. Phagocytosis of bacteria is further impaired by the fluid nature of CSF, which is less conducive to phagocytosis than a solid tissue substrate.

A critical event in the pathogenesis of bacterial meningitis is the inflammatory reaction induced by the invading bacteria. Many of the neurologic manifestations and complications of bacterial meningitis result from the immune response to the invading pathogen rather than from direct bacteria-induced tissue injury. As a result, neurologic injury can progress even after the CSF has been sterilized by antibiotic therapy.

The lysis of bacteria with the subsequent release of cell-wall components into the subarachnoid space is the initial step in the induction of the inflammatory response and the formation of a purulent exudate in the subarachnoid space (Fig. 372-1). Bacterial cell-wall components, such as the lipopolysaccharide (LPS) molecules of gram-negative bacteria and teichoic acid and peptidoglycans of *S. pneumoniae*, induce meningeal inflammation by stimulating the production of inflammatory cytokines and chemokines by microglia, astrocytes, monocytes, microvascular endothelial cells, and CSF leukocytes. In experimental models of meningitis, cytokines including tumor necrosis factor (TNF) and interleukin (IL) 1 are present in CSF within 1 to 2 h of intracisternal inoculation of LPS. This cytokine response is quickly followed by an increase in CSF protein concentration and leukocytosis. Chemokines (cytokines that induce chemotactic migration in leukocytes) and a variety of other proinflammatory cytokines are also produced and secreted by leukocytes and tissue cells that are stimulated by IL-1 and TNF. In addition, bacteremia and the inflammatory cytokines induce the production of excitatory amino acids, reactive oxygen and nitrogen species (free oxygen radicals, nitric oxide, and peroxynitrite), and other mediators that can induce death of brain cells.

Much of the pathophysiology of bacterial meningitis is a direct consequence of elevated levels of CSF cytokines and chemokines. TNF and IL-1 act synergistically to increase the permeability of the blood-brain barrier, resulting in induction of vasogenic edema and the leakage of serum proteins into the subarachnoid space (Fig. 372-1). The subarachnoid exudate of proteinaceous material and leukocytes obstructs the flow of CSF through the ventricular system and diminishes the resorptive capacity of the arachnoid granulations in the dural sinuses, leading to obstructive and communicating hydrocephalus and concomitant interstitial edema.

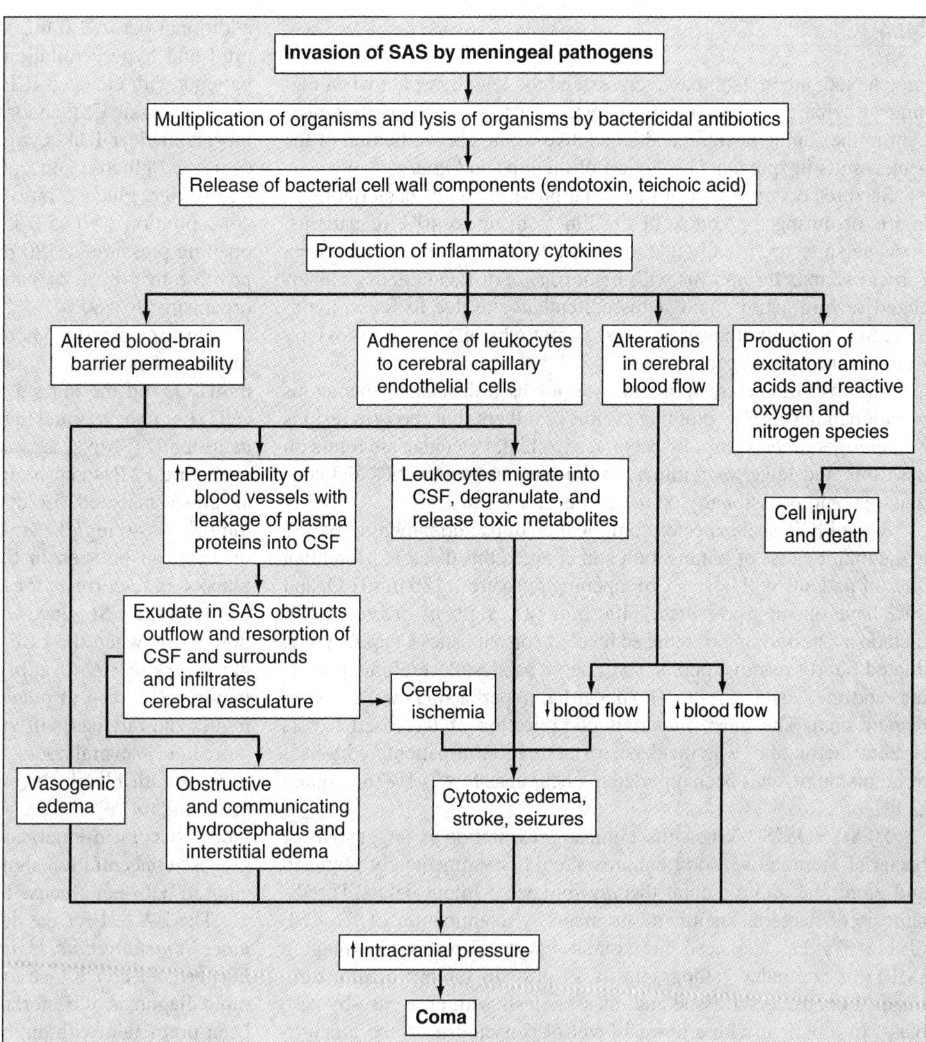

FIGURE 372-1 The pathophysiology of the neurologic complications of bacterial meningitis. SAS, subarachnoid space; CSF, cerebrospinal fluid (©Kroos).

Inflammatory cytokines upregulate the expression of selectins on cerebral capillary endothelial cells and leukocytes, which allows for leukocytes to adhere to vascular endothelial cells and to subsequently migrate into the CSF. The adherence of leukocytes to capillary endothelial cells increases the permeability of blood vessels, allowing for the leakage of plasma proteins into the CSF, which adds to the inflammatory exudate. Neutrophil degranulation results in the release of toxic metabolites that contribute to cytotoxic edema, cell injury, and death. Contrary to previous beliefs, CSF leukocytes probably do little to contribute to the clearance of CSF bacterial infection.

During the very early stages of meningitis there is an increase in cerebral blood flow, soon followed by a decrease in cerebral blood flow and a loss of cerebrovascular autoregulation. Cerebral perfusion pressure (CPP) is defined as the difference between the mean arterial pressure (MAP) and the intracranial pressure (ICP), i.e., CPP = MAP − ICP. CPP is protected by cerebrovascular autoregulation, which dilates or constricts cerebral resistance vessels in response to alterations in CPP, due to changes in either the MAP or the ICP. Loss of cerebrovascular autoregulation means that any increase in systemic blood pressure leads to an increase in cerebral blood flow and ICP. Conversely, a decrease in mean systemic arterial pressure, for example, associated with septic shock, results in a decrease in cerebral blood flow and subsequent cerebral ischemia and infarction. The cerebrovascular complications of bacterial meningitis include not only a loss of autoregulation but also narrowing of the large arteries at the base of the brain due to encroachment on the vessel by the purulent exudate in the subarachnoid space and infiltration of the arterial wall by inflammatory cells with intimal thickening (vasculitis); this may result in ischemia and infarction, obstruction of branches of the middle cerebral artery by thrombosis, thrombosis of the major cerebral venous sinuses, and thrombophlebitis of the cerebral cortical veins. The combination of interstitial, vasogenic, and cytotoxic edema leads to raised ICP and coma. Cerebral edema, either focal or generalized, can lead to cerebral herniation (see below). Focal or diffuse cerebral edema is the most likely cause of meningitis-associated brain herniation; however, hydrocephalus and dural sinus or cortical vein thrombosis may also play a role.

CLINICAL PRESENTATION Meningitis can present as either an acute fulminant illness that progresses rapidly in a few hours or as a subacute infection that progressively worsens over several days. The classic clinical triad of meningitis is fever, headache, and nuchal rigidity ("stiff neck"). Each of these signs and symptoms occurs in >90% of cases. Alteration in mental status occurs in 75% of patients and can vary from lethargy to coma. Nausea, vomiting, and photophobia are also common complaints. Nuchal rigidity is the pathognomonic sign of meningeal irritation and is present when the neck resists passive flexion. Kernig's and Brudzinski's signs are also classic signs of meningeal irritation. Kernig's sign is elicited with the patient in the supine position. The thigh is flexed on the abdomen, with the knee flexed; attempts to passively extend the leg elicit pain when meningeal irritation is present. Brudzinski's sign is elicited with the patient in the supine position and is positive when passive flexion of the neck results in spontaneous flexion of the hips and knees.

Seizures occur as part of the initial presentation of bacterial meningitis or during the course of the illness in up to 40% of patients. Focal seizures are usually due to focal arterial ischemia or infarction, cortical venous thrombosis with hemorrhage, or focal edema. Generalized seizure activity and status epilepticus are due to fever, hyponatremia, or cerebral anoxia or, less commonly, as a result of toxicity from antimicrobial agents.

The rash of meningococcemia begins as a diffuse erythematous maculopapular rash resembling a viral exanthem, but the skin lesions of meningococcemia rapidly become petechial. Petechiae are found on the trunk and lower extremities, in the mucous membranes and conjunctiva, and occasionally on the palms and soles.

Raised ICP is an expected complication of bacterial meningitis and is the major cause of obtundation and coma in this disease. More than 90% of patients will have a CSF opening pressure >180 mmH_2O, and 20% have opening pressures >400 mmH_2O. Signs of increased ICP include a deteriorating or reduced level of consciousness, papilledema, dilated poorly reactive pupils, sixth nerve palsies, decerebrate posturing, and the Cushing reflex (bradycardia, hypertension, and irregular respirations). The most disastrous complication of increased ICP is cerebral herniation. The incidence of herniation in patients with bacterial meningitis has been reported to occur in as few as 1% to as many as 8% of cases.

DIAGNOSIS When the clinical presentation is suggestive of bacterial meningitis, blood cultures should be immediately obtained and empirical antimicrobial therapy initiated without delay. The diagnosis of bacterial meningitis is made by examination of the CSF (Table 372-1). The need for cranial magnetic resonance imaging (MRI) or computed tomography (CT) prior to lumbar puncture remains a controversial issue and must be dealt with on a case-by-case basis. In a patient with a normal level of consciousness and a neurologic examination with no evidence of papilledema or focal deficits, it is safe to perform lumbar puncture without prior neuroimaging studies. If lumbar puncture is delayed in order to obtain neuroimaging studies, empirical antibiotic therapy should be initiated after blood cultures are obtained. Antibiotic therapy for several hours prior to lumbar puncture will not significantly alter the CSF white blood cell count or glucose concentration, nor is it likely to sterilize the CSF so that the organism cannot be identified on Gram's stain. Increased ICP should be treated in patients with clinical signs of increased pressure, and lumbar puncture performed with a 22- or 25-gauge needle. Only a minimum amount of CSF need be removed for analysis; ~3.5 mL of CSF is sufficient to obtain a cell count (1.0 mL), glucose and protein concentrations (1.0 mL), latex particle agglutination (LA) tests (0.5 mL), and Gram's stain and bacterial cultures (1.0 mL). If possible, an additional 0.5 to 1.0 mL should be saved. Preadministration of mannitol and hyperventilation further decrease the risk of herniation in patients with elevated ICP.

Table 372-1 Cerebrospinal Fluid Abnormalities in Bacterial Meningitis

Opening pressure	>180 mmH_2O
White blood cells	>10/μL to <10,000/μL; neutrophils predominate
Red blood cells	Absent, unless traumatic tap
Glucose	<2.2 mmol/L (<40 mg/dL)
CSF serum:glucose ratio	<0.40
Protein	>0.45 g/L (>45 mg/dL)
Gram's stain	Positive in 70–90% of untreated cases
Culture	Positive in 80% of cases
Latex agglutination	Specific for antigens of *S. pneumoniae*, *N. meningitidis*, *E. coli*, *H. influenzae*, type b, and group B streptococcus
Limulus amebocyte lysate assay	Positive in gram-negative meningitis
PCR for bacterial DNA	Specificity and sensitivity unknown

NOTE: PCR, polymerase chain reaction.

The classic CSF abnormalities in bacterial meningitis are: (1) polymorphonuclear leukocytosis (>100 cells per microliter in 90%), (2) decreased glucose concentration [<2.2 mmol/L (<40 mg/dL) and/or CSF/serum glucose ratio of <0.4 in ~60%], (3) increased protein concentration [>0.45 g/L (>45 mg/dL) in 90%], and (4) increased opening pressure (>180 mmH_2O in 90%). CSF bacterial cultures are positive in >80% of patients, and CSF Gram's stain demonstrates organisms in >60%.

Opening pressure should be measured with the patient in the lateral recumbent position. In adults, the normal opening pressure is <180 mmH_2O, and the normal white blood cell count is <5 mononuclear cells (lymphocytes and monocytes) per microliter. Polymorphonuclear neutrophils (PMNs) are not found in cell counts of normal CSF; however, rare PMNs can be found in concentrated CSF specimens, such as those analyzed for cytology. CSF glucose concentrations <2.2 mmol/L (<40 mg/dL) are abnormal, and a CSF glucose concentration of zero can be seen in bacterial meningitis. Use of the CSF/serum glucose ratio corrects for hyperglycemia that may mask a relative decrease in the CSF glucose concentration. The CSF glucose concentration is low when the CSF/serum glucose ratio is <0.6. A CSF/serum glucose ratio <0.40 is highly suggestive of bacterial meningitis but may also be seen in other conditions, including carcinomatous meningitis and rare cases of viral meningitis. It takes at least 30 min, and more likely several hours, for CSF glucose concentration to reach equilibrium with blood glucose concentrations; therefore, administration of 50 mL of 50% glucose (D50) prior to lumbar puncture, as commonly occurs in emergency room settings, is unlikely to alter CSF glucose concentration significantly unless more than a few hours have elapsed between glucose administration and lumbar puncture.

The LA test for the detection of bacterial antigens of *S. pneumoniae*, *N. meningitidis*, *H. influenzae* type b, group B streptococcus, and *Escherichia coli* K1 strains in the CSF is very useful for making a rapid diagnosis of bacterial meningitis, especially in patients who have been pretreated with antibiotics and in whom CSF Gram's stain and culture are negative. The CSF LA test has a *specificity* of 95 to 100% for *S. pneumoniae* and *N. meningitidis*, so a positive test is virtually diagnostic of bacterial meningitis by these organisms. However, the *sensitivity* of the CSF LA test is only 70 to 100% for detection of *S. pneumoniae* and 33 to 70% for detection of *N. meningitidis* antigens, so a negative test does not exclude infection by these organisms. The Limulus amebocyte lysate assay is a rapid diagnostic test for the detection of gram-negative endotoxin in CSF, and thus for making a diagnosis of gram-negative bacterial meningitis. The test has a specificity of 85 to 100% and a sensitivity approaching 100%. Thus, a positive Limulus amebocyte lysate assay occurs in virtually all patients with gram-negative bacterial meningitis, but false-positives may occur. CSF polymerase chain reaction (PCR) tests are not as useful in the diagnosis of bacterial meningitis as they are in the diagnosis of viral CNS infections. A CSF PCR test has been developed for detecting DNA from bacteria in CSF, but its sensitivity and specificity need to be better characterized before its role in diagnosis can be defined.

Almost all patients with bacterial meningitis will ultimately have neuroimaging studies performed. MRI is preferred over CT because of its superiority in demonstrating areas of cerebral edema and ischemia. In patients with bacterial meningitis, diffuse meningeal enhancement is often seen after the administration of gadolinium. Meningeal enhancement is not diagnostic of meningitis but occurs in any CNS disease associated with increased blood-brain barrier permeability.

Petechial skin lesions, if present, should be biopsied. The rash of meningococcemia results from the dermal seeding of organisms with vascular endothelial damage, and biopsy may reveal the organism on Gram's stain.

DIFFERENTIAL DIAGNOSIS Foremost in the differential diagnosis of bacterial meningitis is viral meningoencephalitis, specifically herpes simplex virus (HSV) encephalitis (Chaps. 182, 373). The clinical presentation of HSV encephalitis includes headache, fever, altered consciousness, focal neurologic deficits (e.g., dysphasia, hemiparesis), and focal or generalized seizures. Features that distinguish herpes encephalitis from bacterial meningitis include the findings on CSF studies, neuroimaging, and electroencephalogram (EEG). The classic CSF profile in patients with viral CNS infections is a lymphocytic pleocytosis with a normal glucose concentration, as contrasted with the PMN pleocytosis and hypoglycorrhachia characteristic of bacterial meningitis. MRI abnormalities other than meningeal enhancement are not seen in uncomplicated bacterial meningitis. Patients with HSV encephalitis frequently have MRI abnormalities, including increased signal within the orbitofrontal and medial temporal lobes and insular cortex on T2-weighted and FLAIR images. There is a distinctive EEG pattern in HSV encephalitis consisting of periodic, stereotyped, sharp-and-slow wave complexes originating in one or both temporal lobes and repeating at regular intervals of 2 to 3 s. The periodic complexes are typically noted between the second and the fifteenth day of the illness and are present in two-thirds of pathologically proven cases of HSV encephalitis.

The clinical presentation of encephalitis caused by arthropod-borne viruses (Chap. 198) can also resemble that of bacterial meningitis. Another consideration is rickettsial disease (Chap. 177). Rocky Mountain spotted fever (RMSF) is transmitted by a tick bite and caused by the bacteria *Rickettsia rickettsii*. The disease may resemble bacterial meningitis because of its common presentation with high fever, prostration, myalgia, headache, and nausea and vomiting. Most patients develop a characteristic rash within 96 h of the onset of symptoms. The rash is initially a diffuse erythematous maculopapular rash that may be difficult to distinguish from that of meningococcemia. It progresses to a petechial rash, then to a purpuric rash, and, if untreated, to skin necrosis or gangrene. The color of the lesions changes from bright red to very dark red, then yellowish-green to black. The rash typically begins in the wrist and ankles, and then spreads distally and proximally within a matter of a few hours and involves the palms and soles. Diagnosis is made by immunofluorescent staining of skin biopsy specimens.

Focal suppurative CNS infections (see below), including subdural and epidural empyema and brain abscess, should also be considered. The presence of focal features in a patient with suspected bacterial meningitis should prompt immediate neuroimaging studies; MRI is preferable to CT and is extremely sensitive and specific for diagnosis.

Among noninfectious CNS processes, subarachnoid hemorrhage (SAH; Chap. 361) is generally the major consideration. A classic presentation of SAH is the explosive onset of a severe headache or a sudden transient loss of consciousness followed by a severe headache. Nuchal rigidity and vomiting are frequently present and contribute to the resemblance between SAH and meningitis. CT scan is a sensitive indicator of the presence of SAH and usually allows for prompt diagnosis, although occasional patients with suspected SAH have a normal CT scan. In these patients a lumbar puncture is indicated, and the presence of grossly bloody CSF allows SAH to be immediately distinguished from bacterial meningitis.

℞ TREATMENT **Empirical antimicrobial therapy** (Table 372-2) Bacterial meningitis is a medical emergency. The goal is to begin antibiotic therapy within 60 min of a patient's arrival in the emergency room. Empirical antimicrobial therapy is initiated in patients with suspected bacterial meningitis before the results of CSF Gram's stain and culture are known. *S. pneumoniae* (Chap. 140) and *N. meningitidis* (Chap. 146) are the most common etiologic organisms of community-acquired bacterial meningitis. Due to the emergence of penicillin- and cephalosporin-resistant *S. pneumoniae*, empirical therapy of community-acquired bacterial meningitis in children and adults should include a third-generation cephalosporin (e.g., ceftriaxone or cefotaxime) and vancomycin. Ceftriaxone or cefotaxime provide good coverage for susceptible *S. pneumoniae*, group B streptococci, and *H. influenzae* and adequate coverage for *N. meningitidis*. Ampicillin should be added to the empirical regimen for coverage of *L. monocytogenes* in individuals under three months of age, those over age 55, or those with suspected impaired cell-mediated immunity because of chronic illness, organ transplantation, pregnancy, malignancies, or immunosuppressive therapy. In hospital-acquired meningitis, and particularly meningitis following neurosurgical procedures, staphylococci and gram-negative organisms including *Pseudomonas aeruginosa* are the most common etiologic organisms. In these patients, empirical therapy should include a combination of vancomycin and ceftazidime. Ceftazidime should be substituted for ceftriaxone or cefotaxime in neurosurgical patients and in neutropenic patients, as *P. aeruginosa* may be the meningeal pathogen, and ceftazidime is the only cephalosporin with adequate activity against *P. aeruginosa* in the CNS.

Table 372-2 Antibiotics Used in Empirical Therapy of Bacterial Meningitis and Focal CNS Infections

Indication	Antibiotic
Preterm infants to infants <1 month	Ampicillin + cefotaxime
Infants 1–3 months	Ampicillin + (cefotaxime or ceftriaxone) (consider adjunctive dexamethasone)
Immunocompetent children >3 months, adults <50	(Cefotaxime or ceftriaxone) + vancomycin
Adults >50, individuals with alcoholism or other debilitating illnesses	Ampicillin + vancomycin + (cefotaxime or ceftriaxone)
Hospital-acquired meningitis, meningitis after head trauma or neurosurgery, neutropenic patients	Ceftazidime + vancomycin
Impaired cell-mediated immunity (at any age)	Ceftazidime (in place of cefotaxime or ceftriaxone) + ampicillin

	Total Daily Dose and Dosing Interval	
Antimicrobial Agent	Child (> 1 month)	Adult
Ampicillin	200–300 (mg/kg)/d, q4h	12 g/d, q4h
Cefotaxime	300 (mg/kg)/d, q6h	12 g/d, q4h
Ceftriaxone	100–200 (mg/kg)/d, q12h	4 g/d, q12h
Ceftazidime	150 (mg/kg)/d, q8h	6 g/d, q8h
Metronidazole	30 (mg/kg)/d, q6h	2000 mg/d, q6h
Nafcillin	100–200 (mg/kg)/d, q6h	9–12 g/day, q4h
Vancomycin	60 (mg/kg)/d, q6h	2 g/d, q6h

Specific antimicrobial therapy (Table 372-3) • ***Meningococcal meningitis*** Although ceftriaxone and cefotaxime provide adequate empirical coverage for *N. meningitidis*, penicillin G remains the antibiotic of choice for meningococcal meningitis caused by susceptible strains. Isolates of *N. meningitidis* with moderate resistance to penicillin have been identified, but patients infected with these strains have still been successfully treated with penicillin. CSF isolates of *N. meningitidis* should be tested for penicillin and ampicillin susceptibility, and if resistance is found, cefotaxime or ceftriaxone should be substituted for penicillin. A 7-day course of intravenous antibiotic therapy is adequate for uncomplicated meningococcal meningitis. The index case and all close contacts should receive chemoprophylaxis with a 2-day regimen of rifampin (600 mg every 12 h for 2 days in adults and 10 mg/kg every 12 h for 2 days in children >1 year). Rifampin is not recommended in pregnant women. Alternatively, adults can be treated with one dose of ciprofloxacin (750 mg), one dose of azithromycin (500 mg), or one IM dose of ceftriaxone (250 mg). Close contacts are defined as those individuals who have had contact with oropharyngeal secretions either through kissing or by sharing toys, beverages, or cigarettes.

Pneumococcal meningitis Antimicrobial therapy of pneumococcal meningitis is initiated with a third-generation cephalosporin (ceftriaxone or cefotaxime) and vancomycin (Tables 372-2 and 372-3). All CSF isolates of *S. pneumoniae* should be tested for sensitivity to penicillin and the third-generation cephalosporins. Once the results

Table 372-3 Antimicrobial Therapy of CNS Bacterial Infections Based on Pathogen[a]

Organism	Antibiotic	Total Daily Adult Dose and Dosing Interval
Neisseria meningitidis		
Penicillin-sensitive	Penicillin G	20–24 million U/d, q4h
	or	
	Ampicillin	12 g/d, q4h
Penicillin-resistant	Ceftriaxone	4 g/d, q12h
	or	
	Cefotaxime	12 g/d, q4h
Streptococcus pneumoniae		
Penicillin-sensitive	Penicillin G	20–24 million U/d, q4h
Relatively penicillin-resistant	Ceftriaxone	4 g/d, q12h
	or	
	Cefotaxime	12 g/d, q4h
Penicillin-resistant	Vancomycin	2 g/d, q6h
	plus	
	Ceftriaxone	4 g/d, q12h
	or	
	Cefotaxime	12 g/d, q4h
	±	
	Intraventricular vancomycin	20 mg/d
Gram-negative bacilli (except *P. aeruginosa*)	Ceftriaxone	4 g/d, q12h
	or	
	Cefotaxime	12 g/d, q4h
Pseudomonas aeruginosa	Ceftazidime	6 g/d, q8h
Staphylococci		
Methicillin-sensitive	Nafcillin	9–12 g/d, q4h
Methicillin-resistant	Vancomycin	2 g/d, q6h
Listeria monocytogenes	Ampicillin	12 g/d, q4h
Haemophilus influenzae	Ceftriaxone	4 g/d, q12h
	or	
	Cefotaxime	12 g/d, q4h
Streptococcus agalactiae	Ampicillin	12 g/d, q4h
	or	
	Penicillin G	20–24 million U/d, q4h
Bacteroides fragilis	Metronidazole	2000 mg/d, q6h
Fusobacterium spp.	Metronidazole	2000 mg/d, q6h

[a] All antibiotics are administered intravenously; doses indicated are for patients with normal renal function.

of antimicrobial susceptibility tests are known, therapy can be modified accordingly. For *S. pneumoniae* meningitis, an isolate of *S. pneumoniae* is considered to be susceptible to penicillin with a minimal inhibitory concentration (MIC) < 0.06 μg/mL, to have intermediate resistance when the MIC is 0.1 to 1.0 μg/mL, and to be highly resistant when the MIC > 1.0 μg/mL. Isolates of *S. pneumoniae* that have cephalosporin MICs ≤ 0.5 μg/mL are considered sensitive to the cephalosporins (cefotaxime, ceftriaxone, cefepime). Those with MICs of 1 μg/mL are considered to have intermediate resistance, and those with MICs ≥ 2 μg/mL are considered resistant. Penicillin-resistant strains of *S. pneumoniae* are more common than cephalosporin-resistant strains of *S. pneumoniae*. For meningitis due to pneumococci with cefotaxime or ceftriaxone MICs ≤ 0.5 μg/mL, treatment with cefotaxime or ceftriaxone is usually adequate. If the MIC is ≥ 1 μg/mL, vancomycin is the antibiotic of choice. Rifampin can be added to vancomycin for its synergistic effect but is inadequate as monotherapy because resistance develops rapidly when it is used alone.

Patients with *S. pneumoniae* meningitis should have a repeat lumbar puncture performed 24 to 36 h after the initiation of antimicrobial therapy to document sterilization of the CSF. Failure to sterilize the CSF after 24 to 36 h of antibiotic therapy should be considered presumptive evidence of antibiotic resistance. Patients with penicillin- and cephalosporin-resistant strains of *S. pneumoniae* who do not respond to intravenous vancomycin alone may benefit from the addition of intraventricular vancomycin. The intraventricular route of administration is preferred over the intrathecal route because adequate concentrations of vancomycin in the cerebral ventricles are not always achieved with intrathecal administration. A 2-week course of intravenous antimicrobial therapy is recommended for pneumococcal meningitis.

***L. monocytogenes* meningitis** Meningitis due to this organism is treated with ampicillin for at least 3 weeks (Table 372-3). Gentamicin is often added (2 mg/kg loading dose then 5.1 mg/kg per day given every 8 h and adjusted for serum levels and renal function). The combination of trimethoprim [10 to 20 (mg/kg)/d] and sulfamethoxazole [50 to 100 (mg/kg)/d] given every 6 h may provide an alternative in penicillin-allergic patients.

Staphylococcal meningitis Meningitis due to susceptible strains of *S. aureus* or coagulase-negative staphylococci is treated with nafcillin (Table 372-3). Vancomycin is the drug of choice for methicillin-resistant staphylococci and for patients allergic to penicillin. In these patients, the CSF should be monitored during therapy. If the CSF is not sterilized after 48 h of intravenous vancomycin therapy, then either intrathecal or intraventricular vancomycin, 20 mg once daily, can be added.

Gram-negative bacillary meningitis The third-generation cephalosporins, cefotaxime, ceftriaxone, and ceftazidime, are equally efficacious for the treatment of gram-negative bacillary meningitis, with the exception of meningitis due to *P. aeruginosa*, which should be treated with ceftazidime (Table 372-3). A 3-week course of intravenous antibiotic therapy is recommended for meningitis due to gram-negative bacilli.

Newer antibiotics Cefepime is a broad-spectrum fourth-generation cephalosporin with in vitro activity similar to that of cefotaxime or ceftriaxone against *S. pneumoniae* and *N. meningitidis* and greater activity against *Enterobacter* spp. and *P. aeruginosa*. The dose of cefepime is 2 g intravenously every 12 h in adults. In clinical trials, cefepime has been demonstrated to be equivalent to cefotaxime in the treatment of pneumococcal and meningococcal meningitis, but its efficacy in bacterial meningitis caused by penicillin- and cephalosporin-resistant pneumococcal organisms, *Enterobacter* spp., and *P. aeruginosa* has not been established. Meropenem is a carbapenem antibiotic structurally related to imipenem, but reportedly with less seizure proclivity than imipenem. Meropenem is highly active in vitro against *L. monocytogenes*, has been demonstrated to be effective in cases of meningitis caused by *P. aeruginosa*, and shows good activity against penicillin-resistant pneumococci. In experimental pneumococcal meningitis, meropenem was comparable to ceftriaxone and inferior to vancomycin in sterilizing CSF cultures. The dose of meropenem is 1 to 2 g intravenously every 8 h for adults. The number of patients with bacterial meningitis enrolled in clinical trials of meropenem has not been sufficient to definitively assess the epileptogenic potential of this antibiotic. Firm recommendations regarding the use of cefepime and meropenem in bacterial meningitis await more clinical experience.

Adjunctive therapy The release of bacterial cell-wall components by bactericidal antibiotics leads to the production of the inflammatory cytokines IL-1 and TNF in the subarachnoid space (Fig. 372-1). Dexamethasone exerts its beneficial effect by inhibiting the synthesis of IL-1 and TNF at the level of mRNA, decreasing CSF outflow resistance, and stabilizing the blood-brain barrier. The rationale for giving dexamethasone 20 min before antibiotic therapy is that dexamethasone inhibits the production of TNF by macrophages and microglia only if it is administered before these cells are activated by endotoxin. Dexamethasone does not alter TNF production once it has been induced. The results of clinical trials of dexamethasone therapy in children, predominantly with meningitis due to *H. influenzae* and *S. pneumoniae*, have demonstrated its efficacy in decreasing meningeal inflammation and neurologic sequelae such as the incidence of sensorineural hearing loss. Evidence for efficacy of dexamethasone in other types of bacterial meningitis remains much more limited. The American Academy of Pediatrics recommends the consideration of dexamethasone for bacterial meningitis in infants and children ≥ 2 months. The recommended dose is 0.6 mg/kg per day in four divided doses given intravenously for the first 2 days of antibiotic therapy or

0.8 mg/kg per day in two divided doses given for 2 days. The first dose of dexamethasone should be administered before or at least with the first dose of antibiotic.

The role of dexamethasone in the treatment of bacterial meningitis in adults remains uncertain. In a single clinical trial, dexamethasone was demonstrated to reduce the incidence of mortality in adults from pneumococcal meningitis. Other clinical trials of dexamethasone therapy in adults with bacterial meningitis are in progress. The suggested dose of dexamethasone is 0.6 mg/kg per day in four divided doses for the first 2 to 4 days of antimicrobial therapy. For the reasons cited earlier, dexamethasone should ideally be given 20 min before, or not later than simultaneous with, the first dose of antibiotics. It is unlikely to be of significant benefit if started ≥6h after antimicrobial therapy has been initiated. Dexamethasone may decrease the penetration of vancomycin into CSF, and it delays the sterilization of CSF in experimental models of *S. pneumoniae* meningitis. As a result, its potential benefit should be carefully weighed when vancomycin is the antibiotic of choice. The third-generation cephalosporins and rifampin penetrate the CSF extremely well, even in the presence of dexamethasone, and may provide an alternative when adjunctive dexamethasone is being used to treat *S. pneumoniae* meningitis.

Increased Intracranial Pressure Emergency treatment of increased ICP includes elevation of the patient's head to 30 to 45°, intubation and hyperventilation (Pa_{CO_2} 25 to 30 mmHg), and mannitol. Patients with increased ICP should be managed in an intensive care unit. In these patients, accurate ICP measurements are best obtained with an ICP monitoring device. →***Increased intracranial pressure is discussed in detail in Chap. 376.***

PROGNOSIS Mortality is 3 to 7% for meningitis caused by *H. influenzae*, *N. meningitidis*, or group B streptococci; 15% for that due to *L. monocytogenes*; and 20% for *S. pneumoniae*. In general, the risk of death from bacterial meningitis is significantly associated with (1) decreased level of consciousness on admission, (2) onset of seizures within 24 h of admission, (3) signs of increased ICP, (4) young age (infancy) and age >50, (5) the presence of comorbid conditions including shock and/or the need for mechanical ventilation, and (6) delay in the initiation of treatment. Decreased CSF glucose concentration [<2.2 mmol/L (<40 mg/dL)] and markedly increased CSF protein concentration [>3 g/L (>300 mg/dL)] have been predictive of increased mortality and poorer outcomes in some series. Moderate or severe sequelae occur in ~25% of survivors of bacterial meningitis, although the exact incidence varies with the infecting organism. Common sequelae include decreased intellectual function, memory impairment, seizures, hearing loss and dizziness, and gait disturbances.

BRAIN ABSCESS

DEFINITION A brain abscess is a focal, suppurative process within the brain parenchyma; it begins in an area of devitalized brain tissue as a localized area of cerebritis and develops into a collection of pus surrounded by a well-vascularized capsule.

EPIDEMIOLOGY A bacterial brain abscess is a relatively uncommon intracranial infection, with an incidence of approximately 1 in 100,000 persons per year. Predisposing conditions include paranasal sinusitis, otitis media, and dental infections. Brain abscess is an extremely uncommon complication of these common infections, reflecting the efficiency with which they are treated with oral antimicrobial therapy, thereby minimizing the risk of subsequent intracranial spread of infection. In most modern series, a significant percentage of brain abscesses are not caused by classic pyogenic bacteria, but rather by *Toxoplasmi gondii*, *Aspergillus* spp., *Nocardia* spp., *Mycobacteria* spp., and fungi such as *Cryptococcus neoformans*. This distribution reflects the importance of brain abscesses in hosts whose immune systems are compromised, whether from HIV infection, organ transplantation, cancer, or immunosuppressive therapy. In Latin America and in immigrants from Latin America, the most common cause of brain abscess is *Taenia solium* (neurocysticercosis). The discussion that fol-

lows is limited to bacterial brain abscess; the other etiologies are discussed elsewhere.

ETIOLOGY A brain abscess may develop (1) by direct spread from a contiguous cranial site of infection, such as paranasal sinusitis, otitis media, mastoiditis, or dental infection; (2) following head trauma or a neurosurgical procedure; or (3) as a result of hematogenous spread from a remote site of infection. In 20 to 30% of cases no obvious primary source of infection is apparent (cryptogenic brain abscess).

Abscesses that develop as a result of direct spread of infection from the frontal, ethmoidal, or sphenoidal sinuses and those that occur due to dental infections are usually located in the frontal lobes. The most common pathogens in brain abscesses associated with paranasal sinusitis are microaerophilic and anaerobic streptococci, *Haemophilus* spp., *Bacteroides* spp. (non-*fragilis*), and *Fusobacterium* spp. The most common pathogens in brain abscess from dental infections are streptococci and *Prevotella* and *Porphyromonas* (formerly *Bacteroides*) spp.

The majority of brain abscesses associated with otitis media and mastoiditis occur in the temporal lobe and cerebellum and are caused by streptococci, *Bacteroides* spp. (including *B. fragilis*), *P. aeruginosa*, and Enterobacteriaceae. A brain abscess that is the result of hematogenous spread of infection from a site elsewhere in the body can occur anywhere in the brain but tends to form primarily in areas supplied by the middle cerebral artery (i.e., posterior frontal or parietal lobes). Metastatic abscesses are usually located at the interface of the gray-white matter and are often multiple. The microbiology of these brain abscesses is dependent on the primary source of infection. For example, brain abscesses that develop as a complication of infective endocarditis are often due to viridans streptococci or *S. aureus*; those that follow pyogenic lung infection are often due to *Streptococcus*, *Actinomyces*, or *Fusobacterium* species; those resulting from urinary sepsis are often caused by Enterobacteriaceae or *Pseudomonas aeruginosa*; and those associated with an intraabdominal source are frequently caused by *Streptococcus* spp., Enterobacteriaceae, or anaerobes. Abscesses that follow penetrating head trauma are frequently due to *S. aureus*, *Clostridium* spp., or Enterobacteriaceae, and those following a neurosurgical procedure are usually due to staphylococci, Enterobacteriaceae, or *P. aeruginosa*. Congenital cardiac malformations that produce a right-to-left shunt, such as tetralogy of Fallot, and atrial and ventricular septal defects allow bloodborne bacteria to bypass the pulmonary capillary bed and reach the brain. The decreased arterial oxygenation and saturation from the right-to-left shunt and polycythemia may cause focal areas of cerebral ischemia, thus providing a nidus for microorganisms that bypassed the pulmonary circulation to multiply and form an abscess. Streptococci are the most common pathogens in this setting.

PATHOGENESIS AND HISTOPATHOLOGY Results of experimental models of brain abscess formation suggest that for bacterial invasion of brain parenchyma to occur, there must be preexisting or concomitant areas of ischemia, necrosis, or hypoxia in brain tissue. The intact brain parenchyma is relatively resistant to infection. Once bacteria have established infection, brain abscess formation evolves through four stages, regardless of the infecting organism. The early cerebritis stage (days 1 to 3) is characterized by a perivascular infiltration of inflammatory cells, which surround a central core of coagulative necrosis. Marked edema surrounds the lesion at this stage. In the late cerebritis stage (days 4 to 9), pus formation leads to enlargement of the necrotic center, which is surrounded at its border by an inflammatory infiltrate of macrophages and fibroblasts. A thin capsule of fibroblasts and reticular fibers gradually develops, and the surrounding area of cerebral edema becomes more distinct than in the previous stage. The third stage, early capsule formation (days 10 to 13), is characterized by the formation of a capsule that is better developed on the cortical than on the ventricular side of the lesion. This stage correlates with the appearance of a ring-enhancing capsule on neuroimaging studies. The final stage, late capsule formation (day 14 and be-

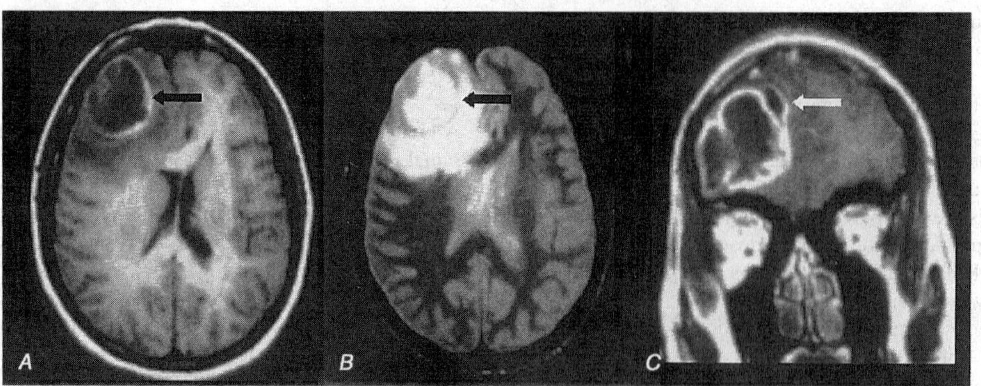

FIGURE 372-2 Pneumococcal brain abscess. Note that the abscess wall has hyperintense signal on the axial T1-weighted image (*A*, black arrow), hypointense signal on the axial proton density images (*B*, black arrow), and enhances prominently after gadolinium administration on the coronal T1-weighted image (*C*). The abscess is surrounded by a large amount of vasogenic edema and has a small "daughter" abscess (*C*, white arrow). *(Courtesy of Joseph Lurito, MD.)*

yond), is defined by a well-formed necrotic center surrounded by a dense collagenous capsule. The surrounding area of cerebral edema has regressed, but marked gliosis with large numbers of reactive astrocytes has developed outside the capsule. This gliotic process may contribute to the development of seizures as a sequelae of brain abscess.

CLINICAL PRESENTATION A brain abscess presents as an expanding intracranial mass lesion, rather than as an infectious process. The most common symptom is headache, occurring in >75% of patients. The headache is often characterized as a constant, dull, aching sensation, either hemicranial or generalized, and it becomes progressively more severe and refractory to therapy. Fever is present in only 50% of patients at the time of diagnosis and is typically low-grade. Thus the absence of fever should not exclude the diagnosis. The new onset of focal or generalized seizure activity is a presenting sign in 25 to 30% of patients. In most large series, a focal neurologic deficit is part of the initial presentation in >60% of patients.

The clinical presentation of a brain abscess depends on its location and on the presence of raised ICP, which develops as edema surrounds the evolving abscess. Hemiparesis is the most common localizing sign of a frontal lobe abscess. A temporal lobe abscess may present with a disturbance of language (dysphasia) or an upper homonymous quadrantanopia. Nystagmus and ataxia are signs of a cerebellar abscess. The earliest signs of increased ICP in a patient with a brain abscess are papilledema, nausea and vomiting, and drowsiness or confusion. Meningismus is not present unless the abscess has ruptured into the ventricle or the infection has spread to the subarachnoid space.

DIAGNOSIS The diagnosis of a brain abscess is made by neuroimaging studies. CT has the advantage of greater feasibility in acutely ill patients, but MRI is better for demonstrating abscesses in the early (cerebritis) stages and is superior to CT for identifying abscesses in the posterior fossa. Cerebritis appears on MRI as an area of low-signal intensity on T1-weighted images with irregular postgadolinium enhancement and as an area of increased signal intensity on T2-weighted images. Cerebritis is often not visualized by CT scan. As the abscess matures, the appearance of the lesion changes. On a contrast-enhanced CT scan, a mature brain abscess appears as a focal area of hypodensity surrounded by ring enhancement. On T1-weighted MRI, a mature brain abscess has the characteristics demonstrated in Fig. 372-2. On T2-weighted MRI, there is a hyperintense central area of pus surrounded by a well-defined hypointense capsule and a hyperintense area of edema.

The microbiologic diagnosis is made by Gram's stain and culture of abscess material obtained by stereotactic needle aspiration. Lumbar puncture should not be performed in patients with known or suspected focal intracranial infections such as abscess or empyema; CSF analysis contributes nothing to diagnosis or therapy, and lumbar puncture increases the risk of herniation.

Additional laboratory studies that may provide clues to the diagnosis of brain abscess in patients with a CNS mass lesion include the peripheral white blood cell count and erythrocyte sedimentation rate; the latter will be elevated in about 60% of patients, and about 50% will have a peripheral leukocytosis.

DIFFERENTIAL DIAGNOSIS Conditions that can cause headache, fever, focal neurologic signs, and seizure activity include brain abscess, subdural empyema, bacterial meningitis, viral meningoencephalitis, superior sagittal sinus thrombosis, and acute disseminated encephalomyelitis. In unusual cases, tumors and, more rarely, cerebral infarction or hematoma can have an MRI or CT appearance resembling brain abscess.

℞ **TREATMENT** Empirical therapy of a brain abscess depends on the source of infection (Table 372-4) and typically includes a third-generation cephalosporin (e.g., cefotaxime) and metronidazole (Table 372-3 for antibiotic dosages). Patients with multiple abscesses, which suggest the possibility of hematogenous spread, or those who develop abscesses following head trauma should have nafcillin added to this regimen for coverage of staphylococci. Patients who develop abscesses following neurosurgical procedures should be treated with vancomycin plus ceftazidime (in place of cefotaxime) for coverage of both staphylococci and *P. aeruginosa.*

Aspiration and drainage of the abscess under stereotactic guidance are beneficial for both diagnosis and therapy. Empirical antibiotic coverage can be modified based on the results of Gram's stain and culture of the abscess contents (Table 372-4). Complete excision of a bacterial abscess via craniotomy or craniectomy is generally reserved for multiloculated abscesses or those in which stereotactic aspiration is unsuccessful. Antibiotic therapy alone is generally not optimal for treatment of brain abscess and should be reserved for patients whose abscesses cannot be surgically aspirated or otherwise drained, for selected patients with multiple abscesses, and in patients whose condition is too tenuous to allow performance of a neurosurgical procedure. All patients should receive a minimum of 6 to 8 weeks of parenteral antibiotic therapy. The role, if any, of supplemental oral antibiotic therapy following completion of a standard course of parenteral therapy has never been adequately studied.

In addition to surgical drainage and antibiotic therapy, patients

Table 372-4 Empirical Therapy of Brain Abscess Based on Source of Infection

Source	Antimicrobial Therapy
Paranasal sinusitis	Penicillin or a third-generation cephalosporin (cefotaxime or ceftriaxone) + metronidazole
Otitis media	Penicillin + metronidazole + ceftazidime
Dental infection	Penicillin + metronidazole
Endocarditis	Nafcillin or vancomycin + metronidazole + third-generation cephalosporin
Lung abscess, urinary sepsis, intra-abdominal source	Ceftazidime + metronidazole + penicillin
Head trauma	Nafcillin or vancomycin + third-generation cephalosporin
Neurosurgical procedure	Vancomycin + ceftazidime
Cyanotic congenital heart disease	Penicillin or third-generation cephalosporin + metronidazole

should receive prophylactic anticonvulsant therapy because of the high risk of focal or generalized seizures. Anticonvulsant therapy is continued for at least 3 months after resolution of the abscess, and decisions regarding withdrawal are then based on the EEG. If the EEG is abnormal, anticonvulsant therapy should be continued. If the EEG is normal, anticonvulsant therapy can be slowly withdrawn, with close follow-up and repeat EEG after the medication has been discontinued.

Glucocorticoids should not be given routinely to patients with brain abscesses. Intravenous dexamethasone therapy (10 mg every 6 h) is usually reserved for patients with substantial periabscess edema and associated mass effect and increased ICP. Dexamethasone should be tapered as rapidly as possible to avoid delaying the natural process of encapsulation of the abscess.

Serial CT or MRI scans should be obtained on a monthly or twice-monthly basis to document resolution of the abscess. More frequent studies (e.g., weekly) are probably warranted in the subset of patients who are receiving antibiotic therapy alone. A small amount of enhancement may remain for months after the abscess has been successfully treated.

PROGNOSIS Bacterial abscess can be successfully treated in the majority of patients. Seizures, however, are a common complication and occur in as many as 70% of patients.

SUBDURAL EMPYEMA

DEFINITION A subdural empyema (SDE) is a collection of pus between the dura and arachnoid membranes (Fig. 372-3).

EPIDEMIOLOGY SDE is a rare intracranial infection. Sinusitis is the most common predisposing condition and typically involves the frontal sinuses, either alone or in combination with the ethmoid and maxillary sinuses. Sinusitis-associated empyema has a striking predilection for young males, possibly reflecting sex-related differences in sinus anatomy and development. SDE may also develop as a complication of head trauma or following neurosurgical drainage of a subdural hematoma. Secondary infection of a subdural effusion may also result in empyema, although secondary infection of hematomas, in the absence of a prior neurosurgical procedure, is rare.

ETIOLOGY Aerobic and microaerophilic streptococci and anaerobic bacteria are the most common causative organisms of sinusitis-associated SDE. Staphylococci and gram-negative bacilli are often the etiologic organisms when SDE follows neurosurgical procedures or head trauma. SDE should be distinguished from subdural effusions that, especially in infants and children, may complicate bacterial meningitis. Subdural effusions are sterile collections of protein-rich fluid that result from increased permeability of the thin-walled capillaries and veins in the inner layer of the dura.

PATHOPHYSIOLOGY Sinusitis-associated SDE develops as a result of either retrograde spread of infection from septic thrombophlebitis of the mucosal veins draining the sinuses or contiguous spread of infection to the brain from osteomyelitis in the posterior wall of the frontal or other sinuses. SDE may also develop from direct introduction of bacteria into the subdural space as a complication of a neurosurgical procedure. The evolution of SDE can be extremely rapid because the subdural space is a large compartment that offers few mechanical barriers to the spread of infection. In patients with sinusitis-associated SDE, suppuration typically begins in the upper and anterior portions of one cerebral hemisphere and then extends posteriorly. SDE is often associated with other intracranial infections including epidural empyema (40%), cortical thrombophlebitis (35%), and intracranial abscess or cerebritis (>25%). Cortical venous infarction produces necrosis of underlying cerebral cortex and subcortical white matter, with focal neurological deficits and seizures (see below).

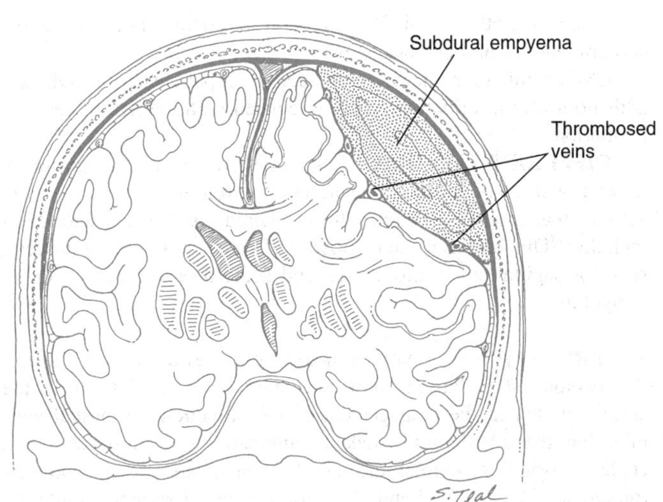

FIGURE 372-3 Subdural empyema is a collection of pus between the dura and arachnoid membranes.

CLINICAL PRESENTATION A patient with SDE typically presents with fever and a progressively worsening headache. Patients may also have signs and symptoms related to sinusitis or other primary sites of intracranial infection. As the infection progresses, focal neurologic deficits, seizures, and signs of increased ICP commonly occur. Headache is the most common complaint at the time of presentation; initially it is localized to the side of the subdural infection but then becomes more severe and generalized. Contralateral hemiparesis or hemiplegia is the most common focal neurologic deficit and can occur from the direct effects of the SDE on the cortex or as a consequence of venous infarction. Seizures begin as partial motor seizures that then become secondarily generalized. Seizures may be due to the direct irritative effect of the SDE on the underlying cortex or result from cortical venous infarction (see above). In untreated SDE, the increasing mass effect and increase in ICP cause progressive deterioration in consciousness, leading ultimately to coma.

DIAGNOSIS Neuroimaging has greatly facilitated the diagnosis of SDE. MRI (Fig. 372-4) is superior to CT in identifying SDE and any associated intracranial infections. The administration of gadolinium greatly improves diagnosis by enhancing the rim of the empyema and allowing the empyema to be clearly delineated from the underlying brain parenchyma. Cranial MRI is also extremely valuable in identi-

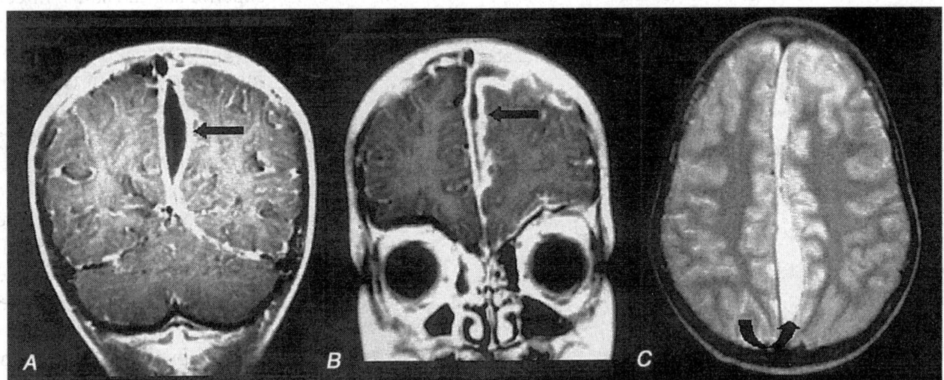

FIGURE 372-4 Subdural empyema. There is marked enhancement of the dura and leptomeninges (*A*, *B*, straight arrows) along the left medial hemisphere. The pus is hypointense on T1-weighted images (*A*, *B*), but markedly hyperintense on the proton density–weighted (*C*, curved arrow) image. *(Courtesy of Joseph Lurito, MD.)*

fying sinusitis, other focal CNS infections, cortical venous infarction, cerebral edema, and cerebritis.

CSF examination should be avoided in all patients with SDE as it adds no useful information and is associated with the risk of cerebral herniation.

DIFFERENTIAL DIAGNOSIS The differential diagnosis of the combination of headache, fever, focal neurologic signs, and seizure activity that progresses rapidly to an altered level of consciousness includes SDE, bacterial meningitis, viral encephalitis, brain abscess, superior sagittal sinus thrombosis, and acute disseminated encephalomyelitis.

℞ TREATMENT Emergent neurosurgical evacuation of the empyema, either through burr-hole drainage or craniotomy, is the definitive step in the management of this infection. Empirical antimicrobial therapy should include a combination of a third-generation cephalosporin (e.g., cefotaxime or ceftriaxone), vancomycin, and metronidazole (Tables 372-3 and 372-4 for dosages). Parenteral antibiotic therapy should be continued for a minimum of 4 weeks. Specific diagnosis of the etiologic organisms is made based on Gram's stain and culture of fluid obtained via either burr holes or craniotomy; the initial empirical antibiotic coverage should be modified accordingly.

PROGNOSIS Prognosis is influenced by the level of consciousness of the patient at the time of hospital presentation, the size of the empyema, and the speed with which therapy is instituted. Long-term neurologic sequelae, which include seizures and hemiparesis, occur in up to 50% of cases.

EPIDURAL ABSCESS

DEFINITION Cranial epidural abscess is a suppurative infection occurring in the potential space between the inner skull table and the dura (Fig. 372-5).

ETIOLOGY AND PATHOPHYSIOLOGY A cranial epidural abscess develops as a complication of a craniotomy or compound skull fracture or as a result of spread of infection from the frontal sinuses, middle ear, mastoid, or orbit. An epidural abscess may develop contiguous to an area of osteomyelitis, when craniotomy is complicated by infection of the wound or bone flap, or as a result of direct infection of the epidural space. Infection in the frontal sinus, middle ear, mastoid, or orbit can reach the epidural space through retrograde spread of infection from septic thrombophlebitis in the emissary veins that drain these areas or by way of direct spread of infection through areas of osteomyelitis. Unlike the subdural space, the epidural space is really a potential rather than an actual compartment. The dura is normally tightly adherent to the inner skull table, and infection must dissect the dura away from the skull table as it spreads. As a result, epidural abscesses are often smaller than SDEs. Cranial epidural abscesses, unlike brain abscesses, only rarely result from hematogenous spread of infection from extracranial primary sites. The bacteriology of a cranial epidural abscess is similar to that of SDE (see above). The etiologic organisms of an epidural abscess that arises from frontal sinusitis, middle ear infections, or mastoiditis are usually streptococci or anaerobic organisms. Staphylococci or gram-negative organisms are the usual cause of an epidural abscess that develops as a complication of craniotomy or compound skull fracture.

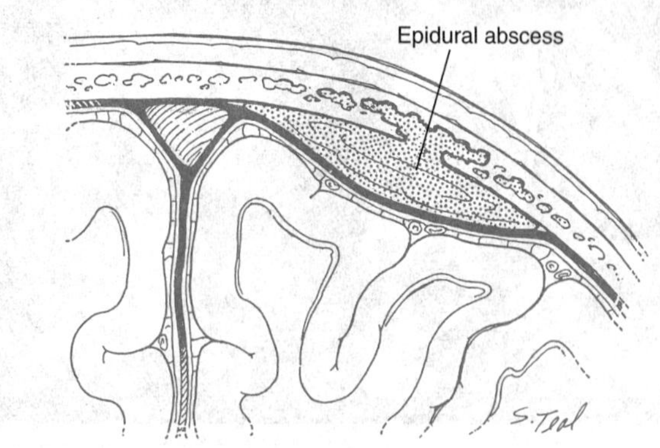

FIGURE 372-5 Cranial epidural abscess is a collection of pus between the dura and the inner table of the skull.

CLINICAL PRESENTATION Patients typically present with severe hemicranial headache and persistent fever. The diagnosis should always be suspected when these symptoms occur following recent head trauma or neurosurgery or in the setting of frontal sinusitis, mastoiditis, or otitis media.

DIAGNOSIS Cranial MRI is the procedure of choice to demonstrate a cranial epidural abscess. The sensitivity of CT is limited by the presence of signal artifacts arising from the bone of the inner skull table. On MRI, an epidural abscess appears as a lentiform or crescent-shaped fluid collection that is hyperintense compared to CSF on T2-weighted images. On T1-weighted images, the fluid collection has a signal intensity that is intermediate between that of brain tissue and CSF. Following the administration of gadolinium, a significant enhancement of the dura is seen on T1-weighted images.

℞ TREATMENT Immediate neurosurgical drainage is indicated. Empirical antimicrobial therapy, pending the results of Gram's stain and culture of the purulent material obtained at surgery, should include a combination of penicillin, a third-generation cephalosporin, nafcillin or vancomycin, and metronidazole (Tables 372-2 and 372-3). When the organism has been identified, antimicrobial therapy can be modified accordingly. Antibiotics should be continued for at least 3 weeks after surgical drainage.

SUPPURATIVE THROMBOPHLEBITIS

DEFINITION Suppurative intracranial thrombophlebitis is septic venous thrombosis of cortical veins and sinuses. This may occur as a complication of bacterial meningitis, SDE, epidural abscess, or infection in the skin of the face, paranasal sinuses, middle ear, or mastoid.

ANATOMY AND PATHOPHYSIOLOGY The cerebral veins and venous sinuses have no valves; therefore, blood within them can flow in either direction. The superior sagittal sinus is the largest of the venous sinuses (Fig. 372-6). It receives blood from the frontal, parietal, and occipital superior cerebral veins and the diploic veins, which communicate with the meningeal veins. Bacterial meningitis is a common predisposing condition for septic thrombosis of the superior sagittal sinus. The diploic veins, which drain into the superior sagittal sinus, provide a route for the spread of infection from the meninges, especially in cases where there is purulent exudate near areas of the superior sagittal sinus. Infection can also spread to the superior sagittal sinus from nearby SDE or epidural abscess. Dehydration from vomiting, hypercoagulable states, and immunologic abnormalities, including the presence of circulating antiphospholipid antibodies, also contribute to cerebral venous sinus thrombosis. Thrombosis may extend from one sinus to another, and often at autopsy thrombi of different histologic ages can be detected in several sinuses. Thrombosis of the superior sagittal sinus is often associated with thrombosis of superior cortical veins and small parenchymal hemorrhages.

The superior sagittal sinus drains into the transverse sinuses (Fig. 372-6). The transverse sinuses also receive venous drainage from small veins from both the middle ear and mastoid cells. The transverse sinus becomes the sigmoid sinus before draining into the internal jugular vein. Septic transverse/sigmoid sinus thrombosis can be a complication of acute and chronic otitis media or mastoiditis. Infection spreads from the mastoid air cells to the transverse sinus via the emissary veins or by direct invasion. The cavernous sinuses are inferior to the superior sagittal sinus at the base of the skull. The cavernous sinuses receive blood from the facial veins via the superior and inferior ophthalmic veins. Bacteria in the facial veins enter the cavernous sinus via these veins. Bacteria in the sphenoid and ethmoid sinuses can spread to the cavernous sinuses via the small emissary veins. The sphenoid and ethmoid sinuses are the most common sites of primary infection resulting in septic cavernous sinus thrombosis.

CLINICAL MANIFESTATIONS *Septic thrombosis of the superior sagittal sinus* presents as headache, nausea and vomiting, confusion, and focal or generalized seizures. There may be a rapid development of stupor and coma. Weakness of the lower extremities with bilateral Babinski signs or hemiparesis is often present. When superior sagittal sinus thrombosis occurs as a complication of bacterial meningitis, nuchal rigidity and Kernig's and Brudzinski's signs may be present.

The oculomotor nerve, the trochlear nerve, the abducens nerve, the ophthalmic and maxillary branches of the trigeminal nerve, and the internal carotid artery all pass through the cavernous sinus. The symptoms of *septic cavernous sinus thrombosis* are fever, headache, frontal and retroorbital pain, and diplopia. The classic signs are ptosis, proptosis, chemosis, and extraocular dysmotility due to deficits of cranial nerves III, IV, and VI. Hypo- or hyperesthesia of the ophthalmic and maxillary divisions of the fifth cranial nerve and a decreased corneal reflex may be detected. There may be evidence of dilated, tortuous retinal veins and papilledema.

Headache and earache are the most frequent symptoms of *transverse sinus thrombosis*. A transverse sinus thrombosis may also present with Gradinego's syndrome characterized by otitis media, sixth nerve palsy, and retroorbital or facial pain. Sigmoid sinus and internal jugular vein thrombosis may present with neck pain.

DIAGNOSIS The diagnosis of septic venous sinus thrombosis is suggested by an absent flow void within the affected venous sinus on MRI and confirmed by magnetic resonance venography or the venous phase of cerebral angiography. The diagnosis of thrombophlebitis of intracerebral and meningeal veins is suggested by the presence of intracerebral hemorrhage but requires cerebral angiography for definitive diagnosis.

℞ **TREATMENT** Septic venous sinus thrombosis is usually treated with antibiotics and hydration. The choice of antimicrobial therapy is based on the bacteria responsible for the predisposing or associated condition. Anticoagulation with dose-adjusted heparin has been reported to be beneficial in patients with aseptic venous sinus thrombosis; it is also used in the treatment of septic venous sinus thrombosis complicating bacterial meningitis in patients who are worsening despite antimicrobial therapy and intravenous fluids. The presence of a small intracerebral hemorrhage from septic thrombophlebitis is not an absolute contraindication to heparin therapy. Successful management of aseptic venous sinus thrombosis has been reported with urokinase therapy and with a combination of intrathrombus recombinant tissue plasminogen activator (rtPA) and intravenous heparin, but there is yet no reported experience with these therapies in septic venous sinus thrombosis.

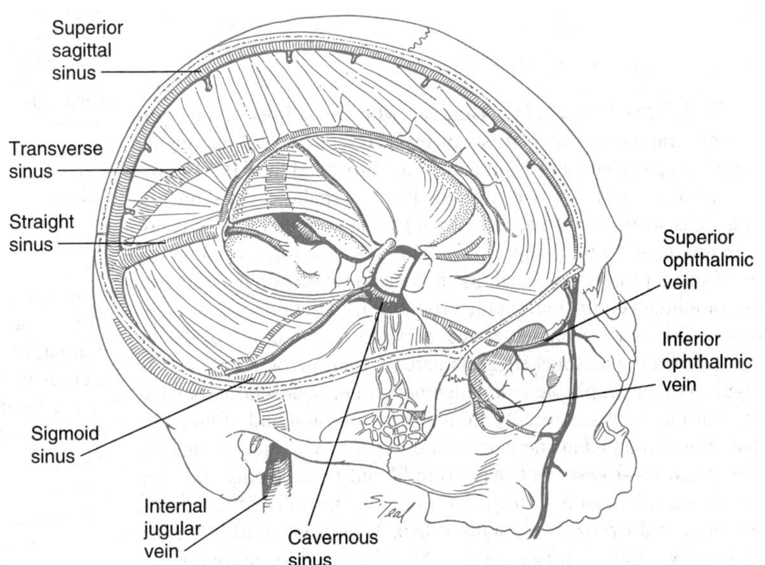

FIGURE 372-6 Anatomy of the cerebral venous sinuses.

BIBLIOGRAPHY

ACUTE BACTERIAL MENINGITIS

COYLE PK: Glucocorticoids in central nervous system bacterial infection. Arch Neurol 56:796, 1999

DURAND ML et al: Acute bacterial meningitis in adults: A review of 493 episodes. N Engl J Med 328:21, 1993

FANG CT et al: Klebsiella pneumoniae meningitis: Timing of antimicrobial therapy and prognosis. QJM 93:45, 2000

PELTOLA H: Prophylaxis of bacterial meningitis. Infect Dis Clin North Am 685, 13 1999

QUAGLIARELLO VJ, SCHELD WM: Treatment of bacterial meningitis. N Engl J Med 336: 708, 1997

ROOS KL: *Meningitis: 100 Maxims in Neurology*. London, Arnold, and New York, Oxford University Press, 1996, 1–208

——— et al: Acute bacterial meningitis in children and adults, in *Infections of the Central Nervous System*, 2d ed, WM Scheld, RJ Whitley, DT Durack (eds). Philadelphia, Lippincott-Raven, 1997, 335–401

SCHUCHAT A et al: Bacterial meningitis in the United States in 1995. N Engl J Med 337: 970, 1997

TAUBER MG, MOSSER B: Cytokines and chemokines in meningeal inflammation: Biology and clinical implications. Clin Infect Dis 28:1, 1999

BRAIN ABSCESS

MAMELAK AN et al: Improved management of multiple brain abscesses: A combined surgical and medical approach. Neurosurg 36:76, 1995

MATHISEN GE, JOHNSON JP: Brain abscess. Clin Infect Dis 25:763, 1997

SUBDURAL EMPYEMA

DILL SR et al: Subdural empyema: Analysis of 32 cases and review. Clin Infect Dis 20: 372, 1995

NATHOO N et al: Intracranial subdural empyema in the era of computed tomography: A review of 699 cases. Neurosurgery 44:529, 1999

CRANIAL EPIDURAL ABSCESS

GELLIN BG et al: Epidural abscess, in *Infections of the Central Nervous System*, 2d ed, WM Scheld, RJ Whitley, DT Durack (eds). Lippincott-Raven, Philadelphia, 1997, 507–522

SILVERBERG AL, DINUBILE MJ: Subdural empyema and cranial epidural abscess. Med Clin North Am 69:361, 1985

SUPPURATIVE THROMBOPHLEBITIS

SOUTHWICK FS et al: Septic thrombosis of the dural venous sinuses. Medicine 65:82, 1986

373

Kenneth L. Tyler

VIRAL MENINGITIS AND ENCEPHALITIS

Hundreds of viruses have been reported to produce acute infection and injury to the central or peripheral nervous systems. Many aspects of the clinical characteristics of these diseases are determined by whether the infection is limited primarily to the meninges (*meningitis*) or extends to involve the parenchyma of the brain (*encephalitis*), spinal cord (*myelitis*), or nerve roots (*radiculitis*). In some cases more than one of these areas can be involved simultaneously (meningoencephalitis, myeloradiculitis, etc.). Viruses can also produce chronic or persistent infections of the central nervous system (CNS). →***Infections caused by HIV are discussed in Chap. 309, human T cell leukemia virus (HTLV) types I and II in Chap. 368, and prions in Chap. 375.***

ACUTE VIRAL INFECTIONS

VIRAL MENINGITIS Clinical Manifestations The syndrome of viral meningitis consists of fever, headache, and meningeal irritation coupled with an inflammatory cerebrospinal fluid (CSF) profile (see below). Fever may be accompanied by malaise, myalgia, anorexia, nausea and vomiting, abdominal pain, and/or diarrhea. It is not uncommon to see a mild degree of lethargy or drowsiness. The presence of more profound alterations in consciousness, such as stupor, coma, or marked confusion, should prompt consideration of alternative diagnoses. Similarly, seizures, cranial nerve palsies, or other focal neurologic signs or symptoms suggests parenchymal involvement and is not typical of uncomplicated viral meningitis. The headache associated with viral meningitis is usually frontal or retroorbital and often associated with photophobia and pain on moving the eyes. Nuchal rigidity is present in most cases but may be mild and present only near the limit of neck anteflexion. Evidence of severe meningeal irritation, such as Kernig's and Brudzinski's signs (Chap. 372), is generally absent.

Etiology Enteroviruses account for 75 to 90% of aseptic meningitis cases in most series (Table 373-1). Viruses belonging to the *Enterovirus* genus are members of the family Picornaviridae and include the coxsackieviruses, echoviruses, polioviruses, and human enteroviruses 68 to 71. Using a variety of diagnostic techniques including CSF polymerase chain reaction (PCR) tests, culture, and serology, a specific viral cause can be found in 75 to 90% of cases of viral meningitis. CSF cultures are positive in 30 to 70% of patients, the frequency of isolation depending on the specific viral agent. Approximately two-thirds of culture-negative cases of aseptic meningitis have a specific viral etiology identified by CSF PCR testing (see below).

Epidemiology The exact incidence of viral meningitis in the United States is impossible to determine since most cases go unreported to public health authorities. In temperate climates, there is a substantial increase in cases during the summer and early fall months, reflecting the seasonal predominance of enterovirus and arthropod-borne encephalitis virus ("arbovirus") infections, with a peak monthly incidence of about 1 reported case per 100,000 population. The dramatic seasonal predilections of some viruses causing meningitis provide a valuable but not always infallible clue to diagnosis (Table 373-2).

Laboratory Diagnosis • *CSF examination* The most important laboratory test in the diagnosis of meningitis is examination of the CSF. The typical profile in cases of viral meningitis is a lymphocytic pleocytosis (25 to 500 cells per microliter), a normal or slightly elevated protein level [0.2 to 0.8 g/L (20 to 80 mg/dL)], a normal glucose level, and a normal or mildly elevated opening pressure (100 to 350 mm H_2O). Organisms *are not* seen on Gram's or acid-fast stained smears or india ink wet mounts of CSF. Rarely, polymorphonuclear neutrophils (PMNs) may predominate in the first 48 h of illness, especially in patients with infections due to echovirus 9 or Eastern equine virus. However, the presence of a persisting PMN pleocytosis should always prompt consideration of bacterial meningitis or parameningeal infections. The total CSF cell count in viral meningitis is typically 25 to 500/μL, although cell counts of several thousand per microliter are occasionally seen, especially with infections due to lymphocytic choriomeningitis virus (LCMV) and mumps virus. The CSF glucose level is typically normal in viral infections, although it may be decreased in 10 to 30% of cases due to mumps as well as in cases due to LCMV. Rare instances of decreased CSF glucose concentration occur in cases of meningitis due to echoviruses and other enteroviruses, herpes simplex virus (HSV) type 2, and varicella-zoster virus (VZV). As a rule, a lymphocytic pleocytosis with a low glucose level should suggest fungal, listerial, or tuberculous meningitis or noninfectious disorders (e.g., sarcoid, neoplastic meningitis).

A number of tests measuring levels of various CSF proteins, enzymes, and mediators, including C-reactive protein, lactic acid, lactate dehydrogenase, neopterin, quinolinate, interleukin (IL) 1β, IL-6, soluble IL-2 receptor, β_2-microglobulin, and tumor necrosis factor (TNF), have been proposed as potential discriminators between viral and bacterial meningitis or as markers of specific types of viral infection (e.g., infection with HIV), but are of limited general use.

Polymerase chain reaction amplification of viral nucleic acid Amplification of viral-specific DNA or RNA from CSF using PCR amplification has become the single most important method for diagnosing CNS viral infections. HSV DNA is frequently amplified from the CSF of patients with herpes simplex encephalitis (HSV-1) and recurrent lymphocytic meningitis (HSV-2), even when standard culture techniques are negative. PCR is also used routinely to diagnose CNS viral infections caused by enteroviruses, cytomegalovirus (CMV), Epstein-Barr virus (EBV), and VZV. Genomic amplification and detection of enteroviral (coxsackie-, polio-, echo-, enterovirus) RNA in the CSF of patients with meningitis is now the diagnostic procedure of choice for this group of viruses.

CSF culture The overall results of CSF culture for the diagnosis of viral infection are disappointing (Table 373-3), presumably because of the generally low concentration of infectious virus present and the need to customize isolation procedures for individual viruses. For viral isolation, 2 mL of CSF should be brought promptly to the microbiology laboratory, where it should be refrigerated and processed as speedily as possible. CSF specimens for viral isolation should never be stored in a −20°C freezer since viruses are often unstable at this temperature, and most freezers have "frostfree" warm-up cycles that are detrimental to viral stability. Storage for >24 h is probably best done in a −70°C freezer.

Other sources for viral isolation Viruses may also be isolated from sites and body fluids other than CSF, including throat swabs, stool, blood, and urine. Enteroviruses and adenoviruses may be found in feces; arboviruses, some enteroviruses, and LCMV, in blood; mumps and CMV, in urine; and enteroviruses, mumps, and adenoviruses, in throat washings. During enteroviral infections, viral shedding in stool may persist for several weeks. The presence of enterovirus in stool is not diagnostic and may result from residual shedding from a

Table 373-1 Viruses Causing Acute Meningitis

Common	Less Common	Rare
Enteroviruses	HSV-1	Adenoviruses
Arboviruses	LCMV	CMV
HIV	Mumps virus	EBV
HSV-2		Influenza A, B; measles; parainfluenza; rubella; VZV

NOTE: CMV, cytomegalovirus; EBV, Epstein-Barr virus; HIV, human immunodeficiency virus; HSV, herpes simplex virus; LCMV, lymphocytic choriomeningitis virus; VZV, varicella-zoster virus.

Table 373-2 Seasonal Prevalence of Viruses Commonly Causing Meningitis

Summer and Early Fall	Fall and Winter	Winter and Spring	Nonseasonal
Arboviruses	LCMV	Mumps	HIV
Enteroviruses			HSV

NOTE: As in Table 373-1.

Table 373-3 Possibility of Culturing Specific Viruses from Cerebrospinal Fluid

Excellent	Fair	Poor or None
Coxsackievirus, echovirus, LCMV, mumps virus	HIV, adenovirus, arboviruses (most), HSV-2, VZV, rabies virus	Poliovirus, HSV-1, EBV, CMV

NOTE: As in Table 373-1.

previous enteroviral infection; it also occurs in some asymptomatic individuals during enteroviral epidemics.

Serologic studies For some viruses, such as the arboviruses, serologic studies remain an important diagnostic tool but are less useful for viruses such as HSV, VZV, CMV, and EBV for which the prevalence of antibody seropositivity in the general population is high. Diagnosis of viral infection can be made by documenting seroconversion between acute-phase and convalescent sera (typically obtained after 2 to 4 weeks), or by demonstrating the presence of virus-specific IgM antibodies. Antiviral antibodies may be measured in CSF (see below). The timing of the antibody response often means that serologic data are useful mainly for the retrospective establishment of a specific diagnosis, and their value in initial diagnosis and management is limited. Most viral infections of the CNS are associated with intrathecal synthesis of antiviral antibody. This results in an elevation in the ratio of antibody in CSF compared to serum (CSF/serum antibody index).

Agarose electrophoresis or isoelectric focusing of CSF γ-globulins may reveal the presence of oligoclonal bands. These bands have been found in association with a number of viral infections, including infections with HIV, HTLV type I, VZV, mumps, subacute sclerosing panencephalitis (SSPE), and progressive rubella panencephalitis. The associated antibodies are often directed against viral proteins. The finding of oligoclonal bands may be of some diagnostic utility, since typically they are not seen with arbovirus, enterovirus, or HSV infections. Oligoclonal bands are also encountered in certain noninfectious neurologic diseases (e.g., multiple sclerosis) and may be found in nonviral infections (e.g., syphilis, Lyme borreliosis).

Other laboratory studies All patients with suspected viral meningitis should have a complete blood count and differential; liver function tests; and measurement of the erythrocyte sedimentation rate (ESR), blood urea nitrogen (BUN), and plasma levels of electrolytes, glucose, creatinine, creatine kinase, aldolase, amylase, and lipase. Abnormalities in specific test results may suggest particular etiologic diagnoses. Magnetic resonance imaging (MRI), computed tomography (CT), electroencephalography (EEG), evoked response studies, electromyography (EMG), and nerve conduction studies are not necessary in most cases. They are best used selectively when atypical presentations or unusual features present diagnostic problems.

Differential Diagnosis The most important issue in the differential diagnosis is the exclusion of nonviral causes that can mimic viral meningitis. The major categories of disease that should always be considered and excluded are (1) bacterial meningitis and other infectious meningidities (e.g., *Mycoplasma*, *Listeria*, *Brucella*, *Coxiella*, and *Rickettsia*); (2) parameningeal infections or partially treated bacterial meningitis; (3) nonviral infectious meningitides where cultures may be negative (e.g., fungal, tuberculous, parasitic, or syphilitic disease); (4) neoplastic meningitis; and (5) meningitis secondary to noninfectious inflammatory diseases such as sarcoid, Behçet's disease, and the uveomeningitic syndromes.

Specific viral etiologies *Enteroviruses* (Chap. 193) are the most common cause of viral meningitis (>75% of cases with etiology identified) and should be considered the leading candidates when a typical case occurs in the summer months, especially in a child (<15 years) (Table 373-4). However, despite their summer prevalence, sporadic cases of enteroviral CNS infection are seen year-round. The physical examination should include a careful search for exanthemata, hand-foot-mouth disease, herpangina, pleurodynia, myopericarditis, and hemorrhagic conjunctivitis, which may be stigmata of enterovirus infections. PCR amplification of enteroviral RNA from CSF has become the diagnostic procedure of choice for these infections.

Table 373-4 Serotypes of Enteroviruses Causing CNS Infections

Frequency as Cause of CNS Infections	Poliovirus	Coxsackievirus	Echovirus	Enterovirus
Frequent	—	B5	7, 9, 11, 30	70, 71
Common	—	A9, B3, B4	4, 6, 18	—
Rare	1–3	B1, B6	2, 3, 12, 22	—

NOTE: CNS, central nervous system.
SOURCE: After Rotbart.

Arbovirus infections typically occur in the summer months, have clear geographic localization, and occur in epidemics, all factors reflecting the ecology of their transmission through infected insect vectors (Fig. 373-1); Table 373-6; Chap. 198). Arboviral meningitis should be considered when clusters of meningitis cases occur in a restricted geographic region during the summer or early fall. A history of tick exposure or travel or residence in the appropriate geographic area should suggest the possibility of Colorado tick fever virus or Powassan virus infection, although nonviral diseases producing meningitis (e.g., Lyme disease) or headache with meningismus (e.g., Rocky Mountain spotted fever) may also present this way.

HSV-2 meningitis (Chap. 182) occurs in approximately 25% of women and 11% of men at the time of an initial (primary) episode of genital herpes. Of these patients, 20% go on to have recurrent attacks of meningitis. In some series, HSV-2 has been the most important cause of aseptic meningitis in adults, especially women, and overall it

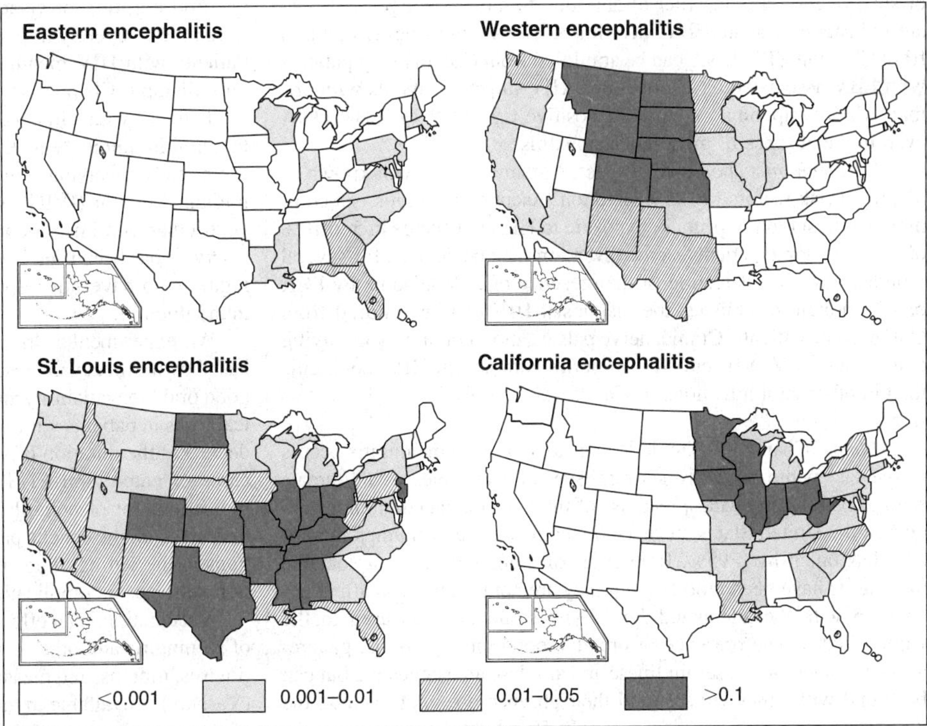

FIGURE 373-1 Incidence of selected forms of arboviral encephalitis in the United States; cases per 10,000 population per year for St. Louis and California encephalitis (bottom maps) and per 100,000 per year for eastern and western encephalitis (top maps). *(Modified from TF Tsai et al.)*

is probably second only to enteroviruses as a cause of viral meningitis. Although HSV-2 can be cultured from CSF during a first episode of meningitis, cultures are invariably negative during recurrent episodes of HSV-2 meningitis. Diagnosis depends on amplification of HSV-2 DNA from CSF by PCR. Almost all cases of recurrent HSV meningitis are due to HSV-2, although rare cases due to HSV-1 have been reported. Most cases of benign recurrent lymphocytic meningitis, including those meeting accepted diagnostic criteria for Mollaret's meningitis, appear to be due to HSV. Genital lesions may not be present, and most patients give no history of genital herpes. CSF cultures are negative, although HSV DNA can be amplified from CSF by PCR during attacks of meningitis but not during symptom-free intervals.

VZV meningitis should be suspected in the presence of concurrent chickenpox or shingles. However, it is important to recognize that in some series up to 40% of VZV meningitis cases have been reported to occur in the absence of rash. The frequency of VZV as a cause of meningitis is extremely variable, ranging from as low as 3% to as high as 20% in different series. The frequency would be expected to decline with the increasing utilization of the live attenuated varicella vaccine (Varivax) in children. In addition to meningitis, encephalitis (see below), and shingles (see below), VZV can also produce acute cerebellar ataxia. This typically occurs in children and presents with the abrupt onset of limb and truncal ataxia. A similar syndrome occurs less commonly in association with EBV and enteroviral infection. PCR has rapidly become a major tool in the diagnosis of VZV CNS infections. In patients with negative CSF PCR results, the diagnosis of VZV CNS infection can be made by the demonstration of VZV-specific intrathecal antibody synthesis and/or the presence of VZV CSF IgM antibodies, or by positive CSF cultures.

EBV infections may also produce aseptic meningitis, with or without accompanying evidence of the infectious mononucleosis syndrome. The diagnosis may be suggested by the finding of atypical lymphocytes in the CSF or an atypical lymphocytosis in peripheral blood. The demonstration of IgM antibody to viral capsid antigen (VCA), antibody to the diffuse (D) component of early antigen (EA), or subsequently a rising titer of antibody to nuclear antigen (EBNA) are indicative of acute EBV infection. EBV is almost never cultured from CSF, but EBV DNA can be amplified from CSF in many patients with EBV-associated CNS infections. HIV-infected patients with primary CNS lymphoma may have a positive CSF PCR for EBV DNA even in the absence of meningoencephalitis.

HIV meningitis should be suspected in any patient with known or identified risk factors for HIV infection. Aseptic meningitis is a common manifestation of primary exposure to HIV and occurs in 5 to 10% of cases. In some patients, seroconversion may be delayed for several months; however, detection of the presence of HIV genome by PCR or p24 protein establishes the diagnosis. HIV can be cultured from CSF in some patients. Cranial nerve palsies, most commonly involving cranial nerves V, VII, or VIII, are more common in HIV meningitis than in other viral infections. →*For further discussion of HIV infection see Chap. 309.*

Mumps (Chap. 196) should be considered when meningitis occurs in the late winter or early spring, especially in males (male/female ratio 3:1). With the widespread use of the live attenuated mumps vaccine in the United States since 1967, the incidence of mumps meningitis has fallen by >95%. Rare cases of mumps vaccine–associated meningitis have been reported, but they are not usually seen after vaccination with the attenuated Jeryl-Lynn strain of virus used in the United States. The presence of orchitis, oophoritis, parotitis, pancreatitis, or elevations in serum lipase and amylase are suggestive but can be found with other viruses, and their absence does not exclude the diagnosis. Clinical meningitis occurs in 5% of patients with parotitis, but only 50% of patients with meningitis have associated parotitis. Mumps infection confers lifelong immunity, so a documented history of previous infection excludes this diagnosis. The presence of hypoglycorrhachia (10 to 30%) may be an additional diagnostic clue, once other causes have been excluded (see above). Up to 25% of patients may have a PMN-predominant CSF pleocytosis, and CSF abnormalities may persist for months. Diagnosis is typically made by isolation of virus from CSF and/or demonstration of seroconversion between acute-phase and convalescent sera.

LCMV infection (Chap. 198) should be considered when aseptic meningitis occurs in the late fall or winter, and in individuals with a history of exposure to house mice (*Mus musculus*), pet or laboratory rodents (e.g., hamsters), or their excreta. Some patients have an associated rash, pulmonary infiltrates, alopecia, parotitis, orchitis, or myopericarditis. Laboratory clues to the diagnosis of LCMV, in addition to the clinical findings noted above, may include the presence of leukopenia, thrombocytopenia, or abnormal liver function tests. Some cases present with a marked CSF pleocytosis (>1000 cells per microliter) and hypoglycorrachia (<30%).

℞ TREATMENT In the usual case of viral meningitis, treatment is symptomatic, and hospitalization is not required. Exceptions include patients with deficient humoral immunity, neonates with overwhelming infection, and patients in whom the clinical or CSF profile suggests the possibility of a bacterial or other nonviral cause of infection. Patients with suspected bacterial meningitis should receive appropriate empirical therapy pending culture results (Chap. 372). Patients usually prefer to rest undisturbed in a quiet, darkened room. Analgesics can be used to relieve headache, which is often reduced by the initial diagnostic lumbar puncture. Antipyretics may help to reduce fever, which rarely exceeds 40°C. Hyponatremia may develop as a result of inappropriate vasopressin secretion (SIADH), so fluid and electrolyte status should be monitored. Repeat lumbar puncture is indicated only in patients whose fever and symptoms fail to resolve after a few days or if there is doubt about the initial diagnosis.

Oral or intravenous acyclovir may be of benefit in patients with meningitis caused by HSV-1 or -2 and in cases of severe EBVor VZV infection. Data concerning treatment of HSV, EBV, and VZV meningitis are extremely limited. Seriously ill patients should probably receive intravenous acyclovir (30 mg/kg per day in three divided doses) for 7 days. Oral acyclovir (800 mg, five times daily), famciclovir (500 mg, tid), or valacyclovir (1000 mg, tid) for a week may be tried in less severely ill patients, although data on efficacy are lacking. Patients with HIV meningitis should receive highly active antiretroviral therapy (Chap. 309).

Patients with viral meningitis who are known to have deficient humoral immunity (e.g. X-linked agammaglobulinemia), and who are not already receiving either intramuscular γ-globulin or intravenous immunoglobulin (IVIG), should be treated with these agents. Intraventricular administration of immunoglobulin through an Ommaya reservoir has been tried in some patients with chronic enteroviral meningitis who have not responded to intramuscular or intravenous immunoglobulin.

An experimental drug, pleconaril (Viropharma Inc., VP 63843), has shown efficacy against a variety of enteroviral infections and has good oral bioavailability and excellent CNS penetration. Ongoing clinical trials in patients with enteroviral meningitis suggest that pleconaril decreases the duration of symptoms compared to placebo. Since most cases of enteroviral CNS infection are benign and self-limited, the indications for pleconaril therapy need to be better defined. Antiviral treatment might benefit patients with chronic CNS enteroviral infections in the setting of agammaglobulinemia or those who develop poliomyelitis as a complication of polio vaccine administration.

Vaccination is an effective method of preventing the development of meningitis and other neurologic complications associated with poliovirus, mumps, and measles infection. A live attenuated VZVvaccine (Varivax) is available in the United States. Clinical studies indicate an effectiveness rate of 70 to 90% for this vaccine. Reduction in primary VZV infection would be expected to reduce the frequency and/or severity both of primary neurologic complications of varicella and of the consequences of later reactivation (e.g., shingles).

Prognosis In adults, the prognosis for full recovery from viral meningitis is excellent. Rare patients complain of persisting headache, mild mental impairment, incoordination, or generalized asthenia for weeks to months. The outcome in infants and neonates (<1 year) is less certain; intellectual impairment, learning disabilities, hearing loss, and other lasting sequelae have been reported in some studies.

VIRAL ENCEPHALITIS **Definition** In distinction to meningitis, where the infectious process and associated inflammatory response is limited largely to the meninges, in encephalitis the brain parenchyma is also involved. Many patients with encephalitis also have evidence of associated meningitis (meningoencephalitis) and, in some cases, involvement of the spinal cord or nerve roots (encephalomyelitis, encephalomyeloradiculitis).

Clinical Manifestations In addition to the acute febrile illness with evidence of meningeal involvement characteristic of meningitis, the patient with encephalitis commonly has an altered level of consciousness, an abnormal mental state, and evidence of either focal or diffuse neurologic signs and symptoms. Any degree of altered consciousness may occur, ranging from mild lethargy to deep coma. Patients with encephalitis are frequently confused, delirious, and disoriented. Mental aberrations may include hallucinations, agitation, personality change, behavioral disorders, and, at times, a frankly psychotic state. Focal or generalized seizures occur in >50% of patients with severe encephalitis. Virtually every possible type of focal neurologic disturbance has been reported in viral encephalitis; the signs and symptoms reflect the sites of infection and inflammation. The most commonly encountered focal findings are aphasia, ataxia, hemiparesis (with hyperactive tendon reflexes and extensor plantar responses), involuntary movements (e.g., myoclonic jerks), and cranial nerve deficits (e.g., ocular palsies, facial weakness). Involvement of the hypothalamic-pituitary axis may result in temperature dysregulation, diabetes insipidus, or the development of SIADH. Despite the clear neuropathologic evidence that viruses differ in the regions of the CNS they injure, it is often impossible to distinguish reliably on clinical grounds alone one type of viral encephalitis (e.g., that caused by HSV) from others (see "Differential Diagnosis," below).

Etiology The number of viruses reported to cause encephalitis is legion. In the United States, there are approximately 20,000 reported cases per year. The same organisms responsible for aseptic meningitis are also responsible for encephalitis, although their relative frequencies differ (Table 373-5; Fig. 373-1). The most important viruses causing sporadic cases of encephalitis in immunocompetent adults are HSV-1, VZV, and, less commonly, enteroviruses. Epidemics of encephalitis are caused by arboviruses, which belong to several different viral taxonomic groups including *Alphavirus* of the family Togaviridae (e.g. Eastern equine encephalitis virus, Western equine encephalitis virus), *Flavivirus* of the family Flaviviridae (e.g., St. Louis encephalitis virus, Powassan virus), and *Bunyavirus* of the family Bunyaviridae (e.g., California encephalitis virus serogroup, LaCrosse virus). In most years, the largest number of cases of arbovirus encephalitis are generally due to St. Louis encephalitis virus and the California encephalitis virus serogroup. New causes of viral encephalitis are constantly appearing, as evidenced by the recent outbreak of ~300 cases of encephalitis with a 40% mortality rate in Malaysia caused by Nipah virus, a new member of the Paramyxovirus family. Similarly, well-known viruses may suddenly appear in unexpected locations, as illustrated by a recent outbreak of encephalitis in New York City due to West Nile virus.

Table 373-5 Viruses Causing Encephalitis

Common	Less Common	Rare
Arboviruses, enteroviruses, HSV-1, mumps	CMV, EBV, HIV, measles, VZV	Adenoviruses, CTFV, influenza A, LCMV, parainfluenza, rabies, rubella

NOTE: As in Table 373-1; also, CTFV, Colorado tick fever virus.

Laboratory Diagnosis • ***CSF examination*** CSF examination should be performed in all patients with suspected viral encephalitis unless contraindicated by the presence of severely increased intracranial pressure (ICP). The characteristic CSF profile is indistinguishable from that of viral meningitis and consists of a lymphocytic pleocytosis, a mildly elevated protein level, and a normal glucose level. A CSF pleocytosis (>5 cells per microliter) occurs in >95% of patients with documented viral encephalitis, and its absence should prompt a careful search for other causes of an encephalopathy. In rare cases, a pleocytosis may be absent on the initial lumbar puncture but present subsequently. Patients who are severely immunocompromised by HIV infection, steroid or other immunosuppressant drugs, chemotherapy, or certain lymphoreticular malignancies may fail to mount a CSF inflammatory response. CSF cell counts exceed 500/μL in only about 10% of patients with encephalitis. Infections with certain arboviruses (e.g., Eastern equine encephalitis or California encephalitis viruses), mumps, and LCMV may occasionally result in cell counts >1000/μL, but this degree of pleocytosis should suggest the possibility of nonviral infections or other inflammatory processes. Atypical lymphocytes in the CSF may be seen in EBV infection and less commonly with other viruses, including CMV, HSV, and enteroviruses. The presence of substantial numbers of PMNs after the first 48 h should prompt consideration of bacterial infection, leptospirosis, amebic infection, and noninfectious processes such as acute hemorrhagic leukoencephalitis. Large numbers of CSF PMNs may be present in patients with viral encephalitis due to Eastern equine encephalitis virus, echovirus 9, and, more rarely, other enteroviruses. About 20% of patients with encephalitis will have a significant number of red blood cells (>500/μL) in the CSF in a nontraumatic tap. The pathologic correlate of this may be the presence of a hemorrhagic encephalitis of the type seen with HSV, Colorado tick fever virus, and occasionally California encephalitis virus. A decreased CSF glucose level is distinctly unusual in viral encephalitis and should suggest the possibility of fungal, tuberculous, parasitic, leptospiral, syphilitic, sarcoid, or neoplastic meningitis. Rare patients with mumps, LCMV, or advanced HSV encephalitis may have low CSF glucose concentrations.

CSF PCR PCR amplification of viral nucleic acid has become the diagnostic procedure of choice for many types of viral encephalitis. Recent studies with HSV encephalitis indicate that the sensitivity (~98%) and specificity (~94%) of CSF PCR equal or exceed those of brain biopsy. Although less detailed specificity and sensitivity data are available for most other viruses, PCR has become the primary diagnostic test for CNS infections caused by CMV, EBV, VZV, and enteroviruses (see "Viral Meningitis," above). Studies of HSV encephalitis indicate that the incidence of positive CSF PCR gradually declines after the second week of illness. PCR results are generally not affected by ≤1 week of antiviral therapy. In one study 98% of CSF specimens remained PCR-positive during the first week of initiation of antiviral therapy, but the numbers fell to ~50% 8 to 14 days, and to ~21% by ≥15 days after initiation of therapy.

Patients suspected of having HSV encephalitis should be started on acyclovir (see below), and their CSF should be assayed for the presence of HSV DNA by PCR. A positive CSF PCR in the appropriate clinical setting is diagnostic of HSV encephalitis. A negative PCR test effectively excludes the diagnosis, unless the test is performed late in the course of illness or following prolonged antiviral therapy (see above). Blood or blood breakdown products may inhibit PCR reactions and generate false-negative results. Nonetheless the negative predictive value of a negative CSF PCR is ~98% and provides sufficient basis to discontinue acyclovir therapy unless mitigating circumstances likely to generate a false-negative PCR are present.

CSF culture Attempts to culture viruses from the CSF in cases of encephalitis are often disappointing (Table 373-3). Cultures are invariably negative in cases of HSV-1 encephalitis.

Serologic studies and antigen detection The basic approach to the serodiagnosis of viral encephalitis is identical to that discussed earlier for viral meningitis. In patients with HSV encephalitis, both antibodies to HSV-1 glycoproteins and glycoprotein antigens have been detected in the CSF. Optimal detection of both HSV antibodies and antigen typically occurs after the first week of illness, limiting the utility of these tests in acute diagnosis. Nonetheless, CSF HSV antibody testing may be of value in selected patients whose illness is >1 week's duration and who are CSF PCR-negative for HSV.

MRI, CT, EEG Patients with suspected encephalitis almost invariably undergo neuroimaging studies and often EEG. These tests help identify or exclude alternative diagnoses and assist in the differentiation between a focal, as opposed to diffuse, encephalitic process. Focal findings in a patient with encephalitis should always raise the possibility of HSV encephalitis. Examples of focal findings include: (1) areas of increased signal intensity in the frontotemporal, cingulate, or insular regions of the brain on T2-weighted spin-echo MRI images (Fig. 373-2); (2) temporoparietal areas of low absorption, mass effect, and contrast enhancement on CT; or (3) periodic focal temporal lobe spikes on a background of slow or low-amplitude ("flattened") activity on EEG. Approximately 10% of patients with PCR-documented HSV encephalitis will have a normal MRI, although nearly 90% will have abnormalities in the temporal lobe. CT is less sensitive than MRI and is normal in up to 33% of patients. EEG abnormalities occur in >90% of PCR-documented cases of HSV encephalitis; they typically involve the temporal lobes but are often nonspecific.

Brain biopsy Brain biopsy is now generally reserved for patients in whom CSF PCR studies fail to lead to a specific diagnosis, who have focal abnormalities on MRI, and who continue to show progressive clinical deterioration despite treatment with acyclovir and supportive therapy. The isolation of HSV from brain tissue obtained at biopsy was once considered the "gold standard" for the diagnosis of HSV encephalitis, although with the advent of CSF PCR tests for HSV it is no longer necessary to perform brain biopsy for this purpose. The need for brain biopsy to diagnose other forms of viral encephalitis has also declined greatly with the widespread availability of CSF PCR diagnostic tests for EBV, CMV, VZV, and enteroviruses. When biopsy is performed, the tissue is cultured for virus and examined histopathologically and ultrastructurally. The biopsy is typically carried out under general anesthesia through a craniectomy. Tissue should be taken from a site that appears to be significantly involved on the basis of clinical and laboratory criteria. Although brain biopsy is not an innocuous procedure, the mortality rate is low (<0.2%). Potential morbidity, in addition to that related to general anesthesia, includes local bleeding and edema, the development of a seizure focus, and wound dehiscence or infection. From a practical viewpoint, the incidence of serious morbidity appears to be between 0.5 and 2%.

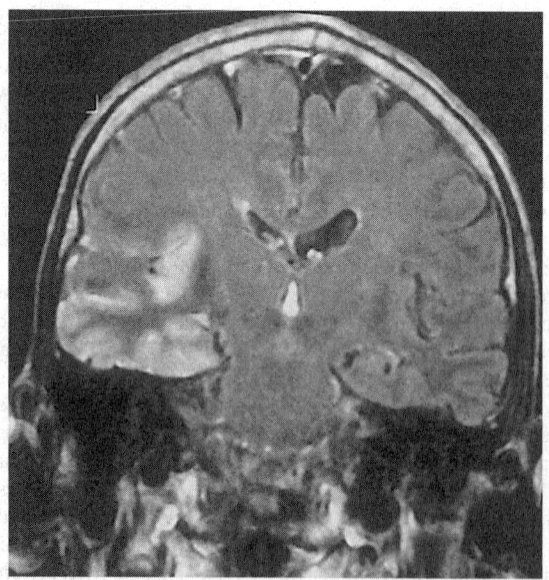

FIGURE 373-2 Coronal FLAIR magnetic resonance image from a patient with herpes simplex encephalitis. Note the area of increased signal in the temporal lobe (left) confined predominantly to the gray matter. This patient had predominantly unilateral disease; bilateral lesions are more common but may be quite asymmetric in their intensity.

Differential Diagnosis The differential diagnosis includes both infectious and noninfectious causes of encephalitis. Some of the most common illnesses masquerading as viral encephalitis, as identified in multicenter clinical trials using brain biopsy as a diagnostic standard, were vascular diseases; abscess and empyema; fungal, parasitic, rickettsial, and tuberculous infections; tumors; Reye's syndrome; toxic encephalopathy; subdural hematoma; and systemic lupus erythematosus. Of the nonviral infections, particular attention should be paid to *Listeria, Mycoplasma, Leptospira, Cryptococcus,* and *Mucor* infections, as well as to toxoplasmosis and tuberculosis.

Once nonviral causes of encephalitis have been excluded, the major diagnostic impetus is to distinguish HSV from other viruses that cause encephalitis. This distinction is particularly important because in virtually every other instance the therapy is supportive, whereas specific and effective antiviral therapy is available for HSV, and its efficacy is enhanced when it is instituted early in the course of infection. HSV encephalitis should be considered when clinical features suggesting involvement of the inferomedial frontotemporal regions of the brain are present, including prominent olfactory or gustatory hallucinations, anosmia, unusual or bizarre behavior or personality alterations, or memory disturbance. HSV encephalitis should always be suspected in patients with focal findings on clinical examination, neuroimaging studies, or EEG. The diagnostic procedure of choice in these patients is CSF PCR analysis for HSV. A positive CSF PCR establishes the diagnosis, and a negative test dramatically reduces the likelihood of HSV encephalitis (see above).

Epidemiologic factors may provide important clues. Particular attention should be paid to the season of the year (Table 373-2), the age of the patient (Table 373-6), the geographic location and travel history (Fig. 373-1; Table 373-6), and possible exposure to animal bites, rodents, and ticks. *Morbidity and Mortality Weekly Reports* provides regular information about the prevalence of particular viruses causing encephalitis by season and region of the country. State public health authorities provide another valuable resource concerning isolation of particular agents in individual regions.

℞ TREATMENT Specific antiviral therapy should be initiated when appropriate. Vital functions, including respiration and blood pressure, should be monitored continuously and supported as required. In the initial stages of encephalitis, many patients will require care in an intensive care unit. Basic management and supportive therapy should include careful monitoring of ICP, fluid restriction and avoidance of hypotonic intravenous solutions, and suppression of fever. Seizures should be treated with standard anticonvulsant regimens, and prophylactic therapy should be considered in view of the high frequency of seizures in severe cases of encephalitis (>50%). As with all seriously ill, immobilized patients with altered levels of consciousness, encephalitis patients are at risk for aspiration pneumonia, stasis ulcers and decubiti, contractures, deep venous thrombosis and its complications, and infections of indwelling lines and catheters.

Acyclovir is of benefit in the treatment of HSV and should be started empirically in all patients with suspected viral encephalitis. Treatment should be discontinued in patients found not to have HSV encephalitis, with the possible exception of patients with severe encephalitis due to VZV or EBV. HSV, VZV, and EBV all encode an enzyme, deoxypyrimidine (thymidine) kinase, that phosphorylates acyclovir to produce acyclovir-5′-monophosphate. Host cell enzymes then phosphorylate this compound to form a triphosphate derivative. It is the triphosphate that acts as an antiviral agent by inhibiting viral DNA polymerase and by causing premature termination of nascent viral DNA chains. The specificity of action depends on the fact that uninfected cells do not phosphorylate significant amounts of acyclovir to acyclovir-5′-monophosphate. A second level of specificity is provided by the fact that the acyclovir triphosphate is a more potent inhibitor of viral DNA polymerase than of the analogous host cell enzymes.

Adults should receive a dose of 10 mg/kg of acyclovir intravenously every 8 h (30 mg/kg per day total dose) for a minimum of 14 days. Although no studies directly addressing this issue are yet available, we suggest repeating the CSF PCR after completion of 14 days of acyclovir therapy, and discontinuing the acyclovir in PCR-negative patients. Patients with a persisting positive CSF PCR for HSV should be treated for an additional 7 days, and the PCR repeated. Neonatal HSV CNS infection is less responsive to acyclovir therapy than HSV encephalitis in adults; it is recommended that neonates with HSV encephalitis receive 20 mg/kg of acyclovir every 8 h (60 mg/kg per day total dose) for a minimum of 21 days.

Table 373-6 Features of Selected Arbovirus Encephalitides

Feature	WEE	EEE	VEE	SLE	CE
Region	West, midwest	Atlantic and Gulf	South	All	East and north-central
Age	Infants, adults >50 years	Children	Adults	Adults >50 years	Children
Deaths	5–15%	50–75%	1%	2–20%	<1%
Sequelae	Low to moderate	80%	Rare	20%	Rare
Vector	Mosquito	Mosquito	Mosquito	Mosquito	Mosquito
Animal host	Birds	Birds	Horses, small mammals	Birds	Rodents

NOTE: CE, California encephalitis virus; EEE, Eastern equine encephalitis virus; SLE, St. Louis encephalitis virus; VEE, Venezuelan equine encephalitis virus; WEE, Western equine encephalitis virus.
SOURCE: After Whitley.

Prior to intravenous administration, acyclovir should be diluted to a concentration ≤7 mg/mL. (A 70-kg person would receive a dose of 700 mg, which would be diluted in a volume of 100 mL.) Each dose should be infused slowly over 1 h rather than by rapid or bolus infusion, to minimize the risk of renal dysfunction. Care should be taken to avoid extravasation or intramuscular or subcutaneous administration. The alkaline pH of acyclovir can cause local inflammation and phlebitis (9%). Dose adjustment is required in patients with impaired renal glomerular filtration. Penetration into CSF is excellent, with average drug levels approximately 50% of serum levels. Complications of therapy include elevations in BUN and creatinine levels (5%), thrombocytopenia (6%), gastrointestinal toxicity (nausea, vomiting, diarrhea) (7%), and neurotoxicity (lethargy or obtundation, disorientation, confusion, agitation, hallucinations, tremors, seizures) (1%). Acyclovir resistance may be mediated by changes in either the viral deoxypyrimidine kinase or DNA polymerase. To date, acyclovir-resistant isolates have not been a significant clinical problem in immunocompetent individuals. However, there have been reports of clinically virulent acyclovir-resistant HSV isolates from sites outside the CNS in immunocompromised individuals, including those with AIDS.

Oral antiviral drugs with efficacy against HSV, VZV, and EBV, including acyclovir, famciclovir, and valacyclovir, have not been evaluated in the treatment of encephalitis either as primary therapy or as supplemental therapy following completion of a course of parenteral acyclovir. An NIAID/NINDS-sponsored phase III trial of supplemental oral valacyclovir therapy (2 g, tid for 3 months) following the initial 14- to 21-day course of therapy with parenteral acyclovir has recently been initiated in patients with HSV encephalitis; it may help clarify the role of extended oral antiviral therapy.

Both ganciclovir and foscarnet have been shown to be effective in the treatment of CMV-related CNS infections. These drugs are often used in combination. Cidofovir (see below) may provide an alternative in patients who fail to respond to ganciclovir and foscarnet, although data concerning its use in CMV CNS infections are extremely limited.

Ganciclovir is a synthetic nucleoside analogue of 2′-deoxyguanosine. The drug is preferentially phosphorylated by virus-induced cellular kinases. Ganciclovir triphosphate acts as a competitive inhibitor of the CMV DNA polymerase, and its incorporation into nascent viral DNA results in premature chain termination. Following intravenous administration, CSF concentrations of ganciclovir are 25 to 70% of coincident plasma levels. The usual dose for treatment of severe neurologic illnesses is 5 mg/kg every 12 h given intravenously at a constant rate over 1 h. Induction therapy is followed by maintenance therapy of 5 mg/kg every day for an indefinite period. Induction therapy should be continued until patients show a decline in CSF pleocytosis and a reduction in CSF CMV DNA copy number on quantitative PCR testing (where available). Doses should be adjusted in patients with renal insufficiency. Treatment is often limited by the development of granulocytopenia and thrombocytopenia (20 to 25%), which may require reduction in or discontinuation of therapy. Gastrointestinal side effects including nausea, vomiting, diarrhea, and abdominal pain occur in ~20% of patients. Some patients treated with ganciclovir for CMV retinitis have developed retinal detachment, but the causal relationship to ganciclovir treatment is unclear.

Foscarnet is a pyrophosphate analogue that inhibits viral DNA polymerases by binding to the pyrophosphate-binding site. Following intravenous infusion, CSF concentrations range from 15 to 100% of coincident plasma levels. The usual dose for serious CMV-related neurologic illness is 60 mg/kg every 8 h administered by constant infusion over 1 h. Induction therapy for 14 to 21 days is followed by maintenance therapy (60 to 120 mg/kg per day). Induction therapy may need to be extended in patients who fail to show a decline in CSF pleocytosis and a reduction in CSF CMV DNA copy number on quantitative PCR tests (where available). Approximately one-third of patients develop renal impairment during treatment, which is reversible following discontinuation of therapy in most, but not all, cases. This is often associated with elevations in serum creatinine and proteinuria and is less frequent in patients who are adequately hydrated. Many patients experience fatigue and nausea. Reduction in serum calcium, magnesium, and potassium occur in approximately 15% of patients and may be associated with tetany, cardiac rhythm disturbances, or seizures.

Cidofovir is a nucleotide analogue that is effective in treating CMV retinitis and equivalent or better than ganciclovir in some experimental models of murine CMV encephalitis, although data concerning its efficacy in human CMV CNS disease are limited. The usual dose is 5 mg/kg intravenously once weekly for 2 weeks, then biweekly for 2 or more additional doses, depending on clinical response. Patients must be prehydrated with normal saline (e.g., 1 L over 1 to 2 h) prior to each dose, and treated with probenecid (e.g., 1 g 3 h before cidofovir and 1 g 2 and 8 h after cidofovir). Nephrotoxicity is common; the dose should be reduced if renal function deteriorates.

Intravenous ribavarin (15 to 25 mg/kg per day in divided doses given every 8 h) has been reported to be of benefit in isolated cases of severe encephalitis due to California encephalitis (LaCrosse) virus. Ribavarin might be of benefit for the rare patients, typically infants or young children, with severe adenovirus or rotavirus encephalitis, and in patients with encephalitis due to LCMV or other arenaviruses. However, clinical trials are lacking. Hemolysis, with resulting anemia, has been the major side effect limiting therapy.

Sequelae There is considerable variation in the incidence and severity of sequelae in patients surviving viral encephalitis. In the case of Eastern equine encephalitis virus infection, nearly 80% of survivors have severe neurologic sequelae. At the other extreme are infections due to EBV, California encephalitis virus, and Venezuelan equine encephalitis virus, where severe sequelae are unusual. For example, approximately 5 to 15% of children infected with LaCrosse virus have a residual seizure disorder, and 1% have persistent hemiparesis. Detailed information about sequelae in patients with HSV encephalitis treated with acyclovir are available from the NIAID-CASG trials. Of 32 acyclovir-treated patients, 26 survived (81%). Of the 26 survivors, 12 (46%) had no or only minor sequelae, 3 (12%) were moderately impaired (gainfully employed but not functioning at their previous level), and 11 (42%) were severely impaired (requiring continuous supportive care). The incidence and severity of sequelae were directly related to the age of the patient and the level of consciousness at the time of initiation of therapy. Patients with severe neurologic impairment (Glasgow coma score 6) at initiation of therapy either died or survived with severe sequelae. Young patients (<30 years) with good neurologic function at initiation of therapy did substantially better (100% survival, 62% with no or mild sequelae) compared with their older counterparts (>30 years); (64% survival, 57% no or mild sequelae). Recent studies using quantitative CSF PCR tests for HSV indicate that clinical outcome following treatment also correlates with the amount of HSV DNA present in CSF at the time of presentation.

ACUTE MYELITIS AND RADICULITIS

Myelitis is a viral infection of the spinal cord, which may occur as an isolated syndrome or in association with encephalitis (encephalomyelitis) or infection involving the nerve roots (myeloradiculitis). Viral infection involving sensory ganglia and nerve roots may also occur as an isolated syndrome, most commonly in the form of shingles.

MYELITIS **Clinical Features and Epidemiology** The prototypical viral myelitis is the syndrome of acute anterior poliomyelitis caused by polioviruses. Paralytic polio (Chap. 193) is a rarity in the United States (four to eight cases per year), although it remains a major problem in some regions of the world. Most cases of paralytic polio in the United States occur as a result of the exceedingly rare reversion of vaccine strains to virulence. The cases are divided among those recently vaccinated and unvaccinated nonimmune adults exposed to recently vaccinated children. Occasional outbreaks have occurred in nonimmunized populations such as the Amish in Pennsylvania. Illness typically begins with prodromal symptoms, including fever, headache, myalgia, pharyngitis, nausea and vomiting, and meningeal signs. These are associated with the typical CSF profile of aseptic meningitis. In some patients these symptoms are followed by the development of muscle weakness resulting from viral injury to the motor neurons in the anterior horn of the spinal cord or in brainstem motor nuclei. The incidence, severity, and pattern of weakness are age-dependent, with more severe disease being seen with increasing age. Young children often develop weakness of one leg, older children weakness of both legs, and adults asymmetric quadriparesis, often with associated urinary retention. Weakness is associated with fasciculations, loss of deep and superficial reflexes, and the development of atrophy. Involvement of the brainstem (bulbar polio) can result in dysphagia, dysarthria, respiratory impairment, and vasomotor disturbances. Although some patients complain of paresthesia, objective sensory loss is not present.

A distinctive polio-like syndrome is produced by enterovirus 70. Patients develop acute hemorrhagic conjunctivitis, followed days to weeks later by a poliomyelitis-like weakness.

Viruses may also affect both the anterior and posterior portions of the spinal cord over a considerable longitudinal extent, producing "transverse" myelitis. The clinical syndrome is one of acute muscle weakness, which may be of the flaccid hyporeflexic type initially but usually develops into spastic paralysis with hyperreflexia and extensor plantar responses. Sensory loss is almost invariably present and typically involves both pain-temperature and position-vibration modalities, producing a sensory level. Urinary symptoms (retention, overflow incontinence, or, in milder cases, hesitancy or decreased voiding sensation) and constipation or even fecal incontinence are present in virtually all patients. Although this syndrome can be caused by a variety of viruses, most cases in immunocompetent patients are due to HSV-2, VZV, or EBV. CMV is an important cause of myelitis in immunocompromised patients, notably those with HIV infection.

A mild form of myelitis predominantly affecting the sacral spinal cord occurs in association with genital HSV-2 infection. At the time of the first episode of genital herpes, about 25% of women, and a smaller percentage of men, develop an aseptic meningitis syndrome. In some individuals this may be associated with urinary retention, dysesthesia, paresthesia, or neuralgia in the legs, buttocks, or genital area, and weakness in one or both legs.

Chronic viral myelitis is associated with advanced HIV infection (vacuolar myelopathy) and with infection due to HTLV-1 (tropical spastic paraparesis and HTLV-I–associated myelopathy). →*For further discussion of these infections see Chap. 309.*

Diagnosis Almost all patients with viral myelitis will have inflammatory changes in the CSF including a lymphocytic pleocytosis and elevated protein; glucose is normal. An exception to this pattern occurs in HIV-associated CMV myeloradiculopathy in which a polymorphonuclear pleocytosis and low CSF glucose are characteristic. For myelitis caused by HSV, EBV, CMV, and VZV, CSF PCR studies may be diagnostic. Some patients show evidence of intrathecal synthesis of antibody or the presence of CSF IgM antibodies, and these studies may be helpful in PCR-negative patients. Viral cultures are frequently positive in patients with CMV myelitis and may be positive in some cases of myelitis due to HSV-2. Neuroimaging studies may be helpful in identifying the site and extent of the myelitis. The usual findings are areas of increased T2 signal within the spinal cord parenchyma. Patients with HIV-associated CMV radiculomyelopathy may show increased signal and enhancement of the nerve roots. Perhaps the most important role of MRI is to exclude compressive lesions and other causes of acute myelopathy.

℞ TREATMENT Reports of treatment of viral myelitis are usually isolated case reports or small series. Patients with myelitis due to HSV, EBV, or VZV should be treated with intravenous acyclovir (10 mg/kg, tid) for 10 to 14 days. Patients with HIV-associated CMV radiculomyelopathy should receive ganciclovir plus foscarnet (see above under CMV encephalitis for dose), although the results of treatment are frequently disappointing.

GANGLIONITIS AND RADICULITIS **Herpes Zoster** (See also Chap. 183) • ***Clinical features*** Reactivation of VZV latent in neurons within the trigeminal or spinal sensory ganglia produces zoster (*shingles*). Zoster is a distinctive clinical syndrome consisting of paresthesia or dysesthesia in a dermatomal distribution followed by a localized cutaneous eruption. Zoster occurs in patients previously infected with chickenpox (varicella). During the initial varicella infection, virus in the skin travels up the sensory nerves to become latent within neurons in the trigeminal and spinal sensory ganglia. Reactivation results in active viral replication in sensory ganglia followed by spread of virus through nerves to the skin, where a dermatomal vesicular eruption occurs. The incidence of zoster increases with age and is higher in patients with compromised cellular immunity. The typical history is one of several days of itching, tingling, burning, or pain in a dermatomal distribution that is followed by a vesicular eruption consisting of clear vesicles on an erythematous base. The vesicles become cloudy, dry, and crust over after 1 to 2 weeks. The lesions are most commonly found in the thoracic dermatomes, with T5-T10 accounting for approximately two-thirds of cases. Most patients will have hypalgesia and hypesthesia in the affected dermatome. About 5% of patients develop motor weakness and atrophy (zoster paresis) in the associated myotome. Rare patients can have zoster-like neuralgic pain in the absence of a cutaneous eruption (*zoster sine herpete*). Diagnosis in these patients depends on serologic studies in serum or CSF or the identification of VZV DNA in CSF by PCR.

Characteristic syndromes result from zoster eruptions involving the trigeminal and geniculate distribution. In 10 to 15% of cases, reactivation of virus in the trigeminal ganglia results in a rash in the distribution of the ophthalmic division of the trigeminal nerve (*ophthalmic zoster*). Vesicular eruption may be conjoined with conjunctivitis, keratitis, ocular muscle palsies, ptosis, and mydriasis. In rare cases, an attack is followed by the development of cerebral angiitis involving the ipsilateral carotid and/or middle cerebral arteries. Vascular compromise may lead to hemiplegia, aphasia, or other focal deficits contralateral to the side of the facial eruption. Reactivation of virus from the geniculate ganglion produces the *Ramsay Hunt syndrome*, consisting of facial palsy often associated with loss of taste in the anterior tongue, tinnitus, hearing loss, and vertigo. Zoster eruptions are found in the external auditory meatus.

Some 45% of patients over age 50 who develop shingles will experience pain persisting for >6 weeks after disappearance of the rash (*postherpetic neuralgia*). Postherpetic neuralgia is almost never seen in children who develop zoster and is rare (6%) in adults younger than 50. (See "Treatment" below, and Chap. 183).

Diagnosis The diagnosis of shingles is generally made on clinical grounds. Recurrent HSV infection may produce a similar syndrome of a cutaneous eruption in a dermatomal distribution associated with paresthesia. Unlike shingles, in which more than two or three recurrences in a lifetime would be virtually unknown, multiple recurrences are characteristic of HSV infection. The presence of VZV can be confirmed by culture or PCR of material obtained from the vesicular lesions. Direct detection of varicella zoster virus antigens in vesicle scrapings by immunocytochemistry or fluorescent microscopy is more sensitive and specific than the traditional Tzanck preparation and more sensitive than culture. A Tzanck preparation is made by smearing material obtained from the base of a vesicle onto a slide, which is then stained with Wright or Giemsa stain. The presence of syncytial giant cells with intranuclear inclusions is typical of a herpesvirus infection but does not distinguish between VZV and HSV.

℞ TREATMENT **Shingles in Immunocompetent Adults** Three antiviral drugs, acyclovir, famciclovir, and valacyclovir, are available for treatment of herpes zoster (shingles). Famciclovir is the diacetyl prodrug form of the nucleoside penciclovir. Following oral administration famciclovir is enzymatically converted to penciclovir (which is not absorbed well orally). Penciclovir acts intracellularly like acyclovir, but its active triphosphate metabolite has an extended half-life compared to acyclovir triphosphate in infected cells. Valacyclovir is the 6-valine ester of acyclovir and is enzymatically converted to acyclovir in the liver. Valacyclovir is better absorbed than acyclovir and allows for significantly (~fourfold) higher serum and CSF acyclovir levels than can be achieved with equimolar doses of oral acyclovir.

Acyclovir, valacyclovir, and famciclovir all produce more rapid resolution of cutaneous lesions and decreased duration of viral shedding compared to placebo if therapy is started within 72 h of rash onset, and decrease the duration of pain. These effects are generally modest, and supportive therapy alone is probably sufficient in immunocompetent patients <50 years who do not have significant pain and whose lesions do not involve the trigeminal dermatome. Immunocompetent patients with trigeminal zoster should be treated with antiviral drugs to reduce the risk of developing keratitis or other ophthalmologic complications of zoster. Patients >50 years should be treated with antiviral drugs in an effort to reduce the risk or duration of postherpetic neuralgia (see below). Typical doses in immunocompetent adults are acyclovir, 800 mg five times per day for 7 to 10 days; famciclovir, 500 mg tid for 7 days; and valacyclovir 1000 mg tid for 7 days.

The role of adjunctive glucocorticoid therapy has not been definitively established. Its use is not recommended in patients <50 or in immunocompromised individuals. In immunocompetent individuals >50, glucocorticoids do not appear to increase complications when used in conjunction with antiviral agents and may reduce the incidence of postherpetic neuralgia. A typical regimen, which should only be used in patients also receiving antiviral therapy, is prednisone, 30 mg bid for 1 week, then 15 mg bid for a second week, and 7.5 mg bid for a final week.

Shingles in Immunocompromised Patients Immunocompromised patients, including those with HIV infection, who have evidence of disease involving more than one dermatome or in the trigeminal distribution should be treated with intravenous acyclovir (10 mg/kg tid for 10 to 14 days). Immunocompromised patients with mild disease limited to a single dermatome (other than the trigeminal) can be treated initially with oral agents. These patients should be closely monitored and switched to intravenous acyclovir if they show any signs of disease progression while receiving oral therapy. Adverse effects of famciclovir, valacyclovir, and acyclovir are generally minor, with headache and nausea being reported in about 8 to 20% of recipients. Patients with renal insufficiency require reduction in dosing.

Postherpetic Neuralgia Controlled trials of both amitriptyline and desipramine have shown these drugs to be of benefit in the treatment of postherpetic neuralgia. Amitriptyline should be started at low dose (12.5 to 25 mg/d) and gradually increased until pain is controlled or side effects prevent further dose increases; the optimal dose is usually in the range of 75 to 150 mg/d. Desipramine is probably equally efficacious; however, selective serotonin reuptake inhibitors appear to be of limited utility. In a controlled study, carbamazepine was shown to be effective in reducing neuropathic lancinating pain but not continuous aching or burning pain. Treatment should be started at 200 mg/d and gradually increased until pain is controlled or side effects limit further therapy. The usual effective dose is ~600 mg/d, but some patients may require up to 1200 mg/d. Gabapentin has also been shown to be effective in a randomized controlled trial. Patients should be started on 300 mg tid, with a gradual increase to a maximum of 1200 mg tid. Phenytoin and valproate sodium may also be effective for neuropathic zoster pain. Topical agents such as 2.5% lidocaine–2.5% prilocaine cream or 5% lidocaine gel may benefit some patients with milder symptoms.

VIRAL INFECTION OF THE PERIPHERAL NERVOUS SYSTEM The distinction between ganglionitis, radiculitis, and neuritis are somewhat arbitrary and depend largely on the whether the brunt of injury involves the ganglia, nerve roots (radiculitis), or peripheral nerves (neuritis). Direct viral infection of peripheral nerves is unusual and should be distinguished from postviral immune-mediated injury to nerves. Many viruses, including CMV, HSV, EBV, VZV, mumps virus, and hepatitis B virus (HBV) have been associated, based predominantly on seroepidemiologic studies, with Guillain-Barré syndrome. It is presumed that the antecedent viral infection triggers an immunologic reaction that subsequently results in damage to peripheral nerve myelin (Chap. 378). A Guillain-Barré–like syndrome can also be seen in association with HIV infection, although these patients typically have a CSF pleocytosis rather than the classic albuminocytologic dissociation (elevated protein, zero or few cells).

Patients with HIV infection may develop CMV infection of peripheral nerves, either alone or in combination with involvement of nerve roots and spinal cord. Patients present with back and leg pain, flaccid paraparesis with areflexia, multimodal sensory loss, and impairment of bowel and bladder function. The CSF shows a polymorphonuclear pleocytosis with an elevated protein and, in some patients, a decreased glucose. As noted earlier, this CSF profile is extremely unusual in viral infections and should suggest the diagnosis of CMV polyradiculopathy in the appropriate clinical setting. CMV inclusions and antigen can be detected in Schwann cells of affected nerves, and CSF cultures or PCR are frequently positive for CMV. Rare cases of CMV-associated multiple mononeuropathy have also been reported. Patients present with radial, peroneal, or sural neuropathies alone or in combination. CMV antigen can be detected in Schwann cells of involved nerves, indicating that the neuropathies are caused by direct viral infection. Evidence of demyelination may be present, and immune mechanisms may contribute to the pathogenesis of the nerve injury.

Viral spread from the site of initial inoculation to the CNS through nerves is integral to the pathogenesis of rabies virus infection (Chap. 197). Rabies virus particles have been detected by electron microscopy and rabies virus antigen by immunocytochemistry in nerves innervating the site of initial viral inoculation. Neural spread of virus is also a central feature of the pathogenesis of shingles (see above) and of recurrent herpes labialis and genitalis (Chap. 182).

Isolated cranial nerve palsies, especially of the facial nerve (Bell's palsy), have been attributed to HSV, VZV (Ramsay Hunt syndrome), HIV, EBV, enteroviruses, and mumps virus, although in many cases the etiologic relationship appears rather tenuous. Pathologic specimens are almost never available from acute cases of Bell's palsy because of the generally benign and self-limited nature of the illness. Virus has never been cultured from the facial nerve, nor have viral antigens or nucleic acid been detected. However, in a study of patients with peripheral facial palsy undergoing decompressive facial nerve surgery, HSV DNA was found by PCR in endoneurial fluid from the facial nerve in ~80% of 14 patients with Bell's palsy, and VZV DNA was found in ~90% of those with Ramsay Hunt syndrome. This represents the strongest evidence to date for the direct role of these viruses in facial palsy.

Auditory and/or vestibular syndromes may also result from viral injury to the eighth cranial nerve. Mumps, measles, and VZV have been associated with cases of unilateral or bilateral nerve deafness. Seroepidemiologic studies also suggest a possible role for parainfluenza viruses, adenoviruses, and HSV in acute hearing loss. HSV has also been suggested to have a role in the pathogenesis of some cases of vestibular neuritis, based on detection of HSV DNA by PCR in vestibular ganglia.

CHRONIC AND PERSISTENT VIRAL CNS DISEASE

PROGRESSIVE MULTIFOCAL LEUKOENCEPHALOPATHY **Clinical Features and Pathology** Progressive multifocal leukoencephalopathy (PML) is a progressive disorder characterized pathologically by multifocal areas of demyelination of varying size distributed throughout the CNS. In addition to demyelination, there are characteristic cytologic alterations in both astrocytes and oligodendrocytes. Astrocytes are tremendously enlarged and contain hyperchromatic, deformed, and bizarre nuclei and frequent mitotic figures. Oligodendrocytes have enlarged, densely staining nuclei that contain viral inclusions formed by crystalline arrays of JC virus particles. Patients often present with visual deficits (45%), typically a homonymous hemianopia, and mental impairment (38%) (dementia, confusion, personality change). Motor weakness may not be present early but eventually occurs in 75% of cases.

Almost all patients (>95%) have an underlying immunosuppressive disorder. Prior to the HIV epidemic, common associated diseases included lymphoproliferative disorders, immune deficiency states, myeloproliferative disease, and chronic infectious or granulomatous diseases. Since 1984, the importance of these associated disorders in PML has been dwarfed by that of AIDS; >60% of currently diagnosed PML cases occur in patients with AIDS. Conversely, it has been estimated that nearly 1% of AIDS patients will develop PML. Early indications suggest that the basic features of AIDS-associated PML do not differ significantly from those of non-AIDS-associated PML.

Diagnostic Studies The diagnosis of PML is frequently suggested by MRI or less commonly CT. MRI is more sensitive than CT and reveals multifocal asymmetric, coalescing white matter lesions located periventricularly, in the centrum semiovale, in the parietal-occipital region, and in the cerebellum. These lesions have increased T2 and decreased T1 signal. The lesions of PML are generally nonenhancing or show only minimal peripheral enhancement and are not associated with edema or mass effect. CT shows hypodense nonenhancing white matter lesions without edema or mass effect.

The CSF is typically normal, although mild elevation in protein and/or IgG may be found. Pleocytosis occurs in <25% of cases, is predominantly mononuclear, and rarely exceeds 25 cells/μL. PCR amplification of JC virus DNA from CSF has become an important diagnostic tool. CSF PCR for JC virus DNA has high specificity, but sensitivity has varied among studies. Rare cases of positive CSF PCR for JC virus DNA in the absence of clinical or radiographic evidence of PML have been described in HIV-infected patients. It remains to be established whether these results are false positives or are indicative of preclinical PML.

The presence of a positive CSF PCR for JC virus DNA in association with typical MRI lesions in the appropriate clinical setting is diagnostic of PML. Patients with negative CSF PCR studies may require brain biopsy for definitive diagnosis. In biopsy or necropsy specimens of brain, JC virus antigen and nucleic acid can be detected by immunocytochemistry, in situ hybridization, or PCR amplification. Detection of JC virus antigen or genomic material should only be considered diagnostic of PML if accompanied by characteristic pathologic changes, since both antigen and genomic material have been found in the brains of normal patients.

℞ **TREATMENT** No effective therapy for PML is available. Intravenous and/or intrathecal cytarabine were not shown to be of benefit in a recent randomized controlled trial. Based on isolated case reports of benefit in some patients, a randomized controlled trial of cidofovir is currently under way. Some patients with HIV-associated PML have shown dramatic clinical improvement associated with improvement in their immune status following institution of highly active antiretroviral therapy.

SUBACUTE SCLEROSING PANENCEPHALITIS **Clinical Features and Epidemiology** SSPE is a rare chronic progressive demyelinating disease of the CNS associated with a chronic nonpermissive infection of brain tissue with measles virus. Fewer than 10 cases per year are reported in the United States. The incidence has declined substantially since the introduction of a measles vaccine. Most patients give a history of primary measles infection at an early age (2 years), which is followed after a latent interval of 6 to 8 years by the development of a progressive neurologic disorder. Some 85% of patients are between 5 and 15 years old at diagnosis. Initial manifestations include poor school performance and mood and personality changes. Typical signs of a CNS viral infection, including fever and headache, do not occur. As the disease progresses, patients develop progressive intellectual deterioration, focal and/or generalized seizures, myoclonus, ataxia, and visual disturbances. In the late stage of the illness, patients are unresponsive, quadriparetic, and spastic, with hyperactive tendon reflexes and extensor plantar responses.

Diagnostic Studies The EEG shows a characteristic periodic pattern with bursts every 3 to 8 s of high-voltage, sharp slow waves, followed by periods of attenuated ("flat") background. The CSF is acellular with a normal or mildly elevated protein level and a markedly elevated γ-globulin level (>20% of total CSF protein). CSF antimeasles antibody levels are invariably elevated, and oligoclonal antimeasles antibodies are often present. CT and MRI show evidence of multifocal white matter lesions, cortical atrophy, and ex vacuo ventricular enlargement. Measles virus can be cultured from brain tissue using special cocultivation techniques. Viral antigen can be identified immunocytochemically, and viral genome can be detected by in situ hybridization or PCR amplification.

℞ **TREATMENT** No definitive therapy for SSPE is available. Treatment with Inosiplex (isoprinosine) (100 mg/kg per day), alone or in combination with intrathecal or intraventricular interferon, has been reported to prolong survival and produce clinical improvement in some patients but has never been subjected to a controlled clinical trial.

PROGRESSIVE RUBELLA PANENCEPHALITIS **Clinical Features and Epidemiology** This is an extremely rare disorder that primarily affects children with congenital rubella syndrome, although isolated cases have been reported following childhood rubella. All the approximately 20 cases reported to date have been in male children. After a latent period of 8 to 19 years, patients develop progressive neurologic deterioration. The initial manifestations are similar to those seen in SSPE and include decline in school performance, behavioral alterations, and seizures, followed by severe progressive dementia, prominent ataxia, pyramidal signs (spasticity, hyperreflexia, extensor plantar responses), and visual deterioration. In the terminal stages of the illness, patients are globally demented, mute, and quadriparetic, often with associated ophthalmoplegia.

Diagnostic Studies CSF shows a mild lymphocytic pleocytosis, slightly elevated protein level, markedly increased γ-globulin, and rubella virus–specific oligoclonal bands. CT scan may show enlarged ventricles, cortical and cerebellar atrophy, and hypodensity in the white matter. Rubella virus has been isolated from explant and cocultivation cultures of brain biopsy material in one reported case.

℞ **TREATMENT** No therapy is currently available. Isoprinosine and amantadine are of no benefit. Universal prevention of both congenital and childhood rubella through the use of the available live attenuated rubella vaccine would be expected to eliminate the disease.

BIBLIOGRAPHY

BALE JF: Viral encephalitis. Med Clin North Am 77:25, 1993

BERGER JR, CONCHA M: Progressive multifocal leukoencephalopathy: The evolution of a disease once considered rare. J Neurovirol 1:5, 1995

CINQUE P et al: The role of laboratory investigation in the diagnosis and management of patients with suspected herpes simplex encephalitis: A consensus report. J Neurol Neurosurg Psychiatr 61:339, 1996

COHEN JI et al: Recent advances in varicella-zoster virus infection. Ann Intern Med 130: 922, 1999

CONNOLLY KJ, HAMMER SM: The acute aseptic meningitis syndrome. Infect Dis Clin North Am 4:599, 1990

DEBIASI R, TYLER KL: Polymerase chain reaction in the diagnosis and management of central nervous system infections. Arch Neurol 56:1215 , 1999

FONG IW, TOMA E: The natural history of progressive multifocal leukoencephalopathy in patients with AIDS. Clin Infect Dis 20:1305, 1995

GILDEN DH et al: Neurologic complications of the reactivation of varicella-zoster virus. N Engl J Med 342:635, 2000

GOH KJ et al: Clinical features of Nipah virus encephalitis among pig farmers in Malaysia. N Engl J Med 342:1229, 2000

JOHNSON RT: Acute encephalitis. Clin Infect Dis 20:971, 1995

———: *Viral Infections of the Nervous System*, 2d ed. Philadelphia, Lippincott Raven, 1998

LANCIOTTI RS et al: Origin of the West Nile virus responsible for an outbreak of encephalitis in the northeastern United States. Science 286:2333, 1999

ROOS KL (ed): Central nervous system infections. Semin Neurol 12:155, 1992

ROTBART HA: Enteroviral infections of the central nervous system. Clin Infect Dis 20: 971, 1995

RUST RS et al: La Crosse and other forms of California encephalitis. J Child Neurol 14: 1, 1999

SCHELD WM et al: *Infections of the Central Nervous System*, 2d ed. New York, Lippincott-Raven, 1997

TSAI TF: Arboviral infections in the United States. Infect Dis Clin North Am 5:73, 1991

TYLER KL, MARTIN JB (eds): Contemporary Neurology Series, vol 41: *Infectious Diseases of the Central Nervous System*. Philadelphia, FA Davis, 1993

374 CHRONIC AND RECURRENT MENINGITIS

Walter J. Koroshetz, Morton N. Swartz

Chronic inflammation of the meninges (pia, arachnoid, and dura) can produce profound neurologic disability and may be fatal if not successfully treated. The condition is most commonly diagnosed when a characteristic neurologic syndrome exists for >4 weeks and is associated with a persistent inflammatory response in the cerebrospinal fluid (CSF) (white blood cell count >5/μL). The causes are varied, and appropriate treatment depends on identification of the etiology. Five categories of disease account for most cases of chronic meningitis: (1) meningeal infections, (2) malignancy, (3) noninfectious inflammatory disorders, (4) chemical meningitis, and (5) parameningeal infections.

CLINICAL PATHOPHYSIOLOGY Neurologic manifestations of chronic meningitis (Table 374-1) are determined by the anatomic location of the inflammation and its consequences. Persistent headache with or without stiff neck and hydrocephalus, cranial neuropathies, radiculopathies, and cognitive or personality changes are the cardinal features. These can occur alone or in combination. When they appear in combination, widespread dissemination of the inflammatory process along CSF pathways has occurred. In some cases, the presence of an underlying systemic illness points to a specific agent or class of agents as the probable cause. The diagnosis of chronic meningitis is usually made when the clinical presentation prompts the astute physician to examine the CSF for signs of inflammation.

CSF is produced by the choroid plexus of the cerebral ventricles, exits through narrow foramina into the subarachnoid space surrounding the brain and spinal cord, circulates around the base of the brain and over the cerebral hemispheres, and is resorbed by arachnoid villi projecting into the superior sagittal sinus. CSF flow provides a pathway for rapid spread of infectious and malignant processes over the brain, spinal cord, and cranial and spinal nerve roots. Spread from the subarachnoid space into brain parenchyma may occur via the arachnoid cuffs that surround blood vessels that penetrate brain tissue (Virchow-Robin spaces).

Intracranial Meningitis Nociceptive fibers of the meninges (Chap. 15) are stimulated by the inflammatory process, resulting in headache or neck or back pain. Obstruction of CSF pathways at foramina or arachnoid villi may produce *hydrocephalus* and symptoms of raised intracranial pressure, including headache, vomiting, apathy or drowsiness, gait instability, papilledema, visual loss, impaired upgaze, or palsy of the seventh cranial nerve (CN) (Chap. 376). Cognitive and behavioral changes during the course of chronic meningitis may also result from vascular damage, which may similarly produce seizures, stroke, or myelopathy.

Inflammatory deposits seeded via the CSF circulation are often prominent around the brainstem and cranial nerves and along the undersurface of the frontal and temporal lobes. Such cases, termed *basal meningitis*, often present as multiple cranial neuropathies, with visual loss (CN II), facial weakness (CN VII), hearing loss (CN VIII), diplopia (CNs III, IV, and VI), sensory or motor abnormalities of the oropharynx (CNs IX, X, and XII), decreased olfaction (CN I), or facial sensory loss and masseter weakness (CN V).

Spinal Meningitis Injury may occur to motor and sensory roots as they traverse the subarachnoid space and penetrate the meninges. These cases present as multiple radiculopathies with combinations of radicular pain, sensory loss, motor weakness, and sphincter dysfunc-

Table 374-1 Symptoms and Signs of Chronic Meningitis

Symptoms	Signs
Chronic headache	+/− Papilledema
Neck or back pain	Brudzinski's or Kernig's sign of meningeal irritation
Change in personality	Altered mental status—drowsiness, inattention, disorientation, memory loss, frontal release signs (grasp, suck, snout), perseveration
Facial weakness	Peripheral seventh CN palsy
Double vision	Palsy of CNs III, IV, VI
Visual loss	Papilledema, optic atrophy
Hearing loss	Eighth CN palsy
Arm or leg weakness	Myelopathy or radiculopathy
Numbness in arms or legs	Myelopathy or radiculopathy
Sphincter dysfunction	Myelopathy or radiculopathy Frontal lobe dysfunction
Clumsiness	Ataxia

NOTE: CN, cranial nerve.

tion. Meningeal inflammation can encircle the cord, resulting in myelopathy. Patients with slowly progressive involvement of multiple cranial nerves and/or spinal nerve roots are likely to have chronic meningitis. Electrophysiologic testing (electromyography, nerve conduction studies, and evoked response testing) may be helpful in determining whether there is involvement of cranial and spinal nerve roots.

Systemic Manifestations In some patients, evidence of systemic disease provides clues to the underlying cause of chronic meningitis. A careful history and physical examination are essential before embarking on a diagnostic workup, which may be costly, prolonged, and associated with risk from invasive procedures. A complete history of travel, sexual practice, and exposure to infectious agents should be sought. Infectious causes are often associated with fever, malaise, anorexia, and signs of localized or disseminated infection outside the nervous system. Infectious causes are of major concern in the immunosuppressed patient, especially in patients with AIDS, in whom chronic meningitis may present without headache or fever. Noninfectious inflammatory disorders often produce systemic manifestations, but meningitis may be the initial manifestation. Carcinomatous meningitis may or may not be accompanied by clinical evidence of the primary neoplasm.

Approach to the Patient

The occurrence of chronic headache, hydrocephalus, cranial neuropathy, radiculopathy, and/or cognitive decline in a patient should prompt consideration of a lumbar puncture for evidence of meningeal inflammation. On occasion the diagnosis is made when an imaging study [computed tomography (CT) or magnetic resonance imaging (MRI)] shows contrast enhancement of the meninges, always an abnormal finding except after a recent neurosurgical procedure. Once chronic meningitis is confirmed by CSF examination, effort is focused on identifying the cause (Tables 374-2 and 374-3) by (1) further analysis of the CSF, (2) diagnosis of an underlying systemic infection or noninfectious inflammatory condition, or (3) pathologic examination of meningeal biopsy specimens.

Two clinical forms of chronic meningitis exist. In the first, the symptoms are chronic and persistent, whereas in the second there are recurrent, discrete episodes of illness. In the latter group, all symptoms, signs, and CSF parameters of meningeal inflammation resolve completely between episodes without specific therapy. In such patients, the likely etiologies include infection with herpes simplex virus (HSV) type 2; chemical meningitis due to leakage into CSF of contents from an epidermoid tumor, craniopharyngioma, or cholesteatoma; primary inflammatory conditions, including Vogt-Koyanagi-Harada syndrome, Behçet's syndrome (Chap. 316), Mollaret's meningitis, and systemic lupus erythematosus (SLE; Chap. 311); and drug hypersensitivity with repeated administration of the offending agent. The duration of chronic meningitis may also be of value in diagnosis; for example, an untreated patient with tuberculous meningitis is unlikely to survive beyond 4 to 6 weeks.

The epidemiologic history is of considerable importance and may provide direction for selection of laboratory studies. Pertinent features include a history of tuberculosis or exposure to a likely case; past travel to areas endemic for fungal infections (the San Joaquin Valley in California and southwestern states for coccidioidomycosis; midwestern states for histoplasmosis, southeastern states for blastomycosis); travel to the Mediterranean region or ingestion of imported unpasteurized dairy products (*Brucella*); time spent in areas endemic for Lyme disease (e.g., Connecticut, New York, Massachusetts); exposure to sexually transmitted disease (syphilis); exposure of an immunocompromised host to pigeons and their droppings (*Cryptococcus*); gardening (*Sporothrix schenkii*); ingestion of poorly cooked meat or contact with a household cat (*Toxoplasma gondii*); residence in Thailand or Japan (*Gnathostoma spinigerum*) or the South Pacific (*Angiostrongylus cantonensis*); rural residence and raccoon exposure (*Baylisascaris procyonis*); and residence in Latin America, the Philippines, or Southeast Asia when eosinophilic meningitis is present (*Taenia solium*).

The presence of focal cerebral signs in a patient with chronic meningitis suggests the possibility of a brain abscess or other parameningeal infection; identification of a potential source of infection (chronic draining ear, sinusitis, right-to-left cardiac or pulmonary shunt, chronic pleuropulmonary infection) supports this diagnosis. In some cases, diagnosis may be established by recognition and biopsy of unusual skin lesions (Behçet's syndrome, cryptococcosis, blastomycosis, SLE, Lyme disease, intravenous drug use, sporotrichosis, trypanosomiasis) or enlarged lymph nodes (lymphoma, tuberculosis, sarcoid, infection with HIV, secondary syphilis, or Whipple's disease). A careful ophthalmologic examination may reveal uveitis [Vogt-Koyanagi-Harada syndrome, sarcoid, or central nervous system (CNS) lymphoma], keratoconjunctivitis sicca (Sjögren's syndrome), or iridocyclitis (Behçet's syndrome) and is essential to assess visual loss from hydrocephalus. Aphthous oral lesions, genital ulcers, and hypopyon suggest Behçet's syndrome. Hepatosplenomegaly suggests lymphoma, sarcoid, tuberculosis, or brucellosis. Herpetic lesions in the genital area or on the thighs suggests HSV-2 infection. A breast nodule, a suspicious pigmented skin lesion, or an abdominal mass directs attention to possible carcinomatous meningitis.

Imaging Once the clinical syndrome is recognized as a potential manifestation of chronic meningitis, proper analysis of the CSF is essential. However, if the possibility of raised intracranial pressure exists, a brain imaging study should be performed before lumbar puncture. In patients with communicating hydrocephalus caused by impaired resorption of CSF, lumbar puncture is safe and may lead to temporary improvement. However, if intracranial pressure is elevated because of a mass lesion, brain swelling, or a block in ventricular CSF outflow (obstructive hydrocephalus), then lumbar puncture carries the potential risk of brain herniation (Fig. 374-1). Obstructive hydrocephalus usually requires direct ventricular drainage of CSF.

Contrast-enhanced MRI or CT studies of the brain and spinal cord can identify meningeal enhancement, parameningeal infections (including brain abscess), encasement of the spinal cord (malignancy or inflammation and infection), or nodular deposits on the meninges or nerve roots (malignancy or sarcoidosis). Imaging studies are also useful to localize areas of meningeal disease prior to meningeal biopsy.

Cerebral angiography may be indicated in patients with chronic meningitis and stroke to identify cerebral arteritis (granulomatous angiitis, infectious arteritis).

Cerebrospinal Fluid Analysis The CSF pressure should be measured and samples sent for bacterial culture, cell count and differential, Gram's stain, and measurement of glucose and protein. In cases without a known cause, CSF should be sent for the Venereal Disease Research Laboratories (VDRL) test, acid-fast bacillus (AFB) stain and culture, fungal wet mount and India ink preparation and culture, culture for fastidious bacteria and fungi, assays for cryptococcal antigen and oligoclonal immunoglobulin bands, and cytology. Other specific CSF tests (Tables 374-2 and 374-3) or blood tests and cultures should be ordered as indicated on the basis of the history, physical examination, or preliminary CSF results (i.e., eosinophilic, mononuclear, or polymorphonuclear meningitis). Rapid diagnosis may be facilitated by polymerase chain reaction (PCR) testing to identify DNA sequences in the CSF that are specific for the suspected pathogenic organism.

In most categories of chronic (not recurrent) meningitis, mononuclear cells predominate in the CSF. When neutrophils predominate after 3 weeks of illness, the principal etiologic considerations are *Nocardia asteroides*, *Actinomyces israelii*, *Brucella*, *Mycobacterium tuberculosis* (5 to 10% of early cases only), various fungi (*Blastomyces dermatitidis*, *Candida albicans*, *Histoplasma capsulatum*, *Aspergillus* species, *Pseudallescheria boydii*, *Cladophialophora bantiana*) and noninfectious causes (SLE, exogenous chemical meningitis). When eosinophils predominate or are present in limited numbers in a primarily mononuclear cell response in the CSF, the differential diagnosis

Table 374-2 Infectious Causes of Chronic Meningitis

Causative Agent	CSF Formula	Helpful Diagnostic Tests	Risk Factors and Systemic Manifestations
COMMON BACTERIAL CAUSES			
Partially treated suppurative meningitis	Mononuclear or mixed mononuclear-polymorphonuclear cells	CSF culture and Gram's stain	History consistent with acute bacterial meningitis and incomplete treatment
Parameningeal infection	Mononuclear or mixed mononuclear-polymorphonuclear cells	Contrast-enhanced MRI or CT to detect parenchymal, subdural, epidural, or sinus infection	Otitis media, pleuropulmonary infection, right-to-left cardiopulmonary shunt for brain abscess, focal neurologic signs; neck, back, ear, or sinus tenderness
Mycobacterium tuberculosis	Mononuclear cells except polymorphonuclear cells in early infection (leukocytes commonly <500/μL); low CSF glucose, elevated protein	Tuberculin skin test may be negative; AFB culture of CSF (sputum, urine, gastric contents if indicated); tuberculostearic acid detection in CSF; identify tubercle bacillus on acid-fast stain of CSF or protein pellicle; PCR	Exposure history; previous tuberculous illness; immunosuppressed or AIDS; young children; fever, meningismus, night sweats, miliary TB on x-ray or liver biopsy; stroke due to arteritis
Lyme disease (Bannwarth's syndrome): *Borrelia burgdorferi*	Mononuclear cells; elevated protein	Serum Lyme antibody titer; western blot confirmation; (patients with syphilis may have false-positive Lyme titer)	History of tick bite or appropriate exposure history; erythema chronicum migrans rash; arthritis, radiculopathy, Bell's palsy, meningoencephalitis–multiple sclerosis-like syndrome
Syphilis (secondary, tertiary): *Treponema pallidum*	Mononuclear cells; elevated protein	CSF VDRL; serum VDRL (or RPR); FTA or MHA-TP; serum VDRL may be negative in tertiary syphilis	Appropriate exposure history; HIV seropositive individuals at increased risk of aggressive infection; ''dementia''; cerebral infarction due to endarteritis
UNCOMMON BACTERIAL CAUSES			
Actinomyces	Polymorphonuclear cells	Anaerobic culture	Parameningeal abscess or sinus tract (oral or dental focus); pneumonitis
Nocardia	Polymorphonuclear cells; occasionally mononuclear cells; often low glucose	Isolation may require weeks; weakly acid fast	Associated brain abscess may be present
Brucella	Mononuclear cells (rarely polymorphonuclear); elevated protein; often low glucose	CSF antibody detection; serum antibody detection	Intake of unpasteurized dairy products; exposure to goats, sheep, cows; fever, arthralgia, myalgia, vertebral osteomyelitis
Whipple's disease: *Tropherema whippelii*	Mononuclear cells	Biopsy of small bowel or lymph node; CSF PCR for *T. whippelii*; brain and meningeal biopsy (with PAS stain and EM examination)	Diarrhea, weight loss, arthralgias, fever; dementia, ataxia, paresis, ophthalmoplegia, oculomasticatory myoclonus
RARE BACTERIAL CAUSES			
Leptospirosis (occasionally if left untreated may last 3–4 weeks); *Pseudoallescheria boydii* (neutrophilic pleocytosis)			
FUNGAL CAUSES			
Cryptococcus neoformans	Mononuclear cells; count not elevated in some patients with AIDS	India ink or fungal wet mount of CSF (budding yeast); blood and urine cultures; antigen detection in CSF	AIDS and immunosuppression; pigeon exposure; skin and other organ involvement due to disseminated infection
Coccidioides immitis	Mononuclear cells (sometimes 10–20% eosinophils); often low glucose	Antibody detection in CSF and serum	Exposure history—southwestern US; increased virulence in dark-skinned races
Candida sp.	Polymorphonuclear or mononuclear cells	Fungal stain and culture of CSF	IV drug abuse; recent surgery; prolonged intravenous therapy; disseminated candidiasis
Histoplasma capsulatum	Mononuclear cells; low glucose	Fungal stain and culture of large volumes of CSF; antigen detection in CSF, serum, and urine; antibody detection in serum, CSF	Exposure history—Ohio and central Mississippi River Valley; AIDS; mucosal lesions
Blastomyces dermatitidis	Mononuclear cells	Fungal stain and culture of CSF; biopsy and culture of skin, lung lesions; antibody detection in serum	Midwestern and southeastern US; usually systemic infection; abscesses, draining sinus, ulcers
Aspergillus sp.	Mononuclear or polymorphonuclear cells	CSF culture	Sinusitis; granulocytopenia or immunosuppression
Sporothrix schenckii	Mononuclear cells	Antibody detection in CSF and serum; CSF culture	Traumatic inoculation; IV drug use; ulcerated skin lesion
RARE FUNGAL CAUSES			
Cladophialophora bantiana (formerly *Cladosporium trichoides*) and other dark-walled (dematiaceous) fungi such as *Curvularia* and *Drechslera*; *Mucor*			

(continued)

Table 374-2 Infectious Causes of Chronic Meningitis—*(continued)*

Causative Agent	CSF Formula	Helpful Diagnostic Tests	Risk Factors and Systemic Manifestations
PROTOZOAL CAUSES			
Toxoplasma gondii	Mononuclear cells	Biopsy or response to empirical therapy in clinically appropriate context (including presence of antibody in serum)	Usually with intracerebral abscesses; common in HIV-seropositive patients
Trypanosomiasis *Trypanosoma gambiense, Trypanosoma rhodesiense*	Mononuclear cells, elevated protein level	Elevated CSF IgM; identification of trypanosomes in CSF and blood smear	Endemic in Africa; chancre, lymphadenopathy; prominent sleep disorder
RARE PROTOZOAL CAUSES			
Acanthamoeba sp. causing granulomatous amebic encephalitis and meningoencephalitis in immunocompromised and debilitated individuals			
HELMINTHIC CAUSES			
Cysticercosis (infection with cysts of *Taenia solium*)	Mononuclear cells; may have eosinophils; glucose level may be low	Indirect hemagglutination assay in CSF; ELISA immunoblotting in serum	Usually with multiple cysts in basal meninges and hydrocephalus; cerebral cysts, muscle calcification
Gnathostoma spinigerum	Eosinophils, mononuclear cells	Peripheral eosinophilia	History of eating raw fish; common in Thailand and Japan; subarachnoid hemorrhage; painful radiculopathy
Angiostrongylus cantonensis	Eosinophils, mononuclear cells	Recovery of worms from CSF	History of eating raw shellfish; common in tropical Pacific regions; often benign
Baylisascaris procyonis (raccoon ascarid)	Eosinophils, mononuclear cells		Infection follows accidental ingestion of *B. procyonis* eggs from raccoon feces; fatal meningoencephalitis
RARE HELMINTHIC CAUSES			
Trichinella spiralis (trichinosis); *Echinococcus* cysts; *Schistosoma* sp. The first may produce a lymphocytic pleocytosis, whereas the latter two may produce an eosinophilic response in CSF associated with cerebral cysts (*Echinococcus*) or granulomatous lesions of brain or spinal cord			
VIRAL CAUSES			
Mumps	Mononuclear cells	Antibody in serum	No prior mumps or immunization; may produce meningoencephalitis; may persist for 3–4 weeks
Lymphocytic choriomeningitis	Mononuclear cells	Antibody in serum	Contact with rodents or their excreta; may persist for 3–4 weeks
Echovirus	Mononuclear cells; may have low glucose	Virus isolation from CSF	Congenital hypogammaglobulinemia; history of recurrent meningitis
HIV (acute retroviral syndrome)	Mononuclear cells	p24 antigen in serum and CSF; high level of HIV viremia	HIV risk factors; rash, fever, lymphadenopathy; lymphopenia in peripheral blood; syndrome may persist long enough to be considered chronic meningitis; or chronic meningitis may develop in later stages (AIDS) due to HIV
Herpes simplex (HSV)	Mononuclear cells	PCR for HSV DNA; CSF antibody	Recurrent meningitis due to HSV-2 (rarely HSV-1) often associated with genital recurrences

ABBREVIATIONS: AFB, acid-fast bacillus stain; CSF, cerebrospinal fluid; ELISA, enzyme-linked immunosorbent assay; EM, electron microscopy; FTA, fluorescent treponemal antibody absorption test; IV, intravenous; MHA-TP, microhemagglutination assay-*Treponema pallidum*; PAS, periodic acid–Schiff; PCR, polymerase chain reaction; RPR, rapid plasma reagin test; TB, tuberculosis; VDRL, Venereal Disease Research Laboratories test.

includes parasitic diseases (*A. cantonensis*, *G. spinigerum*, *B. procyonis*, or *Toxocara canis* infection, cysticercosis, schistosomiasis, echinococcal disease, *T. gondii* infection), fungal infections (6 to 20% eosinophils along with a predominantly lymphocyte pleocytosis, particularly with coccidioidal meningitis), neoplastic disease (lymphoma, leukemia, metastatic carcinoma), or other inflammatory processes (sarcoidosis, hypereosinophilic syndrome).

It is often necessary to broaden the number of diagnostic tests if the initial workup does not reveal the cause. In addition, repeated samples of large volumes of CSF may be required to diagnose certain infectious and malignant causes of chronic meningitis. For instance, lymphomatous or carcinomatous meningitis may be diagnosed by examination of sections cut from a cell block formed by spinning down the sediment from a large volume of CSF. The diagnosis of fungal meningitis may require large volumes of CSF for culture of sediment. If standard lumbar puncture is unrewarding, a cervical cisternal tap to sample CSF near to the basal meninges may be fruitful.

Laboratory Investigation In addition to the CSF examination, an attempt should be made to uncover pertinent underlying illnesses. Tuberculin skin test, chest radiograph, urine analysis and culture, blood count and differential, renal and liver function tests, and measurement of electrolytes (including calcium and phosphate), sedimentation rate, antinuclear antibody, and serum angiotensin-converting enzyme level are often indicated. Liver or bone marrow biopsy may be diagnostic in some cases of miliary tuberculosis, disseminated fungal infection, sarcoidosis, or metastatic malignancy. Abnormalities discovered on chest radiograph or chest CT can be pursued by bronchoscopy or transthoracic needle biopsy.

Meningeal Biopsy A diagnostic meningeal biopsy should be strongly considered in patients who are severely disabled, who need

Table 374-3 Noninfectious Causes of Chronic Meningitis

Causative Agents	CSF Formula	Helpful Diagnostic Tests	Risk Factors and Systemic Manifestations
Malignancy	Mononuclear cells, elevated protein, low glucose	Repeated cytologic examination of large volumes of CSF; CSF exam by polarizing microscopy; clonal lymphocyte markers; deposits on nerve roots or meninges seen on myelogram or contrast-enhanced MRI; meningeal biopsy	Metastatic cancer of breast, lung, stomach, or pancreas; melanoma, lymphoma, leukemia; meningeal gliomatosis; meningeal sarcoma; cerebral dysgerminoma; meningeal melanoma or B cell lymphoma
Chemical compounds (may cause recurrent meningitis)	Mononuclear cells or PMNs, low glucose, elevated protein; xanthochromia from subarachnoid hemorrhage in week prior to presentation with "meningitis"	Contrast-enhanced CT scan or MRI; cerebral angiogram to detect aneurysm	History of recent injection into the subarachnoid space; history of sudden onset of headache; recent resection of acoustic neuroma or craniopharyngioma; epidermoid tumor of brain or spine, sometimes with dermoid sinus tract; pituitary apoplexy
Primary inflammation CNS sarcoidosis	Mononuclear cells; elevated protein; often low glucose	Serum and CSF angiotensin-converting enzyme levels; biopsy of extraneural affected tissues or brain lesion/meningeal biopsy	CN palsy, especially of CN VII; hypothalamic dysfunction, especially diabetes insipidus; abnormal chest radiograph; peripheral neuropathy or myopathy
Vogt-Koyanagi-Harada syndrome (recurrent meningitis)	Mononuclear cells		Recurrent meningoencephalitis with uveitis, retinal detachment, alopecia, lightening of eyebrows and lashes, dysacusis, cataracts, glaucoma
Isolated granulomatous angiitis of the nervous system	Mononuclear cells, elevated protein	Angiography or meningeal biopsy	Subacute dementia; multiple cerebral infarctions; recent zoster ophthalmicus
Systemic lupus erythematosus	Mononuclear or polymorphonuclear cells	Anti-DNA antibody, antinuclear antibodies	Encephalopathy; seizures; stroke; transverse myelopathy; rash; arthritis
Behçet's syndrome (recurrent meningitis)	Mononuclear or polymorphonuclear cells, elevated protein		Oral and genital aphthous ulcers; iridocyclitis; retinal hemorrhages; pathergic lesions at site of skin puncture
Chronic benign lymphocytic meningitis	Mononuclear cells		Recovery in 2–6 months, diagnosis by exclusion
Mollaret's recurrent meningitis	Large endothelial cells and polymorphonuclear cells in first hours, followed by mononuclear cells	PCR for herpes; MRI/CT to rule out epidermoid tumor or dural cyst	Recurrent meningitis; exclude HSV-2; rare cases due to HSV-1; occasional case associated with dural cyst
Drug hypersensitivity	Polymorphonuclear cells; occasionally mononuclear cells or eosinophils		Exposure to ibuprofen, sulfonamides, isoniazid, tolmetin, ciprofloxacin, pyridium; improvement after discontinuation of drug; recurrent episodes with recurrent exposure
Wegener's granulomatosis	Mononuclear cells	Chest and sinus radiographs; urinalysis; ANCA antibodies in serum	Associated sinus, pulmonary, or renal lesions; CN palsies; skin lesions; peripheral neuropathy
Other: multiple sclerosis, Sjögren's syndrome, and rarer forms of vasculitis (e.g., Cogan's syndrome)			

ABBREVIATIONS: ANCA, anti-neutrophil cytoplasmic antibodies; PMN, polymorphonuclear neutrophil; PCR, polymerase chain reaction.

chronic ventricular decompression, or whose illness is progressing rapidly. The activities of the surgeon, pathologist, microbiologist, and cytologist should be coordinated so that a large enough sample is obtained and the appropriate cultures and histologic and molecular studies, including electron microscopic and PCR studies, are performed. The diagnostic yield of meningeal biopsy can be increased by targeting regions that enhance with contrast on MRI or CT. With current microsurgical techniques, most areas of the basal meninges can be accessed for biopsy via a limited craniotomy. In a series from the Mayo Clinic reported by Cheng et al., MRI demonstrated meningeal enhancement in 47% of patients undergoing meningeal biopsy. Biopsy of an enhancing region was diagnostic in 80% of cases; biopsy of nonenhancing regions was diagnostic in only 9%; sarcoid (31%) and metastatic adenocarcinoma (25%) were the most common conditions identified.

Approach to the Enigmatic Case In approximately one-third of cases, the diagnosis is not known despite careful evaluation of CSF and potential extraneural sites of disease. A number of the organisms that cause chronic meningitis may take weeks to be identified by cultures. In enigmatic cases several options are available, determined by the extent of the clinical deficits and rate of progression. It is prudent to wait until cultures are finalized if the patient is asymptomatic or symptoms are mild and not progressive. Unfortunately, in many cases progressive neurologic deterioration occurs, and rapid treatment is required. Ventricular-peritoneal shunts may be placed to relieve hydrocephalus, but the risk of disseminating the undiagnosed inflammatory process into the abdomen must be considered.

Empirical Treatment Diagnosis of the causative agent is essential because effective therapies exist for many etiologies of chronic meningitis, but if the condition is left untreated, progressive damage

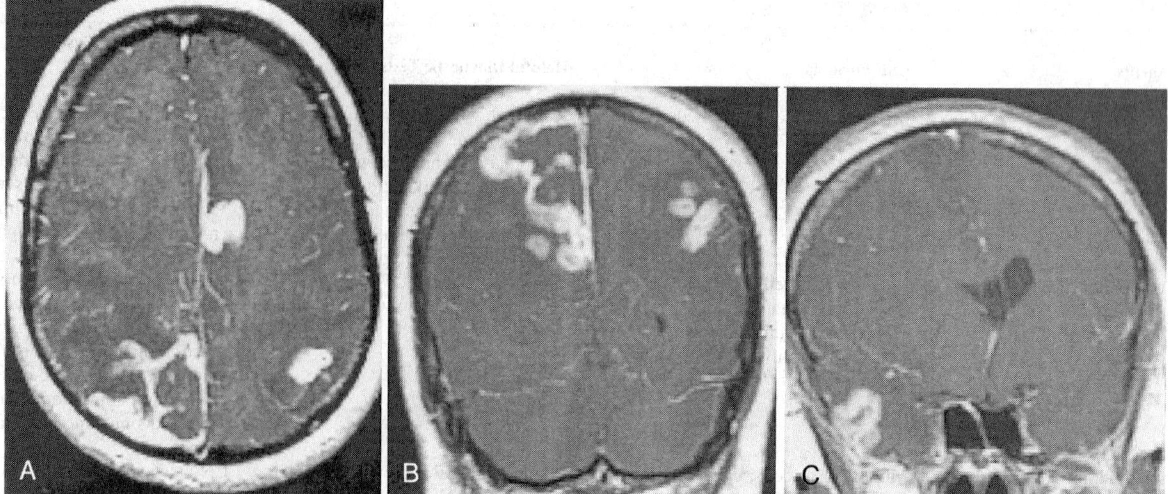

FIGURE 374-1 Tuberculosis. A 38-year-old man presented with a 2-year history of episodic left-sided numbness, transient speech arrest, and a 3-month history of headache with nausea. Axial (*A*) and coronal (*B*, *C*) T_1-weighted gadolinium-enhanced MRI scans showed pial- and dural-based enhancing mass lesions consistent with multiple cerebral tuberculomas; right-to-left horizontal displacement is seen in *C*. The meningeal enhancement indicates complicating tuberculous meningitis due to rupture of a tuberculoma into the subarachnoid space.

to the CNS and cranial nerves and roots is likely to occur. Occasionally, empirical therapy must be initiated when all attempts at diagnosis fail. In general, empirical therapy in the United States consists of antimycobacterial agents, amphotericin for fungal infection, or glucocorticoids for noninfectious inflammatory causes. It is important to direct empirical therapy of lymphocytic meningitis at tuberculosis, particularly if the condition is associated with hypoglycorrhachia and sixth and other CN palsies, since untreated disease is fatal in 4 to 8 weeks. In the Mayo Clinic series, the most useful empirical therapy was administration of glucocorticoids rather than antituberculous therapy. Carcinomatous or lymphomatous meningitis may be difficult to diagnose initially, but the diagnosis becomes evident with time.

THE IMMUNOSUPPRESSED PATIENT Chronic meningitis is not uncommon in the course of HIV infection. Pleocytosis and mild meningeal signs often occur at the onset of HIV infection, and occasionally low-grade meningitis persists. Toxoplasmosis commonly presents as intracranial abscesses and may also be associated with meningitis. Other important causes of chronic meningitis in AIDS include infection with *Cryptococcus*, *Nocardia*, *Candida*, or other fungi; syphilis; and lymphoma. Toxoplasmosis, cryptococcosis, nocardiosis, and other fungal infections are important etiologic considerations in individuals with immunodeficiency states other than AIDS, including those due to immunosuppressive medications. Because of the increased risk of chronic meningitis and the attenuation of clinical signs of meningeal irritation in immunosuppressed individuals, CSF examination should be performed for any persistent headache or unexplained change in mental state.

BIBLIOGRAPHY

ANDERSON NE, WILLOUGHBY EW: Chronic meningitis without predisposing illness. A review of 83 cases. Q J Med 63:283, 1987

BOUZA E et al: Coccidioidal meningitis. Medicine 60:139, 1981

——— et al: Brucellar meningitis. Rev Infect Dis 9:810, 1987

BROSS JE, GORDON G: Nocardial meningitis. Rev Infect Dis 13:160, 1991

CHARLESTON AJ et al: Idiopathic steroid-responsive chronic lymphocytic meningitis—clinical features and long-term outcome in 17 patients. Aust N Z J Med 28:784, 1998

CHENG TM et al: Chronic meningitis: The role of meningeal or cortical biopsy. Neurosurgery 34:590, 1994

JINNAH HA et al: Chronic meningitis with cranial neuropathies in Wegener's granulomatosis: Case report and review of the literature. Arthritis Rheum 40:573, 1997

MAYER SA et al: Biopsy-proven isolated sarcoid meningitis. J Neurosurgery 78:994, 1993

PEACOCK JE et al: Persistent neutrophilic meningitis. Medicine 63:379, 1984

PHILLIPS ME et al: Neoplastic versus inflammatory meningeal enhancement with Gd-DTPA. J Comput Assisted Tomogr 14:536, 1990

REIK L et al: Granulomatous angiitis presenting as chronic meningitis and ventriculitis. Neurology 33:1609, 1983

SCHELD WM et al: *Infections of the Central Nervous System*, 2nd ed. New York, Raven Press, 1997

SMITH JE, AKSAMIT AJ: Outcome of chronic idiopathic meningitis. Mayo Clinic Proc 69:548, 1994

SWARTZ MN: "Chronic meningitis"—many causes to consider. N Engl J Med 317:957, 1987

THWAITS G et al: Tuberculous meningitis. J Neurol Neurosurg Psychiatry 68:289, 2000

WHEAT LJ et al: Histoplasma capsulatum infections of the central nervous system. Medicine 69:244, 1990

375

Stanley B. Prusiner, Patrick Bosque

PRION DISEASES

Creutzfeldt-Jakob disease (CJD) is a degenerative disease of the central nervous system (CNS) that is caused by infectious proteins called *prions*. CJD typically presents with dementia and myoclonus, is relentlessly progressive, and usually results in death within a year of onset. Most patients with CJD are between 50 and 75 years of age; however, patients as young as 17 years and as old as 83 years have been recorded.

In mammals, prions reproduce by binding to the normal, *c*ellular isoform of the *pr*ion *p*rotein (PrP^C) and stimulating its conversion into the di*s*ease-*c*ausing isoform (PrP^{Sc}). PrP^C is rich in α-helix and has little β-sheet, while PrP^{Sc} has less α-helix and a high β-sheet content (Fig. 375-1). This α to β transition in prion protein (PrP) structure is the fundamental event underlying prion diseases, which are disorders of protein conformation (Table 375-1).

Four new concepts have emerged from studies of prions. First, prions are the only known infectious pathogens that are devoid of nucleic acid. All other infectious agents possess genomes composed of either RNA or DNA that direct the synthesis of their progeny. Second, prion diseases may be manifest as infectious, genetic, and sporadic disorders. No other group of illnesses with a single etiology presents with such a wide spectrum of clinical manifestations. Third, prion diseases result from the accumulation of PrP^{Sc}, the conformation of which differs substantially from that of its precursor PrP^C. Fourth, PrP^{Sc} can exist in a variety of different conformations, each of which seems to specify a specific disease phenotype. How a specific conformation of a PrP^{Sc} molecule is imparted to PrP^{C} during prion replication to produce nascent PrP^{Sc} with the same conformation is unknown. Additionally, it is unclear what factors determine where in the CNS a particular PrP^{Sc} molecule will be deposited.

SPECTRUM OF PRION DISEASES The sporadic form of CJD is the most common prion disorder in humans. Sporadic CJD (sCJD) accounts for ~85% of all cases of human prion disease, while inherited prion diseases account for 10 to 15% of all cases (Table 375-2). Familial CJD (fCJD), Gerstmann-Sträussler-Scheinker disease (GSS), and fatal familial insomnia (FFI) are all dominantly inherited prion diseases that are caused by mutations in the PrP gene.

Although infectious prion diseases account for <1% of all cases and infection does not seem to play an important role in the natural history of these illnesses, the transmissibility of prions is an important biologic feature. Kuru of the Fore people of New Guinea is thought to have resulted from the consumption of brains from dead relatives during ritualistic cannibalism. With the cessation of ritualistic cannibalism in the late 1950s, kuru has nearly disappeared with the exception of a few recent patients exhibiting incubation periods of almost 40 years. Iatrogenic CJD (iCJD) seems to be the result of the accidental inoculation of patients with prions. New variant CJD (nvCJD) in teenagers and young adults in Europe is the result of exposure to tainted beef from cattle with bovine spongiform encepalopathy (BSE).

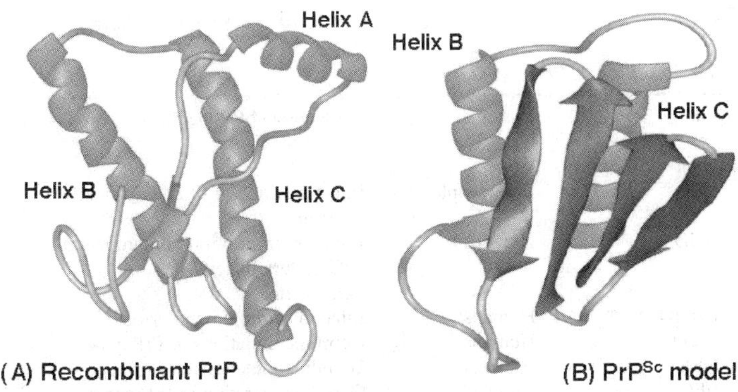

FIGURE 375-1 Structures of prion proteins. *A.* NMR structure of Syrian hamster recombinant (rec) PrP(90–231). Presumably, the structure of the α-helical form of recPrP(90–231) resembles that of PrP^{C}. recPrP(90–231) is viewed from the interface where PrP^{Sc} is thought to bind to PrP^{C}. Shown are: α-helices A (residues 144–157), B (172–193), and C (200–227). Flat ribbons depict B-strands S1 (129–131) and S2 (161–163). *(Reprinted with permission from H Lui et al: Biochemistry 38:5362, 1999.)* *B.* Plausible model for the tertiary structure of human PrP^{Sc}. Shown are α-helices B (residues 178–191) and C (202–218). β-strands are 108–113, 116–122, 128–135 and 138–144. *[Reprinted from Les Prix Nobel T. Frängsmyr (ed), Stockholm, Norstedts Tryckeri, 1998, pp 268–323, with permission.]*

Six diseases of animals are caused by prions (Table 375-2). Scrapie of sheep and goats is the prototypic prion disease. Mink encephalopathy, BSE, feline spongiform encephalopathy, and exotic ungulate encephalopathy are all thought to occur after the consumption of prion-infected foodstuffs. The origin of chronic wasting disease, a prion disease endemic in deer and elk in regions of North America, is uncertain.

EPIDEMIOLOGY CJD is found throughout the world. The incidence of sCJD is approximately one case per million population. Although many geographic clusters of CJD have been reported, each has been shown to segregate with a PrP gene mutation that results in a nonconservative substitution. Attempts to identify common exposure to some etiologic agent have been unsuccessful for both the sporadic and familial cases. Ingestion of scrapie-infected sheep or goat meat as a cause of CJD in humans has not been demonstrated by epidemiologic studies although speculation about this potential route of inoculation continues. Studies with Syrian hamsters demonstrate that oral infection with prions can occur, but the process is inefficient compared to intracerebral inoculation.

PATHOGENESIS The human prion diseases were initially classified as neurodegenerative disorders of unknown etiology on the basis of pathologic changes being confined to the CNS. With the transmission of kuru and CJD to apes, investigators began to view these diseases as CNS infectious illnesses caused by slow viruses. Even though the familial nature of a subset of CJD cases was well described, the significance of this observation became more obscure with the transmission of CJD to animals. Eventually, the meaning of heritable CJD became clear with the discovery of mutations in the *PrP* gene of these patients. The prion concept explains how a disease can manifest as a heritable as well as an infectious illness. Moreover, the hallmark common to all of the prion diseases, whether sporadic, dominantly inherited, or acquired by infection, is that they involve the aberrant metabolism of the prion protein.

A major feature that distinguishes prions from viruses is the finding that both PrP isoforms are encoded by a chromosomal gene. In humans, the *PrP* gene is designated *PRNP* and is located on the short arm of chromosome 20. Limited proteolysis of PrP^{Sc} produces a smaller, protease-resistant molecule of ~142 amino acids designated PrP 27-30; under the same conditions, PrP^{C} is completely hydrolyzed (Fig. 375-2). In the presence of detergent, PrP 27-30 polymerizes into amyloid. Prion amyloid formed by limited proteolysis and detergent extraction is indistinguishable from the filaments that aggregate to form PrP amyloid plaques in the CNS. Both the rods and the PrP amyloid filaments found in brain tissue exhibit similar ultrastructural morphology and green-gold birefringence after staining with Congo red dye.

Species Barrier Studies on the role of the primary and tertiary structures of PrP in the transmission of prion disease have given new insights into the pathogenesis of these maladies. The amino acid sequence of PrP encodes the species of the prion, and the prion derives its PrP^{Sc} sequence from the last mammal in which it was passaged. While the primary structure of PrP is likely to be the most important or even sole determinant of the tertiary structure of PrP^{C}, PrP^{Sc} seems to function as a template in determining the tertiary structure of nascent PrP^{Sc} molecules as they are formed from PrP^{C}. In turn, prion diversity appears to be enciphered in the conformation of PrP^{Sc}, and thus, prion strains seem to represent different conformers of PrP^{Sc}.

In general, transmission of prion disease from one species to another is inefficient, in that not all intracerebrally inoculated animals develop disease, and those that fall ill do so only after long incubation times that can approach the natural lifespan of the animal. This "species barrier" to transmission is correlated with the degree of homology between the amino acid sequence of PrP^{C} in the inoculated host and of PrP^{Sc} in the prion inoculum. The importance of sequence homology

Table 375-1 Glossary of Prion Terminology

Prion	**Pro**teinaceous **in**fectious particle that lacks nucleic acid. Prions are composed largely, if not entirely, of PrP^{Sc} molecules. They can cause scrapie in animals and related neurodegenerative diseases of humans such as Creutzfeldt-Jakob disease (CJD). "Scrapie agent" is a synonym.
PrP^{Sc}	Scrapie isoform of the prion protein. This protein is the only identifiable macromolecule in purified preparations of scrapie prions.
PrP^{C}	Cellular isoform of the prion protein. PrP^{C} is the precursor of PrP^{Sc}.
PrP 27-30	Limited digestion of PrP^{Sc} with proteinase K generates PrP 27-30 by truncation of the N terminus.
PRNP	PrP gene located on human chromosome 20.
Prion rod	An aggregate of prions composed largely of PrP 27-30 molecules. Created by detergent extraction and limited proteolysis of PrP^{Sc}. Morphologically and histochemically indistinguishable from many amyloids.
PrP amyloid	Amyloid containing PrP in the brain of animals or humans with prion disease; often accumulates as plaques.

Table 375-2 The Prion Diseases

Disease	Host	Mechanism of Pathogenesis
Human		
Kuru	Fore people	Infection through ritualistic cannibalism
iCJD	Humans	Infection from prion-contaminated hGH, dura mater grafts, etc.
nvCJD	Humans	Infection from bovine prions?
fCJD	Humans	Germline mutations in PrP gene
GSS	Humans	Germline mutations in PrP gene
FFI	Humans	Germline mutation in PrP gene (D178N, M129)
sCJD	Humans	Somatic mutation or spontaneous conversion of PrP^C into PrP^{Sc}?
sFI	Humans	Somatic mutation or spontaneous conversion of PrP^C into PrP^{Sc}?
Animal		
Scrapie	Sheep	Infection in genetically susceptible sheep
BSE	Cattle	Infection with prion-contaminated MBM
TME	Mink	Infection with prions from sheep or cattle
CWD	Mule deer, elk	Unknown
FSE	Cats	Infection with prion-contaminated beef
Exotic ungulate encephalopathy	Greater kudu, nyala, or oryx	Infection with prion-contaminated MBM

ABBREVIATIONS: BSE, bovine spongiform encephalopathy; CJD, Creutzfeldt-Jakob disease; sCJD, sporadic CJD; fCJD, familial CJD; iCJD, iatrogenic CJD; nvCJD, new variant CJD; CWD, chronic wasting disease; FFI, fatal familial insomnia; sFI, sporadic fatal insomnia; FSE, feline spongiform encephalopathy; GSS, Gerstmann-Sträussler-Scheinker disease; hGH, human growth hormone; MBM, meat and bone meal; TME, transmissible mink encephalopathy.

between the host and donor PrP argues that PrP^C directly interacts with PrP^{Sc} in the prion conversion process.

Prion Strains The existence of prion strains raised the question of how heritable biologic information can be enciphered in a molecule other than nucleic acid. Strains or varieties of prions have been defined by incubation times and the distribution of neuronal vacuolation. Subsequently, the patterns of PrP^{Sc} deposition were found to correlate with vacuolation profiles, and these patterns were also used to characterize strains of prions.

Persuasive evidence that strain-specific information is enciphered in the tertiary structure of PrP^{Sc} comes from transmission of two different inherited human prion diseases to mice expressing a chimeric human-mouse PrP transgene. In FFI, the protease-resistant fragment of PrP^{Sc} after deglycosylation has a molecular mass of 19 kDa, whereas in fCJD and most sporadic prion diseases, it is 21 kDa (Table 375-3). This difference in molecular mass was shown to be due to different sites of proteolytic cleavage at the NH_2 termini of the two human PrP^{Sc} molecules, reflecting different tertiary structures. These distinct conformations were not unexpected because the amino acid sequences of the PrPs differ.

Extracts from the brains of patients with FFI transmitted disease into mice expressing a chimeric human-mouse PrP transgene and induced formation of the 19-kDa PrP^{Sc}, whereas fCJD and sCJD produced the 21-kDa PrP^{Sc} in mice expressing the same transgene. On second passage, these differences were maintained, demonstrating that chimeric PrP^{Sc} can exist in two different conformations based on the sizes of the protease-resistant fragments even though the amino acid sequence of PrP^{Sc} is invariant.

This analysis was extended when patients with sporadic fatal insomnia (sFI) were identified. Although they did not carry a *PrP* gene mutation, the clinical and pathologic phenotype was indistinguishable from that of patients with FFI. Furthermore, 19-kDa PrP^{Sc} was found in their brains, and on passage of prion disease to mice expressing a

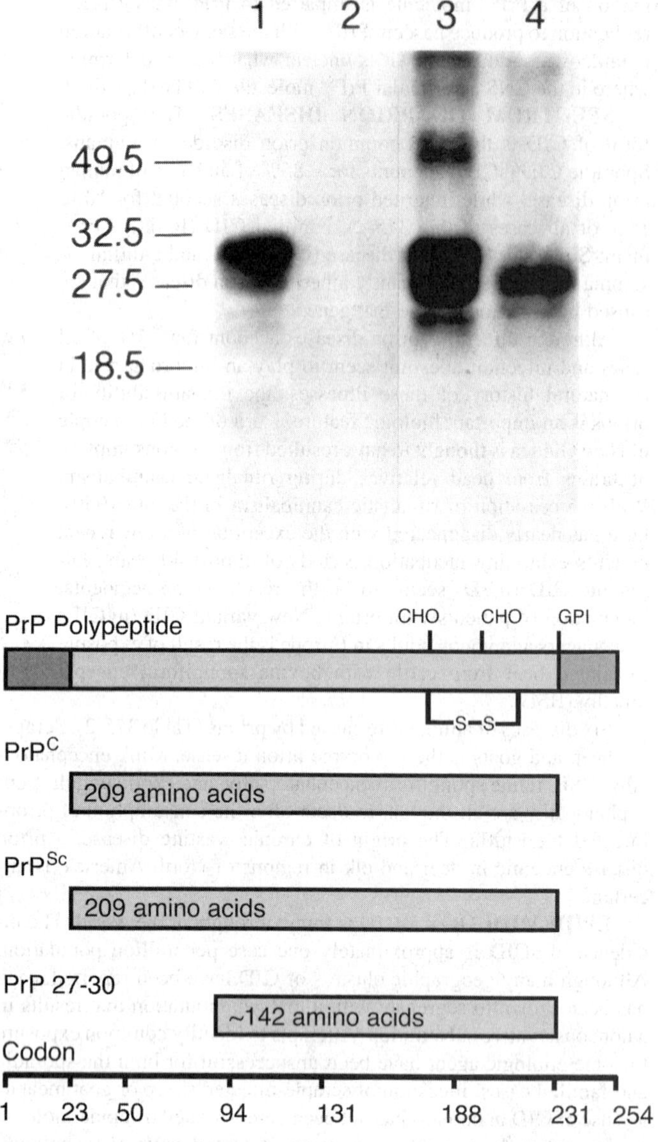

FIGURE 375-2 Prion protein isoforms. *A.* Western immunoblot of brain homogenates from uninfected (lanes 1 and 2) and prion-infected (lanes 3 and 4) Syrian hamsters. Samples in lanes 2 and 4 were digested with proteinase K. PrP^C in lanes 2 and 4 was completely hydrolyzed under these conditions, whereas in PrP^{Sc} (lane 4), approximately 67 amino acids were digested from the NH_2-terminus to generate PrP 27–30. The blot was developed with anti-PrP polyclonal rabbit antiserum. Molecular size markers (*left*) are in kilodaltons. *B.* Bar diagram of Syrian hamster PrP, which consists of 254 amino acids. After processing of the NH_2 and COOH termini, both PrP^C and PrP^{Sc} consist of 209 residues. After limited proteolysis, the NH_2 terminus of PrP^{Sc} is truncated to form PrP 27–30 composed of approximately 142 amino acids. *[Reprinted from Les Prix Nobel T. Frängsmyr (ed), Stockholm, Norstedts Tryckeri, 1998, pp 268–323, with permission.]*

chimeric human-mouse PrP transgene, PrP^{Sc} was also found. These findings indicate that the disease phenotype is dictated by the conformation of PrP^{Sc} and not the amino acid sequence. PrP^{Sc} acts as a template for the conversion of PrP^C into nascent PrP^{Sc}.

SPORADIC AND INHERITED PRION DISEASES

Initiation of sporadic disease may hypothetically follow from a somatic mutation and thus follow a path similar to that for germline mutations in inherited disease. In this situation, the mutant PrP^{Sc} must be capable of targeting wild type PrP^C, a process known to be possible for some mutations but less likely for others. Alternatively, the activation barrier separating wild type PrP^C from PrP^{Sc} could be crossed on rare occasions when viewed in the context of a population. Most individuals would be spared, while presentations in the elderly with an incidence of ~1 per million would be seen.

Twenty different mutations resulting in nonconservative substitutions in the human *PrP* gene have, to date, been found to segregate with inherited human prion diseases. Missense mutations and expansions in the octapeptide repeat region of the gene are responsible for familial forms of prion disease. Five different mutations of the *PrP* gene have been linked genetically to heritable prion disease.

Table 375-3 Distinct Prion Strains Generated in Humans with Inherited Prion Diseases and Transmitted to Transgenic Mice[a]

Inoculum	Host Species	Host PrP Genotype	Incubation Time [days ± SEM] (n/n_0)	PrP^{Sc}(kDa)
None	Human	FFI(D178N, M129)		19
FFI	Mouse	Tg(MHu2M)	206 ± 7 (7/7)	19
FFI → Tg(MHu2M)	Mouse	Tg(MHu2M)	136 ± 1 (6/6)	19
None	Human	fCJD(E200K)		21
fCJD	Mouse	Tg(MHu2M)	170 ± 2 (10/10)	21
fCJD → Tg(MHu2M)	Mouse	Tg(MHu2M)	167 ± 3 (15/15)	21

[a] Tg(MHu2M) mice express a chimeric human-mouse PrP gene.
NOTE: Clinicopathologic phenotype is determined by the conformation of PrP^{Sc} in accord with the results of the transmission of human prions from patients with FFI to transgenic mice.

Although phenotypes may vary dramatically within families, specific phenotypes tend to associate with certain mutations. A clinical phenotype indistinguishable from typical sporadic CJD is usually seen with substitutions at codons 180, 183, 200, 208, 210, and 232. Substitutions at codons 102, 105, 117, 198, and 217 are associated with the GSS variant of prion disease. The normal human PrP sequence contains five repeats of an eight or nine peptide sequence. Insertions from two to nine extra octapeptide repeats are frequently associated with variable phenotypes ranging from a condition indistinguishable from sporadic CJD to a slowly progressive dementing illness of many years duration. A mutation at codon 178 resulting in substitution of asparagine for aspartate produces FFI if a methionine is encoded at the polymorphic 129 residue on the same allele. Typical CJD is seen if a valine is encoded at position 129 of the same allele.

Human *PrP* Gene Polymorphisms Polymorphisms influence the susceptibility to sporadic, inherited, and infectious forms of prion disease. The methionine/valine polymorphism at position 129 not only modulates the age of onset of some inherited prion diseases but also determines the clinical phenotype. The influence of the codon 129 polymorphism iatrogenic and sporadic forms of prion disease has also been documented. The finding that homozygosity at codon 129 predisposes to sCJD supports a model of prion production that favors PrP interactions between homologous proteins.

Substitution of the basic residue lysine at position 219 produced dominant negative inhibition of prion replication in neuroblastoma cells. A lysine at 219 has been found in 12% of the Japanese population, and this group seems to be resistant to prion disease. Dominant negative inhibition of prion replication was also found with substitution of the basic residue arginine at position 171; sheep with arginine are resistant to scrapie.

INFECTIOUS PRION DISEASES

IATROGENIC CJD Accidental transmission of CJD to humans appears to have occurred with corneal transplantation, contaminated electroencephalogram (EEG) electrode implantation, and surgical procedures. Corneas from donors with inapparent CJD have been transplanted to apparently healthy recipients who developed CJD after prolonged incubation periods. The same improperly decontaminated EEG electrodes that caused CJD in two young patients with intractable epilepsy caused CJD in a chimpanzee 18 months after their experimental implantation.

Surgical procedures may have resulted in accidental inoculation of patients with prions during their operations, presumably because some instrument or apparatus in the operating theater became contaminated when a CJD patient underwent surgery. Although the epidemiology of these studies is highly suggestive, no proof for such episodes exists.

Dura Mater Grafts More than 70 cases of CJD after implantation of dura mater grafts have been recorded. All of the grafts were thought to have been acquired from a single manufacturer whose preparative procedures were inadequate to inactivate human prions. One case of CJD occurred after repair of an eardrum perforation with a pericardium graft.

Human Growth Hormone and Pituitary Gonadotropin Therapy The possibility of transmission of CJD from contaminated human growth hormone (hGH) preparations derived from human pituitaries has been raised by the occurrence of fatal cerebellar disorders with dementia in >100 patients ranging in age from 10 to 41 years. These patients received injections of hGH every 2 to 4 days for 4 to 12 years. If it is assumed that these patients developed CJD from injections of prion-contaminated hGH preparations, the possible incubation periods range from 4 to 30 years. Even though several investigations argue for the efficacy of inactivating prions in hGH fractions prepared from human pituitaries with 6 *M* urea, it seems doubtful that such protocols will be used for purifying hGH because recombinant hGH is available. Four cases of CJD have occurred in women receiving human pituitary gonadotropin.

NEW VARIANT CJD The restricted geographic occurrence and chronology of nvCJD have raised the possibility that BSE prions have been transmitted to humans. Approximately 70 cases of nvCJD have been recorded, and the fact that the incidence has remained relatively constant has made establishing the origin of nvCJD difficult. No set of dietary habits distinguishes patients with nvCJD from apparently healthy individuals. Moreover, there is no explanation for the predilection of nvCJD for teenagers and young adults. Epidemiologic studies over the past three decades have failed to find evidence for transmission of sheep prions to humans. Attempts to predict the future number of cases of nvCJD on the basis of possible exposure to bovine prions before the offal ban in 1998 that prevented further feeding of meat and bone meal (MBM) to cattle have been uninformative because so few cases of nvCJD have occurred. Are we at the beginning of a human prion disease epidemic in Great Britain similar to those seen for BSE and kuru, or will the number of nvCJD cases remain small as seen with iCJD caused by cadaveric hGH?

It is possible that a particular conformation of bovine PrP^{Sc} was selected for heat resistance during the rendering process and was then reselected multiple times as cattle infected by ingesting prion-contaminated MBM were slaughtered and their offal rendered into more MBM. Recent studies of PrP^{Sc} from brains of patients who died of nvCJD show a pattern of PrP glycoforms different from those found for sCJD or iCJD. But the usefulness of measuring PrP glycoforms is questionable when trying to relate BSE to nvCJD because PrP^{Sc} is formed after the protein is glycosylated and enzymatic deglycosylation of PrP^{Sc} requires denaturation.

The most compelling evidence that nvCJD comes from BSE prions was obtained from experiments in mice expressing the bovine PrP transgene. Both BSE and nvCJD prions were efficiently transmitted to these transgenic mice. In contrast to sporadic CJD prions, nvCJD did not transmit disease efficiently to mice expressing a chimeric human-mouse PrP transgene. Earlier studies with nontransgenic mice suggested that nvCJD and BSE might be derived from the same source because both sources of inocula transmitted disease with similar but very long incubation periods.

NEUROPATHOLOGY Frequently, the brains of patients with CJD have no recognizable abnormalities on gross examination. Patients who survive for several years have variable degrees of cerebral atrophy.

On light microscopy, the pathologic hallmarks of CJD are spongiform degeneration and astrogliosis. The lack of an inflammatory response in CJD and other prion diseases is an important pathologic feature of these degenerative disorders. Spongiform degeneration is characterized by many 1- to 5-μm vacuoles in the neuropil between nerve cell bodies. Generally, the spongiform changes occur in the cerebral cortex, putamen, caudate nucleus, thalamus, and molecular layer of the cerebellum. Astrocytic gliosis is a constant but nonspecific feature of prion diseases. Widespread proliferation of fibrous astrocytes is found throughout the gray matter of brains infected with CJD prions. Astrocytic processes filled with glial filaments form extensive networks.

Amyloid plaques have been found in ~10% of CJD cases. Purified CJD prions from humans and animals exhibit the ultrastructural and histochemical characteristics of amyloid when treated with detergents during limited proteolysis. In first passage from some human Japanese CJD cases, amyloid plaques have been found in mouse brains. These plaques stain with antisera raised against PrP.

The amyloid plaques of GSS are morphologically distinct from those seen in kuru or scrapie. GSS plaques consist of a central dense core of amyloid surrounded by smaller globules of amyloid. Ultrastructurally, they consist of a radiating fibrillar network of amyloid fibrils with scant or no neuritic degeneration. The plaques can be distributed throughout the brain but are most frequently found in the cerebellum. They are often located adjacent to blood vessels. Congophilic angiopathy has been noted in some cases of GSS.

In nvCJD, a characteristic feature is the presence of "florid plaques." These are composed of a central core of PrP amyloid surrounded by vacuoles in a pattern suggesting petals on a flower.

CLINICAL FEATURES Nonspecific prodromal symptoms occur in about a third of patients with CJD and may include fatigue, sleep disturbance, weight loss, headache, malaise, and ill-defined pain. Most patients with CJD present with deficits in higher cortical function. These deficits virtually always progress over weeks or months to a state of profound dementia characterized by memory loss, impaired judgment, and a decline in virtually all aspects of intellectual function. A few patients present with either visual impairment or cerebellar gait and coordination deficits. Frequently, the cerebellar deficits are rapidly followed by progressive dementia. Visual problems often begin with blurred vision and diminished acuity, rapidly followed by dementia.

Other symptoms and signs include extrapyramidal dysfunction manifested as rigidity, masklike facies, or choreoathetoid movements; pyramidal signs (usually mild); seizures (usually major motor) and, less commonly, hypesthesia; supranuclear gaze palsy; optic atrophy; and vegetative signs such as changes in weight, temperature, sweating, or menstruation.

Myoclonus Most patients (~90%) with CJD exhibit myoclonus that appears at various times throughout the illness. Unlike other involuntary movements, myoclonus persists during sleep. Startle myoclonus elicited by loud sounds or bright lights is frequent. It is important to stress that myoclonus is neither specific nor confined to CJD. Dementia with myoclonus can also be due to Alzheimer's disease (AD) (Chap. 362), to cryptococcal encephalitis (Chap. 204), or to the myoclonic epilepsy disorder Unverricht-Lundborg disease (Chap. 360).

Clinical Course In documented cases of accidental transmission of CJD to humans, an incubation period of 1.5 to 2.0 years preceded the development of clinical disease. In other cases, incubation periods of up to 30 years have been suggested. Most patients with CJD live 6 to 12 months after the onset of clinical signs and symptoms, whereas some live for up to 5 years.

DIAGNOSIS The constellation of dementia, myoclonus, and periodic electrical bursts in an afebrile 60-year-old patient generally indicates CJD. Clinical abnormalities in CJD are confined to the CNS. Fever, elevated sedimentation rate, leukocytosis in blood, or a pleocytosis in cerebrospinal fluid (CSF) should alert the physician to another etiology to explain the patient's CNS dysfunction.

Important variations in the typical course of CJD appear in certain inherited and transmitted forms of the disease. fCJD has an earlier mean age of onset than sCJD. In GSS, ataxia is usually a prominent and presenting feature, with dementia occurring late in the disease course. GSS may present earlier than CJD (mean age, 43 years; range, 24 to 66 years) and is typically more slowly progressive than CJD; death usually occurs within 5 years of onset. FFI is characterized by insomnia and dysautonomia; dementia occurs only in the terminal phase of the illness. Rare sporadic cases have been identified. nvCJD has an unusual clinical course, with a prominent psychiatric prodrome that may include visual hallucinations and early ataxia, while frank dementia usually is a late sign of nvCJD (see below).

DIFFERENTIAL DIAGNOSIS Many conditions may mimic CJD superficially. AD is occasionally accompanied by myoclonus but is usually distinguished by its protracted course and lack of motor and visual dysfunction.

Intracranial vasculitides (Chap. 317) may produce nearly all of the symptoms and signs associated with CJD, sometimes without systemic abnormalities. Myoclonus is exceptional with cerebral vasculitis, but focal seizures may confuse the picture; furthermore, myoclonus is often absent in the early stages of CJD. Stepwise change in deficits, prominent headache, abnormal cerebrospinal fluid, and focal magnetic resonance imaging (MRI) or angiographic abnormalities all favor vasculitis.

Neurosyphilis (Chap. 172) may present with dementia and myoclonus that progresses in a relatively rapid fashion but is easily distinguished from CJD by CSF findings, as is cryptococcal meningoencephalitis. A diffuse intracranial tumor (gliomatosis cerebri; Chap. 370) may occasionally be confused with CJD. In rare cases of CNS neoplasia, neuroimaging studies are normal and there are no signs of increased intracranial pressure; however, CSF protein is usually elevated. Adult onset leukodystrophies (ceroid lipofuscinosis or Kuf's disease) and myoclonic epilepsy with Lafora bodies (Chap. 360) may be responsible for dementia, myoclonus, and ataxia; but the less acute courses and prominent seizures distinguish them from CJD. A number of diseases that may simulate CJD are easily distinguished by noting the clinical setting in which they occur. These diseases include anoxic encephalopathy, subacute sclerosing panencephalitis, progressive rubella panencephalitis, herpes simplex encephalitis (in immunoincompetent hosts), dialysis dementia, uremia, and portasystemic shunt encephalopathy.

When CJD begins atypically, it may for a short time resemble other disorders such as Parkinson's disease, progressive supranuclear palsy (Chap. 363), or progressive multifocal leukoencephalopathy (Chap. 373). However, this resemblance usually fades early in the course of CJD.

Certain drug intoxications, particularly lithium and bismuth, may produce a syndrome with encephalopathy and myoclonus. The rare condition known as Hashimoto's encephalopathy, which presents with a subacutely progressive encephalopathy and myoclonus with periodic triphasic complexes on the EEG should be excluded in every case of suspected CJD. It is diagnosed by the finding of high titers of antithyroglobulin or antithyroid perioxidase (antimicrosomal) antibodies in the blood, and improves with glucocorticoid therapy. Unlike CJD, fluctuations in severity typically occur in Hashimoto's encephalopathy.

The AIDS dementia complex (Chap. 309) may occasionally imitate CJD in onset, early course, physical signs, computed tomography (CT) findings, and lack of abnormalities on routine CSF studies. The few such patients without manifestations of systemic immunodeficiency (<10%) should be questioned about risk factors and should have serum antibodies to HIV determined. Additionally, more specific CSF tests are likely to be abnormal; in one study, CSF oligoclonal bands were present in six of nine patients, and intra-blood-brain barrier synthesis of IgG specific for HIV was elevated in eight of nine.

LABORATORY TESTS With the exception of brain biopsy, there are no specific tests for CJD. If the constellation of pathologic changes frequently found in CJD is seen in a brain biopsy, then the diagnosis is reasonably secure (see Neuropathology, above). The rapid and reliable diagnosis of CJD postmortem can be accomplished with antisera to PrP. Numerous western blotting studies have consistently demonstrated PrP immunoreactive proteins that are proteinase K–resistant in the brains of patients with CJD. Because PrP^{Sc} is not uniformly distributed throughout the CNS, the apparent absence of PrP^{Sc} in a limited sample such as a biopsy does not rule out prion disease. A highly sensitive and quantitative immunoassay was developed based on epitopes that are exposed in PrP^{C} but buried in PrP^{Sc}. Unlike all other immunoassays for PrP^{Sc}, this conformation-dependent immunoassay (CDI) does not require limited proteolysis to hydrolyze PrP^{C} before measurement of the protease-resistant core of PrP^{Sc} (PrP 27-30).

If the patient has a family history suggestive of inherited CJD, sequencing the *PrP* gene may facilitate the diagnosis. Sometimes, the PrP sequence is helpful for even seemingly nonfamilial cases.

CT may be normal or show cortical atrophy. The MRI scan may show a subtle increased intensity in the basal ganglia with T2 or diffusion weighted imaging, but this finding is neither sensitive nor specific enough to make a diagnosis. CSF is nearly always normal but may show a minimal protein elevation. Although the stress protein 14-3-3 is elevated in the CSF of most patients with CJD, similar elevations of 14-3-3 are found in herpes simplex virus encephalitis, multi-infarct dementia, and stroke. In AD, 14-3-3 is generally not elevated. In the serum of some patients with CJD, the S-100 protein is elevated; but like 14-3-3, this elevation is not specific.

The EEG is often useful in the diagnosis of CJD. During the early phase of CJD, the EEG is usually normal or shows only scattered theta activity. In most advanced cases, repetitive, high voltage, triphasic, and polyphasic sharp discharges are seen, but in many cases their presence is transient. The presence of these stereotyped periodic bursts of $<$200 ms duration, occurring every 1 to 2 s, makes the diagnosis of CJD very likely. These discharges are frequently but not always symmetric; there may be a one-sided predominance in amplitude. As CJD progresses, normal background rhythms become fragmentary and slower.

CARE OF CJD PATIENTS It is important to stress that CJD is neither a contagious nor a communicable disease, but it is transmissible. Although the risk of accidental inoculation by aerosols is very small, procedures producing aerosols should be performed in certified biosafety cabinets. Biosafety level 2 practices, containment equipment, and facilities are recommended by the Centers for Disease Control and Prevention and the National Institutes of Health. The primary problem in caring for patients with CJD is the inadvertent infection of healthcare workers by needle and stab wounds, whereas the possible transmission of a contagion through the air has never been documented. Electroencephalographic and electromyographic needles should not be reused after studies on patients with CJD have been performed.

There is no reason for pathologists or morgue dieners to resist performing autopsies on patients whose clinical diagnosis was CJD. Standard microbiologic practices outlined here, along with specific recommendations for decontamination, seem to be adequate precautions for the care of patients with CJD and the handling of infected specimens.

DECONTAMINATION OF CJD PRIONS Prions are extremely resistant to common inactivation procedures, and there is some disagreement about the optimal conditions for sterilization. Some investigators recommend treating CJD-contaminated materials once with 1 *N* NaOH at room temperature, but we believe this procedure may be inadequate for sterilization. Autoclaving at 132°C for 5 h or treatment with 2 *N* NaOH for several hours is recommended for sterilization of prions. The term "sterilization" implies complete destruction of prions; any residual infectivity can be hazardous.

PREVENTION AND THERAPEUTICS There is no known effective therapy for treating or preventing CJD. With one possible exception, there are no well-documented cases of patients with CJD showing recovery either spontaneously or after therapy.

Several compounds have been demonstrated to eliminate prions from prion-infected cultured cells. A class of compounds known as "dendrimers" seems particularly efficacious in this regard. Several drugs delay the onset of disease in animals inoculated with prions if the drugs are given around the time of the inoculation. The most common scenarios in which one would want to treat humans are either patients showing signs of disease or presymptomatic patients carrying mutations predisposing them to develop prion disease. No treatment has shown any efficacy in animal models of these two scenarios.

Structure-based drug design predicated on dominant negative inhibition of prion formation has produced several promising compounds. Whether this approach or that of enhanced clearance of misfolded proteins will provide general methods for developing novel therapeutics for Alzheimer's disease and Parkinson's disease, as well as amyotrophic lateral sclerosis (ALS), remains to be established.

BIBLIOGRAPHY

GAJDUSEK DC: Unconventional viruses and the origin and disappearance of kuru. Science 197:943, 1977

HARRIS DA: *Prions: Molecular and Cellular Biology.* Wymondham, Norfolk, Horizon Scientific Press, 1999

JOHNSON RT, GIBBS CJ JR.: Creutzfeldt-Jakob disease and related transmissible spongiform encephalopathies. N Engl J Med 339:1994, 1998

KIRSCHBAUM WR: *Jakob-Creutzfeldt Disease.* Amsterdam, Elsevier, 1968

PRUSINER SB: Prions. Proc Natl Acad Sci USA 95:13363, 1998

——— (ed): *Prion Biology and Diseases.* Cold Spring Harbor, New York, Cold Spring Harbor Laboratory Press, 1999

SEIPELT M et al: Hashimoto's encephalitis as a differential diagnosis of Creutzfeldt-Jakob disease. J Neurol Neurosurg Psychiatry 66:172, 1999

WILL RG et al: Diagnosis of new variant Creutzfeldt-Jacob disease. Ann Neurol 47:575, 2000

376 CRITICAL CARE NEUROLOGY

J. Claude Hemphill, M. Flint Beal, Daryl R. Gress

Advances in the understanding of the pathophysiology of acute nervous system injury and the development of treatments that target these injury mechanisms have led to the growth of critical care neurology as a discipline. Life-threatening neurologic illness may be caused by a primary disorder affecting any region of the neuroaxis or may occur as a consequence of a systemic disorder such as hepatic failure, multisystem organ failure (MSOF), or cardiac arrest (Table 376-1). Critical care neurology focuses on preservation of neurologic tissue and prevention of secondary brain injury caused by ischemia, edema, and elevated intracranial pressure (ICP).

PATHOPHYSIOLOGY **Brain Edema** Swelling, or edema, of brain tissue occurs with many types of brain injury. The two principal types of edema are vasogenic and cytotoxic. *Vasogenic edema* refers to the influx of fluid and solutes into the brain through an incompetent blood-brain barrier (BBB). In the normal cerebral vasculature, endothelial tight junctions associated with astrocytes create an impermeable barrier (the BBB), through which access into the brain interstitium is dependent upon specific transport mechanisms (Chap. 355). The BBB may be compromised in ischemia, trauma, infection, and metabolic derangements. Typically, vasogenic edema develops rapidly following injury. *Cytotoxic edema* refers to cellular swelling. Originally described as a response to exogenous toxins, cellular swelling occurs in a variety of settings including brain ischemia and trauma. Early astrocytic swelling is a hallmark of ischemia.

Brain edema that is clinically significant usually represents a combination of vasogenic and cellular components. Edema can lead to increased ICP as well as tissue shifts and brain displacement from focal

Table 376-1 Neurologic Disorders in Critical Illness

Localization Along Neuroaxis	Syndrome
Central Nervous System	
Brain: Cerebral hemispheres	Global encephalopathy
	Septic
	Organ failure—hepatic, renal
	Medication related
	Sedative/hypnotics/analgesics
	H_2 blockers, antihypertensives
	Drug overdose
	Electrolyte disturbance—hyponatremia; hypoglycemia
	Hypotension/hypoperfusion
	Hypoxia
	Meningitis
	Subarachnoid hemorrhage
	Wernicke's disease
	Seizure—postictal or nonconvulsive status
	Hypertensive encephalopathy
	Hypothyroidism—myxedema
	Focal deficits
	Ischemic stroke
	Tumor
	Abscess, subdural empyema
	Subdural/epidural hematoma
Brainstem	Mass effect and compression
	Ischemic stroke, intraparenchymal hemorrhage
	Hypoxia
Spinal cord	Mass effect and compression
	Disc herniation
	Epidural hematoma
	Ischemia—hypotension/embolic
	Subdural empyema
	Trauma, central cord syndrome
Peripheral nervous system	
Peripheral nerve	
Axonal	Critical illness polyneuropathy
	Possible neuromuscular blocking agent complication
	Metabolic disturbances, uremia—hyperglycemia
	Medication effects—chemotherapeutic, antiretroviral
Demyelinating	Guillian-Barré syndrome
	Chronic inflammatory demyelinating polyneuropathy
Neuromuscular junction	Prolonged effect of neuromuscular blockade
	Medication effects—aminoglycosides
	Myasthenia-gravis, Lambert-Eaton syndrome
Muscle	Septic myopathy
	Cachectic myopathy—with or without disuse atrophy
	Electrolyte disturbances—hypokalemia/hyperkalemia; hypophosphatemia
	Acute quadriplegic myopathy

processes. These tissue shifts can cause injury by mechanical distraction and compression in addition to the ischemia of impaired perfusion consequent to the elevated ICP.

Cerebral Perfusion and Autoregulation Brain tissue requires constant perfusion in order to ensure adequate delivery of substrate, principally oxygen and glucose. The hemodynamic response of the brain has the capacity to preserve perfusion across a wide range of systemic blood pressures. Cerebral perfusion pressure (CPP), defined as the mean systemic arterial pressure (MAP) minus the ICP, provides the driving force for circulation across the capillary beds of the brain. *Autoregulation* refers to the physiologic response whereby cerebral blood flow (CBF) remains relatively constant over a wide range of blood pressures as a consequence of alterations of cerebrovascular resistance (Fig. 376-1). If systemic blood pressure drops, cerebral perfusion is preserved through vasodilatation of arterioles in the brain; likewise, arteriolar vasoconstriction occurs at high systemic pressures to prevent hyperperfusion. At the extreme limits of MAP or CPP (high or low), flow becomes directly related to perfusion pressure. These autoregulatory changes occur in the microcirculation and are mediated by vessels below the resolution of those seen on angiography. CBF is also strongly influenced by pH and P_{CO_2}. CBF increases with hypercapnia and acidosis and decreases with hypocapnia and alkalosis. This forms the basis for the use of hyperventilation to lower ICP, and this effect on ICP is mediated through a decrease in intracranial blood volume. Cerebral autoregulation is critical to the normal homeostatic functioning of the brain, and this process may be disordered focally and unpredictably in disease states such as traumatic brain injury and severe focal cerebral ischemia.

Cerebrospinal Fluid and Intracranial Pressure The cranial contents consist essentially of brain, cerebrospinal fluid (CSF), and blood. CSF is produced principally in the choroid plexus of each lateral ventricle, exits the brain via the foramina of Luschka and Magendi, and flows over the cortex to be absorbed into the venous system along the superior sagittal sinus. Approximately 150 mL of CSF are contained within the ventricles and surrounding the brain and spinal cord; the cerebral blood volume is also ~150 mL. The bony skull offers excellent protection for the brain but allows little tolerance for additional volume. Significant increases in volume eventually result in increased ICP. Obstruction of CSF outflow, edema of cerebral tissue, or increases in volume from tumor or hematoma may increase ICP. Elevated ICP diminishes cerebral perfusion and can lead to tissue ischemia. Ischemia in turn may lead to vasodilatation via autoregulatory mechanisms designed to restore cerebral perfusion. However, vasodilatation also increases cerebral blood volume, which in turn then increases ICP, lowers CPP, and provokes further ischemia (Fig. 376-2). This vicious cycle is commonly seen in traumatic brain injury, massive intracerebral hemorrhage, and large hemispheric infarcts with significant tissue shift. →*Excitotoxicity and mechanisms of cell death are discussed in Chap. 355.*

Approach to the Patient

Critically ill patients with severe central nervous system dysfunction require rapid evaluation and intervention in order to limit primary and secondary brain injury. Initial neurologic evaluation should be performed concurrent with stabilization of basic respiratory, cardiac, and hemodynamic parameters. Significant barriers may exist to neurologic assessment in the critical care unit. Endotracheal intubation and the

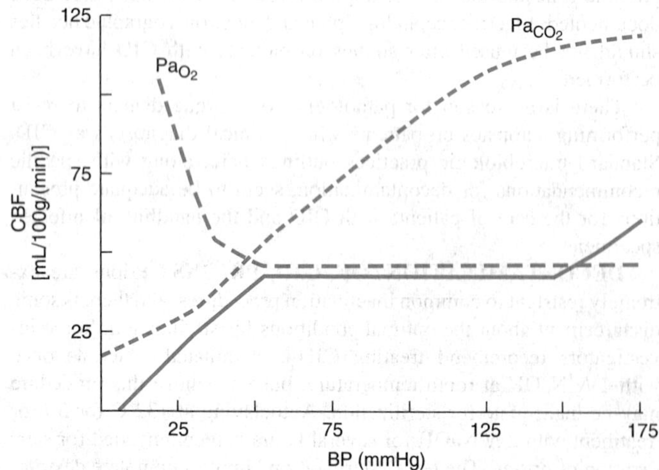

FIGURE 376-1 Cerebral autoregulation curve (solid line). Cerebral perfusion is constant over a wide range of systemic blood pressure. Perfusion is increased in the setting of hypoxia or hypercarbia. BP, blood pressure; CBF, cerebral blood flow. *(Reprinted with permission from Anesthesiology 43:447, 1975. Copyright 1975, Lippincott Company.)*

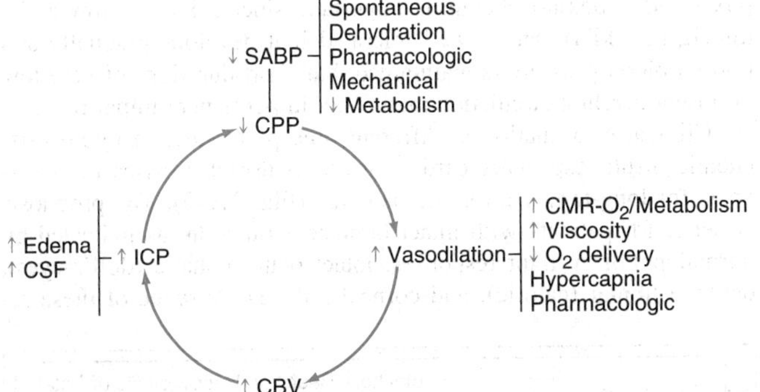

FIGURE 376-2 Ischemia and vasodilatation. Reduced cerebral perfusion pressure (CPP) leads to increased ischemia, vasodilatation, increased intracranial pressure, (ICP) and further reductions in CPP, a cycle leading to further neurologic injury. CBV, cerebral blood volume; CMR, cerebral metabolic rate; CSF, cerebrospinal fluid; SABP, systolic arterial blood pressure. *(From Rosner et al.)*

use of sedative or paralytic agents to facilitate critical care procedures can make clinical assessment challenging.

An impaired level of consciousness is frequent in critically ill patients. The essential first task in assessment is to determine whether the cause of dysfunction is related to a diffuse, usually metabolic, process or whether a focal, usually structural, process is implicated. Examples of diffuse processes include metabolic encephalopathies related to organ failure, drug overdose, or hypoxia-ischemia. Focal processes include ischemic and hemorrhagic stroke and traumatic brain injury, especially with intracranial hematomas. Since these two categories of disorders have fundamentally different causes, treatments, and prognoses, the initial focus is on making this distinction rapidly and accurately. →*The approach to the confused or comatose patient is discussed in Chap. 24; etiologies are listed in Table 24-1.*

Minor focal deficits may be present on the neurologic examination in patients with metabolic encephalopathies. However, the finding of prominent focal signs such as pupillary asymmetry, hemiparesis, gaze palsy, or paraplegia should alert the examiner to the possibility of a structural lesion. All patients with a decreased level of consciousness associated with focal findings should undergo an urgent neuroimaging procedure, as should all patients with coma of unknown etiology. Computed tomographic (CT) scanning is usually the most appropriate initial study because it can be performed quickly in critically ill patients and demonstrates hemorrhage, hydrocephalus, and intracranial tissue shifts well. Magnetic resonance imaging (MRI) may provide more specific information in some situations, such as acute ischemic stroke (diffusion-weighted imaging, DWI) and cerebral venous sinus thrombosis (magnetic resonance venography, MRV). Any suggestion of trauma from the history or examination should alert the examiner to the possibility of cervical spine injury and prompt an imaging evaluation using plain x-rays, MRI, or CT.

Other diagnostic studies are best utilized in specific circumstances, usually when neuroimaging studies fail to reveal a structural lesion and the etiology of the altered mental state remains uncertain. Electroencephalography (EEG) can be important in the evaluation of critically ill patients with severe brain dysfunction. The EEG of encephalopathy typically reveals generalized slowing. One of the most important uses of EEG is to help exclude inapparent seizures, especially nonconvulsive status epilepticus. Untreated continuous or frequently recurrent seizures may cause neuronal injury, making the diagnosis and treatment of seizure crucial in this patient group. Lumbar puncture (LP) may be necessary to exclude infectious processes, and an elevated opening pressure may be an important clue to cerebral venous sinus thrombosis. In patients with coma or profound encephalopathy, it is preferable to perform a neuroimaging study prior to LP. If bacterial meningitis is suspected, an LP may be performed first or antibiotics may be empirically administered before the diagnostic studies are completed. Standard laboratory evaluation of critically ill patients should include assessment of serum electrolytes (especially sodium and calcium), glucose, renal and hepatic function, complete blood counts, and coagulation. Serum or urine toxicology screens should be performed in patients with encephalopathy of unknown cause. EEG, LP, and other specific laboratory tests are most useful when the mechanism of the altered level of consciousness is uncertain; they are not routinely performed in clear-cut cases of stroke or traumatic brain injury.

Monitoring of ICP can be an important tool in selected patients. Indications for ICP monitoring, as well as specific types of monitors, vary. In general, patients who should be considered for ICP monitoring are those with primary neurologic disorders, such as stroke or traumatic brain injury, who are not moribund and who are at significant risk for secondary brain injury due to elevated ICP and decreased CPP. Such patients include those with severe traumatic brain injury resulting in coma [Glasgow Coma Scale (GCS) score of ≤8 (Table 369-1)]; those with large tissue shifts from supratentorial ischemic or hemorrhagic stroke resulting in decreased consciousness; and those with (or at risk for) hydrocephalus from subarachnoid hemorrhage, intraventricular hemorrhage, or posterior fossa stroke. An additional disorder in which ICP monitoring can add important information is fulminant hepatic failure, in which elevated ICP may be treated with barbiturates or, eventually, liver transplantation. In general, ventriculostomy is preferable to ICP monitoring devices that are placed in brain parenchyma, because ventriculostomy allows CSF drainage as a method of treating elevated ICP. However, parenchymal ICP monitoring is most appropriate for patients with diffuse edema and small ventricles (which may make ventriculostomy placement more difficult) or any degree of coagulopathy (in which ventriculostomy carries a higher risk of hemorrhagic complications).

Treatment of Elevated ICP Elevated ICP may occur in a wide range of disorders including head trauma, intracerebral hemorrhage, subarachnoid hemorrhage with hydrocephalus, and fulminant hepatic failure. Because CSF and blood volume can be redistributed initially, by the time elevated ICP occurs intracranial compliance is severely impaired. At this point, small changes in the volume of CSF, intravascular blood, edema, or a mass lesion may result in significant changes in ICP. Elevated ICP then diminishes cerebral perfusion. This is a fundamental mechanism of secondary ischemic brain injury and constitutes an emergency that requires immediate attention. Specific thresholds of ICP vary, but in general, ICP should be maintained at <20 mmHg and CPP should be maintained at ≥70 mmHg.

A number of different interventions may lower ICP, and ideally the selection of treatment will be based on the underlying mechanism responsible for the elevated ICP (Table 376-2). For example, in hydrocephalus from subarachnoid hemorrhage, the principal cause of elevated ICP is impairment of CSF drainage. In this setting, ventricular drainage of CSF is likely to be sufficient and most appropriate. In head trauma and stroke, cytotoxic edema may be most responsible, and the use of osmotic diuretics such as mannitol becomes an appropriate early step. As described above, elevated ICP may cause tissue ischemia, and, if cerebral autoregulation is intact, the resulting vasodilatation can lead to a cycle of worsening ischemia. Paradoxically, administration of vasopressor agents to increase mean arterial pressure may actually lower ICP by improving perfusion, thereby allowing autoregulatory vasoconstriction as ischemia is relieved and ultimately decreasing intracranial blood volume.

Early signs of elevated ICP include drowsiness and a diminished level of consciousness. Neuroimaging studies may reveal evidence of edema and mass effect. Hypotonic intravenous fluids should be avoided, and elevation of the head of the bed is recommended. Patients must be carefully observed for risk of aspiration and compromise of the airway as the level of alertness declines. Coma and unilateral pupillary changes are late signs and require immediate intervention. Emergent treatment of elevated ICP is most quickly achieved by intubation and hyperventilation, which causes vasoconstriction and re-

Table 376-2 Stepwise Approach to Treatment of Elevated Intracranial Pressure (ICP)[a]

Insert ICP monitor—ventriculostomy versus parenchymal device
General goals: maintain ICP < 20 mmHg and CPP > 70 mmHg

For ICP > 20–25 mmHg for >5 min:

1. Drain CSF via ventriculostomy (if in place)
2. Elevate head of the bed
3. Osmotherapy—mannitol 25–100 g q4h as needed
   (maintain serum osmolality <320 mOsm/L)
4. Glucocorticoids—dexamethasone 4 mg q6h for vasogenic edema from tumor, abscess
   (avoid glucocorticoids in head trauma, ischemic and hemorrhagic stroke)
5. Sedation (e.g., morphine, propofol, or midazolam); add neuromuscular paralysis if necessary
   (patient will require endotracheal intubation and mechanical ventilation at this point, if not before)
6. Hyperventilation—to Pa_{CO_2} 30–35 mmHg
7. Pressor therapy—phenylephrine, dopamine, or norepinephrine to maintain adequate MAP to ensure CPP > 70 mmHg,
   (maintain euvolemia to minimize deleterious systemic effects of pressors)
8. Consider second-tier therapies for refractory elevated ICP
   a. High-dose barbiturate therapy ("pentobarb coma")
   b. Aggressive hyperventilation to Pa_{CO_2} < 30 mmHg
   c. Hemicraniectomy

[a] Throughout ICP treatment algorithm, consider repeat head CT to identify mass lesions amenable to surgical evacuation.

NOTE: CPP, cerebral perfusion pressure; MAP, mean arterial pressure; Pa_{CO_2}, arterial partial pressure of carbon dioxide.

duces cerebral blood volume. Because of the concern of provoking or worsening cerebral ischemia, hyperventilation is best used for short periods of time until a more definitive treatment can be instituted. Furthermore, the effects of continued hyperventilation on ICP are short-lived, often only for several hours because of the buffering capacity of the cerebral interstitium, and rebound elevated ICP may accompany abrupt discontinuation of hyperventilation. As the level of consciousness declines to coma, the ability to follow the neurologic status of the patient by examination deteriorates and measurement of ICP must be considered. If a ventriculostomy device is in place, direct drainage of CSF to reduce ICP is possible. Finally, high-dose barbiturates or hypothermia are sometimes used for refractory elevated ICP, although these have significant side effects and have not been shown to improve outcome.

CRITICAL CARE DISORDERS OF THE CENTRAL NERVOUS SYSTEM ASSOCIATED WITH SYSTEMIC DISEASE

HYPOXIC-ISCHEMIC ENCEPHALOPATHY Hypoxic-ischemic encephalopathy occurs from lack of delivery of oxygen to the brain because of hypotension or respiratory failure. The most common causes are myocardial infarction, cardiac arrest, shock, asphyxiation, paralysis of respiration, and carbon monoxide or cyanide poisoning. In some circumstances, hypoxia may predominate. Carbon monoxide and cyanide poisoning are termed *histotoxic hypoxia* since they cause a direct impairment of the respiratory chain.

Clinical Manifestations Mild degrees of pure hypoxia, such as occur at high altitudes, cause impaired judgment, inattentiveness, motor incoordination, and, at times, euphoria. However, with hypoxia-ischemia, such as occurs with circulatory arrest, consciousness is lost within seconds. If circulation is restored within 3 to 5 min, full recovery may occur, but if hypoxia-ischemia lasts beyond 3 to 5 min, some degree of permanent cerebral damage is the rule. Except in extreme cases, it may be difficult to judge the precise degree of hypoxia-ischemia, and some patients make a relatively full recovery after even 8 to 10 min of global cerebral ischemia. The distinction between pure hypoxia and hypoxia-ischemia is important, since a Pa_{O_2} as low as 20 mmHg (2.7 kPa) can be well tolerated if it develops gradually and normal blood pressure is maintained, but short durations of very low or absent cerebral circulation may result in permanent impairment.

Clinical examination at different time points after a hypoxic-ischemic insult (especially cardiac arrest) is useful in assessing prognosis for long-term neurologic outcome (Fig. 376-3). The prognosis is better for patients with intact brainstem function, as indicated by normal pupillary light responses, intact oculocephalic (doll's-eyes), oculovestibular (caloric), and corneal reflexes. Absence of these re-

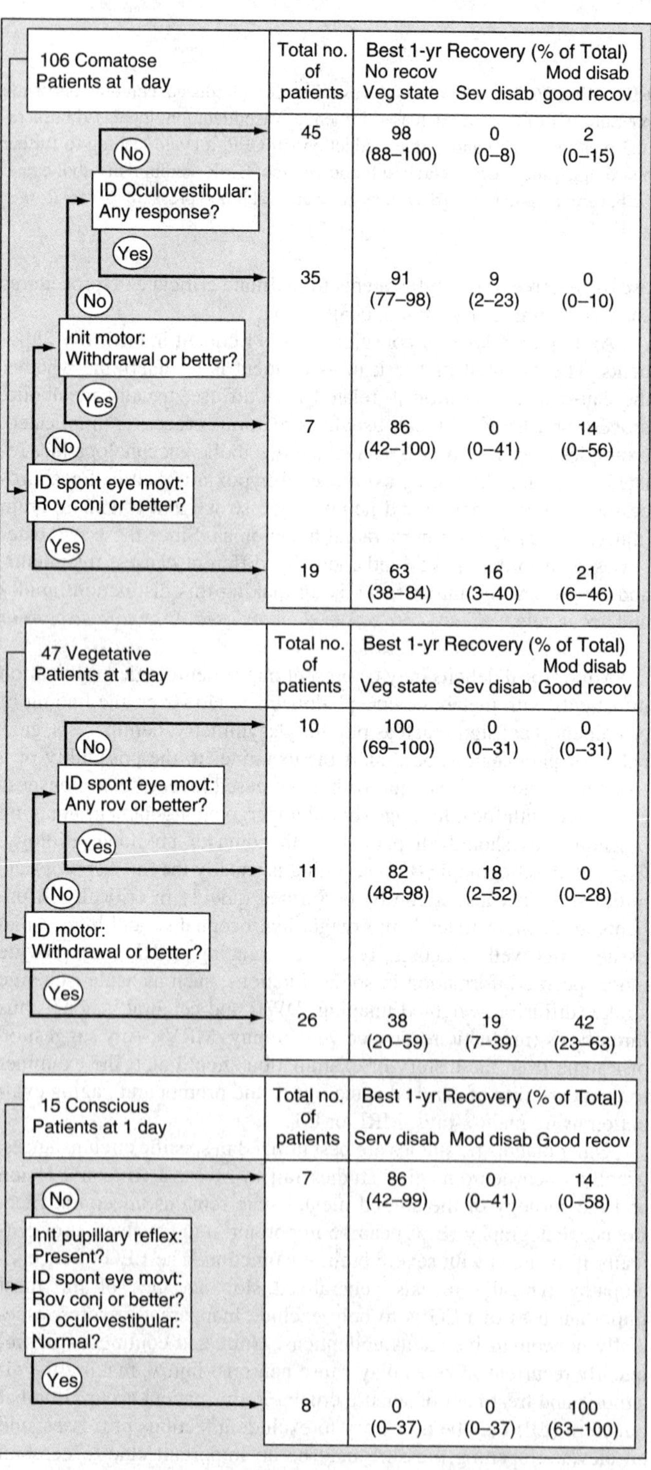

FIGURE 376-3 Clinical examination at day 1 provides useful prognostic information in hypoxic-ischemic encephalopathy. Numbers in parentheses represent 95% confidence intervals. Recov, recovery; veg, vegetative; sev, severe; mod, moderate; spont eye movt, spontaneous eye movement; rov conj, roving conjugate. *(From Levy et al.)*

flexes and the presence of persistently dilated pupils that do not react to light are grave prognostic signs. A uniformly dismal prognosis from hypoxic-ischemic coma is conveyed by the clinical findings of absence of pupillary light reflex or absence of a motor response to pain on day 3 following the injury. Electrophysiologically, the finding of bilateral absence of the early cortical somatosensory evoked response (SSEPs) in the first week also conveys a poor prognosis. Long-term consequences of hypoxic-ischemic encephalopathy include persistent coma or vegetative state (Chap. 24), dementia, visual agnosia (Chap. 25), parkinsonism, choreoathetosis, cerebellar ataxia, myoclonus, seizures, and an amnestic state, which may be a consequence of selective damage to the hippocampus (Chap. 26).

Pathologic Findings Principal histologic findings are extensive multifocal or diffuse laminar cortical necrosis (Fig. 376-4), with almost invariable involvement of the hippocampus. The hippocampal CA1 neurons are vulnerable to even brief episodes of hypoxia-ischemia, perhaps explaining why selective persistent memory deficits may occur after brief cardiac arrest. Scattered small areas of infarction or neuronal loss may be present in the basal ganglia, hypothalamus, or brainstem. In some cases, extensive bilateral thalamic scarring may affect thalamic and extrathalamic pathways that mediate arousal, and this has been suggested as one pathologic explanation for the persistent vegetative state. A specific form of hypoxic-ischemic encephalopathy, so-called watershed infarcts, occurs at the distal territories between the major cerebral arteries and can cause cognitive deficits, including visual agnosia, and weakness that is greater in proximal than in distal muscle groups.

Diagnosis Diagnosis is based upon the history of a hypoxic-ischemic event such as cardiac arrest. Blood pressure <70 mmHg systolic or $Pa_{O_2} < 40$ mmHg is usually necessary, although both absolute levels as well as duration of exposure are important determinants of cellular injury. Occasionally the clinical and radiographic features of a hypoxic-ischemic syndrome are seen without documented profound hypotension or hypoxia. Carbon monoxide intoxication can be confirmed by measurement of carboxyhemoglobin and is suggested by a cherry red color of the skin.

℞ **TREATMENT** Treatment should be directed at restoration of normal cardiorespiratory function. This includes securing a clear airway, ensuring adequate oxygenation and ventilation, and restoring cerebral perfusion, whether by cardiopulmonary resuscitation, fluid, pressors, or cardiac pacing. Hypothermia and neuroprotective agents that target different aspects of the cell injury cascade are experimental approaches that have not yet been shown to have clinical value.

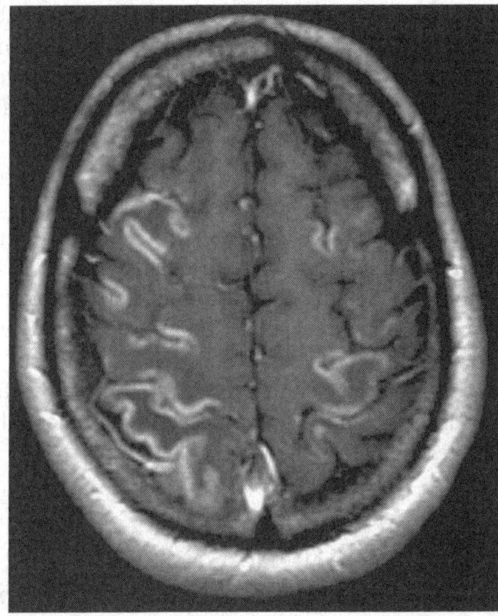

FIGURE 376-4 Cortical laminar necrosis in hypoxic-ischemic encephalopathy. T1-weighted postcontrast magnetic resonance image shows cortical enhancement in a watershed distribution consistent with laminar necrosis.

Severe carbon monoxide intoxication may be treated with hyperbaric oxygen. Anticonvulsants may be needed to control seizures, although these are not usually given prophylactically. Posthypoxic myoclonus may respond to oral administration of clonazepam at doses of 1.5 to 10 mg daily or valproate at doses of 300 mg to 1200 mg daily in divided doses. Myoclonic status epilepticus after a severe hypoxic-ischemic insult portends a universally poor prognosis, even if seizures are controlled.

DELAYED POSTANOXIC ENCEPHALOPATHY Delayed postanoxic encephalopathy is an uncommon phenomenon in which patients appear to make an initial recovery from hypoxic-ischemic insult but then develop a relapse characterized by apathy, confusion, and agitation. Progressive neurologic deficits may include shuffling gait, diffuse rigidity and spasticity, persistent parkinsonism or myoclonus, and, on occasion, coma and death after 1 to 2 weeks. Widespread cerebral demyelination may be present.

Carbon monoxide and cyanide intoxication can also cause a delayed encephalopathy. Little clinical impairment is evident when the patient first regains consciousness, but a parkinsonian syndrome characterized by akinesia and rigidity without tremor may develop. Symptoms can worsen over months, accompanied by increasing evidence of damage in the basal ganglia as seen on both CT and MRI.

METABOLIC ENCEPHALOPATHIES Altered mental states, variously described as confusion, delirium, disorientation, and encephalopathy, are present in many patients with severe illness in an intensive care unit (ICU). Older patients are particularly vulnerable to delirium, a confusional state characterized by disordered perception, frequent hallucinations, delusions, and sleep disturbance. This is often attributed to medication effects, sleep deprivation, pain, and anxiety. The term *ICU psychosis* has been used to describe a mental state with profound agitation occurring in this setting. The presence of family members in the ICU may help to calm and orient agitated patients, and in severe cases, low doses of neuroleptics (e.g., haloperidol 0.5 to 1 mg) can be useful. Ultimately, the psychosis resolves with improvement in the underlying illness and a return to familiar surroundings.

In the ICU setting, several metabolic causes of an altered level of consciousness predominate. Hypercarbic encephalopathy can present with headache, confusion, stupor, or coma. Hypoventilation syndrome occurs most frequently in patients with a history of chronic CO_2 retention who are receiving oxygen therapy for emphysema or chronic pulmonary disease (Chap. 263). The elevated Pa_{CO_2} leading to CO_2 narcosis may have a direct anesthetic effect, and cerebral vasodilatation from increased Pa_{CO_2} can lead to increased ICP. Hepatic encephalopathy is suggested by asterixis and can occur in chronic liver failure or acute fulminant hepatic failure. Both hyperglycemia and hypoglycemia can cause encephalopathy, as can hypernatremia and hyponatremia. Confusion, impairment of eye movements, and gait ataxia are the hallmarks of acute Wernicke's disease (see below).

SEPTIC ENCEPHALOPATHY Pathogenesis In patients with sepsis, the systemic response to infectious agents leads to the release of circulating inflammatory mediators that appear to contribute to encephalopathy. Critical illness, in association with the systemic inflammatory response syndrome (SIRS), can lead to MSOF. This syndrome can occur in the setting of apparent sepsis, severe burns, or trauma, even without clear identification of an infectious agent. Many patients with critical illness, sepsis, or SIRS develop encephalopathy without obvious explanation. This condition is broadly termed *septic encephalopathy*. While the specific mediators leading to neurologic dysfunction remain uncertain, it is clear that the encephalopathy is not simply the result of metabolic derangements of multiorgan failure. The cytokines tumor necrosis factor α, interleukin (IL) 1, IL-2, and IL-6 are thought to play a role in this syndrome.

Diagnosis Septic encephalopathy presents clinically as a diffuse dysfunction of the brain without prominent focal findings. Confusion, disorientation, agitation, and fluctuations in level of alertness are typical. In more profound cases, especially with hemodynamic compromise, the decrease in level of alertness can be more prominent, at times resulting in coma. Hyperreflexia and frontal release signs such as a grasp or snout reflex (Chap. 356) can be seen. Abnormal movements such as myoclonus, tremor, or asterixis can occur. Septic encephalopathy is quite common, occurring in the majority of patients with sepsis and MSOF. Diagnosis is often difficult because of the multiple potential causes of neurologic dysfunction in critically ill patients, and requires exclusion of structural, metabolic, toxic, and infectious (e.g., meningitis or encephalitis) causes. Although the mortality of patients with septic encephalopathy severe enough to produce coma approaches 50%, this reflects the severity of the underlying critical illness and is not a direct result of the septic encephalopathy. Neurologically, successful treatment of the underlying critical illness almost always results in complete resolution of the encephalopathy, without significant residua.

CENTRAL PONTINE MYELINOLYSIS This disorder typically presents in a devastating fashion as quadriplegia and pseudobulbar palsy. Predisposing factors include severe underlying medical illness or nutritional deficiency; most cases are associated with rapid correction of hyponatremia or with hyperosmolar states. The pathology consists of demyelination without inflammation in the base of the pons, with relative sparing of axons and nerve cells. MRI is useful in establishing the diagnosis (Fig. 376-5) and may also identify partial forms that present as confusion, dysarthria, and/or disturbances of conjugate gaze without quadriplegia. Therapeutic guidelines for the restoration of severe hyponatremia should aim for gradual correction, i.e., by ≤10 mmol/L (10 meq/L) within 24 h and 20 mmol/L (20 meq/L) within 48 h.

WERNICKE'S DISEASE Wernicke's disease is a common and preventable disorder due to a deficiency of thiamine (Chap. 75). In the United States, alcoholics account for most cases, but patients with malnutrition due to hyperemesis, starvation, renal dialysis, cancer, or AIDS are also at risk. The characteristic clinical triad is that of ophthalmoplegia, ataxia, and global confusion. However, only one-third of patients with acute Wernicke's disease present with the classic clinical triad. Most patients are profoundly disoriented, indifferent, and inattentive, although rarely they have an agitated delirium related to ethanol withdrawal. If the disease is not treated, stupor, coma, and death may ensue. Ocular motor abnormalities include horizontal nystagmus on lateral gaze, lateral rectus palsy (usually bilateral), conjugate gaze palsies, and rarely ptosis. Gait ataxia probably results from a combination of polyneuropathy, cerebellar involvement, and vestibular paresis. The pupils are usually spared, but they may become miotic with advanced disease.

Wernicke's disease is usually associated with other manifestations of nutritional disease, such as polyneuropathy. Rarely, amblyopia or spinal spastic ataxia occurs. Tachycardia and postural hypotension may be related to impaired function of the autonomic nervous system or to the coexistence of cardiovascular beriberi. Patients who recover show improvement in ocular palsies within hours after the administration of thiamine, but horizontal nystagmus may persist. Ataxia improves more slowly than the ocular motor abnormalities. Approximately half recover incompletely and are left with a slow, shuffling, wide-based gait and an inability to tandem walk. Apathy, drowsiness, and confusion improve more gradually. As these symptoms recede, an amnestic state with impairment in recent memory and learning may become more apparent (*Korsakoff's psychosis*). Korsakoff's psychosis is frequently persistent; the residual mental state is characterized by gaps in memory, confabulation, and disordered temporal sequencing.

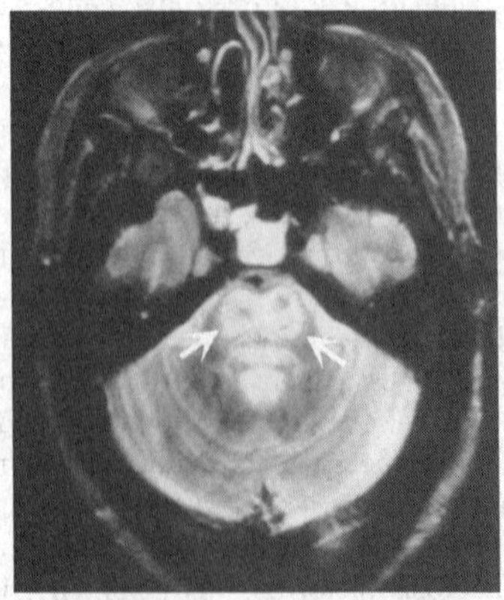

FIGURE 376-5 Central pontine myelinolysis. Axial T2-weighted magnetic resonance scan through the pons reveals a symmetric area of abnormal high signal intensity within the basis pontis (*arrows*).

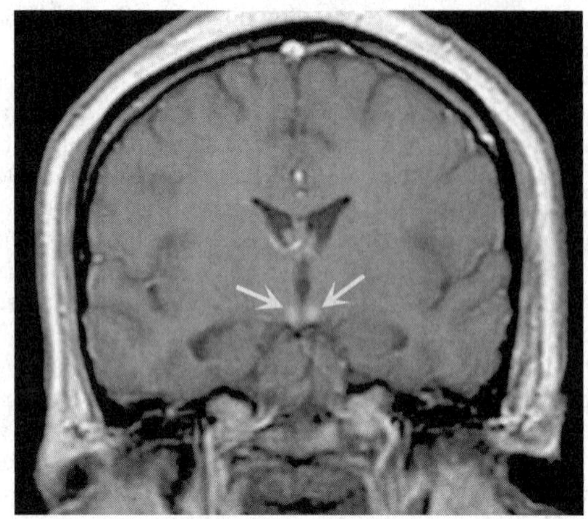

FIGURE 376-6 Wernicke's disease. Coronal T1-weighted postcontrast magnetic resonance image reveals abnormal enhancement of the mammillary bodies (*arrows*), typical of acute Wernicke's encephalopathy.

Pathology Lesions in the periventricular regions of the diencephalon, midbrain, and brainstem as well as the superior vermis of the cerebellum consist of symmetric discoloration of structures surrounding the third ventricle, aqueduct, and fourth ventricle, with petechial hemorrhages in occasional acute cases and atrophy of the mammillary bodies in most chronic cases. There is frequently endothelial proliferation, demyelination, and some neuronal loss. These changes may be detected by MRI scanning (Fig. 376-6). The amnestic defect is related to lesions in the dorsal medial nuclei of the thalamus.

Pathogenesis Thiamine is a cofactor of several enzymes, including transketolase, pyruvate dehydrogenase, and α-ketoglutarate dehydrogenase. Thiamine deficiency produces a diffuse decrease in cerebral glucose utilization and results in mitochondrial damage. Glutamate accumulates owing to impairment of α-ketoglutarate dehydrogenase activity and, in combination with the energy deficiency, may result in excitotoxic cell damage.

℞ TREATMENT Wernicke's disease is a medical emergency and requires immediate administration of thiamine, in a dose of 50 mg either intravenously or intramuscularly. The dose should be given daily until the patient resumes a normal diet and should be begun prior to treatment with intravenous glucose solutions. Glucose infusions may precipitate Wernicke's disease in a previously unaffected patient or cause a rapid worsening of an early form of the disease. For this reason, thiamine should be administered to all alcoholic patients requiring parenteral glucose.

CRITICAL CARE DISORDERS OF THE PERIPHERAL NERVOUS SYSTEM ASSOCIATED WITH SYSTEMIC DISEASE

Critical illness with disorders of the peripheral nervous system (PNS) arises in two contexts: (1) primary neurologic diseases that require critical care interventions such as intubation and mechanical ventilation, and (2) secondary PNS manifestations of systemic critical illness, often involving MSOF. The former include acute polyneuropathies such as Guillain-Barré syndrome (Chap. 378), neuromuscular junction disorders including myasthenia gravis (Chap. 380) and botulism (Chap. 144), and primary muscle disorders such as polymyositis (Chap. 382). The latter result either from the systemic disease itself or as a consequence of interventions.

General principles of respiratory evaluation in patients with PNS involvement, regardless of cause, include assessment of pulmonary mechanics, such as maximal inspiratory force (MIF) and vital capacity (VC), and evaluation of strength of bulbar muscles. Regardless of the cause of weakness, endotracheal intubation should be considered when the MIF falls to <-25 cmH_2O or the VC is <1 L. Also, patients with severe palatal weakness may require endotracheal intubation in order to prevent acute upper airway obstruction or recurrent aspiration. Arterial blood gases and percutaneous oxygen saturation are used to follow patients with potential respiratory compromise from PNS dysfunction; however, intubation and mechanical ventilation should be undertaken long before oxygen saturation drops or CO_2 retention develops from hypoventilation. →*Principles of mechanical ventilation are discussed in Chap. 266.*

NEUROPATHY While encephalopathy may be the most obvious neurologic dysfunction in critically ill patients, dysfunction of the PNS is also quite common. It is typically present in patients with prolonged critical illnesses lasting several weeks and involving sepsis; clinical suspicion is aroused when there is failure to wean from mechanical ventilation despite improvement of the underlying sepsis and critical illness. *Critical illness polyneuropathy* refers to the most common PNS complication related to critical illness; it is seen in the setting of prolonged critical illness, sepsis, and MSOF. Neurologic findings include diffuse weakness, decreased reflexes, and distal sensory loss. Electrophysiologic studies demonstrate a diffuse, symmetric, distal axonal sensorimotor neuropathy, and pathologic studies have confirmed axonal degeneration. The precise mechanism of critical illness polyneuropathy remains unclear, but circulating factors such as cytokines, which are associated with sepsis and SIRS, are thought to play a role. It has been reported that up to 70% of patients with the sepsis syndrome have some degree of neuropathy, although far fewer have a clinical syndrome profound enough to cause severe respiratory muscle weakness requiring prolonged mechanical ventilation or resulting in failure to wean. Treatment is supportive, with specific intervention directed at treating the underlying illness. While spontaneous recovery is usually seen, the time course may extend over weeks to months and necessitate long-term ventilatory support and care even after the underlying critical illness has resolved.

DISORDERS OF NEUROMUSCULAR TRANSMISSION A defect in neuromuscular transmission may be a source of weakness in critically ill patients. Myasthenia gravis (Chap. 380) may be a consideration; however, persistent weakness secondary to impaired neuromuscular junction transmission is almost always due to administration of drugs. A number of medications impair neuromuscular transmission; these include antibiotics, especially aminoglycosides, and beta-blocking agents. In the ICU, the nondepolarizing neuromuscular blocking agents (nd-NMBAs), also known as muscle relaxants, are most commonly responsible. Included in this group of drugs are such agents as pancuronium, vecuronium, rocuronium, and atracurium. They are often used to facilitate mechanical ventilation or other critical care procedures, but with prolonged use persistent neuromuscular blockade may result in weakness even after discontinuation of these agents hours or days earlier. Risk factors for this prolonged action of neuromuscular blocking agents include female sex, metabolic acidosis, and renal failure.

Prolonged neuromuscular blockade does not appear to produce permanent damage to the PNS. Once the offending medications are discontinued, full strength is restored, although this may take days. In general, the lowest dose of neuromuscular blocking agent should be used to achieve the desired result, and, when these agents are used in the ICU, a peripheral nerve stimulator should be used to monitor neuromuscular junction function.

MYOPATHY Critically ill patients, especially those with sepsis, frequently develop muscle wasting, often in the face of seemingly adequate nutritional support. The assumption has been that this represents a catabolic myopathy brought about as a result of multiple factors, including elevated cortisol and catecholamine release and other circulating factors induced by the SIRS. In this syndrome, known as *cachectic myopathy*, serum creatine kinase levels and electromyography (EMG) are normal. Muscle biopsy shows type II fiber atrophy. Panfascicular muscle fiber necrosis may also occur in the setting of profound sepsis. This so-called *septic myopathy* is characterized clinically by weakness progressing to a profound level over just a few days. There may be associated elevations in serum creatine kinase and urine myoglobin. Both EMG and muscle biopsy may be normal initially but eventually show abnormal spontaneous activity and panfascicular necrosis with an accompanying inflammatory reaction.

Acute quadriplegic myopathy describes a clinical syndrome of severe weakness seen in the setting of glucocorticoid and nd-NMBA use. The most frequent scenario in which this is encountered is the asthmatic patient who requires high-dose glucocorticoids and nd-NMBA to facilitate mechanical ventilation. This muscle disorder is not due to prolonged action of nd-NMBAs at the neuromuscular junction but, rather, is an actual myopathy with muscle damage; it has occasionally been described with high-dose glucocorticoid use alone. Clinically this syndrome is most often recognized when a patient fails to wean from mechanical ventilation despite resolution of the primary pulmonary process. Pathologically, there may be vacuolar changes in both type I and type II muscle fibers with evidence of regeneration. Acute quadriplegic myopathy has a good prognosis. If patients survive their underlying critical illness, the myopathy invariably improves and patients usually return to normal. However, because this syndrome is a result of true muscle damage, not just prolonged blockade at the neuromuscular junction, this process may take weeks or months, and tracheostomy with prolonged ventilatory support may be necessary. At present, it is unclear how to prevent this myopathic complication, except by avoiding use of nd-NMBAs, a strategy not always possible. Monitoring with a peripheral nerve stimulator can help to avoid the overuse of these agents. However, this is more likely to prevent the complication of prolonged neuromuscular junction blockade than it is to prevent this myopathy.

BIBLIOGRAPHY

Beal AL, Cerra FB: Multiple organ failure syndrome in the 1990s. Systemic inflammatory response and organ dysfunction. JAMA 271:226, 1994

Bolton CF et al: The neurological complications of sepsis. Ann Neurol 33:94, 1993

Hirano M et al: Acute quadriplegic myopathy: A complication of treatment with steroids, nondepolarizing blocking agents, or both. Neurology 42:2082, 1992

Kimelberg HK: Current concepts of brain edema. Review of laboratory investigations. J Neurosurg 83:1051, 1995

Larsson L et al: Acute quadriplegia and loss of muscle myosin in patients treated with nondepolarizing neuromuscular blocking agents and corticosteroids: Mechanisms at the cellular and molecular levels. Crit Care Med 28:34, 2000

Laureno R: Central pontine myelinolysis following rapid correction of hyponatremia. Ann Neurol 13:232, 1983

Lee JM et al: The changing landscape of ischemic brain injury mechanisms. Nature 399: A7, 1999

Levy DE et al: Predicting outcome from hypoxic-ischemic coma. JAMA 253:1420, 1985

Ropper AH: Neurological intensive care. Ann Neurol 32:564, 1992

Rosner MJ et al: Cerebral perfusion pressure: Management protocol and clinical results. J Neurosurg 83:949, 1995

Segredo V et al: Persistent paralysis in critically ill patients after long-term administration of vecuronium. N Engl J Med 327:524, 1992

The Multi-Society Task Force on PVS: Medical aspects of the persistent vegetative state (2). N Engl J Med 330:1572, 1994

Victor M et al: *The Wernicke-Korsakoff Syndrome and Related Disorders Due to Alcoholism and Malnutrition*. Philadelphia, Davis, 1989

Zandbergen EG et al: Systematic review of early prediction of poor outcome in anoxic-ischemic coma. Lancet 352:1808, 1998

Zochodne DW et al: Critical illness polyneuropathy. A complication of sepsis and multiple organ failure. Brain 110:819, 1987

377 APPROACH TO THE PATIENT WITH PERIPHERAL NEUROPATHY

Arthur K. Asbury

Peripheral neuropathy is a general term indicating peripheral nerve disorders of any cause; the manifestations of neuropathy may be so diverse that it is difficult for the physician to know where to begin and how to proceed.

The clinical and electrodiagnostic (EDX) approach to evaluation and management of a neuropathic disorder is summarized in Fig. 377-1. The EDX approach consists of electrophysiologic examination of nerve and muscle, including nerve conduction studies and electromyography. It is part of the evaluation of any neuropathy and is considered to be an extension of the neurologic examination. Using this scheme, the examiner determines for each patient the tempo, distribution, and severity of the neuropathy and makes a judgment as to whether the problem represents a mononeuropathy, a mononeuropathy multiplex, or a polyneuropathy. Often this distinction is obvious. With the sum of clinical and EDX information in hand, the differential diagnostic possibilities and treatment options are usually narrowed to a manageable number.

MONONEUROPATHY *Mononeuropathy* refers to focal involvement of a single nerve trunk and therefore implies a local cause. Direct trauma, compression, and entrapment are the usual ones. Ulnar neuropathies, due to lesions either at the ulnar groove or in the cubital tunnel, and median neuropathy due to compression in the carpal tunnel constitute the great majority of mononeuropathies encountered in clinical practice. These are described below, and other common mononeuropathies are listed in Table 377-1. EDX examination is part of the evaluation of mononeuropathies, mainly to judge the nature of the focal lesion (demyelinating or axonal degeneration) and, in severe mononeuropathies, to determine whether any nerve fibers remain in continuity.

In the absence of a history of trauma to the nerve trunk, factors favoring conservative management of a mononeuropathy include sudden onset, no motor deficit, few or no sensory findings (even though pain and sensory symptoms may be present), and no evidence of axonal degeneration by EDX criteria. Factors favoring active measures including surgical intervention are chronicity and worsening neurologic deficit on examination, particularly if motor and EDX evidence suggests that the lesion has produced a degree of wallerian degeneration.

Ulnar Neuropathy Complete ulnar paralysis results in a characteristic claw-hand deformity owing to wasting and weakness of many of the small hand muscles and hyperextension of the fingers at the metacarpophalangeal joints and flexion at the interphalangeal joints. The flexion deformity is most pronounced in the fourth and fifth fingers. Sensory loss occurs over the fifth finger, the ulnar aspect of the fourth finger, and the ulnar border of the palm. The superficial location of the nerve at the elbow makes it a common site of pressure palsy. The ulnar nerve may also become entrapped just distal to the

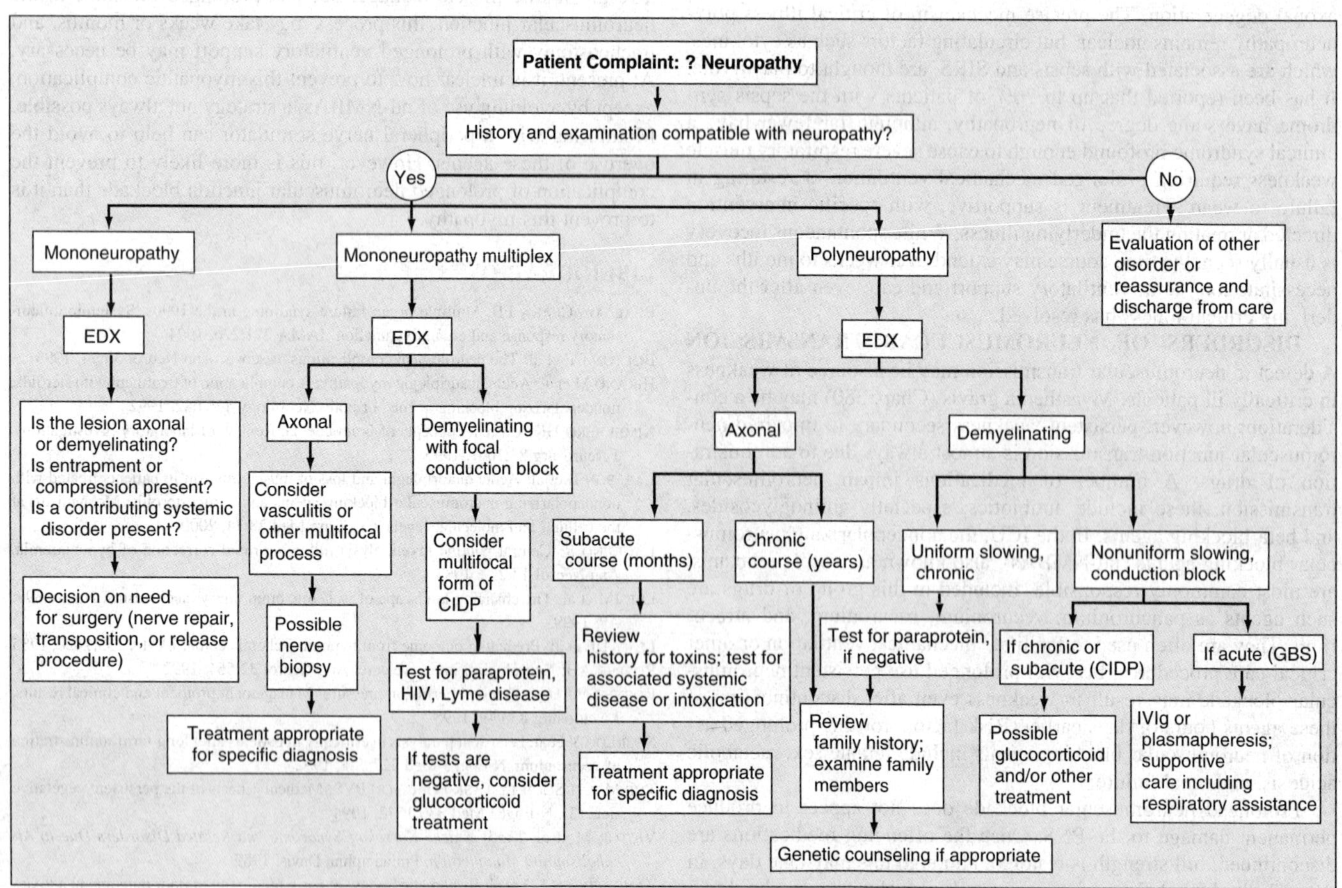

FIGURE 377-1 Approach to the evaluation of peripheral neuropathies. CIDP, chronic inflammatory demyelinating polyradiculoneuropathy; EDX, electrodiagnostic studies; GBS, Guillain-Barré syndrome; IVIg, intravenous immunoglobulin. *(After AK Asbury, in Harrison's Textbook of Internal Medicine, Update IV. New York, McGraw-Hill, 1983.)*

Table 377-1 Common Mononeuropathies

Nerve	Origin (Spinal Segments)	Muscles Innervated	Usual Site of Lesion	Clinical Features	Comments
UPPER EXTREMITY					
Suprascapular	C5, C6	Supraspinatus Infraspinatus	Suprascapular notch of scapula	Weakness of lateral rotation of the humerus	No sensory deficit
Long thoracic	C5–C7	Serratus anterior	Variable	Winging of scapula	No sensory deficit
Axillary	C5, C6	Deltoid, teres minor	Near shoulder joint	Weakness of shoulder abduction; atrophy of shoulder	Sensory deficit similar to C5 dorsal root lesion (See Figs. 23-2 and 23-3)
Radial	C5–T1	Triceps, brachioradialis, wrist, finger, and thumb extensors	Spiral groove of humerus	Wrist drop most obvious, also finger and thumb extensors paralyzed	Saturday night palsy (acute compression) is frequent cause
Posterior interosseous branch	C7, C8	Finger and thumb extensors	Edge of supinator muscle below elbow	Finger drop; wrist relatively spared	No sensory deficit
Ulnar	C8, T1	Ulnar flexor of the wrist, long flexors of 4th and 5th digits, and most intrinsic hand muscles	Ulnar groove at the elbow	Weakness of finger adduction and abduction and thumb adduction (see text); interosseous atrophy, claw-hand	May be acute or insidious; sensory symptoms/signs are distinctive (Figs. 23-2 and 23-3); see also text
			Cubital tunnel	Same as above	Often pain over medial proximal forearm (cubital tunnel)
			Medial base of palm	Intrinsic hand muscles only, interosseous atrophy	No sensory deficit
Median	C6–T1	Abductor pollicis brevis; more proximal muscles include forearm pronator, long finger and thumb flexors	Carpal tunnel	Characteristic sensory symptoms and deficit and inability to make a circle with thumb and index finger	Sensory deficit as per Figs. 23-2 and 23-3 (see text); known as carpal tunnel syndrome
Anterior interosseous branch	C7–T1	Long flexors of thumb and index and middle fingers	Anterior interosseus branch below the elbow	Weakness of pinch; pain in volar forearm	No sensory deficit
LOWER EXTREMITY					
Femoral	L2–L4	Iliopsoas (hip flexor) and quadriceps femoris (knee extensor)	Proximal to inguinal ligament	Knee buckling; absent knee jerk; weak anterior thigh muscles with atrophy	Association with diabetes mellitus; sensory disturbance as per Fig. 23-2
Lateral femoral cutaneous branch	L2, L3	None	Inguinal ligament	Dysesthetic hyperpathia of lateral thigh	Known as meralgia paresthetica
Obturator	L3, L4	Thigh adductors	Intrapelvic or at pubis	Weakness of hip adduction	Sensory deficit on medial thigh
Sciatic	L4–S3	Hamstring muscles, hip abductor, and all muscles below the knee	Near sciatic notch	Severe lower leg and hamstring weakness; flail foot; severe disability	Uncommon except from war wounds
Posterior tibial	L5–S2	Calf muscles (proximally), toe flexors and other intrinsic foot muscles	Tarsal tunnel, near medial malleolus	Pain and numbness of sole, weak toe flexors	Known as tarsal tunnel syndrome (see text)
Peroneal	L4–S1	Dorsiflexors of toes and foot, evertors of foot	At neck of fibula	Foot drop and weakness of foot eversion	Sensory deficit is similar in distribution to L5, S1 sensory roots

elbow in the cubital tunnel formed by the aponeurotic arch linking the two heads of the flexor carpi ulnaris. Also, prolonged pressure on the base of the palm, as occurs with use of hand tools or bicycle riding, may result in damage to the deep palmar branch of the ulnar nerve, causing weakness of the small hand muscles but no sensory loss (Table 377-1).

Carpal Tunnel Syndrome The median nerve in the carpal tunnel lies in close quarters with nine tendons. Entrapment of the nerve at the wrist (*carpal tunnel syndrome*) may be secondary to excessive use of the wrist, tenosynovitis with arthritis, or local infiltration, e.g., by a thickening of connective tissue as in acromegaly or by deposit of amyloid or by one of the mucopolysaccharidoses. Other systemic diseases associated with an increased incidence of carpal tunnel syndrome are hypothyroidism, rheumatoid arthritis, and diabetes mellitus, but underlying diseases account for only a small fraction of all cases. The main symptoms of carpal tunnel syndrome are nocturnal paresthesias of thumb, index, and middle fingers. With worsening, numbness occurs in that distribution, and is demonstrable by pin examination. Eventually weakness and atrophy of the abductor pollicis brevis (thenar eminence) becomes evident. The principal treatment of carpal tunnel syndrome is surgical section of the carpal ligament to relieve entrapment. Incomplete lesions of the median nerve between the axilla and wrist may result in *causalgia* (a particularly severe type of burning pain; Chap. 12; Table 377-1).

Tarsal Tunnel Syndrome The distal tibial nerve, along with several tendons and the posterior tibial artery, lies in the tarsal tunnel just posterior to the medial malleolus. Because of its superficial site, the distal tibial nerve is subject to compression or to direct trauma. Causes include sprain or fracture of the ankle, ill-fitting footwear, post-traumatic fibrosis, cysts, or ganglia adjacent to the nerve, arthritis, and tenosynovitis. Characteristic symptoms are pain in the ankle and the sole of the foot with paresthesias, particularly upon walking. On examination, the tibial nerve trunk in the tarsal tunnel is usually tender to palpation, sensory deficit should be demonstrable on the sole of the foot, and weakness of the toe plantar-flexor muscles may be noted. EDX examination and also nerve block using local anesthetic are useful in establishing the diagnosis. Definitive treatment is extensive surgical decompression of the tibial nerve in the tarsal tunnel. Tarsal tunnel syndrome, in terms of its pathophysiology and management, is similar to carpal tunnel syndrome but is much less common (Table 377-1).

POLYNEUROPATHY The prototypical picture of polyneuropathy occurs with acquired toxic or metabolic neuropathic states. The first symptoms tend to be sensory and consist of tingling, prickling, burning, or bandlike dysesthesias in the balls of the feet or tips of the toes, or in a general distribution over the soles (Chap. 23). Symptoms and findings are usually symmetric and graded distally. If the polyneuropathy remains mild, objective motor or sensory signs may not be detectable.

With progression, dysesthesias spread up the lower legs. Pansensory loss is usually found over both feet, ankle jerks are lost, and weakness of dorsiflexion of the toes, best demonstrated in the great toe, is present. In some instances, the process begins with weakness in the feet, without preceding sensory symptoms. As worsening occurs, sensory loss moves centripetally in a graded "stocking" fashion, and the patient may complain that the feet have a numb or "wooden" feeling or may say "I feel as though I'm walking on stumps." Patients have difficulty walking on their heels during examination, and their feet may slap while walking. Later, the knee jerk reflex disappears and foot drop becomes more apparent. By the time sensory disturbance has reached the upper shin, dysesthesias are usually noticed in the tips of the fingers. The degree of spontaneous pain varies but is often considerable. Light stimuli to hypesthetic areas, once perceived, may be experienced as extremely uncomfortable (*hyperpathia*). Unsteadiness of gait may be out of proportion to muscle weakness because of proprioceptive loss.

Worsening is more severe in the legs than in the arms and proceeds in a centripetal, symmetrically graded manner with pansensory loss, areflexia, and muscle atrophy; motor weakness is usually greater in the extensor muscles than in corresponding flexor groups. When the sensory disturbance reaches the elbows and mid-thighs, a tent-shaped area of hypesthesia may often be demonstrated on the lower abdomen. This area will grow broader, and its apex will extend rostrally toward the sternum as the neuropathy worsens. By this time, patients generally cannot stand or walk or hold objects in their hands.

Overall, nerve fibers are affected according to axon length, without regard to root or nerve trunk distribution—hence the aptness of the term *stocking-glove* to describe the pattern of sensory deficit. In general, the motor deficit is also graded, distal, and symmetric.

Although *polyneuropathy* connotes a widespread symmetric process, usually distal and graded, polyneuropathies are quite diverse because of the variability of tempo, severity, mix of sensory and motor features, and presence or absence of positive symptoms. For instance, a patient with a subacute, severely dysesthetic sensory polyneuropathy and alopecia who is in the early phases of thallium intoxication bears little similarity to the patient with a 40-year history of insidiously progressive clumsiness of gait whose findings are foot drop, lower leg atrophy, pes cavus, and minimal asymptomatic distal sensory deficit due to a hereditary polyneuropathy (Chap. 379). These two patients fall at opposite ends of the spectrum of polyneuropathy.

The classification of peripheral neuropathies has become increasingly complex as the capacity to discriminate new subgroups and identify new associations with toxins and systemic disorders improves. Further, our grasp of the pathophysiologic basis of the clinical phenomena observed in neuropathy has increased rapidly. But these advances are primarily descriptive; little progress has been made in understanding the fundamental pathogenic events in nervous tissue that eventuate in any of the polyneuropathies.

The important features of each major grouping of polyneuropathies are summarized in Table 377-2, and key aspects of specific polyneuropathies are given in Tables 377-3 to 377-6.

MONONEUROPATHY MULTIPLEX (MULTIFOCAL NEUROPATHY) *Mononeuropathy multiplex* refers to simultaneous or sequential involvement of individual noncontiguous nerve trunks, either partially or completely, evolving over days to years. Since the disease process underlying mononeuropathy multiplex involves peripheral nerves in a multifocal and random fashion, progression of the disease involves a tendency for the neurologic deficit to become less patchy and multifocal and more confluent and symmetric. As a result, some patients present with a distal symmetric neuropathy. Attention to the pattern of early symptoms is therefore important in making the judgment that a particular neuropathy is indeed a mononeuropathy multiplex.

ASSESSMENT AND DIAGNOSIS OF POLYNEUROPATHY AND MONONEUROPATHY MULTIPLEX Clues to the diagnosis of these neuropathies often lie in unnoticed or forgotten events occurring weeks or months prior to the onset of symptoms. Inquiry should be made about recent viral illnesses; other systemic symptoms; institution of new medications; exposures to solvents, pesticides, or heavy metals; the occurrence of similar symptoms in family members or coworkers; habits concerning alcohol; and the presence of preexisting medical disorders. Patients should be asked if they would feel well if free of their neuropathic symptoms; answers will suggest the presence or absence of an underlying systemic illness.

Table 377-2 Major Types of Polyneuropathy

Type of Polyneuropathy	Evolution	Causes	Comments
Axonal			
Acute	Days to weeks	Porphyria	See Table 377-3; also Chap. 346
		Massive intoxications (arsenic; inhalants)	See Table 377-4
		Guillain-Barré syndrome—axonal form	See Chapter 378
Subacute	Weeks to months	Mostly toxic or metabolic polyneuropathies; see Tables 377-3 and 377-4	Treatment involves eliminating the toxins or treating the associated systemic disorder
Chronic	Months to years	<5 years, consider toxic/metabolic causes; >5 years, consider hereditary basis, also diabetic and dysproteinemic causes	See Tables 377-3 and 377-4; also Chap. 379 on hereditary neuropathy
Demyelinating			
Acute	Days to weeks	Almost all are the common form of Guillain-Barré syndrome; see Chap. 378	Rare possibilities include diphtheritic polyneuritis or buckthorn berry intoxication
Subacute	Weeks to months	Mostly relapsing form of CIDP (see Chap. 378)	Rarely, toxins mentioned above plus aurothioglucose and taxol (see Table 377-3)
Chronic	Months to years	Many possibilities including hereditary; inflammatory-autoimmune; dysproteinemias, other metabolic and toxic neuropathies	See Chaps. 378 and 379; also Tables 377-3 and 377-4

Table 377-3 Polyneuropathy Associated with Systemic Diseases

Systemic Disease (Occurrence)	Axonal[a]			Demyelinating[a]			Sensory vs. Motor[b]	Autonomic[a]	Comment
	Acute	Subacute	Chronic	Acute	Subacute	Chronic			
Diabetes mellitus (common)	−	±	+	−	±	+	S, SM, rarely M	± to +	See Table 377-5
Uremia (sometimes)	±	+	+	−	−	−	SM	±	Controllable with proper dialysis; curable with successful renal transplant
Porphyria (3 types) (rare)	+	±	−	−	−	−	M or SM	± to +	May be proximal $>$ distal and may have atypical proximal sensory deficits
Hypoglycemia (rare)	±	+	±	−	−	−	M	−	Usually with insulinoma; arms often $>$ legs
Vitamin deficiency, excluding B_{12} (sometimes)	−	+	+	−	−	−	SM	±	Involves thiamine, pyridoxine, folate, pantothenic acid, and probably others
Vitamin B_{12} deficiency (sometimes)	−	±	+	−	−	−	S	−	Neuropathy overshadowed by myelopathy
Critical illness (sepsis) (common)	−	+	±	−	−	−	M $>$ S	−	Sepsis patients severely ill
Chronic liver disease (sometimes)	−	−	−	−	−	+	S or SM	−	Usually mild or subclinical
Primary biliary cirrhosis (rare)	−	±	+	−	−	−	S	−	Intraneural xanthomas; dysesthesia
Primary systemic amyloidosis (rare)	−	±	+	−	−	−	SM	+	Also in amyloidosis with myeloma or macroglobulinemia
Hypothyroidism (rare)	−	−	−	−	±	+	S	−	May respond to thyroid replacement
Chronic obstructive lung disease (rare)	−	±	+	−	−	−	S or SM	−	Severe pulmonary insufficiency
Acromegaly (rare)	−	−	+	−	−	−	S	−	Carpal tunnel syndrome also frequent
Malabsorption (sprue, celiac disease) (sometimes)	−	±	+	−	−	−	S or SM	±	Basis for neuropathy unclear; deficiency?
Carcinoma (sensory) (rare)	−	+	+	−	−	−	Pure S	−	Due to ganglionitis mostly small cell lung or breast carcinoma; paraneoplastic
Carcinoma (sensorimotor) (sometimes)	−	+	+	−	−	−	SM	±	Sensorimotor axonal neuropathy; mostly with lung cancer
Carcinoma (late) (common)	−	+	+	−	−	−	S $>$ M	±	Mild, probably related to weight loss and wasting
Carcinoma (demyelinating) (sometimes)	−	−	−	+	+	±	SM	−	Acute or relapsing demyelinating neuropathy
HIV infection (sometimes)	−	±	+	−	−	−	S $\gg$ M	−	Late stages of AIDS; other neuropathies occur; see text
Lyme disease (sometimes)	−	±	+	−	−	−	S $>$ M	−	Variable picture; see text
Lymphoma, including Hodgkin's (sometimes)	−	+	+	+	+	±	See above	±	Same as with carcinomatous types
Polycythemia vera (rare)	−	±	+	−	−	−	S	−	Also CNS manifestations; often shooting pains in limbs
Multiple myeloma, lytic type (sometimes)	−	±	+	−	−	−	S, M, or SM	±	Symptomatic neuropathy uncommon; subclinical neuropathy frequent
Multiple myeloma, osteosclerotic[c] (sometimes)	−	−	±	−	±	+	SM	−	May show severe slowing of nerve conduction velocity

(continued)

Table 377-3 Polyneuropathy Associated with Systemic Diseases—(*continued*)

Systemic Disease (Occurrence)	Axonal[a] Acute	Axonal[a] Subacute	Axonal[a] Chronic	Demyelinating[a] Acute	Demyelinating[a] Subacute	Demyelinating[a] Chronic	Sensory vs. Motor[b]	Autonomic[a]	Comment
Monoclonal gammopathy of undetermined significance (sometimes):									
IgA	−	±	+	−	−	−	SM	−	IgM_κ mainly; may bind to myelin-associated glycoprotein (MAG) or other glycoconjugates
IgG	−	±	+	−	−	−	SM	−	
IgM	−	−	−	−	±	+	SM or S	−	
Cryoglobulinemia (rare)	−	±	+	−	−	−	SM	−	May be mononeuropathy multiplex in presentation

[a] +, Usually; ±, sometimes; −, rare, if ever.
[b] S, sensory; M, motor; SM, sensorimotor.
[c] Some cases associated with POEMS syndrome (*p*olyneuropathy, *o*rganomegaly, *e*ndocrinopathy, *M* proteins, and *s*kin changes; see Chap. 339).

How did symptoms first appear? Even with distal polyneuropathies, symptoms may appear in the sole of one foot a few days or a week before the other, but usually the patient will describe a distal graded disturbance that moves evenly and symmetrically in centripetal fashion. Symptoms that first appear in the distribution of individual digital nerves, involving only half of a digit at a time, and then gradually spread and coalesce suggest a multifocal process (mononeuropathy multiplex), as might occur with a systemic vasculitis or cryoglobulinemia.

The evolution of neuropathy ranges from rapid worsening over a few days to an indolent process lasting many years. Polyneuropathies that progress slowly, over more than 5 years, are most likely to be genetically determined, particularly if the major manifestations are distal atrophy and weakness with few or no positive sensory symptoms. Diabetic polyneuropathy and paraproteinemic neuropathies also progress insidiously over 5 to 10 years. Axonal degenerations of toxic or metabolic origin tend to evolve over several weeks to a year or more, and the rate of progression of demyelinating neuropathies is highly variable, ranging from a few days in Guillain-Barré syndrome (GBS; Chap. 378) to many years in others.

Major fluctuations in the course of neuropathy raise two possibilities: (1) relapsing forms of neuropathy and (2) repeated toxic exposures. Slow fluctuation in symptoms taking place over weeks or months (reflecting changes in the activity of neuropathy) should not be confused with day-to-day variation or diurnal undulation of symptoms. The latter are common to all neuropathic disorders. An example is carpal tunnel syndrome, in which dysesthesias may be prominent at night but absent during the day.

Palpation of the nerve trunk to detect enlargement is a frequently forgotten part of the neurologic examination. In mononeuropathy or mononeuropathy multiplex, the entire course of the nerve trunk in question should be explored manually for focal thickening, for the presence of neurofibroma, point tenderness, or Tinel's phenomenon (generation of a tingling sensation in the sensory territory of the nerve by tapping along the course of the nerve trunk); and for pain elicited by stretching of the nerve trunk. In leprous neuritis, fusiform thickening of nerve trunks is frequent, and beading of nerve trunks may be encountered in amyloid polyneuropathy. In genetically determined hypertrophic neuropathies, uniform thickening of all nerve trunks may occur, often to the caliber of a clothesline or larger.

Most neuropathies involve nerve fibers of all sizes, but damage is sometimes restricted to either large or small fibers. In a polyneuropathy affecting mainly small fibers, diminished pinprick and temperature sensation, often with painful, burning dysesthesias, will predominate, along with autonomic dysfunction but with relative sparing of motor power, balance, and tendon jerks. Some cases of amyloid and distal diabetic polyneuropathies fall into this category. In contrast, large-fiber polyneuropathy is characterized by areflexia, sensory ataxia, relatively minor cutaneous sensory deficit, and variable degrees of motor dysfunction, sometimes severe.

For patients with polyneuropathy or mononeuropathy multiplex, standard tests should include a complete blood count and measurement of erythrocyte sedimentation rate, urinalysis, chest x-ray, postprandial blood glucose determination, and serum protein electrophoresis. Further tests are dictated by the combined results of the history and the physical and EDX examination (Fig. 377-1).

Electrodiagnosis EDX examination is a key procedure in all patients with suspected neuropathy. It is generally not possible to make the distinction between axonal and demyelinating disorders by clinical examination alone; here EDX analysis is particularly useful. EDX features of demyelination are slowing of nerve conduction velocity (NCV), dispersion of evoked compound action potentials, conduction block (major decrease in amplitude of muscle compound action potentials on proximal stimulation of the nerve, as compared to distal stimulation), and marked prolongation of distal latencies (Chap. 357). In contrast, axonal neuropathies are characterized by a reduction in amplitude of evoked compound action potentials with relative preservation of NCV. The distinction between a primarily demyelinating neuropathy and an axonal neuropathy is crucial because of the differing approaches to diagnosis and management.

EDX studies also help to determine the presence or absence of a sensory involvement when that is not clear by clinical examination alone. It provides information about the distribution of subclinical findings, thus sharpening the diagnostic focus. Other issues that may be clarified by the electrodiagnostician include:

1. The distinction between disorders primary to nerve and to muscle (neuropathy versus myopathy)
2. The distinction between root or plexus involvement and more distal nerve trunk involvement
3. The distinction between generalized polyneuropathic processes and widespread multifocal nerve trunk involvement
4. The distinction between upper and lower motor neuron weakness
5. The distinction, in a given generalized polyneuropathic process, between primary demyelinating neuropathy and axonal degeneration
6. The assessment, in both primary axonal and demyelinating neuropathies, of features bearing on the nature, activity, and likely prognosis of the neuropathy
7. The assessment, in mononeuropathies, of the site of the lesion and its major effect on nerve fibers, especially the distinction between demyelinating conduction block and wallerian degeneration
8. The characterization of disorders of the neuromuscular junction
9. The identification, often in muscle of normal bulk and strength, of important features such as chronic partial denervation, fasciculations, and myotonia
10. The analysis of cramp, and its distinction from physiologic contracture

Table 377-4 Polyneuropathy Associated with Drugs and Environmental Toxins

	Axonal[a]			Demyelinating[a]						
	Acute	Subacute	Chronic	Acute	Subacute	Chronic	Sensory vs. Motor[b]	Autonomic[a]	CNS[a]	Comment
DRUGS[c]										
Amiodarone (antiarrhythmic)	−	−	+	−	−	+	SM	−	−	Dose-dependent neuropathy, reversible by decreasing dose
Aurothioglucose (antirheumatic)	±	±	−	+	+	−	SM	−	−	Idiosyncratic reaction; ? immune-mediated
Cisplatin (antineoplastic)	−	+	+	−	−	−	S	−	−	Severe sensory neuropathy, also ototoxicity; dose-related
Dapsone (dermatologic agent; used, e.g., for leprosy)	−	±	+	−	−	−	M	−	−	Dose-related pure motor neuropathy
Disulfiram (antialcoholism agent)	±	+	+	−	−	−	SM	−	±	Usually occurs after months of treatment
Hydralazine (antihypertensive)	−	±	+	−	−	−	S > M	−	−	A pyridoxine antagonist
Isoniazid	−	±	+	−	−	−	SM	±	−	A pyridoxine antagonist; neurotoxic in slow acetylators
Metronidazole (antiprotozoal)	−	−	±	−	−	−	S or SM	−	+	Dose-related central-peripheral distal axonopathy
Misonidazole (radiosensitizer)	−	±	+	−	−	−	S or SM	−	+	Neurotoxicity is the limiting factor
Nitrofurantoin (urinary antiseptic)	−	±	+	−	−	−	SM	−	−	Generally total dose-related; renal failure enhances toxicity
Nucleoside analogues (ddC, ddI, d4T) (antiretroviral agents)	±	+	+	−	−	−	S ≫ M	−	?	Dose related; painful
Phenytoin (anticonvulsant)	−	−	+	−	−	−	S > M	−	−	After 20–30 years of phenytoin use
Pyridoxine (vitamin)	−	±	+	−	−	−	S	−	−	Occurs with large intake (>300 mg/d)
Suramin (antineoplastic)	+	+	−	+	+	−	M > S	−	−	Related to serum levels 350 μg/mL or above
Taxol (antineoplastic)	±	+	±	±	+	±	S > M	−	−	Dose-related
Vincristine (antineoplastic)	−	+	+	−	−	−	S > M	−	−	Sensory symptoms common, hands > feet; motor signs ominous; should stop treatment
TOXINS[c]										
Acrylamide (flocculant; grouting agent)	−	±	+	−	−	−	S > M	±	+	Large-fiber neuropathy; sensory ataxia
Arsenic (herbicide; insecticide)	±	+	+	−	−	−	SM	±	±	Skin changes, Mees' lines in nails; painful; systemic effects
Diphtheria toxin	−	−	−	+	+	−	SM	−	−	Clinically very rare; can be confused with GBS

(continued)

Table 377-4 Polyneuropathy Associated with Drugs and Environmental Toxins—*(continued)*

	Axonal[a]			Demyelinating[a]						
	Acute	Subacute	Chronic	Acute	Subacute	Chronic	Sensory vs. Motor[b]	Autonomic[a]	CNS[a]	Comment
γ-Diketone hexacarbons (solvents)	−	±	+	−	−	+	SM	±	+	Neurofilamentous swelling of axons; these solvents now in restricted use
Inorganic lead	−	−	+	−	−	−	M > S or M	−	±	Selective motor neuropathy with prominent wrist drop
Organophosphates	−	±	+	−	−	−	SM	−	+	Brain and spinal cord also affected, the latter irreversibly
Thallium (rat poison)	−	+	+	−	−	−	SM	−	+	Also alopecia, Mees' lines in nails; painful

[a] +, Usually; ±, sometimes; −, rare, if ever.
[b] S, sensory; M, motor; SM, sensorimotor.
[c] The following drugs and environmental toxins are also neurotoxic, mainly to the peripheral nervous system:
Drugs: Amitriptyline, chloramphenicol, colchicine, ethambutol, nitrous oxide, perhexiline maleate, sodium cyanate, thalidomide, L-tryptophan.
Environmental toxins: Allyl chloride, buckthorn berry, carbon disulfide, dimethylaminoproprionitrile (DMAPN), ethylene oxide, metallic mercury, methyl bromide, polychlorinated biphenyls, styrene, trichlorethylene, vacor.
NOTE: CNS, central nervous system; GBS, Guillain-Barré syndrome.

If in a particular instance of progressive polyneuropathy of subacute or chronic evolution the EDX findings are those of an axonopathy, a long list of metabolic states and exogenous toxins comes under consideration (Tables 377-3 and 377-4). If the course is protracted over several years, it raises the likelihood of a hereditary neuropathy (Chap. 379); family members must be examined and additional attention given to the family history. If the EDX findings indicate primary demyelination of nerve, the approach is entirely different. The possibilities then include acquired demyelinating neuropathy, thought to be immunologically mediated (Chap. 378), and genetically determined neuropathies, some of which are marked by uniform and drastic slowing of nerve conduction velocities (Chap. 379).

If the clinical features indicate mononeuropathy multiplex, the EDX question is whether the process is primarily axonal or demyelinating. Almost one-third of all adults with the clinical syndrome of mononeuropathy multiplex have a clear-cut picture of a demyelinating disorder, often with foci of persistent conduction block on EDX examination. Multifocal demyelinating neuropathy may represent part of the spectrum of chronic inflammatory demyelinating neuropathy (CIDP), or, if multifocal and only motor, would fit into the related category of multifocal motor neuropathy. →*For further discussion of the management of multifocal motor neuropathy, see Chap. 378.*

The remaining two-thirds of patients with mononeuropathy multiplex have a picture of patchy axonal involvement by EDX examination. Although ischemia should be suspected as the basis of neuropathy in these patients, only about one-half can be shown to have disease of the vasa nervorum, usually vasculitis. Management of those with proven vasculitis of vasa nervorum is often the same as treatment for systemic vasculitis (Chaps. 317 and 378). If the cause of mononeuropathy multiplex remains undiagnosed even on follow-up, management should be conservative. In many patients the disease will stabilize or reverse, at least partially.

Mononeuropathy multiplex syndrome may also be seen as a manifestation of leprosy, sarcoidosis, certain types of amyloidosis, hypereosinophilia syndrome, cryoglobulinemia, neuroAIDs, and multifocal types of diabetic neuropathy.

Nerve Biopsy The sural nerve at the ankle is the preferred site for cutaneous nerve biopsy. There are few indications to employ this invasive technique. The main one is in asymmetric and multifocal neuropathic disorders producing a clinical picture of mononeuropathy multiplex, the basis of which is still unclear after other laboratory investigations are complete. Diagnostic considerations include vasculitis, multifocal demyelinating neuropathies, amyloidosis, leprosy, and occasionally sarcoidosis. Nerve biopsy is also helpful when one or more cutaneous nerves are palpably enlarged. Another clinical application is in establishing the diagnosis in some genetically determined childhood disorders such as metachromatic leukodystrophy, Krabbe's disease, giant axonal neuropathy, and infantile neuroaxonal dystrophy. In all of these recessively inherited diseases, both the central nervous system and the peripheral nervous system are affected.

There is a tendency to carry out sural nerve biopsy in distal symmetric polyneuropathies of subacute or chronic evolution. This practice is discouraged because its yield is low. Nerve biopsy in this situation may be useful as part of an approved research protocol when the biopsy will provide crucial information not otherwise obtainable.

SPECIAL CATEGORIES OF NEUROPATHY Some neuropathies require individual description because of their importance or distinctiveness.

Diabetic Neuropathies The neuropathies of diabetes mellitus are classified in Table 377-5. A limitation of this classification is that most patients do not fit neatly into any single category but instead have overlapping clinical features of several. For instance, many diabetic patients with distal, primarily sensory polyneuropathy can also be shown to have autonomic dysfunction, usually in the form of vasomotor disturbance in the limbs and abnormalities of sweating. Similarly, patients who develop a proximal motor syndrome often have dysautonomic features (including sexual impotence in males) and some degree of distal sensory polyneuropathy. To compound matters, such patients appear at risk of developing a cranial mononeuropathy. Pain is a frequent feature of diabetic neuropathies (Table 377-5) but is variable in incidence and degree.

Table 377-5 Classification of Diabetic Neuropathies

Symmetric
1. Distal, primarily sensory polyneuropathy
   a. Mainly large fibers affected
   b. Mixed[a]
   c. Mainly small fibers affected[a]
2. Autonomic neuropathy
3. Chronically evolving proximal motor neuropathy[a,b]

Asymmetric
1. Acute or subacute proximal motor neuropathy[a,b]
2. Cranial mononeuropathy[b]
3. Truncal neuropathy[a,b]
4. Entrapment neuropathy in the limbs

[a] Often painful.
[b] Recovery, partial or complete, is likely.

Table 377-6 Sensory Neuropathies

Cause or Association	Course	Nerve Fiber Size Affected: Small	Large	Neuronopathy	Comment
TOXINS/DRUGS					
Cisplatin (antineoplastic)	Sub/Chr	+	++	+	Dose-related
Pyridoxine (vitamin, in megadose amounts)	Sub/Chr	+	++	+/−	Dose-related
Taxol (antineoplastic)	Acu/Sub	++	+	−	NGF may be protective
SYSTEMIC DISEASES					
Paraneoplastic	Sub	+	++	++	Most SCLC and breast
Sjögren's syndrome	Sub/Chr	+/−	+	++	Variable presentation
Dysproteinemia (mainly IgM_{κ})	Chr	+	++	−	Demyelinating; may bind to MAG and other myelin glycoproteins
IDIOPATHIC					
Acute sensory neuronopathy	Acu	+/−	++	++	Poor recovery; persistent deficit
Chronic ataxic neuropathy	Chr	+/−	++	Prob.	Gradual progression
HEREDITARY					
Many varieties (see Chap. 379)	Chr	Variable		Some	Progressive

ABBREVIATIONS: ++, most; +, some; ±, occasionally; Prob, probable; Acu, acute; Sub, subacute; Chr, chronic; NGF, nerve growth factor;; MAG, myelin-associated glycoprotein; SCLC, small cell lung carcinoma.

Diabetic neuropathies occur in the setting of long-standing hyperglycemia (decades), whether the diabetes is insulin-dependent or not. By far the most common neuropathies related to diabetes mellitus are the diffuse sensory and autonomic types (categories 1 and 2 under "Symmetric" in Table 377-5). Sensory and autonomic polyneuropathy, chronic and indolent in evolution, may first be noticed in the third to fifth decades in patients with juvenile-onset diabetes but tends to occur after age 50 in patients with adult-onset diabetes. Focal and multifocal types of neuropathy are less common but quite dramatic (categories 1, 2, and 3 under "Asymmetric" in Table 377-5). They rarely occur before the age of 45 and are usually subacute or acute in onset. Cranial mononeuropathies are isolated sixth or third nerve palsies. The latter spares the pupil in three-fourths of cases, and some local pain or headache occurs in one-half. Truncal (thoracoabdominal) neuropathy is painful, involves one or more intercostal or lumbar nerves unilaterally, and frequently coexists with the asymmetric proximal motor neuropathy. In asymmetric proximal motor neuropathy, the most evident features are weakened muscles innervated by the femoral and obturator nerves (quadriceps femoris, iliopsoas, adductor magnus) and ipsilateral loss of the knee jerk reflex. Sensory deficit is minor, but pain in the hip and anterior thigh may be prominent. In all these multifocal and focal neuropathies, the pain usually subsides within weeks to a year, and function is usually partly or completely recovered. The same is true for symmetric proximal motor neuropathy (category 3 under "Symmetric" in Table 377-5).

Focal and multifocal diabetic neuropathies are considered to be ischemic in origin, and ischemia may also underlie symmetric polyneuropathies, which are also thought to involve abnormality of nerve metabolism.

Management of diabetic neuropathies is directed toward optimal glycemic control and symptomatic pain suppression. In the long-term Diabetes Control and Complications Trial, patients who controlled their diabetes meticulously showed significantly less neuropathy. The role of aldose reductase inhibitors in preventing or reversing diabetic complications, including neuropathy, remains unclear. Entrapment neuropathies are frequently amenable to surgical decompression.

Neuropathies with HIV Infection Neuropathies are common in infection with HIV, but different types of neuropathy are seen according to the stage of the disease. GBS or CIDP (Chap. 378) are the neuropathies likely to occur following conversion to seropositivity and during the asymptomatic phase of HIV infection. Treatment is the same as for HIV-negative patients. In later, symptomatic stages, mononeuritis multiplex, axonal in nature, can occur; the course is typically subacute or chronic. In some cases, vasculitis of the vasa nervorum has been demonstrated.

The most common neuropathy is a distal, symmetric, mainly sensory polyneuropathy, which evolves slowly in the late symptomatic stages of HIV infection and frequently coexists with symptomatic encephalopathy and myelopathy (Table 377-3; Chap. 309). Improvement of this polyneuropathy with zidovudine treatment has been claimed. Sensory polyneuropathy of late-stage HIV infection must be distinguished from toxic polyneuropathy that may result from the use of nucleoside analogue treatment (Table 377-4). Also in the late stages, a severe, destructive, subacute, asymmetric polyradiculopathy involving the cauda equina may be seen; it is caused by an opportunistic infection of the nerve roots with cytomegalovirus. Ganciclovir, started early, can arrest the disorder.

Neuropathies with Lyme Disease A focal or multifocal radiculoneuropathy may occur weeks, months, or even years after primary infection by the tick-borne spirochete *Borrelia burgdorferi*. Although usually sensory and either dysesthetic or painful, the neuropathy is variable in distribution, affecting cranial nerves and spinal roots or nerves in a patchy, asymmetric fashion. Neuropathy is often chronic and persistent; cerebrospinal fluid pleocytosis is the rule. In many, improvement occurs spontaneously, but the course is shortened by treatment with antibiotics, usually intravenous ceftriaxone (Chap. 176).

Herpes Zoster This is a sensory neuritis due to infection with varicella-zoster virus and is characterized by acute inflammation of one or more dorsal root ganglia. Lancinating pain and hyperalgesia over the skin surface supplied by the affected roots occur for 3 to 4 days, followed by the appearance in the same segment of a herpetic eruption characterized by painful raised blisters on reddened bases. Pain usually subsides in a few weeks. If the inflammatory process spreads to involve related motor roots, segmental motor weakness and wasting appear. Paralysis of the oculomotor nerves may occur in conjunction with involvement of the ophthalmic division of the trigeminal ganglion (ophthalmoplegic zoster). Facial paralysis may occur with involvement of the geniculate ganglion and herpetic eruption on the ipsilateral tympanic membrane or external ear canal (Ramsay Hunt syndrome).

In fewer than 5% of patients, neuropathic pain persists in the dermatomal distribution of the affected ganglia. This pain, known as *postherpetic neuralgia*, is intense, burning, hyperpathic, and unrelenting; it often dominates the lives of those affected. Advancing age is a risk factor for this outcome. In some patients, blunting of the pain to tolerable levels is achieved by use of carbamazepine or a tricyclic antidepressant such as desipramine (Chap. 12).

Leprous Neuritis This is a major worldwide cause of neuropathy. *Mycobacterium leprae* organisms readily invade Schwann cells in cutaneous nerve twigs, particularly those associated with unmyelinated nerve fibers. *M. leprae* thrives best in the coolest tissues in the body. Two major forms of leprous neuritis are recognized, tuberculoid and lepromatous, which actually represent the ends of a spectrum of disease, the middle of which is called borderline (dimorphous) leprosy (patchy and multifocal involvement of skin and nerve). The treatment of a given case depends on where it falls in this spectrum (Chap. 170). Tuberculoid (high-resistance) leprosy consists of a single patch of hypesthetic or anesthetic skin in any location. The skin patch is frequently thickened, reddened, or hypopigmented. Few or no *M. leprae* bacilli may be demonstrated. If a superficially placed nerve trunk, typically a cutaneous nerve, courses just beneath the area of affected skin, it may be engulfed in the inflammatory reaction, resulting in an associated mononeuropathy. Such a nerve may be palpably enlarged and beaded. Lepromatous (low-resistance) leprosy is marked by immunologic tolerance, numerous bacilli, and widespread skin thickening, cutaneous anesthesia, and anhidrosis, which spare only the warmest parts of the body, notably the axilla, the groin, and beneath the scalp hair. Motor signs (focal weakness and atrophy) result from damage to mixed nerves lying close to the skin, particularly the median, ulnar, peroneal, and facial nerves.

Bell's Palsy This seventh nerve palsy is due to inflammation of the facial nerve in the facial canal, the basis for which remains obscure. Edema may play a part in causing compression of nerve fibers, with resulting acute unilateral paralysis of facial muscles (Chap. 367).

Sarcoidosis This may involve single or multiple peripheral nerves, producing asymmetric mononeuritis or polyneuritis. Unilateral or bilateral facial paralysis is described in association with parotitis and uveitis (Heerfordt's syndrome).

Polyneuritis Cranialis This is a relapsing and remitting mononeuropathy multiplex restricted to cranial nerves (Chap. 367). It is usually associated with indolent tuberculous cervical adenitis (scrofula) or sarcoidosis. Treatment of the underlying condition will halt the cranial nerve palsies.

SPECIAL NEUROPATHIC PRESENTATIONS Some disorders selectively affect the peripheral nervous system, limiting dysfunction to specific systems or sites, such as motor nerves, brachial plexus, or the autonomic nervous system.

Autonomic Neuropathy The autonomic nervous system regulates the visceral organs and vegetative functions (Chap. 366). Many pharmacologic agents modify specific autonomic functions, but autonomic neuropathy (dysautonomia) with structural changes in pre- and postganglionic neurons can also occur. Usually autonomic neuropathy is a manifestation of a more generalized polyneuropathy also affecting somatic peripheral nervous function, as in diabetic neuropathy, GBS, and alcoholic polyneuropathy, but occasionally syndromes of pure pandysautonomia are encountered. Symptoms of dysautonomia are mainly negative (i.e., loss of function) and include postural hypotension with faintness or syncope, anhidrosis, hypothermia, bladder atony, obstipation, dry mouth and dry eyes from failure of salivary and lacrimal glands to secrete, blurring of vision from lack of pupillary and ciliary regulation, and sexual impotence in males. Positive phenomena (hyperfunction) may also occur and include episodic hypertension, diarrhea, hyperhidrosis, and either tachycardia or bradycardia. Management is symptomatic and also directed at the underlying cause, if it can be identified.

Pure Motor Neuropathy Disorder affecting any level of the motor unit—anterior horn cell, motor axon, or neuromuscular junction—can result in a purely lower motor syndrome without sensory disturbance. Distinguishing anterior horn cell disorders (motor neuronopathies) from motor axonopathies may be difficult clinically because they share manifestations (weakness, muscle denervation atrophy, hypo- or areflexia, fasciculations). EDX examination may also fail to localize the primary site of the lesion (neuropathic versus neuronopathic) unless the lesion is demyelinating in nature, in which case it is by definition neuropathic.

Examples of motor neuronopathies include the lower-motor form of amyotrophic lateral sclerosis, poliomyelitis, hereditary spinal muscular atrophies, and adult variant of hexosaminidase A deficiency. Motor neuropathies may be seen with lead or dapsone intoxication, occasionally with porphyria, and also with multifocal motor neuropathy. The latter is a chronic asymmetric disorder of mid-life associated with persistent conduction block on EDX examination, and often high titers of antiganglioside antibodies (particularly anti-GM_1). Neuromuscular junction disorders (e.g., Lambert-Eaton myasthenic syndrome, tick bite paralysis, other types of toxic neuromuscular blockade) are purely motor and can be recognized and localized electrodiagnostically. Some motor-sensory polyneuropathies have predominant motor symptoms and signs, such as hereditary motor-sensory neuropathies, GBS, and CIDP, but the subclinical sensory component is readily demonstrated electrodiagnostically or by quantitative sensory testing.

Pure Sensory Neuropathy Clinical presentations involving primary sensation only (Table 377-6; Chap. 23) are not uncommon. Manifestations may (1) reflect mainly large afferent fiber involvement with deficits of vibratory and proprioceptive sense, areflexia, and sensory ataxia with or without tingling dysesthesias; (2) reflect mainly small afferent fiber involvement with numbness and cutaneous hypesthesia to pin-prick and temperature stimuli, often with painful, burning dysesthesias; or (3) be pansensory, with both large and small fiber manifestations. The pattern of distribution, although variable, is often distal and symmetric, particularly for large-fiber neuropathies.

The most severe and widespread of these pure sensory syndromes exhibit poor or no recovery, suggesting irreversible lesions of nerve cell bodies in dorsal root and trigeminal ganglia. These are referred to as *sensory neuronopathies*. With sensory neurotoxins, moderate doses lead to potentially reversible neuropathy, but high doses appear to cause irreversible neuronopathy (Table 377-6).

Plexopathy This term refers to disorders of either the brachial or the lumbosacral plexus. Lesions of the brachial plexus are characterized by motor and sensory signs different from those expected in either mononeuropathies of the upper limb or polyneuropathies. The usual causes are direct trauma to the plexus, idiopathic brachial neuritis (also called *neuralgic amyotrophy*), cervical rib or band, infiltration by malignant tumor, or prior radiation therapy. When the upper parts of the brachial plexus, arising from cervical roots 5 through 7, are affected, weakness and atrophy of shoulder girdle and upper arm muscles occur. Injuries to the lower brachial plexus, arising from the eighth cervical and first thoracic roots, produce distal arm weakness, atrophy, and focal sensory deficit in the forearm and hand. In general, idiopathic brachial neuritis, irradiation with >60 Gy (6000 rad), and particular types of trauma (arm jerked downward) result in damage to the upper portions of the brachial plexus. In contrast, infiltration by malignant tumor, cervical rib or band, and certain other types of trauma (arm jerked upward) cause damage to the lower brachial plexus. Lumbosacral plexopathies are less common; they may be due to idiopathic lumbosacral plexitis, retroperitoneal hemorrhage, or malignant tumor infiltration or may occur in association with long-standing diabetes mellitus.

Cold Effects Cold exerts direct deleterious effects on peripheral nerve, independent of ischemia. Cold injury to nerve occurs after prolonged exposure, usually of a limb, to moderately low temperatures, as with immersion of the feet in seawater; actual freezing of tissue is not required. Axonal degeneration of myelinated fibers is the pathologic expression of cold injury. Frequently, limbs affected by cold injury to nerve show sensory deficit and dysesthesias, cutaneous vasomotor instability, pain, and marked sensitivity to minimal cold exposure, which persist for many years. The pathophysiology of these phenomena is uncertain.

Trophic Changes The array of observable changes in completely denervated muscle, bone, and skin, including hair and nails, is well known, if incompletely understood. It is unclear what portion of the changes is due purely to denervation versus that caused by disuse, immobility, lack of weight bearing, and particularly recurrent, unnoticed, painless trauma. Considerable evidence favors the view that ulceration of skin, poor healing, tissue resorption, neurogenic arthropathy, and mutilation are the result of repeated unheeded injury to insensitive parts. This sequence of events is avoidable with proper attention to and care of the insensitive parts by both patient and physician.

RECOVERY FROM NEUROPATHY In contrast to axons in the central nervous system, peripheral nerve fibers have an excellent ability to regenerate under proper circumstances. The process of regeneration following axonal degeneration may take from 2 months to more than a year, depending on the severity of the neuropathy and the length of regeneration required. Regeneration can take place when the cause of the neuropathy has been eliminated, such as removal from contact with a neurotoxic substance or correction of an abnormal metabolic state. A deficit secondary to demyelination may recover rapidly, since intact axons may remyelinate in just a few weeks. For example, a patient with GBS, in whom demyelination but no secondary axonal degeneration has occurred, may recover to normal strength from bedfastness and paralysis of arms and legs in as little as 3 to 4 weeks.

PERIPHERAL NERVE TUMORS These tumors are mostly benign and can arise on any nerve trunk or twig. Although peripheral nerve tumors can occur anywhere in the body, including the spinal roots and cauda equina, many are subcutaneous in location and present as a soft swelling, sometimes with a purplish discoloration of the skin. Two major categories of peripheral nerve tumors are recognized: neurilemmoma (schwannoma) and neurofibroma. Neurilemmomas are usually solitary and grow in the nerve sheath, rendering the tumor relatively easy to dissect free. In contrast, neurofibromas tend to be multiple, grow in the endoneurial substance, which renders them difficult to dissect, may undergo malignant changes, and are the hallmark of von Recklinghausen's neurofibromatosis (NF1) (Chap. 370).

BIBLIOGRAPHY

ASBURY AK, THOMAS PK: *Peripheral Nerve Disorders*, 2d ed. Oxford, Butterworth-Heinemann, 1995

BOLTON CF, BREUER AC: Critical illness polyneuropathy. Muscle Nerve 22:419, 1999

CHALK CH: Acquired peripheral neuropathy. Neurol Clin 15:501, 1997

DAWSON DM et al: *Entrapment Neuropathies*, 3d ed. Philadelphia, Lippincott-Raven, 1999

DIABETES CONTROL AND COMPLICATIONS TRIAL RESEARCH GROUP: The effect of intensive diabetes therapy on the development and progression of neuropathy. Ann Intern Med 122:561, 1995

DYCK PJ, THOMAS PK (eds): *Diabetic Neuropathy*, 2d ed, Philadelphia, Saunders, 1999

——— et al (eds): *Peripheral Neuropathy*, 3d ed. Philadelphia, Saunders, 1992

HOLLAND NR et al: Small-fiber sensory neuropathies: Clinical course and neuropathology of idiopathic cases. Ann Neurol 44:47, 1998

MOORE RD et al: Incidence of neuropathy in HIV-infected patients on monotherapy vs those on combination therapy with didanosine, stavudine, and hydroxyurea. AIDS 14:273, 2000

STEWART JD: *Focal Peripheral Neuropathies*, 3d ed. Philadelphia, Lippincott Williams Wilkins, 1999

WARD JD: Improving prognosis in type 2 diabetes. Diabetes Care 22 (Suppl 2): B84, 1999

WOOLF CJ, MANNION RJ: Neuropathic pain: Aetiology, symptoms, mechanisms and management. Lancet 353:1954, 1999

ZOCHODNE DW: Diabetic neuropathies: Features and mechanisms. Brain Pathol 9:369, 1999

378

Arthur K. Asbury, Stephen L. Hauser

GUILLAIN-BARRÉ SYNDROME AND OTHER IMMUNE-MEDIATED NEUROPATHIES

AIDP	acute inflammatory demyelinating polyneuropathy	MAG	myelin-associated glycoprotein
CIDP	chronic inflammatory demyelinating polyneuropathy	MFS	M. Fisher syndrome
CSF	cerebrospinal fluid	MGUS	monoclonal gammopathy of undetermined significance
EAN	experimental allergic neuritis	MMN	multifocal motor neuropathy
GBS	Guillain-Barré syndrome	PAN	polyarteritis nodosa
IVIg	intravenous immune globulin	PE	plasma exchange
		SCLC	small cell lung cancer

GUILLAIN-BARRÉ SYNDROME

Guillain-Barré syndrome (GBS) is an acute, frequently severe, and fulminant polyradiculoneuropathy that is autoimmune in nature. It occurs year-round at a rate of about one case per million per month, or approximately 3500 cases per year in the United States and Canada. Males and females are equally at risk, and in western countries adults are more frequently affected than children.

CLINICAL MANIFESTATIONS GBS manifests as rapidly evolving areflexic motor paralysis with or without sensory disturbance. The usual pattern is an ascending paralysis that may be first noticed as rubbery legs. Weakness typically evolves over hours to a few days and is frequently accompanied by tingling dysesthesias in the extremities. The legs are usually more affected than the arms, and facial diparesis is present in 50% of affected individuals. The lower cranial nerves are also frequently involved, causing bulbar weakness and difficulty with handling secretions and maintaining an airway. Most patients require hospitalization, and almost 30% require ventilatory assistance at some time during the illness. Fever and constitutional symptoms are absent at the onset, and, if present, cast doubt on the diagnosis. Deep tendon reflexes usually disappear within the first few days of onset. Cutaneous sensory deficits, e.g., loss of pain and temperature sensation, are usually relatively mild; but functions subserved by large sensory fibers, such as deep tendon reflexes and proprioception, are more severely affected. Bladder dysfunction may occur in severe cases but is usually transient. If bladder dysfunction is a prominent feature and comes early in the course, possibilities other than GBS should be considered, particularly spinal cord disease. Once clinical worsening stops and the patient reaches a plateau, the crisis is usually past. Improvement may begin within days of the plateau.

Several subtypes of GBS are now recognized, as determined primarily by electrodiagnostic and pathologic distinctions (Table 378-1). In severe cases of GBS requiring critical care management, autonomic involvement is common. Usual features are loss of vasomotor control with wide fluctuation in blood pressure, postural hypotension, and cardiac dysrhythmias. These features require close monitoring and management and can be fatal. Pain is another common feature of GBS; several types are encountered. Most common is deep aching pain in weakened muscles, which patients liken to having over-exercised the previous day. Other pains in GBS include back pain involving the entire spine and sometimes dysesthetic pain in the extremities as a manifestation of sensory nerve fiber involvement. These pains are self-limited and should be treated with standard analgesics.

A range of limited or regional GBS syndromes may be encountered, although uncommonly. These include (1) the M. Fisher syndrome (Table 378-1 and see "Immunopathogenesis," below); (2) pure sensory forms; (3) ophthalmoplegia with anti-GQ1b antibodies (see "Immunopathogenesis," below), as part of severe motor-sensory GBS; (4) GBS with severe bulbar and facial paralysis, sometimes associated

Table 378-1 Subtypes of Guillain-Barré Syndrome (GBS)

Subtype	Features	Electrodiagnosis	Pathology
Acute inflammatory demyelinating polyneuropathy (AIDP)	Adults affected more than children; 90% of cases in western world; recovery rapid; anti-GM1 antibodies (<50%)	Demyelinating	First attack on Schwann cell surface; widespread myelin damage, macrophage activation, and lymphocytic infiltration; variable secondary axonal damage
Acute motor axonal neuropathy (AMAN)	Children and young adults; Prevalent in China and Mexico; May be seasonal; recovery rapid; anti-GD1a antibodies	Axonal	First attack at motor nodes of Ranvier; macrophage activation, few lymphocytes, frequent periaxonal macrophages; extent of axonal damage highly variable
Acute motor sensory axonal neuropathy (AMSAN)	Mostly adults; uncommon; recovery slow, often incomplete; closely related to AMAN	Axonal	Same as AMAN, but also affects sensory nerves and roots; axonal damage usually severe
M. Fisher syndrome (MFS)	Adults and children; uncommon; ophthalmoplegia, ataxia, and areflexia; Anti-GQ1b antibodies (90%)	Demyelinating	Few cases examined; resembles AIDP

with antecedent cytomegalovirus infection and anti-GM2 antibodies; and (5) acute pandysautonomia.

ANTECEDENT EVENTS Seventy-five percent of cases of GBS are preceded 1 to 3 weeks by an acute infectious process, usually respiratory or gastrointestinal. Culture and seroepidemiologic techniques show that 20 to 30% of all cases occurring in North America, Europe, and Australia are preceded by infection or reinfection with *Campylobacter jejuni*. A similar proportion is preceded by a human herpes virus infection, often cytomegalovirus or Epstein-Barr virus. Other viruses and also Mycoplasma pneumoniae have been identified as agents involved in antecedent infections. Recent immunization has also been associated with GBS. The swine influenza vaccine, administered widely in the United States in 1976, is the most notable example; influenza vaccines in use from 1992 to 1994, however, resulted in only one additional case of GBS per million persons vaccinated. Older type rabies vaccine, prepared in nervous system tissue, is implicated as a trigger of GBS in developing countries where it is still used; the mechanism is presumably immunization against neural antigens. GBS also occurs more frequently than can be attributed to chance alone in patients with lymphoma, including Hodgkin's disease (Chap. 112), in HIV-seropositive individuals (Chap. 309), and in patients with systemic lupus erythematosus (Chap. 311).

IMMUNOPATHOGENESIS Several lines of evidence support an autoimmune basis for acute inflammatory demyelinating polyneuropathy (AIDP), the most common and best studied type of GBS; by analogy the concept extends to all of the subtypes of GBS (Table 378-1).

It is likely that both cellular and humoral immune mechanisms contribute to tissue damage in AIDP. T cell activation is suggested by the finding that elevated levels of cytokines and cytokine receptors are present in serum [interleukin (IL)2, soluble IL-2 receptor] and in cerebrospinal fluid (CSF) [IL-6, tumor necrosis factor α, interferon-γ]. AIDP is also closely analogous to an experimental T cell–mediated immunopathy designated experimental allergic neuritis (EAN); EAN is induced in laboratory animals by immune sensitization against protein fragments derived from peripheral nerve proteins, and in particular against the P2 protein. Based on analogy to EAN, it was initially thought that AIDP was likely to be primarily a T cell–mediated disorder, however, abundant data now suggest that autoantibodies directed against nonprotein determinants may be central to many cases.

Circumstantial evidence suggests that all GBS results from immune responses to nonself antigens (infectious agents, vaccines) that misdirect to host nerve tissue through a resemblance-of-epitope (molecular mimicry) mechanism (Fig. 378-1) (Chap. 307). The neural targets are likely to be glycoconjugates, specifically gangliosides (Fig. 378-2). Gangliosides are complex glycosphingolipids that contain one or more sialic acid residues; various gangliosides participate in cell–cell interactions (including those between axons and glia), modulation of receptors, and regulation of growth. They are typically exposed on the plasma membrane of cells, rendering them susceptible to an antibody-mediated attack. Gangliosides and other glycoconjugates are present in large quantity in human nervous tissues and in key sites, such as nodes of Ranvier. Antiganglioside antibodies, most frequently to GM1, are common in GBS (20 to 50% of cases), particularly in those preceded by *C. jejuni* infection. Furthermore, isolates of *C. jejuni* from stool cultures of patients with GBS have surface glycolipid structures that antigenically cross react with gangliosides, including GM1, concentrated in human nerves. Another line of evidence is derived from experience in Europe with parenteral use of purified bovine brain gangliosides for treatment of various neuropathic disorders. Five to 15 days after injection some recipients developed acute motor axonal GBS with high titers of anti-GM1 antibodies that recognized epitopes at nodes of Ranvier and motor endplates.

Particularly noteworthy is the M. Fisher syndrome (MFS), which presents as rapidly evolving ataxia and areflexia of limbs without weakness, and ophthalmoplegia often with pupillary paralysis. The MFS variant accounts for ~5% of all GBS cases. Anti-GQ1b antibodies are found in >90% of patients with MFS (Table 378-1; Fig. 378-2), and titers of IgM and IgG are highest early in the course. Anti-GQ1b antibodies are not found in other forms of GBS unless there is extraocular motor nerve involvement. Of note, extraocular motor nerves are enriched in GQ1b gangliosides in comparison to limb nerves. Further, a monoclonal anti-GQ1b antibody raised against *C. jejuni* isolated from a patient with MFS blocked neuromuscular transmission experimentally.

Taken together, these observations provide strong but still inconclusive evidence that anti-ganglioside antibodies play an important pathogenic role in GBS. Definitive proof requires the passive transfer of GBS with specific antibodies; this procedure has not yet been accomplished, although a single case of apparent maternal-fetal transplacental transfer of GBS has been described.

PATHOPHYSIOLOGY In the demyelinating forms of GBS, the basis for flaccid paralysis and sensory disturbance is conduction block. This finding, demonstrable electrophysiologically, implies that the axonal connections remain intact. Hence, recovery can take place rapidly as remyelination occurs. In severe cases of demyelinating GBS, secondary axonal degeneration usually occurs; its extent can be estimated electrophysiologically. More secondary axonal degeneration correlates with a slower rate of recovery and a greater degree of residual disability. When a primary axonal pattern is encountered electrophysiologically, the implication is that axons have degenerated and become disconnected from their targets, specifically the neuromuscular junctions, and must therefore regenerate for recovery to take place. In motor axonal cases in which recovery is rapid, the lesion is thought to be localized to preterminal motor branches, allowing regeneration and reinnervation to take place quickly.

LABORATORY FEATURES CSF findings are distinctive, consisting of an elevated CSF protein level (100 to 1000 mg/dL) without accompanying pleocytosis. The CSF is often normal when symptoms have been present for ≤48 h; by the end of the first week the level of protein is usually elevated. An increased white cell count in the CSF (10 to 100/μL) in otherwise typical GBS raises the possibility of unrecognized HIV infection (Chap. 309). Electrodiagnostic features are mild or absent in the early stages and lag behind the clinical evolution. In cases with demyelination (Table 378-1) prolonged distal latencies, conduction velocity slowing, evidence of conduction block, and temporal dispersion of compound action potential are the usual features. In cases with primary axonal pathology, the principal electrodiagnostic finding is reduced amplitude of compound action potentials without conduction slowing or prolongation of distal latencies.

DIAGNOSIS GBS is a descriptive entity. The diagnosis is made by recognizing the pattern of rapidly evolving paralysis with areflexia, absence of fever or other systemic symptoms, and characteristic antecedent events (Table 378-2). In the early phases, laboratory tests are helpful only to exclude other disorders that can resemble GBS. Electrodiagnostic features may be minimal, and the CSF protein level may not rise until the end of the first week. If the diagnosis is strongly suspected, treatment should be initiated without waiting for evolution of the characteristic electrodiagnostic and CSF findings to occur. GBS patients with risk factors for HIV or with CSF pleocytosis should have a serologic test for HIV.

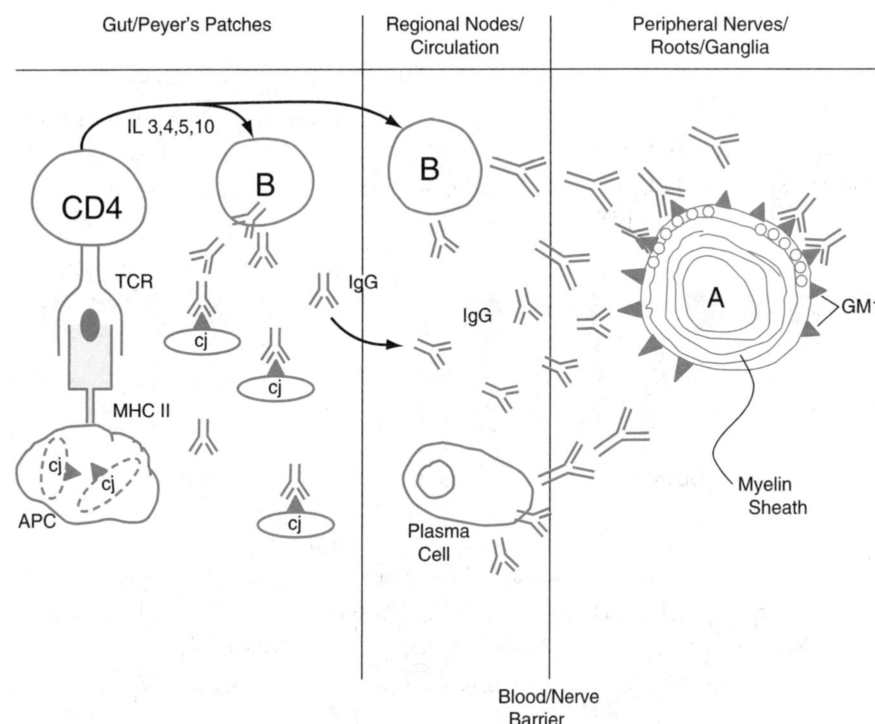

FIGURE 378-1 Postulated immunopathogenesis of GBS associated with *C. jejuni* infection. B cells recognize glycoconjugates on *C. jejuni* (Cj) (triangles) that cross-react with GM1 ganglioside present on peripheral nerve myelin. Some B cells, activated via a T cell–independent mechanism, secrete primarily IgM (not shown). Other B cells (upper left side) are activated via a partially T cell–dependent route and secrete primarily IgG; T cell help is provided by CD4 cells activated locally by fragments of Cj proteins that are presented on the surface of antigen-presenting cells (APC). A critical event in the development of GBS is the escape of activated B cells from Peyers patches into regional lymph nodes. Activated T cells probably also function to assist in opening of the blood-nerve barrier, facilitating penetration of pathogenic autoantibodies. The earliest changes in myelin (right) consist of edema between myelin lamellae and vesicular disruption (shown as circular blebs) of the outermost myelin layers. These effects are associated with activation of the C5b-C9 membrane attack complex and probably mediated by calcium entry; it is possible that the macrophage cytokine tumor necrosis factor (TNF) also participates in myelin damage. B, B cell; MHC II, class II major histocompatibility complex molecule; TCR, T cell receptor; A, axon.

℞ **TREATMENT** Treatment should be initiated as soon after diagnosis as possible. Each day counts; ~2 weeks after the first motor symptoms, immunotherapy is no longer effective. Either high-dose intravenous immune globulin (IVIg) or plasmapheresis can be initiated, as they are equally effective (Table 378-3). A combination of the two therapies is not significantly better than either alone. IVIg is usually administered as five daily infusions for a total dose of 2 g/kg body weight. A course of plasmapheresis, consisting of ~40 to 50 mL/kg plasma exchange (PE) daily for 4 to 5 days, is usually employed. In patients who are treated early in the course of GBS and improve, relapse may occur in the second or third week. Brief treatment with the original therapy is usually effective. Glucocorticoids have not been found to be effective in GBS.

In the worsening phase of GBS, most patients require monitoring in a critical care setting, with particular attention to vital capacity, cardiovascular status, and chest physiotherapy. As noted, ~30% of patients with GBS require ventilatory assistance, sometimes for prolonged periods of time (several weeks or longer). Frequent turning and assiduous skin care are important, as are daily range-of-motion exercises to avoid joint contractures.

PROGNOSIS AND RECOVERY Approximately 85% of patients with GBS achieve a full functional recovery within several months to a year, although minor findings on examination (such as areflexia) may persist. The mortality rate is <5% in optimal settings; death usually results from secondary pulmonary complications. The outlook is worst in patients with severe proximal motor and sensory axonal damage. Such axonal damage may be either primary or secondary in nature (see "Pathophysiology," above), but in either case successful regeneration cannot occur. Other factors that worsen the outlook for recovery are advanced age, a fulminant or severe attack, and a delay in the onset of treatment.

CHRONIC INFLAMMATORY DEMYELINATING POLYNEUROPATHY

Chronic inflammatory demyelinating polyneuropathy (CIDP) is distinguished from GBS by its chronic course. In other respects, this neuropathy shares many features with GBS, including elevated CSF protein levels and the electrodiagnostic findings of acquired demyelination. Most cases occur in adults, and males are affected slightly more often than females. The incidence of CIDP is lower than that of GBS, but due to the protracted course the prevalence is greater.

CLINICAL MANIFESTATIONS Onset is usually gradual, sometimes subacute; and, in a few, the initial attack is indistinguishable from that of GBS. Symptoms are both motor and sensory in most cases. Weakness of the limbs is usually symmetric but can be strikingly asymmetric. There is considerable variability from case to case. Some patients have a chronic progressive course, whereas others, usually younger patients, have a relapsing and remitting course. Some have only motor findings, and a small proportion present with a relatively pure syndrome of sensory ataxia. Tremor occurs in ~10% and may become more prominent during periods of subacute worsening or improvement. A small proportion have cranial nerve findings, including external ophthalmoplegia. CIDP tends to ameliorate over time with

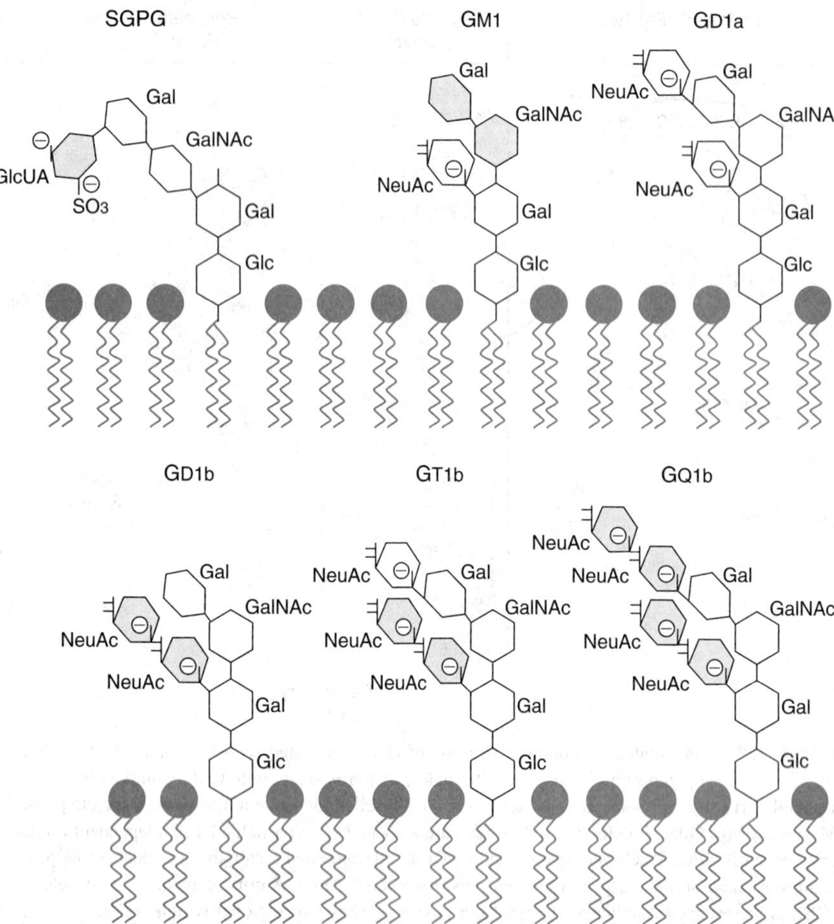

FIGURE 378-2 Glycolipids implicated as antigens in immune-mediated neuropathies. Sulfate-3-glucuronyl paragloboside (SGPG) is the glycolipid sharing a carbohydrate epitope with MAG, and the terminal sulfated glucuronic acid (shaded) is a key part of the epitope. GM1 is the ganglioside implicated in motor nerve disorders, and in most cases the terminal Gal (β1-3) GalNAc epitope (shaded), which is shared with GD1b, is involved. The disialosyl moiety implicated in sensory neuropathies consists of NeuAcα2–8NeuAc- (shaded) and is present in GD1b and GT1b gangliosides, as well as the simpler GD2 and GD3 gangliosides (not shown). GQ1b ganglioside that is an antigen in MFS has two disialoysl moieties. Although GD1a ganglioside has two sialic acid residues, they are not linked to each other, so it usually does not cross-react with the anti-GD1b antibodies. The shaded sugar moieties represent key aspects of the various epitopes, but carbohydrate sequences recognized by the antibodies may include additional sugar residues. GlcUA, glucuronic acid; Gal, galactose; GlcNAc, *N*-acetylglucosamine; Glc, glucose; GalNAc, *N*-acetylgalactosamine; NeuAc, *N*-acetylneuraminic acid (sialic acid). *(From MC Dalakis and RH Quarles: Ann Neurol 39:419, 1996, with permission.)*

treatment; the result is that many years after onset nearly 75% of patients have a reasonable functional recovery with only modest degrees of disability. Death from CIDP is uncommon.

DIAGNOSIS The diagnosis rests on characteristic clinical, CSF, and electrophysiologic findings. The CSF is usually acellular with an elevated protein level, sometimes several times normal. Electrodiagnostically, variable degrees of conduction slowing, prolonged distal latencies, temporal dispersion of compound action potentials, and conduction block are the principal features. In particular, the presence of conduction block is a certain sign of an acquired demyelinating process. Evidence of axonal loss, presumably secondary to demyelination, is present in >50% of patients. In all patients with CIDP, serum protein electrophoresis with immunofixation is indicated to screen for monoclonal gammopathy and associated conditions (see "Monoclonal Gammopathy of Undetermined Significance," below).

PATHOGENESIS Although there is evidence of immune activation in CIDP, the precise mechanisms of pathogenesis are unknown. Biopsy typically reveals little inflammation and onion-bulb thickening of nerves resulting from recurrent demyelination and remyelination. The response to therapy suggests that CIDP is immune-mediated; interestingly, CIDP responds to glucocorticoids (see below), whereas GBS does not. Approximately 25% of patients with clinical features of CIDP also have a monoclonal gammopathy of undetermined significance (MGUS). Cases associated with monoclonal IgA or IgG usually respond to treatment as favorably as cases without a monoclonal gammopathy. Patients with IgM monoclonal gammopathy tend to have more sensory findings, a more protracted course and may have a less satisfactory response to treatment, although this is an area of controversy.

℞ **TREATMENT** Most authorities initiate treatment for CIDP when progression is rapid or walking is compromised. If the disorder is mild, management can be expectant, awaiting spontaneous remission. Controlled studies have shown that high dose IVIg, PE, and glucocorticoids are all more effective than placebo. Initial therapy is usually either IVIg or PE, which appear to be equally effective. IVIg is administered as 0.4 g/kg body weight daily for 5 days; most patients require periodic retreatment at approximately 6-week intervals. PE is initiated at 2 to 3 treatments per week for 6 weeks; periodic retreatment may also be required. Treatment with oral glucocorticoids is another option (60 to 80 mg prednisone daily for 1 to 2 months, followed by a gradual dose reduction of 10 mg per month as tolerated), but long-term adverse effects including bone demineralization, gastrointestinal bleeding, and cushingoid changes are problematic. Approximately one-half of patients with CIDP fail to adequately respond to the initial therapy chosen; a different treatment should then be tried. Patients who fail therapy with IVIg, PE, and glucocorticoids may benefit from treatment with immunosuppressive agents such as azathiaprine, methotrexate, cyclosporine, and cyclophosphamide, either alone or as adjunctive therapy. Use of these therapies requires periodic reassessment of their risks and benefits.

MULTIFOCAL MOTOR NEUROPATHY

Multifocal motor neuropathy (MMN) is a distinctive but uncommon neuropathy that presents as a slowly progres-

Table 378-2 Diagnostic Criteria for Guillain-Barré Syndrome

REQUIRED
1. Progressive weakness of 2 or more limbs due to neuropathy[a]
2. Areflexia
3. Disease course <4 weeks
4. Exclusion of other causes [e.g., vasculitis (polyarteritis nodosa, systemic lupus erythematosus, Churg-Strauss syndrome), toxins (organophosphates, lead), botulism, diphtheria, porphyria, localized spinal cord or cauda equina syndrome]
SUPPORTIVE
1. Relatively symmetric weakness
2. Mild sensory involvement
3. Facial nerve or other cranial nerve involvement
4. Absence of fever
5. Typical CSF profile (acellular, increase in protein level)
6. Electrophysiologic evidence of demyelination

[a] Excluding M. Fisher and other variant syndromes.
SOURCE: Modified from AK Asbury, DR Cornblath: Ann Neurol 27:S21, 1990

Table 378-3 Major Clinical Trials of Treatment for Guillain-Barré Syndrome (GBS)

Trial/Site	Reference	No. Patients (N)/ Follow up (FU)/ Trial Arms	End Points	Results/p value	Comment
GBS Study Group; USA/Canada (18 centers)	Neurology 35:1096, 1985	N = 245 FU 6 months PE vs. none	1. % improved 1 grade at 4 weeks 2. days to improve 1 grade 3. days to reach grade 2	1. 59% (PE) vs. 39% (none) <0.001 2. 19 days (PE) vs. 40 days (none) <0.001 3. 53 days (PE) vs. 85 days (none) <0.001	First major trial showing efficacy—prior smaller trials showed conflicting results
French Coop. Group on PE in GBS; France/Switzerland (28 centers)	Ann Neurol 22:753, 1987; Ann Neurol 32:94, 1992	N = 220 FU = 1 year PE vs. none; Albumin vs. FFP in PE arm	1. days to walk w/ assistance 2. days to positive Δ score 3. Albumin vs. FFP	1. 30 days (PE) vs. 44 days (none) < 0.01 2. 4 days (PE) vs. 12 days (none) <0.001 3. No significant difference	At 1 year, full strength recovery in 71% (PE) vs. 52% (none); p = 0.007
Dutch GB Study Group; The Netherlands (15 centers)	N Engl J Med 326: 1123, 1992	N = 150 FU = 6 months IVIg vs. PE	1. % improved 1 grade at 4 weeks 2. days to reach grade 2	1. 53% (IVIg) vs. 34% (PE) p = 0.024 2. 55 days (IVIg) vs. 70 days (PE) p = 0.07	Patient assignment inadvertently favored IVIg group
Plasma Exchange/ Sandoglobulin GBS Trial (38 centers in 11 countries)	Lancet 349:225, 1997	N = 329 FU = 48 weeks IVIg vs. PE vs. both (3 arms)	1. % improved 1 grade at 4 weeks 2. Secondary end points: days to reach grade 2; days to off-respirator; disability at 48 weeks	No significant difference between the 3 groups for any end points	Nonsignificant trends favoring combined therapy

ABBREVIATIONS: PE, plasma exchange; IVIg, high dose intravenous immunoglobulin; FFP, fresh frozen plasma

NOTE: All studies except the French Coop. Group used the London grade scale: 0, healthy; 1, minor symptoms/signs; 2, walk 5 m unassisted; 3, walk 5 m with assistance; 4, bed/chairbound; 5, requiring assisted respiration; 6, dead.

sive motor weakness and atrophy evolving over years in the distribution of selected nerve trunks, associated with sites of persistent focal motor conduction block in the same nerve trunks. Sensory fibers are relatively spared. The arms are affected more frequently than the legs, and >75% of all patients are male. Some cases have been confused with lower motor neuron forms of amyotrophic lateral sclerosis (Chap. 365). Approximately 50% of patients present with high titers of polyclonal IgM antibody to the ganglioside GM1. It is uncertain how this finding relates to the discrete foci of persistent motor conduction block, but high concentrations of GM1 gangliosides are normal constituents of nodes of Ranvier in peripheral nerve fibers. Pathology reveals demyelination and mild inflammatory changes at the sites of conduction block.

Most patients with MMN respond to high-dose IVIg (dosages as for CIDP, above) and some refractory patients have responded to cyclophosphamide. Glucocorticoids and PE are not effective.

NEUROPATHIES WITH MONOCLONAL GAMMOPATHY

MULTIPLE MYELOMA Clinically overt polyneuropathy occurs in ~5% of patients with the commonly encountered type of multiple myeloma, which exhibits either lytic or diffuse osteoporotic bone lesions. These neuropathies are sensorimotor, are usually mild but may be severe, and generally do not reverse with successful suppression of the myeloma. In most cases, electrodiagnostic and pathologic features are consistent with a process of axonal degeneration.

In contrast, myeloma with osteosclerotic features, although representing only 3% of all myelomas, is associated with polyneuropathy in one-half of cases. These neuropathies, which may also occur with solitary plasmacytoma, are distinct because they (1) are usually demyelinating in nature, (2) often respond to radiation therapy or removal of the primary lesion, (3) are associated with different monoclonal proteins and light chains (almost always lambda as opposed to primarily kappa in the lytic type of multiple myeloma), and (4) may occur in association with other systemic findings including thickening of the skin, hyperpigmentation, hypertrichosis, organomegaly, endocrinopathy, anasarca and clubbing of fingers. These are features of the POEMS syndrome (*p*olyneuropathy, *o*rganomegaly, *e*ndocrinopathy, M protein, and *s*kin changes). The pathogenesis of this uncommon syndrome and the explanation for its association with lambda light chains are unknown.

Neuropathies are also encountered in other systemic conditions with gammopathy including Waldenström's macroglobulinemia, primary systemic amyloidosis, and cryoglobulinemic states (mixed essential cryoglobulinemia, some cases of hepatitis C).

MONOCLONAL GAMMOPATHY OF UNDETERMINED SIGNIFICANCE Chronic polyneuropathies occurring in association with MGUS are usually associated with the immunoglobulin isotypes IgG, IgA, and IgM. From a clinical standpoint, many of these patients are indistinguishable from patients with CIDP without monoclonal gammopathy (see Chronic Inflammatory Demyelinating Polyneuropathy, above), and their response to immunosuppressive agents is also similar. An exception is the syndrome of IgM kappa monoclonal gammopathy associated with an indolent, longstanding, sometimes static sensory neuropathy, frequently with tremor and sensory ataxia. Most patients are male and over age 50. In the majority, the monoclonal IgM immunoglobulin binds to a normal peripheral nerve constituent, myelin-associated glycoprotein (MAG), found in the paranodal regions of Schwann cells. Binding appears to be specific for a polysaccharide epitope that is also found in other normal peripheral nerve myelin glycoproteins, P0 and PMP22, and also in other normal nerve-related glycosphingolipids (Fig. 378-1). In the MAG-positive cases, IgM paraprotein is incorporated into the myelin sheaths of affected patients and widens the spacing of the myelin lamellae, thus producing a distinctive ultrastructural pattern. Demyelination and remyelination are the hallmarks of the lesions. The chronic demyelinating neuropathy appears to result from a destabilization of myelin metabolism rather than activation of an immune response. Therapy with chlorambucil or cyclophosphamide often results in improvement of the neuropathy associated with a prolonged reduction in the levels in the circulating paraprotein; chronic use of these alkylating agents is associated with significant risks (Chap. 84). In a small proportion of patients, MGUS will in time evolve into frankly malignant conditions, such as multiple myeloma (Chap. 113) or lymphoma (Chap. 112).

VASCULITIC NEUROPATHY

Peripheral nerve involvement is common in polyarteritis nodosa (PAN), appearing in half of all cases clinically and in 100% of cases at postmortem studies (Chap. 317). The most common pattern is multifocal (asymmetric) motor-sensory neuropathy (mononeuropathy multiplex) due to ischemic lesions of nerve trunks and roots; however, some cases of vasculitic neuropathy present as a distal, symmetric motor-sensory neuropathy. Symptoms of neuropathy are a common presenting complaint in patients with PAN. The electrodiagnostic findings are those of an axonal process. Small- to medium-sized arteries of the vasa nervorum, particularly the epineural vessels, are affected in PAN, resulting in a widespread ischemic neuropathy. A high frequency of neuropathy is also present in allergic angiitis and granulomatosis (Churg-Strauss syndrome).

Systemic vasculitis should always be considered when a subacute or chronically evolving mononeuropathy multiplex occurs in conjunction with constitutional symptoms (fever, anorexia, weight loss, loss of energy, malaise and nonspecific pains). Diagnosis of suspected vasculitic neuropathy is made by a combined nerve and muscle biopsy, with serial section or skip-serial techniques (Chap. 377).

Approximately one-third of biopsy-proven cases of vasculitic neuropathy are "nonsystemic" in that the vasculitis appears to affect only peripheral nerve. Constitutional symptoms are absent, and the course is more indolent than that of PAN. The erythrocyte sedimentation rate may be elevated, but other tests for systemic disease are negative. Nevertheless, clinically silent involvement of other organs is likely, and vasculitis is frequently found in muscle biopsied at the same time as nerve.

Vasculitic neuropathy may also be seen as part of the vasculitis syndrome occurring in the course of other connective tissue disorders. The most frequent is rheumatoid arthritis, but ischemic neuropathy due to involvement of vasa nervorum may also occur in mixed cryoglobulinemia, Sjögren's syndrome, Wegener's granulomatosis, hypersensitivity angiitis (Chap. 317), and progressive systemic sclerosis (Chap. 313). Management of these neuropathies including the "nonsystemic" vasculitic neuropathy consists of treatment of the underlying condition as well as the aggressive use of glucocorticoids and other immunosuppressant drugs, usually cyclophosphamide.

ANTI-HU PARANEOPLASTIC NEUROPATHY

This uncommon immune-mediated disorder manifests as a sensory neuronopathy, i.e., selective damage to dorsal root ganglia. The onset is often asymmetric with dysesthesias and sensory loss in the limbs that soon progress to affect all limbs, the torso, and face. Marked sensory ataxia, pseudoathetosis, and inability to walk, stand, or even sit unsupported are frequent features and are secondary to the extensive deafferentation. Subacute sensory neuronopathy is often idiopathic, but ~25% of cases are paraneoplastic, primarily related to lung cancer, and most of those are small cell lung cancer (SCLC) (Chap. 101). The gene *HuD*, ordinarily expressed only in neurons, is expressed in SCLC cells; the gene product functions as an RNA binding protein. Host anti-Hu antibodies to this tumor gene product cross-react with the same epitope expressed in dorsal root ganglion neurons, which results in immune-mediated neuronal destruction. An encephalomyelitis may accompany the sensory neuronopathy and presumably has the same pathogenesis. Neurologic symptoms usually precede, by 1 year on average, the identification of SCLC. The sensory neuronopathy runs its course in a few weeks or months and stabilizes, leaving the patient disabled. Most cases are unresponsive to treatment with glucocorticoids, IVIg, PE, or immunosuppressant drugs.

BIBLIOGRAPHY

GENERAL

BENATAR M et al: Immune-mediated peripheral neuropathies and voltage-gated sodium channels. Muscle Nerve 22:108, 1999

GOLD R et al: Mechanisms of immune regulation in the peripheral nervous system. Brain Pathol 9:343, 1999

QUARLES RH, WEISS D: Autoantibodies associated with peripheral neuropathy. Muscle Nerve 22:800, 1999

GUILLAIN-BARRÉ SYNDROME

HO TW et al: Anti-GD1a antibody is associated with axonal but not demyelinating forms of Guillain-Barré syndrome. Ann Neurol 45:168, 1999

JACOBS BC et al: The spectrum of antecedent infections in Guillain-Barré syndrome: A case control study. Neurology 51:1110, 1998

VAN KONINGSVELD R et al: Mild forms of Guillain-Barré syndrome in an epidemiologic survey in the Netherlands. Neurology 54:620, 2000

YUKI N et al: Clinical features and response to treatment in Guillain-Barré syndrome associated with antibodies to GM1b ganglioside. Ann Neurol 47:314, 2000

CHRONIC INFLAMMATORY DEMYELINATING POLYNEUROPATHY

BOUCHARD C et al: Clinicopathologic findings and prognosis of chronic inflammatory demyelinating polyneuropathy. Neurology 52:498, 1999

GORSON K et al: Chronic inflammatory demyelinating polyneuropathy: Clinical features and response to treatment in 67 consecutive patients with and without a monoclonal gammopathy. Neurology 48:321, 1997

MULTIFOCAL MOTOR NEUROPATHY

VAN DEN BERG L et al: The long-term effect of intravenous immunoglobulin treatment in multifocal motor neuropathy. Brain 121:421, 1998

NEUROPATHIES WITH MONOCLONAL GAMMOPATHY

PONSFORD S et al: Long-term clinical and neurophysiological follow-up of patients with peripheral neuropathy associated with benign monoclonal gammopathy. Muscle Nerve 23:164, 2000

ROPPER AH, GORSON KC: Neuropathies associated with paraproteinemia N Engl J Med 338:1601, 1999

VASCULITIC NEUROPATHY

SAID G: Necrotizing peripheral nerve vasculitis. Neurol Clin 15:835, 1997

ANTI-HU PARANEOPLASTIC NEUROPATHY

DALMAU J et al: Anti-Hu-associated paraneoplastic encephalomyelitis/sensory neuronopathy. A clinical study of 71 patients. Medicine 71:59, 1992

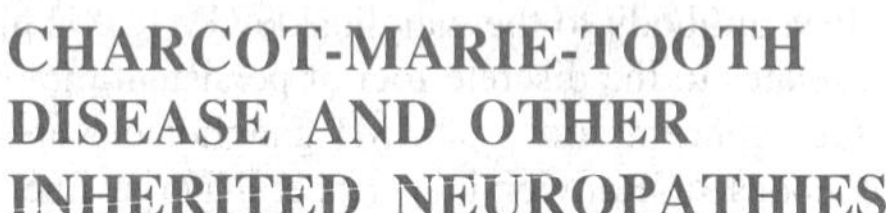

379

Phillip F. Chance, Thomas D. Bird

CHARCOT-MARIE-TOOTH DISEASE AND OTHER INHERITED NEUROPATHIES

CHARCOT-MARIE-TOOTH DISEASE

GENERAL CLINICAL FEATURES Charcot-Marie-Tooth (CMT) neuropathy comprises a heterogeneous group of inherited peripheral nerve diseases (Table 379-1). Transmission is most frequently autosomal dominant but may also be autosomal recessive or X-linked. An estimated 1 in 2500 persons has a form of CMT, making it one of the most frequently encountered inherited neurologic syndromes.

The neuropathy of CMT affects both motor and sensory nerves. Typical features consist of distal muscle weakness and atrophy, impaired sensation, and absent or hypoactive deep tendon reflexes. Common signs and symptoms are related to muscle loss and weakness, initially involving the feet and legs and later progressing to the hands and forearms. A history of an abnormal high-stepped (steppage) gait with frequent tripping and falling is frequently elicited. Complaints related to foot deformity (pes cavus, or high-arched feet) result from loss of intrinsic muscles of the feet. Despite the involvement of sensory nerves in CMT, complaints of limb pain or sensory disturbances are unusual.

Onset is most often during the first or second decade of life, although presentation in mid-adult life is not unusual. The variation in clinical presentation is exceptionally wide, ranging from individuals whose only clinical finding is pes cavus and minimal or no distal muscle weakness to those with severe distal atrophy and marked hand and foot deformity. However, it is unusual for patients with CMT to lose ambulation. There are no therapies that can prevent the onset or

Table 379-1 Genetic Spectrum of Inherited Neuropathies: Forms of Charcot-Marie-Tooth (CMT) Neuropathy/Hereditary Motor and Sensory Neuropathy (HMSN) and Related Disorders

	Locus	Gene	Mechanism
CHARCOT-MARIE-TOOTH TYPE 1			
(HMSNI)			
CMT1A	17p11.2-12	PMP22	Duplication/point mutation
CMT1B	1q22-23	P0	Point mutation
CMT1C	Unknown	Unknown	Unknown
CMT1?	10q21-22	EGR2	Point mutation
CMT4A	8q13-21	Unknown	Unknown
	5q23-33	Unknown	Unknown
CMT4B	11q13	MTMR2	Point mutation
CMTX	Xq13.1	CX32	Point mutation
CHARCOT-MARIE-TOOTH TYPE 2			
(HMSNII)			
CMT2A	1p35-36	Unknown	Unknown
CMT2B	3q13-22	Unknown	Unknown
CMT2C	Unknown	Unknown	Unknown
CMT2D	7p14	Unknown	Unknown
CMT2E	8p21	NF-L	Point mutation
DÉJERINE-SOTTAS			
(HMSNIII)			
DSD (CMT3)	17p11.2-12	PMP22	Point mutation
	1q22-23	P_0	Point mutation
	10q21-22	EGR2	Point mutation
CONGENITAL HYPOMYELINATION			
CH	1q22-23	P_0	Point mutation
	10q21-22	EGR2	Point mutation
HEREDITARY NEUROPATHY WITH PRESSURE PALSIES			
HNPP	17p11.2-12	PMP22	Deletion/point mutation

NOTE: PMP22, peripheral myelin protein 22; P_0, myelin protein zero; Cx32, connexin32; EGR2 (Krox-20) early growth response 2 gene; MTMR2, myotubularin-related protein-2; NF-L, neurofilament-light chain; CH, congenital hypomyelination.

delay progression of disability associated with CMT. Patients frequently benefit from physical therapy, use of ankle-foot orthroses (AFOs) to alleviate foot drop, and, in some cases, surgical procedures to the foot. Surgery should be undertaken only when pain or difficulty walking due to severe foot deformity cannot be managed by more conservative means.

CLASSIFICATION BY PHENOTYPE A widely accepted classification system distinguishes demyelinating forms of CMT (also designated as CMT type 1, or CMT1) from those due to axonal degeneration (CMT type 2, or CMT2). Individuals with CMT1 have electrophysiologic findings of reduced motor and sensory nerve conduction velocities (NCVs; typically <38 to 40 m/s) and pathologic findings of hypertrophic demyelinating neuropathy ("onion bulbs"). By contrast, in CMT2 there is relative preservation of the myelin sheath and these individuals have normal or near-normal NCVs. CMT3 refers to Déjerine-Sottas disease (DSD; see below), CMT4 to autosomal recessive forms of CMT, and CMTX to X-linked varieties.

An alternative classification system designates these disorders as hereditary motor and sensory neuropathies (HMSN); HMSNI refers to CMT1, HMSNII to CMT2, HMSNIII to DSD, and HMSNIV to Refsum disease (see below).

Approach to the Patient

A clinical diagnosis of an inherited peripheral neuropathy consistent with a form of CMT (CMT1 or CMT2) should be established prior to undertaking specific genetic tests. Other causes of peripheral neuropathy (e.g., diabetes mellitus, alcoholism, heavy metal poisoning, immune neuropathies) should also be considered and, if necessary, ruled out. An environmental exposure may affect multiple family members, thereby potentially mimicking a hereditary illness. CMT is usually a chronic, slowly progressive condition. One should be suspicious of cases that seem to have a rapid course of deterioration. As noted above, the neurologic findings show great variability in patients with CMT; mild pes cavus and depressed deep tendon reflexes may be the only signs of disease.

Although symptoms related to sensory disturbances are uncommon in CMT, a careful sensory examination is nonetheless essential. In patients who have no objective signs of sensory impairment and no evidence of sensory nerve dysfunction on electrophysiologic studies, alternative diagnoses including primary motor system disorders (e.g., distal spinal muscle atrophy, juvenile amyotrophic lateral sclerosis) should be considered.

The pedigree is of paramount importance in the diagnosis of CMT. Examination of multiple family members, particularly parents, for subtle signs of neuropathy may help to establish a diagnosis. If possible, it is also important to obtain NCVs and an electromyogram (EMG) from all at-risk family members.

GENETIC CONSIDERATIONS **CMT Neuropathy Type 1A (CMT1A)** The overwhelming majority of autosomal dominant CMT1 pedigrees demonstrate linkage to chromosome 17p11.2-12 (CMT1A) and are most frequently associated with a tandem 1.5-megabase (Mb) DNA duplication in this chromosomal region. The DNA duplication is usually inherited as a stable Mendelian trait; however, it may also arise as a de novo event. The de novo duplication is responsible for most sporadic cases of CMT1 and may also account for some cases of CMT1 previously thought to occur on the basis of an autosomal recessive mode of inheritance. When present as a de novo event, the duplication results more commonly from an error in spermatogenesis; however, ~10% of de novo cases have been found to result from an error in oogenesis.

The critical gene for CMT1A is peripheral myelin protein-22 (PMP22), which is expressed in Schwann cells. The *PMP22* gene encodes a 160-amino-acid protein localized to the compact portion of peripheral nerve myelin; it contains four putative transmembrane domains and is highly conserved in evolution. The level of expression of PMP22 is crucial for proper myelination of peripheral nerves. The neuropathy in patients with the 17p11.2-12 duplication results from the presence of three copies of PMP22 leading to increased expression at this locus. In rare cases, patients homozygous for the CMT1A duplication have been identified, and in some cases these individuals exhibit a more severe phenotype than their heterozygous siblings or parents. As discussed below, monosomic underexpression of PMP22 results in hereditary neuropathy with liability to pressure palsies (HNPP).

Rare CMT1 pedigrees that are linked to chromosome 17p11.2-12 yet lack the DNA duplication may harbor missense mutations within the *PMP22* gene.

Approximately three-quarters of patients with a clinical diagnosis of CMT1 carry the 17p11.2-12 duplication. DNA testing for CMT1A (including the associated chromosome 17 duplication and sequencing to detect point mutations in PMP22) has become available and is now an accepted part of the evaluation of many patients with suspected hereditary neuropathies (see below).

CMT Neuropathy Type 1B (CMT1B) CMT1B is much less common than CMT1A; it results from mutations in the human myelin protein zero gene (*MPZ*, or P_0), which maps to chromosome 1q22-q23. P_0 is the major structural protein component of peripheral nervous system myelin (quantitatively 50% by weight) and represents ~10% of total Schwann cell mRNA. P_0 is a member of the immunoglobulin gene superfamily of cell adhesive molecules and localizes to the compact portion of peripheral nerve myelin. P_0 protein consists of 248 amino acids and contains an intracellular and a glycosylated extracellular domain with a single transmembrane segment. Many different point mutations in the P_0 gene have been found in patients with CMT1B, and these mutations predominately map to the extracellular domain of its gene product.

At the clinical level it is not possible to differentiate patients with CMT1A from those with CMT1B. Molecular genetic testing is available.

Déjerine-Sottas Disease DSD (also called *HMSNIII*) is a severe, infantile or childhood onset, hypertrophic demyelinating polyneuropathy. NCVs are greatly prolonged (typically <10 m/s), and elevations in the cerebrospinal fluid (CSF) protein level are typically present. The clinical features of DSD overlap those of severe CMT1, and for this reason, the continued clinical separation of CMT1 and DSD is perhaps unwarranted. Many cases of DSD appear to be sporadic, occuring in the absence of a family history of neuropathy.

Molecular genetic studies indicate that DSD may be associated with point mutations in the P_0 or the *PMP22* genes, although pedigrees have been described that lack mutations in either the P_0, *PMP22*, or *Cx32* gene (see below). All DSD mutations identified to date appear to function as dominant genetic traits. Recently, a point mutation in the P_0 gene has been proposed as a mechanism for congenital hypomyelinating neuropathy (CHN), likely an even more severe form of DSD.

Hereditary Neuropathy with Liability to Pressure Palsies HNPP (also called *tomaculous neuropathy*) is an autosomal dominant disorder that produces an episodic, recurrent demyelinating neuropathy. HNPP typically develops during adolescence and may cause attacks of numbness, muscular weakness, and atrophy. Peroneal palsies, carpal tunnel syndrome, and other entrapment neuropathies are manifestations of HNPP. Motor and sensory NCVs are mildly reduced in affected patients as well as in asymptomatic gene carriers. Pathologic changes observed in HNPP include segmental demyelination and tomaculous, or sausage-like, formations in peripheral nerves. Because of mild overlap of clinical features with CMT1, HNPP patients may on occasion be misdiagnosed as having CMT1.

The HNPP locus maps to chromosome 17p11.2-12 and is associated with a 1.5-Mb deletion. The duplicated CMT1A chromosome (described earlier) and the deleted HNPP chromosome are the reciprocal products of unequal crossing-over during meiosis. In the case of HNPP, loss of a copy of the *PMP22* gene and underexpression of this critical myelin gene lead to demyelination. Most HNPP patients have the associated chromosome 17 deletion; however, rare patients with HNPP have been found to have point mutations in the *PMP22* gene. Molecular genetic testing is clinically available.

Treatment for HNPP is largely supportive. Surgical decompression of nerves has been proposed but is controversial. There is some evidence that surgical repair of carpal tunnel syndrome in HNPP is of little benefit and that transposition of the ulnar nerve at the elbow may produce poor results because the nerves are especially sensitive to manipulation and minor trauma.

CMT Neuropathy Type 2 CMT2 is less common than CMT1, and less progress has been made towards its molecular understanding. In general, CMT2 has a later age of onset, produces less involvement of the intrinsic muscles of the hands, and lacks palpably enlarged nerves. Extensive demyelination with "onion bulb" formation is not present in CMT2. Motor NCVs are normal or only slightly reduced in affected persons. A CMT2 locus was assigned by linkage studies to the short arm of chromosome 1 (1p35-36) and designated as CMT2A. One CMT2 pedigree was found to demonstrate linkage to markers from chromosome 3q13-q22 and has been designated CMT2B. Further genetic heterogeneity within CMT2 is likely as kindreds with the features of axonal neuropathy, weakness of the diaphragm, and vocal cord paralysis have been described and are designated as having CMT2C. Another form of CMT2, designated CMT2D, has been mapped to chromosome 7p14. More recently, in a large Russian pedigree a CMT2 gene was mapped to chromosome 8p21 (designated CMT2E) and a mutation was found in the neurofilament-light gene. Additionally, certain P_0 or connexin32 (Cx32, see below) mutations have been found to be the underlying genetic defect in a subset of patients with CMT1 or CMTX who were initially thought to have CMT2 because of only mild slowing of NCVs. DNA testing is not available for CMT2.

X-linked CMT Neuropathy The clinical features of X-linked CMT disease (CMTX) include demyelinating neuropathy, absence of male-to-male transmission, and an earlier age of onset and faster rate of progression in males. NCVs vary widely in CMTX from nearly normal to moderately slowed. CMTX accounts for ~10% of all patients thought to have a form of demyelinating CMT (i.e., CMT1). CMTX should be suspected when the commonly associated chromosome 17 duplication is not present and there is no history of father-to-son transmission of the neuropathy.

The gene for CMTX maps to chromosome Xq13-21 and results from point mutations in the connexin32 (*Cx32*) gene. Connexin32 encodes a major component of gap junctions and is expressed in peripheral nerves. Cx32 is structurally similar to PMP22, as both of these proteins contain four putative transmembrane domains in similar orientation. Over 200 different mutations in the *Cx32* gene have been described in patients with CMTX, and the distribution pattern of these mutations suggests that all parts of the connexin32 protein are functionally important. DNA testing is clinically available for Cx32 mutations causing CMTX.

Cx32 has a pattern of expression in peripheral nerve similar to that of other myelin protein genes; however, immunohistochemical studies show a different localization. Unlike PMP22 and P_0, which are present in compact myelin, Cx32 is located at uncompacted folds of Schwann cell cytoplasm around the nodes of Ranvier and at Schmidt-Lanterman incisures. This localization suggests a role for gap junctions composed of Cx32 in providing a pathway for the transfer of ions and nutrients around and across the myelin sheath. Mutations in the Cx32 protein have been suggested to alter its cellular localization and its trafficking and interfere with cell-to-cell communication.

CMT Variants Mutations in the putative zinc finger domain of the early growth response 2 gene (*EGR2*, or *Krox-20*) have been implicated as the underlying defect in CMT1 families that were found to be negative for the CMT1A duplication, as well as for mutations in either PMP22, P_0, or Cx32. Studies have shown that EGR2 acts as a direct transactivator of myelination genes in differentiating Schwann cells. EGR2 mutations have also been reported in a family with CHN.

Rare families with autosomal recessive motor and sensory neuropathy have been reported, particularly Tunisian families with parental consanguinity. Both demyelinating and axonal types of neuropathy have been described and given the designation CMT4. One form of autosomal recessive demyelinating neuropathy has been mapped to chromosome 8q13-q21 (CMT4A). Another form of CMT, characterized by focally folded myelin sheaths (CMT4B), has been mapped to chromosome 11q23 and recently shown to be caused by mutations in MTMR2, a gene encoding myotubularin-related protein-2, which is thought to be a transcriptional regulator. An additional pedigree with phenotypic features of CMT4B did not show linkage to chromosome 11 or to any other known CMT loci, implicating further genetic heterogeneity. Currently, DNA testing is not clinically available for any form of CMT4 or for mutations in EGR2.

Genetic Evaluation of CMT and HNPP An approach for evaluating an individual patient suspected of having an inherited peripheral neuropathy is presented in Fig. 379-1. If a proband has evidence for CMT1, determination of NCVs is a useful screening tool for parents and other at-risk family members. The *CMT1* gene is penetrant in early life, and correct disease status can probably be determined with nerve conduction screening by age 5. However, if a proband's nerve conduction is normal or only mildly prolonged, the diagnosis may be CMT2. In this case the screening examination will need to focus on determination of motor unit amplitudes and other electrical signs of denervation. Rare patients have been found to have point mutations in either P_0 or Cx32 resulting in very mild demyelination and misclassification as CMT2.

The overwhelming proportion of CMT1 and CMT2 pedigrees have autosomal dominant inheritance. In pedigrees lacking male-to-male inheritance and/or those in which males are more severely affected

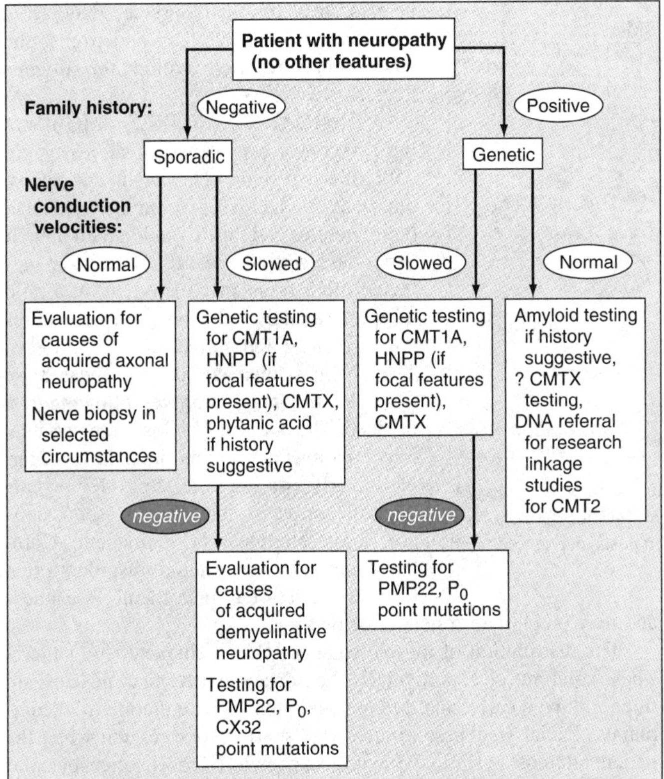

FIGURE 379-1 Evaluation of patients suspected of having an inherited peripheral neuropathy. CMT, Charcot-Marie-Tooth; HNPP, hereditary neuropathy with liability to pressure palsies. *(Modified from Lynch and Chance.)*

than females and have an earlier onset, CMTX should be suspected. Determination of autosomal dominant versus X-linked CMT is important as the genetic counseling for these two modes of inheritance is different. For any form of autosomal dominant CMT, the likelihood of an affected parent (of either sex) having an affected child is 50% for each pregnancy, regardless of the sex of the child. For CMTX, all daughters of an affected father will inherit the gene, and none of the sons will be affected. For a woman with CMTX, there is a 50% likelihood that her children will be affected regardless of their sex.

Sporadic cases in males can be especially difficult to evaluate, as the neuropathy could be nongenetic or the pattern of inheritance could be autosomal dominant, X-linked, or even autosomal recessive. Sporadic cases may also represent de novo duplications (CMT1A) or de novo deletions (HNPP). False paternity is another explanation for apparent sporadic CMT or HNPP.

Molecular genetic testing is currently available for the DNA duplication (or deletion) associated with CMT1A or HNPP and for point mutations in the *PMP22*, P_0 or *Cx32* genes associated with other forms of CMT1 and CMTX. ■

CHEMOTHERAPY IN PATIENTS WITH CMT Chemotherapeutic agents known to affect peripheral nerves should be used with great caution in patients with inherited neuropathies, and in the case of vincristine, total avoidance is strongly advised. A number of reports have documented the serious consequences of vincristine treatment administered in standard oncologic dosages in patients with CMT, including well-documented CMT1A and CMT2. The complications ranged from the precipitation of severe neuropathies in clinically asymptomatic at-risk individuals, through degrees of marked clinical worsening, and even death due to respiratory collapse.

OTHER INHERITED NEUROPATHIES

HEREDITARY SENSORY NEUROPATHIES Hereditary sensory neuropathies (HSN) are a heterogeneous group of disorders affecting sensory neurons. The most common form of HSN, HSN type I, is an autosomal degenerative disorder of sensory and motor neurons. Phenotypically, distal sensory loss, distal muscle wasting and weakness, and variable neural deafness are observed. The disease involves progressive loss of dorsal root ganglion cells and axons in peripheral nerves. Age of onset is the second decade of life or later. The HSN-I locus maps to chromosome 9q22.1-q22.3. Because of the presence of muscular weakness in some patients with HSN, this disorder may be clinically confused with CMT.

FAMILIAL AMYLOID NEUROPATHY Familial amyloid polyneuropathy (FAP) is an autosomal dominant disorder that classically presents as progressive sensory peripheral neuropathy, with early involvement of the autonomic nervous system and an associated cardiomyopathy. Postmortem studies have shown extensive amyloid deposition in multiple organs throughout the body. Transthyretin (TTR) is the most common constituent amyloid fibril protein deposited in FAP. Several different point mutations in the TTR gene have been described in TTR-related FAP, and DNA testing for these mutations is clinically available. →*Amyloidosis is discussed in Chap. 319.*

REFSUM DISEASE This autosomal recessive disorder is characterized by a progressive sensorimotor demyelinating polyneuropathy, associated with cerebellar ataxia and retinitis pigmentosa. Neural deafness, cardiomyopathy, cataracts, and icthyosis are additional features. Onset is in late childhood or early adulthood. Patients often complain of night blindness as the earliest symptom. The CSF protein is typically elevated. Diagnosis is made by demonstration of elevated levels of phytanic acid (a 20-carbon branched-chain fatty acid) in the serum and urine. The disorder appears to be due to a deficiency of a peroxysomal enzyme, phytanic acid oxidase, responsible for alpha oxidation of phytanic acid. Therapy, consisting of avoidance of dietary sources of phytanic acid, and plasmapheresis in some cases, is partially effective.

BIBLIOGRAPHY

BOERKOEL CF et al: Molecular mechanisms for CMT1A duplication and HNPP deletion. Ann NY Acad Sci. 883:22, 1999

CHANCE PF: Overview of hereditary neuropathy with liability to pressure palsies in Charcot-Marie-Tooth Disorders. Ann NY Acad Sci 883:14, 1999

DYCK PJ et al: Hereditary motor and sensory neuropathies, in PJ Dyck et al (eds): *Peripheral Neuropathy*. Philadelphia, Saunders, 1993, pp 1094–1136

KAMHOLZ J et al: Charcot-Marie-Tooth disease type 1: Molecular pathogenesis to gene therapy. Brain 123:222, 2000

KELLER MP, CHANCE PF: Inherited neuropathies: From gene to disease. Brain Pathol 9: 327, 1999

LYNCH D, CHANCE PF: Inherited peripheral neuropathies. *Neurologist* 3:277, 1997

MENSIYANOVA IV et al: A new variant of Charcot-Marie-Tooth disease type 2 is probably the result of a mutation in the neurofilament-light gene. Am J Hum Genet 67:37, 2000

PAREYSON D: Charcot-Marie-Tooth disease and related neuropathies: Molecular basis for distinction and diagnosis. Muscle Nerve 22:1498, 1999

WARNER LE et al: Hereditary peripheral neuropathies: Clinical forms, genetics, and molecular mechanisms. (Review). Annu Rev Med 50:263, 1999

380

Daniel B. Drachman

MYASTHENIA GRAVIS AND OTHER DISEASES OF THE NEUROMUSCULAR JUNCTION

Myasthenia gravis (MG) is a neuromuscular disorder characterized by weakness and fatigability of skeletal muscles. The underlying defect is a decrease in the number of available acetylcholine receptors (AChRs) at neuromuscular junctions due to an antibody-mediated autoimmune attack. Treatment now available for MG is highly effective, although a specific cure has remained elusive.

PATHOPHYSIOLOGY In the neuromuscular junction (Fig. 380-1), acetylcholine (ACh) is synthesized in the motor nerve terminal

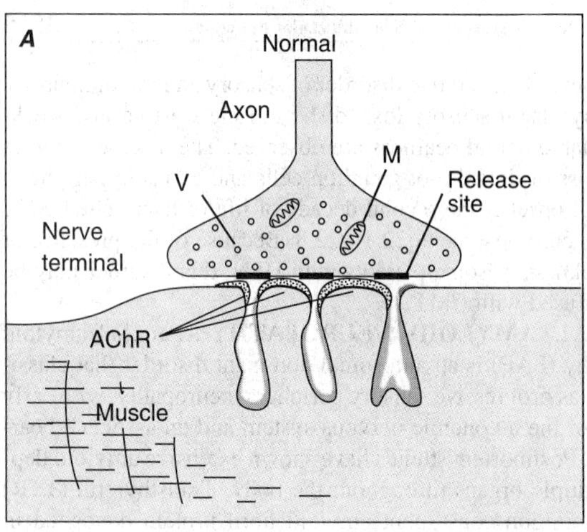

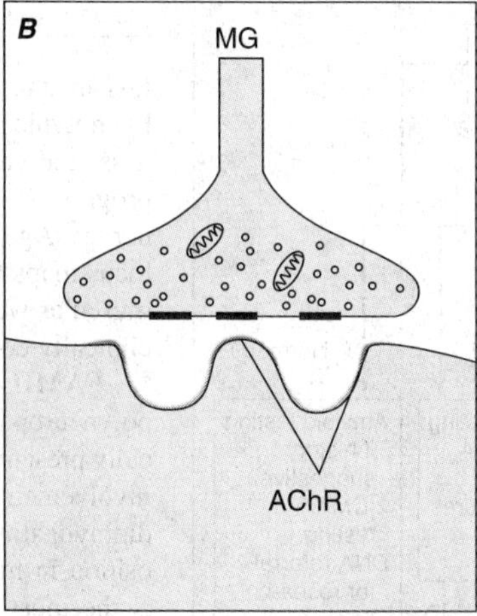

FIGURE 380-1 Diagrams of (*A*) normal and (*B*) myasthenic neuromuscular junctions. V, vesicles; M, mitochondria. See text for description of normal neuromuscular transmission. The MG junction shows a normal nerve terminal; a reduced number of AChRs (stippling); flattened, simplified postsynaptic folds, and a widened synaptic space.

and stored in vesicles (quanta). When an action potential travels down a motor nerve and reaches the nerve terminal, ACh from 150 to 200 vesicles is released and combines with AChRs that are densely packed at the peaks of postsynaptic folds. The structure of the AChR has been fully elucidated; it consists of five subunits (2α, β, δ, and γ or ϵ) arranged around a central pore. When ACh combines with the binding sites on the AChR, the channels in the AChRs open, permitting the rapid entry of cations, chiefly sodium, which produces depolarization at the end-plate region of the muscle fiber. If the depolarization is sufficiently large, it initiates an action potential that is propagated along the muscle fiber, triggering muscle contraction. This process is rapidly terminated by hydrolysis of ACh by acetylcholinesterase (AChE) and by diffusion of ACh away from the receptor.

In MG, the fundamental defect is a decrease in the number of available AChRs at the postsynaptic muscle membrane. In addition, the postsynaptic folds are flattened, or "simplified." These changes result in decreased efficiency of neuromuscular transmission. Therefore, although ACh is released normally, it produces small end-plate potentials that may fail to trigger muscle action potentials. Failure of transmission at many neuromuscular junctions results in weakness of muscle contraction.

The amount of ACh released per impulse *normally* declines on repeated activity (termed *presynaptic rundown*). In the myasthenic patient, the decreased efficiency of neuromuscular transmission combined with the normal rundown results in the activation of fewer and fewer muscle fibers by successive nerve impulses and hence increasing weakness, or *myasthenic fatigue*. This mechanism also accounts for the decremental response to repetitive nerve stimulation seen on electrodiagnostic testing.

The neuromuscular abnormalities in MG are brought about by an autoimmune response mediated by specific anti-AChR antibodies. The anti-AChR antibodies reduce the number of available AChRs at neuromuscular junctions by three distinct mechanisms: (1) accelerated turnover of AChRs by a mechanism involving cross-linking and rapid endocytosis of the receptors; (2) blockade of the active site of the AChR, i.e., the site that normally binds ACh; and (3) damage to the postsynaptic muscle membrane by the antibody in collaboration with complement. The pathogenic antibodies are IgG and are T cell dependent. Thus, immunotherapeutic strategies directed against T cells are effective in this antibody-mediated disease.

How the autoimmune response is initiated and maintained in MG is not completely understood. However, the thymus appears to play a role in this process. The thymus is abnormal in ~75% of patients with MG; in about 65% the thymus is "hyperplastic," with the presence of active germinal centers, while 10% of patients have thymic tumors (thymomas). Muscle-like cells within the thymus (myoid cells), which bear AChRs on their surface, may serve as a source of autoantigen and trigger the autoimmune reaction within the thymus gland.

CLINICAL FEATURES MG is not rare, having a prevalence of at least 1 in 7500. It affects individuals in all age groups, but peaks of incidence occur in women in their twenties and thirties and in men in their fifties and sixties. Overall, women are affected more frequently than men, in a ratio of approximately 3:2. The cardinal features are *weakness* and *fatigability* of muscles. The weakness increases during repeated use (fatigue) and may improve following rest or sleep. The course of MG is often variable. Exacerbations and remissions may occur, particularly during the first few years after the onset of the disease. Remissions are rarely complete or permanent. Unrelated infections or systemic disorders often lead to increased myasthenic weakness and may precipitate "crisis" (see below).

The distribution of muscle weakness has a characteristic pattern. The cranial muscles, particularly the lids and extraocular muscles, are often involved early, and diplopia and ptosis are common initial complaints. Facial weakness produces a "snarling" expression when the patient attempts to smile. Weakness in chewing is most noticeable after prolonged effort, as in chewing meat. Speech may have a nasal timbre caused by weakness of the palate or a dysarthric "mushy" quality due to tongue weakness. Difficulty in swallowing may occur as a result of weakness of the palate, tongue, or pharynx, giving rise to nasal regurgitation or aspiration of liquids or food. In approximately 85% of patients, the weakness becomes generalized, affecting the limb muscles as well. The limb weakness in MG is often proximal and may be asymmetric. Despite the muscle weakness, deep tendon reflexes are preserved. If weakness of respiration becomes so severe as to require respiratory assistance, the patient is said to be in *crisis*.

DIAGNOSIS AND EVALUATION (Table 380-1) The diagnosis is suspected on the basis of weakness and fatigability in the typical distribution described above, without loss of reflexes or impairment of sensation or other neurologic function. The suspected diagnosis should always be confirmed definitively before treatment is undertaken; this is essential because (1) other treatable conditions may

Table 380-1 Diagnosis of Myasthenia Gravis (MG)

History
- Diplopia, ptosis, weakness
- Weakness in characteristic distribution
- Fluctuation and fatigue: worse with repeated activity, improved by rest
- Effects of previous treatments

Physical examination
- Ptosis, diplopia
- Motor power survey: quantitative testing of muscle strength
- Forward arm abduction time (5 min)
- Vital capacity
- Absence of other neurologic signs

Laboratory testing
- Anti-AChR radioimmunoassay: ~90% positive in generalized MG; 50% in ocular MG; definite diagnosis if positive; negative result does not exclude MG
- Edrophonium chloride (Tensilon) 2 mg + 8 mg IV; highly probable diagnosis if *unequivocally* positive
- Repetitive nerve stimulation; decrement of >15% at 3 Hz: highly probable
- Single-fiber electromyography: blocking and jitter, with normal fiber density; confirmatory, but not specific
- For ocular or cranial MG: exclude intracranial lesions by CT or MRI

NOTE: AChR, acetylcholine receptor; CT, computed tomography; MRI, magnetic resonance imaging.
SOURCE: From Drachman, 1994.

closely resemble MG, and (2) the treatment of MG may involve surgery and the prolonged use of drugs with adverse side effects.

Anticholinesterase Test Drugs that inhibit the enzyme AChE allow ACh to interact repeatedly with the limited number of AChRs, producing improvement in the strength of myasthenic muscles. Edrophonium is used most commonly, because of the rapid onset (30 s) and short duration (about 5 min) of its effect. An objective end-point must be selected to evaluate the effect of edrophonium. The examiner should focus on one or more unequivocally weak muscle groups and evaluate their strength objectively. For example, weakness of extraocular muscles, impairment of speech, or the length of time that the patient can maintain the arms in forward abduction may be useful measures. An initial dose of 2 mg of edrophonium is given intravenously. If definite improvement occurs, the test is considered positive and is terminated. If there is no change, the patient is given an additional 8 mg intravenously. The dose is administered in two parts because some patients react to edrophonium with unpleasant side effects such as nausea, diarrhea, salivation, fasciculations, and rarely syncope or bradycardia. Atropine (0.6 mg) should be drawn up in a syringe, ready for intravenous administration if these symptoms become troublesome.

Table 380-2 The Congenital Myasthenic Syndromes

Type	Clinical Features	Electrophysiology	Genetics	Endplate Effects	Treatment
Slow channel	Most common; weak forearm extensors; onset 2d to 3d decade; variable severity	Repetitive muscle response on nerve stimulation; prolonged channel opening and MEPP	Autosomal dominant; α, β, ϵ AChR mutations	Excitotoxic end-plate myopathy; decreased AChRs; postsynaptic damage	Quinidine: decreases end-plate damage; made worse by Anti-AChE
Low-affinity fast channel	Onset early; moderately severe; ptosis, EOM involvement; weakness and fatigue	Brief and infrequent channel openings; opposite of slow channel syndrome	Autosomal recessive; may be heteroallelic	Normal end-plate structure	3,4-DAP; Anti-AChE
Severe AChR deficiencies	Early onset; variable severity; fatigue; typical MG features	Decremental response to repetitive nerve stimulation; decreased MEPP amplitudes	Autosomal recessive; ϵ mutations most common; many different	Increased span of end-plates; variable synaptic folds	Anti-AChE; ?3,4-DAP
AChE deficiency	Early onset; variable severity; scoliosis; may have normal EOM, absent pupillary responses	Decremental response to repetitive nerve stimulation	Mutant gene for AChE's collagen anchor	Small nerve terminals; degenerated junctional folds	Worse with Anti-AChE drugs

ABBREVIATIONS: AChR, acetylcholine receptor; AChE, acetylcholinesterase; EOM, extraocular muscles; MEPP, miniature end-plate potentials; 3,4-DAP, 3-4-Diaminopyridine.

False-positive tests occur in occasional patients with other neurologic disorders, such as amyotrophic lateral sclerosis, and in placebo-reactors. False-negative or equivocal tests also may occur. In some cases it is helpful to use a longer-acting drug such as neostigmine (15 mg given orally), since this permits more time for detailed evaluation of strength. In virtually all instances, it is desirable to carry out further testing to establish the diagnosis of MG definitively.

Electrodiagnostic Testing *Repetitive nerve stimulation* often provides helpful diagnostic evidence of MG. Anti-AChE medication is stopped 6 to 24 h before testing. It is best to test weak muscles or proximal muscle groups. Electric shocks are delivered at a rate of two or three per second to the appropriate nerves, and action potentials are recorded from the muscles. In normal individuals, the amplitude of the evoked muscle action potentials does not change at these rates of stimulation. However, in myasthenic patients there is a rapid reduction in the amplitude of the evoked responses of more than 10 to 15%. As a further test, a single dose of edrophonium may be given to prevent or diminish this decremental reaction.

Antiacetylcholine Receptor Antibody As noted above, anti-AChR antibodies are detectable in the serum of approximately 80% of all myasthenic patients, but in only about 50% of patients with weakness confined to the ocular muscles. The presence of anti-AChR antibodies is virtually diagnostic of MG, but a negative test does not exclude the disease. The measured level of anti-AChR antibody does not correspond well with the severity of MG in different patients. However, in an individual patient, a treatment-induced fall in the antibody level often correlates with clinical improvement.

Inherited Myasthenic Syndromes The *congenital myasthenic syndromes* (CMS) comprise a heterogeneous group of disorders of the neuromuscular junction that are not autoimmune, but rather are due to genetic mutations in which virtually any component of the neuromuscular junction may be affected. Alterations in function of the presynaptic nerve terminal, the various subunits of the AChR or AChE have been identified in the various forms of CMS. These disorders share many of the clinical features of autoimmune MG, including weakness and fatigability of skeletal muscles, in some cases involving extraocular muscles (EOMs), lids, and proximal muscles, similar to the distribution in autoimmune MG. CMS should be suspected when symptoms of myasthenia have begun in infancy or childhood, and AChR antibody tests are consistently negative. Features of four of the most common forms of CMS are summarized in Table 380-2. Although clinical electrodiagnostic and pharmacologic tests may suggest the correct diagnosis, sophisticated electrophysiologic and molecular analysis are required for precise elucidation of the defect; this may lead to helpful treatment as well as genetic counseling. In the forms that involve the AChR, a wide variety of mutations have been identified in each of the subunits, but the ϵ subunit is affected in about 75% of these cases. In most of the recessively inherited forms of CMS, the mutations are heteroallelic; that is, *different* mutations affecting each of the two alleles are present.

Differential Diagnosis Other conditions that cause weakness of the cranial and/or somatic musculature include the nonautoimmune CMS discussed above, drug-induced myasthenia, Lambert-Eaton myasthenic syndrome (LEMS), neurasthenia, hyperthyroidism, botulism, intracranial mass lesions, and progressive external ophthalmoplegia. Treatment with *penicillamine* (used for scleroderma or rheumatoid arthritis) may result in true MG, but the weakness is usually mild, and recovery occurs within weeks or months after discontinuing its use. *Aminoglycoside antibiotics* in very large doses and *procainamide* can cause neuromuscular weakness in normal individuals or exacerbation of weakness in myasthenic patients.

LEMS is a presynaptic disorder of the neuromuscular junction that can cause weakness similar to that of MG. The proximal muscles of the lower limbs are most commonly affected, but other muscles may be involved as well. Cranial nerve findings, including ptosis of the eyelids and diplopia, occur in up to 70% of patients and resemble features of MG. However, the two conditions are readily distinguished, since patients with LEMS have depressed or absent reflexes, show autonomic changes such as dry mouth and impotence, and show incremental responses on repetitive nerve stimulation. It is now known that LEMS is caused by autoantibodies directed against P/Q type calcium channels at the motor nerve terminals, which can be detected in approximately 85% of LEMS patients. These autoantibodies result in impaired release of ACh from nerve terminals. A majority of patients with this syndrome have an associated malignancy, most commonly small cell carcinoma of the lung, which is thought to trigger the autoimmune response. The diagnosis of LEMS may signal the presence of the tumor long before it would otherwise be detected, permitting early removal. Treatment of the neuromuscular disorder involves plasmapheresis and immunosuppression, as for MG.

Neurasthenia may present with weakness and fatigue, but muscle testing usually reveals the "jerky release" or "give-away weakness" characteristic of nonorganic disorders, and the complaint of fatigue in these patients means tiredness or apathy rather than decreasing muscle power on repeated effort. *Hyperthyroidism* is readily diagnosed or excluded by tests of thyroid function, which should be carried out routinely in patients with suspected MG. Abnormalities of thyroid function (hyper- or hypothyroidism) may increase myasthenic weakness. *Botulism* can cause myasthenic-like weakness, but the pupils are often dilated, and repetitive nerve stimulation gives an *incremental* rather than decremental response. Diplopia that mimics the symptoms of MG may occasionally be due to an *intracranial mass lesion* that compresses nerves to the EOMs (e.g., sphenoid ridge meningioma), but magnetic resonance imaging (MRI) of the head and orbits usually reveals the lesion.

Progressive external ophthalmoplegia is a rare condition resulting in weakness of the EOMs, which may be accompanied by weakness of the proximal muscles of the limbs and other systemic features. Most patients with this condition have mitochondrial disorders that can be detected on muscle biopsy (Chaps. 67 and 383).

Search for Associated Conditions (Table 380-3) Myasthenic patients have an increased incidence of several associated disorders. *Thymic abnormalities* occur in ~75% of patients, as noted above. Neoplastic change (thymoma) may produce enlargement of the thymus, which is detected by computed tomography (CT) or MRI scanning of the anterior mediastinum. A thymic shadow on CT scan may normally be present through young adulthood, but enlargement of the thymus in a patient >40 years is highly suspicious of thymoma. *Hyperthyroidism* occurs in 3 to 8% of patients and may aggravate the myasthenic weakness. Tests of thyroid function should be obtained.

Table 380-3 Disorders Associated with Myasthenia Gravis and Recommended Laboratory Tests

Associated disorders
- *Disorders of the thymus:* thymoma, hyperplasia
- *Other autoimmune disorders:* thyroiditis, Graves' disease, rheumatoid arthritis, lupus erythematosus, skin disorders, family history of autoimmune disorder
- *Disorders or circumstances that may exacerbate myasthenia gravis:* hyperthyroidism or hypothyroidism, occult infection, medical treatment for other conditions (aminoglycoside antibiotics, quinine, antiarrhythmic agents)
- *Disorders that may interfere with therapy:* tuberculosis, diabetes, peptic ulcer, gastrointestinal bleeding, renal disease, hypertension, asthma, osteoporosis

Recommended laboratory tests or procedures
- CT or MRI of mediastinum
- Tests for lupus erythematosus, antinuclear antibody, rheumatoid factor, antithyroid antibodies
- Thyroid-function tests
- Tuberculin test
- Chest radiography
- Fasting blood glucose measurement
- Pulmonary-function tests
- Bone densitometry in older patients

SOURCE: From RT Johnson, JW Griffin (eds): *Current Therapy in Neurologic Disease*, 4th ed. St. Louis, Mosby Year Book, 1993, p 379.

Because of the *association of MG with other autoimmune disorders*, blood tests for rheumatoid factor and antinuclear antibodies should be carried out in all patients. Chronic infection of any kind can exacerbate MG and should be sought carefully. Finally, measurements of *ventilatory function* are valuable because of the frequency and seriousness of respiratory impairment in myasthenic patients.

Because of the side effects of glucocorticoids and other immunosuppressive agents used in the treatment of MG, a thorough medical investigation should be undertaken, searching specifically for evidence of chronic or latent infection (such as tuberculosis or hepatitis), hypertension, diabetes, renal impairment, and glaucoma.

℞ TREATMENT (Fig. 380-2) The prognosis has improved strikingly as a result of advances in treatment; virtually all myasthenic patients can be returned to full productive lives with proper therapy. The most useful treatments for MG include anticholinesterase medications, immunosuppressive agents, thymectomy, and plasmapheresis or intravenous immunoglobulin (IVIg).

Anticholinesterase Medications Anticholinesterase medication produces at least partial improvement in most myasthenic patients, although improvement is complete in only a few. There is no substantial difference in efficacy among the various anticholinesterase drugs;

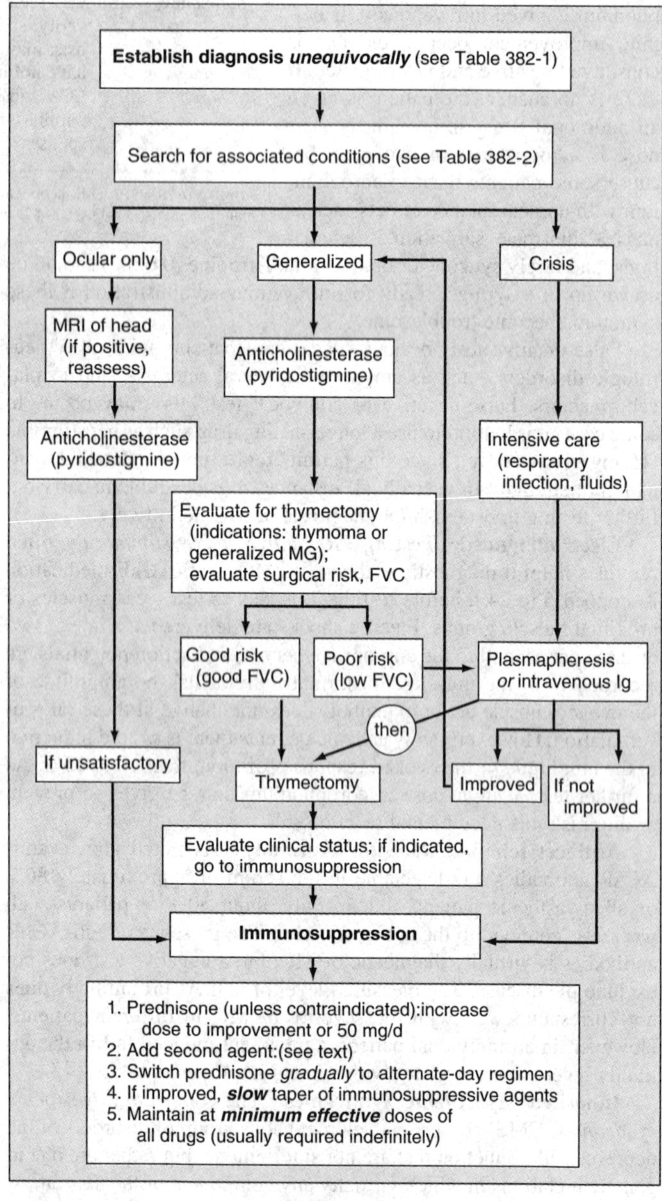

FIGURE 380-2 Algorithm for the management of myasthenia gravis. FVC, forced vital capacity.

oral pyridostigmine is the one most widely used in the United States. As a rule, the beneficial action of oral pyridostigmine begins within 15 to 30 min and lasts for 3 to 4 h, but individual responses vary. Treatment is begun with a moderate dose, e.g., 60 mg three to five times daily. The frequency and amount of the dose should be tailored to the patient's individual requirements throughout the day. For example, patients with weakness in chewing and swallowing may benefit by taking the medication before meals so that peak strength coincides with mealtime. Long-acting pyridostigmine tablets may help to get the patient through the night but should never be used for daytime medication because of their variable absorption. The maximum useful dose of pyridostigmine rarely exceeds 120 mg every 3 h during daytime. Overdosage with anticholinesterase medication may cause increased weakness and other side effects. In some patients, muscarinic side effects of the anticholinesterase medication (diarrhea, abdominal cramps, salivation, nausea) may limit the dose tolerated. In these cases, propantheline bromide may be used to block the autonomic side effects without altering the beneficial effects on skeletal muscle. Loperamide is useful for the treatment of diarrhea.

Thymectomy Two separate issues should be distinguished: (1) surgical removal of thymoma, and (2) thymectomy as a treatment for MG. Surgical removal of a thymoma is necessary because of the possibility of local tumor spread, although most thymomas are benign. In the absence of a tumor, the available evidence suggests that up to 85% of patients experience improvement after thymectomy; of these, ~35% achieve drug-free remission. However, the improvement is typically delayed for months to years. The advantage of thymectomy is that it offers the possibility of long-term benefit, in some cases diminishing or eliminating the need for continuing medical treatment. In view of these potential benefits and of the negligible risk in skilled hands, thymectomy has gained widespread acceptance in the treatment of MG. It is the consensus that thymectomy should be carried out in all patients with generalized MG who are between the ages of puberty and at least 55 years. Whether thymectomy should be recommended in children, in adults >55 years of age, and in patients with weakness limited to the ocular muscles is still a matter of debate. Thymectomy must be carried out in a hospital where it is performed regularly and where the staff is experienced in the pre- and postoperative management, anesthesia, and surgical techniques of total thymectomy.

Myasthenia Gravis Worksheet

History

General	Normal	Good	Fair	Poor
Diplopia	None	Rare	Occasional	Constant
Ptosis	None	Rare	Occasional	Constant
Arms	Normal	Slightly limited	Some ADL impairment	Definitely limited
Legs	Normal	Walks/runs fatigues	Can walk limited distances	Minimal walking
Speech	Normal	Dysarthric	Severely dysarthric	Unintelligible
Voice	Normal	Fades	Impaired	Severely impaired
Chew	Normal	Fatigue on normal foods	Fatigue on soft foods	N-G tube
Swallow	Normal	Normal foods	Soft foods only	N-G tube
Respiration	Normal	Dyspnea on unusual effort	Dyspnea on any effort	Dyspnea at rest

Examination

BP______ Pulse______ Wt______
Vital capacity______
EOMS______
Ptosis time______
Edema______
Face______
Cataracts? R______ L______

Arm abduction R______ L______
Deltoids R______ L______
Biceps R______ L______
Triceps R______ L______
Grip R______ L______
Iliopsoas R______ L______
Quadriceps R______ L______
Hamstrings R______ L______

FIGURE 380-3 Abbreviated interval assessment form for use in evaluating treatment for myasthenia gravis.

Immunosuppression Immunosuppression using glucocorticoids, azathioprine, and other drugs is effective in nearly all patients with MG. The choice of drugs or other immunomodulatory treatments should be guided by the relative benefits and risks for the individual patient and the urgency of treatment. *It is helpful to develop a treatment plan based on short-term, intermediate-term, and long-term objectives. For example, if immediate improvement is essential either because of the severity of weakness or because of the patient's need to return to activity as soon as possible, plasmapheresis should be undertaken or intravenous immunoglobulin (IVIg) administered. For the intermediate term, glucocorticoids and cyclosporine generally produce clinical improvement within a period of 1 to 3 months. The beneficial effects of azathioprine and mycophenolate mofetil usually begin after many months (up to a year), but these drugs have advantages for the long-term treatment of patients with MG.* The side effects of each drug may preclude its use in some patients, as indicated below.

Assessment of patient's status In order to evaluate the effectiveness of treatment as well as drug-induced side effects, it is important to assess the patient's clinical status at baseline and on repeated interval examinations in a systematic manner. Because of the variability of symptoms of MG, the interval history as well as findings on examination must be taken into account. The most useful clinical tests include forward arm abduction time (up to a full 5 min), forced vital capacity, range of eye movements, and time to development of ptosis on upward gaze. Manual muscle testing or, preferably, quantitative dynamometry of limb muscles, especially proximal muscles, is also important. An interval form can provide a succinct summary of the patient's status and a guide to treatment results; an abbreviated form is shown in Fig. 380-3. A progressive reduction in the patient's AChR antibody level also provides clinically valuable confirmation of the effectiveness of treatment; conversely, a rise in AChR antibody levels warns that tapering of immunosuppressive medication may lead to clinical exacerbation. Reliable quantitative measurement of AChR antibody levels provides important information about the results of treatment. It is best to compare antibody levels from prior frozen serum samples with current serum in simultaneously run assays.

Glucocorticoid therapy Glucocorticoids, when used properly, produce improvement in myasthenic weakness in the great majority of patients. The initial dose of prednisone should be relatively low (15 to 25 mg/d) to avoid the early weakening that occurs in about one-third of patients treated initially with a high-dose regimen. The dose is increased stepwise, as tolerated by the patient (usually by 5 mg/d at 2- to 3-day intervals), until there is marked clinical improvement or a dose of 50 mg/d is reached. This dose is maintained for 1 to 3 months and then is gradually modified to an alternate-day regimen over the course of an additional 1 to 3 months; the goal is to reduce the dose to zero or to a minimal level on the "off day." Generally, patients begin to improve within a few weeks after reaching the maximum dose, and improvement continues to progress for months or years. The prednisone dosage may gradually be reduced, but usually months or years may be needed to determine the minimum effective dose, and close monitoring is required by patient and doctor. *Few patients are* *able to do without prednisone entirely.* Patients on long-term glucocorticoid therapy must be followed carefully to prevent or treat adverse side effects. The most common errors in the steroid treatment of myasthenic patients include (1) insufficient persistence—improvement may be delayed and gradual; (2) too early, too rapid, or excessive tapering of steroid dosage; and (3) lack of attention to prevention and treatment of side effects. →*The management of patients treated with glucocorticoids is discussed in Chap. 331.*

Other immunosuppressive drugs Azathioprine, cyclosporine, mycophenolate mofetil, or occasionally cyclophosphamide is effective in many patients, either alone or in combination with glucocorticoid therapy. Azathioprine has been the most widely used of these drugs because of its relative safety in most patients and long track record. Its therapeutic effect may add to that of glucocorticoids and/or allow the steroid dose to be reduced. However, up to 10% of patients are unable to tolerate azathioprine because of idiosyncratic reactions consisting of flulike symptoms of fever and malaise, bone marrow depression, or abnormalities of liver function. An initial dose of 50 mg/d should be used to test for adverse side effects. If this dose is tolerated, it is increased gradually until the white blood count falls to approximately 3000 to 4000/μL. In patients who are receiving glucocorticoids concurrently, leukocytosis precludes the use of this measure. A reduction of the lymphocyte count to <1000/μL and/or an increase of the mean corpuscular volume of red blood cells may be used as indications of adequacy of azathioprine dosage. The typical dosage range is 2 to 3 mg/kg total body weight (including fat in obese patients). The beneficial effect of azathioprine takes at least 3 to 6 months to begin and even longer to peak.

Cyclosporine is approximately as effective as azathioprine and is being used increasingly in the management of MG. Its beneficial effect appears more rapidly than that of azathioprine. It may be used alone but is usually used as an adjunct to glucocorticoids to permit reduction of the steroid dose. The usual dose of cyclosporine is 4 to 5 mg/kg per day, given in two divided doses (to minimize side effects). Side effects of cyclosporine include hypertension and nephrotoxicity, which must be closely monitored. "Trough" blood levels of cyclosporine are measured 12 h after the evening dose. The therapeutic range, as measured by radioimmunoassay, is 150 to 200 ng/L.

Mycophenolate mofetil, which has been used for immunosuppression in transplant patients, is now proving useful in the treatment of MG. A dose of 1 g bid is recommended. Its mechanism of action involves inhibition of purine synthesis by the "de novo" pathway. Since lymphocytes lack the alternative "salvage" pathway that is present in all other cells, mycophenolate inhibits proliferation of lymphocytes but not proliferation of other cells. It does not kill or eliminate preexisting autoreactive lymphocytes, and therefore clinical improvement in autoimmune diseases such as MG may be delayed for many months to a year, until the preexisting autoreactive lymphocytes die spontaneously. The advantage of mycophenolate lies in its relative lack of adverse side effects, with only occasional production of diarrhea and rare development of leukopenia. This drug may become the choice for long-term treatment of myasthenic patients. Unfortunately, the present cost of mycophenolate may be prohibitively high.

Cyclophosphamide is reserved for occasional patients refractory to the other drugs, because of its relatively high risk of adverse side effects, including late development of malignancies.

Plasmapheresis and Intravenous Immunoglobulin Plasmapheresis has been used therapeutically in MG. Plasma, which contains the pathogenic antibodies, is mechanically separated from the blood cells, which are returned to the patient. A course of five exchanges (3 to 4 L per exchange) is generally administered over a 2-week period. Plasmapheresis produces a short-term reduction in anti-AChR antibodies, with clinical improvement in many patients. It is useful as a temporary expedient in seriously affected patients or to improve the patient's condition prior to surgery (e.g., thymectomy).

The indications for the use of IVIg are the same as those for plasma exchange: to produce rapid improvement to help the patient through a difficult period of myasthenic weakness or prior to surgery. This treatment has the advantages of not requiring special equipment or large-bore venous access. The usual dose is 2 g/kg, which is typically administered over 5 days (400 mg/kg/per day). If tolerated, the course of IVIg can be shortened to administer the entire dose over a 3-day period. Improvement occurs in about 70% of patients, beginning during treatment, or within 4 to 5 days thereafter, and continuing for weeks to months. The mechanism of action of IVIg is not known; the treatment has no consistent effect on the measurable amount of circulating AChR antibody. Adverse reactions are uncommon, but include headache, fluid overload, and rarely renal shutdown.

The intermediate and long-term treatment of myasthenic patients requires other methods of therapy outlined earlier in this chapter.

Management of Myasthenic Crisis Myasthenic crisis is defined as an exacerbation of weakness sufficient to endanger life; it usually consists of respiratory failure caused by diaphragmatic and intercostal muscle weakness. Treatment should be carried out in an intensive care unit staffed with physicians experienced in the management of myasthenia gravis, respiratory insufficiency, infectious disease, and fluid and electrolyte therapy. The possibility that the deterioration could be due to excessive anticholinesterase medication ("cholinergic crisis") is best excluded by temporarily stopping anticholinesterase drugs. The most common cause of crisis is intercurrent infection. This should be treated *immediately*, because the mechanical and immunologic defenses of the patient can be assumed to be compromised. The myasthenic patient with fever and early infection should be treated like other immunocompromised patients. Early and effective antibiotic therapy, respiratory assistance, and pulmonary physiotherapy are essentials of the treatment program. As discussed above, plasmapheresis or IVIg is frequently helpful in hastening recovery.

BIBLIOGRAPHY

DRACHMAN DB: Myasthenia gravis: Medical progress. N Engl J Med 330:1797, 1994

———: Myasthenia gravis, in *The Autoimmune Diseases*, 3d ed, N Rose, I Mackay (eds). Orlando, FL, Academic, 1998, pp 637–662

———: The ten most frequently asked questions about myasthenia gravis. Neurologist 5: 350, 1999

ENGEL AG, et al: Congenital myasthenic syndromes: New insights from molecular genetic and patch-clamp studies. Ann N Y Acad Sci, 841:140, 1998

GAJDOS P: Intravenous immune globulin in myasthenia gravis. Clin Exp Immunol 197: 49, 1994

LENNON V: Serologic diagnosis of myasthenia gravis and the Lambert-Eaton myasthenic syndrome, in *Handbook of Myasthenia Gravis and Myasthenic Syndromes*, RP Lisak (ed). New York, Marcel Dekker, 1994, p 149

LINDSTROM JM: Acetylcholine receptors and myasthenia. Muscle Nerve 23:453, 2000

SANDERS DB: *Myasthenia Gravis and Myasthenic Syndromes*. Philadelphia, Saunders, 1994

381 APPROACH TO THE PATIENT WITH MUSCLE DISEASE

Jerry R. Mendell

Skeletal muscle diseases, or myopathies, are defined as disorders with structural changes or functional impairment of muscle. These conditions can be differentiated from other diseases of the motor unit by characteristic clinical and laboratory findings. →*Myasthenia gravis and related disorders are discussed in Chap. 380; inflammatory muscle diseases and inclusion body myositis in Chap. 382; muscular dystrophies and inherited, metabolic, and toxic myopathies in Chap. 383.*

CLINICAL FEATURES **Muscle Weakness** Symptoms of muscle weakness can be either intermittent or persistent. Some patients complain of weakness that physicians more accurately classify as fatigue. Disorders causing intermittent weakness (Fig. 381-1) include myasthenia gravis, periodic paralyses (hypokalemic, hyperkalemic, and paramyotonia congenita), and metabolic energy deficiencies of glycolysis (especially myophosphorylase deficiency) and fatty acid utilization (carnitine palmitoyltransferase deficiency). The states of energy deficiency cause activity-related muscle breakdown accompanied by myoglobinuria, appearing as light-brown- to dark-brown-colored urine. Most muscle disorders cause persistent weakness (Fig. 381-2). In the majority of these, including most types of muscular dystrophy, polymyositis, and dermatomyositis, the proximal muscles are weaker than the distal, and the facial muscles are spared, a pattern referred to as *limb-girdle*. For other patterns of weakness the differential diagnosis is more restricted. Cranial innervated muscle weakness causing ptosis and extraocular muscle weakness without diplopia points to oculopharyngeal muscular dystrophy, mitochondrial myopathies, or myotubular myopathy. Facial weakness (difficulty with eye closure and impaired smile) and scapular winging (Fig. 381-3) are characteristic of facioscapulohumeral dystrophy. Facial and distal limb weakness associated with hand grip myotonia is virtually diagnostic of myotonic dystrophy. A pathognomonic pattern exclusive to inclusion body myositis includes loss of strength in both proximal and distal muscles, handgrip weakness, and wasting of quadriceps muscles. Less frequently, but important diagnostically, is the presence of a dropped head syndrome indicative of selective neck extensor muscle weakness. The most common neuromuscular diseases causing this pattern of weakness include myasthenia gravis, polymyositis, and amyotrophic lateral sclerosis. A final pattern, recognized because of preferential distal extremity weakness, is typical of a unique category of muscular dystrophy, the distal myopathies (Chap. 383).

It is important to examine functional capabilities to help disclose certain patterns of weakness (Table 381-1). The Gowers' sign (Fig. 381-4) is particularly useful. Observing the gait of an individual may disclose a lordotic posture caused by combined trunk and hip weakness, frequently exaggerated by toe walking (Fig. 381-5). A waddling gait is caused by the inability of weak hip muscles to prevent hip drop or hip dip. Hyperextension of the knee (genu recurvatum or backkneeing) is characteristic of quadriceps muscle weakness; and a steppage gait, due to footdrop, accompanies distal weakness.

Any disorder causing muscle weakness may be accompanied by fatigue, referring to an inability to maintain or sustain a force (pathologic fatigability). This condition must be differentiated from asthenia, a type of fatigue caused by excess tiredness or lack of energy (Fig. 381-2). Associated symptoms may help differentiate asthenia and pathologic fatigability. Asthenia is often accompanied by a tendency to avoid physical activities, complaints of daytime sleepiness, necessity for frequent naps, and difficulty concentrating on activities, such as reading. There may be feelings of overwhelming stress and depression. Thus, asthenia is not a myopathy. In contrast, pathologic fatigability occurs in disorders of neuromuscular transmission and in disorders altering energy production, including defects in glycolysis, lipid metabolism, or mitochondrial energy production. Pathologic fatigability also occurs in chronic myopathies because of difficulty accomplishing a task with less muscle. Pathologic fatigability is accompanied by abnormal clinical or laboratory findings. Fatigue without those supportive features almost never indicates a primary muscle disease.

Muscle Pain, Cramps, and Stiffness Muscle pain can be associated with involuntary muscle activity producing cramps, contractures, and stiff or rigid muscles (Chap. 22). In distinction, true myalgia (muscle aching), which can be localized or generalized, has no involuntary activity but may be accompanied by weakness, tenderness to palpation, or swelling. Certain drugs cause true myalgia (Table 381-2).

There are two painful muscle conditions of particular importance, neither of which is associated with muscle weakness. Fibromyalgia is a common, yet poorly understood type of myofascial pain syndrome. Patients complain of severe muscle pain and tenderness and have specific painful trigger points, sleep disturbances, and easy fatigability (Chap. 325). Polymyalgia rheumatica occurs in patients older than 50 years and is characterized by stiffness (without involuntary activity) and pain in the shoulders, lower back, hips, and thighs (Chap. 317). The erythrocyte sedimentation rate is elevated, and temporal arteritis may be present. Polymyalgia rheumatica is important to recognize because treatment with glucocorticoids can relieve discomfort and prevent the associated ischemic arteritis, which threatens vision.

Muscle cramps are painful, involuntary, localized, muscle contractions with a visible or palpable hardening of the muscle. They are abrupt in onset and short in duration, and they may cause abnormal posturing of the joint. The electromyogram (EMG) shows firing of motor units, reflecting an origin from spontaneous neurogenic activity. Muscle cramps are not a feature of most primary muscle diseases, although they occur commonly in Duchenne and related forms of mus-

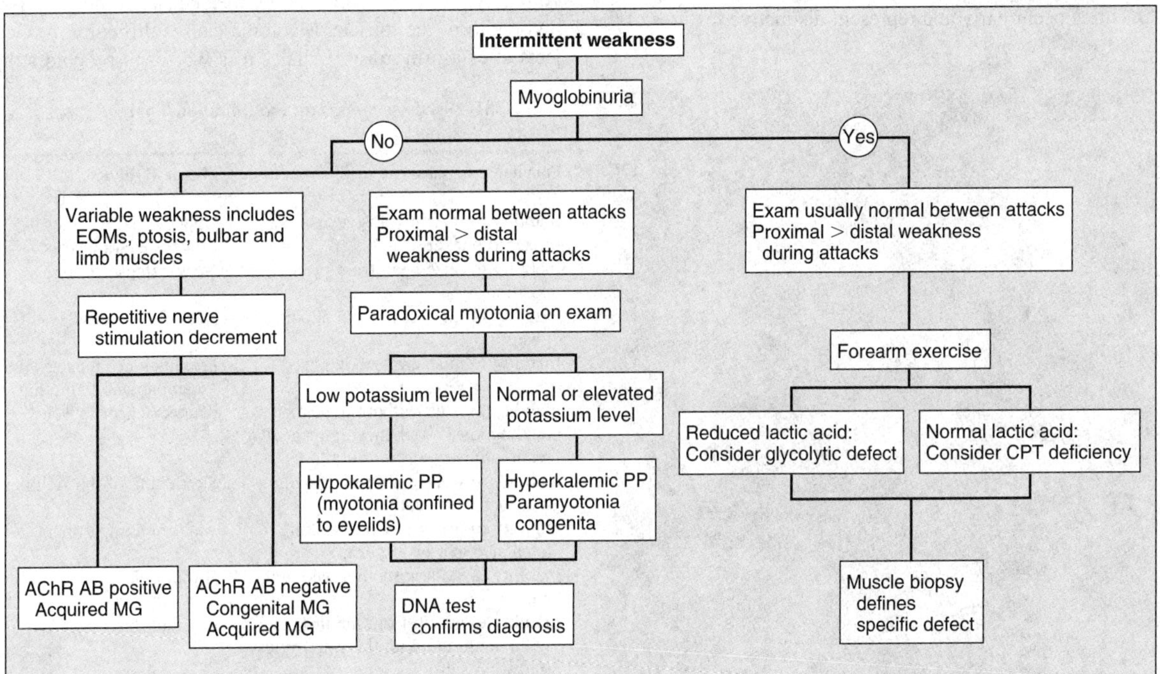

FIGURE 381-1 Diagnostic evaluation for intermittent weakness. EOMs, extraocular muscles; AChR AB, acetylcholine receptor antibody; PP, periodic paralysis; CPT, carnitine palmitoyltransferase; MG, myasthenia gravis.

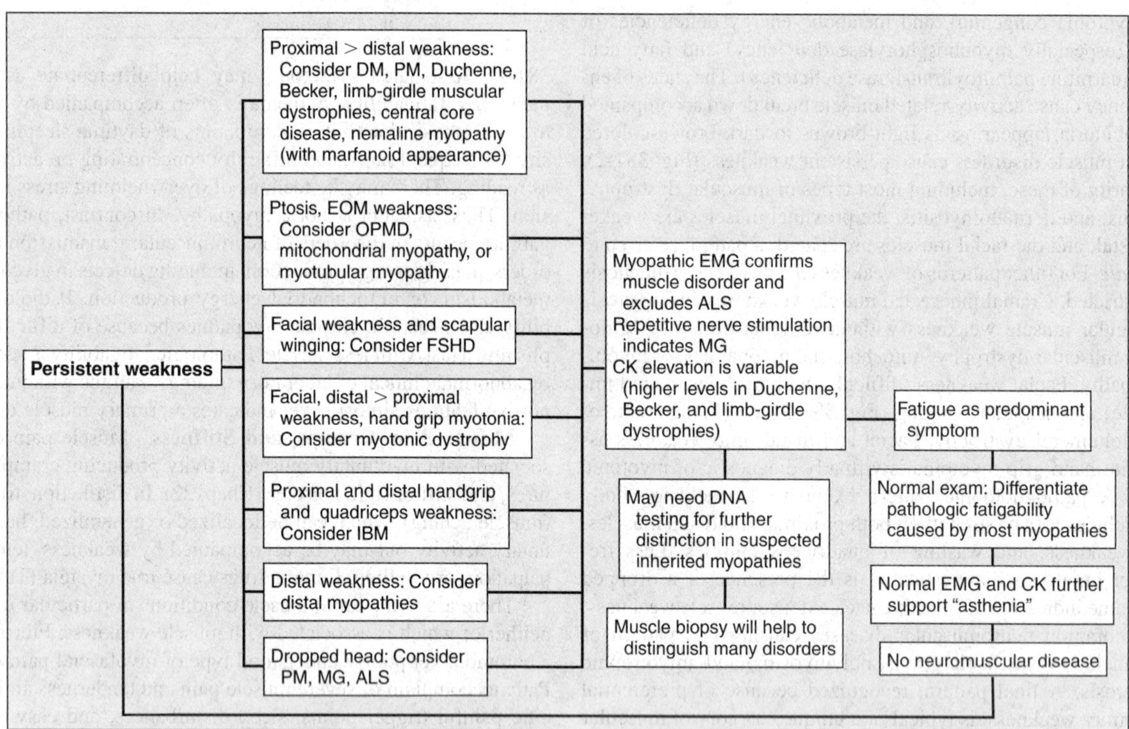

FIGURE 381-2 Diagnostic evaluation for persistent weakness. EOM, extraocular muscle; OPMD, oculopharyngeal muscular dystrophy; FSHD, facioscapulohumeral muscular dystrophy; IBM, inclusion body myositis; DM, dermatomyositis; PM, polymyositis; MG, myasthenia gravis, ALS, amyotrophic lateral sclerosis; CK, creatine kinase.

cular dystrophy (Chap. 383). Muscle cramps more often accompany neurogenic disorders, especially motor neuron disease (Chap. 365), radiculopathies, and polyneuropathies (Chap. 377).

A muscle contracture is different from a muscle cramp. In both conditions, the muscle becomes hard, but a contracture is associated with energy failure in glycolytic disorders. The muscle is unable to relax after an active muscle contraction. The EMG shows electrical silence. Confusion is created because contracture also refers to a muscle that cannot be passively stretched to its proper length (fixed contracture) because of fibrosis. In some muscle disorders, especially Emery-Dreifuss muscular dystrophy and Bethlem myopathy (Chap. 383), fixed contractures occur early and represent distinctive features of the disease.

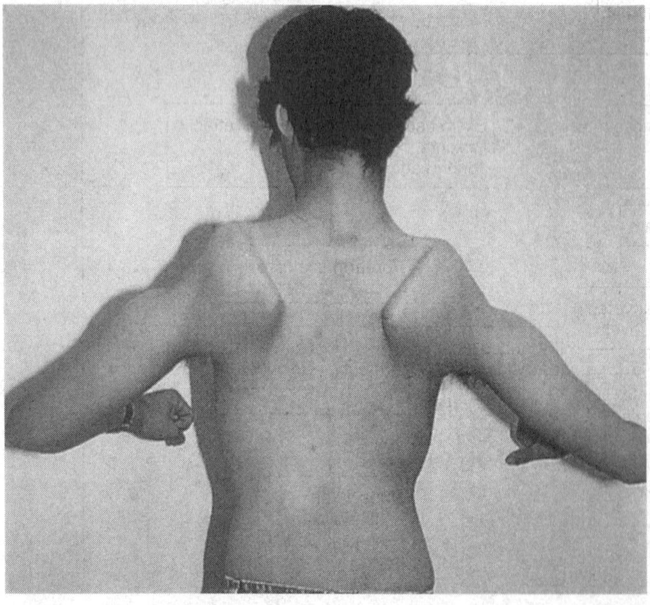

FIGURE 381-3 Facioscapulohumeral dystrophy with prominent scapular winging.

Muscle stiffness can refer to different phenomena. Some patients with inflammation of joints and periarticular surfaces feel stiff. This condition is different from the disorders of hyperexcitable motor nerves causing stiff or rigid muscles (Chap. 22). In *stiff-man syndrome* spontaneous discharges of the motor neuron of the spinal cord cause involuntary muscle contractions mainly involving the axial and proximal lower extremity muscles. Neuromyotonia (Isaac's syndrome) is another cause of motor nerve hyperexcitability.

Myotonia is a condition of prolonged muscle contraction followed by slow muscle relaxation. It always follows muscle activation, usually voluntary, but may be elicited by mechanical stimulation (percussion myotonia) of the muscle. Myotonia causes difficulty in releasing objects after a firm grasp. Usually it is worsened by cold temperatures

Table 381-1 Observations on Examination That Disclose Muscle Weakness

Functional Impairment	Muscle Weakness
Inability to forcibly close eyes	Upper facial muscles
Impaired pucker	Lower facial muscles
Inability to raise head from prone position	Neck extensor muscles
Inability to raise head from supine position	Neck flexor muscles
Inability to raise arms above head	Proximal arm muscles (may be only scapular stabilizing muscles)
Inability to walk without hyperextending knee (backkneeing or genu recurvatum)	Knee extensor muscles
Inability to walk with heels touching the floor (toe walking)	Shortening of the Achilles tendon
Inability to lift foot while walking (steppage gait or footdrop)	Anterior compartment of leg
Inability to walk without a waddling gait	Hip muscles
Inability to get up from the floor without climbing up the extremities (Gowers' sign)	Hip muscles
Inability to get up from a chair without using arms	Hip muscles

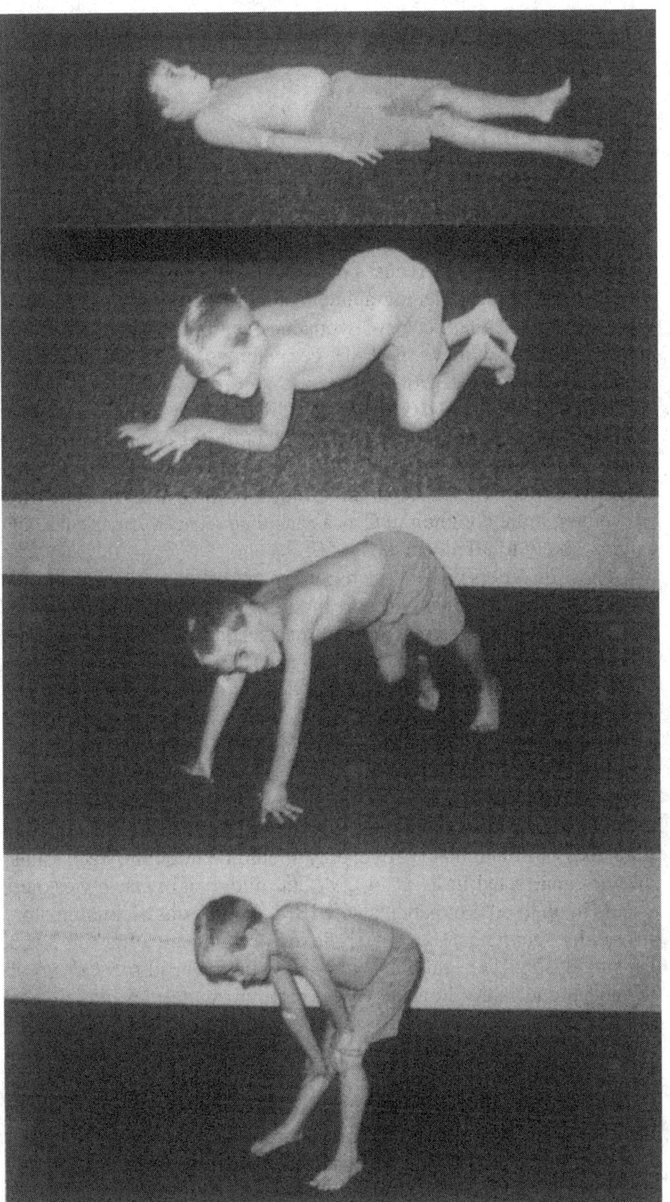

FIGURE 381-4 Gowers' sign showing a patient using arms to climb up the legs in attempting to get up from the floor.

and eases with continued activity. The sodium channelopathies (paramyotonia congenita and hyperkalaemic periodic paralysis) are accompanied by a unique phenomenon, paradoxical myotonia, in which repeated muscle contraction exacerbates the myotonia (Chap. 383). In hypokalemic periodic paralysis, myotonia of the eyelids may be present but limb muscles are usually spared.

Muscle Enlargement and Atrophy In most myopathies muscle tissue is replaced by fat and connective tissue, but the size of the muscle is usually not affected. However, in Duchenne and Becker muscular dystrophies enlarged calf muscles are typical. In the patients with these forms of dystrophy, the enlargement represents true muscle hypertrophy. The calf muscles remain very strong even late in the course of the disease. The term "pseudohypertrophy" should be avoided when referring to these patients. Muscle enlargement can also result from infiltration by sarcoid granulomas, amyloid deposits, bacterial and parasitic infections, and focal myositis. A tendon rupture, especially a biceps brachii tendon, is a common cause of focal muscle enlargement.

LABORATORY EVALUATION A limited battery of tests can be used to evaluate a suspected myopathy. Nearly all patients require serum enzyme level measurements and electrodiagnostic stud-

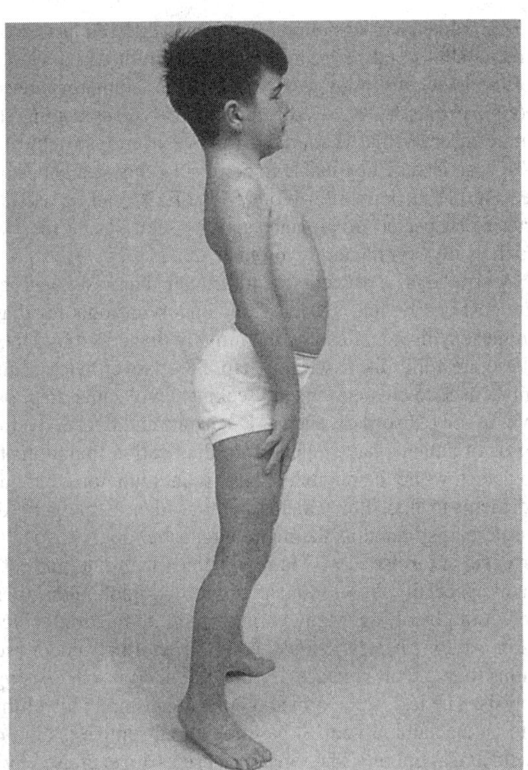

FIGURE 381-5 Lordotic posture, exaggerated by standing on toes, associated with trunk and hip weakness.

ies as screening tools to differentiate muscle disorders from other motor unit diseases. The other tests described—DNA studies, the forearm exercise test, and muscle biopsy—are used to diagnose specific types of myopathies.

Serum Enzymes Creatine kinase (CK) is the preferred muscle enzyme to measure in the evaluation of myopathies. Damage to muscle causes the CK to leak from the muscle fiber to the serum. The MM isoenzyme predominates in skeletal muscle, while CK-MB is the marker for cardiac muscle. Serum CK can be elevated in normal individuals without provocation, presumably on a genetic basis or after strenuous activity, minor trauma (including the EMG needle), a prolonged muscle cramp, or a generalized seizure. Aspartate aminotransferase (AST), alanine aminotransferase (ALT), and lactic dehydrogenase (LDH) are enzymes sharing an origin in both muscle and liver. Problems arise when the levels of these enzymes are found to be elevated in a routine screening battery, leading to the erroneous assumption that liver disease is present when in fact muscle could be the cause. An elevated gamma-glutamyl transferase (GGT) helps to establish a liver origin since this enzyme is not found in muscle. Aldolase is often thought to be a muscle-specific enzyme but is also present in liver.

Electrodiagnostic Studies EMG, repetitive nerve stimulation, and nerve conduction studies (Chap. 357) are essential methods for evaluation of the patient with suspected muscle disease. In combina-

Table 381-2 Drugs That Cause True Myalgia

Clofibrate	Emetine
Lovastatin	Labetalol
Gemfibrozil	Nifedipine
Vincristine	D-Penicillamine
Zidovudine	L-Tryptophan
Cyclosporine	Epsilon aminocaproic acid
Gold	Heroin
Danazol	Cocaine
Cimetidine	Methadone

tion they provide the information necessary to differentiate myopathies from neuropathies and neuromuscular junction diseases. Certain features of the EMG will point to an acquired, inflammatory muscle disorder (e.g., irritability on needle placement) versus a long-standing myopathic disorder that is more suggestive of a dystrophic process. The EMG can also be invaluable in helping to choose an appropriately affected muscle to sample for biopsy. The EMG can be used to fully characterize suspected involuntary activity seen during the examination, such as myokymia and myotonia.

DNA Analysis Advances in molecular diagnosis have evolved over the past decade and now serve as important tools for diagnosis. Certain muscle disorders can be definitively diagnosed by DNA analysis; these are fully discussed in Chap. 383. Nevertheless, important limitations need to be mentioned in seeking a molecular diagnosis. For example, in some disorders, such as Duchenne and Becker dystrophies, two-thirds of patients have deletion- or duplication-mutations that are easy to detect, while the remainder have point mutations that are much more difficult to find. For patients without identifiable gene defects, the muscle biopsy remains the main diagnostic tool.

Forearm Exercise Test In myopathies with intermittent symptoms, and especially those associated with myoglobinuria, there may be a defect in glycolysis. Many variations of the forearm exercise test exist. For safety, the test should not be performed under ischemic conditions to avoid an unnecessary insult to the muscle causing rhabdomyolysis. The test is performed by placing a small indwelling catheter into an antecubital vein. A baseline blood sample is obtained for lactic acid and ammonia. The forearm muscles are exercised by asking the patient to vigorously squeeze a sphygmomanometer bulb for 1 min. Blood is then obtained at intervals of 1, 2, 4, 6, and 10 min for comparison with the baseline sample. Normal controls must be established for each laboratory. A three- to fourfold rise of lactic acid is typical. The simultaneous measurement of ammonia serves as a control, since it should also rise with exercise. In patients with myophosphorylase deficiency or other glycolytic defects (Chap. 383), the lactic acid rise will be absent or below normal, while the rise in ammonia will reach control values. If there is lack of effort, neither lactic acid nor ammonia will rise. Patients with selective failure to increase ammonia may have myoadenylate deaminase deficiency. This condition has been reported to be a cause of myoglobinuria, but deficiency of this enzyme in asymptomatic individuals makes interpretation controversial.

Muscle Biopsy Muscle biopsy analysis is an important step in establishing the final diagnosis of suspected myopathy. The microscopic evaluation uses a combination of techniques—histochemistry, immunocytochemistry with a battery of antibodies, and electron microscopy. Not all techniques need to be used on every case. A specific diagnosis can be established in many disorders. A combination of stains to identify mononuclear cells (polymyositis), complement (dermatomyositis), and amyloid (inclusion body myositis) help to distinguish the inflammatory myopathies. Mitochondrial and metabolic (e.g., myophosphorylase and acid maltase deficiencies) myopathies demonstrate distinctive histochemical and electron microscopic profiles. A battery of antibodies is available for the identification of missing components of the dystrophin-glycoprotein complex and related proteins to help diagnose specific types of muscular dystrophies. In addition, the congenital myopathies have distinctive histologic features essential for diagnosis.

BIBLIOGRAPHY

GRIGGS RC et al: Evaluation of the patient with myopathy, in *Evaluation and Treatment of Myopathies*, RC Griggs et al (eds). Philadelphia, FA Davis, 1995, pp 17–77

KINCAID JC: Muscle pain, fatigue, and fasiculations. Neurol Clin 15:697, 1997

WASIELEWSKI PG et al: Inherited neurologic disorders: Relevant considerations and new aspects, in Clinical Neurology, RJ Joynt, RC Griggs (eds). Philadelphia, Lippincott-Raven, 1996, pp 1–48

ZISMAN DA et al: Sarcoidosis presenting as a tumorlike muscular lesion. Medicine 78: 112, 1983

382

Marinos C. Dalakas, Jr.

POLYMYOSITIS, DERMATOMYOSITIS, AND INCLUSION BODY MYOSITIS

The inflammatory myopathies represent the largest group of acquired and potentially treatable causes of skeletal weakness. On the basis of well defined clinical, demographic, histologic and immunopathological criteria, the inflammatory myopathies can be classified into three major groups: polymyositis (PM), dermatomyositis (DM), and inclusion body myositis (IBM).

GENERAL CLINICAL FEATURES The incidence of PM, DM, and IBM is approximately 1 in 100,000. PM is predominantly a disease of adults. DM affects both children and adults, and women more often than men. IBM is three times more frequent in men than in women, more common in Caucasians than African Americans, and is most likely to affect persons >50.

These disorders present as progressive and often symmetric muscle weakness. Patients usually report increasing difficulty with everyday tasks requiring the use of proximal muscles, such as getting up from a chair, climbing steps, stepping onto a curb, lifting objects, or combing hair. Fine-motor movements that depend on the strength of distal muscles, such as buttoning a shirt, sewing, knitting, or writing, are affected only late in the course of PM and DM, but fairly early in IBM. Falling is common in IBM because of early involvement of the quadriceps muscle with buckling of the knees. Ocular muscles are spared, even in advanced, untreated cases; if these muscles are affected, the diagnosis of inflammatory myopathy should be in doubt. Facial muscles are unaffected in PM and DM, but mild facial muscle weakness occurs in up to 60% of patients with IBM. In all forms of inflammatory myopathy, pharyngeal and neck-flexor muscles are often involved, causing dysphagia or difficulty in holding up the head (*neck drop*). In advanced and rarely in acute cases, respiratory muscles may also be affected. Severe weakness, if untreated, is almost always associated with muscle wasting. Sensation remains normal. The tendon reflexes are preserved but may be absent in severely weakened or atrophied muscles, especially in IBM where atrophy of the quadriceps and the distal muscles is common. Myalgia and muscle tenderness may occur in a small number of patients, usually early in the diseaese and more often in DM than in PM. Weakness in PM and DM progresses subacutely over a period of weeks or months and rarely acutely; by contrast, IBM progresses very slowly, over years, and its course may simulate late-life muscular dystrophies (Chap. 383) or slowly progressive motor neuron disorders (Chap. 365).

SPECIFIC FEATURES (Table 382-1) **Polymyositis** In most patients, the actual onset of PM is not easily determined, and patients typically delay seeking medical advice for several months. This is in contrast to DM, in which the rash facilitates early recognition (see below). PM is a subacute inflammatory myopathy affecting adults, and rarely children, who *do not have* any of the following: rash, involvement of the extraocular and facial muscles, family history of a neuromuscular disease, history of exposure to myotoxic drugs or toxins, endocrinopathy, neurogenic disease, muscular dystrophy, biochemical muscle disorder (deficiency of a muscle enzyme), or IBM as excluded by muscle biopsy analysis (see below). PM may occur either in isolation, in association with a systemic autoimmune or connective tissue disease, or with known viral or bacterial infection. D-Penicillamine and, on occasion, zidovudine (AZT) may also produce an inflammatory myopathy similar to PM.

Dermatomyositis DM is a distinctive entity identified by a characteristic rash accompanying, or more often preceding, muscle weakness. The rash may consist of a heliotrope rash (blue-purple discoloration) on the upper eyelids with edema, a flat red rash on the face and upper trunk, and erythema of the knuckles with a raised violaceous scaly eruption (*Gottron rash*) that later results in scaling of the skin

Table 382-1 Features Associated with Inflammatory Myopathies

Characteristic	Polymyositis	Dermatomyositis	Inclusion Body Myositis
Age at onset	>18 yr	Adulthood and childhood	>50 yr
Familial association	No	No	Yes, in some cases
Associated conditions			
Connective tissue diseases	Yes[a]	Scleroderma and mixed connective tissue disease (overlap syndromes)	Yes, in up to 20% of cases[a]
Other autoimmune diseases[b]	Frequent	Infrequent	Rare, but more frequently recognized
Malignancy	No	Yes, in up to 15% of cases	No
Viruses	Yes, with HIV, HTLV-I;[c] other viruses are uncertain	Unproven	Unproven (rare cases with HIV, HTLV-1)
Drugs[d]	Yes	Yes, rarely	No

[a] Systemic lupus erythematosus, rheumatoid arthritis, Sjögren's syndrome, systemic sclerosis, mixed connective tissue disease.

[b] Crohn's disease, vasculitis, sarcoidosis, primary biliary cirrhosis, adult celiac disease, chronic graft-versus-host disease, discoid lupus, ankylosing spondylitis, Behçet's syndrome, myasthenia gravis, acne fulminans, dermatitis herpetiformis, psoriasis, Hashimoto's disease, granulomatous diseases, agammaglobulinemia, monoclonal gammopathy, hypereosinophilic syndrome, Lyme disease, Kawasaki disease, autoimmune thrombocytopenia, hypergammaglobulinemic purpura, hereditary complement deficiency, IgA deficiency.

[c] HTLV-I, human T cell lymphotropic virus type I.

[d] Drugs include penicillamine (dermatomyositis and polymyositis), zidovudine (polymyositis), and contaminated tryptophan (dermatomyositis-like illness). Other myotoxic drugs may cause myopathy but not an inflammatory myopathy (see text for details).

(see Plates IIE-63 and IIE-65). The erythematous rash can also occur on other body surfaces, including the knees, elbows, malleoli, neck and anterior chest (often in a *V sign*), or back and shoulders (*shawl sign*), and may worsen after sun exposure. In some patients the rash is pruritic, especially on the scalp, chest, and back. Dilated capillary loops at the base of the fingernails are also characteristic. The cuticles may be irregular, thickened, and distorted, and the lateral and palmar areas of the fingers may become rough and cracked, with irregular, "dirty" horizontal lines, resembling *mechanic's hands*. The weakness can be mild, moderate, or severe enough to lead to quadraparesis. At times, the muscle strength appears normal, hence the term *dermatomyositis sine myositis*. When muscle biopsy is performed in such cases, however, significant perivascular and perimysial inflammation is seen. In children, DM resembles the adult disease, except for more frequent extramuscular manifestations, as discussed later. A common early abnormality in children is "misery," defined as an irritable child who appears uncomfortable, has a red flush on the face, is fatigued, does not wish to socialize, and has a varying degree of proximal muscle weakness. A tiptoe gait due to flexion contracture of the ankles is also common.

DM usually occurs alone but may overlap with scleroderma and mixed connective tissue disease. Fasciitis and thickening of the skin similar to that seen in chronic cases of DM have occurred in patients with the *eosinophilia–myalgia syndrome* associated with the ingestion of contaminated L-tryptophan.

Inclusion Body Myositis In patients ≥50, IBM is the most common of the inflammatory myopathies. It is often misdiagnosed as PM and suspected only retrospectively when a patient with presumed PM does not respond to therapy. Weakness and atrophy of distal muscles, especially foot extensors and deep finger flexors, occur in almost all cases of IBM and may be a clue to early diagnosis. Some patients present with falls because their knees collapse due to early quadriceps weakness. Others present with weakness in the small muscles of the hands, especially finger flexors, and complain of inability to hold certain objects, such as golf clubs, or perform certain tasks, such as turning keys or tying knots. On occasion, the weakness and accompanying atrophy can be asymmetric and selectively involve the quadriceps, iliopsoas, triceps, biceps, and finger flexors, resembling a lower motor neuron disease. Dysphagia is common, occurring in up to 60% of IBM patients, and may lead to episodes of choking. Sensory examination is generally normal; some patients have mildly diminished vibratory sensation at the ankles that presumably is age-related. The distal weakness does not represent motor neuron or peripheral nerve involvement but results from the myopathic process affecting distal muscles. The diagnosis is always made by the characteristic findings on the muscle biopsy, as discussed below. Disease progression is slow but steady, and most patients require an assistive device such as cane, walker, or wheelchair within several years of onset.

In at least 20% of cases, IBM is associated with systemic autoimmune or connective tissue diseases. Familial aggregation has also been noted in coaffected siblings with typical IBM; such cases have been designated as *familial inflammatory IBM*. This disorder is distinct from *hereditary inclusion body myopathy* (h-IBM), which describes a heterogeneous group of recessive and less frequently dominant, inherited syndromes. The h-IBMs are noninflammatory myopathies with clinical profiles distinct from sporadic IBM. A subset of h-IBM that spares the quadriceps muscle has emerged as a distinct entity. This disorder, originally described in Iranian Jews and now seen in many ethnic groups, is linked to chromosome 9p1.

ASSOCIATED CLINICAL FINDINGS **Extramuscular Manifestations** In addition to the primary myopathy, a number of extramuscular manifestations may be present to a varying degree in patients with PM or DM:

1. *Systemic symptoms*, such as fever, malaise, weight loss, arthralgia, and Raynaud's phenomenon especially when inflammatory myopathy is associated with a connective tissue disorder.
2. *Joint contractures*, mostly in DM and especially in children.
3. *Dysphagia and gastrointestinal symptoms* due to involvement of the oropharyngeal striated muscles and upper esophagus. Dysphagia may be prominent in the active stages of DM and is frequent in IBM. Gastrointestinal ulcerations due to vasculitis and infection were common in children with DM before the use of immunosuppressive drugs.
4. *Cardiac disturbances*, including atrioventricular conduction defects, tachyarrythmias, dilated cardiomyopathy, and low ejection fraction. Congestive heart failure and myocarditis may also occur, either from the disease itself or from hypertension associated with long-term use of glucocorticoids.
5. *Pulmonary dysfunction*, due to primary weakness of the thoracic muscles, drug-induced pneumonitis (e.g., from methotrexate), or interstitial lung disease may cause dyspnea, nonproductive cough, and aspiration pneumonia. Interstitial lung disease may precede myopathy or occur early in the disease, and develops in up to 10% of patients with PM or DM.
6. *Subcutaneous calcifications*, sometimes extruding on the skin and causing ulcerations and infections, are seen in DM, primarily in children.

Malignancies Although all the inflammatory myopathies can have a chance association with malignant lesions, especially in older age groups, the incidence of malignant conditions appears to be specifically increased only in patients with DM but not PM or IBM. The most common tumors associated with DM are ovarian cancer, breast cancer, melanoma, and colon cancer. The extent of the search that should be conducted for an occult malignant neoplasm in adults with DM depends on the clinical circumstances. Tumors in these patients are usually uncovered by abnormal findings in the medical history and physical examination and not through an extensive radiologic blind search. Thus the weight of evidence argues against performing expensive, invasive, and nondirected tumor searches. When a suspected malignancy is not apparent, a complete annual physical examination with pelvic, breast, and rectal examinations; urinalysis; complete blood count; blood chemistry tests; and a chest film should suffice.

Overlap The term *overlap syndrome* has been used loosely to describe the frequent association of inflammatory myopathies with connective tissue diseases. A well-characterized overlap syndrome occurs in patients with DM who also have manifestations of systemic sclerosis or mixed connective tissue disease, such as sclerotic thickening of the dermis, contractures, esophageal hypomotility, microangiopathy, and calcium deposits (Table 382-1). By contrast, signs of rheumatoid arthritis, systemic lupus erythematosus, or Sjögren's syndrome are very rare in patients with DM. Patients with the overlap syndrome of DM and systemic sclerosis may have a specific antinuclear autoantibody, the anti-PM/Scl, directed against a nucleolar-protein complex.

PATHOGENESIS An autoimmune origin of these disorders is supported by their association with other systemic autoimmune, viral, or connective tissue diseases; the presence of various autoantibodies; their association with histocompatibility genes; the evidence of T cell–mediated myocytotoxicity or complement-mediated microangiopathy; and their response to immunotherapies. However, the specific muscle or capillary target antigens have not been identified, and the agents initiating self-sensitization are still unknown.

Autoantibodies and Immunogenetics Various autoantibodies against nuclear antigens (antinuclear antibodies) and cytoplasmic antigens are found in up to 20% of patients with inflammatory myopathies. The antibodies to cytoplasmic antigens, present in <10% of PM and DM patients, are directed against cytoplasmic ribonucleoproteins, which are involved in translation and protein synthesis. They include antibodies against various synthetases, translation factors, and proteins of the signal-recognition particles. The antibody directed against the histidyl-transfer RNA synthetase, called *anti-Jo-1*, accounts for 75% of all the anti-synthetases and is clinically useful because up to 80% of patients with anti-Jo-1 antibodies have interstitial lung disease. Some patients with the anti-Jo-1 antibody may also have Raynaud's phenomenon, nonerosive arthritis, and the HLA antigens DR3 and DRw52. In both PM and IBM, there is an increased frequency (up to 75%) of haplotypes of DR3 (molecular designation DRB1*0301, DQB1*0201), suggesting that these alleles may be risk factors for the development of these disorders (Chap. 306).

Immunopathologic Mechanisms In DM, the endomysial infiltrates have a higher than normal percentage of B cells, a higher ratio of CD4+ cells (helper cells) to CD8+ cells (suppressor-cytotoxic T cells), proximity of CD4+ cells to B cells and macrophages, and a relative absence of lymphocytic invasion of nonnecrotic muscle fibers, all of which suggest a mechanism mediated primarily by humoral processes. The immune process is directed against microvascular antigens and is mediated by the complement C5b-9 membranolytic attack complex, resulting in necrosis of the endothelial cells, reduced numbers of endomysial capillaries, ischemia, muscle-fiber destruction often resembling microinfarcts, and inflammation. Larger intramuscular blood vessels may also be affected in the same pattern, leading to actual muscle infarction. Residual perifascicular atrophy reflects the endofascicular hypoperfusion that is prominent in the periphery of the fascicles. Complement activation is thought to trigger release of proinflammatory cytokines, induce expression of vascular cell adhesion molecule (VCAM)-1 and intracellular adhesion molecule (ICAM)-1 on endothelial cells, and facilitate migration of activated lymphoid cells to the perimysial and endomysial spaces.

In PM and IBM there is evidence not of microangiopathy and muscle ischemia, as in DM, but of an antigen-directed cytotoxicity mediated by CD8+ cytotoxic T cells. This conclusion is supported by the presence of CD8+ cells, which, along with macrophages, initially surround and eventually invade and destroy healthy, nonnecrotic muscle fibers that aberrantly express class I MHC molecules. MHC-I expression, absent from the sarcolemma of normal muscle fibers, is probably induced by cytokines secreted by activated T cells and macrophages. The cytotoxic autoinvasive CD8+ T cells contain perforin and granzyme granules directed towards the surface of the muscle fibers and capable of inducing cell death. The infiltrating endomysial T cells appear to be clonally restricted, suggesting an antigen-driven T cell response. The putative antigens are more likely to be endogenous sarcolemmal or cytoplasmic self-proteins synthesized within the muscle, rather than endogenous viral peptides, because viruses have not been identified within the muscle fibers.

T cell–derived cytokines (interleukins 2, 4, and 5 and interferon γ), the macrophage-derived cytokines (interleukins 1 and 6 and tumor necrosis factor α), and adhesion molecules on leukocytes (L-selectin and integrins LFA-1, VLA-4) and their respective ligands on endothelial cells (GlyCAM-1, ICAM-1, VCAM-1) in patients with PM, DM, and IBM; these may facilitate the adhesion and transmigration of activated T cells through the endothelial cell wall. T cell metalloproteinases (MMP-2 and MMP-9) are also upregulated and may facilitate adhesion of T cells to muscle, enhancing cytotoxicity.

The Role of Nonimmune Factors in IBM In IBM, the presence of vacuoles, the amyloid-positive deposits within some vacuolated muscle fibers, the abnormal muscle mitochondria with mitochondrial DNA deletions, and the relative resistance of the disease to immunosuppressive therapies suggest that, in addition to the autoimmune component, there is also a degenerative process. Similar to Alzheimer's disease, the amyloid deposits in IBM are immunoreactive against amyloid precurser protein (APP), chymotrypsin, apolipoprotein E, and phosphorylated tau, but it is unclear whether these deposits directly contribute to disease pathogenesis or are secondary phenomena. The same can be said for the mitochondrial abnormalities, which may also be secondary caused by the effects of aging and upregulated cytokines.

Association with Viral Infections and the Role of Retroviruses Several viruses, including coxsackieviruses, influenza, paramyxoviruses, mumps, cytomegalovirus, and Epstein-Barr virus have been indirectly associated with chronic and acute myositis. For the coxsackieviruses, an autoimmune myositis triggered by molecular mimicry has been proposed because of structural homology between histidyl-transfer RNA synthetase that is the target of the Jo-1 antibody (see above) and genomic RNA of an animal picornavirus, the encephalomyocarditis virus. Very sensitive polymerase chain reaction (PCR) studies, however, have repeatedly failed to confirm the presence of such viruses in muscle biopsies from these patients.

The best evidence of a viral connection in PM and IBM is with the retroviruses. Monkeys infected with the simian immunodeficiency virus and humans infected with HIV and human T cell lymphotropic virus (HTLV) develop PM or, rarely, IBM. In humans infected with HIV or HTLV-1, an isolated inflammatory myopathy may occur as the initial manifestation of the retroviral infection or myositis may develop later in the disease course. Retroviral antigens have been detected only in occasional endomysial macrophages and not within the muscle fibers themselves, suggesting that persistent infection and viral replication within the muscle do not occur. Histologic findings in PM and IBM associated with HIV-1 and HTLV-1 infection are identical to retroviral-negative myositis, specifically CD8+ T cells and macrophages that invade or surround MHC-I antigen–expressing nonnecrotic muscle fibers. The development of PM or IBM in HIV-positive patients should be distinguished from a toxic myopathy related to long-term therapy with zidovudine, which is characterized by fatigue, myalgia, mild muscle weakness, and mild elevation of creatine kinase (CK). Zidovudine-induced myopathy, which generally improves when the drug is discontinued, is a mitochondrial disorder characterized histologically by the presence of numerous "ragged-red" fibers. Abnormal muscle mitochondria and depletion of the muscle mitochondrial DNA by zidovudine results from inhibition of γ-DNA polymerase, an enzyme found solely in the mitochondrial matrix.

DIFFERENTIAL DIAGNOSIS The clinical picture of skin rash and proximal or diffuse muscle weakness has few causes other than DM. However, proximal muscle weakness without skin involvement can be due to many conditions other than PM.

Subacute or Chronic Progressive Muscle Weakness This may be due to denervating conditions such as the spinal muscular atrophies or amyotrophic lateral sclerosis (Chap. 365). In addition to the muscle weakness, upper motor neuron signs in the latter aid in the diagnosis. The muscular dystrophies, such as those of Duchenne and Becker and the limb-girdle and facioscapulohumeral types, may be additional considerations (Chap. 383). However, the muscular dystrophies usually develop more slowly (over years rather than weeks or months) and rarely present after the age of 30. In rare patients it may be difficult, even with a muscle biopsy, to distinguish chronic PM from a rapidly advancing muscular dystrophy. This is particularly true of facioscapulohumeral muscular dystrophy, where interstitial inflammatory cell infiltration is commonly found early in the disease. Such doubtful cases should always be given an adequate trial of glucocorticoid therapy. Some metabolic myopathies, including glycogen storage disease due to myophosphorylase or acid maltase deficiency, lipid storage myopathies due to carnitine deficiency, and mitochondrial diseases produce muscle weakness, which is often associated with other characteristic clinical signs (Chap. 383); diagnosis rests upon histochemical and biochemical studies of the muscle biopsy. The endocrine myopathies such as those due to hypercorticosteroidism, hyper- and hypothyroidism, and hyper- and hypoparathyroidism require the appropriate laboratory investigations for diagnosis. Muscle wasting in patients with an underlying neoplasm may be due to disuse, cachexia, or rarely to a paraneoplastic neuromyopathy (Chap. 101).

Diseases of the neuromuscular junction, including myasthenia gravis or the Lambert-Eaton myasthenic syndrome, cause fatiguing weakness that also affects the eye and cranial muscles (Chap. 380). Repetitive nerve stimulation and single-fiber electromyography (EMG) studies aid in diagnosis.

Acute Muscle Weakness This may be caused by an acute neuropathy such as Guillain-Barré syndrome (Chap. 378) or a neurotoxin. When combined with painful muscle cramps, rhabdomyolysis, and myoglobinuria, it may be due to metabolic disorders including some of the glycogen storage diseases, such as myophosphorylase deficiency (McArdle's disease), carnitine palmityltransferase deficiency, and myoadenylate deaminase deficiency (Chap. 383). Acute viral infections may cause a similar syndrome. Several animal parasites, such as protozoa (*toxoplasma*, *trypanosoma*), cestodes (cysticerci), and nematodes (trichinae), may produce a focal or diffuse inflammatory myopathy known as *parasitic polymyositis*. *Staphylococcus aureus*, *Yersinia*, *Streptococcus*, or other anaerobic bacteria may produce a suppurative myositis, known as *tropical polymyositis*, or *pyomyositis*. Pyomyositis, previously rare in the west, is now seen in occasional AIDS patients. Other bacteria, such as *Borrelia burgdorferi* (Lyme disease) and *Legionella pneumophila* (Legionnaire's disease) may infrequently cause myositis.

Chronic alcoholics may develop a painful myopathy with myoglobinuria after a bout of heavy drinking; present with a painless acute hypokalemic myopathy, which is completely reversible; or show an asymptomatic elevation of serum CK and myoglobin. Acute muscle weakness with myoglobinuria may occur with prolonged severe hypokalemia or with hypophosphatemia and hypomagnesemia, often seen in chronic alcoholics and in patients on nasogastric suction receiving parenteral hyperalimentation.

Macrophagic Myofasciitis This distinctive inflammatory muscle disorder, recently described in France, presents as diffuse myalgias, fatigue, and mild muscle weakness. Muscle biopsy reveals pronounced infiltration of the connective tissue around the muscle (epimysium, perimysium, and perifascicular endomysium) by sheets of periodic acid–Schiff-positive macrophages and occasional CD8+ T cells. The CK or erythrocyte sedimentation rate is variably elevated. Most patients respond to glucocorticoid therapy, and the overall prognosis is favorable. Histologic involvement is focal and limited to sites of previous vaccinations, which may have been administered months or years earlier. This disorder, which to date has not been observed outside of France, has been linked to an aluminum-containing substrate used in vaccine preparation.

Drug-Induced Myopathies Penicillamine and procainamide may produce a true myositis resembling PM, and a DM-like illness has been associated with contaminated preparations of L-tryptophan. As noted above, zidovudine causes a mitochondrial myopathy. Other drugs may elicit a toxic noninflammatory myopathy that is histologically different from DM, PM, or IBM. The most common drugs are the cholesterol-lowering agents such as clofibrate, lovastatin, simvastatin, or provastatin, especially when combined with cyclosporine or gemfibrozil. Rhabdomyolysis and myoglobinuria have been associated with amphotericin B, ε-aminocaproic acid, fenfluramine, heroin, and phencyclidine. The use of amiodarone, chloroquine, colchicine, carbimazole, emetine, etretinate, ipecac syrup, chronic laxative use resulting in hypocalcemia, licorice, glucocorticoids, and growth hormone has also been associated with myopathy. Some neuromuscular blocking agents such as pancuronium, in combination with glucocorticoids, may cause the acute critical illness myopathy. A careful drug history is essential for diagnosis of these drug-induced myopathies, which do not require immunosuppressive therapy.

Pain on Movement and Muscle Tenderness A number of conditions including *polymyalgia rheumatica* and arthritic disorders of adjacent joints may enter into the differential diagnosis of inflammatory myopathy, even though they do not cause myositis (Chap. 317). The muscle biopsy is either normal or discloses type II fiber atrophy. Patients with *fibrositis* and *fibromyalgia* complain of focal or diffuse muscle tenderness, fatigue, and aching, which is sometimes poorly differentiated from joint pain. In other patients there may be minor signs of a collagen vascular disorder, such as an increased erythrocyte sedimentation rate, antinuclear antibody, or rheumatoid factor. Occasionally there is slight but transient elevation of the serum CK. The muscle biopsy is usually normal and the prognosis favorable. Many such patients show some response to nonsteroidal anti-inflammatory agents, though most continue to have indolent complaints. *Chronic fatigue syndrome*, which may follow a viral infection, can present with debilitating fatigue, fever, sore throat, painful lymphadenopathy, myalgia, arthralgia, sleep disorder, and headache (Chap. 384). These patients do not have muscle weakness, and the muscle biopsy is usually normal.

DIAGNOSIS The clinically suspected diagnosis of PM, DM, or IBM is confirmed by examining the serum muscle enzymes, EMG findings, and muscle biopsy (Table 382-2).

The most sensitive enzyme is CK, which in active disease can be elevated as much as 50-fold. Although the CK level usually parallels disease activity, it can be normal in some patients with active DM and is frequently normal or only slightly above normal in IBM, even from disease onset. CK may also be normal in patients with untreated, even active, childhood DM and in some patients with DM associated with a connective tissue disease, reflecting the concentration of the pathologic process in the intramuscular vessels and the perimysium. Along with the CK, the serum glutamic-oxaloacetic and glutamate pyruvate transaminases, lactate dehydrogenase, and aldolase may be elevated.

Needle EMG shows myopathic potentials characterized by short-duration, low-amplitude polyphasic units on voluntary activation and increased spontaneous activity with fibrillations, complex repetitive discharges, and positive sharp waves. Mixed potentials (polyphasic units of short and long duration) indicating a chronic process and muscle fiber regeneration are often present in IBM. These EMG findings are not diagnostic of an inflammatory myopathy but are useful to identify the presence of active or chronic myopathy and to exclude neurogenic disorders.

Magnetic resonance imaging is not routinely used for the diagnosis of PM, DM, or IBM. However, it may guide the location of the muscle biopsy in certain clinical settings.

Muscle biopsy is the definitive test for establishing the diagnosis of inflammatory myopathy and for excluding other neuromuscular dis-

Table 382-2 Criteria for Definite Diagnosis of Inflammatory Myopathies

Criterion	Polymyositis	Dermatomyositis	Inclusion Body Myositis
Muscle strength	Myopathic muscle weakness[a]	Myopathic muscle weakness[a,b]	Myopathic muscle weakness with early involvement of distal muscles[a]
Electromyographic findings	Myopathic	Myopathic	Myopathic with mixed potentials
Muscle enzymes	Elevated (up to 50-fold)	Elevated (up to 50-fold) or normal	Elevated (up to 10-fold) or normal
Muscle biopsy findings[c]	Diagnostic[d,e]	Diagnostic or nonspecific	Diagnostic[d,f]
Rash or calcinosis	Absent	Present and diagnostic[d,g]	Absent

[a] Myopathic muscle weakness, affecting proximal muscles more than distal ones and sparing eye and facial muscles, is characterized by a subacute onset (weeks to months) and rapid progression in patients who have no family history of neuromuscular disease, no endocrinopathy, no exposure to myotoxic drugs or toxins, and no biochemical muscle disease (excluded on the basis of muscle-biopsy findings).

[b] In some cases with the typical rash, the muscle strength is seemingly normal (*dermatomyositis sine myositis*); these patients often have new onset of easy fatigue and reduced endurance. Careful muscle testing may reveal mild muscle weakness.

[c] See text for details.

[d] An adequate trial of prednisone or other immunosuppressive drugs is warranted in probable cases. If, in retrospect, the disease is unresponsive to therapy, another muscle biopsy should be considered to exclude other diseases or possible evolution in inclusion body myositis.

[e] Probable polymyositis is present if muscle biopsy shows nonspecific myopathy without inflammation.

[f] Probable inclusion body myositis is present if muscle biopsy shows chronic nonspecific myopathy with inflammation but no vacuoles.

[g] If rash is absent but muscle biopsy findings are characteristic of dermatomyositis, diagnosis is definite.

eases. Inflammation is the histologic hallmark for these diseases; however, additional features are characteristic of each subtype.

In PM there are T cell infiltrates located primarily within the muscle fascicles (endomysially) and surrounding individual, healthy muscle fibers resulting in phagocytosis and necrosis. When the disease is chronic, connective tissue is increased and often reacts positively with alkaline phosphatase.

In DM the endomysial inflammation is predominantly perivascular or in the interfascicular septae and around, rather than within, the muscle fascicles. The intramuscular blood vessels show endothelial hyperplasia with tubuloreticular profiles, fibrin thrombi (especially in children), and obliteration of capillaries. The muscle fibers undergo necrosis, degeneration, and phagocytosis, often in groups involving a portion of a muscle fasiculus in a wedgelike shape or at the periphery of the fascicle, due to microinfarcts within the muscle. This results in perifascicular atrophy, characterized by 2 to 10 layers of atrophic fibers at the periphery of the fascicles. The presence of perifascicular atrophy is diagnostic of DM, *even in the absence of inflammation.*

In IBM, the following occur: (1) intense endomysial inflammation with T cells invading muscle fibers in a pattern identical to (but often more severe) from that seen in PM; (2) basophilic granular deposits distributed around the edge of slitlike vacuoles (rimmed vacuoles); (3) loss of fibers, replaced by fat and connective tissue, and angulated or round fibers, scattered or in small groups; (4) eosinophilic cytoplasmic inclusions; (5) abnormal mitochondria characterized by the presence of ragged-red fibers and cytochrome-oxidase (COX)-negative fibers and supported by the presence of mitochondrial DNA deletions in up to 75% of patients; (6) tiny congophilic amyloid deposits within or next to the vacuoles, best visualized by Texas-red fluorescent optics; and (7) characteristic filamentous inclusions seen by electron microscopy in the vicinity of the rimmed vacuoles. Such filaments can be seen in other vacuolar myopathies; thus they are not unique to IBM. Although demonstration of the filaments by electron microscopy was previously essential for the diagnosis of IBM, currently this is not absolutely necessary if all the other characteristic light-microscopic features, including amyloid deposits, are present.

In some patients with an acquired myopathy that fulfills the clinical criteria for PM or IBM, the muscle biopsy specimen may fail to confirm the suspected diagnosis; in such cases, a diagnosis of probable PM or probable IBM is assigned. An intramuscular inflammatory response around nonnecrotic muscle fibers is an invariable feature of both PM and IBM, and the absence of inflammation raises a critical question about the diagnosis. It is not unreasonable in such cases to obtain another muscle biopsy specimen from a different site. When the patient has the typical clinical phenotype of IBM but the muscle biopsy shows only features of chronic inflammatory myopathy without the typical vacuoles, the diagnosis of probable IBM is also appropriate.

Diagnostic criteria are summarized in Table 382-2. The diagnosis of PM is *definite* if a patient has an acquired, subacute myopathy fulfilling the exclusion criteria noted above, elevated CK levels, and a confirmatory muscle biopsy. The diagnosis of DM is *definite* if the characteristic rash is present, even if there is no inflammation in the muscle biopsy specimen. The diagnosis of IBM is *definite* when the characteristic histologic features are present in the muscle biopsy specimen from a patient with the appropriate clinical characteristics.

℞ **TREATMENT** The goal of therapy is to improve muscle strength, thereby improving function in activities of daily living. When strength improves the serum CK falls concurrently; however, the reverse is not always true. Unfortunately, there is a common tendency to "chase" or treat the CK level instead of the muscle weakness, a practice that has led to prolonged and unnecessary use of immunosuppressive drugs and erroneous assessment of their efficacy. It is prudent to discontinue these drugs if, after an adequate trial, there is no objective improvement in muscle strength whether or not CK levels are reduced. Agents used in the treatment of PM and DM include:

1. *Glucocorticoids.* Oral prednisone is the initial treatment of choice; the effectiveness and side effects of this therapy determine the future need for stronger immunosuppressive drugs. High-dose prednisone, at least 1 mg/kg per day, is initiated as early in the disease as possible. After an initial period of 3 to 4 weeks, prednisone is tapered slowly over a period of 10 weeks to 1 mg/kg every other day. Then, if there is evidence of efficacy and no serious side effects, the dosage is further reduced by 5 or 10 mg every 3 to 4 weeks until the lowest possible dose that controls the disease is reached. The efficacy of prednisone is determined by an objective increase in muscle strength and activities of daily living, which almost always occurs by the third month of therapy. A feeling of increased energy or a reduction of the CK level without a concomitant increase in muscle strength is not a reliable sign of improvement. If prednisone provides no objective benefit after ~3 months of high-dose therapy, the disease is probably unresponsive to the drug and tapering should be accelerated while the next-in-line immunosuppressive drug is started. Although controlled trials have not been performed, almost all patients with true PM or DM respond to glucocorticoids to *some degree and for some period of time*; in general, DM responds better than PM.

The long-term use of prednisone may cause increased weakness associated with a normal or unchanged CK level; this effect is referred to as *steroid myopathy*. In a patient who previously responded to high doses of prednisone, the development of increased weakness may be related to steroid myopathy or to disease activity that either will respond to a higher dose of glucocorticoids or has become glucocorticoid-resistant. In these circumstances, the decision to raise or lower the prednisone dosage may be influenced by reviewing the patient's history of muscle strength (especially with respect to mobility), serum CK levels, and changes in medications during the preceding 2 months. In uncertain cases, the prednisone dosage can be adjusted arbitrarily;

judged by the changes in the patient's strength, the cause of the weakness is usually evident in 2 to 8 weeks.

2. *Immunosuppressive drugs*. Approximately 75% of patients ultimately require treatment with immunosuppressive drugs. Treatment is generally initiated when a patient fails to respond adequately to glucocorticoids after a 3-month trial, the patient becomes glucocorticoid-resistant, glucocorticoid-related side effects appear, attempts to lower the prednisone dose repeatedly result in a new relapse, or rapidly progressive disease with evolving severe weakness and respiratory failure develops.

Drug selection is largely empirical, with choices based on personal experience, relative efficacy, and safety. The following agents are commonly used: (1) *Azathioprine* is well tolerated, has few side effects, and appears to be as effective for long-term therapy as other drugs. The dose is up to 3 mg/kg daily. (2) *Methotrexate* has a faster onset of action than azathioprine. It is given orally starting at 7.5 mg weekly for the first 3 weeks (2.5 mg every 12 h for 3 doses), with gradual dose escalation by 2.5 mg per week to a total of 25 mg weekly. An important side effect is methotrexate pneumonitis, which can be difficult to distinguish from the interstitial lung disease of the primary myopathy associated with Jo-1 antibodies (described above). (3) *Cyclophosphamide* (0.5 to 1 g/m^2 intravenously monthly for 6 months) has limited success and significant toxicity. (4) *Chlorambucil* has variable results. (5) *Cyclosporine* has inconsistent and mild benefit. (6) *Mycophenolate mofetil* has recently shown some effectiveness.

3. *Immunomodulating procedures*. In a double-blind study of patients with refractory DM, intravenous immunoglobulin (IVIg) improved not only the strength and rash but also the underlying immunopathology. The benefit can be impressive but is short-lived (≤8 weeks); repeated infusions every 6 to 8 weeks are required to maintain improvement. A dose of 2 g/kg divided over 2 to 5 days per course is recommended. A controlled double-blind study in PM is not yet completed, but uncontrolled observations suggest that IVIg is beneficial for some patients. Neither plasmapheresis or leukapheresis appears to be effective in PM and DM.

The following sequential empirical approach to the treatment of PM and DM is suggested: *Step 1*: High-dose prednisone; *step 2*: azathioprine or methotrexate; *step 3*: IVIg; *step 4*: a trial, with guarded optimism, of one of the following agents, chosen according to the patient's age, degree of disability, tolerance, experience with the drug, and the patient's general health: cyclosporine, chlorambucil, cyclophosphamide, mycophenolate. Patients with interstitial lung disease may benefit from aggressive treatment with cyclophosphamide.

Common pitfalls leading to failure of steroid or immunosuppressive treatment are inadequate initial dose of prednisone or cytotoxic drugs, short duration of therapy or quick tapering, early development of preventable side effects necessitating early discontinuation of prednisone, and wrong diagnosis. A patient with presumed PM who has not responded to any form of immunotherapy most likely has IBM or another disease. In these cases, a repeat muscle biopsy and a more vigorous search for the putative "other disease" are recommended. In addition to IBM, the most often misdiagnosed disorders are metabolic myopathy such as phosphorylase deficiency, a dystrophic process with endomysial inflammation resembling polymyositis, drug-induced myopathy, or an endocrinopathy.

Calcinosis, a manifestation of DM, is difficult to treat; however, new calcium deposits may be prevented if the primary disease responds to the available therapies. Diphosphonates, aluminum hydroxide, probenecid, colchicine, low doses of warfarin, calcium blockers, and surgical excision have all been tried without success.

IBM is resistant to immunosuppressive therapies. Prednisone together with azathioprine or methotrexate have been disappointing, but most experts try these agents for a few months in newly diagnosed patients. Because occasional patients may feel subjectively weaker after these drugs are discontinued, some clinicians prefer to maintain some patients on low-dose, every-other-day prednisone or weekly methotrexate in an effort to halt disease progression, even though there

is no objective evidence or controlled study to support this practice. In one double-blind study of IVIg in IBM, minimal benefit in up to 30% of the patients was found; the strength gains, however, were not of sufficient magnitude to justify the routine use of this drug. A second controlled trial combining IVIg with prednisone was ineffective in 36 IBM patients. Despite these disappointing results, many experts believe that a 2- to 3-month trial with IVIg may be reasonable for selected patients with IBM who experience rapid progression of muscle weakness or choking episodes due to worsening dysphagia.

PROGNOSIS Although accurate data from large series is not available, it is believed that the 5-year survival rate for treated patients with PM and DM is approximately 80%; death is usually due to pulmonary, cardiac, or other systemic complications. Patients severely affected at presentation or treated after long delays, those with severe dysphagia or respiratory difficulties, older patients, and those with associated cancer have a worse prognosis. DM responds more favorably to therapy than PM and thus has a better prognosis. Most patients improve with therapy, and many make a full functional recovery, which is often sustained with maintenance therapy. Up to 30% may be left with some residual muscle weakness. Relapses may occur at any time.

IBM has the least favorable prognosis of the inflammatory myopathies. Most patients will require the use of an assistive device such as a cane, walker, or wheelchair within 5 to 10 years of onset. In general, the older the age of onset in IBM, the more rapidly progressive is the course.

BIBLIOGRAPHY

ARGOV Z et al: Various types of hereditary inclusion body myopathies map to chromosome 9p1-q1. Ann Neurol 41:548, 1997

CALLEN JP: Dermatomyositis. Lancet 355:53, 2000

DALAKAS MC: Polymyositis, dermatomyositis, and inclusion-body myositis. N Engl J Med 325:1487, 1991

———: Molecular immunology and genetics of inflammatory muscle diseases. Arch Neurol 55:1509, 1998

———: Intravenous immunoglobulin in the treatment of autoimmune neuromuscular diseases: Present status and practical therapeutic guidelines. Muscle Nerve 22:1479, 1999

ENGEL AG et al: The polymyositis and dermatomyositis syndromes, in *Myology*, AG Engel, C Franzini-Armstrong (eds). New York, McGraw-Hill, 1994, pp 1335–1383

GHERARDI RK et al: Macrophagic myofasciitis: An emerging entity. Lancet 352:347, 1998

ILLA I et al: Immunocytochemical and virological characteristics of HIV-associated inflammatory myopathies: Similarities with seronegative polymyositis. Ann Neurol 39: 474, 1991

IOANNOU Y et al: Myositis overlap syndromes. Curr Opin Rheumatol 11:468, 1999

LEON-MONZON DM et al: Polymyositis in patients with HTLV-I: The role of the virus in the cause of the disease. Ann Neurol 36:643, 1994

MILLER FW et al: A randomized double-blind controlled trial of plasma exchange and leukapheresis in patients with polymyositis and dermatomyositis. N Engl J Med 326: 1380, 1992

OLDFORS A, LINDBERG G: Inclusion body myositis. Curr Opin Neurol 12:527, 1999

SIVAKUMAR K et al: An inflammatory, familial, inclusion body myositis with autoimmune features and a phenotype identical to sporadic inclusion body myositis: Studies in three families. Brain 120:653, 1997

383

Robert H. Brown, Jr., Jerry R. Mendell

MUSCULAR DYSTROPHIES AND OTHER MUSCLE DISEASES

The muscle disorders discussed in this chapter include diseases that cause acute, subacute, and chronic muscle weakness. Some cause pain in addition to or instead of weakness. →***Dermatomyositis and polymyositis are discussed in Chap. 382.***

HEREDITARY MYOPATHIES

Muscular dystrophy refers to a group of hereditary progressive diseases. Each type of muscular dystrophy has unique phenotypic and genetic features (Table 383-1).

DUCHENNE MUSCULAR DYSTROPHY This X-linked recessive disorder, sometimes also called *pseudohypertrophic muscular dystrophy*, has an incidence of ~30 per 100,000 live-born males.

Clinical Features Duchenne dystrophy is present at birth, but the disorder usually becomes apparent between ages 3 and 5. The boys fall frequently and have difficulty keeping up with their friends when playing. Running, jumping, and hopping are invariably abnormal. By age 5, muscle weakness is obvious by muscle testing. On getting up from the floor, the patient uses his hands to climb up himself (Gowers' maneuver). Contractures of the heel cords and iliotibial bands become apparent by age 6, when toe walking is associated with a lordotic posture. Loss of muscle strength is progressive, with predilection for proximal limb muscles and the neck flexors; leg involvement is more severe than arm involvement. Between ages 8 and 10 walking may require the use of braces; joint contractures and limitations of hip flexion, knee, elbow, and wrist extension are made worse by prolonged sitting. By age 12, most patients are wheelchair dependent. Contractures become fixed, and a progressive scoliosis often develops that may be associated with pain. The chest deformity with scoliosis impairs pulmonary function, which is already diminished by muscle weakness. By age 16 to 18, patients are predisposed to serious, sometimes fatal pulmonary infections. Other causes of death include aspiration of food and acute gastric dilation.

A cardiac cause of death is uncommon despite the presence of a cardiomyopathy in almost all patients. Congestive heart failure seldom occurs except with severe stress such as pneumonia. Cardiac arrhythmias are rare. The typical electrocardiogram (ECG) shows an increase net RS in lead V_1; deep, narrow Q waves in the precordial leads; and tall right precordial R waves in V_1. Intellectual impairment in Duchenne dystrophy is common; the average intelligence quotient (IQ) is approximately one standard deviation below the mean. Impairment of intellectual function appears to be nonprogressive and affects verbal ability more than performance.

Laboratory Features Serum creatine kinase (CK) levels are invariably elevated to between 20 and 100 times normal. The levels are abnormal at birth but decline late in the disease because of inactivity and loss of muscle mass. Electromyography (EMG) demonstrates features typical of myopathy. The muscle biopsy shows muscle fibers of varying size as well as small groups of necrotic and regenerating fibers. Connective tissue and fat replace lost muscle fibers. A definitive diagnosis of Duchenne dystrophy can be established on the basis of dystrophin deficiency in a biopsy of muscle tissue or mutation analysis on peripheral blood leukocytes as discussed below.

GENETIC CONSIDERATIONS Duchenne dystrophy is caused by a mutation of the gene that encodes dystrophin, a 427-kDa protein localized to the inner surface of the sarcolemma of the muscle fiber. The dystrophin gene is more than 2000 kb in size and thus is one of the largest identified human genes. It is localized to the short arm of the X chromosome at Xp21. At present, mutations of the gene can be identified (in approximately two-thirds of Duchenne patients) with a battery of cDNA probes. Deletions are not uniformly distributed over the gene, but rather are most common near the beginning (5′ end) and middle of the gene. Deletion size does not correlate with severity of disease. Less often, Duchenne dystrophy is caused by a gene duplication or point mutation. Identification of a specific mutation allows for an unequivocal diagnosis, makes possible accurate testing of potential carriers, and is useful for prenatal diagnosis.

A diagnosis of Duchenne dystrophy can also be made by western

Table 383-1 Progressive Muscular Dystrophies

Type	Inheritance	Defective Gene/Protein	Onset Age (years)	Clinical Features	Other Organ Systems Involved
Duchenne	XR	Dystrophin	Before 5	Progressive weakness of girdle muscles Unable to walk after age 12 Progressive kyphoscoliosis Respiratory failure in 2d or 3d decade	Cardiomyopathy Mental impairment
Becker	XR	Dystrophin	Early childhood to adult	Progressive weakness of girdle muscles Able to walk after age 15 Respiratory failure may develop by 4th decade	Cardiomyopathy
Emery-Dreifuss	XR/AD	Emerin/Lamins A/C	Childhood to adult	Elbow contractures, humeral and peroneal weakness	Cardiomyopathy
Limb-girdle	AD/AR	Several (Table 383-2)	Early childhood to early adult	Slow progressive weakness of shoulder and hip girdle muscles	± Cardiomyopathy
Congenital	AR	Several (Table 383-3)	At birth or within first few months	Hypotonia, contractures, delayed milestones Progression to respiratory failure in some; static course in others	CNS abnormalities (hypomyelination, malformation) Eye abnormalities
Myotonic	AD	Expanded non-coding CTG repeat	Usually 2d decade May be infancy if mother affected	Slowly progressive weakness of face, shoulder girdle, and foot dorsiflexion	Cardiac conduction defects Mental impairment Cataracts Frontal baldness Gonadal atrophy
Facioscapulohumeral	AD	Deletion, distal 4q	Before age 20	Slowly progressive weakness of face, shoulder girdle, and foot dorsiflexion	Deafness Coats' (eye) disease
Oculopharyngeal	AD	Expansion, poly-A RNA binding protein	5th to 6th decade	Slowly progressive weakness of extraocular, pharyngeal, and limb muscles	—

ABBREVIATIONS: XR, X-linked recessive; AD, autosomal dominant; AR, autosomal recessive.

blot analysis of muscle biopsy specimens, revealing abnormalities on the quantity and molecular weight of dystrophin protein. In addition, immunocytochemical staining of muscle with dystrophin antibodies can be used to demonstrate absence or deficiency of dystrophin localizing to the sarcolemmal membrane. Carriers of the disease may demonstrate a mosaic pattern, but dystrophin analysis of muscle biopsy specimens for carrier detection is not reliable. ■

Pathogenesis Dystrophin is part of a large complex of sarcolemmal proteins and glycoproteins (Fig. 383-1). Dystrophin binds to F-actin at its amino terminus and to β-dystroglycan at the carboxyl terminus. β-Dystroglycan complexes to α-dystroglycan, which binds to laminin in the extracellular matrix (ECM). Laminin has a heterotrimeric molecular structure arranged in the shape of a cross with one heavy chain and two light chains, β1 and γ1. The laminin heavy chain of skeletal muscle is designated laminin α2. Peripheral to laminin in the ECM are collagen proteins IV and VI. Like β-dystroglycan, the transmembrane sarcoglycan proteins also bind to dystrophin; these five proteins (designated α- through ε-sarcoglycan) complex tightly with each other. More recently, other membrane proteins implicated in muscular dystrophy have been found to be loosely affiliated with constituents of the dystrophin complex. These include caveolin-3 and α7 integrin (Fig. 383-1).

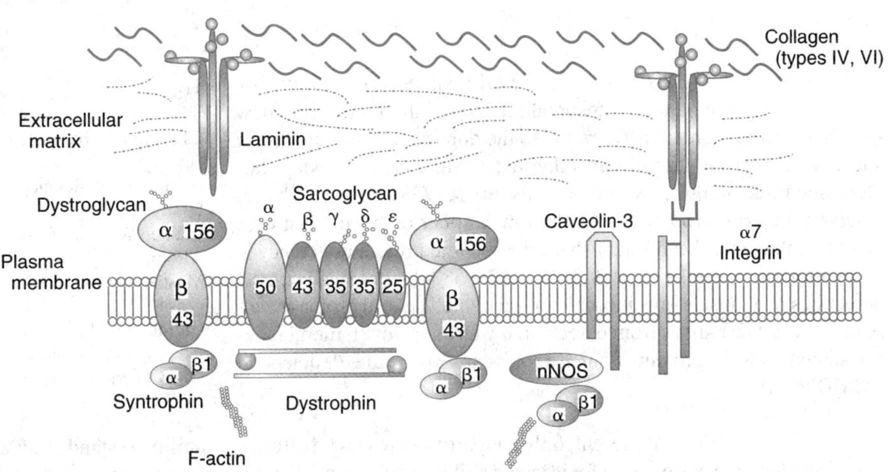

FIGURE 383-1 Dystrophin-associated protein complex. Dystrophin localizes to the cytoplasmic face of the membrane in a subsarcolemmal location. Dystrophin complexes with two transmembrane protein complexes, the dystroglycans and the sarcoglycans. The dystroglycans bind to the extracellular matrix protein laminin. The syntrophin complex and an isoform of nitric oxide synthase (nNOS) are shown in their presumed places in relation to the dystrophin-glycoprotein complex. Also shown are the transmembrane proteins caveolin-3 and α7 integrin that may respectively interact with nNOS and laminin. See text for further explanation.

The dystrophin-glycoprotein complex appears to confer stability to the sarcolemma, although the function of each individual component of the complex is incompletely understood. Deficiency of one member of the complex may cause abnormalities in other components. For example, a primary deficiency of dystrophin (Duchenne dystrophy) may lead to secondary loss of the sarcoglycans and dystroglycan. The primary loss of a single sarcoglycan (see "Limb-Girdle Muscular Dystrophy," below) results in a secondary loss of other sarcoglycans in the membrane without uniformly affecting dystrophin. In either instance, disruption of the dystrophin-glycoprotein complexes weakens the sarcolemma, causing membrane tears and a cascade of events leading to muscle fiber necrosis. This sequence of events occurs repeatedly during the life of a patient with muscular dystrophy.

℞ **TREATMENT** Glucocorticoids, administered as prednisone in a dose of 0.75 mg/kg per day, significantly slow progression of Duchenne dystrophy for up to 3 years. Some patients cannot tolerate glucocorticoid therapy; weight gain in particular represents a significant deterrent for some boys.

BECKER MUSCULAR DYSTROPHY This less severe form of X-linked recessive muscular dystrophy results from allelic defects of the same gene responsible for Duchenne dystrophy. Becker muscular dystrophy is approximately 10 times less frequent than Duchenne, with an incidence of about 3 per 100,000 live-born males.

Clinical Features The pattern of muscle wasting in Becker muscular dystrophy closely resembles that seen in Duchenne. Proximal muscles, especially of the lower extremities, are prominently involved. As the disease progresses, weakness becomes more generalized. Significant facial muscle weakness is not a feature. Hypertrophy of muscles, particularly in the calves, is an early and prominent finding.

Most patients with Becker dystrophy first experience difficulties between ages 5 and 15 years, although onset in the third or fourth decade or even later can occur. By definition, patients with Becker dystrophy walk beyond age 15, while patients with Duchenne dystrophy are typically in a wheelchair by the age of 12. Patients with Becker dystrophy have a reduced life expectancy, but most survive into the fourth or fifth decade.

Mental retardation may occur in Becker dystrophy, but it is not as common as in Duchenne. Cardiac involvement occurs in Becker dystrophy and may result in heart failure.

Laboratory Features Serum CK levels, results of EMG, and muscle biopsy findings closely resemble those in Duchenne dystrophy. The diagnosis of Becker muscular dystrophy requires western blot analysis of muscle biopsy samples demonstrating dystrophin of reduced amount or abnormal size. Mutation analysis of DNA from peripheral blood leukocytes recognizes deletions and duplications of the dystrophin gene in 65% of patients with Becker dystrophy, approximately the same percentage as in Duchenne dystrophy. In both Becker and Duchenne dystrophies, the size of the DNA deletion does not predict clinical severity; however, in ~95% of patients with Becker dystrophy, the DNA deletion does not alter the translational reading frame of messenger RNA. These "in-frame" mutations allow for production of some dystrophin, which accounts for the presence of altered rather than absent dystrophin on western blot analysis.

℞ **TREATMENT** The use of glucocorticoids has not been adequately studied in Becker dystrophy.

LIMB-GIRDLE MUSCULAR DYSTROPHY The syndrome of limb-girdle muscular dystrophy (LGMD) represents more than one disorder.

Clinical Features Muscle weakness affects both males and females, with onset ranging from late in the first decade to the fourth decade. Most LGMDs are progressive and affect primarily the pelvic and shoulder girdle muscles. Respiratory insufficiency from weakness of the diaphragm may occur. The distribution of weakness and rate of progression vary from family to family. Similar to the dystrophinopathies, cardiac involvement may result in congestive heart failure or arrhythmias; occasional patients present with a cardiomyopathy. Intellectual function remains normal.

Laboratory Features An elevated serum CK level, myopathic EMG findings, and muscle biopsy features indicative of myopathy are characteristic. Careful attention is required to exclude phenotypically similar disorders, such as spinal muscular atrophy (Chap. 365), inflammatory myopathies (Chap. 382), and metabolic myopathies (see below). The availability of western blot analysis for dystrophin allows LGMD to be distinguished unequivocally from Becker and Duchenne muscular dystrophies.

GENETIC CONSIDERATIONS LGMD may be transmitted by autosomal dominant or autosomal recessive inheritance. In a new genetic classification, *LGMD1* refers to the dominantly inherited form and *LGMD2* to the recessively inherited form. Genetic linkage has identified three dominantly inherited disorders, LGMD1A–C. The recessively inherited forms of LGMD now number eight. In each case genetic linkage has been established; the specific protein deficiency is known for most forms (Table 383-2 and Fig. 383-1). In LGMD2A the defect lies in a muscle-specific, calcium-activated neutral protease, calpain 3. LGMD2B arises from defects in dysferlin, a novel, membrane-associated muscle protein. Four sarcoglycans (α-δ) are deficient in LGMD2C–F. ■

℞ TREATMENT At present, only supportive care can be offered. Long leg braces are useful for affected children but seldom helpful for adults. Wheelchairs may be essential or may be used to help preserve energy for work or recreational activities. Cardiac or respiratory muscle involvement may require individualized treatment. Studies of primary genetic therapy in LGMD are currently in progress.

EMERY-DREIFUSS MUSCULAR DYSTROPHY This disorder is characterized by childhood onset of contractures at the elbows, weakness in the humeral and peroneal muscles, and cardiomyopathy. The contractures may precede the weakness. As the disease progresses, the weakness may spread to involve the proximal limb-girdle muscles. Perhaps the most critical clinical aspect of Emery-Dreifuss muscular dystrophy (EDMD) is the cardiomyopathy, which may appear as conduction defects of abrupt onset. Sudden death is not uncommon in EDMD, even in otherwise unaffected female carriers; early use of pacemakers may be lifesaving.

Most cases of EDMD are X-linked, arising because of defects in a gene encoding emerin, a nuclear membrane protein. Another group is inherited as autosomal dominant traits. In these instances the molecular defects are in the gene located on chromosome 1, encoding the proteins lamin A and lamin C. These proteins are splice variants that localize to the nuclear envelope where, in some cells, they co-localize with emerin.

CONGENITAL MUSCULAR DYSTROPHY This rare autosomal recessive disorder includes at least six subgroups with overlapping clinical features. Variable involvement of the brain and eyes can help differentiate these conditions; three have been mapped to specific chromosomes, with a specific defect identified in each (Table 383-3). All the forms of congenital muscular dystrophy present at birth or in the first few months of life with hypotonia and proximal limb weakness. Varying degrees of joint contractures at the elbows, hips, knees, and ankles are seen in most patients. Contractures present at birth are referred to as *arthrogryposis*. Weakness of facial muscles may occur, but other cranial nerve musculature is spared. Severity varies greatly, but about half of affected individuals never achieve the ability to stand independently. Death may ensue because of respiratory insufficiency early in life. Some patients learn to walk, although difficulty in motor activities (e.g., running) persists.

Table 383-2 Limb-Girdle Muscular Dystrophies

Disease	Chromosomal Location	Defective Gene/Protein	Protein Size (kDa)
Autosomal Dominant			
LGMD1A	5q	Unknown	Unknown
LGMD1B	1q11–21	Lamins A and C	70
LGMD1C	3p25	Caveolin-3	24
Autosomal Recessive			
LGMD2A	15q15	Calpain-3	95
LGMD2B	2p13	Dysferlin	200
LGMD2C	13q12	γ-Sarcoglycan	35
LGMD2D	17q21	α-Sarcoglycan	50
LGMD2E	4q12	β-Sarcoglycan	43
LGMD2F	5q33	δ-Sarcoglycan	35
LGMD2G	17q11–12	Telethonin	19
LGMD2H	9q31–33	Unknown	Unknown

Table 383-3 Congenital Muscular Dystrophies

Type	Inheritance	Chromosome	Defective Gene/Protein
Laminin α2 chain deficiency	AR	6q22–23	Laminin α2 chain
α7 integrin deficiency	AR	12q13	α7 integrin
Fukuyama CMD	AR	9q31–33	Fukutin
Walker-Warburg syndrome	AR	Unknown	Unknown
Muscle-eye-brain disease	AR	Unknown	Unknown
Unlinked CMD	AR	Unknown	Unknown

ABBREVIATIONS: AR, autosomal recessive; CMD, congenital muscular dystrophy.

In patients with a deficiency of laminin α2 (formerly called merosin), diffuse white matter changes typical of hypomyelination are seen by magnetic resonance imaging. The clinical manifestations of the cerebral hypomyelination are mild, with learning disability as the most severe problem. In *Fukuyama congenital muscular dystrophy*, found mainly in Japan, patients are severely disabled and mentally retarded; most have seizures and die by age 20. Microcephaly and enlarged ventricles occur. Micropolygyria is common. The primary defect in this dystrophy is in the gene encoding fukutin, a secreted protein whose function remains ill-defined. In some patients, the fukutin gene is disrupted by insertion of a transposon, a novel pathogenetic mechanism. Recently, it has been reported that a form of congenital muscular dystrophy arises from the absence of α7 integrin, a muscle membrane protein.

MYOTONIC DYSTROPHY This disorder, the most common adult muscular dystrophy, has an incidence of 13.5 per 100,000 live births and affects males and females equally.

Clinical Features The clinical expression of myotonic dystrophy varies widely and involves many systems other than muscle. Affected patients have a typical "hatchet-faced" appearance due to temporalis, masseter, and facial muscle atrophy and weakness. Neck muscles, including flexors and sternocleidomastoids, and distal limb muscles are involved early. Weakness of wrist extensors, finger extensors, and intrinsic hand muscles impairs function. Ankle dorsiflexor weakness may cause footdrop. Proximal muscles remain stronger throughout the course, although preferential atrophy and weakness of quadriceps muscles occur in many patients. Palatal, pharyngeal, and tongue involvement produce a dysarthric speech, nasal voice, and swallowing problems. Some patients have diaphragm and intercostal muscle weakness, resulting in respiratory insufficiency.

Myotonia, which usually appears by age 5, is demonstrable by percussion of the thenar eminence, the tongue, and wrist extensor muscles. Myotonia causes a slow relaxation of hand grip after a forced voluntary closure. Advanced muscle wasting makes myotonia more difficult to detect.

Congenital myotonic dystrophy is a more severe form of the disease and occurs in ~25% of infants of affected mothers. It is characterized by severe facial and bulbar weakness and transient neonatal respiratory insufficiency.

Cardiac disturbances occur in most patients with myotonic dystrophy. ECG abnormalities are common, including first-degree heart block and more extensive conduction system involvement. Complete heart block and sudden death can occur. Congestive heart failure occurs infrequently but may result from cor pulmonale secondary to respiratory failure. Mitral valve prolapse also occurs commonly.

Other features associated with myotonic dystrophy include intellectual impairment, hypersomnia, posterior subcapsular cataracts, frontal baldness, gonadal atrophy, insulin resistance, and decreased esophageal and colonic motility.

Laboratory Features The diagnosis of myotonic dystrophy can usually be made on the basis of clinical findings. Serum CK levels may be normal or mildly elevated. EMG evidence of myotonia is present in most cases. Muscle biopsy shows muscle atrophy, which selectively involves type 1 fibers in 50% of cases. Typically, increased numbers of central nuclei can be seen. Necrosis of muscle fibers and increased connective tissue, common in other muscular dystrophies, do not usually occur in myotonic dystrophy.

GENETIC CONSIDERATIONS Myotonic dystrophy is an autosomal dominant disorder. New mutations do not appear to contribute to the pool of affected individuals. The disorder is transmitted by an intronic mutation consisting of an unstable expansion of a CTG trinucleotide repeat sequence at 19q13.3. An increase in the severity of the disease phenotype in successive generations (genetic anticipation) is accompanied by an increase in the number of trinucleotide repeats. A similar type of mutation has been identified in fragile X syndrome (Chap. 359). The unstable triplet repeat in myotonic dystrophy can be used for prenatal diagnosis. Congenital disease occurs almost exclusively in infants born to affected mothers; it is possible that sperm with greatly expanded triplet repeats do not function well.

How the CTG expansions impair function of muscle and other cells is not understood. They may alter expression of an adjacent protein kinase gene or of other neighboring genes. Alternatively, the expanded CTG might act as a sink that binds and inactivates important RNA binding proteins.

A subset of patients with multisystemic disease features similar to myotonic dystrophy do not have the diagnostic CTG expansion. Their weakness tends to be proximal rather than distal. This condition, termed proximal myotonic myopathy (PROMM), is genetically distinct from myotonic dystrophy. ■

Rx TREATMENT The myotonia in myotonic dystrophy rarely warrants treatment. Phenytoin is the preferred agent for the occasional patient who requires an antimyotonia drug; other agents, particularly quinine and procainamide, may worsen cardiac conduction. Cardiac pacemaker insertion should be considered for patients with unexplained syncope or advanced conduction system abnormalities with evidence of second-degree heart block, or trifascicular conduction disturbances with marked prolongation of the PR interval. Molded ankle-foot orthoses help prevent footdrop in patients with distal lower extremity weakness.

FACIOSCAPULOHUMERAL MUSCULAR DYSTROPHY This form of muscular dystrophy has an incidence of approximately 1 in 20,000. It is distinct from a similar disorder known as scapuloperoneal dystrophy.

Clinical Features The condition typically has an onset in childhood and young adulthood. In most cases, facial weakness is the initial manifestation, appearing as an inability to smile, whistle, or fully close the eyes. Weakness of the shoulder girdles, rather than the facial muscles, usually brings the patient to medical attention. Loss of scapular stabilizer muscles makes arm elevation difficult. Scapular winging becomes apparent with attempts at abduction and forward movement of the arms. Biceps and triceps muscles may be severely affected, with relative sparing of the deltoid muscles. Weakness is invariably worse for wrist extension than for wrist flexion, and weakness of the anterior compartment muscles of the legs may lead to footdrop.

In most patients, the weakness remains restricted to facial, upper extremity, and distal lower extremity muscles. In 20% of patients, weakness progresses to involve the pelvic girdle muscles, and severe functional impairment and possible wheelchair dependency result.

Characteristically, patients with facioscapulohumeral (FSH) dystrophy do not have involvement of other organ systems, although labile hypertension is common, and there is an increased incidence of nerve deafness. Coats' disease, a disorder consisting of telangiectasia, exudation, and retinal detachment, also occurs.

Laboratory Features The serum CK level may be normal or mildly elevated. EMG usually indicates a myopathic pattern. The muscle biopsy shows nonspecific features of a myopathy. A prominent inflammatory infiltrate, which is often multifocal in distribution, is present in some biopsy samples. The cause or significance of this finding is unknown.

GENETIC CONSIDERATIONS An autosomal dominant inheritance pattern with almost complete penetrance has been established, but each family member should be examined for the presence of the disease, since ~30% of those affected are unaware of involvement. FSH dystrophy is caused by deletions of telomeric heterochromatin at chromosome 4q35. There is a significant correlation between disease severity and the size of the 4q35-associated deletion. Although a specific FSH gene and protein have not been identified, carrier detection and prenatal diagnosis are possible. Most sporadic cases represent new mutations. Genetic heterogeneity has been documented for FSH dystrophy; in occasional families, the disease is linked to chromosome 10. ■

Rx TREATMENT No specific treatment is available; ankle-foot orthoses are helpful for patients with footdrop. Scapular stabilization procedures improve scapular winging but may not improve function.

OCULOPHARYNGEAL DYSTROPHY This form of muscular dystrophy represents one of several disorders characterized by *progressive external ophthalmoplegia*, which consists of slowly progressive ptosis and limitation of eye movements with sparing of pupillary reactions for light and accommodation. Patients usually do not complain of diplopia, in contrast to patients having conditions with a more acute onset of ocular muscle weakness (e.g., myasthenia gravis).

Clinical Features Oculopharyngeal muscular dystrophy has a late onset; it usually presents with ptosis and/or dysphagia in the fourth to sixth decade. The extraocular muscle impairment is less prominent in the early phase but may be severe later. The swallowing problem may become debilitating and result in pooling of secretions and repeated episodes of aspiration. Mild weakness of the neck and extremities also occurs.

Laboratory Features The serum CK level may be two to three times normal. Myopathic EMG findings are typical. On biopsy, muscle fibers are found to contain vacuoles, which by electron microscopy are shown to contain membranous whorls, accumulation of glycogen, and other nonspecific debris related to lysosomes. A distinct feature of oculopharyngeal dystrophy is the presence of tubular filaments, 8.5 nm in diameter, in muscle cell nuclei.

GENETIC CONSIDERATIONS Oculopharyngeal dystrophy has an autosomal dominant inheritance pattern with complete penetrance. The incidence is high in French-Canadians and in Spanish-American families of the southwestern United States. Large kindreds of Italian and of eastern European Jewish descent have been reported. The molecular defect in oculopharyngeal muscular dystrophy is a subtle expansion of a modest polyanine repeat tract in a poly-RNA binding protein (PABP2) in muscle; this disorder maps to chromosome 14q. ■

Rx TREATMENT Dysphagia can cause inanition, making oculopharyngeal muscular dystrophy a potentially life-threatening disease. Cricopharyngeal myotomy may improve swallowing, although it does not prevent aspiration. Eyelid crutches can improve vision in patients in whom ptosis obstructs vision; candidates for ptosis surgery must be carefully selected—those with severe facial weakness are not suitable.

DISTAL MYOPATHIES Patients with predominantly distal weakness usually have a disease of peripheral nerve or anterior horn cells rather than of muscle. There is, however, a heterogeneous group of uncommon disorders of this type with histopathologic and electrophysiologic evidence of myopathy. These distal myopathies can be separated into two types with onset in late adulthood and two types with onset in early adulthood.

The most common late adult–onset form, described by Welander, is inherited as an autosomal dominant condition with onset in the fifth decade. Weakness begins in the hands, and distal anterior-compartment leg muscle involvement occurs later in the course. The serum CK level is either normal or mildly increased. Muscle biopsy shows vacuolated muscle fibers. This disorder genetically maps to chromosome 2p13.

Another late adult–onset form of distal myopathy, also inherited as an autosomal dominant trait, was first recognized in non-Scandinavian patients and also occurs in Finland. Weakness begins in the anterior compartment of the distal lower extremities. The serum CK level is normal or mildly elevated. Muscle fibers often have vacuoles. This disease, sometimes designated "Udd myopathy," maps to the locus for the skeletal muscle protein titin on chromosome 2q31–33.

Both of the distal myopathies with onset in early adulthood have autosomal recessive inheritance. In one type, the weakness usually begins in the anterior compartment of the distal lower extremities, although in some cases it begins in the hands. The serum CK level is moderately elevated (<10 times normal), and muscle biopsies reveal a myopathy with many fibers showing vacuoles. Many of these cases are genetically linked to the centromere on chromosome 9. The other form of early adult–onset distal myopathy (Miyoshi myopathy) is distinguished by weakness beginning in the posterior compartment, i.e., the gastrocnemius muscle. The serum CK level is markedly elevated (>10-fold), and biopsy shows a myopathy without vacuolated fibers. Like LGMB2B, Miyoshi myopathy is caused by defects in the gene encoding the protein dysferlin on chromosome 2p13.

CONGENITAL MYOPATHIES

These rare disorders are distinguished from muscular dystrophies by the presence of specific histochemical and structural abnormalities in muscle. Three major types are described: *central core disease*, *nemaline (rod) myopathy*, and *centronuclear (myotubular) myopathy*. Other rare types, such as multicore disease, fingerprint body myopathy, and sarcotubular myopathy, are not discussed here.

CENTRAL CORE DISEASE Patients with central core disease may have decreased fetal movements and breech presentation. Hypotonia and delay in motor milestones, particularly in walking, are common. Later in childhood, patients develop problems with stair climbing, running, and getting up from the floor. On examination, there is mild facial, neck-flexor, and proximal-extremity muscle weakness. Legs are more affected than arms. Skeletal abnormalities include congenital hip dislocation, scoliosis, and pes cavus; clubbed feet also occur. Most cases are nonprogressive, but exceptions are well documented.

The serum CK level is usually normal. Needle EMG demonstrates a myopathic pattern. Muscle biopsy shows fibers with single or multiple central or eccentric discrete zones (cores) devoid of oxidative enzymes. Cores occur preferentially in type 1 fibers and represent poorly aligned sarcomeres associated with Z disk streaming.

GENETIC CONSIDERATIONS Autosomal dominant inheritance is characteristic; sporadic cases also occur. The disease is caused by point mutations of the ryanodine receptor gene on chromosome 19q, encoding the calcium-release channel of the sarcoplasmic reticulum of skeletal muscle; mutations of this gene also account for some cases of inherited malignant hyperthermia (Chap. 17).

Specific treatment is not required, but establishing a diagnosis of central core disease is extremely important, because these patients have a known predisposition to malignant hyperthermia during anesthesia. ■

NEMALINE MYOPATHY The term *nemaline* refers to the distinctive presence in muscle fibers of rods or threadlike structures (Greek *nema*, "thread"). Nemaline myopathy is clinically heterogeneous. A severe neonatal form presents with hypotonia and feeding difficulties leading to early death. Most commonly, nemaline myopathy presents in infancy or childhood with delayed motor milestones. The course is nonprogressive or slowly progressive. The physical appearance may be striking because of the long, narrow facies, high-arched palate, and open-mouthed appearance due to a prognathous jaw. Other skeletal abnormalities include pectus excavatum, kyphoscoliosis, pes cavus, and clubfoot deformities. Facial and generalized muscle weakness are common. These two early childhood forms of nemaline myopathy are referred to as *congenital nemaline myopathy*, in contrast to an adult-onset disorder with progressive proximal weakness. Myocardial involvement is occasionally present in both the congenital and adult-onset forms of the disease.

The serum CK level is usually normal or slightly elevated. The EMG in weak muscles demonstrates a myopathic pattern with occasional fibrillation potentials. Muscle biopsy demonstrates clusters of small rods (nemaline bodies), which occur preferentially, but not exclusively, in type 1 muscle fibers. The muscle often shows type 1 muscle fiber predominance. Rods originate from the Z disk material of the muscle fiber. In the severe neonatal variant, rods are commonly observed in the nucleus of muscle fibers.

GENETIC CONSIDERATIONS Nemaline myopathy shows at least two patterns of inheritance: autosomal recessive and autosomal dominant with incomplete penetrance. Sporadic cases also occur. Nemaline myopathy is associated with mutations of three genes: TPM3 (α-tropomyosin slow) in both dominant and recessive forms, NEB (encoding nebulin) in the slowly progressive autosomal dominant variant, and ACTA1 (α-actin) in the severe neonatal form. ■

CENTRONUCLEAR MYOPATHY Three distinct variants of centronuclear myopathy occur. A *neonatal form*, also known as myotubular myopathy, presents with severe hypotonia and weakness at birth. The *late infancy–early childhood form* presents with delayed motor milestones. Later, difficulty with running and stair climbing becomes apparent. A marfanoid, slender body habitus, long narrow face, and high-arched palate are typical. Scoliosis and clubbed feet may be present. Most patients exhibit progressive weakness, some requiring wheelchairs. Progressive external ophthalmoplegia with ptosis and varying degrees of extraocular muscle impairment are characteristic of both the neonatal and the late-infantile forms. A third variant, the *late childhood-adult form*, has an onset in the second or third decade. Patients have full extraocular muscle movements and rarely exhibit ptosis. There is mild, nonprogressive limb weakness and no associated skeletal abnormalities.

Normal or slightly elevated CK levels occur in each of the forms. EMG studies often give distinctive results, showing positive sharp waves and fibrillation potentials, complex and repetitive discharges, and rarely myotonic discharges. Muscle biopsy specimens in longitudinal section demonstrate rows of central nuclei, often surrounded by a halo. In transverse sections, central nuclei are found in 25 to 80% of muscle fibers.

GENETIC CONSIDERATIONS A gene for the neonatal form of centronuclear myopathy has been localized to Xq28; this gene encodes myotubularin, a protein tyrosine phosphatase. Missense, frameshift and splice-site mutations predict loss of myotubularin function in affected individuals. Carrier identification and prenatal diagnosis are possible. The inheritance pattern for the late infancy–early childhood disorder is probably autosomal recessive, and for the late childhood–adult form is probably autosomal dominant. ■

DISORDERS OF MUSCLE ENERGY METABOLISM

There are two principal sources of energy for skeletal muscle—fatty acids and glucose. Abnormalities in either glucose or lipid utilization can be associated with distinct clinical presentations that can range from an acute, painful syndrome with rhabdomyolysis and myoglobinuria to a chronic, progressive muscle weakness simulating muscular dystrophy.

GLYCOGEN STORAGE AND GLYCOLYTIC DEFECTS These disorders can be divided into those that can cause exercise intolerance, particularly intermittent muscle pain and myoglobinuria, and those in which fixed muscle weakness is the predominant clinical feature. The latter can mimic LGMD or inflammatory myopathies.

Disorders of Glycogen Storage Causing Fixed Muscle Weakness Three clinical forms of acid maltase deficiency (*type II glycogenosis*) can be distinguished, all of which have autosomal recessive inheritance. The gene for acid maltase is found on the long arm of chromosome 17. The *infantile form* is the most common, with onset of symptoms in the first 3 months of life. Infants develop severe muscle weakness, cardiomegaly, hepatomegaly, and respiratory insufficiency. Glycogen accumulation in motor neurons of the spinal cord and brainstem contributes to muscle weakness. Death usually occurs by 1 year of age. In the *childhood form*, the picture resembles muscular dystrophy. Delayed motor milestones result from proximal limb muscle weakness and involvement of respiratory muscles. The heart may be involved, but the liver and brain are unaffected. The *adult form* begins in the third or fourth decade. Respiratory failure and diaphragmatic weakness are often initial manifestations heralding progressive proximal muscle weakness. The heart and liver are not involved.

In all forms of acid maltase deficiency, the serum CK level is 2 to 10 times normal. EMG examination demonstrates a myopathic pattern, but other features are especially distinctive, including myotonic discharges, trains of fibrillation and positive waves, and complex repetitive discharges. EMG discharges are very prominent in the lumbosacral paraspinal muscles. The muscle biopsy shows vacuoles containing glycogen and the lysosomal enzyme acid phosphatase. Electron microscopy reveals membrane-bound and free tissue glycogen. Definitive diagnosis is established by enzyme determination in muscle.

No satisfactory treatment exists for acid maltase deficiency. A high-protein diet has been advocated, but efficacy has not been documented. Intravenous enzyme replacement has not shown benefit.

In *debranching enzyme deficiency (type III glycogenosis)*, a slowly progressive form of muscle weakness can develop after puberty. Rarely, myoglobinuria may be seen. Patients are usually diagnosed in infancy, however, because of hypotonia and delayed motor milestones, hepatomegaly, growth retardation, and hypoglycemia. *Branching enzyme deficiency (type IV glycogenosis)* is a rare and fatal glycogen storage disease characterized by failure to thrive and hepatomegaly. Hypotonia and muscle wasting may be present, but the skeletal muscle manifestations are minor compared to liver failure.

Disorders of Glycolysis Causing Exercise Intolerance Five glycolytic defects are associated with recurrent myoglobinuria: *myophosphorylase deficiency (type V glycogenosis)*, *phosphofructokinase deficiency (type VII glycogenosis)*, *phosphoglycerate kinase deficiency (type IX glycogenosis)*, *phosphoglycerate mutase deficiency (type X glycogenosis)*, and *lactate dehydrogenase deficiency (glycogensosis type XI)*. Myophosphorylase deficiency, also known as McArdle's disease, is by far the most common of the glycolytic defects associated with exercise intolerance. All are inherited as autosomal recessive traits, except for phosphoglycerate kinase deficiency, which is X-linked recessive. These five glycolytic defects result in a common failure to support energy production at the initiation of exercise, although the exact site of energy failure remains controversial.

Clinical muscle manifestations in these five conditions usually begin in adolescence. Symptoms are precipitated by brief bursts of high-intensity exercise, such as running or lifting heavy objects. A history of myalgia and muscle stiffness usually precedes the intensely painful muscle contractures, which may be followed by myoglobinuria. Acute renal failure accompanies significant pigmenturia. Exercise tolerance can be enhanced by a slow induction phase (warm-up) or brief periods of rest, allowing for the start of the "second-wind" phenomenon (switching to utilization of fatty acids).

Certain features help distinguish some enzyme defects. Varying degrees of hemolytic anemia accompany deficiencies of both phosphofructokinase (mild) and phosphoglycerate kinase (severe). In phosphoglycerate kinase deficiency, the usual clinical presentation is a seizure disorder associated with mental retardation; exercise intolerance is an infrequent manifestation.

In all of these conditions, the serum CK levels fluctuate widely and may be elevated even during symptom-free periods. CK levels >100 times normal are expected, accompanying myoglobinuria. All patients with suspected glycolytic defects leading to exercise intolerance should undergo a forearm exercise test (Chap. 381). An impaired rise in venous lactate is highly indicative of a glycolytic defect. In lactate dehydrogenase deficiency, venous levels of lactate do not increase, but pyruvate rises to normal, after forearm exercise. In all glycolytic defects, a definitive diagnosis is made by muscle biopsy.

Training may enhance the second-wind phenomenon, but attempts to raise blood glucose or to modify these disorders through diet have not proved beneficial.

DISORDERS OF LIPID METABOLISM

Lipid is an important muscle energy source during rest and during prolonged, submaximal exercise. Fatty acids are derived from circulating very low–density lipoprotein (VLDL) in the blood or from triglycerides stored in muscle fibers. Oxidation of fatty acids occurs in the mitochondria. To enter the mitochondria, a fatty acid must first be converted to an "activated fatty acid," acyl-CoA. The acyl-CoA must be linked with carnitine by the enzyme carnitine palmitoyltransferase (CPT) I for transport into the mitochondria. CPT I is present on the inner side of the outer mitochondrial membrane. Carnitine is removed by CPT II, an enzyme attached to the inside of the inner mitochondrial membrane, allowing transport of acyl-CoA into the mitochondrial matrix for β-oxidation.

CARNITINE DEFICIENCY Deficiency of this important substrate results in a myopathic and a systemic disorder.

Myopathic carnitine deficiency is associated with generalized muscle weakness, usually beginning in childhood. The clinical features overlap with those of muscular dystrophy and polymyositis. Patients develop progressive, painless proximal weakness. A severe cardiomyopathy may be present. Serum CK levels may be mildly to markedly (>10-fold) elevated. The muscle biopsy shows striking lipid accumulation. The serum carnitine level is normal. The cause for decreased muscle carnitine is not understood. Most cases are sporadic, but the inheritance pattern is thought to be autosomal recessive. Some patients respond to oral carnitine supplementation; this treatment should be tried in all cases. Other patients have responded to prednisone, riboflavin, or propranolol. A diet substituting medium-chain for long-chain triglycerides has been helpful for some patients.

Systemic carnitine deficiency usually presents in infancy and early childhood and is characterized by progressive weakness and episodes of hepatic encephalopathy with nausea, vomiting, confusion, coma, and early death. Carnitine levels are reduced in muscle, liver, kidney, and heart; but the low serum carnitine levels are especially useful in distinguishing this condition from the myopathic form. No single cause has been identified to explain the low serum carnitine levels. Decreased hepatic synthesis explains some cases, while increased urinary excretion occurs in others. Serum CK levels may be slightly elevated. The muscle biopsy may show lipid storage. In some cases, the liver, heart, and kidney show increased lipid. Treatment with oral carnitine supplementation or glucocorticoids has helped some, but not all, patients.

Secondary carnitine deficiency accompanies a variety of disorders in which carnitine deficiency is caused by decreased synthesis (cirrhosis), insufficient intake (parenteral nutrition), or excessive loss (renal dialysis, Fanconi's syndrome, or organic acidemia). Carnitine deficiency may also be seen in the muscular dystrophies, where it is thought to be a nonspecific result of loss of muscle tissue. Oral carnitine supplementation has not been shown to clearly benefit patients with these secondary syndromes.

CARNITINE PALMITOYLTRANSFERASE DEFICIENCY CPT II deficiency is the most common recognizable cause of recurrent myoglobinuria, more common than the glycolytic defects.

Clinical Features Onset is usually in the teenage years or early twenties. Muscle pain and myoglobinuria occur after prolonged exercise. Fasting predisposes to the development of symptoms. In contrast to disorders caused by defects in glycolysis, in which muscle cramps follow short, intense bursts of exercise, the muscle pain in CPT II deficiency does not occur until the limits of utilization have been exceeded and muscle breakdown has already begun. Episodes of rhabdomyolysis may produce severe weakness. In contrast to carnitine deficiency, strength is normal between attacks.

Laboratory Findings Serum CK levels and EMG findings are both usually normal between episodes. A normal rise of venous lactate during forearm exercise distinguishes this condition from glycolytic defects, especially myophosphorylase deficiency. Muscle biopsy does not show lipid accumulation and is usually normal between attacks. The diagnosis requires direct measurement of muscle CPT.

GENETIC CONSIDERATIONS CPT II deficiency is much more common in men than women (5:1); nevertheless, all evidence indicates autosomal recessive inheritance. A mutation in the gene for CPT II causes the disease in some individuals. ■

℞ TREATMENT It has been suggested that frequent meals and a low-fat, high-carbohydrate diet can prolong exercise tolerance. Others suggest substituting medium-chain triglycerides in the diet. Neither approach has proven beneficial.

MYOADENYLATE DEAMINASE DEFICIENCY The muscle enzyme myoadenylate deaminase converts adenosine 5′-monophosphate (5′-AMP) to inosine monophosphate (IMP) with liberation of ammonia. Myoadenylate deaminase may play a role in regulating adenosine triphosphate (ATP) levels in muscles. Most individuals with myoadenylate deaminase deficiency have no symptoms. Many questions have been raised about the clinical effects of myoadenylate deaminase deficiency, and, specifically, its relationship to exertional myalgia and fatigability; but there is no consensus. There have been a few reports of patients with this disorder who have exercise-exacerbated myalgia and myoglobinuria. The full clinical significance of myoadenylate deaminase deficiency has not been established.

MITOCHONDRIAL MYOPATHIES

In 1972, Olson and colleagues recognized that muscle fibers with significant numbers of abnormal mitochondria could be highlighted with the modified trichrome stain; the term "ragged red fibers" was coined. By electron microscopy, the mitochondria in ragged red fibers are enlarged and often bizarrely shaped and have crystalline inclusions. Since that seminal observation, the understanding of these disorders of muscle and other tissues has expanded (Chap. 67).

Mitochondria play a key role in energy production. Oxidation of the major nutrients derived from carbohydrate, fat, and protein leads to the generation of reducing equivalents. The latter are transported through the respiratory chain in the process known as oxidative phosphorylation. The energy generated by the oxidation-reduction reactions of the respiratory chain is stored in an electrochemical gradient coupled to ATP synthesis.

A novel feature of mitochondria is their genetic composition. Each mitochondrion possesses a DNA genome that is distinct from that of the nuclear DNA. Human mitochondrial DNA (mtDNA) consists of a double-stranded, circular molecule comprising 16,569 base pairs. It codes for 22 transfer RNAs, 2 ribosomal RNAs, and 13 polypeptides of the respiratory chain enzymes. The genetics of mitochondrial diseases differ from the genetics of chromosomal disorders. The DNA of mitochondria is directly inherited from the cytoplasm of the gametes, mainly from the oocyte. The sperm contributes very little of its mitochondria to the offspring at the time of fertilization. Thus, mitochondrial genes are derived almost exclusively from the mother, accounting for maternal inheritance of some mitochondrial disorders.

mtDNA DISORDERS OF MUSCLE Many different classifications of mitochondrial myopathies are possible. A convenient scheme allows for disorders to be grouped by the type of mtDNA mutation: deletions or point mutations.

Disorders Associated with mtDNA Deletions The *Kearns-Sayre syndrome* (KSS) is a sporadic, noninherited disorder with onset before age 20. The characteristic findings include a triad of clinical features: progressive external ophthalmoplegia, pigmentary degeneration of the retina, and heart block. Some patients have only extraocular manifestations. Patients with KSS may also have short stature, ataxia, dementia, sensorineural hearing loss, diabetes, and hypothyroidism. Cerebrospinal fluid (CSF) lactate and pyruvate levels are elevated. The course is progressively downhill, and most patients die in their third or fourth decade. In KSS, two populations of mtDNA, wild type and mutant, are present in the same cell; the mutations in the latter consist of single mtDNA deletions. Heteroplasmy can be recognized on Southern blot analysis. The highest percentage of deleted mtDNA can be detected in postmitotic tissues, especially skeletal muscle. Other tissues can harbor the mutation (e.g., peripheral blood leukocytes, brain, liver, and fibroblasts). The absence of mutant mtDNA reflects both mitotic segregation early in embryogenesis and selection against a mutant cell line in a rapidly dividing tissue. KSS is not inherited, since mutations leading to an affected individual take place in the fertilized ovum.

An *autosomal dominant disorder with progressive external ophthalmoplegia and proximal weakness* shares clinical features with KSS: hearing loss, ataxia, peripheral neuropathy, mental retardation, and hypoparathyroidism. Some of these patients also have weakness of respiratory muscles, exercise intolerance, cataracts, and early death. The patients have ragged red fibers on muscle biopsy and multiple mtDNA deletions, rather than single deletions as in KSS. The mutation accounting for the autosomal dominant inheritance occurs in a nuclear gene that encodes a protein involved in the control of mtDNA replication. A failure or disruption of binding of this nuclear-encoded protein during mtDNA replication results in multiple deletions.

Disorders Associated with mtDNA Point Mutations *Myoclonic epilepsy and ragged red fibers*, called the *MERRF syndrome*, consists of mitochondrial myopathy, myoclonus, generalized seizures, intellectual deterioration, ataxia, and hearing loss. Extraocular movements are normal in MERRF. Onset is often in childhood or early adult life. As with other mitochondrial disorders, individuals display varying manifestations of the disease. Serum and CSF lactate and pyruvate levels are increased. The course is progressively downhill, and most patients die with severe encephalopathy. MERRF syndrome is maternally inherited. Most often, point mutations in the lysine transfer RNA gene of mtDNA can be found. This abnormality can be detected in mtDNA isolated from peripheral blood leukocytes or skeletal muscle and is useful for clinical diagnosis and genetic counseling. These mutations alter the normal conformation of the transfer RNA, impairing translation probably at the ribosomal level.

Mitochondrial myopathy, encephalopathy, lactic acidosis, and stroke-like episodes are referred to by the acronym *MELAS*. This disorder is a multisystem mitochondrial encephalomyopathy that begins in childhood after normal birth and early development. Patients have stunted growth and recurrent stroke-like episodes manifesting as hemiparesis, hemianopia, or cortical blindness. Episodic vomiting may occur, and some patients have hearing loss. Focal or generalized seizures

Table 383-5 Clinical Features of Periodic Paralysis and Nondystrophic Myotonias

	Calcium Channel	Sodium Channel			Chloride Channel
Feature	Hypokalemic PP	Hyperkalemic PP	Paramyotonia Congenita	Sodium Channel Myotonia	Congenital Myotonia
Mode of inheritance	AD	AD	AD	AD	AD or AR
Age of onset	Adolescence	Early childhood	Early childhood	Early childhood	Early childhood
Myotonia[a]	No	Yes	Yes	Yes	Yes
Episodic weakness	Yes	Yes	Yes	No	No
Frequency of attacks of weakness	Daily to yearly	May be 2–3/d	With cold, usually rare	Never	Never
Duration of attacks of weakness	2–12 h	From 1–2 h to >1 day	2–24 h	None	None
Serum K^+ level during attacks of weakness	Decreased	Increased or normal	Usually normal	(No attacks)	(No attacks)
Effect of K^+ loading	No change	Increased myotonia, then weakness	Increased myotonia	Increased myotonia	No change
Effect of muscle cooling	No change	Increased myotonia	Increased myotonia, then weakness	Mild increase in myotonia	Increased myotonia
Fixed weakness	Yes	Yes	Yes	No	No

[a] May be paradoxical.
ABBREVIATIONS: AD, autosomal dominant; AR, autosomal recessive; PP, periodic paralysis.

hypokalemia. The molecular defect in the calcium channel can be defined in many patients. Muscle biopsy often shows the presence of single or multiple centrally placed vacuoles. Patients whose attacks are too infrequent for study of a spontaneous attack to be feasible require provocative testing with glucose and insulin administration. Provocative tests are potentially hazardous and require careful monitoring.

HypoKPP is caused by mutations in a voltage-sensitive, skeletal muscular calcium channel, although details of the pathogenesis are incompletely understood (Fig. 383-2).

The acute paralysis improves after the administration of potassium salts. Oral KCl (0.2 to 0.4 mmol/kg) should be given to patients with severe weakness and repeated at 15- to 30-min intervals depending on the response of the ECG, serum potassium level, and muscle strength. Milder attacks usually resolve spontaneously. When patients are unable to swallow or are vomiting, intravenous therapy may be necessary. Small, repeated boluses of KCl (0.1 mmol/kg) may be administered over 5 to 10 min with careful monitoring of the ECG and serum potassium level. If potassium is administered as a dilute solution (20 to 40 mmol/L) in 5% glucose or in physiologic saline solution, the serum potassium level may decline, and weakness may worsen. Mannitol is the preferred vehicle for administered intravenous potassium in such situations, since it facilitates rapid return of the serum potassium level to normal and does not cause the lowering of the serum potassium level that may be caused by glucose or saline solutions.

The goal of therapy is to eliminate attacks, which also prevents interattack weakness. Before effective means of attack prevention became available, chronic progressive interattack weakness frequently caused serious disability. Prophylactic administration of potassium salts, even in large doses, does not prevent attacks, but acetazolamide (125 to 1000 mg/d in divided doses) or dichlorphenamide (50 to 200 mg/d) abolishes attacks in most cases. The metabolic acidosis induced by acetazolamide may underlie the beneficial effect. Paradoxically, acetazolamide lowers the serum potassium level; to achieve an adequate response in some patients, it may be necessary to give supplementary potassium along with acetazolamide and to avoid high-carbohydrate meals. Chronic acetazolamide treatment may be associated with renal calculi, and patients should be monitored for this complication. In occasional patients, attacks may not respond to or may even be worsened by acetazolamide. In such patients, triamterene (25 to 100 mg/d) or spironolactone (25 to 100 mg/d) may prevent attacks.

SODIUM CHANNEL DISORDERS OF MUSCLE **Hyperkalemic Periodic Paralysis** Hyperkalemic periodic paralysis (hyperKPP) causes episodic weakness of limb muscles; cranial and respiratory muscles are rarely involved. The term "hyperkalemic" is misleading, since patients are often normokalemic during attacks. It is the fact that attacks are precipitated by potassium administration that best defines the disorder. Paresthesias and muscle pain are present during many attacks.

Diagnosis is suggested by a modest elevation of the serum potassium level during attacks in nearly half of patients; at times, however, the serum potassium level is normal or even low. The so-called hyperkalemic and normokalemic forms of this disorder are not separate entities. Intravenous glucose-insulin loading does not precipitate weakness, but potassium-loading tests (0.05 to 0.15 g/kg) do induce weakness in such patients. Potassium-loading tests are potentially hazardous and are contraindicated in patients with renal disease and diabetes. Random serum potassium measurements may suggest the diagnosis, since potassium level elevations are frequent during attack-free intervals. EMG evidence of myotonia and the finding of vacuoles on muscle biopsy provide supporting data.

Like hypoKPP, hyperKPP may also respond to chronic administration of acetazolamide or dichlorphenamide.

Paramyotonia Congenita Paramyotonia congenita (PC) causes attacks of paralysis either spontaneously or with cold provocation. PC with periodic paralysis is similar to hyperKPP, except that paradoxical myotonia (i.e., myotonia worsening with activity) and objective cold sensitivity are more prominent in PC.

In PC, attacks of weakness are seldom severe enough to require emergency treatment and are never fatal. Oral administration of glucose or other carbohydrate hastens recovery. Since interattack weakness may develop after repeated attacks, prophylactic treatment is usually indicated in PC. Thiazide diuretics (e.g., chlorothiazide, 250 to 1000 mg/d) are reported to be effective.

Potassium-Aggravated Myotonia Some patients with muscle sodium channel defects have severe muscle stiffness but no paralytic episodes. The stiffness is accentuated by elevations in serum potassium levels. Mutations in the skeletal muscle voltage-gated sodium channel SCN4A cause hyperKPP, PC and potassium-aggravated myotonia (PAM) (Fig. 383-2). In vitro study of these mutations demonstrates increased conductance through the sodium channels, often because of subnormal, slowed inactivation of the channel after action potential firing.

CHLORIDE CHANNEL DISORDERS OF MUSCLE **Myotonia Congenita** In some families, severe, cold-aggravated muscle stiffness with muscle hypertrophy is transmitted as an inherited trait (dominant or recessive). This problem is usually evident in childhood; symptoms may become less severe in the adult years. This problem is caused by mutations in a skeletal muscle chloride channel resulting in impaired membrane repolarization. Myotonia congenita due to chloride channel defects can be distinguished from sodium channel myo-

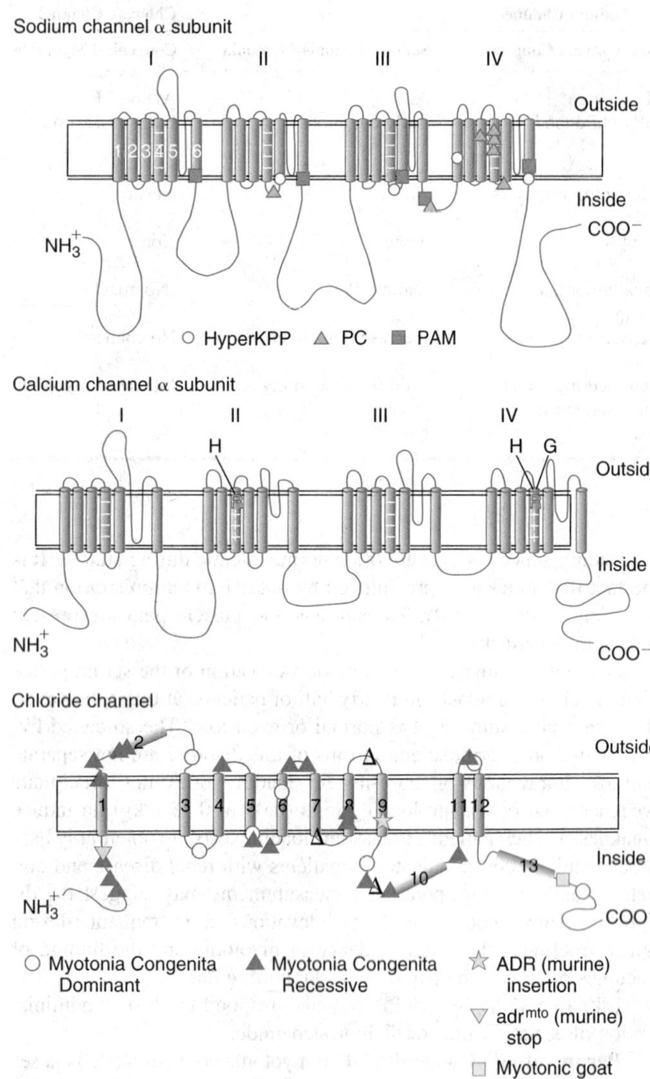

FIGURE 383-2 The sodium and calcium channels are depicted here as containing four homologous domains, each with six membrane-spanning segments. The fourth segment of each domain bears positive charges and acts as the "voltage sensor" for the channel. The association of the four domains is thought to form a pore through which ions pass. Sodium channel mutations are shown along with the phenotype that they confer. HyperKPP, hyperkalemic periodic paralysis; PC, paramyotonia congenita; PAM, potassium-aggravated myotonia. See text for details.

The chloride channel is envisioned to have ten membrane-spanning domains. The positions of mutations causing dominantly and recessively inherited myotonia congenita are indicated, along with mutations that cause this disease in mice and goats.

tonia by the rather striking muscle hypertrophy and by DNA mutational screening.

DISORDERS OF UNKNOWN PATHOGENETIC MECHANISM **Thyrotoxic Periodic Paralysis** This disorder is clinically indistinguishable from hypoKPP. It is common in young Latin American and Asian men, among whom up to 10% of thyrotoxic patients may have this condition. The thyrotoxicosis may be overlooked for many months. Occasionally, the only indication of thyrotoxicosis is a depressed level of thyroid-stimulating hormone. Acute attacks respond to potassium administration. Treatment of the underlying thyrotoxicosis abolishes attacks. β-Adrenergic blocking agents are useful for reducing the frequency and severity of attacks while measures to control thyrotoxicosis are instituted. Acetazolamide is not helpful in preventing attacks. The pathogenesis of thyrotoxic periodic paralysis is uncertain, but there is evidence for a decrease in the activity of the calcium pump.

Andersen's Syndrome In this rare disorder patients manifest periodic paralysis (hyperkalemic or hypokalemic), cardiac dysrhythmias (even when normokalemic), and dysmorphic features (hypertelorism, low set ears, broad nose). Treatment of the episodic weakness is the same as for the other periodic paralyses, although cardiac status must be considered as well.

BIBLIOGRAPHY

ANDERSON LV et al: Dysferlin is a plasma membrane protein and is expressed early in human development. Hum Mol Genet 8:855, 1999

BAROHN RJ: Distal myopathies and dystrophies. Semin Neurol 13:247, 1993

BLAKE DJ, KRÖGER S: The neurobiology of Duchenne muscular dystrophy: Learning lessons from muscle? Trends Neurosci 23:92, 2000

BONNE G et al: Mutations in the gene encoding lamin A/C cause autosomal dominant Emery-Dreifuss muscular dystrophy. Nat Genet 21:285, 1999

CAMPBELL KP: Adhalin gene mutations and autosomal recessive limb-girdle muscular dystrophy. Ann Neurol 38:353, 1995

CANNON SC: Ion-channel defects and aberrant excitability in myotonia and periodic paralysis. Trends Neurosci 19:3, 1996

DIMAURO S et al: Mitochondrial encephalomyopathies, in *The Molecular and Genetic Basis of Neurologic Disease*, RN Rosenberg et al (eds). Boston, Butterworth-Heinemann, 1997

EMERY AEH (ed): *Neuromuscular Disorders: Clinical and Molecular Genetics*. Wiley, Chichester, 1999

GRIGGS RC et al: The muscular dystrophies, in *Evaluation and Treatment of Myopathies*, RC Griggs et al (eds). Philadelphia, FA Davis, 1995

INTERNATIONAL MUSCULAR DYSTROPHY CONSORTIUM (IDMC): The new nomenclature and DNA testing guidelines for myotonic dystrophy type 1 (DM1). Neurology 54:1218, 2000

KISSEL JT et al: Endocrine myopathies, in *Handbook of Clinical Neurology*, vol 19, LP Rowland, S DiMauro (eds). New York, Elsevier, 1992

LIU J et al: Dysferlin, a novel skeletal muscle gene, is mutated in Miyoshi myopathy and limb girdle muscular dystrophy. Nat Genet 20:31, 1998

MINETTI C et al: Mutations in the caveolin-3 gene cause autosomal dominant limb-girdle muscular dystrophy. Nat Genet 18:365, 1998

MOREIRA ES et al: Limb-girdle muscular dystrophy type 2G is caused by mutations in the gene encoding the sarcomeric protein telethonin. Nat Genet 24:163, 2000

TSAO C-Y et al: The childhood muscular dystrophies: Making order out of chaos. Semin Neurol 19:9, 1999

VARDERIO E et al: Carnitine palmitoyltransferase II deficiency: Structure of the gene and characterization of two novel disease-causing mutations. Hum Mol Genet 4:19, 1995

384 CHRONIC FATIGUE SYNDROME

Stephen E. Straus

DEFINITION *Chronic fatigue syndrome* (CFS) is the current name for a disorder characterized by debilitating fatigue and several associated physical, constitutional, and neuropsychological complaints (Table 384-1). This syndrome is not new; in the past, patients diagnosed with conditions such as the vapors, neurasthenia, effort syndrome, hyperventilation syndrome, chronic brucellosis, epidemic neuromyasthenia, myalgic encephalomyelitis, hypoglycemia, multiple chemical sensitivity syndrome, chronic candidiasis, chronic mononucleosis, chronic Epstein-Barr virus infection, and postviral fatigue syndrome may have had what is now called chronic fatigue syndrome. The U.S. Centers for Disease Control and Prevention (CDC) has developed diagnostic criteria for CFS based upon symptoms and the exclusion of other illnesses (Table 384-2).

EPIDEMIOLOGY Patients with CFS are twice as likely to be women as men and are generally 25 to 45 years old, although cases in childhood and in later life have been described.

Cases are recognized in many developed countries. Most arise sporadically, but many clusters have also been reported. The most famous outbreaks of CFS occurred in Los Angeles County Hospital in 1934; in Akureyri, Iceland, in 1948; in the Royal Free Hospital, London, in 1955; in Punta Gorda, Florida, in 1956; and in Incline Village, Nevada, in 1985. While these clustered cases suggest a common environmental or infectious cause, none has been identified.

Estimates of the prevalence of CFS have depended on the case definition used and the method of study. Chronic fatigue itself is a common symptom, occurring in as many as 20% of patients attending general medical clinics; CFS is far less common. Community-based studies find that 100 to 300 individuals per 100,000 population in the United States meet the current CDC case definition.

PATHOGENESIS The diverse names for the syndrome reflect the equally numerous and controversial hypotheses about its etiology. Several common themes underlie attempts to understand the disorder: It is often postinfectious, it is associated with immunologic disturbances, and it is commonly accompanied by neuropsychological complaints and depression.

Table 384-1 Specific Symptoms Reported by Patients with Chronic Fatigue Syndrome

Symptom	Percentage
Fatigue	100
Difficulty concentrating	90
Headache	90
Sore throat	85
Tender lymph nodes	80
Muscle aches	80
Joint aches	75
Feverishness	75
Difficulty sleeping	70
Psychiatric problems	65
Allergies	55
Abdominal cramps	40
Weight loss	20
Rash	10
Rapid pulse	10
Weight gain	5
Chest pain	5
Night sweats	5

SOURCE: From SE Straus: J Infect Diseases 157:405, 1988.

Table 384-2 CDC Criteria for Chronic Fatigue Syndrome

A case of chronic fatigue syndrome is defined by the presence of:

1. Clinically evaluated, unexplained, persistent or relapsing fatigue that is of new or definite onset; is not the result of ongoing exertion; is not alleviated by rest; and results in substantial reduction of previous levels of occupational, educational, social, or personal activities; and
2. Four or more of the following symptoms that persist or recur during six or more consecutive months of illness and that do not predate the fatigue:
   - Self-reported impairment in short-term memory or concentration
   - Sore throat
   - Tender cervical or axillary nodes
   - Muscle pain
   - Multijoint pain without redness or swelling
   - Headaches of a new pattern or severity
   - Unrefreshing sleep
   - Postexertional malaise lasting ≥24 h

SOURCE: Adapted from Fukuda et al.

Many studies in the 1980s and 1990s attempted to link CFS to infection with a persistent virus such as a lymphotropic herpesvirus, retrovirus, or enterovirus. In many patients with chronic fatigue, titers of antibodies to herpesviruses, measles virus, rubella virus, and coxsackievirus B are elevated. Reports that viral antigens and nucleic acids could be specifically identified in patients with CFS have not been confirmed. One study from the United Kingdom failed to detect any association between acute infections and subsequent prolonged fatigue. Another study found that chronic fatigue did not develop after typical upper respiratory infections but did in some individuals after infectious mononucleosis. Thus, while cumulative experience suggests that antecedent viral infections are associated with CFS, a direct viral pathogenesis is unproven.

Changes in immune parameters of uncertain functional significance have been reported in CFS. Modest and nonspecific elevations in titers of antinuclear antibodies, reductions in immunoglobulin subclasses, deficiencies in mitogen-driven lymphocyte proliferation, reductions in natural killer cell activity, disturbances in cytokine production, and shifts in lymphocyte subsets with increases in cells expressing activation markers have been described. None of the immune findings appears in all patients, nor do any correlate with the severity of CFS. None are specific; thus they remain nondiagnostic. In theory, symptoms of CFS could result from excessive production of a cytokine, such as interleukin 1, that induces asthenia and other flulike symptoms; however, conclusive data in support of this long-held hypothesis are lacking.

Disturbances in endocrine function, consistent with reduced production of corticotropin-releasing hormone in the hypothalamus, have been reported in controlled studies of CFS. Mean serum cortisol concentrations were lower in patients than in controls; levels of adrenocorticotropic hormone were correspondingly high. Hypothetically, these neuroendocrine abnormalities could contribute to the impaired energy and depressed mood of patients.

Mild to moderate depression is present in half to two-thirds of patients. Much of this depression may be reactive, but its prevalence exceeds that seen in other chronic medical illnesses. Some propose that CFS is fundamentally a psychiatric disorder and that the various neuroendocrine and immune disturbances arise secondarily.

MANIFESTATIONS Typically, CFS arises suddenly in a previously active individual. An otherwise unremarkable flulike illness or some other acute stress leaves unbearable exhaustion in its wake. Other symptoms, such as headache, sore throat, tender lymph nodes, muscle and joint aches, and frequent feverishness, lead to the belief that an infection persists, and medical attention is sought. Over several weeks, despite reassurances that nothing serious is wrong, the symptoms persist and other features of the syndrome become evident—disturbed sleep, difficulty in concentration, and depression (Table 384-1).

Depending on the dominant symptoms and the beliefs of the patient, additional consultations may be sought from allergists, rheumatologists, infectious disease specialists, psychiatrists, ecologic therapists, homeopaths, or other professionals, frequently with unsatisfactory results. Once the pattern of illness is established, the symptoms may fluctuate somewhat. Many patients report that diverse complaints are linked—that during periods of greatest fatigue they perceive the most pain and difficulty with concentration. Patients also commonly assert that excessive physical or emotional stress may exacerbate their symptoms.

Most patients remain capable of continuing to meet the obligations of family, work, or community despite their symptoms. The discretionary activities are abandoned first. Some feel unable to engage in any gainful employment. A minority of individuals require help with the activities of daily living.

Ultimately, isolation, frustration, and pathetic resignation can mark the protracted course of illness. Patients may become angry at physicians for failing to acknowledge or resolve their plight. Fortunately, CFS does not appear to progress. On the contrary, many patients experience gradual improvement, and a minority recover fully.

DIAGNOSIS Physical examination and routine laboratory tests are required to rule out other causes of the patient's symptoms. Prominent abnormalities argue strongly in favor of alternative diagnoses. No laboratory test, however, can diagnose this condition or measure its severity. In most cases, elaborate, expensive workups are not helpful. Magnetic resonance imaging of the brain may identify small T2 hyperintense signals in a minority of patients, but these findings do not aid diagnosis nor are they prognostic. The dilemma for patient and clinician alike is that CFS has no pathognomonic features and remains a constellation of symptoms and a diagnosis of exclusion. Often the patient presents with features that also meet criteria for other subjective disorders such as fibromyalgia and irritable bowel syndrome.

℞ **TREATMENT** The primary responsibility of a physician confronted with a chronically fatigued patient is to address the cause by taking a thorough history, conducting a complete physical examination, judiciously using the laboratory, and, throughout this process, considering the differential diagnosis. After other illnesses have been excluded, there are several points to address in the long-term care of a patient with chronic fatigue.

The patient should be informed about the illness and what is known of its pathogenesis; its potential impact on the physical, psychological, and social dimensions of life; and its prognosis. Patients are relieved when their complaints are taken seriously. Periodic reassessment is appropriate to identify a possible underlying process that is late in declaring itself and to address intercurrent symptoms that should not be simply dismissed as yet another subjective complaint.

Many symptoms of CFS respond to treatment. Nonsteroidal antiinflammatory drugs alleviate headache, diffuse pain, and feverishness. Allergic rhinitis and sinusitis are common; antihistamines or decongestants may be helpful. Although the patient may be averse to psychiatric diagnoses, depression is often a prominent symptom and, when present, should be treated. Expert psychiatric assessment is sometimes advisable. Nonsedating antidepressants improve mood and disordered sleep and thereby attenuate the fatigue somewhat. Even modest improvements in symptoms can make an important difference in the patient's degree of self-sufficiency and ability to appreciate life's pleasures.

Practical advice should be given regarding lifestyle. Sleep disturbances are common; consumption of heavy meals with alcohol and caffeine at night can make sleep even more elusive, compounding fatigue. Total rest leads to further deconditioning and the self-image of being an invalid, whereas overexertion may worsen exhaustion and lead to total avoidance of exercise. A moderate, carefully graded regimen should be encouraged and has been proven to relieve symptoms and enhance exercise tolerance.

Controlled therapeutic trials have established that acyclovir, intramuscular liver extract–folic acid–cyanocobalamin injections, and intravenous immunoglobulin, among others, are of no value. Two studies showed that low doses of hydrocortisone provide modest benefit, but they may lead to adrenal suppression. Countless anecdotes circulate regarding other traditional and nontraditional therapies. It is important to guide patients away from those therapeutic modalities that are toxic, expensive, or unreasonable.

The physician should promote the patient's efforts toward improvement. Three clinical trials in England showed behavioral therapy to be helpful. This approach aims to dispel misguided beliefs and fears about the illness that can contribute to inactivity and despair. For CFS, as for many other conditions, a comprehensive approach to physical, psychological, and social aspects of well-being is in order.

BIBLIOGRAPHY

Fukuda K et al: The chronic fatigue syndrome: A comprehensive approach to its definition and study. Ann Intern Med 121:953, 1994

Fulcher KY, White PD: Randomised controlled trial of graded exercise in patients with the chronic fatigue syndrome. BMJ 314:1647, 1997

Sharpe MC et al: Cognitive behaviour therapy for the chronic fatigue syndrome: A randomised controlled trial. BMJ 312:22, 1996

Steele L et al: The epidemiology of chronic fatigue in San Francisco. Am J Med 105: 83S, 1998

Straus SE et al: *Chronic Fatigue Syndrome*. New York: Marcel Dekker, 1994

Section 5
PSYCHIATRIC DISORDERS

385 MENTAL DISORDERS

Victor I. Reus

The term "mental disorders," as defined in the 4th edition of the standard psychiatric *Diagnostic and Statistical Manual* (DSM-IV), encompasses a broad range of conditions characterized by patterns of abnormal behavioral and psychological signs and symptoms that result in dysfunction. The implication that mental disorders lack a physical cause is unfortunate and incorrect, and the term survives only for want of a better substitute. Mental disorders are highly prevalent in medical practice and may present either as a primary disorder or as a comorbid condition. The total direct and indirect costs of all mental disorders in the United States has been estimated to be $148 billion dollars, only slightly less than costs incurred by cardiovascular diseases.

The DSM-IV-PC (Primary Care) manual provides a useful synopsis of mental disorders most likely to be seen in primary care practice. The current system of classification is multiaxial and includes the presence or absence of a major mental disorder (axis I), any underlying personality disorder (axis II), general medical condition (axis III), psychosocial and environmental problems (axis IV), and overall rating of general psychosocial functioning (axis V).

Changes in health care delivery underscore the need for primary care physicians to assume responsibility for the initial diagnosis and treatment of the most common mental disorders. Prompt diagnosis is essential to ensure that patients have access to appropriate medical services and to maximize the clinical outcome. Validated patient-based questionnaires have been developed that systematically probe for signs and symptoms associated with the most prevalent psychiatric diagnoses and guide the clinician into a more targeted historic assessment. Prime MD and the Symptom-Driven Diagnostic System for Primary Care (SDDS-PC) are inventories that require only 10 min to complete and link patient responses to the formal diagnostic criteria of anxiety, mood, somatoform, and eating disorders and to alcohol abuse or dependence.

A physician who refers patients to a psychiatrist should know not only when doing so is appropriate but also how to do it, since societal misconceptions and the stigma of mental illness impede the process. Primary care physicians should base referrals to a psychiatrist on the presence of the signs and symptoms of a mental disorder and not simply on the absence of a physical explanation for a patient's complaint. The physician should discuss with the patient the reasons for requesting the referral or consultation and provide reassurance that he or she will continue to provide medical care and work collaboratively with the mental health professional. Consultation with a psychiatrist or transfer of care is appropriate when physicians encounter evidence of psychotic symptoms, mania, severe depression, or anxiety; symptoms of posttraumatic stress disorder (PTSD); suicidal or homicidal preoccupation; or a failure to respond to first-order treatment.→*Eating disorders are discussed in Chap. 78.*

ANXIETY DISORDERS

Anxiety disorders, the most prevalent psychiatric illnesses in the general community, are present in 15 to 20% of medical clinic patients. Anxiety, defined as a subjective sense of unease, dread, or foreboding, can indicate a primary psychiatric condition or can be a component of, or reaction to, a primary medical disease. The primary anxiety disorders are classified according to their duration and course and the existence and nature of precipitants.

When evaluating the anxious patient, the clinician must first determine whether the anxiety antedates or postdates a medical illness or is due to a medication side effect. Approximately one-third of patients presenting with anxiety have a medical etiology for their psychiatric symptoms, but an anxiety disorder can also present with somatic symptoms in the absence of a diagnosable medical condition.

PANIC DISORDER **Clinical Manifestations** Panic disorder is defined by the presence of recurrent and unpredictable panic attacks, which are distinct episodes of intense fear and discomfort associated with a variety of physical symptoms, including palpitations, sweating, trembling, shortness of breath, chest pain, dizziness, and a fear of impending doom or death (Table 385-1). Paresthesias, gastrointestinal distress, and feelings of unreality are also common. Panic attacks have a sudden onset, developing within 10 min and usually resolving over the course of an hour, and they occur in an unexpected fashion. The frequency and severity of panic attacks varies, ranging from once a week to clusters of attacks separated by months of well-being. The first attack is usually outside the home. Onset is usually in late adolescence to early adulthood. In some individuals, anticipatory anxiety develops over time and results in a generalized fear and a progressive avoidance of places or situations in which a panic attack might recur. *Agoraphobia*, which occurs commonly in patients with panic disorder, is an acquired irrational fear of being in places where one might feel trapped or unable to escape (Table 385-2). Typically, it leads the patient into a progressive restriction in life-style and, in a literal sense, in geography. Frequently, patients are embarrassed that they are housebound and dependent on the company of others to go out into the world and do not volunteer this information; thus physicians will fail to recognize the syndrome if direct questioning is not pursued.

Table 385-1 Diagnostic Criteria for Panic Attack

A discrete period of intense fear or discomfort, in which four or more of the following symptoms developed abruptly and reached a peak within 10 min:

1. Palpitations, pounding heart, or accelerated heart rate
2. Sweating
3. Trembling or shaking
4. Sensations of shortness of breath or smothering
5. Feeling of choking
6. Chest pain or discomfort
7. Nausea or abdominal distress
8. Feeling dizzy, unsteady, lightheaded, or faint
9. Derealization (feelings of unreality) or depersonalization (being detached from oneself)
10. Fear of losing control or going crazy
11. Fear of dying
12. Paresthesias (numbness or tingling sensations)
13. Chills or hot flushes

SOURCE: *Diagnostic and Statistical Manual of Mental Disorders*, 4th ed.

Differential Diagnosis A diagnosis of panic disorder is made after a medical etiology for the panic attacks has been ruled out. A variety of cardiovascular, respiratory, endocrine, and neurologic conditions can present with anxiety as the chief complaint. Patients with true panic disorder will often focus on one specific feature to the exclusion of others. For example, 20% of patients who present with syncope as a primary medical complaint have a primary diagnosis of a mood, anxiety, or substance-abuse disorder, the most common being panic disorder. The differential diagnosis of panic disorder is complicated by a high rate of comorbidity with other psychiatric conditions, especially alcohol and benzodiazepine abuse, which patients initially use in an attempt at self-medication. Some 75% of panic disorder patients will also satisfy criteria for major depression at some point in their illness.

When the history is nonspecific, physical examination and focused laboratory testing must be used to rule out medical anxiety states, such as those resulting from pheochromocytoma, thyrotoxicosis, or hypoglycemia. Electrocardiogram (ECG) and echocardiogram may detect some cardiovascular conditions associated with panic, such as paroxysmal atrial tachycardia and mitral valve prolapse. In two studies, panic disorder was the primary diagnosis in 43% of patients with chest pain who had normal coronary angiograms and was present in 9% of all outpatients referred for cardiac evaluation. Panic disorder has also been diagnosed in many patients referred for pulmonary function testing or with symptoms of irritable bowel syndrome.

Etiology and Pathophysiology The etiology of panic disorder is unknown but appears to involve a genetic predisposition, altered

Table 385-2 Diagnostic Criteria for Agoraphobia

1. Anxiety about being in places or situations from which escape might be difficult (or embarrassing) or in which help may not be available in the event of having an unexpected or situationally predisposed panic attack or panic-like symptoms. Agoraphobic fears typically involve characteristic clusters of situations that include being outside the home alone; being in a crowd or standing in a line; being on a bridge; and traveling in a bus, train, or automobile.
2. The situations are avoided (e.g., travel is restricted) or else are endured with marked distress or with anxiety about having a panic attack or panic-like symptoms, or require the presence of a companion.
3. The anxiety or phobic avoidance is not better accounted for by another mental disorder, such as social phobia (e.g., avoidance limited to social situations because of fear of embarrassment), specific phobia (e.g., avoidance limited to a single situation like elevators), obsessive-compulsive disorder (e.g., avoidance of dirt in someone with an obsession about contamination), posttraumatic stress disorder (e.g., avoidance of stimuli associated with a severe stressor), or separation anxiety disorder (e.g., avoidance of leaving home or relatives).

SOURCE: *Diagnostic and Statistical Manual of Mental Disorders*, 4th ed.

Table 385-3 Antidepressants

Name	Usual Daily Dose, mg	Side Effects	Comments
SSRIs			
Fluoxetine (Prozac)	10–80	Headache; nausea and other GI effects; jitteriness; insomnia; sexual dysfunction; can affect plasma levels of other meds (except sertraline); akathisia rare	Once daily dosing, usually in A.M.; fluoxetine has very long half-life; must not be combined with MAOIs
Sertraline (Zoloft)	50–200		
Paroxetine (Paxil)	20–60		
Fluvoxamine (Luvox)	100–300		
Citalopram (Celexa)	20–60		
TCAs			
Amitriptyline (Elavil)	150–300	Anticholinergic (dry mouth, tachycardia, constipation, urinary retention, blurred vision); sweating; tremor; postural hypotension; cardiac conduction delay; sedation; weight gain	Once daily dosing, usually qhs; blood levels of most TCAs available; can be lethal in O.D. (lethal dose = 2 g); nortriptyline best tolerated, especially by elderly
Nortriptyline (Pamelor)	50–200		
Imipramine (Tofranil)	150–300		
Desipramine (Norpramin)	150–300		
Doxepin (Sinequan)	150–300		
Clomipramine (Anafranil)	150–300		
Mixed norepinephrine/serotonin reuptake inhibitors			
Venlafaxine (Effexor)	75–375	Nausea; dizziness; dry mouth; headaches; increased blood pressure; anxiety and insomnia	Bid-tid dosing; lower potential for drug-drug interactions than SSRIs; contraindicated with MAOIs.
Mirtazapine (Remeron)	15–45	Somnolence; weight gain; neutropenia rare	Once daily dosing
Mixed-action drugs			
Bupropion (Wellbutrin)	250–450	Jitteriness; flushing; seizures in at-risk patients; anorexia; tachycardia; psychosis	Tid dosing, but sustained release also available; fewer sexual side effects than SSRIs or TCAs; may be useful for adult ADD
Trazodone (Desyrel)	200–600	Sedation; dry mouth; ventricular irritability; postural hypotension; priapism rare	Useful in low doses for sleep because of sedating effects with no anticholinergic side effects
Nefazodone (Serzone)	300–600	Sedation; headache; dry mouth; nausea; constipation	Once daily dosing; no effect on REM sleep unlike other antidepressants
MAOIs			
Phenelzine (Nardil)	45–90	Insomnia; hypotension; anorgasmia; weight gain; hypertensive crisis; tyramine cheese reaction; lethal reactions with SSRIs; serious reactions with narcotics	May be more effective in patients with atypical features or treatment-refractory depressions
Tranylcypromine (Parnate)	20–50		
Isocarboxazid (Marplan)	20–60		

NOTE: ADD, attention deficit disorder; MAOI, monoamine oxidase inhibitor; REM, rapid eye movement; SSRI, selective serotonin reuptake inhibitor; TCA, tricyclic antidepressant.

autonomic responsivity, and social learning. Panic disorder shows familial aggregation, although concordance in monozygotic twins is only 30%. Acute panic attacks appear to be associated with increased noradrenergic discharge in the locus coeruleus. Intravenous infusion of sodium lactate evokes an attack in two-thirds of panic disorder patients, as do the α_2-adrenergic antagonist yohimbine and carbon dioxide inhalation. It is hypothesized that each of these stimuli activates a neural circuit involving noradrenergic neurons in the locus coeruleus and serotonergic neurons in the dorsal raphe. Agents that block serotonin reuptake are therapeutic in preventing attacks. It is theorized that panic-disorder patients have a heightened sensitivity to somatic symptoms, which triggers increasing arousal, setting off the "panic attack" mechanism. Accordingly, successful therapeutic intervention involves altering the patient's cognitive interpretation of anxiety-producing experiences as well as preventing the attack itself.

℞ **TREATMENT** Achievable goals of treatment are to decrease the frequency of panic attacks and to reduce their intensity. The cornerstone of drug therapy is antidepressant medications (Tables 385-3, 385-4, and 385-5). The tricyclic antidepressant (TCA) agents imipramine and clomipramine can benefit 75 to 90% of panic disorder patients. Low doses (e.g., 10 to 25 mg/d) are given initially to avoid any increased anxiety associated with heightened monoamine levels in the initial stages of treatment. Selective serotonin reuptake inhibitors (SSRIs) are equally effective and do not have the adverse effects of TCAs. SSRIs should be started at one-third to one-half of their usual antidepressant dose (e.g., 5 to 10 mg fluoxetine, 25 to 50 mg sertraline, 10 mg paroxetine). Monoamine oxidase inhibitors (MAOIs) are at least as effective as TCAs and may specifically benefit patients who have comorbid features of atypical depression (i.e., hypersomnia and weight gain). Insomnia, orthostatic hypotension, and the need to maintain a low-tyramine diet (avoidance of cheese and wine) have limited their use, however. Antidepressants typically take 2 to 6 weeks to become effective, and doses may need to be adjusted according to clinical response.

Because of anticipatory anxiety and the need for immediate relief of panic symptoms, benzodiazepines are useful early in the course of treatment and sporadically thereafter (Table 385-6). For example, alprazolam, starting at 0.5 mg qid and increasing to 4 mg/d in divided doses, is effective, but patients must be monitored closely, as some develop dependence and begin to escalate the dose of this medication. Clonazepam, at a final maintenance dose of 2 to 4 mg/d, is also helpful; its longer half-life permits twice-daily scheduling, and patients appear less likely to develop dependence on this agent.

Early psychotherapeutic intervention and psychoeducation aimed at symptom control enhances the effectiveness of drug treatment. Patients can be taught breathing techniques, can be educated about physiologic changes that occur with panic, and can learn to expose themselves voluntarily to precipitating events. Homework assignments and monitored compliance are important components of successful treatment. Once patients have achieved a satisfactory response, drug treatment should be maintained for 1 to 2 years to prevent relapse.

GENERALIZED ANXIETY DISORDER Clinical Manifestations Patients with generalized anxiety disorder (GAD) have persistent, excessive, and/or unrealistic worry associated with other signs and symptoms, which commonly include muscle tension, impaired concentration, autonomic arousal, feeling "on edge" or restless, and insomnia (Table 385-7). Onset is usually before age 20, and a history of childhood fears and social inhibition may be present. The incidence of GAD is increased in first-degree relatives of patients with the diagnosis; family studies also indicate that GAD and panic disorder segregate independently. Over 80% of patients with GAD also suffer from major depression, dysthymia, or social phobia. Comorbid substance abuse is common in these patients, particularly alcohol and/or sedative/hypnotic abuse. Patients with GAD readily admit to worrying excessively over minor matters, with life-disrupting effects; unlike in panic disorder, complaints of symptoms such as shortness of breath, palpitations, and tachycardia are relatively rare.

Table 385-4 Management of Antidepressant Side Effects

Symptoms	Comments and Management Strategies
Gastrointestinal	
Nausea, loss of appetite	Usually short-lived and dose-related; consider temporary dose reduction or administration with food and antacids
Diarrhea	Famotidine, 20–40 mg/d
Constipation	Wait for tolerance; try diet change, stool softener, exercise; avoid laxatives
Sexual dysfunction	Consider dose reduction; drug holiday
Anorgasmia/impotence; impaired ejaculation	Bethanechol, 10–20 mg, 2 h before activity, or cyproheptadine, 4–8 mg 2 h before activity, or bupropion, 100 mg bid or amantadine, 100 mg bid/tid
Orthostasis	Tolerance unlikely; increase fluid intake, use calf exercises/support hose; fludrocortisone, 0.025 mg/d
Anticholinergic	Wait for tolerance
Dry mouth, eyes	Maintain good oral hygiene; use artificial tears, sugar-free gum
Tremor/jitteriness	Antiparkinsonian drugs not effective; use dose reduction/slow increase; lorazepam, 0.5 mg bid, or propranolol, 10–20 mg bid
Insomnia	Schedule all doses for the morning; trazodone, 50–100 mg qhs
Sedation	Caffeine; schedule all dosing for bedtime; buproprion, 75–100 mg in afternoon
Headache	Evaluate diet, stress, other drugs; try dose reduction; amitriptyline, 50 mg/d
Weight gain	Decrease carbohydrates; exercise; consider fluoxetine
Loss of therapeutic benefit over time	Related to tolerance? Increase dose or drug holiday; add amantadine, 100 mg bid, buspirone, 10 mg tid, or pindolol, 2.5 mg bid

Etiology and Pathophysiology In experimental models of anxiety, anxiogenic agents share in common the property of altering the binding of benzodiazepines to the γ-aminobutyric acid (GABA) A receptor/chloride ion channel complex. Benzodiazepines are thought to bind two separate $GABA_A$ receptor sites: type I, which has a broad neuroanatomic distribution, and type II, which is concentrated in the hippocampus, striatum, and neocortex. The antianxiety effects of the various benzodiazepines and side effects such as sedation and memory impairment are influenced by their relative binding to type I and type II receptor sites. Serotonin [5-hydroxytriptamine (5HT)] also appears to have a role in anxiety. Buspirone, a partial $5HT_{1A}$ receptor agonist, and certain $5HT_{2A}$ and $5HT_{2C}$ receptor antagonists (e.g., nefazodone) may also have beneficial effects.

TREATMENT A combination of pharmacologic and psychotherapeutic interventions is most effective in GAD, but complete symptomatic relief is rare. A short course of a benzodiazepine is usually indicated, preferably lorazepam, oxazepam, or temazepam. (The first two of these agents are metabolized via conjugation rather than oxidation and thus do not accumulate if hepatic function is altered.) Administration should be initiated at the lowest dose possible and prescribed on an as-needed basis as symptoms warrant. Benzodiazepines differ in their milligram per kilogram potency, half-life, lipid solubility, metabolic pathways, and presence of active metabolites. Agents that are absorbed rapidly and are lipid soluble, such as diazepam, have a rapid onset of action and a higher abuse potential. Benzodiazepines should generally not be prescribed for >4 to 6 weeks because of the development of tolerance and the risk of abuse and dependence. It is important to warn patients that concomitant usage of alcohol or other sedating drugs may result in neurotoxicity and impair their ability to function. An optimistic approach that encourages the patient to clarify environmental precipitants, anticipate his or her reactions, and plan effective response strategies are essential elements of therapy.

Table 385-5 Possible Drug Interactions with Selective Serotonin Reuptake Inhibitors

Agent	Effect
Monoamine oxidase inhibitors	Serotonin syndrome—absolute contraindication
Serotonergic agonists, e.g., tryptophan, fenfluramine	Potential serotonin syndrome
Drugs that are metabolized by P450 isoenzymes: tricyclics, other SSRIs, antipsychotics, beta blockers, codeine, terfenadine, astemizole, triazolobenzodiazepines, calcium channel blockers	Delayed metabolism resulting in increased blood levels and potential toxicity—possible fatality secondary to QT prolongation with terfenadine or astemizole
Drugs that are bound tightly to plasma proteins, e.g., warfarin, coumadin	Increased bleeding secondary to displacement
Drugs that inhibit the metabolism of SSRIs by P450 isoenzymes, e.g., quinidine	Increased SSRI side effects

NOTE: SSRI, selective serotonin reuptake inhibitor.

Adverse effects of benzodiazepines generally parallel their relative half-lives. Longer-acting agents, such as diazepam, chlordiazepoxide, flurazepam, and clonazepam, tend to accumulate active metabolites, with resultant sedation, impairment of cognition, and poor psychomotor performance. Shorter-acting compounds, such as alprazolam and oxazepam, can result in daytime anxiety, early morning insomnia, and with discontinuation, rebound anxiety and insomnia. Although patients develop tolerance to the sedative effects of benzodiazepines, they are less likely to habituate to the adverse psychomotor effects. Withdrawal from the longer half-life benzodiazepines can be accomplished through gradual, stepwise dose reduction (by ~10% every 1 to 2 weeks) over 6 to 12 weeks. It is usually more difficult to taper patients off shorter-acting benzodiazepines. Physicians may need to switch the patient to a benzodiazepine with a longer half-life or use an adjunctive medication, such as a beta blocker or carbamazepine, before attempting to discontinue the benzodiazepine. Withdrawal reactions vary in severity and duration; they can include depression, anxiety, delirium, lethargy, diaphoresis, tinnitus, autonomic arousal, unusual neuromuscular movements, and, rarely, seizures.

Buspirone, an azaspirone, is a nonbenzodiazepine anxiolytic agent. It is nonsedating, does not lead to tolerance or dependence, does not interact with benzodiazepine receptors or alcohol, and has no abuse or disinhibition potential. However, it requires several weeks to take effect and requires thrice-daily dosing. Patients who were previously responsive to a benzodiazepine are unlikely to rate buspirone as equally effective, but patients with head injury or dementia who have symptoms of anxiety and/or agitation may do well with this agent.

Administration of benzodiazepines to geriatric patients requires special care. Such patients have increased drug absorption; decreased hepatic metabolism, protein binding, and renal excretion; and an increased volume of distribution. These factors, together with the likely presence of comorbid medical illnesses and medication, dramatically increase the likelihood of toxicity. Iatrogenic psychomotor impairment can result in falls and fractures, confusional states, or motor vehicle accidents. If used, agents in this class should be started at the lowest possible dose, and results should be monitored closely. Benzodiazepines are contraindicated during pregnancy and breast-feeding.

PHOBIC DISORDERS Clinical Manifestations The cardinal feature of phobic disorders is a marked and persistent fear of objects or situations, exposure to which results in an immediate anxiety reaction. The patient avoids the phobic stimulus, and this avoidance usually impairs occupational or social functioning. Panic attacks may be triggered by the phobic stimulus or may emerge spontaneously during the course of the illness. Unlike patients with other anxiety disorders, individuals with phobias experience anxiety only in specific situations. Common phobias include fear of closed spaces (claustrophobia), fear of blood, and fear of flying. Social phobia is distinguished

Table 385-6 Anxiolytics

Name	Equivalent PO dose, mg	Onset of Action	Half-life, h	Comments
Benzodiazepines:				
Diazepam (Valium)	5	Fast	20–70	Active metabolites; quite sedating
Flurazepam (Dalmane)	15	Fast	30–100	Flurazepam is a pro-drug; metabolites are active; quite sedating
Triazolam (Halcion)	0.25	Intermediate	1.5–5	No active metabolites; can induce confusion and delirium, especially in elderly
Lorazepam (Ativan)	1	Intermediate	10–20	No active metabolites; direct hepatic glucuronide conjugation; quite sedating
Alprazolam (Xanax)	0.5	Intermediate	12–15	Active metabolites; not too sedating; may have specific antidepressant and antipanic activity; tolerance and dependence develop easily
Chlordiazepoxide (Librium)	10	Intermediate	5–30	Active metabolites; moderately sedating
Oxazepam (Serax)	15	Slow	5–15	No active metabolites; direct glucuronide conjugation; not too sedating
Temazepam (Restoril)	15	Slow	9–12	No active metabolites; moderately sedating
Clonazepam (Klonopin)	0.5	Slow	18–50	No active metabolites; moderately sedating
Non-benzodiazepines				
Buspirone (BuSpar)	7.5	2 weeks	2–3	Active metabolites; tid dosing—usual daily dose 10–20 mg tid; nonsedating; no additive effects with alcohol; useful for agitation in demented or brain-injured patients

by a specific fear of social or performance situations in which the individual is exposed to unfamiliar individuals or to possible examination and evaluation by others. Examples include having to converse at a party, use public restrooms, and meet strangers. In each case, the affected individual is aware that the experienced fear is excessive and unreasonable given the circumstance. The specific content of a phobia may vary across gender, ethnic, and cultural boundaries.

Phobic disorders are common, with a 1-year prevalence rate of 9% and a lifetime rate of 10 to 11%. Onset is typically in childhood to early adulthood. Familial aggregation may occur. In one study of female twins, concordance rates for agoraphobia, social phobia, and animal phobia was found to be 23% for monozygotic twins and 15% for dizygotic twins. Full criteria for diagnosis are usually satisfied first in adulthood, but behavioral avoidance of unfamiliar people, situations, or objects dating from early childhood is common.

Table 385-7 Diagnostic Criteria for Generalized Anxiety Disorder

A. Excessive anxiety and worry (apprehensive expectation), occurring more days than not for at least 6 months, about a number of events or activities (such as work or school performance).
B. The person finds it difficult to control the worry.
C. The anxiety and worry are associated with three (or more) of the following six symptoms (with at least some symptoms present for more days than not for the past 6 months): (1) restlessness or feeling keyed up or on edge; (2) being easily fatigued; (3) difficulty concentrating or mind going blank; (4) irritability; (5) muscle tension; (6) sleep disturbance (difficulty falling or staying asleep, or restless unsatisfying sleep).
D. The focus of the anxiety and worry is not confined to features of an Axis I disorder, e.g., the anxiety or worry is not about having a panic attack (as in panic disorder), being embarrassed in public (as in social phobia), being contaminated (as in obsessive-compulsive disorder), being away from home or close relatives (as in separation anxiety disorder), gaining weight (as in anorexia nervosa), having multiple physical complaints (as in somatization disorder), or having a serious illness (as in hypochondriasis), and the anxiety and worry do not occur exclusively during posttraumatic stress disorder.
E. The anxiety, worry, or physical symptoms cause clinically significant distress or impairment in social, occupational, or other important areas of functioning.
F. The disturbance is not due to the direct physiologic effects of a substance (e.g., a drug of abuse, a medication) or a general medical condition (e.g., hyperthyroidism) and does not occur exclusively during a mood disorder, a psychotic disorder, or a pervasive developmental disorder.

SOURCE: *Diagnostic and Statistical Manual of Mental Disorders*, 4th ed.

℞ **TREATMENT** Recent controlled trials have documented the efficacy of several pharmacologic agents in the treatment of phobic disorders. Beta blockers (e.g., propranolol, 20 to 40 mg orally 2 h before the event) are particularly effective in the treatment of "performance anxiety" (but not general social phobia) and appear to achieve their benefit by preventing the occurrence of peripheral manifestations of anxiety, such as perspiration, tachycardia, palpitations, and tremor. MAOIs alleviate social phobia independently of their antidepressant activity, and SSRIs appear to be effective also. Benzodiazepines can be helpful in reducing fearful avoidance, but the chronic nature of phobic disorders limits their usefulness.

Behaviorally focused psychotherapy is an important component of treatment, as relapse rates are high when medication is used as the sole treatment. Cognitive-behavioral strategies are the cornerstone of treatment; these are based upon the finding that distorted perceptions and interpretations of fear-producing stimuli play a major role in perpetuation of phobias. Individual and group therapy sessions teach the patient to identify specific negative thoughts associated with the anxiety-producing situation and help to reduce the patient's fear of loss of control. In desensitization therapy, hierarchies of feared situations are constructed and the patient is encouraged to pursue and master gradual exposure to the anxiety-producing stimuli.

Patients with social phobia, in particular, have a high rate of comorbid alcohol abuse, as well as of other psychiatric conditions (e.g., eating disorders), necessitating the need for parallel management of each disorder if anxiety reduction is to be achieved.

STRESS DISORDERS **Clinical Manifestations** Patients may develop anxiety after exposure to extreme traumatic events such as the threat of personal death or injury or the death of a loved one. The reaction may occur shortly after the trauma (*acute stress disorder*) or be delayed and subject to recurrence (PTSD) (Table 385-8). In both syndromes, individuals experience associated symptoms of detachment and loss of emotional responsivity. The patient may feel depersonalized and unable to recall specific aspects of the trauma, though typically it is reexperienced through intrusions in thought, dreams, or flashbacks, particularly when cues of the original event are present. Patients often actively avoid stimuli that precipitate recollections of the trauma and demonstrate a resulting increase in vigilance, arousal, and startle response. Patients with stress disorders are at risk for the development of other anxiety, mood, and substance-related disorders. Between 5 and 10% of Americans will at some time in their life satisfy criteria for PTSD, with women more likely to be affected than men.

Risk factors for the development of PTSD include a past psychi-

Table 385-8 Diagnostic Criteria for Posttraumatic Stress Disorder

A. The person has been exposed to a traumatic event in which both of the following were present:
   1. The person experienced, witnessed, or was confronted with an event or events that involved actual or threatened death or serious injury, or a threat to the physical integrity of self or others.
   2. The person's response involved intense fear, helplessness, or horror.
B. The traumatic event is persistently reexperienced in one (or more) of the following ways:
   1. Recurrent and intrusive distressing recollections of the event, including images, thoughts, or perceptions.
   2. Recurrent distressing dreams of the event.
   3. Acting or feeling as if the traumatic event were recurring (includes a sense of reliving the experience, illusions, hallucinations, and dissociative flashback episodes, including those that occur on awakening or when intoxicated).
   4. Intense psychological distress at exposure to internal or external cues that symbolize or resemble an aspect of the traumatic event.
   5. Physiologic reactivity on exposure to internal or external cues that symbolize or resemble an aspect of the traumatic event.
C. Persistent avoidance of stimuli associated with the trauma and numbing of general responsiveness (not present before the trauma), as indicated by three or more of the following:
   1. Efforts to avoid thoughts, feelings, or conversations associated with the trauma
   2. Efforts to avoid activities, places, or people that arouse recollections of the trauma
   3. Inability to recall an important aspect of the trauma
   4. Markedly diminished interest or participation in significant activities
   5. Feeling of detachment or estrangement from others
   6. Restricted range of affect (e.g., unable to have loving feelings)
   7. Sense of a foreshortened future (e.g., does not expect to have a career, marriage, children, or a normal life span)
D. Persistent symptoms of increased arousal (not present before the trauma), as indicated by two (or more) of the following:
   1. Difficulty falling or staying asleep
   2. Irritability or outbursts of anger
   3. Difficulty concentrating
   4. Hypervigilance
   5. Exaggerated startle response
E. Duration of the disturbance (symptoms in criteria B, C, and D) is more than 1 month
F. The disturbance causes clinically significant distress or impairment in social, occupational, or other important areas of functioning.

SOURCE: *Diagnostic and Statistical Manual of Mental Disorders,* 4th ed.

atric history and personality characteristics of high neuroticism and extroversion. Studies of monozygotic and dizygotic twins showed a substantial influence of genetics on all symptoms associated with PTSD, with no evidence for an environment effect.

Etiology and Pathophysiology It is hypothesized that in PTSD there is excessive release of norepinephrine from the locus coeruleus in response to stress. Increased noradrenergic activity at locus coeruleus projection sites in hippocampus and amygdala theoretically facilitates encoding of fear-based memories. Greater sympathetic responses to cues associated with the traumatic event occurs in PTSD.

℞ TREATMENT Acute stress reactions are usually self-limited, and treatment typically involves the short-term use of benzodiazepines and supportive/expressive psychotherapy. The chronic and recurrent nature of PTSD, however, requires a more complex approach employing drug and behavioral treatments. TCAs such as imipramine and amitriptyline, the MAOI phenelzine, and the SSRIs (fluoxetine, sertraline, citalopram, paroxetine) can all reduce anxiety, symptoms of intrusion, and avoidance behaviors. Trazodone, a sedating antidepressant, is frequently used at night to help with insomnia (50 to 150 mg qhs). Carbamazepine, valproic acid, or alprazolam have also independently produced improvement in uncontrolled trials. There is frequent comorbidity with substance abuse, especially alcohol.

Psychotherapeutic strategies are used in treatment of PTSD to help the patient overcome avoidance behaviors and demoralization and master fear of recurrence of the trauma; therapies that encourage the patient to dismantle avoidance behaviors through stepwise focusing on the experience of the traumatic event are the most effective.

OBSESSIVE-COMPULSIVE DISORDER Clinical Manifestations Obsessive-compulsive disorder (OCD) was previously considered a relatively rare condition, but recent epidemiologic data indicate a lifetime prevalence of 2 to 3% worldwide. OCD is characterized by obsessive thoughts and compulsive behaviors that impair everyday functioning. Fears of contamination and germs are common, as are handwashing, counting behaviors, and having to check and recheck such actions as whether a door is locked. The degree to which the disorder is disruptive for the individual varies, but in all cases obsessive-compulsive activities take up >1 h per day and are undertaken to relieve the anxiety triggered by the core fear. Patients often conceal their symptoms, usually because they are embarrassed by the content of their thoughts or the nature of their actions. Physicians must ask specific questions regarding recurrent thoughts and behaviors, particularly if physical clues such as chafed and reddened hands or patchy hair loss (from repetitive hair pulling, or trichotillomania) are present. Tics are sometimes associated with OCD. OCD usually has a gradual onset, beginning in early adulthood, but childhood onset is not rare. The disorder usually has a waxing and waning course, but some cases may show a steady deterioration in psychosocial functioning.

Etiology and Pathophysiology A genetic contribution to OCD is suggested by a higher monozygotic than dizygotic concordance rate and the fact that familial studies show an aggregation with Tourette's disorder. OCD is more common in males and in first-born children.

The anatomy of obsessive-compulsive behavior is thought to involve a frontal-subcortical neural circuit involving the orbital frontal cortex, caudate nucleus, and globus pallidus. Neuroimaging studies have demonstrated a decrease in caudate nucleus volume, abnormalities in frontal lobe white matter, and increases in glucose metabolism in the orbital cortex of the frontal lobes and the head of the caudate nucleus. The caudate nucleus seems particularly involved in the acquisition and maintenance of habit and skill learning, and interventions that are successful in reducing obsessive-compulsive behaviors are paralleled by a comparable decrease in caudate glucose metabolic rate.

℞ TREATMENT Clomipramine, fluoxetine, and fluvoxamine are approved for the treatment of OCD. Clomipramine is a TCA that is often tolerated poorly owing to significant anticholinergic and sedative side effects at the doses required to treat the illness (150 to 250 mg/d). Its efficacy in OCD is unrelated to its antidepressant activity. Fluoxetine (40 to 60 mg/d) and fluvoxamine (100 to 300 mg/d) are as effective as clomipramine and show a more benign side-effect profile. Fluvoxamine, a structurally unique SSRI, is metabolized through the hepatic P450 microsomal system (as is fluoxetine); it appears to inhibit the III A4 isoenzyme specifically and should not be given with other drugs that act on III A4, such as terfenadine and astemizole, because life-threatening cardiac arrhythmias may result. Only 50 to 60% of patients with OCD show an acceptable degree of improvement with pharmacotherapy alone. In treatment-resistant cases, augmentation with other serotonergic agents, such as buspirone, or with a neuroleptic or benzodiazepine may be beneficial. When a therapeutic response is achieved, long-duration maintenance therapy is usually indicated.

For many individuals, particularly those with time-consuming compulsions, behavior therapy will result in as much improvement as that afforded by medication. Effective techniques include the gradual increase in exposure to stressful situations, maintenance of a diary to clarify stressors, and homework assignments that substitute new activities for their compulsive behavior.

MOOD DISORDERS

Mood disorders are characterized by a disturbance in the regulation of mood, behavior, and affect. Mood disorders are subdivided into (1) depressive disorders, (2) bipolar disorders, and (3) depression in association with medical illness or alcohol and substance abuse (Chaps. 387 through 389). Depressive disorders are differentiated from bipolar disorders by the absence of a manic or hypomanic episode. The relationship between pure depressive syndromes and bipolar disorders is not well understood; depression occurs at increased frequency in families of bipolar individuals, but the reverse is not true. Depression in general is associated with high disability and societal cost; in the Global Burden of Disease Study conducted by the World Health Organization, unipolar major depression ranked fourth in percentage of disability-adjusted life years and was projected to rank second in the year 2020.

DEPRESSION IN ASSOCIATION WITH MEDICAL ILLNESS Depression occurring in the context of medical illness is difficult to evaluate. Depressive symptomatology may reflect the psychological stress of coping with the disease, may be caused by the disease process itself or by the medications used to treat it, or may simply coexist in time with the medical diagnosis.

Virtually every class of *medication* includes some agent that can induce depression. Antihypertensive drugs, anticholesterolemic agents, and antiarrhythmic agents are commonly used classes of medications that can trigger depressive symptoms. Among the antihypertensive agents, β-adrenergic blockers and, to a lesser extent, calcium channel blockers are the most likely to cause depressed mood. Iatrogenic depression should also be considered in patients receiving glucocorticoids, antimicrobials, systemic analgesics, antiparkinsonian medications, and anticonvulsants. To decide whether a causal relationship exists between pharmacologic therapy and a patient's change in mood, it is necessary to chart the chronology of symptoms and sometimes to undertake an empirical trial of an alternative medication.

Between 20 and 30% of cardiac patients manifest a depressive disorder; an even higher percentage experience depressive symptomatology when self-reporting scales are used. Depressive symptoms following myocardial infarction impair rehabilitation and are associated with higher rates of mortality and medical morbidity. Depressed patients often show decreased variability in heart rate (an index of reduced parasympathetic nervous system activity), and this has been proposed as one mechanism by which depression may predispose individuals to ventricular arrhythmia and increased morbidity. Although TCAs have been used to treat depression in individuals with cardiac disease for a number of years, and although the quinidine-like effect of tricyclics may be useful in patients with preexisting arrhythmias, TCAs are contraindicated in patients with preexisting bundle branch block. They may also paradoxically precipitate arrhythmias. Tricyclic-induced tachycardia is an additional concern in patients with congestive heart failure. Experience with the SSRIs is more limited, but thus far they appear not to induce ECG changes or adverse cardiac events. SSRIs may interfere with hepatic metabolism of anticoagulants, however, causing increased anticoagulation.

Epidemiologic surveys of depression in patients with cancer show a wide variability in prevalence, as might be predicted by differences in tumor site, severity of illness, and type of medical or surgical intervention. There is an overall mean prevalence of 25%, but depression occurs in 40 to 50% of patients with cancers of the pancreas or oropharynx. Assessment of the validity of prevalence rates is complicated by the fact that extreme cachexia may be misinterpreted as part of the symptom complex of depression. The higher prevalence of depression in patients with pancreatic cancer nevertheless persists when patients are compared to those with advanced gastric cancer. Initiation of antidepressant medication in cancer patients has been shown to improve quality of life as well as mood. Psychotherapeutic approaches, particularly group therapy, may have some effect on short-term depression, anxiety, and pain symptoms and on recurrence rates and long-term survival. In a study of female patients with metastatic breast cancer, patients in group therapy had longer survival than control patients.

Depression occurs frequently in patients with *neurologic disorders*, particularly cerebrovascular disorders, Parkinson's disease, multiple sclerosis, and traumatic brain injury. Left-hemisphere strokes, particularly those involving the dorsal lateral frontal cortex, are most likely to cause depression. Both tricyclic and SSRI antidepressants are effective in the treatment of depression secondary to stroke, as are stimulant compounds and, in some patients, MAOIs.

The reported prevalence of depression in patients with *diabetes mellitus* varies from 8 to 27%, with the severity of the mood state correlating with the physical symptoms of illness and the degree of hyperglycemia. Pharmacologic treatment of depression is complicated by antidepressant effects on the blood glucose level. MAOIs can induce hypoglycemia and weight gain. TCAs can lead to hyperglycemia and carbohydrate craving. SSRIs, like MAOIs, may cause a reduction in fasting plasma glucose, but they are easier to use and may also improve dietary and medication compliance.

Hypothyroidism is frequently associated with features of depression, most commonly depressed mood and memory impairment. Hyperthyroid states may also present in a similar fashion, usually in geriatric populations. Improvement in mood usually follows normalization of thyroid function, but adjunctive antidepressant medication is sometimes required. Patients with subclinical hypothyroidism can also experience symptoms of depression and cognitive difficulty that respond to thyroid replacement.

DEPRESSIVE DISORDERS Clinical Manifestations *Major depression* is defined as depressed mood on a daily basis for a minimum duration of 2 weeks (Table 385-9). An episode may be characterized by sadness, indifference or apathy, or irritability and is usually associated with change in neurovegetative functions, including sleep patterns, appetite and weight, motor agitation or retardation, fatigue, impairment in concentration and decision making, feelings of

Table 385-9 Criteria for Major Depressive Episode

A. Five (or more) of the following symptoms have been present during the same 2-week period and represent a change from previous functioning; at least one of the symptoms is either (1) depressed mood or (2) loss of interest or pleasure. **Note:** Do not include symptoms that are clearly due to a general medical condition, or mood-incongruent delusions or hallucinations.
  1. Depressed mood most of the day, nearly every day, as indicated by either subjective report (e.g., feels sad or empty) or observation made by others (e.g., appears tearful)
  2. Markedly diminished interest or pleasure in all, or almost all, activities most of the day, nearly every day (as indicated by either subjective account or observation made by others)
  3. Significant weight loss when not dieting or weight gain (e.g., a change of >5% of body weight in a month), or decrease or increase in appetite nearly every day
  4. Insomnia or hypersomnia nearly every day
  5. Psychomotor agitation or retardation nearly every day (observable by others, not merely subjective feelings of restlessness or being slowed down)
  6. Fatigue or loss of energy nearly every day
  7. Feelings of worthlessness or excessive or inappropriate guilt (which may be delusional) nearly every day (not merely self-reproach or guilt about being sick)
  8. Diminished ability to think or concentrate, or indecisiveness, nearly every day (either by subjective account or as observed by others)
  9. Recurrent thoughts of death (not just fear of dying), recurrent suicidal ideation without a specific plan, or a suicide attempt or a specific plan for committing suicide

B. The symptoms do not meet criteria for a mixed episode

C. The symptoms cause clinically significant distress or impairment in social, occupational, or other important areas of functioning

D. The symptoms are not due to the direct physiologic effects of a substance (e.g., a drug of abuse, a medication) or a general medical condition (e.g., hypothyroidism)

E. The symptoms are not better accounted for by bereavement; i.e., after the loss of a loved one, the symptoms persist for >2 months or are characterized by marked functional impairment, morbid preoccupation with worthlessness, suicidal ideation, psychotic symptoms, or psychomotor retardation

SOURCE: *Diagnostic and Statistical Manual of Mental Disorders*, 4th ed.

shame or guilt, and thoughts of death or dying. Patients with depression have a profound loss of pleasure in all enjoyable activities, exhibit early morning awakening, feel that the dysphoric mood state is qualitatively different from sadness, and often notice a diurnal variation in mood (worse in morning hours). Paradoxically, these more severe features predict a good response to antidepressant treatment.

Approximately 15% of the population experiences a major depressive episode at some point in life, and 6 to 8% of all outpatients in primary care settings satisfy diagnostic criteria for the disorder. Depression is often undiagnosed, and, even more frequently, it is treated inadequately. If a physician suspects the presence of a major depressive episode, the initial task is to determine whether it represents unipolar or bipolar depression or is one of the 10 to 15% of cases that are secondary to general medical illness or substance abuse. Physicians should also assess the risk of suicide by direct questioning, as patients are often reluctant to verbalize such thoughts without prompting. If specific plans are uncovered or if significant risk factors exist (e.g., a past history of suicide attempts, profound hopelessness, concurrent medical illness, substance abuse, or social isolation), the patient must be referred to a mental health specialist for immediate care. In evaluating suicidal risk the physician should specifically probe each of these areas in an empathic and hopeful manner, being sensitive to denial and possible minimization of distress. The presence of anxiety, panic, or agitation significantly increases near-term suicidal risk. Nearly 15% of patients whose depressive illness goes untreated will commit suicide; most will have sought help from a physician within 1 month of their death.

In some depressed patients, the mood disorder does not appear to be episodic and is not clearly associated with either psychosocial dysfunction or change from the individual's usual experience in life. *Dysthymic disorder* consists of a pattern of chronic (at least 2 years), ongoing, mild depressive symptoms that are less severe and less disabling than those found in major depression; the two conditions are sometimes difficult to separate, however, and can occur together ("double depression"). Many patients who exhibit a profile of pessimism, disinterest, and low self-esteem respond to antidepressant treatment. Dysthymic disorder exists in ~5% of primary care patients.

Studies of various cultures have shown that external manifestations of depression differ but the core symptoms remain the same. The incidence of depression increases with age; the disorder is approximately twice as prevalent in women as in men, regardless of age. These gender differences were previously believed to reflect sociocultural factors, but recent longitudinal twin studies indicate that the liability to major depression in adult women is largely genetic in origin, and that the effect of environmental factors is transitory and does not affect lifetime prevalence. The relationship between psychological stress, negative life events, and the onset of depressive episodes is complex. Negative life events can precipitate and contribute to depression, but recent data indicate that genetic factors influence the sensitivity of individuals to these stressful events. In most cases, both biologic and psychosocial factors are involved in the precipitation and unfolding of depressive episodes. The most potent stressors appear to involve death of a relative, assault, or severe marital or relationship problems.

Unipolar depressive disorders usually have their onset in early adulthood, and recurrences over the course of a lifetime are likely. The best predictor of future risk is the number of past episodes; 50 to 60% of patients who have a first episode have at least one or two more episodes. Some patients experience multiple episodes that become more severe and frequent over time. The duration of an untreated episode varies greatly, ranging from a few months to ≥1 year. The pattern of recurrence and clinical progression in a developing episode is also variable. Within an individual, there is often long-term stability in phenotype (presenting symptoms, frequency and duration of episodes). In a minority of patients, the severity of the depressive episode may progress to psychotic symptomatology; in elderly patients, depressive symptoms may be associated with confusion and mistaken for dementia (i.e., "pseudodementia"). A seasonal pattern of depression, called *seasonal affective disorder*, may manifest with onset and

remission of episodes at predictable times of the year. This disorder is more common in women, whose symptoms are anergy, fatigue, weight gain, hypersomnia, and episodic carbohydrate craving. The prevalence increases with distance from the equator, and mood improvement may occur by altering light exposure.

Etiology and Pathophysiology The neurobiology of unipolar depression is poorly understood. Although evidence for genetic transmission is not as strong as in bipolar disorder, monozygotic twins have a higher concordance rate (46%) than dizygotic siblings (20%), with little evidence for any effect of a shared family environment. Parallels between the affective, motor, and cognitive dysfunctions seen in unipolar depression and those observed in diseases of the basal ganglia have suggested that neural networks involving prefrontal cortex and the basal ganglia may be involved. This hypothesis is supported by positron emission tomography (PET) studies of brain glucose metabolism that show a decrease in metabolic rate in the caudate nuclei and frontal lobes in depressed patients that returns to normal with recovery. Single-photon emission computed tomography (SPECT) studies show comparable changes in blood flow. Magnetic resonance imaging (MRI) findings in some patients include an increased frequency of subcortical white matter lesions. However, because these findings are more prevalent in patients with late onset of depressive illness, their significance remains unproven. A number of studies document increased ventricle-to-brain ratios in some patients with recurrent depression, but whether this finding is state-dependent or represents true cerebral atrophy is controversial.

Postmortem examination of brains of suicide victims suggest altered noradrenergic activity, including increased binding to α_1-, α_2-, and β-adrenergic receptors in the cerebral cortex and a decreased total number and density of noradrenergic neurons in the locus coeruleus. Involvement of the serotonin system is suggested by findings of reduced plasma tryptophan levels, a decreased cerebrospinal fluid level of 5-hydroxyindolacetic acid (the principal metabolite of serotonin in brain), and decreased platelet serotonergic transporter binding. An increase in brain serotonin receptors in suicide victims is also reported. Depletion of blood tryptophan, the amino acid precursor of serotonin, rapidly reverses the antidepressant benefit in depressed patients who have been successfully treated. However, a decrement in mood after tryptophan reduction is considerably less robust in untreated patients, indicating that, if presynaptic serotonergic dysfunction occurs in depression, it likely plays a contributing rather than a causal role.

Neuroendocrine abnormalities that reflect the neurovegetative signs and symptoms of depression include (1) increased cortisol and corticotropin-releasing hormone (CRH) secretion, (2) an increase in adrenal size, (3) a decreased inhibitory response of glucocorticoids to dexamethasone, and (4) a blunted response of thyroid-stimulating hormone (TSH) level to infusion of thyroid-releasing hormone (TRH). Antidepressant treatment leads to normalization of these pituitary-adrenal abnormalities.

Diurnal variations in symptom severity and alterations in circadian rhythmicity of a number of neurochemical and neurohumoral factors suggest that biologic differences may be secondary to a primary defect in regulation of biologic rhythms. Patients with major depression show consistent findings of a decrease in rapid eye movement (REM) sleep onset (REM latency), an increase in REM density, and, in some subjects, a decrease in stage IV delta slow-wave sleep.

Although antidepressant drugs result in a blockade of neurotransmitter uptake within hours, their therapeutic effects typically emerge over several weeks, implicating neuroadaptive changes in second messenger systems and transcription factors as possible mechanisms of action.

℞ TREATMENT Treatment planning requires coordination of short-term symptom remission with longer term maintenance strategies designed to prevent recurrence. The most effective intervention for achieving remission and preventing relapse is medication, but combined treatment, incorporating psychotherapy to help the patient cope with decreased self-esteem and demoralization, improves outcome (Fig. 385-1). About 40% of primary care patients with depression drop out of treatment and discontinue medication if symptomatic improvement is not noted within a month, unless additional support is provided. Outcome improves with (1) increased intensity and frequency of visits during the first 4 to 6 weeks of treatment, (2) supplemental educational materials, and (3) psychiatric consultation as indicated. Despite the widespread use of SSRIs, there is no convincing evidence that this class of antidepressant is more efficacious than TCAs. Between 60 and 70% of all depressed patients respond to any drug chosen, if it is given in a sufficient dose for 6 to 8 weeks. There is no ideal antidepressant; no current compound combines rapid onset of action, moderate half-life, a meaningful relationship between dose and blood level, a low side effect profile, minimal interaction with other drugs, and safety in overdose. A rational approach to selecting which antidepressant to use involves matching the patient's preference and medical history with the metabolic and side effect profile of the drug (Tables 385-4 and 385-5). A previous response, or a family history of a positive response, to a specific antidepressant would suggest that that drug be tried first. Before initiating antidepressant therapy, the physician should evaluate the possible contribution of comorbid illnesses and consider their specific treatment. In individuals with suicidal ideation, particular attention should be paid to choosing a drug with a low toxicity if taken in overdose. The SSRIs and other newer antidepressant drugs are distinctly safer in this regard; nevertheless, the advantages of TCAs have not been completely superseded. The existence of generic equivalents make TCAs relatively cheap, and for several tricyclics, particularly nortriptyline, imipramine, and desipramine, well-defined relationships between dose, plasma level, and therapeutic response exist. The steady-state plasma level achieved for a given drug dose can vary more than tenfold between individuals. Plasma levels may help in understanding resistance to treatment and/or unexpected drug toxicity. The principal disadvantages of TCAs are antihistamine side effects (sedation) and anticholinergic side effects (constipation, dry mouth, urinary hesitancy, and blurred vision). Severe cardiac toxicity due to conduction block or arrhythmias can also occur but is uncommon at therapeutic levels. TCAs are probably contraindicated in patients with cardiovascular risk factors. Tricyclic agents are lethal in overdose, with desipramine carrying the greatest risk. Prescribing only a 10-day supply may be judicious. Most patients require a daily dose of 150 to 200 mg of imipramine or amitriptyline or its equivalent to achieve a therapeutic blood level of 150 to 300 ng/mL and a satisfactory remission; some patients show a partial effect at lower doses. Geriatric patients in particular may require a low starting dose and slow escalation. Ethnic differences in drug metabolism are significant; Hispanic, Asian, and African American patients generally require lower doses than Caucasians to achieve a comparable blood level.

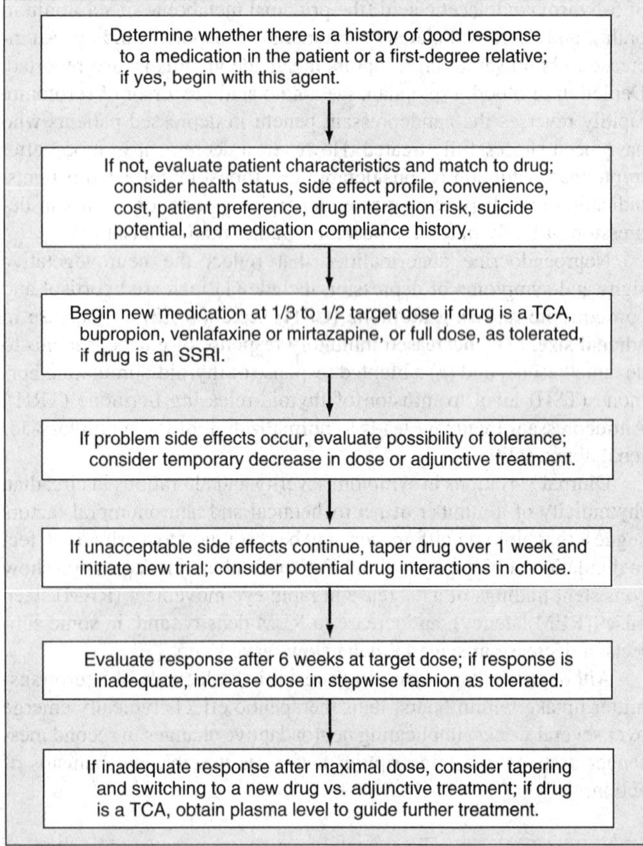

Determine whether there is a history of good response to a medication in the patient or a first-degree relative; if yes, begin with this agent.
If not, evaluate patient characteristics and match to drug; consider health status, side effect profile, convenience, cost, patient preference, drug interaction risk, suicide potential, and medication compliance history.
Begin new medication at 1/3 to 1/2 target dose if drug is a TCA, bupropion, venlafaxine or mirtazapine, or full dose, as tolerated, if drug is an SSRI.
If problem side effects occur, evaluate possibility of tolerance; consider temporary decrease in dose or adjunctive treatment.
If unacceptable side effects continue, taper drug over 1 week and initiate new trial; consider potential drug interactions in choice.
Evaluate response after 6 weeks at target dose; if response is inadequate, increase dose in stepwise fashion as tolerated.
If inadequate response after maximal dose, consider tapering and switching to a new drug vs. adjunctive treatment; if drug is a TCA, obtain plasma level to guide further treatment.

FIGURE 385-1 A guideline for the medical management of major depressive disorder. SSRI, selective serotonin reuptake inhibitor; TCA, tricyclic antidepressant.

Second-generation antidepressants include amoxapine, maprotiline, trazodone, and bupropion. Amoxapine is a dibenzoxazepine derivative that blocks norepinephrine and serotonin reuptake and has a metabolite that shows a degree of dopamine blockade. Long-term use of this drug carries a risk of tardive dyskinesia. Maprotiline is a potent noradrenergic reuptake blocker that has little anticholinergic effect but may produce seizures. Bupropion is a novel antidepressant whose mechanism of action is thought to involve enhancement of noradrenergic function. It has no anticholinergic, sedating, or orthostatic side effects and has a low incidence of sexual side effects. It may, however, be associated with aversive stimulant-like side effects, may lower seizure threshold, and has an exceptionally short half-life, requiring multiple dosing. An extended-release preparation is available.

SSRIs such as fluoxetine, sertraline, paroxetine, and citalopram cause a lower frequency of anticholinergic, sedating, and cardiovascular side effects but a possibly greater incidence of gastrointestinal complaints, sleep impairment, and sexual dysfunction than do TCAs. Akathisia, involving an inner sense of restlessness and anxiety, may also be more common, particularly during the first week of treatment. A serious concern, aside from drug interaction, is the risk of "serotonin syndrome," thought to result from hyperstimulation of brainstem $5HT_{1A}$ receptors and characterized by myoclonus, agitation, abdominal cramping, hyperpyrexia, hypertension, and potentially death. Combinations of serotonergic agonists should be monitored closely for this reason. Considerations such as half-life, compliance, toxicity, and drug-drug interactions may guide the choice of a particular SSRI. Fluoxetine and its principal active metabolite, norfluoxetine, for example, have a combined half-life of almost 7 days, resulting in a delay of 5 weeks before steady-state levels are achieved and a similar delay for complete drug excretion once its use is discontinued. All the SSRIs may impair sexual function, resulting in diminished libido, impotence, or difficulty in achieving orgasm. Sexual dysfunction frequently results in noncompliance and should be asked about specifically in patients using SSRIs. Sexual dysfunction can sometimes be ameliorated by lowering the dose, by instituting drug holidays over the weekend (two or three times a month), or by treatment with amantadine (100 mg tid), bethanechol (25 mg tid), or buspirone (10 mg tid). Paroxetine appears to be more anticholinergic than either fluoxetine or sertraline, and sertraline carries a lower risk of producing an adverse drug interaction than the other two. Rare side effects of SSRIs include vasospastic angina and alterations of prothrombin time. Citalopram is the most specific of currently available SSRIs and appears to have no specific inhibitory effects on the P450 system.

Venlafaxine, like imipramine, blocks the reuptake of both norepinephrine and serotonin, but it produces relatively little in the way of traditional tricyclic side effects. Unlike the SSRIs, it has a relatively linear dose-response curve. Patients should be monitored for a possible increase in diastolic blood pressure, and multiple daily dosing is required because of the drug's short half-life. An extended-release form is available and has a somewhat lower incidence of gastrointestinal side effects. Nefazadone is a selective $5HT_2$ receptor antagonist that also inhibits the presynaptic reuptake of serotonin and norepinephrine. Its side effects are similar to those of the SSRIs, and twice-daily dosing produces a steady state within 4 to 5 days. The drug is related structurally to trazodone, which is currently used more for its sedative than its antidepressant properties. Nefazadone appears to produce a lower incidence of sexual side effects than do the SSRIs. Mirtazapine is a tetracyclic antidepressant that has a comparatively unique spectrum of activity. It increases noradrenergic and serotonergic neurotransmission through a blockade of central α_2-adrenergic auto- and heteroreceptors and postsynaptic $5HT_2$ and $5HT_3$ receptors. It is also strongly antihistaminic and, as such, may produce sedation at lower doses.

With the exception of citalopram, each of the SSRIs, as well as nefazadone, may inhibit one or more cytochrome P450 enzymes (Table 385-5). Depending on the specific isoenzyme involved, the metabolism of a number of concomitantly administered medications can be dramatically affected. Fluoxetine and paroxetine, for example, by inhibiting 2D6, can cause dramatic increases in the blood level of type 1C antiarrhythmics, while sertraline and nefazadone, by acting on 3A4, may alter blood levels of terfenadine, carbamazepine, and astemizole. Because many of these compounds have a narrow therapeutic window and can cause iatrogenic ventricular arrhythmias at toxic levels, the possibility of an adverse drug interaction should be considered.

Other treatment options include the MAOIs and electroconvulsive therapy. The MAOIs are highly effective, particularly in atypical depression, but the risk of hypertensive crisis following intake of tyramine-containing food or sympathomimetic drugs makes them inappropriate as first-line agents. Common side effects include orthostatic hypotension, weight gain, insomnia, and sexual dysfunction. MAOIs should not be used concomitantly with SSRIs, because of the risk of serotonin syndrome, or with TCAs, because of possible hyperadrenergic effects. Electroconvulsive therapy is at least as effective as medication, but its use is reserved for treatment-resistant cases and delusional depressions.

Regardless of the medication chosen, the treatment response should be evaluated after approximately 2 months of therapy. Three-quarters of patients show an adequate response by this time, but if remission is inadequate, the patient should be questioned about medication compliance, and an increase in dose should be considered if side effects are not troublesome. If there is no improvement, consultation with or referral to a mental health specialist is advised. Strategies for treatment then include selection of an alternative drug, combinations of antidepressants, and/or adjunctive treatment with other classes of drugs, including lithium, thyroid hormone, and dopamine agonists. Patients whose response to an SSRI disappears over time may benefit from the addition of buspirone (10 mg tid) or pindolol (2.5 mg tid) or small amounts of a tricyclic antidepressant such as desipramine (25 mg bid or tid). Once significant remission is achieved, drug treatment should be continued for at least 6 to 9 months to prevent relapse. In patients who have had two or more episodes of depression, indefinite maintenance treatment should be considered.

It is essential to counsel patients about depression and the medications they are receiving. An educational approach is best, describing what is known about the depressive syndrome and how the medications may help. Advice about stress reduction, side effects, and expected length of treatment and cautions that alcohol may exacerbate depressive symptoms and impede drug response are helpful. Patients should be given time to describe their experience and the impact it has had on them, their family, and their outlook. Occasional empathic silence may be as helpful for the treatment alliance as verbal reassurance.

BIPOLAR DISORDER **Clinical Manifestations** Bipolar disorder is common, affecting approximately 3 million persons in the United States, but often difficult to diagnose. It is characterized by unpredictable swings in mood from mania (or hypomania) to depression. Some patients suffer only from recurrent attacks of *mania*, which in its pure form is associated with increased psychomotor activity; excessive social extroversion; decreased need for sleep; impulsivity and impairment in judgment; and expansive, grandiose, and sometimes irritable mood (Table 385-10). In severe mania, patients may experience delusions and paranoid thinking indistinguishable from schizophrenia. Half of patients with bipolar disorder present with a mixture of psychomotor agitation and activation with dysphoria, anxiety, and irritability. It may be difficult to distinguish *mixed mania* from *agitated depression*. In some bipolar patients (*bipolar II disorder*), the full criteria for mania are lacking, and the requisite recurrent depressions are separated by periods of mild activation and increased energy (hypomania). In *cyclothymic disorder*, there are numerous hypomanic periods, usually of relatively short duration, alternating with clusters of depressive symptoms that fail, either in severity or duration, to meet the criteria of major depression. The mood fluctuations are chronic and should be present for at least 2 years before the diagnosis is made.

Manic episodes typically emerge over a period of days to weeks, but onset within hours is possible, usually in the early morning hours. An untreated episode of either depression or mania can be as short as several weeks or last as long as 8 to 12 months, and rare patients have an unremitting chronic course. The term *rapid cycling* is used for patients who have four or more episodes of either depression or mania in a given year. This pattern occurs in 15% of all patients, almost all of whom are women. In some cases, rapid cycling is linked to an underlying thyroid dysfunction and, in others, is iatrogenically triggered by prolonged antidepressant treatment.

Although bipolar illness is associated with frequent episodic recurrence, it was once thought to have a favorable prognosis and outcome. More recent data, however, show that approximately half of patients with the disorder have sustained difficulties in work performance and psychosocial functioning. The most frequent age of onset for bipolar disorder is between 20 and 30 years of age, but many individuals report premorbid symptoms in late childhood or early adolescence. The prevalence is similar for men and women; women are likely to have more depressive and men more manic episodes over a lifetime.

Differential Diagnosis The differential diagnosis of mania includes toxic effects of stimulant or sympathomimetic drugs as well as secondary mania induced by hyperthyroidism, AIDS, or neurologic

Table 385-10 Criteria for a Manic Episode

A. A distinct period of abnormally and persistently elevated, expansive, or irritable mood, lasting at least 1 week (or any duration if hospitalization is necessary)
B. During the period of mood disturbance, three (or more) of the following symptoms have persisted (four if the mood is only irritable) and have been present to a significant degree:
   1. Inflated self-esteem or grandiosity
   2. Decreased need for sleep (e.g., feels rested after only 3 hours of sleep)
   3. More talkative than usual or pressure to keep talking
   4. Flight of ideas or subjective experience that thoughts are racing
   5. Distractibility (i.e., attention too easily drawn to unimportant or irrelevant external stimuli)
   6. Increase in goal-directed activity (either socially, at work or school, or sexually) or psychomotor agitation
   7. Excessive involvement in pleasurable activities that have a high potential for painful consequences (e.g., engaging in unrestrained buying sprees, sexual indiscretions, or foolish business investments)
C. The symptoms do not meet criteria for a mixed episode.
D. The mood disturbance is sufficiently severe to cause marked impairment in occupational functioning or in usual social activities or relationships with others, or to necessitate hospitalization to prevent harm to self or others, or there are psychotic features.
E. The symptoms are not due to the direct physiologic effects of a substance (e.g., a drug of abuse, a medication, or other treatment) or a general medical condition (e.g., hyperthyroidism).

Note: Manic-like episodes that are clearly caused by somatic antidepressant treatment (e.g., medication, electroconvulsive therapy, light therapy) should not count toward a diagnosis of bipolar I disorder.

SOURCE: *Diagnostic and Statistical Manual of Mental Disorders*, 4th ed.

disorders, such as Huntington's or Wilson's disease, or cerebrovascular accidents. Comorbidity with alcohol and substance abuse is common, either because of poor judgment and increased impulsivity or because of an attempt at self-medication.

Etiology and Pathophysiology Evidence for a genetic predisposition to bipolar disorder is significant. The concordance rate for monozygotic twin pairs approaches 80%, and segregation analyses are consistent with autosomal dominant transmission. Several chromosomal locations for the gene have been proposed in the past decade on the basis of linkage analysis in affected families. None, however, has yet received convincing confirmation.

The pathophysiologic mechanisms underlying the profound and recurrent mood swings of bipolar disorder remain unknown. Cellular models of changes in membrane Na^+- and K^+-activated ATPase and proposals of disordered signal transduction mechanisms involving the phosphoinositol system and GTP-binding proteins have received the most attention. Alterations in glutamate regulation and in neuroprotective transcription factors are also being investigated as possible explanations for the therapeutic effects of lithium.

Neurophysiologic studies suggest that patients with bipolar disorder have altered circadian rhythmicity. Lithium may exert its therapeutic benefit through a resynchronization of intrinsic rhythms keyed to the light/dark cycle (Chap. 27). Neuroimaging techniques have also identified a higher rate of subcortical white matter abnormalities in patients than in age-matched controls.

℞ TREATMENT (Table 385-11) Lithium carbonate is the mainstay of treatment in bipolar disorder, although sodium valproate is equally effective in acute mania. Carbamazepine is also efficacious. The response rate to lithium carbonate is 70 to 80% in acute mania, with beneficial effects appearing in 1 to 2 weeks. Lithium also has a prophylactic effect in prevention of recurrent mania, and, to a lesser extent, in the prevention of recurrent depression. A simple cation, lithium is rapidly absorbed from the gastrointestinal tract and remains unbound to plasma or tissue proteins. Some 95% of a given dose is excreted unchanged through the kidneys within 24 h.

Serious side effects from lithium administration are rare, but minor complaints such as gastrointestinal discomfort, nausea, diarrhea, polyuria, weight gain, skin eruptions, alopecia, and edema are common. Over time, urine-concentrating ability may be decreased, but significant nephrotoxicity does not occur. In a small subset of patients in whom excessive polyuria occurs (>3000 mL/24 h), dose or schedule adjustments or the adjunctive use of diuretics should be considered. Lithium exerts an antithyroid effect by interfering with the synthesis and release of thyroid hormones. Approximately 5% of patients taking lithium for ≥18 months develop hypothyroidism, with women more likely to be affected than men. Iatrogenic hypothyroidism should be ruled out in any patient who experiences a recurrence of depressive symptomatology during lithium treatment. More serious side effects include tremor, interference with concentration and memory, ataxia, dysarthria, and incoordination. ECG changes of T wave flattening and conduction delays may occur. There is suggestive, but not conclusive, evidence that lithium is teratogenic, inducing cardiac malformations in the first trimester.

In the treatment of acute mania, lithium is initiated at 300 mg bid or tid, and the dose is then increased by 300 mg every 2 to 3 days to achieve blood levels of 0.8 to 1.2 meq/L. Before initiating treatment the physician should obtain baseline measures of electrolytes, creatinine, thyroid function, and a complete blood count (CBC). Because the therapeutic effect of lithium may not appear until 7 to 10 days of treatment, adjunctive usage of lorazepam (1 to 2 mg every 4 h) or clonazepam (0.5 to 1 mg every 4 h) may be beneficial to control agitation. Antipsychotics are indicated in patients with severe agitation who respond only partially to benzodiazepines. These agents should be discontinued in the transition to maintenance lithium therapy. Patients using lithium should be monitored closely, since the blood levels required to achieve a therapeutic benefit are close to those associated with neurotoxicity. Risk factors for neurotoxicity include concomitant medical illness, decrease in salt intake, or concurrent use of medications that may increase the serum level of lithium (neuroleptics, diuretics, and calcium channel blockers). Once stabilization is achieved, the lithium level can be monitored on a bimonthly basis, and thyroid and renal functions on a biannual basis, or more frequently if clinical change occurs.

Valproic acid is an alternative in patients who cannot tolerate lithium or respond poorly to it. Valproic acid may be better than lithium for patients who have a rapid-cycling course (i.e., more than four episodes a year) or who present with a mixed or dysphoric mania. Valproic acid is usually started at 500 to 750 mg/d in divided doses. The dose is increased every several days to achieve blood levels in the range of 50 to 100 μg/mL, which typically are achieved at a dose of 1000 to 2500 mg/d. The most serious adverse effects of valproic acid are hepatoxicity, which may be fatal, and hyponatremia. Such cases are fortunately rare, but periodic monitoring of liver enzymes, particularly during the first 90 days of treatment, is indicated.

Carbamazepine, although not formally approved by the U.S. Food and Drug Administration (FDA) for bipolar disorder, has clinical efficacy in the treatment of acute mania. Carbamazepine is initiated at 400 to 600 mg/d in divided doses, and the dose is increased to achieve a blood level of 4 to 12 mg/L. Carbamazepine may induce a benign leukopenia, but the risk of aplastic anemia is minimal. Nevertheless, it is wise to obtain a CBC periodically.

Preliminary evidence also suggests that other anticonvulsant agents such as gabapentin, lamotrigine, and topiramate may possess some therapeutic benefit.

The recurrent nature of bipolar mood disorder necessitates maintenance treatment. Maintenance of blood lithium levels of at least 0.8 mg/L is important to achieve optimal prophylaxis. Compliance is frequently an issue and often requires enlistment and education of concerned family members to avoid relapse. Efforts to identify and limit psychosocial factors that may trigger episodes are important, as is an emphasis on life-style regularity. Antidepressant medications are sometimes required for the treatment of severe breakthrough depressions, but their use should generally be avoided during maintenance treatment because of the risk of precipitating mania or accelerating the cycle frequency. Loss of efficacy over time may be observed with any of the mood-stabilizing agents. In such situations, an alternative agent or combination therapy is usually helpful.

Table 385-11 Clinical Pharmacology of Mood Stabilizers

Agent and Dosing	Side Effects and Other Effects
Lithium Starting dose: 300 mg bid or tid Therapeutic blood level: 0.8–1.2 meq/L	*Common side effects:* nausea/anorexia/diarrhea, fine tremor, thirst, polyuria, fatigue, weight gain, acne, folliculitis, neutrophilia, hypothyroidism Blood level is increased by thiazides, tetracyclines, and NSAIDs Blood level is decreased by bronchodilators, verapamil, and carbonic anhydrase inhibitors *Rare side effects:* Neurotoxicity, renal toxicity, hypercalcemia, ECG changes
Valproic acid Starting dose: 250 mg tid Therapeutic blood level: 50–125 μg/mL	*Common side effects:* Nausea/anorexia, weight gain, sedation, tremor, rash, alopecia Inhibits hepatic metabolism of other medications *Rare side effects:* Pancreatitis, hepatoxicity, Stevens-Johnson syndrome
Carbamazepine Starting dose: 200 mg bid Therapeutic blood level: 4–12 μg/mL	*Common side effects:* Nausea/anorexia, sedation, rash, dizziness/ataxia Induces hepatic metabolism of other medications *Rare side effects:* Hyponatremia, agranulocytosis, Stevens-Johnson syndrome

NOTE: NSAID, nonsteroidal anti-inflammatory drug; ECG, electrocardiogram.

Table 385-12 Expert Consensus Guidelines on the Drug Treatment of Acute Mania and Bipolar Depression

Condition	Preferred Agents
Euphoric mania	Lithium
Mixed/dysphoric mania	Valproic acid
Mania with psychosis	Valproic acid with olanzapine Conventional antipsychotic or risperidone
Hypomania	Lithium or valproic acid alone
Severe depression with psychosis	Venlafaxine, bupropion, *or* paroxetine *plus* lithium *plus* olanzapine, *or* risperidone; consider ECT
Severe depression without psychosis	Bupropion, paroxetine, sertraline, venlafaxine, *or* citalopram *plus* lithium
Mild to moderate depression	Lithium alone; add bupropion if needed

NOTE: ECT, electroconvulsive therapy.
SOURCE: From GS Sachs et al: Postgrad Med April, 2000.

Consensus guidelines for the treatment of acute mania and bipolar depression are described in Table 385-12.

SOMATOFORM DISORDERS

CLINICAL MANIFESTATIONS Patients with multiple somatic complaints that cannot be explained by a known medical condition or by the effects of alcohol or of recreational or prescription drugs are seen commonly in primary care practice; one survey indicates a prevalence of 5%. The somatoform disorders include a variety of conditions that differ in terms of the specific symptoms that are present and in whether or not the symptoms are intentionally produced. In *somatization disorder*, the patient presents with multiple physical complaints referable to different organ systems (Table 385-13). Onset is usually before age 30, and the disorder is persistent. Formal diagnostic criteria require the recording of at least four pain, two gastrointestinal, one sexual, and one pseudoneurologic symptom. Patients with somatization disorder often present with dramatic complaints, but the complaints are inconsistent. Symptoms of comorbid anxiety and mood disorder are common and may be the result of drug interactions due to regimens initiated independently by different physicians. Patients with somatization disorder may be impulsive and demanding and frequently qualify for a formal comorbid psychiatric diagnosis. In *conversion disorder*, the symptoms focus on deficits that involve voluntary motor or sensory function and on psychological factors that initiate or exacerbate the medical presentation. Like somatization disorder, the deficit is not intentionally produced or simulated, as is the case in factitious disorder (malingering). In *hypochondriasis*, the essential feature is a belief of serious medical illness that persists despite reassurance and appropriate medical evaluation. As with somatization disorder, patients with hypochondriasis have a history of poor relationships with physicians stemming from their sense that they have been evaluated and treated inappropriately or inadequately. Hypochondriasis can be disabling in intensity and is persistent, with waxing and waning symptomatology.

In *factitious illnesses*, the patient consciously and voluntarily produces physical symptoms of illness. The term *Munchausen's syndrome* is reserved for individuals with particularly dramatic, chronic, or severe factitious illness. In true factitious illness, the sick role itself is gratifying. A variety of signs, symptoms, and diseases have been either simulated or caused by factitious behavior, the most common including chronic diarrhea, fever of unknown origin, intestinal bleeding or hematuria, seizures, and hypoglycemia. Factitious disorder is usually not diagnosed until 5 to 10 years after its onset, and it can produce significant social and medical costs. In *malingering*, the fabrication derives from a desire for some external reward, such as a narcotic medication or disability reimbursement.

Table 385-13 Diagnostic Criteria for Somatization Disorder

A. A history of many physical complaints beginning before age 30 years that occur over a period of several years and result in treatment being sought or significant impairment in social, occupational, or other important areas of functioning.
B. Each of the following criteria must have been met, with individual symptoms occurring at any time during the course of the disturbance:
   1. *Four pain symptoms:* a history of pain related to at least four different sites or functions (e.g., head, abdomen, back, joints, extremities, chest, rectum, during menstruation, during sexual intercourse, or during urination)
   2. *Two gastrointestinal symptoms:* a history of at least two gastrointestinal symptoms other than pain (e.g., nausea, bloating, vomiting other than during pregnancy, diarrhea, or intolerance of several different foods)
   3. *One sexual symptom:* a history of at least one sexual or reproductive symptom other than pain (e.g., sexual indifference, erectile or ejaculatory dysfunction, irregular menses, excessive menstrual bleeding, vomiting throughout pregnancy)
   4. *One pseudoneurologic symptom:* a history of at least one symptom or deficit suggesting a neurologic condition not limited to pain (conversion symptoms such as impaired coordination or balance, paralysis or localized weakness, difficulty swallowing or lump in throat, aphonia, urinary retention, hallucinations, loss of touch or pain sensation, double vision, blindness, deafness, seizures; dissociative symptoms such as amnesia; or loss of consciousness other than fainting)
C. Either of the following:
   1. After appropriate investigation, each of the symptoms in criterion B cannot be fully explained by a known general medical condition or the direct effects of a substance (e.g., a drug of abuse, a medication)
   2. When there is a related general medical condition, the physical complaints or resulting social or occupational impairment are in excess of what would be expected from the history, physical examination, or laboratory findings
D. The symptoms are not intentionally produced or feigned (as in factitious disorder or malingering).

SOURCE: *Diagnostic and Statistical Manual of Mental Disorders*, 4th ed.

℞ **TREATMENT** Patients with somatization disorders are frequently subjected to multiple diagnostic testing and exploratory surgeries in an attempt to find their "real" illness. Such an approach is doomed to failure and does not address the core issue. Successful treatment is best achieved through behavior modification, in which access to the physician is tightly regulated and adjusted to provide a sustained and predictable level of support that is less clearly contingent on the patient's level of presenting distress. Visits can be brief and should not be associated with a need for a diagnostic or treatment action. Although the literature is limited, some patients with somatization disorder may benefit from antidepressant treatment. Fluoxetine and MAOIs have both been found to be useful in reducing obsessive ruminations, dysphoria, and anxious preoccupation in patients with multiple somatic complaints.

The treatment of factitious disorder is complicated in that any attempt to confront the patient usually only creates a sense of humiliation and causes the patient to abandon treatment from that caregiver. A better strategy is to introduce psychological causation as one of a number of possible explanations and to include factitious illness as an option in the differential diagnoses that are discussed. Without directly linking psychotherapeutic intervention to the diagnosis, the patient can be offered a face-saving means by which the pathologic relationship with the health care system can be examined and alternative approaches to life stressors developed.

PERSONALITY DISORDERS

CLINICAL MANIFESTATIONS Personality disorders are characteristic patterns of thinking, feeling, and interpersonal behavior that are relatively inflexible and cause significant functional impairment or subjective distress for the individual. The observed behaviors are not secondary to another mental disorder, nor are they precipitated by substance abuse or a general medical condition. This distinction is often difficult to make in clinical practice, as personality change may be the first sign of serious neurologic, endocrine, or other medical illness. Patients with frontal lobe tumors, for example, can present with changes in motivation and personality while the results of the neurologic examination remain within normal limits. Personality traits are stable over time and environmental situation and are recognizable in adolescence or early adult life. Although DSM-IV portrays personality disorders as qualitatively distinct categories, there is an alternative perspective that personality characteristics vary as a continuum between normal functioning and formal mental disorder.

Personality disorders have been grouped into three clusters that share similar attributes. *Cluster A* includes paranoid, schizoid, and schizotypal personality disorders. It includes individuals who are odd and eccentric and who maintain an emotional distance from others. Individuals have a restricted emotional range and remain socially isolated. Patients with schizotypal personality disorder frequently have unusual perceptual experiences and express magical beliefs about the external world. The essential feature of paranoid personality disorder is a pervasive mistrust and suspiciousness of others to an extent that is unjustified by available evidence. *Cluster B* disorders include antisocial, borderline, histrionic, and narcissistic types and describe individuals whose behavior is impulsive, excessively emotional, and erratic. *Cluster C* incorporates avoidant, dependent, and obsessive-compulsive personality types; enduring traits are anxiety and fear. The boundaries between cluster types are to some extent artificial, and many patients who meet criteria for one personality disorder also meet criteria for aspects of another. The risk of a comorbid major mental disorder is increased in patients who qualify for a diagnosis of personality disorder.

℞ TREATMENT Historically, recommended treatment for personality disorders was long-term psychotherapy, in which the pathologic patterns of interaction with the world at large could be relived and examined through the corrective emotional experience of the controlled therapeutic relationship. More recently, the recognition that personality derives in part from biologically determined components of temperament has given rise to the empirical use of drugs to treat specific symptom clusters as well as any coexisting major mental disorder. Antidepressant medications and low-dose antipsychotic drugs have some efficacy in cluster A personality disorders, while anticonvulsant mood-stabilizing agents and MAOIs may be considered for patients with cluster B diagnoses who show marked mood reactivity, behavioral dyscontrol, and/or rejection hypersensitivity. Anxious or fearful cluster C patients often have a response to medication that parallels that for patients with axis I anxiety disorders. In all cases, it is important for both the physician and the patient to have reasonable expectations as to the possible effect of the medication and any associated side effects. Beneficial responses may be subtle and observable only over time.

SCHIZOPHRENIA

CLINICAL MANIFESTATIONS Schizophrenia is a heterogeneous syndrome characterized by perturbations of language, perception, thinking, social activity, affect, and volition. There are no pathognomonic features. The syndrome commonly begins in late adolescence, has an insidious onset, and, classically, a poor outcome, progressing from social withdrawal and perceptual distortions to a state of chronic delusions and hallucinations. Patients may present with positive symptoms (such as conceptual disorganization, delusions, or hallucinations) or negative symptoms (loss of function, anhedonia, decreased emotional expression, impaired concentration, and diminished social engagement) and must have at least two of these for a 1-month period and continuous signs for at least 6 months to meet formal diagnostic criteria. "Negative" symptoms predominate in one-third of the schizophrenic population and are associated with a poor long-term outcome and a poor response to drug treatment. However, marked variability in the course and individual character of symptoms is typical.

Schizophrenia can be classified according to the specific symptomatology present, although such distinctions do not correlate well with either course of illness or response to treatment, and many individuals have symptoms of more than one type. The four main symptom subtypes are catatonic, paranoid, disorganized, and residual. *Catatonic-type* describes patients whose clinical presentation is dominated by profound changes in motor activity, negativism, and echolalia or echopraxia. *Paranoid-type* describes patients who have a prominent preoccupation with a specific delusional system and who otherwise do not qualify as having *disorganized-type* disease, in which disorganized speech and behavior are accompanied by a superficial or silly affect. In *residual-type* disease, negative symptomatology exists in the absence of delusions, hallucinations, or motor disturbance. The diagnosis of *schizophreniform disorder* is reserved for patients who meet the symptom requirements but not the duration requirements for schizophrenia, and that of *schizoaffective disorder* is used for those whose symptoms of schizophrenia are independent of associated periods of mood disturbance. Prognosis depends not on symptom severity but on the response to antipsychotic medication. Patients may present with acute rather than insidious onset of symptoms, and remission without recurrence does occur. About 10% of schizophrenic patients commit suicide. As currently defined, schizophrenia is present in 0.85% of individuals worldwide. Overall, lifetime prevalence is approximately 1 to 1.5%.

The societal costs of schizophrenia are substantial. An estimated 300,000 episodes of acute schizophrenia occur annually, resulting in direct and indirect costs that have been estimated at >$33 billion.

DIFFERENTIAL DIAGNOSIS For a diagnosis of schizophrenia to be made, the symptom complex must cause significant dysfunction in social or occupational domains and last for at least 6 months. The diagnosis is principally one of exclusion, requiring the absence of significant associated mood symptoms, any relevant medical condition, and substance abuse. Drug reactions that cause hallucinations, paranoia, confusion, or bizarre behavior may be dose-related or idiosyncratic; β-adrenergic blockers, clonidine, cycloserine, quinacrine, and procaine derivatives are most commonly associated with these symptoms. Drug causes should be ruled out in any case of newly emergent psychosis. The general neurologic examination in patients with schizophrenia is usually normal, but motor rigidity, tremor, and dyskinesias are noted in one-quarter of untreated patients.

EPIDEMIOLOGY AND PATHOPHYSIOLOGY Epidemiologic surveys identify three principal risk factors for schizophrenia: (1) genetic susceptibility, (2) early developmental insults, and (3) winter birth. Family, twin, and adoption studies show that genetic factors are involved in at least a subset of individuals who develop schizophrenia. Using conservative diagnostic definitions, schizophrenia is observed in approximately 6.6% of all first-degree relatives of an affected proband. If both parents are affected, the risk for offspring is 40%. The concordance rate for monozygotic twins is 50%, compared to 10% for dizygotic twins. Examination of families in which aggregation of schizophrenia occurs has revealed an increased incidence of other psychotic and nonpsychotic psychiatric disorders as well, including schizoaffective disorder and *schizotypal* and *schizoid personality disorders*, the latter terms designating individuals who show a lifetime pattern of social and interpersonal deficits characterized by an inability to form close interpersonal relationships, eccentric behavior, and mild perceptual distortions. Some relatives and individuals with schizophrenia have been found to have distinctive patterns in expressing emotion, most often involving increased criticism, hostility, and emotional overinvolvement.

There is evidence that environmental influences modulate genetic factors in the expression of schizophrenia, and, in sporadic cases, may serve as a sufficient cause. Gestational and birth complications, including Rh factor incompatibility, prenatal exposure to influenza during the second trimester, and prenatal nutritional deficiency have been implicated. Studies of monozygotic twins discordant for schizophrenia have reported neuroanatomic differences between affected and unaffected siblings, supporting a "two-strike" etiology involving both genetic susceptibility and an environmental insult. The latter might involve localized hypoxia during critical stages of brain development.

Neuroimaging and postmortem studies have identified a number of structural and functional abnormalities, including (1) enlargement of the lateral and third ventricles with associated cortical atrophy and sulcal enlargement; (2) volumetric reductions in the amygdala, hippocampus, right prefrontal cortex, and thalamus; (3) altered asymmetry of the planum temporale; and (4) decreases in neuronal metabolism in the thalamus and prefrontal cortex. Some, but not all, prospective studies record progressive reduction in hemispheric volume over years. Neuropathologic studies have reported changes in the size, orientation, and density of cells in the hippocampus and, in the prefrontal cerebral cortex, decreases in neuronal number and the density of interneurons in layer II as well as an increased density of pyramidal cells in layer V. These observations suggest that schizophrenia results from a disturbance in a cortical striatal–thalamic circuit resulting in deficits in sensory filtering and attentional behavior. Although the formal diagnostic requirements for schizophrenia are not usually met until early adult life, children who eventually develop the disorder may exhibit subtle deficits in motor function, cognition, and emotional expression from an early age.

Table 385-14 Antipsychotic Agents

Name	Usual PO Daily Dose, mg	Side Effects	Sedation	Comments
TYPICAL ANTIPSYCHOTICS				
Low-potency				
Chlorpromazine (Thorazine)	100–1000	Anticholinergic effects; orthostasis; photosensitivity; cholestasis	+ + +	EPSEs usually not prominent; can cause anticholinergic delirium in elderly patients
Thioridazine (Mellaril)	100–800		+ + +	
Mid-potency				
Trifluoperazine (Stelazine)	2–15	Fewer anticholinergic side effects; fewer EPSEs than with higher potency agents	+ +	Well tolerated by most patients
Perphenazine (Trilafon)	4–32		+ +	
High potency				
Haloperidol (Haldol)	0.5–10	No anticholinergic side effects; EPSEs often prominent	0/+	Often prescribed in doses that are too high; long-acting injectable forms of haloperidol and fluphenazine available
Fluphenazine (Prolixin)	1–10		0/+	
Thiothixene (Navane)	2–20		0/+	
NOVEL ANTIPSYCHOTICS				
Clozapine (Clozaril)	200–600	Agranulocytosis (1%); weight gain; seizures; drooling; hyperthermia	+ +	Requires weekly WBC
Risperidone (Risperdal)	2–6	Orthostasis	+	Requires slow titration; EPSEs observed with doses >6 mg qd
Olanzapine (Zyprexa)	10–20	Weight gain	+ +	Generally well tolerated
Seroquel (Quetiapine)	300–400	Sedation; weight gain; anxiety	+ + +	Bid dosing

NOTE: EPSEs, extrapyramidal side effects; WBC, white blood count.

The hypothesized alterations in cortical neuronal circuitry are paralleled clinically by impairments in attention and cortical information processing, autonomic nervous system activation, and habituation. Schizophrenic individuals are highly distractible and demonstrate deficits in perceptual-motor speed, ability to shift attention, and filtering out of background stimuli. Event-related evoked potential studies of schizophrenia have defined a specific reduction in P300 amplitude to a novel stimulus, which implicates an impairment in cognitive processing. Impaired information processing is found in unaffected family members.

Despite evidence for a genetic causation, the results of molecular genetic linkage studies in schizophrenia are inconclusive. Reports of linkage of schizophrenia to loci on chromosomes 1, 5, 6, 8, 11, and 22 and other regions have not been formally replicated and have led to larger scale association studies currently underway.

The *dopamine hypothesis* of schizophrenia is based on the serendipitous discovery that agents that diminish dopaminergic activity have beneficial effects in reducing the acute symptoms and signs of psychosis, specifically agitation, anxiety, and hallucinations. Amelioration of delusions and social withdrawal is less dramatic. Thus far, however, evidence for increased dopaminergic activity is indirect. An increase in the activity of nigrostriatal and mesolimbic systems and a decrease in mesocortical tracts innervating the prefrontal cortex is hypothesized, although it is likely that other neurotransmitters, including serotonin, acetylcholine, glutamate, and GABA also contribute to the pathophysiology of the illness. Involvement of excitatory amino acids is postulated, based on the finding that NMDA receptor antagonists and channel blockers, such as phencyclidine (PCP) and ketamine, produce characteristic signs of schizophrenia in normal individuals.

℞ **TREATMENT** Antipsychotic agents (Table 385-14) remain the cornerstone of acute and maintenance treatment of schizophrenia and are effective in the treatment of hallucinations, delusions, and thought disorders, regardless of etiology. The exact mechanism of action remains incompletely understood, but dopaminergic receptor blockade in the limbic system and basal ganglia appears to be an essential element, since the clinical potencies of traditional antipsychotic drugs parallel their affinities for the D_2 receptor, and even the newer "atypical" agents exert some degree of D_2 receptor blockade. All neuroleptics induce expression of the immediate-early gene c-*fos* in the nucleus accumbens, a dopaminergic site connecting prefrontal and limbic cortices. The clinical efficacy of newer atypical neuroleptics, however, may involve D_1, D_3, and D_4 receptor blockade, α_1- and α_2-noradrenergic activity, and/or altering the relationship between $5HT_2$ and D_2 receptor activity.

Conventional neuroleptics differ in their potency and side-effect profile. Older agents, such as chlorpromazine and thioridazine, are more sedating and anticholinergic and more likely to cause orthostatic hypotension, while higher potency antipsychotics, such as haloperidol, perphenazine, and thiothixene, carry a higher risk of inducing extrapyramidal side effects. The model atypical antipsychotic agent is clozapine, a dibenzodiazepine that has a greater potency in blocking the $5HT_2$ than the D_2 receptor and a much higher affinity for the D_4 than the D_2 receptor. Its principal disadvantage is risk of blood dyscrasia, requiring regular monitoring of the CBC. Unlike other antipsychotics, clozapine does not cause a rise in prolactin level. Approximately 30% of patients have a better antipsychotic response to these agents than to traditional neuroleptics, suggesting that they will increasingly displace the older-generation drugs. Clozapine appears to be the most effective member of this class; however, its side-effect profile makes it most appropriate for treatment-resistant cases. *Clozapine* increases the activity of the immediate-early gene c-*fos* in the prefrontal cortex, the neuroanatomic region having the highest concentration of D_4 receptors and an area thought to mediate the specific executive functions that are prominently impaired in schizophrenia. *Risperidone*, a benzisoxazole derivative, is more potent at $5HT_2$ than D_2 receptor sites, like clozapine, but it also exerts significant α_2 antagonism, a property that may contribute to its perceived ability to improve mood and increase motor activity. Risperidone is not as effective as clozapine in treatment-resistant cases but does not carry a risk of blood dyscrasia. *Olanzapine* is more similar neurochemically to clozapine but has a significant risk of inducing weight gain. *Quetiapine* is distinct in having a weak D_2 effect but potent α_1 and histamine blockade.

Conventional antipsychotic agents are effective in ~70% of patients presenting with a first episode. Improvement may be observed within hours or days, but full remission usually requires 6 to 8 weeks. The choice of agent depends principally on the side-effect profile and cost of treatment or on a past personal or family history of a favorable response to the drug in question. Atypical agents appear to be more effective in treating negative symptoms and improving cognitive function. Equivalent treatment response can usually be achieved with relatively low doses of any drug selected, i.e., 4 to 6 mg/d of haloperidol, 10 to 15 mg of olanzapine, or 4 to 6 mg/d of risperidone. Doses in this range result in >80% D_2 receptor blockade, and there is little evidence that higher doses increase either the rapidity or degree of response. Maintenance treatment requires careful attention to the possibility of relapse and monitoring for the development of a movement disorder. Intermittent drug treatment is less effective than regular dosing, but gradual dose reduction is likely to improve social functioning in many schizophrenic patients who have been maintained at high doses. If medications are completely discontinued, however, the relapse rate is ~60% within 6 months. Long-acting injectable preparations (haloperidol decanoate and fluphenazine decanoate) are considered when noncompliance with oral therapy leads to relapses. In treatment-resistant patients, a transition to clozapine usually results in rapid improvement, but a prolonged delay in response in some cases necessitates a 6- to 9-month trial for maximal benefit to occur.

Antipsychotic medications can cause a broad range of side effects, including lethargy, weight gain, postural hypotension, constipation, and dry mouth. Extrapyramidal symptoms such as dystonia, akathisia, and akinesia are also frequent with traditional agents and may contribute to poor compliance if not specifically addressed. Anticholinergic and parkinsonian symptoms respond well to trihexyphenidyl, 2 mg bid, or benztropine mesylate, 1 to 2 mg bid. Akathisia may respond to beta blockers. In rare cases, more serious and occasionally life-threatening side effects may emerge, including ventricular arrhythmias, gastrointestinal obstruction, retinal pigmentation, obstructive jaundice, and neuroleptic malignant syndrome (characterized by hyperthermia, autonomic dysfunction, muscular rigidity, and elevated creatine phosphokinase levels). The most serious adverse effects of clozapine are agranulocytosis, which has an incidence of 1%, and induction of seizures, which has an incidence of 10%. Weekly white blood cell counts are required, particularly during the first 3 months of treatment.

A serious side effect of long-term use of the classic antipsychotic agents is *tardive dyskinesia*, characterized by repetitive, involuntary, and potentially irreversible movements of the tongue and lips (bucco-linguo-masticatory triad), and, in approximately half of cases, choreoathetoid movements of the limbs (Chap. 22). Tardive dyskinesia has an incidence of ~4% per year of exposure, and a maximal prevalence of ~20% in chronic patients treated with high-dose neuroleptics. The risk associated with the newer atypical agents is unknown but expected to be much less. The prevalence increases with age and with total dose and duration of drug administration, but unknown individual factors play the greatest part in determining risk. The cause of tardive dyskinesia is unknown, but evidence suggests that chronic neuroleptic treatment increases the formation of free radicals and perhaps damages mitochondrial energy metabolism. Vitamin E may reduce abnormal involuntary movements if given early in the syndrome.

Drug treatment of schizophrenia is by itself insufficient. Psychoeducational efforts directed towards families and relevant community resources have proven to be necessary to maintain stability and optimize prognosis. A treatment model involving a multidisciplinary case-management team that seeks out and closely follows the patient in the community has proven particularly effective, not only in maintaining pharmacologic adherence but also in facilitating occupational achievement and interactions with welfare, legal, and primary medical care systems.

ASSESSMENT AND EVALUATION OF VIOLENCE

Primary care physicians may encounter situations in which familial, domestic, or societal violence is discovered or suspected. Such an awareness can carry legal and moral obligations; many state laws mandate reporting of child, spousal, and elder abuse. Physicians are frequently the first point of contact for both victim and abuser. Between 1 and 2 million older Americans and 1.5 million U.S. children are thought to experience some form of physical maltreatment each year. Spousal abuse is thought to be even more prevalent. A recent survey of internal medicine practices found that 5.5% of all female patients had experienced domestic violence in the previous year, and that these individuals were more likely to suffer from depression, anxiety, somatization disorder, and substance abuse and to have attempted suicide. When domestic violence is suspected, direct but nonjudgmental questioning should be pursued with each party separately—"Do you feel safe at home?" and "If there's a disagreement or a conflict between the two of you, how is it worked out?" In addition to obvious and suggestive physical injury, individuals who are abused frequently express low self-esteem, vague somatic symptomatology, social isolation, and a passive feeling of loss of control. Although it is essential to treat these elements in the victim, the first obligation is to ensure that the perpetrator has taken responsibility for preventing any further violence. Substance abuse and/or dependence and serious mental illness in the abuser may contribute to the risk of harm and require direct intervention. Depending on the situation, law enforcement agencies, community resources such as support groups and shelters, and individual and family counseling can be appropriate components of a treatment plan. A safety plan should be formulated with the victim, in addition to the provision of information about abuse, its likelihood of recurrence, and its tendency to increase in severity and frequency. Antianxiety and antidepressant medications may sometimes be useful in treating the acute symptoms, but only if independent evidence for an appropriate psychiatric diagnosis exists. Antidepressants are generally not indicated when the diagnosis is linked to the social situation, such as an adjustment disorder with depressed mood. The most important element in treatment is the development of a supportive doctor-patient relationship that avoids further blame of the victim.

In certain circumstances, a significant potential for societal violence may be discovered. Sympathetic, but direct, questioning about potential violent impulses, access to weapons, recreational drug use, and specific homicidal ideation is necessary and is sometimes therapeutic in its own right. The existence and possible contribution of such medical conditions as delirium and/or intoxication should be evaluated. Available disposition options for potentially violent patients include police custody, psychiatric hospitalization, and referral to home care, with involvement of family, friends, and caregivers. In deciding which treatment option is most appropriate, clinicians should endeavor to establish an empathic interaction with the patient, while avoiding interventions or stimuli that might precipitate or increase the risk of violent behavior. Formal verbal limit setting may be necessary if the patient reveals the existence of a weapon or becomes increasingly agitated or verbally abusive. Use of the least restrictive intervention is generally the best approach during the initial evaluation.

MENTAL HEALTH PROBLEMS IN THE HOMELESS

There is a high prevalence of mental disorders and substance abuse among homeless and impoverished people. The total number of homeless individuals in the United States is estimated at 2 to 3 million, one-third of whom qualify as having a serious mental disorder. Poor hygiene and nutrition, substance abuse, psychiatric illness, physical trauma, and exposure to the elements combine to make the provision of medical care a challenging enterprise. Only a minority of individuals receive formal mental health care; the main points of contact are outpatient medical clinics and emergency departments. Primary care settings represent a critical site in which housing needs, treatment of substance dependence, and evaluation and treatment of psychiatric illness can most efficiently take place. Successful intervention is dependent on breaking down traditional administrative barriers to health care and recognizing the physical constraints and emotional costs imposed by homelessness. Simplifying health care instructions and follow-up, allowing frequent visits, and dispensing medications in limited amounts that require ongoing contact are possible techniques for establishing a successful therapeutic relationship. Child neglect, resulting in developmental delay and emotional difficulty in addition to other health problems, is unfortunately common and necessitates an effort to evaluate the well being of any offspring independently.

BIBLIOGRAPHY

GENERAL

AMERICAN PSYCHIATRIC ASSOCIATION: *Diagnostic and Statistical Manual of Mental Disorders*, 4th ed. Washington DC, American Psychiatric Association, 1994

BERRETTINI WH: Genetics of psychiatric disease. Annu Rev Med 51:465, 2000

BROADHEAD WE et al: Development and validation of the SDDS-PC screen for multiple mental disorders in primary care. Arch Fam Med 4:211, 1995

EISENSTAT SA, BANCROFT L: Domestic violence. N Engl J Med 341:886, 1999

FUGH-BERMAN A, COTT JM: Dietary supplements and natural products as psychotherapeutic agents. Psychosom Med 61:712, 1999

PROCTOR R et al: Behavioural management in nursing and residential homes: A randomised controlled trial. Lancet 354:26, 1999

SPITZER RL et al: Utility of a new procedure for diagnosing mental disorders in primary care: The Prime-MD study. JAMA 272:1749, 1994

PSYCHOLOGICAL FACTORS IN MEDICAL ILLNESS

ALI A et al: Emotional abuse, self-blame and self-silencing in women with irritable bowel syndrome. Psychosom Med 62:76, 2000

BLOCK SD: Assessing and managing depression in the terminally ill patient. Ann Intern Med 132:209, 2000

BROERS S et al: Psychological functioning and quality of life following bone marrow transplantation: A 3-year follow-up study. J Psychosom Res 48:11, 2000

CARNEY RM et al: Can treating depression reduce mortality after an acute myocardial infarction? Psychosom Med 61:666, 1999

DROSSMAN DA: Presidential address: Gastrointestinal illness and the biopsychosocial model. Psychosom Med 60:258, 1998

MCDANIEL JS et al: Cancer and depression: Theory and treatment. Psychiat Ann 27:360, 1997

ROBINSON RG, YATES WR (eds): *Psychiatric Treatment of the Medically Ill*. New York, Marcel Dekker, 1999

SELNES OA et al: Neurobehavioural sequelae of cardiopulmonary bypass. Lancet 353: 1601, 1999

ANXIETY DISORDERS

BARTOW DH et al: Cognitive-behavioral therapy, imipramine, or their combination for panic disorder. A randomized controlled trial. JAMA 283:2529, 2000

STOUDEMIRE A: Epidemiology and psychopharmacology of anxiety in medical patients. J Clin Psychiatry 57:64, 1996

MOOD DISORDERS

BALDESSARINI RJ, TONDO L: Does lithium treatment still work? Arch Gen Psychiatry 57:187, 2000

BALLENGER JC, et al: Consensus statement on the primary care management of depression from the International Consensus Group on Depression and Anxiety. J Clin Psychiatry 60:54, 1999

CASE DB, SLABY AE: The suicidal patient in family practice. Primary Psychiatry 3:30, 1996

DORIS A et al: Depressive illness. Lancet 354:1369, 1999

FRANK E, THASE ME: Natural history and preventative treatment of recurrent mood disorders. Annu Rev Med 50:453, 1999

IRWIN M et al: Screening for depression in the older adult. Arch Intern Med 159:1701, 1999

KELLER MB et al: A comparison of nefazodone, the cognitive behavioral-analysis system of psychotherapy, and their combination for the treatment of chronic depression. N Engl J Med 342:1462, 2000

KENT JM: SNaRIs, NaSSAs, and NaRIs: New agents for the treatment of depression. Lancet 355:911, 2000

LEIBENLUFT E, SUPPES T: Treating bipolar illness: Focus on treatment algorithms and management of the sleep-wake cycle. Am J Psychiatry 156:1976, 1999

PERSONS JB et al: The role of psychotherapy in the treatment of depression. Arch Gen Psychiatry 53:283, 1996

SOMATOFORM DISORDERS, PERSONALITY AND BEHAVIORAL DISORDERS

KEELEY R et al: Somatoform symptoms and treatment nonadherence in depressed family medicine outpatients. Arch Fam Med 9:46, 2000

SIMON GE et al: An international study of the relation between somatic symptoms and depression. N Engl J Med 341:1329, 1999

SCHIZOPHRENIA

BRZUSTOWICZ LM et al: Location of a major susceptibility locus for familial schizophrenia on chromosome 1q21-22. Science 288:678, 2000

LAURIELLO J et al: A critical review of research on psychosocial treatment of schizophrenia. Biol Psychiatry 46:1409, 1999

MCEVOY JP et al (eds): The expert consensus guideline series: Treatment of schizophrenia 1999. J Clin Psychiatry (Suppl) 60:1, 1999

PULVER AE: Search for schizophrenia susceptibility genes. Biol Psychiatry 47:221, 2000

SCHULTZ SK, ANDREASEN NC: Schizophrenia. Lancet 353:1425, 1999

Section 6
ALCOHOLISM AND DRUG DEPENDENCY

386 BIOLOGY OF ADDICTION

Robert O. Messing

Drug addiction is a chronic, relapsing disorder characterized by compulsion to take a drug and loss of self-control in limiting drug intake. The American Psychiatric Association (*DSM-IV*) uses the term *substance dependence* instead of drug addiction and requires at least three of the following symptoms to be present for diagnosis: (1) tolerance; (2) withdrawal; (3) persistent desire or unsuccessful attempts to reduce use; (4) use in larger amounts than intended; (5) reduction in important social, occupational, or recreational activities because of drug use; (6) considerable time spent obtaining the substance; and (7) continued use despite health, social, or economic problems resulting from substance use. *Substance abuse* is a milder disorder characterized by repetitive drug use that results in social or economic distress. Experimental studies in humans and in animal models (rodents and also simpler organisms such as flies and worms) have begun to elucidate the cellular and molecular mechanisms that mediate the loss of control in drug taking that is the hallmark of addiction. This chapter will review current understanding of the neurobiology of drug abuse relevant to the specific substances discussed in subsequent chapters, namely alcohol (Chap. 387), opioids (Chap. 388), cocaine and marijuana (Chap. 389), and nicotine (Chap. 390).

BEHAVIORAL RESPONSES TO DRUGS OF ABUSE Drugs of abuse produce *euphoria*, which is an emotional state characterized by intensely pleasant feelings. A major reason why users are motivated to seek and take more of a drug is because they perceive

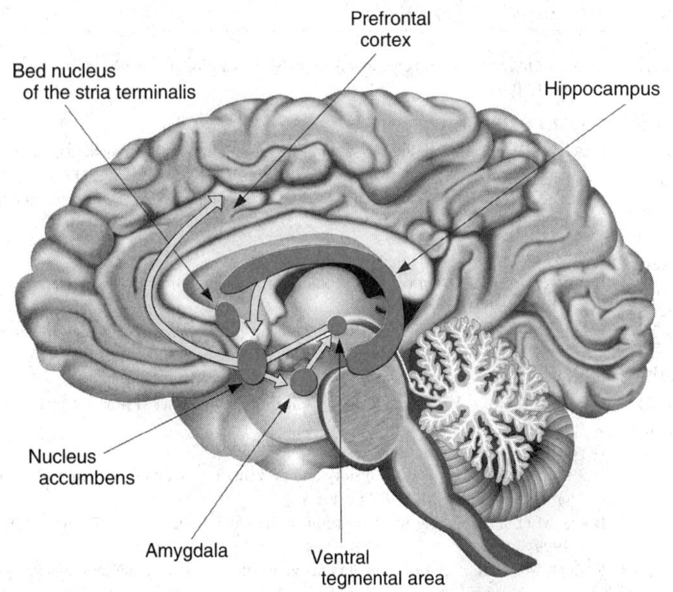

FIGURE 386-1 Mid-sagittal section of the human brain demonstrating limbic structures involved in brain reward pathways.

the experience as *rewarding*. *Reinforcement* refers to the ability of a drug to produce a pleasurable response that motivates the user to take the drug repeatedly. The powerful reinforcing and rewarding properties of abusable drugs can be measured by the tremendous effort experimental animals will expend, e.g., by pressing a lever multiple times, to obtain an oral or intravenous dose of a drug.

Tolerance is a reduction in response to a drug after repeated use and is a normal, adaptive, physiologic response. *Pharmacokinetic tolerance* may arise through an increase in the rate of metabolism. For example, barbiturates induce hepatic microsomal enzymes resulting in more rapid metabolism. *Pharmacodynamic tolerance* results from drug-induced changes in cell signaling and gene expression. Behavioral *sensitization* is a process whereby repeated administration of a drug leads to a progressively stronger behavioral response. Sometimes called "reverse tolerance," it is often measured by examining drug-induced locomotor activation. It generally requires longer intervals between doses to develop than does tolerance. Both tolerance and sensitization can promote repeated drug use. Tolerance develops to the rewarding properties of most abusable drugs, requiring the user to employ higher doses to achieve a euphoric effect. Sensitization also promotes drug self-administration, since rodents will expend greater effort in lever-pressing for drugs to which they are sensitized.

Physical dependence is an adaptive state that develops through resetting of homeostatic mechanisms to permit normal function despite the continued presence of a drug. When drug intake is abruptly terminated in a physically dependent individual, a withdrawal syndrome emerges. The symptoms of withdrawal tend to be opposite to those seen during acute drug exposure. Thus, abstinence from alcohol and other sedative-hypnotics causes nervous system hyperactivity, whereas withdrawal from cocaine and other stimulants is characterized by fatigue, sedation, and depression. Withdrawal symptoms are the principal evidence for physical dependence. Like tolerance, physical dependence is a normal physiologic response to repeated drug exposure and does not necessarily indicate drug abuse or addiction. However, withdrawal can cause intensely negative, unpleasant emotions such as dysphoria, anxiety, and irritability. In animal studies employing intracranial self-stimulation, withdrawal is also associated with reduced brain reward function. Thus, it appears that drug withdrawal can act as a negative reinforcer that contributes to repeated drug use.

Human patients prescribed opioids for treatment of pain may develop tolerance and physical dependence but rarely become addicted. Likewise, in experimental animals, establishing physical dependence is not sufficient to induce voluntary drug self-administration. Instead, it appears that animals and humans seek abusable drugs mainly for their positive reinforcing properties. In susceptible persons, repeated use of abusable drugs induces drug *craving*, a powerful motivational state in which the addict seeks the drug to the exclusion of other activities. Craving is a manifestation of *psychological dependence* on a drug and is most severe during acute abstinence. It is a long-lasting, conditioned response that may be evoked by environmental cues such as sights, smells, or situations associated with previous drug use, even after long periods of drug abstinence. Understanding the mechanisms that underlie susceptibility to drug craving is a critical task in addiction research.

GENETIC FACTORS IN ADDICTION Genetic factors have been studied most extensively in alcoholism (Chap. 387). Patterns of inheritance in humans are most consistent with alcoholism being a polygenic disorder. Some genes confer a reduced risk for alcoholism. Approximately half of all individuals in Asian populations carry an allele of aldehyde dehydrogenase that encodes an isozyme with reduced enzymatic activity. After ingesting alcohol, they have increased blood levels of acetaldehyde and experience vasodilatation, tachycardia, hot sensations, and hypotension. They also report feeling intoxicated at very low doses of alcohol. Individuals expressing this isoenzyme rarely abuse alcohol. Other genetic factors predispose individuals to increased risk for alcoholism. A recent multicenter study of 105 families of alcoholics revealed evidence for susceptibility loci for alcohol dependence on chromosomes 1, 7, and possibly 2. An additional study of a Southwestern Native American population found evidence for genetic linkage to alcohol dependence on chromosomes 4 and 11. The identity of the genes associated with increased risk is not yet known.

NEUROANATOMY OF DRUG REWARD Early studies of intracranial electrical self-stimulation in rodents identified key structures involved in drug reward and motivational aspects of drug dependence (Fig. 386-1). These include the midbrain ventral tegmental area (VTA), median forebrain bundle (MFB), nucleus accumbens, medial frontal cortex, amygdala, and lateral hypothalamus. Many of these structures are key components of a *mesocorticolimbic dopamine system* that is now a principal focus of addiction research. Dopaminergic neurons in the VTA project axons via the MFB to the nucleus accumbens, amygdala, and frontal cortex. Reciprocal projections from γ-aminobutyric acid (GABA)-containing neurons in the nucleus accumbens project back through the MFB onto VTA neurons. Other brain regions modulate this system through opioid peptide, GABA, serotonin, and glutamate inputs that interact with the VTA, nucleus accumbens, and other structures within the system.

Certain nuclei within the mesocorticolimbic dopamine system share similarities in architecture, receptor expression, and connectivity with other brain regions. These related structures reside in the basal forebrain and include the central medial amygdala, bed nucleus of the stria terminalis, and shell of the nucleus accumbens. They appear to constitute a functional entity that has been called the "extended amygdala." The extended amygdala receives inputs from the hippocampus, basolateral amygdala, midbrain, and lateral hypothalamus and sends efferents to the ventral pallidum, VTA, and lateral hypothalamus.

MOLECULAR TARGETS OF ABUSED DRUGS Dopamine released from presynaptic terminals of VTA neurons in the nucleus accumbens is a major mediator of drug reward and reinforcement (Fig. 386-2*A*). Acute administration of all abusable drugs increases extracellular levels of dopamine in the shell of the nucleus accumbens. In addition, dopamine receptor antagonists injected into this region reduce drug self-administration in animals. Dopamine binds to a family of five G protein–coupled, seven-transmembrane receptors that can be grouped into two major classes, D_1-like (D_1 and D_5 receptors) and D_2-like (D_2, D_3, and D_4 receptors). D_1-like receptors activate adenylyl cyclase by coupling to the stimulatory G protein G_s, whereas D_2-like

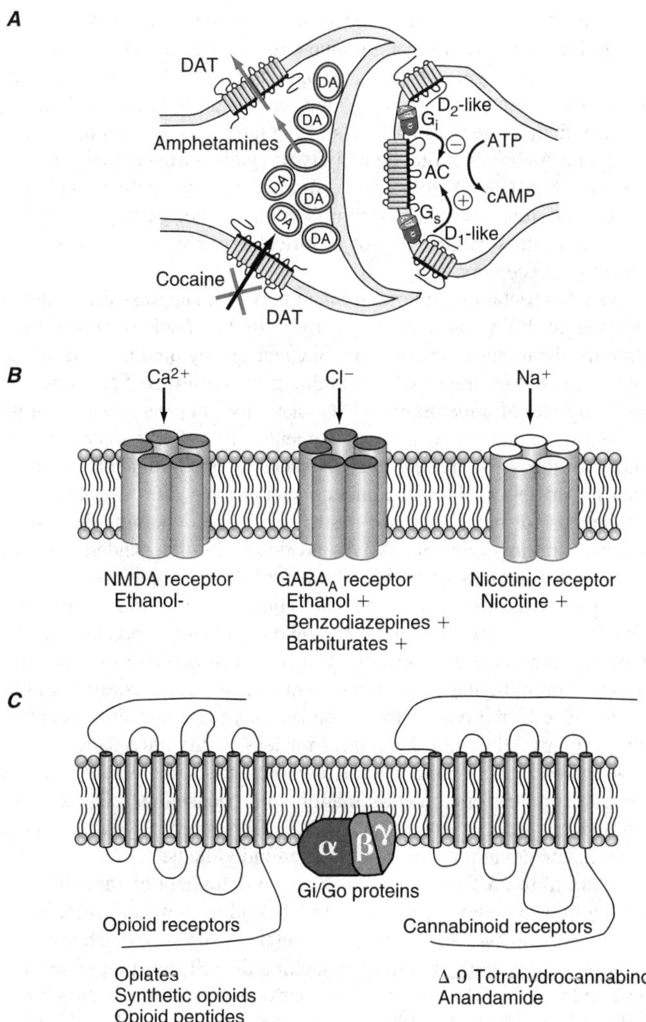

FIGURE 386-2 Schematic representation of molecular targets for drugs of abuse. *A*. Dopaminergic synapse showing a presynaptic axon terminal of a ventral tegmental area dopaminergic neuron (*left*). Dopamine (DA) released from synaptic vesicles in the terminal bind to dopamine D_1-like and D_2-like receptors that regulate the activity of adenylyl cyclase (AC) in the dendritic terminal of a medium spiny GABA-ergic neuron (*right*) in the nucleus accumbens shell. *B*. Neurotransmitter receptor–gated ion channels (ionotropic receptors) regulated by ethanol, benzodiazepines, barbiturates, and nicotine. Stimulatory (+) and inhibitory (−) effects of these drugs on these channels are indicated. *C*. Seven-transmembrane receptors coupled to $G_{i/o}$ proteins (metabotropic receptors) that mediate actions of opioids and cannabinoids.

receptors inhibit adenylyl cyclase by coupling to inhibitory G_i proteins. Despite opposing actions on adenylyl cyclase, both classes of dopamine receptors appear to mediate drug reinforcement. Experimental animals will self-administer D_1-like and D_2-like receptor agonists, and antagonists of D_1, D_2, and D_3 receptors decrease the reinforcing properties of cocaine. These receptor-specific responses most likely result from dopamine actions on different subpopulations of cells in the nucleus accumbens.

Opioids, nicotine, psychostimulants, barbiturates, benzodiazepines, and cannabinoids elicit their acute behavioral effects by binding to specific seven-transmembrane neurotransmitter receptors (opioids and cannabinoids), neurotransmitter receptor–gated ion channels (nicotine, barbiturates, and benzodiazepines), or transporters (cocaine and amphetamines) on the plasma membrane of neuronal cells (Fig. 386-2). Ethanol interacts with several signaling proteins including serotonin 5HT-3 receptors, nicotinic receptors, voltage-gated calcium channels, and sodium-independent purine transporters, but $GABA_A$ receptors and the *N*-methyl-D-aspartate (NMDA) subtype of glutamate receptors appear to be most sensitive to intoxicating concentrations of ethanol. As discussed below, drug actions at these targets lead to elevation of extracellular dopamine levels in the nucleus accumbens. This appears to be extremely important for the reinforcing properties of psychostimulants. For several other drugs of abuse, dopamine-independent pathways also contribute.

Dopamine Transporter Much evidence indicates that the rewarding properties of cocaine and amphetamine are due primarily to their ability to elevate extracellular dopamine levels in the nucleus accumbens. Specific populations of neurons within the nucleus accumbens are activated during cocaine self-administration in rodents. In addition, selective destruction of dopaminergic terminals within the nucleus accumbens or administration of dopamine receptor antagonists into that region eliminates cocaine self-administration. Cocaine and amphetamines act by altering transport of dopamine through plasma membrane dopamine transporters (DATs) in presynaptic nerve terminals (Fig. 386-2*A*). Reuptake of dopamine through DATs is the major mechanism for termination of dopaminergic neurotransmission. DAT is a 12-transmembrane glycoprotein and a member of the large sodium- and chloride-dependent transporter family, which also includes carriers for GABA, glycine, serotonin, norepinephrine, and other organic molecules. Cocaine binds to DATs and inhibits dopamine reuptake. Amphetamine causes intracellular release of dopamine from vesicles and reverse transport of dopamine through DATs. These actions serve to elevate levels of extracellular dopamine at dopaminergic synapses.

Recent studies of mice lacking the DAT gene have revealed redundancy in systems mediating cocaine reinforcement. Psychostimulants fail to alter extracellular dopamine levels or induce locomotor activity in these mice. However, DAT-null mice can still be trained to press a lever to receive intravenous cocaine, suggesting that other genes can also mediate the reinforcing properties of cocaine. In addition to inhibiting DAT function, cocaine blocks reuptake of serotonin and norepinephrine. In DAT-null mice, residual binding of a cocaine analogue can be displaced by serotonin reuptake inhibitors, and cocaine stimulates neurons in brain regions with a high density of serotonergic fibers. Therefore, inhibition of serotonin uptake through plasma membrane serotonin transporters may also contribute to psychostimulant reward.

$GABA_A$ Receptors The major inhibitory neurotransmitter in the nervous system is GABA. Binding of GABA to $GABA_A$ receptors activates a Cl^- current that is enhanced by benzodiazepines, barbiturates, and ethanol (Fig. 386-2*B*). Activation of this current maintains the neuronal plasma membrane close to its resting potential and thereby inhibits the generation of action potentials. $GABA_A$ receptors appear to be pentameric membrane glycoproteins composed of α, β, γ, and possibly δ peptide subunits. Fifteen subunits are known to be expressed in the mammalian central nervous system (six α, three β, three γ, one δ, one ϵ, one θ) and RNA splice variants have been identified. In rodents, the $GABA_A$ receptor agonist muscimol substitutes for ethanol in tests of drug discrimination; when injected into the nucleus accumbens, muscimol terminates ethanol self-administration. These results suggest that the reinforcing properties of ethanol are mediated in part by ethanol's actions at $GABA_A$ receptors in the nucleus accumbens.

NMDA Receptors In the nervous system, excitatory synaptic activity evoked by glutamate and aspartate is mediated by neurotransmitter receptor–gated ion channels (ionotropic receptors) that regulate cation conductances and by G protein–coupled receptors (metabotropic receptors) that stimulate phosphoinositide hydrolysis. Ionotropic glutamate receptors have been subclassified based on activation by selective agonists into three groups: NMDA receptors, high-affinity kainate receptors, and α-amino-3-hydroxy-5-methyl-4-isoxazole propionic acid (AMPA) receptors. There is a rich glutamatergic projection from neurons in the frontal cortex to the nucleus accumbens where fibers terminate mainly on medium spiny GABA-ergic neurons. NMDA receptors in the nucleus accumbens appear to play a role in the rewarding properties of several drugs. Thus, phencyclidine and other NMDA antagonists have rewarding actions when administered in the nucleus accumbens. The rewarding properties of ethanol may also be partly due to inhibition of NMDA-activated calcium currents. In addition, NMDA receptors modulate responses to psychostimulants since administration of the NMDA receptor antagonist MK-801 prior to cocaine or amphetamine prevents sensitization to these drugs.

Nicotinic Receptors Like other drugs of abuse, nicotine elicits dopamine release in the nucleus accumbens, and intravenous self-administration of nicotine is blocked by dopamine antagonists and by neurochemical lesions that destroy dopaminergic fibers in the nucleus accumbens. Nicotine increases dopamine release by activating nicotinic acetylcholine receptors (nAChRs) on cell bodies and nerve terminals of dopaminergic VTA neurons. Neuronal nAChRs are receptor-gated ion channels that allow entry of sodium into cells when acetylcholine is present. They appear to be pentameric complexes composed of different combinations of at least 10 different subunits. Targeted disruption of the β_2 subunit gene eliminates most high-affinity nicotine binding in the brain and prevents nicotine-induced dopamine release in the nucleus accumbens. In addition, mice that lack the β_2 subunit show attenuated nicotine self-administration, indicating that β_2-containing nAChRs mediate the reinforcing properties of nicotine.

Opioid Receptors Morphine and other opioids activate opioid receptors, which are a family of seven-transmembrane, G protein–coupled receptors (Figs. 386-2C and 386-3). Three classes, μ, δ, and κ, have been identified. The rewarding action of opioids appears to be mediated by activation of μ receptors since opioid reinforcement is blocked by selective μ receptor antagonists and by targeted disruption of the μ receptor gene. Binding of opioid agonists to μ receptors activates the G proteins G_i and G_o. This results in inhibition of adenylyl cyclase, thereby decreasing levels of the intracellular second messenger cyclic AMP and reducing activity of cyclic AMP–dependent protein kinase A (PKA). In addition, these G proteins activate voltage-gated potassium channels and inhibit voltage-gated calcium channels. The net result is suppression of electrical excitability in neurons expressing μ receptors.

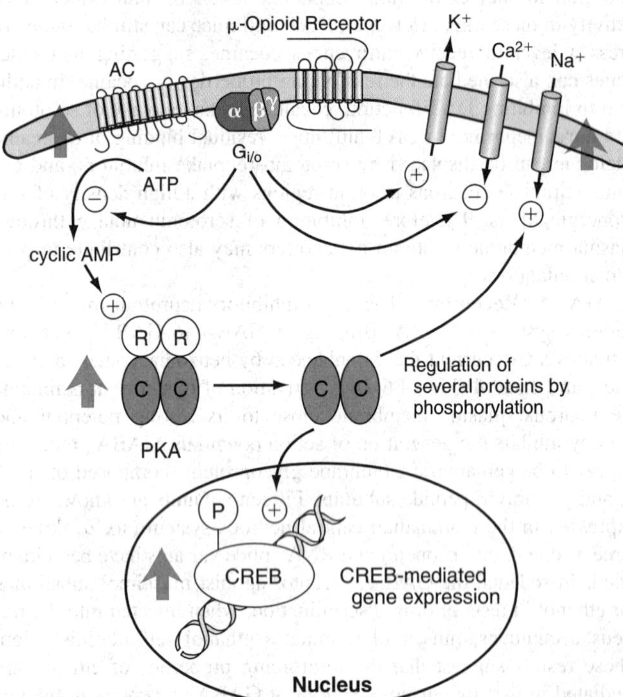

FIGURE 386-3 Schematic representation of opioid signaling in the locus coeruleus. Brief exposure to opioids activates μ-opioid receptors leading to G protein dissociation and $G\alpha_i$-mediated inhibition of adenylyl cyclase (AC), cyclic AMP formation, and protein kinase A (PKA). In addition, the $\beta\gamma$ subunits of the dissociated G proteins inhibit presynaptic voltage-gated Ca^{2+} channels and enhance the function of G protein–gated, inwardly rectifying K^+ channels, leading to a decrease in cell excitability. Bold arrows indicate compensatory increases in AC, PKA, and cyclic AMP response element binding protein (CREB) levels, and increased function of Na^+ channels following chronic exposure to opioids. This leads to increased neuronal activity, thereby contributing to opioid tolerance and to hyperexcitability during acute opioid withdrawal. Increases in CREB-mediated gene expression may also lead to long-term changes in neuronal function that contribute to addiction.

GABA-containing interneurons in the VTA suppress firing of dopaminergic VTA neurons that project to the nucleus accumbens. Opioids disinhibit these dopaminergic neurons by binding to μ receptors expressed by the GABA-containing interneurons. This increases the firing rate of dopaminergic VTA neurons and promotes dopamine release in the nucleus accumbens. Rodents will self-administer opioids into both the VTA and the nucleus accumbens. Opioid self-administration into the nucleus accumbens occurs even after dopaminergic projections to that region are destroyed. Thus, dopamine-dependent mechanisms involving the VTA and dopamine-independent mechanisms in the nucleus accumbens both contribute to opioid reward.

Opioid receptors also regulate ethanol consumption. Ethanol acutely inhibits opioid binding to δ-opioid receptors, and chronic ethanol exposure increases the density of μ- and δ-opioid receptors. Nonselective opioid antagonists reduce ethanol self-administration in animals. Several regions of the extended amygdala appear to mediate this response, although the central nucleus of the amygdala appears most important. In two independent clinical trials, the opioid receptor antagonist naltrexone, in combination with counseling, reduced craving and relapse in abstinent alcoholics. Thus, opioid systems appear to modulate ethanol craving in addicted individuals.

Cannabinoid Receptors The active ingredient of cannabis, Δ^9-tetrahydrocannabinol (Δ-9-THC), and the endogenous cannabinoid anandamide bind two subtypes of G protein–coupled cannabinoid receptors. Studies with mutant mice lacking the CB_1 receptor gene have revealed that the CB_1 receptor is responsible for the reinforcing properties of cannabinoids. When administered intravenously, Δ-9-THC increases dopamine levels in the nucleus accumbens. This is blocked by cannabinoid receptor antagonists and by μ-opioid receptor antagonists administered into the VTA. Conversely, morphine reinforcement and the severity of opioid withdrawal are reduced in mice that lack CB_1 receptors. These results suggest that opioids and cannabinoids share common signaling pathways in the brain and can interact to promote each other's reinforcing properties.

ADAPTATION TO CHRONIC DRUG USE Repeated drug exposure elicits changes in neural function that lead to drug dependence and craving. Several mechanisms are being elucidated, including drug-induced alterations in receptor and ion channel function, intracellular signal transduction, gene expression, and synaptic connectivity.

Chronic exposure to drugs of abuse can change the function of receptors and ion channels by altering their density, subunit composition, or coupling to signal transduction cascades. For example, chronic exposure to ethanol increases the density of NMDA receptors and L-type voltage-gated calcium channels in the brain. These changes contribute to neuronal hyperactivity observed during alcohol withdrawal since NMDA and L-type channel antagonists reduce signs of withdrawal in alcohol-dependent rodents deprived of ethanol. In addition, chronic exposure to ethanol decreases $GABA_A$ receptor function and abolishes potentiation by ethanol. Downregulation of $GABA_A$ receptor function contributes to manifestations of alcohol withdrawal since benzodiazepines and barbiturates, which activate $GABA_A$ receptors, are very helpful in reducing alcohol withdrawal symptoms.

Chronic exposure to many drugs of abuse induces adaptive changes in neuronal signal transduction pathways. This has been most clearly demonstrated for opioids, which increase cyclic AMP signaling in the locus coeruleus after chronic administration (Fig. 386-3). The locus coeruleus is the principal adrenergic nucleus in the brain and regulates attention states and the autonomic nervous system. Hyperactivity of this nucleus has been implicated in opioid withdrawal. Chronic opioid exposure increases expression of adenylyl cyclase, PKA, and the cyclic AMP response element binding protein, CREB, which mediates cyclic AMP–dependent gene expression. These changes increase the intrinsic firing rate of neurons in the locus coeruleus, in part through activation of an inward sodium current. Thus, upregulation of cyclic AMP signaling opposes the acute inhibitory action of opioids on this pathway.

Chronic exposure to cocaine, opioids, or ethanol upregulates cyclic AMP–mediated signaling in other brain regions, including the VTA and the nucleus accumbens. Upregulation of cyclic AMP signaling in the nucleus accumbens contributes to psychostimulant tolerance since pharmacologic inhibition of PKA or overexpression of CREB in the nucleus accumbens decreases the rewarding properties of cocaine. Upregulation of cyclic AMP signaling may also account for supersensitivity of neurons in the nucleus accumbens to D_1 receptor agonists following chronic cocaine administration. Additional neuroadaptive changes in dopamine signaling can modify drug-seeking behavior in rodents. Rats can be readily trained to voluntarily self-administer intravenous cocaine for several hours. If during a course of self-administration, saline is substituted for cocaine, the rate of self-administration declines dramatically. However, exposure to a single intraperitoneal priming injection of cocaine or a D_2-like receptor agonist causes the animal to resume lever pressing. In contrast, treatment with a D_1-like receptor agonist blocks the ability of cocaine to reinstate drug-seeking behavior. It appears that D_1-like agonists inhibit relapse in drug seeking. Therefore, they may prove to be useful in treatment of cocaine addiction.

A current hypothesis views addiction as a form of learning mediated by maladaptive recruitment of memory systems involving limbic structures. Mechanisms that could contribute to such learned, long-term adaptation include drug-induced gene expression and synaptic reorganization. For example, the transcription factor CREB, which is activated by chronic drug use, has been implicated in models of learning. Repeated exposure to many drugs of abuse also causes prolonged activation of another transcription factor, *Fos*-related antigen, in the nucleus accumbens. Ethanol increases the number of dendritic spines on hippocampal pyramidal cells and somatosensory cortical neurons, whereas amphetamine increases dendritic length and the density of dendritic spines on neurons in the nucleus accumbens and prefrontal cortex. Such drug-induced changes in gene expression and neuronal connectivity could lead to long-term alterations in brain reward pathways that may underlie drug addiction in humans.

BIBLIOGRAPHY

AMARA SG, SONDERS MS: Neurotransmitter transporters as molecular targets for addictive drugs. Drug Alcohol Depend 51:87, 1998

BERKE JD, HYMAN SE: Addiction, dopamine, and the molecular mechanisms of memory. Neuron 25:515, 2000

CRABBE JC et al: Identifying genes for alcohol and drug sensitivity: Recent progress and future directions. Trends Neurosci 22:173, 1999

KANDEL ER et al (eds): *Principles of Neural Science*. 4th ed, New York, McGraw-Hill, 2000

KOOB GF et al: Neuroscience of addiction. Neuron 21:467, 1998

LEDENT C et al: Unresponsiveness to cannabinoids and reduced addictive effects of opiates in CB1 receptor knockout mice. Science 283:401, 1999

MESSING RO, DIAMOND I: Molecular biology of alcohol dependence, in *The Molecular and Genetic Basis of Neurological Disease*, 2d ed, R Rosenberg et al (eds). Boston, Butterworth-Heinemann, 1997, pp 1109–1126

NESTLER EJ: Molecular mechanisms of opiate and cocaine addiction. Curr Opin Neurobiol 7:713, 1997

ROBINSON TE, KOLB B: Persistent structural modifications in nucleus accumbens and prefrontal cortex neurons produced by previous experience with amphetamine. J Neurosci 17:8491, 1997

ROCHA BA et al: Cocaine self-administration in dopamine-transporter knockout mice [see comments]. Nat Neurosci 1:132, 1998

SELF DW et al: Opposite modulation of cocaine-seeking behavior by D1- and D2-like dopamine receptor agonists. Science 271:1586, 1996

387 ALCOHOL AND ALCOHOLISM

Marc A. Schuckit

The yearly cost of alcohol-related problems in the United States is as much as $300 billion, including accidents, health problems, lost productivity, crime, and treatment. There are more than 22,000 deaths from alcohol-related auto accidents per year, as well as almost 2 million nonfatal injuries and damage to almost 5 million vehicles. In addition, alcohol is responsible for almost 5% of missed work time, with a 25% decrease in work performance among heavy drinkers. Men and women who fulfill criteria for alcohol use disorders decrease their life span by approximately 15 years, with abuse and dependence responsible for almost 25% of premature deaths in men and 15% in women, figures that represent a three- to sixfold odds ratio of early death even among people with higher levels of education and socioeconomic functioning.

PHARMACOLOGY AND NUTRITIONAL IMPACT OF ETHANOL Ethanol is a weakly charged molecule that moves easily through cell membranes, rapidly equilibrating between blood and tissues. The effects of drinking depend in part on the amount of ethanol consumed per unit of body weight; the level of alcohol in the blood is expressed as milligrams or grams of ethanol per deciliter (e.g., 100 mg/dL or 0.10 g/dL). A level of 0.02 to 0.03 results from the ingestion of one to two typical drinks. In round figures, 340 mL (12 oz) of beer, 115 mL (4 oz) of nonfortified wine, and 43 mL (1.5 oz) (a shot) of 80-proof beverage each contain approximately 10 g of ethanol; 0.5 L (1 pint) of 86-proof beverage contains approximately 160 g, and 1 L of wine contains approximately 80 g of ethanol. Congeners found in alcoholic beverages may contribute to body damage with heavy drinking; these include low-molecular-weight alcohols (e.g., methanol and butanol), aldehydes, esters, histamine, phenols, tannins, iron, lead, and cobalt.

Ethanol is a central nervous system (CNS) depressant that decreases activity of neurons, although some behavioral stimulation is observed at low blood levels. This drug has cross-tolerance and shares a similar pattern of behavioral problems with other brain depressants, including the benzodiazepines and barbiturates. Alcohol is absorbed from mucous membranes of the mouth and esophagus (in small amounts), from the stomach and large bowel (in modest amounts), and from the proximal portion of the small intestine (the major site). The rate of absorption is *increased* by rapid gastric emptying; by the absence of proteins, fats, or carbohydrates (which interfere with absorption); by the absence of congeners; by dilution to a modest percentage of ethanol (maximum at about 20% by volume); and by carbonation (e.g., champagne).

Between 2% (at low blood alcohol concentrations) and about 10% (at high blood alcohol concentrations) of ethanol is excreted directly through the lungs, urine, or sweat, but the greater part is metabolized to acetaldehyde, primarily in the liver. At least two metabolic routes, each with different optimal concentrations of ethanol (K_m), result in the metabolism of approximately one drink per hour. The most important pathway occurs in the cell cytosol where alcohol dehydrogenase (ADH) produces acetaldehyde, which is then rapidly destroyed by aldehyde dehydrogenase (ALDH) in the cytosol and mitochondria. Each of these steps requires nicotinamide adenine dinucleotide (NAD) as a cofactor, and it is the increased ratio of the reduced cofactor (NADH) to NAD (NADH:NAD) that is responsible for many of the metabolic derangements observed after drinking. A second pathway occurs in the microsomes of the smooth endoplasmic reticulum (the microsomal ethanol-oxidizing system, or MEOS), which is responsible for 10% or more of ethanol oxidation at high blood alcohol concentrations.

One gram of ethanol has approximately 29.7 kJ (7.1 kcal) of energy, and a drink contains between 293.0 and 418.6 kJ (70 and 100 kcal) from ethanol and other carbohydrates. However, these are "empty" of nutrients such as minerals, proteins, and vitamins. In addition, alcohol interferes with absorption of vitamins in the small intestine and decreases their storage in the liver. These actions affect folate (folacin or folic acid), pyridoxine (B_6), thiamine (B_1), nicotinic acid (niacin, B_3), and vitamin A. Heavy drinking can also produce low blood levels of potassium, magnesium, calcium, zinc, and phosphorus as a consequence of dietary deficiency and acid-base imbalances during excess alcohol ingestion or withdrawal.

An ethanol load in a fasting, healthy individual is likely to produce transient hypoglycemia within 6 to 36 h, secondary to the acute actions of ethanol on gluconeogenesis. This can result in glucose intolerance until the alcoholic has abstained for 2 to 4 weeks. Alcohol ketoacidosis, probably reflecting a decrease in fatty acid oxidation coupled with poor diet or recurrent vomiting, should not be misdiagnosed as diabetic ketosis. With the former, patients show an increase in serum ketones along with a mild increase in glucose but a large anion gap, a mild to moderate increase in serum lactate, and a β-hydroxybutyrate/lactate ratio of between 2:1 and 9:1 (with normal being 1:1).

BEHAVIORAL EFFECTS, TOLERANCE, AND DEPENDENCE The effects of any drug depend on the dose, the rate of increase in plasma, the concomitant presence of other drugs, and the past experience with the agent. With alcohol, an additional factor is whether blood alcohol levels are rising or falling; the effects are more intense during the former period.

Even though "legal intoxication" requires a blood alcohol concentration of at least 80 to 100 mg/dL, behavioral, psychomotor, and cognitive changes are seen at levels as low as 20 to 30 mg/dL (i.e., after one to two drinks). Deep but disturbed sleep can be seen at twice the legal intoxication level, and death can occur with levels between 300 and 400 mg/dL. Beverage alcohol is probably responsible for more overdose deaths than any other drug.

The intoxicating effects of alcohol appear to be due to actions at specific neurotransmitter receptors and transporters. Alcohol enhances γ-aminobutyric acid A ($GABA_A$) receptors, and inhibits *N*-methyl-D-asparate (NMDA) receptors (Chap. 386). In vitro studies suggest that additional effects involve inhibition of adenosine uptake and a translocation of the cyclic AMP–dependent protein kinase catalytic subunit from the cytoplasm to the nucleus. Neurons adapt quickly to these actions, and thus different effects may be present during chronic administration and withdrawal.

At least three types of compensation develop after repeated exposure to the drug, producing tolerance of higher ethanol levels. First, after 1 to 2 weeks of daily drinking, *metabolic or pharmacokinetic tolerance* develops, with a 30% increase in the rate of hepatic ethanol metabolism. This alteration disappears almost as rapidly as it develops. Second, *cellular or pharmacodynamic tolerance* develops through neurochemical changes that may also contribute to physical dependence. Third, individuals can learn to adapt their behavior so that they can function better than expected under drug influence (*behavioral tolerance*).

The cellular changes caused by chronic ethanol exposure may not resolve for several weeks or longer following cessation of drinking. In the interim, the neurons require ethanol to function optimally, and the individual can be said to be physically dependent. This physical condition is distinct from psychological dependence, a concept indicating that the person is psychologically uncomfortable without the drug.

THE EFFECTS OF ETHANOL ON BODY SYSTEMS

While one to two drinks per day in an otherwise healthy and nonpregnant individual can have some beneficial effects, at higher doses alcohol is toxic to most body systems. Knowledge about the deleterious effects of alcohol helps the practicing physician to identify alcoholic patients. Signs and symptoms of ethanol abuse can be used to help motivate the patient to abstain. It is important to remember that the typical white- or blue-collar alcoholic functions at a fairly high level for years, and that not everyone develops each problem.

CENTRAL NERVOUS SYSTEM Approximately 35% of drinkers may experience a *blackout*, an episode of temporary anterograde amnesia, in which the person forgets all or part of what occurred during a drinking evening. Another common problem, one seen after as few as one or two drinks, is that while alcohol can help someone to fall asleep, it also "fragments" the sleep pattern causing alterations between sleep stages and a deficiency in deep sleep. At the same time, alcohol diminishes rapid eye movement (REM) or dream sleep early in the evening, with resulting prominent and sometimes disturbing dreams later in the night. Finally, alcohol relaxes muscles in the pharynx, which can cause snoring and exacerbate sleep apnea, with symptoms of the latter in 75% of alcoholic men over age 60.

An additional problem related to the acute effects of alcohol on most drinkers is the impairment in judgment, balance, and motor coordination that contributes to the high incidence and severity of accidents. At least half of individuals who experience severe physical trauma in an accident have evidence of substance-related impairment, a finding that is consistent with the fact that 40% of drinkers in the United States have at some time driven while intoxicated with alcohol and that 15% of flight crews have evidence of repeated heavy drinking. Regarding the latter, at least one study noted that pilot performance is still impaired 14 h after a blood alcohol concentration of 100 mg/dL, despite subsequent abstinence.

The effect of alcohol on the nervous system is even more pronounced among alcohol-dependent individuals. Chronic intake of high doses of ethanol causes *peripheral neuropathy* in 5 to 15% of alcoholics, which is possibly related to thiamine deficiency. Patients complain of bilateral limb numbness, tingling, and paresthesias; symptoms are more pronounced distally than proximally. The treatment is abstinence and thiamine supplementation.

Wernicke's syndrome (ophthalmoparesis, ataxia, and encephalopathy) and *Korsakoff's syndrome* (alcohol-induced persisting amnestic disorder), are seen in the United States at a rate of approximately 50 per million people per year. These disorders are the result of thiamine deficiency in vulnerable individuals, possibly owing to interaction with a genetic transketolase deficiency. Korsakoff's syndrome presents as profound and persistent anterograde amnesia (inability to learn new material) and a milder retrograde amnesia. Additional symptoms can include impairment in visuospatial, abstract, and conceptual reasoning but with a normal intelligence quotient (IQ). Some patients demonstrate an acute onset of Korsakoff's syndrome in association with the neurologic stigmata seen with Wernicke's syndrome (e.g., sixth nerve palsy and ataxia), whereas others have a more gradual onset. With oral thiamine replacement (50 to 100 mg/d), only one-quarter of Korsakoff's patients achieve full recovery, one-half experience partial improvement, and one-quarter show no improvement, even after many months of supplementation. →***Wernicke's syndrome is discussed in detail in Chap. 376.***

About 1% of alcoholics develop *cerebellar degeneration*, a syndrome of progressive unsteady stance and gait often accompanied by mild nystagmus. Atrophy of the cerebellar vermis is seen on brain computed tomography and magnetic resonance imaging scans, but the cerebrospinal fluid is usually normal. Treatment consists of abstinence and multiple vitamin supplementation, although improvement is often minimal.

Alcoholics can show severe *cognitive* problems and impairment in recent and remote memory for weeks to months after an alcoholic binge. Increased size of the brain ventricles and cerebral sulci are seen in 50% or more of chronic alcoholics, but these changes are often reversible, returning toward normal after a year or more of abstinence. Permanent CNS impairment (alcohol-induced persisting dementia) can develop and accounts for up to 20% of chronically demented patients. There is no single alcoholic dementia syndrome; rather, this label is used to describe patients who have apparently irreversible cognitive changes (possibly from diverse causes) in the midst of chronic alcoholism.

Finally, almost every psychiatric syndrome can be seen temporarily during heavy drinking or subsequent withdrawal. These include intense *sadness* lasting for days to weeks in the midst of heavy drinking in 40% of alcoholics, which is classified as an alcohol-induced mood disorder in the *Fourth Diagnostic and Statistical Manual* of the American Psychiatric Association (DSM-IV); severe *anxiety* in 10 to 30% of alcoholics, often beginning during alcohol withdrawal and which can persist for many months after cessation of drinking (alcohol-induced anxiety disorder); and auditory *hallucinations* and/or *paranoid delusions* in the absence of any obvious signs of withdrawal—a state now called *alcohol-induced psychotic disorder*—and reported at sometime in 1 to 10% of alcoholics. Treatment of all forms of alcohol-induced psychopathology includes abstinence and supportive care, with the likelihood of full recovery within several days to 6 weeks. A history of alcohol intake is an important consideration in *any* patient with one of these psychiatric symptoms.

THE GASTROINTESTINAL SYSTEM **Esophagus and Stomach** Acute alcohol intake can result in inflammation of the esophagus (possibly secondary to reflux of gastric contents) and stomach (resulting from both an increase in acid production and damage to the gastric mucosal barrier). Esophagitis can cause epigastric distress, and gastritis, the most frequent cause of gastrointestinal bleeding in heavy drinkers, can present as anorexia and/or abdominal pain. Chronic heavy drinking, if associated with violent vomiting, can produce a longitudinal tear in the mucosa at the gastroesophageal junction—a Mallory-Weiss lesion. Although many gastrointestinal problems are reversible, two complications of chronic alcoholism, esophageal varices secondary to cirrhosis-induced portal hypertension and atrophy of the gastric mucosa, may be irreversible.

Pancreas The incidence of acute pancreatitis in alcoholics (about 25 per 1000 per year) is almost threefold higher than in the general population, accounting for an estimated 10% or more of the cases of this disorder (Chap. 304).

Liver Ethanol absorbed from the small bowel is carried directly to the liver, where it becomes the preferred fuel; NADH accumulates and oxygen utilization escalates; gluconeogenesis is impaired (with a resulting fall in the amount of glucose produced from glycogen); lactate production increases; and there is a decreased oxidation of fatty acids in the citric acid cycle with an increase in fat accumulation within liver cells. In the healthy individual taking no medications, these changes are reversible, but with repeated exposure to ethanol, more severe changes in liver functioning are likely to occur. These include, in overlapping stages, fatty accumulation, alcohol-induced hepatitis, perivenular sclerosis, and cirrhosis, with the latter observed in an estimated 15 to 20% of alcoholics (Chap. 298).

CANCER As discussed briefly below, the leading cause of death in alcoholics is cardiovascular disease, but cancer occupies a solid second place. Women drinking as few as 1.5 drinks per day increase their risk of breast cancer 1.4-fold. For both genders, four drinks per day increases the risk for oral and esophageal cancers by approximately threefold and rectal cancers by a factor of 1.5, whereas seven to eight or more drinks per day enhances the risks for many of these cancers by a factor of five. Overall, it has been estimated that alcoholics have a rate of carcinoma 10 times higher than the general population.

HEMATOPOIETIC SYSTEM Ethanol exerts multiple reversible acute and chronic effects on all blood cells. The impact on red blood cells (RBC) is an increase in size (mean corpuscular volume, MCV), usually without anemia. This change appears to reflect the effect of alcohol on stem cells. If heavy drinking is accompanied by folic acid deficiency, there can also be hypersegmented neutrophils, reticulocytopenia, and hyperplastic bone marrow; if malnutrition is present, sideroblastic changes can also be observed. Chronic heavy drinking can also decrease production of most white blood cells (WBCs), decrease granulocyte mobility and adherence, and impair the delayed-hypersensitivity response to new antigens (with a possible false-negative tuberculin skin test). Finally, many alcoholics present with mild thrombocytopenia. When due to repeated intoxication, the low platelet count usually resolves within a week of abstinence. Thrombocytopenia can also occur secondary to hepatic cirrhosis and congestive splenomegaly (increased destruction) or to folic acid deficiency (decreased production). Ethanol itself might not have a major effect on platelet function, but polyphenols and other constituents of some alcoholic beverages, particularly wine, may interfere with platelet aggregation.

CARDIOVASCULAR SYSTEM Acutely, ethanol decreases myocardial contractility and causes peripheral vasodilation, with a resulting mild decrease in blood pressure and a compensatory increase in cardiac output. Exercise-induced increases in cardiac oxygen consumption are higher after alcohol intake. These acute effects have little clinical importance for the average healthy drinker but can produce problems in men and women with cardiac disease.

Chronic intake of even modest doses of alcohol can have both deleterious and beneficial effects. Regarding the latter, a maximum of one to two drinks per day over long periods may decrease the risk for cardiovascular death, perhaps through an increase in high-density lipoprotein (HDL) cholesterol or changes in clotting mechanisms. In one large national study, cardiovascular mortality was reduced by 30 to 40% among individuals reporting one or more drinks daily compared to nondrinkers, with overall mortality lowest among those consuming approximately one drink per day. Recent data have also corroborated the decreased risk for ischemic, but not hemorrhagic, stroke associated with regular light drinking.

The consumption of three or more drinks per day results in a dose-dependent increase in blood pressure, which returns to normal within weeks of abstinence. As a result, heavy drinking is an important contributor to mild to moderate hypertension. Chronic heavy drinking can cause cardiomyopathy, with symptoms ranging from unexplained arrhythmias in the presence of left ventricular impairment to heart failure with dilation of all four heart chambers and hypocontractility of heart muscle. Perhaps one-third of cases of cardiomyopathy are alcohol-induced. Mural thrombi can form in the left atrium or ventricle, while heart enlargement exceeding 25% can cause mitral regurgitation. Atrial or ventricular arrhythmias, especially paroxysmal tachycardia, can also occur after a drinking binge in individuals showing no other evidence of heart disease—a syndrome known as the "holiday heart."

GENITOURINARY SYSTEM CHANGES, SEXUAL FUNCTIONING, AND FETAL DEVELOPMENT Acutely, modest ethanol doses (e.g., blood alcohol concentrations of 100 mg/dL or even less) can both increase sexual drive and decrease erectile capacity in men. Even in the absence of liver impairment, a significant minority of chronic alcoholic men may show irreversible testicular atrophy with concomitant shrinkage of the seminiferous tubules, decreases in ejaculate volume, and a lower sperm count (Chap. 335).

The repeated ingestion of high doses of ethanol by women can result in amenorrhea, a decrease in ovarian size, absence of corpora lutea with associated infertility, and spontaneous abortions. Heavy drinking during pregnancy results in the rapid placental transfer of both ethanol and acetaldehyde, which may have serious consequences for fetal development. The *fetal alcohol syndrome* can include any of the following: facial changes with epicanthal eye folds, poorly formed concha, and small teeth with faulty enamel; cardiac atrial or ventricular septal defects; an aberrant palmar crease and limitation in joint movement; and microcephaly with mental retardation. The specific amount of ethanol and/or specific time of vulnerability during pregnancy have not been defined, making it advisable for pregnant women to abstain completely.

OTHER EFFECTS OF ETHANOL Between one-half and two-thirds of alcoholics have evidence of decreased skeletal muscle strength caused by acute *alcoholic myopathy*, a condition that improves but which might not disappear with abstinence. Effects of repeated heavy drinking on the *skeletal system* include alterations in calcium metabolism, lower bone density, and less growth in the epiphyses, with an increased risk for fractures and osteonecrosis of the femoral head. *Hormonal changes* include an increase in cortisol levels, which can remain elevated during heavy drinking; inhibition of vasopressin secretion at rising blood alcohol concentrations and the opposite effect at falling blood alcohol concentrations (with the final result that most alcoholics are likely to be slightly overhydrated); a modest and reversible decrease in serum thyroxine (T_4); and a more marked decrease in serum triiodothyronine (T_3).

ALCOHOLISM (ALCOHOL ABUSE OR DEPENDENCE)

Because many drinkers occasionally imbibe to excess, temporary alcohol-related pathology is common in nonalcoholics. The period of heaviest drinking is usually the late teens to the late twenties. This is also a time of high risk for temporary alcohol-related social, occupational, or driving difficulties. These phenomena are often isolated events or self-limited, but when repeated problems in multiple life areas develop, the person is likely to meet criteria for alcohol abuse or dependence.

DEFINITIONS AND EPIDEMIOLOGY DSM-IV defines alcohol dependence as repeated alcohol-related difficulties in at least three of seven areas of functioning that cluster together over any 12-month period. These problems include any combination of tolerance, withdrawal, taking larger amounts of alcohol over longer periods than intended, an inability to control use, spending a great deal of time associated with alcohol use, giving up important activities to drink, and continued use of alcohol despite physical or psychological consequences. In this diagnosis a special emphasis is placed on evidence of tolerance and/or withdrawal, a condition referred to as "dependence with a physiological component" and which is associated wtih a more severe clinical course. Dependence occurs in both men and women, in individuals from all socioeconomic strata, and in people of all racial backgrounds. The diagnosis predicts a course of recurrent problems with the use of alcohol and the consequent shortening of the life span by a decade or more. In the absence of alcohol dependence, an individual can be given a diagnosis of *alcohol abuse* if he or she demonstrates *repetitive* problems with alcohol in any one of four life areas: an inability to fulfill major obligations, use in hazardous situations such as driving, legal problems, or use despite social or interpersonal difficulties.

The clinical diagnosis of alcohol abuse or dependence rests on the documentation of a pattern of *difficulties associated with alcohol use*; the definition is *not* based on the quantity and frequency of alcohol consumption. Thus, in screening for alcohol abuse or dependence, it is important to probe for life problems and then attempt to tie in use of alcohol or another substance. Information regarding marital or job problems, legal difficulties, histories of accidents, medical problems, evidence of tolerance, etc., is an important component of all evaluations and yields data that are of use even for nonalcoholic individuals.

The lifetime risk for alcohol dependence in most western countries is about 10 to 15% for men and 5% for women. When alcohol abuse is also considered, the rates are even higher. The typical alcoholic is a blue- or white-collar worker or homemaker and thus does not fit the common stereotype.

GENETICS OF ALCOHOLISM Alcoholism is a multifactorial disorder in which both environmental and biologic factors contribute. The importance of genetic influences in alcoholism is supported by the higher risk for this disorder in the identical versus fraternal twin of an alcoholic and the fourfold increased risk for children of alcoholics even if adopted at birth and raised without knowledge of the problems of their biologic parents.

The evidence supporting genetic influences in alcoholism has stimulated a search for trait markers of a vulnerability toward the disorder. A 15-year follow-up of 453 men originally studied at age 20 has shown that subjects with alcoholic fathers demonstrated relatively lower levels of response to alcohol, including less intense subjective feelings of intoxication, less alcohol-related impairment in cognitive and psychomotor tests, and less intense alcohol-related changes in prolactin and cortisol secretion. This low level of response to alcohol at around age 20 was a powerful predictor of later alcoholism, explaining most of the relationship between a family history of this disorder and later alcohol problems. Additional genetically influenced characteristics that contribute to the risk of alcoholism appear to include some personality traits such as higher levels of impulsivity and sensation seeking, and several electrophysiologic measures such as the P300 wave of the event-related potential (Chap. 357), which might relate to cognitive styles or evidence of CNS disinhibition. All the genetic factors combined appear to explain up to 60% of the risk, with environmental influences contributing at least 40%.

NATURAL HISTORY For the "average" alcoholic, the age of first drink and first minor problems (e.g., an argument with a friend while drunk or an alcoholic blackout) are similar to those in the general population. However, by the early to mid-twenties, most men and women moderate their drinking (perhaps learning from minor problems), whereas difficulties for alcoholics are likely to escalate, with the first major life problem from alcohol appearing in the mid-twenties to early forties. Once established, the course of alcoholism is likely to be one of exacerbations and remissions. As a rule, there is remarkably little difficulty in stopping alcohol use when problems develop, and this step is often followed by days to months of carefully controlled drinking. Unfortunately, these periods are almost inevitably followed by escalations in alcohol intake and subsequent problems. The course is not hopeless, because between half and two-thirds of alcoholics maintain abstinence for extended periods after treatment. Even without formal treatment or self-help groups there is at least a 20% chance of long-term abstinence. However, should the alcoholic continue to drink, the life span is shortened by an average of 15 years, with the leading causes of death, in decreasing order, being heart disease, cancer, accidents, and suicide.

IDENTIFICATION OF THE ALCOHOLIC AND INTERVENTION Physicians even in affluent areas should recognize that approximately 20% of patients have alcoholism. Therefore, it is important to pay attention to the alcohol-related symptoms and signs described above as well as laboratory tests that are likely to be abnormal in the context of regular consumption of 6 to 8 or more drinks per day. These include a high-normal or slightly elevated MCV (e.g., ≥91 fL), γ-glutamyl transferase (GGT) (≥30 units), serum uric acid [>416 μmol/L (7 mg/dL)], carbohydrate-deficient transferrin (CDT) (≥20 g/L), and triglycerides [≥2.0 mmol/L (180 mg/dL)]. Mild and fluctuating hypertension (e.g., 140/95), repeated infections such as pneumonia, and otherwise unexplained cardiac arrhythmias should also raise the possibility that the patient is an alcoholic. Other disorders suggestive of alcoholism include cancer of the head and neck, esophagus, or stomach as well as cirrhosis, unexplained hepatitis, pancreatitis, bilateral parotid gland swelling, and peripheral neuropathy.

Once the likelihood of alcoholism is established, only a few moments are needed to gather the history of alcohol-related life problems. The patient and the spouse or another close family member should be asked about patterns of accidents, relationship difficulties, problems on the job, and driving-related difficulties, after which the role played by alcohol should be identified. All physicians should be able to take the time needed to gather such information. In addition, a simple 25-item form to be answered by the patient, the Michigan Alcohol Screening Test (MAST), is available to aid in identifying alcoholics. However, this is only a screening tool, and a careful face-to-face interview is still required for a meaningful diagnosis. The CAGE, which consists of asking about alcohol-related trouble *c*utting down on intake, being *a*nnoyed by criticisms, *g*uilt, or use of an "*e*ye-opener," can also be helpful as an initial screen.

After alcoholism is identified, the diagnosis must be shared with the patient. The presenting complaint can be used as an entrée to the alcohol problem. For instance, the patient complaining of insomnia or hypertension could be told that these are clinically important symptoms and that physical findings and laboratory tests indicate that alcohol appears to have contributed to the complaints and is increasing the risk for further medical and psychological problems. The physician should share information about the course of alcoholism and explore possible avenues of attacking the problem. Some patients and family members will benefit from the opportunity to read additional material (see "Bibliography").

The process of intervention is rarely accomplished in one session. For the person who refuses to stop drinking at the first intervention, a logical step is to "keep the door open," establishing future meetings so that help is available as problems escalate. In the meantime the family may benefit from counseling or referral to self-help groups such as Al-Anon (the Alcoholics Anonymous group for family members) and Alateen (for teenage children of alcoholics). The patient should be reminded that driving while intoxicated is dangerous and illegal.

THE ALCOHOL WITHDRAWAL SYNDROME Once the brain has been repeatedly exposed to high doses of alcohol, any sudden decrease in intake can produce symptoms of withdrawal. As with all CNS depressants, the symptoms are generally the opposite of those produced by intoxication. Features include tremor of the hands (shakes or jitters); agitation and anxiety; autonomic nervous system overactivity such as an increase in pulse, respiratory rate, and body temperature; insomnia, possibly accompanied by bad dreams; and gastrointestinal upset. These withdrawal symptoms generally begin within 5 to 10 h of decreasing ethanol intake, peak in intensity on day 2 or 3, and improve by day 4 or 5. Anxiety, insomnia, and mild levels of autonomic dysfunction may persist at decreasing levels for 6 months or more as a protracted abstinence syndrome, which may contribute to the tendency to return to drinking.

At some point in their lives, between 2 and 5% of alcoholics experience withdrawal seizures ("rum fits"), usually within 48 h of stopping drinking. These are usually generalized (unless there is an underlying focal lesion), and any electroencephalographic abnormalities are mild and generally return to normal within several days.

The term *delirium tremens* (DTs) refers to delirium (mental confusion with fluctuating levels of consciousness) along with a tremor, severe agitation, and autonomic overactivity (e.g., marked increases in pulse, blood pressure, and respirations). Fortunately, this serious and potentially life-threatening complication of alcohol withdrawal is rare. Only 5 to 10% of alcohol-dependent individuals ever experience DTs; the chance of DTs during any single withdrawal is less than 1% but is higher if there has been a withdrawal seizure. DTs are most likely to develop in patients with concomitant severe medical disorders or evidence of underlying brain damage, and thus can usually be avoided if the underlying medical problems can be identified and treated.

℞ TREATMENT **Acute Intoxication** The first priority is to be certain that the vital signs are relatively stable without evidence of respiratory depression, cardiac arrhythmia, or potentially dangerous changes in blood pressure. Life-threatening problems require appropriate emergency care and hospitalization. The clinician must recognize that a variety of causes may produce obtundation or coma in the alcoholic patient. The possibility of intoxication with other drugs should be considered, and a blood or urine sample is indicated to screen for opioids or other CNS depressants such as benzodiazepines or barbiturates. A coexisting seizure disorder, head injury, meningitis, brain abscess, or other potentially life-threatening neurologic disorder may be present. Other medical conditions that must be considered include hypoglycemia, hepatic failure, or diabetic ketoacidosis.

Patients who are medically stable should be placed in a quiet environment and asked to lie on their side if fatigued in order to minimize the risk of aspiration. When the behavior indicates an increased likelihood of violence, hospital procedures should be followed, including planning for the possibility of a show of force with an intervention team. In the context of aggressiveness, patients should be clearly reminded in a nonthreatening way that it is the goal of the staff to help them to feel better and to avoid problems. If the aggressive behavior continues, relatively low doses of a short-acting benzodiazepine such as lorazepam (e.g., 1 mg by mouth) may be used and can be repeated as needed, but care must be taken so that the addition of this second CNS depressant does not destabilize vital signs or worsen confusion. An alternative approach is to use an antipsychotic medication (e.g., 5 mg of haloperidol liquid), but this has the potential danger of lowering the seizure threshold. If aggression escalates, the patient might require a short-term admission to a locked ward, where medications can be used more safely and vital signs more closely monitored.

Withdrawal The first, and most important, step is to perform a *thorough* physical examination in all alcoholics who are considering stopping drinking. It is necessary to evaluate organ systems likely to be impaired, including a search for evidence of liver failure, gastrointestinal bleeding, cardiac arrhythmia, and glucose or electrolyte imbalance.

The second step in treating withdrawal for even the typical well-nourished alcoholic is to give patients adequate nutrition and rest. All patients should be given oral multiple B vitamins, including 50 to 100 mg of thiamine daily for a week or more. Most patients enter withdrawal with normal levels of body water or mild overhydration, and intravenous fluids should be avoided unless there is evidence of significant recent bleeding, vomiting, or diarrhea. Medications can usually be administered orally.

The third step in treatment is to recognize that most withdrawal symptoms are caused by the rapid removal of a CNS depressant. Therefore, patients can be weaned by administering any drug of this class and gradually decreasing the levels over 3 to 5 days. While many CNS depressants are effective, the *benzodiazepines* have the highest margin of safety and are, therefore, the preferred class of drugs in the treatment of alcohol withdrawal. Benzodiazepines with short half-lives (Chap. 385) are especially useful for patients with serious liver impairment or evidence of preexisting encephalopathy or brain damage. On the other hand, short-half-life benzodiazepines, e.g., oxazepam or lorazepam, result in rapidly changing drug blood levels and must be given every 4 h to avoid abrupt fluctuations in blood levels that may increase the risk for seizures. Therefore, most clinicians use drugs with longer half-lives, such as diazepam or chlordiazepoxide. The goal is to administer enough drug on day 1 to alleviate most of the symptoms of withdrawal (e.g., the tremor and elevated pulse), and then to decrease the dose by 20% on successive days over a period of 3 to 5 days. The approach is flexible; the dose is increased if signs of withdrawal escalate, and the medication is withheld if the patient is sleeping or shows signs of increasing orthostatic hypotension. The average patient requires 25 to 50 mg of chlordiazepoxide or 10 mg of diazepam given orally every 4 to 6 h on the first day.

For the patient with DTs, treatment can be difficult and the condition is likely to run a course of 3 to 5 days regardless of the therapy employed. The focus of care is to identify medical problems and correct them and to control behavior and prevent injuries. Many clinicians recommend the use of high doses of benzodiazepine (doses as high as 800 mg/day of chlordiazepoxide have been reported), a treatment that will decrease the agitation and raise the seizure threshold but probably does little to improve the confusion. Other clinicians recommend the use of antipsychotic medications, such as 20 mg or more per day of haloperidol, an approach less likely to exacerbate confusion but which may increase the risk of seizures. Antipsychotic drugs have no place in the treatment of mild withdrawal symptoms.

Generalized wtihdrawal seizures rarely require aggressive pharmacologic intervention beyond that given to the usual patient undergoing withdrawal, i.e., adequate doses of benzodiazepines. There is little evidence that anticonvulsants such as phenytoin are effective in drug-withdrawal seizures, and the risk of seizures has usually passed by the time effective drug levels are reached. →***The rare patient with status epilepticus must be treated aggressively, as outlined in Chap. 361, initially with intravenous lorazepam.***

While alcohol withdrawal is often treated in a hospital, efforts at reducing costs have resulted in the development of outpatient detoxification for relatively mild abstinence syndromes. This is appropriate for patients in good physical condition who demonstrate mild signs of withdrawal despite low blood alcohol concentrations and for those without prior history of DTs or withdrawal seizures. Such individuals still require a careful physical examination, evaluation of blood tests, and vitamin supplementation. Benzodiazepines can be given *in a 1- to 2-day supply* to be administered to the patient by a spouse or other family member four times a day. Patients are asked to *return daily* for evaluation of vital signs and to come to the emergency room if signs and symptoms of withdrawal escalate.

Rehabilitation of Alcoholics After completing alcoholic rehabilitation, 60% or more of middle-class alcoholics maintain abstinence for at least a year, and many for a lifetime. As is true for any long-term disorder for which treatment requires changes in life-style (e.g., diabetes or hypertension), therapeutic approaches include general supports that meet commonsense guidelines. Considering the lack of evidence for the superiority of any specific treatment type, it is best to keep interventions simple.

Maneuvers in rehabilitation fall into two general categories. First are attempts to help the alcoholic achieve and maintain a high level of motivation toward abstinence. These include education about alcoholism and instructing family and/or friends to stop protecting the person from the problems caused by alcohol. The second step is to help the patient to readjust to life without alcohol and to reestablish a functional lifestyle through counseling, vocational rehabilitation, and self-help groups such as Alcoholics Anonymous. The third component, called *relapse prevention*, helps the person to identify situations in which a return to drinking is likely, formulate ways of managing these risks, and develop coping strategies that increase the chances of a return to abstinence if a slip occurs.

There is no convincing evidence that inpatient rehabilitation is always more effective for the average alcoholic than is outpatient care. However, more intense interventions work better than those that are less intensive, and some alcoholics do not respond to outpatient care. The decision to hospitalize can be made if (1) the patient has medical problems that are difficult to treat outside a hospital; (2) depression, confusion, or psychosis interferes with outpatient care; (3) the patient has such a severe life crisis that it is difficult to get his or her attention as an outpatient; (4) outpatient treatment has failed; or (5) the patient lives far from the treatment center. In any setting, the best predictors of continued abstinence include evidence of higher levels of life stability (e.g., supportive family and friends) and higher levels of functioning (e.g., job skills, higher levels of education, and absence of crimes unrelated to alcohol).

Whether the treatment begins in an inpatient or an outpatient setting, subsequent outpatient contact should be maintained for a minimum of 6 months and preferably a full year after abstinence is achieved. Counseling with an individual physician or through groups focuses on day-to-day living—emphasizing areas of improved functioning in the absence of alcohol (i.e., why it is a good idea to continue to abstain) and helping the patient to manage free time without alcohol, develop a nondrinking peer group, and handle stresses on the job without alcohol.

The physician serves an important role in identifying the alcoholic, treating associated medical or psychiatric syndromes, overseeing detoxification, referring the patient to rehabilitation programs, and providing counseling. The physician is also responsible for selecting which (if any) medication might be appropriate during alcoholism rehabilitation. Patients often complain of continuing sleep problems or anxiety when acute withdrawal treatment is over, problems that may be a component of protracted withdrawal. Unfortunately, there is no place for hypnotics or antianxiety drugs in the treatment of most alcoholics after acute withdrawal has been completed. Regarding insomnia, patients should be reassured that the trouble in sleeping is normal after alcohol withdrawal and will improve over the subsequent weeks and months. They should then follow a rigid bedtime and awakening schedule and avoid any naps or the use of caffeine in the evenings. The sleep pattern will improve rapidly. Anxiety can be approached by helping the person to gain insight into the temporary nature of the symptoms and to develop strategies to achieve relaxation as well as using forms of cognitive therapy.

In addition, while the mainstay of alcoholic rehabilitation involves counseling, education, and cognitive techniques, several interesting medications are under active evaluation and might prove to be useful. The first is the opioid-antagonist drug naltrexone, which has been reported in several small-scale, short-term studies to decrease the probability of a return to drinking and to shorten periods of relapse. While this medication looks promising, longer-term large-scale trials in more diverse clinical settings will be required before the cost-effectiveness of naltrexone can be established. A second medication, acamprosate, has been tested in over 5000 patients in Europe, with results that appear similar to those reported for naltrexone. Currently, acamprosate is not available in the United States, although a long-term, trial of naltrexone, acamprosate, and their combination is in progress. A third medication, which has historically been used in the treatment of alcoholism, is the ALDH inhibitor disulfiram. Taken in doses of 250 mg/day, this drug produces an unpleasant (and potentially dangerous) reaction in the presence of alcohol, a phenomenon related to rapidly rising blood levels of the first metabolite of alcohol, acetaldehyde. However, few adequate double-blind controlled trials have demonstrated the superiority of disulfiram over placebo. Disulfiram has many side effects, and the reaction with alcohol can be dangerous, especially for patients with heart disease, stroke, diabetes mellitus, and hypertension. Thus, most clinicians reserve this medication for patients who have a clear history of longer-term abstinence associated with prior use of disulfiram and for those who might take the drug under the supervision of another individual (such as a spouse), especially during discrete periods that they have identified as representing high-risk drinking situations for them (such as the Christmas holiday).

More data are required before any medication can be recommended for routine use in alcohol rehabilitation. However, additional support for alcoholics is available through Alcoholics Anonymous in almost every community. Alcoholics Anonymous is a self-help group of recovering alcoholics (men and women who have stopped drinking, perhaps many years ago) that offers an effective model of abstinence, provides a sober peer group, and makes crisis intervention available when the urge to drink escalates. No matter what type of rehabilitation program is planned, the alcoholic should be offered the option of joining Alcoholics Anonymous.

BIBLIOGRAPHY

LIEBER C: Medical disorders of alcoholism. N Engl J Med 333:1058, 1995

PRESCOTT CA, KENDLER KS: Genetic and environmental contributions to alcohol abuse and dependence in a population-based sample of male twins. Am J Psychiatry 156: 34, 1999

PROJECT MATCH RESEARCH GROUP: Matching alcoholism treatments to client heterogeneity. J Stud Alcohol 58:7, 1997

SACCO RL et al: The protective effect of moderate alcohol consumption on ischemic stroke. JAMA 281:53, 1999

SCHUCKIT MA: Biological, psychological, and environmental predictors of the alcoholism risk: A longitudinal study. J Stud Alcohol 59:485, 1998

———: *Educating Yourself About Alcohol and Drugs: A People's Primer*. New York, Plenum, 1995

——— et al: Clinical implications for four drugs of the DSM-IV distinction between substance dependence with and without a physiological component. Am J Psychiatry 156:41, 1999

———: *Drug and Alcohol Abuse: A Clinical Guide to Diagnosis and Treatment*, 5th ed. New York, Plenum, 2000

——— et al: The clinical course of alcohol-related problems in alcohol dependent and nonalcohol dependent drinking women and men. J Stud Alcohol 59:581, 1998

THUN MJ et al: Alcohol consumption and mortality among middle aged and elderly U.S. adults. N Engl J Med 337:1705, 1997

WIESE JG et al: The alcohol hangover Ann Int Med 132:897, 2000

388 OPIOID DRUG ABUSE AND DEPENDENCE

Marc A. Schuckit, David S. Segal

The principal effects of the opioids (opiate-like drugs) are a damping of pain perception along with modest levels of sedation and euphoria. Drugs in this category include heroin, morphine, and codeine as well as many prescription analgesics and antitussive agents. Opioid drugs are widely used in medical practice, and, thus, dependence and abuse are not limited to the classic opiod-dependent person on the street.

Tolerance to any one opioid is likely to extend to the others (i.e., cross-tolerance is likely), and all opioids are associated with a similar pattern of drug-related problems. Each is capable of producing dependence as defined in the *Fourth Diagnostic and Statistical Manual* of the American Psychiatric Association (DSM-IV), including evidence of physical dependence, a diagnosis made in the context of a history of tolerance and/or withdrawal. The abstinence syndrome from any of the substances can be treated with administration of any of the others.

PHARMACOLOGY The prototypic opiates, morphine and codeine (3-methoxymorphine), are taken directly from the milky juice of the poppy *Papaver somniferum*. The semisynthetic drugs produced from the morphine or thebane molecules include hydromorphone, diacetylmorphine (heroin), and oxycodone. The purely synthetic opioids, sharing many of the basic properties of opium and morphine, include meperidine, propoxyphene, diphenoxylate, fentanyl, buprenorphine, methadone, and pentazocine. Despite claims to the contrary, all these substances (including almost all prescription analgesics) are capable of producing euphoria as well as psychological and physical dependence when taken in high enough doses over prolonged periods.

The opioids produce their effects by binding to different types of opioid receptors throughout the body, including the central nervous system (CNS). Endogenous opioid peptides (i.e., enkephalins, endorphins, dynorphins, and others) have been identified that appear to be natural ligands for opioid receptors. These peptides have a distinct distribution in the CNS. The receptors with which opioid peptides interact are differentially engaged in production of the various opiate effects, such as analgesia, respiratory depression, constipation, and euphoria. Substances capable of antagonizing one or more of these actions include nalorphine, levallorphan, cyclazocine, butorphanol, buprenorphine, and pentazocine, each of which has mixed agonist and antagonist properties, as well as naloxone, nalmefene, and naltrexone, which are pure opiate antagonists. All antagonist drugs (including those with mixed agonist properties), can precipitate withdrawal symptoms if administered to a patient who is physically dependent on other opioids. The availability of relatively specific antagonists has helped identify different receptor subtypes, including μ receptors, which influence some of the more classic opioid actions such as pain control, reinforcement, constipation, hormone levels, and respiration; κ receptors, with possible similar functions along with sedation and effects on hormones; and δ receptors, thought to relate mostly to analgesia, mood, reinforcement, and breathing. The major features of tolerance, dependence, and withdrawal are thought to be mediated primarily by μ receptors. All opioid receptors are coupled to inhibitory G proteins, which mediate their actions within cells (Chap. 386).

Opioid drugs are absorbed from the gastrointestinal system, the lungs, and/or the muscles. The most rapid and pronounced effects occur following intravenous administration, with only slightly less efficient absorption after smoking or inhaling the vapor ("chasing the dragon"), and the least intense actions are seen after absorption from the digestive tract. Most of the metabolism of opioids occurs in the liver, primarily through conjugation with glucuronic acid, and only small amounts are excreted directly in the urine or feces. The plasma half-lives of these drugs range from 2.5 to 3 h for morphine to more than 22 h for methadone and even longer for levomethadyl acetate (LAAM).

Street heroin is typically only 5 to 10% pure. The remainder consists of materials such as lactose and fruit sugars, quinine, powdered milk, phenacetin, caffeine, antipyrine, and strychnine, which are used to "cut" the drug and increase the profit margin. Any marked, unexpected increase in the purity of street drugs is likely to cause unintentional lethal overdoses in users expecting less effect from a "hit."

THE ACUTE AND CHRONIC EFFECTS OF OPIOID DRUGS With the exception of overdose and physical dependence, most opioid effects are relatively benign and rapidly reversible. A major danger, however, comes through the use of contaminated needles by intravenous users, which increases the risk of hepatitis B and C, bacterial endocarditis, and infection with HIV (Chap. 309).

Effects on Body Systems Acute changes in the *gastrointestinal system* are the result of decreased motility with resulting constipation and anorexia. Chronic gastrointestinal problems in opioid-dependent individuals typically occur as a consequence of hepatitis in injection drug users.

Effects of opiods in the CNS include intoxication-induced nausea and vomiting (medulla), decreased pain perception (spinal cord, thalamus, and periaqueductal gray region), euphoria (limbic system), and sedation (reticular activating system). The adulterants added to street drugs may contribute to some of the more permanent nervous system damage, including peripheral neuropathy, amblyopia, myelopathy, and leukoencephalopathy. One study revealed abnormalities in cognitive function and brain computed tomography scans of opioid-dependent subjects; whether these abnormalities are due to the opioid itself, the adulterants, the consequences of dirty needles, or an unhealthy lifestyle is unknown. Acute opioid administration decreases levels of luteinizing hormone, with a subsequent reduction in testosterone, which might contribute to the decreased sex drive reported by most opioid-dependent people. Other hormonal changes include a decrease in the release of thyrotropin and increases in prolactin and possibly growth hormone (Chap. 328).

Acute changes in the *respiratory system* include respiratory depression, which results from a decreased response of the brainstem to carbon dioxide tension, a component of the drug overdose syndrome described below. At even low drug doses, this effect can be clinically significant in individuals with underlying pulmonary disease. *Cardiovascular* changes tend to be relatively mild, with no direct opiate effect on heart rhythm or myocardial contractility, but there is a potential problem from orthostatic hypotension, probably secondary to dilation of peripheral vessels. Bacterial infections of the lungs and heart valves can occur from contaminated needles; the latter can result in emboli and thus an increased risk for stroke.

The Toxic Reaction or Overdose Syndrome High doses of opioids can result in a potentially lethal toxic reaction or overdose syndrome. While toxic reactions are seen with all opioids, the more potent drugs such as fentanyl (80 to 100 times more powerful than morphine) are especially dangerous. The typical syndrome, which occurs immediately with intravenous overdose, includes shallow respirations at a rate of two to four per minute, pupillary miosis (with mydriasis once brain anoxia develops), bradycardia, a decrease in body temperature, and a general absence of responsiveness to external stimulation. If this medical emergency is not treated rapidly, respiratory depression, cyanosis, cardiorespiratory arrest, and death can ensue. Postmortem examination reveals few specific changes except for diffuse cerebral edema. An "allergic-like" reaction to intravenous heroin, perhaps in part related to adulterants, can also occur and is characterized by decreased alertness, a frothy pulmonary edema, and an elevation in the blood eosinophil count.

The first step in managing overdose is to provide any needed respiratory or cardiovascular support including intubation for airway protection if needed. Definitive treatment for the typical opioid overdose is the administration of a narcotic antagonist such as naloxone in an initial dose of 0.4 mg to 2 mg intravenously, expecting a response in 1 to 2 min. This dose can be repeated every 2 to 3 min up to a dose of 10 mg. With the exception of overdoses with buprenorphene, if no response is seen after 10 mg, it is unlikely that an opioid overdose is responsible for the respiratory depression or coma. If an intravenous line is not available, the drug can be given intramuscularly. It is important to titrate the dose relative to the patient's symptoms. The goal is to ameliorate the respiratory depression but not provoke a severe withdrawal state. Because the effects of this drug diminish within 2 to 3 h, the individual must be monitored for at least 24 h after a heroin overdose and 72 h after an overdose of a longer-acting drug such as methadone. If there is little response to naloxone alone, the possibility of a concomitant overdose with a benzodiazepine should be considered and a challenge with intravenous flumazenil, 0.2 mg/min up to a maximum of 3 mg in an hour, might be used. Patients who are physically dependent on an opioid may experience a precipitous onset of an abstinence syndrome after administration of the opioid antagonist, but aggressive treatment of this syndrome is not appropriate until all vital signs are relatively stable.

As with any drug overdose, treatment of either the typical or the "allergic" type of opioid toxic reaction often requires continued supportive care until the drug effect subsides. Patients may require respiratory support (often with oxygen supplementation and positive-pressure breathing for the "allergic" type of overdose), intravenous fluids perhaps accompanied by pressor agents to support blood pressure, and gastric lavage to remove any remaining drug with care taken to use a cuffed endotracheal tube to prevent aspiration if the patient is not alert. It is important to evaluate and treat any possible anaphylactic reactions. Cardiac arrhythmias and/or convulsions, especially likely to be seen with codeine, propoxyphene, or meperidine, also need to be treated.

OPIOID ABUSE AND DEPENDENCE **Definition and Epidemiology** Repeated opioid use to the point of developing multiple problems is a good indicator that future abuse and dependence are likely. DSM-IV criteria for opioid dependence are the same as those for alcohol dependence (Chap. 387). An individual is dependent if within a 12-month period repeated difficulties occur in any three areas of functioning, including tolerance, withdrawal, use of greater amounts of opiates than intended, and use despite consequences. Patients who do not have dependence but demonstrate repeated difficulties with the law, impaired ability to meet obligations, use in hazardous situations, or continued use despite problems can be labeled as having abuse.

The use of opioids for intoxication is less prevalent than the use of alcohol, marijuana, and several other drugs. A 1997 national survey reported that almost 5% of men and women age 12 or above in the United States had used an opioid for intoxication, including almost 2% in the prior year and slightly less than 1% in the prior month. Focusing specifically on heroin, the lifetime prevalence was approximately 1%, with 0.3% having taken the drug in the prior year. Use patterns of these drugs were almost twice as high in another 1997 survey sampling 12th graders in high school. In all studies, prevalence rates were higher in males than females. None of the national surveys offered data regarding the prevalence of dependence.

Genetics While most data on the importance of genetic influences in substance use disorders apply to alcoholism, there are interesting findings regarding other drugs. One large study of over 3000 male twin pairs reported that there are genetic influences that relate uniquely to heroin dependence and also noted additional genetic factors related to an overall vulnerability toward substance-related problems. The genetic influences operate in the context of additional environmental factors that are likely to relate both to the family of upbringing and the general environment. Genetic factors might influence personality characteristics such as impulsivity and sensation-seeking or susceptibility to develop antisocial personality disorder. Genes relating to the actions of the drug on specific neurochemical systems such as dopamine are also potential candidates for an enhanced vulnerability toward developing opioid dependence.

Natural History Dependence on or abuse of opioids can be seen in at least three types of patients. First, a minority of people with nonfatal *chronic pain syndromes* (e.g., back, joint, and muscle disorders) misuse their prescribed drugs. If physical dependence is established, abstinence syndromes can then intensify the pain, promoting continued drug intake. Physicians can avoid contributing to physical dependence by helping the patient to accept the goal of minimization rather than disappearance of the pain and to recognize that discomfort may not be completely eliminated (Chap. 12). Analgesic medication should be only one component of treatment and limited to the oral administration of the least potent analgesic that is able to "take the edge off" the pain (e.g., ibuprofen or, if needed, propoxyphene). Behavior modification techniques, such as muscle relaxation and meditation, and carefully selected exercises should be used as appropriate to help increase function and decrease pain. Finally, nonmedicinal approaches, including electrical transcutaneous neurostimulation for muscle and joint disease, may be useful.

The second group at high risk are *physicians*, *nurses*, and *pharmacists*, primarily because of their easy access to substances of abuse. Physicians may begin to use opioids to help them sleep or to reduce stress or physical aches and pains. This group appears to be at especially high risk for developing dependence on the highly potent drugs such as fentanyl. Because of the growing awareness of these problems, impaired-physician programs have been established in many hospitals and by most state medical societies. Such groups attempt to identify and aid substance-impaired physicians, giving them peer support and education to help them achieve abstinence before problems escalate to the point of licensure revocation. All doctors are advised never to prescribe opioids for themselves or for members of their family—physicians deserve the same level of care and protection from future problems as their patients.

The third and most obvious group are those who buy street drugs to get high. While some of these men and women have prior histories of severe antisocial problems, most have a relatively high level of premorbid functioning. The typical person begins using opioids occasionally, often after experimenting with tobacco, then alcohol, then marijuana, and then brain depressants or stimulants. Occasional opiate use, or "chipping," might continue for some time, and some individuals never escalate their intake to the point of developing dependence.

Of course, opiate-dependent individuals are likely to continue to have experience with many other drugs. At least three of these often remain as problems during the course of opioid dependence. First, alcohol is typically used to moderate withdrawal problems, to enhance the opioid high, and as a substitute when the preferred drug is not readily available, including during methadone and other treatments. This pattern of problematic drinking, often meeting criteria for alcohol dependence, is present at some time in approximately half of opioid-dependent persons. The second drug, cocaine, appears to be taken for many of the same reasons as alcohol, and is often administered intravenously with the opioid in a mixture known as a "speedball." The third class of drugs misused in combination with opioids consists of the benzodiazepines, especially among people in methadone maintenance.

Once persistent opioid use is established, severe problems are likely to develop. At least 25% die within 10 to 20 years from suicide, homicide, accidents, or infectious diseases such as tuberculosis, hepatitis, or AIDS. The mortality rate has escalated in recent years in response to the AIDS epidemic among injection drug users, with an estimated 60% of these men and women carrying HIV (Chap. 309). At the same time, while the majority of opioid-dependent persons show frequent exacerbations and remissions, it is important to remember that approximately 35% achieve long-term, often permanent, abstinence. This remission is probably most often seen after the age of 40 but can occur at any point in the clinical course. While this favorable outcome can be observed in any opioid-dependent person, as is true with most drugs of abuse a better prognosis is associated with prior histories of marital and employment stability and fewer criminal activities unrelated to drugs.

℞ TREATMENT The key to diagnosis is to discard the erroneous stereotype that opioid-dependent men and women are always unemployed and homeless. Abuse or dependence is possible in any patient who demonstrates symptoms of what might be opioid withdrawal; anyone who has a chronic pain syndrome; physicians, nurses, and pharmacists or others with easy access to opioids; and all patients who repeatedly seek out prescription analgesics. Therefore, it is important to take the time with *every* patient, especially those with complaints of pain, to gather a history that includes the patterns of opioid use and the list of doctors and clinics from which they have received prescriptions. If the chronic use of opioids is suspected, gathering further data from an additional informant such as a relative or close friend can be essential. Another indicator of an enhanced risk for opioid dependence is a history of pervasive antisocial problems beginning in the preteen years. Blood and urine screens can be used to identify opioids in patients in whom misuse is suspected, and clinicians should search for physical stigmata of misuse (e.g., needle marks).

After identifying opioid dependence, the next step is intervention. The need for active treatment of the abstinence syndrome can be presented, and the availability of help in establishing a drug-free life-style can be emphasized. The final decision, of course, rests with the patient. This approach to intervention is presented in relation to alcoholism in Chap. 387.

The Symptoms of Withdrawal Withdrawal symptoms, usually the opposite of the acute effects of the drug, include nausea and diarrhea, coughing, lacrimation, mydriasis, rhinorrhea, profuse sweating, twitching muscles, piloerection (or "goose bumps") as well as mild elevations in body temperature, respiratory rate, and blood pressure. In addition, diffuse body pain, insomnia, and yawning occur, along with intense drug craving. Drugs with a short half-life, such as morphine or heroin, cause symptoms typically within 8 to 16 h of the last dose (thus, many dependent individuals awake in mild withdrawal every morning); symptom intensity peaks within 36 to 72 h after discontinuation of the drug, and the acute syndrome disappears within 5 to 8 days. However, a protracted abstinence phase of mild symptoms (e.g., moodiness, slight changes in pupillary size, autonomic dysfunction, changes in sleep pattern) may persist for 6 or more months. These lingering symptoms, which can be relieved by administering an opioid, probably contribute to relapse.

Treatment of the Withdrawal Syndrome A thorough physical examination, including an assessment of neurologic function and a search for local and systemic infections, especially abscesses, is mandatory. Laboratory testing generally includes assessment of liver function and, in intravenous users, HIV status. Proper nutrition and rest must be initiated as soon as possible.

Optimal treatment of withdrawal requires administration of sufficient opioid medication on day 1 to decrease symptoms, followed by a more gradual withdrawal of the drug, usually over 5 to 10 days. Any opioid will work (all have some level of cross-tolerance), but for ease of administration, many physicians prefer to use a long-acting drug such as methadone. To estimate the first day's dose from the patient's history, 1 to 2 mg of methadone can be considered approximately equivalent to 3 mg of morphine, 1 mg of heroin, or 20 mg of meperidine. Most patients require between 10 and 25 mg of methadone orally twice on day 1, with higher doses given if prominent symptoms of withdrawal are not dampened. After several days of a stabilized drug dose, the opioid is then decreased by 10 to 20% of the original day's dose each day.

However, most states restrict the prescription of opioids to dependent persons, and, in the absence of special permits, detoxification with opioids is often proscribed or limited. Thus, pharmacologic treatments often center on relief of symptoms of diarrhea with Imodium or a nonopioid drug, of "sniffles" with decongestants, and pain with nonopioid analgesics (e.g., ibuprofen). Comfort can be enhanced with the α_2-adrenergic agonist clonidine to decrease sympathetic nervous system overactivity. Given at doses of approximately 5 μg/kg (up to 0.3 mg given two to four times a day), clonidine decreases autonomic nervous system dysfunction and produces sedation. Blood pressure should be monitored closely. Some clinicians augment this regimen with low to moderate doses of benzodiazepines for 2 to 5 days to decrease agitation.

A special case of opioid withdrawal is seen in the newborn made passively dependent through the mother's drug abuse during pregnancy. Some level of withdrawal develops in 50 to 90% of children of heroin-dependent mothers. As few as 25% of infants of methadone-maintenance mothers show clinically relevant withdrawal symptoms, probably because of the longer half-life of this drug. The syndrome consists of irritability, crying, a tremor (in 80%), increased reflexes, increased respiratory rate, diarrhea, hyperactivity (in 60%), vomiting (40%), and sneezing/yawning/hiccuping (in 30%). The child usually has a low birth weight but may be otherwise unremarkable until the second day, when symptoms are likely to begin.

The treatment follows the same general steps used in the treatment of the physically dependent adult. The child must be carefully evaluated to rule out medical problems such as hypoglycemia, hypocalcemia, infections, and trauma; general support in a warm, quiet environment and regulation of electrolytes and glucose are also required. The infant with moderate to severe symptoms can be treated with any of the following: paregoric (0.2 mL orally every 3 to 4 h), methadone (0.1 to 0.5 mg/kg per day), phenobarbital (8 mg/kg per day), or diazepam (1 to 2 mg/kg every 8 h). Medication should be given in decreasing levels for 10 to 20 days. Dependent infants of mothers on methadone maintenance also benefit by breast feeding while the mother continues to take methadone.

Rehabilitation of Opioid-Dependent Persons Despite some differences in demographics, the same general rules for rehabilitation apply to opioid-dependent persons as to alcoholics. The basic strategy includes detoxification and family support, and the process can benefit from the use of reading materials or referral to self-help groups. It is also important to establish realistic patient goals and a program of counseling and education to increase motivation toward abstinence. A long-term commitment to rebuilding a life-style without the substance is essential for preventing recidivism.

Most rehabilitation approaches have common elements, regardless of the drug involved. Patients are educated about their responsibility for improving their lives, and *motivation for abstinence* is increased by providing information about the medical and psychological problems that can be expected if dependence continues. Patients and families are encouraged to *establish an opioid-free life-style* by learning to cope with chronic pain and develop realistic vocational planning (e.g., for pharmacists, physicians, and nurses). The dependent person is also encouraged to establish a drug-free peer group and to participate in self-help groups such as Narcotics Anonymous. Another important treatment component is *relapse prevention* aimed at identifying triggers for a return to drugs and developing appropriate coping strategies.

Much of this advice and counseling can be given by the physician, but many clinicians refer patients to more formal drug programs, including methadone maintenance clinics, programs using narcotic antagonists, and therapeutic communities. Long-term follow-up of treated patients indicates that approximately one-third were completely drug free in the previous year; 60% were no longer using opioids, although some were misusing other substances. Individuals who stay in methadone maintenance or in therapeutic communities show significant improvement in antisocial behavior and employment status. In general, the best prognosis is for those individuals who are employed, who have higher levels of education, and who remain in treatment for at least 2 months. Dependence among health care providers, such as physicians, is treated similarly, but in addition a closely supervised "diversion" procedure is usually instituted and carried out for 1 to 2 years or more.

Methadone maintenance Maintenance programs with methadone and the even longer-acting agent LAAM should only be used in combination with education and counseling. It is important to note that drug maintenance is not aimed at "curing" opioid dependence; rather, it provides a substitute drug that is legally accessible, safer, can be taken orally, and has a long half-life so that it can be taken once a day. The goal is to help persons who have repeatedly failed in drug-free programs to improve functioning within the family and job, to decrease legal problems, and to improve health.

Methadone is a long-acting opioid that possesses almost all the physiologic properties of heroin. The recipient, who has been carefully screened to rule out prior psychiatric disorders, may be maintained on a relatively low dose (e.g., 30 to 40 mg/d); a better approach is to use a higher dose (80 to 120 mg/d), because it may be more effective in blocking heroin-induced euphoria and decreasing craving. There is some evidence that the higher methadone doses result in greater retention in treatment and consequently in lower levels of arrest and relapse to street drugs. Three-quarters or more of patients, especially those receiving the higher doses, are likely to remain heroin-free for 6 months or longer. Methadone is administered as an oral liquid given once a day at the program, with weekend doses taken by the patient at home. The longer-acting analogues, such as LAAM, can be given two or three times a week, with the dose of LAAM increased to as high as 80 mg three times a week if needed. After a period of maintenance (usually 6 months to 1 year or longer), the clinician can work closely with the patient to regulate the rate of drug decrease (by about 5% per week) if possible.

In the past, the British have used heroin maintenance with goals and guidelines similar to those of current methadone programs. There is no evidence that heroin maintenance has any advantages over methadone maintenance, but the heroin approach does add the risk that the drug will be easily sold on the streets. Treatment with mixed agonists-antagonists such as buprenorphine also appears beneficial, although results are not as good as with methadone.

Opioid antagonists The opiate antagonists (e.g., naloxone) compete with heroin and other opioids for receptors, reducing the effects of the opioid agonists. Administered over long periods with the intention of blocking the "high" produced if the patient takes opioids, these drugs can be useful as part of an overall treatment approach that includes counseling and support. The most widely used antagonist in rehabilitation is naltrexone; 50 mg per day antagonizes 15 mg of heroin for 24 h, and higher doses (125 to 150 mg) block the effects of 25 mg of intravenous heroin for up to 3 days. Naltrexone is free of agonist properties, produces no known withdrawal symptoms when stopped, and its side effects tend to be mild. To avoid precipitating a withdrawal syndrome, patients should be free of opioids for a minimum of 5 days before beginning treatment with this medication. In addition, they should first be challenged with 0.4 or 0.8 mg of the shorter-acting agent naloxone to be certain they are able to tolerate the long-acting antagonist. Following this procedure, a test dose of 10 mg of naltrexone can be given, with the expectation that any withdrawal symptoms will be seen in 0.5 to 2 h. Several variations of this approach can be used with detoxification from methadone maintenance, including a fairly rapid, medically supervised plan. Over a 10-day period, the daily dose should be increased to about 100 mg on Mondays and Wednesdays and 150 mg on Fridays. Unfortunately, despite the apparent advantages of this treatment approach, some patients are resistant to continuing care. In one study, only about 60% of the patients completed 6 days of naltrexone induction, and only 10% remained in the program at the end of 6 months. However, another study reported much higher rates of compliance, with almost a third achieving continuous abstinence for at least a year.

Drug-free programs Most existing halfway houses and recovery centers for opioid-dependent persons use some variant of the therapeutic community approach. This is an exception to the general preference for short-term residential (as opposed to outpatient) rehabilitation, since care can last a year or more while the person is taken out of the street culture and given a new life within the group. In this structure, members, including leaders who are themselves in the process of recovery, help participants gain insights into more successful strategies for coping with problems.

As is true for treatments of all substance-use disorders, it is likely that counseling, behavioral treatments, and relatively simple approaches to psychotherapy add significantly to a positive outcome. Most approaches focus on teaching participants to cope with stress, enhancing their understanding of personality attributes, teaching better cognitive styles, and, through the process of relapse prevention, addressing issues that might contribute to increased craving, easy access to drugs, or periods of decreased motivation. A combination of these therapies with the approaches described above appears to give the best results.

Finally, it is important to discuss prevention. Except for the terminally ill, physicians should carefully monitor opioid drug use in their patients, keeping doses as low as is practical and administering them over as short a period as the level of pain would warrant in the average person. Physicians must be vigilant regarding their own risk for opioid abuse and dependence, *never* prescribing these drugs for themselves. For the nonmedical intravenous drug–dependent person, all possible efforts must be made to prevent AIDS, hepatitis, bacterial endocarditis, and other consequences of contaminated needles both through methadone maintenance and by considering needle-exchange programs.

BIBLIOGRAPHY

AHMED SH, KOOB GF: Transition from moderate to excessive drug intake: Change in hedonic set point. Science 282:298, 1998

AMERICAN PSYCHIATRIC ASSOCIATION: Practical guidelines for the treatment of substance use disorders. Am J Psychiatry 52(Suppl):1, 1995

BALL J, ROSS A: *The Effectiveness of Methadone Maintenance Treatments*. New York, Springer-Verlag, 1991

CORNISH JW et al: Naltrexone pharmacotherapy for opioid dependent federal probationers. J Subst Abuse Treat 14:529, 1997

GOLDMAN D, BERGEN A: General and specific inheritance of substance abuse and alcoholism. Arch Gen Psychiatry 55:964, 1998

JONES JE et al: Induction with levomethadyl acetate. Arch Gen Psychiatry 55:729, 1998

KLEE H, MORRIS J: The role of needle exchanges in modifying sharing behavior: Cross-study comparisons 1989–1993. Addiction 90:1635, 1995

MAGURA S et al: Pre- and in-treatment predictors of retention in methadone treatment using survival analysis. Addiction 93:51, 1998

MANFREDINI R et al: Emergency admissions of opioid drug abusers for overdose: A chronobiological study of enhanced risk. Ann Emerg Med 24:615, 1994

MORRISON J, WICKERSHAM P: Physicians disciplined by a state medical board. JAMA 279:1889, 1998

SCHOTTENFELD RS et al: Buprenorphine vs methadone maintenance treatment for concurrent opioid dependence and cocaine abuse. Arch Gen Psychiatry 54:713, 1997

SCHUCKIT MA: *Educating Yourself about Alcohol and Drugs: A People's Primer*. New York, Plenum, 1998

———: *Drug and Alcohol Abuse: A Clinical Guide to Diagnosis and Treatment*, 5th ed. New York, Plenum, 2000

——— et al: Clinical implications for four drugs of the DSM-IV distinction between substance dependence with and without a physiological component. Am J Psychiatry 156:41, 1999

SEES KL et al: Methadone maintenance vs 180-day psychosocially enriched detoxification for treatment of opioid dependence. A randomized controlled trial. JAMA 283:1303, 2000

TSUANG MT et al: Co-occurrence of abuse of different drugs in men: The role of drug-specific and shared vulnerabilities. Arch Gen Psychiatry 55:967, 1998

389

Jack H. Mendelson, Nancy K. Mello

COCAINE AND OTHER COMMONLY ABUSED DRUGS

The abuse of cocaine and other psychostimulant drugs appears to be increasing in many metropolitan and rural areas throughout the world, according to a year 2000 report by the National Institute on Drug Abuse (NIDA). The number of deaths associated with these drugs has also increased. In several urban areas of the United States, use of these drugs has increased more sharply among women than men. Although enhanced legal enforcement as well as educational prevention procedures have attenuated, in part, the increase in psychostimulant abuse among youths in the United States, there appears to be an enhanced worldwide risk for psychostimulant abuse and dependence.

The initiation and continuation of drug abuse are determined by a complex interaction of the pharmacologic properties and relative availability of each drug, the personality and expectations of the user, and the environmental context in which the drug is used. Polydrug abuse, the concurrent use of several drugs with different pharmacologic effects, is increasingly common among individuals from all socioeconomic strata. There has been an alarming increase in particularly dangerous forms of polydrug abuse, such as the combined use of heroin and cocaine intravenously. There is no simple explanation for this change in polydrug use patterns. Drug abusers may attempt to attenuate one drug effect with another, as when heroin or alcohol is used to modulate the cocaine high. Sometimes one drug is used to enhance the effects of another, as with benzodiazepines and methadone, or cocaine plus heroin in methadone-maintained patients.

Chronic cocaine and psychostimulant abuse may cause a number of adverse health consequences, ranging from pulmonary disease to reproductive dysfunction. Preexisting disorders such as hypertension and cardiac disease may be exacerbated by drug abuse, and the combined use of two or more drugs may accentuate medical complications associated with abuse of one of them. The adverse health consequences of drug abuse are further complicated by AIDS.

Drug abuse increases the risk of exposure to HIV. Cocaine and psychostimulant abuse contribute to the risk for HIV infection in part by the adverse immunomodulatory effects of these drugs. In addition, concurrent use of cocaine and opiates (the "speedball") is frequently associated with needle-sharing by intravenous drug users. These individuals continue to represent the largest single group of persons with HIV infection in several major metropolitan areas in the United States as well as in urban areas in Scotland, Italy, Spain, Thailand, and China.

COCAINE Cocaine is a stimulant and local anesthetic with potent vasoconstrictor properties. The leaves of the coca plant (*Erythroxylon coca*) contain approximately 0.5 to 1% cocaine. The drug produces physiologic and behavioral effects when administered orally, intranasally (snorting), intravenously, or via inhalation following pyrolysis (smoking). Cocaine increases synaptic concentrations of the monoamine neurotransmitters dopamine, norepinephrine, and serotonin by binding to transporter proteins in presynaptic neurons and blocking reuptake. The reinforcing effects of cocaine are related to effects on dopaminergic neurons in the mesolimbic system (Chap. 386).

Prevalence of Cocaine Use Cocaine has become widely available throughout the United States, and cocaine abuse occurs in virtually all social and economic strata of society. The prevalence of cocaine abuse in the general population has been accompanied by an increase in cocaine abuse by heroin-dependent persons, including those in methadone maintenance programs. Intravenous cocaine is often used concurrently with intravenous heroin—a combination that purportedly attenuates the postcocaine "crash" and substitutes a cocaine "high" for the heroin "high" blocked by methadone.

Acute and Chronic Cocaine Intoxication There has been an increase in both intravenous administration and inhalation of pyrolyzed cocaine via smoking. Following intranasal administration, changes in mood and sensation are perceived within 3 to 5 min, and peak effects occur at 10 to 20 min. The effects rarely last >1 h. Inhalation of pyrolyzed materials includes inhaling crack/cocaine or smoking coca paste, a product made by extracting cocaine preparations with flammable solvents, and cocaine free-base smoking. Free-base cocaine, including the free base prepared with sodium bicarbonate (crack), is becoming increasingly popular because of the relative high potency of the compound and its rapid onset of action (8 to 10 s following smoking).

Cocaine produces a brief, dose-related stimulation and enhancement of mood and an increase in cardiac rate and blood pressure. Body temperature usually increases, and high doses of cocaine may induce

lethal pyrexia or hypertension. Because cocaine inhibits reuptake of catecholamines at adrenergic nerve endings, the drug potentiates sympathetic nervous system activity. Cocaine has a short plasma half-life of approximately 45 to 60 min. Cocaine is metabolized primarily by plasma esterases, and cocaine metabolites are excreted in urine. The very short duration of euphorigenic effects of cocaine observed in chronic abusers is probably due to both acute and chronic tolerance. Frequent self-administration of the drug (two to three times per hour) is often reported by chronic cocaine abusers. Alcohol is used to modulate both the cocaine high and the dysphoria associated with the abrupt disappearance of cocaine's effects. A metabolite of cocaine, cocaethylene, has been detected in blood and urine of persons who concurrently abuse alcohol and cocaine. Cocaethylene induces changes in cardiovascular function similar to those of cocaine alone, and the pathophysiologic consequences of alcohol abuse plus cocaine abuse may be additive when both are used together.

The prevalent assumption that cocaine inhalation or intravenous administration is relatively safe is contradicted by reports of death from respiratory depression, cardiac arrhythmias, and convulsions associated with cocaine use. In addition to generalized seizures, neurologic complications may include headache, ischemic or hemorrhagic stroke, or subarachnoid hemorrhage. Disorders of cerebral blood flow and perfusion in cocaine-dependent persons have been detected with magnetic resonance spectroscopy (MRS) studies. Severe pulmonary disease may develop in individuals who inhale crack cocaine; this effect is attributed both to the direct effects of cocaine and to residual contaminants in the smoked material. Hepatic necrosis has been reported to occur following crack cocaine use.

Although men and women who abuse cocaine may report that the drug enhances libidinal drive, chronic cocaine use causes significant loss of libido and adversely affects reproductive function. Impotence and gynecomastia have been observed in male cocaine abusers, and these abnormalities often persist for long periods following cessation of drug use. Women who abuse cocaine have reported major derangements in menstrual cycle function including galactorrhea, amenorrhea, and infertility. Chronic cocaine abuse may cause persistent hyperprolactinemia as a consequence of disordered dopaminergic inhibition of prolactin secretion by the pituitary. Cocaine abuse by pregnant women, particularly the smoking of crack, has been associated with both an increased risk of congenital malformations in the fetus and perinatal cardiovascular and cerebrovascular disease in the mother. However, cocaine abuse per se is probably not the sole cause of these perinatal disorders, since many problems associated with maternal cocaine abuse, including poor nutrition and health care status as well as polydrug abuse, also contribute to risk for perinatal disease.

Protracted cocaine abuse may cause paranoid ideation and visual and auditory hallucinations, a state that resembles alcoholic hallucinosis. Psychological dependence on cocaine, as manifested by inability to abstain from frequent compulsive use, has also been reported. Although the occurrence of withdrawal syndromes involving psychomotor agitation and autonomic hyperactivity remains controversial, severe depression ("crashing") following cocaine intoxication may accompany drug withdrawal.

℞ **TREATMENT** Treatment of cocaine overdose is a medical emergency that is often best managed in an intensive care unit. Cocaine toxicity produces a hyperadrenergic state characterized by hypertension, tachycardia, tonic-clonic seizures, dyspnea, and ventricular arrhythmias. Intravenous diazepam in doses up to 0.5 mg/kg administered over an 8-h period has been shown to be effective for control of seizures. Ventricular arrhythmias have been managed successfully by administration of 0.5 to 1.0 mg of propranolol intravenously. Since many instances of cocaine-related mortality have been associated with concurrent use of other illicit drugs (particularly heroin), the physician must be prepared to institute effective emergency treatment for multiple drug toxicities.

Treatment of chronic cocaine abuse requires combined efforts by primary care physicians, psychiatrists, and psychosocial care providers. Early abstinence from cocaine use is often complicated by symptoms of depression and guilt, insomnia, and anorexia, which may be as severe as those observed in major affective disorders. Individual and group psychotherapy, family therapy, and peer group assistance programs are often useful for inducing prolonged remission from drug use. A number of medications used for the treatment of various psychiatric disorders have been administered to reduce the duration and severity of cocaine abuse and dependence. However, no available medication is both safe and highly effective for either cocaine detoxification or maintenance of abstinence. Some psychotherapeutic interventions are occasionally effective; however, no specific form of psychotherapy or behavioral modification is uniquely beneficial.

MARIJUANA AND CANNABIS COMPOUNDS *Cannabis sativa* contains >400 compounds in addition to the psychoactive substance, delta-9-tetrahydrocannabinol (THC). Marijuana cigarettes are prepared from the leaves and flowering tops of the plant, and a typical marijuana cigarette contains 0.5 to 1 g of plant material. Although the usual THC concentration varies between 10 and 40 mg, concentrations >100 mg per cigarette have been detected. Hashish is prepared from concentrated resin of *C. sativa* and contains a THC concentration of between 8 to 12% by weight. "Hash oil," a lipid-soluble plant extract, may contain a THC concentration of 25 to 60% and may be added to marijuana or hashish to enhance its THC concentration. Smoking is the most common mode of marijuana or hashish use. During pyrolysis, >150 compounds in addition to THC are released in the smoke. Although most of these compounds do not have psychoactive properties, they do have potential physiologic effects.

THC is quickly absorbed from the lungs into blood and is then rapidly sequestered in tissues. It is metabolized primarily in the liver, where it is converted to 11-hydroxy-THC, a psychoactive compound, and >20 other metabolites. Many THC metabolites are excreted through the feces at a rate of clearance that is relatively slow in comparison to that of most other psychoactive drugs.

Specific cannabinoid receptors (CB_1 and CB_2) have been identified in the central nervous system, including the spinal cord, and in the peripheral nervous system. High densities of these receptors have been found in the cerebral cortex, basal ganglia, and hippocampus. B lymphocytes also appear to have cannabinoid receptors. A naturally occurring THC-like ligand has been identified in the nervous system, where it is widely distributed.

Prevalence of Marijuana Use Marijuana is the most commonly used illegal drug in the United States. Use is particularly prevalent among adolescents; studies suggest that ~40% of high school students in the United States have used marijuana. Marijuana is relatively inexpensive and is considered by many persons to be less hazardous than the use of other controlled drugs and substances. Very potent forms of marijuana (sinsemilla) are now available in many communities, and concurrent use of marijuana with crack/cocaine and phencyclidine is increasing. Marijuana abuse by individuals from all social strata has been increasing.

Acute and Chronic Marijuana Intoxication Acute intoxication from marijuana and cannabis compounds is related to both the dose of THC and the route of administration. THC is absorbed more rapidly from marijuana smoking than from orally ingested cannabis compounds. Acute marijuana intoxication usually consists of a subjective perception of relaxation and mild euphoria resembling mild to moderate alcohol intoxication. This condition is usually accompanied by some impairment in thinking, concentration, and perceptual and psychomotor function. Higher doses of cannabis may produce behavioral effects analogous to severe alcohol intoxication. Although the effects of acute marijuana intoxication are relatively benign in normal users, the drug can precipitate severe emotional disorders in individuals who have antecedent psychotic or neurotic problems. As with other psychoactive compounds, both set (user's expectations) and setting (environmental context) are important determinants of the type and severity of behavioral intoxication.

As is true of alcoholics, chronic marijuana abusers may lose interest in common socially desirable goals and steadily devote more time to drug acquisition and use. However, THC does not cause a specific and unique "amotivational syndrome." The range of symptoms sometimes attributed to marijuana use is difficult to distinguish from mild to moderate depression and the maturational dysfunctions often associated with protracted adolescence. Chronic marijuana use has also been reported to increase the risk of psychotic symptoms in individuals with a past history of schizophrenia.

Physical Effects of Marijuana Conjunctival injection and tachycardia are the most frequent immediate physical concomitants of smoking marijuana. Tolerance for marijuana-induced tachycardia develops rapidly among regular users; angina may be precipitated by marijuana smoking in persons with a history of coronary insufficiency. Exercise-induced angina may be increased after marijuana use to a greater extent than after tobacco cigarette smoking. Patients with cardiac disease should be strongly advised not to use cannabis compounds.

Significant decrements in pulmonary vital capacity have been found in regular daily marijuana smokers. Because marijuana smoking typically involves deep inhalation and prolonged retention of marijuana smoke, marijuana smokers may develop chronic bronchial irritation. Impairment of single-breath carbon monoxide diffusion capacity (DL_{co}) is greater in persons who smoke both marijuana and tobacco than in tobacco smokers. Despite the well-documented association between tobacco smoking and lung cancer, at present there is no direct evidence that marijuana smoking induces lung cancer. However, heavy marijuana use among Americans may be too recent to permit detection of this problem.

Although marijuana has also been associated with adverse effects on a number of other systems, many of these studies await replication and confirmation. A reported correlation between marijuana use and decreased testosterone levels in males has not been confirmed. Decreased sperm count and sperm motility and morphologic abnormalities of spermatozoa following marijuana use have also been reported. Administration of high doses of marijuana to female rhesus monkeys suppresses pituitary gonadotropins and gonadal steroids. Prospective studies demonstrated a correlation between impaired fetal growth and development and heavy marijuana use during pregnancy. Marijuana has also been implicated in derangements of the immune system; in chromosomal abnormalities; and in inhibition of DNA, RNA, and protein synthesis; however, these findings have not been confirmed or related to any specific physiologic effect in humans.

Tolerance and Physical Dependence Habitual marijuana users rapidly develop tolerance to the psychoactive effects of marijuana and often smoke more frequently and try to secure more potent cannabis compounds. Tolerance for the physiologic effects of marijuana develops at different rates; e.g., tolerance develops rapidly for marijuana-induced tachycardia but more slowly for marijuana-induced conjunctival injection. Tolerance to both behavioral and physiologic effects of marijuana decreases rapidly upon cessation of marijuana use.

Withdrawal signs and symptoms have been reported in chronic cannabis users, with the severity of symptoms related to dosage and duration of use. These include tremor, nystagmus, sweating, nausea, vomiting, diarrhea, irritability, anorexia, and sleep disturbances. Withdrawal signs and symptoms observed in chronic marijuana users are usually relatively mild in comparison to those observed in heavy opiate or alcohol users and rarely require medical or pharmacologic intervention. More severe and protracted abstinence syndromes may occur after sustained use of high potency cannabis compounds.

Therapeutic Use of Marijuana Marijuana, administered as cigarettes or as a synthetic oral cannabinoid (dronabinol), has been proposed to have a number of properties that may be clinically useful in some situations. These include antiemetic effects in chemotherapy recipients, appetite-promoting effects in AIDS, reduction of intraocular pressure in glaucoma, and reduction of spasticity in multiple sclerosis and other neurologic disorders. With the possible exception of AIDS-related cachexia, none of these attributes of marijuana compounds is clearly superior to other readily available therapies. Furthermore, any therapeutic benefit of marijuana must be balanced against the many unhealthy psychoactive effects associated with its use.

METHAMPHETAMINE The abuse of methamphetamine, also referred to as "meth," "speed," "crank," "chalk," "ice," "glass," or "crystal," has been declining in many metropolitan areas and communities throughout the United States. This decrease is attributed in part to drug seizures and the closures of clandestine laboratories that produce methamphetamine illegally. Prevention programs focusing upon methamphetamine abuse have also increased.

Most persons who abuse amphetamine self-administer the drug orally, although there have been reports of methamphetamine administration by inhalation and intravenous injection. Individuals who abuse or become dependent upon methamphetamine state that use of this drug induces feelings of euphoria and decreases fatigue associated with aversive life situations. Adverse physiologic effects observed as a consequence of methamphetamine abuse include headache, difficulty concentrating, diminished appetite, abdominal pain, vomiting or diarrhea, disordered sleep, paranoid or aggressive behavior, and psychosis. Severe, life-threatening toxicity may present as hypertension, cardiac arrythmia or failure, subarachnoid hemorrhage, ischemic stroke, intracerebral hemorrhage, convulsions, or coma. Amphetamines increase the release of monoamine neurotransmitters (dopamine, norepinephrine, and serotonin) from presynaptic neurons. It is thought that the euphoric and reinforcing effects of this class of drugs are mediated through dopamine and the mesolimbic system, whereas the cardiovascular effects are related to norepinephrine. Magnetic resonance spectroscopy studies suggest that chronic abuse may injure the frontal areas and basal ganglia of the brain.

Therapy of acute methamphetamine overdose is largely symptomatic. Ammonium chloride may be useful to acidify the urine and enhance clearance of the drug. Hypertension may respond to sodium nitroprusside or α-adrenergic antagonists. Sedatives may reduce agitation and other signs of central nervous system overactivity. Treatment of chronic methamphetamine dependence may be accomplished in either an inpatient or outpatient setting using strategies similar to those described above for cocaine abuse.

MDMA (3,4-methylenedioxymethamphetamine), or *Ecstasy*, is a derivative of methamphetamine. Ecstasy is usually taken orally but may be injected or inhaled. In addition to amphetamine-like effects, MDMA can induce vivid hallucinations and other perceptual distortions. These toxicities are similar to those of lysergic acid diethylamide (LSD) and may be mediated through the release of serotonin.

LYSERGIC ACID DIETHYLAMIDE The discovery of the psychedelic effects of LSD in 1947 led to an epidemic of LSD abuse during the 1960s. Imposition of stringent constraints on the manufacture and distribution of LSD (classified as a Schedule I substance by the U.S. Food and Drug Administration), as well as public recognition that psychedelic experiences induced by LSD were a health hazard, have resulted in a reduction in LSD abuse. The drug still retains some popularity among adolescents and young adults, however, and there are indications that LSD use among young persons has been increasing in some communities in the United States.

LSD is a very potent drug; oral doses as low as 20 μg may induce profound psychological and physiologic effects. Tachycardia, hypertension, pupillary dilation, tremor, and hyperpyrexia occur within minutes following oral administration of 0.5 to 2 μg/kg. A variety of bizarre and often conflicting perceptual and mood changes, including visual illusions, synesthesias, and extreme lability of mood, usually occur within 30 min after LSD intake. The action of LSD may persist for 12 to 18 h, even though the half-life of the drug is only 3 h.

Tolerance develops rapidly for LSD-induced changes in psychological function when the drug is used one or more times per day for 4 or more days. Abrupt abstinence following continued use does not produce withdrawal signs or symptoms. There have been no clinical reports of death caused by the direct effects of LSD.

The most frequent medical emergency associated with LSD use is panic episode (the "bad trip"), which may persist up to 24 h. Management of this problem is best accomplished by supportive reassurance ("talking down") and, if necessary, administration of small doses of anxiolytic drugs. Adverse consequences of chronic LSD use include risk for schizophreniform psychosis and derangements in memory function, problem solving, and abstract thinking. Treatment of these disorders is best carried out in specialized psychiatric facilities.

PHENCYCLIDINE Phencyclidine (PCP), a cyclohexylamine derivative, is widely used in veterinary medicine to briefly immobilize large animals and is sometimes described as a dissociative anesthetic. PCP binds to ionotropic *n*-methyl-*d*-aspartate (NMDA) receptors in the nervous system, blocking ion current through these channels. PCP is easily synthesized; its abusers are primarily young people and polydrug users. It is used orally, by smoking, or by intravenous injection. It is also used as an adulterant in THC, LSD, amphetamine, or cocaine. The most common street preparation, *angel dust*, is a white granular powder that contains 50 to 100% of the drug. Low doses (5 mg) produce agitation, excitement, impaired motor coordination, dysarthria, and analgesia. Users may have horizontal or vertical nystagmus, flushing, diaphoresis, and hyperacusis. Behavioral changes include distortions of body image, disorganization of thinking, and feelings of estrangement. Higher doses of PCP (5 to 10 mg) may produce hypersalivation, vomiting, myoclonus, fever, stupor, or coma. PCP doses of $\geq$10 mg cause convulsions, opisthotonus, and decerebrate posturing, which may be followed by prolonged coma.

The diagnosis of PCP overdose is difficult because the patient's initial symptoms may suggest an acute schizophrenic reaction. Confirmation of PCP use is possible by determination of PCP levels in serum or urine; PCP assays are available at most toxicologic centers. PCP remains in urine for 1 to 5 days following high-dose intake.

PCP overdose requires life-support measures, including treatment of coma, convulsions, and respiratory depression in an intensive care unit. There is no specific antidote or antagonist for PCP. PCP excretion from the body can be enhanced by gastric lavage and acidification of urine. Death from PCP overdose may occur as a consequence of some combination of pharyngeal hypersecretion, hyperthermia, respiratory depression, severe hypertension, seizures, hypertensive encephalopathy, and intracerebral hemorrhage.

Acute psychosis associated with PCP use should be considered a psychiatric emergency since patients may be at high risk for suicide or extreme violence toward others. Phenothiazines should not be used for treatment because these drugs potentiate PCP's anticholinergic effects. Haloperidol (5 mg intramuscularly) has been administered on an hourly basis to induce suppression of psychotic behavior. PCP, like LSD and mescaline, produces vasospasm of cerebral arteries at relatively low doses. Chronic PCP use has been shown to induce insomnia, anorexia, severe social and behavioral changes, and, in some cases, chronic schizophrenia.

POLYDRUG ABUSE Although drug abusers often report a preference for a particular drug, such as alcohol or opiates, the concurrent use of other drugs is common. Multiple drug use often involves substances that may have different pharmacologic effects from the preferred drug. Concurrent use of dissimilar compounds such as stimulants and opiates or stimulants and alcohol is not unusual. The diversity of reported drug use combinations suggests that achieving some perceptible change in state, rather than any particular direction of change (stimulation or sedation), may be the primary reinforcer in polydrug use and abuse. There is also evidence that intoxication with alcohol or opiates is associated with increased tobacco smoking. There is relatively little systematic information available about multiple drug abuse interactions. However, the combined use of cocaine, heroin, and alcohol increases the risk for toxic effects and adverse medical consequences over risks associated with use of a single drug. One determinant of polydrug use patterns is the relative availability and cost of the drugs. There are many examples of situationally determined drug-use patterns. For example, alcohol abuse, with its attendant medical complications, is one of the most serious problems encountered in former heroin addicts participating in methadone maintenance programs.

The physician must recognize that perpetuation of polydrug abuse and drug dependence is not necessarily a symptom of an underlying emotional disorder. Neither alleviation of anxiety nor reduction of depression accounts for initiation and perpetuation of polydrug abuse. Severe depression and anxiety are as frequently the consequences of polydrug abuse as they are the antecedents. There is also evidence that some of the most adverse consequences of drug use may be reinforcing and contributing to the continuation of polydrug abuse.

℞ **TREATMENT** Adequate treatment of polydrug abuse, as well as other forms of drug abuse, requires innovative programs of intervention. The first step in successful treatment is detoxification, a process that may be difficult because of the abuse of several drugs with different pharmacologic actions (e.g., alcohol, opiates, and cocaine). Since patients may not recall or may deny simultaneous multiple drug use, diagnostic evaluation should always include urinalysis for qualitative detection of psychoactive substances and their metabolites. Treatment of polydrug abuse often requires hospitalization or inpatient residential care during detoxification and the initial phase of drug abstinence. When possible, specialized facilities for the care and treatment of chemically dependent persons should be used. Outpatient detoxification of polydrug abuse patients is likely to be ineffective and may be dangerous.

As in the treatment of alcohol abuse, no single therapeutic modality has been shown to be uniquely effective in inducing remission. Polydrug abuse is a chronic disorder with an unpredictable pattern of remission and recrudescence. Even temporary remissions with attendant physical, social, and psychological improvements are preferable to the continuation or progressive acceleration of polydrug abuse and its related adverse medical and interpersonal consequences. In polydrug abuse, as in many chronic disorders, definitive "cures" rarely occur. The concerned physician should continue to assist polydrug abuse patients throughout the cyclic oscillations of this complex behavior disorder, recognizing that resumption of drug use may be the rule rather than the exception.

BIBLIOGRAPHY

ERNST T et al: Evidence for long-term neurotoxicity associated with methamphetamine abuse: A 1H MRS study. Neurology 54:1344, 2000

KAUFMAN MJ et al: Cocaine-induced cerebral vasoconstriction detected in humans with magnetic resonance angiography. JAMA 279:376, 1998

MENDELSON JH, MELLO NK: Drug therapy: Management of cocaine abuse and dependence. N Engl J Med 334:965, 1996

——— et al: Cocaine pharmacokinetics in men and in women during the follicular and luteal phase of the menstrual cycle. Neuropsychopharmacology 21:294, 1999

NAHAS GG et al: *Marihuana and Medicine*. Totowa, NJ, Humana Press, 1999

NATIONAL INSTITUTE ON DRUG ABUSE: *Epidemiologic Trends in Drug Abuse, Advance Report*. NIH Publication No. 00-4738, 2000

SCHUCKIT MA: *Drug and Alcohol Abuse: A Clinical Guide to Diagnosis and Treatment*, 5th ed. New York, Kluwer Academic/Plenum, 2000

SIEGEL AJ et al: Cocaine-induced erythrocytosis and increase in Von Willebrand factor. Arch Intern Med 159:1925, 1999

390 NICOTINE ADDICTION

David M. Burns

The use of tobacco leaf to create and satisfy nicotine addiction was introduced to Columbus by Native Americans and spread rapidly to Europe. The use of tobacco as cigarettes, however, is predominantly a twentieth century phenomenon, as is the epidemic of disease caused by this form of tobacco.

Nicotine is the principal constituent of tobacco responsible for its addictive character. Addicted smokers regulate their nicotine intake and blood levels by adjusting the frequency and intensity of their tobacco use both to obtain the desired psychoactive effects and avoid withdrawal.

Unburned cured tobacco contains nicotine, carcinogens, and other toxins capable of causing gum disease and oral cancer. When tobacco is burned, the resultant smoke contains, in addition to nicotine, carbon monoxide and >4000 other compounds that result from volatilization, pyrolysis, and pyrosynthesis of tobacco and various chemical additives used in making different tobacco products. The smoke is composed of a fine aerosol, with a particle size distribution predominantly in the range to deposit in the airways and alveolar surfaces of the lungs, and a vapor phase. The bulk of the toxicity and carcinogenicity of the smoke resides in the aerosolized particulate phase, which contains a large number of toxic constituents and >40 carcinogenic compounds. The aggregate of particulate matter, after subtracting nicotine and moisture, is referred to as tar. The vapor phase contains carbon monoxide, respiratory irritants, and ciliotoxins as well as many of the volatile compounds responsible for the distinctive smell of cigarette smoke.

The alkaline pH of smoke from blends of tobacco utilized for pipes and cigars allows sufficient absorption of nicotine across the oral mucosa to satisfy the smoker's need for this drug. Therefore, smokers of pipes and cigars tend not to inhale the smoke into the lung, confining the toxic and carcinogenic exposure (and the increased rates of disease) largely to the upper airway for most users of these products. The acidic pH of smoke generated by the tobacco used in cigarettes dramatically reduces absorption of nicotine in the mouth, necessitating inhalation of the smoke into the larger surface of the lungs in order to absorb quantities of nicotine sufficient to satisfy the smoker's addiction. The shift to using tobacco as cigarettes, with resultant increased deposition of smoke in the lung, has created the epidemic of heart disease, lung disease, and lung cancer that dominates the current disease manifestations of tobacco use.

DISEASE MANIFESTATIONS OF CIGARETTE SMOKING Over 400,000 individuals die prematurely each year in the United States from cigarette use; this represents approximately one out of every five deaths in the United States. Approximately 40% of cigarette smokers will die prematurely due to cigarette smoking unless they are able to quit.

The major diseases caused by cigarette smoking are listed in Table 390-1, with the relative risks for each disease listed for male and female current smokers. The incidence of smoking-related diseases is proportionately greater in younger than in older smokers, particularly for coronary artery disease and stroke. At older ages, the background rate of disease in nonsmokers increases, diminishing the fractional contribution of smoking and the relative risk; however, absolute excess rates of disease mortality found in smokers compared to nonsmokers increase with increasing age. The organ damage caused by smoking and the number of smokers who die from smoking are both greater among the elderly, as one would expect from a process of cumulative injury.

Cardiovascular Diseases Cigarette smokers are more likely than nonsmokers to develop large vessel atherosclerosis as well as small vessel disease. Approximately 90% of peripheral vascular disease in the nondiabetic population can be attributed to cigarette smoking, as can approximately 50% of aortic aneurysms. In contrast, 20 to 30% of coronary artery disease and approximately 10% of occlusive cerebrovascular disease are caused by cigarette smoking. There is a

Table 390-1 Relative Risks for Current Smokers of Cigarettes

Disease or Condition	Relative Risk Males	Relative Risk Females
All causes of death	2.3	1.9
Coronary heart disease		
Age 35–64	2.8	3
Age >64	1.6	1.6
Cerebrovascular lesions		
Age 35–64	3.7	4.8
Age ≥65	1.9	1.5
Aortic aneurysm	4.7	3.9
Peripheral vascular disease	13.5	2.2
Chronic obstructive pulmonary disease	9.7	10.4
Cancer		
Lip, oral cavity, pharynx	27.5	5.6
Esophagus	7.6	10.3
Pancreas	2.1	2.3
Larynx	10.5	17.8
Lung	22.4	11.9
Kidney	3.0	1.4
Bladder, other urinary organs	2.9	2.6
Complications of pregnancy		1.4
Perinatal complications		1.3
Low birth weight		2.1

multiplicative interaction between cigarette smoking and other cardiac risk factors such that the increment in risk produced by smoking among individuals with hypertension or elevated serum lipids is substantially greater than the increment in risk produced by smoking for individuals without these risk factors.

In addition to its role in promoting atherosclerosis, cigarette smoking also increases the likelihood of myocardial infarction and sudden cardiac death by promoting platelet aggregation and vascular occlusion. Reversal of these effects may explain the rapid benefit of smoking cessation for a new coronary event demonstrable among those who have survived a first myocardial infarction. This effect may also explain the substantially higher rates of graft occlusion among continuing smokers following vascular bypass surgery for cardiac or peripheral vascular disease, as well as the high failure rate of angioplasty procedures among continuing smokers.

Cessation of cigarette smoking reduces the risk of a second coronary event within 6 to 12 months after quitting, and rates of first myocardial infarction or death from coronary heart disease also decline within the first few years following cessation. After 15 years of cessation, the risk of a new myocardial infarction or death from coronary heart disease in former smokers is similar to that in those who have never smoked.

Cancer Cancers of the lung, larynx, oral cavity, esophagus, pancreas, kidney, and urinary bladder are caused by cigarette smoking. In addition, there is evidence suggesting that cigarette smoking may play a role in increasing the risk of cervical and stomach cancer. There is conflicting evidence on the relationship of cigarette smoking and cancer of the breast, but overall there does not appear to be a causal link. There is a lower risk of uterine cancer among postmenopausal women who smoke.

The risks of cancer increase with the increasing number of cigarettes smoked per day and the duration of smoking, and there are synergistic interactions between cigarette smoking and alcohol use for cancer of the oral cavity, esophagus, and possibly lung. Several occupational exposures also synergistically increase lung cancer risk among cigarette smokers, most notably occupational asbestos and radon exposure.

Cessation of cigarette smoking reduces the risk of developing cancer relative to continuing smoking, but even 20 years after cessation there is a modest persistent increased risk of developing lung cancer.

Respiratory Disease Cigarette smoking is responsible for >90% of chronic obstructive pulmonary disease. Within 1 to 2 years of beginning to smoke regularly, many young smokers will develop inflammatory changes in their small airways, although lung function measures of these changes do not predict development of chronic airflow obstruction. After ≥20 years of smoking, pathophysiologic changes in the lungs develop and progress proportional to smoking intensity and duration. Chronic mucous hyperplasia of the larger airways results in a chronic productive cough in as many as 80% of smokers over age 60. Chronic inflammation and narrowing of the small airways and/or enzymatic digestion of alveolar walls resulting in pulmonary emphysema can result in reduced expiratory airflow sufficient to produce clinical symptoms of respiratory limitation in approximately 15% of smokers.

Changes in the small airways of young smokers will reverse after 1 to 2 years of cessation. There may also be a small increase in measures of expiratory airflow following cessation among individuals who have developed chronic airflow obstruction, but the major change following cessation is a slowing of the rate of decline in lung function with advancing age rather than a return of lung function toward normal.

Pregnancy Cigarette smoking is associated with several maternal complications of pregnancy: premature rupture of membranes, abruptio placentae, and placenta previa; there is also a small increase in the risk of spontaneous abortion among smokers. Infants of smoking mothers are more likely to experience preterm delivery, have a higher perinatal mortality, are small for their gestational age, are more likely to die of sudden infant death syndrome, and appear to have a developmental lag for at least the first several years of life.

Other Conditions Smoking delays healing of peptic ulcers; increases the risk of osteoporosis, senile cataracts, and macular degeneration; and results in premature menopause, wrinkling of the skin, gallstones and cholecystitis in women, and male impotence.

Environmental tobacco smoke Long-term exposure to environmental tobacco smoke increases the risk of lung cancer and coronary artery disease among nonsmokers. It also increases the incidence of respiratory infections, chronic otitis media, and asthma in children as well as causing exacerbation of asthma in children.

PHARMACOLOGIC INTERACTIONS Cigarette smoking may interact with a variety of other drugs in ways that may have clinically significant implications (Table 390-2). Cigarette smoking induces the cytochrome P450 system, which may alter the metabolic clearance of drugs such as theophylline. This effect may result in more drug toxicity among nonsmokers on fixed drug dosage schedules and in inadequate serum levels in smokers as outpatients when the dosage is established in the hospital under nonsmoking conditions. Correspondingly, serum levels may rise when smokers are hospitalized and not allowed to smoke. Smokers may also have higher first-pass clearance for drugs such as lidocaine, and the stimulant effects of nicotine may reduce the effect of benzodiazepines or beta blockers.

Table 390-2 Interactions of Smoking and Prescription Drugs

Drug	Interaction
Benzodiazepines	Less sedation
Beta blockers	Reduced lowering of heart rate and blood pressure
Caffeine	Faster metabolic clearance
Chlorpromazine	Decreased serum concentrations of uncertain clinical implications
Dextropropoxyphene	Less analgesia
Flecainide	Increased first-pass clearance
Fluvoxamine	Decreased serum concentrations of uncertain clinical implications
Haloperidol	Decreased serum concentrations of uncertain clinical implications
Heparin	Faster clearance
Imiprimine	Decreased serum concentrations of uncertain clinical implications
Insulin	Delayed absorption due to skin vasoconstriction
Lidocaine	Increased first-pass clearance
Mexiletine	Increased first-pass clearance
Pentazocine	Less analgesia, possibly increased clearance
Propranolol	Increased first-pass clearance
Tacrine	Faster metabolic clearance
Theophylline	Faster metabolic clearance

OTHER FORMS OF TOBACCO USE Other major forms of tobacco use are moist snuff deposited between the cheek and gum, chewing tobacco, pipes and cigars, and recently bidi (tobacco wrapped in tendu or temburni leaf and commonly used in India) and clove cigarettes. Oral tobacco use leads to gum disease and can result in oral cancer. All forms of burned tobacco generate toxic and carcinogenic smoke similar to that of cigarette smoke. The differences in disease consequences of use relate to frequency of use and depth of inhalation. The risk of upper airway cancers is similar among cigarette and cigar smokers, while those who have smoked only cigars have a much lower risk of lung cancer, heart disease, and chronic obstructive pulmonary disease. However, cigarette smokers who switch to pipes or cigars do tend to inhale the smoke, increasing their risk; and it is likely that comparable inhalation and frequency of exposure to tobacco smoke from any of these forms of tobacco use will lead to comparable disease outcomes.

Recent prevalence-of-use data have suggested a resurgence of cigar and bidi use among adolescents of both genders, raising concerns that these older forms of tobacco use are once again causing a public health concern.

LOWER TAR AND NICOTINE CIGARETTES Since the bulk of the toxicity of cigarette smoke is contained in the tar, and since nicotine is the principal addictive agent in cigarettes, it has been suggested that cigarettes that deliver less tar and nicotine to the smoker might be safer. Studies of smokers of low-yield cigarettes suggest that there may be a 10 to 20% reduction in the risk of developing lung cancer among those who reduce the nominal tar yield of their cigarettes by ≥50%. However, this benefit is only evident if smokers do not compensate for the lower nicotine delivery with an increased intensity of smoking, and most studies show that smokers of low-yield cigarettes do compensate. Because of their addiction to nicotine, most smokers tend to preserve their intake of nicotine, and correspondingly their tar intake, when they shift to lower nicotine cigarettes.

Newer, very low yield cigarettes commonly use vents in the filters or other engineering designs to reduce the tar and nicotine when the cigarette is smoked by machine. However, the delivery of tar and nicotine is much higher when these cigarettes are smoked by actual smokers. Current evidence suggests that if there is any disease-reduction benefit for smokers of low-yield cigarettes, it is too small to be clinically meaningful, and individuals should be discouraged from thinking of low-yield cigarettes as a substitute for cessation.

CESSATION The process of stopping smoking is often a cyclical one, with the smoker sometimes making multiple attempts to quit and failing before finally being successful. Approximately 70 to 80% of smokers would like to quit smoking, approximately one-third of current smokers attempt to quit each year, and ≥90% of these unassisted quit attempts fail. Smokers have been categorized into those who are not thinking about quitting (precontemplation), those who are thinking about quitting (contemplation), and those who are in the action phase of quitting. A useful conceptualization of the cessation process is one where smokers cycle through the stages of cessation; each time smokers go around the cycle, a few more smokers become successful in their cessation efforts. One goal of clinician-based smoking interventions then becomes moving smokers from one stage of the cessation cycle to another, and efforts can be focused on moving the smoker to the next stage rather than focusing exclusively on immediate cessation.

The move from thinking about quitting to making a quit attempt is often triggered by a variety of environmental stimuli independent of physician control. The cost of cigarettes can be a powerful trigger for cessation attempts. Media campaigns, particularly when coupled with cessation events, are also able to trigger cessation attempts in large numbers of smokers. Changes in workplace rules to restrict smoking in the workplace have been associated with quit attempts in substantial numbers of workers. However, physician advice to quit, particularly around an acute illness, is also a powerful trigger for cessation activity, with up to half of patients who are advised to quit making a cessation effort.

Telephone counseling and nicotine-replacement therapy are all useful enhancers of long-term cessation success. Clinic-based cessation programs have a substantial benefit for long-term cessation for those who can be recruited to participate, and physician recommendation can double the fraction of smokers who are willing to participate in these programs.

PREVENTION Approximately 90% of individuals who will become cigarette smokers initiate the behavior during adolescence. Factors that promote adolescent initiation are parental or older generation cigarette smoking, tobacco advertising and promotional activities, the availability of cigarettes, and the social acceptability of smoking. The need for an enhanced self-image and to imitate adult behavior is greatest for those adolescents who have the least external validation of their self-worth, which may explain in part the enormous differences in adolescent smoking prevalence by socioeconomic and school performance strata.

Prevention of smoking initiation must begin early, preferably in the elementary school years. Physicians who deal with adolescents should be sensitive to the prevalence of this problem in their patient population. Effective physician-based interventions for adolescent smokers remain to be developed, but current clinical guidelines suggest that physicians should ask all adolescents whether they have experimented with tobacco or currently use tobacco, reinforce the facts that most adolescents and adults do not smoke, and explain that all forms of tobacco are both addictive and harmful.

GENETIC CONSIDERATIONS Several genes have been associated with nicotine addiction. Some reduce the clearance of nicotine, and others have been associated with an increased likelihood of becoming dependent on tobacco and other drugs as well as a higher incidence of depression. Genetic alterations that involve the neurotransmitter dopamine, and possibly the serotoninergic and cholinergic neuroregulatory pathways, are being explored for their contribution to development of addiction to tobacco and other substances. The precise role these genetic differences play in development and maintenance of nicotine addiction remains to be determined, but it is unlikely that genetic factors are the principal determinants of addiction. Rates of smoking initiation among males, and corresponding rates of nicotine addiction, have dropped by almost 50% since the mid-1950s, suggesting that factors other than genetics are the principal determinants of whether individuals will become addicted. It is more likely that genetic polymorphism represents a range of biologic susceptibility conditioning the intensity of cigarette use and the probability that experimentation with tobacco as an adolescent leads to addiction as an adult. ■

PHYSICIAN INTERVENTION Physicians can make a clear difference in promoting successful cessation among their smoking patients, and the Agency for Health Care Policy and Research (AHCPR) has developed clinical guidelines for health care system–based smoking cessation (Table 390-3). All patients should be asked whether they smoke, their past experience with quitting, and whether they are currently interested in quitting. Those who are not interested in quitting should be encouraged and motivated to quit; provided a clear, strong, and personalized physician message that smoking is an important health concern; and offered assistance if they become interested in quitting in the future. There is a relationship between the amount of assistance a patient is willing to accept, and the success of the cessation attempt. A quit date should be negotiated, usually not the day of the visit but within the next few weeks, and a follow-up contact by office staff around the time of the quit date should be provided.

There are a variety of nicotine-replacement products, including over the counter nicotine patch and gum, as well as nicotine nasal and oral inhalers available by prescription. Clonidine and, more recently, antidepressants such as bupropion have also been shown to be effective; some evidence supports the combined use of nicotine-replacement therapy and antidepressants. Nicotine-replacement therapy is provided in different dosages for use with smokers of different numbers of cigarettes per day. Antidepressants are more effective in those with a history of depression symptoms. At this time there are few clear

Table 390-3 Clinical Practice Guidelines

Physician Actions	Effective Pharmacologic Interventions	Other Effective Interventions
Ask: systematically identify all tobacco users at every visit	Nicotine patch or gum	Physician or other medical personnel counseling (10 min)
Advise: strongly urge all smokers to quit	Nicotine nasal inhaler	Intensive smoking cessation programs[a]
Identify smokers willing to quit	Nicotine oral inhaler	Clinic-based smoking status identification system
Assist the patient in quitting	Clonidine	Counseling by nonclinicians and social support by family and friends
Arrange follow-up contact	Bupropion	Telephone counseling

[a] At least four to seven sessions of 20- to 30-min duration, lasting at least 2 weeks, preferably 8 weeks.

indications favoring the use of one agent over another as initial therapy. Current recommendations are to offer pharmacologic treatment to all who will accept it and to provide counseling and other support to the patient as a part of the cessation attempt. Cessation advice alone is likely to increase success by 50% compared with no intervention; a more comprehensive approach with advice, pharmacologic assistance, and counseling can increase cessation success by almost threefold.

In order for physicians to incorporate cessation assistance into their practice successfully, it is essential to change the infrastructure in which the physician practices. The following are simple changes: (1) including questions on smoking and interest in cessation on patient-intake questionnaires, (2) asking patients whether they smoke as part of the initial vital sign measurements made by office staff, (3) listing smoking as a problem in the medical record, and (4) automating follow-up contact with the patient on their quit date. These changes are essential to institutionalizing smoking intervention within the practice setting; without this institutionalization, the best intentions of physicians to intervene with their patients who smoke are often lost in the time crush of a busy practice.

BIBLIOGRAPHY

National Cancer Institute: *Changes in Cigarette-Related Disease Risks and Their Implication for Prevention and Control.* Smoking and Tobacco Control Monograph No. 8, USDHHS NIH NCI, (NIH) Publication 97-4213, 1997

Prochazka AV: New developments in smoking cessation. Chest 17:169S, 2000

US Department of Health and Human Services: *The Health Benefits of Smoking Cessation: A Report of the Surgeon General.* DHHS (CDC) Publication 90-8416, 1990

———: *Women and Tobacco. A Report of the Surgeon General.* DHHS (CDC), National Center for Chronic Disease Prevention and Health Promotion, Office on Smoking and Health, in press

———: *Smoking Cessation and Prevention.* Clinical Practice Guideline Number 18, Agency for Health Care Policy and Research Publication, Public Health Service, DHHS, 2000

Zevin S, Benowitz NL: Drug interactions with tobacco smoking: An update. Clin Pharmacokinet 36:426, 1999

NOBEL PRIZE IN PHYSIOLOGY OR MEDICINE, 1924

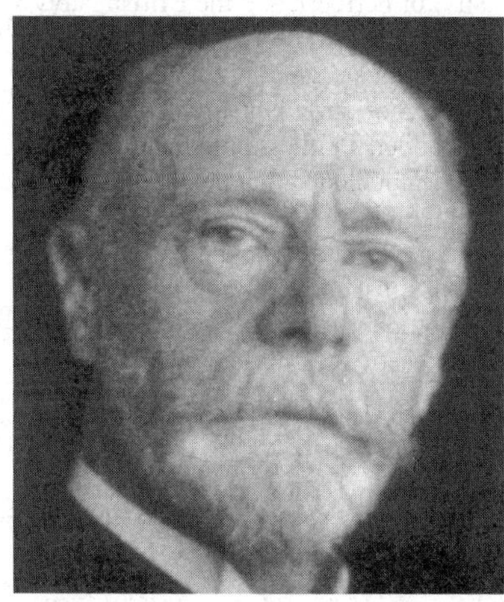

Willem Einthoven was born on May 16, 1860, in Semarang, Java, in the Dutch East Indies (Indonesia) to Jacob Einthoven and Louise de Vogel. He was the third of six children and his father was a practicing physician who died when Willem was only 10 years old. After his father's death, the family returned to the Netherlands. Einthoven attended the University of Utrecht where he received his B.S. degree in 1878, and then studied medicine at the same institution. During his medical studies, he undertook a number of research projects with outstanding investigators at Utrecht University that culminated in scientific publications, particularly in the area of eye physiology. On receiving his medical degree in 1885 and based on his scientific contributions, at the age of 25 years he was appointed a Professor of Physiology at the University of Leiden. In addition to his work in the physiology of the eye, he also studied the nervous control of bronchial vessels. He then commenced his work on the electrophysiology of the heart. The first study of the electrical deflections of the heart was by Augustus Waller, a friend of Einthoven, who used the capillary ergometer to show the electrical changes associated with the heartbeat. Waller rejected any importance of these electrical changes and did not pursue the work further. Einthoven, however, was convinced of the importance of these electrical impulses, but the capillary electrometer was too sensitive to be reliable. To counter this problem, Einthoven made a hole some 3.0 to 4.5 m (10 to 15 ft) below his laboratory and lined it with rocks to insulate the capillary ergometer from the vibrations caused by horse-drawn trucks as they passed the wooden building of his laboratory. Nevertheless, Einthoven's efforts with the capillary ergometer were still unsuccessful, so he turned to another device. He began working with the d'Arsonval galvanometer and replaced the silver-plated quartz coil with a wire, which was much lighter than the coil. This change allowed not only increased sensitivity but also more rapid response time for recording the electrical potentials from the heart.

Using this string galvanometer, Einthoven demonstrated that there was a characteristic electrocardiogram for each individual. He labeled the waves of this electrocardiogram P, Q, R, S, and T—the nomenclature still used in electrocardiography. Einthoven then connected his laboratory to the hospital a mile away using a transmission wire owned by the telephone company. With this approach he could study the electrocardiograms of patients in the hospital from his own laboratory. This was the first instance of the development and use of the telecardiogram. Einthoven showed that patients with different heart diseases had different electrocardiograms including cardiac enlargement secondary to valvular problems, premature contractions, and heart block. He also described the electrical axis of the heart that correlated with the anatomical axis, another observation that is still key in cardiogram interpretation a century later. Einthoven also recognized that electrical deflection varied based on the position of the electrodes and therefore proposed a standardized system for placing the electrodes and gave the leads their current names I, II, and III. Throughout his career, Einthoven combined his knowledge of physiology and physics as he laid the groundwork for modern electrocardiography. Einthoven clearly deserves to be the "Father of Electrocardiography." For his accomplishments, he was awarded the Nobel Prize in Physiology or Medicine in 1924. Einthoven, however, received little public recognition during his lifetime for his contributions in electrocardiography; awareness of the value of the electrocardiogram in clinical medicine came later.

REFERENCES

1. Magill FN (ed): *Nobel Prize Winners: Physiology or Medicine*, vol 1. Pasadena, Salem Press, 1993
2. Schrier RW: *A Salute to Nobel Laureates in Physiology and Medicine*, Proceedings of the Association of American Physicians 108(1): Jan 1996
3. Sourkes TL: *Nobel Prize Winners in Medicine and Physiology 1901–1965*. London, Abelard-Schuman, 1967

Robert W. Schrier, MD

NOBEL PRIZE IN PHYSIOLOGY OR MEDICINE, 1929

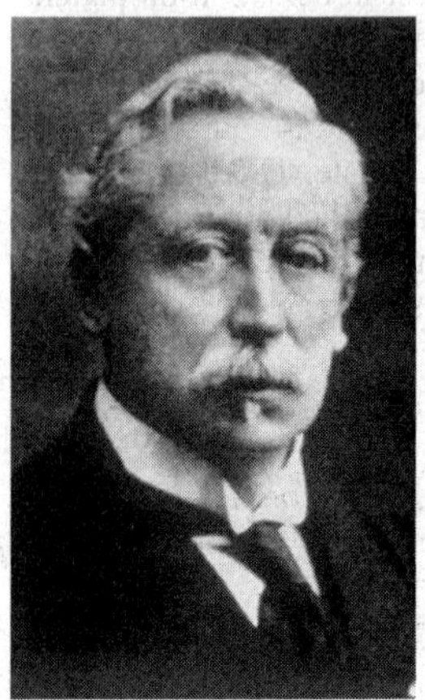

Christiaan Eijkman, Jr., was born in Nijerk, the Netherlands, on August 11, 1858, the seventh child of a schoolteacher. His family moved to Amsterdam where he received his early schooling and then entered the University of Amsterdam. The government paid for his tuition in medical school in exchange for his agreement to be an army physician. Thus, after graduation from medical school in 1883 he was sent to the Dutch East Indies, where he spent 2 years in Java and Sumatra. Eijkman had become quite interested in bacteriology and went to study this field in Berlin with Robert Koch.

While in Berlin, Eijkman met the members of a two-man commission being sent by the Dutch government to the Dutch East Indies to discover the cause of beriberi, then epidemic in tropical and subtropical countries. They went to Koch's laboratory before departing for the East Indies because they thought that bacteria must be causing beriberi. Beriberi was characterized by a polyneuritis with resulting paralysis of the lower extremities (*dry beriberi*) as well as respiratory and cardiac failure with edema (*wet beriberi*). Eijkman volunteered to accompany the team to help in isolating the proposed causative bacteria and then to implement sterilization techniques. The team at first believed that they had identified a bacterium as the cause of beriberi, and the other members of the team then returned to The Netherlands. Applying Koch's principles for proving a bacterial cause of beriberi, however, frustrated Eijkman since he could not document the transmission of the disease in any manner.

The investigation appeared to be at a dead end when a coincidence put Eijkman "on the right track." A disease quite similar to beriberi broke out among chickens in the Djakarta laboratory of a military hospital. The chickens had muscular weakness, could not use their wings or raise their heads, and died of respiratory failure. Microscopic examination demonstrated degeneration of the chickens' peripheral nerves. Eijkman attempted to pass the disease from one chicken to another and was unsuccessful. Again, there seemed to be an impasse in Eijkman's research, but suddenly the affected chickens began to improve and there were no new cases. Eijkman then focused on the chickens' food and found that they had been receiving leftover polished rice from the officers' dining room from June 17th to November 27th. Then a new cook took over, and the chickens again were fed with unpolished rice. The chickens' beriberi had commenced on July 10th and subsided during the last part of November. Eijkman was able to reproduce the symptoms of beriberi by again feeding the chickens polished rice and to reverse the disease by feeding the chickens unpolished (whole-grain) rice. Eijkman was then able to extract an active substance from the inner hull (pericarp) of the rice grain that could be administered either by mouth or by injection.

The final proof came when Eijkman learned that some prison inmates on the island of Java were fed polished rice and others were fed unpolished rice. Epidemiologic studies demonstrated a 300 times greater incidence of beriberi in those prisons using polished rice. The essential substance in the rice husk was found to be an amine, and thus the term *vital amine* was coined, later shortened to *vitamin*. Eijkman's discovery of the water-soluble vitamin, thiamine saved thousands of lives and opened the era whereby vitamins were recognized as essential elements of the diet.

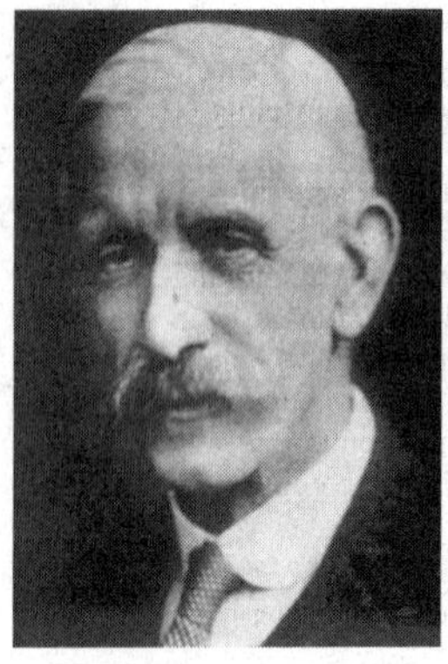

Frederick Gowland Hopkins was born on June 20, 1861, at Eastbourne, England. He became interested in science at an early age with the worlds revealed by a microscope given to him by his father. He later said that the observations that he made at home with his microscope, ". . .were something very important—the most important thing that I had come against; so much more important than anything I was being taught in school." Although he received a "first class" in chemistry at the City of London School, he left school at 17 and became a bank clerk. However, after 6 months at that job he became an assistant to an analytic chemist. This work led him ultimately to a university degree in chemistry and finally a medical degree at age 32—quite an old age to become a physician in that era.

Hopkins clearly made up for any "lost time." In 1898 he moved to Cambridge University to teach the chemical aspects of physiology, became a Reader, and ultimately, in 1914, Professor of a new Department of Biochemistry at Cambridge. His Department of Biochemistry attracted some of the brightest young minds. He was one of the first to teach the dynamics of biochemistry; he thus not only observed what chemical substances are in living cells but what they do in the life of the living cell. Hopkins discovered tryptophan and glutathione but rather than pursue their structure, he immediately sought what they were doing in the body. On the background of Eijkman's discovery of thiamine deficiency as the cause of beriberi, and the British Navy's cure of scurvy by dietary means, Hopkins studied the factors involved in animal growth. He found that adequate amounts of fat, carbohydrates, proteins, and minerals were not sufficient to sustain normal animal growth. It was not until he added a milk supplement to the diet that normal growth was restored. He concluded that the failure to grow was not due to a lack of food intake but rather to an inability to use the food optimally. In his classic paper published in 1912, Hopkins concluded that milk and other foods must contain important accessory food factors. While Hopkins did not identify these factors, his studies were important in future discoveries of the roles of vitamin C and vitamin B complex (see figure).

REFERENCES

1. Aaseng N: *The Disease Fighters*. Minneapolis, Lerner Publications, 1987
2. Magill FN (ed): *Nobel Prize Winners: Physiology or Medicine*, vol. 1. Pasadena, Salem Press, 1993
3. Schrier RW: *A Salute to Nobel Laureates in Physiology and Medicine*, Proceedings of the Association of American Physicians 108(1): 1996.
4. Sourkes TL: *Nobel Prize Winners in Medicine and Physiology 1901-1965*. London, Abelard-Schuman, 1967

Robert W. Schrier, MD

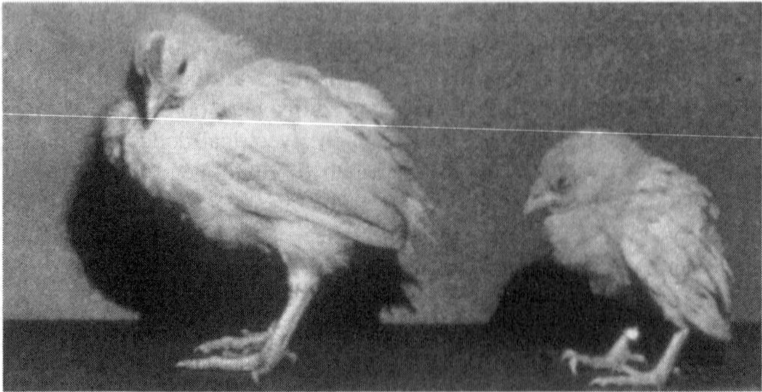

The chicken on the left was fed a normal diet, whereas the chicken on the right was fed a diet lacking in vitamins B and C. (Reprinted with permission from Ref. 1.)

PART FIFTEEN

ENVIRONMENTAL AND OCCUPATIONAL HAZARDS

Section 1
SPECIFIC ENVIRONMENTAL AND OCCUPATIONAL HAZARDS

391

Howard Hu, Frank E. Speizer

SPECIFIC ENVIRONMENTAL AND OCCUPATIONAL HAZARDS

It cannot be overemphasized that an appropriate environmental/occupational history is an essential part of the medical workup of many chronic diseases. The general approach to the patient whose illness may have been caused or exacerbated by environmental or occupational hazards is detailed in Chap. 5.

The term *hazards* in this context is generally synonymous with *toxins* and *toxic exposures* and encompasses chemical factors as well as other risks posed by the physical environment and by selected natural phenomena. These hazards may exist in the general environment or in the workplace. Strictly speaking, smoking, alcohol ingestion, nutritional factors, and infectious agents can also be considered chemical or environmental hazards.

Once a specific hazard has been identified as a factor in the pathogenesis of an illness or as an imminent threat, the clinical approach must include the development of a strategy for preventing further exposure and for treating the specific manifestations of the illness, using antidotes and supportive measures. In the following chapters, specific hazards are considered, including acute poisoning and drug overdose; heavy metal poisoning; disorders caused by venoms, bites, and stings; drowning and near-drowning; electrical injuries; and radiation injury. The health effects of ambient air pollution, occupational respiratory exposures, passive smoking, and assorted toxic air pollutants are discussed briefly in Chap. 254. Space does not allow specific discussion in this text of many other important categories of hazards, such as organic solvents; chemicals used in the plastics, synthetic textiles, and rubber industries; and pesticides. The reader should consult other detailed texts or electronic information sources for clinical data on these topics. In this volume, however, brief attention is focused on several selected issues in light of recent developments in research that have enhanced our understanding of the way these hazards may interact with human behavior and consequently pose increased risks to both individuals and society.

HAZARDOUS WASTE AND GROUNDWATER CONTAMINATION The term *hazardous waste* embodies toxic chemicals, radioactive materials, and biologic or infectious wastes. In many communities, hazardous waste has emerged as a major public health concern. In the United States, some 50,000 sites (defined by specific criteria) have been estimated to contain hazardous chemicals; 1000 or so of these have been included as "Superfund sites" on a National Priority List drawn up by the Environmental Protection Agency (EPA). New or unrecognized sites are likely to exist as well. These sites may require long-term remedial action. The spectrum of substances contained at the sites is wide and theoretically may include any of some 30,000 chemicals that are commonly used in commerce. However, the EPA keeps fewer than 200 chemicals on a special hazardous substance list in light of their toxicity, the frequency with which they are encountered, and other factors. One difficulty in anticipating risks associated with hazardous waste sites is that the substances are usually present in mixtures whose composition is seldom fully known. In addition, with respect to toxicity, chemicals may interact with one another in an additive, protective, or synergistic fashion, and little knowledge exists on which to base predictions regarding the interactions of these complex mixtures.

Waste-site employees and the surrounding community can incur hazardous exposures through the inhalation of toxic vapors or dusts emanating directly from a waste site or an on-site incinerator; the ingestion of water contaminated by surface runoff or by material leaching through soil into surface water or groundwater; the ingestion of contaminated plants, fish, or other wildlife; or direct contact. This last risk is particularly likely for children, who may enter a poorly secured site. Perhaps the exposure of greatest concern to community residents has been the contamination of groundwater by volatile organic compounds or solvents (VOCs); together, the widespread detection of low levels of VOCs in groundwater and the several studies suggesting an association between heavy VOC contamination of drinking water and cancer probably account for the high priority given in public opinion polls to avoiding cancer risks. A 1983 study found that 11 of the 20 chemicals most commonly detected at National Priority List waste sites were VOCs (Table 391-1).

Current regulatory policy rests on the assumption that there is no threshold below which a carcinogen exerts no effect or risk. Thus, once a substance is identified as a probable carcinogen (see below), it is regulated to a concentration that is believed to be accompanied by an acceptable level of risk. Clearly, great uncertainty exists regarding methods used to classify drinking-water carcinogens and to extrapolate the risks related to exposure to these substances. Regardless, VOC contamination in groundwater is likely to continue to be a high-priority issue in the public arena.

ENVIRONMENTAL CARCINOGENS Based on studies and reviews of the literature by the International Agency for Research on Cancer, enough evidence exists to classify around 60 substances and processes as probably or definitely carcinogenic in humans (Table 391-2). Some processes are deemed carcinogenic on the basis of epidemiologic evidence, even though the specific causative agent cannot always be clearly identified. Tumor promoters are not distinguished from tumor initiators in this listing, and the chemical structures and modes of action are diverse. Around 150 additional agents and processes have been designated as possibly carcinogenic on the basis of studies of bacteria and animals as well as human epidemiologic studies. The

Table 391-1 Volatile Organic Compounds Most Frequently Detected in 1983 at National Priority List Hazardous Waste Sites (in Order of Frequency and Detection) and (When Known) Associated Cancer Risks

Chemical	Risk Level[a]
Trichloroethylene	3.0
Toluene	
Benzene	1.0
Chloroform	0.43
Tetrachloroethylene	0.7
1,1,1-Trichloroethane	
Ethylbenzene	
Trans-1,2-dichloroethane	0.4
Xylene	
Dichloromethane	
Vinyl chloride	0.02

[a] Concentration in water (μg/L) equivalent to a lifetime cancer risk of 1×10^{-6}. Risk estimates used in these calculations were derived from the U.S. Environmental Protection Agency (1990).

Table 391-2 Substances and Processes Classified as Definitely or Probably Carcinogenic by the International Agency for Research on Cancer

AGENTS AND GROUPS OF AGENTS	MIXTURES
Aflatoxins, naturally occurring [1402-68-2][a]	Alcoholic beverages
4-Aminobiphenyl [92-67-1]	Analgesic mixtures containing phenacetin
Arsenic [7440-38-2] and arsenic compounds	Betel quid with tobacco
Asbestos [1332-21-4]	Coal-tar pitches [65996-93-2]
Azathioprine [446-86-6]	Coal tars [8007-45-2]
Benzene [71-43-2]	Mineral oils, untreated and mildly treated
Benzidine [92-87-5]	Salted fish (Chinese style)
Beryllium [7440-41-7] and beryllium compounds	Shale oils [68308-34-9]
N,N-Bis(2-chloroethyl)-2-naphthylamine (chlornaphazine) [494-03-1]	Soots
Bis(chloromethyl)ether [542-88-1] and chloromethyl methyl ether [107-30-2]	Tobacco products, smokeless
1,4-Butanediol dimethanesulfonate (busulfan; Myleran) [55-98-1]	Tobacco smoke
Cadmium [7440-43-9] and cadmium compounds	Wood dust
Chlorambucil [305-03-3]	**EXPOSURE CIRCUMSTANCES**
1-(2-Chloroethyl)-3-(4-methylcyclohexyl)-1-nitrosourea (methyl-CCNU; Semustine) [13909-09-6]	Aluminum production
Chromium [VI] compounds	Auramine manufacturing
Cyclosporine [79217-60-0]	Boot and shoe manufacture and repair
Cyclophosphamide [50-18-0] [6055-19-2]	Coal gasification
Diethylstilbestrol [56-53-1]	Coke production
Erionite [66733-21-9]	Furniture and cabinet making
Ethylene oxide [75-21-8]	Hematite mining (underground) with exposure to radon
Melphalan [148-82-3]	Iron and steel founding
δ-Methoxypsoralen (methoxsalen) [298-81-7] plus ultraviolet radiation	Isopropanol manufacturing (strong-acid process)
MOPP and other combined chemotherapy including alkylating agents	Magenta manufacturing
Mustard gas (sulfur mustard) [505-60-2]	Painting (occupational exposure)
2-Naphthylamine [91-59-8]	Rubber industry
Nickel compounds	Strong-inorganic-acid mists containing sulfuric acid (occupational exposure)
Estrogen therapy, postmenopausal	
Radon [10043-92-2] and its decay products	
Silica [14808-60-7], crystalline	
Solar radiation	
Talc-containing asbestiform fibers (tamoxifen) [10540-29-1][b]	
2,3,7,8-Tetrachlorodibenzo-*para*-dioxin [1746-01-6]	
Thiotepa [52-24-4]	
Treosulfan [299-75-2]	
Vinyl chloride [75-01-4]	

[a] Numbers in brackets are Chemical Abstract Service Registration Numbers.
[b] There is also conclusive evidence that tamoxifen reduces the risk of contralateral breast cancer.

extent to which inferences can be made from nonhuman studies is controversial but certainly depends on minimal standards in the execution of such studies. For example, the Interagency Regulatory Liaison Group recommends that for a carcinogen assay to be considered positive, the test must have been performed on at least 50 animals of each sex in two different species with at least three dose groups (control and two dose levels) over the lifetime of the animals.

BUILDING-RELATED ILLNESSES Reports of discomfort and symptoms in relation to office environments began in the United States in the 1970s. Research has led to the recognition that some building-related illnesses have a clear etiology; these illnesses include hypersensitivity diseases, infections, and exacerbations of asthma due to airborne irritants. However, the majority of such complaints, particularly those of mucous membrane irritation, fatigue, and headache, have no clear etiology. Terms such as *sick-building syndrome* (SBS; also called *tight-building syndrome*) and *nonspecific building-related illnesses* have been used to designate this constellation of symptoms, which have been found in most investigations to occur most often in sealed buildings with centrally controlled mechanical ventilation. Early characterizations of SBS as mass psychogenic illness have not been borne out in the majority of cases by subsequent epidemiologic investigations. Since indoor air-exchange rates were sharply reduced in the 1970s to conserve energy, current hypotheses focus on inadequate dilution of irritants arising from building materials (such as formaldehyde-containing particle board), office supplies (such as carbonless copy paper and photocopy developer solution), toxins from mold and bacterial endotoxin, and personal care products used by occupants as risk factors for SBS. Confirmation of these hypotheses and further characterization of SBS await additional research.

MULTIPLE-CHEMICAL SENSITIVITY The multiple-chemical sensitivity (MCS) syndrome is a diagnosis that has increasingly been given to patients with a wide variety of symptoms that they attribute to exposure at very low levels to a number of commonly encountered chemicals. The syndrome usually begins after a well-defined environmental event, such as a reaction to a more clearly toxic dose of an organic solvent, pesticide, or respiratory irritant. Some cases of MCS begin as SBS. Affected persons commonly report symptoms such as fatigue, malaise, headache, dizziness, lack of concentration, memory loss, and "spaciness"—symptoms that overlap somewhat with those of other diagnoses of uncertain etiology, such as chronic fatigue syndrome. The pathogenesis of MCS is obscure, and no proven methods exist for its diagnosis, evaluation, and treatment. Case series suggesting a high prevalence of affective disorders indicate that psychological factors may play a role in causing MCS and/or in determining its severity; however, evidence does not support MCS as a purely psychogenic illness. A few studies of MCS patients suggest that the biologic mechanism of MCS may involve neurogenic inflammation of the nasal mucosa (as indicated by abnormal rhinolaryngoscopic findings) linked to central nervous system dysfunction (as indicated by alterations seen on single photon emission computed tomography); however, well-controlled research remains sparse, and no firm conclusions can be drawn. Other than the ruling out of other treatable conditions and the avoidance of exacerbating exposures, no specific recommendations for the management of MCS patients can yet be made. A panel of European scientists convened by the World Health Organization recommended that the designation *MCS* be replaced by the term *idiopathic environmental illness* (IEI).

PERSISTENT ORGANIC POLLUTANTS Persistent organic pollutants (POPs) are a class of chemical compounds that tend to travel thousands of miles if released into the atmosphere, to accumulate in the food chain, and to persist in the environment as well as in human tissues (principally fat cells). Although the list of POPs is long, 12 have been identified as particularly important: nine pesticides (aldrin, chlordane, DDT, dieldrin, endrin, heptachlor, hexachlorobenzene, mirex, and toxaphene), dioxins and furans (byproducts of incineration), and polychlorinated biphenyls (PCBs, fluids used mainly as dielectrics in transformers). The persistence and lipid solubility of these compounds allow them to bioconcentrate several thousand-fold as they are passed up the food chain to humans. High levels of exposure to a number of POPs have been shown to contribute to birth defects, infertility, immunosuppression, impaired cognitive development, and some types of cancers. These effects have been linked to the potential of POPs to act as endocrine disruptors—i.e., hormonal mimics. The further production and use of most POPs have been banned, but concern remains over the possible low-level effects of POPs that persist in the environment and in human tissues. Concern has been raised, for example, that population exposures to POPs are contributing to worldwide declines in sperm density and increased rates of congenital hypospadias and testicular and breast cancer; epidemiologic studies testing these theories have yielded mixed results, however, and more research is needed.

GLOBAL CLIMATIC CHANGES An increasing body of evidence indicates that human activities are responsible for global climatic changes, which, in turn, may be directly or indirectly increasing human exposure to environmental hazards. The depletion of stratospheric ozone by chlorinated fluorocarbons, with a consequent increase in ultraviolet radiation exposure, has been firmly established. Increased risks of skin cancers and cataracts are accepted as results of this phenomenon. Less clear is whether the immunosuppressive effects of ultraviolet radiation detected in animals and in vitro have significant clinical impacts on human resistance to infection. Although uncertainties in climate modeling persist, an increasing if not overwhelming amount of evidence indicates that anthropogenic greenhouse gases are fostering global warming. A prominent concern is that global warming can abet the introduction and dissemination of serious infectious diseases, such as mosquito-borne infections (malaria, dengue, and viral encephalitis) and waterborne infectious and toxin-related illnesses (cholera, shellfish poisoning). The World Health Organization has identified global warming as one of the largest public health challenges facing the twenty-first century.

BIBLIOGRAPHY

BARTHA L et al: Multiple chemical sensitivity: A 1999 consensus. Arch Environ Health 54:147, 1999

DOLK H et al: Risk of congenital anomalies near hazardous-waste landfill sites in Europe: The EUROHAZCON Study. Lancet 352:423, 1998

FISHER BE: Most unwanted—persistent organic pollutants. Environ Health Perspect 107: A18, 1999

GRAVELING RA et al: A review of multiple chemical sensitivity. Occup Environ Med 56: 73, 1999

JOHNSON BL, DEROSA C: The toxicologic hazard of Superfund hazardous-waste sites. Rev Environ Health 12:235, 1997

MCMICHAEL AJ, HAINES A: Global climate change: The potential effects on health. BMJ 315:805, 1997

MENZIES D, BOURBEAU J: Building-related illness. N Engl J Med 337:1524, 1997

PATZ JA et al: Global climate change and emerging infectious diseases. JAMA 275:217, 1996

392

Jerome H. Modell

DROWNING AND NEAR-DROWNING

It is an unexpected tragedy when a previously healthy person dies or is exposed to severe cerebral hypoxia and suffers permanent brain damage. For many years, drowning was considered a "fight for survival": Arms flailing and screaming for help, a person who could not swim struggled to remain on the surface of the water to reach safety. This situation, however, is rarely reported by persons at the scene of aquatic emergencies. Furthermore, no single set of circumstances comprises drowning or near-drowning. It may be a secondary event following such precursors as head or spinal trauma; hypoxia-induced unconsciousness; or unconsciousness due to preexisting cardiovascular disease, sudden cardiac death, or myocardial infarction. The initiating event is usually unknown, so the drowned or near-drowned victim must be treated based on probable physiologic effects of the near-drowning itself. If survival with normal brain function is to occur, a thorough understanding of the pathophysiology of drowning and an organized approach to therapy are imperative.

PATHOPHYSIOLOGY OF DROWNING Approximately 90% of near-drowning victims aspirate fluid into their lungs. In those who do not aspirate fluid, hypoxemia results simply from breath holding, laryngospasm, or apnea. In those who do aspirate, the volume and the composition of the fluid determine the physiologic basis of the hypoxemia. Freshwater aspiration alters the surface tension properties of pulmonary surfactant and makes alveoli unstable, which causes a decreased ventilation/perfusion ratio. Some alveoli collapse and become atelectatic, which produces a true or absolute intrapulmonary shunt, while others are poorly ventilated and produce a relative shunt; in either case, significant pulmonary venous admixture occurs. Fresh water in the alveoli is hypotonic and is rapidly absorbed and redistributed throughout the body. While some have proposed that water continues to enter the lungs after death, at autopsy the lungs of victims who died in the water frequently contain little water. Also, it has been shown experimentally that if a dead body is submerged in tagged or colored water, water is not found in the lungs at autopsy. These findings support the premise that active respiration determines the volume of water aspirated.

Hypertonic seawater pulls additional fluid from the plasma into the lungs, and thus the alveoli are fluid-filled but perfused, which causes substantial pulmonary venous admixture. With both types of water, pulmonary edema may occur secondary to events such as fluid shifts, a change in capillary permeability, or cerebral hypoxia, which causes neurogenic pulmonary edema. Regardless of the cause, pulmonary edema adds to the ventilation/perfusion abnormality.

Water that is grossly contaminated with bacteria or that contains particulate matter may complicate the picture. Particulate matter can obstruct the smaller bronchi and respiratory bronchioles. Grossly contaminated water increases the risk of severe pulmonary infection. Neither problem is sufficiently common, however, to justify recommending specific therapy routinely for all victims.

At least 85% of near-drowned victims are thought to aspirate 22 mL/kg of water or less, which does not result in a clinically significant alteration of blood volume or serum electrolyte concentrations. After resuscitation, by the time blood is analyzed, serum electrolyte concentrations are usually normal or close to normal. Significant changes are documented in only approximately 15% of those who cannot be resuscitated and only rarely in those who are resuscitated. These findings suggest that either a small amount of water was aspirated, fluid was rapidly redistributed, or both. Therefore, electrolyte disturbance rarely needs treatment. When a large quantity of water is aspirated, seawater causes hypovolemia, which concentrates extracellular electrolytes, and fresh water causes acute hypervolemia. If enough water is aspirated that plasma becomes severely hypotonic and the patient is hypoxemic, red cell membranes can rupture, and plasma hemoglobin and serum potassium concentrations increase significantly. However, this development has been reported only rarely. With rapid redistribution of fluid and development of pulmonary edema, even freshwater victims frequently demonstrate hypovolemia by the time they reach the hospital.

Hypercarbia, which is associated with apnea and/or hypoventilation, is less often documented by blood gas analysis than is hypoxemia. While hypoxemia due to pulmonary venous admixture persists in all near-drowned victims who aspirate water, hypercarbia is usually corrected sooner with artificial mechanical ventilation and improved minute ventilation and, thus, is reported in only a small percentage of victims evaluated at the hospital. Besides hypoxemia, metabolic acidosis also persists in most patients. Abnormal cardiovascular function, usually ascribed to hypoxemia, is brief with effective, timely therapy. Abnormality in renal function is uncommon, but when it does occur, it too is secondary to hypoxemia, altered renal perfusion, or, in extremely rare circumstances, significant hemoglobinuria.

℞ **TREATMENT** The first step is retrieving the victim from the water, and, if necessary, performing artificial ventilation and circulation. The American Heart Association recommends that an ab-

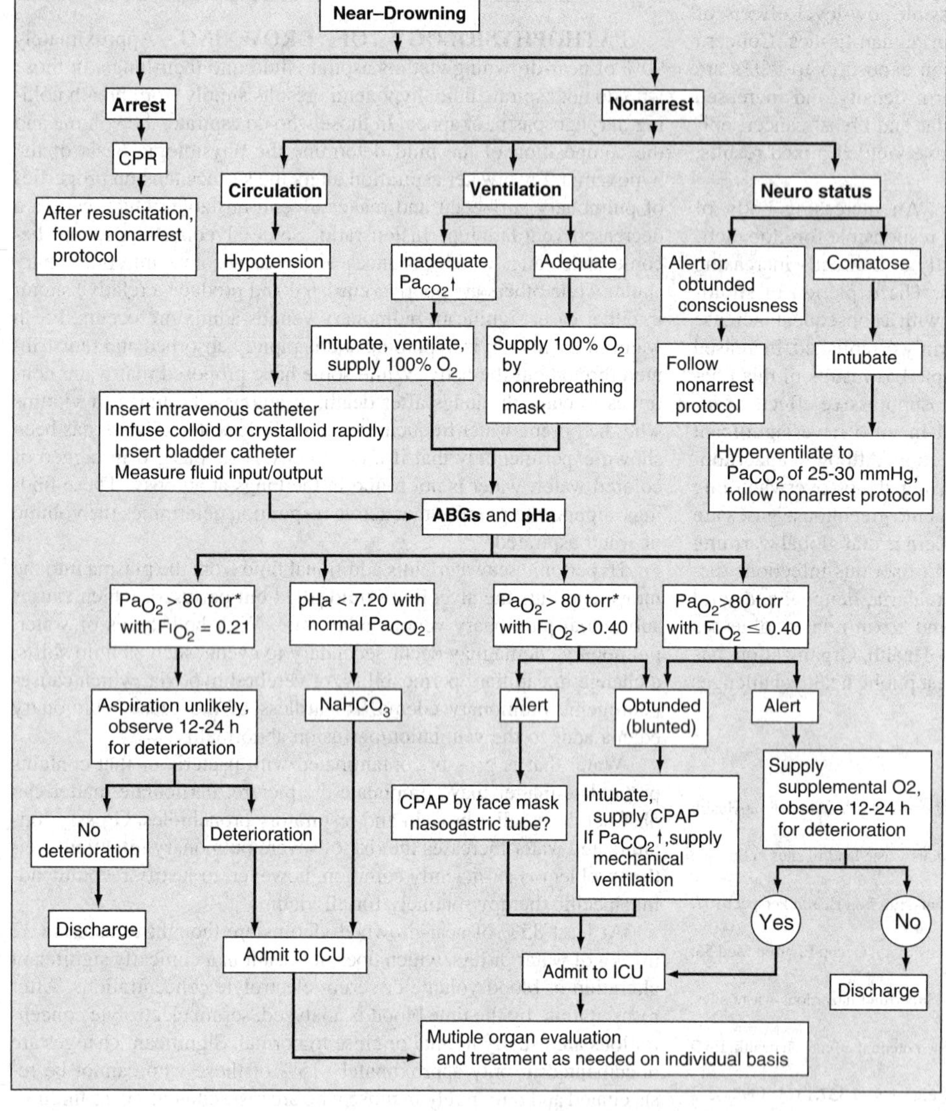

FIGURE 392-1 Treatment of a near-drowned victim should follow a sequence of priorities. *Guidelines only; assumes victim had normal arterial blood gas values (ABGs) before near-drowning. Abbreviations/definitions: CPAP, continuous positive airway pressure; CPR, cardiopulmonary resuscitation; FI_{O_2}, fraction of inspired oxygen; intubate: endoctracheal intubation; ICU, intensive care unit; $NaHCO_3$, bicarbonate; Pa_{O_2}/Pa_{CO_2}, arterial oxygen/carbon dioxide tension; pHa, arterial pH. *(Modified from Graves and Layon.)*

dominal thrust not be used routinely in victims of submersion. This recommendation was upheld by a special committee of the Institute of Medicine convened in 1994 specifically to evaluate the efficacy of an abdominal thrust in the treatment of near-drowned victims. In these patients, an abdominal thrust may lead to regurgitation of gastric contents and, thus, to aspiration of the vomitus. Further, an abdominal thrust may delay ventilatory or circulatory resuscitation. Therefore, an abdominal thrust should be used only when the airway is obstructed with a foreign body or when the victim fails to respond to mouth-to-mouth ventilation.

Because emergency services and intensive pulmonary and cardiovascular care have improved during the past 25 years, central nervous system depression now presents the major therapeutic challenge in near-drowning. The rate of survival with normal cerebral function varies considerably in retrospective studies. Some factors that adversely influence survival are prolonged submersion, delay in initiation of effective cardiopulmonary resuscitation, severe metabolic acidosis (pH < 7.1), asystole upon arrival at a medical facility, fixed dilated pupils, and a low Glasgow coma score (<5). None of these predictors is absolute, however, and, when maximally treated, normal survivors have been reported in all of the above categories. Absence of cortical evoked potentials does indicate irreversibility of the cerebral hypoxic lesion; this test, however, cannot be done in the field to guide rescuers. A comparison of outcomes between one institution that added brain preservation techniques to intensive pulmonary and circulatory treatment and another institution that did not found no significant differences.

Hypothermia appears to be protective, but only if it occurs early, at the time of the accident, in which case it increases the victim's chance of cerebral salvage after relatively long periods of acute hypoxia and cardiac arrest. While hypothermia prolongs tolerance to hypoxia, it also can precipitate fatal cardiac arrhythmia; thus, its occurrence can be helpful on the one hand and harmful on the other. The diving reflex produces bradycardia, breath holding, and circulatory redistribution when the face is submerged in cold water. However, the effect of the diving reflex in explaining cerebral recovery after prolonged immersion has not been specifically documented.

Significant pulmonary venous admixture usually persists even after successful resuscitation; therefore, supplemental oxygen should be administered until arterial blood gas analysis confirms that oxygen is no longer needed. Intravenous access should be established as soon as possible. The trachea should be intubated if necessary for airway maintenance or to facilitate mechanical ventilatory support. Electrocardiographic monitoring will facilitate prompt treatment of cardiac arrhythmia.

Victims should be transported to a hospital for definitive testing of the adequacy of ventilation and blood gas exchange, cardiac activity, and effective circulating blood volume. Other variables, such as serum electrolyte concentrations, renal function, and cerebral status, should be analyzed as indicated.

The single most effective treatment for hypoxemia, regardless of cause, is mechanical ventilatory support including continuous positive airway pressure (CPAP). After freshwater aspiration, improvement in ventilation/perfusion matching is more consistent when CPAP is combined with mechanical inflation of the lung than with spontaneous respiration. The question of whether CPAP should be combined with spontaneous respiration or with mechanical ventilation should be decided by whether the specific patient can perform the necessary work of breathing, adequately eliminate carbon dioxide, and adequately match ventilation/perfusion ratios. Positive airway pressure should be withdrawn gradually as the lungs stabilize and ventilation/perfusion ratio returns toward normal.

The pH in near-drowned victims is commonly significantly acidotic, which, in turn, can depress cardiac function. The metabolic component of the acidosis, if it results in a pH < 7.20, should be corrected pharmacologically, although there is some disagreement on this point. With cardiovascular instability, cannulation of the pulmonary artery with a Swan-Ganz catheter or evaluation by transesophageal echocardiography is indicated. Many patients will be hypovolemic from loss of fluid into the lung as pulmonary edema or from decreased venous return secondary to increased intrathoracic pressure during mechanical ventilatory support.

Because recovery after long periods of submersion under frigid conditions has been reported, body temperature should be taken into account before a decision is made to terminate therapy. The body temperature of victims depends not only on the temperature of the water from which they are retrieved but also on how well they were insulated by clothing. The volume of water actually aspirated is also important, because a large volume, if distributed before cardiac arrest occurs, can produce rapid central cooling. Thus, cold water can be protective when it produces total-body hypothermia, which decreases metabolic oxygen requirement. On the other hand, cold water may also contribute to the accident if hypothermia occurs before total submersion, and severe, or even fatal, cardiac arrhythmia results. Several methods of rewarming hypothermic victims have been advocated, but any technique that increases oxygen utilization, such as shivering, should be avoided.

Regardless of the conditions surrounding a drowning or near-drowning, treatment should adhere to the following sequence of priorities (Fig. 392-1):

1. Remove the victim from the water as soon as possible and stabilize the patient's head and neck if trauma is suspected.
2. Immediately follow the ABCs of cardiopulmonary resuscitation—even in the water if this does not endanger the rescuer.
3. If the patient is unconscious, protect the airway as needed with endotracheal intubation.
4. Establish venous access as soon as possible.
5. Provide supplemental oxygen and ventilatory support until each is no longer needed. This can be judged from analysis of arterial blood for oxygen tension, carbon dioxide tension, and pH.
6. Monitor cardiac rhythm with an electrocardioscope as soon as possible.
7. Monitor body temperature and restore it to normal.
8. If the patient has persistent respiratory insufficiency, provide intensive pulmonary support with CPAP and mechanical ventilation therapy as necessary.
9. If the patient has cardiovascular instability, evaluate cardiac output and effective circulatory volume by invasive monitoring, and measure serum electrolyte concentrations. Intravenous fluid replacement should be provided as necessary.
10. Evaluate and treat renal function and cerebral status as indicated.

Glucocorticoid therapy, prophylactic antibiotic therapy, and monitoring of intracranial pressure are no longer recommended.

ACCIDENT PREVENTION Because drowning begins as an accident that results in a medical problem, the definitive strategy is to prevent the accident. For those victims in whom the accident is secondary to a medical condition, as in persons susceptible to syncope or seizure, the only way to prevent the accident is to identify those who ought to avoid the water or to encourage them to use the buddy system. For young children, early swimming lessons, vigilant caretakers, and stringent laws governing pool enclosures are needed. Those who teach parenting classes should routinely warn parents about the risk of toddlers' drowning in such household fixtures as toilets, buckets of water, and even washing machines. Preventing accidents during boating, athletics, and other water-related recreational activities requires public education. Rules associated with these activities to maximize safety and judicious, responsible behavior should be portrayed as life-saving measures. Similarly, drinking alcohol, a "ubiquitous catalyst" to drowning, should be portrayed as life-threatening whenever water is nearby.

BIBLIOGRAPHY

AMERICAN HEART ASSOCIATION: Guidelines for cardiopulmonary resuscitation and emergency cardiac care. JAMA 268:2171, 1992

BOHN DJ et al: Influence of hypothermia, barbiturate therapy, and intracranial pressure monitoring on morbidity and mortality after near-drowning. Crit Care Med 14:529, 1986

GRAVES SA, LAYON AJ: Drowning and near-drowning, in *Emergency Medicine: A Comprehensive Review*, 3d ed, TC Kravis et al (eds). New York, Raven, 1993, pp 689–700

LAYON AJ, MODELL JH: Drowning and near drowning, in *The Lung at Depth*, C Lundgren, JH Miller (eds). New York, Marcel Dekker, 1999, pp 395–415

MODELL JH: Drowning. N Engl J Med 328:253, 1993

———, GOODWIN SR: Drowning and near-drowning, in *Kendig's Disorders of the Respiratory Tract in Children*, 6th ed, V Chernick, TF Boat (eds). Philadelphia, Saunders, 1998, pp 572–584

——— et al: Drowning without aspiration: Is this an appropriate diagnosis. J Foren Sci. 44:1119, 1999

——— et al: Clinical course of 91 consecutive near-drowning victims. Chest 70:231, 1976

ROSEN P et al (eds): *The Use of the Heimlich Maneuver in Near-Drowning*. Committee on the Treatment of Near-Drowning Victims, Institute of Medicine, Washington, DC, 1994

SWANN HG et al: Freshwater and seawater drowning: A study of the terminal cardiac and biochemical events. Texas Rep Biol Med 5:423, 1947

393

Raphael C. Lee

ELECTRICAL INJURIES

EPIDEMIOLOGY Electrical injury occurs when the body experiences levels of current that alter electrophysiologic function or cause tissue damage. Most commonly, such injuries result from contact with commercial electrical power sources in the home and workplace. Microwave, radiofrequency, light irradiation, and other injuries are less common. Ionizing electromagnetic fields (radiation) involve atomic absorption and free radical production, leading to biochemical alterations.

Electrical shock is one of the leading causes of work related injury, comprising 7% of all workplace fatalities. The exact incidence is unknown because many victims don't report minor injuries. The economic impact of industrial electrical injury in the United States is estimated to be in excess of $1 billion annually. Approximately one-third of high-power electrical injuries occur in the construction industry, one-third occur in the utility and petrochemical industries, and one-third are non-work related. More than 90% of the injuries occur in males, most commonly between the ages of 20 and 34. The extremities are nearly always involved, and limb amputation may be required.

Most injuries are due to low-voltage (<1000 V) electrical shock. Low-voltage power-frequency electrical shocks usually occur in and around the home. The household electric power in the United States is 120 V, AC 60-cycle current. In Europe it is 220 V. Low-voltage shocks carry a significant risk of electrocution due to cardiac arrest because they may cause muscle spasm that results in prolonged contact. Roughly 3 to 4% of all United States hospital burn unit admissions are for electrical injury, mostly a result of high-voltage (>1000 V) shocks. Extensive tissue damage, rather than electrocution, is characteristic of high-voltage shocks.

PATHOPHYSIOLOGY The term *direct current* (DC) is used to indicate a field frequency of zero (i.e., constant voltage gradient), and *alternating current* (AC) indicates that the field is changing direction (i.e., alternating polarity) with time. DC electrical power passes through the body on direct electrical contact. AC current can be carried by direct contact, capacitive coupling, and magnetic induction.

Tissue damage can result from exposure to harmful levels of current at any frequency in the electromagnetic spectrum that ranges from DC to ζ-hertz (ionizing irradiation). The tissue effects of electricity depend as much on the frequency as on the magnitude of current. Table 393-1 presents a classification of electrical injury according to fre-

Table 393-1 Electrical Injuries by Frequency Range

Frequency Range	General Applications	Harmful Tissue Effects
Low (DC–10 KHz)	Commercial electrical power, batteries	Joule heating, cell membrane electroporation
Radiofrequency (10 KHz–10 MHz)	Radiocommunication, diatherm, electrocautery	Joule heating, dielectric heating of proteins
Microwave (10 MHz–10 GHz)	Microwave heating	Dielectric heating of water
Light and ionizing ($\geq 10^{15}$ Hz)	Photooptical and ionizing irradiation (ultraviolet, x-ray, gamma)	Reactive oxygen intermediates production

quency range. Commercial electrical power operates in the narrow frequency range of DC to 150 Hz in the low frequency regime. An electrical shock in this frequency range is most common.

When the voltage is <1000 V, direct mechanical contact is usually required for electrical contact. For high voltages (>1000 V), arcing usually initiates the electrical contact. On direct electrical contact, the electron flow in the metal conductor or arc is converted at the skin surface into electrolyte ions that carry the current through the body. This electrochemical process generates heat and toxic chemical byproducts that contribute to contact area injury. In high-voltage contacts, exposure to the expanding arc, an excellent conductor, brings the victim into the electrical circuit. The arc can reach very high temperatures, leading to skin burns or clothing ignition. At higher frequencies (>10 MHz) electrical power can couple electrical energy across an air gap into the body without charge transport across the skin surface (capacitive coupling).

Low-frequency electricity causes tissue injury primarily by permeabilizing cell membranes, electroconformational denaturation of cell membrane proteins, and thermal denaturation of tissue proteins. Factors that determine the anatomic pattern, the extent of tissue injury, and the relative contribution of heat versus direct electrical damage include the amount of current, anatomic location, and the contact duration. The type of clothing, the use of protective gear, and the power capability of the electrical source also contribute to the wide range of clinical manifestations in victims of electrical shock. In addition, a very high-energy electrical arc can produce a strong thermoacoustic blast force leading to barotrauma. Associated falls and skin burns are frequent, exacerbating the injury. Cataracts characteristically occur after rapid and brief exposure of the eyes to hot gases and arc-mediated electrical current. The latency period for development of cataracts averages approximately 6 months.

Peripheral nerve and skeletal muscle tissues are most vulnerable to membrane damage by applied electrical currents. The "no-let-go" phenomenon results from the passage of more than 14 to 16 mA longitudinally through the forearm that induces tetanic contractions of muscles controlling handgrip. The resulting involuntary muscle spasm may lead to joint dislocations and spine fractures. When current of >50 mA is passed hand-to-hand or hand-to-foot, there is enough induced depolarization of myocardial membranes to cause cardiac arrhythmias, particularly if the induced depolarization occurs during early myocardial repolarization. Disruption of extremity skeletal muscle and nerve cell membranes by the process of electroporation results when more than 0.5 to 1 A is passed through the extremity. Electroporation damage accumulates on the time scale of milliseconds, leading to lethal cellular injury. With more prolonged contacts in the range of seconds, thermal damage in the subcutaneous tissues becomes substantial. Because the vulnerability to supraphysiologic temperature exposure is similar regardless of tissue type, all tissues in the current path are burned when pathologic levels of heating occur. Extensive disruption of cell membranes leads to release of myoglobin and hemoglobin, which enter the circulation. Acute renal failure can result from intrarenal crystalization of these molecules. Acute renal failure superimposed on extensive tissue injury has a very high mortality rate.

DIAGNOSIS For the more common low-frequency electrical injuries, at least two skin contact wounds are present. Differences in wound size and topography are largely determined by the surface contact area, the shape of the objects that conducted the current through the victim, and the duration of contact.

Cardiac arrhythmias and most respiratory disturbances must be rapidly detected by examination of the pulse, chest, and electrocardiogram. The next priority is to determine the location and extent of tissue damage. Injured skeletal muscle and nerves are often found beneath undamaged skin. Lateral spine x-rays or computed tomography (CT) are needed to rule out unstable spine fracture patterns. X-ray images of the extremities involved are also important to rule out skeletal fractures or joint dislocations. Blood chemistries should be immediately evaluated and monitored. Metabolic acidosis and elevated serum potassium levels may exist as consequences of extensive skeletal muscle injury. Serum CPK levels will rise over several hours if there is significant rhabdomyolysis.

Tissue edema begins to form because of increased vascular permeability and the release of intracellular contents into the extravascular space. Muscle compartment syndrome and compression neuropathies are common manifestations. If available, magnetic resonance imaging (MRI) scans can rapidly localize tissue edema. Where severe heating has coagulated the blood vessels, tissue injury may exist in the absence of edema. Muscle compartment fluid pressures should be measured where edema is present. If MRI is not available, then the muscle compartments in the current path between contact points should be monitored for elevated interstitial fluid pressure. Elevated compartment pressures may evolve during resuscitation. Muscle compartment fluid pressures >30 cmH_20 are indications for fasciotomy. It may be necessary to check the pressures every 8 h for 24 h. Radionucleotide scanning with ^{99m}Tc-pyrophosphate can also be useful to detect tissue damage. These scans, however, take 4 to 6 h to complete and are mostly useful in the less severe injuries. If there is a history of loss of consciousness, CT of the head is indicated.

℞ **TREATMENT** The first priority is to disconnect the patient from the electrical power source. When high-capacity circuits are involved, disconnection must not be attempted before the circuit is deenergized. Cervical spine fracture should be assumed until proven otherwise. Critical initial considerations are evaluation and support of vital organ function and, secondarily, assessment of the extent of injury. After very-high voltage trauma, prolonged cardiopulmonary resuscitation (CPR) may be necessary before the stunned myocardium regains the ability to sustain a coordinated rhythm.

Patients with significant wounds and tissue injury as well as those with vital organ injury require hospital admission. It is unlikely for cardiac arrhythmias to develop if cardiac injury is not detectable on initial presentation. Peripheral nerve injury invariably occurs even in minor shocks and usually resolves over several days. If symptoms persist, however, they may be controlled with cyclooxygenase inhibitors alone or with antioxidants. Small wounds can be managed by cleaning and applying topical antibiotics. Major neuropsychological and stress disorders often follow a terrifying "no-let-go" experience. Management often involves psychiatric consultation.

For more substantial trauma, a Foley catheter and large bore peripheral intravenous lines delivering normal saline at a rate sufficient to generate a 30 to 50 mL/h urine output are essential. If the urine is visibly pigmented with myoglobin or hemoglobin, the output should be doubled and alkalinized to a pH >6 by adding bicarbonate to the intravenous solutions until the urine has cleared. In the most severe injuries, hyperpermeability of peripheral capillaries may result in rapid interstitial (third space) fluid accumulation. In such cases, it may be necessary to increase blood oxygen levels and add dextran to resuscitation fluids.

Cardiac arrhythmias must be immediately controlled by antiarrhythmic drugs simultaneously with the correction of serum pH and electrolyte abnormalities. Brain injury–related seizures must be controlled with antiepileptic agents. Patients who have lost central nervous system (CNS) control of respiration or airways should be intubated and mechanically ventilated. A paralyzed ventilated patient may need monitoring by electroencephalogram (EEG) to assess seizure control. Appropriate management of corneal burns or abrasions, tympanic membrane rupture, and closed head injury should be instituted.

Large skin burn wounds are often present because of arc-mediated contacts and clothing ignition. Care should be taken to prevent rapid loss of body heat through open wounds. Tetanus prophylaxis should be administered.

Perfusion of devascularized tissue must be quickly restored. Diminished pulses or decreased tissue oxygen by transcutaneous pulse oximetry are indications for escharotomy releases. Fasciotomy is often required. The classic clinical signs of pain in acute compartment syndrome cannot be relied on because of associated nerve injury. In addition to decompression of extremity muscle compartments, decompression of nerve within edematous fibrous and osseous conduits (e.g., carpal tunnel, Guyon's canal, and tarsal tunnel) should be carried out to help prevent compression neuropathy. Care to avoid tissue drying or desiccation is important. Debridement of nonviable subcutaneous tissue should be performed as soon as a general anesthetic can be safely administered.

Anaerobic bacterial infection of devascularized skeletal muscle is a common complication. Intravenous penicillin G and/or hyperbaric oxygen as prophylactic antibiotics are sometimes utilized but have unproven value. Radiographs taken to rule out fractures may reveal air bubbles in the subcutaneous tissues. This gas results from tissue boiling when prolonged Joule heating has occurred.

Rehabilitation into society and gainful employment are the ultimate objectives. For severely injured victims these goals require functional muscle and nerve reconstruction as well as correction of scar contractures. Psychological and neurocognitive problems are expected and require treatment by experts. Persistent peripheral neurologic problems are also common and often require detailed evaluation and therapeutic intervention.

LIGHTNING INJURIES

Lightning injury is a powerful manifestation of arc-mediated electrical contact. Arcing occurs when the voltage gradient in air exceeds 2 million V/m. The arc consists of a hot ionized gas of subatomic particles that is highly conductive. Peak lightning currents reach into the range of 30,000 to 50,000 A for a duration of 5 to 10 μs. Lightning arc temperatures reach up to 30,000°K, which generates thermoacoustic blast waves, commonly called thunder. Peak blast pressures reach 4 or 5 atm in the immediate vicinity of a lightning strike, and up to 1 or 2 atm 1 m away. Substantial barotrauma can result.

Like radiofrequency current, lightning current flows along the surfaces of conducting objects. Initially, the flow of an enormous current through the lightning strike generates a very large surrounding magnetic field pulse. This magnetic field pulse can induce current flow in the body, enough to disrupt cardiac and CNS function. When lightning current enters the ground, it spreads out radially, which sets a large current traveling along the surfaces of the ground. A substantial voltage drop can occur between the feet of a nearby individual. The voltage drops between widely separated feet can reach 1500 to 2000 V and can induce a 2 to 3 A current flow in the legs for a 10-μs period.

Victims of direct lightning strikes experience a multimodal injury. Superficial burns on the skin represent the current path along the skin surface. The intense brief shock pulse seems to arrest all electrophysiologic processes. The victim appears lifeless. Prolonged CPR may be necessary. Muscle and nerve necrosis is rare in survivors. Deeper injury results when the victim is in contact with a large conducting object such as a truck or fence that has been struck by lightning, which then discharges over several milliseconds through the victim.

Delay in resuscitation is the most common cause of death. Bystanders are usually afraid to touch the victim while precious minutes pass. However, unless the victim is on an insulating platform, there is no residual electric charge on the body afer several milliseconds. When needed, CPR should be given without hesitation. Victims should be cared for in an intensive care unit until life-threatening CNS and cardiac injuries are ruled out. Late neurologic and ophthalmologic sequelae often develop.

BIBLIOGRAPHY

DeBono R: A histological analysis of a high voltage electric current injury to an upper limb. Burns 25:541, 1999

Lederer W et al: Electricity-associated injuries II: Outdoor management of lightning-induced casualties. Resuscitation 43:89, 2000

Lee RC: Injury by electrical forces: Pathophysiology, manifestations, and therapy. Curr Probl Surgery 34(9):677–764, 1997

Lee RC, Capelli-Schellpfeffer M, Kelley KM (eds): *Electrical Injury: A Multidisciplinary Approach to Therapy, Prevention and Rehabilitation.* Ann NY Acad Sci vol. 720, 1994

Luce EA: Electrical burns. Clin Plast Surg 27:133, 2000

394

Stephen M. Hahn, Eli Glatstein

RADIATION INJURY

All human beings are constantly exposed to ionizing radiation. Environmental sources include the cosmic radiation from space and radiation from the ground and from inhaled and ingested materials. Airline travel and mining both increase exposure to the background radiation. For example, air travel at 30,000 ft exposes individuals to a dose equivalent of 0.5 mrem/h. Radiation originating in the body comes mainly from radioactive potassium, which emits beta and gamma rays. Lungs are exposed to irradiation from inhaled air, which contains small amounts of radioactive radon. The cosmic exposure contributes approximately 28 mrem per year. The ground and internal sources contribute approximately 26 and 27 mrem per year, respectively. The most prominent man-made sources of radiation include x-ray equipment, nuclear weapons, and radioactive medications.

TERMINOLOGY AND DEFINITIONS

The first major unit of radiation exposure was the roentgen (R), defined as an amount of x-rays or gamma rays that produces a specific amount of ionization in a unit of air under standard temperature and pressure (Table 394-1); this quantity can be measured directly in an ionization chamber. The rad, or *r*adiation *a*bsorbed *d*ose, is defined as 100 ergs/g of tissue. Thus, the rad represents a net deposition of energy in a three-dimensional volume, because x-rays attenuate as they traverse tissue. The rad has been replaced by the Système Internationale (SI)

Table 394-1 Units and Definitions

Unit	Quantity Measured	Definition
Roentgen (R)	Exposure	Amount of x-rays or gamma rays that produces a specific amount of ionization in a given volume of air
Rad	Dose	100 ergs deposited per gram of tissue
Gray (Gy)	Dose	SI unit of dose; equals 100 rad
Rem	Dose equivalence	Unit that reflects the biologic response. It is used to compare various types of radiation
Sievert (Sv)	Dose equivalence	SI unit of dose equivalence; equals 100 rem

unit of the gray (Gy), which represents 100 rad. Roentgens and rads can be converted by means of various tables; the relation between them depends on photon energy.

The above definitions reflect physical variables. The unit that reflects the biologic response and that can be used to compare the effects of various types of radiation is the unit of *dose equivalence*, the rem (*r*oentgen *e*quivalent in *m*an). The rem has been replaced by the SI unit, the sievert (Sv), which equals 100 rem. These units reflect the exposure or absorption dose multiplied by a biologic factor that represents the biologic effectiveness of the specific type of radiation (see below).

TYPES OF IONIZING RADIATION

The absorption of energy from radiation in tissue often leads to excitation or ionization. Excitation involves elevation of an electron in an atom or molecule to a higher energy state without actual ejection of the electron. Ionization involves actual ejection of one or more electrons from the atom. Ionizing radiation is subclassified as electromagnetic (photon) or particulate radiation (Table 394-2). X-rays and gamma rays are examples of electromagnetic photon radiation. They differ only in their source: X-rays are produced mechanically, by making electrons strike a target, which causes the electrons to give up their kinetic energy as x-rays, while gamma rays are produced by nuclear disintegration of radioactive isotopes.

X-rays can be thought of as packets of energy, or photons. X-rays have no mass or charge, travel in straight lines, and attenuate continuously as they traverse tissue. Gamma rays have similar properties. Each photon contains an amount of energy equal to $h\nu$, where h is Planck's constant. The critical difference between nonionizing and ionizing radiation is the energy of individual photons, not the energy of the total dose.

Types of *particulate radiation* include electrons, protons, alpha particles, neutrons, negative pi-mesons, and heavy charged ions; these have discrete mass and charge (except for neutrons, which lack charge; Table 394-2). *Electrons*, or *beta particles*, are small and negatively charged and can be accelerated to close to the speed of light. They decelerate fairly rapidly in tissue and penetrate it to only a limited depth. Thus, electron beams are often used to treat superficial problems. *Protons* are positively charged and have a mass about 2000 times that of an electron. Protons stop abruptly, depending on their energy; in the process of sudden deceleration, most of their energy is given up, which tends to cause ionization just before the proton stops. This region of enhanced ionization, sometimes called the Bragg peak, means that proton beams exert their effects in a relatively compact region. *Alpha particles* are helium nuclei, consisting of two protons and two neutrons. The mass and charge are great enough that these particles do not penetrate far through matter unless they have tremendous energy; even a piece of paper is enough to protect against most alpha particles. Because these particles are charged, they can be accelerated in electrical fields.

Neutrons are similar in mass to protons (having an atomic mass of 1), but they are not charged and therefore cannot be accelerated in an electrical field. Neutron beams are produced by colliding charged particles into a suitable target or are emitted as a fission product of heavy radioactive atoms. *Heavy charged ions* are nuclei of heavier elements that have a positive charge owing to the stripping away of some or all of the orbiting electrons.

Equal doses of different types of radiation do not necessarily produce equal biologic effects; thus 1 Gy of neutrons produces a greater biologic effect than 1 Gy of x-rays. The biologic effects produced by a given dose of radiation can be quantified by the relative biologic effectiveness (RBE) value, which relates them to the effects produced by 250-kV photon radiation as a standard. In general, the greater the RBE value for a given type of radiation, the greater the biologic effect. The RBE value will be greater for more densely ionizing radiation, such as neutrons. The RBE value depends on the linear energy transfer (see below), the dose, the dose rate, and the nature of the biologic system.

The linear energy transfer (LET) is the amount of ionization occurring per unit length of the radiation track. It is usually expressed as kilovolts per micron and increases with the square of the charge of the incident particle. High-LET radiation is biologically different from low-LET (i.e., conventional) radiation: Hypoxic and oxygenated cells respond similarly to high-LET irradiation, whereas it takes about three times as much low-LET radiation to produce a given killing effect in hypoxic cells as in oxygenated cells. It is thought that low-LET radiation must produce multiple hits on DNA to destroy a cell, whereas high-LET radiation need produce only a single hit on DNA to kill a cell. Representative values of LET and RBE are given in Table 394-3.

Radiation, especially x-rays, is absorbed and causes ionization in three major ways: the *photoelectric effect*, the *Compton effect*, and *pair production*. At low energies (30 to 100 keV), as in diagnostic radiology, the photoelectric effect is important. In this process, the incident photon interacts with an electron in one of the outer shells of an atom (typically K, L, or M). If the energy of the photon is greater than the binding energy of the electron, then the electron is expelled from the orbit with a kinetic energy that is equal to the energy of the incident photon minus the binding energy of the electron. The photoelectric effect varies as a function of the cube of the atomic number of the material exposed (Z^3); this fact explains why bone is visualized much better than soft tissue on radiographs.

At higher energies, as used in therapeutic radiology, the Compton effect dominates. In this process, the incident photon interacts with an electron in an orbital shell. Part of the incident photon energy appears as kinetic energy of electrons, and the residual energy continues as a less energetic deflected photon.

At energy levels above 1.02 MeV, the photons may be absorbed

Table 394-2 Common Types of Ionizing Radiation

Type	Mass	Charge	Comment
Electromagnetic			
X-ray	0	0	X-rays and gamma rays do not differ except in the source. Gamma rays are produced intranuclearly, and x-rays are produced extranuclearly (i.e., mechanically).
Gamma ray	0	0	
Particulate			
Electron (e)	9.1×10^{-31} kg	−1	—
Proton (p)	2000 × e	+1	Exhibits a Bragg peak
Neutron (n)	2000 × e	0	Cannot be accelerated by an electrical field
Alpha particle	2p + 2n ~8000 × e	+2	Helium nucleus

Table 394-3 Linear Energy Transfer (LET) and Relative Biologic Effectiveness (RBE) Values

Type of Radiation	LET Values, keV/μm
Cobalt-60 gamma rays	0.2
250-keV x-rays	2.0
10 MeV protons	4.7
Type of Radiation	**RBE Values (Quality Factors)**
X-rays, gamma rays, and electrons	1
Neutrons	3–20
Heavy particles	1–20

through pair production. In this process, both a positron and an electron are produced in the absorbing material. A positron has the same mass as an electron but has a positive instead of a negative charge. The positron travels a very short distance in the absorbing medium before it interacts with another electron. When that happens, the entire mass of both particles is converted to energy, with the emission of two photons in exactly opposite directions.

BIOLOGIC EFFECTS OF RADIATION

Radiation must produce double-strand breaks in DNA to kill a cell, owing partly to the high capacity of mammalian cells for repairing single-strand damage. Radiation can also produce effects indirectly by interacting with water (which makes up approximately 80% of a cell's volume) to generate free radicals, which can damage the cell. Free radicals are highly reactive chemical entities that lack a stable number of outer-shell electrons. A free radical is not stable and has a life span of a fraction of a second. It is estimated that most x-ray-induced cell damage is due to the formation of hydroxyl radicals, as follows:

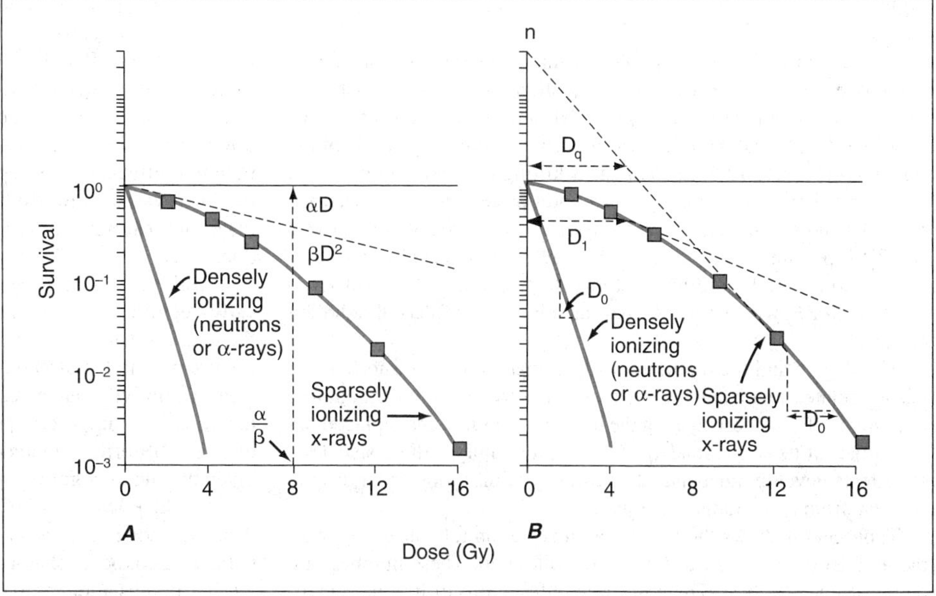

FIGURE 394-1 Shape of survival curve for mammalian cells exposed to radiation. The fraction of cells surviving is plotted on a logarithmic scale against dose on a linear scale. For alpha particles or low-energy neutrons (said to be densely ionizing) the dose-response curve is a straight line from the origin (i.e., survival is an exponential function of dose). The survival curve can be described by just one parameter, the slope. For x-rays or gamma rays (said to be sparsely ionizing), the dose-response curve has an initial linear slope, followed by a shoulder; at higher doses the curve tends to become straight again. *A*. The experimental data are fitted to a linear-quadratic function. There are two components of cell killing: one is proportional to dose (αD), while the other is proportional to the square of the dose (βD^2). The dose at which the linear and quadratic components are equal is the ratio α/β. The linear-quadratic curve bends continuously but is a good fit to experimental data for the first few decades of survival. *B*. The curve is described by the initial slope (D_1), the final slope (D_0), and a parameter that represents the width of the shoulder, either n or D_q. *(From Hall, with permission.)*

$$\text{Ionizing radiation} + H_2O \rightarrow H_2O^+ + e^-$$
$$H_2O^+ + H_2O \rightarrow H_3O^+ + OH\bullet$$
$$OH\bullet \rightarrow \text{Cell damage}$$

The result of radiation damage is cell death. The biologic effects on epithelial cell reproduction are typically expressed only when the damaged cells attempt to divide. Another biologic effect is the induction of cancerous growth by mutation many years after radiation exposure. Patients who receive radiation have a significant risk of neoplasm two to three decades after their exposure; this risk is significantly higher than that of the population as a whole.

RADIATION-INDUCED CHROMOSOME ABERRATIONS Chromosome breaks can occur when cells are irradiated. The broken ends of chromosomes can combine with broken ends of different chromosomes. These abnormal combinations are most readily seen during mitosis. Chromosome abnormalities typically occur in cells irradiated in the G1 phase of the cell cycle, before the doubling of genetic material. If cells are irradiated in the G2 phase, chromatid aberrations may result. The frequency of chromosomal aberrations in peripheral circulating lymphocytes correlates with the dose received. The dose can be estimated by comparing the chromosomal changes to in vitro cultures exposed to controlled doses of irradiation. The minimum dose that can be detected by peripheral lymphocyte analysis is about 0.1 to 0.2 Sv (10 to 20 rem). Lymphocyte analysis may provide evidence of recent total-body exposure.

CELL SURVIVAL CURVE The dose-response curve for all mammalian cells appears to have a linear-quadratic relationship. In simple terms, the mathematical model that explains the relationship between the dose and the fraction of surviving cells has both linear and exponential components. The linear component results from double-stranded chromosomal breaks produced by single hits. The exponential component represents breaks produced by multiple hits. Figure 394-1 shows the shape of a typical survival curve for mammalian cells exposed to radiation. The fraction of cells surviving is plotted on a semilogarithmic scale. For x-rays or gamma rays, the dose-response curve has a shoulder that is followed by a straight line curve as the dose is increased. The shoulder represents the cell's ability to repair sublethal injury. For alpha particles or lower energy neutrons, the dose-response curve is a straight line from the origin. Thus, the survival rate is an exponential function of the dose.

In all mammalian cell lines studied, increases in the radiation dose decrease the survival rate of cells. However, a number of factors may contribute to a relative resistance to radiation in human tumors in vivo, including hypoxia and expression of particular oncogenes, such as *ras*. The biologic basis for radiation resistance has not been fully defined.

Four important processes that occur after radiation exposure can be summarized as the "four R's" of radiobiology. The first is *repair*. Repair is temperature dependent and is thought to represent the enzymatic mechanisms for healing intracellular injury. The second R is *reoxygenation*, a process whereby oxygen (and other nutrients) are actually better distributed to viable cells following radiation injury and cell killing. The third R is *repopulation*, the ability of the cell population to continue to divide and to replace dying and dead cells. The fourth R is *redistribution*, which reflects the variability of a cell's radiosensitivity over the cell cycle. Radiosensitivity can vary through the cell cycle by as much as a factor of 3. The G1 phase has the most variable length of all the phases of the cell cycle. For most cell lines, cells that have a short G1 period are most sensitive at the G2/mitosis interface, less sensitive in G1, and most resistant toward the end of the synthesis (S) period.

Radiation therapy is effective in cancer treatment when it exerts greater cytotoxic effects on tumor cells than on normal tissues. A major determinant of the therapeutic index is exploiting differences in the four R's between tumor cells and normal tissues by delivering the radiation in dose fractions.

CLINICAL FINDINGS ON FRACTIONATION The clinical radiation response may be related to the interactions of various growth factors and cytokines. For example, radiation can induce growth factors and cytokines such as tumor necrosis factor (TNF), interleukin (IL) 1. TNF can induce proliferation of fibroblasts and enhance the inflammatory response. TNF and IL-1 have been shown to radioprotect hematopoietic cells in vitro by increasing the D_0 of the cell survival curve. TNF also enhances killing of a human tumor cell line by irradiation. TNF may produce radioprotection or radiosensitization depending on the cell type. Efforts to modulate radiation effects with TNF remain experimental. Other factors implicated in the radiation response are basic fibroblast growth factor and platelet-derived growth factor β, which may be associated with late effects of radiation on vessels.

The degree and the duration of functional recovery of normal tissues are related to the number of stem cells surviving after irradiation. If the stem cells are destroyed in the irradiated volume and replacement from adjacent tissues is inadequate, radiation injury will persist. True late effects develop independent of early reactions; they occur despite recovery from acute radiation injury.

Table 394-4 shows the frequency of radiation tolerance seen with fractionated radiotherapy at 5 years of follow-up. These numbers are rough estimates at best. The clinical manifestations of irradiation will depend on the volume of the organ irradiated, the total dose, the dose per fraction, and the length of time taken to deliver the dose. Dose per fraction is the most important factor determining normal tissue effects. In addition, the cellular consequences of treatment can be progressive over time. Thus, length of follow-up is also crucial in judging clinical sequelae.

Central Nervous System Traditionally, the central nervous system (CNS) has been described as relatively resistant to radiation-induced changes. When the human brain is treated with standard fractionation (1.8 to 2.0 Gy/d), acute reactions are seldom observed.

Subacute CNS reactions to radiation treatment are more common. The clinical manifestations may include *Lhermitte's sign*, which is a self-limited paresthesia occurring with flexion of the neck. It is believed to be due to transient demyelination of the spinal cord following significant radiation exposure. It can be seen 1 to 3 months after completion of radiation treatment to the spinal cord. The frequency of Lhermitte's sign varies according to the type of radiation therapy and

Table 394-4 Class 1 Organs: Fatal or Severe Morbidity Following Cumulative Doses of Radiation Delivered with Standard Fractionation

Organ	Injury	$TD_{5/5}$[a]	$TD_{50/5}$[b]	Whole or Partial Organ (Field Size or Length)
Bone marrow	Aplasia, pancytopenia	250	450	Whole
		3000	4000	Segmental
Liver	Acute and chronic hepatitis	2500	4000	Whole
		1500	2000	Whole (strip)
Stomach	Perforation, ulcer, hemorrhage	4500	5500	100 cm
Intestine	Ulcer, perforation, hemorrhage	4500	5500	400 cm
		5000	6500	100 cm
Brain	Infarction, necrosis	5000	6000	Whole
Spinal cord	Infarction, necrosis	4500	5500	10 cm
Heart	Pericarditis, pancarditis	4500	5500	60%
		7000	8000	25%
Lung	Acute and chronic pneumonitis	3000	3500	100 cm
		1500	2500	Whole
Kidney	Acute and chronic nephrosclerosis	1500	2000	Whole (strip)
		2000	2500	Whole
Fetus	Death	200	400	Whole

[a] $TD_{5/5}$ is the minimal tolerance dose—the dose that, when administered to a given patient population under a standard set of treatment conditions, results in a rate of severe complications of 5% or less within 5 years of treatment.

[b] $TD_{50/5}$ is the maximal tolerance dose—the dose that, when administered to a given population of patients under a standard set of treatment conditions, results in a rate of severe complications of 50% within 5 years of treatment.

SOURCE: From P Rubin et al (eds): *Radiation Biology and Radiation Pathology Syllabus*, set RT 1: *Radiation Oncology*. Chicago, American College of Radiology, 1975.

can be as high as 15% after mantle-field radiation. Mild encephalopathy and focal neurologic changes can occur after irradiation limited to the cranium. If radiation treatments to the brain are given at the same time that chemotherapeutic agents are administered, the effects can be more severe, presumably reflecting altered permeability to the drugs. The effect of cranial irradiation is believed to be secondary to radiation effects on the replicating oligodendrocytes and possibly on the microvasculature. Both clinical and radiologic changes may simulate tumor progression and can often pose diagnostic and treatment dilemmas.

Postirradiation pathology and associated clinical symptoms typically begin 6 to 36 months after radiation therapy and are related to the total dose and volume treated. Fraction size appears to be the most important variable affecting the rate of postirradiation brain necrosis. Neurocognitive changes can also be seen in children after cranial irradiation. The important pretreatment factors that predict the degree of late CNS effects include the age at which cranial irradiation was given and neurocognitive functional level at the time of treatment.

A unique late effect of cranial irradiation combined with chemotherapy, known as *leukoencephalopathy*, has been described in some patients. Leukoencephalopathy is a necrotizing reaction usually noted 4 to 12 months after combined treatment with methotrexate and cranial irradiation. Dementia and dysarthria may progress to seizures, ataxia, or death.

Transverse myelitis after radiation treatment is a spinal cord reaction similar to cerebral necrosis. This syndrome consists of progressive and irreversible leg weakness and loss of bladder function and sensation referrable to a single spinal cord level. Flaccid paralysis eventually occurs. Symptoms can occur as early as 6 months after radiation treatment, but the usual time to onset is 12 to 24 months. Lhermitte's sign does not correlate with transverse myelitis.

Skin Skin reaction can be seen within 2 weeks of fractionated radiotherapy, a delay that correlates with the time required for cells to move from the basal to the keratinized layer of skin. The severity of the reaction depends on the skin dose per fraction and the total dose delivered to an area of skin. Erythema is observed, soon followed by dry desquamation. The skin at this time can be erythematous, warm, and sometimes edematous. The vessels in the upper dermis are dilated, and inflammatory infiltration with granulocytes, macrophages, eosinophils, plasma cells, and lymphocytes is noted.

When a severe skin reaction occurs, it is usually located where the beam strikes the skin tangentially. *Moist desquamation* consists of eruption of the epidermal layer. Healing is through reepithelialization from cells of less affected basal layers. When skin reactions are severe, treatment interruptions are needed to permit healing.

Dry desquamation is treated conservatively. Symptoms of dryness can be alleviated by advising the patient to wear only cotton fabric next to the affected skin and to refrain from the use of irritants of any kind. If treatment becomes necessary, hydrophilic agents that do not contain heavy metals are recommended. Petroleum jellies should not be used, as they may trap bacteria and increase the chance of infection. Moist desquamation is best managed by leaving the affected area dry and open to air.

A chronic reaction to radiation can be seen starting 6 to 12 months after irradiation. The epidermis is usually atrophic and may be more easily injured than normal skin. Interstitial fibrosis may also be increased. Hyperpigmentation of irradiated skin outlining the treatment field can be seen within a couple of months after completion of irradiation. This will fade gradually. The skin becomes thin, and hair loss may be permanent. Radiation therapy can induce second malignancies, which tend to be more aggressive than cancers arising in patients without significant radiation exposure.

Heart and Blood Vessels When cardiac disease appears after radiation treatment, it is often difficult to tell to what extent the radiation treatment was causative. The pathogenesis of atherosclerotic heart disease is multifactorial. Exposure of a large heart volume to high-dose radiation therapy accelerates the development of coronary artery disease. Acute "pericarditis" may result from cardiac irradiation.

The symptoms may include chest pain and fever, with or without pericardial effusion. This syndrome is usually self-limited and typically manifests itself a few months after treatment. Asymptomatic pericardial effusion may be the most common manifestation of radiation-induced heart disease. It is usually detected by chest x-ray and confirmed by an echocardiogram.

Most patients with symptomatic radiation-induced constrictive pericarditis will have received more than 40 Gy to a large portion of the heart. The risk increases significantly with cardiac doses greater than 50 Gy.

Chronic cardiac changes may have their onset from 6 months to several years after irradiation. The clinical symptoms may indicate chronic constrictive disease due to pericardial, myocardial, and endocardial fibrosis—a pancarditis. The clinical signs may include dyspnea, chest pain, venous distention, pleural effusion, and paradoxical pulse.

Lung The clinical symptoms of radiation pneumonitis can be separated into early and late phases. During the early phase, clinical manifestations may include dyspnea, cough, and fever. Shortness of breath is relatively infrequent. It is more common to observe only the radiologic changes on a chest x-ray, without clinical symptoms. The clinical signs and symptoms of radiation pneumonitis may appear in 3 to 6 weeks if a large region of lung is irradiated to a dose above 25 Gy. An infiltrate outlining the treatment field may become evident on the chest x-ray. Radiation changes should not occur outside the treated field. Computed tomography can often help in distinguishing radiation pneumonitis from other causes of the infiltrate. The incidence of radiation pneumonitis can be reduced with careful treatment planning designed to lower the total dose given to the treated lung volume. Permanent scarring that results in respiratory compromise may develop if the dose and the volume of lung irradiated are excessive. Dyspnea and cough may be severe and debilitating.

Patients with symptoms of radiation pneumonitis may respond rapidly to glucocorticoids, but the medication has little effect on fibrotic changes. Glucocorticoids must be tapered very slowly to avoid rebound exacerbation of symptoms, which can prove lethal for some patients. Prophylactic administration of glucocorticoids is of no proven merit. Supportive care includes bronchodilators and oxygen at the lowest possible FI_{O_2}.

Digestive Tract Pathologic changes of the epithelial layer occur early during radiation treatments. The underlying submucosa may become edematous, with dilation of capillaries. Recovery from radiation damage can be expected within a few weeks after completion of radiation therapy, provided that sufficient numbers of stem cells are left. The radioresponsiveness of the aerodigestive tract, like that of other structures, is not uniform but varies according to the location.

Patients often have symptoms from radiation exposure that are similar to other forms of acute gastritis. The clinical signs include epigastric pain, loss of appetite, nausea, and vomiting. Decreased gastric acidity is observed after 15 to 20 Gy of fractionated radiation therapy. The tolerance of the stomach to radiation is also aggravated by addition of systemic chemotherapy, such as 5-fluorouracil.

The germinal centers of the bowel mucosa are in the crypts of Lieberkühn. Newly formed cells move upward along the walls of the crypts as transitional cells, undergoing maturation. The epithelial lining of the small bowel is the most rapidly renewed system in the human body and is completely renewed in 3 to 6 days. Within 12 to 24 h after the first dose of radiation therapy, pathologic evidence of dead cells are seen in the mucosal lining. Complete denudation of the mucosal surface rarely occurs during a regular course of radiation treatment because of the high capacity of the mucosa for regeneration. However, a focal area of erosion may be seen. The histologic appearance may be nearly normal within 2 to 3 weeks after radiation therapy.

Clinical manifestations of acute radiation enteropathy are nausea and vomiting, diarrhea, and cramping pain. Relevant factors contributing to the pathogenesis of diarrhea include malabsorption and alterations in the intestinal bacterial flora. The severity of symptoms, as in other anatomic areas, is proportional to the irradiated volume and the total dose.

Symptoms of chronic radiation enteropathy include diarrhea, abdominal cramping, nausea, malabsorption, vomiting, and obstruction. Progressive fibrosis, perforation, fistula formation, and stenosis of the irradiated portion of the bowel can occur during the chronic phase of radiation enteropathy. Most clinical manifestations of chronic changes occur between 6 months and 5 years after radiation therapy.

Conservative noninvasive treatment can frequently control gastrointestinal symptoms. A low-residue or elemental diet may be beneficial. When nonsurgical treatment fails to relieve severe symptoms, surgical intervention is often indicated.

Bladder Radiation injury to the bladder generally becomes symptomatic 3 to 6 weeks after the start of treatment, and symptoms usually subside 3 to 4 weeks after completion of radiation therapy. Patients often complain of increased frequency and dysuria. Cystoscopy often shows diffuse mucosal changes similar to those of acute cystitis. Sometimes desquamation and ulceration can be seen. Without infection, urinary symptoms are managed symptomatically. Concurrent chemotherapy with cytotoxic agents such as cyclophosphamide increases the severity of the acute bladder reaction.

The late effects of high radiation doses to the bladder may include interstitial fibrosis, telangiectasia, and ulceration. The blood vessels may be dilated and prone to rupture, resulting in painless hematuria. These changes are often difficult to distinguish from tumor recurrence and progression. A contracted bladder may result from doses in excess of 60 Gy.

Testes and Ovaries In general, type B spermatogonia are exquisitely sensitive to the effects of radiation. The type A spermatogonia are thought to be more resistant because their longer cell cycle time allows considerable variation in radiosensitivity among different phases of the cell cycle. Sertoli cells and Leydig cells are less radiosensitive than the spermatogonia. Elevated levels of follicle-stimulating hormone (FSH) and luteinizing hormone (LH) have been observed after as little as 75 cGy. Doses as low as 10 cGy to the testicles may result in injury to the type B spermatogonia. The single dose required for permanent sterilization on normal human males is believed to be between 6 and 10 Gy. In normal human males, sperm count recovery requires 9 to 18 months after a fractionated dose of 8 to 100 cGy.

The radiation dose necessary to induce ovarian failure is age-dependent. A single dose of 3 to 4 Gy can induce amenorrhea in almost all women over 40 years of age. In young women, oogenesis is much less sensitive to radiation than is spermatogenesis in men.

ACUTE TOTAL-BODY IRRADIATION The data regarding the acute effects of total-body irradiation on humans come primarily from Japanese survivors of the atomic bomb, Marshallese exposed to radioactive fall-out in 1954, and persons exposed to radiation from the Chernobyl nuclear accident. Early symptoms of acute total-body irradiation, known as the *prodromal radiation syndrome*, last for a limited time. Clinical manifestations depend on the total-body dose. At doses $>$100 Gy, death usually occurs 24 to 48 h later from neurologic and cardiovascular failure. This is known as the *cerebrovascular syndrome*. Because cerebrovascular damage causes death very quickly, the failures of other systems do not have time to develop.

At doses between 5 and 12 Gy, death may occur in a matter of days as a result of the *gastrointestinal syndrome*. The symptoms during this period may include nausea, vomiting, and prolonged diarrhea for several days leading to dehydration, sepsis, and death. A total-body dose $>$10 Gy is uniformly fatal unless supportive therapy (fluid, electrolytes, blood products, and antibiotics) is given. The process of intestinal denudation depends on the dose and may take between 3 and 120 days. Death from intestinal denudation usually occurs before the full effects of radiation on the blood-forming elements are seen.

At total-body doses between 2 and 8 Gy, death may occur 2 to 4 weeks after exposure from bone marrow failure, the *hematopoietic syndrome*. The full effect of radiation is not apparent until the mature

Table 394-5 Examples of Radiation-Induced Cancers

Types of Exposure	Types of Cancer Observed
Neck irradiation during infancy for benign conditions	Thyroid carcinoma
Radiation therapy for other malignant tumors	Thyroid carcinoma Breast cancer Gastric cancer Melanoma Lung cancer Sarcomas in the field
Cranial irradiation	Central nervous system tumors
Breast irradiation for postpartum mastitis	Breast cancer
Brush-licking by radium dial painters	Bone sarcomas
Uranium mining	Lung cancer
In utero exposure	Leukemia

hematopoietic cells are depleted. Clinical symptoms during this period may include chills, fatigue, and petechial hemorrhage. Peripheral blood lymphopenia develops during the first 12 to 48 h after any significant exposure. Beyond 5 to 6 Gy, the rate and magnitude of the drop are not well correlated to radiation exposure. Some stem cells may survive acute exposure to ≥10 Gy. Death is from infection or bleeding and usually occurs before anemia can develop (red blood cell half-life is 100 to 120 days).

The $LD_{50/60}$ (the dose at which 50% of the population is dead by 60 days) is around 3.25 Gy if support is not given. There is considerable variability in the total-body dose tolerated. The very young and the old are more radiosensitive than middle-aged and young adult individuals. Females in general appear to be more tolerant of radiation than males. Persons exposed to <2 Gy will require little or no therapy but should probably be observed closely with daily blood counts for a few days.

The role of bone marrow transplantation for patients exposed to acute total-body irradiation is debated. At doses <8 Gy, the patient is likely to survive with supportive care. Most people exposed to doses higher than 10 Gy will die from the gastrointestinal syndrome. Therefore, 8 to 10 Gy may be the dose range in which bone marrow transplantation could have a role, although the Chernobyl experience did not confirm this prediction. Estimating the dose received by a given patient after radiation exposure is difficult. However, exposure estimation must be done quickly because bone marrow transplantation is most effective if it is performed within the first 3 to 5 days after exposure.

RADIATION AND CANCER INDUCTION Some nonlethal changes in DNA sequences caused by irradiation may cause malignant transformations. Thus, it is not surprising that second neoplasms can be caused by exposure to ionizing radiation. However, paradoxically, this risk is actually less with doses above a certain level. Whether there is a "safe" dose that will not have any adverse biologic effect is unclear. Estimates of the risk of developing cancer after low-level exposure to ionizing radiation are often derived by extrapolation from the risks for higher doses and acute exposures. Predicted risks of cancer are, therefore, prone to modification depending on the assumptions made about the data available for analysis.

Throughout the history of human exposure to ionizing radiation, increased rates of cancer have been noted after exposure to radiation. The populations studied include survivors of the atomic bomb during World War II; radium watch-dial painters who shaped their brush tips with their tongues; and patients who underwent multiple fluoroscopic examinations for tuberculosis, received spinal irradiation for ankylosing spondylitis, and received breast irradiation for postpartum mastitis; and others. Exposure to ionizing radiation at an earlier age appears to increase the chance of developing radiation-induced carcinomas. However, the radiation-induced cancers have an age of onset similar to that of the native cancers, and the available data argue against radiation as the only cause of the increased incidence of cancers seen after exposure to radiation. Table 394-5 shows examples of cancer observed in specific situations.

Because a safe dose of radiation is unknown at present, it is prudent to avoid routine exposures to ionizing irradiation.

ACKNOWLEDGMENT

The authors wish to acknowledge Dr. L. Chinsoo Cho for his contribution to this chapter in the 14th edition.

BIBLIOGRAPHY

HALL EJ: *Radiobiology for the Radiologist*, 4th ed. Philadelphia, Lippincott, 1994

METTLER FA JR, UPTON AC: *Medical Effects of Ionizing Radiation*, 2d ed, Philadelphia, Saunders, 1995

MOSS WT, COX JD: *Moss' Radiation Oncology: Rationale, Technique, Results*, 7th ed. St. Louis, Mosby, 1994

PEREZ CP, BRADY LW: *Principles and Practice of Radiation Oncology*, 3d ed. Philadelphia, Lippincott-Raven, 1998

RUBIN P: Late effects of normal tissues consensus conference. Int J Radiat Oncol Biol Phys 31:5, 1995

RUIFROK ACC, MCBRIDE WH: Growth factors: Biological and clinical aspects. Int J Radiat Oncol Biol Phys 43:877, 1999

395 HEAVY METAL POISONING

Howard Hu

Metals constitute a major category of toxins that pose a significant threat to health through occupational as well as environmental exposures. One indication of their importance relative to other potential hazards is their ranking by the U.S. Agency for Toxic Substances and Disease Registry, which lists all hazards present in toxic waste sites according to their prevalence and the severity of their toxicity. The first, second, third, and sixth hazards on the list are heavy metals: lead, mercury, arsenic, and cadmium, respectively. This chapter offers specific information on the sources and metabolism of each of these metals as well as on the toxic effects produced by each and the appropriate treatment for poisoning by each.

The intrinsic atomic stability of metals allows their relatively easy tracing and measurement in biologic material, although the clinical significance of the levels measured is not always clear. Metals are inhaled primarily as dusts and fumes (the latter defined as tiny particles generated by combustion). Metal poisoning can also result from exposure to vapors (e.g., mercury vapor in the manufacture of fluorescent lamps). When metals are ingested in contaminated food or drink or through hand-to-mouth activity (implicated especially often in children), their gastrointestinal absorption varies greatly with the specific chemical form of the metal and the nutritional status of the host. Once a metal is absorbed, blood is the main medium for its transport, with the precise kinetics dependent on diffusibility, binding forms, rates of biotransformation, availability of intracellular ligands, and other factors. Some organs (such as bone, liver, and kidney) sequester metals in relatively high concentrations for years. Most metals are excreted through renal clearance and gastrointestinal excretion; some proportion is also excreted through salivation, perspiration, exhalation, lactation, skin exfoliation, and loss of hair and nails.

Some metals, such as copper and selenium, are essential to normal metabolic function as trace elements (Chap. 75) but are toxic at high levels of exposure. Others, such as lead and mercury, are xenobiotic and theoretically are capable of exerting toxic effects at any level of exposure. Indeed, much research is currently focused on the contribution of low-level xenobiotic metal exposure to chronic diseases and to subtle changes in health that may have significant public health consequences.

The most important component of treatment for metal toxicity is the termination of exposure. Another component is the use of *chelating agents*, which are used to bind metals into stable cyclic compounds with relatively low toxicity and to enhance their excretion. The principal chelating agents are dimercaprol (British Anti-Lewisite, BAL), edetate (EDTA), succimer (DMSA, dimercaptosuccinic acid), and penicillamine; their specific use depends on the metal involved and the clinical picture. Activated charcoal does not bind metals and thus is of limited usefulness in cases of acute metal ingestion.

Besides the four metals discussed in detail in this chapter, several others deserve mention. *Aluminum* contributes to the encephalopathy occurring in patients with severe renal disease who are undergoing dialysis (Chap. 341). High levels of aluminum are found in the neurofibrillary tangles in the cerebral cortex and hippocampus of patients with Alzheimer's disease as well as in the drinking water and soil of areas with an unusually high incidence of Alzheimer's disease. The experimental and epidemiologic evidence for the aluminum–Alzheimer's disease link is so far relatively weak, however, and it cannot be concluded that aluminum is a causal agent or a contributing factor in neurodegenerative disease. Hexavalent *chromium* is corrosive and sensitizing. Workers in the chromate and chrome pigment production industries have consistently had an excess risk of lung cancer. The introduction of *cobalt* chloride as a fortifier in beer led to outbreaks of fatal cardiomyopathy among heavy consumers. Occupational exposure (e.g., of some miners, dry-battery manufacturers, and arc welders) to *manganese* can cause a Parkinsonian syndrome within 1 to 2 years, including gait disorders; postural instability; a masked, expressionless face; tremor; and psychiatric symptoms. With the introduction of methylcyclopentadienyl manganese tricarbonyl (MMT) as a gasoline additive, concern has arisen over the toxic potential of environmental manganese exposure. *Nickel* exposure induces an allergic response, and inhalation of nickel compounds with low aqueous solubility (such as nickel subsulfide and nickel oxide) in occupational settings is associated with an increased risk of cancer of the lung. Overexposure to *selenium* may cause local irritation of the respiratory system and eyes, gastrointestinal irritation, liver inflammation, loss of hair, depigmentation, and peripheral nerve damage. Workers exposed to certain organic forms of *tin* (particularly trimethyl and triethyl derivatives) have developed psychomotor disturbances, including tremor, convulsions, hallucinations, and psychotic behavior.

Finally, *thallium*, which is a component of some insecticides, metal alloys, and fireworks, is absorbed through the skin as well as through ingestion and inhalation. Severe poisoning follows a single ingested dose of >1 g or >8 mg/kg. Nausea and vomiting, abdominal pain, and hematemesis precede confusion, psychosis, organic brain syndrome, and coma. Thallium is radiopaque. Induced emesis or gastric lavage is indicated within 4 to 6 h of acute ingestion; Prussian blue prevents absorption and is given orally at 250 mg/kg in divided doses. Unlike other types of metal poisoning, thallium poisoning may be less severe when activated charcoal is used to interrupt its enterohepatic circulation. Other measures include forced diuresis, treatment with potassium chloride (which promotes renal excretion of thallium), and peritoneal dialysis.

LEAD

SOURCE Lead has been mined and used in industry and in household products for centuries. The dangers of lead toxicity, the clinical manifestations of which are termed *plumbism*, have been known since ancient times. The twentieth century saw both the greatest-ever exposure of the general population to lead and an extraordinary amount of new research on lead toxicity.

Populations are exposed to lead chiefly via paints, cans, plumbing fixtures, and leaded gasoline. The intensity of these exposures, while decreased by regulatory actions, remains high in some segments of the population because of the deterioration of lead paint used in the past and the entrainment of lead from paint and vehicle exhaust into soil and house dust. Many other environmental sources of exposure exist, such as leafy vegetables grown in lead-contaminated soil, improperly glazed ceramics, lead crystal, and certain herbal folk remedies. Many industries, such as battery manufacturing, demolition, painting and paint removal, and ceramics, continue to pose a significant risk of lead exposure to workers and surrounding communities.

New research on lead toxicity has been stimulated by advances in toxicology and epidemiology as well as by a shift of emphasis in toxicology away from binary outcomes (life/death; 50% lethal dose) to grades of function, such as neuropsychological performance, indices of behavior, blood pressure, and kidney function.

Tests for levels of lead in blood have facilitated both research on lead and surveillance of individuals at risk. Blood lead is now measured with stringent quality controls in commercial laboratories throughout the United States. Measurement of the blood lead levels of children 6 months to 5 years of age is mandated by some states, and the U.S. Occupational Safety and Health Administration (OSHA) requires the testing of workers who may be exposed to lead in the course of their jobs.

METABOLISM Elemental lead and inorganic lead compounds are absorbed through ingestion or inhalation. Organic lead (e.g., tetraethyl lead, the lead additive to gasoline) is absorbed to a significant degree through the skin as well. Pulmonary absorption is efficient, particularly if particle diameters are <1 μm (as in fumes from burning lead paint). Children absorb up to 50% of the amount of lead ingested, whereas adults absorb only ~10 to 20%. Gastrointestinal absorption of lead is enhanced by fasting and by dietary deficiencies in calcium, iron, and zinc; such absorption is minimal, however, for lead in the form of lead sulfide, a common constituent of mining waste. Lead is absorbed into blood plasma, where it equilibrates rapidly with extracellular fluid, crosses membranes (such as the blood-brain barrier and the placenta), and accumulates in soft and hard tissues. In the blood, ~95 to 99% of lead is sequestered in red cells, where it is bound to hemoglobin and other components. As a consequence, lead is usually measured in whole blood rather than in serum. The largest proportion of absorbed lead is incorporated into the skeleton, which contains >90% of the body's total lead burden. Lead is excreted mainly in the urine (in a process that depends on glomerular filtration and tubular secretion) and in the feces. Lead also appears in hair, nails, sweat, saliva, and breast milk. The half-life of lead in blood is ~25 days; in soft tissue, ~40 days; and in the nonlabile portion of bone, >25 years. Thus, blood lead levels may decline significantly while the body's total burden of lead remains heavy.

The toxicity of lead is probably related to its affinity for cell membranes and mitochondria, as a result of which it interferes with mitochondrial oxidative phosphorylation and sodium, potassium, and calcium ATPases. Lead impairs the activity of calcium-dependent intracellular messengers and of brain protein kinase C. In addition, lead stimulates the formation of inclusion bodies that may translocate the metal into cell nuclei and alter gene expression.

CLINICAL TOXICOLOGY Symptomatic lead poisoning in childhood generally develops at blood lead levels >3.9 μmol/L (80 μg/dL) and is characterized by abdominal pain and irritability followed by lethargy, anorexia, pallor (resulting from anemia), ataxia, and slurred speech. Convulsions, coma, and death due to generalized cerebral edema and renal failure occur in the most severe cases. Subclinical lead poisoning [blood lead level >1.4 μmol/L (> 30 μg/dL)] can cause mental retardation and selective deficits in language, cognitive function, balance, behavior, and school performance despite the lack of discernible symptoms. Epidemiologic studies and meta-analyses of studies regarding lead's effect on the intellectual function of children indicate that cognition is probably impaired in a dose-related fashion at blood lead levels well below 1.4 μmol/L (30 μg/dL) and that no threshold for this effect is likely to exist above the lowest measurable blood lead level of 0.05 μmol/L (1 μg/dL). The impact is greatest when the exposure is of long duration and has been most apparent when it takes place around the age of 2 years; however, the impact of fetal lead exposure remains to be clarified, particularly in view of the observation that maternal bone lead stores can be mobilized to a significant degree during pregnancy, with consequent exposure of the fetus.

In adults, symptomatic lead poisoning, which usually develops when blood lead levels exceed 3.9 μmol/L (80 μg/dL) for a period of weeks, is characterized by abdominal pain, headache, irritability, joint pain, fatigue, anemia, peripheral motor neuropathy, and deficits in short-term memory and the ability to concentrate. Encephalopathy is rare. A "lead line" sometimes appears at the gingiva-tooth border after prolonged high-level exposure. Some individuals develop these symptoms and signs at lower blood lead levels [1.9 to 3.9 μmol/L (40 to 80 μg/dL)] and/or with briefer periods of exposure. Chronic subclinical lead exposure is associated with interstitial nephritis, tubular damage (with tubular inclusion bodies), hyperuricemia (with an increased risk of gout), and a decline in glomerular filtration rate and chronic renal failure. Epidemiologic evidence also suggests that blood lead levels in the range of 0.34 to 1.7 μmol/L (7 to 35 μg/dL) are associated with increases in blood pressure, decreases in creatinine clearance, and decrements in cognitive performance that are too small to be detected as a lead effect in individual cases but nevertheless may contribute significantly to the causation of chronic disease.

An additional issue for both children and adults is whether lead that has accumulated in bone and lain dormant for years can pose a threat later in life, particularly at times of increased bone resorption such as pregnancy, lactation, and senile osteoporosis. Elevation of the bone lead level appears to be a risk factor for anemia, hypertension, cardiac conduction delays, and impairment of cognitive function. Hyperthyroidism has been reported to cause lead toxicity in adults by mobilizing stores of bone lead acquired during childhood.

Genetic polymorphisms, such as variants of the gene that codes for aminolevulinic acid dehydratase (a critical enzyme in the production of heme) or the C282Y hemochromatosis gene, may confer differences in susceptibility to lead retention and toxicity; ~15% of Caucasians have a variant form of one of these genes. This issue is the focus of continued research.

LABORATORY FINDINGS In 1991, the Centers for Disease Control and Prevention designated 0.48 μmol/L (10 μg/dL) as the blood lead level of concern in children. A specific set of interventions is recommended when the level exceeds this value. OSHA requires the regular measurement of blood lead in lead-exposed workers and the maintenance of blood lead levels <1.9 μmol/L (40 μg/dL). Concentrations of heme precursors (such as δ-aminolevulinic acid) in plasma and urine are sometimes increased at blood lead levels as low as 0.73 μmol/L (15 μg/dL). Levels of protoporphyrin (free erythrocyte or zinc) rise—although not consistently—once blood lead levels have exceeded 1.2 μmol/L (25 μg/dL) for several months. Lead-associated anemia is usually normocytic and normochromic and may be accompanied by basophilic stippling. Lead-induced peripheral demyelination is reflected by prolonged nerve conduction time and subsequent paralysis, usually of the extensor muscles of the hands and feet (wristdrop and footdrop). An increased density at the metaphyseal plate of growing long bones (lead lines) can develop in children and resemble those seen in rickets. Children with high-level lead exposure sometimes develop Fanconi's syndrome, pyuria, and azotemia. Adults chronically exposed to lead can develop elevated serum creatinine levels, decreased creatinine clearance rates, and chronic changes and intranuclear inclusion bodies (detected at renal biopsy). Deficits may be apparent in neuropsychometric tests of both children and adults; these abnormalities by themselves are not pathognomonic. Bone lead levels measured in vivo by K-x-ray fluorescence, a technique adapted for this purpose, are more sensitive than blood lead levels as a predictor of hypertension, cognitive impairments, and reproductive toxicity in epidemiologic studies; however, measurement of bone lead levels has not yet been shown to be of clinical value and is not widely available.

℞ **TREATMENT** It is absolutely essential to prevent further exposure of affected individuals to lead. Cases of lead poisoning should be reported to OSHA (if the exposure is occupational) and to local boards of health so that home evaluations can be performed. Pharmacologic treatment for lead toxicity entails the use of chelating agents, principally edetate calcium disodium (CaEDTA), dimercaprol, penicillamine, and succimer, which is given orally and has relatively few side effects. Chelation is recommended for the treatment of all children whose blood lead levels are >2.7 μmol/L (55 μg/dL), with the addition of dimercaprol if lead encephalopathy is found. Chelation is also recommended for children if blood lead levels are between 1.2 and 2.7 μmol/L (25 and 55 μg/dL) and the total amount of lead excreted in urine during the 8 h after a single dose of edetate calcium disodium exceeds 9.7 μmol/L (200 μg/dL). Chelation is recommended for adults if blood lead levels exceed 3.9 μmol/L (80 μg/dL) or if these levels exceed 2.9 μmol/L (60 μg/dL) and symptoms have developed. The ability of chelation to improve subclinical outcomes (such as performance on psychometric testing) at lower levels of blood lead in both children and adults is the subject of current research.

MERCURY

SOURCE Metallic mercury (Hg^0) is used in thermometers, dental amalgams, and some batteries. Mercurous mercury (Hg^+) and mercuric mercury (Hg^{2+}) can be combined with other chemicals, such as carbon, chlorine, or oxygen, to form inorganic or organic mercury compounds. All three forms of mercury are toxic to various degrees. Organic mercury compounds are slowly broken down into inorganic compounds; conversely, inorganic mercury can be converted by microorganisms in soil and water into the organic compound methyl mercury. Fish, particularly tuna and swordfish, can concentrate methyl mercury at high levels; such contamination of fish by industrial runoff and their subsequent ingestion was responsible for the Minamata Bay epidemic of mercury poisoning in Japan in 1955. Occupational exposure to inorganic mercury compounds continues in some chemical, metal-processing, electrical-equipment, automotive, and building industries and in medical and dental services. Environmental exposure probably takes place most commonly through ingestion of contaminated fish and through inhalation of the vapor generated by ordinary dental amalgam, which typically contains ~50% metallic mercury. There is also concern about exposure to drinking water contaminated by toxic waste sites included on the National Priority List, almost half of which contain mercury, and about the inhalation of fumes from incinerators burning mercury-contaminated waste products. Such incineration can also lead to environmental mercury contamination, methylation of the contaminating mercury by environmental bacteria, concentration of the resultant organic mercury compounds up the food chain, and consequent human exposure (particularly to contaminated fish). Ironically, the medical/hospital industry has been identified as a major incinerator of mercury-contaminated waste.

METABOLISM Elemental mercury is not well absorbed by the gastrointestinal tract and is excreted almost entirely in the feces after being ingested; however, when left standing, mercury is volatilized at room temperature into a vapor that is well absorbed by the lungs. Once absorbed, mercury in this form is lipid soluble, crosses the blood-brain barrier and the placenta, and can be oxidized by catalase and hydrogen peroxide into mercuric chloride, which is retained by the kidney and brain for years. Elemental mercury in blood has a half-life of ~60 days and is excreted mainly in the urine and feces.

The gastrointestinal and dermal absorption of inorganic mercury is significant. Large overdoses disrupt gastrointestinal barriers, further enhancing absorption. Once absorbed, inorganic mercury breaks down into metallic and mercuric mercury. Relatively little of this mercury crosses the blood-brain barrier; most is excreted in the urine or feces, with a half-life of 40 days, or is retained by the kidneys as mercuric mercury.

Organic mercury, particularly methyl mercury, can evaporate and undergo pulmonary absorption. Forms that are ingested (e.g., in contaminated fish) are well absorbed. Only small amounts are absorbed through the skin. Absorbed organic mercury is lipid soluble, readily crosses the blood-brain barrier and the placenta, appears in breast milk, and concentrates in the kidneys and central nervous system. Methyl mercury is acetylated in the liver, excreted in bile, reabsorbed, and then excreted in urine. Methyl mercury can also be conjugated with cysteine or glutathione. Only 1% of organic mercury is excreted unchanged into urine. The half-life of organic mercury compounds is in the range of 70 days. Exposure to mercury in any form stimulates the kidney to produce metallothionein, a metal-binding protein that affords partial protection against mercury toxicity.

CLINICAL TOXICOLOGY Inhalation of metallic mercury vapor is the form of mercury exposure that has been best studied in terms of toxicity. High levels of exposure are most likely in an occupational setting in which mercury vapors are generated by heat-induced volatilization of metallic mercury. Cough, dyspnea, and tightness or burning pain in the chest are common symptoms that may be accompanied by diffuse infiltrates or a pneumonitis-like appearance on chest x-ray. Respiratory distress, pulmonary edema, lobar pneumonia, fibrosis, and desquamation of the bronchiolar epithelium can occur in relatively severe cases and have sometimes led to death. Acute inhalation of mercury vapor can also cause neurologic toxicity manifested by tremors (beginning in the hands), emotional lability, headaches, and polyneuropathy. Chronic exposure to metallic mercury produces a characteristic intention tremor and mercurial *erethism*, a constellation of findings including excitability, memory loss, insomnia, timidity, and sometimes delirium that was described in workers with occupational exposure in the felt-hat industry—hence the expression "mad as a hatter." Dentists with occupational exposure to mercury score below normal on neurobehavioral tests of motor speed, visual scanning, verbal and visual memory, and visuomotor coordination. Low-level exposure from dental amalgams may also be associated with adverse immunologic reactions in individuals with certain major human leukocyte antigen genotypes; further research is needed in this area.

Acute high-dose ingestion of inorganic mercury causes severe gastrointestinal corrosion with nausea, vomiting, hematemesis, and abdominal pain; acute renal failure, cardiovascular collapse, and shock may ensue. The lethal dose of inorganic mercury is estimated to be in the range of 10 to 42 mg/kg. Lower levels of exposure cause milder forms of gastrointestinal inflammation, gingivitis and loosening of the teeth, increased blood pressure and tachycardia, and the nephrotic syndrome. Symptoms similar to erethism may develop. Skin exposure to mercuric salts can cause exfoliative dermatitis.

Ingestion of organic mercury compounds is followed by diarrhea, tenesmus, and blisters of the upper gastrointestinal tract. The fatal dose of organic mercury is estimated at 10 to 60 mg/kg. People who ingested flour contaminated with *N*-(ethylmercuri)-*p*-toluenesulfonanilide developed bradycardia, QT prolongation, ST-segment depression, and T-wave inversions. The neurotoxicity resulting from organic mercury exposure is characterized by paresthesia; impaired peripheral vision, hearing, taste, and smell; slurred speech; unsteadiness of gait and limbs; muscle weakness; irritability; memory loss; and depression. In general, such symptoms begin at doses >1.7 mg/kg. Autopsy findings suggest that lesions in the basal ganglia and gray matter of the cortex and cerebellum are chiefly responsible for these symptoms. Organic mercury exposure, primarily through the ingestion of grain treated with mercuric fungicides or of contaminated fish, is also associated with an increased risk of fetal toxicity. After the 1955 mercury poisoning outbreak in Minamata, Japan, exposed mothers gave birth to infants with mental retardation; retention of primitive reflexes; cerebellar symptoms; dysarthria; hyperkinesia; hypersalivation; atrophy of the cerebral cortex, corpus callosum, and cerebellum; and abnormal neuronal cytoarchitecture. This last change may reflect derangement of neuronal migration during fetal development.

Worthy of special note is dimethylmercury, a "supertoxic" compound encountered exclusively in laboratory settings. The physical properties of dimethylmercury permit transdermal absorption (against which latex gloves do not afford protection) as well as volatilization with inhalation. Exposure to ~400 mg (an amount equivalent to a few drops) is lethal, with cerebellar degeneration as a prominent feature.

Exposure of children to mercury in any of its forms can cause a particular syndrome known as *acrodynia*, or pink disease. This condition is characterized by flushing, itching, swelling, tachycardia, elevated blood pressure, excessive salivation or perspiration, irritability, weakness, morbilliform rashes, and desquamation of the palms and soles.

LABORATORY FINDINGS Levels of mercury in blood and urine should not exceed 180 nmol/L (3.6 μg/dL) and 0.7 μmol/L (15 μg/L), respectively. Symptoms may develop when blood and urine mercury levels exceed 1 μmol/L (20 μg/dL) and 3 μmol/L (60 μg/L), respectively. If a baseline 24-h urinary mercury value is low, repetition of the measurement after a single 2-g oral dose of succimer may be useful in documenting elevated renal mercury burdens in retired mercury-exposed workers; an increase of >20 μg in a 24-h urine sample suggests previous exposure. Levels in hair may be used as a dosimeter for chronic organic mercury exposure; neurobehavioral dysfunction in children may occur if the maternal mercury concentration in hair exceeds 30 nmol/g (6 μg/g).

℞ **TREATMENT** Acute ingestion of mercuric salts can be treated by induced emesis or gastric lavage. Polythiol resins can be administered orally to bind mercury in the gastrointestinal tract. The most effective chelating agents are dimercaprol, succimer, and penicillamine, which have active mono- or dithiol groups. Acute inorganic mercury poisoning can be treated with dimercaprol at a dose not exceeding 24 mg/kg per day and given intramuscularly in divided doses. Therapy is usually given in 5-day courses separated by several days of rest. The *N*-acetyl form of penicillamine is also useful at a dose of 30 mg/kg per day in divided doses. Peritoneal dialysis, hemodialysis, and extracorporeal regional complexing hemodialysis with succimer have all been used with some success in the treatment of patients with renal failure.

Chronic inorganic mercury poisoning is best treated with *N*-acetyl penicillamine.

ARSENIC

SOURCE Significant exposure to arsenic occurs through both anthropogenic and natural sources. Arsenic is released into the air by volcanoes and is a natural contaminant of some deep-water wells. Occupational exposure to arsenic is common in the smelting industry (in which arsenic is a byproduct of ores containing lead, gold, zinc, cobalt, and nickel) and is increasing in the microelectronics industry (in which gallium arsenide is responsible). Low-level arsenic exposure continues to take place in the general population (as do some cases of high-dose poisoning) through the commercial use of inorganic arsenic compounds in common products such as wood preservatives, pesticides, herbicides, fungicides, and paints; through the consumption of foods and the smoking of tobacco treated with arsenic-containing pesticides; and through the burning of fossil fuels in which arsenic is a contaminant. Arsenic was also a major ingredient of Fowler's solution and continues to be found in some folk remedies.

METABOLISM The toxicity of an arsenic-containing compound depends on its valence state (zero-valent, trivalent, or pentavalent), its form (inorganic or organic), and the physical aspects governing its absorption and elimination. In general, inorganic arsenic is more toxic than organic arsenic, and trivalent arsenite is more toxic than pentavalent and zero-valent arsenic. The normal intake of arsenic by adults occurs primarily through ingestion and averages ~50 μg/d (range, 8 to 104 μg/d). Most (~64%) of this amount is accounted for by organic arsenic from fish, seafood, and algae; the specific arsenic compounds obtained from these sources are arsenobentaine and arsenocholine, which are relatively nontoxic and are rapidly excreted in unchanged form in the urine. After absorption, inorganic arsenic accumulates in the liver, spleen, kidneys, lungs, and gastrointestinal tract. It is then rapidly cleared from these sites but leaves a residue in keratin-rich tissues such as skin, hair, and nails. Arsenite (+5) undergoes biomethylation in the liver to the less toxic metabolites methylarsenic acid and dimethylarsenic acid; biomethylation can quickly become saturated, however, and the result is the deposition of increasing doses of inorganic arsenic in soft tissues. Arsenic, particularly in its trivalent form, inhibits critical sulfhydryl-containing enzymes. In the pentavalent form, the competitive substitution of arsenic for phosphate can lead to rapid hydrolysis of the high-energy bonds in compounds such as ATP.

CLINICAL TOXICOLOGY Acute arsenic poisoning from ingestion results in increased permeability of small blood vessels and inflammation and necrosis of the intestinal mucosa; these changes manifest as hemorrhagic gastroenteritis, fluid loss, and hypotension. Delayed cardiomyopathy accompanied by electrocardiographic abnormalities may develop. Symptoms include nausea, vomiting, diarrhea, abdominal pain, delirium, coma, and seizures. A garlicky odor may be detectable on the breath. Acute tubular necrosis and hemolysis may develop. The reported lethal dose of arsenic ranges from 120 to 200 mg in adults and is 2 mg/kg in children. Arsine gas causes severe hemolysis within 3 to 4 h of exposure and can lead to acute tubular necrosis and renal failure.

In chronic arsenic poisoning, the onset of symptoms comes at 2 to 8 weeks. Typical findings are skin and nail changes, such as hyperkeratosis, hyperpigmentation, exfoliative dermatitis, and Mees' lines (transverse white striae of the fingernails); sensory and motor polyneuritis manifesting as numbness and tingling in a "stocking-glove" distribution, distal weakness, and quadriplegia; and inflammation of the respiratory mucosa. Epidemiologic evidence has linked chronic consumption of water containing arsenic at concentrations in the range of 10 to 1820 ppb with diabetes, vasospasm, and peripheral vascular insufficiency culminating in "blackfoot disease," a gangrenous condition affecting the extremities. Chronic arsenic exposure has also been associated with a greatly elevated risk of skin cancer and possibly of cancers of the lung, liver (angiosarcoma), bladder, kidney, and colon.

LABORATORY FINDINGS When acute arsenic poisoning is suspected, an x-ray of the abdomen may reveal ingested arsenic, which is radiopaque. The serum arsenic level may exceed 0.9 μmol/L (7 μg/dL); however, arsenic is rapidly cleared from the blood. Electrocardiographic findings may include QRS complex broadening, QT prolongation, ST-segment depression, T-wave flattening, and multifocal ventricular tachycardia. Urinary arsenic should be measured in 24-h specimens collected after 48 h of abstinence from seafood ingestion; normally, levels of total urinary arsenic excretion are <0.67 μmol/d (50 μg/d). Arsenic may be detected in the hair and nails for months after exposure. Abnormal liver function, anemia, leukocytosis or leukopenia, proteinuria, and hematuria may be detected. Electromyography may reveal features similar to those of Guillain-Barré syndrome.

℞ **TREATMENT** Vomiting should be induced with ipecac in the alert patient with acute arsenic ingestion. Gastric lavage may be useful; activated charcoal with a cathartic (such as sorbitol) may be tried, although its efficacy is not clear. Aggressive therapy with intravenous fluid and electrolyte replacement in an intensive-care setting may be life-saving. Dimercaprol is the chelating agent of choice and is administered intramuscularly at an initial dose of 3 to 5 mg/kg on the following schedule: every 4 h for 2 days, every 6 h on the third day, and every 12 h thereafter for 10 days. (An oral chelating agent may be substituted.) Succimer is sometimes an effective alternative, particularly if adverse reactions to dimercaprol develop (such as nausea, vomiting, headache, increased blood pressure, and convulsions). In cases of renal failure, doses should be adjusted carefully, and hemodialysis may be needed to remove the chelating agent–arsenic complex. Arsine gas poisoning should be treated supportively with the goals of maintaining renal function and circulating red-cell mass. Other than the avoidance of additional exposure, specific treatment is not of proven benefit in chronic arsenic toxicity. Recovery, particularly from the resulting peripheral neuropathy, may take months and may never be complete.

CADMIUM

SOURCE Environmental exposure to cadmium can result from the ingestion of basic foodstuffs, especially grains, cereals, and leafy vegetables, which readily absorb cadmium occurring naturally or in soil contaminated by sewage sludge, fertilizers, and polluted groundwater. Serious cadmium poisoning can follow the contamination of food and water by mining effluents, as took place in the 1946 outbreak of *itai-itai* ("ouch-ouch") disease (so named because cadmium-induced bone toxicity caused painful bone fractures) in the Jintzu River basin in Japan. Airborne cadmium can be released during smelting or during the incineration of municipal waste containing plastics and nickel-cadmium batteries. Cigarette smoke contains cadmium. Occupational exposure takes place in the metal-plating, pigment, battery, and plastics industries.

METABOLISM The normal daily intake of cadmium through ingestion or inhalation is from 20 to 40 μg, although only 5 to 10% of this amount is absorbed. Most absorbed cadmium is concentrated in the liver and kidneys. In erythrocytes and soft tissues, cadmium is bound to metallothionein, a low-molecular-weight protein that mitigates the toxicity of the unbound ion. This complex is filtered at the glomerulus but is then reabsorbed by the proximal tubules. The lack of an effective elimination pathway is responsible for cadmium's biologic half-life of 10 to 30 years. The toxicity of cadmium may involve its binding to key cellular sulfhydryl groups, its competition with other metals (zinc and selenium) for inclusion in metalloenzymes, and its competition with calcium for binding sites on regulatory proteins such as calmodulin.

CLINICAL TOXICOLOGY Acute high-dose cadmium inhalation can cause severe respiratory irritation with pleuritic chest pain, dyspnea, cyanosis, fever, tachycardia, nausea, and life-threatening noncardiogenic pulmonary edema. The onset of symptoms may be delayed from 4 to 24 h. Acute exposure through ingestion can cause severe nausea, vomiting, salivation, abdominal cramps, and diarrhea. Single lethal oral doses have reportedly ranged from 350 to 8900 mg. Chronic effects of cadmium exposure are dose-dependent and include anosmia, yellowing of the teeth, emphysema, minor changes in liver function, microcytic hypochromic anemia unresponsive to iron therapy, renal tubular dysfunction characterized by proteinuria and increased urinary excretion of β_2-microglobulin, and (with prolonged poisoning) osteomalacia leading to bone lesions and pseudofractures. In follow-up studies of occupationally exposed workers, β_2-microglobulinuria was found to be irreversible. Associations with hypertension, prostate cancer, and lung cancer have been suggested by some studies but await confirmation. In one study of men and women living in an area moderately contaminated with cadmium, higher body cadmium burdens were found to be a significant risk factor for lower bone density, a higher incidence of fractures, and a faster decline in height. These changes may be related to cadmium's calciuric effect on the kidney.

LABORATORY FINDINGS The daily level of excretion of cadmium by persons without known cadmium exposures is usually <10 nmol/L (1 μg/L or 1 μg/g of creatinine). This level increases somewhat with age and smoking. Toxicity, including renal dysfunction, is considered unlikely until the urinary cadmium level exceeds 100 nmol/L (10 μg/g of creatinine). Serum cadmium levels reflect recent rather than chronic exposure and generally are <30 nmol/L (0.3 μg/dL) in unexposed persons. A blood level >500 nmol/L (5 μg/dL) is considered toxic. An increased urinary concentration of β_2-microglobulin is the most sensitive indicator of an elevated cadmium dose and of nephropathy but may also be detected in other renal diseases, such as chronic pyelonephritis.

℞ **TREATMENT** There is no effective treatment for cadmium poisoning. Chelation therapy is not useful, and dimercaprol is contraindicated as this agent may exacerbate nephrotoxicity. Avoidance of further exposure and supportive therapy (including vitamin D if osteomalacia exists) are the mainstays of management.

BIBLIOGRAPHY

GENERAL

APOSHIAN HV et al: Mobilization of heavy metals by newer, therapeutically useful chelating agents. Toxicology 97:23, 1995

GOYER RA: Nutrition and metal toxicity. Am J Clin Nutr 61:646S, 1995

LYZNICKI JM et al: Manganese in gasoline. J Occup Environ Med 41:140, 1999

ROELS HA et al: Usefulness of biomarkers of exposure to inorganic mercury, lead, or cadmium in controlling occupational and environmental risks of nephrotoxicity. Ren Fail 21:251, 1999

LEAD

GONZÁLEZ-COSSÍO T et al: Decrease in birth weight in relation to maternal bone lead burden. Pediatrics 100:856, 1997

HU H et al: The relationship of blood and bone lead to hypertension among middle-aged to elderly men. JAMA 275:1171, 1996

KIM R et al: A longitudinal study of low-level lead exposure and renal function in men from the Normative Aging Study. JAMA 275:1177, 1996

KORRICK SA et al: Lead and hypertension in a sample of middle-aged women. Am J Public Health 89:330, 1999

STEWART WF et al: Neurobehavioral function and tibial and chelatable lead levels in 543 former organolead workers. Neurology 52:1610, 1999

MERCURY

CLARKSON TW: Mercury: Major issues in environmental health. Environ Health Perspect 100:31, 1993

NIERENBERG DW et al: Delayed cerebellar disease and death after accidental exposure to dimethylmercury. N Engl J Med 338:1672, 1998

ROELS HA et al: Urinary excretion of mercury after occupational exposure to mercury vapour and influence of the chelating agent meso-w,e-dimercaptosuccinic acid (DMSA). Br J Ind Med 48:247, 1991

ARSENIC

ABERNATHY CO et al: Arsenic: Health effects, mechanisms of actions, and research issues. Environ Health Perspect 107:593, 1999

ÇÖL M et al: Arsenic-related Bowen's disease, palmar keratosis, and skin cancer. Environ Health Perspect 107:687, 1999

CADMIUM

LAUWERYS RR et al: Cadmium: Exposure markers as predictors of nephrotoxic effects. Clin Chem 40:1391, 1994

STAESSEN JA et al: Environmental exposure to cadmium, forearm bone density, and risk of fractures: Prospective population study. Lancet 353:1140, 1999

Section 2
ILLNESSES DUE TO POISONS, DRUG OVERDOSAGE, AND ENVENOMATION

396 *Christopher H. Linden, Michael J. Burns*

POISONING AND DRUG OVERDOSAGE

ARDS adult respiratory distress syndrome	G6PD glucose-6-phosphate dehydrogenase
AV atrioventricular	MAO monoamine oxidase
BUN blood urea nitrogen	NAC *N*-acetylcysteine
CNS central nervous system	NAPQI *n*-acetyl-*p*-benzoquinoneimine
COX cyclooxygenase	PEMA phenylethylmalonamide
ECG electrocardiogram	SA sinoatrial
EEG Electroencephalographic	SSRIs Selective serotonin reuptake inhibitors
GABA γ-aminobutyric acid	TCAs Tricyclic antidepressants
GBL γ-butyrolactone	
GHB γ-hydroxybutyrate	

Poisoning refers to the development of dose-related adverse effects following exposure to chemicals, drugs, or other xenobiotics. To paraphrase Paracelsus, the dose makes the poison. In excessive amounts, substances that are usually innocuous, such as oxygen and water, can cause poisoning. Conversely, in small doses, substances commonly regarded as poisons, such as arsenic and cyanide, can be consumed without ill effect. There is, however, substantial individual variability in the response to, and disposition of, a given dose (Chaps. 70 and 71). Some of this variability is genetic, and some is acquired on the basis of enzyme induction, inhibition, or because of tolerance. Poisoning may be local (e.g., skin, eyes, or lungs) or systemic depending on the chemical and physical properties of the xenobiotic, its mechanism of action, and the route of exposure. The severity and reversibility of poisoning also depend on the functional reserve of the individual or target organ, which is influenced by age and preexisting disease. All of these factors must be considered when attempting to predict the effects of a particular exposure.

EPIDEMIOLOGY

In the United States, exposure to xenobiotics results in over 5 million requests for medical advice or treatment each year. Most exposures are acute, accidental, involve a single agent, occur in the home, result in minor or no toxicity, and involve children under 6 years of age. Common routes of exposure are ingestion (74%), dermal (8.2%), inhalation (6.7%), ocular (6%), bites and stings (3.9%), and parenteral injections (0.3%). Exposures most frequently involve cleaning agents, analgesics, cosmetics, plants, cough and cold preparations, and bites and envenomations (Chaps. 397 and 398). Pharmaceuticals are involved in 41% of exposures and 75% of serious or fatal poisonings.

Accidental exposures can result from the improper use of chemicals at work or play; product mislabeling; label misreading; mistaken identification of unlabeled chemicals; uninformed self-medication; and dosing errors by nurses, parents, pharmacists, physicians, and the elderly. Excluding the recreational use of ethanol, attempted suicide is the most common reason for intentional exposure. Unintended poisonings may result from the intentional use of drugs for psychotropic effects (abuse) or excessive self-dosing (misuse).

About 5% of exposures require hospitalization. They account for 5 to 10% of all ambulance transports, emergency room visits, and intensive care unit admissions. Up to 30% of psychiatric admissions are prompted by attempted suicide via overdosage.

Overall, the mortality rate is low: 0.03% of all exposures. It is much higher (1 to 2%) in hospitalized patients with nonaccidental (suicidal) overdose, who account for the majority of serious poisonings. Carbon monoxide poisoning is the leading cause of death; patients with such poisoning are typically dead when discovered and are included in medical examiner but not hospital or poison center statistics. Drug-related fatalities are most commonly due to analgesics, antidepressants, sedative-hypnotics, neuroleptics, stimulants and street drugs, cardiovascular drugs, anticonvulsants, antihistamines, and asthma therapies. Nonpharmaceutical agents most often implicated in

Table 396-1 Differential Diagnosis of Poisoning Based on Physiologic Status as Determined by Vital Signs and CNS Activity

Excited	Depressed	Discordant	Normal
Sympathomimetic syndrome Amphetamines Bronchodilators (β_2-adrenergic agonists) Caffeine Cocaine Decongestants (α-adrenergic agonists) Ergot alkaloids MAO inhibitors Theophylline Thyroid hormones **Anticholinergic syndrome** Antidepressants (tricyclic) Antihistamines Antiparkinsonian agents Antispasmodics (GI, GU) Belladonna alkaloids Cyclobenzaprine Mydriatics (topical) Orphenadrine Plants/mushrooms Phenothiazines **Hallucinogenic syndrome** LSD and its analogues Marijuana Mescaline and its analogues Phencyclidine **Withdrawal syndrome** Antidepressants β-Adrenergic blockers Clonidine Ethanol Opioids Sedative-hypnotics	**Sympatholytic syndrome** α-Adrenergic blockers Angiotensin-converting enzyme inhibitors Antiarrhythmics Antidepressants (tricyclic) β-Adrenergic blockers Calcium channel blockers Clonidine Decongestants (imidazolines) Digitalis **Cholinergic syndrome** Bethanechol Carbamate insecticides Echothiophate Myasthenia gravis drugs (e.g., pyridostigmine) Organophosphate insecticides Physostigmine Pilocarpine Urecholine **Opioid syndrome** Analgesics Antidiarrheal agents Antispasmodics (GI) Heroin Opium **Sedative-hypnotic syndrome** Alcohols Anticonvulsants Barbiturates Benzodiazepines Bromide Ethchlorvynol γ-Hydroxybutyrate Hydrocarbons Glutethimide Methyprylon Muscle relaxants	**Asphyxiants** Carbon monoxide Cyanide Hydrogen sulfide Inert gases Irritant fumes, gases, vapors Methemoglobinemia Nitrophenol herbicides **CNS syndromes** Disulfiram Dystonic/extrapyramidal reactions Isoniazid Neuroleptic malignant syndrome Serotonin syndrome Strychnine Volatile hydrocarbon inhalation **Membrane-active agents** Amantadine Antiarrhythmic agents Antidepressants (cyclic) β-Adrenergic blockers Fluorides Heavy metals Lithium Local anesthetics Meperidine Neuroleptic agents Propoxyphene Quinine and related antimalarial agents **Metabolic acidosis (low lactate; high anion gap)** Alcoholic ketoacidosis Ethylene glycol Methanol Formaldehyde/paraldehyde Salicylate Sulfur/sulfate Toluene Valproic acid	**Agents with slow absorption** Carbamazepine Digitalis preparations Dilantin Kapseals Enteric-coated pills Lomotil Salicylates Sustained-release preparations **Agents with slow distribution** Digitalis preparations Heavy metals Lithium Salicylates **Agents that are activated metabolically** Acetaminophen Chloramphenicol Chlorinated hydrocarbons Ethylene glycol L-thyroxine Methanol Paraquat Certain methemoglobin inducers **Inhibitors of metabolic pathways** Disulfiram Inhibitors of thyroid hormone synthesis MAO inhibitors Salicylates **Inhibitors of nucleic acid synthesis** Anticancer agents Antiviral agents Immunosuppressive drugs Mushrooms (amatoxins) Podophylline **Nontoxic exposure** **Psychogenic illness**

NOTE: CNS, central nervous system; MAO, monoamine oxidase; GI, gastrointestinal; GU, genitourinary; LSD, lysergic acid diethylamide.

fatal poisoning include alcohols and glycols, gases and fumes, chemicals, cleaning substances, pesticides, and automotive products.

DIAGNOSIS

Although poisoning can mimic other illnesses, the correct diagnosis can usually be established by the history, physical examination, routine and toxicologic laboratory evaluations, and characteristic clinical course. The *history* should include the time, route, duration, and circumstances (location, surrounding events, and intent) of exposure; the name and amount of each drug, chemical, or ingredient involved; the time of onset, nature, and severity of symptoms; the time and type of first aid measures provided; and the medical and psychiatric history.

In many cases the victim is confused, comatose, unaware of an exposure, or unable or unwilling to admit to one. Suspicious circumstances include unexplained illness in a previously healthy person; a history of psychiatric problems (particularly depression); recent changes in health, economic status, or social relationships; and onset of illness while working with chemicals or after ingesting food, drink (especially ethanol), or medications. Patients who become ill soon after arriving from a foreign country or being arrested for criminal activity should be suspected of "body packing" or "body stuffing" (ingesting or concealing illicit drugs in a body cavity). Relevant history may be available from family, friends, paramedics, police, pharmacists, physicians, and employers, who should be questioned regarding the patient's habits, hobbies, behavior changes, available medications, and antecedent events. A search of clothes, belongings, and place of discovery may reveal a suicide note or a container of drugs or chemicals. The imprint code on pills and the label on chemical products may be used to identify the ingredients and potential toxicity of a suspected poison by consulting a reference text, a computerized database, the manufacturer, or a regional poison information center.

In the absence of a history of exposure, the *clinical course* may suggest a diagnosis of poisoning. Poisoning typically evolves and resolves more rapidly than other disorders. Signs and symptoms characteristically develop within an hour of acute exposure, peak within several hours, and resolve over hours to days. However, the absence of signs and symptoms soon after an overdose does not rule out a poisoning.

The *physical examination* should focus initially on the vital signs, cardiopulmonary system, and neurologic status. On the basis of the pulse, blood pressure, respiratory rate, temperature, and mental status, the physiologic state can be characterized as excited, depressed, discordant, or normal. A differential diagnosis can then be formulated (Table 396-1). Examination of the eyes (for nystagmus, pupil size and reactivity), abdomen (for bowel activity and bladder size), and skin (for burns, bullae, color, warmth, moisture, pressure sores, and puncture marks) may narrow the diagnosis to a particular disorder. Grading the severity of poisoning (Table 396-2) is useful for assessing the clinical course and response to treatment.

The patient should also be examined for evidence of trauma and underlying illnesses. Except with carbon monoxide, theophylline, and drugs that cause hypoglycemia or hypoxia, seizures and neurologic manifestations of poisoning are nonfocal. Hence, focal findings should prompt evaluation for a structural central nervous system (CNS) lesion. When the history is unclear, all orifices should be examined for the presence of chemical burns and drug packets. The odor of breath or vomitus and the color of nails, skin, or urine may provide diagnostic clues.

Laboratory assessment may be helpful in the differential diagnosis

Table 396-2 Severity of Physiologic Stimulation and Depression in Poisoning and Drug Withdrawal

PHYSIOLOGIC STIMULATION	
Grade 1	Anxious, irritable, tremulous; vital signs normal; diaphoresis, flushing or pallor, mydriasis, and hyperreflexia may be present
Grade 2	Agitated; may have confusion or hallucinations but is able to converse and follow commands; vital signs mildly to moderately increased
Grade 3	Delirious; unintelligible speech, uncontrollable motor hyperactivity; moderately to markedly increased vital signs; tachyarrhythmias possible
Grade 4	Coma, seizures, cardiovascular collapse
PHYSIOLOGIC DEPRESSION	
Grade 1	Awake, lethargic, or sleeping but arousable by voice or tactile stimulation; able to converse and follow commands; may be confused
Grade 2	Responds to pain but not voice; can vocalize but not converse; spontaneous motor activity present; brainstem reflexes intact
Grade 3	Unresponsive to pain; spontaneous motor activity absent; brainstem reflexes depressed; motor tone, respirations, and temperature decreased
Grade 4	Unresponsive to pain; flaccid paralysis; brainstem reflexes and respirations absent; cardiovascular vital signs decreased

of poisoning (Fig. 396-1). An increased anion-gap metabolic acidosis is characteristic of advanced methanol, ethylene glycol, and salicylate intoxication but can occur with other agents (Table 396-1) and in any poisoning that results in hepatic, renal, or respiratory failure, seizures, or shock. The serum lactate concentration is low (less than the anion gap) in the former and high (nearly equal to the anion gap) in the latter. An abnormally low anion gap can be due to elevated blood levels of bromide, calcium, iodine, lithium, magnesium, or nitrate. An increased osmolal gap—the difference between the serum osmolality (measured by freezing point depression) and that calculated from the serum sodium, glucose, and blood urea nitrogen (BUN) of >10 mmol/L—suggests the presence of a low-molecular-weight solute such as an alcohol, glycol, or ketone or an unmeasured electrolyte or sugar. The osmolal gap can also provide an estimate of the amount of anion present (Table 396-3). Ketosis suggests acetone, isopropyl alcohol, or salicylate poisoning. Hypoglycemia may be due to poisoning with β-adrenergic blockers, ethanol, insulin, oral hypoglycemic agents, quinine, and salicylates, whereas hyperglycemia can occur in poisoning with acetone, β-adrenergic agonist, calcium channel blockers, iron, theophylline, or Vacor. Hypokalemia can be caused by barium, a β-adrenergic agonist, a diuretic, theophylline, or toluene; hyperkalemia suggests poisoning with an α-adrenergic agonist, a β-adrenergic blocker, cardiac glycosides, or fluoride.

Radiologic studies may also be useful for diagnostic purposes. Pulmonary edema (adult respiratory distress syndrome, or ARDS) can be caused by poisoning with carbon monoxide, cyanide, an opioid, paraquat, phencyclidine, a sedative-hypnotic, or salicylate; by inhalation of irritant gases, fumes, or vapors (ammonia, metal oxides, mercury); or by prolonged anoxia, hyperthermia, or shock. Aspiration pneumonia is common in patients with coma, seizures, and petroleum distillate ingestion. Radiopaque densities may be visible on abdominal x-rays following the ingestion of calcium salts, chloral hydrate, chlorinated hydrocarbons, heavy metals, illicit drug packets, iodinated compounds, potassium salts, psychotherapeutic agents, lithium, phenothiazines, enteric-coated tablets, or salicylates.

The electrocardiogram (ECG) can be useful to assist with the differential diagnosis and to guide treatment. Bradycardia and atrioventricular (AV) block may occur in patients poisoned by α-adrenergic agonists, antiarrhythmic agents, beta blockers, calcium channel blockers, cholinergic agents (carbamate and organophosphate insecticides), cardiac glycosides, lithium, magnesium, or tricyclic antidepressants. QRS- and QT-interval prolongation may be caused by hyperkalemia and by membrane-active drugs (Table 396-1). Ventricular tachyarrhythmias may be seen in poisoning with cardiac glycosides, fluorides, membrane-active drugs, sympathomimetics, or agents that cause hyperkalemia or potentiate the effects of endogenous catecholamines (e.g., chloral hydrate, aliphatic and halogenated hydrocarbons).

Analysis of urine and blood (and occasionally of gastric contents and chemical samples) may be useful to confirm or rule out suspected poisoning. Interpretation of laboratory data requires knowledge of the tests used for screening and confirmation (thin-layer, gas-liquid, or high-performance liquid chromatography; colorimetric and fluorometric assays; enzyme-multiplied and radioimmunoassays; gas chromatography; mass spectrometry), their sensitivity (limit of detection) and specificity, the preferred biologic specimen for analysis, and the optimal time of specimen sampling. Personal communication with the laboratory is essential. A negative result on a screen may mean the substance is not detectable by the test used or that its concentration is too low for detection at the time of sampling. In the latter case, repeating the test at a later time may yield a positive result.

Although some rapid screening tests for a limited number of drugs of abuse are available, comprehensive screening tests require 2 to 6 h for completion, and immediate management must be based on the history, physical examination, and routine ancillary tests. In addition,

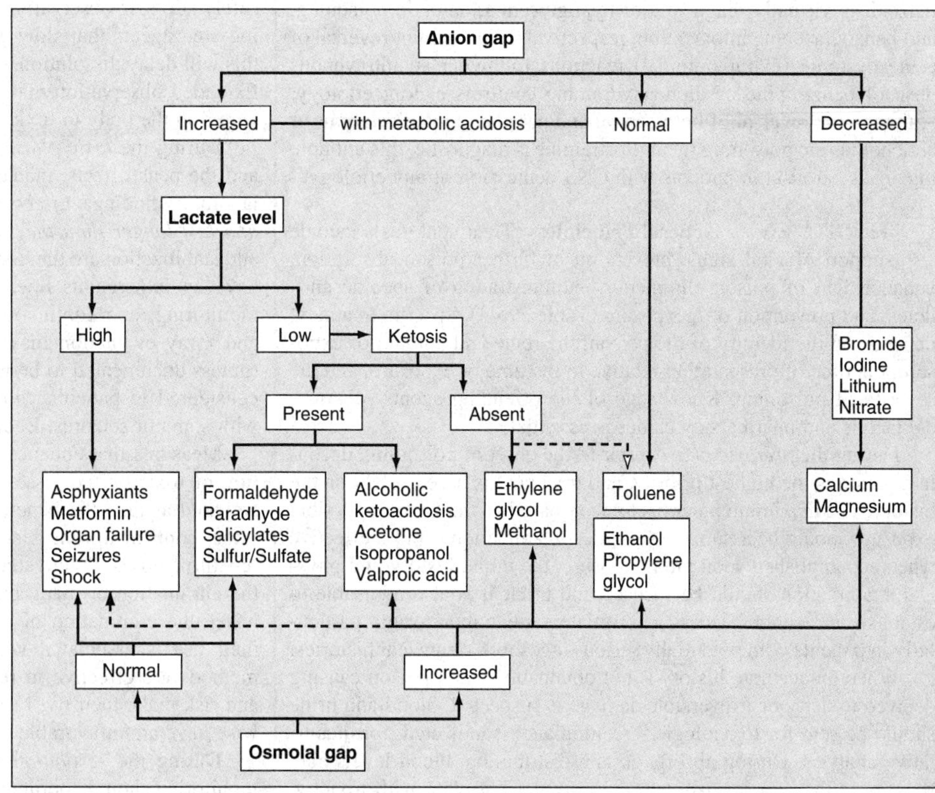

FIGURE 396-1 Differential diagnosis of poisoning based on the results of routine laboratory tests. Dashed lines indicate possible pathways.

Table 396-3 Solute Effects on Serum Osmolality

Agent	Approximate Serum Concentrations (mg/dL) of Solute That Will Increase the Serum Osmolality by 1 mmol/kg[a]
Alcohols	
Ethanol	4.6
Isopropanol	6.0
Methanol	2.6
Glycols	
Ethylene glycol	5.2
Propylene glycol	7.6
Ketones	
Acetone	5.8
Electrolytes	
Calcium	4
Magnesium	2.4
Sugars	
Mannitol	18
Sorbitol	18

[a] Equivalent to 2 mmol/L of calcium and magnesium and 1 mmol/L of all other compounds.

when the patient is asymptomatic, or when the clinical picture is consistent with the reported history, qualitative screening is neither clinically useful nor cost-effective. It is of greatest value in patients with severe or unexplained toxicity who have coma, seizures, cardiovascular instability, metabolic or respiratory acidosis, and nonsinus cardiac rhythms. Quantitative analysis is useful for poisoning with acetaminophen, acetone, alcohol (including ethylene glycol), antiarrhythmics, anticonvulsants, barbiturates, digoxin, heavy metals, lithium, paraquat, salicylate, and theophylline, as well as for carboxyhemoglobin and methemoglobin. Results can often be available within an hour.

The *response to antidotes* may be useful for diagnostic purposes. Resolution of altered mental status and abnormal vital signs within minutes of intravenous administration of dextrose, naloxone, or flumazenil is virtually diagnostic of hypoglycemia, narcotic poisoning, and benzodiazepine intoxication, respectively. The prompt reversal of acute dystonic (extrapyramidal) reactions following an intravenous dose of benztropine or diphenhydramine confirms a drug etiology. Although the reversal of both central and peripheral manifestations of anticholinergic poisoning by physostigmine is diagnostic, this antidote may cause arousal in patients with CNS depression of any etiology.

℞ TREATMENT **General Principles** Treatment goals include support of vital signs, prevention of further poison absorption, enhancement of poison elimination, administration of specific antidotes, and prevention of reexposure (Table 396-4). Specific treatment depends on the identity of the poison, the route and amount of exposure, the time of presentation relative to the time of exposure, and the severity of poisoning. Knowledge of the offending agents' pharmacokinetics and pharmacodynamics is essential.

During the *pretoxic phase*, prior to the onset of poisoning, decontamination is the highest priority, and treatment is based solely on the history. The maximum potential toxicity based on the greatest possible exposure should be assumed. Since decontamination is more effective when accomplished soon after exposure, the initial history and physical examination should be focused and brief. It is also advisable to establish intravenous access and initiate cardiac monitoring, particularly in patients with potentially serious ingestions or unclear histories.

When an accurate history is not obtainable, and a poison causing delayed toxicity or irreversible damage is suspected, blood and urine should be sent for toxicologic screening and, if indicated, for quantitative analysis. During absorption and distribution, blood levels may be greater than those in tissue and may not correlate with toxicity. However, high blood levels of agents whose metabolites are more toxic than the parent compound (acetaminophen, ethylene glycol, or

Table 396-4 Fundamentals of Poisoning Management

SUPPORTIVE CARE	
Airway protection	Treatment of seizures
Oxygenation/ventilation	Correction of temperature abnormalities
Treatment of arrhythmias	Correction of metabolic derangements
Hemodynamic support	Prevention of secondary complications
PREVENTION OF FURTHER POISON ABSORPTION	
Gastrointestinal decontamination	Decontamination of other sites
Syrup of ipecac–induced emesis	Eye decontamination
Gastric lavage	Skin decontamination
Activated charcoal	Body cavity evacuation
Whole-bowel irrigation	
Catharsis	
Dilution	
Endoscopic/surgical removal	
ENHANCEMENT OF POISON ELIMINATION	
Multiple-dose activated charcoal	Extracorporeal removal
Forced diuresis	Peritoneal dialysis
Alteration of urinary pH	Hemodialysis
Chelation (Chap. 395)	Hemoperfusion
	Hemofiltration
	Plasmapheresis
	Exchange transfusion
	Hyperbaric oxygenation
ADMINISTRATION OF ANTIDOTES	
Neutralization by antibodies	Metabolic antagonism
Neutralization by chemical binding	Physiologic antagonism
PREVENTION OF REEXPOSURE	
Adult education	Notification of regulatory agencies
Child-proofing	Psychiatric referral

methanol) may indicate the need for additional interventions (antidotes, dialysis).

Most patients who remain or become asymptomatic 4 to 6 h after ingestion will not develop subsequent toxicity and can be discharged safely. Longer observation may be necessary for patients who have ingested agents that slow gastric emptying and intestinal motility as this will delay dissolution, absorption, and distribution characteristics. Extended observation may also be indicated for agents that are converted in the body to toxic metabolites (Table 396-1).

During the *toxic phase*, the time between the onset of poisoning and the peak effects, management is based primarily on clinical and laboratory findings. *Effects after an overdose begin sooner, peak later, and last longer than they do after a therapeutic dose.* Resuscitation and stabilization are the first priority. All symptomatic patients should have an intravenous line, oxygen saturation determination, cardiac monitoring, and continuous observation. Baseline laboratory, ECG, and x-ray evaluation may also be appropriate. Intravenous glucose (unless documented to be normal), naloxone, and thiamine should be considered in patients with altered mental status, particularly those with soma or seizures. Decontamiation may also be appropriate.

Measures that enhance poison elimination may shorten the duration of toxicity and lessen its severity. However, the risks must be weighed against the benefits. Diagnostic certainty (usually via laboratory confirmation) is generally a prerequisite. Intestinal dialysis with repetitive doses of activated charcoal is usually safe and can enhance the elimination of many poisons. Diuresis and chelation therapy enhance the elimination of a relatively small number of poisons, and their use is associated with potential complications. Extracorporal methods are effective in removing many poisons, but their expense and risk make their use reasonable only in patients who would otherwise have an unfavorable outcome.

During the *resolution phase* of poisoning, supportive care and monitoring should continue until clinical, laboratory, and ECG abnormalities have resolved. Since chemicals are eliminated from the blood before tissues, blood levels are usually lower than tissue levels during this phase and may not correlate with toxicity. This is particularly true when extracorporeal elimination procedures are used. Redistribution from tissues may cause a rebound increase in the blood level after termination of these procedures. When a metabolite is responsible for toxic effects, continued treatment of an asymptomatic patient might be necessary because of a potentially toxic blood level (acetaminophen, ethylene glycol, and methanol).

Supportive Care The goal of supportive therapy is to maintain physiologic homeostasis until detoxification is accomplished and to prevent and treat secondary complications such as aspiration, bedsores, cerebral and pulmonary edema, pneumonia, rhabdomyolysis, renal failure, sepsis, thromboembolic disease, and generalized organ dysfunction due to prolonged hypoxia or shock.

Admission to an intensive care unit is indicated for the following: patients with severe poisoning (coma, respiratory depression, hypotension, cardiac conduction abnormalities, cardiac arrhythmias, hypothermia or hyperthermia, seizures); those needing close monitoring, antidotes, or enhanced elimination therapy; those showing progressive clinical deterioration; and those with significant underlying medical problems. Patients with mild to moderate toxicity can be managed on a general medical service, intermediate care unit, or emergency department observation area, depending on the anticipated duration and level of monitoring needed (intermittent clinical observation versus continuous clinical, cardiac, and respiratory monitoring). Patients who have attempted suicide require continuous observation and measures to prevent self-injury until they are thought unlikely to make further attempts.

Respiratory care Endotracheal intubation for protection against the aspiration of gastrointestinal contents is of paramount importance in patients with CNS depression or seizures as this complication can increase morbidity and mortality. Mechanical ventilation may be necessary for patients with respiratory depression or hypoxia and to facilitate therapeutic sedation or paralysis in order to prevent hyperthermia, acidosis, and rhabdomyolysis associated with neuromuscular hyperactivity. Since clinical assessment of respiratory function is often inaccurate, the need for oxygenation and ventilation is best determined by oximetry or arterial blood gas analysis. The gag reflex is not a reliable indicator of the need for intubation. A patient may maintain airway patency while being stimulated but not if left unattended. Those who cannot respond to voice or who are unable to sit and drink fluids without assistance are best managed by prophylactic intubation.

Drug-induced pulmonary edema is usually noncardiac rather than cardiac in origin. Profound CNS depression and cardiac conduction abnormalities suggest the latter etiology. Measurement of pulmonary artery pressure may be necessary to establish etiology and direct appropriate therapy. Extracorporeal measures (membrane oxygenation, venoarterial perfusion, cardiopulmonary bypass), partial liquid (perfluorocarbon) ventilation, and hyperbaric oxygen therapy may be appropriate for severe but reversible respiratory failure.

Cardiovascular therapy Maintenance of normal tissue perfusion is critical to allow for complete recovery once the offending agent has been eliminated. If hypotension is unresponsive to volume expansion, treatment with norepinephrine, epinephrine, or high-dose dopamine may be necessary (Chap. 38). Intraaortic balloon pump counterpulsation and venoarterial or cardiopulmonary perfusion techniques should be considered for severe but reversible cardiac failure. Bardyarrhythmias associated with hypotension generally should be treated as described in Chap. 229. Glucagon and calcium may be effective in both beta blocker and calcium channel blocker poisoning. Antibody therapy may be indicated for cardiac glycoside poisoning.

Supraventricular tachycardia associated with hypertension and CNS excitation is almost always due to agents that cause generalized physiologic excitation (Table 396-1). Most cases are mild or moderate in severity and require only observation or nonspecific sedation with a benzodiazepine. For cases that are severe or associated with hemodynamic instability, chest pain, or ECG evidence of ischemia, specific therapy is indicated. For patients with sympathetic hyperactivity, treatment with a combined alpha and beta blocker (labetalol), a calcium channel blocker (verapamil or diltiazem), or a combination of a beta blocker and a vasodilator (esmolol and nitroprusside) is preferred. For those with anticholinergic poisoning, physostigmine is the treatment of choice. Supraventricular tachycardia without hypertension is generally secondary to vasodilation or hypovolemia and responds to fluid administration.

Lidocaine and phenytoin are generally safe for ventricular tachyarrhythmias, but beta blockers can be hazardous unless the arrhythmia is clearly due to sympathetic hyperactivity. For ventricular tachyarrhythmias due to tricyclic antidepressants and probably other membrane-active agents (Table 396-1), class IA, IC, and III antiarrhythmic agents are contraindicated (because of similar electrophysiologic effects), but sodium bicarbonate may be helpful. Magnesium sulfate and overdrive pacing (by isoproterenol or a pacemaker) may be useful in patients with torsade de pointes and prolonged QT intervals. Magnesium and antidigoxin antibodies should be considered in patients with severe cardiac glycoside poisoning. Invasive (esophageal or intracardiac) ECG recording may be necessary to determine the origin (ventricular or supraventricular) of wide-complex tachycardias (Chap. 230). If the patient is hemodynamically stable, however, it may be prudent to observe rather than to treat with another potentially proarrhythmic agent. Arrhythmias may be resistant to drug therapy until underlying acid-base, electrolyte, oxygenation, and temperature derangements are corrected.

Central nervous system therapies Neuromuscular hyperactivity and seizures can lead to hyperthermia, lactic acidosis, and rhabdomyolysis, with their attendant complications, and should be treated aggressively. Seizures caused by excessive stimulation of catecholamine receptors (sympathomimetic or hallucinogen poisoning and drug withdrawal), or decreased activity of γ-aminobutyric acid (GABA) (isoniazid poisoning) or glycine (strychnine poisoning) receptors are best treated with enhancers of GABA effects such as benzodiazepines or barbiturates. Since benzodiazepines and barbiturates act by slightly different mechanisms (the former increases the frequency and the latter increases the duration of chloride channel opening in response to GABA), therapy with both may be effective when neither is effective alone. Seizures caused by isoniazid, which inhibits the synthesis of GABA, may require high doses of pyridoxine (which facilitates the synthesis of GABA). Seizures resulting from membrane destabilization (beta blocker or cyclic antidepressant poisoning) may require a membrane-active anticonvulsant such as phenytoin as well as GABA enhancers. For poisons with central dopaminergic effects (phencyclidine), an agent with opposing activity, such as haloperidol, may be useful. In anticholinergic and cyanide poisoning, specific antidotal therapy may be necessary. The treatment of seizures secondary to ischemia, edema, or metabolic abnormalities should include correction of the underlying cause. Neuromuscular paralysis is indicated in refractory cases. Electroencephalographic (EEG) monitoring and continuing treatment of seizures are necessary to prevent permanent neurologic damage.

Other measures Temperature extremes, metabolic abnormalities, hepatic and renal dysfunction, and secondary complications should be treated by standard therapies.

Prevention of Poison Absorption • ***Gastrointestinal decontamination*** Whether or not to perform gastrointestinal decontamination, and which procedure to use, depends on the time since ingestion; the existing and predicted toxicity of the ingestant; the availability, efficacy, and contraindications of the procedure; and the nature, severity, and risk of complications. In animal and human volunteer studies, the efficacy of activated charcoal, gastric lavage, and syrup of ipecac decreases with time, and there are insufficient data to support or exclude a beneficial effect when they are used more than 1 h after ingestion. Due to the lack of clinical studies using control groups without treatment, the efficacy of these procedures for improving the outcome of overdose patients has not been established.

The average time from ingestion to presentation for treatment is over 1 h for children and over 3 h for adults. Most patients will recover from poisoning uneventfully with good supportive care alone, but complications of gastrointestinal decontamination, particularly aspiration, can prolong this process. Hence, gastrointestinal contamination should be performed selectively, not routinely, in the management of overdose patients. It is clearly unnecessary when predicted toxicity is minimal or the time of expected maximal toxicity has passed without significant effect.

Activated charcoal has comparable or greater efficacy, fewer contraindications and complications, is less aversive and invasive than ipecac or gastric lavage, and is the preferred method of gastrointestinal decontamination in most situations.

Activated charcoal is prepared as a suspension in water, either alone or with a cathartic. It is given orally via a nippled bottle (for infants), or via a cup, straw, or small-bore nasogastric tube. The recommended dose is 1 g/kg body weight, using 8 mL of diluent per gram of charcoal if a premixed formulation is not available. Palatability may be increased by adding a sweetener (sorbitol) or a flavoring agent (cherry, chocolate, or cola syrup) to the suspension. Charcoal adsorbs ingested poisons within the gut lumen, allowing the charcoal-toxin complex to be evacuated with stool. The complex can also be removed from the stomach by induced emesis or lavage. In vitro, charcoal adsorbs ≥90% of most substances when given in an amount equal to 10 times the weight of the substance. Charged (ionized) chemicals such as mineral acids, alkalis, and highly dissociated salts of cyanide, fluoride, iron, lithium, and other inorganic compounds are not well adsorbed by charcoal. In animal and human volunteer studies, charcoal decreases the absorption of ingestants by an average of 73% when given within 5 min of ingestant administration, 51% when given at 30 min, and 36% at 60 min. Charcoal is at least equally as effective as ipecac syrup or gastric lavage. Experimentally, lavage followed by charcoal is more effective than charcoal alone, and charcoal before and after lavage is more effective than charcoal alone or charcoal after lavage. In the treatment of poisoned patients, however, charcoal alone generally results in a better clinical outcome than either treatment with ipecac followed by charcoal or lavage followed by charcoal. Side effects of charcoal include nausea, vomiting, and diarrhea or constipation. Charcoal may also prevent the absorption of orally administered therapeutic agents. Complications include mechanical obstruction of the airway, aspiration, vomiting, and bowel obstruction and infection caused by inspissated charcoal. Charcoal is not recommended for patients who have ingested corrosives because it obscures endoscopy.

Gastric lavage is performed by sequentially administering and aspirating about 5 mL fluid per kilogram of body weight through a no. 28 French orogastric tube in children and a no. 40 French tube in adults. Except for infants, tap water is acceptable. The patient should be placed in Trendelenburg and left lateral decubitus positions to prevent aspiration (even if an endotracheal tube is in place). Lavage decreases ingestant absorption by an average of 52% if performed within 5 min of ingestion administration, 26% if performed at 30 min, and 16% if performed at 60 min. Its efficacy is similar to that of ipecac. Significant amounts of ingested drug are recovered in one-tenth of patients. Aspiration is a common complication (occurring in up to 10% of patients), especially when lavage is perfomed improperly. Serious complications (tracheal lavage, esophageal and gastric perforation) occur in approximately 1% of patients. For this reason, the physician should personally insert the lavage tube and confirm its placement, and the patient must be cooperative or adequately restrained (with pharmacologic sedation if necessary) during the procedure. Gastric lavage is contraindicated in corrosive or petroleum distillate ingestions because of the respective risks of gastroesophageal perforation and aspiration-induced hydrocarbon pneumonitis.

Syrup of ipecac can be used for the home management of patients with accidental ingestions, reliable histories, and mild predicted toxicity. It may delay the administration and decrease the effectiveness of activated charcoal, oral antidotes, and whole-bowel irrigation and is very rarely appropriate for patients treated at a health care facility. It is administered orally in a dose of 30 mL for adults, 15 mL for children, and 10 mL for small infants. Clear liquids should also be given. Ipecac irritates the stomach and stimulates the central chemoreceptor trigger zone. Vomiting usually occurs about 20 min after administration. The dose may be repeated if vomiting does not occur. In animal and human volunteer studies, ipecac decreases ingestant absorption by an average of 60% if given within 5 min of ingestant administration, 32% if given at 30 min, and 30% if given at 60 min. Side effects include lethargy in children (12%) and protracted vomiting (8 to 17%). Chronic ipecac use (by patients with anorexia nervosa or bulimia) may cause electrolyte and fluid abnormalities, cardiac toxicity, and myopathy. Except for aspiration, serious complications are rare. Gastric or esophageal tears and perforations and stroke have been reported. Ipecac is contraindicated in patients with recent gastrointestinal surgery, CNS depression, or seizures, and in those who have ingested corrosives or rapidly acting CNS poisons (camphor, cyanide, tricyclic antidepressants, propoxyphene, strychnine).

Whole-bowel irrigation is performed by administering a bowel-cleansing solution containing electrolytes and polyethylene glycol (Golytely, Colyte) orally or by gastric tube at a rate of up 0.5 L/h in children and 2.0 L/h in adults until rectal effluent is clear. The patient must be in a sitting position. Although data are limited, whole-bowel irrigation may be at least equally as effective as other decontamination procedures. It may be appropriate for those who have ingested foreign bodies, packets of illicit drugs, slow-release or enteric-coated medications, and agents that are poorly adsorbed by charcoal (e.g., heavy metals). It is contraindicated in patients with bowel obstruction, ileus, hemodynamic instability, and compromised unprotected airways.

Cathartic salts (disodium phosphate, magnesium citrate and sulfate, sodium sulfate) or *saccharides* (mannitol, sorbitol) promote the rectal evacuation of gastrointestinal contents. The most effective cathartic is sorbitol in a dose of 1 to 2 g/kg of body weight. Alone, cathartics do not prevent ingestant absorption and should not be used as a method of gut decontamination. Their primary use is to prevent constipation following charcoal administration. Abdominal cramps, nausea, and occasional vomiting are side effects. Complications of repeated dosing include hypermagnesemia and excessive diarrhea. Cathartics are contraindicated in patients who have ingested corrosives and in those with preexisting diarrhea. Magnesium-containing cathartics should not be used in patients with renal failure.

Dilution (i.e., drinking 5 mL/kg of body weight of water or another clear liquid) should be accomplished as soon as possible after the ingestion of corrosives (acids, alkali). However, it may increase the dissolution rate (and hence absorption) of capsules, tablets, and other solid ingestants and should *not* be used in these circumstances.

Endoscopic or surgical removal of poisons may be useful in rare situations, such as ingestion of a potentially toxic foreign body that fails to transit the gastrointestinal tract, a potentially lethal amount of a heavy metal (arsenic, iron, mercury, thallium), or agents that have coalesced into gastric concretions or bezoars (barbiturates, glutethimide, heavy metals, lithium, meprobamate, sustained-release preparations). Patients who become toxic from cocaine due to its leakage from multiple ingested drug packets require immediate surgical intervention.

Decontamination of other sites Immediate, copious flushing with water, saline, or another available clear, drinkable liquid is the initial treatment for topical exposures (exceptions include alkali metals, calcium oxide, phosphorus). Saline is preferred for eye irrigation. A triple wash (water, soap, water) may be best for dermal decontamination. Inhalational exposures should be treated initially with fresh air or oxygen. The removal of liquids from body cavities such as the vagina or rectum is best accomplished by irrigation. Solids (drug packets, pills) should be removed manually, preferably with visual guidance.

Enhancement of Poison Elimination Although the elimination of most poisons can be accelerated by therapeutic interventions, the pharmacokinetic efficacy (removal of drug at a rate greater than that accomplished by intrinsic elimination) and clinical benefit (in terms of a shortened duration of toxicity or improved outcome) of such interventions are often more theoretical than proven. Hence, the decision to use such measures should be based on the actual or predicted toxicity and the potential efficacy, cost, and risks of therapy.

Multiple-dose activated charcoal Repetitive oral dosing with charcoal can enhance the elimination of previously absorbed substances by binding them within the gut as they are excreted in the bile, secreted by gastrointestinal cells, or passively diffuse into the gut lumen (reverse absorption or enterocapillary exsorption). Doses of 0.5 to 1 g/kg body weight every 2 to 4 h, adjusted downward to avoid regurgitation in patients with decreased gastrointestinal motility, are generally recommended. Experimentally, this treatment enhances the elimination of nearly all substances tested. Pharmacokinetic efficacy approaches that of hemodialysis for some agents (e.g., phenobarbital, theophylline). Multiple-dose therapy is not effective in accelerating elimination of chlorpropamide, tobramycin, or agents that adsorb poorly to charcoal. Complications include intestinal obstruction, pseudoobstruction, and nonocclusive intestinal infarction in patients with decreased gut motility.

Forced diuresis and alteration of urinary pH Diuresis and ion trapping via alteration of urine pH may prevent the renal reabsorption of poisons that undergo excretion by glomerular filtration and active tubular secretion. Since membranes are more permeable to nonionized molecules than to their ionized counterparts, acidic (low-pK_a) poisons are ionized and trapped in an alkaline urine, and basic poisons are ionized and trapped in an acid urine. Saline diuresis can enhance the renal excretion of alcohols, bromide, calcium, fluoride, lithium, meprobamate, potassium, and isoniazid. Alkaline diuresis (a urine pH ≥7.5 and a urine output of 3 to 6 mL/kg body weight per hour) enhances the elimination of chlorphenoxyacetic acid herbicides, chlorpropamide, diflunisal, fluoride, methotrexate, phenobarbital, sulfonamides, and salicylates. Contraindications include congestive heart failure, renal failure, and cerebral edema. Acid-base, fluid, and electrolyte parameters should be monitored carefully. Acid diuresis enhances the renal elimination of amphetamines, chloroquine, cocaine, local anesthetics, phencyclidine, quinidine, quinine, strychnine, sympathomimetics, tricyclic antidepressants, and tocainide. Its use, however, has been largely abandoned because of potential complications and lack of clinical efficacy.

Extracorporeal removal Peritoneal dialysis, hemodialysis, charcoal or resin hemoperfusion, hemofiltration, plasmapheresis, and exchange transfusion are capable of removing any toxin from the bloodstream. Agents most amenable to enhanced elimination by dialysis have low molecular mass (<500 Da), high water solubility, low protein binding, small volumes of distribution (<1 L/kg body weight), prolonged elimination (long half-life), and high dialysis clearance relative to total-body clearance. Molecular weight, water solubility, or protein binding do not limit the efficacy of the other forms of extracorporeal removal.

Dialysis should be considered in cases of severe poisoning due to barbiturates, bromide, chloral hydrate, ethanol, ethylene glycol, isopropyl alcohol, lithium, methanol, procainamide, theophylline, salicylates, and possibly heavy metals. Although hemoperfusion may be more effective in removing some of these poisons, it does not correct associated acid-base and electrolyte abnormalities. Hemoperfusion should be considered in cases of severe poisoning due to carbamazepine, chloramphenicol, disopyramide, and hypnotic-sedatives (barbiturates, ethchlorvynol, glutethimide, meprobamate, methaqualone), paraquat, phenytoin, procainamide, theophylline, and valproate. Both techniques require central venous access and systemic anticoagulation and often result in transient hypotension. Hemoperfusion may also cause hemolysis, hypocalcemia, and thrombocytopenia. Peritoneal dialysis and exchange transfusion are less effective but may be used when other procedures are either not available, contraindicated, or technically difficult (e.g., in infants). Exchange transfusion removes poisons affecting red blood cells (as in methemoglobinemia or arsine-induced hemolysis). The roles of hemofiltration and plasmapheresis are not yet defined.

Candidates for these treatments include patients with severe toxicity who deteriorate despite aggressive supportive therapy; those with potentially prolonged, irreversible, or fatal toxicity; those with dangerous blood levels of toxins; those who lack the capacity for self-detoxification because of liver or renal failure; and those with a serious underlying illness or complication that will adversely affect recovery.

Other techniques The elimination of heavy metals can be enhanced by chelation, and the removal of carbon monoxide can be increased by hyperbaric oxygenation as discussed in sections on specific poisons.

Administration of Antidotes Antidotes counteract the effects of poisons by neutralizing them (e.g., antibody-antigen reactions, chelation, chemical binding) or by antagonizing their physiologic effects (e.g., activation of opposing nervous system activity, provision of competitive metabolic or receptor substrate). Poisons or conditions with specific antidotes include acetaminophen, anticholinergic agents, anticoagulants, benzodiazepines, beta blockers, calcium channel blockers, carbon monoxide, cardiac glycosides, cholinergic agents, cyanide, drug-induced dystonic reactions, ethylene glycol, fluoride, heavy metals, hydrogen sulfide, hypoglycemic agents, isoniazid, methemoglobinemia, narcotics, sympatomimetics, Vacor, and a variety of evenomations. Antidotes can significantly reduce morbidity and mortality, but most are potentially toxic. Since their safe use requires correct identification of a specific poisoning or syndrome, details of antidotal therapy are discussed with the conditions for which they are indicated.

Prevention of Reexposure Poisoning is a preventable illness. Unfortunately, some adults and children are poison-prone, and recurrences are common. Adults with accidental exposures should be instructed regarding the safe use of medications and chemicals (according to labeling instructions). Confused patients may need assistance with the administration of medications. Errors in dosing by health care providers may require educational efforts. Patients should be advised to avoid circumstances that result in chemical exposure or poisoning. Appropriate agencies and health departments should be notified in cases of environmental or workplace exposure. The best approach with young children and patients with intentional overdose is to limit access to poisons. In households where children live or visit, alcoholic beverages, medications, household products (automotive, cleaning, fuel, pet-care, toiletry products), nonedible plants, and vitamins should be kept out of reach or in locked or child-proof cabinets. Depressed or psychotic patients should receive psychiatric assessment, disposition, and follow-up. They should be given prescriptions for a limited supply of drugs and with a limited number of refills and be monitored for compliance and response to therapy.

SPECIFIC POISONS

The following discussion focuses on poisonings that are common, produce life-threatening toxicity, or require unique therapeutic interventions. Poisonings not covered here are described in the referenced texts. →***Alcohol, cocaine, hallucinogens, and opioids are discussed in Chaps. 386 to 389, and heavy metal poisoning is discussed in Chap. 395.***

ACETAMINOPHEN Acetaminophen is absorbed rapidly and has a volume of distribution of 1 L/kg body weight. Plasma concentrations range from 160 to 660 μmol/L (5 to 20 μg/mL) following therapeutic doses. Most acetaminophen is metabolized by hepatic conjugation with sulfate and glucuronide to form nontoxic metabolites, with minor amounts being excreted unchanged or oxidized by hepatic cytochrome P450 enzymes (primarily CYPIIE1) to form a highly reactive, electrophilic, and potentially toxic intermediary metabolite *n*-acetyl-*p*-benzoquinoneimine (NAPQI). After therapeutic doses, NAPQI is rapidly detoxified by conjugation with glutathione and excreted as cysteine and mercapturic acid conjugates. Following an acute ingestion of ≥140 mg/kg body weight, sulfate and glucuronide pathways become saturated, resulting in an increased fraction and amount of acetaminophen metabolized to NAPQI and eventual glutathione depletion. When this occurs, free NAPQI binds covalently to hepatocytes and causes their lysis (centrilobular necrosis). Less often, hepatotoxicity develops following the chronic ingestion of therapeutic or slightly greater amounts in conditions associated with decreased glutathione reserves (e.g., alcoholism, childhood, acute starvation, chronic malnutrition) and possibly in conditions with enhanced P450 enzyme activity (e.g., anticonvulsant and antitubercolosis drug use). The plasma half-life is usually 2 to 4 h but may be prolonged if hepatotoxicity develops.

Clinical Toxicity Early manifestations of poisoning are nonspecific and not predictive of subsequent hepatotoxicity. Within 2 to 4 h of acute overdose, nausea, vomiting, diaphoresis, and pallor may develop. CNS depression is typically absent unless massive doses are ingested. Within 24 to 48 h, hepatotoxicity is evidenced by right upper quadrant tenderness and mild hepatomegaly. Renal function may also be impaired. Laboratory evidence of hepatic toxicity includes prolongation of the prothrombin time and elevation of serum bilirubin and transaminase activity (aspartate transaminase, alanine transaminase). Severe poisoning may cause hepatic failure. Greater than twofold prolongation of prothrombin time, a serum bilirubin level >68 μmol/L (4 mg/dL), pH <7.30, serum creatinine >3.3, and a high-grade encephalopathy indicate a poor prognosis. In patients who recover, liver function returns to normal within 1 week, and liver histology returns to normal within 3 months. Chronic poisoning is usually similar, but alcoholics may present with a syndrome of severe combined hepatic and renal insufficiency with dehydration, jaundice, coagulopathy, hypoglycemia, and acute tubular necrosis.

Diagnostic Evaluation A serum acetaminophen level should be obtained between 4 and 24 h after ingestion. A level above the lower line on the Rumack-Matthew nomogram (Fig. 396-2) indicates possible hepatotoxicity and the need for antidote therapy.

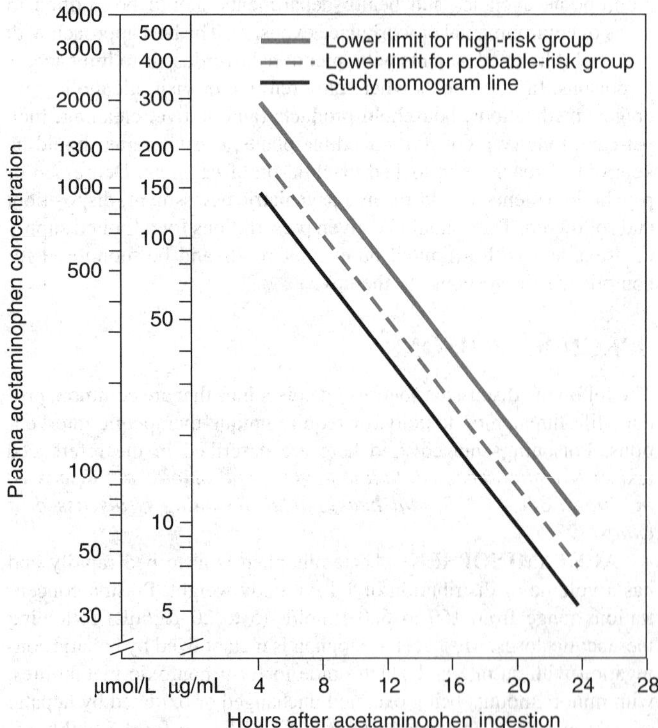

FIGURE 396-2 Nomogram to define risk according to initial plasma acetaminophen concentration. *(After BH Rumack, H Matthew: Pediatrics 55:871, 1975.)*

℞ **TREATMENT** Activated charcoal is recommended for patients who present within 4 h of ingestion. (Charcoal does not interfere significantly with acetylcysteine therapy.) Antidotal therapy consists of oral *N*-acetylcysteine (NAC), diluted 3:1 with a nonalcoholic, nondairy beverage. It is given at a loading dose of 140 mg/kg body weight, followed by a maintenance dose of 70 mg/kg body weight every 4 h for 17 additional doses. Treatment is most effective if started within 8 to 10 h of an overdose and should be administered before the serum level is known. If the level is subsequently shown to be nontoxic, therapy may be discontinued. Side effects of NAC include nausea, vomiting, and epigastric discomfort. The dose should be repeated if vomiting occurs within an hour of dosing. Antiemetics (metoclopramide, droperidol, odansetron) may be necessary. Liver and renal function should be monitored during therapy. Patients with severe hepatotoxicity should be considered for liver transplantation.

ACIDS AND ALKALI Common alkaline products include ammonia, bleach (sodium hypochlorite), drain cleaners (sodium hydroxide), surface cleaners (phosphates), laundry and dishwasher detergents (phosphates, carbonates), disk batteries, denture cleaners (borates, phosphates, carbonates), and Clinitest tablets (sodium hydroxides). Acids are used in toilet bowl cleaners (hydrofluoric, phosphoric, and sulfuric acids), soldering fluxes (hydrochloric acid), antirust compounds (hydrofluoric and oxalic acids), automobile battery fluid (sulfuric acid), and stone cleaners (hydrofluoric and nitric acids). Other corrosives include hydrogen peroxide, hydrazine, and phenol.

Alkalis produce liquefactive necrosis with rapidly penetrating tissue injury and a higher risk of perforation of the esophagus and stomach than do acids. Acids produce coagulative necrosis. Both may burn the mouth, esophagus, stomach, and proximal small bowel. Liquids tend to produce superficial, often circumferential burns over a larger surface area, while solids and tablets cause localized but deeper burns. The severity of the burn relates to the contact time, the amount ingested, and the pH (especially if <2 or >12) of the ingested product.

Clinical Toxicity Burns of the mouth result in excess salivation, pain, dysphonia, and dysphagia and are manifested by erythema, edema, ulceration, and necrosis. Deep burns may destroy mucosal nerve endings and produce anesthesia. Lack of oral findings does not rule out esophageal or gastric injury. Esophageal symptoms and signs include drooling, painful swallowing, retrosternal pain, and neck tenderness. Vomiting of blood and mucus may occur. Esophageal perforation is suggested by increased severity of chest pain, often with respiratory distress. Epigastric pain, vomiting, and tenderness may occur with burns to the stomach. Aspiration of acids and alkalis may cause fulminant tracheitis and bronchial pneumonia. In severe cases, hypotension, shock, metabolic acidosis, liver and renal dysfunction, hemolysis, and disseminated intravascular coagulation may be seen. Deep burns, particularly if extensive or circumferential, may be followed by fibrosis with stricture formation and obstruction of the esophagus (alkalis) or of the gastric outlet (acids).

Diagnosis Endoscopy, best performed 12 to 24 h after ingestion, is used to document the site of injury and its severity and should be performed in symptomatic patients. Chest and abdominal x-rays and routine laboratory testing should be obtained to evaluate for aspiration, perforation, and organ dysfunction. Residual effects of the ingestion can be assessed by barium swallow.

℞ **TREATMENT** Treatment includes immediate dilution with milk or water. Administration of a weak acid (carbonated beverage or citrus juice) or base (antacid) is also acceptable. Glucocorticoids and esophageal stents have traditionally been used for alkali burns to prevent esophageal stricture formation, but their efficacy is not proven. Animal studies suggest that glucocorticoids may be effective if begun immediately on presentation. If used, a dose of 1 to 2 mg of methylprednisolone per kilogram every 4 to 6 h for at least 2 weeks is suggested. Concomitant prophylactic broad-spectrum antibiotic use is also recommended. Glucocorticoids are not useful for acid burns. Antacids should be used for burns of the stomach. Esophageal stricture or gastric outlet obstruction may require subsequent dilatation and bouginage or surgical reconstruction.

ANTIARRHYTHMIC DRUGS Class IA (disopyramide, moricizine, procainamide, and quinidine), IB (lidocaine, mexiletine, phenytoin, and tocainide), and IC (encainide, flecainide, propafenone) antiarrhythmics block myocardial cell membrane fast sodium channels and slow cardiac conduction, whereas class III agents (amiodarone, bretylium, ibutilide, and sotalol) block potassium currents and prolong refractoriness. These agents are rapidly absorbed (except for disopyramide and sustained-release formulations), have volumes of distribution ranging from 1 to 10 L/kg, have half-lives of 3 to 16 h, and are eliminated mainly by hepatic metabolism.

Clinical Toxicity The acute ingestion of more than twice the usual daily dose is potentially toxic. Effects generally begin within 1 h and peak within several hours. Toxicity may also develop during chronic therapeutic use. Manifestations include nausea, vomiting, and diarrhea, followed by lethargy, confusion, ataxia, bradycardia, hypotension, and cardiovascular collapse. Anticholinergic effects (blurred vision, dry mucosae) may be seen in disopyramide poisoning. Quinidine and class IB agents may cause agitation, dysphoria, and seizures. ECG findings include bradycardia with AV block, ventricular tachycardia, ventricular fibrillation (including the polymorphous form, torsade de pointes), and QT-interval prolongation. More specifically, class IA agents prolong the PR, QRS, and JT intervals, class IC agents prolong the QRS interval, and class III agents prolong the JT interval. Class IB agents have little or no effects on conduction intervals. Depressed myocardial contractility and arrhythmias may lead to decreased cardiac output and pulmonary edema. Hypoglycemia and mild hypokalemia may be seen with disopyramide and quinidine intoxication, respectively.

Diagnosis Comprehensive toxicology screening will detect most of these agents. Measurement of serum levels are used for monitoring therapy and for confirmation of overdose.

℞ TREATMENT Activated charcoal is the procedure of choice for gastrointestinal decontamination. Hypotension, bradyarrhythmias, and seizures are treated with standard measures. Patients with persistent hypotension may benefit from pulmonary arterial pressure measurement. Cardiac pacing, intraaortic balloon pump counterpulsation, and cardiopulmonary bypass may be necessary. Ventricular tachyarrhythmias that cause hemodynamic instability should be treated with lidocaine. Bretylium is probably also safe. Sodium bicarbonate (0.5 to 1 mmol/kg by intravenous bolus) may be effective for tachyarrhythmias due to class IA or IC agents. Mild hypokalemia may be protective, and potassium levels as low as 3.0 mmol/L may be best treated by watchful waiting. Magnesium sulfate (4 g or 40 mL of a 10% solution given intravenously as an initial dose) and overdrive pacing (with isoproterenol or electricity) are used for torsade de pointes. Hemodialysis and hemoperfusion may enhance the elimination of disopyramide, the active procainamide metabolite *N*-acetylprocainamide, and possibly other agents.

ANTICHOLINERGIC AGENTS Agents that can competitively block the binding of acetylcholine to CNS and parasympathetic postganglionic muscarinic neuroreceptors include antihistamines (H_1 blockers), belladonna alkaloids and related agents (atropine, glycopyrrolate, homatropine, hyoscine, ipratropium, scopolamine), drugs for Parkinson's disease (benztropine, biperiden, trihexyphenidyl), topical mydriatics (cyclopentolate, tropicamide), neuroleptics (clozapine, olanzepine, phenothiazines), skeletal muscle relaxants (cyclobenzaprine, orphenadrine), smooth-muscle relaxants (clidinium, dicyclomine, isometheptene, oxybutynin), tricyclic antidepressants, and some plants (e.g., *Datura stramonium*, or jimson weed) and mushrooms. Their absorption can be delayed following an overdose. Most are weak bases, exhibit variable binding to plasma proteins (18 to 98%), and have moderate volumes of distribution (2 to 6 L/kg). They are eliminated primarily by hepatic metabolism and have half-lives ranging from 2 to 24 h or more.

Clinical Toxicity Manifestations usually begin within an hour of acute overdosage and 1 to 3 days after beginning treatment in cases of chronic poisoning. Toxic doses are only slightly greater than therapeutic ones. CNS manifestations include agitation, ataxia, confusion, delirium, hallucinations, and movement disorders (choreoathetoid and picking movements). Lethargy, respiratory depression, and coma may occur. Peripheral nervous system findings include decreased or absent bowel sounds, dilated pupils, dry skin and mucosal surfaces, urinary retention, and increases in pulse rate, blood pressure, respiratory rate, and temperature. Neuromuscular hyperactivity may lead to rhabdomyolysis and hyperthermia. First-generation H_1 blockers (diphenhydramine and probably others) can sometimes cause tricyclic antidepressant–like cardiotoxicity and seizures. Because of class III antiarrhythmic activity, original nonsedating or second-generation antihistamines (astemizole, terfenadine) caused QT-interval prolongation with subsequent ventricular tachyarrhythmias, especially torsade de pointes, and were withdrawn from U.S. markets.

Diagnosis The diagnosis is supported by detecting these agents in the urine. It can be confirmed by demonstrating resolution of anticholinergic toxicity in response to physostigmine.

℞ TREATMENT Activated charcoal adsorbs these agents effectively and is the preferred method of gastrointestinal decontamination. Agitation may respond to benzodiazepines, and comatose patients may require intubation and mechanical ventilation. Cardiovascular toxicity and arrhythmias should be treated as described for antiarrhythmics and tricyclic antidepressants. Physostigmine, an acetylcholinesterase inhibitor, reverses anticholinergic toxicity. It is indicated primarily for uncontrolled agitation and delirium. The dose is 1 to 2 mg given intravenously over 2 to 5 min; the dose can be repeated if there is an incomplete response or recurrent toxicity. If signs of cholinergic poisoning occur (see "Organophosphate and Carbamate Insecticides," below), they can be reversed by atropine in half the amount of physostigmine given. Physostigmine should not be given for seizures or for coma; its arousal effects are nonspecific and cannot be used for diagnostic purposes. Physostigmine is contraindicated in the presence of cardiac conduction defects or ventricular arrhythmias because it can cause asystole in such patients.

ANTICONVULSANTS Carbamazepine, lamotrigine, phenytoin and other hydantoins, topiramate, and valproate act primarily to limit the spread of a seizure from its focus by inhibiting the passive influx of sodium through voltage-dependent sodium channels in neuronal membranes, an activity analogous to that of class I antiarrhythmics (see above). This action, and the resultant inhibition of the release of excitatory neurotransmitters (e.g., aspartate, glutamate), limits posttetanic potentiation of synaptic transmission. Like the barbiturates and benzodiazepines (see below), felbamate, gabapentin, and the investigational agents tiagabine and vigabatrin enhance synaptic transmission of the inhibitory neurotransmitter GABA. The succimides ethosuximide and methsuximide elevate the seizure threshold by reducing calcium conduction through T-type calcium channels. Valproate also inhibits GABA metabolism and calcium conductance. Valproate and its metabolites interfere with enzymes involved in fatty acid synthesis and oxidation, gluconeogenesis, and the urea cycle. Carbamazepine is structurally similar to the tricyclic antidepressants and can cause similar toxicity (see "Cyclic Antidepressant," below) in overdose.

Anticonvulsants are well absorbed after oral administration. Phenytoin is also available for intravenous use, both as phenytoin and the prodrug phosphenytoin. A prodrug formulation of valproate, divalproex, a molecule of which dissociates into two molecules of valproate, is also marketed. Gastrointestinal absorption is prolonged with regular and sustained-release formulations of carbamazepine, extended-release phenytoin, and enteric-coated divalproex, particularly following overdose. The volume of distribution is small for valproate (0.1 to 0.4 L/kg); moderate for phenytoin (0.5 to 0.8 L/kg); large for carbamazepine, felbamate, gabapentin, and lamotrigine (≥1 L/kg); and unknown for other agents. All are eliminated primarily by hepatic metabolism. Carbamazepine has an active (10,11-epoxide) metabolite. Half-lives, therapeutic doses, serum concentrations, adverse effects, and drug interactions are listed in Table 360-9. The half-life of phenytoin, valproate, and possibly carbamazepine and other agents is prolonged following overdose.

Clinical Toxicity Anticonvulsants primarily cause CNS depression (Table 396-2). Cerebellar and vestibular function are affected first, with cerebral depression occurring later. Effects are the same and occur at similar blood levels, regardless of whether overdose is acute or chronic. Ataxia, blurred vision, diplopia, dizziness, nystagmus, slurred speech, tremors, and nausea and vomiting are common initial manifestations. Paradoxical excitation can occur, and membrane-active agents can sometimes cause de novo seizures and exacerbation of epilepsy. Coma with respiratory depression usually occurs at serum carbamazepine concentrations >20 μg/mL, serum phenytoin levels >60 μg/mL, and serum valproate levels >180 μg/mL. Anticholinergic effects (see above) may be present in carbamazepine poisoning, and tricyclic antidepressant–like cardiotoxicity (see below) can occur at drug levels >30 μg/mL.

Hypotension and arrhythmias (e.g., bradycardia, conduction disturbances, ventricular tachyarrhythmias) can occur during the rapid infusion of phenytoin. Although these effects have been attributed to its propylene glycol diluent, they have also been reported with rapid infusions of phosphenytoin, which does not contain this solvent. Cardiovascular toxicity after oral phenytoin overdose, however, is essentially nonexistent. Extravasation of phenytoin can result in local tissue necrosis due to the high pH of this formulation. Intravenous phenytoin may also cause the "purple glove syndrome" (limb edema, discoloration, and pain). This can occur hours after infusion and without signs of extravasation. A compartment syndrome with limb ischemia and muscle necrosis is a potential complication. Multiple metabolic abnormalities, including anion-gap metabolic acidosis, hyperosmolality, hypocalcemia, hypoglycemia, hypophosphatemia, hypernatremia, and hyperammonemia (with or without other evidence of hepatotoxicity), can occur in valproate poisoning. Three or more days may be required for resolution of toxicity in severe carbamazepine, phenytoin, and valproate poisoning.

Diagnosis The diagnosis of carbamazepine, phenytoin, and valproate poisoning can be confirmed by measuring serum drug concentrations. Serial drug levels should be obtained until a peak is observed following acute overdose. Quantitative serum levels of other agents are not generally available. Most anticonvulsants can be detected by comprehensive urine screening tests.

℞ TREATMENT Activated charcoal is the method of choice for gastrointestinal decontamination. Multiple-dose charcoal therapy can enhance the elimination of carbamazepine, phenytoin, valproate, and perhaps other agents. Airway protection and support of respiration with endotracheal intubation and mechanical ventilation, if necessary, are the mainstays of treatment. Seizures should be treated with benzodiazepines or barbiturates. Physostigmine (see "Anticholinergic Agents," above) should be considered for anticholinergic poisoning due to carbamazepine. The treatment of carbamazepine-induced hypotension, cardiac conduction disturbances, and ventricular tachyarrhythmias should include sodium bicarbonate (see "Antiarrhythmic Drugs," above). Phenytoin and phosphenytoin cardiotoxicity usually resolves promptly upon discontinuation of the infusion. Crystalloids and lidocaine can be given if necessary. Tissue injury secondary to phenytoin extravasation should be treated by standard wound care measures. Treatment of the purple glove syndrome includes elevation of the affected extremity. A vascular surgeon should evaluate this condition, if signs of ischemia are present. Occasionally, CNS depression due to valproate will respond to naloxone (2 mg intravenously). Metabolic derangements should be corrected. Hemodialysis and hemoperfusion can enhance the elimination of valproate and its metabolites. Hemodialysis can also correct associated metabolic disturbances. Hemoperfusion only modestly increases carbamazepine elimination. These procedures should be reserved for patients with persistently high drug levels (e.g., carbamazepine ≥40 μg/mL and valproate ≥1000 μg/mL) who do not respond to supportive care.

BARBITURATES Barbiturates bind to the GABA receptor complex and prolong the opening of the chloride channels in response to GABA, thereby inhibiting excitable cells of the CNS and other tissues. They can be classified as long-acting (6 to 12 h; mephobarbital, barbital, phenobarbital, primidone), intermediate-acting (3 to 6 h; amobarbital, aprobarbital, butabarbital, butalbital), short-acting (1 to 3 h; hexobarbital, pentobarbital, and secobarbital), and ultrashort-acting (<30 min; methohexital, thiamylal, and thiopental).

Barbiturates are weak acids with pK_a values ranging from 7.2 to 8.5, volumes of distribution of 0.8 to 1.5 L/kg of body weight, and 45 to 70% protein binding in the plasma. With therapeutic doses, plasma concentrations generally peak in 1 to 4 h (earlier for short-acting agents than for long-acting ones). Most barbiturates are metabolized by the liver. Some are converted to active metabolites: mephobarbital to barbital, and primidone to phenobarbital and phenylethylmalonamide (PEMA). In contrast to short-acting agents, long-acting ones also undergo significant renal excretion: 95% for barbital, 25 to 33% for phenobarbital, 15 to 42% for primidone, and 95% for PEMA. Half-lives range from 1 h for ultrashort-acting agents to 6 d for long-acting ones.

Clinical Toxicity Barbiturates cause CNS depression (Table 396-2). Hypothermia, hypotension, pulmonary edema, and cardiac arrest may occur in severe cases. Pressure sores, bullous skin lesions, and rhabdomyolysis can develop with prolonged coma. Maximal toxicity usually occurs within 4 to 6 h but may be delayed to 10 h or more after overdosage with long-acting barbiturates.

Diagnosis Serum drug levels can confirm the diagnosis. Significant toxicity is usually apparent when serum concentrations of long-acting barbiturates exceed 170 μmol/L (4 mg/dL) and those of short-acting barbiturates exceed 88 μmol/L (2 mg/dL). Because of tolerance, the degree of CNS depression relative to dose and drug level is dependent on prior exposure to the drug.

℞ TREATMENT Activated charcoal effectively adsorbs barbiturates and is the method of choice for gastrointestinal decontamination. Hemodynamic and respiratory support and correction of temperature and electrolyte derangements may be necessary. Renal elimination of phenobarbital (and probably other long-acting agents) is enhanced by alkalinization of urine to a pH of 8 (by giving intravenous sodium bicarbonate) and by saline diuresis. Elimination can also be enhanced by repeated doses of activated charcoal. Since short-acting barbiturates are predominantly metabolized by the liver, diuresis is ineffective. Hemodialysis and hemoperfusion are effective in removing both long- and short-acting barbiturates, but their use should be reserved for patients with refractory hypotension.

BENZODIAZEPINES Benzodiazepines potentiate the inhibitory effect of GABA on CNS neurons by binding to the GABA receptor complex and increasing the frequency of opening of chloride channels in response to GABA stimulation. They can be classified as long-acting (chlordiazepoxide, clonazepam, clorazepate, diazepam, flurazepam, prazepam, quazepam), short-acting (alprazolam, flunitrazepam, lorazepam, and oxazepam), and ultrashort-acting (estazolam, midazolam, temazepam, and triazolam). Benzodiazepines are readily absorbed, exhibit 85 to 99% protein binding in the plasma, are lipid soluble, and have an apparent volume of distribution of 0.3 to 2 L/kg body weight. They are weak acids with pK_a values ranging from 1.3 to 6.2 and are eliminated mainly by hepatic metabolism. Some have active metabolites. Half-lives range from 2 h for short-acting agents to 8 days for long-acting ones.

Clinical Toxicity CNS depressant effects (Table 396-2) begin within 30 min of acute overdose. Coma and respiratory depression are rare but can occur with ultrashort-acting agents and when benzodiazepines are combined with other CNS depressants. Paradoxical excitation may occur early in the course of poisoning.

Diagnosis The diagnosis is supported by identification of benzodiazepine metabolites in urine. Since immunoassays do not detect all benzodiazepines, a negative result does not exclude the diagnosis. A response to flumazenil confirms the diagnosis.

℞ TREATMENT Activated charcoal adsorbs benzodiazepines and is the method of choice for gastrointestinal decontamination. Respiratory support should be provided as necessary. Flumazenil, a competitive benzodiazepine receptor antagonist, can reverse CNS and respiratory depression and obviate the need for endotracheal intubation. Doses of 0.1 mg should be given intravenously at 1-min intervals until the desired effect is achieved or a cumulative dose of 3 mg has been given. Since flumazenil has a relatively short duration of action, patients must be monitored carefully for relapse. Should relapse occur, treatment can be repeated (at intervals of 20 min with a maximum dose of 3 mg/h). Flumazenil can cause seizures in patients who have coingested stimulants and tricyclic antidepressants or who are physically dependent on benzodiazepines as a result of chronic use. It should not be used in patients with ECG evidence of tricyclic antidepressant cardiotoxicity.

β-ADRENERGIC BLOCKING AGENTS β-Adrenergic blocking agents act by competitively inhibiting β-adrenergic neurohumoral receptors. This activity defines them as class II antiarrhythmics. At therapeutic doses, some beta blockers act at both β_1 and β_2 receptors and are "nonselective" (carvedilol, labetalol, nadolol, pindolol, propranolol, timolol); some act predominantly on β_1 receptors and are "cardioselective" (acebutolol, atenolol, betaxolol, bisoprolol, esmolol, metoprolol). Certain beta blockers have partial agonist or sympathomimetic activity (acebutolol, carteolol, pindolol, and possibly penbutolol), some have an α_1 blocking activity and the additional property of vasodilation (carvedilol, labetalol), and some have quinidine-like antiarrhythmic effects (acebutolol, metoprolol, pindolol, propranolol, sotalol, and possibly betaxolol). Antiarrhythmic effects are due to a reduction of sodium and calcium influx during membrane depolarization (phase 0) as a consequence of decreased production of cyclic AMP by adenylate cyclase. Decreased cardiac contractility results from inhibition of calcium influx into cells and the release of calcium from sarcoplasmic reticulum.

Beta blockers are readily absorbed and exhibit variable protein binding (5 to 93%), water solubility, and volumes of distribution (0.23 to 10.0 L/kg body weight). Most beta blockers are eliminated predominantly by hepatic metabolism. Atenolol, nadolol, and sotalol are eliminated primarily by renal excretion, and esmolol is metabolized by erythrocyte esterases.

Clinical Toxicity Effects usually begin within 1/2 h following an overdose and peak within 2 h. Onset may be delayed with the ingestion of sustained-release preparations. Findings include nausea and vomiting followed by bradycardia, hypotension, and CNS depression. However, agents with sympathomimetic activity can cause hypertension and tachycardia. CNS effects can include seizures and tend to be more pronounced with highly lipophilic agents (penbutolol, propranolol). The skin is often pale and cool. Bronchospasm and pulmonary edema are uncommon unless there is a history of asthma, chronic obstructive pulmonary disease, or congestive heart failure. Metabolic abnormalities include hyperkalemia and hypoglycemia (as a direct result of β-adrenergic receptor blockade) and metabolic acidosis (due to seizures, shock, or respiratory depression). ECG manifestations include all degrees of AV block, bundle branch block, prolonged QRS duration, and asystole. Sotalol may cause QT-interval prolongation with ventricular tachycardia, ventricular fibrillation, and torsade de pointes occurring up to 20 h after overdose. Patients with mild poisoning usually recover within 6 to 12 h, whereas those with severe poisoning and ingestions of sustained-release preparations may be symptomatic for 24 to 48 h.

Diagnosis The diagnosis is primarily based on the clinical presentation. Urine toxicology screening may identify the presence of beta blockers, but blood levels are neither generally available nor helpful in guiding therapy.

℞ TREATMENT Activated charcoal adsorbs these agents effectively and is the preferred method of gastrointestinal decontamination. Gastric emptying procedures may produce vagal stimulation and exacerbate bradyarrhythmias. Bradycardia associated with hypotension will sometimes respond to atropine, isoproterenol, and vasopressors (amrinone, dopamine, dobutamine, epinephrine, and norepinephrine have been used with variable success, alone or in combination). With severe poisoning, these agents may be ineffective, and glucagon, calcium, cardiac pacing (external or internal), and intraaortic balloon pump support may be necessary. Glucagon, which stimulates adenylate cyclase by a nonadrenergic mechanism, is given at an initial dose of 5 to 10 mg. Patients who respond favorably can be treated with an infusion of 1 to 5 mg/h. Calcium and high-dose insulin can be given with glucose and potassium to reverse negative inotropic effects, as described for calcium channel blocker poisoning. Bronchospasm may be treated with an inhaled beta agonist, subcutaneous epinephrine, and intravenous aminophylline. Lidocaine, magnesium (as for antiarrhythmic poisoning), or overdrive pacing may be used for sotalol-induced ventricular tachyarrhythmias. Extracorporeal elimination procedures are probably not of benefit, except possibly for atenolol, metoprolol, nadolol, and sotalol.

CALCIUM CHANNEL BLOCKERS Bepridil, diltiazem, verapamil, and the dihydropyridine derivatives amlodipine, felodipine, isradipine, nicardipine, nifedipine, nimodipine, and nisoldipine decrease the influx of calcium across slow (L-type) calcium channels in the membranes of myocardial and vascular smooth-muscle cells during phases 2 (plateau) and 4 (spontaneous depolarization) of the action potential. These actions define them as class IV antiarrhythmics. Bepridil also has class I antiarrhythmic activity. Electrophysiologic effects include decreased cardiac contractility, heart rate [sinoatrial (SA) node rate], and AV nodal conduction. At therapeutic doses, all calcium channel blockers cause vasodilation. Diltiazem and verapamil also have significant negative inotropic and chronotropic activity.

Calcium channel blockers are well absorbed and exhibit high (80 to 99%) plasma protein binding. Most have distribution volumes ranging from 1 to 8 L/kg body weight. They are eliminated mainly by hepatic metabolism, and the half-lives typically range from 1 to 24 h.

Clinical Toxicity Toxic effects begin within 2 h of ingestion of immediate-release preparations but may be delayed up to 18 h following overdoses of sustained-release preparations. Manifestations include nausea, vomiting, bradycardia, hypotension, and CNS depression (Table 396-2). Hypotension caused by diltiazem and verapamil is usually due to myocardial depression (decreased cardiac output), whereas that caused by the dihydropyridine derivatives is usually due to low peripheral vascular resistance. Reflexive tachycardia is sometimes seen in dihydropyridine poisoning. Seizures can occur and are the result of direct membrane effects as well as cerebral hypoperfusion. Hypotension may precipitate mesenteric or myocardial ischemia or infarction, and depression of cardiac function may lead to pulmonary edema. ECG findings include all degrees of AV block, prolonged QRS and QT intervals (mainly with verapamil), evidence of ischemia or infarction, and asystole. Metabolic acidosis (secondary to shock) and hyperglycemia (resulting from the inhibition of insulin release) may be present. Serum calcium levels, however, remain normal.

Diagnosis These agents can be detected by comprehensive urine screening tests. Serum levels are not generally available or helpful in guiding therapy.

TREATMENT Activated charcoal is preferred for gastrointestinal decontamination. Symptomatic bradycardia should be treated with atropine, calcium, isoproterenol, glucagon, and electrical (external or internal) pacing. Restoring perfusion is particularly important in patients with organ ischemia. The initial dose of calcium is 10 mL of 10% calcium chloride or 30 mL of the 10% gluconate solution intravenously over 2 min. This dose may be repeated up to four times in patients with a partial, transient, or absent response. High serum calcium levels may be required for a therapeutic effect. A continuous calcium infusion (0.2 mL/kg body weight per hour up to a maximum of 10 mL/h) may be appropriate when relapse occurs after an initial bolus. Although electrical pacing may be required, glucagon, in the same dose as for beta blocker poisoning, may also be effective. High-dose insulin (0.1–0.2 units/kg body weight of regular insulin as a bolus followed by 0.1–1 units/kg per hour) along with glucose (25-g bolus followed by 1 g/kg per hour of a 20% infusion) and potassium to maintain euglycemia and normokalemia should also be considered. This treatment enhances myocardial metabolism and improves myocardial contactility. It may be particularly effective in verapamil poisoning. Hypotension that persists despite resolution of bradycardia should initially be treated with fluids. Amrinone, dopamine, dobutamine, glucagon, and norepinephrine, alone or in combination, have also been used with success. Intraaortic balloon pump support should be used in patients with refractory shock. Patients with mild toxicity usually recover within a few hours, whereas those with severe toxicity or overdose with sustained-release preparations may remain symptomatic for 24 h or longer.

CARBON MONOXIDE Carbon monoxide is produced in large amounts in industrial processes as well as by internal combustion engines, fossil-fueled home appliances (generators, heaters, stoves), and the incomplete combustion of nearly all natural materials and synthetic products. Methylene chloride, a solvent in paint removers, is metabolized to carbon monoxide.

Carbon monoxide is absorbed rapidly through the lungs and binds to hemoglobin (forming carboxyhemoglobin) with an affinity 210 times that of oxygen. Its binding reduces oxygen transport by hemoglobin and also decreases the release of oxygen in tissues (the oxygen dissociation curve shifts to the left). Carbon monoxide also binds to myoglobin, decreasing its oxygen-carrying capacity, and to mitochondrial cytochrome oxidase, inhibiting cellular respiration. The net effect is tissue hypoxia with anaerobic metabolism, lactic acidosis, lipid peroxidation, and free radical formation. Once carbon monoxide exposure is discontinued, dissociation of the hemoglobin–carbon monoxide complex occurs, and carbon monoxide is excreted through the lungs. At atmospheric pressure, the carboxyhemoglobin half-life is 4 to 6 h. It decreases to 40 to 80 min when breathing 100% oxygen and to 15 to 30 min with hyperbaric oxygen therapy. The apparent half-life after methylene chloride exposure is considerably longer.

Clinical Toxicity Manifestations of carbon monoxide poisoning include shortness of breath, dyspnea, tachypnea, headache, emotional lability, confusion, impaired judgment, clumsiness, and syncope. Nausea, vomiting, and diarrhea may also occur. Cerebral edema, coma, respiratory depression, and pulmonary edema may be seen in severe poisoning. Cardiovascular manifestations include ischemic chest pain, arrhythmias, heart failure, and hypotension. In comatose patients, blisters and bullae may develop over pressure points. Serum creatine kinase and lactate dehydrogenase levels may be elevated. Myoglobinuria secondary to muscle necrosis may result in renal failure. Visual field defects, blindness, and venous engorgement with papilledema or optic atrophy may be noted. Arterial blood gas analysis may reveal metabolic acidosis, a normal P_{O_2}, decreased oxygen saturation (when measured by CO-oximetry, but not when calculated from the P_{O_2} or measured by pulse oximetry), and a variable P_{CO_2}. Oxygen saturation measured by pulse oximetry will be falsely elevated but less than normal. A cherry-red color of skin and mucous membranes is rare, and cyanosis is usual.

After brief exposure, carboxyhemoglobin fractions of 15 to 20% are associated with mild symptoms, 20 to 40% with moderate symptoms, and 40 to 50% with severe symptoms. Fractions >60% are often fatal. With prolonged exposure, toxicity occurs at lower fractions. Patients with loss of consciousness are at risk for developing neuropsychiatric sequelae 1 to 3 weeks after exposure. Manifestations vary from subtle personality changes and intellectual impairment to gross neurologic deficits such as blindness, deafness, incoordination, and parkinsonism.

Diagnosis An elevated carboxyhemoglobin fraction confirms exposure, but the result must be interpreted with respect to the time elapsed from exposure to sampling. If the carboxyhemoglobin fraction cannot be measured directly, the difference between the oxygen saturation calculated from the P_{O_2} and that measured by CO-oximetry can be used to estimate the carboxyhemoglobin fraction.

TREATMENT In conscious patients, oxygen should be administered by a non-rebreather mask at 10 L/min until carboxyhemoglobin fraction is <10% and symptoms have resolved. Infants and pregnant women require treatment for several more hours, because fetal hemoglobin has a higher affinity for carbon monoxide than adult hemoglobin. Endotracheal intubation and mechanical ventilation with 100% oxygen are indicated in patients with coma, seizures, or cardiovascular instability. Arrhythmias and hypotension are treated by usual measures. Although hyperbaric oxygen therapy is often recommended for patients with coma, syncope, seizures, and cardiovascular instability, for those with less severe neurologic or cardiovascular dysfunction that does not resolve with oxygen and supportive measures, and for those who develop neurologic sequalae, recent data suggest that it is no more effective than prolonged high-flow normobaric oxygen in reversing acute toxicity and preventing sequelae.

CARDIAC GLYCOSIDES Poisoning with digitalis and other cardiac glycosides occurs most often during therapeutic or suicidal use of digoxin. It can also occur when plants (foxglove, oleander, squill) or the skin (venom) of *Bufo* toads (Colorado River, Asian, Chinese, European) are ingested. Toad venom also contains hallucinogens and accounts for the practice of toad licking as a form of recreational drug abuse. At therapeutic doses, cardiac glycosides inhibit the enzyme Na^+, K^+-ATPase, leading to increased intracellular levels of Na^+ and Ca^{2+} and decreased intracellular K^+ levels. Increased cytosolic Ca^{2+} enhances the excitation-contraction coupling of actin and myosin during systole and improves myocardial contractility. Electrophysiologic effects are due to indirect sympatholytic and vagotonic effects and to direct effects on cardiac muscle, pacemaker, and conduction cells (reduced action potential duration and AV node resting potential, prolongation of the refractory period). ECG manifestations include prolongation of the PR interval, shortening of the QT interval, scooping and depression of the ST segment, and decreased T-wave amplitude. In toxic doses, SA node automaticity and AV nodal conduction are decreased. Sympathetic tone; automaticity in muscle, AV nodal, and conduction cells; and afterdepolarizations are increased. ECG manifestations include bradydysrhythmias as well as triggered tachydysrhythmias. Hypokalemia potentiates the electrophysiologic effects of cardiac glycosides, increases their tissue binding, and decreases their renal excretion. Magnesium blocks calcium channels and modulates their sympathetic effects, whereas calcium and hypoxia enhance their activity.

Digoxin is absorbed and distributed slowly. Serum levels may not correlate with clinical effect for up to 8 h following a dose. Digoxin is 25 to 30% protein bound in the plasma, has a large volume of distribution of 5 to 6 L/kg body weight, and is eliminated primarily by renal excretion. The half-life ranges between 36 and 45 h, is prolonged in hepatic failure and in renal failure, and may be shortened in overdose. Therapeutic serum concentrations range from 0.6 to 2.5 nmol/L (0.5 to 2.0 ng/mL).

Clinical Toxicity Symptoms include vomiting, confusion, delirium, and occasionally hallucinations, blurred vision, photophobia, scotomata, and chromotopsia (disturbed color perception). Cardiac manifestations include sinus arrhythmia, sinus bradycardia, and all degrees of AV block. Premature ventricular contractions, bigeminy, ventricular tachycardia, and fibrillation also occur. The combination of a supraventricular tachyarrhythmia and AV block (e.g., paroxysmal atrial tachycardia with second-degree AV block, atrial fibrillation with third-degree AV block) or the presence of bidirectional ventricular tachycardia is highly suggestive of cardiac glycoside poisoning. Bradyarrhythmias and hypokalemia are common with chronic intoxication, whereas tachyarrhythmias and hyperkalemia are generally seen with acute poisoning. Similarly, serum digoxin levels may be minimally elevated or even therapeutic in chronic toxicity, whereas they are usually markedly elevated following acute overdose. Since chronic poisoning occurs almost exclusively in patients with underlying heart disease, the incidence, variety, and severity of dysrhythmias tend to be greater than with acute poisoning. In patients taking digoxin, poisoning should be suspected when a normal or fast heart rate becomes slow or the rhythm becomes regularly irregular.

Diagnosis The diagnosis is confirmed by measuring the serum digoxin level. Levels must be interpreted with respect to the time of the last dose. Digoxin assays may cross-react with nondigoxin glycosides and produce a false-positive result. Toxicology screening tests do not detect cardiac glycosides.

℞ **TREATMENT** Activated charcoal is preferred for gastrointestinal decontamination. Emesis and gastric intubation may cause vagal stimulation and precipitate or worsen conduction disturbances. Repeated doses of charcoal can enhance the elimination of digoxin. Potassium, magnesium, and calcium abnormalities and hypoxia should be corrected. Sinus bradycardia and second- and third-degree heart block resulting in hypotension can be treated with atropine, dopamine, epinephrine, and possible phenytoin (100 mg intravenously every 5 min up to 15 mg/kg) and isoproterenol. Magnesium sulfate (as for antiarrhythmic poisoning), phenytoin, lidocaine, bretylium, and amiodarone may be given for ventricular tachyarrhythmias. Antidotal therapy with digoxin-specific Fab-fragment antibodies should be administered for potentially life-threatening dysrhythmias. A serum potassium level ≥5.5 meq/L following acute overdose is associated with severe poisoning and is an indication for antibody therapy in the absence of dysrhythmias. Electrical pacing may be necessary as a temporizing measure. Prophylactic pacing is not recommended, as the pacing wire may increase ventricular irritability and precipitate tachydysrhythmias. If defibrillation is necessary, a low energy level (e.g., 50 W·s) should be used initially as the electrical shock may precipitate arrhythmias, which are more malignant and refractory to treatment. Digoxin-specific Fab-fragment antibodies are given intravenously over 15 to 30 min, unless cardiac arrest has occurred, in which case the solution is given as a bolus. Effects are usually apparent within an hour. The drug-antibody complex is excreted in the urine with a half-life of 16 to 20 h. In patients with renal failure, the drug-antibody complex is metabolized over a period of days to weeks. Although free digoxin levels decrease rapidly to zero following antibody administration, routine methods used to measure digoxin do not differentiate between bound and unbound drug, so that drug levels do not correlate with toxicity after antibody therapy.

Each vial (40 mg) of digoxin antibody fragments can neutralize 0.6 mg of digoxin. Formulas and tables for calculating the dose of antibody are available in the package insert. Unfortunately, toxicity may occur before distribution is complete or before levels are available. In addition, the amount of an acute overdose may be unknown, and calculated doses often exceed the effective dose (leading to costly overtreatment). The following empirical dosing guidelines are therefore offered. With chronic intoxication, the total-body drug load and serum drug levels only slightly exceed therapeutic amounts, patients may be dependent on inotropic effects, and a dose of 1 to 4 vials is usually effective. In acute poisoning, drug load is generally quite high, and 5 to 15 vials are usually required. Initial doses can be on the low side and repeated as necessary. Antibodies cross-react with other cardiac glycosides, but larger doses may be needed for toxicity not involving digoxin.

CYANIDE Cyanide salts are used in photography, metallurgy, electroplating, metal cleaning, and ore refining. Hydrogen cyanide gas, which is used as a fumigant rodenticide and in chemical syntheses, is liberated when they are combined with acids. Cyanide is also produced during the decomposition and metabolism of nitroprusside. Organic cyanides (nitriles) are used in making rubber, in artificial nail removers, and as rodenticides. Cyanogenic glycosides are present in the seeds of the chokeberry, cherry, plum, peach, apricot, pear, bean, apple, and crabapple.

Cyanide inhibits mitochondrial cytochrome oxidase, thereby blocking electron transport and preventing oxygen utilization and oxidative metabolism. Lactic acidosis occurs as a consequence of anaerobic metabolism. Cyanide is rapidly absorbed from the stomach, lungs, mucosal surfaces, and unbroken skin. Ingested salts react with gastric hydrochloric acid to form hydrocyanic acid, which is then absorbed. A dose of 200 mg of potassium or sodium cyanide, or 50 mg of hydrocyanic acid, is potentially lethal. Cyanide is 60% protein bound, concentrated in red cells, and has a volume of distribution of 1.5 L/kg body weight. Mitochondrial rhodanase mediates the transfer of sulfur from thiosulfate to the cyanide ion and converts it to less toxic thiocyanate, which is excreted in the urine. Cyanide poisoning during nitroprusside therapy can be prevented by the prophylactic administration of thiosulfate.

Clinical Toxicity Effects begin within seconds of inhalation and within 30 min of ingestion. Initial manifestations of cyanide poisoning include a burning sensation in the mouth and throat, agitation, anxiety, faintness, headache, nausea, vomiting, diaphoresis, dyspnea, tachycardia, and hypertension. A bitter almond odor may be detected on the breath. Later effects include coma, convulsions, opisthotonus, trismus, paralysis, respiratory depression, pulmonary edema, arrhythmias, bradycardia, and hypotension. A rough correlation exists between blood cyanide levels and symptoms: Levels <8 μmol/L (0.02 mg/L) are associated with no symptoms; 20 to 40 μmol/L (0.05 to 0.1 mg/dL) with flushing and tachycardia; 40 to 100 μmol/L (0.1 to 0.25 mg/dL) with obtundation; 100 to 200 μmol/L (0.25 to 0.3 mg/dL) with coma and respiratory depression; and levels >120 μmol/L (0.3 mg/dL) with death. With significant poisoning, lactic acidosis is invariably present. ECG abnormalities include both tachyarrhythmias and bradyarrhythmias.

Diagnosis The diagnosis is based on the history and physical examination. Although measurement of the whole-blood cyanide level will confirm the diagnosis, cyanide assays are not routinely available and treatment decisions must be based on clinical findings. Lactate levels have been used as a surrogate marker.

℞ **TREATMENT** Management involves supportive therapy, gastrointestinal decontamination, high-dose oxygen, and antidotal therapy with amyl nitrite, sodium nitrite, and sodium thiosulfate (the Lilly cyanide antidote kit). Nitrites convert hemoglobin to methemoglobin, which has a higher affinity for cyanide than does cytochrome oxidase and thus promotes its dissociation from this enzyme. Thiosulfate reacts with cyanide, which is slowly released from cyanomethemoglobin, to form thiocyanate. Oxygen reverses the binding of cyanide to cytochrome oxidase sites and enhances the efficacy of sodium nitrite and sodium thiosulfate, in addition to acting as a substrate for metabolism.

Indications for antidotal therapy include altered mental status, abnormal vital signs, and metabolic acidosis. Amyl nitrite, administered for 30 s of each minute and using a fresh ampule every 3 min, is a first-aid measure and is omitted when intravenous sodium nitrite is available or the patient has been intubated. The ampule is broken between two pads of gauze and placed over the airway while the patient breathes spontaneously or is ventilated by a bag-mask unit. Sodium nitrite is administered as a 3% solution at a dose of 10 to 15 mL (300 to 450 mg) over 1 to 2 min. Sodium thiosulfate is also administered intravenously, as a 25% solution at a dose of 50 mL (12.5 g) given over 1 to 2 min. With recurrent or persistent symptoms, doses of sodium nitrite and sodium thiosulfate can be repeated. Hyperbaric oxygen therapy should be considered in patients who fail to respond to antidotal therapy. Hydroxycobalamin, a vitamin B_{12} precursor that also binds cyanide ion, is an alternative antidote that is not yet widely available.

CYCLIC ANTIDEPRESSANTS Tricyclic antidepressants (TCAs) such as amitriptyline, imipramine (and their respective active metabolites nortriptyline and desipramine), chlomipramine, doxepin, protriptyline, and trimipramine and polycyclic agents such as amoxapine, bupropion, maprotiline, mirtazepine, and trazodone (and its metabolite nefazodone) act primarily by blocking the presynaptic reuptake monoamine neurotransmitters in the CNS, most importantly norepinephrine and serotonin, but also dopamine. They also have anticholinergic, α-adrenergic receptor blocking, and quinidine-like (class IA antiarrhythmic) effects as well as variable and selective blocking activity at histamine and monoamine receptors. Bupropion, nefazodone, and trazodone have serotonin agonist activity. Selective serotonin reuptake inhibitors (SSRIs) such as fluoxetine, paroxetine, sertaline, citalopram, and fluvoxamine can enhance the presynaptic release of serotonin and block its receptors in addition to inhibiting its reuptake. The nonselective serotonin reuptake inhibitors such as venlafaxine also inhibit norepinephrine reuptake.

Cyclic antidepressants are well absorbed. Peak serum levels usually occur within 2 to 6 h of ingestion but can sometimes occur later. These agents exhibit high (about 95%) protein binding in the plasma, have large volumes of distribution (20 to 45 L/kg body weight), and are eliminated mainly by hepatic metabolism, with half-lives of 24 h or more.

Clinical Toxicity Effects generally develop within 30 min of ingestion and peak within 6 h. Following low overdosage (about 10 mg/kg) of TCAs, anticholinergic effects predominate (see "Anticholinergic Agents," above). With larger doses, marked CNS depression (Table 396-2), cardiotoxicity, seizures, and hypotension occur. Ventricular tachyarrhythmias, atrioventricular and intraventricular conduction delays, terminal bradycardia, decreased cardiac output, and pulmonary edema may be seen. Death can occur within 6 h of ingestion from cardiovascular effects or much later from multiple organ failure or pulmonary complications. Terminal (last 40 ms) QRS right-axis deviation, an R wave greater than the S wave or >3 mm in lead aV_R, and prolongation of the QRS complex (>100 ms) of the ECG are sensitive indicators of TCA cardiotoxicity. Increasing duration of the QRS complex correlates with an increased risk of cardiac arrhythmias and seizures.

Although seizures can occur, CNS depression is typically mild with SSRIs and moderate with the polycyclic agents. Sinus tachycardia is common, but life-threatening cardiovascular effects are virtually nonexistent. An exception is trazodone, which can cause QT-interval prolongation and ventricular tachycardia. The serotonin syndrome (discussed separately) is also a potential complication of SSRI overdose.

Diagnosis The diagnosis is supported by the presence of these drugs in the urine on comprehensive screening tests. TCA serum levels are diagnostic and generally correlate with severity. Serum levels of active metabolites should be summed with that of the parent compound when estimating the serum concentration. Levels $\leq$1000 nmol/L (300 ng/mL) are therapeutic. Levels $>$3300 nmol/L (1000 ng/mL) are associated with severe poisoning.

℞ **TREATMENT** Activated charcoal is the preferred method of gastrointestinal decontamination. Repeated doses may enhance the elimination of some agents. Physostigmine (see "Anticholinergic Agents," above) can reverse anticholinergic effects due to low-dose TCA poisoning and may be used if the ECG is normal and deterioration has been excluded by a suitable period of observation. For other toxicity, treatment includes support of respiration and volume expansion and norepinephrine or high-dose dopamine for hypotension. Seizures should be treated with benzodiazepines and barbiturates. Phenytoin is of uncertain benefit. Acidemia increases the likelihood of arrhythmias and should be corrected. Sodium bicarbonate should be given as a bolus following a seizure and as an infusion to maintain a serum pH of 7.45 to 7.50 in patients with QRS prolongation. Treatment of ventricular tachyarrhythmias is similar to that described for antiarrhythmic agents and should include sodium bicarbonate. Phenytoin is often recommended, but its efficacy is not established. β-Adrenergic blockers and class IA, IC, and III antiarrhythmics should be avoided. Cardiac pacing and invasive hemodynamic support may be necessary for severe cardiovascular depression.

ETHYLENE GLYCOL Ethylene glycol is a colorless, odorless, sweet-tasting, water-soluble liquid used as a solvent for paints, plastics, and pharmaceuticals; in the manufacture of explosives, fire extinguishers, and foams; and as an ingredient in hydraulic fluids, windshield cleaners, radiator antifreeze, and de-icer solutions.

Ethylene glycol produces intoxication similar to that caused by ethanol but is more potent. Peak blood levels occur approximately 2 h after ingestion. The volume of distribution is 0.6 to 0.8 L/kg body weight. Ethylene glycol is oxidized by alcohol dehydrogenase to glycoaldehyde, which is metabolized successively to glycolic acid, glyoxylic acid, and oxalic acid. Pyridoxine and thiamine are cofactors in degradation pathways. As much as 20% is excreted unchanged in the urine. The half-life ranges from 3 to 8 h. Metabolites, primarily glycolic acid, cause CNS depression, metabolic acidosis with an increased anion gap, and interstitial and tubular damage to the kidney. Oxalic acid may precipitate as calcium oxalate in the brain, heart, kidney, lung, pancreas, and urine and cause hypocalcemia.

Ethanol and fomepizole bind to alcohol dehydrogenase with a higher affinity than ethylene glycol and hence block the production of toxic metabolites. Ethanol is metabolized by alcohol dehydrogenase, but fomepizole is not. Ethanol and fomepizole prolong the half-life of ethylene glycol to 15 to 20 h.

Clinical Toxicity As little as 120 mg/kg body weight or 0.1 mL/kg body weight (one swallow) of pure ethylene glycol can result in a potentially toxic serum concentration of 3 mmol/L (20 mg/dL). Effects begin about 30 min after ingestion and include nausea, vomiting, slurred speech, ataxia, nystagmus, and lethargy. A faint, sweet aromatic odor may be detected on the breath, and the serum osmolality may be elevated. Effects caused by metabolites begin 3 to 12 h after ingestion (longer if ethanol has also been ingested) and include tachypnea, agitation, confusion, lethargy, back pain, hypotension, coma, and seizures. In severe cases, ARDS, cyanosis, pulmonary edema, and cardiomegaly may be seen. Laboratory findings include metabolic acidosis, an increased anion gap (low bicarbonate and chloride), hypocalcemia, leukocytosis, increased BUN and creatinine, calcium oxalate crystalluria, and proteinuria. Acute tubular necrosis with oliguria or anuria typically becomes evident 12 to 24 h following ingestion. Renal failure is usually reversible but may last days to weeks.

Diagnostic Evaluation The diagnosis is established by measuring serum ethylene glycol and glycolate levels. The diagnosis is suggested by an elevated serum osmolality and ethanol-like effects soon after ingestion and by an increased anion-gap metabolic acidosis and crystalluria later on. If laboratory confirmation is not immediately available, the osmolal gap can also be used to estimate the serum ethylene glycol concentration (Table 396-3).

℞ **TREATMENT** Gastric aspiration is the decontamination procedure of choice. Activated charcoal should also be administered. Supportive measures include protection of the airway, ventilatory and circulatory support, and anticonvulsants for seizures. Metabolic acidosis will not resolve spontaneously and should be corrected with sodium bicarbonate; large doses may be required. Sodium bicarbonate should also be given to alkalinize the urine as this will enhance the excretion of acid metabolites. Fluids and diuretics can be used to treat oliguria but they do not increase the excretion of ethylene glycol. Hypocalcemia is treated with intravenous calcium salts. Supplemental pyridoxine (50 mg qid) and thiamine (100 mg qid) may be beneficial.

Indications for ethanol or fomepizole therapy include an ethylene glycol concentration >3 mmol/L (20 mg/dL); an elevated osmolal gap, an increased anion-gap metabolic acidosis, back pain, laboratory evidence of renal toxicity, or ethanol-like intoxication in a patient with a history of ethylene glycol ingestion and a low or undetectable ethanol level; an elevated osmolal gap not accounted for by the presence of ethanol, isopropyl alcohol, acetone, or propylene glycol in a patient with ethanol-like intoxication; and an increased anion-gap metabolic acidosis with a low lactate level not explained by alcoholic or diabetic ketoacidosis, uremia, or salicylate, formaldehyde, paraldehyde, or toluene exposure. A serum ethanol level of ≥20 mmol/L (100 mg/dL) is required to inhibit the metabolism of ethylene glycol (higher levels may be needed with very high ethylene glycol concentrations). The loading dose of ethanol is 10 mL/kg of 10% ethanol intravenously or 1 mL/kg of 95% ethanol by mouth; the maintenance dose is 1.5 mL/kg per hour of 10% ethanol intravenously or 3 mL/kg per hour of 10% ethanol intravenously during hemodialysis. Maintaining a therapeutic concentration is often difficult; levels must be monitored frequently and the dose adjusted as necessary. Ethanol induces its own metabolism and progressively higher doses may be required as time passes. Fomepizole is diluted in 100 mL of intravenous fluid and administered over 30 min in a loading dose of 15 mg/kg followed by 10 mg/kg every 12 h for four doses and 15 mg/kg thereafter. Additional doses are required in patients undergoing dialysis. Although expensive (about $1000 U.S. per 1.5-g vial), fomepizole has a number of advantages over ethanol: it does not cause CNS depression, hypoglycemia, or fluid, electrolyte, and serum osmolality derangements; it has a longer duration of action; and does not require monitoring of serum drug levels. Although seizures have occurred after fomepizole, their etiology is unclear, and side effects have generally been limited to headache, nausea, dizziness, rash, eosinophilia, and mild self-limited hepatotoxicity. Serum ethylene glycol concentrations should be monitored frequently. Ethanol or fomepizole should be continued until the ethylene glycol level falls below 1.5 mmol/L (10 mg/dL).

Hemodialysis enhances the elimination of ethylene glycol and its toxic metabolites so that it is complete in about 3 h. Indications for hemodialysis include an ethylene glycol concentration >8 mmol/L (50 mg/dL) and metabolic acidosis not readily correctable with bicarbonate and antidotal therapy, lack of clinical improvement despite treatment, and laboratory evidence of renal toxicity (regardless of the ethylene glycol level). This therapy should be continued (repeated intermittently) until acidemia resolves and the ethylene glycol level is <3 mmol/L (20 mg/dL).

HYDROCARBONS Aromatic hydrocarbons, such as xylene and toluene, halogenated hydrocarbons, such as carbon tetrachloride and trichloroethane, and petroleum distillate hydrocarbons, such as gasoline, lacquer thinner, mineral seal oil, kerosene, and lighter fluid, are CNS depressants and gastrointestinal and respiratory tract irritants. They are absorbed rapidly following inhalation or pulmonary aspiration. Aromatic and halogenated hydrocarbons are also absorbed following ingestion and are toxic to the heart, liver, and kidneys. Aromatic hydrocarbons can cause bone marrow suppression and skeletal muscle damage. Petroleum distillate hydrocarbons are poorly absorbed following ingestion.

Clinical Toxicity Hydrocarbons produce CNS excitation in low doses and depression in high doses. Rarely, coma and seizures occur. Psychosis, cerebral and cerebellar atrophy, encephalopathy, and peripheral neuropathy can result from chronic inhalation. Other effects include nausea, vomiting, abdominal pain, hepatitis, renal tubular acidosis, acute hepatic or renal failure, and rhabdomyolysis. Sudden death due to myocardial irritability and ventricular fibrillation may occur following hydrocarbon sniffing. After ingestion, hydrocarbons cause burning of the mouth and throat with subsequent nausea, vomiting, and diarrhea. Aspiration into the lungs may occur with ingestion or as a result of vomiting and cause pneumonia. Following aspiration, chest x-ray abnormalities include infiltrates, atelectasis, effusions, pneumothorax, and pneumatoceles. Renal tubular acidosis with decreased serum bicarbonate, calcium, phosphate, and potassium and increased serum chloride may result from chronic aromatic hydrocarbon inhalation.

Diagnosis The diagnosis is based on the clinical presentation. Assays for hydrocarbons are not routinely available.

℞ TREATMENT The ingestion of aromatic and halogenated hydrocarbons requires prompt gastric lavage. More than one episode of ipecac-induced emesis is contraindicated, and the role of activated charcoal is controversial. Since the ingestion of other types of hydrocarbons is unlikely to result in systemic toxicity and since the risk of aspiration during gastric decontamination is greater than the potential benefit, decontamination is contraindicated for these ingestions. Supportive therapy includes oxygen, respiratory support, and monitoring of liver, renal, and myocardial function. Metabolic abnormalities should be corrected, and patients with aspiration pneumonitis should be monitored for superimposed bacterial infection. Glucocorticoids are ineffective.

HYDROGEN SULFIDE Hydrogen sulfide is a rapidly acting, malodorous ("rotten eggs"), colorless, irritating gas. It is encountered in the petroleum and mining industries, tanning of leather, vulcanization of rubber, the production of synthetic fabrics, metal refining, the production of heavy water for atomic reactors, and glue and felt manufacturing. It is also found in sewers, sulfur springs, and the holds of fishing vessels and as a byproduct of manure storage.

Sulfide anion inhibits electron transport in the cytochrome oxidase system, thereby inhibiting aerobic metabolism with resultant cellular anoxia and lactic acidosis. Hydrogen sulfide is rapidly detoxified by oxidation to sulfate products, which are excreted by the kidneys.

Clinical Toxicity Exposure to low concentrations of hydrogen sulfide results in rhinitis, conjunctivitis, and pharyngitis. Inhalation of large amounts causes headache, vertigo, nausea, vomiting, confusion, seizures, and coma. Hypoventilation, hypoxia, cyanosis, metabolic acidosis, pneumonia, and pulmonary edema can occur.

Diagnosis The diagnosis is based on the characteristic clinical features, including the characteristic odor, exposure setting, and rapidity of onset. Sulfide levels have been used to confirm the diagnosis but are not routinely available.

℞ TREATMENT Treatment includes prompt removal of the victim from the site of exposure, assisted ventilation, and 100% oxygen. Although controversial, amyl and sodium nitrite, in the same dose as for cyanide poisoning, should be considered for patients with coma or cardiac arrest who fail to respond to oxygen therapy. Nitrites promote the dissociation of sulfide ions from cytochrome oxidase by providing an alternative binding site (methemoglobin). They also enhance detoxification by acting as a catalyst for sulfide oxidation. Hyperbaric oxygen should be considered in patients who do not respond to the preceding measures.

IRON Non-transferring-bound plasma iron catalyzes the formation of free radicals, which then cause mitochondrial injury, lipid peroxidation, increased capillary permeability, vasodilation, and intestinal, renal, hepatic, myocardial, and pulmonary toxicity. Ingestion of 20 mg/kg body weight of elemental iron typically produces gastrointestinal symptoms, and 60 mg/kg body weight may cause systemic toxicity. Ferrous sulfate, fumarate, gluconate, and succinate contains 20, 33, 12, and 35% elemental iron, respectively.

Ferrous iron is absorbed by duodenal and jejunal cells, oxidized to ferric iron, and bound to ferritin. It is then slowly released, binds to plasma transferrin (an iron-specific globulin) and other proteins, and is transported to tissues. Serum iron levels usually peak 4 to 6 h after overdosage (later for delayed-release formulations). Iron bound to transferrin is nontoxic.

Clinical Toxicity Initial manifestations include vomiting and diarrhea (often bloody). X-rays may reveal iron tablets in the stomach or small bowel. Systemic effects include lethargy, hypotension, and metabolic acidosis. Seizures, coma, pulmonary edema, and vascular collapse may occur with severe poisoning. Jaundice, elevated hepatic enzyme levels, prolongation of prothrombin time, and hyperammonemia are indicative of liver injury. Proteinuria and cells in the urine indicate renal injury. In the recovering patient, gastric ulcerations and scars may cause outlet obstruction. Overgrowth of *Yersinia enterocolitica* with sepsis is a rare complication of iron overload.

Diagnosis The diagnosis is primarily based on clinical findings. A serum iron concentration >50 μmol/L (300 μg/dL) is potentially toxic. A positive x-ray, fever >38.5°C, hyperglycemia >8.5 mmol/L (150 mg/dL), and leukocytosis (white blood cell count >15,000/μL) have also been associated with potential toxicity. Serious poisoning is generally associated with levels >80 μmol/L (500 μg/dL). A positive urine deferoxamine provocative challenge test (see below) is also diagnostic.

℞ TREATMENT Gastric lavage and whole-bowel irrigation are the preferred methods of gastrointestinal decontamination. When iron tablets are visible on x-ray, serial films can be used to assess their success. Endoscopic removal and gastrostomy may be necessary when these procedures are ineffective (e.g., large ingestions, concretions). Complexation of ingested iron with orally administered activated charcoal, bicarbonate, phosphate, deferoxamine, or magnesium hydroxide has not been shown to reduce toxicity.

Intravenous sodium bicarbonate should be used to correct metabolic acidosis. Nearly all patients are volume depleted and should be given intravenous crystalloid. Coagulation abnormalities should be treated with vitamin K or blood products.

Parenteral deferoxamine should be given to patients with elevated serum iron levels or clinical manifestations of poisoning. If the iron level is mildly elevated or not immediately available or if the patient has mild clinical toxicity, an intravenous challenge dose of 15 mg/kg per hour can be given. Urine becomes a vin rosé or rusty orange color in the presence of the iron-deferoxamine complex (ferrioxamine), indicating that free iron is present. Patients with a positive challenge test or significant clinical toxicity should be given intravenous deferoxamine at a rate of 10 to 15 mg/kg per hour. When iron levels exceed 180 μmol/L (1000 μg/dL), larger deferoxamine doses (up to 30 mg/kg per hour) can be given initially. Once the patient is asymptomatic or improved, deferoxamine therapy should be discontinued. Rapid infusion of deferoxamine can cause hypotension. Pulmonary edema is a complication of prolonged, high-dose therapy, and renal failure can occur if it is administered to hypovolemic patients. Exchange transfusion or plasmapheresis should be reserved for patients with renal failure or who fail to respond to the preceding therapy.

ISONIAZID Toxic doses of isoniazid decrease the synthesis of the inhibitory CNS neurotransmitter GABA by interfering with the activation and supply of pyridoxal-5-phosphate, a cofactor for the enzyme glutamic acid decarboxylase, which converts glutamic acid to GABA. Isoniazid also causes pyridoxine depletion by complexing with pyridoxine to form hydrazides that are then excreted, and it forms hydrazones that inhibit the production and activity of pyridoxal phosphate enzymes. The resultant decrease in GABA can cause seizures with increased lactate production by muscle. Since isoniazid also inhibits the metabolism of lactate to pyruvate, profound and intractable lactic acid acidosis may ensue.

Isoniazid is rapidly absorbed, with peak serum concentrations noted within 1 to 2 h. The volume of distribution is approximately 0.7 L/kg body weight. Serum protein binding is slight. Elimination is primarily by hepatic acetylation to acetylisoniazid followed by hydrolysis to isonicotinic acid. The rate of acetylation is genetically determined and characterized as either slow or fast with corresponding half-lives of 0.5 to 1.5 and 2 to 4 h.

Clinical Toxicity Nausea, vomiting, dizziness, slurred speech, lethargy, and confusion begin within 30 min of ingestion of doses greater than 20 mg/kg body weight. Severe poisoning results in coma, respiratory depression, generalized seizures, and lactic acid acidosis. Seizures may be protracted and relatively unresponsive to standard anticonvulsant therapy. Acidosis does not occur when seizures are prevented.

Diagnosis The diagnosis is primarily based on clinical findings. It can be confirmed by measuring isoniazid in blood, but isoniazid assays are not routinely available. Urine screening tests do not detect the drug.

℞ TREATMENT Activated charcoal adsorbs isoniazid quite well and is the preferred method of gastrointestinal decontamination. Ipecac-induced vomiting should be avoided because of the potential for rapid deterioration with coma and seizures. Seizures are sometimes responsive to benzodiazepines and barbiturates, but pyridoxine (vitamin B_6), which reverses isoniazid-induced enzyme inhibition, is often also necessary. Diazepam and pyridoxine are synergistic. Bicarbonate may be necessary to correct acidosis. Intravenous pyridoxine is given intravenously (over 5 min in patients with seizures and over 30 min in those without) in an amount equal to the ingested dose of isoniazid. When the ingested dose is not known, 5 g of pyridoxine should be administered. Seizures are usually promptly controlled, but the patient may not awake for several hours. The dose may be repeated if the response is partial or if symptoms recur. Saline diuresis enhances the excretion of isoniazid, and the drug is efficiently removed by hemodialysis. Because pyridoxine therapy is highly effective, these procedures are rarely necessary.

ISOPROPYL ALCOHOL AND ACETONE Isopropyl alcohol is a component of rubbing alcohol, solvents, aftershave solutions, antifreeze, and window cleaners. Acetone is found in cleaners, solvents, and nail polish removers. Both are absorbed rapidly from the stomach and the lungs and distributed in body water with volumes of distribution of about 0.6 L/kg body weight. Isopropyl alcohol is metabolized to acetone in the liver by the enzyme alcohol dehydrogenase. Up to 20% is excreted unchanged in urine. Its half-life ranges from 3 to 6 h. Acetone is excreted by the kidneys and lungs with a half-life of 20 to 30 h. Isopropyl alcohol and acetone are CNS depressants and have about twice the potency of ethanol.

Clinical Toxicity Effects begin within 30 min of ingestion and include vomiting, abdominal discomfort, and sometimes hematemesis as well as headache, dizziness, and ethanol-like intoxication. Obtundation, coma, respiratory depression, hypothermia, and hypotension may be seen with severe poisoning. Their characteristic odors may be detected on the breath or gastric contents. Both hypoglycemia and hyperglycemia can occur. Increased serum osmolality, mild ketoacidosis, and a falsely elevated serum creatinine with a normal BUN (due to the interference with creatinine assays by acetone) may be present.

Diagnosis Characteristic clinical and laboratory findings suggest the diagnosis. Direct measurement of serum levels will confirm it. Routine urine screening tests do not detect these agents. If laboratory confirmation is not readily available, the osmolal gap can be used to estimate the serum concentration (Table 396-3).

℞ TREATMENT Gastric aspiration is the preferred method of gastrointestinal decontamination. Activated charcoal is ineffective. Intravenous fluids and possibly bicarbonate should be given for dehydration, hypotension, and acidosis. Ventilatory support may be necessary. Hemodialysis is effective for removing isopropyl alcohol and acetone and should be considered in patients with high serum levels who do not respond to conservative therapy.

LITHIUM Lithium, an alkali metal like sodium and potassium, appears to act by substituting for endogenous cations, thereby intefering with cell membrane ion transport and excitability, adenylate cyclase activation, neurotransmitter (norepinephrine) release, and Na^+, K^+-ATPase activity. It is available as the carbonate salt in pill form and as the liquid citrate salt. These preparations contain 8 mmol (meq) of lithium per 300 mg and 5 mL, respectively.

Lithium is absorbed slowly, with peak serum levels occurring 2 to 4 h after ingestion (later with overdosage and with sustained-release preparations). Lithium is not bound to plasma proteins. It has an initial volume of distribution of 0.3 to 0.4 L/kg body weight and a final one of 0.7 to 1 L/kg. Therapeutic serum levels are 0.6 to 1.2 mmol/L. An increase in the postdistribution lithium level of 1 to 1.5 mmol/L for each mmol/kg ingested can be predicted following acute overdose. Levels obtained prior to complete distribution will be higher than those in tissue and not correlate with clinical effects. Elimination is primarily (95%) by renal excretion (glomerular filtration with significant reabsorption in the proximal tubule). Renal excretion is increased by diuresis and urinary alkalinization and decreased by hypovolemia and hyponatremia. The serum half-life ranges from 18 to 36 h and can be prolonged in patients with chronic intoxication.

Clinical Toxicity Effects begin 1 to 4 h after acute ingestion. Onset can be delayed following overdose of sustained-release preparations. It typically occurs insidiously during chronic therapy, often resulting from an intercurrent illness that causes dehydration and decreased lithium elimination. Gastrointestinal effects include nausea, vomiting, and diarrhea; neuromuscular effects include weakness, confusion, ataxia, tremors, fasciculations, myoclonus, choreoathetosis, coma, and seizures; and cardiovascular effects include arrhythmias and hypotension. Hyperthermia can occur. Leukocytosis, hyperglycemia, albuminuria, glycosuria, nephrogenic diabetes insipidus, and a falsely elevated serum chloride level (due to interference by lithium with its assays) resulting in a low anion-gap may be present. ECG changes include sinus tachycardia or bradycardia, flattened or inverted T waves, AV block, and a prolonged QT interval. Prolonged or permanent encephalopathy and movement disorders can occur in patients with severe poisoning.

Diagnosis Since lithium is not detected by routine screening tests, a serum level must be requested specifically. Because of slow absorption and distribution, serial drug levels should be obtained following acute overdosage. In chronic poisoning, severe toxicity may occur at serum levels of 3 to 4 mmol/L. Following acute overdose, only mild effects may be present despite serum levels that rise to $\geq$8 mmol/L. As distribution occurs and levels fall, progressive toxicity may ensue.

℞ TREATMENT Gastric lavage and whole-bowel irrigation are the procedures of choice for gastrointestinal decontamination. Whole-bowel irrigation is preferred for sustained-release formulations because intact pills will not fit through a lavage tube. Endoscopy should be considered if a concretion is suspected (persistently high or rising drug levels 2 or more days following ingestion). Activated charcoal does not adsorb lithium. Experimentally, oral administration of the ion-exchange resin sodium polystyrene sulfonate (Kayexalate) can bind lithium, prevent its absorption, and enhance its elimination, but the clinical effectiveness of this therapy is unproven. Supportive therapy includes standard treatments for seizures, CNS depression, hypotension, and arrhythmias. Symptomatic patients should be given an intravenous saline bolus and infusion to correct dehydration, to achieve a normal urine output, and to replace fluid losses in those with diabetes insipidus. Although diuresis can enhance renal excretion of lithium, there is little evidence that this therapy is more effective than simply maintaining a normal urine output. Hemodialysis, however, is highly effective in enhancing lithium elimination. It is recommended for patients with coma, seizures, and severe, persistent or progressive confusion, CNS depression, or movement disorders; lesser toxicity in the presence of renal failure; and when the peak lithium level exceeds 8 mmol/L following acute overdose (because of the likelihood of severe postdistribution toxicity). Because of slow redistribution, drug levels typically rise following dialysis. Dialysis should be repeated until the postredistribution level is <1 mmol/L. Despite dialysis, clinical recovery may take days to weeks. There is no conclusive evidence that dialysis decreases the incidence of permanent sequelae.

METHANOL Methanol is a component of shellacs, varnishes, paint removers, canned fuel (Sterno), windshield-washer solutions, and copy machine fluid. It is also used to denature ethanol and render it unfit for consumption. It is a CNS depressant with a potency about half of that of ethanol. Methanol is initially metabolized by alcohol dehydrogenase to formaldehyde, with subsequent oxidation to formic acid, and then to carbon dioxide and water. Formic acid is responsible for metabolic acidosis and retinal toxicity. Its detoxification utilizes tetrahydrofolate as a cofactor.

Methanol is readily absorbed, with peak serum levels occurring 1 to 2 h after ingestion. It is distributed throughout body water, with a volume of distribution of 0.7 L/kg body weight. Protein binding is negligible. Elimination occurs mainly by hepatic metabolism, with up to 10% excreted unchanged by the lungs and kidneys. Elimination follows first-order kinetics, with a half-life of 2 to 4 h at low serum levels ($\leq$9 mmol/L or 30 mg/dL). At higher levels, it changes to zero-order kinetics, with an elimination rate of about 3 mmol/L per hour (10 mg/dL per hour) and an apparent half-life of up to 30 h. As with ethylene glycol, ethanol and fomepizole block the production of methanol metabolites, by competitively inhibiting alcohol dehydrogenase, and increase its elimination half-life to 30 to 60 h.

Clinical Toxicity As with ethylene glycol, as little as one swallow of pure methanol is potentially toxic. Effects begin within an hour of ingestion. Initial manifestations are caused by methanol itself and include nausea, vomiting (sometimes bloody), abdominal pain, headache, vertigo, and an ethanol-like intoxication. An increased osmolal gap may be present. Pancreatitis has been reported. Later effects are due to formic acid and include coma, seizures, an increased anion-gap metabolic acidosis, and retinal injury. Ophthalmologic manifestations occur 15 to 30 h after ingestion and include clouding and diminished vision, dancing and flashing spots, dilated or fixed pupils, hyperemia of optic disks, retinal edema, and blindness. These changes are potentially reversible with prompt institution of therapy. With severe poisoning, myocardial depression, bradycardia, and shock may occur.

Diagnosis The diagnosis is confirmed by measurement of serum methanol and formate levels. Early in the course, the diagnosis is suggested by ethanol-like intoxication and an elevated serum osmolality. Later, the diagnosis is suggested by an increased-anion-gap metabolic acidosis and visual complaints. If laboratory confirmation is not immediately available, the osmolal gap can also be used to estimate the serum methanol concentration (Table 396-3).

℞ TREATMENT Gastric aspiration is the treatment of choice for gastrointestinal decontamination. Supportive measures should include volume replacement, respiratory care, and treatment of seizures. Acidosis should be corrected with sodium bicarbonate; large amounts may be required. Sodium bicarbonate should also be given to alkalinize the urine as this will enhance the excretion of formic acid. Supplemental folate (50 mg qid) is recommended.

Indications for ethanol or fomepizole therapy include a methanol concentration >6 mmol/L (20 mg/dL); an elevated osmolal gap, an increased anion-gap metabolic acidosis, visual symptoms, or ethanol-like intoxication in a patient with a history of methanol ingestion and a low or undetectable ethanol level; an elevated osmolal gap not accounted for by the presence of ethanol, isopropyl alcohol, acetone, or propylene glycol in a patient with ethanol-like intoxication; and an increased anion-gap metabolic acidosis with a low lactate level not explained by alcoholic or diabetic ketoacidosis or uremia or by salicylate, formaldehyde, paraldehyde, or toluene exposure. Doses and treatment considerations are the same as for ethylene glycol. Serum methanol concentrations should be monitored frequently. Ethanol or fomepizole should be continued until the methanol level falls below 3 mmol/L (10 mg/dL).

Hemodialysis enhances the elimination of methanol and formic acid. Indications for hemodialysis include methanol levels >15 mmol/L (50 mg/dL) and metabolic acidosis not readily correctable with bicarbonate and antidotal therapy, lack of clinical improvement despite treatment, or visual symptoms (regardless of the methanol level). This therapy should be continued or repeated intermittently until acidemia resolves and the methanol level is <6 mmol/L (20 mg/dL).

METHEMOGLOBINEMIA Methemoglobinemia results from exposure to chemicals that oxidize the ferrous (Fe^{2+}) iron in hemoglobin to the ferric (Fe^{3+}) state. Concomitant oxidation of hemoglobin protein may cause its precipitation in erythrocytes and consequent hemolytic anemia, manifest as Heinz bodies and "bite cells," respectively, on peripheral blood smear. Oxidizing agents include aniline and its derivatives, aminophenols, aminophenones, chlorates, dapsone, local anesthetics (particularly benzocaine), nitrites, nitrates, naphthalene, nitrobenzene and related chemicals, oxides of nitrogen, phenazopyridine, primaquine and related antimalarials, and sulfonamides.

Methemoglobin (ferric hemoglobin) cannot carry oxygen and causes a functional anemia. It also shifts the oxygen-dissociation curve to the left, limiting the release of oxygen to tissues. Symptoms are due to hypoxia and anaerobic metabolism.

Various systems normally operate to keep methemoglobin at physiologic levels (1% of the total hemoglobin concentration). Oxidizing agents are inactivated by enzymes that utilize ascorbic acid and sulfhydryl agents such as glutathione. Methemoglobin is reduced to hemoglobin by NADH-methemoglobin reductase (responsible for 95% of baseline reducing capacity), NADPH-methemoglobin reductase, and the ascorbic acid and glutathione enzyme systems. When supplied with the cofactor methylene blue, the activity of NADPH-methemoglobin reductase is greatly increased. Because this enzyme is dependent on NADPH, individuals with glucose-6-phosphate dehydrogenase (G6PD) deficiency have profound impairment in the ability to reduce methemoglobin after oxidant exposure.

Clinical Toxicity Onset may be immediate or delayed depending on whether the parent compound or a metabolite is the oxidant. Cyanosis with a gray-brown hue that is unresponsive to oxygen occurs when the fraction of hemoglobin existing as methemoglobin exceeds 15% (about 15 g/L or 1.5 g/dL of absolute methemoglobin). Most patients are asymptomatic until the methemoglobin fraction is >20 to 30%, at which point fatigue, headache, tachycardia, dizziness, and weakness develop. At fractions >45%, dyspnea, bradycardia, hypoxia, metabolic (lactic) acidosis, seizures, coma, and cardiac arrhythmias may occur. Fractions >70% are rapidly fatal. Hemolytic anemia is typically delayed in onset and may cause hyperkalemia and renal failure.

Diagnosis The diagnosis is confirmed by measuring the methemoglobin level by CO-oximetry. If CO-oximetry is not available, the methemoglobin fraction can be estimated by the difference between the oxygen saturation calculated from the P_{O_2} and that measured directly. Oxygen saturation measured by pulse oximetry will be subnormal but either falsely depressed or elevated with respect to the true value. Blood with high levels of methemoglobin is chocolate-colored when placed on filter paper and compared with normal blood. Urine toxicology testing may detect the oxidizing agent.

℞ TREATMENT Activated charcoal is the preferred method of gastrointestinal decontamination. Supplemental oxygen should be administered. Methylene blue is indicated for methemoglobin fractions >30% and at lower fractions in patients with anemia or cardiovascular disease, particularly if manifestations of hypoxia or organ ischemia are present. Methylene blue is given at a dose of 1 to 2 mg/kg body weight as a 1% solution over 5 min. If a clinical response is not observed within 1 h, the dose may be repeated. As long as the oxidizing agent is present, methemoglobin will continue to be generated, and additional doses may be necessary. Side effects of methylene blue include anxiety, dysuria, precordial pain, and blue or green discoloration of the urine. It is contraindicated in patients with G6PD deficiency in whom it may induce hemolysis. In doses >7 mg/kg of body weight, methylene blue itself can cause methemoglobinemia. Exchange transfusion and hyperbaric oxygen therapy may be of benefit in patients with very high methemoglobin fractions or severe clinical toxicity that is refractory to the above and those with G6PD deficiency. Erythrocyte transfusion may be necessary if hemolysis is severe. Hemodialysis may be useful for removing the offending agent.

MONOAMINE OXIDASE INHIBITORS The antidepressants isocarboxazid, phenelzine, and tranylcypromine and the chemotherapeutic agent procarbazine irreversibly and nonselectively block monoamine oxidase (MAO) isoenzymes in the brain, gut, and liver, thus inhibiting the catabolism of endogenous MAO substrates such as epinephrine, dopamine, norepinephrine, and serotonin and exogenous ones such as ingested tyramine. Clorgyline and moclobemide selectively inhibit MAO-A, which preferentially deaminates serotonin, and pargyline and selegiline selectively inhibit MAO-B. Toxicity results from the accumulation and effects of MAO substrates. A tyramine reaction can occur when foods with high tyramine content such as aged cheese, aged, pickled, or smoked meat and fish, and red wine are ingested by individuals taking MAO inhibitors. Interactions with sympathomimetics can result in exaggerated sympathetic effects, and interactions with serotonergic agents can cause the serotonin syndrome (discussed subsequently).

MAO inhibitors are absorbed and appear to have relatively large volumes of distribution (>1 L/kg body weight). They are eliminated primarily by hepatic metabolism and have half-lives ranging from several hours to >24 h.

Clinical Toxicity Onset following overdose is typically delayed and insidious. Effects may not begin until 6 to 24 h after ingestion and progress slowly. Initial manifestations include dilated pupils, agitation, diaphoresis, tachycardia, hypertension, and tachypnea. Nausea and vomiting may also occur. Later, confusion, CNS depression, fasciculations, twitching, tremor, muscle rigidity, rhabdomyolysis, hyperthermia, and lactic acidosis may be noted. Terminal bradycardia and cardiovascular collapse may ensue.

Tyramine and sympathomimetic reactions occur within 30 to 90 min of food or drug ingestion and resolve within a few hours. Manifestations are similar to overdose. Reflex bradycardia, seizures, and intracranial hemorrhage have also been described.

Diagnosis The diagnosis is based on the history and clinical presentation. Serum assays are not available, and urine screening tests do not usually detect these agents.

℞ TREATMENT Activated charcoal is the preferred method of gastrointestinal decontamination. Benzodiazepines should be given for neuromuscular hyperactivity. Therapeutic paralysis is recommended for refractory or progressive neuromuscular hyperactivity, particularly if concomitant rhabdomyolysis and hyperthermia are present. The treatment of hyperthermia should include external cooling measures. Replacement of insensible fluid losses is also important. Severe hypertension and tachycardia should be treated with labetalol or nitroprusside and esmolol. Hypotension should first be treated with intravenous fluids and then with pressors. Pressors should initially be given at lower than normal doses because of the possibility of an exaggerated response. In fact, before any drug is given, potential interaction with MAO inhibitors should be investigated. Because MAO inhibition may persist for up to 2 weeks after discontinuing therapy, drug and dietary precautions should be maintained during this period.

MUSCLE RELAXANTS AND MISCELLANEOUS SEDATIVE-HYPNOTICS Muscle relaxants (baclofen, carisoprodol, chlorphenesin, chlorzoxazone, cyclobenzaprine, methocarbamol, and orphenadrine) and nonbarbiturate, nonbenzodiazepine sedative-hypnotics (buspirone, chloral hydrate, ethchlorvynol, glutethimide, meprobamate, methaqualone, methyprylon, zolpidem) including the street drugs γ-butyrolactone (GBL) and its metabolite γ-hydroxybutyrate (GHB) are primarily CNS depressants. Most interact with GABA receptor complexes, enhancing the effects of this inhibitory neurotransmitter. Some muscle relaxants also depress spinal synaptic reflexes. Cyclobenzaprine and orphenadrine have anticholinergic activity. Orphenadrine also has sodium channel blocking activity.

These agents are readily absorbed, with peak blood levels occurring 1 to 2 h after ingestion. They are eliminated primarily by hepatic metabolism. Baclofen, an exception, is largely excreted unchanged in the urine. Chloral hydrate is rapidly metabolized to trichloroethanol, an active compound with a much longer half-life than the parent drug. Carisoprodol is metabolized to meprobamate. Glutethimide also has an active metabolite. Half-lives are >20 h for cyclobenzaprine, ethchlorvynol, and methaqualone; 10 to 20 h for glutethimide, meprobamate, methyprylon, and orphenadrine; and <6 h for other agents.

Clinical Toxicity Effects begin within an hour of ingestion. All muscle relaxants cause CNS depression (Table 396-2). Nystagmus is usually present. Carisoprodol, chloral hydrate, chlorphenesin, chlorzoxazone, and methocarbamol also cause nausea and vomiting. Cyclobenzaprine and orphenadrine cause anticholinergic toxicity, and orphenadrine can cause ventricular tachyarrhythmias, including torsades de pointes. Baclofen can produce hypothermia, excitability, delirium, myoclonus, seizures, cardiac conduction abnormalities, tachycardia, bradycardia, and hypotension. Intrathecal baclofen overdose can lead to precipitous and profound effects. Supraventricular and ventricular tachycardia can occur in chloral hydrate poisoning. GBL and GHB can cause paradoxical agitation, seizures, miosis, and bradycardia in addition to CNS depression. The effects of GBL and GHB typically last only a few hours; the duration of toxicity from other agents is substantially longer. Coma from ethchlorvynol and glutethimide, which are highly lipophilic, and from meprobamate, which can form concretions, can last for several days. With glutethimide, erratic absorption can result in cyclic coma.

Diagnosis The clinical diagnosis is supported by detecting the drugs on comprehensive urine screening. Quantitative measurements of serum levels are not routinely available.

Rx TREATMENT Activated charcoal is preferred for gastrointestinal decontamination. Repetitive doses may enhance their elimination. The treatment of anticholinergic poisoning is discussed in the section pertaining to these agents. Although arrhythmias due to orphenadrine have responded to physostigmine, they are more likely due to sodium channel blockade than to anticholinergic effects and should probably be treated as described above for class I antiarrhythmics. Cerebrospinal fluid drainage may enhance the elimination of intrathecal baclofen. CNS depression from zolpidem may respond to flumazenil (see "Benzodiazepines," above). Treatment is otherwise supportive. Extracorporeal hemodynamic support and enhanced elimination procedures should be considered for patients with cardiovascular depression unresponsive to standard therapy.

NEUROLEPTIC AGENTS Clozapine, chlorprothixene, droperidol, haloperidol, loxapine, molindone, olanzapine, pimozide, quetiapine, risperidone, sertindole, thiothixene, trimethobenzamide, ziprasidone, and the phenothiazines (chlorpromazine, fluphenazine, perphenazine, prochlorperazine, promazine, promethazine, thiethylperazine, thioridazine and its metabolite mesoridazine, trifluoperazine, triflupromazine, trimeperazine) primarily act by blocking type 2 dopamine receptors in the CNS. They also have variable inhibitory activity at α-adrenergic, histaminergic, muscarinic, serotonergic, and other dopamine receptor subtypes. Some phenothiazines have a quinidine-like activity. Acute extrapyramidal effects (dystonia, akathisia, Parkinsonism) result from an imbalance of cholinergic and dopaminergic activity in the basal ganglia. These effects are idiosyncratic rather than dose-related and can be delayed in onset. The neuroleptic malignant syndrome (Chaps. 17 and 363) rarely, if ever, occurs following acute overdose.

Neuroleptic agents are well absorbed, exhibit 90 to 95% protein binding in plasma, have large apparent volumes of distribution (10 to 40 L/kg body weight), and are eliminated slowly by hepatic metabolism with half-lives of 10 to 40 h.

Clinical Toxicity Toxic effects begin within 30 to 60 min of ingestion and include CNS depression (Table 396-2), respiratory depression, hypotension, pulmonary edema, and hypothermia. Pupils are often constricted, and the skin is usually warm and dry. Anticholinergic manifestations may be the predominant effect of low overdosage (see "Anticholinergic Agents," above). Cardiac effects include tachycardia, atrioventricular block, and atrial and ventricular arrhythmias. Torsade de pointes; prolonged PR, QRS, and QT intervals; and U- and T-wave abnormalities may be seen with pimozide, mesoridazine, respiridone, thioridazine ingestions and high-dose intravenous droperidol and haloperidol.

Acute dystonic reactions are characterized by sustained muscle contractions resulting in abnormal posturing of the eyes, face, tongue, jaw, neck, back, abdomen, and pelvis. Akathisia is the subjective sensation of motor restlessness, and Parkinsonism is manifest by akinesia and rigidity. Patients may be anxious but remain alert and oriented during these reactions.

Diagnosis The diagnosis is supported by detecting the presence of these agents on toxicologic screening of the urine. Quantitative measurement is not helpful.

Rx TREATMENT Activated charcoal is the preferred method of gastrointestinal decontamination. Supportive care includes airway protection and mechanical ventilation for CNS and respiratory depression, fluid resuscitation followed by pressors for hypotension, and anticonvulsants for seizures. Diuresis and dialysis are ineffective. Seizures should be treated with benzodiazepines, and hypotension should be managed with volume expanders and pressor agents. Physostigmine may be useful for anticholinergic toxicity (see "Anticholinergic Agents," above). Treatment of ventricular dysrhythmias is the same as described above for class I antiarrhythmics.

Acute extrapyramidal reactions usually respond rapidly to antimuscarinic therapy such as intravenous diphenhydramine (1 mg/kg body weight given over 2 min) or benztropine (1 to 2 mg). Doses may be repeated in 20 min if the response is incomplete. Treatment should be continued with an oral formulation for 2 to 3 days since these reactions can recur in the absence of additional exposure.

NONSTEROIDAL ANTI-INFLAMMATORY DRUGS Diclofenac, diflunisal, etodolac, fenoprofen, flurbiprofen, ibuprofen, indomethacin, ketoprofen, ketorolac, meclofenamate, mefenamic acid, naproxen, oxaprozin, piroxicam, phenylbutazone, sulindac, and tolmetin inhibit prostaglandin and thromboxane synthesis by blocking cyclooxygenase (COX) isoenzymes: COX-1, the constitutive form in the gastrointestinal tract, kidney, and platelets, and COX-2, an inducible form that becomes expressed in response to bacterial toxins and cytokines (tissue inflammation). They are absorbed rapidly, and blood concentrations peak 1 to 2 h after ingestion. They are highly protein bound (>90%) and have volumes of distribution of less than 1.0 L/kg body weight. They are primarily eliminated by hepatic metabolism. Half-lives range from 1 to 16 h except for phenylbutazone, which has a half-life of 2 to 4 days.

Clinical Toxicity Effects are usually mild and include nausea, vomiting, abdominal pain, drowsiness, headache, glycosuria, hematuria, and proteinuria. Acute renal failure and hepatitis occur rarely. Diflunisal can cause hyperventilation, tachycardia, and sweating. Coma, respiratory depression, seizures, and cardiovascular collapse may occur with mefenamic acid and phenylbutazone. Ibuprofen can cause metabolic acidosis, coma, and seizures. Metabolic acidosis is relatively common in phenylbutazone poisoning and occurs rarely with naproxen. Seizures can also occur with ketoprofen and naproxen. Preliminary data indicates that selective COX-2 inhibitors, such as celecobix and rofecobix, do not share the toxicity of these nonselective inhibitors.

Diagnosis Comprehensive toxicology screening will identify these drugs in the urine, but quantitative analysis is not useful.

℞ TREATMENT Activated charcoal is the preferred method of gastrointestinal decontamination. Repeated doses may enhance the elimination of indomethacin, phenylbutazone, and piroxicam. Renal excretion is not increased by diuresis, and protein binding limits the efficacy of hemodialysis. Hemoperfusion might be useful in patients with hepatic or renal failure and severe clinical toxicity. Treatment is otherwise supportive.

ORGANOPHOSPHATE AND CARBAMATE INSECTICIDES Organophosphorus compounds such as the insecticides chlorpyrifos, phosphorothioic acid (Diazinon), dichlorvos, fenthion, malathion, and parathion and the chemical warfare "nerve gases" such as sarin irreversibly inhibit acetylcholinesterase and cause accumulation of acetylcholine at muscarinic and nicotinic synapses and in the CNS. Carbamates such as the insecticides aldicarb, propoxur (Baygon), carbaryl (Sevin), and bendiocarb (Ficam) and the therapeutic agents ambenonium, neostigmine, physostigmine, and pyridostigmine reversibly inhibit this enzyme. Agents that directly stimulate cholinergic receptors such as arecholine (from betel nuts), bethanechol, pilocarpine, and urecholine have the same effect.

Organophosphates are absorbed through the skin, lungs, and gastrointestinal tract; are distributed widely in tissues; and are slowly eliminated by hepatic metabolism. Oxidative metabolites of parathion and malathion (paraoxon, malaoxon) are the active forms of these agents. Carbamates are eliminated rapidly by serum and liver enzymes.

Clinical Toxicity The time from exposure to the onset of toxicity varies from minutes to hours but is usually between 30 min and 2 h. Muscarinic effects include nausea, vomiting, abdominal cramps, urinary and fecal incontinence, increased bronchial secretions, cough, wheezing, dyspnea, sweating, salivation, miosis, blurred vision, lacrimation, and urinary frequency and incontinence. In severe poisoning, bradycardia, conduction block, hypotension, and pulmonary edema may occur. Nicotinic signs include twitching, fasciculations, weakness, hypertension, tachycardia, and in severe cases paralysis and respiratory failure. CNS effects include anxiety, restlessness, tremor, confusion, weakness, seizures, and coma. Toxicity due to carbamates is shorter in duration and usually less severe than that due to organophosphates. Most patients recover within 24 to 48 h, but fat-soluble organophosphates may cause effects for weeks to months. Death is most often due to pulmonary toxicity.

Diagnosis A reduction of cholinesterase activity in plasma and in red blood cells to <50% of normal confirms the diagnosis. A reduction in red blood cell cholinesterase activity is more specific; however, this test is less readily available, and some organophosphates inhibit only one type of cholinesterase. With carbamates, depression in plasma or red blood cell cholinesterase levels is transient because of the rapid reversibility of the inhibition. Since cholinesterase assays are not routinely or rapidly available, the initial diagnosis is clinical.

℞ TREATMENT Contaminated clothing should be removed, and the skin should be washed with soap and water. Gastrointestinal decontamination should include use of activated charcoal. Supportive measures include oxygen administration, ventilatory assistance, and treatment of seizures. Atropine, a muscarinic receptor antagonist, should be administered for muscarinic effects. A dose of 0.5 to 2 mg is given intravenously every 5 to 15 min until bronchial and other secretions have dried. Repeated doses or a constant infusion may be necessary for recurrent toxicity. Pralidoxime (2-PAM) reactivates cholinesterases and is indicated for nicotinic symptoms due to organophosphate poisoning. The use of pralidoxime in carbamate poisoning is controversial. It is usually unnecessary, but its use is safe, particularly if it is administered in conjunction with atropine. A dose of 1 to 2 g is given intravenously over 5 to 30 min (depending on severity). It can be repeated in 30 min if the response is incomplete. Rapid injection can cause tachycardia, laryngospasm, muscle rigidity, and weakness. Repeated doses (every 4 to 6 h) or a continuous infusion (500 mg/h) are indicated for recurrent effects. Neither atropine nor pralidoxime is particularly effective at reversing CNS effects; seizures should be treated aggressively with benzodiazepines.

SALICYLATES Aspirin (acetylsalicyclic acid) and salicylate salts have activity similar to that of other nonsteroidal anti-inflammatory drugs described above. Aspirin, but not other salicylates, also inhibits platelet aggregation. Toxic doses increase the sensitivity of respiratory centers in the brain to changes in oxygen and carbon dioxide concentrations. They also uncouple oxidative phosphorylation, increase the rate of metabolism (oxygen consumption, glucose utilization, and carbon dioxide and heat production), and inhibit the Krebs cycle and carbohydrate and lipid metabolism. Metabolic effects lead to respiratory center stimulation and respiratory alkalosis early in the course of poisoning and lactic and ketoacidosis in later stages. Salicylates can also inhibit the hepatic synthesis of clotting factors.

With therapeutic doses, peak serum levels of 0.7 to 1.4 mmol/L (10 to 20 mg/dL) occur 1 to 2 h after ingestion, 50 to 80% is bound to albumin, the volume of distribution is small (0.2 L/kg body weight), and the half-life is 2 to 3 h. Being a weak acid, the unbound portion in the serum exists mainly in an ionized state. Elimination occurs primarily by hepatic metabolism, with about 10% being excreted unchanged.

Although salicylates are absorbed rapidly, absorption may continue for 24 h or longer after an overdose. Acidosis increases the nonionized (diffusable) fraction, and unbound salicylate promotes its tissue distribution (i.e., increases the volume of distribution). Saturation of metabolic pathways results in a prolonged half-life (20 to 36 h), and renal excretion becomes the most important route of elimination. Alkalinization of the urine enhances renal excretion by converting urinary salicylate to the ionized form, which cannot be reabsorbed.

Clinical Toxicity Initial manifestations occur 3 to 6 h after an overdose of ≥150 mg/kg and include vomiting, sweating, tachycardia, hyperpnea, fever, tinnitus, lethargy, confusion, respiratory alkalosis with compensatory bicarbonate excretion resulting in an alkaline urine (pH >6). Increases in the rate or depth of respirations may be subtle. Vomiting, diaphoresis, and hyperventilation may lead to dehydration and decreased renal function. As acid products of intermediary metabolism accumulate, increased anion-gap metabolic acidosis and ketosis develop, and their excretion results in the urine becoming acidic (pH <6). In moderate poisoning, both respiratory alkalosis and metabolic acidosis are present, usually with alkalemia and paradoxical aciduria, although the serum pH can be normal. Elevation of the hematocrit, white blood cell count, and platelet count; hypernatremia; hyperkalemia; hypoglycemia; and prolongation of the prothrombin time may be seen. Severe poisoning is manifest by coma, respiratory depression, seizures, cardiovascular collapse, and cerebral and pulmonary edema (both noncardiogenic and cardiogenic). At this stage, metabolic evaluation reveals acidemia (metabolic acidosis with respiratory alkalosis or acidosis) and aciduria.

Diagnosis The diagnosis should be suspected in anyone with an unexplained acid-base disorder. Salicylates are identified by a positive urine ferric chloride test (purple color), which is usually included in routine screening procedures, or quantitative serum analysis. Following acute overdose, a peak level of <2.2 mmol/L (30 mg/dL) is associated with little or no toxicity, one of 2.2 to 7 mmol/L (30 to 100 mg/dL) with mild to moderate effects, and one of >7 mmol/L (100 mg/dL) with severe poisoning. Because of delayed and prolonged absorption, serial levels should be obtained. In chronic poisoning, symptoms may occur at levels only slightly above the therapeutic range.

℞ TREATMENT Activated charcoal is the preferred method of gastrointestinal decontamination. Repeated doses may enhance elimination. Because of delayed absorption, decontamination may be helpful 12 to 24 h after ingestion. Gastric lavage and whole-bowel irrigation should be considered in patients with ingestions of >500 mg/kg, particularly when toxicity progresses and drug levels continue to rise following charcoal administration. Endoscopy may be useful for the diagnosis and removal of gastric bezoars. A bedside glucose level should be determined in patients with altered mental status. Intravenous saline should be given to replace fluid losses and to produce a brisk urine flow. The degree of dehydration is often underestimated; several liters or more may be necessary. Supplemental glucose and oxygen should also be given. Electrolyte and metabolic abnormalities should be corrected. Coagulopathy should be treated with intravenous vitamin K. Seizures and heart failure are treated with standard therapies. Saline diuresis and urinary alkalinization (to a pH of 8) enhance the elimination of salicylate and should be instituted in symptomatic patients and those with salicylate levels >2.2 mmol/L (30 mg/dL). Depending on severity, 50 to 150 mmol of bicarbonate (along with potassium) can be added to a liter of dextrose-containing saline solution (such that the final sodium concentration is nearly isotonic) and administered at a rate of 2 to 6 mL/kg per hour. Electrolytes, calcium, acid-base status, urine pH, and fluid balance must be monitored carefully during such therapy. When acidemia is present, bicarbonate should also be given to correct the serum pH, increase the ionization of serum salicylate, and limit its tissue distribution. Diuresis is contraindicated when cerebral or pulmonary edema and renal failure are present. Salicylates are effectively removed by hemodialysis. Indications for hemodialysis include severe clinical toxicity, levels that approach or exceed 7 mmol/L (100 mg/dL) following acute overdose, and contraindications or failure to respond to other treatment modalities.

SEROTONIN SYNDROME This syndrome is due to excessive CNS and peripheral serotonergic (5HT-1a and possibly 5HT-2) activity and results from the concomitant use of agents that promote the release of serotonin from presynaptic neurons (e.g., amphetamines, cocaine, codeine, methylenedioxy-methamphetamine or MDMA, reserpine, some MAO inhibitors), inhibit its reuptake (e.g., cyclic antidepressants, particularly the SSRIs, ergot derivatives, dextromethorphan, meperidine, pentazocine, sumatriptan and related agents, tramadol, some MAO inhibitors) or metabolism (e.g., cocaine, MAO inhibitors), or stimulate postsynaptic serotonin receptors (e.g., bromocryptine, bupropion, buspirone, levodopa, lithium, L-tryptophan, lysergic acid diethylamide or LSD, mescaline, trazodone). Less often, it results from the use or overdose of a single serotonergic agent or when one agent is taken soon after another has been discontinued (up to 2 weeks for some agents). Serotonergic effects also appear to have been responsible for pulmonary hypertension and valvulopathy associated with the anorexiants dexfenfluramine and fenfluramine (withdrawn from U.S. markets in 1997).

Clinical Toxicity Onset occurs as early as an hour after single or multiple drug overdose or the addition of another serotonergic agent to current therapy and as a long as several days after increasing the dose of one or more agents. Manifestations include altered mental status (agitation, confusion, delirium, mutism, coma, and seizures), neuromuscular hyperactivity (restlessness, incoordination, hyperreflexia, myoclonus, rigidity, and tremors), and autonomic dysfunction (abdominal pain, diarrhea, diaphoresis, fever, elevated and fluctuating blood pressure, flushed skin, mydriasis, tearing, salivation, shivering, and tachycardia). Complications include hyperthermia, lactic acidosis, rhabdomyolysis, kidney and liver failure, ARDS, and disseminated intravascular coagulation. Effects last from 6 to 48 h, depending on severity.

Diagnosis The diagnosis is based on clinical manifestations and the history of drug exposure. Toxicology testing is useful only for confirming an exposure or detecting an unsuspected one. In contrast to the neuroleptic malignant syndrome (Chap. 363), with which its shares many features, the serotonin syndrome becomes maximal and later resolves over a period of hours rather than days, and there is myclonus and hyperreflexia in contrast to "lead-pipe" rigidity.

℞ TREATMENT Gastrointestinal decontamination may be indicated for acute overdose. Supportive measures include hydration with intravenous fluids, airway protection and mechanical ventilation, benzodiazepines (and paralytics, if necessary) for neuromuscular hyperactivity, and mechanical cooling measures for hyperthermia.

The administration of serotonin-receptor antagonists may hasten the resolution of this syndrome. Cyproheptadine (Periactin), an antihistamine with 5HT-1a and 5HT2 receptor blocking activity, and chlorpromazine (Thorazine), a nonspecific serotonin receptor antagonist, have been used with success. Cyproheptadine is given orally or by gastric tube in an initial dose of 4 to 8 mg and repeated as necessary every 2 to 4 h up to a maximum of 32 mg in 24 h. A response is usually noted in 1 to 2 h but may be absent in severe cases. Chlorpromazine has the advantage that it can be given parenterally (intramuscularly or by slow intravenous injection in doses of 50 to 100 mg). Since it can cause hypotension, its use should be preceded by adequate fluid hydration. The use of chlorpromazine for the neuroleptic malignant syndrome misdiagnosed as the serotonin syndrome, and conversely, the use of bromocriptine for the serotonin syndrome misdiagnosed as the neuroleptic malignant syndrome may result in worsening of symptoms. Other medications with variable success in treating the serotonin syndrome include propranolol, methysergide, and dantrolene.

SYMPATHOMIMETICS Amphetamines (amphetamine itself, benzphetamine, dextroamphetamine, diethylpropion, methamphetamine, phendimetrazine, phentermine), cathinone (from khat, or the plant *Catha edulis*), ephedrine, mazindol, methylphenidate, and pemoline directly stimulate α- and β-adrenergic receptors. Some also induce the release of dopamine and norepinephrine. Phenylephrine, pseudoephedrine, and phenylpropanolamine primarily stimulate α receptors, whereas mephentermine and bronchodilators such as albuterol, bitoterol, isoetherine, etaproterenol, pirbuterol, and salmeterol primarily stimulate β receptors.

These agents are readily absorbed, with peak serum levels occurring 1 to 2 h after ingestion (sooner after nasal insufflation and with the "ice" or crystalline form of methamphetamine, which, like crack cocaine, can be smoked). They are weak bases with volumes of distribution of 2 to 6 L/kg body weight. Elimination occurs by a combination of hepatic metabolism and renal excretion of unchanged drug. Half-lives range from 2 to 34 h. Excretion is enhanced in an acid urine and slowed in an alkaline one.

Clinical Toxicity Effects are seen within 30 to 60 min after ingestion and include nausea, vomiting, abdominal cramps, and headache as well as manifestations of adrenergic and CNS stimulation (Table 396-2). Although hypertension and tachycardia occur with nonselective agents, hypertension with reflex bradycardia, and even AV block, may occur with agents that have predominantly alpha effects. Tachycardia with hypotension (as a result of vasodilation) can be seen with selective β agonists. Other findings may include combativeness, auditory and visual hallucinations, dilated pupils, dry mouth, pallor, and tachypnea. Complications include lactic acidosis, rhabdomyolysis, and intracranial hemorrhage. β-Adrenergic stimulation causes potassium to move into cells and may result in hypokalemia.

Diagnosis The diagnosis is supported by finding these agents in the urine by toxicology screening. Quantitative measurement is not useful.

℞ **TREATMENT** Activated charcoal is the preferred method of gastrointestinal decontamination. Benzodiazepines or barbiturates should be used to control neuromuscular hyperactivity and to treat seizures. A nonselective adrenergic blocker such as labetalol or the selective α-adrenergic antagonist phentolamine (1 to 5 mg intravenously every 5 min until the desired response is achieved) with or without a cardioselective beta blocker such as esmolol are recommended for severe or symptomatic hypertension; propranolol or a cardioselective beta blocker is recommended for severe or symptomatic tachycardia. Lidocaine and propranolol are preferred for the treatment of ventricular tachyarrhythmias. Hyperthermia should be treated with external cooling measures along with sedation and, if necessary, paralyzing agents. Although theoretically effective for enhancing drug elimination, acid diuresis is not recommended due to lack of documented clinical efficacy and risks of side effects such as worsening of acidosis and potential triggering of myoglobinuric renal failure.

THEOPHYLLINE Theophylline, caffeine, and other methylxanthines are phosphodiesterase inhibitors that reduce the degradation of intracellular cyclic AMP, thereby enhancing the actions of endogenous catecholamines and leading to β-adrenergic stimulation. Theophylline is absorbed rapidly from the stomach and upper small bowel. Following overdose, serum levels peak 1 to 2 h after ingestion of liquid preparations, 2 to 4 h after ingestion of tablets, and 6 to 24 h after ingestion of sustained-release preparations. Theophylline is approximately 60% bound to albumin and has a low volume of distribution (0.6 L/kg body weight). Therapeutic serum levels are 55 to 110 μmol/L (10 to 20 mg/L). Elimination occurs primarily by hepatic metabolism, which is saturable at levels in the high therapeutic range. The serum half-life, normally 4 to 6 h, is therefore prolonged in overdoses. Elimination is also decreased with impaired liver function, congestive heart failure, viral infections, and concomitantly administered drugs such as cimetidine, erythromycin, fluoroquinolones, and tetracycline.

Clinical Toxicity Effects begin 30 min to 2 h following overdose and include nausea, vomiting, psychomotor excitation, pallor, diaphoresis, tachypnea, tachycardia, and muscle tremors. Severe poisoning is characterized by coma, seizures, respiratory depression, cardiac arrhythmias, hypotension, and rhabdomyolysis. Seizures can be focal and are often protracted, repetitive, and resistant to therapy. Both atrial and ventricular tachyarrhythmias, including ventricular fibrillation, can occur. Hypotension develops only after acute overdose. Ketosis, metabolic acidosis, hyperamylasemia, hyperglycemia, hypokalemia, hypocalcemia, and hypophosphatemia may also be seen in acute poisoning.

Diagnosis The diagnosis is confirmed by measuring a serum drug level. Theophylline is not readily detected by routine urine screening. Wtih chronic exposure, arrhythmias and seizures occur at lower serum levels (200 to 300 μmol/L, or 40 to 60 mg/L) than the levels seen after acute overdose (400 to 500 μmol/L, 80 to 100 mg/L). Because of prolonged and delayed absorption after overdosage, particularly with sustained-release preparations, levels should be measured serially to determine the peak concentration.

℞ **TREATMENT** Activated charcoal is the preferred method of gastrointestinal decontamination. With sustained-release forms, whole-bowel irrigation should also be considered. Antiemetics are often required for vomiting. Seizures and neuromuscular hyperactivity should be treated with benzodiazepines and barbiturates and pharmacologic paralysis in refractory cases; phenytoin is ineffective. Intravenous propranolol is preferred for the treatment of tachyarrhythmias. It can also reverse hypotension, which results from β_2-adrenergic stimulation. Although β_2 receptor blockade can potentially cause bronchospasm in those with reactive or obstructive airway disease, this has not been reported when propranolol has been used in this setting. The selective beta$_1$ blocker esmolol can also be used for supraventricular tachycardias, and ventricular tachycardias can be treated with lidocaine or other antiarrhythmics. Volume expansion and an α agonist such as norepinephrine can be given for hypotension. Repeated doses of charcoal shorten the serum half-life of theophylline by approximately 50% and are recommended for all patients. Hemodialysis and hemoperfusion are effective in removing theophylline and are indicated for patients with severe clinical toxicity or a serum drug level equal to or greater than that associated with such toxicity.

BIBLIOGRAPHY

General Principles

Hardman JD et al (eds): *Goodman and Gilman's The Pharmacologic Basis of Therapeutics*, 9th ed. New York, McGraw-Hill, 1996

Klaassen CD (Ed): *Casarett and Doull's Toxicology: The Basic Science of Poisons*, 5th ed. New York, McGraw-Hill, 1996

Epidemiology

Henderson A et al: Experience with 732 acute overdose patients admitted to an intensive care unit over 6 years. Med J Austral 158:28, 1993

Litovitz TL et al: 1997 Annual Report of the American Association of Poison Control Centers Toxic Exposure Surveillance System. Am J Emerg Med 16:443, 1998

Diagnosis

Aabakken et al: Osmolal and anion gaps in patients admitted to an emergency medical department. Hum Exp Toxicol 13:131, 1994

Bradberry SM, Vale JA: Disturbances of potassium homeostasis in poisoning. Clin Toxicol 33:295, 1995

Chan TC et al: Drug-induced hyperthermia. Crit Care Clin 13:785, 1997

Council on Scientific Affairs, American Medical Association: Scientific issues in drug testing. JAMA 257:3110, 1987

Curry SC et al: Drug- and toxin-induced rhabdomyolysis. Ann Emerg Med 18:1068, 1989

Hoffman RS, Goldfrank LR: The poisoned patient with altered consciousness: Controversies in the use of the "coma cocktail." JAMA 274:562, 1995

Olson KR et al: Physical assessment and differential diagnosis of the poisoned patient. Med Toxicol 2:52, 1987

Zaccara G et al: Clinical features, pathogenesis, and management of drug-induced seizures. Drug Safety 5:109, 1990

Treatment

American Academy of Clinical Toxicology/European Association of Poisons Centers and Clinical Toxicologists: Position Statements on Gastrointestinal Decontamination: Introduction, ipecac syrup; gastric lavage; Single-dose activated charcoal; Cathartics; Whole bowel irrigation. Clin Toxicol 35: 695, 699, 711, 721, 743, 753, 1997

———: Multi-dose activated charcoal. Clin Toxicol 37:731, 1999

Brett AS et al: Predicting the clinical course of intentional drug overdose: Implications for utilization of the intensive care unit. Arch Intern Med 147:133, 1987

Burgess JL et al: Emergency department hazardous materials protocol for contaminated patients. Ann Emerg Med 34:205, 1999

Cooney DO: *Activated Charcoal in Medical Applications*. New York, Marcel Dekker, 1995

Garrettson LK, Geller RJ: Acid and alkaline diuresis: When are they of value in the treatment of poisoning? Drug Safety 5:220, 1990

Manoguerra AS: Gastrointestinal decontamination after poisoning: Where is the science. Crit Care Clin 13:709, 1997

Minocha A, Spyker DA: Acute overdose with sustained-release drug formulations: Perspectives in treatment. Med Toxicol 1:300, 1986

Neuvonen PJ, Olkkola KT: Oral activated charcoal in the treatment of intoxications: Role of single and repeated doses. Med Toxicol 3:33, 1988

Pond SM: Diuresis, dialysis and hemoperfusion: Indications and benefits. Emerg Med Clin North Am 2:29, 1984

Stead AH, Moffat AC: A collection of therapeutic, toxic and fatal blood drug concentrations in man. Hum Toxicol 3:437, 1983

397

Robert L. Norris, Paul S. Auerbach

DISORDERS CAUSED BY REPTILE BITES AND MARINE ANIMAL EXPOSURES

Few topics in medicine are as controversial or as influenced by tradition as the management of bites and stings from venomous creatures. Because the incidence of serious bites and stings is relatively low in developed nations, there remains a paucity of relevant clinical research and literature, and therapeutic decision-making is often based on anecdotal information. Furthermore, the responses of different species to various toxins make it difficult to extrapolate data from animal studies to clinical application. This chapter outlines general principles for the evaluation and management of victims of venom poisoning or intoxication by certain reptiles and marine creatures and presents a clinical approach to these emergencies.

VENOMOUS SNAKEBITE

EPIDEMIOLOGY The venomous snakes of the world are grouped into the families Viperidae (subfamily Viperinae: the Old World vipers; subfamily Crotalinae: the New World and Asian pit vipers), Elapidae (including the cobras, coral snakes, and all Australian venomous snakes), Hydrophiidae (the sea snakes), Atractaspididae (the burrowing asps), and Colubridae (a large group of which only a few species are dangerously toxic to humans). The highest bite rates occur in temperate and tropical regions where people subsist by manual agriculture. Global estimates suggest that 30,000 to 40,000 persons die each year from venomous snakebite, but this range is likely an underestimate because of incomplete reporting.

SNAKE ANATOMY/IDENTIFICATION The typical snake-venom apparatus consists of bilateral venom glands—one on each side of the head, below and behind the eye—connected by ducts to hollow, anterior maxillary teeth. In viperids (vipers and pit vipers), these teeth are long, mobile fangs that retract against the roof of the mouth when the animal is at rest. In elapids and sea snakes, the fangs are less enlarged and are fixed in an erect position. Venomous snakes can bite without injecting venom. Approximately 20% of pit viper bites and an even higher percentage of bites inflicted by some other snake families (e.g., up to 75% for sea snakes) are "dry."

Differentiation of venomous from nonvenomous snake species can be difficult. Viperids are characterized by somewhat triangular heads (a feature shared with many harmless snakes); elliptical pupils (also seen in some nonvenomous snakes, such as boas and pythons); enlarged maxillary fangs; subcaudal scalation that involves a single scale running the full width of the ventral surface of the tail for several rows just distal to the anal plate (as opposed to two scales in each subcaudal row for most nonvenomous snakes); and, in the case of pit vipers, the heat-sensing pits (foveal organs located slightly inferior and anterior to the eyes on each side) for which they are named. Color pattern is notoriously misleading in identifying most venomous snakes except for the coral snakes, whose other body characteristics are similar to those of harmless colubrids. The American coral snakes can be identified by red, yellow (or white), and black bands completely encircling the body; a few species have red and black bands only. North of Mexico City, the immediate contiguity of red and yellow bands is fairly reliable for distinguishing a coral snake from its many harmless mimics. Further south, differentiation by color pattern is more problematic.

In many areas of the world, enzyme-linked immunoassay (ELISA) kits are available to aid in determining the specific snake species involved in a bite. These kits identify venom in the victim's blood, urine, or wound aspirate. No such kit is commercially available in the United States, however.

VENOMS AND CLINICAL MANIFESTATIONS Snake venoms are complex mixtures of enzymes, low-molecular-weight polypeptides, glycoproteins, and metal ions. Among the deleterious components are hemorrhagins that promote vascular leaking and cause both local and systemic bleeding. Various proteolytic enzymes cause local tissue necrosis, affect the coagulation pathway at various steps, and impair organ function. Myocardial depressant factors reduce cardiac output, and neurotoxins act either pre- or postsynaptically to inhibit peripheral nerve impulses. Most snake venoms have multisystem effects in their victims.

℞ TREATMENT **Field Management** Initial (prehospital) measures should focus on rapidly delivering the victim to definitive medical care while keeping him/her as inactive as possible to limit systemic spread of venom. Any other measures employed should at least do no further harm to the victim.

After viperid bites, local mechanical suction applied to the site within 3 to 5 min may remove a small percentage of deposited venom. A useful device is the Extractor (Sawyer Products, Safety Harbor, FL), which delivers one atmosphere of negative pressure to the wound. Suction should be continued for at least 30 min. Mouth suction should be avoided as it inoculates the wound with oral flora and theoretically can also result in the absorption of venom by the rescuer through lesions of the upper digestive tract. If the victim is >60 min from medical care, a proximal lympho-occlusive constriction band may limit the spread of venom when applied within 30 min. To avoid worsening tissue damage, however, the band should not interrupt arterial blood flow. The bitten extremity should be splinted if possible and kept at approximately heart level. Measures to be avoided include incising or cooling the bite site, giving the victim an alcoholic beverage, or applying electric shocks.

For elapid or sea snake bites, the Australian pressure-immobilization technique, in which the entire bitten extremity is wrapped with an elastic or crepe bandage and then splinted, is highly effective. The bandage is applied with the same snugness used for a sprained ankle. This technique greatly restricts absorption and circulation of venom. The utility of this method in viperid poisoning requires further research, as it theoretically could compound local tissue damage by restricting venom to the local tissues.

Hospital Management In the hospital, the victim should be closely monitored (vital signs, cardiac rhythm, and oxygen saturation) while a history is quickly obtained and a brief but thorough physical examination is performed. The level of erythema and/or swelling in a bitten extremity should be marked and limb circumferences measured in several locations every 15 min until swelling has stabilized. Large-bore intravenous access in unaffected extremities should be established. Early hypotension is due to pooling of blood in the pulmonary and splanchnic vascular beds. Hours later, hemolysis and loss of intravascular volume into soft tissues may play important roles. Fluid resuscitation with normal saline or Ringer's lactate should be initiated for clinical shock. If the blood pressure response is inadequate after administration of 20 to 40 mL/kg of body weight, then a trial of 5% albumin (10 to 20 mL/kg) is in order. If tissue perfusion fails to respond to volume resuscitation and antivenom infusion (see below), vasopressors (e.g., dopamine) should be administered. Invasive hemodynamic monitoring (central venous and/or pulmonary arterial pressures) can be helpful in such cases, although obtaining access is riskier if coagulopathy is present.

Blood should be drawn for laboratory evaluation as soon as possible. Blood typing and cross-matching procedures can be affected over time by circulating venom. Also important are a complete blood count to evaluate the degree of hemorrhage or hemolysis, studies of renal and hepatic function, coagulation studies to identify signs of consumptive coagulopathy, and testing of urine for blood or myoglobin. In severe cases or in the face of significant comorbidity, arterial blood gas studies, electrocardiography, and chest radiography are indicated.

Attempts to locate a source of appropriate antivenom should begin early in all cases of known venomous snakebite, regardless of symptoms. In the event that signs and symptoms progress rapidly, any delay in the administration of antivenom is dangerous. Antivenoms rarely offer cross-protection against snake species other than those used in their production unless the species are closely related. An example of good cross-protection is that of Australian tiger snake (*Notechis scutatus*) antivenom for sea snake bites (see below). The package insert accompanying a particular antivenom should be consulted for information regarding the spectrum of coverage. In the United States, assistance in finding antivenom can be obtained 24 hours a day from the University of Arizona Poison and Drug Information Center (telephone: 520-626-6016).

Rapidly progressive or severe local findings (soft tissue swelling, ecchymosis, petechiae, etc.) or manifestations of systemic toxicity (signs and symptoms or laboratory abnormalities) are indications for the administration of intravenous antivenom. The package insert outlines techniques for reconstitution of antivenom (when necessary), skin-testing procedures (for potential allergy), and appropriate starting doses. Most commercial antivenoms are of equine origin and carry a risk of anaphylactic, anaphylactoid, and delayed-hypersensitivity reactions. Skin testing does not reliably predict which patients will have an allergic reaction to equine antivenom; false-negative and false-positive results are common. Before antivenom infusion, the patient should receive appropriate loading doses of intravenous antihistamines (e.g., diphenhydramine, 1 mg/kg to a maximum of 100 mg; and cimetidine, 5 to 10 mg/kg to a maximum of 300 mg) in an effort to limit acute reactions. Modest expansion of the patient's intravascular volume with crystalloids may also be beneficial in this regard. Epinephrine should be immediately available, and the antivenom dose to be administered should be diluted (e.g., in 1000 mL of normal saline for adults or in 20 mL/kg for children). This volume can be decreased if necessary (e.g., if the victim has a history of congestive heart failure). The antivenom should be started slowly, with the physician at the bedside to intervene in the event of an acute reaction. The rate of infusion can be increased gradually in the absence of allergic phenomena until the total starting dose has been administered (over a total period of 1 to 4 h). Further antivenom may be necessary if the patient's clinical condition worsens. Laboratory values should be rechecked hourly, particularly if abnormal, until stability is apparent.

The management of a life-threatening envenomation in a victim with an apparent allergy to antivenom requires significant expertise. Consultation with a poison specialist, an intensive care specialist, and/or an allergist is recommended. Often antivenom can still be administered in these situations under closely controlled conditions and with intensive premedication (e.g., with epinephrine, antihistamines, and steroids).

Care of the bite wound should include application of a dry sterile dressing and splinting of the extremity with padding between the digits. Once the administration of an indicated antivenom has been initiated, the extremity should be elevated above heart level to relieve edema. Tetanus immunization should be updated as appropriate. The use of prophylactic antibiotics is controversial, as the incidence of secondary infection following venomous snakebite appears to be low. Many authorities, however, prescribe a broad-spectrum antibiotic (such as ampicillin or a cephalosporin) for the first few days.

If swelling in the bitten extremity raises concern that subfascial muscle edema may be impeding tissue perfusion (muscle-compartment syndrome), intracompartmental pressures should be checked by any minimally invasive technique (e.g., the wick catheter). If pressures are elevated and remain so despite antivenom administration, prompt surgical consultation for possible fasciotomy should be obtained. This complication, fortunately, is rare after snakebites.

Whether or not antivenom is given, any patient with signs of venom poisoning should be observed in the hospital for at least 24 h. A patient with an apparently "dry" bite should be watched for at least 6 to 8 h before discharge, as significant toxicity occasionally develops after a delay of several hours. The onset of systemic symptoms is commonly delayed for a number of hours after bites by several of the elapids (including the coral snakes) and sea snakes. Patients bitten by these reptiles should be observed in the hospital for 24 h.

Significant work is being done in several regions of the world to produce safer, more effective antivenoms. Much of this work involves production of ovine-based antivenoms that are further purified and enzymatically cleaved to yield functional F(ab) fragments of the immunoglobulin molecules. These antivenoms are currently in clinical use in many countries, and trials of one product are under way in the United States.

MORBIDITY AND MORTALITY The overall mortality rates for venomous snakebite are low in areas of the world with rapid access to medical care and appropriate antivenom. In the United States, for example, the mortality rate is <1% for victims who receive antivenom. Eastern and western diamondback rattlesnakes (*Crotalus adamanteus* and *C. atrox*, respectively) are responsible for most snakebite deaths in the United States. Snakes responsible for large numbers of deaths in other regions of the world include the cobras (*Naja* spp.) of Asia and Africa, the carpet and saw-scaled vipers (*Echis* spp.) of the Middle East and Africa, Russell's viper (*Daboia russelli*) of the Middle East and Asia, the large African vipers (*Bitis* spp.), and the lancehead pit vipers (*Bothrops* spp.) of Central and South America.

The incidence of morbidity in terms of permanent functional loss in a bitten extremity is difficult to estimate but is probably substantial. Such loss may be due to muscle, nerve, or vascular injury or to scar contracture. In the United States, such loss due to snakebite tends to be much more common and severe after rattlesnake bites than after bites by copperheads or water moccasins.

LIZARD BITES

Bites from the two species of venomous lizards (the gila monster, *Heloderma suspectum*, of the southwestern United States and the Mexican beaded lizard, *H. horridum*) are infrequent and usually follow attempts to capture or handle these creatures. The wounds are characterized by soft tissue trauma with surrounding local edema and occasionally local cyanosis and ecchymosis. Broken teeth may be embedded in the wounds. The venom contains proteases and phospholipases. Systemic effects may include hypotension, weakness, dizziness, and diaphoresis.

Prehospital care measures for these bites should follow the guidelines listed above for viperid bites. If the biting lizard is still attached to the victim, its jaws may need to be manually pried apart for removal.

The sparseness of data on the pathophysiologic effects of helodermatid venom precludes specific recommendations regarding laboratory evaluation, but routine studies (complete blood count, coagulation studies, electrolyte analysis, blood typing and cross-matching, urinalysis, and electrocardiography) are prudent in anything other than a trivial bite. Wounds should be cleansed thoroughly and irrigated when possible. Tetanus immunization should be updated as indicated. Soft tissue radiography of the bite site and sterile probing under local anesthesia may identify retained teeth. The extremity should be splinted and elevated, but antibiotic treatment is not usually required. Systemic care is supportive (e.g., crystalloid infusion for hypotension). No commercial antivenom exists. Pain due to local venom effects and mechanical trauma can be treated with opiates and regional nerve blocks. The mortality rate is extremely low.

MARINE ENVENOMATIONS

Management of venom poisoning by marine creatures is similar to that of venomous snakebite in that much of the treatment administered is supportive in nature. A few specific marine antivenoms can be used when appropriate.

INVERTEBRATES *Hydroids, fire coral, jellyfish, Portuguese man-of-war,* and *sea anemones* possess specialized stinging cells called nematocysts. The venoms from these organisms are mixtures of proteins, carbohydrates, and other components. The clinical syndrome following envenomation by any of these species is similar but of variable severity. Victims usually report immediate prickling or burning, pruritus, paresthesia, and painful throbbing with radiation. A legion of neurologic, cardiovascular, respiratory, rheumatologic, gastrointestinal, renal, and ocular symptoms have been described. Victims in unstable condition with hypotension or respiratory distress should be treated supportively. During stabilization, the skin should be immediately decontaminated with a forceful jet of vinegar (5% acetic acid) or rubbing alcohol (40 to 70% isopropyl alcohol), which inactivates nematocysts. For the venomous *box-jellyfish* (*Chironex fleckeri*; **Plate**

IID-53), vinegar should be used. Perfume, aftershave lotion, and high-proof ethanol are less efficacious and may be detrimental. Shaving the skin helps remove remaining nematocysts. Freshwater irrigation and rubbing lead to further stinging by adherent nematocysts and should be avoided. After decontamination, application of anesthetic ointments (lidocaine, benzocaine), antihistamine creams (diphenhydramine), or steroid lotions (hydrocortisone) may be helpful. Persistent pain following decontamination may be treated with morphine or meperidine. Muscle spasms may respond to 10% calcium gluconate (5 to 10 mL) or diazepam (2 to 5 mg, titrated upwards as necessary) given intravenously. An antivenom is available from Commonwealth Serum Laboratories (see section on antivenom sources, below) for stings from the box-jellyfish found in Australian waters.

Touching a *sea sponge* may result in dermatitis. If contact occurs, the skin should be gently dried and adhesive tape used to remove embedded spicules. Vinegar should be applied immediately and then for 10 to 30 min three or four times a day. Rubbing alcohol may be used if vinegar is unavailable. After spicule removal and skin decontamination, a steroid or antihistamine cream may be applied to the skin. Severe vesiculation should be treated with a 2-week course of systemic glucocorticoids.

Annelid worms (bristleworms) possess rows of soft, cactus-like spines capable of inflicting painful stings. Contact results in symptoms similar to those of nematocyst envenomation. Without treatment, pain usually subsides over several hours, but inflammation may persist for up to a week. Victims should resist the urge to scratch, since scratching may fracture retrievable spines. Visible bristles should be removed with forceps and adhesive tape, a commercial facial peel, or a thin layer of rubber cement. Use of vinegar, rubbing alcohol, or dilute ammonia or a brief application of unseasoned meat tenderizer (papain) may provide additional relief. Local inflammation should be treated with topical or systemic glucocorticoids.

Sea urchins possess either hollow, venom-filled, calcified spines or triple-jawed, globiferous pedicellariae with venom glands. Their venom contains several toxic components, including steroid glycosides, hemolysins, proteases, serotonin, and cholinergic substances. Contact with either venom apparatus produces immediate and intensely painful stings. The affected part should be immersed immediately in hot water (see below). Accessible embedded spines should be removed but may break off and remain lodged in the victim. Residual dye from the surface of a spine remaining after the spine's removal may mimic a retained spine but is otherwise of no consequence. Soft tissue radiography or magnetic resonance imaging can confirm the presence of retained spines; this finding may warrant referral for attempted surgical removal if the spines are located near vital structures (e.g., joints, neurovascular bundles). Retained spines may cause the formation of granulomas that are amenable to excision or to intralesional injection with triamcinolone hexacetonide (5 mg/mL).

Cone shells are predatory, carnivorous mollusks. The most dangerous of these creatures are found in the Indian and Pacific oceans. A neurotoxic venom comprising multiple peptides is delivered through harpoon-like darts propelled from an extensible proboscis. Clinically, the sting is like that of a bee. The victim may report wound, perioral, and generalized paresthesias. Bulbar dysfunction and systemic muscular paralysis indicate severe envenomation. The sting of the geographer cone (*Conus geographus*) can cause cerebral edema, coma, and death due to respiratory or cardiac failure. Immediately after envenomation, a circumferential pressure-immobilization dressing 15 cm wide should be applied over a gauze pad measuring approximately $7 \times 7 \times 2$ cm that has been placed directly over the sting. The dressing should be applied at venous-lymphatic pressure with the preservation of distal arterial pulses. Once the victim has been transported to the nearest medical facility, the bandage can be released. Provision should be made for cardiovascular and respiratory support.

Serious envenomations and deaths have followed bites of the *Australian blue-ringed octopuses* (*Octopus maculosus* and *O. lunulata*). Although these animals rarely exceed 20 cm in length, their venom contains a potent neurotoxin (maculotoxin) that inhibits peripheral nerve transmission by blocking sodium conductance. Within several minutes of a serious envenomation, oral and facial numbness develops and rapidly progresses to total flaccid paralysis, including failure of respiratory muscles. If respirations are assisted, the victim may remain awake although completely paralyzed. Since there is no antidote, treatment is supportive. Immediately after envenomation, attempts should be made to limit the dispersion of venom by application of a pressure-immobilization or venous-lymphatic pressure dressing. Hot-water immersion and cryotherapy are ineffective. Artificial respiration should be provided. Even with serious envenomations, significant recovery often takes place within 4 to 10 h. Sequelae are uncommon unless related to hypoxia.

VERTEBRATES A number of marine vertebrates, including stingrays, scorpionfish, catfish, surgeonfish, and weeverfish, can envenom humans. The management of most of these stings is similar.

A *stingray* injury is both an envenomation and a traumatic wound. The venom, which contains serotonin, 5′-nucleotidase, and phosphodiesterase, causes immediate and intense pain that may last up to 48 h. Systemic effects include weakness, diaphoresis, nausea, vomiting, diarrhea, dysrhythmias, syncope, hypotension, muscle cramps, fasciculations, paralysis, and (in rare cases) death.

The designation *scorpionfish* encompasses members of the family Scorpaenidae and includes not only scorpionfish but also lionfish and stonefish. A complex venom with neuromuscular toxicity is delivered through 12 or 13 dorsal, two pelvic, and three anal spines. Pectoral spines do not contain venom. The severity of envenomation depends on the species of fish, the number of stings, and the amount of venom released. In general, the sting of a stonefish is regarded as the most serious (severe to life-threatening); that of the scorpionfish is of intermediate seriousness; and that of the lionfish is the least serious. Like that of a stingray, the sting of a scorpionfish is immediately and intensely painful. Pain from a stonefish envenomation may last for days. The systemic manifestations are similar to those of stingray envenomations but may be more pronounced, particularly in the case of a stonefish sting. The rare deaths following stonefish envenomation usually occur within 6 to 8 h.

Two species of marine *catfish*, *Plotosus lineatus* (the oriental catfish) and *Galeichthys felis* (the common sea catfish), as well as several species of freshwater catfish are capable of stinging humans. Venom is delivered through a single dorsal spine and two pectoral spines. Clinically, a catfish sting is comparable to that of a stingray, although marine catfish envenomations are generally more severe than those of their freshwater counterparts. *Surgeonfish* (doctorfish, tang), *weeverfish*, and *horned venomous sharks* have also been implicated in human envenomations.

The stings of all these marine vertebrates are treated in a similar fashion. Except for stonefish and serious scorpionfish envenomations (see below), no antivenom is available. The affected part should be immersed immediately in nonscalding hot water (113°F/45°C) for 30 to 90 min or until there is significant relief of pain. This measure also helps inactivate the heat-labile components of the venoms. Recurrent pain may respond to repeated hot-water treatment. Cryotherapy is contraindicated. Opiates will help alleviate the pain, as will local wound infiltration or regional nerve block with 1% lidocaine, 0.5% bupivacaine, and sodium bicarbonate mixed in a 5:5:1 ratio. After soaking and anesthetic administration, the wound must be explored and debrided. Radiography may be helpful in the identification and location of foreign bodies. After exploration and debridement, the wound should be vigorously irrigated with warm sterile water, saline, or 1% povidone-iodine in solution. Bleeding can usually be controlled by sustained local pressure for 10 to 15 min. In general, wounds should be left open to heal by secondary intention or be treated by delayed primary closure. Tetanus immunization should be updated. Antibiotic treatment should be considered for serious wounds and for envenomation in immunocompromised hosts. The initial antibiotics should cover *Staphylococcus* and *Streptococcus* spp. If the victim is immunocompromised or an infection develops, antibiotic coverage should be broadened to include *Vibrio* spp.

Approach to the Patient

It is not uncommon for a physician to encounter a patient who has been envenomed by a marine creature that cannot be positively identified at the scene of the envenomation. Therefore, it is useful to be familiar with the local marine fauna and to recognize patterns of injury.

A large puncture wound or jagged laceration, particularly on the lower extremity, that is more painful than one would expect from the size and configuration of the wound is likely a stingray envenomation. Smaller punctures, as described above, represent the activity of a sea urchin or starfish. Stony corals cause rough abrasions and, in rare instances, lacerations or puncture wounds.

Coelenterate (marine invertebrate) stings sometimes create diagnostic skin patterns. A diffuse urticarial rash on exposed skin is often indicative of exposure to fragmented hydroids or larval anemones. A linear, whiplike print pattern appears where a jellyfish tentacle has contacted the skin. In the case of the dreaded box-jellyfish (**Plate IID-53**), a frosted cross-hatched appearance followed by dark purple coloration within a few hours of the sting heralds skin necrosis. An encounter with fire coral causes immediate pain and a red, swollen skin irritation in the pattern of contact, similar to but more severe than the imprint left by exposure to an intact feather hydroid. Seabather's eruption, caused by thimble jellyfishes and larval anemones, may cause a diffuse rash that consists of clusters of erythematous macules or raised papules, accompanied by intense itching. Toxic sponges (exposure to which usually occurs during handling) create a burning and painful red rash on exposed skin, which may blister and later desquamate. Virtually all marine stingers invoke the sequelae of inflammation, so that local erythema, swelling, and adenopathy are fairly nonspecific.

SOURCES OF ANTIVENOMS AND OTHER ASSISTANCE An antivenom for stonefish (and severe scorpionfish) envenomation, made in Australia by the Commonwealth Serum Laboratories (CSL; 45 Poplar Road, Parkville, Victoria, Australia 3052; 61-3-389-1911; fax: 61-3-389-1434), is available in the United States through the pharmacies of Sharp Cabrillo Hospital Emergency Department, San Diego, CA, at (619) 221-3429, and Community Hospital of Monterey Peninsula (CHOMP) Emergency Department, Monterey, CA, at (408) 625-4900.

Polyvalent sea snake antivenom is available from CSL or CHOMP. If sea snake antivenom is unavailable, tiger snake (*N. scutatus*) antivenom should be used.

Divers Alert Network, a nonprofit organization designed to assist in the care of injured divers, may also help with the treatment of marine injuries. The network can be reached 24 h a day at (919) 684-8111 or on the Internet at www.dan.ycg.org.

MARINE POISONINGS

CIGUATERA Ciguatera poisoning is the most common nonbacterial food poisoning associated with fish in the United States. The poisoning involves almost exclusively tropical and semitropical marine coral reef fish. Of reported cases, 75% (except in Hawaii) involve the barracuda, snapper, jack, or grouper. The ciguatera syndrome is associated with at least five toxins, all of which are unaffected by freeze-drying, heat, cold, and gastric acid and none of which affects the odor, color, or taste of fish.

The onset of symptoms may come within 15 to 30 min of ingestion and typically takes place within 1 to 3 h. Symptoms then increase in severity over the ensuing 4 to 6 h. Most victims develop symptoms within 12 h of ingestion, and virtually all are afflicted within 24 h. The more than 150 symptoms reported include abdominal pain, nausea, vomiting, diarrhea, chills, paresthesias, pruritus, tongue and throat numbness or burning, sensation of "carbonation" during swallowing, odontalgia or dental dysesthesias, dysphagia, dysuria, dyspnea, weakness, fatigue, tremor, fasciculations, athetosis, meningismus, aphonia, ataxia, vertigo, pain and weakness in the lower extremities, visual blurring, transient blindness, hyporeflexia, seizures, nasal congestion and dryness, conjunctivitis, maculopapular rash, skin vesiculations, dermatographism, sialorrhea, diaphoresis, headache, arthralgias, myalgias, insomnia, bradycardia, hypotension, central respiratory failure, and coma. Death is rare.

Diarrhea, vomiting, and abdominal pain usually develop 3 to 6 h after ingestion of a ciguatoxic fish. Symptoms may persist for 48 h and then generally resolve (even without treatment). A pathognomonic symptom is the reversal of hot and cold tactile perception, which develops in some persons after 3 to 5 days and may last for months. Tachycardia and hypertension have been described, in some cases after potentially severe transient bradycardia and hypotension. More severe reactions tend to occur in persons previously stricken with the disease. Persons who have ingested parrotfish (scaritoxin) may suffer from classic ciguatera poisoning as well as a "second-phase" syndrome (after 5 to 10 days' delay) of disequilibrium with locomotor ataxia, dysmetria, and resting or kinetic tremor. This affliction may persist for 2 to 6 weeks.

The differential diagnosis of ciguatera includes paralytic shellfish poisoning, eosinophilic meningitis, type E botulism, organophosphate insecticide poisoning, tetrodotoxin poisoning, and psychogenic hyperventilation. At present, the diagnosis of ciguatera poisoning is made on clinical grounds because no routinely used laboratory test detects ciguatoxin in human blood. A ciguatoxin enzyme immunoassay or radioimmunoassay may be used to test small portions of the suspected fish.

Therapy is supportive and based on symptoms. Although not of proven efficacy, gastric lavage or syrup of ipecac–induced emesis followed by the administration of a slurry of activated charcoal (100 g) in sorbitol may be of limited value if performed within 3 h after ingestion. Nausea and vomiting may be controlled with an antiemetic, such as prochlorperazine (2.5 to 5 mg intravenously). Hypotension may require the administration of intravenous crystalloid and, in rare cases, a pressor drug. Bradyarrhythmias that lead to cardiac insufficiency and hypotension generally respond well to atropine (0.5 mg intravenously, up to 2 mg). Cool showers or the administration of hydroxyzine (25 mg orally every 6 to 8 h) may relieve pruritus. Amitriptyline (25 mg orally twice a day) reportedly ameliorates pruritus and dysesthesias. In three cases unresponsive to amitriptyline, tocainide appeared to be efficacious. Intravenous infusion of mannitol may be beneficial in moderate or severe cases, particularly for the relief of distressing neurologic or cardiovascular symptoms. The infusion is rendered initially as 1 g/kg per day over 45 to 60 min during the acute phase (days 1 to 5). The mechanism of the benefit against ciguatera intoxication is hyperosmotic water-drawing action, which reverses ciguatoxin-induced Schwann cell edema. Mannitol may also act in some fashion as a "hydroxyl scavenger."

During recovery from ciguatera poisoning, the victim should exclude the following from the diet: fish (fresh or preserved), fish sauces, shellfish, shellfish sauces, alcoholic beverages, and nuts and nut oils. Consumption of fish in ciguatera-endemic regions should be avoided. All oversized fish of any predacious reef species should be suspected of harboring ciguatoxin. Neither moray eels nor the viscera of tropical marine fish should ever be eaten.

PARALYTIC SHELLFISH POISONING Paralytic shellfish poisoning (PSP) is induced by the ingestion of any of a variety of feral or aquacultured filter-feeding organisms, including clams, oysters, scallops, mussels, chitons, limpets, starfish, and sand crabs. The origin of their toxicity is the chemical toxin they accumulate and concentrate by feeding on various planktonic dinoflagellates and protozoan organisms. The unicellular phytoplanktonic organisms form the foundation of the food chain, and in warm summer months these organisms "bloom" in nutrient-rich coastal temperate and semitropical waters. A number of dinoflagellates produce a variety of toxins. These planktonic species can release massive amounts of toxic metabolites into the water and cause enormous mortality in bird and marine populations. The paralytic shellfish toxins are water-soluble as well as heat- and acid-stable; they cannot be destroyed by ordinary cooking. The best-characterized and most frequently identified paralytic shellfish toxin is saxitoxin, which takes its name from the Alaska butter clam *Saxidomus giganteus.* A toxin concentration of >75 μg/100 g of foodstuff is considered hazardous to humans. In the 1972 New England "red tide," the concentration of saxitoxin in blue mussels exceeded 9000 μg/100 g of foodstuff. Saxitoxin appears to block sodium conductance, inhibiting neuromuscular transmission at the axonal and muscle membrane levels.

Within minutes to a few hours after ingestion of contaminated shellfish, there is the onset of intraoral and perioral paresthesias, notably of the lips, tongue, and gums, that progress rapidly to involve the neck and distal extremities. The tingling or burning sensation later changes to numbness. Other symptoms rapidly develop and include lightheadedness, disequilibrium, incoordination, weakness, hyperreflexia, incoherence, dysarthria, sialorrhea, dysphagia, thirst, diarrhea, abdominal pain, nausea, vomiting, nystagmus, dysmetria, headache, diaphoresis, loss of vision, chest pain, and tachycardia. Flaccid paralysis and respiratory insufficiency may follow 2 to 12 h after ingestion. In the absence of hypoxia, the victim often remains alert but paralyzed.

Treatment is supportive and based on symptoms. If the victim comes to medical attention within the first few hours after poison ingestion, the stomach should be emptied by gastric lavage and then irrigated with 2 L (in 200-mL aliquots) of a solution of 2% sodium bicarbonate. The administration of activated charcoal (50 to 100 g) and a cathartic (sorbitol, 20 to 50 g) makes empirical sense but has not been proved effective. Some authors advise against administration of magnesium-based solutions, such as certain cathartics, cautioning that hypermagnesemia may contribute to suppression of nerve conduction.

The most serious problem is respiratory paralysis. The victim should be closely observed in a hospital for at least 24 h for respiratory distress. With prompt recognition of ventilatory failure, endotracheal intubation and assisted ventilation prevent anoxic myocardial and brain injury.

DOMOIC ACID INTOXICATION In late 1987 in eastern Canada, an outbreak of gastrointestinal and neurologic symptoms (amnestic shellfish poisoning) occurred after consumption of mussels found to be contaminated with domoic acid. A heat-stable neuroexcitatory amino acid whose biochemical analogs are kainic acid and glutamic acid, domoic acid binds to the kainate type of glutamate receptor with three times the affinity of kainic acid and is 20 times as powerful a toxin. Mussels can be tested for domoic acid by mouse bioassay and high-performance liquid chromatography. The regulatory limit for domoic acid in shellfish is 20 parts per million.

The abnormalities noted within 24 h of ingesting contaminated mussels *(Mytilus edulis)* include arousal, confusion, disorientation, and memory loss. The median time of onset is 5.5 h. Other prominent symptoms include severe headache, nausea, vomiting, diarrhea, abdominal cramps, hiccoughs, arrhythmias, hypotension, seizures, ophthalmoplegia, hemiparesis, mutism, grimacing, agitation, emotional lability, coma, copious bronchial secretions, and pulmonary edema. Histologic study of brain tissue taken at autopsy has shown neuronal necrosis or cell loss and astrocytosis, most prominently in the hippocampus and the amygdaloid nucleus—findings similar to those in animals poisoned with kainic acid. Several months after the primary intoxication, victims still demonstrate chronic residual memory deficits and motor neuronopathy or axonopathy. Nonneurologic illness does not persist.

Therapy is supportive and based on symptoms. Since kainic acid neuropathology seems to be nearly entirely seizure mediated, an emphasis should be placed on anticonvulsive therapy, for which diazepam appears to be as effective as any other drug.

SCOMBROID Scombroid (mackerel-like) fish include the albacore, bluefin, and yellowfin tuna; mackerel; saury; needlefish; wahoo; skipjack; and bonito. Nonscombroid fish that produce scombroid poisoning include the dolphinfish (mahimahi, *Coryphaena*), kahawai, sardine, black marlin, pilchard, anchovy, herring, amberjack, and Australian ocean salmon. In the northeastern and mid-Atlantic United States, bluefish has been linked to scombroid poisoning. Because greater numbers of nonscombroid fish are being recognized as scombrotoxic, the syndrome may more appropriately be called *pseudoallergic fish poisoning.*

Under conditions of inadequate preservation or refrigeration, the musculature of these dark- or red-fleshed fish undergoes bacterial decomposition, which includes the decarboxylation of the amino acid L-histidine to histamine, histamine phosphate, and histamine hydrochloride. Histamine levels of >20 to 50 mg/100 g are noted in toxic fish, with levels in excess of 400 mg/100 g on occasion. The toxin is heat stable and is not destroyed by domestic or commercial cooking. Affected fish typically have a sharply metallic or peppery taste; however, they may be normal in appearance, color, and flavor.

Symptoms occur within 15 to 90 min of ingestion and include flushing (sharply demarcated; exacerbated by ultraviolet exposure; particularly pronounced on the face, neck, or upper trunk), a sensation of warmth without elevated core temperature, conjunctival hyperemia, pruritus, urticaria, angioneurotic edema, bronchospasm, nausea, vomiting, diarrhea, epigastric pain, abdominal cramps, dysphagia, headache, thirst, pharyngitis, burning of the gingiva, palpitations, tachycardia, dizziness, and hypotension. Without treatment, the symptoms generally resolve within 8 to 12 h. The reaction may be more severe in a person who is concurrently ingesting isoniazid because of blockade of gastrointestinal tract histaminase.

Therapy is directed at reversing the histamine effect with antihistamines, either H-1 or H-2. If bronchospasm is severe, an inhaled bronchodilator—or in rare, extremely severe circumstances, injected epinephrine—may be used. Glucocorticoids are of no proven benefit. Protracted nausea and vomiting, which may empty the stomach of toxin, may be controlled with a specific antiemetic, such as prochlorperazine. The persistent headache of scombroid poisoning may respond to cimetidine or a similar antihistamine if standard analgesics are not effective.

PFIESTERIA In the summer of 1997, reports of adverse reactions after casual exposure to Maryland waters infested with the fish-eating dinoflagellate *Pfiesteria* prompted the Centers for Disease Control and Prevention (CDC) to undertake multistate surveillance and to establish a case definition. As defined by the CDC, the human disease syndrome associated with *Pfiesteria* is characterized by either of two groups of signs and symptoms: (1) memory loss, confusion, or acute skin burning on direct contact with infested water; or (2) at least three of the following: headache, rash (flat red sores), eye irritation, upper respiratory irritation, muscle cramps, and gastrointestinal symptoms. Since the initial reports from Maryland, many such cases have followed both casual exposure to infested water and laboratory work with *Pfiesteria* (which is currently conducted in biohazard III facilities).

Research on *Pfiesteria* has been complicated by a variety of factors, including the lack of a test for detection of its toxins, which have yet to be purified, and the organism's complex life cycle, which includes at least two dozen stages. In nature, the proximity of a school of fish elicits *Pfiesteria's* transformation into a flagellated zoospore that releases at least two toxins: a water-soluble, neuroactive toxin that kills fish within minutes, and a fat-soluble toxin that causes epidermal delamination. Polluted environments appear to favor *Pfiesteria.*

For the treatment of *Pfiesteria*-associated syndromes, one teaspoon of milk of magnesia followed by one scoop of cholestyramine in 8 ounces of water and 70% sorbitol solution is administered daily for 2 weeks.

BIBLIOGRAPHY

Snakes and Lizards

Dart RC et al: Affinity-purified, mixed monoclonal specific crotalid antivenom ovine Fab for the treatment of crotalid venom poisoning. Ann Emerg Med 30:33, 1997

Meyer WP et al: First clinical experiences with a new ovine Fab *Echis ocellatus* snake bite antivenom in Nigeria: Randomized comparative trial with Institute Pasteur Serum (IPSER) Africa antivenom. Am J Trop Med Hyg 56:291, 1997

Minton SA, Norris RL: Non-North American venomous reptile bites, in *Wilderness Medicine: Management of Wilderness and Environmental Emergencies,* 3d ed, PS Auerbach (ed). St. Louis, Mosby, 1995, pp 710–730

Russell FE: *Snake Venom Poisoning.* New York, Scholium International, 1983

Sullivan JB et al: North American venomous reptile bites, in *Wilderness Medicine: Management of Wilderness and Environmental Emergencies,* 3d ed, PS Auerbach (ed). St. Louis, Mosby, 1995, pp 680–709

Marine Creatures

Auerbach PS: Marine envenomation, in *Wilderness Medicine: Management of Wilderness and Environmental Emergencies,* 3d ed, PS Auerbach (ed). St. Louis, Mosby, 1995, pp 1327–1374

Auerbach PS: Marine envenomations. N Engl J Med 325:486, 1991

Brown CK, Shepherd SM: Marine trauma, envenomations, and intoxications. Emerg Med Clin North Am 10:385, 1992

Burnett JW et al: Coelenterate venom research 1991–1995: Clinical, chemical and immunological aspects. Toxicon 34:1377, 1996

Halstead BW, Auerbach PS: *Dangerous Aquatic Animals of the World: A Color Atlas: With Prevention, First Aid, and Emergency Treatment Procedures.* Princeton, Darwin Press, 1992, pp 29–124, 241–252

Meier J, White J (eds): *Handbook of Clinical Toxicology of Animal Venoms and Poisons.* Boca Raton, FL, CRC Press, 1996, pp 89–176

Mines D et al: Poisonings: Food, fish, and shellfish. Emerg Med Clin North Am 15:157, 1997

Stewart MPM: Ciguatera fish poisoning: Treatment with intravenous mannitol. Trop Doct 21:54, 1991

Teitelbaum JS et al: Neurologic sequelae of domoic acid intoxication due to the ingestion of contaminated mussels. N Engl J Med 322:1781, 1990

398

James H. Maguire, Andrew Spielman

ECTOPARASITE INFESTATIONS, ARTHROPOD BITES AND STINGS

Ectoparasites are arthropods or helminths that *infest* the skin of other animals from which they derive sustenance. They may penetrate beneath the surface of the host or attach superficially by their mouthparts. These organisms damage their hosts by inflicting direct injury, by eliciting a hypersensitivity reaction, or by inoculating toxins or pathogens. The main medically important ectoparasites are arachnids (including mites and ticks), insects (including lice, fleas, and flies), pentastomes (tongue worms), and leeches. Arthropods may also harm humans through brief encounters in which they take a blood meal or attempt to defend themselves by biting, stinging, or inoculating venoms. Various arachnids (spiders, scorpions), insects (including bees, hornets, wasps, ants, flies, bugs, caterpillars, and beetles), millipedes, and centipedes produce ill effects in this manner, as do certain ectoparasites of animals, including ticks, biting mites, and fleas (discussed in this chapter as biting arthropods). More people in the United States die each year as a consequence of arthropod stings than from poisonous snake bites.

ECTOPARASITE INFESTATIONS

SCABIES The human itch mite, *Sarcoptes scabiei,* which infests some 300 million persons each year, is one of the most common causes of itching dermatoses throughout the world. Gravid female mites measuring 0.3 to 0.4 mm in length burrow superficially beneath the stratum corneum for a month, depositing two or three eggs a day. Nymphs that hatch from these eggs mature in about 2 weeks through a series of molts and then emerge as adults to the surface of the skin, where they mate and subsequently reinvade the skin of the same or another host. Transfer of newly fertilized female mites from person to person occurs by intimate personal contact and is facilitated by crowding, uncleanliness, and multiple sexual partners. Medical practitioners are at particular risk of infestation. Transmission via sharing of contaminated bedding or clothing is infrequent because these mites cannot survive much more than a day without host contact. In the United States, scabies may account for 2 to 5% of visits to dermatologists; involved particularly often are children, immigrants from developing countries, and close household contacts. Outbreaks occur in nursing homes, mental institutions, and hospitals.

The itching and rash associated with scabies derive from a sensitization reaction directed against the excreta that the mite deposits in its burrow (**Plate IID-52**). For this reason, an initial infestation remains asymptomatic for 4 to 6 weeks, and a reinfestation produces a hypersensitivity reaction without delay. Scratching generally destroys the burrowing mite, but symptoms remain even in its absence. Burrows become surrounded by infiltrates of eosinophils, lymphocytes, and histiocytes, and a generalized hypersensitivity rash later develops in remote sites. By destroying these pathogens, immunity and associated scratching limit most infestations to fewer than 15 mites per person. Hyperinfestation with thousands or millions of mites, a condition known as *crusted scabies* or *Norwegian scabies,* may result from glucocorticoid use, immunodeficiency diseases (including AIDS and infection with human T-lymphotropic virus type I), and neurologic and psychiatric illnesses that interfere with itching and scratching.

Patients with scabies report intense itching that worsens at night and after a hot shower. Typical burrows may be difficult to find because they are few in number and may be obscured by excoriations. Burrows appear as dark wavy lines in the epidermis, measure 3 to 15 mm, and end in a small pearly bleb that contains the female mite. Such lesions generally develop on the volar wrists, between the fingers, on the elbows, and on the penis. Small papules and vesicles, often accompanied by eczematous plaques, pustules, or nodules, are symmetrically distributed in these sites and in skin folds under the breasts and around the navel, axillae, belt line, buttocks, upper thighs, and scrotum. Except in infants, the face, scalp, neck, palms, and soles are spared. Burrows and other typical lesions may be sparse in persons who wash frequently, and topical glucocorticoid treatment and bacterial superinfection may alter the appearance of the rash. Atypical presentations of scabies include bullous lesions, which resemble those of bullous pemphigoid, and vesicular lesions, which resemble those of dermatitis herpetiformis. Superinfection with nephritogenic strains of streptococci has led to acute glomerulonephritis. Crusted scabies resembles psoriasis in its typical widespread erythema, thick keratotic crusts, scaling, and dystrophic nails. Characteristic burrows are not seen in crusted scabies, and patients usually do not itch, although their infestations are highly contagious and have been responsible for outbreaks of classic scabies in hospitals. Bacteremia occurs frequently in AIDS patients with crusted scabies and prominent fissures. Persons with massive infestations occasionally present with diffuse pruritus and generalized papules or with minimal or no cutaneous signs.

A diagnosis of scabies should be considered in patients with pruritus and symmetric polymorphic skin lesions in characteristic locations, particularly if there is a history of household contact with a case. Burrows should be sought and unroofed with a sterile needle or scalpel blade, and the scrapings should be examined microscopically for the mite, its eggs, and its fecal pellets. A drop of mineral oil facilitates removal of the sample. Biopsies or scrapings of papulovesicular lesions may also be diagnostic. In the absence of identifiable mites or mite products, the diagnosis is based on clinical presentation and history. The possibility of other sexually transmitted diseases should be excluded in adults with scabies.

℞ **TREATMENT** For the treatment of scabies, 5% permethrin cream is less toxic than the once commonly used 1% lindane preparations and is effective against lindane-tolerant infestations. Both scabicides are applied thinly but thoroughly behind the ears and from the neck down after bathing and are removed 8 h later with soap and water. Lindane is absorbed through the skin, and its overuse has led to seizures and aplastic anemia. It should not be applied to pregnant women or infants. Alternatives include topical crotamiton cream, benzyl benzoate, and sulfur ointments. Successful treatment of crusted scabies requires the application first of a keratolytic agent such as 6% salicylic acid (to improve the penetration of scabicides) and then of scabicides to the scalp, face, and ears (with care to avoid the eyes). Repeated treatments or the sequential use of several agents may be necessary. A single oral dose of ivermectin (200 μg/kg) effectively treats scabies in otherwise healthy persons. Patients with crusted scabies may require two or more doses of ivermectin. Although ivermectin may become the agent of choice for treating crusted scabies, it has not yet received approval by the U.S. Food and Drug Administration (FDA) for any form of scabies. Its use should be reserved for persons who fail to respond to topical scabicides, the elderly, persons with generalized eczema, and other persons who may not tolerate topical therapy.

Although effectively treated scabies infestations become noninfectious within a day, itching and rash due to hypersensitivity frequently persist for weeks or months. Unnecessary re-treatment of the affected patients may provoke contact dermatitis. Antihistamines, salicylates, and calamine lotion relieve itching during treatment, and topical glucocorticoids are useful for the pruritus that lingers after effective treatment. An oral antibiotic may be necessary for bacterial superinfections that fail to resolve with antiscabietic therapy. Relapses of scabies may be due to infestations of the scalp when topical therapy is applied only from the neck down. To prevent reinfestations, bedding and clothing should be washed in hot water, and close contacts, even if asymptomatic, should be treated simultaneously.

OTHER MITE INFESTATIONS Species of *Demodex*, the follicle mite, live in hair follicles and sebaceous glands of the face and ears. The wormlike mites measure up to 0.4 mm in length and, if carefully sought, can be found on almost all persons. They appear not to cause disease, although their density is high in persons with rosacea. House dust mites of the genus *Dermatophagoides* infest houses throughout the world, living on furniture and rugs and feeding on shed human dander. Exposure to their allergens causes asthma, rhinitis, conjunctivitis, and eczema in persons with house dust allergies. Management includes immunotherapy with mite extracts and environmental interventions such as frequent vacuuming and removal of rugs from bedrooms to reduce mite density.

PEDICULOSIS (LOUSE INFESTATIONS) All three species of human louse feed at least once a day on human blood. *Pediculus humanus* var. *capitis* infests the head, *P. humanus* var. *corporis* the clothing, and *Phthirus pubis* mainly the hair of the pubis. Females cement their eggs (nits) firmly to hair or clothing. The saliva of lice produces an intensely irritating maculopapular or urticarial rash in sensitized persons.

Head lice, which infest an estimated 6 to 12 million people in the United States, are transmitted directly from person to person and occasionally by shared headgear and grooming implements. The prevalence is highest among school-aged girls who wear long hair; in the United States, black children are less frequently infested than other children. Excoriations of pruritic lesions on the scalp, neck, and shoulders lead to oozing, crusting, matting of hair, bacterial infections, and regional lymphadenopathy. Adult lice are frequently seen crawling in the hair with a velocity that approaches 25 mm/min.

Body lice remain in clothing except when feeding and cannot survive more than a few hours away from the human host. It follows, therefore, that *P. humanus* var. *corporis* mainly infests disaster victims or indigent persons who do not change their clothes. Transmission by direct contact or by sharing of clothing and beds is enhanced under crowded conditions. The fact that the body louse leaves febrile persons or corpses as they become cold facilitates the transmission of typhus, louse-borne relapsing fever, and trench fever (Chap. 177). Trench fever and endocarditis due to *Bartonella quintana* have emerged as diseases of homeless persons living in large cities of the United States and Europe. Pruritic lesions are particularly common around the neckline. Chronic infestations result in the postinflammatory hyperpigmentation and thickening of skin known as *vagabonds' disease*.

The cosmopolitan crab or pubic louse is transmitted mainly by sexual contact but can infest eyelashes, axillary hair, and hair in other sites as well as pubic hair. Children with pubic lice generally acquire their infestations from parents rather than via sexual transmission. Polymerase chain reaction (PCR) analysis of the blood meal of lice permits identification of host DNA in cases of child abuse or rape. Intensely pruritic lesions and 2- to 3-mm blue macules (maculae ceruleae) develop at the site of bites. Blepharitis commonly accompanies infestations of the eyelashes.

A suspected diagnosis of pediculosis is confirmed by the finding of nits or adult lice on hairs or in clothing. The dorsoventrally flattened adult lice measure 2 to 4 mm in length and have three pairs of legs ending in claws that enable them to grasp hair shafts or clothing. Oval nits measure 0.8 mm in length and are opaque white or cream-colored (body and head lice) or dark brown (pubic lice).

℞ **TREATMENT** The preferred treatment is a 10-min application of 1% permethrin creme rinse, which kills both lice and eggs and is available without prescription. An alternative, 0.5% malathion, requires a prescription and must be left in place for 8 to 12 h. Other agents, such as the more toxic 1% lindane and pyrethrins with piperonyl butoxide, are not ovicidal and require a second application 1 week after the first to kill hatching nymphs. Dead or hatched nits, which remain attached to hair sheaths and become translucent or opalescent, may falsely suggest an active infection. Resistance of head lice to permethrin, malathion, and lindane has been reported. When a properly applied treatment fails, a higher concentration (5%) of permethrin may be tried or the class of pediculicide changed (e.g., by switching from permethrin to malathion). Ivermectin may be useful in cases of resistance to both malathion and permethrin but has not been approved for this purpose by the FDA.

After louse infestations have been treated with insecticide, the hair should be combed with a fine-toothed nit comb to remove nits. Combs and brushes should be disinfected in hot water at 65°C for 5 min or soaked in insecticide for 1 h. Body lice can be eliminated by bathing and application of topical pediculicides from head to foot. Clothes and bedding are deloused by heat sterilization in a dryer at 65°C for 30 min or by fumigation. Infestations with pubic lice are treated with topical pediculicides except for eyelid infestations (*phthiriasis palpebrum*), which respond to a coating of petroleum applied for 3 to 4 days or 1% yellow oxide of mercury ointment applied four times daily for 2 weeks.

TUNGIASIS *Tunga penetrans*, like other fleas, is a wingless, laterally flattened insect measuring 2 to 4 mm in length that feeds on blood. Also known as the chigoe flea, sand flea, or jigger, it occurs in tropical regions of Africa and the Americas. Adults live in sandy soil and burrow under the skin between toes, under nails, or on the soles of bare feet. The fleas engorge on blood and grow from pinpoint to pea size over a 2-week period. The lesions resemble a white pustule with a central black depression and may be pruritic or painful. Occasional complications include tetanus, bacterial infections, and autoamputation of toes. Tungiasis is treated by removal of the intact flea with a sterile needle or scalpel, tetanus vaccination, and topical antibiotics.

MYIASIS *Myiasis* refers to infestations by maggots, mainly due to the larvae of metallic-colored screw-worm flies or botflies. Maggots invade living or necrotic tissue or body cavities and produce different clinical syndromes depending on the species of fly.

Furuncular Myiasis In forested parts of Central and South America, larvae of *Dermatobia hominis* (the human botfly) produce boil-like subcutaneous nodules 2 to 3 cm in diameter. The adult female captures a mosquito or other bloodsucking insect and deposits her eggs beneath its abdomen. When the carrier insect attacks a human or bovine host several days later, the warmth and moisture of the host's surface stimulate the larvae to hatch and penetrate the skin. After 6 to 12 weeks, the larvae mature and drop to the ground, where they pupate. The African tumbu fly, *Cordylobia anthropophaga*, produces similar lesions. Dozens of eggs are deposited on sand or drying laundry that is contaminated with urine or sweat. Larvae hatch on contact with the body, penetrate the skin, and produce boils from which they emerge 8 or 9 days later. A diagnosis of furuncular myiasis is suggested by uncomfortable lesions with a central breathing pore that emits bubbles when submerged in water. There is often a sensation of movement under the skin that may lead to severe emotional distress. Tumbu fly larvae can be removed by manual expression after the air pore is coated with petroleum to suffocate the larvae and induce them to emerge. Removal of *Dermatobia* larvae is facilitated by injection of a local anesthetic into the surrounding tissue, but surgical excision is often necessary because up-pointing spines hold the larva firmly in place.

Creeping Dermal Myiasis Maggots of the horse botfly, *Gasterophilus intestinalis*, do not mature after penetrating human skin but migrate for weeks in the epidermis. The resulting pruritic and serpiginous eruption resembles cutaneous larva migrans caused by *Ancylostoma braziliense*. Horseback riders become infested when eggs deposited on the flank of the horse hatch against their bare legs. The black spines of the larvae can be identified after mineral oil is smeared over the lesion. Larva are removed with a needle. The larvae of the cattle botfly (*Hypoderma* species) invade more deeply and produce boil-like swellings.

Wound and Body Cavity Myiasis Certain flies are attracted to blood and pus, and their newly hatched larvae enter wounds or diseased skin. Larvae of species such as *Phaenicia sericata*, the greenbottle fly, remain superficial and confined to necrotic tissue and were used in the past to debride purulent wounds. Other species, including the screw-worms (*Chrysomyia bezziana* in Asia and Africa and *Cochliomyia hominivorax* in Latin America) and the flesh fly (*Wohlfahrtia vigil* in northern North America), invade more deeply into viable tissue and produce large suppurating lesions. Larvae that infest wounds also may infest body cavities such as the mouth, nose, ears, sinuses, anus, vagina, and lower urinary tract, particularly in unconscious or otherwise debilitated patients. The consequences range from harmless colonization to destruction of the nose, meningitis, and deafness. Treatment involves removal of maggots and debridement of tissue.

Other Forms of Myiasis The maggots responsible for furuncular and wound myiasis may also cause ophthalmomyiasis. Sequelae include nodules in the eyelid, retinal detachment, and destruction of the globe. In addition, the adult sheep botfly, *Oestrus ovis*, may deposit larvae in the eyes of persons tending sheep and goats, and the larvae may produce a conjunctival infestation and acute conjunctivitis. True intestinal myiasis occurs when eggs or larvae of the drone fly (*Eristalis tenax*) are ingested with contaminated food, mature in the gut, and cause enteritis. Most instances in which maggots are found in human feces are the result of larviposition by flesh flies on recently passed stools.

PENTASTOMIASIS Pentastomids, or tongue worms, are parasites with characteristics of both helminths and arthropods and are classified in a separate phylum. The wormlike adults inhabit the respiratory passages of reptiles and carnivorous mammals. Human infestation with *Linguatula serrata* is common in the Middle East and occurs in the Sudan following ingestion of encysted larval stages in raw liver or lymph nodes of sheep and goats, the intermediate hosts. The larvae migrate to the nasopharynx and produce an acute self-limiting syndrome known as *halzoun* (*Marrara* in the Sudan), which is characterized by pain and itching of the throat and ears, coughing, hoarseness, dysphagia, and dyspnea. Severe edema may cause obstruction and necessitate tracheostomy, and ocular invasion has been described. Diagnostic larvae measuring 5 to 10 mm in length are found in the copious nasal discharge or vomitus. Human beings become infected with *Armillifer armillatus* by ingesting eggs in contaminated food or drink or after handling the definitive host, the African python. Larvae encyst in various organs but rarely cause symptoms unless they compress vital structures or perforate an organ during migration. Cysts occasionally require surgical removal as they enlarge during molting, but they are usually encountered as an incidental finding at autopsy. There are reports of the cutaneous larva migrans syndrome due to other pentastomes (*Reighardia* and *Sebekia* species) in Southeast Asia and Central America.

LEECH INFESTATIONS Medically important leeches are annelid worms that attach to their hosts with chitinous cutting jaws and draw blood with muscular suckers. The medicinal leech, *Hirudo medicinalis*, is still used occasionally to reduce venous congestion in surgical flaps or replanted body parts. This practice has been complicated by wound infections, myonecrosis, and sepsis due to *Aeromonas hydrophila*, which colonizes the gullets of commercially available leeches.

Ubiquitous aquatic leeches that parasitize fish, frogs, and turtles readily attach to the skin of human beings and avidly suck blood. More notorious are the land leeches (*Haemadipsa*) that live in moist vegetation of tropical rain forests. Attachment is usually painless. Hirudinin, a powerful anticoagulant secreted by the leech, causes continued bleeding after the leech has detached. Healing of the wound is slow, and bacterial infections are not uncommon. Several species of aquatic leeches in Africa, Asia, and southern Europe can enter through the mouth, nose, and genitourinary tract and attach to mucosal surfaces at sites as deep as the esophagus and trachea. Bleeding may be intense. Externally attached leeches are removed by steady gentle traction. Removal is hastened by application of alcohol, salt, vinegar, or a flame to the leech. Internally attached leeches may detach on exposure to gargled saline or may be removed by forceps.

DELUSIONAL INFESTATIONS The groundless conviction that one is infested with arthropods or other parasites is an extremely difficult disorder to treat and unfortunately is not rare. Patients report infestations of their skin, clothing, or homes and describe sensations of something moving in or on their skin. Excoriations often accompany complaints of pruritus or insect bites. Patients bring in as evidence of infestation specimens that are identified microscopically as plant-feeding or peridomestic arthropods, pieces of skin, vegetable matter, or inanimate objects. In suspected cases, it is imperative to rule out true infestations and neuropathies, environmental irritants such as fragments of fiberglass, and other causes of tingling or prickling sensations. Pharmacotherapy with pimozide, which blocks dopamine receptors, has been more helpful than psychotherapy in treating this disorder.

ARTHROPOD BITES AND STINGS

SPIDER BITES Of the >30,000 recognized species of spider, only about 100 defend themselves aggressively and have fangs sufficiently long to penetrate human skin. The venom that spiders use to immobilize and digest their prey can cause necrosis of skin and systemic toxicity. While the bites of most spiders are painful but not harmful, envenomations of the brown or fiddle spiders (*Loxosceles* species), widow spiders (*Latrodectus* species), and other species may be life-threatening. Identification of the offending spider should be attempted, since specific treatments exist for bites of widow and brown recluse spiders and since injuries attributed to spiders are frequently due to other causes.

Recluse Spider Bites and Necrotic Arachnidism Severe necrosis of skin and subcutaneous tissue follows envenomation by *Loxosceles reclusa*, the brown recluse spider, and by at least four other species of *Loxosceles* in the southern and midwestern United States. Other spiders that produce necrotic ulceration include the hobo spider (*Tegenaria agrestis*) in the Pacific Northwest, the sac spiders (*Chiracanthium* species) throughout the United States and abroad, the South American brown spider *Loxosceles laeta* in Central and South America, and other *Loxosceles* species in Africa and the Middle East. All these spiders measure 7 to 15 mm in body length and 2 to 4 cm in leg span. Recluse spiders are brown and have a dark violin-shaped spot on their dorsal surface; hobo spiders are brown with gray markings; and sac spiders may be pale yellow, green, or brown.

These spiders are not aggressive toward human beings and bite only if threatened or pressed against the skin. They hide under rocks and logs or in caves and animal burrows, and they emerge at night to hunt other spiders and insects. They invade homes, particularly in the fall, and seek dark and undisturbed hiding spots in closets, in folds of clothing, or under furniture and rubbish in storage rooms, garages, and attics. Bites often occur while the victim is dressing and are sustained primarily to the arms, neck, and lower abdomen.

The clear viscous venoms of these spiders contain an esterase, alkaline phosphatase, protease, and other enzymes that produce tissue necrosis and hemolysis. Sphingomyelinase B, the most important dermonecrotic factor, binds cell membranes and promotes chemotaxis of neutrophils, leading to vascular thrombosis and an Arthus-like reaction. Initially, the bite is painless or produces a stinging sensation. Within the next few hours, the site becomes painful and pruritic, with central induration surrounded by a pale zone of ischemia and a zone of erythema. In most cases, the lesion resolves without treatment over 2 to 3 days. In severe cases, the erythema spreads, and the center of the lesion becomes hemorrhagic and necrotic with an overlying bulla. A black eschar forms and sloughs several weeks later, leaving an ulcer that may be ≥25 cm in diameter and eventually a depressed scar. Healing usually takes place within 3 to 6 months but may take as long as 3 years if adipose tissue is involved. Local complications include injury to nerves and secondary infection. Fever, chills, weakness, headache, nausea, vomiting, myalgia, arthralgia, maculopapular rash, and leukocytosis may develop within 72 h of the bite. In rare instances, acute complications such as hemolytic anemia, hemoglobinuria, and renal failure are fatal.

℞ TREATMENT Initial management includes local cleansing, application of sterile dressings and cold compresses, and elevation and loose immobilization of the affected limb. Analgesics, antihistamines, antibiotics, and tetanus prophylaxis should be administered if indicated. Within the first 48 to 72 h, the administration of dapsone, a leukocyte inhibitor, may halt the progression of lesions that are becoming necrotic. Dapsone is given in oral doses of 50 to 100 mg twice daily after glucose-6-phosphate dehydrogenase deficiency has been ruled out. The efficacy of locally or systemically administered glucocorticoids has not been demonstrated, and a potentially useful *Loxosceles*-specific antivenin has not been approved for use in the United States. Debridement and later skin grafting may be necessary after signs of acute inflammation have subsided, but immediate surgical excision of the wound is detrimental. Patients should be monitored closely for signs of hemolysis, renal failure, and other systemic complications.

Widow Spider Bites The bite of the female widow spider is notorious for the effect of its potent neurotoxin. *Latrodectus mactans*, the black widow, has been found in every state of the United States except Alaska and is most abundant in the southeast. It measures up to 1 cm in body length and 5 cm in leg span, is shiny black, and has a red hourglass marking on the ventral abdomen. Other dangerous North American *Latrodectus* species include *L. geometricus* (the brown widow), *L. bishopi* (the red widow), *L. variolus*, and *L. hesperus*, and there are related species in other temperate and subtropical parts of the world.

Widow spiders spin their webs under stones, logs, plants, or rock piles or in dark spaces in barns, garages, and outhouses. Bites are most common in the summer and early autumn and occur when the web is disturbed or when the spider is trapped or provoked. The buttocks or genitals are sites of bites incurred by humans while sitting in an outdoor privy.

The initial bite goes unnoticed or is perceived as a sharp pinprick. Two small red marks, mild erythema, and edema develop at the fang entrance site. The oily yellow venom that is injected does not produce local necrosis, and some persons experience no other symptoms. However, α-latrotoxin, the most active component of the venom, binds irreversibly to nerves and causes release and eventual depletion of acetylcholine, norepinephrine, and other neurotransmitters from presynaptic terminals. Within 30 to 60 min, painful cramps spread from the bite site to large muscles of the extremities and the trunk. Extreme rigidity of the abdominal muscles and excruciating pain may suggest peritonitis, but the abdomen is not tender on palpation. Other features include salivation, diaphoresis, vomiting, hypertension, tachycardia, labored breathing, anxiety, headache, weakness, fasciculations, paresthesia, hyperreflexia, urinary retention, uterine contractions, and premature labor. Rhabdomyolysis and renal failure have been reported, and respiratory arrest, cerebral hemorrhage, or cardiac failure may end fatally, especially in very young, elderly, or debilitated persons. The pain begins to subside during the first 12 h but may recur during several days or weeks before resolving spontaneously.

℞ TREATMENT Treatment consists of local cleansing, application of ice packs, and tetanus prophylaxis. Hypertension that does not respond to analgesics and antispasmodics, such as benzodiazepines or methocarbamol, requires specific antihypertensive medication. Intravenous administration of one or two vials of a widely available equine antivenin rapidly relieves pain and can be life-saving. Because of the risk of anaphylaxis and serum sickness, antivenin should be reserved for severe cases involving respiratory arrest, uncontrollable hypertension, seizures, or pregnancy.

Envenomations by Tarantulas and Other Spiders Tarantulas are long-lived, hairy spiders of which 30 species are found in the United States, primarily in the southwest. The tarantulas that have become popular household pets are usually imported species with bright colors and a leg span of up to 25 cm. Tarantulas bite only when threatened and cause no more harm than a bee sting, but the venom occasionally provokes deep pain and swelling. Several species are covered with urticating hairs that are launched in the thousands when a threatened spider rubs its hind legs across the dorsal abdomen. These hairs penetrate human skin and produce pruritic papules that last for weeks. Failure to wear gloves or to wash the hands after handling the Chilean Rose tarantula, the most popular pet spider, has resulted in transfer of hairs to the eye and devastating ocular inflammation. Treatment of bites includes local washing and elevation of the bitten area, tetanus prophylaxis, and analgesic administration. Antihistamines and topical or systemic glucocorticoids are given for exposure to urticating hairs.

Atrax robustus, the Sydney funnel-web spider of Australia, and *Phoneutria* species, the South American banana spiders, are among the most dangerous spiders in the world because of their aggressive behavior and potent neurotoxins. Envenomation by *A. robustus* causes a rapidly progressive neuromotor syndrome that can be fatal within 2 h. The bite of the banana spiders causes severe local pain followed by profound systemic symptoms and respiratory paralysis that can lead to death within 2 to 6 h. Specific antivenins for envenomation by each of these spiders are available. *Lycosa* species (wolf spiders) are found throughout the world and may produce painful bites and transient local inflammation.

SCORPION STINGS Scorpions are crablike arachnids that feed on ground-dwelling arthropods and small lizards, which they grasp with a pair of frontal pinchers and paralyze by injecting venom from a stinger on the tip of the tail. Painful but relatively harmless scorpion stings need to be distinguished from the potentially lethal envenomations that are produced by about 30 of the approximately 1000 known species and cause more than 5000 deaths worldwide each year. Scorpions feed at night and remain hidden during the day in crevices or burrows or under wood, loose bark, or rocks on the ground.

They seek cool spots under buildings and often enter houses, where they get into shoes, clothing, or bedding or enter bathtubs and sinks in search of water. Scorpions sting human beings only when disturbed.

Scorpions of the United States Of the 40 or so scorpion species in the United States, only the bark scorpion (*Centruroides sculpturatus* or *C. exilicauda*) produces a venom that can be lethal. Stings of the other species, such as the common striped scorpion *C. vittatus* and the large *Hadrurus arizonensis*, cause immediate sharp local pain followed by edema, ecchymosis, and a burning sensation. Symptoms typically resolve within a few hours, and skin does not slough. Allergic reactions to the venom sometimes develop.

The deadly *C. sculpturatus* of the southwestern United States and northern Mexico measures about 7 cm in length and is yellow-brown in color. Its venom contains neurotoxins that cause sodium channels to remain open and neurons to fire repetitively. In contrast to the stings of nonlethal species, *C. sculpturatus* envenomations are usually associated with little swelling, but prominent pain, paresthesia, and hyperesthesia can be accentuated by tapping on the affected area (the tap test). These symptoms soon spread to other locations; dysfunction of cranial nerves and hyperexcitability of skeletal muscles develop within hours. Patients present with restlessness, blurred vision, abnormal eye movements, profuse salivation, lacrimation, rhinorrhea, slurred speech, difficulty in handling secretions, diaphoresis, nausea, and vomiting. Muscle twitching, jerking, and shaking may be mistaken for a seizure. Complications include tachycardia, arrhythmias, hypertension, hyperthermia, rhabdomyolysis, and acidosis. Symptoms progress to maximal severity in about 5 h and subside within a day or two, although pain and paresthesia can last for weeks. Fatal respiratory arrest is most common among young children and the elderly.

Other Dangerous Scorpions Envenomations by *Leiurus quinquestriatus* in the Middle East and North Africa, by *Mesobuthus tamulus* in India, by *Androctonus* species along the Mediterranean littoral and in North Africa and the Middle East, and by *Tityus serrulatus* in Brazil cause massive release of endogenous catecholamines with hypertensive crises, arrhythmias, pulmonary edema, and myocardial damage. Acute pancreatitis occurs with stings of *Tityus trinitatis* in Trinidad, and central nervous toxicity complicates stings of *Parabuthus* and *Buthotus* scorpions of South Africa. Tissue necrosis and hemolysis may follow stings of the Iranian *Hemiscorpius lepturus*.

℞ **TREATMENT** Identification of the offending scorpion aids in planning therapy. Stings of nonlethal species require at most ice packs, analgesics, or antihistamines. Because most victims of dangerous envenomations (such as those produced by *C. sculpturatus*) experience only local discomfort, they can be managed at home with instructions to return to the emergency department if signs of cranial-nerve or neuromuscular dysfunction develop. Aggressive supportive care and judicious use of antivenin can reduce or eliminate mortality from more severe envenomations. Keeping the patient calm and applying pressure dressings and cold packs to the sting site decrease the absorption of venom. A continuous intravenous infusion of midazolam controls the agitation, flailing, and involuntary muscle movements produced by scorpion stings. Close monitoring during treatment with this drug and other sedatives or narcotics is necessary for persons with neuromuscular symptoms because of the risk of respiratory arrest. Hypertension and pulmonary edema respond to nifedipine, nitroprusside, hydralazine, or prazosin, and bradyarrhythmias can be controlled with atropine.

Commercially prepared antivenins are available in several countries for some of the most dangerous species. A caprine *C. sculpturatus* antivenin (not yet FDA approved) is available as an investigational drug from the Arizona State University for use only in Arizona. Because of the risk of anaphylaxis or serum sickness following administration of goat serum, use of the antivenin is controversial. Intravenous administration of antivenin rapidly reverses cranial-nerve dysfunction and muscular symptoms but does not affect pain and paresthesia. The benefit of scorpion antivenin has not been established in controlled trials.

Prevention In scorpion-infested areas, shoes, clothing, bedding, and towels should be shaken and inspected before being used. Removal of wood, stones, and debris from yards and campsites eliminates hiding places for scorpions, and household spraying of insecticides can deplete their source of food.

CHIGGERS AND OTHER BITING MITES Chiggers are the larvae of trombiculid (harvest) mites that normally feed on mice in grassy or brush-covered sites in the tropics and subtropics and (less frequently) in temperate areas during warm months. They wait for hosts on low vegetation and attach themselves to passing animals or to people. The larva then pierces the skin of its host and deposits a tubelike structure in the dermis through which it imbibes lymph and tissue juices. This highly antigenic "stylostome" serves as the focus of an exceptionally pruritic papular, papulovesicular, or papulourticarial lesion that may be 2 cm in diameter and that develops within hours of attachment in persons previously sensitized to mite antigen. Feeding mites appear as tiny red vesicles in hair follicles. Scratching invariably destroys the body of a mite attached to a person. These lesions generally vesiculate and develop a hemorrhagic base. Itching and burning last for weeks. The rash is most common on the ankles or near tight-fitting clothes that obstruct the mites' movements. Chiggers are the vectors of scrub typhus in tropical and subtropical parts of Asia. Repellents are useful for preventing chigger bites.

Certain mesostigmatid mites that infest the nests of mice or birds feed on human beings when their usual hosts have been displaced. For example, intense episodes of itching dermatitis in humans may follow the removal of trash from a human residence or the departure of pigeons that have been nesting on a window air-conditioner. Other mites that infest grain, straw, cheese, or other animal products occasionally produce similar episodes. Persons who have close contact with dogs—and, to a lesser extent, cats—may develop a self-limited pruritic papulovesicular rash from bites of cheyletiellid mites that cause a mangelike condition in these animals. Mouse mites are the vectors of rickettsialpox in cities of the northeastern United States. Fowl and chicken mites transmit the viruses of St. Louis encephalitis and western equine encephalitis. Although sanitary measures effectively prevent rickettsialpox, removal of accumulated refuse may result in a transient period of elevated risk.

Diagnosis of mite-induced dermatitides (including those caused by chiggers) relies heavily on a history of exposure to the source of the mite, since the tiny mite may escape notice or may already have fallen off or been scratched off the lesions. Antihistamines or topical steroids effectively reduce mite-induced pruritus.

HYMENOPTERA STINGS Insects that sting to defend their colonies or subdue their prey belong to the order Hymenoptera, which includes apids (bees and bumblebees), vespids (wasps, hornets, and yellow jackets), and ants. Their venoms contain a wide array of amines, peptides, and enzymes that are responsible for local and systemic reactions. Although the toxic effect of multiple stings can be fatal, nearly all of the 50 or more deaths due to hymenopteran stings in the United States each year are the result of allergic reactions.

Bee and Wasp Stings Bees lose their venom apparatus in the act of stinging and subsequently die, while vespids can sting numerous times in succession. The familiar honeybees (*Apis mellifera*) and bumblebees (*Bombus* and other genera) attack when a colony is disturbed, but the extremely aggressive Africanized honeybees respond to minimal intrusions rapidly and in large numbers. Since their introduction into Brazil in 1957, these "killer bees" have spread through South and Central America to the southern and western United States.

The common vespids in the United States include the yellow jacket, notable for the yellow and black bands on its abdomen; the bald-faced hornet, with a black body and a white face; the brown hornet, measuring 2.5 to 3.5 cm in length; and the paper wasps, which have variously colored elongate bodies. Vespids sting in defense of their nests, which they often build near human dwellings and suspend from eaves or shubbery, plaster onto walls, or burrow into wood or soil. Yellow jackets feed on sugary substances and decaying meat and are annoyingly abundant at recreation sites and around garbage, particularly in the late summer and fall.

Venom is produced in glands at the posterior end of the abdomen and is expelled rapidly by contraction of muscles of the venom sac, which has a capacity of up to 0.1 mL in large insects. The venoms of different species of hymenopterans are biochemically and immunologically distinct. Direct toxic effects are mediated by mixtures of low-molecular-weight compounds such as serotonin, histamine, and acetylcholine and several kinins. Polypeptide toxins in honeybee venom include mellitin, which damages cell membranes; mast cell–degranulating protein, which causes histamine release; apamin, a neurotoxin; and adolapin, which has anti-inflammatory action. Enzymes in venom include hyaluronidase, which allows the spread of other venom components, and phospholipases, which may be among the major venom allergens. There appears to be little cross-sensitization between honeybee and wasp venoms.

Uncomplicated stings cause immediate pain, a wheal-and-flare reaction, and local edema and swelling that subside in a few hours. Stings from accidentally swallowed insects may induce life-threatening edema of the upper airways. Multiple stings can lead to vomiting, diarrhea, generalized edema, dyspnea, hypotension, and collapse. Rhabdomyolysis and intravascular hemolysis may cause renal failure. Death from the direct effects of venom has followed 300 to 500 honeybee stings.

Large local reactions that spread ≥10 cm around the sting site over 24 to 48 h are not uncommon. These reactions may resemble cellulitis but are caused by hypersensitivity rather than secondary infection. Such reactions tend to recur on subsequent exposure but are seldom accompanied by anaphylaxis and are not prevented by venom immunotherapy.

An estimated 0.4 to 4.0% of the U.S. population exhibits clinical immediate-type hypersensitivity to insect stings, and 15% may have asymptomatic sensitization manifested by positive skin tests. Persons who experience severe allergic reactions are likely to have similar reactions after subsequent stings; occasionally, adults who have had mild reactions later experience serious reactions. Mild anaphylactic reactions from insect stings, as from other causes, consist of nausea, abdominal cramping, generalized urticaria, flushing, and angioedema. Serious reactions, including upper airway edema, bronchospasm, hypotension, and shock, may be rapidly fatal. Severe reactions usually begin within 10 min of the sting and only rarely develop after 5 h. Unusual complications, including serum sickness, vasculitis, neuritis, and encephalitis, develop several days or weeks after a sting.

℞ **TREATMENT** Stingers embedded in the skin should be scraped or brushed off with a blade or a fingernail but not removed with forceps, which may squeeze more venom out of the venom sac. The site should be cleansed and disinfected and ice packs used to slow the spread of venom. Elevation of the affected site and administration of analgesics, oral antihistamines, and topical calamine lotion relieve symptoms; application of meat tenderizer containing papain is of no proven value. Large local reactions may require a short course of oral therapy with glucocorticoids. Patients with numerous stings should be monitored for 24 h for evidence of renal failure or coagulopathy.

Anaphylaxis is treated with subcutaneous injection of 0.3 to 0.5 mL of epinephrine hydrochloride in a 1:1000 dilution; treatment is repeated every 20 to 30 min if necessary. Intravenous epinephrine (2 to 5 mL of a 1:10,000 solution administered by slow push) is indicated for profound shock. A tourniquet may slow the spread of venom. Parenteral antihistamines, fluid resuscitation, bronchodilators, oxygen, intubation, and vasopressors may be required. Patients should be observed for 24 h for recurrent anaphylaxis.

Prevention Persons with a history of allergy to insect stings should carry a sting kit with a preloaded syringe containing epinephrine for self-administration in case of a sting. These patients should seek medical attention immediately after using the kit. To avoid stings when outdoors, individuals can wear shoes and protective clothing and avoid attracting insects with sweet foods, bright-colored clothes, perfumes, or cosmetics.

Venom Immunotherapy Repeated injections of purified venom produce a blocking IgG antibody response to venom and reduce the incidence of recurrent anaphylaxis from between 50 and 60% to <5%. Honeybee, wasp, yellow jacket, and mixed vespid venoms are commercially available for desensitization and for skin testing. Adults with a history of anaphylaxis should undergo desensitization. Results of skin tests and venom-specific radioallergosorbent tests aid in the selection of patients for immunotherapy and guide the design of such treatment. The risk of a systemic reaction to a sting is ~5 to 10% after discontinuation of a ≥5-year course of immunotherapy.

Stings of Fire Ants and Other Ants All ants that are large enough can bite human beings, and some can secrete repugnant substances when handled. Stinging fire ants are an important medical problem in the United States. The imported fire ants *Solenopsis richteri* and *S. invicta* were introduced from South America into Alabama in 1918 and now infest urban and rural areas of southern states from Texas to North Carolina, with colonies in California, New Mexico, Arizona, and Virginia. They excavate open fields and yards to build tall mounds that can harbor 200,000 worker ants. Slight disturbances of the mounds have provoked massive outpourings of ants and as many as 10,000 stings on a single person. Each year fire ants sting up to 60% of the inhabitants of some cities. Waterborne ants bite on contact during times of flooding. The elderly and immobile persons are at high risk for attacks when fire ants invade dwellings.

Red-brown or brown-black fire ants attach to human skin with powerful mandibles and rotate their bodies around their heads while repeatedly injecting venom with posteriorly situated stingers. The alkaloid venom consists of cytotoxic and hemolytic piperidines and several proteins with enzymatic activity. The initial wheal-and-flare reaction, burning, and itching resolve in about 30 min, and a sterile pustule develops within 24 h. The pustule ulcerates over the next 48 h and then heals a week or 10 days later unless it becomes secondarily infected. Large areas of erythema and edema lasting several days are not uncommon and in extreme cases may compress nerves and blood vessels. Anaphylaxis occurs in ~1 to 2% of persons, and seizures and mononeuritis have been reported. Stings are treated with ice packs, topical glucocorticoids, and oral antihistamines. Covering pustules with bandages and antibiotic ointment may prevent bacterial infection. Epinephrine and supportive measures are indicated for anaphylactic reactions. Whole-body extracts are available for skin testing and immunotherapy, which appears to lower the rate of anaphylactic reactions.

The western United States is home to harvester ants (*Pogonomyrmex* species) as well as to less aggressive fire ants not yet displaced by the introduced species. The painful local reaction following harvester ant stings often extends to lymph nodes and may be accompanied by anaphylaxis. Large Australian bulldog ants and the aggressive South American *Paranopera* ants deliver extremely painful stings and may cause systemic symptoms. Velvet ants that inhabit sandy beaches in the United States and sting the bare feet of bathers are actually wingless female wasps of the genus *Dasymutilla*.

TICK BITES AND TICK PARALYSIS In the United States, hard ticks (Ixodidae) have increased in abundance since the mid-1900s to become the most common carriers of vector-borne diseases. Deer ticks of the genus *Ixodes* transmit the pathogens of Lyme disease, babesiosis, and human granulocytic ehrlichiosis. Other ticks, such as *Dermacentor variabilis* (the dog tick), *D. andersoni* (the wood tick), and *Amblyomma americanum* (the Lone Star tick), are vectors of tularemia, Rocky Mountain spotted fever, Colorado tick fever, and human monocytic ehrlichiosis. Outside the United States, hard ticks transmit pathogenic rickettsiae and arboviruses as well. Soft ticks (Argasidae) of the genus *Ornithodoros* transmit tick-borne relapsing fever

(Chap. 175). Except in parts of Africa, soft ticks rarely attack human beings, and relapsing fever occurs only sporadically in the United States. Hard ticks differ from soft ticks by virtue of a dorsal scutum or plate and their preference for wooded, brushy, or weedy habitats. Soft ticks, which are nonscutate and leathery, are generally found in animal burrows and bird nests.

Ticks attach and feed painlessly; blood is their only food. Their secretions, however, produce local reactions, a febrile illness, or paralysis. Soft ticks attach for <1 h and produce erythematous macular lesions up to 2 to 3 cm in diameter. Some species in Africa, the western United States, and Mexico produce painful hemorrhagic lesions. At the site of hard-tick bites, small areas of induration with surrounding erythema and occasionally necrotic ulcers develop. Chronic nodules, or "tick granulomas," reach several centimeters in diameter and may require surgical excision. Tick-induced fever, associated with headache, nausea, and malaise, usually resolves within 24 to 36 h after the tick is removed. Tick paralysis is an ascending flaccid paralysis believed to be caused by a toxin in tick saliva that causes neuromuscular block and decreased nerve conduction. Throughout the world, this rare complication has followed the bites of more than 40 kinds of tick—most commonly, dog and wood ticks in the United States. Children, especially girls with long hair, are most often affected. Weakness begins in the lower extremities 5 to 6 days after the tick's attachment and ascends symmetrically over several days to result in complete paralysis of the extremities and cranial nerves. Deep tendon reflexes are diminished or lacking altogether, but sensory examination and findings on lumbar puncture are typically normal. Removal of the tick results in improvement within a few hours and usually in complete recovery after several days. Failure to remove the tick may lead to dysarthria, dysphagia, and ultimately death from aspiration or respiratory paralysis. Diagnosis depends on finding the tick, which often is hidden beneath hair and which, when engorged, may resemble a pedunculated nevus.

An antiserum to the saliva of *Ixodes holocyclus*, the usual cause of tick paralysis in Australia, effectively reverses paralysis caused by these ticks. Ticks should be removed by firm traction with a forceps placed near their point of attachment. The site of attachment should be disinfected (e.g., with tincture of iodine). Mouthparts remaining in the skin may cause persistent irritation or lead to secondary infection. Removal of ticks during the first 48 h of attachment nearly always prevents transmission of the agents of Lyme disease, babesiosis, and erhlichiosis. Gentle handling to avoid rupture of ticks and use of gloves may avert accidental contamination with tick fluids containing pathogens. Protective measures against ticks include avoidance of brushy vegetation, removal of ticks from pet dogs and cats, use of protective clothing sprayed with 0.5% permethrin, and application of a repellent containing *N,N*-diethyl-*m*-toluamide (DEET). The cuffs of trousers should be tucked inside the socks.

OTHER ARTHROPOD BITES AND ENVENOMATIONS

Dipteran (Fly and Mosquito) Bites In the process of feeding on vertebrate blood, adults of certain fly species inflict painful bites, produce local allergic reactions, or transmit infectious diseases. Unlike insect stings, insect bites rarely cause anaphylaxis. Mosquitoes are ubiquitous pests and are the vectors of malaria, filariasis, yellow fever, dengue, and viral encephalitides. Female mosquitoes require a blood meal to produce eggs and an environment of standing water in which to deposit them. Their bite typically produces a wheal and later a pruritic papule. In the United States, a similar reaction follows the bite of tiny but aggressive midges known as "no-see-ums," which attack in swarms during warm months, or of other *Culicoides* species that transmit "nonpathogenic" filariae in tropical climates. Nodular lesions at the site of midge bites may last for months. The bite of the small humpbacked blackfly of the genus *Simulium* leaves a large bleeding puncture and painful and pruritic sores that are slow to heal; regional lymphadenopathy, fever, or anaphylaxis occasionally ensues. Blackflies are common summertime nuisances in the United States and Canada and are vectors of onchocerciasis in Africa and Latin America. The widely distributed tabanids, including deerflies (*Chrysops* species) and horseflies (*Tabanus* species), are stout flies measuring 10 to 25 mm in length that attack during the day and produce large and painful bleeding punctures. Deerflies transmit loiasis in African equatorial rain forests and tularemia in the United States and elsewhere. Tsetse flies of the genus *Glossina* transmit African trypanosomiasis in sub-Saharan Africa. Tiny phlebotomine sandflies are the vectors of leishmaniasis, bartonellosis (Carrión's disease), sandfly fever, and other arboviral infections in warm climates. *Stomoxys calcitrans*, the stable fly, which resembles a large housefly, is a fierce biter of human beings and domestic animals and a major pest in seacoast areas. Houseflies do not bite.

℞ **TREATMENT** Treatment of fly bites is symptom-based. Topical application of antipruritic agents, glucocorticoids, or antiseptic lotions may relieve the itching and pain. Allergic reactions may require oral antihistamines. Antibiotics may be necessary for large bite wounds that become secondarily infected. Personal protection measures against biting flies include avoidance of infested areas, application of a DEET-containing repellent to exposed skin, and use of protective clothing and bed nets treated with permethrin. Higher concentrations of DEET provide longer-lasting protection, and 10 to 35% DEET provides adequate protection under most conditions. Repellents used on children should contain ≤10% DEET to avoid absorption of toxic levels that provoke encephalopathy and seizures. Permethrin applied to clothing maintains its potency for at least 2 weeks, even with laundering. It should not be applied to the skin.

Flea Bites Common human-biting fleas include the dog and cat fleas (*Ctenocephalides* species) and the rat flea (*Xenopsylla cheopis*), which inhabit the nests and resting sites of their hosts. Larval fleas feed on pellets of dried host blood that the adult fleas eject from their rectums while feeding. The high-jumping adults attack human beings or other available warm-bodied animals when the usual host abandons or is driven from its nest. The human flea (*Pulex irritans*) infests human bedding and furniture but mainly in relatively humid buildings that lack central heating. Sensitized persons develop erythematous pruritic papules, urticaria, and occasionally vesicles and bacterial superinfection at the site of the bite. Treatment consists of antihistamines and antipruritics.

Fleas transmit plague, murine typhus, a typhus-like illness due to *Rickettsia felis*, the rat and dog tapeworms, and *B. henselae*. Flea infestations are eliminated by frequent cleaning of the nesting sites and bedding of the host or judicious dusting or spraying of insecticides such as pyrethrin, DDT, or malathion.

Hemipteran (True Bug) Bites Several true bugs of the family Reduviidae inflict bites that produce allergic reactions and are sometimes painful. The cosmopolitan bedbug (*Cimex* species) hides in mattresses, behind bedboards, and under loose wallpaper during the day and takes its blood meal at night. The bite is painless, but sensitized persons develop erythema, itching, and wheals around a central hemorrhagic punctum. The cone-nose bugs, so called because of their elongated heads, include the assassin and wheel bugs, which feed on other insects and bite human beings only in self-defense, and the kissing bugs, which routinely feed on vertebrate blood. Assassin and wheel bugs inhabit many parts of the world, including the southwestern and southern United States, where they are notorious for their painful bites. The bites of the nocturnally feeding kissing bugs are painless and occur commonly in groups on the face and other exposed parts of the body. Reactions to such bites depend on prior sensitization and include tender and pruritic papules, vesicular or bullous lesions, giant urticaria, fever, lymphadenopathy, and anaphylaxis. *Triatoma infestans* and other species of kissing bug are the vectors of *Trypanosoma cruzi* in South and Central America and Mexico, but transmission of *T. cruzi* to human beings by species indigenous to the United States is exceedingly rare. Bug bites are treated with topical antipruritics or oral antihistamines. Persons with anaphylactic reactions to reduviid bites should keep an epinephrine kit available.

Centipede Bites and Millipede Dermatitis The fangs of centipedes of the genus *Scolopendra* can penetrate human skin and deliver a venom that produces intense burning pain, swelling, erythema, and lymphangitis. Dizziness, nausea, and anxiety are occasionally described, and rhabdomyolysis and renal failure have been reported. Treatment includes washing of the site, application of cold dressings, oral analgesic administration or local lidocaine infiltration, and tetanus prophylaxis. Species of *Scolopendra*, measuring up to 25 cm, occur widely in the southern United States and other areas with warm climates worldwide. The smaller house centipede *Scutigera coleopatrata*, which is common throughout the United States, is harmless.

Millipedes, unlike centipedes, do not bite but rather secrete and in some cases eject defensive fluids that burn and discolor human skin. Affected skin turns brown overnight and may blister and exfoliate. Secretions in the eye cause intense pain and inflammation that may lead to corneal ulceration and blindness. Management includes irrigation with copious amounts of water or saline, use of analgesics, and local care of denuded skin. Millipedes are found throughout the world in leaf litter and under rocks.

Caterpillar Stings and Dermatitis The surface of caterpillars of several moth species is covered with hairs or spines that produce mechanical irritation and may contain or be coated with venom. Contact with these caterpillars causes an immediate burning sensation followed by local swelling and erythema and occasionally by regional lymphadenopathy, nausea, vomiting, and headache; shock, seizures, and coagulopathy are rare complications. In the United States, stings are most often caused by io moth larvae and puss as well as saddleback and brown-tail moth caterpillars as they cling to leaves and branches. Contact with even detached hairs of other caterpillars, such as gypsy moth larvae (*Lymantria dispar*) in the northeastern United States, can produce a pruritic urticarial or papular rash hours later. Spines may be deposited on tree trunks and drying laundry or may be airborne and cause irritation of the eyes and upper airways. Treatment of caterpillar stings consists of repeated application of adhesive or cellophane tape to remove the hairs, which can then be identified microscopically. Local ice packs, topical steroids, and oral antihistamines relieve symptoms.

Beetle Vesication When disturbed, blister beetles extrude cantharidin, a low-molecular-weight toxin that produces thin-walled blisters measuring up to 5 cm in diameter 2 to 5 h after contact with the beetle. The blisters are not painful or pruritic unless broken, and they resolve without treatment in a week to 10 days. Nephritis may follow unusually heavy cantharidin exposure. In the southern United States, blister beetles of several *Epicauta* species are abundant in the summer months. Contact occurs when people sit on the ground, work in the garden, or deliberately handle the beetles. In other countries, different species of beetle produce different vesicants. No treatment is necessary, although ruptured blisters should be kept clean and bandaged until healing is complete.

BIBLIOGRAPHY

AUERBACH PS (ed): *Wilderness Medicine*, 3d ed. St. Louis, Mosby, 1995

DESHAZO RD et al: Fire ant attacks on residents in health care facilities: A report of two cases. Ann Intern Med 131:424, 1999

DOWNS AM et al: Head lice: Prevalence in schoolchildren and insecticide resistance. Parasitol Today 15:1, 1999

FRADIN MS: Mosquitoes and mosquito repellents: A clinician's guide. Ann Intern Med 128:931, 1998

GODDARD J: *Infectious Diseases and Arthropods*. Totowa, NJ, Humana, 2000

HAWDON GM, WINKEL KD: Spider bite. A rational approach. Aust Fam Physician 26: 1380, 1997

KING MS: Pathogenesis of envenomation. Ann Emerg Med 34:411, 1999

LAVARDE V, FORNES P: Lethal infection due to *Armillifer armillatus* (*Porocephalida*): A snake-related parasitic disease. Clin Infect Dis 29:1346, 1999

MILLIKAN LE: Myiasis. Clin Dermatol 17:191, 1999

PETERS W: *A Colour Atlas of Arthropods in Clinical Medicine*. London, Wolfe, 1992

NOBEL PRIZE IN PHYSIOLOGY OR MEDICINE, 1977

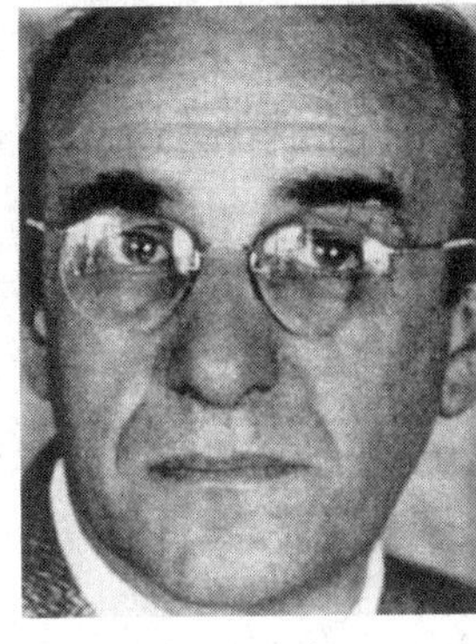

Roger Guillemin was born on January 11, 1924, in Dijon, France. His early education was in the public schools in Dijon after which he received his B.A. and B.S. degrees there in college. In 1943 he pursued a medical degree in a joint program at the School of Medicine in Dijon and the University of Lyon. At the same time he also served in the French Resistance from 1940 to 1944. For his degree in medicine, Guillemin desired to write his thesis on hormonal adaptation to alarm reactions after meeting Dr. Hans Selye during his visit to Paris. Selye invited Guillemin to work at the new Institute of Experimental Medicine and Surgery at Montreal University in Canada. With this background in medicine and hormonal research, he began his search for the chemical structure of peptide hormones. Geoffrey W. Harris in England had provided anatomical evidence that the brain hypothalamus controlled the pituitary and suggested that this control was not by nerve impulses, but rather hormones that flowed through a capillary network connecting the hypothalamus and the pituitary.

Guillemin became a professor of physiology at the Baylor College of Medicine where in 1955 he demonstrated, in a co-culture experiment, the regulatory effect of the hypothalamus on the pituitary. Between 1960 and 1963 Guillemin held a temporary associate director position at the Laboratory of Experimental Endocrinology, Collège de France, where he collected from slaughterhouses, 5 million pieces of sheep hypothalamus weighing about 50 tons. From this material he and his collaborator, R. Burgus, isolated 1 mg of thyrotropin-releasing factor (TRF) from 300,000 sheep hypothalami. In 1969 he established the primary structure to be a tripeptide composed of three amino acids and demonstrated the hormone's stimulating effect on thyroid-stimulating hormone (TSH). In 1920 Guillemin, Burgus, and colleagues isolated luteinizing hormone–releasing factor (LHRF) from sheep hypothalami. LHRF was found to stimulate both luteinizing and follicle-stimulating hormones of the pituitary. The structure of LHRF was then determined in 1971. At the same time, Andrew Schally's group independently identified the structures of TRF and LHRF at Tulane University.

In 1970 Guillemin moved his neuroendocrinology laboratory from Baylor to the Salk Institute in La Jolla, California. After his identification of LHRF, Guillemin demonstrated an inhibitory effect of the hypothalamus on pituitary growth hormone and eventually identified the substance to be somatostatin or somatotrophin-release inhibiting factor. Guillemin did not stop there. In 1976, from 25,000 swine hypothalami, he isolated and purified a group of opiate-like substances called endorphins (endogenous morphine).

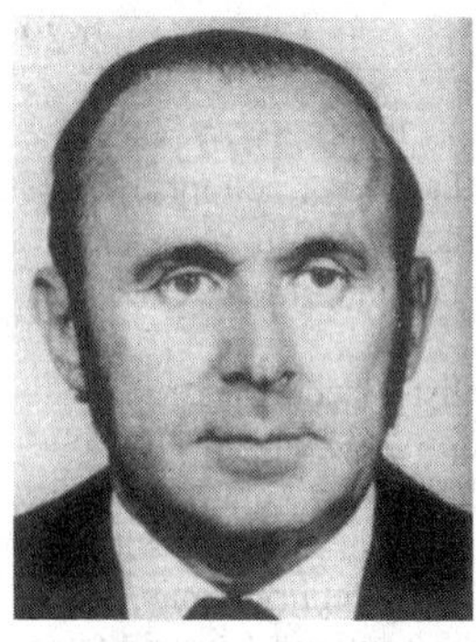

Andrew Victor Schally was born on November 30, 1926, in Wilno, Poland. His family fled Poland when Germany occupied it, and his father became a major general with the allied forces in World War II. After the war he moved to Scotland where he finished high school. Schally then became a research laboratory technician at the National Institute for Medical Research in London, but ultimately moved to Montreal where in 1957 he received his Ph.D. at McGill University. At McGill he worked with Murray Saffran, who was pursuing the possibility of hypothalamic hormones. In 1954 he joined Roger Guillemin's laboratory at Baylor University in Houston, but ultimately, they became scientific competitors rather than collaborators. In 1962 Schally became Chief of the Endocrine and Polypeptide Laboratory at the New Orleans Veterans Administration Hospital and a professor at Tulane University School of Medicine. Schally was successful in isolating TRF, but falsely concluded that the structure was not a peptide. He had worked a total of 11 years in his search of hypothalamic hormones and their structure. The National Institutes of Health Endocrine Study Section was considering terminating funding for the project. Both Schally and Guillemin had mistaken impurities for the TRF compound. However, Guillemin's colleague, Roger Burgus, finally purified the material and demonstrated that TRF was a tripeptide. There was, however, still another barrier since differing sequences of the amino acids demonstrated no biological activity until the cap at the end of the TRF molecule was found to curl back and create an internal loop in the molecule. The publisher received Schally's paper five weeks before Guillemin's paper, which arrived at a similar conclusion. Although the papers were published only a few days apart, Schally's was given credit for identifying the first hypothalamic hormone because of his earlier submission. Schally's team next turned to defining the structure of LHRF. From 160,000 pig brains, Schally extracted 250 μg of LHRF. Schally's colleague, Hisayuko Matsuo, knew that this amount of LHRF was not enough to determine the structure by standard means. Using the Yalow and Berson radioimmunoassay technique, he demonstrated that LHRF stimulated release of reproductive hormones, namely the luteinizing and follicle-stimulating hormones. The Schally team also isolated and identified somatostatin, an inhibitory hormone. Although rivals, Guillemin and Schally opened the era of hypothalamic hormones that was to have an enormous impact on the future of neuroendocrinology.

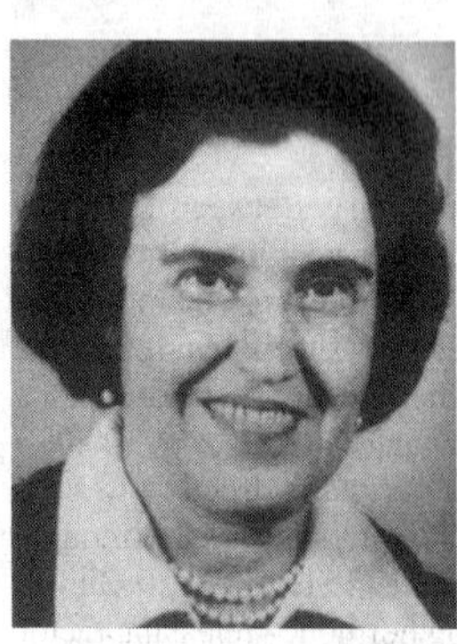

Rosalyn Sussman Yalow was born in the South Bronx, New York, the second child of Simon and Clara Sussman. Clara had emigrated from Germany at the age of four, and Simon ran a paper and twine business in the Bronx. Although neither parent finished high school, they instilled in their children the importance of education. Rosalyn Yalow graduated from Walton Public High School and attended Hunter College where she was the first ever to be graduated from that institution with a physics major. Her professors convinced her that as a woman she could never obtain a physics position in graduate school, but they were wrong. She was offered a teaching assistant position at the University of Illinois and she entered the College of Engineering as the only woman among 400 graduate students. She obtained her Ph.D. in nuclear physics in 1945. She met and married another physics graduate student, Aaron Yalow, and they had two children. During her graduate studies she learned laboratory techniques for measuring radioactivity, including constructing the necessary apparatus. This experience would become invaluable in her future work. During her free summer from teaching, however, she volunteered to work in Edith Quimby's laboratory at Columbia College of Physicians and Surgeons in order to obtain experience in using radioisotopes in medical research. This experience enabled her to obtain a part-time position at the Bronx Veterans Administration Hospital (VAH). She began to establish a radioisotope service and to conduct research out of a converted janitor's closet at the VAH. She then resigned her teaching position at Hunter College, accepted a full-time staff position at the Veterans Hospital, and was joined by a physician trained at New York University, Solomon Berson. Berson brought the clinical insights to this remarkable team, which spanned the disciplines of biochemistry, medicine, and nuclear physics. Their pivotal work began with an interest in adult-onset diabetes (type 2), where a hypothesis was proposed that insulin was being removed from the body too rapidly. Berson and Yalow, therefore, injected ^{131}I-labeled insulin into normal individuals and adult-onset diabetic patients and surprisingly found the opposite result. The insulin disappearance was slower in the diabetic patients. Further analysis of the data revealed that those diabetic patients who had been treated previously with insulin demonstrated the slowest disappearance of the hormone. Yalow and Berson then hypothesized that antibodies had developed against the bovine or pork insulin that the diabetic patients had received. They realized that the amount of injected labeled insulin that was bound by the antibody was dependent on the amount of endogenous insulin present in the body at the time of the injected radiolabeled insulin. This observation led to the development of the radioimmunoassay (RIA) that revolutionized medicine. This technique allowed the measurement of proteins in concentrations as small as 0.05 pmol, which was a million times smaller than any technique available at that time. The Yalow and Berson team extended their RIA technique from insulin to growth hormone, corticotropin, parathyroid hormone, and gastrin.

In 1977, Yalow was the second woman to receive the Nobel Prize in Physiology or Medicine, an award that would, no doubt, have been shared with Solomon Berson had it not been for his untimely death in 1972. In her Nobel lecture on receiving the award in Stockholm, Yalow concluded that, like the microscope, the RIA allowed for new avenues of biology to be explored. At the formal Nobel dinner she rose to speak on behalf of equal opportunities for women, stating that, "The world cannot afford the loss of talents of half of its people."

REFERENCES

1. Magill FN (ed): *Nobel Prize Winners: Physiology or Medicine*, vol 3. Pasadena, Salem Press, 1993
2. Schrier RW: *A Salute to Nobel Laureates in Physiology and Medicine*, Proceedings of the Association of American Physicians 108(1): Jan 1996

Robert W. Schrier, MD

APPENDICES

LABORATORY VALUES OF CLINICAL IMPORTANCE

INTRODUCTORY COMMENTS

All laboratory appendices should be interpreted with caution since normal values differ widely among clinical laboratories. The values given in this Appendix are meant primarily for use with this text. In preparing the Appendix, the editors have taken into account the fact that the system of international units (SI, système international d'unités) is now used in most countries and in most medical and scientific journals.[1] However, clinical laboratories in many countries continue to report values in traditional units. Therefore, both systems are used in the Appendix. Values in SI units appear first and traditional units appear in parentheses after the SI units. The dual system is also used in the text except for (1) those instances in which the numbers remain the same but only the terminology is changed (mmol/L for meq/L or IU/L for mIU/mL), when only the SI units are given; and (2) most pressure measurements (e.g., blood and cerebrospinal fluid pressures), when the traditional units (mmHg, mmH_2O) are used. In all other instances in the text the SI unit is followed by the traditional unit in parentheses. The SI base units, SI derived units, other units of measure referred to in Appendix A, and SI prefixes are listed in Tables A-1 to A-3. Conversions from one system to another can be made as follows:

$$\text{mmol/L} = \frac{\text{mg/dL} \times 10}{\text{atomic weight}}$$

$$\text{mg/dL} = \frac{\text{mmol/L} \times \text{atomic weight}}{10}$$

TABLE A-1 RADIATION-DERIVED UNITS

Quantity	Old Unit	SI Unit	Name for SI Unit (and Abbreviation)	Conversion
Activity	curie (Ci)	Disintegrations per second (dps)	becquerel (Bq)	1 Ci = 3.7 × 10^{10} Bq 1 mCi = 37 mBq 1 μCi = 0.037 MBq or 37 GBq 1 Bq = 2.703 × 10^{-11} Ci
Absorbed dose	rad	joule per kilogram (J/kg)	gray (Gy)	1 Gy = 100 rad 1 rad = 0.01 Gy 1 mrad = 10^{-3} cGy
Exposure	roentgen (R)	coulomb per kilogram (C/kg)	—	1 C/kg = 3876 R 1 R = 2.58 × 10^{-4} C/kg 1 mR = 258 pC/kg
Dose equivalent	rem	joule per kilogram (J/kg)	sievert (Sv)	1 Sv = 100 rem 1 rem = 0.01 Sv 1 mrem = 10 μSv

[1]Young DS: Implementation of SI units for clinical laboratory data. Ann Intern Med 106:114, 1987

TABLE A-2 BODY FLUIDS AND OTHER MASS DATA

	Reference Range	
	SI Units	**Conventional Units**
Ascitic fluid: See Chap. 46		
Body fluid, total volume (lean) of body weight	50% (in obese) to 70%	
Intracellular	0.3–0.4 of body weight	
Extracellular	0.2–0.3 of body weight	
Blood		
Total volume		
Males	69 mL per kg body weight	
Females	65 mL per kg body weight	
Plasma volume		
Males	39 mL per kg body weight	
Females	40 mL per kg body weight	
Red blood cell volume		
Males	30 mL per kg body weight	1.15–1.21 L/m² of body surface area
Females	25 mL per kg body weight	0.95–1.00 L/m² of body surface area

TABLE A-3 CEREBROSPINAL FLUID[a]

	Reference Range	
Constituent	**SI Units**	**Conventional Units**
Osmolarity	292–297 mmol/kg water	292–297 mOsm/L
Electrolytes		
Sodium	137–145 mmol/L	137–145 meq/L
Potassium	2.7–3.9 mmol/L	2.7–3.9 meq/L
Calcium	1.0–1.5 mmol/L	2.1–3.0 meq/L
Magnesium	1.0–1.2 mmol/L	2.0–2.5 meq/L
Chloride	116–122 mmol/L	116–122 meq/L
CO_2 content	20–24 mmol/L	20–24 meq/L
P_{CO_2}	6–7 kPa	45–49 mmHg
pH	7.31–7.34	
Glucose	2.2–3.9 mmol/L	40–70 mg/dL
Lactate	1–2 mmol/L	10–20 mg/dL
Total protein	0.2–0.5 g/L	20–50 mg/dL
Albumin	0.066–0.442 g/L	6.6–44.2 mg/dL
IgG	0.009–0.057 g/L	0.9–5.7 mg/dL
IgG index[b]	0.29–0.59	
Oligoclonal bands (OGB)	<2 bands not present in matched serum sample	
Ammonia	15–47 μmol/L	25–80 μg/dL
Creatinine	44–168 μmol/L	0.5–1.9 mg/dL
Myelin basic protein	<4 μg/L	
CSF pressure		50–180 mmH_2O
CSF volume (adult)	~150 mL	
Leukocytes		
Total	<5 per μL	
Differential:		
Lymphocytes	60–70%	
Monocytes	30–50%	
Neutrophils	None	

[a] Since cerebrospinal fluid concentrations are equilibrium values, measurements of the same parameters in blood plasma obtained at the same time are recommended. However, there is a time lag in attainment of equilibrium, and cerebrospinal levels of plasma constituents that can fluctuate rapidly (such as plasma glucose) may not achieve stable values until after a significant lag phase.

[b] $\text{IgG index} = \frac{\text{CSF IgG(mg/dL)} \times \text{serum albumin(g/dL)}}{\text{Serum IgG(g/dL)} \times \text{CSF albumin(mg/dL)}}$

TABLE A-4 CHEMICAL CONSTITUENTS OF BLOOD

Constituent	Specimen	Reference Range: SI Units	Reference Range: Conventional Units
Acetoacetate	P	<100 μmol/L	<1 mg/dL
Albumin	S	35–55 g/L	3.5–5.5 g/dL
Aldolase		0–100 nkat/L	0–6 U/L
Alpha$_1$ antitrypsin	S	0.8–2.1 g/L	85–213 mg/dL
Alpha fetoprotein (adult)	S	<30 μg/L	<30 ng/mL
Aminotransferases	S		
Aspartate (AST, SGOT)		0–0.58 μkat/L	0–35 U/L
Alanine (ALT, SGPT)		0–0.58 μkat/L	0–35 U/L
Ammonia, as NH_3	P	6–47 μmol/L	10–80 μg/dL
Amylase	S	0.8–3.2 μkat/L	60–180 U/L
Angiotensin-converting enzyme (ACE)		<670 nkat/L	<40 U/L
Anticonvulsant drug levels: see Table 360-8			
Arterial blood gases			
$[HCO_3^-]$		21–28 mmol/L	21–30 meq/L
P_{CO_2}		4.7–5.9 kPa	35–45 mmHg
pH		7.38–7.44	
P_{O_2}		11–13 kPa	80–100 mmHg
β-Hydroxybutyrate	P	<300 μmol/L	<3 mg/dL
Bilirubin, total	S (Malloy-Evelyn)	5.1–17 μmol/L	0.3–1.0 mg/dL
Direct	S	1.7–5.1 μmol/L	0.1–0.3 mg/dL
Indirect	S	3.4–12 μmol/L	0.2–0.7 mg/dL
Calcium, ionized		1.1–1.4 mmol/L	4.5–5.6 mg/dL
Calcium	P	2.2–2.6 mmol/L	9–10.5 mg/dL
Carbon dioxide content	P (sea level)	21–30 mmol/L	21–30 meq/L
Carbon dioxide tension (P_{CO_2})	Arterial blood (sea level)	4.7–5.9 kPa	35–45 mmHg
Carbon monoxide content	Blood	Symptoms with 20% saturation of hemoglobin	
Chloride	S (as Cl^-)	98–106 mmol/L	98–106 meq/L
Cholesterol: see Table A-9			
Complement	S		
C3		0.55–1.20 g/L	55–120 mg/dL
C4		0.20–0.50 g/L	20–50 mg/dL
Coproporphyrins (types I and III)	U	150–460 μmol/d	100–300 μg/d
Creatine kinase	S (total)		
Females		0.17–1.17 μkat/L	10–70 U/L
Males		0.42–1.50 μkat/L	25–90 U/L
Creatine kinase-MB		0–7 μg/L	
Creatinine	S	<133 μmol/L	<1.5 mg/dL
Erythropoietin	S	5–36 U/L	
Fatty acids, free (nonesterified)	P	180 mg/L	<18 mg/dL
Ferritin	S		
Women		10–200 μg/L	10–200 ng/mL
Men		15–400 μg/L	15–400 ng/mL
Fibrinogen: See "Hematologic Evaluations: Platelets and Coagulation Parameters"			
Fibrinogen split products: See "Hematologic Evaluations: Platelets and Coagulation Parameters"			
Glucose (fasting)	P		
Normal		4.2–6.4 mmol/L	75–115 mg/dL
Diabetes mellitus		>7.8 mmol/L	>140 mg/dL
Glucose, 2 h postprandial	P		
Normal		<7.8 mmol/L	<140 mg/dL
Impaired glucose tolerance		7.8–11.1 mmol/L	140–200 mg/dL
Diabetes mellitus		>11.1 mmol/L	>200 mg/dL
Hemoglobin	B (sea level)		
Male		140–180 g/L	14–18 g/dL
Female		120–160 g/L	12–16 g/dL
Hemoglobin A_{1c} Up to 6% of total hemoglobin			
Iron	S	9–27 μmol/L	50–150 μg/dL
Iron-binding capacity	S	45–66 μmol/L	250–370 μg/dL
Saturation		0.2–0.45	20–45%
Lactate dehydrogenase	S	1.7–3.2 μkat/L	100–190 U/L
Lactate dehydrogenase isoenzymes	S (agarose)		
Fraction 1 (of total)		0.14–0.25	14–26%
Fraction 2		0.29–0.39	29–39%
Fraction 3		0.20–0.25	20–26%
Fraction 4		0.08–0.16	8–16%
Fraction 5		0.06–0.16	6–16%

(continued)

Constituent	Specimen	Reference Range	
		SI Units	Conventional Units
Lactate	P, venous	0.6–1.7 mmol/L	5–15 mg/dL
Lipase	S	0–2.66 μkat/L	0–160 U/L
Lipids: see Table A-9			
Lipids, triglyceride: S see "Triglycerides"			
Lipoprotein: see Table A-9			
Lipoprotein (a)	S	0–300 mg/L	0–3 mg/dL
Magnesium	S	0.8–1.2 mmol/L	1.8–3 mg/dL
Myoglobin	S		
Male		19–92 μg/L	
Female		12–76 μg/L	
Osmolality	P	285–295 mmol/kg serum water	285–295 mosmol/kg serum water
Oxygen content	B, arterial (sea level)		17–21 vol%
	B, venous arm (sea level)		10 to 16 vol%
Oxygen percent saturation (sea level)	B, arterial	0.97 mol/mol	97%
	B, venous, arm	0.60–0.85 mol/mol	60–85%
Oxygen tension (P_{O_2})	Blood	11–13 kPa	80–100 mmHg
pH	B	7.38–7.44	
Phosphatase, acid	S	0.90 nkat/L	0–5.5 U/L
Phosphatase, alkaline	S	0.5–2.0 nkat/L	30–120 U/L
Phosphorus, inorganic	S	1.0–1.4 mmol/L	3–4.5 mg/dL
Porphobilinogen	U	None	None
Potassium	S	3.5–5.0 mmol/L	3.5–5.0 meq/L
Prostate-specific antigen (PSA)	S		
Female		<0.5 μg/L	<0.5 ng/mL
Male: <40 years		0.0–2.0 μg/L	0.0–2.0 ng/mL
≥40 years		0.0–4.0 μg/L	0.0–4.0 ng/mL
PSA, free, in males 45–75 years, with PSA values between 4 and 20 μg/mL	S	>0.25 associated with benign prostatic hyperplasia	>25% associated with benign prostatic hyperplasia
Protein, total	S	55–80 g/L	5.5–8.0 g/dL
Protein fractions	S		
Albumin		35–55 g/L	3.5–5.5 g/dL (50–60%)
Globulin		20–35 g/L	2.0–3.5 g/dL (40–50%)
Alpha$_1$		2–4 g/L	0.2–0.4 g/dL (4.2–7.2%)
Alpha$_2$		5–9 g/L	0.5–0.9 g/dL (6.8–12%)
Beta		6–11 g/L	0.6–1.1 g/dL (9.3–15%)
Gamma		7–17 g/L	0.7–1.7 g/dL (13–23%)
Pyruvate	P, venous	60–170 μmol/L	0.5–1.5 mg/dL
Sodium	S	136–145 mmol/L	136–145 meq/L
Transferrin	S	2.3–3.9 g/L	230–390 mg/dL
Triglycerides	S	<1.8 mmol/L	<160 mg/dL
Troponin I	S	0–0.4 μg/L	0–0.4 ng/mL
Troponin T	S	0–0.1 μg/L	0–0.1 ng/mL
Urea nitrogen	S	3.6–7.1 mmol/L	10–20 mg/dL
Uric acid:	S		
Men		150–480 μmol/L	2.5–8.0 mg/dL
Women		90–360 μmol/L	1.5–6.0 mg/dL
Urobilinogen	U	1.7–5.9 μmol/d	1–3.5 mg/d

NOTE: B, blood; P, plasma; S, serum; U, urine.

TABLE A-5 DRUG LEVELS

Drug	Therapeutic Range		Toxic Level	
	Conventional Units	**SI Units**	**Conventional Units**	**SI Units**
Acetaminophen	10–30 μg/mL	66–199 μmol/L	>200 μg/mL	>1324 μmol/L
Amikacin				
Peak	25–35 μg/mL	43–60 μmol/L	>35 μg/mL	>60 μmol/L
Trough	4–8 μg/mL	6.8–13.7 μmol/L	>10 μg/mL	>17 μmol/L
Amitriptyline	120–250 ng/mL	433–903 nmol/L	>500 ng/mL	>1805 nmol/L
Amphetamine	20–30 ng/mL	148–222 nmol/L	>200 ng/mL	>1480 nmol/L
Barbiturates, most short-acting			>20 mg/L	>88 μmol/L
Bromide			>1250 μg/mL	>15.6 mmol/L
Carbamazepine	6–12 μg/mL	26–51 μmol/L	>15 μg/mL	>63 μmol/L
Chlordiazepoxide	700–1000 ng/mL	2.34–3.34 μmol/L	>5000 ng/mL	>16.7 μmol/L
Clonazepam	15–60 ng/mL	48–190 nmol/L	>80 ng/mL	>254 nmol/L
Clozapine	200–350 ng/mL	0.6–1 μmol/L		
Cocaine	100–500 ng/mL	330–1650 nmol/L	>1000 ng/mL	>3300 nmol/L
Desipramine	75–300 ng/mL	281–1125 nmol/L	>400 ng/mL	>1500 nmol/L
Diazepam	100–1000 ng/mL	0.35–351 μmol/L	>5000 ng/mL	>17.55 μmol/L
Digoxin	0.8–2.0 ng/mL	1.0–2.6 nmol/L	>2.5 ng/mL	>3.2 umol/L
Doxepin	30–150 ng/mL	107–537 nmol/L	>500 ng/mL	>1790 nmol/L
Ethanol			>300 mg/dL	>65 mmol/L
Behavioral changes	>20 mg/dL	>4.3 mmol/L		
Legal intoxication	>80 mg/dL	>17 mmol/L		
Ethosuximide	40–100 μg/mL	283–708 μmol/L	>150 μg/mL	>1062 μmol/L
Flecainide	0.2–1.0 μg/mL	0.5–2.4 μmol/L	>1.0 μg/mL	>2.4 μmol/L
Gentamicin				
Peak	8–10 μg/mL	16.7–20.9 μmol/L	>10 μg/mL	>21μmol/L
Trough	<2–4 μg/mL	<4.2–8.4 μmol/L	>4 μg/mL	>8.4 μmol/L
Imipramine	125–250 ng/mL	446-893 nmol/L	>500 ng/mL	>1784 nmol/L
Lidocaine	1.5–6.0 μg/mL	6.4–26 μmol/L		
CNS or cardiovascular depression			6–8 μg/mL	26–34.2 μmol/L
Seizures, obtundation, decreased cardiac output			>8 μg/mL	>34.2 μmol/L
Lithium	0.6–1.2 meq/L	0.6–1.2 nmol/L	>2 meq/L	>2 mmol/L
Methadone	100–400 ng/mL	0.32–1.29 μmol/L	>2000 ng/mL	>6.46 μmol/L
Methotrexate	Variable	Variable		
Low-dose (1–2 weeks)			>9.1 ng/mL	>20 nmol/L
High-dose (48 h)			>227 ng/mL	>0.5 μmol/L
Morphine	10–80 ng/mL	35–280 μmol/L	>200 ng/mL	>700 nmol/L
Nitroprusside (as thiocyanate)	6–29 μg/mL	103–499 μmol/L		
Nortriptyline	50–170 ng/mL	190–646 nmol/L	>500 ng/mL	>1.9 μmol/L
Phenobarbital	10–40 μg/mL	43–170 μmol/L		
Slowness, ataxia, nystagmus			35–80 μg/mL	151–345 μmol/L
Coma with reflexes			65–117 μg/mL	280–504 μmol/L
Coma without reflexes			>100 μg/mL	>430 μmol/L
Phenytoin	10–20 μg/mL	40–79 μmol/L	>20 μg/mL	>79 μmol/L
Procainamide	4–10 μg/mL	17–42 μmol/L	>10–12 μg/mL	>42–51 μmol/L
Quinidine	2–5 μg/mL	6–15 μmol/L	>6 μg/mL	>18 μmol/L
Salicylates	150–300 μg/mL	1086–2172 μmol/L	>300 μg/mL	>2172 μmol/L
Theophylline	8–20 μg/mL	44–111 μmol/L	>20 μg/mL	>110 μmol/L
Thiocyanate				
After nitroprusside infusion	6–29 μg/mL	103–499 μmol/L		
Nonsmoker	1–4 μg/mL	17–69 μmol/L	>120 μg/mL	>2064 μmol/L
Smoker	3–12 μg/mL	52–206 μmol/L		
Tobramycin				
Peak	8–10 μg/mL	17–21 μmol/L	>10 μg/mL	>21 μmol/L
Trough	<4 μg/mL	<9 μmol/L	>4 μg/mL	>9 μmol/L
Valproic acid	50–150 μg/mL	347–1040 μmol/L	>150 μg/mL	>1040 μmol/L
Vancomycin				
Peak	18–26 μg/mL	12–18 μmol/L		
Trough	5–10 μg/mL	3–7 μmol/L	>80–100 μg/mL	>55–69 μmol/L

TABLE A-6 CIRCULATORY FUNCTION TESTS

Test	Results: Reference Range	
	SI Units (Range)	Conventional Units (Range)
Arteriovenous oxygen difference	30–50 mL/L	30–50 mL/L
Cardiac output (Fick)	2.5–3.6 L/m² of body surface area per min	2.5–3.6 L/m² of body surface area per min
Contractility indexes		
Max. left ventricular *dp/dt*	220 kPa/s (176–250 kPa/s)	1650 mmHg/s (1320–1880 mmHg/s)
(*dp/dt*)/DP when DP = 5.3 kPa (40 mmHg)(DP, diastolic pressure)	(37.6 ± 12.2)/s	(37.6 ± 12.2)/s
Mean normalized systolic ejection rate (angiography)	3.32 ± 0.84 end-diastolic volumes per second	3.32 ± 0.84 end-diastolic volumes per second
Mean velocity of circumferential fiber shortening (angiography)	1.66 ± 0.42 circumferences per second	1.66 ± 0.42 circumferences per second
Ejection fraction: stroke volume/end-diastolic volume (SV/EDV)	0.67 (0.55–0.78)	0.67 (0.55–0.78)
End-diastolic volume	75 mL/m² (60–88 mL/m²)	75 mL/m² (60–88 mL/m²)
End-systolic volume	25 mL/m² (20–33 mL/m²)	25 mL/m² (20–33 mL/m²)
Left ventricular work		
Stroke work index	30–110 (g·m)/m²	30–110 (g·m)/m²
Left ventricular minute work index	1.8–6.6 [(kg·m)/m²]/min	1.8–6.6 [(kg·m)/m²]/min
Oxygen consumption index	110–150 mL	110–150 mL
Maximum oxygen uptake	35 mL/min (20–60 mL/min)	35 mL/min (20–60 mL/min)
Pulmonary vascular resistance	2–12 (kPa·s)/L	20–120 (dyn·s)/cm⁵
Systemic vascular resistance	77–150 (kPa·s)/L	770–1500 (dyn·s)/cm⁵

TABLE A-7 NORMAL VALUES OF DOPPLER ECHOCARDIOGRAPHIC MEASUREMENTS IN ADULTS

	Range	Mean
RVD (cm)	0.9 to 2.6	1.7
LVID (cm)	3.5 to 5.7	4.7
Posterior LV wall thickness (cm)	0.6 to 1.1	0.9
IVS wall thickness (cm)	0.6 to 1.1	0.9
Left atrial dimension (cm)	1.9 to 4.0	2.9
Aortic root dimension (cm)	2.0 to 3.7	2.7
Aortic cusps separation (cm)	1.5 to 2.6	1.9
Percentage of fractional shortening	34 to 44%	36%
Mitral flow (m/s)	0.6 to 1.3	0.9
Tricuspid flow (m/s)	0.3 to 0.7	0.5
Pulmonary artery (m/s)	0.6 to 0.9	0.75
Aorta (m/s)	1.0 to 1.7	1.35

NOTE: RVD, right ventricular dimension; LVID, left ventricular internal dimension; LV, left ventricle; IVS, interventricular septum.

SOURCE: From H Feigenbaum, *Echocardiography*, 5th ed, Philadelphia. Lea & Febiger, 1994

TABLE A-8 GASTROINTESTINAL TESTS. SEE ALSO "STOOL ANALYSIS"

Test	Results	
	SI Units	Conventional Units
Absorption tests		
D-Xylose: after overnight fast, 25 g xylose given in oral aqueous solution		
Urine, collected for following 5 h	33–53 mmol (or >20% of ingested dose)	5–8 g (or >20% of ingested dose
Serum, 1 h after dose	1.7–2.7 mmol/L	25–40 mg/dL
Vitamin A: a fasting blood specimen is obtained and 200,000 units of vitamin A in oil is given orally	Serum level should rise to twice fasting level in 3–5 h	Serum level should rise to fasting level in 3–5 h
Bentiromide test (pancreatic function): 500 mg bentiromide (chymex) orally; *p*-aminobenzoic acid (PABA) measured		
Plasma		>3.6 (±1.1) μg/mL at 90 min
Urine	>50% recovered in 6 h	>50% recovered in 6 h
Gastric juice		
Volume		
24 h	2–3 L	2–3 L
Nocturnal	600–700 mL	600–700 mL
Basal, fasting	30–70 mL/h	30–70 mL/h
Reaction		
pH	1.6–1.8	1.6–1.8
Titratable acidity of fasting juice	4–9 μmol/s	15–35 meq/h
Acid output		
Basal		
Females (mean ± 1 SD)	0.6 ± 0.5 μmol/s	2.0 ± 1.8 meq/h
Males (mean ± 1 SD)	0.8 ± 0.6 μmol/s	3.0 ± 2.0 meq/h
Maximal (after SC histamine acid phosphate, 0.004 mg/kg body weight, and preceded by 50 mg promethazine, or after betazole, 1.7 mg/kg body weight, or pentagastrin, 6 μg/kg body weight)		
Females (mean ± 1 SD)	4.4 ± 1.4 μmol/s	16 ± 5 meq/h
Males (mean ± 1 SD)	6.4 ± 1.4 μmol/s	23 ± 5 meq/h
Basal acid output/maximal acid output ratio	≤0.6	≤0.6
Gastrin, serum	40–200 μg/L	40–200 pg/mL
Secretin test (pancreatic exocrine function): 1 unit/kg body weight, IV		
Volume (pancreatic juice) in 80 min	>2.0 mL/kg	>2.0 mL/kg
Bicarbonate concentration	>80 mmol/L	>80 meq/L
Bicarbonate output in 30 min	>10 mmol	>10 meq

TABLE A-9 METABOLIC AND ENDOCRINE TESTS

Substance	Specimen	Reference Range: SI Units	Reference Range: Conventional Units
Adrenocorticotropin (ACTH), 8 A.M.	P	1.3–16.7 pmol/L	6.0–76.0 pg/mL
Aldosterone, 8 A.M., (patient supine, 100 mmol/L Na and 60–100 mmol/L K intake)	P	<220 pmol/L	<8 ng/dL
Aldosterone	U	14–53 nmol/d	5–19 μg/d
Androstenedione	P		
Women		3.5–7.0 nmol/L	1–2 ng/mL
Men		3.0–5.0 nmol/L	0.8–1.3 ng/mL
Angiotensin II, 8 A.M.	P	10–30 nmol/L	10–30 pg/mL
Arginine vasopressin (AVP), random fluid intake	P	1.4–5.6 pmol/L	1.5–6.0 ng/L
Calciferols (vitamin D)	P		
1,25-dihydroxyvitamin D [1,25$(OH)_2$D]		40–160 pmol/L	16–65 pg/mL
25-hydroxyvitamin D [25(OH)D]		20–200 nmol/L	8–80 ng/mL
Calcitonin	P		
Women		≤8 ng/L	≤8 pg/mL
Men		≤4 ng/L	≤4 pg/mL
Catecholamines			
Epinephrine	U	<275 nmol/d	<50 μg/d
Free	U	<590 nmol/d	<100 μg/d
Metanephrine	U	<7 μmol/d	<1.3 mg/d
Norepinephrine	U	89–473 nmol/d	15–80 μg/d
Vanillylmandelic acid (VMA)	U	<40 μmol/d	<8 mg/d
Chorionic gonadotropin, β subunit (β-hCG), men and nonpregnant women	P	<3 IU/L	<3 mIU/mL
Cortisol			
Free	U	25–140 nmol/d	10–50 μg/d
8 A.M.	P	140–690 nmol/L	5–25 μg/dL
4 P.M.	P	80–330 nmol/L	3–12 μg/dL
Dehydroepiandrosterone (DHEA)	P	7–31 nmol/L	2–9 ng/dL
11-Deoxycortisol (compound S)	P	<30 nmol/L	<1 μg/dL
DHEA sulfate	P	1.3–6.8 μmol/L	500–2500 μg/dL
Estradiol	P		
Women (higher at ovulation)		70–220 pmol/L	20–60 pg/mL
Men		<180 pmol/L	<50 pg/mL
Gastrin	S	40–200 ng/L	40–200 pg/mL
Glucagon	P	50–100 ng/L	50–100 pg/mL
Gonadotropins			
Follicle-stimulating hormone (FSH)	P		
Women			
Mature, premenopausal, except at ovulation		1.4–9.6 IU/L	1.4–9.6 mIU/mL
Ovulatory surge		2.3–21 IU/L	2.3–21 mIU/mL
Postmenopausal		34–96 IU/L	34–96 mIU/mL
Men		0.9–15 IU/L	0.9–15 mIU/mL
Luteinizing hormone (LH)	P		
Children, prepubertal		1.0–5.9 IU/L	1.0–5.9 mIU/mL
Women			
Mature, premenopausal, except at ovulation		0.8–26 IU/L	0.8–26 mIU/mL
Ovulatory surge		25–57 IU/L	25–57 mIU/mL
Postmenopausal		40–104 IU/L	40–104 mIU/mL
Men		1.3–13 IU/L	1.3–13 mIU/mL
Growth hormone, after 100 g oral glucose		<2 μg/L	<2 ng/mL
Hemoglobin A_{1c}	WB	0.038–0.064	3.8–6.4%
17-Hydroxycorticosteroids	U	5.5–28 μmol/d	2–10 mg/d
5-Hydroxyindoleacetic acid (5-HIAA)	U	≤31.4 μmol/d	≤6 mg/d
17-Hydroxyprogesterone	P		
Women			
Follicular phase		0.6–3 nmol/L	0.2–1.0 μg/L
Luteal phase		1.5–10.6 nmol/L	0.5–3.5 μg/L
Men		0.2–9.0 nmol/L	0.06–3.0 μg/L
Insulin, fasting	S, P	43–186 pmol/L	6–26 μU/mL
Insulin-like growth factor (somatomedin C, IGF-1/SM C)	S		
16–24 years		182–780 μg/L	182–780 ng/mL
25–39 years		114–492 μg/L	114–492 ng/mL
40–54 years		90–360 μg/L	90–360 ng/mL
>54 years		71–290 μg/L	71–290 ng/mL
17-Ketosteroids	U		
Women		20–59 μmol/d	6–17 mg/d
Men		20–69 μmol/d	6–20 mg/d
Oxytocin			
Random		1–4 pmol/L	1.25–5 ng/L
Ovulatory peak in women		4–8 pmol/L	5–10 ng/L
Parathyroid hormone	S	10–60 ng/L	10–60 pg/mL
Parathyroid hormone–related protein	P	<1.3 pmol/L	<1.3 pmol/L
Progesterone	P		
Women, luteal, peak		6–60 nmol/L	2–20 ng/mL
Men, prepubertal girls, preovulatory women, postmenopausal women		<6 nmol/L	<2 ng/mL
Prolactin	S	2–15 μg/L	2–15 ng/mL
Radioactive iodine uptake, 24 h (range varies in different areas due to variations in iodine intake)			5–30%
Renin (adult, normal-Na diet)	P		
Supine		0.08–0.83 ng/(L·s)	0.3–3.0 ng/(mL/h)
Upright		0.28–2.5 ng/(L·s)	1.0–9.0 ng/(mL/h)
Resin triiodothyronine (T_3)		0.25–0.35	25–35%
Reverse T_3 (rT_3)	P	0.15–0.61 nmol/L	10–40 ng/dL
Semen analysis: see Chap. 335			
T_3	P	1.1–2.9 nmol/L	70–190 ng/dL
Testosterone	P		
Women		<3.5 nmol/L	<1 ng/mL
Men		10–35 nmol/L	3–10 ng/mL
Prepubertal boys and girls		0.17–0.7 nmol/L	0.05–0.2 ng/mL
Thyroglobulin	S	0–60 μg/L	0–60 ng/mL
Thyroid stimulating hormone (TSH)		0.4–5.0 mU/L	0.4–5.0 μU/mL
Thyroxine (T_4)	SR	64–154 nmol/L	5–12 μg/dL

NOTE: P, plasma; S, serum; SR; serum radioimmunoassay; U, urine; WB, whole blood.

TABLE A-10 CLASSIFICATION OF TOTAL CHOLESTEROL, LDL-CHOLESTEROL, AND HDL-CHOLESTEROL VALUES

	Total Plasma Cholesterol		LDL-Cholesterol		HDL-Cholesterol	
	SI, mmol/L	C, mg/dL	SI, mmol/L	C, mg/dL	SI, mmol/L	C, mg/dL
Desirable	<5.2	<200	<3.36	<130	>1.55	>60
Borderline	5.20–6.18	200–239	3.36–4.11	130–159	0.9–1.55	35–60
Undesirable	≥6.21	≥240	≥4.14	≥160	<0.9	<35

NOTE: LDL, low-density lipoprotein; HDL, high-density lipoprotein; SI, SI units; C, conventional units

SOURCE: Modified from the report of the Expert Panel on Detection, Evaluation, and Treatment of High Blood Cholesterol in Adults: Second Report of the National Cholesterol Education Program (NCEP) expert panel on detection, evaluation, and treatment of high blood cholesterol (Adult Treatment Panel II). Circulation 89:1329, 1994.

TABLE A-11 VITAMINS AND TRACE MINERALS

	Specimen	Reference Range SI Units	Reference Range Conventional Units
Carotenoids	S	0.9–5.6 μmol/L	50–300 μg/dL
Ceruloplasmin	S	270–370 mg/L	27–37 ng/dL
Copper	S	11–22 μmol/L	70–140 μg/dL
Folic acid	RC	340–1020 nmol/L cells	150–450 ng/mL cells
Folic acid	S	7–36 nmol/L cells	3–16 ng/mL cells
Lead	S	<1 μmol/L	<20 μg/dL
Vitamin A	S	0.7–3.5 μmol/L	20–100 μg/dL
Vitamin B_1 (thiamine)	S	0–75 nmol/L	0–2 μg/dL
Vitamin B_2 (riboflavin)	S	106–638 nmol/L	4–24 μg/dL
Vitamin B_6	P	20–121 nmol/L	5–30 ng/ml
Vitamin B_{12}	S	148–443 pmol/L	200–600 pg/mL
Vitamin C (ascorbic acid)	S	23–57 μmol/L	0.4–1.0 mg/dL
Vitamin D_3, 1,25-dihydroxy	S	60–108 pmol/L	25–45 pg/mL
Vitamin D_3, 25-hydroxy	P		
Summer		37.4–200 nmol/L	15–80 ng/mL
Winter		34.9–105 nmol/L	14–42 ng/mL
Vitamin E	S	12–42 μmol/L	5–18 μg/mL
Zinc	S	11.5–18.5 μmol/L	75–120 μg/dL

NOTE: P, plasma; RC, red cells; S, serum.

TABLE A-12 PULMONARY FUNCTION TESTS

See Table A-19: Summary of Values Useful in Pulmonary Physiology

TABLE A-13 RENAL FUNCTION TESTS

	Reference Range SI Units	Reference Range Conventional Units
Clearances (corrected to 1.72 m^2 body surface area):		
Measures of glomerular filtration rate:		
Inulin clearance (Cl)		
Males (mean ± 1 SD)	2.1 ± 0.4 mL/s	124 ± 25.8 mL/min
Females (mean ± 1 SD)	2.0 ± 0.2 mL/s	119 ± 12.8 mL/min
Endogenous creatinine clearance	1.5–2.2 mL/s	91–130 mL/min
Urea	1.0–1.7 mL/s	60–100 mL/min
Measures of effective renal plasma flow and tubular function:		
p-Aminohippuric acid clearance (Cl_{PAH}):		
Males (mean ± 1 SD)	10.9 ± 2.7 mL/s	654 ± 163 mL/min
Females (mean ± 1 SD)	9.9 ± 1.7 mL/s	594 ± 102 mL/min
Concentration and dilution test:		
Specific gravity of urine:		
After 12-h fluid restriction	≥1.025	≥1.025
After 12-h deliberate water intake	≤1.003	≤1.003
Protein excretion, urine	<0.15 g/d	<150 mg/d
Males	0–0.06 g/d	0–60 mg/d
Females	0–0.09 g/d	0–90 mg/d
Specific gravity, maximal range	1.002–1.028	1.002–1.028
Tubular reabsorption, phosphorus	0.79–0.94 of filtered load	79–94% of filtered load

TABLE A-14 HEMATOLOGIC EVALUATIONS. SEE ALSO "CHEMICAL CONSTITUENTS OF BLOOD"

	Reference Range	
	SI Units	Conventional Units
Bone marrow: see Table A-6		
Carboxyhemoglobin		
Nonsmoker	0–0.023	0–2.3%
Smoker	0.021–0.042	2.1–4.2%
Erythrocyte		
Count	4.15–4.90 $\times 10^{12}$/L	4.15–4.90 $\times 10^6$/mm^3
Distribution width	0.13–0.15	13–15%
Glucose-6-phosphate dehydrogenase	0.78 $\pm$ 0.13 MU/mol Hb	12.1 $\pm$ 2 IU/g Hb
Life span		
Normal survival	120 days	120 days
Chromium-labeled, half-life ($t_{1/2}$)	28 days	28 days
Mean corpuscular hemoglobin (MCH)	28–33 pg/cell	28–33 pg/cell
Mean corpuscular hemoglobin concentration (MCHC)	320–360 g/L	32–36 g/dL
Mean corpuscular volume (MCV)	86–98 fl	86–98 μm^3
Ham's test (acid serum)	Negative	Negative
Haptoglobin (serum)	0.5–2.2 g/L	50–220 mg/dL
Hematocrit		
Males	0.42–0.52	42–52%
Females	0.37–0.48	37–48%
Hemoglobin		
Plasma	0.01–0.05 g/L	1–5 mg/dL
Whole blood		
Males	8.1–11.2 mmol/L	13–18 g/dL
Females	7.4–9.9 mmol/L	12–16 g/dL
Hemoglobin A_2 (HbA_2)	0.015–0.035	1.5–3.5%
Hemoglobin, fetal (HbF)	<0.02	<2%
Leukocytes		
Alkaline phosphatase (LAP)	0.2–1.6 μkat/L	13–100 μ/L
Count	4.3–10.8 $\times 10^9$/L	4.3–10.8 $\times 10^3$/mm^3
Differential		
Neutrophils	0.45–0.74	45–74%
Bands	0–0.04	0–4%
Lymphocytes	0.16–0.45	16–45%
Monocytes	0.04–0.10	4–10%
Eosinophils	0–0.07	0–7%
Basophils	0–0.02	0–2%
T cells: see Chap. 309		
Methemoglobin: <2 mg/L (<2 μg/mL)		
Osmotic fragility		
Slight hemolysis		0.45–0.39%
Complete hemolysis	0.33–0.30%	
Platelets and coagulation parameters:		
Alpha$_2$ antiplasmin		70–130%
Antithrombin III		80–120%
Bleeding time (Simplate)	<7 min	<7 min
Euglobulin lysis time	>2 h	>2 h
Factor II		60–100%
Factor V		60–100%
Factor VII		60–100%
Factor IX		60–100%
Factor X		60–100%
Factor XI		60–100%
Factor XII		60–100%
Factor XIII		60–100%
Fibrinogen	2–4 g/L	200–400 mg/dL
Plasminogen		2.4–4.4 CTA U/mL
Protein C (antigenic assay)		58–148%
Protein S (antigenic assay)		58–148%
Partial thromboplastin time (activated PTT) comparable to control		
Prothrombin time (quick one-stage) control $\pm$ 1 s		
Platelets	130–400 $\times 10^9$/L	130,000–400,000/mm^3
Thrombin time control $\pm$ 3 s		
von Willebrand's antigen		60–150%
Protoporphyrin, free erythrocyte (FEP)	0.28–0.64 μmol/L of red blood cells	16–36 μg/dL of red blood cells
Red cells: see "Erythrocytes"		
Schilling test, orally administered vitamin B_{12} excreted in urine		7–40%
Sedimentation rate		
Westergren, <50 years of age		
Males		0–15 mm/h
Females		0–20 mm/h
Westergren, >50 years of age		
Males		0–20 mm/h
Females		0–30 mm/h
Sucrose hemolysis	Negative	Negative
Viscosity		
Plasma	1.7–2.1	1.7–2.1
Serum	1.4–1.8	1.4–1.8
White blood cells: see "Leukocytes"		

TABLE A-15 DIFFERENTIAL NUCLEATED CELL COUNTS OF BONE MARROW

	Normal, Mean %[a]	Range, %[b]
Myeloid	56.7	
Neutrophilic series	53.6	
Myeloblast	0.9	0.2–1.5
Promyelocyte	3.3	2.1–4.1
Myelocyte	12.7	8.2–15.7
Metamyelocyte	15.9	9.6–24.6
Band	12.4	9.5–15.3
Segmented		
Eosinophilic series	3.1	1.2–5.3
Basophilic series	<0.1	0–0.2
Erythroid	25.6	
Pronormoblasts	0.6	0.2–1.3
Basophilic normoblasts	1.4	0.5–2.4
Polychromatophilic normoblasts	21.6	17.9–29.2
Orthochromatic normoblasts	2.0	0.4–4.6
Megakaryocytes	<0.1	
Lymphoreticular	17.8	
Lymphocytes	16.2	11.1–23.2
Plasma cells	2.3	0.4–3.9
Reticulum cells	0.3	0–0.9

[a] From MM Wintrobe et al, *Clinical Hematology*, 8th ed. Philadelphia, Lea & Febiger, 1981.

[b] Range observed in 12 healthy men.

TABLE A-16 IMMUNOLOGY

	Specimen	Reference Range	
		SI Units	Conventional Units
α_2 Antitrypsin (adult)	S	0.76–1.89 g/L	76–189 mg/dL
Antiglomerular basement membrane antibodies	S		
Qualitative		Negative	Negative
Quantitative		<5 kU/L	<5 U/mL
Antineutrophil cytoplasmic autoantibodies, cytoplasmic (C-ANCA)	S		
Qualitative		Negative	Negative
Quantitative (antibodies to proteinase 3)		<2.8 kU/L	<2.8 U/mL
Antineutrophil cytoplasmic autoantibodies, perinuclear (P-ANCA)	S		
Qualitative		Negative	Negative
Quantitative (antibodies to myeloperoxidase)		<1.4 kU/L	<1.4 U/mL
Autoantibodies			
Antiadrenal antibody	S	NA	Negative at 1:10 dilution
Anti-double-stranded (native) DNA	S	NA	Negative at 1:10 dilution
Antigranulocyte antibody	S	NA	Negative
Anti-Jo-1 antibody	S	NA	Negative
Anti-La antibody	S	NA	Negative
Antimitochondrial antibody	S	NA	Negative
Antinuclear antibody	S	NA	Negative at 1:40 dilution
Antiparietal cell antibody	S	NA	Negative at 1:20 dilution
Anti-Ro antibody	S	NA	Negative
Anti-RNP antibody	S	NA	Negative
Anti-Scl-70 antibody	S	NA	Negative
Anti-Smith antibody	S	NA	Negative
Anti-smooth-muscle antibody	S	NA	Negative at 1:20 dilution
Antithyroglobulin antibody	S	NA	Negative
Antithyroid antibody	S	<0.3 kIU/L	<0.3 IU/mL
Bence Jones protein	S	NA	None detected
Qualitative	U	NA	None detected in a 50-fold concentration
Quantitative	U		
Kappa		<0.03 g/L	<2.5 mg/dL
Lambda		<0.05 g/L	<5.0 mg/dL
C1 esterase-inhibitor protein	S		
Antigenic		0.12–0.25 g/L	12.4–24.5 mg/dL
Functional		Present	Present
Complement			
C3 (adult)	S	0.86–1.84 g/L	86–184 mg/dL
C4 (adult)	S	0.20–0.58 g/L	20–58 mg/dL
Total complement (adult)	S	63–145 kU/L	63–145 U/mL
Factor B	S	0.17–0.42 g/L	17–42 mg/dL
Cryoproteins	S	NA	None detected
CSF	CSF		
Agarose electrophoresis		NA	No banding seen in an 80-fold concentration
Quantitation of albumin (adult)		0.11–0.51 g/L	11.0–50.9 mg/dL
Quantitation of IgG (adult)		0.0–0.08 g/L	0.0–8.0 mg/dL
Immunoglobulins	S		
IgA		0.9–3.2 g/L	90–325 mg/dL
IgD		0–0.08 g/L	0–8 mg/dL
IgE		<0.00025 g/L	<0.025 mg/dL
IgG		8.0–15.0 g/L	800–1500 mg/dL
IgM		0.45–1.5 g/L	45–150 mg/dL
Rheumatoid factor	S, JF	<30 kIU/L	<30 IU/mL
Serum protein electrophoresis	S	NA	Normal pattern
T cells: see Chap. 309			
Viscosity	S	1.4–1.8 relative viscosity units, as compared with water	1.4–1.8 relative viscosity units, as compared with water

NOTE: CSF, cerebrospinal fluid; JF, joint fluid; S, serum; U, urine; NA, not applicable.

SOURCE: Adapted from A Kratz, KB Lewandrowski: N Engl J Med 339:1063, 1998.

TABLE A-17 STOOL ANALYSIS

	Reference Range	
	SI Units	Conventional Units
Bulk		
Wet weight	<197.5 (115 ± 41)g/d	<197.5 (115 ± 41) g/d
Dry weight	<66.4 (34 ± 15) g/d	<66.4 (34 ± 15) g/d
α_1 Antitrypsin	0.98 (±0.17) mg/g dry weight	0.98 (±0.17) mg/g dry weight
Coproporphyrin	600–1500 nmol/d	400–1000 μg/d
Fat (on diet containing at least 50 g fat), measured on a ≥ 3-day collection		
Fat		
Percent of dry weight	<0.30	<30.4%
Coefficient of fat absorption	>0.95	>95%
Fatty acid		
Free	0.01–0.10	1–10% of dry matter
Combined as soap	0.005–0.12	0.5–12% of dry matter
Nitrogen	<1.7 (1.4 ± 0.2) g/d	<1.7 (1.4 ± 0.2) g/d
Protein content	Minimal	Minimal
Urobilinogen	68–470 μmol/d	40–280 mg/d
Water	~0.65	~65%

TABLE A-18 URINE ANALYSIS

	Reference Range	
	SI Units	Conventional Units
Acidity, titratable	20–40 mmol/d	20–40 meq/d
Ammonia	30–50 mmol/d	30–50 meq/d
Amylase		4–400 U/L
Amylase/creatinine clearance ratio $[(Cl_{am}/Cl_{cr}) \times 100]$	1–5	1–5
Calcium (10 meq/d or 200-mg/d dietary calcium)	<7.5 mmol/d	<300 mg/d
Creatine, as creatinine		
Women	<760 μmol/d	<100 mg/d
Men	<380 μmol/d	<50 mg/d
Creatinine	8.8–14 mmol/d	1.0–1.6 g/d
Glucose, true (oxidase method)	0.3–1.7 mmol/d	50–300 mg/d
5-Hydroxyindoleacetic acid (5-HIAA)	10–47 μmol/d	2–9 mg/d
Protein	<0.15 g/d	<150 mg/d
Potassium (varies with intake)	25–100 mmol/d	25–100 meq/d
Sodium (varies with intake)	100–260 mmol/d	100–260 meq/d

TABLE A-19 SUMMARY OF VALUES USEFUL IN PULMONARY PHYSIOLOGY

		Typical Values	
	Symbol	Man Aged 40, 75 kg, 175 cm Tall	Woman Aged 40, 60 kg, 160 cm Tall
PULMONARY MECHANICS			
Spirometry—volume-time curves			
Forced vital capacity	FVC	4.8 L	3.3 L
Forced expiratory volume in 1 s	FEV_1	3.8 L	2.8 L
FEV_1/FVC	FEV_1%	76%	77%
Maximal midexpiratory flow	MMF (FEF 25–27)	4.8 L/s	3.6 L/s
Maximal expiratory flow rate	MEFR (FEF 200–1200)	9.4 L/s	6.1 L/s
Spirometry—flow-volume curves			
Maximal expiratory flow at 50% of expired vital capacity	V_{max} 50 (FEF 50%)	6.1 L/s	4.6 L/s
Maximal expiratory flow at 75% of expired vital capacity	V_{max} 75 (FEF 75%)	3.1 L/s	2.5 L/s
Resistance to airflow:			
Pulmonary resistance	RL (R_L)	<3.0 (cmH_2O/s)/L	
Airway resistance	Raw	<2.5 (cmH_2O/s)/L	
Specific conductance	SGaw	>0.13 cmH_2O/s	
Pulmonary compliance			
Static recoil pressure at total lung capacity	Pst TLC	25 ± 5 cmH_2O	
Compliance of lungs (static)	CL	0.2 L cmH_2O	
Compliance of lungs and thorax	C(L + T)	0.1 L cmH_2O	
Dynamic compliance of 20 breaths per minute	C dyn 20	0.25 ± 0.05 L/cmH_2O	
Maximal static respiratory pressures:			
Maximal inspiratory pressure	MIP	>90 cmH_2O	>50 cmH_2O
Maximal expiratory pressure	MEP	>150 cmH_2O	>120 cmH_2O
LUNG VOLUMES			
Total lung capacity	TLC	6.4 L	4.9 L
Functional residual capacity	FRC	2.2 L	2.6 L
Residual volume	RV	1.5 L	1.2 L
Inspiratory capacity	IC	4.8 L	3.7 L
Expiratory reserve volume	ERV	3.2 L	2.3 L
Vital capacity	VC	1.7 L	1.4 L
GAS EXCHANGE (SEA LEVEL)			
Arterial O_2 tension	Pa_{O_2}	12.7 ± 0.7 kPa (95 ± 5 mmHg)	
Arterial CO_2 tension	Pa_{CO_2}	5.3 ± 0.3 kPa (40 ± 2 mmHg)	
Arterial O_2 saturation	Sa_{O_2}	0.97 ± 0.02 (97 ± 2%)	
Arterial blood pH	pH	7.40 ± 0.02	
Arterial bicarbonate	HCO_3^-	24 + 2 meq/L	
Base excess	BE	0 ± 2 meq/L	
Diffusing capacity for carbon monoxide (single breath)	DL_{CO}	0.42 mLCO/s/mmHg (25 mL CO/min/mmHg)	
Dead space volume	V_D	2 ml/kg body wt	
Physiologic dead space; dead space-tidal volume ratio	V_D/V_T		
Rest		≤35% V_T	
Exercise		≤20% V_T	
Alveolar-arterial difference for O_2	$P(A - a)_{O_2}$	≤2.7 kPa ≤20 kPa (≤20 mmHg)	

B

INSTRUCTIONS FOR COLLECTION AND TRANSPORT OF SPECIMENS FOR CULTURE

It is absolutely essential that the microbiology laboratory be informed of the site of origin of the sample to be cultured and of the infections that are suspected. This information determines the selection of culture media and the length of culture time.

Type of Culture (Synonyms)	Specimen	Minimum Volume	Container	Other Considerations
BLOOD				
Blood, routine (blood culture for aerobes, anaerobes, and yeasts)	Whole blood	10 mL in each of 2 bottles for adults and children; 5 mL, if possible, in each of 2 bottles for infants; less for neonates	See below.[a]	See below.[b]
Blood for fungi/*Mycobacterium* spp.	Whole blood	10 mL in each of 2 bottles, as for routine blood cultures, or in Isolator tube requested from laboratory	Same as for routine blood culture	Specify "hold for extended incubation," since fungal agents may require 4 weeks or more to grow.
Blood, Isolator (lysis centrifugation)	Whole blood	10 mL	Isolator tubes	Use mainly for isolation of fungi, *Mycobacterium,* or other fastidious aerobes and for elimination of antibiotics from cultured blood in which organisms are concentrated by centrifugation.
RESPIRATORY TRACT				
Nose	Swab from nares	1 swab	Sterile culturette or similar transport system containing holding medium	Swabs made of calcium alginate may be used.
Throat	Swab of posterior pharynx, ulcerations, or areas of suspected purulence	1 swab	Sterile culturette or similar swab specimen collection system containing holding medium	See below.[c]
Sputum	Fresh sputum (not saliva)	2 mL	Commercially available sputum collection system or similar sterile container with screw cap	*Cause for rejection:* Care must be taken to ensure that the specimen is sputum and not saliva. Examination of Gram's stain, with number of epithelial cells and PMNs noted, can be an important part of the evaluation process. Induced sputum specimens should not be rejected.
Bronchial aspirates	Transtracheal aspirate, bronchoscopy specimen, or bronchial aspirate	1 mL of aspirate or brush in transport medium	Sterile aspirate or bronchoscopy tube, bronchoscopy brush in a separate sterile container	Special precautions may be required, depending on diagnostic considerations (e.g., *Pneumocystis*).
STOOL				
Stool for routine culture; stool for *Salmonella, Shigella,* and *Campylobacter*	Rectal swab or (preferably) fresh, randomly collected stool	1 g of stool or 2 rectal swabs	Plastic-coated cardboard cup or plastic cup with tight-fitting lid. Other leak-proof containers are also acceptable.	If *Vibrio* spp. are suspected, the laboratory must be notified, and appropriate collection/transport methods should be used.
Stool for *Yersinia, E. coli* O157	Fresh, randomly collected stool	1 g	Plastic-coated cardboard cup or plastic cup with tight-fitting lid	*Limitations:* Procedure requires enrichment techniques.
Stool for *Aeromonas* and *Plesiomonas*	Fresh, randomly collected stool	1 g	Plastic-coated cardboard cup or plastic cup with tight-fitting lid	*Limitations:* Stool should not be cultured for these organisms unless also cultured for other enteric pathogens.
UROGENITAL TRACT				
Urine	Clean-voided urine specimen or urine collected by catheter	0.5 mL	Sterile, leak-proof container with screw cap or special urine transfer tube	See below.[d]
Urogenital secretions	Vaginal or urethral secretions, cervical swabs, uterine fluid, prostatic fluid, etc.	1 swab or 0.5 mL of fluid	Transwab containing Amies transport medium or similar system containing holding medium for *Neisseria gonorrhoeae;* modified Todd-Hewitt broth for group B *Streptococcus* surveillance cultures	Vaginal swab samples for "routine culture" should be discouraged whenever possible unless a particular pathogen is suspected. For detection of multiple organisms (e.g., group B *Streptococcus, Trichomonas, Chlamydia,* or *Candida* spp.), 1 swab per test should be obtained.

(continued)

BODY FLUIDS, ASPIRATES, AND TISSUES

Cerebrospinal fluid (lumbar puncture)	Spinal fluid	1 mL for routine cultures; ≥5 mL for *Mycobacterium*	Sterile tube with tight-fitting cap	Do not refrigerate; transfer to laboratory as soon as possible.
Body fluids	Aseptically aspirated body fluids	1 mL for routine cultures	Sterile tube with tight-fitting cap. Specimen may be left in syringe used for collection if the syringe is capped before transport.	For some body fluids (e.g., peritoneal lavage samples), increased volumes are helpful for isolation of small numbers of bacteria.
Biopsy and aspirated materials	Tissue removed at surgery, bone, anticoagulated bone marrow, biopsy samples, or other specimens from normally sterile areas	1 mL of fluid or a 1-g piece of tissue	Sterile "culturette"-type swab or similar transport system containing holding medium. Sterile bottle or jar should be used for tissue specimens.	Accurate identification of specimen and source is critical. Enough tissue should be collected for both microbiologic and histopathologic evaluations.
Wounds	Purulent material or abscess contents obtained from wound or abscess without contamination by normal microflora	2 swabs or 0.5 mL of aspirated pus	Culturette swab or similar transport system or sterile tube with tight-fitting screw cap. For simultaneous anaerobic cultures, send specimen in anaerobic transport device or closed syringe.	*Collection:* Abscess contents or other fluids should be collected in a syringe (see above) when possible to provide an adequate sample volume and an anaerobic environment.

SPECIAL RECOMMENDATIONS

Fungi	Specimen types listed above may be used. When urine or sputum is cultured for fungi, a first morning specimen is usually preferred.	1 mL or as specified above for individual listing of specimens. Large volumes may be useful for urinary fungi.	Sterile, leak-proof container with tight-fitting cap	*Collection:* Specimen should be transported to microbiology laboratory within 1 h of collection. Contamination with normal flora from skin, rectum, vaginal tract, or other body surfaces should be avoided.
Mycobacterium (acid-fast bacilli)	Sputum, tissue, urine, body fluids	10 mL of fluid or small piece of tissue. Swabs should not be used.	Sterile container with tight-fitting cap	Detection of *Mycobacterium* spp. is improved by use of concentration techniques. Smears and cultures of pleural, peritoneal, and pericardial fluids often have low yields. Multiple cultures from the same patient are encouraged. Culturing in liquid media shortens the time to detection.
Legionella	Pleural fluid, lung biopsy, bronchoalveolar lavage fluid, bronchial/transbronchial biopsy. Rapid transport to laboratory is critical.	1 mL of fluid; any size tissue sample, although a 0.5-g sample should be obtained when possible	—	—
Anaerobic organisms	Aspirated specimens from abscesses or body fluids	1 mL of aspirated fluid or 2 swabs	An appropriate anaerobic transport device is required.[e]	Specimens cultured for obligate anaerobes should be cultured for facultative bacteria as well.
Viruses[f]	Respiratory secretions, wash aspirates from respiratory tract, nasal swabs, blood samples (including buffy coats), vaginal and rectal swabs, swab specimens from suspicious skin lesions, stool samples (in some cases)	1 mL of fluid, 1 swab, or 1 g of stool in each appropriate transport medium	Fluid or stool samples in sterile containers or swab samples in viral culturette devices (kept on ice but not frozen) are generally suitable. Plasma samples and buffy coats in sterile collection tubes should be kept at 4 to 8°C. If specimens are to be shipped or kept for a long time, freezing at −80°C is usually adequate.	Most samples for culture are transported in holding medium containing antibiotics to prevent bacterial overgrowth and viral inactivation. Many specimens should be kept cool but not frozen, provided they are transported promptly to the laboratory. Procedures and transport media vary with the agent to be cultured and the duration of transport.

[a] For samples from adults and children, two bottles (smaller for pediatric samples) should be used: one with dextrose phosphate, tryptic soy, or another appropriate broth and the other with thioglycollate or another broth containing reducing agents appropriate for isolation of obligate anaerobes. For special situations (e.g., suspected fungal infection, culture-negative endocarditis, or mycobacteremia), different blood collection systems may be used (Isolator systems; see table).

[b] *Collection:* An appropriate disinfecting technique should be used on both the bottle septum and the patient. Do not allow air bubbles to get into anaerobic broth bottles. *Special considerations:* There is no more important clinical microbiology test than the detection of blood-borne pathogens. The rapid identification of bacterial and fungal agents is a major determinant of patients' survival. Bacteria may be present in blood either continuously (as in endocarditis, overwhelming sepsis, and the early stages of salmonellosis and brucellosis) or intermittently (as in most other bacterial infections, in which bacteria are shed into the blood on a sporadic basis). Most blood culture systems employ two separate bottles containing broth medium: one that is vented in the laboratory for the growth of facultative and aerobic organisms and a second that is maintained under anaerobic conditions. In cases of suspected continuous bacteremia/fungemia, two or three samples should be drawn before the start of therapy, with additional sets obtained if fastidious organisms are thought to be involved. For intermittent bacteremia, two or three samples should be obtained at least 1 h apart during the first 24 h.

[c] Normal microflora includes alpha-hemolytic streptococci, saprophytic *Neisseria* spp., diphtheroids, and *Staphylococcus* spp. Aerobic culture of the throat ("routine") includes screening for and identification of beta-hemolytic *Streptococcus* spp. and other potentially pathogenic organisms. Although considered components of the normal microflora, organisms such as *Staphylococcus aureus, Haemophilus influenzae,* and *Streptococcus pneumoniae* will be identified by most laboratories, if requested. When *Neisseria gonorrhoeae* or *Corynebacterium diphtheriae* is suspected, a special culture request is recommended.

[d] (1) Clean-voided specimens, midvoid specimens, and Foley or indwelling catheter specimens that yield ≥50,000 organisms/mL and from which no more than three species are isolated should have organisms identified. (2) Straight-catheterized, bladder-tap, and similar urine specimens should undergo a complete workup (identification and susceptibility testing) for all potentially pathogenic organisms, regardless of colony count. (3) Certain clinical problems (e.g., acute dysuria in women) may warrant identification and susceptibility testing of isolates present at concentrations of <50,000 organisms/mL.

[e] Aspirated specimens in capped syringes or other transport devices designed to limit oxygen exposure are suitable for the cultivation of obligate anaerobes. A variety of commercially available transport devices may be used. Contamination of specimens with normal microflora from the skin, rectum, vaginal vault, or another body site should be avoided. Collection containers for aerobic culture (such as dry swabs) and inappropriate specimens (such as refrigerated samples; expectorated sputum; stool; gastric aspirates; and vaginal, throat, nose, and rectal swabs) should be rejected as unsuitable.

[f] Laboratories generally use diverse methods to detect viral agents, and the specific requirements for each specimen should be checked before a sample is sent.

INDEX

Bold number indicates the start of the main discussion of the topic; numbers with "f" and "t" refer to figure and table pages; italic roman numerals refer to the Color Atlas plates.